Pediatric Dermatology

THIRD EDITION

Commissioning Editor: **Sue Hodgson**
Project Development Manager: **Tim Kimber**
Project Manager: **Camilla Rockwood**
Design Manager: **Jayne Jones**
Illustration Manager: **Mick Ruddy**
Illustrator: **Marion Tasker**

Pediatric Dermatology

THIRD EDITION

Edited by

Lawrence A Schachner MD
Professor of Dermatology and Cutaneous Surgery
Professor of Pediatrics
Director, Division of Pediatric Dermatology
University of Miami School of Medicine
Miami, Florida
USA

Ronald C Hansen MD
Chief, Pediatric Dermatology, Phoenix
Children's Hospital
Professor, Departments of Medicine
(Dermatology) and Pediatrics
University of Arizona School of Medicine
Tucson, Arizona
USA

Associate Editors

Rudolf Happle MD
Professor and Chairman, Department of Dermatology
Philipp University of Marburg, Faculty of Medicine
Marburg
Germany

Bernice R Krafchik MB ChB FRCPC
Professor, Departments of Paediatrics and Medicine
University of Toronto
Head, Section of Dermatology, Division of Paediatric Medicine
Hospital for Sick Children
Toronto, Ontario
Canada

Anne W Lucky MD
Volunteer Professor of Dermatology and Pediatrics
The University of Cincinnati College of Medicine
and
The Cincinnati Children's Hospital Medical Centre
Cincinnati, Ohio
USA

Amy S Paller MD
Professor of Pediatrics and Dermatology
Northwestern University Medical School
Head, Pediatric Dermatology
Children's Memorial Hospital
Chicago, Illinois
USA

Maureen Rogers MB BS FACD
Head, Department of Dermatology
Children's Hospital at Westmead
Sydney
Australia

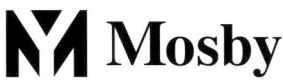

Mosby

Edinburgh London New York Oxford Philadelphia St Louis Sydney Toronto 2003

MOSBY
An affiliate of Elsevier Limited

' Churchill Livingstone Inc. 1988
' Churchill Livingstone Inc. 1995
' 2003, Elsevier Limited. All rights reserved.

First edition 1988
Second edition 1995
Third edition 2003

ISBN 0 323 02611 7

British Library Cataloguing in Publication Data
A catalogue record for this book is available from the British Library

Library of Congress Cataloging in Publication Data
A catalog record for this book is available from the Library of Congress

Notice
Medical knowledge is constantly changing. Standard safety precautions must be followed, but as new research and clinical experience broaden our knowledge, changes in treatment and drug therapy may become necessary or appropriate. Readers are advised to check the most current product information provided by the manufacturer of each drug to be administered to verify the recommended dose, the method and duration of administration, and contraindications. It is the responsibility of the practitioner, relying on experience and knowledge of the patient, to determine dosages and the best treatment for each individual patient. Neither the publishers nor the editors assume any liability for any injury and/or damage to persons or property arising from this publication.

Printed in Spain

The
publisher's
policy is to use
**paper manufactured
from sustainable forests**

Contents

List of Contributors

Robert Baran MD
Head, Nail Disease Centre
Cannes
France

Nancy K Barnett MD
Associate Clinical Professor of Dermatology and
Pediatrics
University of California at San Francisco
Director of Pediatric Dermatology
Children's Hospital of Central California
Madera, CA
USA

Christine Bodemer MD PhD
Professor of Pediatric Dermatology
Hôpital Necker Enfants Malades
Paris
France

Lesley V Boyer MD
Associate Professor of Clinical Pediatrics
University of Arizona Health Sciences Center
Medical Director
Arizona Poison and Drug Information Center
Tucson, AZ
USA

Alanna F Bree MD
Department of Dermatology
St Louis University
St Louis, MO
USA

Walter C Burgdorf MD
Clinical Lecturer
Department of Dermatology
Ludwig Maximilian University
Munich
Germany

Hector W Caceres-Rios MD
Professor of Pediatric Dermatology
Peruvian University Cayetano Heredia
Instituto de Salud del Niño
Lima
Peru

Bari B Cunningham MD
Assistant Professor, Pediatrics and Medicine
University of California at San Diego
Children's Hospital and Health Center
San Diego, CA
USA

Mark V Dahl MD
Professor and Chairman
Department of Dermatology
Mayo Clinic Scottsdale
Scottsdale, AZ
USA

Gary L Darmstadt MD MS
Division of Health Systems
Department of International Health
Bloomberg School of Public Health
The Johns Hopkins University
Baltimore, MD
Senior Research Advisor
Saving Newborn Lives Initiative
Save the Children Federation USA
Washington, DC
USA

Zoe Diana Draelos MD
Clinical Associate Professor
Department of Dermatology
Wake Forest University School of
Medicine
Winston-Salem, NC
USA

Ana Duarte MD FAAP FAAD
President, Children's Skin Center
Pediatric Dermatologist
Division of Dermatology
Miami Children's Hospital
Miami, FL
USA

Robin Anthony Jeffery Eady DSc FRCP FMedSci
Professor of Experimental Dermatopathology and
Consultant Dermatologist
St John's Institute of Dermatology
Guy's, King's and Thomas' School of Medicine
St Thomas' Hospital
London
UK

Lawrence F Eichenfield MD
Chief, Division of Pediatric and Adolescent
Dermatology
Professor of Pediatrics and Medicine
(Dermatology)
Children's Hospital and Health Center
San Diego, CA
USA

Odile Enjolras MD
Pediatric Dermatologist
Director, *Consultation des Angiomes*
Hôpital Lariboisière
Assistance Publique Hôpitaux de Paris
France

Nancy Esterly MD
Professor of Dermatology and
Pediatrics
Pediatric Dermatology
Medical College of Wisconsin
Milwaukee, WI
USA

Rafael Falabella MD
Professor and Chairman
Department of Dermatology
School of Medicine
Universidad Del Valle
Cali
Colombia

Gayle Olivia Fischer MBBS FACD
Visiting Dermatologist
The Children's Hospital, Westmead
Visiting Dermatologist
The Royal North Shore Hospital
St Leonards
Australia

Ilona J Frieden MD
Clinical Professor of Dermatology and Pediatrics
Chief, Division of Pediatric Dermatology
University of California School of
Medicine
San Francisco, CA
USA

Sheila Friedlander MD
Associate Clinical Professor
School of Medicine and Children's
Hospital
San Diego, CA
USA

Wesley King Galen MD
Professor, Louisiana State University School of
Medicine
Associate Clinical Professor, Tulane University
School of Medicine
Staff Dermatologist, Children's Hospital
New Orleans, LA
USA

Edith Garcia-Gonzales MD
Section of Immunodermatology
Instituto Nacional de Perinatologica
Mexico City
Mexico

Maria Garzon MD
Assistant Professor of Dermatology and Pediatrics
Columbia University
Director, Pediatric Dermatology
Children's Hospital of New York
New York Presbyterian Hospital
New York, NY
USA

Carlo Gelmetti MD
Professor of Dermatology and Venereology,
University of Milan
Head, Unit of Pediatric Dermatology
IRCCS "Ospedale Maggiore" di Milano
Milano
Italy

Lowell Goldsmith MD
Professor of Dermatology
University of North Carolina Chapel Hill
Chapel Hill, NC
USA

Anne Halbert FACD
Head, Department of Pediatric Dermatology
Princess Margaret Hospital for Children
Perth
Australia

Henning Hamm MD
Professor of Dermatology
Department of Dermatology
University of Würzburg
Würzburg
Germany

Eckart Haneke MD PhD
Professor of Dermatology
Klinikk Bunas
Sandvika
Norway

Rudolf Happle MD
Professor and Chairman, Department of
Dermatology
Philipp University of Marburg, Faculty of Medicine
Marburg
Germany

Adelaide A Hebert MD
Professor of Dermatology and Pediatrics
Vice Chairman, Department of Dermatology
University of Texas Medical School - Houston
Houston, TX
USA

Peter A Hogan MB BS BMedSc DCH FACD
Department of Dermatology
Children's Hospital at Westmead
Sydney
Australia

Karen A Holbrook BS MS PhD
President
The Ohio State University
Columbus, OH
USA

Peter H Itin MD
Head of Department of Dermatology
Kantonsspital Aarau
Aarau
Switzerland

Michael Steven Jellinek MD
Chief, Child Psychiatry Service
Massachusetts General Hospital
Boston, MA
USA

Robert Johr MD
Associate Clinical Professor of Dermatology and
Pediatrics
Director, Pigmented Lesion Clinic
University of Miami School of Medicine
Boca Raton, FL
USA

Tomisaku Kawasaki MD
Director, Japan Kawasaki Disease Research
Center
Tokyo
Japan

Sandra R Knowles MD
Glaxo Drug Safety Clinic
Sunnybrook & Women's College Health Sciences
Centre
Toronto, Ontario
Canada

Arne König MD
Senior Physician/Specialist Dermatology
Department of Dermatology
Philipp University of Marburg
Marburg
Germany

Bruce Korf MD PhD
Wayne H and Sara Crews Finley Professor of
Medical Genetics
Chair, Department of Genetics
University of Alabama
Birmingham, AL
USA

Bernice R Krafchik MB ChB FRCPC
Professor, Departments of Paediatrics and
Medicine
University of Toronto
Head, Section of Dermatology, Division of
Paediatric Medicine
Hospital for Sick Children
Toronto, Ontario
Canada

Walter Krause MD
Professor of Dermatology
Department of Andrology and Venerology
University Hospital
Philipp University
Marburg
Germany

Alfons Krol MD FRCPC
Professor of Dermatology and
Pediatrics
Director of Pediatric Dermatology
Doernbecher Children's Hospital
Department of Dermatology
Oregon Health and Science University
Portland, OR
USA

Daniel P Krowchuk MD
Professor of Pediatrics and Dermatology
Wake Forest University Health Sciences
Winston-Salem, NC
USA

Margarita Mirta Larralde MD PhD
Associate Professor of Dermatology
University of Buenos Aires
Chief, Pediatric Dermatology Section
Hospital Ramos Mejia
Buenos Aires
Argentina

Stephen Lauer PhD MD
Clinical Assistant Professor of
Pediatrics
Department of Pediatrics
University of Kansas Medical Center
Kansas City, KS
USA

Stephan Lautenschlager MD
Associate Professor of Dermatology and
Venereology
University of Zurich
Head, Outpatient Clinic of Dermatology and
Venereology Triemli
Zurich
Switzerland

Patsy Lenane MB BCH BAO MRCPI
Fellow in Paediatric Dermatology
The Hospital for Sick Children
Toronto, Ontario
Canada

Norman Levine MD
Professor and Chief of Dermatology
University of Arizona
Tucson, AZ
USA

Anne W Lucky MD
Volunteer Professor of Dermatology and
Pediatrics
The University of Cincinnati College of Medicine
and
The Cincinnati Children's Hospital Medical Center
Cincinnati, OH
USA

Susan Bayliss Mallory MD
Professor of Dermatology and Pediatrics
Washington University School of Medicine
Director, Pediatric Dermatology
St Louis Children's Hospital
St Louis, MO
USA

Anthony J Mancini MD
Associate Professor of Pediatrics and
Dermatology
Northwestern University Feinberg School of
Medicine
Children's Memorial Hospital
Chicago, IL
USA

Johannes Mayer MD
Department of Dermatology
University of Würzburg
Würzburg
Germany

John Alexander McGrath MB BS MD FRCP
Professor of Molecular Dermatology
St John's Institute of Dermatology
The Guy's, King's College and St Thomas'
Hospitals Medical School
St Thomas' Hospital
London
UK

Teřri Meinking BA
Research Assistant Professor
Field Epidemiology Survey Team
Department of Dermatology
University of Miami School of Medicine
Miami, FL
USA

Joseph Morelli MD
Associate Professor of Dermatology and
Pediatrics
University of Colorado School of Medicine
Denver, CO
USA

Celia Moss MB BS DM FRCP MRCPCH
Consultant Dermatologist
Department of Dermatology
Birmingham Children's Hospital
Birmingham
UK

Amy Jo Nopper MD
Chief, Section of Pediatric Dermatology
Children's Mercy Hospital
Associate Professor of Pediatric Dermatology
University of Missouri
Kansas City, MO
USA

David Orchard MBBS FACD
Paediatric Dermatologist
Department of Dermatology
Royal Children's Hospital
Victoria
Australia

Seth J Orlow MD PhD
Professor of Dermatology, Cell Biology and
Pediatrics
Director of Pediatric Dermatology
New York University School of Medicine
New York, NY
USA

Amy S Paller MD
Professor of Pediatrics and Dermatology
Northwestern University Medical School
Head, Division of Dermatology
Children's Memorial Hospital
Chicago, IL
USA

Adrián-Martín Pierini MD
Professor of Dermatology
Faculty of Medicine
University of Buenos Aires
Chairman, Service of Dermatology
Hospital de Pediatria Prof. Juan P Garrahan
Buenos Aires
Argentina

Mark R Pittelkow MD
Professor, Departments of Dermatology,
Biochemistry and Molecular Biology
Mayo Medical School
Mayo Clinic and Foundation
Rochester, MN
USA

Julie Powell MD FRCPC
Clinical Associate Professor of Paediatrics
(Dermatology)
University of Montreal
Chief, Division of Dermatology
Sainte-Justine Hospital
Montreal, Quebec
Canada

Julie Prendiville MB MRCPI FRCPC
Clinical Associate Professor in Paediatrics
University of British Columbia
Head, Division of Paediatric Dermatology
British Columbia's Children's Hospital
Vancouver, BC
Canada

Chulabhorn Pruksachatkunakorn MD
Associate Professor
Chief, Division of Dermatology
Department of Pediatrics
Chiang Mai University
Chiang Mai
Thailand

Ben Raimer MD
Professor of Pediatrics and Family Medicine
University of Texas Medical Branch
Galveston, TX
USA

Sharon S Raimer MD
Professor of Dermatology and Pediatrics
Chairman of Dermatology
University of Texas Medical Branch
Galveston, TX
USA

Paula K Rauch MD
Chief, Child Psychiatry Consultation Service
Massachusetts General Hospital
Assistant Professor
Harvard Medical School
Boston, MA
USA

Gabriele Richard MD
Associate Professor of Dermatology and Genetics
Department of Dermatology and Cutaneous
Biology
Thomas Jefferson University and Jefferson
Medical School
Philadelphia, PA
USA

Maureen Rogers MB BS FACD
Head, Department of Dermatology
Children's Hospital at Westmead
Sydney
Australia

Ramon Ruiz-Maldonado MD
Professor of Dermatology and Pediatric
Dermatology
Department of Dermatology
National Institute of Pediatrics
Mexico

Rikako Sasaki MD
Director, Division of Dermatology
National Center for Child Health and
Development
Tokyo
Japan

Lori E Shapiro MD
Department of Medicine
Glaxo Drug Safety Clinic
Sunnybrook & Women's College Health Sciences
Centre
Toronto, Ontario
Canada

Neil H Shear MD FRCPC FACP
Professor and Chief of Dermatology
University of Toronto
Chief of Dermatology
Sunnybrook & Women's Medical Center
Toronto, Ontario
Canada

Elaine C Siegfried MD
Associate Clinical Professor of Pediatrics and
Dermatology
Saint Louis University School of Medicine
Saint Louis, MO
USA

Robert A Silverman MD
Clinical Associate Professor
Departments of Dermatology and Pediatrics
The University of Virginia
Georgetown University
Washington, DC
USA

Mary K Spraker MD
Associate Professor of Dermatology and
Pediatrics
Emory University School of Medicine
Atlanta, GA
USA

Stephanie Swords DO
Medicine/Pediatrics Resident
Children's Mercy Hospital
University of Missouri-Kansas City
Kansas City, MO
USA

Alain Taieb MD
Professor and Chair
Service de Dermatologie et Unité de
Dermatologie Pédiatrique
Centre Hospitelier et Universitaire
Bordeaux
France

Lourdes Tamayo MD
Professor of Pediatric Dermatology
Servicio de Dermatologia
Instituto Nacional de Pediatria, SS
Mexico City
Mexico

David Taplin MD
Professor, Departments of Dermatology and
Cutaneous Surgery and Epedimology and Public
Health
University of Miami Medical School
Miami, FL
USA

Yong-Kwang Tay MD
Consultant Dermatologist
Dermatology Service
Changi General Hospital
Singapore

Michael Tidman MD FRCP (Edin)
Consultant Dermatologist
Department of Dermatology
The Royal Infirmary
Edinburgh
UK

Gail Todd FFDerm (SA) MBChB PhD BSc
Associate Professor and Head
Division of Dermatology
University of Cape Town
South Africa

Heiko Traupe MD
Associate Professor of Dermatology
University of Munster Medical School
Munster
Germany

Patricia Treadwell MD
Professor of Dermatology and Pediatrics
Indiana University School of Medicine
Indianapolis, IN
USA

Annette Wagner MD
Attending Physician
Children's Memorial Hospital
Departments of Pediatrics and Dermatology
Northwestern University
Chicago, IL
USA

William L Weston MD
Professor of Dermatology and Pediatrics
Section Head, Dermatology
Department of Dermatology
University of Colorado Medical Center
Denver, CO
USA

Dowain A Wright MD PhD
Clinical Assistant Professor in Pediatrics
University of California, San Francisco
Medical Director of Immunology
Children's Hospital, Central California
Madera, CA
USA

Kazuya Yamamoto MD
Professor and Chairman
Department of Dermatology
Allku Hospital
Japan

Acknowledgements

This book would not exist without the
excellent contributions to the first and second
editions made by the following authors:

Michelle A Bene-Bain
Joel H Berg
Carl Bigler
Raymond V Caputo
Bernard A Cohen
Irwin Cohen

Jo-David Fine
Joan Guitart
Sidney Hurwitz
Alfred T Lane
Moise L Levy
Giuseppe Micali
Neal S Penneys
Neil Prose
Thomas T Provost
Linda G Rabinowitz

Steven D Resnick
Findlay E Russell
Tor A Schwayder
Edward M Sills
Margaret H D Smith
Lawrence M Solomon
David H Stein
Virginia P Sybert
Ronald G Wheeland
Mary L Williams

Preface

The third edition of *Pediatric Dermatology* represents a major change from the first and second editions. While those editions stood as the first encyclopedic texts in the field, they did not fully achieve our goals of international authorship and color photography. Those goals are achieved in the third edition. Through the years we have been gratified when pediatric dermatologists around the globe have thanked us for making available a resource they needed. We feel the third edition will prove an even more useful resource.

This project could not have been completed with only two senior editors, as was the case in our previous editions. Accordingly, five associate editors were chosen, and they in fact did the lion's share of the editing. Without Drs. Rudi Happle, Bernice Krafchik, Anne Lucky, Amy Paller, and Maureen Rogers, we could never have achieved our objectives. Our goal has always been to have close editorial scrutiny of each chapter, and we feel this has been achieved by our combined editorship. While no text is perfect, we have endeavored to have each segment approved by the author, associate editor, and senior editor. While not wishing to stifle controversy and personal opinion, we feel such close oversight encourages a discriminating product with collective wisdom and collaborative merit. It also ensures broad coverage while minimizing overlap.

Every chapter has been extensively revised. Chapter writing is a difficult, tedious and often thankless task. We cannot be more pleased with the authors' work for this edition. Thirty-three authors from the previous edition have once again graciously contributed to the third edition. The previous editions have been largely written by North Americans from the USA, Canada and Mexico. For this effort, we have added fifty-two new authors including experts from Europe, South America, Asia, Africa and Australia. Our international colleagues have greatly enriched the textbook.

We are also excited about the new design layout presented by Mosby. Tables are crisply displayed with color separation; interspersed color photographs add to the attractiveness and teaching value of the text; and the unique same-page referencing style allows easier reading and eliminates page flipping to identify cited references. These features, plus the close coordination of the project by our Mosby colleagues, Sue Hodgson and Tim Kimber, have allowed us to produce a textbook we can all be proud of.

We trust that the third edition will be helpful to physicians interested in the skin problems of children. We thank our families and office staff for once again enduring the prolonged process involved in the development of this textbook. We specifically thank Myrian Baker, Charlotte Cohen and Lynne Morrison for their invaluable assistance. We thank our patients, whose problems first have stimulated us to attempt this work. We trust that this effort will in turn positively influence the quality of care for other children.

Lawrence A Schachner MD
Ronald C Hansen MD

2003

Structure and Function

Robin Eady, Lowell Goldsmith, Mark Dahl

SKIN DEVELOPMENT

In order to interpret the structural and functional properties of the skin in children, it is helpful to know how the skin develops in the embryo and fetus. Skin development will constitute the initial section of this chapter. Skin structure, composition, and function in the adult will follow. Comparisons of mature skin with newborn and infant skin will be included where appropriate.

EMBRYOGENESIS OF THE SKIN

Robin Eady and Karen Holbrook

The embryonic and fetal periods are the two major stages of development of the organism. The embryo becomes a fetus at the end of the second month of gestation, coincident with the onset of bone marrow function. Within each period, specific stages of skin development can be defined by biochemical, immunohistochemical, and morphologic characteristics of epidermal cells.[1] There is a clear distinction between the structure of the embryonic skin compared with all of the stages thereafter. Skin development in the fetus is separated into stages that correlate with major events in epidermal differentiation: stratification, follicular keratinization, and keratinization of the interfollicular epidermis. The final stage of fetal skin development occurs in the third trimester, and corresponds to the skin of the premature infant. A generalized scheme for the stages of skin development is shown in Fig. 1.1.

The germ layers that give rise to the epidermis, dermis, and hypodermis organize very early in development. Ectoderm (origin of the epidermis) and the endoderm are formed at 10 to 12 days estimated gestational age (EGA) and the mesoderm (origin of the dermis) forms around 18 to 19 days EGA. All the major organs and organ systems become established (organogenesis) between 20 and 50 days EGA; the organs of ectodermal origin (e.g., brain and eyes), in particular, develop very early during that period. Studies of skin development in humans have been performed only on embryos older than 30 days, because tissue younger than this is rarely available. By this age the epidermis, dermal–epidermal junction (DEJ), dermis, and hypodermis are defined. By 40 days it is already possible to recognize in the skin certain structural and biochemical markers characteristic for each of these zones.

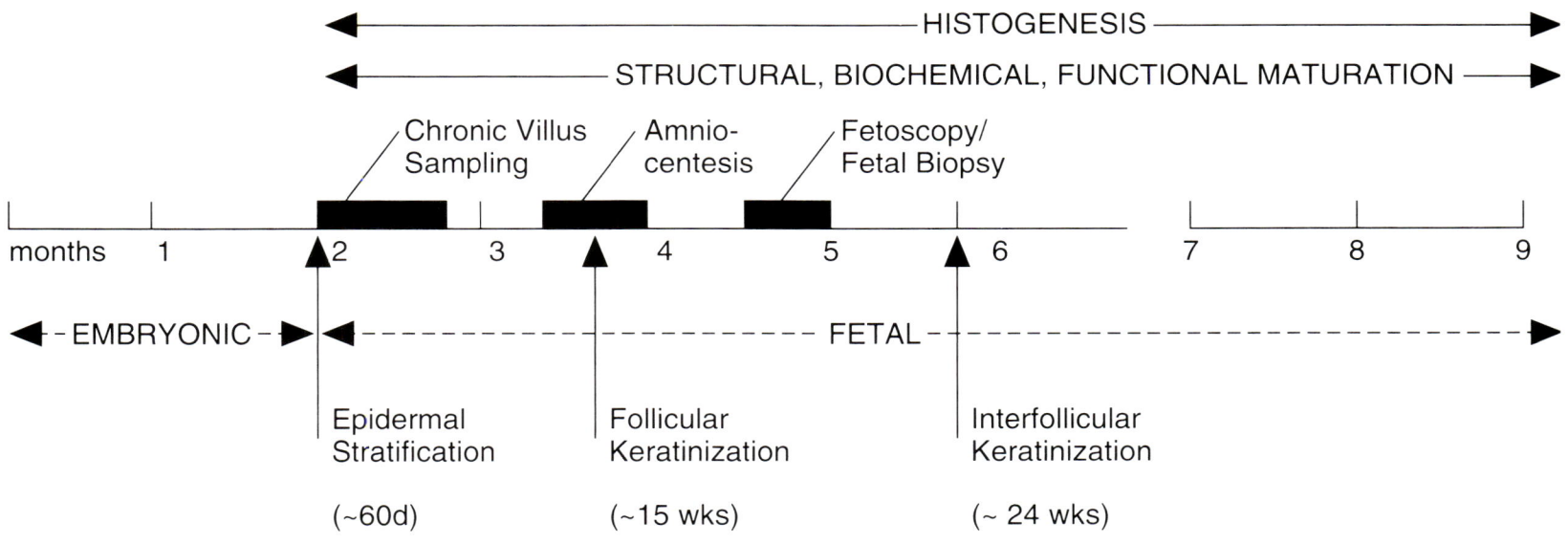

Fig. 1.1   Landmarks in epidermal development.

1. Holbrook KA (1991) Structure and function of the developing human skin. In: Physiology, Biochemistry and Molecular Biology of the Skin, 2nd edn Vol. 1, Goldsmith LE, ed. New York: Oxford University Press, p. 63.

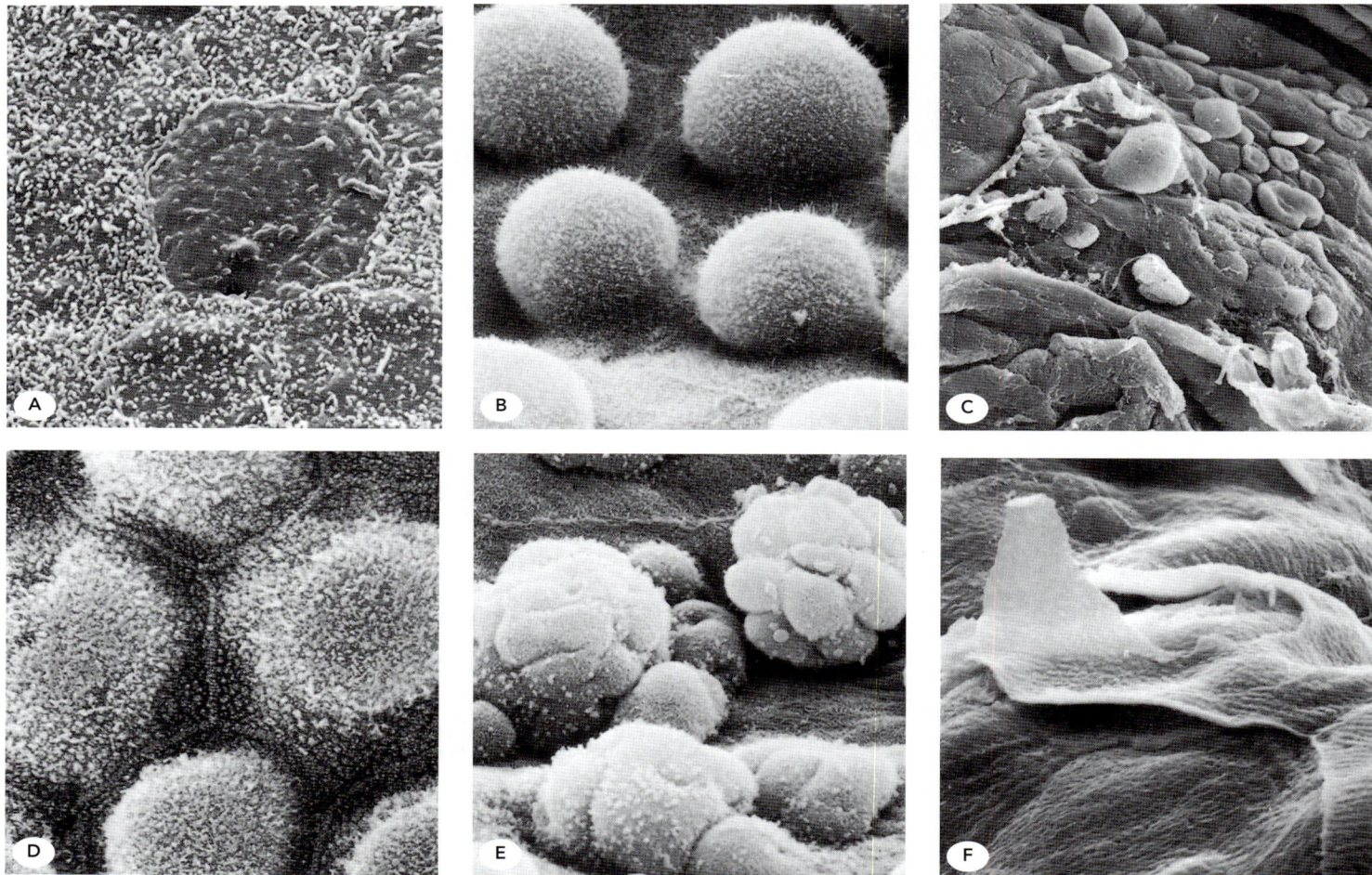

Fig. 1.2 Scanning electron micrographs of the surface (periderm) of human (A) embryonic and (B–F) fetal skin of 70, 100, 112, 140, and 160 days EGA. Note the microvilli and blebs in **A–D**, regression of the blebs in E, and the keratinized surface in F. (A) × 4000; (B) × 2650; (C) × 2500; (D) × 2100; (E) × 1000; (F) × 2750.

UNIQUE PROPERTIES OF PRENATAL SKIN

Some of the properties of adult skin (e.g., expression of cell-layer specific epidermal keratins) are also prominent features of developing skin. Other characteristics of fetal skin are unique.

ASSEMBLY AND DIFFERENTIATION OF THE SKIN OCCUR IN PARALLEL

In both the fetus and the adult, the epidermis is organized into layers that correlate with stages of keratinocyte differentiation. Basal layer keratinocytes divide and at least one of the daughter cells moves upward through the strata, ultimately becoming a terminally differentiated, nonviable cell of the stratum corneum. At each stage, which corresponds to an epidermal layer, the cells become more specialized structurally, synthesize new gene products, and perform new functions. The end point of epidermal differentiation in both the fetus and the adult is keratinization, but there are differences in how this is accomplished by each. In the adult, keratinization requires a relatively short time. A cell that leaves the basal layer moves into the lowest cornified cell layer in about 14 days. The fetal epidermis requires 22 to 24 weeks to keratinize. New layers of cells are established as cells move upward from the basal layer and undergo differentiation. Thus, the fetal epidermis acquires the pattern of the adult tissue concurrent with stratification and differentiation. Keratinization in the adult epidermis occurs in a dry environment; the epidermis of the fetus is exposed to amniotic fluid as it differentiates.

THE PERIDERM

The periderm is a characteristic found only in developing skin. It is the transient outermost layer of the embryonic and fetal epidermis. Periderm is ectodermal in origin, contains a single population of cells, and is either the first layer of the skin (perhaps the "true" primordial epidermis that divides and gives rise to the single layer of the epidermis proper), or it is derived secondarily from cells that divide in the basal layer. Similarities in the cytoplasmic keratins, cell surface morphology, and antigens of periderm and amnion cells[2–5] support the first hypothesis even though this is the reverse of our way

2. Dale BA, Holbrook KA, Kimball JR et al. (1985) Expression of the epidermal keratins and filaggrin during fetal human development. **J Cell Biol** 101:1257.
3. Moll R, Moll I, Wiest W (1982) Changes in the pattern of cytokeratin polypeptides in epidermis and hair follicles during skin development in human fetuses. **Differentiation** 23:170.
4. Regauer S, Franke WW, Virtanen I (1985) Intermediate filament cytoskeleton of amnion epithelium and cultured amnion epithelial cells: expression of epidermal cytokeratins in cells of a simple epithelium. **J Cell Biol** 100:997.
5. Nanbu Y, Fujii S, Konishi I et al. (1989) CA 125 in the epithelium closely related to the embryonic ectoderm: the periderm and the amnion. **Am J Obstet Gynecol** 161:462.

of thinking about the directionality of epidermal cell division and migration. Alternatively, the periderm may be formed from cells of the amnion that grow over the developing, single-layered epidermis.[6] Studies in the mouse embryo using a retroviral vector with a marker gene have provided some evidence for the origin of periderm from the epidermis proper.[7] Ultrastructural studies of embryonic mouse skin show that the periderm is established in patches, also arguing against a migrating sheet of amnion as the precursor to the periderm.[8] Regardless of its origin, the periderm persists as a single layer of cells that remains on the surface of the developing skin until keratinization of cells in the underlying epidermal layers is complete.[9] At that point, the periderm is sloughed in sheets and as individual cells from the skin surface into the amniotic fluid. Loss of a certain number of periderm cells occurs throughout the second trimester, as determined from the composition of cells in the amniotic fluid.

The periderm cells cease to divide during the first trimester and do not appear to undergo any further steps in differentiation, but they continue to expand markedly in size and volume as the embryo/fetus grows. Characteristic changes in morphology (e.g., blebbing) and expression of markers characteristic of apoptotic cells (e.g., transglutaminases and DNA fragmentation) suggest that the periderm undergoes a sequence of programmed cell death.[10] The shape and surface characteristics of periderm cells are so consistent for the specific, progressive stages of gestation that these features have been used to define stages of epidermal development[9] (Fig. 1.2). Monoclonal antibodies have been made that recognize only the periderm cells among the epidermal cell populations;[6,11] some of them recognize stage-specific periderm cells. These antibodies may be helpful in sorting this population of cells and establishing them in culture, both in isolation and in association with developing keratinocytes.

Further evidence in support of the concept that periderm cells are a unique epidermal cell population comes from studies of fetuses affected with two genetic diseases, bullous congenital ichthyosiform erythroderma (BCIE) and epidermolysis bullosa simplex Dowling–Meara (EBS D–M), that affect the epidermis. Abnormal aggregations of keratin filaments occur in fetal basal (EBS D–M) or intermediate cells (BCIE), but in neither case are keratins of the periderm cells altered from normal. Moreover, the periderm remains as a single layer in harlequin ichthyosis, lamellar ichthyosis, and Sjögren–Larsson syndrome even though the underlying fetal epidermal layers are excessive.

The function of the periderm is unknown, but it has been suggested that in early stages of development it protects the basal epidermal layer. The extensive microvilli and blebbing of the periderm cell surfaces that face the amniotic cavity suggest that these cells play a role in some type of exchange between the fetus and the amniotic fluid. Evidence for this function includes: (1) the observation that periderm cells share antigens (epitopes) in common with other absorptive fetal and adult epithelial cells; (2) the demonstration that periderm in the sheep fetus is involved in the uptake of substances from the amniotic fluid;[12] and (3) the observation that the plasma membrane of human periderm cells has the morphologic characteristics of epithelia involved in water transport.[13,14] The periderm may also be a secretory epithelium, contributing material to the amniotic fluid.[15]

SKIN DEVELOPMENT DURING THE EMBRYONIC PERIOD

At 30 to 40 days gestation, the skin consists of an epidermis, DEJ, dermis, and subcutaneous connective tissue (Fig. 1.3).

THE EPIDERMIS

The epidermis includes basal (the epidermis proper) and periderm layers. From the surface, the periderm is seen as a simple, pavement epithelium composed of hexagonally shaped, microvilli-covered cells (Fig. 1.3A). In sectioned specimens periderm and basal cells are similar morphologically; both contain large amounts of glycogen, few organelles, and small quantities of keratin filaments that are organized into fine networks and associated with desmosomes (Fig. 1.3B). The species of keratins in periderm and basal cells are unique and overlapping, and include keratins that are characteristic of simple and glandular epithelia K19, K18, and K8.[2,3,16] K18 is found only in periderm cells (and in Merkel cells, see below); basal cells contain the keratins that are markers of epithelia that will stratify and are those of the basal layer keratinocytes of adult epidermis K5 and K14.[2,3,17] A planar, microfilamentous network is present internal to the plasma membrane of basal cells adjacent to the basement membrane. This assembly may promote adhesion and reinforce the cell before hemidesmosomes are organized in sufficient numbers to maintain the structural integrity of the dermal–epidermal interface. The composition of this network and its relationship with the junctions between the basal keratinocyte and the basement membrane zone are discussed below (see The Dermal–Epidermal Junction). There is no morphologic evidence that epidermal appendages have begun to form in embryonic skin.

Other populations of cells within the epidermis (Langerhans cells, melanocytes, and Merkel cells), some of them immigrant cells (Langerhans cells and melanocytes), are recognized in sections of embryonic epidermis by their nuclear morphology, cytoplasmic density, and orientation in the tissue; they are identified more precisely in both tissue sections and epidermal sheets using immunocytochemistry to identify cell-specific, antigenic markers. Langerhans cells are evident in embryonic epidermis as early as 43 days EGA. They are dendritic and react positively for cytoplasmic Mg^{2+}-dependent-ATPase and with antibodies to HLA-DR.[18,19] The appearance of Langerhans cells before the onset of bone marrow function suggests that the first Langerhans cells in the embryonic epidermis are derived from the yolk sac or fetal liver. The density of these cells is low (65 cells/mm²) in the epidermis during both the first and second trimesters of development.[19,20]

Melanocytes migrate from the neural crest into the embryonic epidermis around 50 days EGA. Although they do not contain melanosomes at this age, they are easily detected using the HMB-45 monoclonal antibody that recognizes an antigen common to melanoma and embryonic/fetal melanocytes. Even at this early age, melanocytes are dendritic, high in density (~1000 cells/mm²), and distributed uniformly throughout the epidermal tissue.[21]

6. Lane AT, Negi M, Goldsmith LA (1987) Human periderm: a monoclonal antibody marker. **Curr Probl Dermatol** 16:83.

7. Sanes JR, Rubenstein JLR, Nicolas J-F (1986) Use of a recombinant retrovirus to study post-implantation cell lineage in mouse embryos. **EMBO J** 5:3133.

8. M'Boneko V, Merker H-J (1988) Development and morphology of the periderm of mouse embryos (days 9–12 of gestation). **Acta Anat** 133:325.

9. Holbrook KA, Odland GF (1975) The fine structure of developing human epidermis: light, scanning and transmission electron microscopy of the periderm. **J Invest Dermatol** 65:16.

10. Polakowska RR, Piacentini M, Bartlett R et al. (1994) Apoptosis in human skin development: morphogenesis, periderm and stem cells. **Dev Dynam** 199:176.

11. Schofield OMV, McDonald JN, Fredj-Reygrobellet D et al. (1990) Common antigen expression between human periderm and other tissues identified by GB1-monoclonal antibody. **Arch Dermatol Res** 282:143.

12. Mears GJ, Van Petten GR (1977) Fetal absorption of drugs from the amniotic fluid. **Proc West Pharmacol Soc** 20:109.

13. Parmely TH, Seeds AE (1970) Fetal skin permeability to isotopic water (THO) in early pregnancy. **Am J Obstet Gynecol** 108:128.

14. Riddle CV (1985) Intramembranous response to cAMP in fetal epidermis. **Cell Tissue Res** 241:687.

15. Lind T, Kendal A, Hytten FE (1972) The role of the fetus in the formation of amniotic fluid. **J Obstet Gynaecol Br Commonw** 79:289.

16. Moll R, Franke WW, Schiller DL (1982) The catalog of human cytokeratins: patterns of expression in normal epithelia, tumors and cultured cells. **Cell** 31:11.

17. Tseng SCG, Jarvinen M, Nelson WG et al. (1982) Correlation of specific keratins with different types of epithelial differentiation: monoclonal antibody studies. **Cell** 30:361.

18. Foster CA, Holbrook KA, Farr AG (1986) Ontogeny of Langerhans cells in human embryonic and fetal skin: expression of HLA-DR and OKT-6 determinants. **J Invest Dermatol** 86:240.

19. Drijkoningen M, DeWolf-Peeters C, VanDerSteen K et al. (1987) Epidermal Langerhans cells and dermal dendritic cells in human fetal and neonatal skin: an immunohistochemical study. **Pediatr Dermatol** 4:11.

20. Foster CA, Holbrook KA (1989) Ontogeny of Langerhans cells in human embryonic and fetal skin: expression of HLA-DR and OKT6 determinants. **Am J Anat** 184:157.

21. Holbrook KA, Underwood RA, Vogel AM et al. (1989) The appearance, density and distribution of melanocytes in human embryonic and fetal skin revealed by the anti-melanoma monoclonal antibody, HMB-45. **Anat Embryol** 180:443.

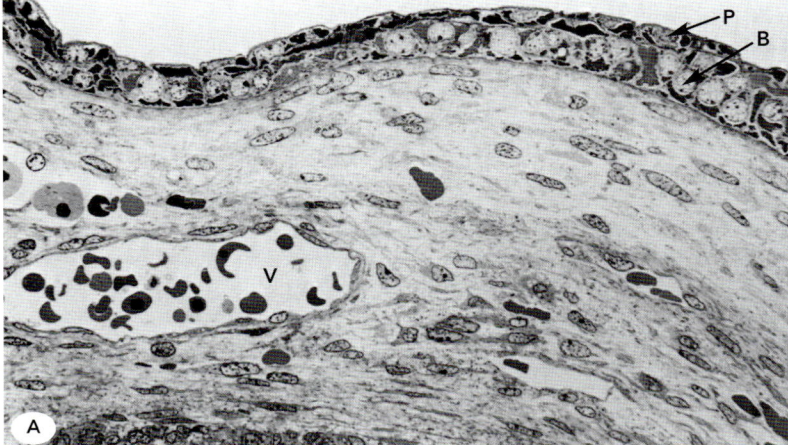

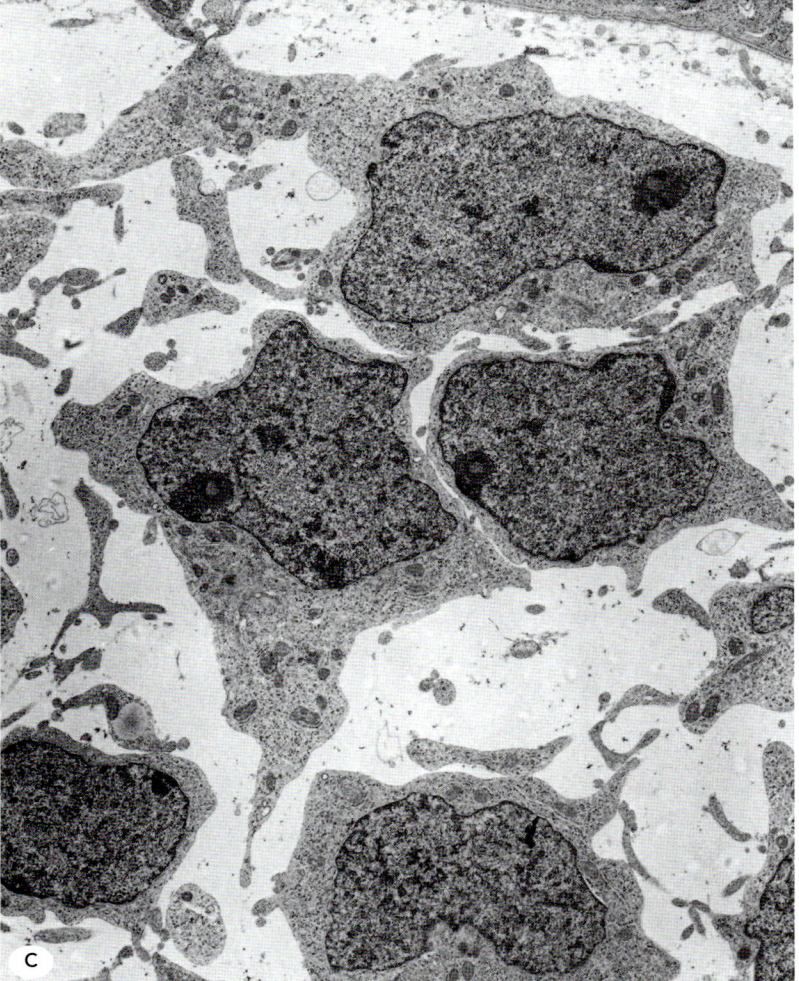

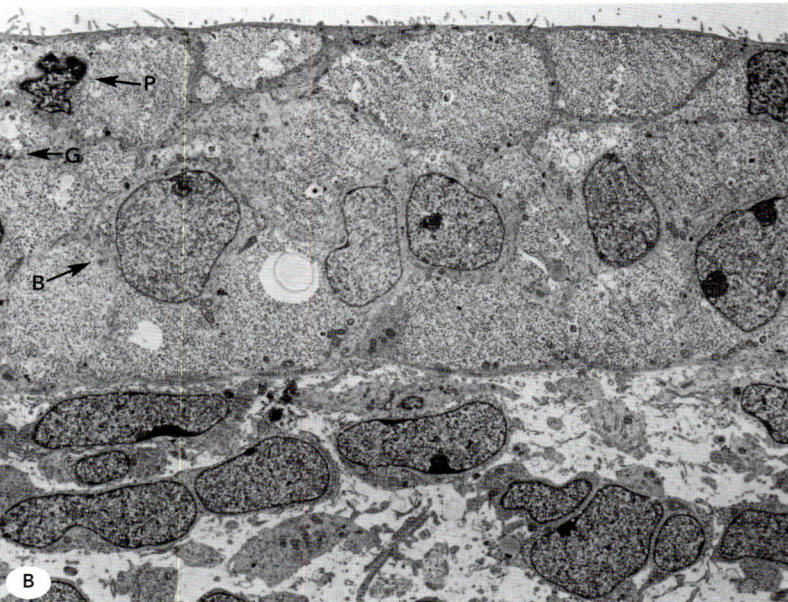

Fig. 1.3   Light and transmission electron micrographs of human embryonic skin. (**A** and **B**) The two-layered epidermis consists of glycogen-filled (G) basal (B) and periderm (P) cells. In **A** the presumptive dermis is delineated by large vascular channels (V). (**C**) The dermis is largely cellular with little fibrous connective tissue. (A) × 350; (B) × 3500; (C) × 5300.

It is now generally agreed that Merkel cells originate *in situ* from epidermal keratinocytes.[22–27] Both cells contain keratins and form desmosomes with adjacent cells. Adult Merkel cells are easily recognized by characteristic neuropeptides, but in the fetal epidermis detection of these cells relies on the presence of keratins that are unique to Merkel cells (K8, K18, and K20). Merkel cells are known to be plentiful in adult palmar skin. Antibodies to K20[28] have been used to recognize Merkel cells as early as 56 days EGA[26] or week 8.[25] No other morphologic markers (e.g., dense-core granules) are apparent at this stage.

THE DERMAL–EPIDERMAL JUNCTION

The epidermis is associated with a basement membrane at the DEJ at all embryonic and fetal ages. Ultrastructural images of this region show the basal keratinocytes physically separated from the lamina densa by a clear zone known as the lamina lucida. Several molecules and antigens that are characteristic of all basement membranes (e.g., type IV collagen, laminin, heparan sulfate proteoglycan, nidogen/entactin), regardless of the epithelia with which they are associated, are also present in the embryonic DEJ. Skin-specific antigens are added to various regions of the DEJ coincident with epidermal

22. Moll I, Moll R, Franke W (1986) Formation of epidermal and dermal Merkel cells during human fetal skin development. **J Invest Dermatol** 87:779.

23. Moll R, Moll I, Franke W (1984) Identification of Merkel cells in human skin by specific cytokeratin antibodies: changes in cell density and distribution in fetal and adult plantar epidermis. **Differentiation** 28:136.

24. Moll I, Lane A, Franke W et al. (1990) Intraepidermal formation of Merkel cells in xenografts of human fetal skin. **J Invest Dermatol** 94:359.

25. Moll I, Moll R (1992) Early development of human Merkel cells. **Exp Dermatol** 1:180.

26. Kim D-G, Holbrook KA (1995) The appearance, density and distribution of Merkel cells in human embryonic and fetal skin: their relation to sweat gland and hair follicle development. **J Invest Dermatol** 104:241.

27. Narisawa Y, Hashimoto K (1991) Immunohistochemical distribution of nerve–Merkel cell complex in fetal human skin. **J Dermatol Sci** 2:361.

28. Moll R, Schiller D, Franke W (1990) Identification of protein IT of the intestinal cytoskeleton as a novel type I cytokeratin with unusual properties and expression patterns. **J Cell Biol** 111:567.

stratification at the embryonic–fetal transition of development.[29] Early stages of hemidesmosome formation are evident morphologically but these structures are sparse and incomplete in structure.[30] Occasional strands of fine filamentous material (anchoring filaments) can be seen crossing the lamina lucida.[30]

THE DERMIS

The embryonic dermis is a loose network of mesenchymal cells with little intervening fibrous connective tissue matrix.[31–33] The high water content and hyaluronic-acid rich environment promotes cell migration during all phases of active tissue morphogenesis.[34] Types I, III, V, and VI interstitial collagens are present in the earliest embryonic skin samples obtainable, but the fiber bundles contain few fibrils and are associated primarily with the surfaces of fibroblastic cells and in the zone subjacent to the DEJ.[16,32,33] The latter zone, sometimes called the compact mesenchyme, is also a site that contains sulfated proteoglycans and is rich in growth factors.[35] At later stages the collagens become distributed in accord with the adult pattern of deposition.[32] Elastic fibers are not present in embryonic dermis although both fibrillin and elastin proteins of the elastic fiber have been identified immunohistochemically and visualized by confocal microscopy (Smith and Sakai, unpublished observations), and microfibrillar structures are seen by electron microscopy.[1]

Small capillary-like vessels are evident in the embryonic dermis.[36] They are sparse and do not appear to be organized as yet into patterns. Nerve fibers are recognized by immunostaining embryonic skin with antibodies to the p75 low-affinity nerve growth factor receptor. Fine fibers in the dermis connect with large nerve trunks located at the dermal–subcutaneous junction.

THE HYPODERMIS

It is difficult to distinguish subcutaneous tissue from dermis in the embryonic skin because the cells are quite similar and adipose tissue is synthesized considerably later in development. There is frequently, however, a difference in the density and/or orientation of the mesenchymal cells in the two regions, and, large, dilated channels (presumptive lymphatics), organized in the plane of the skin form an arbitrary boundary (Fig. 1.3A). In some regions of the body there is also a greater density of fibrous connective tissue in the subcutaneous tissue compared with the dermis.

THE POTENTIAL OF EMBRYONIC SKIN TO DIFFERENTIATE

The potential of embryonic skin to differentiate apart from systemic influences has been studied using suspension organ culture and raft organ culture systems. Samples of skin placed into suspension organ culture form closed spherules within the first few days after explantation. The epidermis is on the external surface and the dermis and subcutaneous tissue are internal. The spherules grow in diameter and can be maintained for as long as 60 days *in vitro*.[35,37] The epidermis stratifies into several layers but, except for a few isolated cells, it does not keratinize and further events of morphogenesis such

as follicle formation are not initiated. Epidermal and dermal integrity are maintained. In contrast, embryonic skin in raft organ culture shows changes in the epidermis that mimic differentiation but the dermis degenerates rather rapidly *in vitro* and the epidermis and dermis separate at the DEJ. Without the dermal support (influence) the epidermis stratifies, keratinizes, and dies at a rate that reflects the age of the tissue.[38,39] Younger samples of skin survive longer in culture before undergoing terminal differentiation.[38] Maintenance of a healthy dermis and dermal–epidermal adhesion appear to regulate the development of the epidermis in organ culture and to maintain it in the state at which it existed when explanted. Not surprisingly, samples of embryonic skin were maintained and proceeded toward normal differentiation when they were explanted into the kidney capsule, anterior chamber of the eye, or subcutaneously into the nude mouse.[40,41]

SKIN DEVELOPMENT AT THE EMBRYONIC–FETAL TRANSITION THROUGH THE END OF THE FIRST TRIMESTER

Remarkable changes in the structure and biochemistry of the skin occur around 60 days EGA when the embryo becomes a fetus (Fig. 1.2), a period that is defined by the onset of bone marrow function. From this time to the end of the first trimester all regions of the skin acquire features that establish a template of adult skin.

THE EPIDERMIS

The first obvious change in the structure of the skin at the embryonic–fetal transition is the stratification of the epidermis to basal, intermediate, and periderm cell layers. The cells of the first intermediate layer show little difference in morphology from the basal cells; they have a high glycogen content (Fig. 1.4B) and the few organelles are positioned around the nucleus and at the cell borders. There are larger and more densely staining bundles of keratin filaments located in the peripheral cytoplasm where they are associated with desmosomes (Fig. 1.4B). Intermediate cells stain with antibodies that recognize the higher molecular weight, differentiation-specific keratins (K1 and K10) of the adult stratified, keratinized epidermis.[2,3] This indicates that as soon as the basal keratinocytes divide and a layer of intermediate cells is added, the tissue is "differentiated" in terms of the expression of adult epidermal keratins. Other markers of differentiation are present in the intermediate layer cells (e.g., involucrin, keratolinin, loricrin).[1,31] Once the intermediate layer is formed, the basal layer begins to lose some of its glycogen content and thus appears to begin to acquire more of the adultlike features of basal keratinocytes. Glycogen is common in cells of fetal tissues where it may serve as an energy source; it occupies a significant volume of fetal keratinocytes and fibroblasts through the first and second trimester but diminishes in later stages of development toward birth.

The epidermis continues to stratify by additional intermediate cell layers during the second trimester of development (Fig. 1.4A and B). All cells of the fetal epidermis, including the periderm, can divide during the first trimester, but around the end of month 3 this ability appears to become restricted primarily to basal keratinocytes.[39,42]

29. Fine J-D, Smith LT, Holbrook KA et al. (1984) The appearance of four basement membrane zone antigens in developing human fetal skin. J Invest Dermatol 83:66.
30. McMillan JR, Eady RAJ (1996) Hemidesmosome ontogeny in human fetal skin. Arch Dermatol Res 288:91–97.
31. Holbrook KA (1991) Structural and biochemical organogenesis of skin and cutaneous appendages in the fetus and neonate. In: Neonatal and Fetal Medicine, Physiology and Pathophysiology, Polin RA, Fox WW, eds. New York: Grune & Stratton, p. 527.
32. Smith LT, Holbrook KA, Madri JM (1986) Collagen types I, III and V in human embryonic and fetal skin. Am J Anat 175:501.
33. Smith LT (1994) Patterns of type VI collagen compared to types I, III and V collagen in human embryonic and fetal skin and in fetal-skin derived cell cultures. Matrix Biol 14:159.
34. Breen M, Weinstein HG, Johnson RL et al. (1970) Acid glycosaminoglycans in human skin during fetal development and in adult life. Biochim Biophys Acta 201:54.
35. Holbrook KA, Smith LT, Kaplan ED et al. (1993) Expression of morphogens during human follicle development *in vivo* and a model for studying follicle morphogenesis *in vitro*. J Invest Dermatol 101:39S.

36. Johnson CL, Holbrook KA (1989) Development of human embryonic and fetal dermal vasculature. J Invest Dermatol 93:10S.
37. Holbrook KA, Minami SA (1991) Hair follicle morphogenesis in the human: characterization of events *in vivo* and *in vitro*. NY Acad Sci 642:167.
38. Fisher C, Holbrook KA (1987) Cell surface and cytoskeletal changes associated with epidermal stratification in organ cultures of embryonic human skin. Dev Biol 119:231.
39. Bickenbach JR, Holbrook KA (1986) Proliferation of human embryonic and fetal epidermis in organ culture. Am J Anat 177:97.
40. Holbrook KA, Fisher C, Dale BA et al. (1988) Morphogenesis of hair follicles during ontogeny of the human skin. In: The Biology of Wool and Hair, Rogers GE, Reis PJ, Ward KA, Marshall RC, eds. New York: Chapman & Hall, p. 15.
41. Lane AT, Scott GA, Day KH (1989) Development of human fetal skin transplanted to the nude mouse. J Invest Dermatol 93:787.
42. Bickenbach JR, Holbrook KA (1987) Label-retaining cells in human embryonic and fetal epidermis. J Invest Dermatol 88:42.

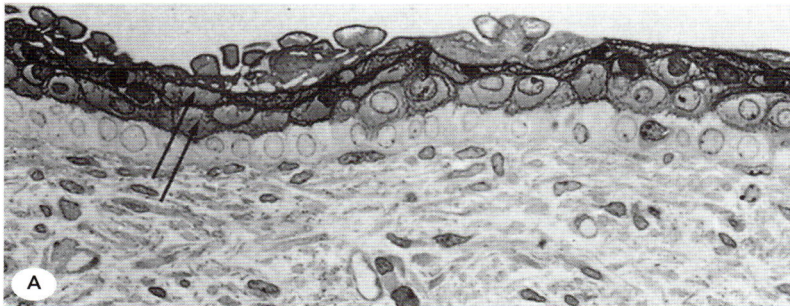

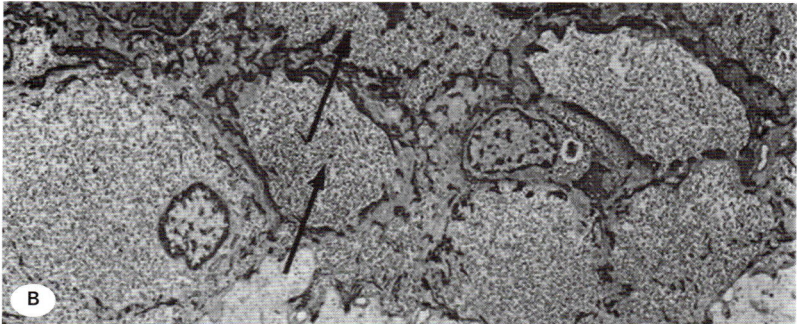

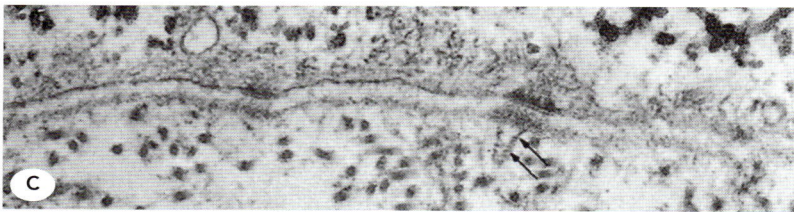

Fig. 1.4   Light and electron micrographs of human fetal skin (**A** and **B**) after epidermal stratification starts (13 to 15 weeks EGA). New intermediate layer cells are present between the basal and periderm layers. These cells (**B**) contain abundant glycogen (arrows) and keratin filaments are evident at the periphery of the cell. (**C**) Note the presence of complete hemidesmosomes and anchoring fibril-like structures (arrows) at the dermal epidermal junction of skin from a 70-day EGA fetus. (**A**) × 350; (**B**) × 3500; (**C**) × 38 000. (B with permission from Holbrook KA (1983) The biology of human total skin at ages related to prenatal diagnosis. **Ped Dermatol** 1:99.)

Periderm cells at this stage have a large volume of cytoplasm and appear rounded in surface view. At later ages within the same period one or more blebs project from the surfaces of periderm cells[5] (Figs 1.2C and 1.4A, B); they remain densely covered by microvilli and retain in their cytoplasm the same keratin proteins that were recognized earlier.

The nonkeratinocytes of the epidermis are easily distinguished from one another in the stratified epidermis by their morphologic and antigenic properties. Langerhans cells are recognized both by the same surface markers expressed in embryonic epidermis and now also by CD1a expression,[19–21] which appears rather abruptly around 80 days EGA. The number of Langerhans cells in the epidermis does not increase significantly until the third trimester and after birth.[20,21] Langerhans cell granules are evident in the cytoplasm, suggesting that the cells already may be involved in antigen procession and presentation.

Melanocytes reach a remarkably high density (~3000 cells/mm²) in the fetal epidermis of about 80 days EGA.[21] The labeling index of epidermal keratinocytes is also high at this stage.[39,42] The rise in both cell populations may be coordinated; they may respond to a common influence that stimulates proliferation or one may influence the other. Alternatively, there may be a time-specific new influx of neural crest cells. The uniformly regular distribution of melanocytes in epidermal sheet preparations[21] suggests that the relationship between keratinocytes and melanocytes does not occur by chance.

Melanosomes first appear in the cytoplasm of melanocytes around 65 days EGA depending on the region of the body and the race of the fetus. The eyelids, external auditory meatus, and labial mucosa appear to have melanin-producing melanocytes before they are evident in the skin in other regions,[43,44] but the cells are present only transiently in these structures. Stage I premelanosomes or stage II melanosomes, in which the internal filamentous structure is evident, are evident in general body epidermal melanocytes in the first trimester; there is little if any melanin synthesis. Melanocytes begin to transfer melanosomes to keratinocytes in the fifth month of gestation. Studies of HMB-45 immunostained, epidermal sheets have revealed that the density of immunopositive cells decreases toward birth, probably reflecting the growth of the fetus. The total cutaneous numbers at this time appear to be similar to the total numbers of the melanocytes in newborn epidermis.[45]

Merkel cells have been demonstrated at 8 weeks EGA in fetal palmar and plantar skin,[23,26] although the density of cells at this stage was low and quite variable.[26] By 80 to 90 days EGA, the density was as great as 1400 cells/mm³,[26] and by 22 to 24 weeks EGA 1700 cells/mm² were measured in the tissue.[23] At both ages, the cells were organized specifically along the primary epidermal ridges. This is the expected location because Merkel cells in adult skin are commonly found in association with hair follicles and sweat glands and both of these appendages are beginning to form during this stage of fetal development. Merkel cells were first seen in hairy skin at 75 days EGA where they were located in the infundibulum and bulge regions of the developing hair pegs and bulbous hair pegs.[26,46] Merkel cells are frequently associated with nerve fibers. They may serve as target structures for the ingrowth of nerve fibers, possibly through the synthesis and use of nerve growth factor, or they may attract other cells (e.g., smooth muscle cells of the arrector pili muscle[46,47]) that are associated with nerve fibers in the skin.

INITIATION OF EPIDERMAL APPENDAGES

The basal epidermal cells give rise not only to cells of the intermediate layer, but also form the epidermal appendages. In accord with this activity, they store less glycogen in their cytoplasm and assume a more adultlike basal cell morphology.[47] At approximately 80 days EGA, the pilosebaceous structures begin to form, first as hair germs that are recognized as groups of basal cells that bulge into the dermis.[1,35,48] Hair germs are distributed in regular patterns depending on the body region. Follicle formation begins on the head and proceeds in a cephalocaudal direction. Collections of fibroblasts associate closely with the developing germs to become cells of both the dermal papilla that will influence the formation of the hair fiber and the connective tissue sheaths that surround the follicle. The interchange of messages between the epithelial and mesenchymal cells of the follicle induce and promote follicle morphogenesis, then maintain the fully formed follicle and regulate certain aspects of the hair cycle. There has been considerable descriptive and experimental work to investigate the nature of the inductive signals between these two populations of cells at all stages.[35,49] Hair germs grow into the dermis over the next several weeks *in utero* as elongated cords of cells from

43. Becker SW, Zimmerman AA (1955) Further studies on melanocytes and melanogenesis in human fetus and newborn. J Invest Dermatol 25:103.
44. Barla-Szabo L (1970) Ejection of melanocytes and melanin from fetuses and newborn mammalian animals. Acta Morphol Acad Sci Hung 18:213.
45. Hamada H (1970) Age changes in melanocyte distribution of the normal, human epidermis. Jpn J Dermatol 82:223.
46. Narisawa Y, Hashimoto K, Nakamura Y et al. (1993) A high concentration of Merkel cells in the bulge prior to the attachment of the arrector pili muscle and the formation of the perifollicular nerve plexus in human fetal skin. Arch Dermatol Res 285:261.
47. Sharp F (1971) A quantitative study of the glycogen content of human fetal skin in the first trimester. J Obstet Gynaecol Br Commonw 78:981.
48. Pinkus H (1958) Embryology of Hair. In: The Hair Growth, Montagna W, Ellis RA, eds. New York: Academic Press, p. 1.
49. Kaplan ED, Holbrook KA (1994) Dynamic expression patterns of tenascin, proteoglycans and cell adhesion molecules during human hair follicle morphogenesis. Dev Dynam 199:141.

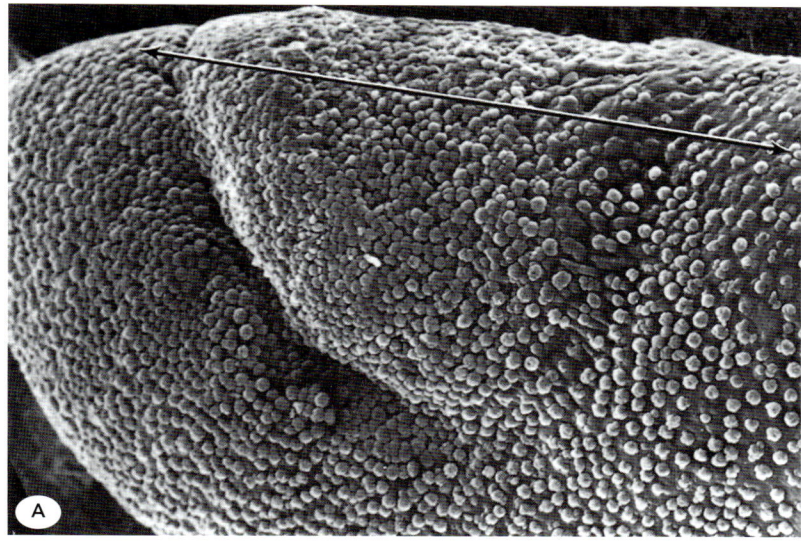

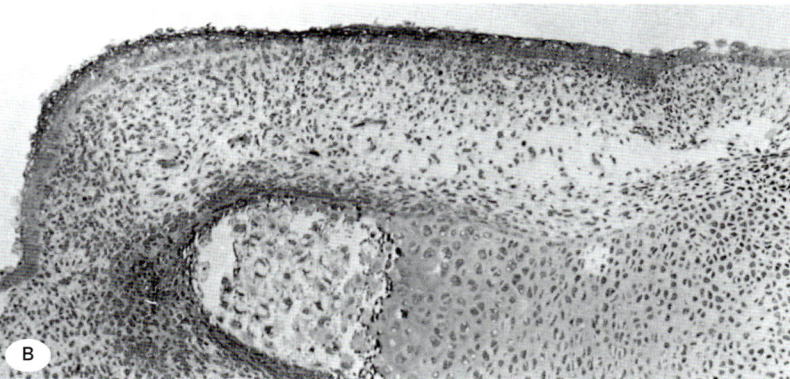

Fig. 1.5   Scanning and light micrographs of the developing nail. In (**A**) the boundaries of the nail field are marked by folds. In (**B**) note the differentiation of the epidermis of the presumptive nail plate. (A) × 150; (B) × 125.

which the primordia of the apocrine gland, sebaceous gland, and the "bulge" develop. The bulge marks the approximate site for the attachment of the arrector pili muscle and, in terminal hairs, the level where the proximal, permanent portion of the follicle ends and the distal, transient portion begins. It is also the presumptive location of follicle stem cells.[50,51] Details of follicle development are reviewed elsewhere.[2,35,49]

The suspension organ culture system mentioned earlier offers an opportunity to learn more about the regulation of hair follicle morphogenesis. Tissue sampled from a fetus during a critical window of time (60–80 days EGA) will initiate follicle morphogenesis *in vitro*. Follicle germs will continue to develop to the hair peg stage before arresting this process. Various factors can be tested in the culture to determine if/how they may influence the process.[35,37]

Tooth buds and nails also begin to form around 10 to 11 weeks EGA.[52] The boundaries of the presumptive nail field are delineated on the dorsal surface of the digit by lateral and proximal grooves that define the position and shape of the nail bed (Fig. 1.5A) and the distally located, dorsal ridge. The nail fold is evident in sectioned specimens (Fig. 1.5B). The ventral portion of the fold, the nail matrix, will contribute cells to the nail plate. The dorsal ridge keratinizes around 11 weeks EGA;[52] keratinization then spreads over the nail bed toward the nail fold. The first, soft nail is easily sloughed and is replaced in the fourth month by the hard nail that is synthesized from cells of the ventral matrix.[52,53] The nails are the earliest structures of the skin to keratinize *in utero*. The role of the mesenchyme in supporting epithelial morphogenesis associated with nail formation has not received much investigation, but because this tissue plays a significant role in the morphogenesis of other epithelial derivatives, it is likely that it is critical in nail formation as well.

Sweat gland formation is initiated on the palms and soles around 10 to 12 weeks EGA (Fig. 1.6). Primary epidermal ridges organize from the basal epidermal layer. Sweat gland formation elsewhere on the body does not begin until several weeks later. Mounds of mesenchyme that underlie the epidermis accumulate on the ventral surface of the digits. The shape and composition of these volar pads are thought to influence the dermatoglyphic patterns.[54] The volar pads are transient during early stages of digit morphogenesis and are largely gone by the end of the first trimester.[55]

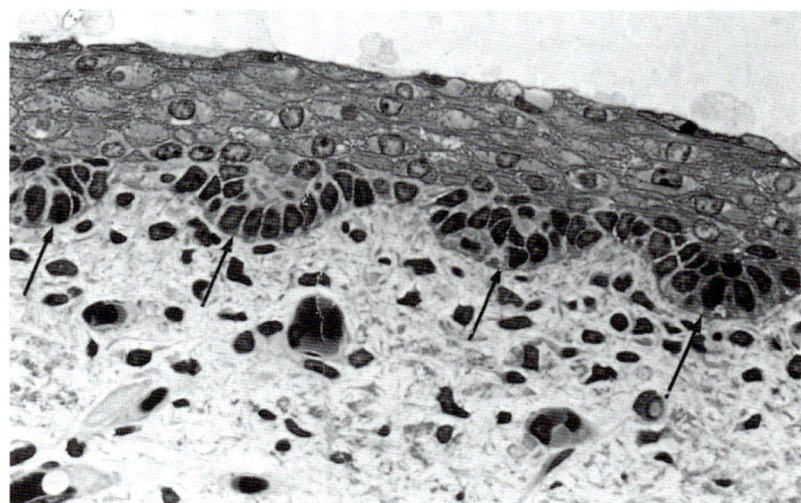

Fig. 1.6   Light micrograph of the epidermis from the plantar surface of a digit of a late first trimester human fetus. Note the thickness of the epidermis and the primary epidermal ridges (arrows) that mark the onset of development of the sweat ducts and glands (× 350).

THE DERMAL–EPIDERMAL JUNCTION

Changes in the structure and composition of the DEJ parallel epidermal stratification. The basal keratinocytes synthesize the components of the hemidesmosomes, anchoring filaments, and anchoring fibrils. Fibroblasts of the papillary dermis contribute collagens and components of elastic fibrils (e.g., oxytalan fibers) to the connective tissue matrix of the sublamina densa.[31] Hemidesmosomes are now complete in structure and anchoring filaments and anchoring fibrils organize in relation to these sites.[30] It has been suggested from studies of chick cornea that there may be an interdependent relationship

50. Cotsarelis G, Sun TT, Lavker RM (1990) Label-retaining cells reside in the bulge area of pilosebaceous unit: implications for follicular stem cells, hair cycle and skin carcinogenesis. **Cell** 61:1329.
51. Lavker RM, Miller S, Wilson C et al. (1993) Hair follicle stem cells: their location, role in hair cycle, and involvement in skin tumor formation. **J Invest Dermatol** 101:16S.
52. Zaias N (1963) Embryology of the human nail. **Arch Dermatol** 87:37.
53. Hashimoto K, Gross BG, Nelson R et al. (1966) The ultrastructure of the skin of human embryos. III. The formation of the nail in the 16–18 weeks old embryo. **J Invest Dermatol** 47:205.
54. Mulvihill JJ, Smith DW (1969) The genesis of dermatoglyphics. **J Pediatr** 75:597.
55. Hirsch W, Schweichel JU (1973) Morphological evidence concerning the problem of skin ridge formation. **J Ment Defic Res** 17:58.

between hemidesmosomes and anchoring fibrils during morphogenesis.[56] If this is correct, it cannot be a dependent relationship because patients with junctional epidermolysis bullosa (EB) who lack hemidesmosomes do not lack anchoring fibrils,[57] and vice versa in the case of individuals with recessive dystrophic EB who do not have anchoring fibrils but whose hemidesmosomes assemble normally.[58] Several of the antigens that correlate with these structures are expressed in the DEJ at the time of the embryonic fetal transition.[59,60]

THE DERMIS

During the remainder of the first trimester, the mesenchymal cells differentiate into fibroblastic cells and the dermis becomes less cellular and watery as more fibrous connective tissue accumulates in the interstitial spaces. By the end of this period, papillary and reticular regions can be distinguished on the basis of differences in cell density (higher in the papillary dermis) and orientation, fibril diameter (smaller in the papillary dermis), and fiber bundle size (smaller in the papillary dermis).[31,32,61] Approximate boundaries between the two regions are also created by the organization of the subpapillary, horizontal vascular plane. A decrease in hyaluronic acid parallels the transition of the dermis from a cellular to a fibrous tissue; the water content of the dermis still remains greater than 80%.[62] Like adult dermis, the proteoglycan composition favors the sulfated molecules.

Around 70 days EGA the basic pattern of the adult vasculature is evident in fetal dermis, in simple organization.[36] Horizontal plexuses are present within the dermis (subpapillary plexus) and separate the dermis from the subcutaneous tissue. The structure of the vessel wall is simple, making identification of vascular segments difficult. Nerve patterns are also well developed by the mid- to later first trimester and generally follow the vascular pattern, although the nerve fibers appear to be a little more "aggressive" in their ascent toward the epidermis.

Thus, the beginning of the fetal period is characterized by epidermal stratification and the histogenesis of various tissues of the skin. Epidermal stratification coincides with the onset of tooth, nail, and follicle morphogenesis, the addition of antigens and adhesive structures at the DEJ, regionalization of the dermis via the organization of fibrous extracellular matrix and patterns of nerves and vessels, and the expression of surface and cytoplasmic markers by melanocytes and Langerhans cells. Merkel cells are established in both hairy and glabrous skin.

SKIN DEVELOPMENT DURING THE SECOND TRIMESTER: LANDMARKS OF FOLLICULAR AND INTERFOLLICULAR KERATINIZATION

THE EPIDERMIS

By 15 weeks' gestation, the interfollicular epidermis is stratified further with one or two additional layers of intermediate cells, but until the end of the second trimester there is no evidence of keratinization (Fig. 1.7). The adult pattern of keratin polypeptides is maintained in the basal cells (K5 and K14) and the suprabasal keratinocytes of all intermediate layers express K1 and K10. Keratin filaments have continued to increase in quantity in the intermediate layers. Glycogen remains a significant component (Fig. 1.8).

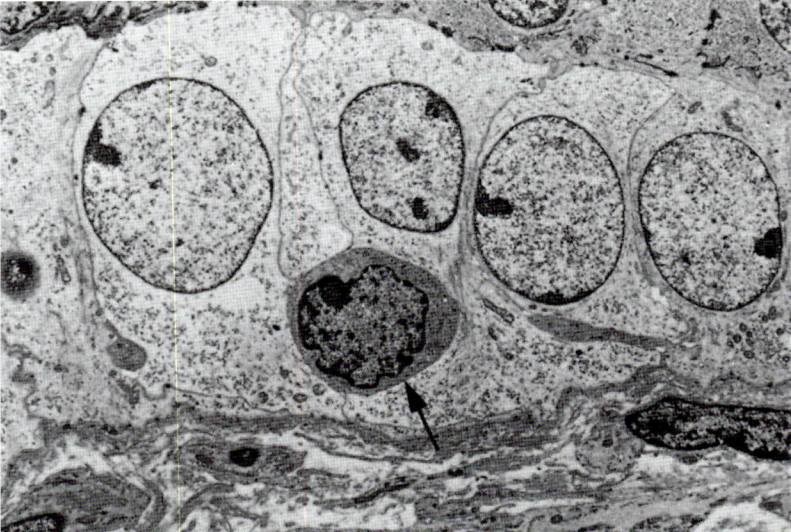

Fig. 1.7 Electron micrograph of the skin at the time of follicular keratinization. The epidermis is several layers in thickness. An accumulation of keratin filaments at the periphery of the intermediate cells is evident. Note the melanocyte (arrow) among keratinocytes of the basal layer (× 3500) (From Holbrook K (1983) The biology of human total skin at ages related to prenatal diagnosis. **Ped Dermatol** 1:99. with permission.)

The surface of the skin is still covered by a complete layer of periderm. The nondividing, periderm cells have attained a peak stage of structural modification in which one or more simple or complex blebs project from the surface; all portions of the periderm cells facing the amniotic cavity are covered with microvilli[5] (Figs 1.2D and 1.7). Both of these features serve to increase the external surface area of the skin markedly, suggesting a role for the periderm (skin) in the exchange of substances between the fetus and the amniotic fluid. The internal morphology of the cells, however, is variable. Some of the cells contain the organelles associated with active metabolic processes (e.g., mitochondria, rough endoplasmic reticulum, Golgi, etc.); others have few organelles and are filled with filaments (Fig. 1.7). The latter cells also have a thickened cell envelope, which is morphologically and biochemically equivalent to the cornified cell envelope. Involucrin, keratolinin, and loricrin have been identified at the boundary of the periderm cell[63] and an active epidermal transglutaminase is present that appears able to cross-link the envelope proteins.[9,63] It is not certain if these molecules are expressed as markers of differentiation or of a dying cell. At later stages of this period (~18 weeks) the periderm cells flatten, the blebs regress to small, buttonlike protrusions,[9] and the subcellular morphology is indicative of a nonfunctional, perhaps nonviable, apoptotic remnant of this tissue[10] (Fig. 1.2E).

Between 22 and 24 weeks EGA the interfollicular epidermis begins to keratinize; the exact timing depends on the region of the body.[64] Early evidence for keratinization is the appearance of lamellar granules and small keratohyalin granules in the uppermost intermediate cell layer. This is the first age at which filaggrin is expressed in the fetal interfollicular epidermis,[2] thus the onset of filaggrin synthesis appears to correlate precisely with the mor-

56. Gipson IK, Spurr-Michaud SJ, Tisdale AS (1988) Hemidesmosomes and anchoring fibril collagen appear synchronously during development and wound healing. **Dev Biol** 126:253.

57. Tidman MJ, Eady RAJ (1986) Hemidesmosome heterogeneity in junctional epidermolysis bullosa revealed by morphometric analysis. **J Invest Dermatol** 86:51–56.

58. Tidman MJ, Eady RAJ (1985) Evaluation of anchoring fibrils and other components of the dermal-epidermal junction in dystrophic epidermolysis bullosa by a quantitative ultrastructural technique. **J Invest Dermatol** 84:374–377.

59. Fine J-D, Horiguchi Y, Couchman JR (1989) 19-DEJ-1, a hemidesmosomal-anchoring filament complex associated monoclonal antibody: definition of a new skin basement membrane antigenic defect in junctional and dystrophic epidermolysis bullosa. **Arch Dermatol** 125:520.

60. Smith LT, Sakai LY, Burgeson RE et al. (1988) Ontogeny of structural components at the dermal-epidermal junction in human embryonic and fetal skin: the appearance of anchoring fibrils and type VII collagen. **J Invest Dermatol** 90:480.

61. Smith LT, Holbrook KA, Byers PH (1982) Structure of the dermal matrix during development and in the adult. **J Invest Dermatol** 79:93S.

62. Widdowson EM (1969) Changes in the extracellular compartment of muscle and skin during normal and retarded development. **Bibl Nutr Dieta** 13:60.

63. Holbrook KA, Underwood RA, Dale BA et al. (1991) Cornified cell envelope (CCE) in human fetal skin: involucrin, keratolinin, loricrin and transglutaminase expression and activity, abstracted. **J Invest Dermatol** 96:542.

64. Holbrook KA, Odland GF (1980) Regional development of the human epidermis in the first trimester embryo and the second trimester fetus (ages related to the timing of amniocentesis and fetal biopsy). **J Invest Dermatol** 80:161.

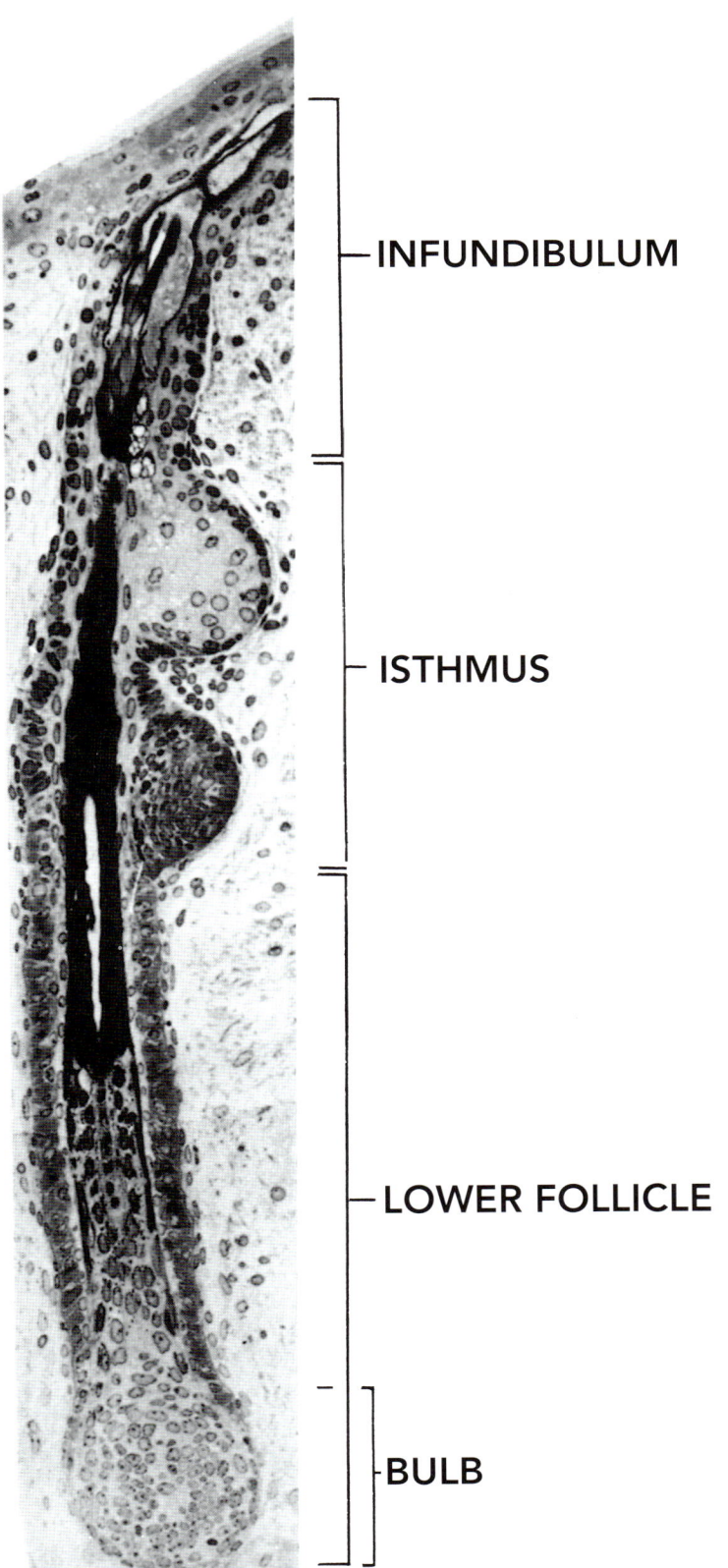

INFUNDIBULUM

ISTHMUS

LOWER FOLLICLE

BULB

Fig. 1.8   Light micrograph of a developing hair follicle from a 15-week EGA human fetus. The regions of the follicle and the sebaceous gland (SG) and bulge (B) are identified. Note keratinization of the developing hair and of the lining of the hair canal in the region of the infundibulum and within the epidermis (× 400). (Holbrook K (1983) The biology of human total skin at ages related to prenatal diagnosis. **Ped Dermatol** 1:99.)

phologic appearance of keratohyalin granules. The first few layers of cells that keratinize are a combination of "regressed" periderm cells (cells that contain primarily filaments and have a cornified cell envelope) and incompletely keratinized keratinocytes; the latter cells are characterized by a condensed nucleus, dense organelles, cornified cell envelope, and flattened shape of the stratum corneum cell. The numbers of layers of keratinized cells and the size of keratohyalin granules gradually increase so that the epidermis of the third trimester fetus appears similar to that of the neonate and adult with the exception that glycogen remains in the cytoplasm of the keratinocytes. Coincident with keratinization, the periderm is sloughed from most of the skin surface revealing the underlying keratinized epidermis.

The surface of the skin is coated with the lipid–rich material of the vernix caseosa, a combination of sebum secreted from the sebaceous gland of the follicle, epidermal lipids, desquamated cells, hair and other tissue debris, and certain other lipids that are unique to this material alone.[65,66] Like sebum, the vernix contains a significant level of triglycerides and wax esters, and like cornified cells it has a high proportion of sterols. Other lipids that are not characteristic of either of these sources contribute to the unique content of this material.[65] Vernix caseosa is often apparent on the skin at birth. It is not clear if there is a benefit from this substance to the fetal skin in its late stages of development or to the neonatal skin. In the premature infant, it is suggested to augment the as yet poorly established barrier properties of the epidermis or to serve as a natural emollient. The skin of the premature infant is more resistant to desquamation than that of the term newborn and has a more gelatinous quality. Both of these properties may be a consequence of the vernix.

HAIR FOLLICLE MATURATION

There can be a hiatus of as much as 10 weeks between keratinization of structures of the epidermal appendages and keratinization of the interfollicular epidermis. Keratinization of the follicle begins around 15 weeks EGA.

At the beginning of the second trimester, the follicle is an elongated cord of cells consisting of a cellular core and an outer cellular layer. In general, the core cells are similar to intermediate layer epidermal cells and the cells of the external layer are more like cells of the basal epidermal layer. The hair peg grows and differentiates to become the bulbous hair peg (a structure named for the terminal bulb of the follicle)[37,48] (Fig. 1.7), around 12 to 14 weeks EGA when primordia of the sebaceous gland, bulge, and the apocrine gland are recognized (Fig. 1.8).[37,48] Lipid is synthesized in the sebaceous gland around 15 weeks EGA. Simultaneously smooth muscle cells of the arrector pili muscle grow toward and attach to the follicle in the region of the bulge.[67] The bulge is an exceptionally large structure in the developing and lanugo follicle and thus potentially available for extirpation and analysis of the cells *in vitro*. The apocrine gland grows as a short cord of cells that originates from the infundibular portion of the follicle; apocrine glands persist and continue

65. Kurkkainen J, Nikkari T, Ruponen S et al. (1965) Lipids of the vernix caseosa. J Invest Dermatol 44:333.

66. Nazarro-Porro M, Possi S, Boniforti L et al. (1979) Effects of aging on fatty acids in skin surface lipids. J Invest Dermatol 73:112.

67. Akiyama M, Dale BA, Sun TT, Holbrook KA (1995) Characterization of hair follicle bulge in human fetal skin: the human fetal bulge is a pool of undifferentiated keratinocytes. J Invest Dermatol 105:844–850.

to develop only in specialized regions of the body. The mechanisms for establishing these precisely positioned structures are unknown. The terminus of the bulbous hair peg has a concavity within which cells of the dermal papilla are sequestered.

Regulation of the exquisite differentiation of regions of the follicle is of great interest. Remarkable changes in cytoplasmic proteins and the surface receptors of the follicle cells and in the cells and matrix surrounding the follicle occur during this period of differentiation.[9,35,49] The differences in expression of these molecule factors, matrix proteins, growth factors, and receptors in the cells of the follicle, the basement membrane zone of the follicle, and the dermal papilla and cells and sheaths surrounding the follicle provide some level of understanding of the complexity of this molecular signaling during development. They may also provide some clues about the regulation of the hair cycle after birth.

Cells that form the hair and the hair canal begin to keratinize about 15 weeks EGA.[2,35,68] Hair canals are channels through which hairs extend as they grow toward the skin surface.[68] They are recognized in sections through the epidermis as tangential channels surrounded by concentric layers of granular and cornified cells. These are the only keratohyalin-containing (and filaggrin-positive) cells within the epidermis at 15 to 17 weeks EGA. Expression of

filaggrin by cells of the follicle allows the follicle to be evaluated in the skin of a fetus at risk for a disorder of keratinization (e.g., lamellar ichthyosis). At later stages (18 to 21 weeks EGA) the hair canals can be seen as elongated ridges visible at the epidermal surface. The integrity of the periderm is disrupted along the tops of the ridges where the hair canal will rupture and open to the surface. The length of the canals, the time of hair release, and the density of the hair is dependent on the region of the body.[31,68] The position of eyebrow and scalp hairs can be recognized as early as 15 weeks EGA by the presence of short, closely positioned, periderm-covered hair canals. At 21 weeks the hair canals on the trunk begin to rupture, interrupting the continuity of the periderm over the body surface and releasing a fully elongated hair.[68]

THE DERMIS

The second trimester dermis contains an extensive amount of fibrous connective tissue, including elastic fibers. The elastic microfibrils are synthesized early in development but, based on studies in which fetal skin fibroblasts of this age were assayed for elastin mRNA expression,[69] the elastin gene does not appear to be expressed until approximately 15 weeks

---

TABLE 1.1   A comparison of the structural features of premature, newborn, and adult skin

	Premature[a]	Newborn	Adult
Full thickness skin	0.9mm	1.2mm	2.1mm
Epidermal surface	Vernix ("gelatinous")	Vernix	Dry
Epidermal thickness	20–25µm	~40–50µm	~50µm
Stratum corneum thickness	4–5µm 5–6 cell layers	9–10µm 15+ cell layers	9–15µm 15+ cell layers
Spinous cell content	Glycogen	Little or no glycogen	No glycogen
Melanocytes	Numbers of cells; few mature melanosomes	Similar to number of cells in young adult; low melanin production	Numbers decrease with age; melanin production depends on the individual, region, etc.
Dermal–epidermal junction	Structural components similar to adult although the number and size of hemidesmosomes is less than the adult; all known adult antigens expressed	Structural features and antigens similar to those of the adult	Well-developed attachment and adhesive structures; large number of antigens expressed that may be markers for disease
Papillary dermis			
Boundary with the reticular dermis	Present but not marked	Present but not marked	Marked
Size of collagen fiber bundles	Small	Small	Small
Density of cells	Abundant	Abundant	Abundant
Reticular dermis			
Boundary with the hypodermis	Marked	Marked	Marked
Size of collagen fiber bundles	Small	Small–intermediate	Large
Density of cells	Abundant	Moderately abundant	Sparse
Elastic fibers	Tiny, immature in structure and sparse	Small size and immature in structure; distribution similar to adult	Large in reticular dermis, small and immature in papillary and intermediate dermis; network
Hypodermis	Well-developed fatty layer	Well-developed fatty layer	Well-developed fatty layer

[a] Features are more similar to newly keratinized fetal skin than to newborn or adult.

---

68. Holbrook KA, Odland GF (1978) Structure of the hair canal and the initial eruption of hair in the human fetus. J Invest Dermatol 71:385.

69. Sephel GC, Buckley A, Davidson JM (1987) Developmental initiation and elastin gene expression by human fetal skin fibroblasts. J Invest Dermatol 88:732.

EGA. Elastic fiber networks are seen in the skin by histochemical and immunohistochemical methods around 20 weeks EGA.[61,70] These fibers are immature in structure, more similar to adult elaunin fibers, and thus it is unrealistic to consider using the structure of the elastic fibers to identify a fetus at risk of a genetic disorder of elastic connective tissue such as cutis laxa. Even at birth the amount of elastin associated with elastic fibers is minimal.

THE HYPODERMIS

Coarse fiber bundles of the deep dermis clearly distinguish it from the fine connective tissue of the hypodermis. This pattern is reversed from the situation in younger skin where the density of matrix in the subcutaneous tissue is greater than that of the dermis. The organization of the hypodermis is readily apparent at 15 weeks EGA, and by 18 weeks EGA there is a small accumulation of subcutaneous fat.

INITIATION OF SWEAT GLANDS ON THE BODY

The eccrine sweat glands develop on the body late in the second trimester, more than 2 months after they were initiated on the palms and soles. Assuming that epithelial–mesenchymal interactions are responsible for induction of such structures, one must surmise that the signals to initiate sweat glands on the body are different from those at earlier stages of gestation when the skin composition was significantly different. This aspect of development has not been investigated.

SKIN DEVELOPMENT IN THE THIRD TRIMESTER: IMMATURE/PREMATURE SKIN

The skin of the premature infant is that of the third trimester fetus. During this period the skin increases in bulk, primarily by the addition of connective tissue to the dermis, the epidermis is keratinized, all of the adnexae are formed, and the dermis contains all of the matrix proteins characteristic of the newborn and adult. Nonetheless, the skin is still immature in both structural and physiologic properties. Table 1.1 compares structural properties of premature, newborn, and adult skin.

THE EPIDERMIS

The epidermis has all of the layers of the adult epidermis, but it is thinner. The cells retain a substantial amount of glycogen, and the stratum corneum forms a less formidable barrier. The relatively poor barrier properties of the preterm infant are of great importance when considering topical application of various pharmacologic and cleansing compounds.[71–73] In some cases, failure to consider the enhanced permeability of the premature skin has led to systemic poisoning. The uptake of pharmacologic compounds applied topically to the skin is much more rapid in the 28- to 34-week premature newborn than in older newborns[71–73] and the loss of water through the skin and evaporative water loss from the surface decreases exponentially with increasing gestational age.[74–75] The amount of transepidermal water loss

through the skin of a 25- to 30-week EGA infant can be so substantial that death can result from dehydration.

THE DERMAL–EPIDERMAL JUNCTION

The structure of the DEJ of the premature infant correlates with the gestational age. As the age increases, the contours (rete ridges and dermal papillae) become more prominent. In the youngest (26 to 34 weeks EGA) premature infants, the DEJ is relatively flat, although the structural components of the DEJ that anneal the epidermis and dermis are well established. The papillary dermis immediately underlying the DEJ is edematous and the bundles of collagen fibrils are smaller and more widely spaced than those of the term newborn or adult, and thus the epidermal–dermal integrity might be expected to be more easily compromised than in the term newborn.[76]

The dermis of the premature infant is approximately three-quarters of the thickness of adult dermis and comparable in connective tissue organization. Fine collagen fibrils and the small-sized collagen fiber bundles give the dermis a highly cellular and delicate appearance. The water content of the dermis remains high in premature babies, but this, like many properties of the premature and newborn skin, depends on the nutritional status of the fetus in additional to gestational age.

All of the adult epidermal appendages are established in premature skin. The fully formed, hair-synthesizing lanugo follicles of fetal skin are equivalent to those of the term newborn or adult; however, the eccrine sweat glands have formed only a few coils of the glandular segment and the light and dark cells (see below) are not easily distinguishable.[76] Sweat ducts are partially occluded until the end of the seventh month.[77] The sweating response is limited or absent in premature infants[78,79] and appears to have a strong correlation with gestational age; there is a tendency toward total anhidrosis in the premature neonate,[80] although this dysfunction rapidly resolves after a few days of extrauterine life.

STRUCTURAL AND FUNCTIONAL PROPERTIES OF SKIN OF INFANTS, CHILDREN, AND ADULTS

Lowell Goldsmith

INTRODUCTION

Understanding the structure of the skin is essential for understanding the functions of skin and the alterations in skin causing disease and caused by disease. Modern molecular and biophysical techniques make the segueing from structure to function and back to structure more informative than ever before. The presumed function of skin components is often derived from comparative studies from other species, genetically constructed knockout or transgenic animals or human genetic and nongenetic diseases. All of these "functions" must be evaluated critically.

70. Deutsch TA, Esterly NB (1975) Elastic fibers in fetal dermis. **J Invest Dermatol** 65:320.
71. Nachman RL, Esterly NB (1971) Increased skin permeability in preterm infants. **J Pediatr** 79:628.
72. Webster RC, Maibach HI (1981) Comparative percutaneous absorption. In: Neonatal Skin, Maibach HI, Boisits EK, eds. New York: Marcel Dekker, p. 137.
73. West DP, Worobec S, Solomon LM (1981) Pharmacology and toxicology of infant skin. **J Invest Dermatol** 76:147.
74. Hammarlund K, Sedin G (1979) Transepidermal water loss in newborn infants. **Acta Paediatr Scand** 68:795.
75. Faranoff AA, Wald M, Gruber HS et al. (1972) Insensible water loss in low birth weight infants. **Pediatrics** 50:236.

76. Holbrook KA (1981) A histologic comparison of infant and adult skin. In: Neonatal Skin, Maibach HI, Boisits EK, eds. New York: Marcel Dekker, p. 3.
77. Borsetto PL (1951) Observazioni sullo sviluppo delle ghiandole sudoripare nelle diverse regioni della cute umana. **Arch Ital Anat Embriol** 56:332.
78. Foster KG, Hey EN, Katz G (1969) The response of sweat glands of the newborn baby to the thermal stimuli and to intradermal acetylcholine. **J Physiol (Lond)** 203:13.
79. Sinclair JC (1972) Thermal control in premature infants. **Annu Rev Med** 23:129.
80. Green M (1981) Comparison of adult and neonatal skin eccrine sweating. In: Neonatal Skin, Maibach HI, Boisits EK, eds. New York: Marcel Dekker, p. 35.

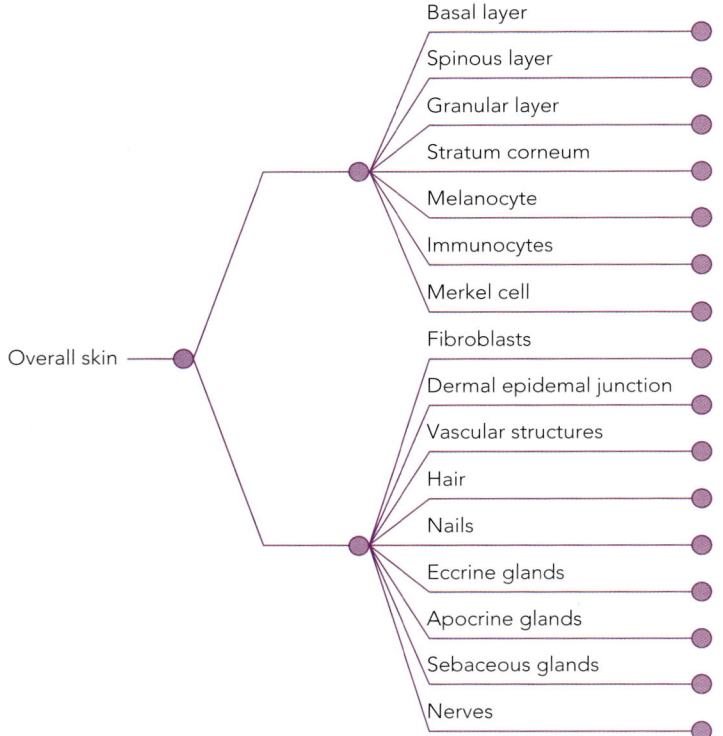

Fig. 1.9   Organization of the sections in this chapter.

This section of the text is highly structured and can be read by itself and easily referenced when tissue, cells and molecules are considered in other sections of this text. Figure 1.9 shows the outline of this main section. Subsections combine illustrative materials and text and are organized in a similar format to enhance comparisons. The alterations in disease are discussed in detail elsewhere in this book.

OVERALL SKIN STRUCTURE AND FUNCTION
(Fig. 1.10)

TISSUES

The epidermis is a highly cellular layer atop the relatively acellular dermis, which is rich in secreted extracellular molecules. The functioning of the skin is dependent on these two tissues, which contain a variety of epidermal appendages and the blood vessels and nerves, which support the nutrition, and integration of these tissues. The epidermis has a very effective strategy to make a continually regenerating living barrier, which can continuously respond to the numerous diverse external and internal stimuli that bombard the skin daily.

CELLS

Cell types in the epidermis consist of keratinocytes, including stem cells and cells at various stages of differentiation, Merkel cells, melanocytes and two cells of the immune system, Langerhans cells (antigen presentation) and γ-δ T cells (immunoregulation). The DEJ is a complex acellular structure with multiple secreted macromolecules, which support the epidermal structure and the transmittal of cells and molecules in a bidirectional fashion between the epidermis and the dermis. The dermis has a complex structure: fibroblasts in the two portions of the dermis, the papillary and the reticular dermis; mast cells; blood and lymphatic vessels; hairs; eccrine sweat glands; sebaceous glands; apocrine sweat glands; and the hair-associated arrector pili muscles. The vascular system has a number of modifications within the skin for thermoregulation; in addition, the skin is richly innervated, and has nerve endings secreting sympathetic and the parasympathetic mediators as well as other neurotransmitters.

Layer	Cellular and molecular characteristics	Function
Stratum corneum	Cell envelope assembly extracellular lipids	Epidermal barrier to diffusion
Granular layer	Filaggrin synthesis and degradation Urocanic acid synthesis	Early cell envelope
Spinous layer	Site for Langerhans cells, keratin 1 and 10 synthesis	Antigen processing Bulk of keratins synthesized Vitamin D synthesis
Basal layer	Site for melanocytes and Merkel cells Keratin 5 and 14 synthesis	UV light protection mechanoreceptor Site of keratinocyte stem cells Synthesis of dermal-epidermal junction molecules
Dermal–epidermal layer	Site for laminin 5, collagen IV, V, and VII, proteoglycans	Attaches epidermis to rest of body Differential barrier to molecular diffusion and cell migration

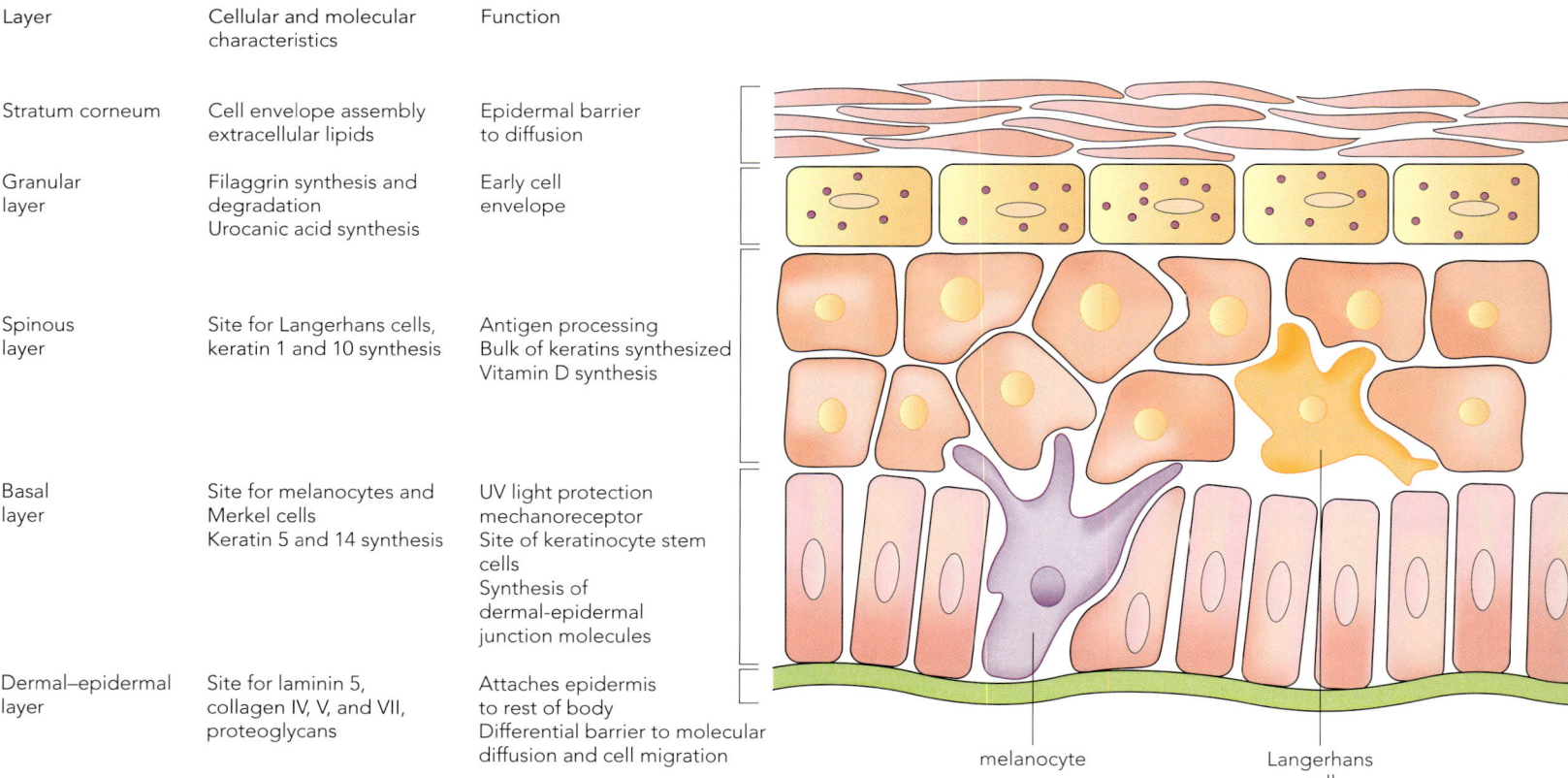

melanocyte   Langerhans cell

Fig. 1.10   Schematic diagram of the overall organization of the epidermis and dermal–epidermal junction.

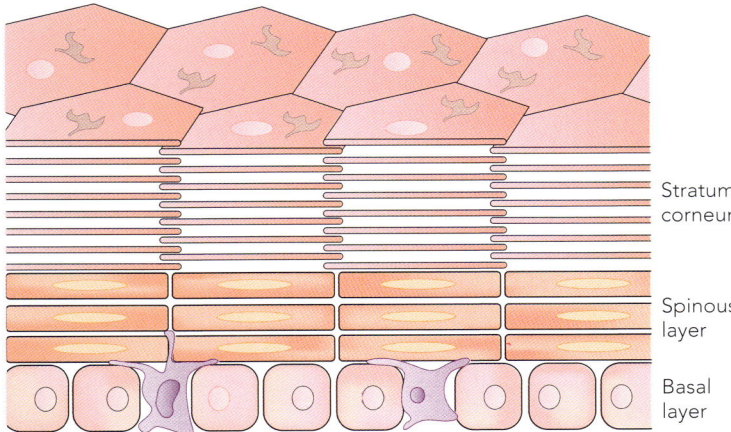

Fig. 1.11   **The epidermis is organized in functional units best visualized in monkey palm and mouse general body epidermis.** Columns of proliferating and differentiating cells are capped by closely interdigitated layers of stratum corneum cells. (Modified from Freedberg et al. (1999) Fitzpatrick's Dermatology in General Medicine, McGraw-Hill, with permission).

SUMMARY OF BIOLOGICAL MECHANISMS

The cells of the skin communicate with each other through paracrine, autocrine, and endocrine messages. In the epidermis, cells may contact each other physically, leading to interaction through cell surface molecules, some of which remain on the cell surface and some of which are internalized. External agents, such as organisms, may interfere with these functions. Internal and secreted cytokines may also interact with cell surface molecules. The skin is also the site of interaction with physical and biological agents from the external environment. Physical agents include ultraviolet light, visible light, and infrared radiation, in addition to heat and moisture. Biological agents include endogenous cytokines and organisms and their products. The details of the interaction of the skin are essential for understanding normal physiology and the altered physiology associated with disease.

EPIDERMAL STRUCTURE AND FUNCTION
(Figs 1.11, 1.12)

TISSUES

The epidermis is a complex tissue in which the keratinocytes comprise more than 90% of the cells. Cells from other embryonic origins are regularly dispersed through the epidermis and have specialized epidermal functions, which are integrated with the keratinocytes. The epidermis rests on a complex basement membrane (DEJ), which is derived from macromolecular components of epidermal and dermal origins. There is a rich, full and complex traffic of cells, macromolecules and micromolecules across the basement membrane zone. Epidermal cells are stacked in a multicellular array capped by a stratum corneum cell. This structure is dependent on an orderly process of differentiation; when that is altered by disease, the epidermal structure is disarrayed and its barrier function may be compromised.

SUMMARY OF FUNCTIONS

Mechanical, physical (e.g., ultraviolet light), chemical and immunological protection from the external environment, maintaining a homeostatic internal environment for the body and from the skin's components, synthesis of essential nutrients (e.g., vitamin D), are the general functions of the skin.

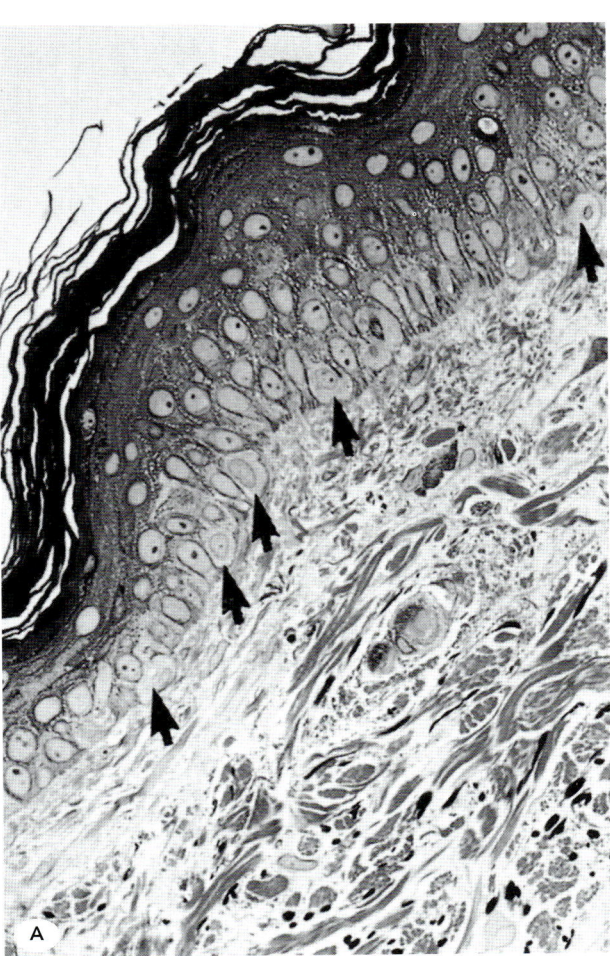

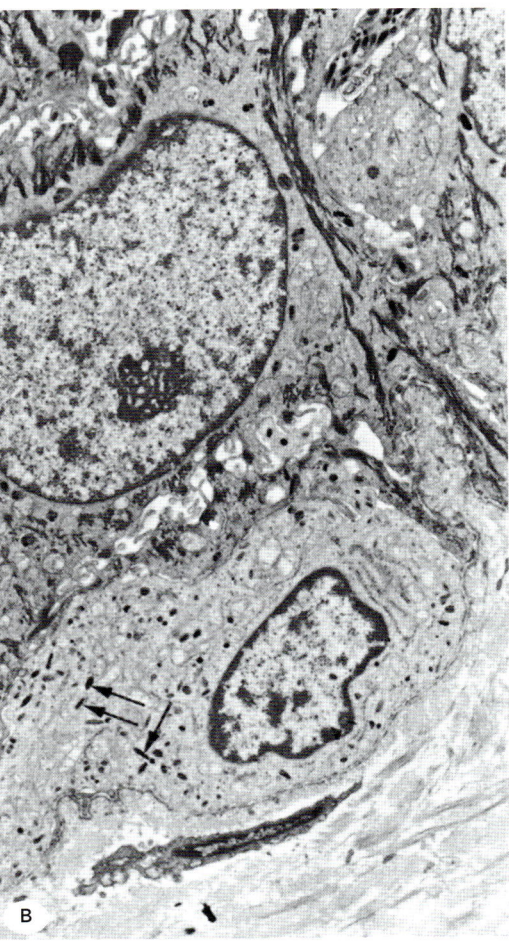

Fig. 1.12   **Light micrographs of melanocytes in adult epidermis.** Note their position among cells of the basal layer (arrows), their pale cytoplasm compared with the keratinocytes, and in (**B**) the presence of individual melanosomes (compared with melanosome complexes in keratinocytes) in the cytoplasm (arrows). (A) × 400; (B) × 6000. (From Holbrook and Sybert, 1995, with permission)

CELLS

Keratinocytes are the major epidermal cells and are derived originally from the embryonic ectoderm. The stem cells are in the basal layer of the epidermis; cells in the basal layer include both stem cells and cells that are destined for terminal differentiation. The fate of the individual cell is determined by its interaction with matrix molecules of the basement membrane zone and a large number of growth factors. The individual cell layers and their spatial orientations are discussed as separate sections based on their anatomical location: cells that actively divide (basal cells); cells that actively synthesize and process multiple biological macromolecules (spinous cells, granular cells, and intermediate cells); and stratum corneum cells that are anucleate in normal epidermis but retain rich sets of active biomolecules, and distinctive biological functions. These individual layers have many common characteristics but distinctive structural and functional consequences.

Melanocytes are derived from the neural crest and produce melanin, a complex biopolymer that absorbs wavelengths between ultraviolet and near infrared, including the visible spectrum. Melanin is synthesized in organelles called melanosomes, which aggregate in melanocytes and are also transferred to keratinocytes where they are photoprotective.

Langerhans cells are part of the afferent limb of the immune system and, through their class II HLA receptors, process predominantly exogenous antigens. The γ-δ-T cells are a resident population of T cells that function predominantly in immunoregulation.

The *Merkel cell* is a population of individual and grouped mechanical receptors, which respond to changes in movement and also may respond to changes in osmotic pressure.

SUMMARY OF FUNCTIONS

Keratinocytes form the stratum corneum and regulate solute, water, and gas interchange across the epidermis. Synthesis of previtamin D, the precursor of active vitamin D intermediates, occurs in the basal and spinous layer.

SUMMARY OF BIOLOGICAL MECHANISMS

Basal keratinocytes maintain a continually renewing population of keratinocyte cells in association with the basement membrane and then begin a

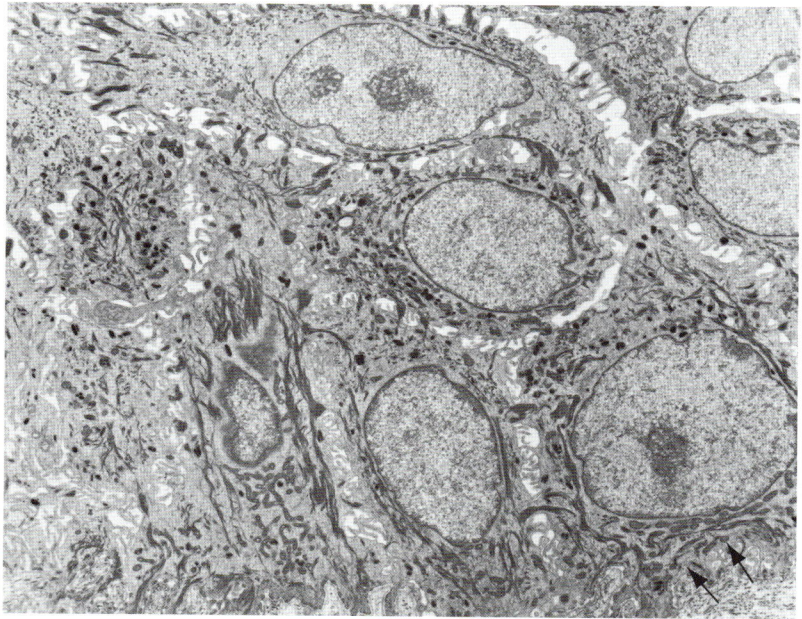

Fig. 1.13   Transmission electron micrograph of basal and suprabasal spinous layers of epidermal keratinocytes. Note the extensive network of keratin filaments, desmosomes, and vacuoles containing melanosomes in these cells. The dermal–epidermal junction is indicated (arrows) (× 6000). (From Holbrook and Sybert, 1995, with permission)

stereotypic program of terminal differentiation. The skin retains the life-long ability for epidermal wound healing by the close regulation of a program of epidermal repair, which is coordinated with the dermal repair processes as well as the ability to restore epidermal structure and function after epidermal damage from physical, biological, or immunologically mediated damage. Gap junctions composed of connexins are important for cell–cell communication.

BASAL KERATINOCYTE STRUCTURE AND FUNCTION

TISSUES

The basal layer of cells is known as the stratum germinativum (Fig. 1.13).

CELLS

The basal keratinocyte is a columnar cell, which rests on the basement membrane with a specialized modification, the hemidesmosome. It has desmosomal junctions, gap junctions, and adherens junctions with other basal keratinocytes and spinous keratinocytes, and desmosomal junctions with Merkel cells. It also borders on Langerhans cells and melanocytes. The melanosomes, transferred to keratinocytes from melanocytes, are often localized to a supranuclear cap.

MOLECULAR

Keratin filaments are the hallmark of the basal keratinocytes, and are members of the large family of the intermediate filaments that includes vimentin, desmin and neurofilaments. These 8–10-nm diameter molecules are arranged in regions: An N-terminal random region, a central helical region, and a C-terminal random region. The helical regions allow interactions within the keratin filaments and the formation of larger intracellular aggregates of molecules; the N- and C-terminal portions of the molecules allow interactions with other intracellular macromolecules, including molecules forming cell attachments within cells to the nuclear envelope and between cells and the basement membrane zone. Keratins can be divided into an acidic subclass (type I keratins), K9–19, and a basic subclass (type II keratins), K1–8. Keratins form heterodimers (20–30μm long) of type I and type II keratin pairs, which in turn form tetramers. The basic keratin is usually 5kDa heavier than their acidic partner and hence longer than their natural partners, forming heterodimers with an intrinsic asymmetry, which affects their biological interactions. Keratins have cysteine (—SH) residues, which can form intermolecular cysteine (S—S) disulfide bonds, stabilizing the molecules and decreasing the susceptibility of keratins to proteolytic enzyme degradation. Keratins are glycosylated and also phosphorylated.

The basal keratins, K5 and K14, 30% of the basal cell mass, are restricted to the basal layer. Other keratins such as K15, in the basal layer, are found in small amounts but may have functional significance when K14 is absent or severely impaired as in the Dowling–Meara form of EB simplex. The basal border of the keratinocyte has sugar molecules that are not present on the apical or lateral borders and has hemidesmosomes, which connect the cell to the basement membrane. The hemidesmosome contains plectin, integrin α6β4, and two bullous pemphigoid antigens, BP 230, and BP180 (collagen XVII). Microfilaments (containing actin, α-actinin, and myosin) associate with the integrin receptor at the basal border. The keratinocyte also has cytoskeletal components, such as F-actin, α-actinin, tubulins, and others, which are found in many other cell types.

SUMMARY OF FUNCTIONS

The essential function of the basal keratinocyte is to supply a renewing source of cells to populate the epidermis for the lifetime of the individual. If the epidermis is destroyed by a burn or radiation, the epidermis can regenerate from extraepidermal components, including precursor cells in the skin appendages,

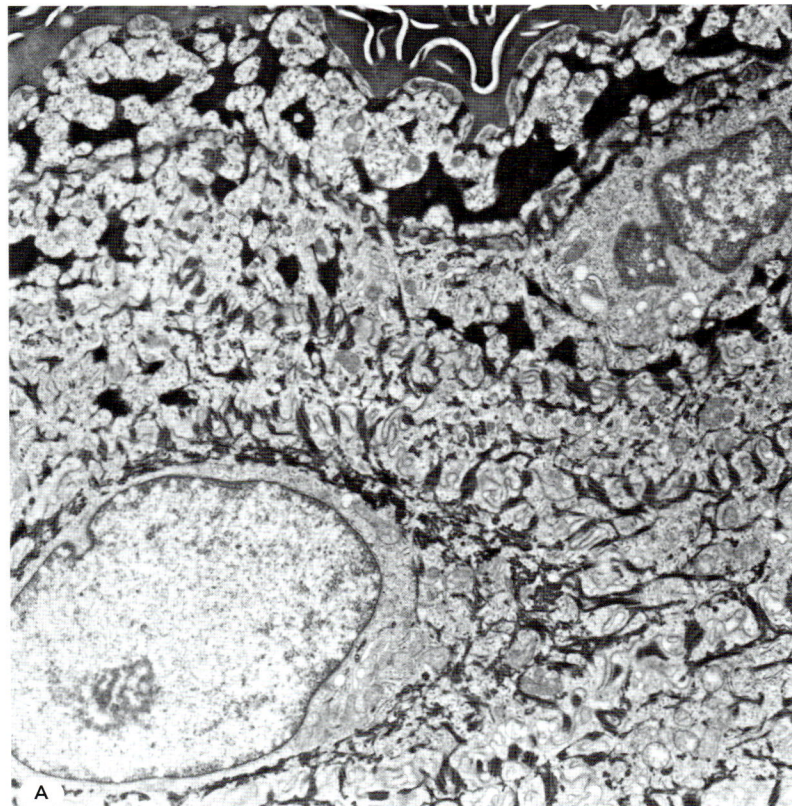

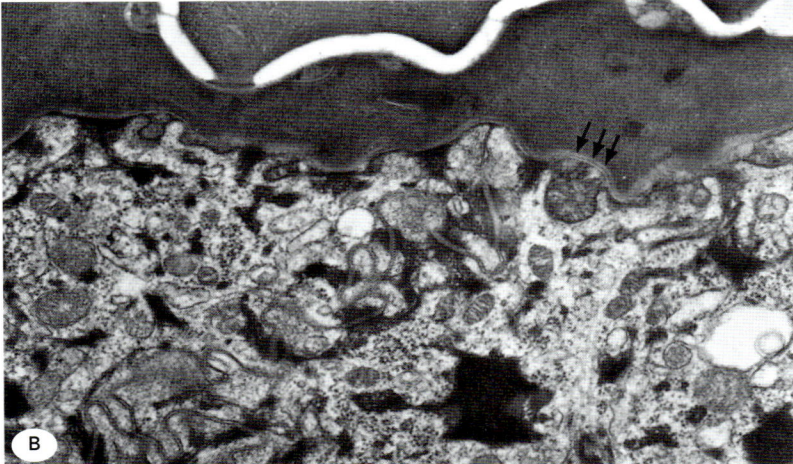

Fig. 1.14   Transmission electron micrographs of the upper spinous and granular layer cells of the epidermis. (**A**) Note the three layers of cells that contain keratohyalin granules. (**B**) Lamellar granules are evident within the cytoplasm and at the boundaries of the granular cells. Note the abrupt change in morphology between the upper granular layer cell and the first cornified cell layer. The cornified cell envelope in the first cornified cell is marked (arrows). (A) × 13 000; (B) × 36 000. (From Holbrook and Sybert, 1995, with permission)

such as the sweat glands and the hair follicles, and possibly by lateral migration from other sites. There is no evidence of formation of this destroyed epidermis from nonectodermally derived sources. To maintain this proliferative capacity the epidermis has 10% stem cells and 50% transient amplifying cells; 40% of cells have left the cell cycle and are postmitotic. The stem cells can be identified by the long-term retention of ^{3}H–thymidine after labeling ("label-retaining cells"), their location at the base of the deep rete ridges of the palm, their prominent long membrane modifications ("non-serrated cells"), and their

increased levels of α6β4 and β$_1$ integrins. Those interested in gene therapy envision stem cells as an important site for gene transfer.

SUMMARY OF BIOLOGICAL MECHANISMS

Postmitotic cells are identified by the synthesis of the intracellular protein involucrin, an early protein to be cross-linked into the cell envelope, and by the expression of spinous layer keratins, K1 and K10. When epidermis is stressed, K6 and K16 are produced, for example during wound healing, and in patients with hyperproliferative epidermal disorders (psoriasis, epidermolytic hyperkeratosis). The keratins form a dense cytoskeleton in the cell. Mechanical properties are imputed to this structure, which may allow the tissue to withstand the stress of shearing. The cytoskeleton may also have critical roles in the compartmentalization of metabolic pathways and the process of conveying of extracellular signals from the cell surface to the nucleus. In the upper epidermal cell layers keratins may be incorporated into the cell envelope. Other proteins that associate with keratins include the lamins of the nuclear envelope and the desmoplakins of the desmosome; in higher cell layers, filaggrin associates with keratins, and in hair keratin interacts with a variety of hair proteins. The keratinocyte is also capable of producing a variety of growth factors and cytokines, which are important in wound healing and in inflammatory responses.

SPINOUS KERATINOCYTE STRUCTURE AND FUNCTION

TISSUE

The epidermis is organized into multicellular units. Disturbances in epidermal kinetics perturb the coordination of multicellular function and interfere with the structure and thus the function of all epidermal layers (Fig. 1.15).

CELLS

There are three to four layers of spinous cells and the individual cells undergo change from a plump polyhedral shape to a flatter shape. Prominent bundles of keratin filaments are present and multilayered lamellar granules are seen in the upper spinous layers. *Lamellar granules* are 300–500μm intracellular components, which are Golgi-derived membrane-bound organelles. They have disk-like lipid bilayers (with alternate thick and thin lamellae), which will form the cell envelope. They eventually fuse with the cell membrane and their components are extruded to form the physiological basis of the epidermal barrier to diffusion.

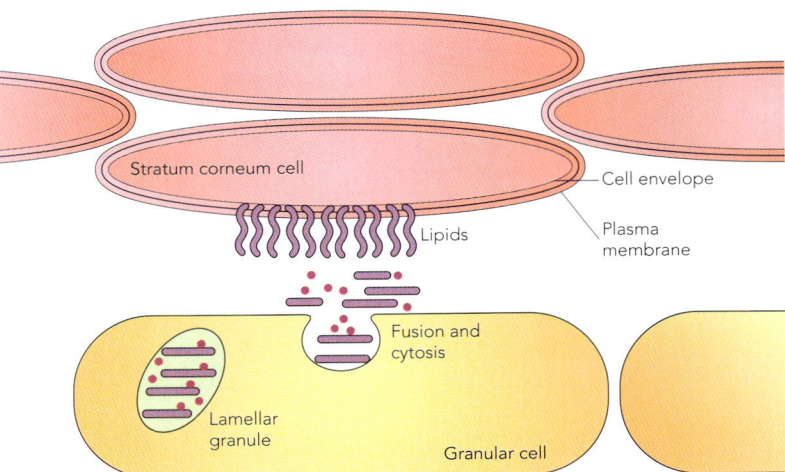

Fig. 1.15   Schematic diagram of extracellular lipid deposition for barrier function and enzyme deposition for desquamation in the stratum corneum. (Modified from Freedberg et al. (1999) Fitzpatrick's Dermatology in General Medicine, McGraw-Hill with permission)

MOLECULAR

The mRNAs for K1 and K10 are most prominent in all sites of epidermis, as are K1 and K10 proteins. In palmar and plantar epidermis K9 predominates. K2e, which is related to K1 and pairs with K10, is expressed in the upper half of the epidermis. K6/K16 are synthesized during wound healing and with hyperproliferation, as occurs in psoriasis.

The "spines" of the spinous level are *desmosomes*, which have not retracted during the process of preparing the cell for light microscopy. Desmosomes are reversible cell adhesion complexes composed of three main portions: an intracellular portion, a transmembrane portion, and an external extracellular portion. On the inner surface of the plasma membrane are plakoglobin, plakophilin 1, 2 and 3, desmoplakin 1 and 2, keratocalmin, desmoyokin, a calmodulin binding protein, and keratocalmin (desmocalmin), at the site of the filament insertion of the plaque. Transmembrane molecules include desmoglein 1 and 3, and desmocalmin 1, 2, and 3. The extracellular cadherin family components of two adjacent cells interact. Desmoglein 1 and desmoglein 3 form part of this complex; more desmoglein 1 is present on the cell of higher cell layers and more desmoglein 3 is present on basal cells than on higher epidermal cells. Only desmoglein 3 is found on mucosal surfaces.

Adherens junctions are located between epidermal cells and between basal keratinocytes and the DEJ. Integrins, vinculin, and talin link microfibrils to these attachments. E-cadherins, desmogleins (1–2) and desmocollins (1–3) are also associated with these junctions. The cell surface is rich in glycosylated molecules, as measured by lectin binding.

The formation of the cell envelope is anticipated by synthesis of its major precursor loricin; involucrin may be the earliest component to be crosslinked. Lamellar granules contain phospholipids, glycosphingolipids, ceramides and proteolytic enzymes, such as ceramidases, proteases, lipases, and glycosidases. Glucosylceramides are precursors to the ceramides, which are found in the extracellular space in the stratum corneum.

SUMMARY OF FUNCTIONS

There is coordinated movement of cells through the epidermis, which involves breaking and reformation of cell junctional components.

Vitamin D synthesis occurs in the spinous layer and the basal layer. Under the influence of ultraviolet light (290–315nm) from sunlight, 7-dehydrocholesterol is converted to previtamin D_3 and, in a heat-dependent step Vitamin D_3 then leaves the cell, enters the circulation, and is 25-hydroxylated in the liver and 1-hydroxylated in the kidney to form 1,25-dihydroxyvitamin D_3. Synthesis decreases with age and is less in the Northern hemisphere during winter. Receptors for 1,25-dihydroxyvitamin D_3 are in the epidermis, external root sheath and cells of the dermal papillae. When the receptor is absent due to an autosomal recessive genetic disease, in addition to clinical rickets, anagen is not initiated and universal persistent alopecia occurs, beginning in early infancy.

GRANULAR CELLS

CELLS

These postmitotic cells comprise two to three layers in normal epidermis and have been recognized for more than a century by distinctive keratohyalin granules, which stain strongly with basophilic stains (Fig. 1.16). Between the granular layer and the stratum corneum, lamellar granules fuse and aggregate with the plasma membrane.

Transitional cells are a rarely recognized component of the epidermis and are at the border between the uppermost granular cells and the first stratum corneum cell. They have the heavily convoluted nucleus characteristic of a cell in the early stages of apoptosis. Dense keratin filaments are present. Other granules contain loricin, the cysteine-rich protein that is the major component (by mass) of the cell envelope.

MOLECULAR

Profilaggrin is a histidine-rich, very basic protein, which is highly phosphorylated and forms a large (~400kDa) polymer. Filaggrin forms in the granular layer, aggregates with keratin, and may have a role in forming keratin filaments in upper layers of the epidermis. With proteolysis filaggrin releases histidine, which then is deaminated by a histidase present in the stratum corneum and forms *trans*-urocanic acid. *Trans*-urocanic acid is converted to *cis*-urocanic acid by UVB. Glutamic acid released from filaggrin is converted to *pyroglutamic acid* and may function as a natural moisturizing agent in the epidermis. Keratins are both phosphorylated and subject to proteolytic degradation in this layer. Pre-desquamin in the transitional layer may facilitate apoptosis.

SUMMARY OF FUNCTIONS

In the cells of the granular layer, lamellar granules are extruded, apoptosis is initiated, the nucleus and other cellular contents susceptible to proteolysis are destroyed, and the potential for protein synthesis is lost.

SUMMARY OF BIOLOGICAL MECHANISMS

Many pathological conditions involving the epidermis show parakeratosis (retention of nuclei in the outermost epidermal layers) and are associated with increased epidermal turnover and abnormal barrier function.

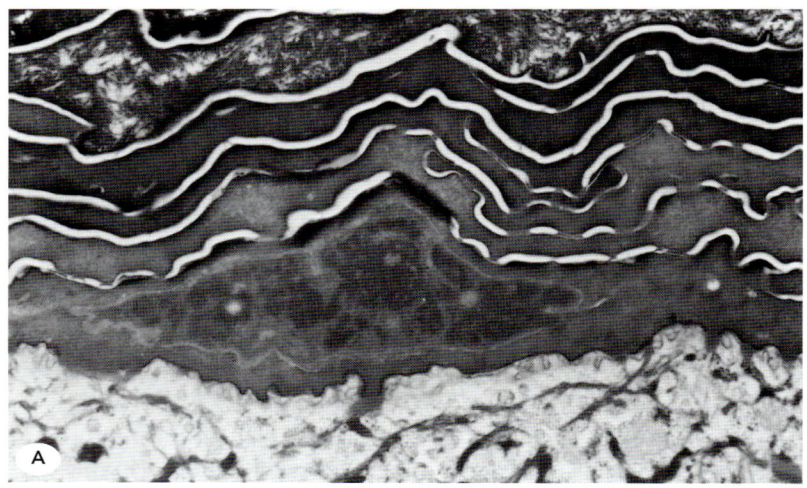
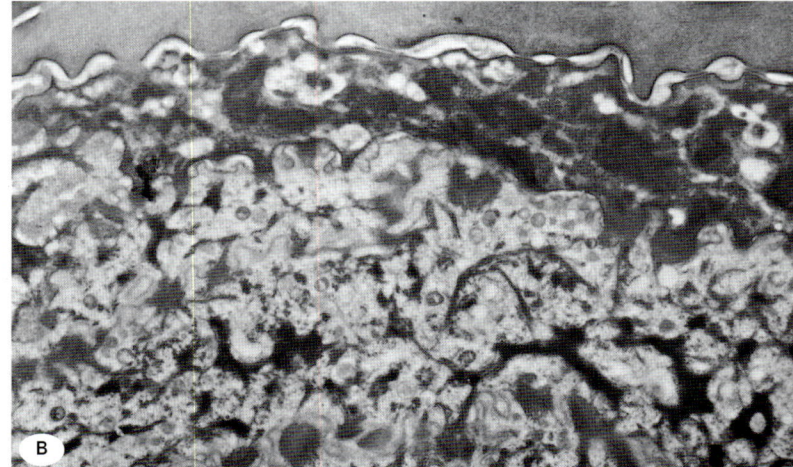

Fig. 1.16   Electron micrograph of transitional cells that show morphology intermediate between that of granular and cornified cells. (**A**) The nucleus is retained, and (**B**) some of the organelles (ribosomes and keratohyalin granules) are evident. (A) × 12 000; (B) × 13 000. (From Holbrook and Sybert, 1995, with permission)

STRATUM CORNEUM

TISSUE

The innermost cells and a denser keratin pattern seem more compact (*stratum compactum*) and have more desmosomal attachments. The superficial cells (*stratum corneum dysjunctum*) have fewer attachments, and a less organized keratin pattern.

CELLS

There is a large difference in the number of cell layers of the so-called dead epidermis. It is about 15 layers thick on the general body skin, and hundreds of layers thick on the palms and soles. Stratum corneum thickness is similar in children and in adults (Figs 1.17 and 1.18).

Within a thinned plasma membrane (with a 5nm lipid layer) is a very highly crosslinked structure, the cell envelope, which is 7–15nm in thickness. This structure is formed by progressive post-translational crosslinking by the calcium-dependent enzyme epidermal transglutaminase I of involucrin, then loricin (a cysteine, glycine/serine rich protein which comprised 75% of the envelope mass), and then several other proteins, including keratins, pancornulin, cornifins, elafins (a serine proteinase), envoplakin (a desmoplakin homolog), and filaggrin linker segment peptide, to form an insoluble, highly crosslinked structure (Fig. 1.19). The γ-glutamyl-ε lysine cross-links formed are very resistant to the usual proteolytic enzymes of the human cell and to organisms, which may attack the epidermis. Epidermal ceramides are crosslinked across the cell membrane to the envelope, which may stabilize the extracellular lipid layer.

MOLECULAR

Disulfide bonded keratins make up 80% of the mass of stratum corneum cells. The hydrophobic nature of the extracellular lipid chains, glycolipids, free sterol and phospholipids explains why lipophilic molecules pass through the epidermis more easily than hydrophilic molecules. Ceramides are the most abundant lipid in the extracellular space.

SUMMARY OF FUNCTIONS

The stratum corneum is the ultimate structural fate for the keratinocyte. Although dead, the cell contains a large number of enzymes and DNA that

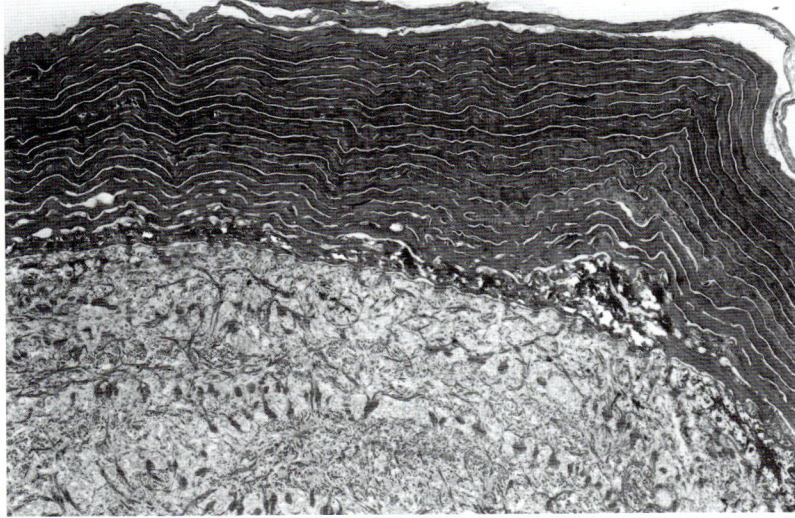

Fig. 1.17   Transmission electron micrographs show flattened cell layers of the stratum corneum from the trunk (× 6100). (From Holbrook and Sybert, 1995, with permission)

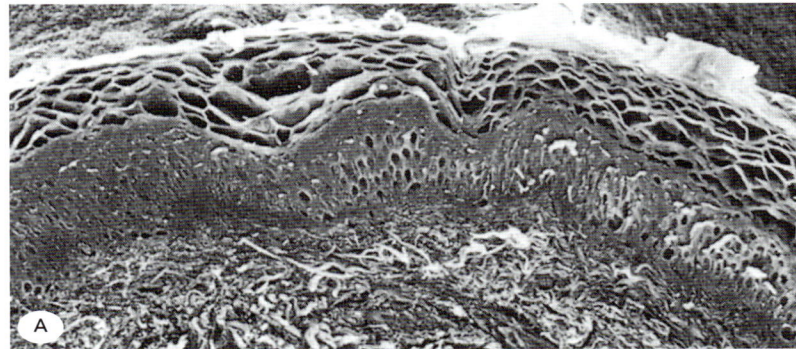

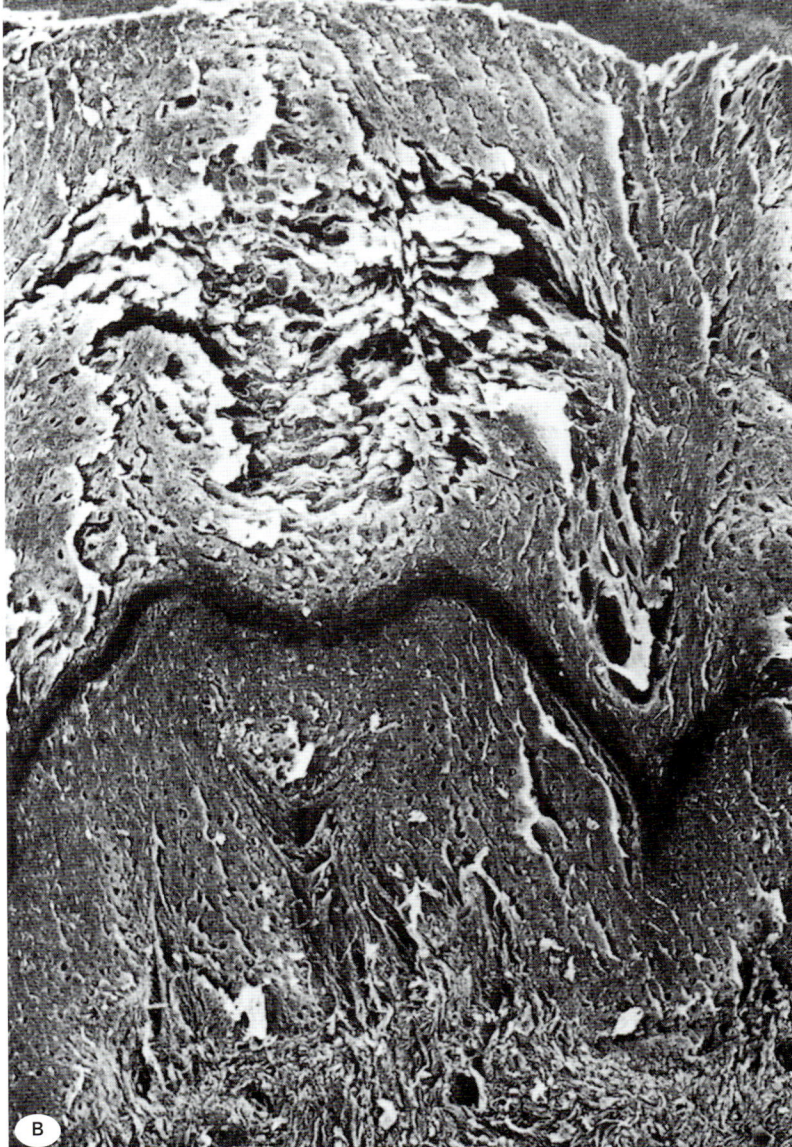

Fig. 1.18   Scanning electron micrographs comparing the thickness of the stratum corneum from (**A**) the arm and (**B**) the palm of an adult. (A) × 200; (B) × 200. (From Holbrook and Sybert, 1995, with permission)

has been amplified by the polymerase chain reaction. The corneocyte has a highly structured cell surface and extracellular lipid coat forming the barrier against water loss, which prevents a large number of small and medium-sized molecules from passively passing through the epidermis.

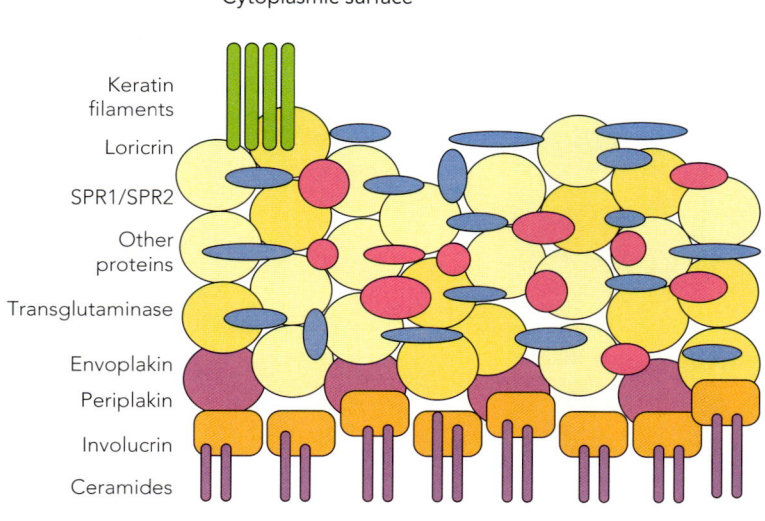

Cytoplasmic surface

Keratin filaments
Loricrin
SPR1/SPR2
Other proteins
Transglutaminase
Envoplakin
Periplakin
Involucrin
Ceramides

Exterior surface of cornified cell

Fig. 1.19   The cell envelope is formed by sequential incorporation of several structural proteins and extracellular lipids across the plasma membrane. (From Steinert, 2000; reproduced with permission.)

EPIDERMAL MELANOCYTES

TISSUE

Melanocytes are derived from neural crest cells, which are usually singly disposed in the epidermal basal layer and rest on the basement membrane; they are located in the spinous layer during fetal life. Through dendrites melanocytes have a close relationship with approximately 36 basal and spinous cells ("epidermal melanin unit"). There are 1220 melanocytes/mm² by age 16, but the highest melanocyte density is actually at birth. Melanocyte is highest on the face and genital region, and lowest on the abdomen. Melanocytes are also present in the nail matrix and hair cortex.

CELLS

The melanocyte is a round to oval cell with refractile brown granules in the cytoplasm. It contains prominent intermediate filaments composed of vimentin, which forms homopolymers and not to the heteropolymers of keratin. Melanocytes have integrin receptors (α6β4), receptors for fibronectin and laminin that may attach melanocytes to the dermal–epidermal junction, and E- and P-cadherins that may attach melanocytes to keratinocytes. Silver nitrate stains melanin-containing cells; dopamine is oxidized by tyrosinase and stains cells with enzymatically active tyrosinase.

Melanosomes are complex organelles and the site of melanin production. The tyrosinase containing part of the melanosome is thought to develop from the trans-Golgi network with saccules, and the premelanosome portion is thought to develop from the smooth endoplasmic reticulum. Melanosomes have lysosomal enzymes, such as acid phosphatase, and β glucuronidase, and lysosomal markers such as Lamp-1, CD63, and specific enzymes and structural proteins related to the synthesis of melanin. Melanosomes less than 1µm in diameter are packaged multiply; those larger than 1µm are packaged singly. Keratinocytes have a role in regulating whether melanosomes are distributed individually or clustered. Dark-skinned African-Americans have 450–600 melanosomes per melanocyte and light-skinned Europeans and Americans have 2–12 melanosomes per melanocyte.

The four stages of melanosome development include: stage I, premelanosome; stage II, no pigment but some internal structure; stage III, moderate pigment; stage IV, extensive pigment. Melanosomes are transferred from melanocyte dendritic structures in basal keratinocytes and even into Langerhans cells. The melanosomes are distributed in clusters above the nucleus in basal keratinocytes and more diffusely in keratinocytes higher in the epidermis.

SUMMARY OF FUNCTIONS

Melanocytes synthesize melanin, which absorbs and scatters ultraviolet light, visible light, and near infrared radiation. Melanin is a free radical, functions as part of an antioxidant pathway, and may bind metals. Tyrosine is a major amino acid of melanin, and forms relatively insoluble oligomers within elliptical eumelanosomes, with internal filamentous structures; pheomelanin contains tyrosine and cysteine with spheroidal melanosomes. Melanin formation is catalyzed by tyrosinase, a transmembrane glycoprotein with an essential copper cofactor that catalyzes the oxidation of tyrosine within the melanosome. Tyrosine is oxidized to dopaquinone, which then forms dopachrome and eventually melanin. Tyrosine-related proteins (TRP-1 and TRP-2) with sequence homology to tyrosinase, function as Dopachrome tautomerase and dihyroxyindole 2-carboxylic acid oxidase, respectively, in the early stages of melanin formation.

CELL REGULATION AND SIGNALING

Proopiomelanocortin is the precursor of adrenocorticotrophic hormone α-melanocyte stimulating hormone (MSH), and β-MSH (in addition to other molecules). These peptides interact with a family of cell surface MSH receptors that functions with G-proteins, the cAMP pathway and protein kinase A. The agouti protein blocks MSH binding to its receptor. Frequent polymorphisms in the MSH receptor include mutations associated with red hair. Endothelin is a 21-amino acid peptide, which is increased after ultraviolet exposure, and functions via the protein kinase C pathway and tyrosine phosphorylation. Melanocytes produce growth factors and are greatly influenced by melanocortin and its derived factors.

IMMUNOCYTES IN THE EPIDERMIS (LANGERHANS CELLS AND γ–δ T CELLS)

CELLS

Langerhans cells are derived from the bone marrow and comprise 2–5% of epidermal cells; they do not have junction structures with other epidermal cells. They are regularly distributed, usually in a suprabasal location, at a density of 460–1000 cells/mm². They have a convoluted nucleus and a characteristic granule, the *Birbeck granule*. The granule represents an infolding of the plasma membrane related to the processing of an immunogenic peptide. Vimentin intermediate filaments are present (Fig. 1.20).

Cutaneous nerves that secrete calcitonin gene-related peptide (CGRP) join Langerhans cells and are a potential structural link between the nervous system and the immune system. Thy-1+ dendritic cells (γ–δ cells) are well described in mice and are located between basal keratinocytes; their functional presence in normal human epidermis is still under investigation.

MOLECULAR

Langerhans cells have several surface markers that relate to its function as an antigen-presenting cell. These include class I and II HLA-antigens, S-100 protein, receptors for the Fc region of IgG, a high affinity receptor for IgE (FcϵR1), and a receptor to complement (C3bi/CR-III). The CD1a receptor distinguishes LCs from other antigen-processing dendritic cells. Langerhans cells secrete interleukin (IL)-6, tumor necrosis factor (TNF)-α amd IL-1.

SUMMARY OF FUNCTIONS

Langerhans cells are the antigen-presenting cells for the epidermis. Adhesion molecules of the integrin and intracellular adhesion molecule (ICAM-1) family mediate Langerhans cell–T-cell interactions. Langerhans cells are destroyed by irradiation or ultraviolet light, but can be replenished from bone marrow by circulating (CD45+) cells that enter the epidermis. Lower ultraviolet doses incapacitate, but do not kill Langerhans cells.

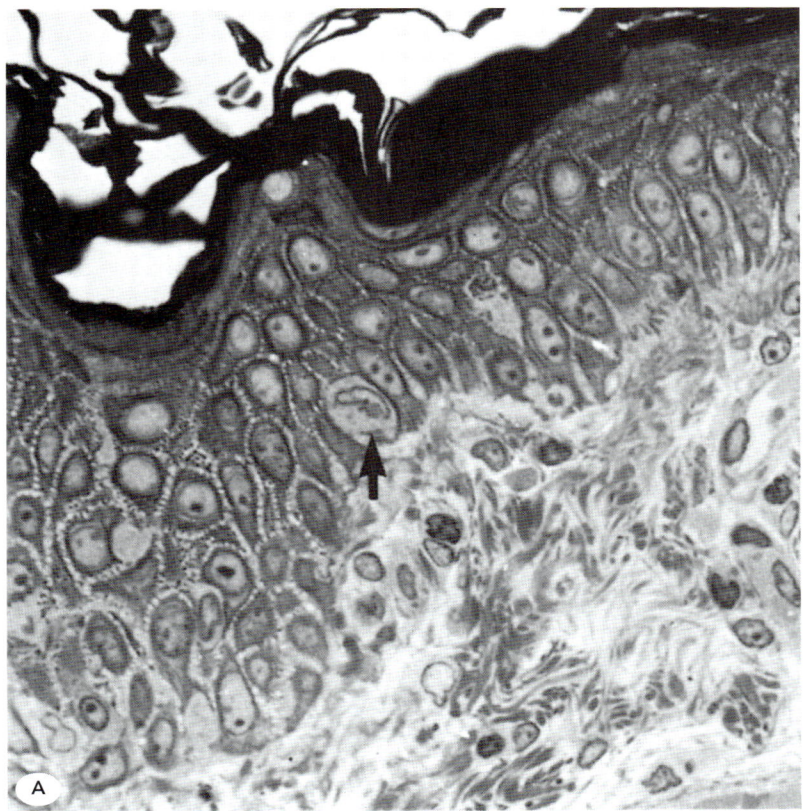
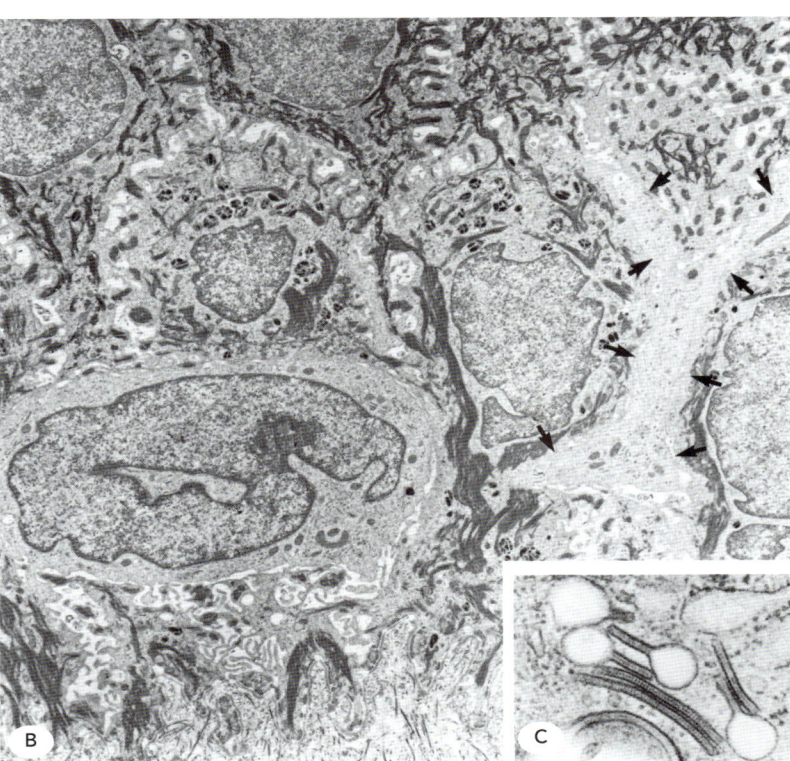

Fig. 1.20   (A and B) Light and electron micrographs of Langerhans cells in the epidermis. Note the pale staining cytoplasm, the convoluted nucleus, and the dendritic nature of the cell (dendritic process indicated with arrows in **B**). Several Langerhans cell granules (Birbeck granules) are enlarged in **C**. (A) × 400; (B) × 6000; (C) 50 000 (From Holbrook and Sybert, 1995, with permission)

MERKEL CELLS

CELLS

Merkel cells are epithelial-derived cells that are individually disposed in the basal layer or arranged in larger groups (up to 50) as tactile disc or touch domes with an associated myelinated nerves in epidermis, hairs (Haarssheiben and the bulge region) and mucosae. Merkel cells have desmosomal connections. Dense bands of Merkel cells are in the isthmus and infundibulum of the hair follicle. They are associated with nerve fibers except in the bulge region. Merkel cells are located on the palms and soles, where eccrine ducts penetrate the epidermis. They contain Golgi-derived membrane *dense core granules* that are bound 80–100nm in diameter. The contacting membrane between a neurite and a Merkel cell resembles a synapse (Fig. 1.21).

MOLECULAR

Merkel cells contain simple keratins (K8 and K18) and K20, a mucosal keratin largely found in urothelial and intestinal epithelial cells, which is relatively specific for Merkel cells in the skin. High levels of bcl-2 are present in Merkel cells, and may interfere with apoptosis induced by traditional chemotherapeutic regimens.

SUMMARY OF FUNCTIONS

The Merkel cell is a type I slow-adapting mechanosensory receptor for touch. Its granules are similar to monoamine granules of the diffuse neuroendocrine system (APUD) system. The granules stain for CGRP, substance P, neuron-specific enolase, bombesin, chromogranin A, acetylcholine and synaptophysin. It is hypothesized that the release of neuromodulatory compounds could modulate the threshold of the sensory terminal.

THE DERMIS

TISSUES

The dermis is predominantly composed of extracellular matrix molecules with fibroblasts, blood and lymph vessels, mast cells, appendages, glands, nerves, sensory receptors and wandering cells of the immune system, which are constant visitors and sometimes long-term guests in the dermis. Melanocytes are rare in Caucasian dermis but not uncommon in blacks and Asians, in whom they may aggregate and appear as dark blue patches (e.g., Mongolian spots).

Overall the dermis has two main zones – the *papillary dermis* and the *reticular dermis* (Fig. 1.22). The papillary dermis is uppermost and adjacent to the DEJ. It is not more than twice the width of the epidermis and resembles the dermis around the appendages. The *reticular lamina* is a sublamina densa zone in the superior papillary dermis with fine but dense collagen, sometimes called the "compact zone". It contains anchoring plaques and the ends of the anchoring fibrils. The subpapillary vascular plexus defines the border between the reticular and papillary dermis. This border is less prominent in young infants compared with adults. The reticular dermis has collagen bundles that are thicker than those of the papillary dermis, a higher density of vessels, is more cellular and contains oxytalan elastic fibers.

The thicker collagen bundles and elastic fibers of the reticular dermis increase in size as the reticular dermis reaches its border with the subcutaneous tissue of the hypodermis. Based on fiber diameter, the reticular dermis may be divided into an upper "intermediate zone" and a "deeper zone".

The *hypodermis* begins relatively sharply where the fibrous dermis transitions into a fat containing tissue. The hypodermis contains anagen follicles, and in its deeper portions apocrine and eccrine glands. It contains types I, III and V collagen. There is a relatively sharp border between the hypodermis and the reticular dermis because the connective tissue of hypodermis is more adipose than fibrous.

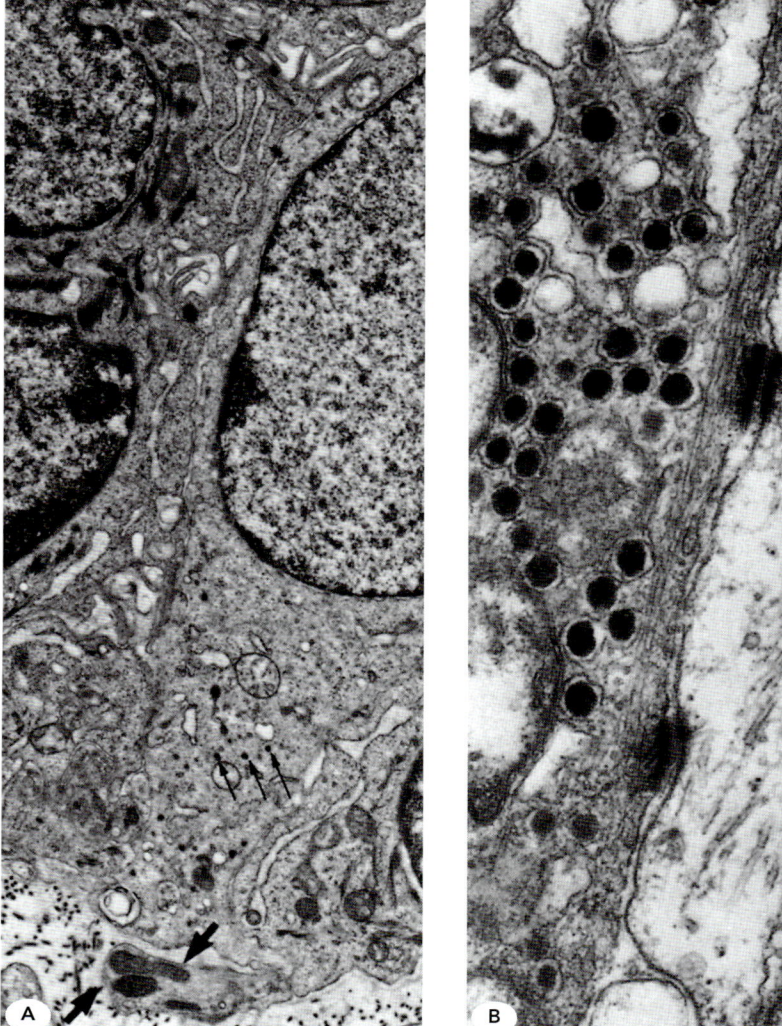

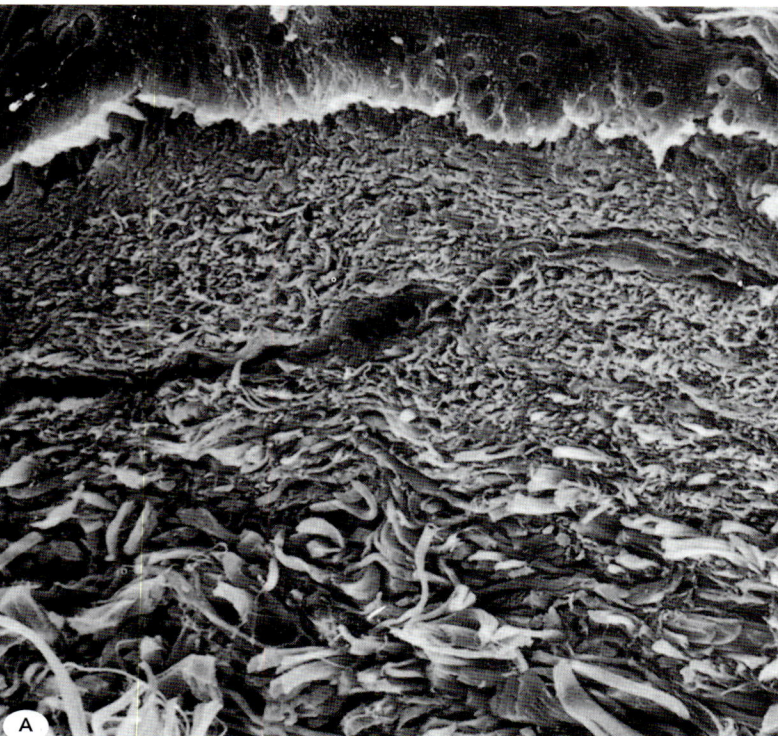

Fig. 1.21   (**A**) Transmission electron micrographs of a Merkel cell and (**B**) the dense-core granules from the skin of a premature infant. Small arrows point to a few granules in the cell and the larger arrows indicate the neurite. (A) × 9000; (B) × 51 000. (From Holbrook and Sybert, 1995, with permission)

CELLS

Fibroblasts are the source of the extracellular structural molecules of the dermis. Many of these dermal elements are highly glycosylated as a post-translational structural modification prior to secretion from the fibroblast.

Dermal dendrocytes are CD45+, dendritic, highly phagocytic, and are abundant in the papillary dermis and upper reticular dermis. They bear the markers of antigen-presenting cells and express a subunit of plasma blood coagulation factor, factor XIII. They are thought to be part of the afferent limb of the immune response.

SUMMARY OF FUNCTIONS

The dermis gives the skin most of its mechanical properties, and is involved in expansion or regression of the skin. Type I collagen is responsible for the tensile strength and pliability of the skin. Type III collagen is more prominent where compliance of the skin is important, such as in the superficial papillary dermis and around vessels. The hypodermal fat provides reserve energy, cushioning, mobility over the underlying bony structure, and molding of body contours.

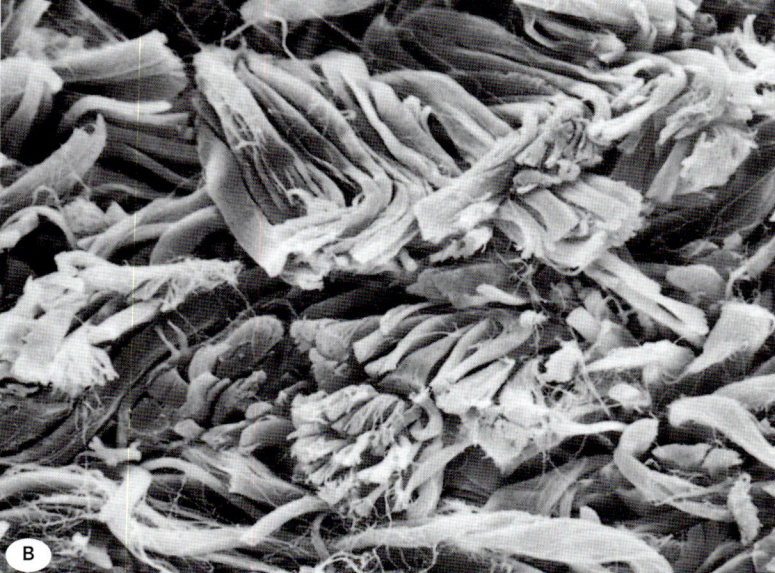

Fig. 1.22   Scanning electron micrographs of (A) papillary and (A and B) reticular dermis. In (A) note the small size of the collagen bundles in the papillary dermis in contrast to the larger bundles at the upper limit of the reticular dermis, called the intermediate dermis. The "cleft" corresponds to a horizontal vessel of the subpapillary plexus. Fig. B shows the large collagen fiber bundles of the reticular dermis. (A) × 550; (B) × 550. (From Holbrook and Sybert, 1995, with permission)

FIBROBLASTS

TISSUES

Mature elastin fibrils comprise about 1–2% of the fibrillar proteins of the dermis. They are flat branching structures that contain up to 90% elastin and they are frequently at the periphery of collagen fibers. They are assembled into bundles, beginning at the *microfibrils* (10–12nm in diameter), where the early elastic fibrils are called *oxytalan*, and run perpendicularly from the DEJ through the papillary dermis to the upper dermis. There they network with *elaunin fibers*, which form a horizontal plexus of fibers. Oxytalan fibers are covered with soluble elastin. Eventually, a mature elastic fiber is formed in the reticular dermis.

MOLECULAR

Collagen has many of its prolines hydroxylated and this allows the formation of the collagen triple helix; some of the lysines are hydroxylated and this allows the formation of new cross-links intermolecularly between collagen molecules (Fig. 1.23). These hydroxylations require ascorbic acid and separate and specific hydroxylating enzymes for proline and lysine. Collagen is glycosylated with galactosyl or glucosyl-galactosyl residues covalently bound to hydroxylysine. Collagen is a major component (72–75% of the dry weight) of the dermis. Eighty to 85% of the dermal collagen is type I and 10–15% is type III. Less than 5% is type V collagen. Type III fibers frequently form thinner fibrils. Type IV collagen is in the DEJ and around appendages and blood vessels. Type VI collagen is found throughout the dermis.

Elastin, which is 0.6–1.2% of the dry weight of the skin, is synthesized as a soluble precursor, tropoelastin. Tropoelastin contains lysine residues that are covalently cross-linked throughout their hydroxyl groups forming desmosine and isodesmosine.

Microfibrils are secreted by fibroblasts and elastin is deposited on them; these two molecules constitute 90% of the mature elastic fibers. Other matrix components are proteoglycans and glycosaminoglycans. *Fibrillin*, a 350kDa glycoprotein, is a major component of the elastic fibers, as are other microfibrillar associated proteins, including fibulin, MP70/78 and MFMP1, 3 and 4.

Proteoglycans are comprised of a protein core with 1–100 linked glycosaminoglycan (GAG) chains and are large molecules (100–2500kDa). Hyaluronic acid (hyaluronate) is a GAG. Proteoglycans include chondroitin sulfate/dermatan sulfate (biglycan, decorin, and versican); heparan/heparan sulfate proteoglycans (HSPG, perlecan, and syndecan) and chondritin-6-sulfate proteoglycan (CSPG) in the DEJ. Decorin is most abundant in the papillary dermis. Versican has 12–15 GAG chains and forms large aggregates. It is upregulated by transforming growth factor-β. Syndecan-4, which is less prominent in fetal life, is a proinflammmatory and profibrotic molecule. Hyaluran, present in fetal life, is associated with the absence of scarring of the fetal skin. Proteoglycans are gel-like, highly glycosylated and sulfated, and retain large amount of water.

Tenascin is abundant in developing skin and present at sites of epithelial–mesenchymal interactions, which influence appendage development. Other dermal macromolecules include fibronectin, vitronectin, thrombospondin and epibolin. These molecules interact with each other and with the GAGs. They influence migration, inflammation, and wound healing and have major roles in embryonic development.

SUMMARY OF FUNCTIONS

The elastin fibers give the elastic recoil of the dermis. GAGs are associated with proteoglycans or occur as free hyaluronic acid, which is thought to allow

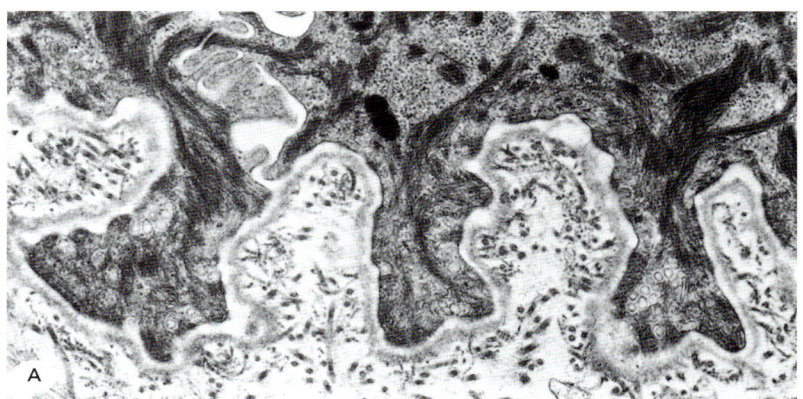

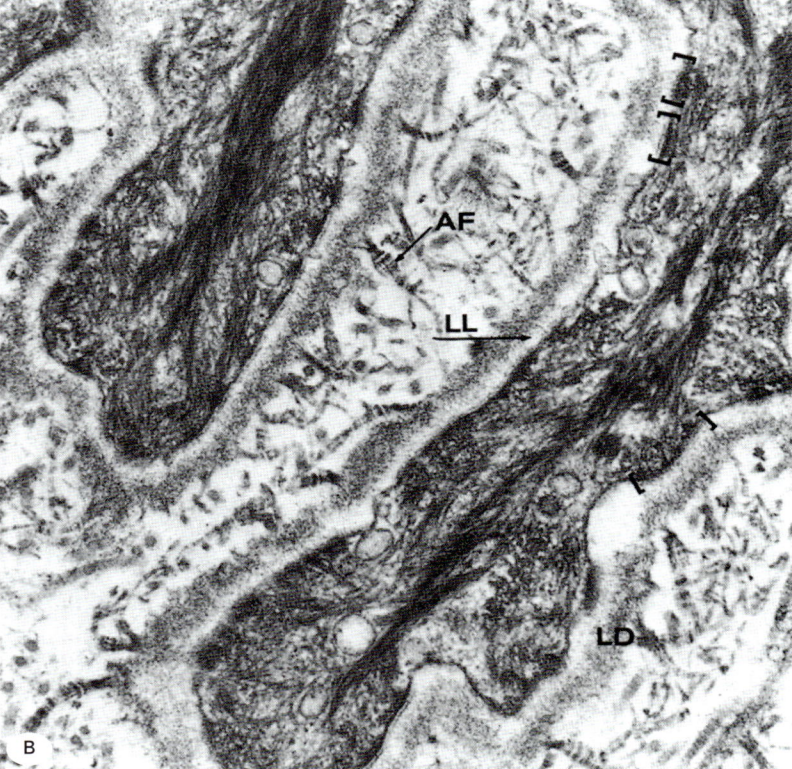

Fig. 1.24   (A and B) Transmission electron micrographs of the structural components of the dermal–epidermal junction. Portions of basal keratinocytes are shown. Hemidesmosomes are bracketed and the lamina densa (LD), lamina lucida (LL), and anchoring fibrils (AF) are evident. (A) × 31 000; (B) × 70 000. (From Holbrook and Sybert, 1995, with permission)

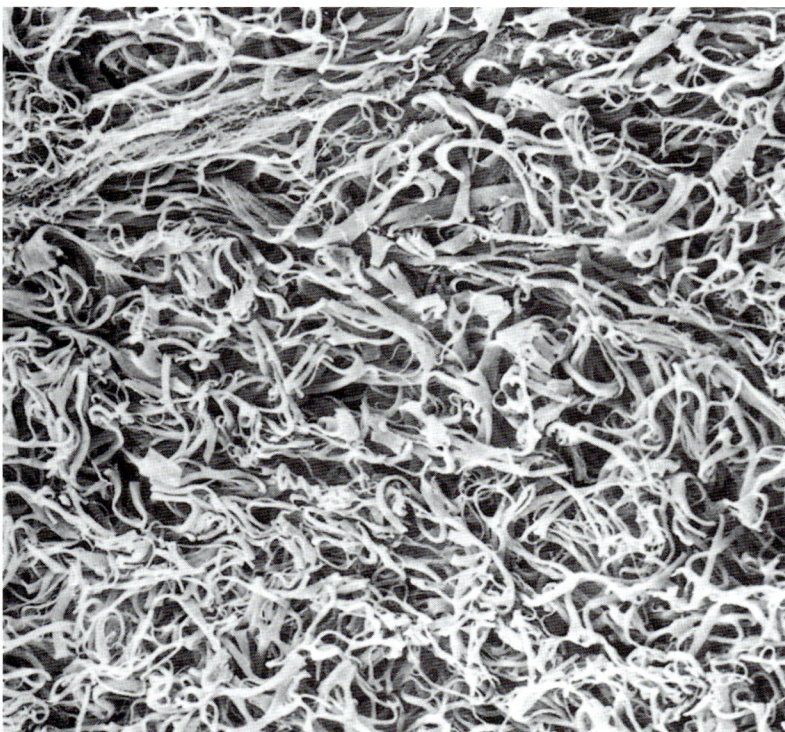

Fig. 1.23   Scanning electron micrograph of elastic fibers of the dermis after the tissue has been digested and autoclaved. Note the extensive network of branching fibers (× 600). (From Holbrook and Sybert, 1995, with permission)

cell separation and migration. Proteoglycans bind water and, by regulating compressibility and rigidity of the dermis, determine its limits of deformability.

DERMAL–EPIDERMAL JUNCTION (BASEMENT MEMBRANE ZONE)

TISSUES

The DEJ is composed of the basal border of the keratinocyte and many molecules, which forms a barrier regulating the passage of large molecules and cells. The border is undulating. Projections of dermis reach upward (dermal ridges and dermal papillae) and mesh with downward epidermal projections (rete ridges and rete pegs). This undulating pattern is most prominent on the palms and soles and is decreased or lost with some inflammatory diseases of the DEJ. It is also decreased during physiological aging after the pediatric age group.

As viewed by transmission electron microscopy (Fig. 1.24), the DEJ shows an electron clear zone (*lamina lucida*), a denser zone (*lamina densa*), anchoring filaments, anchoring fibrils, the reticular lamina and the subepidermal region of the papillary dermis. The regions have distinctive molecular constituents and organization.

Hemidesmosomes are structures at the plasma membrane of the keratinocyte and the DEJ, and include the cytoplasm of the keratinocyte and portions of the lamina lucida (Fig. 1.25). The plaque of the hemidesmosome includes the 180 and 230-kDa bullous pemphigoid antigens, α6β4 and α3β1 (a laminin receptor) integrins and plectin. The 180-kDa bullous pemphigoid antigen (type XVII collagen) is both within the epidermal cells and extends into the lamina lucida where is accessible to autoantibodies that cause bullous pemphigoid, a disorder seen rarely in the pediatric age group. Integrin receptors co-localize with focal adhesions between the keratinocytes actin–stress fibers and laminin in the lamina lucida.

MOLECULAR

Type VII collagen, produced predominantly by keratinocytes, is the major component of the anchoring fibrils. The fibrils extend from the lamina densa into the papillary dermis, where they interact via their NC-1 terminal portion with other anchoring fibrils and type IV collagen to form a complex structure, the attachment plaque. The triple helical collagens (middle section is 424nm long) laterally associate as antiparallel dimers, which are stabilized by disulfide bonds. GDA-J/F3 is an asialoglycoprotein located where the anchoring fibrils fan out and insert into the lamina densa.

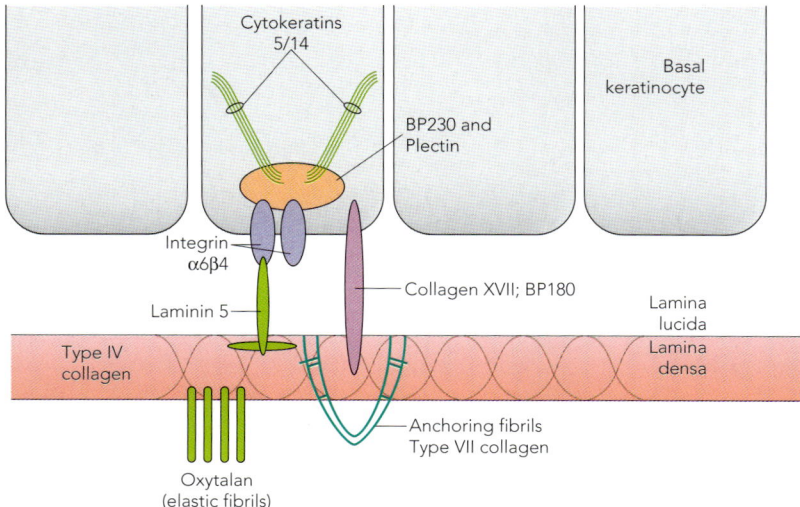

Fig. 1.25 Schematic representation of hemidesmosomes and other components of the DEJ.

Anchoring filaments are composed of laminin type 5, which is formed by three distinct chains, each separately encoded. These structures extend from the hemidesmosome across the lamina lucida to the lamina densa.

The lamina lucida contains laminin, entactin/nidogen and fibronectin. These molecules self-aggregate and also associate with other matrix molecules.

The lamina densa contains the ends of anchoring fibrils and the elastic oxytalan fibers. Type IV collagen, type V collagen and heparan sulfate proteoglycan, all products of keratinocytes, are also within the lamina densa. In the DEJ collagen types IV and collagen type V co-distribute. Fibronectin binds to the dermal side of the lamina densa.

SUMMARY OF FUNCTIONS

Sulfated proteoglycans in the lamina densa restrict passage of cationic macromolecules. Molecules less than 40kDa can cross the basement membrane zone. Other cells, such as Langerhans cells, regularly cross the DEJ as part of their physiological functioning. Other cells, such as malignant cells, cross the barrier by modification and proteolysis of the DEJ components. In wound healing, inflammation and certain skin disease there is dramatic and continual remodeling of the DEJ. Genetic diseases of DEJ components and autoimmune diseases with antibodies to DEJ molecules have provided important demonstrations of DEJ function.

VASCULAR STRUCTURES (BLOOD VESSELS AND LYMPHATICS)

TISSUES

Musculocutaneous vessels start from the muscle of the body wall, penetrate the subcutaneous tissue and, in the deep reticular dermis, branch and form a deep horizontal plexus with arterioles that rise toward the epidermis. There are valves in the venules in the hypodermal–subcutaneous plexus. Upper dermal vessels are highly branching and anastomosing; their roughly vertical loops in the dermal papillae have been compared to candelabra. A second horizontal plexus (subpapillary plexus) forms at the border of the papillary and reticular dermis. The vessels of the subpapillary plexus are terminal arterioles, arterial and venous capillaries, and postcapillary venules. Capillary loops ascend into the dermal papillae from this subpapillary plexus and descend to rejoin the plexus. The organization and patterns of the vascular system are complete by one and one-half years of life (Figs 1.26 and 1.27).

Glomus bodies are direct connections between arterioles and venous vessels without capillaries, allowing for vascular shunting. The glomi occur mainly in the reticular dermis of the nail bed, pads of the volar tissue, on ears and the central face. The arteriole portion of this channel is the Suquet–Hoyer canal and is 20–40μm in diameter. The vascular endothelium has a periodic acid–Schiff-positive basement membrane, which is surrounded by four to five layers of glomus cells, which are epithelioid smooth muscle cells. These cells are surrounded by large numbers of non-myelinated nerves.

The *lymphatic system* is organized in synchronization with the venous system. There are two lymphatic plexuses: a horizontal plexus of lymphatic vessels that is deep to the subpapillary vascular plexus, and a deeper plexus at the subcutaneous–hypodermal boundary. Lymph vessels have valves, a larger diameter than the corresponding blood vessels, and a thin endothelial wall with minimal collagen but more fine elastic fibers. In the deeper reticular dermis (hypodermis) vessels with flattened endothelial cells and smooth muscle cells surrounding the vessel walls are present.

CELLS

Endothelial cells form a continuous monolayer less than 10μm thick with a 1000μm² surface area. They contain characteristic granules, the Weibel–Palade body, which contains von Willebrand factor. The cells have gap, occludens, and adherens junctions.

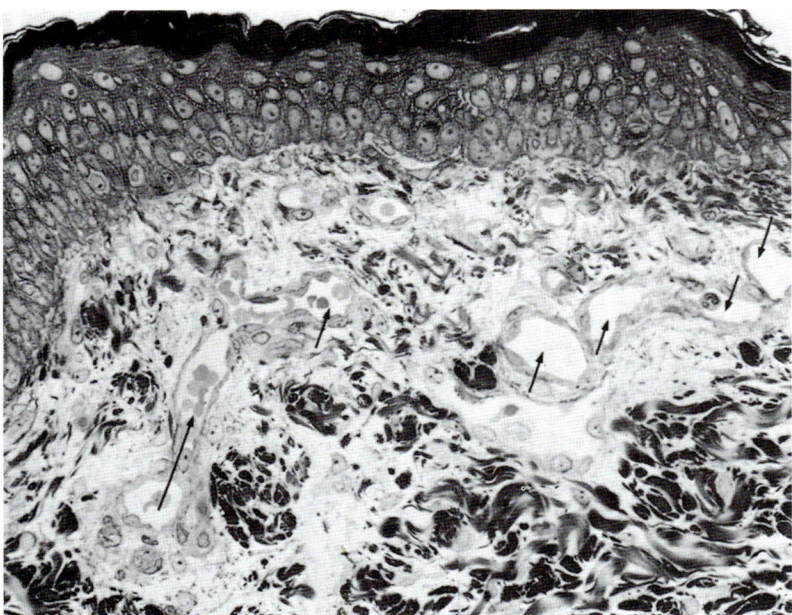

Fig. 1.26   Light micrograph of the upper region of the skin showing the vessels of the subpapillary plexus (arrows) marking the approximate boundary between the papillary and reticular dermis (× 350). (From Holbrook and Sybert, 1995, with permission)

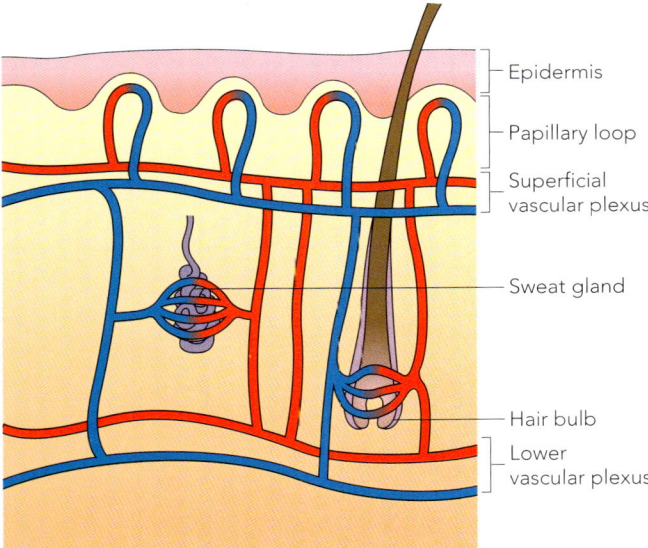

- Epidermis
- Papillary loop
- Superficial vascular plexus
- Sweat gland
- Hair bulb
- Lower vascular plexus

Fig. 1.27   Schematic representation of the superficial and deep vascular plexuses – arterial portions (red) and venous portions (blue), and the blood supply of eccrine glands and hair follicles. The vascular loop in the dermal papilla consists of terminal arterioles, arterial capillaries, venous capillaries, and postcapillary venules.

Veil cells are in the adventia external to the vessel. They are flat, have factor XIII activity and are part of the dermal dendrocyte system.

Mast cells are derived from CD34+ bone marrow cells. Their density is highest in the papillary dermis near the DEJ, and in the sheaths of the appendages and blood vessels. They are round to spindle-shaped and up to $25\mu m$ in their largest dimension. There are 7000–20 000 mast cells per mm³. They are associated with neuropeptide containing sensory nerves. These have metachromatic red–purple granules $(0.3–0.8\mu m)$ that stain with Alcian Blue and or with Giemsa stain.

SUMMARY OF FUNCTIONS

The vasculature functions in the transport of metabolites, temperature regulation, wound repair, and scaffolding for cutaneous immune responses. The highly anastomosing nature of vessels allows shunting and temperature control. Lymphatics return the flow of solute and enable cellular migration. Mast cells contain the c-kit receptor, which responds to the stem cell factor ligand through the tyrosine kinase signaling pathway. Mast cells are active participants in allergic reactions through their receptors for IgE.

Mast cells have preformed inflammatory mediators and can synthesize inflammatory mediators. Preformed mediators include histamine, tryptase, heparin, chymase, neutrophilic and eosinophilic chemotactic factors. Mast cells can synthesize IL-1, IL-2, IL-3, IL-4, IL-5, GM-CSF, TNF-α, leukotrienes, and platelet-activating factors.

HAIR

TISSUES

The first hair begins in fetal life and is called *lanugo hair*, which is fine, silky, nonmedullated, and lightly pigmented. Fine intermediate hairs are on the scalp until about age 2 when terminal hairs erupt. *Vellus hairs* are short, soft, fine, nonmedullated and have less pigment than terminal hairs. *Terminal hairs* are long, coarse, and pigmented.

The hair is usually associated with the sebaceous gland. Hair emerges from the skin surface at an angle. The tip of the growing hair is tapered.

The hair follicle can be conceptualized as a set of concentric sheaths with different functions and characteristics. These include supportive sheaths that surround and stabilize the growing hair, and then the final multilayered hair itself (Fig. 1.28). The hair follicle is divided into four segments.

The *infundibulum* is uppermost and is defined by the skin surface and the junction of the sebaceous duct (Fig 1.29). The duct in the infundibulum is lined by a stratified keratinized epithelium. The apocrine gland also empties into the follicle in this zone. The *isthmus* is between the opening of the sebaceous duct and the bulge. The bulge is at the site of expansion of outer root sheath cells and is at the insertion of the *arrector pili muscle*. The bulge is the site of the stem cell population for the follicle. The cells in this region have high levels of β1 integrin and low levels of E-cadherin, β- and γ-catenin. They show an undifferentiated morphology. The *lower follicle* is between the bulge and the bulb. It contains those portions of the follicle that proliferate or regress, depending on the hair cycle. The *bulb* contains the germinative cells of the follicle and other cells including melanocytes, Langerhans cells and Merkel cells. The bulb for terminal hairs contains the germinal matrix cells at the end of the follicle. The bulb is in the dermis for vellus hairs, but is located in the subcutaneous tissue for the terminal hair follicle. Within a concavity in the bulb is the dermal papillae, a collection of special fibroblasts, which are related to follicle differentiation and maintenance; the size of the hair is related to the volume of the dermal papilla. Each follicle has a smooth muscle, the arrector pili muscle, which attaches to the bulge at one end and originates with subepidermal elastic fibers. It contracts with cold or fright producing pebbly skin, "goose bumps".

CELLS

The *outer root sheath* is the outermost cell layer of the follicle. It does not keratinize and its basement membrane thickens in the region of the isthmus ("glassy membrane"). The outer root sheath contains K6 and K16 keratins and is several cell layer thick above the isthmus but only one to two layers thick below the isthmus.

The *inner root sheath* has several components. Most peripheral is the layers of Henle, then the layers of Huxley and innermost the cuticle. The inner root sheath ends at the junction between the isthmus and the infundibulum and forms some of the desquamated keratinized cells, which adhere to the hair when it emerges from the scalp. The cells of the innermost sheath cells synthesize trichohyalin, which is a matrix protein (Fig. 1.30).

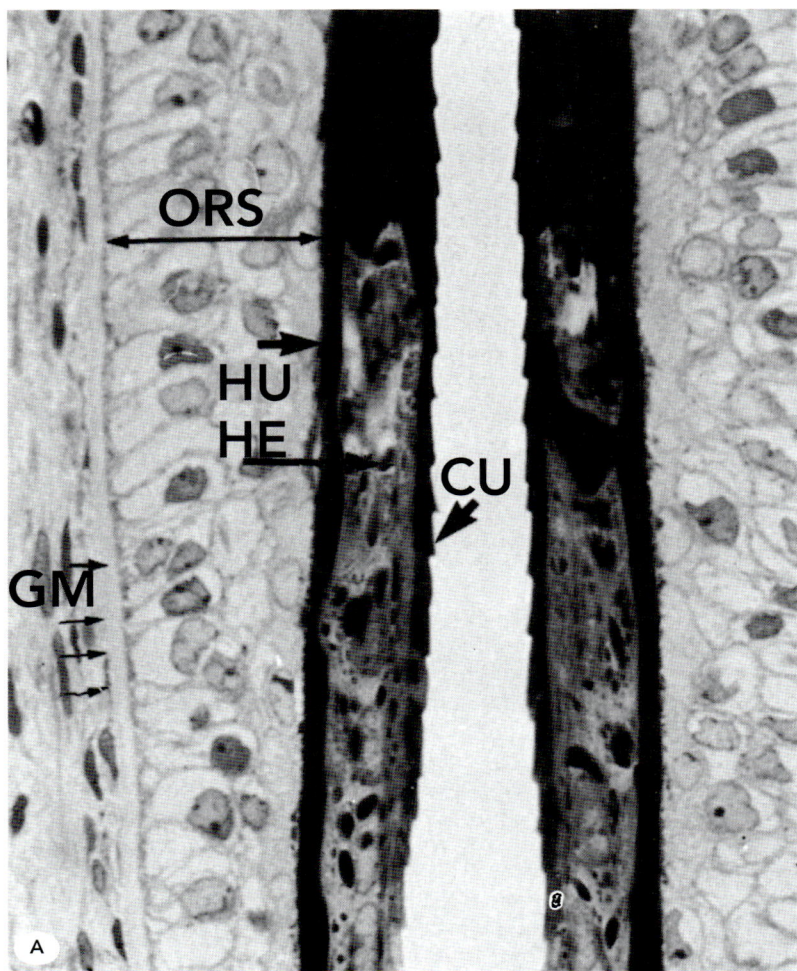

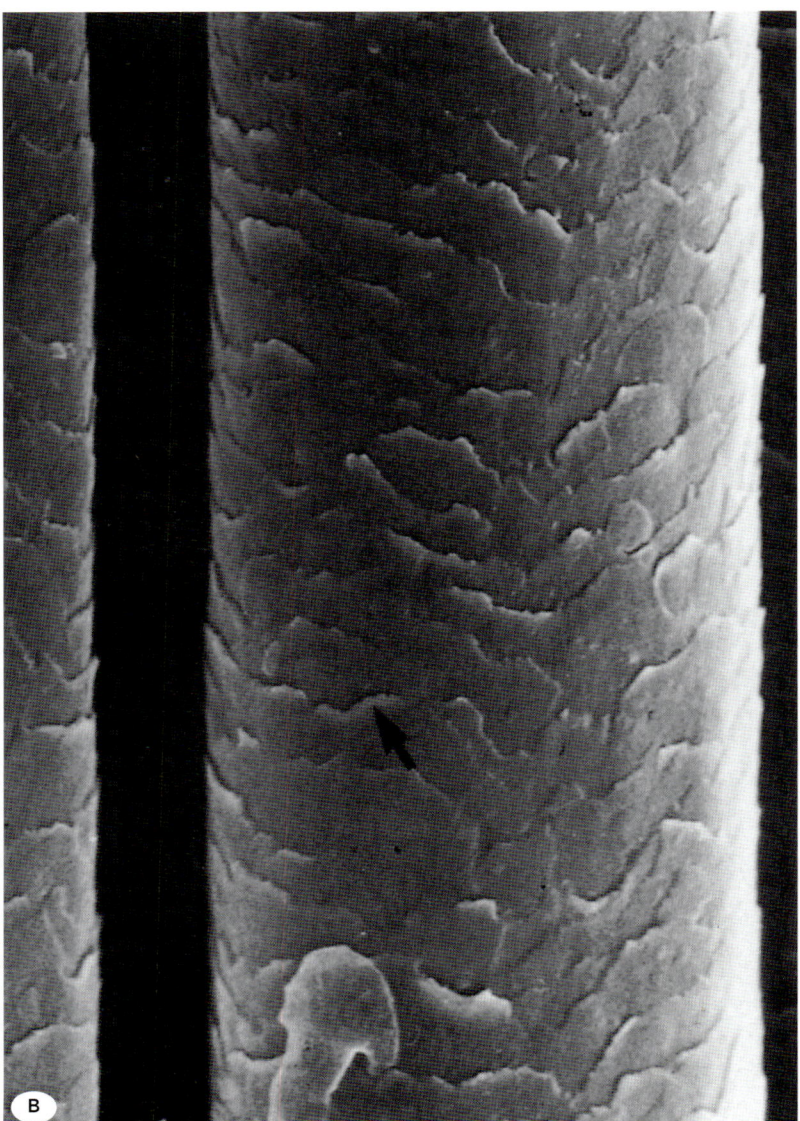

Fig. 1.28   Light and scanning electron micrographs of the (A) follicle and (B) hair. The cells of the outer root sheath (ORS) are surrounded by the glassy membrane (GM). Huxley (HU), Henle (HE), and cuticular (CU) layers of the inner root sheath are also shown. Note that the direction of the cuticular scales is opposite that of the cuticle of the hair. (A) × 350; (B) × 600. (From Holbrook and Sybert, 1995, with permission)

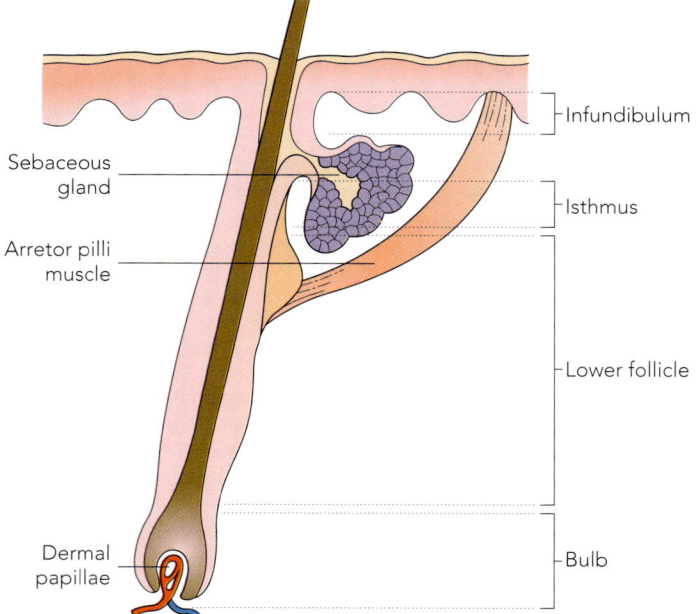

Fig. 1.29   Diagram of the hair and its related structures. The bulb of the hair follicle (lowest portion) often extends into the subcutaneous tissue.

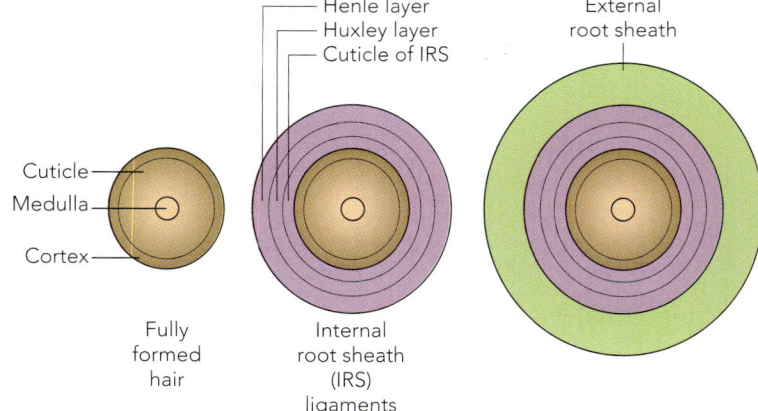

Fig. 1.30   Transverse sections of the hair and hair follicles at different levels emphasizing three main components; fully formed terminal hair, the inner root sheath system and the outer (external root) sheath.

The fully formed hair has outer and inner cuticular layers which have overlapped and interdigitated cells. The cortex forms the bulk of the hair and is composed of keratinized cells, which contain pigment from the bulb melanocytes. Innermost is the medulla, which has a set of type I and type II keratins, a unique set of high-glycine, high-tyrosine proteins, and abundant high-sulfur matrix proteins. The medullary proteins are crosslinked with γ-ε(-glutamyl) lysine peptide bonds.

SUMMARY OF FUNCTIONS

The hair provides protection (eyelashes, nasal hair), sensory perception, and especially adornment. In humans hair does not have the important role in thermoregulation it has in other mammals.

NAILS

TISSUES

The *nail plate* is a keratinized structure, which is continually growing throughout life. Its germinative cells are located in the proximal portion of the nail bed and underneath the nail fold. The white *lunula* visible under most nails is the nail's germinative population. The *nail bed* beneath the nail plate contains longitudinally arrayed vascular loops, which is the basis of longitudinal hemorrhages in the nails with disease or after trauma. The *lateral nail fold* and the *proximal nail fold* (*epionychium*) protects and seals the bed and plate from the environment and organisms. The cuticle is stratum corneum extending from the proximal nail fold (Figs 1.31–1.33).

The *nail matrix* is a keratinizing tissue, which differs from epidermis and hair in not synthesizing keratohyalin; the cells retain their nuclei (parakeratotic cells) similar to the oral mucosa or the skin of aquatic mammals. The proliferative component of the matrix determines the thickness of the nail and its growth rate. *Melanocytes* are in the lower two to five layers of the matrix and contribute to the pigmented bands in some nails and to the general dark hue of the nail plate in heavily pigmented individuals.

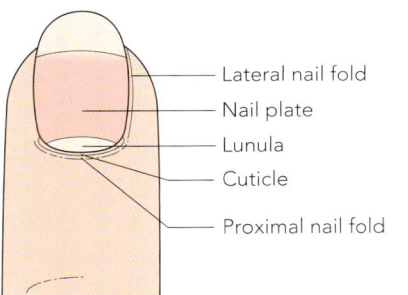

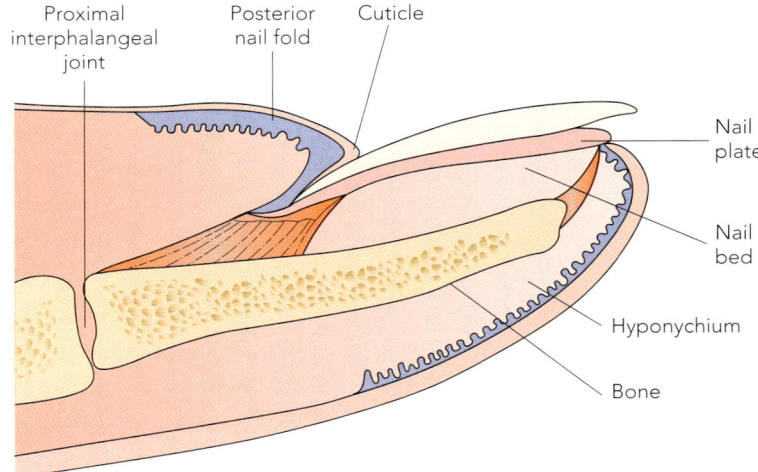

Fig. 1.33   Lateral section of the nail and its underlying structures.

The nail bed is beneath the matrix and the *hyponychium*. This epithelium has a corrugated appearance reflecting the underlying vascular bed. There are prominent arteriovenous anastomoses including glomus cells, which are smooth muscle in origin, and may form benign but painful tumors. As distinct from other portions of the integument there is no subcutaneous tissue in the dermis under the nails, which allows this tissue to reflect changes in serum albumin clinically as paleness of the nail bed, the half-and-half nail and parallel pale lines in the nail bed. The nail plate is attached to the nail bed tightly through unknown mechanisms. Distally the nail plate is attached by the hyponychium, which is the only portion of the nail that is keratinized with a granular layer and a true stratum corneum. This is a common site for dermatophyte infection.

SUMMARY OF FUNCTIONS

In addition to protecting the soft tissue of the finger and toes the nail enhances dexterity and can be used for protection and for scratching. Nails

Fig. 1.31   Boundaries and landmarks of the nail.

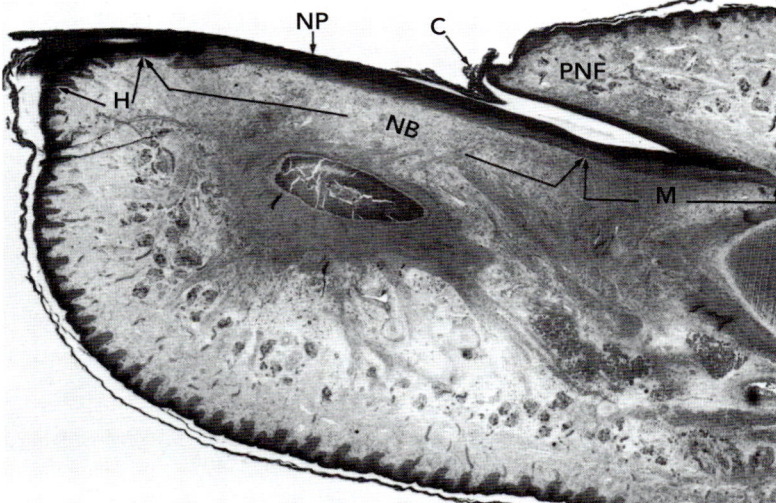

Fig. 1.32   Light micrograph of a longitudinal section through the nail of a newborn illustrating the regions of the nail unit. C, cuticle; PNF, proximal nail fold; M, matrix; NB, nail bed; NP, nail plate; H, hyponychium (× 30). (From Holbrook and Sybert, 1995, with permission)

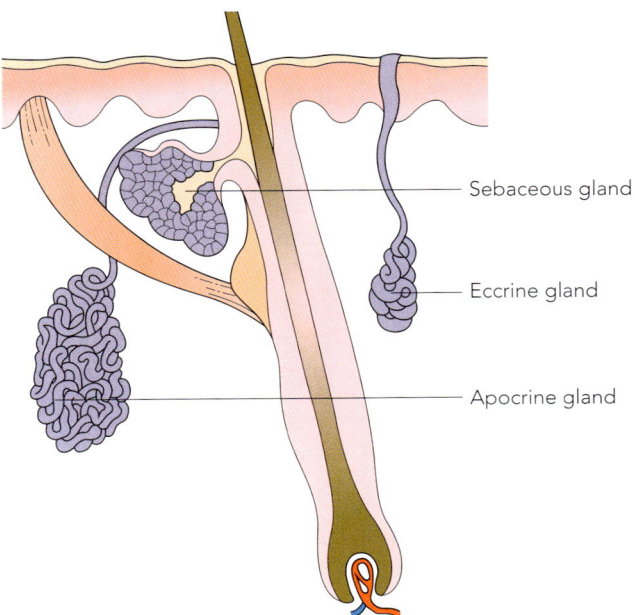

Fig. 1.34   The glands of the skin. The apocrine gland is deeper than the eccrine gland and its duct empties into the follicular canal. Sebaceous gland products are discharged into the sebaceous duct which is connected to the hair canal. Eccrine gland ducts exit directly on the skin surface independent of the hair follicle.

are translucent. They block UVB light, but UVA light readily passes through the nail plate, allowing for phototoxic subungal reactions with administration of some drugs, e.g., tetracyclines.

ECCRINE GLANDS

TISSUES

Eccrine glands first develop in the axilla associated with apocrine glands. They are distributed over the body generally. The tubular mass of the eccrine sweat glands is 100g. The total number of eccrine glands does not increase postnatally. There are 2–5 million glands per individual. The highest density of eccrine glands is on the palms, soles (620/cm²), and forehead in the adult. The secretory coil is deep in the reticular dermis or subcutaneous fat. The sweat duct opens directly at the skin surface. The gland and duct are surrounded by circumferential fibroblasts, collagen and elastic microfibrils (Fig. 1.34).

CELLS

Secretory region

The *pyramidal cells* have a broad base, narrow luminal surface, and serous cells with no secretory granules; dark mucous cells face the lumen. *Clear cells* with interdigitating peripheral villi and intercellular canniculi have abundant glycogen, and discharge material into the glandular lumen. These clear cells are the source of the secretion of water and electrolytes. *Dark cells* (broad luminal surface, small base) have mucous-containing, periodic acid–Schiff-positive secretory granules, many ribosomes, and lipid droplets. The function of dark cells is uncertain. *Myoepithelial cells* are discontinuous, peripherally joined by desmosomes, and contain myofilaments and keratins. The basement membrane of the eccrine gland is distal to the myoepithelial cell (Fig. 1.35).

Ducts

The eccrine duct has two layers in the dermis. The intraepidermal portion of the duct lining is keratinized at the outermost sweat pore. The outer cells have prominent microvilli and mitochondria for reabsorption. The innermost

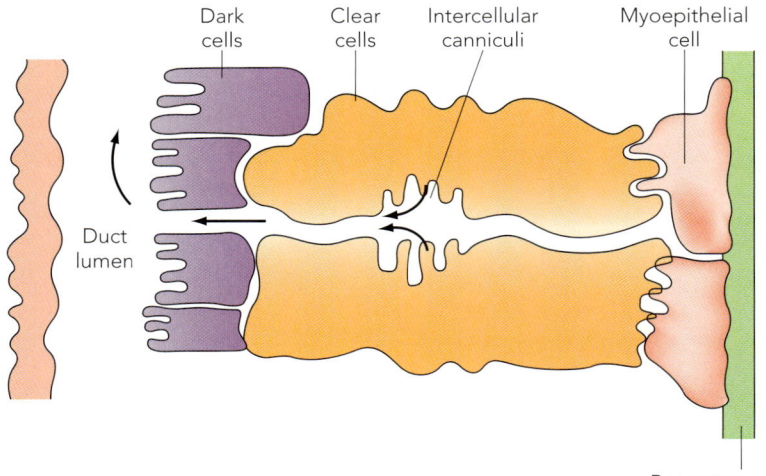

Fig. 1.35 The secretory coil of the eccrine gland. Sweat is secreted (arrows) into intracellular canniculi and then proceeds to the ductal lumen (Modified from Freedberg et al. (1999) Fitzpatrick's Dermatology in General Medicine, McGraw-Hill, with permission.)

cells form a "cuticular border" with microvilli, microfilaments and intermediate filaments – these features are more developed as the duct approaches the epidermal surface (Fig. 1.36).

MOLECULAR

Sodium pumps along basal lateral plasma membrane transport sodium from the duct lumen to the plasma. Glycogen in clear cells is metabolized to lactate which is secreted with water, sodium, potassium and chloride into the canniculi. The concentration of sweat when first secreted is close to isotonic concentration.

SUMMARY OF FUNCTIONS

The eccrine glands secrete water, which is brought to the surface by ducts. At the surface, it can evaporate, decreasing excessive body temperature. Glands are functional by late in the third trimester, but clinical sweating does not start until one day after birth, beginning on the face. Isotonic sweat becomes hypotonic as ions and water are resorbed along duct. Myoepithelial cells may strengthen the cell wall. Dark cells secrete a glycoprotein of unknown function.

SUMMARY OF BIOLOGICAL MECHANISMS

A well-acclimatized individual can sweat 10l/day. The ducts concentrate and modify sweat. Absorption is higher when closer to the secretory coil. Basal cells reabsorption through microvilli. Sweat contains large amounts of lactate, especially at low rates of sweating, drugs, enzymes including lysosomal enzymes, histamine, prostaglandins, immunoglobulins and kallikrein. Sweat occurs in response to peripheral receptors in skin and muscle via the hypothalamic temperature-regulated center. The response is by sympathetic (cholinergic) via postganglionic fibers that surround the gland. Acetylcholine may stimulate calcium transport and adrenergic stimulation increases cellular cAMP to decrease the permeability to calcium. Adrenergic drugs induce sweating in children; adults need higher dosages for a response. Neurological control of sweating is not complete until age 2–3 years. Myoepithelial cells respond to acetylcholine and contract. Botulinum toxin A blocks acetylcholine, the mediator of sympathetic stimulation to eccrine sweat glands, and is an effective treatment for palmar hyperhidrosis. The concentration of sodium chloride in sweat of adults is higher than in children.

APOCRINE GLANDS (Figs 1.37, 1.38)

TISSUES

Apocrine glands are blind ended with large coiled tubular glands deep in the dermis. They are deeper than eccrine glands and limited to face, scalp, axilla and anogenital regions. Modified apocrine glands are in eyelids (Moll's gland), ear canal and areolar glands of the breast. The duct opens into the infundibulum of the hair follicle. Sebum and apocrine material merge at this site.

CELLS

The *secretory cell* contains several kinds of granules. The "true" secretory granule is small, periodic acid–Schiff-positive, and contains lipids and particulate material. Smaller dense core granules are presumed precursors of true granules. In addition, the cells have rod-like granules containing ferritin, lipid and pigment. *Myoepithelial cells* are contractile and responsible for the pulsatile nature of secretion. The *duct* contains three cell layers. The cuticular borders on the cells of the lumen and is similar to that of the eccrine duct.

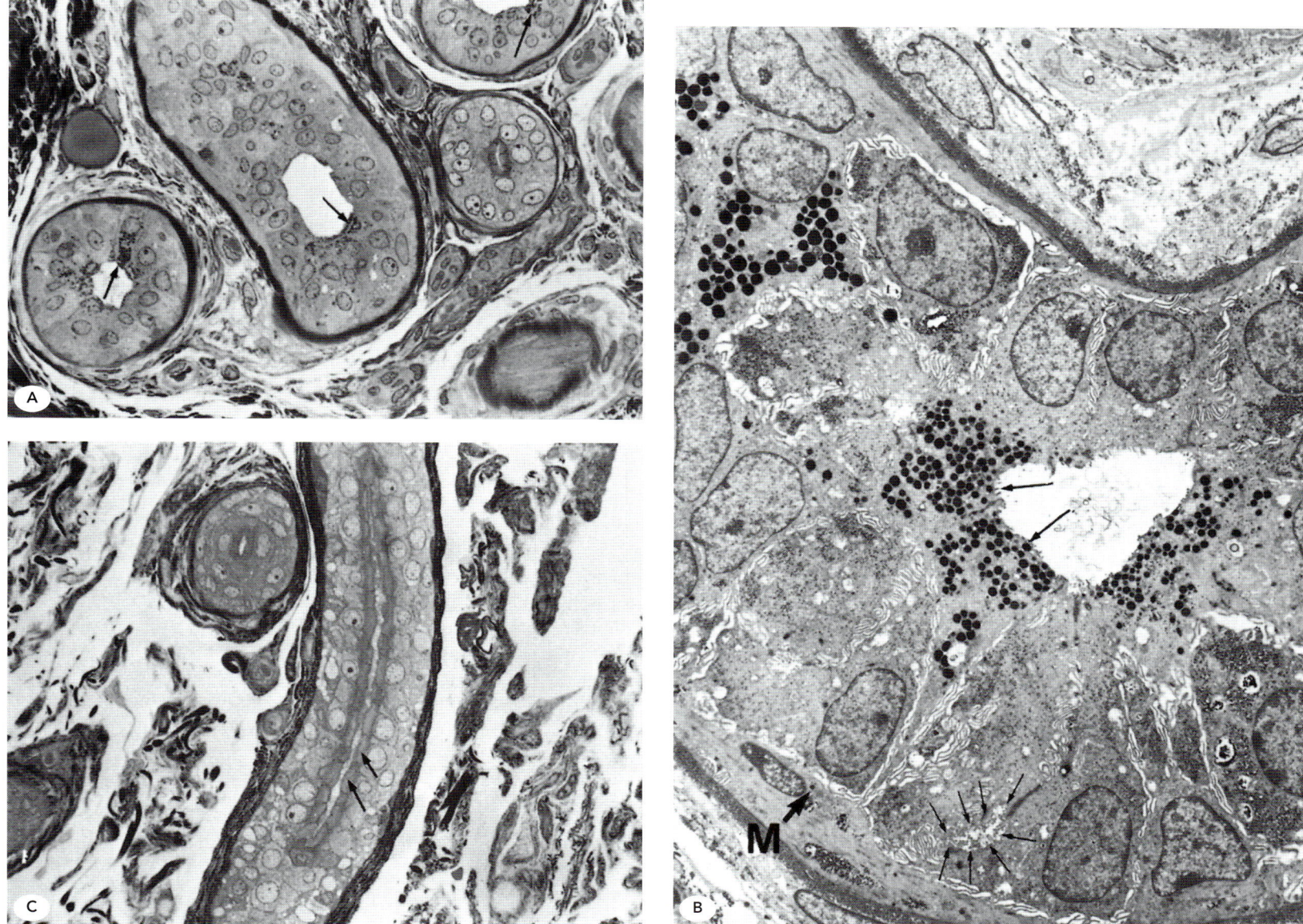

Fig. 1.36   Light and transmission electron micrographs of (A and B) eccrine sweat gland coils, (A, C and D) the dermal portion of a sweat duct, and (E and F) the intraepidermal sweat duct and sweat pore. In (A), three segments of a sweat gland are shown in cross-section. Note the secretory granules in the dark cells (arrows). In (B) of the electron micrograph, light cells are identified by the absence of granules, and dark cells are filled with electron-dense granules at their luminal borders. Myoepithelial cells (M) lie along the basal lamina. Note the extensive interdigitations of the intercellular borders. An intercellular canniculus is demonstrated by a series of small arrows. In (C) the two layers of the wall and the cuticular borders (arrows) of the inner ductal cells are evident.

SUMMARY OF FUNCTIONS

In humans, apocrine glands are not important for thermoregulation and their true functions remain uncertain.

SUMMARY OF BIOLOGICAL MECHANISMS

Holocrine secretion with loss of apical projection of secretory cells forms the secreted material. The periodicity of secretion may be related to myoepithelial cell contraction. Strong emotion or pain but not exposure to heat, causes secretion. Secretion is controlled by alpha adrenergic stimulation and possibly by cholinergic stimulation. There is no resorption of secreted materials. Local or systemic administration of epinephrine causes secretion. Secretion is inhibited by botulinum toxin.

SEBACEOUS GLANDS

TISSUES

Sebaceous glands develop from a collection of outer root sheath cells of the hair peg early in the second trimester of fetal life. They are unilobular when small; when follicles are large and dense the sebaceous glands are multilobular with multiple acini with connective tissue separations. The innermost cells and secretions are released into the sebaceous duct (keratinized) and then into the hair follicle.

The sebaceous glands are largest on the face, scalp, and upper chest. Sebaceous follicles are defined as those with prominent glands and tiny or absent hair. Specialized sebaceous glands are found in the eyelid (Moll and Zeis), lips and buccal mucosa (Fordyce spots), nipple, glans penis and prepuce (Figs 1.37–1.39).

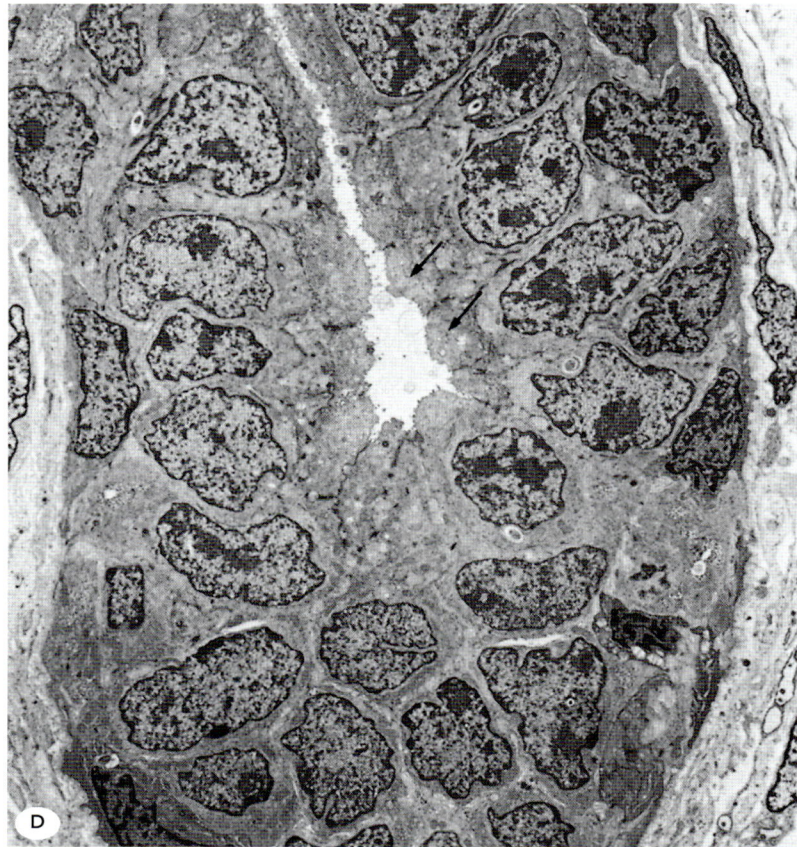

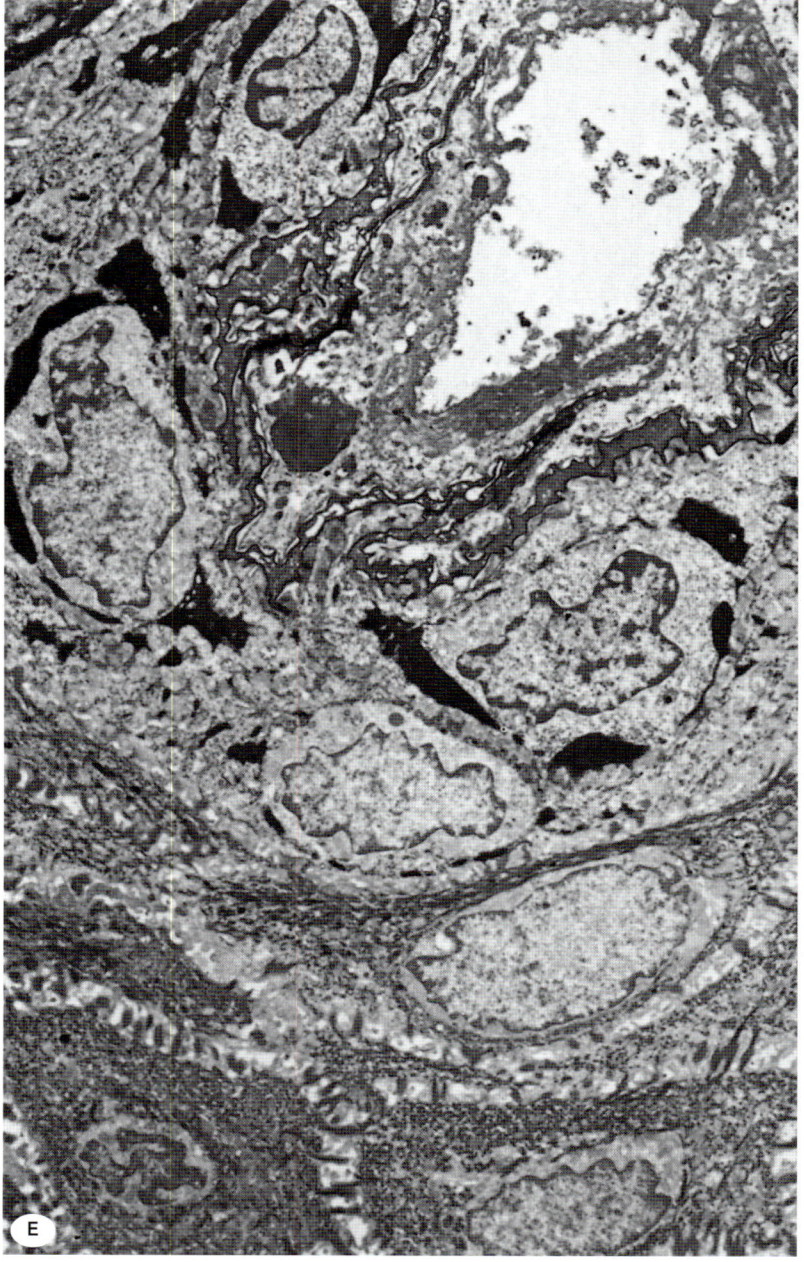

Fig. 1.36 The similarity of cells of both layers is evident in (D). In (E) circumferentially organized cells form a keratinized lining of the duct within the epidermis.

CELLS

Peripheral cells can divide. Intracellular lipid synthesis occurs in cells beyond the basal layer.

SUMMARY OF FUNCTIONS

Holocrine secretion without neural stimulation begins by 8 months' gestation, and regresses between 6 and 12 months. Increased sebum secretion may occur as early as 6–7 years of age, and is initiated by adrenal androgens. Subsequently, gonadal androgens which are increased in secretion at puberty and during late teenage years also stimulate sebum production. Sebaceous lipids contain squalene, cholesterol, cholesterol esters and triglycerides. Sapienic acid (palmitic acid with a delta–six double bond, 16:1Δ6) is the major fatty acid of sebum. Wax esters and squalene in skin surface lipids are uniquely derived from sebum.

SUMMARY OF BIOLOGICAL MECHANISMS

Androgens are the primary stimulators of sebaceous glands enlargement and secretion whether in the fetus, newborn, or postpubertally.

CUTANEOUS NERVES

TISSUES

Nerves follow the pattern of vessels and are derived from large segmental musculocutaneous spinal nerve branches and branches of cranial nerve V to form a deep and superficial plexus. Autonomic motor fibers innervate eccrine sweat glands, sebaceous glands, vessels and the arrector pili muscle. Up to 1000 afferent nerves innervate an area of 100cm² (Figs 1.40–1.43).

Bare nerve cell endings are ensheathed by a basal lamina and Schwann cell processes. They are common in the papillary dermis close to the lamina densa and intraepidermally. They have large numbers of vesicles and mitochondria at their terminals. Penicillate fibers are free nerve endings in hairy skin, which respond to touch, pain, temperature and itch.

Arrector pili smooth muscles have adrenergic and cholinergic innervation with motor fibers that course along with the sensory fibers to the follicle. Meissner's corpuscles and the Pacinian corpuscle are corpuscular receptors with a capsule and inner core and have both neuronal and non-neuronal components. Meissner's corpuscles are individually situated within a dermal papillae with the endings of myelinated axons ensheathed with Schwann cells. The endbulbs of Krause on the lip, eyelid, perianal canal, clitoris and glans penis have a similar structure. The Pacinian corpuscle is a rapidly adapting pressure receptor in subcutis and at arteriovenous anastomoses. It has 30 or more layers (onion skin pattern) of perineurium and connective tissue surrounding the single axon of a digital nerve.

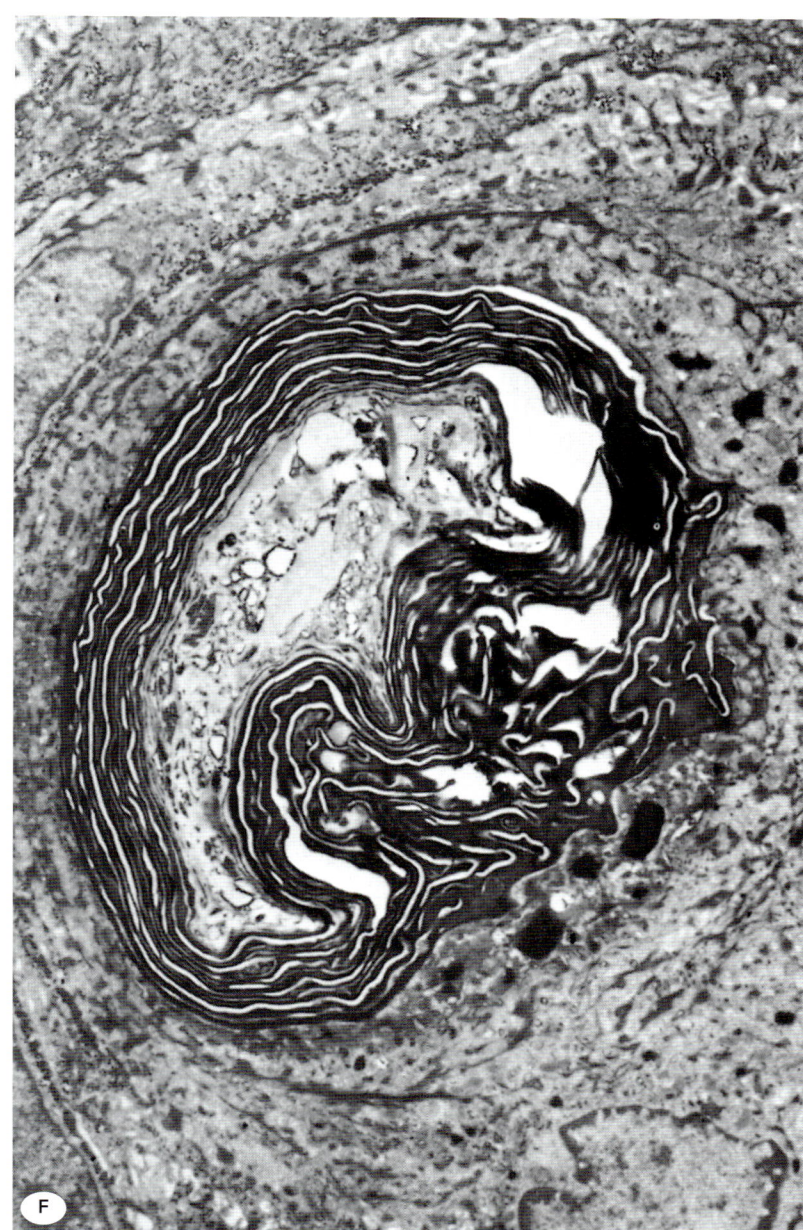

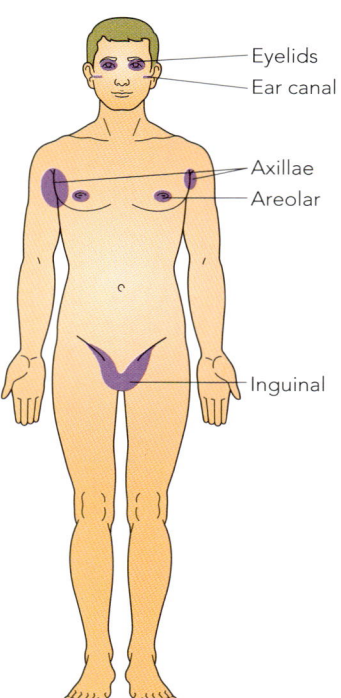

Fig. 1.37   Distribution of human apocrine glands (total = 100 000).

Eyelids

Ear canal

Axillae

Areolar

Inguinal

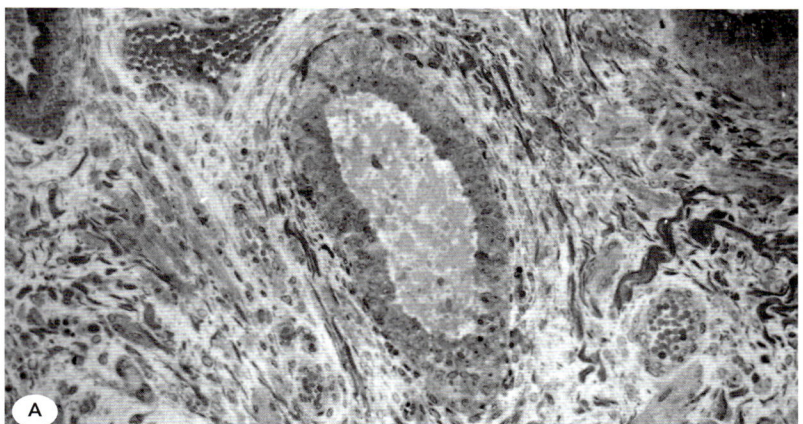

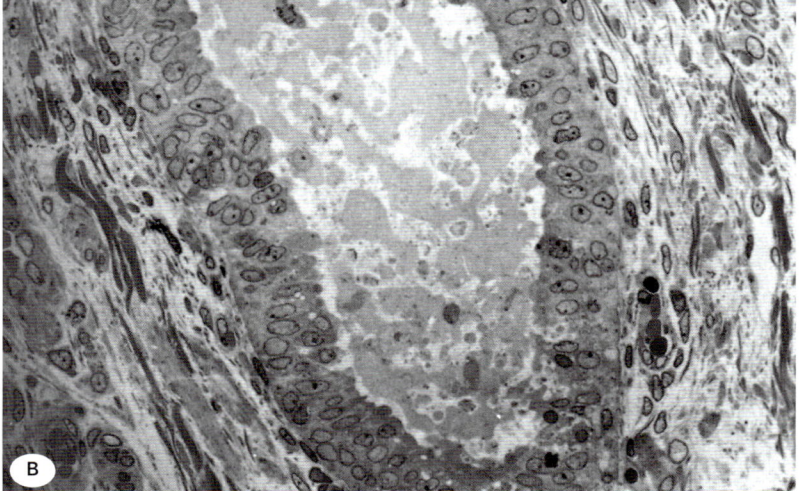

Fig. 1.36   (F) shows several layers of cornified cells at the level of the sweat pore. (A) × 350; (B) × 2500 (C) × 350; (D) × 2600; (E) × 2800; (F) × 3200. (From Holbrook and Sybert, 1995, with permission)

Hair follicles have free nerve endings (papillary nerve endings) just below the entrance of the sebaceous gland and are slowly adapting mechano-receptors. Nerves of hair follicles have a basket-like arrangement around the hairs; in addition, there are specific mechanoreceptors (Merkel cells) in the hair bulb (see Merkel cells).

SUMMARY OF FUNCTIONS

Afferent impulses originate in epidermal and hair follicle mechanoreceptors (Merkel cells), and in deeply situated pressure and vibration receptors, especially on the ridged skin of the palms and soles (Pacinian corpuscles), encapsulated superficial receptors (Meissner's corpuscles), and the "bare" nerve cell endings. Free nerve endings in nonhairy skin enter dermal papillae indi-vidually and can provide precise discrimination. Receptors are densely dispersed in three hairless areas: the areola, labia and glans penis.

Karen Holbrook is acknowledged as the original author of this section.

Fig. 1.38   (A and B) Light micrographs of an apocrine sweat gland from the areola of a newborn infant. Note the apparent homogeneity of cell types, the absence of large, distinguishable secretory granules, and the bulging of the luminal borders of the cells. (A) × 140; (B) × 350. (From Holbrook and Sybert, 1995, with permission)

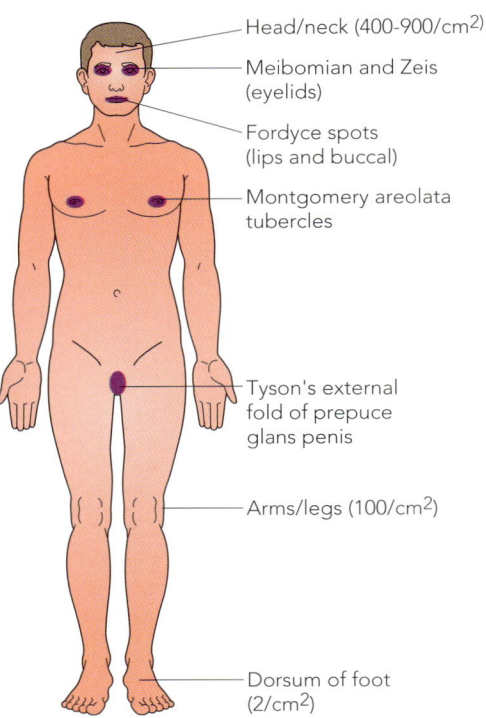

Head/neck (400-900/cm²)

Meibomian and Zeis
(eyelids)

Fordyce spots
(lips and buccal)

Montgomery areolata
tubercles

Tyson's external
fold of prepuce
glans penis

Arms/legs (100/cm²)

Dorsum of foot
(2/cm²)

Fig. 1.39   Distribution of human sebaceous glands.

BASIC IMMUNOLOGY

Mark Dahl

INTRODUCTION

The immune system can evoke inflammation, ward off infectious organisms, protect against cancer, and induce or elicit allergic and hypersensitive skin diseases. The immune system in children is much like the immune system in adults, although there are some differences. The mechanisms of immunity are the same and the immune systems of children are usually efficient and work better than the immune systems of adults, especially older adults. Nonetheless, children have not been exposed to as many antigens as adults and therefore normally have increased susceptibility to common infectious organisms. An increased incidence of infections also occurs in children with primary deficiencies of the immune system. These defects in the immune system often cause non-infectious health problems as well.

The immune system is composed of a number of elements. These include lymphocytes, immunoglobulins, lymphokines, complement, inflammatory mediators, phagocytes, and lymphoid organs such as lymph nodes, the spleen, and the thymus. To discuss the immune system, one must discuss each component individually; however, the immune system generally functions as a complete and integrated whole. When a reaction occurs in one arm of the immune system, a reaction is often occurring simultaneously in another. Each area of the immune system normally interacts with the others.

Sometimes the immune system does not act correctly, or all its parts do not work in harmony. For example, the immunity may be adequate, but if the

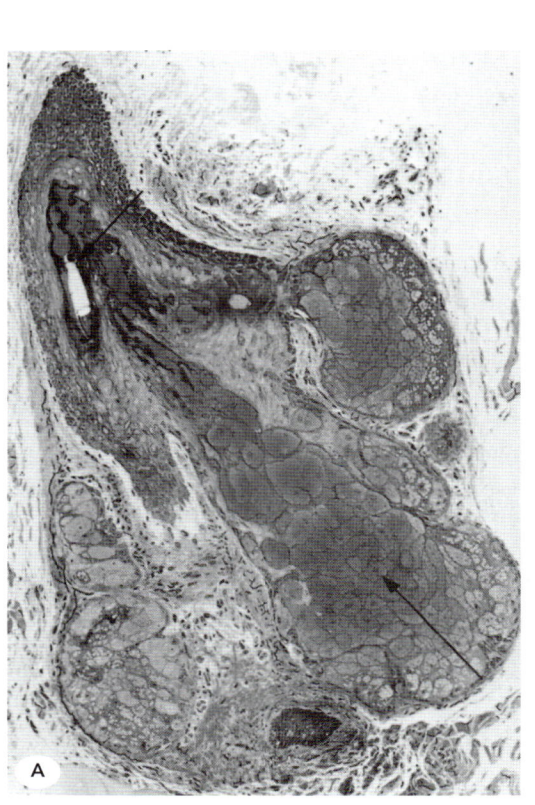

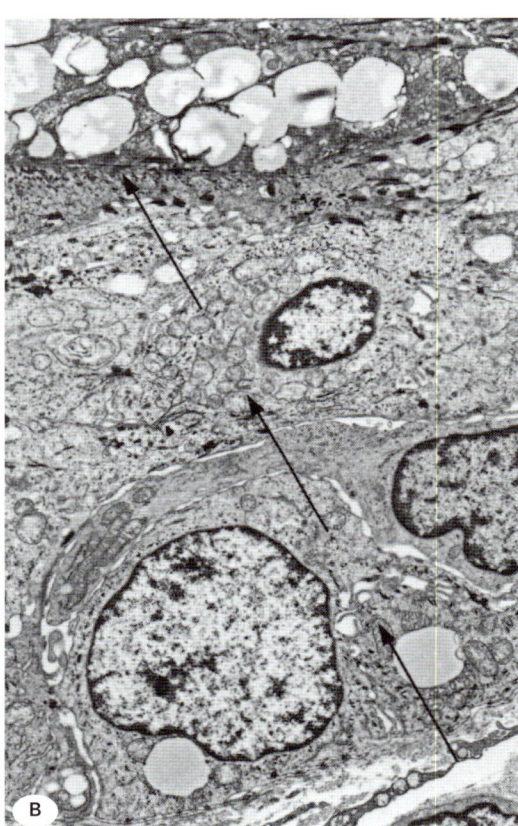

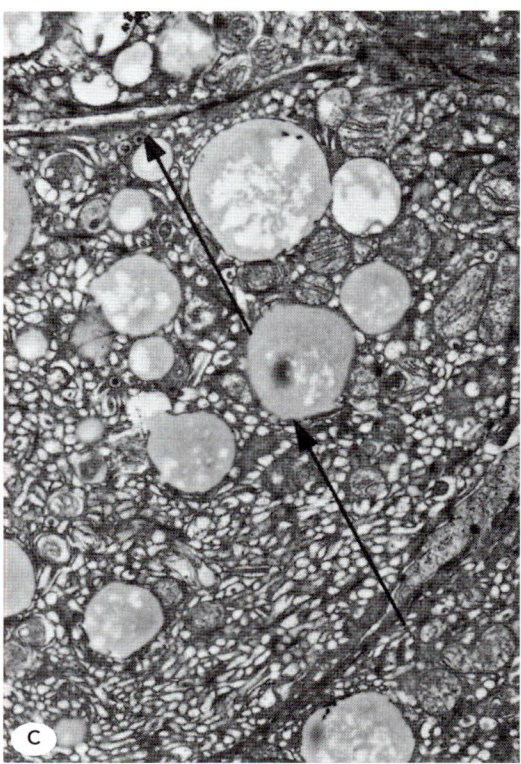

Fig. 1.40   Light and transmission electron micrographs of sebaceous glands (A and B). The gland is organized in acini with the least differentiated cells positioned peripherally. (C) The more differentiated cells are filled with sebaceous lipids, which are released via a keratinized duct (seen in A) into the infundibulum of the follicle. The arrows indicate the direction of lipid synthesis and secretion. (A) × 100; (B) × 4800; (C) × 4800. (From Holbrook and Sybert, 1995, with permission)

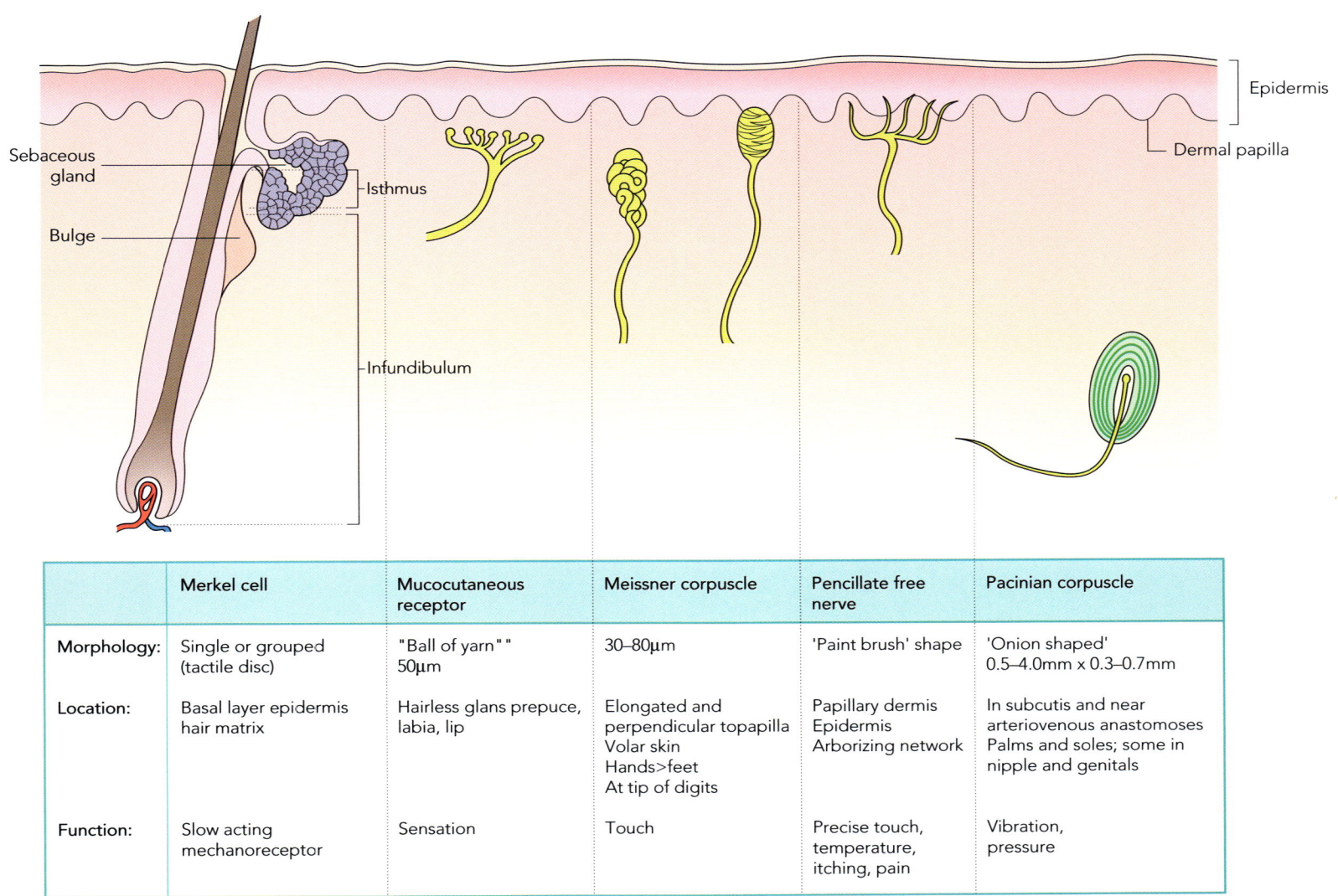

	Merkel cell	Mucocutaneous receptor	Meissner corpuscle	Pencillate free nerve	Pacinian corpuscle
Morphology:	Single or grouped (tactile disc)	"Ball of yarn"" 50μm	30–80μm	'Paint brush' shape	'Onion shaped' 0.5–4.0mm x 0.3–0.7mm
Location:	Basal layer epidermis hair matrix	Hairless glans prepuce, labia, lip	Elongated and perpendicular topapilla Volar skin Hands>feet At tip of digits	Papillary dermis Epidermis Arborizing network	In subcutis and near arteriovenous anastomoses Palms and soles; some in nipple and genitals
Function:	Slow acting mechanoreceptor	Sensation	Touch	Precise touch, temperature, itching, pain	Vibration, pressure

Fig. 1.41　Schematic representation of the location, overall morphology and function of the cutaneous receptors.

inflammatory response is insufficient, the child is predisposed to infection. In other instances the inflammatory response may be too great or may be directed against host tissues leading to tissue damage and autoaggressive disorders.

HUMORAL IMMUNITY

Humoral immunity is immunity mediated by immunoglobulins and the cells that produce them, namely B and plasma cells. An antigen is a chemical substance that can induce an immune response. It may be a polysaccharide such as a bacterial cell wall, a polypeptide, glycoprotein, or other material. An antibody is an immunoglobulin that can specifically combine with the antigen that stimulated its production. Although all antibodies are immunoglobulins, not all immunoglobulins are antibodies because the antigen specificity of an immunoglobulin may be unknown.

There are five major types of immunoglobulin, namely IgG, IgM, IgA, IgD, and IgE. All immunoglobulin molecules have a similar structure consisting of large and small polypeptide (Fig. 1.46). The large polypeptide chain is called a heavy or H chain. The smaller polypeptide chain is called an L or light chain. The sequence of amino acids within about three-quarters of the heavy chain determines its immunoglobulin class (e.g., IgG). Although there are five major types of heavy chains (designated γ, μ, α, δ, and ε), there are only two major types of light chains, namely κ and λ. The light chains and the heavy chains each have long sequences of amino acids that are relatively constant for each immunoglobulin class, regardless of the antigen specificity. This portion of the immunoglobulin molecule is called the *constant region* and its end is called the *Fc end*. Phagocytes and some other cells have on their surface Fc receptors that can bind this "back end" of the immunoglobulin molecule, for example, as an initial step toward phagocytosing an immune complex. The sequence of amino acids at the other end (the Fab end) of the immunoglobulin molecule is highly variable. This portion is called the *variable region*, and differences here determine differences in antigen binding (antigen specificity). A typical immunoglobulin molecule is composed of two heavy chains of identical amino acid composition and two light chains of identical amino acid composition. One light chain is associated with one heavy chain by disulfide bonds, which hold them together.

IMMUNOGLOBULIN G

Immunoglobulin G is responsible for long-lasting immunity. Of all the immunoglobulins, it is the one present in the highest concentration in plasma. There are four subclasses of IgG based on subtle structural differences in the constant portion of the heavy chain. These subclasses are designated IgG1, IgG2, IgG3, and IgG4. IgG (except IgG4) can activate complement by the classical pathway and can enter the fetal circulation by passing across the placental barrier *in utero*.

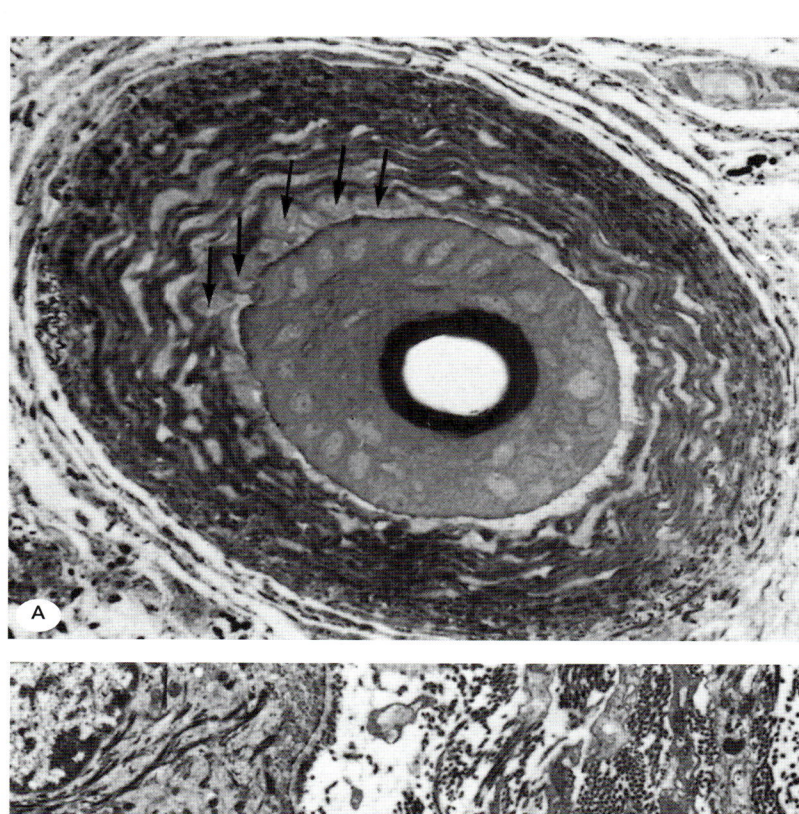

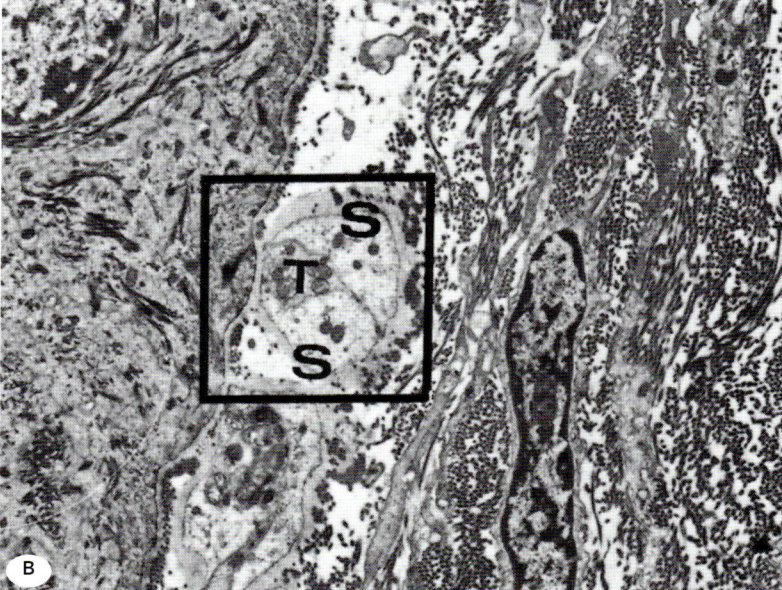

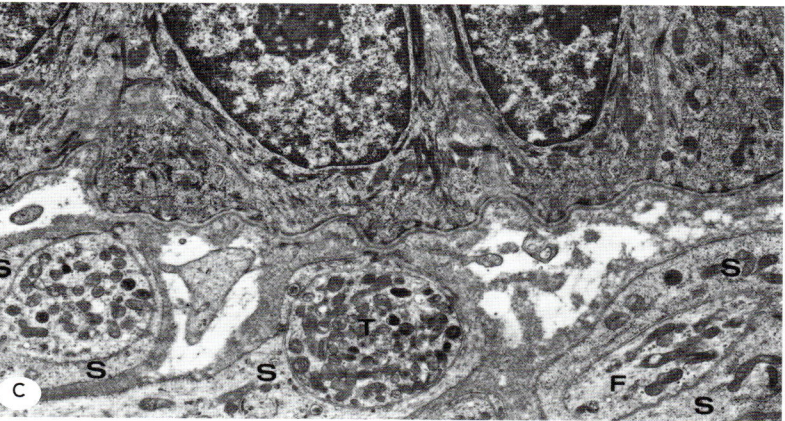

Fig. 1.42   Light and transmission electron micrographs of the bare nerve terminals that innervate the follicle (arrows). Note the position and structure of the terminals (T) and Schwann cells (S) just outside the basement membrane of the outer root sheath. A nerve fiber (F) surrounded by Schwann cells is also shown. (From Holbrook and Sybert, 1995, with permission)

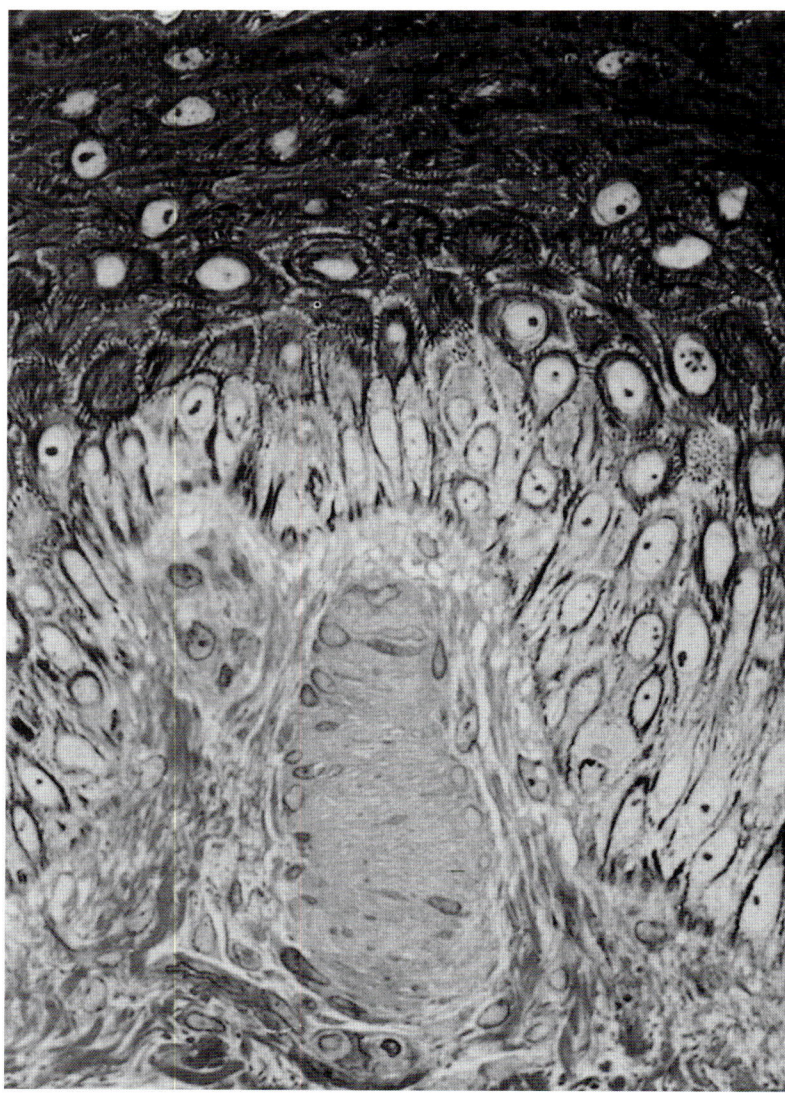

Fig. 1.43   Light micrograph of a Meissner corpuscle in the palm (× 350). (From Holbrook and Sybert, 1995, with permission)

IMMUNOGLOBULIN M

The basic structure of IgM is composed of two heavy and two light chains, but usually IgM exists in serum as a pentamer of 10 heavy chains and 10 light chains. Its molecular weight is about 900 000Da, about five times heavier than IgG. IgM is the first antibody detected after antigenic stimulation, and therefore IgM constitutes the first line of antibody defense against infectious organisms. Because it has 10 antibody–antigen binding sites, there is a great opportunity for it to combine with antigens. Furthermore, IgM can activate complement by the classical pathway, but unlike IgG it cannot cross the placental barrier. Its half-life in plasma is about 5 days, which is about 1/10 that of IgG and so IgM plays little role in long-lasting immunity.

IMMUNOGLOBULIN A

Like IgG, the basic structural IgA molecule is composed of two heavy chains and two light chains, but unlike IgG it usually exists in polymeric form, usually a dimer or trimer. Although some IgA is present in plasma, much IgA is secreted into the respiratory tract or the gastrointestinal tract where it functions to neutralise infectious agents and toxins before they can be absorbed into the body. Therefore IgA serves as a sort of protective coating to limit attachment of these molecules to the mucosal cells of the respiratory or gastrointestinal tract.

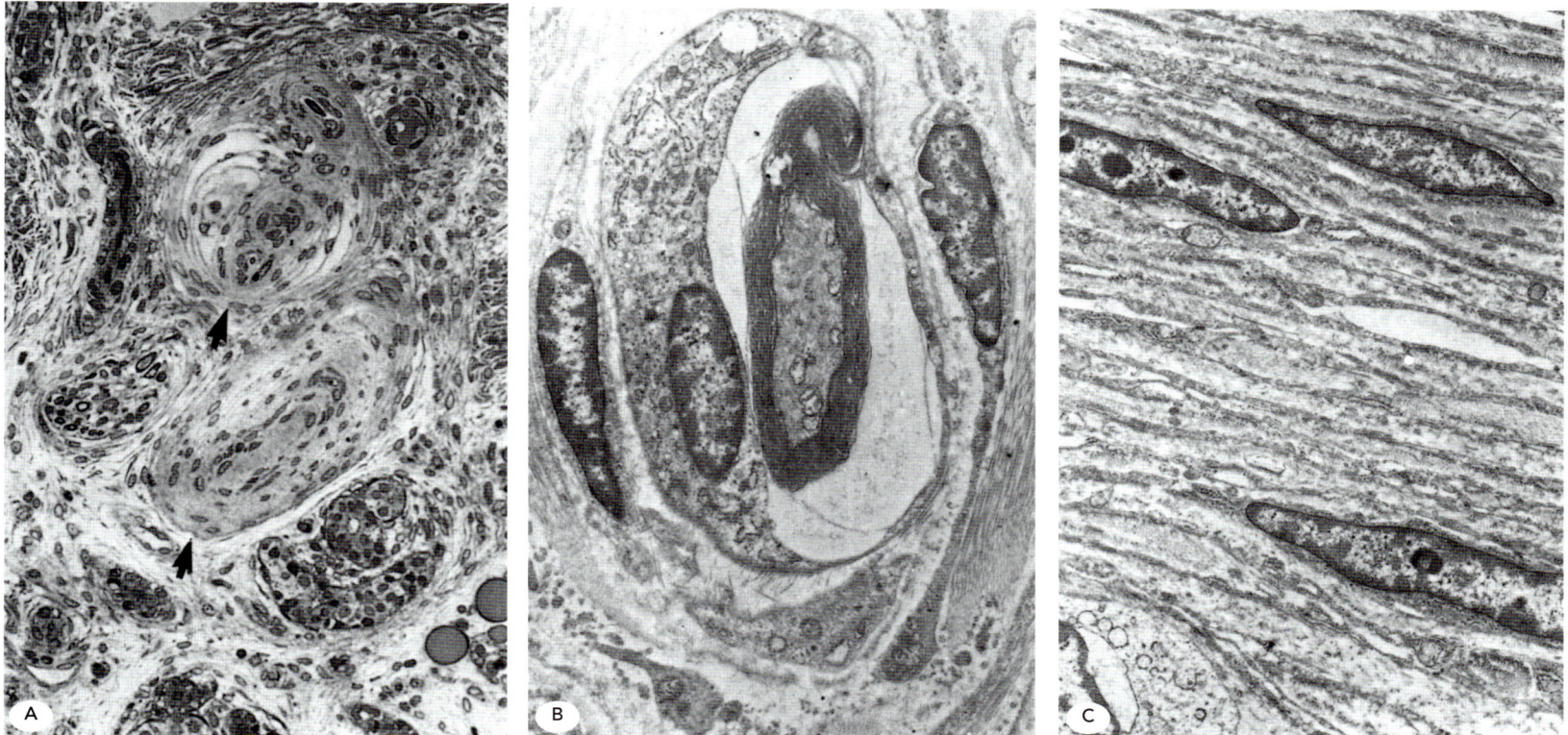

Fig. 1.44   Light and transmission electron micrographs of Pacinian corpuscles in the palm. Note the position of the corpuscles (arrows) at the border of the deep dermis and the hypodermis adjacent to eccrine sweat gland and ducts. (From Holbrook and Sybert, 1995, with permission)

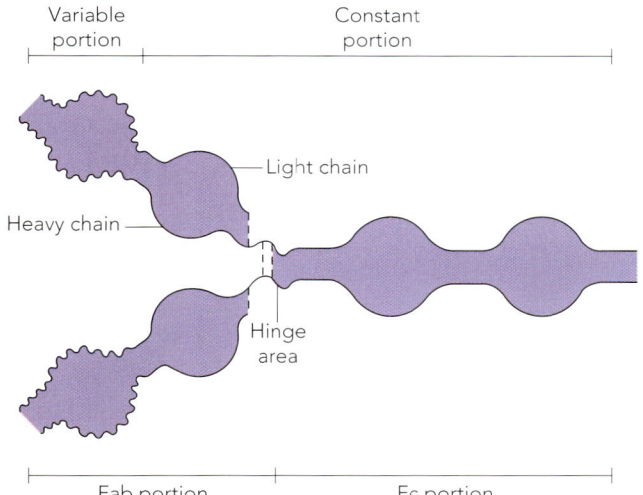

Fig. 1.45   A molecule of IgG is composed of two heavy chains and two light chains. The antibody specificity is determined by the sequence of amino acids at the Fab (antigen combining) end.

IgA cannot pass across the placental membrane and its half-life in plasma is about 6 days. Aggregated IgA activates complement by means of the alternative pathway.

IMMUNOGLOBULIN E

IgE consists of two heavy chains and two light chains, but very little IgE can be found circulating in plasma. The half-life is about 2 days, and the concentration of IgE in plasma is about 0.0001 that of IgG. Instead of circulating, most IgE is bound to mast cells in tissue where its half-life is much longer. Each mast cell has a receptor for the Fc end of IgE (i.e., the end of the immunoglobulin opposite the antigen-binding sites). Therefore, mast cells in tissue capture IgE molecules in such a way that the antibody-combining ends of IgE extend outward from the mast cell membrane. When an antigen bridges across two IgE molecules with specificity for that antigen, the entire mast cell is triggered to degranulate and release histamine and other mediators. IgE is therefore involved in the anaphylactic type of immune responses. These are reactions that develop rapidly and elicit vasodilatation and tissue edema.

IMMUNOGLOBULIN D

IgD is present in plasma in minute quantities. IgD is found on lymphocytes especially at times early in lymphocytic development, where it functions as a cell-membrane receptor. A lymphocyte is triggered to mature and divide after the IgD molecule combines with antigen. The function of IgD in plasma, if any, is entirely unknown.

B CELLS

B lymphocytes are involved in antibody production. They make up approximately 10–20% of lymphocytes in peripheral blood, but they are present in much higher percentages in certain organs such as the spleen. Precursor B cells have IgD or monomeric IgM molecules on their surfaces, which serve as receptors for antigens. When an antigen binds to these immunoglobulin receptors, the lymphocyte is then stimulated to undergo differentiation and proliferation. As the lymphocyte divides, a family of daughter cells is created all of which express IgM and IgD of identical specificity. Eventually these cells differentiate to a point where receptor immunoglobulins disappear and specific antibodies of only one type are synthesized (i.e., IgG, IgM, IgA, or IgE). The antigenic specificity of these antibodies is identical to the specificity of the receptor IgD or monomeric IgM molecules that initiated B-cell proliferation and differentiation. B lymphocytes secrete these antibodies into the plasma. They also differentiate into plasma cells that are specifically designed for copious antibody production.

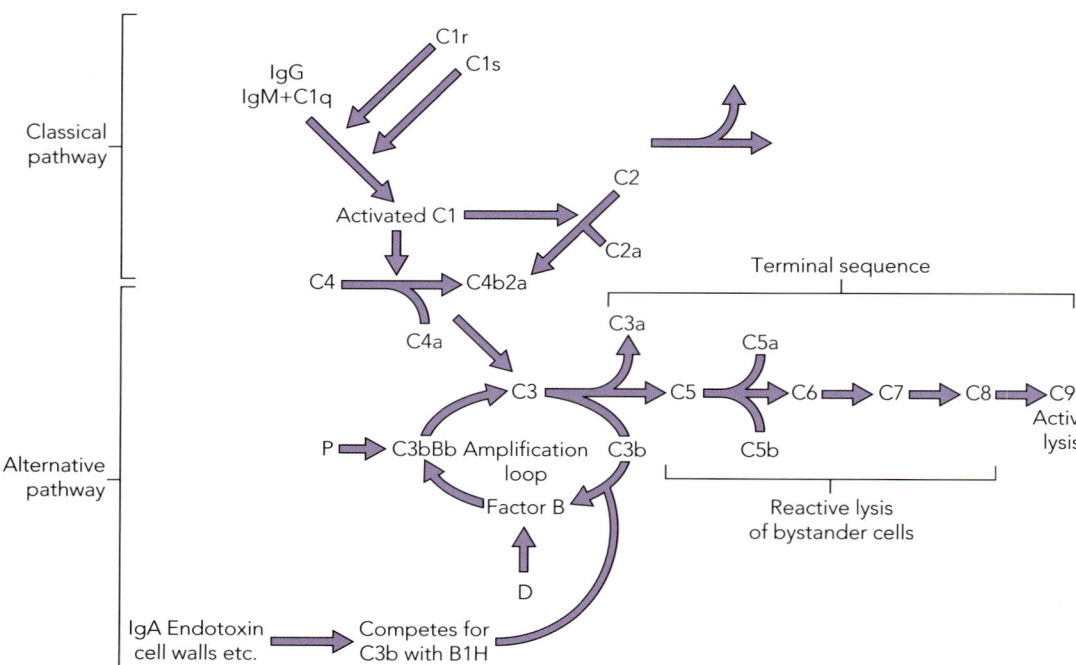

Fig. 1.46 The four divisions of complement activation are the classical pathway, the alternative pathway, the amplification the alternative pathway, the amplification loop, and the terminal sequence.

In order for B cells to differentiate, they must interact with cytokines produced by a subset of T cells called *T-helper cells*. As discussed below, there are two subsets of these: type 1 (Th1) and type 2 (Th2). It is the Th2 CD4 cell that fosters differentiation of B cells and antibody production. In other words, production of antibodies and other immunoglobulins is controlled by T lymphocytes.

COMPLEMENT

In order for an IgG or IgM antibody to work, usually it must interact with complement in some way. Complement is actually a series of plasma enzymes and structural proteins that are activated in sequence by antigen–antibody reactions. There are four basic arms of the complement system: the classical pathway, alternative pathway, terminal sequence, and C3b amplification loop (Fig. 1.47).

The classical pathway is activated when IgG or IgM combine with an antigen. A portion of C1 called C1q interacts with the Fc portion of the antibody, and after a series of sequential enzymatic steps, C3 is cleaved.

The alternative pathway has no initiating factor. C3–cleaving enzyme (C3bBb) is continuously formed and cleaves C3 until inhibitors such as C3b inactivator (C3b INA) or B1h globulin inactivates it. Various chemicals, toxins, bacterial cell walls, and aggregated immunoglobulins shield C3b from these inactivators, allowing more to be cleaved (i.e., complement is activated). Alternative pathway components factor D and factor B are components of the C3Bb. Properdin is a factor that stabilizes this complex. Like the classical pathway, the alternative pathway also leads to cleavage of C3.

The terminal sequence is the sequence of steps from cleavage of C3 to stacking of C9. C3 is cleaved into C3a and C3b. C3b binds to cell surfaces and acts as an opsonin to coat a particle for subsequent phagocytosis. C3b receptors on phagocytes bind to particles opsonized by C3b. C3b also is involved in immune adherence, the complement amplification loop, and the cleavage of C5 to C5a and C5b. Although complement activation very typically ends with phagocytosis, C5 can combine with C6 and C7 to form C567, which is also chemotactic, and which leads to the further assembly of C8 and C9, eventually leading to lysis of membranes. The combined molecule C5, 6, 7, 8 is called the *membrane attack complex* or *C5b678*. Once formed, membrane attack complex allows stacking of many molecules of C9 to form

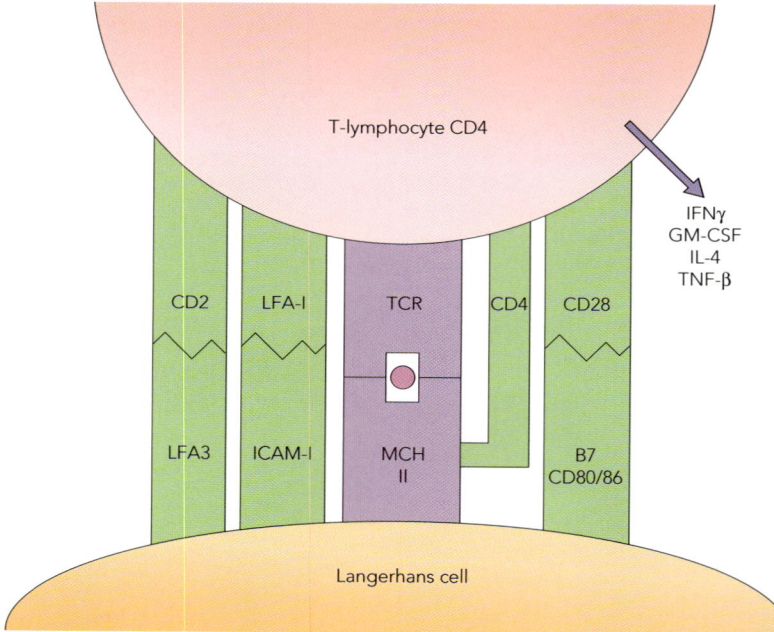

Fig. 1.47 Presentation of an antigen to a T cell by a Langerhans cell requires interactions not only of the T cell receptor (TCR) with antigen, but also with the major histocompatibility (MHC) molecule holding the antigenic peptide between its two peptide chains. Activation of the T cell requires participation of various accessory molecules such as CD80/86 to costimulate the T cell, and adhesion molecules to hold the T cell and Langerhans cell together. ICAM-1, intercellular adhesion molecule-1; LFA-1, Leukocyte function-associated antigen-1.

a sort of tube that pokes through a cell membrane leading to fluid fluxes and cell lysis.

When C3b cleaves C5, C5a is generated. C5a is a potent chemotactic factor, which attracts phagocytes from blood vessels to the area where the C5a is being generated, often the site of early bacterial invasion. When the neutrophils arrive, they ingest the opsonized particles, thereby limiting infection.

TABLE 1.2   Cytokine classes

Cytokines	Examples
Interleukins	IL-1, IL-2
Interferons	IFN-α, IFN-γ
Tumor necrosis factors	TNF-α
Growth factors	EGF
Colony-stimulating factors	GM-CSF
Chemokines	RANTES

EGF, epidermal growth factor; GM-CSF, granulocyte-macrophage colony-stimulating factor; RANTES, regulated by activation, normal T-cell expressed and secreted.

The C3b amplification loop is actually a part of the alternative pathway. It is an amplification loop because C3b can cleave many molecules of C3, all of which can form more C3b to amplify the process.

CELL-MEDIATED IMMUNITY

Cell-mediated immunity is different from humoral immunity because immunoglobulins are not directly involved. Cell-mediated immunity is mediated by T lymphocytes. These constitute 80–90% of circulating lymphocytes in the peripheral blood, and also a majority of the lymphocytes that traffic through the skin.

When T lymphocytes encounter an antigen, they undergo a blastogenic response, birthing numerous daughter cells with similar antigenic specificity. However, instead of secreting antibody, the T lymphocytes elaborate mediators called cytokines (lymphokines, interleukins, colony-stimulating factors, interferons, etc.). These factors influence inflammation by recruiting other lymphocytes and macrophages to the area. They work as local hormones to upregulate and downregulate various cell functions. Some cytokines increase selectin and integrin molecules leading to increased adherence and diapedisis of leukocytes from blood vessels into skin. Other cytokines stabilize the macrophage at the site of inflammation, while still others activate the macrophage and cause it to secrete mediators. Cytokines can also kill tumor cells and inhibit viral replication (Table 1.2).

MACROPHAGES AND LANGERHANS CELLS

Before a lymphocyte can respond to an antigen, antigen-presenting cells of the mononuclear phagocyte system (i.e., a macrophage, Langerhans cell, or dermal dendrocyte) usually must process the antigen. Extracellular antigens are engulfed and partially degraded. Portions of them are reexpressed on the surface of the antigen-presenting cell, locked in a groove between the two chains of class II HLA molecule. T cells have a receptor for antigen called the *T-cell receptor* (TCR). The sequence of amino acids in the distal portion of the TCR determines which antigen it can bind and also how strongly the TCR can bind it (avidity).

The process of antigen recognition involves intimate contact between the T cell and the antigen-presenting cell. The TCR binds to antigen on the antigen-presenting cell. The TCR also binds to part of the class II molecule holding the antigen. During this interaction, the T cell and antigen-presenting cell are held together by adhesion molecules such as intercellular adhesion molecule 1 (ICAM-1) and lymphocyte function-associated antigens-1 and –3 (LFA-1, LFA-3; Fig. 1.47). Before transduction of the signal to the T cell to replicate and secrete cytokines, the Langerhans cell ligand B7 (CD80/86) must bind with costimulatory molecule CD28 elsewhere on the T-cell surface or the immune system will become tolerant to the antigen (i.e., unable to elicit an immune response against it).

Once triggered by this complex but necessary process, the T cell secretes cytokines and builds DNA in preparation for cell division. T-cell proliferation is driven by interaction of IL-2 (T-cell growth factor) produced by activated

T cells with specific receptors (IL-2R) expressed on the surfaces of T cells, especially when activated. Proliferation leads to a family of T cells with TCR specific for the stimulating antigen. When enough are present, patients have cell-mediated immunity.

T cells eliminate antigen by secreting cytokines that attract and activate inflammatory cells such as neutrophils, macrophages, basophils, and eosinophils. These cells not only are directed into the inflammatory arena by these cytokines, but also are controlled locally by them. As such, the cell-mediated immune system is capable of a much finer degree of tuning, whereas humoral immunity is a systemic reaction irrespective of antigen site. In other words, reexposure or continued exposure to antigen in tissue elicits a cell-mediated immunoreaction. Specific T cells collect at the sites of antigen and secrete cytokines that attract and activate phagocytes and other cells. The intensity and character of the cell-mediated immune response is regulated by the type of T cell interacting with the antigen and the amount and type of cytokine the lymphocyte produces in response to it.

CD8 lymphocytes are cytotoxic. Sometimes a cell becomes infected with an intracellular pathogen such as a virus. Luckily, the presence of the virus is usually heralded by the appearance of processed viral antigens on HLA-A, B, or C molecules on the surface of a cell. CD8 cells are trained to recognize these antigens and kill the cell (Fig. 1.48). CD8 cells are generated during an induction response. CD8 cells can also kill certain cancerous cells and allograft cells.

Helper T cells express CD4 molecules on their surfaces and build immunity as discussed above. CD4 type 1 (Th1) and CD4 type 2 (Th2) cells are phenotypically identical, but differ by the cytokines they produce in culture (Fig. 1.49). Th1 CD4 lymphocytes mediate cell-mediated immunity and delayed hypersensitivity. They secrete large amounts of IL-2 and interferon-γ. Th2 cells, in contrast, secrete large amounts of IL-4 that serves to enhance antibody synthesis by B cells, especially IgE. Interferon-γ produced by Th1 cells can inhibit Th2 cells, and IL-10 produced by Th2 cells can inhibit Th1 cells. Thus, lymphocytes regulate the type and amount of immune response. Of course, genes ultimately regulate this process, as all processes.

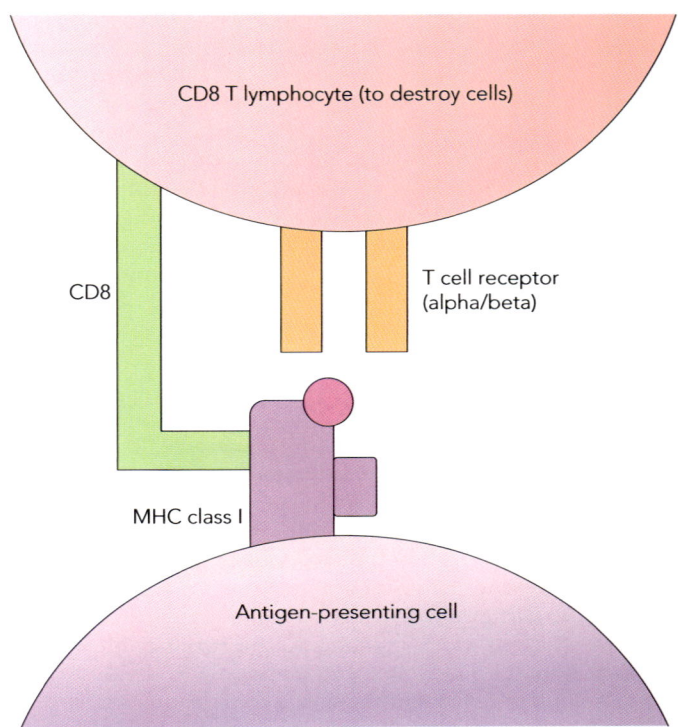

Fig. 1.48   CD8 cytotoxic T lymphocytes target cells for destruction by recognizing antigens presented to them by class I major histocompatibility (MHC) molecules.

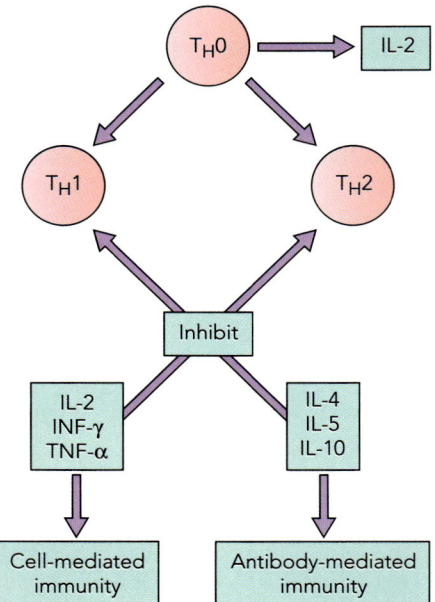

Fig. 1.49 T cells can become type 1 lymphocytes that work for cell-mediated immune responses and delayed hypersensitivity, or type 2 lymphocytes that work for humoral immunity, B-cell differentiation, and antibody synthesis.

PHAGOCYTES

Whether immunity is humoral, cell-mediated, or both, phagocytes are the cells that most commonly rid the body of antigen. B cells and plasma cells make antibodies and T cells make cytokines. Antibodies can neutralize certain toxins and infectious agents and lymphocytes can kill certain cells (e.g., allogenic grafts) directly, but phagocytes such as neutrophils and monocytes destroy most bacteria and immune complexes.

Neutrophils are the professional phagocytes whose sole purpose is to go to an area of infection and control it, usually by ingesting and killing the infecting organisms, especially bacteria. Neutrophils migrate through blood vessel walls and move directionally through tissue in response to chemotactic factors. Among the most important chemotactic factors are polypeptides elaborated by bacteria during replication, components of complement such as C5a, denatured protein, proteases derived from the clotting system, IL-8, and derivatives of prostaglandins.

Basophils and eosinophils are also polymorphonuclear leukocytes. Eosinophils can respond to chemotactic factors, although these may be different from those recruiting neutrophils. The function of eosinophils in tissue is unknown. However, one component of the eosinophilic granule (major basic protein) can kill certain parasites, and many other components directly antagonize or destroy products released by mast cells or basophils.

THE SKIN AS AN IMMUNOLOGIC ORGAN

The skin can act as an immunologic organ because it contains all the components necessary for a cell-mediated response. Furthermore, cells of the skin can control immune reactions and inflammation and selectively recruit "skin homing lymphocytes" into the skin. Macrophages, Langerhans cells, and dermal dendrocytes represent the skin's mononuclear phagocyte system. Langerhans cells are dendritic cells located within the epidermis capable of performing such tasks as phagocytosis, antigen processing, antigen presentation, and interaction with lymphocytes. Langerhans cells can also release IL-1 to help chemotaxis and lymphocyte activation.

The first line of host defense of the skin is the stratum corneum and keratinocyte wall making up the epidermis. If an antigen such as an infectious agent manages to penetrate the barrier, an immune response may be induced. Meanwhile, the skin's "native immune system" seeks to hold the pathogen in check. For example, many bacterial and fungal cells walls active complement

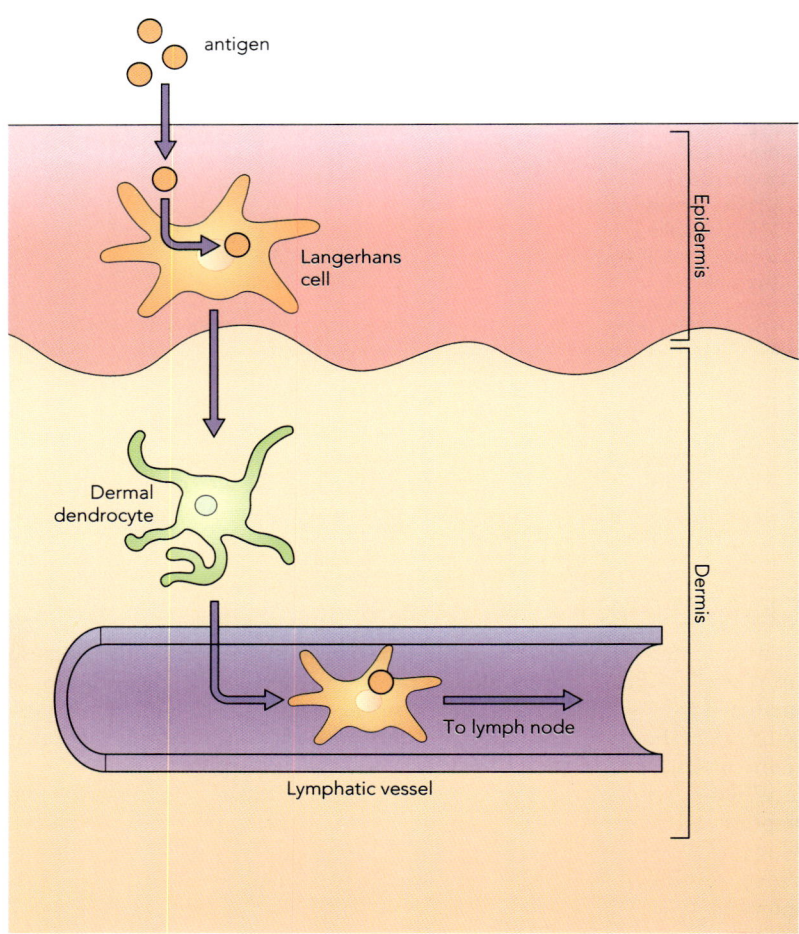

Fig. 1.50 In the induction phase of an immune response, antigen is trapped by Langerhans cells in the epidermis and carried inside them to the regional lymph nodes. In the nodes, the Langerhans cells present antigen to appropriate T cells leading to clonal proliferations and cell-mediated immunity.

by the alternative pathway leading to destruction of the pathogen by opsonization, chemotaxis, engulfment, and neutrophil or macrophage-directed killing. The epidermis contains some primitive lymphocytes called T-γ-δ cells. As their name implies, their TCR has a different sequence of amino acids in the constant region. The antigenic specificity of T-γ-δ cells is very limited. Injury to a cell such as a keratinocyte may liberate heat-shock protein or other substance recognized by the T-γ-δ cell leading to its activation and more-or-less nonspecific immune response. In effect, these cells say: "I don't know what's wrong, but something is, and I'm going to fight it off."

Meantime, the body begins to prepare a specific immune response (Fig. 1.50). Langerhans cells are intraepidermal macrophages. Their dendrites form an antigen-trapping net among keratinocytes. Antigens are internalized, and the Langerhans cell then somehow leaves the epidermis, finds a regional lymphatic vessel, and moves to the regional lymph node. Here in the paracortical area, it intermingles with numbers of lymphocytes of various specificities. Now renamed an "interdigitating reticulum cell," the Langerhans cell looks for T cells with receptors that can bind to the antigen, which it is expressing as a processed peptide on the Langerhans cell surface. Once found, that lymphocyte undergoes clonal proliferation to produce very many T cells with T-cell receptors specific for the antigen that stimulated the clone.

Now the lymphocytes return to the skin (Fig. 1.51). Traffic is partially directed, i.e., lymphocytes reactive to skin-encountered antigens tend to "home" back to the skin. They do this because they express certain molecules on their surfaces (addressins) that bind to specific receptors (selectins) on skin endothelial cells. After binding to the blood vessel, the T cells migrate out of it. Biopsies of normal skin show scattered lymphocytes, especially around

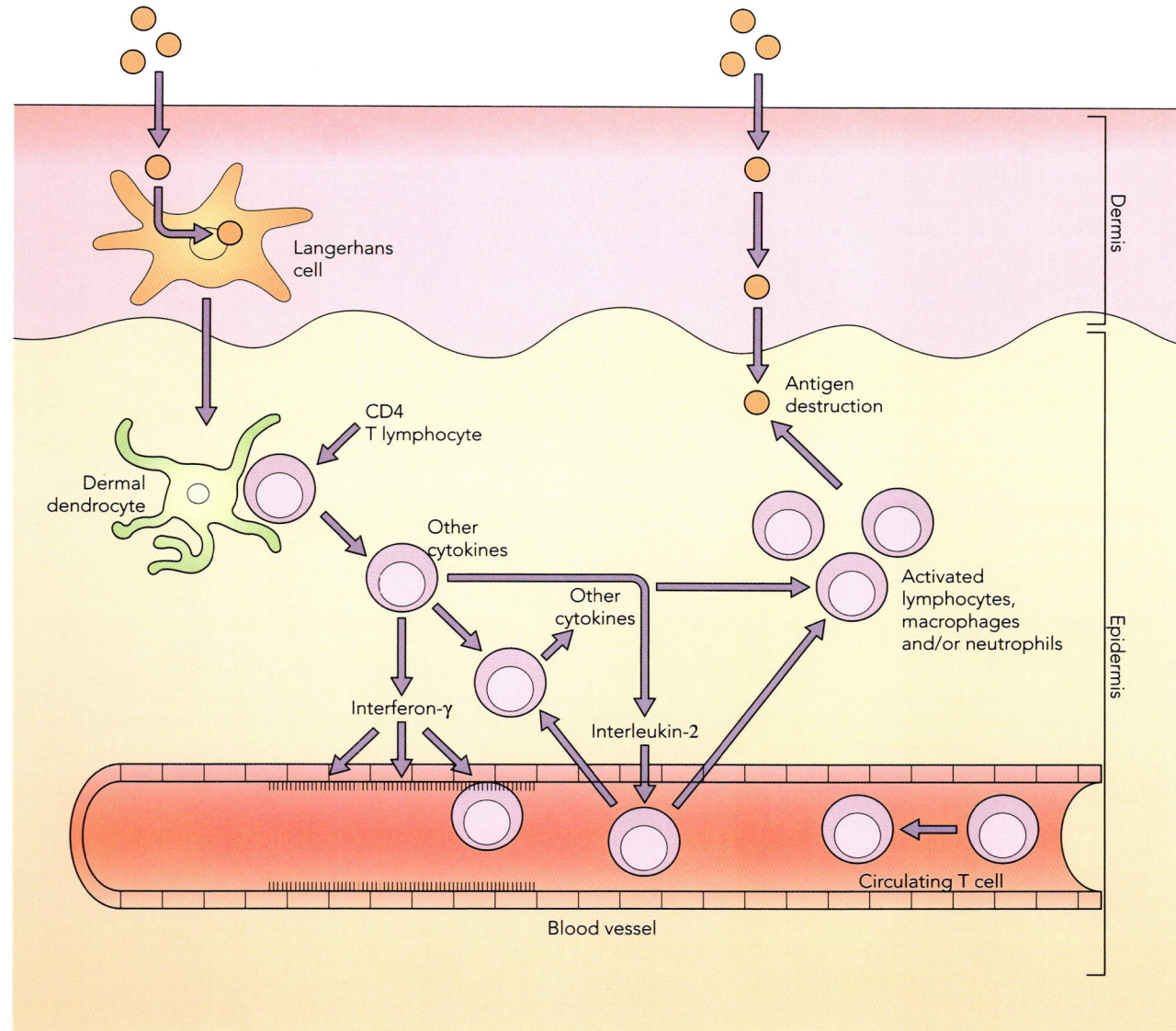

Fig. 1.51 **In the elicitation phase of an immune response, antigen is again trapped by Langerhans cells in the epidermis.** Because cell mediated immunity is present, T cells with appropriate specificities are present in the dermis. Presention of antigen to them leads to elaboration of cytokines and an inflammatory response.

blood vessels. These are sentinel "homed" lymphocytes hunting for their antigen in skin. If the antigen is still present, an immunologically mediated immune response can occur.

If antigen is still present, or if antigen is encountered again at some later time after immunity has been induced, lymphocytes react with it in the skin to create inflammation or kill an infected or cancerous cell. To elicit an inflammatory response to antigen, Langerhans cells, macrophages, and dermal dendrocytes again capture the antigens, process them, and present them to the T cells. This process can occur in the dermis or epidermis. In the elicitation response, Langerhans cells find appropriate lymphocytes in the skin rather than in the draining lymph nodes. In response, they secrete cytokines into the skin leading to inflammation there. Some lymphokines stop circulating lymphocytes in adjacent capillaries by upregulating vascular selectins and integrins. Lymphocytes adhere to the vessel wall, and roll along it as they are gradually dragged to a stop. Other lymphokines (called chemokines) now attract lymphocytes. For example, RANTES (regulated on activation, normal T-cell expressed, and secreted) liberated by lymphocytes reacting to antigen in the skin attracts lymphocytes from the circulation. Only 2–4% of lymphocytes in the skin arena of inflammation are actually reacting to specific antigens. The others recruited there are programmed to react to other antigens, but participate in the cytokine-producing party by themselves producing cytokines in response to cytokine signals from antigen-driven lymphocytes.

Under certain circumstances, keratinocytes may act as antigen-presenting cells. Interferon-γ is produced by activated T cells and causes keratinocytes to express antigen-presenting molecules on their surfaces. Keratinocytes can also mediate inflammation and immunity by secreting cytokines such as IL-1, IL-3 (a growth factor for mast cells), IL-8 (a chemotactic factor), and a growth factor for T cells (Table 1.2). More often these keratinocyte-derived cytokines function to augment or suppress immune and inflammatory responses of lymphocytes, or help direct traffic within the epidermis.

Delayed hypersensitivity is a special form of cell-mediated immunoreaction of skin. It peaks about 48h after intradermal injection or deposition of antigens into skin. Examples of delayed hypersensitivity reactions in skin are recall intradermal antigen skin tests (e.g., purified protein derivative test for tuberculosis) and allergic contact dermatitis (e.g., poison ivy).

TYPES OF IMMUNOREACTIONS

There are a number of different types of immunoreactions. Four types are commonly discussed.

Type I reactions involve IgE and mast cells. When antigen bridges across the IgE molecules attached by their Fc ends to a mast cell, the mast cell degranulates and liberates vasoactive materials such as histamine, leukotrienes, and neutrophil chemotactic factor of anaphylaxis. These factors cause edema and vasodilatation in the area around the degranulated mast cell leading to skin diseases such as urticaria and anaphylaxis.

Type II reactions are cytotoxic reactions requiring the participation of complement. Normally IgG or IgM antibodies bind to antigen and initiate complement activation through the classic pathway, although aggregated immunoglobulins can also activate complement to cause cytotoxic reactions. Assembly of the membrane attack complex of complement (C5, 6, 7, 8, and 9), leads to the formation of small channels in cell membranes, osmotic leakage, and disruption and lysis of cells. The cell target could be a tissue cell such as a blood cell, but it could also be a bacterium, virus, parasite, infectious agent, or structural protein such as an antigen in the basement membrane zone. The antibody- and complement-mediated engulfment and destruction of antigens by phagocytes is usually considered a type II reaction. So is the immune reaction of bullous pemphigoid. Although the antibasement membrane antibodies associated with bullous pemphigoid do assemble membrane attack complex, dermal–epidermal separation usually results from complement-mediated attraction and activation of eosinophils.

Type III reactions are immune complex reactions. Antigens combine with antibodies to form lattices. Lattice formation can occur in the wall of the blood vessel such as occurs in the Arthus reaction, or it can occur in the circulation such as occurs in serum sickness. If these circulating immune complexes then lodge in the vessel wall, complement activation can lead to an influx of inflammatory cells such as neutrophils. Release of catalytic proteins from neutrophils can damage vessel walls. An example of a type III reaction in the skin is vasculitis.

Type IV reactions are cell-mediated immunoreactions as discussed above. Examples in the skin are allergic contact dermatitis and recall skin test reactions. Here, lymphocytes rather than immunoglobulins are primary, and the mechanism of antigen destruction is by way of a phagocyte or a direct toxic effect of a lymphokine.

There are other ways that immunoglobulins can directly cause tissue reactions. For example, antibody can combine with a cell and stimulate it to release a hormone-like product. Long-acting thyroid stimulator is an immunoglobulin that causes the thyroid cell to produce thyroglobulin. Similarly pemphigus antibody may cause epidermal cells to change adhesion functions or release a proteolytic enzyme that decreases epidermal cell adhesion.

Cells can also be destroyed by immunoglobulins cooperating with a cytotoxic lymphocyte. In antibody-mediated cellular cytotoxicity, an immunoglobulin such as IgG combines with an antigen, for example, on the surface of a cell. A lymphocyte (K cell) with a Fc receptor can then bind to the Fc end (i.e., the non–antibody combining end) of that immunoglobulin and destroy the cell to which the immunoglobulin is attached. Natural killer (NK) cells are lymphocytes that kill cells directly (without antibody) by pumping a cytotoxic material (granzyme) through cell membranes that the NK cells first puncture with perforin.

IMMUNOGENETICS

All the events of the immune system are under direction of genes and chromosomes. Many genetic influences are involved in a properly timed and tuned immune response, but many of the genes controlling these functions lie within a small area of the short arm of the sixth human chromosome, which is called the major histocompatability complex (MHC). Genes within the MHC cause specific proteins to appear on the membrane of cells. These proteins are called HLA antigens and are denoted by the name of the genetic locus that stimulated their production (i.e., HLA-A, HLA-B, HLA-C, HLA-D, HLA-DR, HLA-DP, and HLA-DQ). HLA-DR, DP, and DQ antigens are called "class II molecules" (two heavy chains) and are the molecules that hold peptides for presentation to lymphocytes. HLA-A, B, and C are "class I molecules" (one heavy chain) that hold antigens on cell membranes to mark them for destruction by cytotoxic lymphocytes. Other genes mediate production of immunologic factors such as components of complement: C2, C4, and factor B. Still other gene products control cytokine production (especially tumor necrosis factor), the activity of cells, and the ability or nonability of the cell to respond to an antigen. These genes relate to helper and suppressor function as well as to the quantity of immune response.

In summary, the immune response is an integrated and complicated system involving a variety of cells such as lymphocytes, macrophages, and phagocytes, and a variety of soluble chemicals such as complement components, cytokines, lymphokines, interleukins, histamine, and other mediators. Like many complex biologic systems, the immune response is directed and controlled by numerous augmenting and feedback loops, and on-site control mechanisms. Normally these function well to rid the organism of infectious agents or toxins and yet control the immune response so that tissue destruction is minimized. If control mechanisms are lacking or deficient, then infection can often gain a foothold. On the other hand, if inflammation is too vigorous, actual tissue injury can occur and produce an inflammatory skin disease.

Because the skin acts as the interface between the changing environment and the constant milieu of body organs, it is often the site where immune and inflammatory reactions are manifest. Infections of the skin are common and the immune system plays a great role in preventing infection, and preventing or limiting the spread of infection. The immune system also participates in wound healing and tissue repair, and in inflammatory responses of noninfectious skin diseases, as well. The exact sequence of events is variable.

LABORATORY TESTS FOR IMMUNOLOGIC DISORDERS

The laboratory can aid the physician in determining the ability of the immune response to react to antigens and infectious agents. One common use of the laboratory in pediatric dermatology is the systematic evaluation of children suspected of being immunodeficient. As might be anticipated because the immune system is so complicated, many of the tests are complex and must be performed in special laboratories. However, some tests are simple and more widely available. Only the more common, readily available tests will be discussed here.

QUANTITATIVE IMMUNOGLOBULINS

The absolute levels of each immunoglobulin class can be determined. Approximate concentrations of IgG, IgM, and IgA are determined by radial immunodiffusion. Because serum IgE is present in such low concentrations, it must be quantitated by radioimmunoassay.

Each laboratory has its own normal laboratory values. Furthermore, the values for children differ from those of adults. Low levels of immunoglobulins in serum or plasma may reflect a genetic inability to make immunoglobulins of one or all classes. But low levels can also be found in diseases with increased metabolism or abnormal immunoglobulin loss. If low levels of serum immunoglobulins are accompanied by low levels of serum albumin, the latter is more likely.

COMPLEMENT

A total hemolytic complement level (CH50) can determine the integrity of the classical complement pathway. This functional assay indicates the amount of complement present in serum. Because congenital complement deficiency states usually involve absence of complement components of the classical pathway or terminal sequence, the CH50 determination is an excellent test to screen patients for possible complement deficiency. If the CH50 level is zero or very low, there may be a deficiency of one component. Alternatively, the complement system could be intact but in an activated state such that components of complement pathway are being consumed. In order to distinguish whether a very low CH50 is due to consumption or deficiency, serum levels of individual complement components can be obtained. The most useful complement components to study are C3 and C4 because they are most widely available and rather easily quantitated. If the CH50 is low because a complement component such as C2 is absent, then the C4 level will be normal, as complement is not being consumed abnormally under these circumstances. Thus if the C4 level is normal and the CH50 level is low, then each individual component of the classical pathway must be quantitated in order to learn exactly which component is lacking. Alternatively, if the CH50 is low because complement consumption is ongoing (e.g., in active systemic lupus erythematosus), then the C4 and often the C3 levels will usually be low as well, reflecting consumption of C4 and C3 by the activating process.

C1-esterase inhibitor is a controlling protein that normally inactivates C1qrs when it is acting as an esterase to cleave C2 and C4. Patients with hereditary angioedema are either deficient in this esterase inhibitor or have it in a dysfunctional form. In the former case, the absence of C1-esterase inhibitor can be detected chemically. In the latter case, functional assays are necessary. Determination of a serum C4 level is a useful test to screen for a deficiency or dysfunctional C1-esterase inhibitor because in either case the complement system is activated and C4 is consumed. Therefore most patients with hereditary angioedema have low levels of serum C4 regardless of whether they have C1-esterase deficiency or C1-esterase dysfunction. Functional tests of complement consumption are available in special laboratories to confirm the diagnosis.

OTHER TESTS RELATING TO HUMORAL IMMUNITY

Some patients with agammaglobulinemia and severe combined immunodeficiency lack adenoid tissue, and this can be detected in a lateral radiograph of the pharynx. They may also lack hilar adenopathy on chest radiographs. In a similar way, lymph nodes are often not palpable, although in some patients with agammaglobulinemia, enough histiocytes infiltrate nodes to allow them to be felt.

Specific antibodies can be measured. Streptococci have infected most children, so that antibodies to streptococcal antigens are usually present. The ASO titer reflects the serum level of IgG antibodies reactive against streptolysin-O antigen. These antibodies will only be present if the child has been exposed to streptococci. Low levels may therefore reflect a defect in antigen recognition, memory, or IgG production, but also may reflect lack of exposure. The same is true of antibody titers to other infectious organisms or toxins.

Patients who have blood type O normally have isohemagglutinins in their serum. Isohemagglutinins are IgM antibodies that react with blood group substances A and B. Patients with deficiencies of IgM antibody production will have absent or extremely low titers of isohemagglutinins, but so will patients with AB blood type. Furthermore, many normal children do not develop isohemagglutinins until they are about 2 years old.

Some patients have normal levels of immunoglobulins and normal titers of antibodies to previously encountered infectious agents, but are unable to mount antibody responses to new antigens. To test this, sometimes the patient can be immunized with typhoid or paratyphoid vaccines and then have their serum tested for antibodies to these agents. Many children have been immunized with diphtheria, rubella, varicella, mumps, or tetanus toxoids. Booster immunizations normally increase antibody titers to these agents several-fold. In order to test the ability of patients to produce additional antibody following booster challenge, repeat immunization can be followed with serial antibody titers. It is best to obtain serum before immunization and weekly thereafter. Submitting the specimens together minimizes laboratory variation. Immunization with live viruses such as polio, rubella, varicella, or measles is not recommended in a patient with suspected immunodeficiency.

Because B cells constitute only about 10–20% of peripheral blood lymphocytes, an isolated deficiency of B cells will not normally be detected by counting peripheral blood lymphocytes. The percentage of B cells in peripheral blood can be quantitated using monoclonal antibodies directed against specific B-cell antigens such as CD19, CD20, or CD21, or by using antibodies directed against surface immunoglobulins, which are attached to the surface of B cells. These tests are now widely available.

Ultimately antibodies are produced by plasma cells. Most patients with agammaglobulinemia lack plasma cells in their bone marrow or rectal tissue so that the performance of a biopsy of each of these organs is sometimes helpful. If agammaglobulinemia is suspected, biopsy of a lymph node may reveal the lack of lymphocytes in the follicular areas of nodes themselves.

Sometimes special laboratory tests are necessary to evaluate humoral immunity. Cells in tissue culture can produce antibodies. Pokeweed mitogen or a specific antigen is usually added to stimulate B lymphocytes *in vitro*. Elicited antibodies can be measured by radioimmunoassay. These tests require sophisticated laboratory support.

In order to provoke a normal antibody response, T-helper cells must cooperate with B cells. Occasionally a deficiency of T-helper cells will cause hypogammaglobulinemia. Therefore, quantitation of CD4 T-helper cells using monoclonal antibodies and peripheral blood lymphocytes helps evaluate a patient with suspected deficiency of humoral immunity.

CELL-MEDIATED IMMUNITY

Cell-mediated immunity is more difficult to evaluate than humoral immunity. One simple test counts small lymphocytes in the peripheral blood. Because 80–90% of lymphocytes are T cells, a deficiency of T lymphocytes is usually reflected as lymphocytopenia. However, the percentage of T cells in the peripheral blood of children may be lower than that of adults, particularly when the total lymphocyte count is high.

To confirm a possible deficiency of T cells, monoclonal antibodies can be used. These react with receptors present on T cells but not B cells so that lymphocytes with monoclonal antibody attached to them are T cells. Using other monoclonal antibodies, the type of T cells can be determined, not only in blood, but also in tissue. In particular, monoclonal antibodies can identify helper cells (CD4) and cytotoxic cells (CD8), and lymphocytes in early stages of differentiation. Type 1 and type 2 CD4 cells are identified by the cytokines they produce *in vitro*.

Functional aspects of cell-mediated immunity can be evaluated using intradermal skin tests to tuberculin, trichophytin, candidin, or even tetanus toxoid. Patients who have previously encountered these antigens develop erythema and induration at the injection site within 48h. A positive test indicates that a patient has processed an antigen, committed it to memory, reprocessed it when it was reintroduced by the test intradermal injection, recognized it, and responded appropriately. Bacterial contamination may cause false-positive reactions. If a child fails to respond to all of these antigens, that child may have a defect in his or her cell-mediated immune system. However, young children and infants often have not encountered these antigens and hence have negative tests. There are other causes of false-negative reactions as well. These include subcutaneous injection of antigen, loss of antigenic potency over time, concomitant viral infection, concomitant vaccination, or concomitant administration of immunosuppressive agents. Therefore, repeat testing is often worthwhile, sometimes with higher concentrations of antigens.

In order to test the ability of the cell-mediated immune system to respond to new antigens, patients may be induced (sensitized) to dinitrochlorobenzene (DNCB). An alcoholic solution containing 60μg of DNCB is placed on a 10mm diameter filter paper disk, applied to the skin, and occluded for 6h. Redness at the site is normally observed 1–2 days later. This is a normal irritant response and should not be mistaken for an allergic response. Many patients spontaneously develop an allergic reaction at the test site about 14 days after the induction. To prove a cell-mediated immune response has been induced, a patch test with a more dilute nonirritating concentration of DNCB (15μg) is placed on the skin for 24h and checked for inflammation 24–48h later. Using this controlled application procedure, at least 90% of people will become allergic to DNCB.

Deficiency of cell-mediated immune response can also be caused by congenital absence of thymus (DiGeorge syndrome). This is often suspected by careful evaluation of a lateral chest X-ray film. In adults the thymic shadow is normally absent.

Lymphocytes can be tested *in vitro* using nonspecific mitogens. Peripheral blood lymphocytes are incubated with chemicals such as phytohemagglutinin or concanavalin A. Most of the T cells will undergo a proliferative response where they synthesize protein, incorporate nucleotides into new DNA, and divide. Using radioactive thymidine, this blastogenic response can be measured. Most, if not almost all, T cells respond to these mitogenic substances. However cell-mediated immunity to a specific antigen may be lacking, despite an otherwise normal overall cell-mediated immune response (e.g., specific tolerance). To identify this, very sophisticated laboratory tests are required.

Lymphocytes are stimulated with specific antigens, but because only a small number of lymphocytes normally respond, detection is difficult. Mixed lymphocyte cultures are also a measure of lymphocyte activity for responding to specific antigen, but also require rather sophisticated laboratory support.

The effector chemicals generated by lymphocytes participating in a cell-mediated immune response are called lymphokines. Enzyme-linked immunosorbent assays can assess secreted cytokines. Of the many lymphokines, the one most usually assayed is interferon-γ.

PHAGOCYTIC CELL FUNCTION

Defects of phagocyte function are often included among the immunodeficiency disorders since patients with deficiencies are prone to infection. A routine white blood cell count with differential smear quantitates the number of neutrophils and often provides useful information. Many clinical problems of phagocytic cell function are associated with neutropenia.

In order to test the function of phagocytes, sophisticated laboratory tests are usually needed. However, the Rebuck skin window technique is a simple method that assesses leukocyte locomotion. In this test, the skin is gently abraded and covered with a microscope coverslip. At various times thereafter, the coverslip is removed and the cells adhering to it are stained and counted. Adequate polymorphonuclear leukocyte response is usually followed by mononuclear cell accumulation in healthy people. Modifications of the Rebuck skin window have utilized plastic chambers applied either to abraded or to tape-stripped skin. Using these plastic chambers, the response to specific chemotactic factors can be assayed.

The chemotactic response of neutrophils can be quantitated *in vitro* by using the "under agarose" technique. Here, neutrophils are placed in a well cut into agarose gel, and the distance that the fastest neutrophils migrate out from the well underneath the agarose toward a well containing chemotactic factor is measured. The Boyden chamber technique measures the number of neutrophils that migrate through a filter separating a chamber containing a suspension of neutrophils from one containing chemotactic factors. Responses can be compared to normal values and to simultaneous controls in order to determine if chemotaxis is deficient.

The nitroblue tetrazolium dye reduction (NBT) test measures the oxidative metabolism of neutrophils. A small amount of yellow soluble NBT is added to whole blood, and incubated for 30 min. Activated neutrophils reduce NBT to a blue–black insoluble formazan precipitate. One counts the number of neutrophils containing black pigment by examining a smear of cells. Normally, 5–15% of neutrophils contain the pigment. Patients with systemic infections have higher counts, whereas patients with chronic granulomatous disease have lower ones. Chemiluminescence is an important test of neutrophil function. Normally after phagocytosis, a neutrophil emits a small amount of light as it undergoes its respiratory burst. This small amount of light can be detected using a scintillation counter. A normal chemiluminescence response indicates that the phagocyte is able to attach to an opsonized particle, engulf it, stimulate a respiratory burst, and probably kill the organism. Chemiluminescence is the test of choice for detecting patients with chronic granulomatous disease.

DIRECT IMMUNOFLUORESCENCE

Direct immunofluorescence uses fluorescent antibodies to stain human antibodies in tissue. Specificity of the stain is determined by the specificity of the antibody. Typically a skin biopsy is snap frozen in liquid nitrogen or placed in special preservative media. Ten percent formalin usually denatures antigens so that tissue biopsies preserved in formalin cannot be used. Sections of frozen tissue are placed on microscope slides and overlaid with a solution of fluorescein-labeled antibody. If antigen is present in the tissue section, the fluorescent antibody will bind to it and an area of fluorescence will mark the site of antibody deposition when the tissue section is subsequently viewed under fluorescence microscopy. Immunocytochemistry is similar, but the marker is not fluorescent and the presence of antigen can be determined using an ordinary light microscope.

INDIRECT IMMUNOFLUORESCENCE

Whereas direct immunofluorescence is a histologic technique, indirect immunofluorescence is a serologic technique that is used to detect specific antibodies in serum or tissue fluids. Serum is incubated with frozen tissue sections of normal tissue. If the serum contains antibody to a component of the normal tissue substrate, the antibody will bind to it. After washing, the section is incubated with fluorescein-labeled antihuman antibody and washed again. If antibody bound to the tissue in the first steps, then the anti–antibody will bind to it in the second step and can be detected by examining the tissue under the fluorescence microscope. By diluting the serum, the titer of antibody can be determined. The titer is the most dilute serum specimen that shows fluorescence.

SUMMARY

The clinical laboratory is essential for evaluating children with suspected immunodeficiency states. The exact laboratory findings associated with each of these states are reviewed elsewhere in this chapter. Some of these tests are readily available whereas others require sophisticated testing in medical centers. Regardless of where the tests are performed, correct interpretation of results is critical. Children are often different from adults, so normal values in children may not be comparable to normal adult values. Furthermore, each laboratory has its own way of performing each test and its own normal laboratory values. The normal values for each laboratory must be known in order to properly interpret the results.

FURTHER READING

Aiba S, Tagami H (1999) Dendritic cells play a crucial role in innate immunity to simple chemical. J Invest Dermatol Symp Proc 4:158–163.

Arm MJ, Longley MA, Scoff G et al. (1999) A novel mutation in the IA domain of keratin 2e in ichthyosis bullosa of Siemens. J Invest Dermatol 112:380–382.

Asahina A, Hosoi J, Grabbe S et al. (1995) Modulation of Langerhans cell function by epidermal nerves. J Allergy Clin Immunol 96:1178–1192.

Bergman E, Ulfhake B, Fundin BT et al. (2001) Regulation of NOF-family ligands and receptors in adulthood and senescence: correlation to degenerative and regenerative changes in cutaneous innervation. Eur J Neurosci 12:2694–2706.

Borradori, L, Sonnenberg A (1999) Structure and function of hemidesmosomes: more than simple adhesion complexes. J Invest Dermatol 112:411–418.

Borradori L, Chanas S, Calafat J et al. (1998) Role of the bullous pemphigoid antigen (BP 180) in the assembly of hemidesmosomes and cell adhesion-reexpression of BP 180 in generalized atrophic benign epidermolysis bullosa keratinocytes. Exp Cell Res 239:463–476.

Bruckner-Tuderman L (1999) Hereditary skin diseases of anchoring fibrils. J Dermatol Sci 20:122–133.

Bruckner-Tuderman L, Bruckner P (1998) Genetic diseases of the extracellular matrix: more than just connective tissue disorders. J Mol Med 76:226–237.

Byers HR, Yaar M, Gilchrest BA et al. (2000) Role of cytoplasmic dynein in melanosome transport in human melanocytes. J Invest Dermatol 114:990–997.

Chen M, Marinkovich MP et al. (1997) Interactions of the amino-terminal noncollagenous (NC1) domain of type VII collagen with extracellular matrix components: a potential role in epidermal–dermal adherence in human skin. J Biol Chem 272:14516–14522.

Chudnow RS, Wolfe GI, Roach ES et al. (2000) Abnormal sudomotor function in the hypomelanotic macules of tuberous sclerosis complex. J Child Neurol 15:529–532.

Compensatory mechanism maintaining skin barrier function in the absence of a major cornified envelope protein. J Cell Biol 151:389–400.

Corsini E, Galli CL (2000) Epidermal cytokines in experimental contact dermatitis. Toxicology 142:203–211.

Cumberbatch M, Dearman RJ, Griffiths CE, Kimber I (2000) Langerhans cell migration. Clin Exp Dermatol 25:287–290.

Dahi MV (1996) Clinical Immunodermatology, 3rd edn. Chicago: Mosby-Yearbook, Inc.

Delves PJ, Roitt IM (2000) The immune system. N Engl J Med 343:37–49.

Detmar M (2000) The role of VEGF and thrombospondins in skin angiogenesis. J Dermatol Sci 24(Suppl 1):S78–84.

Diaz LA, Giudice GJ (2000) End of the century overview of skin blisters. Arch Dermatol 136:106–112.

Eckes B, Zigrino P, Kessler D et al. (2000) Fibroblast–matrix interactions in wound healing and fibrosis. Matrix Biol 19:325–332.

Freedberg IM, Eisen AZ, Wolff K et al. (1999) Fitzpatrick's Dermatology in General Medicine, 5th edn. New York: McGraw-Hill.

Freinkel RK, Woodley DT (2001) The Biology of the Skin. New York: Parthenon.

Fuchs E, Segre, JA (2000) Stem cells: a new lease on life. Cell 100:143–155.

Garg A, Chren MM, Sands, LP et al. (2001) Psychological stress perturbs epidermal permeability barrier homeostasis: implications for the pathogenesis of stress-associated skin disorders. Arch Dermatol 137:53–59.

Goldsmith LA (1991) The Physiology, Biochemistry and Molecular Biology of the Skin, New York: Oxford University Press.

Hanley K, Komuves LG, He Y et al. (1999) Fetal epidermal differentiation and barrier development in vivo is accelerated by nuclear hormone receptor activators. J Invest Dermatol 113:788–795.

Hasegawa K, Pereira BP, Pho RW et al. (2001) The microvasculature of the nail bed, nail matrix and nail fold of a normal human fingertip. **J Hand Surg (Am)** 26:283–290.

Hatta N, Ray AJ, Dixon C et al. (2001) Expression, candidate gene and population studies of the melanocortin S receptor. **J Invest Dermatol** 116:564–570.

Heckmann M, Ceballos-Baumaim AO, Plewig O et al. (2001) Botulinum toxin A for axillary hyperhidrosis (excessive sweating). **N Engl J Med** 344:488–493.

Hilliges M, Wang L, Johansson O et al. (1995) Ultrastructural evidence for nerve fibers within all vital layers of the human epidermis. **J Invest Dermatol** 104:134–137.

Holbrook KA, Sybert VP (1995) Basic science. In Pediatric Dermatology, 2nd edn, LA Schachner, RC Hansen, eds. New York: Churchill Livingstone, pp. 1–70.

Iozzo RV (1998) Matrix proteoglycans: from molecular design to cellular function. **Ann Rev Biochem** 67:609–652.

Ishida-Yamamoto A, Kato H, Eady RA et al. (2000) Mutant loricin is not crosslinked into the cornified cell envelope but is translocated into the nucleus in loricin keratoderma. **J Invest Dermatol** 115:1088–1094.

Kamradi T, Mitchison NA (2001) Tolerance and autoimmunity. **N Engl J Med** 344:655–664.

Koch PJ, De Viragh PA, Suga Y et al. (2000) Lessons from loricin-deficient mice: compensatory mechanisms maintaining skin barrier function in the absence of a major cornified envelope protein. **J Cell Biol** 15:389–400.

Kuechle MK, Thulin CD, Dale BA et al. Profilaggrin requires both linker and filaggrin peptide sequences to form granules: implications for profilaggrin processing *in vivo*. **J Invest Dermatol** 112:843–852.

Lavker R, Sun TT (1995) Hair follicle stem cells: present concept. **J Invest Dermatol** 104:385–395.

Lavker, RM, Sun, TT (2000) Epidermal stem cells: properties, markers, and location. **Proc Natl Acad Sci USA** 97:13473–13475.

Madison KVC (2000) Barrier function of the skin: la raison d'etre of the epidermis. **Progr Dermatol** 34:1–12.

Mecklenburg L, Tobin DJ, Pohi S et al. (2000) Active hair growth (anagen) is associated with angiogenesis. **J Invest Dermatol** 114(5):909–916.

Minwalla L, Zhao Y, LePoole C et al. (2001) Keratinocytes play a role in regulating distribution patterns of recipient melanosomes *in vitro*. **J Invest Dermatol** 117:341.

Nemes Z, Steinert PM (1999) Bricks and mortar of the epidermal barrier. **Exp Mol Med** 31:5–19.

Nemes Z, Marekov LN, Fesus L, Steinert PM (1999) A novel function for transglutaminase 1: attachment of long-chain omega-hydroxyceramides to involucrin by ester bond formation. **Proc Natl Acad Sci USA** 96:8402–8407.

Nordlund JJ, Boissy RE, Hearing V et al. (1998) The Pigmentary System: Physiology and Pathophysiology. New York: Oxford.

Numahara T, Tanemura M, Nakagawa T et al. (2001) Spatial data analysis by epidermal Langerhans cells reveals an elegant system. **J Dermatol Sci** 25:219–228.

Odderson IR (1998) Hyperhidrosis treated by botulinum A exotoxin. **Dermatol Surg** 24:1237–1241.

Olsen EA (2002) Disorders of Hair Growth. New York: McGraw-Hill.

Paus R, Cotsarelis O (1999) The biology of hair follicles. **N Engl J Med** 341:491–497.

Porter AM (2001) Why do we have apocrine and sebaceous glands? **J Roy Soc Med** 94:236–237.

Raghunath M, Unsold C, Peters R et al. (1998) The cutaneous microfibrillar apparatus contains transforming growth factor-beta binding protein and is a repository for latent TGF-beta 1. **J Invest Dermatol** 111:528–533.

Rassner U, Feingold KR, Elias PM et al. (1999) Coordinate assembly of lipids and enzyme proteins into epidermal lamellar bodies. **Tissue Cell** 31:489–498.

Rothnagel JA, Roop DR (1995) Hair follicle companion layer: reacquainting an old friend. **J Invest Dermatol** 104:42S–43S.

Sakai Y, Kishimoto J, Demay MB et al. (2001) Metabolic and cellular analysis of alopecia in vitamin D receptor knockout mice. **J Clin Invest** 107:961–966.

Schinelz M., Schmidt R, Bickel A et al. (1997) Specific C-receptors for itch in human skin. **J Neurosci** 17:8003–8008.

Skobe M, Detmar M (2000) Structure, function and molecular control of the skin lymphatic system. **J Invest Derm Symp Proc** 5:14–19.

Steinert PM (2000) The complexity and redundancy of epithelial barrier function. **J Cell Biol** 151:FS–8.

Steinert PM, Marekov LN (1999) Initiation of assembly of the cell envelope barrier structure of stratified squamous epithelia. **Mol Biol Cell** 10:4247–4261.

Streilein JW, Alard P, Nuzeki H et al. (1999) Neural influences on induction of contact hypersensitivity. **Ann NY Acad Sci** 885:196–208.

Swensson O, Langbein L, Leigh I et al. (1998) Specialized keratin expression pattern in human ridged skin as an adaptation to high physical stress. **Br J Dermatol** 139:767–775.

Tani H, Morris RJ, Kaur P (2000) Enrichment for murine keratinocyte stem cells based on cell surface phenotype. **Proc Natl Acad Sci USA** 97:10960–10965.

Uchi H, Terao H, Koga T, Furue M (2000) Cytokines and chemokines in the epidermis. **J Dermatol Sci** Suppl 1:S29–38.

Wood JM, Jimbow K, Tosk J et al. (1999) What's the use of generating melanin. **Exp Dermatol** 8:153–164.

Yano K, Brown LF, Detmar M et al. (2001) Control of hair growth and follicle size by VEGF-mediated angiogenesis. **J Clin Invest** 107:409–417.

Psychosocial Development in Children with Cutaneous Disease

CHAPTER 2

Paula K. Rauch and Michael S. Jellinek

Children with dermatologic complaints are seen by pediatricians and dermatologists in settings characterized by large numbers of patients, short individual visits, and many weeks elapsing between appointments. An estimated 60 percent of patients in a pediatric dermatology clinic are seen only once.[1] Clinicians are under pressure to keep the flow of patients moving. They must contend with restless patients and families in the waiting room, unexpectedly lengthy office procedures, and unscheduled visits. Insurance reimbursements reward short, frequent visits over lengthier encounters. All of these factors may encourage the pediatric dermatologist to focus attention solely on the parade of dermatologic lesions, with little attention to psychosocial considerations. In this chapter we discuss how an understanding of psychosocial issues potentially can increase efficiency and improve the quality of care.

Larry is a cherubic blond, 4½-year-old boy, who presents in the clinic with two warts on his hand and one on his foot. Quick cryosurgical treatment with liquid nitrogen is planned. As Larry enters the examining room, the dermatologist notices he is looking increasingly frightened. The doctor smiles. He makes an effort to cheer Larry up by splashing liquid nitrogen over the office floor. As the smoke rises off the carpet, Larry begins to wail. He desperately tries to squirm off his mother's lap. The doctor and Mrs Scott, Larry's mother, try unsuccessfully to hold Larry still. They struggle to pry open his fist in order to apply the liquid nitrogen. Neither the doctor's reassurances nor Mrs Scott's promises of candy seem to help. The procedure takes three times as long as anticipated and fewer than the optimum number of applications are administered to the warts.

On a chance meeting with the primary pediatrician, the dermatologist learned Larry had had several nightmares following the wart removal.

To understand why the treatment resulted in a losing battle, it is helpful to view the same appointment through Larry's 4½-year-old eyes. To him adults, like the dermatologist, have superhuman powers far exceeding his cognitive understanding. Although the powers are reassuring when an adult is protecting him, the same imagined powers become frightening when Larry feels threatened by a stranger in a new setting. From his young vantage point, any injury to his body must be an angry attack directed against him. The seemingly magical smoke of liquid nitrogen reinforces Larry's propensity to imagine scary fantasies. He imagines his hand going up in smoke, or worse his arm, or perhaps all of his leg burning and disappearing. An adult might view this as Larry's imagination running wild, but to the 4½-year-old the possibility is real, impending, and terrifying. From his perspective, he is struggling against being badly hurt, so a fierce battle seems the appropriate response.

Similarly frustrating clinical vignettes could describe a school-age child or a teenager. Ten-year-old Doug adamantly refused to expose his psoriatic skin to the healing summer sun. The dermatologist did not know that Doug

worried about being teased by his peers. Ann presented as an intelligent 14-year-old who seemed, during her appointments, to understand her acne medication plan, yet returned every 6 weeks without having carried out the treatment at home. The physician was surprised to learn that Ann feared becoming "addicted" to her antibiotics.

No physician wishes to scare a young child, and non-compliant patients are time-consuming and do not benefit from their medical treatment. The compliance and satisfaction of the three patients described above could be improved by addressing the developmental concerns of the children and adolescents involved. A pediatrician or dermatologist who practices without a developmental perspective practices with an unnecessarily narrow focus.

The meaning attached to the state of a person's skin is multifaceted, ranging from a broad cultural perspective to the individual's very personal experience. The dermatologist's challenge is to consider the complexity of meanings and offer treatment that tries to integrate medical and psychological perspectives.[2]

The cultural significance of skin goes beyond style or beauty. Clean white skin has long been used to symbolize purity. Perhaps the "Ivory girl" best typifies the Madison Avenue image of wholesomeness and virtue associated with flawless skin. Advertising agencies capitalize on an association that dates back to the Old Testament. Of the 10 plagues God delivered against the ancient Egyptians, only one organ system was assaulted, the skin, with the affliction of boils.

The mass media reflect the current societal emphasis on appearance. Consumers are exposed to a barrage of advertisements for a vast array of skin care products. There are countless cleansers, moisturizers, toners, soaps, creams, powders, and pastes. They feature a multitude of ingredients: honey, oatmeal, aloe, estrogen, protein, and vitamins, to name only a few. Advertisements touting the appeal of these products used to be directed exclusively at women, but today men as consumers represent a growing proportion of the billion-dollar beauty aid industry. Adolescents, too, are spending millions on over-the-counter products to fight acne and clean, moisturize or decorate skin and hair.

First impressions and attraction are often based on superficial appearance. However, what sustains enduring interpersonal relationships are the characteristics of sympathy and empathy with another person. In a study of adult psoriasis sufferers, 88 percent reported that the worst feature of their disease was the embarrassment caused by their appearance.[3] Among patients' most common concerns were that they would be viewed as infectious and be stared at or ostracized in social situations. Unless physicians question patients directly about their inner experience, significant psychological morbidity is likely to go undetected. This is well demonstrated in a study of port-wine stain (facial nevus flammeus) patients who only revealed their feelings of stigmatization when asked probing questions.[4]

1. Schachner L, Ling NS, Press S (1983) A statistical analysis of a pediatric dermatology clinic. **Pediatr Dermatol** 1:2.
2. Czyzewski DI, Lopez M (1998) Clinical psychology in the management of pediatric skin disease. **Dermatologic Clinics** 6:619–629.
3. Stankler L (1981) The effect of psoriasis on the sufferer. **Clin Exp Dermatol** 6:303.
4. Lanigan SW, Cotterill JA (1989) Psychological disabilities amongst patients with port wine stains. **Br J Dermatol** 121:2.

Although adolescents are particularly sensitive about how they appear to others, even younger children associate popularity with an attractive appearance.[5,6] Data on children disfigured by burns[7] suggest that the change in appearance seriously affects their subsequent peer relationships. Observable skin disorders cause stress for the sufferer, especially during initial meetings with others. In a large-scale, multicenter study of psychosocial adjustment in school-age children (6 to 12 years old) seen in pediatric dermatology clinics, the dermatology patients screened positively for psychosocial distress at rates similar to that found in general pediatric office patients when matched for socio-economic status. In that study, children judged to have substantial alteration of their appearance by their skin condition were also more likely to show significant psychosocial distress when compared with those rating the impact on appearance as minimal. Further, the parental ratings of impact on appearance were surprising. Nearly one-quarter of all parents indicated that their child's appearance was affected "a lot" (the highest rating) by the presenting skin condition.[8]

In addition to the role of appearance, or perceived appearance, subjective life experience and family environment play roles in the expression of skin conditions. In a study of children with atopic dermatitis, increased individual stress and family discord correlated with increased symptom severity.[9] Literature review suggests that psychological morbidity is a complex function of diagnosis, impact on appearance, family context, and subjective experience.[10] Atopic dermatitis in childhood highlights the interplay of family or caretaker stress and psychological symptomatology in a child.[11,12] When this condition interferes with an infant's sleep, the parent's sleep is also compromised and the result is often an irritable infant and an exhausted parent.[13]

More basic than the cultural or interpersonal associations, skin has primary psychological significance as the sensory organ through which the developing infant first experiences the world. It defines newborns' boundaries as they discover their separateness from the mother and the pleasures of her touch. It signals danger in the form of pain to the inquisitive toddler exploring the environment. It is the human armor of 4 and 5 year olds who admire superheroes and fear their own vulnerability. It is the outer layer that the adolescent recognizes as "me" in the mirror. It is suntanned, tattooed, scarred, and decorated. It is imbued with sexuality and intimacy. It heralds the onset of old age with telltale signs of wrinkling and discoloration, and finally loses its color in death.

The skin is an integral part of every step of development. Acting in the cultural, interpersonal, and personal arenas, it is crucial to self-esteem and identity formation that individuals be comfortable in their skin.

A single disorder takes on many different meanings throughout the phases of its development. Progressive phases in the development of the condition are characterized by new capacities to understand different interpersonal situations. The experience of having eczema, for example, is different at age 2, age 10, and age 17.

PSYCHOLOGICAL RESPONSES TO DERMATOLOGIC DISEASE

A mild, a moderate, and a severe dermatologic condition (a small facial port-wine stain, atopic dermatitis, and epidermolysis bullosa, respectively) have been chosen to illustrate dominant developmental issues in an effort to emphasize how the age of the child alters the way an illness is experienced. It is now possible to treat a facial port-wine stain with laser, largely obliterating the impact of the condition. We have elected to use it as an example through childhood development nonetheless, as the age for laser treatment is under discussion in the literature,[14,15] and thus a developmental understanding of a cosmetic problem, with or without solution, remains clinically germaine. We are not suggesting that dermatologic conditions cause psychopathology, but rather that there is a wide range of responses to an illness that can be better understood from a developmental perspective.

THE RELATIONSHIP OF INFANT AND PARENT

Parental expectations of their child begin at inception. In concert with intrauterine growth, parental hopes and dreams for the unborn child are an expression of the parents' own wishes and aspirations. They are often humorously expressed during pregnancy in discussions about the football players and doctors still *in utero*. The best and worst combinations of maternal and paternal family traits are considered, along with wishes for a preferred eye color, complexion, or profile.

At the core of these rising hopes is the process of attachment, a biologically determined mechanism to ensure the survival of the vulnerable, dependent infant. This is symbolic of the increasing emotional attachment and the preparation for the demanding caretaking work to come.

Port-wine stain

When an infant is born with any defect, regardless of how minor, it is a disappointment to the parents. Their disappointment in the child's appearance is often transformed into blaming themselves for the child's defect. The actual infant in front of them differs from the expectation of a perfect, imagined one. Parents' capacity to adjust to the reality of their infant's appearance and the extent of their disappointment is based on multiple factors related to the seriousness of the defect and to the parents' capacities to tolerate stress and loss.

An infant with a port-wine stain is likely to evoke a combination of parental feelings, including shock, embarrassment, fear, and guilt. The parents' awareness that their child is in some way defective is exacerbated by the constant reminder of the nevus on the child's face. As the parents find their attention focused on the birthmark, feelings of embarrassment are aroused. Their own disappointment about the nevus raises concerns about whether other people will find their infant attractive.

All physicians need to be aware of the anxiety generated by confusing medical terminology. Medical jargon should be avoided whenever possible. What is unfamiliar is likely to be frightening, so that even a "benign" port-wine stain arouses potential fear. The word "benign," although intended to reassure, may be associated in a parent's mind with a dreaded cancer. Common parental worries include potential danger to the infant's health, the possibility of the nevus enlarging, and the concern that the nevus overlies a more serious illness. The port-wine stain on the cheek is "benign" but the parental fear that it is cancer or another life-threatening condition can seriously interfere with the development of the critical process of attachment.

Birth defects commonly arouse parental guilt. Regardless of the medical etiology, one or both parents may feel responsible for causing the infant's problem. A mother may worry particularly that during pregnancy her child was exposed to potentially harmful agents such as cigarettes, medication, or alcohol, and therefore feels guilty about the infant's defect. Even a mother who tried to maintain exemplary behavior during pregnancy may have deeply held notions of how she caused her infant's defect.

5. Porter J, Nordlund JJ, Beuf AH (1979) Psychological reactions to chronic skin disorders: a study of patients with vitiligo. **Gen Hosp Psychiatry** 4:73.
6. Dion KK, Berscheid E, Walster E (1966) What is beautiful is good. **J Pers Soc Psychol** 24:285.
7. Molinaro JR (1978) The social fate of children disfigured by burns. **Am J Psychiatry** 135:8.
8. Rauch PK, Jellinek MS, Murphy JM et al. (1991) Screening for psychosocial dysfunction in pediatric dermatology practice. **Clin Pediatr** 30:8.
9. Gil KM, Keefe FJ, Sampson HA et al. (1987) The relation of stress and family environment to atopic dermatitis symptoms in children. **J Psychosom Res** 31:6.
10. Howlett S (1999) Emotional dysfunction, child–family relationships and childhood atopic dermatitis. **Br J Dermatol** 140:381–384.

11. Lawson V, Lewis-Jones MS, Finlay AY, Reid P, Owens RG (1998) The family impact of childhood atopic dermatitis: the Dermatitis Family impact Questionaire. **Br J Dermatol** Jan;138:107–113.
12. Absolon CM, Cottrell D, Eldridge SM, Glover MT (1997) Psychological disturbance in atopic eczema: the extent of the problem in school-aged children. **Br J Dermatol** Aug; 137:241–245.
13. Pauli-Pott U, Darui A, Beckmann D (1999) Infants with atopic dermatitis: maternal hopelessness, child-rearing attitudes and perceived infant temperament. **Psychotherapy & Psychosomatics** 68:39–45.
14. Trolius A, Wrangsjo B, Ljunggren B (2000) Patients with port-wine stains and their psychosocial reactions after photothermolytic treatment. **Dermatologic Surgery** Mar; 26:190–196.
15. Miller AC, Pit-Ten Cate IM, Watson HS, Geronemus RG (1999) Stress and family satisfaction in parents of children with facial port-wine stains. **Pediatric Dermatology** May–June; 16:190–197.

The experience of disappointment and mixed feelings about the infant are often in themselves very upsetting. The parents have imagined feeling unequivocal delight at seeing their infant and instead may feel more distant than expected.

The capacity to negotiate through a disappointment about the infant and the ease with which it is put into perspective will depend on the relationship between the parents, their individual maturity, and the severity of past losses or experiences. It is easier if the decision to have a child was shared equally by the parents and the anticipation during pregnancy was enjoyed together.

Mutually supportive parents can more easily focus on the attributes of their joint product. Conversely, in the setting of marital discord, an imperfection in the infant's appearance may become more ammunition for fighting. A typical scenario would be one parent blaming the other for the existence of the nevus, or the more distressed parent being belittled by the other for experiencing such distress because of the defect.

Parents with greater individual maturity, particularly in terms of their sense of self-worth, adapt more easily to an infant that differs from their original expectation. Parents who rely heavily on the attributes of the infant to enhance their own sense of self-worth will experience the infant's defect in a more stress-causing manner. A parent's own past experiences with attractiveness will affect how the infant's facial imperfection is viewed. A parent whose childhood appearance has little memorable impact will ascribe less significance to the nevus than the parent who remembers being teased or feeling socially handicapped by, for example, a misshaped nose or a strabismus.

Atopic dermatitis

The bonding between mother and child depends on many factors, including the five senses. The importance of the experience of touching in the development of mother–infant attachment was first highlighted in Harlow's research with rhesus monkeys. He offered isolated newborn monkeys the choice of two types of surrogate mothers. One surrogate was made out of wire-mesh with a bottle; the other surrogate was wire-mesh covered in a soft material but without a bottle. The infants spent most of their time clinging to the soft mother, ignoring the uncovered wire-mesh mother except at feeding times.[16] This behavior challenged the earlier hypothesis that the bond of attachment occurred on the basis of satisfying hunger, and highlighted the role touch plays in attachment.

It is easy to imagine that a red, scaly, weepy dermatitis alters the relationship between mother and infant by affecting the mother's spontaneous touching of her infant. More spontaneous and soothing touching may be replaced by hesitancy and regimented medication applications, especially if the mother attempts to restrict scratching. Affected infants often are irritable and appear uncomfortable. This behavior challenges the mother's confidence in her caretaking skills and can lead to feelings of inadequacy and self-doubt.

Attachment is in part biologically determined, but the individual infant–mother relationship is shaped by the intensity or temperament of the infant, and the mother's comfort with the infant's style. In pioneering research, Chess and Thomas[17] suggested that infants demonstrate variability in temperament from birth. They differ in their intensity of responses and thresholds of irritability. This variability in temperament influences the broad range of infant reactions seen with equally severe cases of atopic dermatitis. A mother's relative comfort and ease in adaptation to her infant's temperament allows greater leeway to accommodate stress caused by the condition. Fortunately, most mothers and infants attach well in spite of the challenges imposed by skin sensitivity. However, a combination of an infant with a difficult temperament, an irritating skin condition, and a less well-attuned mother may lead to attachment problems.

A mother's frustration, guilt, and sense of inadequacy in her mothering skills adversely affect her relationship with her infant. A stressed mother is more vulnerable to withdrawal or overinvolvement. For example, a mother may withdraw when she feels her best efforts at soothing her infant seem to only result in continued crying, believing the less she handles her infant the happier the infant will be. At the opposite end of the spectrum, it is the overinvolved mother who responds to her infant's irritability with constant anxious attentiveness, repeatedly offering the infant food and diaper changes without waiting for or discerning the cues from the infant.

The father's role is also important during the attachment phase. Depending on how the couple divides the parenting duties, the father may be called on to negotiate the same issues previously ascribed to the mother. However, the father who assumes less of the primary caretaking role with his infant may be vulnerable to feeling excluded by the intense relationship between the mother and the infant. He may feel less important to his wife because she is focusing most of her attention on the infant. Even a mild case of atopic dermatitis may be problematic for such a father because of his increasing awkwardness in handling his infant. A willing father can be included in the caretaking process of treating the skin condition, thus offering him more involvement with both the wife and the child.

Epidermolysis bullosa

The birth of an infant with a potentially severely disfiguring or life-threatening disorder intensifies previously outlined parental stresses.

The maternal response to an infant that may be dying is one of distance and premature mourning, a reaction that inevitably causes severe guilt. Attachment is further inhibited when touching the infant is prevented by the risk of infection, while recurrent medical crises add the additional emotional burden of uncertainty.

The postpartum period in general is a vulnerable time for maternal depression. When the infant is critically ill, the physician needs to be alert to changes that suggest the parent's grief is evolving into a clinically significant depression. It is common for a grief-stricken individual to have some symptoms associated with depression, such as appetite loss, insomnia, and less interest in previously pleasurable activities. The parent who demonstrates persistent feelings of worthlessness, severe guilt, difficulty functioning at home and work, or psychomotor retardation may be experiencing more than uncomplicated grief, and should be referred for psychiatric evaluation.

The stress of a prolonged acute illness or chronic disease may become manifest in the relationship between the parents. Ideally, each parent will be emotionally available and supportive of the other in their sadness. However, rate and style of grieving is an individualized process. It is likely that the parents will use different coping styles and proceed at somewhat different rates. For example, one parent (commonly the mother) may feel the need to review repeatedly the circumstances of the infant's illness and treatment, while the other parent may find such discussions painful and frustrating, perhaps preferring to return to work with an extra determination that comes from the grief. The risk is that one parent will feel that the other does not appreciate his or her sense of loss. Struggles can arise over whose sadness is greater or whose response is more reasonable. In some inherited forms of epidermolysis bullosa, an additional conflict can arise between the parents. The genetic responsibility can be used as a weapon by one parent against the other in marital fights.

A terminally ill infant may have a profound effect on the other children in the family. Children of all ages are vulnerable to the withdrawal of grief-stricken parents. In their sadness the parents may find it difficult to react in the usual ways to their other children's relatively less serious daily concerns. The more support the parents have, including that from each other and from available relatives and friends, the greater the likelihood that they will have more of a reservoir to draw upon to nurture the other children in the family.

Preschoolers and early school-age children are particularly vulnerable to feeling responsible for the death of a sibling. Children at this age cannot distinguish between "wishing" and "causing." The preschooler is likely to have felt jealous of the sickly infant, wished the infant would disappear or die, thereby not taking so much of the parents' attention. The child then worries that the wish actually caused the infant to die. Young children can be reassured by verbalizing their fear and by the parents explaining the reality of the

16. Harlow HF (1959) Love in infant monkeys. **Sci Am** 200:68.

17. Chess S, Thomas A (1977) Temperament and Development. New York: Brunner//Mazel.

situation by explaining, for example, "It's not your fault that the baby died. You are a good boy. The baby died because he was born sick."

Summary

The dermatologist can play an important role in facilitating parents' adjustment to dermatologic conditions, ranging from minor to severe, and therefore support the developmental task of attachment in infancy. It is helpful for the dermatologist to offer a simple description of the skin problem, highlighting etiology, natural history, treatment, and prognosis.

By inviting the parents to ask questions, even ones viewed by the parents as silly, the dermatologist gives them permission to verbalize their mixed feelings. Explaining that it is common for loving parents to also feel disappointment, embarrassment, or distance from their infant, depending on the severity of the infant's illness, may help the parents to recognize that such feelings are not unusual and do not make them bad parents. The physician may want to inquire specifically about whether each parent feels responsible for causing the problem, and if so in what way. Alternatively, parental guilt can be addressed indirectly by describing the etiology of the condition.

Dermatologists cannot avert marital discord, but by taking a stance that is considerate of each parent's experience of the skin disorder, they can model an attitude that will perhaps leave the infant's condition out of the center of the marital fighting, and may be able to make an early referral for counseling.

In the event that either parent presents with clinically significant depression or intense discord, dermatologists are in a position to make a psychiatric referral because of their role as trusted caretaker of the infant. The dermatologist may also discuss a potential psychiatric referral with the infant's pediatrician or family practitioner.

DERMATOLOGIC CONDITIONS IN PRESCHOOLERS

The preschool child, 3 to 5 years of age, has developed a new awareness of his body and its parts. This emerging sense of self includes a pride in physical capability and fear about bodily injury. Preschoolers express many of their feelings through their imaginative play (fantasy), becoming such characters as superheroes, tea party hostesses, and wild animals. They charm adults with their uniquely unscientific explanations for why things happen and how they work. Children at this age have an extreme sense of self-importance; they believe they are responsible for all the things that happen around them.

Port-wine stain

Preschoolers have developed the cognitive capacity to examine their physical appearance and thus to become aware of their port-wine stain. Children at this age are curious about their bodies and will commonly raise questions about their port-wine stains. The nevus now gains a personal meaning for the child. At earlier ages, its meaning derived exclusively from the parents' response. The preschooler is usually spending a significant part of the day out of the home for the first time in a nursery school or preschool setting. The reactions of nonparental adults, especially teachers and peers, are added to the children's own view of themselves. There is now research to suggest that laser treatment of port-wine stain during these early years may benefit the child's later adjustment.

Preschoolers' interest in the different parts of their body carries with it a heightened concern about bodily injury. By adult standards children often overreact to minor cuts and bruises. Preschoolers commonly present small "boo boos" with tearful requests for Band-Aids, while hardly seeming to react to more painful injuries, such as hitting their heads, if there is no visible wound. The combination of fantasy and age-appropriate concern about bodily injury makes surgery particularly frightening to preschoolers (see Surgery for dermatologic problems).

When a 4-year-old makes a new discovery, such as the port-wine stain on his cheek, he arrives at an intermingling of reality based and fantasy based conclusions. For example, having been told he was born with the nevus flammeus, he might explain, "There was a fire when I was born and it got on my face," or, "I was sleeping when I was born and my brother hit me." Preschoolers do not understand the concept of chance occurrences.

Without the mediating influence of adult explanations, they invent their own etiologies, some of which are frightening. In the second explanation above, for example, the child may be frightened of what might happen to him while he sleeps or if his brother hits him. The pediatrician or dermatologist is helping the child by eliciting the fantasy "how do you think you got that spot?," reassuring the child if the fantasy is anxiety provoking, and offering a simply worded statement that people are born different (freckles, eye color, etc.).

Atopic dermatitis

Every preschooler is moving along a continuum toward increasing independence while maintaining the wish to remain close to and be cared for by the parental figure. An expected balance between independence (leaving the parent) and dependence (checking back for security) is commonly seen. The relative balance varies with different children and varies over time with respect to the same child. It is expected, for example, that 5-year-olds may want to shampoo their hair without their mother's help one day and request her assistance from start to finish of the bath on another day of the same week.

An acute illness results in a predictable, temporary return to a more dependent state (regression). A chronic illness, such as atopic dermatitis, by virtue of its persistent presence, becomes a part of the hour-to-hour parent–child interaction. Most children and parents adapt relatively easily to the chronic dermatitis, especially when mild. Treatments are applied as needed and the usual state of the dermatitis is accepted as normal for the child. The child is able to continue the expected course toward independence with little tension between parent and child in regard to the dermatitis. However, some children may respond to the condition with increasing dependence, for example, claiming they are unable to dress themselves because it itches too much, or needing a parent to stay at the bedside with them every night until they fall asleep to help keep them from scratching. Other children may adopt an overly independent stance, such as resisting prescribed treatments applied by parents or refusing to permit parents to view elbows, knees, and other affected areas. The temperament of the child and the caretaking style of the parent may contribute to the development of equally problematic patterns of overdependence or a false independence.

A developmentally appropriate task for the preschooler is to begin to express feelings with words. Young children may use words on one occasion and body actions on another. For example, a 4-year-old who is prevented from getting a cookie may angrily and say, "I want that cookie and I hate you," or may walk around the kitchen stomping his feet and kicking the cabinets.

Children with an itchy dermatitis may find an outlet for a range of feelings by scratching instead of using words to express themselves. The scratching may initially elicit a pleasurable sensation that only becomes painful with continued scratching. Aggravating the relentless itching by continued scratching may become an expression of frustration and irritability. Scratching may also be a weapon to remind parents of their relative powerlessness against the child's discomfort.

The preschooler's understanding of events is a mixture of reality and fantasy. Hence, uncomfortable or painful experiences, like itching, burning skin are often construed to be punishment for bad thoughts or behaviors, and raise concerns about the body's vulnerability. Itching is affected by fantasy, mood, temperament, and anxiety. Intensity and tolerance of itching vary between children and with regard to different contexts for the same child. Like an adult who reaches for a cigarette in certain situations, the preschooler may begin scratching at the dermatitis when stressed. For example, a shy 5-year-old girl scratches her arm furiously as her mother drives her to a classmate's birthday party in an unfamiliar house. When she sees her best friend from school at the party, she takes the friend's hand and stops scratching. In anticipating the party her anxiety heightened her sensation of itchiness, which declined when she was more relaxed. Similarly, a child happily involved in play may be oblivious to the itchiness and later be acutely aware of it when trying to fall asleep.

The impact of scratching on the interaction between parent and child is influenced by how the scratching is viewed. Most parents encourage their children to try not to scratch, but recognize that some scratching is inevitable. Children at this age have little self-control. They are more likely to stop scratching when distracted by other interests rather than by parental rules, particularly at the times when the parent is not present. Problems commonly occur when parents expect complete control (i.e., no scratching). The behavior may be seen as either the child's being bad or the parent's own failure to exert control. Some children respond to unreasonable expectations with a sense of shame at their own lack of control, while others respond by open defiance, expressing their anger at their parents by increased scratching. The latter response is problematic for treatment, but both extremes cause injury to the child.

The dermatologist can help this difficult interaction between parent and child by sharing reasonable expectations for the child with the parent. This helps both the parent and child to feel less burdened by an expected response to an itchy dermatitis.

Epidermolysis bullosa

Independence is particularly problematic for a child with epidermolysis bullosa because minor injuries may result in dramatic blistering. This adds a painful reality to the age-appropriate fears about bodily integrity and physical vulnerability.

Parents are likely to have more difficulty allowing a child with epidermolysis bullosa to determine a balance between dependence and independence as suited to the child's particular temperament. Motivated by the wish to protect their child, the parents may find it difficult to foster her emerging independence. By creatively seeking safe ways for the child to express her independence, such as picking her own clothes each day, choosing her dessert, or painting her room the color of her choice, parents can facilitate the developmental task of increased independence.

A tendency to be overprotective would be further complicated by parental guilt. Such feelings are often especially intense in a genetically transmitted illness because the parent feels so responsible for the child's suffering. If the parent has the disorder, his or her attitude will be influenced by personal experiences with the illness during childhood. The personal memories may be so powerful that the parent has difficulty seeing the ways the child's experience differs from his or her own. Alternatively, for some parents, personal knowledge of the disorder can be positive by enhancing their sensitivity to the child's needs.

Most preschoolers are spending more time with a number of different adults, primarily at school. These new adults are likely to be unfamiliar with the illness and may be overly cautious and restricting. It is important to foster a relatively safe environment, but also one that interferes as little as possible with the child's relationship with peers in order that the developmentally important process of playing can occur.

Surgery for dermatologic problems

Because preschoolers are normally preoccupied with body injury and tend to understand all events based on fantasy and the power of their own actions, surgery is a particularly frightening prospect, which is often experienced as a punishment for "bad" thoughts or behavior.

When surgery is indicated for the preschooler, preparation of the child and taking additional history from the parents are essential.

Preoperative preparation

In preparation for surgery, it is important for the physician to discuss the following with the patient and the parents:

1. Describe the procedure, including both painful and pain-free steps.
2. Visit the office or hospital where the procedure is to take place.
3. Supply the names of appropriate books and videos.[18]
4. Ensure the presence of parents throughout the awake portions of the procedure.

Preschoolers can benefit from simple education as preparation for the surgery. The dermatologist should describe each step of the procedure. A tour of the hospital or outpatient setting, with an explanation of what will happen where, will also decrease the anxiety associated with the uncertainties. Parents should be encouraged by the dermatologist to give their children ample opportunity to explain their understanding of the procedure as a way of uncovering their misconceptions and offer them the opportunity to ask questions. Children will want to know where their parents will be before, during, and after the procedure. Following the procedure, the child should be encouraged to continue to ask questions both in the hospital and at home. Questions can be followed up and facilitated at home with hospital play. Many children will enjoy being the doctor to their dolls or stuffed animals, especially if Band-Aids, gauze, or other medical supplies are offered.

Preoperative history

Five considerations represent major stressful events for the young child that can be expected to increase preoperative anxiety. They include:

1. previous injuries or surgeries;
2. previous hospitalizations or other separation from the family;
3. illnesses of family members;
4. deaths in the family; and
5. family discord.

Preschoolers are likely to generalize from previous experience and therefore assume their upcoming surgery and/or hospitalization will be like their past experiences. This can be especially frightening if the earlier experiences are remembered as unpleasant or there is a physical reminder from a previous injury. If children have experienced a family illness or death, they are likely to assume their fate will be like that of their relative. In cases of family discord or divorce, preschoolers are vulnerable to seeing the surgery as punishment for the trouble they believe they have caused in the family, and they may be very frightened about their safety.

Postoperative considerations

Postoperative symptoms of difficulty include recurrent nightmares and prolonged regression with such symptoms as enuresis, baby talk, and needing more help with activities such as dressing. It is normal for these symptoms to occur transiently after the stress of surgery, but if they persist for more than a few weeks, psychiatric referral is indicated.

Summary

Children age 3 to 5 years do not understand the concept of chance, nor do they understand the difference between wishing something would happen and making it happen. They are preoccupied with concerns about body injury and are likely to view an accidental injury or surgical procedure as punishment for bad thoughts or behavior.

The dermatologist can ease the preschooler's anxiety about treatments and procedures by collaborating with parents to provide simple explanations for what to expect prior to treatment. Children with reasons to feel more insecure, such as previous experiences with painful procedures, frightening accidents, or stressful family situations will need more preparation and support. Common symptoms of stress, as mentioned above, should be noted. If symptomatology persists more than a few weeks after surgery, psychiatric attention is warranted.

SCHOOL-AGE CHILDREN

The school-age child is developing new skills in all areas such as sports, academics, and the arts. The peer group takes on new significance as children compare their own performance with that of their friends. Status within the group becomes important with fighting, teasing, and scapegoating as ways of establishing the social hierarchy.

18. Rey HA, Rey M (1966) Curious George Goes to the Hospital. Boston: Houghton Mifflin.

Port-wine stain

School-age children look for acceptance from their peer group and for a sense that their various skills compare favorably with those of their peers. A port-wine stain has the potential to be used as an instrument for teasing. Some children, however, are more vulnerable than others. The child who has an area of competence that is valued by the peer group is likely to withstand teasing and aggression better than a less capable child who is more apt to become the scapegoat. For example, the 10-year-old star pitcher of his minor league baseball team is less likely to be teased about a port-wine stain than his unathletic teammate in the outfield who strikes out whenever he is up at bat.

Parents play a key role in supporting the child's appreciation of emerging skills. But some children expect themselves to be the best in all arenas, and thus it is the responsibility of the parents to help them set more reasonable expectations.

The distressed parent and child may present to the dermatologist's office requesting treatment of the port-wine stain because the child is being teased. The parent and child may view the nevus as an isolated problem, without recognizing that some teasing is a part of life for the school-age child. For less fortunate children who become the frequent scapegoat because of lesser skills in particular areas such as athletics, it is helpful to find another peer setting in which their competencies are supported. Organized groups such as photography or computer clubs can serve this function.

Atopic dermatitis

Most children adapt well and are more interested in mastering new activities within the peer group than they are preoccupied with or limited by their skin disorder. School-age children are most likely to be concerned with how the atopic dermatitis affects their image among their peers. It is common for children to attempt to conceal the affected skin under long sleeves, long pants, and high collars. Some children will restrict their activities, for example, not swimming because of embarrassment about the dermatitis. Children who limit their activities in order to hide the dermatitis miss developmentally important experiences with other children.

The increased cognitive capacity of children at this age enables them to conceptualize the dermatitis as an isolated entity that affects their skin. This contrasts with the earlier experience, where affected younger children viewed themselves as broadly damaged. School-age children are less worried about their physical vulnerability and more confident about their ability to take charge of their environment.

The dermatitis may perpetuate existing parent–child struggles, but new struggles are less likely if children are involved as collaborators in their own treatment. With encouragement, they can communicate their concerns, such as if the dermatitis or the treatment is interfering in their important peer activities. The demonstration of motivation and capability for assuming more responsibility for self-care suggests better adjustment.

Epidermolysis bullosa

Epidermolysis bullosa presents many challenges to the developing school-age child. The self-image at this age is based on the mastery of new skills, many of which depend on physical capacities such as speed, strength, and coordination. To the extent that the epidermolysis bullosa limits the child's liberty to join in age-appropriate activities and to play one's hardest, it may challenge the child to find other arenas of accomplishment in order to build a positive self-image.

Many children with epidermolysis bullosa will find safe activities that permit the development of a sense of competency and peer group connectedness. Appropriate choices include such activities as swimming, bowling, nature study, action movies, and video games.

Some children are not able to take advantage of the safe activities available to them, and feel isolated from their peer group and personally inadequate. Of equal concern are the children who engage in reckless contact sports or other self-injurious activities in defiance of their illness. They are eager to prove themselves to the peer group in ways that are self-destructive. The extremes of inactivity and recklessness are maladaptive and warrant psychiatric consultation.

Summary

The school years represent an important period for the acquisition of new athletic, academic, artistic, and social skills. Teasing and fighting are an expected part of peer group interaction, but may be particularly painful for the child with an apparent dermatologic problem.

The dermatologist can help the parents support the child's emerging competencies and if necessary direct the child toward particular activities that foster a positive self-image and do not aggravate the skin disorder. The pride in mastering a task provides a good context for encouraging children to take increasing responsibility for their own treatment.

ADOLESCENCE

Adolescents are establishing a sense of autonomy by scrutinizing, modifying, or rejecting their parents' values and identifying with the standards of their peer group. An example of this is seen in adolescent fashion trends that appear extreme in comparison with adult clothing fashions. However, within the adolescent peer group, every member dresses almost alike. The adolescent has an internal struggle between the wish to be both independent and dependent at the same time. For some teenagers, this internal struggle, which they are not consciously aware of, gets acted out in control struggles with parents. The emphasis on autonomy and sexuality makes these years exciting and anxiety provoking.

Adolescents can be challenging patients to treat. They often question rules in the developmental context of resenting authority figures (including physicians). Noncompliance with medical regimes poses a significant problem for this age group.

Acne

In large part, adolescents' self-esteem depends on their own sense of attractiveness. Teenagers are both vain and self-conscious. Most are dissatisfied with their appearance, and acne increases this dissatisfaction more than one might predict. From the adolescents' perspective acne is as stressful as asthma, epilepsy or diabetes.[19] Some of this impact may be lessened by education directed at misconceptions about the causes of acne, but the cosmetic impact remains significant.[20] Some adolescents look into the mirror and actually see only their pimples, not their faces.

Adolescents are particularly sensitive to peer rejection, especially when it involves the opposite sex. The considerable variability in physical maturity among teenagers of the same age results in many feeling inadequate in comparison with their friends.

The self-consciousness associated with appearance makes the adolescent with acne more vulnerable to interpreting behavior, such as a classmate's unenthusiastic greeting, as further evidence of being unattractive. In some teenagers, these feelings lead to social withdrawal and isolation. For example, it is common for adolescents to worry before a party that no one will want to dance with them. Usually, however, they are able to bear this concern and go to the party. Some adolescents with acne use their skin condition as an excuse to avoid such social situations, feeling that the acne makes them too unattractive to make it worthwhile to go to a party. It is easy to identify the acne as the source of social frustration. The short-term satisfaction of attacking the frustrating pimples results in continued aggravation and worsening of the acne.

It is difficult for adolescents to be patient and passively wait for the dermatologist's treatment to work. Acne, like atopic dermatitis, is a chronic dermatologic condition that the adolescent must learn to live with, at least for

19. Mallon E, Newton JN, Klassen A, Stewart-Brown SI, Ryan TJ, Fainlay AY (1999) The quality of life in acne: a comparison with general medical conditions using generic questionnaires. **Br J Dermatol** 140:672–676.

20. Pearl A, Arroll B, Lello L, Birchall NM (1998) The impact of acne: A study of adolescents' attitudes, perception and knowledge. **New Zealand Med Journ** 111:269–270.

some time. As one pimple clears up, another one appears. Passivity is a particularly difficult stance for adolescents who want to be actively in control in all aspects of their lives. The impulsive and at times short-sighted perspective of the adolescent is reflected in the high incidence of accidents in this age group. Similarly, allowing pimples to heal untouched requires a future-oriented perspective more characteristic of an adult, not an adolescent.

Addressing the frustration and temptation to attack the pimples may help the adolescent to choose to "tough it out" and wait for a medication to take action. The dermatologist can present potential benefits of the treatment along with presenting the risks of self-inflicted scarring, but the ultimate decision to implement treatment is up to the adolescent.

Often, parents seek treatment for their adolescent child's acne. In this situation it is easy to fall into the trap of negotiating a treatment plan with the parent instead of with the teenager. It is key that the dermatologist establish an alliance with the teenager around the wish to improve the acne. Without establishing a relationship with the patient around a shared treatment goal, dermatologists are likely to find themselves in the middle of a parent–adolescent struggle. In other words, adolescents may assert their independence from their parents by defying the treatment plan endorsed by them. The struggle is manifest by noncompliance.

Port-wine stain

Issues of sexual attractiveness may arouse insecurities that make a life-long nevus take on new significance at this age. The teenager's style of coping depends largely on earlier emotional development. Some social withdrawal is commonly seen as a technique for coping with adolescent social awkwardness, but when the birthmark becomes an excuse for exaggerated withdrawal and isolation, psychiatric consultation is indicated.

Epidermolysis bullosa

Adolescents live in the present and tend not to worry about their future. They tend not to fear death and enjoy showing off with daredevil antics. They engage in a range of reckless activities from cigarette smoking to diving off bridges.

It is difficult for the adolescent with epidermolysis bullosa to confront the physical limitations and consider the long-term effects of current behavior. Overreaction to physical restrictions imposed by the epidermolysis bullosa may be maladaptively expressed as rigid limitation of all activities at one extreme and careless disregard for potential risk at the other. Overreaction in either direction is reason for psychiatric consultation.

Sexually transmitted diseases

Over 12 million adolescents in the United States are sexually active by age 18;[21] however, the meaning of the sexual contact varies. Common motivations include curiosity, peer pressure, a wish for intimacy or companionship, and rebellion against parental or religious rules. Usually the choice to engage in sexual activity is determined by a number of factors. The experience arouses many feelings that may interfere with seeking appropriate treatment for sexually transmitted diseases. Sexual activity is often so important to the adolescent's self-image that appropriate precautions against transmitting these illnesses to others and protecting against acquired immunodeficiency syndrome (AIDS) are not exercised.

The discovery of skin lesions on the genitals is likely to frighten adolescents regardless of the etiology. They may not know who to turn to in order to get answers to questions about a condition. Peers may be the easiest to approach but are unlikely to have accurate information. Fear of parental discovery and punishment or parental rejection may inhibit seeking medical advice, as well as treatment. Fear of AIDS may not lead adolescents to practice "safe sex," and may accentuate the fear of seeking medical help once they are aware of a problem. Acknowledging a sexually transmitted disease to peers may arouse concerns about peer rejection from angry previous contacts and about future sexual isolation.

Some adolescent fears and misconceptions may respond to simple education. Patients may be too shy to express their actual fears. The dermatologist's careful explanation of how diseases are transmitted, the symptoms, the treatment, and the prevention of transmittal may answer many important, yet unexpressed questions, and may make it easier for some teenagers to ask their remaining questions. The physician can invite adolescents to share their own understanding of the disease as a way of ascertaining any additional confusion.

It is important that the dermatologist knows the statutes concerning confidentiality, the reporting of sexually transmitted illnesses, and the notification of sexual partners.

Summary

Noncompliance is a significant problem in treating adolescents. It can be decreased by establishing an alliance with the patient around the goal of therapy. Although the parent may have brought the teenager to the physician, the success of treatment depends on the patient. The adolescent is most likely to follow through if the dermatologist presents the pros and cons of the treatment and explicitly leaves the choice and responsibility of implementation up to the adolescent. Parents who confidently offer to make sure the adolescent follows through on the treatment may only increase noncompliance by placing the treatment in the middle of existing parent–child struggles.

For a variety of reasons, adolescents are hesitant to ask the dermatologist questions, but this is especially true in sexually transmitted conditions. Teenagers may turn to each other and receive inaccurate information unless the physician actively invites their questions. In sexually transmitted diseases, including AIDS, lack of accurate information is a public health hazard. In all dermatologic conditions this may adversely affect compliance.

Conclusion

The psychological meaning of a dermatologic condition changes according to the development stage of the affected child. In infancy, a skin disorder is viewed in terms of how it affects survival of the newborn and the mother–infant attachment. In the preschool years attention is focused on the fears about body injury and consideration is given to the important role of fantasy. During the school-age period, a dermatologic condition will be most significant in terms of its effect on the child's status in the peer group and any limitations it puts on new skills. In adolescence, skin disorders increase the normal self-consciousness about appearance. Successful treatment requires establishing a doctor–patient alliance sensitive to developmental and family issues.

THE PSYCHOSOCIAL INTERVIEW

The focus of this chapter thus far has been on the potential impact at different developmental points of dermatologic disorders. In cases where psychosocial concerns become evident, either in the distress of the patient or family, or as an interference with optimal therapy, the dermatologist needs a strategy for evaluating the underlying problem.[22] The fundamental skills necessary for this process are expressed in the evaluation interview. The goal of the interview is to elucidate the problem and assess the need for further treatment by the dermatologist or by a consultant.

After identifying a psychosocial concern, dermatologists must consciously change their mindset temporarily from the usual rapid pace and style of routine office practice to one that is slower and more reflective. Obviously there are time constraints for the dermatologist based on the economics of practice and the pressure of knowing other patients are waiting. A psychosocial

21. Teenage pregnancy. The problem that hasn't gone away. Alan Guttmacher Institute, 1981.

22. Hack S, Jellinek M (1998) Early identification and behavioral problems in a primary care setting. In: Adolescent Medicine, State of the Art Reviews, S Friedman, D DeMaso eds. Philadelphia: Hanley and Belfus, Inc., pp. 335–350.

evaluation does take more time, for which hopefully the physician can be at least partially compensated. At the minimum, the dermatologist must allot 10 minutes for this purpose.

Once the initial decision is made, it should be communicated to the patient and family, for example, "I am concerned about Billy giving you a hard time about the medicine. I would like to take the next 10 minutes to talk with you about this. If we need more time, I will set up a follow-up appointment sooner than usual." Communicating the time constraints serves multiple purposes. The physician has set clear limits as to the amount of time available; this protects against feeling pressured by thoughts about the interview going on indefinitely, and making the remainder of the day impossibly rushed. It lets the patient and family know that the time is limited, so an effort will be made to focus and prioritize concerns. When the time ends, they are prepared and are less likely to feel hurt that the physician has interrupted them in the middle of the discussion or is rushing them out. In addition, the potential for further discussion at another appointment has been offered at the outset.

The next step in the interview process is to communicate interest by relaxing and assuming a listening posture. Communicating this change in mindset can be accomplished by sitting down in a relaxed posture at eye level with the child or lower, and putting down pens and other equipment. This conveys an intent to engage the child in a true dialogue. Asking, if possible, not to be interrupted by phone calls or by staff walking into the room indicates that this communication is important. Thinking about the likely area of concern given the disorder, age of the child, and family situation, the dermatologist must decide which of two types of interviews will be conducted. One type gives information and the other tries to gain an understanding of psychosocial concerns.

The major goal of an interview that attempts to communicate information is to be sure that both the parent and the patient have a reasonably accurate understanding of the issues being presented. For example, do they understand the seriousness of the illness? Underestimating the seriousness will possibly result in noncompliance or later anger and disappointment. Overestimating will likely result in unnecessary anguish and possible withdrawal of the parent from the child or physician. It is common for parents to distort or "not hear" bad news. Some studies of parents remembering medical information suggest that well over half of the factual information is rapidly forgotten.

The dermatologist giving worrisome or complex information should present the material in clear, easily understood terms, and then ask the patient or parent to give a brief summary of what is understood to be the nature, treatment, and prognosis of the disorder. It is often useful to make quite clear the etiology of the illness in a manner that relieves that parent as much as possible of guilt feelings for having caused the child's problem.

If the child is very ill, it is especially important for physicians to be certain that the parents understand the critical nature of the situation with as little distortion as possible. The physician could ask for example, "Now that you have heard my summary of the current problem, could you tell me on a scale of 1 to 10, with 1 being complete recovery and 10 being a child near death, what number you feel is appropriate given what I have said?" Parents will usually be able to give a numerical assessment, which physicians can then compare with their own in a way that results in congruence with the parents in understanding the situation.

The second type of interview is designed to elicit information in order to gain an understanding of a psychosocial problem or noncompliance with treatment recommendations. The opening question is especially important. When physicians are in a hurry, there is a tendency to ask questions that both in number and grammatical structure must be answered yes or no. The purpose of a psychosocial evaluation interview is to help the patient paint as detailed a picture as possible of the current problem. Questions in this type of interview are most effective if they cannot be answered with a yes or no response. Some examples of such questions include: "How do you feel it is

reasonable to deal with your child's constant desire to scratch his eczema?," "Do you and your spouse agree on how to handle this problem?," "What seems to be most difficult about taking (or giving) the medicine?" These types of questions encourage the patient or parent to describe specific problems in their own words.

Interviews that give information or attempt an understanding of the problem serve a therapeutic function. An interview that accurately gives information to parent and patient will help forge the doctor–patient and doctor–parent relationships, increase compliance with medical regimens, and in serious disorders support the parents' intellectual attempts to cope with the illness.

Interviews that give information to children, such as pre-procedure or pre-surgical preparation, will build an alliance with the child, reduce anxiety before the procedure, increase cooperation, and possibly reduce post-procedure stress. Preparing or giving information to adolescents is especially important in order to build a relationship with the patient somewhat independent of the parents, and thus increase compliance.

The interview that elicits a deeper understanding of a problem is intrinsically therapeutic. The dermatologist's questions should convey many implicit messages, such as that the patient's experience of the disorder is important, the parents are not to blame, they are not alone or unique in blaming themselves, treatment complications are not their fault, and chronic diseases are stressful for families. By making the effort to ask about these problems, some tension is relieved and a process of attempting solutions can begin.

Beyond the immediate benefit of relieving guilt and isolation, the interview will likely result in the physician giving additional reassurance, correcting misperceptions about etiology or prognosis, and possibly adapting medical regimens to the family's pattern.

If the issues presented are complex and cannot be understood in the 10 minutes of available time, then the physician can consider an additional appointment. If the family's or child's health or age-appropriate functioning is adversely affected, then a child psychiatric referral is indicated.

SCREENING FOR PEDIATRIC PSYCHOSOCIAL DYSFUNCTION IN THE DERMATOLOGIST'S OFFICE

Given the barriers of time and complexity, a number of questionnaires are available to assess psychosocial functioning. The best validated, and most convenient to use, focus on children 4 to 16 years of age. At the ages of 4 and below the questionnaires are not as effective, because of the child's limited school experiences. Above age 14 these parent-completed questionnaires cannot identify, as successfully, adolescent depression. With these caveats in mind the two best questionnaires are the Child Behavior Checklist (CBCL), which is comprehensive and takes 20 to 30 minutes to complete and score, and the Pediatric Symptom Checklist (PSC),[23–25] which is shorter and takes 3 to 5 minutes.

The PSC is a 35-item single-page questionnaire (Table 2.1) that parents typically complete in the waiting area prior to their child's appointment. Office staff scores the PSC by assigning one point for any questions answered "sometimes" and two points for "often" (zero points for "never"). If the total number of points is equal to or above 24 for 4 to 5 year olds or equal to or above 28 for children 6 to 16, there is a high probability that the child has substantial psychosocial dysfunction. The PSC can be used as a screening tool for all patients, or selectively if the physician suspects psychosocial difficulties, especially those that might interfere with treatment or overall psychosocial development. A positive score could then lead the dermatologist to pursue a more in-depth interview or refer the child for mental health consultation.

23. Jellinek MS, Murphy JM (1990) The recognition of psychosocial disorders in pediatric office practice: the current status of the pediatric symptom checklist. **J Dev Behav Pediatr** 11:273.

24. Jellinek MS, Murphy JM, Robinson J et al. (1988) The pediatric symptom checklist: screening school age children for psychosocial dysfunction. **J Pediatr** 112:201.

25. Jellinek MS, Murphy JM, Pagano ME, Comer D, Kelleher K (1999) Use of the pediatric symptom checklist (PSC) to screen for psychosocial problems in pediatric primary care: A national feasibility study. **Arch Peds Adol Med** 153:254–260.

TABLE 2.1   Pediatric symptom checklist

Please mark under the heading that best fits your child:

	Never	Sometimes	Often
1. Complains of aches or pains	——	——	——
2. Spends more time alone	——	——	——
3. Tires easily, little energy	——	——	——
4. Fidgety, unable to sit still	——	——	——
5. Has trouble with a teacher	——	——	——
6. Less interested in school	——	——	——
7. Acts as if driven by a motor	——	——	——
8. Daydreams too much	——	——	——
9. Distracted easily	——	——	——
10. Is afraid of new situations	——	——	——
11. Feels sad, unhappy	——	——	——
12. Is irritable, angry	——	——	——
13. Feels hopeless	——	——	——
14. Has trouble concentrating	——	——	——
15. Less interest in friends	——	——	——
16. Fights with other children	——	——	——
17. Absent from school	——	——	——
18. School grades dropping	——	——	——
19. Is down on him or herself	——	——	——
20. Visits doctor with doctor finding nothing wrong	——	——	——
21. Has trouble with sleeping	——	——	——
22. Worries a lot	——	——	——
23. Wants to be with you more than before	——	——	——
24. Feels he or she is bad	——	——	——
25. Takes unnecessary risks	——	——	——
26. Gets hurt frequently	——	——	——
27. Seems to be having less fun	——	——	——
28. Acts younger than children his or her age	——	——	——
29. Does not listen to rules	——	——	——
30. Does not show feelings	——	——	——
31. Does not understand other people's feelings	——	——	——
32. Teases others	——	——	——
33. Blames others for his or her troubles	——	——	——
34. Takes things that do not belong to him or her	——	——	——
35. Refuses to share	——	——	——

In a multicenter pediatric dermatology study, 377 6- to 12-year-old patients were screened using the PSC. The results parallel those found in primary care settings in that 13 percent of all children screened positive. Social class, as in other epidemiologic samples, had a major impact, with poor children having approximately twice the positive rate (9 percent versus 19 percent) compared with those from the middle class. Of note is that children whose dermatologic disorder was perceived to have a greater impact on their appearance were at higher risk for psychosocial dysfunction.

This study highlighted the convenience of using the PSC in a dermatology office setting, parental acceptance, and the sensitivity parents feel concerning their child's appearance. Thus the PSC may be appropriate for general screening, but particularly so if the dermatologist suspects parental or patient concerns about appearance, if there is poor compliance with treatment, or if there is a clinical sense that psychosocial issues are impairing the child's functioning and development.

PSYCHOSOCIAL CONCERNS AND PSYCHIATRIC ILLNESS

Dermatologists and pediatricians are in a particularly challenging setting for identifying children at risk for psychiatric illness. The high volume of patients, short visit lengths, and extended periods between appointments necessitate setting priorities about what can realistically be accomplished in a brief visit. In this section we highlight for the dermatologist and pediatrician psychiatric symptomatology that can be appreciated within these office constraints and addressed when psychiatric consultation can be most useful.

A common inhibition to requesting psychiatric consultation is concern about the patient's or family's reaction to the referral. Often a physician fears that asking for a psychiatric consultation will be viewed as tantamount to calling the patient crazy, and therefore will result in the patient angrily leaving treatment. The patient and family are likely to respond to a psychiatric referral in concordance with the attitude of the dermatologist and the explanation for why a consultation is being requested.

It is best to first identify the symptoms of concern, such as, "I noticed Jane is losing weight, and I am concerned about the sleep difficulties and school problems you have described." It can then be helpful to let the patient and family know that it is a common practice to make psychiatric referrals, saying, for example, "When I see patients with symptoms like Jane's, I like to consult Dr A, a child psychiatrist, to see if he has some ideas about what might make her feel better." In this context, the parents and the patient can be asked permission for the requested consultation: "Mr and Mrs Smith, would that be all right with you?" and, "Jane, I think you will like Dr A, he is a doctor who talks to children about their worries. Would you be willing to talk with him?" This is an appropriate way of asking permission for a younger child. A teenager's permission should be asked first, and then the permission of the parent asked thereafter.

An alternative approach, if child psychiatric consultation is available, is to develop protocols with specific criteria for referrals, such as having all patients with potentially disfiguring disorders be evaluated by a psychiatrist as part of the initial workup, or referring any patient who is noncompliant after three visits. Such an approach is used at the Massachusetts General Hospital, with all pediatric oncology patients and cystic fibrosis patients referred for child-psychiatric evaluation at the time of initial diagnosis. The majority of patients and families appreciate the referral and several request or need follow-up services.

Psychiatric consultation is most useful when the dermatologist develops a working relationship with one or two child psychiatrists who can become familiar with the particular needs of the dermatologist. This allows the dermatologist and psychiatrist to determine what information or interventions prove most useful.

The most relevant psychosocial issues in dermatologic practice are noncompliance, parent–child interaction, and the psychiatric diagnoses of depression and anxiety. Although there is a broad range of other issues, many of these will be discovered by pediatricians and schools. The two relatively uncommon entities of trichotillomania and factitial skin ulcers are also presented in this section, because although somewhat rare, they often present to the dermatologist first, and pose particular challenges to treatment.

NONCOMPLIANCE

Noncompliance is discussed at the outset, because it interferes dramatically with providing quality care. Also, it often does not occur to the dermatologist to refer these patients for a psychiatric evaluation. Several common etiologies leading to noncompliance are described here.

Sometimes noncompliance is due to treatment regimens that are too complicated for the child and family to manage, are poorly communicated, or are not understood. Reviewing the essential features of the treatment and/or modifying the times or frequency of applications to accommodate the child's and family's schedule will often improve compliance in these cases.

Some patients or parents equate treatment with illness, as if ignoring the treatment would negate the existence of the illness. These patients benefit from exploring in a psychiatric interview their denial of the illness, which often comes from unexpressed fears and past experiences.

At times, noncompliance is a symptom of a larger problem with the parent–child relationship. In these cases, the treatment may become one more opportunity for a struggle. Unfortunately, these occur at the expense of the child's skin condition and the dermatologist's valuable time. The psychiatric consultant may be able to determine what role the noncompliance serves in the ongoing struggle between parent and child, and work toward separating the treatment goal from the ongoing struggle.

Adolescent rebellion is a developmentally based etiology for noncompliance and is described more fully in the section on adolescence. Some adolescents may require more time to develop a reasonable treatment alliance with the dermatologist, who is viewed as suspect either as an authority figure or because treatment has not been quickly successful. A psychiatric consultant may be helpful if the dermatologist is having difficulty establishing a treatment alliance.

Another etiology for noncompliance is as a symptom of family problems such as marital discord, alcoholism, or parental depression. The child's non-compliance or worsening of the skin condition may serve any one of a number of functions, such as temporarily uniting the parents or focusing the parents' attention on the child instead of on the more threatening family issues. The dermatologist can make a referral to the child psychiatrist to have the role of the family stress evaluated as it affects the treatment noncompliance.

Case study

Carrie is a 12-year-old with atopic dermatitis. She has been seen on a twice-yearly basis for a mild to moderate condition, up until the previous 6 months, during which time her dermatitis took a turn for the worse. For this period she was being seen on a monthly basis, and despite topical steroids, her skin was more red and raw at each visit. Carrie's mother was becoming more irritable with the dermatologist, asserting that an improvement should have occurred by this time. She complained of the daily struggles with Carrie surrounding the application of the medicine, as well as the scratching. In the office Carrie always agreed with the medication regimen eagerly, but at home she was increasingly noncompliant.

Carrie and her mother were referred for psychiatric consultation. What the psychiatrist learned was that Carrie's parents, who had been separated for several years, were now getting divorced. Because her mother could not drive, Carrie's father always drove them to all of her doctor's appointments. He would wait in the car reading, and his presence was unknown to the derma-tologist. Carrie's secret hope was that all these car rides would result in reuniting her parents. The psychiatrist recommended to the parents that someone other than the father drive Carrie to her appointments. He also scheduled a session with Carrie, where she could talk about how sad she was feeling about her parents' divorce. At the 6-month follow-up visit, Carrie's dermatitis was markedly improved, as was her compliance.

PARENT–CHILD RELATIONSHIP DIFFICULTIES

Some pediatric dermatology patients present in the dermatologist's office demonstrating a disquieting relationship between the mother and child. The dermatologist may recognize that the parent's expectation of the child is not in keeping with the child's age. At one extreme the parent may describe her implementation of a treatment plan as a battle in which compliance is demanded of the child without allowing for age-appropriate initiative or flexibility in the regimen.

Often the child is described as becoming either increasingly obstinate or increasingly passive and dependent. It is common for a child to adopt either stance in response to the parent's over-control. At the other extreme are underinvolved parents who expect their children to be responsible for their own treatment beyond what is developmentally appropriate. A mother may report, for example, that her son is not disciplined. Therefore, she reports her 6-year-old's steroid cream is left with his toothbrush and toothpaste each night, and she does not remind him or help him with its application.

In some cases the child is in control and resistant. The mother is afraid or unable to enforce the dermatologist's recommendation except on the days when the child accepts the treatment. Often these patients, even young children, are more in control of their treatment regimen than are their parents. This control is of concern in view of the child's inability to appreciate the usefulness of the treatment, and because it signals a broader parent–child problem.

Case study

Willie is an 11-year-old fifth grader with severe atopic dermatitis. He is seen routinely in the clinic, and the receptionist has learned to tell his mother to bring him at least an hour earlier than needed, so that he may arrive on time. His mother always complains to her about how hard it is to get Willie to come to the clinic.

In the dermatologist's office, Willie's mother described her daily struggles over getting Willie to take his baths and apply his topical medication. She highlights struggles such as the time Willie threatened to break her most expensive bottle of perfume if she added his medication to the bath water, to let the doctor know how impossible Willie has become. Willie smiles mischievously through the diatribes and then flatly denies that they occurred.

Willie sat next to his mother during his appointment, episodically scratching furiously. When he would scratch, his mother would grab his hand and force it down to his side. After a few seconds he would begin scratching with his heel in exaggerated motions. His mother would glare at Willie, repeat his name in a threatening voice, and slap his knee. Willie would appear worried for an instant, then smile and wait two minutes to begin the scratching cycle again. Willie's mother reported to the derma-tologist, "I don't think it even itches. He only scratches to aggravate me." Willie responded with, "How would you know?" His mother then shook her head and said, "He's like this about everything. I keep trying to help him, but he doesn't appreciate it. He is impossible."

Willie is a frustrating patient for dermatologists to attempt to treat. He would benefit from the usual treatment for atopic dermatitis, especially if he was not scratching himself so aggressively, but he and his mother are locked in a struggle over who is in control. Their adversarial relationship prevents successful treatment.

A psychiatric consultant would take a detailed developmental history on Willie, looking for indications of how the relationship between mother and son developed. He would inquire about the child's behavior in other settings, such as at school, with friends, at home with his siblings, and with other adults. Depending on the scope of the problem, a short-term therapy primarily addressing the skin condition and its treatment, or more comprehensive long-term treatment could be initiated. The psychiatrist, through an understanding of the mother–son relationship, will be able to make some suggestions about how the destructive pattern of their interaction can be altered to allow good dermatologic treatment.

DEPRESSION

Adults view childhood as such a happy time that the depressed child is frequently overlooked. Young children in particular do not have the capacity to express in words their feelings of sadness. A depressed child is likely to present in the dermatologist's office as glum, irritable, or apathetic. It is often difficult to engage these children in conversation or to arouse their curiosity about the office and its contents, or even about an upcoming procedure.

The key symptoms for dermatologists to consider in the diagnosis of depression come from questioning the patient and the parent.[26] They should inquire about appetite disturbance (either extreme increases or decreases), sleep disturbance (insomnia or hypersomnia), psychomotor alteration as either retardation or agitation, and loss of pleasure in previously enjoyable pastimes.

Case study

Louis is a 10-year-old fourth grader who attends a Catholic school. He was seen in the clinic on two previous occasions about a year earlier for treatment of his atopic dermatitis. He and his mother arrived late for this appointment and the doctor noticed he was scheduled for two previous appointments that were cancelled. Louis looks thinner and is unusually silent. His dermatitis appears mild. The doctor inquires about how he has been feeling lately, but Louis remains silent.

His mother responds to the doctor's questions by saying that Louis is not himself of late. He is scratching more than he used to and even crying. Over the past six weeks, Louis's grades have gone down at school, he refuses to play with his friends, and it is a struggle to get him to go to soccer practice, which he used to love. He complains of headaches and stomachaches that keep him out of school and were the reason why they had to cancel their previous two appointments.

When the dermatologist inquires about sleep and appetite, Louis tells him he lies in bed awake until after his parents are asleep each night and wakes up very early in the morning. He used to love hamburgers and french fries, but lately eating is a chore. Louis blames his dermatitis, saying he is in a bad mood because it itches and looks ugly. His mother wonders how the skin condition could be responsible for the change in her son's behavior.

Louis presents as a depressed child. He has a persistent mood change of more than two weeks' duration, with sleep and appetite disturbance, as well as loss of interest in a favorite activity. It interferes with his schoolwork, his peer relationships, and, as is often seen in children, is associated with somatic complaints such as headaches or stomachaches.

When Louis is seen by a child psychiatrist, he will take a detailed history including his current symptoms, and his functioning at home, at school, and with peers. A family history will be gathered to assess stressors that may be affecting Louis's presentation, and to learn if there is a family history for affective illness.

Louis's presentation suggests the possibility of treatment with an antidepressant. Prior to initiating treatment, baseline blood work and a cardiogram are indicated. Regular monitoring of the cardiogram, antidepressant blood levels, and blood pressure are indicated for the duration of treatment. In the hands of an experienced psychiatrist, antidepressants can be safe and effective for use in children. Untreated depression leads to a child missing out on important age-appropriate experiences.

ANXIETY DISORDERS

The anxious child is likely to present in the dermatologist's office as agitated, often crying and clinging to the parent, overactive, or fretful. The dermatologist is usually aware that a level of anxiety exists exceeding what might be expected, or that social reticence is present. During the exam, anxious school-aged children may refuse to sit on the examining table without a parent holding them. The children may verbalize extreme fears that neither respond to the dermatologist's reassurances nor are appropriate to the treat-

ment at hand such as, "I know he is going to hurt me," or, "Don't let him touch me!" while the dermatologist is not even near the child.

It is important to get a history from the parent about how the child's behavior in the office compares with behavior at home and at school. The dermatologist can inquire whether the child has excessive worries about his parents dying or about his own behavior being acceptable. Anxious children often fear being away from their parents. Key times to ask about include going to school in the morning, going to sleep at night, and being left at home with a babysitter when the parents go out. The child's anxiety is considered significant if it interferes with peer relationships, school functioning, or comfort at home. (Psychiatrists divide childhood anxiety disorders into three major diagnostic categories: separation anxiety, avoidant disorder, and overanxious disorder. The specific criteria for these categories are beyond the scope of this discussion and we refer readers to the *Diagnostic and Statistical Manual for Primary Care (DSM-PC) child and adolescent version*.[27]

Case study

In the dermatologist's office, it was difficult to coax 9-year-old Max into allowing his foot to be examined. The doctor remembered him from his previous appointment. Max had hopped out without his shoe on when his mother stepped outside the office to talk with the nurse. On this visit, Max sat tearfully in his mother's lap worrying aloud about the dermatologist hurting him. His nervousness was striking since only a painless examination of a nevus was being done on this appointment and the previous ones.

Perplexed by Max's fearfulness and his clinging to his mother, the dermatologist asked Max what he was scared about. Max was silent, but his mother, Mrs Roth, responded for him. Max had told her he thought the dermatologist did not like him and he worried before every visit that he would get yelled at. The doctor knew he had never spoken harshly to Max. Mrs Roth said Max was always worrying. He hated his parents going out at night because he worried they would get into an accident and die. He routinely thought his teacher and his friend's mother were angry at him despite his exemplary behavior.

Mrs Roth had hoped Max would outgrow his anxiety. She knew he was more nervous than her other two children, but she was embarrassed about considering a psychiatric evaluation.

Max presents with an anxiety disorder that warrants a psychiatric evaluation. Anxious but well-behaved children are less likely to be noted and referred by their school. When the child psychiatrist sees Max, he will explore the symptoms of distress. He will look for separations or losses, such as a death in the family, a move, or a relative leaving. He will take a detailed history of Max's early development with special attention to difficulties starting preschool. It will be important to assess the family looking for possible sources of stress.

Treatment approaches may include individual or family psychotherapy. Psychopharmacologic agents may offer some benefit for anxiety disorders in childhood. Antianxiety drugs, such as benzodiazepines, may be helpful in children or they may act as disinhibiting agents and result in overly silly or impulsive behavior. Antidepressants may be effective in some cases of separation anxiety and in teenagers with panic attacks. Childhood depression may present with symptoms of anxiety and should be considered in the differential diagnosis.

CHILD ABUSE

Child abuse is not a childhood psychiatric illness, but psychiatrists are often asked to evaluate and treat children and families with this problem. Physical and sexual abuse of children is unfortunately a common problem. Abusing parents often bring the abused child to a physician with genuine concern for

26. Snyder J, Jellinek MS (1998) Depression and suicide in children and adolescents. **Pediatrics in Review** 19:255–264.

27. The American Academy of Pediatrics. The classification of child and adolescent mental diagnoses in primary care. Diagnostic and statistical manual for primary care (DSM-PC) child and adolescent version. Illinois: Elk Grove Village, 1996.

the well-being of the child. It is the moral and legal responsibility of health professionals to educate themselves about the symptoms of abuse and to notify the appropriate agency as determined by the site in which they practice when there is suspected abuse.

Case study

Marcia is a 3-year-old who was brought in by her mother to have a facial nevus evaluated for possible excision. In examining Marcia, the doctor found 10 partially healing or healed small circular burns extending over her back and buttocks. When the doctor asked Marcia's mother about the burns, she hesitatingly reported that they were from a pot of boiling water, which splashed accidentally on Marcia. Noting the old burns, she reported that Marcia had been born with them. The scars seemed too round for scalding and the dermatologist suspected that they were cigarette burns.

The process for reporting suspected child abuse cases varies among locations, but the key word is *suspected*. If a physician believes there is a possibility of abuse, the appropriate agency should be notified. It is not the responsibility of the doctor to determine whether it is actual abuse that has occurred, but only to report the possibility.

TRICHOTILLOMANIA

Case studies

Debbie is a 5-year-old brought to the dermatology clinic because she pulls out her hair during temper tantrums. She has an obvious bald patch on the right side of her head. Although previously Debbie had occasional temper tantrums without pulling out her hair, the trichotillomania began approximately six months ago while her mother was hospitalized for several weeks with hepatitis.

Rachelle is a 16-year-old who presents with no eyelashes and few eyebrow hairs. With obvious embarrassment she explains how she pulls out her eyelashes and eyebrow hairs especially at bedtime. She has tried many times to make herself stop, but at the moments she pulls out the hairs the feeling of needing to do so is just too strong to stop. She finds her habit repugnant, and fears her friends will learn of it and view her as bizarre. On careful history, she has other compulsive behaviors. The other behaviors are of little concern to her; they include needing to touch certain objects in her room before going to school and needing to arrange her books in alphabetical order in her locker.

Trichotillomania is a perplexing condition. It has been reported in association with a wide array of psychiatric disorders (autism, obsessive-compulsive disorder, depression, schizophrenia, borderline personality disorder), mental retardation, and as an isolated symptom with no clinical significance.[28] Some patients will respond to a combined treatment of cognitive behavioral therapy and medication.[29] Anecdotally, it has been associated with actual or feared loss of an important person in the patient's life. Debbie's experience of her mother's absence during her prolonged illness seems consistent with this etiology while Rachelle's trichotillomania is more suggestive of obsessive-compulsive disorder. Rachelle finds her own behavior alien, yet is unable to stop it. She has other compulsive, ritualized behavior.

Each child was referred to a child psychiatrist. Debbie benefited from a short-term play psychotherapy. Rachelle had a psychopharmacologic trial of a specialized antidepressant, fluoxetine, which is very effective in the treatment of obsessive-compulsive disorder (*see* Pediatric psychopharmacology).

FACTITIAL SKIN ULCERS (MÜNCHAUSEN'S SYNDROME)

Case study

Tracy is a 15-year-old who was followed in the dermatology clinic for several months with progressively worsening circular lesions on her abdomen and thighs. Over the months of care in the clinic, the lesions increased in number and size until there was hardly any unaffected skin on her abdomen, but no lesions on her back. The etiology of the condition remained unclear despite careful history taking and two skin biopsies.

Tracy's mother, a single parent and a registered nurse, was distraught over her only child's escalating illness. At her request, Tracy was admitted to the hospital for closer observation.

On the third hospital day, Tracy was inadvertently discovered applying cream depilatory to her abdomen to cause a chemical burn. Tracy initially denied the etiology of her lesions, but later admitted that after accidentally discovering her skin sensitivity to the depilatory, she began causing the skin lesions as a way to get her mother's attention and the sympathy of her friends.

Tracy was referred for a psychiatric evaluation, which she refused, but her mother prevailed upon her. After the evaluation, she began a course of psychotherapy.

Factitial disease is perplexing and often provokes anger from the physicians caring for the patient. Commonly, the factitious etiology is discovered after the physician has invested many hours and performed numerous unnecessary procedures. Discovery is the result of good detective work in addition to good medical care. Suspected cases often require an in-hospital evaluation during which the patient can be carefully observed. Many patients escape close scrutiny by switching from doctor to doctor.

Although psychiatric intervention is the only treatment for this condition, it is difficult to get these patients to accept referral. There are differing views on whether it is preferable for the dermatologist (or primary physician) to confront the patient or to defer to the psychiatrist.[30] This decision is best made in a consultation between the primary physician and the psychiatrist prior to recommending the psychiatric referral to the patient.

MÜNCHAUSEN'S BY PROXY SYNDROME

Münchausen's By Proxy syndrome must be in the differential diagnosis of a suspicious illness in a younger child. This is a condition in which a parent either makes a child ill or makes a child appear to be ill. This uncommon entity carries a high risk of child mortality.[31] Children should be carefully monitored medically as long as they are cared for by the parents, and the appropriate agencies, as in child abuse cases, should be alerted. The parents should be referred for psychiatric treatment, but they are likely to be resistant unless it is mandated by court action.

PEDIATRIC PSYCHOPHARMACOLOGY

Pediatric psychopharmacology is an exciting new frontier. With the advent of effective pharmacotherapies, the importance of accurate diagnosis of psychiatric illness is crucial. Most of the experience with psychopharmacologic agents is in adults[32] but increasing numbers of children are benefitting from these treatments. The dermatologist is likely to see three categories of psychiatric conditions. There are primary psychiatric entities (such as

28. Krishnan KR, Davidson JR, Guajardo C (1985) Trichotillomania: a review. **Compr Psychiatry** 26:123.
29. Keuthen NJ, Stein DJ, Christenson GA (2001) Help for Hair Pullers. Oakland, CA: New Harbinger.
30. Fras I (1978) Factitial disease: an update. **Psychosomatics** 19:119.
31. Waller DA (1983) Obstacles to the treatment of Münchausen by Proxy syndrome. **J Am Acad Child Psychiatry** 22:80.
32. Koo JY, Pham CT (1992) Psychodermatology. Practical guidelines on pharmacotherapy. **Arch Dermatol** 128:3.

trichotillomania of obsessive-compulsive disorder,[33] neurotic excoriations, and delusional disorders). There are comorbid psychiatric illnesses such as depression and anxiety that may aggravate primary dermatologic disorders such as eczema, psoriasis, alopecia areata, and acne. Finally, there are the disorders of conduct or attention not directly related to a skin disorder, but of importance because of the impact on compliance. Each diagnosis carries with it potentially appropriate pharmacotherapy. Trichotillomania may respond to the specific antidepressants, selective seretonin reuptake inhibitors, or clomipramine,[32] delusional disorders to antipsychotics, depression to tricyclic antidepressants such as desipramine and doxepin (the latter with evidence of additional antipruritic effects[32]), anxiety disorders to clonazapam and other benzodiazepines, and attentional difficulties to methylphenidate and clonidine.

The decision to medicate children with psychoactive drugs demands a risk-benefit assessment, a thorough premedication workup, informed consent by parents, and careful monitoring of levels and potential side effects during use. Antipsychotic use warrants particular caution, because of the risk of tardive dyskinesia, an irreversible movement disorder. The full benefit of psychoactive drug use in children is best achieved by a partnership between child psychiatrist and pediatric dermatologist.[34]

CONCLUSION

The high volume and fast pace of pediatric and dermatology practices can encourage a narrow perspective that focuses on the skin only as an organ, rather than reflective of a whole person and thus imbued with many personal, interpersonal, and cultural meanings. Especially for children, understanding these many meanings within a developmental context can be valuable, or even critical, for patients, families, and physicians. Surgery can be made less anxiety provoking, compliance with medical regimens improved, parents' tendency toward guilt and/or marital discord at least moderated, and psychological damage to the child kept to a minimum. Lastly, a fuller appreciation of the developmental, psychological, and familial implications of dermatologic disorders will enrich the physician's professional life as the repetitious nature of evaluating lesions is replaced by a sensitivity toward treating the child as a whole person.

33. Koo JY, Smith LL (1991) Obsessive compulsive disorders in the pediatric dermatology practice. **Pediatr Dermatol** 8:2.

34. Wozniak J, Biederman J, Spencer T, Wilens T (1988) Pediatric Psychopharmacology. In: The Practioner's Guide to Psychoactive Substances, Gelenberg A and Bassuk E, eds, 4th ed. Washington DC: American Psychiatric Press, pp. 385–416.

Principles of Diagnosis in Pediatric Dermatology

Henning Hamm, Robert Johr and Johannes Mayer

INTRODUCTION

Diagnosis in dermatology is, just as in other clinical disciplines, based on three pillars: careful history, thorough examination, and various diagnostic methods. Among them, the observation of individual lesions is commonly of greatest significance. The morphology of skin lesions, their arrangement, and distribution will often lead to a suspected diagnosis or at least allow for a differential diagnosis to be generated.

There is a wealth of diagnostic aids – non-invasive, little invasive and invasive – with the help of which a suspected diagnosis may be confirmed or a differential diagnosis may be excluded. In pediatric dermatology, particularly in young children, doctors will try to get as much information as possible from non-invasive diagnostic methods and to confine themselves to a minimum of invasive diagnostic procedures to arrive at the correct diagnosis.

This chapter summarizes an approach to the clinical diagnosis of pediatric skin disease including history taking and refined dermatological examination and gives an overview on the most important diagnostic aids available to the dermatologist and pediatrician.

HISTORY

PRELIMINARY REMARKS

The joint effort of patient and physician towards solving a medical problem usually begins with history taking. However, in pediatric dermatology, there are two peculiarities. First, in younger children the history has to be obtained from the parents or other caretakers. Of course, the older the children the more they will be able to participate in the review of the problem under consideration and the more they should be involved.[1] This will also create a level of confidence which is useful for the following examination. Second, the pathology is easily accessible to the eyes. The pediatric dermatologist may take advantage of this fact since, for estimation of the scope of the history and for putting more tailored questions, it is often worthwhile to start with a brief look at the skin lesions.

The history has two main parts, namely the special history focusing on the presenting complaint, and the general history giving information about other medical or personal problems that may be of influence on the current or future diseases. The more unclear or complex the problem the more important is a detailed history. For instance, a full medical history is useless in a school boy with a single finger wart whereas a detailed history is essential in a toddler with atopic dermatitis or an adolescent with systemic lupus erythematosus. These examples also show that the aim of the history is not only to arrive at a clear or suspected diagnosis but also to evaluate etiological or worsening factors. The skill of the pediatric dermatologist consists in putting all questions relevant to the problem and, because of time limitations, leaving out irrelevant ones. To avoid unintentional omissions it is prudent to adapt to an orderly and logical framework in history-taking,[2] as proposed in the following. Some key questions are summarized in Table 3.1.

SPECIAL HISTORY

As the patient mostly presents or is presented with a concrete problem it seems reasonable to start with the special history. Time and site(s) of onset of the skin lesions should be accurately determined. Patients or parents should be asked to describe the initial lesions and whether they have changed in appearance or character.[3] Further evolution of the lesions in terms of extension, exacerbations, remissions and recurrences should be recorded. In conditions limited to short episodes their frequency and duration have to be ascertained. Assessment of the duration of individual lesions may be a valuable clue. Moreover, it is important to note whether the parents or the patient are aware of any provoking or aggravating factors, such as food, sunlight, cold, heat, physical activities, contact with animals, or exposure to topical agents or chemicals.

Symptoms are often reported by the parents or patients themselves. However, the severity and periodicity of itch, pain, burning, stinging, or other

TABLE 3.1 Ten basic questions for a dermatological history (modified from du Vivier[6])	
Special history	• When, where and how did it start?
	• Has it occurred anywhere else?
	• How does it behave?
	• What affects it?
	• Does it itch, hurt, burn, or anything else?
General history	• Do you/does your child suffer from any symptoms not related to the skin?
	• Have you/has your child been ill recently or previously?
	• Have you/has your child been treated topically or systemically, and if so how?
	• Are there or have there been similar problems in other family members?
	• What are your thoughts about the cause of the problem?

1. Levy ML (1995) Principles of diagnosis. In: Pediatric Dermatology. 2nd edn. Schachner LA, Hansen RC, eds. New York: Churchill Livingstone, pp. 139–163.
2. MacKie RM (1991) The dermatological history: examination and investigations frequently used in dermatology. In: Clinical dermatology. An illustrated textbook. Oxford: Oxford Medical Publications, pp. 1–15.
3. Champion RH, Burton JL (1998) Diagnosis of skin disease. In: Rook/Wilkinson/Ebling Textbook of Dermatology, 6th edn. Champion RH, Burton JL, Burns DA, Breathnach SM, eds. Oxford: Blackwell, pp. 157–170.

sensations have to be asked for. Information about the complaints is particularly helpful for confirmation of a suspected diagnosis since subjective symptoms are often characteristic of specific dermatoses.[4] Thus, for example, scabies, urticaria, atopic and contact dermatitis can be excluded in non-itching conditions.

Previous therapies of the condition in question, whether topical or systemic, have to be recorded including the duration of use, tolerance, and efficacy.[4] They may grossly influence the actual presentation of a skin disease. In such cases, it may be inevitable to stop every kind of treatment and to make an appointment one or two weeks later. Furthermore, knowledge about previous treatments helps to avoid repeated prescription of ineffective agents.

GENERAL HISTORY

The skin disorder may be related to a prior or current systemic disease. Therefore, associated extracutaneous symptoms, such as fever, fatigue, sore throat, joint pain, or seizures, and previously diagnosed chronic illnesses, hospitalizations, or surgeries have to be precisely recorded. Of special importance are metabolic and endocrine disorders, chronic infections, and states of congenital or acquired immunodeficiency. Suspected syndromes, congenital anomalies or infections afford a detailed review of the prenatal history, the delivery and the postnatal mental and motor development. When considering a genetically determined dermatosis, family history taking including a diagram of the pedigree may disclose the pattern of transmission and support the suspected diagnosis.

The past history of skin and related disorders may be a great help for the classification of the actual problem. Of special importance is the recognition of an atopic diathesis (atopic dermatitis including cradle's cap and flexural eczema, hay fever and bronchial asthma) in the background of the patient and the family.[5] Since many systemic agents can cause diverse cutaneous side effects, the current and previous drug therapies including over-the-counter medications have to be noted. Knowledge about the medication may also uncover a medical problem which was not otherwise mentioned by the parents.[5] Immunosuppressive agents predispose to skin infections, especially viral diseases and mycoses. Furthermore, information about known adverse reactions to drugs, such as an allergy to penicillin, or to food has to be obtained. A question about dietary and nutritional habits, whether on health, religious or other grounds, should not be missing when dealing with an unexplained skin disorder.

The ethnic background of a child may provide information on a certain genetic predisposition and pattern of reaction.[3] Asking about past holidays in foreign countries may disclose the decisive factor in uncommon skin infections. Contact with animals, particularly pets, is often more intense in children than in adults and may be the cause for certain infections, infestations or allergies.

Occupational history plays an important role only in adult dermatological patients. However, enquiry about hobbies and other leisure activities may uncover exposure to sunlight, contact allergens, or irritant chemicals in older children and adolescents, as well.[3]

The social history deals with the living conditions of the patient, the socio-economic, nutritional and health status of the family, and includes knowledge about further persons of close relation. This kind of information is particularly helpful in children with chronic skin diseases, also in estimating the compliance and prognosis of a patient.

Finally, the physician should try to get an idea about the psychological effects of the disease on the patient and family and about the patient's or parents' thoughts on its cause, respectively.[2,6] Domestic conflicts caused or triggered by the disease and difficulties in coping with it may have extremely negative repercussions on the condition. On the other hand, a chronic skin disorder may not improve because the child is fearful of losing the increased

attention and affection associated with it. The consequences on the quality of life have also to be considered for the choice of treatment. Inept worries about infectivity or malignancy may be easily dispelled, and exaggerated expectations have to be cautiously lowered by the doctor. Fortunately, a time-consuming history comprising all of the items addressed above will rarely be necessary. However, in complex problems, such as inherited disorders with extracutaneous involvement, allergological questions and conditions related to physical or chemical agents, as well as in difficult patients or parents, a very detailed or even repeated enquiry may be indispensible.

Patients and parents should feel as comfortable as possible in a given clinical setting. The physician should mainly be seated, move cautiously within the examination room, speak to the child in an understandable language and be careful not to touch the patient early or to speak loudly, particularly with young children.[1] This simple code of conduct will usually enable the physician to gain the child's confidence, which is essential for the realization of the following examination.

DERMATOLOGICAL EXAMINATION

PROCEDURE AND TECHNICAL CONSIDERATIONS

The first step in a dermatological examination is to gain a preliminary impression of the pattern of involvement by inspecting the skin lesions from a distance. The subsequent close examination aims at the analysis of the type and morphology of primary and secondary skin lesions, their arrangement, and involved sites, as explained in detail below. Afterwards, the distribution over the body has to be assessed. For this purpose, the entire skin surface should be examined, especially in all patients attending for the first time. Infants and toddlers should be totally undressed including removal of the diapers, whereas older children may keep their underwear on, except for inspection of the genitoanal area. The examination should be performed in an orderly sequence and include the hair, eyebrows and eyelashes, nails, adjacent mucous membranes, and teeth as well as the palpation of the cervical, axillary and inguinal lymph nodes. The latter is particularly required if acute infections, chronic inflammations, and malignant conditions are suspected. Total skin examination may reveal unchanged lesions which are more characteristic than those presented by the patient or parents but may also disclose potentially harmful findings, such as congenital abnormalities.

The examination room should be well lit with natural light being best. Additional lighting by high-intensity examination lamps and magnification of skin lesions by hand-held magnifying glasses are very useful.

The realization of the examination mainly depends on the age of the child. For example, special precautions have to be followed when examining newborn infants in hospital nurseries. Examination of toddlers and pre-school children may be facilitated by distracting them with small toys, keeping them seated on the parent's lap, or the promise of a reward.[1] In contrast, many adolescents will prefer to be examined in the absence of their parents.

DESCRIPTION AND TERMINOLOGY OF SKIN DISEASES

Introductory remarks

The majority of skin diseases can be diagnosed by appropriate history taking and proper examination alone. Diagnostic accuracy may be further improved by repeated examination since the actual state represents only a snapshot of a dynamic process. In spite of the wealth of dermatological conditions considered in this textbook the pediatric dermatologist is usually dealing with a reasonable number of diagnoses only. Among them, atopic dermatitis, viral warts, impetigo, scabies, acquired melanocytic nevi, and alopecia areata may be the most common ones. Interestingly, Schachner *et al.* found 25

4. Braun-Falco O, Plewig G, Wolff HH, Winkelmann RK (1991) Principles of dermatological diagnosis. In: Dermatology. Berlin: Springer, pp. 1–12.
5. Lynch PJ (1996) Principles of diagnosis. In: Principles and Practice of Dermatology, 2nd edn, Sams WM, Lynch PJ eds. New York: Churchill Livingstone, pp. 23–32.
6. Du Vivier A (1990) The dermatological diagnosis. In: Dermatology in Practice. Philadelphia: JB Lippincott, pp. 1–14.

diagnoses to account for approximately 82 percent and 50 diagnoses for more than 91 percent of all skin disorders seen in a pediatric dermatology clinic.[7]

Correct recognition of the morphological features is an essential prerequisite to diagnosis of a given skin disorder and, for obvious reasons, a basic vocabulary of well-defined terms is indispensible for a proper description. However, differences in terminology become evident when comparing standard dermatological textbooks and noting continuing discussions in dermatological journals.[8,9] For example, there is considerable inconsistency with regard to the minimum or maximum size of some primary skin lesions. Exanthem and erythroderma are further examples of often-used but ill-defined expressions. The following definitions partly keep to the glossary of basic dermatology lesions that was published by the committee on nomenclature of the International League of Dermatological Societies in 1987[10] but also reflect recent recommendations.[8,9]

Dermatologists will be glad to confirm the Chinese proverb saying that a picture may be worth more than a thousand words. Therefore, photographic documentation of skin lesions is often expedient, especially if the diagnosis is unclear or unusual, if changes or courses are to be monitored, and for teaching and publication purposes. Skin tumors of uncertain origin should likewise be documented prior to excision or biopsy. Moreover, pictures offer the possibility to send them to expert colleagues via common or electronic mail ("teledermatology") and seek their advice. With increasing spreading and simplification of technical requirements, teledermatology will undoubtedly be used more and more frequently as a powerful diagnostic tool in the future.

Primary skin lesions

Those fundamental morphological changes that appear first on formerly unchanged skin are called primary skin lesions. Secondary lesions usually do not develop on uninvolved skin but mostly arise from alteration of primary lesions. They can provide clues as to the primary lesions if these are absent.[1] However, as secondary lesions, such as scales or excoriations, may also occur on clinically unchanged skin the limits between primary and secondary lesions are somewhat blurred. Nonetheless, the following list of basic terms keeps this differentiation.

MACULE

A circumscribed, flat area of skin different in color or texture from the surrounding (normal) skin (Fig. 3.1). By definition, a macule does not exceed 1cm in greatest diameter.

PATCH

A large macule, more than 1cm in diameter (Fig. 3.2).

A macule or patch can result from:

● deposition of endogeneous (hemosiderin) or exogeneous products (tattooing, ingrained dirt, topical agents, systemic drugs),
● extravasation of blood (petechiae, purpura, sugillations, ecchymoses, hematoma),
● changes in melanin content of the epidermis or dermis (hyper- and hypo- or depigmentation, melanoderma and leukoderma),
● active (erythema) and passive hyperemia (cyanosis),
● diminished blood supply and vasoconstriction.[4]

Occasionally, macules and patches may be slightly depressed below the skin surface (atrophic macules) or show minor surface changes, such as scaling.

PAPULE

A circumscribed solid elevation of the skin up to 1cm in diameter. It is mostly caused by tissue proliferation or cell infiltration (Fig. 3.3).

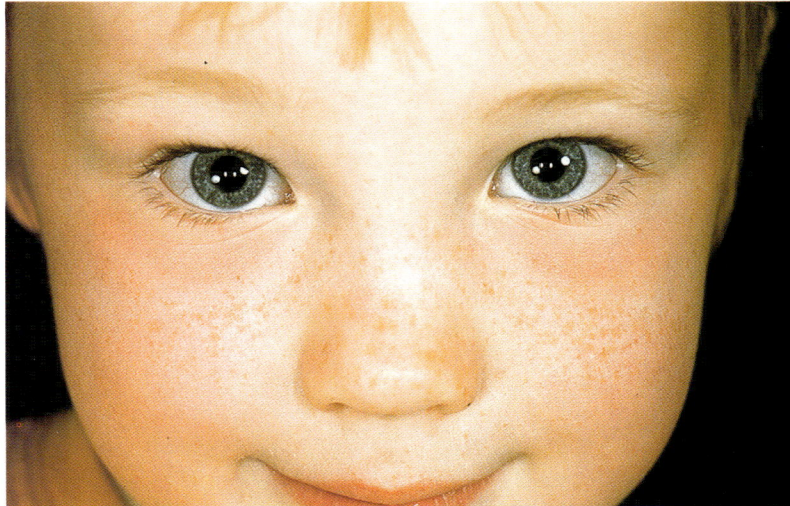

Fig. 3.1   Macules. Multiple small hyperpigmentations on nose and cheeks of the fair-skinned son of the author (freckles).

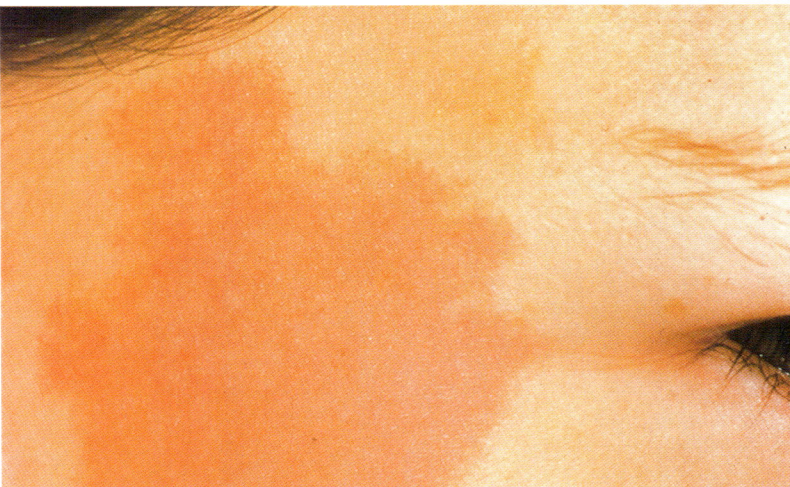

Fig. 3.2   Patch. A large, red, flat area of irregular shape on the right temple (port-wine stain).

The following types of papules can be distinguished:

● An *epidermal papule* is composed of localized thickening of the epidermis or of the stratum corneum.
● A *dermal papule* is composed of a localized, solid thickening of the upper dermis produced by hyperplasia of dermal structures, deposition of metabolic products, concentration of cells, or other pathologic changes.
● *Dermoepidermal papules* are formed by both epidermal and dermal abnormalities.

Caused by an abundance of different pathological processes, papules may show a considerable variety of shapes, colors, and surface qualities.

PLAQUE

A circumscribed, superficial, solid elevation of the skin greater than 1cm in diameter (Fig. 3.4).

Some intracutaneous plaques may not be visibly raised, as in morphea.[5] Plaques may occur as primary lesions but may also result from coalescence

7. Schachner L, Ling NS, Press S (1983) A statistical analysis of a pediatric dermatology clinic. **Pediatr Dermatol** 1:157–164.
8. Lewis EJ, Dahl MV (1997) On standard definitions: 33 years hence. **Arch Dermatol** 133:1169.
9. Reisfeld PL (1998) On standard dermatologic definitions. **Arch Dermatol** 134:635–636.
10. Winkelmann RK (1987) Glossary of basic dermatology lesions. The International League of Dermatological Societies Committee on Nomenclature. **Acta Derm Venereol** Suppl 130:1–16.

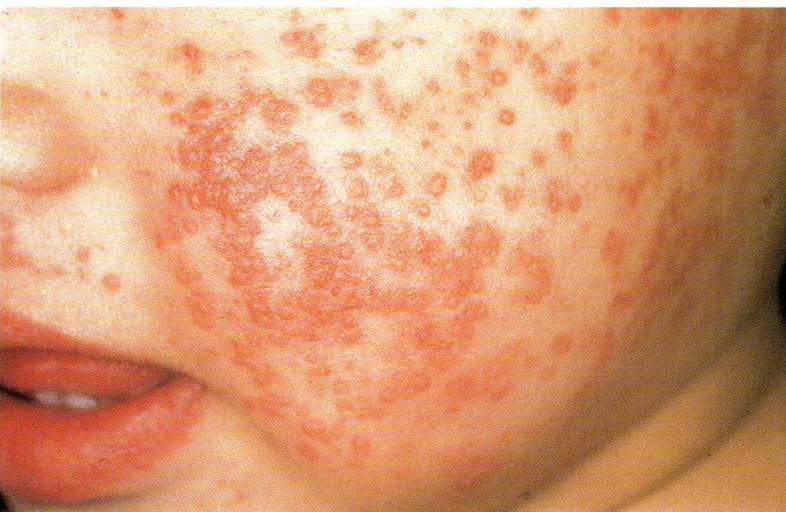

Fig. 3.3   Papules. Multiple small red solid elevations on the left cheek (Gianotti-Crosti syndrome).

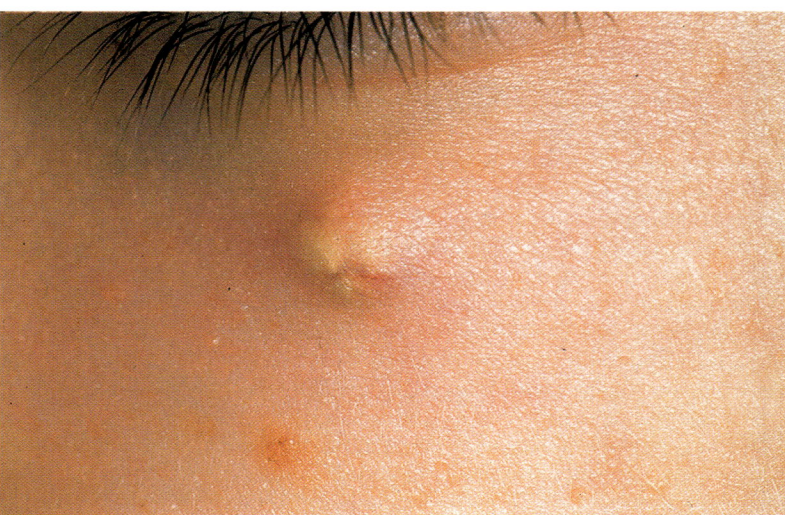

Fig. 3.5   Nodule. A solid lobulated elevation with depth less than 1cm in size below the left eye (pilomatricoma).

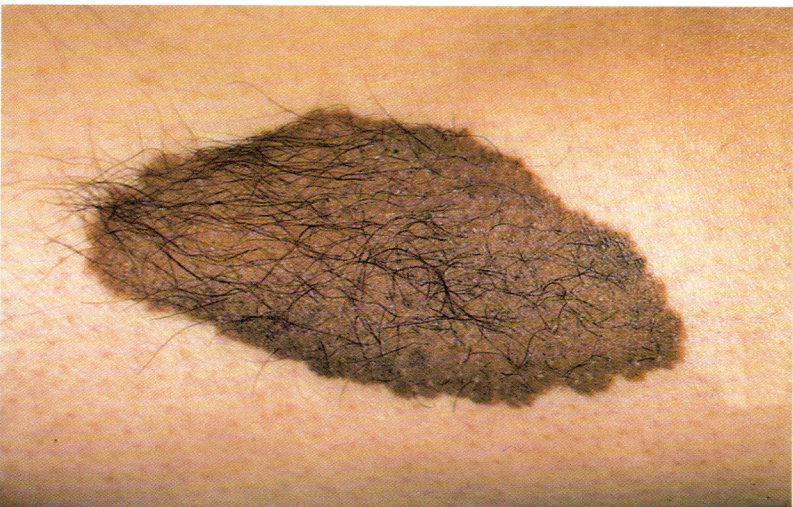

Fig. 3.4   Plaque. A large, solid hyperpigmented elevation with hypertrichosis on the lower leg (congenital melanocytic nevus).

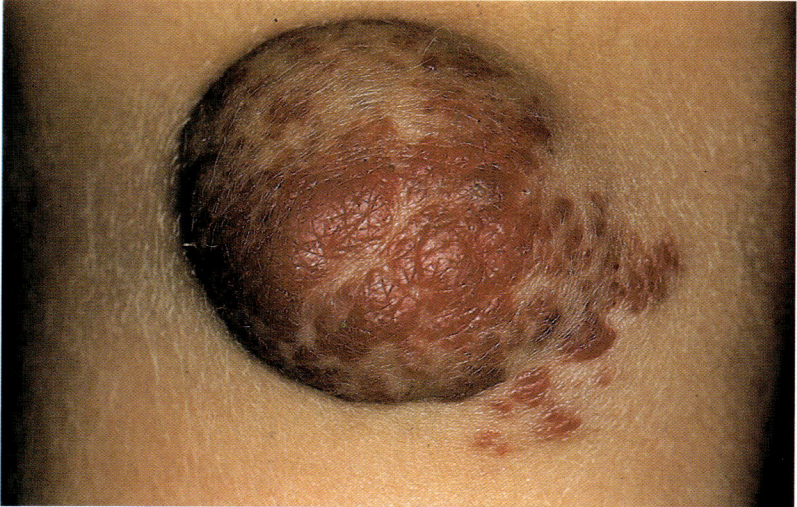

Fig. 3.6   Tumor. A large red, markedly elevated mass with skin-colored portions (deep hemangioma with signs of partial regression).

of papules and then, strictly speaking, represent secondary lesions. Plaques may have the same subdivisions as papules.

NODULE

A circumscribed solid lesion of the skin up to 1cm in size with depth (Fig. 3.5). It may not absolutely present as an elevation but can always be palpated. The distinction between papule and nodule depends essentially on extension to the depth. Nodules may be located deep–dermally, dermal–subdermally or solely in the subcutaneous fat.

TUMOR (MASS)

A solid lesion of the skin greater than 1cm in diameter with more than superficial height or palpable depth (Fig. 3.6). Tumors differ from papules and nodules by size, from plaques by endophytic or exophytic extension. A tumor may be inflammatory or non–inflammatory, benign or malignant.

WHEAL

An elevated, transient dermal edema, varied in size (Fig. 3.7).

Wheals are characteristically evanescent, disappearing within up to 24 hours.[11] The changeability is due to the fact that they are mostly made up of a circumscribed, rapidly resorbed accumulation of interstitial fluid in the upper dermis and hardly of cellular components. Their color is pale red if the capillaries are dilated, or whitish if the dermal edema is heavy enough to compress the blood vessels. Wheals typically cause itching which is answered by rubbing. They are the characteristic lesion of urticaria. Whether a wheal should be regarded as a basic dermatologic lesion or better described as a type of papule or plaque is disputed.[9]

VESICLE (SMALL BLISTER)

A circumscribed elevation of the skin up to 1cm in diameter and containing a fluid (Fig. 3.8).

11. Fitzpatrick TB, Bernhard JD, Cropley TG (1999) The structure of skin lesions and fundamentals of diagnosis. In: Fitzpatrick's Dermatology in General Medicine, 5th edn, Freedberg IM, Eisen AZ, Wolff K et al. New York: McGraw-Hill, pp. 13–41.

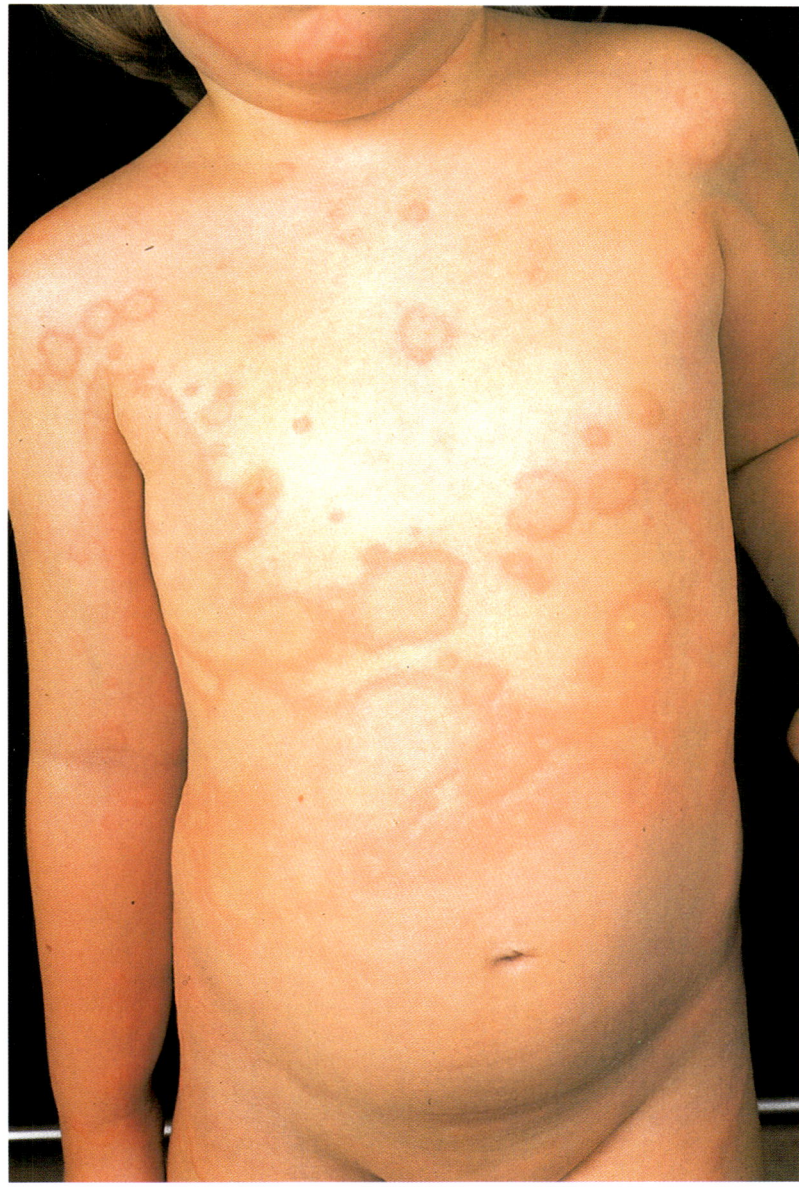

Fig. 3.7   Wheals. Multiple coalescing marginated lesions on the trunk (acute urticaria).

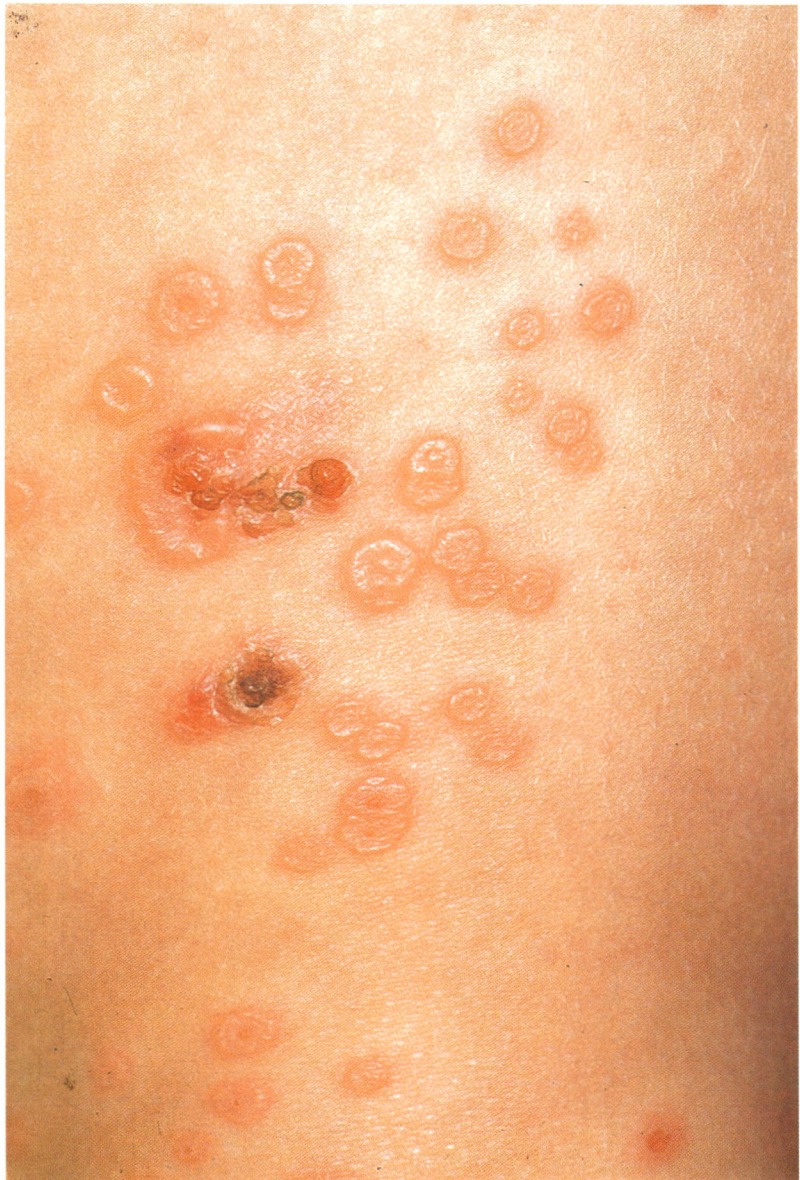

Fig. 3.8   Vesicles and bullae (blisters). Multiple fluid-containing elevations of varying size (linear IgA disease). Some blisters are eroded.

BULLA (LARGE BLISTER)

A circumscribed elevation of the skin greater than 1cm in diameter containing a fluid (Fig. 3.8).

The distinction between vesicle and bulla depends only on size. The term *blister* unites vesicles and bullae. The following types of vesicles and bullae can be distinguished:

- A *subcorneal vesicle or bulla* is formed by exudate beneath the stratum corneum, as in bullous impetigo.
- *Intraepidermal vesicles or bullae* are located within the epidermis. The three main pathogenetic principles include spongiosis (collection of fluid between individual keratinocytes), ballooning (collection of fluid within individual keratinocytes), and acantholysis (separation of keratinocytes by loss of intercellular adhesion).[12]

- *Subepidermal vesicles and bullae* develop by cleavage of the dermo–epidermal junction. The roof of the bulla is composed of the entire epidermis.
- A *dermal vesicle or bulla* is caused by separation of tissue components of the dermis.

Blisters may house serum, blood, lymph, or a mixture of these fluids. Depending on their pathogenesis, they may consist of a single chamber (unilocular blisters) or of multiple compartments (multilocular blister). Vesicles are almost always tense, bullae may be either tense or flaccid. Their stability towards physical forces allows some conclusions with regard to pathogenesis and plane of cleavage. Intraepidermal blisters caused by spongiosis and ballooning, and subepidermal blisters tend to be tense whereas subcorneal and acantholyic blisters are mostly flaccid.[12]

12. Cockerell CJ (1996) How are abnormalities of the skin described? In: Cutaneous Medicine and Surgery. An Integrated Program in Dermatology, Arndt KA, Robinson JK, LeBoit PE, Wintroub BU, eds. Philadelphia: WB Saunders, pp. 84–110.

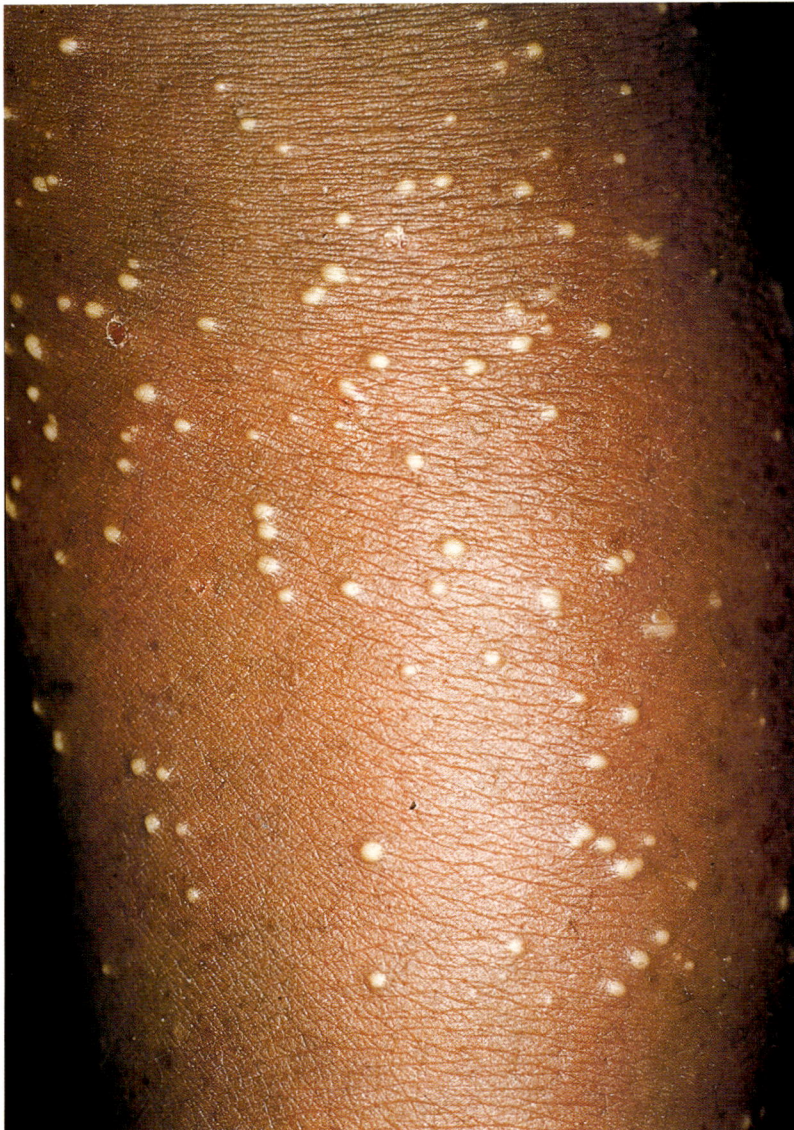

Fig. 3.9   Pustules. Multiple small whitish elevations containing pus (beginning staphylococcal scalded skin syndrome).

PUSTULE

A circumscribed superficial elevation of the skin filled with pus (Fig. 3.9).

Pus is composed of leukocytes, mostly neutrophils, with or without cellular debris. Pustules are white or yellow in color. They may occur within the epidermis, for example in intracorneal or subcorneal sites, within a pilosebaceous follicle or, much more rarely, in an eccrine duct.[13] Important to differentiate, they may be sterile or contain microorganisms. They do not always occur primarily but may also develop from vesicles or bullae (secondary pustules).

Secondary skin lesions

SCALE

A perceptible flat plate or flake of stratum corneum.

The abnormal shedding or accumulation of stratum corneum in perceptible flakes (scales) is called desquamation (scaling). Several types of scales can be distinguished, among them:

- *collarette scales*: fine, ruff-like scales surrounding inflammatory lesions,
- *exfoliative scales*: large, sheet-like scales,
- *furfuraceous/pityriasiform scales*: fine, loose, bran-like scales,
- *ichthyosiform scales*: large, polygonal, fish-like scales,
- *lamellar scales*: thin, relatively large scales,
- *psoriasiform scales*: coarse, non-adherent, silvery-white scales.[4,11]

KERATOSIS

A horny thickening that firmly adheres to the skin.

Keratoses may be epidermal or follicular, they may be arranged either horizontally, such as scales, or vertically, such as spines and horns.[12]

EROSION

A loss of the epidermis or a viable part of it that heals without scarring. It usually results from rupture of vesicles and bullae or from superficial trauma to the skin.

EXCORIATION

Any loss of substance of skin produced by scratching.

Usually, the papillary dermis is reached resulting in bleeding, crust formation, and healing with formation of a superficial scar. Excoriations often have a linear arrangement. They point to the severe pruritus associated with the skin disease.

FISSURE, RHAGADE

Any linear gap or slit in the skin surface reaching into the dermis.

Fissures usually develop in hyperkeratotic or excessively dry skin over flexural creases, especially of hands and feet, and may be painful.

ULCER

A deep defect or loss of the entire epidermis and at least the upper (papillary) dermis which heals with scarring.

Since dermal damage is present, ulcers are usually accompanied by vessel disruption, bleeding and the formation of hemorrhagic crusts which, by enrichment of fibrin, form dark-colored, difficult-to-remove, so-called *eschars*.[5] The pathogenesis of ulcers is variform. Ulcers may result from the enlargement of erosions and excoriations, they may be due to venous insufficiency, occlusive arterial disease, vasculitis, infections, injuries, artifacts, or other causes. Moreover, nodules and tumors, especially malignant ones, may ulcerate.

CRUST

An outer layer from the drying of exudate, secretion, pus, or hemorrhage.

Correspondingly, the color of crusts can vary considerably.

SCAR

The fibrous tissue replacing normal tissues destroyed by injury or disease.

A scar is the irreversible end stage of many inflammatory and destructive processes. Clinically, the normal skin markings and appendages are lacking, hyper- or hypopigmentation may be evident. Scars may be smooth or sclerotic, they may lie in the level of the skin, be depressed and wrinkled (atrophic scar) or firm and elevated (hypertrophic scar).

Some common terms used in clinical dermatology

The following list includes a number of specific terms which make a short, apt description of a dermatological condition much easier and help to avoid longwinded phrasings.

ABSCESS

A localized collection of pus in a cavity formed by disintegration or necrosis of tissues.

13. Ackerman AB, Chongchitnant N, Sanchez J et al. (1997) Definition of terms. In: Histologic Diagnosis of Inflammatory Skin Diseases. An Algorithmic Method based on Pattern Analysis, 2nd edn. Baltimore: Williams & Wilkins, pp. 75–98.

ALOPECIA
Absence or reduction of hair from normally hairy areas.

APHTHA
A small ulcer of the mucous membranes.

ATROPHY
A diminution in the size of a tissue.

This is a broadly used term applicable in pathology and many clinical disciplines. In dermatology, the following types of atrophy may be distinguished:[11,12]

- In *superficial cutaneous atrophy*, usually both epidermis and dermis are involved. The skin appears thinned and finely wrinkled reminiscent of cigarette paper. Loss of skin markings and epidermal appendages produces a shiny appearance. Pigmentary disturbances and telangiectasias may be present. Deep veins and tendons are perceptible through the transparent skin.
- *Deep cutaneous atrophy* is caused by the loss of connective tissue in the reticular dermis. The skin appears normal in color and markings, but is depressed. If extensive, eversion of the skin caused by herniations of fat may occur.
- *Lipoatrophy*: Atrophy of the subcutaneous tissue usually results in deep depressions of the body surface without textural changes of the skin.

BURROW
A narrow, elevated passage or tunnel in the skin produced by a parasite, particularly the scabies mite.

COMEDO
A plug of cornified cells, sebum, and microorganisms in a dilated orifice (infundibulum) of a pilosebaceous follicle. The follicular orifice may be dilated ("open" comedo, blackhead) or narrowed ("closed" comedo, whitehead).

CORD
A string- or rope-like structure in or beneath the surface of the skin.[12] Most often, they represent thickened, indurated blood vessels or nerves.

CYST
Any closed cavity with an epithelial, endothelial or membraneous lining containing fluid or soft material.

ENANTHEM
See *exanthem*.

ERUPTION
See rash.

ERYTHEMA
Transient redness of the skin produced by vascular congestion or increased perfusion.[3]

ERYTHRODERMA
Generalized redness associated with infiltration and desquamation of the skin.

EXANTHEM
Generalized or widespread rash of similar skin lesions with a dynamic course (acute onset, temporary persistence, spontaneous regression). *Enanthem* is the corresponding term for mucosal lesions.

FISTULA
An abnormal passage from a deep structure to the skin surface or between two deep structures, often lined with squamous epithelium or endothelium.

GANGRENE
Severe necrotizing process resulting from arterial occlusion or infection.[11]

IMPETIGINIZATION
Impetigo-like secondary infection of an initially nonbacterial skin disorder by bacteria.[4]

INFILTRATION
Thickening of the skin by cellular elements over a relatively large area, generally associated with inflammation and redness.[4]

LICHENIFICATION
Thickening of the skin with accentuation and coarsening of the skin markings usually induced by habitual rubbing.[5]

MILIUM
Tiny, white cyst containing lamellated keratin.

PETECHIA
An isolated punctate hemorrhagic spot.

POIKILODERMA
A combination of atrophy, telangiectasia, and variegated pigmentary changes (hyper- and hypopigmentation).

PURPURA
An eruption of many small circumscribed extravasations of blood (*petechiae*). *Vibices* are streaky, *sugillations* coin-sized, and *ecchymoses* extensive, bruise-like purpuric lesions.[4]

RASH
In a broader sense, the totality of multiple skin lesions, corresponding to the term *eruption*. In the narrower sense, rash is applied to a widespread skin disease with red and only slightly elevated lesions,[5] similar to an *exanthem*.

SCAB
A devitalized integral portion of the skin resulting from necrosis.

SCLEROSIS
A circumscribed or diffuse induration or hardening of the skin often due to fibrosis. Due to loss of skin markings and reduction of hair follicles, the skin looks shiny and often ivory-colored. On palpation, it is hard and tight, often adheres to deeper structures and cannot be raised or folded.

SINUS
An epithelium-lined channel that permits, via an ostium, the escape of fluid or pus onto the skin surface.

TELANGIECTASIA
A visible dilation of small cutaneous blood vessels.

VEGETATION
A growth of pathologic tissue consisting of multiple closely set papillary elevations, often in intertriginous areas.

Further morphological characteristics

Size
The size of individual lesions is already roughly determined by the description of the type of primary lesion. In most instances, particularly in tumors and ulcers, the size should be noted more exactly by indicating the greatest diameter and that at right angles. Metric measures are preferable to terms of comparable objects.

Color
Skin lesions may take on a variety of colors with red, brown and white being probably the most relevant ones in pediatric dermatology. However, just red

and brown have many different shades which should be realized as exactly as possible since many dermatoses have their own typical color. Of course, the influence of the patient's complexion and intensity of circulation on the color of the lesional skin has to be taken into consideration. The darker the skin the less informative is the color of the lesions.

Common colors and causes are put together in Table 3.2.

Shape/configuration

The shape of an individual lesion may be characteristic enough to inform about its evolution or even to make a diagnosis. Many lesions are roundish or oval and may be, for example, guttate (drop-shaped), nummular (coin-shaped) or discoid. Others are polygonal (with several sides) or serpiginous (wavy, snake-like). An annular (ring-like) shape often emerges from peripheral extension and central healing of a lesion. If parts of the ring clear, a circinate/arcuate (arc-like) shape may also result. The characteristic target lesion (iris lesion) of erythema multiforme is a cocardiform macule or small plaque that has a dusky center and an erythematous border with an eventual vesicle in the midst. Patches may have leaf-like, linear, whorled, phylloid (like large leafs), or checkerboard configurations. Linear and whorled patches may follow the lines of Blaschko representing the outgrowth of a different cell population during early embryogenesis.

TABLE 3.2	Common colors and causes in dermatology (modified from Braun-Falco *et al.*[4] and Fritsch[14])
Color	**Causes**
Red	Hyperemia, erythema Telangiectasia Recent extravasation of blood (purpura)
White	Absence of melanin Anemia Vascular spasm Hyperkeratosis Fibrosis of the upper dermis
Grey	Melanin in the dermis Early necrosis Arsenic, silver, mercury, exogeneous pigments, some drugs
Brown	Melanin in the epidermis Hemosiderin Granulomas Serous crust
Black	Melanin in the epidermis Old blood crust Old necrosis
Blue	Cyanosis Stasis Hematoma Melanin in the dermis Arsenic, silver, mercury, exogeneous pigments, some drugs
Yellow	Pus Carotene Lipids Bile pigments Infiltrates of mast cells Senile elastosis
Green	Old hemosiderin

Contour

This criterion only applies to solid elevated lesions. They may be flat-topped or dome-shaped, slightly elevated or acuminate, papillated/papillomatous (nipple-like), digitated (finger-like) or umbilicated.[12]

Surface characteristics

If secondary lesions are lacking the surface texture of a lesion should be checked for roughness or smoothness, shine or dullness, verrucous, papillomatous, and other changes of unevenness.

Margins

Skin lesions may be regularly or irregularly, sharply or indistinctly marginated.

Consistency

In contrast to all other criteria mentioned above, the consistency of a lesion can only be assessed by palpation. Therefore, it is the last element in the description of an individual lesion.

Terms suited for the description of the consistency of a lesion are soft, pasty, firm, hard, fluctuating, compressible, lobulated, and so on. Consistencies may also be compared with natural objects.

Number

Low numbers of lesions, around up to 10, should be counted. Higher numbers may be estimated or called multiple, numerous, countless.

Arrangement

Turning away from the individual lesion, the relationship of different lesions to each other has to be assessed. Sometimes, their arrangement is so characteristic, such as in herpes zoster, that a diagnosis is readily enabled.

Table 3.3 summarizes the most relevant patterns in which skin lesions may be arranged. The terms circinate/arcuate, gyrate/polycyclic, and serpiginous are applicable both to the shape of a single and the arrangement of multiple lesions. Individual lesions arranged in these irregular forms may occur. More often, however, a single lesion may take on this shape by extension, confluence and partial recession of several annular lesions.

Linearity of skin lesions is particularly ambiguous. Underlying causes may be:

- the contact with exogeneous agents and artificial influences,
- physical trigger factors, as defined by the Köbner phenomenon,
- the course of blood vessels or lymphatics involved in a disease process,
- a genetic mosaic state visualizing the lines of Blaschko,
- further factors not satisfactorily explained.[3]

Köbner phenomenon (isomorphic effect)

A nonspecific external or internal trauma, such as physical damage, infection, or irritant/allergic reactions, may provoke the occurrence of disease-specific new lesions in the traumatized skin after an average of 10 to 14 days.[15] This observation is particularly striking when the lesions show a linear arrangement. The Köbner phenomenon is often seen in psoriasis (Fig. 3.10), lichen planus, and vitiligo but can also occur in many other dermatoses.

Distribution

The distribution and sites of involvement of a skin disease can only be assessed if the entire integument including adnexal structures and mucous membranes are inspected. Remote or hidden lesions may be more characteristic than those demonstrated by the patient or parents and may provide the decisive diagnostic clue. Furthermore, the distribution itself may be very informative with regard to the cause. It should be noted whether the skin lesions show a localized, regional, generalized, or universal, uni- or bilateral, symmetric

14. Fritsch P (1998) Dermatologischer Untersuchungsgang. In: Dermatologie und Venerologie. Lehrbuch und Atlas. Berlin: Springer, pp. 99–115.

15. Boyd AS, Neldner KH (1990) The isomorphic response of Koebner. **Int J Dermatol** 29:401–410.

TABLE 3.3   Types of arrangement of skin lesions

Term	Explanation	Examples
Disseminated	Nongrouped, randomly distributed	Exanthemas
Grouped	Clustered, located close together	Viral warts
Herpetiform	Tightly grouped, touching, partly confluent	Herpes simplex, Herper zoster
Corymbiform	Central lesion or cluster of lesions surrounded by scattered smaller lesions	Melanoma with satellite metastases
Agminate	Grouped without touching	Multiple Spitz nevi
Linear	Following a line (see text)	Phytophotodermatitis, urticaria factitia
Blaschkoid	Following the lines of Blaschko	Linear nevi
Sporotrichoid	Separated but in line	Sporotrichosis
Segmental/zosteriform	Following a dermatome	Herpes zoster
Systematized	Following an overriding principle, such as the vascular system, the nervous system, or lines of embryonal development	Widespread linear nevi
Annular	Ring-like, active margin with clear center	Granuloma annulare
Circinate/arcuate	Arc-like, semicircular	Erythema arciforme et palpabile migrans
Gyrate/polycyclic	Winding, curved, joined annular and arcuate lesions	Erythema annulare centrifugum
Serpiginous	Wavy, snake-like	Creeping eruption
Follicular	Bound to openings of hair follicles	Folliculitis
Reticular	Net-like	Livedo reticularis

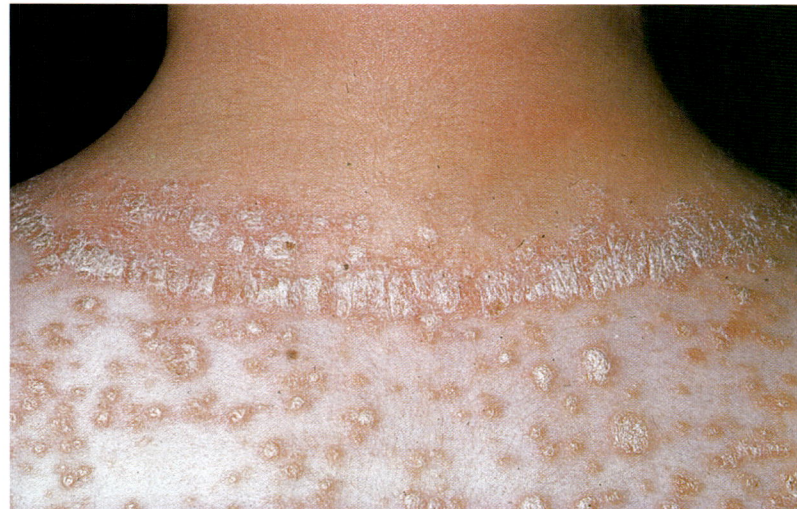

Fig. 3.10   Köbner phenomenon. Psoriatic lesions around the neck provoked by a necklace.

or asymmetric distribution. Bilateral and symmetric rashes are often caused by endogeneous or systemic agents via hematogeneous spread.[11] External influences may tend to provoke more focal, unilateral or asymmetrical findings.

In most cases, the distribution is not random but certain areas are preferentially involved. These sites of predilection are characteristic of many dermatoses but their origin is often not understood. However, in a number of conditions, the pattern of distribution may be explained, for example, by exposure to sunlight, chemical agents, or mechanical forces, or the blood or nerve supply of the involved areas may be the underlying principle.

The documentation of the distribution is often more accurate and rapid in standardized drawings of the body than in wordy records, especially in widespread conditions.

SIMPLE CLINICAL TESTS

PALPATION AND MANIPULATION

The first clinical test is usually to prove the consistency of a lesion (see above). The palpating finger or fingers can also serve to assess whether, for example, a lesion is slightly raised or in the level of the skin, whether the skin is foldable or sclerotic, whether a swelling is dentable ("pitting edema") or fluctuating (both pointing to fluids), whether the skin is movable over a nodule or a nodule is fixed to underlying structures, whether a swelling, nodule or tumor is painful to palpation, whether a patch is anesthetic, or whether arteries or cords are pulsatile. The skin temperature which is cool in ischemia and cyanosis and warm in acute inflammation is best percieved with the dorsa of the fingers. The vasal reaction after a short pressure exerted on the skin is different in erythemas and cyanosis from normal skin in that the pale macule is filled from the periphery to the center, similar to the aperture of a lens. Rubbing on the skin may help to differentiate between patches due to hypopigmentation and vasoconstriction (nevus anemicus) since the latter fail to redden intensively. After putting on gloves, it can be determined whether a secretion or pasty material can be expressed from a cyst or sinus.

Nikolski signs

When exerting gentle tangential pressure on apparently normal skin, particularly near vesicles, the epidermis or parts of it may be detached in certain

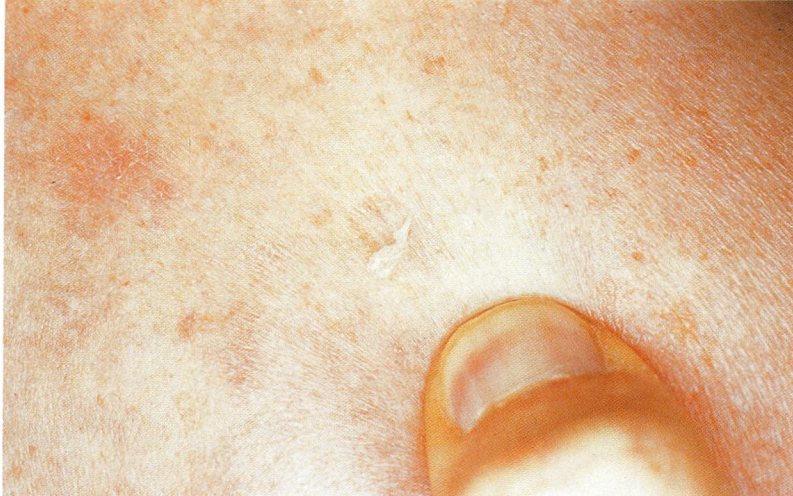

Fig. 3.11   Nikolski (I) sign. Induction of a small erosion by tangential pressure.

bullous diseases, such as pemphigus vulgaris and toxic epidermal necrolysis (Nikolski I, "direct" Nikolski sign, Fig. 3.11). Vertical pressure on the top of a blister may spread the contents laterally (Nikolski II, "indirect" Nikolski sign). The latter test is less specific and positive in many bullous diseases.

Simple aids for clinical tests

Apart from the indispensable magnifying glass there are some simple readily disposable diagnostic aids.

Exact sizes of lesions can be measured by dermatometers with millimeter scales. Some of them also have round punches of growing diameters.

With the help of a cotton bud one can examine whether a coating on the tongue can be wiped off, as is the case in oral candidiasis. It may also serve to test the fragility of tissues, such as the margins of an ulcer.

A probe is used to check the length of a sinus or fistula and whether the margins of an ulcer are undermined.

A wooden spatula serves to examine the oral mucosa and to remove or better visualize inconspicuous scaling, such as in pityriasis versicolor.

Dermographism

This term refers to the cutaneous response to a firm stroke applied with a wooden spatula to the back. In normal subjects, a bright-red non-raised line due to vasodilation occurs after 3 to 15 seconds (*red dermographism*). It is usually followed by a reflex erythema. After a few to 10 minutes, a wheal due to the release of histamine may occur in predisposed individuals (*urticarial dermographism*, Fig. 3.12). Only if itching and otherwise matching the history, urticaria factitia can be diagnosed. In most patients with atopic dermatitis and other atopic diseases, the vascular response to the stroke is paradoxically anemic (*white dermographism*). However, it has a longer time to onset and shorter duration than red dermographism in non-atopic subjects.[16] Interestingly, a marked age-dependent increase of the demonstrability of white dermographism in patients with infantile eczema was reported.[17] According to personal experience, the type of dermographism also depends on the strength of the applied mechanical pressure and on the site where it is studied. Therefore, the use of dermographometers seems reasonable in controlled studies. Rarely, *delayed urticarial dermographism* occurring in pressure urticaria 3–6 hours after the stroke and *hemorrhagic dermographism* in hemorrhagic diatheses can be observed.

Psoriasis phenomena

The following three phenomena typical for psoriasis vulgaris can be studied with a wooden spatula in unclear cases:

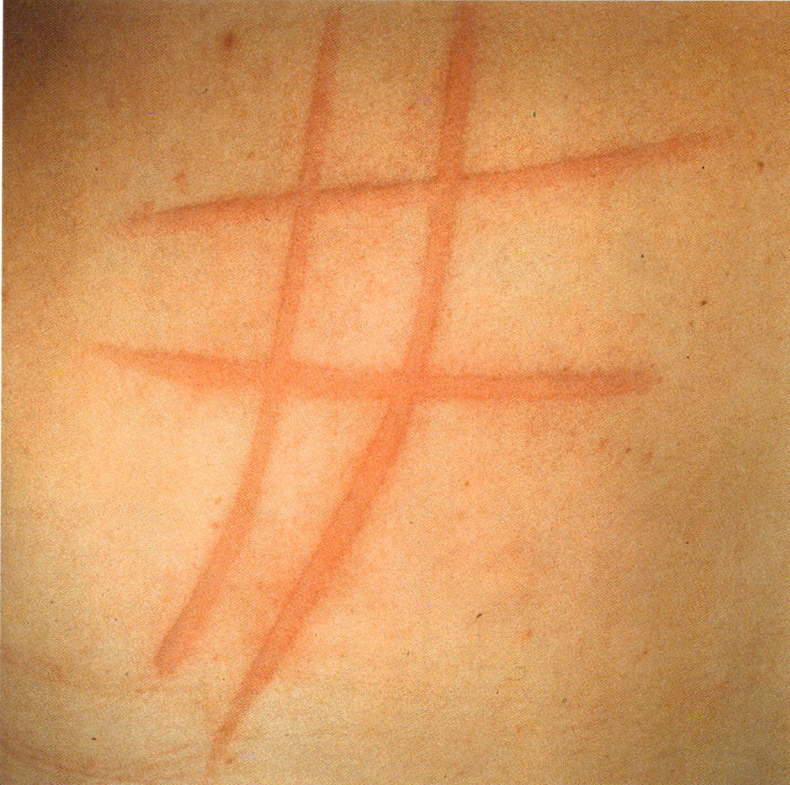

Fig. 3.12   Urticarial dermographism induced by firm strokes with a wooden spatula.

- *Candle sign*. If the silvery-white scales are scraped off, they detach from the lesion as small flakes, similar to wax flakes scraped from a candle.
- *Last cuticle sign*. With continuing scraping one can remove a coherent moist sheet from the lesion corresponding to the lowest layers of the epidermis.
- *Auspitz sign*. After removal of the last cuticle, spotty bleeding ("bloody dew") occurs indicating that the dilated capillaries in the papillary dermis are ruptured.[4]

Although best known, the Auspitz sign is not sensitive or specific for psoriasis. The last cuticle sign has the greatest diagnostic value.

Darier sign

Heavy rubbing with a spatula or the round end of a pen induces after some minutes an urticarial swelling in a mastocytoma (Fig. 3.13) and in lesions of urticaria pigmentosa. Occasionally, even a blister may occur.

Diascopy

Firm pressure of a hard, transparent instrument, such as a plastic or glass spatula or two microscope slides, may be used to temporarily blanch the skin. By this simple procedure, an erythema can be distinguished from a purpura. The erythema subsides whereas extravasations remain visible. Moreover, the brownish color compared to apple jelly of certain granulomatous infiltrates may be recognized, such as in sarcoidosis, tuberculosis, and foreign body granulomas (Fig. 3.14).

DERMOSCOPY

Dermoscopy (also, known as dermatoscopy, epiluminescence microscopy, ELM and skin surface microscopy) is the cutting edge of technology to

16. Wong RC, Fairley JA, Ellis CN (1984) Dermographism: a review. **J Am Acad Dermatol** 11:643–652.

17. Aizawa H, Tagami H (1989) Inability to produce white dermographism in the early stage of infantile eczema. **Pediatr Dermatol** 6:6–9.

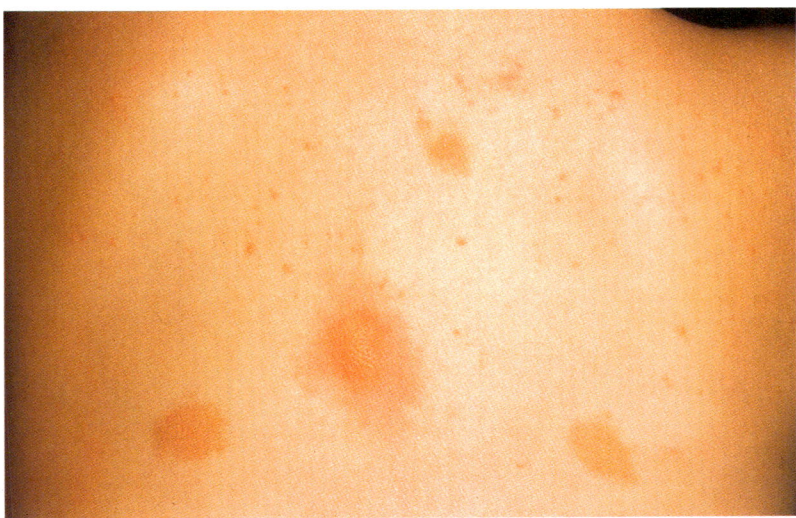

Fig. 3.13   Darier sign. Redness and urticarial swelling after rubbing of a mastocytoma in urticaria pigmentosa.

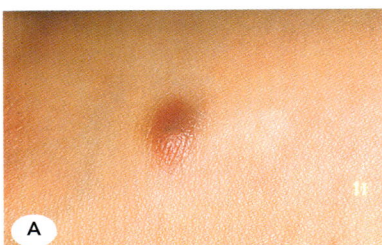
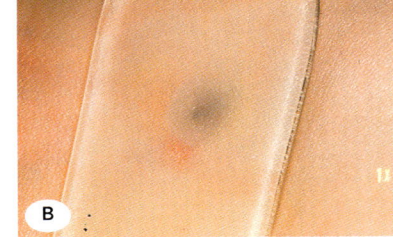

Fig. 3.14   Diascopy. (A) A purple papule showing **(B)** central bluish discoloration after pressure with a glass spatula corresponding to a broken cactus prickle.

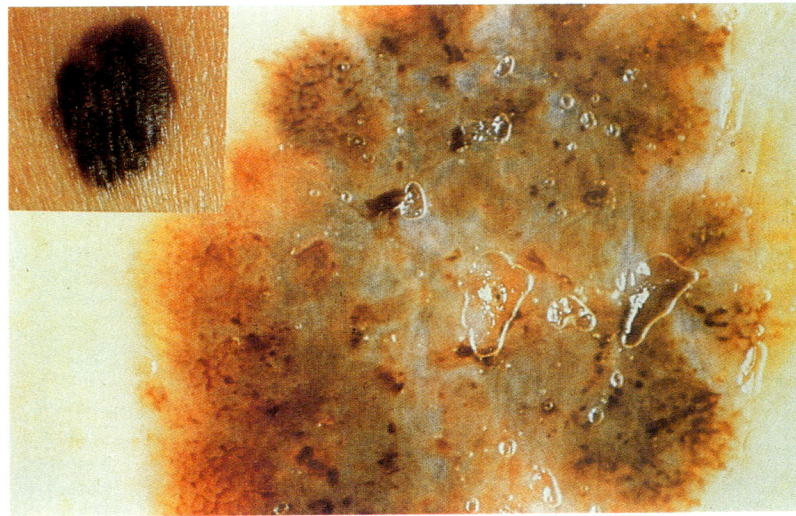

Fig. 3.15   Both clinical and dermoscopic images of the same invasive melanoma. The clinical image (insert) lacks the ABCD criteria suggestive of a melanoma. With dermoscopy there is a great deal of asymmetry of colors and structures diagnostic of melanoma. (*Image courtesy of Wilhelm Stolz, Regensburg, Germany.*) (*Reprinted with permission from Dermoscopy of Pigmented Skin Lesions. An Atlas based on the Consensus Net meeting on Dermoscopy 2000. EDRA Medical Publishing and New Media, Milan, 2001.*)

TABLE 3.4   Pattern analysis criteria

Pigment network – honeycomb-like pattern of line segments
Diffuse pigmentation – unstructured pigmentation without other criteria seen
Depigmentation (regression areas) – whitish and/or bluish-white color
Dots/globules – globular pigment aggregations
Streaks (pseudopods and radial streaming) – finger-like or radially oriented extensions of the pigment network at the periphery of a lesion
Blue-whitish veil – areas with the appearance of ground glass

---

evaluate pigmented skin lesions. It is an *in vivo* non-invasive technique that magnifies the skin in such a way that colors and structures in the epidermis, dermoepidermal junction and papillary dermis become visible. These are colors and structures that cannot be seen with the typical magnification clinicians use (Fig. 3.15). With training and experience,[18] the analysis of this extra criteria has been shown to significantly improve the clinical diagnosis of pigmented skin lesions.

Instrumentation available includes the hand-held dermatoscope (different models and manufacturers are available) with a 10 × magnification and digital computer systems. With the dermatoscope, some type of oil or fluid (mineral oil, immersion oil, K–Y jelly, alcohol or water) is placed over the lesion to be examined. Liquid eliminates reflection of light from the surface of the skin and renders the stratum corneum transparent allowing visualization of subsurface colors and structures. The dermatoscope is then placed directly over the lesion to be examined. One variation on the theme of the dermatoscope is the Dermlite which utilizes a polarizing system; therefore, fluid is no longer needed to perform the technique.

Dermoscopic analysis is a two-step process. Step one is to determine if a lesion is melanocytic or non-melanocytic, and there are primary criteria to do this. Step two is to determine if a melanocytic lesion is benign or malignant. Based on the recently completed Internet international consensus meeting of dermoscopy 2000, there are four algorithms to analyze a melanocytic lesion;

pattern analysis, Menzies scoring system, the ABCD rule of dermatoscopy and the 7-point checklist.[19,20,21]

Pattern analysis

With pattern analysis, one has to identify eight criteria and at least 28 variables of those criteria (Table 3.4). The criteria identified in a lesion are put into patterns, and patterns correlate with specific pathology. For example, there are patterns of criteria suggestive of different types of melanoma (superficial spreading, nodular, lentigo maligna and lentigo maligna melanoma), and different types of melanocytic nevi (common, blue, dysplastic and Spitz).

If a pigment network can be identified, then it is necessary to determine if it is regular or irregular, prominent or subtle, and whether it thins gradually at the periphery or ends abruptly. The more prominent and irregular the pigment network is, the greater the chance that the lesion is malignant (Fig. 3.16).

If dots and/or globules are present, are they regular, or irregular in size, shape and distribution in the lesion? As a general rule, symmetrical and uniform criteria favor a benign diagnosis, and asymmetry of colors and

---

18. Binder M, Schwarz M et al. (1997) Epiluminescence microscopy of small pigmented skin lesions: short-term training improves the diagnostic performance of dermatologists. **J Am Acad Dermatol** 36:197–202.

19. Argenziano G, Soyer HP et al. (2001) Dermoscopy of pigmented skin lesions. An atlas based on the consensus net meeting on dermoscopy 2000. Milan: EDRA Medical Publishing and New Media.

20. Menzies SW, Crotty KA et al. (1996) An Atlas of Surface Microscopy of Pigmented Skin Lesions. Sydney, Australia: McGraw-Hill.

21. Stolz W, Braun-Falco O et al. (1994) Color Atlas of Dermatoscopy. Oxford, England: Blackwell Scientific Publications.

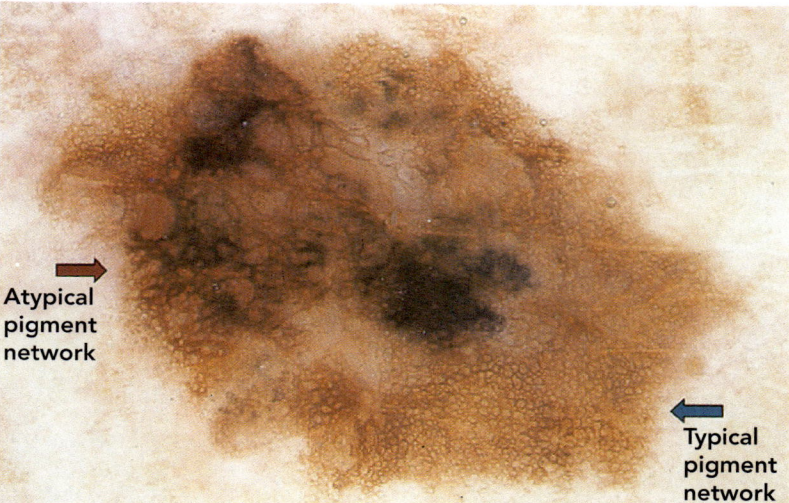

Fig. 3.16   A typical/regular pigment network is characterized by regularly meshed and narrowly spaced line segments that gradually thin at the periphery. The atypical pigment network is thickened and branched, usually ending abruptly at the periphery. (*Reprinted with permission from Dermoscopy of Pigmented Skin Lesions. An Atlas based on the Consensus Net meeting on Dermoscopy 2000. EDRA Medical Publishing and New Media, Milan, 2001.*)

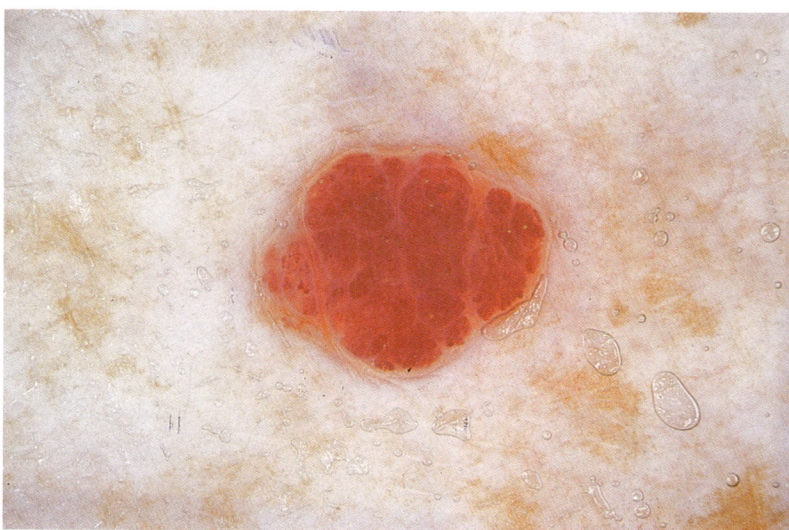

Fig. 3.17   The saccular pattern diagnostic of a hemangioma. (*Reprinted with permission from Dermoscopy of Pigmented Skin Lesions. An Atlas based on the Consensus Net meeting on Dermoscopy 2000. EDRA Medical Publishing and New Media, Milan, 2001.*)

structures, plus the presence of melanoma-specific criteria, are suggestive but not 100% diagnostic of melanoma.

Menzies scoring method

Menzies scoring method is a variation on the theme of pattern analysis in an attempt to simplify the process. If a lesion demonstrates symmetry of pattern within the lesion (not necessarily symmetry of contour) and the presence of a single color, then in most cases it would not be a melanoma. On the other hand, if a lesion demonstrates asymmetry of pattern and more than one color, and if one or more of 9 positive features can be identified, then the lesion should be considered a melanoma (Table 3.5).

ABCD rule of dermatoscopy

With the ABCD rule of dermatoscopy, four criteria were found to be significant cofactors for diagnosing melanoma and they include asymmetry (A), borders (B), colors (C) and the presence of different structural components (D). It is semi-quantitative mathematical approach that gives points for the criteria identified in a lesion and a formula to determine the total dermatoscopy score (TDS) for each lesion. A TDS less than 4.75 in most cases would be benign. A TDS of 4.75 to 5.45 is suggestive of melanoma, and a TDS greater than 5.45 is highly suspicious but not 100% diagnostic of

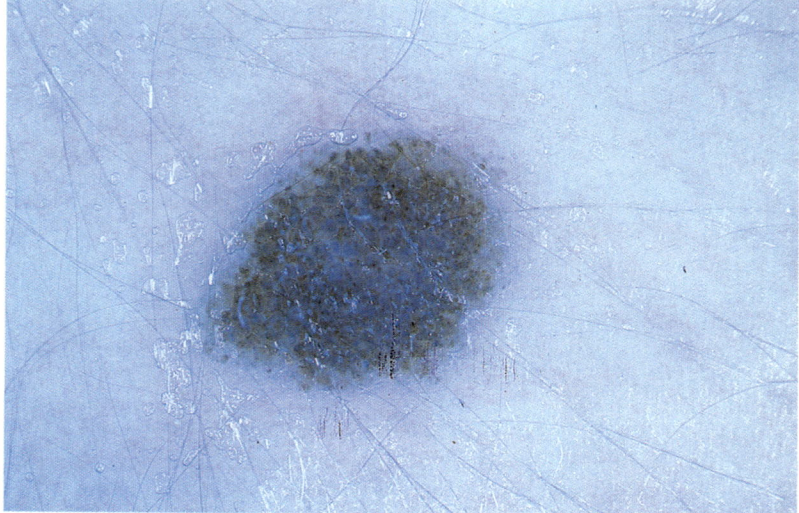

Fig. 3.18   A globular pattern with uniform brown globules indicating a low risk melanocytic lesion. This pattern is commonly seen in children in lesions that clinically look atypical; however, excision is not indicated. (*Reprinted with permission from Dermoscopy of Pigmented Skin Lesions. An Atlas based on the Consensus Net meeting on Dermoscopy 2000. EDRA Medical Publishing and New Media, Milan, 2001.*)

melanoma. A false high total dermatoscopy score (TDS) is possible with a benign lesion.

By definition, there are some lesions that always have a pattern recognition diagnosis, and the ABCD rule of dermatoscopy should not be applied. Hemangiomas (Fig. 3.17), some compound nevi (Fig. 3.18), and Spitz nevus (Fig. 3.19) are examples of that dermoscopic concept.

Asymmetry (A) of contour, color, or structural components

The lesion is visually divided into two 90 degree right angle axes, then assigned a score ranging from zero for a lesion that is completely symmetrical in contour, color or structure, to one point for a lesion that is asymmetrical in one axis and a maximum of two points for a lesion that is asymmetrical in both axes (Figs 3.20, 3.21, 3.22).

TABLE 3.5   Menzies scoring method

- symmetry of pattern
- presence of a single color   } benign
- asymmetry of pattern, more than one color plus 1 to 9 positive features = melanoma

Positive features
- blue-white veil
- multiple brown dots
- pseudopods
- radial streaming
- scar-like depigmentation
- peripheral black dots/globules
- multiple colors (5 or 6)
- multiple blue/gray dots
- broad pigment network

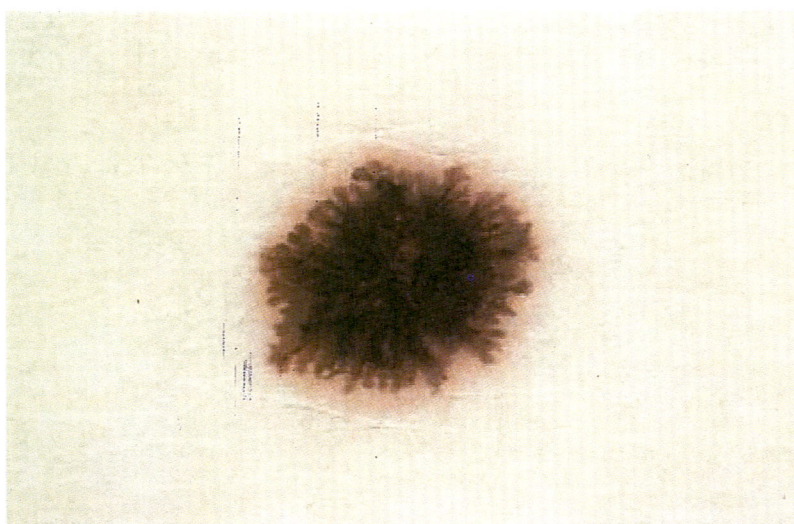

Fig. 3.19   The starburst pattern in a Spitz nevus demonstrating a symmetrical lesion with a rim of psuedopods radially oriented at the periphery of the lesion. (*Reprinted with permission from Dermoscopy of Pigmented Skin Lesions. An Atlas based on the Consensus Net meeting on Dermoscopy 2000. EDRA Medical Publishing and New Media, Milan, 2001.*)

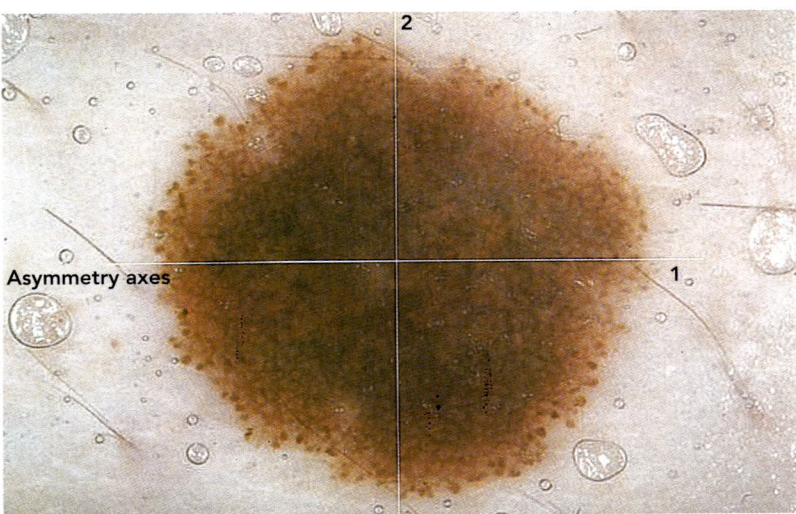

Fig. 3.20   A = 0 (× 1.3) = 0,
B = 8 (0 × 0.1) = 0.8,
C = 2 (light and dark brown) (× 0.5) = 1
D = 2 (network, globules) (× 0.5) = 1
TDS = 2.8 (benign)
(*Reprinted with permission from Dermoscopy of Pigmented Skin Lesions. An Atlas based on the Consensus Net meeting on Dermoscopy 2000. EDRA Medical Publishing and New Media, Milan, 2001.*)

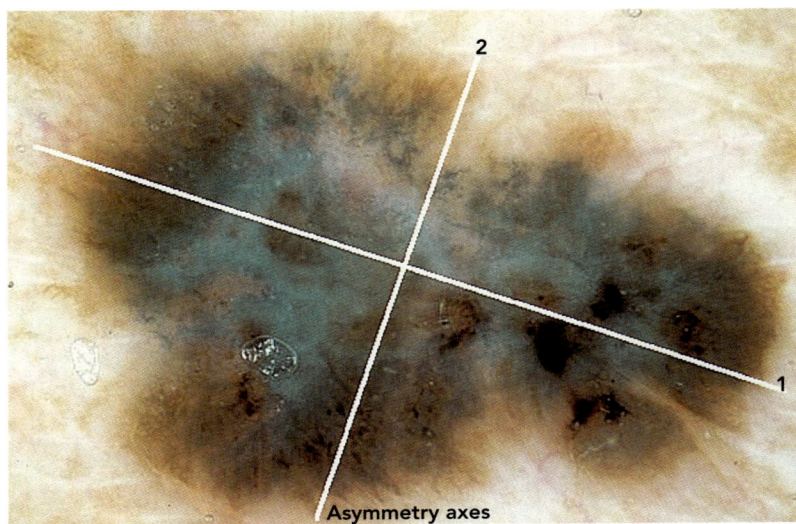

Fig. 3.21   A=2 (× 1.3) = 2.6
B = 5 (× 0.1) = 0.5
C = 5 (light and dark brown, blue-gray, black, white) × (0.5) = 2.5
D = 4 (homogeneous areas, streaks, dots, globules) × (0.5) = 2
TDS = 7.6 (malignant)
(*Reprinted with permission from Dermoscopy of Pigmented Skin Lesions. An Atlas based on the Consensus Net meeting on Dermoscopy 2000. EDRA Medical Publishing and New Media, Milan, 2001.*)

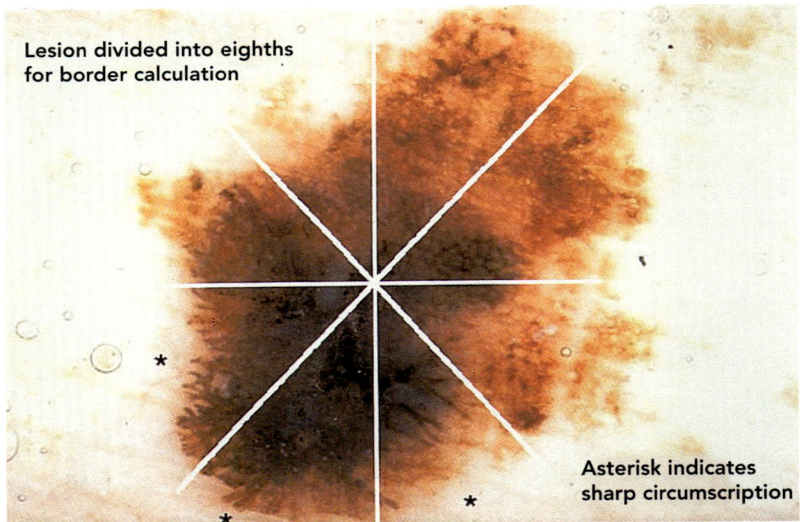

Fig. 3.22   A=2 (× 1.3) = 2.6
B = 3 (× 0.1) = 0.3
C = 4 (light and dark brown, blue-gray, black) × (0.5) = 2.0
D = 4 (network, streaks, dots, globules) × (0.5) = 2
TDS = 6.9 (malignant)
(*Reprinted with permission from Dermoscopy of Pigmented Skin Lesions. An Atlas based on the Consensus Net meeting on Dermoscopy 2000. EDRA Medical Publishing and New Media, Milan, 2001.*)

Borders (B)

To determine the border score, the lesion is visually divided into eight pie-shaped segments, and then the number of segments is counted in which there is an abrupt cutoff at the margins of identifiable criteria (pigment network, branched streaks, dots, globules or diffuse pigmentation). The score can range from zero to eight (Figs 3.20, 3.21, 3.22).

Color (C)

Colors to look for include red, white (white color should be lighter than the surrounding skin. Do not confuse the white color of a regression area with hypopigmentation commonly seen in melanocytic lesions), light and dark brown, blue-gray and black. Each color gets a point and the total score ranges from one to six. A lesion with 5 or 6 bright and distinct colors is a significant clue that the lesion is a melanoma (Figs 3.20, 3.21, 3.22).

Different structural components (D)

Look for a pigment network, branched streaks (thickened and branched pigment network), structureless areas (color, but no structures such as pigment network, branched streaks, dots or globules) dots and globules. The total different structural component score ranges from one to five (Figs 3.20, 3.21, 3.22). After all of the criteria have been identified, the total dermatoscopy score is calculated by multiplying the points by conversion factors (A × 1.3 + B × 0.1 + C × 0.5 + D × 0.5 = TDS).

The 7-point checklist

This is another variation on the theme of pattern analysis with a point system. The major and minor criteria within a lesion are identified. Major criteria receive two points each and minor criteria receive one point. A score of three or greater has a 95% sensitivity of being a melanoma (Figs 3.23, 3.24 and Table 3.6).

Dermoscopy with all of the extra criteria seen, criteria that cannot be seen with the naked eye or typical magnification clinicians use, should be put together with the patient's personal and family history plus the history and

TABLE 3.6   7-point checklist

Criteria	7-point score
Major Criteria	
1. Atypical pigment network	2
2. Atypical vascular pattern (linear-irregular and/or dotted)	2
3. Blue-whitish veil	2
Minor Criteria	
4. Irregular streaks (pseudopods/radial streaming)	1
5. Irregular pigmentation	1
6. Irregular dots/globules	1
7. Regression areas	1
7-point total score <3 non-melanoma	
>3 melanoma	

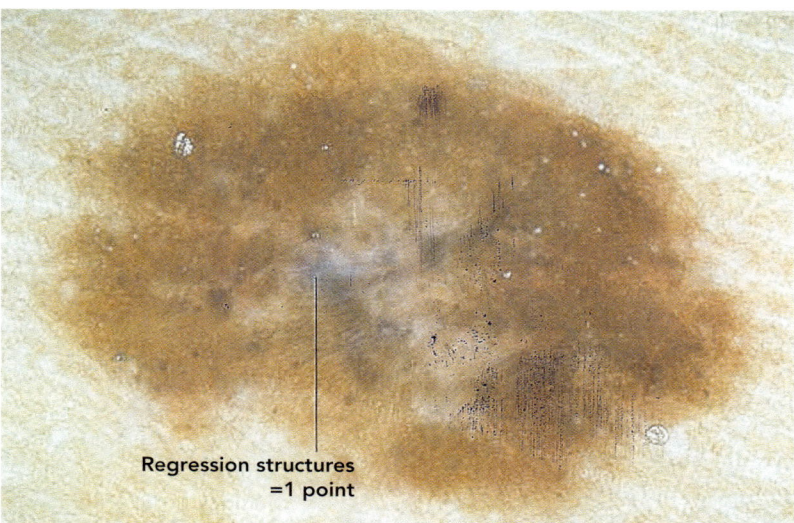

Regression structures
=1 point

Fig. 3.23   Analysis using the 7-point checklist with only one point in a benign nevus. (*Reprinted with permission from Dermoscopy of Pigmented Skin Lesions. An Atlas based on the Consensus Net meeting on Dermoscopy 2000. EDRA Medical Publishing and New Media, Milan, 2001.*)

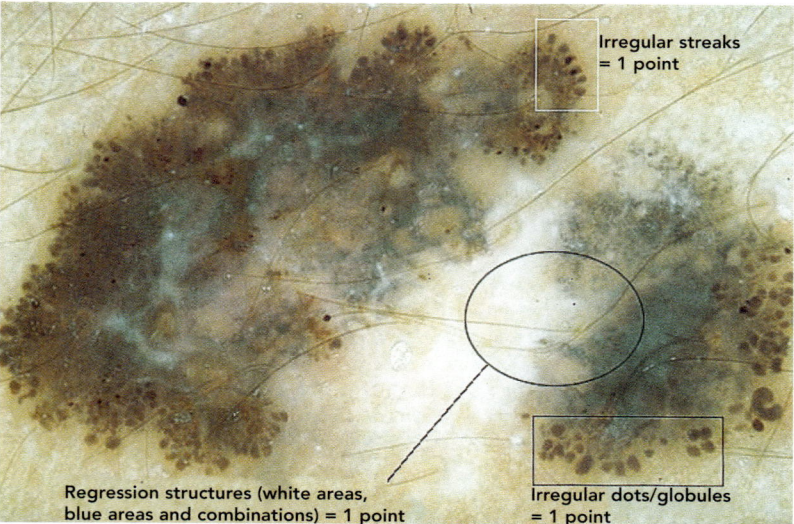

Irregular streaks
= 1 point

Regression structures (white areas,
blue areas and combinations) = 1 point

Irregular dots/globules
= 1 point

Fig. 3.24   A melanoma getting 3 points using the 7-point checklist. (*Reprinted with permission from Dermoscopy of Pigmented Skin Lesions. An Atlas based on the Consensus Net meeting on Dermoscopy 2000. EDRA Medical Publishing and New Media, Milan, 2001.*)

appearance of a lesion before a decision for or against an excision is made. The technique is not 100% diagnostic of melanoma or other pigmented skin lesions. However, it has many advantages over the clinical evaluation of a skin lesion by other methods and is especially helpful for patients with many atypically pigmented skin lesions which are not uncommonly seen in children.[22]

WOOD'S LIGHT EXAMINATION

Wood's lamp is a high-pressure mercury lamp with a special filter that allows the emission of a largely monochromatic UV light with a wavelength of 365nm. It is especially useful in the diagnostics of certain fungal and bacterial diseases and in the assessment of pigmentary disorders. For examination, the room has to be completely darkened and the patient should be totally undressed. Lesions caused by *Microsporum audouinii*, *M. canis* and *M. ferrugineum* can be identified by their blue-green fluorescence. *Trichophyton schoenleinii* may show a bright green to yellow color. Otherwise inapparent tinea versicolor may be detected by a yellow–white or copper-orange hue. Wood's light is also suited to diagnose skin infections that are clinically similar to mycoses but are caused by bacteria, e.g. erythrasma due to *Corynebacterium minutissimum* (coral–red fluorescence). *Pseudomonas aeruginosa* colonization gives rise to a blue fluorescence.[23]

Furthermore, conditions characterized by hypopigmentation or depigmentation, such as the ash leaf macules of tuberous sclerosis, hypopigmented patches in hypomelanosis of Ito type, vitiligo, and piebaldism, can be more easily detected with the aid of the Wood's lamp. Subtle areas of hyperpigmentation can also be highlighted. Compared to normal skin, the pigmentation difference is more enhanced in epidermal than in dermal melanocytoses.[11] Lastly, urine, stool, and red blood cells of patients suspected of having porphyria can be screened with the Wood's lamp, provoking a characteristic orange-red fluorescence.

TZANCK TEST

The Tzanck test is a simple and rapid cytodiagnostic method used to examine cells from blistering conditions, particularly in infections induced by herpes simplex viruses and in autoimmune bullous diseases of the pemphigus group. For this, the roof of an intact blister is removed with a scissors. Excess blister fluid is cautiously absorbed at an edge of the blister with a gauze or cotton bud. Subsequently, the blister base is gently scraped with a round scalpel blade. The specimen is smeared on a microscope slide, allowed to air-dry for some minutes, stained with Giemsa or another rapid stain used in hematological cytodiagnosis, and examined under the light microscope.[24]

22. Johr R, Izakovic J (2000) Should you be using epiluminescence microscopy? **Skin and Aging** Mar:28–38.

23. Jillson OF (1981) Wood's light: an incredibly important diagnostic tool. **Cutis** 28:620–626.
24. Pariser DM, Caserio RJ, Eaglstein WH (1986) Techniques for Diagnosing Skin and Hair Disease, 2nd edn. New York: Thieme.

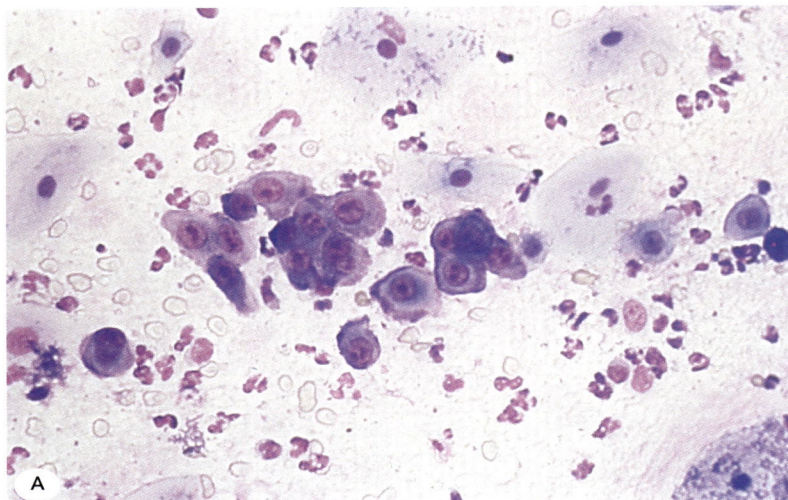

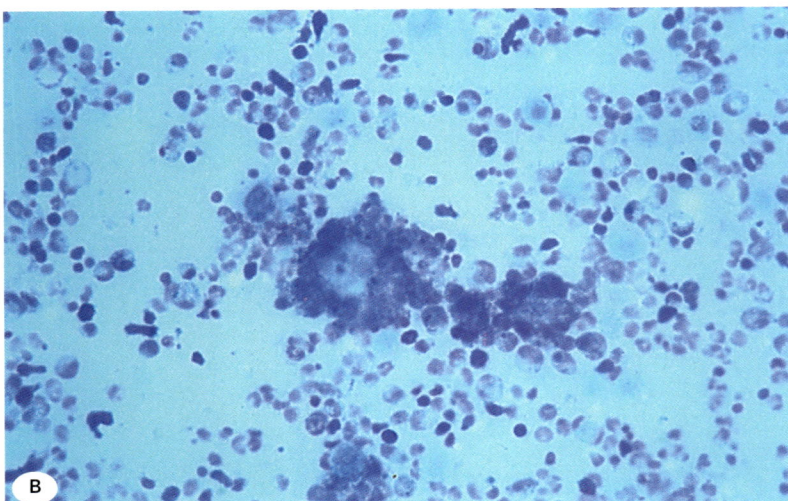

Fig. 3.25 Tzanck test. (A) Rounded acantholytic keratinocytes in pemphigus vulgaris (courtesy of D. Zillikens, Würzburg). (B) Multinucleated giant cells in herpes zoster. Giemsa × 200.

In all forms of pemphigus many rounded epidermal cells, the so-called Tzanck cells, are seen (Fig. 3.25A). They have small amounts of dark-staining, peripherally concentrated cytoplasm and are not attached to one another. In contrast, normal keratinocytes are polygonal in shape and often aggregate to clumps. In subepidermal bullous diseases many inflammatory cells and fibrin threads can be noticed but epidermal cells are lacking.

Multinucleated giant cells and some acantholytic epidermal cells are the diagnostic finding in herpes simplex, herpes zoster, and varicella (Fig. 3.25B). These infections cannot be further distinguished by the Tzanck test.[24]

The Tzanck test may also be helpful in neonatal vesicular and pustular lesions to mark the presence of neutrophils in transient neonatal pustular melanosis and acropustulosis of infancy, or eosinophils in erythema toxicum neonatorum and eosinophilic pustulosis of infancy. It has also been used to help determine staphylococcal scalded skin syndrome from toxic epidermal necrolysis with a large nuclear to cytoplasmic ratio in the latter and a small one in the former.

DIAGNOSTIC METHODS IN BACTERIAL DISEASES

Gram stain

Gram stain is the most common stain used in microbiology. A thin smear made from inflammatory exudates is air-dried on a microscope slide. The slide is fixed by passing it through a flame and flooded with crystal violet

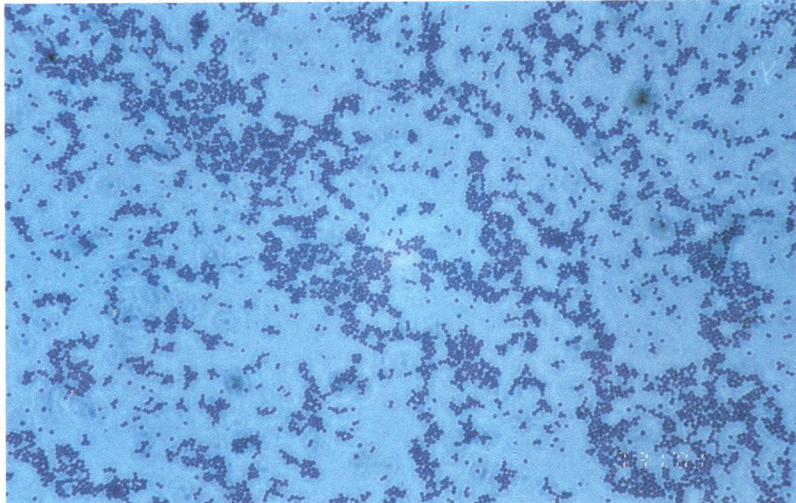

Fig. 3.26 Gram stain showing gram-positive *Stapholococcus aureus*. Germs occur singly, in pairs and in irregular grape-like clusters. × 1000.

solution for two minutes. After gentle washing with tap water the slide is flooded with iodine solution for one minute and washed again with water. Decolorization is done with acetone-alcohol. The slide is briefly washed again, counterstained with safranin for 10 seconds, washed again, blot dry, and now ready for examination.

With the Gram stain gram-positive bacteria, e.g., staphylococci and streptococci, and gram-negative bacteria, e.g., *E. coli*, can be differentiated (Fig. 3.26). Stain of material from a suspected skin infection can guide decisions on early antibiotic therapy many hours before cultural diagnosis is available.

Cultures

Many bacterial diseases are encountered in pediatric dermatology, staphylococci and streptococci being the most common causes of superficial pyodermas. The most important diagnostic test for any suspected bacterial infection is a culture. Material can be obtained:

- by swabbing representative lesions with a swab or brush;
- by scraping skin, hair, mucosa, or nails with a sterile curette or scalpel;
- by aspiration of a pustule or an abscess; or
- by biopsy of a suspicious-looking lesion.

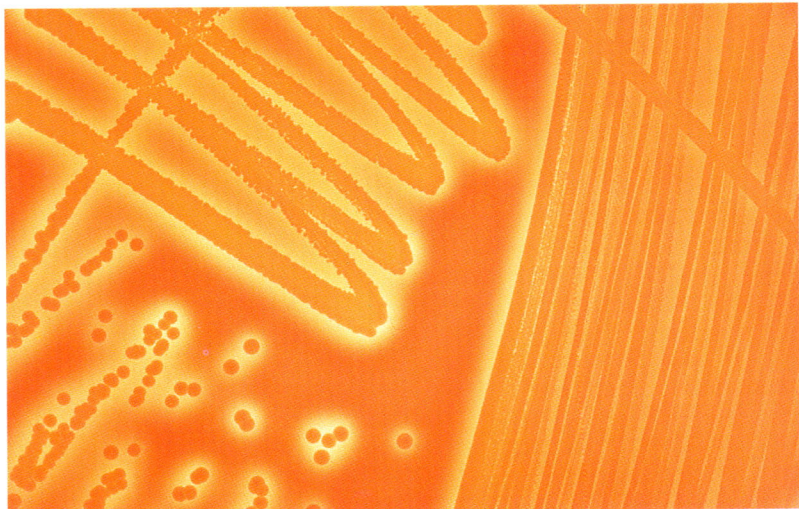

Fig. 3.27 Bacterial colony morphology on blood agar. Colonies of *Staphylococcus aureus* are 1–3mm in diameter within 24 hours of incubation at 37°C and grow with hemolysis.

Sterile culturettes are especially suited for transportation to the laboratory. All samples for culture should be immediately planted on blood agar. Blood agar is routinely used for identification of streptococci or staphylococci because of their characteristic hemolysis (Fig. 3.27). More selective media should be used as indicated by clinical findings and evaluation of the gram-stained smear. For example, the MacConkey plate is suited for isolation of gram-negative bacteria. Pathogenic organisms such as *S. aureus* can be submitted to dilution susceptibility testing methods, in most cases after 24 hours of culture. These tests are used to determine the minimal concentration of an antimicrobial agent required to inhibit the growth of a microorganism. Mycobacterial cultures can be retrieved in the same manner as described above for routine bacterial cultures (mostly biopsy material). Clinicians should consult their own laboratories regarding requirements for obtaining samples for mycobacterial cultures.

DIAGNOSTIC METHODS IN MYCOSES

The clinical diagnosis of cutaneous fungal infections should be supported by light microscopic examination of clinical material and confirmed by culture on suitable mycological media.[25] Specimens are collected from scaling skin lesions, nails, and hairs.

Sampling

SKIN

Prior to taking of material, skin lesions should be superficially sterilized with 70% alcohol solution. Small scales are scraped off from the margin of the lesion using a sterile scalpel blade or edge of a glass microscope slide. The instrument should be angled with the sharp edge away from the direction in which the skin is being scraped. This will minimize any chance of cutting the skin and drawing blood which is not desirable for successfully obtaining a sample. The material is placed onto a clean glass slide for examination under the microscope or can be applied directly on Sabouraud glucose agar in a Petri dish. Note that the causative agent in the central portion of the lesion has mostly died off and, therefore, the scaling margin of a lesion is more suited for evaluation.

NAIL

For obtaining fingernail or toenail samples for mycological examination, a scalpel blade or curette can be used. In the case of a suspected superficial white onychomycosis, samples can be easily obtained by gently scraping the surface of the nail plate. To confirm the more common distal lateral subungual onychomycosis, nail fragments and debris should be gently collected from the distal lateral nail bed or underside of the nail.

HAIR

Hair samples are obtained for examination in the case of suspected fungal infection of the scalp or beard region. Fungi are particularly grown from the hair bases. Therefore, epilation of broken hairs with a needle holder or forceps is most promising for the proof of fungi. Suitable amounts of scales from the scalp can also be used to reveal fungal elements.

Direct light microscopy

Potassium hydroxide (5–20% KOH solution) examination is widely used for confirmation of dermatophytes. KOH digests the proteins, lipids, and most of the other epithelial debris present in the samples. Clinical specimens are placed on microscope slides and a few drops of KOH are supplied. After a coverslip is placed, the slide may be gently heated with a match or a small Bunsen flame to facilitate examination. Alternatively, the keratin may be dissolved by waiting 15–20 minutes without heating. Staining is usually not necessary but sometimes helpful. For this, Parker ink No. 51 (blue-black ink/30% KOH 1:1) may be used. Slides prepared in this manner are examined for suspected fungi by routine microscopy at 20× power with the condenser

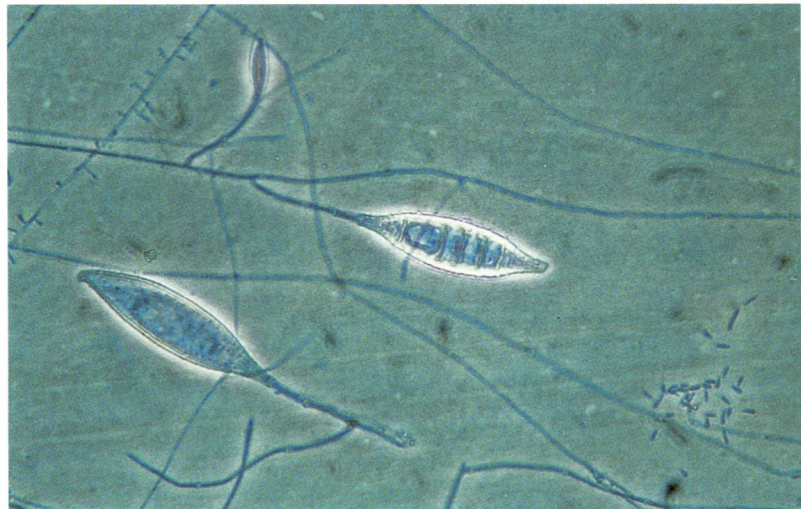

Fig. 3.28 Direct light microscopy of *Microsporum canis* causing tinea capitis. The spindle-shaped macroconidia are rough-walled and 6–12 celled. × 400.

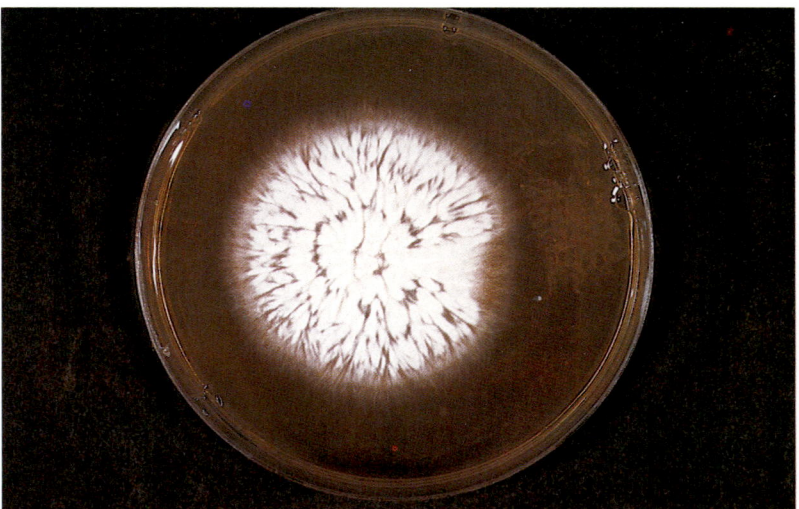

Fig. 3.29 Fungal culture morphology of *Microsporum canis* on Sabouraud glucose agar. Colonies are fast growing, thin, fluffy, and tannish white; reverse orange.

in the lowest position. Dermatophytes are recognized as septate, tube-like structures (hyphae or mycelia) or as chains of rounded cells (Fig. 3.28).

Fungal cultures

Specimens should always be cultivated, regardless of the results of direct microscopy. Skin, hair, or nail samples obtained by the means described above can be applied directly to appropriate fungal culture media (Sabouraud glucose agar and malt extract agar) supplemented with antibiotics in a Petri dish.[25] Antibiotics are chloramphenicol 1mg/ml or penicillin 20 units/ml and streptomycin 40 units/ml. Clinical material is pressed into the agar to increase contact with the medium. Contamination with saprophytic fungi can be reduced by addition of cycloheximide (Actidione 0.5mg/ml) to the medium. Cultures with presumptive dermatophytes are incubated for at least 2 up to 6 weeks at 24°C to 28°C (Fig. 3.29). Purchasable dermatophyte test media have a dye indicator that turns the normal golden hue of the Taplin agar red in the presence of a dermatophyte. However, this unspecific method is hardly

25. Tan CS, Hoekstra ES, Samson RA (1994) Fungi that cause superficial mycoses. Baarn: Centraalbureau voor Schimmelcultures and Beerse: Dr. Paul Janssen Medical Institute.

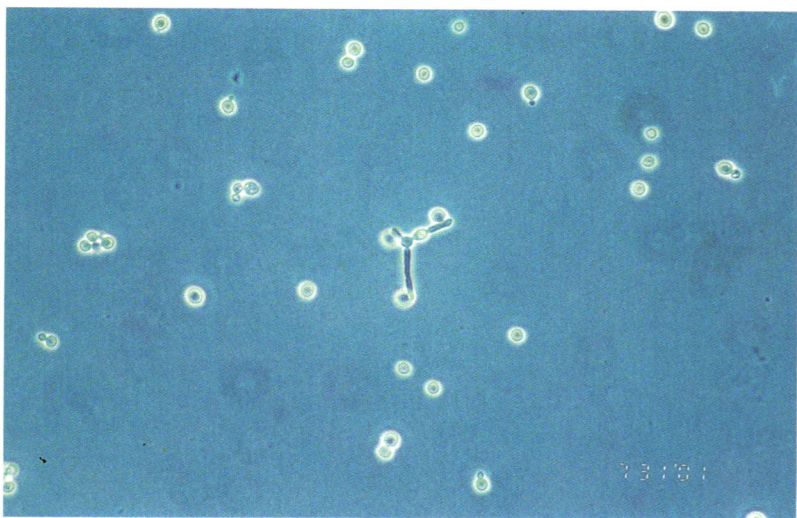

Fig. 3.30   Germ tube formation for rapid recognition of *Candida albicans*. Yeast cells are roundish and begin to produce germ tubes (center of figure) after 2–3 hours of incubation at 37°C in human serum. × 400.

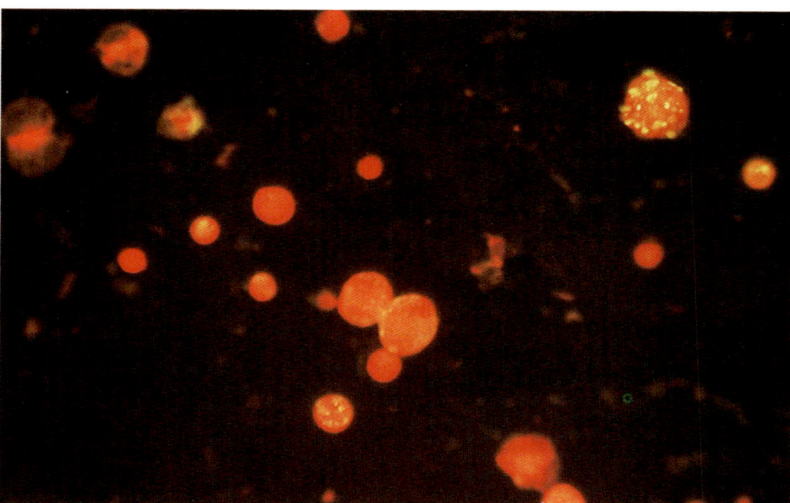

Fig. 3.31   Detection of Herpes simplex virus type 2 (HSV-2) in clinical specimen by fluorescent antibody staining. HSV-2 infected cells show a speckled distribution of intense fluorescent staining in cytoplasm and nucleus. × 400.

suited to distinguish between different dermatophyte species and, therefore, not generally recommended. For this purpose, yeasts need only 24–48 hours of culture until interpretation. For therapeutic purposes it is important to distinguish between the different yeasts since some Candida species are highly resistant to antimycotic treatment. *C. albicans* accounts for 80–90% of all Candida infections and is frequently isolated from skin lesions, vaginal and oral mucosa. The species can be rapidly recognized by production of germ tubes when incubated for 2–3 hours at 37°C in human serum (Fig. 3.30).

Identification and specification of fungi with clinical relevance require careful observation, properly prepared samples and a lot of experience.

DIAGNOSTIC METHODS IN VIRAL DISEASES

Numerous methods are used to diagnose viral infections including virus tissue culture, transmission electron microscopy, demonstration of viral nucleic acids by polymerase chain reaction or ligase chain reaction, and detection of viral antigens by enzyme-linked immunosorbent assay (ELISA), immuno-fluorescence microscopy, and serological tests.[26,27] Growth in tissue culture cells represents the gold standard for virus diagnosis, but molecular methods play a more and more important role in detection and identification of pathogens. Material for viral culture requires inoculation into special transport media for delivery to the laboratory. In vesicular conditions, a firm swab from the basis of an early vesicle is often a good virus source. Susceptible culture cells infected by Herpes simplex viruses (HSV) usually demonstrate a typical cytopathic effect within 1–4 days. Immunologic assays, such as the ELISA, immunoperoxidase staining, and fluorescent antibody staining, can be used to identify and type HSV isolates following growth in culture. More relevant to daily routine, diagnosis may also be made by means of the latter methods directly from the sample without cell culture amplification, if adequate numbers of infected cells are available (Fig. 3.31). Clinicians should be informed which diagnostic tests are offered by their local laboratories and what kind of material is needed for examination.

Cytodiagnosis of molluscum contagiosum

If mollusca contagiosa cannot be diagnosed clinically with certainty, simple cytodiagnosis may be helpful. A selected lesion is punctured centrally and the "core" is loosened and extracted with a large needle. A comedone extractor may be used to squeeze out the central debris. Small lesions may be

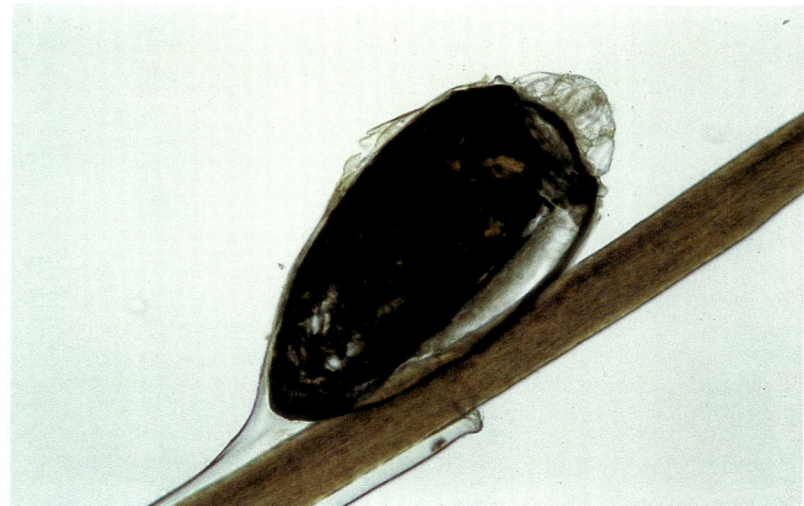

Fig. 3.32   Light microscopy of an egg sticked on to a hair shaft in pediculosis capitis. × 200.

completely scraped off with a curette. The specimen is crushed between two microscope slides, stained with Wright's or Giemsa stain, and examined under the light microscope. Distinctive alterations of epidermal cells infected by the causing virus, the so-called molluscum bodies, are looked for. They stain dark and have a flattened peripherally displaced nucleus.[24]

DIAGNOSTIC METHODS FOR DETECTION OF OTHER MICROORGANISMS

In suspected cases of *pediculosis capitis*, the diagnosis can be confirmed by witness of a live organism on the scalp. When the parasite is not directly noticeable ova or nits firmly attached to the hair shaft are looked for (Fig. 3.32). Affected hairs should be cut with scissors and applied to glass slides. It may be useful to apply some plastic mounting medium such as Permount to stabilize the hair. A coverslip is then applied and the hair is examined under the light microscope.

26. Goldstein LC, Corey L, McDougall JK et al. (1993) Monoclonal antibodies to herpes simplex virus: use in antigenic typing and rapid diagnosis. **J Infect Dis** 16:130–132.

27. Mayer J, Schwarzmann F, Wolf H. (1995) Herpes-Viren, virologische Grundlagen. In: Diagnostik und Therapie von Herpesvirus-Infektionen, Ring J, Zander AR, Malin JP, eds. Karlsruhe: Braun, pp. 7–30.

For suspected *scabies* lesions, whether crusted papules, vesicles, pustules, or linear burrows, dermatoscopy of the skin with a drop of immersion oil is very useful. The highest yield in identifying a mite is in typical burrows on the finger webs, flexor aspects of wrists, and penis.

Parasites, ova, and scybala of scabies mites can also be seen when the burrow is scraped off with a scalpel blade or lancet and the sample is placed on a microscope slide. A drop of immersion oil is placed on the scraping which is then covered with a coverslip. The scraping material is examined microscopically under low power. By this method ectoparasites such as *demodex* mites can also be detected.

SKIN TESTS IN IMMEDIATE TYPE ALLERGY

Skin testing is a useful method in conditions caused or complicated by immediate-type allergy, such as atopic disorders, allergic urticaria, certain oral and gastrointestinal symptoms, and anaphylactic shock. The most relevant allergen sources in IgE-mediated reactions include pollen, molds, house dust mites, domestic and laboratory animals, food, insect venoms, and drugs.[28]

All immediate-type skin testing aims at introducing the allergen into the upper dermis and inducing the release of histamin and other mediators from mast cells in a sensitized individual. For this purpose, watery solutions with standardized allergen concentrations are used. Noteworthy, solutions for prick testing have 100- to 1000-fold strength compared to solutions for intradermal testing. Every test series has to include a negative control performed with physiological NaCl solution as well as a positive control with 0.1% histamin dihydrochloride. The volar aspect of the forearm is commonly used as test site. As severe systemic reactions may rarely occur in sensitivity testing, emergency medication and equipment should be at the physician's disposal. In children with severe symptoms of immediate-type allergy written informed consent from the parents may be wise before testing.

Prick test

A drop of the test solution is placed on the skin and a superficial prick is made through it with the tip of a small lancet (Fig. 3.33). Bleeding should be avoided. Firm cleaning of the lancet is essential between each prick. On account of good reproducibility, favourable correlation with the clinical symptoms, and low risk of systemic reactions the prick test is considered the skin test of first choice in immediate-type allergies.[28]

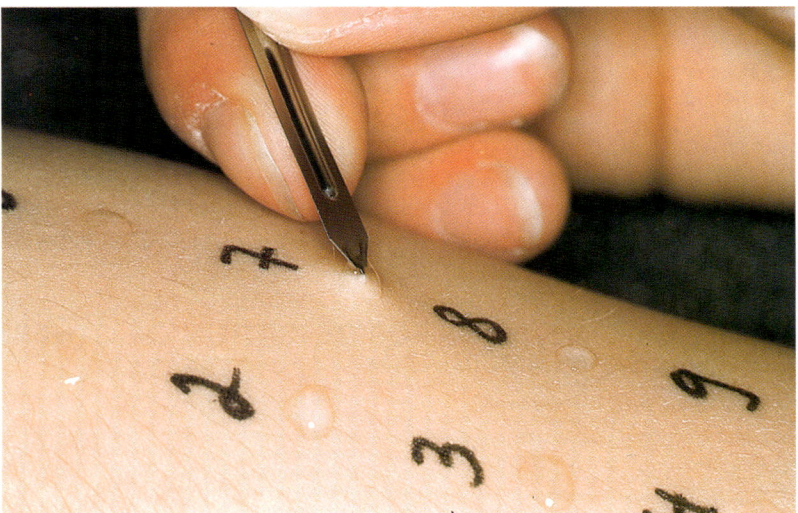

Fig. 3.33   Prick test.

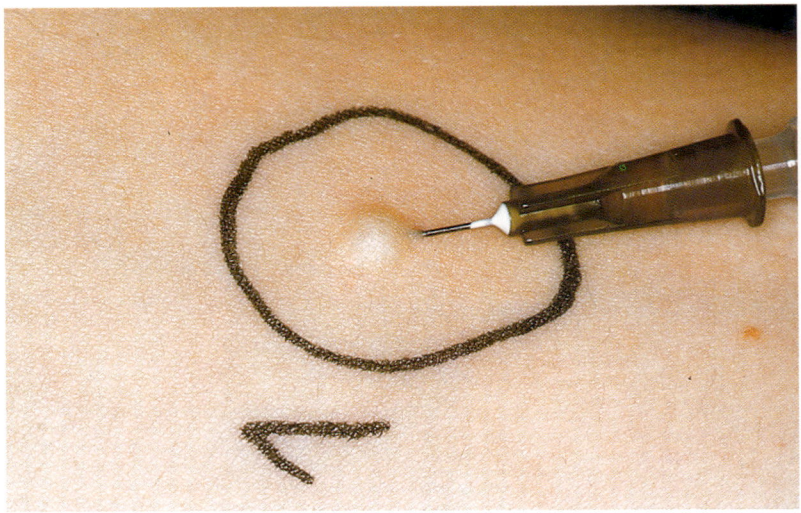

Fig. 3.34   Intracutaneous test.

Intradermal test

In this test, 0.02–0.05ml of the test solution are injected into the superficial dermis through a thin needle with its bevel pointing upwards.[3] The injection, if properly done, leads to a wheal of about 3mm size (Fig. 3.34). For each test solution, new syringes and needles have to be used. Intradermal testing is more sensitive than prick testing but is also more painful and associated with a higher risk of systemic side effects.

Scratch test

After applying the test solution a 5–10mm long, non-bleeding scarification is made through the epidermis. Compared to the prick test, results are less standardized and reproducible. Therefore, the scratch test is only rarely applied.

Rub test

This test mainly serves in the diagnosis of contact urticaria. Native material, such as fruits, vegetables or animal hairs, are rubbed about ten times with slight pressure in a circular way onto a coin-sized area of the skin. The skin is not injured, which is an important advantage in testing children.

Reading and interpretation

A positive test reaction develops within minutes and appears as a wheal with a surrounding flare. By agreement, results are read after (15–) 20 minutes measuring the size of the wheal and the flare separately. A 5-point scale from 0 (negative) to 4+ (wheal >6mm, flare >20mm in prick test; wheal >15mm, flare >40mm in intradermal test) is widely used. Further readings after 6–8, 24 and 48 hours may be required to identify delayed or late reactions.

Tests may reveal false positive results in urticarial dermographism or due to technical mistakes. Taking of antihistamines, corticosteroids and tricyclic antidepressive agents, as well as the application of topical corticosteroids at the test site has to be stopped before testing. The interval depends on the individual drug.[28] Important to note for pediatric patients, the use of an anesthetic cream like EMLA® may inhibit the flare response of a positive test reaction.

In any case test results have to be interpreted by an experienced allergist. Correlation with the history, signs and symptoms, and the results of *in vitro* tests, such as determination of total and specific serum IgE, is essential to arrive at reasonable conclusions.

28. Ruëff F, Przybilla B (1997) Hauttests bei Soforttyp-Allergie. In: Diagnostische Verfahren in der Dermatologie, Korting HC, Sterry W, eds. Berlin: Blackwell, pp. 87–98.

ORAL PROVOCATION TEST

Oral provocation tests are used to disclose any individual hypersensitivity, whether allergic or pseudo-allergic, to foods and oral drugs if skin tests and *in vitro* tests have failed to reveal conclusive results. Oral testing may help to identify certain food allergens, such as cow's milk, hen's egg, soybean, and peanut, that provoke exacerbations in infants with severe atopic dermatitis. Because of the risk of intense, at times threatening effects, and complex design, oral provocation testing is limited to special circumstances.[29]

PATCH TEST

The patch test is a valuable diagnostic tool for the proof of delayed-type hypersensitivity in patients with allergic contact dermatitis.

Most allergens are diluted in petrolatum whereas watery solutions of allergens have to be absorbed onto filter paper. In children the same concentrations are used as in adults. Test substances are placed into small round aluminium chambers (Finn chambers) fixed to special plaster that is applied to the upper quadrants of the back (Fig. 3.35).[30] Alternatively, there are ready-to-apply systems with incorporated allergens, such as the TRUE test, which may facilitate the procedure in young children. Commonly, a set of standard substances, such as the European standard series (Table 3.7), is tested and is eventually completed by additional allergen series or single allergens according to the patient's history. As the spectrum of relevant allergens is more limited in infancy and childhood, a shortened standard series of patch tests may be sufficient for pediatric patients.[31]

The chambers with the allergens are left on the skin for 48 hours, and the first reading is made 20–30 minutes after removal. A second reading is definitely necessary 72 hours after application, and a 96-hour-reading is recommendable. Readings are recorded in a standardized way, as follows:

- −   negative;
- ?×   erythema without infiltrate; allergic vs. irritant reaction cannot be differentiated;
- ?a   erythema without infiltrate, estimated as being an allergic reaction;
- +   erythema and infiltrate, possibly tiny papules;

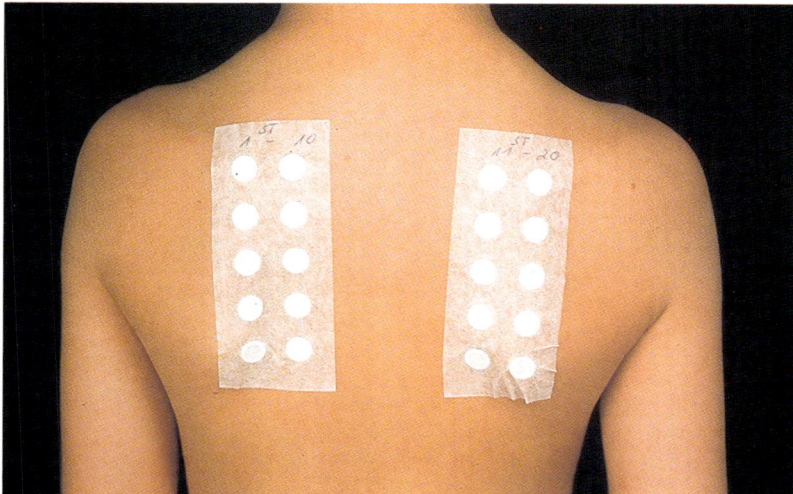

Fig. 3.35   Patch test.

TABLE 3.7   The European standard series of contact allergens

Substance	Concentration (%)
Potassium dichromate	0.5
Neomycin sulfate	20
Thiuram mix	1
Para-phenylenediamine (free base)	1
Cobalt chloride (6H$_2$O)	1
Benzocaine	5
Formaldehyde (in water)	1
Colophony	20
Clioquinol	5
Balsam of Peru	25
N-isopropyl-N'-phenyl para-phenylenediamine	0.1
Wool alcohols	30
Mercapto mix	2
Epoxy resin	1
Paraben mix	16
Para-tertiary butyl phenol formaldehyde resin	1
Fragrance mix	8
Quaternium-15	1
Nickel sulfate (6H$_2$O)	5
Methylchloroisothiazolinone/methylisothiazolinone (in water)	0.01
Mercaptobenzothiazole	2
Sesquiterpene lactone mix	0.1
Primin (important only in some countries)	0.01

- ++   erythema, infiltrate, papules and vesicles;
- +++ erythema, infiltrate and confluent vesicles.[32]

The main challenge is to differentiate allergic from irritant reactions. For distinction, not only morphologic criteria but also the course of the reaction ("crescendo" vs. "decrescendo" pattern) is important. Nevertheless, observer's variability is high.[32] Besides, there are many other sources of interference in patch testing. Skin reactivity may be increased if the dermatitis is still florid ("angry back") and decreased after UV exposure or under immunosuppressive drugs. Skin lesions should have ceased for at least two weeks before testing. It is the allergist's duty to judge the clinical relevance of the test results and to inform patients and parents about the identified allergens and their avoidance.

The most important risk of patch testing is the possibility of induction of a new sensitization. This may be the main reason for the common restraint of patch testing in childhood. However, many studies have found allergic contact sensitivity to be rather frequent even in pre-school children. Nickel sulfate, mercury compounds as thiomersal, fragrance allergens, kathon CG, neomycin, wool alcohols, and rubber chemicals are among the commonest allergens in infancy and childhood.

ATOPY PATCH TEST

Patch testing with aeroallergens known to elicit IgE-mediated reactions can provoke eczematous skin lesions in patients with atopic dermatitis. This so-called atopy patch test is increasingly applied to identify sensitized individuals who can benefit from avoidance measures. For house dust mite, cat dander, and grass pollen the test had a higher specificity with regard to clinical relevance than the prick test and radio-allergosorbent test.[33,34] Recently, the atopy patch test has also been claimed to be a useful tool for the diagnosis of

29. Przybilla B, Ruëff F (1997) Oraler Provokationstest. In: Diagnostische Verfahren in der Dermatologie, Korting HC, Sterry W, eds. Berlin: Blackwell, pp. 123–131.
30. White IR (2000) Allergic contact dermatitis. In: Textbook of Pediatric Dermatology, Harper J, Oranje A, Prose N, eds. Oxford: Blackwell, pp. 287–294.
31. Roul S, Ducombs G, Taïeb A (1999) Usefulness of the European standard series for patch testing in children. A 3-year single-center study of 337 patients. **Contact Dermatitis** 40:232–235.

32. Schnuch A, Martin V (1997) Epikutantest. In: Diagnostische Verfahren in der Dermatologie, Korting HC, Sterry W, eds. Berlin: Blackwell, pp. 99–116.
33. Darsow U, Vieluf D, Ring J (1999) Evaluating the relevance of aeroallergen sensitization in atopic eczema with the atopy patch test: a randomized, double-blind multicenter study. Atopy patch test group. **J Am Acad Dermatol** 40:187–193.
34. Darsow U, Ring J (2000) Airborne and dietary allergens in atopic eczema: a comprehensive review of diagnostic tests. **Clin Exp Dermatol** 25:544–551.

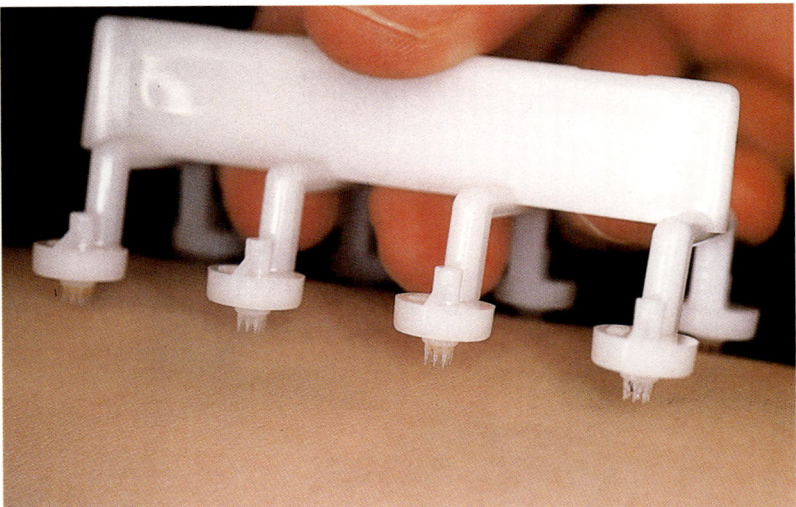

Fig. 3.36 **Delayed-type antigen test.** Disposable test stamp applied to the volar aspect of the forearm.

food allergy in children with atopic dermatitis.[35] Due to difficulties in standardization, the test has not yet entered clinical routine.

INTRADERMAL DELAYED-TYPE ANTIGEN TEST

Delayed-type hypersensitivity can be evoked by a variety of antigens, such as contact allergens and many microorganisms. It often represents the major immunologic defense mechanism in the development of acquired resistance to pathogens. Sensitization is mostly induced by standardized antigens that can be used for general determination of the actual cellular immune response. Intradermal injection of standard antigens often leads to a local reaction which usually reaches its maximum intensity after 48 hours. It consists of a sharply circumscribed area of erythema and induration. Disposable testing devices preloaded with 7 antigens (tetanus, diphtheria, streptococcus, tuberculin, candida, trichophyton, and proteus antigens) and a negative control are commercially available for intracutaneous application on the volar aspect of the forearm (Fig. 3.36). For calculation of the test result the mean diameters of the individual indurations are measured and added up 48 hours later. As T-cell immunity is still immature in infants under one year of age, testing in this age group would not only be painful but also meaningless. Examples of circumstances under which the cellular immune response may be temporarily depressed or even fail completely include the following:

- during or after a disease accompanied by fever (e.g., virus infection);
- after immunization with live vaccines (e.g., measles, rubella);
- during a treatment with corticosteroids or other immunosuppressive drugs;
- during or after radiation therapy;
- in septicemia;
- after major surgery or polytrauma

PHOTOTESTING

Phototesting may be indicated if the diagnosis of a photosensitive disorder cannot be made on the patient's history alone or if additional information is required for adequate treatment. In particular, it may be performed:

- to confirm a suspected diagnosis by provoking lesions,
- to establish the degree of photosensivity,
- to determine the action spectrum that provokes the lesions,
- to evaluate the effect of a treatment, and
- to follow the evolution of a photodermatosis over time.[36]

There are essentially three diagnostic methods suited to clarify a photosensitive condition:

- determination of the minimal erythema dose (MED),
- photoprovocation of pathologic lesions, and
- photopatch testing.

Minimal erythema dose (MED)

The MED is defined as the weakest dose necessary to induce a perceptible erythema 24 hours after ultraviolet (UV) light irradiation. For testing, six skin squares of 1.5×1.5cm on the sacral or gluteal area are irradiated with increasing doses of mono- or polychromatic UV-B and another six areas in a parallel row with polychromatic UV-A. UV-B doses are adjusted to the skin phototype of the patient (Table 3.8): doses of 25 to 150mJ/cm² for phototypes I and II, and doses of 75 to 200mJ/cm² for phototypes III and IV.[38] UV-A doses of 10 to 80J/cm² are applied irrespectively of the phototype. MEDs are read 24 hours after the test. In addition, the threshold dose of the immediate pigment darkening can be assessed straightaway after UV-A exposure and the minimal tanning dose 24 hours later.

Photoprovocation of pathologic lesions

The MEDs are only a rough measure of the sensitivity of a patient to UV rays, and their validity for the diagnosis of a photodermatosis is limited. For this purpose, photoprovocation tests are performed. Single provocations with 10, 30, and 60J/cm² UV-A (phototypes I and II) or 30, 60, and 100J/cm² UV-A (phototypes III and IV) each and with the 1.5-fold MED dose of UV-B are sufficient to induce photodermatoses which occur shortly after UV

TABLE 3.8 Skin phototypes according to Fitzpatrick, from Hornung[37]

Skin phototype	Skin color/characteristics	Reaction to sun exposure[a]
I	White/red hair, freckles	Always burns, never tans
II	White/light hair, blue eyes	Usually burns, sometimes tans
III	White/brown to light hair	Sometimes burns, usually tans
IV	Light brown	Minimally burns, always tans
V	Brown/brown to black hair	Rarely burns, tans profusely
VI	Dark brown or black	Never burns, tans deeply

[a] Based on the first significant (45–60min) sun exposure following an interval without sun exposure (e.g., the winter season).

35. Niggemann B, Reibel S, Wahn U (2000) The atopy patch test (APT) – a useful tool for the diagnosis of food allergy in children with atopic dermatitis. **Allergy** 55:281–285.
36. Roelandts R (2000) The diagnosis of photosensitivity. **Arch Dermatol** 136:1152–1157.
37. Hornung R (2000) Photoprotection. In: Textbook of Pediatric Dermatology, Harper J, Oranje A, Prose N, eds. Oxford: Blackwell, pp. 921–934.
38. Neumann NJ, Fritsch C, Lehmann P (2000) Photodiagnostische Testverfahren. Teil 1: Die Lichttreppe und der Photopatch-Test. **Hautarzt** 51:113–125.

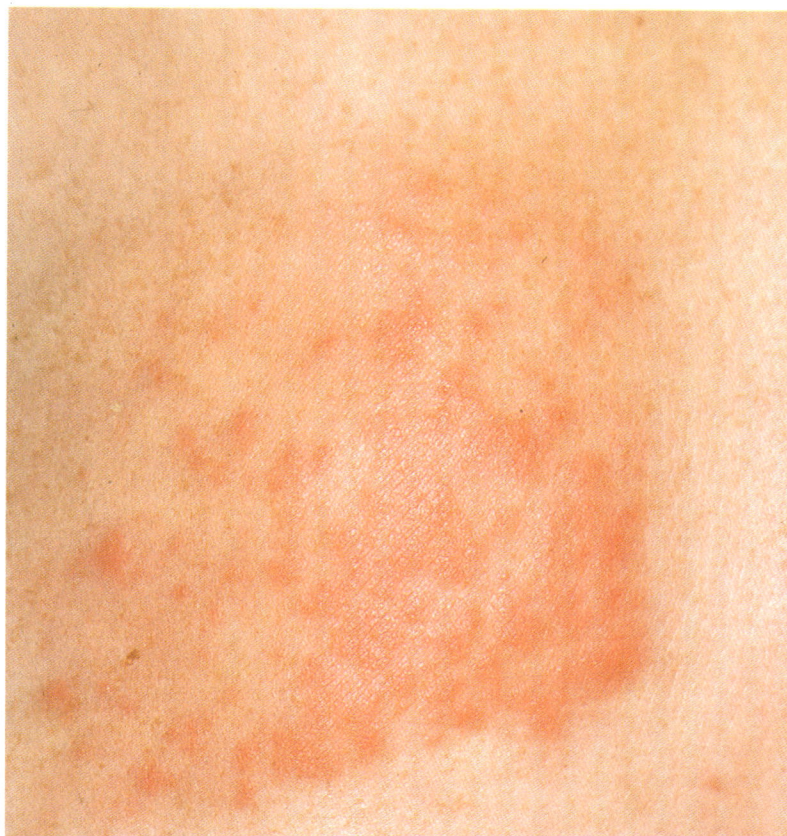

Fig. 3.37   Photoprovocation of subacute cutaneous lupus erythematosus one week after repeated UV-A exposure.

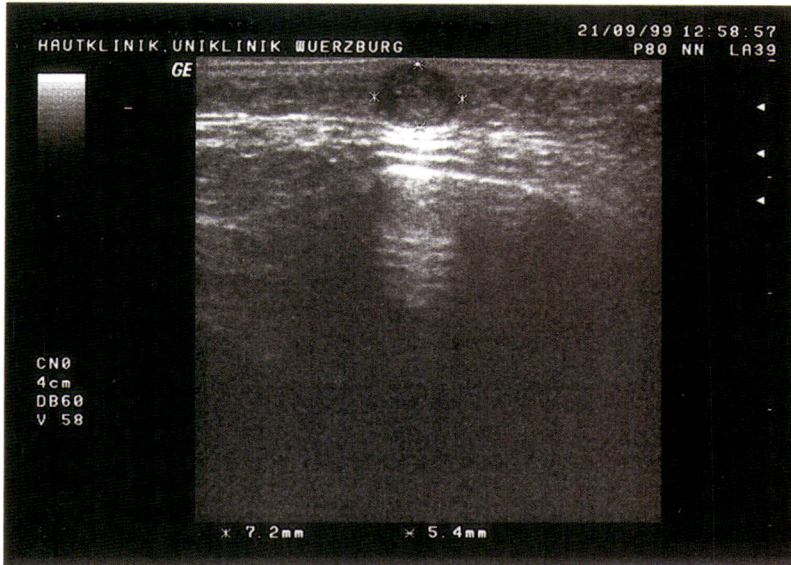

Fig. 3.38   A 13MHz sonographic picture of a pilomatricoma. The tumor is hypoechoic, ovally shaped, 7.2 × 5.4mm in size and shows dorsal echo enhancement.

exposure, such as solar urticaria, actinic prurigo, chronic actinic dermatitis, and erythropoetic protoporphyria.[39] Repeated photoprovocations on three consecutive days are performed if polymorphous light eruption, hydroa vacciniforme or lupus erythematosus (Fig. 3.37) are suspected.[36,39] Test protocols and times of reading may be modified according to the photodermatosis in question.[39] For example, it has to be considered that lupus erythematosus lesions may occur up to three weeks after photoprovocation.

Photopatch testing

The photopatch test is a diagnostic method for the detection of photosensitizing agents in patients with photodermatoses. Tedious attempts have been made to standardize this procedure.[40] A duplicate set of test substances is placed in small Finn chambers on aluminium disks, and the disks are fixed to the patient's back. The photopatch test material is removed after 24 hours, and the skin is irradiated with 10J/cm² UV-A (320–400nm). The test sites are evaluated before, immediately after, and 24, 48, and 72 hours after UV-A irradiation. The unirradiated control test sites are left on the skin for 24 or 48 hours and are read immediately after patch test removal, as well as 24, 48, and 72 hours later.[38,40] Test reactions are graded according to a 5-point scale as follows:

- 0 = no reaction;
- 1 = erythema;
- 2 = erythema and dermal infiltrate;
- 3 = erythema and papulovesicles; and
- 4 = erythema and blisters or erosions.

The interpretation of the patch test requires experience since contact reactions, phototoxic and photoallergic reactions have to be differentiated. Nonsteroidal anti-inflammatory drugs, disinfectants, phenothiazines, and UV filters represent the most common photoallergens, at least in central Europe.[38]

ULTRASOUND

Dermatosonography allows assessment of skin morphology at an intermediate level between clinical and microscopic examination.[41] It has become a standard diagnostic method, at least in Europe, since the advantages of a non-invasive, painless, in vivo imaging technique with relatively low costs are obvious. In dermatology, ultrasound essentially serves for detection and verification of tumors and other morphological changes in the skin, the subcutaneous tissue and in lymph node basins.[42]

The frequency of the ultrasound determines both penetration and resolution of the imaging system. Consequently, high frequencies over 20MHz are used for examination of the skin, whereas medium-sized frequencies between 7.5 and 15MHz are suited for subcutaneous lesions and lymph nodes. Most scans in routine use work in a so-called brightness mode (B-mode, B-scan) creating a two-dimensional image. Main applications of high-frequency sonography are tumors, inflammatory and sclerotic changes of the skin. The method does not allow a definite tumor diagnosis but is well suited for preoperative assessment of the thickness and size of a cutaneous tumor (Fig. 3.38).[41] In scleroderma, psoriasis, and dermatitis it can be used for follow-up recording of changes in the echogenicity and thickness of the dermis. Medium-sized frequencies allow determination of the exact position of a deep-dermal or subcutaneous tumor, the dimension of the lesion in two perpendicular diameters, the echo pattern, the distance from the skin surface, and the relation to surrounding anatomical structures.[42] Ultrasound is highly effective in discriminating roundish, hypoechoic to echo-free lymph node metastases and subcutaneous malignant lesions from longitudinally shaped, more hyperechoic innocent nodes. Another important indication is the assessment and monitoring of hemangiomas.

39. Lehmann P, Fritsch C, Neumann NJ (2000) Photodiagnostische Testverrfahren. Teil 2: Die Photoprovokationstestungen. **Hautarzt** 51:449–459.
40. Neumann NJ, Hölzle E, Plewig G et al. (2000) Photopatch testing: the 12-year experience of the German, Austrian, and Swiss photopatch test group. **J Am Acad Dermatol** 42:183–192.
41. Jemec GBE, Gniadecka M, Ulrich J (2000) Ultrasound in dermatology, part I. High frequency ultrasound. **Eur J Dermatol** 10:492–497.
42. Ulrich J, Voit C (2001) Ultrasound in dermatology, part II. Ultrasound of regional lymph node basins and subcutaneous tumours. **Eur J Dermatol** 11:73–79.

DIAGNOSTIC METHODS IN HAIR DISEASE

History taking and clinical examination of hair and scalp are of paramount importance in diagnosing hair disease. The physician has to pay attention to density, distribution, length, structure and color of the hair. If alopecia is evident, a diffuse form has to be differentiated from a focal type, and a scarring from a non-scarring type. For detailed examination, there are quite a number of diagnostic aids to evaluate hair loss, hair growth and hair abnormalities.

Hair counts

To objectify the assumption of excessive hair loss, patients or parents may be advised to collect all shed hairs over a period of 10–14 consecutive days in a clear plastic sandwich bag. Of course, hairs that fall out during combing and washing have to be included. At the end of the period all hairs are counted and divided by the number of days. Daily loss should not exceed 100 hairs.

Hair pull test

This clinical test allows a gross estimate of the quantity of hair loss. Sixty adjacent hairs are counted and grasped with thumb and index finger close to the scalp. A slow constant moderate tension is exerted while moving the fingers towards the distal ends of the hair shafts. The procedure is repeated in 2–3 other areas. More than six epilated hairs per area is suggestive of increased hair loss.[24] The hair bulbs can be examined under a magnifying glass or a light microscope to differentiate telogen from anagen hairs.

Hair feathering

If abnormal fragility of the ends of the hairs is suspected, such as in trichorrhexis nodosa, the distal 2–3cm of the hairs are grasped between thumb and index finger and the fingers are briskly pulled to the tips of the hair. After repeating the procedure in other affected areas the finger tips are examined. Presence of short hair fragments indicates hair shaft abnormality with increased friability.[24]

PART WIDTH ASSESSMENT
A series of parts over the vertex, the occipital and temporal scalp made with the patient's comb reveals the overall density of the scalp hair.

Hair growth window

This simple test, suited to record the hair growth rate, is indicated in factitial hair loss, as trichotillomania, and in complaints of slow growth or hair loss without regrowth. The hairs in a 2 × 2cm square area of the scalp are cut short and subsequently shaved. This "hair growth window" is covered with an occlusive dressing to avoid manipulation by the patient. One week later, the dressing is removed by the physician and the length of the regrowing hair is measured with a ruler or caliper. Measurements can be repeated in weekly intervals. Normal hair growth is at least 2.5mm for one week and 1cm for one month.[24]

Trichogram

The trichogram or hair pluck is a semi-invasive method widely used to objectify and differentiate several types of hair loss. In childhood, it essentially serves to diagnose anagen-dystrophic and telogen effluvium, loose anagen syndrome, and trichotillomania. As the method is painful it should be well indicated, especially in children. Four to five days after the last hair wash, 50–60 hairs in a row are firmly clamped with the rubber-armed tips of a robust hemostat or surgical needle holder as close to the scalp as possible. Subsequently, they are briskly plucked out of the scalp in hair growth direction.[24,43] The distal ends of the hairs are cut off, the bulb ends are placed on a microscope slide and prepared for examination. In diffuse effluvium or alopecia, a frontal and an occipital standard epilation site 2cm

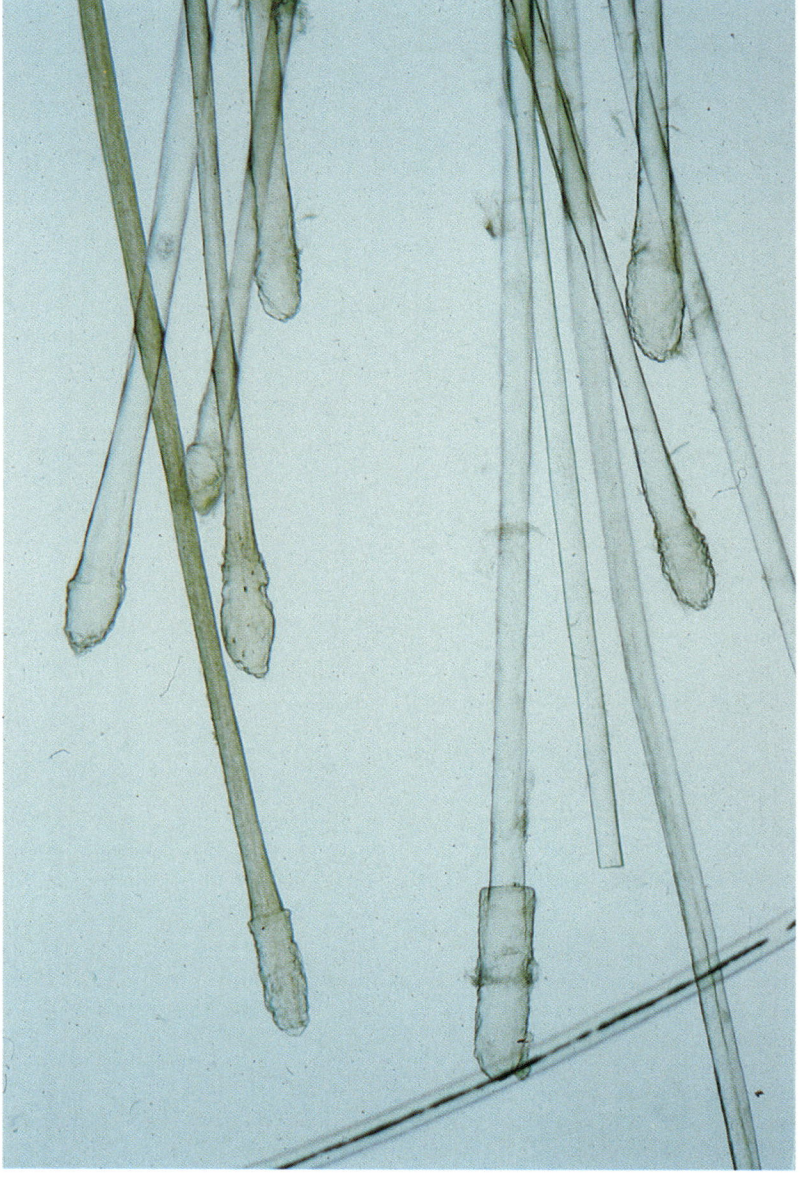

Fig. 3.39 Trichogram showing telogen hair bulbs in telogen effluvium. × 50.

from the midline are chosen for sampling; in focal alopecia, hairs are plucked from the margin of an active lesion and from the normal-appearing contralateral side.

The hair roots are assigned to the anagen, telogen and catagen phase of hair growth under the light microscope. Normal counts are around 85–90% anagen hairs, 10–15% telogen hairs (Fig. 3.39), and 0–2% catagen hairs. So-called dystrophic hairs point to serious damage of the hair or to inappropriate pluck technique. Some characteristic trichogram findings are summarized in Table 3.9.

Phototrichogram

This elegant non-invasive technique allows the *in vivo* determination of the anagen/telogen ratio with greater reliability than the ordinary trichogram.[44] It can also provide information about total hair density and thickness of the hair shafts. The same area of the scalp can be re-examined often. Due to the

43. Barth JH, Messenger AG (1997) Measurement of hair growth and investigation of hair disease. In: Diseases of the Hair and Scalp, 3rd edn, Dawber R, ed. Oxford: Blackwell, pp. 564–579.

44. D'Amico D, Vaccaro M, Guarneri F et al. (2001) Phototrichogram using videomicroscopy: a useful technique in the evaluation of scalp hair. **Eur J Dermatol** 11:17–20.

TABLE 3.9   Characteristic trichogram patterns in some important hair diseases of childhood and adolescence

Diagnosis	Trichogram findings
Alopecia areata	Dystrophic hairs and/or raised telogen rate at margin of an active lesion (not diagnostic)
Androgenetic alopecia, androgenetic effluvium	Raised telogen rate on frontal epilation site, normal anagen/telogen ratio on occipital epilation site
Anagen-dystrophic effluvium	Many dystrophic hairs on frontal and occipital epilation site
Telogen effluvium	Raised telogen rate on frontal and occipital epilation site
Loose anagen syndrome	Almost only anagen hairs without inner root sheath on frontal and occipital epilation site
Trichotillomania	Almost only anagen hairs with often preserved inner root sheath at margin of an active lesion

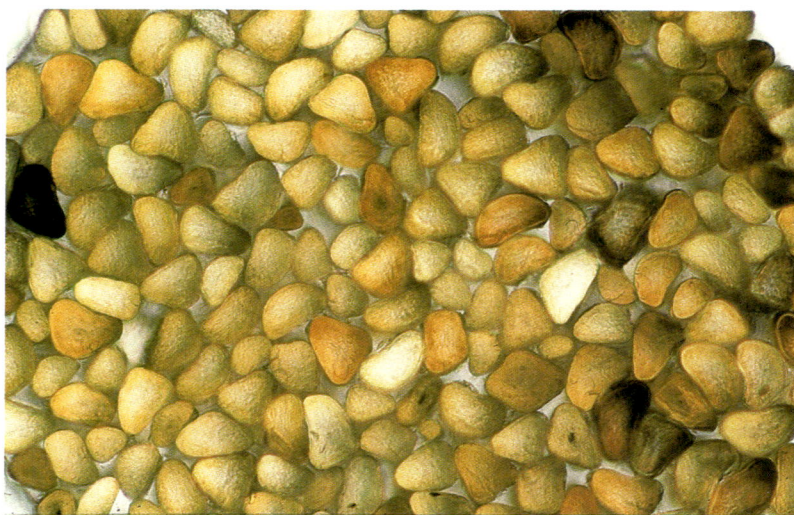

Fig. 3.41   **Shrinking tube technique**. Many cross-sections of hair fibers show triangular shapes, as typical for uncombable hair syndrome. × 50.

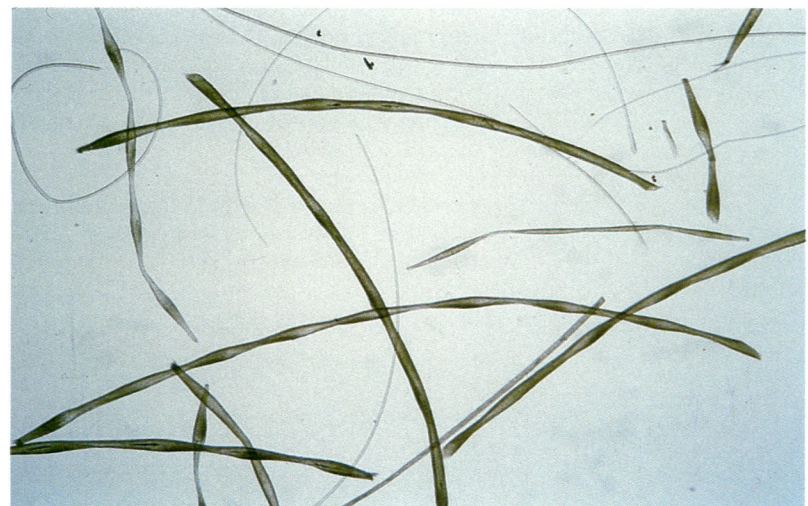

Fig. 3.40   **Light microscopy of hair shafts**. The sample shows variations of shaft diameters in regular intervals characteristic for monilethrix. × 25.

high cost of videomicroscope and computer-assisted image analysis, it is mainly used for trichologic studies.

Light microscopic evaluation of hair shafts

Light microscopy is of utmost importance in the diagnosis of structural abnormalities of the hair shaft. For this purpose, it is essential to cut the hairs from involved areas as close to the scalp as possible. Short hairs have to be sampled with a razor. The hairs are placed on microscope slides, embedded in a suited medium, such as Eukitt®, and examined along their entire length under low and, if conspicuous, under high power.[24] Fractures and diameter variations (Fig. 3.40) are more easily noticed than slight longitudinal torsions or irregular shapes. Moreover, the light microscope serves to examine the hair root morphology of trichogram and shed hairs and the distal tip morphology (tapered tips, cut ends, or split ends).

Polarizing light microscopic evaluation of hair shafts

For this, the light microscope has to be fitted with polarizing lenses that are permanently turned during microscopic examination. The most important indication is the proof of short, alternating dark and bright bands (tiger tail pattern) in sulfur-deficient hairs in trichothiodystrophy.

Shrinking tube technique

The purpose of this rather simple but little-known method is to study cross-configurations of hair shafts in a larger sample (Fig. 3.41). Hair tufts are pulled into a plastic tube of small caliber. On heating, the tube begins to shrink which fixes the hair fibers. After reaching room temperature again, thin cross-sections of 0.1 to 0.2mm thickness are cut with the aid of a razor blade and mounted on a glass microscope slide. Usually, more than 90% of hair shafts show oval or round shapes.[45]

Scanning electron microscopic evaluation of hair shafts

Scanning electron microscopy of hair shafts allows a more accurate three-dimensional view on abnormalities of the configuration and the cuticula of individual hair shafts. It is reserved for scientific questions.

SWEAT TESTING

The Minor iodine-starch test is used to visualize an area of hyperhidrosis or to prove absence or abnormal distribution of sweat glands. After cleaning the skin, a solution containing 2g of iodine in 10ml of castor oil and 90ml of ethanol is painted with large cotton wool swabs onto the test area. After drying of the solution, potato starch powder is uniformly sprinkled onto the area with a fine sieve. Sweat causes the mixture to turn dark blue. For quantification, the sweat production in a defined time interval is assessed gravimetrically. For this purpose, a filter paper is weighed on an electronic precision scale, placed on the dried test area and re-weighed immediately after the test period (usually 1 to 5 minutes). The weight difference is taken as the amount of sweat secreted during the collection period.

In females affected with X-linked hypohidrotic ectodermal dysplasia, sweat testing on the back discloses alternately sweating and non-sweating areas following the lines of Blaschko (Fig. 3.42).

45. Hamm H, Traupe H (1989) Loose anagen hair of childhood: The phenomenon of easily pluckable hair. **J Am Acad Dermatol** 20:242–248.

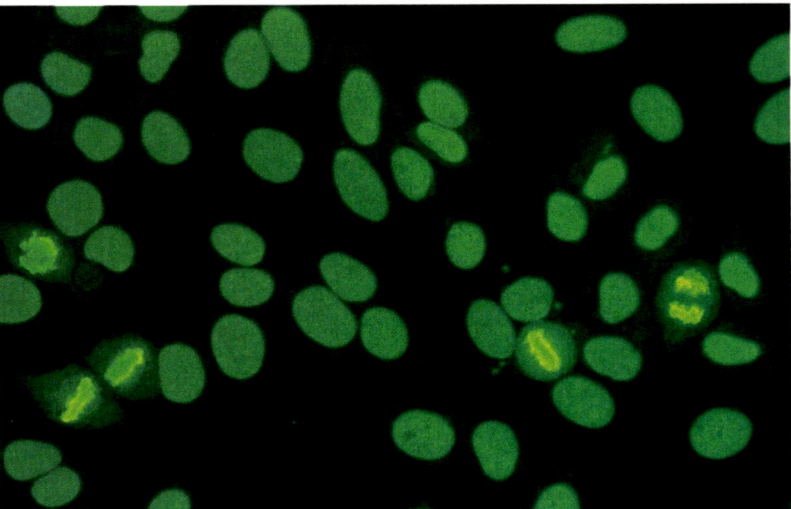

Fig. 3.42 **Minor iodine-starch test for detection of sweat glands.** Alternately sweating and non-sweating streaks following the lines of Blaschko on the back of a female with X-linked hypohidrotic ectodermal dysplasia.

Fig. 3.43 **Detection of antinuclear antibodies by indirect immunofluorescence on HEp-2 cells.** Nuclei are homogeneously stained (homogeneous pattern). Some of them show mitoses in different stages. × 400.

LABORATORY TESTS

Clinical chemistry

Clinical chemical assays are almost exclusively performed on serum or plasma. Serum is obtained from spontaneously coagulated whole blood, plasma via the addition of anticoagulants, such as ethylene diamine tetra-acetate (EDTA), citrate, oxalate, and heparinate. Differences between serum and plasma are generally only observed in the determination of potassium, inorganic phosphate, lactate dehydrogenase, and in electrophoresis of fibrinogen. Since the rate of glycolysis is around 7% per hour, a glycolysis inhibitor, e.g., sodium fluoride, mannose or iodoacetate, must be added to the blood sample prior to determination of the glucose concentration. Centrifugation should generally take place no more than one hour after sample collection. Compared to the values of adults, the reference values of almost all parameters are different in children.[46]

Hematology

In the vast majority of hematological analyses venous blood treated with EDTA is used. In isolated cases, EDTA-induced pseudothrombocytopenia can develop which is of no clinical significance. Use of citrated blood returns cell numbers to normal. Blood treated with EDTA cannot be used for coagulation assays since these substances may cause more rapid inactivation of clotting factors V and VIII, for example.

Serology

A wide variety of assays is available for the detection of antibodies to infectious agents. All these assays make use of a similar basic reaction, namely the binding of the patient's immunoglobulin to a defined microbiological antigen. Current assay methods vary considerably in their ability to detect specific antibodies and in their sensitivity and specificity. In general, the solid-phase enzyme immunoassays, also known as *enzyme-linked immunosorbent assays* (ELISA, EIA), offer the highest degree of sensitivity and specificity. Older techniques, such as complement fixation, agglutination, and immunofluorescence, are also very common but less sensitive.

Antinuclear antibodies (ANA)

ANA are a group of antibodies that react with various nuclear antigens, e.g., DNA, RNA, desoxyribonucleoprotein, smooth muscle antigen, and many others. The determination of ANA is a screening test and is mainly performed in the serum of patients by fluorescent antibody techniques using HEp-2 cells (a human laryngeal cell line) as human standard substrate.[47] ANA are found in most patients with systemic lupus erythematosus (SLE) but also in many other collagen vascular and connective tissue diseases, including juvenile rheumatoid arthritis, dermatomyositis, and progressive systemic scleroderma (PSS). Important to emphasize, ANA are neither entirely diagnostic nor specific for any of these diseases. They are found in 10% of the general population.

Some distinct patterns of ANA can be differentiated:

- The often non-specific *speckled pattern* shows minute points of fluorescence scattered all over the nucleus;
- in the *homogeneous pattern*, which is often seen in patients with SLE, the nuclei are stained all over (Fig. 3.43);
- the *nucleolar pattern* commonly detected in patients with PSS shows uniform staining of each nucleolus; and
- the *peripheral pattern* is associated with the presence of anti-nDNA antibodies.[47]

A significant ANA titer in children should prompt complete history taking and clinical examination in combination with complementary serologic tests. For example, serum should be tested for the presence of double-stranded DNA antibodies which are highly specific for SLE.

Radioallergosorbent test (RAST)

As an alternative or supplement to skin testing, the RAST measures specific serum IgE antibodies to a particular antigen.[48] Today, it is mostly performed with purified allergen attached to a solid-phase immunosorbent which is usually a cellulose disc. However, a negative RAST does not exclude the possibility of anaphylactic reactions to certain allergens. Specific IgE antibodies to house dust mites, pollen, or animal hair proteins can be ruled out with this test.

46. Heil W, Koberstein R, Zawta B (1997) Reference ranges for adults and children. Pre-analytical considerations. Mannheim: Boehringer.

47. Casiano CA, Tan EM (1996) Recent developments in the understanding of antinuclear autoantibodies. **Int Arch Allergy Immunol** 111:308–313.

48. Ishizaka K, Ishizaka T (1978) Mechanisms of reaginic hypersensitivity and IgE antibody response. **Immunol Rev** 41:109–148.

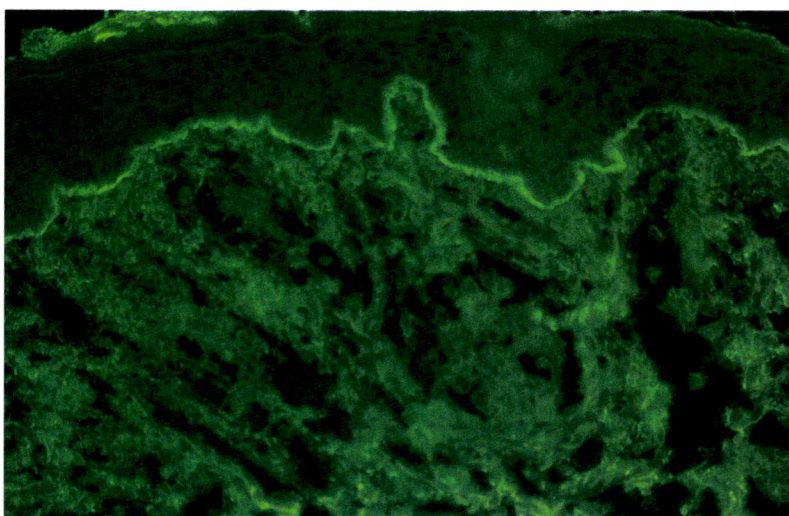

Fig. 3.44 Direct immunofluorescence demonstrating linear IgA deposits in linear IgA disease (Courtesy of D. Zillikens, Würzburg). × 160.

IMMUNOFLUORESCENCE MICROSCOPY

Immunofluorescence (IF) microscopy is a laboratory technique for demonstrating the presence of antibodies in tissues or body fluids.[49] It has become indispensable in the diagnosis of autoimmune, especially bullous dermatoses. Two basic types of IF techniques can be distinguished: direct IF and indirect IF microscopy.

Direct immunofluorescence microscopy

This one-step procedure serves to detect antibodies bound to tissue *in vivo*.[49,50] The substrate of the test is a skin biopsy of the patient. The most suitable site of the biopsy depends on the disease under evaluation. For example, the biopsy should be taken from normal-appearing skin adjacent to a blister in autoimmune bullous dermatoses, such as linear IgA disease, and from an early erythematous or purpuric lesion in Schönlein-Henoch purpura. If direct IF microscopy is performed at the institution where the biopsy is taken, it should be immediately snap-frozen in liquid nitrogen and stored at −70° until used. Otherwise, it is placed in a special liquid fixative (Michel's medium), which prevents degradation of tissue including immunoreactants,[51] and sent at ambient temperature to a specialized laboratory. On processing, cryostat sections of the biopsy specimen are incubated with fluorescein-labeled antibodies against human immunoglobulins G, A, and M, complement C3, and fibrinogen. Sections are read under the fluorescent microscope where the sites of the antigen can be identified from the apple-green color of the fluorescein (Fig. 3.44).[49,50] Table 3.10 gives some examples of typical direct IF microscopy patterns in various dermatoses.

Indirect immunofluorescence microscopy

Unlike direct IF microscopy, indirect IF microscopy is a two-step serologic test for the detection of circulating autoantibodies in serum or other fluid.[49,50] Sera to be analysed by indirect IF microscopy can be sent by regular mail without freezing or special preservatives; they are stored at +4°C until examined. Normal tissue, preferably monkey esophagus and normal human skin, is used as substrate. Frozen sections of tissue substrate are placed on microscope slides and incubated with serially diluted patient's serum so that the antibodies can bind to the normal tissue components of the substrate. Subsequently, specimens are washed to remove excess antibodies that are not specifically bound, reincubated with fluorescein-labeled antihuman immunoglobulin or complement, and washed again. The binding sites are identified under the fluorescence microscope. Typical findings are summarized in Table 3.10. Usually, antibody reactivity is expressed as serum titers. The titer is the highest dilution of serum still resulting in a detectable labeling of the antibody.[49]

Complement indirect immunofluorescence microscopy

This three-step technique is a modification of indirect IF microscopy suited for demonstrating whether circulating antibodies in the patient's serum are capable of binding complement.[49,50] It may be more sensitive than common IIF and is used particularly in the diagnostic of pemphigoid gestationis.

Split-skin indirect immunofluorescence microscopy technique

This indirect IF microscopy method is used for differentiation of acquired bullous dermatoses with circulating IgG antibodies against antigens of the

TABLE 3.10   Typical patterns of direct and indirect immunofluorescence microscopy in some important dermatoses

Disease	Direct immunofluorescence	Indirect immunofluorescence
Pemphigus vulgaris	Intercellular IgG, C3	Intercellular IgG, C3
Bullous pemphigoid	Linear IgG, C3 at BMZ	Linear IgG, C3 at BMZ
Dermatitis herpetiformis	Granular IgA in dermal papillae	IgA antibodies to endomysium
Linear IgA disease	Linear IgA at BMZ	Linear IgA at BMZ
Schönlein-Henoch purpura	IgA, C3 and fibrinogen at superficial and deep dermal vessels	Negative
Lichen planus	Colloid bodies coated with IgM; fibrinogen at BMZ	Negative
Discoid lupus erythematosus	Granular or linear IgG, IgM, IgA, or C3 at BMZ	Negative
Subacute cutaneous lupus erythematosus Systemic lupus erythematosus	Granular IgG, IgM, C3, fibrinogen at BMZ Linear IgG, IgM, C3 at BMZ	Ro/SSA, La/SSB High titer of antinuclear antibodies

BMZ: basement membrane zone

49. Dahl MV (1996) Immunofluorescence in dermatology. In: Clinical Immunodermatology. St. Louis: Mosby, pp. 417–445.
50. Bhogal BS, Black MM (1990) Diagnosis, diagnostic and research techniques. In: Management of Blistering Diseases, Wojnarowska F, Briggaman RA, eds. London: Chapman and Hall, pp. 15–34.
51. Mutasim DF, Pelc NJ, Supapannachart N (1993) Established methods in the investigation of bullous diseases. **Dermatol Clin** 11:399–418.

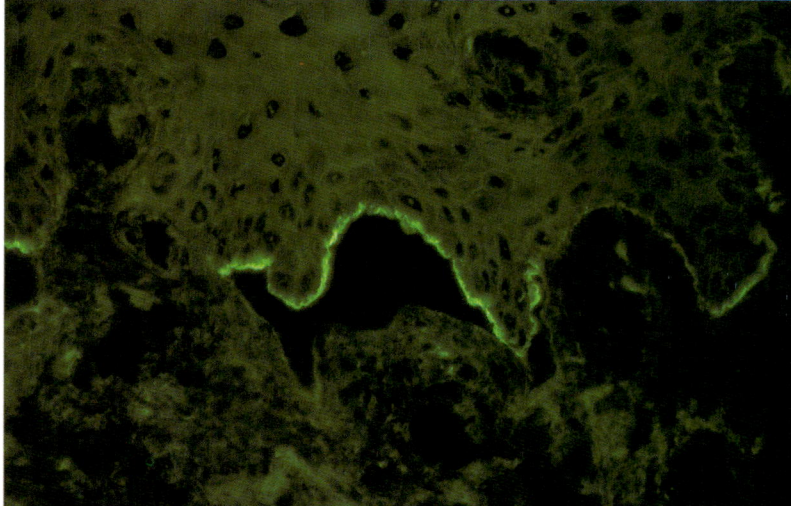

Fig. 3.45 Indirect immunofluorescence visualizing binding of circulating IgA antibodies of the patient to the epidermal roof of a split-skin cleavage in linear IgA disease (Courtesy of D. Zillikens, Würzburg). × 400.

TABLE 3.11 Staining patterns of antibodies to bullous pemphigoid antigen 180 (BP 180) and type IV collagen in the three major types of epidermolysis bullosa (EB)

EB type	Binding pattern of antibody to	
	BP 180	Type IV collagen
EB simplex	Floor	Floor
Junctional EB	Roof	Floor
Dystrophic EB	Roof	Roof

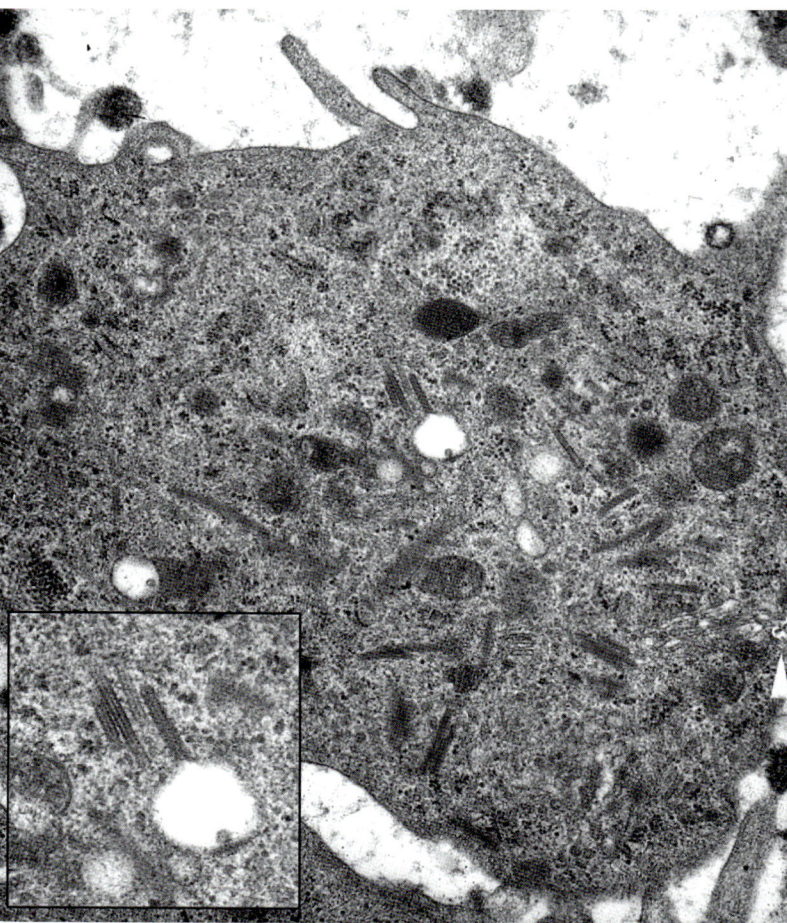

Fig. 3.46 **Electron microscopy**. Detection of Birbeck granules in the cytoplasm of a Langerhans cell in Langerhans cell histiocytosis. × 18 000.

basement membrane zone. Split skin with the plane of cleavage in the lamina lucida is produced by incubation with cold 1M NaCl solution and then used as a substrate for the IIF technique (Fig. 3.45). Antibodies in bullous pemphigoid, pemphigoid gestationis, and in a subgroup of cicatrical pemphigoid bind to the epidermal roof of the split whereas antibodies to type VII collagen or laminin 5 in epidermolysis bullosa acquisita or in another subgroup of cicatrical pemphigoid bind to the dermal side.[50]

Antigen mapping

This rapid, elegant IF microscopy method serves to assign an inherited bullous disease to one of the three main types of epidermolysis bullosa (EB), namely EB simplex, junctional EB, and dystrophic EB. Sections of an excisional skin biopsy of a freshly induced blister are stained with mono- or polyclonal antibodies against bullous pemphigoid antigen, laminin 5, and type IV collagen. The level of blister formation and, thus, the EB type can be determined by evaluation of whether a given reagent stains the roof or the floor of the blister (Table 3.11).[49]

ELECTRON MICROSCOPY

Electron microscopic examination is a sumptuous method requiring great experience in preparation and evaluation. It is not available in most dermatology departments and, therefore, is not suited for routine use. However,

it may be extremely helpful in the diagnostics of some special questions. These mainly include:

- the rapid diagnosis of infections by herpes, parapox, and orthopox viruses through negative-contrast staining;
- the definite diagnosis of Langerhans cell histiocytosis by proof of Birbeck granula in the cytoplasm of histiocytic cells (Fig. 3.46);
- important contribution in the diagnosis of many genodermatoses, such as epidermolysis bullosa, ichthyoses, collagen and storage diseases.[52]

MOLECULAR METHODS

In situ hybridization

In situ hybridization techniques allow specific nucleic acid sequences to be detected in morphologically preserved chromosomes, cells or tissue sections.[53,54] In combination with immunocytochemistry, *in situ* hybridization can give microscopic topological information about gene activity at the DNA, mRNA, and protein level. Though gene probe hybridization technology is capable of detecting as few as about 10^3 pathogens (e.g., viruses or bacteria), there was still an urgent need to detect even lower numbers of target organisms. The advantage of nucleic acid amplification tests (e.g., polymerase chain reaction or ligase chain reaction) is the potential ability to detect very low amounts of specific target DNA in the midst of a large number of non-target sequences within a short period of time.

52. Schaller M, Korting HC (1997) Elektronenmikroskopie. In: Diagnostische Verfahren in der Dermatologie, Korting HC, Sterry W, eds. Berlin: Blackwell, pp. 177–181.
53. Reischl U, Wolf H (1998) The use of molecular methods in infectious diseases. **Biotest Bulletin** 6:3–20.
54. Pardue ML, Gall JG (1969) Molecular hybridisation of radioactive DNA to the DNA of cytological preparations. **Proc Natl Acad Sci USA** 64:600–604.

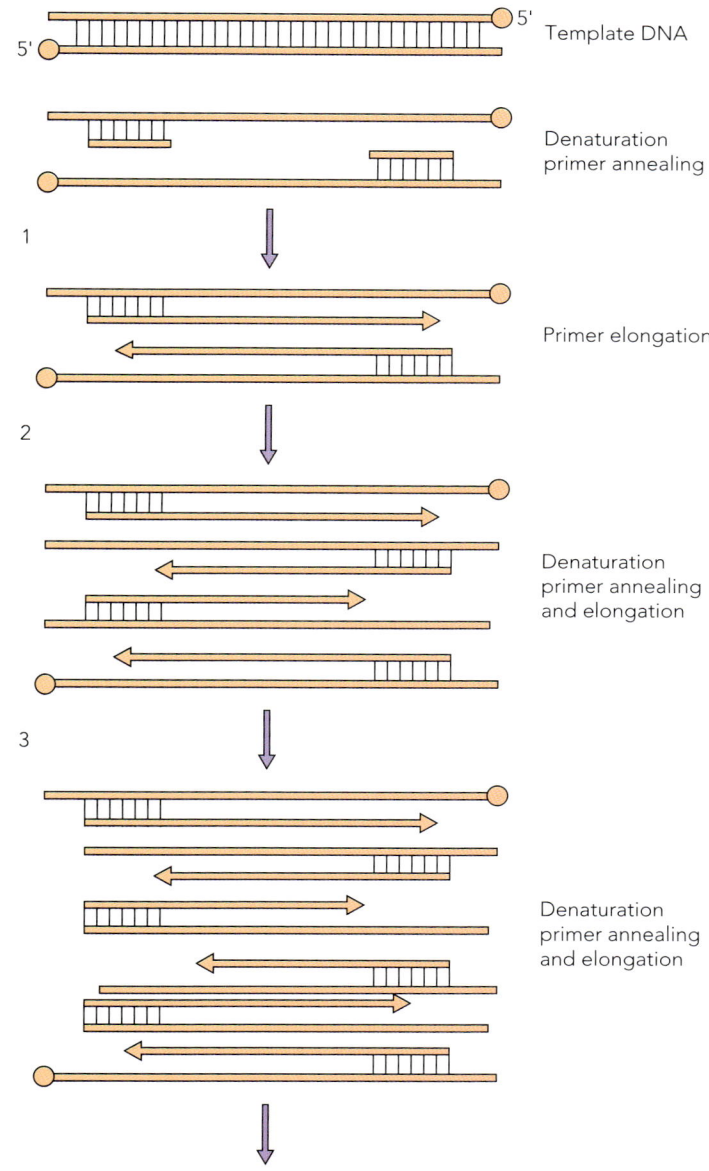

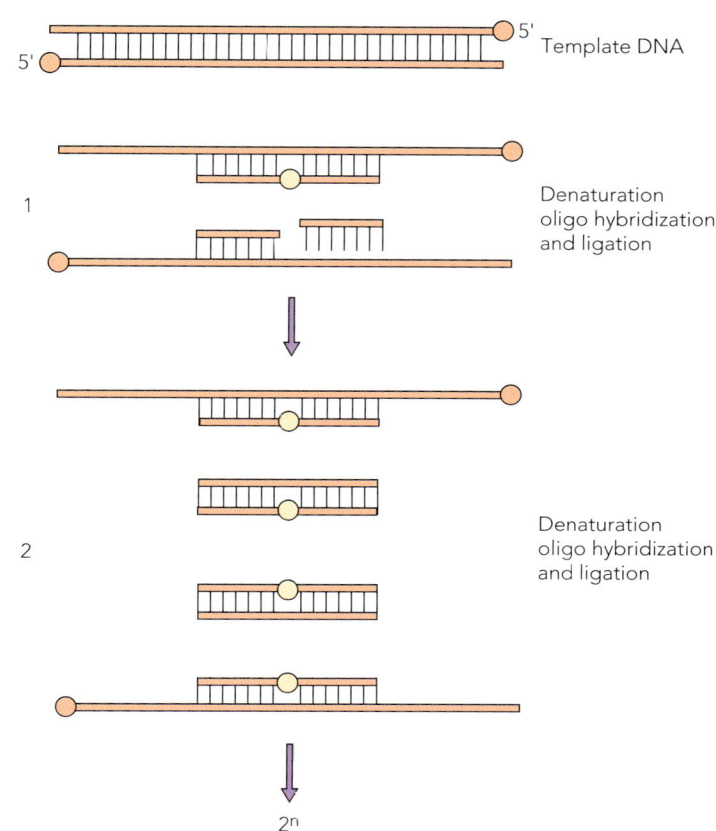

Fig. 3.47   Polymerase chain reaction (PCR). PCR uses a thermostable DNA polymerase to amplify a specific target segment of the DNA defined at each end by a specific primer.

Fig. 3.48   Ligase chain reaction (LCR). LCR uses a thermostable DNA ligase to link two adjacent oligonucleotide probes on each strand of the target DNA.

Polymerase chain reaction (PCR)

The PCR is an *in vitro* technique for enzymatically synthesizing defined sequences of DNA. For example, it can be used to find very low quantities of an infectious agent present in clinical samples by exponentially increasing the quantity of a specific nucleotide sequence of the pathogen.[55] The patented PCR technology uses two primers that hybridize to opposite strands and flank the target DNA sequence to be amplified. The primer pair consists of short oligonucleotides (15–25 bases) chosen from known nucleic acid sequences of the target and corresponding to complementary DNA strands. The elongation of the primers is catalyzed by a heat-stable DNA polymerase, such as Taq DNA polymerase. The reaction is accomplished by a series of temperature changes that consist mainly of three steps (Fig. 3.47):

● *denaturation* (DNA strand separation at 95°C);
● *annealing* (primer attachment to a complementary strand at 55–60°C); and
● *extension* (3'-DNA strand synthesis starting at the 5'–3'-end of each primer molecule at 72°C).

Because the primer extension products synthesized in a given cycle can serve as a template in the next cycle, the number of target DNA copies approximately doubles every cycle. Thus, 20 cycles of PCR yield about a million copies (2^{20}) of the target DNA. Detection of the amplificate is mostly performed by hybridization with labeled probes. Recently, ultra-rapid real-time cycling techniques, such as the LightCycler System™ (Roche Molecular Biochemicals), have been developed to complete PCR in 20 minutes due to very rapid air heating and cooling.

Ligase chain reaction (LCR)

The LCR is another technique for detecting or amplifying a target sequence. Unlike PCR, LCR uses a thermostable DNA ligase to link two adjacent oligonucleotide probes on each strand of the target DNA.[53,55] After ligation and denaturation, the joined fragments serve as templates for further rounds of thermocyclic amplification which, like in PCR, proceeds exponentially (Fig. 3.48). In clinical tests (e.g., Abbott LCx™ Probe System) capture and detection ligands are attached to the opposite ends of probe fragments so that only ligated products are both captured and detected. Current applications include the direct detection of *Mycobacterium tuberculosis*, *Neisseria gonorrhoae* and *Chlamydia trachomatis* in clinical specimens.

PRENATAL DIAGNOSIS

Prenatal diagnosis in pregnancies at particular risk for recurrence of severe hereditary skin diseases, such as severe types of epidermolysis bullosa and ichthyosis, started in the early 1980s by submitting mid-trimester fetal skin biopsies to ultrastructural and immunohistological evaluation. In the last decade remarkable progress has been made in elucidating the molecular basis

55. Reischl U, Mayer J (1993) Modern methods in nucleic acid-based diagnostics. **Lab Med** 17:456–464.

of many genodermatoses. As a result, DNA-based prenatal diagnosis in chorionic villus samples during the first trimester of pregnancy has become available for more and more inherited conditions.[56,57] More recently, pre-implantation diagnosis has become possible using *in vitro* fertilization techniques. In this case, DNA analysis is performed from a blastomere biopsy of the 6–10-cell embryo, thereby avoiding the need for later termination of a fetus found to be affected by conventional methods.[56] Of course, the severity of the clinical phenotype has to justify the effort of prenatal diagnosis, and the parents should be willing to bear the consequences of positive results. The current status of prenatal diagnosis is discussed in more detail in the chapter on neonatal skin disorders.

56. Shimizu H, Suzumori K (1999) Prenatal diagnosis as a test for genodermatoses: its past, present and future. **J Dermatol Sci** 19:1–8.

57. Ashton GH, Eady RA, McGrath JA (2000) Prenatal diagnosis for inherited skin diseases. **Clin Dermatol** 18:643–648.

Principles of Treatment in Pediatric Dermatology

CHAPTER 4

Elaine Siegfried, Amy Jo Nopper, Zoe Draelos, Alanna Bree,

Stephanie Swords and Stephen J. Lauer

TOPICAL TREATMENT

Elaine Siegfried and Alanna Bree

INTRODUCTION

Each physician's approach to therapy is tailored to the individual patient based on collective experience and accumulated research data. Unfortunately, accumulated research data have been less than adequate for pediatric patients. Children have been referred to as "therapeutic orphans" because the majority of commercially available medications have never been studied in pediatric patients, and clinical trials for new drugs are also limited in this age group.[1,2] This chapter is an introduction to the basic principles of dermatologic treatment for children, intrinsically biased by the personal experiences of the authors.

For hundreds of years, until more specific pharmacologic agents became available, variations of salicylic acid, zinc oxide, tar, sulfur, phenol, mercury, boric acid and iodine were the mainstays of therapy for a wide variety of skin problems. The therapeutic and safety profiles of many of these older drugs have not been subjected to the rigorous scrutiny required for today's approval by the United States Food and Drug Administration (FDA). Long-term and widespread use confer a degree of confidence for a few of these compounds, but many have been responsible for under-appreciated toxicity in vulnerable infants.[3]

Newer approaches to treatment are so much more effective and specific that old cliches have lost their meanings: "If it's wet, dry it…" is still true, but the improved dermatologic armamentarium now includes a variety of topical and systemic antibacterials, antifungals, antivirals, retinoids, vitamin D analogs, corticosteroids and a host of nonsteroidal biologic immune response modifiers.

Making the correct diagnosis is the most important step in prescribing effective treatment. The wrong treatment will not only fail to improve the primary problem but may also cause side effects that can further complicate the process.

GUIDELINES FOR AGE-APPROPRIATE TREATMENT OF PEDIATRIC PATIENTS

Pediatricians are well aware that children are not merely "small adults." Their presentation and spectrum of diseases as well as range of treatment options and responses to medical intervention are unique. For practitioners who have not received specific training in pediatrics, we present guidelines for evaluating and treating children and for educating their parents.

HIGHLIGHTS OF THE HISTORY

Almost all children are accompanied by a caregiver; usually a parent. Although the primary focus of the visit is the child and his or her dermatologic problem, the physician's relationship with each caregiver is an important component of the therapeutic process. It must be recognized that many parents have anxiety and guilt about possible contributions to the child's problem. Physicians should avoid accusatory questions; open-ended questions are nonthreatening and leave options that may help clarify the chief complaint. For example, for problems that seem subtle or ill-defined, the question, "What bothers you the most about this?" will often reveal essential background information. A child whose parents are at ease will usually feel secure. However, the physician must also establish a good rapport with the child. The type of interaction should be age appropriate[4] (Table 4.1).

Taking the time to become familiar with the broad range of parents' and children's responses to a routine history and physical examination will also help the physician recognize abnormal responses. This skill is critical when suspicions of abuse or neglect are raised.

HIGHLIGHTS OF THE PHYSICAL EXAMINATION

The most reliable indicators of a child's well-being are normal growth and development. Updated, standardized growth charts for infants and children are available through the Centers for Disease Control (http://www.cdc.gov/growthcharts/). Height, weight and head circumference are easily obtained and are extremely useful health parameters. Growth charting is mandatory for children receiving prolonged courses of corticosteroids (topical or systemic), cytotoxic agents or immunomodulating drugs. Monitoring for accelerated growth, as a sign of precocious puberty, is important in children with early onset acne. Age-related milestones for fine motor skills, gross motor skills, expressive and receptive language, problem-solving and psychosocial development have also been defined for children up to 6 years of age. The most widely used assessment is the Denver II Developmental Test.[5] This easy-to-administer screening tool is only one of several such development tests, all of which have inherent shortcomings.[6] The main criticism of the original Denver Developmental Screening Test was its emphasis on motor, rather than

1. Blumer JL (ed.) (1999) The Therapeutic Orphan. A Joint Conference of the Pediatric Pharmacology Research Unit Network, the European Society of Developmental Pharmacology, and the National Institute of Child Health and Human Development, held in Washington DC May 2 1997. **Pediatrics** 104(3):581–645.
2. Rowell M, Zlotkin S (1997) The ethical boundaries of drug research in pediatrics. **Pediatr Clin North Am** 1997 Feb; 44(1):27–40.
3. Spray A, Siegfried E (2001) Dermatologic toxicology in children. **Pediatr Ann** 30(4):197–202.
4. Piedalue RJ, Millnes A (1990) An overview of non-pharmacological pedodontic behaviour management techniques for the general practitioner. **Can Dent Assoc J** 56:137.
5. Frankenburg WK, Dodds J, Archer P, et al. (1992) The Denver II: a major revision and restandardization of the Denver Development screening test. **Pediatrics** 89:91.
6. Adesman A (1992) Is the Denver II Developmental Test worthwhile? **Pediatrics** 90:1009.

TABLE 4.1   Age-appropriate interactions with children

Age	Age-appropriate behaviors	Interview/examination techniques	Procedure techniques
<6mo	Watches faces	Approach slowly	Allow parents to hold, and encourage them to talk
	Dislikes sudden movements Poor short-term memory	Speak softly	
6–16mo 1½–4yr	Stranger anxiety Seeks caregivers and favorite objects for comfort	Offer toys Give directed attention Use simple language	Distract Allow them to see and touch instruments
	Tantrums Magical thinking	Provide a safe environment	Demonstrate Be truthful Look to parents for help with tantrums Give unconditional rewards
5–12yr	Fears physical harm and loss of control	Speak to the child Answer questions	Explain first Allow choices Give positive reinforcement
	Coping strategies reflect past experiences Ability to reason Conscious of peer pressure		
Adolescent	Attempts self-control Seeks independence	Provide privacy Use open-ended questions	Expect temporary regression

language, skills. (The Denver II was standardized in 1989 and has 86 percent more language skills than the DDST). Early language development is probably the best predictor of intelligence in the infant and young child, with problem-solving skills the second best predictor. Attainment of motor milestones is the worst predictor of below-average intelligence.[7] Screening for developmental delay is important when evaluating a child with a suspected metabolic abnormality, dysmorphic features, phakomatosis or genodermatosis. Within this context, any suspicion of abnormal development should prompt appropriate referral for a more detailed examination.

The physical examination, as with simple verbal and non-verbal communication, should be age appropriate (Table 4.1). In all cases, the goal is to gain trust. A physician should neither lie to, nor threaten, a child. "This won't hurt," is never appropriate before an injection or other painful procedure, but "this will hurt" could accentuate pain perception.[8] Other accurate descriptors (e.g., "pinch" or "sting," or "bite") are suitable. Unnecessary fear and discomfort should be avoided, but if an uncomfortable examination or procedure is necessary, it should not be omitted. Demonstration is a valuable way to alleviate fear. For example, a mock skin scraping can be done first on a parent or an extremity so the child can see what you are doing. A puppet or doll can also help to demonstrate a procedure and displace fear.[9] Sometimes gentler techniques are just as effective as painful ones: using a toothbrush or cotton swab, instead of a blade, to obtain a sample of tinea capitis for culture;[10] applying silver nitrate, suction, catharidin or nail polish to molluscum instead of freezing or curetting.[11,12] Procedures can almost always be done in the presence of parents, often with the child sitting in a parent's lap. Parent, patient and physician must be securely positioned to avoid a "moving target." Some parents and children prefer to be separated and should always be offered the option. For fast but uncomfortable procedures, especially for very young children and/or anxious parents, it may be most useful to excuse the caregiver and then return the child for solace after the fact.[13]

DOCUMENTATION

It is always important to document significant psychosocial factors and unusual emotional overlay during a visit (see Ch. 2). Most infants and young children are seen by their primary physician at frequent, regular intervals; therefore, it is extremely important to communicate with the primary physician about any child with a chronic or unusual problem. The primary physician can also serve as a source of vital information about the unique aspects of the child and address concerns that have been raised in consultation.

THERAPEUTICS APPROPRIATE FOR AGE AND FAMILY

A family visit is an excellent opportunity to provide anticipatory guidance, particularly during a follow-up visit or after an acute problem has been addressed. Most parents will appreciate information about the principles of good skin care and sun protection in children, as outlined in the sections below.

If a treatment cannot be delivered, it will not work. This is an obvious fact that emphasizes the need to consider several variables when prescribing therapy for children. The form and taste of a medication will strongly influence the successful completion of a course of therapy. For example, the antistaphylococcal antibiotic, dicloxacillin, is bitter and poorly tolerated in liquid form. Better-tasting alternatives are erythromycin preparations (also available in chewable form), trimethoprim/sulfamethoxazole, or first-generation cephalosporins. Prednisone, available in a concentration of 5mg/5ml (tsp), is also very bitter. Prednisolone, with equivalent glucocorticoid activity, is commercially available at three times the concentration and allows for a smaller volume per dose. In general, medications required once or twice a day will be given more reliably than those prescribed three or four times a day, especially by working parents and/or to children in day care. For adolescents, compliance can be improved by allowing them to choose when possible. For example, the

7. Blasco P (1993) Early developmental indicators of intellectual deficit. **Pediatr Rounds** 2(4):1.
8. Olness K (1991) Cyberphysiologic strategies in pediatric practice (biofeedback, self-hypnosis, and relaxation training). **Pediatr Ann** 3:115, 119.
9. Rothman K, Nutile A, Appel C (1990) The use of dolls as a teaching aid for children undergoing treatment with the flashlamp-pulsed tunable dye laser. **J Am Acad Dermatol** 22(5 Pt 1):854.
10. Hubbard TW, de Triquet JM (1992) Brush-culture method for diagnosing tinea capitis. **Pediatrics** 90:416.
11. Epstein E (1989) Cantharidin treatment of molluscum contagiosum. **Acta Derm Venereol (Stockh)** 69:91.
12. Blum E (1993) Glue for fissures, conservative treatment for molluscum contagiosum in children. **Schoch Lett** 43(12):48.
13. Gonzalez JC, Routh DK, Saab PG et al. (1989) Effects of parent presence on children's reactions to injections: behavioral, physiological, and subjective aspects. **J Pediatr Psychol** 14:449.

question, "Would it be more convenient for you to take your medication on a full or empty stomach?" is a valuable guide to selecting antibiotic therapy for these patients. Costs, insurance coverage and limitations of managed-care formularies must also be considered. If the prescribed treatment has failed due to "poor compliance," the physician should not immediately blame the patient or parents. Rather, the type and frequency of required therapy should be reconsidered. One should be as flexible as possible; working with the family to minimize their guilt and designing the most acceptable therapeutic regimen will undoubtedly increase compliance. It is well to remember that an anxious parent will hear and retain only a fraction of the information given at the clinic. Detailed written instructions and handouts are very helpful and minimize later phone calls.

Several poorly understood pediatric dermatologic diseases do not have a uniformly safe and effective therapy (e.g., lichen sclerosus, morphea, urticaria pigmentosa, alopecia areata, and vitiligo). It is prudent to begin with inexpensive, safe and painless therapy that may offer some benefit. For example, topical corticosteroids provide symptomatic relief for childhood lichen sclerosus; but topical testosterone, commonly advocated for the treatment of lichen sclerosus in adults, can cause significant androgenization in girls. Potent topical corticosteroids (with or without occlusion) are preferred initially or as adjunct therapy[14] to corticosteroid injections for children with alopecia areata, although the efficacy of topical therapy may not be equal to that achieved with injections.

Many common pediatric skin problems are benign and self-limited, but they can be distressing to parents. Examples are mollusca, verruca vulgaris, acute urticaria and pityriasis alba. In many cases, a supportive, but non-therapeutic, approach is an appropriate alternative to intervention. Recognize that a parent's degree of concern may greatly differ from that of the child. Parental anxiety must be evaluated separately from the patient's signs and symptoms. Unrecognized, a parent's angst can influence a physician's perception of a problem or can prompt a more aggressive workup and/or treatment. For several skin problems, very aggressive, painful evaluation or treatment may be appropriate only if the child assents.

Despite the best efforts of the most experienced clinician, children can be uncooperative. Occasionally, scary or painful intervention is unavoidable. In the past, the subject of pain control in infants and children was largely ignored. Recently, much more attention has been given to the development of safe and effective strategies to minimize and control the apprehension, fear and pain that destroy a child's cooperation.[15–17] Some of these are behavioral tactics suitable for children in specific age groups. For children of all ages, a few guidelines are essential (Table 4.1).

Physical strategies may also be helpful. These include the application of heat, cold (e.g., ice cubes, a chilled can of cola, ethyl chloride spray)[18,19] or vibration, as well as the use of small (30-gauge) flexible siliconized needles. There are also several improved pharmacologic approaches to pediatric analgesia and anesthesia. Commercially available lidocaine hydrochloride has a pH value of 3.3 to 5.5. The acidic pH is responsible for the pain associated with infiltration.[20,21] This may be reduced by buffering 9ml of 1 percent lidocaine with 1ml of sodium bicarbonate (75mg/ml).[22] Warming the anesthetic solution to body temperature may also reduce the pain associated with local injection.[23,24]

ANESTHETICS

Eutectic mixture of local anesthetics (EMLA cream) received FDA approval in 1993. A eutectic mixture is a unique combination of ingredients whose melting point is lower than that of either pure chemical alone and allows for oil formation at room temperature. EMLA cream is a 1:1 oil-in-water emulsion of lidocaine and prilocaine hydrochloride bases. Unlike either single anesthetic agent, the combination is effective on intact skin and especially after application under an occlusive dressing for 1–2h. EMLA can reduce or eliminate the pain of curettage, visible-light laser or injections.[4] Anesthetic agents have an especially narrow margin of safety; the appropriate dose for a child must always be calculated on a milligram-per-kilogram (mg/kg) basis. The maximum recommended dose of topical viscous or subcutaneously injected plain lidocaine is 5mg/kg given every 2–3h. A 2% gel or solution contains 20mg/ml. For an infant weighing 5kg, the maximum dose is only 1.25ml. When epinephrine is added, local vasoconstriction will limit systemic absorption, and the dose can be safely increased to 7mg/kg. EMLA cream contains 25mg/g of prilocaine and an equal amount of lidocaine. The maximum recommended dose for an infant under 1 year of age is 2g (less than half a tube). Methemoglobinemia is a rare adverse effect from prilocaine. EMLA cream is not recommended in pediatric patients at increased risk of this problem: infants under 3 months of age or children receiving sulfonamides.

Despite all of these tactics, fear of pain, especially from "shots," remains overwhelming in some children. Young children can safely be restrained and will calm easily when they realize that the injection was not as uncomfortable as feared. However, avoid revealing the needle and syringe to older children unless they want to see it. When an older child develops irrational fear, physical restraint will only exacerbate the problem. Infrequently, a procedure must be rescheduled.

A discussion of safe, effective alternatives for office sedation in children is a very important evolving subject. Comparative data on the safety and efficacy of sedatives in children are limited. Pediatric biological responses and risks of analgesics, anxiolytics and anesthetics vary from those of adults. Children have increased oxygen requirements, decreased functional residual capacity and decreased oxygen reserves leading to a resting oxygen consumption twice that of adults. Children also have a central respiratory drive that is less responsive to hypoxemia. These factors lead to a more rapid onset of hypoxia and a greater degree of respiratory depression in children who are given sedative and anesthetic agents. Children also have comparatively hyperreactive airway reflexes with increased risk of laryngospasm. This tendency can be exacerbated by inadequate pain control in sedated patients.

The degree of cooperation required and expected level of pain will define the level of pharmacologic support. Conscious sedation causes drowsiness without loss of airway control. Deep sedation is needed for more invasive procedures. At this level, loss of respiratory drive and airway reflexes may unpredictably occur.[25] Sedating antihistamines, such as hydroxyzine, can be safely and sometimes successfully used to achieve conscious sedation. Chloral hydrate is one of the most widely used drugs for this purpose because it has a relatively wide margin of safety. Given orally, this drug is rapidly metabolized to trichloroethanol which has pharmacologic effects similar to those of ethanol.[26] An appropriate starting dose is 75mg/kg given

14. Phairas D (1992) Wrongful birth and birth injury claims: new risks for oral surgeons. **J Mass Dent Soc** 41(2):82.
15. Agency for Health Care Policy and Research (1992) Acute pain management in infants, children and adolescents: operative and medical procedures. **Am Fam Physician** 46:469.
16. Anonymous (1992) Guidelines for monitoring and management of pediatric patients during and following sedation for diagnostic and therapeutic procedures. **Pediatrics** 89(6 Pt 1):1110.
17. French G, Painter E, Coury D (1994) Blowing away shot pain: a technique for pain management during immunization. **Pediatrics** 93:384.
18. Gedaly-Duff V, Burns C (1992) Reducing children's pain-distress associated with injections using cold: a pilot study. **J Am Acad Nurse Pract** 4:95.
19. Maikler V (1991) Effects of a skin refrigerant/anesthetic and age on the pain responses of infants receiving immunizations. **Res Nurs Health** 14:397.
20. Bartfield J, Ford D, Homer P (1993) Buffered versus plain lidocaine for digital nerve blocks. **Ann Emer Med** 22:216.
21. Wheeland R (1988) Surgical Techniques. In: Pediatric Dermatology, Schachner L, Hansen R, eds. New York: Churchill Livingstone, p. 209.
22. Stewart JH, Cole G, Klein J (1989) Neutralized lidocaine with epinephrine for local anesthesia. **J Dermatol Surg Oncol** 15:1081.
23. Alonso PE, Perula LA, Rioja LF (1993) Pain-temperature relation in the application of local anesthesia. **Br J Plast Surg** 46:76.
24. Maikler V (1991) Effects of a skin refrigerant/anesthetic and age on the pain responses of infants receiving immunizations. **Res Nurs Health** 14:397.
25. American Academy of Pediatrics Committee on Drugs (1992) Guidelines for monitoring and management of pediatric patients during and after sedation for diagnostic and therapeutic procedures. **Pediatrics** 89:1110.
26. Anonymous (1993) American Academy of Pediatrics Committee on Drugs and Committee on Environmental Health: use of chloral hydrate for sedation in children. **Pediatrics** 92:471.

30–60min before the procedure. If the child is not drowsy after 30min, an additional 25–30mg/kg may be given to a maximum total dose of 1g. Responses to chloral hydrate are extremely variable. An idiosyncratic reaction to this and other sedatives is not uncommon in children, causing agitation, rather than drowsiness. In addition, the half-life of trichloroethanol can be as long as 40h. Prolonged drowsiness requiring extended postoperative monitoring can occur. Chronically administered chloral hydrate is carcinogenic in mice, leading to concern about its use in humans;[26] however, epidemiologic data have not supported this risk.

Midazolam is a short-acting, sedating benzodiazepine that has the added advantage of amnesia.[27] It can be given orally or intranasally at 0.5–0.75mg/kg with rapid onset of action.[28] Sublingual or oral administration of the injectable solution (5mg/ml) mixed in fruit juice concentrate is much more easily accomplished than intranasal administration. Respiratory depression can rarely occur with the use of midazolam as a single agent.

Low-level (less than 50%) inhaled nitrous oxide is anxiolytic, sedating and mildly analgesic. Given as a sole agent with at least 20% oxygen, it is extremely safe, has a rapid onset, rapid recovery time and does not cause respiratory depression. However, face mask administration of nitrous oxide can be as challenging as an anesthetic injection in an uncooperative child. For these difficult patients, and for up to 15% of the general population, a concentration of less than 50% nitrous oxide as a sole agent is less likely to be effective. Higher doses of nitrous oxide increase the risks of agitation, laryngospasm and diffusion hypoxia.[29] Nitrous oxide has been widely used in children undergoing dental procedures. It has an excellent safety profile; but, in combination with narcotics for deep sedation, there is a significant risk of cardiorespiratory depression. Portable nitrous oxide units cost $1000 to $2000, not including the monitoring equipment. Specialized training is also important for physicians. Information on training courses can be obtained from the American Dental Association at (800) 621-8099 ext. 2869.

Another cocktail, given orally or intramuscularly, that has been widely used for conscious and deep sedation consists of variable mixtures of meperidine hydrochloride, promethazine hydrochloride and chlorpromazine. This combination has a slow onset and long recovery time. Life-threatening adverse reactions include respiratory depression, significant hypotension, lowered seizure threshold and the neuroleptic malignant syndrome.[21] Other regimens that have not been well studied or widely used in children include mild sedative/analgesic combinations such as hydroxyzine or codeine with acetaminophen, aspirin, ibuprofen or ketorolac and more deeply sedating anesthetic agents including fentanyl, ketamine and methohexital.[30,31]

Specific guidelines for monitoring and management of pediatric patients under conscious and deep sedation have been defined.[25,32] Normally healthy children or those with only mild systemic disease are candidates for office sedation. Sedative medication should not be administered before the patient arrives at the health care facility. Presedation dietary precautions should be followed. The patient must be accompanied by a responsible caregiver. The office must be properly furnished, including personnel and equipment to manage emergency situations such as a positive-pressure oxygen delivery system, suction apparatus, sphygmomanometer with pediatric cuffs, a pulse oximeter and a crash cart. After the procedure, the patient must be observed in a suitably equipped facility.

General anesthesia, as supervised by trained personnel, is necessary when a procedure mandates deep sedation with loss of reflexes. There is a 1:10 000 risk of mortality from general anesthesia in healthy children. This risk is somewhat increased in infants less than 1 year old. Fortunately, deep sedation is rarely needed for pediatric dermatologic procedures.

PRESCRIBING PEARLS

Escalating costs of health care are a major concern for everyone. The cost of medication is a significant out-of-pocket expense that can be prohibitive. It is difficult to generalize about the consumer cost of any medication; retail prices vary according to the buying power and profit margin of the retail outlet. However, for particular brand-name drugs, the price of different forms (e.g., liquid versus tablet) may vary greatly. The prices are similar for 1-, 2.5-, 5-, and 10-mg tablets of prednisone. Per milligram, 10-mg capsules of 13-*cis*-retinoic acid (Accutane) cost two to three times as much as 40-mg tablets. In general, liquid forms of medication are more costly than equivalent doses in capsule or tablet form. Liquid medication may also have altered bioavailability, significantly shortened shelf-life and require refrigeration. Milligram for milligram, cimetidine syrup and griseofulvin suspension cost almost three times more than equivalent doses in tablet form. However, cefadroxyl (Duricef) liquid, 500mg/5ml, is one-half the price of 500-mg tablets. Methotrexate can be purchased in injectable form (25mg/ml) and taken orally with careful measurement at a small fraction of the cost of 2.5-mg tablets.

Generic medications are almost always less costly and in many cases can be substituted for brand-name drugs. Benadryl (diphenhydramine hydrochloride) costs 10 times more than its generic equivalent. An affordable midpotency topical steroid may be compounded by adding 5ml (200mg) of generic triamcinolone acetonide, 40mg/ml, to 1lb of white petrolatum or vegetable shortening. It is mixed in a bowl and kept in the refrigerator. This is a 0.045% triamcinolone ointment and is intermediate to the commercially available 0.1% and 0.025% preparations. Generic preparations may not perform as consistently as the brand-name equivalent, particularly in the category of topical corticosteroids.[33]

Costs also vary greatly for over-the-counter products including dressing materials, cleansers, emollients, sunscreens, topical wart therapies and antiseborrheic shampoos. Simple soap-and-water baths will sanitize, wet and gently debride the skin just as well as a host of more expensive chemical baths. Discarded, clean towels can fulfill the need for dressings just as well as any commercially available dry gauze material. White petrolatum is the least irritating and most cost-effective emollient available (see sections on emollients, baths, and dressing, below).

When the cost of medication is a family burden, or if more convenient, readily available therapy has failed, the use of time-honored preparations may be considered. Many of these compounds have predated requirements for rigorous testing of safety and efficacy but have survived decades, or even centuries, of use with good reputations. Salicylic acid is a good example. This agent has recently enjoyed a renaissance in popularity and is commercially available in a variety of nonprescription topical products. However, simple formulations may also be compounded. Three to 6% salicylic acid in isopropyl alcohol is inexpensive and useful for the treatment of acne, seborrheic dermatitis and tinea. If this mixture is too drying, glycerin may be added to the solution as follows: 10% in the summer, 15% in the winter and 20–40% for xerotic skin. In an effort to stop itching, 0.25% menthol can be added if desired. This mixture can also be used to treat itchy, scaly, dry skin; however, it burns when applied to open wounds, cuts, or scrotal skin. Forty to 70% salicylic acid is an effective agent for debriding warts. Salicylic acid may be systemically absorbed and could lead to salicylism; therefore, it should not be used on infants or extensively on children with widespread skin disease.

Topical phenol, at a concentration of 0.5–2%, has been popular since the early 20th century. It has been an active ingredient in many widely used over-the-counter preparations (e.g., Noxzema, Ungentine, Sarna Carmex and

27. Sievers TD, Yee JD, Foley ME et al. (1991) Midazolam for conscious sedation during pediatric oncology procedures: safety and recovery parameters. **Pediatrics** 88:1172.
28. Wilton NT, Leigh J, Rosen D et al. (1988) Preanesthetic sedation of pre-school children using intranasal midazolam. **Anesthesiology** 69:972.
29. Weber P, Weber M, Dzubow L (1989) Sedation for dermatologic surgery. **J Am Acad Dermatol** 20:815.
30. Laub M, Sjogren P, Holm-Knudsen R et al. (1990) Lytic cocktail in children. Rectal versus intramuscular administration. **Anaesthesia** 45:110.
31. Schwanda AE, Freyer DR, Sanfilippo DJ et al. (1993) Brief unconscious sedation for painful pediatric oncology procedures. Intravenous methohexital with appropriate monitoring is safe and effective. **Am J Pediatr Hematol Oncol** 15:370.
32. Committee on Drugs (1985) Guidelines for the elective use of conscious sedation, deep sedation, and general anesthesia in pediatric patients. **Pediatrics** 76:317.
33. Jackson D, Thompson C, McCormack J et al. (1989) Bioequivalence of generic corticosteroids. **J Am Acad Dermatol** 20:791.

Chloraseptic) for its bacteriostatic and anesthetic properties. Other phenolic compounds include hexachlorophene (pHisoHex), triclosan (the active ingredient in many liquid deodorant soaps) and resorcinol. In addition to its antimicrobial properties, application of a phenolated material for 1h is believed to augment the antipruritic and anti–inflammatory effects of a subsequently applied topical corticosteroid. In concentrations above 5%, phenol may be a tumor promoter. Use in infants under 6 months of age should be avoided due to associated neonatal hyperbilirubinemia, seizures and death.[34,35] Phenol has recently been eliminated from Sarna and Chloraseptic preparations because of concerns about toxicity.

A very effective swish-and-swallow oral preparation can be custom compounded for patients with extensive oral erosions from a varity of non-infectious disease such as Stevens–Johnson syndrome, epidermolysis bullosa, lichen planus and aphthous stomatitis. Given the name Magic Mouthwash, it is administered up to four times a day in divided doses of up to 4ml/kg/day. It contains 120ml nystatin suspension (100 000U/ml), 480ml diphen-hydramine elixir (12.5mg/5ml) and 240mg hydrocortisone powder (USP) mixed in 720ml of 2% sodium carboxymethylcellulose. Two hundred and forty ml (125mg/ml) of either erythromycin (for children under age 8) or tetracycline suspension (for older children) may be added. Two percent viscous lidocaine may also be added with caution (see below).

DRUG TOXICITIES: SPECIAL CONSIDERATIONS FOR PEDIATRIC PATIENTS

POISONING

Infants and children have unique risks of drug toxicities. Poisoning by accidental ingestion, most often in children under 5 years of age, almost always occurs in the home. Topical agents are not among the most common substances ingested, but a few are extremely toxic. These products are not routinely packaged in childproof containers and may not be as closely guarded as other medications. Systemic signs of toxicity associated with several topical preparations are listed in Table 4.2.

RISKS DUE TO INCREASED BODY SURFACE AREA

Compared with adults, infants and children have an increased ratio of skin surface area to body weight. This increases the potential for significant systemic absorption of topically applied medications. Controlled percutaneous absorption is the basis for transdermal drug delivery. However, for local–acting topical medications, systemic absorption can be a danger. For drugs with a narrow margin of safety, the appropriate dose must always be calculated on a mg/kg basis. For example, the maximum recommended dose of topical viscous or subcutaneously injected lidocaine is 5mg/kg. A 2% gel or solution contains 20mg/ml; therefore, the maximum dose for an infant weighing 4kg is approximately 0.5ml. Orally applied lidocaine in subtoxic doses includes the additional risk of aspiration. Lindane (γ-benzene hexachloride) toxicity of the hematologic and central nervous system (CNS) is also much greater in infants because of their proportionately greater body surface area; thus, permethrin is a safer alternative.[36,37]

Alterations in the stratum corneum can increase skin permeability. Premature infants of less than 32 weeks' gestation and those less than 2 weeks old have a relatively deficient stratum corneum. Infants and children with ichthyosis, extensive burns, or widespread eczematous or papulosquamous conditions also have impaired skin barrier function. Topical corticosteroids

TABLE 4.2 Systemic toxicity to be expected from commonly used topical agents following ingestion

Chemical	Sites/toxicity[a]
Extremely toxic	
Ammoniated mercury	GI tract, CNS
Phenylmercuric acids	GI tract, CNS
Lindane	CNS
Very toxic	
Boric acid	GI tract, CNS, renal, liver, skin
Coal tars	GI tract, CNS, CV
Hexachlorophene	GI tract, CNS
Methylasalicylate	CNS
Phenol	CNS, GI tract, CV
Potassium permanganate	GI tract
Resorcinol	CNS (CNS and anemia)
Thimerosal	CNS
Thioglycolic acid	CNS
Moderately toxic	
Acetone	CNS
Benzoyl peroxide	GI tract (?)
Denatured alcohol	CNS, hypoglycemia
Metallic hair dyes	HTN, asthma, CNS, methemoglobinemia
Selenium sulfide	Renal, cardiopulmonary, spleen, GI tract
Sodium thiosulfate	Osmotic catharsis
Sulfur	GI tract, gas production
Undecylenic acid	GI tract, CNS, fever, urticaria
Zinc oxide	GI tract
Low toxicity	
Aluminum acetate	GI tract (mild symptoms)
Petrolatum	Mild laxative
Propylene glycol	CNS depression

GI, gastrointestinal; CNS, central nervous system; CV, cardiovascular.
[a] Toxicity ratings and sites of action are those reported in references 15, 16, and 312.
From Battan FK, Dart RC, Rumack BH (1997) Emergencies, Injuries & Poisoning. In: Current Pediatric Diagnosis & Treatment, 13th Led. Chap. 12, Hay WW et al. ed. Stamford, Appleton & Lange, pp. 308–329.

are much more efficiently absorbed through eczematous skin compared to intact skin,[38] with increased risk of adrenal suppression and growth failure if chronically applied. Growth parameters should be routinely monitored for all children requiring this type of therapy. In infants, topical corticosteroids applied once in the morning may be the safest regimen.[39]

Liberal use of any topical agent should be recommended with caution to children who have an impaired skin barrier. Excessive absorption of the sulfa component of silver sulfadiazine can cause hyperbilirubinemia in infants, and argyria has resulted from percutaneous absorption of the silver component in at least one adult.[40] Liberal use of topical urea on a collodion baby has been associated with an elevated blood urea nitrogen (BUN).[41] In these patients, there is a theoretical risk of lactic acidosis following excessive use of topical ammonium lactate, or of salicylism following excessive use of topical salicylic acid. Other topically applied agents that should be used with caution in infants are propylene glycol (systemic administration has been associated with CNS toxicity), povidone–iodine (excessive topical application has resulted in hyper-thyroidism and goiter) and clioquinol (peripheral and optic neuopathy following topical application).

34. West DP, Worobec S, Solomon LM (1994) Pharmacology and toxicology of infant skin. **J Invest Dermatol** 76:147.

35. Adams R (1971) Principles in practice of topical therapy. **Pediatr Clin North Am** 18:685.

36. Taplin D, Meinking T (1987) Pyrethrins and pyrethroids for the treatment of scabies and pediculosis. **Semin Dermatol** 6:125.

37. Schultz M, Gomez M, Hansen RC et al. (1990) Comparative study of 5% permethrin cream and 1% lindane lotion for the treatment of scabies. **Arch Dermatol** 126:167.

38. Bronaugh R, Weingarten D, Lowe N (1986) Differential rates of percutaneous absorption through the eczematous and normal skin of a monkey. **J Invest Dermatol** 87:45.

39. Turpein M, Salo O, Leista S (1986) Effect of percutaneous absorption of hydrocortisone on adrenocortical responsiveness in infants with severe skin disease. **Br J Dermatol** 115:475.

40. Payne CM, Bladin C, Colchester AC et al. (1992) Argyria from excessive use of topical silver sulphadiazine. **Lancet** 340(8811):126.

41. Anonymous (1987) High plasma urea concentrations in collodion babies. **Arch Dis Child** 62:212.

ABSOLUTE AND RELATIVE CONTRAINDICATIONS

When prescribing for children, it is important to be aware of medications that are contraindicated as well as those that are not FDA approved for pediatric use. In children under 8 years of age, the use of tetracycline and doxycycline is contraindicated. These agents cause irreversible dysgenesis of dental enamel and depressed bone growth due to formation of a tetracycline–calcium orthophosphate complex in growing osseous tissue. Increased tendency to caries and staining of permanent teeth occur in children treated before the age of 8 years. These antibiotics are also contraindicated during pregnancy but will not interfere with dental bud formation until after the third month of gestation when hard tissue formation begins.[42] Taken during the second or third trimesters, the infant's deciduous, but not permanent, teeth will be affected. Aspirin must be used with caution in children under age 16 who have no history of chickenpox or who have signs and symptoms of influenza due to the associated risk of Reye syndrome. H_1-antihistamines are contraindicated in newborns and premature infants due to the risk of central nervous system (CNS) toxicity.

Eighty percent of FDA-approved drugs listed in the *Physician's Desk Reference* lack a pediatric indication. There are many reasons why safety and efficacy of drugs has not been established for children, but stronger arguments support an increased need to collect this data.[1] As an example, FDA labeling for ciprofloxacin includes a warning against using the drug in patients under age 18 because of the associated arthropathy documented in juvenile animals. However, published data show no significant risk of arthropathic toxicity with the use of ciprofloxacin and other quinolones in children.[43] Among the drugs commonly prescribed off-label to children include: Phenergan, Lotrisone, Tavist and Tagamet. Dermatop and Cutivate cream preparations are the only topical corticosteroids that have FDA approval for use in infants with the mandated disclaimer warning against use in the diaper area.[44] Federal legislation first addressed the issue of children as "therapeutic orphans" with a 1994 Final Rule. The 1997 Modernization Act created an incentive with extended patent protection in exchange for pediatric studies. The 1998 Final Rule finally required pharmaceutical manufacturers to study all newly developed drugs likely to be used in children.[45] Nevertheless, it remains important to be cautious and vigilant when prescribing any new drug.

DRUG INTERACTIONS

A few important pharmacokinetically based drug reactions should be kept in mind for combinations that are commonly prescribed in children. Erythromycin will increase serum levels of several other drugs that have narrow margins of safety. These include theophylline, phenytoin, carbamazepine and cyclosporine. Cimetidine can also increase the serum level of theophylline and phenytoin. Fluconazole and ketoconazole will increase serum levels of co-administered phenytoin, rifampin or cyclosporine.[46] Children who are allergic to penicillin may have cross-reactivity to griseofulvin. Nonsteroidal anti-inflammatory drugs including ibuprofen as well as TMP/sulfamethoxazole will interfere with methotrexate metabolism and lead to elevated, potentially toxic blood levels.

Antimicrobial agents, especially ampicillin and amoxicillin, but also tetracyclines, sulfonamides, metronidazole, erythromycin and other antibiotics alter colonization by gastrointestinal (GI) flora. This interferes with the enterohepatic recirculation of ethinylestradiol and theoretically reduces the efficacy of oral contraceptives. Griseofulvin, rifampin and fluconazole potentiate the activity of hepatic enzymes that increase the metabolism of estrogens and progestogens with similar effects on the efficacy of oral contraceptives.[43,47,48] Patients using low-dose estrogen birth control pills (35µg or less of ethinylestradiol) may be at higher risk of unsuppressed ovulation than those on high-dose estrogen. Large studies documenting actual effects of these drugs on the metabolism of oral contraceptives are lacking, and a meaningful prospective trial looking at the incidence of pregnancy in women taking the combinations will probably never be done for ethical and practical reasons.[49] Oral contraceptives, as a sole form of birth control, have a predictable failure rate of 1 percent; however, a small number of published reports of alleged antibiotic-oral contraceptive failures have led to wrongful birth and birth-injury claims.[50] All female patients of childbearing age who are receiving long-term treatment with any of these antimicrobial drugs should be informed of this potential risk. Treatment should be designed to address individual concerns.

ADVERSE REACTIONS

The use of any sedating H_1-antihistamine in young children, while not contraindicated, may have an idiosyncratic stimulatory effect. This may be a mild manifestation of central anticholinergic syndrome which has been reported in associated with excessive topical and oral administration of diphenhydramine and also after therapeutic doses of cyproheptadine.[3] All parents should be warned of the possibility of antihistamine-associated agitation, and the first dose should be given during the child's waking hours. Increased appetite and weight gain are common side effects of cyproheptadine in children, which may be advantageous for children with atopic dermatitis complicated by failure-to-thrive. A characteristic serum sickness-like reaction has been described in association with penicillins and cephalosporins, especially cefaclor (Ceclor).[51] Other drugs that have precipitated a similar reaction include sulfonamides, isoniazid, minocycline, thyroid preparations, phenytoin and nonsteroidal anti-inflammatory drugs.[52,53] Symptoms usually develop 4 to 12 days after starting the drug and include rash, fever, malaise, arthralgias and lymphadenopathy. Laboratory findings are nonspecific and inconsistent, but they may include elevated erythrocyte sedimentation rate, eosinophilia, presence of cryoglobulins, C3 and C4 complement depression and positive rheumatoid factor. Children who have developed the characteristic hypersensitivity to phenytoin, manifesting with rash, fever, leukocytosis and hepatitis, are likely to have a similar reaction to phenobarbitol and carbamazepine; valproic acid and ethosuximide do not carry this risk.[54–56]

Topical benzoyl peroxide, although not mutagenic, is a tumor promoter in the skin of certain strains of mice. This is presumably mediated by benzoyloxyl free radicals.[57] However, epidemiologic studies in humans have not shown any association between treatment with benzoyl peroxide and skin cancer.[58] Topical tacrolimus was associated with an increased risk of photocarcinogenicity in mice, thereby prompting the recommendation to minimize sun exposure with use of this drug. Dinitrochlorobenzene (DNCB) is mutagenic

42. Lunt R, Lawd A (1974) A review of the chronology of the eruption of deciduous teeth. **J Am Dent Ass** 89:872.
43. Schaad UB, Stoupis C, Wedgwood J et al. (1991) Clinical, radiologic and magnetic resonance monitoring for skeletal toxicity in pediatric patients with cystic fibrosis receiving a three-month course of ciprofloxacin. **Pediatr Infect Dis** 10(10):723.
44. Rainer SS (2001) The safe use of topical corticosteroids in children. **Pediatr Ann** 30(4):225–229.
45. Ward RM (2001) Children, drugs and the Food and Drug Administration: studies of pediatric drugs are beginning to catch up. **Pediatr Ann** 30(4):189–194.
46. Sanford J (1992) Drug interactions with antifungals, antivirals, and other anti-infectives. **J Crit Illness** 7:605.
47. van Dijke C, Weber J (1984) Interaction between oral contraceptives and griseofulvin. **Br Med J** 288(6424):1125.
48. Fleischer AB, Resnick SD (1989) The effect of antibiotics on the efficacy of oral contraceptives. A controversy revisited. **Arch Dermatol** 125:1562.
49. Shenfield GM (1993) Oral contraceptives. Are drug interactions of clinical significance? **Drug Saf** 9:21.
50. Phairas D (1992) Wrongful birth and birth injury claims: new risks for oral surgeons. **J Mass Dent Soc** 41:82.
51. Herbert A, Sigman E, Levy M (1991) Serum sickness-like reactions from cefaclor in children. **J Am Acad Dermatol** 25:805.
52. Eichenfield AH (1999) Minocyclin and autoimmunity. **Curr Opin Pediatr** 11(5):447.
53. Knowles SR (2000) Idiosyncratic drug reactions: the reactive metabolite syndromes. **Lancet** 356(9241):1587–1591.
54. Reents S, Luginbuhl W, Davis S (1989) Phenytoin–carbamazepine cross sensitivity. **Ann Pharmacother** 23:235.
55. Shear N, Spielberg S (1988) Anticonvulsant hypersensitivity syndrome in vitro assessment of risk. **J Clin Invest** 82:1826.
56. Gennis M, Vemuri R, Burns E et al. (1991) Familial occurrence of hypersensitivity to phenytoin. **Am J Med** 91:631.
57. Swauger J, Dolan P, Zweier J et al. (1991) Role of the benzoyloxy radical in DNA damage mediated by benzoyl peroxide. **Chem Res Toxicol** 4:223.
58. Hogan D, Wilson E, To T et al. (1991) A study of acne treatment as risk factors for skin cancer of the head and neck. **Br J Dermatol** 125:343.

by the Ames test, although no association has been made between use of DNCB and carcinogenesis in humans. Potentially safer alternatives have been developed and include squaric acid dibutylester and diphenylcyclopropenone (see the section on Topical Sensitizers, below).[59,60]

GENERAL PRINCIPLES OF SKIN CARE IN CHILDREN

BATHING, SOAPS, AND CLEANSERS

The skin of infants and children does not differ significantly from that of adults in regard to cleaning. Skin thickness and epidermal barrier function are mature by 32 weeks' gestation. The skin surface lipids of neonates are similar to those of adults, with an increased ratio of sebum lipids (triglycerides, wax esters and squalene) to lipids derived from keratinocytes (cholesterol, ceramides and fatty acids). By comparison, sebum lipids are proportionately diminished in children.[61] Similar to its role in adolescent acne, the increased ratio of sebum in infants may influence the pathogenesis of neonatal acne. Otherwise, the presence or absence of sebum has not been shown to significantly contribute to basic skin integrity or cutaneous disease in pediatric patients.[62]

Cleansing agents lower the surface tension of water emulsifying and trapping oil and dirt. Classic soaps are derived from animal fat (tallow) or vegetable fat (e.g., coconut oil) processed with lye (sodium or potassium hydroxide) to yield alkali or metallic salts of fatty acids. They are by nature alkaline in solution (pH 9.5 to 10.5), with superfatted soaps at the lower end of this range; in comparison, the pH value of normal skin is approximately 4 to 5.5. Synthetic detergents, or "syndets," are synthetically derived organic quaternary ammonium compounds or fatty acids that have been polymerized or sulfonated. Syndets can be buffered to a neutral or slightly acidic pH.[63] Many claims have been made about the importance of using neutral or cationic cleansers to avoid interruption of epidermal barrier function and to prevent skin irritation. However, the pathogenesis of skin irritation is complex, and pH alone probably does not play the primary role.[64] Bar soaps tend to be more irritating than liquid cleansers, but liquids can be easily over-dispensed. Excessive amounts of cleanser, scrubbing and incomplete rinsing will contribute to irritation. Hundreds of millions of dollars are spent annually on the products manufactured and marketed for the care of infant's skin. These products have more stringent standards for purity, potential toxicity and irritancy. However, for infants and children with normal skin there is no need to use special cleansing products. The best soap for normal skin is the one the buyer likes best.

"Soapless cleansers" are lotions that are primarily composed of either glycerin (Aquanil) or propylene glycol (Cetaphil) and cetyl/steryl alcohols. They are hygroscopic, lubricating agents that work by hydrating insoluble molecules. When applied to skin, they produce a foam that can be wiped off with a humectant residue. Propylene glycol has additional antimicrobial properties but is a more common sensitizer than glycerin.

A wide variety of "medicated soaps" are available. Those containing antimicrobial agents are used as deodorants, antiseptics and to augment therapy for bacterial folliculitis (see section on Antimicrobial Agents). Triclosan, a popular antimicrobial agent found in a variety of liquid deodorant cleansers, is a phenolic compound that should be avoided on infants.

Other types of additives (e.g., benzoyl peroxide, tar, salicylic acid, sulfa) probably do not stay on the skin long enough to have a therapeutic effect. These, as well as fragrances and dyes, may act as primary irritants or allergens in susceptible individuals.

A self-cleansing mechanism is inherent in skin; thus, daily bathing is more a pleasurable ritual than a necessity. Regional cleansing is necessary only in areas that accumulate waste and dirt. Frequent bathing in tepid water can be helpful in debriding wounds, controlling pruritus and hydrating xerotic skin. Colloidal oatmeal or cornstarch added to bathwater can also be soothing. The addition of oil to bath water does not effectively moisturize skin, but it can transform the bathtub into a slippery hazard.[65] Immediate application of an ointment or cream emollient after bathing is a safe and effective method to maintain skin hydration.

Percutaneous penetration is enhanced through warm, wet skin. Emollients and topical corticosteroids are best applied after bathing while skin is damp. Irritating or potentially toxic topical medications (e.g., topical retinoids, vitamin D analogs, DEET and lindane) should be not be applied until at least 20min after bathing when the skin has thoroughly dried.

SHAMPOOS

Shampoos are liquid soaps or detergents. Baby shampoos are more tolerable for infants and children because they are isotonic to tears and less irritating to the eye. Baby shampoos generally contain fragrances and dyes, but trigger allergic contact dermatitis only in very susceptible individuals. Shampoo can be an effective vehicle for applying anti-inflammatory and antimicrobial agents to the scalp. A variety of medicated shampoos are available. Coal tar shampoo is relatively inexpensive and effective, but its odor is offensive to some and repeated use can discolor blonde hair. Shampoo containing fluocinolone acetonide (Dermasmoothe) is a more cosmetically acceptable anti-inflammatory alternative. Shampoos that contain anti-pityrosporium agents, including salicylic acid, urea, ketoconazole, zinc pyrithione and selenium sulfide, are also effective in the treatment of psoriasis and seborrheic dermatitis. Many active ingredients in medicated shampoos are substantive (with residual adherence to the scalp after rinsing). To maximize efficacy, shampoos should be applied before a bath and left on for 10–20min under a towel before washing and rinsing. Shampooing twice a week controls normal flaking. There is no harm in daily shampooing.

EMOLLIENTS

Dry skin is manifest by diminished pliability, scaling and mechanical cracking. Appropriate water balance (neither under- nor overhydration, as described in the section on Care of the Diaper Area below) is the most important factor in maintaining barrier homeostasis. Several humidity-dependent enzymatic catabolic pathways mediate normal stratum corneum development.[65] Balanced ratios of ceramide, fatty acids and cholesterol (the three major stratum corneum lipids) also play an important role in barrier function. Emollients are lipid-containing substances that soften the skin and influence epidermal homeostasis by preventing transepidermal water loss and facilitating corneocyte sloughing at the level of the stratum corneum. Evidence suggests that changes in hydration and corneocyte adhesion at the stratum corneum affects the growth and development of the entire epidermis.[66] Ointment emollients are primarily occlusive. Cream emollients often contain hygroscopic agents that attract environmental moisture to the skin. A wide variety of skin moisturizers are available (see below and Table 4.3). Petrolatum, a non-physiologic mineral lipid, is an ointment that consists of long-chain aliphatic hydrocarbons. It has been considered the gold standard of emollients. It is non-sensitizing and provides an effective barrier to transepidermal water loss for 4–6h. Other nonphysiologic lipids from animals (e.g., lanolin) or plants (e.g., vegetable shortening) may be more sensitizing. Unfortunately, many

59. Happle R, Kalveram K, Buchner U et al. (1980) Contact allergy as a therapeutic tool for alopecia areata: application of squaric acid dibutylester. **Dermatologica** 161:289.
60. van der Steen P, van Baar H, Perret C et al. (1991) Treatment of alopecia areata with diphenylcyclopropenone **J Am Acad Dermatol** 24:253.
61. Ramassastry P, Downing D, Pochi P et al. (1970) Chemical composition of human skin surface lipids from birth to puberty. **J Invest Dermatol** 54:139.
62. Pochi P (1982) The sebaceous gland. In: Neonatal Skin: Structure and Function, Ch. 3. Maibach H, Boisits EK, eds. New York: Marcel Dekker.
63. Strube D, Nicoll G (1987) The irritancy of soaps and syndets. **Cutis** 39:544.
64. Murahata R, Toton-Quinn R, Finkey M (1988) Effect of pH on the production of irritation in a chamber irritation test. **J Am Acad Dermatol** 18:62.
65. Hills RJ, Unsworth A, Ive FA (1994) A comparative study of the frictional properties of emollient bath additives using porcine skin. **Br J Dermatol** 130:37.
66. Imayame S, Ueda S, Isoda M (2000) Histologic changes in the skin of hairless mice following peeling with salicylic acid. **Arch Dermatol** 136(11):1390–1395.

TABLE 4.3   Classification of moisturizing ingredients

Ingredient type	Mechanism of action	Examples
Lubricating agents	Occlusion	Petrolatum Mineral oil Lanolin Silicones
Humectants	Absorption of moisture from the air	Glycerin Propylene glycol Ethylene glycol Sorbitol
Tissue-derived compounds	Unclear	Hyaluronic acid Collagens Elastin Lecithins Polycationic resins
Keratin softeners	Alters keratin to produce a softening effect	Urea Lactic acid[a] Glycolic acids[a]
Polyamino sugar condensate (keratin-binding factor)	Binds keratin	Pen-Kera Creme

[a] alpha-Hydroxy acids have both exfoliant and humectant properties. (Modified from Grove GL (1991) The effects of moisturizers on skin surface hydration as measured *in vivo* by electrical conductivity. Curr Ther Res 50:712, with permission.)

adults have a tactile aversion to the thick, sticky texture of ointments. Occlusive ointments may exacerbate some children with atopic dermatitis in hot or humid environments, and may exacerbate pruritus especially in children with atopic dermatitis or miliaria. The use of ointments may also exacerbate acne and folliculitis. Mineral oil is a similar product with a lower melting point that provides a less effective artificial barrier, but it may be more cosmetically acceptable.

In attempts to create products that spread more easily and that feel and smell better, the cosmaceutical industry continues to develop cream and lotion formulations. These oil-and-water emulsions contain many other active and inactive ingredients. Inactive ingredients, including preservatives, emulsifiers, dyes and fragrances, are common causes of allergic contact dermatitis in susceptible children. Active ingredients include humectants, exfoliants and physiologic lipids. Humectants, such as propylene glycol and glycerin, are hygroscopic compounds. Exfoliants decrease corneocyte adhesion and result in superficial sloughing. α- and β-hydroxy acids have both humectant and exfoliant properties. Many new emollients containing α-hydroxy acids (e.g., lactic acid or glycolic acid) have recently been popularly marketed, while β-hydroxy acid (a.k.a. salicylic acid) has enjoyed a resurgence in popularity. The efficacy of these compounds compared to occlusive moisturizers is currently under investigation.[67] Exfoliants are useful in the treatment of scaling conditions; however, these compounds can be quite irritating in higher concentrations. Excessive absorption can lead to systemic acidosis after topical application to large surface areas on infants or on compromised skin (e.g., icthyoses).[45] Topical application of an optimized ratio of exogenous physiologic stratum corneum lipids (cholesterol, free fatty acids and ceramide) offers a safe, new approach to barrier repair for xerosis and atopic dermatitis.[68]

For children with normal skin, the best moisturizer is the one that the patient prefers. For children with xerosis and/or a tendency toward atopic, irritant or allergic dermatitis, ointment or simple (fragrance and preservative-free) cream emollients are the most effective, safest and usually least costly.

The efficacy of any emollient can be optimized by applying it to damp skin immediately after bathing. To maximize hydration at localized areas of xerosis, such as the hands, feet or knees, emollients can be applied overnight under vinyl occlusion with polyethylene film (e.g., Saran Wrap). "Moist vinyl occlusion" is achieved using a layer of warm, damp white cotton under secured plastic wrap. The wrap technique is appropriate only beyond toddler age to avoid the risk of inadvertent asphyxiation. Suggestions for wrapping specific body areas include: footless sock bands with the plastic sleeves from newspapers for arms and legs, long underwear with plastic dry-cleaning bags for the trunk, socks with baggies for the feet and white cotton gloves with vinyl examination gloves for the hands. To hold plastic dressings in place, pantyhose and snug T-shirts can be used. The edges should be sealed with tape. After removal of the occlusive dressing, the emollient should be immediately reapplied to moist skin.

ANTIPRURITICS

The pathophysiology of pruritus is complex and is not well understood.[69] Histamine is the primary stimulus of the pruritus associated with urticaria. Other chemical stimuli that provoke itch include opioids and enkephalins. Pruritus may be associated with a wide variety of skin disease, or it may be "essential" – a nagging primary symptom without obvious skin lesions. Everyone's itch threshold is different, so the presence or absence of pruritus may not be a diagnostic clue. The most important steps in relieving itch are to find and treat the underlying cause. Several nonspecific measures can also be helpful to all patients that itch: avoiding physical stimuli such as vigorous scratching and rubbing, heat, hot water, wool and tight-fitting clothing. Scratching, in particular, will induce skin changes that itch and perpetuate a vicious "itch–scratch" cycle. A behavior modification technique that works well for some children is to teach them to squeeze or pat the itchy area rather than scratch. Tepid to cool bath water with colloidal oatmeal added may be soothing. It is important to follow the above recommendations for moisturizing in all patients with a tendency toward xerosis.

Topical antipruritic agents include anesthetics and products that mask itch. Pramoxine hydrochloride is a nonirritating, rarely sensitizing, topically applied anesthetic agent, commercially available over-the-counter with or without hydrocortisone in cream, lotion and gel formulations. Topical 5% doxepin hydrochloride cream (Zonalon) is FDA approved for the short-term management of pruritus in adults, and has a very low incidence of sensitization.[70] Excessive absorption can cause drowsiness. Other antipruritic ingredients are potentially irritating and/or sensitizing and should be avoided. Topically applied diphenhydramine has been such a common cause of allergic contact dermatitis that it is no longer the active ingredient in topical Benadryl. Given the popularity of oral diphenhydramine, it has surprisingly not been reported to provoke systemic contact dermatitis. Camphor and menthol are over-the-counter agents that mask itch by promoting a cooling or tingling sensations. Coal tar has anti-inflammatory properties. These agents are minimally irritating, have a low potential for sensitization and are available as gels, lotions, creams, foams and ointments. Menthol and gel vehicles are only appropriate for use on intact skin. Phenol has anesthetic properties, but carries a risk of percutaneous toxicity and should be avoided in infants and small children.

Systemic type 1 antihistamines are widely used as a nonspecific treatment for pruritis in infants and children. Even at therapeutic doses, they carry the adverse CNS effects of idiosyncratic agitation, dyskinesia and even anticholinergic syndrome. Long-acting, nonsedating antihistamines have been available since 1990. The first of these, astemizole and terbinafine, were associated with the development of hemodynamically significant cardiac tachyarrhythmias in adults. An overdose of astemizole resulted in multiple cardiac

67. Bernstein EF, Lee J, Brown DB et al. (2001) Glycolic acid treatment increases type I collagen mRNA and hyaluronic acid content of human skin. **Dermatol Surg** 27(5):429–433.
68. Chamlin SL, Frieden IJ, Fowler A et al. (2001) Ceramide-dominant, barrier-repair lipids improve childhood atopic dermatitis. **Arch Dermatol** 137:1110–1112.
69. Denman S (1986) Review of pruritus. **J Am Acad Dermatol** 14:375.
70. Drake L, Breneman D, Phillips S, Monroe C (1993) Topical doxepin hydrochloride provides an increased clinical benefit when added to topical corticosteroid treatment for atopic dermatitis. Presented at the AAD Annual Meeting, Washington DC, December 1993.

arrhythmias in a 3-year-old.[71] These medications are no longer marketed. Newer agents have not been associated with similar adverse effects. FDA approval for safety and efficacy has been demonstrated for non-sedating antihistamines, fexofenadine (down to age 12), loratadine (to age 3), and cetirizine to age 2.

Systemic antihistamines are the drugs of choice for treating itch associated with urticaria and dermatographism. For patients with these histamine-mediated conditions, nonsedating agents are an effective but expensive option[72] that will interfere with skin allergy testing for up to 1 month after discontinuation. For other types of pruritus, antihistamines are used primarily for their sedative effects. Nonsedating antihistamines are widely used to help control the pruritus associated with atopic dermatits, but only a few small randomized, double-blind, placebo-controlled (RDBPC) clinical studies have evaluated their efficacy.[72] Of these, only cetirizine yielded a marginally significant improvement compared to placebo at the highest, sedating dose (40mg/d).[73] Recent basic science data support a possible adverse effect of H1 blockade, and beneficial effect of H2 blockade on the atopic immune response. This information should give pause to clinicians who routinely prescribe diphenhydramine and hydroxyzine for children with atopic dermatitis.[74]

CARE OF THE DIAPER AREA

Many aspects of this common condition have been studied for well over a century, but the etiology, true prevalence and optimal treatment of diaper dermatitis are still issues of debate. Diaper dermatitis typically occurs at 6 to 12 months of age.[75] The condition was once attributed to the effects of ammonia; however, objective studies did not support this theory.[76,77] Many factors contribute to the pathogenesis of diaper dermatitis, but the nidus of the problem begins with excessive hydration, maceration and friction.[78] Once skin barrier function has been compromised, irritants (e.g., urine, fecal lipases, proteases, bile salts) and microorganisms (urease-splitting bacteria, *Staphylococcus aureus*, β–hemolytic streptococcus, *Pseudomonas* spp., *Candida albicans*) can exacerbate the problem. Exogenous irritants or potential allergens in cleansers, commercial diaper wipes and a myriad of over-the-counter topical products can perpetuate the process in susceptible infants.

The most important steps in preventing diaper dermatitis are maintaining good hygiene, preserving skin barrier function and preventing irritation. Traditionally, an effective but labor-intensive approach has been frequent diaper changes with gentle cleansing, thorough drying and limited use of vapor-impermeable plastic or rubber diaper covers. This practice has been greatly simplified by the introduction of disposable diapers.

The first disposable diapers (Pampers; Proctor & Gamble Co., Cincinatti, OH, USA) were marketed in 1963. For 20 years, the absorbent core was composed primarily of cellulose fluff. During that time, several conflicting studies compared the incidence of diaper dermatitis in infants using cloth diapers versus infants using disposable diapers.[75] In the mid-1980s, a super-absorbant core material was developed. It was composed of a cross-linked sodium polyacrylate that transforms to hold a proportionately large amount of fluid within a gel substance. Several studies have concluded that super-absorbant diapers are superior to cloth diapers in preventing diaper dermatitis.[79] In addition, superabsorbant diapers may prevent occult fecal contamination of clothing and fomites in daycare settings.[80] Another diaper

innovation was first marketed in 2000 as Pampers Rash Care diapers. An incorporated inner layer continuously deposits a petroleum-based barrier product to the skin. Limited trials with normal infants demonstrated a reduction in skin microtopography and erythema when compared to controls.[81]

Routine use of topical preparations to prevent diaper dermatitis is not necessary for infants with normal skin. Some of these products have additional risks. Additives have the potential to cause contact sensitization, irritation and/or percutaneous toxicity. Powders applied vigorously enough to aerosolize pose an aspiration risk. This is especially true for talc (mainly hydrous magnesium silicate) powders which can cause irritant pneumonitis. Talc may also cause granulomatous reactions when applied to wounds. Contrary to previous theory, cornstarch does not enhance the growth of *C. albicans* on the skin.[82] Boric acid, once popular as a diaper rash treatment and still an ingredient in some diaper care products, is a cause of diarrhea, erythroderma and failure to thrive.[3]

Appropriate treatment of diaper dermatitis begins with correct diagnosis of the underlying cause. Most infants develop acute diaper dermatitis as a result of the factors described above. However, other primary pathologic processes must be considered for any infant with chronic, severe and/or recurrent diaper rash. Primary cutaneous diseases that may present with diaper rash include contact dermatitis, seborrheic dermatitis, psoriasis and candidiasis. Infants with atopic dermatitis may be more susceptible to irritants, and diaper dermatitis was common in this group prior to the availability of super-absorbent diapers. Since that time, the diaper area of atopic infants is most often dramatically spared, an important diagnostic and therapeutic sign. Several uncommon causes of diaper dermatitis have serious, or even life-threatening,

---

TABLE 4.4   Uncommon causes of diaper dermatitis

Acrodermatitis enteropathica
Bullous pemphigoid
Cutaneous signs of child abuse – ecchymoses, scald injury
Chronic bullous dermatosis of childhood
Congenital syphilis
Dermatitis herpetiformis
Enterobius (pinworm) infestation
Epidermolysis bullosa
Granuloma gluteale infantum
Herpes simplex
Histiocytosis X
Incontinentia pigmenti
Kawasaki disease
Papular urticaria
Perianal streptococcal dermatitis
Post-scarlet fever desquamation
Psoriasis
Scabies
Staphylococcal scalded skin syndrome
Tinea inguinalis
Wiskott–Aldrich syndrome

(Modified from Schaad *et al.*[43] with permission.)

---

71. Tobin J, Doyle T, Ackerman A et al. (1991) Astemizole-induced cardiac conduction disturbances in a child. **JAMA** 266:2727.
72. Wahlgren C, Hagermark O, Bergstrom R (1990) The antipruritic effect of a sedative and a non-sedative antihistamine in atopic dermatitis. **Br J Dermatol** 122:545.
73. Klein PA, Clark RA (1999) An evidence-based review of the efficacy of antihistamines in relieving pruritus in atopic dermatitis. **Arch Dermatol** 135:1522.
74. Jutel M, Watanabe T, Klunkel S et al. (2001) Histamine regulates T-cell and antibody responses by differential expression of H1 and H2 receptors. **Nature** 413:420.
75. Overgaard Olsen L, Jemec GB (1993) The influence of water, glycerin, paraffin oil and ethanol on skin mechanics. **Acta Dermat-Venereol** 73:404.
76. Jordan W, Blaney T (1982) Factors influencing infant diaper dermatitis. In: Neonatal Skin: Predisposition, Structure and Function, Vol. 1. Maibach H, Boisits EK, eds. New York: Marcel Dekker.
77. Leyden J, Katz S, Stewart R et al. (1977) Urinary ammonia and ammonia-producing microorganisms in infants with and without diaper dermatitis. **Arch Dermatol** 113:1678.
78. Elias M, Feingold KR (2001) Does the tail wag the dog? Role of the barrier in the pathogenesis of inflammatory dermatoses and therapeutic implications. **Arch Dermatol** 2001 137(8):1079–1081.
79. Lane A, Rehder P, Helm K (1990) Evaluation of diapers containing absorbent gelling material with conventional disposable diapers in new-born infants. **Am J Dis Child** 144:315.
80. Rory V, Wun C, Morrow A et al. (1991) The effect of diaper type and overclothing on fecal contamination in day-care centers. **JAMA** 265:1840.
81. Odio MR, O'Connor RJ, Sarbaugh F, Baldwin S (2000) Continuous topical administration of a petroleum formulation by a novel disposable diaper. 1. Effect on skin surface microtopography. 2. Effect on skin condition. **Dermatology** 200(3):232–234.
82. Leyden J (1984) Corn starch, *Candida albicans*, and diaper rash. **Pediatr Dermatol** 1:322.

implications[83] (Table 4.4). These conditions should always be considered in infants presenting in the first month of life and those who are not otherwise thriving.

Mild to moderately irritant diaper dermatitis should be treated initially by reminding caregivers of the importance of avoiding excessive wetness and exposure to feces. This can be achieved with traditional frequent diaper changes and the use of superabsorbent diapers. Leaving the area open is impractical; a hair dryer used only on the cool setting may be useful. All potential irritants or sensitizers, including often-overlooked commercial diaper wipes, should be discontinued. Water-dampened soft cloths or paper towels, or mineral-oil-soaked cotton pledgettes are safe alternatives. Zinc oxide, in ointment or paste formulation, is an inexpensive, bland protective agent with antiseptic and astringent properties. Zinc may also play a role in wound healing.[84–86] This is an ideal first-line therapy for diaper dermatitis, applied liberally with each diaper change. Adherent zinc oxide need not be removed, but it wipes away easily with mineral oil to allow skin examination. If there is no objective evidence of candidiasis, a short course of a topical low-potency corticosteroid may be beneficial. When potassium hydroxide (KOH) preparation or culture supports the diagnosis of a yeast infection, initiate treatment with a topical antiyeast agent. However, the majority of topical antifungals are inheritantly irritating and may exacerbate the dermatitis. Nystatin ointment and Loprox cream are the least irritating products. Gentian violet is another effective alternative that requires only one to two applications. Combination products containing potent topical corticosteroids and antifungal agents are less effective than an antifungal agent used alone.[87] One such product that combines the potent class I topical steroid of 0.05% betamethasone diproprionate with 1% clotrimazole (Lotrisone, Schering-Plough, Kenilworth, NJ) has resulted in reports of skin atrophy, striae and even adrenal suppression when applied under the occlusion of a diaper.[88] Lotrisone as well as the similar product combining 0.1% triamcinolone acetonide and nystatin (Mycolog II, Bristol-Myers Squibb, Princeton, NJ, USA) are contraindicated for diaper dermatitis.

COSMETICS

Many cosmetics and personal grooming products are now produced and marketed specifically for children and adolescents. In many cases, only the packaging distinguishes these products from those marketed for adults. Products marketed specifically for infants may contain minimally irritating ingredients or feature safety packaging. Adverse reactions from these products have not been reported, but cosmetics should be considered as a possible cause in children with dermatitis.[89]

Contrary to popular belief, cosmetics do not cause or exacerbate acne. Many cosmetologists and dermatologists recommend the use of specific "non-comedogenic" products in their patients with acne. This practice is based on the concept of comedogenesis as a primary process in the pathogenesis of acne. The rabbit ear assay has been a widely used test to evaluate comedogenicity. The predictive value of this model is not necessarily a reliable model for humans, and the association between acne and cosmetics is currently over-marketed.[90] Therefore, it is difficult to predict whether a cosmetic will exacerbate acne for a given patient based on industry standards for product testing.

Rarely, cosmetic products are associated with two distinct types of adverse cutaneous reactions in people with acne. One is a rapid-onset irritant folliculitis. The other develops slowly following chronic use of a truly comedogenic product and is known as acneigenesis. There are industrial acneigens that cause occupational acne, but most cosmetics available today do not promote the formation of comedones. With few exceptions, notably hair pomades and some petrolatum products, it is not necessary to recommend restricted cosmetic products for patients with acne.

SUNLESS TANNING PRODUCTS

For adolescents who insist on a tanned appearance, sunless tanning is a safe and often cosmetically acceptable alternative. The active ingredient in self-tanning or sunless products is dihydroxyacetone (DHA).[91] DHA is a three-carbon sugar and is a white, crystalline powder that is stable between a pH of 4 to 6. It reacts with the free amino acid group of amino acids, peptides and proteins found in sweat and stratum corneum keratinocytes to form melanoidin, the brown substance that mimics a suntan. Most over-the-counter products contain 3–5% DHA. Some also contain sunscreen. Higher concentrations of DHA and body areas with increased keratin (e.g., elbows, knees) will stain a darker color. Patients should be informed that skin coloration from sunless tanners provides only minimal, unsubstantial sun protection.

SUN PROTECTION

The overall density of melanocytes in skin is greater in children than in adults, but melanin production in infants is probably limited (see Ch. 1). In addition, infants and children have not had the gradual ultraviolet (UV) exposure that stimulates facultative pigmentation. For these reasons, pediatric patients are more susceptible to the damaging effects of excessive exposure to sunlight. The adverse consequences of excessive doses of UV light are acute and cumulative. Acute overexposure results in erythema and skin necrosis. Acute photoallergic and phototoxic reactions occur in susceptible individuals. The effects of long-term excessive exposure may not become apparent for decades. The skin changes that were previously believed to be due to chronologic aging are now referred to as "dermatoheliosis" because UV exposure plays a primary role in their pathogenesis. These changes include mottled pigmentation, coarseness, wrinkling, telangiectasia and purpura, as well as the development of premalignant and malignant neoplasms.[92] Eighty percent of lifetime sun exposure occurs in childhood.[93]

More than 500 000 new cases of skin cancer are diagnosed in the United States every year. Among these is melanoma, whose incidence is increasing more rapidly than any other type of cancer. A child born in 1935 had a 1 in 1500 chance of developing a melanoma. A child born today has a projected risk of 1 in 71. Factors that significantly increase that risk include red or blonde hair, marked freckling on the upper back, multiple nevi, blistering sunburns in childhood, an outdoor summer job for at least 3 years during adolescence and a family history of melanoma. A routine visit to the dermatologist is a perfect opportunity to provide parents, children and adolescents with this information, as well as strategies to minimize the risks of excessive sun exposure (Table 4.5).

A sunscreen is a compound that absorbs, reflects or scatters the harmful spectrum of ultraviolet light (290–400nm). An increasingly wide variety of sunscreen products are available. Marketing claims have been a source of confusion for consumers. In 1999, the FDA reviewed sunscreens and published a final monograph, *Final Rule*. This was implemented in May 2001 to define conditions under which over-the-counter sunscreens are deemed

83. Lane A (1988) Diaper rash: causes and cures. **Patient Care.**
84. Maitra A, Dorani B (1992) Role of zinc in post-injury wound healing. **Arch Emerg Med** 9:122.
85. Okada A, Takagi Y, Nezu R et al. (1990) Zinc in clinical surgery – a research review. **Surg Today** 20:635.
86. Rackett S, Rothe M, Grant-Kels J (1993) Diet and dermatology – The role of dietary manipulation in the prevention and treatment of cutaneous disorders. **J Am Acad Dermatol** 29:447.
87. Gange RW, Soparkar A, Matzinger E et al. (1986) Efficacy of a sunscreen containing butylmethoxydibenzoylmethane against ultraviolet a radiation in photosensitized subjects. **J Am Acad Dermatol** 15:494.
88. Barkley W (1987) Striae and persistent tinea corporis related to prolonged use of betamethasone diproprionate. **J Am Acad Dermatol** 17:518.

89. Draelos Z (1992) Preadolescent cosmetics may cause dermatologic problems and misconceptions. **Cosmet Dermatol** 5(12):14.
90. Nelson F, Rumsfield J (1988) Cosmetics: content and function. **Int J Dermatol** 27:665.
91. Levy SB (1992) Dihydroxyacetone-containing sunless or self-tanning lotions. **J Am Acad Dermatol** 27:989–993.
92. Taylor C, Stern R, Leyden J et al. (1990) Photoaging/photodamage and photoprotection. **J Am Acad Dermatol** 22:1.
93. Stern RS, Weinstock MC, Baker SG (1986) Risk reduction for non-melanoma skin cancer with childhood sunscreen use. **Arch Dermatol** 122:537.

TABLE 4.5   Strategies to minimize sun exposure in children

Keep infants and young children out of the sun.
Avoid exposure between 10 AM and 2 PM; be aware that clouds scatter
    only 20% of the UV light.
Use protective clothing and hats.
Use the appropriate sunscreen.
Beware of reflected light from water, sand, snow, and cement.
Use extra protection at high altitudes and low latitudes.
Avoid artificial tanning devices.
Be aware of photosensitizing medications and diseases.
Do regular skin self-examination.
Set an example for children.

(Modified from Hurwitz S, Rhodes A, Wiley H (1986) For Every Child Under the Sun.
New York: Skin Cancer Foundation. with permission.)

safe and effective and are not misbranded.[94] Relative sunscreen efficacy, as originally defined, is the ability to prevent UVB-induced erythema and is expressed as a number known as the "sun protection factor" (SPF). SPF is measured and calculated under standardized conditions using a solar simulator (290–400 nm) to determine the minimal dose of UVB needed to produce erythema (MED) with protection compared to the MED without protection. Prior to the *Final Rule*, sunscreens labelled with SPF values greater than 30 overemphasized the benefits of using these products. Under the new regulations, labelling may indicate a qualitative degree of protection against sunburn: minimal (SPF 2–12), moderate (SPF 12–<30) or high (≥30). Products proven to maintain their SPF value after two 20-min swim–dry cycles may advertise "water-resistance" while "very water-resistant" products have preserved SPF protection after four cycles. Eighteen active ingredients, alone or in combination, are approved. Ingredients that reflect and scatter a large portion of the solar spectrum, including UVB, UVA and visible light, are zinc oxide and titanium dioxide. Each of the remaining approved active sunscreen ingredients absorbs a narrower range of ultraviolet light.[95] A combination of ingredients can yield "broad spectrum" protection including some degree of UVA absorption (see below). UV absorbing dyes and rinses have also been developed for fabrics, including Tinosorba FB (CIBA Specialty Chemicals, Inc. now marketed as Rit Sun Guard; Bestfoods Products; Indianapolis, IN, USA). The UV protective factor of clothing is increased with use of these products as well as with increased fabric weight, increased thickness, decreased porosity, darker color and repeated washing; it is decreased with stretch and wetness.[96] Specially tested, tightly woven sun protective fabrics are commercially available (Solumbra, Solarweave), but less expensive fabrics (Hanes Beefy-T) have been found to provide comparable SPF.[97]

UVA is 1000 times less erythemogenic than UVB. Standardized methods are still being developed to quantify a product's relative ability to absorb UVA.[98,99] UVA exposure plays an important role in the pathogenesis of photosensitivity disorders (e.g., polymorphous light eruption, solar urticaria, lupus erythematosus) and the majority of phototoxic and photoallergic drug reactions. UVA exposure will also exacerbate postinflammatory pigment change as well as primary disorders of pigmentation (e.g., melasma, café-au-lait spots, vitiligo). Agents that block the UVA spectrum can minimize the disfigurement associated with these conditions.[100] Individuals exposed to excessive sunlight while using UVB-absorbing sunscreens or those with

frequent tanning booth use will receive large doses of UVA. The role of UVA in the development of skin cancers is controversial. However, UVA exposure (e.g., from tanning booths) probably increases the risk of skin cancer in people with a history of excessive exposure to UVB.[101]

The selection of an appropriate vehicle is just as important as the active ingredient. Variables include degree of water resistance, ease of application, emollient versus drying properties and the number of potentially irritating or sensitizing additives. Frequent application of most topical sunscreens is a difficult task for caregivers of active children. Products in the form of sprays and solid sticks with incorporated colors have been developed and are fun for children to apply. Adverse reactions developed in 19% of patients in one longitudinal prospective study,[102] including subjective irritation, irritant and allergic contact dermatitis, contact urticaria, photosensitivity and acne.[103] Patients with acne usually prefer liquid or gel preparations; those with dry skin prefer an emollient base. Individuals susceptible to allergic and/or irritant reactions should be aware of the spectrum of active and inactive ingredients in the products they choose. For infants under 6 months of age, the safety of topically applied sunscreens has not been established, but the theoretical risk of toxicity is low and the American Academy of Pediatrics has recently approved sunscreen use in infants under 6 months. Concerns have focused on neonatal metabolism of *p*-aminobenzoic acid (PABA), a folic acid analog with structural similarities to those of the sulfonamides. The safest first-line strategy for sun protection in infants is sun avoidance followed by the use of appropriate clothing and/or zinc oxide-containing sunscreens. In general, the best sunscreens for recreational use are those labelled "highly water-resistant" with a "high level" of protection. For optimal efficacy, sunscreens must be applied liberally according to package directions and reapplied every 40 min if swimming or perspiring.

INSECT REPELLANTS

Arthropod-borne diseases, most commonly transmitted via mosquitoes and ticks, can be fatal and are luckily rare in the United States. Also rare are anaphylactic and systemic arthus reactions. The more common reaction to an arthropod bite is the localized cutaneous response. This can be an immediate type I, or a delayed type IV hypersensitivity reaction.[104] Avoiding exposure and wearing protective clothing reduces the risk of bites, as does proven effective chemical methods including N, N, diethyl-*m*-toluamid (DEET) and permethrin. Plant-derived repellents, including citronella, are of limited effectiveness.

DEET is the most effective topical insect repellant available. It repels mosquitoes, chiggers, ticks, fleas and biting flies; no topical repellant is effective against Hymenoptera.[105] Only products with <10% DEET are safe for children. A product containing only 6% DEET in a controlled-release vehicle (e.g., Skedaddle) has been marketed as longer lasting but safe for children. Other commercially available preparations contain up to 33% DEET. High-concentration products containing up to 95% DEET (e.g., Ultrathon, Muskol) are for adults only. Concentrated formulations provide longer-lasting protection, greater efficacy in highly infested areas and enhanced potency against more resistant insects (e.g., blackflies). DEET should only be used on intact exposed skin or clothing. Frequent reapplication as well as use around the mouth, eyes and hands of young children should be avoided. Pretreatment of clothing with permethrin spray (e.g., Permanone Tick Repellant) which is a contact insecticide and repellant will augment the efficacy of DEET

94. Sunscreen drug products for over-the-counter human use; final monograph. Food and Drug Administration, HHS. Final rule. **Fed Regist** 1999 May 21; 64(98):27666–27693.
95. Lowe N (1990) Photoprotection. **Semin Dermatol** 9:78.
96. Hoffman K, Laperre J, Avermaete A, Altmeyer P, Gambichler T (2001) Defined UV protection by apparel textiles. **Arch Dermatol** 137:1089–1092.
97. Consumer Reports, May 1998, p. 2.
98. Sayre R, Again P (1990) A method for the determination of UVA protection for normal skin. **J Am Acad Dermatol** 23:429.
99. Agin P (1992) Broad-spectrum protection in sunscreen products. **J Am Acad Dermatol** 27:648.
100. Farr P, Diffey B (1993) Adverse effects of sunscreens in photosensitive patients. **Lancet** 341(885b):347.

101. Anonymous (1991) Sunscreen protection controversy heats up. **JAMA** 265:3218.
102. Foley P, Nixon R, Marks R et al. (1993) The frequency of reactions to sunscreens: results of a longitudinal population-based study on the regular use of sunscreens in Australia. **Br J Dermatol** 128:512–518.
103. Schauder S, Ippen H (1997) Contact and photocontact sensitivity to sunscreens. Review of a 15-year experience and of the literature. **Contact Dermatitis** 37(5):221–232.
104. Reunala T, Brummer-Korvenkontio H, Lappala nen P et al. (1990) Immunology and treatment of mosquito bites. **Clin Exp Allergy** 20(Suppl 4):19–24.
105. Magnon G, Kline D, Roberts L et al. (1991) Repellency of two DEET formulations and Avon Skin-So-Soft against biting midges (Diptera: Ceratopogonidae) in Honduras. **J Am Mosquito Control Assoc** 7:80.

applied to skin. Products containing a combination of DEET and sunscreen, or dual application of both products diminishes the sun protection.[106]

The most common adverse reactions to DEET are eye irritation and skin sensitivity. However, DEET can be percutaneously absorbed. Severe CNS toxicity has been reported following excessive or prolonged use especially in infants and children.[107] Ingestion of DEET can be fatal. More information about DEET may be obtained from Chemical Specialties Manufacturers Association; 1913 Eye St., NW; Washington, DC 20006; telephone (216) 872-8110.

Avon's Skin-So-Soft is a product initially marketed as a bath oil, but popularized as an insect repellant. A modified formulation containing oil of citronella is now marketed as an insect repellant. It was found to be less effective at repelling mosquitoes than DEET, but significantly more effective than placebo in one study.[105] However, the duration of this action is probably less than 30min. Additional Skin-So-Soft products contain additional ingredients including sunscreen and common sensitizers (imidazolidinyl urea, parabens and fragrance). The efficacy of these have not been studied, and the safety of widespread repeated application of Skin-So-Soft on infants and children is unknown.

Once established, type I hypersensitivity bite reactions are difficult to treat. Potent topical corticosteroids may reduce the inflammation. Over-the-counter products with menthol or camphor sooth the skin by masking the itch; those with pramoxine provide temporary local anesthesia; astringents minimize erythema. Topically applied diphenhydramine is a common contact allergen that should be avoided, but systemic antihistamines can provide symptomatic relief. Children who present with recurrent, exuberant bite reactions may benefit from prophylactic cetirizine.[108]

CLOTHING

Clothes insulate and protect the skin from dirt and excessive sunlight (see the section on Sun Protection). Normal skin can tolerate almost any type of clean outer garment. Finely woven cotton, silk, rayon and other similar natural or synthetic fibers are comfortable next to the skin; wool and other coarse fabrics have barbed fibers that can prickle or itch. Nylon does not wick moisture, can be uncomfortable with heavy perspiration and can trigger miliaria. Allergic clothing dermatitis is unusual in children. The most common clothing allergen is nickel. It is easily identified from the configuration and distribution of dermatitis from snaps on infant sleepers, belt buckles and rivets or zippers on jeans. Rubber and elastomers characteristically cause dermatitis at the site of waistbands and shoulder straps. Chlorine bleach can potentiate rubber allergy by releasing reaction products.[109] Durable-press finishes that reduces wrinking and shrinkage can be responsible for a more widespread clothing dermatitis from formaldehydes. Contrary to marketing implications for fragrance and color "free" products, the majority of laundry detergent is rinsed away from fabric and rarely causes contact dermatitis. In contrast, residue from fabric softeners and dryer sheets adhere to clothing and may provoke contact dermatitis in susceptible individuals. Washing infant clothes separately will not prevent exposure from a contaminated dryer or close contact with garments of other family members. Percutaneous toxicity from contact with diapers and blankets was reported in 1967 after an industrial laundry product containing pentachlorophenol was identified as the cause of an epidemic of diaphoresis, fever, tachycardia, tachypnea, acidosis and death in a newborn nursery. Phenolic detergents are contraindicated for cleaning infants' diapers, linens and clothing. Otherwise, only tradition and marketing

have conditioned some clinicians to recommend the use of certain brands, such as Ivory Snow and Dreft, for children.

For infants, quantity of clothing is a more significant problem than quality. Many caregivers have a tendency to overbundle infants. Although the total number of normal-appearing sweat glands is present at birth, their ability to produce sweat in response to thermal stimulation is diminished during the first $2\frac{1}{2}$ years of life.[110] Excessive bundling and warm environments can promote fever in neonates[111] and may contribute to the pathogenesis of miliaria. Infants should be dressed with no more insulation than adults in a similar environment.

WOUND CARE

PRINCIPLES OF WOUND HEALING

The ability of a wound to heal is based on the microenvironment of the wound, which is influenced by the local wound care, as well as the general health of the patient including nutritional status, metabolic abnormalities, concurrent illnesses and genetically inherited traits. The healing of a wound is a continuous process, but has been divided into three phases: inflammation; proliferation including reepithelialization, granulation tissue formation and angiogenesis; and extracellular matrix remodeling.[112] These phases are modulated by the complex interactions of myriad cells and soluble mediators. The inflammatory phase is divided into the early stage with accumulation of neutrophils from days 0–3 and the late stage with accumulation of macrophages from days 0.3–10. Reepithelialization begins within 24h and may be completed within 72h. Granulation tissue formation, including fibroplasia and neovascularization, occurs on days 3–21. Wound contraction occurs during this phase, typically from days 7–10, after granulation tissue is well established. During the final phase of matrix formation and remodeling, the provisional matrix of fibronectin and hyaluronan is replaced by the deposition of proteoglycans and collagen. This phase typically begins on about day 5 with maximal collagen synthesis from days 14–21, but continued remodeling with improved orientation and crosslinking of collagen fibrils and reduction in cellularity continues for 2 or more years. When any of these phases is disrupted, usually due to underlying pathology, a chronic would may develop. Appropriate wound care may help prevent disruption of healing and even aid in its progression. This concept, along with the significant morbidity and associated health care costs of chronic wounds, has lead to considerable research in improved wound management.

SOAKS AND BATHS

Bathing is the most convenient method of treating soiled, xerotic or pruritic skin. Water, regardless of its method of application, hydrates and gently debrides the outer layers of the skin. The penetration of topically applied medication is also enhanced when the epidermis is well hydrated. The method and materials are simple. Soaking in a tapwater bath at a comfortable temperature is the easiest method to soothe and cleanse. Whirlpool therapy is also beneficial and aids in nontraumatic debridement of widespread dermatoses and wounds. Other direct techniques to facilitate debridement include; irrigation, utilizing direct pouring, bulb syringe, angiocatheter-fitted syringes or battery-powered systems and wet-to-dry compresses. The selected garments for the compress should be soft (e.g., laundered sheets, towels, T-shirts), moistened to the point of dampness but not saturation, and then applied to

106. Montemarano AD, Gupta RK, Burge JR, Klein K (1997) Insect repellants and the efficacy of sunscreens. **Lancet** 349:1670–1671.
107. Lipscomb J, Kramer J, Leikin J (1992) Seizure following brief exposure to the insect repellent N,N-diethyl-m-toluamide. **Ann Emerg Med** 21:315.
108. Reunala T, Brummer-Korvenkontio H, Karpinnen A et al. (1993) Treatment of mosquito bites with cetirizine. **Clin Exp Allergy** 23:72–75.
109. Jordan WP Jr, Bourlas MC (1975) Allergic contact dermatitis to underwear elastic chemically transformed by laundry bleach. **Arch Dermatol** 111(5):593–595.
110. Flesch P (1963) Chemical basis of emollient function in horny layers. **Toilet Goods Assoc** 40:12.
111. Cheng T, Partridge J (1993) Effect of bundling and high environmental temperature on neonatal body temperature. **Pediatrics** 92:238.
112. Clark RAF (1996) The Molecular and Cellular Biology of Wound Repair, 2nd edition. New York: Plenum.

the affected lesions in one or two layers. The wet garment should be covered with a dry towel or plastic wrap to minimize contamination and leaking. Vinyl "sauna suits" are commercially available in a variety of sizes, down to those for older children (Sleep Sauna®; 1-800-229-5210). Cotton and vinyl gloves are also available to treat problems localized to hands (Allerderm Laboratories, Inc. Petaluma, CA, USA; 1-800-365-6868). Most children can tolerate compresses for 10–60min three to four times a day, if engaged in distracting activities.

Medication added during or after bathes or soaks can provide supplemental therapy. Chlorhexidine, dilute acetic acid, dilute aluminum acetate (Burow's solution), LCD or other antimicrobial agents added to the water may be beneficial for infected lesions (see Topical Antimicrobial Agents, below). Once cleansed and hydrated, the skin can more effectively absorb topically applied medications. Ideally, the skin should be patted dry and remain damp when the topical therapy is applied. To further maximize effectiveness, moist vinyl occlusion following application of the topical medication can be employed (see Emollients, above).

DRESSINGS

From sesame oil used by the Babylonians in 2250 BC and honey used by Egyptians in 2000 BC to the currently available polymeric films, hydrocolloids, vacuum-assisted devices, growth-factors and tissue engineered skin, the evolution of wound care products over the millennia has been influenced by our expanding understanding of wound healing. Many intrinsic and extrinsic factors influence wound healing; some of these have been elucidated, while others have yet to be discovered. Control of infection was once thought to be the primary factor for successful wound healing. Other factors now known to prolong healing time include: altered arterial or venous circulation; diabetes mellitus; excessive use of topical corticosteroids; immunosuppression; malignancy; inflammatory disorders; advanced age; malnutrition; and exposure to pressure or shear forces.

The ancient Babylonians and Egyptians must have observed that covered, moist wounds heal more rapidly than open, dry wounds. Investigational support of this concept emerged from landmark studies, initially in pigs and later in humans, that demonstrated faster reepithelialization of wounds under occlusion.[113,114] More recent studies focused on the growth factors, including transforming growth factor beta (TGF-β), platelet derived growth factor, fibroblast growth factor, insulin-like growth factor, epidermal growth factor, colony-stimulating factor and hepatocyte growth factor, all of which have been identified in wounds and may signal and/or coordinate the cellular events of the wound healing process.

The observation that fetal tissues can heal without scarring, as well as the observation that prolonged wound healing occurs in patients with advanced age, inspired studies of age-related differences in growth factors, hormones, receptor expression and extracellular matrix proteins.[115,116] TGF-β plays a major role in scar formation. The production of TGF-β isoforms and expression of their receptors is decreased in fetal wounds compared to those in adults, possibly contributing to the scarless-healing observed in fetal tissue.[117,118]

These collective observations stimulated development of a plethora of commercially available dressing materials.[119,120] Occlusive dressings are the most well known and readily available. They enable a moist wound environ-ment to aid keratinocyte migration, accelerate the dermal inflammatory and proliferative phases, produce a delicate oxygen balance for enhanced angiogenesis, protect wounds from outside contamination, and permit accumulation of transudate that facilitates autodebridement, enhanced reepithelialization and retention of growth factors. Occlusive dressings can be left in place for several days which minimizes the pain, wound bed disruption and labor required with traditional dressing changes. They are very helpful in managing chronic, noninfected wounds and ulcerated hemangiomas. Occlusive dressings also enhance percutaneous absorption of topically applied medications and guard against continued trauma to the skin. These properties are especially useful for treating neurotic excoriations, prurigo nodules and lichen simplex chronicus, but should be recognized when applied to infants who are at higher risk for percutaneous toxicity.

Each category of occlusive dressing material has unique properties with respect to adhesiveness, absorbancy and transparency (Table 4.6). Each of these properties is suitable for different kinds of wounds. Adhesive dressings (e.g., polyurethanes and hydrocolloids) are easy to apply and remain secure for long periods of time. However, adherent dressings, removed prematurely, can strip away newly formed epidermis.[121] Transparent dressings (e.g., polyurethane and hydrogel) allow some visualization of the wound although this may be obscured by exudate. Contact-layer dressings are thin, non-adherent, porous sheets designed to protect tissue from direct contact with other agents and allow wound fluid to pass through for absorption by an overlying dressing. Contact-layer and hydrogels are the most appropriate choices for the fragile skin of premature infants and patients with mechanobullous diseases. Dressings with a capacity to absorb excess wound fluid, foams and hydrocolloids, are appropriate for very transudative wounds. The absorptive capacity of hydrocolloid dressings can be augmented by the supplementary use of pectin-based absorbent granules or paste, or calcium alginate. Caregivers should be informed that nonexcessive accumulation of wound fluid is a normal beneficial part of wound healing. This accumulated material can be malodorous and appear purulent but does not indicate infection without accompanying increases in redness, swelling, warmth and/or tenderness.

Skin substitutes, in the form of xenografts or cadaveric skin, have been used for decades to treat large and chronic wounds. Bioengineered skin substitutes have recently been developed. Several products are commercially available: Epicel (Genzyme Tissue Repair); Dermagraft (Smith & Nephew); TransCyte (Advanced Tissue Science); Apligraft (manufactured by Organogenesis and marketed in US by Novartis). Epicel is based on autologous cells. The others are allogeneic, without the potential for long-term survival and integration. Apligraf is a skin bilayer consisting of stratified human keratinocytes over a a bovine collagen and fibroblast matrix, FDA approved for the treatment of chronic venous ulcers. It provides temporary wound coverage and has been reported to accelerate wound healing for a variety of other applications, including burns and epidermolysis bullosa.[122,123]

Tissue glue is a specialized wound care product FDA approved for approximation of skin edges that are not under tension. It can also be used to help heal chronic fissures. Medical-grade tissue adhesives are similar to short-chain methyl cyanoacrylate (Super Glue), but are less toxic to tissue. Octyl-2-cyanoacrylate, (DermaBond; Biersdorf), is a long-chain acrylate. It polymerizes to form an adhesive film in the presence of moisture. This product functions as a hemostatic agent and possibly reduces infection rates via antimicrobial properties. It has been shown to produce good cosmesis for

113. Winter GD (1962) Formation of a scab and the rate of epithelialization of superficial wounds in the skin of the young domestic pig. **Nature** 193:293.
114. Hinman CD et al. (1963) Effect of air exposure and occlusion on experimental human skin wounds. **Nature** 200:377.
115. Ballas CD, Davidson JM (2001) Delayed wound healing in aged rats is associated with increased collagen gel remodeling and contraction by skin fibroblasts, not with differences in apoptotic or myofibroblast cell populations. **Wound Repair Regeneration** 9(3):223–227.
116. Moulin V, Tam BY, Castilloux G et al. (2001) Fetal and adult human skin fibroblasts display intrinsic differences in contractile capacity. **J Cell Physiol** 188(2):211–222.
117. O'Kane S, Ferguson MWJ (1997) Transforming growth factor betas and wound healing. **Int J Biochem Cell Biol** 29:63–78.
118. Cowin AJ, Holmes TM, Brosnan P, Ferguson MW (2001) Expression of TGF-beta and its receptors in murine fetal and adult dermal wounds. **Eur J Dermatol** 11(5):424–431.

119. Reed B, Clark RF (1985) Cutaneous tissue repair: practical implications of current knowledge. II. **J Am Acad Dermatol** 13:919.
120. Helfman T, Ovington L, Falanga V (1994) Occlusive dressings and wound healing. **Clin Dermatol** 12:121.
121. Dykes PJ, Hill SA (2001) Effects of adhesive dressings on the stratum corneum of the skin. **J Wound Care** 10(2):7.
122. Kolokol'chikova EG, Budkevich LI, Bobrovnikov AE et al. (2001) Morphologic changes in burn wounds after transplantation of allogeneic fibroblasts. **Bull Exp Biol Med** 131(1)89–93.
123. Falabella AF, Valencia IC, Eaglstein WH, Schachner LA (2000) Tissue-engineered skin (Apligraf) in the healing of patients with epidermolysis bullosa wounds. **Arch Dermatol** 136(10):1225–1230.

TABLE 4.6   Occlusive and semiocclusive wound dressings

Dressing	Composition	Properties		
		Adhesive	Absorbent	Transparent
Polyurethane membranes Bioclusive, Select Opsite Tegaderm Acu-Derm Epiview Mefilm Polyskin II Blisterfilm Proclude	0.2-mm polyurethane with an adhesive backing	++	−	++
Hydrocolloids Duoderm Comfeel Cutinova Hydro Restore Ultec Replicare Tegasorb Mitraflex	Carboxymethyl cellulose with an adhesive backing	+	+	−
Hydrogels Vigilon Second Skin Nugel Clearsite Intrasite Gel Flexiderm Tegagel Normigel	Polyethylene oxide-and-saline gel sandwiched between polyethylene sheets	−	++	+
Alginates Sorbsan Kaltostat Algosteril Curasorb Algisite Tegagen Melgisorb	Alginic acid, mixed calcium and sodium salts	−	++++	−

repair of lacerations and incisions, but it compares less favorably than standard suture for higher-tension closure of skin biopsies and excisional wounds.[124,125] Newer formulation of octyly-2-cyanoacrylate has been studied as a "liquid dressing" that yielded instantaneous hemostasis and enhanced wound healing of partial thickness wounds in pigs.[126]

Topical and dressing-impregnated growth factors are subjects of long-term investigation. Becaplermin (Reganex) is a recombinant, human platelet-derived growth factor, FDA approved in gel formulation to speed healing of lower extremity, diabetic and neuropathic ulcers.[127] Reganex has been anecdotally reported to speed healing of a refractory ulcerated hemangioma.[128] Epidermal growth factor-loaded microspheres incorporated into a polymeric

bilayer dressing has also been developed as a novel approach to enhance wound healing.[129]

Silicone gel sheeting was first reported as an effective treatment for burn scars in 1983.[130] Since that time, a variety of silicone-based dressing materials have been marketed to prevent and treat hypertrophic scars.[131,132] Although the mechanism of action is unclear, these products are thought to work by generating and maintaining a field of static electricity to prevent surface friction.[133] The dressings are self-adherent, durable and flexible. They are designed to be applied and left in place for 12–24h/day, and be removed daily for cleansing for a treatment period of 2 to 7 months. Compared to repeated injection of steroids, this treatment option is safe, painless, relatively cost

124. Quinn J, Wells G, Sutcliffe T et al. (1997) A randomized trial comparing octylcyanoacrylate tissue adhesive and sutures in the management of lacerations. **JAMA** 277:1527–1530.
125. Quinn JV, Osmond MH, Yurack JA, Moir PJ (1995) N-2-butylcyanoacrylate: risk of bacterial contamination with appraisal of its antimicrobial effects. **J Emerg Med** 13:581–585.
126. Davis SC, Eaglstein WH, Cazzaniga AL, Mertz PM (2001) An octyl-2-cyanoacrylate formulation speeds healing of partial thickness wounds. **Dermatol Surg** 27:783–788.
127. Smiell JM, Wieman TJ, Steed DL et al. (1999) Efficacy and safety of becaplermin in patients with non-healing, lower extremity diabetic ulcers; a combined analysis of four randomized studies. **Wound Rep Regen** 7:335–346.
128. Sugarman JL, Mauro TM, Frieden IJ (2002) Treatment of an ulcerated hemangioma with recombinant platelet-derived growth factor. **Arch Dermatol** 138(3):314–316.

129. Ulubayram K, Nur Cakar A, Korkusuz P et al. (2001) EGF containing gelatin-based wound dressings. **Biomaterials** 22(11):1345–1356.
130. Perkins K, Davey RB, Wallis KA (1983) Silicone gel: a new treatment for burn scars and contractures. **Burns Incl Therm Inj** 9(3):201–204.
131. Ahn S, Monafo W, Mustoe T (1991) Topical silicone gel for the prevention and treatment of hypertrophic scar. **Arch Surg** 126:499.
132. Poston J (2000) The use of silicone gel sheeting in the management of hypertrophic and keloid scars. **J Wound Care** 9(1):10–16.
133. Hirschowitz B, Alimna Y (1993) Silicone occlusive sheeting is recommended for the treatment of hypertrophic and keloid scars. **Eur J Plast Surg** 16:5.

TABLE 4.6   Occlusive and semiocclusive wound dressings—con't

Dressing	Composition	Properties		
		Adhesive	Absorbent	Transparent

Foams
  Lyofoam
  Cutinova Plus
  Curaforam
  Allevyn
  Sof-Foam
  Mepilex
	Synthetic polymers and copolymers	−	+ + + + + +	−

Foam Gel
  Mitraflex
  Epilock				

Contact Layer
  Silon TSR
  N-Terface
  Mepitel
  TelfaClear
  Drynet
  Tegapore
	Transparent, non-adherent, porous, protective sheet	−	−	+ + + +

(Modified from Helfman T, Oringtan L, Falanga V (1994) Occlusive dressings and wound healing. Clin Dermatol 12:121; and Falanga V, Eaglstein WH (1987) Wound healing: practical aspects. Prog Dermatol 22(3):1, with permission.)

effective and especially appropriate for children. Several variants of this product are commercially available (e.g., Topigel, CUI Corporation [Carpenteria, CA, USA]; Epi-Derm, Biodermis [Las Vegas, NV, USA]. A more recent comparative trial demonstrated that silicone and nonsilicone gel occlusive dressings are equally effective in the treatment of keloids and hypertrophic scars.[134]

Other modalities used for wound healing and treatment of hypertrophic scars and keloids include: hyperbaric oxygen therapy, vacuum-assisted closure pumps, pharmacologic approaches to delay or inhibit synthesis and cross-linking of collagen (e.g., β-aminoproprionitrile, D-penicillamine, calcium-channel antagonists), immunomodulators (e.g., imiquimod, intreferon-γ cyclosporin), specific antigrowth factor therapy (e.g., neutralizing antibodies to TGF-β) and even gene therapy.[135]

TOPICAL TREATMENT

PRINCIPLES

Vehicles

Successful topical therapy depends not only on selection of the most appropriate pharmacologically active ingredient but also on the most optimal vehicle for delivery. Vehicles include water-soluble liquids, gels and foams, powders and lipid-based ointments, creams and lotions. A variety of other ingredients are added to improve the odor, texture, color, and shelf life. Liquid bases include water, alcohol, glycerin and propylene glycol. Glycerin is hygroscopic, humectant and soluble in water and alcohol. Propylene glycol is more widely used than glycerin. It is not only miscible with water, alcohol, acetone and essential oils, but it is also a preservative and possesses *in vivo* antimicrobial activity against certain bacteria, dermatophytes and pityrosporium. Propylene glycol in concentrations of greater than 5% may irritate

the skin; allergic contact dermatitis is uncommon, but important to recognize because of its prevalence in foods, medications, industrial products and a wide variety of topical preparations.[136] Used as a vehicle for orally administered vitamins or intravenous medications, propylene glycol has been associated with CNS toxicity in premature infants.[137] Adverse reactions to glycerin are much less common.[138]

A popular line of emollient products (Biersdorf) illustrates the relationship between ointment, cream and lotion: Aquaphor is petrolatum, mineral oil, mineral wax and wool wax alcohols; Eucerin Creme is Aquaphor with water, emulsifiers and preservatives; Nivea Creme is Eucerin with more water, glycerin plus additional emulsifiers, stabilizers, solvents and fragrance. The preservative used in the cream and lotion products (methylisochlorothiazolinone/isothiazolinone or Kathon CG) is a common cause of allergic contact dermatitis in adults and children.[139]

Propellants

Propellants are rapid but less cost-effective vehicles for topical medication. Sprays require extra effort to avoid the eyes and direct the medication to where it is needed. Alcohol-based vehicles can cause stinging and irritation when applied to compromised skin. Commercially available petrolatum-based emollients sprays include Dermamist (Ferndale Laboratories), with 10% petrolatum in a mineral oil, coconut oil, butane, isobutene, propane vehicle, and Diaper Rash with Vitamins A&D Spray (Touchless Care Concepts, LLC), with 50% mineral oil, 15% petrolatum, cyclomethicone, cod liver oil, lanolin, microcrystalline wax, lemon oil. Moisture Barrier Spray with Zinc Oxide (Touchless Care Concepts, LLC), is a similar product that also contains 25% zinc oxide. Sprays are a fast and effective means of applying sunscreen to children. Foam is another rapid and well-accepted vehicle that is more easily directed to the application site. Alcohol-based foams (e.g., Luxiq, Connetics) are especially useful to treat hair-bearing areas.

134. de Oliveira GV, Nunes TA, Magna LA et al. (2001) Silicone versus nonsilicone gel dressings: a controlled trial. **Dermatol Surg** 27(8):721–726.
135. Cherry GW, Hughes AM et al. (2000) Wound healing. In Oxford Textbook of Surgery, Chapter 6, Vol. 1, 2nd edition, Morris PJ, Wood WC, eds. New York: Oxford University Press, pp. 131–159.
136. Catanzaro J, Smith J (1991) Propylene glycol dermatitis. **J Am Acad Dermatol** 24:90.
137. MacDonald MG, Getson PR, Glaogow AM et al. (1987) Propylene glycol: increased incidence of seizures in low birth weight infants. **Pediatrics** 79:622.
138. Fischer AA (1986) In: Contact Dermatitis, Ch. 17, 3rd edn. Philadelphia: Lea & Febiger.
139. Manzini BM, Fewrdani G, Simonetti V et al. (1998) Contact sensitization in children. **Pediatr Dermatol** 15(1):12.

Gels

Gels are popular astringent vehicles for people with oily skin and are well suited for acne medications and sunscreens. They are colloidal dispersions in a semisolid base that liquify on contact and dry to a greaseless film. Most gels are composed primarily of water, acetone, alcohol or propylene glycol suspended with organic polymers such as agar, gelatin, hydroxypropyl cellulose, carbomer methylcellulose, pectin and polyethylene glycol. Gels also enhance penetration through the epidermis, so they are useful for the delivery of corticosteroids especially in hair-bearing areas. In some cases, initial treatment with a gel-based exfolliant will thin psoriatic plaques prior to topical corticosteroid therapy and allow increased absorption. Disadvantages of gels include lack of emollient properties, burning and stinging on application and in some cases, ready dissolution after washing or perspiring.

Lotions

Lotions are suspensions of powder or other material in liquid. They offer the convenience of easy spreadability over large areas. They can be rubbed into almost any surface, even hair-bearing and intertriginous areas. Lotions containing alcohols are cooling, antiseptic and astringent, but they often sting or burn when applied to compromised skin which limits their use in eczematous conditions.

A "shake lotion" is a powder-in-water suspension that requires mixing immediately before application. Shake lotions have been historically useful as protective, drying and soothing treatments for subacute inflammatory processes. Basic shake lotion contains zinc oxide, talc, glycerin and water. Calamine lotion is basic shake lotion plus ferric oxide, bentonite magma and calcium hydroxide.

"Soapless cleansers" are lotions primarily composed of either glycerin (Aquanil) or propylene glycol (Cetaphil) and fatty alcohols. These products were originally designed to limit skin drying from frequent bathing with hot water and harsh soaps. When applied to dry skin, these products produce a foamy film that can be wiped off, leaving a humectant lubricating residue. However, frequent, short, tepid water baths with limited use of gentle cleansing products has many benefits including skin debridement, fun, and relaxation. Immediately after bathing, application of a bland emollient will limit evaporative dessication and enhance skin hydration.

Creams

Creams are emulsions of oil (hydrophobic hydrocarbons, animal or vegetable fats) and water; the ratio of these ingredients determines the texture, emollient and occlusive properties of the product. The less greasy, washable oil-in-water emulsions have been referred to as "hydrophilic ointment" or "vanishing cream." The more lubricating, occlusive products are also known as "cold cream." Formulation of creams requires the addition of emulsifiers, stabilizers and preservatives. Humectants, perfumes, and coloring agents are often added. Cream is the most popular vehicle for topical medications. As a generalization, the number of ingredients in a cream is proportional to the risk of contact irritation or sensitization, but specific ingredients such as wool wax alcohols, formaldehyde, formaldehyde releasers, parabens and Kathon CG are particularly common sensitizers. Other limitations of creams are poor retention on oozing surfaces, matting of hairy areas and diminished efficacy compared to ointments for maintaining stratum corneum hydration or promoting penetration of an active ingredient.

Ointments

Ointments are water-insoluble occlusive mixtures of animal, vegetable or mineral lipids. White petrolatum, a mineral-based hydrocarbon, is a purified and bleached or more often synthethic mixture of high-molecular-weight alkanes. This inexpensive ointment is widely used because it is odorless, colorless and rarely sensitizing. Anhydrous lanolin is a natural product derived from sheep's wool. It contains sterols (cholesterol, lanosterol), fatty alcohols (steryl and cetyl alcohol) and fatty acids with varying composition. Lanolin is rarely sensitizing in people with normal skin, but it is a cause of allergic contact dermatitis in those with chronic skin problems. Ointments impart a greasy–tacky feel to the skin and can exacerbate miliaria, acne and folliculitis in some patients.

The commercial division separating ointments from creams is blurred, and the nomenclature can be confusing. Many prescription "ointment" vehicles are greasy water-in-oil creams (e.g., Westcort, hydrocortisone valerate ointment). "Hydrophilic ointment" is an oil-in-water cream that contains a high proportion of water to make it washable and easily spreadable. While plain white petrolatum is a pure hydrocarbon grease, hydrophilic petrolatum (e.g., Aquaphor, Beiersdorf) is a mixture of pure petrolatum, beeswax, alcohols, cholesterol and a little water, formulated to facilitate compounding with hydrophilic ingredients.

Powders

Powders are finely pulverized, hygroscopic agents that dry and minimize friction of the skin surface. Examples include zinc oxide, zinc stearate, magnesium stearate, talc, cornstarch, and precipitated calcium carbonate. Applied to intertriginous areas, powders absorb body fluids to prevent maceration and irritation, but caking is often a problem. Powder should be administered gently and directly to the skin, not shaken or dusted so as to avoid inhalation of the material. Contrary to popular belief, cornstarch does not encourage bacterial, yeast, or fungal over-growth. Some commercially available powders contain other active ingredients (e.g., antimicrobial agents) for use in the treatment of tinea pedis or as deodorants/antiperspirants.

Pastes

Pastes are a mixture of powder and ointment. They are used as protectants against external irritants and sunlight. Lassar's Plain Zinc Paste is a historically compounded 1:1:4 mixture of zinc oxide, starch and white petrolatum. Variants of this recipe are useful for diaper dermatitis and intertrigo. Pastes are opaque and are best applied liberally, obscuring the underlying skin from inspection. However, ointment-based pastes are easily removed with mineral oil and gentle wiping. Zinc oxide-based pastes may be used as broad-spectrum sunscreen. Opaque products were popularized by the addition of day-glo coloring. Micronized zinc oxide is a more cosmetically acceptable alternative, transparent to visible light, but effectively blocks UVA and UVB.

TOPICAL ANTIMICROBIALS

Minor skin infections are best treated with cleansing, gentle debridement and occlusive dressings. Many antimicrobial cleansers are available, but there is limited data to support the clinical efficacy of these products compared to plain soap and water. Five percent acetic acid is readily available as white vinegar. Diluted to 0.25% in water (approximately one tablespoon per quart (per liter)), it makes an effective, nonirritating antiseptic soak. Three percent hydrogen peroxide solution is another inexpensive and readily available antiseptic for minor skin wounds; it can also be diluted to 1% as a mouthwash. It interacts with serum catalases to produce free oxygen and water. The effervescence gently debrides devitalized tissue. Intrinsic hydrogen peroxide released from neutrophils in a wound stimulates production of macrophage vascular endothelial growth factor (VEGF), which is crucial for wound healing.[140] Seventy percent isopropyl alcohol is bactericidal, but it will not reliably destroy fungus or virus. It is not recommended for wound cleansing because it is irritating and can coagulate protein. Elemental tincture of iodine and iodophors provide broad-spectrum, substantive antimicrobial activity. Povidone–iodine is an iodophor comprised of iodine and an organic nonsurfactant polymer that acts to release the iodine slowly so it is less irritating and less toxic than elemental iodine solutions. However, iodine-containing antimicrobial agents should be avoided in infants and children.

140. Cho M, Hunt TK, Hussain MZ (2001) Hydrogen peroxide stimulates macrophage vascular endothelial growth factor release. **Am J Physiol – Heart Circ Physiol** 280(5):H2357–2363.

Povidone–iodine has been associated with impaired wound healing and reduced wound strength.[141] The use of povidone–iodine is a routine practice in many newborn and neonatal intensive care nurseries that deserves reconsideration. Adverse effects of topically applied iodine antiseptics in infants have been recognized for at least 20 years. Skin necrosis has been documented by case report, an injury most likely to occur when an excess amount of solution is inadvertently left in contact with the skin for a prolonged period of time. Exposure to iodine in the perinatal or neonatal period has been associated with dramatic, prolonged elevation in plasma and urinary iodine, transient hypothyroxinemia, hypothyroidism and goiter.

The most convenient antimicrobial products are widely available in a variety of bar and liquid cleansers: triclocarban (e.g., Coast, Dial, Safeguard, Zest), chlorhexidine (Hibiscrub, Hibiclens, Hibistat), triclosan (Lever 2000, liquid Dial, pHisoderm) and hexachlorophene (pHisoHex). These agents have antibacterial and antifungal properties. Chlorhexidine has the broadest spectrum, the most substantivity and a low potential for producing contact sensitivity.[142] Its substantivity enhances the efficacy of chlorhexidine and minimizes the risk of percutaneous absorbtion. No toxic systemic effects have been attributed to chlorhexidine alone, even after massive oral ingestion (Zenca Pharmaceuticals, personal communication). In addition, it is rapid acting, and has low potential for producing contact sensitivity even with long term contact. Triclocarban is a carbanilamide and is effective against Gram-positive organisms. Triclosan and hexachlorophene are phenolic compounds with Gram-positive and Gram-negative antimicrobial activity. Triclosan has also been shown to have anti-inflammatory properties.[143] Hexachlorophene is a phenolic compound well known for its anti-staphylcoccal properties and found in 3% concentration in pHisoHex® (Sterling Winthrop Inc). pHisoHex® is an antiseptic cleanser popularized for bathing infants until its neurotoxic properties were recognized in the early 1970s. Percutaneous absorption resulted in an acute encephalopathy, seizures, and death. Phenolic compounds should be avoided in pediatric patients with poor skin barrier function (e.g., preterm infants and children with severe dermatitis).[144]

Gentian violet is a time-honored antimicrobial agent, effective against some Gram-positive and Gram-negative bacteria as well as some pathogenic *Candida* spp.[145] It has been widely used to treat thrush, and is a simple, single application treatment for secondary candidiasis complicating irritant diaper dermatitis. Gentian violet is infamous for transient deep purple staining of the skin, and permanent accidental staining of clothing. Prolonged use has been associated with nausea, vomiting, diarrhea, and ulceration of mucous membranes; carcinogenicity in mice has been reported. However, this compound has enjoyed decades of widespread use with very few reported adverse events.

A number of over-the-counter topical antibiotics are available for initial treatment of superficial injuries. The most widely used product, Neosporin, contains neomycin sulfate, zinc bacitracin, and polymyxin sulfate with broad-spectrum activity against *Staphylococcus*, *Streptococcus* and many Gram-negative bacteria. However, neomycin is a potent topical sensitizer affecting 1% of the general population and a much higher percentage of individuals with chronic eczematous conditions.[146] Polysporin is an alternative product, containing only bacitracin and polymyxin. However, the use of Neosporin can cosensitize

some individuals to bacitracin as well; bacitracin-containing antibiotics are not an acceptable alternative in these patients.[147] Bacitracin monotherapy has also been associated with contact dermatitis and rare cases of septic shock.[148] Cost was the only difference found in a comparative trial of bacitracin and white petrolatum in the treatment of surgical wounds. Healing time and infection rates were similar.[149]

Silver sulfadiazine is the active component of Silvadene® (Hoechst Marion Roussel) a topical antibiotic commonly applied to second- and third-degree burns to prevent and/or treat wound sepsis. It has a broad spectrum of activity against Gram-positive bacteria including *S. aureus* and methicillin–resistant *S. aureus* (MRSA), Gram-negative bacteria including *Pseudomonas* and yeast including *C. albicans*.[150] In addition, both the vehicle (white petrolatum, stearyl alcohol, isopropyl myristate, sorbitan monooleate, polyoxyl 40 stearate, propylene glycol, water and methylparaben) and the active ingredient speed epidermal migration and wound healing.[151] Reported percutaneous toxicities include kernicterus and agranulocytosis related to the sulfa component, and argyria.[21,23,24] Children with large surface area burns are at highest risk and should be monitored closely. This and other sulfa drugs should be used with caution in newborns. Increased absorption of the silver moiety has been associated with argyria. Hyperbilirubinemia is a well-recognized complication of systemic sulfa drugs in neonates.

Topical gentamicin is an aminoglycoside antibiotic and is bactericidal against Gram-negative bacteria including *Pseudomonas aeruginosa* as well as some Gram-positive organisms, including *S. aureus*. Although it is available in ointment, cream and ophthalmic solution, the latter form is most useful for the treatment of paronychia complicated by *Pseudomonas*. Associated allergic contact dermatitis is rare, but cross-sensitization between gentamicin and neomycin can occur.

For the past three decades, systemic antibiotics have been the gold standard for the treatment of primary or secondary bacterial skin infections. However, the development of 2% mupirocin ointment (Bactroban) has allowed safe and effective topical therapy for cutaneous staphylococcal and streptococcal infections. This antibacterial compound is produced by the saprophyte *Pseudomonas fluorescens*.[152] Several comparative studies have established that mupirocin ointment and oral erythromycin are equally effective in the treatment of outpatient impetigo.[153] Topical therapy may also improve compliance in the treatment of infants and children. *S. aureus* nasal and hand carriage has been a significant, difficult-to-treat epidemiologic problem. Intranasally applied mupirocin ointment will safely and effectively eliminate *S. aureus* nasal colonization after 5 days with lasting effects for at least 3 months.[154] Recurrent staphylococcal skin infections can be minimized with monthly 5-day courses of nasal mupirocin.[155] Mupirocin can also effectively treat MRSA but chronic and widespread use has resulted in *S. aureus* resistance reported as early as 1990 in as series of patients with epidermolysis bullosa and in 65% of MRSA strains.[156,157]

Novel antimicrobial alternatives are being investigated to address emergence of multiple-agent resistant organisms. Tea tree oil has been shown to be active against staphylococi, streptococci, bacteroides, coliforms and fungus via its terpene constituents which disrupt the bacterial cell wall. In a study comparing mupirocin and tea tree oil in conjunction with triclosan washes

141. Kramer SA (1999) Effect of povidone-iodine on wound healing: a review. **J Vasc Nursing** 17(1):17–23.
142. Wade J, Casewell M (1991) The evaluation of residual antimicrobial activity on hands and its clinical relevance. **J Hosp Infect, Suppl B** 18:23.
143. Gaffar A, Scherl D, Afflitto J et al. (1995) The effect of triclosan on mediators of gingival inflammation. **J Clin Periodontol** 22:480–484.
144. Lester R (1983) Topical formulary for the pediatrician. **Pediatr Clin North Am** 30:749.
145. Anonymous (1997) Gentian violet. In Martindale: The Extra Pharmacopoeia (electronic version), Reynolds J, ed. Englewood, CO.
146. Patrick J, Panzer J, Derbes V (1970) Neomycin sensitivity in the normal individual. **Arch Dermatol** 102:532.
147. Binnick A, Clendenning W (1978) Bacitracin contact dermatitis. **Contact Dermatitis** 4:180.
148. Elsner P, Pevney I, Burg G (1990) Anaphylaxis induced by topically applied bacitracin. **Am J Contact Dermat** 1:162–164.
149. Smack DP, Harrington AC, Dun C et al. (1996) Infection and allergy incidence in ambulatory surgery patients using white petrolatum vs bacitracin ointment. A randomized controlled trial. **JAMA** 276:972–977.
150. Marone P, Monzillo V, Perversi L et al. (1998) Comparative *in vitro* activity of silver sulfadine, alone and in combination with cerium nitrate against staphtlococci and Gram-negative bacteria. **J Chemother** 10:17–21.
151. Alvarez O, Goslen J, Eaglstein W et al. (1987) Wound healing. In: Dermatology in General Medicine, 3rd ed. Fitzpatrick TB, Eisen AZ, Wolff K, ed. eds. New York: McGraw-Hill.
152. Leyden J (1990) Mupirocin: a new topical antibiotic. **J Am Acad Dermatol** 22:879.
153. McLinn S (1990) A bacteriologically controlled randomized study comparing the efficacy of 2% mupirocin ointment with oral erythromycin in the treatment of patients with impetigo **J Am Acad Dermatol** 22(5 Pt 1):883.
154. Reagan D, Doebbeling B, Pfaler M et al. (1991) Elimination of coincident *Staphylococcus aureus* nasal and hand carriage with intranasal application of mupirocin calcium ointment. **Ann Intern Med** 114:101.
155. Raz R, Miron D, Colodner R et al. (1996) A 1-year trial of mupirocin in the prevention of recurrent staphylococcal nasal colonization and skin infection. **Arch Intern Med** 156:1109–1112.
156. Moy J, Caldwell-Brown D, Lin A et al. (1990) Mupirocin-resistant *Staphylococcus aureus* after long-term treatment of patients with epidermolysis bullosa. **J Am Acad Dermatol** 22:893.
157. Miller AM, Dascal A, Portnoy J et al. (1996) Development of mupirocin resistance among methicillin-resistant *Staphylococcus aureus* after widespread use of nasal mupirocin ointment. **Infect Control Hosp Epidemiol** 17:811–813.

for the treatment of MRSA carriers, mupirocin cleared 13%, while tea tree oil cleared 33%.[158] Additional studies evaluating *Ocimum gratissimum* essential oil have also demonstrated remarkable *in vitro* antibacterial effects.[159]

A variety of topical antibiotics have been approved to treat acne, including benzoyl peroxide, azelaic acid, clindamycin, erythromycin, metronidazole, tetracycline and sodium sulfacetamide. Benzoyl peroxide (BP) has broad-spectrum bactericidal activity as well as exfoliant and comedolytic effects.[160] These two actions make it a useful first-line drug in the management of patients with mild inflammatory and comedonal acne. Clinical improvement may be seen in several days. BP is available with or without a prescription in a variety of vehicles (creams, lotions, washes or gels) in concentrations ranging from 2.5% to 10%. Increasing the concentration of BP to 10% does not greatly enhance the therapeutic effect but does increase the likelihood of drying, erythema and burning.[161] Adverse reactions include irritation, and rarely contact sensitization. It will bleach dark clothing.

Azelaic acid is a naturally occurring saturated dicarboxylic acid, bactericidal against *Pityrosporum acnes*, but also toxic to functionally abnormal melanocytes. Topical azalaic acid cream is an indicated treatment for acne vulgaris, and is a logical choice for patients with associated postinflammatory hyper-pigmentation. In addition, azelaic acid has an antiproliferative and cytotoxic effect on the human malignant melanocyte. Preliminary findings suggest an inhibitory effect on the progression of cutaneous malignant melanoma. The mechanism of this selective cytotoxic action of azelaic acid is unclear, but may possibly be related to its inhibition of mitochondrial oxidoreductase activity and DNA synthesis.[162]

Products containing clindamycin or erythromycin have comparable efficacy and are commercially available in a variety of vehicles. Clindamycin is effective against Gram-positive and anaerobic bacteria including *P. acnes*. Erythromycin has good Gram-positive coverage and anti-inflammatory properties, but it is a weak sensitizer.[163,164] Topical tetracycline is effective against staphylococci, streptococci and *P. acnes*, but may cause faint yellowing of the skin. Combination products that are more effective than either drug alone include those combining BP and erythromycin (Benzamycin) or clindamycin (Benzaclin), and a formulation of erythromycin and zinc. The disadvantages of combination preparations are cost, a need for refrigeration in some cases, and short shelf life.

Emergence of resistant *P. acnes* is a concern.[165] The percentage of patients attending a dermatology clinic in the UK who harbored antibiotic-resistant organisms rose from 34.5% to 60% between 1991 and 1996.[166] The majority of strains resistant to erythromycin exhibited cross-resistance to clindamycin and other macrolide, lincosamide and streptogamin antibiotics. *P. acnes* resistance to minocycline is least common, followed by doxycycline, tetracycline, and erythromycin. There is an association between carriage of erythromycin-resistant propionibacteria and poor clinical response to oral treatment with this agent.[167]

Metronidazole is active against Gram-positive, Gram-negative, anaerobic, and even some parasitic organisms. It is available in cream, lotion and gel formulations, useful in the treatment of acne vulgaris and rosacea, and with antedoctal success for ulcerated hemangiomas.[168] Sodium sulfacetamide is active against *P. acnes* via inhibition of proinflammatory enzymes.[169] A topical formulation of dapsone in 5% gel (Artisone) is currently under investigation for the treatment of acne vulgaris. Along with its potent anti-inflammatory properties, it has been found to be active against *P. acnes*. It is reportedly well tolerated with no local irritation, and systemic absorption appears to be minimal.[170]

Topical antifungal agents

More than $150 million is spent annually on topical antifungal agents.[171] Several products are available without a prescription, including less expensive, less specific, time-honored products. Whitefield's ointment contains 12% benzoic acid, which is fungistatic, and 6% salicyclic acid to enhance penetration. Castellani's paint is an astringent with antimicrobial properties that contains 10% ethyl alcohol, 10% resorcinol, 5% acetone, 1% boric acid, 0.3% basic fuchsin, and sometimes phenol. This combination stains the skin red and includes several compounds with the potential for percutaneous toxicity that should not be used on large surface areas or on infants. Gentian violet is another stain with activity against *Candida* as well as *S. aureus in vitro* (see the section on Topical Antibiotics, above).[172] Zinc pyrithione and selenium sulfide are available as a 1–2.5% shampoos. They both possess cytostatic activities, and have good residual adherence to skin after rinsing.

Nonprescription drugs include compounded undecylenic acid (e.g., Cruex, Desenex), available for more than 30 years, and tolnaftate (e.g., Tinactin, Aftate), was approved for use in 1963. These agents have been formulated in a wide variety of vehicles. Undecylenic acid is a fatty acid fungistatic against dermatophytes. It is well tolerated and more effective than placebo, but it is inferior to prescription medications. Tolnaftate is a thiocarbamate that inhibits fungal squalene epoxidase, and it is effective against dermatophytes and pityrosporum but not *Candida*. Clotrimazole (Lotrimin, Mycelex) and miconazole (Monistat) were the first imidazoles introduced during the early 1970s. These preparations have been available without prescription since 1990. They are broad-spectrum agents with fungicidal activity against dermatophytes, pityrosporum and *C. albicans*. Although they are effective against a wider range of organisms and for a greater percentage of users, local irritation or contact sensitization is more common with the use of these products than with the other nonprescription agents.

Many more antifungal agents, available by prescription, have been synthesized to specifically attack important sites of fungal metabolism. These can be grouped according to their pharmacologic activities. The major categories are Polyenes, Imidazoles, Triazoles and Allylamines/Benzylamines (Table 4.7). Certain agents claim both fungistatic and fungicidal activity. There are no standard models to compare efficacy of various preparations, but higher concentrations are generally more potent. Clinical studies are of importance in comparing the relative antifungal action of these products.[173,174]

A major problem in the development of safe antifungal agents is the similarities between the synthetic pathways that yield fungal ergosterol and mammalian cholesterol. Polyenes are naturally occurring products of *Streptomyces* species that alter fungal membrane integrity by irreversibly binding to ergosterol. Imidazoles alter fungal membrane permeability by blocking the synthesis of ergosterol through interaction with ^{14}C-α-demethylase, a cytochrome P450-dependent enzyme, not specific for fungi. This leads to

158. Allen P (2001) Tea tree oil: the science behind the antimicrobial hype. **Lancet** 358(9289):1245.
159. Orafidiya LO, Oyedele AL, Shittu A, Elujoba AA (2001) The formulation of an effective topical antibacterial product containing *Ocimum gratissimum* leaf essential oil. **Int J Pharm** 224(1–2):177–183.
160. Oh CW, Myung KB (1996) Tetention hyperkeratosis of experimentally induce comedones in rabbits: the effects of three comedolytics. **J Dermatol** 23:169–180.
161. Mills OH Jr, Kligman AM, Pochi P et al. (1986) comparing 2.5%, 5%, and 10% benzoyl peroxide on inflammatory acne vulgaris. **Int J Dermatol** 25:664.
162. Nguyen QH, Bui TP (1995) Azelaic acid: pharmacokinetic and phamacodynamic properties and its therapeutic role in hyperpigmentary disorders and acne. **Int J Dermatol** 34:75–84.
163. Ianaro A, Ialenti A, Maffia P et al. (2000) Anti-inflammatory activity of macrolide antibiotics. **J Pharmacol Exp Ther** 292(1):156–163.
164. Martins C, Freitas JD, Goncalo M et al. (1995) Allergic contact dermatitis from erythromycin. **Contact Dermatitis** 33:360.
165. Eady EA, Jones CE, Tipper JL et al. (1993) Antibiotic resistant propionibacteria in acne: need for policies to modify antibiotic usage. **Br Med J** 306:555–556.
166. Eady EA (1998) Bacterial resistance in acne. **Dermatology** 196:59.
167. Eady EA, Cove JH, Holland KT et al. (1989) Erythromycin resistant propionibacteria in antibiotic treated acne patients. Association with therapeutic failure. **Br J Dermatol** 121:51.
168. Witkowski JA, Parish LC (1991) Topical metronidazole gel. The bacteriology of decubitus ulcers. **Int J Dermatol** 30(9):660–661.
169. Breneman DL, Ariano MC (1993) Successful treatment of acne vulgaris in women with a new topical sodium sulfacetamide/sulfur lotion. **Int J Dermatol** 32:365–367.
170. Guttman C (2001) Topical dapsone gel offers dual mode of action in phase III studies. **Dermatol Times** November:22–23.
171. Chren MM (1994) Costs of therapy for dermatophyte infections. **J Am Acad Dermatol** 31:5103.
172. Brockow K, Grabenhorst P, Abeck D et al. (1999) Effect of gentian violet, corticosteroid and tar preparations in *Staphylococcus aureus* colonized atopic eczema. **Dermatology** 199(3):231–236.
173. Elewski BE (1993) Mechanisms of action of systemic antifungal agents. **J Am Acad Dermatol** 28:S28.
174. Ablon G, Rosen T, Spedale J (1996) Comparative efficacy of naftifine, oxiconazole and terbinafine in short-term treatment of tinea pedis. **Int J Dermatol** 35:591–593.

TABLE 4.7 Antifungal agents

Drug	Routes of administration	Spectrum of activity	Special considerations
Undecylenic acid (Desenex, Cruex)	Topical 10–22% powder, cream, ointment, spray, foam	Dermatophytes, ± *Candida*	Available OTC
Tolnaftate (Tinactin, Aftate)	Topical 1% cream, gel, spray, and powder	Dermatophytes	Available OTC
Ciclopirox olamine (Loprox)	Topical 1% cream, gel, lotion, solution; 8% nail lacquer	Dermatophytes, yeasts	Lower incidence of dermatitis than imidazoles May cause irritant and rarely allergic contact dermatitis; available OTC
Imidazoles			
Clotrimazole (Lotrimin, Mycelex, Micatin)	Topical 1% cream, 1% lotion, 2% spray, vaginal tablets Oral troches	Dermatophytes, yeasts	Available OTC Available OTC
Miconazole nitrate (Monistat)	Topical 2% cream, vaginal tablets Intravenous solution	Dermatophytes, yeasts	
Econazole nitrate (Spectazole)	Topical 1% cream	Dermatophytes, yeasts	
Sulconazole (Exelderm)	Topical 1% cream, 1% solution	Dermatophytes, yeasts	
Ketoconazole (Nizoral)	Topical 2% cream, 2% shampoo Oral 200mg tablets	Dermatophytes, *Candida*, Pityrosporum, systemic mycoses with oral form	
Oxiconazole (Oxistst)	Topical 1% cream, 1% lotion	Dermatophytes, yeasts (weak), Pityrosporum	
Triazoles			
Itraconazole (Sporanox)	Oral 100-mg capsules	Dermatophytes, *Candida*, Pityrosporum, *Sporothrix*, systemic mycoses	Extensive hepatic metabolism and excretion, highly lipophilic, does not penetrate CSF
Fluconazole (Diflucan)	Oral 50-, 100-, and 200-mg tablets Intravenous solution	Dermatophytes, *Candida*, Pityrosporum, *Sporothrix*, systemic mycoses	A bis-triazole compound, low lipophilicity, penetrates CSF, concentrates in urine

depletion of ergosterol and accumulation of lanosterol. Triazoles, like imidazoles, inhibit the cytochrome P450-dependent pathway but have a much higher relative affinity for the fungal, rather than the mammalian, enzyme system.[173] Allylamines/benzylamines also block the synthesis of ergosterol, but they do so by selectively inhibiting the fungal enzyme squalene epoxidase without affecting the cytochrome P450 pathway. This leads to accumulation of squalene rather than lanosterol. The importance of the sterol-to-squalene ratio is not clear.[175]

Ketoconazole is an imidazole that has been available since 1987 in topical form as a cream or shampoo. It has broad-spectrum fungistatic activity against dermatophytes and yeasts. It also has anti-inflammatory properties, proven in the treatment of seborrheic dermatitis, due to its ability to inhibit 5-lipoxygenase which decreases leukotriene B4.[176,177]

The allylamines, naftifine and terbinafine, have been developed and formulated as topical antifungal preparations. Butenafine, the most recently approved, is structurally and functionally similar to the allylamines, but a butylbenzyl group replaces the allylamine group. It has been used to successfully treat tinea pedis, tinea corporis and tinea cruris with activity against *Trichophyton mentagrophytes*.[178,179] Naftifine has shown broad-spectrum activity against most fungi *in vitro*; however, clinical studies have demonstrated efficacy only against the common causes of tinea cruris and tinea pedis. These do not include yeasts or dermatophytes commonly seen in childhood infections, *Trichophyton tonsurans* and *Microsporum* species, with reports of naftifine-unresponsive cases of tinea corporis due to *T. tonsurans* in children.[180] In addition to its inhibitory activity against fungal squalene epoxidase, naftifine has also been shown to inhibit the chemotaxis and respiratory burst of human polymorphonuclear leukocytes *in vitro*. In comparative studies with the azoles, the allylamine/benzylamines were shown to have a greater degree of direct anti-inflammatory properties.[181] Terbenafine, also useful in its spray formulation, has *in vitro* inhibitory activity against Gram-positive and Gram-negative organisms including *S. aureus*, *S. faecalis*, *Propionibacterium acnes*, and *Pseudomonas aeruginosa*.[182]

Ciclopirox, unlike many of the other antifungals that alter sterol biosynthesis, is a hydroxypyridone that interferes with cellular transport of essential precursors, membrane integrity and respiratory pathways.[183] It is effective for the treatment of tinea corporis, tinea cruris, tinea pedis, tinea versicolor. Effective against *C. albicans* and less irritating than the imidazoles, ciclopirox cream is a reasonable choice for candida diaper dermatitis. However, the commercially available cream and lotion formulations (Loprox, Medicis) contain 1% benzyl alcohol as a preservative. Benzyl alcohol has been

175. Georgopapadakou NH, Bertasso A (1992) Effects of squalene epoxidase inhibitors on *Candida albicans*. **Antimicrob Agents Chemother** 36:1779.
176. Beetens JR, Loots W, Somers T et al. (1986) Ketoconazole inhibits the biosynthesis of leukotrienes *in vitro* and *in vivo*. **Biochem Pharmacol** 35:883–891.
177. Taieb A, Legrain V, Palmier C et al. (1990) Topical ketoconazole for infantile seborrhoeic dermatitis. **Dermatologica** 181:26–32.
178. Savin R, De Villez RL, Elewski B et al. (1997) One-week therapy with twice butenafine 1% cream versus vehicle in the treatment of tinea pedis. **J Am Acad Dermatol** 36:S15–19.
179. Arika T, Hase T, Yokoo M (1993) Anti-*Trichophyton mentagrophytes* activity and percutaneous permeation of butenafine in guinea pigs. **Antimicrob Agents Chemother** 37:363–365.

180. Rabinowitz L, Esterly N (1992) Naftifine (Naftin) in pediatrics. **Pediatrics** 90:652.
181. Rosen T, Schell BJ, Orngo I (1997) Anti-inflammatory activity of antifungal preparations. **Int J Dermatol** 36:788–792.
182. Nolting S, Brautigam M (1992) Clinical relevance of the antibacterial activity of terbinafine: a contralateral comparison between 1% terbinafine cream and a 0.1% gentamicin sulphate cream in pyoderma. **Br J Dermatol** 126(Suppl 39):56–60.
183. Abrams B, Heinz H, Hoehler T (1992) Ciclopirox olamine. A hydroxypyridone antifungal agent. **Clin Dermatol** 9:471–477.

TABLE 4.7   Antifungal agents—con't

Drug	Routes of administration	Spectrum of activity	Special considerations
Allylamines/benzylamines		Dermatophytes ± *Candida*, *Pityrosporum*, systemic mycoses with oral form	May not be as effective for *T. tonsurans* or *Microsporum*
Naftifine (Naftin)	Topical 1% cream, 1% gel		
Terbinafine (Lamasil)	Topical 1% cream, 1% solution, 1% spray		
	Oral 250-mg tablets		Contraindicated in preexisting renal and/or liver disease
Butenafine (Mentax)	Topical 1% cream		
Polyenes		*Candida*, systemic mycoses	
Amphotericin B (Fungizone)	Topical 3% cream, 3% lotion, 3% ointment		
	Powder for injection		
Nystatin (Mycostatin, Mytrex)	Topical Cream, ointment, powder (100 000U/g)	*Candida*	
	Oral		
	Suspension (100 000U/ml)		
	Tablets (500 000 units)		
	Pastilles (200 000 units)		
Griseofulvin	Oral	Dermatophytes	*T. tonsurans* resistance has been reported
	Microsize 250–500-mg tablets; 125–250-mg capsules; 125-mg/tsp susp.		
	Ultramicrosize 125-, 165-, 250-, 330-mg tablets		

CSF, cerebrospinal fluid; OTC, over the counter.

associated with kernicterus and intraventricular hemorrhage in premature infants treated with intravenous flush solutions containing the preservative in low concentrations.[184] As a nail lacquer, it is a less effective, but safer alternative for onychomycosis than systemic therapy.[185] Ciclopirox has been shown to have superior *in vitro* activity against *T. mentagrophytes* and *C. albicans* compared to other antifungals, as well as additional antibacterial activity against Gram-positive organisms, *Mycoplasma* sp. and *Trichomonas vaginalis*.[183] Anti-inflammatory properties have also been demonstrated via inhibition of both 5-lipoxygenase and cyclooxygenase.[186]

Topical antiviral agents

The most common cutaneous viral infections are molluscum contagiosum, caused by a poxvirus, verruca vulgaris and condyloma acuminatum caused by human papillomavirus (HPV), and herpes labialis caused by herpes simplex virus (HSV). Several topical treatments have been described for these generally self-limited infections. Categories include cytodestructive agents, immunomodulating medications (see below, Immunomodulating Agents and Topical Sensitizers), antiviral drugs, and active nonintervention.

Studies of both common and anogenital warts have shown that the majority of lesions resolve without treatment within 2 years.[187,188] This high rate of spontaneous regression supports the use of conservative therapy. Active nonintervention is a reasonable initial approach to asymptomatic, focal warts that have been present for less than 2 years. Adhesiotherapy (occlusion with tape) is an inexpensive, noninvasive alternative aimed at preventing the spread of lesions while providing a proactive approach for parents and patients.

Although safety and efficacy have not been studied in children, several topical viricidal medications are commercially available. The majority of these products have been studied for the treatment of herpes labialis. For maximum efficacy, most require impractically frequent application, four to six times a day, beginning at the earliest onset of symptoms. Acyclovir is available in a 5% ointment and is active against HSV1, HSV2 and varicella zoster virus (VZV). It is FDA approved in adults for the treatment of herpes labialis when applied six times per day for 7 days. Penciclovir (Denavir) is available in a 1% cream and is active against HSV1, HSV2, VZV and EBV. Compared to placebo, penciclovir was shown to decrease healing time from 5.5 days to 4.8 days in herpes labialis.[189] *n*-Docosanol promotes resistance against a variety of lipid-enveloped viruses including the herpesviruses by inhibiting fusion of the HSV envelope with the plasma membrane.[190] Docosanol (Abreva), available over-the-counter as a 10% cream for the treatment of herpes labialis, was shown to reduce symptoms and healing time by 18 hours.[191] Although this difference is statistically significant, it is not clinically significant. A comparative topical trial concluded that penciclovir was more effective than acyclovir, which was more effective than docosanal in a guinea pig model of

184. Cronin CM, Brown DR, Ahdab-Barmada M (1991) Risk factors associated with kernicterus in the newborn infant: importance of benzyl alcohol exposure. **Am J Perinatol** 8(2):80–85.
185. Ceschin-Roques CG, Hanel H, Pruja-Bouret SM et al. (1991) Cicolpirox nail lacquer in onychomycosis: *in vivo* penetration into and through nails and *in vitro* effect on pig skin. **Skin Pharmacol** 4:89–94.
186. Hanel H, Smith-Krutz E, Pastowsky S (1991) Therapy of seborrheic eczema with an antifungal agent with an antiphlogistic effect. **Mycoses** 34(Suppl 1):91–93.
187. Massing AM, Estonia WL (1963) Natural history of warts. **Arch Dermatol** 87:306–310.
188. Allen AL, Siegfried EC (1998) The natural history of condyloma in children. **J Am Acad Dermatol** 39:951–955.
189. Spruance SL, Rea TL, Thoming C et al. (1997) Penciclovir cream for the treatment of herpes simplex labialis. A randomized, multicenter, double-blind, placebo-controlled trial. **JAMA** 277:1374–1379.

cutaneous HSV. Docosanal was no more effective than vehicle.[192] S-1-(3-hydroxy-2-phosphonyl methoxypropyl) cytosine (HPMPC), also known as cidofovir, is an acyclic nucleoside phosphonate with antiviral activity against DNA viruses. An injectable formulation is FDA approved for intravenous treatment of cytomegalovirus retinitis in patients with AIDS. Cidofovir is an investigational antiviral agent available in a 1% gel and 3% cream, anecdotally reported to be effective for molluscum contagiosum, condyloma acuminatum and verruca vulgaris.[193–195] Although topical cidofovir is potentially effective against a number of viral infections, it is not commercially available and remains an investigational drug. Further product development has been curtailed due to its high cost and potential carcinogenic effects.

Imiquimod (Aldara) is an immune response modifier that acts by inducing production of cytokines, especially alpha interferon. Imiquimod has been shown to decrease viral DNA and gene transcription of proteins that aid in cellular proliferation, and reduce the HPV load at the site of application.[196] It is formulated as a 5% patient-applied cream (used three times weekly) that is FDA approved for treatment of genital warts in adults. Imiquimod cream has been useful for treating molluscum contagiosum,[197] but common warts do not respond as well as condylomata. However, the use of imiquimod cream applied to common warts under tape occlusion has become popular. Imiquimod cream has demonstrated efficacy in the treatment of actinic keratoses and superficial basal cell carcinoma. It has been anecdotally used to treat infantile hemangiomas.

Topically applied cytotoxic agents are time-honored alternatives for the treatment of molluscum contagiosum, condyloma and verruca vulgaris. Cytotoxic agents that require in-office application and include podophyllin and cantharidin. Podophyllin is a crude resin of the May apple plant and is commercially available in 10 to 50% solutions in alcohol or benzoin. It exerts its cytotoxic effects by interfering with the microtubule during metaphase. Several local and systemic reactions have occurred with use over large areas. In-office application of podophyllin has been largely replaced by self-application of purified podophyllotoxin because it offers the convenience of home use and greater safety. Purified 0.5% podophyllotoxin solution (Condylox) has been FDA approved for treatment of condyloma in adults. It is applied twice daily to the warts and a surrounding rim of normal skin in cycles of 3-days-on, 4-days-off. Purified podophyllotoxin is more effective than placebo in treating condylomata in adults, with clearance rates as high as as 77% after 16 weeks of therapy; however, high relapse rates diminish the long-term efficacy to 30%.[198] Although safety and efficacy have not been studied in children, purified podophyllotoxin can be considered for treatment of symptomatic, persistent anogenital warts in this population. Local pain and erosions occur in three-quarters of treated patients.

Cantharidin is a chemical extracted from the "blister beetle" Lytta vsicatoria that interferes with keratinocyte mitochondrial activity leading to cell death with suprabasal blistering. A 1% formulation of cantharidin in flexible collodion is commercially available for in-office use (Canthacur, Pharmascience, Montreal, Quebec, Canada, or Delasco Dermatologic Lab and Supply, Inc., Council Bluffs, IA, USA). Like many other destructive therapies, the efficacy of cantharadin has not been studied in controlled trials. Molluscum can be treated by applying a small drop to each lesion using the wooden end of a cotton-tipped applicator. After application site has been allowed to dry, tape may be applied to prevent the medication from being spread to other sites. Cantharadin

should be washed off after 4–12h, or sooner if pain occurs. The response to treatment is variable; there may be no reaction, crusting, blistering or hemorrhagic blistering. Anticipatory guidance and instructions for blister debridement and wound care should be provided.

A commercially available combination product containing 30% salicylic acid, 2% podophyllin, and 1% cantharidin in flexible collodion is also available (Canthacur PS, Pharmascience, Montreal, Quebec, Canada, or Cantharone 1; Dormer Labs, Rexdale, Ontario, Canada). Combination cantharidin is usually reserved for the treatment of nonmucosal, nonfacial warts. It is particularly valuable for children and caregivers that prefer in-office treatment but cannot tolerate cryotherapy. A thin coat is applied to the lesion and allowed to dry; the area is then occluded with tape. Anticipatory guidance must be given with regard to blister formation and care. Blister formation usually occurs 24–48h after application and is usually more dramatic than with cantharadin alone. In addition, ring warts are more likely to occur following combination therapy. Timely removal of the blister roof may help prevent this complication. Warm soaks and acetaminophen or EMLA cream (see above) can be used for any associated pain. After the treated site has healed, repeated applications at 2–4-week intervals may be indicated.

Antiviral treatments aimed at nonspecific tissue destruction do not carry a risk of systemic toxicity in children, but are painful and best reserved for assenting children. Destructive methods include liquid nitrogen, curetting, excision, electrosurgery and laser treatment, all of which are no more effective than less painful alternatives.

Antiparasitic agents

Scabies and lice are very common infestations in school-aged children. Permethrin and lindane are the most readily used medication for treatment, with other non-prescription therapies available including benzyl benzoate and precipitated sulfur.

Permethrin is a synthetic pyrethroid available in a 5% cream (Elimite) or a 1% cream rinse (Nix). It is FDA approved for the first line therapy of scabies and lice, and it acts by interfering with the arthropod's neuromembrane sodium channels causing paralysis. It is the treatment of choice in children due to its relative safety and is approved for use in patients 2 months or older. In the treatment of scabies, the cream should be applied on the patient from neck to toes, as well as on involved areas of the face and scalp with full application repeated in one week. All family members should also be treated with the same regimen. The cream rinse is available over-the-counter for the treatment of head lice, and should be applied twice with applications one week apart. Permethrin resistance has been reported.[199] Treatment failures may respond to 5% cream, addition of oral trimethorim/sulfamethoxazole,[200] or oral ivermectin.

Lindane is an organochloride insecticide available in 1% lotion and 1% shampoo. It is FDA approved for the treatment of scabies and lice that is unresponsive to other therapies, and it inhibits neurotransmission with subsequent paralysis of the arthropod. Its use should be avoided in infants and children due to its toxicity. Serum levels, when compared to permethrin, are 40 times higher with wide distribution, slow metabolism and storage in the brain and fatty tissues.[201,202] It is also associated with hematologic abnormalities and neurotoxicity including seizures.[203]

Benzoyl benzoate, used in animals and internationally in humans for the treatment of scabies, can be compounded in a 20–25% solution. Precipitated

190. Pope LE, Marcelletti JF, Katz LR et al. (1998) The anti-herpes simplex virus activity of n-docosanol includes inhibition of the viral entry process. Antiviral Res 40(1–2):85–94.
191. Sacks SL, Thisted RA, Jones TM (2001) Clinical efficacy of topical docosanol 10% cream for herpes simplex labialis: a multicenter, randomized, placebo-controled trial. J Am Acad Dermatol 45(2):222–230.
192. McKeough MB, Spruance SL (2001) Comparison of new topical treatments for herpes labialis: efficacy of penciclovir cream, acyclovir cream and n-docosanol cream against experimental cutaneous herpes simplex virus type 1 infection. Arch Dermatol 137(9):1153–1158.
193. Meadows KP, Tyring SK, Pavia AT et al. (1997) Resolution of recalcitrant molluscum contagiosum virus lesions in human immunodeficiency virus-infected patients treated with cidofovir. Arch Dermatol 133:987–990.
194. Snoeck R, VnRanst M, Anderi G et al. (1995) Treatment of anogenital papillomavirus infections with an acyclic nucleoside phosphaonate analogue (letter). N Engl J Med 333:943–944.
195. Zabawski EJ, Sand B, Goetz D et al. (1997) Treatment of verruca vulgaris with topical cidofovir (letter). JAMA 278:1236.
196. Perry CM, Lamb HM (1999) Topical imiquinod: a review of its use in genital warts. Drug 58:375–390.
197. Syed TA, Goswami J, Ahmadour OA, Ahmad SA (1998) Treatment of molluscum contagiosum in males with an analog of imiquinod 1% cream: a placebo-controlled, double-blind study. J Dermatol 25:309–312.
198. Link MR (1992) Therapy of genital human papillomavirus infections. II Methods of treatment. Int J Dermatol 31:769–776.
199. Burgess IF, Peock S, Brown CM (1995) Head lice resistant to pyrethroid insecticides in Britain. Br Med J 311:752.
200. Hippolito RB, Mallorca FG, Zuniga-Macaraig ZO (2001) Head lice infestation: single drug versus combination therapy with one percent permethrin and trimethoprim/sulfamethoxasole. Pediatrics 107(3):E30.

sulfur, the treatment of choice for scabies before development of insecticides, can be compounded in 6% cream or ointment. The safety or efficacy of these two therapies has not been established in children.

Malathion is an organothiophosphate insecticide. USP grade malathion is US FDA approved for the treatment of tinea capitis (Ovide® Lotion, 0.5%). Technical grade malathion can contain impurities such as isomalathion, malaoxon, and trimethyl phosphothioate, which were implicated as a cause of a variety of illnesses after exposure aimed at eradicating a 1998 Medfly infestation in Florida.[204] The level of these impurities in USP grade malathion is low, and the product has no demonstrable carcinogenic or mutagenic activity.

An *in vitro* trial in Florida demonstrated pediculocidal efficacy (from most to least effective) as follows: 0.5% malathion, A-200 shampoo (a natural pyrethrin product synergized with piperonyl butoxide), undiluted 1% permethrin, diluted permethrin, RID (a natural pyrethrin product synergized with piperonyl butoxide), and 1% lindane shampoo.[205] An evidence-based systematic review of the literature concluded that permethrin, synergized pyrethrin and malathion were all effective in the treatment of head lice, while physical lice removal was a relatively ineffective treatment.[206] Emerging drug resistance means there is no direct contemporary evidence of the comparative effectiveness of these products. The "best" choice depends on local resistance patterns.

Exfolliants

This category of active ingredients was formally identified by the misnomer, "keratolytics." These agents do not lyse keratin, but do alter thickened stratum corneum to allow enhanced hydration, desquamation and percutaneous penetration of other active ingredients. Water is the most basic exfolliant. The pharmacologic properties of most products can be enhanced by first hydrating the skin with water.

Salicylic acid was the first identified exfolliant agent, and it has been in use for the treatment of skin disorders for over 2000 years.[207] It can be considered a β-hydroxy acid or a phenolic aromatic acid and is lipid-soluble allowing interactions with keratinocytes in the epidermis and hair follicles.[208] Salicylic is exfolliant, comedolytic and promotes desquamation, in part, by decreasing cell–cell adhesion.[209] In one study of hairless mice, 30% salicylic acid caused loss of cornified cells with subsequent activation of epidermal basal cells and fibroblasts.[210] Formulations containing salicylic acid are still used to treat a wide variety of skin disorders. Low-potency 3–6% ointments or propylene glycol-based salicylic acid lotions (e.g., Keralyt, Saligel) augment therapy for psoriasis, seborrheic dermatitis, icthyoses and other scaling dermatoses. Five to 40% salicylic acid together with equal parts of lactic acid in a flexible collodion or compounded in Aquaphor can be used on a daily basis as a convenient relatively painless treatment for warts or calluses. Six percent salicylic acid with 12% benzoic acid (e.g., Whitfield's ointment or tincture) is a time-honored treatment for superficial fungal infections. Salicylic acid is also anti-inflammatory. Adverse reactions are infrequent. Salicylic acid is a weak sensitizer.[211] Systemic toxicity is rare but can occur after prolonged and/or extensive use of topical salicylic acid, especially in children.[212] The initial symptoms are headache, dizziness, and tinnitus, which might be inappropriately treated with salicylates, converting a precarious situation into a grave one.

α-Hydroxy acids are carboxylic acids derived from natural plant sources. Glycolic acid and lactic acid have recently gained popularity in the treatment of a wide range of hyperkeratotic conditions as well as in the cosmetics industry as a skin rejuvenating agent. Use of α-hydroxy acids causes detachment of keratinocytes with normalization of keratinization and an increase in epidermal thickness, collagen, elastin and glycosaminoglycans.[213,214] These agents also act as humectants and free-radical scavengers.[215] Many different over-the-counter products are available either directly to patients or marketed exclusively through physician's offices. Formulations of less than 12% concentration have been used effectively for xerosis, icthyoses, keratosis pilaris and palmoplantar keratodermas.[216–218] Twelve percent ammonium lactate (e.g., Lac-Hydrin) has been shown to mitigate the adverse local effects of potent topical corticosteroids without decreasing their anti-inflammatory activity.[212] At higher concentrations, glycolic acid has been used for chemical peeling, in the treatment of acne scarring and photoaging. Adverse effects are limited to irritation. There is a theoretical risk of lactic acidosis following prolonged or excessive use of lactic acid products in infants and/or children with poor skin barrier function (e.g., those with icthyosis).

Propylene glycol, alone in a 40–60% aqueous solution or compounded in Aquaphor as a 25% ointment, is an effective humectant and exfolliant agent with antimicrobial properties. Its efficacy is boosted when used under occlusion. It can also augment the exfolliant activity of salicylic acid (see above). Irritant and/or allergic contact dermatitis can occur following topical application of propylene glycol. Systemic administration has resulted in CNS toxicity.[137]

Urea is a hygroscopic and proteolytic agent with exfolliant activity. It increases skin hydration, decreases transepidermal water loss and enhances penetration of topical medications.[219] Forty percent urea ointment applied under occlusion can effectively dissolve thickened nails. In lower concentrations of 2–20% it causes desquamation of keratinocytes and has been used to treat the same spectrum of scaling dermatoses as lactic and glycolic acid preparations. Urea may be slightly more irritating.

Tars

Tar is produced following distillation of organic materials. Coal tars, wood tars and shale tars (ichthammol) have therapeutic uses in psoriasis, atopic dermatitis, seborrheic dermatitis, tinea versicolor, yeast/dermatophyte infections, vitiligo and pruritis. Tars are antipruritic and are believed to decrease epidermal proliferation and inflammation, although, the mechanism of action is unclear. Suppression of DNA synthesis[220] and prevention of the development of parakeratosis[221] by tar products have been demonstrated. Anti-inflammatory activity via inhibition of leukotriene B4, C5a and prevention of neutrophil chemotaxis has been shown.[222] A more recent study in patients with atopic dermatitis has shown tar to decrease the influx of T cells, eosinophils, CD1(+)/IFN-γ(+)/IL-4(+) cells as well as decrease vascular

201. Franz TJ, Lehman PA, Franz SF et al. (1997) Comparative percutaneous absorption of lindane and permethrin. **Arch Dermatol** 132:901–905.
202. Ginsburg CM, Loury W, Reisett JS (1997) Absorption of lindane in infants and children. **J Pediatr** 91:353–357.
203. Boffa MJ, Brough PA, Ead RD (1995) Lindane neurotoxicity. **Br J Dermatol** 133:1013.
204. Anonymous (1999) Surveillance for acute pesticide-related illness during the Medfly eradication program – Florida 1998. **MMWR – Morbidity & Mortality Weekly Report** 48(44):1015–1018, 1027.
205. Meinking TL, Serrano L, Hard B et al. (2002) Comparative *in vitro* pediculicidal efficacy of treatments in a resistant head lice population in the United States. **Arch Dermatol** 138(2):220–224.
206. Dodd CS (2001) Interventions for treating head lice. **Cochrane Database Syst Rev** 3:CD001165. Review.
207. Lin AN, Nakatsui T (1998) Salicylic acid revisited. **Int J Dermatol** 37:335–342.
208. Brackett W (1997) The chemistry of salicylic acid. **Cosmet Derm** 10(Suppl 4):5–6.
209. Roberts D, Marshall R, Marks R (1980) Detection of the action of salicylic acid on the normal stratum corneum. **Br J Dermatol** 103:191.
210. Imayama S, Ueda S, Isoda M (2000) Histologic changes in the skin of hairless mice following peeling with salicylic acid. **Arch Dermatol** 136(11):1390–1395.
211. Goh CL, Ng SK (1986) Contact allergy to salicylic acid. **Contact Dermatitis** 14:114.

212. Pascher F (1978) Systemic reactions to topically applied drugs. **Int J Dermatol** 17:768.
213. Hood HL, Kraeling ME, Robl MG, Bronaught RL (1999) The effects of an alpha hydroxy acid (glycolic acid) on hairless guinea pig skin permeability. **Food Chem Toxicol** 37(11):1105–1111.
214. Bernstein EF, Underhill CB, Lakkaakorpi J et al. (1997) Citric acid increases viable epidermal thickness and glycosaminoglycan content of sun-damaged skin. **Dermatol Surg** 23:689–694.
215. Elson M (1993) The molecular structure of glycolic acid and its importance in dermatology. **Cosm Dermatol** 6:31.
216. Vilaplana J, Coll J, Trullas C, Azon A, Pelejero C (1992) Clinical and non-invasive evaluation of 12% ammonium lactate emulsion for the treatment of dry skin in atopic and non-atopic subjects. **Acta Derm Venereol (Stockh)** 72:28.
217. Dahl M, Dahl A (1983) 12% lactate lotion for the treatment of xerosis. **Arch Dermatol** 119:27.
218. Buxman M, Hickman J, Ragsdale W (1986) Therapeutic activity of lactate 12% lotion in the treatment of ichthyosis. **J Am Acad Dermatol** 15:1253.
219. Loden M (1996) Urea-containing moisturizers influence barrier properies of normal skin. **Arch Dermatol Res** 288:103–107.
220. Lowe N (1982) New coal tar extract and coal tar shampoos: evaluation by epidermal cell DNA synthesis suppression assay. **Arch Dermatol** 118:487.

expression of vascular cell adhesion molecule-1; this effect was similar to the effect seen with topical corticosteroids.[223]

Crude coal tar is a nonuniform mixture of 10 000 chemicals including polycylic aromatic hydrocarbons (benzol, naphthalene, anthracene), nitrogens and phenolic compounds produced by the distillation of coal. The active ingredient(s) have not been identified. An alcohol extract of coal tar is also produced as a 20% solution called liquor carbonis detergens (LCD) and is cosmetically more acceptable product, available in several formulations: bath oils (25% Polytar bath, 30% Zetar emulsion), ointments (5% Unquentum Bossi, Elta Tar), creams (5% Tarbonis) and shampoos (4.3% Pentrax, 1% Zetar). Formulations containing tar, salicylic acid and/or sulfur are also available for hyperkeratotic dermatoses of the scalp (e.g., Sebutone and T-Sal shampoos). The most recently marketed tar products are gels (5% Estar, 7.5% psoriGel). They are not as odorous or staining as previous preparations; however, they sting when applied to nonintact skin.

Wood tars are products derived from pine, beech, birch and juniper ("oil of Cade"). Topical preparations are most commonly used in the Scandinavian countries. Wood tars are also present in cough syrups, disinfectants and insecticides.

Ichthammol is a bituminous tar derived from shale deposits containing fossilized fish. The crude distillate contains at least 10% sulfur and 5–7% ammonium sulfate. It is slightly analgesic and antiseptic and is believed to be anti-inflammatory. It is inexpensive and time tested as a safe and well-tolerated product sometimes referred to as "drawing salve." The associated odor may be unacceptable to some, and patients should be warned that it can stain clothing. In the United States, ichthammol is commercially available as a 10% or 20% product in lanolin and petrolatum. It may also be compounded to lower, more cosmetically acceptable, concentrations in zinc oxide ointment.

Serious adverse reactions from coal tar are few. It has an unpleasant odor and can stain clothing. Tar shampoo can leave an orange discoloration on blonde hair. Tars can produce irritant, contact and photoallergic/photoallergic reactions as well as folliculitis, acne and keratoses. Only coal tar is phototoxic ("tar smarts") and can be irritating, but it rarely causes allergic reactions. Wood tars are more sensitizing and can cross-react with Balsum of Peru and terpentine. Wood tars also have associated toxic potential due to the phenol content, but this has been reduced in newer formulations.[224] More than two centuries ago, scrotal cancer in chimney sweeps was linked to coal soot. Coal tar agents (polycyclic aromatic hydrocarbons, anthracene and pyridines) are also carcinogenic in experimental animals. Isolated reports of malignancy in humans treated with coal tars and with coal tars plus UV light has prompted concern. However, a 25-year follow-up study found no increased incidence of skin cancers in psoriatics treated with the Goeckerman regimen.[225] The safety of topically applied tar has been best demonstrated after a century of widespread use, and its use has subsequently been deemed safe and effective by the FDA.[226]

Anthralin

Anthralin (dithranol) is a stable synthetic derivative of chrysarobin, a natural product that comes from the South American Araroba tree. Anthralin is an anthracene, consisting of three fused benzene rings with a methylene group, that is easily oxidized by oxygen, alkali and light. The mechanism of action is poorly understood. It inhibits DNA synthesis in vitro[227] as well as Langherhans cell-mediated responses.[228] Anthralin also stimulates monocyte proinflammatory mediators and induces oxygen free radicals.[229] The associated irritation seen with anthralin was found to be inhibited by local antioxidants, and irritation after application was coincident with elevated expression of interleukin-6, granulocyte–macrophage colony-stimulating factor, macrophage inflammatory protein-2 and TNF-α mRNA.[230]

Anthralin is available in a cream at varying concentrations from 0.1 to 1.0% (Drithrocreme, Drithroscalp) and also encapsulated in a matrix of semicrystalline monoglycerides that protect it from oxidation (Micanol). Anthralin was developed for the treatment of psoriasis, but it has been used to treat alopecia areata with 25% of patients experiencing significant regrowth over 6 months in one study.[231,232] Traditional therapy is with daily application, increasing in duration as tolerated up to several hours or overnight. A more convenient, and equally effective, "short-contact" regimen was designed to minimize irritation. This approach begins with a brief application, washed off after 10 to 60min, beginning every other day and increasing to every day as tolerated. After maximal exposure time is achieved, increasing concentrations can be prescribed. Anthralin is a strong irritant but a rare sensitizer. Formulations of dithranol cream that had salicylic acid as a stabilizer produced 42% more irritation when compared to formulations with only sorbic acid or no stabilizers.[233] Common adverse effects are erythema, scaling, pruritus, folliculitis, regional lymphadenopathy and staining of skin and clothing. Stains on white fabrics may be removed with chlorine bleach.

Calcipotriol

Calcipotriene (calcipotriol, MC903) is a synthetic vitamin D_3 analog with potent effects on cell proliferation and differentiation, as well as inflammation,[234,235] but it has negligible effects on calcium metabolism. Topical 0.005% calcipotriene ointment (Dovonex) was FDA approved in 1994. Large clinical trials comparing topical calcipotriene to topical steroids have demonstrated the efficacy of calcipotriene with a more favorable side effect profile in the treatment of plaque-type psoriasis in adults. Clinical trials have also proven it to be a safe and effective alternative therapy for childhood, and even infantile, psoriasis.[236–238] Favorable results have also been shown in the the treatment of morphea and linear scleroderma,[239,240] confluent and reticulated papillomatosis,[241] inflammatory linear verrucous epidermal nevus,[242] congenital icthyoses,[243,244] and vitiligo.[245] Irritation is the most common side effect but allergic contact dermatitis can occur.[246] Hypercalcuria may also occur, and isolated cases of hypercalcemia have been reported. Twenty-four hour urine collections for elevated ratios of calcium to creatinine

221. Wrench S (1981) Scale prophylaxis. **Arch Dermatol** 117:213.
222. Czarnetzki B (1988) Inhibitory effect of shale oils (ichthyols) on the secretion of chemotactic leukotrienes from human leukocytes and on leukocyte migration. **J Invest Dermatol** 87:694–697.
223. Langeveld-Wildschut EG, Riedl H, Thepen T et al. (2000) Modulation of the patch test reaction by topical corticosteroids and tar. **J Allergy Clin Immunol** 106(4):737–743.
224. Schmid MH, Korting HC (1996) Coal tar, pine tar and sulfonated shale oil preparations: comparative activity, efficacy and safety. **Dermatology** 193:1–5.
225. Pittelkow K, Perry H, Muller S et al. (1981) Skin cancer in patients with psoriasis treated with coal tar. **Arch Dermatol** 117:465.
226. Final Rule (1991) Dandruff, seborrheic dermatitis and psoriasis drug products for over-the-counter human use. **Fed Regist** 56:63554–63569.
227. Griffiths WAD, Ive FA, Wilkinson JD (1986) Topical therapy. In: Textbook of Dermatology, 4th ed. Vol. 3. Rook A, Ebling FJ, Wilkinson DS et al. eds. Oxford: Blackwell Scientific.
228. Morhenn VB, Orenberg EK, Kaplan J et al. (1983) Inhibition of a Langerhans cell-mediated immune response by treatment modalities useful in psoriasis. **J Invest Dermatol** 81:23–27.
229. Mrowietz U, Falsafi M, Schroder JM et al. (1992) Inhibition of human monocyte functions by anthralin. **Br J Dermatol** 127:382–387.
230. Lange RW, Germolec DR, Foley JF, Luster MI (1998) Antioxidants attenuate anthralin-induced skin inflammation in BALB/c mice: role of specific proinflammatory cytokines. **J Leukoc Biol** 64(2):170–176.

231. Fiedler-Weiss VC, Buys CM (1987) Evaluation of anthralin in the treatment of alopecia areata. **Arch Dermatol** 123:1491–1493.
232. Li LF, Fiedler VC, Kumar R (1999) Induction of hair growth by skin irritants and its relation to skin protein kinase C isoforms. **Br J Dermatol** 140(4):616–23.
233. Prins M, Swinkels OQ, Kolkman EG et al. (1998) Skin irritation by dithranol cream. A blind study to assess the role of the cream formulation. **Acta Dermato-Venereolog** 78:262–265.
234. van der Kerkhof PCM (1998) An update on vitamin D3 analogues in the treatment of psoriasis. **Skin Pharmacol Appl Skin Physiol**, 11:2–10.
235. Nissen JB, Avrach WW, Hansen ES et al. (1999) Decrease in enkephalin levels in psoriatic lesions after calcipotriol and mometasone furoate treatment. **Dermatology** 198(1):11–7.
236. Darley CR, Cunliffe WJ, Green CM et al. (1996) Safety and efficacy of calcipotriol ointment in treating children with psoriasis. **Br J Dermatol** 135:390–393.
237. Oranje AP, Marcoux D, Svensson A et al. (1997) Topical calcipotriol in childhood psoriasis. **J Am Acad Dermatol** 36:203–238.
238. Travis LB, Silverberg NB. (2001) Psoriasis in infancy: Therapy with calcipotriene ointment. **Cutis** 68(5):341–344.
239. Cunningham BB, Landells IDR, Langman C et al. (1998) Topical calcipotriene for morphea/linear scleroderma. **J Am Acad Dermatol** 39:211–215.
240. Kreuter A, Gambichler T, Avermaete A et al. (2001) Combined treatment with calcipotriol ointment and low-dose ultraviolet A1 phototherapy in childhood morphea. **Pediatr Dermatol** 18(3):241–245.

is a useful parameter for safety monitoring in infants and small children requiring treatment of large body surface areas.

Retinoids

Vitamin A (retinol) is a fat-soluble vitamin. It is essential for growth, bone development, night vision and skin integrity. It was the first retinoid to be used therapeutically. Beta carotene is a precursor molecule that is available from green and yellow vegetables and metabolized to vitamin A in humans. All-*trans*-retinol is the natural alcohol form of vitamin A that binds to retinol-binding proteins for transport from hepatic storage to target tissues. All-*trans*-retinol is oxidized in the basal keratinocytes to all-*trans*-retinoic acid (tretinoin). All-*trans*-retinoic acid can then isomerize to form 9-*cis*-retinoic acid.[247] The biological effects are mediated via intracellular receptors. Two families of retinoic acid receptors each have three subtypes. Retinoic acid receptors (RARs) interact with all-*trans*-retinoic acid and retinoid X receptors (RXRs) interact with 9-*cis*-retinoic acid. The acid–receptor complex acts in the cell nucleus to alter gene transcription with target cell-specific changes. These changes include alterations in cell growth, differentiation and apoptosis[248–250] as well as alterations in cellular receptors, integrins and cytokines of the skin.[251–254]

Topical retinoids have been used since the 1970s. All-*trans*-retinol is available in multiple over-the-counter products in the cosmeceutical market, and all-*trans*-retinoic acid (tretinoin) is availabe in several prescription formulations. These products are naturally occuring retinoids. Since the introduction of all-*trans*-retinol and all-*trans*-retinoic acid, synthethic retinoids including adapalene and tazarotene have been developed with significant structural differences and more selective retinoid receptor interactions. The first topical RXR-selective receptor agonist, bexarotene (Targretin gel), is approved for the treatment of cutaneous T-cell lymphoma.[255]

Topical retinoids were first used in the treatment of acne vulgaris as a comedolytic agent and currently provide a mainstay of acne treatment. During the past decade, the FDA-approved indications have expanded to include the treatment of photodamage, psoriasis,[256] and refractory early-stage cutaneous T-cell lymphoma.[256,257] Clinical uses also include actinic keratoses,[258] striae,[259] melasma and postinflammatory hyperpigmentation, verruca,[260] Darier disease,[261] vellus hair cysts,[262] inflammatory linear verrucous epidermal nevus,[263] epidermolytic hyperkeratosis,[264] and many other cutaneous conditions.[265]

Topical sensitizers

Dinitrochlorobenzene (DNCB), diphenylcyclopropenone (diphencyprone, DCP) and squaric acid dibutylester (SADBE) are chemically distinct, potent contact allergens used in the treatment of diverse and therapeutically challenging conditions.[266] They are most commonly used for the treatment of alopecia areata and refractory verruca vulgaris, but have also been used in limited cases of atopic dermatitis, lichen nitidus, chronic nodular prurigo, systemic lupus erythematosus, HIV and cutaneous cancers.[267–270]

Dinitrochlorobenzene (DNCB) was the first compound used, but concerns about potential for carcinogenesis stimulated development of DCP and SADBE. These agents promote a reaction in 95% of immunocompetent patients, do not occur naturally in the environment, are inexpensive and have few side effects, although a severe allergic contact dermatitis may occur. Contact immunotherapy stimulates Th1-mediated delayed-type hypersensitivity. This cellular immune response may act against a complex of the contact agent hapten bound to either viral or human protein. It has been postulated that an immune response to one antigen may prevent a reaction to a second unrelated antigen via competition or immune distraction.[271] Sensitizers may also act by altering the ratio of T-cell subsets in the area or by modulation of local cytokines.[272,273] Alterations in levels of protein kinase C has also been demonstrated in mouse models and pretreatment with granulocyte–macrophage colony-stimulating factor has been found to modify responses to subsequent contact sensitization in humans.[274,275] The use of these agents is currently limited because they have not been subjected to the stringent testing required for FDA approval and commercial availability.

DNCB, commercially used as an algicide in water cooling systems, was the first agent studied. Although several reports have shown clinical efficacy,

241. Kurkcuoglu N, Celebi CR (1995) Confluent and reticulated papillomatosis: response to topical calcipotriol. **Dermatology** 191:341–345.
242. Micali G, Nasca MR, Musumeci ML (1995) Effect of topical calcipotriol on inflammatory linear verrucous epidermal nevus. **Pediatr Dermatol** 12:386–387.
243. Lucker GPH, van de Kerhof PCM, van Dijk MR et al. (1994) Effect of topical calcipotriol on congenital ichthyoses. **Br J Dermatol** 131:546–550.
244. Kragballe K, Steijlen PM, Ibsen HH et al. (1995) Efficacy, tolerability and safety of calcipotriol ointment in disorders of keratinization. **Arch Dermatol** 131:556–560.
245. Parsad D, Saini R, Verma N (1998) Combination of PUVAsol and topical calcipotriol in vitiligo. **Dermatology** 197:167–170.
246. Frosch PJ, Rustemever T (1999) Contact allergy to calcipotriol does exist. **Contact Dermatitis** 40:66–71.
247. Kurlandsky SB, Duell EA, Kang S et al. (1996) Autoregulation of retinoic acid biosynthesis through regulation of retinol esterification in human keratinocytes. **J Biol Chem** 271:15346–15352.
248. Boehm MF, Heyman RA, Nadzan AM (1997) A new generation of retinoid drugs for the treatment of dermatological diseases. **Emerging Drugs** 2:287–303.
249. van Rossum MM, Mommers JM, van de Kerkhof PC (2000) Coexpression of keratins 13 and 16 in human keratinocytes indicates association between hyperproliferation-associated and retinoid-induced differentiation. **Arch Dermatol Res** 292(1):16–20.
250. Virtanen M, Torma H, Vahiquist A (2000) Keratin 4 upregulation by retinoic acid *in vivo*: a sensitive marker for retinoid bioactivity in human epidermis. **J Invest Dermatol** 114(3):487–493.
251. Stoll SW, Elder JT (1998) Retinoid regulation of heparin-binding EGF-like growth factor gene expression in human keratinocytes and skin. **Exp Dermatol** 7(6):391–397.
252. Jansens S, Bols L, Vandermeeren M et al. (1999) Retinoic acid potentiates TNF-alpha-induced ICAM-1 expression in normal human epidermal kerationocytes. **Biochem Biophys Res Commun** 255(1):64–69.
253. Kligman LH, Yang S, Schwartz E (1999) Steady-state mRNA levels of interleukin-γ, integrins, cJun and cFos in hairless mouse skin during short-term chronic UV exposure and the effect of topical tretinoin. **Photodermatol Photoimmunol Photomed** 15(5):198–204.
254. Diaz BV, Lenoir MC, Ladoux A et al. (2000) Regulation of vascular endothelial growth factor expression in human keratinocytes by retinoids. **J Biol Chem** 275(1):642–650.
255. Liu HL, Kim YH (2002) Bexarotene gel: a Food and Drug Administration-approved skin-directed therapy for early-stage cutaneous T-cell lymphoma. **Arch Dermatol** 138(3):398–399.
256. Krueger GG, Drake LA, Elias PM et al. (1998) The safety and efficacy of topical tazarotene gel, a topical acetylenic retinoid, in the treatment of psoriasis. **Arch Dermatol** 134:57–60.
257. Henney JE (2000) New drug for refractory cutaneous T-cell lymphoma. **JAMA** 283(9):1131.
258. Alirezai M, Dupuy P, Amblard P et al. (1994) Clinical evaluation of topical isotretinoin in the treatment of actinic keratoses. **J Am Acad Dermatol** 30:447–451.
259. Kim KJ, Griffiths CEM et al. (1996) Topical tretinoin (retinoic acid) improves early stretch marks. **Arch Dermatol** 132:519–26.
260. Leaman JA, Benton EC (2000) Veruccas. Guidelines for management. **Am J Clin Dermatol** 1(3):143–149.
261. Thappa PM, Jeevankumar B (2000) Darier's disease with multiple verrucae. **J Dermatol** 10:682–684.
262. Fischer DA (1984) Retinoic acid in the treatment of eruptive vellus hair cysts. **J Am Acad Dermatol** 2:221–222.
263. Rulo HF, van de Kerkhof PC (1991) Treatment of inflammatory linear verrucous epidermal nevus. **Dermatologica** 182(2):112–114.
264. Virtanen M, Gedde-Dahl T Jr, Mork NJ et al. (2001) Phenotypic/genotypic correlation in patients with epidermolytic hyperkeratosis and the effects of retinoid therapy on keratin expression. **Acta Derm Venereol** 81(3):16370.
265. Orfanos CE, Zouboulis CC, Almond-Roesler B et al. (1997) Current use and future potential role of retinoids in dermatology. **Drugs** 53:358–538.
266. Buckley DA, DuVivier AW (2001) The therapeutic use of topical contact sensitizers in benign dermatoses. **Br J Dermatol** 145(3):385–405.
267. Yoshizawa Y, Matsui H, Izaki S et al. (2000) Topical dinitrochlorobenzene therapy in the treatment of refractory atopic dermatitis: systemic immunotherapy. **J Am Acad Dermatol** 42:258–262.
268. Kano Y, Otake Y, Shiohara T (1998) Improvement of lichen nitidus after topical dinitrochlorobenzene application. **J Am Acad Dermatol** 39:305–308.
269. Yoshizawa Y, Kitamura K, Maibach HL (1999) Successful treatment of chronic nodular prurigo with topical dinitrochlorobenzene. **Br J Dermatol** 141:387–389.
270. Stricker RB, Goldberg B, Mills BL et al. (1995) Improved results of delayed-type hypersensitivity skin testing in HIV-infected patients treated with topical dinitrochlorobenzene. **J Am Acad Dermatol** 33:608–11.
271. Happle R (1980) Antigenic competition as a therapeutic concept for alopecia areata. **Arch Dermatol Res** 267:109–114.
272. Happle R, Klein HM, Macher E (1986) Topical immunotherapy changes the composition of the peribulbar infiltrate in alopecia areata. **Arch Dermatol Res** 278:214–218.
273. Hoffmann R, Wenzel E, Huth A et al. (1994) Cytokine mRNA levels in alopecia areata before and after treatment with the contact allergen diphenylcyclopropenone. **J Invest Dermatol** 103(4):530–533.

DNCB is mutagenic by the *Salmonella typhimurium* bacterial plate incorporation assay (Ames test) and is toxic via chromatid exchange in fibroblasts.[276] SADBE is an organic compound requiring refrigeration that can be purchased in 97% pure solution (Acros Organics, Fair Lawn, NJ, USA). SADBE is not mutagenic, but it is expensive and has a short shelf life. DCP is a substituted cyclopropenone organic compound. It decomposes on exposure to ultraviolet A light, but is stable when shielded from light in acetone solution. DCP has no identified industrial or commercial uses, is expensive, is not mutagenic by the Ames test, is not teratogenic or organ toxic by the hen's egg and mouse teratogenicity tests, is not detectable in the serum or urine of treated patients[277] and is stable in acetone for up to 6 months if shielded from light. Commercial grade DCP can be purchased (Sigma Chemical Co., St. Louis, MO, USA), but must be properly purified; a possible contaminant, dibromobenzylketone, is a potent mutagen.[278]

Sensitization is achieved by initial application of a 2% solution at an accessible location such as the hip or in the arm to receive future topical therapy. In most cases one application is sufficient to induce sensitization. Following sensitization, a lower concentration is applied weekly or, for the treatment of warts, as often as necessary to the affected area(s) to achieve and/or maintain mild erythema and/or pruritus. The appropriate concentration is selected based on patient response and is usually 0.0001–1.0% Contact sensitization is convenient, painless and safe, but requires experience and patient education. Many clinicians limit use to in-office application, although SADBE has been shown to be effective as an at-home treatment for warts with minimal adverse effects.[279]

Adverse effects include the possibility of severe allergic contact reactions that can occur at the sensitization site, treatment site or rarely as a disseminated process. Postinflammatory pigment change may also occur. Choosing a discrete location will minimize any distress from this possible side effect. Flare-up reactions at the site of initial sensitization are also common. Erythema and pruritus can usually be controlled by adjusting the concentration of the solution and the interval between applications. Regional lymphadenopathy almost always occurs but is occasionally tender. Fever, arthralgia, contact urticaria, erythema multiforme and vitiligo have been reported.[227] Tolerance and loss of efficacy may occur after prolonged therapy.

Topical corticosteroids

In 1952, Sulzberger and Witten published their observation on the efficacy of topical hydrocortisone in the treatment of atopic dermatitis. Since then, hydrocortisone, followed soon by more potent analogs, has been used extensively for the treatment of inflammatory dermatoses in children. The effects of corticosteroids are exerted at the transcriptional level with immediate and delayed effects on a myriad of cytokines, immune, epidermal and dermal cellular components making them useful in the treatment of a wide variety of inflammatory and/or immune-mediated dermatologic conditions, but responsible for associated local and systemic side effects.

Hydrocortisone, the biologically active 11-hydroxyl analog of cortisol, was the first topical corticosteroid to be developed. The design and synthesis of chemical variations on the hydrocortisone molecule have yielded a multitude of products with increasing potency. This potency can be influenced by increasing the concentration of the active ingredient, optimizing the vehicle, hydrating the skin before application and/or applying under prolonged occlusion (see the section on emollients). Penetration is also enhanced through thin (e.g., facial, genital or atrophic) and/or inflamed skin.

Altering the structure of the steroid molecule by fluorination, methylation or acetylation, esterification, and double-bond induction can also increase the anti-inflammatory activity of the glucocorticoids. Fluorinated or halogenated corticosteroids are often assumed to be more potent and to have greater risks for side effects than nonhalogenated preparations, but molecular variants lacking these modifications are not always safer. For example, hydrocortisone esters, such as hydrocortisone butyrate (Locoid) or hydrocortisone valerate (Westcort), belong in the moderately potent group of steroids with risk/benefit ratios similar to other mid-potency topical corticosteroids and are not equivalent to the least potent (Class VII) hydrocortisone formulations.

TABLE 4.8 Ranking of topical corticosteroids

Class	Brand name[a]	Active ingredient
I	Diprolene ointment	0.05% betamethasone dipropionate[b]
	Diprolene AF cream	
	Psorcon ointment	0.05% diflorasone diacetate
	Temovate ointment	0.05% clobetasol proprionate
	Temovate cream	
	Ultravate ointment	0.05% halobetasol proprionate
	Ultravate cream	
II	Cyclocort ointment	0.1% amcinonide
	Diprosone ointment	0.05% betamethasone diproprionate[b]
	Elocon ointment	0.1% mometasone fuorate
	Florone ointment	0.05% diflorasone diacetate
	Halog ointment	0.1% halcinonide
	Halog cream	
	Halog solution	
	Lidex ointment	0.05% fluocinonide
	Lidex cream	
	Lidex gel	
	Lidex solution	
	Maxiflor ointment	0.05% diflorasone diacetate
	Maxivate ointment	0.05% betamethasone diproprionate[b]
	Maxivate cream	
	Topicort ointment	0.25% desoximetasone
	Topicort cream	
	Topicort gel	0.05% desoximetasone
III	Aristocort A ointment	0.1% triamcinolone acetonide
	Cutivate ointment	0.005% fluticasone propionate
	Cyclocort cream	0.1% amcinonide
	Cyclocort lotion	
	Diprosone cream	0.05% betamethasone dipropionate[b]
	Flurone cream	0.05% diflorosone diacetate
	Lidex E cream	0.05% fluocinonide
	Maxiflor cream	0.05% diflorosone diacetate
	Maxivate lotion	0.05% betamethasone dipropionate[b]
	Topicort LP cream	0.05% desoximetasone
	Valisone ointment	0.1% betamethasone valerate
IV	Aristocort ointment	0.1% triamcinolone acetoninide
	Cordran ointment	0.05% flurandrenolide
	Elocon cream	0.1% mometasone furoate
	Elocon lotion	
	Kenalog ointment	0.1% triamcinolone acetonide
	Kenalog cream	
	Synalar ointment	0.025% fluocinolone acetonide
	Westcort ointment	0.2% hydrocortisone valerate

274. Li LF; Fiedler VC, Kumar R (1999) The potential role of skin protein kinase C isoforms alpha and delta in mouse hair growth induced by diphencyprone-allergic contact dermatitis. **J Dermatol** 26(2):98–105.
275. Kremer IB, Stevens SR, Gould JW (2000) Intradermal granulocyte-macrophage colony-stimulating factor alters cutaneous antigen-presenting cells and dffrentially affects local versus distant immunization in humans. **Clin Immunol** 96(1):29–37.
276. DeLeve LD (1996) Diinitrochlorobenzene is genotoxic by sister chromatid exchange in human skin fibroblasts. **Mutation Res** 371:105–108.
277. Berth-Jones J, McBurney A, Hutchinson PE (1994) Diphencyprone is not detected in serum or urine following topical application. **Acta Derm Venereol** 74:312–313.
278. Wilkerson M, Connor T, Henkin J (1987) Assessment of DCP for photo-chemically induced mutagenicity in the Ames assay. **J Am Acad Dermatol** 17:606.
279. Silverberg NB, Lim JK, Paller AS, Mancini AJ (2000) Squaric acid immunotherapy for warts in children. **J Am Acad Dermatol** 42:803–808.

TABLE 4.8   Ranking of topical corticosteroids—con't

Class	Brand name[a]	Active ingredient
V	Cordran cream	0.05% flurandrenolide
	Cutivate cream	0.05% fluticasone propionate
	Dermatop cream	0.1% prednicarbate
	Diprosone lotion	0.05% betamethasone dipropionate[b]
	Kenalog lotion	0.1% triamcinolone acetonide
	Locoid ointment	0.1% hydrocortisone butyrate
	Locoid cream	
	Synalar cream	0.025% fluocinolone acetonide
	Tridesilon ointment	0.05% desonide
	Valisone cream	0.1% betamethasone valerate
	Westcort cream	0.2% hydrocortisone valerate
VI	Aclovate ointment	0.05% alclometasone
	Aclovate cream	
	Aristocort cream	0.1% triamcinolone acetonide
	DesOwen cream	0.05% desonide
	Kenalog cream	0.025% triamcinolone acetonide
	Kenalog lotion	
	Locoid solution	0.1% hydrocortisone butyrate
	Snyalar cream	0.01% fluocinolone acetonide
	Snyalar solution	
	Tridesilon cream	0.05% desonide
	Valisone lotion	0.1% betamethasone valerate
VII	Topical agents with hydrocortisone, dexamethasone, flumethalone, prednisolone, and methylprednisolone	

[a] Class I is the most potent, and potency descends with each group to Class VII, which is least potent. There is no significant difference of agents within any given class; within each class, the compounds are arranged alphabetically.

[b] Betamethasone dipropionate (0.05%) is the active ingredient in topical products, with relative potencies ranging from class I to class V, demonstrating the important role of the vehicle. Topical corticosteroids with similar ranges in bioavailability include diflorasone diacetate and triamcinolone acetonide.

The list of different topical corticosteroids available in the United States today is so long that few practitioners are familiar with the unique properties of each product. In an effort to simplify comparison of these products, a scale was created based on the vasoconstrictor assay as a measure of potency.[280,281] In most, but not all, cases, this bioassay corresponds with clinical efficacy.[282] Products are ranked into one of seven categories (Table 4.8). These lists are commonly published by pharmaceutical companies on convenient pocket-size cards and are provided to practitioners on a complementary basis. Relative rankings vary based on modifications of the assays used. Although the vaso-constrictor assay is the most widely utilized, there are multiple assays used and developed by the pharmaceutical industry.[283]

For most products, the vehicle has a significant effect on the bioavailability of the topical corticosteroid. Hence, chemical equivalence (concentration of the pharmacologically active ingredient) does not always reflect therapeutic equivalence (clinical efficacy). For example, 0.05% betamethasone dipropionate

in different vehicles is ranked in class I (Diprolene gel and ointment), class II (Diprolene AF cream and Diprosone ointment), class III (Diprosone cream) and class V (Diprosone lotion). Similar examples are given in Table 4.8. Additives that augment potency are propylene glycol, hexylene glycol urea and salicylic acid. This concept is especially important when considering generic substitutions which frequently do not have bioequivalence to trade name topical corticosteroid products.[33,284]

Observing a few simple guidelines will facilitate safe and effective topical therapy with corticosteroids. It is important to choose the correct vehicle (see below). The lowest-strength product that will clear an eruption in the shortest period of time should be chosen. Patient compliance is maximal when progress is rapid, and strong steroids do have a place in pediatric therapy with important restrictions. In general, more potent corticosteroids should be used for shorter periods of time. Tapering from a class I to a less potent topical product, rather than abruptly discontinuing, will minimize the problem of rebound flare. Penetration is increased on the face, skinfolds and diaper area; therefore, preparations from classes V, VI or VII are usually sufficient for these sites. Eyelids have the thinnest skin on the body, and treatment should be for less than 30 days because of the additional risk of direct ocular absorption and glaucoma. If long-term eyelid therapy is absolutely necessary, ophthalmologic follow-up with tonometry is indicated. A single daily application of a topical corticosteroid followed by frequent application of emollient is often equally effective, safer and less costly than application of the corticosteroid several times a day.[285] Weekly application of a corticosteroid under an occlusive dressing is another strategy to limit the quantity of medication used without sparing efficacy.[286] A sufficient amount of medication should be prescribed. Small sample tubes usually contain 1.5g. For children and adolescents, one application to the hands, face, head or groin requires 2g of medication and equals 56 total grams for application two times per day for 2 weeks. Three g per dose or 84g for 2 weeks is sufficient medication for one arm or for one-half a trunk. Therapy for an entire leg requires 4g per dose or 112g for 2 weeks.[287] Quantification by "fingertip units" is a practical and easy way to describe adequate dosing to patients and caregivers.[288]

The following guidelines are useful for choosing an appropriate corticosteroid preparation in selected dermatitic conditions:

1. *Lesions on the face, skinfolds, and diaper area*: low-potency cream or ointment.
2. *Widespread lesions with minimal symptoms*: low-potency cream or ointment.
3. *Lesions of hair-bearing areas*: moderate-potency gels, foams or alcohol-based lotions if no open lesions exist; otherwise, nonalcohol-based lotions; occlusion of the scalp is best achieved with a snug-fitting swim cap.
4. *Secondarily infected lesions*: systemic antibiotic therapy and wet-to-damp compresses initiated for 2 to 5 days before beginning topical corticosteroids under occlusive wet dressings.
5. *Thickened dry lesions*: ointments in combination with exfoliant agents; intermediate to high potency for the first week and strength decreased accordingly as improvement occurs.
6. *Insect bites*: ointments with tape occlusion over individual lesions (scratching over the tape causes the medication to penetrate deeper and makes it more effective).
7. *Intraoral lesions*: topical corticosteroids available in orabase or oral troches; beclomethasone dipropionate nasal spray is a convenient and effective preparation for oral lesions as well.

280. McKenzie A (1962) Percutaneous absorption of steroids. **Arch Dermatol** 86:611.
281. Guin J, Wallis M, Walls R et al. (1993) Quantitative vasoconstrictor assay for topical corticosteroids: the puzzling case of fluocinlone acetonide. **J Am Acad Dermatol** 29:197.
282. Cornell RA, Stoughton R (1985) Correlation of the vasoconstriction assay and clinical activity on psoriasis. **Arch Dermatol** 121:63.
283. Kukutsch NA, Coors EA, Gruschwitz MS et al. (1999) Modulation of irritation-induced increase of E-selectin mRNA *in vivo* by topically applied corticosteroids. **J Invest Dermatol** 113(2):170–174.
284. Olsen E (1991) A double-blind controlled comparison of generic and trade-name topical steroids using the vasoconstrictor assay. **Arch Dermatol** 127:197.

285. Turpeinen M (1991) Absorption of hydrocortisone from skin reservoir in atopic dermatitis. **Br J Dermatol** 124:358.
286. Volden G (1992) Successful treatment of therapy-resistant atopic dermatitis with clobetasol propinate and a hydrocolloid occlusive dressing. **Acta Derm Venereol (Stock), suppl.** 176:126.
287. Weston W, Lane A (1989) The use and abuse of topical steroids in children. Scientific exhibit. **Am Acad Pediatr.**
288. Long CC, Mills CM, Finlay AY (1998) A practical guide to topical therapy in children. **Br J Dermatol** 138(2):293–296.

Children are more susceptible to local and systemic effects of topical corticosteroids than are adults (see the section on drug toxicities). Several types of adverse reactions are possible following the use of topical corticosteroids. Telangiectasia, striae, atrophy and purpura are common problems when potent corticosteroids are used for more than 4 weeks on the face and in intertriginous areas. Atrophy, which typically resolves 1–4 weeks after discontinuation of therapy, has been correlated with a decrease in type I and type III mRNA and propeptides.[289] Striae do not resolve with discontinuation of therapy. Perioral dermatitis in children and granuloma gluteale infantum are iatrogenic conditions associated with prolonged use of topical corticosteroids.[290] Glaucoma can occur after excessive or prolonged periocular application. The symptoms and clinical appearance of impetigo, scabies, and dermatophytoses will initially improve after the use of topical corticosteroids. This condition, referred to as tinea or scabies "incognito," is more difficult to diagnose. The infection is ultimately potentiated by corticosteroid therapy leading to a delay in appropriate antimicrobial therapy and sometimes precipitating serious consequences.[88] Contrary to this phenomenon, skin colonization with *S. aureus* is actually decreased after topical corticosteroid therapy in patients with atopic dermatitis.[291,292] Barrier function is affected by topical corticosteroid use as evidenced by increased transepidermal water loss, augmented whealing to dimethyl sulfoxide, enhanced sodium hydroxide erosion formation and decreased ceramides, cholesterol and free fatty acids.[293] Allergic contact dermatitis can also occur following sensitization to topical steroids with a prevalence of 0.2–4.8%, although allergy to a component of the vehicle (including emollients, emulsifiers, humectants, stabilizers, preservatives, antioxidants and solvents) is more common. This should be suspected in patients who are not responding well to therapy. Patch testing, despite its limitations, should be considered if clinical suspicion is high for an associated allergic contact dermatitis. Tixocortol pivolate and budesonide, representing two of the four cross-reaction groups of topical corticosteroids, have proved to be important markers for identifying allergic contact dermatitis.[294] Tachyphylaxis is also encountered with chronic topical corticosteroid use.

Intermittent, long-term use of high- to mid-potency steroids has proven beneficial, with no associated side effects, in adults with atopic dermatitis allowing a maintained level of control and a reduced risk and delayed time to relapse.[295] In contrast, short-term use of high-potency preparations and chronic use of even low-potency preparations can cause systemic side effects in children. These include suppression of the pituitary–adrenal axis, weight gain, poor linear growth, glycosuria, full-blown Cushing syndrome, and posterior subcapsular cataracts (see section on systemic steroids, below).

Cimetidine

Cimetidine (Tagamet, Smith-Kline) was granted FDA approval in 1977 for the treatment of acid-peptic disorders in adults. It has been one of the most widely prescribed medications, and is now available over-the-counter. While cimetidine has not received specific FDA approval for children under 12 years old, it has enjoyed over 2 decades of widespread use for a variety of pediatric indications without significant adverse reactions.[296] A few pediatric dermatologic conditions that may benefit from cimetidine therapy include urticaria, cutaneous mastocytosis, widespread molluscum and refractory verruca vulgaris. However, objective data supporting the efficacy of treating these conditions with cimetidine is lacking.

Cimetidine is a type 2 histamine (H_2) receptor antagonist. H_2-receptors are also present on T-suppressor cells, playing a role in cell-mediated immune response. Experimental data have demonstrated *in vitro* increases in cell-mediated immunity, principally via blockade of H_2-receptors on T-suppressor cells.[297–299] Other H_2-antagonists, ranitidine and famotidine, have no such action.[300] In addition to its effects on gastric acid secretion, cimetidine also acts as an immunomodulating agent by blocking histamine-mediated inhibition of T helper 1 (Th1) cells and preventing histamine-mediated enhancement of Th2 cells *in vitro* in a dose-dependant manner.[301] Cimetidine has been used successfully to treat common variable hypogammaglobulinemia,[302] chronic mucocutaneous candidiasis,[303] hyperimmuno-globulinemia E, and severe mucocutaneous herpes simplex virus (HSV) infections in immunocompromised patients.[304,305]

Open-label studies of cimetidine treatment for children with common warts documented cure rates of up to 82%.[306] However, small controlled trials failed to demonstrate a statistically significant success rate compared to placebo. Most of these studies lacked stringent enrollment and outcome criteria. One study revealed a trend towards efficacy in younger patients, receiving the highest dose, 40mg/kg/day.[307] The popularity of cimetidine treatment for warts despite a lack of objective data supporting its efficacy reflects the dearth of innocuous and successful treatments for this common condition. The controversy generated by the widespread use of cimetidine for warts[308] can only be settled by a carefully designed and executed study. The optimal study must: anticipate a low response rate and enroll enough subjects to generate the power to accept or reject the null hypothesis; control for confounding factors of age and gender; and maximize the dose to 40mg/kg/day. Duration of disease should be greater than 2 years to minimize the effect of spontaneous resolution.

H_1-receptor antagonists are first-line therapy for acute allergic reactions and chronic urticaria. However, for patients who do not respond to standard treatment, the addition of an H_2-antagonist will often control the disease. This has been demonstrated in several double-blind placebo-controlled trials of H_1-antihistamines with and without cimetidine for the treatment of chronic urticaria.[309,310] Case reports have also supported the efficacy of H_1 plus H_2-antihistamine therapy in the control of physical urticarias.[309,310] H_2-receptor blockade is the assumed mechanism of action behind these observations. However, cimetidine interferes with the metabolism of several

289. Oikarinen A, Haapasaari KM, Suinen M, Tasanen K (1998) The molecular basis of glucocorticoid-induced skin atrophy: topical glucocorticoid apparently decreases both collagen synthesis and the corresponding collagen mRNA level in human skin *in vivo*. Br J Dermatol 139(6):1106–1110.
290. Manders S, Lucky A (1992) Perioral dermatitis in childhood. J Am Acad Dermatol 27:688.
291. Burden A, Beck M (1992) Contact hypersensitivity to topical corticosteroids. Br J Dermatol 127:497.
292. Nilsson E, Henning C, Magnusson J (1992) Topical corticosteroids and *Staphylococcus aureus* in atopic dermatitis. J Am Acad Dermatol 27:29.
293. Kolbe L, Kligman AM, Schreiner V, Stoudemayer T (2001) Corticosteroid-induced atrophy and barrier impairment measured by non-invasive methods in human skin. Skin Res Technol 7(2):73–77.
294. Devos SA, Van Der Valk PG (2001) Relevance and reproducibility of patch-test reactions to corticosteroids. Contact Dermatitis 44(6):362–365.
295. Van Der Meer JB, Glazenburg EJ, Mulder PG et al. (1999) The management of moderate to severe dermatitis in adults with topical fluticasone propionate. The Netherlands Adult Atopic Dermatitis Study Group. Br J Dermatol 140(6):1114–1121.
296. O'Mara NB, Nahata MC (1994) Parenteral histamine2 receptor antagonists in the pediatric population. J Pharm Technol 10:53–57.
297. White W, Ballow M (1985) Modulation of suppressor-cell activity by cimetidine in patients with common variable hypogammaglobulinemia. N Engl J Med 198:198.
298. Fraser I, Bell P (1981) Cimetidine, the immune system, and cancer. Lancet 1(8218):900.
299. Gifford R, Ferguson R, Voss B (1981) Cimetidine reduction of tumour formation in mice. Lancet 1(8221):638.
300. Feldman M, Burton M (1990) Histamine 2-receptor antagonists. N Engl J Med 323:1749.
301. Elenkov IJ, Webster E, Papanicolaou DA et al. (1998) Histamine potently suppresses human IL-2 and stimulates IL-10 production via H2 receptors. J Immunol 161(5):2586–2593.
302. Segal R, Dayan M, Epstein N et al. (1989) Common variable immunodefiency: a family study and therapeutic trial with cimetidine. J Allergy Clin Immunol 84:753.
303. Jorizzo J, Sama W, Jegasothy B et al. (1980) Cimetidine as an immunomodulator: chronic mucocutaneous candidiasis as a model. Ann Intern Med 92:192.
304. Cohen P, Kurzrock R (1987) Herpes simplex virus infections and cimetidine therapy. J Am Acad Dermatol 17:845.
305. Ershler WB, Hacker MP, Burroughs BJ et al. (1983) Cimetidine and the immune response: *in vivo* augmentation on non-specific and specific immune response. Clin Immunol Immunopathol 26:10–17.
306. Orlow SJ, Paller A (1993) Cimetidine therapy for multiple viral warts in children. J Am Acad Dermatol 28:794–796.
307. Rogers CJ, Gibney MD, Siegfried EC et al. (1999) Cimetidine therapy for warts: is it any better than placebo? J Am Acad Dermatol 41:123–127.
308. Bigby M (1998) Snake oil for the 21st century. Arch Dermatol 134:1512–1514.
309. Frieri M, Alling DW, Metcalfe DD (1985) Comparison of the therapeutic efficacy of cromolyn sodium with that of combined chlorpheniramine and cimetidine in systemic mastocytosis. Results of a double-blind clinical trial. Am J Med 78:9.
310. Fenske NA, Lober CW, Pautler SE (1985) Congenital bullous urticaria pigmentosa. Treatment with concomitant use of H1- and H2-receptor antagonists. Arch Dermatol 121:115.

TABLE 4.9   Acyclovir

Condition	Dose	Route	Duration
Primary episode of genital HSV	Adult:1000mg–1200mg/day in 3–5 divided doses Children: 40–80mg/kg/day divided in 3–4 doses	Oral	5–10 days
Genital Herpes simplex virus (HSV) primary episode	15mg/kg/d in 3 divided doses	IV	5–7 days
Recurrent genital HSV	Adult: 1000–1200mg/day in 3–5 divided doses	Oral	5 days
Chronic suppressive therapy	Adult: 400–1200mg/day in 3–5 divided doses Adult: 400mg bid	Oral Oral	Up to 12 months Up to 12 months
HSV in immunocompromised host (localized, progressive, or disseminated)	15–30mg/kg/day in 3 divided doses	IV	7–14 days
Prophylaxis of HSV in an immunocompromised patient	Adult: 600–1000mg/day in 3–5 doses	Oral	During periods of risk
HSV Encephalitis	30mg/kg/day in 3 divided doses	IV	Minimum of 14–21 days
Neonatal HSV	60mg/kg/day in 3 divided doses	IV	14–21 days
Varicella in the immunocompromised host	<1 year of age: 30mg/kg/day divided in 3 doses >1 year of age: 1500mg/m^2 in 3 times daily	IV	7–10 days
Varicella in the immunocompetent host	80mg/kg/day divided in 4 doses with maximum of 3200mg/day	Oral	5 days
Zoster in an immunocompetent host	Adult: 4000mg/day in 5 divided doses Children: 80mg/kg/day in 4–5 divided doses	Oral	5–7 days

Table adapted from the RedBook 2000.

concommitantly administered drugs, including some H$_1$-antihistamines. Relatively increased blood levels of H$_1$-antihistamines could account for the enhanced efficacy of combination therapy, in some cases.

The efficacy of combination antihistamine therapy in mast cell disease has been less well studied, but there have been reports of symptomatic relief from treatment with cimetidine plus chlorpheniramine or cyproheptadine for bullous urticaria pigmentosa and systemic mastocytosis.[309,310]

It is important to remember, when prescribing long-term high-dose therapy, that cimetidine will increase the blood levels of several concomitantly administered drugs. Theophylline, cyclosporine and phenytoin are important examples. Baseline and follow-up levels of these drugs should be closely monitored in children taking cimetidine.

SYSTEMIC TREATMENT

Stephanie Swords, Stephen J. Lauer and Amy Jo Nopper

ACYCLOVIR

Acyclovir (Zovirax) is a synthetic purine nucleoside analog. It is taken up by virus-infected cells, where it is then phosphorylated by viral thymidine kinase, inhibiting viral DNA polymerase and viral replication in infected cells, without adversely affecting normal cells. Acyclovir was first synthesized in 1977. The oral preparation was approved by the FDA for use in 1985. It is active against herpes viruses, especially herpes simplex virus (HSV) and varicella-zoster virus (VZV). Acyclovir is effective and well tolerated and has a very high margin of safety. It is the treatment of choice for primary and frequently recurrent labial and genital herpes simplex and herpes zoster in adults.[311] In 1992 acyclovir was FDA approved to treat varicella infections in pediatric patients.[311–313] It is also recommended as first-line therapy for neonatal HSV[314] and herpes simplex encephalitis in children.[315] Acyclovir has other controversial, but potentially important uses in pediatric dermatology. It has been used to treat herpes zoster[316,317] and recurrent erythema multiforme.[318] It has also been used as a prophylactic agent against recurrent HSV in children and against varicella in exposed sick neonates,[319] immuno-compromised children, and even healthy siblings of children with chickenpox[313] (Table 4.9).

Acyclovir is available in capsules, tablets, and suspension for oral use (200mg/5ml), as a sterile powder, reconstituted for intravenous administration, and as a 5% ointment for topical use. Acyclovir dosing and preferred route of delivery is dependent on the type of viral infection (HSV or VZV), the status of the immune system of the patient, and the age of the patient.[320,321] A delay in initiation of systemic therapy, more than 24h after the appearance of skin lesions, will significantly decrease efficacy.[312] Topically applied acyclovir may decrease the duration of viral shedding in immunocompetent patients with recurrent HSV infections. However, this formulation is not as effective as systemic acyclovir in decreasing symptoms, probably because epidermal penetration does not very effectively extend to basal keratinocytes.[322]

Acyclovir is well tolerated. Side effects include nausea in less than 8% and vomiting in less than 3% of patients, and lower incidences of diarrhea, headache, and rash. Overdosage or dehydration can lead to precipitation of

311. Whitley R (1992) Therapeutic approaches to varicella-zoster virus infections. **J Infect Dis** (suppl 1) 166:S51.
312. Dunkle E (1991) A controlled trial of acyclovir for chickenpox in normal children. **N Engl J Med** 325:1539.
313. Anonymous (1992) American Academy of Pediatrics Committee on Infectious Diseases: the use of oral acyclovir in otherwise healthy children with varicella. **Pediatrics** 91:674.
314. Englund J, Fletcher C, Balfour H (1991) Acyclovir therapy in neonates. **J Pediatr** 119(Pt 1):129.
315. Committee on Infectious Diseases (1991) American Academy of Pediatrics: Red Book. p. 576, 22nd ed. American Academy of Pediatrics.

316. Rothe M, Feder H, Grant-Kels J (1991) Oral acyclovir therapy for varicella and zoster infections in pediatric and pregnant patients: a brief review. **Pediatr Dermatol** 8:236.
317. Martin J (1988) Efficacy of oral acyclovir treatment of acute herpes zoster. **Am J Med** (suppl 2A) 85:79.
318. Brice S, Huff J, Weston W (1991) Erythema multiforme minor in children. **Pediatrician** 18:188.
319. Lipton S, Brunell P (1989) Management of varicella exposure in a neonatal intensive care unit. **JAMA** 261:1782.
320. American Academy of Pediatrics (2002) RedBook 2002. Practice Management Information Corp.
321. Wolverton S (ed.) (2001) Dermatologic Drug Therapy. Philadelphia: WB Saunders.
322. Parry G, Dunn P, Shah V, et al. (1992) Acyclovir bioavailability in human skin. **J Invest Dermatol** 98:856.

drug in the renal tubules. It is especially important to monitor renal function and adjust the dosage in young premature infants.[314]

The potential for widespread use of acyclovir, including otherwise healthy children with VZV, raises several concerns.[313,323,324] First, do the benefits of treatment outweigh the costs? When looking at data on how treatment affects the disease course, it has been shown that acyclovir use decreased the time off work, and out of school, by 2 days. Regarding the effects of therapy on herd immunity, it is postulated that if the appearance of lesions initiates treatment, viral replication has been ongoing for at least 2 weeks. This is sufficient time for the immune system to generate a response and should not interfere with long-term immunity.[321] Will treated children have an increased susceptibility to recurrent chickenpox or zoster? Will widespread resistance and/or more virulent strains emerge? These questions remain unanswered and further studies are needed.

In 1992, the American Academy of Pediatrics established a set of guidelines to promote the safe and practical use of oral acyclovir in children.[313]

1. Oral acyclovir is not recommended *routinely* for uncomplicated varicella in otherwise healthy children.
2. For children at increased risk of severe varicella or its complications (older than 13 years, those receiving chronic corticosteroid or aspirin therapy, those with chronic cutaneous or pulmonary diseases), oral acyclovir should be considered, if it can be initiated within 24h of the appearance of this rash.
3. When given, oral acyclovir should be administered for 5 days. The patient must maintain adequate fluid intake.
4. Primary varicella or recurrent zoster in immunocompromised children and virus-mediated complications of varicella in normal hosts should be treated with intravenous acyclovir.
5. Oral treatment is not recommended in pregnant adolescents with uncomplicated disease.
6. Oral acyclovir may be considered for household contacts, because they usually have more severe illness.

Although acyclovir is the most commonly used antiviral drug in pediatrics, other antivirals are emerging for the treatment of herpes simplex and herpes zoster. These agents, valacyclovir and famciclovir, were approved for use in these conditions due to their ease in dosing and increased bioavailability. Valacyclovir is a prodrug with the active metabolite being acyclovir. Famciclovir is a prodrug of penciclovir (PCV) and like acyclovir must be phosphorylated to PCV triphosphate to become active. It is this form that allows famciclovir to have a prolonged intracellular half-life (10–20h) within HSV infected cells when compared to acyclovir (less than 1h).[321] Famciclovir has been found to be effective in the treatment of patients with human immunodeficiency virus (HIV) and concomitant recurrent genital HSV infections and was the first oral drug approved by the FDA for this use. Both drugs have similar side effect profiles when compared to acyclovir with the exception of the pregnancy classification. Acyclovir carries a pregnancy class C where Famciclovir and Valacyclovir carry a class B rating. None of the antivirals is metabolized by the hepatic microsomal system. These drugs are not yet approved by the FDA for treatment in pediatrics (Tables 4.10 and 4.11).

ANTIMALARIALS

Antimalarial agents have been used for more than a century in the treatment of dermatologic disorders. The prototype is quinine, a naturally occurring 4-aminoquinoline compound, derived from the bark of the South American cinchona tree. Quinine has been used since the early 1800s to treat malaria. It was first used in 1894 to treat discoid lupus erythematosus. Synthetic antimalarial agents were developed when shortages of quinine occurred during World War I. These include quinacrine (Atabrine), chloroquine (Aralen), and hydroxychloroquine (Plaquenil).

More than four decades ago, quinacrine was recognized as an effective drug in the treatment of discoid lupus erythematosus. However, during the next

TABLE 4.10 Systemic antivirals

Drug	Bioavailability	Indications	Contraindications	Half-life
Acyclovir	15–30%	HSV infections (primary, recurrent, or suppressive therapy) Varicella-zoster infections Off label uses: Erythema multiforme Other subset of HSV infections (whitlow, eczema herpeticum, etc)	Hypersensitivity to acyclovir Hypersensitivity to formulation Pregnancy C	1.3–1.5 hours
Valacyclovir	54.5%	Same as acyclovir	Hypersensitivity to valacyclovir Hypersensitivity to formulation Pregnancy B	2.5–3.3 hours
Famciclovir	77%	HSV infections (primary, recurrent, or suppressive therapy) HSV in immunocompromised patients (HIV) Varicella-zoster infections Off-label uses-subset HSV infections, primary varicella	Hypersensitivity to famciclovir Hypersensitivity to formulation Pregnancy B	2.3–3.0 hours

HSV, herpes simplex virus.

323. Brunell P (1991) Chickenpox – examining our options. N Engl J Med 325:1577.
324. Hirsch M, Schooley R (1989) Resistance to antiviral drugs: the end of innocence. N Engl J Med 320:313.

TABLE 4.11   Regimens for human herpes virus infections

Viral Infection/ Immune Status	Valacyclovir	Famciclovir
Herpes simplex-primary	1000mg po BID for 10 days	250mg po TID for 10 days
Recurrent herpes simplex	500mg po BID for 5 days	125mg po BID for 5 days
Suppressive therapy for herpes simplex	500mg po QD	250mg po BID
Herpes zoster-acute	1000mg po TID for 7–10 days	500mg po TID for 7 days
Primary varicella in children	Not well evaluated or FDA approved	Not well evaluated or FDA approved
Recurrent herpes simplex in the immunocompromised patient	Studies pending	500mg po BID for 7 days
Suppressive therapy for herpes simplex	Studies pending	500mg po BID
Herpes zoster in the immunocompromised patient	Studies pending	500mg po TID for 10 days

From ref 321.

20 years, reports of retinal toxicity dampened enthusiasm for this class of drugs in the long-term management of chronic diseases.

Several mechanisms of action have been proposed to explain the efficacy of antimalarial agents in inflammatory skin diseases. These drugs are easily absorbed from the gastrointestinal (GI) tract and have high affinities for several tissues, resulting in prolonged and concentrated tissue levels. Excretion, primarily through the kidneys, and to a lesser extent in feces, can take years. Antimalarial agents bind DNA, lysosomes, and melanin. They accumulate in the uvea, adrenals, spleen, lungs, liver, and kidney, with levels up to several thousand times higher than in plasma. Leukocytes and epidermis are lesser foci. *In vitro*, antimalarial agents have been shown to inhibit DNA replication and transcription and to stabilize lysosomal membranes, which could have profound anti–inflammatory effects.[325,326]

While all the antimalarial agents are FDA approved for use in children, hydroxychloroquine is the only antimalarial agent with FDA approval for use in dermatology. It is indicated for the treatment of chronic cutaneous and discoid lupus erythematosus. Antimalarial agents have also been shown to be effective in the treatment of several other skin diseases including porphyria cutanea tarda,[327] sarcoidosis,[328] polymorphous light eruption,[329] dermatomyositis,[330] pseudopelade of Brocq,[331] Weber–Christian panniculitis,[331] and reticular erythematous mucinosis.[332] Anecdotal reports have documented successful treatment of lupus profundus, morphea, and disseminated granuloma annulare with antimalarial therapy.[333–335] Other disease processes in which antimalarial agents may be potentially effective include solar urticaria, lymphocytic infiltration of the skin, Meischer's granuloma, lichen sclerosis et atrophicus, acrodermatitis chronica atrophicans, epidermolysis bullosa, and hypocomplementemic urticarial vasculitis.[336]

Despite the fact that antimalarial agents have been widely used in the treatment of rheumatoid arthritis and parasitic diseases in children, the dermatologic literature contains warnings against the use of these drugs for pediatric skin diseases.[336] These warnings are based on reports of ingestions, rather than an increased incidence of subacute or chronic toxicities. Antimalarial agents have relatively narrow margins of safety and are quickly and completely absorbed, so overdose can be rapidly toxic in children. Ingestion of as little as 70mg/kg, 10 to 15 times the recommended therapeutic dose, or only four to five tablets of hydroxychloroquine for an average 2-year-old, can be fatal. Poisoning resembles salicylism, with vomiting, tinnitus, and vertigo, followed by seizures and cardiac and respiratory arrest.[337] Treatment of antimalarial ingestions is controversial. Ipecac is recommended within 30min of ingestion and has been used with antimalarial overdoses. Newer literature supports the use of activated charcoal if the ingestion has occurred within 1h of seeking treatment. It is postulated that the rapid absorption from the gastrointestinal tract that occurs with antimalarials is slowed and can be ultimately decreased with the use of charcoal. Furthermore, one of the signs of antimalarial toxicity is seizures, which is a relative contraindication for using ipecac. Parents of young children in households in which antimalarial drugs are used should be warned about the potential for poisoning and informed about safety guidelines. With the appropriate precautions and monitoring, antimalarial agents can be used with equal safety in the pediatric and adult populations.[336,337]

Antimalarial side effects can involve the skin, gastrointestinal tract, hematopoietic system, and eyes. All side effects are seen less often with hydroxychloraquine than with the other antimalarial agents. Mucocutaneous staining is the most frequent side effect, occurring in up to one-third of patients receiving therapy for more than 3 months. Quinacrine is associated with yellow discoloration; the other agents can turn skin and mucous membranes blue–gray. These changes are usually reversible within several months after discontinuation of the drug.[337] Nausea and vomiting from gastric irritation can be minimized by giving smaller doses more frequently, or administering with meals. Leukopenia and thrombocytopenia have been reported to occur in a small percentage of patients receiving chloroquine. Aplastic anemia is a rare side effect in patients on quinacrine. Hemolytic anemia can occur in treated patients with glucose-6-phosphate dehydrogenase (G6PD) deficiency. Reversible agranulocytosis has been reported with all antimalarial agents.

The ophthalmologic toxicities have been well described, and are most often associated with chloroquine use. These ocular effects are often asymptomatic

325. Weiss JS (1991) Antimalarial medications in dermatology. A review. **Dermatol Clin** 9:377.
326. Salmeron G, Lipsky P (1983) Immunosuppressive potential of antimalarials. **Am J Med** 75:19.
327. Grossman M, Poh-Fitzpatrick M (1986) Porphyria cutanea tarda. **Dermatol Clin** 4:297.
328. Jones E, Callen J (1990) Hydroxychloroquine is effective therapy for control of cutaneous sarcoidal granulomas. **J Am Acad Dermatol** 23:487.
329. Murphyy G (1987) Hydroxychloroquine in polymorphous light eruption: a controlled trial with drug and visual sensitivity monitoring. **Br Med J** 116:379.
330. Woo T (1984) Cutaneous lesions of dermatomyositis are improved by hydroxychloroquine. **J Am Acad Dermatol** 4:592.
331. Ziering C, Rabinowitz L, Esterly N (1993) Antimalarials for children: indications, toxicities, and guidelines. **J Am Acad Dermatol** 8:764–770.
332. Braddock S (1988) Reticular erythematous mucinosis and thrombocytopenic purpura. **J Am Acad Dermatol** 19:859.
333. Carlin M (1987) A case of generalized granuloma annulare responding to hydroxychloroquine. **Cleve Clin J Med** 54:229.
334. Fox J (1987) Lupus profundus in children: treatment with hydroxychloroquine. **J Am Acad Dermatol** 16:839.
335. Wuthrich R, Roenigk H, Steck W (1975) Localized scleroderma. **Arch Dermatol** 111:98.
336. Thiers BH (1991) Isoprinosine treatment of dopecia areata. **J Invest Dermatol** 96(5):725–735.
337. Rasmussen J (1983) Antimalarials – are they safe to use in children? **Pediatr Dermatol** 1:89.

TABLE 4.12   Recommended baseline and monitoring laboratory tests for antimalarials

Laboratory Test	Baseline Study	Monitoring Laboratory
Complete blood count	Yes	Yes: monthly for 6 months and then every 3–6 months
Liver function tests	Yes	Yes: every 4–6 months
BUN, creatinine	Yes	Yes: every 3–6 months
Ophthalmologic tests	Yes	Yes: every 3–6 months Visual fields Amsler grids (home monitoring every 2 weeks in older children) Color vision testing Fundoscopic examination Slit lamp examination
24h urine test for porphyrins	Yes	Yes: at 1 month when indicated
Serum pregnancy test in females of childbearing age	Yes	Yes: with every prescription
Electrocardiogram	Yes	No: unless abnormal baseline ECG
G6PD level	Yes	No

BUN, blood urea nitrogen; G6PD, glucose 6-phosphate dehydrogenase.

TABLE 4.13   Side effects of antimalarial drugs

Gastrointestinal: nausea, vomiting, diarrhea, hepatotoxicity
Skin: discoloration, pruritus, acromotrichia, exfoliative dermatitis
Hematologic: aplastic anemia, hemolysis, pancytopenia, thrombocytopenia, agranulocytosis
Central nervous system: tinnitus, seizures, irritability
Cardiovascular: depressed cardiac activity with overdose
Ophthalmologic: corneal deposits, diplopia, retinopathy

but can cause blurred vision, halos around objects, and photophobia. Therapy can be continued in patients who develop corneal deposits, as this problem is completely reversible within 2 months after drug discontinuation. Retinopathy is a rare but serious and irreversible side effect. Several retrospective studies have been reviewed in the literature to determine whether the daily dose per total body weight or the cumulative dose are more indicative of the risk of developing retinopathy. Most studies support using the daily dose per body weight as a guideline to avoid this irreversible side effect.[331] Recommended doses of chloroquine should not exceed 3.5mg/kg/day and hydroxychloroquine should not exceed 6.5mg/kg/day. Regular ophthalmologic examinations should be obtained in patients receiving antimalarial medications.[331]

Hydroxycholorquine is the preferred antimalarial agent for use in pediatric dermatology. To maximize efficacy and minimize side effects, the recommended initial dose is 6.5mg/kg/day for 6–8 weeks. The dose should be adjusted every 3 to 6 months, to reach a minimum effective level, usually 4–5mg/kg/day. Hydroxychlorquine is only available in the tablet form. More precise and easier administration in children can be achieved by prescribing pulverized individually weighed doses. These can be mixed with jelly or applesauce.[338]

Pretreatment baseline evaluations should include a glucose-6-phosphate dehydrogenase (G6PD) level and electrocardiogram. A baseline and monthly complete blood count should be obtained for the first 6 months to follow cell count stability. Once stable, cell counts can be followed every 3–6 months thereafter depending upon the clinical course and dosing changes. Baseline renal and liver function tests should be evaluated and repeated every 4–6 months. A direct ophthalmologic examination for signs of toxicity should be performed within 1 month of initiating therapy and repeated every 3–6 months. These tests should include visual fields, amsler grids for the detection of macular injury (in children older than 2 years of age), color vision testing, fundoscopic examination, and slit lamp examination to evaluate for corneal deposits.[331] Patients should also wear ultraviolet filtering sunglasses while outdoors. When treating patients with porphyria cutanea tarda, a 24 hour urine for porphyrin excretion should be evaluated initially and after 1 month of therapy. To avoid toxicity, the urinary excretion of porphyrins should be less than 75mg/24 hours[339] (Tables 4.12 and 4.13).

Contraindications to using antimalarial drugs include retinal disease, visual field changes or a known hypersensitivity to 4-aminoquinolone compounds. Relative contraindications include pregnancy (as chloroquine is known to cross the placenta), liver disease, alcoholism, administration of hepatotoxic drugs, and renal disease.[331] Use of the antimalarial medications in conditions such as porphyria cutanea tarda (PCT) and G6PD deficiency must be undertaken with extreme caution as reports of toxicity have been reported in PCT as well as significant hemolysis in G6PD deficiency.[331] Furthermore, exacerbations of myasthenia gravis, multiple sclerosis, and psoriasis have been reported with the use of antimalarial medications, which should be used with caution in patients with these conditions.[336]

ANTI-TUMOR NECROSIS FACTOR-α THERAPY

In recent years, our understanding of the molecular mechanisms of the inflammatory cascade has increased dramatically.[340] Numerous immune cell types, including T cells, B cells, natural killer cells, monocyte/macrophages and neutrophils, have been shown to play a role in initiating, maintaining, and/or suppressing the inflammatory response. These various cells secrete a multitude of cytokines, chemokines, metalloproteinases and other soluble factors that modulate the inflammatory process. While the exact role of many of these factors has yet to be elucidated, it has become clear that tumor necrosis factor-α (TNF-α) plays a central role in the initiation of the response to immunologic and inflammatory stimuli.[341–344]

TNF-α is produced primarily by monocyte/macrophages but is also made by keratinocytes, melanocytes, mast cells and Langerhans cells. TNF-α is initially synthesized as a transmembrane protein that is subsequently cleaved to produce the soluble plasma protein. Both the membrane-bound and soluble factors can interact with one of two TNF-α receptors. One of the receptors, p55, is ubiquitous while the p75 receptor is found primarily on hematopoietic and endothelial cells. In addition, the extracellular domain of each receptor can be cleaved to generate a soluble factor that can act to modulate TNF-α activity. Binding of TNF-α to its receptors leads to the activation of a number of transcription factors that control expression of inflammatory cascade genes. Synthesis and secretion of IL-1, IL-6, IL-8, granulocyte–monocyte colony-stimulating factor (GM-CSF), intercellular adhesion molecule 1 as well as several metalloproteinases are increased after cellular exposure to TNF-α. In turn, these factors stimulate the activation or recruitment of various cells, ultimately leading to activation of the inflammatory pathway.[341,344,345]

338. Ziering C, Rabinowitz L, Esterly N (1993) Antimalarials for children: indications, toxicities, and guidelines. J Am Acad Dermatol 28:764.
339. Weiss, Jonathan S (1991) Antimalarial medications in dermatology. Dermatol Clin 9(2):377–385.
340. Gallen JL, Snyderman R (1999) In: Inflammation, 3rd edn, Gallin JI, ed. Baltimore: Lippincott Williams & Wilkins.
341. LaDuca JR, Gaspari AA (2001) Targeting tumor necrosis alpha. Dermatol Clin 19:617–635.
342. Choy EHS, Panayi GS (2001) Cytokine pathways and joint inflammation in rheumatoid arthritis. N Engl J Med 34:907–916.
343. Luster AD (1988) Chemokines – chemotactic cytokines that mediate inflammation N Engl J Med 338:436–445.
344. Krueger JG (2002) The immunologic basis for the treatment of psoriasis with new biologic agents J Am Acad Dermatol 46:1–23.

Tumor necrosis factor-α has been implicated in many inflammatory disease processes including Crohn's disease, rheumatoid arthritis, sepsis, as well as congestive heart failure. It has become clear that many dermatologic diseases, including atopic dermatitis and psoriasis, are the result of abnormalities in the response of immune cells, especially T and B cells. The clinical manifestations of these diseases are modulated by many of the soluble factors listed above, including TNF-α. Thus, they may be responsive to therapies aimed at disrupting the effects of TNF-α.[344,345]

Recent advances in molecular biology and biotechnology have led to the development of specifically targeted molecules aimed at interrupting the inflammatory cascade in a more specific way than traditional drugs. Not only are natural products now able to be produced in therapeutic quantities, but new biologically active molecules not found in nature have been engineered and synthesized and are now being used to treat disease. Two hybrid antibody molecules, infliximab and etanercept, designed to block the activity of TNF-α are currently available and are being used to treat a variety of inflammatory conditions, including several dermatologic processes. Both hybrid molecules are thought to work by reducing the ability of TNF-α to stimulate the production of proinflammatory cytokines such as IL-1 and IL-6. In addition, the secretion of chemokines such as IL-8 and monocyte chemoattractant protein-1 is also reduced, leading to a reduction in the recruitment of new inflammatory cells (neutrophils, monocyte/macrophages) to a site.[340,341,345]

INFLIXIMAB

Infliximab (Remicade) is a humanized, chimeric anti-TNF-α monoclonal IgG1 antibody. In the final product, the constant region of a human antibody is fused to a murine antibody variable region that is specific for TNF-α.[345,346] Generation of the humanized, chimeric antibody results in a protein that is less antigenic in human subjects and thus may be able to be used for longer periods of time.

Infliximab was first tested in patients with rheumatoid arthritis. It has since been shown, in several studies, to be an effective therapy for rheumatoid arthritis, especially in patients with persistent active disease that had been refractory to other therapies. Studies showed both a clinical response, as evidenced by improved patient activity, and a slowing of joint damage as found in radiographic studies.[346,347] Infliximab has also been found to be effective in treating refractory Crohn's disease in both adults and children.[348,349] There is now evidence that infliximab may be useful as treatment for plaque-type psoriasis, indicating that TNF-α plays a key role in the pathogenesis of this disease.[350] Dosing regimens have varied in these studies; usually 5–10mg/kg of infliximab has been administered intravenously every 4–8 weeks. The length of treatment has varied with the studies. It is likely the exact dosing of infliximab will be dependent upon the disease being treated and the response of the individual patient.

Immediate side effects of infliximab have generally been minimal. There have been reports of infusion reactions, usually presenting as flushing,

headache, and skin rash, in approximately 5% of patients.[351] In addition, there is a report of a severe anaphylactic reaction in a patient receiving a fourth infusion of infliximab.[352] While anaphylactic reactions are rare with infliximab infusions, any setting in which infliximab is being administered should be prepared to handle a severe reaction. Patients may develop anti-dsDNA antibodies and new ANA antibodies after initiation of infliximab therapy; however, only rarely have the presence of these antibodies been associated with clinical symptoms.[353] However, there are reports of reactivation of granulomatous diseases, including tuberculosis and histoplasmosis, after treatment with infliximab.[354,355] Given the immunosuppressive activity of TNF-α therapies, it is perhaps not surprising that reactivation of latent disease could occur. However, prior to use of infliximab, patients should be screened for latent tuberculosis; prophylactic treatment of tuberculosis should be considered prior to initiation of infliximab therapy in patients found to have latent disease.[354] There have been reports of lymphoma and myeloma in patients being treated with infliximab, but currently there does not appear to be an increased risk of developing malignancy with infliximab therapy as compared to the untreated control groups.[345,353]

ETANERCEPT

Etanercept (Enbrel), like infliximab, is a genetically engineered chimeric protein. Etanercept contains an Fc portion of human IgG1 linked to two chains of the soluble, extracellular portion of the p75 TNF-α receptor. This fusion protein contains only human sequences and thus should prove to be less immunogenic when used in humans. In addition, the binding portion of the protein, the fragment of the p75 TNF-α receptor, is able to bind both TNF-α and TNF-β (or lymphotoxin). TNF-β is a member of the TNF-α gene family and has many proinflammatory characteristics in common with TNF-α. Thus, etanercept may be able to block activation of the inflammatory cascade in a more complete way than can infliximab.[345]

The efficacy of etanercept in the treatment of several inflammatory diseases has been tested in a recent series of clinical trials. Adult patients with rheumatoid arthritis responded well to etanercept with improvements in clinical scores and significant delays in the radiographic progression of their disease.[356] Children with juvenile rheumatic arthritis also showed a significant response, with the average number of days between disease flares increasing from 28 to 116 days after administration of etanercept as compared to placebo.[357] In a second study, there was a significant reduction in the erythrocyte sedimentation rate as well as improvement in disease-related anemia.[358]

While only a few trials have been completed to date, the usefulness of etanercept in the treatment of Crohn's disease remains unclear. One report suggested that etanercept may be effective in the treatment of this chronic inflammatory bowel disease,[359] while a second study failed to show an effect of etanercept in signs and symptoms of the disease.[360]

TNF-α levels are increased in the serum of patients with congestive heart failure. Studies in animal models have shown that TNF-α is able to reduce

345. Taylor PC (2001) Anti-tumor necrosis factor therapies. **Curr Opin Rheumatol** 13:164–169.
346. Maini R, St Clair EW, Breedveld F et al. (1999) Infliximab (chimeric anti-tumor necrosis factor α monoclonal antibody) versus placebo in rheumatoid arthritis patients receiving concomitant methotrexate: a randomized phase III trial. **Lancet** 354:1932–1939.
347. Lipsky PE, van der Heijde DM, St Clair EW et al. (2000) Infliximab and methotrexate in the treatment of rheumatoid arthritis. **N Engl J Med** 343:1594–1602.
348. Hyams JS, Markowitz J, Wyllie R (2000) Use of infliximab in the treatment of Crohn's disease in children and adolescents. **J Pediatr** 137:192–196.
349. Present DH, Rutgeerts P, Targan S et al. (1999) Infliximab for the treatment of fistulas in patients with Crohn's disease. **N Engl J Med** 340:1398–1405.
350. Chaudhari U, Romano P, Mulcahy LD et al. (2001) Efficacy and safety of infliximab monotherapy for plaque-type psoriasis: a randomized trial. **Lancet** 357:1842–1847.
351. Maini RN, Taylor PC (2000) Anti-cytokine therapy for rheumatoid arthritis **Annu Rev Med** 51:207–229.
352. Soykan I, Ertan C, Ozden A (2000) Severe anaphylactic reaction to infliximab: report of a case. **Am J Gastroenterol** 95:2395–2396.
353. Blam ME, Stein RB, Lichtenstein GR (2001) Integrating anti-tumor necrosis factor therapy in inflammatory bowel disease: current and future perspectives. **Am J Gastroenterol** 96:1977–1997.
354. Keane J, Gershon S, Wise RP et al. (2001) Tuberculosis associated with infliximab, a tumor necrosis factor α-neutralizing agent. **N Engl J Med** 345:1098–1104.
355. Makelchik M, Mangino JE (2002) Reactivation of histoplasmosis after treatment with infliximab need reference. **Am J Med** 112:78.
356. Bathon JM, Martin, RW, Fleischmann RM et al. (2000) A comparison of etanercept and methotrexate in patients with early rheumatoid arthritis. **N Engl J Med** 343:1586–1593.
357. Lovell DJ, Giannini EH, Reiff A et al. (2000) Etanercept in children with polyarticular juvenile rheumatoid arthritis. **N Engl J Med** 342:763–769.
358. Keitz DA, Pepmueller PH, Moore TL (2000) Clinical response to etanercept in polyarticular course juvenile rheumatoid arthritis. **J Rheumatol** 28:360–362.
359. D'Haens G, Swijsen C, Noman M et al. (2001) Etanercept in the treatment of active refractory Crohn's disease: a single-center pilot trial. **Am J Gastroenterol** 96:2564–2568.
360. Sandborn WJ, Hanauer SB, Katz S et al. (2001) Etanercept for active Crohn's disease: a randomized, double-blind placebo-controlled trial. **Gastroenterology** 121:1088–1094.

myocardial contractility and that this effect is at least partly mediated via the nitric oxide system. In addition, TNF-α is associated with the development of a dilated cardiomyopathy.[361] A recent study provided preliminary data showing that patients with congestive heart failure treated with etanercept had significant improvement in left ventricular function and left ventricular remodeling; in addition, there was a trend toward improvement in a clinical composite score.[362]

More recently, the utility of etanercept has been tested in dermatologic disease. Psoriasis is now recognized as a T-cell mediated epidermal hyperplasia. Many of the inflammatory cells and mediators, including TNF-α, that have been identified as playing a key role in such diseases as rheumatoid arthritis and Crohn's disease have also been found in the lesions of psoriasis.[344] A clinical trial[363] has shown a dramatic response to etanercept treatment in patients with psoriasis and/or psoriatic arthritis. In the clinical trial, 87% of patients showed an improvement in symptoms versus only 23% of those in the placebo group. These results, as well as results from other unpublished trials, led to the recent approval by the FDA of etanercept as a treatment for psoriatic arthritis.[364]

In most of the etanercept trials, the dose used in adults was 25mg given subcutaneously twice a week, while children have been treated with 0.4mg/kg subcutaneously twice a week. In general, etanercept has been well tolerated. Injection site reactions have been reported in 20–40% of patients,[345,365] but these reactions generally resolve quickly. The induction of anti-dsDNA antibodies has been noted in patients treated with etanercept and there has been a report of a patient who developed subacute cutaneous lupus erythematosus while being treated for rheumatoid arthritis.[366] To date, anaphylactic reactions and reactivation of granulomatous disease have not been noted in patients treated with etanercept, but its use has been more limited than infliximab. Given the similar mechanisms of action of the two drugs, it may be wise to consider using the precautions mentioned for infliximab prior to initiating etanercept therapy. Because these drugs may reduce the ability of the inflammatory/immune response to respond to an infectious challenge, all patients receiving these medications should be carefully monitored for signs of infection.

Overall, these early studies suggest that biologic agents that target TNF-α may have a significant role to play in several inflammatory dermatologic conditions. As more is learned of the exact molecular pathways involved in the pathophysiology of skin diseases, additional therapies directed at specific steps of the inflammatory cascade will be developed and should allow for a more specific approach to therapy.

CALCITRIOL AND CALCIPOTRIOL

Vitamin D is synthesized in several steps beginning with the conversion of 7-dehydrocholesterol to vitamin D3 (cholecalciferol) in the skin after exposure to ultraviolet light. This prohormone is then converted to the active hormone by subsequent hydroxylations to form 25-hydroxyvitamin D3 and ultimately 1,25-dihydroxyvitamin D3 (1,25(OH)D3), the predominant active form of the vitamin. The initial hydroxylation step occurs in the liver while the second step occurs mainly in the kidney and to a lesser degree in skin,

activated T lymphocytes and other tissues.[367,368] Vitamin D3 and vitamin D2 (ergocalciferol) are also available in the diet and are metabolized as described above.

Multiple biologic effects have been defined for 1,25(OH)D3. Perhaps best understood is its role in regulating calcium metabolism in the parathyroid glands, kidney, bone and intestine. It has multiple effects on epithelial cell growth and differentiation. In the skin, the net result of 1,25(OH)D3 action is the inhibition of basal cell and dermal fibroblast proliferation as well as keratinocyte terminal differentiation. In addition, 1,25(OH)D3 has been found to be active as an immunomodulator, suppressing the activity of Langerhans cells. Effects of 1,25(OH)D3 on pancreatic function, reproduction and embryologic maturation have also been described.[368,369] These effects are modulated by a specific 1,25(OH)D3 receptor (D3R) that is a member of the same nuclear receptor gene family as are the receptors for glucocorticoids and retinol. The D3R forms a nuclear complex with one of the retinoic acid receptors, the RXR-α receptor; after binding to 1,25(OH)D3, this complex interacts with a vitamin D3 response element in the promoter region of a 1,25(OH)D3-responsive gene. Subsequent recruitment of additional transcription factors as well as alterations in the local chromatin structure result in the activation of the responsive gene.[369,370]

Because of its multiple *in vivo* effects, 1,25(OH)D3 and its analogs have been used to treat a variety of disease. Initially, calcitriol was used for renal transplant patients and for those with hypoparathyroidism to stabilize their calcium status. In dermatology, the effect of 1,25(OH)D3 analogs on the psoriatic diseases, especially plaque-type psoriasis, has been most extensively studied. While oral calcitriol was found to be useful in the treatment of plaque-type psoriasis, concerns about hypercalcemia and renal toxicity were raised with systemic use of the drug. Because the effectiveness of calcitriol in the treatment of psoriasis does not appear to involve the calcium homeostasis effects of the hormone, attempts were made to synthesize compounds that worked primarily to effect cellular differentiation without impacting calcium metabolism. Calcipotriol (also called calciptriene) is the most extensively tested of the second generation 1,25(OH)D3 analogs and topical calcipotriol has replaced topical calcitriol in the clinical setting. Calcipotriol has relatively minor effects on calcium metabolism as compared to 1,25(OH)D3 but retains much of the growth and differentiation effects of the parent compound.

Numerous trials investigating the efficacy of topical calcipotriol (0.005% ointment; Dovonex) on psoriasis have been carried out, although to date, most of these trials have not involved children. A recent review[371] of many of these trials concluded that calipotriol is as effective as potent topical corticosteroids in the treatment of mild to moderate chronic plaque psoriasis and is well tolerated. Two small studies to assess the use of calcipotriol in childhood psoriasis have likewise found the drug to be effective.[372,373] However, in one of these studies, the mean serum values of 1,25(OH)D3 were decreased in patients although serum calcium levels remained within the normal range.[373] Monitoring of serum calcium levels in childhood is prudent.

Both oral calcitriol and topical calcipotriol have been used with mixed results in small studies for the treatment of morphea. In one study of topical calcipotriol, 12/12 patients reported improvement in their symptoms with BID use under occlusion for 3 months.[372A] In contrast, a study of oral

361. Blum A, Miller H (2001) Pathophysiological role of cytokines in congestive heart failure. **Annu Rev Med** 52:15–27.
362. Bozkurt B, Torre-Amione G, Warren MS et al. (2001) Results of targeted anti-tumor necrosis factor therapy with etanercept (Enbrel) in patients with advance heart failure. **Circulation** 103:1044–1048.
363. Mease PJ, Goffe BS, Metz J et al. (2000) Etanercept in the treatment of psoriatic arthritis and psoriasis: a randomised trial. **Lancet** 356:385–390.
364. Schwetz BA (2002) Treatment for psoriatic arthritis. **JAMA** 287:1103.
365. Bleumink GS, ter Borg EJ, Ramselaar CG, Stricker BH (2001) Etanercept-induced subacute cutaneous lupus erythematosus. **Rheumatology** 40:1317–1319.
366. Zeltser R, Valle L, Tanck C et al. (2001) Clinical, histological, and immunophenotypic characteristics of injection site reactions associated with etanercept **Arch Dermatol** 137:893–899.
367. Zehnder D, Bland R, Williams MC et al. (2001) Extrarenal expression of 25-hydroxyvitamin D3-1alpha-hydroxylase. **J Clin Endocrinol Metab** 86:888–894.
368. Kragballe K (1997) The future of vitamin D in dermatology. **J Am Acad Dermatol** 37:S72–S76.

369. Jones G, Strugnell SA, DeLuca HF (1998) Current understanding of the molecular action of vitamin D. **Physiol Rev** 78:1193–1231.
370. Carlberg C, Saurat J-H (1996) Vitamin D-retinoid association: molecular basis and clinical applications. **J Invest Dermatol Symp Proc** 1:82–86.
371. Ashcroft DM, Po ALW, Williams HC, Griffiths CEM (2000) Systematic review of comparative efficacy and tolerability of calcipotriol in treating chronic plaque psoriasis. **Br Med J** 320:963–967.
372. Cunningham BB, Landells ID, Langman C (1998) Topical calcipotriene for morphea/linear scleroderma. **J Am Acad Dermatol** 39:211–215.
372A. Oranje AP, Marcoux D, Svensson A et al. (1997) Topical calcipotriol in childhood psoriasis. **J Am Acad Dermatol** 36 (2 Pt 1): 203–208.
373. Hulshof MM, Bouwes Bavinck JN, Bergman W et al. (2000) Double-blind, placebo-controlled study of oral calcitriol for the treatment of localized and systemic scleroderma. **J Am Acad Dermatol** 43:1017–1023.
373A. Park SB, Suh DH, Youn JI (1999) A pilot study to assess the safety and efficacy of topical calcipotriol treatment in childhood psoriasis. **Pediatr Dermatol** 16:321–325.

calcitriol (0.75μg per day for 6 months, then 1.25μg per day for 3 months) found calcitriol to be no more effective than placebo in the treatment of localized and systemic scleroderma.[373A] Vitiligo responded well to topical calcipotriol in several clinical trials, including one pediatric trial.[374–376] It has been suggested that 1,25(OH)D3 analogs may be useful in a variety of keratinization disorders characterized by hyperproliferation but definitive studies remain to be completed.[377] While indications for the use of 1,25(OH)D3 analogs may well expand in the future, careful consideration will have to be given to potential side effects, especially with extensive or long-term use.

COLCHICINE

Colchicine, extracted from the seeds and tubers of *Colchicum autumnale*, continues to be used for a variety of dermatologic disorders. The *Colchicum* species has been used in to treat acute attacks of gout since the 6th century AD. Colchicine remains the therapy of choice for acute gout as well as familial Mediterranean fever and is used primarily in dermatology for the treatment of disorders with significant neutrophilic inflammation.[378,379]

Colchicine's primary mechanism of action is the prevention of microtubule assembly. The drug binds to tubulin dimers and prevents their association with a growing microtubule chain. The disruption of microtubules interferes both with mitosis and with cellular migration. Colchicine appears to be especially active in neutrophils, where it has been shown to inhibit cellular adherence, motility, and chemotaxis.

The adult dose of colchicine is typically 0.6mg two to three times daily as tolerated. It comes in both 0.5 and 0.6mg tablets. Colchicine alters jejunal and ileal function and may cause significant diarrhea and abdominal cramping. Colchicine dosing is often limited by these commonly observed gastrointestinal side effects and many patients may tolerate only twice daily dosing.

Off-label dermatologic uses of colchicine include various neutrophilic dermatoses such as Behçet's disease,[380] recurrent apthous stomatitis,[381] dermatitis herpetiformis,[382] and linear IgA disease.[383–385] The effectiveness of colchicine therapy in leukocytoclastic vasculitis remains controversial. While one prospective, randomized controlled study of 41 patients showed no statistically significant therapeutic efficacy there were 3 complete responders to colchicine who experienced relapse of disease upon its discontinuation. This suggests there may be individuals in whom colchicine therapy is effective[386]

for the treatment of cutaneous vasculitis. In addition, colchicine has been used with variable efficacy in a variety of other dermatoses including psoriasis, dermatomyositis, scleroderma, and Sweet's syndrome.

Gastrointestinal toxicity is the most commonly observed adverse effect with colchicine therapy. Overdosage of colchicine can be life threatening. Manifestations of colchicine intoxification include electrolyte disorders (decreased sodium, potassium, calcium) metabolic acidosis, renal failure, respiratory distress syndrome, disseminated intravascular coagulation, bone marrow failure, central nervous system disorders and myopathy. Because chronic colchicine adminstration at recommended doses can result in leukopenia, aplastic anemia, and megaloblastic anemia it is recommended to perform a complete blood count at least every 3 months on chronic therapy and it is advisable to monitor counts monthly during the first few months of therapy. Due to the low risk of electrolyte disturbances, hepatic and renal effects, it is also suggested to monitor electrolytes, hepatic and renal function at least every 3 months with long–term therapy.[387]

CYCLOSPORINE

Cyclosporine is a neutral lipophilic peptide with a unique cyclic structure that was first isolated in 1972, a product of the fungal species *Tolypocladium inflatum* Gams.[388] Although it had no antifungal properties, cyclosporine was found to be a potent immunosuppressant, with a selective inhibitory effect on T-helper cells. Cyclosporine is FDA approved for the prevention and treatment of organ transplant rejection in adults and children. It has been studied in the treatment of many other diseases whose pathogenesis may include T-helper cell dysfunction. In adults, it is effective for several cutaneous diseases, including psoriasis,[389,390] alopecia areata,[391] atopic dermatitis,[392,393] lichen planus, Behçet's disease,[394] and pyoderma gangrenosum.[388] Documented pediatric uses include dermatomyositis,[395,396] pemphigus vulgaris,[397] Langerhans cell histiocytosis,[398,399] and atopic dermatitis.[400–402] Cyclosporine is approved by the United States FDA for treatment of severe psoriasis in adults and is approved for the treatment of atopic dermatitis in Australia.

The mechanism by which cyclosporine works has been well described. When T cells become activated, a tyrosine kinase cascade is initiated that results in an increase in intracellular calcium and 1,2-diacylglycerol. The increased intracellular levels of calcium catalyze the formation of a calmodulin–calcineurin complex; activated calcineurin is a serine–threonine

374. Ameen M, Exarchou V, Chu AC (2001) Topical calcipotriol as monotherapy and in combination with psoralen plus ultraviolet A in the treatment of vitiligo. **Br J Dermatol** 145:476–479.

375. Ermis O, Alpsoy E, Cetin L, Yilmaz E (2001) Is the efficacy of psoralen plus ultraviolet A therapy for vitiligo enhanced by concurrent topical calcipotriol? A placebo-controlled double-blind study. **Br J Dermatol** 145:472–475.

376. Parsad D, Saini R, Nagpal R (1999) Calcipotriol in vitiligo: a preliminary study. **Pediatr Dermatol** 16:317–320.

377. Thiers BH (1997) The use of topical calcipotriene/calcipotriol in conditions other than plaque-type psoriasis. **J Am Acad Dermatol** 37 (3 Pt 2): S69–71.

378. Famaey JP (1988) Colchine in therapy: state of the art and new perspectives for an old drug. **Clin Exp Rheumatol** 6:305–317.

379. Harper RM, Allen BS (1982) Use of colchine in the treatment of Behçet's disease. **Int J Dermatol** 21:551–554.

380. Jorizzo JL, Hudson RD, Schmalstieg FC et al. (1984) Behçet's syndrome: immune regulation, circulating immune complexes, neutrophil migration, and colchicine therapy. **J Am Acad Dermatol** 10:205–214.

381. Ruah CB, Stram JR, Chasin WD (1988) Treatment of severe recurrent apthous stomatitis with colchicine. **Arch Otolaryngol Head Neck Surg** 114:671–675.

382. Silvers DN, Jahlin EA, Berczeller PH et al. (1980) Treatment of dermatitis herpetiformis with colchicine. **Arch Dermatol** 116:1373–1384.

383. Banodkar DD, al-Suwaid AR (1997) Colchicine as a novel therapeutic agent in chronic bullous dermatosis of childhood. **Int J Dermatol** 36(3):213–216.

384. Ang P, Tay YK (1999) Treatment of linear IgA bullous dermatosis of childhood with colchicine. **Pediatr Dermatol** 16 (1):50–52.

385. Zeharia A, Hodak E, Mukamel M et al. (1994) Successful treatment of chronic bullous dermatosis of childhood with colchicine. **J Am Acad Dermatol** 30:660–661.

386. Sais G, Vidaller A, Jucgla, Gallardo F, Peyri J (1995) Colchicine in the treatment of cutaneous leukocytoclastic vasculitis. Results of a prospectie, randomized controlled trial. **Arch Dermatol** 131:1399–1402.

387. Davis LS (2001) Newer uses of older drugs – an update In: Comprehensive Dermatologic Drug Therapy, Wolverton SE, ed. Philadelphia: WB Saunders.

388. Gupta A, Brown M, Ellis C et al. (1989) Cyclosporin in dermatology. **J Am Acad Dermatol** 21:1245.

389. Ellis C, Fradin M, Messana J et al. (1991) Cyclosporin for plaque-type psoriasis. **N Engl J Med** 324:277.

390. Fradin M, Ellis C, Voorhees. J (1990) Rapid response of von Zumbusch psoriasis to cyclospor n **J Am Acad Dermatol** 23 (5 Pt 1):925.

391. Gupta A, Ellis C, Cooper K et al. (1990) Oral cyclosporine for the treatment of alopecia areata. A clinical and immunohistnochemical analysis. **J AM Acad Dermatol** 22(2 Pt 1):242.

392. Sepp N, Fritsch P (1993) Can cyclosporin A induce permanent remission of atopic dermatitis? **Br J Dermatol** 128:213.

393. DeProst Y (1992) Management of severe atopic dermatitis. **Acta Derm Venereol** 72:117.

394. Groisser D, Griffiths C, Ellis C et al. (1991) A review and update of the clinical uses of cyclosporine in dermatology. **Dermaotol Clin** 9:805.

395. Kavanagh G, Ross J, Black M (1991) Dermatomyositis treated with cyclosporine. **J R Soc Med** 84:306.

396. Heckmatt J, Hasson N, Saunders C et al. (1989) Cyclosporine in juvenile dermatomyositis. **Lancet** I (8646):1063.

397. Alijotas J, Pedragosa R, Bosch J et al. (1990) Prolonged remission after cyclosporine therapy in pemphigus vulgaris: report of two young siblings. **J AM Acad Dermatol** 23(4 pt 1):701.

398. Arico M (1991) Cyclosporine therapy for refractory Langerhans cell histiocytosis. **Blood** 78:1540.

399. Mahmoud H, Wang W, Murphy S (1991) Cyclosporine therapy for advanced Langerhans cell histiocytes. **Blood** 77:721.

400. Zaki I, Emerson R, Allen BR (1996) Treatment of severe atopic dermatitis in childhood with cyclosporin. **Br J Dermatol** 135(Suppl 48):21–24.

401. Harper JI, Ahmed I, Barclay G et al. (2000) Cyclosporin for severe childhood atopic dermatitis: short course versus continuous therapy. **Br J Dermatol** 142(1):52–58.

402. Berth-Jones J, Finlay AY, Aaki I et al. (1997) Cyclosporine in severe childhood atopic dermatitis: a multicenter study. **J Am Acad Dermatol** 36(6 pt 1):1029–1030.

phosphatase that dephosphorylates NF-AT, a transcription factor found in an inactive form in the cytoplasm. This dephosphorylated factor is able to enter the nucleus where it functions to initiate a transcriptional cascade that results in increased production of numerous immunomodulatory molecules, including IL-2, IL-4, GM-CSF and interferon-γ.[403] These newly synthesized factors are secreted by activated T cells and activate the inflammatory/immune cascade. Cyclosporine acts to interfere with this pathway by first binding with its cellular receptor cyclophilin PA; this complex then binds to the calmodulin-calcineurin complex, blocks the phosphatase activity and prevents the activation of NF-AT.[404] Thus, the production of the factors noted above, most importantly IL-2, is blocked and the immune response is blunted. Other important immunosuppressant drugs, including FK506 and rapamycin, work through similar mechanisms.

While cyclosporine is only FDA approved in the USA for the treatment of severe psoriasis, its best studied off-label uses are atopic dermatitis and pyoderma gangrenosum. Psoriasis patients receiving cyclosporine should have severe disease which has not responded to at least one systemic therapy such as retinoids, methotrexate, or PUVA or have contraindications or intolerance of other forms of sytemic therapy. Patients generally require 3–5mg/kg/day, and experts disagree on dosing strategies. Some recommend starting with maximum therapy and titrating the dose downward as tolerated while others advocate starting with more moderate doses of 2.5–3mg/kg/day and gradually increasing the dose as needed to achieve an adequate clinical response. Cyclosporine is available commercially as Sandimmune or Neoral, a microemulsion preparation. Neoral appears to have greater bioavailability than Sandimmune and thus may require dosing adjustments in selected cases.

There are several studies demonstrating the effectiveness of cyclosporine in the treatment of childhood atopic dermatitis. In an open-label multicenter study, Berth-Jones and colleagues[402] concluded that cyclosporine was a safe and effective short-term treatment for children with severe atopic dermatitis. Twenty-seven children were treated and 22 patients showed either complete clearing or marked clinical improvement. No patient experienced a persistent increase in blood pressure or serum creatinine. Another study of 18 children treated with cyclosporine for severe atopic dermatitis yielded similar results. Sixteen of the 18 patients had a good or excellent response to therapy and there were no serious adverse effects observed during 6 weeks of treatment.[400] Starting doses of approximately 5mg/kg/day were administered in these studies. Unfortunately, relapse was observed within several weeks of discontinuing therapy in most patients. On the other hand, there were a few individuals who obtained more long-term control. Harper and colleagues evaluated the effects of continuous versus short-course cyclosporine therapy on the control of childhood atopic dermatitis. Their open-label study of 40 patients compared continuous cyclosporine therapy with doses of 5mg/kg/day for 1 year to intermittent therapy with multiple courses of 12 weeks. While there were no clinically significant changes in either blood pressure or serum creatinine levels, the group receiving continuous therapy demonstrated more consistent control of their atopic dermatitis.[401]

It is imperative to monitor closely for potential drug interactions in patients receiving cyclosporine therapy. As the medication is metabolized by the hepatic cytochrome P450 (CYP) 3A4 enzyme system, concurrent administration of medications which compete for or induce cytochrome P450 3A4 activity may significantly alter the serum level of cyclosporine. CYP 3A4 inhibitors increase cyclosporine levels and include macrolide and fluoroquinolone antibiotics, azole antifungal agents, H$_2$ antihistamines, corticosteroids and several other classes of medications. Aromatic anticonvulsants and antituberculous drugs, in contrast, are CYP 3A4 inducers which decrease cyclosporine drug levels. Care should also be taken when giving concomitant medications which may

potentiate renal toxicity such as aminogylcosides, amphoteracin, and non-steroidal anti-inflammatory drugs (Tables 4.14 and 4.15).

Cyclosporine has many side effects, particularly at high doses and for long-term therapy. The most significant adverse effects are hypertension and nephrotoxicity; these occur on low-dose (less than 7mg/kg/day) therapy in adults[404–406] and in children.[407] Baseline laboratory studies should include two baseline creatinine levels as well as a BUN and urinalysis with microscopic examination. If at any time during therapy the creatinine level increases to more than 25% above baseline, then the dose of cyclosporine should be temporarily reduced by 1mg/kg/day for 2–4 weeks and the creatinine level should be rechecked. If it does not return to within 25% of baseline, then cyclosporine should be discontinued. If, however, the creatinine decreases to within 25% of baseline, the cyclosporine may be continued at the lower dose. There have been no reports in the world literature of clinically significant kidney damage occurring when following these guidelines.[321]

Hypertension occurs in about one-quarter of psoriasis patients treated with cyclosporine. The development of renal dysfunction may play a role in this complication. While blood pressure should be monitored closely during cyclosporine therapy, development of hypertension is not an indication for drug discontinuation if blood pressure can be satisfactorily controlled with appropriate antihypertensive agents.

Patients receiving prolonged high-dose therapy (7–15mg/kg/day) also have an increased risk of subsequent malignancies, an especially worrisome prospect for children. However, the risk of malignancy does not appear to be increased

TABLE 4.14   Cyclosporine drug interactions

Drugs that increase cyclosporine levels via cytochrome P-3A4 inhibition	Drugs that decrease cyclosporine levels via cytochrome P-3A4 induction
Calcium channel blockers (diltiazem, nicardipine, verapamil)	Antibiotics (nafcillin, rifampin)
Azole antifungals (itraconazole, fluconazole ketoconazole)	Anticonvulsants (carbamazapine, phenobarbital, valproate, phenytoin)
Macrolide antibiotics (erythromycin> clarithromycin>azithromycin)	Octreotide
Methylprednisolone	Ticlopidine
Allopurinol	
Bromocriptine	
Danazol	
Metoclopramide	
Androgens	
Amiodarone	
Other antibiotics (ciprofloxacin, doxycycline, cephalosporins)	
HIV protease inhibitors	
Food: grapefruit or grapefruit juice	
Diuretics (thiazides, furosemide)	
H2 antihistamines	

403. Koo JY, Lee CS, Maloney JE (2001) Cyclosporine and related drugs. In: Comprehensive Dermatologic Drug Therapy, Wolverton SE, ed. Philadelphia: WB Saunders.

404. Gothel SF, Marahiel MA (1999) Peptidyl-prolyl cis-trans isomerases, a superfamily of ubiquitous folding catalysts. Cell Mol Life Sci 55:423–436.

405. Deray G, Benmida M, LeHoang P et al. (1992) Renal function and blood pressure in patients receiving long-term, low-dose cyclosporin therapy for idiopathic autoimmune uveitis. Ann Int Med 117:578.

406. Powels A, Cook T, Hulme B et al. (1993) Renal function and biopsy findings after 5 years' treatment with low-dose cyclosporin for psoriasis. Br J Dermatol 128:159.

407. Peters A, Heckmatt J, Hasson N et al. (1991) Renal haemodynamics of cyclosporine A nephrotoxicity in children with juvenile dermatomyositis. Clin Sci 81:153.

TABLE 4.15   Other cyclosporine drug interactions

Drug	Adverse effect
Nonsteroidal anti-inflammatory agents	May potentiate renal dysfunction
Methotrexate	Increases levels of serum methotrexate
Digoxin	Reduce clearance of digoxin with reports of digoxin toxicity
Prednisone/prednisolone	Cyclosporine reduces clearance
Lovastatin	As above
Potassium sparing diuretics	Hyperkalemia
Antibiotics (gentamicin, tobramycin, vancomycin, trimethoprim/sulfamethoxazole)	May potentiate renal dysfunction
Antineoplastic agents	As above
Antifungals (amphotericin B, ketoconazole)	As above
H2 antihistamines	As above
Immunosuppressive agents (tacrolimus)	As above
ACE inhibitors	May increase incidence of hyperkalemia and renal dysfunction
Alfentanil	Regular doses may increase risk of prolonged respiratory and CNS depression after anesthesia with alfentanil
Fentanyl	Lower doses encouraged as cyclosporine may reduce hepatic metabolism of fentanyl and prolong sedation
Metformin	Increased risk of renal dysfunction and lactic acidosis
Potassium supplements	Increased risk of hyperkalemia

in patients receiving cyclosporine doses of 5mg/kg/day or less for dermatologic conditions who are not on concomitant immunosuppressives.

Neurologic effects including tremor, headache, and paresthesia are the most common side effects noted in the first two months of cyclosporine therapy.[403] Lymphoproliferative disorders are well-known complications of immunosuppressive therapy, including cyclosporine. This has been reported primarily in solid organ transplant recipients and in patients being treated for rheumatologic diseases, particularly those with high-dose therapy.[408–410] Hypertrichosis can be a disfiguring problem that occurs in up to 95 percent of patients, usually within the first few months of therapy.[388] These adverse reactions increase the risk–benefit ratio for cyclosporine beyond acceptability for all but the most serious skin diseases. Topical and intralesional cyclosporine have been studied in small numbers of patients with skin diseases.[388,411,412]

including oral lichen planus, psoriasis, and atopic dermatitis. Although safer than systemic therapy, the cost of this form of therapy is likely to be prohibitive.

Contraindications to cyclosporine include significant renal insufficiency, uncontrolled hypertension, clinically cured or persistent malignancy with the exception of nonmelanoma skin cancers, and hypersensitivity to cyclosporine or its formulation ingredients.

SULFONES AND SULFONAMIDES

The sulfa drugs, sulfones and sulfonamides, are related compounds with a broad spectrum of pharmacological activity. Sulfones have a sulfoxide core with two symmetrically attached aminophenyl groups. Dapsone, 4.4′-diaminodiphenylsulfone, is the only sulfone available in the United States. Sulfonamides have a similar structure, with an aminophenylsulfone core. Of this group, sulfapyridine differs from dapsone only by the substitution of a pyridine group for one aminophenyl group. The prototype compound was first synthesized in Germany in 1908 for industrial use. A quarter-century later, the sulfones' antibacterial properties were realized. By the 1940s, their therapeutic spectrum was expanded to include a variety of dermatologic disorders. Currently, dapsone is the only drug in this class commonly used in dermatology. Sulfapyridine is no longer available in the United States, except on a compassionate basis.

Dapsone has both antimicrobial and anti-inflammatory actions. The antimicrobial effects are due to the reduction of dihydrofolate synthesis by competitive inhibition of the enzyme dihydropteroate synthase.[413] The anti-inflammatory effects of the drug have been more difficult to define. However, disease processes that respond to dapsone generally are associated with neutrophil infiltrations in the affected tissues. Studies have shown that treatment of neutrophils *in vitro* with dapsone results in a decrease in integrin-mediated adherence of neutrophils to target cells as well as a reduction in myeloperoxidase activity. It appears that dapsone is able to reduce the ability of neutrophils to respond to chemotactic stimuli, possibly by disrupting the G-protein associated signal transduction pathway.[414] Potential uses of dapsone in dermatology are shown in Table 4.16.

Dapsone, when orally ingested, is well absorbed from the gastrointestinal tract with bioavailability approaching 86%. Gastrointestinal absorption is reduced in severe leprosy. Peak serum concentrations are reached quickly within 0.5 to 4h of ingestion and the elimination half-life ranges from 12 to 30h. After absorption, dapsone is taken up by the portal circulation and transported to the liver. Here, dapsone is metabolized by acetylation or N-hydroxylation. This dual metabolic pathway produces either toxic hydroxylamines via the N-hydroxylation pathway or nontoxic acetyl-dapsone via the acetylation pathway. Both metabolites are then conjugated with glucuronic acid and excreted.[415]

The N-hydroxylation pathway has been extensively evaluated in the literature as this pathway produces dapsone's toxic metabolite, hydroxylamine, via the CY P450 enzyme system. Although it is not known exactly which enzyme within this system is responsible for metabolism of dapsone, studies using low molecular weight inhibitors suggest that CYP2E and CYP2C are involved in dapsone hydroxylation. In Caucasion populations, dapsone N-hydroxylation was extremely variable making predictability of toxicity very difficult. It was also noted within this Caucasion population that increasing age was associated with decreased incidence of hydroxylation.[415] Dapsone is highly protein bound and is distributed throughout the body to all major

408. Kamel OW (1997) Iatrogenic lymphoproliferative disorders in nontransplantation settings. **Semin Diagn Pathol** 14:27–34.
409. Tanner JE, Alfieri C (2001) The Epstein–Barr virus and post-transplant lymphoproliferative disease interplay of immunosuppression, EBV, and the immune system in disease pathogenesis. **Trans Infect Dis** 3:60–69.
410. Trofe J, Buell JF, First MR et al. (2002) The role of immunosuppression in lymphoma. **Recent Research Cancer Res** 159:55–66.
411. Mizoguchi M, Kawaguchu K, Ohsuga Y et al. (1992) Cyclosporine ointment for psoriasis and atopic dermatitis. **Lancet** 339:1120.

412. Burns M, Ellis C, Eisen D et al. (1992) Intralesional cyclosporine for psoriasis. Relationship of dose, tissue levels, and efficacy. **Arch Dermatol** 128:786.
413. Coleman MD (1993) Dapsone: modes of action toxicity and possible strategies for increasing patient tolerance. **Br J Dermatol** 129:507–513.
414. Debol SM, Herron MJ, Nelson RD (1997) Anti-inflammatory action of dapsone: inhibition of neutrophil adherence is associated with inhibition of chemoattractant-induced signal transduction. **J Leukoc Biol** 62:827–836.
415. Zhu I, Stiller M (2001) Dapsone and sulfones in dermatology: Overview and update. **J Am Dermatol** 45(3):420–428.

TABLE 4.16   Potential uses of dapsone in dermatology

Acne fulminans	Actinomycetoma
Brown recluse spider bites	Lichen planus
Cicatricial pemphigoid	Linear IgA disease (chronic bullous disease of childhood)
Dermatitis herpetiformis*	Pemphigus vulgaris
Eosinophilic cellulitis	Pustular psoriasis
Erythema elevatum diutinum	Pyoderma gangrenesum
Granuloma annulare	Relapsing polychondritis
Granuloma faciale	Rheumatoid arthritis Sneddon–Wilkinson disease
IgA pemphigus	Sweet's syndrome
Leprosy*	Systemic lupus (bullous SLE)

* FDA approved.

TABLE 4.17   Adverse reactions to dapsone

Pharmacologic/predictable	Allergic/idiosyncratic
	Hepatitis: cholestatic or hepatocellular disease or both
Hemolytic anemia	Agranulocytosis
Methemoglobinemia	Cutaneous: exanthematous eruption, Stevens–Johnson syndrome, toxic epidermal necrolysis
Nonspecific: Nausea, vomiting, fatigue, dizziness, weakness, nervousness, shortness of breath, headache	Nephritis Pneumonitis Hypothyroidism Dapsone hypersensitivity syndrome Psychosis Peripheral neuropathy

organ systems including the skin. Dapsone also crosses the blood–brain barrier, the placenta, and is found in breast milk.[415]

The mechanisms by which dapsone interferes with the inflammatory process are still under investigation. It is clear that dapsone disrupts neutrophil chemotactic migration which further suppresses neutrophil recruitment and local production of toxic respiratory and secretory products. Dapsone also appears to bind irreversibly to myeloperoxidase in neutrophils and eosinophil peroxidase and convert these enzymes to inactive compounds. Little is known about the mechanism of dapsone in antibody-mediated diseases such as bullous dermatoses, but some research suggests a dose-dependent inhibition of neutrophilic adherence to basement zone antibody.[415]

Dapsone is approved for use in children and is available in tablet, and in some institutions suspension form. The suspension concentration is 2mg/ml and is currently under investigation as to the absorption and pharmacokinetics compared to the tablet form. The starting dose is variable depending on the disease to be treated and the comorbidities involved. Often physicians start with 0.5–2.0mg/kg/day, and adjust to the lowest effective amount, to minimize side effects. Tablets may be ground into a suspension and refrigerated, maintaining potency for a minimum of 3 months.

The most common adverse effects of dapsone therapy are hemolysis and methemoglobinemia (see Table 4.17). Most patients on dapsone will have some hemolysis, but patients with hereditary G6PD deficiency are at greatest risk of clinically significant hemolytic anemia. Idiosyncratic reactions, unrelated to dosage, including cholestasis, nephrotoxicity, agranulocytosis, and motor neuropathy have been reported.

The "sulfone syndrome" is a well-described idiosyncratic mononucleosis-like hypersensitivity reaction, occurring in less than 1% of patients, which may result in multiorgan disease. This syndrome is similar to other hypersensitivity syndromes that can occur with anticonvulsants, allopurinol, non-steroidal anti-inflammatory medications, and sulfonamide antibiotics. Typically this syndrome appears 4 or more weeks after initiation of dapsone therapy and carries a higher risk of liver involvement than other hypersensitivity syndromes. The pathogenesis of dapsone hypersensitivity syndrome, as with other drug hypersensitivity syndromes, is not well understood and the treatment is controversial and dependent on the severity of symptoms and prescence of end organ involvement. Systemic glucocorticoid therapy has been used in anecdotal reports of dapsone hypersensitivity syndrome with varied results. When steroid therapy is initiated, it should be slowly tapered over 1 to 2 months as dapsone persists for up to 35 days in organs via protein binding and enterohepatic circulation.[416] A late finding in some patients with dapsone hypersensitivity syndrome is hypothyroidism, which may occur up to 3 or more months after the onset of the reaction.[415]

Agranulocytosis, another rare life-threatening idiosyncratic reaction associated with dapsone, remains poorly understood. It is postulated that the mechanism by which dapsone affects the bone marrow could be erythrocyte-mediated. *In vitro*, erythrocytes exposed to hydoxylamine and repeatedly washed may still be capable of releasing this metabolite in sufficient amounts to kill mononuclear leukocytes *in vitro*. By this pathway, these erythrocytes may serve as a conduit to reach the bone marrow. Once in the marrow, this toxic metabolite could bind to hematopoietic precursors and trigger an immune response, leading to this potentially fatal agranulocytosis.[417]

Pretreatment screening should include a G6PD level, complete blood count, renal and liver function tests, and urinalysis. During the first 3 months of therapy, the hematocrit should be closely monitored until a stable level is reached. A recommended schedule is a weekly complete blood count for the first month, bimonthly for the next 2 months, then every 3 months. Patients who have tolerated dapsone for 6 to 12 months are unlikely to develop problems, unless the dose is changed.

TABLE 4.18   Drug interactions with dapsone

Drug	Interaction
Antacids	Reduces absorption
Interferons, didanosine, zidovudine, cytotoxic chemotherapy, and clozapine	Bone marrow suppression
Probenecid	Increases dapsone levels by decreasing renal excretion
Trimethoprim, trimethoprim/sulfamethoxazole	Increased risk of hemolysis (especially in G6PD patients), increased risk of methemoglobinemia, increases plasma concentrations
Rifampin	Induces dapsone metabolism and enhances urinary excretion of dapsone
Cimetidine	Inhibits formation of the toxic hydroxylamine metabolite of dapsone
Omeprazole	Inhibits cytochrome enzymes and decreases the rate of hydroxylamine formation

416. Prussick R, Shear NH (1996) Dapsone hypersensitivity syndrome. J Am Acad Dermatol 35:346–349.

417. Remlinger, KA (2001) Hematologic toxicity of drug therapy. In: Comprehensive Dermatologic Drug Therapy, Wolverton SE, ed. Philadelphia: WB Saunders, pp. 798–811.

Dapsone tolerance may be improved by simultaneous use of cimetidine. Cimetidine reduces the hepatic oxidation of dapsone to hydroxylamine which decreases the amount of side effects reported including headache, methemoglobin production, and lethargy. Furthermore, concomitant use of Vitamin C and E in the role of antioxidants may also be helpful in reduction of side effects, but further studies are needed.[415]

The use of dapsone in pregnancy is generally considered safe for the mother and fetus, but carries a pregnancy category C rating. There have been a few reports of neonatal complications linked to maternal dapsone use such as hemolytic anemia, methemoglobinemia, and hyperbilirubinema. Dapsone can cross the placenta and is found in limited concentrations in human breast milk. As always, potential risks to mother and fetus verses benefit of therapy should be weighed when trying to decide whether dapsone therapy should be initiated or continued during pregnancy. This is particularly true of pregnant women with leprosy. It has been shown that 20% of children born to women with leprosy will develop leprosy by puberty. In this situation, these women often require treatment.[415]

Dapsone therapy is contraindicated in patients with a history of hypersensitivity reactions to dapsone including agranulocytosis. Dapsone should be used with caution when other potentially hemolytic drugs are being used especially if those patients are G6PD deficient. These drugs should be used with extreme caution if an allergy exists to another drug in the sulfa family (trimethoprim-sulfamethoxazole, sulfasalazine). Also, starting dapsone in patients with signs of megaloblastic anemia should be delayed until folic acid replacement is adequate or the cause of the hemopoietic disturbance is discovered and addressed.

There are several potential drug interactions with the use of dapsone. First, dapsone should not be given with antacids as they decrease its absorption. One should also try to avoid use of dapsone with other medications that are potentially toxic to bone marrow such as clozapine, certain chemotherapeutics, didanosine, zidovudine, and interferons. If avoidance of dual therapy is not possible, cell counts should be checked weekly for signs of bone marrow suppression. The concomitant use of other sulfa drugs with dapsone increases the risk of hemolysis and methemoglobinemia. Finally, due to the hepatic metabolism of dapsone, any drug which is metabolized by the cytochrome P450 system may also influence dapsone metabolism.

GAMMAGLOBULIN

Gammaglobulin is a fraction of human serum pooled from at least 1000 donors that contains a high concentration of antibodies. It was first purified and administered to provide passive immunity for the prevention and treatment of certain viral diseases. It is now FDA approved for the treatment of primary antibody immunodeficiency diseases, immune thrombocytopenic purpura (ITP), Kawasaki's disease, and various inflammatory diseases where intravenous immunoglobulin (IVIG) serves as an immunomodulator.[418]

The first form of pooled gammaglobulin was human serum immunoglobulin (HSIG). HSIG contains 95–99% IgG with specificity for a wide spectrum of antigens. It is purified of infectious particles and most other serum proteins. However, this preparation contains high-molecular-weight complexes of IgG that tend to aggregate *in vitro*. Given intravenously, these complexes can activate complement and cause severe anaphylactic reactions. HSIG is safe only for subcutaneous or intramuscular injection, a painful process. A safe IVIG, free of high-molecular-weight complexes and preservatives, has been available in the United States since 1981, largely replacing the use of HSIG.

IVIG is a relatively safe form of therapy, but it is very expensive to manufacture and administer. Adverse reactions, including back and abdominal pain, headache, nausea, and vomiting, can occur during infusion. Early

preparations of IVIG were associated with a 10–15% incidence of adverse reactions. With newer preparations of IVIG, reported reactions have declined to 2–6%. These reactions are generally rate-related and often resolve after slowing the rate of infusion.[419] Chills, fever, headache, myalgia, and fatigue can persist after infusion. These side effects can be prevented or treated with acetaminophen, diphenhydramine, or oral hydrocortisone. Anaphylaxis, although rare, is reported in the use of IVIG, particularly in those IgA-deficient patients with anti-IgA antibodies; such patients should receive and IgA-depleted preparation of IVIG.[418]

As with any blood product, there are concerns about the transmission of infectious agents. In 1994, a small group of hepatitis C cases was reported to the FDA.[418] All but one case was related to a certain batch of IVIG by one manufacturer. To ensure the safety of the patient population, a solvent-detergent process was added to the preparation to inactivate lipid-enveloped viruses. This process, in addition to careful donor screening and meticulous clinical guidelines, should help prevent further transmission. There are no documented cases of hepatitis B transmission. Furthermore, the human immunodeficiency virus (HIV) is effectively inactivated during the manufacturing process itself and HIV transmission has not been reported with IVIG.[419]

As several methods of manufacturing processes are used, varying degrees of IVIG purity may result. In an attempt to standardize the various preparations, the World Health Organization suggested the following criteria for the production of IVIG

1. Each batch should be prepared from plasma pooled from at least 1000 donors.
2. Each batch should contain at least 90% intact IgG with a subclass distribution that closely approximates that in normal serum.
3. All IgG molecules should retain their biological activity, such as the ability to fix complement.
4. The preparation should be free of vasoactive substances such as prekallikrein activator, kinins, plasmin, and preservatives.
5. The preparation should as far as possible be free of aggregates.
6. The preparation should be free of infective agents and other potentially harmful contaminants.[419]

The mechanisms by which IVIG are effective in both replacement therapy and immunomodulatory therapy are different as are the doses of IVIG required (Table 4.19). Therapy in immunodeficiency conditions probably depends on straightforward replacement of missing antibodies. The effective dosages range from 0.2g/kg per month to 0.8g/kg per month, depending on the extent of failure of antibody production and the increased susceptibility to infection as a result of damage following previous infections.

Administration of IVIG has multiple, generally anti-inflammatory, effects on the immune system. Anti-inflammatory or immunomodulatory doses of IVIG for autoimmune conditions are considerably larger; cumulative doses of 2g/kg or more are given over 1–4 days. Several different pathways of activity have been proposed to play a role in the response of disease states to IVIG therapy. IVIG can interfere with the interaction of circulating antigen–antibody complexes and Fc receptors on the surface of various immune cells; this interaction is important in the activation of cell-mediated immunity. IVIG provides naturally occurring anti-idiotypic antibodies that may act to neutralize pathogenic autoantibodies.[420,421] IVIG also has a direct anti-inflammatory effect, in part mediated by its ability to bind complement factors C3b and C4b. IVIG interferes with endothelial and monocyte cell activation, leading to reduced production of IL-1 and TNF-α. IVIG can directly bind to pathogenic autoimmune antibodies, preventing their interaction with their target antigen. Similarly, IVIG may be able to bind to and inactivate bacterial toxins and superantigens. Finally, IVIG may have direct

418. Anderson, M (1999) Intravenous gammaglobulin for pediatric infectious diseases. **Pediatr Ann** 28:8.

419. Misbah SA, Chapel HM (1993) Adverse effects of intravenous immunoglobulin. **Drug Saf** 9(4):254–262.

420. Jolles S, Hughes J, Whittaker S (1998) Dermatological uses of high-dose intravenous immunoglobulin. **Arch Dermatol** 134:80–86.

421. Kazatchkine MD, Kaveri SV (2001) Immunomodulation of autoimmune and inflammatory diseases with intravenous immune globulin. **N Engl J Med** 345:747–753.

TABLE 4.19 Recognized indications for IVIG

Replacement Therapy	Immunomodulatory
Primary antibody deficiencies	Immune thrombocytopenia purpura
X-linked agammaglobulinemia	Kawasaki disease
X-linked immunodeficiency with hyperimmunoglobulin M	Guillain–Barré syndrome
Common variable immunodeficiency	Chronic inflammatory demyelinating neuropathy
Immunoglobulin G subclass deficiencies with infections	Acquired hemophilia
Severe combined immunodeficiency (SCID) prior to bone marrow transplantation	Juvenile dermatomyositis
Failure of B cell engraftment after bone marrow transplantation for SCID	Toxic epidermal necrolysis
Selected cases of secondary antibody deficiency Intestinal lymphangiectasia	
Chronic lymphocytic leukemia and B cell lymphoma with hypogammaglobulinemia	
Myeloma with specific antibody deficiency	
Low birth weight babies at risk of sepsis	
Infants and children with HIV	

TABLE 4.20 Complications of IVIG therapy

Hematological	Renal	Neurological
Hemolysis (Coombs' positive)	Transient rise in serum creatinine	Aseptic meningitis
Neutropenia	Acute renal failure in mixed cryoglobulinemia	
Rise in plasma viscosity		

From Mishah and Chapel 1993[419]

TABLE 4.21 Cautions and contraindications in the use of IVIG

Cautions	Contraindications
Renal insufficiency Rapidly progressive renal disease (30% rise in creatinine in the previous 2 weeks)	Cryoglobulinemia
Acute infection	Anaphylaxis (relative)
Hyperviscosity or conditions associated with hyperviscosity/thromboembolic events	
HIV	
IgA autoantibodies/IgA deficiency	
History of hemolysis	
Systemic lupus erythematous	

immunomodulatory effects on B and T lymphocytes. These pathways are not mutually exclusive and the importance of each in the response of different disease states to IVIG administration remains to be elucidated.[421,422]

Aside from adverse effects relating to the immediate infusion, other complications have been reported which may be related to immune complex formation or other secondary effects. These complications have been noted in several organ systems and are shown in Table 4.20.[419]

In a few patient populations, IVIG should be used with extreme caution (Table 4.21). Patients with anti-IgA antibodies or a history of anaphylaxis to IVIG should be treated with IVIG only when other alternatives have been exhausted and they should be monitored closely for any reaction. IgA deficient IVIG and prophylactic medications should be used in these settings. Due to the possibility of renal compromise, patients with documented renal disease should be treated with extreme caution, especially when using high-dose IVIG. Similarly, the use of IVIG in patients with systemic lupus erythematosus (SLE) is controversial. There have been reports of worsening nephritis in the setting of SLE which may further decrease clearance of immune complexes and predispose a patient to sepsis. Other reports have documented acute renal failure in patients treated with IVIG (cryoglobulinemia) due to a paraprotein with rheumatoid factor. This condition has been reported in the literature as a contraindication for IVIG therapy.[419,420]

It is also important to remember in the pediatric population that the use of IVIG often impacts immunization schedules and the level of immunity achieved by an immunization. This is particularly relevant when administering live-virus vaccines (measles, mumps, rubella, varicella) It is generally recommended that the period between immunization and the initiation of therapy with IVIG be at least 14 days for the vaccine to establish a sufficient immune response.[320] If this time period is not attained, serum testing for specific antibody titers is appropriate to document an adequate immune response. If an immune response to the vaccine is not mounted, then readministration of the vaccine is warranted following the use of IVIG therapy. This timing, however, is variable and depends upon the indication for therapy,

as well as the dose of IVIG given. It is prudent for every physician to instruct the patient on these gudielines for live-virus vaccinations to ensure adequate and safe use of vaccinations in patient populations.

While the use of IVIG is expanding, it is not without substantial cost. Prices of each preparation of IVIG are different and also depend on the contractual stipulations between production companies and various organizations. The approximate cost of IVIG has been reported to be $25.00 per gram.[420] For treatment of a 25-kg child with dermatomyositis at a dose of 2g/kg per month, the monthly cost would average $1250.00, with yearly cost projecting nearly $15 000.00 per year.[420]

The use of IVIG in the last several years has been expanded to include several dermatologic condtions. Use of IVIG in the treatment of penphigus vulgaris has been recently studied. Ahmed and colleagues studied patients with recalcitrant disease not responding to high-dose corticosteroids or other immunomodulators and also followed patients in whom other treatments were contraindicated. IVIG infusions were begun at various doses ranging of 500–2000mg/kg per cycle (total dose of IVIG divided equally between three doses and infused daily) and continued at four-week intervals until all lesions had healed. The infusion intervals were then gradually extended to six, eight, ten, twelve, fourteen, and sixteen weeks, respectively, with the dose of each infusion remaining constant. This trial demonstrates the potential use of IVIG in pemphigus vulgaris patients as a monotherapy and steroid-sparing agent. Compared to other treatment modalities, IVIG in this study was associated with fewer recurrences and relapses of pemphigus vulgaris. All 21 patients in the study were weaned off corticosteroids as well as other immunomodulators while on the IVIG infusion protocol. The lowest effective dose of IVIG was

422. Colsky AS (2000) Intravenous immunoglobulin in autoimmune and inflammatory dermatoses. Dermatol Clin 18:447–457.

noted to be 2g/kg/cycle. No patient in this study was hospitalized during the infusion protocol with diagnoses related to either pemphigus or IVIG infusion complications.[423]

Recent investigations suggest that IVIG may also hold promise in the treatment of other autoimmune bullous disorders, including pemphigus foliaceous and oral pemphigoid.[423,424] A review by Jolles[425] of 62 reported patients who received IVIG for treatment of immunobullous disorders between 1966 and 2000 suggests that IVIG may be more helpful as adjunctive therapy. Analysis of these case reports and uncontrolled trials showed a 91% response rate when IVIG was used as adjunct therapy as compared to a response rate of 56% when IVIG was used as monotherapy.[425] IVIG may also be useful as adjunct therapy in the management of severe atopic dermatitis, although results of small case series have been inconsistent.[426,427] Several recent case reports and case series suggest that IVIG may be useful in the treatment of Stevens–Johnson syndrome, anticonvulsant hypersensitivity syndromes and toxic epidermal necrolysis.[428–430] Viard et al. treated 10 patients with histologically confirmed toxic epidermal necrolysis with IVIG and reported rapid recovery in all 10 patients.[430]

GLUCOCORTICOIDS

Systemic glucocorticoids are widely used for their potent immunosuppressive, anti–inflammatory, and vasoconstrictive effects in the management of many dermatologic diseases, including severe eczematous and papulosquamous dermatoses, autoimmune diseases, and proliferative hemangiomas. These drugs have greater suppressive effects on cell–mediated than on antibody–mediated immune responses, and on monocyte more than polymorphonuclear leukocyte function. The potency of each glucocorticoid preparation is determined by tissue and plasma half–lives and by their relative glucocorticoid versus mineralocorticoid activities (Table 4.22). Hydrocortisone and cortisone are the lowest-potency preparations with the shortest half–lives. Prednisone, prednisolone, and triamcinolone are midpotency and dexamethasone and betamethasone are the longest-acting and highest-potency agents. All dermatologists must be aware of the wide range of side effects and complications of intralesional and systemic glucocorticoid therapy. In general, the longer acting steroids have greater suppression of growth and the integrity of hypothalamic–pituitary–adrenal (HPA) axis function. The use of these medications in children presents special problems.[431]

Corticosteroids are 21-carbon aromatic compounds, consisting of a core of three hexane and one pentane ring. Modification of this basic structure enhances the pharmacologic effects of the various corticosteroid preparations. Dermatologic diseases are best treated with corticosteroid preparations that have predominantly, or exclusively, glucocorticoid activity, with little or no mineralocorticoid activity. Cortisol (or hydrocortisone) is the physiologically secreted glucocorticoid, with equal glucocorticoid and mineralocorticoid effects. It is the prototype for all synthetic corticosteroids. Prednisolone is an analog of cortisol, with a 5:1 predominant glucocorticoid activity. Prednisone is a similar preparation, with a keto group at C–11, another site that determines glucocorticoid potency. In the liver, prednisone is transformed to prednisolone by conversion of an inactive 11-keto to an active 11-hydroxy configuration. These preparations are most often used in pediatric dermatology because they are short acting and have a relatively low potency, allowing for easy dosing manipulation. Substitution of a halide molecule (chlorine or fluorine) at C–9 enhances anti–inflammatory activity. In the halogenated compounds, additional modification at C–16 reduces mineralocorticoid activity. Thus, the 9-fluoro-16-hydroxy compound is triamcinolone, 9-fluoro-16-methyl substitutions make dexamethasone, and the 9-fluoro-16-methyl compound is betamethasone.

The glucocorticoids have been studied intensively for over 50 years and much has been learned about how they work at the cellular and molecular level. However, we still do not have a complete understanding of their mechanism of action. It is clear that many of the effects of glucocorticoids are mediated by a nuclear receptor that acts as a ligand–dependent transcription factor. This receptor is a member of the nuclear receptor superfamily, as are the receptors for retinoic acid, thyroid hormone, and vitamin D3.

The glucocorticoid receptor (GCR) normally resides in the cytoplasm in a complex with heat-shock proteins and immunophilins. In this state, it is inactive. When a glucocorticoid diffuses across the cell membrane and binds to the GCR, the receptor dissociates from the heat shock proteins and immunophilin and is translocated into the nucleus. Here the glucocorticoid–GCR complex interacts with specific DNA-sequences, called glucocorticoid response elements or GREs, that are found in the promoter regions of glucocorticoid-responsive genes. Depending upon the specific gene and the available positive and negative transcriptional cofactors, the targeted gene may be activated or repressed. While the complete pathway has yet to be elucidated, it is clear that the genes for IL-1, IL-2, IFN-γ and TNF-α are all

---

TABLE 4.22   Half-lives and potencies of corticosteroids

Biologic corticosteroids	Approximate equivalent dose	Relative glucocorticoid potency	Relative mineralocorticoid potency	Half-life (hours)
Cortisone	25mg	0.8	0	8–12
Hydrocortisone	20mg	1	2	8–12
Prednisolone	5mg	4	1	18–36
Prednisone	5mg	4	1	18–36
Methylprednisolone	4mg	5	0	18–36
Triamcinalone	4mg	5	0	18–36
Dexamethasone	0.75mg	20–30	0	36–54
Betamethasone	0.6–0.75mg	20–30	0	36–54

423. Ahmed A (2001) Intravenous immunoglulin therapy in the treatment of patients with pemphigus vulgaris unresponsive to conventional immunosuppressive treatment. **J Am Acad Dermatol** 45(6):825–835.
424. Ahmed AR, Sami N (2002) Intravenous immunoglobulin therapy for patients with pemphigus foliaceus unresponsive to conventional therapy. **J Am Acad Dermatol** 46:42–49.
425. Jolles S (2001) A review of high-dose intravenous immunoglobulin (hdIVIg) in the treatment of the autoimmune blistering disorders. **Clin Exp Dermatol** 26:127–131.
426. Wakim M, Alazard M, Yajima A et al. (1998) High dose intravenous immunoglobulin in atopic dermatitis and hyper-IgE syndrome. **Ann Allergy Asthma Immunol** l 81:153–158.

427. Jolles S, Hughes H, Rustin M (2000) The treatment of atopic dermatitis with adjunctive high-dose intravenous immunoglobulin: a report of three patients and review of the literature. **Br J Dermatol** 142:551–554.
428. Morici MV, Galen WK, Shetty AK et al. (2000) Intravenous immunoglobulin therapy for children with Stevens–Johnson syndrome **J Rheumatol** 27:2494–2497.
429. Scheuerman O, Nofech-Moses Y, Rachmel A, Askenazi S (2001) Successful treatment of antiepileptic drug hypersensitivity syndrome with intravenous immune globulin. **Pediatrics** 107:e14.
430. Viard I, Wehrli P, Bullani R et al. (1998) Inhibition of toxic epidermal necrolysis by blockade of CD95 with human intravenous immunoglobulin. **Science** 282:490–493.
431. Lucky A (1984) Principles of the use of glucocorticosteroids in the growing child. **Pediatr Dermatol** 3:226.

repressed in the presence of glucocorticoids, resulting in a damping of the inflammatory response.[432]

Besides regulating specific cytokine genes, glucocorticoids are also able to initiate the apoptosis pathway in lymphocytes. Again, the precise sequence of events that occurs when apoptosis is activated is unclear, but the end result is the activation of a series of proteolytic enzymes known as caspases and ultimately the orderly death of the cell.[432,433]

There are many levels of control of the glucocorticoid response in inflammatory or immune cells. For instance, there is a second form of the GCR, known as GCR-β, which may act as a negative regulator of GCR function. The GCR is multiply phosphorylated and its activity is likely to be regulated in this manner. In addition, it is becoming more clear that there are nongenomic effects of glucocorticoids, but it is not yet clear how this is accomplished.[434]

INTRALESIONAL GLUCOCORTICOIDS

Injectable corticosteroid preparations (triamcinolones, betamethasone acetate) are formulated in suspensions. They are insoluble in water and form cloudy solutions when shaken. Suspensions are intended only for intralesional or intramuscular injection where the drug is deposited as a particulate reservoir. This form has a more sustained local effect than that of a glucocorticoid in solution (e.g., dexamethasone, methylprednisolone, hydrocortisone). Triamcinolone acetonide (Kenalog) or diacetate (Aristocort) suspensions are most often used by dermatologists. Betamethasone suspension (Celestone Soluspan) may also be used when a higher-potency preparation is required.

Triamcinolone suspensions are available in concentrations of 10 and 40mg/ml. These can be diluted with lidocaine solution or normal saline to the appropriate strength for the nature and site of the lesion. For acne cysts, 1 to 2mg/ml is usually sufficient. Keloids and hypertrophic scars on the trunk or extremities may require 10 to 40mg/ml. Intralesional injections are best given by using a siliconized sharp needle securely attached to a Luer-lock syringe. A 30-gauge needle can be used with suspensions of less than 10mg/ml. More concentrated solutions require a larger bore. The needle should be quickly inserted through the greatest diameter of the lesion. As it is withdrawn, the steroid solution is injected until the lesion blanches. Care must be taken to ensure that the injection is not intravascular by asserting backpressure on the syringe before injecting the medication. Thick hypertrophic scars and keloids can be difficult to penetrate. A 5 to 10s freeze with liquid nitrogen performed 10min prior to injection will generate local edema and facilitate injection of a larger volume of material.

Intralesional injections may cause local side effects of tissue atrophy, hypopigmentation or depigmentation, and sterile abscess formation. Local atrophy can occur when the material is deposited too deeply into the subcutis or when higher concentrations are used. Atrophy and depigmentation last several months but are usually not permanent. Hypopigmentation may occur when an injection is too superficial, lodging the material in the lower epidermis.

Accidental embolization of the retinal artery with resulting blindness has been reported following intralesional corticosteroid injection of periorbital hemangiomas in infancy. This tragic adverse effect can occur ipsilaterally, contralaterally, or bilaterally.[435] Many clinicians consider systemic corticosteroid therapy a much safer alternative for periorbital hemangiomas that require treatment.

The total dose of an intralesional corticosteroid injection is systemically available. Systemic side effects, as described below, can result from intralesional administration when injections are given frequently, in high concentrations, and/or large quantities. Clinicians should know the dose equivalence of the preparations they use: 0.6mg of betamethasone is equivalent to 4mg of triamcinolone or 5mg of prednisone. Total and mg/kg dosage must always be calculated and recorded. As a reference point, the maximum recommended anti-inflammatory dose of prednisone in children is 2mg/kg/day. Due to the long half-life of most injected corticosteroids, intralesional steroid injections are likely to result in more pronounced suppression of the HPA axis as compared with oral prednisone or prednisilone.

SYSTEMIC GLUCOCORTICOIDS

The decision to use a systemic corticosteroid must be based on a risk–benefit analysis for each patient. Alternative forms of therapy should always be considered, especially for chronic conditions. As a general rule, it is best to begin with a high enough dose to control the disease, tapering to the lowest possible dose for the shortest period of time. However, under special circumstances, systemic corticosteroids can be used successfully for conditions such as atopic dermatitis, psoriasis, seborrheic dermatitis, and hand ezema.

The dose and dosage schedule must be designed to optimize the therapeutic effect and minimize adverse side effects. Systemic corticosteroids are best administered in the early morning, (approximately 8 a.m.) as this correlates with the normal daily physiologic surge of cortisol. Higher doses given more than once a day will have maximal anti-inflammatory activity but will also have maximal side effects. The physiologic equivalent of 0.125 to 0.16mg/kg of prednisone is secreted daily. Higher daily doses of medication, commonly given for dermatologic diseases, will suppress the HPA axis[436] and growth in children.[431] The average systemic dose varies from 0.5 to 2mg/kg/day for most dermatologic conditions although higher doses may be required for the treatment of serious proliferating hemangiomas. The glucocorticoid dose should be based upon the size of the patient, the type and severity of disease, and the urgency for improvement. Generally, the starting dose is high, with gradual tapering as the condition improves. For acute conditions, especially severe eczematous processes, premature discontinuation or overly rapid tapering can result in a rebound flare.

Prednisone tablets are relatively inexpensive. The cost of 1-, 5-, 10-, and 20-mg tablets are comparable, so 20-mg tablets are the least expensive form per milligram. A suspension containing 5mg/5ml (Pediapred) is also available commercially. Prednisolone syrup (Prelone) is available in a more concentrated form, 15mg/5ml allowing for a smaller volume per dose (see Prescribing Pearls). Unfortunately, most oral preparations of prednisone and prednisolone are foul tasting and administration in infants and toddlers can be extremely challenging. A newer preparation of prednisolone (Orapred) 15mg/5ml is reportedly more palatable and may provide another dosing option.

Regimens with multiple daily doses maximally suppress the HPA axis and should be prescribed only for acute management of severe inflammatory conditions, such as pyoderma gangrenosum or pemphigus vulgaris. Once-a-day dosing, between 6 and 8 a.m., will minimize HPA axis suppression. An alternate-day dosage regimen will have the least amount of HPA axis suppression and will minimize other adverse effects, such as weight gain and growth retardation.[437] However, some patients placed on an alternate-day regimen will experience relapse of their disease and/or suffer withdrawal symptoms. This can usually be avoided by a gradual conversion from daily to alternate-day dosing: a small incremental decrease in the dose taken every other day is prescribed, with dosage adjustments made at weekly intervals, until the medication is taken every 48 hours (e.g., 40mg on day 1, 35mg on day 2 for the first week; 40mg on day 1, 30mg on day 2 for the second week). An alternative method to shift from daily to alternate-day therapy is to triple

432. Ashwell JD, Lu FWM, Vacchio MS (2000) Glucocorticoids in T cell development and function. **Annu Rev Immunol** 18:309–345.

433. Planey SL, Litwack G (2000) Glucocorticoid-induced apoptosis in lymphocytes. **Biochem Biophys Res Comm** 279:307–312.

434. Refojo D, Liberman AC, Holsboer F, Arzt E (2001) Transcription factor-mediated molecular mechanisms involved in the functional cross-talk between cytokines and glucocorticoids. **Immunol Cell Biol** 79:385–397.

435. Ruttum M, Abrams G, Harris G, Ellis M (1993) Bilateral retinal embolization associated with intralesional corticosteroid injection for capillary hemangioma of infancy. **J Pediatr Ophthalmol Strabismus** 30.

436. Gallant C, Kenny P (1986) Oral glucocortisteroids and their complications. **J Am Acad Dermatol** 14:161.

437. Kimura Y, Fieldston E, Devries-Vandervlugt B, Li S, Imundo L (2000) High dose, alternate day corticosteroids for systemic onset juvenile rheumatoid arthritis. **J Rheumatol** 27:2018–2024.

the daily dose (e.g., from 10mg/day to 30mg every other morning). The degree of HPA axis suppression for 30mg of prednisone taken every other morning is less than that for 5mg given three times a day.[438]

HPA axis response will recover promptly following short-term therapy (less than 2 weeks). However, prolonged therapy, over 1 month, will result in HPA axis suppression for up to 1 year. Patients who require prolonged therapy should be slowly tapered off medication, as above, and instructed in the details of stress–dose replacement therapy.[439] Morning cortisol levels may be obtained to assess basal HPA axis function although the low-dose ACTH stimulation test has become the gold standard in the assessment of HPA axis suppression and need for stress doses of steroids. In this study, a baseline cortisol level is obtained and 1μg of ACTH (cosyntropin) is administered intravenously. Follow-up cortisol levels are then obtained at 10, 20, and 30min following the infusion of ACTH.[440,441] An increase in cortisol level of >10μg/dl indicates normal function of the HPA axis under conditions of stress. Patients receiving long-term systemic corticosteroids should be gradually tapered off of therapy after reaching physiologic doses in order to prevent steroid withdrawal syndrome. If testing of the HPA axis is not performed, clinicians should presume the HPA axis is suppressed for approximately one year and should administer stress doses of steroids accordingly for major surgeries, trauma or illness.

Intramuscular administration should not be used in pediatric dermatology for several reasons. It is unnecessarily painful and medication is erratically absorbed. If adverse sequelae develop following injection (e.g., stress, infectious illness, local ulceration), there is no way to remove the long-acting depot of medication. In addition, the long-acting preparations do not provide flexibility in dosage titration. Furthermore, the longer-acting injections result in significantly greater suppression of the HPA axis and growth.

Large-bolus intermittent-dose intravenous therapy has been used in selected pediatric cases of aggressive inflammatory disease.[442] It is a theoretical alternative therapy for children with steroid-responsive dermatoses that are refractory to standard doses. This form of steroid administration may be especially beneficial in juvenile dermatomyositis.[443] Serious risks are associated with this form of therapy, including altered electrolyte balance, cerebrovascular accidents, and cardiac arrhythmias. Most clinicians advocate inpatient administration and close cardiac monitoring during intravenous pulse corticosteroid administration.

The following side effects are among those associated with systemic administration of corticosteroids:

1. Suppression of the HPA axis.
2. Cutaneous effects (acne, striae, hirsutism, easy bruisability).
3. Altered body habitus (truncal obesity, moon face, buffalo hump).
4. Hypertension.
5. Hyperglycemia.
6. Growth suppression in children.
7. Osteoporosis.
8. Aseptic necrosis of bone.
9. Ocular effects (posterior subcapsular cataracts, glaucoma).
10. Decreased cell-mediated immunity, increased risk of infections.
11. Hematologic abnormalities (neutrophilia, lymphocytopenia, monocytopenia).
12. Delayed wound healing.
13. Behavioral and personality changes (increased appetite, insomnia, nervousness, euphoria, hyperkinesia).
14. Myopathy.
15. Pseudotumor cerebri.

Children are more susceptible than adults to growth suppression and to posterior subcapsular cataracts. Both adverse effects are associated with prolonged corticosteroid therapy.[444] Patients expected to receive systemic corticosteroids for more than 1 month should be closely monitored, including baseline purified protein derivative of tuberculin (PPD) skin test and interval urine and blood sugars, blood pressure, growth parameters, and ophthalmologic examinations. It may be necessary to treat certain adverse sequelae, such as diabetes and high blood pressure, concomitantly. Aseptic necrosis is a serious irreversible side effect that is not necessarily dose related that has been reported as early as 6 weeks after beginning therapy.[445] If significant side effects are noted, alternative steroid-sparing forms of therapy should be considered, including IVIG, immunosuppressive agents, antimalarial agents, and sulfones, whenever medically indicated. If a susceptible child receiving long-term therapy with corticosteroids is exposed to varicella, prophylactic therapy with varicella zoster immunoglobulin (VZIG) should be promptly administered and treatment with acyclovir should be initiated if cutaneous manifestations of varicella develop. Patients receiving long-term (>14 days) high-dose glucocorticoid therapy (>2mg/kg/day) should not receive live vaccines (varicella-zoster, measles, mumps, rubella). Specific vaccine recommendations can be found in the American Academy of Pediatrics Red Book.[320]

One of the more important uses of systemic corticosteroids in pediatric dermatology is in the management of serious infantile hemangiomas. The treatment is generally most effective during the proliferative phase of the hemangioma and may result in shrinkage of the lesion or prevention of further growth. Systemic corticosteroid therapy should be reserved for the treatment of significant hemangiomas in high-risk clinical locations such as the periorbital region. Other problematic lesions likely to necessitate therapy include large lesions on the nose or lip, hemangiomas in the beard distribution with increased risk of airway involvement, or massive lesions with the potential for high-output congestive heart failure. Multiple small hemangiomas with visceral involvement and vascular tumors such as Kaposi-form hemangioendothelioma with coagulopathy are additional special situations requiring more aggressive management. Generally, standard daily doses of 2–3mg/kg/day are initiated and continued for 4–6 weeks until stabilization or shrinkage of the hemangioma is observed.[446,447] Occasionally, higher doses of 3–5mg/kg/day are necessary during initial therapy and are generally well tolerated.[448] Duration of therapy depends upon the age of the infant at initiation of therapy and the corresponding growth phase of the hemangioma. Gradually tapering therapy is often required for 6–8 months when systemic steroids are started in early infancy.

While the side effect profile of glucocorticoid therapy is well described, there is minimal literature addressing the safety of long-term therapy in infants with hemangiomas. In a study by Boon and colleagues,[449] a retrospective review was performed on infants who had received glucocorticoid therapy for management of problematic hemangiomas. Information was obtained via a parental questionnaire on 62 of 80 patients treated. The initial dose of cor-

438. Morris H, Neuman I, Ellis E (1974) Plasma steroid concentrations during alternate-day treatment with prednisone. **J Allergy Clin Immunol** 54:350.
439. Fass B (1979) Glucocorticoid therapy for nonendocrine disorders: withdrawal and "coverage". **Pediatr Clin North Am** 26:251.
440. Tordjman K, Jaffe A, Grazas N et al. (1995) The role of low dose (1 microgram) adrenocorticotropin test in the evaluation of patients with pituitary disease. **J Clin Endocrinol Metab** 80:1301–1305.
441. Dickstein G, Spigel D, Arad E et al. (1997) One microgram is the lowest ACTH dose to cause a maximal cortisol response. There is no diurnal variation of cortisol response to submaximal ACTH stimulation. **Eur J Endocrinol** 137:172–175.
442. Job D, Menkes C (1991) Administration of methylprednisolone pulse in chronic arthritis in children. **Clin Exp Rheum**, 9 (suppl) 6:15.
443. Lang B, Laxer R, Murphy G et al. (1991) Treatment of dermatomyositis with intravenous gammaglobulin. **Am J Medi** 91:169.
444. Bhagat G, Chai H (1974) Development of posterior sub-capsular cataracts in asthmatic children. **Pediatrics** 73:626.
445. Gallant C, Kenny P (1986) Oral glucocorticoids and their complications. **J Am Acad Dermatol** 14:161.
446. Frieden IJ (1997) Management of hemangiomas. **Pediatr Dermatol** 14:757–783.
447. Frieden IJ, Eichenfield LF, Esterly NB et al. (1997) Guidelines Outcomes Committee. Guidelines of care of hemangiomas of infancy. **J Am Acad Dermatol** 37:631–637.
448. Sadan N, Wolach B (1996) Treatment of hemangiomas of infants with high doses of prednisone. **J Pediatr** 128(1):141–146.
449. Boon LM, MacDonald DM, Mulliken JB (1999) Complications of systemic therapy for problematic hemangiomas. **Plast Reconstr Surg** 104:1616–1622.

ticosteroid varied from 2 to 3mg/kg/day and mean duration of therapy was 7.9 months. The most commonly observed side effects included cushingoid facies (71%), personality changes (29%) and gastric irritation (21%). While a deceleration in both vertical growth and weight gain was observed in approximately one-third of patients, catch-up growth occurred and more than 90% of treated infants had returned to their pre-treatment percentile for both height and weight by 24 months of age. The potential adverse effects of hypertension or adrenal suppression were not addressed in this study.

In a recent retrospective review of 22 infants (mean age 13 weeks at beginning of therapy) treated with systemic steroids for their hemangiomas, elevated blood pressures were observed in the majority (82%) of patients during steroid therapy. The mean initial prednisolone dose was 2.23mg/kg/day which was gradually tapered over several months. The average duration of therapy was 28 weeks. Forty-five percent (10 patients) were noted to have elevated blood pressures on at least three separate occasions and 8 of the 22 (36%) patients were treated with hydrochlorothiazide for persistent hypertension. Other commonly observed side effects included irritability (73%), gastric irritation (32%), and decreased morning cortisol levels in 13 of 15 infants evaluated.[450]

When treating serious infantile hemangiomas with systemic steroids, the lowest therapeutically effective dose should be used and given as a single morning dose. Occasionally, alternate-day dosing is sufficient for stabilization of growth and should be considered in less urgent situations. Due to the frequency of subjective and objective gastrointestinal side effects, it is the author's practice to use ranitidine prophylactically in infants receiving steroid doses of 2–3mg/kg/day. After stabilization of the hemangioma has occurred (usually after 4–6 weeks) the clinician may begin to gradually taper the glucocorticoid dose. There are many approaches to the steroid taper, but it is our practice to gradually taper the dose every other day with the goal of achieving alternate-day therapy as soon as possible to minimize side effects of growth and HPA axis suppression. HPA axis integrity may be evaluated once the infant is on physiologic doses of steroids in order to determine the need for stress doses of steroids as well as to determine the rapidity at which the infant may be weaned from physiologic doses of systemic steroids. If it is not possible to perform this evaluation, then the clinician should presume the infant to be adrenally compromised for approximately 6 to 12 months after cessation of steroid therapy and parents should be educated on the appropriate use of stress doses of glucocorticoids.

AZATHIOPRINE (IMURAN)

Azathioprine is a synthetic purine analog that has been available for over 30 years and is commonly used for immunomodulatory therapy in dermatology. It continues to be used because of its favorable therapeutic index as well as its role as a steroid-sparing agent. As an imidazole derivative of 6-mercaptopurine, azathioprine has many biological effects similar to the parent compound. This drug is FDA approved for the treatment of severe rheumatoid arthritis and for chronic immunosuppression in renal transplant patients to prevent organ rejection. In dermatology, azathioprine has been used in the treatment of numerous disorders with varied success for over 30 years. Immunobullous disorders, such as bullous pemphigoid, pemphigus vulgaris, and cicatricial pemphigoid are some of the more common dermatologic disorders treated with azathioprine

Azathioprine is well absorbed after oral administration but is rapidly metabolized after three hours. Drug metabolites linger for hours after administration allowing for a once daily dosing advantage. The drug is metabolized hepatically and excreted via the renal system, requiring dosage adjustment with renal insufficiency.[451] Hepatic dysfunction does not necessitate the alteration of dosing, but does require vigilant monitoring for toxicity.[452] If liver enzymes continue to increase or impaired synthetic function is noted, azathioprine should be discontinued.

Initially, azathioprine is converted to 6-mercaptopurine (6-MP) by glutathione-S-transferase. Three competing pathways are known to participate in the metabolism of 6-MP (Fig. 4.1). The first enzymatic pathway noted in the metabolism of 6-MP involves thiopurine methyltransferase (TPMT). Through this reaction TPMT catalyzes S-methylation to generate 6-methyl mercaptopurine which is an inactive compound. The second pathway involves oxidation of 6-MP by xanthine oxidase to another inactive compound, 6-thiouric acid. The last competing pathway is the conversion of 6-mercaptopurine by hypoxanthine–guanine phosphoribosyl transferase (HGPRT) to active 6-thioguanine metabolites. These enzymes vary from patient to patient in both their quantity and their level of activity. It is this difference in the patient population that contributes to the variability to which azathioprine is metabolized and therefore mediates its effectiveness as well as its toxicity. Thus, serum azathioprine levels are inadequate to measure the true effectiveness of this drug.[452,454]

Studies have shown that there are genetic determinants that affect the level of TPMT and its activity. In mainly Caucasian patient populations it is recognized that 89% are homozygous for high TPMT activity with 0.5% being homozygous for low TPMT activity along with approximately 10% of patients falling in the intermediate range.[452,454] Those patients with a low level of TPMT activity are more likely to develop leukopenia (1 in 300 patients), while patients with higher levels of TPMT activity experience less immunosuppression and may require higher doses of azathioprine.[452] A correlation has also been made among patients with intermediate range levels of TPMT and development of late-onset neutropenia.[452] Checking pre-treatment TPMT activity may predict those patients at increased risk for early-onset neutropenia. Leukopenia may also be associated with variations in the enzyme glutathione-S-transferase.[452] This enzyme converts azathioprine to 6-MP and differences in enzyme activity may generate varying levels of 6-MP. With various mechanisms contributing to the etiology of leukopenia, it is always important to monitor blood counts regularly in patients taking azathioprine.

After azathioprine is metabolized by multiple competing enzymes, numerous active metabolites are generated which orchestrate immunosuppression. These metabolites prevent cell growth by inhibiting the synthesis and interconversion of purine bases. Other postulated mechanisms are interference with: natural killer T-cell function, T-cell cytolytic activity, prostaglandin production, and neutrophil activity.[452]

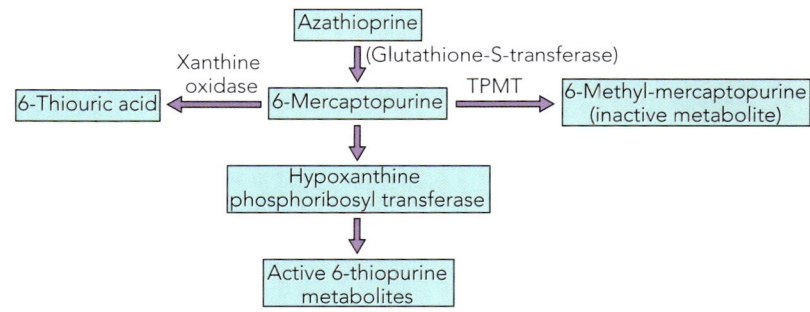

Fig. 4.1   The metabolism of azathioprine.

450. George ME, Simon S, Jacobson J, Sharma V, Nopper AJ (2002) Personal communication.
451. Physician's Desk Reference 2000.
452. Dutz JP, Ho VC (1988) Immunosuppressive agents in dermatology. An update. **Dermatol Clin** 16(2):235–251.
453. Wolverton SE (1991) In: Systemic Drugs for Skin Diseases, Wolverton SE. Wilkin JK, eds. Philadelphia: WB Saunders.
454. Flores F, Kerdel FA (2000) Other novel immunosuppressants. **Dermatol Clin** 18(3):475–483.

TABLE 4.23   Potential side effects of azathioprine

	Side effects
Hematologic	Pancytopenia
	Leukopenia
	Anemia
	Coagulopathy
Gastrointestinal	Nausea
	Vomiting
	Liver enzyme elevation
Dermatologic	Rash
	Increased squamous cell carcinoma
Idiosyncratic	Azathioprine hypersensitivity syndrome
Renal	Renal insufficiency
Infectious disease	Opportunistic infections
Pregnancy	Immunosuppression during pregnancy
	Birth defects

Azathioprine can adversely affect multiple organ systems (Table 4.23). Myelosuppression can occur with various cell lines being affected. As noted earlier, measurement of TPMT activity may help predict the severity of the leukopenia, but all patients should be closely monitored. Late-onset myelosuppression can occur years after therapy is initiated. More commonly observed side effects include nausea and vomiting. There have also been reported cases of hepatoxicity, most notably in bullous pemphigoid patients receiving combination azathioprine and prednisolone therapy.[452]

Immunosuppression may lead to a predisposition for opportunistic infections. The likelihood is in part dependent upon the degree of immunosuppression as well as environmental factors. It has been documented that patients receiving azathioprine and corticosteroids are at an increased risk for these infections even in the absence of leukopenia.[455] Chronic therapy is also associated with an increased risk of developing certain malignancies, possibly due to a disruption of immunosurveillance. This risk increases with prolonged therapy and high doses of azathioprine but may be influenced by additional host and environmental factors. Reported malignancies observed more commonly in association with long-term azathioprine therapy include Kaposi's sarcoma, lymphoproliferative disorders, carcinoma of the cervix, and various skin cancers.[456]

There is a well-described hypersensitivity syndrome associated with azathioprine, but the mechanism by which this reaction occurs is not well understood. This syndrome manifests with multiorgan system involvement and signs and symptoms may include hypotension, fever, shock, maculopapular skin eruption, nephritis, pneumonitis, hepatitis, pancreatitis, and rarely, rhabdomyolysis.[452] This rare syndrome may occur within a few hours of beginning therapy up to several weeks after initiation, most commonly developing 14 days after azathioprine therapy is started.[452] At least 50 case reports of suspected azathioprine hypersensitivity syndrome have been reported in various patient populations.

The use of azathioprine in dermatology as a steroid-sparing agent is increasing. This drug is commonly used in immunobullous disorders in combination with corticosteroids. Several studies have been undertaken looking at the effectiveness of azathioprine in treating these diseases. Of these studies, few considered the impact of enzyme variability on the metabolism of azathioprine which led to fixed dosing regimens that were often inadequate. In one large, randomized, controlled study, this aspect of TPMT variability was again omitted from the study design making it unclear whether azathioprine had a steroid-sparing effect in bullous pemphigoid patients due to the possibility of under-dosing.[457] The general consensus clinically among dermatologists is that azathioprine does show therapeutic efficacy in immunobullous disorders but further studies are needed to quantify this as well as to better define the side effects associated with azathioprine use.

Other reported uses of azathioprine in dermatology include dermatomyositis, pyoderma gangrenosum, systemic lupus erythematosus, lichen planus, psoriasis, Behçet's disease, prurigo nodularis, cutaneous lupus erythematosus, atopic dermatitis, vasculitis, sarcoidosis, and subcorneal pustular dermatosis. Although azathioprine is widely used and is a generally accepted form of treatment, few studies exist that support its use in dermatology. Few studies show a benefit for the use of azathioprine as a steroid-sparing agent for generalized lichen planus.[458] Conflicting evidence exists as to the efficacy of azathioprine for dermatomyositis–polymyositis, severe systemic lupus, and immunobullous disorders.[455,459,460] Efficacy as well as long-term benefit has been shown with the use of azathioprine in Behçet's disease for both ocular and extraocular manifestations.[461]

The typical starting dose for azathioprine is 1–2mg/kg/day in either the intravenous or oral forms given once or twice daily. Doses as high as 3mg/kg/day have been used, but exceeding this dose is not recommended. The dose should be adjusted based upon the patient's clinical response as well as hematologic tolerance as documented by frequent monitoring. Renal and liver function tests should be followed and the dose adjusted when evidence of renal insufficiency exists. Use of azathioprine is contraindicated in pregnancy as the drug and its metabolites cross the placenta and may act as teratogens.[462] There is no data known that documents gonadotoxicity and infertility with azathioprine.[452]

Potential drug interactions with azathioprine may occur when allopurinol is used concomitantly. This agent, often used in gout or tumor lysis prophylaxis inhibits the activity of xanthine oxidase, one of the major competing enzymes that metabolizes 6-MP. The dual use of these drugs should be avoided, but if concomitant use is necessary, the dose of azathioprine should be decreased by at least two-thirds. Although this might reduce the possibility of myelotoxicity, it does not completely prevent its occurrence.[463] Angiotensin-converting enzyme (ACE) inhibitors used in the treatment of hypertension and nephropathy have been noted to potentiate anemia in patients on azathioprine due to decreased erythropoietin production. While anemia is not a contraindication to initiating azathioprine therapy, its presence warrants caution and close monitoring. It has been shown that sulfa drug metabolites in conjunction with azathioprine work synergistically to suppress bone marrow function.[464] Pancuronium, a neuromuscular blocker, is also metabolized by the liver and has been documented to compete with the metabolism of azathioprine.[453] See Table 4.24 for drug interactions with azathioprine.

While there are no specific guidelines for hematological monitoring in dermatology, in other medical arenas initial screening often includes a complete blood cell count, liver function tests, renal function tests, urine pregnancy tests when appropriate, and a urinalysis. Evaluating the activity of thiopurine methyltransferase (TPMT) in patients prior to initiating therapy is not standard but is often recommended as the incidence of severe early

455. Dutz J, Ho V (1996) Immunosuppressive agents in skin disorders. Clin Immunother 5:268–293.
456. Penn I (1996) Cancers in cyclosporine-treated versus azathioprine-treated patients. Transplantation 28:876–878.
457. Anstey (1995) Azathioprine in dermatology. J Roy Soc Med 88:155–160.
458. Lear JT, English JS (1986) Erosive and generalized lichen planus responsive to azathioprine. Clin Exp Dermatol 21:56–57.
459. Guillaume JC, Vaillant L, Bernard P et al. (1993) Controlled trial of azathioprine and plasma exchange in addition to prednisolone in the treatment of bullous pemphigoid. Arch Dermatol 129:49–53.
460. Villalba L, Adams EM (1996) Update on therapy for refractory dermatomyositis and polymyositis. Curr Opin Rheumatol 8:544–551.
461. Yazici H, Pazarli H, Barnes CG et al. (1990) A controlled trial of azathioprine in Behçet's syndrome. N Engl J Med 322:281–285.
462. Briggs GG, Freeman RK, Yaffe SJ (1994) Drugs in Pregnancy and Lactation, a Reference Guide to Fetal and Neonatal Risk, 4th edn. Baltimore: Williams & Wilkins.
463. Cummins D, Sekar M, Halil O et al. (1996) Myelosuppression associated with azathioprine–allopurinol interaction after heart and lung transplantation. Transplantation 61:1661–1662.
464. Bradley PP, Warden GD, Maxwell JG et al. (1996) Neutropenia and thrombocytopenia in renal allograft recipients in Queensland, Australia. A follow-up study. Transplantation 61:715–721.

TABLE 4.24 Drug interactions with azathioprine

Drug	Mechanism of action
Allopurinol	Inhibits xanthine oxidase increasing the risk of myelosuppression
Sulfa antibiotics	Increase risk of myelosuppression via synergistic effect of drug metabolites
Warfarin	Warfarin resistance documented with concomitant use of azathioprine
Sulfasalazine	Potentiates azathioprine toxicity via inhibition of TPMT activity
Angiotension converting enzyme inhibitors	Increase risk of anemia secondary to erythropoietin suppression
Pancuronium	Competes with azathioprine for metabolism, often increased doses of pancuronium are needed for paralysis

TPMT, thiopurine methyltransferase.

neutropenia is 1 in 300 patients.[451] These tests, excluding TPMT levels, should be repeated every 1–2 weeks for the first 1–2 months and then monthly if stable. The dose should be decreased if the white blood cell count is less than 4×10^9/l or if platelets are less than 1×10^{11}/l. Azathioprine should be completely discontinued if white blood cell count falls below 2.5×10^9/l. Doses can be increased after 6–8 weeks of therapy by 0.5mg/kg if hematologic indices are acceptable. If no clinical response is noted after 12–16 weeks of therapy, azathioprine should be discontinued.[452]

INTERFERONS

Interferons are a family of low-molecular-weight glycoproteins produced by different cell types that inhibit viral replication and tumor growth. Interferons have been classified into three groups, based primarily on their cell of origin. Interferon-α (IFN-α) is produced mainly by leukocytes, IFN-β by fibroblasts and epithelial cells, and IFN-γ by lymphocytes. IFN-α and -β share a common receptor and have a spectrum of biologic effects that differs from those of IFN-γ.[465] Purified human interferons are increasingly available through improved production techniques, but less expensive recombinant forms are also manufactured. There are several forms of IFN-α. The products obtained from cultured human cells are usually a mixture of different subtypes of IFN-α. There are also different forms of recombinant IFN-α, the α_2 family. The formation of neutralizing antibodies is more common in those receiving the recombinant products.[466] Interferons are inactivated in the stomach. Therefore, they must be locally or systemically injected. Much like insulin administration, interferon injections are minimally painful and are generally well tolerated by children. Side effects include flu-like symptoms, fever, and transient leukopenia.

There are several FDA approved uses for interferon therapy (Table 4.25). IFN-α is approved for the treatment of hairy cell leukemia, condyloma acuminata, Kaposi's sarcoma in AIDS, and hepatitis C. IFN-γ is approved for the treatment of chronic granulomatous disease. IFN-β has been approved for the treatment of multiple sclerosis.[467] The list of potential therapeutic uses for interferons is growing to include treatment of a wider variety of virally mediated conditions, including hepatitis C-associated cryoglobulinemia,[468] benign and malignant neoplasms, and inflammatory and immunodeficiency diseases.[465,470] With several available forms of the interferons, and several possible doses and dosage regimens, optimal treatment in each of these conditions has not yet been determined. Potential uses of interferons in pediatric dermatology may be adjunct therapy for widespread condyloma acuminata, treatment of alarming hemangiomas in infancy, Kasabach–Merritt phenomena, and atopic dermatitis.

Adults with condyloma acuminatum have been treated with injected and topically applied IFN-α, -β, and -γ, with variable responses. Complete remission has been reported in some studies where interferon is used systemically and intralesionally.[472] Use of both IFN-α, at low doses (1×10^6 units) subcutaneously and IFN-β, intramuscularly has resulted in significant responses.[472] Adjunctive treatment, using interferon and ablative therapy, may prove to be the most successful.[473,474] Small studies of topically applied interferon preparations in women and children have been disappointing.[469] Administration by injection limits the practicality of interferon therapy for anogenital condyloma in children.

Imiquimod or Aldara is a topical immunomodulator that is FDA approved for the treatment of condyloma acuminata. Imiquimod alters the immune response by inducing the release of IFN-α, along with other cytokines. It is currently being studied in a variety of disorders including resistent herpes

TABLE 4.25 FDA approved uses of interferon therapy

Interferon-α	Interferon-β	Interferon-γ
Kaposi's sarcoma (2α)		Chronic granulomatous disease of childhood
Condyloma acuminata	Multiple sclerosis	Kaposi's sarcoma
Hairy cell leukemia		
Hepatitis C		
Melanoma		Melanoma

Potential uses of interferon therapy

Atopic dermatitis	Basal cell carcinoma
Squamous cell carcinoma	Melanoma
Cutaneous T-cell lymphoma	Keratoacanthoma
Herpes simplex	Varicella zoster
Verruca vulgaris/bowenoid papulosis	Discoid lupus erythematosus
Life threatening hemangiomas	Follicular mucinosis
Behçet's disease	Psoriatic arthritis
Fibrotic disease (systemic sclerosis, keloids, morphea)	Mycosis fungoides
Kasabach–Merritt phenomena	

465. Luger T, Schwarz T (1991) Therapeutic use of cytokines in dermatology. **J Am Acad Dermatol** 24:915.
466. Finter N, Chapman S, Dowd P et al. (1991) The use of interferon-alpha in virus infections. **Drugs** 42:749.
467. Thiers P (1995) Pediatric oncology. Family admission. **Soirs Pediatr Pueric** 166:15–16 (in French).
468. Misiani R, Bellayita T, Fenili D et al. (1993) Interferon alpha 2A therapy in cryoglobulinemia associated with hepatitis C virus. **N Engl J Med** 330:751.
469. Tamayo L, Ortiz D, Orozoco-Covarrubias L et al. (1997) Therapeutic efficacy of interferon alfa-2b in infants with life-threatening hemangiomas. **Arch Dermatol** 133:1567–1571.
470. Berman B, Sequeira M (1995) Dermatologic uses of interferons. **Dermatol Clin** 13(3):699–711.

471. Borden E (1992) Interferons – expanding therapeutic roles. **N Engl J Med** 326:1491.
472. Creagan ET, Schaid DJ, Ahmann DL, Frytak S (1990) Disseminated malignant melanoma and recombinant interferon: analysis of seven consecutive phase II investigations. **J Invest Dermatol** 95(6 suppl):188S–192S.
473. Davis B, Noble M (1992) Initial experience with combined interferon-alpha 2B and carbon dioxide laser for the treatment of condylomata acuminata. **J Urol** 147:627.
474. Fierlbeck G, Rassner G, Pfister H (1992) Condylomata acuminata in children – detection of HPV 6/11 and 2. Local therapy with interferon-beta hydrogel. **Hautarzt** 43:148.
475. Keay S, Teng N, Eisenberg M et al. (1988) Topical interferon for treating condyloma acuminata in women. **J Infect Dis** 158:934.

simplex virus infections, resistant leishmaniasis, lentigo maligna,[476] actinic keratosis, molluscum contagiosum,[477] basal cell carcinoma, and high-grade cervical intraepithelial neoplasia among others. While early studies of imiquimod in the treatment of anogenital warts were initially unimpressive, recent studies have shown imiquimod to be modestly successful in the treatment of anogenital warts. Most treatment modalities recommend using imiquimod topically three to five times per week for 8–12h for a time period of up to 16 weeks. In a recent multicenter trial, a sustained clearance rate was observed in approximately 42 and 33% of study patients at 3 and 6 months post-treatment, respectively. In the treatment group the most common side effect was local inflammation and irritation at the application site (67% of patients).[478] The use of this product requires adequate patient instruction and compliance with therapy as imiquimod is self-applied.

Both IFN-α and –γ have been used in the treatment of atopic dermatitis, with some success.[479–482] However, studies of the basic immunomodulatory defects in atopic dermatitis suggest that IFN-γ may be the more useful form of therapy. Circulating and tissue-based lymphocytes of patients with atopic dermatitis have been shown to produce excessive amounts of IL-4 and reduced levels of IFN-γ. These data support a hypothesis about the basic immune dysregulation causing atopic dermatitis. The theory assumes an imbalance of T-cell subsets, with inhibition of the cells that produce IFN-γ (Th1 T cells), and a relative activation of the cells that produce IL-4 (Th2 T cells). This is thought to potentiate a vicious circle of enhanced production of IgE, eosinophilia, mast cell proliferation, release of histamine by basophils and mast cells, and further expansion of Th2 cells.[483] Various studies with IFN-γ showed marked improvement in patients with atopic dermatitis. Improvement was judged by physicians' examination and based on at least 50% improvement. This study was a randomised, placebo-controlled, double-blind study in which 78 patients were treated with subcutaneous IFN-γ for 12 weeks ($50\mu g/m^2$) versus placebo. Interestingly, there were also significant reductions of systemic symptoms such as pruritus, erythema, and conjunctivitis reported by patients. On further study, circulating IgE was unchanged but a marked reduction of serum eosinophils was noted.[470] Other studies have been undertaken to evaluate the efficacy of IFN-α in the treatment of atopic dermatitis with conflicting results.

The success of IFN-α therapy in the treatment of Kaposi's sarcoma suggested that it may be beneficial in the treatment of other forms of proliferative vascular disease. Several anecdotal reports, and various prospective and retrospective studies have documented the efficacy of daily subcutaneous injections of IFN-α for alarming hemangiomas, Kasabach–Merritt syndrome, and diffuse hemangiomatosis in infants.[483–487] The recombinant preparation, IFN-α$_{2a}$ was used in most of these reports. Interferon efficacy in the treatment of these conditions is thought to be related to the antiangiogenic effects of interferon.[468] Often, large life-threatening hemangiomas that are refractory to other forms of treatment (systemic and intralesional glucocorticoids, carbon dioxide laser, and pentoxifylline) or are causing a consumptive coagulopathy, are stabilized and show significant improvement on interferon therapy.[488]

Side effects from interferon therapy most often resemble a flu-like illness but can affect many organ systems (Table 4.26). Symptoms include fever, myalgias, anemia, generalized gastrointestinal complaints, depression, thrombocytosis, anorexia, chills, and elevated liver enzymes. An uncommon complication from use of interferon therapy is spastic diplegia. In a study by Barlow and colleagues,[489] of 26 infants receiving interferon for serious hemangiomas, five developed spastic diplegia. In three of the five infants, these neorological changes persisted.

Another study in which 48 newborns, infants, and children with similar life-threatening hemangiomas were treated with IFN-α showed no significant neurologic sequelae.[490] It is postulated that the difference in outcomes may be due to the formulation differences of interferon. One preparation is processed as a sterile powder which is then reconstituted with sterile normal saline, while other preparations contain alcohol as a preserving agent. Alcohol-induced toxicity and neuropathy is well documented in infants and children. Thus, it is recommended to watch patients, especially young infants, closely for neurotoxicity. Further studies are needed in this area to uncover the true mechanism associated with neurotoxicity associated with interferon use.

Contraindications for using interferon vary depending upon the type of interferon being used (Table 4.27). All types of interferon are contraindicated when patients have a history of hypersensitivy to either interferon or the preparation. Caution should be used when the patient has any underlying debilitating medical condition, including diabetes mellitus predisposed to ketoacidosis, coagulation disorders, cardiovascular disease, thyroid dysfunction,

TABLE 4.26   Side effects of interferon

Influenza-like	Fever
	Chills
	Headache
	Fatigue
	Myalgia
Gastrointestinal	Nausea
	Vomiting
	Diarrhea
	Anorexia
CNS	Dizziness
	Decreased mental status
	Depression
	Paresthesias
	Spastic diplegias
Skin	Partial alopecia
	Rash
Cardiovascular	Hypotension
	Syncope
	Arrhythmias

476. Ahmed I, Berth-Jones J (2000) Imiquimod: a novel treatment for lentigo maligna. **Br J Dermatol** 143(4):843–846.
477. Barba AR, Kapoor S, Berman B (2001) An open label safety study of topical imiquimod 5% cream in the treatment of molluscum contagrosum in children. **Dermatol Online J** 7(1):20.
478. Garland SM, Sellors JW, Wikstrom A, Petersen CS et al. (2001) Imiquimod 5% cream is a safe and effective self-applied treatment for anogenital warts – results of an open-label, multicentre Phase IIIB trial. **Int J Sex Transm Dis** 12(11):722–729.
479. Gruner S, Liebenthal C, Heusser C et al. (1990) The influence of interferon-gamma and interleukin-4 on IgE production in B lymphocytes of patients with atopic dermatitis. **Acta Derm Venereol** 71:484.
480. Hanifin J, Schneider L, Leung D et al. (1993) Recombinant interferon gamma therapy for atopic dermatitis. **J Am Acad Dermatol** 28:189.
481. Mackic R (1990) Interferon-α for atopic dermatitis. **Lancet** 335:1282.
482. Torrelo A, Harto A, Sendagorta E et al. (1992) Interferon-a therapy in atopic dermatitis. **Acta Derm Venereol** (Stock) 72:370.
483. Orchard P, Smith CM III, Woods WG et al. (1989) Treatment of haemangioendotheliomas with alpha interferon. **Lancet** 2(8662):565.
484. Ezekowitz R, Mulliken J, Folkman J (1992) Interferon alpha-2a therapy for life threatening hemangiomas of infancy. **N Engl J Med** 326:1456.
485. Blei F, Orlow S, Geronemus R (1993) Interferon alpha-2a therapy for extensive perianal and lower extremity hemangioma. **J Am Acad Dermatol** 29:98.
486. Illum N (1992) Treatment of hemangioma in children with recombinant interferon. **Ugeskri Laeger** 154:3408.
487. Spiller J, Sharma V, Woods G et al. (1992) Diffuse neonatal hemangiomatosis treated successfully with interferon alpha. **J Am Acad Dermatol** 27:102.
488. Ezekowitz RA, Mulliken JB, Folkman J (1992) Interferon alfa-2a therapy for life-threatening hemangiomas of infancy. **N Engl J Med** 326(22):1456–1463.
489. Barlow C, Priebe C, Mulliken J et al. (1998) Spastic diplegia as a complication of interferon a lfa-2a treatment of hemangiomas of infancy. **J Pediatr** 132:527–530.
490. Deb G, Jenker A, Donfrancesco A (1999) Spastic diplegia and interferon. **J Pediatr** 134(3):324–332.

TABLE 4.27   Interferon contraindications

IFN-α2b	IFN-α2a	IFN-αn3	IFN-γ
Hypersensitivity to α-IFN or components of the injections	Hypersensitivity to α-IFN, mouse immunoglobulin, or components of the injection	Hypersensitivity to α-IFN, mouse immunoglobulin, egg protein, or neomycin	Hypersensitivity to γ-IFN, E coli products, or components of the injection

autoimmune diseases, transplant patients, depression (particularly with suicidal ideation), or hepatic disorders. Interferon is relatively contraindicated in pregnant or nursing women and carries a class C pharmacologic rating. It should only be given in those circumstances when the benefits of therapy clearly outweigh the risks of treatment.

POTASSIUM IODIDE

Potassium iodide has been used in medicine for approximately 150 years, and it remains an effective therapy for several dermatologic conditions such as sporotrichosis and several hypersensitivity reactions. Potassium iodide is a combination of iodine (76% by weight) and potassium (23% weight), an alkali metal. It comes in the form of a saturated solution (SSKI) with a concentration of 47mg/drop. Because this solution can cause gastrointestinal irritation, it is best administered in combination with water, juice or milk.

The dosage of potassium depends upon the condition being treated. For treatment of inflammatory dermatoses, an oral dose of 300mg or six drops of SSKI administered three times daily would be an appropriate starting dose for adults. This dose can then be gradually increased as tolerated to achieve the desired anti-inflammatory response. In contrast, the treatment of fungal infections, including sporotrichosis, usually requires substantially higher doses. Adult antimycotic doses typically begin at 600mg (about 12 drops) three times daily and may be increased if tolerated to doses as high as 6g daily. Most conditions respond promptly within 2 to 4 weeks of SSKI therapy.

A study by Cabezas and colleagues concluded that SSKI could be given daily rather than three times daily with comparable results in the pediatric population in order to improve patient compliance.[491] Special caution should be taken to avoid concomitant administration of other potassium or iodide containing medications (see Table 4.28).

While potassium iodide is not FDA approved specifically for any dermatologic conditions, it has been used in the management of many cutaneous disorders including various fungal infections (excluding the mucormycoses), granulomatous dermatoses, panniculitis, and neutrophilic dermatoses.[492] The specific mechanisms by which potassium iodide exerts its effects remain poorly understood. Honma and colleagues demonstrated that KI inhibits neutrophil chemotaxis in peripheral blood.[493] Others speculate that KI

TABLE 4.28   Potential dermatologic uses of potassium iodide

Fungal infections: Sporotrichosis, Cryptococcosis, *Nocardia*
Neutrophilic dermatoses: pyoderma gangrenosum, Sweet's syndrome
Panniculitis: erythema nodosum, nodular vasculitis, subacute migratory panniculitis
Granulomatous dermatoses: Wegener's granulomatosis, granuloma annulare
Hypersensitivity reactions: erythema multiforme
Behçet's syndrome

TABLE 4.29   Concurrent medications to avoid with potassium iodide therapy

Potassium-containing medications
Potassium-sparing diuretics
Angiotensin-converting enzyme inhibitors
Iodine containing medications (amiodarone)
Drugs that inhibit thyroid function (lithium, phenothiazone)

suppresses the generation of inflammatory oxygen intermediates from activated PMNs while some postulate that KIs effect in hypersensitivity disorders is secondary to an immunosuppressive effect mediated through heparin.

While potassium iodide is generally considered quite safe, there are myriad potential systemic and cutaneous adverse effects with which the treating physician should be familiar. Many of these side effects are dose-related and observed more often with chronic therapy. Common systemic side effects include diarrhea, nausea, vomiting, and abdominal pain. Signs of iodine toxicity include a metallic taste and/or burning sensation of the mouth, soreness of the gingiva and teeth, headache, and enlargement or tenderness of the parotid and submaxillary glands. Potassium toxicity may cause cardiac arrhythmias, confusion, parasthesias, and weakness. As with any iodide, chronic use of SSKI can often lead to a variety of skin problems including acneiform eruptions, vasculitis, dermatitic eruptions and iododerma (a distinct vegetating eruption).

Potential effects on the thyroid gland should also be considered with chronic potassium iodide therapy. Depending upon the underlying functional integrity of the thyroid gland, excess iodine administration can result in either hypothyroidism and goiter or hyperthyroidism. Patients should be questioned prior to initiating therapy regarding any previous history of thyroid disease and baseline thyroid function tests including thyroid-stimulating hormone (TSH), T4, antithyroglobulin and antimicrosomal antibodies should be obtained in patients if there is a suspicion of underlying thyroid abnormalities. All patients should have a follow-up TSH obtained after the first month of therapy. Potassium iodide-induced thyroid abnormalities are usually reversible upon discontinuation of therapy.

Potassium iodide should not be used in individuals with known hypersensitivity to iodides. Special caution should be taken in patients with underlying thyroid disease, renal insufficiency, Addison's disease, and cardiac disease. Because KI crosses the placenta and is distributed in breast milk, it should not be used in pregnant or breastfeeding females. Table 4.29 shows medications that should be avoided while taking potassium iodide.

METHOTREXATE

Methotrexate is a folic acid analog that acts by inhibiting dihydrofolate reductase and subsequently interfering with DNA, RNA, and protein synthesis. Its efficacy in the treatment of psoriasis was discovered serendi-

491. Cabezas C, Bustamante B, Holgado W, Begue RE (1996) Treatment of cutaneous sporotrichosis with one daily dose of potassium iodide. **Pediatr Infect Dis** 15(4):352–354.

492. Heymann WR (2000) Potassium iodide and the Wolff Chaikoff effect: relevance for the dermatologist. **J Am Acad Dermatol** 42:490–492.

493. Honma K, Saga K, Onodera H, Takahashi M (1990) Potassium iodide inhibits neutrophil chemotaxis. **Acta Derm Venereol** 70:247–249.

pitously during studies investigating the effects of the related aminopterin on rheumatoid arthritis by Gubner and colleagues more than 50 years ago. Methotrexate became FDA approved for the treatment of psoriasis nearly 20 years later and approval for treatment of rheumatoid arthritis followed in the late 1980s. The daily schedule used for treatment of psoriasis in the 1960s was associated with frequent toxicity and was replaced with weekly dosing in the 1970s.

While methotrexate has been utilized most frequently in dermatology for the treatment of adult psoriasis patients, it has been used increasingly over the past 2 decades for a growing number of inflammatory skin diseases (Table 4.30). Its use in pediatric dermatology has been more limited due to the potential for systemic toxicity; however, there is extensive experience in the pediatric rheumatologic population in the treatment of juvenile rheumatoid arthritis. There is also considerable experience with methotrexate in the treatment of pediatric malignancies, especially acute lymphocytic leukemia. The use of this drug in pediatric dermatology has been greatest in severe, recalcitrant pustular or erythrodermic psoriasis, pityriasis rubra pilaris, pemphigus vulgaris, morphea and dermatomyositis.[493A] However, methotrexate is rarely indicated as a primary therapy in any of these conditions, because of the possibility of several serious side effects.

Methotrexate may be administered either orally, intramuscularly, or intravenously. It is well absorbed via the gastrointestinal tract with peak levels occurring approximately 1h after ingestion; however, absorption of higher doses orally is more variable. In children, the bioavailability of methotrexate may be reduced by the concurrent intake of food, especially when milk-based. Some experts prefer the intramuscular route of administration when higher doses of methotrexate are deemed necessary. In children, it is appropriate to start with a lower dose of 0.2mg/kg per week, if possible. If toxicity is not detected, the dose can be gradually increased, to achieve therapeutic efficacy, up to 0.7mg/kg per week. Methotrexate is available as a 2.5mg scored tablet that can be divided, crushed, and mixed in a non-milk food.[494] Alternatively, the injectable preparation can be given orally, mixed in juice, at a fraction of the cost (available in 2ml vials in concentrations of 2.5mg/ml or 25mg/ml).

Methotrexate is a folic acid analog that is metabolized to a polyglutamate form after absorption from the gastrointestinal tract. The polyglutamate form of the drug has a long intracellular half-life, allowing for once weekly dosing of the drug. Methotrexate is a competitive inhibitor of dihydrofolate reductase (DHFR) and acts to reduce *de novo* synthesis of purines, pyrimidines and polyamines; in addition, trans-methylation of phospholipids and proteins is inhibited.[495] Cumulatively, inhibition of these various metabolic pathways is thought to reduce the ability of various cells, e.g., T cells and B cells, to mediate a continued inflammatory response. How methotrexate can be therapeutic even when given with folate supplements is poorly understood.

An alternative mechanism for the anti-inflammatory effects of methotrexate has been proposed. Methotrexate-polyglutamate, the intracellular form of the drug, has been shown to inhibit AICAR transformylase, an enzyme that catalyzes an early step in *de novo* purine synthesis.[496] It has been shown that this inhibition leads to an increase in production and secretion of adenosine, a potent immunomodulator. Adenosine has at least four receptors and exerts multiple effects in different cell types. *In vitro* studies have shown that increased adenosine levels can result in a decrease in the production of reactive oxygen species, leukotriene B4 production and TNF-α as well as increases in IL-1 receptor antagonist protein and IL-10; each of these would be expected to have anti-inflammatory effects *in vivo*. More importantly, use of an adenosine receptor antagonist in a mouse model of inflammation reversed the anti-inflammatory effects of methotrexate. An inhibitor of adenosine production, ecto-5′-nucleotidase, abrogated the anti-inflammatory effects of methotrexate in a mouse model as did adenosine deaminase, an enzyme that degrades adenosine.[495]

These studies indicate that at least part of the effect of methotrexate in inflammation is mediated by an increased production of adenosine. It is possible that therapies specifically targeted to increasing adenosine levels may prove beneficial in the treatment of multiple dermatologic conditions in the near future.

Methotrexate is FDA approved for treatment of adults with psoriasis, Sezary syndrome and rheumatoid arthritis. Methotrexate therapy in childhood psoriasis should be reserved for the most recalcitrant of cases including patients with erythrodermic psoriasis, psoriatic arthritis nonresponsive to traditional therapy, pustular psoriasis which is generalized or debilitating, or in patients with extensive plaque psoriasis (>20% surface involvement) nonresponsive to more conservative therapy.[321] Methotrexate has many additional off-label uses including other proliferative dermatoses such as pityriasis rubra pilaris and pityriasis lichenoides, immunobullous disorders, autoimmune connective tissue diseases, vasculitides and neutrophilic dermatoses, as well as sarcoidosis and lymphomatoid papulosis. There have been recent reports advocating the use of methotrexate therapy in the treatment of widespread morphea/localized scleroderma.[497,498] Yet to date there are no prospective double-blind placebo–controlled studies to evaluate its efficacy.

Nausea, anorexia, and fatigue are the most commonly observed side effects of methotrexate therapy. Diarrhea, vomiting, and stomatitis are seen less frequently but when severe, warrant a decrease in methotrexate dosage or discontinuation of therapy. Alopecia may be seen in as many as 6% of treated patients.[499] Other rare cutaneous effects include acral erythema, vasculitis, epidermal necrosis, and an unusual "recall" reaction that may follow preceding sunburn or radiation therapy (see Table 4.31).

Hepatotoxicity resulting from long-term methotrexate therapy is the adverse effect of most concern. There are minimal data on the incidence of fibrosis and cirrhosis in children, but it appears to be less commonly reported as compared to the adult population. Known risk factors for the development of methotrexate-associated hepatotoxicity include diabetes, obesity, and alcoholism. Unfortunately, hematologic indices of liver function including transaminase levels may be normal even in the setting of significant hepatic fibrosis and/or cirrhosis and are not highly sensitive screening measures. The risk of hepatic toxicity appears to be greater with higher cumulative doses of methotrexate (>1.5g total dose). While baseline and follow-up liver biopsies are advocated in adult patients treated for psoriasis, standards of care are not well established in the pediatric dermatology setting. A recent survey of pediatric dermatologists indicated that the majority of clinicians do not routinely obtain baseline liver biopsies and that only a minority obtain follow-up biopsies in the setting of psoriasis (after doses of >1.5g) (personal communication).

TABLE 4.30 Potential uses for methotrexate in pediatric dermatology

Atopic dermatitis	Pityriasis rubra pilaris
Behçet's disease	Psoriasis/psoriatic arteritis
Bullous pemphigoid	Pyoderma gangrenosum
Cutaneous polyarteritis nodosa	Reiter's disease
Juvenile dermatomyositis	Sarcoidosis
Leukocytoclastic vasculitis	Scleroderma
Morphea	Sezary syndrome/mycosis fungoides
Pemphigus vulgaris	Systemic lupus erythematosus
Pityriasis lichenoides	

493A. Paller A (1985) Dermatologic uses of methotrexate in children: indications and guidelines. **Pediatr Dermatol** 23:238.

494. Zachariae H (1993) Methotrexate therapy. **J Clin Dermatol**, November/December:14.

495. Cronstein BN (1997) The mechanism of action of methotrexate. **Rheum Clin NA** 23.4.739–755.

496. Allegra CJ, Drake JC et al. (1985) Inhibition of phosphoribosylaminoimidazolecarboxamide transformylase by methotrexate and dihydrofolic acid polyglutamates. **Proc Natl Acad Sci USA** 82:4881–4885.

497. Swyger MMB, van den Hoogen FHJ, de Boo T, de Jong EMGJ (1998) Low-dose methotrexate in the treatment of widespread morphea. **J Am Acad Dermatol** 39:220–225.

498. Uziel Y, Feldman BM, Krafchik BR, Yeung RSM, Laxer RM (2000) Methotrexate and corticosteroid therapy for pediatric localized scleroderma. **J Pediatr** 136:91–95.

499. Olson EA (1991) The pharmacology of methotrexate. **J Am Acad Dermatol** 25:306–318.

TABLE 4.31   Methotrexate adverse effects

Hematologic	Gastrointestinal	Central nervous system	Respiratory	Dermatology	Ophthalmic	Cardiovascular	Immunology	Renal	Reproductive/ Hormonal	Other
Thrombo-cytopenia	Hepatotoxicity	Leuko-encephalo-pathy	Pneumonitis	Stevens–Johnson syndrome/ toxic epidermal necrolysis	Vision changes	Pericarditis	Opportunistic infections	Renal failure	Teratogen	Anaphylaxis
Leukopenia	Hepatitis	Fever	Pulmonary fibrosis	Exfoliative dermatitis	Conjunctivitis	Thrombotic events		Nephropathy	Abortive effects	Osteoar-thropathy
Aplastic anemia	Nausea and vomiting	Dizziness		Photosensitivity		Pericardial effusion		Hematuria		
				Alopecia		Hypotension		Azotemia	Transient oliogospermia	
				Radiation/sunburn "recall"					Infertility	
				Acral erythema					Gynecomastia	
									Menstrual irregularities	

Pulmonary toxicity is a rare adverse effect reported with methotrexate therapy. Pulmonary effects are idiosyncratic, may be either acute or chronic in nature, and are potentially life threatening. A prevalence of up to 5% has been reported in the adult rheumatologic literature but may be less frequent in children. Patients may develop either an acute pneumonitis or chronic pulmonary fibrosis. Evaluation including chest X-ray is warranted in patients receiving methotrexate who present with respiratory symptoms.

Hematologic side effects include megaloblastic anemia and leukemia. Pancytopenia represents the adverse effect with greatest potential for increased mortality. This risk is reported more commonly in the rheumatologic literature than in dermatology. This toxicity is observed more frequently in elderly patients and individuals with impaired renal function. It is usually seen within the first 4–6 weeks of therapy. The risk is also greater in patients receiving concomitant therapy with trimethoprim/sulfamethoxazole or non-steroidal anti-inflammatory agents. The potential risk of hematotoxicity can be reduced with administration of folic acid at doses of 1–5mg/day while methotrexate efficacy is not adversely affected.[500] In patients with evidence of methotrexate-induced hematotoxicity, leukovorin (folinic acid) should be administered and will allow for normal cell division to return. Methotrexate should be discontinued or dosage should be reduced when leukocyte counts drop below 3500/mm^3 or platelets fall below 100 000/mm^3.

Other potential toxicities include renal impairment due to precipitation of methotrexate in renal tubules with high dose therapy, potential induction of malignancy, and rare neurologic side effects including acute chemical arachnoiditis which can be observed in 5–50% patients within hours of intrathecal methotrexate injections.

The majority of safety data in children can be found in the rheumatology literature pertaining to treatment of juvenile rheumatoid arthritis (JRA). In a study of 62 children treated with methotrexate for JRA,[501] no patients experienced significant pulmonary or hepatotoxicity. A liver biopsy was performed in 12 of the 62 patients and there were no findings of fibrosis or cirrhosis. Transient elevation in transaminases was observed in 9 of the 62 patients and only 1 patient who was receiving concurrent therapy with trimethoprim–sulfamethoxasole developed a macrocytic anemia. The most commonly observed side effects included nausea (14), elevated aminotransferases (9), and peptic ulcer disease (4). Their findings suggest that methotrexate may be better tolerated in children. In another study of 29 patients with JRA,[502] there were no manifestations of hematologic, pulmonary, renal or cutaneous toxicity. Two patients developed moderate gastrointestinal upset, 1 patient stomatitis, and 1 had transient elevations of hepatic transaminase levels. Finally, in a multicenter study of 127 children with JRA,[503] doses of 5–10mg/m^2 per week were associated with no severe toxicities.

In higher doses, methotrexate is an abortifacient as well as a potential teratogen. In female patients of childbearing age, pregnancy should be ruled out before initiating therapy, and conception should be avoided for at least 3 months after discontinuation. However, women who have become pregnant while receiving methotrexate therapy for psoriasis have delivered normal infants.[504] Male patients should also be counseled not to impregnate their female partners until 3 months after methotrexate therapy is discontinued.

Baseline evaluation should include a careful history and physical examination as well as laboratory studies: CBC with differential and platelet count, liver function tests including transaminases, serology for hepatitis A, B, and C antibodies, and renal function tests. Follow-up laboratory tests should include CBC, platelet count and liver function tests weekly for 2–4 weeks and with dosing increases, then every 3 months during long-term therapy. Renal function tests should be monitored 1 to 2 times yearly. Chest radiographs should be obtained in the setting of pulmonary symptoms. The necessity of baseline and follow-up liver biopsy remains controversial and no standard recommendations exist for the pediatric population. Patients should be counseled on the importance of avoiding other medications with the potential for liver toxicity including alcohol consumption. Patients receiving methotrexate should also be warned about the potential for toxicity from concomitantly administered drugs that impair methotrexate clearance, including trimethoprim–sulfamethoxazolc, many nonsteroidal anti-inflammatory drugs, and salicylates.[504]

500. Morgan SL, Baggott JE, Vaughn WH et al. (1990) The effect of folic acid supplementation on the toxicity of low-dose methotrexate in patients with rheumatoid arthritis. **Arthritis Rheum** 33(1):9–18.
501. Graham LD, Myones BL, Rivas-Chacon RF, Pachman LM (1992) Morbidity associated with long-term methotrexate therapy in juvenile rheumatoid arthritis. **J Pediatr** 120:468–473.
502. Rose C, Singsen BH, Eichenfield AH, Goldsmith DP, Athreya BH (1990) Safety and efficacy of methotrexate therapy for juvenile rheumatoid arthritis. **J Pediatr** 117:653–659.
503. Giannini EH, Brewer EJ, Kuzmina N et al. (1992) Methotrexate in resistant juvenile rheumatoid arthritis. **N Engl J Med** 326:1043–1049.
504. McDonald C (1985) Cytotoxic agents for use in dermatology. I. **J Am Acad Dermatol** 12:753.

MINOCYCLINE

Minocycline, a semisynthetic tetracycline derivative, was first introduced in 1972. It is discussed in this chapter due to its potential for many uncommon yet clinically important adverse reactions which have been reported increasingly over the past decade. Because minocycline is the most commonly prescribed antibiotic in the treatment of acne vulgaris,[505] clinicians should be familiar with these reactions and their associated morbidities.

Tetracyclines bind to the 30S ribosomal subunit and inhibit protein synthesis resulting in antibacterial activity against both Gram-positive and Gram-negative bacteria. They also have antimicrobial activity against mycoplasma, *Chlamydia* organisms, Rickettsia organisms, spirochetes, and some parasites. Tetracyclines have greater Gram-positive activity than Gram-negative in general and minocycline and doxycycline are usually more effective in treating *Staphylococcus aureus* as compared to tetracycline. Furthermore, there is less *Propionibacterium acnes* resistance with minocycline than with tetracycline or erythromycin making it more effective in the management of acne. Minocycline is usually dosed at 50 to 200mg daily and can be taken with or without food once to twice daily. Tetracyclines increase the levels of digoxin, lithium and warfarin which may lead to potential toxicity. It is believed that concurrent use of the tetracyclines with isotretinoin therapy may increase the risk of pseudotumor cerebri and this combination is not recommended.

The tetracycline family can cause gastointestinal side effects of nausea, vomiting, abdominal pain, and epigastric burning. They have the potential for hepatotoxicity and should be used carefully in high-risk individuals or in combination with other medications which may damage the liver. Tetracyclines, in particular doxycycline, cause photosensitivity and photo-toxicity with or without onycholysis. This family of antibiotics should not be administered to children less than 9 years of age as they may cause brown discoloration of the teeth and delayed bone growth.

In a recent comparison of the tetracyclines, minocycline was more commonly associated with several potentially serious adverse reactions including hypersensitivity syndrome, serum-sickness-like reaction, and drug-induced lupus.[506] Hepatotoxicity may also be more commonly reported in association with minocycline.[507]

Over the past several years there have been several reports of serum-sickness-like reaction (SSLR) in patients taking minocycline.[508,509] SSLR manifestations usually present after 10–30 days of minocycline therapy. Typically, SSLR is characterized by fever, rash (often urticarial), and arthralgia/arthritis. The condition is self-limited and has a favorable prognosis.

There have been multiple case reports and small patient series of minocycline hypersensitivity syndrome, especially over the past decade. This unusual and poorly understood reaction is similar to the hypersensitivity syndrome associated with the aromatic anticonvulsants and sulfonamide antibiotics. This potentially life-threatening reaction usually presents with the triad of fever, rash, and lymphadenopathy in addition to internal organ involvement. Its initial manifestations usually appear after 2 to 4 weeks of therapy and fever is often the first sign of the hypersensitivity syndrome followed by rash. Cutaneous manifestations may be nonspecific early on and resemble a viral exanthem. Progression to more severe eruptions, including Stevens–Johnson syndrome and toxic epidermal necrolysis, may occur. Erythroderma and exfoliative dermatitis are often observed later in the clinical course. Hematologic changes are commonly seen, especially atypical lymphocytosis and/or eosinophilia. This hypersensitivity reaction can also lead to significant

leukopenia, anemia, and/or thrombocytopenia. Internal organ involvement most commonly affects the liver and fatal cases of hepatic failure have been reported.[507] While any organ system can be affected, special attention should be directed toward the possible renal and pulmonary toxicity. Hypothyroidism has been described late in the clinical course. Treatment includes prompt discontinuation of minocycline and supportive care. Systemic glucocorticoids, immunosuppressive agents, and/or intravenous immunoglobulin may be warranted in severe hypersensitivity reactions, however treatment modalities remain poorly defined and controlled outcome studies are lacking.

In 1992, Matsuura and colleagues first described a case of drug-induced lupus related to minocycline,[510] and over the past decade there have been numerous additional reports. Sturkenboom demonstrated that the relative risk of developing drug-induced lupus in patients receiving chronic minocycline therapy for acne is increased 8.5-fold as compared to patients receiving other tetracyclines or no antibiotic therapy.[511] The risk of drug-induced lupus was not significantly increased with either tetracycline or doxycycline.

Minocycline-induced lupus is defined as having at least one clinical feature of systemic lupus, positive ANA titers, and a temporal association with the use of minocycline. This condition is observed most commonly in young female patients (mean age of 17 in one recent analysis) receiving long-term minocycline therapy for acne. In a recent review of minocycline-induced autoimmune syndromes, the average duration of therapy in 36 patients who developed minocycline-induced lupus was 30 months at doses of 50–200mg daily. Arthralgia was reported in all 36 patients and synovitis in 26 of the 36 patients. Fever and rash were less commonly observed (12 and 7 patients, respectively).[512] Laboratory studies in this analysis of patients revealed a positive ANA in all patients, dsDNA in 4 patients, anti-histone antibodies in 4 patients, and anti-cardiolipin in 10 individuals. Ten of 13 patients evaluated were positive for pANCA antibodies. An additional study revealed positive p-ANCA antibodies in 14 of 14 patients evaluated as well as elevated antimyeloperoxidase antibodies in 11 of 14 patients and 10 of 14 patients with anti-elastase antibodies.[513] Major histocompatability complex class II testing revealed 9 of 13 patients to be HLA-DR4 positive while 4 of 13 patients were HLA-DR2 positive, suggesting a genetic susceptibility to this sydrome.[513] The outcome is favorable in the majority of patients with spontaneous remission usually occurring within several weeks after discontinuation of minocycline therapy.

A systematic review of the literature and pharmacovigilance data addressing liver damage associated with minocycline use in acne was published in 2000. The authors identified 65 reported cases of hepatitis or liver damage. Ninety-four percent of the cases occurred in patients less than 40 years of age and 58% of the cases were in females. For 45 of the 65 reports, it was possible to classify the event into one of two categories: autoimmune hepatitis associated with lupus-like symptoms occurring after long-term therapy (29) and hypersensitivity reactions which were associated with eosinophilia and exfoliative dermatitis occurring within 35 days of minocycline treatment (16). There were four deaths among the 65 cases reported in association with minocycline hepatotoxicity.[507]

It is not well understood why hepatotoxicity and hypersensitivity reactions have been reported more frequently with minocycline as compared with the other tetracyclines. One factor may be that minocycline metabolism may generate a reactive metabolite (an iminoquinone derivative) which can act as a foreign antigen and trigger an immune reaction.[508] Interestingly, in the review by Lawrenson and colleagues, 6 of the 16 cases of hepatotoxicity associated with hypersensitivity reactions occurred in patients of African-

505. Eichenfield AH (1999) Minocycline and autoimmunity. **Curr Opin Pediatr** 11:447–456.
506. Shapiro LE, Knowles SR, Shear NH (1997) Comparative safety of tetracycline, minocycline, and doxycycline. **Arch Dermatol** 133(10):1224–1230.
507. Lawrenson RA, Seaman HE, Sundstrom A, Williams TJ, Farmer RD (2000) Liver damage associated with minocycline use in acne. A systematic review of the published literature and pharmacovigilance data. **Drug Saf** 23(4):333–349.
508. Knowles SR, Shapiro L, Shear NH (1996) Serious adverse reactions induced by minocycline. Report of 13 patients and review of the literature. **Arch Dermatol** 132:934–939.
509. Harel L, Amir J, Livni E, Straussberg R, Varsano I (1996) Serum-sickness-like reaction associated with minocycline therapy in adolescents. **Ann Pharmacother** 30:481–483.

510. Matsuura T, Shimizu Y, Fujimoto H et al. (1992) Minocycline-related lupus (letter). **Lancet** 340:1553.
511. Sturkenboom MC, Meier CR, Jick H, Stricker BH (1999) Minocycline and lupuslike syndrome in acne patients. **Arch Intern Med** 159:493–497.
512. Elkayam O, Yaron M, Caspi D (1999) Minocycline-induced autoimmune syndromes: an overview. **Semin Arthritis Rheum** 28:392–397.
513. Dunphy J, Oliver M, Rands AL, Lovell CR, McHugh NJ (2000) Antineutrophil cytoplasmic antibodies and HLA class II alleles in minocycline-induced lupus-like syndrome. **Br J Dermatol** 142:461–467.

Caribbean descent suggesting that genetic factors likely have a role in the minocycline hypersensitivity syndrome. Because of possible cross-reactivity between the tetracyclines and the potential seriousness of the adverse reactions, it is prudent not to use the other tetracycline antibiotics when there is the suspicion of minocycline-related reactions.

MYCOPHENOLATE

Mycophenolic acid (MPA) was originally used in the 1970s for the treatment of severe psoriasis. While it was shown to be effective in the management of recalcitrant psoriasis, concerns of potential immunosuppression and carcinogenicity led to a decline in its clinical use. However, in 1995 a morpho-linoester of MPA, mycophenolate mofetil (MMF, CellCept) was approved by the FDA for prevention of renal allograft rejection. Pharmacologic studies showed that MMF has improved bioavailability compared to MPA. In recent years, there has been renewed enthusiasm for this agent as a treatment of psoriasis as well as other inflammatory rheumatologic and dermatologic conditions.

After absorption from the gastrointestinal tract, MMF is metabolized to MPA. MPA is a weak organic acid which inhibits *de novo* purine synthesis via its noncompetitive inhibition of inosine monophosphate dehydrogenase. It preferentially affects cells which rely upon *de novo* purine synthesis rather than the purine salvage pathway. An important example of such cells are proliferating T and B lymphocytes.[514]

In 1993, Goldblum reported the use of MMF in greater than 600 patients with rheumatoid arthritis. In the past several years, there has been a growing number of case reports and small patient series suggesting that MMF is effective in the therapy of autoimmune bullous disorders including bullous pemphigoid, pemphigus vulgaris, and pemphigus foliaceous. In 1999, Enk and Knop described their use of MMF in the treatment of 12 patients with pemphigus vulgaris.[515] These patients were treated concomitantly with systemic glucocorticoids; however, steroid doses were tapered from an initial 2mg/kg/day to a median dose of 2.5mg/day after 9 months of mycophenolate therapy.[515] Grundmann-Kollmann and colleagues reported the successful use of mycophenolate as monotherapy in 2 patients with bullous pemphigoid and 1 patient with pemphigus vulgaris at doses of 2g/day.[516] Thus far, there are no reports of MMF use in the pediatric population for autoimmune bullous disorders.

One report has described the treatment of 10 adult patients with severe atopic dermatitis using mycophenolate. Patients were given 1g per day for the first week and then 2g per day for 11 weeks. The drug was well tolerated and the median disease score improved by 68%.[517] Other small studies have reported varying degrees of success treating severe atopic dermatitis with mycophenolate.[518–521] Significant side-effects have been noted in two patients treated with mycophenolate. One developed herpetic retinitis[518] while another developed *Staphylococcus* endocarditis and septicemia.[522]

On average, the usual dose of MMF in the treatment of dermatologic conditions is approximately 1 to 2g/day although some clinicians report the need for higher doses in the treatment of pemphigus vulgaris.[523] The most common adverse effects of MMF are gastrointestinal symptoms including nausea, diarrhea, soft stools, abdominal cramps, vomiting, anorexia, and anal tenderness. Less frequently observed is urinary frequency or urgency, dysuria, and sterile pyuria.

Overall, MMF is very well tolerated and does not appear to cause significant renal or hepatic toxicity. Hematologic abnormalities are occasionally observed, most commonly lymphopenia. Complete blood count with platelets and differential should be monitored every 1 to 2 weeks during the first month of therapy and biweekly during the second and third months of therapy. MMF doses should be decreased or the medication discontinued if the leukocyte count falls below 4000 cells/mm^3. Occasional elevations in liver transaminases may be observed and liver function tests should be followed monthly early in therapy. The potential for carcinogenicity with MMF therapy remains uncertain.

PHOTOTHERAPY

UV light is the 200–400-nm portion of the electromagnetic spectrum between visible light and X-rays. Each portion of the UV light spectrum has unique photobiologic characteristics. UVA is the long-wavelength portion of the UV light spectrum, ranging from 320 to 400nm, closest to visible light. The primary cutaneous effect of UVA is tanning. UVB ranges from 290 to 320nm. This portion of the spectrum plays the greatest role in sunburn and is 1000 times more erythemogenic than UVA. UVC, at 200 to 290nm, is absorbed by the atmospheric ozone and does not reach the earth. Erythema and superficial desquamation occur after exposure to artificial UVC (see Table 4.32). High dose UVA therapy, known as UVA-1, selectively emits ultraviolet light greater than 340nm wavelength. Narrow-band UVB phototherapy at 311 nm is becoming widely used, often replacing conventional broad-band UVB therapy.

The therapeutic benefits of natural sunlight were recognized in ancient Greece. In modern times, natural and artificial light has been used since the early twentieth century, beginning with use of the Nobel-prize-winning discovery of carbon arc lamp treatment for lupus vulgaris.[524] The high-pressure mercury vapor "hot quartz" lamp, emitting UVB, was developed during the 1920s and used in combination with topical tar (Goeckerman regimen) or anthralin (Ingram regimen) for the treatment of psoriasis. The low-pressure mercury vapor "cold quartz" lamp, emitting UVC, has been used since the 1930s to treat acne. Visible light phototherapy, using fluorescent white or narrow-band blue light, has been used since the 1950s for the treatment of neonatal jaundice. During the 1970s, oral psoralen + UVA (PUVA) photochemotherapy was developed. Broad-band and narrow-band UVB and oral or topical PUVA, alone or in combination with other forms of therapy, are currently used routinely and investigationally to treat a wide variety of dermatoses.[525]

TABLE 4.32   Wavelengths and sites of action of ultraviolet light used in phototherapy

Ultraviolet Radiation (UV)	Wavelength	Site of action
UVA	320–400nm	Epidermis and dermis
UVA-1	>340nm	Epidermis and dermis
UVB (broadband)	290–320nm	Epidermis
UVB (narrowband)	311nm	Epidermis
UVC	200–290nm	N/A

514. Silverman Kitchin JE, Pomeranz MK, Pak G, Washenik K, Shupack J (1997) Rediscovering mycophenolic acid: a review of its mechanism, side effects and potential uses. **J Am Acad Dermatol** 37:445–449.

515. Enk AH, Knop J (1999) Mycophenolate is effective in the treatment of pemphigus vulgaris. **Arch Dermatol** 135:54–56.

516. Grundmann-Kollmann M, Korting HC, Behrens S et al. (1999) Mycophenolate mofetil: a new therapeutic option in the treatment of blistering autoimmune disease. **J Am Acad Dermatol** 40:957–960.

517. Neuber K, Schwartz I, Itschert G, Dieck AT (2000) Treatment of atopic eczema with oral mycophenolate mofetil. **Br J Dermatol** 143:385–391.

518. Grundmann-Kollmann M, Korting HC et al. (1999) Successful treatment of severe refractory atopic dermatitis with mycophenolate mofetil. **Br J Dermatol** 141:175–176.

519. Grundmann-Kollmann M, Podda M, Ochsendorf F et al. (2001) Mycophenolate mofetil is effective in the treatment of atopic dermatitis. **Arch Dermatol** 137:870–873.

520. Benez A, Fierlbeck G (2001) Successful long-term treatment of severe atopic dermatitis with mycophenolate mofetil. **Br J Dermatol** 144:638–639.

521. Hansen ER, Buus S, Deleuran M, Andersen KE (2000) Treatment of atopic dermatitis with mycophenolate mofetil. **Br J Dermatol** 143:1324–1325.

522. Satchell AC, Barnetson RStC (2000) Staphylococcal septicaemia complicating treatment of atopic dermatitis with mycophenolate. **Br J Dermatol** 141:202–203.

523. Nousari HC, Anhalt G (1999) (Letter) The role of mycophenolate mofetil in the management of pemphigus. **Arch Dermatol** 135:853–854.

524. Anderson T (1983) Pediatric phototherapy. **Pediatr Clin North Am** 30:701.

525. Green C, Diffey B, Hawk J (1992) Ultraviolet radiation in the treatment of skin disease. **Phys Med Biol** 37:1.

Of the dozens of skin diseases that benefit from UV phototherapy, several are seen in the pediatric population: vitiligo, psoriasis, acne, atopic dermatitis, pityriasis rubra pilaris, pityriasis lichenoides, solar urticaria, urticaria pigmentosa, and chronic graft-versus-host disease.[524] However, the administration of UV light phototherapy to children requires special precautions. Cooperation is essential. Parents and children must be informed about the problems associated with cumulative UV light exposure. UV light-induced cataracts, skin pigment and textural changes, and skin cancers have a delayed onset of many years (see the section on sun protection). UV light therapy should be reserved for stubborn and/or severe childhood skin diseases that are recalcitrant to others forms of therapy, and treatment courses should be as short as possible.

Phototherapy can be administered by simple outdoor exposure, home-based light units, or office/hospital-based treatment centers. Outdoor exposure is cost free and convenient but nonspecific and unpredictable. Home-based light units can be costly. This form of therapy is difficult to monitor, often resulting in suboptimal dosing or more severe side effects. Although it is not the preferred form of phototherapy, it may be the only alternative for some. Explicit guidelines for home-based phototherapy can be obtained from the National Psoriasis Foundation; 6600 S.W. 92nd Avenue, Suite 300, Portland OR 97223 USA. The most precise, most successful, and safest form of phototherapy is at a medical center, where the correct wavelength and dosage can be administered and the cumulative dose can be monitored. Office-based phototherapy is time consuming, often inconvenient, and costly, but it is the recommended site for administering pediatric phototherapy.

Ultraviolet phototherapy has numerous effects on the immunologic response of the skin. Production of IL-10, α-MSH, prostaglandin E2 and matrix metalloproteinases, all of which have immunosuppressive activities, is increased in keratinocytes that have been exposed to UV light. Levels of ICAM-1 and IFN-γ, which are generally proinflammatory, are reduced in UV light-exposed keratinocytes.[526] In addition to these specific effects, exposure of keratinocytes, monocytes and T lymphocytes to UV light can result in the activation of apoptotic pathways, leading ultimately to programmed cell death. The exact mechanism of this activation is not yet fully understood, but the formation of UV light-induced DNA-crosslinks is thought to play an important role in the process.[527] Psoralens act by intercalating into DNA and then forming psoralen-DNA crosslinks after exposure to UV light. These crosslinks interfere with DNA replication and lead to the arrest of cell division. In addition, PUVA may affect the cytokine profile of exposed cells and well as inducing apoptosis.[528]

Artificial sources of UVC radiation are "cold-quartz" germicidal lamps. These are low-pressure mercury lamps with a monochromatic emission at 254nm. They are inexpensive and relatively simple to operate. They do not need time to warm up or cool off. UVC is mutagenic *in vitro*, effectively killing microorganisms in the immediate vicinity. Brief skin exposure has not been associated with a high incidence of carcinogenesis, probably because it does not penetrate beyond the stratum corneum. Cold quartz lamps have been used to promote a sterile environment in operating rooms and, although no controlled studies have been done, the antimicrobial properties and desquamating effects of UVC have been used to treat acne patients. UVC does not promote skin pigmentation, but it does cause an immediate burning sensation and desquamation 24 to 48h after treatment. Exposure for only a few seconds can cause a painful keratitis; the use of protective eyewear is mandatory.[524]

UVB therapy has classically been the most frequently recommended form of phototherapy, but is being rivaled by combined UVA/UVB and narrow-band therapy. The first artificial source of UVB was the high-pressure mercury vapor "hot-quartz" lamp. Fluorescent bulbs with more specific emission spectra and total body cabinet phototherapy units are now available for rapid and precise delivery of measured doses of UVB. UVB phototherapy is a recommended alternative in severe cases of psoriasis, atopic dermatitis, and pityriasis lichenoides et varioliformis acuta (PLEVA) in children. Actinic damage is to be expected following prolonged therapy with UVB, but 25-year follow-up studies have not found an alarming risk of carcinogenesis.[524] Narrow-band UVB is superior to broad-band UVB treatment in regards to both the degree of clearing as well as duration of remission.[528,529] In fact, narrow-band UVB phototherapy may be almost as effective as PUVA therapy in the management of psoriasis.[530,531] Narrow-band UVB therapy also shows promise in the treatment of vitiligo in small case series of both children and adults with a more rapid response rate as compared with previous reports with PUVA therapy.

Patients undergoing UV therapy must wear eye protection during treatment to avoid the potential long-term risk of cataracts. Pediatric patients must be closely monitored, because of their urge to "peek." Lips, nipples, genitalia, and unaffected areas should be shielded with sunscreen or UV-protective clothing. Short-term adverse effects of phototherapy include xerosis, pruritus, erythema, blistering and precipitation of herpes simplex virus infections. Potential adverse effects of long-term ultraviolet therapy include accelerated photoaging of the skin and carcinogenesis.

UVA alone has little effect on skin disease.[532] Artificial UVA is commercially used for tanning, because it is minimally erythemogenic; however, many tanning salons are now using both UVA and UVB lights. Excessive tanning causes actinic skin damage, such as wrinkling, atrophy, and freckling; the precise association with development of skin cancer is less clear. Psoralens, also known as furocoumarins, are a family of photoactive compounds. Furocoumarins derived from plant sources were used in ancient Egypt and India to treat depigmenting skin diseases. Topical or orally administered psoralens and sunlight have been used empirically to treat vitiligo in children and adults since the mid-1900s. During the 1970s, PUVA therapy was defined after *in vitro* and clinical studies found that psoralens greatly enhance skin response to UVA in hyperproliferative skin conditions. Beginning in the late 1980s, the technique of extracorporeal photopheresis was developed, using systemic psoralens and plasmapharesis with selective exposure of circulating cells to UVA, in the treatment of T-cell-mediated malignant and inflammatory diseases.[534]

Bioavailable psoralens are taken up by rapidly proliferating cells. UVA radiation promotes covalent bonding between psoralen and DNA, inhibiting cell proliferation. Erythema induced by PUVA differs from sunburn in several ways. UVA penetrates the skin more deeply than does UVB.[535] UVA erythema has a delayed onset and longer duration, peaking at 48h rather than 24h after exposure. The damage to DNA induced by PUVA is much different and more lethal than UVB-induced cell injury. Although the long-term consequences of these observations are unknown, they raise serious concerns about the use of PUVA in children.

PUVA photochemotherapy has been strongly opposed for children under the age of 12 by the American Academy of Pediatrics,[536] and is not FDA approved for that age group, because of theoretical concerns about cumulative toxicity. However, PUVA has been used with caution for several

526. Krutmann J, Morita A (1999) Mechanisms of ultraviolet (UV) B and UVA phototherapy. **J Invest Dermatol Symp Proc** 4:70–72.
527. Godar DE (1999) Light and death: photons and apoptosis phototherapy. **J Invest Dermatol Symp Proc** 4:17–23.
528. Green C, Ferguson J, Lakshmipathi T, Johnson BE (1988) 311nm UVB phototherapy – an effective treatment for psoriasis. **Br J Dermatol** 119:691–696.
529. Van Weelden H, De La Faille HB, Young E, Van der Leun IC (1988) A new development in UVB phototherapy of psoriasis. **Br J Dermatol** 119:11–19.
530. Van Weelden H, Baart de la Faille H, Young E, Van der Leun JC (1990) Comparison of narrow-band UV-B phototherapy and PUVA photochemotherapy in the treatment of psoriasis. **Acta Derm Venereol** 70:212–215.
531. Tanew A, Radakovic-Fijan S, Schemper M, Honigsmann H (1999) Paired comparison study on narrow-band (TL-01) UVB phototherapy versus photochemotherapy (PUVA) in the treatment of chronic plaque type psoriasis. **Arch Dermatol** 135:519–524.
532. Scherschun L, Kim JJ, Lim HW (2001) Narrow-band ultraviolet B is a useful and well-tolerated treatment for vitiligo. **J Am Acad Dermatol** 44:999–1003.
533. Njoo MD, Bos JD, Westerhof W (2000) Treatment of generalized vitiligo in children with narrow-band (TL-01) UVB radiation therapy. **J Am Acad Dermatol** 42:245–253.
534. Pathak M, Fitzpatrick T (1992) The evolution of photochemotherapy with psoralens and UVA (PUVA): 2000 BC to 1992 AD. **J Photochem Photobiol** 14:3.
535. Diffey B (1993) Ultraviolet radiation in medicine. In: Medical Physics Handbook II, Diffey B, ed. Bristol: Adam Hilger, p. 886.
536. Anonymous (1978) PUVA: a caution. **Pediatrics** 62:253.

TABLE 4.33 Skin disorders treated with PUVA

FDA indications	Neoplastic conditions	Dermatitis/ papulosquamous	Photosensitivity dermatoses	Pruritic dermatoses	Immunologic dermatoses	Miscellaneous
Psoriasis	CTCL	Atopic dermatitis	PMLE	Chronic urticaria	Alopecia areata	Grover's disease
Vitiligo	LCH	Seborrheic dermatitis	EPP	Polycythemia vera	Graft vs. host disease	Pigmented purpura
		Chronic hand dermatitis	Solar urticaria	Prurigo nodularis	Morphea	Icthyosis linearis circumflexa
		Palmoplantar pustulosis	Chronic actinic dermatitis	Idiopathic pruritus		Scleromyxedema
		Pityriasis lichenoides		Urticaria pigmentosa		Generalized granuloma annulare
		Lymphomatoid papulosis				

PMLE, polymorphous light eruption; EPP, erythropoetic protoporphyria; LCH, Langerhans cell hystiocytosis; CTCL, cutaneous T-cell lymphoma.

inflammatory and hyperproliferative childhood dermatoses, without reports of significant adverse effects to date. Cooperative children with skin diseases unresponsive to other forms of therapy are candidates for PUVA (see Table 4.33). These include vitiligo, psoriasis, atopic dermatitis, generalized lichen planus, urticaria pigmentosa, graft-versus-host disease and polymorphous light eruption.[534]

Psoralen is commercially available in two forms: trioxsalen and methoxsalen. Trioxsalen (Trisoralen) is a synthetic psoralen derivative. It is a potent drug, but has a LD_{50} six times that of methoxsalen, permitting a larger dose with a higher margin of safety. When used in conjunction with measured exposure to UVA, trioxsalen is FDA approved for repigmentation of vitiligo and for increasing a patient's tolerance to sunlight. Trioxsalen is not approved for use in patients under 12 years old, but it has been used to treat vitiligo in children, with better results than in adults.[534] It is available in 5mg tablets. An appropriate initial oral dose is 0.3mg/kg taken 2–3h before light exposure. Standard dosage is 0.6mg/kg 2h before UVA exposure in long-term therapy.[537] Trioxsalen can also be compounded into a liquid vehicle for topical use.[538] Treatments can be given three times a week, but not on consecutive days. The dose of UVA radiation can be increased every week as tolerated to produce minimal erythema at the affected areas. Severe burns have resulted from misuse of this technique.

8-Methoxypsoralen (Methoxsalen, 8-MOP), is a naturally occurring compound derived from the seeds of the Egyptian *Ammi majus* plant. 8-MOP is FDA approved for the treatment of severe psoriasis that is unresponsive to other forms of therapy. It is available in two oral preparations in addition to Oxsoralen Lotion (a 1% lotion formulated for topical use). The 10mg Oxsoralen capsules are no longer manufactured. Oxsoralen-Ultra is a newer formulation, made available in 1987, as 10mg soft capsules. Compared to Oxsoralen, the Ultra preparation has enhanced bioavailability and a faster onset of activity, with blood levels peaking at 1.8h, compared to 3h. Appropriate initial doses are determined for each individual, based on a minimal erythema response. The standard dose of Oxsoralen Ultra is 0.4mg/kg given 1h before UVA exposure. The other oral option is Methoxsalen 10mg capsules dosed at 0.6mg/kg 2h before UVA exposure. Food intake, especially that with a high fat content, slows absorption of the psoralens and decreases the peak levels. There is large inter- and intraindividual variation in absorption of the oral psoralens which may have clinical implications in the therapeutic response.

As an alternative to systemic therapy, Oxsoralen lotion may be diluted in bathwater, or as a 1:100 solution, cream or ointment, for topical application. This form of therapy decreases the total surface area treated and avoids possible ocular toxicity compared to systemic PUVA. However, in the treatment of vitiligo, topical therapy can actually accentuate affected areas, if not applied precisely, by stimulating hyperpigmentation at the border.[536] It is also associated with an increased risk of unpredictable phototoxic reactions. 5-Meth-oxypsoralen (5-MOP, bergapten) is another naturally occurring furocoumarin, currently under investigation and not available in the United States. A higher dose of 5-MOP is required for therapeutic efficacy, but this form appears to stimulate melanogenesis better and to have a wider margin of safety, with less nausea and fewer phototoxic reactions than occur with 8-MOP.[534]

PUVA treatment protocols are complex and should be directed only by physicians experienced with them; comprehensive guidelines were established by the American Academy of Dermatology in 1993.[539] Two deaths have occurred in patients prescribed oral psoralens and referred for light treatment at a commercial tanning booth.[540] Successful systemic or topical PUVA requires extreme cooperation and diligence, making it a most difficult therapy in children. Adverse effects of PUVA include nausea, pruritus, hypertrichosis, the acute risk of severe phototoxic reactions, and the potential cumulative risks of actinic damage, cataracts, and skin cancers. Candidates for PUVA photochemotherapy should have a thorough history and physical examination with emphasis on potentially worrisome/premalignant skin lesions and actinic damage which may be apparent even in older children and teenagers. A baseline ophthalmologic examination should include gross examination of the eye, slit lamp exam of the lens and cornea, fundoscopic exam of the retina, and assessment of visual acuity. Examinations should be repeated at least yearly or more frequently if abnormal findings are noted. Some experts advocate that potential PUVA patients also be screened with serum ANA, and renal and liver function tests.

Contraindications to PUVA therapy include various skin conditions which increase the risk of phototoxicity such as pemphigus and bullous pemphigoid, lupus erythematosus, xeroderma pigmentosa, or a history of idiosyncratic reaction to a psoralen compound. PUVA should not be used in breast-feeding mothers and the psoralens are classified as pregnancy class C drugs. Relative contraindications for the use of PUVA include concomitant use of photosensitizing drugs such as doxycycline and fluoroquinolones and prior exposure

537. Morison WL (2001) PUVA photochemotherapy. In: Comprehensive Dermatologic Drug Therapy, Wolverton SE, ed. Philadelphia: WB Saunders.
538. Africk J, Fulton J (1971) Treatment of vitiligo with topical trimethylpsoralen and sunlight. Br J Dermatol 84:151.
539. Task Force (1994) Guidelines of care for phototherapy and photochemotherapy. J Am Acad Dermatol 31:643.
540. Potter B (1993) Another iatrogenic death from ultra-violet light and psoralens. Schoch Lett 43(11):41.

to ionizing radiation or arsenic. If baseline physical examination or laboratory studies are abnormal, therapy should be pursued with extreme caution and lab values followed closely. Young patients should enter into PUVA therapy educated on the long-term risk of cumulative photodamage and the increased risk of cutaneous malignancy. During therapy, patients must wear special UV-blocking glasses for 24h after receiving the medication. This requirement alone may make it difficult or impossible to provide safe PUVA therapy for all but the most cooperative children.

RETINOIDS

The term retinoids refers to all natural and synthetic compounds which produce effects like that of vitamin A. The term vitamin A does not refer to one single compound but rather a family of naturally occurring chemicals including retinal, retinol, and retinoic acid. Similar to other vitamins, vitamin A cannot be synthesized *in vivo* and humans are dependent upon dietary consumption for adequate levels of vitamin A. Dietary vitamin A is primarily derived from retinyl esters found in meat, eggs and milk as well as from beta-carotene present in green leafy and yellow vegetables. Vitamin A plays a role in many physiologic processes including vision, morphogenesis, growth, reproduction, epithelial differentiation, and immunologic responses. Clinical manifestations of vitamin A deficiency include epidermal hyperkeratosis and a variety of keratinization disorders, some precancerous conditions as well as squamous metaplasia of mucous membranes.

Of the naturally occurring forms of vitamin A, retinol (vitamin A alcohol) is the most potent and the main form of vitamin A in the human diet. It was first synthesized *in vitro* in 1946. Retinoic acid (RA) is a byproduct of retinol and is the most oxidized and water soluble of the three naturally occurring compounds. It was first synthesized *in vitro* in 1947 and is far less toxic than retinol. Finally, retinal (vitamin A aldehyde) plays an important role in the visual cycle. Vitamin A was initially used clinically for the treatment of ance in 1943 by Straumfjord.[541] Approximately two decades later, topical tretinoin (All-*trans* retinoic acid) had been synthesized. This first generation retinoid was initially used in the 1960s and 1970s for the treatment of both acne as well as disorders of keratinization including ichthyoses, pityriasis rubra pilaris, and actinic keratoses.[541,542]

In 1972, isotretinoin (13-*cis*-retinoic acid) was used in clinical trials for the treatment of disorders of keratinization,[543] and it was noted serendipitously that study patients with nodulocystic acne experienced marked clinical improvement while on isotretinoin therapy. Subsequently, isotretinoin was confirmed in the late 1970s to be effective in the treatment of severe acne vulgaris and approved by the FDA in 1982 for acne therapy.[544] In 1986, etretinate (Tegison) was released in the USA for treatment of psoriasis. This second generation (monoaromatic) retinoid was later replaced in 1998 in the USA by its active metabolite acitretin (Soriatane), while etretinate had been phased out approximately one decade earlier in Europe.

There is also a third generation (polyaromatic) retinoid, bexarotene, which has been recently FDA approved for the treatment of cutaneous T-cell lymphoma. The scope of this chapter, however, will focus on the clinical uses of isotretinoin and acetretin in pediatric dermatology.

PHARMACOLOGY

Isotretinoin (Accutane) is available in 10, 20 and 40mg capsules and the standard dose is 0.5-2mg/kg/day or 45mg/m^2/day. However, lower doses are sometimes effective in the treatment of acne vulgaris. Similar to the other retinoids, isotretinoin's oral bioavailability is significantly enhanced when administered with food. Acitretin (Soriatane), which comes in 10 and 25mg tablets, is given at doses of 25–50mg/day in adults and 0.5 to 1.0mg/kg per day in smaller children. Both synthetic retinoids have significant accumulation in the liver similar to vitamin A storage.

Isotretinoin and acitretin are both water soluble and have minimal lipid deposition in contrast to etretinate which is 50 times more lipophilic and is stored in greater quantity in adipose tissue.[545] Because etretinate is very slowly released from the adipose tissue, serum etretinate levels may be detectable for 2 to 3 years after discontinuation of therapy in contrast with the more water-soluble retinoids (isotretinoin and acitretin) which are undetectable in serum within one month of cessation of therapy. The terminal elimination half-life of isotretinoin is 10–20h and approximately 50h for acitretin as compared with 80–160 days with etretinate.

However, the re-esterification of acitretin to etretinate may be indirectly enhanced by the consumption of alcohol[546] resulting in a prolonged elimination half-life. Therefore, women with child bearing potential who are treated with acitretin should be instructed to avoid alcohol intake and are counseled to use contraception for 3 years after cessation of therapy (guidelines are 2 years in Europe). In an analysis of male patients taking acitretin or etretinate, the equivalent of only 1/200 000 of a 25mg capsule was detectable in seminal fluid. Because small amounts of acitretin (about 1.5% of maternal dose consumed by breast-feeding infant) are detected in breast milk, retinoid therapy should be avoided in breast-feeding women.

MECHANISM OF ACTION/RECEPTORS

The retinoids, primarily retinoic acid, act through a family of receptors that are ligand-dependent transcriptional activators. Three retinoic acid receptors (RAR) have been found and their genes have been sequenced. These receptors are members of a large gene family (at least 48 members) that contains the receptors for steroid hormones, thyroid hormone and vitamin D as well as receptors for which natural ligands have not yet been identified. The three RAR variants (α, β and γ) bind all-*trans* retinoic acid and are expressed in tissue-specific and developmentally-specific patterns.[547,548] An RAR molecule forms a 1:1 heterodimer with a member of a second group of receptors, termed the retinoid X receptors (RXR). As with the RARs, there are three forms of the RXRs (α, β and γ), all of which have been cloned and sequenced. The physiologic ligand for these receptors is 9-*cis*-retinoic acid. An RAR–RXR heterodimer binds to a specific DNA sequence, known as a retinoic acid response element (RARE), in the promoter region of a retinoic acid-responsive gene. In the absence of retinoic acid, the heterodimer, in association with several other nuclear factors, acts to suppress transcription from that specific gene. However, when all-*trans* retinoic acid interacts with the RAR protein of the heterodimer, a conformational change in the protein occurs leading to a reorganization of the local chromatin structure and to the recruitment of transcriptional activators to the promoter region of the gene. The net result of this process is to activate the target gene.[541] Multiple genes are controlled in this manner and their activation can lead to changes in cellular metabolism or differentiation, including apoptosis, depending upon the specific cellular environment.[549]

Given the large number of related receptors in this receptor gene family and their ability to interact to varying degrees with each other, the complexity of the retinoid response is only beginning to be appreciated. Several new

541. Wolverton SE (1991) Retinoids. In: Systemic Drugs for Skin Diseases, Wolverton SE, Wilkin JK, eds. Philadelphia: WB Saunders, pp. 187–218.
542. Bollag W (1983) The development of retinoids in experimental and clinical oncology and dermatology. **J Am Acad Dermatol** 9:797–805.
543. Peck GL, Yoder FW (1976) Treatment of lamellar ichthyosis and other keratinizing dermatoses with a synthetic retinoid. **Lancet** 2:1172–1174.
544. Peck GL, Olsen TG, Yoder FW et al. (1979) Prolonged remissions of cystic and conglobate acne with 13-*cis* retinoic acid. **N Engl J Med** 300:329–333.

545. Wiegand UW, Chou RC (1998) Pharmacokinetics of acitretin and etretinate. **J Am Acad Dermatol** 39:S25–33.
546. Koo J, Nguyen Q, Gambla C (1997) Advances in psoriasis therapy. **Adv Dermatol** 12:47–72.
547. Piedrafita FJ, Pfahl M (1999) Nuclear retinoid receptors and mechanisms of action. **Handbook Exp Pharmacol** 139:153–184.
548. Chawla A, Repa JJ, Evans RM, Mangelsdorf DJ (2001) Nuclear receptors and lipid physiology: opening the X-files. **Science** 294:1866–1870.
549. Orfanos CE, Zouboulis CC, Almond-Roesler B, Geilen CC (1997) Current use and future potential role of retinoids in dermatology. **Drugs** 53:358–388.

therapeutic agents have been generated that are targeted specifically to the RAR or RXR receptors. For instance adapalene, a synthetic drug that binds to an RAR-β/RXR-γ heterodimer,[547] has been approved for the treatment of acne vulgaris. However, the precise mechanism by which these newer drugs affect the retinoic acid-responsive pathway remains to be fully elucidated.

CLINICAL USE

There are three FDA approved uses of retinoids in dermatology: (1) isotretinoin for acne vulgaris; (2) acitretin for psoriasis; and (3) bexarotene for mycosis fungoides. However, retinoids have been used in many additional dermatologic conditions including disorders of cornification such as the ichthyoses and pityriasis rubra pilaris. Retinoids have also been used with some success in the chemoprevention of certain malignancies and in the management of several inflammatory dermatoses including lupus erythematosus and lichen planus.

The most common use of oral retinoids in pediatric dermatology is by far isotretinoin therapy for severe acne vulgaris. Isotretinoin is usually initiated at doses of 0.5–1.0mg/kg/day, while some experts recommend starting at lower doses especially in males with severe nodulocystic acne at risk for development of acne fulminans. This latter condition may be precipitated rarely with isotretinoin therapy. The average treatment course is approximately 20 weeks; however, more recalcitrant acne may require several additional months of isotretinoin therapy especially when lower doses are initiated and increased gradually as tolerated. Some experts advocate continuing therapy until a cumulative dose of 120mg/kg has been given.[321] Initial improvement is usually observed within 8 weeks of therapy.

While acitretin therapy is approved for the treatment of psoriasis in adults, it is to be reserved for the management of severe subtypes including erythrodermic psoriasis, generalized pustular psoriasis, severe plaque-type psoriasis, and severe recalcitrant psoriasis. In an analysis of 385 patients with generalized pustular psoriasis, retinoid therapy proved to be superior to methotrexate, cyclosporine, and oral psoralen plus ultraviolet A therapy.[550] Adult doses are usually initiated at 25mg/day of acitretin and often maintained between 20–75mg/day.[321] Once the psoriasis is well controlled, attempts can be made to gradually taper acitretin doses to as low as 10–25mg daily or every other day.

While not FDA approved for treatment of disorders of cornification, after acne and psoriasis this is the next most common indication for retinoid therapy. For many years etretinate was successsfully used in the treatment of the ichthyoses, especially lamellar ichthyosis. Etretinate was subsequently replaced by acitretin therapy and doses of 0.5 to 1.0mg/kg/day result in significant clinical improvement, usually apparent within 2 months of therapy. One must consider the potential benefits of therapy versus the potential for adverse effects in the pediatric population. Treatment should be reserved for more severe ichthyosis subtypes and the lowest dose possible should be used for the shortest practical period of time.

Ruiz-Maldonado reported the Mexican experience with treatment of children with severe keratinization disorders with etretinate.[551] Thirty–nine patients were treated, six of whom had long-term follow-up of 8–9 years. These six patients were started on oral retinoids between 2.75 and 11 years of age and were treated with doses between 0.5 and 1.0mg/kg/day. Therapy was continuous except for interruptions of no longer than 3 months (no longer than 12 months total) While etretinate was well tolerated in most patients, skeletal side effects were observed in all six patients on prolonged treatment. In two of the six patients, osseous reabsorption of the distal phalanges was observed after 8 and 9 years of retinoid therapy. Skeletal abnor-

malities were usually asymptomatic and not associated with any laboratory alterations of calcium, phosphate, or alkaline phosphatase. The authors recommend radiology studies of the long bone epiphysis yearly during the duration of retinoid therapy and close monitoring of the growth parameters in the pediatric population.[551]

More recently, (1996) Lacour and colleagues[552] published the English experience with acitretin therapy in children with disorders of keratinization. They had treated 46 children since 1992; 29 of these patients were treated for disorders of keratinization while the remaining patients were treated for psoriasis (16) and extensive viral warts (1). Analysis of these 29 patients revealed the mean optimal acetretin dosage was 0.47mg/kg/day ± 0.17mg/kg/day. They did not observe significantly different dosing requirements between the treated disorders including lamellar ichthyosis (9), non-bullous ichthyosiform erythroderma (5), bullous ichthyosiform erythroderma (4) or Sjögren–Larsson syndrome. Therapy was well tolerated and 26 of the 29 children were reported to demonstrate considerable clinical improve-ment on retinoid therapy. The most commonly observed side effects were mucocutanous (see below) in nature with only 1 patient developing lipid abnormalities and 4 patients with elevation in liver enzymes, not requiring discontinuation of therapy. The only patient with Netherton's syndrome worsened significantly while on acitretin. These authors conclude that for treatment of disorders of keratinization, the optimal starting dose of acitretin is 0.5mg/kg/day.

ADVERSE EFFECTS

Mucocutaneous side effects are by far the most commonly experienced adverse effects with the oral retinoids. Virtually all patients experience chapped lips and some degree of dry skin. Nose bleeds are observed in approximately one-half of patients and over 40% experience dry eyes at some point during therapy.[553] Other mucocutaneous effects include hair loss, nail fragility, pyogenic granulomas, excessive granulation tissue blepharoconjunctivitis, increased colonization with Staphylococcus aureus,[554,555] and paronychia. Some experts advocate more aggressive antimicrobial therapy in patients with cardiac valve disease who develop staphylococcal infections while on oral retinoids.

Musculoskeletal effects are also commonly observed with oral retinoid therapy. Myalgias are reported in approximately 15% of patients treated with isotretinoin, most often in patients with increased physical exertion. While elevations in creatine phosphokinase levels have been observed, rhabdomyolysis has not been reported.

While neurologic side effects are uncommonly observed, all patients treated with oral retinoids should be counseled regarding the small risk of pseudotumor cerebri and depression. Mild headaches are not unusual with isotretinoin, especially early during the treatment course but accompanying symptoms of nausea, vomiting or visual changes should raise suspicion of possible pseudotumor cerebri. The concomitant use of isotetinoin with tetracycline, doxycycline or minocycline may increase the patient's risk of this unusual complication.[556]

The issue of isotretinoin related depression has received much media attention in recent years and its true association remains controversial. Since its initial marketing in 1982 until May 2000, the FDA received 37 reports of suicide in patients in the United States receiving isotretinoin therapy. An additional 110 patients were hospitalized for suicidal attempt or ideation or depression. There were also 284 reports of depression which did not result in hospitalization. Based on this reporting system, isotretinoin is ranked within the top 10 of FDA approved drugs for number of reports of suicide attempts and depression.[557]

550. Ozawa A, Ohkido M, Haruki Y et al. (1999) Treatment of generalized pustular psoriasis: a muticenter study in Japan. **J Dermatol** 26:141–149.
551. Ruiz-Maldonado R, Tamayo L (1987) Retinoids in disoorders of keratinization: their use in children. **Dermatologica** 175(Suppl. 1):125–132.
552. Lacour M, Mehta-Nikhar B, Arhertan DJ, Harper JI (1996) An appraisal of acitretin therapy in children with inherited disorders of keratinization. **Br J Dermatol** 134(6):1023–1029.
553. Mclane J (2001) Analysis of common side effects of isotretinoin. **J Am Acad Dermatol** 45:S188–194.
554. Lianou P, Bassaris H, Vlachodimitropoulos D et al. (1989) Acitretin induces an increased adherence of S. aureus to epithelial cells. **Acta Derm Venereol** 69:330–332.
555. Williams RE, Doherty VR, Perkins W et al. (1992) Staphylococcus aureus and intranasal mupirocin in patients receiving isotretinoin for acne. **Br J Dermatol** 126:362–366.
556. Andersen WK, Feingold DS (1995) Adverse drug interactions clinically important for the dermatologist. **Arch Dermatol** 131:468–473.
557. Wysowski DK, Pitts M, Beitz J (2001) An analysis of reports of depression and suicide in patients treated with isotretinoin. **J Am Acad Dermatol** 45:515–519.

However, there have been no large comparative trials which substantiate this association. In fact, the Jick study, a large Canadian population-based cohort study, revealed no statistically significant increase in the relative risk of depression and suicide in acne patients treated with isotretinoin as compared to those receiving systemic antibiotic therapy for acne. Nor were significant differences noted in patients before, during, or following isotretinoin therapy using patients as their own comparison.[558]

Most likely, depression is an idiosyncratic reaction which may occur in a small minority of patients receiving isotretinoin therapy. Nevertheless, it is critical to educate patients and families about this rare adverse effect and screen for its development during and following retinoid therapy. In fact, a standardized consent form has been created by the drug manufacturer (Roche) and should be obtained before initiating therapy in all patients. Patients with a personal or family history of serious depression may have an increased risk of depression during isotretinoin therapy.

Ocular side effects are a serious and potentially irreversible complication of isotretoin therapy. Retinoid related ocular changes include abnormal meibomian gland secretion, blepharoconjunctivitis, corneal opacities, decreased dark adaptation, decreased tolerance of contact lenses, reduced vision, keratitis, myopia, meibomian gland atrophy, photophobia, ocular sicca and increased tear osmolarity. It is also likely that a reversible decrease in color vision and permanent loss of dark adaptation may occur secondary to isotretinoin therapy.[559] Because night blindness may be an irreversible complication, it is prudent to discontinue therapy at the first sign of decreased dark adaptation and seek ophthalmologic consultation. Ophthalmologic evaluation for decreased night vision should include dark-adaptation testing and consideration of an electroretinogram or electrooculogram.[541]

Alterations in lipid levels are the most commonly observed laboratory abnormality in patients receiving retinoid therapy. Triglyceride levels are elevated in one-half of patients taking isotretinoin, etretinate or acetretin while 30% of patients experience elevation in cholesterol levels. These alteration are observed more frequently with isotretinoin than with etretinate or acetretin; however lipid abnormalities are seen even more commonly with the third generation retinoid bexarotene. Fortunately, these lipid alterations are reversible upon discontinuation of retinoid therapy. This risk is increased in obese patients and those with a history of diabetes or hyperlipidemia.

While retinoid-induced hepatotoxicity is rare, transient elevation in hepatic transaminase levels are not infrequently observed. These changes are seen more commonly with acitretin (13–16%) and etretinate (20–30%) therapy and are seen in less than 10% of patients receiving isotretinoin (Bexarotene package insert).[546,560,561] Most mild changes will reverse spontaneously despite continuation of retinoid therapy. However, for transaminase elevations of more than 3-fold, retinoid therapy should be promptly discontinued. For elevations of 2- to 3-fold, treatment should be stopped but may be reintroduced at a lower dose upon normalization of laboratory parameters.

Bone effects have been observed with isotretinoin, etretinate, and acitretin therapy.[561A] These skeletal effects can occur with both short- and long-term retinoid therapy and may be irreversible. The most commonly observed retinoid bone toxicities are hyperostotic changes or calcification of tendons and ligaments which resemble changes observed in the condition diffuse idiopathic skeletal hyperostosis (DISH). DISH is characterized by the development of osteophytes and bony bridge formation that occurs most commonly in the spine. In addition, tendons and ligaments may undergo calcification and bone formation. Risk of DISH-like changes are probably greater in elderly patients and those with arthritis.

A report from 1983 raised concern about the risk of hyperostosis with long-term isotretinoin therapy. Four patients receiving isotretinoin from 2 to 6 years at doses of 3–4mg/kg/day developed hyperostosis.[562] The following year four of eight patients receiving 2 years of isotretinoin developed osteophytes at two or more vertebral levels as compared with 9% of age-matched controls. The incidence was only 11% (4 of 37) in those receiving 2 years of etretinate therapy. In a prospective study in 1984, baseline radiographs were obtained prior to initiating therapy with isotretinoin. In patients with disorders of cornification receiving an average dose of 2mg/kg/day, two of eight patients had hyperostosis on radiographs obtained after 6 months of therapy while hyperostosis was observed radiographically in six of eight patients after 1 year of isotretinoin. When the films obtained after 6 months of retinoid therapy were reexamined retrospectively, subtle early changes of hyperostosis were noted in an additional three patients. These findings suggest that bone changes can be seen after only 6 months of isotretinoin therapy.[563]

This leads to the question of whether there is a substantial risk of DISH-like skeletal changes in the doses and duration of therapy used to treat acne patients. In a prospective study of acne patients treated with 1–2mg/kg/day of isotretinoin, 10 patients developed "minimal spinal hyperostosis."[564] Even very low-dose isotretinoin therapy may result in bone toxicity over time. Of 139 patients receiving only 10mg/day of isotretinoin over 3 years it was noted that 40% of patients (vs. 18% in the placebo group) experienced progression of existing hyperostosis of the vertebra while 8% of treated patients were noted to develop new sites of hyperostosis. The clinical significance of these radiographic findings remains unknown.

Long-term etretinate therapy likewise appears to carry a risk of hyperostosis. DiGiovanna and colleagues found radiographic evidence of calcification of the tendons and ligaments at extraspinal locations in 84% of 38 patients treated with etretinate for an average of 5 years at doses of 0.8mg/kg/day on average. The radiographic findings did not correlate well with the location of symptoms. Since etretinate is converted to acitretin upon ingestion, it is likely that therapy with acitretin will result in the same bone toxicity.

Because hyperostotic changes may precede retinoid therapy, clinicians should consider obtaining baseline X-rays of the wrists, ankles, or thoracic spine prior to initiating long-term therapy. Yearly follow-up films may be helpful in monitoring for hyperostotic changes and radiographic studies should be obtained on significantly symptomatic joints.

While hyperostosis is of greater risk in older patients, children have the unique risk of premature epiphyseal closure. There have been only a handful of cases reported with both isotretinoin and etretinate.[541,565–567] This complicaton has been observed with prolonged and very high-dose therapy and closure is usually partial. Height and knee X-ray should be monitored closely in children treated with high doses of retinoids for long periods of time.

Osteoporosis is yet another skeletal concern with etretinate therapy. In addition to anecdotal reports of retinoid induced bone demineralization and osteoporosis, a study of 15 patients receiving an average of 10 years' treatment with etretinate therapy showed a decrease in bone mineral density as

558. Jick SS, Kremers HM, Vasilakis-Scaramozza C (2000) Isotretinoin use and risk of depression, psychotic symptoms, suicide, and attempted suicide. **Arch Dermatol** 136:1231–1236.
559. Fraunfelder FT, Fraunfelder FW, Edwards R (2001) Ocular side effects possibly associated with isotretinoin usage. **Am J Ophthalmol** 132:299–305.
560. Bexarotene (Targretin) package insert and product monograph. San Diego, CA. Ligand Pharmaceuticals, 2000.
561. David M, Hodak E, Lowe NJ (1988) Adverse effects of retinoids. **Med Toxicol** 3:273–288.
561A. DiGiovanna JJ (2001) Isotretinoin effects on bone. **J Am Acad Dermatol** 45:S176–182.
562. Pittsley RA, Yoder FW (1983) Retinoid hyperostosis. Skeletal toxicity associated with long-term administration of 13-cis-retinoic acid for refractory ichthyosis. **N Engl J Med** 308(17):1012–1014.

563. Pennes DR, Ellis CN, Madison KC, Voorhees JJ, Martel W (1984) Early skeletal hyperostoses secondary to 13-cis-retinoic acid. **AJR Am J Roentgenol** 142:979–983.
564. Kilcoyne RF, Cope R, Cunningham W et al. (1986) Minimal spinal hyperostosis with low-dose isotretinoin therapy. **Invest Radiol** 21:41–44.
565. Nishimura G, Mugishima H, Hirao J et al. (1997) Generalized metaphyseal modification with cone-shaped epiphyses following long-term administration of 13-cis-retinoic acid. **Eur J Pediatr** 156:432–435.
566. Prendiville J, Bingham EA, Burrows D (1986) Premature epiphyseal closure – a complication of etretinate therapy in children. **J Am Acad Dermatol** 15:1259–1262.
567. Milstone LM, McGuire J, Ablow RC (1982) Premature epiphyseal closure in a child receiving oral 13-cis-retinoic acid. **J Am Acad Dermatol** 7:663–666.

compared with age and sex-matched controls as well as with an isotretinoin treated group.[568] One final skeletal abnormality reported with vitamin A toxicity as well as in children receiving long-term etretinate therapy for disorders of cornification is the radiologic finding of slender long bones.[568]

In summary, patients receiving oral retinoids are at risk for several skeletal complications including hyperostosis and DISH-like changes, osteoporosis, slender long bones and premature closure of the epiphysis. These risks appear to be greatest with higher doses and more prolonged therapy. Individual risk factors including patient sex, age, medication history, and concurrent medical problems should all be taken into consideration when deciding how to monitor for potential bone toxicity.

Of greatest concern with retinoid therapy is its teratogenicity. Retinoids have known toxic effects on cephalic neural crest development during the first trimester, especially weeks 3 to 6.[561] Some of the more common targets of teratogenicity include the cardiovascular system with resultant congenital heart defects as well as many craniofacial abnormalities. Ocular, auditory, central nervous system, and bone abnormalities are other common sites of retinoid birth defects. In fact, these congenital defects are seen in almost one-half of full-term pregnancies with a known first trimester exposure to retinoids. Spontaneous abortions and stillbirths are also seen more commonly in pregnancies with retinoid exposure.[541]

For these reasons, it is imperative that women of child-bearing potential are appropriately counseled regarding the importance of contraception and that two reliable measures of contraception are used in all sexually active women. The manufacturer (Roche) has implemented a comprehensive pregnancy prevention program which has been in place for several years yet there are continued reports of unplanned pregnancies during retinoid therapy, especially with isotretinoin. The manufacturer's program (the SMART program) has recently been modified and all prescribers are to have company distributed stickers that indicate that the prescriber and the patient have been

TABLE 4.35   Retinoid drug interactions

Drugs with potential to increase retinoid levels/toxicity	Drugs with potential to decrease retinoid levels via CYP3A4 induction
• Vitamin A • Tetracycline family • Gemfibrozil • Macrolides, azoles, other CYP3A4 inhibitors	Antituberculosis drugs • Rifampin • Rifabutin Anticonvulsants • Phenobarbital • Phenytoin • Carbamazepine
Drug levels which may be increased by retinoid treatment	**Drug levels which may be decreased by retinoid therapy**
Cyclosporine	Progestin-only contraceptives

Adapted from Table 13-E, Retinoid drug interactions (Wolverton 2001).[321]

TABLE 4.34   Laboratory/radiographic retinoid monitoring guidelines

Baseline	Follow-up
Laboratory • Pregnancy tests (2) within 1 week of initiating therapy for women of childbearing potential • CBC/platelets • Renal function tests (BUN/creatinine) • Liver profile (AST, ALT, alkaline phosphatase, bilirubin) • Fasting lipid profile (cholesterol, HDL, LDL, triglycerides) • Optional urinalysis	*Laboratory* • Monthly serum/urine pregnancy test • Monthly CBC with platelets • Monthly renal function Consider checking every other month if stable • Monthly liver profile (AST, ALT) • Monthly fasting lipid studies (cholesterol, triglycerides)
X-rays • Consider X-rays of wrists, ankles, knees or thoracic spine if long-term therapy anticipated	*X-rays* • Consider yearly radiographs of wrists, ankles, knees or thoracic spine with long-term retinoid therapy. • Radiographs of symptomatic joints

CBC, complete blood count; BUN, blood urea nitrogen; AST, aspartate aminotransferase; ALT, alanine aminotransferase.

educated on the pertinent steps of pregnancy prevention and that they are compliant with the manufacturer's contraception recommendations. This includes obtaining two negative pregnancy tests within the week of initiating isotretinoin therapy. Isotretinoin therapy should be initiated on the second day of the next normal menstrual cycle or more than 11 days after the last unprotected sexual intercourse. Pregnancy tests should be followed monthly during therapy.

Appropriate contraceptive measures should be initiated at least one month prior to retinoid therapy and throughout the treatment regimen. Contraception needs to be continued for an additional month after cessation of therapy with isotretinoin or bexarotene. However, with acetretin therapy contraception is required for three years after cessation of therapy due to the conversion of acitretin to etretinate with alcohol consumption.

While the retinoids have been found to be effective in the treatment of many dermatologic disorders, they should be used judiciously. Due to the extensive side effects associated with retinoid therapy, the clinical monitoring guidelines detailed in Table (4.34) should be adhered to closely. In addition, concurrent therapy with the medications listed in Table (4.35) should be avoided to minimize the risk of a serious drug interaction.

COSMETIC TREATMENT

Zoe Draelos

Cosmetic treatment serves two purposes in pediatric patients: adornment and camouflage. This section addresses both issues by focusing on the dermatologic problems associated with cosmetic use in the female pediatric patient and the use of camouflaging cosmetics to minimize the appearance of acne, vitiligo, pigmentation anomalies, tumors, and hair loss.

COSMETICS FOR CHILDREN

Cosmetics for children can be divided into the following product categories: aesthetic, personal grooming, and colored. Aesthetic products are those designed to impart a taste or fragrance to the skin, while personal grooming aids are designed to impart a feeling of cleanliness. Finally, colored products are designed to adorn to the face, eyes, and lips.

568. DiGiovanna JJ, Sollitto RB, Abangan DL, Steinberg SM, Reynolds JC (1995) Osteoporosis is a toxic effect of long-term etretinate therapy (see comments). **Arch Dermatol** 131:1263–1267.

AESTHETIC PRODUCTS

Aesthetic products, designed to impart taste or fragrance to the body, are popular among pre-adolescent girls, as they are a combination of candy and perfume with youthful appeal. The most popular of these products is lip gloss, designed to impart shine and taste to the lips. Lip gloss is a common cause of vermilion border comedones, irritant contact dermatitis, or allergic contact dermatitis in young girls due to the essential flavoring oils combined with petrolatum and mineral oil.[569]

PERSONAL GROOMING PRODUCTS

Personal grooming products for children include soaps, deodorants, antiperspirants, shampoos, conditioners, and styling aids. In most cases, these products are identical in formulation to those marketed for adults, except the packaging appears to be more colorful, and the products generally have a youthful fragrance.

COLORED PRODUCTS

Colored cosmetics are available for young girls to adorn the face, eyelids, eyelashes, lips and cheeks. Most pre-adolescent and early adolescent girls do not want to "look like they wear makeup" but still want to go through the motions of applying cosmetics to their face.

Popular cosmetics in this age group include transparent lipsticks and lip glosses, transparent facial color gels, rouges, and mascaras. Transparent facial color gels and teenage rouges are similar in formulation except that color gels are more lightly colored for all-over application to the face, while the rouge is brightly colored and is only applied to the upper cheeks. Both contain a polymer to which a synthetic stain is added. The product must be applied evenly and quickly to avoid streaking; unfortunately, it stains everything it contacts, including fingertips.

Mascaras for young girls are identical in formulation to those for women except that colors besides the traditional black, brown, and navy are available. Yellow, orange, red, pink, purple, and royal blue mascaras are designed to coordinate with clothing.

COSMETICS SELECTION

Cosmetic products selected for the pediatric patient should ideally be hypoallergenic, noncomedogenic, and nonacneigenic. There are no industry standards regarding product testing prior to placing these labels on a given formulation. Unfortunately, these words must be viewed only as marketing claims.

It is inaccurate to assume that a cosmetic lacking any of the ingredients on standard dermatologic patch testing trays is hypoallergenic. Furthermore, it is inaccurate to assume that a cosmetic lacking any substances found on a standard list of comedogenic chemicals is noncomedogenic. The entire finished cosmetic, along with the concentration of individual ingredients, must be evaluated in statistically significant use testing.[332] Nevertheless, some valuable general cosmetic recommendations can be given to pediatric patients with dermatitis or acne.

DERMATITIS (TABLE 4.36)

Dermatitic skin is more susceptible to both allergic and irritant contact dermatitis than healthy skin because of stratum corneum barrier deficits. Pediatric patients should be discouraged from wearing cosmetics until the skin is completely healed. Complete healing may require an additional 2 weeks beyond the time cutaneous signs of inflammation have resolved.

TABLE 4.36   Cosmetics and skin care product recommendations for the pediatric atopic patient

1. Cleanser: Select a lipid-free cleanser without detergents to provide mild cleansing morning and evening.
2. Moisturizer: Select a bland cream facial moisturizer without fragrance or other additives.
3. Facial foundation: Select a moisturizing facial foundation with mineral oil.
4. Colored cosmetics: Select fragrance free powdered colored cosmetics for their low concentration of preservatives in light colors to minimize pigment concentration in a matte finish.

Cosmetic selection in pediatric patients with eczema or atopic dermatitis should avoid fragrances, the most common cause of cutaneous problems in cosmetics. Products should be labeled "fragrance free" or "without perfume" and not "unscented," as these products may contain a masking scent. Additionally, formulations containing preservatives of low allergenicity, such as the parabens, should be selected over preparations with formaldehyde, formaldehyde releasers (quaternium-15 and imidazolidinyl urea), and cutaneous irritants (Kathon CG). It may be wise to avoid lanolin and its derivatives as well.

ACNE (TABLE 4.37)

Pediatric patients with acne should be encouraged to avoid thick creamy facial cosmetics, which are generally high in oils and petrolatum that may be comedogenic. This means cream facial foundations and cream rouges should be avoided. Liquid facial foundations containing silicones, such as cyclomethicone or dimethicone, are an excellent choice, as these oils are nongreasy, hypoallergenic, noncomedogenic, and nonacneigenic. All other colored facial cosmetics should be powdered.

It is important to emphasize to the pediatric patient that cosmetics should only be worn when necessary and always removed prior to sleeping. To prevent secondary infection, cosmetics should not be shared with friends or other family members.

There are a variety of acne treatment cosmetics designed to prevent and treat comedonal acne that may be of value. These products contain 2% or less salicylic acid, a potent comedolytic and United State, over-the-counter drug monographed ingredient. Two percent salicylic acid is incorporated into face washes, astringents, moisturizers, and facial foundations, and can exfoliate both

---

TABLE 4.37   Cosmetics and skin care product recommendations for the pediatric acne patient

1. Cleanser: Select a 2% salicylic acid-containing face wash for morning cleansing as a comedolytic. Use a facial exfoliating cloth to remove cosmetics for bedtime cleansing. The goal is to achieve cleansing without irritation.
2. Moisturizer: Select an oil-free moisturizer containing zinc oxide to provide broad-spectrum sun protection and absorb excess sebum.
3. Facial foundation: Select oil-free facial foundations with a water and silicone base, which are noncomedogenic and nonacnegenic.
4. Colored cosmetics: Select powdered blush and eye shadow, pencil lipsticks, and avoid flavored cosmetics to minimize oils and comedone formation.

---

569. Benmaman O, Sanchez JL (1988) Treatment and camouflaging of pigmentary disorders. *Clin Dermatol* 6:50.

TABLE 4.38 Cosmetic application for cutaneous defects

Cutaneous defect	Color anomaly	Color of corrective cosmetic	Comments
Portwine stain	Purplish red	Green	Green cream complementary-colored cosmetic applied over red lesion
Acne	Red	Tan	Tan coverstick applied to obscure underlying acne lesion
Vitiligo	White	Brown	Water proof surgical brown makeup applied to conceal underlying hypopigmentation
Hyperpigmentation	Brown	Light brown	Skin colored water resistant cream makeup to blend hyperpigmentation

the skin surface and within the pores due to its phenolic, hydrophobic nature. These treatment products can be added to benzoyl peroxide or retinoid therapy to accelerate comedone resolution. Unfortunately, many acne treatment products produce xerosis and the resultant unattractive peeling of the facial skin. This can be avoided through the use of zinc oxide-based oil-free moisturizers that provide broad-spectrum sun protection while smoothing the facial skin scale.

SKIN CAMOUFLAGE TECHNIQUES

Cosmetics can also be valuable in the pediatric patient to camouflage skin deformities of both color and contour. These deformities may be due to congenital anomalies (e.g., port-wine stain, extensive nevocytic nevus), hyperpigmentation, vitiligo, or acne lesions (Table 4.38).

COLOR DEFORMITIES

Color deformities can be camouflaged through the use of two differnt cosmetics: opaque cover foundations and color correctors. Opaque cover foundations provide complete masking of any underlying pigment abnormality, while color correctors are thin lotions tinted in a color that is complimentary to the lesion.

Opaque cover foundations

Opaque cover foundations are valuable in covering skin discolorations, such as congenital nevi, nevus flammeus, and vitiligo. Any colored defect can be effectively camouflaged, as none of the underlying skin can be seen.[570] Table 4.39 lists some of the manufacturers of surgical camouflage products.

Opaque cover foundations are available for both the face and body in a variety of types. Some are thick waterproof creams in several standard colors that must be mixed to the patient's skin color, while others are available in tubes or sticks of premixed colors. Some are not waterproof and are available in a compressed compact that is wiped with a damp sponge.

Formulation considerations

The formulation of all waterproof cover products is similar. Generally, mineral oil blended with petrolatum, lanolin oil, or other emollients is mixed with a combination of waxes to achieve the final product consistency. Titanium dioxide pigmented with iron oxides provides both coverage and color. Because of the high oil content of these products, they are recommended for children with normal to dry skin.

Children with acne and/or oily complexions should be advised to use a pancake-style cover cosmetic that is mixed with water prior to facial application with a sponge. This product consists of mineral and vegetable oils combined with triethanolamine soap as an emulsifier. Titanium dioxide pigmented with iron oxides again provides the coverage and color. Both talc

and titanium dioxide provide oil control required for long wear on an oily complexion, but they also leave the face with a dull or matte finish.

Products appropriate for covering pigmentation defects on the body are also available. The easiest products to apply are creams that can be squeezed from a tube. These products are thinner than the facial products and spread better over larger areas. They may incorporate both zinc oxide and titanium

TABLE 4.39 Camouflage cosmetics manufacturers

Camouflage cosmetic	Address
Corrective Concepts	Pattee Products European Crossroads 2829 West Northwest Highway Dallas, TX 75220
Coverette	Ben Nye Company, Inc. 5935 Bowcroft Street Los Angeles, CA 90016
Covermark	Lyda O'Leary 1 Anderson Avenue Moonachie, NJ 07074
Cover Tone	Fashion Fair Cosmetics 820 South Michigan Avenue Chicago, IL 60605
Cream Makiage	Il-Makiage P.O. Box 1064 Long Island City, NY 11101
Dermablend	Dermablend Corrective Cosmetics P.O. Box 3008 Lakewood, NJ 08701
Dermaceal	Joe Blasco Cosmetics 1708 Hillhurst Avenue Hollywood, CA 90027
Dermacolor	Kryolan Corporation 132 Ninth Street San Francisco, CA 94103
Natural Cover	LS Cosmetics P.O. Box 32203 Baltimore, MD 21208
Veil	Atelier Esthetique Suite 209 386 Park Avenue South New York, NY 10016

(Adapted from Draelos,[570] with permission.)

570. Draelos ZK (1990) Cosmetics in Dermatology. Edinburgh: Churchill Livingstone, p. 30.

dioxide for coverage, iron pigments for color, methylcellulose or other waxes for viscosity, and glycerin or other nonevaporating substances for increased adherence of the product to the skin.

Application technique

It takes practice to develop application skill and speed with opaque cover cosmetics. Application can be facilitated by selecting the proper color, which minimizes the need for blending.

The cream opaque cover foundations are firm and should be warmed in the hand before application. The cosmetic is best applied with a sponge or the fingertips and dabbed, not rubbed, onto the face. Dabbing will ensure that the product is pushed into the pores and allows more even application. Rubbing the foundation, especially over scarred areas, will remove the cover cosmetic.[571]

The cover cosmetic should be allowed to set 5min on the skin prior to finishing with a loose translucent powder. Powder should be pressed, not rubbed, into the foundation with a puff or sponge and allowed to set 5min. Excess powder can be dusted away with a fluffy powder brush. The powder is necessary to set the foundation and improve waterproof characteristics.

TABLE 4.40   Camouflaging techniques for pigmentary abnormalities

Color of lesion	Example lesions	Color corrector hue
Red	Nevus flammeus, cherry angioma, capillary hemangioma, etc.	Green
Blue	Laser purpura, venous lake, blue nevus, etc.	Peach
Purple	Postsurgical purpura, mature nevus flammeus, etc.	Greenish yellow
Yellow	Hemosiderin staining, jaundice, xanthomas, etc.	Purple
Brown	Nevi, nevus spilus, postinflammatory hyperpigmentation, etc.	White
White	Vitiligo, mature scar tissue, etc.	Brown

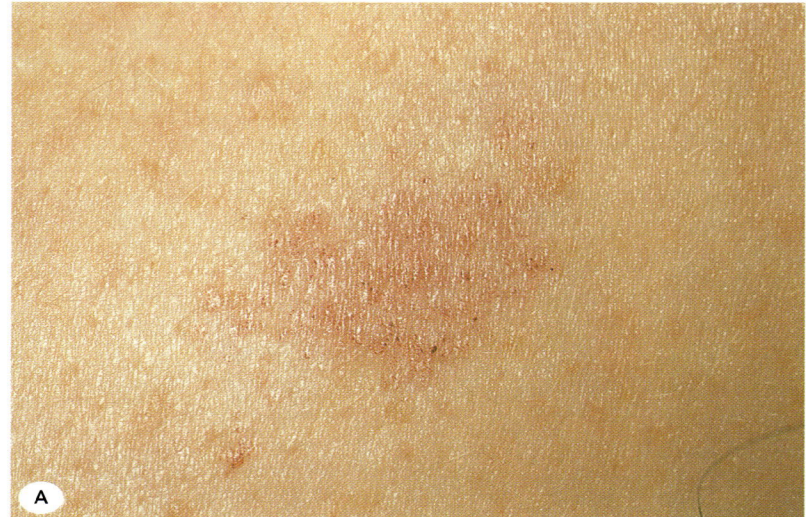

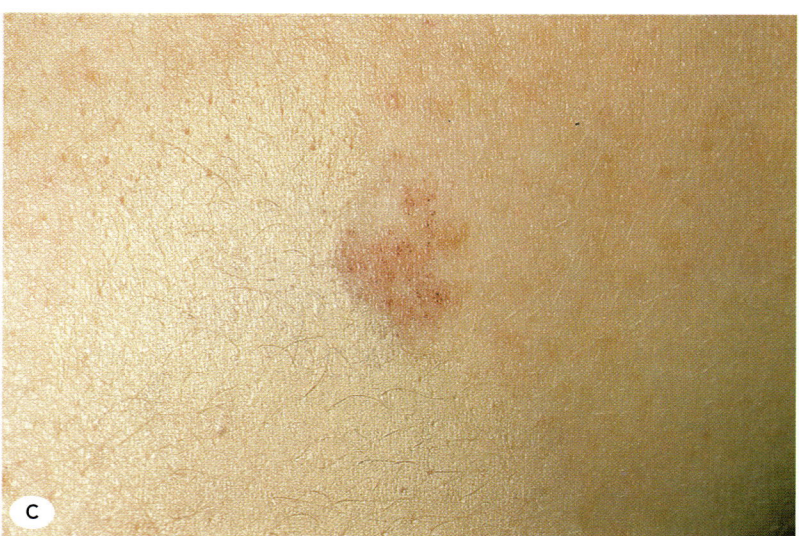

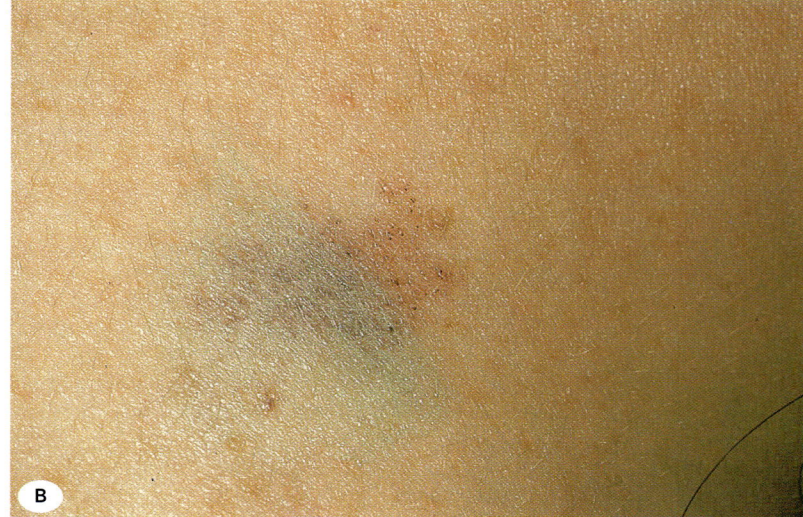

Fig. 4.2   (A) A green color corrector can be used to camouflage reddish lesions of the skin such as seen in nevus flammeus. To demonstrate the technique, only the lower part of the lesion is camouflaged. (B) A green lotion or cream is dabbed over the lesion, providing the complementary color to red. (C) Lastly, a brown facial foundation is applied to complete the camouflage technique. This technique can be used on any body area.

Since cover cosmetics are designed for long wear, they can also be difficult to remove. The cosmetic should be removed completely prior to bed each night or when it is no longer necessary to wear the cosmetic. Most products have a specially designed cleanser for their removal.

Color correctors

Another method of camouflaging color abnormalities of the skin is the use of color correctors. Color correctors are thin lotions selected in a color that is complementary to the skin defect (Table 4.40). For example, a red nevus

571. Helland JR, Schneider MR (1985) Special Features Technique for One-of-a-Kind Beauty. M Evans, New York, p. 41.

flammeus can be camouflaged with a standard nonsurgical moderate to heavy coverage facial foundation, if a green-colored corrector lotion or cream is applied prior to the foundation (Fig. 4.2). The combination of the green-colored corrector and red skin lesion yields a brown hue that can be covered easily, eliminating the need for a surgical cover product. Further more, yellow pigmentation present following hematoma resolution can be blended with a complimentary colored purple foundation, also to yield brown tones. Bluish bruising, commonly seen following certain types of laser surgery, can be camouflaged through the use of a peach or orange-colored corrector.

Sometimes color correction must be used in conjunction with medical treatment such as is the case in the pediatric patient with hyperpigmentation (Table 4.41).

CONTOUR DEFORMITIES

Contour deformities represent areas of cutaneous atrophy (e.g., morphea, facial hemiatrophy, depressed surgical scar) or hypertrophy (e.g., hypertrophic scar, exophytic nevus). Usually, most cutaneous defects contain both contour and color deformities, necessitating the need to combine both camouflaging techniques.

Camouflaging of contour deformities is based on the principle that lighter colors appear to project, while darker colors appear to recede. For example, skin affected by morphea or hemiatrophy appears to be darker than the surrounding unaffected skin, but adequate lighting to eliminate shadows may show that no color defect is present. The darkness is simply due to the presence of shadows from the atrophy. This can be corrected by applying a lighter shade of powdered blush or cream rouge to the atrophic skin, thereby preventing shadows.[572,573]

Similarly, hypertrophic scars may appear lighter than the surrounding skin due to the absence of shadows. A darker shade or powdered blush or cream rouge can minimize the appearance of the skin protuberance.

HAIR CAMOUFLAGE TECHNIQUES

Camouflaging hair loss in children due to congenital anomaly, surgical scarring, or alopecia areata presents a challenge because of high activity level of children and their inability to sit still for long periods while a hair prosthesis is attached. A decision must be made by the parents and the child as to which prosthesis, if any, is most appropriate. It is also important to determine whether the hair loss bothers mostly the child or the parent, thus illuminating any underlying motives.

TABLE 4.41   Cosmetics and skin care product recommendations for the pediatric patient with cutaneous hyperpigmentation

1. Cleanser: Select a foaming face wash to remove oils prior to medication and cosmetic application.
2. Medication: 3–4% hydroquinone cream, 0.025% tretinoin cream, 1% hydrocortisone cream applied in succession to areas of hyperpigmentation morning and bedtime.
3. Moisturizer: No moisturizer may be necessary after using the 1% hydrocortisone cream in a moisturizing base.
4. Facial foundation: Apply a liquid oil-containing facial foundation to the entire face followed by application of a powder facial foundation to match the normal skin color.
5. Colored cosmetics: Liberally brush light pink powder matte-finish blush on the central forehead, nasal tip, central chin, and lateral cheekbones to minimize the dyspigmentation while maintaining a youthful face.

Methods of camouflaging hair loss include wigs, hairpieces, hair integration systems, hair additions, and scalp coloring. The replacement method selected depends on the age of the child, extent of hair loss, permanence of hair loss, and financial resources.

WIGS

Wigs are the least time-consuming method of camouflaging scalp hair loss in children. A wig is designed to cover the entire scalp and can be purchased through a wig shop or custom made. Mass-produced wigs are available with synthetic fibers or natural human hairs sewn to a fenestrated cap meshwork that is fit to the scalp with adjustable elastic bands. Clips are used to fasten the wig to any remaining hair. Table 4.42 lists several wig manufacturers and their company addresses in the USA.

Children who have complete hair loss that is likely to be longstanding may have difficulty keeping a standard wig in place. Vacuum wig prostheses provide a more secure attachment. This custom-made wig is constructed by making a plaster mold of the scalp that is transformed into an acrylic piece to which hair is glued. The accurate fit between the acrylic mold and the scalp provides a secure attachment. These wigs are generally cut and styled on the child's head, giving a more natural appearance than mass-produced wigs. Custom-made wigs are expensive and must be remade as the child's head enlarges.

HAIRPIECES

Hairpieces do not cover the entire scalp and are designed only to supplement localized hair loss. Premade standard hair pieces are available for individuals with a mature head size, but they are not appropriate for younger children. By contrast, custom-made hair pieces can be designed in any style required. The hairpiece can cover only the posterior scalp or a localized surgical scar or can reconstruct the entire anterior hairline. The hairpieces, made from synthetic or natural human hair, are attached either through the use of clips or adhesives. Table 4.42 lists some of the manufacturers of hairpieces.

Most children seem to adapt better to a hairpiece emotionally than to a wig, as they are easier to wear and allow any existing hair to be seen. They also permit more flexibility as the child's head enlarges.

HAIR INTEGRATION SYSTEMS

Hair integration is a wig variant employing a custom-made net fit to the entire scalp. Individual synthetic or human hair fibers are then tied to the netting in the appropriate color, curl, and amount.[337] The child then pulls remaining hair through the holes in the net to anchor the hairpiece. This method allows hair to be supplemented more heavily in the areas where needed while providing tremendous flexibility in hairstyle, as well as head circumference.

HAIR ADDITIONS

Hair additions involve the use of existing scalp hair to anchor synthetic or natural human hair fibers. The added fibers may be affixed by braiding, sewing, bonding, or gluing. The attachment method selected depends on the amount of natural hair and the number or length of fibers to be added.[571]

Hair additions are worn continually for a period of 8 weeks, at which time they must be removed. The additions are shampooed along with the child's existing hair using the same cleansing products and cleansing frequency. Many parents are afraid to wash the additions, as they fear that loosening will occur, but good hygiene is important to prevent seborrheic dermatitis and bacterial folliculitis. The main concern with long-term use of hair additions is the development of traction alopecia.

---

572. Draelos ZD (1994) Camouflage cosmetics and techniques. **Cosmetics Toiletries** 109:75.

573. Pivot Point International: Educational brochure: Designing Hair Additions.

TABLE 4.42   Wig and hairpiece manufacturers

Company Name	Address	Comments
American Hairlines	1808 Jerome Avenue Brooklyn, NY 11235	Manufacture medical hair prostheses for adults and children
Editch Imre	8 West 56th Street New York, NY 10024	Manufacture medical hair prostheses for adults and children
Eva Gobor Wigs	55 West 39th Street New York, NY 10018	Sell ready-made synthetic wigs to local wig outlets
Louis Feder	14 East 38th Street New York, NY 10016	Custom-made human hair wigs
Jacques Darcel	50 West 57th Street New York, NY 10019	Custom-styled and ready-made wigs of synthetic and human
Knight and Day Hair Products	P.O. Box 849 Corte Madera, CA 94925	Manufacture custom-made vacuum hair prostheses for adults and children
Nisus Concepts, Inc.	2315 Fairplay Drive Loveland, CO 80538	Manufacture custom-made vacuum hair prostheses for adults and children
Top Priority	174 Fifth Avenue New York, NY 10011	Custom-design and manufacture synthetic wigs and hairpiece for adults and children
The Wig Company	P.O. Box 12950 Pittsburgh, PA 15241	Premade synthetic wigs available for mail order purchase
Wilshire Wigs	13213 Saticyo Street Hollywood, CA 91605	Manufacture synthetic and human premade and custom hairpieces, including eyelashes, eyebrows, and other facial hair

Braiding on the scalp

Braiding on the scalp is performed in rows, also known as "cornrowing." Synthetic or human hair fibers that have been wefted, or sewn together, are affixed with a needle and thread to the braids. This is a rapid method of adding large amounts of hair; however, traction alopecia is a side effect if the hair is braided with excessive tension or if the hair addition is too heavy.

Braiding off the scalp

Braiding off the scalp employs a standard braiding or plaiting technique to which individual synthetic or natural human hair fibers are added. The fibers are attached by working them securely into the braids while leaving the loose ends free to be curled or styled as desired. This method is best for supplementing areas of hair thinning, but it is not appropriate for areas of total loss.

Bonding

Bonding employs a heat gun to bond clumps of synthetic hair fibers to the base of clumps of existing scalp hair. Only a few fibers can be attached at a time due to the weight of the additions. This technique, while popular in adults, is not recommended for children.

Adhesives

Finally, adhesives can be used to attach wefted hair to braids formed on the posterior scalp in concentric arcs, known as "tracks." These tracks serve as anchors to which the added hair is glued with a cold latex-based glue. This method allows the rapid addition of large amounts of synthetic or natural human hair. However, removal of the adhesive from the child's natural hair can be somewhat difficult.

SCALP COLORING

The absence of scalp hair is more obvious in children with dark hair and white scalp skin because of the color contrast. This contrast can be minimized by darkening the scalp in the areas of hair loss with a specially formulated wax crayon. The crayon is water soluble and must be reapplied daily.

SUMMARY

Cosmetics can be used by children for both adornment and camouflage purposes. The physician should be able to identify problems attributable to cosmetic use, such as comedogenicity and contact dermatitis. Furthermore, the physician should be able to provide basic information on the camouflage of cutaneous pigmentation and contour deformities, as well as hair loss abnormalities.

Surgical Techniques

Bari Cunningham and Annette M. Wagner

Dermatologic procedures in children can range from simple cryosurgery of warts to complex excisional surgery and repair. These procedures may be more challenging to perform in children due to their heightened fear, anxiety, and pain perception. The astute physician will tailor his surgical approach to the needs and age of each pediatric patient. Historically, painful procedures were performed on infants without regard to anesthesia or techniques to reduce the perception of pain. This lack of regard for pain control was due to the incorrect belief that infants had limited nerve tract myelinization and no recollection of previous painful experiences. It has now been clearly documented that pain in infants is a fully developed physiologic response due to intact neural circuits leading to predictable hormonal and metabolic responses.[1,2] The ill-prepared child who suffers unnecessary anxiety or pain will likely bear psychological scars that may lead to difficulty in their future dealings with physicians and other paramedical personnel (see Table 5.1). [3] Ensuring a child's positive experience may foster healthy coping skills for future medical procedures.[4,5] To obtain the best results, an extraordinary amount of patience, support, and communication are required to put the child at ease. The use of selected behavioral interventions, sedatives, analgesics, and a thorough understanding of developmental pediatrics will result in pediatric dermatologic procedures which are executed with minimal anxiety and pain.

THE SURGICAL CONSULTATION

The child's initial impressions of the physician begin long before the physician actually meets the patient. The office should be as child centered and "kid friendly" as possible with waiting rooms stocked with toys and reading material for all pediatric ages. Children feel more comfortable in examination rooms which are decorated with bright, friendly colors and juvenile themes.

TABLE 5.1   Factors that may influence children's pain perception

1. Age
2. Cognitive development
3. Fear
4. Anxiety
5. Personal history (eg., prior painful procedures)
6. Family support/interaction
7. Office environment/staff interaction

With permission Current Problems in Dermatology Jan/Feb 1999.

The physician should be conscious of his or her body language and the message it sends to anxious and potentially fearful children. Seating oneself at or below the level of the child is preferred to standing above a frightened child, which can be intimidating and anxiety producing. If possible, small infants and toddlers should be examined while seated in their parent's lap. For self-conscious adolescents, it is often helpful to examine them early in the patient encounter and then allow them to get dressed as soon as the examination is over. This way, patient counseling and discussion can proceed in a more relaxed and comfortable fashion. Additionally, it is important to talk to the patient even if they are young children. It is often helpful to ask them why they came to the dermatologist. Their understanding of the reason for the visit can help to establish how much about the procedure needs to be explained to the child. Allowing the child's input will validate them and their needs.

Age, by necessity, becomes an important factor in considering the proper timing for performing any surgical procedure on a child or adolescent. There are no hard and fast rules regarding the appropriate age at which to safely and efficiently perform surgery under local anesthesia. Some 5-year-olds are ready to cooperate, while the occasional 15-year-old is not. There are, however, tools one can use to assess a child's level of maturity and likelihood of cooperating with a surgical procedure. Much can be concluded from the physician's initial impression and interaction with the child. A child found cowering under the examination table or laying in the fetal position when the dermatologist enters the room is unlikely to cooperate with the requirements of a surgical office procedure without a great deal of effort and coercion. Similarly, specific questions can be helpful in planning one's approach to a procedure with a child. It's often helpful to ask, "If you have a Band-Aid to take off, do you like to do it or do you like Mommy or Daddy to do it? Do you like them to rip it off fast or slowly?" Asking the same type of questions about splinter removal can also help assess the child's nature and appropriate surgical approach.

In addition to evaluating the child's maturity and emotional status, the consultation visit gives the physician the opportunity to observe the parental interaction with the child as well as the emotional state of the parents.[6] It is not uncommon for parents to harbor significant guilt, whether appropriate or not, over their child's surgical problem. Perhaps they feel responsible for something that they did or did not do during the pregnancy that caused their child's current problem, and that they are somehow to blame. These feelings may make the parents unusually anxious and unable to comprehend the therapeutic options available and the relative risks and benefits of each proposed treatment. Parental anxiety can have a profound effect on the fearful child leading to undo stress and poor surgical outcomes. Children use their

1 Anand KJS, Hickey PR (1987) Pain and its effects in the human neonate and fetus. **N Engl J Med** 317:1321–1329.
2 Anand KJS, Jickey PR (1992) Halothane-morphine compared with high dose sufentanil for anesthesia and postoperative analgesia in neonatal cardiac surgery. **N Engl J Med** 326:1–9.
3 Gabriel HP (1997) A practical approach to preparing children for dermatologic surgery. **J Dermatol Surg Oncol** 3:523.
4 Hays RM, Hackworth SR, Speltz ML et al. (1992) Exploration of variables related to children's behavioral distress during electrodiagnosis. **Arch Phys Med Rehabil** 7:1160–1162.
5 Zelter LK, Altman A, Cohen D et al. (1990) Report on the subcommittee on the management of pain associated with procedures in children with cancer. **Pediatrics** 36:826–831.
6 Schechter NL, Bernstein BA, Beck A, Hart L, Scherzer L (1991) Individual differences in children's response to pain: role of temperament and parental characteristics. **Pediatrics** 87(2):171–177.

parents as vital cues for their behavior. Children of highly anxious mothers are similarly less relaxed during procedures than children of calm mothers.[7] Excessive apologies, reassurance and criticism from parents are associated with increased distress for the child undergoing a medical procedure[8] and should be discouraged. On the other hand, parents who understand the medical necessity of the procedure and act accordingly can be a tremendous help for the fearful child.

It is often reassuring to the patient to review the procedure, step by step, on the initial consultation visit. When explaining a procedure to a child it is crucial that enough time is taken to properly prepare them for the impending events. The extra minute or two taken to explain all of the necessary elements of a procedure can save a tremendous amount of time overall and avoid the need for excessive bargaining on the part of the physician and parent. The child should always be involved in the preoperative discussion with the family. Sending the child out of the room only adds to their lack of control and understanding. It is especially important to use age-appropriate descriptions of the procedure and to use terms like "it might feel like," etc. Children should not be lied to about the likelihood that the procedure will involve pain. Nothing will destroy a doctor–patient relationship more rapidly and lead to an out-of-control encounter than dishonesty. The physician should never hesitate to correct a well-meaning parent who tells the child that a painful procedure will not hurt, especially if it is likely to uncomfortable. On the other hand, hurtful words, themselves, should be avoided. For example, when describing local anesthetic infiltration words like "prick," "stick," "needle," "shot," "beesting" or other words which conjure painful, frightening images are best avoided. It is best to liken the process to something the child has experienced without a great deal of fear. For example, a pinch can appropriately describe local lidocaine injection. Telling the child all of the steps involved with the procedure in gentle, easy to understand terms will go a long way to make the entire process smooth and atraumatic. Similarly, the physician should not be afraid to set boundaries and rules in advance of the procedure. It often helps to reassure the child that they will be told when the painful part is coming and that it's okay to scream and cry as long as they do not kick or bite anyone (see Table 5.2).[9]

The consultation visit permits the dermatologic surgeon to obtain vital information about the overall health of the patient, more specifically, information regarding any medical conditions or medications that may influence the proposed surgical procedure. A history should include any previous surgery or accidental injuries to the child and the quality of the ensuing scar (eg., keloid or hypertrophic scarring, etc.). Prior experience with lacerations or minor surgical procedures will give the physician an idea how the patient tolerated the experience and may be used to modify the proposed procedure if necessary. Written instructions are provided to the parents describing all preoperative precautions to take for their child. The use of sal-

icylates and other non-steroidal anti-inflammatory agents that inhibit platelet function should be stopped for a two week period prior to the proposed surgery. Postoperative activity restriction should be thoroughly reviewed at this time and included in the written instructions sent home with the family. The dermatologic surgeon must be sympathetic and cognizant of the adolescent's sports schedule and be flexible and accommodating when planning for the impending surgery. Noncompliance with postoperative activity and bathing restrictions will lead to poor wound healing and a suboptimal surgical scar.

INTRAOPERATIVE TECHNIQUES FOR PAINFUL PROCEDURES IN THE PEDIATRIC PATIENT

Children do not naturally have good pain control strategies, but by adhering to principles of child development we can foster healthy coping skills. One method to reduce anxiety is to enhance a child's sense of control of the medical environment.[10] Simple techniques such as allowing the patient to select the radio station, color of suture or postoperative dressing can go a long way in allaying the child's fears. The physician should talk to the patient as much is as comfortable; the surgeon should not spend excessive time discussing personal issues with the nurse or assistant. However, some adolescents prefer to distract themselves with the use of music on a personal stereo which should be readily available in any dermatologic surgery suite. The benefit of this form of distraction has been validated in younger children undergoing immunizations. Those children who were listened to lullabies experienced less pain than those who were not exposed to music during the painful procedure.[11]

For most simple procedures in children, parents should be seated at the head of the table distracting the child with books or activities (Fig. 5.1). Parents should never be used as assistants and should not be used to restrain the young child. There should be sufficient skilled paramedical personnel to perform that role. If the caregiver wishes to observe the procedure, he or she should be allowed to watch while seated out of the surgeon's way. The surgical

TABLE 5.2   Preoperative techniques for pediatric patients
1. Office should be child-centered.
2. Physician should be at or below patient level.
3. Talk to the patient and involve them. Never have child leave the room.
4. Explain impending procedure carefully and thoroughly. There should be no surprises.
5. Do not lie.
6. Avoid hurtful words.
7. Set boundaries and rules.

With permission Current Problems in Dermatology Jan/Feb 1999.

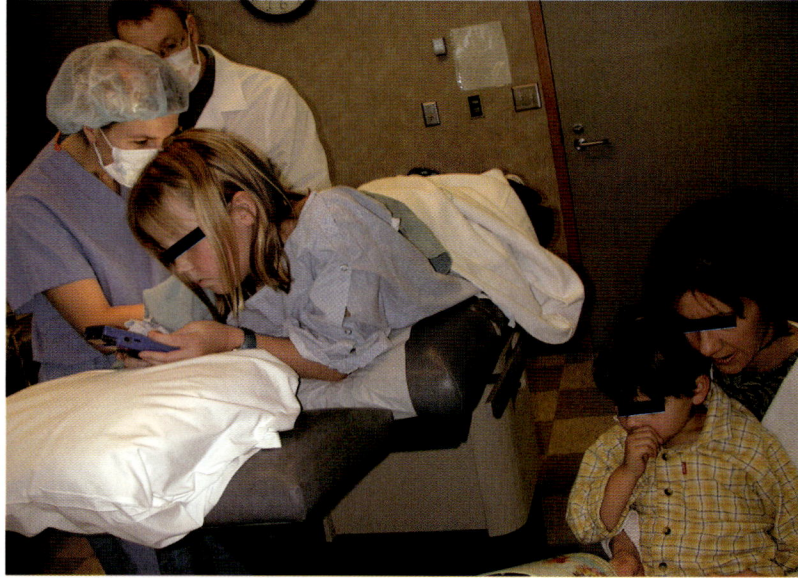

Fig. 5.1   For most dermatologic procedures in children, parents should be seated at the head of the procedure table, distracting the child.

7. Fishman BE, Cook EW, Hammock et al. (1989) Familial transmission of fear: effects of maternal anxiety and presence of children's response to dental treatment. Presented at the Conference on Child Health Psychology. Gainsville FL.
8. Blount RL, Davis N, Powers SW, Roberts MC (1991) The influence of environmental factors and coping style on children's coping and distress. Clin Psychol Rev 11:93–116.
9. Rothman KF (1995) Pain management for dermatologic procedures in children. Adv Dermatol 10:287–307.
10. Zelter LK, Bush JP, Chen E, Riveral A (1997) Psychobiologic approach of pediatric pain, II: prevention and treatment. Curr Probl Pediatr 27:264–284.
11. Megel ME, Houser CW, Gleaves LS (1998) Children's responses to immunizations: lullabies as a distraction. Issues Compr Pediatr Nurs Jul–Sep;21(3):129–145.

site, however, should be placed out of the child's view using surgical drapes in the fashion of a cesarean section. Surgical trays should be covered with drapes prior to the start of the procedure in order to obscure anxiety producing needles and instruments. Furthermore, blood-soaked material should be hidden from view at the completion of the surgery as well.

A variety of distraction techniques can be employed when painful procedures are performed on children. The young child can be given bubbles to blow[12,13] while older children are often distracted from the discomfort by engaging in conversation about music, movies, or school or by using handheld electronic games or toys. A more involved technique using visual imagery can be an extremely effective tool to help a child through a painful procedure.[14,15,16] Children have a shorter attention span than adults and distraction techniques of nonimagery and simple cognitive information may not be as effective in children as they are older patients.[17] It is often helpful to engage children in active imagery and fantasy to help them become lost in their imagination. This type of "hypnotic" distraction has been compared with nonhypnotic forms of simple distraction techniques such as squeezing mother's hands, focusing on objects in the room, deep breathing, etc., with regard to pain reduction during medical procedures. Although both forms of distraction are effective in reducing pain and anxiety associated invasive procedures, active visual imagery is more effective.[18]

The positive effect of distraction on pain perception can be seen even in the very young. In a study of 54 infants, Blass et al.[19] found that a simple pacifier given to babies undergoing routine heel stick resulted in 35% less crying, while those babies who were given sugar and a pacifier cried 69% less.

SKIN PREPARATIONS

The type of skin preparation required is dependent upon the type of procedure performed. For some superficial shave-biopsy procedures, a simple cleansing of the skin with 70% alcohol will destroy more than 90% of the surface bacteria within two minutes.[20,21,22] However, for more extensive procedures, such as excisions with intermediate repair, a more thorough and effective technique is required.

The agents commonly used for topical antisepsis are a povidone-iodine[23] solution and 4% chlor-hexidine.[24,25] When either of these agents is applied to the skin surface for 3–5 minutes, a sufficient reduction in the number of Gram-negative and Gram-positive organisms present will allow aseptic surgery to be performed. These agents should be applied first to the center of the surgical field. With a circular motion, the antiseptic agent is applied in a centrifugal fashion with gradually enlarging diameters until the treatment site and an area of normal surrounding tissue is cleansed.

Povidone-iodine solution

Povidone-iodine is one of the most commonly used antiseptics and is widely available in 10% solution, 2% detergent, and 2% ointment or wash. It is active against Gram-positive and Gram-negative organisms and yeast. The iodophor-containing solutions should be used with caution in atopic individuals since iodine sensitivity may occur. Also, iodophors do not bind well to skin, making povidone-iodine less effective for longer procedures. The use of iodine-containing antiseptics in neonates deserves special consideration. Povidone-iodine should be used cautiously, if at all, in the neonatal intensive care unit and newborn nursery. Adverse effects of iodine-containing antiseptics have been recognized for at least 20 years.[26] Exposure to iodine in the neonatal period has been associated with dramatic elevation in plasma and urinary iodine, leading to transient hypothyroxinemia, hypothyroidism, and concern over the possibility of an increased subsequent risk of cerebral palsy.[27,28,29] Because of these concerns regarding the increased toxicity of povidone-iodine in neonates, it should be used cautiously, if at all, in this age group.

Chlorhexidine gluconate

Chlorhexidine gluconate is the preferred skin antiseptic for use in children. This agent has broad-spectrum activity against Gram-positive and Gram-negative bacteria and yeast.[23,24,30] One-half percent chlorhexidine gluconate is superior to 10% povidone-iodine in reducing the risk of colonization of peripheral intravenous catheterization.[31] Chlorhexidine offers several advantages over iodine-containing antiseptics including better substantivity leading to increased efficacy and less risk of percutaneous absorption. Topical application of chlorhexidine appears very safe even in neonates and no toxic systemic effects have been documented from this agent even after massive oral ingestion.[32,33] Caution must be taken when this agent is used near the ear or eye as pluronics, added for lathering purposes, are toxic to the cornea and middle ear and may cause serious damage to these structures.

HAIR-BEARING SKIN PREPARATION

The preparation of hair-bearing skin is a matter of some controversy. There is good evidence showing a greater risk of postoperative wound infection in patients who have been shaved preoperatively.[34,35] As a consequence, most surgeons prefer merely to trim the hair prior to the procedure or, if shaving is considered important, to shave immediately beforehand. Chemical depilatories have also been advocated for this purpose and also seem to offer an advantage over shaving.[36] In any event, the child who is required to have hair removed before any surgical procedure should be told that the area being prepped is the smallest possible.[37] Keeping in mind the concerns of the child or adolescent regarding personal appearance, the physician should also provide

12. Manne SL, Bakeman R, Jacobsen PB, Gorfinkle K, Redd WH (1994) An analysis of behavioral intervention for children undergoing venipuncture. **Health Psychol** 13:556–566.
13. French GM, Painter EC, Coury DL (1994) Blowing away shot pain: a technique for pain management during immunization. **Pediatrics** 93:384–388.
14. Zelter LK (1994) Pain and symptom management. In: Pediatric Psychooncology, Bearison DJ, Mulhern RK, eds. New York: Oxford University Press, pp. 9–34.
15. Olness K (1989) Hypnotherapy: A cyberphysiologic strategy in pain management. **Pediatr Clin North Am** 36:873–884.
16. Kuttner L (1988) Favorite stories: a hypnotic pain-reduction technique for children in acute pain. **Am J Clin Hypnosis** 289–295.
17. Zelter L, LeBaron S (1982) Hypnosis and nonhypnotic techniques for reduction of pain and anxiety during painful procedures in children and adolescents with cancer. **J Pediatr** 101:1032–1035.
18. Olness K (1989) Hypnotherapy: a cyberphysiologic strategy in pain management. **Pediatr Clin North Am** 36:873–884.
19. Blass EM, Hoffmayer LB (1991) Sucrose as an analgesia for newborn infants. **Pediatrics** 87:215–218.
20. Groschel DHH (1985) Surgical antisepsis. **JAMA** 254:1234.
21. Mertz PM, Alvarez OM, Smerbeck RV et al. (1984) A new in vivo model for the evaluation of topical antiseptics on superficial wounds. **Arch Dermatol** 120:58.
22. Sebben JE (1983) Surgical antiseptics. **J Am Acad Derm** 9:759.
23. Hair BM, Garcia RL (1984) The effect of a 15-second povidone-iodine scrub on resident skin flora. **J Assoc Mil Dermatol** 10:16.
24. Peterson AF, Rosenberg A, Alatary SD (1978) Comparative evaluation of surgical scrub preparations. **Surg Gynecol Obstet** 146:63.

25. McManus AT, Denton CL, Mason AD (1984) Topical chlorhexidine diphosphanilate (WB-973) in burn wound sepsis. **Arch Surg** 119:206.
26. Pyati SP, Ramamurthy RS, Krauss MT et al. (1977) Absorption of iodine in the neonate following topical use of povidone iodine. **J Pediatr** 91:825–828.
27. Gordon CM, Rowitch DH, Mitchell ML et al. (1995) Topical iodine and neonatal hypothyroidism. **Arch Pediatr Adolesc Med** 149:1336–1339.
28. Parravincini E, Fontana C, Giuseppe L et al. (1996) Iodine, thyroid function, and very low birth weight infants. **Pediatrics** 98:730–734.
29. Reuss ML, Paneth N, Pinto-Martin JA et al. (1996) The relation of transient hypothroxinemia in preterm infants to neurologic development at two years of age. **N Engl J Med** 334:821–858.
30. Reynolds J, ed. (1996) Chlorhexidine. Englewood CO: Micromedex.
31. Garland JS, Buck RK, Maloney P et al. (1995) Comparison of 10% povidone-iodine and 0.5% chlorhexidine gluconate for the prevention of peripheral intravenous catheter colonization in neonates: a prospective trial. **Pediatr Infect Dis** 14:510–516.
32. Ruttner N (1987) Percutaneous drug absorption in the newborn: Hazards and uses. **Clin Perinatol** 14:911–930.
33. Zenca Pharmaceuticals, Wilmington Delaware. Personal Communication.
34. Seropian R, Reynolds BM (1971) Wound infections after preoperative depilatory versus razor preparation. **Am J Surg** 121:251.
35. Alexander JW, Fischer JE, Boyajian M et al. (1983) The influence of hair-removal methods on wound infections. **Arch Surg** 118:347.
36. Prigot A, Garnes AL, Nwagbo U (1962) Evaluation of a chemical depilatory for preoperative preparation of 515 surgical patients. **Am J Surg** 104:900.
37. Kretschmer T, Braun V, Richter HP (2000) Neurosurgery without shaving: indications and results. **Br J Neurosurg** Aug;14(4):341–344.

the child with reassurance that the trimmed hair will grow back to its previous length and density with time.

INSTRUMENT PREPARATION

In order to minimize the chance of postoperative infection, the instruments used during the procedure must be carefully prepared. Each time an instrument is used, blood and tissue debris must be removed at the completion of the procedure. This can be accomplished either manually or with use of an ultrasonic cleanser. To eliminate bacterial spores and viral particles, steam autoclaving of instruments remains the best method for most office-based physicians.[38,39] While gas sterilization is equally effective, the equipment required for this procedure is generally too expensive and bulky for the office setting; for that reason, this technique remains largely limited to hospital settings. While dryheat sterilization of instruments[40] is also effective, the potential for contamination during storage is too great, limiting the potential value of this technique.

ANESTHESIA

A variety of topical and systemic agents may induce cutaneous anesthesia and decrease the pain of dermatologic procedures. The use of EMLA and other newer topical anesthetics is invaluable for the pediatric dermatologist performing painful procedures on children. Appropriately used, these agents may make certain pediatric procedures painless or minimally uncomfortable. For younger children or more lengthy procedures such as pulsed dye laser treatment of a hemifacial port–wine stain, additional techniques including general anesthesia may be required.

TOPICAL AND LOCAL NONINJECTABLE ANESTHETICS

Eutectic mixture of local anesthetics (EMLA)

Since its approval by the Federal Drug Administration (FDA) in December 1992, EMLA has gained popularity for minimizing the pain of certain dermatologic procedures and has particular appeal for use in children. The anesthetic components of this oil-in-water emulsion are 2.5% prilocaine and 2.5% lidocaine. Though the eutectic preparation melts at a lower temperature than its individual components, the mixture remains stable at room temperature. Proper use of this agent requires that it be occluded for 60–120 minutes, usually with a Tegaderm polyurethane film (Fig. 5.2). Simple plastic wrap with enough adhesive tape to ensure occlusion without extrusion is an economical and effective alternative. Longer application times may be used to increase the depth of anesthesia, as both the duration and depth of pain blockade are each a direct function of application time.[41] Shorter application times are indicated for broken, non-intact skin, genitalia and mucosal surfaces, due to faster absorption rates.

EMLA, originally proven effective for minimizing the pain of venipuncture,[42] has proven to be effective as a local anesthetic for numerous dermatologic procedures including laser therapy for port-wine stains, intralesional

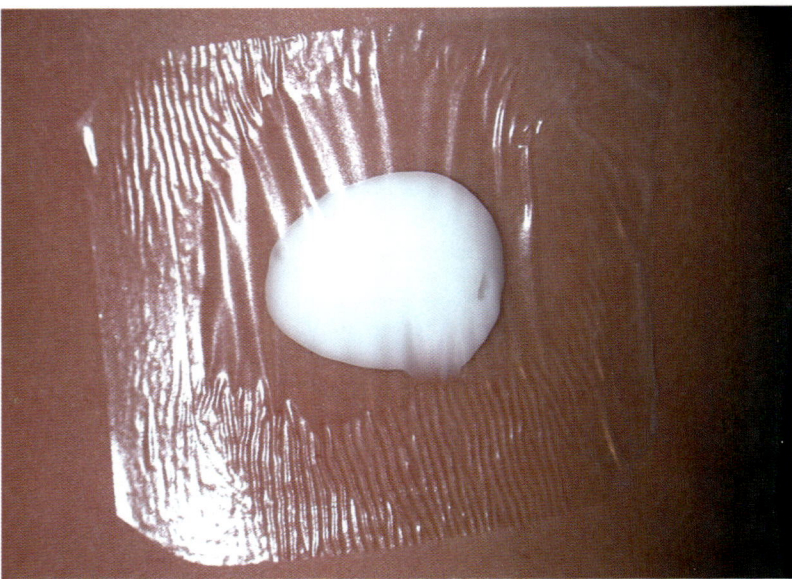

Fig. 5.2 Proper application of EMLA with clear adhesive tape as occlusion.

injections for keloids, cysts and hemangiomas, and in the paring of verruca vulgaris lesions, among others.[41,43] While EMLA alone does not provide adequate anesthesia for more invasive procedures such as skin biopsies and excisions in children, it is useful as a "prenumbing" agent, prior to the infiltration of local injectable anesthetics.[44]

Parental application of EMLA one to two hours prior to outpatient dermatologic procedures has been shown to be no less effective than that administered by trained medical personnel.[45] The list of potential applications for EMLA is growing but the clinician should be reminded that EMLA alone is appropriate only for relatively superficial procedures and is perhaps best reserved for use prior to infiltration with local anesthetic.

The EMLA disk is an anesthetic patch that administers the same formulation of prilocaine and lidocaine, and has proven to be equally effective as EMLA cream.[46] Though convenient and quick to apply, its small size (contact surface area measuring only 10cm²) limits this product's utility for many dermatologic procedures. It is also relatively inefficient for use in highly contoured areas such as fingers or nose.

Potential complications and caveats with the application of EMLA

When used appropriately, EMLA is usually well tolerated and considered safe in most children. Methemoglobinemia remains the most concerning and potentially life-threatening complication of EMLA use, particularly in neonates. Premature neonates are at greatest risk of this complication, though term newborns under 3 months of age are also more susceptible than older infants.[47–49] Methemoglobinemia has occurred in infants and neonates with EMLA use in the treatment of hemangiomas, for heel lancing/venipuncture, and during circumcision.[50,51] Signs of this condition include mottling and

38. Sebben JE (1984) Sterilization and care of surgical instruments and supplies. **J Am Acad Dermatol** 11:381.
39. Sebben JE (1989) Sterile technique and the prevention of wound infection in office surgery – Part II. **J Dermatol Surg Oncol** Jan;15(1):38–48.
40. Pollack SV (1990) Rapid instrument sterilization. **J Dermatol Surg Oncol** May;16(5):438–439.
41. Arendt-Nielson L, Bjerring P (1988) Laser-induced pain for evaluation of local analgesia: a comparison of topical application (EMLA) and local injection (lidocaine). **Anesth Analg** 67:115–123.
42. Choy L, Collier J, Watson AR (1999) Comparison of lidocaine-prilocaine cream and amethocaine gel for local analgesia before venipuncture in children. **Acta Paediatr** Sep;88(9):961–964.
43. Gupta AK, Sibbald RG (1996) Eutectic lidocaine/prilocaine 5% cream and patch may provide satisfactory analgesia for excisional biopsy or curettage with electrosurgery of cutaneous lesions: a randomized, controlled, parallel group study. **J Am Acad Dermatol** 35:419–423.
44. De Waard-van der Spek FB, Mulder PG, Oranje AP (1997) Prilocaine/lidocaine patch as a local premedication for skin biopsy in children. **J Am Acad Dermatol** 37:418–421.

45. Koh JL, Fanurik D, Stoner PD et al. (1999) Efficacy of parental application of eutectic mixture of local anesthetics for intravenous insertion. **Pediatrics** 103(6):e79.
46. Chang PC, O'Connor G, Rogers PJC et al. (1994) A multicentre randomized study of single-unit dose package of EMLA patch vs. EMLA cream 5% for venipuncture in children. **Can J Anesth** 41:59–63.
47. Jakobson B, Nilsson A (1985) Methaemoglobinemia in children treated with prilocaine-lidocaine cream and trimethoprim-sulphamethoxazole: a care report. **Acta Anesth Scand** 29:453–455.
48. Kumar AR, Dunn N, Naqvi M (1997) Methemoglobinemia associated with a prilocaine-lidocaine cream. **Clin Pediatri** 36:239–240.
49. Frayling IM, Addison GM, Chattergee K, Meakin G (1990) Methaemoglobinaemia in children treated with prilocaine-lignocaine cream. **BMJ** 301:153–154.
50. Elsner P, Dummer RS (1997) Signs of methaemoglobinaemia after topical application of EMLA cream in an infant with haemangioma. **Dermatology** 195:153–154.
51. Couper RTL (2000) Methaemoglobinaemia secondary to topical lignocaine/prilocaine in a circumcised neonate. **J Paediatr Child Health** 36:406–407.

pallor of the skin, perioral cyanosis, and clinical evidence of acral cyanosis even hours after EMLA has been removed from the skin surface. The reaction results from deficient methemoglobin reductase in the setting of a prilocaine-induced methemoglobin stress.[52] 4 hydroxy-2 methylaniline and o-toluidine are the oxidizing metabolites of prilocaine responsible for the development of methemoglobinemia.[53] Other oxidizing agents known to increase the risk of EMLA-associated methemoglobinemia and whose concomitant use, therefore, should be avoided include benzocaine, sulfonamides, phenytoin, dapsone, phenobarbital and chloroquine.[54]

Methemoglobin levels of 70% are associated with a high incidence of mortality. If symptomatic, drug-induced methemoglobinemia can be treated with iv methylene blue or ascorbic acid.[55] Because of the real risk of methemoglobinemia from EMLA in children less than 3 months of age, such use is controversial and cannot be recommended.[56] Though the relative risk of this complication with EMLA use is greater in children less than 3 months of age, methemoglobinemia clearly can occur in older children as well. A recent report describes a 3-year-old child who presented with signs and symptoms of methemoglobinemia 2.5 hours after her caregiver applied approximately 25mg of EMLA.[57] Practitioners are advised, in general, to limit application times and the quantity of EMLA applied, to lower the risk of EMLA-associated methemoglobinemia in all children. ELA-max, a relatively new liposomal lidocaine product without prilocaine may represent an effective alternative for use in the young infant.

Although usually safe and effective in older infants and children, local side effects have been reported with EMLA, including a temporary erythema or blanching, edema, eye irritation especially with periorbital applications, and an allergic contact dermatitis.[58,59] There has been one reported case of 90% corneal de-epithelialization from EMLA application.[60] Localized purpura has developed with the application of as little as one gram of EMLA and for as short a time period as 30 minutes in children, with complete resolution over several days.[61,62] The purpura may occur more commonly in premature infants and in children with atopic dermatitis.[63] The mechanism is thought to involve toxicity to the capillary endothelium rather than an allergic response. As with any form of lidocaine use, seizures may occur following prolonged application of EMLA, especially when applied under occlusive dressings.[64,65]

ELA-max

ELA-max (liposomally encapsulated 4% or 5% lidocaine) is a newer topical anesthetic than EMLA with a competitive safety profile. In comparative trials,

ELA-max and EMLA were deemed equally effective in minimizing the pain associated with simple dermatologic procedures.[66–68] There have been no reports of serious adverse effects with the topical use of ELA-max, though data regarding its use currently are limited. Further studies are warranted to evaluate this potentially useful topical anesthetic, especially in neonates, due to the theoretic diminished risk of methemoglobinemia.

Tetracaine formulations

Amethocaine, a 4% tetracaine gel, offers a more rapid onset (40 minutes) and longer duration of action than EMLA cream.[69] This topical anesthetic is widely used in Europe, but is not currently FDA approved in the United States. Topical amethocaine gel may be superior to EMLA and has been proved effective in reducing the pain of venous cannulation and pulsed dye laser treatment of vascular lesions in children, without significant side effects.[70] Investigators also have examined the use of amethocaine gel to reduce procedural pain in neonates, though the data regarding efficacy is preliminary.[71] Amethocaine offers the advantage of less vasoconstriction than EMLA, which may be beneficial for venous cannulation.[72] Local effects include transient erythema, edema, and pruritus.[73] A combination of 0.5% tetracaine, 1:1000 epinephrine, and 11.8% cocaine (TAC) has been a useful preparation for the exploration and repair of lacerations, but poor transdermal absorption limits its utility for most dermatologic procedures in children. The substitution of lidocaine for cocaine (LAT preparations) may be preferable to injectable lidocaine for laceration repair.[74] Use of liposome-encapsulated tetracaine (LET) may be more effective than EMLA for topical analgesia, but has not yet been studied in pediatric patients and is not available for use in the United States.[75]

Iontophoresis

Iontophoresis was first described in 1747 but its mechanism of action was not understood until the twentieth century. With this technique, any drug that ionizes in solution, such as 1 to 4 percent lidocaine, can be delivered painlessly into the superficial layers of the skin by the use of a 1-milliamp (mA) galvanic current for 3 to 5 minutes.[76] Advantages of this technique include a needle-free process and a rapid onset of anesthesia (within 10 minutes). Lidocaine iontophoresis has been proven effective in decreasing the pain of iv cannulation, as premedication before propofol injection and for anesthesia during the pulsed-dye lasering of port-wine stains.[77–79] A superficial burn at the application site has been reported.[80] Iontophoresis has not been

52. Nilsson A, Engberg G, Henneberg S, Danielson K, De Verdier CH (1990) Inverse relationship between age-dependent erythrocyte activity of methaemoglobin reductase and prilocaine-induced methaemoglobinaemia during infancy. Br J Anaesth 64:72–76.
53. Frey B, Kehrer B (1999) Toxic methaemoglobin concentrations in premature infants after application of a prilocaine-containing cream and peridural prilocaine. Eur J Pediatr 158(10):785–788.
54. EMLA prescribing information (1998) Westborough (MA): Astra Pharmaceutical Products.
55. Hall AH, Kulig KW, Rumack BH (1986) Drug and chemical induced methaemoglobinaemia. Clinical features and management. Toxicology 1:253–260.
56. Essink-Tebbes CM, Wuis EW, Liem KD, van Dongen RT, Hekster YA (1999) Safety of lidocaine-prilocaine cream application four times a day in premature neonates: a pilot study. Eur J Pediatr 158(5):421–423.
57. Touma S, Jackson JB (2001) Lidocaine and prilocaine toxicity in a patient receiving treatment for mollusca contagiosa. J Am Acad Dermatol 44:399–400.
58. Suhonen R, Kanerva L (1997) Contact allergy and cross-reactions caused by prilocaine. Am J Contact Dermat 8:231–235.
59. Le Coz CJ, Cribier BJ, Heid E (1996) Patch testing in suspected allergic contact dermatitis due to EMLA cream in haemodialyzed patients. Contact Dermatitis 35:316–317.
60. McKinlay JR, Hofmeister E, Ross EV (1999) EMLA cream-induced eye injury. Arch Dermatol July;135:855–856.
61. DeWaard-van der Spek FB, Oranje AP (1997) Purpura caused by EMLA is of toxic origin. Contact Dermatitis 36:11–13.
62. Calobrisi SD, Drolet BA, Esterly NB (1998) Petechial eruption after the application of EMLA cream. Pediatrics 101:471–473.
63. DeWaard-van der Spek FB, Oranje AP (1997) Purpura caused by EMLA is of toxic origin. Contact Dermatitis 36:11–13.
64. Rincon E, Baker RL, Iglesias AJ, Duarte A (2000) CNS toxicity after topical application of EMLA cream on a toddler with molluscum contagiosum. Pediatr Emerg Care 16(4):252–254.
65. Boulinguqz, S, Sparsa A, Gauthier-Bouyssou ML, Bedane C, Bonnetblanc JM (2000) Adverse effects associated with EMLA cream used as topical anesthetic for the mechanical debridement of leg ulcers. J Am Acad Dermatol 42(1 Part 1):146–148.
66. El-Rady MS, Khalil RM (1999) Free versus liposome-encapsulated lignocaine hydrochloride topical applications. Pharmazie 54(9):682–684.
67. Friedman PM, Fogelman JP, Nouri K, Levine VJ, Ashinoff R (1999) Comparative study of the efficacy of four topical anesthetics. Dermatol Surg Dec;25(12):950–954.
68. Koppel RA, Coleman KM, Coleman WP (2000) The efficacy of EMLA versus ELA-Max for pain relief in medium-depth chemical peeling: a clinical and histopathologic evaluation. Dermatol Surg 26(1):61–64.
69. Huang W, Vidimos A (2000) Topical anesthetics in dermatology. J Am Acad Dermatol 43:286–298.
70. McCafferty DF, Woolfson AD, Handley J, Allen G (1997) Effect of percutaneous local anaesthetics on pain reduction during pulse dye laser treatment of portwine stains. Br J Anaesth 78(3):286–289.
71. Jain A, Rutter N (2000) Local anaesthetic effect of topical amethocaine gel in neonates: randomised controlled trial. Arch Dis Child Fetal Neonatal Ed Jan;82(1):F42–45.
72. Browne J, Awad I, Plant R, McAdoo J, Shorten G (1999) Topical amethocaine (Ametop) is superior to EMLA for intravenous cannulation. Eutectic mixture of local anesthetics. Can J Anaesth Nov;46(11):1014–1018.
73. O'Connor B, Tomlinson AA (1995) Evaluation of the efficacy and safety of amethocaine gel applied topically before venous cannulation in adults. Br J Anaesth 74:706–708.
74. Smith GA, Strausbaugh SD, Harbeck-Weber C et al. (1997) New non-cocaine-containing topical anesthetics compared with tetracaine-adrenaline-cocaine during repair of lacerations. Pediatrics 100:825–830.
75. Fisher R, Hung O, Mezei M, Stewart R (1998) Topical anaesthesia of intact skin: liposome-encapsulated tetracaine vs EMLA. Br J Anaesth 81(6):972–973.
76. Maloney JM, Bezzant JL, Stephen RL, Petelenz TJ (1992) Iontophoretic administration of lidocaine anesthesia in office practice: an appraisal. J Dermatol Surg Oncol 18(11):937–940.
77. Sadler PJ, Thompson HM, Maslowski P (1999) Iontophoretically applied lidocaine reduces pain on propofol injection. Br J Anaesth 82(3):432–434.
78. Squire SJ, Kirchhoff KT, Hissong K (2000) Comparing two methods of topical anesthesia used before intravenous cannulation in pediatric patients. J Pediatr Health Care 14(2):68–72.
79. Nunez M, Miralles ES, Boixeda P et al. (1997) Iontophoresis for anesthesia during pulsed dye laser treatment of port-wine stains. Pediatr Dermatol 14(5):397–400.
80. DeCou JM, Abrams RS, Hammond JH et al. (1999) Iontophoresis: a needle-free, electrical system of local anesthesia delivery for pediatric surgical office procedures. J Pediatr Surg 34(6):946–949.

widely used in dermatologic practice for a variety of reasons. In addition to its prohibitive cost, its use is limited to small surface areas and most patients dislike the tingling sensation associated with the use of an electric current. Furthermore, the wires and electrodes associated with this unit often appear threatening to an apprehensive young child.

Topical anesthesia for mucosal surfaces

Topical cetacaine, benzocaine, and viscous lidocaine are effective topical agents for mucosal anesthesia. The onset of action of these agents is very rapid with anesthesia occurring virtually upon application of the agent. When using cetacaine or benzocaine in neonates, the volume of anesthetic should be limited due to the risk of anesthetic induced methemoglobinemia.[81–85]

Techniques to decrease the pain of injection of local anesthetics

Sodium bicarbonate buffering of lidocaine

Despite its efficacy as a local anesthetic, injection of lidocaine with epinephrine is painful. Buffering of commercially available lidocaine may diminish the pain of its injection.[86,87] In order to neutralize the acidic pH of lidocaine with epinephrine solution, 1ml of 8.4% sodium bicarbonate is added to every 10ml of anesthetic solution. Addition of bicarbonate results in the degradation of epinephrine at approximately 25% per week so that it is generally recommended that the neutralized solutions be discarded after 1 week. Refrigeration at a temperature of 0–4 degrees C, however, maintains the epinephrine in the lidocaine at 90% of its initial concentration.[88]

Several studies have shown that buffered lidocaine has antibacterial activity *in vitro.*[89–91] One study compared the growth of six species of bacteria incubated with plain versus buffered lidocaine. Incubation with buffered lidocaine resulted in a 99% decrease in all bacteria tested. Plain lidocaine, bupivacaine, and mepivicaine have bacteriocidal activity. Sodium bicarbonate has broad antimicrobial properties, including antifungal and antibacterial effects.[92] Theoretically these effects may help to minimize the risk of postoperative wound infections. Exposure to local anesthetics, especially buffered lidocaine, may inhibit recovery of bacteria from biopsy specimens sent for culture. Unbuffered lidocaine is, therefore, recommended for use in biopsy specimens sent for culture.

Warming of lidocaine and rate of injection

Warming of lidocaine to body temperature has been shown to decrease infiltration associated pain,[93,94] without a decrement in efficacy.[95] Rate of administration is also of great importance in pain of local anesthetics, with one blinded study finding that administration rate had a greater impact on perceived pain of lidocaine subcutaneous infiltration than did buffering. Slowly infiltrated, buffered solution was judged least painful in several studies.[96,97] Optimally, local anesthetics are buffered, warmed to body temperature, and infiltrated slowly.

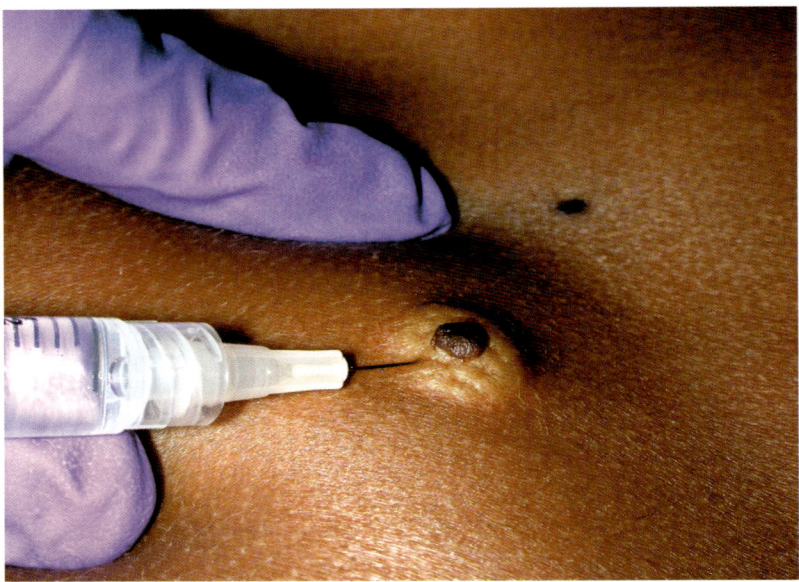

Fig. 5.3 Local infiltration of lidocaine with small 30-gauge needle.

Size of the needle

Obviously, injection of local anesthetic with a large-gauge needle hurts more than a small needle.[98] For most lesions encountered in pediatric dermatology, 0.5-inch silicon-coated disposable 30-gauge needles are utilized for injection of intradermal local anesthetics (Fig. 5.3).[99] The small size of this needle permits the surgeon to introduce the bevel of the needle into a follicular orifice in many situations to minimize the initial pricking sensation of the injection. This will result in less discomfort than that produced by a fast stabbing or jabbing injection through intact normal skin. By slowly advancing the needle deeper into the skin and at the same time injecting small quantities of local anesthetic, the procedure can be accomplished almost painlessly.[100] For larger lesions, longer 1-inch, 30-gauge needles are preferred. Prefrozen needles stored at −7 degrees Celsius have led to significantly less pain than room-temperature needles of the same caliber.[101] Some authors advocate their use as another technique to diminish the pain of injection of local anesthetic in children.

Nerve blocks

When performing large surgical procedures on the face or when operating on the fingers or toes, the pain from injection of local anesthetics can be minimized by use of various types of nerve blocks.[102–104] While these blocks frequently provide anesthesia of longer duration than a traditional cutaneous field block, they offer additional benefits as well. Four nerve blocks are

81. Vessely MB, Zitsch RP III (1993) Topical anesthetic-induced methemoglobinemia: a case report and review of the literature. **Otolaryngol Head Neck Surg** 108:763–767.
82. Nguyen ST, Cabrales RE, Bashour A et al. (2000) Benzocaine-induced methemoglobinemia. **Anesth Analg** 90:369–371.
83. Gupta PM, Lala DS, Asura EL (2000) Benzocaine-induced methemoglobinemia. **South Med J** 93(1):83–86.
84. Wurdeman RL, Mohiuddin SM, Holmberg MJ, Shalaby A (2000) Benzocaine-induced methemoglobinemia during an outpatient procedure. **Pharmacotherapy** Jun;20(6):735–738.
85. Donnelly GB, Randlett D (2000) Images in clinical medicine. Methemoglobinemia. **N Engl J Med** Aug 3;343(5):337.
86. McKay W, Morris R, Mushlin P (1987) Sodium bicarbonate attenuates pain on the skin infiltration with lidocaine, with or without epinephrine. **Anesth Analg** 66:572.
87. Stewart JH, Cole GW, Klein JA (1989) Neutralized lidocaine with epinephrine for local anesthesia. **J Dermatol Surg Oncol** 15:1081.
88. Holmes SG (1994) Choosing a local anesthetic. **Dermatol Clin** 12:817–823.
89. Thompson KD, Welykyj S, Massa MC (1993) Antibacterial activity of lidocaine in combination with a bicarbonate buffer. **J Dermatol Surg Oncol** Mar;19:216–220.
90. Williams BJ, Hanke CW, Bartlett M (1997) Antimicrobial effects of lidocaine, bicarbonate, and epinephrine. **J Am Acad Dermatol** Oct;37:662–664.
91. Aydin ON, Eyigor M, Aydin N (2001) Antimicrobial activity of ropivacaine and other local anaesthetics. **Eur J Anaesthesiol** Oct;18(10):687–694.
92. Sakuragi T, Ishino H, Dan K (1996) Bactericidal activity of clinically used local anesthetics on Staphylococcus aureus. **Reg Anesth** May;21(3):239–242.

93. Mader TJ, Playe SF, Garb JL (1994) Reducing the pain of local anesthetic infiltration: Warming and buffering have a synergistic effect. **Ann Emerg Med** 23:550–554.
94. Bainbridge LC (1991) Comparison of room temperature and body temperature local anesthetic solutions. **Br J Plast Surg** 44:147–148.
95. Brogan Jr, GX, Giarusso E, Hollander JE et al. (1995) Comparison of plain, warmed and buffered lidocaine for anesthesia of traumatic wounds. **Ann Emerg Med** 26:121–125.
96. Scarfone RJ, Jasani M, Gracely EJ (1998) Pain of local anesthetics: Rate of administration and buffering. **Ann Emerg Med** 31:36–40.
97. Colaric KB, Overton DT, Moore K (1998) Pain reduction in lidocaine administration through buffering and warming. **Am J Emerg Med** Jul;16(4):353–356.
98. Palmon SC, Lloyd AT, Kirsch JR (1998) The effect of needle gauge and lidocaine pH on pain during intradermal injection. **Anesth Analg** Feb;86(2):379–381.
99. Robinson JK (1979) Advantages and technique of inducing local anesthesia with a small-bore, angled needle. **J Dermatol Surg Oncol** 5:465.
100. Arndt KA, Burton C, Noe JM (1983) Minimizing the pain of local anesthesia. **Plast Reconstr Surg** 72:676.
101. Denkler K (2001) Pain associated with injection using frozen vs room-temperature needles. **JAMA** 286:1578.
102. Leversee JH, Bergman JJ (1981) Wrist and digital nerve blocks. **J Fam Pract** 13:415.
103. Abadir A (1976) Use of local anesthetics in dermatology. **J Dermatol Surg** 2:63.
104. Panje W (1979) Local anesthesia of the face. **J Dermatol Surg Oncol** 5:311.

generally used in dermatologic surgery. The first nerve block, and probably the one most commonly used, is the digital block for fingers and toes.[105] This block is technically easy to perform and highly successful in producing anesthesia of the affected digit.[106] With the use of plain 1% lidocaine and a 0.5-inch 30-gauge needle, approximately 1ml is injected on both sides of the proximal digit, at the superior aspect of the interphalangeal crease. The needle is directed both dorsally and ventrally, and a small wheal is raised. The areas of injection are then softly massaged in an attempt to diffuse the anesthetic throughout the soft tissue. Complete anesthesia is usually obtained within four to five minutes. However, if incomplete anesthesia is present after that interval, additional local anesthetic can be infiltrated in the surgical field.

The remaining three nerve blocks share a common anatomic position. The mental nerve, infraorbital nerve, and supraorbital and supratrochlear nerves are responsible for providing sensation to the central chin and lower lip, upper lip and medial cheek, and mid-forehead, respectively. These four nerves all lie along a vertical line that crosses the midpupil, approximately 2.5cm from the midline. If the various bony foramina cannot be palpated, using these anatomic reference points can usually result in performing successful nerve blocks.

The mental nerve block is not commonly used in dermatologic surgery but may prove beneficial for surgical procedures of the lower lip or chin, as in laser surgery.[107] Pretreating the mucosa with benzocaine, cetacaine or viscous lidocaine can ameliorate the discomfort of this block. Using a cotton-tipped applicator, a small quantity of anesthetic agent is introduced into the sulcus of the mandibular–buccal junction at the bases of the first and second lower premolars. After several minutes, a 1-inch 30-gauge needle can be painlessly introduced through this zone of anesthesia and advanced to the depth of the mandibular periosteum. At this point, 1 to 2ml of 1% plain lidocaine is injected near the mental foramen. To prevent prolonged anesthesia, the anesthetic should not be injected directly into the nerve itself. Within five minutes, the effect of the nerve block should be complete.

A similar approach is used to inject the infraorbital nerve to obtain anesthesia of the medial cheek.[108] Topical anesthetic is applied to the labial sulcus superior to the canine fossa. After several minutes, a 1-inch 30-gauge needle can be painlessly advanced superiorly 1 to 2cm to the infraorbital foramen, where 1 to 2ml of 1% plain lidocaine is injected.

To obtain anesthesia of the forehead, both the supraorbital and supratrochlear nerves must be blocked. Using a 0.5-inch 30-gauge needle, a small intradermal wheal is raised overlying the foramen. This is massaged with the finger for one to two minutes; the needle is then advanced in a vertical fashion through this zone of anesthesia down to the frontal periosteum. At this point, 1 to 2ml of 1% plain lidocaine is injected. Again, after four to five minutes, complete anesthesia of the ipsilateral forehead can be expected. With practice, these blocks can be used to reduce the pain of injection.

Preoperative sedation

In almost all cases, even in the uncooperative infant or extremely apprehensive child, preoperative sedation and slow gentle injection of local anesthetics will permit the physician to operate without the need for restraints. The use of restraints has never proved a satisfactory method to deal with uncooperative children when performing procedures. Not infrequently, the degree of immobility obtained with these devices is still insufficient to perform the surgical procedure satisfactorily with the normal level of safety of the customary expertise that would otherwise be expected. In addition, in many cases, the act of forcibly restraining a child serves to increase the level of

agitation in all those involved including the surgeon, the assistant, and the parents. Although the actual extent of permanent psychological harm caused by the use of restraints is unknown, it is probably preferable to use additional sedation or postpone the procedure rather than resort to this type of practice. When performing longer operative procedures, such as pulsed dye laser surgery for port-wine stains or surgical excision of a congenital nevus on the face, it may be necessary to employ use of general anesthesia.

No one sedative is suitable for all pediatric dermatologic procedures.[109,110] Furthermore, pure sedatives do not inhibit pain perception. They can block sensory input through a decrease in consciousness and can decrease anxiety, making them useful for use in conjunction with analgesics. They should not be used as single agents for painful procedures. In general, proper sedative use for pediatric dermatologic procedures will involve concomitant analgesic or anesthetic agents. Combining drugs from different classes can be used to produce desired effects not induced by either drug alone. The combination use of codeine, a narcotic, and midazolam, a sedative, is an example of a combined drug regimen for painful procedures in children. Caution must be taken with drug combinations, however, as they may potentiate adverse reactions.[111,112]

GENERAL ANESTHESIA

The services of an anesthesiologist are frequently enlisted for procedures involving children too young to fully cooperate with the requirements of local anesthesia. There are many factors that determine if, and when, a child is mature enough to cooperate with a procedure using only a local anesthetic. As a general rule, girls are often able to tolerate procedures under local anesthesia at 8 or 9 years of age, whereas boys may be ready by 10 or 11 years. Obviously, there is marked variability in development and personality and therefore each child must be assessed individually. When possible, elective procedures are delayed until pre-adolescence in an attempt to avoid the risks of general anesthesia. Certain clinical situations, however, may warrant the assumption of these risks.

General anesthesia: assessing the risks

Historically, the following myths have resulted in limited use of general anesthesia for pediatric dermatologic procedures: 1) general anesthesia is too dangerous for elective procedures, 2) multiple surgeries under general anesthesia are associated with increased cumulative risk, 3) infants and small children do not remember the pain of procedures if anesthesia is not administered.

The potential long-term effects of repeated painful procedures under restraint should not be underestimated. Infants are capable of painful memories following procedures and these may significantly impact a child's response to future painful stimuli.[113] In answering the question "what are the risks of general anesthesia?" several factors must be taken into consideration. The risk of a serious complication or death from anesthesia has fallen significantly in the past few decades as a result of improved training and education of anesthesiologists as well as the availability of safer anesthetic agents. The American Society of Anesthesiologists states that the risk of an anesthetic complication for a healthy child is 1:20 000 to 80 000 or less.[114] Large, prospective studies of pediatric dermatologic procedures under general anesthesia have not been performed. However, a multicenter retrospective review of the risk and complication rate of general anesthetics in children undergoing dermatologic procedures demonstrated a very low complication rate. This study evaluated

105. Abadir A (1975) Use of local anesthetics in dermatology. J Dermatol Surg 1:68.
106. Wagner AM, Suresh S (1998) Peripheral nerve blocks for warts: taking the cry out of cryotherapy and laser. Pediatr Dermatol 15(3):238–241.
107. Gormley DE (1981) A simplified, painless method of anesthetizing the lower lip. J Dermatol Surg Oncol 7:963.
108. Goldberg MP (1979) Induction of anesthesia in portions of the skin of the face by intraoral injections. J Dermatol Surg Oncol 5:570.
109. Selbst SM (1989) Managing pain in the pediatric ED. Pediatr Emerg Care 5:56–61.
110. Van der Bijl P (1991) Disinhibitory reactions to benzodiazipines: A review. J Oral Maxillofac Surg 49:519–120.

111. Yaster M, Nichols Dg, Deshpande JK (1990) Midazolam-fentanyl intravenous sedation in children: Case report of respiratory arrest. Peciatrics 86:463–466.
112. Hartwig S, Roth B, Theisohn M (1991) Clinical experience with continuous intravenous sedation using midazolam and fentanyl in the paediatric intensive care unit. Eur J Pediatr 150:784–788.
113. Taddio A, Goldback M, Ipp M, Stevens B, Koren G (1995) Effect of neonatal circumcision on pain responses during vaccination in boys. Lancet 345:291–292.
114. Tiret L, Nivoche Y, Hatton F, Desmonts JM, Vourc'h G (1988) Complications related to anaesthesia in infants and children. Br J Anaesth 61:263–269.
Wagner AM, Suresh S (1998) Peripheral nerve blocks for warts: taking the cry out of cryotherapy and laser. Pediatr Dermatol 15(3):238–241.

over 800 infants, children, and young adults undergoing surgical and laser procedures under general anesthesia.[115] Overall, less than 5% of children experienced a minor complication, with nausea and vomiting the most commonly reported event. There were no serious complications or deaths. When counselling parents regarding the risk of general anesthesia for pediatric dermatologic surgery, the physician should emphasize the following points whenever possible: 1) short procedure duration, 2) elective nature of the procedure, 3) good baseline health, 4) use of pediatric anesthesiologists (if applicable). In summary, general anesthetic use for elective pediatric dermatologic procedures is typically associated with few comorbid factors, making it relatively safe, especially when administered by physicians trained in pediatric anesthesia.

WOUND CLOSURE MATERIALS

TAPES VS. STAPLES

Before a wound is created, the physician must be aware of the different methods used to close the defect. One of the simplest techniques in treating the apprehensive child who is afraid of needles, is to coapt the edge of the wound using sterile adhesive skin tapes. These tapes are available in various sizes from 0.5 inch to 1.5 inch and are useful for closing small wounds, wounds that are not subject to high tension, and wounds that can be easily reapproximated. They are also used to support wounds after the sutures have been removed, in order to maintain precise epidermal apposition and lessen the chance of wound dehiscence or spreading of the scar. The security with which they can be used is dependent on the quality of the adherence to the skin surface. This, is turn, is dependent on the type of adhesive used and on the volume of sebum produced by the skin. One effective technique to add to the security of the tape closure is to first vigorously cleanse the skin surface with 70% alcohol to remove all oil and debris that might otherwise interfere with adhesion. A light film of tincture of benzoin or Mastisol™ is then applied to the margins of the wound and given sufficient time to become tacky. Once this has occurred, the tapes can be applied on the surface (Fig. 5.4). The initial tapes can be either replaced or reinforced when they begin to lift off while the patient is at home.

An alternative to suture materials is stainless steel staples.[116] Several companies now market disposable staple guns preloaded with one to 35 prepackaged sterile stainless steel staples.[117] The nonreactive staples are used quite effectively to evert the skin edges after placement of appropriate absorbable buried sutures.[118] The staples, which can be positioned very rapidly, can be left in place for longer periods than standard suture material without producing much inflammation. They can also be removed rapidly and painlessly with use of a specially designed extractor. Staples are less appropriate for use in the pediatric patient, however, as children are not likely to accept the look of metal on their skin or the Frankenstein-esque appearance.

SUTURE MATERIALS

When traditional suture materials are used to repair a defect or close a wound, there are two types of materials from which to choose: absorbable and non-absorbable. Absorbable sutures are generally used for buried suturing, to reduce tension on the skin surface and to ligate any arteriolar bleeding that cannot be controlled with electrosurgical devices. On occasion, an absorbable suture, most often 6–0 chromic gut, may be used as a skin closure, especially in the

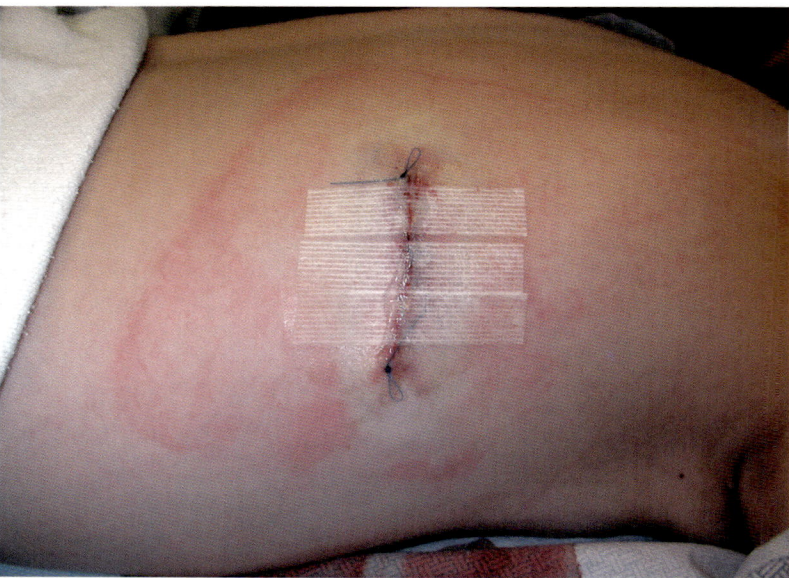

Fig. 5.4   Adhesive tape applied to wound postoperatively.

infant or young child, where the anticipated level of cooperation for suture removal is low.

Absorbable suture materials

The suturing of wounds is an ancient art that dates to 3500 BC.[119] Mummies in ancient Egypt were found with body cavities closed with sutures made of braided horsehair, leather strips and vegetable fibers.[120] Galen, physician to the Roman gladiators, first documented the use of silk and hemp sutures for hemostasis in 400 BC.[121]

The five types of absorbable suture materials that are currently in common use are surgical gut, copolymers of glycolic and lactic acids, polyglycolic acid, and synthetic polydioxanone and poliglecaprone. The desirable properties of absorbable sutures are high knot security, high tensile strength, easy handling, and lack of tissue inflammatory response.

Surgical gut

Gut material was derived from oxen or sheep intestinal material. It was originally used for violin strings and obtained at musical instrument shops that provided "kits," hence the terms "kitgut" or "catgut."[122] Current day surgical gut, prepared from sheep or cow intestinal collagen, is usually treated with chromate salts or chromic acid before it is spun into monofilament fibers to prolong tensile strength. This type of material passes easily through tissue, ties easily and has good knot security. However, it maintains its tensile strength for only seven to 12 days and is removed by foreign body granuloma formation, which limits its potential usefulness in many cosmetic surgical procedures.

Polyglycolic acid

Dexon, a polymer of polyglycolic acid, is a multifilament, absorbable, braided synthetic suture that is stiff. This agent has a higher tensile strength than catgut and minimal tissue reactivity.

115. Cunningham BB (2000) Complications of general anesthesia in pediatric dermatologic surgery (abstract). **Am Soc Derm Surg** annual general meeting, Denver.
116. Stillman RM, Marino CA, Seligman SJ (1984) Skin staples in potentially contaminated wounds. **Arch Surg** 119:821.
117. Johnson A, Rodeheaver GT, Durant LS et al. (1981) Automatic disposable stapling devices for wound closure. **Ann Emerg Med** 10:631.
118. Campbell JP, Swanson NA (1982) The use of staples in dermatologic surgery. **J Dermatol Surg Oncol** 8:680.

119. Margotta R (1968) The Story of Medicine. New York: Golden Press.
120. Sabiston DC (1991) Textbook of Surgery, 14th ed, Philadelphia: WB Saunders, pp. 115–220.
121. Snyder CC (1976) On the history of suture. **Plast & Reconstr Surg** 58:1087–1093.
122. LaBagnara J Jr (1995) A review of absorbable suture materials in head & neck surgery and introduction of monocryl: a new absorbable suture. **ENT Journal** 74:409–415.

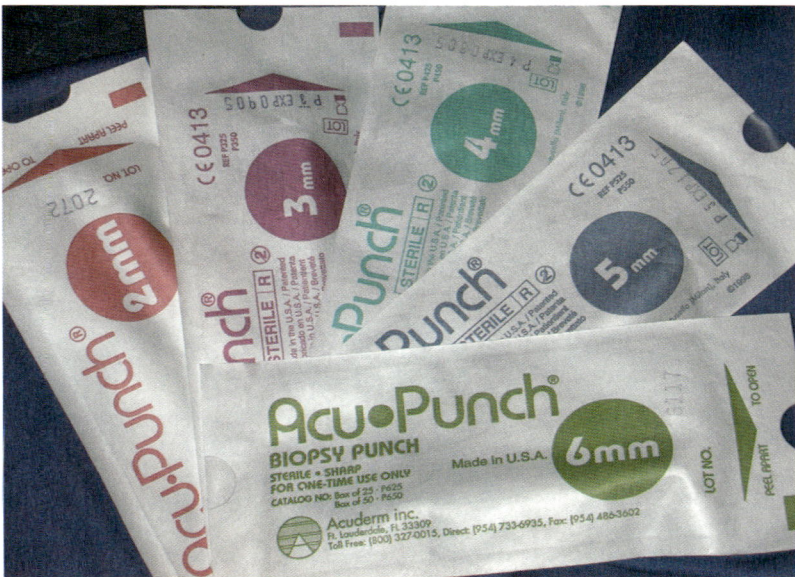

Fig 5.8   Various sizes of disposable biopsy punches available.

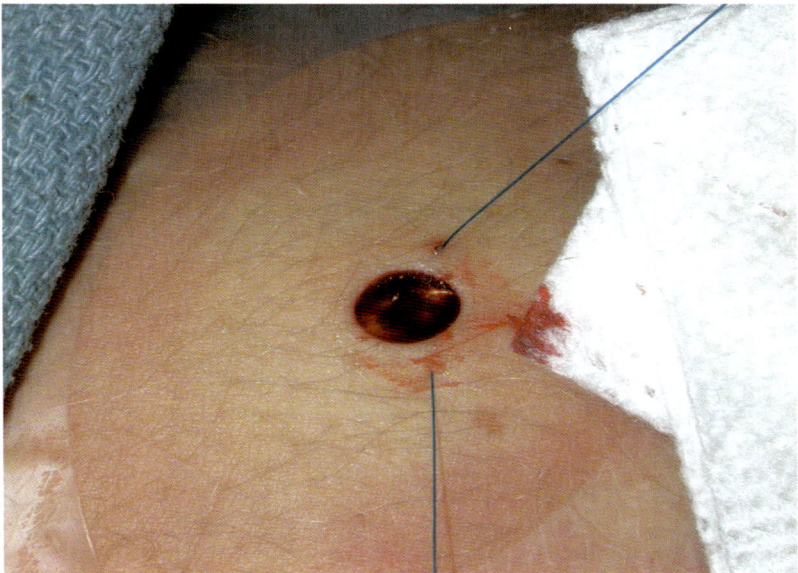

Fig. 5.10   The punch biopsy site is closed using a single nonabsorbable simple interrupted suture.

In children with a suspicious pigmented lesion,[138] such as a Spitz nevus, malignant melanoma, or dysplastic nevus, punch biopsies are not recommended, as the size of the specimen obtained may not provide an adequate amount of tissue for accurate pathologic diagnosis or determination of an accurate depth of invasion. Whenever possible, a lesion suspected of being a malignant melanoma or a Spitz nevus should be completely excised with narrow margins and submitted in its entirety for complete histologic analysis. If required, additional surgery can be performed after the pathologic diagnosis has been made.

Although still very controversial, some believe that due to the theoretical possibility that a biopsy could cause dissemination of melanoma cells through vascular spaces, performing a punch biopsy on a pigmented lesion is inappropriate.[139] While evidence for this theory remains scant, it does seem

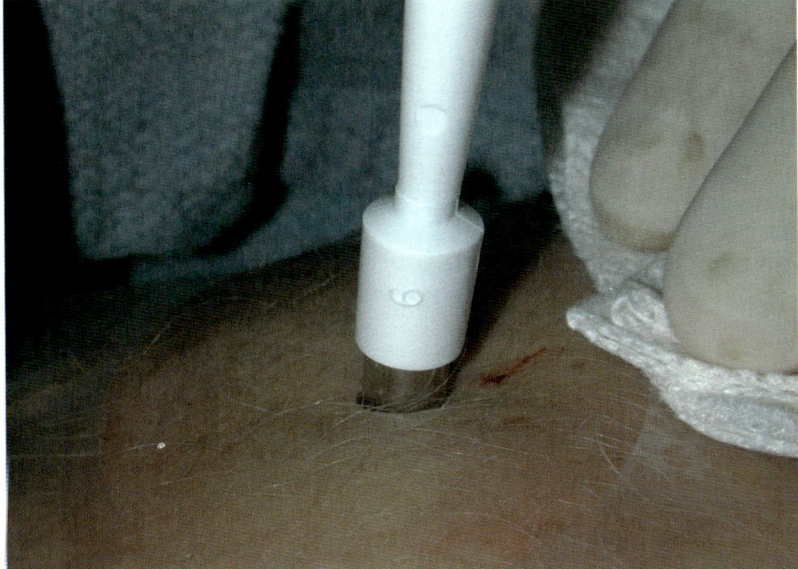

Fig. 5.9   Punch biopsy is performed using slight downward pressure and rotation simultaneously.

prudent to remove the entire pigmented lesion at the time of the initial biopsy if this can be done without creating a disfiguring scar.

After the appropriate lesion has been chosen for biopsy and the proper size punch instrument selected, the skin is cleansed with a suitable antiseptic. The punch biopsy instrument is held between the thumb and forefinger perpendicular to the surface of the skin (Fig. 5.9). Using a slight downward pressure, the punch is rotated approximately one complete turn, until it pops through the dermis into the subcutaneous fatty layer. When the punch is removed, the specimen will frequently protrude through the hole. If the specimen does not come through the wound spontaneously, it can be carefully lifted out by gently grabbing one epidermal edge with a pair of fine-toothed forceps. Bleeding is usually minimal and can be controlled, in most cases, with light external finger pressure for one to two minutes.

If the biopsy is being performed for the purpose of histologic diagnosis and a second, more definitive, procedure is likely to follow, the wound may be allowed to heal by secondary intention. In many cases on the trunk this may give extremely good cosmetic results.[140] In this situation, hemostasis can be achieved using topical application of aluminum chloride or Monsel's (ferric subsulfate) solution to the biopsy site with a cotton-tipped applicator. Both solutions provide rapid hemostasis, but on occasion a semi-permanent iron tattoo can result from the use of Monsel's solution and thus should be avoided in Caucasian skin types. This solution should be used with extra caution in the periorbital area, especially in active children, because inadvertent splattering or dripping of this material into the eyes can be a potential problem.

Wound care for an open biopsy site is relatively simple. The wound should be cleansed twice daily using a wet cotton ball that has been soaked in 3% hydrogen peroxide. This is followed with application of a thin film of antibacterial ointment and a simple spot Band-Aid dressing. The central crust that forms usually separates in eight to 10 days, and restrictions on bathing and physical activities are not required.

If the punch biopsy completely removes a small lesion, or if the surgeon wishes to speed wound healing and provide the best cosmetic results possible, the punch biopsy site can be surgically closed with suture. The requirements for performing this procedure are changed only slightly to accomplish this closure. The skin is prepared in the usual fashion. Before obtaining the

138. Harris MN, Gumport SL (1975) Biopsy technique for malignant melanoma. **J Dermatol Surg** 1:24.
139. Rampen FHJ, van der Esch EP (1985) Biopsy and survival of malignant melanoma. **J Am Acad Dermatol** 12:385.
140. Barnett R, Stranc M (1979) A method of producing improved scars following excision of small lesions of the back. **Ann Plast Surg** 3:391.

specimen, however, the skin is stretched slightly, 90 degrees away from the line of anticipated closure. This is accomplished by stretching the skin between the thumb and index finger of the surgeon's opposite hand. While the skin is being stretched in this fashion, the punch biopsy is performed in the same fashion as previously described. This maneuver results in the creation of an oval defect, not a round one, greatly facilitating linear closure of the wound.

The suture material used for this type of closure is frequently a function of the child's age and the size of the biopsy performed. The use of an absorbable suture may be preferable when treating small children who are apprehensive about the discomfort of having sutures removed. This could include polyglactin and polyglycolic acid suture materials, or mild chromic gut, which is less reactive than the normal chromic gut sutures. The 6–0 size will predictably dissolve in five to seven days (Fig. 5.10). For adolescents or other patients in whom suture removal does not present a problem, it is preferable to use 4–0 or 5–0 monofilament nylon sutures and remove them after seven to eight days. For added support after the sutures have been removed, reinforcing adhesive skin strips can be applied on the surface for an additional seven to 10 days.

SHAVE BIOPSY

Another common and simple biopsy procedure is the superficial shave biopsy.[141] This technique is usually employed in the rapid removal of benign exophytic lesions such as molluscum contagiosum, verruca vulgaris, intradermal nevocellular nevi and acrochordons. This procedure is also helpful in the removal of dome-shaped lesions from anatomic locations, such as the nose, where excisional removal might create an unacceptable scar. In addition, it is often useful in children presenting with a large number of lesions since it can provide a rapid and inexpensive form of treatment with minimal scarring or pain, and rapid healing.

For this biopsy, after local anesthesia has been obtained and the skin suitably prepped, a #15 Bard-Parker blade attached to a scalpel handle is used in a sawing back-and-forth motion to remove the lesion flush with the surrounding skin. When the lesion has been nearly completely severed, the free edge of the specimen is held with a pair of fine-toothed forceps to stabilize the specimen and provide counteraction. Hemostasis is obtained using topical application of aluminum chloride. Wound care is identical to that required for punch biopsies and complete re-epithelialization usually occurs within seven to 10 days.

With practice, an alternate method of performing shave biopsies can be performed using a sterilized razor blade (Fig. 5.11). With this technique, the blade is first broken into halves longitudinally. The sharp edge of one-half of the blade is bent into a semicircular shape between the thumb and forefinger. Alternatively, a similar procedure may be performed using a specialized instrument called a Dermablade™. Using a sawing, back-and-forth motion, the lesion is removed completely flush with the surrounding skin.

SCISSOR BIOPSY

Scissor biopsies are generally reserved for removing small pedunculated lesions, such as acrochordons and intradermal nevi. These types of lesions can often be removed without local anesthesia, even in children, using small, sharp, curved iris scissors. If no anesthesia is used, however, the application of a hemostatic agent will result in a significant amount of burning pain that is not well tolerated, even by adults. If a larger lesion is to be removed with this technique, the use of local anesthetic is recommended. The technique employed for scissor biopsies consists of holding the pedunculated lesion with a pair of fine-toothed forceps while the lesion is snipped flush with the surrounding skin using iris scissors. There is usually minimal bleeding and postoperative wound care is minimal. Complete healing is usually accomplished within seven to 10 days.

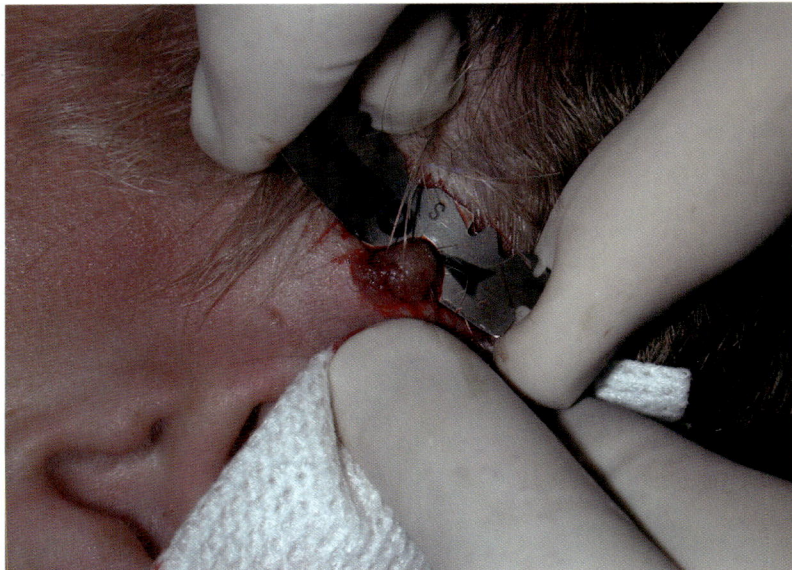

Fig. 5.11 Shave biopsy is performed using the sharp edge of a razor blade and a sawing, back-and-forth motion.

EXCISIONAL BIOPSY

Excisions or excisional biopsies are used for complete removal of lesions that are too large or deep to remove comfortably with either the punch- or shave-biopsy techniques. The main principle in planning excisions is to attempt to place the resultant scar within or parallel to natural body folds, creases, or relaxed skin-tension lines.[142] If no lines or creases are present, which is commonly the case in children and adolescents, the incision line should be placed at a right angle to the pull of the underlying muscles. The location of these lines can be relatively well predicted to occur in certain directions and form with age due to the intrinsic effects of ultraviolet, aging and muscular activity. The presence of these lines was first described in 1886 by Langer,[143] and they still bear his name (Fig. 5.12). While not constant in all patients, these lines frequently offer some guidance in determining the best placement of surgical incisions.

An alternative method to determine proper orientation of incision lines in children is the squeeze-and-pinch method. In this procedure, the skin surrounding the excision site is compressed between the thumb and forefinger in all directions. Pinching in one direction will usually demonstrate greater laxity than the others, which becomes the direction in which the incision line should be placed.

Slightly curved, crescent-shaped, or S-shaped lines are more often anatomically correct and are therefore less noticeable than straight lines. Regardless of age, the child can often assist the surgeon in determining the proper alignment of an incision line by exaggerating certain facial expressions, such as squinting, smiling, frowning, or pursing the lips. Every effort should be made for the healed incision line to simulate a natural fold, crease, or line.[144]

Once the correct orientation for an excision has been established, the proper length must also be determined. This is usually dependent on the size of the lesion to be removed, the anatomic location, the elasticity and thickness of the skin, and the type of lesion present. Generally, benign lesions can be removed with very narrow margins of 0.5 to 1.0mm and still ensure adequate removal. The length of the incision is then determined by the width and is usually in the ratio of 3:1. This length-to-width ratio will create a fusiform excision with 30-degree angles at both ends in most cases.

141. Kopf AW, Popkin GL (1974) Shave biopsies for cutaneous lesions. **Arch Dermatol** 110:637.
142. Borges AF (1984) Relaxed skin tension lines (RSTL) versus other skin lines. **Plast Reconstr Surg** 73:144.
143. Rubin LR (1958) Langer's lines and facial scars. **Plast Reconstr Surg** 3:147.
144. Kraissl CJ (1951) The selection of appropriate lines for elective surgical incisions. **Plast Reconstr Surg** 8:1.

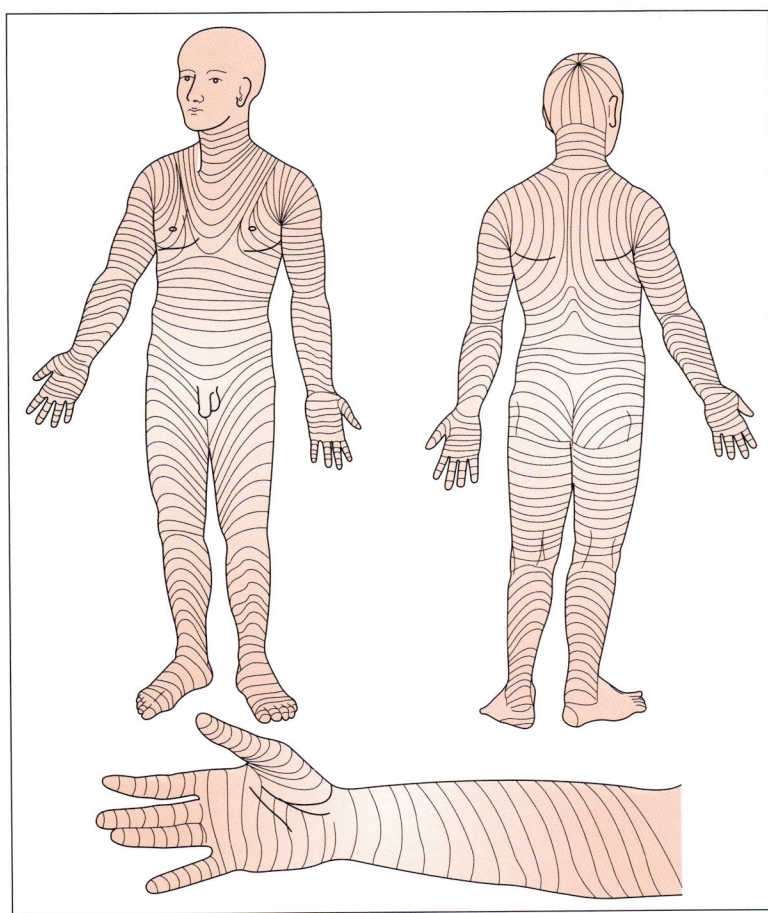

Fig. 5.12   Langer's lines offer guidance when determining the best placement of surgical incisions.

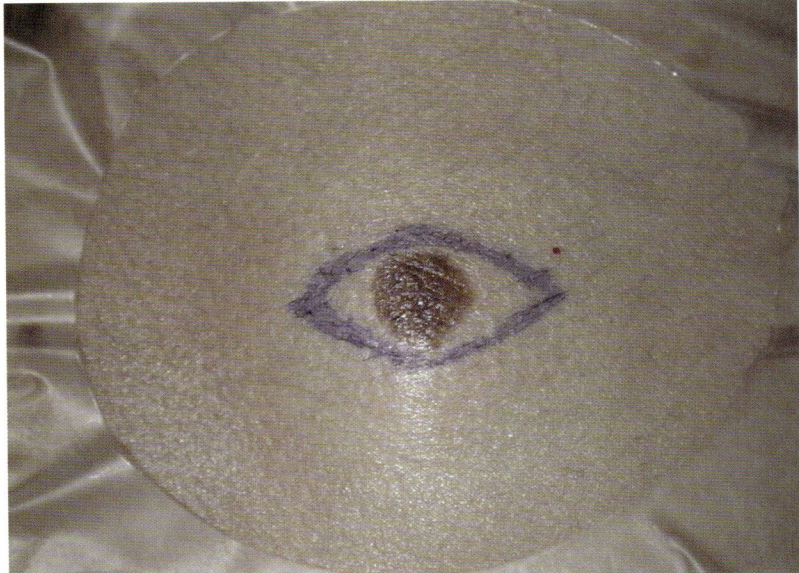

Fig. 5.13   Preoperative appearance of a nevus with planned excision lines in place.

This has been shown to yield the most satisfactory cosmetic and functional result.

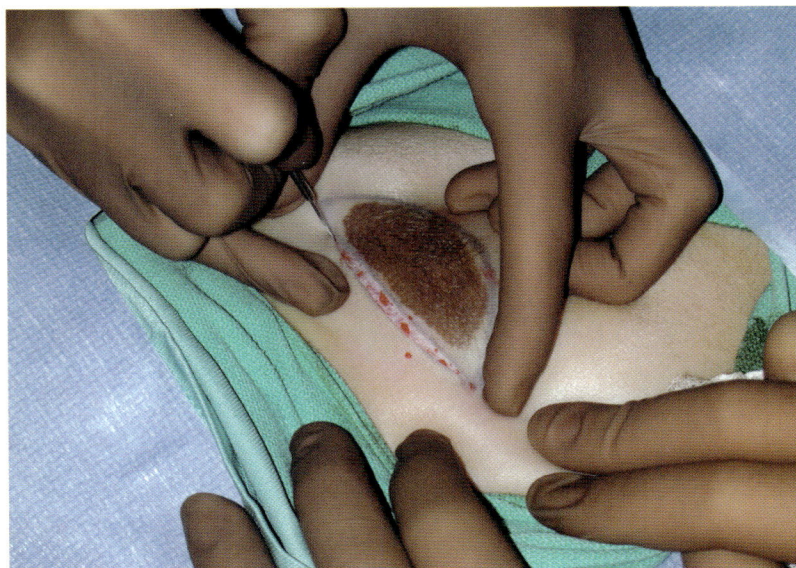

Fig. 5.14   The fusiform specimen is sharply excised using a #15 Bard-Parker blade held perpendicular to the skin.

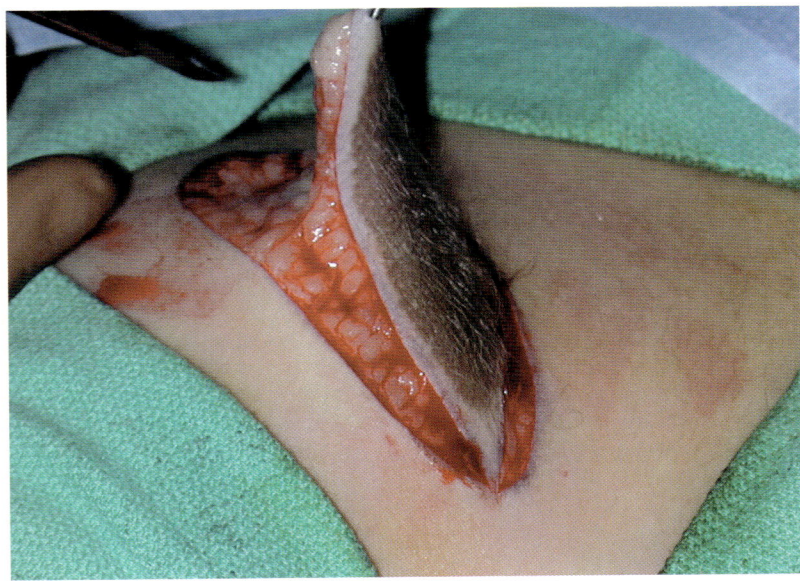

Fig. 5.15   The fusiform specimen is freed from attached deeper structures using a scalpel or iris scissor.

The planned excision lines are marked with a skin-marking pen usually containing gentian violet (Fig. 5.13). The skin is then prepped in the standard fashion with chlorhexidine or povidone-iodine. After placing sterile towels around the planned excision site, the fusiform specimen is sharply excised using a #15 Bard-Parker blade, which is held perpendicular to the skin (Fig. 5.14).[145] The ellipse is freed from attached deeper structures using a scalpel or iris scissors, and the specimen is submitted for histopathologic examination (Fig. 5.15).

The wound is prepared for closure by first controlling any minor bleeding that is present with either electrosurgical instrumentation or suture ligatures. Undermining is performed with blunt-tipped dissection scissors by lifting up each edge of the excision with skin hooks[146] to minimize trauma, or fine-

145. Robinson JK (1982) Some tips on wound closure. **J Dermatol Surg Oncol** 8:698.

146. Stegman SJ (1978) Suturing techniques for dermatologic surgery. **J Dermatol Surg Oncol** 4:63.

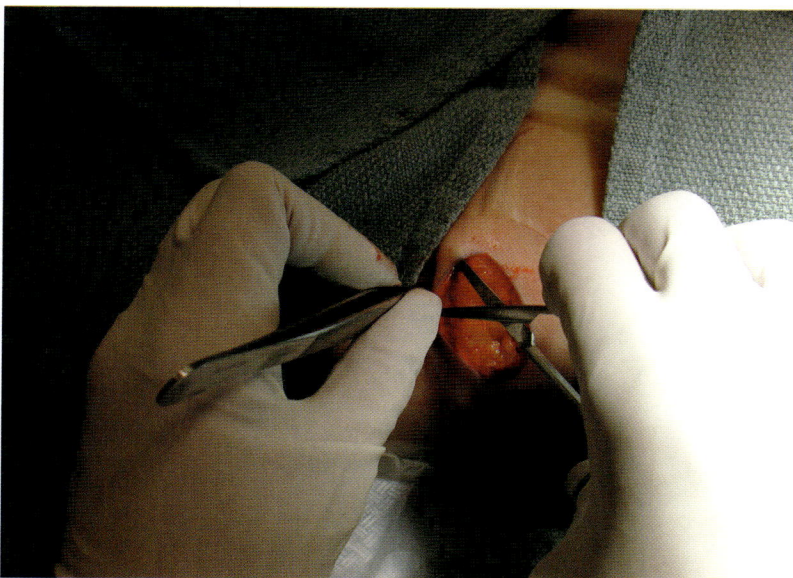

Fig. 5.16 Undermining is performed with blunt-tipped dissection scissors.

toothed forceps and inserting the scissors with the blades closed (Fig. 5.16). Once they have been sufficiently inserted, the blades are opened to loosen the soft tissue attachments gradually. After sufficient laxity of tissue has been created to permit easy closure, the wound is rechecked for any residual bleeding. If none is found, the wound is ready for closure.

Wound closure techniques for excisional biopsies

Wound closure is usually performed in layers.[147,148] If a large dead-space has been created by the removal of a large cyst, for example, the dead space should be closed to minimize the risk of postoperative hematoma or seroma formation. This can best be accomplished by using a pursestring type of closure with absorbable suture. This type of suture placement will pull the deep tissues together from all sides. More commonly, however, buried absorbable sutures may be used to close the dermal defect. This suturing technique reduces tension so epidermal sutures will not cause cross-hatched scarring. By starting the passage of the needle in the middle of the wound at its greatest depth, the knot, when tied, will end up being buried at the depth of the tissue. This lessens the possibility of suture material spitting through the incision line before it has been completely absorbed. Depending on the size of the excision and the amount of tension present, several buried sutures may be necessary to close the excision without tension at the surface.[149]

The surface of the wound may be closed with any number of different methods.[150] The simplest and most common method is to use interrupted monofilament nylon sutures. Interrupted sutures will permit fine adjustments to give precise coaptation of wound edges and give equal tension across the incision line even when edges are of unequal thickness. If tension is present, the epidermal suture is tied with a surgeon's knot. This is done by double-looping the first throw and then tying the second knot square. Interrupted sutures can also be used as the preliminary approximation sutures in accurately coating edges of large wounds or flaps.

If there is much tension across a wound, even after placement of buried sutures, two other types of suturing techniques may be required. The first is the vertical mattress. This technique acts to evert the wound edges by creating two loops with the needle. The first loop is the far one and is made 5 to 10mm from the incision line. The second loop is the near one made inside the first one, 1 to 2mm from the incision line. The other tension-relieving suturing technique is the horizontal mattress. This box type of suturing places all entrance and exit wounds equidistant from the incision line, approximately 5 to 10mm from the edge. Both techniques permit satisfactory closure of wounds with tension but may increase the risk of cross-hatched scarring and are usually removed four to five days postoperatively to minimize that risk.

Another epidermal closure technique that is especially advantageous in the closure of long wounds is the running or running-locked suturing technique. In this procedure, a single knot is tied at one end of the incision line, as is normally done for simple interrupted suturing, but the suture is not cut. Instead, the suture is run the entire length of the incision by repeatedly passing it from side to side in continuous fashion. For wounds which are highly vascular and hemostasis is difficult to achieve, the needle can be passed through each loop, which results in the locking of the stitch in place and prevents slippage of the entire chain of knots. With practice, this technique can substantially shorten the time required to close a long wound.

Another technique to close a wound is the running subcuticular suturing method,[151] using 4–0 monofilament suture made from either polypropylene or polybutester. While this technique is more difficult to perform, and the surgeon must still first close the dead-space in the standard manner, it can serve several useful purposes. The first is to avoid the frequent cosmetic problem of cross-hatching that results from the tension created by interrupted epidermal sutures. The second is that this type of suturing technique allows the sutures to remain in place for a longer period of time without resulting in much tissue reactivity. This in turn permits the development of greater tensile strength in the healing wound prior to suture removal. Lastly, since very little suture material is left exposed with this technique, there is little chance the child will subject the wound to undue manipulation or surface trauma.

With the subcuticular closure technique, care must be taken to keep the suture in the same plane from one side of the incision to the other in order to achieve accurate wound edge approximation (Fig. 5.17). If any small gaps or irregularities are present after completion of this stitch, they can be corrected by the placement of several small superficial epicuticular sutures. For long wounds, eg., wounds greater than 3 or 4cm, a loop of suture should

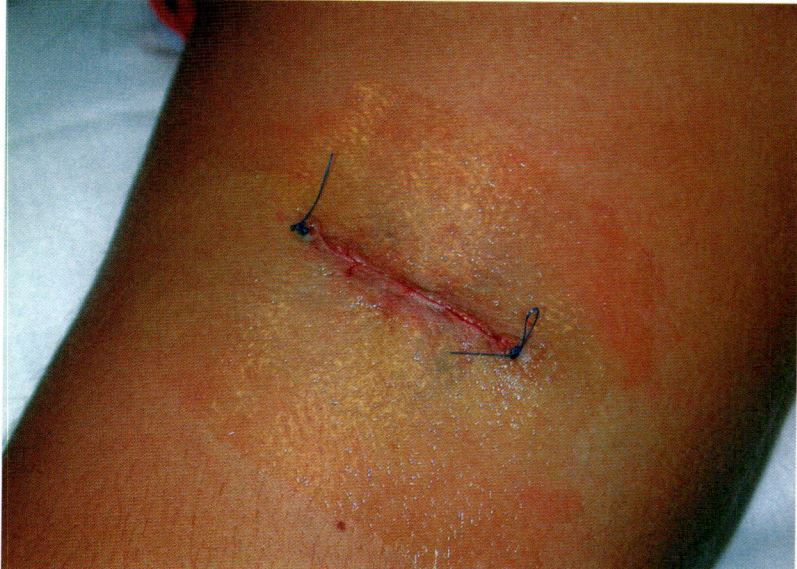

Fig. 5.17 Running subcuticular suture in place on an extremity. This suture may be left in place for several weeks, allowing wounds under tension to heal maximally prior to suture removal.

147. Stegman SJ (1975) Fifteen ways to close surgical wounds. **J Dermatol Surg** 1:25.
148. Stegman SJ (1978) Suturing techniques for dermatologic surgery. **J Dermatol Surg Oncol** 4:63.
149. Sauter E, Thibodeaux K, Myers B (1985) Effect of high tension and relaxing incisions on wound healing in rats. **South Med J** 78:1451.
150. Wagner AM (1998) Slick suturing for impatient patients. **Pediatr Dermatol** 15(1):62–64.
151. Sanders RJ (1975) Subcuticular skin closure description of technique. **J Dermatol Surg** 1:61.

be left exposed every inch to facilitate removal without suture breakage, the so-called "escape stitch." Alternatively, the subcuticular suture can be periodically tied with a short piece of silk suture, which protrudes through the incision, the spider stitch,[152] so called due to the silk sutures that resemble the legs of a spider that emanate from the wound. In this way, the long subcuticular suture may be removed painlessly and without the risk of suture breakage common in longer incisions.

Sutures are left in place for variable periods of time, depending on the anatomic location, size of excision, amount of tension under which the wound was closed, and the type of closure that was used. In general, sutures used to close excisions performed on the trunk are left in place for 10 to 14 days; for the extremities for seven to 10 days; and for the face five to seven days. Regardless of the anatomic site, once the sutures have been removed, it is worthwhile to place supportive adhesive strips on the surface for an additional week, to minimize the possibility of dehiscence of the wound by reducing tension on the surface.

INCISIONAL BIOPSY

The incisional biopsy is usually reserved for obtaining tissue from large lesions for histologic confirmation of a clinical diagnosis. It is also used when complete surgical removal of a lesion is not feasible as a primary procedure, and a more definitive procedure is anticipated at a later date. This technique is commonly used in the diagnosis of inflammatory and infiltrative disorders of the dermis, or subcutaneous tissue. Incisional biopsy is the most efficient method to diagnose panniculitis and other disorders of adipose tissue.

On occasion, serial-staged excision of large solitary lesions may be used to minimize the scarring that would result from a single-stage procedure. The most common situation in which this type of surgical procedure is used is with medium-sized congenital nevocellular nevi on the face. This technique uses an incisional biopsy to remove only the central portion of the nevus (Figs 5.18, 5.19). The wound is closed in standard fashion and allowed to heal for two to three months. After that interval, a second incisional biopsy procedure is performed to remove both the first surgical scar as well as an additional portion of the center of the nevus. This serial process is continued until the entire lesion has been removed, which for some larger lesions may require one year or more. The main advantage of this technique is in minimizing anatomical distortion by keeping the scar as small as possible. By removing only small portions of the lesion at a time and allowing the body to adjust to the new tension and relax sufficiently to permit removal of additional portions of the lesion, this procedure can be truly beneficial. The technique for incisional biopsy is identical to that described for excisions, except that only a portion of the lesion is removed at a time.

COMPLICATIONS

When performing surgical biopsies of any type, it is important for the surgeon to remember that there are certain danger areas where there is a risk of inadvertent injury to sensory or motor nerves. One commonly overlooked danger area is lateral to the eyebrow, which is the location of the temporal branch of the facial nerve. This nerve gives motor innervation to the forehead and lies at a relatively superficial level in the skin. Most surgeons are acquainted with the location of the facial nerve found in the preauricular area, so this is not a common problem. Also, the facial nerve lies relatively deep within the mass of the parotid gland in most individuals so the risk of injury is relatively small. However, the 11th cranial (spinal accessory) nerve is not deeply located. It lies superficially within the posterior triangle of the neck, bordered by the sternocleidomastoid and trapezius muscles and clavicle. Injury to this nerve will result in shoulder drop. The final nerve which may be inadvertently injured because of its superficial location is the common

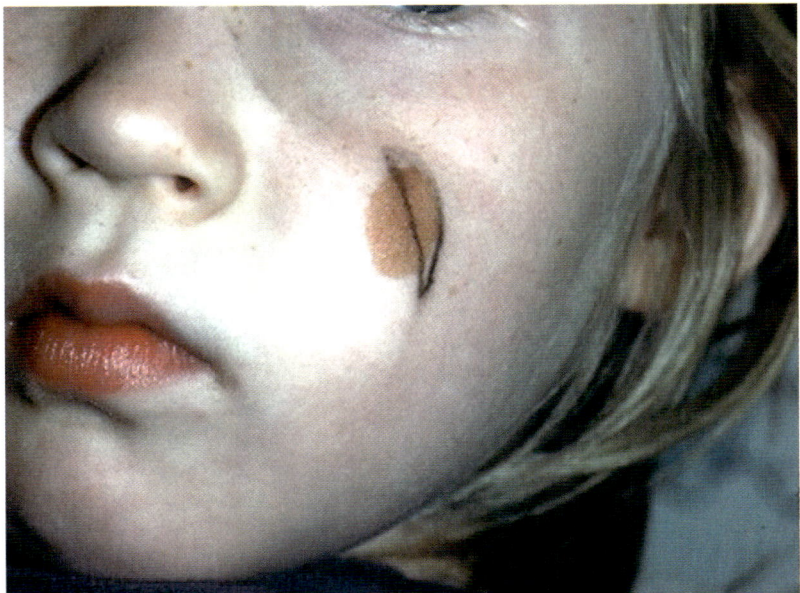

Fig. 5.18 Preoperative appearance of young child with a facial congenital melanocytic nevus before a two-staged excision.

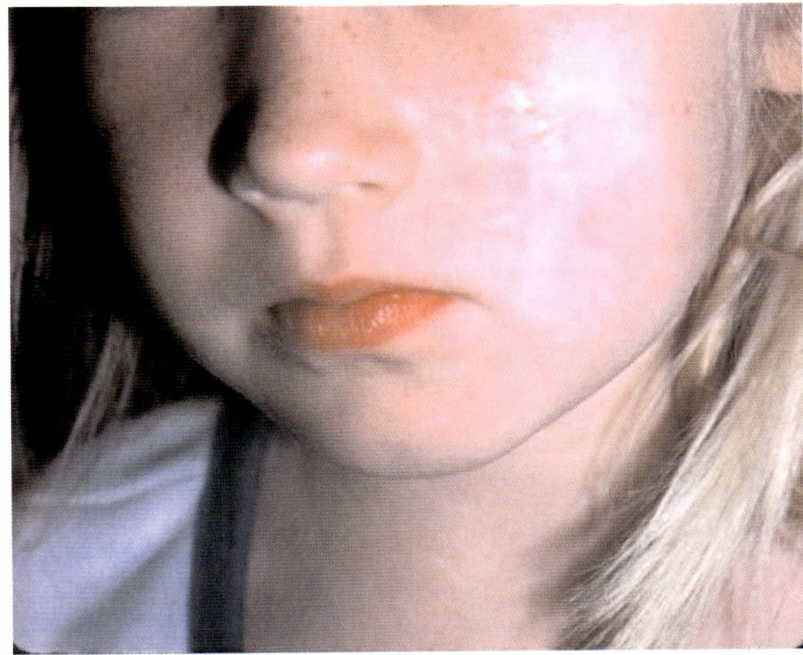

Fig. 5.19 Postoperative appearance after two-staged excision of facial nevus.

peroneal nerve. This nerve is found on the lateral aspect of the proximal lower leg. If damaged, foot drop will likely result.

When the dermatologic surgeon is working in one of these high-risk areas, it may be prudent to perform a more superficial biopsy than normal. To add an additional measure of safety, local infiltration of sterile saline into the biopsy area following injection of local anesthetic will bulge the skin and subcutaneous tissue up away from the deeper nerves. This effectively increases the amount of tissue that must be transected before reaching the level of the motor nerves.

152. Bickel KD, Gibbs NF, Cunningham BB (1998) The subcuticular "spider" stitch: a simple solution to suture breakage and patient discomfort in long incisions. **Pediatr Dermatol** Nov–Dec;15(6):480–481.

The only arterial structure likely to be damaged by surgical biopsies is the temporal artery. This vessel takes a variably circuitous route within or slightly anterior to the temporal hairline. Before performing biopsies in this location, especially punch biopsies, care should be taken to palpate for the location of this vascular structure. If this vessel is accidentally severed, the wound should be explored, and the proximal end of the vessel should be suture-ligated with polyglycolic acid suture to prevent postoperative bleeding.

The diagnostic or therapeutic biopsy techniques used by dermatologists are relatively simple to learn and safe to perform. By following some simple guidelines and taking some precautions, uncomplicated surgical skin biopsies can be performed even in infants and small children.

DRESSINGS

With little doubt, no aspect of dermatologic surgery has undergone more recent change than wound care and surgical dressings (Table 5.3). This is largely the result of the recognition that of all the local factors that can favorably influence wound healing, maintaining the surface humidity of the wound is the most important consideration.[153–155] A demonstrable reduction in the rate and quality of healing has been proved in association with wound desiccation.[156,157] Wound desiccation, occurring with an air exposure time of only two to three hours, can result in the creation of additional necrosis at the base of the wound which can delay healing by up to 50%.[158] Despite our increased knowledge of the pathophysiology of the healing wound, a number of wound care practices that have been shown to be ineffective or harmful are still widely used. This includes the repeat application of toxic wound cleansing agents, inappropriate use of antibiotics, and the practice of wet-to-dry dressings.[159]

The traditional technique that has been used for years to prevent wound desiccation consisted of the application of a thin layer of occlusive antibacterial ointment, followed by the application of a nonadherent sterile gauze dressing. An absorptive cotton gauze layer, placed on the surface for protection against

external trauma, was held in place with slight compression using paper tape. Dressings were typically changed once or twice a day following interval cleansing of the wound surface with a 3% solution of hydrogen peroxide. Although effective, dressings of this type were particularly unsuitable for pediatric patients. They were bulky and difficult to maintain with the high activity level of a child. In addition, frequent dressing changes were traumatic and painful for both parent and child.

Fortunately, many new synthetic surgical dressings have been introduced over the past several years. These dressings were developed in an attempt to reduce the amount of wound care required by the patient, while simultaneously maximizing the opportunity for rapid wound healing through the creation of the moist ideal environment for the wound healing processes to occur. While the precise indications for many of these dressings have not been unequivocally established, they usually are interchangeable to reduce postoperative wound care, minimize pain and swelling,[156] speed healing,[157] and prevent desiccation.[160] The first two types of surgical dressings to be developed were made from polyurethane and hydrocolloid materials. These dressings have been shown to be very useful in treating children with small sutured wounds because of their shared features of relative water impermeability and self-adherence. When treating small sutured wounds, either type of dressing can be applied directly to the surface of the wound immediately after completion of the procedure and left in place until suture removal.[161] A small pressure dressing can be placed over the hydrocolloid dressing for the first 48 hours if the suspected activity level of the child will increase the risk for postoperative bleeding. This can be removed in 48 hours if the dressing is too bulky, maintaining the wound sterility and avoiding exposure to the air. These techniques reduce the amount of wound care required by the patient or by parents while protecting the wound from dust, dirt and bacterial invasion.[162–164] The dressings also speed the rate of wound healing by maintaining the surface humidity of the wound.[165–167] The disadvantage of these dressings lies in the misconception by parents that children can continue normal bathing habits and physical activities.

Synthetic polyurethane and hydrocolloid dressings have also revolutionized the care of ulcerated hemangiomas.[168] The use of these dressings can markedly reduce the pain, risk of infection, and rate of time to healing in these open wounds. Dressings can be kept in place for several days at a time and the dressing adhesives are less irritating to infant skin than standard tape adhesive. The hydrocolloid dressings and hydrogel dressings are particularly effective when there is significant exudate from the wounds since they are able to absorb many times their weight in exudative fluid. Dressings can be applied immediately post-laser treatment for these ulcerated wounds and the infrequent need for the dressing changes minimizes the pain and trauma, both for the infant and parents.

Synthetic polyurethane and hydrocolloid surgical dressings have also been used with great success in the management of split-thickness skin graft donor sites where they simultaneously reduce pain and speed the rate of re-epithelialization.[169,170] The hydrocolloid dressings are also effective in debriding ulcers[171] and for treating superficial burns.[172] For patients who are susceptible to friction blisters, the hydrocolloid dressings may be used prophylactically at predisposed sites on the heels or toes before engaging in physical activity.

TABLE 5.3	Common types of surgical dressings
Impregnates	Adaptic, Vaseline Gauze, Biobrane Gauze, Xeroflo, Jelonet, Aquaphor Gauze
Polyurethane films	Op-Site, Bioclusive, Tegaderm, Ensure-It, ACU-derm, Polyskin, Uniflex, Omiderm, Mefilm
Hydrocolloids	Duoderm, Comfeel, Ulcus, J&J Ulcer Dressing, Actiderm, Restore, Ultec, Duoderm-CGF, Hydrapad, Intrasite, Tegasorb, Granuflex, Coloplast
Hydrogels	Vigilon, Spenco Second Skin, Geliperm, Elastogel, Cutinova Gelfolie, Cutinova-Thin
Alginates	Algiderm, Kaltostat, Seasorb, Tegagen, Sobsan, Melgisorb
Foams	Synthaderm, LYOfoam, Allevin, Epigard
Miscellaneous	N-terface, Biobrane, Mepitel

153. Ladin DA (1998) Understanding dressings. **Clinics in Plastic Surgery** 25:433.
154. Aubock J (1999) Synthetic dressings. **Current Problems in Dermatology** 27:26.
155. Bello YM, Phillips TJ (2000) Therapeutic dressings. **Advances in Dermatol** 16:253.
156. Eaglstein WH (1985) Experiences with biosynthetic dressings. **J Am Acad Dermatol** 12:434.
157. Eaglstein WH (2001) Moist wound healing with occlusive dressings: a clinical focus. **Dermatologic Surgery** 27:175.
158. Hinman CD, Maibach H (1963) Effect of air exposure and occlusion on experimental human skin wounds. **Nature** 200:377.
159. Nwomeh BC, Yager DR, Cohen LK (1998) Physiology of the chronic wound. **Clinics in Plastic Surg** 25:341.
160. Winter GD, Scales JT (1963) Effect of air drying and dressings on the surface of a wound. **Nature** 197:191.
161. Hunt TK, Hopf H, Hussain Z (2000) Physiology of wound healing. **Advances in Skin and Wound Care** 135:6.
162. Mertz PM, Marshall DA, Eaglstein WH (1985) Occlusive wound dressings to prevent bacterial invasion and wound infection. **J Am Acad Dermatol** 12:662.
163. Smith DJ, Thomson PD, Garner WL, Rodriguez JL (1994) Donor site repair. **Am J Surg** 167:495.
164. Newman JP, Fitzgerald P, Koch RJ (2000) Review of closed dressings after laser resurfacing. **Dermatologic Surgery** 26:562.
165. Lui HT (2000) Wound care following CO_2 laser resurfacing using Kaltostat, Duoderm and Telfa for dressings. **Dermatologic Surgery** 26:341.
166. Hien NT, Prawer SE, Katz HI (1988) Facilitated wound healing using transparent film dressing following Mohs micrographic surgery. **Arch Dermatol** 124:903.
167. Viclano V, Castera JE, Medrano J et al. (2000) Effect of hydrocolloid dressings on healing by second intention. **European Journal of Surgery** 166:229.
168. Freiden IJ (1997) Special symposium: management of hemangiomas. **Pediatric Dermatology** 14:57.
169. Barnett A, Berkowity RL, Mills R, Vistnes LM (1983) Comparison of synthetic adhesive moisture vapor permeable and fine mesh gauze dressings for split-thickness skin graft donor sites. **Am J Surg** 145:379.
170. Persson K, Salemark L (2000) How to dress split thickness skin grafts: a prospective randomized study of four dressings. **Scand J of Plastic & Reconstr Surg and Hand Surg** 34:55.
171. Handfield-Jones SE, Grattan CE, Simpson RA, Kennedy CT (1988) Comparison of a hydrocolloid dressing and paraffin gauze in the treatment of venous ulcers. **Br J Dermatol** 118:425.
172. Hermans MH (1987) Hydrocolloid dressing (Duoderm) for the treatment of superficial and deep partial thickness burns. **Scand J Plast Reconstr Surg Hand Surg** 21:283.

Several unique synthetic surgical dressings have also been introduced with very specific indications.[173] One of these, N-Terface, is constructed as a porous monofilament fabric from high-density plastic. It is used as an interpositional membrane on the surface of skin graft recipient sites, as it allows the passage of surface exudate from the wound without becoming adherent to it. This permits dressings to be changed in an atraumatic fashion without disturbing the graft. Another unique dressing, Biobrane, has been used successfully in managing dermabrasion wounds and skin graft donor sites. This dressing is composed of a nylon mesh that is bound to dimethylsiloxane and purified type 1 porcine skin collagen polypeptides. The dressing adheres to the surface of the wound to provide a flexible covering that maintains the humidity by reducing the amount of water lost from the skin. In this fashion, Biobrane has been used successfully in managing dermabrasion wounds,[174] skin graft donor sites,[175] burns, Stevens–Johnson syndrome and toxic epidermal necrolysis.[176]

For more exudative wounds, the hydrogel dressings are most effective. These are nonadherent, gas-permeable, and largely composed of water and polyethylene oxide or polyvinyl alcohol.[177] This group of synthetic surgical dressings has the remarkable ability to absorb one to two times their weight in exudative fluid while maintaining the surface humidity of the wound. Because of these properties, dressings in this group have been used to manage dermabrasion wounds[178] and superficial open wounds following carbon dioxide laser surgery[164] or pulsed dye laser surgery for ulcerated hemangiomas.[168]

BIOLOGICAL DRESSINGS

In the past decade, tremendous progress has been made in the development of biologic dressings.[155] Many of these skin substitutes have been approved by the United States Food and Drug Administration (FDA) in the treatment of chronic wounds such as burns and venous leg ulcers (Table 5.4). Although these are rare problems in the pediatric dermatology population, the benefit of these systems is apparent for wound healing problems such as epidermolysis bullosa or surgical wounds.

Three types of grafts have been developed over the last 25 years since Rheinwalt and Green first developed a method that made cultivation of human keratinocytes *in vitro* possible in 1975.[179] The original grafts were epidermal in nature and derived from either the patient's own skin (autografts) or from allogenic donors (allografts).[180] Success in the pediatric population in treatment of giant congenital nevi[181] and epidermolysis bullosa[182] has been seen with autografts. Although they provided the benefit of coverage of large areas, they required skin biopsy, considerable time for graft cultivation and were quite fragile as well as very costly. Currently, cultured epidermal allografts that derive from neonatal foreskin are being developed, but are not yet commercially available. They have been successfully used in treating epidermolysis bullosa[183] and dermabrasion wounds.[184]

The second group of skin substitute products that have been developed is dermal replacement products: AlloDerm, Integra, and TransCyte (formerly Dermagraft-transitional covering). AlloDerm is a chemically treated human cryopreserved de-epidermalized allograft that forms an acellular dermal matrix

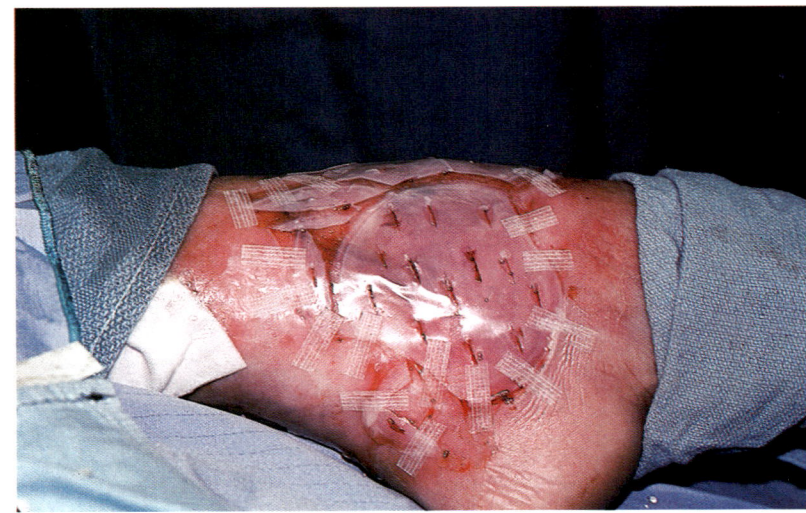

Fig. 5.20 Placement of *Apligraf*™ on epidermolysis bullosa patient with chronic wound.

TABLE 5.4   Pediatric applications of skin substitutes

Substitute	Tissue type	Pediatric use
Epidermal Grafts: Cultured epidermal autographs, allografts (Epicel)	Living keratinocyte sheets	Congenital nevi, EB, vitiligo, burns
Dermal Substitutes: Nonliving dermal replacements (Alloderm, Integra, TransCyte)	Extracellular matrix allogenic, acellular chondroitin-6-sulfate with silicone backing generated by allogeneic human dermal fibroblasts	Surgical wounds, EB Burns Burns
Composite Grafts: Human skin equivalent Apligraf	Living allogeneic bilayered construct of keratinocytes, fibroblasts and bovine type 1 collagen	EB, chronic wounds, excisional wounds

173. Salasche SJ, Winton GB (1986) Clinical evaluation of a nonadhering wound dressing. **J Dermatol Surg Oncol** 12:1220.
174. Pinski JB (1987) Dressings for dermabrasion: new aspects. **J Dermatol Surg Oncol** 13:673.
175. Prasad JK, Feller I, Thomson PD (1987) A prospective controlled trial of Biobrane versus scarlet red on skin graft donor areas. **J Burn Care Rehabil** 8:384.
176. Bradley T, Brown RE, Kucan JO, Smoot EC, Hussmann J (1995) Toxic epidermal necrolysis: a review and report of the successful use of Biobrane for early wound coverage. **Annals of Plastic Surgery** 35:124.
177. Mandy SH (1983) A new primary wound dressing made of polyethylene oxide gel. **J Dermatol Surg Oncol** 9:153.
178. Geronemus RG, Robins P (1982) The effect of two new dressings on epidermal wound healing. **J Dermatol Surg Oncol** 8:850.

179. Rheinwald J, Green H (1975) Serial cultivation of strains of human epidermal keratinocytes: Formation of keratinizing colonies from single cells. **Cell** 6:331–344.
180. Philips TJ (1998) New skin for old: Developments in biological skin substitutes (editorial; comment). **Arch Dermatol** 134:344–349.
181. Gallico GI, O'Connor N, Compton C et al. (1989) Cultured epithelial autografts for giant congenital nevi. **J Plast Reconstr Surg** 84:1–9.
182. Carter D, Lin A, Varghese M et al. (1987) Treatment of junctional epidermolysis bullosa with epidermal autografts. **J Am Acad Dermatol** 17:246–250.
183. Witt PD, Cohen DT, Mallory S (1999) Use of a permanent acellular dermal allograft in recessive dystrophic epidermolysis bullosa involving the hands. **Arch Dermatol** 135:503–506.
184. Arambula H, Sierra-Martinez E, Gonzalez-Aguirre N et al. (1999) Frozen human epidermal allogeneic cultures promote rapid healing of facial dermabrasion wounds. **Dermatol Surg** 25:708–712.

with an intact basement membrane complex. Integra is a bovine collagen and chondroitin-6-sulfate dermal matrix backed by a removable silicon rubber membrane. TransCyte is an extracellular matrix generated by human newborn fibroblasts cultured on a nylon mesh with a silicon epidermal layer, and Dermagraft is a biodegradable fibroblast polygalactic acid mesh without the silicon membrane. All of these have been used to accelerate the healing of diabetic ulcers,[185] in the treatment of burn injuries,[186] and in some patients with epidermolysis bullosa.[187]

More recently a third skin substitute product has been developed in the form of composite grafts, also known as Human Skin Equivalent or *Apligraf™* (Fig. 5.20). This dressing is a bilayered living construct that is composed of cultured human neonatal foreskin keratinocytes, fibroblasts and bovine type 1 collagen.[186] *Apligraf™* is approved by the FDA for use in venous ulcers and has been used in the treatment of patients with epidermolysis bullosa with successful wound healing.[187–190] Studies have shown that the use of *Apligraf™* for chronic venous ulcers is superior to compression alone and results in much more rapid healing.[191] A multicenter study looking at the efficacy of *Apligraf™* for the treatment of partial- and full-thickness surgical wounds has also been undertaken, demonstrating safe and satisfactory cosmetic results that were the same or better than what would be expected with split-thickness autografts in half of the patients.[192,193]

Composite grafts offer an advantage in that the construct acts as a barrier against infection and mechanical damage by providing structural support while secreting cytokines that can interact with the underlying tissue to promote wound repair.[187] Further studies will be needed to define the place of this composite graft in the treatment of pediatric surgical wounds and chronic wound patients with epidermolysis bullosa.

PEDIATRIC SURGICAL DRESSINGS: POSTOPERATIVE WOUND CARE

Success in pediatric surgery requires the use of patient-friendly dressings and postoperative wound care instructions that address the level of activity and special needs of the pediatric patient. Wound care instructions and post-operative restrictions must be reviewed with the pediatric patient prior to scheduling the surgery and again at the time of surgery. Written postoperative instructions are essential (Table 5.5). There are two important premises to caring for the postoperative wounds in the pediatric patient. The first is to minimize manipulation of the wound and thereby maintain wound integrity and sterility, and the second is to minimize postoperative activity thereby decreasing the postoperative complication rate.

Punch biopsy sites

Punch biopsy sites should be kept dry for 48 hours following the biopsy. Topical antibiotic ointment and adhesive tape changed on a daily basis subsequent until suture removal is recommended. Scalp biopsy sites should be covered with ointment only. Facial biopsy sites can be covered with hydrocolloid or poly-urethane dressings and left untouched until suture removal at five to seven days.

Shave biopsy sites

Wounds left to heal by second intention require specialized care in the pediatric patient to monitor for signs of infection. The most important aspect of postoperative care is preventing wound desiccation. This can be accomplished with the liberal application of topical antibiotic ointment and fresh adhesive tape on a daily basis or with the use of polyurethane or

TABLE 5.5   Post-operative instructions

- Keep bulky dressings in place for a minimum of 48 hours.
- DO NOT remove Steri-Strips from the wound. If Strips are lifting off, secure these with additional tape or Band-aids.
- Keep the wound dry until suture removal.
- Blood staining on the Steri-Strips is expected when the pressure dressing is removed. You may cover these, but do not remove them.
- Tylenol for pain; avoid ibuprofen (Motrin or Advil). Most pain results from excessive activity. If pain occurs, restrict activities.
- Physical activity, including but not limited to the following, should be restricted for four weeks following surgery:
- *No sports activities* including swimming, bicycle, scooter, skateboard or roller blade riding, dance, karate, horseback riding, frisbee, golf, tennis bowling, lasertage.
  - No gym at school for four weeks.
  - No sleepovers.
  - Avoid excessive walking (including shopping and "walking the mall" with friends).
  - No tumbling, pillow fights or wrestling.
- For bleeding or drainage from the wound, tenderness or pain (especially after 48°) contact:_____
- Follow-up suture removal:_____

hydrocolloid surgical dressings. The latter is preferable and can be changed every 2–3 days to speed healing. Dressings kept on longer will increase the risk of infection. Bathing daily will require daily dressing changes since even polyurethane dressings become dislodged with exposure to water.

It is typical for a rim of erythema to develop surrounding the second intention wound. Healing typically takes two to three weeks, depending on the size of the wound. Exudate from the wound and pain are signs of infection and should be brought to the attention of the surgeon immediately.

Sutured wounds

In general, wound dressings that minimize the necessity of wound care by parents will be most successful in the pediatric population. It is impossible to keep wound dressings intact with daily bathing, even when extraordinary attempts are made to use polyurethane dressings and to cover the affected area during the shower. I usually recommend that bathing be limited to hair washing and sponging the child until suture removal. This routine works best for pre-adolescents. For adolescent-age patients, the routine can be modified to allow for more age-appropriate personal hygiene.

The appropriate timing for suture removal depends on the type of suture placed and the location of the wound. (Table 5.6) In general, suture puncture

TABLE 5.6   Recommended timing of suture removal

Face	5–7 days
Trunk or extremities	10 days (interrupted sutures)
	14–21 days (running subcuticular sutures)
Scalp	12–14 days
Palms and soles	10–12 days

185. Gentzkow GD, Jensen JL, Pollak RA et al. (1999) Improved healing of diabetic foot ulcers after grafting with a living human dermal replacement. **Wounds** 11:77–84.
186. Purdue G (1996) Dermagraft-TC pivotal safety and efficacy study. **J Burn Care Rehabil** 18:13S–14S.
187. McGuire J, Birchall N, Cuono C et al. (1987) Successful engraftment of allogeneic keratinocytes in recessive dystrophic epidermolysis bullosa. **Clin Res** 35:720A.
188. Falabella A, Schachner L, Valencia I et al. (1999) The use of tissue engineered skin (Apligraf) to treat a newborn with epidermolysis bullosa. **Arch Dermatol** 135:1219–1222.
189. Falabella AF, Valencia IC, Eaglstein WH, Schachner LA (2000) Tissue-engineered skin (Apligraf) in the healing of patients with epidermolysis bullosa wounds. **Arch Dermatol** 136:1225.
190. Fine JD (2000) Skin bioequivalents and their role in the treatment of inherited epidermolysis bullosa. **Arch Dermatol** 136:1259.
191. Falanga V, Margolis D, Alvarez O et al. (1998) Rapid healing of venous ulcers and lack of clinical rejection with an allogeneic cultured human skin equivalent. Human Skin Equivalent Investigators Group [see comments]. **Arch Dermatol** 134:293–300.
192. Eaglstein WH, Alvarez OM, Auletta M et al. (1999) Acute excisional wounds treated with a tissue-engineered skin (Apligraf). **Dermatol Surg** 25:195–201.
193. Phillips T (1999) Tissue engineered skin. **Arch Dermatol** 135:977–978.

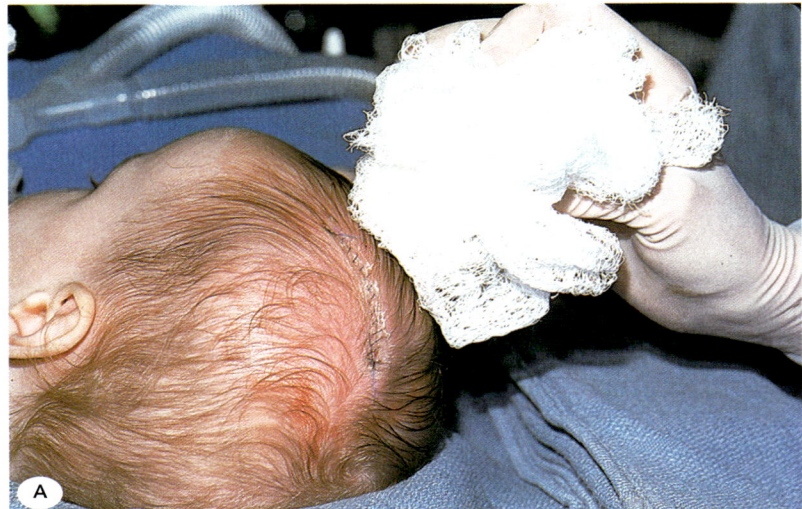

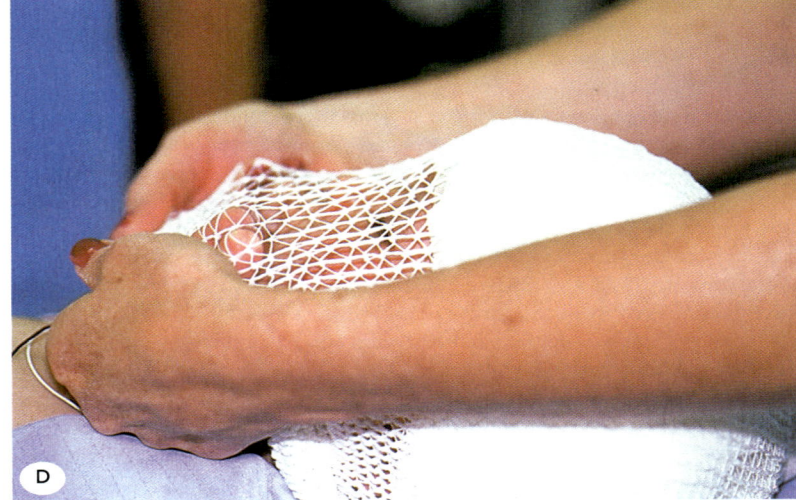

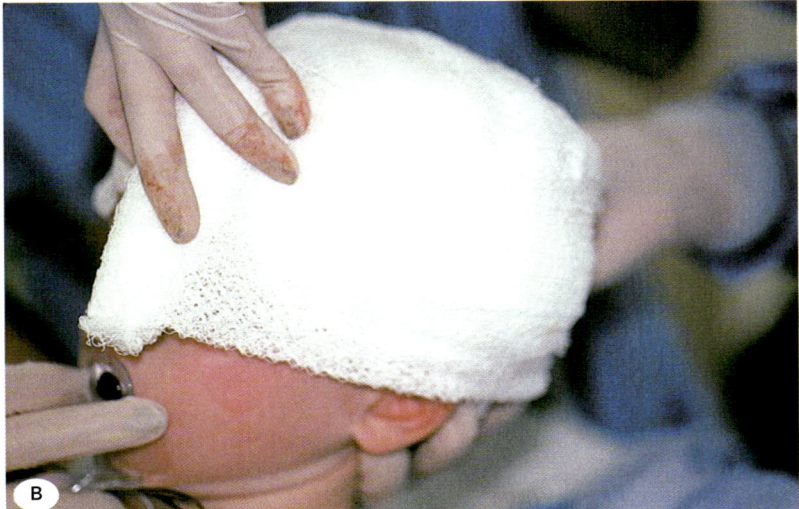

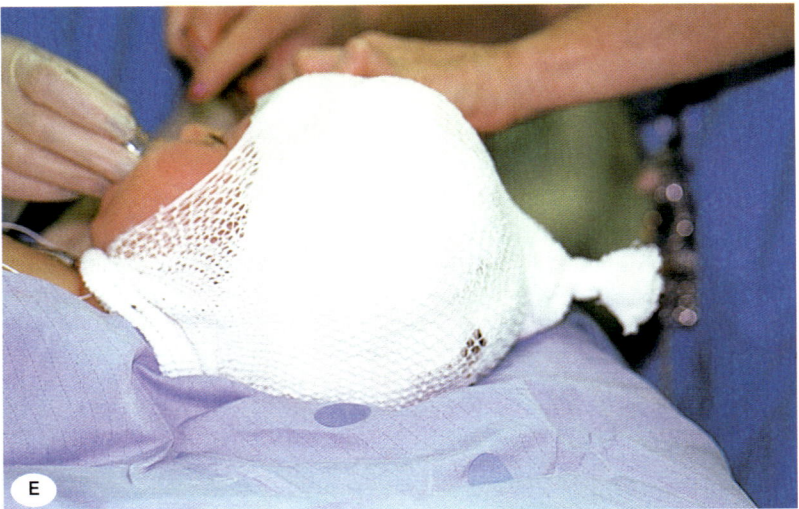

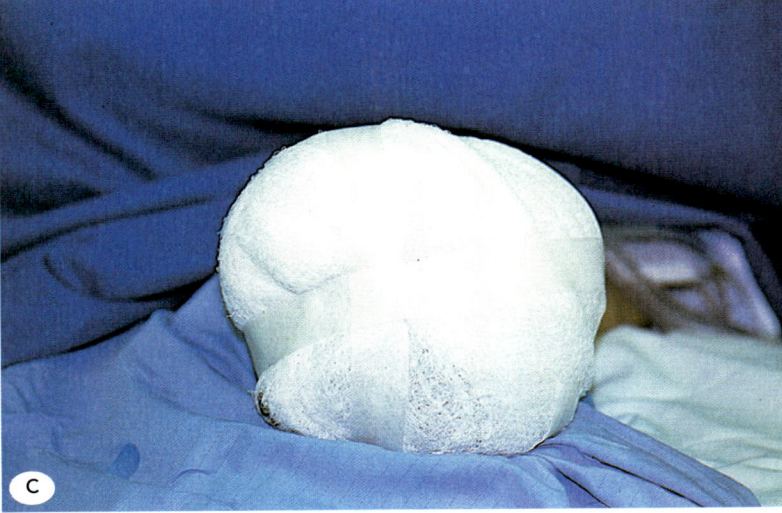

Fig. 5.21 Postoperative pressure dressing for the scalp. **(A)** Bulky dressing is used to cover the excision site. **(B)** Roll of gauze is wrapped around the head to keep dressing in place. **(C)** Silk tape is applied to surface of rolled gauze and along the forehead skin and posterior neck skin to secure dressing in place. **(D)** Tube bandage is pulled over the dressing. **(E)** Patient's face and ears are cut out of the tube bandage.

cuticular suture offers a great advantage in that it can be safely left in place for much longer without running the risk of producing suture marks. (See previous section.)

Scalp dressings

The pediatric dermatologic surgeon is frequently called upon to remove lesions from the scalp including nevus sebaceous, congenital nevi, and aplasia cutis. Wound dressings are particularly challenging here. For any dressing to be adherent to the scalp, the scalp must be shaved. Unfortunately a shaved scalp is more traumatic for a child than the procedure itself and is not recommended. Since scalps are highly vascular and therefore at the greatest risk of bleeding of all body sites, a modified scalp dressing is recommended that will avoid the need for removing scalp hair in larger wounds. Wounds of 1 cm or less in the scalp can usually be managed with antibiotic ointment only, without the need for any dressing. Wounds should be absolutely dry *before* suture closure. The ointment should be applied regularly several times per day to minimize crusting of the scalp wound and facilitate removal of the sutures with minimal discomfort. For prepubertal children, I recommend no

sites will re-epithelialize in approximately 10 days. For areas on the body that heal rapidly, such as the face and genital skin, removal of interrupted sutures at seven days is highly unlikely to leave noticeable suture marks. Unfortunately, the trunk, extremities, and scalp require longer for complete healing, especially in an active child. Interrupted sutures removed at 10 days may even result in suture marks on the trunk and extremities. Here, a running sub-

hair washing until suture removal. For adolescents, bathing is restricted for 48 hours and then permitted daily with liberal application of antibiotic ointment to the wound after the shower.

For larger scalp wounds, a pressure dressing can be used on the scalp for 48 hours (Fig. 5.21). Liberal antibiotic ointment is applied to the sutures on the scalp surface and nonadherent dressing is applied over the antibiotic ointment. Fenestrated gauze is placed over the nonadherent dressing and a roll of gauze is used in a turban fashion to hold the fenestrated gauze in place. Silk tape is used along the forehead and the posterior neck, avoiding contact with hair, to keep the turban in place and an elastic tube bandage is placed on top of the dressing.[194] At 48 hours, the dressing can be snipped under the chin and the tape removed from the forehead and posterior scalp. The entire dressing will come off without trauma and ointment can be applied on a daily basis to the exposed sutures to prevent crusting.

Facial wounds

Polyurethane and hydocolloid wound dressings are most useful on the face. These can be applied directly to the sutured wound and left in place until suture removal. If necessary, a small pressure dressing can be made out or gauze and a polyurethane dressing or tape placed over the wound for the first 48 hours. Most facial wounds do not require pressure dressing. The new synthetic dressings hasten healing and reduce the risk of infection by maintaining the integrity of the wound until suture removal.[5] It is recommended that wounds closed with skin adhesive should be steri-stripped before covering with a polyurethane dressing to increase the security of the closure in children.

Extremity and trunk wounds

Although the simplest to perform, extremity and trunk surgery can be most frustrating for the dermatologic surgeon because these scars spread significantly in the pediatric age group, due to the elasticity of tissue and the activity level in this patient population. The use of running subcuticular sutures, which can be kept in place for longer and nonabsorbable suture material in the deep dermis, can minimize spreading of the wound. However, restriction of activity in the postoperative period is essential to maximize the appearance of postoperative scarring in these locations. Wounds closed with a running subcuticular suture should be steri-stripped before covering with a polyurethane dressing to improve wound edge apposition (Fig. 5.22). Steri-strips stay on better if extra adhesive is applied to the skin surface.[195] This should be kept dry and intact until suture removal. The use of bulky pressure dressings on extremities can be helpful in reminding the pediatric patient that a procedure was done and that activities should be restricted. Since there is minimal postoperative pain, most children are ready to resume normal activity within 24 hours of a procedure. The bulkier dressing is visible and can restrict activity over joints, reminding the child of the need to modify activity level. In general, for pre-adolescents, the bulkier and more colorful the dressing, the happier the patient. Wraps cross joints are especially helpful on extremities

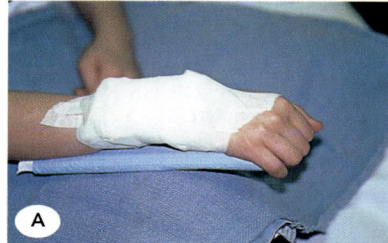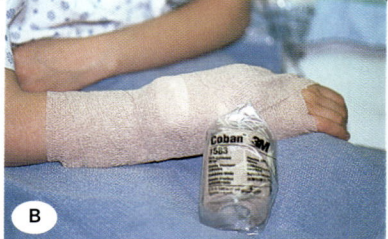

Fig. 5.23 Extremity wounds over joints should be immobilized to decrease movement of the wound in the immediate postoperative period in children.

when excision lines (Fig. 5.23). The use of soft splints (*Velcro*™ closure joint immobilizers) or casting material molded to the ankle and wrapped to limit movement can also be helpful. These do not fully restrict movement around the joints, but they do restrict movement significantly. For lesions around the knee or on the ankle and foot, crutches can be helpful for patients 8 years of age and older. Younger patients are not coordinated well enough to use these and they should be avoided.

Palms and soles

Excisions on the palms and soles or between the toes and fingers are particularly prone to infection, especially in the pediatric population. A running suture technique should be avoided in these locations. The wound in this location should be cleansed on a daily basis after 48 hours and examined by the parent for evidence of drainage, erythema, or wound dehiscence. Any evidence of erythema, pain or exudate should be treated with oral antibiotics such as cephalexin for a 10-day period. Since maceration of the skin in the web spaces contributes to an increased risk of infection, these wounds should be covered only with antibiotic ointment. Hydrocolloid and polyurethane dressings are of limited use on the palms and soles since they do not adhere well. Postoperative complications on the foot in the pediatric population are proportionate to the activity level of the child. Restricting ambulation is essential for good wound healing in this location. The thickness of the statum corneum on the palms and soles results in hydration and maceration of the skin that can be mistaken for partial dehiscence. It is worthwhile to review with the parent the expected appearance of the wound to avoid unnecessary concern in the postoperative period.

POSTOPERATIVE FOLLOW-UP-DRESSINGS CONCERNS

It is important to maintain close contact with families in the postoperative period. Most parents are extraordinarily concerned about pain and postoperative care. A quick phone call the day after a procedure is very reassuring for families and helps minimize complications. Be sure to provide families with phone numbers to call for any problems. Wound infection is rare in the first five postoperative days. Yet parents, and even health care providers, will immediately assume that a fever after surgery is most likely related to wound infection. I insist that families call me before allowing anyone to remove a wound dressing. Fever resulting from a skin surgery is highly unlikely unless there is obvious wound infection saturating the dressing with surrounding cellulitis. All other sources of fever should be addressed before attributing the fever to a wound infection.

Many parents are concerned about their inability to "see" the wound to properly evaluate it. Reassurance that wound dehiscence and infection are preceded by pain is very helpful. A painless wound is highly unlikely to be a

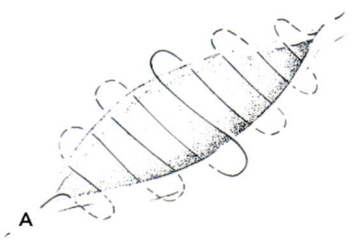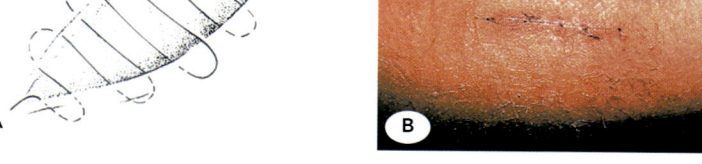

Fig. 5.22 Running subcuticular suture.

194. Wagner AM, Listina K (1999) The ultimate dressing: No mess, no fuss, no phone calls. **Pediatr Dermatol** 16:62.

195. Carrington PR (2000) Tacky but refined: A "slick" technique for dressings that hold better. **Dermatol Surg** 26:929.

problem. In sites where infection is more likely, such as the feet, hands and groin, the liberal use of antibiotic ointment as the only dressing allows for ready access to the wound for evaluation and cleansing.

Parents are frequently concerned that the dressing will fall off. Careful application of the steri-strips, hydrocolloid, or polyurethane dressing with skin adhesive is usually sufficient to prevent this complication.[195] Despite parental concerns, most infants leave their dressings alone. If the pressure dressing falls off inadvertently in the first 48 hours, there is no need to replace it. It functions only to prevent bleeding and trauma. If the dressing immediately covering the wound becomes loose, it should be reinforced, but not replaced. Blood-stained dressings can be covered with adhesive tapes or gauze if the parents prefer not to see the soiled areas. Some blood-staining on the dressing is normal and parents should be alerted to this likelihood. Unless blood is seeping through or around the dressing, there is no cause for concern. The risk of infection is reduced if the initial wound dressing remains intact.

HYPERTROPHIC SCAR DRESSINGS

The incidence of hypertrophic scarring is increased in the pediatric population. This is probably due to the markedly increased activity level of young children. It is therefore essential that close postoperative follow-up is obtained for all patients. Facial wounds should be examined one month postoperative and wounds in all other locations should be examined three months' postoperatively. Parents should be alerted to the appearance of a hypertrophic scar (Fig. 5.24). Although spreading of the scar on a trunk or extremity is quite likely in the first three postoperative months, the tissue should not become firm or raised above the skin. In the likelihood that this occurs, it is important to begin treatment early. Numerous silicone scar patch systems have been developed for this purpose.[196] Although the mechanism of action of these patches is not well understood, it is felt by most that applying firm pressure to the wound surface and maintaining a moist environment with the use of these dressing result in a favorable improvement in scar hypertrophy.[197] The remodeling phase of scars is a full year and the use of these dressings is most effective during this remodeling period.[198] Patches are typically worn for many months during the first postoperative year (Fig. 5.25). The longer the patch is in place, the greater the effect of minimizing scar hypertrophy.

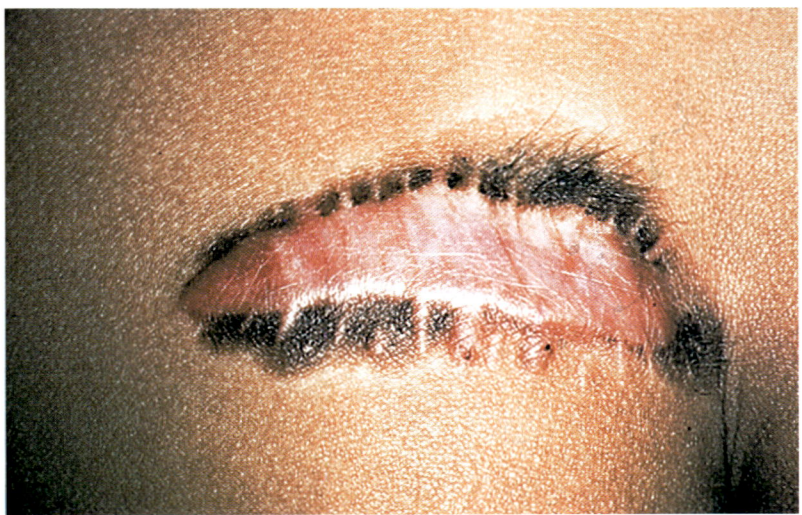

Fig. 5.24   Hypertrophic scar following 1st stage excision of large congenital nevus.

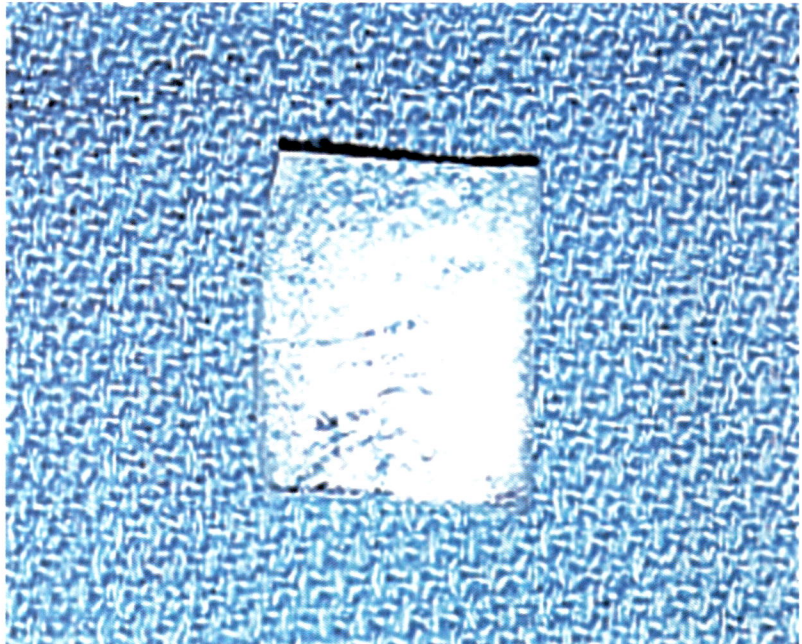

Fig. 5.25   Silicone scar patch.

For adolescents, nighttime use of these patches may be reasonable. For younger children, wearing these patches 24 hours each day is recommended. The most effective patch systems come with cleansers to allow cleaning of the patch on a daily basis. Each patch lasts approximately three weeks using this method. For patients who are unable to afford the costly scar patch systems, stretch foam tape can be helpful. Once hypertrophy has been identified in a healing wound, follow-up should be every two months until the physician and parents are content with the appearance of the scar or the hypertrophy has resolved.

In addition to scar patching systems, injection of triamcinolone acetate 20–40mg/cc into the hypertrophic areas of the scar at monthly intervals can be very effective. This can be readily accomplished in most children over the age of 8 with the use of a topical anesthetic cream prior to the procedure. The pulsed dye laser has also been shown to be effective in reducing scar hypertrophy and erythema, and this can also be used as an adjunct to reduce scar overgrowth. For the majority of children, however, the patch system is sufficient and painful procedures can be averted.

SPECIALIZED FORMS OF DERMATOLOGIC SURGERY IN CHILDREN

CRYSOSURGERY

Cryosurgery is one of the most common procedures performed in pediatric dermatology. Liquid nitrogen (−195.8°C) is the cryogenic agent that is used most commonly. The ready availability of this inexpensive agent makes this form of therapy very popular even among primary care physicians. It is important to understand the mechanism of action of cryogenic agents, the types of lesions that are amenable to treatment, the appropriate method of application, and the potential complications with this therapy in the pediatric population.

196. Berman B, Flores F (1999) Comparison of a silicone gel-filled cushion and silicone gel sheeting for the treatment of hypertrophic or keloid scars. **Dermatol Surg** 25(6):484–486.
197. Suetak T, Sasai S, Zhen YX, Tagami H (2000) Effects of silicone gel sheet on the stratum corneum hydration. **Br J Plastic Surg** 53(6):503–507.
198. Fulton JE Jr. (1995) Silicone gel sheeting for the prevention and management of evolving hypertrophic and keloid scars. [see comments]. **Dermatol Surg** (Nov;) 21(11):947–951.

TABLE 5.7   Lesions treated with cryotherapy in pediatric patients

Verruca vulgaris
Verruca plana
Verruca plantaris
Condyloma acuminatum
Keloids
Hypertrophic scars
Molluscum contagiosum
Acrochordon
Dermatofibroma
Hemangioma (controversial)
Granuloma annulare

Cryosurgery is the production of localized areas of frostbite on the skin. With application of liquid nitrogen to the skin surface intracellular and extracellular ice crystals form within the tissue. This may cause direct injury to the cell membranes or cause cell death indirectly through changes in electrolytes and osmotic pressure. The cold injury to cutaneous blood vessels also accounts for part of the clinical effectiveness of the cryosurgical procedure. Cutaneous injury and cell death occur during the rewarming phase *after* application of the cryogen as the tissue returns to room temperature.[199] The depth of injury with cryosurgery is severe with prolonged application or repeat freeze/thaw cycles. It is this property that allows for effective treatment of cutaneous malignancy. Unfortunately, it is also this property that leads to inadvertent complications with incorrect use in pediatric patients.

Cryotherapy in the pediatric population is used to remove benign cutaneous lesions.[200] The goal of the therapy is to minimize the discomfort and side effects while maximizing treatment efficacy. Many cutaneous lesions are amenable to cryotherapy. The lesions most commonly treated in children are listed in Table 5.7. Acne is no longer treated with cryotherapy. All atypical or unusual lesions should be biopsies prior to treatment with cryotherapy. Cutaneous viral skin infections account for the vast majority of cryotherapy treatments in pediatric patients. Superficial application of cryotherapy is used to treat these lesions. The method used and duration of application of liquid nitrogen will depend on the size, type and location of the lesion being treated.

Cryotherapy is a first-line treatment for single or small numbers of verruca vulgaris in the pediatric population. Patients under the age of 8 years with multiple lesions should be treated with other modalities. The pain of cryotherapy applied repeatedly to multiple warts is too severe for young children. Children should not be restrained for wart treatment. There are

multiple, effective medical therapies available that are better alternatives in this population including cimetidine,[201] topical imiquimod,[202] topical retinoinds, salicylic acid plasters, or immunotherapy.[203]

Liquid nitrogen is commonly applied to the surface of the verruca using a cotton-tipped applicator. To maximize efficacy, it is recommended that extra cotton be rolled onto the end of the applicator. The lesion is touched gently allowing the ice ball to spread through the verruca by convection rather than pressure. When the entire lesion is white and a 1–2mm rim of white appears on the normal skin, the lesion has been adequately treated. The depth of the freeze is equal to the size of the white rim on the normal skin. Cryotherapy applied in this manner is unlikely to cause scarring. Application of the cryogen with pressure or repeat freeze/thaw cycles is not routinely recommended. For smaller lesions, treatment will take seconds. For larger planter warts, treatment of each wart will take 45–60 seconds. Mosaic planter warts may require two freeze/thaw cycles and repeat application at two week intervals for several treatments. Most flat and filiform warts require a single treatment only. Fifty percent of common warts will require two treatments for complete resolution.

Liquid nitrogen can also be applied to the skin with a spraying device or a solid brass probe. Most children are frightened by the appearance and noise of these systems. For older children, the cryogen spray unit is a rapid means of applying liquid nitrogen to larger palm and sole lesions. The more rapidly the infected tissue is frozen and the slower the thawing, the better the degree of necrosis, and the more effective the therapy.

Cryotherapy is the most painful procedure performed by a pediatric dermatologist. It is inappropriate to use this therapy on children who are unwilling or unable to tolerate the discomfort. All lesions treated with cryotherapy are benign. Often the parental concern is much greater than that of the patient, especially in younger children. The severity of the treatment should fit the severity of the problem. It is important to keep this in mind when treating patients for benign lesions. Sixty-five percent of all verruca spontaneously involute in two years. The insistence of a parent that a child be treated does not justify psychologic damage to the patient.

The pain of cryotherapy can be minimized with some simple techniques.[204] Topical anesthetic agents are not very effective in this procedure, but they are excellent at hydrating the skin overlying the verruca and facilitating paring without discomfort (Fig. 5.26A,B).[205] The smaller the wart, the shorter the duration of cryotherapy and pain for the child. Children returning for a second treatment should be premeditated with acetomenophen or ibuprofen 30 minutes before the next appointment. The least painful areas should be treated first. For multiple periungal warts, digital blocks are an excellent solution in patients over 10 years of age (Fig. 5.27A,B).[206] Topical anesthetic

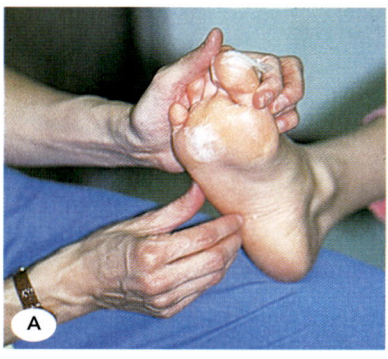
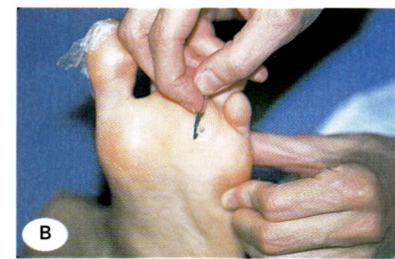

Fig. 5.26A,B   Topical anesthetic cream is applied under occlusion prior to paring of warts.

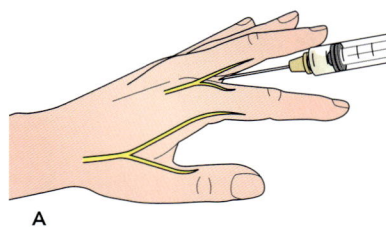
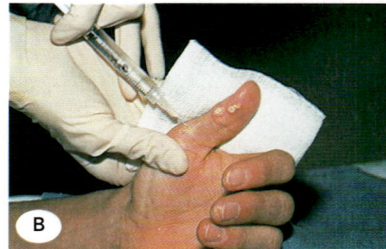

Fig. 5.27A,B   Digital blocks are helpful to control the pain of cryotherapy or laser in the treatment of warts.

199. Torre D (1973) Dermatological cryotherapy: a progress report. **Cutis** 11:782.
200. Babich D, Crollick JS (1998) Pediatric dermatologic surgery for the primary care pediatrician [Review] [47 refs]. **Pediatr Clins of N Am** 45(6):1437–1453.
201. Parsad D, Pandhi R, Juneja A, Negi KS (2002) Cimetidine and levamisole versus cimetidine alone for recalcitrant warts in children. [Clinical Trial. Journal Article. Randomized Controlled Trial]. **Pediatr Dermatol** Jul-Aug;18(4):349–352.
202. Oster-Schmidt C (2001) Imiquimod: a new possibility for treatment-resistant verrucae plana. **Arch Dermatol** May;137(5):666–667.
203. Micali G, Nasca MR, Tedeschi A, Dall'Oglio F, Pulvirenti N (2000) Use of squaric acid dibutylester (SADBE) for cutaneous warts in children. **Pediatr Dermatol** Jul-Aug;17(4):315–318.
204. Wagner AM (1998) Pain control in the pediatric patient. [Review] [41 refs]. **Dermatologic Clinics** Jul;16(3):609–617.
205. Gupta AK, Koren G, Shear NH (1998) A double-blind, randomized, placebo-controlled trial of eutectic lidocaine/prilocaine cream 5% (EMLA) for analgesia prior to cryotherapy of warts in children and adults. **Pediatr Dermatol** Mar-Apr;15(2):129–133.
206. Wagner AM, Suresh S (1998) Peripheral nerve blocks for warts, taking the cry out of cryotherapy and laser. [Review] [8 refs]. **Pediatr Dermatol** May-Jun;15(3):238–241.

can be applied to the web spaces prior to the visit. The pain of the injections is preferable to the discomfort during and after cryotherapy. Injection of local anesthetic under the verruca to minimize pain is not recommended. Saturation of the tissue with fluid before freezing can result in the production of an ice ball deeper within the normal tissue than desired and extension of the field of necrosis increasing the risk of scarring. All patients should be offered acetomenophen after therapy if it has not been previously administered. Throbbing occurs in the area for an average of 20 minutes after treatment. Patients should be instructed to keep the treated limbs elevated and avoid "flicking" the hands. Finally, distraction is a powerful tool in the pediatric population. Pouring the remaining liquid nitrogen on the floor or in the basin with the water for soaking is both fun and therapeutic for the patient. Covering the lesions with adhesive dressing is also recommended.

Molluscum contagiousum is another lesion commonly treated with cryotherapy in the pediatric population. Larger lesions on the trunk and extremities that do not respond to topical cantharidin[207] can be effectively removed with light freezing. It is usually sufficient to hold the cryotherapy on the lesion for 3–5 seconds only. Even minimal inflammation, regardless of the nature of the injury, can cause these lesions to involute.[208] Cryotherapy can also be used to treat molluscum on the orbital rim or upper eyelid where cantharidin is contraindicated. For extensive lesions, alternate medical therapies are preferred such as cimetidine,[209] topical retinoids, or topical 5% imiquimod.[210,211]

Condyloma acuminatum is an increasing problem in the pediatric population due to the high rate of adult infection and ascending viral infection at the time of birth. Condyloma on moist skin responds well to chemodestruction with podophyllin and trichloracetic acid, but lesions on glaberous skin require alternate therapy. Liquid nitrogen can be used effectively to treat these patients.[212] As with molluscum contagiosum, short 3–5 second applications of cryotherapy are usually effective. Antibiotic ointment and daily bathing is recommended to minimize the risk of infection in the blistered skin after treatment.

Cryotherapy has also been used to treat early capillary hemangiomas, predominantly in Europe.[213,214] Contact cryosurgery using an applicator tip that is a constant −32 degrees Centigrade is an effective method to induce remission and regression of superficial lesions with minimal side effects.[215] The pulsed dye laser is largely used for this purpose in North America. Treatment of superficial hemangiomas is controversial using any method.

Other benign cutaneous lesions can be effectively treated with cryotherapy including acrocordons, granuloma annulare,[216] hypertrophic scars,[217] keloids, and dermatofibromas. With the exception of acrocordons, it is unusual to treat these lesions in the pediatric population.

The use of cryotherapy in children is associated with numerous complications, especially when inappropriately applied. The most common complications of liquid nitrogen cryotherapy are postoperative pain, hypopigmentation, atrophic scarring, permanent nail dystrophy and inadvertent nerve injury. Transient hypopigmentation is common in pigmented races. Melanocytes exhibit extreme sensitivity to cold resulting in significant injury with treatment. Extreme caution should be used in the treatment of any facial lesions in dark-skinned patients. Cryotherapy is NOT recommended to treat flat warts on the face of a pigmented child. The high risk of pigment loss will make the areas treated more visible than the lesions themselves.

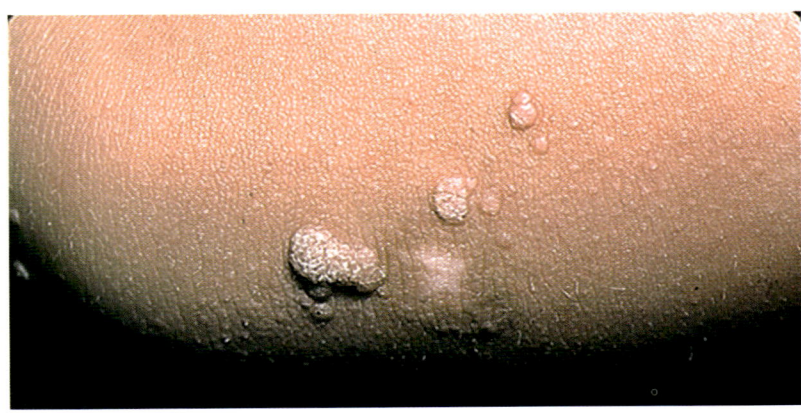

Fig. 5.28   Scarring of knee from repeat cryotherapy for warts.

Permanent hypopigmentation can result in all patients from aggressive therapy. Atrophic scarring and hypopigmentation are most common when treating lesions overlying joints, especially the knees (Fig. 5.28) and elbows.[218] Hypertrophic, painful scarring can result from aggressive cryotherapy for planter warts. A painful scar on the sole of the foot is disabling. Nail dystrophy frequently results from repeat application of liquid nitrogen to periungal warts. It is not uncommon to see recurrence of the verruca at the proximal nail fold of a dystrophic nail treated repeatedly with cryotherapy. Cryotherapy to the cuticle area is especially likely to produce permanent nail changes and alternative therapies may be preferable for persistent periungal warts.

The lateral digits are also a common site for inadvertent nerve injury.[219] It is important to be aware of the location of superficial nerves when applying cryotherapy to the skin surface. The lateral aspects of the fingers and toes, the volar aspect of the wrist and the olecranon fossa of the elbow are areas particularly susceptible to nerve injury with cryotherapy. Lighter applications of liquid nitrogen should be used in all of these areas.

Successful use of cryotherapy in the pediatric population requires knowledge of the risk and benefits of this therapy. It is also important to inform parents of the risks and the limitations of treatment. It is a common misconception that one treatment with liquid nitrogen will be sufficient to cause resolution of a wart and that the procedure is painless. Education of parents and patients is crucial to minimize morbidity and increase patient satisfaction.

CURETTAGE

Curettage or superficial scraping of cutaneous lesions is a dermatologic practice used much more commonly in adult patients. Despite this, there are several benign cutaneous lesions that are encountered in the pediatric population that respond well to curettage. Molluscum contagiosum, a benign viral skin infection, is commonly treated with topical cantharidin. This produces a superficial blister with resolution of the lesions. Cantharidin is not very effective for larger molluscum contagiosum lesions and should not be used on the face due to the increased risk of scarring. Persistent and troublesome lesions can be effectively treated with cryotherapy (see previous section) or with gentle curettage. It is important to pre-treat the lesions to be

207. Silverberg NG, Sidbury R, Mancini AJ (2000) Childhood molluscum contagiosum: experience with cantharidin therapy in 300 patients [Clinical Trial. Journal Article]. **J Am Acad Dermatol** Sep;43(3):503–507.

209. Yashar SS, Shamiri B (1999) Oral cimetidine treatment of molluscum contagiosum [Letter]. **Pediatr Dermatol** Nov–Dec;16(6):493.

210. Barba AR, Kapoor S, Berman B (2001) An open label safety study of topical imiquimod 5% cream in the treatment of Molluscum contagiosum in children [Clinical Trial. Journal Article]. **Dermatology Online Journal** Feb;7(1):20.

211. Skinner RB Jr., Ray S, Talanin NY (2000) Treatment of molluscum contagiosum with topical 5% imiquimod cream [Letter]. **Pediatr Dermatol** 17(5):420.

212. Boyd AS (1990) Condylomata acuminata in the pediatric population [see comments] [Review] [84 refs]. **A Jour of Diseas Child** 144(7):817–824.

213. Cremer H (1998) Cryosurgery for hemangiomas [letter; comment]. **Pediatr Dermatol** 15(5):410–411.

214. Cremer JH, Djawari D (1995) Fruhtherapie der kutanen hamangiome mit der kontaktkryochirurgie. **Chir Praxis** 49:295–312.

215. Reischle S, Schuller-Petrovic S (2000) treatment of capillary hemangiomas of early childhood with a new method of cryosurgery. **J Am Acad Dermatol** 42(5 Pt 1):809–813.

216. Blume-Peytavi U, Zouboulis CC, Jacobi H, Scholz A, Bisson S, Orfanos CE (1994) Successful outcome of cryosurgery in patients with granuloma annulare. **Br J Dermatol** 130(4):494–497.

217. Zouboulis CC, Blume U, Buttner P, Orfanos CE (1993) Outcomes of cryosurgery in keloids and hypertrophic scars. A prospective consecutive trial of case series. **Arch Dermatol** 129(9):1146–1151.

218. Yaffe B, Shafir R, Tsur H, Shewach-Millet M (1986) Complications of liquid nitrogen cryosurgery for verrucae over bony prominences. **Ann Plastic Surg** 16(2):146–149.

219. Nix TE Jr (1965) Liquid nitrogen neuropathy. **Arch Dermatol** 92:185.

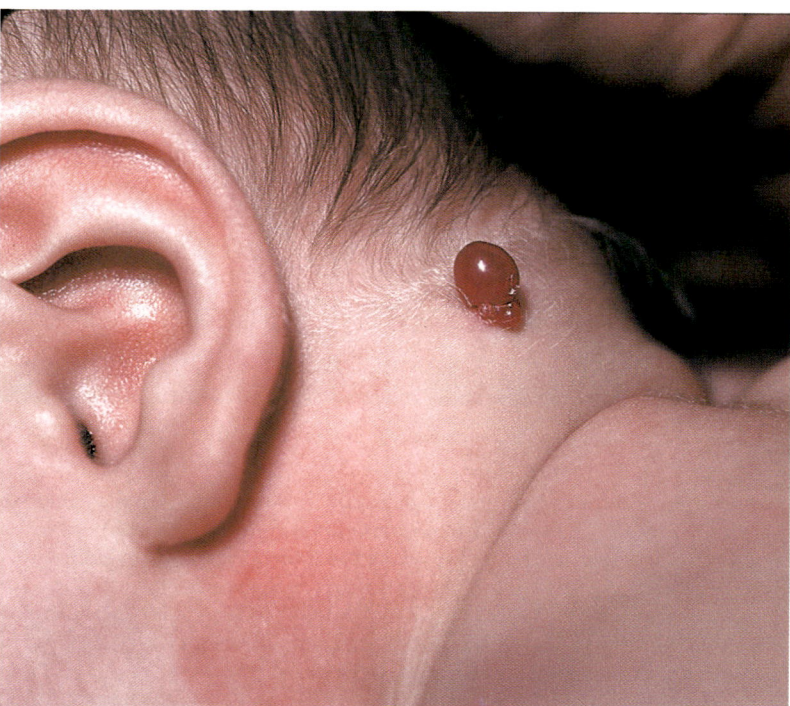

Fig. 5.29 Pyogenic granuloma on the neck of an infant.

curetted with topical anesthetic cream 30–60 minutes prior to the procedure to minimize the discomfort. A disposable curette is preferable to the reusable intruments commonly used by adult dermatologists to curette small skin cancers. The former are sharper, requiring less pressure for effective removal. Lesions are easily and painlessly removed by gentle scraping with a low risk of scarring. Antibiotic ointment can be used to cover the abraded areas after curettage to minimize the risk of infection. Curetting molluscum has the added advantage of removing the lesion while the patient is in the clinic. Parent satisfaction is increased when they can see that the lesions are gone.

Pyogenic granulomas are also treated with curettage. These are benign eruptive vascular tumors that occur commonly in children (Fig. 5.29). The cause is unknown although trauma may play a role in the production of these tumors which have occurred at sites of minor skin injury or in response to superficial laser treatment of vascular lesions on the skin. Typical lesions are 6–12mm and pedunculated with a prominent collarette. Bleeding is a usual complication and patients often present to the emergency room for evaluation and treatment of these bleeding lesions. Often a large portion of the tumor will fall off during these episodes only to grow back over the next several days.

Pyogenic granulomas are usually treated by shave or snip excision at the base where the tumor attaches to the skin surface. Any remaining vascular tissue is then curetted and light electrodessication of the base is accomplished using a hyfrecator. The resulting wound is covered with antibiotic ointment and a dressing to prevent dessication and crust formation. Pyogenic granulomas treated in this manner rarely recur and the scar that is produced is small and round corresponding to the stalk of the pedunculated lesion. Lesions can also be removed by excision but curettage is the preferred method to minimize the size of the resultant scar. Pulsed dye laser has also been used and will be discussed later in this chapter.

Small verruca plana can also be effectively treated with curettage. This is a simple method to remove troublesome facial lesions in adolescents. Lesions should be treated with topical retinoids for several weeks prior to curettage. Spontaneous involution of lesions is common in this period. Remaining lesions can be covered with topical anesthetic cream 30–60 minutes before the procedure and lightly curetted. Lesions readily peel from the skin when treated in this manner. This procedure is only recommended for Type I-III Caucasians since curettage will remove pigmentation in the upper layer of the skin, which can make the areas more visible in darker skinned patients.

ELECTROSURGICAL PROCEDURES

Electrosurgery has long been used in the treatment of dilated cutaneous blood vessels, removal of unwanted hair, and superficial destruction of benign cutaneous tumors.[220] Visible light lasers have largely supplanted the use of electrosurgery for these purposes. This is especially true in the pediatric population where the pain associated with electrosurgery is poorly tolerated and inappropriate for such cosmetic concerns. Removal of dilated cutaneous blood vessels and spider angiomas can be readily accomplished with minimal discomfort using the pulsed dye laser and topical anesthetic creams.[221] Unwanted hair removal in adolescents or in congenital nevi or Becker's nevus is more successfully and less painfully approached with hair removal lasers and intense light systems. The risk of unacceptable scarring is markedly reduced with these new approaches.[222,223] Electrosurgery is no longer the treatment of choice for removal of flat or filiform warts. These can be approached less painfully and more effectively with lasers or cryotherapy.

Electrosurgery is still used in the treatment of pyogenic granulomas and in the control of minor bleeding during surgical excisions.[224] Superficial vessels can be treated with electrocautery, electrodessication or electocoagulation. In electrocautery, an exposed hot wire tip is held in direct contact with the blood vessel producing hemostasis. This method works poorly in a wet field and is difficult to do with precision. Electrodessication is the most common form of electosurgery used in the pediatric population. Here, a monopolar surgical electrode is used to dessicate the tissue at the site of contact using heat generated from a monoterminal electrosurgical device. For larger procedures, biterminal electrosurgical devices are needed to produce electrocoagulation. Patients must be grounded to use this system where current flows out of the surgical electrode, through the patient, into the indifferent electrode (grounding pad) and directly back to the unit's power generator. The advantage of the biterminal electrosurgery unit is that tissue can be both coagulated and cut. In addition, the energy can be delivered with bipolar electrodes using a small forceps allowing for precise destruction of blood vessels and hemostasis.[225]

It is important that special attention be paid to electrosurgery during excisional surgery in the pediatric population. The activity of patients in the immediate postoperative period is significant despite efforts by the parents and surgeon at enforcing restrictions. The wise surgeon will insure that the wound is completely dry before closing to minimize the liklihood of a post-operative hematoma or bleeding from the excision site.

ACNE SURGERY AND SCAR REVISION

Acne surgery is not performed commonly in a pediatric dermatology practice. The mainstay of acne treatment is medical and adolescents are not eager to undergo procedures that may require the use of needles or sharp objects. There are three basic procedures that are infrequently offered to pediatric acne patients: comedone extraction, injection of intralesional steroids into cysts or deep inflammatory papules, and scar revision. Superficial peeling

220. Blankenship ML (1979) Electrosurgery, electrocautery and electrolysis. **Int J Dermatol** 18:443.
221. Richards KA, Garden JM (2000) The pulsed dye laser for cutaneous vascular and nonvascular lesions. **Seminars in Cutaneous Medicine & Surgery** 19:276.
222. Dierickx C, Alora MB, Dover JS (1999) A clinical overview of hair removal using lasers and light sources. **Dermatol Clin** 17:357.
223. Olsen EA (1999) Methods of hair removal. **J Am Acad Dermatol** 40:143.
224. Sebben JE (1984) Electrocoagulation in a sterile surgical field. **J Dermatol Surg Oncol** 10:603.
225. Pollack SV, Grekin RC (1996) Electrosurgery and Electroepilation in Roenigk & Roenigk's Dermatologic Surgery, 2nd ed. New York: Marcel Dekker, p. 219.

with glycolic acid may also be offered to select patients as an adjunct to conventional medical therapy.[226]

When sebaceous material and keratin debris fill the follicular orifice, it may become desiccated and result in the formation of an open comedone. To improve the cosmetic appearance, as well as attempt to reestablish the normal transfollicular elimination of sebum, this blockage must be removed with only minimal trauma to the adjacent tissue. This can usually be accomplished with use of a comedone extractor.[227] Many different types of comedone extractors are available, but all share the common feature of having a slot or hole in one end of a relatively flat bladelike instrument. To use this instrument, the hole is placed directly over the comedone and pressed downward. This creates peripheral pressure around the comedone causing it to be extruded upwards without rupturing or damaging the follicle. If material is not readily expressed, a small beveled needle or #11 blade scalpel can be used to dislodge the keratin plug in the top of the pore. Comedone extraction will be more successful if the patient used a topical retinoid on a regular basis. The effects of the retinoid on comedone formation facilitates extraction of the keratin plug minimizing trauma.

Closed comedones appear as small 1–3mm, white milial lesions. To prevent inadvertent injury during the extraction process, a very superficial stab wound is made into the comedome using a #11 scalpel blade or a small-caliber beveled needle. This acts to guide the direction of the sebum and keratin upward through the incision and without rupturing laterally through the wall of the follicle or down into the skin, as the extractor exerts lateral pressure and minimizes injury to the normal surrounding tissue.

Occasionally, large inflammatory papules and cysts develop despite compliant oral antibiotic therapy. Deep inflammatory acne lesions have a high risk of scarring. For more mature adolescents, relief can be obtained with intralesional injections of the fluorinated corticosteroid, triamcinolone. A con-

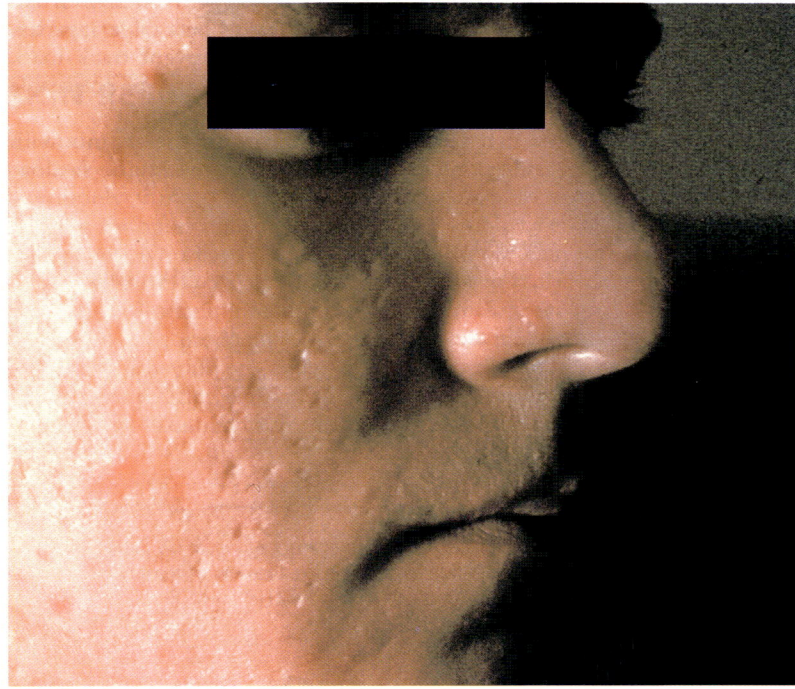

Fig. 5.30 Acne scarring in adolescent that is amenable to surgical treatment.

centration of 2.5 to 5mg/ml and a dosage of 0.1–0.2ml per cyst is usually all that is required. Application of topical anesthetic cream can decrease the pain of the needle stick, although burning is still present when the triamcinalone is injected. The injection of more concentrated or larger volumes of steroid solution should be done with caution, since hypopigmentation and atrophy can result.

Despite the development of excellent medical therapies for acne, a significant number of patients will develop scarring from adolescent acne (Fig. 5.30). Various forms of treatment have been developed to improve the cosmetic appearance of acne scars.[228,229] However, a conservative approach is often the most appropriate choice in the treatment of an adolescent or teenager who has a mild form of acne scarring, as significant spontaneous improvement may occur over time, obviating the need for any form of corrective surgery. As a minimum, the treatment of acne scarring should be postponed in adolescents until the skin has been clear of new acne lesions for a minimum of six months.

Approaches to acne scar revision differ depending on the type of scars that are present. Scars in acne can be hypertrophic or atrophic. Hypertrophic scars that commonly form on the face and trunk following severe cystic acne can also be successfully treated with injections of small quantities of intralesional fluorinated corticosteroids. Usually this is performed using a concentration of 2.5 to 10mg/ml of triamcinolone, and less than 0.5ml is injected into any single scar. Light freezing of a scar before injection may produce slight edema of the fibrous tissue to permit a more uniform distribution of the steroid suspension throughout the scar, providing a better effect. Atrophic scars cause contour defects in the skin surface. Numerous procedures, both surgical and non-surgical, have been used to improve the appearance of these controur defects.

Non-surgical approaches to atrophic scar correction include the use of subcutaneous or dermal fillers such as autologous fat, bovine collagen, human collagen, hyaluranonic acid derivatives, and poly-methyl-methacrylate microspheres with collagen. The elevation of the depressed scars occurs as a result of the intradermal or subcutaneous implantation of these substances. One of the most commonly used materials is a biologic material made from purified bovine collagen.[230–232] This material is used to elevate depressed, soft, distensible scars to the level of the surrounding skin. In order to properly determine which scars are likely to be improved with this type of treatment, slight traction is placed with the surgeon's fingers on opposite sides of a scar. If the central portion of the scar rises with this minimal amount of tension, it can most likely be elevated with collagen injections. If thick or fibrotic scar tissue is present, tension across a depressed scar will not result in elevation, and it is unlikely to be improved with intradermal injection of collagen. While other types of acne scars may also respond to this type of treatment, accurate assessment in advance is impossible.

The collagen products that are currently available for intradermal injection are of bovine derivation and come in purified sterile suspensions of 30% and 60%. Because of the known 1–3% incidence of transient allergic reaction to this material,[233] a 0.1ml test dose is injected into the forearm as a trial. If no swelling, pruritus, or inflammatory reaction has been detected after four weeks, the actual treatment injections can begin. Some physicians, concerned with the potential for allergic reactions, perform a second test dose of 0.1ml, usually done as a very small treatment at the site of the scarring process, to identify those allergic patients who did not react with the initial test dose. After the two test injections, treatments are usually performed at 2- to 3-week intervals until complete correction has been accomplished.[234] Patients with a history of autoimmune disorders[235] or those who develop a reaction to the

226. Atzori L, Brundu MA, Orru A, Biggio P (1999) Glycolic acid peeling in the treatment of acne. **J Euro Acad Dermatol & Venereol** 12(2):119–122.

227. Shalita AR (1975) Surgical procedures for the treatment of acne vulgaris. **J Dermatol Surg** 1:46.

228. Orentreich N, Durr NP (1982) Acne scars. In: Male Aesthetic Surgery, Courtiss EH, ed. St. Louis: CV Mosby.

229. Jacob CJ, Dover JS, Kramerer MS (2001) Acne scarring: a classification system and review of treatment options. **J Am Acad Dermatol** 45:109.

230. Alster TS, West TB (1997) Treatment of scars: a review. **Ann Plast Surg** 39:418–432.

231. Stegman SJ, Tromovitch TA (1980) Implantation of collagen for depressed scars. **J Dermatol Surg Oncol** 6:450.

232. Parrish LC, Witkowski JA (1985) Collagen implants soft tissue augmentation. **Int J Dermatol** 24:499.

233. Barr RJ, Stegman SJ (1984) Delayed skin test reaction to injectable collagen implant (Zyderm). **J Am Acad Dermatol** 10:652.

234. Monheit G (1989) Surgical treatment of acne scars. **Cosmet Dermatol** 2:17.

235. Castrow FF, Krull EA (1983) Injectable collagen implant-update. **J Am Acad Dermatol** 9:889.

longer the treatment of choice for removal of cutaneous skin lesions or scarring in children due to the unacceptable high risk of residual scarring.

Recent technology has allowed for refinement of the CO_2 laser that minimizes thermal injury and the risk of scarring. The new resurfacing CO_2 laser systems use high-energy, short pulses or use a focused continuous wave CO_2 beam with a rapid beam scanner system that moves the laser spot at constant velocity but dwells for less than 1msec on any tissue area.[267] By pulsing or quickly moving the laser beam, there is maximal vaporization with minimal diffusion of the thermal energy that produces scarring. Results with these systems are excellent since they allow for precise control of the amount of tissue that is removed.[264,275–277] Used improperly, disastrous scarring can result, however, so operator experience is paramount when recommending or performing this procedure in children. The disadvantage of CO_2 laser resurfacing lies in the prolonged postoperative recovery period. Re-epithelialization can take 10 to 14 days and during this period synthetic biologic membrane dressings must be used to speed the healing time and minimize postoperative discomfort. Once the skin has re-epitheliazed, it will remain erythematous for an additional 6–12 weeks.[267] Caution must be taken with any sunlight exposure, since irregular hyperpigmentation may develop and affect the overall cosmetic results.

The Er:YAG resurfacing laser has also been used for skin resurfacing. This laser emits light at 2940nm, the wavelength that is most strongly absorbed by water. Light energy penetrates 1μm rather than 20μm for the CO_2 laser, which allows for more precise ablation with less thermal injury and shorter healing times. The disadvantage of this system is failure to cause hemostasis which makes the field difficult to evaluate between laser passes. In addition, the benefit of skin tightening that is seen with CO_2 resurfacing is not present with this system. Few studies have directly compared results using these two laser systems.[259,278,279] Excellent results have been reported in the treatment of acne scarring with Er:YAG resurfacing.[262,280–282]

Combinations of CO_2 and Er:YAG laser resurfacing have been used to take advantage of the properties of both systems. A full face treated with CO_2 laser resurfacing will heal faster if a pass of Er:YAG laser is performed at the end of treatment.[267,283,284] For resurfacing of an entire face, Jacob[284] recommends an initial pass with the CO_2 laser using the computer pattern generator (CPG) at 300mJ/pulse, 60W, and CPG pattern settings of 2 (parallelogram), 9 (the largest size) and a density of 5. The mandibular area is feathered at lower energies to reduce the risk of scar or pigmentary changes (250 mJ/pulse, 50W). Two to four additional passes are recommended over the scarred areas until dermal tightening and effacement of the scars is observed. The Er:YAG laser is used over the full face with a fluence of 5.2J/cm² (7mm handpiece, 2J) overlapping 50% with each spot. This removes some of the residual damage from the CO_2 laser to hasten healing and diminish the risk for prolonged erythema.

During the first 72 hours, silicone sheeting, gauze and tube netting are used to cover the wounds. Soaking with cold water for 20 minutes every 2–4 hours while awake is recommended. The skin is well lubricated with occlusive ointment and the dressing replaced. The original silicone is kept in place for 72 hours; the gauze and tube netting are changed as needed. After 72 hours the dressing is completely removed and occlusive ointment is used as the only cover. Continued soaking is recommended until epithelialization is complete, typically by 7–10 days. Sun protection is essential after epithelialization is complete. Improvement is noted at two weeks but continued improvement occurs for 18 months after laser resurfacing for acne scars.[264]

LASERS

Since the development of the first functional laser system in 1960, the laser has changed from initially being considered an expensive esoteric gadget to an extremely valuable, as well as versatile, instrument for the successful treatment of numerous skin conditions for which previous therapy had either not existed or offered such poor results that it was not considered useful.[285,286] Lasers have become increasingly widespread over the past decade. Most patients can now be effectively treated with the latest equipment available in

TABLE 5.8 Currently available lasers			
Laser system	**Wavelength output (nm)**	**Mode of emmision**	**Absorption characteristics**
Visible (400–700nm)			
Argon	488–514 (blue-green)	CW	Hemoglobin, melanin
Dye	510	Q-switch	Melanin
Krytpon	521, 530 (green)	CW	Hemoglobin, melanin
Nd:YAG	532 (green)	Q-switch	Melanin, tattoos (red)
Copper	511 (green)	Pulsed	Hemoglobin, melanin
Krypton	568 (yellow)	CW	Hemoglobin
Copper	578 (yellow)	Pulsed	Hemoglobin
Dye	585–595	CW, pulsed	Hemoglobin
Ruby	694	Q-switch	Melanin, tattoos
Alexandrite	755	Q-switch	Tattoos
Infrared (700–100 000nm)			
Nd:YAG	1064	CW, Q-switch	Protein, tattoos
CO_2	10 600	CW, SP	H_2O

CW = Continuous wave
SP = Short pulse

275. West TB (1997) Laser resurfacing of atrophic scars [Review] [45 refs]. **Dermatologic Clinics** 15(3):449–457.
276. Ross EV, McKinlay JR, Anderson RR (1999) Why does carbon dioxide resurfacing work? **Arch Dermatol** 135:444–454.
277. Ratner D, Tse Y, Marchell N et al. (1999) Cutaneous laser resurfacing. **J Am Acad Dermatol** 41:367–389.
278. Khatri K, Ross E, Grevelink J, Anderson R (1997) Comparison of Er:YAG and CO₂ lasers in skin resurfacing. **Lasers Surg Med** (Supple.):37 (Abstr.).
279. McDaniel DH, Lord J, Ash K, Newman J (1999) Combined CO₂/erbium:YAG laser resurfacing of peri-oral rhytides and side by side comparison with carbon dioxide laser alone. **Dermatol Surg** 25:285–293.
280. Jeong JT, Kye YC (2001) Resurfacing of pitted facial acne scars with a long-pulsed Er:YAG laser. **Dermatol Surg** 27(2):107–110.
281. Kye YC (1997) Resurfacing of pitted facial scars with the pulsed Er:YAG laser. **Dermatol Surg** 23:880–883.
282. Teikemier G, Goldberg DJ (1997) Skin resurfacing with the erbium:YAG laser. **Dermatol Surg** 23:685–687.
283. Weinstein C (1999) Modulated dual mode erbium/CO₂ lasers for the treatment of acne scars. **J Cutan Laser Ther** 1(4):204–208.
284. Jacob CI, Dover JS, Kaminer MS (2001) Acne scarring: a classification system and review of treatment options [Review] [26 refs]. **J Am Acad Dermatol** 45(1):109–117.
285. Arndt KA, Noe JM (1982) Lasers in dermatology. **Arch Dermatol** 118:293.
286. Acland KM, Barlow RJ (2000) Lasers for the dermatologist. **Br J Dermatol** 143:244.

various ambulatory laser surgical centers across the country (Table 5.8). Since lasers offer significant opportunities to manage a variety of vascular and pigmented conditions found in infants, children, adolescents, and teenagers, it is certainly appropriate for dermatologists to become familiar with their indications, to permit thoughtful consideration of all possible forms of treatment for managing their patients' conditions.

The word laser is an acronym, which stands for light amplification through the stimulated emission of radiation. These instruments are capable of producing extremely intense and precisely controlled light that has three unique characteristics. First, laser light is of single wavelength or is monochromatic. Second, it is temporally and spatially in phase or coherent. Finally, it is highly collimated, so that it can be propagated over long distances with little divergence of the beam.[285,287]

All laser systems are composed of the same four components. The first is the laser medium, which determines the wavelength of the emitted laser light and also generally gives each laser its name. The laser medium may be composed of a solid (e.g., ruby, Nd:YAG, or Alexandrite lasers), a liquid (e.g., dye lasers), or a gas (e.g., argon, krypton, and carbon dioxide lasers). The laser medium is contained within an optical cavity that serves as a resonator in which the laser process occurs. This usually has the configuration of a tube with mirrors at either end, one of which is only partially reflective to allow the beam of light to emerge. The third component is the pump or power source, which is used to energize the system. The power source may be electrical or radiofrequency energy, but photo-optical energy, as in the argon dye laser or flashlamp dye laser, or even mechanical or chemical energy, may also be employed. The fourth component of all laser systems is the delivery system, which may be an articulated arm having mirrored joints or fiberoptics.

Laser energy is produced when the pump energizes the atoms or molecules of the laser medium and creates a condition known as population inversion. This condition occurs when there are more atoms or molecules existing in a higher unstable energy state than in the normal resting energy state. Once this critical energy level is created, stimulated emission of energy occurs. As an energized atom or molecule returns or decays to its stable resting energy state, it releases a photon of energy. If this photon strikes another energized molecule or atom, it results in the release of two photons of energy of precisely the same wavelength and traveling in exactly the same direction in phase with one another. As this cascade process continues, energy amplification occurs, with more and more photons traveling together within the optical cavity or resonator. As the photons travel back and forth between the two parallel mirrored ends, the amplification process continues to build.

Only a small portion of the photons are permitted to exit as a laser beam through the partially reflective mirrored end of the optical cavity. This beam of light may be released as a single pulse, as with the ruby laser, as a chain of pulses, as in the copper vapor laser, or in continuous fashion, as with the carbon dioxide, krypton, and argon lasers. Laser systems that have continuous discharge patterns can be gated with a mechanical or electronic shuttering mechanism to produce individual pulses of energy of variable duration or broken into a predetermined computerized geometric pattern, using a robotic scanning device. These scanners act to separate adjacent pulses from one another temporally and spatially, reducing the potential for thermal damage and the unwanted scarring that may result from it.[288,289]

More than a dozen different laser systems are currently available for the treatment of a host of different skin conditions. New technological developments occur so rapidly in the laser field that the indications and benefits offered by the various laser systems also change with great rapidity. The different applications of the laser systems are generally determined as functions of their wavelengths, the amount of energy delivered to the tissue, the length of time the light has contact with the skin, and the optical characteristics of the tissue.

The power density or irradiance (IR) is a measure of the brightness or intensity of the laser beam:

$$IR = \frac{\text{laser output (watts)}}{\pi r^2}$$

where r = the radius of the laser beam. This factor can be precisely determined based on the size of the laser beam and the power setting of the laser. In general, the higher the irradiance, the greater the effect will be on the tissue.[290] The energy fluence (EF) is a measure of the quantity of energy delivered by a single pulse to a target tissue:

$$EF = \frac{\text{laser output (W)} \times \text{exposure time (sec)}}{\pi r^2} = J/cm^2$$

The shorter the exposure, the less the tissue will be heated. The longer the exposure to laser energy, the greater the tissue heating and the greater will be the possibility of nonspecific thermal injury to the surrounding tissues. Poor precision or reduced specificity of the laser–tissue interaction will increase the chance of unwanted additional tissue damage, prolonging the time required for healing, and reducing the quality of the cosmetic result. Improved understanding of these principles has changed the manner in which many cutaneous disorders are now treated with lasers, improving the results and allowing the treatment of many conditions earlier in life, with fewer complications than before.

In addition to IR and EF, the optical characteristics of the target tissue can also play a major role in determining the effect produced by laser energy, a concept generally known as laser–tissue interaction. If light is reflected from the surface of the target or transmitted completely through it, the energy does not interact with the tissue, so no effect will result. In order for light to have any effect on tissue, it must be absorbed by some cellular component, tissue chromophore, or protein. The two main chromophores of skin are melanin and hemoglobin; both have absorption peaks that are within the visible portion of the electromagnetic spectrum. This knowledge allows the laser surgeon to select a laser system with the appropriate emission to treat both melanocytic and vascular lesions of the skin with relative selectivity because of the precise absorption. Conversely, the mid-infrared energy from the carbon dioxide laser is absorbed by intracellular and extracellular water and not by a specific chromophore. As a consequence, this laser lacks color specificity and produces the same effects in all soft tissues, regardless of their color, since they are composed of 70 to 90 percent water.

In order to control the laser–tissue interaction, a specific laser must emit sufficient energy to injure the target and the energy that is emitted must be selectively absorbed in the skin by the desired target without injuring the surrounding tissue. Newer laser systems accomplish this in three ways. First, the wavelength emitted by the laser must be absorbed primarily by the skin component that is being targeted. Second, the duration of the laser impulse must be adjusted to match the thermal relaxation time of the tissue chromophore, a theory known as selective photothermolysis. This theory, introduced by Anderson and Parrish in 1983, is the basis for many advancements in dermatological lasers.[290] When light is absorbed by a target tissue in the skin, it heats up the tissue and immediately diffuses away. The thermal relaxation time of any tissue is the time it takes for that tissue to cool and is roughly proportional to the square of the diameter of the target in millimetres.[291] By limiting the exposure duration to the thermal relaxation time, the spread of thermal damage to the surrounding tissue and therefore the risk of scarring can be reduced. Finally, since most laser targets are components of the dermis, chromophores that are present within the epidermis must be minimized to reduce thermal injury to the upper layers of the skin during treatment of deeper layers. Pigmented and vascular lesions in the dermis are therefore optimally treated when the epidermis is unpigmented (tanning is

287. Wheeland RG, Walker NPJ (1986) Lasers – twenty-five years later. **Int J Dermatol** 25:209.
288. Mordon S, Rotteleur G, Buys B et al. (1989) Comparative study of the "point by point" technique and the "scanning" technique for laser treatment of port-wine stains. **Lasers Surg Med** 9:398.
289. McDaniel DH, Modron S (1990) Hexascan: a new robotized scanning laser handpiece. **Cutis** 45:300.

290. Anderson RR, Parrish JA (1983) Selective photothermolysis: precise microsurgery by selective absorption of pulsed radiation. **Science** 220:524–527.
291. Alova MBT, Anderson RR (2000) Recent developments in cutaneous lasers. **Lasers in Surg & Medicine** 26:108.

minimal) to avoid inadvertent injury to the epidermis and resultant post-inflammatory hyper- or hypopigmentation or scarring. In addition, the use of cryogen spray units to cool the epidermis during laser treatment minimizes the thermal injury to the epidermis.[291–293]

LASER TREATMENT OF VASCULAR LESIONS IN CHILDREN

The treatment of vascular birthmarks and acquired vascular lesions in children is by far the widest use of laser surgery in the pediatric population. Port-wine stains were the lesions originally targeted for treatment by these lasers, but as the technology has improved the spectrum of vascular lesions amenable to treatment with laser has expanded (Table 5.9).

The argon laser was the first laser system to become available for the treatment of port-wine stains. Because the two primary emission energy peaks from this laser occurred at wavelengths that overlapped the absorption spectrum for oxyhemoglobin, it was assumed that very precise and selective damage to blood vessels with a minimal amount of injury to non-vascular

tissues would be possible.[294–297] However, the existence of a number of side effects and complications, such as textural changes, hypertrophic scarring,[298,299] and permanent hypopigmentation,[300] proved that there were a significant number of limitations, including the inability to treat children effectively.[301–304]

All undesired effects are due to a lack of precision in the laser–tissue interaction, which results from the fact that the argon laser emits its energy at a trough in the absorption spectrum for oxyhemoglobin. This fails to restrict the thermal injury to blood vessels, permitting wide distribution of the heat throughout the dermis. In addition, there is inadvertent absorption by melanin in the overlying epidermis,[305] which not only causes damage to the epidermis but also reduces the amount of energy available to reach the blood vessels.

In an attempt to minimize the side effects of these laser systems, yellow light lasers were developed. Yellow light, with an approximate wavelength of 577nm, was chosen because it closely matches one of the major absorption peaks for oxyhemoglobin.[306,307] This wavelength is preferable to the strongest absorption peak for oxyhemoglobin at 418nm because the major competing chromophore in skin, melanin, absorbs energy significantly at this lower wavelength. In addition, this longer wavelength of light is also capable of penetrating deeper into the dermis and is not absorbed as well as argon laser light by melanin in the epidermis. The argon-pumped tunable dye laser delivered light with a wavelength of 577 or 585nm released in a continuous fashion. The light was mechanically or electronically shuttered to deliver pulses of light[308,309] in a polka-dot or pointilistic technique delivered through a robotic optical scanning device.[310–312] The pulse duration with this system was still substantially longer than the thermal relaxation time of the small vascular channels that make up port-wine stains, however, and there was still a significant risk of complications with this system.

The first laser system developed for the treatment of port-wine stains in children that utilized the priniciple of selective photothermolysis[313] was the flashlamp-pumped pulsed dye laser. Although modifications of this laser system have occurred in the past 15 years to optimise treatment outcome, the pulsed dye laser remains the laser of choice in the treatment of vascular lesions in children. Like the argon dye laser, the pulsed dye laser also uses an organic dye, energized by short pulses of white light from a flashlamp, to produce yellow light with a wavelength of 577 to 600nm. It differs from the argon dye laser in that the energy is released in short pulses (Fig. 5.32).[305,314] For the ideal treatment of port-wine stains, pulse durations are in the 1–10ms range and vary depending on the size of the vessels.[315] The original pulsed dye laser had a pulse duration of 450μs. Pulsed dye laser systems have now been developed that allow for adjustment of the pulse duration and wavelength. The spot size has increased from 3mm to 10mm and the power emitted by the lasers has increased by 50%.[316] Cryogen units are attached to

TABLE 5.9 Vascular lesions amendable to laser in children

	Comment*
Port-wine stains	Average 8 treatments Recurrence likely especially on face
Hypertrophic port-wine stains	Pulsed KTP 532nm (1–200ms) or IPLS 515–1200 (2–20ml)
Ulcerated and superficial hemangiomas	Risk of scarring high in rapid proliferative phase
Spider angiomas	Removes pigment in tanned patients
Facial telangiectasias	PDL 595nm (1.5msec) most effective but purpura × 1 Pulsed KTP 532nm (1–200ms) or IPLS 515–1200 (2–20ml) – no purpura
Pyogenic granuloma	Effective only if lesion small (<3mm depth)
Vascular angiofibromas	Reduces erythema only
Warts	Requires general anesthetic for extensive warts
Scars	Most effective on face in scars < 1 year old
Vascular malformations angiokeratomas	Decreases bleeding but full resolution rare

* Unless indicated recommended treatment is with pulsed dye laser 585–595nm (0.5–1.5msec pulse duration).

292. Nelson JS, Milner TE, Anvari B et al. (1995) Dynamic epidermal cooling during pulsed laser treatment of port-wine stain, a new methodology with preliminary clinical evaluation. **Arch Dermatol** 131:695–700.
293. Waldorf HA, Alster TS, McMillan K et al. (1997) Effect of dynamic cooling on 585-nm pulsed dye laser treatment of port-wine stain birthmarks. **Dermatol Surg** 23:657–662.
294. Goldman L (1980) The argon laser and the port wine stain. **Plast Reconstr Surg** 65:137.
295. Cosman B (1980) Experience in the argon laser therapy of port wine stains. **Plast Reconstr Surg** 65:119.
296. Apfelberg DB, Maser MR, Lash H et al. (1981) The argon laser for cutaneous lesions. **JAMA** 245:2073.
297. Arndt KA (1982) Argon laser therapy of small cutaneous vascular lesions. **Arch Dermatol** 118:220.
298. Cotterill JA (1982) Laser treatment of portwine stains. **BMJ** 284:766.
299. Dixon JA, Huether S, Rotering R (1984) Hypertrophic scarring in argon laser treatment of port wine stains. **Plast Reconstr Surg** 73:771.
300. Landthaler M, Haina D, Waidelich W, Braun-Falco O (1984) A three-year experience with the argon laser in dermatotherapy. **J Dermatol Surg Oncol** 10:456.
301. Arndt KA, Noe JM, Northam DBC, Itzkan I (1981) Laser therapy: basic concepts and nomenclature. **J Am Acad Dermatol** 5:649.
302. Noe JM, Barsky SH, Geer DE et al. (1980) Port-wine stains and the response to argon laser therapy: successful treatment and the predictive role of color, age, and biopsy. **Plast Reconstr Surg** 65:130.
303. Brauner GJ, Schliftman A (1987) Laser surgery for children. **J Dermatol Surg Oncol** 13:178.
304. Dixon JA, Rotering RH, Huether SE (1984) Patients' evaluation of argon laser therapy of port-wine stain, decorative tattoo, and essential telangiectasia. **Lasers Surg Med** 4:181.
305. Dorer JS, Arndt KA (2000) New approaches to the treatment of vascular lesions. **Lasers in Surg and Med** 26:158.
306. Greenwald J, Rosen S, Anderson RR et al. (1981) Comparative histological studies of the tunable dye (at 577nm) laser and argon laser: the specific vascular effects of the dye laser. **J Invest Dermatol** 77:305.
307. Landthaler M, Haina D, Brunner R et al. (1986) Effects of argon, dye and Nd:YAG lasers on epidermis, dermis and venous vessels. **Lasers Surg Med** 6:87.
308. Scheibner A, Wheeland RG (1989) Argon-pumped tunable dye laser therapy for facial port-wine stain hemangiomas in adults – a new technique using small spot size and minimal power. **J Dermatol Surg Oncol** 15:277.
309. Scheibner A, Wheeland RG (1991) Use of the argon-pumped tunable dye laser for port-wine stains in children. **J Dermatol Surg Oncol** 17:735.
310. Wheeland RG, Walker NPJ (1986) Lasers – twenty-five years later. **Int J Dermatol** 25:209.
311. Mordon S, Rotteleur G, Buys B et al. (1989) Comparative study of the "point by point" technique and the "scanning" technique for laser treatment of port-wine stains. **Lasers Surg Med** 9:398.
312. McDaniel DH, Mordon S (1990) Hexascan: a new robotized scanning laser handpiece. **Cutis** 45:300.
313. Anderson RR, Parrish JA (1983) Selective photothermolysis: precise microsurgery by selective absorption of pulsed radiation. **Science** 220:524.
314. Garden JM, Tan OT, Kerschmann R et al. (1986) Effect of dye laser pulse duration on selective cutaneous vascular injury. **J Invest Dermatol** 87:653.
315. Dierickx CC, Casparian JM, Venugopaban V et al. (1995) Thermal relaxation of port-wine stain vessels probed in vivo: the need for 1–10ms laser pulse treatment. **J Invest Dermatol** 105:709–714.
316. Richards KA, Garden JM (2000) The pulsed dye laser for cutaneous vascular and nonvascular lesions. **Seminars in Cutaneous Med and Surg** 19:276.

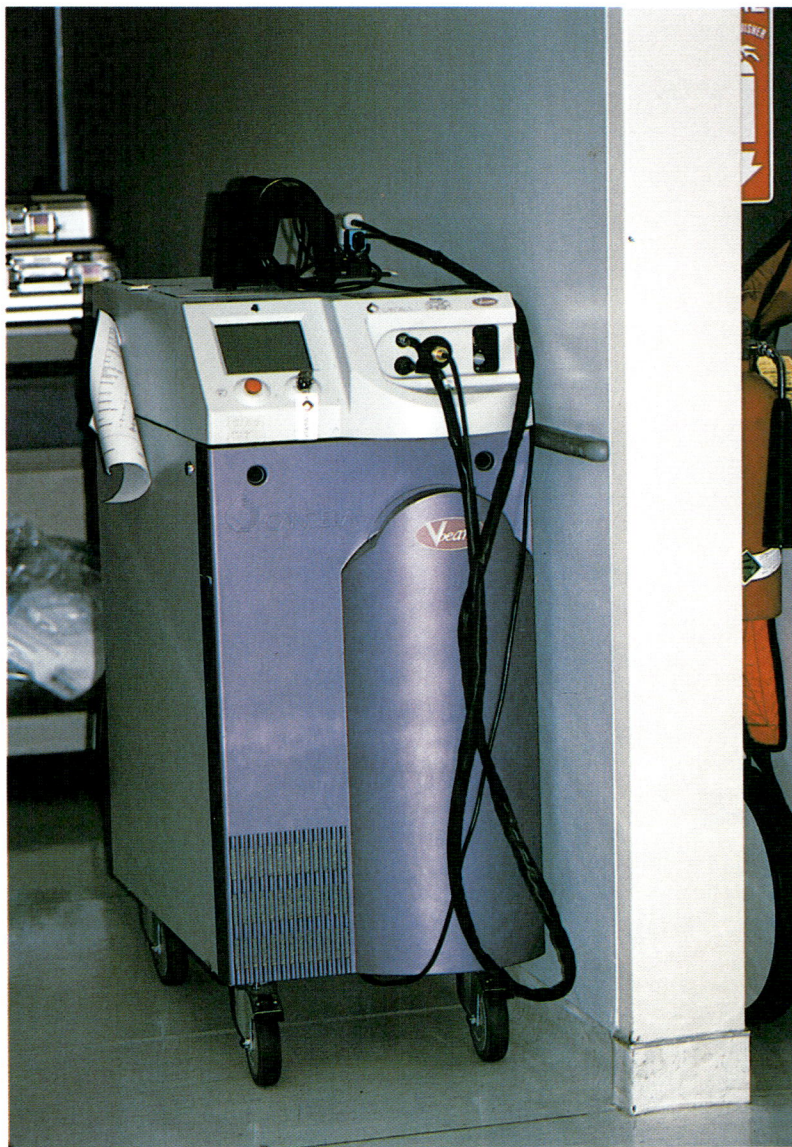

Fig. 5.32   Pulsed dye laser (595nm, V-Beam, Candela).

Port-wine stains

The pulsed dye laser system is the optimal laser in the treatment of port-wine stains (PWS) in children. Current pulsed dye laser systems deliver wavelengths from 585 to 600nm, pulse duration from 0.45 to 20ms and energy ranging from 3–15joules per square centimeter. Spot sizes of 7–10mm are generally used.[316] The disadvantages of the current systems are discomfort with use, the production of bruising or PWS darkening for 7–21 days following laser impact and the need for retreatment at 2–3 month intervals for many treatment sessions to produce maximal lesional lightening. The average PWS is treated 8–10 times, although even after 20 treatment sessions further lightening may be achieved. After resolution of the purpura, the lesion often appears redder for several weeks, then unchanged for four to six weeks. Lightening is noted for up to three months subsequent to treatment. It is important to maintain strict protection from the sun during this period to allow for the maximal effects from the laser. The percentage of lightening with each treatment decreases and eventually the effects of the laser become inapparent and therapy should be suspended.

The final outcome of pulsed dye laser treatment for PWS ranges from total clearance to little change. Most of the studies that have evaluated the efficacy of lesional lightening with the pulsed dye laser have demonstrated superior lightening in children over adults. Adult studies predict 36–44% of patients will have >75% lightening, and >75% of patients will have >50% lightening after 4 treatments (Fig. 5.33).[318,319] Patients who continued beyond nine treatments who had not obtained >75% clearance had more significant clearing after 10–25 treatments.[320] In children, studies demonstrate >50% lightening in 87% of patients[321] with many studies predicting almost 100% clearance.[322,323] Treatment in early infancy may also offer some advantage.[324] Although no differences have been noted between children treated at 9–16 years versus >16 years,[325,326] this authors experience suggests that very early treatment (under 3 months) may reduce the number of treatments necessary for maximum clearance as well as improve final outcome. The more superficial, smaller caliber, tortuous vessels with slow blood flow respond the best to laser therapy.[327] Redder stains predict a better response than pink stains since vessels are more superficial.[316]

Different anatomical areas also respond differently to laser treatment. PWS of the central cheeks, the upper lip or those with a V2 distribution are less responsive.[328] Lower extremities and more distal extremities, especially on the palmar or plantar surfaces, respond poorly. The best results are seen in periorbital, lateral face, post-auricular and neck areas, and on the upper chest and arms.[328,329] Larger stains do less well than smaller stains.[330]

Recurrence of PWS in children, especially those in highly sun-exposed areas, is expected. An estimated rate of recurrence of 50% between 3–4 years is typical.[331] After a primary treatment series that averages 8–10 treatments, most children return annually or every several years for a "tune up" treatment to restore the clearance of the stain to its best appearance.

Side effects of pulsed dye laser treatment are minimal. In a large series of 701 patients, 9.1% developed hyperpigmentation which resolved over 6–12 months; 1.4% developed hypopigmentation; blistering and crusting, which did not usually result in an undesirable outcome, occurred in 5.9% and 0.7%, respectively; and atrophic scarring occurred in 4.3%.[332] These results

the laser systems to allow protection of the epidermis during laser treatment at these higher energies and to reduce the discomfort of treatment.[315] It is hoped that these new laser systems will be more effective in the treatment of deep and nodular port-wine stains and may reduce the number of total treatment sessions for maximum improvement.[317]

317. Kauvar AWB (1997) Long-pulse high energy pulsed dye laser treatment of port wine stains and hemangiomas. **Laser Surg Med** (Suppl); 9:36.
318. Garden JM, Polla LL, Tan OT (1988) The treatment of portwine stains by the pulsed dye laser: analysis of pulse duration and long-term therapy. **Arch Dermatol** 124:889–896.
319. Glassberg E, Lask GP, Tan EML et al. (1988) The flashlamp-pumped 577nm pulsed tunable dye laser: clinical efficacy and in vitro studies. **J Dermatol Surg Oncol** 14:1200–1208.
320. Kauvar ANB, Geronemus RG (1995) Repetitive pulsed dye laser treatments improve persistent port wine stains. **Dermatol Surg** 21:515–521.
321. Reyes BA, Geronemus R (1990) Treatment of portwine stains during childhood with the flashlamp-pumped pulsed dye laser. **J Am Acad Dermatol** 23:1142–1148.
322. Tan OT, Sherwood K, Gilchrest BA (1989) Treatment of children with portwine stains using the flashlamp-pumped tunable dye laser. **N Engl J Med** 320:416–421.
323. Garden JM, Burton CS, Geronemus R (1989) Dye laser treatment of children with portwine stains. **N Engl J Med** 321:901–902.
324. Nguyen CM, Yohn JJ, Huff C (1998) Facial port wine stains in childhood: prediction of the rate of improvement as a function of the age of the patient, size and location of the port wine stain and the number of treatments with the pulsed dye (585nm) laser. **Br J Dermatol** 138:821–825.
325. Alster TS, Wilson F (1994) Treatment of port wine stains with the flashlamp pumped pulsed dye laser: extended clinical experience in children and adults. **Ann Plast Surg** 32:478–484.
326. Van der Horst C, Koster PHL, DeBorgre CAJM et al. (1998) Effect of the timing of treatment of port wine stains with the flash-lamp-pumped pulsed dye laser. **N Engl J Med** 338:1028–1033.
327. Fiskarstrand EJ, Svaasand LO, Kopstad G et al. (1996) Photothermally induced vessel-wall necrosis after pulsed dye laser treatment: lack of response in PWS with small sized or deeply located vessels. **J Invest Dermatol** 107:671–674.
328. Renfro L, Geronemus R (1993) Anatomical differences of portwine stains in response to treatment with the pulsed dye laser. **Arch Dermatol** 128:182–188
329. Holy A, Geronemus RG (1992) Treatment of periorbital portwine stains with the flashlamp-pumped pulsed dye laser. **Arch Ophthalmol** 110:793–797.
330. Morelli JG, Weston WL, Huff JC (1995) Initial lesion size as a predictive factor in determining the response of port-wine stains in children treated with the pulsed dye laser. **Arch Pediatr Adolesc Med** 149:1142–1144.
331. Orten SS, Warner M, Flock S (1996) Port wine stains: an assessment of 5 years of treatment. **Arch Otolaryngol Head Neck Surg** 122:1174–1179.
332. Seukeran DC, Collins P, Sheehan-Dare RA (1997) Adverse reactions following pulsed tunable dye laser treatment of port wine stains in 701 patients. **Br J Dermatol** 136:725–729.

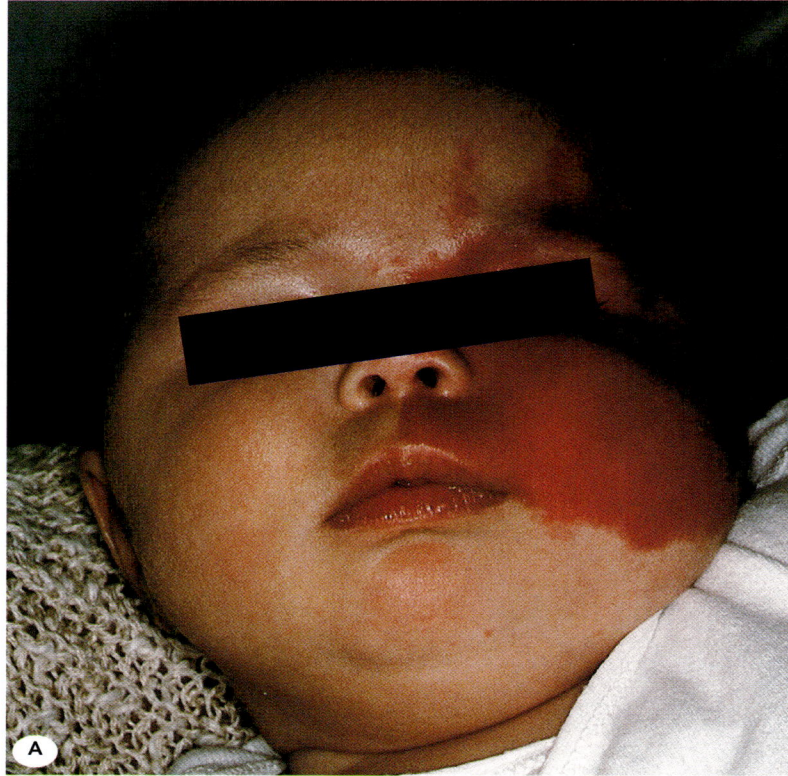

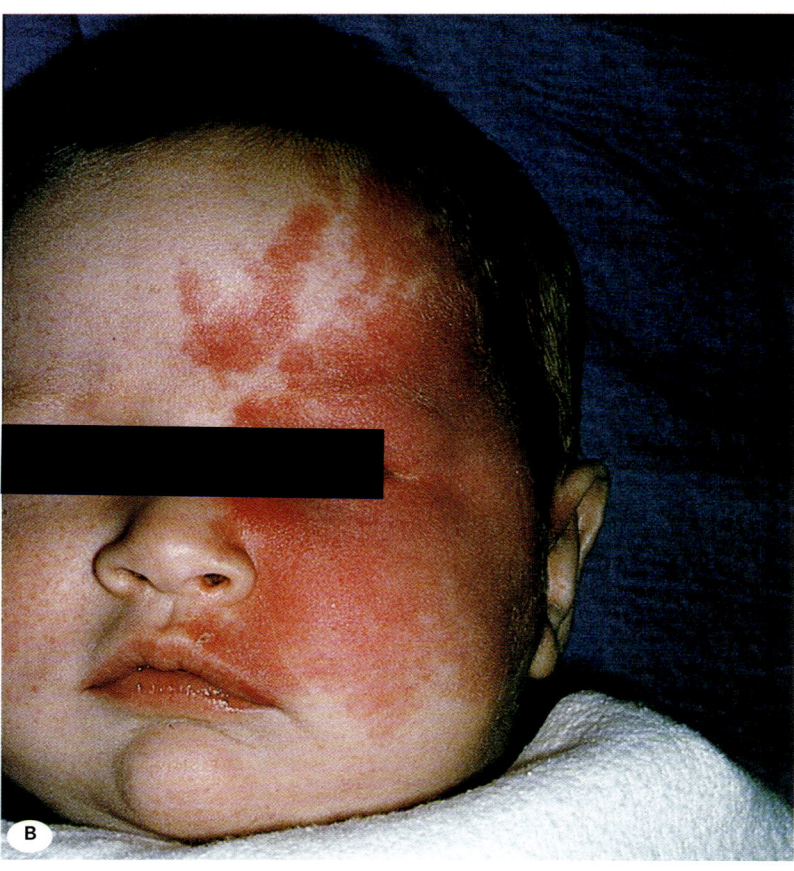

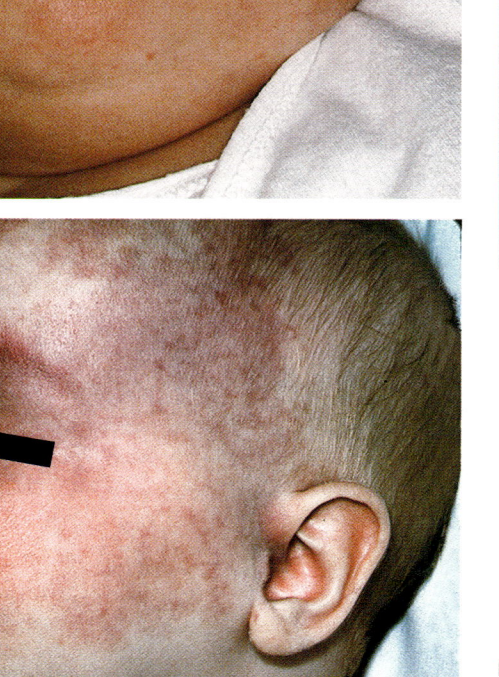

Fig. 5.33 Treatment of a patient with pulsed dye laser for port-wine stain of the face. **(A)** Pre-laser treatment at six weeks. **(B)** After three laser treatments. **(C)** After six laser treatments.

have been confirmed in other studies.[333,334] A low incidence of atrophic and hypertrophic scarring has been reported by many authors.[335–337] Textural changes appear to occur more frequently in the pediatric population and it is recommended that lower energies be used initially with cryogen spray or other epidermal cooling systems to minimize these side effects. Patients with more melanin pigmentation in their skin are more susceptible to post-inflammatory changes following laser. Effective treatment in this population

requires greater care due to the absorption of laser energy by melanin. Longer intervals between treatments are required to allow for resolution of the post-inflammatory changes. The results with dark-skinned patients are less impressive and patients have an increased risk of permanent pigmentary abnormalities and atrophic scarring.[338] Despite this, patients with Type V skin can be treated with pulsed dye laser with proper caution, provided that treatment expectations and risks are fully discussed.

333. Levine VJ, Geronemus RG (1995) Adverse effects associated with the 577 and 585-nanometer pulsed dye laser in the treatment of cutaneous vascular lesions: a study of 500 patients. **J Am Acad Dermatol** 32:613–617.
334. Boixeda P, Nunez M, Perez B et al. (1997) Complications of 585nm pulsed dye laser therapy. **Int J Dermatol** 36:393–397.
335. Sommer S, Sheehan-Dare RA (1999) Atrophie blanche-like scarring after pulsed dye laser treatment. **J Am Acad Dermatol** 41:100–102.

336. Gaston DA, Clark DP (1998) Facial hypertrophic scarring from pulsed dye laser. **Dermatol Surg** 24:523–525.
337. Buscaglia DA (1999) Hypertrophic scarring from pulsed dye laser treatment. **Dermatol Surg** 25:75.
338. Sommer S, Sheehan-Dare RA (2000) Pulsed dye laser treatment of port-wine stains in pigmented skin. **J Am Acad Dermatol** 42:667–671.

Protective goggles should be worn by the patient and operator to avoid eye injury. For treatment around the eye, non-plastic eye shields are required. Ethyl chloride cryogen spray, supplemental oxygen, and green vinyl tubing should be avoided to reduce the risk of flash fires.[339,340]

One of the greatest challenges in pulsed dye laser in the pediatric population is providing an adequate level of comfort for the patient during treatment. The laser light impact on the skin is analogous to the snap of a small rubber band. With the use of a cryogen spray or cooling system and the topical application of anaesthetic creams such as EMLA or 4% lidocaine gel, most pediatric patients will tolerate up to 50 pulses.[341,342] Treatment of facial stains is more painful than stains on the chest or extremities. Hands, feet, the upper lip, and periorbital areas are the most painful. Iontophoresis of lidocaine 4–5% is effective but impractical in children.[343] Chloral hydrate or other mild sedatives are not recommended since they do not provide analgesia and the degree of sedation and cooperation that is attainable after administration of these agents is unpredictable and often detrimental to the procedure. Most pediatric patients will require a form of general anesthetic to safely and adequately control pain during extensive pulsed dye laser treatment. Intravascular propofol, ketamine or combinations of versed and fentanyl can be used effectively, but should only be administered by well-trained pediatric anesthetists. All of these agents can induce serious complications including respiratory arrest. Ketamine does not cause respiratory depression but is associated with hallucinations in many patients. The most effective anesthetic for infants and young children are inhalent agents such as halothane or sevoflurane.[344,345] These agents can be rapidly administered by mask without the need for intubation in most patients. Recovery is quick and side effects are minimal. An experienced pediatric anesthesiologist should be on hand to administer these agents.

PWS undergo a natural history of thickening and darkening with time. It is not uncommon to see hypertrophy of stain with the development of vascular blebs in older adolescents and adults. The frequency of these changes is reduced by early treatment of the PWS in the pediatric population. Although the development of the longer wavelength and more energetic pulsed dye laser systems with epidermal cooling units has improved the clearance of these thicker stains, most are poorly responsive to pulsed dye laser. For these resistant PWS, the use of continuous wave or quasi-continuous wave laser systems, such as the Nd:YAG, copper-vapor, krypton, or argon lasers may offer benefit.[346] Recently, a high-intensity pulsed noncoherent light source (IPLS) was developed that emits single, double or triple pulses of broadband light from 515 to 1200nm in pulses of 2–20ms duration. This new light system shows promise in the treatment of resistant PWS.[347,348]

Hemangiomas

Most hemangiomas do not require treatment of any kind. A small subset of hemangiomas respond well to pulsed dye laser therapy (Fig. 5.34).[349–353] There have been no double-blind placebo-controlled trials evaluating the efficacy of laser therapy in the treatment of hemangiomas. Studies fail to address response variability between sites or according to age at the onset of treatment or the stage of growth of the tumor. Laser fluences and the interval between treatments is highly variable. In addition, the natural history of spontaneous involution of superficial hemangiomas with excellent cosmetic outcomes complicates outcome measures.

All authors report improvement in the appearance of superficial and thin plaque hemangiomas (3mm or less) with multiple laser treatments. It is recommended that treatment be used early, before or immediately at the onset of the rapid proliferative stage.[316] It should be cautioned, however, that the surface of an early proliferating hemangioma is fragile and the risk of causing ulceration and potential scarring is considerable when lasering at this time. This is especially concerning since it is often too early in the natural history of the hemangioma to predict how much growth will occur. Left alone, small superficial hemangiomas undergo natural involution leaving completely normal skin; therefore scarring from early intervention with laser is unacceptable.

When treating hemangiomas, low fluences are used every three weeks. The use of epidermal cooling units is recommended to reduce the risk of skin texture changes including atrophic scarring and hyper- or hypopigmentation. Table 5.10 provides some clinical criteria for consideration of the use of pulsed dye laser in the treatment of early hemangiomas. Based on the limited data that are currently available, the risk of scarring appears to be in the 4–6% range.[350,352] No improvement has been demonstrated in deeper hemangiomas or in the deep component of mixed hemangiomas using laser therapy. Three-month follow-up of >550 patients treated during the first year of life demonstrated 67% complete or marked regression in flat and superficial hemangiomas with 87% patient satisfaction.[352]

The use of pulsed dye laser for treatment of ulcerated hemangiomas is recommended for those lesions that do not respond to appropriate wound care and oral antibiotics (Fig. 5.35). Morelli reported a series of 37 patients with ulcerated hemangiomas presenting during the proliferative phase (2–6 months) whose ulcers healed in 1–3 treatments with the pulsed dye laser

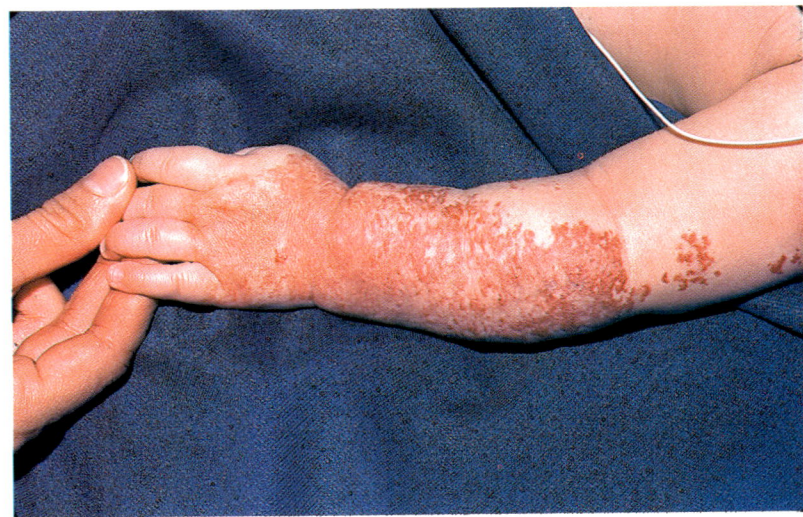

Fig. 5.34 Superficial hemangioma that could be effectively treated with pulsed dye laser.

339. White J-M, Siegfried E, Boulder M et al. (1999) Possible hazards of cryogen use with pulsed dye laser. **Dermatol Surg** 25:250–253.
340. Waldorf HA, Kauvar ANB, Geronemus RG et al. (1996) Remote fire with the pulsed dye laser – risk and prevention. **J Am Acad Dermatol** 34:503–506.
341. Tan OT, Stafford TJ (1992) EMLA for laser treatment of portwine stains in children. **Lasers Surg Med** 12:543–548.
342. Mallory SB, Lehman PA, Vanderpcol DR et al. (1993) Topical lidocaine for anesthesia in patients undergoing pulsed dye laser treatment for vascular malformations. **Pediatr Dermatol** 10:370–375.
343. Nunez M, Mirolles ES, Boirelos P et al. (1997) Iontophoresis for anesthesia during pulsed dye laser treatment of port-wine stains. **Pediatr Dermatol** 14:397–400.
344. Rabinowitz L, Esterly N (eds) (1992) Anesthesia and/or sedation for pulsed dye laser therapy: special symposium. **Pediatr Dermatol** 9:132–153.
345. Grevelink JM, White VR, Bonodr R et al. (1997) Pulsed laser treatment in children and the use of anesthesia. **J Am Acad Dermatol** 37:75–81.
346. Kane KS, Smoller BR, Fitzpatrick RE et al. (1996) Pulsed dye laser-resistant port-wine stains. **Arch Dermatol** 132:839–844.

347. Raulin C, Schroeter CA, Weiss RA, Keiner MN, Werner S (1999) Treatment of port wine stains with a non-coherent pulsed light source: a retrospective study. **Arch Dermatol** 135:679–683.
348. Dover JS, Arndt KA (2000) New approaches to the treatment of vascular lesions. **Lasers in Surgery and Medicine** 26:158.
349. Ashinoff R, Geronemus RG (1991) Capillary hemangiomas and treatment with the flashlamp pumped dye laser. **Arch Dermatol** 127:202–205.
350. Garden JM, Bakus AD, Paller AS (1992) Treatment of cutaneous hemangiomas by the flashlamp-pumped pulsed dye laser: prospective analysis. **J Pediatr** 120:555–560.
351. Poetke M, Philipp C, Berlien HP (2000) Flashlamp-pumped pulsed dye laser for hemangiomas in infancy. **Arch Dermatol** 136:628–632.
352. Hohenleutner S, Badur-Ganter E, Landthaler M et al. (2001) Long-term results in the treatment of childhood hemangioma with the flashlamp-pumped pulsed dye laser: an evaluation of 617 cases. **Lasers Surg Med** 28:273–277.
353. Achauer BM, Change CJ, VanderKam VM (1997) Management of hemangioma of infancy: review of 245 patients. **Plast Reconstr Surg** 99:1301–1308.

TABLE 5.10 Clinical criteria for considering pulsed dye laser in the treatment of superficial hemangiomas

Functional impairment or potential functional impairment
Ulceration or area at high risk for ulceration (groin, lip)
Rapid enlargement or large surface area
Cosmetic disfigurement*
Recurrent bleeding or trauma

* with parental knowledge of risk of scarring

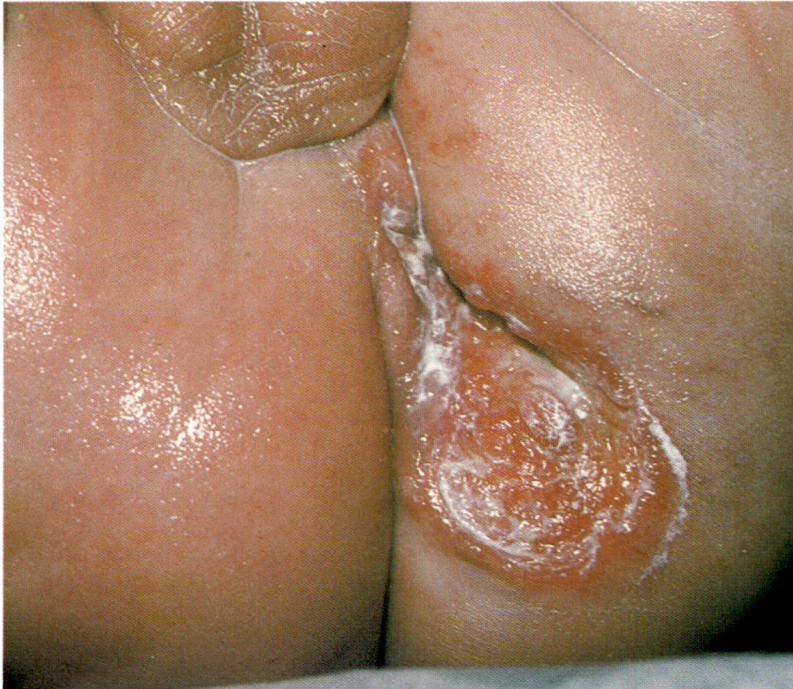

Fig. 5.35 Ulcerated hemangioma on the buttock.

after unsuccessful healing for 1–12 weeks.[354,355] Laser treatment was done at 2–4 week intervals using laser fluences of 6–6.5 joules per square centimeter to the entire surface of the hemangioma. Seventy-six percent of lesions treated were in the diaper area. Ulcerations >2cm required multiple treatments for complete healing but subjective pain improvement was noted after the first

treatment. Other studies have confirmed the benefit of laser in reduction of pain and increasing the rate of healing of ulcerated hemangiomas.[356,357] No epidermal cooling units were used for the treatment of patients in these reports.

The treatment of deep hemangiomas has been undertaken using ultrasound or nuclear magnetic resonance guided interstitial Nd:YAG or KTP laser therapy.[358–363] Laser energy is applied directly to the deep hemangioma tissue using a bare fiber inserted through a cannula or catheter. The position of the tip of the fiber is changed when increased sonographic density of the vascular tissue is noted until all areas are dense. Several treatments are required (average 2–3) in most patients and surface ulceration occurs in 17–30% of patients. Reduction in the size of these large, often inoperable hemangiomas is 50–90% over 3–9 months. This may provide an effective therapy to control the growth of rapidly enlarging, disfiguring or ulcerated deep hemangiomas, especially those that are potentially functionally impairing and poorly responsive to oral steroids.

Other vascular and nonvascular lesions

Many cutaneous vascular lesions repond well to pulsed dye laser therapy. Spider angiomas and benign facial telangiectasias can readily be treated with this laser system with minimal side effects.[364–368] One or two treatments is usually adequate to cause resolution of these more tortuous and superficial vessels. Larger vessels do not resolve with this treatment and may require other light systems, such as the IPLS or the longer-pulsed 532nm laser,[348,369] or combination laser therapy and sclerosis. Since treatment areas are usually smaller and the children presenting with these problems are usually older, topical anesthetic creams are effective. Retreatment of persisting lesions after two or three months is recommended along with the judicial use of sunscreen to try to prevent recurrence.

Pyogenic granulomas have been successfully treated with pulsed dye laser[370–372] but multiple treatments are required and lesions raised more than 3–4mm above the skin are best treated by conventional methods. Laser does offer the advantage of a very low risk of scarring and is an appropriate option for early pyogenic granulomas on the face.

Vascular malformations, other than superficial PWS, are not usually amenable to treatment with the pulsed dye laser. The exception to that is small angiokeratomas or the superficial angiokeratoma-like vascular blebs that develop on the surface of extremities in Klippel–Trenauney syndrome. Bleeding from these lesions is readily treated by this laser. Resolution of the more keratotic plaque is unusual.

Non-vascular cutaneous lesions with prominent erythema and significant vascularity can also be treated with pulsed dye laser. Vascular angiofibromas are an example of a cutaneous lesion that is not primarily vascular in origin, but whose vascular component is very amenable to treatment with this laser system. The laser removes the erythema associated with early central facial lesions effectively.[373] It does not, however, remove the underlying fibrous

354. Morelli JG, Tan OT, Weston WL (1991) Treatment of ulcerated hemangiomas with the pulsed tunable dye laser. **AJDC** 145:1062–1064.
355. Morelli JG, Tan OT, Yohn JJ et al. (1994) Treatment of ulcerated hemangiomas in infancy. **Arch Pediatr Adolesc Med** 148:1104–1105.
356. Scheepers JH, Quaba AA (1995) Does the pulsed tunable dye laser have a role in the management of infantile hemangiomas? Observations based on 3 years' experience. **Plast Reconstr Surg** 95:305–312.
357. Kim HJ, Colombo M, Frieden IJ (2001) Ulcerated hemangiomas: clinical characteristics and response to therapy. **J Amer Acad Dermatol** 44:962–972.
358. Werner JA, Lippert BM, Hoffman P et al. (1995) Nd:YAG laser therapy of voluminous hemangiomas and vascular malformations. **Adv Otorhinolaryngol** 49:75–80.
359. Apfelberg DB, Maser MR, White DN et al. (1990) Combination treatment for massive cavernous hemangioma of the face: YAG laser photocoagulation plus direct steroid injection followed by YAG laser resection with sapphire scalpel tips, aided by superselective embolization. **Lasers Surg Med** 10:217–223.
360. Werner JA, Lippert BM, Gottschlich S et al. (1998) Ultrasound-guided interstitial Nd:YAG laser treatment of voluminous hemangiomas and vascular malformations in 92 patients. **Laryngoscope** 108:463–470.
361. Achauer BM, Celikoz B, VanderKam VM (1998) Intralesional bare fiber laser treatment of hemangioma of infancy. **Plast Reconstr Surg** 5:1212–1217.
362. Achauer BM, Chang CJ, VanderKam VM et al. (1999) Intralesional photocoagulation of periorbital hemangiomas. **Plast Reconstr Surg** 103:11–19.

363. Burstein FD, Simms C, Cohen SR et al. (2000) Intralesional laser therapy of extensive hemangiomas in 100 consecutive pediatric patients. **Ann Plast Surg** 44:188–194.
364. Polla LL, Tan OT, Garden JM et al. (1987) Tunable pulsed dye laser for the treatment of benign vascular ectasia. **Dermatologica** 174:11–17.
365. Swinehart JM (1999) Textural change following treatment of facial telangiectasis with the tunable pulsed-dye laser. **Arch Dermatol** 135:472–473.
366. Garden JM, Geronemus RG (1990) Dermatologic laser surgery. **J Dermatol Surg Onc** 16:156–168.
367. Garden JM, Bakus AD (1993) Clinical efficacy of the pulsed dye laser in the treatment of vascular lesions. **J Dermatol Surg Oncol** 19:321–326.
368. Geronemus RG (1993) Pulsed dye laser treatment of vascular lesions in children. **J Dermatol Surg Oncol** 19:303–310.
369. West TB, Alster TS (1998) Comparison of the long-pulsed dye and KTP lasers in the treatment of facial and leg telangiectasia. **Dermatol Surg** 24:221–226.
370. Goldberg DJ, Sciales CW (1991) Pyogenic granulomas in children: treatment with the flashlamp-pumped pulsed dye laser. **J Dermatol Surg Oncol** 17:960.
371. Gonzalez S, Vibnagool C, Folo LD et al. (1996) Treatment of pyogenic granulomas with the 585nm pulsed dye laser. **J Am Acad Dermatol** 35:428–431.
372. Tay YK, Weston WL, Morelli JG (1997) Treatment of pyogenic granuloma in children with the flashlamp-pumped pulsed dye laser. **Pediatrics** 99:368.
373. Morelli JG (1998) Use of lasers in pediatric dermatology. **Pediatr Dermatol** 16:489.

papule. Adolescents often opt for initial treatment with pulsed dye laser since it is the erythema that is most noticeable during early development of angiofibromas. More definitive treatment can be obtained with the carbon dioxide and copper vapor lasers.[374,375]

Warts, like angiofibromas, have a prominent vascularity that can readily be targeted by the pulsed dye laser. Since warts are common in the pediatric population, pulsed dye laser is used with some frequency to treat symptomatic warts.[376,377] Recent studies suggest that this laser offers no advantage over conventional therapy with liquid nitrogen in the treatment of warts.[378] Patients in this study, however were treated at one month intervals and optimal treatment of warts using the pulsed dye laser requires treatment at 2–3 week intervals to avoid regrowth of the warts between treatment sessions.

The pulsed dye laser is not recommended as a first line treatment for warts in children. However, for some children who have failed conventional therapy, especially those who have more than 20 warts on the hands or on the plantar surface of the feet, the pulsed dye laser is a good alternative (Fig. 5.36). This author reserves the use of laser in the treatment of warts for those patients who have failed treatment with cimetidine and squaric acid therapy. Extensive warts cannot be treated in most children without some form of anesthetic. For acral warts in adolescents, digital blocks can be helpful. For younger children, however, the use of a general anesthetic will be necessary, since topical anesthetics are not sufficient to reduce the pain of pulsed dye laser or cryotherapy for wart treatment.

Flat warts respond the best to the pulsed dye laser, requiring one or two treatments only in most cases. Caution must be taken in the treatment of facial lesions on pigmented skin because the transient post-inflammatory hypopigmentation is more noticeable and disfiguring than the warts themselves. For larger, periungal or plantar warts, 3–4 treatments is more typical for resolution. It is recommended that the warts be aggressively pared prior to laser treatment to allow better penetration of the tissue for vascular injury. High fluence (8.5–10J/cm²) and multiple pulses to each wart to produce purpura are recommended. A minimum of three pulses is usually required per wart. The risk of scarring and the pain and length of postoperative healing is markedly reduced with the pulsed dye laser compared to the carbon dioxide laser. The latter is no longer considered an appropriate treatment in the pediatric population because of the associated morbidity and availability of superior treatments.

The pulsed dye laser has also been used in the treatment of scars and keloids. Persistent erythema in a scar is readily improved with pulsed dye laser therapy. The texture of scars[379] and striae[380] may also improve with this treatment. These cosmetic procedures are rarely performed in children.

VASCULAR LESIONS

Laser treatment of pigmented lesions and tattoos in children

Pigmented lesions are also amenable to laser treatment in children, although the use of these lasers is generally deferred until adolescence. Melanin, the main chromophore of the epidermis, is the target of these lasers. It absorbs energy from about 300 to 1000nm. For this reason, a number of different lasers can be used for selective treatment of a multitude of benign pigmented

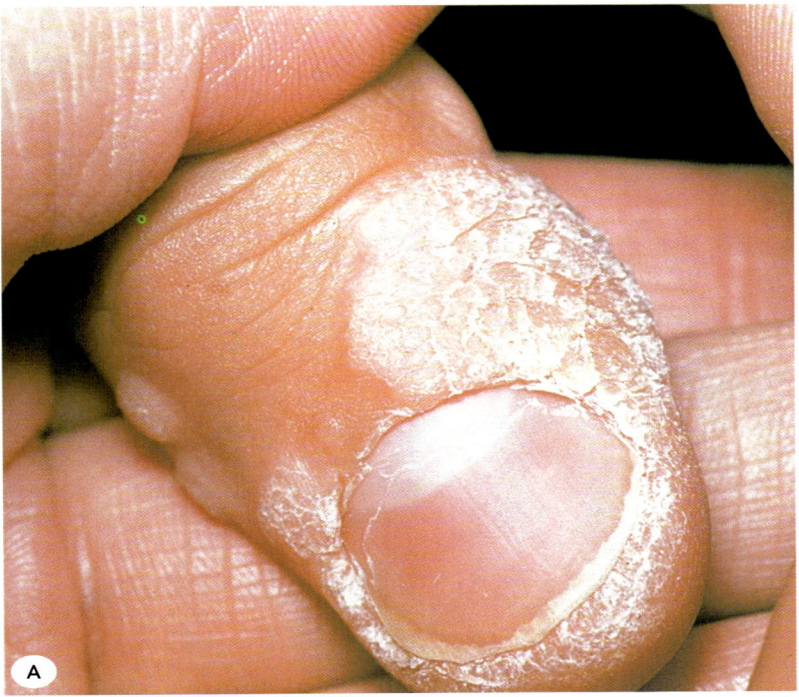
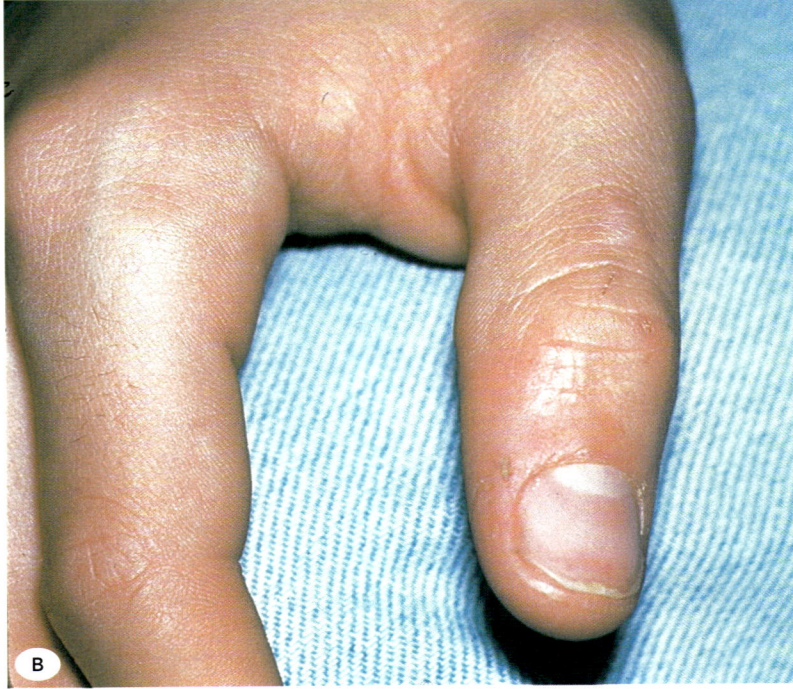

Fig. 5.36 Periungal wart (**A**) before treatment with pulsed dye laser. (**B**) After two treatments with pulsed dye laser.

374. Weston J, Apfelberg DB, Maser MR et al. (1985) Carbon dioxide laserbrasion for the treatment of adenoma sebaceum in tuberous sclerosis. **Ann Plast Surg** 15:132.
375. Kaufman AJ, Grekin RC, Geisse JK et al. (1994) Treatment of adenoma sebaceum with the copper vapor laser. **J Am Acad Dermatol** 33:770.
376. Tan OT, Hurwitz RM, Stafford TJ (1993) Pulsed dye laser treatment of recalcitrant verrucae: a preliminary report. **Lasers Surg Med** 13:127–137.
377. Ross BS, Levine VJ, Nehal K et al. (1999) Pulsed dye laser treatment of warts: an update. **Dermatol Surg** 25:377–380.
378. Kauver AN, Geronemus RG (2001) Pulsed-dye laser versus conventional therapy in the treatment of warts. **J Am Acad Dermatol** 45:151.
379. Alster TS, McMeekin TO (1996) Improvement of facial acne scars by the 585nm flashlamp-pumped pulsed dye laser. **J Am Acad Dermatol** 35:79–81.
380. McDaniel DH, Ash K, Zukowski M (1996) Treatment of stretch marks with the 585nm flashlamp-pumped pulsed dye laser. **Dermatol Surg** 22:332–337.

lesions.[381] Two types of pigmented laser systems are available to treat pigmentary lesions: highly selective lasers, and nonselective or somewhat selective lasers. In general, the highly selective laser systems are preferred for treatment in children. Like the pulsed dye laser, these lasers have pigmentary specificity based on the theory of selective photothermolysis. The target of selective pigmentary lasers is melanin in melanosomes. Selective injury to melanosomes and pigment cells occurs with high-intensity light at short pulse durations of <1 microsecond. The thermal relaxation time of a melanosome, which ranges in size from 0.5–1.0 micrometer, is between 250 and 1000 nanoseconds. For laser injury to be specific for melanin and avoid injury to the surrounding tissue, short impulses of light in these ranges must be used.[382] The pigment-specific lasers are listed in Table 5.11. The longer the wavelength, the deeper the laser penetrates into the skin. Lasers with longer wavelengths are preferred for lesions that have dermal melanin. The choice of pigmentary laser depends on the pigmented lesion being targeted and the depth of melanin in the lesion.

The spectrum of pigmentary lesions amenable to laser in children includes epidermal pigmented lesions (café-au-lait macules, nevus spilus, ephelides and lentigines), dermal pigmented lesions (Nevus of Ota, Nevus of Ito and tattoos) and lesions with combination of epidermal and dermal components (Becker's nevus, congenital pigmented nevi, junctional or compound acquired melanocytic nevi and epidermal nevi) (Table 5.12). Despite this, the treatment of pigmented lesions in the pediatric population is not commonplace.[383] With the exception of Nevus of Ota, complete recurrence of congenital pigmented lesions after multiple laser treatments is a frequent occurrence. Availability of these laser systems in a setting that can provide adequate anesthesia for the pediatric patient is also limited. Most treatment is deferred until adolescence or young adulthood, when the patient is invested in the removal of the lesion, usually for cosmetic purposes. Patients with epidermal nevi often note overgrowth of these lesions, especially on the neck or in intertriginous areas, as they progress through puberty. Successful treatment of these lesions is also difficult due to the depth of penetration of the nevus.[384] Fortunately, occurrence of these lesions on the face is uncommon.

Café-au-lait macules

Café-au-lait macules (CALMs) are common, occurring in 10–20% of patients. Most are small and inconspicuous. Facial lesions are most likely to present for laser therapy, especially when they are large, such as those seen in McCune–Albright syndrome. The pigment is CALMs is present at the basal layer in giant macromelanosomes. Several lasers have been used to treat these lesions, including the Q-switched ruby laser, the frequency-doubled neodymium YAG laser, and the pulsed dye laser at 510 or 504nm, all of which can penetrate to the basal layer.[381] Response to laser treatment is variable, however, and similar lesions treated with the same laser can lighten, clear with recurrence, remain unchanged or be transiently or permanently

---

TABLE 5.11   Highly selective lasers for treating pigmented lesions in children

Laser	Wavelength (nm)	Pulse duration (ns)	Location of targeted pigment
Flashlamp pumped pulsed dye (PDL)	504, 510	300–500	Epidermis, superficial dermis
QSNd:YAG	532	5–20	Epidermis, superficial dermis
QS Ruby (QSR)	694	20–40	Epidermis, dermis
QS Alexandrite	755	50–100	Epidermis, dermis
QS Nd:YAG	1064	5–20	Deep dermis
Long-pulsed Ruby (LPR)	694	300–3000	Dermis (larger targets)
Long-pulsed alexandrite (QSA)	755	200–20 000	Dermis (larger targets)

Freq	frequency
QSNd:YAG	Q-switched, neodymium-yttrium, aluminum-garnet laser
QS	Q-switched

TABLE 5.12   Pigmented lesions amenable to laser in children

Lesion	Laser of Choice	Other Laser Options	Comments
Café au lait	PDL 510/504 (300–500ns)	QSR 694 (20–40ns) QSNd:YAG 532 (5–20ns)	Recurrence rate high
Small congenitalnevi	LPR 694 (0.3–3μs)	QSR 694 (20–40ns) QSA 755 (50–100ns)	Does not eliminate risk of malignancy
Nevus spilus	QSR 694 (20–40ns)	QSNd:YAG 532 (5–20ns) PDL 504/510 (300–500ns)	Recurrence rate high for café au lait pigmentation
Nevus of Ota or Ito Tattoos	QSR 694 (20–40ns)	QSA 755 (50–100ns) QSNd:YAG 1064 (10ns)	
Lentigenes	QSNd:YAG 532 (5–20ns)	QSR 694 (20–40ns) PDL 510/504 (300–500ns)	Equal efficacy noted with all lasers listed
Becker's Nevus	LPR 694 (0.3–3μs) with QSR 694 (20–40ns)	Nd:YAG 532 (5–20ns) PDL 510/504 (300–500ns)	LPR most effective on hair removal; QSR? effective for pigment removal

See abbreviations Table 5.11.

---

381. Carpo BG, Grevelink JM, Grevelink SV (1999) Laser treatment of pigmented lesions in children. **Semin Cutan Med Surg** 18(3):233–243.
382. Anderson RR (2000) Lasers in dermatology – a critical update. **J Dermatol** 27(11):700–705.

383. Morelli JG (1998) Use of lasers in pediatric dermatology. **Pediatr Dermatol** 16:489–495.
384. Michel JL, Has C, Has V (2001) Resurfacing CO_2 laser treatment of linear verrucous epidermal nevus. **Eur J Dermatol** 11(5):436–439.

darkened.[385,386] Side effects of treatment such as transient hyper- and hypopigmentation, prolonged hyperpigmentation, scarring and recurrence of the entire lesion are common.[381,385] The best results have been reported with the pulsed dye laser at 510 or 504nm. Alster successfully cleared 34 CALMs in an average of 8.4 treatments with no recurrence at one year with the 510nm pulsed dye laser.[387] Tan reported similar findings with the 504nm pulsed dye laser in 18 CALMs.[388] Facial lesions may be more responsive to laser treatment than lesions in other areas. It is essential to discuss the limitations of treatment and the potential darkening of lesions that can occur with the patient and parents prior to undergoing any laser therapy for CALMs in the pediatric population.

Nevus spilus

Nevus spilus is a congenital or acquired pigmented lesion that frequently begins as a CALM that becomes studded with smaller more darkly hyperpigmented macules that histologically consist of lentiginous melanocytic hyperplasia or lentiginous junctional, dermal or compound nevi, or Spitz nevi. Lesions can range in size of 1–20cm and are most frequently found on the trunk or extremities. Although rare, malignant melanoma has developed within these lesions and any suspicious area should be biopsied.[389,390] Moreover, lesions treated with laser should be followed indefinitely for any recurrence and suspicious areas immediately biopsied.

Numerous lasers have been used in the treatment of nevus spilus. Like other CALMs, the background pigmentation is the most difficult to eradicate completely. Most reports demonstrate successful removal of the junctional nevi within the plaques using Q-switched ruby laser or the frequency-doubled Q-switched neodymium YAG laser.[391,392] Removal of the background pigmentation is less predictable. Reports indicate that 1–7 treatments are needed for maximum improvement or clearance.[1]

Lentigines can also be treated with the Q-switched ruby,[393,394] frequency-doubled neodynium YAG[395,396] and pulsed dye laser (510nm).[1] Similar efficacy is noted with all of these lasers and results are preferable to those obtained with liquid nitrogen[395] or trichloroacetic acid (35%) peels.[396] Children with Peutz–Jeghers, Laugier–Hunziker syndrome, or other multiple lentigines syndromes can be effectively treated with these lasers.

Congenital nevi

The treatment of congenital nevi with laser is controversial. Congenital nevi of all sizes have an increased risk of malignant melanoma. Treatment with lasers alters the clinical appearance of these nevi by lightening or removing the superficial cutaneous pigment without destroying the melanocytes deeper within the skin.[397–400] Histologic evidence of persistent melanocytes has been demonstrated following laser treatment with the normal–mode ruby laser, the QS ruby laser, and the QS neodymium YAG laser (1064nm).[398,399] Moreover, recurrence of pigmentation occurs in most treated lesions.[400] Laser therapy of congenital nevi carries the risk of altering the clinical appearance of the nevus in a manner that may lead to the delayed recognition of malignant change. Laser does *not* remove the malignant risk since there is histologic evidence that even in the absence of clinically detectable pigmentation following laser, S–100, HMB-45 and Masson–positive cells persist deep in the dermis and around adnexal structures.[401] For these reasons, the author feels that laser treatment of congenital nevi in pediatric patients is ***contraindicated***.

Becker's nevus

A Becker's nevus is a hamartoma of smooth muscle that develops in adolescence. It occurs more frequently in males than females (4:1) and is typically a unilateral, hyperpigmented patch on the shoulder, anterior chest or scapular region with hypertrichosis. Smooth muscle hamartoma is considered by most to be the congenital variant of this benign entity.

Successful treatment of Becker's nevus has been accomplished with the long–pulsed ruby laser.[402] This laser penetrates to the deeper hair follicles eliminating the hyperhidrosis. Injury to the epidermal melanin decreases the pigmentation. Ideal therapy then involves the use of the Q-switched ruby laser to target the epidermal pigment that persists.[403] The frequency–doubled neodymium YAG laser also improves the appearance of this lesion, but the superficial penetration of the laser does not allow for effective treatment of the hypertrichosis.[392] Similarly the PDL at 504 and 510nm can reduce the pigmentation but the risk of recurrence is higher since the pigmented keratinocytes and melanocytes of the deep hair follicle act as a resevoir for repigmentation.[388]

Epidermal nevus

Epidermal nevi are benign hamartomas of the epidermis. They are usually congenital, but delayed appearance and extension throughout the early childhood years is common. Typical lesions are flat and velvety at birth with gradual increase in thickness and hyperpigmentation with time. The most dramatic changes are usually noted around adolescence when filiform and warty papules develop in many patients. Lesions are most symptomatic in the intertrigenous areas where the thickened plaques harbor bacteria and become malodorous. For solitary small plaques, or symptomatic lesions such as the inflamed linear verrucous epidermal nevus (ILVEN) variant, surgical resection is often the treatment of choice and the small scar that results is usually considered a good trade by the pediatric patient.[404] For larger areas, this is not practical.

385. Grossman MC, Anderson RR, Farinelli W et al. (1995) Treatment of café-au-lait macules with lasers: A clinicopathologic correlation. Arch Dermatol 131:1416–1420.
386. Shimbashi T, Kamide R, Hashimoto T (1997) Long-term follow-up in treatment of solar lentigo and café-au-lait macules with Q-switched ruby laser. Aesth Plast Surg 21:445–448.
387. Alster TS (1995) Complete elimination of large café-au-lait birthmarks by the 510-nm pulsed dye laser. Plast Reconstr Surg 96:1660–1664.
388. Tan OT, Morelli JG, Kurban AK (1992) Pulsed dye laser treatment of benign cutaneous pigmented lesions. Laser Surg Med 12:538–542.
389. Rhodes AR (1996) Nevus spilus: A potential precursor of cutaneous melanoma worthy of aggressive surgical excision? Pediatr Dermatol 13:250–252.
390. Weinberg JM, Schutzer PJ, Harris RM et al. (1998) Melanoma arising in nevus spilus. Cutis 61:287–289.
391. Grevelink JM, Gonzalez S, Bonoan R et al. (1997) Treatment of nevus spilus with the Q-switched ruby laser. Dermatol Surg 23:365–370.
392. Tse Y, Levine VJ, McClain SA et al. (1994) The removal of cutaneous pigmented lesions with the Q-switched ruby laser and the Q-switched neodymium:yttrium-aluminum-garnet laser. J Dermatol Surg Oncol 20:795–800.
393. Kato S, Takeyama J, Tanita Y, Ebina K (1998) Ruby laser therapy for labial lentigines in Peutz–Jeghers syndrome. Eur J Pediatrics 157(8):622–624.
394. Kopera D, Hohenleutner U, Landthaler M (1997) Quality-switched ruby laser treatment of solar lentigines and Becker's nevus: a histopathological and immunohistochemical study. Dermatology 194(4):338–343.
395. Todd MM, Rallis TM, Gerwels JW, Hata TR (2000) A comparison of 3 lasers and liquid nitrogen in the treatment of solar lentigines: a randomized, controlled, comparative trial [see comments]. Archives of Dermatology 136(7):841–846.
396. Li YT, Yang KC (1999) Comparison of the frequency-doubled Q-switched Nd:YAG laser and 35% trichloroacetic acid for the treatment of face lentigines. Dermatologic Surgery 25(3):202–204.
397. Imayama S, Ueda S (1999) Long- and short-term histological observations of congenital nevi treated with the normal-mode ruby laser. Archives of Dermatology 135(10):1211–1218.
398. Duke D, Byers HR, Sober AJ, Anderson RR, Grevelink JM (1999) Treatment of benign and atypical nevi with the normal-mode ruby laser and the Q-switched ruby laser: clinical improvement but failure to completely eliminate nevomelanocytes. Archives of Dermatology 135(3):290–296.
399. Grevelink JM, van Leeuwen RL, Anderson RR, Byers HR (1997) Clinical and histological responses of congenital melanocytic nevi after single treatment with Q-switched lasers. Archives of Dermatology 133(3):349–453.
400. Waldorf HA, Kauvar AN, Geronemus RG (1996) Treatment of small and medium congenital nevi with the Q-switched ruby laser. Archives of Dermatology 132(3):301–304.
401. Kopera D, Hohenleutner U, Stolz W, Landthaler M (1997) Ex vivo quality-switched ruby laser irradiation of cutaneous melanocytic lesions: persistence of S-100-, HMB-45- and Masson-positive cells. Dermatology 194(4):344–450.
402. Nanni CA, Alster TS (1998) Treatment of a Becker's nevus using a 694-nm long-pulsed ruby laser. Dermatol Surg 24:1032–1034.
403. Kopera D, Hohenleutner U, Landthaler M (1997) Quality-switched ruby laser treatment of solar lentigines and Becker's nevus. Dermatology 194:338–343.
404. Lee BJ, Mancini AJ, Renucci J, Paller AS, Bauer BS (2001) Full-thickness surgical excision for the treatment of inflammatory linear verrucous epidermal nevus [Review][23 refs]. Annals of Plastic Surgery 47(3):285–292.

Laser therapy of epidermal nevi has not been very successful. Recurrence is common and scarring is a frequent side effect.[381,384] The thickness of the lesion usually precludes effective use of the pulsed laser systems that do not penetrate deeply enough into the skin to eradicate the lesion. Occasionally, in more darkly pigmented lesions, the long-pulsed ruby laser has been effective.[405] The newer pulsed and scanned CO_2 and Erbium:YAG lasers allow for more precise control of the depth of tissue ablation.[406] This reduces the risk of scarring, but also results in a higher rate of recurrence than the older continuous wave CO_2 and argon lasers. Careful use of the continuous wave lasers has been successful in treatment without significant scarring in some patients.[407]

Nevus of Ota and Ito

Nevus of Ota (Nevus fuscocuruleus ophthalmomaxillaris) is the presence of deep dermal melanocytosis, typically in an irregular patch along the distribution of the first and second divisions of the trigeminal nerve. Patchy blue-gray or greenish pigmentation elsewhere on the skin (excluding the transient Mongolian spots seen in pigmented races) is termed Nevus of Ito. In both cases, lesions can be congenital or acquired and histologically demonstrate pigment laden, spindle-shaped dendritic melanocytes deep in the dermis.[408]

Laser treatment of Nevus of Ota is accomplished with Q-switched lasers that have longer wavelengths to target the dermal melanin. Early studies demonstrated efficacy of the Q-switched ruby laser in effective treatment of these lesions. Typically several treatments (3–7) at 4–8 week intervals are required.[409,410] A recent retrospective study of long-term complications of treatment with this laser demonstrated a 16.8% incidence of persistant hypopigmentation and a 5.9% incidence of persistent hyperpigmentation. Recurrence of the lesion was noted in only 1% of treated patients.[411]

The Q-switched alexandrite and neodymium YAG (1064nm) are also effective in the treatment of Nevus of Ota.[412,413] Chen has demonstrated a slightly increased efficacy of the QS-neodymium YAG over the QS-alexandrite[414] but a patient preference for use of the QS-alexandrite,[415] a difference which may be more relevant in pediatric patients. Transient hyperpigmentation is noted in 50% of patients lasting 4–6 months that is usually treated with hydroquinone and tretinoin cream.[412] Persistent hypopigmentation and hyperpigmentation was seen in 3% of patients treated with both lasers. Texture changes and scarring occurred in 2.9% and 1.9%, respectively.[413] Recurrence was seen in <1% of patients.

Incomplete and poor responses are noted in a significant number of patients (10–20%). Some authors feel that this is related to the color of the lesions with browner lesions responding better than more violaceous lesions.[416] Others feel that response to laser treatment is determined by the depth of

pigment rather than the color, with lesions containing melanocytes to the depth of 1mm or less achieving the best results.[408]

Tattoos

An increasing number of pediatric patients are obtaining tattoos in late adolescence and early adulthood. Studies of adults who return for tattoo removal have shown that most obtained their tattoos impulsively and cite poor decision making and personal regret as their main reasons for seeking removal.[417] This highlights the importance of educating adolescents to dissuade them from tattoo placement. Tattoo removal is painful, costly and frequently incomplete and accompanied by undesirable scarring. It is important to emphasize these facts to our adolescents whom we see for unrelated issues.

Traumatic tattoos are the most common form of tattoo encountered in younger pediatric patients. Tattoo with lead from pencils, or foreign body materials such as metal, glass, dirt, sand, and ashphalt are common. Pencil point tattoos typically clear with one treatment with QS ruby,[418] QS alexandrite[419] or QS neodymium YAG.[420,421] More treatments are needed for most other forms of traumatic tattoo removal but all of these lasers have demonstrated effective treatment.

Decorative tattoos are more difficult to remove than most traumatic tattoos. Amateur tattoos are usually easier to treat since they generally consist of a single pigment at variable depths in the skin.[422] Older tattoos are also easier to clear probably due to the migration of pigment particles deeper into the skin or out of the dermis by the action of phagocytic cells.[420] For professional decorative tattoos many treatments are generally required. In recent prospective trials of the QS Nd:YAG (532 and 1064nm) vs. QS ruby laser and QS alexandrite laser in the treatment of decorative tattoos the QS ruby produced the greatest degree of lightening.[423,424] However, treatment with this laser is also associated with a higher risk of permanent hypopigmentation

TABLE 5.13 **Lasers for tattoo removal**

Color of tattoo	Optimal laser	Alternative lasers
Blue-black	QSR (694 nm)	QSA QSNd:YAG (1064nm)*
Green	QSA (755nm)	QSR (694nm) QSNd:YAG
Red, orange, yellow	PDL (510nm)	QSNd:YAG (532nm)

* Recommended as treatment of choice for all dark complected patients.
See abbreviations Table 5.11.

405. Baba T, Narumi H, Hanada K et al. (1995) Successful treatment of dark-colored epidermal nevus with ruby laser. **J Dermatol** 22:567–570.
406. Losee JE, Serletti JM, Pennino RP (1999) Epidermal nevus syndrome: a review and case report [Review][9 refs]. **Ann Plastic Surg** 43(2):211–214.
407. Hohenleutner U, Wlotzke U, Konz B et al. (1995) Carbon dioxide laser therapy of a widespread epidermal nevus. **Lasers Surg Med** 16:288–291.
408. Kang W, Lee E, Choi GS (1999) Treatment of Ota's nevus by Q-switched alexandrite laser: therapeutic outcome in relation to clinical and histopathological findings. **Eur J Dermatol** 9(8):639–643.
409. Geronemus RG (1992) Q-switched ruby laser therapy of nevus of Ota. **Arch Dermatol** 128:1618–1622.
410. Watanabe S, Takahashi H (1994) Treatment of nevus of Ota with the Q-switched ruby laser. **N Engl J Med** 331:1745–1750.
411. Kono T, Nozaki M, Chan HH, Mikashima Y (2001) A retrospective study looking at the long-term complications of Q-switched ruby laser in the treatment of nevus of Ota. **Lasers in Surgery & Medicine** 29(2):156–159.
412. Lam AY, Wong DS, Lam LK, Ho WS, Chan HH (2001) A retrospective study on the efficacy and complications of Q-switched alexandrite laser in the treatment of acquired bilateral nevus of Ota-like macules. **Dermatologic Surgery** 27(11):937–941; discussion 941–942.
413. Chan HH, Leung RS, Ying SY et al. (2000) A retrospective analysis of complications in the treatment of nevus of Ota with the Q-switched alexandrite and Q-switched Nd:YAG lasers. **Dermatologic Surgery** 26(11):1000–1006.
414. Chan HH, Ying SY, Ho WS (2000) An in vivo trial comparing the clinical efficacy and complications of Q-switched 755nm alexandrite and Q-switched 1064nm Nd:YAG lasers in the treatment of nevus of Ota. **Dermatologic Surgery** 26(10):919–922.

415. Chan HH, King WW, Chan ES et al. (1999) In vivo trial comparing patients' tolerance of Q-switched Alexandrite (QS Alex) and Q-switched neodymium:yttrium-aluminum-garnet (QS Nd:YAG) lasers in the treatment of nevus of Ota. **Lasers in Surgery & Medicine** 24(1):24–28.
416. Ueda S, Isoda M, Imayama S (2000) Response of naevus of Ota to Q-switched ruby laser treatment according to lesion colour. **Br J Dermatol** 142(1):77–83.
417. Armstrong ML, Stuppy DJ, Gabriel DC, Anderson RR (1996) Motivation for tattoo removal. **Archives of Dermatology** 132(4):412–416.
418. Knoell KA, Schreiber AJ, Kutenplon M et al. (1997) Q-switched ruby laser treatment of traumatic tattooing induced by pencil point puncture in children. **Pediatr Dermatol** 14:325–326.
419. Moreno-Arias GA, Casals-Andreu M, Camps-Fresneda A (1999) Use of Q-switched alexandrite laser (755nm, 100nsec) for removal of traumatic tattoo of different origins. **Lasers in Surgery & Medicine** 25(5):445–450.
420. Troilius AN (1998) Effective treatment of traumatic tattoos with a Q-switched Nd:YAG laser. **Lasers Surg Med** 22:103–108.
421. Suzuki H (1996) Treatment of traumatic tattoos with the Q-switched neodymium:YAG laser. **Arch Dermatol** 132:1226–1229.
422. Alster TS (1997) Laser treatment of tattoos. In: Alster TS (ed). Manual of Cutaneous Laser Techniques, Philadelphia, PA: Lippincott-Raven, pp. 64–68.
423. Goyal S, Arndt KA, Stern RS et al. (1997) Laser treatment of tattoos: A prospective, paired, comparison study of the Q-switched Nd:YAG (1064nm), frequency doubled Q-switched Nd:YAG, and Q-switched ruby lasers. **J Am Acad Dermatol** 36:122–125.
424. Leuenberger ML, Mulas MW, Hata TR et al. (1999) Comparison study of the Q-switched alexandrite, Nd:YAG, and ruby lasers in treating blue-black tattoos. **Dermatologic Surgery** 25(1):10–14.

and textural changes. This is especially true in darkly pigmented patients who should optimally be treated with the QS Nd:YAG to minimize side effects.

Although the QS ruby laser is the most effective overall in removing decorative tattoos, the laser of choice depends to some degree on the colors present in the tattoo. Red, yellow or orange pigment is not effectively removed by either the QS ruby or the QS alexandrite lasers (Table 5.13). Additionally, some pigment that cannot be removed by the QS ruby laser may be effectively treated with the longer wavelength of the QS Nd:YAG, which can clear deeper pigment particles.

Complications of laser removal of tattoos are frequent. Transient or long-lasting hypopigmentation, transient post-inflammatory hyperpigmentation, textural changes and atrophic scarring can be seen.[420,422] Immediate post-treatment pigment darkening may occur in tattoos with skin-colored tones containing iron or titanium dioxide through reduction of ferric oxide to ferrous oxide. This darkening can be very difficult to remove.[381]

Prior to the development of pigment-selective lasers, the carbon dioxide laser (10 600nm) was used in the treatment of tattoos.[425] This non-specific laser targets intra- and extracellular water and vaporizes tissue. In the defocused mode many benign cutaneous lesions including warts, epidermal nevi, vascular lesions, and adenoma sebaceum were frequently treated with this destructive laser.[426,427] Injury from this laser always produces scarring and healing, especially on the lower extremities where it was used to treat plantar warts was prolonged and painful. It did not prevent recurrence of these lesions.[428] The use of this laser in the pediatric population is inappropriate. There is no benign cutaneous lesion for which there is not an alternative laser or excisional therapy that has a better outcome. Use of this laser should be limited to the second-line treatment of lesions resistant to these better therapies with a full discussion of the scarring that will result. One area where this laser may continue to offer advantages is in the treatment of smaller areas of epidermal nevi on the neck or in intertrigenous regions. Here the scarring may be preferable to the high rate of recurrence with other lasers.

Hair removal lasers

Unfortunately, the amount and distribution of hair plays an important role in the cultural definition of beauty. Having plentiful scalp hair is desirable. Conversely, the presense of hair on the face, axillae and legs is often deemed socially unacceptable in women. Adolescents are often severely emotionally distressed by the presence of excessive hair in certain body regions and seek advice about hair removal. The pediatric dermatologist is wise to keep abreast of the rapid progress in laser technology that is ongoing as this cosmetic market is being aggressively developed by laser companies.

Traditional approaches to hair removal have been primarily temporary. Shaving, plucking, waxing, chemical depilatories, and bleaching remain the methods used most frequently by adolescents to control unwanted hair growth. Electrolysis, the use of a direct current or electrothermolysis, the use of a radiofrequency current, were the only methods available to provide permanent hair removal prior to the use of laser systems. Unfortunately, these techniques were inconvenient, painful, operator-dependent and carried a significant risk of scarring. In addition, they were impractical for removal of large numbers of hair.

Improved hair removal can now be provided with the use of lasers and xenon flashlamps, but there remains little scientific evidence that any of the currently available systems is effective in permanent hair removal for the majority of patients. Aggressive marketing has led to public belief that this is a reasonable goal and many adolescents approach laser treatment with false expectations of treatment outcome. It is the pediatric dermatologist's job to ensure that the expectation of the patient is consistent with the limitations of currently available treatments.

Adolescents seeking permanent hair removal should be informed that long-standing hair removal is only possible for patients with dark hair. Moreover, those patients with dark hair and dark skin are unlikely to achieve good results since the target of most laser systems is melanin, and the use of sufficient energy to permanently destroy the hair follicles in these patients can cause permanent injury to the skin pigment. Individuals with blonde, red, gray or white hair should understand that laser treatment is unlikely to effect permanent hair removal. If the adolescent is willing to undergo repeat laser treatments at 2–4 month intervals, temporary hair removal is attainable and may be a more acceptable alternative to traditional hair removal methods. Even for those ideal patients with dark hair and light skin, treated at high fluences ($>$30joules/cm^2) using a large spot size (7mm diameter), the average long-term hair loss per treatment is only 20–30%.[429–433]

There are multiple hair removal systems now commercially available and FDA approved for hair removal. Table 5.14 lists the properties of the currently available systems. No one system is optimal for removal of hair in all patients. The first laser system that was FDA approved for hair removal was the Nd:YAG laser that was used with the application of carbon particles to the skin surface.[434] This laser system provides little permanent hair removal although it can be used safely in patients with pigmented skin with 3–6 month delay in hair regrowth.[435] Lasers that target melanin, including the long-pulsed ruby laser, the alexandrite laser and the diode laser, offer more permanent benefit but all require multiple treatments for a low percentage yield of permanent removal with each treatment.[436,437] The intense pulsed light system offers an advantage in patients with darker skin pigment although hyperpigmentation has been reported.[438]

Optical hair removal is painful and adolescents should be prepared for discomfort when they seek this treatment. Satisfaction with therapy is possible, but only with realistic expectations.

TISSUE EXPANDERS

A relatively new technique, known as tissue expansion, uses the gradual expansion of normal skin and soft tissue to develop excess material for the repair of an anticipated defect.[439,440] This technique uses one or more sterile inflatable silicone bags placed beneath the adjacent normal skin surface near the anticipated surgical site or defect. Each expander, which is capable of massive inflation two or three times its normal volume, its attached to a self-sealing injection port by way of silicone tubing.

After an incision is made under local anesthesia, the expander is placed in proper position and the wound is sutured closed (Fig. 5.37). Once this heals,

425. Bailin PL, Ratz JL, Levine HL (1980) Removal of tattoos by CO₂ laser. J Dermatol Surg Oncol 6:997.
426. Wheeland RG, Bailin PL, Kantor GR et al. (1985) Treatment of adenoma sebaceum with carbon dioxide laser vaporization. J Dermatol Surg Oncol 11:861.
427. Sloan K, Haberman H, Lynde CW (1998) Carbon dioxide laser-treatment of resistant verrucae: retrospective analysis. J Cutan Med Surg 2(3):142–145.
428. Mixter RC, Carson LV, Walton BJ, Gerson RW (1997) Treatment of recalcitrant verrucae with both the ultrapulse CO₂ and PLDL pulsed dye lasers. Plast Reconstr Surg 100(6):1612–1613.
429. Ort RJ, Anderson RR (1999) Optical hair removal. Semin Cutan Med Surg 18(2):149–158.
430. Olsen EA (1999) Methods of hair removal. J Am Acad Dermatol 40:143–155.
431. Dierickx C, Aora MB, Dover JS (1999) A clinical overview of hair removal using lasers. Dermatol Clin 17(2):357–366, ix.
432. Liew SH (1999) Unwanted body hair and its removal: a review. Dermatol Surg 25(6):431–439.
433. Kierickx CC (2000) Hair removal by lasers and intense pulsed light. Semin Cutan Med Surg 19(4):267–275.

434. Nanni CA, Alster TS (1997) Optimizing treatment parameters for hair removal using a carbon-based solution and a 1064nm Q-switched neodymium:YAG laser energy. Arch Dermatol 133:1546–1549.
435. Nanni CA, Alster TS (1998) A practical review of laser-assisted hair removal using the Q-switched Nd:YAG, long-pulsed ruby, and long-pulsed alexandrite lasers. Dermatol Surg 24:1–7.
436. Finkel B, Eliezri YD, Waldman A, Slatkine M (1997) Pulsed alexandrite laser technology for noninvasive hair removal. J Clin Laser Med Surg 15:225–229.
437. Dierickx CC, Grossman MC, Farinelli WA, Anderson RR (1998) Permanent hair removal by normal mode ruby laser. Arch Dermatol 134:837–842.
438. Gould MH, Bell MW, Foster TD, Street (1997) Long term epilation using the Epilight broad band, intense pulsed light hair removal system. Dermatol Surg 23:909–913.
439. Unlu RE, Sensoz O, Uysal AC (2001) Re: the use of serial tissue expansion in pediatric plastic surgery. Annals of Plastic Surgery 47(6):679.
440. Hudson DA, Lazarus D, Silfen R (2000) The use of serial tissue expansion in pediatric plastic surgery. Annals of Plastic Surgery 45(6):589–593; discussion 593–594.

TABLE 5.14   Lasers and lightsources for hair removal

Type	Wavelength (nm)	Pulse duration (ms)	Fluence (J/cm²)	Spot size (mm)	Commercial name	Comment
Neodynium-YAG laser	1064	10–20	2–3	7–10	Softlight	? Permanent hair removal; carbon solution unnecessary, less painful, less skin pigmentation injury
Long-pulsed Ruby Laser	694	1.2–3	10–40	4–6 7–10	Epitouch Epilaser	Slow
Alexandrite Laser	755	2 3 5, 10, 20	5–50 10–100 5–20	5–10 7–15 7–10	Epitouch Alex Gentle lase PhotoGenic a LPIR	Fast Slow Requires multiple pulses
Diode laser	800	5–30	10–40	9×9	Light Sheer	Fewer side effects
Intense Xenon flashlamp	550–1200	Variable	Variable	10×45	Epilight	Slow Multiple pulses Operator experience Need for efficiency May be safe for dark skin

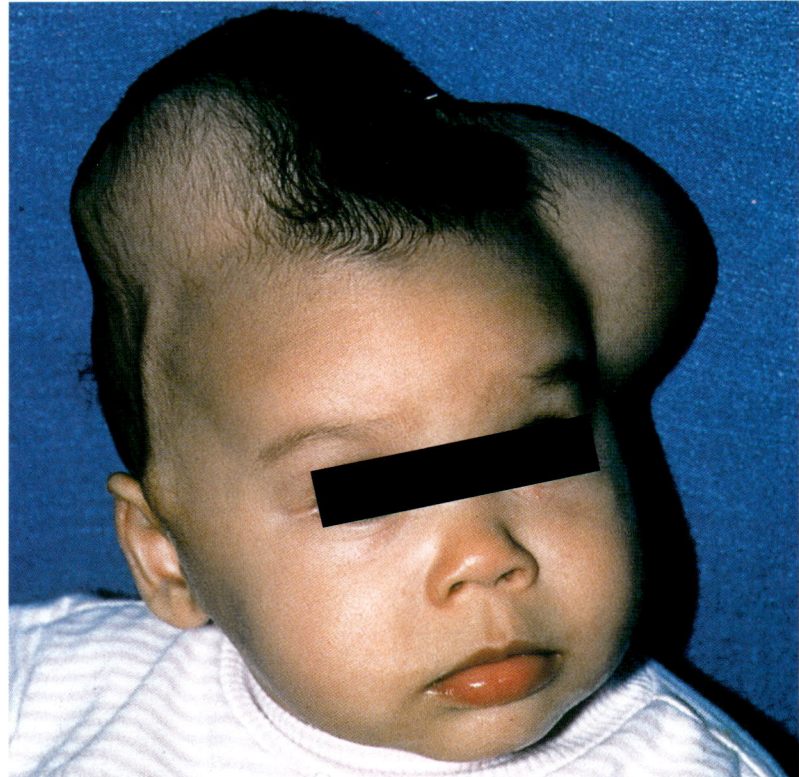

Fig. 5.37   Tissue expansion for excision of a large congenital nevus of the scalp.

the expander. Usually the quantity injected at each visit is 10–20% of the total volume of the expander. This sequential injection process gradually expands the silicone bag and results in a slow stretching of the overlying soft tissue and skin to accommodate the increase in size. This injection and expansion process is continued until sufficient excess soft tissue has been created to cover the proposed surgical defect. In most cases, this can be accomplished within six to eight weeks.

This process stimulates the growth of new skin from the adjacent normal tissue. The resulting advancement flap that is created provides an ideal color-and-texture match with the surrounding skin, and normal sensation is also maintained. None of this is true for either skin grafts or local cutaneous flap surgery, which are commonly used in similar situations. In addition, tissue expansion eliminates the need for extensive grafting and the resultant care of the donor site, since the expanded tissue is sufficient to cover both the primary and secondary defects at one time. Also, since hair-bearing tissue can be expanded in a similar fashion, tissue expanders can be used to provide an excellent cosmetic result not obtainable with either skin grafts or flaps for treatment of scalp defects. Placement of tissue expanders in children is generally accomplished with an outpatient anesthetic. All expansion injections are carried out in a painless manner with topical anesthetic cream placed over the injection port one hour before the time of injection.

This procedure has been successfully employed in the treatment of burn wounds, removal of large congenital nevi,[441,442] nevus sebaceous, aplasia cutis, hemangiomas,[443] lymphangiomas, linear epidermal nevi,[444] and scarring alopecia. Serial expansions can be performed to allow for removal of extremely large lesions covering large areas of the trunk and extremities. Since pre-expanded skin is under less tension, scars heal with minimal spreading. The potential uses for tissue expansion techniques are continuing to be explored.

Tissue expanders should not be used where primary closure in one or two stages is possible, however. The complication rate of tissue expansion is significant. It has been calculated in two recent studies at 18–19%.[445,446] The most common complications are infection 6%, deflation 3% and exposure 2%. Complications are greatest in older patients, burn patients, with the use of internal expander ports and for serial expansion patients.[446]

usually after seven to 10 days, the expansion process can begin. At weekly intervals, sterile saline is injected without anesthesia into the buried injection port. The volume injected is dependent on the anatomic location and size of

441. Bauer BS, Few JW, Chavez CD, Galiano RD (2001) The role of tissue expansion in the management of large congenital pigmented nevi of the forehead in the pediatric patient. **Plastic & Reconstr Surgery** 107(3):668–675.

442. Perlyn C, Meara JG, Smith JD, Breuing KH, Bartlett R (1999) Secondary reconstruction of a giant congenital lentiginous dermal nevus with serial, large-volume tissue expansion. **Ann Plastic Surgery** 43(5):546–550.

443. Chang CJ, Achauer BM, VanderKam VM (1997) Reconstruction of head and neck hemangiomas with tissue expansion in the pediatric population. **Ann Plastic Surgery** 38(1):15–18.

444. Lee BJ, Mancini AJ, Renucci J, Paller AS, Bauer BS (2001) Full-thickness surgical excision for the treatment of inflammatory linear verrucous epidermal nevus [Review][23 refs]. **Ann Plastic Surgery** 47(3):285–292.

445. Gibstein LA, Abramson DL, Bartlett RA et al. (1997) Tissue expansion in children: a retrospective study of complications. **Ann Plastic Surgery** 38(4):358–364.

446. Friedman RM, Ingram AE Jr., Rohrich RJ et al. (1996) Risk factors for complications in pediatric tissue expansion. **Plastic & Reconstr Surgery** 98(7):1242–1246.

SKIN GRAFTS

Skin grafting is not a common procedure performed by office-based dermatologic surgeons, especially when treating children. However, a brief review of the various skin grafting techniques may serve as useful information for the physician caring for patients who may require this type of procedure for the correction of some cutaneous condition or defect. Skin grafts are used to provide closure of those defects where primary closure cannot be accomplished because of size or limited quantity of adjacent tissue. Grafts may also be used to protect deeper underlying structures from desiccation or to prevent contraction of soft tissues around the mouth, eyes, nose, or on the extremities. Split-thickness skin grafts are used most often to repair larger defects resulting from ablative surgery, burns, or other injuries. Tissue expansion techniques together with composite grafts of Human Skin Equivalent (see previous sections) have markedly reduced the need for these procedures in young children.

Split-thickness grafts

The traditional split-thickness skin graft employs the use of a sharp knife, or dermatome, to remove large thin sheets of tissue.[447] One instrument, the Davol dermatome, is a rechargeable battery-powered dermatome that will harvest medium-thickness grafts of 0.015 inch in thickness and $1\frac{5}{16}$ inch in width. This is frequently adequate for the treatment of many dermatologic conditions. Other instruments used to harvest split-thickness skin grafts include the Brown and Padgett dermatomes; these electrically powered machines are capable of harvesting grafts of variable thickness and width.

Regardless of the instrument chosen, the technique used to harvest split-thickness grafts is essentially the same. The donor site may be any part of the body, but most commonly the anterior thigh, buttocks, abdomen, and back are used.[448] After infiltration with a local anesthetic agent, the area to be removed is coated with mineral oil or sterile surgical ointment to facilitate the harvesting of tissue. For larger grafts, tumescent anesthesia may offer a benefit, especially in children where the amount of local anesthetic that can be safely administered is limited.[449] A graft of suitable length and width is cut using a dermatome. It is then laid into the recipient area and sewn or stapled into place and covered with a suitable dressing, to immobilize it and prevent shearing forces that could disrupt the new blood vessels that are growing into the graft.[450] The donor site is covered with a synthetic surgical dressing and allowed to heal by second intention.

Most split-thickness skin grafts develop a sufficient vascular supply within two weeks to permit limited function by the patient. Over a period of several months, the graft gradually begins repigmenting to provide a more satisfactory cosmetic result. Since the texture of a split-thickness graft almost never is an ideal match with the normal skin, and the sensation of the graft is abnormal, this type of graft may always remain visible and produce cosmetic difficulties.

In cases in which a large defect is present, like a burn wound in a small child or infant, and there is only a limited amount of donor area available, meshed split-thickness grafts are often used.[451] The mesher mechanically cross-hatches a standard split-thickness skin graft to increase the area over which it can be placed. Meshed grafts can be used to double, triple, or increase the surface even ninefold over the original size of the split-thickness skin graft. While the cosmetic appearance from this process is inferior to that obtained with a regular split-thickness graft, it does permit coverage of large areas with greater ease and will generally improve satisfactorily with time.

When large defects are present, ultra-thin or meshed split-thickness grafts can be used in combination with artificial skin.[452] Non-healing skin defects in dystrophic epidermolysis bullosa have been successfully treated with a combination of autologous meshed split-thickness grafts from the non-involved skin that was covered with allogeneic keratinocytes.[448] More recently, tissue-engineered skin alone has been successfully used in these patients with improved cosmesis obviating further the need for split-thickness grafts.[453,454]

Full-thickness grafts

Full-thickness skin grafts are used to cover small defects that cannot be closed primarily without creating tension on the wound edges or distorting the adjacent normal anatomy. This type of graft has a much higher nutritional requirement and has a higher failure rate than that of split-thickness grafts. However, since a full thickness of soft tissue is transferred from one site to another, the improved color, texture, and presence of appendageal structures will normally provide an improved cosmetic result over that obtained with other grafts.[455,456]

The key to performing ideal full-thickness skin grafting is the proper selection of the donor tissue.[450,457] The closer the donor site resembles the recipient site in color, texture, hair, and sebaceous gland activity, the better will be the final cosmetic result. With that in mind, the surgeon can select the best possible match from a number of available donor sites. The most common sites used for this purpose include the supraclavicular area, pre- and postauricular skin, upper eyelid, glabella, posterior neck, inguinal fold, and antecubital fossa. It is crucial to remember that skin taken from below the mammary line will not blush when placed on the face. As a consequence of this, if the primary defect is located on the face, the best donor site should be superior to this line.

The technique for full-thickness skin grafting begins with the creation of a template that is based upon the actual size of the defect. Since some shrinkage of the graft is expected after harvesting, the template is placed on the appropriate donor tissue and a fusiform excision is designed to remove an adequate amount of tissue that can be used as the graft. Once the excision has been made, the graft is defatted and cut to fit the size of the defect precisely. It is then sutured into place, and a large immobilizing bulky dressing is tied over the surface to prevent any inadvertent shearing action from disrupting the normal healing process. The donor site is then repaired in a simple linear manner with appropriate suture material.

To prevent injury to the full-thickness skin graft, most surgeons do not examine it for two to seven days. When examined, there is almost always some vascular congestion present that results in a cyanotic appearance. Sometimes the epidermis becomes blistered and separates from the graft with the first dressing change. Neither of these findings is indicative of graft failure; rather, they are normal expected changes.[458] The sutures are usually removed from the graft at nine to 10 days, but diligent wound care is required for an additional 10 days, to ensure graft survival. If there is a suboptimal cosmetic result due to poor color or texture match, additional improvement can often be obtained by lightly dermabrading the surface at the end of eight weeks. Relatively normal sensation and color can be expected in most cases within four to six months.

Composite skin grafts

Composite skin grafts that contain cartilage in addition to skin and subcutaneous tissue are primarily used for reconstruction of defects on the nose and ear. While no more difficult to perform than standard skin-grafting

447. Rosenberg L (1985) A new system of dermatomes. **Plast Reconstr Surg** 75:743.
448. Verplancke P, Beele H, Monstrey S, Naeyaert JM (1997) Treatment of dystrophic epidermolysis bullosa with autologous meshed split-thickness skin grafts and allogeneic cultured keratinocytes. **Dermatology** 194(4):380–382.
449. Field LM, Hrabovszky T (1997) Harvesting split-thickness grafts with tumescent anesthesia. **Dermatol Surg** 23(1):62.
450. Rudolph R, Fisher JC, Ninnemann JL (1979) Skin Grafting. Bosto:, Little Brown.
451. Kirsner RS, Eaglstein WH, Kerdel FA (1997) Split-thickness skin grafting for lower extremity ulcerations. **Dermatol Surg** 23(2):85–91.
452. Thomas WO, Rayburn S, LeBlanc RT et al. (2001) Artificial skin in the treatment of a large congenital nevus. **South Med J** 94(3):325–328.
453. Falabella AF, Valencia IC, Eaglstein WH, Schachner LA (2000) Tissue engineered skin (Apligraf) in the healing of patients with epidermolysis bullosa wounds. **Arch Dermatol** 136:1225.
454. Fine JD (2000) Skin bioequevalants and their role in the treatment of inherited epidermolysis bullosa. **Arch Dermatol** 136:1259.
455. Ratner D (1998) Skin grafting. From here to there. **Dermatologic Clinics** 16(1):75–90.
456. Valencia IC, Falabella AF, Eaglstein WH (2000) Skin grafting. **Dermatologic Clinics** 18(3):521–532.
457. Gloster HM Jr (2000) The use of full thickness skin grafts to repair nonperforating nasal defects. **J Amer Acad Dermatol** 42(6):1041–1050.
458. Mast BA (1997) Healing in other tissues. **Surgical Clinics of North America** 77(3):529–547.

procedures, failure of this graft is not uncommon, due to the tremendous nutritional requirements. This is especially common when grafts are larger than 2cm in diameter. The donor area for this procedure is most often the superior or anterior helical rim of the ear.

SIMPLE CUTANEOUS FLAPS

The alternatives to wound closure for those defects that cannot be closed primarily in a simple side-to-side fashion include both skin grafting and skin flaps. The prime advantage of skin flaps over grafting is the improved final cosmetic result. Since simple skin flaps move adjacent loose tissue into a defect, the color match, texture, sensation, and presence of appendageal structures tend to be much closer to that of the original tissue than can be obtained with use of skin grafts of any type.

Common simple skin flap

The common simple skin flaps consist of advancement, rotation, transposition, and rhomboid flaps.[459,460] Each derives its name from the type of motion involved in the transfer of adjacent tissue to fill the primary defect. Each flap has some unique properties that may give certain advantages and disadvantages. In performing proper flap surgery, the surgeon must be familiar with each type of flap in order to select the most appropriate one to use in any given situation.

Rotation flap

The appearance of a rotation flap suggests that the movement consists entirely of rotation about a given pivot point. However, there is also a component of

transposition and advancement involved (Fig. 5.38). This flap is intrinsically safe to perform, even in the movement of large amount of tissue, due to the maintenance of a large pedicle through which the vascular structures remain intact. This flap can be used to mobilize the entire cheek to close a large nasal defect, or much of the scalp may be mobilized with this flap to close a forehead or temple defect. At the same time, a much smaller version of this flap can also be successfully used to close defects of lesser size. The curved lines that are created in the movement of this type of flap are often beneficial in that they are easier to conceal by placing them within one of the naturally curved folds or creases, which will improve the cosmetic results that are obtained.

Advancement flap

The advancement flap uses a sliding movement of tissue to fill a void (Fig. 5.39). This flap is probably the easiest one to plan and perform in a satisfactory manner. However, because of the design of this flap, necrosis of the tip may occur if the vascular supply, determined by the width of the flap, is impaired by excessive stretching or if the metabolic demands, determined by the length of the flap, outstrip the supply. The linear nature of this flap creates straight lines that may, in certain areas of the body, be obvious. When used on the forehead, where naturally straight lines exist, the cosmetic result can be exceptionally good. Advancement flaps can also be used to reduce the contraction of scars that have adversely distorted normal anatomy. This type of advancement flap is known as the V–Y flap; it is used to lengthen a scar and reduce tension.[461,462] This is commonly used for scars on the eyelids where ectropion has resulted from previous injury or surgery.

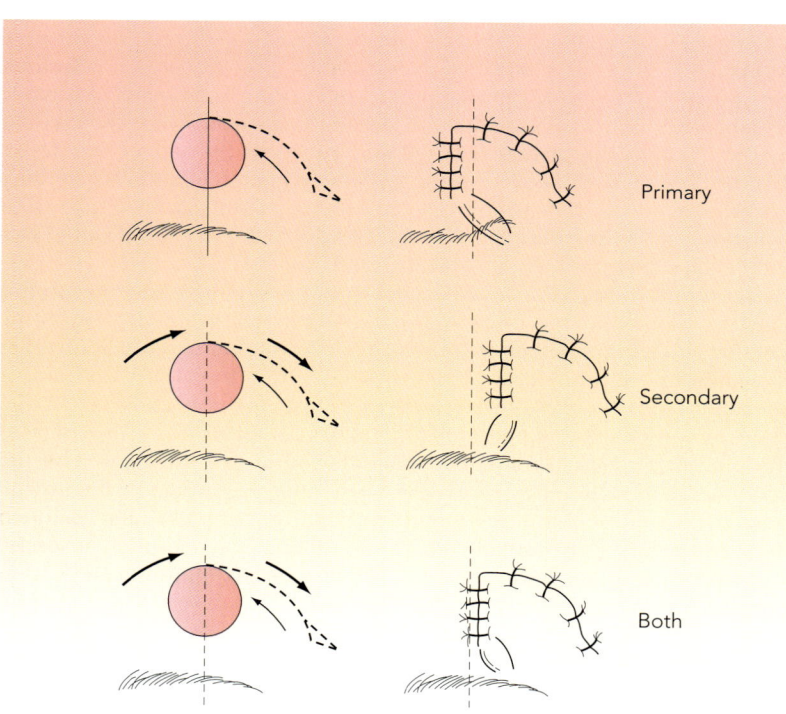

Fig. 5.38   Schematic drawing of a rotation flap showing its three separate movements. The pucker that is formed by the rotation of the skin is shown on the pedicle of the flap nearest the defect. The size and direction of this pucker change depending on the amount of primary and secondary movement (*Schachner and Hansen, 2nd edition*).

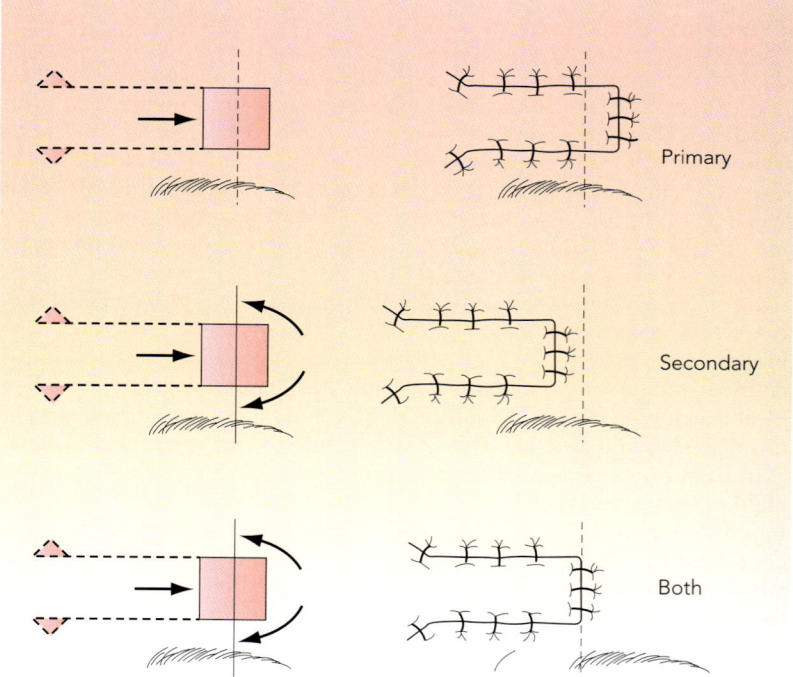

Fig. 5.39   Schematic drawing of an advancement flap showing its three movements. The vertical line indicates the center of the defect, while the eyebrow is also shown as a fixed anatomical structure to compare how the various movements of the flap alter the location of each. The darker sutures represent key stitch placement (*Schachner and Hansen, 2nd edition*).

459. Stegman SJ (1980) Principals of design and the dynamics of movement of flaps. **J Dermatol Oncol** 6:182.
460. Heniford BW, Bailin PL, Marsico RE Jr. (1998) Field guide to local flaps. **Dermatol Clinics** 16(1):65–74.

461. Peled IJ, Wexler MR (1983) The usefulness and versatility of V-Y advancement flaps. **J Dermatol Surg Oncol** 9:1003.
462. Clark JM, Wang TD (2001) Local flaps in scar revision. **Facial Plastic Surgery** 17(4):295–308.

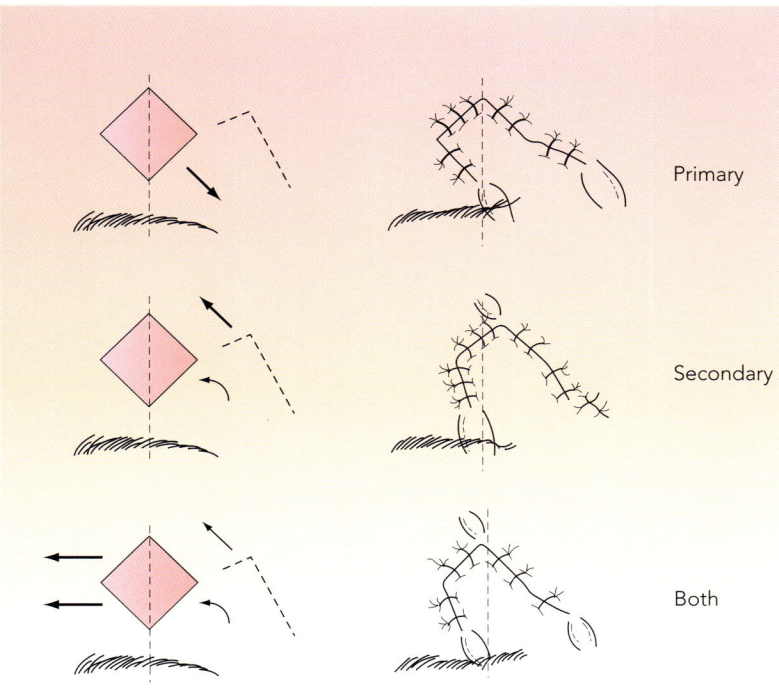

Fig. 5.40 Schematic drawing of a rhomboid flap showing its three separate movements. It should be noted that the flap and the triangle of skin created by the flap interchange with one another in a similar manner to that in a Z-plasty (*Schachner and Hansen, 2nd edition*).

Primary

Secondary

Both

Transposition flap

The transposition flap can be characterized by the most common type, the Z-plasty.[463] This type of flap is used to change the directions of a scar by reversing or transposing the two arms of the flap. It is often used for long linear scars to break up the line and make it more cosmetically acceptable, by reducing its visibility. This flap also can be used to effectively lengthen a scar. If tension across a joint or other mobile part of the body, like the neck, has resulted from a linear incision, by using a series of small Z-plasties the direction and length of the scar can be changed to reduce the tension.

Rhomboid flap

Without doubt, the rhomboid flap is the most difficult flap to visualize as far as the movement of tissue is concerned (Fig. 5.40). However, once the proper geometric shape of this flap has been designed, it offers significant advantages over the other flaps. This has to do with its versatility, since any one of four different quadrants around the original defect can be rotated into position to close the defect.

Before flap surgery is performed for wound closure, the physician must have a thorough knowledge of the procedure. The best results will only be obtained when the dynamics of flap movement are understood. With this knowledge the correct decision can be made as to whether or not a flap should be used, and which type of flap is the best choice to provide the most satisfactory technique for wound repair.

SPECIAL EQUIPMENT

Since most dermatologists perform minor surgical procedures routinely, even on a daily basis, very little additional equipment is required for the effective treatment of children. Certain types of dermatologic surgical procedures require the purchase of special instruments, but few other tools are necessary for their adaptations to treat children, since virtually all the surgical instruments and local anesthetics used in the surgical treatment of children and adolescents are identical to those used in the treatment of adults. For those physicians who like to employ restraints, the purchase of a papoose board or similar restraining device might be worthwhile, but this is certainly not mandatory. More humane methods of restraining children, such as wrapping with an office sheet, are effective and far less traumatic than commercially available restraining devices (Fig. 5.41). If the surgical procedure takes longer than five minutes, the use of restraining devices is contraindicated. Excisional surgery should never be performed using restraints. Children too young to cooperate during these procedures should have the benefit of outpatient anesthesia.

When purchasing surgical instruments, it is important to keep in mind that pediatric patients are smaller than adult patients. Closing wounds in confined spaces in children can be facilitated by the use of smaller instruments. Pick-ups that are three inches long and shorter needle holders allow for more precise control in small spaces. The use of a 15-C blade or a Beaver blade can facilitate small excisions (Fig. 5.42). Availability of proper suture removal equipment is also essential since pediatric patients are often uncooperative at suture removal. Suture removal sissors with fine but blunt tips are ideal for removing 6–0 suture on the face (Fig. 5.43).

Since all invasive surgical procedures are associated with some risk of secondary infection, the physician performing proper dermatologic surgery must use strict aseptic technique, and this requires the use of sterile instruments. The most ideal method for sterilizing surgical tools is steam heat with pressurization. This can best be achieved for the office-based physician with an autoclave, which becomes an important piece of equipment essential for performing surgery on the skin.

In order for the surgeon to perform the best possible technical procedure, comfort is a requirement. An electrically powered adjustable surgical table facilitates positioning of the patient for maximum exposure and greatest comfort possible. An adjustable stool can also make a long procedure more tolerable for the surgeon. Adequate lighting is also a requirement for performing cutaneous surgical procedures. Additional lighting can be suspended from the ceiling, attached to the surgical table, or mounted on rollers, depending upon the space available in the operating room suite.

It is equally important during surgery to keep the patient comfortable. Pediatric patients are most comfortable surrounded by familiar objects: a pillow or blanket from home, a parent, a stuffed animal and a television. There is no more effective distraction than a movie. A television with a VCR or DVD player is a worthwhile investment in the pediatric surgery suite.

One area of common neglect in many physicians' offices is an emergency kit. Prepackaged kits are now widely available and come stocked with the necessary medications to handle various levels of office emergencies. The types and kinds of emergency medications and intravenous fluids included in the emergency kits should be determined by the training and expertise of the personnel in the office and the availability of emergency technicians in the community. Dosages of all medications for both adults and children should be placed in the emergency kit for immediate use. All medications contained in the kits should be checked periodically to ascertain that they have not become outdated. At a minimum, all office personnel should be familiar with basic cardiopulmonary resuscitation emergency techniques, as well as the necessary steps to take in the event of an emergency.

In addition to the emergency kit, an emergency supply of oxygen and ventilation breathing bags fitted with both pediatric and adult sizes of masks should be available. Plastic oralpharyngeal airways and endotracheal tubes in a full range of sizes should also be present. Infant and child-sized blood pressure cuffs and a stethoscope with pediatric head should also be available. If conscious sedation is carried out, a cardiac moniter and pulse oxymeter should be used.

463. Mandy SH (1985) The practical use of Z-plasty. **J Dermatol Surg Oncol** 11:745.

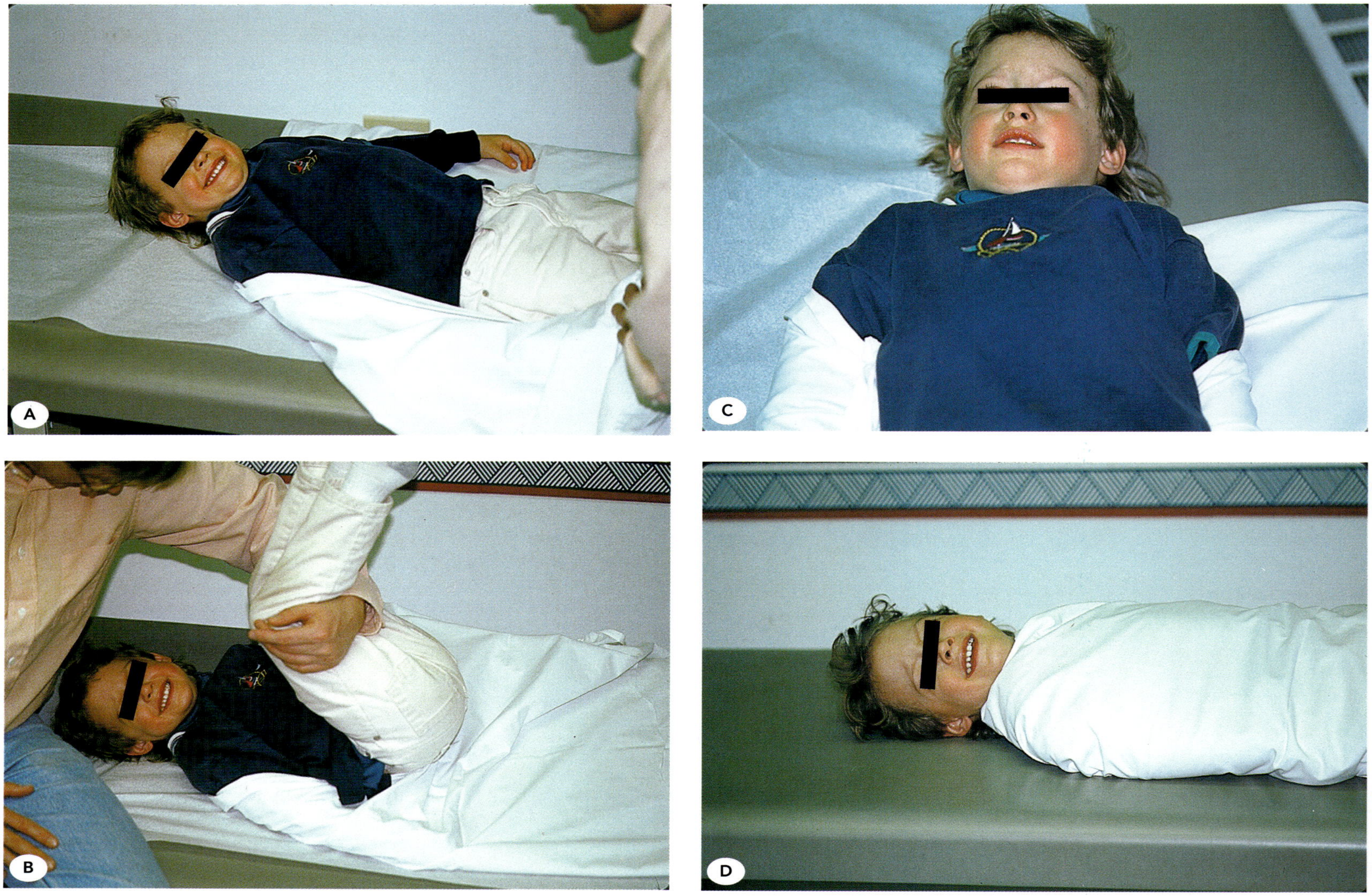

Fig. 5.41   Immobilization of a child using a sheet. (**A**) The child is place on a sheet folded in half on the table. One half of the sheet is wrapped around the arm. (**B**) The child is lifted and the sheet is wound behind the back. (**C**) The sheet is passed beneath the second arm and wrapped over the arm and under the back again as in A and B. (**D**) The other edge of the sheet is wrapped around the child to secure the restraint.

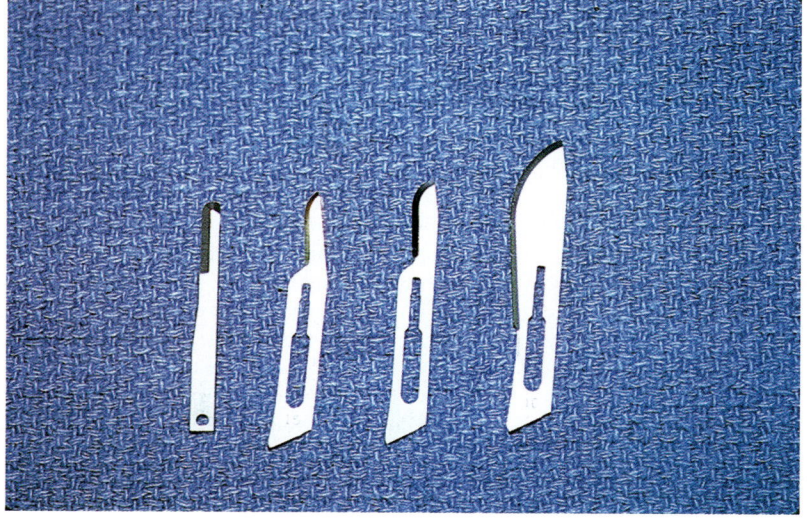

Fig. 5.42   Comparison of blade types. 1) Beaver blade 2) 15-C blade 3) 15 blade 4) 10 blade.

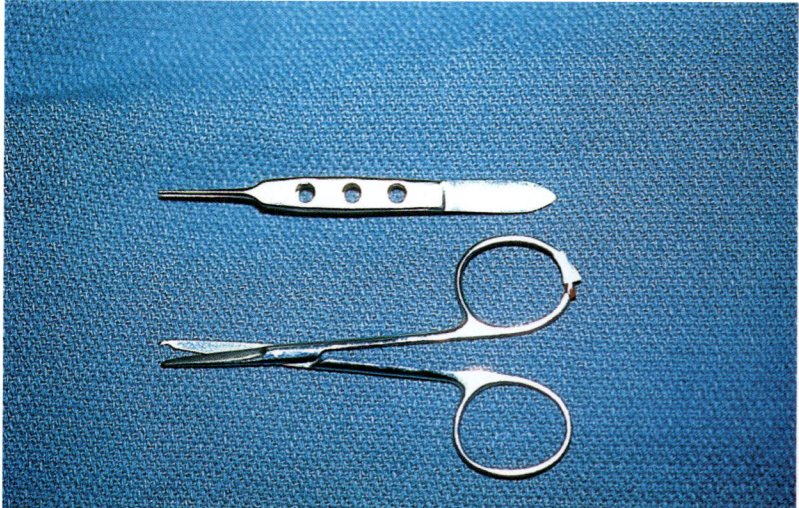

Fig. 5.43   Suture removal sissor with small pick-up.

SPECIAL DERMATOLOGIC SURGERY PROBLEMS

The pediatric dermatologic surgeon is rarely called upon to excise skin cancers. Most excisional surgery in this field is performed because of the risk of malignant transformation that is present in some birthmarks or to improve the cosmetic appearance of a child by removing the birthmark. These surgeries are elective and therefore choosing the optimal time for excision is important. Many factors enter into a decision to perform an elective surgery in a child.

The goal of every procedure is to minimize surgical risk while providing the best surgical outcome. For many lesions, postponement until the age of pre-adolescence is recommended when excisions can be accomplished readily with a local anesthetic. For some lesions, such as large congenital nevi, the risk of malignancy is sufficiently great that earlier intervention is usually recommended. In addition, in some body locations, such as the scalp and face, early excision is advisable to maximize the cosmetic appearance of the resultant scar. Table 5.15 outlines the recommended timing of surgical excision

TABLE 5.15 Recommended timing of surgical excision

Lesion	Location	Size	Age	Comments
Nevus sebaceous	Scalp	<1cm	7–10 years	Excise if alopecia is visible – local anesthetic
		>1cm	6–12 months	1° excision, staged excision or tissue expansion under general anesthetic
	Face	all	6–12 months	early excision recommended
Congenital nevi	All locations	Small <1cm	7–10 years	Observation unless atypical or changing
	Scalp or face, palms, soles, any body location requiring staged excision or expansion	medium 1.5–20cm		Early staged excision and expansion results in better scars
	Body	1.5–20cm	7–10 years	Excision under local anesthetic
	Scalp	>20cm	>6 months	Tissue expansion <6 months causes skull deformity
	All other locations	>20cm	3–6 months	Tissue expansion
Aplasia cutis	All	>1cm	6–12 months	For cosmetic improvement
		<1cm	7–10 years	For cosmetic improvement
Pilomatricoma	Face	All	When diagnosed	Early removal decreases size of scar
	Body	All	7–10 years	Excision only recommended if large and visible, painful, or symptomatic
Dermoid cysts	Lateral eyebrow or scalp	visible	6–12 months	General anesthetic early to minimize scars
		invisible	7–10 years	Defer or remove under local anesthetic at age 7–10 years
	Midline face	all	6–12 months	Need MRI prior to removal
Giant JXG	Face, scalp or ulcerated	>4cm	6–12 months or preschool	Large JXG's leave fibrofatty deposition with involution
	Body	>4cm	7–10 years	
Giant solitary mastocytomas	Face, scalp	>3cm	6–12 months	Excision for symptoms of severe recurrent blistering or pain or if lesion fails to involute by > age 7
	Body	>3cm	7–10 years	
Ulcerated hemangioma	All	Amenable to 1° closure	Infancy	Consider excision when significant scarring or if failure of medical therapy to heal ulcer
Non-ulcerated hemangioma	All	>1cm	>4 years	For cosmetic improvement of fibrofatty deposition
Pyogenic granulomas	All	<6mm	When diagnosed	Pulsed dye laser can be effective
	All	>7mm	When diagnosed	Electrodesiccation with curretage for pedunculated lesion; if base ≥8mm excision is preferred
Epidermal nevi	Face	>1cm	6–12 months	Excision for cosmetic purposes only
		<1cm	7–10 years	
Acquired nevi	Face	All	>16 years	Cosmetic removal should be deferred in early adolescence
Atypical nevi	All	All	When diagnosed	Excision for changes
Spitz nevi	Face	>2mm	When diagnosed	Early excision improves scar
	Body	>6mm	When diagnosed	Observation unless atypical appearance Excision for changes when they occur
Vascular malformation Angiokeratoma				Larger lesions more likely to recur Excise early if painful or enlarging
Lymphangioma circumscriptum	All	<3cm	7–10 years	May recur

in the pediatric dermatologic population. This section reviews the more common pediatric dermatologic surgery entities, indications for treatment of these conditions, and surgical treatment options.

NEVUS SEBACEOUS OF JADASSOHN

The nevus sebaceous of Jadassohn is an uncommon congenital hamartoma of the skin and adnexa with a predominance of sebaceous glands, abortive hair follicles, and ectopic apocrine glands. It is most commonly located on the scalp and face where sebaceous elements are present in the greatest abundance.[464,465] Lesions are usually solitary and range in size from several millimeters to large hemifacial plaques (Fig. 5.44). Extensive areas of nevus sebaceous can be associated with multiple systemic manifestations that are not impacted by treatment of the nevus.

Surgical indications

Although nevus sebaceous is a benign lesion, it undergoes a natural history of transformation and has the potential for development within it of both benign and malignant neoplasms, typically after puberty. Although the risk of malignant degeneration has been estimated to be as high as 31% by some authors,[464] recent studies suggest that many of the tumors that develop within nevus sebaceous are basaloid hamartomas, most commonly trichoblastomas rather than basal cell carcinoma.[466-468]

At birth, the nevus sebaceous is often more erythematous, thickened and impressive in appearance. This results because of stimulation of the sebaceous elements of this hamartoma by the hormones of pregnancy from the mother and typically persists for about three months. The lesion then becomes less erythematous and flattens. Many parents feel that the lesion is self-resolving due to the improvement in appearance noted at this time. Despite this, the underdeveloped hair follicles result in persistant alopecia and it is this that typically causes the parent to seek medical attention. Changes during early childhood are rare, but with the approach of puberty it is typical to see a wart-like thickening of the plaques of nevus sebaceous as well as the development of tumors within it. A large percentage of patients (46.8%) will develop benign tumors within nevus sebaceus, predominantly in the adult years.[469] In addition, basal cell carcinoma, squamous cell carcinoma, apocrine carcinoma, and other adnexal carcinomas have all been reported to arise in nevus sebaceous.[469-471] Recently a defect in the PTCH gene has been elucidated in nevus sebaceous.[472] This is the same defect that is seen in basal cell nevus syndrome and some basal cell carcinomas. Mice that have a knockout of the PTCH gene develop both trichoblastomas and basal cell carcinomas with UV and ionizing radiation.[473] Whether nevus sebaceous in humans is subject to malignant deterioration with UV exposure remains to be determined. However, it seems prudent to approach these lesions with surgical excision. Excision allows for improvement in the cosmetics of the area by removing an area of alopecia on the scalp or a disfiguring facial lesion. It also eliminates the risk of malignant degeneration within the tumor. This author feels that prophylactic excision of nevus sebaceus should continue to be the standard of care.

For lesions that are larger than 1cm on the scalp or for any obvious lesion of cosmetic importance on the face, removal of nevus sebaceous under a general anesthesia in infancy may be preferred. Scalp flexibility is maximal in the first year of life and large areas can be primarily resected without the need of tissue expansion and with decreased spreading of the scars in this period (Fig. 5.45). Most small areas of nevus sebaceous can be readily approached in

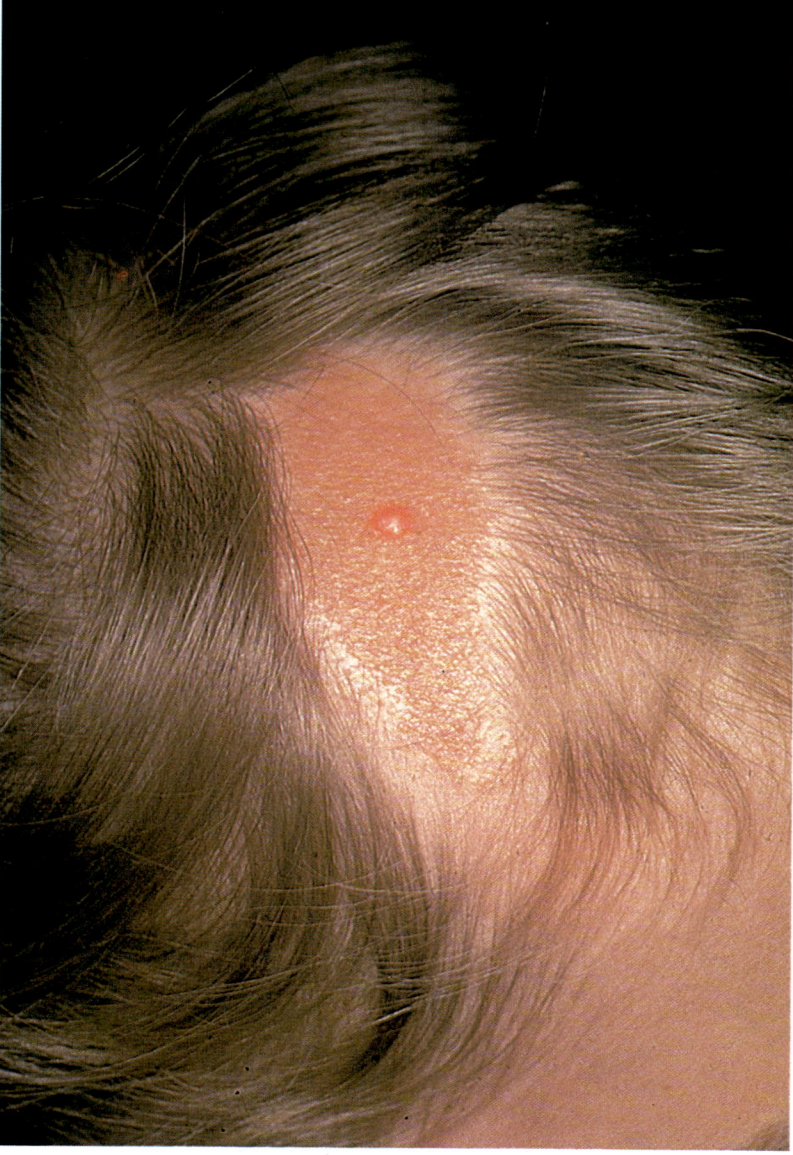

Fig. 5.44   Nevus sebaceous of the scalp with a new papule. (Biopsy demonstated benign trichoblastoma.)

the pre-adolescent years using a local anesthetic in the clinic. All excisional surgery leaves a scar that will not grow hair and significant spreading of scars can occur in certain locations on the scalp, especially the occiput. The parents should be informed of this prior to making a decision to proceed with excision or to postpone excision in early infancy. Laser destruction of nevus sebaceous is not recommended. There is a high rate of recurrence of these lesions when treated with more superficial laser systems and the risk of malignancy is not altered by this therapy due to the failure of the laser systems to penetrate deeply and fully remove the tumor.

464. Wilson Jones E, Heyl T (1970) Nevus sebaceous. Br J Dermatol 82:99.
465. Mehregan AH, Pinkus H (1965) Life history of organoid nevi: special reference to nevus sebaceous of Jadassohn. Arch Dermatol 91:574.
466. Cribier B, Scrivener Y, Grosshans E (2000) Tumors arising in nevus sebaceous. J Am Acad Derm 42(2pt1):263–268.
467. Jaqueti G, Requena L, Sanchez Yis E (2000) Trichoblastoma is the most common neoplasm developed in nevus sebaceous of Jadassohn; a clinicopathologic study of a series of 155 cases. Am Journal of Dermatopath 22(2):108–118.
468. Kaddu S, Schaeppi H, Kerl H, Soyer HP (2000) Basaloid neoplasms in nevus sebaceous. Journal of Cutaneous Pathology 27(7):327–337.

469. Beer GM, Widder W, Cierpka K, Kompatscher P, Meyer VE (1999) Malignant tumors associated with nevus sebaceous:therapeutic consequences. Aesthet Plast Surg 23:224.
470. Turner CD, Shea CR, Rosoff PM (2001) Basal cell carcinoma originating from a nevus sebaceous on the scalp of a 7-year-old boy. Jour Pediatric Hematology Oncol 23(4):247–249.
471. Rinaggio J, McGuff HS, Otto R, Hickson C (2002) Postauricular sebaceous arising in association with nevus sebaceous. Head and Neck 24(2):212–216.
472. Xin H, Matt D, Burg G, Boni R (1999) Deletions of the PCTH gene in sebaceous nevi. J Invest Dermatol 112:587.
473. Aszterbaum M, Epstein J, Oro A, Douglas V et al. (1999) Ultraviolet and ionizing radiation enhance the growth of BCC's and trichoblastomas in patched heterozygous knockout mice. Nat Med 11:1285.

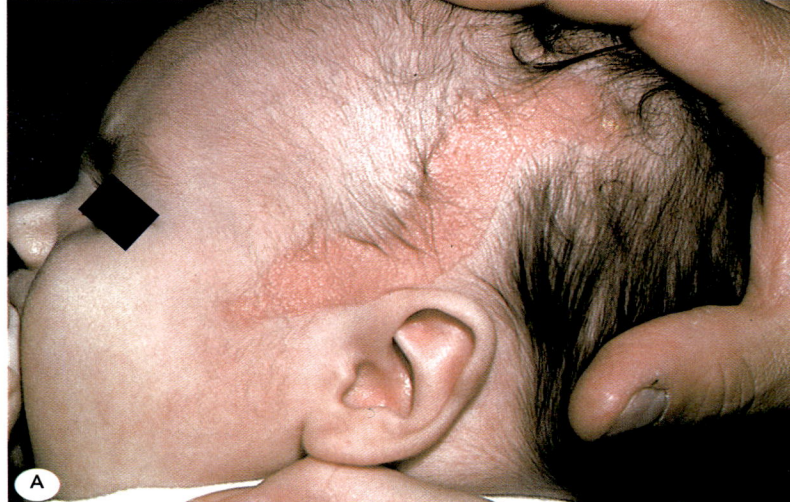

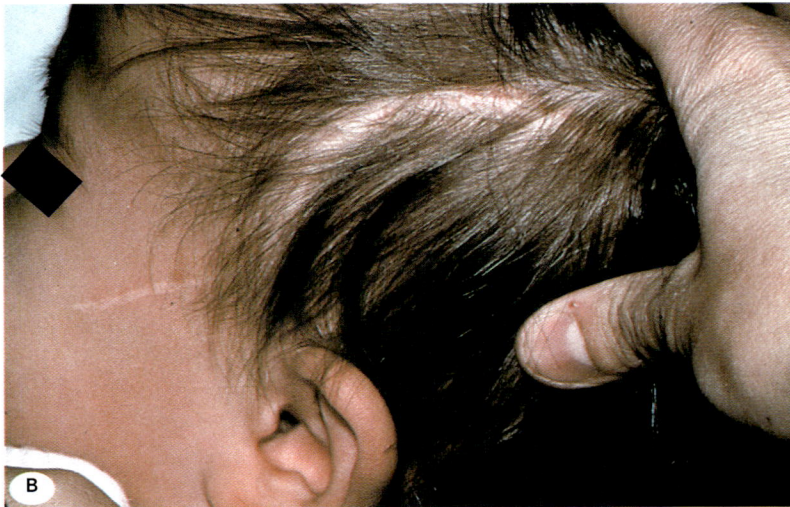

Fig. 5.45 (A) Pre-op appearance of large nevus sebaceous of the scalp and face. (B) Post-op appearance of the scar one year after resection.

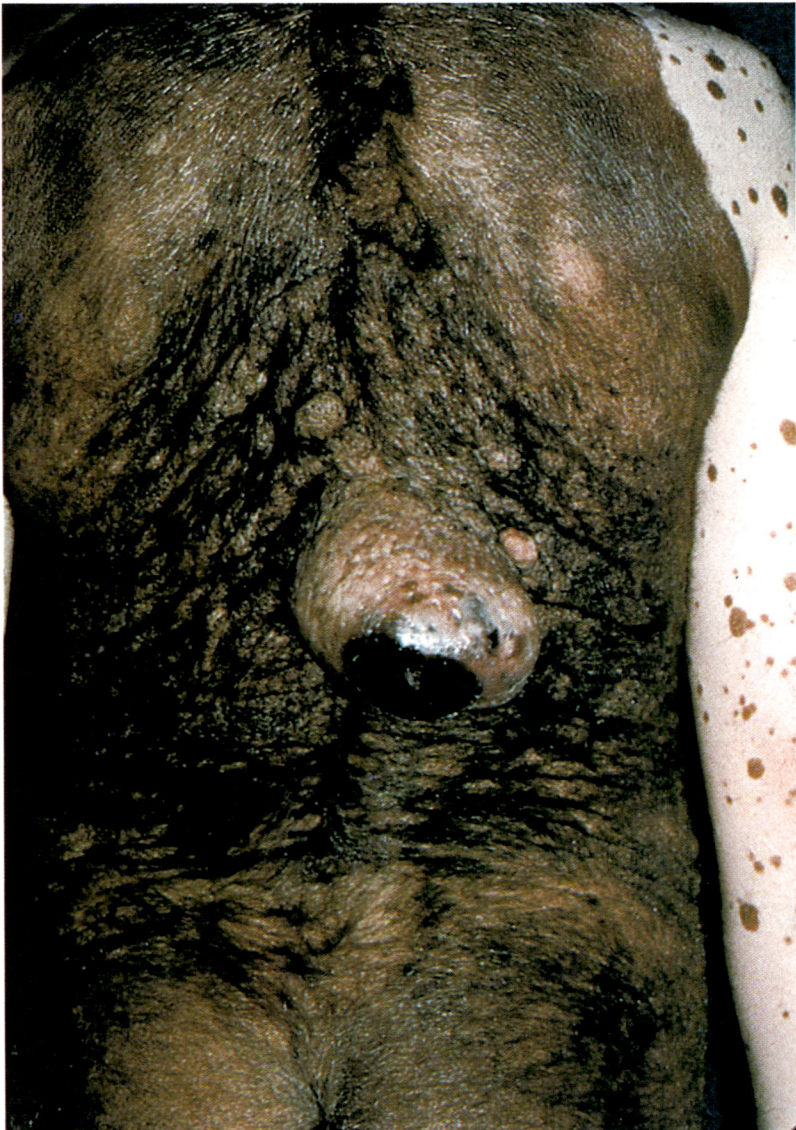

Fig. 5.46 Malignant melanoma in a garment-type, giant congenital nevus.

Patients who have undergone surgical resection of nevus sebaceous in the early years of life require close follow-up until puberty. Extension of nevus sebaceous with skip areas is a commonly described occurrence. If new areas of nevus sebaceous develop after primary surgical resection, these can be approached as an outpatient local procedure in a pre-adolescent.

Larger areas of nevus sebaceous should be excised with the aid of tissue expansion techniques to minimize the spreading of the postoperative scar. For intermediate size nevi, staged excisions can also be beneficial.

CONGENITAL NEVUS

Nevocellular nevi are present at birth in 1% of the population. The risk of development of malignant melanoma in a congenital nevus is unknown, but clearly increased over acquired nevocellular nevi.[474,475] Removal of congenital nevi to prevent malignant deterioration is therefore controversial. Studies are

ongoing to better define the risk of melanoma in these lesions. It appears that the size of the congenital nevus is the most important contributing factor to increased risk (Fig. 5.46). Risk estimations in large congenital nevi (more than 20cm in an adult) have been estimated at 4.6–12%.[476,477] For small congenital nevi, the risk is estimated as 1% or less. Nonetheless, histologic evidence of malignant melanoma occurring in small pre-existing nevi that have features of congenital nevi continue to be reported.[478–480] Intermediate-size nevi are extrapolated to have an intermediate risk, although little data is available looking at this subset of nevi.[474,481] There is some racial variation in the risk of malignant deterioration. Patients of African-American descent with small congenital nevi are believed to have a much lower risk than Caucasian patients. The risk has been estimated at 1 in 20 000 in this population.[482]

474. Kanzler MH, Mraz-Fernhard S (2001) Primary cutaneous malignant melanoma and its precursor lesions: diagnostic and therapeutic overview. **J Am Acad Dermatol** 45(2):260–276.
475. Chamlin SL, Williams ML (1998) Moles and melanoma. **Current Opinion on Pediatrics** 10(4):398–404.
476. Egan CL, Oliveria SA, Elenitsa R et al. (1998) Cutaneous melanoma risk and phenotypic changes in large congenital nevi: a follow up study of 46 patients. **J Am Acad Dermatol** 39(6):923–932.
477. Aron MS, Hurwortz S (1983) Longenital melanocytic nevi. A review of the treatment controversy and report of 46 cases. **Plast Reconstr Surg** 12:355.
478. Mackie RM, Watt D, Doherty V, Aitchison T (1991) Malignant melanoma occurring in those aged under 30 in the west of Scotland 1979–1986: a study of incidence, clinical features, pathological features and survival. **Br J Dermatol** 124(6):560–564.

479. Harley S, Walsh N (1996) A new look at nevus-associated melanomas. **Am J Dermatopathol** 18(2):137–141.
480. Betti R, Inselvini R, Crosti C (2000) Small congenital nevi associated with melanoma: case reports and considerations. **J Dermatol** 27(9):583–590.
481. De Raeve L, Danau W, DeBacker A, Otten J (1993) Prepubertal melanoma in a medium sized congenital naevus. **Eur J Pediatr** 152(9):734–736.
482. Shpall S, Frieden I, Chesney M, Newman T (1994) Risk of malignant transformation of congenital melanocytic in nevi in blacks. **Pediatr Dermatol** 11(3):204–208.

Surgical indications

Many congenital nevi are excised to prevent deterioration into malignancy, although the exact risk is unknown. Congenital nevi are flat at birth, but develop a carpet-like thickness or a cerebriform surface texture with time. In addition, hypertrichosis is common within these. Variation in pigmentation and in nodularity can make observation difficult. The cosmetic appearance of large congenital nevi may also contribute to the decision for removal as well as the appropriate timing of surgical excision when excision is desired.

Most pediatric dermatologists recommend observation of small congenital nevi rather than excision. Exceptions to this include nevi in cosmetically disfiguring areas such as the central face, nevi in locations that are difficult to follow such as the scalp, groin, palms or soles, or nevi that have atypical features that make elective observation difficult and risky. Any small congenital nevus that undergoes a clinical change in color, shape, or nodularity should be evaluated by a pediatric dermatologist. Changes that are concerning for malignancy should precipitate full excision of the nevus when they occur. In the absence of concerning changes all small congenital nevi should be observed at least until puberty. A decision to remove a small congenital nevus for cosmetic or prophylactic reasons at this time will allow for the use of a local anesthetic. The exception to this is lesions on the face where early surgical excision in the first year of life may improve the final appearance of the scar.

For medium-sized congenital nevi, a larger proportion of practicing pediatric dermatologists recommends excision. This relates to a perceived increase in the risk for malignancy as well as an increased concern for the cosmetics of these lesions. Many factors enter into recommendations for excision and the timing of recommended excision of medium-sized congenital nevi. Lesions that are present in areas with minimal skin mobility such as the anterior lower legs or forearms, the palms and soles, and the scalp are generally recommended for early excision in the first year of life. The flexibility of tissue is greatest at this time and excision during the active period of pre-adolescence and adolescence results in poor cosmetic results due to a high level of activity. This also eliminates the need for two-staged procedures in many nevi. The risk of developing a poor scar must be balanced against the risk of developing melanoma in larger nevi.

For large congenital nevi, most practitioners recommend early excision when this is possible. Plastic surgical techniques including partial-thickness skin grafting and tissue expansion have allowed for complete removal of giant congenital nevi in many patients.[483] This requires many procedures and is best approached early in life. The risk of malignancy in giant congenital nevi is greatest in the first five years of life. For nevi that cannot be completely excised, a discussion of partial removal is indicated to improve the cosmesis of these disfiguring lesions. The risks and benefits of undergoing multiple procedures, the scars that ensue, and the appearance with and without treatment should all be considered in decisions to proceed with aggressive intervention in this setting. Families must be informed that failure to fully remove a congenital nevus does not eliminate the risk of malignancy. It is also recommended that children who have extensive scalp nevi or nevi overlying the spinal column have an MRI to look for evidence of neurocutaneous melanosis. The prognosis for patients with this disorder is very poor, and surgery is not recommended in this subset of patients.

The standard of care in the removal of congenital nevi is full-thickness excision. Other treatment modalities that have been employed include dermabrasion,[484] shave excision and curettage, and laser removal.[485–487] All of these treatments remain extremely controversial and are not recommended in giant congenital nevi where the risk of malignancy is significant and the ability to recognize a malignant change may be altered by the partial removal technique. Successful laser removal of small congenital nevi has been reported.[486] Most small nevi treated with lasers undergo partial repigmentation with time.[487]

ACQUIRED NEVI

Acquired nevi occur in all races and typically begin to develop after the age of 18 months. In the Caucasian population, approximately 30 acquired nevi are average. These occur in two peaks: in the preschool years, and in the preadolescent years. More-pigmented races have fewer nevi on average, although the expected number of nevi in an individual is very familial.

The development of acquired nevi on the face is a typical source of referral for the pediatric dermatologic surgeon. As children approach adolescence and become self-conscious, lesions on the face are a common source of concern. It is also usual to see changes in acquired nevi around adolescence. Parents note increase in size, thickness, and often changes in characteristics of nevi at this time. It is important to review the ABCDs of atypical nevi with parents who present for evaluation of acquired nevi in their adolescents and to reassure them that lesions that are growing and raising above the skin are not concerning for malignancy. These changes are part of the benign natural evolution of acquired nevi.

Surgical indications

Cosmetic removal of benign acquired nevi on the face is not recommended in early adolescence unless there is a medical indication to pursue removal.[488] Many adolescents are unhappy with the appearance of their facial nevi. It is important to understand that this degree of concern is transient. Replacing benign acquired nevi with facial scars is not a good choice for most patients unless the scars can be concealed in the melolabial crease or made faintly visible in the preauricular area. Young adolescents may have false expectations of what can be accomplished with plastic surgery. Before proceeding with excision for cosmetic reasons, it is essential that the nature and degree of scarring be demonstrated to the patient and family. Most facial nevi are more noticeable to the adolescent than to others. The scars that result from excision are more noticeable and attract more attention than the nevus itself. It is important to make the adolescent aware of this prior to proceeding with any facial nevus removal for cosmetic reasons. Some small and flat lesions can be removed with pigmented lasers.[489] The larger, more raised lesions do not respond well to laser therapy.

Beyond the age of 16 years, with a reasonable discussion of the outcome of the procedure, cosmetic removal can be approached in adolescents as in the adult population with the higher likelihood of satisfactory outcome.

Although melanoma is an uncommon entity in the pediatric population, any concerning changes within an acquired nevus should be biopsied for diagnosis. Children with atypical nevi should be followed closely due to an increased risk of the development of melanoma.[490]

SPITZ NEVUS

A Spitz nevus, or a spindle and epithelial nevus, is a benign melanocytic tumor that is unique to children and adolescents. Lesions are usually solitary and the face is a common location. Most lesions develop between the ages of 3 and

483. Gosain AK, Santoro TD, Larson DL, Gingrass RP (2001) Giant congenital nevi: a 20-year experience and an algorithm for their management. **Plastic and Reconstr Surgery** 108(3):622–636.

484. Rompel R, Moser M, Petres J (1997) Dermabrasion of congenital nevocellular nevi: experience 215 patients. **Dermatology** 194(3):261–267.

485. Ueda S, Imayama S (1997) Normal-mode ruby laser for treating congenital nevi. **Archives of Dermatology** 133(3):355–359.

486. Grevelink JM, VanLeeuwen RL, Anderson RR, Buyers HR (1997) Clinical and histological responses of congenital melanocytic nevi after a single treatment with Q-switched lasers. **Archives of Dermatology** 133(3)349–353.

487. Waldorf HA, Kauvar AN, Geronemus RG (1996) Treatment of small and medium congenital nevi with the Q-swtiched ruby laser. **Archives of Dermatology** 132(3):301–304.

488. Eichenfield LF, Honig PJ (1991) Difficult diagnostic and management issues in pediatric dermatology. **Pediatr Clin N Am** Jun;38(3):687–710.

489. Morelli JG (1998) Use of lasers in pediatric dermatology. **Dermatol Clin** Jul;16(3):489–495.

490. Williams ML, Sagebiel RS, Soloman AR, Spraker MK (1990) Dysplastic nevi in children. **Pediatr Dermatol** Sep;7(3):218–234.

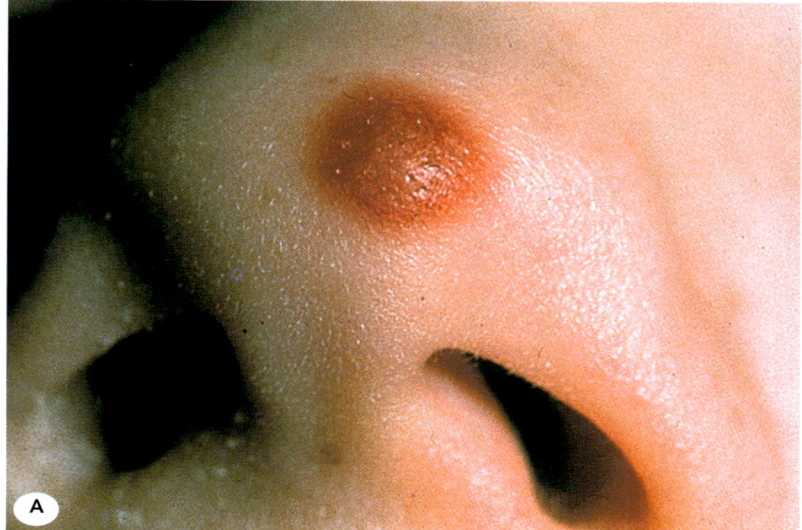

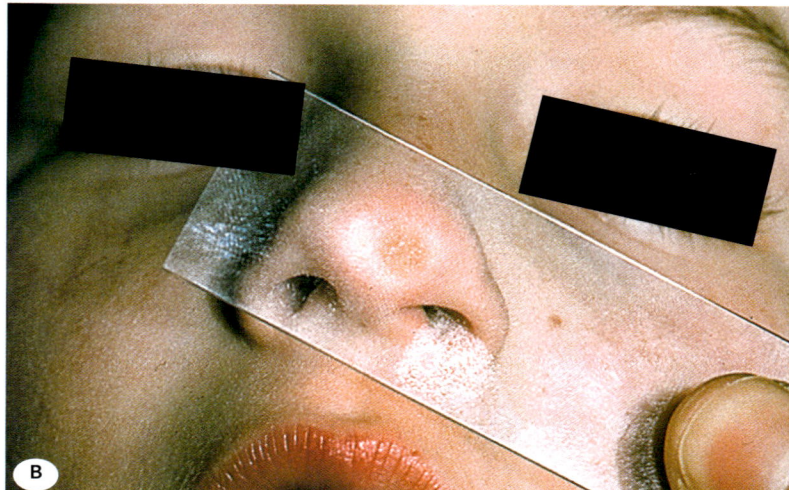

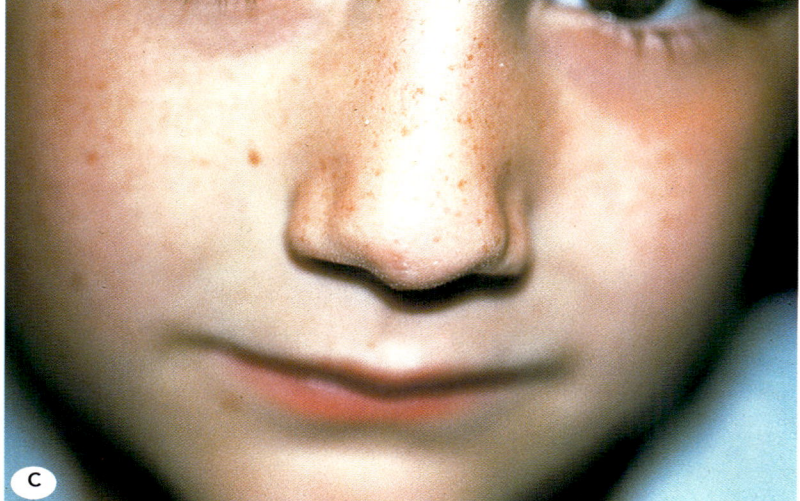

Fig. 5.47 (A) Pre-op appearance of a Spitz nevus on the nose. (B) Vascularity of Spitz nevus is demonstrated using diascopy. (C) Post-op appearance of the scar three months after resection.

13 as solitary reddish-brown or brown-black papules, ranging in size from 5 to 10mm. Spitz nevi grow more rapidly than normal acquired nevi. They can be mistaken for pyogenic granulomas because of their vascular appearance. The rapidity of growth can be concerning for malignant melanoma. The natural history of Spitz nevi is similar to other benign compound nevi. They persist into adult life, becoming intradermal in many cases. Histologically the diagnosis of a Spitz nevus relies heavily on architecture. The nevus cells are spindle shaped and pleomorphic, often with evidence of upward migration into the epidermis. These features can be mistaken for malignant melanoma in the hands of an inexperienced pathologist.[491] In addition, recent authors have defined subsets of Spitz nevi with varying degrees of atypia in an attempt to distinguish those lesions most likely to have malignant potential.[492–494] Although most Spitz nevi are benign, metastasis of Spitz nevi have been reported.[495,496]

Surgical indications

Excision of Spitz nevi is controversial.[497] Undoubtedly the majority of these will remain benign and the malignant risk is low in the pediatric population. Barnhill[493] has recently described a grading system for Spitz nevi in an attempt to identify those lesions at greatest risk for malignant change. Any nevus displaying clinical atypia should be excised to confirm its benign nature. In addition, Spitz nevi tend to occur in cosmetically important areas such as the central face and nose. They frequently grow rapidly to a significant size, typically reaching 8 to 10mm over a six-month period. For this reason, cosmetic removal of Spitz nevi on the face is recommended at the time of diagnosis to minimize scarring and improve appearance (Fig. 5.47). For Spitz nevi in less cosmetically concerning locations such as the trunk or extremities, observation is recommended unless atypical features develop within these lesions. Any change in a Spitz nevus should result in rapid excision.

491. Leboit P (2000) Spitz nevus: a look back and a look ahead. Advances in Dermatology 16:81–109; discussion 110.
492. Spatz A, Calonje E, Handfield-Jones S, Barnhill RL (1999) Spitz tumors in children: a grading system for risk stratification. Arch Dermatol 135(3):2282–2285.
493. Barnhill RL, Argenyi ZB, From L et al. (1999) Atypical Spitz nevi/tumors:lack of consensus for diagnosis, discrimination, discrimination from melanoma and prediction of outcome. Human Pathol 30(5):513–520.
494. Barnhill RL (2000) Malignant melanoma, dysplastic melanocytic nevi, and spitz tumors. Histologic classification and characteristics. Clinics in Plastic Surgery 27(3):331–360.
495. Fabrizi G, Massi G (2001) Spitzoid malignant melanoma in teenagers: an entity with not better prognosis than that of other forms of melanoma. Histopathology 38(5):448–453.
496. Mooi WJ (2001) Histopathology of Spitz naevi and "spitzoid" melanomas. Current Topics in Pathology 94:65–77.
497. Spatz A, Barnhill RL (1999) The spitz tumor 50 years later: revisiting a landmark contribution and unresolved controversy. J Am Acad Dermatol 40(2 Pt 1):223–228.

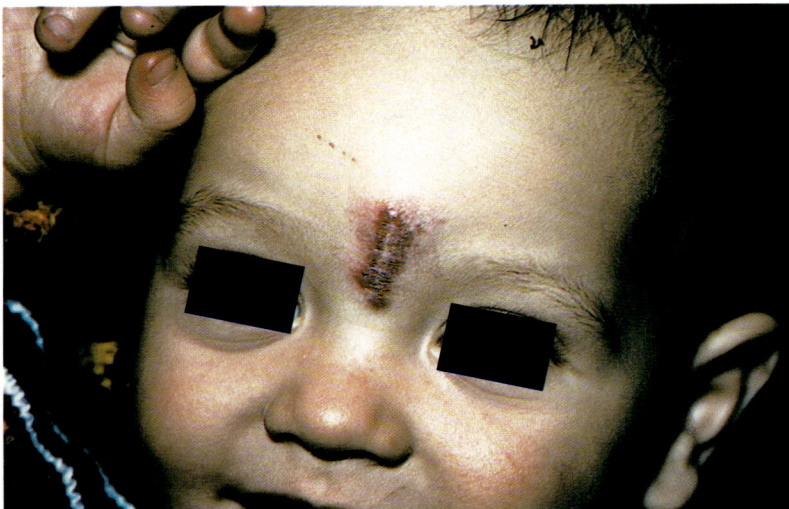

Fig. 5.48 Recurrence of hemangioma after resection at 4 months of age. Note significant glabellar scarring.

The pediatric dermatologic surgeon is often referred patients who have undergone biopsies of their Spitz nevi with incomplete removal. The histologic appearance of a Spitz nevus is often concerning to an inexperienced skin pathologist and many patients are referred for re-excision based on these features. In general, if the majority of the lesion has been removed by punch biopsy, the risk of recurrence with positive surgical margins appears to be low, and a full-thickness excision is not recommended. A conservative full-thickness excision is recommended if the histopathology demonstrates clearly that only a small portion of the nevus has been removed, if the nevus was biopsied using a shave technique, or if significant atypia is identified within the lesion. Residual nevus is removed due to the high likelihood of recurrence and the histologic difficulty of identifying the characteristic architectural features of a Spitz nevi in a recurrent lesion. Often multiple histopathologic opinions must be sought to assist the surgeon in a decision to proceed with a more extensive excision of a Spitz nevus in a cosmetically important area. This is one area in pediatric dermatology where the opinion of an experienced dermatopathologist is critical to prevent unnecessary morbidity in pediatric patients.

HEMANGIOMAS

Hemangiomas are benign vascular proliferative lesions of infancy. They are typically not present at birth, appear at several weeks of life, and enlarge rapidly for four months with slower growth to eight to 12 months. Involution occurs slowly. Half of these are gone by the age of 5. Superficial or strawberry hemangiomas, deep or cavernous hemangiomas, and mixed lesions are all common. Since natural involution for the majority of patients with hemangiomas results in acceptable cosmesis, surgical intervention is not recommended for the majority of these tumors.[498–500]

Surgical indications

The surgical indications for removal and treatment of hemangiomas are controversial. There is no doubt that aggressive surgical intervention early will result in unnecessary scarring for some patients (Fig. 5.48). There are also circumstances, however, under which surgical excision may be preferable to awaiting natural involution to minimize the morbidity of these lesions or to impact functional impairment. Current recommendations for primary excision of hemangiomas are: 1) removal of all functionally impairing hemangiomas that are nonresponsive to medical therapy; 2) removal of tissue redundancy and fibrofatty residual that remains after involution of hemangiomas; 3) removal of ulcerated hemangiomas that are amenable to primary closure and poorly responsive to medical therapy and pulsed dye laser therapy; 4) removal of significant lip and nasal tip hemangiomas that fail to respond to medical therapy; and 5) removal of large and disfiguring hemangiomas in cosmetically important areas to decrease the psychologic morbidity of growing up with these lesions, including non-involuting congenital hemangiomas (controversial) (Table 5.16).

For larger lesions on the face and scalp, where residual tumor and tissue redundancy is assured, it is recommended that excision be accomplished in the preschool years, optimally between the ages of 4 and 5.[501,502] Finn et al. demonstrated in a retrospective review that only 50% of hemangiomas completely involuted by 6 years of age.[503] Of the remaining 50% that did not involute, 80% left a substantial residual cosmetic deformity. Of the 50% that were completely involuted by age 6 years, 38% left a substantial cosmetic residual. These statistics have led to a more aggressive surgical approach by some physicians who advocate surgical excision in the second year of life, or even during the proliferative phase.[501,504,505] Delaying excision until age 4 to 7 allows the surgeon to take advantage of the benefit of natural involution. Intervention is critical before age 7, since children suffer severe psychosocial trauma once they reach the developmental stage where they identify body image and distinguish differences between themselves and others.[506] Preschoolers are curious; first-graders are mean. Resection before age 7 allows for as much natural involution as possible and minimizes the extent of the surgical procedure that is undertaken. Care should be taken to resect only the abnormal skin in early resection. Staged excision with pursed string closure can markedly decrease the size of the final scar (Fig. 5.49). Laser treatment can be used as an adjunct to surgical excision after debulking of large tumors to improve the cosmetic appearance.[501,507,508]

For tumors on the trunk and extremities that are asymptomatic, postponement of resection until the age of 7 to 10 years, when this can be accomplished as a local procedure without the need for a general anesthetic, is recommended. Early excision of hemangiomas in the rapid proliferative phase of the first year of life can result in partial resection and recurrence. The best surgical results are obtained when the proliferative phase has ended and the tumors have entered involution. Excision is not recommended for small superficial hemangiomas on the face or scalp where early intervention will result in unnecessary scarring. Three important exceptions to this are significant lip hemangiomas, nasal tip hemangiomas and non-involuting congenital hemangiomas (NICH). Rapidly enlarging hemangiomas of the

---

TABLE 5.16 **Indications for surgical excision of hemangiomas**

Functionally impairing lesion nonresponsive to medical therapy
Postinvolution fibrofatty tissue or tissue redundancy
Ulcerated hemangiomas nonresponsive to medical or laser therapy
Significant lip or nasal tip hemangiomas nonresponsive to medical therapy
Large disfiguring hemangiomas (controversial)

498. Bowers RE, Graham EA, Tomlinson KM (1960) The natural history of the strawberry nevus. **Arch Dermatol** 59–71.
499. Wallace HJ (1953) The conservative treatment of hamangiomatous nevi. **Br J Plast Surg** 6:78–82.
500. Rogers M (2000) Treatment of "angiomas": a modern commentary. **Australas J Dermatol** Nov;41 Suppl S89–91.
501. Wiliams EF 3rd, Stanislaw P, Dupree M et al. (2000) Hemangiomas in infants and children. An algorithm. **Arch Facial Plast Surg** 2(2):103–111.
502. Demiri EC, Pelissier P, Genin-Etcheberry T et al. (2001) Treatment of facial hemangiomas: the present status of surgery. **Br J Plast Surg** 54(8):665–674.
503. Finn MC, Glowacki J, Mullikan JB (1983) Congenital vascular lesions: clinical application of a new classification. **J Pediatr Surg** 18:894–900.

504. Waner M, Suen JY, Dinehart S (1992) Treatment of hemangiomas of the head and neck. **Laryngoscope** 102(10):1123–1132.
505. Waner M, Suen JY (1995) Management of congenital vascular lesions of the head and neck. **Oncology** 9(10):989–994, 997.
506. Tanner JL, Dechert MP, Frieden IJ (1998) Growing up with a facial hemangioma: parent and child coping and adaptation. **Pediatrics** 101:446–452.
507. Poetke M, Philipp C, Berlien HP (2000) Flashlamp-pumped pulsed dye laser for hemangiomas in infancy. **Arch Dermatol** 136:628–632.
508. Hohenleutner S, Badur-Ganter E, Lanthaler M (2001) Long-term results I the treatment of childhood hemangioma with the flashlamp-pumped pulse dye laser: and evaluation of 617 cases. **Laser Surg Med** 28:273–277.

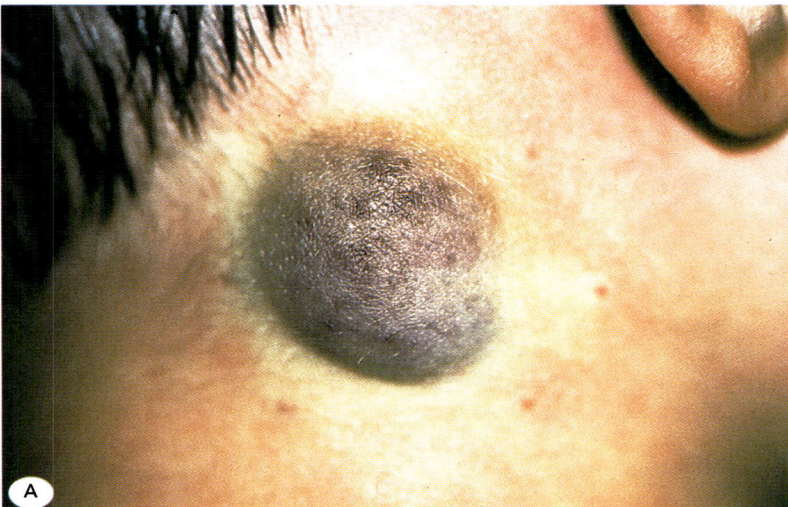

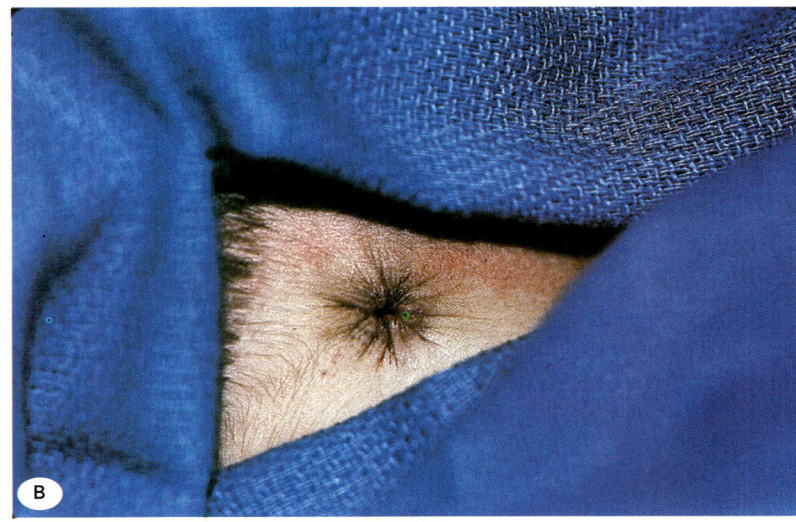

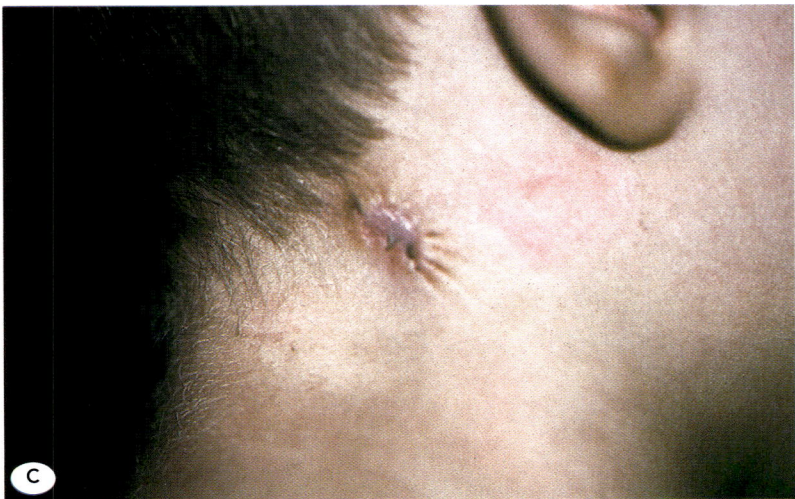

Fig. 5.49 (A) Appearance of a hemangioma in a 7-year-old boy. (B) Purse-string closure. (C) Scar one month after surgery demonstrating reduced scar length possible with this stage closure. Final scar will be formed by second stage fusiform closure at 3–6 months after first surgery.

early proliferative phase of hemangioma growth.[508,514] Although cosmetic improvement in the superficial component of hemangiomas can be accomplished with pulsed dye laser, this laser does not impact the development of the deeper component of the hemangioma or the natural history of these lesions, which is one of spontaneous involution. It remains unclear whether superficial hemangiomas treated with pulsed dye laser aggressively in the first year of life have a final outcome that is superior to what is expected from observation alone. Most superficial hemangiomas have undergone involution by the age of 5 and therefore the psychologic effects of attending school with these are minimal. The parents should be informed of the limited benefit of laser treatment for these lesions.

For deep hemangiomas in functionally impairing locations that are poorly responsive to medical therapy, there have been recent reports of the use of bare-fiber laser to reduce the size of lesions. Ultrasound or MR-guided interstitial Nd:YAG or KTP laser therapy has been undertaken.[515–517] Laser energy is applied directly to the deep hemangioma tissue using a bare fiber inserted through a cannula or catheter. With these treatments, a reduction in the size of large hemangiomas of 50 to 90% is seen over three to nine months with a 20% risk of scarring. Laser intervention can be used as the primary treatment or to facilitate rapid reduction in size, allowing surgical resection in an otherwise inoperable severe hemangioma. Further investigation into the efficacy of these techniques is needed.

PYOGENIC GRANULOMAS

Pyogenic granulomas are benign acquired vascular lesions that are common in childhood. The majority occurs between the ages of 1 and 4 on the face and neck. The etiology is unknown, but trauma may play a role. Most lesions begin as small vascular papules that rapidly enlarge to 5 to 8mm over a several-week period. They are usually solitary and often pedunculated with a dis-

lip and nasal tip can have devastating cosmetic outcomes if not approached early.[509,510] Medical intervention is always the recommended first-line approach. Frequently, however, multiple surgical procedures are needed to reduce the deformity of hemangiomas in these locations. Early surgical intervention, within the first year of life, may be indicated. For NICH, early surgical resection will yield the best outcome.[511]

In addition to primary excision, hemangiomas can be approached with the pulsed dye laser. The indications for the use of pulsed dye laser in the treatment of hemangiomas is limited to effecting more rapid healing of ulcerated hemangiomas that are poorly responsive to good topical wound care.[512,513] The pulsed dye laser can diminish the pain in these ulcerated hemangiomas and decrease the risk of infection by facilitating earlier healing. The pulsed dye laser is ineffective in treatment of hemangiomas with a deep component. Treatment of superficial hemangiomas results in early involution in the superficial layers of the skin.[507,508] Multiple treatments are required. There is a higher risk of scarring in pulsed dye laser treatment during the

509. McCarthy JG, Borud LJ, Schreiber JS (2002) Hemangiomas of the nasal tip. **Plat Reconstr Surg** 109(1):31–40.
510. Warren SM, Longaker MT, Zibe BM (2002) The subunit approach to nasal tip hemangiomas. **Plast Reconstr Surg** 109(1):25–30.
511. North PE, Waner M, James CA et al. (2001) Congenital nonprogressive hemangioma: a distinct clinicopathologic entity unlike infantile hemangioma. **Arch Dermatol** 137(12):1607–1620.
512. Kim HJ, Colomo M, Frieden IJ (2001) Ulcerated hemangiomas: clinical characteristics and response to therapy. **J Amer Acad Dermatol** 44:962–972.
513. Morelli JG, Tan OT, Yohn JJ (1994) Treatment of ulcerated hemangiomas in infancy. **Arch Pediatr Adolesc Med** 148:1104–1105.

514. Garden JM, Bakus AS, Paller AS (1992) Treatment of cutaneous hemangiomas by the flashlamp-pumped pulse dye laser: prospective analysis. **J Pediatr** 120:555–560.
515. Werner JA, Lippert BM, Gottschlich S (1998) Ultrasound-guided interstitial Nd;YAG laser treatment of voluminous hemangiomas and vascular malformations in 92 patients. **Laryngoscope** 108:463–470.
516. Achauer BM, Celikoz B, VanderKam VM (1998) Intralesional bare fiber laser treatment of hemangioma of infancy. **Plast Reconstr Surg** 5:1212–1217.
517. Burstein FD, Simms C, Cohen SR (2000) Intralesional laser therapy of extensive hemangiomas in 100 consecutive pediatric patients. **Ann Plast Surg** 44:188–194.

cernable rim of scale or epidermal collarette. The surface becomes superficially crusted and bleeds easily. Left untreated, they continue to enlarge slowly and are likely to ulcerate and bleed. Spontaneous involution has been reported.[518]

Surgical indications

Most pyogenic granulomas cause considerable morbidity due to repeated episodes of bleeding and crusting. Infection can also occur. In addition, since the majority of these are located on the face and neck, they are a considerable cosmetic issue. Surgical removal is therefore recommended for all symptomatic pyogenic granulomas. If lesions are smaller than 6mm and relatively flat (less than 3mm in thickness), pyogenic granulomas can be effectively treated with the pulsed dye laser.[519–521] Multiple treatments are required, but provide the benefit of a nonscarring treatment alternative.

For lesions that are larger, thicker, or pedunculated, pulsed dye laser is ineffective. Treatment options include electrodesiccation with curettage, primary excision with two-layered closure, shave excision and laser photocoagulation of the base,[522] and combined continuous-wave/pulsed carbon dioxide laser.[523] When the base of the pyogenic granuloma is 8mm or less, electrodesiccation and curettage, or carbon dioxide laser therapy are the preferred procedures. A small scar results and recurrence is uncommon. For larger lesions, electrodesiccation results in an unfavorable cosmetic outcome. Here, carbon dioxide laser[523] or primary excision with two-layered closure is recommended. Recurrence and the development of satellite lesions of pyogenic granuloma have been described in the literature.[524,525] These are rare events and should not deter surgical treatment of these lesions. Electrodesiccation, cryotherapy and shave removal without curettage or electrodesiccation have all been attempted and result in higher rates of recurrence. These techniques are therefore not recommended.

VASCULAR MALFORMATIONS

Vascular malformations are aberrant vascular channels present in the skin that typically present early in life. Unlike hemangiomas, these are nonproliferative lesions. They are malformations of lymphatic and blood vessels within the skin. Small vascular malformations tend to be asymptomatic and to present minimal cosmetic problems. Larger malformations may require intervention with sclerotherapy for recurrent thrombotic or infectious episodes. Malformations that contain a large percentage of lymphatic channels can result in swelling and leakage of lymphatic and vascular fluid through blebs in the skin surface. Vascular malformations on the extremities are associated with the Klippel–Trenaunay syndrome with overgrowth. Most malformations are not amenable to surgical resection due to their extent and the high risk of recurrence with partial excision.

Surgical indications

There are two subsets of vascular malformations that commonly present to the dermatologic surgeon for evaluation and consideration of excision. One is an angiokeratoma and the second is lymphangioma circumscriptum. These are more localized malformations that become keratotic on the skin surface.

Smaller lesions that are less than 5cm can often be primarily excised to improve the cosmetic appearance and decrease leakage and crusting on the skin surface.[526] The larger the lesion, the more likely that the surrounding skin is also affected with the vascular defect and the higher likelihood of recurrence. Many of these lesions overly deep malformations that extend to subcutaneous tissue and muscle.[527,528] Excision of localized lesions can usually be accomplished in the 7–10-year-old range with a local anesthetic unless repeated episodes of pain or infection occur earlier in life to precipitate removal at an earlier age. Occasionally, pulsed dye laser can be helpful when superficial lesions are more vascular.[529]

Larger vascular and lymphatic malformations may require surgical intervention that is beyond the scope of the pediatric dermatologist. These lesions are difficult to fully excise and recurrence is common. Where possible, less aggressive intervention with sclerotherapy is usually recommended.[530,531] Partial resection of symptomatic areas may also be helpful. Percutaneous and bare-fibre neodymium:YAG laser have also been used with some success.[532] Compression garments or pneumatic pumps are the mainstay of therapy for these lesions. Small dilated areas (blebs) on the skin surface that bleed and leak serosanguinous or lymphatic fluid are amenable to treatment with pulsed dye laser. Although symptoms improve, new lesions usually develop with time, especially on the lower extremities.

EPIDERMAL NEVUS

Epidermal nevi are hamartomas of cutaneous elements. The majority is present at birth, although some extension can be seen up to the years of puberty. Many lesions follow the lines of Blaschko and are believed to arise as a result of mosaicism.[533] Extensive variants of this have been observed. Most epidermal nevi are solitary and small. They do not require treatment unless they are in cosmetically important areas. Malignant change in these lesions is extremely rare.[534]

Surgical indications

Most epidermal nevi are treated to improve the cosmesis of the lesion. The natural history of an epidermal nevus is one of thickening and progressive hyperkeratosis that is most marked around puberty. This can be particularly problematic in nevi located along the neck or in the axilla.

Excision of epidermal nevi on the face and scalp that are more than 1cm in size is usually recommended early in life. Clinical confusion with nevus sebaceous, which has malignant potential, can occur in these locations due to the larger number of sebaceous glands that are present within the skin. In addition, scarring in these locations is best when surgical excision is accomplished in the first year of life. For smaller lesions, approach at age 7–10 under a local anesthetic is reasonable. Larger areas of epidermal nevus on the extremities causing morbidity can also be approached surgically. The risks and benefits of these procedures must be discussed at some length with the family prior to excision. It is difficult to remove the entire nevus in many patients with extensive disease. Localized excision results in spread scars and scar hypertrophy around joints, which are the areas most problematic in adolescents.

518. Requena L, Sangueza OP (1997) Cutaneous vascular proliferation. Part II Hyperplasias and benign neoplasms. **J Am Acad Dermatol** 37(6):887–919;920–922.
519. Morelli JG (1998) Use of lasers in pediatric dermatology. **Dermatol Clin** 16(3):489–495.
520. Tay KY, Weston WL, Morelli JG (1997) Treatment of pyogenic granuloma in children with the flashlamp-pumped pulsed dye laser. **Pediatrics** 99(3):368–370.
521. Gonzalez S, Vibhagool C, Falo LD Jr et al. (1996) Treatment of pyogenic granulomas with the 585nm pulsed dye laser. **J Am Acad Dermatol** 35(3pt1):428–431.
522. Kirschner RE, Low DW (1999) Treatment of pyogenic granuloma by shave excision and laser photocoagulation. **Plast Reconst Surg** 104(5):12346–12349.
523. Raulin C, Greve B, Hammes S (2002) The combined continuous-wave/pulsed carbon dioxide laser for treatment of pyogenic granuloma. **Arch Dermatol** 138(1):33–37.
524. DeAloe G, Rubengni P, Pacenti L et al. (2001) Human herpesvirus type 8 is not associated with pyogenic granulomas with satellite recurrence. **Br J Dermatol** 144(1):202–203.
525. Blickenstaff RD, Roenigk RK, Peters MS, Goellner JR (1989) Recurrent pyogenic granuloma with satellitosis. **J Am Acad Dermatol** 21(6):1241–1244.
526. Wentscher U, Happle R (2000) Linear verrucous hemangioma. **J Am Acad Dermatol** 42(3):516–518.

527. Kraus MD, Lind AC, Adler SL, Dehner LP (1999) Angiomatosis with angiokeratoma-like features in children: a light microscopic and immunophenotypic examination of four cases. **Am J Dermatopathol** 21(4):350–355.
528. Latifoglu O, Yavuzer R, Demir Y et al. (1999) Surgical management of penoscrotal lymphangioma circumscriptum. **Plast Reconstr Surg** 103(1):175–178.
529. Lai CH, Hanson SG, Mallory SB (2001) Lymphangioma circumscriptum treated with pulsed dye laser. **Pediatric Dermatol** 18(6):509–510.
530. Lee BB, Kim Di, Hutt S et al. (2001) New experiences with absolute ethanol sclerotherapy in the management of a complex form of congenital venous formation. **J Vasc Surg** 33:764–772.
531. Lewin JS, Merkle EM, Duert JL, Tarr RW (1999) Low-flow vascular malformation in the head and neck: safety and feasibility of MR imaging-guided percutaneous sclerotherapy—preliminary experience with 14 procedures in three patients. **Radiology** 211:566–570.
532. Wimmershoff MB, Lanthaler M, Hohenleutner U (1999) Percutaneous and combined percutaneous and intralesional Nd:YAG-laser therapy for vascular malformations. **Acta Dermato-Venereologica** 79:71.
533. Happle R (1995) Epidermal nevus syndromes. **Semin Dermatol** 14(2):111–121.
534. Ichikawa T, Saiki M, Kaneko M, Saida T (1996) Squamous cell carcinoma arising in a verrucous epidermal nevus. **Dermatology** 193(2):135–138.

Multiple alternative destructive and surgical techniques have been used in the treatment of these lesions, including pulsed carbon dioxide laser,[535,536] ruby laser,[537] dermabrasion, partial thickness excision, and some chemical peeling.[538] Recurrence is frequent with most of these modalities.

A subset of patients has a form of epidermal nevus termed the ILVEN or inflamed linear verrucous epidermal nevus (Fig. 5.50). This nevus is characterized by extreme pruritus and inflammation, and these symptoms can be intractable and poorly responsive to medical therapy.[539] Topical and intralesional steroids can provide temporary relief, but excision is often necessary since these lesions respond incompletely to these therapies.[540] The pulsed dye laser has been effective in diminishing pruritis, but these symptoms usually recur.[541] The timing of surgical excision for ILVEN should be determined by the degree of symptoms that are present. Excision is not recommended unless topical therapies are ineffective.

APLASIA CUTIS

Aplasia cutis is a congenital defect that results in a localized absence of skin. All components of the skin can be involved including the epidermis, dermis, and sometimes subcutaneous tissues as well as an underlying bony defect. Lesions are quite typical on the scalp but can occur anywhere on the trunk or extremities. Most lesions are solitary and small. The occiput is the most common location. The cause of this defect is unknown. At birth, lesions are often ulcerated or eroded with a punched-out appearance. The overlying skin heals as an atrophic membrane-like scar, although hypertrophic scars can also occur (Fig. 5.51). Many malformation syndromes and chromosomal defects have been reported in association with aplasia cutis.[542] For the majority of patients, however, this is a cosmetic issue only.

Surgical indications

Aplasia cutis heals as a scar and when present on the scalp results in a localized area of alopecia. This is the most common reason for resection of aplasia cutis. Removal of the area of aplasia cutis essentially replaces one scar with another and it is important to notify the parents that there will be an area of alopecia postoperatively from this procedure. The location of the area of aplasia cutis and its size are very important in the surgical approach and the timing of surgical resection. For lesions that are smaller than 1cm on the scalp, resection in the pre-adolescent years if alopecia is cosmetically apparent is very reasonable. For lesions larger than 1cm or lesions located on the vertex of the scalp, especially those with a surrounding hair whorl, earlier resection is important to minimize the postoperative scarring. Flap procedures such as O-to-Zs can be helpful in redirecting the hair growth around the vertex of the scalp to minimize the postoperative alopecia and improve the cosmetic appearance post-resection. Any patient with a marked hair whorl or "hair collar sign" should undergo MRI imaging to look for an underlying developmental anomaly of the brain to rule out the possibility of an encephalocele. Large irregular and stellate scalp defects can also occur with aplasia cutis, most commonly along the midline of the scalp. These larger lesions are more typically accompanied by bony defects, some of which may require replacement of the bony table. Here, serial tissue expansion with skin flaps can be used to minimize spreading of the scar with surgical excision.[543] Aplasia cutis has no malignant potential.

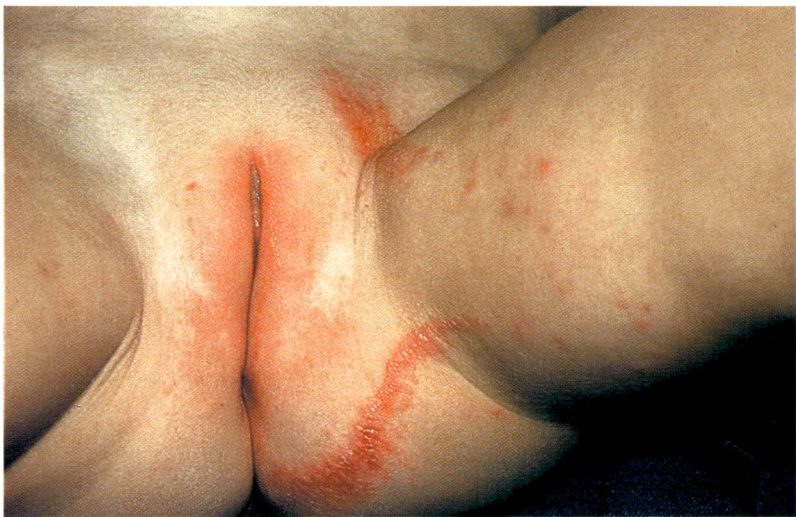

Fig. 5.50   Inflamed linear verrucous epidermal nevus.

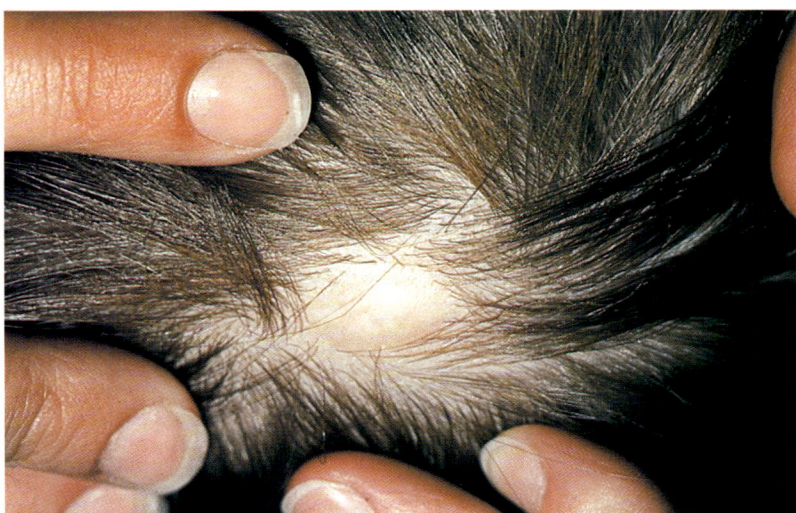

Fig. 5.51   Aplasia cutis healed with a hypertrophic scar.

DERMOID CYSTS

Dermoid cysts are ectodermal growths that occur at the site of closure of embryonic clefts. Most are manifest at birth and 70% are visible by the age of 5. They are usually soft, round, and rubbery subcutaneous tumors between 1 and 4cm. They are normally fully moveable. Sometimes there is a sinus

535. Alam M, Arndt KA (2002) A method for pulsed carbon dioxide laser treatment of epidermal nevi. **J Am Acad Dermatol** 46(4):554–556.
536. Michel JL, Has C, Has V (2001) Resurfacing CO₂ laser treatment of linear verrucous epidermal nevus. **Eur J Dermatol** 11:436.
537. Baba T, Narumi H, Hashimoto I (1995) Successful treatment of dark-colored epidermal nevus with ruby aser. **J Dermatol** 22(8):567–570.
538. Bazex J, el Sayed F, Sans B et al. (1995) Shave excision and phenol peeling of generalized verrucous epidermal nevus. **Dermatol Surg** 21:719–722.
539. Kim JJ, Chang MW, Shwayder T (2000) Topical tretinoin and 5-fluorouracil in the treatment of linear verrucous epidermal nevus. **J Am Acad Dermatol** 43(1pt1):129–132.
540. Lee BJ, Mancini AJ, Renucci J et al. (2001) Full-thickness surgical excision for the treatment of inflammatory linear verrucous epidermal nevus. **Ann Plast Surg** 47:285.
541. Alster TS (1994) Inflammatory linear verrucous epidermal nevus: successful treatment with the 585nm flashlamp-pumped pulse dye laser. **J Am Acad Dermatol** 31(3pt1):513–514.
542. Frieden IJ (1986) Aplasia cutis congenital: a clinical review and proposal for classification. **J Am Acad Dermatol** 14(4):646–660.
543. Kruk-Jeromin J, Janik J, Rykala J (1998) Aplasia cutis congenital of the scalp. Report of 16 cases. **Dermatologic Surgery** 24(5):549–553.

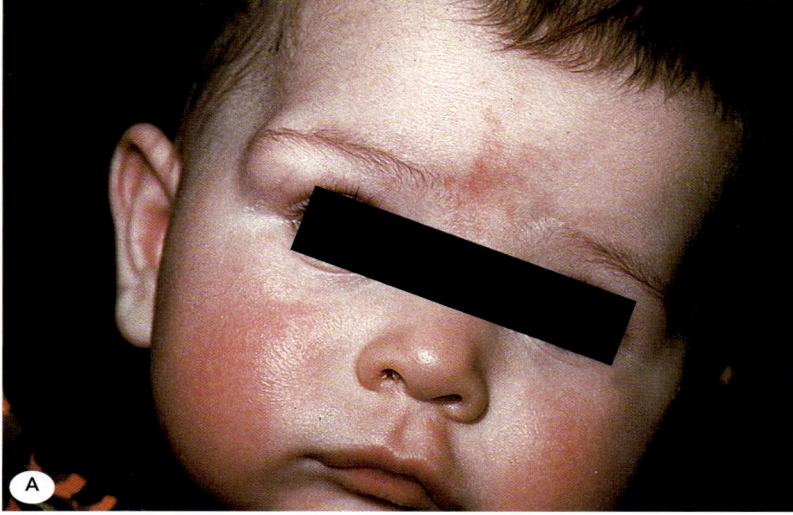

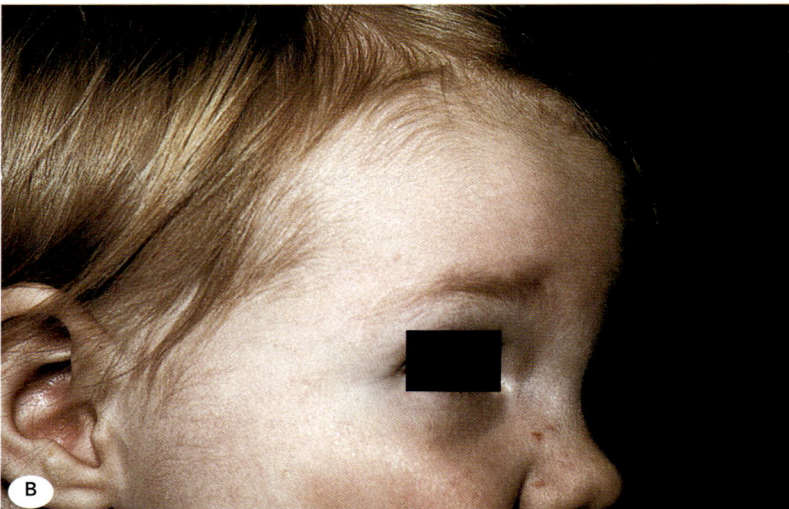

Fig. 5.52   (A) Lateral eyebrow dermoid cyst. (B) Postoperative appearance of scar place above the brow.

opening from which hairs may project.[544] The majority of cysts are located on the temporal forehead at the lateral eyebrow or lateral canthus,[545] with a predilection for the last third of the eyebrow and the midline nasal bridge (Fig. 5.52). They can also occur on the anterior lateral neck, the sternum, scrotum, perineal raphe, sacral area, and the postauricular area.[546]

Surgical indications

Up to 45% of dermoid cysts are associated with intracranial connections. This is most common when a sinus pit is present. All midline facial lesions should be evaluated with MRI or axial CT prior to excision.[547] The midline lesion that has an intracranial connection should be surgically excised to avoid the risk of local or ascending infection. This should be accomplished in the hands of an experienced pediatric otolaryngologist, a neurosurgeon, or a plastic surgeon. An external rhinoplasty approach can be used to improve the cosmetic approach by avoiding the standard vertical midline scar.

The more common dermoid cysts, located at the lateral eyebrow, rarely have intracranial connections.[548,549] Imaging is not routinely performed in this location unless the presentation or clinical appearance is unusual. Excision of these lesions can usually be accomplished at any age. If the lesions are more than 1cm in size and visible in the first several years of life, a general anesthetic at this time will minimize the final scar. For lesions that are invisible or barely visible, waiting until the age of 7 to 10 to approach these surgically is recommended. At that time a local anesthetic can be used. Most lateral brow dermoid cysts are removed through a primary incision. When dermoid cysts are located inferior and lateral to the eyebrow, or within the brow itself, it is sometimes possible, in the hands of an experienced plastic surgeon, to remove these without a cutaneous scar. Such an approach requires skill and experience to avoid injury to the ocular muscles. The subtarsal approach is important to avoid placing the scar line in the eyebrow itself. Endoscopic excision through a small incision at the hairline of the scalp has also been successful but has an increased risk of nerve injury for periorbital lesions.[550] Placement of the incisional line immediately above or below the brow is optimal for cutaneous approaches. The scar does not grow hair, and eyebrow scars are very visible.

PILOMATRICOMA

A pilomatricoma or calcifying epithelioma of Malherbe is a benign calcified tumor of hair matrix origin that most commonly occurs on the face of a child.[551,552] The cause of these is unknown, but tumors may develop due to mutations in beta-catenin/LEF genes.[553] This tumor accounts for 15% of all

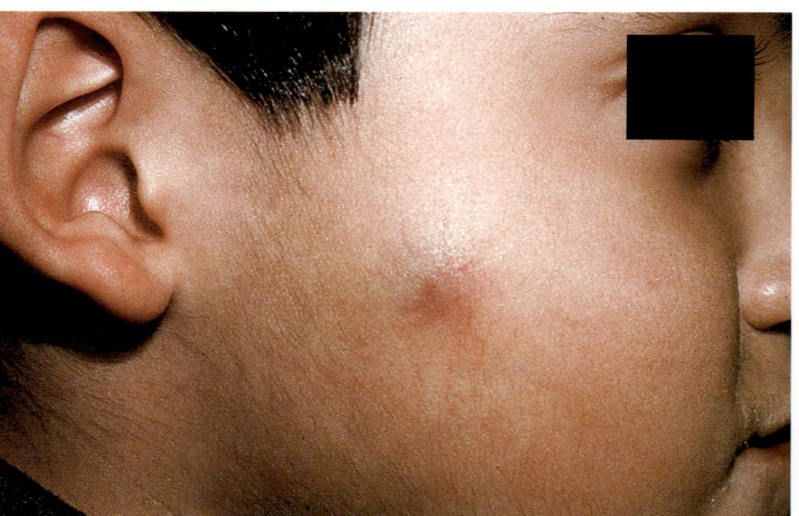

Fig. 5.53   Pilomatricoma of the cheek demonstrating overlying telangiectasia and bluish skin discoloration.

544. Fitzpatrick E, Miller RH (1996) Congenital midline nasal masses: dermoids, gliomas, and encephaloceles. Jour Louisiana State Med Soc 148(3):93–96.
545. Chawda SJ, Moseley IF (1999) Computed tomography of orbital dermoids: a 20-year review. Clinical Radiology 54(12):821–825.
546. Rosen D, Wirtschafter A, Rao VM, Wilcox TO Jr (1998) Dermoid cyst of the lateral neck: a case report and literature review. Ear, Nose, & Throat Journal 77(2):125, 129–132.
547. Paller AS, Pensler JM, Tomita T (1991) Nasal midline masses in infants and children. Arch Dermatol 127:362.
548. Niederhagan B, Reich RH, Zentner J (1998) Temporal dermoid with intracranial extension: report of a case. Journal of Oral & Maxillofacial Surgery 56(11):1352–1354.

549. Hong SW (1998) Deep frontotemporal dermoid cyst presenting as a discharging sinus: a case report and review of literature. Br J Plast Surg 51(3):255–257.
551. Yencha MW (2001) Head and neck pilomatricoma in the pediatric age group: a retrospective study and literature review. Internat J Pediatric Otorhinolaryngology 57(2):123–128.
552. Julian CG, Bowers PW (1998) A clinical review of 209 pilomatricomas. J Am Acad Dermatol 39:191–195.
553. Chan EF, Gat U, McNiff JM, Fuchs E (1999) A common human skin tumour is caused by activating mutations in beta-catenin. Nat Genet 21(4):410–413.

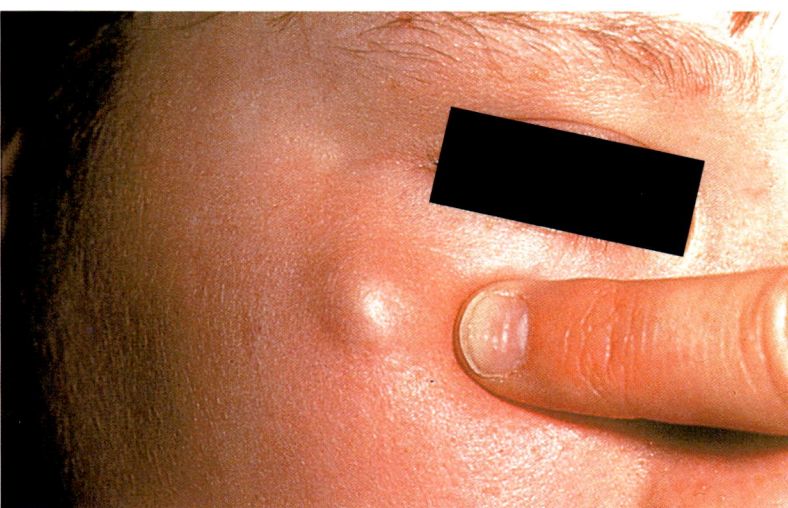

Fig. 5.54 Pilomatricoma of the cheek with plate-like calcification.

Surgical indications

The natural history of pilomatricomas is one of slow enlargement over months. Surgical intervention is recommended as soon as possible in locations where the development of this lesion will be of cosmetic importance.[551] There are rare reports of malignancy in pilomatricoma.[556,557] Lesions undergoing this change would be expected to display rapid and atypical growth patterns. Surgical excision is the only available treatment and is performed for cosmetic improvement. Lesions can be easily dissected through a small cutaneous incision. If the overlying skin is affected with telangiectasias, a larger excision with a small ellipse may be preferable. Pulsed dye laser can be used to treat the telangiectasias in the postoperative period if they are persistent. Occasionally, lesions are firmly adherent to the overlying epidermis resulting in anetodermatous changes. These lesions are also better treated with excision of the overlying skin rather than incision and dissection.

Smaller lesions on the body or subcutaneous lesions on the face that are not visible or symptomatic can be observed. Surgical removal is recommended when lesions become visible, tender, when there is perforation or drainage, or for rapid enlargement. After removal, the subcutaneous fat should be lavaged with saline to prevent leaving behind any small, calcified areas, especially if the tumor is not removed intact. These can result in poor wound healing with foreign body reaction and inflammation in the postoperative period. Recurrence is rare and recurrent lesions should be re-excised to rule out malignancy.

the cutaneous nodules in childhood and has a slight female preponderance. Most cases are sporadic, although familial occurrence has been reported[554] and an association with multiple polyposis syndrome has recently been noted.[555] Pilomatricomas typically arise as subcutaneous, firm, slow-growing papules on the head or neck. They are usually solitary and the overlying epidermis moves freely. Most are less than 1cm in size. As lesions grow, it is typical to see telangiectasias and a bluish hue to the overlying skin (Fig. 5.53). The calcification results in a rock-hard firmness on palpation (Fig. 5.54) Occasionally, lesions perforate and drain a chalky calcium-containing material. Inflammation is less common in pilomatricomas than in epidermoid cysts. Because of the calcification, spontaneous regression of these lesions is not seen.

GIANT JUVENILE XANTHOGRANULOMAS

Juvenile xanthogranuloma is the most common non-Langerhans cell histiocytosis of childhood. These are benign tumors. They commonly appear in infancy and undergo involution in the early childhood years.[558,559] There is a low risk of intraoccular xanthogranuloma[559] and systemic forms.[560] Excision of these is not recommended since spontaneous involution occurs and rarely leaves behind any significant cutaneous defect.

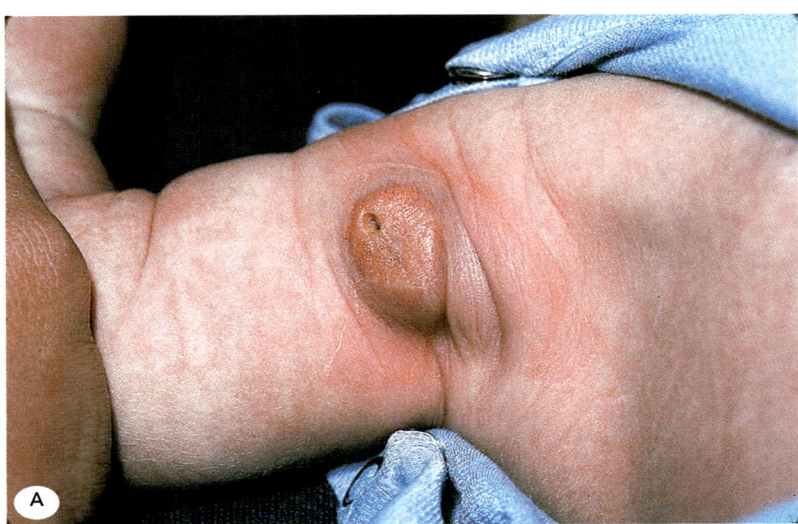

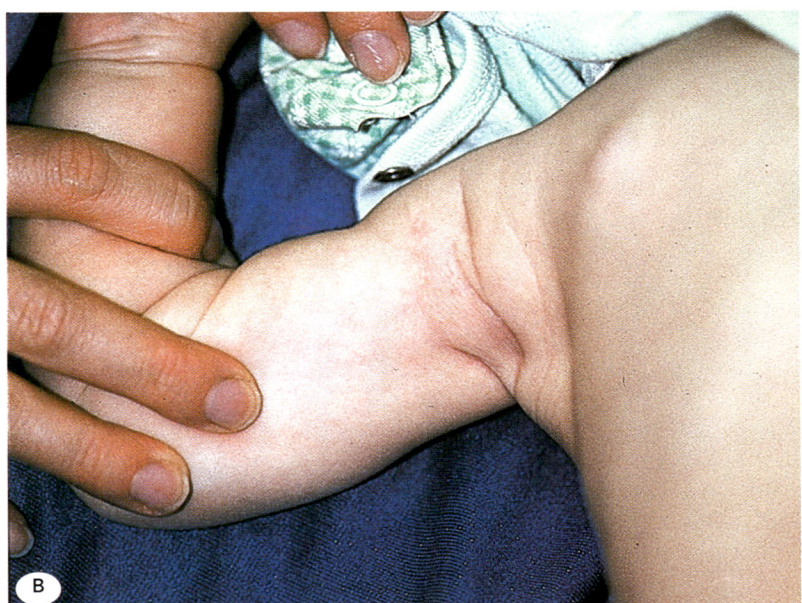

Fig. 5.55 (A) Giant juvenile xanthogranuloma of the axilla in a 4-month-old infant. (B) Postoperative appearance after resection of lesion at six months.

554. Dermircan M, Balik E (1997) Pilomatricoma in children: a prospective study. **Ped Derm** 14(6):430–432.

555. Pujol RM, Casanova JM, Egido R et al. (1995) Multiple familial pilomatricomas: a cutaneous marker for Gardner syndrome? **Pediatr Dermatol** 12(4):331–335.

556. DeGalvez-Aranda MV, Herrera-Ceballos E, Sanchez-Sanchez P et al. (2002) Pilomatrix carcinoma with lymph node and pulmonary metasis: report of a case arising on the knee. **Am J Dermatopathol** 24(2):139–143.

557. Hardisson D, Linares MD, Cuevas-Santos J, Contreras F (2001) Pilomatrix carcinoma: a clinicopathologic study of six cases and review of the literature. **Am J Dermatopathol** 23(5):304–401.

558. Henandez-Martin A, Baselga E, Drolet BA, Esterly NB (1997) Juvenile xanthogranuloma. **J Am Acad Dermatol** 36(3 Pt 1):355–367; quiz 368–369.

559. Chang MW, Frieden IJ, Good W (1996) The risk of intraocular juvenile xanthogranuloma: survey of current practices and assessment of risk. **J Am Acad Dermatol** 34(3):445–449.

560. Chang MW (1999) Update on juvenile xanthogranuloma: unusual cutaneous and systemic variants. **Seminars in Cutaneous Medicine & Surgery** 18(3):195–205.

Surgical indications

Rarely, giant juvenile xanthogranuloma occur.[561,562] They typically are solitary and measure 4–10cm. A diagnostic biopsy is recommended for large and atypical lesions. Like other involuting tumors of infancy such as hemangiomas, when involution of a giant juvenile xanthogranuloma occurs, a fibrofatty tumor often remains in the skin. For these giant lesions, many of which ulcerate, early surgical intervention is preferred on the face and scalp or if ulcerations occur that are difficult to heal or manage (Fig. 5.55). Larger lesions are best approached at 6 to 12 months, when primary closures are still possible on the scalp and to minimize the facial scarring. It is also recommended that these tumors be excised no later than the preschool years due to the psychologic impact of attending school with a deforming tumor on the face or scalp.

For giant juvenile xanthogranulomas on the body, a more conservative approach can be taken. Unless these are symptomatic, they can be left alone to involute until the early school years. If there is a significant cosmetic defect due to fibrofatty deposition or skin redundancy at the age of 7 to 10 years, the remaining tumor can be primarily excised.

GIANT SOLITARY MASTOCYTOMAS

Mast cell disease is a benign group of childhood diseases characterized by mast cell hamartomas in the skin. Multiple clinical presentations of this disease have been described. The most common is urticaria pigmentosa where multiple hyperpigmented macules and papules develop shortly after birth and involute in the early school years.[563] The second most common form in childhood is solitary mastocytomas.[564] These are nodular lesions that may be present at birth or develop early in infancy. Lesions are most common on the neck, arms and trunk, are typically oval, and range in size from 1 to 5cm. The surface color is brown or yellow-brown and the texture is often pebbly with a thickened or rubbery consistency. For most infants, this is a benign disease. Involution occurs in the early school years. Smaller lesions leave behind no cutaneous residual. No surgical treatment is recommended for these lesions.

Surgical indications

In a subset of patients, giant solitary mastocytomas form. These lesions are 3–10cm in size and commonly located on the scalp and trunk. Severe recurrent blistering, often with episodes of superinfection, can occur in these lesions.[565] Episodes are provoked by minimal trauma and are difficult to control with antihistamine therapy. For patients with these problematic lesions, primary excision is a recommended solution. Lesions that are present on the face or scalp should be approached early to allow for primary closure with the best cosmetic outcome. Lesions may become symptomatic later in the childhood years and can be approached surgically at any time that the severity of symptoms warrants intervention.[566]

Like other benign tumors of infancy and childhood that undergo spontaneous involution, larger lesions can leave behind fibrofatty deposition and a tumor that is persistent. If this occurs, the residual tumor can be excised for cosmetic purposes at the age of 7 to 10 years, avoiding the need for a general anesthetic and allowing the maximum time for spontaneous involution.

SUMMARY

The role of dermatologic surgery in caring for the pediatric dermatology patient is ever expanding. The new techniques, like tissue expansion and various forms of laser surgery, allow the dermatologic surgeon to treat a variety of disorders for which either no therapy or only poor therapy previously existed. With only a minimum number of changes in the normal procedures and standard equipment, the physician can provide quality care for the child or teenager who may require some form of cutaneous surgical intervention. While some additional discussion and patience may be necessary, the caring physician can expect to obtain excellent results in spite of the youthful age of the patient. Knowledge of the various types of surgical procedures, and the modifications required to perform them safely and expertly in children, will be beneficial to both patient and physician.

561. Bazan A, Lasso JM, Elejabeitia J, Garcia Tutor E (1998) Giant juvenile xanthgranuloma present since birth. **Annals of Plastic Surgery** 41(3):335–337.
562. Shapiro NL, Malis DJ, Charon CC et al. (1999) Giant juvenile xanthogranuloma of the tongue. **Am J Otolaryngology** 20(4):241–244.
563. Hannaford R, Rogers M (2001) Presentation of cutaneous mastocytosis in 173 children. **Australas J Dermatol** 42(1):15–21.
564. Kacker A, Huo J, Huang R, Hoda RS (2000) Solitary mastocytoma in an infant-case report with a review of literature. **Internat J Pediatric Otorhinolaryngology** 52(1):93–95.
565. Munro CS, Farr PM (1992) Solitary mastocytoma causing recurrent blistering in infancy. **Arch Dis Child** 67(8):1038–1039.
566. Ashinoff R, Soter NA, Freedberg IM (1993) Solitary mastocytoma in an adult. Treatment by excision. **J Dermatol Surg Oncol** 19(5):487–488.

Neonatal Skin and Skin Disorders

CHAPTER

6

Lawrence Eichenfield and Margarita Larralde

FETAL AND NEONATAL SKIN DEVELOPMENT

Embryonic and fetal skin development is a carefully controlled process that can be divided into three overlapping stages: organogenesis, histogenesis, and maturation.[1] The stages correspond roughly to the embryonic period (0–60 plus days), the early fetal period (60 days to 5 months) and late fetal period (5–9 months) of development. During organogenesis ectoderm lateral to the neural plate develops into epidermis, while sets of mesenchymal and neural crest cells develop into the dermis. Tremendous morphologic changes occur during histogenesis, when epidermis stratifies and epidermal appendages differentiate, and dermis and hypodermis become demarcated. Vascular neogenesis is important during histogenesis as well. The functional evolution of skin including barrier function and tensile strength during maturation is key to the transition from *in utero* existence to postnatal life.

NEONATAL SKIN STRUCTURE AND FUNCTION

There are many structural differences among adult, term, and preterm infants' skin (Table 6.1).[2] By 22 to 24 weeks gestation, the anatomic elements are essentially present, while functional, biochemical, and even structural maturity is delayed for years.

Skin immaturity has significant clinical consequences in the care of preterm and newborn infants. Fragility of the epidermis is marked in preterm infants, necessitating special care in the use of adhesives and their removal. Chemical burns from topical alcohol swabs and thermal burns from transcutaneous monitors are recognized problems, necessitating limited use or rotation of sites to decrease the occurrence of burns. The use of topical agents is limited because of potential local and systemic toxicity. These and other skin complications unique to the neonatal intensive care setting are addressed in greater detail later in this chapter.

Neonatal skin has different absorbtion characteristics than adult skin, first demonstrated by blanching responses after topical application of phenylephrine hydrochloride. Transcutaneous absorption is increased, especially in premature infants,[3] and may be a route for toxic effects from many topical agents.[4] Among those recognized to produce physiologic abnormalities, neurotoxicity, structural damage, and even death are iodine-containing soaps,[5,6] analine dyes,[7–9] hexachlorophene,[10,11] gamma-benzene hexachloride (lindane),[12] phenol,[13–15] pentachlorophenol,[16] and benzyl alcohol.[17]

Although exposure to most of these substances is unique to the neonatal intensive care setting, potential toxicity of topically applied substances is of equal concern outside of this environment. A study of parents of 1-month-old neonates reported that the average newborn had 48 different chemicals applied to the skin in the form of over-the-counter skin care products.[18] Many of these products contain alcohol and fatty acids. This is particularly concerning because *in vitro* studies have demonstrated marked increase in permeability to these substances in neonatal skin as compared with adult skin.[19]

Conversely, the increased skin permeability of premature infants can be exploited, clinically, as a useful alternative method of drug administration. *In vivo* and *in vitro* studies have demonstrated therapeutic levels of percutaneously applied caffeine[20] and diamorphine,[21] respectively, with an inverse relationship between gestational age and skin absorption.

The dramatic increase in percutaneous absorption observed in neonatal versus adult skin reflects differences in the structural and biochemical properties of neonatal skin. The stratum corneum and its thickness are the key factors responsible for exclusion or absorption of substances applied to the skin. In preterm infants, the stratum corneum thickness is markedly less than that of normal term infant or adult skin. Defective stratum corneum function, manifested as reduced water-holding capacity, has been measured in newborn skin and probably contributes to the observed xerosis as well as the increased permeability.[22]

The presence of skin surface lipids may also contribute significantly to the barrier properties of the epidermis. The development of the epidermal barrier in the neonatal rat is associated with increasing thickness of the stratum

1. Holbrook KA (1998) Structural and biochemical organogenesis of skin and cutaneous appendages in the fetus and newborn. In: Fetal and Neonatal Physiology, Polin RA, Fox WW, eds. Philadelphia: WB Saunders, pp. 729–752.
2. Holbrook KA (1982) A histological comparison of infant and adult skin. In: Neonatal Skin Structure and Function, Maibach HI, Boisits EK, eds. New York: Marcel Dekker, p. 3.
3. Nachman RL, Esterly NB (1971) Increased skin permeability in preterm infants. J Pediatr 79:628.
4. Harpin VA, Rutter N (1983) Barrier properties of the newborn infant's skin. J Pediatr 102:419.
5. Chabrolle JP, Rossier A (1978) Goitre and hypothyroidism in the newborn after cutaneous absorption of iodine. Arch Dis Child 53:495.
6. Mitchell IM, Pollock JC, Jamieson MP et al. (1991) Transcutaneous iodine absorption in infants undergoing cardiac operation. Ann Thorac Surg 52:1138.
7. Scott EP, Prince GE, Rotondo CC (1946) Dye poisoning in infancy. J Pediatr 28:713.
8. Kagan BM, Mirman B, Calvin J et al. (1949) Cyanosis in premature infants due to aniline dye intoxication. J Pediatr 34:574.
9. Fisch RO, Berglund EB, Bridge AG et al. (1963) Methemoglobinemia in a hospital nursery. JAMA 185:760.
10. Shuman RM, Leech RW, Acvord EC Jr. (1975) Neurotoxicity of hexachlorophene in the human. J Pediatr 54:689.
11. Greaves SJ, Ferry DG, McQueen EG et al. (1975) Serial hexachlorophene blood levels in the premature infant. NZ Med J 81:334.
12. Solomon LM, Fahrner L, West DP (1977) Gamma benzene hexachloride toxicity: a review. Arch Dermatol 113:353.
13. Thiemes C, Haley T (1972) Clinical Toxicology, 5th ed. Philadelphia: Lea & Febiger, p. 267.
14. Ruedemann R, Diechmann WB (1953) Blood phenol level after topical application of phenol-containing preparations. JAMA 142:506.
15. Brown BW (1970) Fatal phenol poisoning from improperly laundered diapers. Am J Public Health 60:901.
16. Robson AM, Kissane JM, Elvick NH et al. (1969) Pentachlorophenol poisoning in a nursery for newborn infants. Clinical features and treatments. J Pediatr 75:309.
17. Gershanik J, Boecler B, Ensley H et al. (1982) The gasping syndrome and benzyl alcohol poisoning. N Engl J Med 307:1384.
18. Cetta F, Lambert GH, Ros SP (1991) Newborn chemical exposure from over-the-counter skin care products. Clin Pediatr 30:286.
19. McCormack JJ, Boisits EK, Fisher LB (1982) An in vitro comparison of the permeability of adult versus neonatal skin. In: Neonatal Skin Structure and Function, Maibach HI, Boisits EK, eds. New York: Marcel Dekker, p. 149.
20. Amato M, Huppi P, Isenschmid M et al. (1992) Developmental aspects of percutaneous caffeine absorption in premature infants. Am J Perinatol 9:431.
21. Barrett DA, Rutter N, Davis SS (1993) An in vitro study of diamorphine permeation through premature human neonatal skin. Pharm Res 10:583.
22. Saijo S, Tagami H (1991) Dry skin of newborn infants: functional analysis of the stratum corneum. Pediatr Dermatol 8:155.

TABLE 6.1 Structural comparison of adult, term, and preterm infant skin (30 to 32 weeks)

Structure	Adult	Term	Preterm
Epidermal thickness	50µm	50µm	27.4µm
Stratum corneum thickness	15 cell	15 cell	Few cells
	9.3µm	9.3µm	4.1µm
Density of keratin filaments	Normal	Normal	Smaller bundles
Frequency of desmosomes	Normal	Normal	Fewer
Melanosomes	Normal	Fewer	One-third of term infant
Dermal-epidermal junction	Ridged	Flat but complete	Flat but complete
Anchoring filaments	Normal	Normal	Fewer and smaller
Anchoring fibrils	Normal	Normal	Fewer and smaller
Hemidesmosomes	Normal	Normal	Fewer and smaller
Papillary dermal collagen	Normal	Normal	Edematous, loosely organized
Reticular dermal collagen	Normal	Smaller bundles	Much smaller bundles
Reticular dermal elastic fibers	Normal	Finer, less mature	Visible only by electron microscopy
Reticular dermal cellularity	Few fibroblasts	More fibroblasts	Most fibroblasts
Components of basement membrane	Present	Present	Present

corneum and progressive accumulation of neutral lipids, particularly cholesterol, as well as nonpolar ceramides.[23] Lipid production is minimal in the premature infant's skin, reflecting immature epidermal and sebaceous gland function. Changes in surface lipids are well documented in the adult during starvation and have been previously seen in the neonate with essential fatty acid deficiency receiving incomplete parenteral nutrition.[24–26] Impaired barrier function and xerosis are clinical features of these conditions, which are characterized by defective sebaceous gland function.

Other structural parameters that affect percutaneous absorption and dermal clearance include epidermal thickness, the basement membrane zone, the vasculature of the papillary dermis, and dermal thickness and organization. In the premature infant, all these parameters are less well developed, facilitating increased absorption of topically applied chemicals.

The risk of toxicity from cutaneous absorption in premature infants is compounded by the fact that neonatal skin is also less effective in detoxifying these substances. Adult epidermal cells have the metabolic potential to activate enzyme systems to detoxify, deactivate, or modify chemicals by means of enzymes that oxidate, hydrolyze, hydroxylate, reduce, deaminate, or conjugate. The enzymatic activity in the epidermis of preterm viable infants is limited; therefore, deactivation and detoxification of applied compounds are similarly limited. Potentially harmful substances applied to neonatal skin may pass directly into the bloodstream unchanged.[27]

The potential for toxicity of percutaneously applied compounds also relates to body surface area. Term infants have three times more surface area per unit weight as compared with an adult and the premature infant may have seven times more surface area per unit weight.

The poor barrier function of neonatal skin permits not only absorption of substances from the external environment, but also tremendous transepidermal water and heat losses from the internal environment. This necessitates close attention to fluid and temperature control. The rate of heat loss by evaporation can exceed the baby's resting rate of heart production. Lack of subcutaneous fat for insulation, poor autonomic control of cutaneous vessels, and functionally reduced sweating in the preterm infant all contribute to poor thermal

regulation.[28,29] Maintaining a moist environment can dramatically reduce insensible water losses and assist in skin hydration, as can application of petrolatum-based ointments or semi-permeable dressings.[30] Caution must be taken with these approaches, since the preterm infant is at risk of sepsis from skin-associated organisms (see Skin care of newborn infants).

Although inroads are being made toward our understanding of the structure, function, and biochemistry of fetal skin, its function and biochemistry during neonatal illness have not been studied or quantitated for various degrees of maturity. Surely hypoxia, hypothermia, hypoglycemia, central nervous system (CNS) hemorrhage, congenital heart disease, perinatal malnutrition, and viremia may modify skin cell function, absorption, metabolic capabilities, and drug clearance. These modifications may in turn reflect changes in function of other tissues, especially those of neuroectodermal origin.

TRANSIENT PHYSIOLOGIC CHANGES AND CUTANEOUS LESIONS IN THE NEWBORN

Neonatal skin displays many unique characteristics that reflect immaturity and the transition from intrauterine life. These conditions and normal processes should be recognized and differentiated from pathologic processes.

VERNIX CASEOSA

Vernix caseosa is a chalky-white, greasy, slippery substance, composed of shed epithelial cells, sebaceous secretions, and shed lanugo hair. It lubricates the skin and facilitates passage through the birth canal. Little vernix is present in premature infants, and it becomes thicker with gestational age with substantial coverage of near-term infants. Interestingly, postmature infants are usually devoid of vernix. After birth, the vernix disappears over several days.

The lipid composition of vernix has been measured and is highly variable, including cholesterol, free fatty acids, and ceramide.[31] In general, vernix from term infants contains more squalene and a higher wax ester to sterol ester ratio than vernix from preterm infants.[32] Since wax esters are produced only

23. Aszterbaum M, Gopinathan MK, Feingold KR et al. (1992) Ontogeny of the epidermal barrier to water loss in the rat: correlation of function with stratum corneum structure and lipid content. **Pediatr Res** 31:308.
24. Friedman Z (1980) Essential fatty acids revisited. **Am J Dis Child** 134:397.
25. Friedman Z, Danon A, Stahlman MT (1976) Rapid onset of essential fatty acid deficiency in the newborn. **Pediatrics** 58:649.
26. Downing DT, Strauss JS, Pochi PE (1972) Changes in skin surface lipid composition induced by severe caloric restriction in man. **Am J Clin Nutr** 25:365.
27. Noonan PK, Wester RC (1987) Cutaneous biotransformations and some pharmacological and toxicological implications. In: Dermatoxicology, 3rd ed, Marzulli FN, Maibach HI, eds. Washington, DC: Hemisphere, p. 71.

28. Harpin VA, Rutter N (1982) Sweating in preterm infants. **J Pediatr** 100:614.
29. Smales ORC, Kime R (1978) Thermoregulation in babies immediately after birth. **Arch Dis Child** 53:58.
30. Vermon HJ (1990) The effect of semipermeable dressings on transepidermal water loss in premature infants. **Pediatrics** 86:357.
31. Hoeger PH, Schreiner V, Klaassen IA et al. (2002) Epidermal barrier lipids in human vernix caseosa: corresponding ceramide pattern in vernix and fetal skin. **Br J Dermatol** 146:194–201.
32. Wysocki SJ, Grauaug A, O'Neill G et al. (1981) Lipids in forehead vernix from newborn infants. **Biol Neonat** 39:300.

by sebaceous glands, this change reflects increased sebaceous function in fetal skin as term approaches.[33]

The biologic role of vernix has long been disputed. Histochemical and ultrastructural studies have demonstrated great variability among cells. Activity of acid phosphatase, an enzyme that shows a marked increase in amniotic fluid toward term, is found both in intracytoplasmic granules and as amorphous material between the vernix caseosa cells.[34] It has been suggested that vernix is antibacterial, since it contains sebum, which has some antibacterial and antifungal properties.[35] There is little evidence to support a direct antimicrobial role of vernix, but studies have demonstrated that it provides a mechanical barrier to bacterial passage; these studies are the basis for recommendation that vernix be left on the newborn until it is spontaneously shed.[36]

The color of vernix can reflect intrauterine problems. Yellow-brown discoloration is frequently seen in post-term infants, with bile staining from meconium passage, and with hemolytic disease of the newborn. Vernix can also be colonized with bacteria during intrauterine infections. Infected vernix has an odor that is easily recognized as a sign of neonatal sepsis.

RUBOR AND ACROCYANOSIS

Both rubor and acrocyanosis are physiologic findings seen in most newborns during the neonatal period, representing manifestations of vasomotor instability, as the infant adjusts from intra-amniotic to extrauterine life. Generalized rubor is often present in the first several hours of life and reflects cutaneous vasodilation and hyperemia (Fig. 6.1). This can be in striking contrast to the peripheral acrocyanosis that is also seen.

Acrocyanosis is characterized by bilateral and symmetric bluish discoloration of the hands and feet that is intermittent and variable in intensity. It gradually remits by several weeks of age and has no pathologic significance. The epidermis is normal without induration or edema. The coloration of the acral surfaces may be blanched with pressure and is ameliorated by warming of the extremities. Acrocyanosis is more pronounced in hypothermia, polycythemia, and other hyperviscosity syndromes.

The pathogenesis of these entities is not well understood. Studies of skin blood flow in term infants, during the first several weeks of life, have shown delayed and prolonged cutaneous vasodilation in response to normal or increased core temperature. Increased sympathetic tone is considered responsible for the delayed vasodilation response.[37] This is in contrast to the exaggerated vasomotor response to hypothermia, discussed below. The rhythmic periodic oscillations of skin blood flux, observed using laser Doppler in mature skin, are absent in newborns. Oscillation patterns reach the lower range of adult values by the end of the first week in term infants but remain below this range for prolonged periods in preterm infants.[38]

The mechanism of rubor or erythema neonatorum is thought to be a reflex vasodilation of cutaneous capillaries perhaps related to decreased sympathetic tone present at birth. The hyperemic flush that occurs appears bright red through the thin skin of the newborn.

Acrocyanosis is thought to result from dilation of the subpapillary and papillary venous plexuses. Blood flow in the dilated structures is significantly reduced, allowing time for greater release of oxygen and the formation of desaturated hemoglobin, which is responsible for the cyanotic appearance.[39]

Cyanosis due to cardiovascular or respiratory problems is central or generalized cyanosis, rather than in the acral distribution of acrocyanosis. Ecchymoses and nevoid lesions on the acral surfaces may be similar in appearance, but are unlikely to be bilateral, symmetric, intermittent, or blanchable with pressure. There is no pathologic significance to acyrocyanosis and no therapy is required.

CUTIS MARMORATA

A transient, benign reticulate, mottled bluish discoloration of the skin that may last minutes to hours, is termed cutis marmorata (Fig. 6.2). Both full-term and preterm infants may be affected.[40]

Cutis marmorata is thought to be an exaggerated vasomotor response to hypothermia. In neonatal vascular reaction studies using heated thermocouple techniques, environmental temperature changes produce cutaneous vasomotor responses, with marked vasoconstriction occurring at temperatures

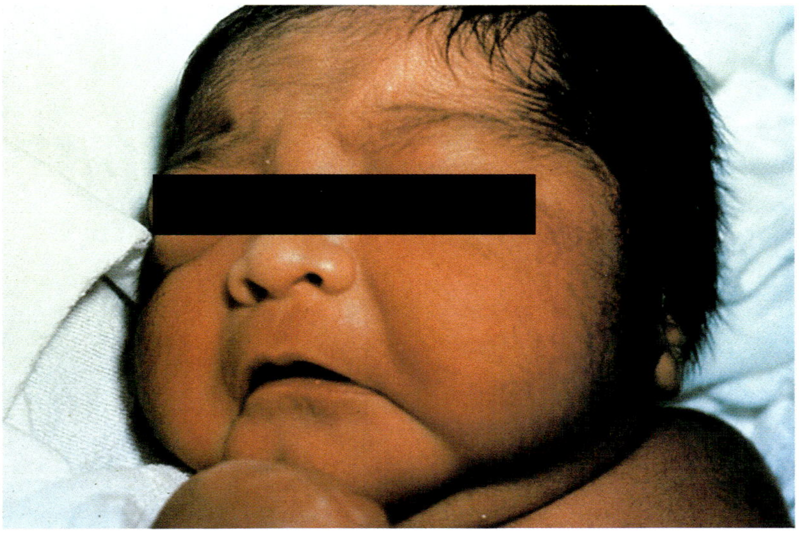

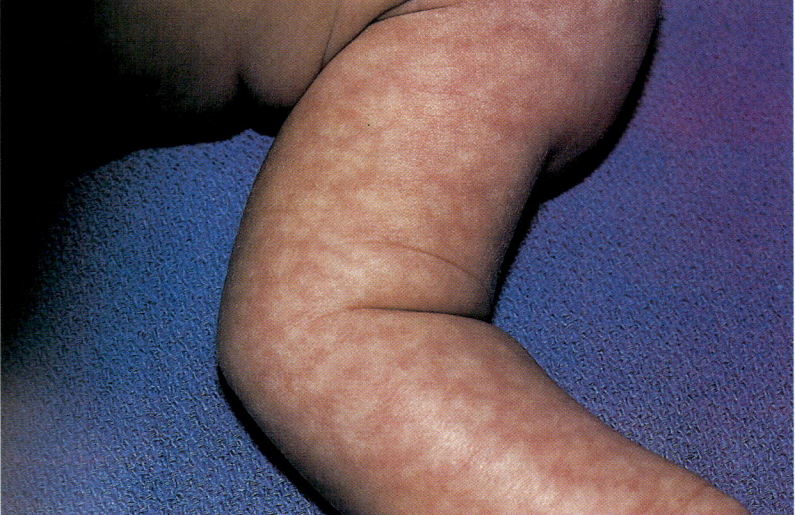

Fig. 6.1   Rubor. Transient erythema of newborn due to vasodilation.

Fig. 6.2   Mottling, cutis marmorata in premature infant.

33. Stewart ME, Quinn MA, Downing DT (1982) Variability in the fatty acid composition of wax esters from vernix caseosa and its possible relation to sebaceous gland activity. **J Invest Dermatol** 78:291.

34. Agorastos T, Hollweg G, Grussendorf EL et al. (1988) Features of vernix caseosa cells. **Am J Perinatol** 5:253.

35. Aly R, Maibach HI, Rahman R et al. (1975) Correlation of human in vivo and in vitro cutaneous antimicrobial factors. **J Infect Dis** 131:579.

36. Joglekar VM (1980) Barrier properties of vernix caseosa. **Arch Dis Child** 55:817.

37. Brüuck K (1978) Heat production and temperature regulation. In Stave U (ed): Perinatal Physiology. Plenum, New York, p. 455.

38. Poschl J, Weiss T, Diehm C et al. (1991) Periodic variations in skin perfusion in full-term and preterm neonates using laser Doppler technique. **Acta Paediatr Scand** 80:999.

39. Ryan TJ (1983) Cutaneous circulation. In Goldsmith LA (ed): Biochemistry and Physiology of the Skin. Oxford University Press, New York, p. 817.

40. Lucky AW (2001) Transient benign cutaneous lesions in the newborn. In: Textbook of Neonatal Dermatology. Eichenfield LF, Frieden IJ, Esterly NB, eds. Philadelphia, PA: WB Saunders, pp. 98–99.

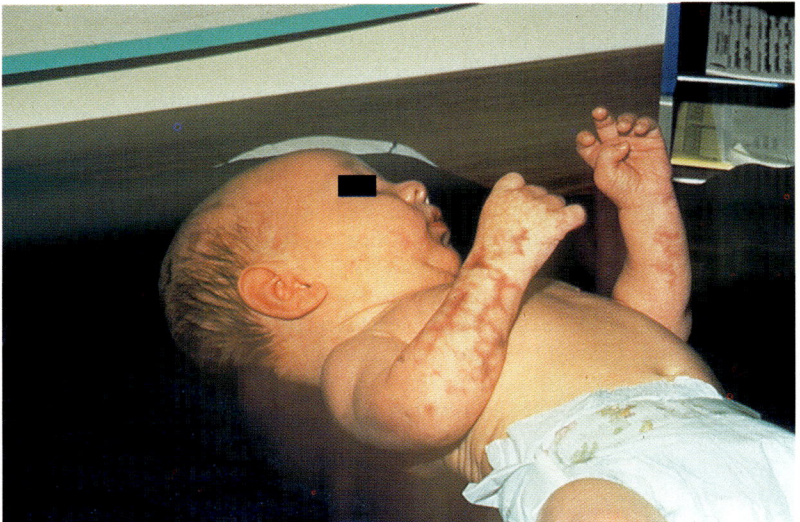

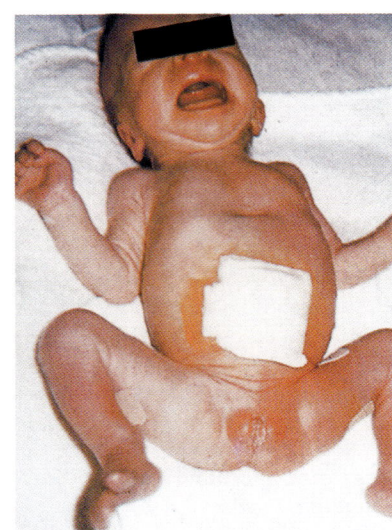

Fig. 6.4 Harlequin color change: premature infant with striking midline color change.

Fig. 6.3 Cutis marmorata telangiectatica congenita. Note bilateral dusky reticulate pattern, unaffected by temperature.

below the thermoneutral zone (32° to 35°C). Rhythmic changes in blood flow to the skin surfaces can be created by environmental temperature changes, even thought the core temperature is stable. When core temperatures are below normal (36.5° to 37.5°C) and subsequently increased to become normal, cutaneous vasodilation is delayed, presumably because of increased sympathetic tone. In cutis marmorata, warming the infant causes the skin to regain a normal or near-normal appearance.[41] Profound or persistant cutis marmorata has been reported with Downs syndrome, trisomy 18, hypothyroidism, and the Cornelia de Lange syndrome.

Physiologic cutis marmorata is distinguishable from cutis marmorata telangiectatica congenita (CMTC), a persistent vascular anomaly that presents at birth (Fig. 6.3). CMTC presents with a pronounced reticulate purple discoloration that may be localized, segmental or diffuse.[42–45] The mottling of the skin in CMTC does not resolve with warming of the skin. Telangiectasias, phlebectasias, atrophy, and ulcerations may be seen in addition to mottling. Verrucous or hyperkeratotic lesions may appear later. Although as many as two-thirds of infants with CMTC have been reported to have associated abnormalities,[46] other series have noted a much lower frequency.[47] Reported abnormalities have included defective bony and soft tissue growth,[46–48] congenital heart disease,[47] glaucoma,[49,50] branchial cleft cysts,[47] and other vascular malformations.

Another cause of a mottled appearance that does not respond to rewarming is livedo reticularis seen in collagen vascular disease, such as neonatal lupus.

In cutis marmorata, no specific therapy is required, but warming may be needed if environmental temperatures and core body temperatures are not appropriate.

HARLEQUIN COLOR CHANGE

Differential coloration of the newborn on the left and right side was first described by Neligan and Strange in 1952 (Fig. 6.4).[51] Originally noted in

preterm infants and estimated to occur in as many as 15% of these infants, it may be seen at a lower frequency in term infants, especially those of low birth weight. The harlequin color change occurs, with axial rotation, commonly when infants are being turned. If the infant is lying on its side, the dependent side of the body shows profound vasodilation, in marked contrast to the pale upper half of the body. The head and genitalia may be spared, and mucous membranes are not involved. Reversal of the perfusion pattern can occur when the infant is placed on the opposite side.[52]

Although reported to occur shortly after birth or up to 3 weeks of age, the harlequin color change is most frequently seen at age 3 to 4 days. About 50% of affected infants will have repeated episodes, the duration of which may be seconds or up to 20 minutes.

There are no cutaneous histologic findings; therefore, skin biopsy is not indicated. There are usually no cardiovascular abnormalities, infections or other pathologic conditions associated with the color change. However, harlequin color change has been reported in association with tricuspid atresia in a 3½-month-old infant.[53] The pathophysiologic basis for this transient vascular abnormality is not well understood. Since it has been seen in infants with intracranial hemorrhage, it is thought to be related to immaturity or dysfunction of the hypothalamic centers responsible for peripheral vascular tone.[54]

No therapy is required, and increased activity such as crying usually ablates the color change. The harlequin color change is quite distinct from the lower body and acral cyanosis seen in infants with congenital heart disease. The latter is bilateral and predominantly involves the lower extremities rather than being a vertical unilateral midline change seen with harlequin vasomotor instability. It is tempting to speculate that these early signs of vasomotor instability reflect adaptation of neonatal skin to the dry, extrauterine environment. While *in utero*, the amniotic fluid helps regulate temperature. There are no insensible water losses, and sweating is not an important thermoregulatory function of the skin. The increased transepidermal water loss, large body surface area, defective and immature sweat glands, and vasomotor instability of neonatal skin make temperature regulation difficult. As the skin matures, becoming

41. Smales ORC, Kime R (1978) Thermoregulation in babies immediately after birth. **Arch Dis Child** 53:58.
42. Suarez SM, Grossman ME (1991) Localized cutis marmorata telangiectatica congenita. **Pediatr Dermatol** 8:329.
43. Moroz PK (1993) Cutis marmorata telangiectatica congenita: long-term follow-up, review of the literature, and report of a case in conjunction with congenital hypothyroidism. **Pediatr Dermatol** 10:6–11.
44. Devillers ACA, de Waard-Van der Spek, Oranje AP (1999) Cutis marmorata telangiectatica congenita. Clinical features in 35 cases. **Arch Dermatol** 135:34–38.
45. Kennedy C, Oranje AP, Keizer K et al. (1992) Cutis marmorata telangiectatica congenita. **Int J Dermatol** 31:249–252.
46. Pehr K, Moroz B (1993) Cutis marmorata telangiectatica congenita: long-term follow-up, review of the literature, and report of a case in conjunction with congenital hypothyroidism. **Pediatr Dermatol** 10:6.
47. Picascia DD, Esterly NB (1988) Cutis marmorata telangiectatica congenita: report of 22 cases. **J Am Acad Dermatol** 20:1098–1104.
48. Dutkowsky JP, Kasser JR, Kaplan LC (1993) Leg length discrepancy associated with vivid cutis marmorata. **J Pediatr Orthop** 13:456.
49. Weilepp AE and Eichenfield LF (1996) Association of glaucoma with cutis marmorata telangiectatica congenita: A localized anatomic malformation. **J Am Acad Dermatol** 35:276–278.
50. Lynch PJ (1990) Cutis marmorata telangiectatica congenita associated with congenital glaucoma. **J Am Acad Dermatol** 22:857.
51. Neligan GA, Strange LB (1952) A "harlequin" colour change in the newborn. **Lancet** 2:1005.
52. Selimoglu MA, Dilmen U, Karakelleoglu C et al. (1995) Harlequin color change. **Arch Pediatr Adolesc Med** 149:1171–1172.
53. Pearson HA, Cone TE (1957) Harlequin color change in a young infant with tricuspid atresia. **J Pediatr** 50:609.
54. Herlitz G (1953) Unilateral skin vessel crises in the newborn. **Acta Pediatr Scand** 42:506

more adept at temperature control, these transient cutaneous vascular phenomena disappear.

PHYSIOLOGIC JAUNDICE

Neonatal skin frequently acquires a yellow coloration in the first few days of life. Physiologic jaundice, or icterus neonatorum, is observed in 60% of term infants and in 80% of preterm infants. Relative intrauterine hypoxemia results in polycythemia in newborns. After birth, the increased oxygen tension stimulates a spontaneous breakdown of the increased red blood cell mass. Bilirubin, the pigment comprising hemoglobin, is released into the circulation, where it is conjugated to the direct form in the liver, and eliminated in the stool. Hepatic immaturity results in excess unconjugated bilirubin that accumulates in the skin, producing physiologic jaundice.

In the absence of exacerbating conditions, such as dehydration, hemolysis, sepsis, or extensive hematoma or ecchymosis resorption, jaundice peaks on the fourth day and gradually resolves. Premature infants have higher peak levels of bilirubin and more persistent hyperbilirubinemia lasting into the second week of life. Early appearing or persistent jaundice suggests infection, blood group incompatibility, Crigler–Najjar syndrome, or other liver disease. Some breast-fed infants have prolonged low-grade hyperbilirubinemia beginning late in the first week of life and persisting for up to 10 weeks. A factor in human milk increases the enterohepatic circulation of bilirubin, and insufficient caloric intake may increase unconjugated bilirubin levels.[55]

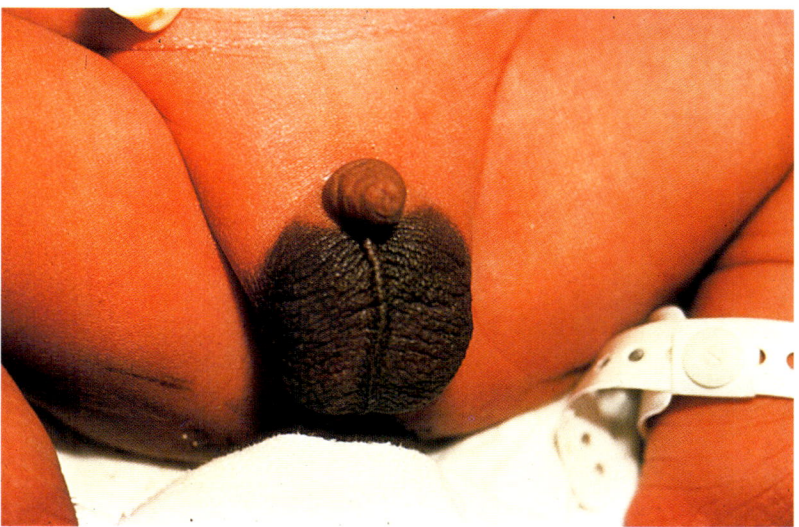

Fig. 6.5   Hyperpigmentation of genitalia and linea nigra in normal newborn male.

PIGMENTARY CHANGES

Another common variation in skin color observed in newborns is skin hyperpigmentation in a pattern similar to that seen during pregnancy and, to a lesser degree, at puberty. This is believed to result from the influences of maternal and placental hormones, as part of the "mini puberty" of the newborn (see below). Darkly pigmented external genitalia and hyperpigmentation of the linea alba are especially prominent in dark-skinned races (Fig. 6.5). This pigmentation is common in newborns and may persist for two or three months. Pigment dilution at birth, in non-Caucasian infants, also occurs. The basis for this is unknown, but it may also be hormonally mediated.

SKIN FRAGILITY

Neonatal skin exhibits a fragility that is not present in mature skin. There appear to be weakened attachments between the epidermis and dermis that are easily severed by physical or chemical trauma. This leads to iatrogenic abrasion from adhesive tape and other mild forms of trauma. Fragility is pronounced in preterm infants (Fig. 6.6) and special care must be taken even with routine handling in the neonatal intensive care setting to avoid skin injury. Frequent positioning, the use of emollients, and strict avoidance of harsh soaps and adhesives, can reduce the trauma.

PEELING

Desquamation of neonatal skin is present in most term neonates in the first few days of life.[56] It is most pronounced in infants born at 40 to 42 weeks gestation but occurs to some extent in all newborns. Shedding is commonly localized to the hands, ankles and feet in term infants. Postmature infants (more than 42 weeks gestation) have a more widespread general desquamation (Fig. 6.7), accompanied by other cutaneous signs of their gestational age, including absence of vernix, long nails and hair, and decreased subcutaneous fat. Scaling is most prominent on the hands, feet, and lower trunk in these infants.

The differential diagnosis of neonatal desquamation is presented in Table 6.2. Distinction among severe physiologic desquamation, X-linked ichthyosis, ichthyosis vulgaris and the continual peeling skin syndrome can

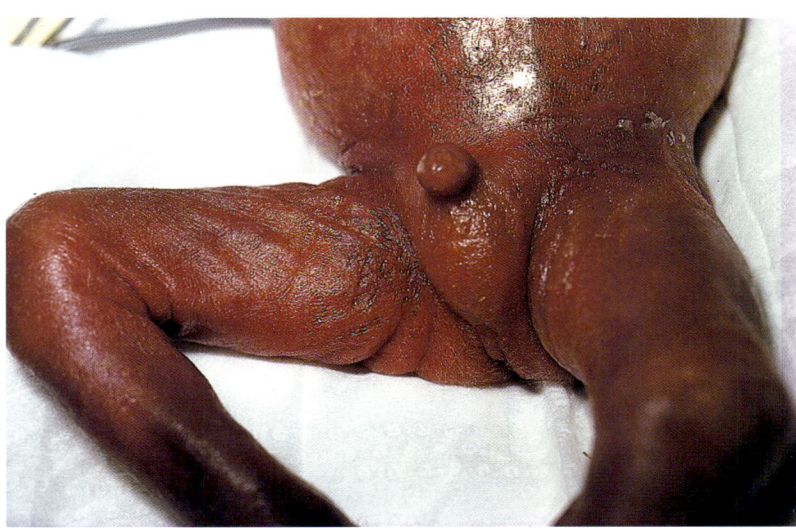

Fig. 6.6   Fissures and skin fragility in premature infant.

be difficult in the first several days of life. Persistence of scaling beyond the first few weeks, combined with family history, distribution, and appearance of the scale, usually lead to a correct diagnosis of ichthyosis shortly after birth. The rare familial continual peeling skin syndrome is characterized by superficial sheet-like skin peeling and pruritus.[57]

Other inherited conditions, including disorders of lipid metabolism such as Refsum disease, Rud disease, and neutral lipid storage disease, essential fatty acid deficiency, amino acid deficiencies and Sjögren–Larsson syndrome, can also present with desquamation at birth, as can congenital infections such as congenital syphilis. Fortunately, other features of these rare conditions are usually present to aid in the diagnosis.

LANUGO

Newborns are covered with silky, fine unmedullated hairs called lanugo. This hair is more prominent in preterm infants, as the first coat of it is normally shed *in utero* during the last trimester and replaced with a second coat of shorter lanugo hairs.[58] Shoulders and posterior trunk generally will have

55. Gartner LM (2001) Breastfeeding and jaundice. **J Perinatol** 21:Supp 1:S25–9;discussion S35–9.
56. Lucky AW (2001) Transient benign cutaneous lesions in the newborn. In Textbook of Neonatal Dermatology. Eichenfield LF, Frieden IJ, Esterly NB, eds. WB Saunders Company. Philadelphia, PA. 98–99.
57. Janin A, Copin M-C, Dubos JP et al. (1996) Familial peeling skin syndrome with eosinophilia: clinical, histologic, and ultrastructural study of three cases. **Arch Pathol Lab Med** 120:662–665.
58. Kligman AM (1961) Pathological diagnosis of human hair loss. **Arch Dermatol** 83:175.

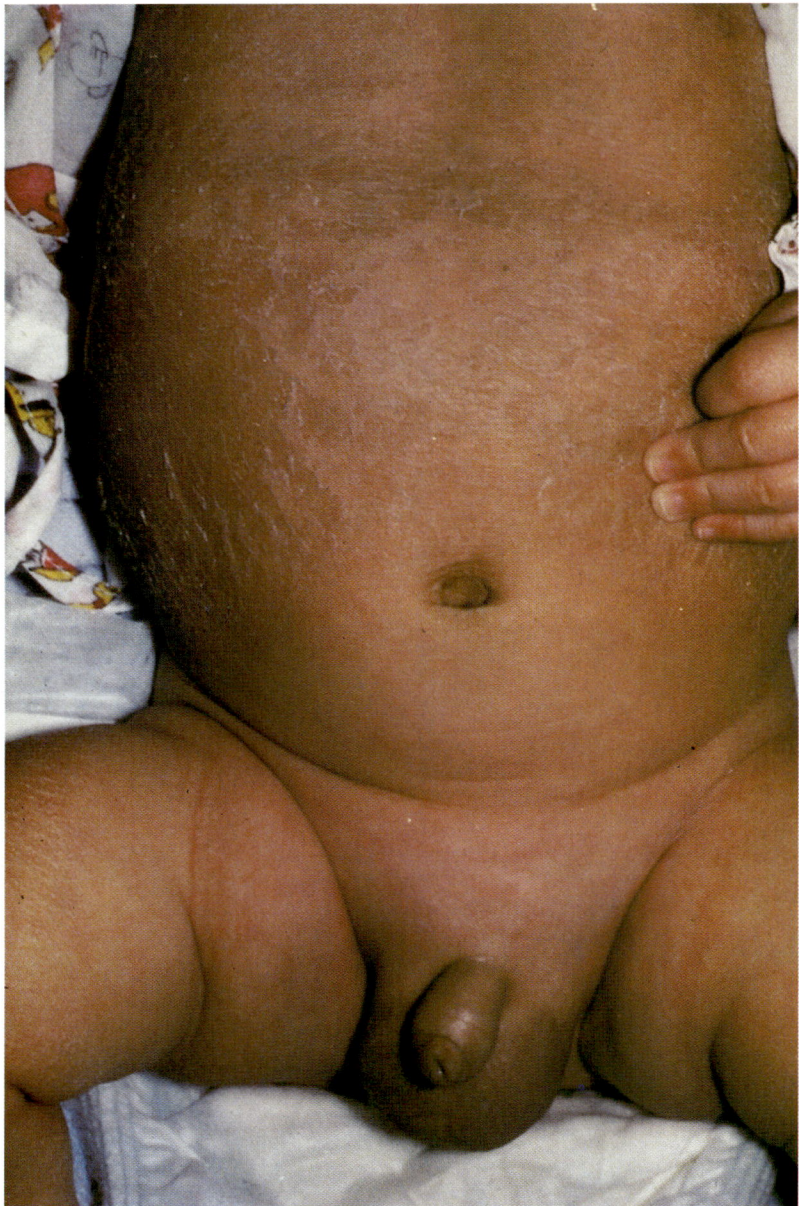

Fig. 6.7   Desquamation in post-term infant.

the most pronounced hair, lateral cheek involvement may be extensive and distal limbs generally have less hair (Fig. 6.8).[59] Lanugo hairs are usually unpigmented and are replaced by vellus hairs during the first few months of life.

Congenital hypertrichosis lanuginosa is a rare, inherited disorder that can be mistaken for normal lanugo hair growth in the neonate. In this condition the newborn is covered with profuse, light-colored lanugo hair several centimeters

in length. Historically, affected children were exhibited and referred to as "monkey men" or "human Skye Terriers." Autosomal dominant inheritance pattern is well documented, though sporadic cases are common and a family with possible autosomal recessive inheritance has been reported.[60–62] Long lanugo hair may be present on all body parts, except for the palms, soles, prepuce, glans penis, labia minora, and dorsal terminal phalanges. There may be regional variability of hairiness with localized sparing and often accentuation over the spine and pinnae. Examination of the mucous membranes, teeth, nails, and skin is otherwise normal. Most patients are otherwise well, though some congenital anomalies may occur with this disorder, including dental defects, physical and mental retardation, and glaucoma.[63,64] Improvement with time is seen in some patients, while persistence or worsening is reported by others. The pubic, axillary, and beard areas retain the lanugo hair at puberty, without conversion to terminal hair.

The mechanism of hair growth in congenital hypertrichosis lanuginosa is not understood. The number of hair follicles has been reported to be greater than normal, but histologic and biochemical abnormalities have not been well studied. No endocrine and metabolic abnormalities have been found to date. Treatments for congenital hypertrichosis lanuginosa are all unsatisfactory. Shaving or depilatory therapy is preferred to treatment with oral or topical antiandrogens. A case of spontaneous hair loss following infrequent shaving during infancy has been reported.[64]

The differential diagnosis of increased neonatal hair is fairly broad and should include hypertrichosis observed with other genetically determined disorders including congenital lipodystrophy, leprechaunism, Cornelia de Lange syndrome, gingival fibromatosis, Coffin–Siris syndrome, Rubenstein–Taybi syndrome, and Barber–Say syndrome. In mucopolysaccharidoses, hypertrichosis may not be evident until beyond the neonatal period.[64–66]

HAIR PATTERNS, HAIR CYCLE CHANGES, AND POSTNATAL ALOPECIA

Terminal hairs are present on the scalp of most neonates at birth, though the pattern of hair growth is distinctive. The hairline of newborns is lower and less sharply defined than in older children, with the terminal hairs on the border converting to hypopigmented vellus hairs during the first year of life.[67] In addition, eyebrows are poorly demarcated, and eyelashes are commonly absent or scant at birth. Mature terminal hair growth patterns are generally established by the second half of the first year of life.

Scalp hair can be abundant or sparse at birth. The former is more common in pigmented races, although patterns also tend to be familial. The normal fetus undergoes synchronous shedding of scalp hair in the fifth month of fetal life. The regrown hair then enters telogen in a wave from front to back, starting about 12 weeks before term (Fig. 6.9). Most hair roots have entered anagen phase again before delivery.[68,69] Occipital alopecia is often observed in infants in the first few months of life (Fig. 6.10). It is commonly but incorrectly, attributed to the trauma of rubbing the posterior scalp on the bed covers. In fact, the occipital area is the last area on the scalp to enter the telogen wave and does not do so until birth.[67] Although trauma may result in earlier loss of the posterior scalp hair, shedding of these telogen hairs is inevitable.

The normal post-delivery hair cycle consists of waves of hair loss and regrowth from front to back (Fig. 6.11) until the childhood pattern of hair growth is established, usually by the end of the first year.[70] Occasionally, there

59. Heyl T (1986) The skin of the pre-term baby: a visual appraisal. **Clin Exp Dermatol** 11:584.
60. Kint AH, Vermander FR, Decroix JM (1985) Congenital hypertrichosis lanug nosa. **Hautarzt** 36:423.
61. Felgenhauer WR (1969) Hypertrichosis lanuginosa universalis. **J Genet Hum** 17:1–44.
62. Freire-Maia M, Felizali J, de Figueiredo AC et al. (1976) Hypertrichosis lanuginosa in a mother and son. **Clin Genet** 10:303–306.
63. Judge MR, Khaw PT, Rice NS et al. (1981) Congenital hypertrichosis lanugir osa and congenital glaucoma. **Br J Dermatol** 124:495.
64. Partridge JW (1987) Congenital hypertrichosis lanuginosa: neonatal shaving. **Arch Dis Child** 62:623–625.

65. Baumeister FAM, Schwartz HP, Stengel-Rutkowski S (1995) Childhood hypertrichosis: diagnosis and management. **Arch Dis Child** 72:457–459.
66. Rogers M (2001) Hair disorders. In: Textbook of Neonatal Dermatology, Eichenfield LF, Frieden IJ, Esterly NB, eds. Philadelphia, PA: WB Saunders, pp. 487–503.
67. Rogers M (2001) Hair disorders. In: Eichenfield LF, Frieden IJ, Esterly NB, eds. Philadelphia, PA: WB Saunders, pp. 487–503.
68. Barman JM, Pecoraro V, Astore I et al. (1967) The first stage in the natural history of the human scalp hair cycle. **J Invest Dermatol** 48:138.
69. Pecoraro V, Astore I, Barman JM (1964) Cycle of the scalp hair of the newborn child. **J Invest Dermatol** 43:145.
70. Barth JH (1987) Normal hair growth in children. **Pediatr Dermatol** 4:173.

TABLE 6.2 Differential diagnosis of desquamation at birth

Condition	Sites of predilection	Type of scale	Inheritance	Distinguising features	Course and prognosis
Physiologic desquamation	Ankles, feet, and hands	Noninflammatory, white, thin fine scale	None	Distribution, lack of erythema, mild nature, and resolution	Resolves within days to 2 weeks of birth
Postmature desquamation	Hands, ankles, feet, lower trunk	Noninflammatory white, thin fine scale	None	Postmature infant with other signs of postmaturity, such as long nails and absent vernix	Resolves within days to 2 weeks of birth
Postinflammatory desquamation	Trunk more common than extremities	Erythematous base with fine white scale	None	History of clinical evidence of preceding inflammation; no scale on noninflamed skin	Resolves within days to 2 weeks of inflammatory insult
Continual peeling skin syndrome	Generalized, including face; spares palms and soles	Noninflammatory, large, poorly adherent sheets, and fine scale	Familial (some autosomal recessive)	Widespread distribution and persistence; ability to peel away large sheets of skin atraumatically; biopsy is helpful	Persists for life with seasonal variation in some patients
Ichthyosis vulgaris	Face, trunk, extensor extremities	Noninflammatory, fine, white adherent scale	Autosomal dominant	Hyperlinearity of palms, family history, presence of atopy in 50%	Improves with age and humidity
X-linked ichthyosis	Prominence in neck folds, ears, popliteal fossa, abdomen, and lower legs	Large dark brown "dirty"-appearing scale	X-linked	Associated with steroid sulfatase deficiency; fine collodion membrane rarely present at birth	Persists for life but waxes and wanes with seasons
Lamellar ichthyosis	Generalized	Thick yellow brown adherent platelike scales	Autosomal recessive	Erythroderma or collodion membrane at birth: may have ectropion hyperlinear palms and nail changes	Severe, unremitting course
Congenital ichthyosiform erythroderma	Generalized	Fine white scale overlying erythroderma	Autosomal recessive	May be indistinguishable from lamellar ichthyosis at birth	Mild erythroderma may persist, scaing persists for life but less severe than lamellar ichthyosis

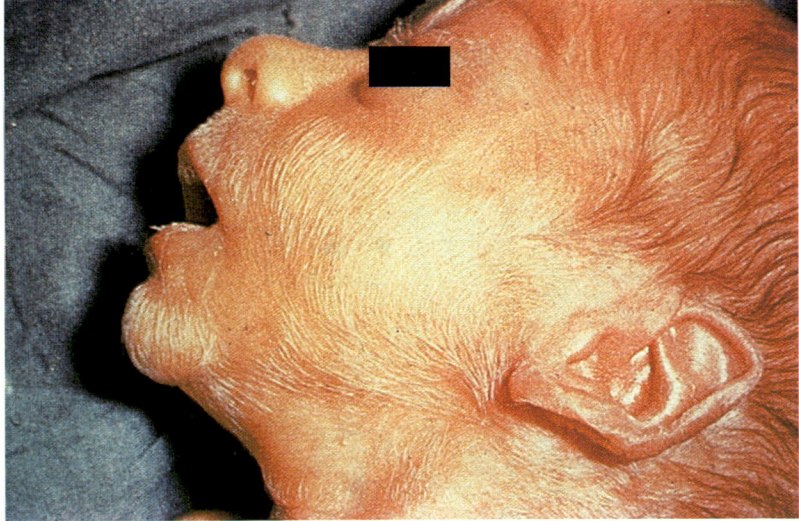

Fig. 6.8   Lanugo facial hair in premature infant.

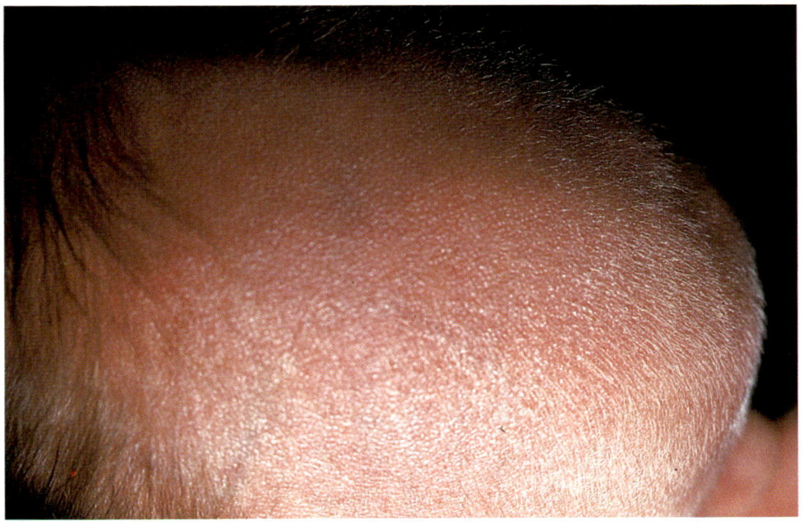

Fig. 6.9   Alopecia, front to back sequence shown in full-term infant at birth. Right is front; retained hair noted posteriorly.

is synchronous loss of nearly all hair during the neonatal period, resulting in diffuse alopecia or telogen effluvium of the newborn. More commonly, the cycle of hair loss and regrowth is so subtle that parents do not perceive the loss at all.

ORAL LESIONS

A number of benign lesions are present in the oral cavity of newborns. These are discussed also in Chapter 9.

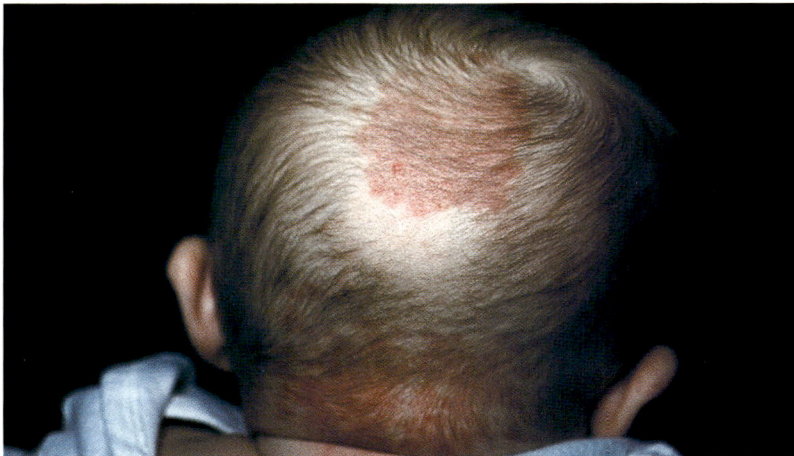

Fig. 6.10 Occipital post-neonatal alopecia (plus occipital and nuchal salmon patch/stork bite telangiectatic changes).

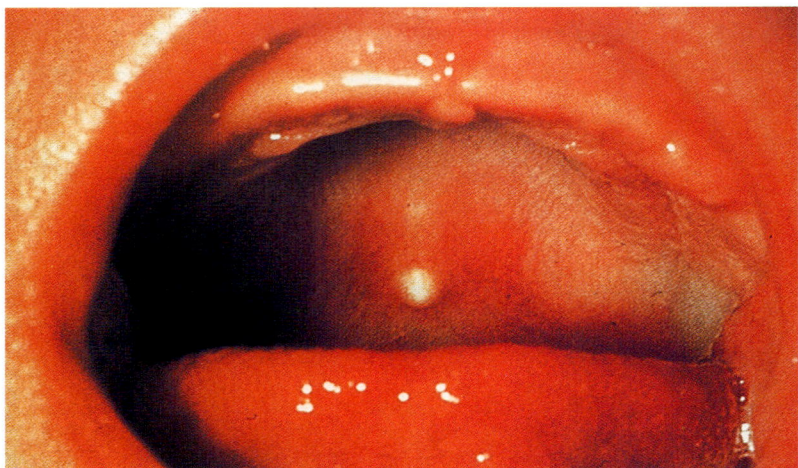

Fig. 6.12 Epstein's pearl: palatal, milium-like.

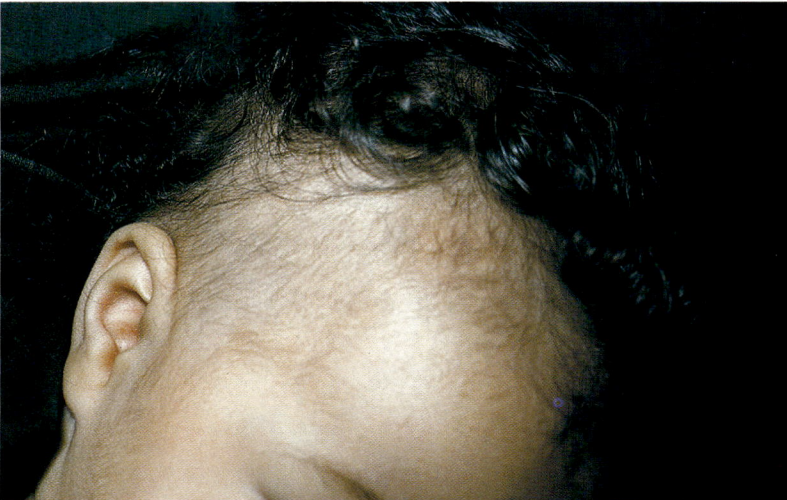

Fig. 6.11 Frontotemporal post-neonatal alopecia, age 2 months.

EPSTEIN'S PEARLS

Epstein's pearls are benign, cystic lesions, which occur along the median palatal raphe, most commonly at the junction of the hard and soft palate (Fig. 6.12). Lesions are multiple and small, ranging in size from less than a millimeter to several millimeters in diameter. The overall appearance is similar to the Bohn nodule, but the location and etiology makes this a distinct entity. Epstein's pearls are common, occurring in 60 to 85% of newborn infants. Japanese newborns are most commonly affected (up to 92%), followed by Caucasians and African-Americans.[71,72] They are epidermal inclusion cysts formed during the fusion of the soft and hard palates, and contain desquamated keratin within their lumens. They are considered the counterpart of milia, which are commonly seen on the faces of neonates. No therapy is indicated; most lesions spontaneously rupture within the first few weeks to months of life.

BOHN'S NODULES

Bohn's nodules are multiple, small cystic structures found along the lingual or buccal surfaces of the alveolar ridges and the lateral palate. These lesions

are common, being found in up to 85% of newborn infants. Bohn's nodules most likely develop from epithelial remnants of salivary gland tissue or from remnants of the dental lamina. However, some authors refute this idea because mucinous glands are rarely found on the lateral surfaces of the alveolar ridges. Therapy for Bohn's nodules is unnecessary as spontaneous involution or shedding is the rule. Sometime the lesions are very prominent and the diagnosis is difficult.[71,72]

ERUPTION CYSTS

An eruption cyst (or eruption hematoma) is a circumscribed fluctuant swelling, which develops over the site of an erupting tooth. Lesions in the newborn may occur secondary to natal or neonatal teeth, but these cysts are more commonly associated with the eruption of deciduous or permanent teeth. Eruption cysts most commonly develop on the alveolar ridge of the maxilla or mandible. Size varies with the type of tooth overlaid, but most lesions are approximately 0.6cm in diameter. The surface of the cyst may appear flesh-colored or have a bluish-red to blue-black color if the cyst cavity contains blood. Although removal of the tissue overlying the tooth may aid in its eruption, most eruption cysts resolve spontaneously within several weeks without treatment.

Dental lamina cysts

These are rare lesions of the oral cavity of the newborn. In the sixth week *in utero*, a U-shaped thickening, the dental lamina, is present along each alveolar ridge. Small buds of dental lamina form below the surface to become the ectodermal portion of developing teeth. As the enamel and dentine of the tooth buds calcify, the connecting bridge of dental lamina to the overlying epithelium degenerates. Remnants may be trapped in place and later manifest as dental lamina cysts.[73] These rare cysts are found only in the crests of the alveolar ridges. They may be single or multiple, are filled with keratin, and are lined with stratified squamous epithelium.[73]

CONGENITAL RANULA

The congenital ranula is very rare type of mucocele, which results from an obstructed, imperforate, or atretic sublingual or submandibular salivary gland duct.[74] Lesions are found specifically on the anterior floor of the mouth, lateral to the lingual frenulum. The overlying mucosa may be normal in color or have a translucent blue hue. Ranulas do not generally resolve without

71. Larralde de Luna, M (1995) Dermatosis neonatales. In: Dermatologia neonatal y pediatrica, 1 era ed, Larralde de Luna M, ed. Edimed, Bs.As. pp. 8–29.
72. Peters R, Schock RK (1971) Oral cysts in newborn infants. **Oral Surg** 7:10–14.
73. Cohen RL (1984) Clinical perspectives on premature tooth eruption and cyst formation in neonates. **Ped Dermatol** 1:301–306.
74. Steelman R et al. (1998) Congenital ranula. **Clin Pediatr** 37:205–206.

intervention. Although some investigators continue to recommend simple marsupialization with packing,[75] recurrences are frequent. Definitive therapy involves meticulous dissection of the thin wall of the cyst in continuity with the sublingual gland of origin.[76]

CONGENITAL EPULIS

Gingival granular cell tumor (CGCT), also known as congenital epulis (CE) or granular cell epulis of infancy, typically occurs as a tumor of the upper alveolar mucosa in newborns. It is an uncommon, benign lesion of unknown etiology. It usually presents as a pedunculated tumor located on the alveolar ridge, most frequently involving the maxilla.[77,78] It can cause feeding and breathing as well as cosmetic problems. Although the tumor is most often solitary, multiple CE lesions have been reported. There are no associations with other congenital malformations. Females are affected more than males in an 8:1 ratio.[79] The histologic features of CE are distinctive and consist of large polyhedral cells with pale cytoplasm and coarse granules that are PAS-positive and diastase resistant. The nuclei are small and centrally located. These cells are arranged in nests that can infiltrate collagen and skeletal muscle bundles.[80]

The histogenesis of CE remains unclear. There has been some controversy as to whether CE and granular cell tumor are the same or separate entities. However, the hypothesis that CE and granular cell tumor exhibit similar reactivity for macrophage markers was recently accepted: both tumors were reactive with anti-CD68 and KIMIP, and nonreactive with anti-MAC387, antilysozyme, and 3ª5 antibodies.[80] Both show intracytoplasmic staining for fibronectin, laminin, CD49E, neuron-specific enolase (NSE), and vimentin; interstitial cells are positive for S-100 protein. These findings indicate that there could be an alteration in synthesis and secretion of extracellular matrix proteins or a problem with their receptor system.[81]

Since lesions cannot resolve spontaneously, the treatment is by simple excision. Early diagnosis and intervention are important to prevent any destruction of the surrounding structures. Recurrence is uncommon if excision is adequate.

NATAL TEETH

Natal teeth are defined as teeth present at birth. Natal teeth are to be differentiated from neonatal teeth, which erupt during the first month of life. Both may occur in either premature or term infants. The reported incidence of both natal and neonatal teeth varies widely but the conditions are decidedly rare. However, natal teeth occur three times more often than neonatal teeth. Natal teeth are twice as common in females. Two-thirds of natal teeth occur in pairs. The most common location for natal teeth is at the sites of the central mandibular incisors (85%), followed by the maxillary incisors (11%).[73]

Although the exact etiology for natal teeth remains unknown, it appears that the primary tooth bud develops in a more superficial location than normal, and therefore erupts prematurely. Many syndromes have been associated with natal teeth (Table 6.3).

Natal teeth usually represent deciduous rather than supernumerary teeth, which can be distinguished by radiography. Supernumerary teeth are extraneous teeth, which should be extracted, as they may interfere with normal tooth eruption. The lower central incisors are normally the first teeth in the oral cavity to erupt.

Treatment of natal teeth is dependent upon morphology, amount of root development, and mobility. If the tooth is only minimally loose, it will tend

TABLE 6.3   Syndromes associated with natal teeth[16]
Syndrome
◆ Ellis–van Creveld (chondroectodermal dysplasia)
◆ Hallermann–Streiff
◆ Pachyonychia congenita (Jadassohn–Lewandowsky or Jackson–Lawler)
◆ Pallister–Hall (hypothalamic hamartoblastoma)
◆ Weidemann–Rautenstrauch
◆ Natal teeth, patent ductus arteriosus, intestinal pseudo-obstruction

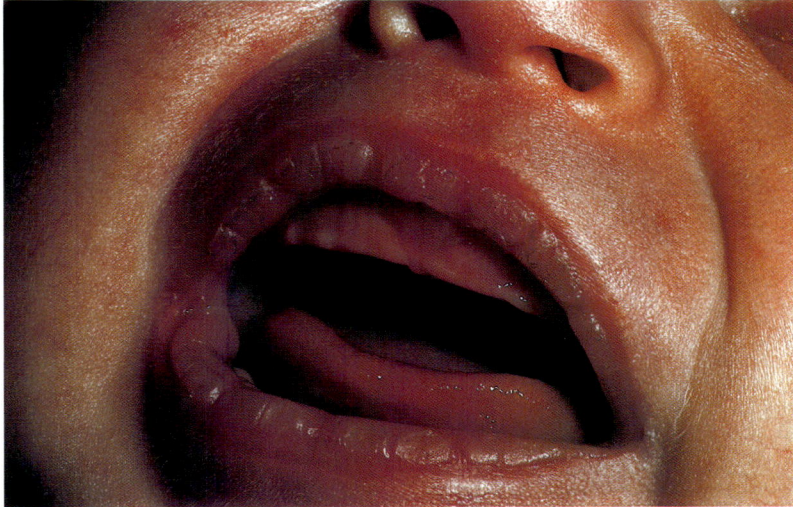

Fig. 6.13   Sucking callus: diffuse pale thickening of vermilion border in a 4-week-old breast-fed infant.

to stabilize over time and can be left in place. Problematic teeth should be extracted to prevent trauma or aspiration.

SUCKING CALLUSES

Sucking calluses (or sucking pads) develop on the lips or buccal mucosa as solitary, oval thickenings or extensive vermilion thickening (Fig. 6.13). When these lesions are congenital, they are indicative of vigorous sucking *in utero*. Presentation after birth is more common in breast-fed, black infants. Histology reveals a thickened epidermis secondary to intracellular edema and hyperkeratosis (leukoedema). Sucking calluses involute spontaneously within a few days or weeks after birth or upon cessation of breast-feeding.

LYMPHATIC MALFORMATIONS

Lymphatic malformations of the alveolar ridge have also been described in neonates and may mimic other cystic lesions.[82] These present as blue-domed and fluid-filled cysts on the alveolar mucosa. They are present in 3.7% of black neonates. Lymphatic malformations may also be seen on lips, buccal

75. Baurmash HD (1992) Marsupialization for treatment of oral ranula: a second look at the procedure. **J Oral Maxillofac Surg** 50:1274.
76. Takimoto T, Ishikawa S, Nishimura T et al. (1989) Fibrin glue in the surgical treatment of ranulas. **Clin Otolaryngol** 14:429.
77. Zuker RM et al. (1993) Congenital epulis: review of the literature and case report. **J Oral Maxillofac Surg** 51:1040–1043.
78. Larralde de Luna M, Santos Muñoz A, Martin de Kramer N et al. (1998) Gingival tumor in a newborn. **Pediatr Dermatol** 15:318–320.

79. Junquera LM et al. (1997) Granular-cell tumours: an immunohistochemical study. **Br J Oral Maxillofac Surg** 35:180–184.
80. Billeret-Lebranchu V, Martin de la Salle E, Vandenhaute B et al. (1999) Granular cell tumor and congenital epulis. Histochemical and immunohistochemical study of 58 cases. **Arch Anat Cytol Pathol** 47:31–37.
81. Lapid O, Shaco Levy R, Krieger J et al. (2001) Congenital epulis. **Pediatrics** 107:1–3.
82. Levin LS, Jorgenson RJ, Jarvey BA (1976) Lymphangiomas of the alveolar ridges in neonates. **Pediatrics** 58:881.

mucosa, and palate, and have been described on the floor of the mouth in continuity with cervical lymphatic malformations.[83,84] They also occur on the tongue, causing macroglossia. Airway compromise can occur with these larger malformations, as well as disfigurement of the maxilla and mandible.[85]

MUCOCOELES OR SALIVARY RETENTION CYSTS

These can occasionally be found in the oral cavity or on the lower lip of the newborn. They result from extravasation or retention of salivary gland contents (see Chapter 9).[84]

Median alveolar notch is a midline notch in the upper alveolar ridge seen in many neonates. This has been reported in 26% of black infants and in 12% of white infants.[85] The tectolabial frenulum is a soft connective tissue structure in the anterior midline of the maxillary arch in continuity with the labial frenulum. When pronounced, this frenulum causes a fissure in the alveolus, producing the median alveolar notch. As teeth erupt, the connective tissue septum and frenular plate ordinarily resorb, and the notch is reduced in size. Occasionally, the notch persists and may contribute to a space between the central incisors.[86]

OTHER DISORDERS

SUCKING BLISTERS AND EROSIONS

Sucking blisters, erosions, or calluses are present at birth, usually located on the fingers, wrists or forearms (Fig. 6.14).[86,87] The primary lesion is a tense vesicle or bulla on noninflamed skin, though erosions may result from blister rupture. Calluses may be seen from chronic sucking. These lesions appear to be the result of vigorous sucking *in utero*.[87] They spontaneously resolve without sequelae, usually by two weeks of life.[88] These erosions and blisters may be confused with more serious diseases in the newborn, such as herpes simplex, bullous impetigo, bullous mastocytosis, or epidermolysis bullosa. The focal presentation, characteristic morphology, and failure to develop other blisters during the first few days of life should allow correct diagnosis.

SEBACEOUS GLAND HYPERPLASIA

Sebaceous gland hyperplasia occurs in more than 50% of term newborns and less commonly in preterm infants.[89,90] Multiple, pinpoint, white-yellowish papules are seen at the opening of each pilosebaceous follicle in areas in which sebaceous glands are abundant, such as the nose (Fig. 6.15), cheeks, upper lip and forehead. There is no surrounding redness.

Sebaceous hyperplasia results from the influences of maternal androgens on the pilosebaceous follicle. This stimulation occurs during the final month of gestation resulting in an increase in sebaceous cell number and volume.[91] Biopsy of these lesions reveals large sebaceous glands with prominent secretory cells surrounding the pilosebaceous follicles. Milia papules, which are inclusion cysts, are differentiable as they are often solitary, discrete, and whiter in color. Milia may accompany sebaceous gland hyperplasia in approximately half of affected infants.

No treatment is necessary for sebaceous hyperplasia. Lesions resolve spontaneously in the first few months of life.

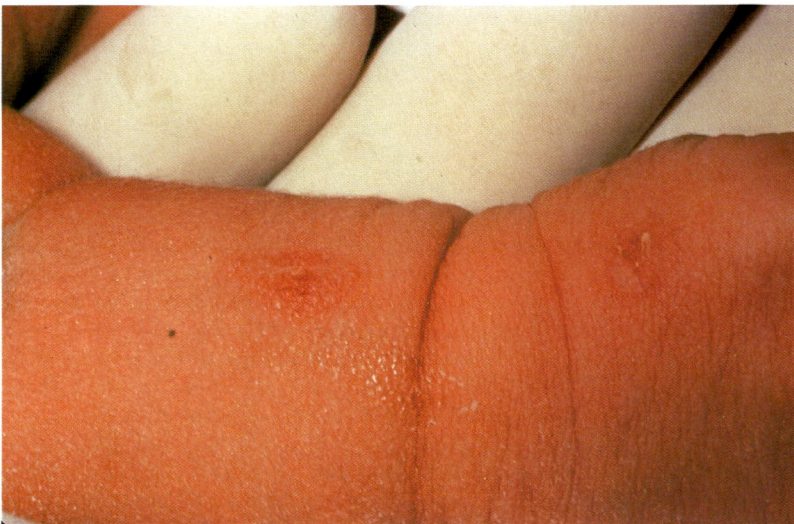

Fig. 6.14   Sucking blisters: two erosions (wrist and base of thumb) in a well, full-term newborn.

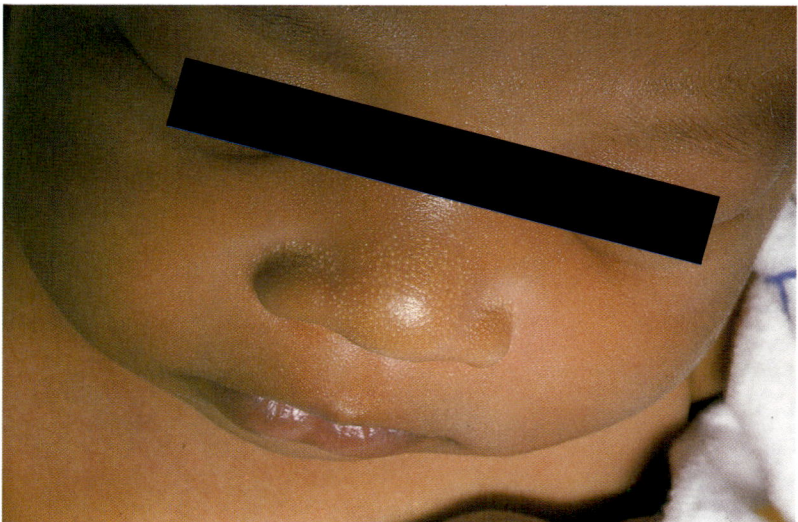

Fig. 6.15   Sebaceous gland hyperplasia: yellowish closely set nasal papules in a neonate.

MILIA

Milia are tiny inclusion cysts commonly found on the face and scalp skin of newborns. These white, pearly, firm 1–2mm globular papules occur prominently on the nose, cheeks, chin and foreheads in 40% of term newborns.[92,93] The number of milia present can vary from a few to a few hundred. Larger, solitary lesions can be seen on the foreskin, areolae, scrotum, and labia majora. Lesions may appear at birth or in later infancy, but usually appear and disappear spon-

83. Ikemura K, Hidaka H, Fujiwara I et al. (1987) A case of cystic lymphangioma extending from the neck to the tongue. Management of the lesion remaining after surgery. **J Craniomaxillofac Surg** 15:369.
84. Jasper RD, Goldberg MH, Zborowski RG (1989) Lymphangioma and cystic hygroma. Correction of facial growth disharmony and obstructive sleep. **Int J Oral Maxillofac Surg** 18:152.
85. Bodner L, Tal H (1991) Salivary gland cysts of the oral cavity: clinical observation and surgical management. **Compendium** 12:150.
86. Jorgenson RJ, Shapiro SD, Salinas CF et al. (1982) Intraoral findings and anomalies in neonates. **Pediatr** 69:577.
87. Murphy WF, Langley AL (1963) Common bullous lesions – presumably self-inflicted – occurring in utero in the newborn infant. **Pediatrics** 32:1099.

88. Lucky AW (2001) Transient benign cutaneous lesions in the newborn. In: Eichenfield LF, Frieden IJ, Esterly NB, eds. Philadelphia, PA: WB Saunders, pp. 88–102.
89. Rivers JK, Frederiksen PC, Dibdin C (1990) A prevalence survey of dermatoses in the Australian neonate. **J Am Acad Dermatol** 23:77–81.
90. Nanda A, Kaur S, Bhakoo ON, Dhall K (1989) Survey of cutaneous lesions in indian newborns. **Pediatr Dermatol** 6:39–42.
91. Holbrook KA, Smith LT (1981) Ultrastructural aspects of human skin during the embryonic, fetal, premature, neonatal and adult periods of life. **Birth Defects** 1:9.
92. Lucky AW (2001) Transient benign cutaneous lesions in the newborn. In Eichenfield LF, Frieden IJ, Esterly NB, eds. WB Saunders Company. Philadelphia, PA. 88–102.
93. Gordon I (1949) Miliary sebaceous cysts and blisters in the healthy newborn. **Arch Dis Child** 24:286.

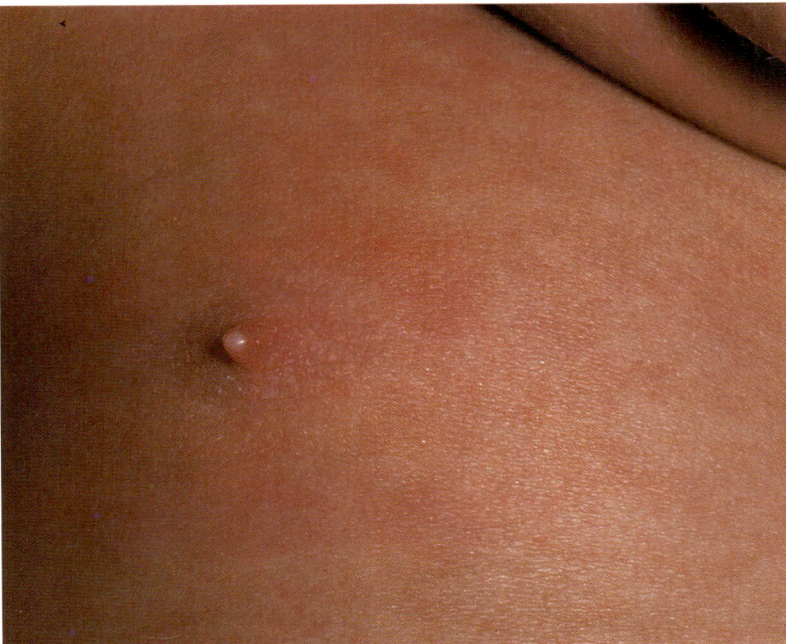

Fig. 6.16   Milium: isolated truncal lesion in a 4-week infant.

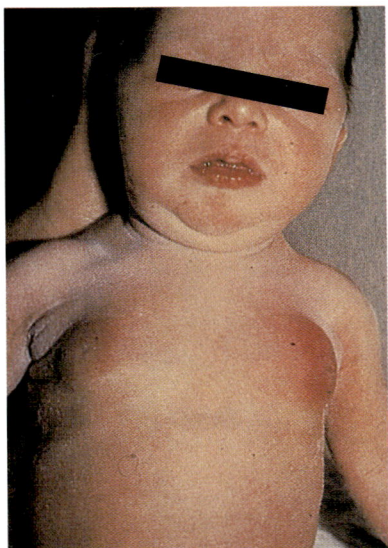

Fig. 6.17   Neonatal mastitis.

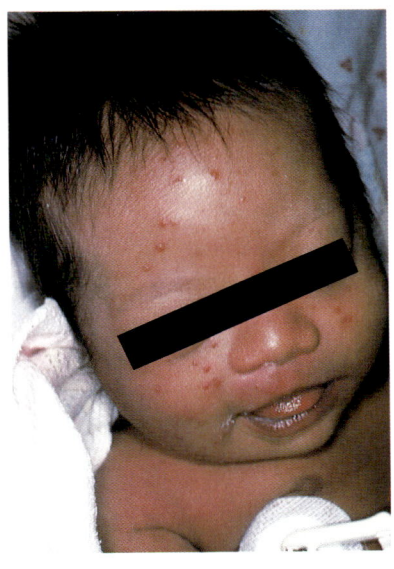

Fig. 6.18   Neonatal acne/cephalic pustulosis.

taneously during the first month (Fig. 6.16). In some cases, milia may persist for several months.

The tiny epidermal inclusion cysts originate from the pilosebaceous apparatus of vellus hair, and contain concentric layers of keratinized stratum corneum. Secondary milia may appear after trauma and may originate from epithelial structures such as sweat ducts, hair follicles, or sebaceous ducts. Milia are numerous and persistent in several syndromes, such as junctional and dystrophic epidermolysis bullosa, oral-facial-digital syndrome (type I),[94] pachyonychia congenital and hereditary trichodysplasia (Marie Unna hypotrichosis). Milia generally resolve spontaneously over several weeks to months. Incision and expression of keratinous contents is rarely necessary.

MATERNAL AND PLACENTAL HORMONAL EFFECTS – "MINIATURE PUBERTY" OF THE NEWBORN

A number of phenomena occur during the newborn period as a result of the influence of placental and maternal hormones. These have been collectively called "miniature puberty of the newborn." Hyperpigmentation of the linea alba (linea nigra), scrotum, and external genitalia is frequent and pronounced in dark-skinned newborns. Female genitalia may appear swollen, with an enlarged clitoris. A whitish, creamy vaginal discharge, indistinguishable on vaginal smear from that of a pregnant woman, is common. Within days of birth, desquamation of the hyperplastic vaginal mucosa occurs, leaving a more normal infantile mucosa. Rarely, frank withdrawal bleeding may occur on the third or fourth day of life, lasting several days as a "miniature menses."

Male genitalia appear similarly enlarged and well developed during the newborn period, and both males and females can undergo hypertrophy of the mammary glands. Palpable breast tissue hypertrophy is typical of term infants and is used as a measure of gestational maturity in the neonatal Dubowitz scale. The engorged breast tissue can secrete a colostrum-like substance termed "witches milk" late during the first week of life. This swelling subsides rapidly and is gone by the end of the first month.

Infrequently, stagnant milk in the breast of infants can become infected leading to mastitis or abscess formation (Fig. 6.17). Staphylococcus aureus is the usual infecting agent. The bacteria are thought to enter the breast tissue through the hypertrophied ducts. Abscess formation is heralded by the development of redness, swelling, and fluctuance in one breast from 5 to 20 days after birth. Fever is rare, but systemic antibiotic therapy in this setting is indicated, since unrecognized infection can lead to bacterial sepsis.[95]

Neonatal acne (Fig. 6.18) and perhaps malassezia colonization, associated with neonatal cephalic pustulosis may also be influenced by maternal and fetal hormones.[96]

CONGENITAL INGROWN TOENAILS

Due to the relative hypoplasia of the nail plates, especially noticeable on the toes, embedding of the distal free margin of the nail plate into the hyponychium is not uncommon.[97] The bulbous distal phalanx surrounding a diminutive nail plate gives the impression of an ingrown toenail. Most neonatal nails grow out normally without discomfort during the first year of

94. Larralde de Luna M, Raspa ML, Ibargoyen J (1992) Oral-Facial-Digital Type 1 Syndrome of Papillon-Leage and Psaume. **Pediatr Dermatol** 9:52–56.
95. Rudoy RC Nelson JD (1975) Breast abscess during the neonatal period. A review. **Am J Dis Child** 129:1031.
96. Bergman JN, Eichenfield LF (2002) Neonatal acne and cephalic pustulosis: is malassezia the whole story? **Arch Dermatol** 138:255–7.
97. Honig PJ, Spitzer A, Bernstein R, Leyden JJ (1982) Congenital ingrown toenails. **Clin Pediatr** 21:424–426.

life and assume the more typical childhood appearance. Conditions to be distinguished from this common finding are congenital hypertrophy of the lateral hallux nailfolds, which presents with firm, red tissue masses, and congenital malalignment of the great toe nails, which appears with a trapezoid-shaped nail plate with lateral deviation (see also Chapter 12).[98]

BIRTHMARKS

Most birthmarks are collections of highly differentiated cells of one or more of the normal components of the skin. Any of the skin elements can produce a birthmark: melanocytes, blood vessels, lymphatics, the epidermis, sebaceous glands, hair follicles, connective tissue, collagen, elastin, and smooth muscle. The congenital malformations produced by these tissue components vary in frequency and importance. Some are associated with an increased incidence of malignancy. Some are cutaneous hallmarks of congenital syndromes. Some improve or disappear with age; most are persistent with a predictable evolution. Some can be disfiguring. This section outlines the most common birthmarks seen in the neonatal period. Readers are referred to the various chapters listed for a more in-depth discussion of these entities.

Recent studies have shown that birthmarks are extremely common, occurring in more than 99% of newborns.[99–101] The most frequently observed birthmark is the telangiectatic nevus, or salmon patch, present in 60–70% of all infants. Oriental and black babies have an even higher frequency of mongolian spots, (91% and 80%, respectively). These two skin lesions are 100 times more common than all other birthmarks. They are so common that they are frequently overlooked by parents and caregivers.

Several important syndromes are associated with vascular anomalies, including capillary malformations (port-wine stains).[102,103] Sturge–Weber syndrome occurs in 8% of patients with facial capillary malformations, specifically when staining is in the distribution of the ophthalmic (first) branch of the trigeminal (fifth cranial) nerve. Bilateral staining in this distribution or involvement of the upper eyelids is strongly associated with this syndrome.[102] In Sturge–Weber syndrome, associated ocular and intracranial vascular anomalies can produce seizures, mental retardation, and glaucoma. Vascular anomalies are discussed in Chapter 20.

HYPERPIGMENTED BIRTHMARKS

Hyperpigmented lesions are commonly present at birth. The most common hyperpigmented birthmarks are presented in Tables 6.4A–6.6. Skin hyperpigmentation in the neonate can result from the accumulation of melanin in melanocytes or keratinocytes, the presence of nevus cells in the epidermis or dermis, from incontinence of melanin or melanin in macrophages in the dermis, or from a thickened hyperplastic epidermis. Some lesions are frequently seen in newborns and are of little significance, such as Mongolian spots, while others may be associated with systemic diseases and genetic syndromes. Some lesions with specific neonatal aspects are discussed below; many other hyperpigmented birthmarks are discussed as distinct entities in other chapters (see also Chapter 10).

Mongolian spots

The Mongolian spot is a brownish, blue-gray or blue-black patch usually located over the sacrogluteal area. It is the most common of all birthmarks in pigmented races, being present at birth in 91% of Orientals, 80% of blacks and 46% of Hispanics but occurring in only 10% of white infants.[104–107] The sacrogluteal area is most often affected, though lesions may occur also on the dorsal trunk and extremities and even the scalp (Fig. 6.19).[108] Typically, the irregular patch increases in size over the first year of life and then fades in early childhood. A small percentage (3–4%) persist beyond age 5.[106]

Deep elongated, spindle shaped dermal melanocytes scattered between collagen bundles are evident on histological specimens. The blue color results from the absorption pattern of dermal melanin. The pathogenesis of the Mongolian spot is not well understood. It is thought that arrest of melanocyte migration from the neural crest to the skin during fetal life may be responsible for these lesions. It is not known why these lesions resolve or why there is a predisposition to the development of these patches in the sacrogluteal area. There are no known extracutaneous findings. They may be associated with with capillary malformations in phakomatosis pigmentovascularis, and extensive atypical Mongolian spots may be seen with GM1 gangliosidosis[109] and Hunter syndrome.[110]

Café-au-lait spots

Café-au-lait spots are light brown, oval macules with distinct margins ranging in size from a few millimeters to 20 centimeters in diameter. They are present in 0.3–18% of all newborns, with racial and ethnic variation.[111,112] Café-au-lait macules may be present at birth or develop in the first few months of life, and may increase in number and size with age.[113] They may be present anywhere on the body and grow commensurate with the child. In neonates, some flat congenital nevi may be indistinguishable from café-au-lait macules, though clinical differentiation is obvious with time. On biopsy, café-au-lait macules have increased melanin in both melanocytes and keratinocytes, without melanocytic proliferation, readily distinguishing them from melanocytic nevi. Most children with these lesions have no other associated abnormalities. However, the presence of multiple larger hyperpigmented macules and patches should alert the clinician to the possibility of several syndromes associated with café-au-lait spots, most commonly neurofibromatosis type I.[113–115] The presence of five or more café-au-lait spots greater than 5mm at 5 years is suggestive of this disease. Large unilateral café-au-lait spots with irregular borders (coast of Maine) that usually do not cross the midline are typical of McCune–Albright syndrome. These patients have fewer, larger, darker café-au-lait spots, in addition to polyostotic fibrous dysplasia of the bones, precocious puberty, and multiple endocrine abnormalities.

Congenital melanocytic nevi

Congenital melanocytic nevi are proliferations of nested melanocytes present at birth or appearing in the first few months of life. They occur in 1% of newborns, and may range in size from a few millimeters to greater than

98. Silverman RA (2001) Nail Defects. In: Textbook of Neonatal Dermatology. Eichenfield LF, Frieden IJ, Esterly NB, eds. WB Saunders Company. Philadelphia, PA, 504–516.
99. Dohil MA, Baugh WP, Eichenfield LF (2000) Vascular and pigmented birthmarks. **Pediatr Clin North Am** 47:783–812.
100. Mallory SB (1991) Neonatal skin disorders. **Pediatr Clin North Am** 38:745.
101. Alper JC, Holmes LB (1983) The incidence and significance of birthmarks in a cohort of 4,641 newborns. **Pediatr Dermatol** 1:58.
102. Tallman B (1991) Location of port-wine stain and the likelihood of ophthalmologic or CNS complications. **Pediatrics** 87:323.
103. Silverman RA (1991) Hemangiomas and vascular malformations. **Pediatr Clin North Am** 38:811.
104. Mallory SB (1991) Neonatal skin disorders. **Pediatr Clin North Am** 38:745.
105. Alper JC, Holmes LB (1983) The incidence and significance of birthmarks in a cohort of 4,641 newborns. **Pediatr Dermatol** 1:58.
106. Cordova A (1981) The Mongloian spot. **Clin Pediatr** 20:714.
107. Leung AK (1988) Mongolian spots in Chinese children. **Int J Dermatol** 27:106.
108. Leung AKC, Kao CP (1999) Extensive Mongolian spots with involvement of the scalp. **Pediatr Dermatol** 16:371.

109. Tang TT, Esterly NB, Lubinsky MS et al. (1993) GM1-gangliosidosis type 1 involving the cutaneous vascular endothelial cells in a black infant with multiple ectopic Mongolian spots. **Acta Derm Venereol** 73:412–415.
110. Sapadin AN, Friedman IS (1998) Extensive Mongolian spots associated with Hunter syndrome. **J Am Acad Dermatol** 39:1013–1014.
111. Alper J, Holmes LB, Mihm MC Jr. (1979) Birthmarks with serious medical significance: nevocellular nevi, sebaceous nevi, and multiple café-au lait spots. **J Pediatr** 95:696.
112. Alper JC, Holmes LB (1983) The incidence and significance of birthmarks in a cohort of 4,641 newborns. **Pediatr Dermatol** 1:58.
113. Landau M, Krafchik B (1999) The diagnostic value of café-au-lait macules. **J Amer Acad Dermatol** 40:877–890.
114. Crowe FW, Schull WJ (1993) Diagnostic importance of cafe-au-lait spots in neurofibromatosis. **Arch Intern Med** 91:758–766.
115. Korf BR (1992) Diagnostic outcome in children with multiple cafe au lait spots. **Pediatrics** 90:924–927.

TABLE 6.4A   Hyperpigmented birthmarks by description

Description of lesions		Location	Possible diagnoses
Blue-gray/blue-black patches	Dermal melanocytosis	Torso Face Shoulder/neck Torso, in association with port-wine stain	Mongolian spot Nevus of Ota Nevus of Ito Phakomatosis pigmentovascularis
Labial macules	Involving mucosa	Perioral More widespread facial	Peutz–Jeghers syndrome Carney syndrome
	More widespread, not involving mucosa	Face/trunk	LEOPARD syndrome
	Central face, not involving mucosa	Face	Carney syndrome Centrofacial lentiginosis
Brown sharply-defined patches or plaques	Patch		Congenital nevus Café-au-lait macule
	Plaque		Congenital nevus
Small brown macules		Perioral/mucosal Widespread, non mucosal	Peutz–Jeghers syndrome LEOPARD syndrome Generalized lentiginosis Inherited patterned lentiginosis Carney syndrome
		Central face/widespread Involves mucosa Axilla/groin/neck only Central face only, not mucosa Clustered in a defined body area or segment. Background skin color normal Clustered in a defined body area or segment. Background skin color darker Single	Carney syndrome Neurofibromatosis Centrofacial lentiginosis Segmental lentiginosis Mosaicism Speckled lentiginous nevus Nevus spilus Congenital nevus
Linear hyperpigmentation in swirled or Blaschko pattern		Flat	Linear and whorled nevoid hyperpigmentation[1,2] Epidermal nevus Incontinentia pigmenti Goltz syndrome Conradi–Hünermann syndrome Mosaicism
		Raised	Epidermal nevus Incontinentia pigmenti

[1] Harre J, Millikan LE, Linear and Whorled Pigmentation. *Intern J Dermatol* 33: 529–537, 1994.
[2] Nehal KS, PeBenito R, Orlow SJ, Analysis of 54 cases of hypopigmentation and hyperpigmentation along the lines of Blaschko. *Arch Dermatol* 132: 1167–1170, 1996.

20 centimeters, termed large or giant nevi.[116,117] Congenital nevi may be tan or brown plaques, papules or nodules. Nevus cells at the dermo–epidermal junction produce dark brown or black regularly bordered macules. Raised nevi result from dermal nevus cells and are more common in black neonates.

Large or giant congenital nevi may involve large segments of the trunk (garment type) scalp, or extremities, and numerous satellite lesions distinct from the main nevus are common. Hair may be present or develop within congenital nevi, and its presence or absence has no impact on the development of malignancy. Lesions overlying the spinal column and multiple lesions can have significant associations including spinal dysraphism, leptomeningeal melanosis, posterior cranial fossa malformations and hydrocephalus. Giant nevi may be severely disfiguring and have a risk as well of malignant change. Smaller congenital nevi are associated with a much lower risk of melanoma, especially in the prepubertal period.

Nevus of Ota and Ito

The nevus of Ota is a blue-gray or gray-brown patch in the distribution of the ophthalmic or maxillary branches of the facial nerve. It is usually unilateral, and ipsilateral scleral pigmentation is common. Approximately one-half of these lesions present at birth with presentation around puberty for the remainder. There is female predominance (75%), and they are more common in black and Asian infants.[118] The nevus of Ito is a similar-appearing hyperpigmented patch of the trunk. It is commonly unilateral over the scapula or deltoid region, in the approximate distribution of the posterior supraclavicular and lateral brachial cutaneous nerves.[118] Both lesions are similar to Mongolian spots, with histologic findings of dermal melanocytosis. While the pathogenesis is considered to be similar to Mongolian spots, related to a defect in neural crest cells embryogenesis, these patches do not involute with time. Nevus of Ota has been associated with glaucoma secondary to melanocytes

116. Walton RG, Jacobs AH, Cox A (1976) Pigmented lesions in newborn infants. **Br J Dermatol** 95:389.
117. Eichenfield LF and Gibbs NF (2001) Hyperpigmented disorders. In: Textbook of Neonatal Dermatology, Eichenfield LF, Frieden IJ, Esterly NB, eds. Philadelphia, PA: WB Saunders, pp. 370–394.
118. Mishima Y, Mevorah B (1961) Nevus of Ota and nevus of Ito in American Negroes. **J Invest Dermatol** 36:133.

TABLE 6.4B   Hyperpigmented birthmarks by diagnosis

Association	Shape	Location	Color	Size	Frequency	Features	Associations
Café-au-lait macule	Round or oval	Trunk, extremities	Tan	2–20mm	1.9% (12% blacks)	Increased epidermal melanin, enlarge in proportion to body growth. Histology: No surface change	Neurofibromatosis (coast of Cal), Albright's (coast of Maine, respect midline), Watson's, Ring chromosome 2
Congenital nevus	Oval or irregular; large nevi have satellite lesions; flat or raised	Tan to dark brown irregular pigmentation	All	Variable	1%	May have hypertrichosis or verrucous surface; may darken with age. Histology: nevus cells may infiltrate appendageal structures	Melanoma risk; vertebral column defects; neurocutaneous melanocytosis
Mongolian spot	Irregular patch	Sacrogluteal location or posterior trunk	Blue-green or blue-gray	2–10cm	96% blacks; 10% whites	<90% resolve by age 4 years. Histology: deep dermal melanocytes	Extensive atypical MS with GM1 gangliosidosis and Hunter syndrome
Nevus spilus	Round	Trunk, proximal extremities	Light brown patch may contain or acquire dark brown macules	5mm–>10cm	Unknown	Speckled appearance. Histology: lentigo with junctional nevi	Rare melanoma
Nevus of Ito or Ota	Irregular	Ito: supraclavicular or scapular blue brown Ota: periocular	Blue brown	1–>10cm	More common in Asians and blacks	May follow the lines of Blaschko on trunk; may be acquired after birth, 75% females. Histology: dermal melanocytes	Glaucoma and melanoma reported in nevus of Ota
Nevoid hyper-melanosis (mosaic hyper-pig-mentation)	Swirls that follow Blaschko's lines	Segmental may be widespread: asymmetric	Speckled light brown	10–20cm	Relatively common	Sharp midline cutoff and pattern. Histology: basilar hyperpigmentation	Chromosomal mosaicism
Congenital smooth muscle hamartoma	Oval	Trunk and extremities	Skin-colored to tan	3–10cm	Rare	Increased vellus or terminal hair. Histology: hyperplasia of smooth muscle bundles	None
Epidermal nevus	Oval or linear; raised	Trunk and extremities in Blaschko's lines	Hyper-pigmented or skin colored	2–3cm	<1	Velvety or verrucous surface. Histology: hyperkeratosis, acanthosis, papillomatosis	Extensive forms associated with epidermal nevus syndrome: CNS, ocular, skeletal, cardiovascular and skin malformations possible
Lentigo	Round or oval	All locations	Medium brown	2–3mm	Common	Histology: lentiginous hyperplasia	Multiple lentigines associated with some congenital syndromes (see Tables 6.6, 6.7)
Plexiform neurofibroma	Irregular	Trunk and extremities	Tan or skin colored	5–>20cm	Rare	Doughy consistency on palpitation. Histology: basilar hyperpigmentation overlying spindle cell tumor	Nearly diagnostic of neurofibromatosis; association with hypertrophy of underlying tissue; rare development of neurofibrosarcoma
Post-inflammatory[a] hyper-pigmentation	Poorly marginated	All locations	Tan to dark brown	Variable	Very common	Sites of previous inflammation, complete resolution occurs. Histology: incontinent pigment	Seen intrauterine transient neonatal pustular melanosis

[a] Although this may present at birth, it is acquired and not a true birthmark.

TABLE 6.5   Syndromes associated with café-au-lait spots

Strong association
Neurofibromatosis
Ring chromosome Type I and II
McCune–Albright syndrome

Less strong association
Bloom syndrome
Ataxia telangiectasia
Fanconi anemia
Russell–Silver syndrome
Watson syndrome
Jaffe–Campanacci syndrome
Basal cell nevus syndrome
Gaucher disease
Turner syndrome
Hunter syndrome

TABLE 6.6   Syndromes associated with multiple lentigines

Syndrome	Features
LEOPARD	Lentigines, ECG abnormalities, ocular hypotelorism, pulmonic stenosis, abnormal genitalia, growth retardation, deafness (LEOPARD)
Peutz–Jegher	Periorificial, mucosal, and acral lentigines; gastrointestinal polyposis
Carney[a]	Myxomas, spotty pigmentation, endocrine hyperactivity
NAME[a]	Nevi, atrial myxomas, myxoid neurofibromas, ephelides (NAME)
LAMB[a]	Lentigines, atrial myxomas, mucocutaneous myxomas, blue nevi (LAMB)
Xeroderma pigmentosa	Lentigines, basal cell CA, squamous cell CA, melanoma, UV light sensitivity

[a] NAME and LAMB syndromes are now considered variants of Carney syndrome.

in the ciliary body of the anterior chamber of the eye,[119] and there are rare reports of melanoma within a nevus of Ota.[120]

Nevoid hypermelanosis and segmental hyperpigmentation

Macular hyperpigmentation that presents in a segmental pattern, or a whorled pattern following the lines of Blaschko may be considered a physical representation of mosaicism.[121] This may be an isolated cutaneous condition, or be part of a more significant genetic disease. Linear and whorled nevoid hypermelanosis is a term that has been used to describe asymmetric hyperpigmented patches occurring in streaky configurations along Blaschko's lines.[122,123] The onset of lesions is usually during the first few weeks of life with no preceding inflammation. Pigmentation gradually spreads until the second year of life, when it stabilizes, occasionally becoming less prominent with time.

In many infants with lentiginous hyperpigmentation, the pattern does not display well-developed whorls and swirls of Blaschko's lines. Lesions may be segmental, discontinuous, cross the midline, and there are speckles as well as areas of more homogeneous pigmentation.

Other conditions with segmental hyperpigmented lesions such as incontinentia pigmenti, Conradi–Hünermann syndrome, Goltz syndrome, Naegeli–Franceschetti–Jadassohn syndrome, and linear epidermal nevus should be considered in the differential diagnosis. It may be difficult to separate nevoid hypermelanosis from widespread Blaschko-distributed hypopigmentation.

Postinflammatory hyperpigmentation

Postinflammatory hyperpigmentation is rarely congenital. Some black infants who have transient neonatal pustular melanosis are born with speckled hyperpigmentation resulting from the resolution of intrauterine lesions (Fig. 6.20).[124] These lesions demonstrate pigment incontinence as evidence of previous inflammation.

The intensity of postinflammatory hyperpigmentation depends on racial and genetic factors (i.e., pigmented races have more persistent and intense pigmentation) and on the nature of the inflammatory insult. For example, interface lichenoid inflammatory conditions produce dramatic pigmentation. Any inflammatory insult to the skin that occurs during the neonatal period can produce hyperpigmentation as part of the resolution phase.

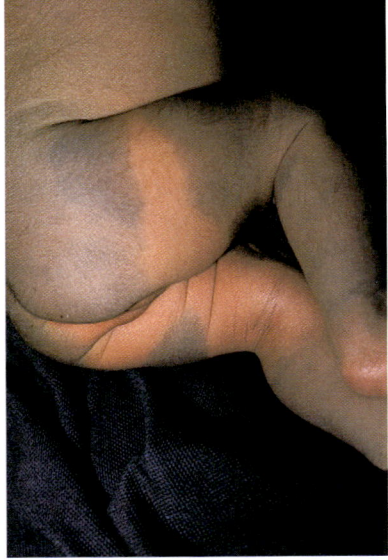

Fig. 6.19   Mongolian spot, extensive in Native American infant.

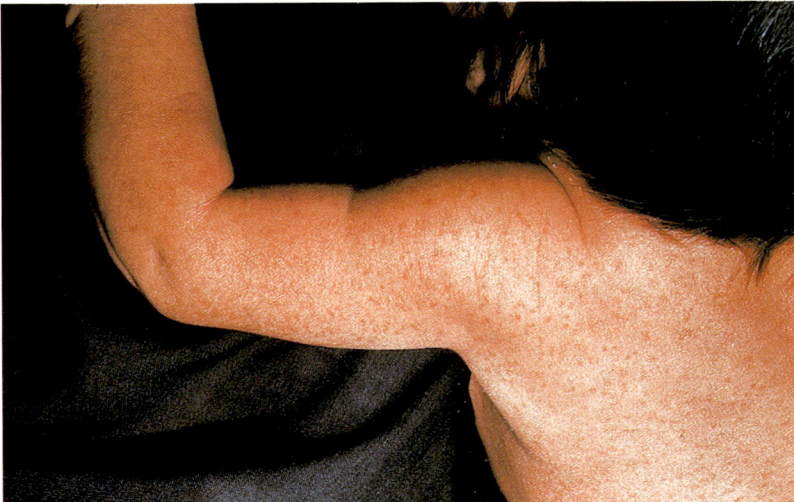

Fig. 6.20   Congenital speckled hyperpigmentation of transient neonatal pustular melanosis (prenatal healing of pustular lesions).

119. Lui JC, Ball SF (1991) Nevus of Ota with glaucoma: report of three cases. **Ann Ophthalmol** 23:286.
120. Shaffer C, Walker K, Weiss GR (1992) Malignant melanoma in a Hispanic male with nevus of Ota. **Dermatology** 1:146.
121. Eichenfield LF, Gibbs NF (2001) Hyperpigmented disorders. In: Textbook of Neonatal Dermatology, Eichenfield LF, Frieden IJ, Esterly NB, eds. Philadelphia, PA: WB Saunders, 370–394.
122. Kalter DC, Griffiths WA, Atherton DJ (1988) Linear and whorled nevoid hypermelanosis. **J Am Acad Dermatol** 19:1037–1044.
123. Alvarez J, Peteiro C, Toribio J (1993) Linear and whorled nevoid hypermelanosis. **Pediatr Dermatol** 10:156–158.
124. Ramamurthy RS, Riveri M, Esterly NB et al. (1979) Transient neonatal pustular melanosis. **J Pediatr** 88:636.

Other congenital lesions that can appear hyperpigmented include epidermal nevi, congenital smooth muscle hamartoma, and plexiform neurofibromas (Table 6.4B).

HYPOPIGMENTED BIRTHMARKS

Although less common than hyperpigmented birthmarks, a number of hypopigmented lesions present in the newborn period. These are listed in Table 6.7. In addition to these, more generalized hypopigmentation can occur at birth in a variety of congenital syndromes. These are listed in Table 6.8 (for a more detailed discussion see Ch. 10). Some specific neonatal conditions are highlighted below.

Nevus depigmentosus, nevoid hypomelanosis, hypomelanosis of Ito

The term nevus depigmentosus or achromic nevus is often used for a congenital well-circumscribed, oval or irregularly shaped, solitary, hypopigmented patch that usually does not cross the midline. The term "depigmentosus" is, in fact, a misnomer, as the lesions are actually hypopigmented rather than depigmented. Nevus depigmentosus lesions are usually located on the trunk or proximal extremities. These lesions do not involute but grow commensurate with the patient.[125] Skin is normal on histologic examination, but electron microscopic examination demonstrates a defect in transfer of pigment between the melanocyte and the keratinocyte, producing the hypopigmentation.[126]

Linear lesions with bands or bizarre streaks that resemble splashed paint can occur (Figs 6.7–6.16), often covering large body segments.[127,128] These can clearly be seen to follow the lines of Blaschko, which may not be as evident with the solitary lesions.

These lesions represent cutaneous manifestations of mosaicism. The vast majority of infants with this disorder are otherwise normal but in some cases there are associated abnormalities, in particular ocular, skeletal, or neurological.

The so-called "hypomelanosis of Ito," where there is extensive Blashko-distributed hypopigmentation with multiple systemic associations, was previously thought to be a distinct disease, but is now recognized as a manifestation of a variety of types of mosaicism – chromosomal, genomic and functional X-chromosome – or of chimerism.[129]

Ash leaf spots

Ash leaf spots are 2–12mm hypopigmented macules and patches that classically have a lance-ovate shape. They are usually present at birth and may represent the earliest sign of tuberous sclerosis (TS), though they are more commonly a normal variant in unaffected infants.[130] Ash leaf spots in TS are most commonly located on the trunk and extremities. On the trunk, they are often transversely oriented (Fig. 6.21), whereas on the extremities, the long axis is up and down. Perifollicular pigmentation can be seen within the spots. Once present, they do not change in size or shape with time. Occasionally in TS confetti-like 2–4mm macules are also seen covering the trunk or extremities.

The differential diagnosis of ash leaf spots includes nevus anemicus and nevus depigmentosus. Nevus anemicus can be excluded by diascopy, which obscures the border, or by stroking where no erythema can be elicited within the lesion. Nevus depigmentosus may be indistinguishable

---

TABLE 6.7 **Hypopigmented birthmarks**

Type	Shape	Location	Frequency	Size	Distinguishing features	Important association
Ash leaf macule	Lance ovate	Trunk or extremities	Rare	1–3cm	>1 lesion at birth is concerning for tuberous sclerosis	Present at birth in 70–90% of patients with tuberous sclerosis
Nevus depigmentosus, nevoid hypopigmentation, hypomelanosis of Ito (mosaic hypopigmentation)	Blaschko-distributed	Trunk or extremities	Uncommon	Small and localized to very extensive	Splashed paint appearance; hypopigmented not depigmented	Association, when extensive, with mental retardation, seizures, skeletal asymmetry and ocular abnormalities
Piebaldism	Poorly defined patches, containing macules of normally pigmented skin	Trunk, extremities, spares hands and feet	1/20 000	Variable	White forelock; depigmentation	Woolf syndrome: neurologic deficits with piebaldism. Waardenburg syndrome: heterochromia of iris, hearing deficit with piebaldism
Nevus anemicus	Sharp margination, may be surrounding vasodilation	Trunk	Uncommon	1–3cm	Disappears with blanching does not flare with stroking; no reflex vasodilation after cold	None
Postinflammatory hypopigmentation[a]	Variable, poorly defined	All	Common	Variable	Sites of previous inflammation; complete resolution with time	None

[a] Although this may be present shortly after birth, it is acquired and is not a true birthmark.

---

125. Pinto FJ, Bolognia JL (1991) Disorders of hypopigmentation in children. **Pediatr Clin North Am** 38:991.
126. Jimbow K, Fitzpatrick TB, Szabo G et al. (1975) Congenital circumscribed hypomelanosis: a characterization based on electron microscopic study of tuberous sclerosis, nevus depigmentosus and piebaldism. **J Invest Dermatol** 64:50.
127. Harre J, Millikan LE (1994) Linear and whorled pigmentation. **Intern J Dermatol** 33:529–537.
128. Nehal KS, PeBenito R, Orlow SJ (1996) Analysis of 54 cases of hypopigmentation and hyperpigmentation along the lines of Blaschko. **Arch Dermatol** 132:1167–1170.
129. Chitayat D, Friedman JM, Johnston MM (1990) Hypomelanosis of Ito – a nonspecific marker of somatic mosaicism. **Am J Med Genet** 35:422.
130. Vanderhooft SL, Francis JS, Pagon RA et al. (1996) Prevalence of hypopigmented macules in a healthy population. **J Pediatr** 129:355–361.

TABLE 6.8 Syndromes associated with generalized hypopigmentation at birth

Syndrome	Associated findings
Albinism	Strabismus, decreased visual acuity
Hermansky–Pudlak	Bleeding diathesis, visual abnormalities, pulmonary fibrosis, inflammatory bowel disease
Chediak–Higashi	Silver-gray hair, recurrent infection, seizures, pancytopenia, lymphoreticular malignances
Prader–Willi[a]	Neonatal hypotonia, hyperphagia, developmental delay, mental retardation, ocular abnormalities
Angelman[a]	Abnormal facies, developmental delay, mental retardation, neurologic abnormalities, ocular abnormalities
Griscelli	Silver-gray hair, T- and B-cell immunodeficiency, recurrent pyogenic infections, hepatosplenomegaly, neutropenia, thrombocytopenia
Cross	Mental retardation, spastic diplegia, ocular abnormalities
Zyorowski–Margolis syndrome	Heterochromic irides, congenital nerve deafness, mutism

[a] Skin pigment dilution present, not true depigmentation.

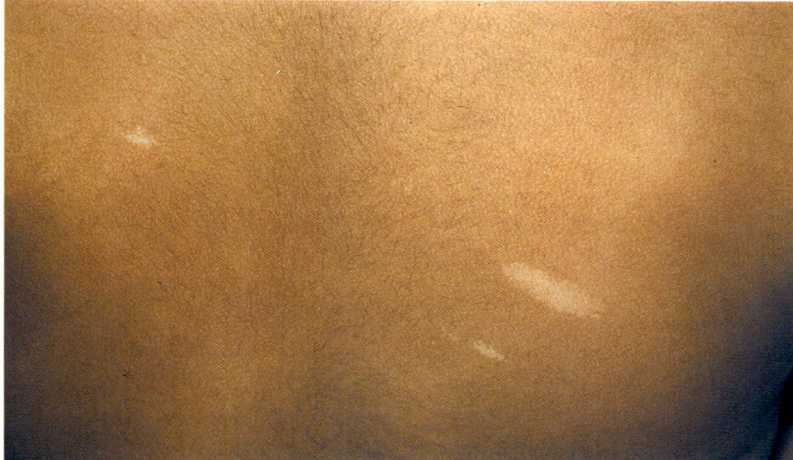

Fig. 6.21 Ash leaf spots on back of an infant with tuberous sclerosis.

from ash leaf spots. One study using electron microscopy demonstrated a decrease in the size of the melanosomes in ash leaf spots compared with nevus depigmentosus.[131] However, there is no consensus on the reliability of this study.

Strong consideration should be given to tuberous sclerosis in infants with three or more hypopigmented macules, even if they are not classic in shape.

A Wood's light examination may reveal subtle areas of pigment loss that are not readily appreciated in ambient light. Examination of the parents and other family members may also aid in the diagnosis, since this autosomal dominant disease can be manifested in asymptomatic individuals as cutaneous signs only.

Piebaldism

Piebaldism is a rare autosomal dominant congenital disorder characterized by a white forelock and large hypopigmented patches over the head, neck, anterior trunk, flanks, and midportion of the extremities. Normally pigmented or hyperpigmented macules are common within or at the lateral edges of the hypopigmented patches. Electron microscopic examination of the hypopigmented areas demonstrates absence of melanocytes.[131] Piebaldism is caused by mutations of the c-KIT gene on chromosome 4q12.[132,133] The c-KIT gene is involved in melanocytic proliferation and mutations impact on tyrosine kinase transmembrane receptors, causing abnormal melanocyte embryogenesis.

Nevus anemicus

Nevus anemicus is a congenital vascular anomaly that appears as a hypopigmented patch at or soon after birth. The affected pale macules are hypersensitive to the effects of vasoconstricting catecholamines.[134] The border of these lesions can be obscured by gentle pressure with a glass slide (diascopy), and rubbing of the skin or heat application causes reflex hyperemia and erythema of the surrounding skin, but not within the lesion.[135,136]

Postinflammatory hypopigmentation

Like postinflammatory hyperpigmentation, postinflammatory hypopigmentation is an acquired disorder. It can present in the newborn period in the aftermath of inflammation, especially in infants with genetically darker pigmentation. Common precursor inflammatory conditions include diaper dermatitis, seborrheic dermatitis, irritant contact dermatitis, and infectious or inflammatory papules.

EPIDERMAL NEVI

Epidermal nevi arise from the embryonic ectoderm which differentiates into both keratinocytes and the cells forming the epidermal appendages. Although epidermal nevi may show a mixture of components,[137] these nevi are best classified according to their predominant component into keratinocytic (non-organoid) nevi and organoid nevi such as sebaceous, follicular, and sweat gland naevi. The general term epidermal nevus is often, however, still used for simplicity.[138] It is now accepted that each type of epidermal nevus represents the cutaneous manifestation of a different mosaic phenotype.[139–141]

Nevus sebaceus

Nevus sebaceous (of Jadassohn) is an organoid epidermal nevus estimated to occur in 0.3% of births.[142] It is always present at birth and is typically a pink-yellow or yellow-orange plaque, frequently recognized as a patch of localized alopecia (Fig. 6.22).[143] It may be smooth, slightly raised, or verrucous. Rarely, pedunculated lesions occur. Multiple small underdeveloped sebaceous glands are almost always present in association with immature hair follicles.[144]

131. Jimbow K, Fitzpatrick TB, Szabo G et al. (1975) Congenital circumscribed hypomelanosis: a characterization based on electron microscopic study of tuberous sclerosis, nevus depigmentosus and piebaldism. J Invest Dermatol 64:50.
132. Spritz RA, Ho L, Strunk KM (1994) Inhibition of proliferation of human melanocytes by a KIT antisense oligodeoxynucleotide: implications for human piebaldism and mouse dominant white spotting (W). J Invest Dermatol 103:148–150.
133. Spritz RA (1997) Piebaldism, Waardenburg syndrome, and related disorders of melanocyte development. Sem Cutan Med Surg 16:15–23.
134. Requena L, Sangueza OP (1997) Cutaneous vascular anomalies. Part I. Hamartomas, malformations, and dilation of preexisting vessels. J Am Acad Dermatol 37:523–549.
135. Mountcastle EA, Distelmeier MR, Lupton GP (1986) Nevus anemicus. J Am Acad Dermatol 14:628.
136. Dohil MA, Baugh WP, Eichenfield LF (2000) Vascular and pigmented birthmarks. Pediatr Clin North Am 47:783–812.

137. Solomon LM, Esterly NB (1975) Epidermal and other congenital organoid nevi. Curr Probl Pediatr 1:3–56.
138. Rogers M (1999) Epidermal naevi. In: Textbook of Pediatric Dermatology, Harper J, Oranje AP, Prose N, eds. Oxford, England: Blackwell Sciences, pp. 955–956.
139. Happle R (1987) Lethal genes surviving by mosaicism: A possible explanation for sporadic birth defects involving the skin. J Am Acad Dermatol 25:550–556.
140. Happle R (1991) How many epidermal nevus syndromes exist? A clinicogenetic classification. J Am Acad Dermatol 25:550–556.
141. Paller AS, Syder AJ, Chan Y-M et al. (1994) Genetic and clinical mosaicism in a type of epidermal nevus. New Engl J Med 331:1408–1415.
142. Alper J, Holmes LB, Mihm MC (1979) Birthmarks with serious medical significance: nevocellular nevi, sebaceous nevi, and multiple cafe au lait spots. J Pediatr 95:696–700.
143. Weng CJ, Tsai YC, Chen TJ (1990) Jadassohn's nevus sebaceous of the head and face. Ann Plast Surg 25:100.
144. Pinkus P (1978) Organoid nevus. Mod Probl Paediatr 20:50.

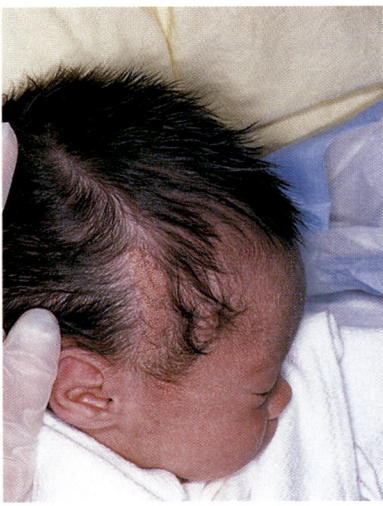

Fig. 6.22 Nevus sebaceous: congenital salmon-colored plaque over temporal scalp of a newborn.

The nevus sebaceus is most commonly an isolated lesion with no extra-cutaneous findings. Large lesions and ones involving the centrofacial area may be associated with other abnormalities including mental retardation and seizures, skeletal abnormalities and ophthalmologic problems including eyelid coloboma and conjunctival lipodermoid.[145–147]

The differential diagnosis includes other causes of focal alopecia. Aplasia cutis congenita displays atrophy, scarring or ulceration at birth, and may display surrounding dark terminal hair. Neural tube defects, meningoceles, encephaloceles, and rests of heterotopic meningeal or brain tissue may also mimic nevus sebaceus.

Nevus comedonicus

Nevus comedonicus is a rare organoid nevus of follicular origin, present at birth in about half of the affected patients. It usually presents as a well-circumscribed group of firm, dark, hyperkeratotic papules with central horny plugs, most commonly on the face, neck, chest, abdomen, or upper arms.[137] Plaques are usually several centimeters in size but more extensive and clearly Blaschko-distributed lesions can be seen.[138,148]

Histology reveals patulous, widely dilated, keratin-filled invaginations of the epidermis with hyperkeratosis and acanthosis and cyst formation. In some cases systemic associations occur including particularly skeletal and ocular.

Differential diagnosis includes nevus sebaceus, acne neonatorum, and grouped comedonal acne.

Non-organoid or keratinocytic epidermal nevus

Keratinocytic nevi occur mainly on the trunk and limbs. They consist of gray, brown, or black verrucous or velvety, Blaschko-distributed lines or plaques.[138]

There is a rarer inflammatory variant that most often involves the lower limb with or without adjacent groin or buttock area.[149,150] Some lesions occur in association with other abnormalities particularly of the skeletal system but occasionally elsewhere. An epidermal nevus may be one feature of Proteus syndrome[151,152] and CHILD syndrome.[153–156]

Congenital smooth muscle hamartoma

Congenital smooth muscle hamartoma is a benign proliferation of smooth muscle within the skin, usually present at birth although often fairly subtle. The estimated prevalence of these lesions is 1:2600 live newborns with a slight male predominance.[157]

Congenital smooth muscle hamartomas present as skin-colored or lightly hyperpigmented patches, or mildly elevated plaques, often with overlying vellus hypertrichosis. They are commonest in the lumbosacral area (67%) or proximal limbs, and may measure several centimeters in diameter.[156] Follicular papules are often present within the plaque.[158,159] Firm rubbing of the lesion may cause fasciculation of the skin or a "gooseflesh-appearance" (pseudo-Darier's sign), due to stimulation of the arrector pili muscles within the tumor. Multiple lesions or linear configurations are rare presentations.[160] There is no associated systemic involvement, except in children with extensive hamartomas as part of the Michelin tire baby syndrome,[161] or risk of malignant transformation.

The histology of smooth muscle hamartoma demonstrates well-defined smooth muscle bundles in the reticular dermis, often associated with hair follicles.

The differential diagnosis can include Becker nevus (and there is some controversy about whether the two conditions are in the same spectrum), congenital melanocytic nevus, plexiform neurofibroma, leiomyoma and solitary mastocytoma (see also Chapter 21).

DEVELOPMENTAL ANOMALIES

A number of errors of fetal embryogenesis result in developmental anomalies that are first recognized during the newborn period. This section discusses the clinical and histologic appearance, pathologic mechanisms, and differential diagnosis of some of the more common abnormalities that result from errors in morphogenesis.

BRANCHIAL CLEFTS AND AURICULAR SINUSES

The development of the branchial system begins in the fourth and fifth embryonic weeks with the formation of four paired pouches in the lateral pharyngeal wall. At the same time four grooves, the pharyngeal or bronchial clefts, appear in direct apposition on the external surface of the embryo.[162,163] In fish and amphibians, these two structures meet to form open communications known as gills, hence the term branchial.[164] However, in the human embryo, only the first cleft and pouch remain in direct approximation,

145. Baker RS, Ross PA, Baumann RJ (1987) Neurologic complications of the epidermal nevus syndrome. **Arch Neurol** 44:227–232.
146. Pavone L, Curatolo P, Rizzo R et al. (1991) Epidermal nevus syndrome: a neurologic variant with hemimegalencephaly, gyral malformation, mental retardation, seizures, and facial hemihypertrophy. **Neurol** 41:266.
147. Palazzi P, Artese O, Paolini A et al. (1996) Linear sebaceous nevus syndrome: report of a patient with unusual associated abnormalities. **Pediatr Dermatol** 13:22–24.
148. Patrizi A, Neri I, Fiorentini C, Marzaduri S (1998) Nevus comedonicus syndrome: a new pediatric case. **Pediatr Dermatol** 15:304–306.
149. de Jong E, Rulo HF, van de Kerkhof PC (1991) Inflammatory linear verrucous epidermal naevus (ILVEN) versus linear psoriasis. A clinical, histologic and immunohistochemical study. **Acta Derm Venereol** (Stockh) 71:343.
150. Lee SH, Rogers M (2001) Inflammatory linear verrucous naevi: a review of 25 cases. **Australas J Dermatol** 42:252–256.
151. Wiedemann HR, Burgio GR, Aldenhoff P et al. (1983) The Proteus syndrome. **Eur J Pediatr** 140:5–12.
152. Biesecker LG, Happle R, Mulliken JB et al. (1999) Proteus syndrome: diagnostic criteria, differential diagnosis, and patient evaluation. **Am J Med Genet** 84:389–395.
153. Happle R, Koch H, Lenz W (1980) The CHILD syndrome. Congenital hemidysplasia with ichthyosiform erythroderma and limb defects. **Eur J Pediatr** 134:27–33.
154. Hebert AA, Esterly NB, Holbrook KA et al. (1987) The CHILD syndrome. **Arch Dermatol** 123:503–509.
155. König A, Happle R, Bornholdt D et al. (2000) Mutations in the NSDHL gene, encoding for 3-beta hydroxysteroid dehydrogenase, cause CHILD syndrome. **Am J Med Genet** 90:339–346.
156. Happle R, König A, Grzeschik K-H (2000) Behold the CHILD, its only one. **Am J Med Genet** 94:341–343.
157. Zvulunov A, Rotem A, Merlob P, Metzker A (1990) Congenital smooth muscle hamartoma: prevalence, clinical findings, and follow-up in 15 patients. **AJDC** 144:782–784.
158. Prigent F (1992) Smooth muscle hamartoma and congenital hypertrichosis. **Ann Dermatol Venereol** 119:489.
159. Johnson MD, Jacobs AH (1989) Congenital smooth muscle hamartoma. **Arch Dermatol** 125:820–822.
160. Guillot B, Huet P, Joujoux JM, Lorette G (1998) Multiple congenital smooth muscle hamartomas. **Ann Derm Venereol** 125:118–120.
161. Schnur RE, Herzberg AJ, Spinner N et al. (1993) Variability in the Michelin tire syndrome: a child with multiple anomalies, smooth muscle hamartoma, and familial paracentric inversion of chromosome 7q. 102. **J Am Acad Dermatol** 28:364–370.
162. Langman J (1990) Head and neck. In: Medical Embryology, 6th ed, Baltimore: Williams & Wilkins, p. 297.
163. Ford GR, Balakrishnan A, Evans JN, Bailey CM (1992) Branchial cleft and pouch anomalies. **J Laryngol Otol** 106:137.
164. Willshaw HE, Al-Ashkar F (1983) The branchial arch syndromes. **Trans Ophthalmol Soc UK** 103:331.

forming the tympanic membrane; the remaining ectodermal clefts are separated from the endodermal pouches by mesodermal tissue.[163,165]

As a result of the cleft formation, five ridges become apparent on the lateral surface of the embryo; these are known as the branchial arches. Each arch is composed of a cartilaginous core surrounded by components that subsequently develop into the muscular, vascular and neural components of the ear, lower face and neck. During the sixth embryonic week, the second branchial arch grows caudally over the third and fourth arches, fusing with the epipericardial ridge of the lower neck. Remnants of these lower arches form the cervical sinus.[162–165]

The first pharyngeal pouch becomes the eustachian tube and the middle ear cavity, while the corresponding branchial cleft remains as the external ear canal. Most of the second pouch is obliterated; the rest forms the palatine tonsil. The third and fourth pouches lose their connections with the pharynx, forming tissue of the thymus and parathyroid gland; the fifth pouch is retained as part of the thyroid gland.[162–165]

Abnormalities of the branchial system occur whenever a cleft or pouch fails to obliterate, as a result of toxic, mechanical or vascular insults to the 4- to 8-week-old embryo.[164,166,167] The branchial fistulae and cysts are lined with stratified or pseudostratified ciliated columnar epithelium and/or stratified nonkeratinizing squamous epithelium.[167] Those lined with squamous epithelium become symptomatic earlier in life. Most complete fistulae and some external sinuses are diagnosed during the newborn period. Internal sinuses, although presumably present at birth, are usually discovered later in life.[166,168]

Defects of the second cleft are the most common.[163] Incomplete fusion of the second arch as it overgrows the third and fourth arches leaves a tract connecting the cervical sinus to the external surface of the embryo. This fistulous opening is usually found anterior to the lower sternocleidomastoid muscle and may provide drainage for a persistent cervical sinus. Such a remnant is called a **lateral cervical cyst** and is commonly located below the angle of the jaw.[169,170] While these are congenital malformations, they often present in the first to third decade of life. Infection is the most frequent complication of this lesion.[169]

In addition to lateral cervical cysts, **sinuses and fistulae of the second branchial cleft** can occur.[171] An incomplete external fistula with a blind inner pouch is most frequently found.[169,170,172] These sinuses present at birth as pits or blind-ending tracts in the lower third of the neck, along the anterior border of the sternocleidomastoid muscle. A skin tag, sometimes containing cartilage, can occur at the site of the opening, and the entire tract may be palpable beneath the skin. A discharge frequently occurs if the fistula is complete, and there is risk of infection similar to that seen with the branchial cysts. About 33% of these developmental defects are bilateral.[169]

Anomalies of the first branchial cleft are less common but have been reported as **preauricular cysts or sinuses**. They occur more commonly in females and may occur alone or in conjunction with hearing loss.[163,173] The cleft extends along the superior anterior border of the sternocleidomastoid muscle, ending in or near the external ear canal or the middle ear.[163,173] Presentation at birth is as a progressively enlarging mass or draining sinus in the preauricular (rarely retroauricular) area or in the anterior superior neck. The combination of a sinus in the upper neck with discharge from the ear in the absence of otitis media

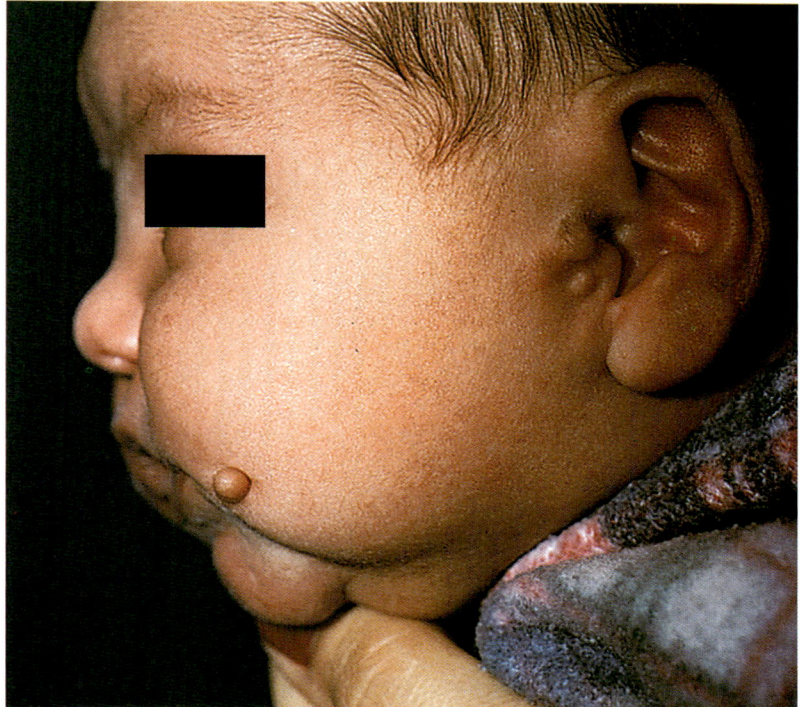

Fig. 6.23 Accessory tragus.

should suggest this diagnosis.[169] The diagnosis can be delayed in cases of first branchial cleft anomalies.[163] It is facilitated by the use of CT, which demonstrates the bony structures and the cystic nature of these lesions better than MRI.[174]

A more common anomaly found in the preauricular area is the **accessory tragus** (Fig. 6.23). The tragus is derived from the dorsal portion of the first branchial arch. As the arches grow ventrally to join in the midline during embryogenesis, accessory tragi can be found along the entire course of migration. Clinically, this path is reflected by a line drawn between the tragus and the corner of the mouth or on the neck at the anterior edge of the sternocleidomastoid muscle.

Accessory tragi can be unilateral, bilateral, singular, or multiple.[175] Vellus hairs are often present. They can be soft but are usually firm, due to the presence of cartilage.[176] Excision should involve careful dissection of the underlying cartilage, which can extend deeply. Rarely, accessory tragi are associated with other defects of the branchial arches in complex syndromes, such as Goldenhar syndrome (see below). Familial occurrence also occurs.[177]

Congenital midline cervical clefts, with or without other associated midline defects, such as cleft tongue, lip, mandible, or sternum, are also thought to arise from the first branchial arch as a result of imperfect fusion during embryogenesis.[178] They may be associated with skin tags or sinus tracts of the anterior lower midline neck.[179]

Persistent second, third, or fourth pouches have been misdiagnosed in the neonate as acute suppurative thyroiditis,[180] cysts,[168] neck abscesses,[181–183]

165. Al-Fallouji MAR, Butler MF (1983) First branchial cleft anomaly. **Postgrad Med J** 59:447.
166. Burge D, Middleton A (1983) Persistent pharyngeal pouch derivatives in the neonate. **J Pediatr Surg** 18:230.
167. Takimoto T, Itoh M, Furukawa M et al. (1991) Branchial cleft (pouch) anomalies: a review of 42 cases. **Auris Nasus Larynx** 18:87.
168. Lin JN, Wang KL (1991) Persistent third brachial apparatus. **J Pediatr Surg** 26:663.
169. Bill AH, Vadheim JL (1955) Cysts, sinuses and fistulas of the neck arising from the first and second branchial clefts. **Ann Surg** 142:904.
170. Kenealy JF, Torsiglieri AJ, Tom LW (1990) Branchial cleft anomalies: a five-year retrospective review. **Trans Penn Acad Ophthalmol Otolaryngol** 42:1022.
171. Maran AGD, Buchanan DR (1978) Branchial cysts, sinuses and fistulae. **Clin Otolaryngol** 3:77–92.
172. Agaton-Bonilla FC, Gay-Escoda C (1996) Diagnosis and treatment of branchial cleft cysts and fistulae. A retrospective study of 183 patients. **Int J Oral Maxillofac Surg** 25:449–452.
173. Cavo JW, Pratt LL, Alonso SA (1976) First branchial cleft syndrome and associated congenital hearing loss. **Laryngoscope** 86:739.
174. Mukherji SK, Tart RP, Slattery WH et al. (1993) Evaluation of first branchial anomalies by CT and MR. **J Comput Assist Tomogr** 17:576.

175. Cosman BC (1993) Bilateral accessory tragus. **Cutis** 51:199.
176. Satoh T, Tokura Y, Katsumata M et al. (1990) Histological diagnostic criteria for accessory tragi. **J Cutan Pathol** 17:206.
177. Tadini B, Cambiaghi S, Scarabelli G et al. (1993) Familial occurrence of isolated accessory tragi. **Pediatr Dermatol** 10:26.
178. Bergevin MA, Sheft S, Myer C, McAdams AJ (1989) Congenital midline cervical cleft. **Pediatr Pathol** 9:731.
179. Elgart GW, Patterson JW (1990) Congenital midline hamartoma: case report with histochemical and immunohistochemical findings. **Pediatr Dermatol** 7:199.
180. Abe K, Fujita H, Matsuura N et al. (1981) A fistula from pyriform sinus in recurrent acute suppurative thyroiditis. **Am J Dis Child** 135:178.
181. Takimoto T, Yoshizaki T, Ohoka H et al. (1990) Fourth branchial pouch anomaly. **J Laryngol Otol** 104:905.
182. Rosenfeld RM, Biller HF (1991) Fourth branchial pouch sinus: diagnosis and treatment. **J Laryngol Otol** 105:44.
183. Miller MB, Cohn AS (1993) Case report: fourth branchial pouch sinus. **Ear Nose Throat** 72:356.

cervical lymphadenitis,[184] cystic hygroma,[166] or malignant tumors.[170] Presentation in the newborn or young child is that of an acute painful swelling in the thyroid region, often with accompanying sore throat or fever. Later in childhood, a fistula in the lower neck or suppurative thyroiditis may be present if the fistula ends in the thyroid gland.[180] Interestingly, these have mainly been located on the left side of the neck,[180] although right-sided fistulae are rarely reported.[182]

Barium swallow (esophagram),[183,185] endoscopy,[185] CT,[181,186] and MRI have all been used to aid in the diagnosis of these anomalies. A simple diagnostic test is a plain radiography of the neck, revealing an air–fluid level in the lesion.[166] Once identified, fistulography can be used to demonstrate the communication between the pyriform sinus and the cystic mass.[185,187]

Definitive treatment of all these cysts and fistulae consists of careful and complete surgical removal,[167,184] although endoscopy with laser has been reported to be an effective alternative.[188] Initial drainage and marsupialization may be adequate,[166] but recurrences are common unless the tract is completely destroyed.[182]

In addition to these abnormalities, several syndromes of aberrant branchial arch development deserve mention: (1) Treacher–Collins syndrome (mandibulofacial dysostosis), characterized by malformed ears, a beaked nose, facial dysostosis, and deafness; (2) Goldenhar syndrome (oculoauricular vertebral dysplasia), which involves ocular lipodermoids, accessory tragi, and mandibular and vertebral abnormalities;[189] (3) Hallerman–Strieff syndrome (oculomandibular dyscephaly), exhibiting dwarfism, hypotrichosis, atrophic skin, a beaked nose, and abnormal dentition; (4) Pierre–Robin syndrome, presenting with micrognathia, glossoptosis, and neonatal respiratory distress;[164] (5) Branchio-otorenal syndrome, an autosomal dominant disorder recently localized to chromosome 8q[190] that accounts for 2% of profoundly deaf children, combining renal anomalies with hearing impairment, as well as preauricular pits, branchial cleft sinus tracts or other branchial pouch anomalies;[191] and (6) Branchio-oculofacial syndrome, also autosomal dominant, characterized by branchial cleft sinuses, ocular anomalies including coloboma, cataracts, and microphthalmia, pseudocleft or cleft lip and palate, and unusual facies.[192,193]

THYROGLOSSAL DUCT CYSTS

Thyroglossal duct cysts are relatively common, sporadic developmental anomalies of the anterior neck. They are infrequently familial in occurrence.[194,195] The cysts result from a failure to obliterate the embryonic thyroglossal duct. They can be found anywhere along the length of this duct, which corresponds clinically to the midline of the neck.[196] The diagnosis of thyroglossal duct cysts usually occurs during the first 5 years, but may be delayed until adulthood. They present as small 1–3cm, soft, midline anterior neck masses over the hyoid bone that move upward on swallowing or protrusion of the tongue (Fig. 6.24). Occasionally, they open into the mouth, producing an unpleasant taste.[196]

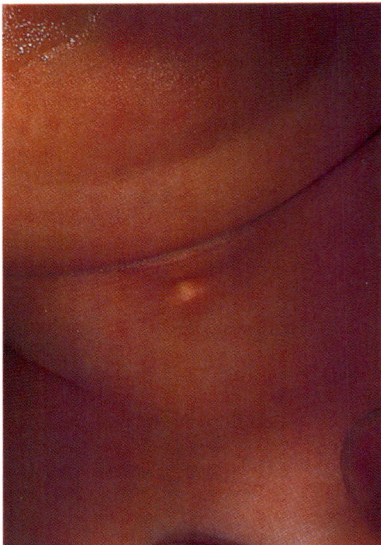

Fig. 6.24   Thyroglossal duct cyst.

Multiple complications of these cysts have been described, including thyroiditis, thyrotoxicosis, infection, and airway obstruction.[197] Malignant degeneration of these embryologic remnants occurs in less than 1% of cases. Papillary thyroid adenocarcinoma,[198] thyroid adenoma,[197] Hürthle cell adenoma,[199] and squamous cell carcinoma[200] have all been reported. The prognosis is usually good after excision of these tumors.

Thyroglossal duct cysts are the most common cause of midline anterior neck swelling in children. The differential diagnosis includes ectopic thyroid gland, enlarged lymph nodes, dermoid cysts, and bronchogenic cysts.[201] Treatment is by complete excision. It is imperative that a correct diagnosis is made prior to surgery since inadvertent removal of an ectopic thyroid gland may result in removal of the only functional thyroid tissue in the patient. Preoperative evaluation by ultrasound or nuclear scanning is recommended.[200]

BRONCHOGENIC CYSTS

Bronchogenic cysts are rare congenital anomalies that usually occur in the chest or mediastinum, but occasionally in the skin. Cutaneous bronchogenic cysts are characteristically located close to the suprasternal notch or over the manubrium sternum.[202] They are thought to develop from abnormal budding of the ventral segment of the primitive foregut at division of the foregut into its tracheal and esophageal components in the fifth or sixth week of gestation, before the sternum has fused.[203,204]

Bronchogenic cysts of the skin are usually present at birth as asymptomatic nodules that enlarge and discharge mucoid fluid through a skin fistula.[205–207]

184. Nonomura N, Ikarashi F, Fujisaki T et al. (1993) Surgical approach to pyriform sinus fistula. **Am J Otolaryngol** 14:111.

185. Godin MS, Kearns DB, Pransky SM et al. (1990) Fourth branchial pouch sinus: principles of diagnosis and management. **Laryngoscope** 100:174.

186. Herman TE, McAlister WH, Siegel MJ (1992) Branchial fistula: CT manifestations. **Pediatr Radiol** 22:152.

187. Feldman JI, Kearns DB, Pransky SM et al. (1990) Catheterization of branchial sinus tracts. A new method. **Int J Pediatr Otorhinolaryngol** 20:1.

188. Vermeire V, Moreau P (1993) A case of 3rd pharyngeal pouch sinus. **Acta Oto-Rhino-Laryngologica Belg** 47:55.

189. Zelante L, Gasparini P, Scanderbeg AC et al. (1997) Goldenhar complex: a further case with uncommon associated anomalies. **Am J Med Genet** 69:418–421.

190. Smith RJ, Coppage KB, Ankerstjerne JK et al. (1992) Localization of the gene for branchio-otorenal syndrome to chromosome 8q. **Genomics** 14:841.

191. Chitayat D, Hodgkinson KA, Chen MF (1992) Branchio-oto-renal syndrome: further delineation of an underdiagnosed syndrome. **Am J Med Genet** 43:970.

192. Hing AV, Torack R, Dowton SB (1992) A lethal syndrome resembling branchio-oculo-facial syndrome. **Clin Genet** 41:74.

193. Lin AE, Losken HW, Jaffe R (1991) The branchio-oculo-facial syndrome. **Cleft Palate Craniofac J** 28:96.

194. Klin B, Serour F, Fried K et al. (1993) Familial thyroglossal duct cyst. **Clin Genet** 43:101.

195. Issa MM, de Vries P (1991) Familial occurrence of thyroglossal duct cyst. **J Pediatr Surg** 26:30.

196. Heymann WR (1992) Cutaneous manifestations of thyroid disease. **J Am Acad Dermatol** 26:885.

197. Colohan DP, Hillborn M (1993) An unusual case of intermittent upper airway obstruction. **J Emerg Med** 11:157.

198. Vincent SD, Synhorst JB 2d (1989) Adenocarcinoma arising in a thyroglossal duct cyst: report of a case and literature review. **J Oral Maxillofac Surg** 47:633.

199. Lyos AT, Schwartz MR, Malpica A et al. (1993) Hürthle cell adenoma arising in a thyroglossal duct cyst. **Head Neck** 15:348.

200. Yanagisawa K, Eisen RN, Sasaki CT (1992) Squamous cell carcinoma arising in a thyroglossal duct cyst. **Arch Otolaryngol Head Neck Surg** 118:538.

201. Radkowski D, Arnold J, Healy GB et al. (1991) Thyroglossal duct remnants. Preoperative evaluation and management. **Arch Otolaryngol Head Neck Surg** 117:1378.

202. Patterson JW, Pittman DL, Rich JD (1984) Presternal ciliated cyst. **Arch Dermatol** 120:240.

203. Kuhn C, Kuhn JP (1992) Coexistence of bronchial atresia and bronchogenic cyst: diagnostic and embryologic considerations. **Pediatr Radiol** 22:568.

204. Lazar RH, Younis RT, Bassila MN (1991) Bronchogenic cysts: a cause of stridor in the neonate. **Am J Otolaryngol** 12:117.

205. Miller OF, Tyler W (1984) Cutaneous bronchogenic cyst with papilloma and sinus presentation. **J Am Acad Dermatol** 11:367.

206. Muramatsu T, Shirai T, Sakamoto K (1990) Cutaneous bronchogenic cyst. **Int J Dermatol** 29:143–144.

207. Jona JZ (1995) Extramediastinal bronchogenic cysts in children. **Pediatr Dermatol** 12:304–306.

Cysts of the mediastinum can present as stridor in the newborn.[203] Histologically, they are composed of a mucosal lining consisting of lamina propria and a pseudostratified columnar ciliated epithelium with goblet cells. The cyst wall contains smooth muscle, mucous glands, and occasionally cartilage.

The differential diagnosis includes anomalies of the branchial arches, thyroglossal duct cysts, and teratomas. Nuclear imaging or ultrasound can aid in the diagnosis.[202] There are rare reports of malignant degeneration of these cysts.[208] Treatment is by surgical excision.

APLASIA CUTIS CONGENITA

Aplasia cutis is a focal, congenital, localized absence of skin. It is reported to occur in approximately 1 in 10 000 births.[209,210] A variety of *in utero* events associated with several pathogenetic mechanisms are presumed responsible for aplasia cutis, and several classifications have been proposed incorporating disease and syndrome associations.[210,211] Clinical findings including morphology and distribution may be helpful in determining etiology, pathogenesis, systemic associations and prognosis.

The most common type of aplasia cutis congenita is membranous aplasia cutis, which usually appears as small sharply defined, oval or round lesions (Fig. 6.25). The surface is atrophic and the lesion appears to be covered with a thin membrane; rarely the lesion is apparently bullous with fluid which drains and refills. Occasionally there is a peripheral collar of hypertrophic hair. Involvement may include subcutaneous fat or underlying bony structures. Mature scar appearance is more common in older children. They may be single or often multiple. The commonest position is on the midline vertex of the scalp but they also occur 1–2cm off the midline on the parietal scalp and extending down onto the brow in a line from the lateral forehead to the lateral eyebrows.[211] Rarely, they occur on the face in a line from the preauricular area to the angle of the mouth, a condition termed focal facial dermal hypoplasia.[212]

Another type of aplasia cutis is as often large irregular or stellate scalp defects, again often along the midline of the scalp. These may be associated with significant skull defects and underlying vascular anomalies and malformations (Fig. 6.26).[213]

Histologically in aplasia cutis there is absence of the epidermis and dermal appendages and decreased dermal elastic tissue. Healed areas show an atrophic epidermis, dermal fibrosis, and absence of adnexal structures.[210,214] Hypertrophic scars can occur.

The etiology of scalp aplasia cutis is uncertain and may be heterogeneous. The location, morphology and distribution suggests incomplete closure of the neural tube for midline lesions and incomplete closure of embryonic fusion lines for lateral lesions.[209,210,215]

While membranous aplasia cutis is usually sporadic, autosomal dominant and autosomal recessive patterns of inheritance of aplasia cutis have been reported.[216–219] Amniotic membrane adhesions, intrauterine infections and teratogenic agents have also been implicated. Because of the heterogeneity of associated findings, a single cause is unlikely.

Adams–Oliver syndrome is an autosomal dominant condition described with scalp aplasia cutis congenita associated with limb defects and cranial bone defects.[220–223] Multiple other syndromes and chromosomal anomalies have been associated with aplasia cutis (Table 6.9). Aplasia cutis congenita also occurs on the extremities and the trunk. Lesions that occur in areas other than the scalp are often multiple and symmetric.[209]

Truncal lesions and limb lesions have been associated with fetus papyraceus, and appear as linear or stellate erosions or scars, often strikingly symmetric.[224–226]

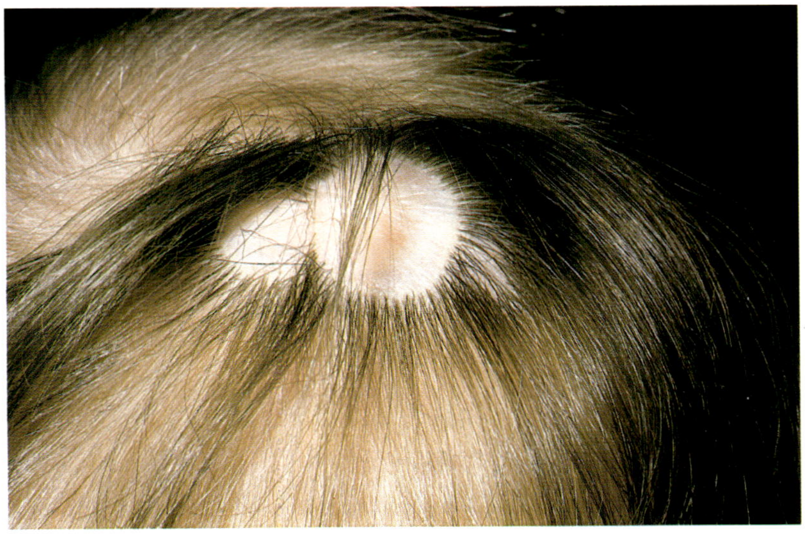

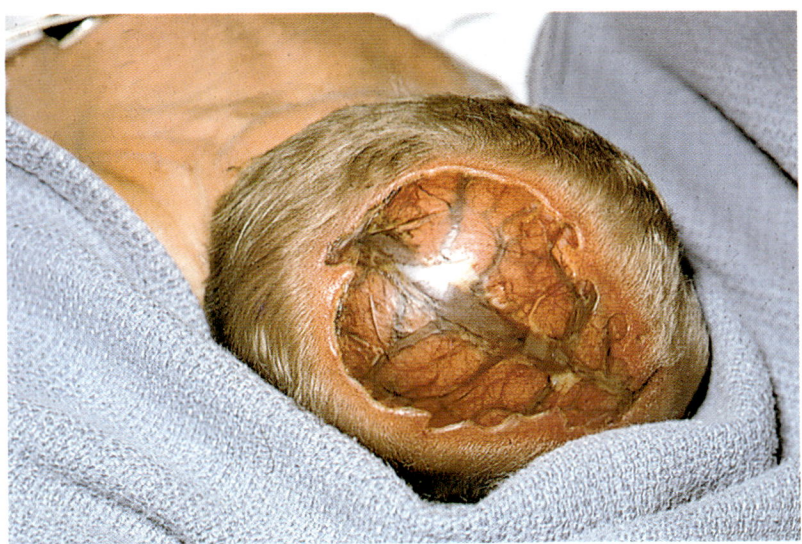

Fig. 6.25 Membranous aplasia cutis with hair collar.

Fig. 6.26 Aplasia cutis, with underlying skull defect.

208. Szram S, Zalewski P, Buczylko K et al. (1992) On primarily bifocal laryngeal carcinoma and bronchogenic cyst of the neck. **Otolaryngol Pol** 46:488.
209. Guillen P, Pichardo A, Martinez F (1985) Aplasia cutis congenita. **J Am Acad Dermatol** 13:429.
210. Frieden IJ (1986) Aplasia cutis congenita: a clinical review and proposal for classification. **J Am Acad Dermatol** 14:646.
211. Drolet BA (2001) Developmental abnormalities. In: Textbook of Neonatal Dermatology, Eichenfield LF, Frieden IJ, Esterly NB, eds. Philadelphia, PA: WB Saunders, pp. 126–130.
212. Drolet BA, Baselga E, Gosain AK et al. (1997) Preauricular skin defects: a consequence of a persistent ectodermal groove. **Arch Dermatol** 133:1551–1554.
213. Singman R, Asaikan S, Hotson G, Prose N (1990) Aplasia cutis congenita and arterialvenous fistula. **Arch Neurol** 47:1255–1258.
214. Lever WF (1997) Congenital diseases (genodermatoses). In: Histopathology of the Skin, 8th ed. Philadelphia: JB Lippincott, p. 127.
215. Stratis JP, Ramer JC, Manders EK et al. (1992) Cutaneous scar at anterior hair line in mother and child with associated frontal bone defect in child. **Am J Med Genet** 44:197.
216. Pap GS (1970) Congenital defect of the scalp and skull in three generations of one family. **Plast Reconst Surg** 46:194–196.
217. Sybert V (1985) Aplasia cutis congenita. A report of 12 new families and review of the literature. **Pediatr Dermatol** 3:1–14.
218. Lin YJ, Chen HC, Jee SH et al. (1993) Familial aplasia cutis congenita associated with limb anomalies and tetralogy of Fallot. **Int J Dermatol** 32:52.
219. Gucuyener K, Tunaoglu FS, Demirsoy S et al. (1992) Aplasia cutis congenita of the scalp without other defects in three siblings. **Acta Paediatr** 81:182.
220. Whitley CB, Gorlin RJ (1991) Adams–Oliver syndrome revisited. **Am J Med Genet** 40:319.
221. Jaeggi E, Kind C, Morger R (1990) Congenital scalp and skull defects with terminal transverse limb anomalies (Adams–Oliver syndrome): report of three additional cases. **Eur J Pediatr** 149:565.
222. Bork K, Pfeifle J (1992) Multifocal aplasia cutis congenita, distal limb hemimelia, and cutis marmorata telangiectatica in a patient with Adams–Oliver syndrome. **Br J Dermatol** 127:160.
223. Chitayat D, Meunier C, Hodgkinson KA et al. (1992) Acrania: a manifestation of the Adams–Oliver syndrome. **Am J Med Genet** 44:562.
224. Mannino F, Jones K, Benirschke K (1977) Congenital skin defects and fetus papyraceus. **J Pediatr** 91:559–564.
225. Saier F, Burden L, Cavanagh D (1975) Fetus papyraceus: an unusual case with congenital anomaly of the surviving fetus. **Obstet Gynecol** 45:217–220.
226. Leaute-Lebreze C, Depaire-Duclos F, Sarlangue J et al. (1998) Congenital cutaneous defects as complications of surviving co-twins; aplasia cutis congenita and neonatal Volkmann ischemic contracture of the forearm. **Arch Dermatol** 134:1121–1124.

TABLE 6.9   Associated malformations and chromosomal defects reported with aplasia cutis

Syndrome	Clinical phenotype	Associated features	Inheritance
Opitz syndrome	Membranous aplasia cutis	Hypertelorism, cleft lip/palate, hypospadias, cryptorchidism	
Adams–Oliver syndrome	Large, ill-defined, irregular scalp defects	Distal limb reduction abnormalities	Autosomal dominant
Oculocerebrocutaneous syndrome	Membranous aplasia cutis	Orbital cysts, cerebral malformations, facial skin tags, seizures, developmental delay	
Trisomy D (13–15)	Membranous aplasia cutis	Holoprosencephaly, seizures, ocular abnormalities, deafness, neural tube defects	
4p(−) syndrome	Not specified	Mental retardation, deafness, seizures, ocular abnormalities	
Johanson–Blizzard syndrome	Small stellate defects of frontal scalp and membranous aplasia cutis	Dwarfism, mental retardation, deafness, hypothyroidism, pancreatic insufficiency	
X-p22 microdeletion syndrome	Bilateral linear reticulated defects of the malar region of the face	Microphthalmia, sclerocornea	
Chromosome 16–18 defect	Large scalp defects	Scalp arteriovenous malformation with underlying bony defect	

With permission: Drolet BA (2001) Developmental Abnormalities. In: Textbook of Neonatal Dermatology, Eichenfield LF, Frieden IJ, Esterly NB, eds. Philadelphia, PA: WB Saunders, 126–130.

It is theorized that the skin lesions are secondary to placental vascular disruption after the death of a twin fetus, with skin infarction.

Defects of the extremities and trunk with blistering of the skin has been called Bart syndrome, now considered to be a form of epidermolysis bullosa.[227–230] These cases may be associated with pyloric atresia and other abnormalities.

Linear skin defects of the malar facial area have been reported with Xp22 microdeletion syndrome, which is also associated with microphthalmia and scelerocornea.[231,232]

Aplasia cutis congenita can usually be diagnosed clinically. Ultrasound is a useful investigation to identify the presence of underlying skull defects. Skull radiographs may be helpful in assessing the extent of the defect for larger lesions.

Most cases of aplasia cutis congenita heal without complication. Trauma and secondary infection should be avoided. Superficial ulcerations usually heal in several months, with small bony defects usually ossifying without treatment in five to seven months.[209] Meningitis and exsanguination from rupture of the superior sagittal sinus have occurred with large scalp defects, and careful imaging is recommended before any surgical correction due to risks of intracranial vascular anomalies.[233,234] Grafts of skin and/or bone may be necessary in the larger defects.[233,234] After healing, defects often become inconspicuous, though larger lesions may be surgically excised in later life.

Aplasia cutis congenita should be distinguished from iatrogenic injury caused by a scalp electrodes[209] or forceps delivery, congenital varicella syndrome, focal dermal hypoplasia (Goltz syndrome), Volkmann's ischemic contracture,[226,235] and epidermolysis bullosa in the absence of aplasia cutis.

Examination of the placenta and the umbilical cord may aid in the diagnosis. For medicolegal reasons, it is important to recognize this as an intrauterine event unrelated to birth trauma or forceps delivery.

FOCAL DERMAL HYPOPLASIA

Focal dermal hypoplasia (Goltz syndrome) is characterized by congenital absence of skin. This rare hereditary disorder presents at birth with widespread linear areas of dermal hypoplasia, herniation of the underlying subcutaneous tissue (resembling striae distensae), telangiectasia, and linear or reticulated areas of hyperpigmentation or hypopigmentation.[236,237] Abnormalities of skeletal and ocular structures may also be seen at birth.[235,236] Almost 90% of cases occur in females, suggesting an X-linked dominant mode of inheritance with lethality in the male. A few affected males have been described and are believed to have resulted from postzygotic mutations of the gene or occurrence in the setting of Klinefelter syndrome. Studies have suggested that genes for Goltz syndrome lie on the terminal end of the short arm of the X chromosome (Xp22.31), though the gene has not been identified.[238,239]

AMNIOTIC BAND SYNDROME

The amniotic band syndrome is an uncommon constellation of congenital deformities presumably due to fetal entanglement in strands of ruptured amniotic sac. The approximate incidence is of 1 in 10 000 births[240] and although some familial cases have been reported, it is usually sporadic. Abdominal trauma, connective tissue disorders,[241] epidermolysis bullosa,

227. Bart B, Gorlin R, Anderson V, Lynch F (1966) Congenital localized absence of skin and associated abnormalities resembling epidermolysis bullosa. **Arch Dermatol** 93:296.
228. Kanzler MH, Smoller B, Woodley DT (1992) Congenital localized absence of the skin as a manifestation of epidermolysis bullosa. **Arch Dermatol** 128:1087.
229. Jones EM, Hersh JH, Yusk JW (1992) Aplasia cutis congenita, cleft palate, epidermolysis bullosa, and ectrodactyly: a new syndrome? **Pediatr Dermatol** 9:293.
230. Lestringant GG, Akel SR, Qayed KI (1992) The pyloric atresia–junctional epidermolysis bullosa syndrome. Report of a case and review of the literature. **Arch Dermatol** 128:1083.
231. Al-Gazali LI, Mueller RF, Caine A et al. (1990) Two 46, xxt(X:Y) females with linear skin defects and congenital microphthalmia: a new syndrome at Xp2.3. **J Med Genet** 27:59–63.
232. Temple K, Hurst JA, Hings S et al. (1990) De novo deletion of Xp22.2pter in a female with linear skin lesions on the face and neck, microphthalmia, and anterior chamber eye anomalies. **J Med Genet** 27:56–58.
233. Abbott R, Cutting CB, Wisoff JH (1991–92) Aplasia cutis congenita of the scalp: issues in its management. **Pediatr Neurosurg** 17:182.
234. Sargent LA (1990) Aplasia cutis congenita of the scalp. **J Pediatr Surg** 25:1211.
235. Caouette-Laberge L, Bortoluzzi P, Egerszegi EP et al. (1992) Neonatal Volkmann's ischemic contracture of the forearm: a report of five cases. **Plast Reconstr Surg** 90:621.
236. Pereyo NG, Lugo-Janer GJ, Sanchez JL (1993) Atrophic macules in an infant. Goltz syndrome (focal dermal hypoplasia [FDH] syndrome). **Arch Dermatol** 129:897.
237. Landa N, Oleaga JM, Raton JA et al. (1993) Focal dermal hypoplasia (Goltz syndrome): an adult case with multisystemic involvement. **J Am Acad Dermatol** 28:86.
238. Burgdorf W, Dick G, Soderberg M, Goltz R (1981) Focal dermal hypoplasia in a father and daughter. **J Am Acad Dermatol** 4:273.
239. Ishii N, Baba N, Kanaizuka I et al. (1992) Histopathological study of focal dermal hypoplasia (Goltz syndrome). **Clin Exp Dermatol** 17:24.
240. Foulkes GD, Reinker K (1994) Congenital constriction band syndrome: a seventy years experience. **J Pediatr Orthop** 14:242–248.
241. Young ID, Lindenbaum RH, Thompson EM et al. (1985) Amniotic bands in connective tissue disorders. **Arch Dis Child** 60:1061–1063.

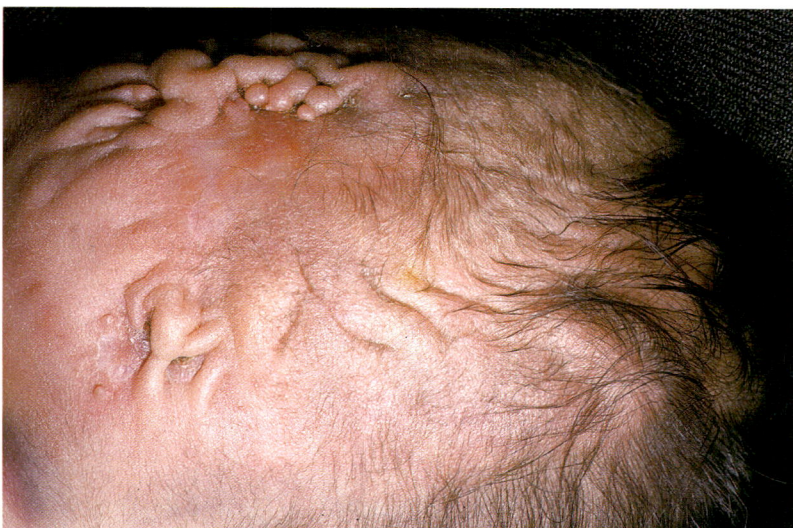

Fig. 6.27   Amniotic band sequence: major scalp malformation.

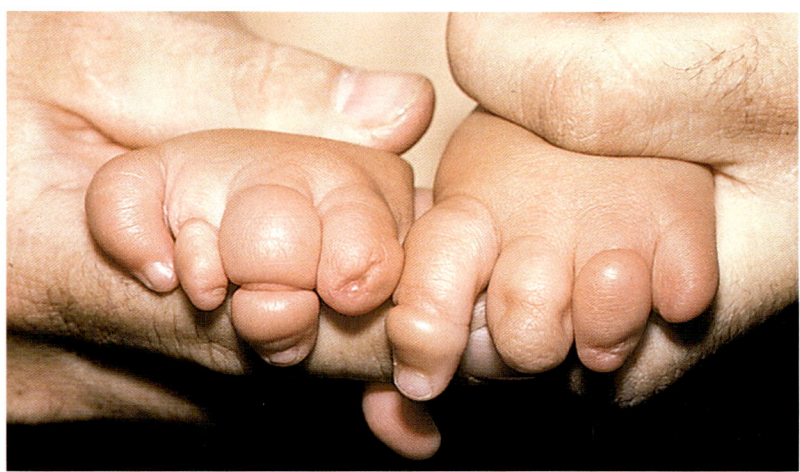

Fig. 6.28   Amniotic band sequence: multiple anomalies of the feet.

uterine malformations, first gestation in mothers younger than 25 years, and amniocentesis[242] are the most frequently fetomaternal risk factors described.[243] It is widely accepted that amniotic bands derive from early amniotic rupture; this rupture permits fluid leakage, leading to the introduction of the fetus into the chorionic cavity. The chorion reabsorbs this fluid, stimulating the proliferation of mesodermal strings that envelop and compress fetal structures giving rise to malformations of variable severity depending on the gestational period. This hypothesis is based in large part in the observations of Torpin.[244] It has been suggested that craniofacial (Fig. 6.27) and abdominal wall closure malformations arise as a consequence of earlier amniotic sac rupture and extremity malformations result from later sac rupture.[245]

The most classic cutaneous finding is a constriction band of a distal extremity. The band is usually circumferential (Fig. 6.28) and may cause lymphedema or even amputation, syndactyly, pseudosyndactyly, and acro-syndactyly. Aplasia cutis of stellate morphology, irregular patches of alopecia, altered dermal pattern, lack of normal hair whorl, and abnormal hand creases are dermatologic defects that can also be found.[240,243,246]

Extracutaneous findings include multiple malformations such as clubfoot, and scoliosis can result from the compression due to the oligohydramnios. A rupture early in gestation during organogenesis will lead to the most severe deformities like neural tube defects, and facial, chest and abdominal wall clefts.[246]

Surgical correction of the deformities is the only treatment option and is very difficult. Recently, prenatal surgical interventions have been successfully performed to treat constricting amniotic bands to avoid amputation or severe dysfunction of the limb.[247]

CONGENITAL LIP PITS (FISTULAE LABII CONGENITA)

Three types of congenital lip pits have been described. The most common of these are commissural lip pits, found in about 2% of neonates, with increased frequency in blacks.[248] They are usually bilateral involving the lower lip and are frequently inherited in an autosomal dominant fashion.[249] Although typically asymptomatic, they occasionally drain small amounts of salivary secretions.[250] Commissural pits are actually sinuses that end blindly within a few millimeters of their opening. Rare association with preauricular sinuses or communication with the parotid duct have been reported.[251] These pits have rarely been described in association with other ectodermal disorders.[252,253] Histologically, the sinuses are composed of stratified squamous epithelium identical to that of the vermilion border. Ducts with cuboidal epithelium have been identified opening into the sinuses.[250]

Midline cysts of the upper lip have also been reported, although they are very rare.[254,255] A blind-ended sinus tract is found in the midline of the upper lip philtrum. It has been proposed that these pits form by a burrowing process analogous to that which occurs during the development of the nasal cavities. The upper lip and nasal cavities form at the same stage in embryogenesis, and both are lined with stratified squamous epithelium, in support of this theory.[255] A third type of congenital lip pit is located on the paramedian lower lip. These can be sporadic, but they are more commonly familial. Pits are usually bilateral, but solitary pits can occur and are more frequent on the left side.[250] A variety of names have been applied to these uncommon congenital defects. They have been reported as paramedian sinuses of the lower lip, humps of the lower lip, labial cysts, labial fistulae, accessory salivary glands, mucoceles, and dermoid cysts of the lip.[256]

In 1954, Van der Woude[257] noted the association of these labial fistulae with cleft lip and/or palate (Van der Woude syndrome). This autosomal dominant

242. Kohn G (1987) The amniotic band syndrome. A possible complication of amniocentesis. Prenat Diagn 7:303–305.
243. Bower C, Norwood F, Knowles S et al. (1993) Amniotic band syndrome: a population-based study in two Australian states Pediatr Perinat Epidemiol 7:395–403.
244. Torpin R (1965) Amniochorionic mesoblastic fibrous strings and amniotic bands. Am J Obstet Gynecol 91:65–75.
245. Kalousek DK, Bamforth S (1988) Amnion rupture sequence in previable fetuses. Am J Med Genet 31:63–73.
246. Ray M, Hendrick SJ, Raimer SS et al. (1988) Amniotic band syndrome. Int J Dermatol 27:312–314.
247. Quintero RA, Morales WJ, Phillips J et al. (1997) In utero lysis of amniotic bands. Ultrasound Obstet Gynecol 10:316–320.
248. Jorgenson RJ, Shapiro SD, Salinas CF et al. (1982) Intraoral findings and anomalies in neonates. Pediatrics 69:577.
249. Everett FG, Wescott WB (1961) Commissural lip pits. Oral Surg 14:202.
250. Soricelli DA, Bell L, Alexander WA (1966) Congenital fistulas of the lower lip. Oral Surg Oral Med Oral Pathol 21:511.
251. Arriaga MA, Dindzans LJ, Bluestone CD (1990) Parotid duct communicating with a labial pit and ectopic salivary cyst. Arch Otolaryngol Head Neck Surg 116:1445.
252. Ohishi M, Kai S, Ozeki S et al. (1991) Alveolar synechia, ankyloblepharon, and ectodermal disorders: an autosomal recessive disorder? Am J Med Genet 38:13.
253. Marres HA, Cremers CW (1991) Congenital conductive or mixed deafness, preauricular sinus, external ear anomaly, and commissural lip pits: an autosomal dominant inherited syndrome. Ann Otol Rhinol Laryngol 100:928.
254. Holbrook LA (1970) Congenital midline sinus of the upper lip. Br J Plast Surg 23:155.
255. Miller CJ, Smith JM (1980) Midline sinus of the upper lip and a theory concerning etiology. Plast Reconstr Surg 65:674.
256. Cheney ML, Cheney WR, LeJeune FE (1986) Familial incidence of labial pits. Am J Otolaryngol 7:311.
257. Van der Woude A (1954) Fistula labii inferioris congenita and its association with cleft lip and palate. Am J Hum Genet 6:244.

syndrome, with variable expressivity and high penetrance (80%), has been localized to chromosome 1q.[258,259] It accounts for 2% of all cases of cleft lip and palate. An infant with Van der Woude syndrome may exhibit any or none of the signs (lip pits, cleft lip, or cleft palate) and may transmit any or all of the anomalies to offspring.[257] Lip pits in this syndrome are usually bilateral, symmetric depressions on the vermilion border of the lower lip, just lateral to the midline.[258,259] All types and degrees of clefts are seen in Van der Woude syndrome, including complete or incomplete, unilateral or bilateral clefts in the lip or palate, or both.[259] Up to 50% of the patients with congenital lip pits have cleft palate; 33% have cleft lip and palate; and only 10–20% have no cleft at all.[256,259] The conical elevations are also specific, being present in 40% of patients with cleft palate and in fewer than 1% of patients with cleft lip or no cleft.[260] Other syndromes associated with congenital pits of the lip, usually in combination with cleft lip or palate, include the popliteal pterygia syndrome[261] and the orofacial digital syndrome.[262]

The only successful treatment for symptomatic or unsightly fistulae is surgical excision.

CUTANEOUS SIGNS OF SPINAL DYSRAPHISM

Spinal dysraphism (SD) is a term coined by Lichtenstein in 1940 to refer a group of congenital malformations or incomplete fusion of the posterior midline embryonic structures. This failure is thought to be produced by a delay or alteration in the sequence of closure, a reopening or an incomplete regression of the caudal end of the neural tube. A multifactorial etiology is reported. It may occur in various genetic and malformation syndromes or as a result of nutritional and teratogenic factors.[263]

Skin and nervous system are intimately related by their common ectodermal origin; by the third and fifth week of intrauterine life the neural groove separates from the ectodermal epithelium and is surrounded by mesodermal structures to form the cererebrospinal axis. Hence, it is not unexpected that an abnormal event in some part of this process produces simultaneous malformations.

Spinal dysraphism may be grouped into four types depending on the developmental anomaly: 1) a simple incomplete fusion of the elements, e.g., spina bifida; 2) a failure of separation of germinal layers, e.g., a dimple; 3) abnormal growth of cell nests of one germinal layer remaining among the cells of another, e.g., dermoid or epidermoid cyst; 4) a disturbance in the growth of normal tissue leading to the formation of intraspinal or intramedullary tumours, e.g., lipoma.[264] Combinations of these anomalies are often found.

When overt, SD is easily recognized; but occult forms may be unnoticed until neurological symptoms become apparent. In more than 50% of these cases, cutaneous markers are present,[265,266] usually already evident at birth, which can point to the underlying pathology. These are most important to recognize as a delay in diagnosis increases the child's risk of progressive neurologic and urologic deterioration.

The cutaneous stigmata of SD are located on or near midline and include depressed lesions, dermal lesions, dyschromic lesions, hairy lesions, neoplasms, polypoid lesions, subcutaneous nodules and vascular lesions (Table 6.10).[266–268] Most spinal deformities are in the lumbosacrococcygeal region.

TABLE 6.10   **Cutaneous lesions associated with spinal dysraphism**

High index of suspicion	Low index of suspicion
Hypertrichosis	Telangiectasia
Dimples (large, >2.5cm from the anal verge, atypical)	Capillary malformation (port-wine stain)
Acrochordons/pseudo-tails/true tails	Hyperpigmentation
Lipomas	Melanocytic nevi
Hemangiomas	Teratomas
Aplasia cutis or scar	
Dermoid cyst or sinus	

After Drolet BA (2001) Developmental Abnormalities. In: Textbook of Neonatal Dermatology, Eichenfield LF, Frieden IJ, Esterly NB, eds. Philadelphia, PA: WB Saunders, 126–130.

Skin dimples are round depressions with a frequency that ranges from 4% to 23% in different series.[265] Most commonly they are isolated phenomena but they can point to underlying neurological pathology, particularly when they are deep or wide, occur above the gluteal crease or are associated with other markers. These larger lesions usually represent fixation of the skin to bony or fibrous structures.[266]

Dermal sinus tracts are often associated with **dermoid or epidermoid cysts**. The sinus may connect the skin directly with the spinal cord and hence there is a significant risk of infection, including meningitis, epidural, subdural or spinal cord abscesses.[267] Large cysts may cause neurological compromise because of compression.[268] When the tract is superficial to the sacral fascia and contains hairs, is called a pilonidal sinus, and is almost never accompanied by neurological damage.[268]

Aplasia cutis is only rarely located in the lumbosacral area; in some of these cases underlying pathology has been reported. It presents as a congenital scar-like defect.

A **hairy patch** is the most common cutaneous sign of SD evident at birth and can point to skeletal abnormalities at various levels of the cord.[269] It may comprise long silky hair (the faun tail), a broad lozenge-shaped patch of long coarse terminal hair, a discrete midline patch of soft vellus or lanugo hair; and localized hypertrichosis, a patch of normal appearing hair, over the lower part of midline.[268]

Congenital **lipomas** are manifested as soft swellings consisting of a mass of adipose tissue. They mostly occur in the midline of the lower cervical, upper thoracic and lumbar spine, regions that correspond to the last sites of closure of the embryonic neural arch.[270] In some instances, the lipoma may be slightly lateral to the spinal column. The overlying skin may be normal in appearance, or may be marked by dimpling, abnormal hair, or a vascular lesion.[264,267] Congenital lipomas are histologically non-encapsulated and are finely lobulated. They may be superficially located or may penetrate into the intraspinal space; frequently they are attached to the dura by a fibrous stalk and on some occasions, particularly when placed lateral to the midline (Fig. 6.29), they are associated with a meningocele (lipomyelomeningocele).[271] Intraspinal lipomas are a marker of a tethered cord.

258. Murray JC, Nishimura DY, Buetow KH et al. (1990) Linkage of an autosomal dominant clefting syndrome (Van der Woude) to loci on chromosome 1q. **Am J Hum Genet** 46:486.
259. Sander A, Moser H, Liechti-Gallati S et al. (1993) Linkage of Van der Woude syndrome (VWS) to REN and exclusion of the candidate gene TGFB2 from the disease locus in a large pedigree. **Hum Genet** 91:55.
260. Ranta R, Rintala AE (1983) Correlations between microforms of the Van der Woude syndrome and cleft palate. **Cleft Palate J** 20:158.
261. Hammer J, Klausler M, Schinael A (1989) The popliteal pterygium syndrome: distinct phenotypic variation in two families. **Helv Paediatr Acta** 43:507.
262. Salinas CF, Pai GS, Vera CL (1991) Variability of expression of the orofaciodigital syndrome type I in black females: six cases. **Am J Med Genet** 38:574.
263. Van Allen M, Kalousek D, Chernoff G et al. (1993) Evidence for multi-site closure of the neural tube in humans. **Am J Med Genet** 47:723–743.
264. Tavafoghi V, Ghandchi A, Hambrick G et al. (1978) Cutaneous signs of spinal dysraphism. **Arch Dermatol** 114:573–578.
265. Harrist T, Gang D, Kleinman G et al. (1982) Unusual sacrococcygeal embryologic malformations with cutaneous manifestations. **Arch Dermatol** 118:643–648.
266. Hamm H (2000) Cutaneous signs of occult spinal dysraphism. In: Textbook of Pediatric Dermatology, Harper J, Orange A, Prose N, eds. Oxford: Blackwell Scientific, pp. 86–88.
267. Hebert H, Miller F (1976) Midline cutaneous and spinal defects. **Arch Dermatol** 112:1724–1728.
268. Davis D, Cohen P, George R (1994) Cutaneous stigmata of occult spinal dysraphism. **J Am Acad Dermatol** 31:892–896.
269. Herane M, Apt P, Perez L et al. (1997) Hipertricosis localizada: Sindrome de la cola de fauno. Caso clinico y estudio de signos cutáneos de disrrafismo espinal. Rev. **Chilena Dermatol** 13(1):11–15.
270. Lambram E, El-Shunnar K, Hilton D et al. (1999) Revisited: Spinal angiolipoma. Three additional cases. **Br J Neurosurg** 13(1):25–30.
271. Goldberg N, Hebert A, Esterly N (1986) Sacral hemangiomas and multiple congenital abnormalities. **Arch Dermatol** 122:684–687.

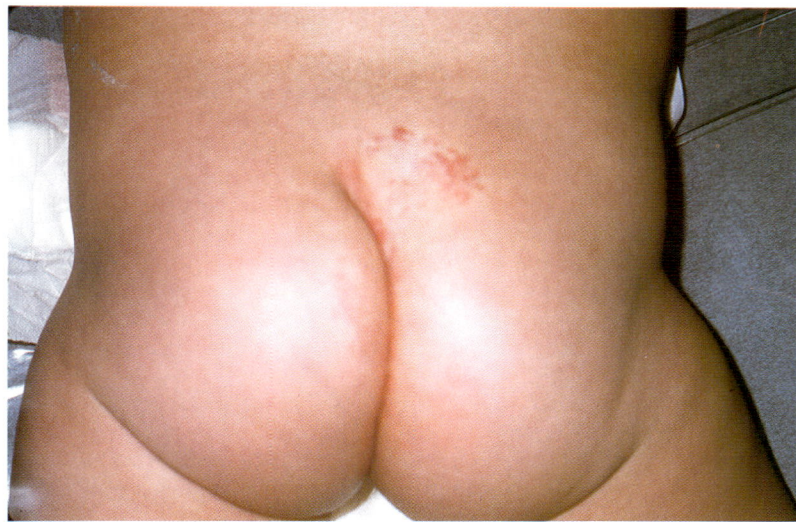

Fig. 6.29 Lipoma associated with meningocele (lipomeningocele). Note papular hemangioma as well.

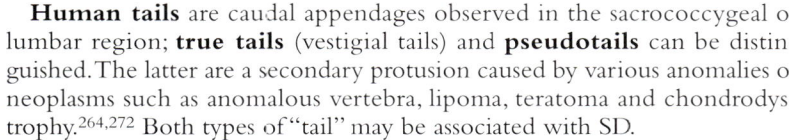

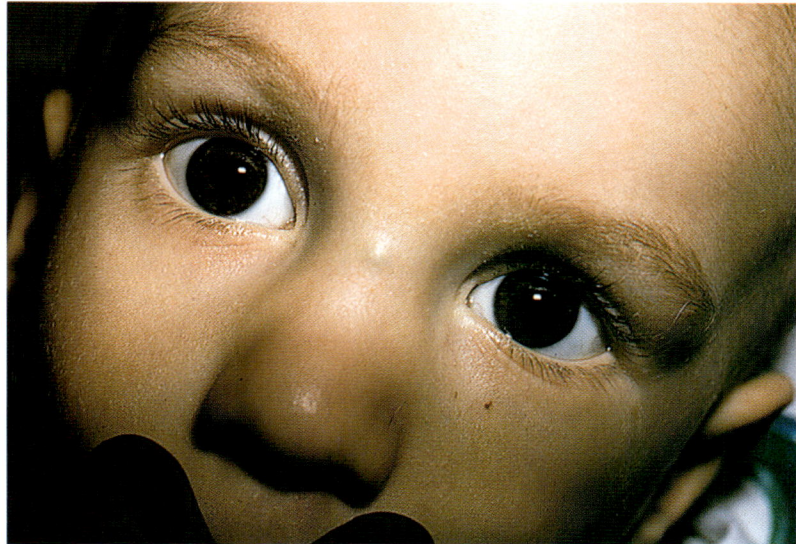

Fig. 6.30 Small midline nasal dermoid cyst.

Human tails are caudal appendages observed in the sacrococcygeal or lumbar region; **true tails** (vestigial tails) and **pseudotails** can be distinguished. The latter are a secondary protusion caused by various anomalies or neoplasms such as anomalous vertebra, lipoma, teratoma and chondrodystrophy.[264,272] Both types of "tail" may be associated with SD.

Vascular lesions such as sacral **hemangiomas** are also described in association with spinal lesions;[271] they are usually larger than 4cm, overlie the midline and may have a central scar-like lesion associated.[273]

Capillary malformations in the lumbosacral area are usually unassociated with SD,[274] but there are rare reports of the association.[275]

Other skin lesions such as pigmented macules, congenital melanocytic nevi, hamartomas and neurofibromas, may also occur in association with SD and sacrococcygeal teratomas.

Several methods of investigation must be done prior to embarking upon a surgical procedure. These include high resolution ultrasonography of the lesion and spinal cord which is particularly useful in infants under 3–4 months of age because until then the posterior bony elements of the spine are not yet fused.[276,277] MR imaging provides the most accurate information in a noninvasive manner; CT myelography may be required in the more complex abnormalities.[277]

The removal of the skin lesions that are suspected to be associated with spinal dysraphism without a previous diagnostic evaluation is contraindicated; doing a biopsy is hazardous because of the risk of introduction of infection into the spinal canal.[278] When a skin lesion that may be related to an underlying spinal dysraphism is detected, referral to a neurosurgeon should occur.

DERMOID CYSTS

Dermoid cysts are congenital subcutaneous ectodermal growths that occur along embryonic fusion lines. They are unrelated to benign cystic teratomas, which are also referred to as dermoids. While dermoid cysts are congenital, they may not be noted until early childhood; 40% manifest at birth, and 70% by age 5. If small, they may not be noticed until they become inflamed in later life. Lesions present as soft or rubbery, round, subcutaneous tumors measuring 1–4cm in diameter.[279,280] They are noncompressible and do not transilluminate or enlarge with Valsalva maneuvers. They are most common on the upper lateral region of the forehead within or near the outer third of the eyebrow, overlying the anterior fontanel, in the midline nasal bridge (Fig. 6.30) and the submental region, though they may occur anywhere on the scalp, face, or spinal axis.[280–283] The epidermis is clinically normal and freely moveable over the cyst. There is often a sinus opening from which hairs may project. In the periorbital areas they can cause proptosis and eyelid displacement. The anterior or lateral neck is another common location, but cysts may also occur on the sternum, scrotum, perineal raphe and sacral areas. It is more common for one cyst to be present, but more than one may occur. They represent faulty development and may include both epidermal and dermal elements.

Although most dermoid cysts are superficial, dermal sinuses within these defects can extend intracranially to the extradural or intradural compartments. Up to 45% of cysts have been associated with intracranial connections.[282,284] Such connections are more frequent in the presence of a sinus pit. There is also increased association with other anomalies in children with this defect.[284] Histologically, dermoid cysts are encapsulated and differ from other types of cysts in that the wall is composed of keratinizing, stratified, squamous epithelium, complete with hair follicles, sebaceous glands, and frequently eccrine and apocrine glands.[285] The lumen contains lipid, keratin and hair.

Although these cysts are usually asymptomatic, recurrent infections can occur, including periorbital or nasal cellulitis or abscesses, with rare osteomyelitis or meningitis.[284] Pressure erosion of bone is another occasional complication.[286]

272. Aso M, Kawaguchi T, Mihara M et al. (1987) Pseudotail associated with spinal dysraphism. Dermatologia 174:45–48.
273. Albright AL, Gartner JC, Weiner GS (1989) Lumbar cutaneous hemangiomas as indicators of tethered spinal cords. Pediatrics 31:63–70.
274. Patrizi A, Neri I, Orlandi C, Marini R (1996) Sacral medial telangiectatic vascular nevus: A study of 43 children. Dermatol 192:301–306.
275. Ben-Amitai D, Davidson S, Schwartz M et al. (2000) Sacral nevus flammeus simplex: The role of imaging. Ped Dermatol 178&9:469–471.
276. Kriss V, Kriss T (1995) Occult spinal dysraphism in the infant. Clin Ped 34(12):650–655.
277. Steinbok P, Cochrane D (1991) The nature of congenital posterior cervical or cervicothoracic midline cutaneous mass lesions. Report of eight cases. J Neurosug 75:206–212.
278. Larralde M (1998) Dermatological lesions in the midline. In: Dermatology at the Millennium, Dyall Smith D, Marks R. ed. New York: The Parthenton Publishing Group; 1998, p. 470–473.

279. Brownstein MH, Helwig EB (1973) Subcutaneous dermoid cysts. Arch Dermatol 107:237.
280. Paller As, Pensler J, Tomita T (1991) Nasal midline masses in infants and children. Dermoids, encephaloceles, and nasal gliomas. Arch Dermatol 127:362–366.
281. Nocini P, Barbaglio A, Dolci M et al. (1996) Dermoid cyst of the nose: A case report and review of the literature. J Oral Maxillofac Surg 54:357–362.
282. Peter J, Sinclair-Smith C, deVillies J (1991) Midline dermal sinuses and cysts and their relationship to the central nervous system. Eur J Pediatr Surg 1:73–79.
283. Hattori H, Higuchi Y, Tashiro Y (1999) Dorsal dermal sinus and dermoid cysts in occult spinal dysraphism. J Pediatr 134:793.
284. Wardinsky TD, Poagon RA, Kropp RJ et al. (1991) Nasal dermoid sinus cysts: association with intracranial extension and multiple malformations. Cleft Palate Craniofac J 28:87.
285. Lever WF (1997) Tumors and cysts of the epidermis. In: Histopathology of the Skin, 8th ed. Philadelphia: JB Lippincott, p. 698.
286. Pensler JM, Baur BS, Naidich TP (1988) Craniofacial dermoids. Plast Reconstr Surg 82:953.

TABLE 6.11   Differential diagnosis of midline facial lesions

Tumor	Clinical features
Dermoid cyst	Mobile, solid, skin-colored tumor May have sinus and hair Does not transilluminate Nonpulsatile Frequent infection
Encephalocele	Blue, soft, pulsatile, compressible tumor Enlarges with crying and compression of jugular veins May transilluminate
Nasal glioma	Mobile, red-blue, firm tumor Noncompressible Does not transilluminate Nonpulsatile
Hemangioma	Mobile, red-blue, doughy tumor Noncompressible
Epidermoid cyst	Mobile, cystic, skin-colored to yellow tumor May have sinus opening
Infiltrative tumors	Firm, fixed tumor Irregular shaped Skin-colored

Adapted from Paller et al., with permission. Paller AS, Pensler JM, Tomita T (1991) Nasal midline masses in infants and children. Arch Dermatol 127:362.

The differential diagnosis of these lesions varies with anatomic location. When located on the neck, thyroglossal duct cyst, branchial cyst, submaxillary cyst, and ectopic thyroid tissue should be considered. For this reason, all patients with a midline anterior cervical mass should be evaluated, with thyroid function tests and ^{99m}Tc or ^{123}I scintillation scanning, to identify any possible ectopic thyroid tissue.[287] Nuclear imaging can be used for positive identification and delineation of these anomalies prior to surgery.

Central facial lesions raise a differential diagnosis of hemangioma, encephalocele, nasal glioma, epidermoid cysts and infiltrative tumors (Table 6.11). Midline lesions on the face should be evaluated with MRI or axial CT; MRI has greater sensitivity, while CT may be superior for delineation of bony defects.[288,289] High-resolution ultrasound with Doppler has also been used successfully to delineate subtle structural abnormalities of the midline face.[290] Biopsy of midline nasal masses should be avoided until intracranial connections are ruled out. The imaging studies may show intracranial masses or bony distortion; the former confirms the presence of an intracranial connection, but in patients with the latter there may be no evidence of a connection on surgical exploration.

Surgery is essential for all lesions with intracranial connections to avoid the risk of local or ascending infection. Removal may be difficult if the cyst has extended into surrounding structures through the cranial sutures and the patient should be managed by an experienced pediatric otolaryngologist, neurosurgeon, or plastic surgeon.[281] An external rhinoplasty approach can be used to improve the final cosmetic result by avoiding the standard vertical midline scar.[291]

NASAL GLIOMA

Nasal gliomas are rare tumors that present at birth or shortly thereafter as firm bluish or red swellings of the nasal root.[292] They are composed of ectopic neural tissue and can be regarded as a variant of encephalocele (see below). Unlike true encephaloceles, however, they do not always have an intracranial connection. They are usually more firm on palpation, and do not increase in size with crying or the Valsalva maneuver.[293] The pathogenesis of the nasal glioma is thought to involve evagination of neuroectodermal tissue through the nasofrontal fontanelle during development. Normally, this tissue retracts with formation of the dura, but failure of complete retraction can lead to amputation of tissue with closure of the craniofrontal sutures. A stalk of fibroglial tissue can connect these tumors to the underlying brain through the foramen caecum.[294]

Nasal gliomas are usually external, but 30% are intranasal or extend into the oropharynx.[293] The latter tumors can be a cause of upper respiratory obstruction in the newborn.[295] Histologic examination of these lesions shows collections of astrocytes embedded in dense connective tissue trabeculae. Striated muscle can also be found in the dermis.[296]

The differential diagnosis of nasal gliomas includes encephaloceles, hemangiomas, nasal dermoids, lacrimal duct cysts, neuroblastoma, or rhabdomyosarcoma. They are most commonly mistaken for hemangiomas, as they are often bluish in appearance with overlying telangiectasias.[297] Evaluation should include a CT or MRI;[298] the latter is more sensitive for soft tissue imaging.[294] Treatment of these lesions is surgical and should involve experienced pediatric otolaryngologists, often in collaboration with neurosurgeons.[293]

ENCEPHALOCELE

An encephalocele is a true herniation of brain tissue through the skull. By definition, all encephaloceles connect with the underlying brain tissue. The most common is the frontal midline encephalocele. These lesions can be fronto-ethmoid, with herniation through the ethmoid plate behind the crista galli, or nasofrontal, with herniation anterior to the crista galli.[299] Frontal midline encephaloceles are usually diagnosed in the newborn period. They commonly present as nasal broadening (67%) or as a blue pulsatile mass of the nasal bridge that transilluminates (Fig. 6.31). Unlike nasal gliomas, these masses are soft and increase in size with Valsalva maneuvers, crying, or compression of the jugular veins.[300] Histologically, they are indistinguishable from a nasal glioma. Both contain astrocytes and interweaving strands of fibrous tissue. Occasionally, neurons or muscle fibers are also present.

Differential diagnosis of these lesions includes hemangioma, nasal glioma and dermoid cyst. The deformity of the nasal root may be erroneously interpreted as hypertelorism. Infants should undergo a thorough evaluation for other associated anomalies, especially in the midline. Facial clefting is the most common association. Unsuspected encephaloceles have been reported in cases of median cleft face syndrome after CT or MRI.[301]

Infection and bony atropy or distortion can result if these lesions are not surgically excised early in life. CT and MRI are recommended to define the extent of the complex tumor mass.[302] The combined efforts of a pediatric otolaryngologist and neurosurgeon are usually required for removal of both intracranial and extracranial portions of these developmental defects. Complete

287. Conklin WT, Davis RM, Dabb RW et al. (1981) Hypothyroidism following removal of a "thyroglossal duct cyst." **Plast Reconstr Surg** 68:930.
288. Goffin J, Plets C, Van Calenbergh F et al. (1993) Posterior fossa dermoid cyst associated with dermal fistula: report of 2 cases and review of the literature. **Childs Nerv Syst** 9:179.
289. Barkovich AJ, Vandermarck P, Edwards MS et al. (1991) Congenital nasal masses: CT and MR imaging features in 16 cases. **Am J Neuroradiol** 12:105.
290. Glasier CM, Brodsky MC, Leithiser RE et al. (1992) High resolution ultrasound with Doppler: a diagnostic adjunct in orbital and ocular lesions in children. **Pediatr Radiol** 22:174.
291. Morrisey MS, Bailey CM (1991) External rhinoplasty approach for nasal dermoids in children. **Ear Nose Throat J** 70:445.
292. Kennard CD, Rasmussen JE (1990) Congenital midline nasal masses: diagnos s and management. **J Dermatol Surg Oncol** 16:1025.
293. Paller AS, Pensler JM, Tomita T (1991) Nasal midline masses in infants and children. **Arch Dermatol** 127:362.
294. Whitaker SR, Sprinkle PM, Chou SM (1981) Nasal glioma. **Arch Otolaryngol** 107:550.
295. Puppala B, Mangurten HH, McFadden J (1990) Nasal glioma. Presenting as neonatal respiratory distress. Definition of the tumor mass by MRI. **Clin Pediatr** 29:49.
296. Fletcher CDM, Carpenter C, McKee PH (1986) Nasal glioma: a rarity. **Am J Dermatopathol** 8:341.
297. Levine MR, Kellis A, Lash R (1993) Nasal glioma masquerading as a capillary hemangioma. **Ophthalmol Plast Reconstruct Surg** 9:132.
298. Barkovich AJ, Vandermarck P, Edwards MS et al. (1991) Congenital nasal masses: CT and MR imaging features in 16 cases. **Am J Neuroradiol** 12:105.
299. Paller AS, Pensler JM, Tomita T (1991) Nasal midline masses in infants and children. **Arch Dermatol** 127:362.
300. Bagger-Sjoback, Bergstrand G, Edner G et al. (1983) Nasal meningoencephalocele: a clinical problem. **Clin Otolaryngol** 8:329.
301. Moore MH, Lodge ML, David DJ (1993) Basal encephalocoele: imaging and exposing the hernia. **Br J Plast Surg** 46:497.
302. Barkovich AJ, Vandermarck P, Edwards MS et al. (1991) Congenital nasal masses: CT and MR imaging features in 16 cases. **Am J Neuroradiol** 12:105.

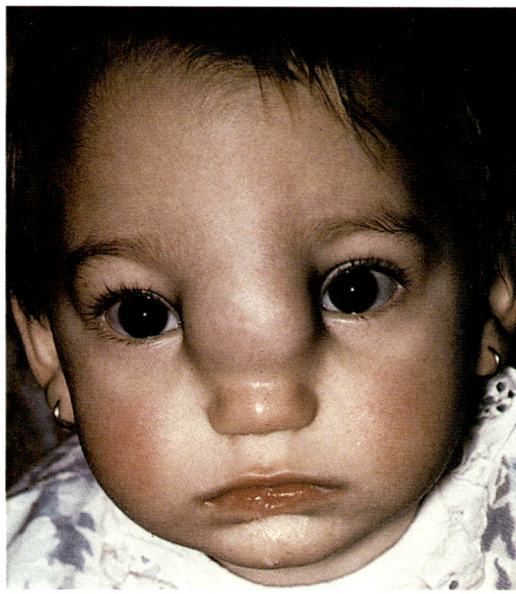

Fig. 6.31 Frontal encephalocele (courtesy Odile Enjolras, MD).

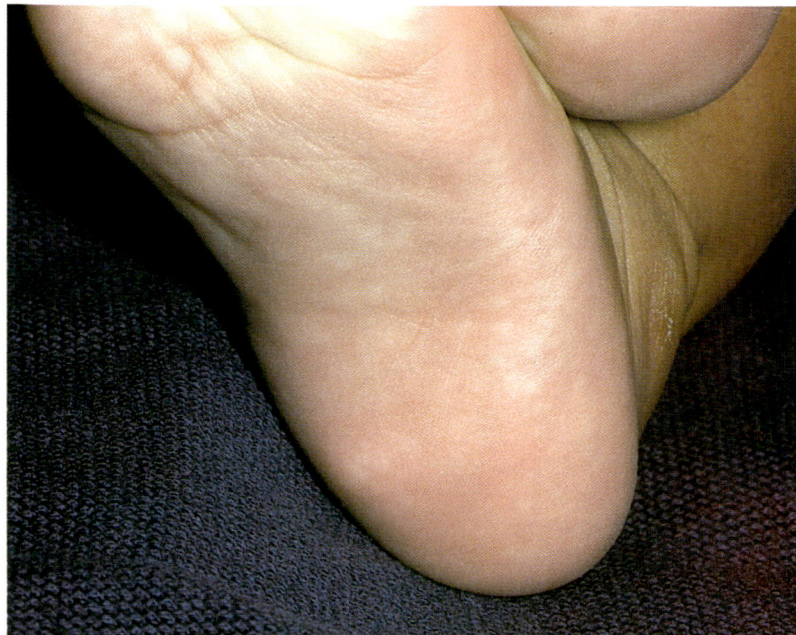

Fig. 6.32 Congenital pedal papules. These were bilateral and biopsy confirmed lipomatous nature.

excision is essential to prevent recurrence; obliteration of the bone and dural defects is necessary to prevent ascending infections.[303]

CONGENITAL PEDAL PAPULES IN THE NEWBORN

Congenital pedal papules are congenital, bilateral and symmetrical, subcutaneous nodules on the plantar surfaces of the heels, usually in the midline. The condition was first described by Larralde *et al.* in 1990,[304] reporting four cases and describing their similarity to adult piezogenic papules. Subsequently, more cases have been reported.[305–307] They present as 0.5–1cm diameter, skin-colored, non-inflammatory, asymptomatic, soft lesions on the plantar surface of each heel (Fig. 6.32). They tend to persist and grow in proportion to the growth of the child. Rarer variants are unilateral lesions and those which develop several weeks after birth.

The exact pathogenesis of these lesions is unclear but incomplete regression of fetal tissue has been suggested.[305] Histopathological examination demonstrates mature adipose tissue in the reticular dermis and subcutis, enveloped in predominantly collagenous fibrous sheaths.[307] The epidermis is normal and no inflammatory changes are observed.

In the literature they can be found under a variety of different names including congenital fibrolipomata,[307] podalic papules in the newborn,[308] bilateral congenital fatty heel pads, precalcaneal congenital fibrolipomatous hamartoma,[305] bilateral congenital adipose plantar nodules,[309] and congenital piezogenic-like pedal papules.[306]

Though this is a uncommon benign condition it is important to separate it from more serious entities such as juvenile fibromatosis, particularly plantar aponeurotic fibroma and childhood fibrous hamartoma.[307]

UMBILICAL POLYPS

Umbilical polyp is an uncommon condition present at birth or arising during infancy, that consists of umbilical remnants of ectopic gastrointestinal mucosa caused by incomplete closure of the omphalomesenteric duct.[310] This omphalomesenteric (vitelline) duct, which connects the mid gut with the yolk sac of the embryo, usually disappears during the seventh week of embryonic life. A remnant of the duct may persist anywhere along its embryonic course from the skin to the intestine, and may give rise to the formation of polyps, sinuses, or cysts with or without connection to the intestine or to the skin surface.[311]

Nix and Young[312] classified the conditions as:

(1) complete patency (umbilical–enteric fistula)
(2) partial patency
    (a) peripheral portion (umbilical sinus)
    (b) intermediate portion (vitelline cyst)
    (c) enteric portion (Meckel's diverticulum)
(3) mucosal remnant at the umbilicus (umbilical polyp)
(4) congenital band (obliterated vitellointestinal duct)

Meckel's diverticulum is the most common anomaly and occurs in 1–3% of the population.[310,312,313] Umbilical polyp is less common and it may occur alone or it may be associated with other omphalomesenteric duct anomalies including Meckel's diverticulum, a fibrous band from the umbilicus to the intestine, or a vitelline cyst. As a consequence, it may be associated with significant complicating features such as intestinal obstruction, gastrointestinal bleeding, perforation, intussusception, diverticulitis, or abdominal masses.[310,313,314,315]

The umbilical polyp is a reddish tumor of a few millimeters; it seldom bleeds or is exudative and typically does not disappear after silver nitrate cauterization. Histopathology shows ectopic gastrointestinal epithelium with the appearance of gastric, intestinal or colonic mucosa, and in rare instances pancreatic tissue can be seen.

303. Kennard CD, Rasmussen JE (1990) Congenital midline nasal masses: diagnosis and management. **J Dermatol Surg Oncol** 16:1025.
304. Larralde de Luna M, Ruiz León J, Cabrera HN (1990) Papulas podálicas en el recién nacido. **Med Cut ILA** 18:9–12.
305. Larregue M, Vabres P. Echard P et al. (1996) Precalcaneal congenital fibrolipomatous hamartoma. Presented at the V International Congress of Pediatric Dermatology, Rótterdam.
306. Eichenfield LF, Cunningham BC, Friedlander SF (1998) Congenital piezogenic-like pedal papules. Presented at the VIII Congress of Pediatric Dermatology, Paris.
307. Ortega Monzó C, Molina-Gallardo I, Monteagudo-Castro C et al. (2000) Precalcaneal congenital fibrolipomatous hamartoma: a report of four cases. **Pediatr Dermatol** 17:429–431.
308. Larralde de Luna M (1995) Dermatosis neonatales. In: Dermatología Neonatal y Pediátrica, Larralde de Luna, ed. Argentina: Buenos Aires, pp. 8–29.
309. Pujol RM, Idoate MA, Vazquez Doval J, Romani J (2000) Bilateral congenital adipose plantar nodules. **Br J Dermatol** 142:1262–1264.
310. Larralde M, Rossito A, Santos Muñoz A et al. (2000) Pólipos umbilicales y otras anomalías del conducto onfalomesentérico. **Med Cut ILA** 28:326–330.
311. Steck Wb, Heiwig EB (1964) Cutaneous remnant of the omphalomesenteric duct. **Arch Dermatol** 90:463–470.
312. Nix TE, Young JC (1964) Congenital umbilical anomalies. **Arch Dermatol** 90:160–165.
313. Armstrong DKB, Thomton C, Bingham A (1998) Infantile umbilical polyp: important diagnostic considerations. **Dermatology** 197:94.
314. Moore TC (1956) Omphalomesenteric duct anomalies. **Surgery Gynec Obstet** 103:569–580.
315. Larralde M, Ciccioni V, Herrera A et al. (1987) Umbilical polyps. **Pediatr Dermatol** 4:341–343.

The management of this lesion varies depending on whether or not it communicates with the bowel. If there is no communication, surgical resection of the lesion can be performed. If a fistula is present, it must be investigated carefully with invasive radiographic studies to exclude other underlying embryologic anomalies.

The parents must be educated regarding the possibility of persistent intra-abdominal remnants. Internal omphalomesenteric duct polyps have been found in up to 60% of the patients with umbilical polyps who had undergone surgical exploration, although the actual frequency is unknown. If significant abdominal symptoms develop during the patient's lifetime, immediate surgical evaluation is needed.[310]

CONGENITAL EROSIVE AND VESICULAR DERMATOSIS

Congenital erosive and vesicular dermatosis is a rare disorder of unknown etiology that presents at birth, with extensive ulcerations, intact vesicles, crusts, and fissures covering as much as 75 percent of the cutaneous surface (Fig. 6.33A). Lesions heal in the first month of life without progression producing supple and reticulate scarring (Fig. 6.33B).[316–318] Infants affected with this condition are usually premature and may have underlying neurologic defects, including mental and motor retardation, seizures, cerebral palsy and microcephaly. The face, palms, and soles are characteristically spared. Nails are absent or hypoplastic (Fig. 6.33C) and patchy alopecia is seen on the scalp.

Histology of chronic scarred lesions demonstrates a normal appearing epidermis and a dermis with minimally increased collagen, a decrease in hair follicles and absent eccrine glands. The histology of acute lesions is not well defined, with only several cases studied, with a predominantly neutrophilic infiltrate in one child, and an eosinophil-rich infiltrate and subepidermal split in another.[319,320] The cause of this disorder is unknown; an intrauterine event, such as an infection, amniotic adhesions, or a developmental defect, with unusual healing in premature skin, have been postulated.[316,317,318,319]

The differential diagnosis at birth includes congenital absence of skin (aplasia cutis), Goltz syndrome, epidermolysis bullosa, staphylococcal scalded skin and other congenital infections.

Care for these infants is supportive. Like infants with epidermolysis bullosa, they are susceptible to contractures and infection. Insensible water losses are increased, necessitating close attention to hydration status. Close pediatric follow-up evaluation for evidence of developmental delay or neurologic impairment is recommended.[316–318]

VESICULOPUSTULAR AND BULLOUS DISEASES OF THE NEWBORN

Vesiculopustular and bullous disorders are common in neonates.[321–324] Many of the conditions are benign, innocuous and self-limited, while others are life threatening. Prompt and accurate diagnosis is necessary. This section, and

Tables 6.12, 6.13, present some of the conditions that may cause vesicles, pustules, bullae or erosions and/or ulcerations in the newborn period. Detailed discussions of many of these diseases are presented in other sections of this textbook. Several are discussed below.

Causes of vesiculopustular eruptions include transient phenomena such as erythema toxicum, transient neonatal pustular melanosis, miliaria, acne neonatorum, cephalic pustulosis and infantile acropustulosis. Infectious causes include localized bacterial infections (commonly *Staphylococcus aureus* or *Streptococcus pyogenes*), systemic bacterial infections (*Listeria monocytogenes*, *Escherichia coli*, and group B *streptococcus*), viral infections (Herpes simplex or varicella), treponenal infection (syphilis) fungal infections (such as congenital or neonatal candidiasis) or parasitic infestations (scabies). Several systemic diseases may present with vesiculopustules, bullae or erosions, such as Langherhan's cell histiocytosis, incontinentia pigmenti, hyperimmunoglobulin E syndrome, and focal dermal hypoplasia. Cutaneous diseases such as mastocytosis, epidermolysis bullosa, pustular psoriasis and bullous ichythyosis may also present with these findings in the neonatal period (Table 6.12). The characteristics of some of these entities and the features that aid in their distinction are discussed below.

ERYTHEMA TOXICUM NEONATORUM (TOXIC ERYTHEMA OF THE NEWBORN)

Erythema toxicum neonatorum is a benign, self-limited condition of the neonatal period. It was probably first described by Metlinger in 1472.[325] It is very common in term infants, but is rare in preterm infants and infants with less than 2500g birth weight.[326–328] Most lesions appear during the second 24 hours of life, but they may begin any time from birth to 2 weeks of age,[329–332] lasting several days or rarely persisting for several weeks.[333,334] Recurrences during the first 2 weeks have been reported.

Erythema toxicum presents as erythematous macules, papules, pustules or wheals that can be found on any body surface, though palms and soles are rarely affected (Fig. 6.34). The sites of predilection include the face, trunk, proximal arms, and buttocks. Red macular areas and wheals range from a few millimeters to several centimeters with superimposed 1–2mm papules and pustules. Lesions present at birth are likely to be more pustular, but erythematous macules, papules, and pustules may be present singularly or in combination. The lesions may be few in number but more often are present in large numbers. Individual lesions are discrete, but adjacent macules of erythema may become confluent. Vesicles may be seen occasionally before becoming pustular. An estimated 10% of newborns will develop pustules on macular lesions within 24 hours. The eruption may evolve with crops of lesions waxing and waning, with spontaneous resolution of individual lesions within hours to days. The infant with erythema toxicum neonatorum is asymptomatic and usually well, although the disorder may occur in infants with other neonatal illnesses.

The etiology of erythema toxicum neonatorum remains unknown, and its appearance is unrelated to prenatal or perinatal events. Intestinal toxins, allergic reactions, mechanical or chemical irritation, hormonal influences on the

316. Cohen BA, Esterly NB, Nelson PF (1985) Congenital erosive and vesicular dermatosis healing with reticulated scarring. **Arch Dermatol** 121:361.
317. Gupta AK, Rasmussen JE, Headington JT (1987) Extensive congenital erosions and vesicles healing with reticulate scarring. **J Am Acad Dermatol** 17:369.
318. Plantin P, Delaire P, Guillois B et al. (1990) Congenital erosive and vesicular dermatosis with reticulated supple scarring: first neonatal report. **Arch Dermatol** 126:544.
319. Cohen B (1999) Congenital erosive and vesicular dermatosis. In: Textbook of Pediatric Dermatology, Harper J, Oranje AP, Prose N, eds. Oxford, England: Blackwell Sciences. pp. 120–124.
320. Sadick NS, Shea CR, Schlessel JS (1995) Congenital erosive and vesicular dermatosis with reticulate, supple scarring: a neutrophilic dermatosis. **J Am Acad Dermatol** 32:203–206.
321. Frieden IJ and Howard R (2001) In: Textbook of Neonatal Dermatology. Eichenfield LF, Frieden IJ, Esterly NB, eds. WB Saunders Company: Philadelphia, PA.
322. Frieden IJ (1992) The dermatologist in the newborn nursery: approach to the neonate with blisters, pustules, erosions, and ulcerations. **Current Problems in Dermatology** 4:123–68.
323. Wagner A (1997) Distinguishing vesicular and pustular disorders in the neonate. **Curr Opin Pediatr** 9:396–405.
324. van Praag MC, van Rooij RW, Folkers E, Spritzer R, Menke HE, Oranje AP (1997) Diagnosis and treatment of pustular disorders in the neonate. **Pediatr Dermatol** 14:131–143.

325. Lehndorff H (1951) Bartholomaeus Metlinger: a fifteenth century pediatrician. **Arch Pediatr** 68:322.
326. Prigent F, Vige P, Martinet C (1991) Cutaneous lesions during the 1st week of life in 306 consecutive newborn infants. **Ann Dermatol Venereol** 118:697.
327. Plantin P, Delaire P, Gavanou J et al. (1990) Benign cutaneous lesions observed within the 1st 48 hours of 847 infants born at a maternity ward of a university hospital. **Ann Dermatol Venereol** 117:181.
328. Berg FJ, Solomon LM (1987) Erythema neonatorum toxicum. **Arch Dis Child** 62:327–328.
329. Leung AC, Wheeler BH, Robson WL et al. (1992) Erythema toxicum present at birth. **Pediatr Dermatol** 9:162.
330. Levy HL, Cothran F (1962) Erythema toxicum neonatorum present at birth. **Am J Dis Child** 103:125.
331. Carr JA, Hodgman JE, Freedman RI et al. (1966) Relationship between toxic erythema and infant maturity. **Am J Dis Child** 112:129–134.
332. Marino LJ (1965) Toxic erythema present at birth. **Archives of Dermatology** 92:402–403.
333. Chang M, Jiang S, Orlow S (1999) Atypical erythema toxicum neonatorum of delayed onset in a term infant. **Pediatr Dermatol** 16:137–141.
334. Luder D (1960) Histologic observations in erythema toxicum neonatorum. **Pediatrics** 26:219.

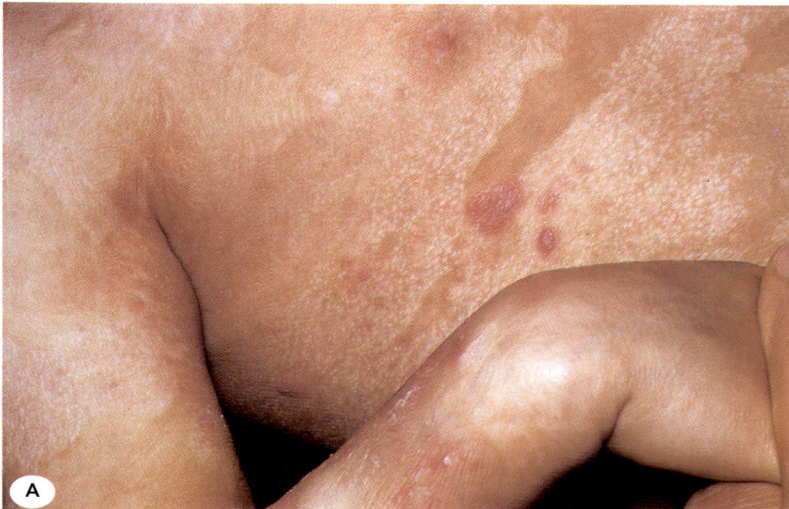

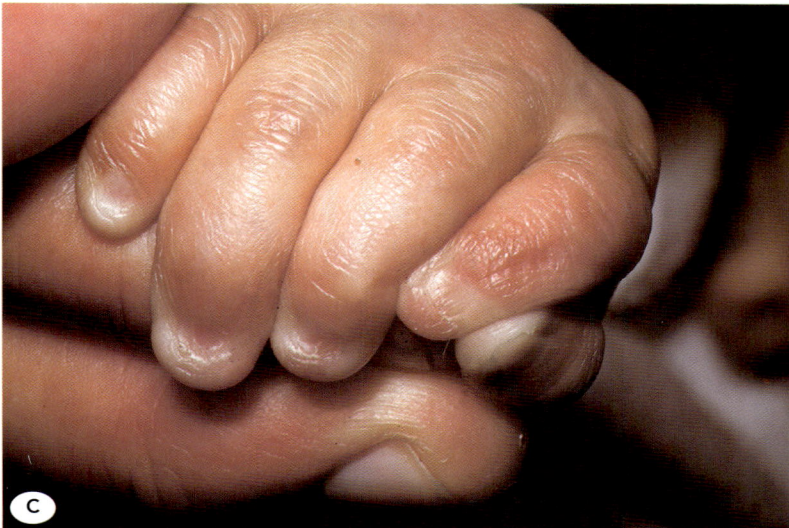

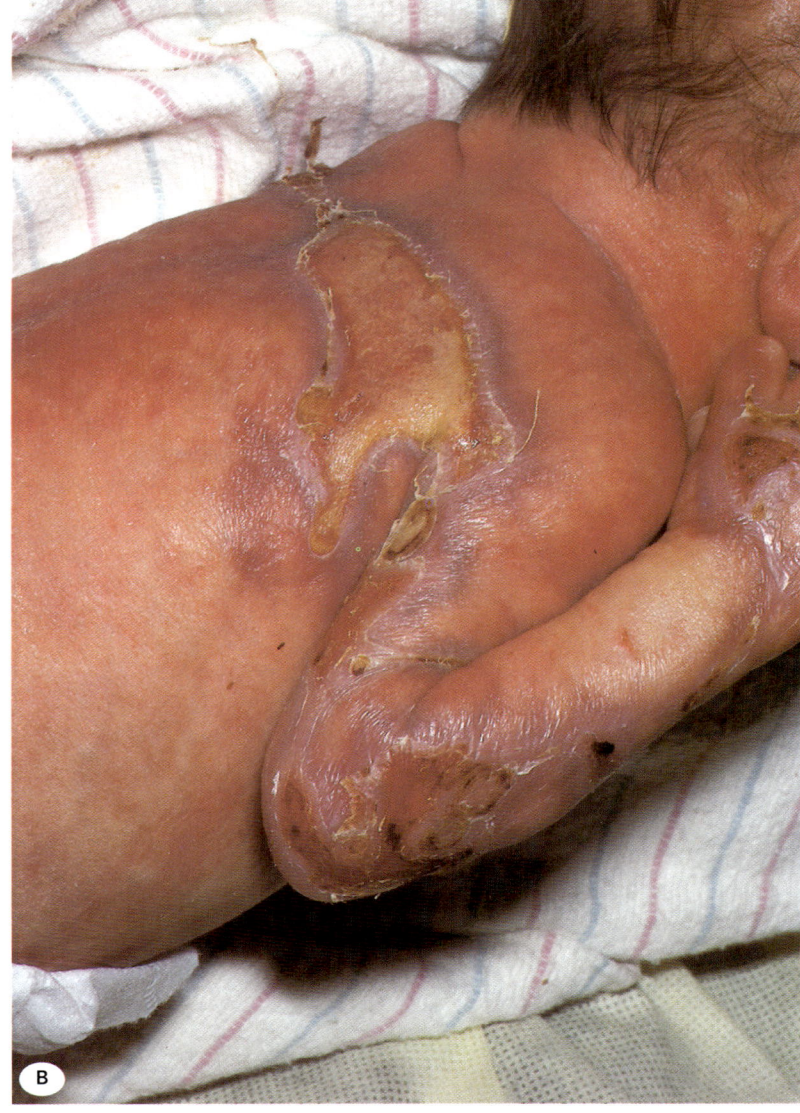

Fig. 6.33 (A) Congenital erosive and vesicular dermatosis: newborn with extensive symmetrical ulcerative and erosive changes. (B) Supple reticulate scarring at age 4 months. (C) Hypoplastic nails at birth.

extracellular matrix, and a transient graft–versus–host reaction from maternal lymphocytes have been suggested as possible causes, but none has been confirmed.[335,336]

Diagnosis is usually made by clinical appearance. Microscopic examination of a Wright stain of pustular contents will show large numbers of eosinophils, frequently in sheets, and is useful for diagnostic confirmation. Peripheral blood eosinophilia is seen in some cases.[334] While biopsy is not usually necessary, histologic examination of erythematous macular lesions shows a perivascular accumulation of eosinophils in the upper dermis. Papular lesions are characterized by upper dermal eosinophils. In addition, an accumulation of eosinophils and some neutrophils is found around the outer root sheath of hair follicles extending into the epidermis. In pustular lesions, intrafollicular subcorneal eosinophilic pustules are present.[334]

The differential diagnosis should include transient neonatal pustular melanosis, congenital candidiasis, miliaria, bacterial infections, Herpes simplex infection, incontinentia pigmenti, scabies, eosinophilic pustular folliculitis (Ofuji disease), and acropustulosis of infancy.[337] Erythema and postnatal onset may distinguish erythema toxicum from pustular melanosis, though both are common and can occur simultaneously.[338,339] Pustular bacterial infections are usually due to *Staphylococcus aureus*, but occasional neonatal infections with group B *streptococcus*, *Pseudomonas aeruginosa*, *Listeria monocytogenes*, *Haemophilus influenzae*, and *Klebsiella pneumoniae* have occurred with pustules. These infections are characterized by the presence of large numbers of neutrophils on Wright stain, the presence of organisms on Gram stain, and a positive bacterial culture. Candidiasis may be differentiated on the basis of a positive potassium hydroxide preparation. Miliaria may be excluded on the basis of its extrafollicular location and the presence of lymphocytes on Wright stain.

As erythema toxicum is self-limiting, no treatment is necessary other than parental reassurance.

335. Stone OJ (1990) High viscosity of newborn extracellular matrix is the etiology of erythema toxicum neonatorum: neonatal jaundice? hyaline membrane disease? **Med Hypoth** 33:15.
336. Bassukas ID (1992) Is erythema toxicum neonatorum a mild self-limited acute cutaneous graft-versus-host-reaction from maternal-to-fetal lymphocyte transfer? **Med Hypoth** 38:334.
337. Schachner L, Press S (1983) Vesicular, bullous and pustular disorders in infancy and childhood. **Pediatr Clin North Am** 3C:609.
338. Coroleu LW, Natal PA, Ferrandez FC et al. (1990) Transient neonatal pustular melanosis. **Ann Espanol Pediatr** 33:117.
339. Ferrandiz C, Coroleu LW, Ribera M et al. (1992) Sterile transient neonatal pustulosis is a precocious form of erythema toxicum neonatorum. **Dermatology** 185:18.

TABLE 6.12　Differential diagnosis of neonatal vesiculopustular diseases

Noninfectious: benign
　Acropustulosis of infancy
　Eosinophilic pustular folliculitis
　Erythema toxicum
　Miliaria crystallina, rubra, profunda
　Transient neonatal pustular melanosis

Noninfectious: potentially serious
　Acrodermatitis enteropathica
　Epidermolysis bullosa
　Epidermolytic hyperkeratosis (congenital ichthyosiform erythroderma)
　Herpes gestationis – neonatal
　Incontinentia pigmenti
　Pemphigus vulgaris – neonatal
　Urticaria pigmentosa

Infectious: usually mild
　Candidiasis – neonatal
　Impetigo neonatorum
　Scabies

Infectious: serious
　Bacterial infections
　　Chlamydia trachomatis
　　Escherichia coli
　　Hemophilus influenzae
　　Klebsiella pneumoniae
　　Listeria monocytogenes
　　Pseudomonas aeruginosa
　　Staphylococcus aureus
　　Streptococcus (group A β-hemolytic)
　　Syphilis
　　Candidiasis: congenital
　　Staphylococcal scalded skin syndrome
　Viral infections
　　Cytomegalic
　　Herpes
　　Varicella

From Schachner and Press, with permission. Schachner L, Press S (1983) Vesicular, bullous and pustular disorders in infancy and childhood. Pediatr Clin North Am 30:609.

TRANSIENT NEONATAL PUSTULAR MELANOSIS (TRANSIENT NEONATAL PUSTULAR DERMATOSIS)

Transient neonatal pustular melanosis (TNPM) is a benign condition of term neonates. It was described by Ramamurthy et al in 1976,[340] and occurs in approximately 0.2–4% of all term newborn infants and is more commonly seen in black infants.[340–342] It is characterized by the presence at birth of neutrophil-containing pustules or vesicles without surrounding erythema (Fig. 6.35). Lesions may measure 1–5mm and are found in clusters or singly. After birth, new lesions usually do not develop, but existing vesicular or pustular lesions may progress to produce a brownish crust, or rupture, leaving a fine white collarette of scale. Vesicopustules resolve within several days leaving hyperpigmented macules in darker-skinned individuals. As pigmentation is not usually a feature in white infants it has been suggested that transient neonatal pustular dermatosis may be a better terminology. Most commonly affected areas include the forehead, posterior ears, chin, neck, upper chest, back, buttocks, abdomen, and thighs, but all areas may be affected, including the palms and soles. In fact all types of lesion – vesicles, intact pustules, crusted lesions, ruptured pustules with a collarette of scale, and pigmented macules – may be present singly or in combination at birth, suggesting their *in utero* formation and evolution. When present, macular pigmentation fades within weeks to months.

The cause of transient neonatal pustular melanosis is unknown. Maternal infection, drug use, and primary fetal infection have no influence on its occurrence. Some investigators have proposed that it is a variant eruption of erythema toxicum neonatorum while others have suggested that this condition is actually a precocious form of erythema toxicum.[343] Nonetheless, transient neonatal pustular melanosis is nonfollicular and noneosinophilic, lacks the erythematous wheal of erythema toxicum neonatorum, is present at birth, and infrequently affects the palms and soles.

Wright staining of pustular contents show neutrophils and occasional eosinophils. No organisms are observed. Skin biopsy shows pustules displaying intracorneal or subcorneal aggregates of neutrophils. There may also occasionally be a predominantly neutrophilic dermal infiltrate. Eosinophils may be present in limited numbers in the dermis as well as in the epidermal infiltrate.[344] Biopsy of pigmented macules shows increased basilar melanocytes.[342]

The differential diagnosis includes erythema toxicum, staphylococcal pustulosis and other bacterial, viral, and candidal infections, miliaria, and acropustulosis of infancy. Onset, morphology, and characteristics of Wright and Gram stain and KOH should allow confirmation of clinical suspicions. However, a clear-cut differentiation between transient neonatal pustular melanosis and erythema toxicum is not always possible.

No therapy is necessary.

MILIARIA

Miliaria is a term used to descrbe obstructions of the eccrine duct resulting in rupture of the ducts and sweating into the skin. The level of obstruction determines the clinical manifestations. It can be seen in up to 15% of neonates, occurring more commonly in warm climates, in nurseries without air-conditioning and in febrile infants.[345,346]

Miliaria crystallina (sudamina) is the most common type of miliaria in the newborn period, manifested by fragile, 1–2mm clear, non-inflammatory vesicles without surrounding inflammation. These superficial, asymptomatic lesions may appear like dewdrops on the skin (Fig. 6.36), and reflect superficial obstruction of the eccrine duct at the level of the stratum corneum. Slight pressure will generally rupture miliaria crystallina lesions. Miliaria crystallina is most common in the first week of life, with some reports of congenital lesions.[347–350] Lesions are most common on the forehead and upper trunk.

Miliaria rubra (prickly heat, or "heat rash") is due to intraepidermal obstruction of the sweat duct with sweat leakage around the ducts. A secondary local inflammatory response is responsible for the erythema

340. Ramamurthy RS, Reveri M, Esterly NB et al. (1976) Transient neonatal pustular melanosis. J Pediatr 88:830.
341. Merlob P, Metzker A, Reisner SH (1982) Transient neonatal pustular melanosis. Am J Dis Child 136:521.
342. Coroleu LW, Natal PA, Ferrandiz C et al. (1990) Transient neonatal pustular melanosis. Ann Espanol Pediatr 33:117.
343. Ferrandiz C, Coroleu W, Ribera M et al. (1992) Sterile transient neonatal pustulosis is a precocious form of erythema toxicum neonatorum. Dermatology 185:18–22.
344. Cohen LM, Skopicki BK, Harrist TJ et al. (1997) Noninfectious vesiculobullous and vesiculopustular diseases. In: Lever's Histopathology of the Skin, Elder D, Eleritsas R, Jaworsky C, Johnson B, eds. Philadelphia: Lippencott-Raven, pp. 209–252.

345. Hidano A, Purwoko R, Jitsukawa K (1986) Statistical survey of skin changes in Japanese neonates. Pediatr Dermatol 3:140–144.
346. Nanda A, Kaur S, Bhakoo ON, Dhall K (1989) Survey of cutaneous lesions in Indian newborns. Pediatr Dermatol 6:39–42.
347. Straka BF, Cooper PH, Greer KE (1991) Congenital miliaria crystallina. Cutis 47:103–106.
348. Arpey CJ, Nagashima-Whalen LS, Chren MM, Zain MT (1992) Congenital miliaria crystallina: case report and literature review. Pediatr Dermatol 9:283–287.
349. Lucky AW (2001) Transient benign cutaneous lesions in the newborn. In: Textbook of Neonatal Dermatology, Eichenfield LF, Frieden IJ, Esterly NB, eds. Philadelphia, PA: WB Saunders, pp 98–99.
350. Holzle E, Kligman A (1978) The pathogenesis of miliaria rubra. Role of the resident microflora. Br J Dermatol 99:117.

TABLE 6.13   Comparison of the benign vesiculopustular diseases of the neonate and young infant

Disease	Incidence	Usual age of onset	Duration	Lesions	Distribution	Pathology	Stains	Treatment
Acropustulosis of infancy	Incidence <1 percent, possibly increased in blacks and males	Hours after birth to 10 months	2–3 years	Red papules evolving into pustular and vesicular lesions in 1 day	Hands, feet, both surfaces	Subcorneal pustules with neutrophils and occasionally eosinophils	Gram: neutrophils, no bacteria KOH: negative Wright and Giemsa: neutrophils	Potent topical steroids, oral antihistamines; dapsone 2 mg/kg/day for severe cases
Candidiasis, congenital	Incidence <1 percent, equal among sexes	Birth to 24hr	2 weeks	Pink to red macules and papules evolving into pustules and vesicles	Diffuse, generalized	Subcorneal pustules with pseudohyphae and spores	KOH: pseudohyphae and spores Others: negative	Topical anticandidal agent (e.g., nystatin, clotrimazole, or miconazole) preparation for 10 days: oral fluconazole if severe cancer for candida sepsis in premature
Candidiasis, neonatal	Incidence approximately 4 to 5 percent	After the first week of life	2 weeks	Pink to red macules and papules evolving into pustules and vesicles	Oral mucosa, diaper area	Subcorneal pustules with pseudohyphae spores	KOH: pseudohyphae and spores Others: negative	Topical anticandidal agent (e.g., nystatin, clotrimazole, or miconazole for 10 days: nystatin suspension/oral fluconazole for persistent thrush
Erythema toxicum neonatorum	Approximately 1/3 of full-term newborns	24–72hr	1 week	Red macules and papules; white to pink pustules, vesicles	Trunk, extremities, face	Subcorneal pustules with eosinophils associated with pilosebaceous system	Gram: eosinophils, no bacteria KOH: negative; Wright and Giemsa: eosinophils	None
Eosinophilic pustular folliculitis	Very rare	Birth to 1 year	Years	Crops of papules, vesicles, and pustules that crust	Primarily scalp with some trunk and extremity lesions	Epidermal and dermal infiltrates of eosinophils associated with hair folicles	Gram: eosinophils no bacteria KOH: negative Wright and Giemsa: eosinophils	Questionable benefit of topical corticosteroid preparation
Impetigo neonatorum	<1 percent	Second day to second week	5–10 days	Vesicles, pustules, plus bullae on an erythematous base	Diaper area, neck, groin, axilla	Subcorneal pustules with Gram-positive cocci in clusters and neutrophils	Gram: Gram-positive cocci in clusters and neutrophils KOH: negative Wright and Giemsa: neutrophils	Dicloxacillin, 12.5–25mg/kg/day; cephalexin, 40mg/kg/day; for 10-day course
Millaria crystallina	Equal among sexes and races	First weeks of life	Hours to days	Miliaria crystallina, clear vesicles	Generalized with intertriginous increase	Subcorneal vesicles associated with sweat ducts	All stains negative	Cooling baths, air conditioning, removal of excess clothing
Miliaria rubra	Equal among sexes and races	First weeks of life	Hours to days	Miliaria rubra, grouped erythematous papules	Generalized with intertriginous increase	Intraepidermal spongiosis and vesicles associated with sweat ducts	All stains negative	Cooling baths, air conditioning, removal of excess clothing

TABLE 6.13   Comparison of the benign vesiculor pustular diseases of the neonate and young infant—cont'd

Disease	Incidence	Usual age of onset	Duration	Lesions	Distribution	Pathology	Stains	Treatment
Neonatal scabies	Rare	2–4 weeks	Until treated	Vesicles and papules; rare burrows	Hands, feet, trunk, genitalia	Subcorneal burrow with mite, eggs, scyballa	Oil prep: mite, eggs, scyballa	5% permethrin cream overnight
Transient neonatal pustular melanosis	5 percent of all black neonates; <1 percent in Caucasians	Birth, indicative of intrauterine involvement	Pustules; days; macules: 3 months	Vesicles and pustules desquamate leaving brown macules	Chin, neck, palms, soles	Macules: basilar hyperpigmentation; Pustule: intracorneal and subcorneal neutrophils and rare eosinophils	Gram: neutrophils, no bacteria, rare eosinophils KOH: negative Wright and Giemsa: neutrophils, rare eosinophils	None

From Schachner and Press with permission. Schachner L, Press S (1983) Vesicular, bullous and pustular disorders in infancy and childhood. Pediatr Clin North Am 30:609.

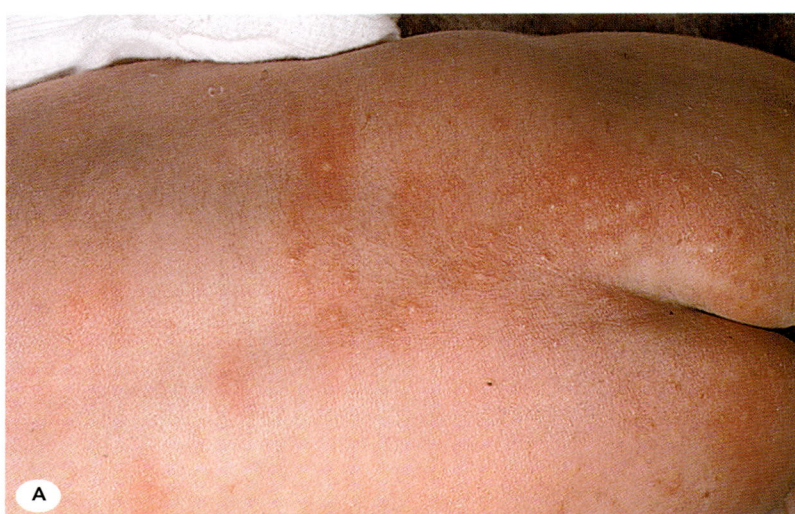

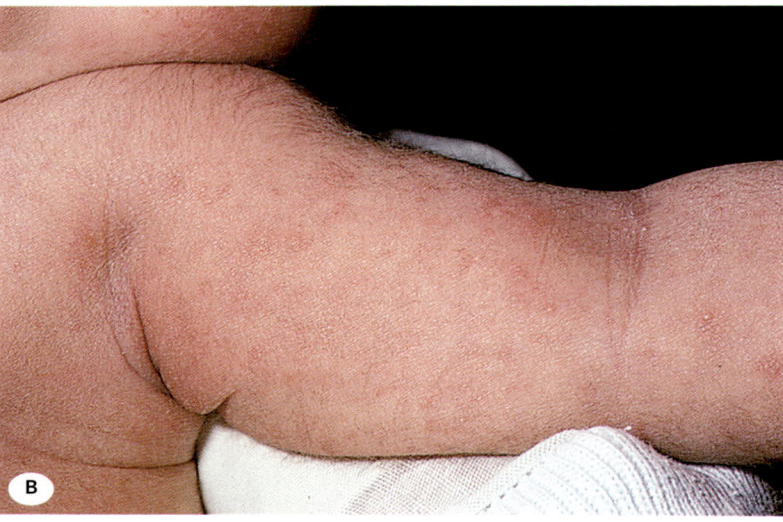

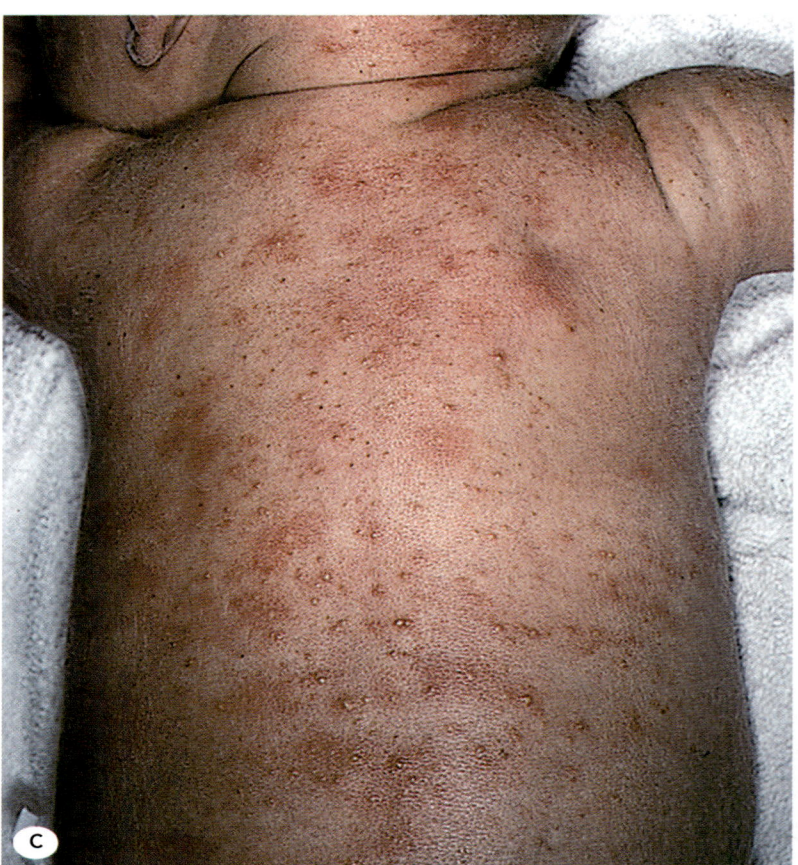

Fig. 6.34   Erytema toxicum. Erythematous macules and wheals may predominate (**A**). In some cases pustules are sparse (**B**), whereas in others extensive white to yellow papulovesicles with flares of erythema are noted (**C**).

associated with the papules and vesicles. Lesions are 1–3mm erythematous non-follicular papules, vesicles, or pustules (Fig. 6.37). Common sites are the face, neck, and trunk. Miliaria rubra occurs later than miliaria crystallina, usually beyond the first week of life and often in the second.

Miliaria profunda is rare in neonates. This disorder presents as a non-erythematous papulopustular eruption, most prominent on the trunk and

extremities, and reflects eccrine ductal occlusion at the dermo-epidemal junction.

Histologic examination of miliaria crystallina shows subcorneal vesicles adjacent to underlying sweat ducts, often with a keratotic plug overlying the duct. A biopsy of miliaria rubra shows intraepidermal vesicles contiguous with a sweat duct, with an intravesicular and/or dermal chronic inflammatory

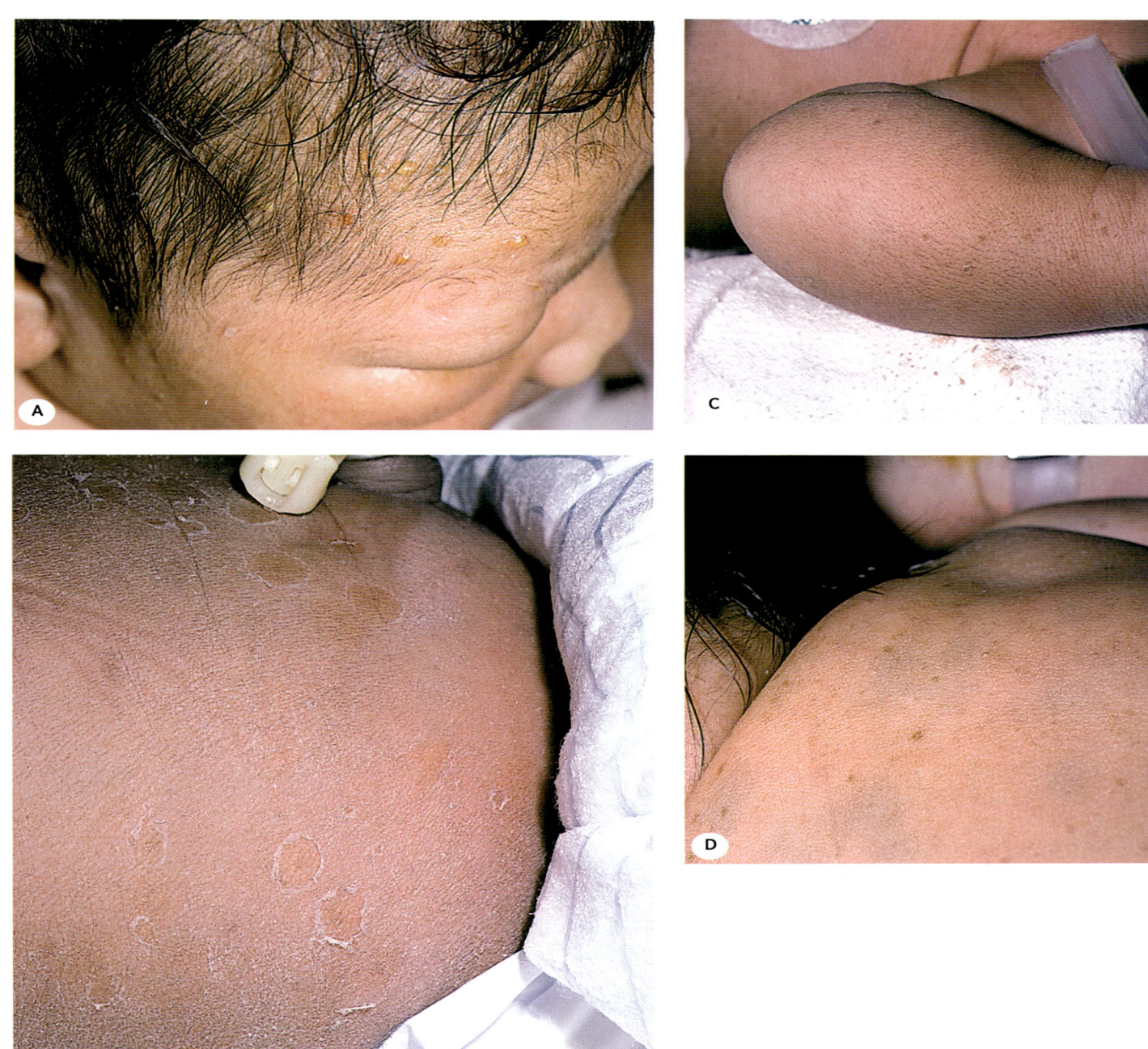

Fig. 6.35 Transient neonatal pustular melanosis first appears as small superficial pustules without inflammation (A). Collarettes of scale, typical of the second stage, are occasionally seen at birth without pustules evident (B) or may develop after pustules have ruptured (C). The final stage is that of small hyperpigmented macules resembling lentils, which gradually fade over weeks to months (D).

infiltrate.[351,352] With special stains, Gram-positive cocci may be seen beneath and within the keratinous plug in miliaria rubra and profunda.[350] The precise cause of miliaria is not known. There is some support for an extracellular polysaccharide substance produced by some strains of Staphylococcus epidermidis being involved in sweat duct obstruction and poral occlusion by epidermal cellular edema may be an initial event.[353]

The differential diagnosis includes erythema toxicum, transient neonatal pustular melanosis, candidiasis, HSV infection, neonatal acne/cephalic pustulosis, and bacterial folliculitis. Skin scrapings of vesicular contents and of the base of the vesicle may be examined for hyphae, multinucleated giant cells, eosinophils, bacteria, and neutrophils to help support the diagnosis of miliaria.

351. Feng E, Janniger C (1995) Miliaria. **Cutis** 55:213–216.
352. Cohen LM, Skopicki BK, Harrist TJ et al. (1997) Noninfectious vesiculobullous and vesiculopustular diseases. In: Lever's Histopathology of the Skin, Elder D, Elenitsas R, Jaworsky C, Johnson B, eds. Philadelphia: Lippencott-Raven, 209–252.
353. Mowad CM, McGinley KJ, Foglia A, Leyden JJ (1995) The role of extracellular polysaccharide substance produced by Staphylococcus epidermidis in miliaria. **J Am Acad Dermatol** 33:729–733.

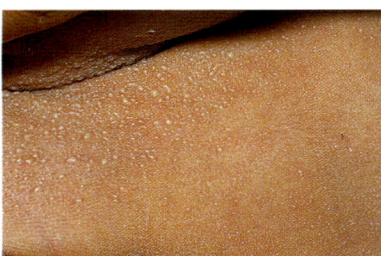

Fig. 6.36 Miliaria crystallina (courtesy Dr. Libby Edwards).

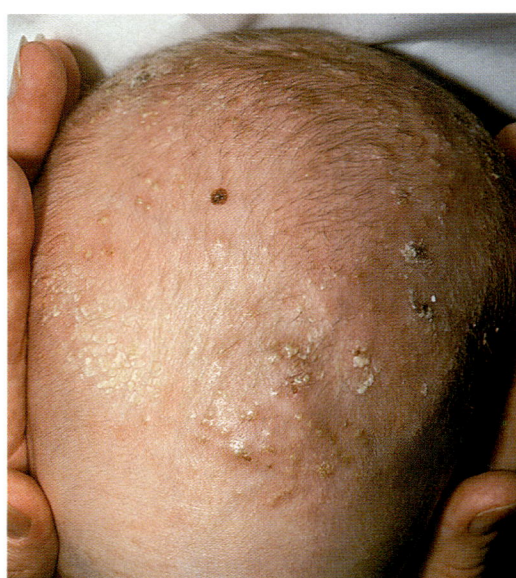

Fig. 6.38 Eosinophilic pustular folliculitis on the scalp.

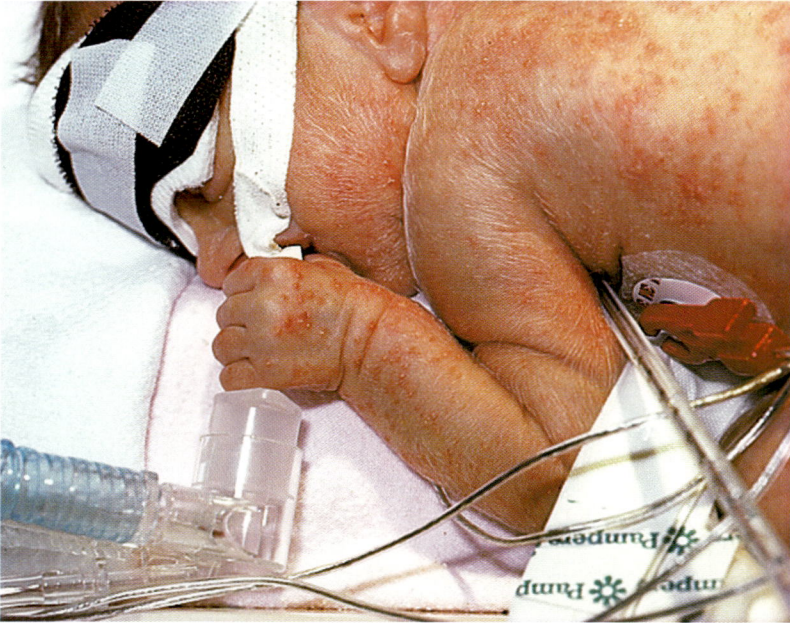

Fig. 6.37 Miliaria rubra/pustulosa in premature infant.

Minimizing overheating of the infant is the only necessary treatment. Cool baths and air-conditioning are useful. Lesions usually resolve rapidly with no other intervention.

EOSINOPHILIC PUSTULAR FOLLICULITIS

Eosinophilic pustular folliculitis (or eosinophilic pustulosis), is an uncommon condition first described in infants by Lucky *et al.* in 1984.[354] It may present at birth or in the first few days of life with yellowish pustules predominately on the scalp and face (Fig. 6.38), but also on trunk and extremities.[354–360]

Pustules range from 1 to 3mm in size and generally crust within two or three days of onset. Pustules may recur in crops, with a waxing and waning course that may last days to weeks, with some reports of relapses over a number of years.[357] Pruritus or irritability in younger infants is common. Peripheral eosinophilia is present in many patients. Pustular smears display eosinophils with occasional neutrophils without organisms, and cultures for bacteria, fungus, and viruses are all negative.[359]

Histopathologic examination of scalp lesions demonstrates eosinophilic spongiosis with an occasional subcorneal pustule. A dense mixed dermal infiltrate with many eosinophils, as well as lymphocytes and histiocytes, is variably perifollicular[356,357] or interfollicular.[354,357,359] The etiology of this condition is unknown. It has been suggested that it may represent a more persistent form of erythema toxicum, based on the histopathologic similarities.[359] Clinical similarities also exist with acropustulosis of infancy.

Differential diagnosis includes scalp pyoderma, erythema toxicum, transient neonatal pustular melanosis, acropustulosis of infancy, bacterial or fungal folliculitis, scabies, candidiasis, and Langerhans cell histiocytosis. The clinical presentation, location, and histology of these lesions allow differentiation from all these entities. This disease appears to be quite different from the adult form of eosinophilic pustular folliculitis (Ofuji disease), which is more widespread in distribution and tends toward the formation of confluent polycyclic plaques with central healing and peripheral extension, unlike the pattern seen in infants. The strong association with human immunodeficiency virus (HIV) seen in adult patients with Ofuji disease is not seen in infants with eosinophilic pustular folliculitis, though immunodeficiency has been described.[361–363] Secondary infection resulting in localized pyoderma or sepsis has been observed.[360]

Treatment of eosinophilic pustular folliculitis in infancy is moderately successful with low- or midpotency topical corticosteroids and/or antibiotic therapy.[359] Antihistamines may be useful in controlling the pruritus. Other therapies that may be useful include dapsone,[357] oral cimetidine,[364] and systemic prednisone.

ACROPUSTULOSIS OF INFANCY

Acropustulosis of infancy (infantile acropustulosis) is a chronic or recurrent benign condition of very pruritic vesicles and pustules occurring on the hands and feet. It was first described in 1979 by Kahn and Rywlin[365] and by Jarrett and Ramsdell,[366] and its etiology is unknown.[366] It may be present at birth,

354. Lucky AW, Esterly NB, Heskel N et al. (1984) Eosinophilic pustular folliculitis in infancy. **Pediatr Dermatol** 1:202–206.

355. Colton AS, Schachner LA, Kowalczyk AP (1986) Eosinophilic pustular folliculitis. **J Am Acad Dermatol** 14:469.

356. Giard F, Marcoux D, McCuaig C et al. (1991) Eosinophilic pustular folliculitis (Ofuji disease) in childhood: a review of 4 cases. **Pediatr Dermatol** 8:189.

357. Taieb A, Bassan-Andrieu L, Maleville J (1992) Eosinophilic pustulosis of the scalp in childhood. **J Am Acad Dermatol** 27:55.

358. Darmstadt GL, Tunnessen WW Jr, Swerer RJ (1992) Eosinophilic pustular folliculitis. **Pediatrics** 89:1095.

359. Duarte AM, Kramer J, Yusk JW et al. (1993) Eosinophilic pustular folliculitis in infancy and childhood. **Am J Dis Child** 147:197.

360. Larralde M, Morales S, Munoz AS et al. (1999) Eosinophilic pustular folliculitis in infancy: Report of two new cases. **Pediatr Dermatol** 16:118–120.

361. Soeprono F, Schinella R (1986) Eosinophilic pustular folliculitis in patients with acquired immunodeficiency syndrome. **J Am Acad Dermatol** 14:1020.

362. Buchness M, Lim H, Hatcher V et al. (1988) Eosinophilic pustular folliculitis in the acquired immunodeficiency syndrome. **N Engl J Med** 318:1183.

363. Rybojad M, Guibai F, Vignon-Pennamen MD et al. (1999) Eosinophilic pustulosis in an infant accompanied by immune deficit. **Ann Dermatol Venerol** 126:29–31.

364. Rogers M (1999) Successful treatment of eosinophilic pustulosis with oral cimetidine. **Pediatr Dermatol** 16:335–336.

365. Kahn G, Rywlin AM (1979) Acropustulosis of infancy. **Arch Dermatol** 115:831.

366. Jarrett M, Ramsdell W (1979) Infantile acropustulosis. **Arch Dermatol** 115:834.

but more commonly develops in the first several weeks to months of life, and may continue throughout infancy and early childhood.[365,367] Acropustulosis was originally reported to be more common in males and in blacks,[368] but other studies do not support sexual or racial predominance.[369–371] Infants and children often present with severe pruritus, sleep disturbance, fretfulness and appetite loss. Early lesions are 1–2mm papules or distinct vesicles that rapidly evolve into larger vesicopustules measuring up to 4mm in diameter. Characteristic lesions are on the palms, soles, dorsal hands and feet, and sides of fingers and toes (Fig. 6.39). Occasional lesions on the ankles, wrists, proximal limbs, and trunk may be seen, but mucosal surfaces are spared. Postinflammatory hyperpigmentation can be observed. Crops of lesions appear in cycles of two to four weeks, with individual lesions lasting three to seven days. The number of lesions is greatest in the early episodes, becoming less with subsequent episodes until permanent resolution occurs at 2 to 3 years of age.

The etiology remains unknown. Theories include a reaction pattern in predisposed individuals to infection or infestation.[369] A history of scabies preceding the diagnosis of infantile acropustulosis is common, though the relationship between the two remains unclear, as often the diagnosis of scabies is made without microscopic confirmation.[372,373] It is clear, however, that some infants, after eradication of documented scabies infection, may have a condition with clinical manifestations, course, and histologic features identical to those of infantile acropustulosis (see below).[372,373]

Clinical characteristics and microscopic evaluation of smears or skin biopsies can confirm the diagnosis. Laboratory studies are usually normal in infantile acropustulosis, but peripheral blood eosinophilia has been reported.[374] Pustule contents may show prominent neutrophils and occasional eosinophils, without mites, eggs, ova, or feces as seen with scabies.[367,370] Skin biopsy shows intra-epidermal or subcorneal pustules filled with neutrophils or eosinophils. Focal vesiculation and degeneration of keratinocytes with cell necrosis may also be seen.[365,366,367]

The differential diagnosis should include scabies, eosinophilic pustulosis, candidiasis, erythema toxicum, transient neonatal pustular melanosis, bacterial pustulosis, dyshidrotic eczema, and pustular palmoplantar psoriasis. Multiple skin scrapings are necessary to differentiate active scabies. Smears for Gram and Wright stains, and potassium hydroxide (KOH) preparations should help eliminate candidiasis, impetigo, VZV, and HSV. Erythema toxicum and transient neonatal pustular melanosis may be confused, but both are non-pruritic and transient conditions making differentiation easier. Pustular psoriasis is very rare in neonates; the morphology, distribution, and histology will help distinguish it. Similarly, the histology of eosinophilic pustulosis is distinct and will separate it from infantile acropustulosis.

Acropustulosis of infancy will spontaneously remit over one to two years. Treatment with very potent topical corticosteroids is usually successful for control of outbreaks.[373] Oral antihistamines may be useful to minimize symptoms of pruritus. Oral dapsone in a dosage of 1 to 3mg/kg per day speeds pustule resolution within 2–3 days[365,374,375] and has been used as intermittent therapy during pustular phases to control the disease until spontaneous resolution occurs at two to three years of age. This therapy should be reserved for severe cases unresponsive to potent topical steroids. Baseline glucose-6-phosphate dehydrogenase (G6PD) levels and close monitoring of complete blood counts and platelets are appropriate as well as clinical assessment for methemoglobinemia, fever, jaundice, pallor or purpura.[365,374,375]

NEONATAL ACNE AND TRANSIENT NEONATAL CEPHALIC PUSTULOSIS

There is some degree of controversy regarding the etiology and nomenclature of neonatal acne and what has been termed transient neonatal cephalic pustulosis. Neonatal acne has been described as usually beginning at a few weeks of life and manifested by multiple, inflammatory, erythematous papules, comedones, and pustules (Fig. 6.40). Investigators have proposed that much of what has been termed neonatal acne is in fact not an acneiform condition but a superficial pustular infection caused by Malassezia species.[376–378] *Malassezia sympodialis*, and less commonly *Malassezia furfur*, have been cultured from subsets of facial pustules. However, since these organisms may be found

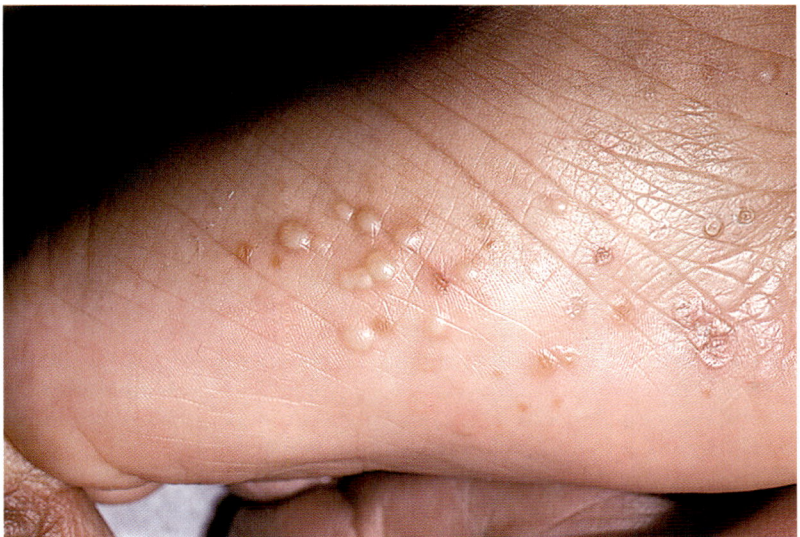

Fig. 6.39   Acropustulosis of infancy.

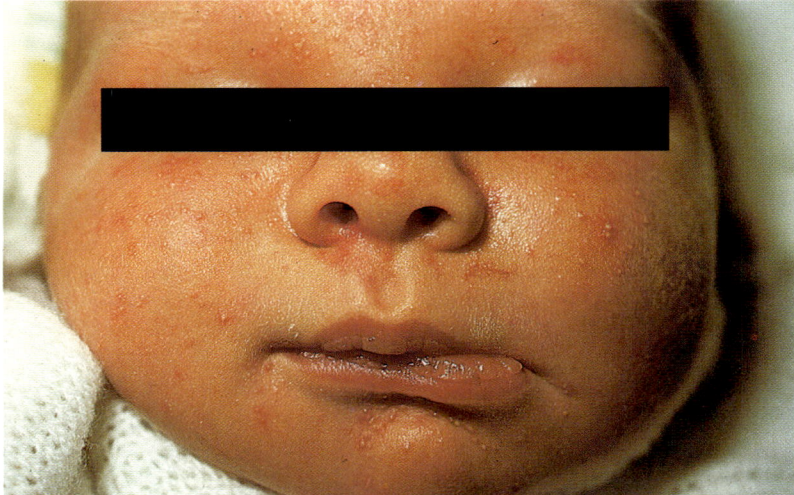

Fig. 6.40   Neonatal acne/transient neonatal cephalic pustulosis. Polymorphous inflammatory papules and pustular.

367. Lucky AW, McGuire JS (1982) Infantile acropustulosis with eosinophilic pustules. **J Pediatr** 100:428.
368. Palungwachira P (1989) Infantile acropustulosis. **Aust J Dermatol** 30:97.
369. Dromy R, Raz A, Metzker A (1991) Infantile acropustulosis. **Pediatr Dermatol** 8:284.
370. Jennings JL, Burrows WM (1983) Infantile acropustulosis. **J Am Acad Dermatol** 9:733–738.
371. Lowy G, Serapiaao CJ, Oliveira MM (1986) Childhood acropustulosis. A study of 10 cases. **Med Cutan Ibero Lat Am** 14:171–176.
372. Nguyen J, Strobel M, Arnaud JP et al. (1991) Infantile acropustulosis: unusual manifestation of scabies in the infant? **Ann Pediatr** 38:479.
373. Mancini AJ, Frieden IJ, Paller AS (1998) Infantile acropustulosis revisited: history of scabies and response to topical corticosteroids. **Pediatr Dermatol** 15:337–341.

374. Bundino S, Zina AM, Ubertalli S (1982) Infantile acropustulosis. **Dermatologica** 165:615.
375. Findlay RF, Odom RB (1983) Infantile acropustulosis. **Am J Dis Child** 137:455.
376. Rapelanoro R, Mortureux P, Couprie B et al. (1996) Neonatal Malassezia furfur pustulosis. **Arch Dermatol** 132:190–193.
377. Niamba P, Weill FX, Sarlangue J et al. (1998) Is common neonatal cephalic pustulosis (neonatal acne) triggered by Malassezia sympodialis? **Arch Dermatol** 134:995–998.
378. Bernier V, Weill FX, Hirigoyen V et al. (2002) Skin colonization by Malassezia species in neonates: a prospective study and relationship with neonatal cephalic pustulosis. **Arch Dermatol** 138(2):215–218.

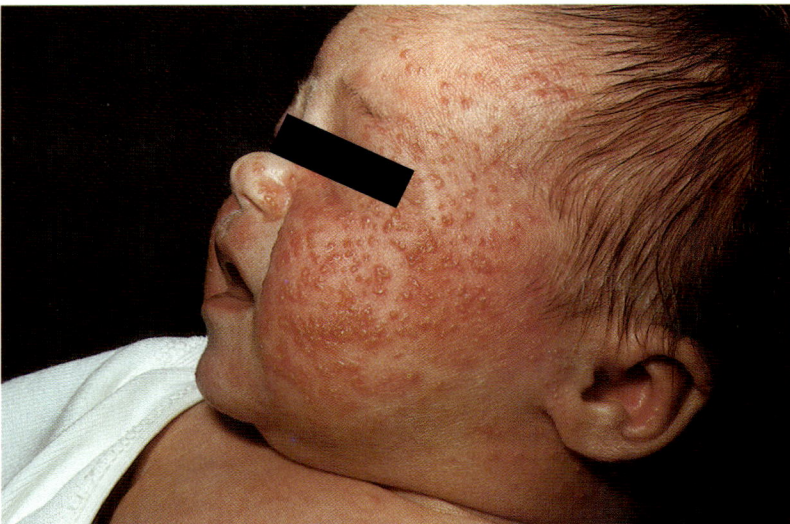

Fig. 6.41 Neonatal acne/transient neonatal cephalic pustulosis. Eruptive monomorphous papulopustular disorder.

on the skin as commensal organisms, their etiologic role in the facial eruption is uncertain.[379] Like previously described neonatal acne, TNCP onset usually occurs at a few weeks with multiple, inflammatory, erythematous papules and pustules and resolves in several months (Fig. 6.41). Comedonal lesions are rare, and treatment is rarely needed, though it has been stated that topical anti-yeast agents speed resolution. Stimulation of the sebaceous glands by maternal and neonatal hormones may influence comedone formation as well as malassezia colonization.

Neonatal papulopustular eruptions are quite common on the face, neck, chest and back at several weeks of age. Neonatal acne and cephalic pustulosis may be accompanied by, and should be distinguished from, sebaceous hyperplasia, pustular miliaria and milia. The differential diagnosis includes transient neonatal pustular melanosis, erythema toxicum, candidiasis, eosinophilic pustular folliculitis, staphylococcal folliculitis, scabies, and other infections. Pustule smears may be Giemsa stained to look for fungal spores. Neonatal acne and cephalic pustulosis are self-limited processes. Malassezia associated pustules may respond to topical imidizaole creams.

INCONTINENTIA PIGMENTI

Incontinentia pigmenti, or Bloch–Sulzberger syndrome, is a rare, X-linked, dominant genodermatosis that is usually lethal in males. It has been associated with mutations in the NEMO (IKK-gamma) gene.[380] There are four distinct stages of which the first is seen in the neonatal period. Cutaneous lesions are present at birth in 50% of cases, with onset within the first few weeks of life in another 40% of affected neonates. The usual presenting skin findings are firm yellow vesicles in linear streaks following the lines of Blaschko.[381–383] Vesicles are most common on the limbs but occur also on trunk and scalp and may occur in crops. Seizures may occur in the neonatal period in this condition and these patients should be carefully observed.

While characteristic linearly grouped vesicles may support a clinical diagnosis, a skin biopsy is appropriate for confirmation of this potentially serious disorder. Findings are eosinophilic spongiosis with eosinophilic infiltration, eosinophilic microabcesses and dyskeratosis.[384] The vesicular phase of incontinentia pigmenti is usually accompanied by peripheral eosinophilia.

The differential diagnosis of the first stage of incontinentia pigmenti includes neonatal HSV infection, erythema toxicum, bullous impetigo, epidermolysis bullosa, Herpes zoster, focal dermal hypoplasia, and diffuse cutaneous mastocytosis. IP is discussed in detail in Chapter 10.

HYPERIMMUNOGLOBULIN E SYNDROME (JOB'S SYNDROME)

Vesicular eruptions in newborns with hyperimmunoglobulin E syndrome have been reported.[385,386] Lesions include single, grouped, and confluent tense and umbilicated vesicles on inflamed skin, located on the face, scalp, ears, and shoulders. Blood eosinophilia is variable in the infantile period, and IgE levels may not be significantly elevated until later life. Biopsy displays intraepidermal vesicles with eosinophils. Other features of hyper-IgE syndrome (which generally develop after the neonatal period) include recurrent staphylococcal infections, cold abscesses, eczematous rashes (with a predominance of facial inflammatory papules), recurrent pneumonia, osteomyelitis and recurrent fractures, retained primary teeth, a characteristic facies, and mucocutaneous candidiasis. IgE levels are usually greater than 2000IU/ml, but may not rise until after one year of age.[387–389]

BULLOUS DISEASES IN THE NEWBORN

A number of conditions, both infectious and noninfectious, present during the newborn period with prominent bullae. Occasionally, the vesiculopustular diseases of the newborn will produce similar appearing bullae, but these diseases are characterized by smaller, less impressive lesions. The differential diagnosis of predominantly bullous diseases in the newborn is presented in Table 6.14. An in-depth discussion of these clinical entities can be found in various individual chapters.

NEONATAL HERPES GESTATIONIS

Although the name suggests a relationship to HSV infection, neonatal herpes gestationis is an acquired autoimmune disorder affecting neonates of mothers with this condition, which is completely unrelated to the herpes virus. Herpes gestationis was named by Milton in 1872 and is estimated to occur in 1 in 10 000 pregnancies.

Maternal disease may be acquired at any time during pregnancy or during the postpartum period, but it is most common during the second trimester. It may occur during subsequent pregnancies. Once manifested, maternal disease may last for the duration of the pregnancy or for up to two years after delivery, but remission usually occurs during pregnancy or shortly thereafter. Even though mothers may have extensive disease, only a small percentage of their babies (2–11%) will develop cutaneous manifestations.[390–392]

Transplacental passage of maternal immunoglobulins formed against the maternal basement membrane zone (lamina lucida) is responsible for the

379. Bergman JN and Eichenfield LF (2002) Neonatal acne and cephalic pustulosis: is malassezia the whole story? **Arch Dermatol** 138(2):255–257.
380. Smahi A, Courtois G, Vabres P et al. (2000) Genomic rearrangement in NEMO impairs NF-kappaB activation and is a cause of incontinentia pigmenti. The International Incontinenia Pigmenti (IP) Consortium. **Nature** 25:466–472.
381. Cohen BA (1987) Incontinentia pigmenti. **Neurol Clin** 5:361–377.
382. Carney RJ (1976) Incontinentia pigmenti: a world of statistical analysis. **Arch Dermatol** 112:535–542.
383. Landy SJ, Donnai D (1993) Incontinentia pigmenti (Bloch–Sulzberger syndrome). **J Med Genet** 30:53.
384. Cohen LM, Skopicki BK, Harrist TJ et al. (1997) Noninfectious vesiculobullous and vesiculopustular diseases. In: Lever's Histopathology of the Skin, Elder D, Elenitsas R, Jaworsky C, Johnson B, eds. Philadelphia: Lippencott-Raven, pp. 209–252.

385. Kamei R, Honig PJ (1988) Neonatal Job's syndrome featuring a vesicular eruption. **Pediatr Dermatol** 5:75–82.
386. Blum R, Geller G, Fish LA (1977) Recurrent severe staphylococcal infections, eczematoid rash, extreme elevations of IgE, eosinophilia, and divergent chemotactic responses in two generations. **J Pediatr** 90:607–609.
387. Grimbacher B, Holland SM, Gallin JI et al. (1999) Hyper-IgE syndrome with recurrent infections – an autosomal dominant multisystem disorder. **N Engl J Med** 340:692–702.
388. Wellington GB, Hensley T, Carey JC et al. (1998) The face of Job. **J Pediatr** 133: 303.
389. Donabedian H, Gallin JI (1983) The hyperimmunoglobulin E recurrent-infection Job's syndrome. A review of the NIH experience and the literature. **Medicine Baltimore** 62:195–208.
390. Shornick JK (1993) Herpes gestationis. **Dermatol Clin** 11:527.
391. Karna P, Broecker AH (1991) Neonatal herpes gestationis. **J Pediatr** 119:299.
392. Lawley TJ, Stingl G, Katz SI (1978) Fetal and maternal risk factors in herpes gestationis. **Arch Dermatol** 114:552.

TABLE 6.14 Differential diagnosis of prominent bullae in newborn

Disorder	Chapter(s)
Bullous impetigo	24
Neonatal herpes gestationis	16
Bullous mastocytosis	17
Epidermolysis bullosa	16
Neonatal pemphigus vulgaris	16
Epidermolytic hyperkeratoses (bullous congenital icthyosiform erythroderma)	8
Congenital syphilis	6, 28

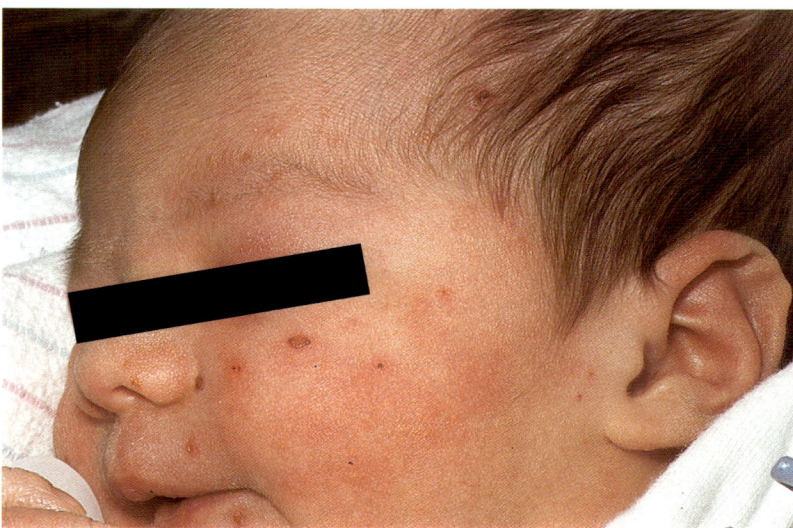

Fig. 6.42 Langerhans cell histiocytosis in newborn. Hemorrhagic vesicales mimic a herpes-group viral infection.

neonatal disease.[393] Maternal autoantibodies include two immunoglobulin G (IgG) antibodies: one a circulating anti-basement membrane antibody, and the other an IgG antibody, called the herpes gestationis (HG) factor, capable of fixing C3 at the basement membrane of human skin and detectable by complement indirect immunofluorescence.[391–394]

Neonatal disease may be evident at birth or within several hours. Erythematous macules, papules, vesicles, and frank bullae up to several centimeters in diameter may be present. Lesions may progress from papular to vesicular or bullous forms. Occasionally, lesions are grouped in a herpetiform pattern. The trunk, head, and extremities are most often involved. Spontaneous resolution usually occurs by 1 month of age.[394]

No visceral complications are associated with neonatal herpes gestationis, but 25% of all infants born to affected mothers are small for gestational age and 20% or more are born before 37 weeks gestation.[391,394,395] For these reasons, all affected mothers must be considered at high risk and delivered at a perinatal center with the capability to monitor and treat such infants. Although Lawley's studies suggested increased fetal mortality,[392] subsequent reports have found no evidence of fetal death and minimal morbidity.[395] Fetal complications may be increased with maternal eosinophilia greater than 10% and with titers of at least 1:80 of circulating anti-basement membrane antibodies.[392]

The diagnosis is suggested by the maternal history, but it is established on the basis of histopathology and immunofluorescence. Blood eosinophilia may be present initially,[395] and Wright stain of vesicular or bullous fluid shows a predominance of eosinophils. Histologic examination of perilesional skin shows dermal–epidermal separation with a mixed perivascular infiltrate that includes many eosinophils. There may be necrosis of the basal cells.[394] Direct immunofluorescent studies demonstrate C3 in a band-like pattern along the basement membrane in most patients and may show IgG antibodies in this area as well. The HG factor, IgG, may be present in the infant's serum and demonstrable on indirect immunofluorescence by its ability to fix C3 at the basement membrane area.[392]

The differential diagnosis should include bullous impetigo, epidermolysis bullosa, HSV infection, and neonatal syphilis. Wright stain demonstrating neutrophils and a positive Gram stain will help identify bullous impetigo. Viral culture, immunofluorescence studies for HSV, electron microscopic evaluation of viral particles, and a Tzanck preparation from the base of a lesion for multinucleated giant cells will identify HSV infection. Syphilis is ruled out by the presence of a normal IgM level, negative VDRL, or negative IgM fluorescent treponemal antibody absorption test (FTA-ABS).

Epidermolysis bullosa may be excluded by history, but skin biopsy and electron microscopy are occasionally needed. Elevated IgM levels were reported by Bonifazi et al.[394] in one neonatal case of herpes gestationis without evidence of congenital infection. Therapy is symptomatic and includes wet compresses, topical antibiotics, and prevention of secondary infection.

LANGERHANS CELL HISTIOCYTOSIS

Congenital Langerhans cell histiocytosis can present in neonates with vesicles and bullae (Fig. 6.42), as well as pustules, papules, nodules and crusts.[396–398] Hemorrhagic bullae, as well as petechiae, atrophy and milia may be present. The disease can be limited to skin or be multisystemic, and skin lesion morphology does not correlate with extracutaneous disease.[399] Diagnosis requires biopsy, which shows mid-dermal histiocytes with large cells, irregularly shaped vesicular nuclei and eosinophilic cytoplasm.[400] S-100 stain and immunohistochemical stains and/or electron microscopy to delineate Langerhans cells are useful for specific diagnosis.[401] Tzanck preparation can show histiocytes with uniform nuclei and abundant cytoplasm, which may be incorrectly interpreted as suggestive of herpes by inexperienced personnel.[400] Systemic work–up is appropriate in all infants. The term "self-healing Langerhans cell histiocytosis" has been used for neonatal cases presenting with skin lesions that spontaneously resolve. Extracutaneous disease or cutaneous relapse may occur months to years later, so ongoing monitoring is necessary.[402] Diabetes insipidus may occur as a sequel of neonatal presentations of Langerhans cell histiocytosis in over 20% of patients.[399]

EPIDERMOLYSIS BULLOSA

Neonatal vesicles, bullae, and denuded skin, with friction and trauma induced blistering are the hallmark of all subtypes of epidermolysis bullosa (EB). The term comprises a set of diseases with various presentations and genetic

393. Dahl MV (1988) The bullous diseases: Peraphigus, pemphigoid and others. In: Clinical Immunodermatology, 2nd ed. Chicago: Year Book Medical, p. 206.
394. Bonifazi E, Meneghini CL (1984) Herpes gestationis with transient bullous lesions in the newborn. **Pediatr Dermatol** 1:215.
395. Shornick JK, Black MM (1992) Fetal risks in herpes gestationis. **J Am Acad Dermatol** 26:63.
396. Hertz CG, Hambrick GW, Jr. (1968) Congenital Letterer–Siwe disease. A case treated with vincristine and corticosteroids. **Am J Dis Child** 116:553–556.
397. Valderrama E, Kahn LB, Festa R et al. (1985) Benign isolated histiocytosis mimicking chicken pox in a neonate: report of two cases with ultrastructural study. **Pediatr Pathol** 3:103–113.
398. Herman LE, Rothman KF, Harawi S et al. (1990) Congenital self-healing reticulohistiocytosis. A new entity in the differential diagnosis of neonatal papulovesicular eruptions. **Arch Dermatol** 126:210–212.
399. Stein SL, Paller AS, Haut PR et al. (2001) Langerhans cell histiocytosis presenting in the neonatal period: a retrospective case series. **Arch Pediatr Adolesc Med** 155(7):778–783.
400. Colon-Fontanes F, Eichenfield LF, Krous HF et al. (1998) Congenital Langerhans cell histiocytosis: the utility of the Tzanck test as a diagnostic screening tool. **Archiv Dermatology** 134:1039–1040.
401. Rowden G, Connelly EM, Winkelmann RK (1983) Cutaneous histiocytosis X. The presence of S-100 protein and its use in diagnosis. **Arch Dermatol** 119:553–539.
402. Longaker MA, Frieden IJ, LeBoit PE et al. (1994) Congenital "self-healing" Langerhans cell histiocytosis: the need for long-term follow-up. **J Am Acad Dermatol** 31:910–916.

etiologies. The clinical presentation and course of EB is quite variable, and depends on the specific subtype. EB is classified by the clinical extent and ultrastructural level of blistering, by inheritance pattern and, more recently, by specific molecular defect[403–406] with EB simplex, junctional EB, and dystrophic EB being the major subgroups. Because infants with all subtypes can present with marked blistering in the newborn period, predicting specific EB subtypes based on clinical findings can be difficult in the first weeks of life. The scalp and face may blister due to the trauma of vaginal birth. The depth of blistering depends on EB subtype. More superficial blisters may rupture easily, while deeper blisters may be tense or hemorrhagic. Some EB subtypes tend to be severe in the neonatal period and may be fatal in the first few weeks of life.

EB should be in the differential diagnosis of neonatal localized or diffuse vesicles and bullae, or localized or generalized skin denudation or scarring. Biopsy diagnosis is appropriate, and may be aided by electron microscopy (see also Chapter 16).

INFECTIOUS DISEASES OF THE NEWBORN

Congenital infections usually present during the newborn period and are often recognized by their cutaneous manifestations. This section describes the most common congenital infections and their associated skin findings.

NEONATAL SCABIES

Scabies, a cutaneous infestation caused by *Sarcoptes scabiei*, is rare in the neonatal period.[407] Congenital scabies has not been reported. Clinical manifestations may occur from postnatal exposure in the early weeks of life and evidence of disease in infants as young as 9 days has been reported.[408,409] Neonates do not have a coordinated scratch response, and they may have no observable symptoms, or be irritabile, restless, or feed poorly as signs of pruritus.[410]

Vesicles, papules, pustules, and excoriations may be present anywhere on the body, often with a generalized pattern. Palm and sole lesions are very common in infants. While the face and scalp are commonly spared in older children and adults, infants and young children will commonly have scabies lesions in these locations. Burrows, thin lines with tiny black dots at one end indicating the location of the female mite, are pathognomonic for scabies, but are often not found because of excoriation or eczematous changes.[411,412] Nodular lesions are common in infants, and scabies mites may be found from scrapings of these. Bullae or honey-colored crusting should raise suspicion of bacterial superinfection.

Diagnosis should be suspected based upon rash morphology and distribution, strengthened by a family history of itching or rash. The diagnosis is confirmed by a skin scraping of a fresh vesicle, pustule, or burrow demonstrating mite parts, larva, or fecal material. Fluorescence-microscopy or dermatoscopy has been reported as helpful in identifying scabies.[413] Infants are infested with many mites; careful selection of the lesion to examine will usually demonstrate evidence of infestation. Biopsy shows a spongiotic dermatitis and is nonspecific unless a mite or mite parts are seen. The differential diagnosis and management are discussed in detail elsewhere. Permethrin 5% cream is the treatment of choice in infants, although some prefer to use precipitated sulphur in the very early weeks or in low birth weight infants.[414]

IMPETIGO NEONATORUM (BULLOUS IMPETIGO) AND STAPHYLOCOCCAL SCALDED SKIN SYNDROME

The neonate, especially when premature, is particularly susceptible to nosocomial infection with *Staphylococcus aureus*. This organism produces a wide variety of skin infections as well as systemic infection in the neonatal intensive care unit (NICU). The most common of these infections is impetigo neonatorum, and the neonate is especially liable to develop bullous impetigo, perhaps due to the lack of good adhesion between the epidermis and dermis seen in immature skin. Group II strains of *Staphylococcus aureus*, phage type 55 and 71, are most commonly responsible for this presentation and have caused epidemics of methicillin-resistant strains in many nurseries.[415]

Lesions of impetigo neonatorum usually appear during the second week of life. The neck creases, periumbilical area, and perineum are most commonly involved (Fig. 6.43). Bullae enlarge rapidly and spread quickly, and may potentially be complicated by fatal infections such as pneumonia, septicemia, and osteomyelitis.[416] Hence, early aggressive treatment of neonatal impertigo is imperative.

Although rare, staphylococcal scalded skin syndrome (SSSS) has also been described in neonates. This begins as a scarlatiniform eruption with rapid progression to deep, confluent erythroderma and edema, followed by wrinkling and sheet-like desquamation of the skin. Most infants have impetiginous crusting around the nose and mouth. Distinction from toxic epidermal necrolysis is critical, since the latter has an extremely poor prognosis. Treatment is with systemic antistaphylococcal antibiotics. Systemic steroids should not be used in these infants.[417]

The differential diagnosis of bullous impetigo neonatorum and SSSS includes epidermolysis bullosa, incontinentia pigmenti, bullous mastocytosis, bullous congenital ichthyosiform erythroderma, neonatal herpes gestationis, and VZV and HSV infections. The site of predilection of lesions and other clinical features together with appropriate culture and Gram stain, can help distinguish these entities.

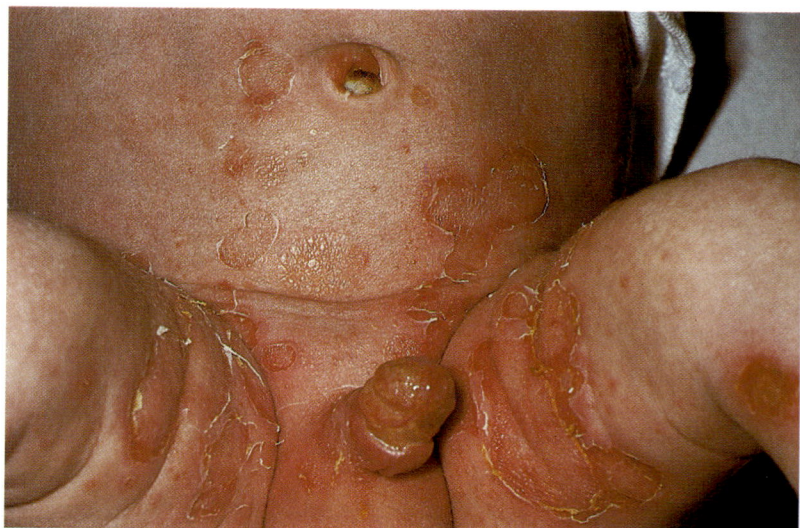

Fig. 6.43 Bullous impetigo in a neonate.

403. Fine J, Bauer EA, Briaggaman RA et al. (1991) Revised clinical and laboratory criteria for subtypes of inherited epidermolysis bullosa. **J Am Acad Dermatol** 24:119–135.
404. Fine J, Bauer E, McGuire J et al. (1999) Epidermolysis Bullosa: Clinical, Epidermiologic, and Laboratory Advances and the Findings of the National Epidermolysis Bullosa Registry. Baltimore: Johns Hopkins University Press.
405. Marinkovich M. (1999) Update on inherited bullous dermatoses. **Dermatologic Clinics** 17:473–485.
406. Horn HM, Tidman MJ (2002) The clinical spectrum of dystrophic epidermolysis bullosa. **Br J Dermatol** 146(2):267–274.
407. Sterling GB, Janniger CK, Kihiczak G (1990) Neonatal scabies. **Cutis** 45:229.
408. Quarterman MJ, Lesher JL (1994) Neonatal scabies treated with permethrin 5% cream. **Pediatr Dermatol** 11:264–266.
409. Paller AS (1993) Scabies in infants and small children. **Semin Dermatol** 12:3.

410. Peterson CM, Eichenfield LF (1996) Scabies. **Pediatr Ann** 25:97–100.
411. Hurwitz S (1973) Scabies in babies. **Am J Dis Child** 126:226–228.
412. Camassa F, Fania M, Ditano G et al. (1995) Neonatal scabies. **Cutis** 56:210–212.
413. Bhutto AM, Honda M, Kudo Y et al. (1993) Introduction of fluorescence-microscopic technique for the detection of eggs, egg shells, and mites in scabies. **J Dermatol** 20:122.
414. Committee on infectious Disease, American Academy of Pediatrics (2000) Red Book: Report of the Committee on Infectious Disease. p. 583–584. 25th ed. American Academy of Pediatrics.
415. Aihara M, Sakai M, Iwasaki M et al. (1993) Prevention and control of nosocomial infection caused by methicillin-resistant *Staphylococcus aureus* in a premature infant ward – preventive effect of a povidone-iodine wipe of neonatal skin. **Postgrad Med J** suppl 3. 69:S117.
416. Dancer SJ, Simmons NA, Poston SM et al. (1988) Outbreak of staphylococcal scalded skin syndrome among neonates. **J Infect** 16:87.
417. Rasmussen JE (1975) Toxic epidermal necrolysis: a review of 75 cases in children. **Arch Dermatol** 111:1135.

CONGENITAL AND NEONATAL CANDIDIASIS

Candida is the most common fungal pathogen in neonates.[418] Infection may be acquired vertically from the mother or horizontally by nosocomial transmission in the nursery. Several types of infection with Candida spp. are seen during the neonatal period.

Congenital candidiasis is acquired *in utero*, presents in the first few days of life, and may be responsible for premature labor and delivery or rarely intrauterine death. There is a broad spectrum of disease, from congenital cutaneous candidiasis with a diffuse skin eruption with or without systemic symptoms, to severe life-threating candidal systemic infection without cutaneous findings.[419]

Candidiasis acquired during passage through an infected birth canal and presenting after the first few days of life is called neonatal candidiasis. Perinatal and postnatal acquisition of candida may be:

1. Localized as thrush or diaper dermatitis;
2. Invasive fungal dermatitis in which primary candidial species skin infec-tion presents with erosive, crusted plaques which may lead to systemic disease;
3. Systemic infection associated with central catheters, chronic antibiotic therapy, hyperalimentation, or other invasive procedures with candidal contamination.[420–422]

Candida parapsilosis, Candida tropicalis, and Candida stellatoidea can cause congenital or neonatal candidiasis, but Candida albicans is isolated in 95% of cultures from neonates. The prevalence of candida is significantly higher among infants of gestational age less than 28 weeks (65%).[423,424]

Congenital candidiasis

Congenital candidiasis generally presents in the first day of life as a diffuse eruption of erythematous macules, papulovesicles, and pustules 2–4mm in size (Fig. 6.44) commonly on a 5–10mm erythematous base. Lesions develop anywhere on the body surface including palms, soles, and nails but the diaper area and oral cavity (thrush) are usually spared. Congenital candidiasis confined to the nail plates only has been described.[425] Pustular lesions sometimes coalesce and slough, leaving denuded weeping areas. In other cases, pustular or papular lesions fade within four to seven days, leaving post-inflammatory desquamation.[423–426] The presence of cutaneous candidiasis at birth is not diagnostic of systemic disease. In fact, most infants with congenital cutaneous candidiasis do not develop systemic disease, and respond rapidly to topical treatment or oral fluconazole.[419,427–429]

In very low birth weight infants (VLBW) (<1000g) congenital candidiasis most often presents with a widespread desquamating dermatitis, sometimes with a scald-like appearance. Ecchymoses and necrosis may also be seen in these infants. These patients have a higher risk of systemic candidal infection and fatal outcome.[419,430,431] Invasive disease correlates with prolonged broad-spectrum antibiotic therapy or prolonged endotracheal intubation. Any premature infant with a widespread rash or ill appearance should prompt con-sideration of systemic candidiasis.[430,431] Systemic manifestations warrant intravenous therapy.

Risk factors for congenital cutaneous candidiasis include presence of an intrauterine device or of a cervical suture during pregnancy.[419,423] Candida

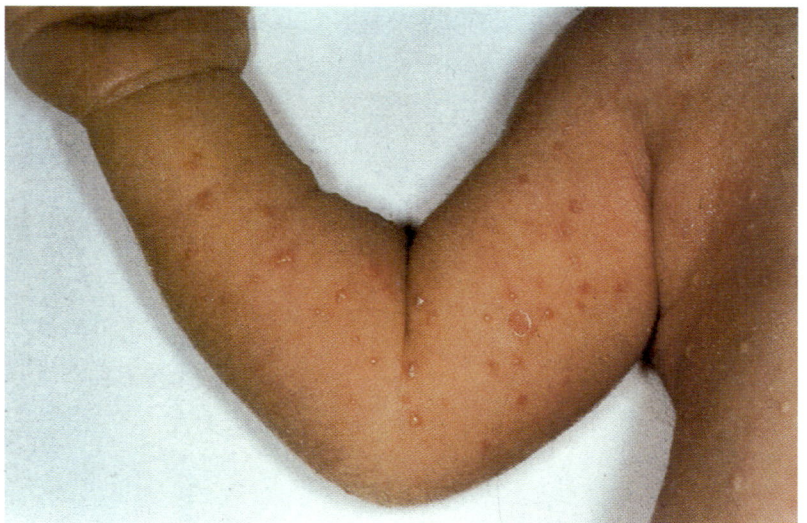

Fig. 6.44 Congenital candidiasis.

organisms are unable to pass the placental barrier; congenital infection is acquired by ascending vaginal or cervical infection. Amniotic membrane rupture is not required for fetal infection; fetal involvement has been reported in an infant delivered by cesarean section without rupture of membranes.[432] The proposed route of infection is via ascending organisms from the vagina that penetrate macro- or microamniotic tears and infect amniotic fluid. The infected amniotic fluid produces numerous cutaneous fetal lesions. Upon swallowing or aspirating the infected fluid, the fetus becomes infected, resulting in severe gastrointestinal and respiratory involve-ment. The presence of microruptures in the amniotic lining is assumed but has not been proved. However, the rarity of congenitally acquired candidiasis as compared with the frequency of vaginal candidiasis mitigates against the penetration of completely intact membranes.[432] Candida spp. grow well in amniotic fluid, and organisms are present in the gastric aspirate of most infants with congenital or neonatal infection.

Systemic candidiasis

Candida infection in an otherwise sterile body fluid, such as blood, urine or cerebrospinal fluid, is termed systemic candidiasis. These infections can be acquired *in utero* or postnatally. Systemic candidiasis affects 2–4% of very low birth weight infants, with 50–60% displaying skin manifestations.[431,433] VLBW infants with systemic candidiasis can present with an extensive burn-like dermatitis (Fig. 6.45) followed by desquamation, progressive diaper dermatitis involving papules and pustules, and isolated diaper rash with or without thrush.[433] Systemic signs include apnea, bradycardia, hypotension, abdominal distension, hyperglycemia, temperature instability, guaiac positive stools, and a leukemoid reaction.[420,422]

Oral therapy of mucocutanous candidiasis with nystatin or other topical anticandidal agents does not influence the progression to systemic disease.[434]

418. Ruiz-Diez B, Martinez V, Alvarez M et al. (1997) Molecular tracking of Candida albicans in a neonatal intensive care unit: long-term colonizations versus catheter-related infections. **J Clin Microbiol** 35:3032–3036.
419. Darmstadt GL, Dinulos JG, Miller Z (2000) Congenital cutaneous candidiasis: Clinical presentation, pathogenesis, and management guidelines. **Pediatrics** 105:438–444.
420. Pong AL, McCuaig, CC (2001) Fungal infections, infestations and parasitic infections in neonates. In: Textbook of Neonatal Dermatology, Eichenfield LF, Frieden IJ, Esterly NB, eds. Philadelphia, PA: WB Saunders, pp. 223–240.
421. Rowen JL, Atkins JT, Levy ML et a . (1995) Invasive fungal dermatitis in the <1000-gram neonate. **Pediatr** 95:682–687.
422. Pradeepkumar VK, Rajadurai VS, Tan KW (1998) Congenital candidiasis: varied presentations. **J Perinatology** 18:311–316.
423. Whyte RK, Hussain Z, deSa D (1982) Antenatal infections with Candida species. **Arch Dis Child** 57:528.
424. Sharp AM, Odds FC, Evans EG (1992) Candida strains from neonates in a special care baby unit. **Arch Dis Child** 67:48.
425. Arbegast KD, Lamberty LF, Koh JK et al. (1990) Congenital candidiasis limited to the nail plates. **Pediatr Dermatol** 7:310.
426. Delaplane D, Wiringa KS, Shulman ST et al. (1983) Congenital mucocutaneous candidiasis following amniocentesis. **Am J Obstet Gynecol** 147:342.
427. Glassman BD, Muglia JJ (1993) Widespread erythroderma and desquamation in a neonate. Congenital cutaneous candidiasis (CCC). **Arch Dermatol** 129:899.
428. Almeida Santos L, Beceiro J, Hernandez R et al. (1991) Congenital cutaneous candidiasis: report of four cases and review of the literature. **Eur J Pediatr** 150:336.
429. Broberg A, Thiringer K (1989) Congenital cutaneous candidiasis. **Int J Dermatol** 28:464.
430. Cosgrove BF, Reeves K, Mullins D et al. (1997) Cutaneous congenital candidiasis associated with respiratory distress and elevation of liver function tests: A case report and review of the literature. **J Am Acad Dermatol** 37:817–823.
431. Santos LA, Beceiro J, Hernandez R et al. (1991) Congenital cutaneous candidiasis: report of four cases and review of the literature. **Eur J Pediatr** 150:336–338.
432. Dvorak AM, Gavaller B (1966) Congenital systemic candidiasis. **N Engl J Med** 274:540.
433. Baley JE, Silverman RA (1988) Systemic candidiasis: cutaneous manifestations in low birth weight infants. **Pediatrics** 82:211–215.
434. Faix RG, Kovarik SM, Shaw TR et al. (1989) Mucocutaneous and invasive candidiasis among very low birth weight (less than 1,500 grams) infants in intensive care nurseries: a prospective study. **Pediatr** 83:101.

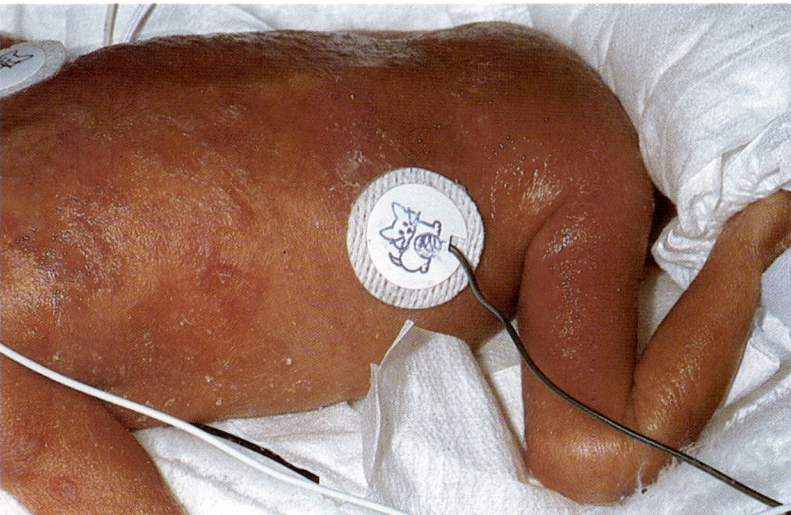

Fig. 6.45 Systemic candidiasis with burn-like changes of buttock and thigh.

Attempts to identify those infants most at risk for systemic candidiasis have not been very successful. Stool cultures have been systematically examined for evidence of colonization with Candida in VLBW infants, but the presence of colonization, detected in 11%, did not correlate with clinical infection.[435] Similarly, the presence of candida antigen in serum was not predictive of systemic infection, although this antigen was not detected in full-term neonatal controls.[435] Cellular and tissue defense mechanisms appear to be particularly important in preventing tissue invasion in experimental models.[436] This may partly explain the prevalence of systemic disease in VLBW premature infants.

Localized neonatal candidiasis

This occurs as a result of passage through an infected birth canal or postnatal infection and appear some days or weeks after birth. This includes oral candidiasis or thrush and candida diaper dermatitis. Lesions of similar morphology to those in classic congenital candidiasis can occur in the diaper or intertriginous areas in neonatal candidiasis. Erythematous weeping patches with satellite papulopustular lesions and peripheral scaling are more common, however. Thrush is present in most cases. Autoinoculation of the hand or wrist due to repeated sucking can result in unilateral pustules of neonatal candidiasis.[437]

Invasive fungal dermatitis

Invasive fungal dermatitis (IFD) is a term used for primary cutaneous erosive crusting lesions in VLBW infants due to Candida species or other fungal organisms, including Aspergillus, *Trichosporum beigelii*, and a Curvularia species. Risk factors are extreme prematurity, vaginal delivery, hyperglycemia, and steroid administration. Fungal invasion into the epidermis and even into the dermis may be seen on skin biopsy, and secondary systemic disease results.[421]

Investigation

Potassium hydroxide (KOH) preparations of skin pustules or scales are positive for pseudohyphae and spores in these infants. When disease is limited to the skin, microscopic examination shows the primary lesion to be a subcorneal pustule. In some cases, a subcorneal or spongiform pustule is located within the spinous layer of the epidermis similar to lesions seen in pustular psoriasis. In systemic disease, histologic examination of biopsy specimens may show subcorneal pustules as well as focal perivascular damage in the dermis with aggregates of pseudohyphae and spores visible with periodic acid–Schiff (PAS) or silver stains. Histopathologic examination of umbilical cord vessels may also provide early evidence of organ dysfunction disease.[438]

Dissemination of candidiasis may present with subtle signs and symptoms in these infants, making early recognition difficult.[439] Ultrasound of the kidneys and head may display characteristic fungal balls that cause hydronephrosis and fungal strands may be seen in the cerebral ventricles before clinical or laboratory evidence of organ dysfunction.[440]

Recognition of asymptomatic intra-amniotic infection with Candida in the setting of premature rupture of membranes can facilitate prompt aggressive neonatal treatment, improving significantly the poor outcome of these pregnancies.[436,441,442] Funisitis, characterized by yellow discrete plaques, develops on the umbilical cord and placenta in infants with intra-amniotic infection.[438] Yeast and pseudohyphae can be seen when the plaques are examined microscopically.[438] In the presence of proven antenatal Candida chorio-amnionitis and funisitis, systemically ill infants demonstrate hematologic evidence of infection even in the face of negative blood and cerebrospinal fluid (CSF) cultures.[443] For infants suspected of having systemic involvement, repeated cultures should be made of their urine, CSF, and blood. Periodic endotracheal tube and umbilical vessel catheter cultures should be done to monitor pulmonary infection and appliance colonization.

Differential diagnosis

The differential diagnosis of candidiasis includes bacterial pustulosis, transient neonatal pustular melanosis, erythema toxicum, and HSV infection. Gram stain, Wright stain, and bacterial culture of lesions will permit differentiation of candidiasis from other dermatoses that can occur during the early neonatal period (see Table 6.13).

Management

For oral thrush nystatin solution (100 000 units/ml) can be applied to the oral mucosa four times per day for at least one week for oral thrush. Resistant thrush may respond to oral fluconazole or itraconazole,[444] particularly in immunocompromised children.

Appropriate therapy for cutaneous disease includes topical antifungal agents and oral nystatin or fluconazole to decrease the number of organisms on the skin and in the gastrointestinal tract.[445] The use of barrier creams, such as zinc oxide, seems to afford some protection against local maceration induced by occlusion, which predisposes the infant to increased severity of infection.[446] Most infants do well without systemic therapy when infection is limited to the skin, placenta, or umbilical cord.

Systemic therapy is indicated if systemic cultures are positive, or if respiratory distress or laboratory signs of neonatal sepsis are present. Birthweight of less than 1500g, prolonged rupture of membranes, evidence of chorioamnionitis, extensive manipulation during the delivery, the necessity of

435. Ormala T, Korppi M, Katila ML et al. (1992) Fungal gut colonization with Candida or Pityrosporum sp. and serum Candida antigen in preterm neonates with very low birth weights. **Scand J Infect Dis** 24:781.
436. Bykov VL (1991) Velocity of Candida albicans invasion into host tissues. **Mycoses** 34:293.
437. Resnick SD, Greenberg RA (1989) Autoinoculated palmar pustules in neonatal candidiasis. **Pediatr Dermatol** 6:206.
438. Schwartz DA, Reef S (1990) Candida albicans placentitis and funisitis: early diagnosis of congenital candidemia by histopathologic examination of umbilical cord vessels. **Pediatr Infect Dis J** 9:661.
439. Baley JE (1991) Neonatal candidiasis: the current challenge. **Clin Perinatol** 18:263.
440. Currie JL (1989) Ultrasound appearances of systemic candidiasis in the neonate. **Radiogr Today** 55:20.
441. Reid M, Rollins N, Halliday H et al. (1991) Systemic neonatal candidiasis. **Ulster Med J** 60:35.
442. Mazor M, Chaim W, Shinwell ES (1992) Asymptomatic amniotic fluid invasion with Candida albicans in preterm premature rupture of membranes. Implications for obstetric and neonatal management. **Acta Obstet Gynecol Scand** 24:781.
443. Wolach B, Bogger-Goren S, Whyte R (1991) Perinatal hematological profile of newborn infants with candida antenatal infections. **Biol Neonate** 59:5.
444. Crutchfield CE, Lewis EJ (1997) The successful treatment of oral candidiasis (thrush) in a pediatric patient using itraconazole. **Pediatr Dermatol** 14:246.
445. Dhondt F, Ninane J, DeBeule K et al. (1992) Oral candidosis: treatment with absorbable and non-absorbable antifungal agents in children. **Mycoses** 35:1.
446. Auger P, Colin P, Joly J et al. (1989) Treatment of cutaneous candidosis in guinea pigs: effect of zinc oxide on the antifungal efficacy of nystatin. **Mycoses** 32:455.

performing invasive procedures, or the use of prolonged antibiotic therapy, intubation, or hyperalimentation should increase suspicion for systemic infection with candida.[428,434,447] Systemic therapy has traditionally been amphotericin B, 0.5mg/kg per day, increasing to 1mg/kg per day for 14–21 days, with or without 5-flucytosine.[448] Fluconazole is an alternative therapy that may be considered.[449–451]

CONGENITAL TOXOPLASMOSIS

Congenital infection with the intracellular protozoan *Toxoplasma gondii* was recognized by Wolf *et al.* in 1939.[452] Infection commonly occurs through consumption of undercooked meats containing toxoplasma cysts or oocysts excreted by cats.[453] Congenital toxoplasmosis is a sequel of acute maternal infection or reactivation, with risk of transmission being 15% in the first trimester, 30% in the second and 60% in the third.[454,455] Severity of fetal disease varies inversely with gestational age at the time of infection, with early infection more likely to lead to fetal death or severe neurologic and ophthalmologic disease.[456] Most newborns infected in the second or third trimester have mild or subclinical manifestations. Infection is discovered late in at least 40% of cases, manifesting as chorioretinitis, visual impairment, and neurologic sequelae.[455] Risk of fetal infection is estimated to be 1 per 1000 to 8000 live births.[453]

Eighty percent of affected infants are asymptomatic at birth.[455,457] The cutaneous findings of congenital toxoplasmosis are non-specific. These skin manifestations occur in 14–25% of symptomatic neonates.[458] A maculopapular or punctate eruption is most frequent, while petechiae, ecchymoses, "blueberry muffin" lesions, hemorrhages, and calcification of the skin occur. The skin lesions may be present on the day of birth or may first appear at several weeks of age. All body areas, including the scalp, palms, and soles, may be affected, while the mucous membranes are usually spared. Skin lesions gradually fade but may last for up to three weeks. With resolution, desquamation, or exfoliation occurs, which may leave postinflammatory pigmentation changes.[459] Classical systemic findings of congenital toxoplasmosis are chorioretinitis, hydrocephalus, seizures, microcephaly and intracerebral calcifications. Generalized disease can also cause prematurity, cataracts, optic atrophy, glaucoma, microphthalmia, hepatosplenomegaly, hyperbilirubinemia, lymphadenopathy, jaundice, anemia, eosinophilia, thrombocytopoenia, vomiting, and diarrhea.

Infection of the fetus occurs when the mother acquires toxoplasmosis during pregnancy, either by eating inadequately cooked meat or after contact with cat feces or contaminated soil containing the toxoplasma oocysts.[455] Sporozoites penetrate the gastrointestinal mucosa, and tachyzoites are released into the bloodstream. Maternal parasitemia occurs and placental involvement develops, with subsequent fetal vascular invasion by trophozoites. Infection of fetal endothelial cells and vascular wall damage produce vasculitis and perivasculitis. Trophozoites are released into the fetal tissue, leading to dysmorphogenesis.

The diagnosis of congenital toxoplasmosis in the neonate is made through a combination of serologic testing, parasite isolation, detection of Toxoplasma antigens in tissue or body fluid, or detection of Toxoplasma nucleic acid by polymerase chain reaction (PCR).[460] An attempt should be made to isolate *Toxoplasma gondii* from placenta, cord, WBCs, and buffy coat, if the diagnosis has not already been established. *Toxoplasma gondii* has been isolated from 95% of the placentas of congenitally infected newborns when the mother has not been treated and from approximately 81% when the mother has been treated. The definitive diagnosis relies on demonstration of the parasite in blood or tissue or on serologic evidence in the form of IgM- or IgG-specific antibodies. Due to delay in antibody response and the presence of maternal IgG, early serologic diagnosis may be difficult. Both the enzyme linked immunosorbent assays (ELISA) and immunosorbent agglutination assays (ISAGA) are useful tests.[455] PCR testing of amniotic fluid has now replaced cordocentesis for the prenatal diagnosis of fetal infection.[461] Nonspecific laboratory findings suggesting the diagnosis include anemia, thrombocytopenia, eosinophilia, hyperbilirubinemia, elevated CSF protein, and WBC counts.

Histopathologic examination of the maculopapular eruption of congenital toxoplasmosis has not been reported, but organisms have been found in the subcutaneous tissue in the absence of a rash.[462]

Prognosis of congenital toxoplasmosis has improved with therapy. However many cases of congenital toxoplasmosis are not recognized in the newborn period[456] and so go untreated. Without treatment, chorioretinitis and mental retardation develop in most patients, including those with asymptomatic infections at birth.[463]

Therapy for infants with congenital toxoplasmosis has never been well studied in controlled clinical trials. The most commonly used regimen is pyrimethamine (1mg/kg per day), sulfadiazine (100mg/kg per day), and folic acid (2mg/kg per day), given for three weeks, followed by four to five weeks of spiramycin (50 to 100mg/kg per day).[454] In some cases, vertical transmission has been prevented by administration of spiramycin to the mother.[464] Corticosteroids have been advised by some for early initial improvement of chorioretinitis but must be used concurrently with anti-toxoplasmotic drugs to prevent exacerbation of infection.[464]

The differential diagnosis includes congenital CMV infection, syphilis, HSV, rubella, erythroblastosis, and congenital leukemia. Although special studies, including serologic studies and cultures, are required to confirm the diagnosis, characteristics of certain associated findings may be helpful. Cortical calcifications, macular or central chorioretinitis, the absence of cataracts, and the infrequency of heart disease substantiate the clinical impression of Toxoplasma infection when attempting to distinguish toxoplasmosis from rubella or CMV.

RUBELLA

Neonatal disease produced by the rubella virus is characterized by intrauterine growth retardation (43%), microcephaly (39%), microphthalmia (20%), visceral abnormalities (50–75%), and cutaneous manifestations (20–50%), somewhat similar to the picture for congenital CMV infection.[465] Rubella infections of the embryo or fetus occur equally in all races and sexes, and infants affected with this syndrome have a decreased life span.[466] Not all infants exposed *in utero* acquire the infection, nor do all infected infants manifest disease during the neonatal period. Infection may be limited only to certain organs. In studies

447. Johnson DE, Thompson TR, Ferrieri P (1981) Congenital candidiasis. Am J Dis Child 135:273.
448. Butler KM, Rench MA, Baker CJ (1990) Amphotericin B as a single agent in the treatment of systemic candidiasis in neonates. Pediatr Infect Dis 9:51.
449. Fasano C, O'Keeffe J, Gibbs D (1994) Fluconazole treatment of neonates and infants with severe fungal infections not treatable with conventional agents. Eur J Clin Microbiol Infect Dis 13:351–354.
450. Schwarze R, Penk A, Pittrow L (1998) Administration of fluconazole in children below 1 year of age – review. Mycoses 41:61–70.
451. Aleck KA, Bartley DL (1997) Multiple malformation syndrome following fluconazole use in pregnancy. Report of an additional patient. Am J Med Genet 72:253–256.
452. Wolf A, Cowen D, Paige BH (1939) Toxoplasmic encephalomyelitis. Am J Pathol 15:657.
453. Remington JS, McLeod R, Desmonts G (1995) Toxoplasmosis. In: Infectious Disease of the Fetus and Newborn Infant, 4th ed, Remington JS, Klein JO, eds. Philadelphia: WB Saunders, pp. 140–267.
454. Bakht FR, Gentry LO (1992) Toxoplasmosis in pregnancy: an emerging concern for family physicians. Am Fam Physician 45:1683.
455. Lynfield R, Guerina NG (1997) Toxoplasmosis. Pediatr Rev 18:75–83.
456. Remington JS (1990) The tragedy of toxoplasmosis. Pediatr Infect Dis J 9:762.

457. Boyer KM (1996) Diagnosis and treatment of congenital toxoplasmosis. Adv Pediatr Infect Dis 11:449–467.
458. Roizen N, Swisher CN, Stein MA et al. (1995) Neurologic and developmental outcome in treated congenital toxoplasmosis. Pediatrics 95:11–20.
459. Pong AL, McCuaig, CC (2001) Fungal infections, infestations and parasitic infections in neonates. In: Textbook of Neonatal Dermatology, Eichenfield LF, Frieden IJ, Esterly NB, eds. Philadelphia, PA: WB Saunders, pp. 223–240.
460. Cazenave J, Forestier F, Bessieres MH et al. (1992) Contribution of a new PCR assay to the prenatal diagnosis of congenital toxoplasmosis. Prenat Diagn 12:119.
461. Alger LS (1997) Toxoplasmosis and parvovirus B19. Infect Obstetr 11:55–75.
462. Dische MR, Gooch WM 3rd (1981) Congenital toxoplasmosis. In: Perspectives in Pediatric Pathology, vol. 6, Rosenberg HS, Bernstein J, eds. New York: Masson USA, p. 83.
463. Committee on Infectious Disease, American Academy of Pediatrics (2000) Red Book: Report of the Committee on Infectious Disease. p. 583–584. 25th ed. American Academy of Pediatrics.
464. Wilson CB (1990) Treatment of toxoplasmosis. Ped Infect Dis J 9:682.
465. Friedlander SF, Bradley JS (2001) Viral Infections. In: Textbook of Neonatal Dermatology, Eichenfield LF, Frieden IJ, Esterly NB, eds. Philadelphia, PA: WB Saunders, pp. 201–222.
466. McIntosh ED, Menser MA (1992) A fifty-year follow-up of congenital rubella. Lancet 340:414.

reporting observations made in the rubella epidemic of 1964, only 30% of affected neonates had clinical manifestations at birth, and nearly 70% had subclinical infections.[467] Severely affected infants have been born to mothers who had asymptomatic rubella infection in pregnancy and documented pre-existing antibody.[468]

During the immediate neonatal period, the most common cutaneous manifestation is areas of extramedullary hematopoiesis called blueberry muffin spots, though hemorrhagic changes secondary to thrombocytopenia may give these lesions a more "cranberry muffin" appearance.[465] These occur in 20–50% of affected infants.[466] Lesions are initially dark blue, dark red, or blue-gray and are usually present at birth, although they may appear during the first 48 hours of life. They begin as macules but may develop into papules measuring 7–8mm in diameter, and can persist for up to eight weeks before fading.

The morbilliform macular rash characteristic of rubella infection in older children has not been found to occur in neonates but has been recognized in older infants known to be suffering from congenital infection.[469] Cutaneous abnormalities not seen during the immediate neonatal period, but noted in congenitally infected infants with encephalitis at 3 to 9 months of age, include recurrent urticaria, cutis marmorata, seborrhea, and hyperpigmentation.[469] The nails, hair, and mucous membranes of affected infants are normal, but necrosis of the inner enamel epithelium of the teeth has been described.[470]

Infection is most severe in the embryonic and early fetal period before 12 weeks gestation. Infection after 20 weeks gestation probably occurs but may not produce dramatic clinical findings during the neonatal period. Systemic manifestations include anemia and thrombocytopenia, present in 20% of congenitally infected infants, and visceral abnormalities, reported in up to 75% of symptomatic neonates.[465] Although these manifestations may aid in the diagnosis of congenital rubella infection, many are nonspecific. The "salt-and-pepper" unilateral retinopathy present in congenitally infected infants is a helpful diagnostic clue.[471] Other ocular findings include congenital cataracts, microphthalmos, strabismus, and glaucoma, but none is diagnostic.[471] Other associated findings include congenital heart disease (patent ductus arteriosus, pulmonic stenosis, and aortic stenosis) and pneumonitis.

The most reliable laboratory tests for confirmation of the diagnosis are viral cultures; culture of the pharynx is the definitive test, while CSF, urine, and conjunctival cultures might also be obtained.[466] Detection of viral antigen by direct immunoflorescence of pharyngeal swabs is helpful if positive, but it is negative in a significant proportion of affected infants.[472] Culture of tissue obtained by lesional skin biopsy has grown the rubella virus in older infants but this has not been reported in the neonate.[469] Viral excretion decreases during infancy; sampling should therefore be done as soon as rubella infection enters the differential diagnosis.

The detection of rubella-specific antibodies of the IgM class at levels greater than 20mg/dl is specific for rubella infection. False-positive tests for the presence of IgM-specific rubella antibodies can be produced by rheumatoid factor. Detection of IgM in cord blood makes the diagnosis of infection *in utero* possible.[473,474] Caution should be used in interpretation of these data, since both false-positive[473] and false-negative[474] results have been reported. Persistence of IgG antibodies beyond 6 months of age in infants suspected of having congenital rubella is presumptive evidence for intrauterine infection.[466]

Histologic examination of blueberry muffin lesions shows evidence of extramedullary hematopoeisis and the appearance is not specific for congenital rubella.[475] The clinical differential diagnosis should include metastatic tumors, toxoplasmosis, vascular nevi and CMV infection. Clinical findings as well as ophthalmologic, radiographic, histologic, and immunologic studies will help substantiate the diagnosis. In infants suspected of having subclinical infection, neuroimaging may be helpful. Ultrasonic evidence of subependymal cysts, calcification, and vascular changes in the basal ganglia support this diagnosis. MRI is the most sensitive test to identify the minor atrophic changes and white matter lesions seen in congenital infection.[472]

There is no specific therapy for congenital rubella infections. Supportive care should include thermal, nutritional, and cardiovascular needs. Affected infants excrete the virus for a prolonged time and are considered infective until 6 months of age, although virus can be isolated from infants past 1 year.[465]

CYTOMEGALOVIRUS DISEASE

Cytomegaloviral infection of the newborn is common, and may be acquired congenitally, perinatally or postnatally. It is the most commonly recognized cause of congenital infection, seen in 1% to 2% of births.[476] Of susceptible mothers who are infected, approximately 40% will deliver infants with congenital CMV infection.[477] Only 5–10% of affected infants are symptomatic at birth, with the classical findings of petechiae or purpura (50%), hepatosplenomegaly (50%), intrauterine growth retardation, hyperbilirubinemia, thrombocytopenia (43%), chorioretinitis, deafness, microcephaly, and ultimately mental retardation.[478] Extramedullary hematopoiesis ("blueberry muffin spots") (Fig. 6.46) similar to congenital rubella may be seen.[479] Petechiae usually develop within the first 48 hours after birth but may not appear until later. Intermittent showers of petechiae occur during early childhood, usually when the spleen is enlarged. Lesions of extramedullary erythropoiesis resolve slowly, as in congenital rubella. Although rare, vesicular lesions present at birth on the forehead of a neonate with CMV infection have been reported.[480] No new

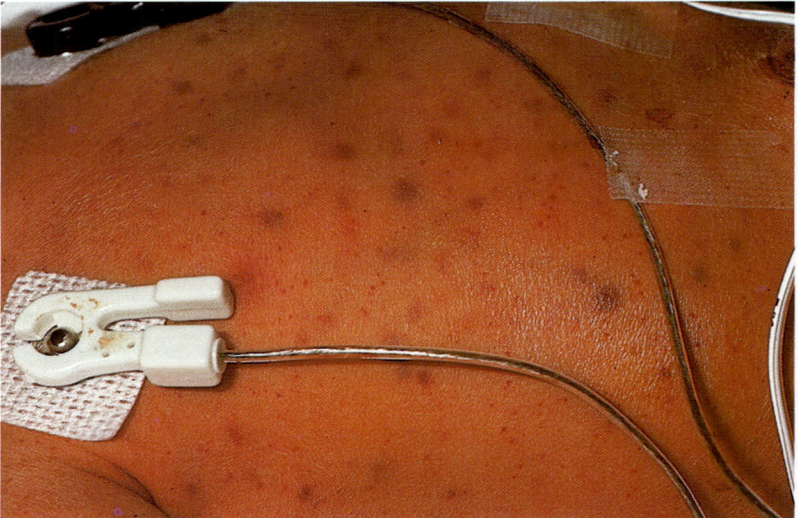

Fig. 6.46 Congenital cytomegalovirus infection. "Blueberry muffin spots" plus petechiae.

467. Schiff GM, Sutherland J, Light I (1971) Congenital rubella. In: Prenatal Infections, Thalhammer O, ed. International Symposium of Vienna. Stuttgart: Georg Thieme, p. 31.
468. Das BD, Lakhani P, Kurtz JB et al. (1990) Congenital rubella after previous maternal immunity. **Arch Dis Child** 65:545.
469. Marshall WL, Trompeter RS, Risdon RA (1975) Chronic rashes in congenital rubella: Isolation of virus from skin. **Lancet** 1:1349.
470. Tondury G, Smith DW (1992) Fetal rubella pathology. **J Pediatr** 68:867.
471. Armstrong NT (1992) The ocular manifestations of congenital rubella syndrome. **Insight** 17:14.
472. Yamashita Y, Matsuishi T, Murakami Y et al. (1991) Neuroimaging findings (ultrasonography, CT, MRI) in 3 infants with congenital rubella syndrome. **Pediatr Radiol** 21:547.
473. Kunakorn M, Petchclai B, Liemsuwan C (1992) Laboratory diagnosis of congenital and maternal rubella infection: a review. **J Med Assoc Thai**, suppl 1 75:282.
474. Suzumori K, Iida T, Adachi R et al. (1991) Prenatal diagnosis of rubella infection by fetal blood sampling. **Asia Oceania J Obstet Gynaecol** 17:113.
475. Esterly JR, Oppenheimer EH (1973) Intrauterine rubella infection. In: Perspectives in Pediatric Pathology, vol. 1. Rosenberg HS, Bolande RP, eds. Chicago: Year Book Medical, p. 313.
476. Saigal S, Luny KO, Larke R et al. (1982) The outcome in children with congenital cytomegalovirus infection. **Am J Dis Child** 136:896–901.
477. Peckham CS (1991) Cytomegalovirus infection: congenital and neonatal disease. **Scand J Infect Dis** suppl. 80:82.
478. Dobbins JG, Stewart JA, Demmler GJ (1992) Surveillance of congenital cytomegalovirus disease, 1990–1991. Collaborating Registry Group. **MMWR CDC Surveill Summ** 41:35.
479. Groark SP, Jampel RM (1989) Violaceous papules and macules in a newborn. Dermal erythropoiesis associated with congenital cytomegalovirus infection. **Arch Dermatol** 125:114.
480. Blatt J, Kastner O, Hodes DS (1978) Cutaneous vesicles in congenital cytomegalovirus infection. **J Pediatr** 92:509.

vesicular lesions appeared after birth. The hair, nails, and teeth are normal in congenitally infected infants.

Ninety percent of congenitally infected infants are asymptomatic at birth, but approximately 5% of these asymptomatic infants will develop sequelae of infection in later infancy, most commonly sensorineural hearing loss.[481,482] Other subtle neuroradiologic and neurodevelopmental abnormalities are also detectable in this group. The presence of high levels of IgG antibodies reactive with envelope glycoprotein gB early in pregnancy in women whose asymptomatic infants later developed hearing impairment suggests that early viral acquisition is the important factor in determining the likelihood of these sequelae of congenital infection.[483,484] Infants who developed late-onset hearing loss and who were more disabled were also more likely to have abnormalities on CT or MRI scan of the brain.[482,485]

CMV is a DNA virus of the herpesvirus group. The mechanism of embryo or fetal infection is unclear but is most likely by infection of endometrial vessels or trophoblast cells prior to placental development or by later transplacental transmission of the virus.[486] Severe sequelae of infection relate to the time of acquisition of infection, with infections early in gestation having a poorer prognosis than those from later exposure.[478] Seronegative mothers who acquire primary CMV infection during pregnancy have a greater incidence of symptomatic neonates.[487] Intrauterine transmission of CMV can occur whether the pregnant woman has prior immunity or acquires CMV for the first time during pregnancy. However, the presence of maternal antibody to CMV before conception provides substantial protection against damaging congenital CMV infection in the newborn. Infants have less sensorineural hearing loss, no mental retardation, and no bilateral hearing loss, and are more likely to be unaffected.[488]

Viral culture of urine or saliva is widely available and highly reliable if the specimen is cultured promptly. Culture positivity is reduced to 93% after storage for one week and 77% after two weeks.[489] These should be obtained within the first two weeks of life to diagnose congenital infection, as cultures after this time period will not be able to differentiate perinatal CMV infection. Spun urine samples will demonstrate viral inclusions in tubular epithelial cells in up to 50% of culture-positive samples, and electron microscopy findings in up to 93%.[490] Specific neonatal CMV-IgM antibody, or a persistent, increasing titer of IgG antibody during the first four to six months of life may also be used to diagnose CMV. While the presence of specific CMV-IgM in cord blood will verify congenital infection, the sensitivity of this test as currently performed in reference laboratories may be less than 50%.[491] Polymerase chain reaction (PCR) for CMV-DNA in plasma is a sensitive test and may be useful for evaluation of newborns.[492]

Despite the focus on congenital infections, perinatal infections resulting from transmission during birth, through breast milk, and by blood transfusion are much more prevalent than congenital infections.[486] Fortunately, the vast majority of these infants are intellectually and physically normal.

The differential diagnosis of CMV includes congenital rubella, toxoplasmosis, HSV infection, and syphilis. Unlike rubella, CMV is rarely associated with cataracts, congenital heart disease, or generalized retinitis. Toxoplasma infection is very similar to CMV and requires more specific antibody tests to separate it. However, Toxoplasma infections sometimes manifest a rash that is more maculopapular than purpuric in character. Congenital HSV infections may present with petechiae and purpura, but extramedullary hematopoiesis is rare, and vesicles and erosions are more common. In congenital syphilis, cartilage and bone inflammation, diffuse scaling, or a papulosquamous rash, and mucous membrane involvement are more common. Intrauterine growth retardation, intracranial calcifications, and visceral involvement occur in nearly all congenital infections, and other studies are essential to pinpoint the diagnosis.

Ganciclovir, a nucleoside analog with potent CMV activity, may be used as a treatment for CMV infection, but is associated with significant bone marrow toxicity. Unfortunately, congenital CMV infections cannot be cured, but only suppressed during the period of antiviral administration. It should be noted that while congenitally infected children continue to excrete the virus in either their urine or saliva, or both, for many years, this is also true of up to 20% of healthy 1-year-olds. Isolation of these children is therefore neither recommended nor necessary. It may be useful to obtain urine cultures every 12 months to document cessation of viral shedding.

NEONATAL HERPES SIMPLEX VIRUS INFECTION

Herpes simplex (HSV) infection is one of the most feared diseases in the newborn.[493–495] Subtle or inconspicuous skin lesions may herald the onset of this potentially devastating infection. Neonates may be infected with HSV in several ways. Intrauterine infection, resulting in congenital infection, can occur through viremic transplacental seeding from an infected mother or from ascending infection through apparently intact membranes.[496] With neonatal herpes simplex infection, most infants are presumed to be infected around the time of delivery, either by exposure to the virus in infectious secretions or lesions in the birth canal. Postnatal exposure to HSV can lead to neonatal infection, with exposure from maternal, nongenital sites as well as from nonmaternal sources, including family members and healthcare workers.[497] Neonatal herpes is estimated to occur at a rate of 1–2.5 per 5000 live births.[498]

Intrauterine HSV infections occur infrequently as a consequence of primary or recurrent genital HSV, comprising about 4–5% of all babies with neonatal HSV infection.[496,499,500] Infection becomes apparent within 24 to 48 hours of life. In addition to the characteristic vesicles, widespread bullae and erosions resembling epidermolysis bullosa,[501–503] absence of skin on the scalp (resembling aplasia cutis congenita), and scars on the scalp, face, trunk or extremities have been reported (Fig. 6.47).[496] Affected infants are often premature, weighing less than 2500g. Affected organs include brain (microcephaly, hydrocephalus, hydranencephaly), eye (chorioretinitis, microphthalmia), and skin. Infection can occur in the presence of intact membranes and with cesarean delivery. Immunohistochemistry using herpes-specific antibodies, coupled with routine histologic examination has enabled

481. Williamson WD, Percy AK, Yow MD et al. (1990) Asymptomatic congenital cytomegalovirus infection. Audiologic, neuroradiologic, and neuro-developmental abnormalities during the first year. **Am J Dis Child** 144:1365.
482. Williamson WD, Demmler GJ, Percy AK et al. (1992) Progressive hearing loss in infants with asymptomatic congenital cytomegalovirus infection. **Pediatrics** 90:862.
483. Boppana SB, Pass RF, Britt WJ (1993) Virus-specific antibody responses in mothers and their newborn infants with asymptomatic congenital cytomegalovirus infections. **J Infect Dis** 167:72.
484. Britt WJ, Vugler LG (1990) Antiviral antibody responses in mothers and their newborn infants with clinical and subclinical congenital cytomegalovirus infections. **J Infect Dis** 161:214.
485. Sugita K, Ando M, Makino M et al. (1991) Magnetic resonance imaging of the brain in congenital rubella and cytomegalovirus infections. **Neuroradiology** 33:239.
486. Alford CA, Stagno S, Pass RF et al. (1990) Congenital and perinatal cytomegalovirus infections. **Rev Infect Dis** 12 Supp 7:S745.
487. Stagno S, Pass RF, Dworsky ME et al. (1982) Congenital cytomegalovirus infection: The relative importance of primary and recurrent maternal infection. **N Eng J Med** 306:945–949.
488. Fowler KB, Stagno S, Pass RF et al. (1992) The outcome of congenital cytomegalovirus infection in relation to maternal antibody status. **N Engl J Med** 326:663.
489. Stagno S, Pass RF, Reynolds DW et al. (1980) Comparative study of diagnostic procedures for congenital cytomegalovirus infection. **Pediatrics** 65:251.
490. Demmler GJ (1991) Summary of a workshop on surveillance for congenital cytomegalovirus disease. **Reviews of Infectious Disease** 13:315–329.
491. Friedlander SF, Bradley JS (2001) Viral Infections. In: Textbook of Neonatal Dermatology, Eichenfield LF, Frieden IJ, Esterly NB, eds. Philadelphia, PA: WB Saunders, pp. 201–222.
492. Nelson CT, Istas AS, Wilkerson MK et al. (1995) Polymerase chain reaction detection of cytomegalovirus DNA in serum as a diagnostic test for congenital cytomegalovirus infection. **J Clin Microbiol** 33:3317–3318.
493. Jacobs RF (1998) Neonatal herpes simplex virus infections. **Semin Perinatol** 22:64–71.
494. Kohl S (1997) Neonatal herpes simplex virus infection. **Clin Perinatol** 24:129–150.
495. Riley LE (1998) Herpes simplex virus. **Semin Perinatol** 22:284–292.
496. Hutto C, Arvin A, Jacobs R et al. (1987) Intrauterine herpes simplex virus infections. **J Pediatr** 110:97.
497. Jenkins M, Kohl S (1992) New aspects of neonatal herpes. **Infect Dis Clin North Am** 6:57.
498. Friedlander SF, Bradley JS (2001) Viral Infections. In: Textbook of Neonatal Dermatology, Eichenfield LF, Frieden IJ, Esterly NB, eds. Philadelphia, PA: WB Saunders, pp. 201–222.
499. Overall JC (1994) Herpes simplex virus infection of the fetus and newborn. **Pediatr Ann** 23:131–136.
500. Baldwin S, Whitley RJ (1989) Intrauterine herpes simplex virus infection. **Teratology** 39:1.
501. Sarkell B, Blaylock WK, Vernon H (1992) Congenital neonatal herpes simplex virus infection. **J Am Acad Dermatol** 27:817.
502. Harris HH, Foucar E, Andersen RD et al. (1986) Intrauterine herpes simplex infection resembling mechanobullous disease in a newborn infant. **J Am Acad Dermatol** 15:1148–1155.
503. Honig PJ, Brown D (1982) Congenital herpes simplex virus infection initially resembling epidermolysis bullosa. **J Pediatr** 101:958–960.

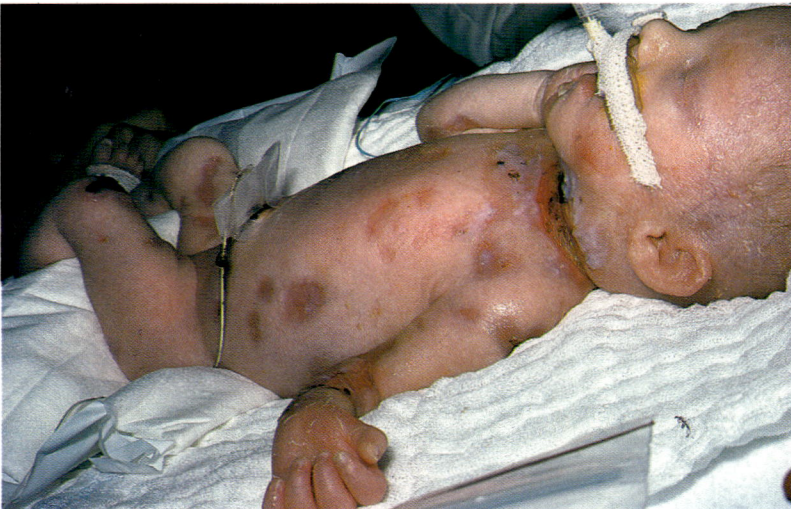

Fig. 6.47   Intrauterine HSV infection. Deep atrophic/ulcerative lesions suggesting epidermolysis bullosa or aplasia cutis.

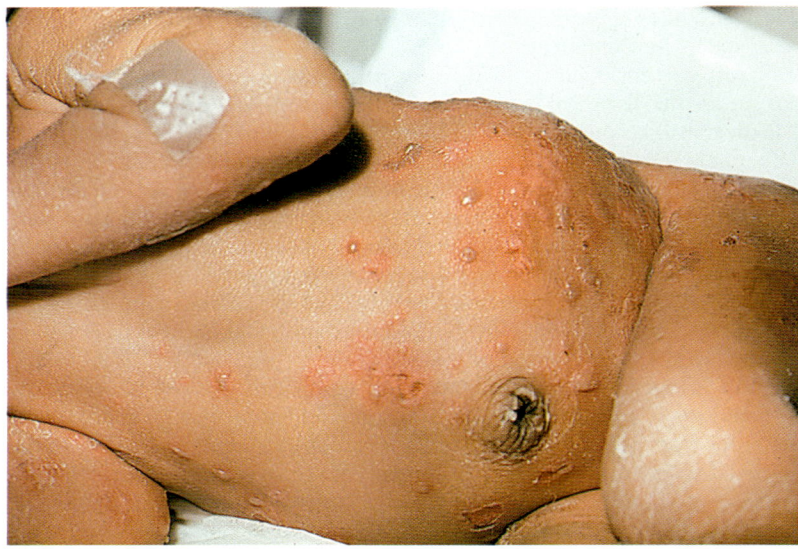

Fig. 6.48   Neonatal herpes simplex with multiple vesicles.

documentation that congenital HSV infection usually occurs by an ascending route.[504]

Neonatal HSV infection acquired around the time of delivery manifests in three general patterns of disease with overlapping features: (1) mucocutaneous infection (limited to skin, eye or mouth); (2) disseminated infection, with evidence of visceral organ involvement including lungs, liver, and CNS; and (3) central nervous system infection (CSF or brain abnormalities with or without mucocutaneous disease but with no visceral organ involvement).[497,505]

Skin disease is the most characteristic finding in neonatal HSV infection, but often lags behind other symptoms. The most common skin lesion seen in neonatal HSV is the vesicle, measuring 1–2mm in diameter, usually on an erythematous base. A single vesicle may be the only cutaneous finding, but multiple discrete vesicles are more common (Fig. 6.48). Occasionally, clusters of five or six vesicles are seen. Although grouped vesicles on an erythematous base are a hallmark of herpetic infection, lesions in neonatal herpes frequently lack such grouping, and in some cases, a widespread vesicular exanthem or zoster–like blistering localized to one or two dermatomes may occur. Vesicles may be easily denuded and erosions may be present. Vesicles may become pustular after 24 to 48 hours and ultimately become crusted or ulcerated. The initial site of involvement is frequently the area that first comes into contact with the maternal HSV lesions (i.e., face or scalp lesions for neonates in the cephalic presentation, and buttock lesions for those in the breech presentation). Initial cutaneous involvement has been reported at the site of fetal scalp electrode implantation.[506] Oral ulcerations are present in nearly one-third of cases.[494] Vesicles may be absent at presentation in 17% of mucocutaneous disease, 32% of CNS disease, and 39% of disseminated disease patients.[507] All newborns with skin or mucosal lesions of HSV, even without extracutaneous symptoms, should be evaluated to rule out disseminated or CNS disease.

Erythematous macular lesions, usually few in number, have been reported; these ultimately develop vesicular lesions within the macule within several days.[508] The histopathologic pattern seen in these macular lesions sometimes demonstrates intranuclear inclusions in the epidermal keratinocytes as well as multinucleated giant cells, even though the more recognized vesicular lesion associated with HSV infections has not yet occurred. Exanthems without vesicles, pustules, or erosions have been reported, but the histopathologic findings in such cases are unclear. Presumably, multinucleated giant cells and intranuclear inclusions might be detected.

Nonspecific symptoms suggesting CNS or systemic illness, such as fever, lethargy, irritability, poor feeding, or poor muscle tone, are as suggestive as skin lesions as the presenting signs of HSV infection.[497,509] The average time period of onset of symptoms is in the first week of life; 39% of infants had symptoms within the first five days of life in one study.[507]

The risk of acquiring neonatal HSV infection is related to the nature of the maternal genital HSV infection.[510] Reactivation of maternal HSV-2 at the time of delivery has about a 5% rate of transmission to the neonate, while primary infection has about a 50% rate of infection.[511–513] The lower risk of HSV infection among infants whose mothers have recurrent genital infection is likely due, in part, to the transplacental passage of type-specific or other functional antibodies to HSV.[494] Antibodies may protect the fetus through neutralizing activity or through antibody–dependent cellular cytotoxicity (ADCC).[514] In one study, approximately 10% of pregnant women were at risk of acquiring a primary infection from their partners.[515] Although HSV-2 is thought to account for 80% of neonatal infections, there are no discernible differences in the cutaneous or visceral manifestations with HSV-1 or HSV-2 neonatal infections. Disease onset during the first 28 days of life is associated with a higher incidence of dissemination and visceral complications than disease acquired in older infants, children, or adults.

In addition to primary HSV infection in the mother, prematurity may be an independent risk factor for HSV infection in the neonate.[516] Premature delivery may be precipitated by ascending infection with HSV. Alternatively, premature infants may lack the protective transplacental antibody, usually

504. Hyde SR, Giacoia GP (1993) Congenital herpes infection: placental and umbilical cord findings. **Obstet Gynecol** 81:852.
505. Whitley R, Arvin A, Prober C et al. (1991) Predictors of morbidity and mortality in neonates with herpes simplex virus infections. The National Institute of Allergy and Infectious Diseases Collaborative Antiviral Study Group. **N Engl J Med** 324:450–454.
506. Amann ST, Fagnant RJ, Chartrand SA et al. (1992) Herpes simplex infection associated with short-term use of a fetal scalp electrode. A case report. **J Reprod Med** 37:372.
507. Kimberlin DW. Lin C-Y. Jacobs RF et al. (2001) Natural history of neonatal herpes simplex virus infections in the acyclovir era. **Pediatrics** 108:223–229.
508. Sieber OF, Fulginiti VA, Brazie J et al. (1966) In utero infection of the fetus by herpes simplex virus. **J Pediatr** 69:30.
509. Koskiniemi M, Happonen JM, Jarvenpaa AL et al. (1989) Neonatal herpes simplex virus infection: a report of 43 patients. **Pediatr Infect Dis J** 8:30.

510. Riley LE (1998) Herpes simplex virus. **Semin Perintol** 22:284–292.
511. Prober CG, Sullender WM, Yasukawa LL et al. (1987) Low risk of herpes simplex virus infections in neonates exposed to the virus at the time of vaginal delivery to mothers with recurrent genital herpes simplex virus infections. **N Engl J Med** 316:240.
512. Kulhanjian JA, Soroush V, Au DS et al. (1992) Identification of women at unsuspected risk of primary infection with herpes simplex virus type 2 during pregnancy. **N Engl J Med** 326:916.
513. Brown ZA, Ashley R, Douglas J et al. (1991) Neonatal herpes simplex virus infection in relation to asymptomatic maternal infection at the time of labor. **N Engl J Med** 324:1247.
514. Kohl S (1991) Role of antibody-dependent cellular cytotoxicity in neonatal infection with herpes simplex virus. **Rev Infect Dis**, suppl 11, 13:S950.
515. Ashley RL, Dalessio J, Burchett S et al. (1992) Herpes simplex virus-2 (HSV-2) type-specific antibody correlates of protection in infants exposed to HSV-2 at birth. **J Clin Invest** 90:511.
516. Prober CG, Arvin AM (1989) Prematurity and risk of herpes simplex infection. **Pediatr Infect Dis J** 8:660.

acquired during the third trimester, resulting in predisposition to more severe infection.[516,517] Prematurity in infants with CNS disease is also associated with an increased mortality risk with HSV infection.[507] Other risk factors for mortality include lethargy at the time of the initiation of treatment in infants with disseminated disease, and AST elevations of equal to greater than 10 times normal at the time of treatment initiation in infants with disseminated disease treated with acyclovir.[507] Morbidity has been associated with the extent of disease and with seizures at the time of initiation of treatment in infants with CNS disease.

Cutaneous lesions can recur up to 5 years of age in the same anatomic site as the original lesions or in different areas of the skin. Dissemination in otherwise healthy infants and children beyond the neonatal period usually does not occur, and systemic therapy is generally not required. It is controversial as to whether recurrences should be treated orally. Long-term follow-up evaluation has, however, demonstrated that multiple (greater than three) cutaneous recurrences are associated with an increased risk of neurologic impairment.[505] Relapses of CNS infection up to one year later have been reported, making additional therapy necessary in these cases.

The broad differential diagnosis of vesicular, bullous, macular, or petechial lesions includes infectious and noninfectious entities. The infectious entities include neonatal enteroviral infections, bullous impetigo, syphilis, scabies, candidiasis, rubella, CMV infections, congenital varicella, and sepsis with a bleeding diathesis. In many instances, the acute onset and rapid progression of skin signs point to HSV infection. Noninfectious etiologies that should be considered are erythema toxicum, transient neonatal pustular melanosis, miliaria, epidermolysis bullosa, Langerhans cell histiocytosis, incontinentia pigmenti, bullous mastocytosis, pemphigus vulgaris, herpes gestationis, and neonatal acropustulosis. A maternal history of HSV infection may be helpful, though at least 50% of mothers having neonates with HSV infection have no history, signs, or symptoms suggestive of current or previous herpes infection.[513]

If skin lesions suggest herpes infection, prompt diagnosis and institution of treatment is imperative.[518] Skin scrapings for Tzanck stains should be obtained. The Tzanck test is a rapid and useful test for early diagnosis of HSV. Morphologic changes characterized by multinucleated giant cells (representing damaged epidermal cells that have coalesced) and intranuclear inclusions can be seen on microscopic examination of material obtained by scraping the base or floor of the vesicle, pustule, erosion, or crusted lesion. Tzanck test results of vesicular lesions are more likely to be positive (67%) than those of pustular (55%) or ulcerated lesions (17%). A specific diagnosis of herpes simplex virus can be obtained rapidly by antibody-specific stains (such as direct fluorescent antibody for HSV-1 or HSV-2). Immunoperoxidase antigen detection and PCR are other rapid ways to obtain preliminary confirmation of HSV infection.[519] False-positive immunofluorescence has been reported.[520] Viral cultures remain the gold standard of diagnosis, and cultures of the skin vesicular fluid and epidermal cells, conjunctiva, throat, cerebrospinal fluid, and urine should be obtained.[494] Gentle aspiration of vesicular fluid is ideal but, if the lesion is eroded, a swab of the base may be adequate. Cultures taken of vesicular or pustular lesions are positive in 73–100% of cases.[521] If the lesions are vesicular, and pustular lesions are not included, the viral culture is positive in nearly 100% of cases. Cytopathic

effects of the virus on tissue culture cells may be evident within 24 to 48 hours; otherwise, seven to 10 days may be required to fully evaluate positive or negative culture results. PCR for HSV may be equivalent to culture.[522,523] Identification of HSV in neonatal infection as type 1 (20%) or as type 2 (80%) is possible and important for epidemiologic studies, but is is not essential for diagnostic or therapeutic considerations.

The histologic findings of HSV lesions are specific in most instances. The early vesicle is intraepidermal, and ballooning degeneration at the base of the vesicle is associated with the formation of multinucleated giant cells. Since intercellular bridges are lost, acantholysis occurs. Intranuclear inclusions can be seen in the epithelial balloon cells. These changes are more likely to be found at the margins of ulcerated lesions. A dermal inflammatory infiltrate suggestive of leukocytoclastic vasculitis may be present in severe reactions. Histologically, HSV lesions can be confused with pemphigus vulgaris, but the presence of primarily basal layer degeneration and intranuclear inclusions should permit differentiation. Neonatal pemphigus vulgaris is rare, and the infant is not systemically ill.[524]

The treatment of choice for neonatal herpes infections of all types is intravenously administered acyclovir.[525] The dose of acyclovir originally studied for skin or mucosal surface infection was 15mg/kg per d divided into 8-hourly doses, though data have shown the safety and a small increase in efficacy of 30mg/kg per d in mild to moderate neonatal infection.[526] Clinical trials of 60mg/kg per d for dissemination and encephalitis suggest a small incremental improvement in efficacy, with safety that is equivalent to the 30mg/kg per d dose.[527] In infants with renal failure, the doses should be adjusted.

The prognosis for neonates with HSV infection is related to the pattern of disease evident in the first few weeks of life. Outcome in the congenital HSV syndrome resulting from intrauterine infection is universally poor, with high mortality rates and severe impairments, including mental retardation, seizure disorders, blindness, and deafness, in all survivors. Infants with localized mucocutaneous infections do very well if treated early with antiviral therapy. Deaths are rare, and progression to the more severe forms of disease occurs in only 2% of infants.[526] More than 90% of these infants are developmentally normal. Morbidity, in the form of subtle hearing loss or language delay, is confined to the subset of infants who go on to have multiple recurrences of vesicles, seen exclusively with HSV-2 infection. Among neonates with disseminated infection, mortality is high, with a high incidence of morbidity in survivors.

CONGENITAL AND NEONATAL VARICELLA

Three distinct disorders occur following intrauterine or neonatal exposure to VZV: the fetal varicella syndrome, neonatal varicella and infantile herpes zoster. Approximately 95% of women have acquired varicella infection prior to pregnancy, rendering themselves and their fetus immune. The exact incidence of varicella during pregnancy is unknown; there is a range of 1–10 cases per 10 000 pregnancies reported in the US.[528–530] Fetal and congenital disease occur much less often. Maternal infection early in pregnancy may cause the congenital varicella syndrome, whereas late gestational infection causes perinatal varicella within the first 10 days after delivery. The risk of neonatal chickenpox when maternal chickenpox occurs in the 21 days

517. Harger JH, Guevarra L, Armstrong JA (1990) Neutralizing antibody to herpes simplex virus in pregnant women and their neonates. **J Perinatol** 10:16.
518. Elder DE, Minutillo C, Pemberton PJ (1995) Neonatal herpes simplex infection: keys to early diagnosis. **J Paediatr Child Health** 31:307–311.
519. Cohen PR (1994) Tests for detecting herpes simplex virus and varicella-zoster virus infections. **Dermatol Clin** 12:51–68.
520. Detlefs RL, Frieden IJ, Berger TG et al. (1987) Eosinophil fluorescence: a cause of false positive slide tests for herpes simplex virus. **Pediatr Dermatol** 4:129–133.
521. Solomon AR, Rasmussen JE (1983) Correlation of Tzanck preparation and viral cultures in cutaneous herpes simplex. **Clin Res** 31:922.
522. Nahass GT, Goldstein BA, Zhu WY et al. (1992) Comparison of Tzanck smear, viral culture, and DNA diagnostic methods in detection of herpes simplex and varicella-zoster infection. **JAMA** 268:2541.
523. Kimura H, Futamura M, Kito H et al. (1991) Detection of viral DNA in neonatal herpes simplex virus infections: frequent and prolonged presence in serum and cerebrospinal fluid. **J Infect Dis** 164:289.

524. Storer JS, Galen WK, Nesbitt LT (1982) Neonatal pemphigus vulgaris. **J Am Acad Dermatol** 6:929.
525. Englund JA, Fletcher CV, Balfour HH (1991) Acyclovir therapy in neonates. **J Pediatr** 119:129–135.
526. Whitley R, Arvin A, Prober C et al. (1991) A controlled trial comparing vidarabine with acyclovir in neonatal herpes simplex virus infection. **N Engl J Med** 324:444.
527. Kimberlin DW, Jacobs RF, Powell DA et al. (2001) The safety and efficacy of high dose acyclovir in neonatal herpes simplex virus. **Pediatrics** 108:230–238.
528. Dufour P, de Bievre P, Vinatier D et al. (1996) Varicella and pregnancy. **Eur J Obstet Gynecol Reprod Biol** Jun; 66(2):119–123.
529. McIntosh D (1993) Varicella-zoster virus infection in pregnancy. **Arch Dis Child** 68:1–2.
530. Brunell PA (1992) Varicella in pregnancy, the fetus, and the newborn: problems in management. **J Infect Dis**, suppl 1, 166:S42.

preceding delivery has been estimated at 25–60%.[531,532] Varicella infections after 10 days of age are considered acquired as a result of a postnatal exposure.

Fetal varicella syndrome

Fetal varicella syndrome, also known as congenital varicella syndrome or varicella embryopathy, was described by La Foret and Lynch.[533] Affected infants have an unusual pattern of congenital defects that includes skin lesions, neurologic abnormalities (encephalitis, hydrocephalus, seizures, mental retardation, microcephaly, nerve palsies), eye anomalies (chorioretinitis, microphthalmia, nystagmus, cataracts), musculoskeletal anomalies (hypoplastic extremities; abnormalities of scapula, ribs or mandible), gastrointestinal anomalies (duodenal stenosis, colonic atresia), and genitourinary anomalies (hydronephrosis, absence of kidney). Skin lesions are cicatrical areas that correspond to a dermatome, often accompanied by hypoplasia of an ipselateral extremity (Fig. 6.49).[534–536] Sometimes the affected areas are denuded at birth with scarring occurring subsequently. The segmental nature of the anomalies is thought to be a manifestation of the neurotropism of the varicella virus, and it has been proposed that it may result from reactivation of primary varicella in the developing fetus at a time when the immune system is not sufficiently developed to modify the severity of infection.

Retrospective studies estimate an incidence of up to 9% of fetal varicella syndrome after maternal infection, with a 2.2% first trimester attack rate.[534,537,538] The risk period for fetal varicella syndrome is generally in the first 20 weeks of gestation, with the highest risk between 13 and 20 weeks gestation (2%).[539] A lower rate before 13 weeks gestation (0.4%) may reflect underreporting or a higher rate of spontaneous abortion. Reports of congenital varicella syndrome in infants exposed as late as 25 weeks gestation have appeared.[540] Maternal zoster does not carry the same risks as maternal primary varicella. No cases of congenital varicella were observed in 366 women with zoster during pregnancy studied prospectively, and there was no serological evidence of transplacental transmission.[539] Approximately 18 cases of congenital anomalies occurring in association with maternal herpes zoster infection have been reported, though it is uncertain if these resulted from maternal zoster.[534] One case of maternal herpes zoster at 12 weeks gestation was associated fetal skin lesions lesions and limb hypoplasia.[541]

The differential diagnosis of congenital denuded or scarred areas includes aplasia cutis congenita and epidermolysis bullosa (including the Bart syndrome presentation of EB simplex). Other congenital viral infections should be considered in any infant presenting with microcephaly, ophthalmologic or neurologic abnormalities. Prenatal diagnosis of fetal varicella syndrome using viral or immunologic methods may not be reliable.[542] IgM may be undetectable, even in infants with classic clinical findings. Cordocentesis, amniocentesis or chorionic villus sampling may aid prenatal diagnosis, with viral culture from amniotic fluid or blood and DNA detection of blood or placental tissue.[542–544] Transplancental viral transfer, however, can occur without fetal involvement. Ultrasonography at 20–22 weeks may be useful to observe for microcephaly, limb hypoplasia, fetal hydrops, polyhydramnios, and liver abnormalities.[545]

Neonatal varicella

Transmission of the virus to the fetus shortly before birth may cause severe systemic illness without congenital defects. Neonatal varicella may result if a mother develops chickenpox prior to or immediately following delivery. Neonates in whom chickenpox develops within 10 days of birth are considered to have acquired the infection transplacentally, since the incubation period of chickenpox is 10 to 21 days. If the mother develops varicella five days before to two days after delivery, or the infant develops disease between five and 10 days of life then the child is at high risk for severe disease. The disease is less severe if the onset of the infant's rash occurs before five days of age or if the mother's rash developed five or more days before delivery, allowing adequate time for maternal antibody to form and to be transmitted to the fetus.

Neonatal varicella may present with widespread skin disease, respiratory distress, hepatitis, or encephalitis. Overall mortality is estimated at 5–30%, though the latter figure is probably overstated.[531–532]

The usual time of onset of rash is nine to 15 days after onset of maternal rash but administration of VZIG may prolong the incubation period to 28 days.[546] Vesicles develop in any location and may be few in number, occur in crops, or coalesce (Fig. 6.50). Hemorrhagic vesicles can be seen in severe cases. In most cases, healing is complete in 10 days, but in severe cases several weeks may be required. Lesions may involve the lungs, liver, brain, kidneys, adrenals, and the myocardium.

Diagnosis may be made by Tzanck smears of vesicles, direct fluorescent antibody testing, viral culture, and PCR detection. Fluorescent antibody tests are occasionally false positive in incontinentia pigmenti and Langerhans cell histiocytosis.[547]

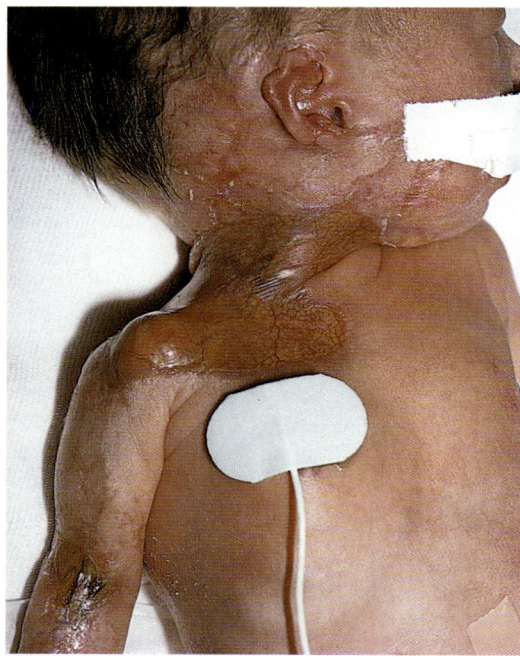

Fig. 6.49 Fetal varicella syndrome. Segmental deep scars, dermatomal distribution.

531. Whitley RJ (1990) Epidemiology. In: Infectious Diseases of the Fetus and Newborn Infant, Remington JS, Klein JO, eds. Philadelphia: WB Saunders, p. 285.
532. Miller E, Cradock-Watson JE, Ridenhalgh MK (1989) Outcome in newborn babies given anti-varicella-zoster immunoglobulin after perinatal maternal infection with varicella-zoster virus. **Lancet** 2:371.
533. La Foret E, Lynch FL (1947) Multiple congenital defects following maternal varicella. **N Engl J Med** 236:534.
534. Paryani SG, Arvin AM (1986) Intrauterine infection with varicella-zoster virus after maternal varicella. **N Engl J Med** 314:1542.
535. Alkalay AL, Pomerance JJ, Rimoin D (1987) Fetal varicella syndrome. **J Pediatr** 111:320.
536. Kellner B, Kitai I, Krafchik B (1996) What syndrome is this? Congenital varicella syndrome. **Pediatr Dermatol** 13:341–344.
537. Enders G (1984) Varicella-zoster virus infection in pregnancy. **Prog Med Virol** 29:166–196.
538. Patstuszak AL LM, Schick B et al. (1994) Outcome after maternal varicella infection in the first 20 weeks of pregnancy. **N Engl J Med** 330:901–905.
539. Enders G ME, Craddock-Watson J et al. (1994) Consequences of varicella and Herpes zoster in pregnancy: Prospective study of 1739 cases. **Lancet** 343:1547–1550.
540. Salzman MB, Sood SK (1992) Congenital anomalies resulting from maternal varicella at 25 1/2 weeks of gestation. **Pediatr Infect Dis J** 11:504.
541. Enders G (1984) Varicella-zoster virus infection in pregnancy. **Prog Med Virol** 29:166–196.
542. Chapman SJ (1998) Varicella in pregnancy. **Semin Perinatol** 22:339–346.
543. Hartung J, Enders G, Chaoui R et al. (1999) Prenatal diagnosis of congenital varicella syndrome and detection of varicella-zoster virus in the fetus: a case report. **Prenat Diagn** Feb;19(2):163–166.
544. Mouly F, Mirlesse V, Meritet JF et al. (1997) Prenatal diagnosis of fetal varicella-zoster virus infection with polymerase chain reaction of amniotic fluid in 107 cases. **Am J Obstet Gynecol** 177:894–898.
545. Pretorius DH, Hayward I, Jones KL et al. (1992) Sonographic evaluation of pregnancies with maternal varicella infection. **J Ultrasound Med** 11(9):459–463.
546. Prober CG, Gershon AA, Grose C et al. (1990) Consensus: varicella-zoster infections in pregnancy and the perinatal period. **Pediatr Infect Dis J** 9:865–869.
547. Frieden IJ, Berger TG, Westrom D (1987) Eosinophil fluorescence: A cause of false positive slide tests for herpes simplex virus. **Pediatr Dermatol** 4:129–133.

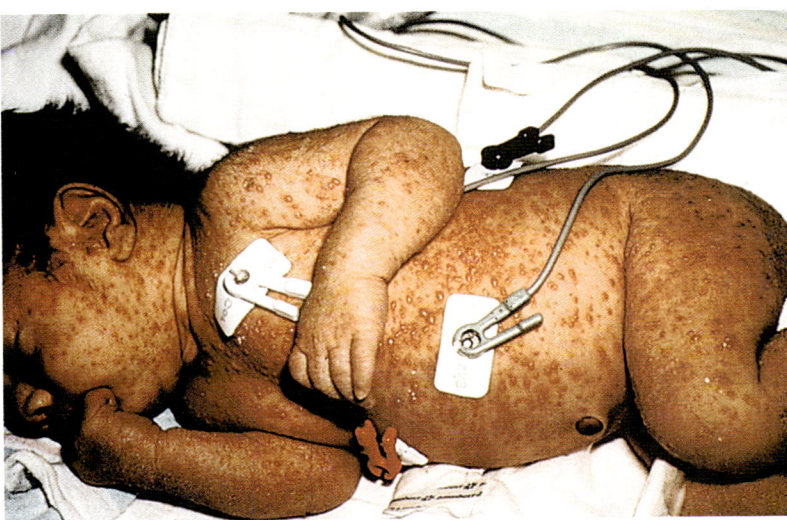

Fig. 6.50   Neonatal varicella: generalized crusted papules and vesicles. (Courtesy Gerald Goldberg, MD).

Neonates born to mothers who have developed varicella from five days before to two days after delivery should receive VZIG at a dose of 125 units.[546] Even with VZIG, approximately 50% of at-risk infants will develop varicella though the disease is generally milder.[532] Mothers should avoid direct lesional contact with the infant. Breast-feeding is permitted if lesional contact can be avoided. Intravenous acyclovir 20mg/kg every eight hours for a minimum of five days and aggressive supportive therapy are indicated for neonatal varicella.

NEONATAL CONGENITAL SYPHILIS

Congenital syphilis (CS) is a rare infection occuring in infants born to mothers infected with the spirochete *Treponema pallidum*. The clinical manifestations of congenital syphilis are multisystemic, though they are often absent at birth. Congenital syphilis is divided into early and late disease. Early disease usually presents before 3 months of age, although signs can appear any time in the first two years of life. Late disease appears after age 2 years. Episodic epidemics of congenital syphilis are observed, reflecting varying community prevalences of syphilis and influenced by poor prenatal care.[548]

T. pallidum infects the fetus through placental invasion at any time during pregnancy, with bloodborne spread to multiple organs. Spirochetes induce vasculitis through endothelial cell adherence.[549] There is a high incidence of *in utero* death, and prematurity.[550] Neonates infected during the third trimester are usually normal at birth, becoming ill during the first weeks of life, particularly weeks 2 to 6.

The most common clinical manifestations of symptomatic infants are mucocutaneous lesions (40–50%), prematurity (39%), growth failure (38%), hepatosplenomegaly (40–70%), bony involvement (78%), and jaundice (15%), although lymphadenopathy, severe pneumonia, nephritis, enteritis, pancreatitis, and hematologic abnormalities may be present in severely ill infants.[551,552]

Approximately 50–60% of infants with congenital syphilis are asymptomatic at birth, with cutaneous findings in 38%.[553] Maculopapular or papulosquamous lesions are the most common lesions found on the skin of the neonate. These lesions are similar to those seen in the adult with secondary syphilis and are most pronounced on the face, posterior trunk, palms, soles, and diaper area. Lesions may be annular in configuration. The rash gradually appears over one week and may remain for several months if left untreated, changing from

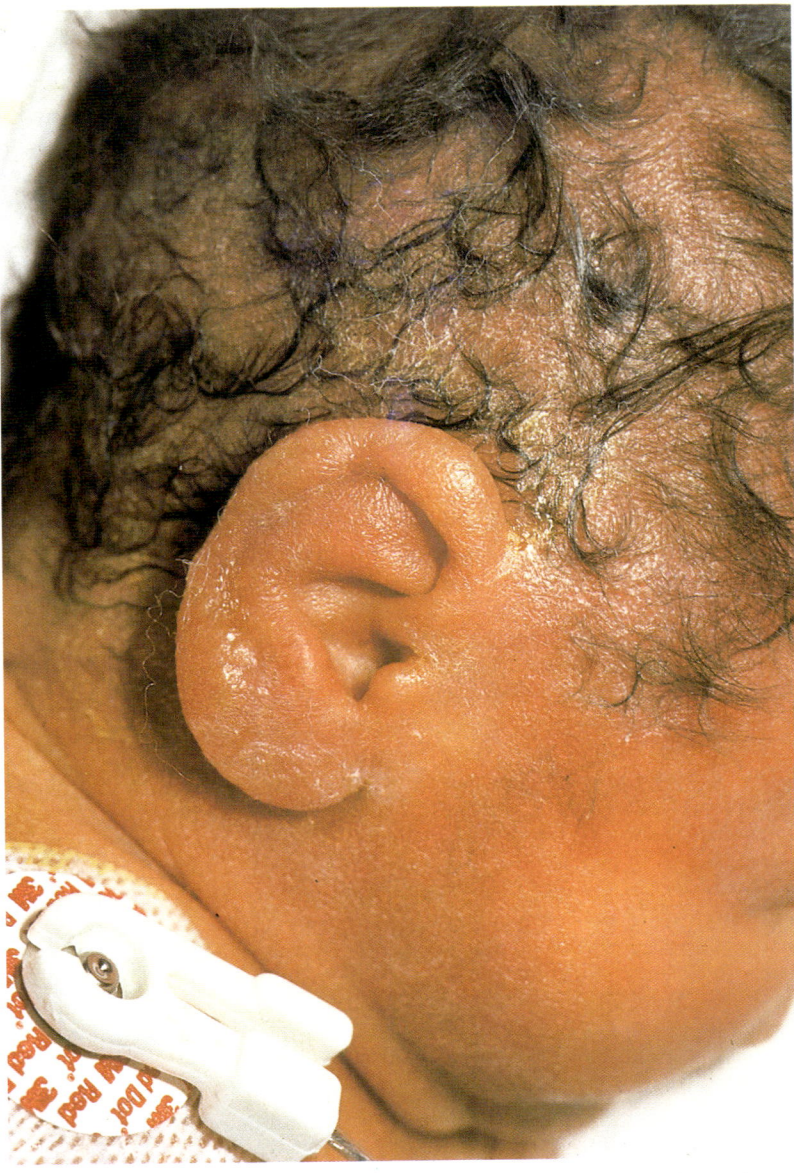

Fig. 6.51   Congenital syphilis with desquamative dermatitis, ear vesicles, and moth-eaten alopecia.

pink or red to copper-brown, ultimately leaving pigmentary changes in some cases.

Infants can also present with a desquamative dermatitis.[554] Other less common skin findings in neonatal congenital syphilis include vesicles (Fig. 6.51), bullae (pemphigus syphiliticus), pustules, erosions, ulcerations, and thrombocytopenia-induced petechiae. Hemorrhagic vesicobullous lesions, when present on the palms and soles, are considered diagnostic of congenital syphilis. More commonly, the palms and soles demonstrate oval ham-colored macules and papules that acquire a coppery-brown color as they age or are swollen and erythematous, causing fissuring. Pemphigus syphiliticus is unique to the newborn. Bullae form on an indurated, red base, and rupture easily to leave a macerated area that may form a crust. Nail deformities, paronychia, and alopecia may occur.

548. Congenital syphilis New York City. 1986–1988. **MMWR Morb Mortal Wkly Rep** 1989; 38:825.
549. Darmstadt GL, Dinulos JG (2001) Bacterial infections. In: Textbook of Neonatal Dermatology, Eichenfield LF, Frieden IJ, Esterly NB, eds. Philadelphia, PA: WB Saunders, pp. 103–116.
550. Guidelines for the prevention and control of congenital syphilis. **MMWR Morb Mortal Wkly Rep** 1988; 37 Suppl 1:1.
551. Mascola L, Pelosi R, Blount JH et al. (1985) Congenital syphilis revisited. **Am J Dis Child** 139:575.
552. Lowy G (1992) Sexually transmitted diseases in children. **Pediatr Dermatol** 9:329.
553. Chawla V, Pandit P, Nkrumah F (1988) Congenital syphilis in the newborn. **Arch Dis Child** 63:1393.
554. Wood VD, Rana S (1992) Congenital syphilis presenting as desquamative dermatitis. **J Fam Pract** 35:327.

Neonatal mucocutaneous lesions include rhinitis ("snuffles"), condylomata, mucous membrane patches, maculopapular lesions, erosions, and hemorrhagic bullae. These lesions may be present at birth but are more likely to appear between the second and sixth weeks of life. Syphilitic rhinitis is often the initial sign of CS, beginning as a clear nasal discharge often mistakenly thought to be a viral upper respiratory infection. The discharge may be profuse and occasionally hemorrhagic. It may be destructive, causing ulcers of the nasal mucosa, performation of the nasal septum, and nasal cartilage changes (saddle nose deformity).[555] Small, round, moist, raised lesions may be present on mucosal surfaces (mucous patches) including lips, tongue and palate. Flat wart-like lesions, condylomata lata, occur in moist areas of the body, particularly the anogenital area, nares, and the angles of the mouth. These lesions are highly infective and are the most characteristic of the early lesions seen in neonatal syphilis. Lesions at the angle of the mouth frequently fissure and ulcerate, producing fibrosis.

Systemic findings of congenital syphilis include low birthweight, hepatomegaly, splenomegaly, jaundice, periostitis, generalized lymphadenopathy, respiratory distress, hydrops fetalis, meningitis, meningoencepahalitis, chorioretinitis, nephrotic syndrome, anemia, and thrombocytopenia.[553]

Other extracutaneous findings manifest later, after 2 years of age. These include disorders of central nervous system (neurosyphilis, which may be asymptomatic), skeleton (frontal bossing, saddle nose, concave central face, sabre tibias, Clutton's joints), teeth (Hutchinson teeth – peg-shaped notched central incisors, mulberry molars – multicuspid), eyes (interstitial keratitis, optic atrophy), and ears (eighth nerve deafness).[556] Hutchinson's triad of incisor defects, interstitial keratitis, and sensorineural hearing loss is pathognomonic.

With the variety of presentations and lesional morphology, syphilis has been called "the great imitator." Vesiculobullous lesions of CS should be considered in the broad differential diagnosis of blistering eruptions. Other conditions with blisters on the palms and soles include congenital candidiasis, scabies, acropustulosis of infancy, and epidermolysis bullosa.

The most effective way to identify newborns at risk of congenital syphilis is through maternal serologic diagnosis during pregnancy and testing of maternal and neonatal sera at delivery.[557] Positive IgG serology in a neonate is not sufficient to make the diagnosis of congenital syphilis, as IgG will be transferred through the placenta even if the mother was adequately treated during pregnancy. Serum should be taken from the infant, rather than from cord blood, to increase the accuracy of serologic test results.[558] Passive transfer of maternal IgG antibody cannot be distinguished by comparison of titers, but most agree that a fourfold titer increase in the infant's blood is diagnostic of congenital infection and not merely reflective of passively transferred antibody. Falsely negative non-treponemal tests in both an infected mother and her congenitally infected infant may occur if the mother acquired the disease late in pregnancy or in the case of a prozone phenomenon. False positive reactivity of non-treponemal tests can be caused by infectious diseases (e.g., varicella, measles, hepatitis, infectious mononucleosis, tuberculosis, malaria, endocarditis), malignancies (e.g., lymphoma), and connective tissue disease (e.g., systemic lupus erythematosus). The IgM FTA-ABS is the best specific test that is currently widely available to identify infant infection. The

rate of false-positive (10%) and false-negative (35%) results may require the use of serial reagin tests in uncertain cases.[559] False-positive tests are seen in the presence of IgM RF and with competitive inhibition by IgG.[560] A VDRL test on cerebral spinal fluid should be performed on all neonates evaluated for CS.[551] Negative results do not exclude neurosyphilis, however, and, false-positive results can occur in an uninfected newborn with a high serum VDRL titer acquired transplacentally.

Darkfield examination or direct fluorescent microscopy for spirochetes from infant lesions are easily done by experienced technicians. Nasal discharge or scrapings from moist lesions are most likely to reveal *Treponema pallidum*. Histopathologic examination of the placenta and umbilical cord with specific fluorescent antitreponemal antibody staining also is recommended. A skin biopsy is helpful in the evaluation of CS and shows swelling and proliferation of endothelial cells, and a predominantly perivascular infiltrate composed of lymphoid cells and plasma cells. PCR, a highly sensitive test that detects *Treponema pallidum* DNA, has been used on amniotic fluid, neonatal sera, and neonatal cerebrospinal fluid (CSF) with a specificity of 100% compared to the rabbit infectivity test.[561] Radiographic findings may be helpful, seen in up to 95% of symptomatic and 20% of asymptomatic neonates.[562,563]

Treatment for infants with proven or probable CS is a 10 to 14 day course of parenteral aqueous crystalline penicillin G.[564] A fourfold decrease in non-treponemal test titers is indicative of successful treatment, and these tests usually become nonreactive within two years. Follow-up examinations at 1, 2, 4, 6, and 12 months of age are recommended, with nontreponemal tests at 3, 6, and 12 months after treatment or until they become nonreactive. Empiric treatment is recommended if an infant cannot be fully evaluated, or if adequate follow-up is uncertain. Transplacentally acquired maternal antibody in an uninfected infant should decline in titer by 3 months of age and be nonreactive at age 6 months. CSF examinations at six-month intervals are recommended for treated infants until the examination becomes nonreactive. Positive MHA-TP and FTA-ABS treponemal tests usually remain reactive for life despite successful treatment (see also Chapter 28).

NEONATAL HIV DISEASE

The acquired immunodeficiency syndrome (AIDS) is caused by infection with human immunodeficiency virus-1 (HIV-1). Perinatal transmission from infected mothers is the most common cause of childhood infection.[565] There is a variable latency period, and a high mortality rate. While most infants are asymptomatic in the first few months of life, severe disease can be seen and cutaneous abnormalities may be early findings.

Skin and mucous membrane disease is very common in infants with symptomatic HIV infection.[566–568] Frequently the first indication that an infant is infected is the development of a severe or recurrent bacterial or fungal infection. In other instances, widespread and protracted seborrheic dermatitis may be the first clue to the patient's underlying immunodeficiency. Cutaneous infections that are extensive, progressive, or difficult to treat should raise suspicion of HIV infection.[569,570] The type of cutaneous involvement that occurs with the disease is generally related to the degree of immunosuppression.

555. Hurwitz S (1993) Cutaneous disorders of the newborn. In: Clinical Pediatric Dermatology. Philadelphia: WB Saunders, p. 6.
556. Darmstadt G, Harris J (1989) Luetic hearing loss: clinical presentation, diagnosis, and treatment. **Am J Otolaryngol** 10:410.
557. Chabra RS, Brion LP, Castro M et al. (1993) Comparison of maternal sera, cord blood, and neonatal sera for detecting presumptive congenital syphilis: relationship with maternal treatment. **Pediatrics** 91:88.
558. Rawstron S, Bromberg K (1991) Comparison of maternal and newborn serologic tests for syphilis. **Am J Dis Child** 145:1383.
559. Bromberg K, Rawstron S, Tannis G (1993) Diagnosis of congenital syphilis by combining Treponema pallidum-specific IgM detection with immunofluorescent antigen detection for T. Pallidum. **J Infect Dis** 168:238.
560. Stoll B, Lee F, Larsen S et al. (1993) Clinical and serologic evaluation of neonates for congenital syphilis: a continuing diagnostic dilemma. **J Infect Dis** 167:1093.
561. Grimprel E, Sanchez PJ, Wendel GD et al. (1991) Use of polymerase chain reaction and rabbit infectivity testing to detect Treponema pallidum in amniotic fluid, fetal and neonatal sera, and cerebrospinal fluid. **J Clin Microbiol** 29:1711.
562. Brion LP, Manuli M, Rai B et al. (1991) Long bone radiographic abnormalities as a sign of congenital syphilis in asymptomatic newborns. **Pediatr** 88:1037.
563. Greenberg SB, Bernal DV (1992) Are long bone radiographs necessary in neonates suspected of having congenital syphilis? **Radiology** 182:637.
564. American Academy of Pediatrics (2000) Syphilis. In: 2000 Red Book: Report of the Committee on American Academy of Pediatrics, 25th edition, Pickering LK, ed. Elk Grove Village, IL: American Academy of Pediatrics, pp. 547–559.
565. Friedlander SF, Bradley JS. (2001) Viral infections. In: Textbook of Neonatal Dermatology, Eichenfield LF, Frieden IJ, Esterly NB, eds. Philadelphia, PA: WB Saunders, pp. 201–222.
566. Pahwa S, Kaplan M, Fikrig S et al. (1986) Spectrum of human T-cell lymphotropic virus type III infection in children. Recognition of symptomatic, asymptomatic, and seronegative patients. **JAMA** 255:2299–2305.
567. Prose NS (1991) Mucocutaneous disease in pediatric human immunodeficiency virus infections. **Pediatr Clin North Am** 38:977.
568. Straka BF, Whitaker DL, Morrison SH et al. (1988) Cutaneous manifestations of the acquired immunodeficiency syndrome in children. **J Am Acad Dermatol** 18:1089–1102.
569. Nair P, Alger L, Lines S (1993) Maternal and neonatal characteristics associated with HIV infection in infants of seropositive women. **J Acquir Immun Defic Syndr** 6:298.
570. Aiken CG (1992) HIV-1 infection and perinatal mortality in Zimbabwe. **Arch Dis Child** 67:595.

Cutaneous findings of HIV in neonates include bacterial infections (impetigo, folliculitis, cellulitis, abcesses), viral infections (atypical varicella and herpes simplex, frequent and/or severe molluscum or papillomavirus infection), fungal and yeast infections (thrush, tinea, opportunistic infections),[571] scabies (including crusted scabies), neoplastic diseases (Kaposi's sarcoma),[572,573] and inflammatory diseases (seborrheic dermatitis, drug eruptions).

Reports of a craniofacial syndrome have appeared, but have not been substantiated.[574–576] Prospective studies have noted a statistically increased incidence in low birthweight and intrauterine growth retardation in these infants.[569,577]

Serologic evidence of neonatal infection is problematic, as infants born to HIV-positive mothers will be seropositive for months due to transplacentally acquired antibodies.[578] Positive viral cultures are seen in 25–50% of infected children. PCR is very sensitive and widely available for HIV detection.[579] If initial tests are negative in the first two days, repeat tests are recommended at 1–2 and at 4–6 months.

Cesarean section may reduce the risk of transmission of HIV to the infant, presumably because of a lesser exposure to maternal secretions and blood.[580]

Antiviral therapy for HIV-infected pregnant women and infected children, with agents such as zidovudine, continues to evolve, and can greatly decrease infection rates and clinical disease symptoms.[581–583]

PRENATAL INJURY, BIRTH TRAUMA AND INJURY IN THE NEONATAL PERIOD

The transition from intrauterine life to extrauterine life, whether passage through the birth canal or by cesarean section, is one of unavoidable trauma to the newborn infant. Fortunately, most of this trauma results in no lasting sequelae, though the extent of this trauma is often dramatically reflected in neonatal skin.

PRENATAL INJURY
Chorionic villus sampling
Scarring as well as limb and jaw malformations have been reported following chorionic villus sampling.[584–586]

Fetal skin biopsy
Scarring can also result from damage from fetal skin biopsies.

Fig. 6.52   Amniocentesis scar, dimple-like.

Amniocentesis
Especially when performed before 11 weeks gestation, amniocentesis has been associated with severe malformations resulting from intra-amniotic bleeding.[587] The organizing blood clots on the surface of the skin influence the growth of underlying tissues. Unusual facial clefts, microphthalmia and micrognathia have resulted. *In utero* perforation of the globe has resulted in unilateral microphthalmia,[588] congenital iris cysts,[589] or uniocular blindness.[590] Needle puncture sites on the skin produce single or multiple, depressed, 1–5mm dimplelike scars (Fig. 6.52) that may be mistaken for focal dermal hypoplasia, aplasia cutis and congenital sinus tracts.[591–595] Amniocentesis scars are more common when the procedure has been performed in the first and third trimesters; mid-trimester amniocentesis has the lowest risk, as the fetus occupies a lower percentage of the amniotic cavity.

Fetal heart monitoring
Fetal heart monitoring is frequently used during uterine contractions in labor to monitor fetuses at risk of hypoxia. This can be performed by an ultrasonic transducer placed on the maternal abdominal wall or by a spiral electrode attached to the presenting vertex of the fetus; the latter one may lead to a scalp lesion. Although it is a nontraumatic procedure, if the electrode is abruptly detached, a mild laceration, ulcer or abscess may result and scarring may follow.[596,597] Lesions can vary in number, from single to multiple. Multiple lesions are observed when electrodes accidentaly separate because of the mother's movements and are subsequently reapplied.[598] Scalp abscesses are mostly noticed on the first or fourth day of life, but sometimes can be evident about the third week. In neonatal herpes simplex infection lesions are more prominent in areas of injury from scalp electrodes.[599,600]

571. Shetty D, Giri N, Gonzalez CE et al. (1997) Invasive aspergillosis in human immunodeficiency virus-infected children. **Pediatr Infect Dis J** 16(2):216–221.
572. Guiterrez-Ortega P, Hierro-Orozoco S, Sanchez-Cisneros R et al. (1989) Kaposi's sarcoma in a 6-day-old infant with human immunodeficiency virus. **Arch Dermatol** 125:432.
573. Athale UH, Patil PS, Chintu C et al. (1995) Influence of HIV epidemic on the incidence of Kaposi's sarcoma in Zambian children. **J Acquir Immune Defic Syndr Hum Retrovirol** 8:96–100.
574. Marion RW, Wiznia AA, Hutcheon RG et al. (1987) Fetal AIDS syndrome score. Correlation between severity of dysmorphism and age at diagnosis of immunodeficiency. **Am J Dis Child** 141(4):429–431.
575. Quazi QH, Sheikh TM, Fikrig S et al. (1988) Lack of evidence for craniofacial dysmorphism in perinatal human immunodeficiency virus infection. **J Pediatr** 112:7.
576. Semprini AE, Ravizza M, Bucceri A et al. (1990) Perinatal outcome in HIV-infected pregnant women. **Gynecol Obstet Invest** 30:15.
577. Hand LL, Wiznia A, Checola RT et al. (1992) Human immunodeficiency virus seropositivity in critically ill neonates in the South Bronx. **Pediatr Infect Dis J** 11:39.
578. Andiman WA, Simpson BJ, Olson B et al. (1990) Rate of transmission of human immunodeficiency virus type 1 infection from mother to child and short-term outcome of neonatal infection. Results of a prospective cohort study. **Am J Dis Child** 144:758.
579. Pappaioanou M, Kashamuka M, Behets F et al. (1993) Accurate detection of maternal antibodies to HIV in newborn whole blood dried on filter paper. **AIDS** 7:483.
580. Gelber RD, Shapiro DE (1999) Mode of delivery and the risk of vertical transmission of HIV-1. **N Engl J Med** 15;341(3):206–207
581. Culnane M, Fowler M, Lee SS et al. (1999) Lack of long-term effects of in utero exposure to zidovudine among uninfected children born to HIV-infected women. Pediatric AIDS Clinical Trials Group Protocol 219/076 Teams. **JAMA** 13;281(2):151–157.
582. Pizzo PA, Eddy J, Falloon J et al. (1988) Effect of continuous intravenous injection of zidovudine (AZT) in children with symptomatic HIV infection. **N Engl J Med** 319:889.
583. Levin BW, Driscoll JM Jr, Fleischman AR (1991) Treatment choice for infants in the neonatal intensive care unit at risk for AIDS. **JAMA** 265:2976.
584. Froster UG (1996) Limb defects and chorionic villus sampling: results from an international registry, 1992–94. **Lancet** 347:489–494.
585. Firth H, Boyd PA, Chamberlain P et al. (1996) Limb defects and chorionic villus sampling. **Lancet** 347:1406.
586. Mastroiacovo P, Botto LD (1996) Limb defects and chorionic villus sampling. **Lancet** 347:1406–1407.
587. Jauniaux E, Rodeck C (1995) Use, risks and complications of amniocentesis and chorionic villus sampling for prenatal diagnosis in early pregnancy. **Early Pregnancy: Biology and Medicine** 1:245–252.
588. BenEzra D, Sela M, Peer J (1989) Bilateral anophthalmia and unilateral microphthalmia in two siblings. **Ophthalmologica** 198:140.
589. Rummelt V, Rummelt C, Naumann GO (1993) Congenital nonpigmented epithelial iris cyst after amniocentesis. Clinicopathologic report on two children. **Ophthalmology** 100:776.
590. Merin S, Beyth Y (1980) Uniocular congenital blindness as a complication of midtrimester amniocentesis. **Am J Ophthalmol** 89:299.
591. Karp LE, Hayden PW (1977) Fetal puncture during midtrimester amniocentesis. **Obstet Gynecol** 49:115–117.
592. Epley SL, Hanson JW, Cruikshank DP (1979) Fetal injury with mid-trimester diagnostic amniocentesis. **Obstet Gynecol** 53:77–80.
593. Cambiaghi S, Restano L, Cavalli R et al. (1998) Skin dimpling as a consequence of amniocentesis. **J Am Acad Dermatol** 39:888–890.
594. Bruce S, Duffy JO, Wolf Jr JE (1984) Skin dimpling associated with mid-trimester amniocentesis. **Pediatr Dermatol** 2:140–142.
595. Raimer SS, Raimer BG (1984) Needle puncture scars from midtrimester amniocentesis. **Arch Dermatol** 120:1360–1362.
596. Wagener M, Rycheck R, Yee R et al. (1984) Septic dermatitis of the neonatal scalp and maternal endomyometritis with intrapartum internal fetal monitoring. **Pediatr** 74(1):81–85.
597. Ashkenazi S, Metzker A, Merlob P et al. (1985) Scalp changes after fetal monitoring. **Arch Dis Child** 60(3):267–269.
598. Metzker A, Brenner S, Merlob P (1999) Iatrogenic cutaneous injuries in the neonate. **Arch Dermatol** 135:697–702.
599. Esterly N (2001) Iatrogenic and traumatic injuries. In: Textbook of Neonatal Dermatology, Eichenfield LF, Frieden IJ, Esterly NB, eds. Philadelphia, PA: WB Saunders, pp. 103–116.
600. Guill M, Aton J, Rogers R (1982) Neonatal herpes simplex associated with fetal scalp monitoring. **J Am Acad Dermatol** 7(3):408–409.

Fetal scalp blood sampling

This is a procedure performed by puncture to establish acid–base status and may cause lacerations and subsequent scarring.

INJURIES DURING DELIVERY

Erythema

Although newborn skin is normally plethoric, marked erythema commonly occurs at sites of pressure during delivery, such as the face and scalp. Shoulders and buttocks may also appear erythematous, as these areas comprise the widest diameters that must pass through the birth canal. Erythema usually resolves spontaneously within the first day of life. Rarely, it persists for two or three days.

Skin and soft tissue injury

Skin and soft tissue trauma at birth are more common in the setting of a prolonged labor because of cephalopelvic disproportion, and when intervention with instruments is necessary. Ecchymoses can occur in areas traumatized by application of forceps or vacuum extractors in assisted deliveries.[601] Forceps-aided deliveries may produce erythema or hematomas, ecchymosis and deep erosions, especially on temples and cheeks (Fig. 6.53). When vacuum extractors are applied, mild ecchymoses, severe purpura, hematomas, or edema (chignon or artificial captum succedaneum)[599] a rare but important complication. Alopecia is also a rare but important complication. Subaponeurotic haemorrhage may also occur in association with vacuum or forceps delivery. This bleeding is present at birth and is not confined to a single cranial bone, but spreads quickly over the head. It usually disappears spontaneously after 7–10 days. The application of pads to standard forceps and the use of pliable-cup vacuum extractors have diminished the frequency and severity of these skin findings.[602,603]

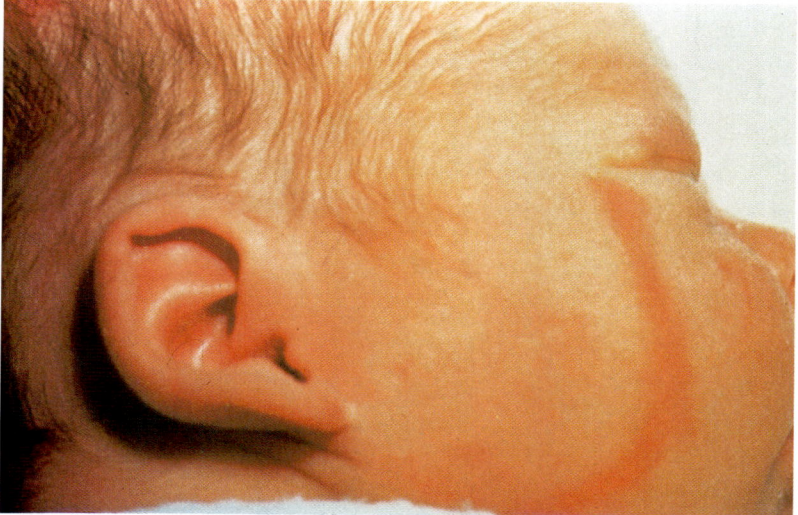

Fig. 6.53   Forceps injury (ecchymosis).

Difficult deliveries in vertex presentation or extended arms in breech deliveries may lead to clavicular fracture. Skin over the osseous defect may be edematous with a hematoma making it impossible to feel the margins of the affected clavicle.

Interestingly, even premature infants, despite their smaller size and birth weight, are occasionally born with ecchymoses for no discernible reason. This may relate to the increased skin fragility that is known to occur in these neonates.

Caput succedaneum and edema

During normal or difficult deliveries, a diffuse edematous swelling without sharp borders of the presenting part, known as captum succedaneum, may develop. Mostly observed in scalp, it appears at birth or within hours after delivery and is due to pressure of the uterus, cervix, and the vaginal wall on the infant. It can be ecchymotic but is rarely associated with any significant blood loss. Caput is frequently accompanied by molding of the scalp that becomes more apparent when the edema disappears over the first few days of life. More severe caput occurs with prolongation of the second stage of labor and with the use of vacuum extractors. Severe caput has rarely been associated with scalp necrosis[604] and scarring (Fig. 6.54). Annular alopecia, usually located over the vertex, is known as halo scalp ring and can follow a caput succedaneum.[605–607]

This swelling can be distinguished from a cephalhematoma (see below) as it extends across suture lines and across the midline. Skin findings resolve within several days, and treatment is not necessary except in rare instances when severe hemorrhage requires blood transfusions.

Cephalhematoma

Cephalhematoma is a subperiosteal hemorrhage that presents with an impressive swelling overlying the neonatal scalp. Cephalhematoma is usually unilateral, as the hemorrhage is confined by the periosteal margin of the bone. If bilateral, the affected areas are separated by a midline depression corresponding to the intervening suture line. Ecchymosis and epidermal discoloration is not seen with these lesions, which develop after several hours to days postdelivery. Subperiosteal bleeding is a slow process, so several hours or days are needed for it to become apparent. Cephalhematomas are caused by the rupture of the diploic veins of the skull and are associated with prolonged or difficult labor and delivery, especially vaginal deliveries using vaccum extractors.[599,608–611] Occasionally cephalhematomas overlie a linear skull fracture. An underlying fracture is more likely when the swelling is massive; ordinary cephalhematomas do not require routine radiographs.

Rarely, cephalhematomas are complicated by secondary bacterial infection and cellulitis. Most commonly, the fluctuant cystic nature of the lesion is mistaken for an underlying bacterial abscess. Culture of aspirated material will confirm the benign nature of this swelling but is rarely needed. Distinction from an encephalocele or meningocele is important.[612] These are often associated with pulsation, increased pressure with crying, and radiographic evidence of an underlying bony defect.

No treatment for cephalhematomas is necessary unless substantial blood resorption results in hyperbilirubinemia.[613] Resorption occurs over weeks to months and is often accompanied by calcification of the organized rim that

601. Broekhuezen FF, Washington JM, Johnson F et al. (1987) Vacuum extraction versus forceps delivery: indications and complications, 1979 to 1984. **Obstet Gynecol** 69:338.
602. Kuit JA, Eppinga HG, Wallenburg HC et al. (1993) A randomized comparison of vacuum extraction delivery with a rigid and a pliable cup. **Obstet Gynecol** 82:280.
603. Hebertson RM, Sanders MS, Warenski JC et al. (1985) Obstetric forceps pad designed to reduce infant trauma. **Obstet Gynecol** 65:275.
604. Morykwas MJ, Beason ES, Argenta LC (1991) Scalp necrosis in a neonate treated with cultured autologous keratinocytes. **Plast Reconstr Surg** 87:549.
605. Beutner KR (1985) Halo ring scarring alopecia. **Pediatr Dermatol** 3:83.
606. Neal PR, Merk PF, Norins AL (1984) Halo scalp ring: A form of localized scalp injury associated with caput succedaneum. **Pediatr Dermatol** 2:52–54.
607. Prendiville JS, Esterly NB (1987) Halo scalp ring: A cause of scarring alopecia. **Arch Dermatol** 123:992–993.

608. Bofill JA, Rust OA, Davidas M et al. (1997) Neonatal cephalohematoma from vacuum extraction. **J Reprod Med** 42:565–569.
609. Kendall N, Woolshin H (1952) Cephalhematoma associated with fracture of the skull. **J Pediatr** 41:125–127.
610. Zelson C, Lee SJ, Pearl M (1974) The incidence of skull fractures underlying cephalhematomas in newborn infants. **J Pediatr** 85:371–373.
611. Benjamin B, Khan MR (1993) Pattern of external birth trauma in south-western Saudi Arabia. **J Trauma** 35:737.
612. Winter TC, Mack LA, Cyr DR (1993) Prenatal sonographic diagnosis of scalp edema/cephalohematoma mimicking an encephalocele. **Am J Roentgenol** 161:1247–1248.
613. Tan KL, Lim GC (1995) Phototherapy for neonatal jaundice in infants with cephalhematomas. **Clin Pediatr** 34:7–11.

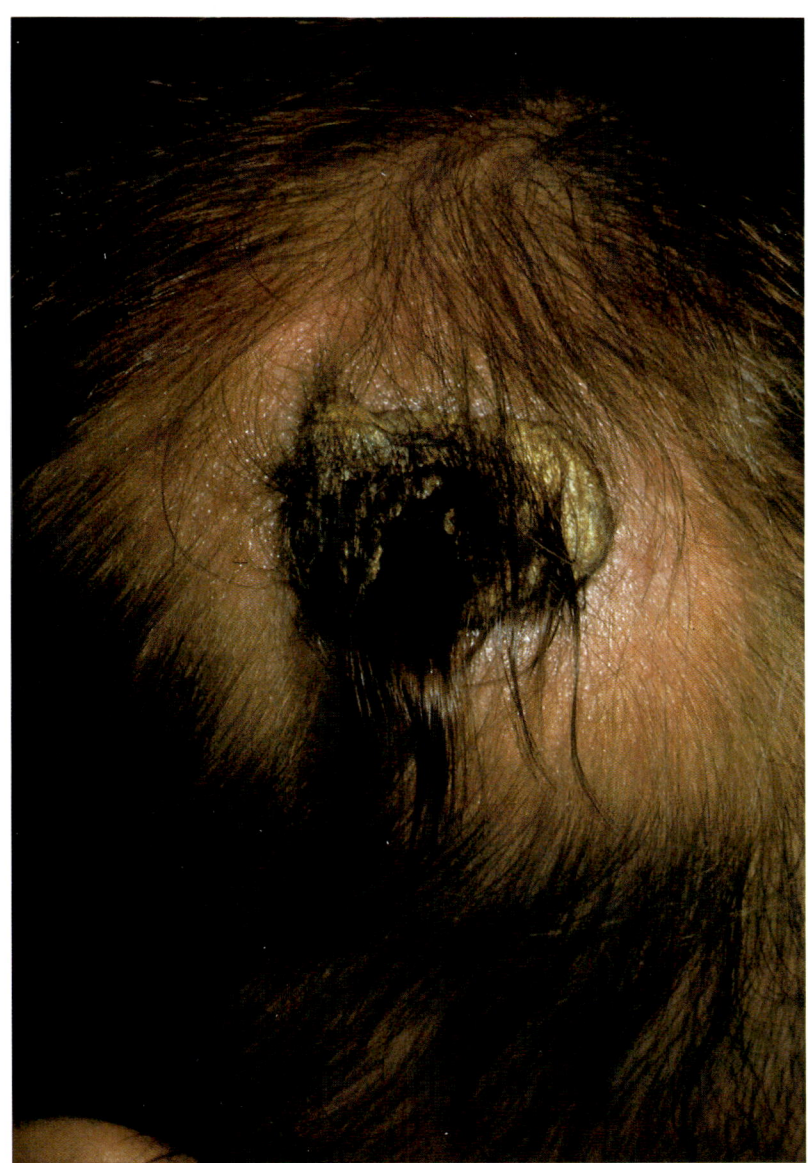

Fig. 6.54 Scalp necrosis, post-vacuum extraction (resulted in scarring alopecia).

is easily palpable. Residual calcification of cyst-like defects that are visible on skull radiograph can persist for years.

Petechiae and subconjunctival hemorrhage

Subconjunctival hemorrhages and petechiae, especially of the scalp, face, and upper trunk, can be seen following prolonged labor or breech delivery. Cutaneous compression combined with the increased intrathoracic and venous pressures of delivery, causes leakage of red blood cells from superficial blood vessels into the skin.

The differential diagnosis of traumatic petechiae in the newborn includes hematologic disorders and infection. Petechiae or purpura accompanying disseminated intravascular coagulation (DIC) or coagulation abnormalities, such

as protein C deficiency, hemophilia, or vitamin K, tend to be localized and asymmetric and accompanied by diffuse mucous membrane bleeding. Platelet abnormalities, such as those seen in idiopathic thrombocytopenic purpura (ITP), neonatal lupus erythematosus, or Wiskott–Aldrich syndrome, can also present with petechiae during the first few days of life. In addition, thrombocytopenia or platelet dysfunction, secondary to maternal ITP or maternal medications, may occasionally cause widespread petechiae. Infections associated with petechiae and purpura include congenital infection with toxoplasmosis, syphilis, rubella, herpes simplex virus (HSV), or cytomegalovirus. Appearance of these lesions, especially in a preterm or small-for-gestational-age (SGA) infant, should warrant examination for other signs of congenital infection.

Treatment of traumatic petechiae and purpura is rarely necessary unless sufficient hemorrhage has occurred to elevate bilirubin levels, requiring phototherapy.

Intrapartum lacerations

Occasionally, lacerations from scalpel blades are seen following cesarean section delivery. These are more common in deliveries in which amniotic fluid is minimal, since this fluid provides a natural cushion to help prevent such injury to the underlying fetus. In vaginal deliveries, when amniotomy or episiotomy takes place, deep penetration of the scissors may lacerate the presenting part of the neonate. It may be necessary to suture lacerations if they are unusually deep, but steri-strips usually suffice to approximate wound edges.

POSTNATAL INJURY

Endotracheal intubation

Prolonged endotracheal intubation is occasionally used to treat respiratory distress in infants. Possible complications of intubation include laryngeal or tracheal ulceration and perforation, subglottic edema, granuloma formation, vocal cord damage, acquired palatal groove[614] and cleft palate,[615] erosions and necrosis in skin and mucosa of mouth or nose. Mid-facial hypoplasia may occur following prolonged intubation.[616] There may be a late fibrotic reaction with stenosis of larynx or of nasal passages following damage during nasotracheal intubation.[617] Both mechanical and chemical factors are important in leading to complications, with the fixation of the tube probably being the most important factor. Recent tubing material, less likely to produce chemical injury, has become available.[614]

Pneumothorax treatment

Treatment of pneumothorax includes prompt placement of chest tubes for drainage. The superior approach (through the first, second, or third intercostal space, or just lateral to the mid-clavicular line) yields fewer complications than the lateral approach (through the fourth, fifth, or sixth space, or just lateral to anterior axillary line),[618] but the residual scar may be more evident with the former. Permanent breast tissue damage is the most serious complication of superior chest drains.[619]

Arterial catheterization

Catheterization of the umbilical artery is a common procedure performed in critically ill neonates giving easy accessibility to large vessels, enabling assessment of oxygenation and administration of fluid and medications.

Thrombosis in the abdominal aorta or iliac arteries is the most frequent problem. Other complications include bacterial or fungal infection, vasospasm, embolism, perforation of the vessels, vascular damage from hypertonic solutions and hemorrhage.[620] The skin is usually the first organ to show

614. Saunders B, Easa D, Slaughter R (1976) Acquired palatal groove in neonates. A report of two cases. **J Pediatr** 89:988–989.
615. Duke P, Coulson J, Santos J et al. (1976) Cleft palate associated with prolonged orotracheal intubation in infancy. **J Pediatr** 89:990–991.
616. Rotshchild A, Dison P, Chitayat D et al. (1990) Midfacial hypoplasia associated with long-term intubation for bronchopulmonary dysplasia. **AJDC** 144:1302–1306.
617. Jung A, Thomas G (1974) Stricture of the nasal vestibule: A complication of nasotracheal intubation in newborn infants. **J Pediatr** 85(3):412–414.
618. Allen R, Jung A, Lester P (1981) Effectiveness of chest tube evacuation of pneumothorax in neonates. **J Pediatr** 99(4):629–634.
619. Maalouf E, Harvey D (2000) Iatrogenic skin disorders. In: Textbook of Pediatric Dermatology, Harper J, Oranje A, Prose N, eds. Oxford: Blackwell Scientific Publications, pp. 125–135.
620. Ortonne J, Jeune R, Souteyrand P et al. (1978) Cutaneous and urinary complications of central umbilical artery injection. **Arch Dermatol** 114:286–287.

evidence of catheter problems. Vasospasm or ischemia can lead to necrosis of the overlying skin. This is especially frequent in the gluteal region and progression to gangrene may occur.[621] Major aortic compromise with embolization or thrombosis may lead to infarcts of the toes or gangrene of limbs, respectively. Early ischemia responds favorably to prompt removal of catheter and heparinization.[622] Severe cases may need surgical intervention.[623]

In cases of peripheral catheterization, similar lesions may appear. Brachial artery catheterization may lead to ischemia or gangrene of the lower limb, radial artery cannulation may cause reversible gangrene of the hand, and posterior tibial artery catheterization may produce reversible cyanosis of the toes.[619]

Transcutaneous oxygen and carbon dioxide monitoring

Transcutaneous measurements of oxygen and carbon dioxide partial pressures using skin surfaces monitoring has become routine practice in the neonatal intensive care unit. A circumscribed first-degree burn usually resolving in 2–3 days may occur as a result of the heat of the electrodes (42–45 degrees C). With prolonged application of the monitors, severe burns with vesiculation and subsequent dyspigmentation may occur (Fig. 6.55). In addition, the skin surrounding the electrode may be damaged by removal of the adhesive ring

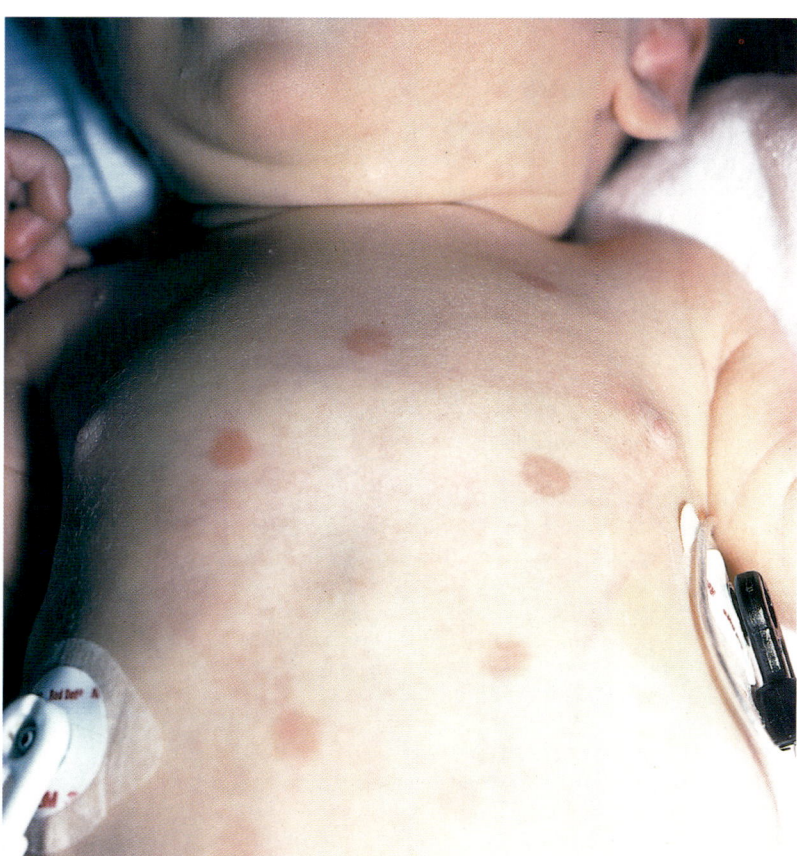

Fig. 6.55 Monitor burns (transcutaneous O_2/CO_2 electrodes).

that secures the sensor in place. Frequent changing of the electrode site and the use of a copolymer acrylic dressing for adherence can reduce the skin damage without interfering with the transcutaneous measurements.[599]

Pulse oximetry is gradually replacing transcutaneous PO_2 monitoring. This sensor does not need to be heated, and may be wrapped around a hand, foot, or finger, thus reducing the risks.

Transillumination

Transillumination with a high-intensity fiberoptic light source is an effective means of diagnosing pneumothoraces and localizing arteries and veins for blood sampling, as well as detecting hydrocephalus, subdural effusion, or macrocystic lymphatic malformation. Thermal burns may be a complication, appearing as small, round, discrete blisters with a necrotic base. The damage is believed to be produced by specific wavelengths of the high-intensity fiberoptic light which transform into heat energy in the skin. The use of infrared and ultraviolet filters within the light source reduce the risk.[624]

Anetoderma of prematurity

This is a recently described entity of unknown etiology that was reported to occur in extremely premature newborns that spend several months in a neonatal intensive care unit.[625] Atrophic, depressed, skin-colored or violaceous patches, measuring from several millimeters to centimeters, may be seen on the trunk and proximal limbs. At least half of the reported infants have no previous preceding inflammatory lesions, whereas the others are reported to develop the anetoderma at sites of application of adhesives and placement of monitoring devices. It has been postulated that the decrease in the elastic tissue may be due to a change in flow of ions or water under those devices or adhesives, causing a subclinical inflammatory reaction.[625]

Chemical injury

Infants of any gestational age are vulnerable to local and systemic effects of various chemicals because of their immature, thin, and poorly keratinized skin and their increased surface area:body weight ratio.[626] Potassium permanganate used in the bath can cause tiny, deep, localized areas of necrosis because of the presence of undissolved crystals. The paste used for electroencephalography and electrocardiography can act as a local irritant. Second- or third-degree chemical burns can occur from prolonged contact with cleansers, such as isopropyl alcohol, when used as preoperative cleanser or as skin preparation for sterile procedures such as umbilical artery catheterization. Excess alcohol inadvertently soaked the diaper under one infant resulting in prolonged exposure.[627] Topical iodine or povidone-iodine application may cause both burns and transient hypothyroidism.[628] Topical chlorhexidine has also caused superficial necrosis. Clearly, the use of disinfectants in preterm neonates necessitates extreme caution and sparse quantities.

Phototherapy

Hyperbilirubinemia affects nearly half of all newborns in some degree, but only about 10% require treatment.[629] Phototherapy with visible light in the absorption band (450–490nm) of bilirubin, has become standard therapy for neonatal jaundice.

The most commonly reported cutaneous side effect is the development of a transient, dark gray-brown discoloration known as the bronze baby syndrome (Fig. 6.56). This occurs almost exclusively in newborns with primary hepatocellular dysfunction.[630,631] Although the exact nature of the pigment is unknown, it is supposed to be a photo-oxidation product of bilirubin or a

621. Meneghini C (1998) Some guidelines in neonatal care. **Eur J Pediatr** 8:229–232.
622. Alpert J, O'Donnell J, Parsonnet V et al. (1980) Clinically recognized limb ischemia in the neonate after umbilical artery catheterization. **Am J Surg** 140(3):413–418.
623. O'Neill J, Neblettt W, Born M (1981) Management of major thromboembolic complications of umbilical artery catheters. **J Pediatr Surg** 16:972–978.
624. Sajben F, Gibbs N, Friedlander S (1999) Transillumination blisters in a neonate. **J Am Ac Dermatol** 41(2):264–265.
625. Prizant T, Lucky A, Frieden I et al. (1996) Spontaneous atrophic patches in extremely premature infants. Anetoderma of prematurity. **Arch Dermatol** 132:671–674.
626. Lane A (1987) Development and care of the premature infant's skin. **Pediatr Dermatol** 4(1):1–5.
627. Harpin VA, Rutter N (1982) Percutaneous alcohol absorption and skin necrosis in a premature infant. **Arch Dis Child** 57:477.
628. Pyat SP, Ramamurthy RS, Krauss MT et al: (1979) Absorption of iodine in the neonate following topical use of providone-iodine. **J Pediatr** 91:825.
629. Sisson T (1981) Molecular basis of hyperbilirubinemia and phototherapy. **J Invest Dermatol** 77:158–161.
630. Ashley J, Littler C, Burgdorf W et al. (1985) Bronze baby syndrome. **J Am Acad Dermatol** 12:325–328.
631. Rodot S, Lacour C, Dageville C et al. (1994) Le syndrome du "bebe de coleur bronze." **Ann Dermatol Venereol** 121:568–570.

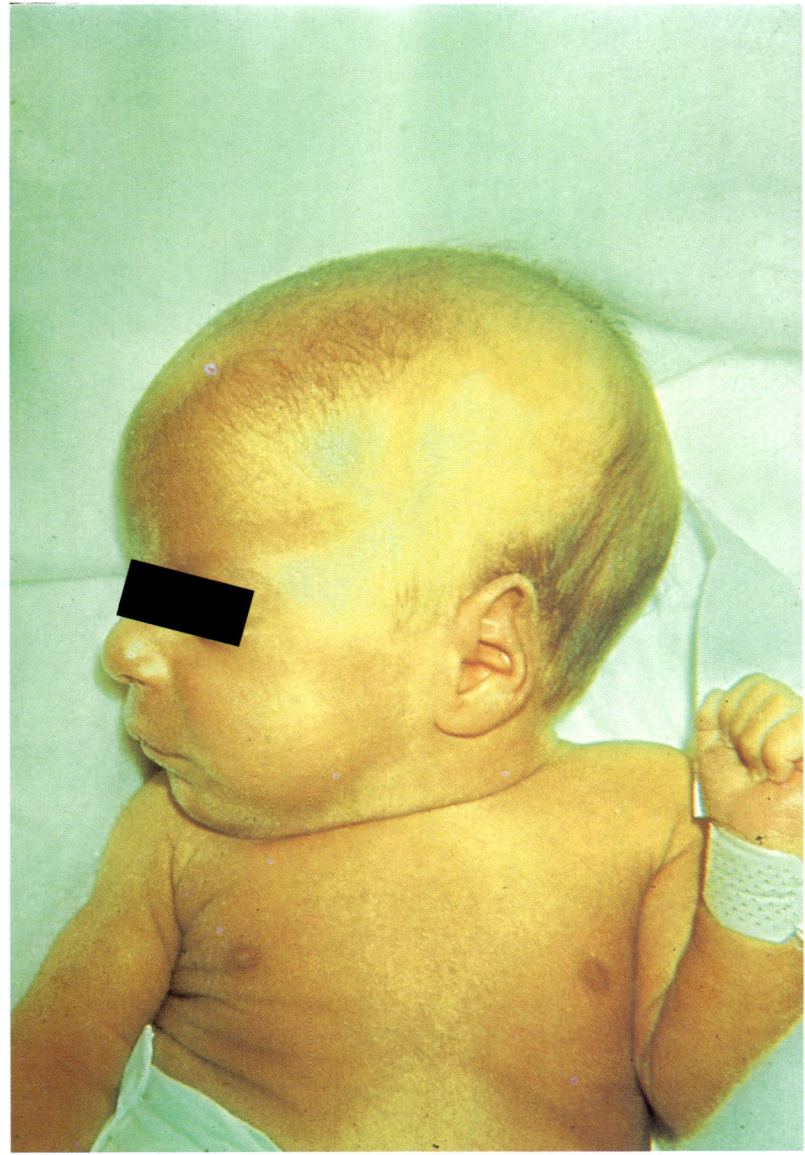

Fig. 6.56   Bronze baby syndrome.

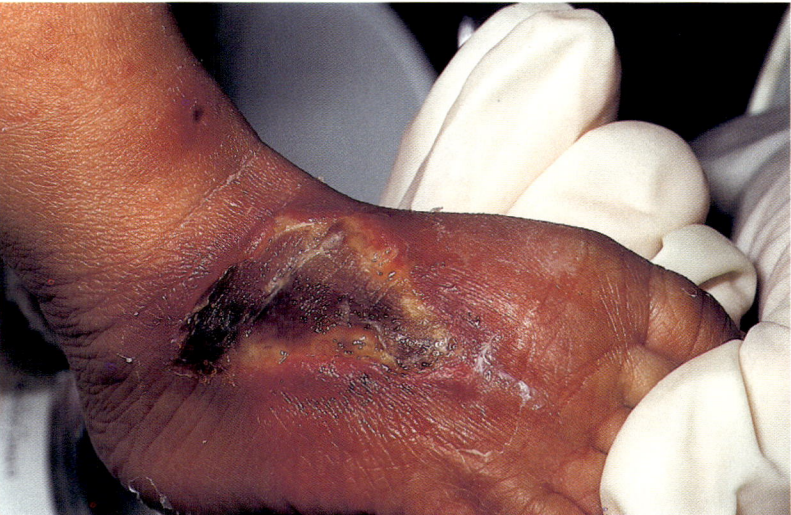

Fig. 6.57   Extravasation injury (calcium infiltration) resulting in ulcer.

Pressure ulcerations

Scarring has been reported with the resolution of pressure ulcerations in sick neonates with poor skin perfusion secondary to hypoxemia and acidosis. All had disrupted cardiac circulation and required vasopressor treatment. The institution of a positioning schedule and the use of a thermostable Spenco gel pad subsequently eliminated the occurrence of pressure ulceration and resultant scarring alopecia.[636]

Extravasation injuries

Leakage of cytotoxic drugs, parenteral nutrition, or maintenance intravenous solutions containing calcium, potassium, 10% dextrose, or bicarbonate, into the dermis or subcutaneous tissue, is relatively common in the NICU. Superficial sloughing or deep necrosis of the skin can occur around the involved vessels (Fig. 6.57).[637] Thrombophlebitis, abscess formation, and gangrene have been seen following extravasation of total parenteral nutrition in newborns.[638] Extravasation can result in scarring around tendons, nerves, and joints that requires extensive reconstruction. Lower limb shortening and deformity secondary to direct epiphyseal damage following extravasation of calcium and dextrose from a peripheral venous line has been reported.[639]

Most intravenous infiltrations are minor and have no sequelae other than transient edema and erythema. A recent report has demonstrated a beneficial effect of saline flushout or liposuction in the early stages following extravasation of noxious substances. The majority (86%) of children treated in this manner had no soft tissue loss and conservation of the overlying skin.[640]

Calcinosis cutis

Calcinosis cutis, the cutaneous deposition of calcium salts in the dermis, can occur through a variety of pathogenetic mechanisms, and can be associated with normal and elevated calcium levels. Heterotopic calcification may be subclassified as: idiopathic, with normal tissue and calcium phosphorus ratio; dystrophic, with damaged tissue and normal calcium phosphorus ratio; and metastatic, with normal tissue and abnormal calcium phosphorus ratio.[641] Calcinosis cutis in neonates is usually dystrophic calcification.

photoproduct of copper-porphyrin metabolism; it is also related to biliverdin pigment.[632] Another side effect is ultraviolet burn when using daylight fluorescent bulbs. This can be avoided by using plexiglass covers over the banks of bulbs, which interfere with the UVA transmission.[633]

Minor cutaneous side effects are tanning or darkening of the skin, which are thought to result from immediate pigment darkening induced by long wavelength UV light.

Blistering associated with phototherapy can occur with congenital erythropoietic porphyria and erythropoietic protoporphyria as well as with a transient porphyrinemia reported in neonates in the setting of alloimmune hemolytic disease.[634,635]

632. Purcell S, Wians F, Ackerman N et al. (1987) Hyperbiliverdinemia in the bronze baby syndrome. J Am Acad Dermatol 16:172–177.
633. Siegfried E, Stone M, Madison K (1992) Ultraviolet light burn: a cutaneous complication of visible light phototherapy of neonatal jaundice. Pediatr Dermatol 9(3):278–282.
634. Mallon E, Wojnarowska F, Hope P et al. (1995) Neonatal bullous eruption as a result of transient porphyrinemia in a premature infant with hemolytic disease of the newborn. J Am Acad Dermatol 33:333–336.
635. Crawford RI, Lawlor ER, Wadsworth LD (1996) Transient erythroporphyria of infancy. J Am Acad Dermatol 35:833–834.

636. Gershan LA, Esterly NB (1993) Scarring alopecia in neonates as a consequence of hypoxaemia-hypoperfusion. Arch Dis Child 68:591.
637. Hironaga M, Fujigaki T, Tanaka S (1982) Cutaneous calcinosis in a neonate following extravasation of calcium gluconate. J Am Acad Dermatol 6:392.
638. Vaidya UV, Hedge VM, Bhave SA et al. (1991) Reduction in parenteral nutrition related complications in the newborn. Indian Pediatr 28:477.
639. Guy RL, Holland JP, Shaw DG et al. (1990) Limb shortening secondary to complications of vascular cannulae in the neonatal period. Skel Radiol 19:423.
640. Gault DT (1993) Extravasation injuries. Br J Plast Surg 46:91.
641. Kagen M, Bansal M, Grossman M (2000) Calcinosis cutis following the administration of intravenous calcium therapy. Cutis 65:193–194.

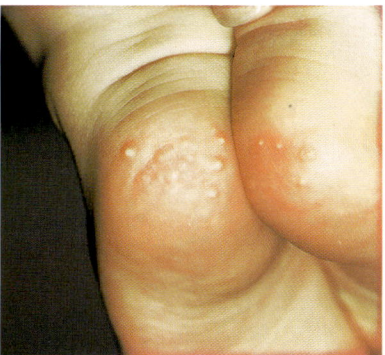

Fig. 6.58 Calcified heel nodules.

The most common cause of iatrogenic calcinosis cutis is calcified heel nodules. It consists of a self-limited, dystrophic calcinosis affecting neonates receiving many heel sticks to obtain blood for examination.[642–644] The disorder usually begins at 4 to 12 months of age as tiny depressions in the lateral heel. Over a period of four to 12 months, tiny yellow papules develop within the depressions, slowly enlarging to form heel nodules (Fig. 6.58). These nodules are usually asymptomatic, although some children have discomfort with walking in shoes. Lesions appear to resolve spontaneously by 2 to 3 years of life, probably by transepithelial elimination. Symptomatic children can be treated with curettage or light cryosurgery until spontaneous resolution.

Calcinosis cutis has also been reported at the sites of lead placement for electroencephalography or electrocardiography or electromyography.[645–647] Affected infants develop calcification following the use of electrode paste containing calcium chloride. A history of skin abrasion at the site of the electrode placement is usually obtained. Lesions typically occur within 24 hours to several days after exposure, are asymptomatic and last two to six months before spontaneous resolution.

Calcinosis cutis can occur following intramuscular or intravenous administration of calcium gluconate or calcium chloride for the treatment of symptomatic hypocalcemia in the neonate. It occurs particularly when sodium bicarbonate is also being administered.[648] The usual appearance is a linear arrangement of firm, yellow-white papules or plaques following an earlier transient erythema. When extravasation is massive, there may be a marked erythema with swelling and subsequent soft tissue necrosis appearing several days after the calcium administration.[637,649,650] Several theories have been proposed to explain the pathogenesis of this entity including tissue damage and transient elevation of the local calcium concentration.[650,651] These lesions usually resolve by transepidermal elimination in about two or three months.[636]

ADVERSE DRUG REACTIONS

Neonates are potentially at significant risk for adverse drug reactions because of underdeveloped mechanisms and systems for handling drugs.

The gray baby syndrome is a potentially fatal syndrome that results from chloramphenicol intoxication. Affected infants develop irregular respirations, progressive pallid cyanosis (gray color), hypothermia, and abdominal distension and vomiting, with eventual vasomotor collapse and even death.[652,653] Susceptibility in infants results from immature liver function. Chloramphenicol is metabolized to chloramphenicol glucuronide by the liver. Decreased hepatic glucuronidation results in elevated serum levels, since only the metabolized form is effectively excreted by the kidneys. Administration of the usual doses of chloramphenicol to preterm infants results in gray baby syndrome. Chloramphenicol can be used effectively in this population if the dose is appropriately adjusted to compensate for the diminished metabolism. Doses of 15 to 50mg/kg per day (less than one-half of the usual dose), provide beneficial therapeutic effects in a nontoxic range.[654]

Other complications related to drug reactions have been reported, including: metahemoglobinemia from aniline dye absorption; deafness from percutaneous absorption of neomycin; metabolic acidosis, hypernatremia, renal dysfunction and transient hypothyroidism from systemic absorption of iodine compounds; and spongiform changes in the newborns' brains from hexachlorophene.[619]

NOSOCOMIAL INFECTION

Nosocomial infection within the NICU is a constant source of anxiety among caregivers. Reports of multiple cases within a nursery of group B *streptococcus*, *Staphylococcus aureus*, Pseudomonas, candidiasis, or HSV can be found in the literature. An unusual case of nosocomial dermatophyte infection with *Microsporum canis* in six infants in the intermediate-case nursery was recently reported.[655] A nurse with an indolent infection was identified as the source. Human-to-human transmission of *Microsporum canis* is rare, suggesting increased susceptibility in neonates.

SUBCUTANEOUS FAT NECROSIS

Subcutaneous fat necrosis is idiopathic necrosis of the panniculus of the neonate, manifested as indurated plaques or nodules beneath the skin. Some affected infants have been subjected to perinatal asphyxia, peripheral hypoxemia meconium aspiration, hypothermia, or other forms of trauma during labor and delivery.[656–659] However, infants with uncomplicated obstetric histories or atraumatic cesarean deliveries have also been reported with this condition.[660,661] In general, affected infants have been born at term or later and are otherwise healthy.

Most commonly, lesions are located on the buttocks, cheeks, posterior trunk, arms, and legs, with sparing of the anterior trunk. Involved areas may be colorless, red (Fig. 6.59), or hemorrhagic in appearance and are characteristically painful when palpated. The overlying skin may be attached to the subcutaneous lesions, but it is frequently freely movable.[656] Fluctuance is occasionally observed.

Lesions appear in the first or second month of life, resolving within several weeks to months, although resolution has been reported to take as long as six

642. Sell EJ, Hansen RC, Struck-Pierce S (1980) Calcified nodules on the heel: a complication of neonatal intensive care. **J Pediatr** 96:473.
643. Cambiaghi S, Restano L, Imondi D (1997) Calcified nodule of the heel. **Ped Dermatol** 14(6):494.
644. Cambiaghi S, Imondi D, Gangi S et al. (2000) Fingertip calcinosis cutis. **Cutis** 66:465–467.
645. Wiley HE III, Eaglstein WE (1979) Calcinosis cutis in children following electroencephalography. **JAMA** 242:455.
646. Johnson R, Fitzpatrick J, Hahn D (1993) Calcinosis cutis following electromyographic examination. **Cutis** 52:161–164.
647. Mancuso G, Tosti A, Fanti P et al. (1990) Cutaneous necrosis and calcinosis following electroencephalography. **Dermatological** 181:324–326.
648. Speer M, Rudolph A (1983) Calcification of superficial scalp veins secondary to intravenous infusion of sodium bicarbonate and calcium chloride. **Cutis** 32:65–66.
649. Goldminz D, Raymond B, McGuire J et al. (1988) Calcinosis cutis following extravasation of calcium chloride. **Arch Dermatol** 124:922–925.
650. Millard T, Harris A, MacDonald D (1999) Calcinosis cutis following intravenous infusion of calcium gluconate. **Br J Dermatol** 140:184–186.
651. Sahn E, Smith D (1992) Annular dystrophic calcinosis cutis in an infant. **J Am Acad Dermatol** 26:1015–1017.
652. Craft AW, Broklebank JT, Jackson RH (1974) The "gray toddler": chloramphenicol toxicity. **Arch Dis Child** 49:235.
653. Krasinki K, Perkin R, Rutledge J (1982) The grey baby syndrome revisited. **Clin Pediatr** 21:571.
654. Reed MD (1992) Principles of drug therapy. In: Nelson Textbook of Pediatrics, 14th ed, Behrman RE, Kliegman RM, Nelson WE, Vaughan VC III, eds. Philadelphia, PA: WB Saunders, p. 255.
655. Snider R, Landers S, Levy ML (1993) The ringworm riddle: an outbreak of Microsporum canis in the nursey. **Pediatr Infect Dis J** 12:145.
656. Thomsen RJ (1980) Subcutaneous fat necrosis of the newborn and idiopathic hypercalcemia. **Arch Dermatol** 116:1155.
657. Katz DA, Huerter C, Bogard P et al. (1984) Subcutaneous fat necrosis of the newborn. **Arch Dermatol** 120:1517.
658. Mogilner BM, Alkalay A, Nissim F et al. (1981) Subcutaneous fat necrosis of the newborn. **Clin Pediatr** 20:748.
659. Chen TH, Shewmake SW, Hansen DD et al. (1981) Subcutaneous fat necrosis of the newborn. **Arch Dermatol** 117:36.
660. Cunningham K, Paes BA (1991) Subcutaneous fat necrosis of the newborn with hypercalcemia: a review. **Neonatal Network** 10:7.
661. Yasuda T, Sunami S, Ogura N et al. (1986) Infantile hypercalcemia with subcutaneous fat necrosis. **Acta Paediatr Scand** 75:1042.

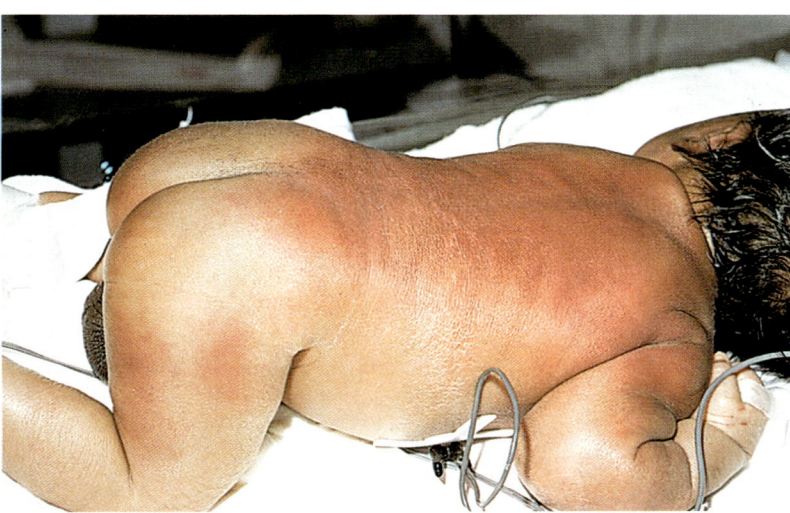

Fig. 6.59 Subcutaneous fat necrosis. Extensive erythema and induration of back, proximal arms and thighs.

months.[656] Lesions may calcify.[656,662] They may appear progressively, rather than all at one time, suggesting differences in the degree of tissue damage that has occurred.[658] Slight atrophy of the epidermis may occur with resolution.

The underlying mechanism of subcutaneous fat necrosis remains obscure. Antecedent obstetric trauma, neonatal hypoxemia, and hypothermia in predisposed neonates are postulated to contribute to the production of panniculitis and thrombocytopenia. In perinatal asphyxia, physiologic shunting from the skin surfaces produces a compensatory ischemia that may result in fat necrosis. Hypothermia has been thought by some to be a cause of fat necrosis, for this too would produce physiologic shunting away from the skin surfaces.[663] These hypotheses do not explain the absence of necrosis at the skin surface itself, the site where ischemia would be most marked under these circumstances.

Hypercalcemia has been documented to occur during the resolution phase in some affected infants.[656,650,662–667] The mechanism of hypercalcemia is not understood. Several investigators have noted unregulated, inappropriately increased levels of extrarenal $1,25(OH)_2D_3$.[666–669] They postulate that this hypervitaminosis D is produced by the granulomatous infiltrate of the necrotic cutaneous fat in a manner analogous to that observed in other granulomatous conditions, such as sarcoidosis or tuberculosis. Increased intestinal absorption of calcium in response to this elevated $1,25(OH)_2D_3$ results in hypercalcemia. Vomiting, failure to thrive, irritability, seizures, and even death can result from unrecognized hypercalcemia.[665]

Laboratory tests are usually normal in healthy infants with active subcutaneous fat necrosis, but metabolic and electrolyte abnormalities are present in those infants with respiratory failure, sepsis, and perinatal asphyxia.[670] Transient thrombocytopenia has been reported in several asphyxiated infants with subcutaneous fat necrosis.[658,663,671]

Biopsy of early subcutaneous fat necrosis demonstrates perivascular inflammation and endothelial cell swelling in the subcutaneous tissues. Later,

necrosis of fat and a granulomatous infiltrate with multinucleated giant cells are present. Doubly refractile crystals, thought to represent triglycerides, are visible within the macrophages and the damaged fat cells on frozen section, when examined with polarized light microscopy.[672]

The differential diagnosis should include sclerema neonatorum, lipogranulomatosis, deep tissue infection, or nodular panniculitis. The clinical appearance, general well-being in most infants, and histology are distinctive features that can be used to differentiate the infant with subcutaneous fat necrosis from the infant with sclerema. Infants with lipogranulomatosis (Farber disease) are usually hoarse and have tender nodules, predominant on the wrists and ankles. Deep tissue infection is usually accompanied by signs of systemic illness, whereas infants with subcutaneous fat necrosis appear otherwise well. Primary hyperparathyroidism, osteoma cutis and dermal calcifications associated with Albright hereditary osteodystrophy (pseudo-hypoparathyroidism) should be ruled out when calcification or hypercalcemia are present.

Observation is the key to therapy. Aspiration of fluctuant areas is appropriate when they occur.[673] Serum calcium levels need to be monitored for potential hypercalcemia for the first six weeks of life.[666] If hypercalcemia occurs, initial therapy includes hydration and furosemide for diuresis. A low-calcium, low-vitamin-D diet is recommended. Occasionally, corticosteroids, and possibly calcitonin, are necessary.[665,666] Parental reassurance is important in regard to the transient, self-healing nature of the condition.

SCLEREMA NEONATORUM

Sclerema neonatorum is a diffuse, symmetric, woody induration of the skin and subcutaneous tissues affecting sick neonates and infants up to 4 months of age. Typical infants are small and debilitated and have serious underlying diseases. The skin rapidly becomes taut and waxy with a yellowish-white, cadaver-like appearance. On palpation it feels bound down and hard. Perfusion of the involved sites is decreased. In early sclerema, the buttocks, cheeks, thighs, and lower legs become involved before the skin and subcutaneous tissues of the trunk. Small preterm infants are subject to total body involvement.

Sclerema occurs more frequently in preterm infants, but its exact frequency in neonates and young infants is unknown. Three term neonates have been described with sclerema and joint contractures present at birth following chronic intrauterine hypoxia.[674]

The etiology of sclerema neonatorum is unknown. The myriad of serious associated underlying conditions, such as hypothermia, sepsis, glucose or electrolyte imbalance, cardiovascular disease, or CNS dysfunction from hemorrhage, suggests that this may represent an end-stage common pathway indicating grave prognosis.

Biochemical findings may include elevated serum potassium and decreased sodium levels, metabolic acidosis, hypoglycemia, and azotemia. Histologic studies demonstrate epidermal thinning with loss of the rete pegs and increased collagen deposition in the dermis. The subcutaneous tissue appears thickened with edema and fibrosis of the connective tissue septae causing marked lobulation of the fat.[675] Occasionally, fat necrosis and crystalized clefts are seen, as in subcutaneous fat necrosis, but this is not a conspicuous feature. Vasculitis and giant cell infiltration are absent.[675] Electron microscopic

662. Cunningham K, Atkinson SA, Paes BA (1990) Subcutaneous fat necrosis with hypercalcemia. **Can Assoc Radiol J** 41:158.
663. Glover MT, Catterall MD, Atherton DJ (1991) Subcutaneous fat necrosis in two infants after hypothermic cardiac surgery. **Pediatr Dermatol** 8:210.
664. Lewis A, Cowen P, Rodda C et al (1992) Subcutaneous fat necrosis of the newborn complicated by hypercalcaemia and thrombocytopenia. **Australas J Dermatol** 33:141.
665. Fernandez-Lopez E, Garcia-Dorado J, de Unamuno P et al. (1990) Subcutaneous fat necrosis of the newborn and idiopathic hypercalcemia. **Dermatologica** 180:250.
666. Cook JS, Stone MS, Hansen JR (1992) Hypercalcemia in association with subcutaneous fat necrosis of the newborn: studies of calcium-regulating hormones. **Pediatrics** 90:93.
667. Finne PH, Sanderrud J, Aksnes L et al. (1988) Hypercalcemia with increased and unregulated 1,25-dihydroxyvitamin D product on in a neonate with subcutaneous fat necrosis. **J Pediatr** 112:792.
668. Norwood-Galloway A, Lebwohl M, Phelps RG et al. (1987) Subcutaneous fat necrosis of the newborn with hypercalcemia. **J Am Acad Dermatol** 16:435.
669. Kruse K, Irle U, Uhlig R (1993) Elevated 1,25-dihydroxyvitamin D serum concentrations in infants with subcutaneous fat necrosis. **J Pediatr** 122:460.
670. Vonk J, Janssens PM, Demacker PN et al. (1993) Subcutaneous fat necrosis in a neonate, in association with aberrant plasma lipid and lipoprotein values. **J Pediatr** 123:462.
671. Wolach B, Raas-Rothschild A, Vogel R et al. (1990) Subcutaneous fat necrosis with thrombocytopenia in a newborn infant. **Dermatologica** 181:54.
672. Friedman SJ, Winkelmann RK (1989) Subcutaneous fat necrosis of the newborn: light, ultrastructural and histochemical microscopic studies. **J Cutan Pathol** 16:99.
673. Walker WP, Smith RJ, Cohen MB (1993) Fine-needle aspiration biopsy of subcutaneous fat necrosis of the newborn. **Diagn Cytopathol** 9:329.
674. Molteni RA, Ames MR (1986) Sclerema neonatorum and joint contractures at birth as a potential complication of chronic in utero hypoxia. **Am J Obstet Gynecol** 155:380.
675. Dasgupta A, Ghosh RN, Pak RK et al. (1993) Sclerema neonatorum—histopathologic study. **Indian J Pathol Microbiol** 36:45.

studies of fat cells demonstrate destruction of cell membranes and damage to cytoplasmic organelles and nuclei. The interlobular fat septae have thick, tightly bound collagen bundles alternating with loosely bound bands. Ultrastructurally, collagen fibers split to form microfibrils. Vascular endothelial cells have damaged cell membranes, but this may be a nonspecific finding related to hypoxia or post-mortem autolysis.[676]

The biochemical basis for sclerema neonatorum is unclear, but studies suggest a decrease in the enzymatic desaturation of triglycerides, hence reduced production of fatty acids in the infant's subcutaneous tissues.[677,678] This most likely represents lipid metabolic or cell wall dysfunction as a component of sick cell syndrome. Norepinephrine, the major mediator for lipolysis resulting in heat production in infants, is decreased in the urine of infants exposed to hypothermia sufficient to cause sclerema.[679] These levels increase after recovery and correlate with increased lipolysis.

Visceral fat may be involved in severely ill infants or in infants in whom sclerema develops, leading to death. Perinephric and retroperitoneal fat, as well as other body fat, may be affected.[680]

The differential diagnosis is limited. Scleredema has not been reported to occur in neonates; it differs histologically in that the fat is unaffected other than being quantitatively decreased and replaced by collagen. Classically, in scleredema, the collagen bundles are thickened and fenestrated with hyaluronic acid present between the bundles. Sclerodermoid skin changes in neonates have not been described. Subcutaneous fat necrosis may be differentiated by the presence of erythema, bluish discoloration of the skin, focal distribution, and the histologic presence of inflammatory cells, giant cells, and calcium crystals. A newborn with clinical and histologic evidence of both sclerema neonatorum and subcutaneous fat necrosis has been described.[681]

Therapy for sclerema has included systemic steroids,[682] supplemental intravenous calcium, and exchange transfusion.[683,684] Systemic steroids alone do not appear to be beneficial in infants with sclerema. Their use, coupled with systemic antibiotics, has been advocated, despite the lack of controlled trials demonstrating their efficacy, because mortality is extremely high in this condition. Polymorphonuclear leukocyte transfusions as well as steroids given in conjunction with exchange transfusion have been reported to increase survival in septic infants with sclerema.[684,685] Adequate nutritional support, correction of acid–base imbalance, antimicrobial agents, thermal control, and supportive care are perhaps more responsible for survival than any one specific medication or procedure. Because death is likely, but not inevitable, the prognosis for an infant with sclerema is guarded, and the parents should be so informed. Realistic expectations for survival should not exceed 40%, but 70% survival in cases of sclerema associated with sepsis have been reported.[684]

PRENATAL DIAGNOSIS

Genodermatoses contribute significantly to the daily practice of the pediatric dermatologist. Most genetic skin diseases are severe chronic disorders for which a specific treatment is not yet available.[686] Several of these have a poor and often lethal prognosis and others result in highly morbid conditions. Prenatal diagnosis (PD) of several devastating hereditary skin disorders has become available as a preventive method of remarkable importance for families at risk for genetic skin diseases,[687] and may be an option for such families with the possibility of ending a pregnancy if shown to carry an affected fetus. In the past, many healthy fetuses have been aborted only because of statistical risks of recurrence.

There has been considerable progress in gene identification in severe hereditary skin diseases. Gene therapy may become available for specific genodermatoses,[688,689] and prenatal intrauterine interventions may be possible. New molecular, enzymatic, and ultrastructural markers will be available in the future, which will aid in the accuracy and utility of *in utero* or preimplantation diagnosis. Readers are referred to their local genetic centers for information regarding prenatal diagnosis of specific genetic diseases. The human genome contains approximately 100 000 individual genes, many of which have been identified through the Human Genome Project and other molecular cloning studies, which are available on the Internet. It is a valuable resource for current information on specific dermatologic conditions and their prenatal diagnosis. The Online Mendelian Inheritance in Man website, http://www.ncbi.nlm.nih.gov/Omim, is a database of human genes and genetic disorders. The database contains textual information and pictures, and is a valuable reference.[690–692]

Some disorders in which karyotype analysis and cytogenetics are uninformative may still be able to be diagnosed prenatally. Some inborn errors of metabolism, such as X-linked ichthyosis with steroid sulfatase deficiency, or Fabry disease with lack of alpha galactosidase, can be diagnosed from the amniotic fluid.

Ultrastructural abnormalities are well known for many genodermatoses such as epidermolisis bullosa (EB) and some inherited ichthyoses,[693] and can be looked for on fetal skin samples obtained *in utero* via fetoscopy under sonographic control.[694,695]

Since early 1980,[695,696] many genodermatoses have been shown to express markers early enough during fetal skin development that they can be safely prenatally diagnosed from fetal skin samples.[697] Advances in understanding the molecular basis of several serious, often life-threatening, skin diseases have provided the basis for early DNA-based prenatal diagnosis during first trimester of gestation. This approach will replace the invasive fetal skin biopsy in cases in which candidate genes or specific genetic mutations have been identified, such as recessive dystrophic EB.[698] Presently, this kind of PD, based on the specific mutation analysis of DNA, is still restricted to those families in whom the underlying basic abnormalities have been determined.

Knowledge of specific gene defects for many genodermatoses has led to the development of DNA-based prenatal diagnosis, which has largely superceded older techniques such as fetoscopy and fetal skin biopsy. DNA may be derived through chorionic villus sampling at 10–15 weeks gestation

676. Pasyk K (1980) Sclerema neonatorum, light and electron microscopic studies. **Virchows Archiv Abteilung a Pathologische Anatomie** 388:87.
677. Horsfield GI, Yardley HJ (1965) Sclerema neonatorum. **J Invest Dermatol** 44:326.
678. Kellum RE, Ray TL, Brown GR (1968) Sclerema neonatorum. **Arch Dermatol** 97:372.
679. Anagnostakis D, Economou-Mavrou C, Agathopoulos H et al. (1974) Neonatal cold injury: Evidence of defective thermogenesis due to impaired norepinephrine release. **Pediatr** 53:24.
680. Zeek P, Madden EM (1946) Sclerema adiposum neonatorum of both internal and external adipose tissue. **Arch Pathol Lab Med** 41:166.
681. Jardine D, Atherton DJ, Trompeter RS (1990) Sclerema neonatorum and subcutaneous fat necrosis of the newborn in the same infant. **Eur J Pediatr** 150:125.
682. Milansky A, Levin SE (1966) Sclerema neonatorum: a clinical study of 79 cases. **S Afr Med J** 40:638.
683. Narayanan I, Mitter A, Gujral VV (1982) A comparative study on the value of exchange and blood transfusion in the management of severe neonatal septicemia with sclerema. **Indian J Pediatr** 49:519.
684. Vain NE, Mazlumain JR (1980) Role of exchange transfusion in the treatment of severe septicemia. **Pediatrics** 66:693.
685. Laurenti F, Ferro R, Isacchi G et al. (1981) Polymorphonuclear leukocyte transfusion for the treatment of sepsis in the newborn infant. **J Pediatr** 98:118.
686. Anton-Lamprecht I (2000) Prenatal diagnosis of inherited skin disorders. In: Text Book of Pediatric Dermatology, Harper J, Oranje A, Prose N, eds. London: Blackwell Science, pp. 1358–1389.
687. Blanchet-Bardon C, Nazzaro V (1986) Diagnosi antenatale in dermatologia. **Giorn It Derm Vener** 121:161–168.

688. Taichman LB (1994) Epithelial gene therapy. In: The Keratinocyte Handbook, Leigh IM, Watt FM, eds. Cambridge: Cambridge University Press, pp. 543–551.
689. Greenhalgh DA, Rothnagel JA, Roop DR (1994) Epidermis. An attractive target tissue for gene therapy. **J Invest Dermatol** 103:63s–69s.
690. Cunningham BB, Wagner AM (2001) Diagnostic and therapeutic procedures. In: Textbook of Neonatal Dermatology, Eichenfield LF, Frieden IJ, Esterly NB, eds. Philadelphia, PA: WB Saunders, pp. 73–87.
691. McGrath JA, Handyside AH (1998) Preimplantation genetic diagnosis of severe inherited skin diseases. **Exp Dermatol** 7:65–72.
692. Hadj-Rabia S, Bodemer C, De Prost Y et al. (1999) Diagnostic prenatal en dermatologie. **Ann Dermatol Venereol** 126:981–991.
693. Anton-Lampretcht I (1978) Electron microscopy in the early diagnosis of genetic disorders of the skin. **Dermatologica** 157:65–85.
694. Anton-Lamprecht I (1983) Genetically induced abnormalities of epidermal differentiation and ultrastructure in ichthyoses and epidermolyses: pathogenesis, heterogeneity, fetal manifestation, and prenatal diagnosis. **J Invest Dermatol** 81:149s–156s.
695. Anton-Lamprecht I (1981) Prenatal diagnosis of genetic disorders of the skin by means of electron microscopy. **Hum Genet** 59:392–405.
696. Elias S, Mazur M, Sabaggha R et al. (1980) Prenatal diagnosis of harlequin ichthyosis. **Clin Genet** 17:275–280.
697. Brusasco A, Nicolini U, Cavalli R et al. (1994) Diagnosi prenatale mediante biopsia cutanea fetale. Esperienza di 12 casi. **G Ital Dermatol Venereol** 129:135–142.
698. Christiano AM, Uitto J (1993) DNA-based prenatal diagnosis of heritable skin diseases. **Arch Dermatol** 129:1455–1459.

or by amniocentesis at 12–15 weeks gestation in families at risk for recurrence of EB, for example. Periumbilical vein blood samples during the early weeks of pregnancy may provide an even earlier source of fetal DNA without any increased fetal risk.[699] In most cases, fetal cells are also cultured, and the test can be confirmed approximately two weeks later. Thus, DNA-based prenatal diagnosis offers an early, expedient, and accurate method of prenatal testing for genodermatoses with known underlying disorders.

It must be emphasized, however, that use of molecular techniques for prenatal diagnosis requires that the molecular defect is known. Although prenatal cytogenetic diagnosis based on amniocytes or chorionic villus cells is accurate, the procedure carries a risk of miscarriage. Because of this iatrogenic risk, CVS or amniocentesis-based prenatal testing should be reserved for women at high risk for chromosomal abnormalities.

Preimplantation genetic diagnosis (PGD) is an alternative to conventional approaches to prenatal diagnosis. With this technique, the genetic abnormality in question is diagnosed prior to implantation of the fetus, allowing selection of nonaffected, normal fetuses. DNA analysis and *in vitro* fertilization are utilized to select for a normal genotype prior to implantation. At the 6–10 cell stage, one cell is removed for DNA extraction and PCR amplification. Removal of one or two cells at this stage does not affect viability or the rate of development of the embryo. After analysis of DNA, only embryos with normal DNA are implanted, theoretically assuring that the implanted fetus will be normal. This technique has been used in families at risk for cystic fibrosis[700] and EB.

Present technology and ethical perspectives do not warrant PD of genodermatoses as a screening method, and it is only performed if the severity of the disorder at risk justifies termination of pregnancy in case of affected fetus. Mild diseases with good postnatal treatment response are not an indication for PD, even with a high risk of recurrence.

Extensive counseling of the at-risk family and detailed information is necessary on the severity and prognosis of the condition, and the risks and reliability of PD in the specific case, to enable them to decide early enough about whether they can accept termination of the pregnancy if their baby is found to be affected.[686]

SKIN CARE OF NEWBORN INFANTS

Skin care of newborn infants must focus on the following critical issues: (1) prevention of physical injury to the skin, (2) minimizing insensible water losses, (3) maintaining thermal stability, and (4) minimizing infection. This section focuses on our current knowledge of neonatal skin physiology and applications for skin care.

Standards of routine skin care of premature or term neonates have not been established. New information is available on the physiology of infant's skin, but concrete data on what to do are not available.[701] The full-term infant has skin that is considerably more mature than that of a preterm infant, displaying normal barrier function and less fragility.[702] All neonates have a large skin surface area in proportion to body mass, providing an increased risk for systemic toxicity from topically applied substances.[703] This, combined with the poor barrier function of immature skin, leaves the preterm infant at great risk for iatrogenic complications from topically applied soaps, cleansing solutions, or lotions.

The skin of the full-term infant is soft and supple. The smooth texture and softness reflect a well-hydrated epidermis overlying newly formed dermal collagen and dermal matrix substances.[704] The premature infant's skin does not have this supple quality. The dermis and subcutaneous tissue are thin, and the skin is frequently dry, scaly, and fissured.[701] The markedly increased fragility leads to abrasions and trauma, even in the course of careful routine handling.

The goal of all infant skin care is to maintain the soft flexible texture of the skin by providing lubrication and hydration. For the term infant, moisturizers can be used to attain this goal, even in a dry environment, but for the preterm infant, skin care is more difficult and complex.

Preterm infants should be handled with the utmost care to prevent physical injury to the skin. Caution should be taken to account for all limbs and the head with any movements to avoid unnecessary trauma from inadvertent dangling or rubbing of body parts on the infant warmer. Routine handling can produce significant cutaneous pain in these infants, who generally have multiple areas of epidermal and dermal skin injury. Steps should be taken to minimize movements by thoughtful preparation prior to any procedure. Rotation of severely ill, paralyzed neonates is essential to prevent the development of pressure-related ulcerations. These most commonly occur on the occiput due to the proportionately larger percentage of body weight of the head in the neonate. Scarring alopecia has been reported in infants from ulcerations due to pressure necrosis.[705]

Adhesive tape should be used sparingly and removed gently by peeling with one hand, while holding the underlying skin with a finger. If tape is very adherent, a small amount of soap or glue solvent on a cotton-tipped swab can enable removal without tearing of the underlying fragile skin. The use of a pectin-based barrier under tape to minimize the trauma of stripping when the tape is removed has been described.[706] Diminished irritation, erythema, and maceration of the underlying skin is observed.

Cardiac monitor leads should be replaced only when they are no longer functional to reduce skin trauma. The use of karaya electrodes has been demonstrated to be effective in cardiorespiratory monitoring with decreased trauma to neonatal skin.[708] Placement of electrodes on the limbs, especially in VLBW infants, can eliminate the need to frequently remove these pads to facilitate auscultation or other assessment of the chest wall.[709]

All antiseptic solutions used to prepare the skin for sterile procedures should be applied only to the immediate skin area and in very small amounts. Such solutions should be removed with water-soaked gauze when the procedure is complete to prevent unnecessary absorption due to prolonged exposure. Serious complications of systemic absorption of these substances has occurred.[710–712] Alcohol should be avoided, as it is drying and painful to superficially abraded skin, in addition to being toxic when systemically absorbed.[710,711]

If transcutaneous oxygen monitors are necessary, electrodes should be adjusted to the lowest effective heat and positions changed every four hours to prevent skin burns.[713] Where possible, pulse oximetry is a better alternative for oxygen monitoring in these infants. Close attention to these measures can dramatically reduce routine trauma to neonatal skin.

Minimizing insensible water losses is essential for overall hydration and for maintaining hydration of neonatal skin. Insensible water losses are substantial in preterm infants, especially when they are exposed to ambient, nonhumidified air in an open warmer. Frequent assessment of hydration is critical to their care. Accurate measurement of fluid intake and output along

699. Bianchi DW (1995) Prenatal diagnosis using fetal cells in maternal blood. **J Pediatr** 127:847–856.
700. Handyside AH, Lesko JG, Tain JJ et al. (1992) Birth of a normal girl after in vitro fertilization and preimplantation diagnostic testing for cystic fibrosis. **N Engl J Med** 327:905–909.
701. Lane AT (1987) Development and care of the premature infant's skin. **Pediatr Dermatol** 4:1.
702. Lane AT (1986) Human fetal skin development. **Pediatr Dermatol** 3:487.
703. Smales ORC, Kime R (1978) Thermoregulation in babies immediately after birth. **Arch Dis Child** 53:58.
704. Holbrook KA, Smith LT (1981) Ultrastructural aspects of human skin during the embryonic, fetal, premature, neonatal and adult periods of life. **Birth Defects** 1:9.
705. Gersham IA, Esterly NB (1993) Scarring alopecia in neonates as a consequence of hypoxaemia-hypoperfusion. **Arch Dis Child** 68:591.
706. Lund C, McManus-Kuller J, Tobin C (1986) Evaluation of a pectin-based barrier under tape to protect neonatal skin. **JOGN Nurs** 15:39.

707. Ching D, Mell DL (1990) Use of adhesive dressings in skin care: Duoderm Extra Thin. **J Pediatr Health Care** 4:155.
708. Scholz D (1984) EKG electrodes and skin irritation. **Neonat Network** 3:46.
709. Malloy MB, Perez-Woods RC (1991) Neonatal skin care: prevention of skin breakdown. **Pediatr Nurs** 17:41.
710. Haprin Va, Rutter N (1982) Percutaneous alcohol absorption and skin necrosis in a premature infant. **Arch Dis Child** 57:477.
711. Ruschell K (1981) Percutaneous alcohol intoxication. **Eur J Pediatr** 136:317.
712. Fyat SP, Ramamurthy RS, Krauss MT et al. (1979) Absorption of iodine in the neonate following topical use of povidine-iodine. **J Pediatr** 91:825.
713. Evans NJ, Rutter N (1986) Reduction of skin damage from transcutaneous oxygen electrodes using a spray on dressing. **Arch Dis Child** 61:881.

with daily weights are critical to evaluate the state of hydration. Maintaining a humid environment by using a thin plastic tent beneath the warmer will decrease transepidermal water loss and improve skin hydration. Petroleum-based ointments applied gently to the skin will reduce scaling and fissuring as well as increase skin hydration. The improved wound care and decreased fragility afforded by emollients serves to protect these infants from skin trauma, in addition to diminishing insensible losses and improving skin hydration.[714]

The use of paraffin as an occlusive barrier to diminish insensible water losses has been tried with limited success.[715] Infants often develop rashes beneath the barrier.[716] More recent studies using semipermeable membranes on premature infant skin show promise in diminishing these losses.[717] Reports of increased bacterial growth beneath semipermeable dressings necessitate caution in their use.[718] The limited application of such dressings to traumatized skin facilitates rapid wound healing and is probably safe. Transparent barriers have also been used as "knee pads" to protect reddened, irritated knees from trauma due to rubbing on the bed sheets.[718] Such dressings can be allowed to slough off naturally or can be removed carefully by pulling the edges laterally while maintaining traction on the opposite lateral edge.

Maintaining thermal stability is another challenge in the neonate. Heat losses through the skin are considerable, due to increased body surface area and poorly developed mechanisms of thermal regulation. Sweating is functionally reduced, contributing to this poor regulation.[719] In addition, there is a lack of subcutaneous fat for insulation and poor autonomic control of cutaneous vessels.[720] Evaporation, radiation, conduction, and convection losses are all increased in the preterm infant. The servo control probe is frequently used to maintain a preset abdominal temperature in the radiant warmer. Placement in a temperature and humidity controlled isolette at the earliest possible opportunity minimizes radiation, conduction, and convection losses in addition to allowing improved control of humidity to diminish insensible water losses.

Finally, minimizing infection in the preterm infant is critical, and necessitates maintaining the integrity of the skin. Although the newborn infant's skin is relatively sterile at birth, colonization with bacteria occurs rapidly during the first week of life. Antibiotic-resistant strains of coagulase-negative staphylococci, similar to those found on adult skin, are found in significant numbers shortly after birth.[721] These organisms are a frequent cause of neonatal septicemia, most likely resulting from innoculation at the sites of skin trauma or intravenous placement. The mainstay of infection prevention is frequent handwashing by the nursery staff and avoidance of skin trauma.

Bathing is a standard practice done in most nurseries and has thousands of years of tradition. Bathing should never be done during the immediate neonatal period until temperature stability and successful transition from the intrauterine environment have been accomplished. Infrequent bathing with water only, or with a low-alkaline soap once or twice weekly, is sufficient in preterm infants. If a product other than water is used for bathing, one must be aware of the chemical ingredients.[722] The use of hexachlorophene in bathwater to prevent colonization of the skin by Staphylococcus has been associated with systemic absorption and neurotoxicity.[723] This should be avoided. Replacement of skin moisture by the liberal use of petroleum-based emollients after bathing is recommended. Water-in-oil emollient creams decrease dermatitis in premature neonates without changing the microbiologic flora.[698]

Further research is needed to develop methods of protecting the integrity and barrier function of premature infant skin and to determine the most appropriate topical skin care for term and premature infants.

714. Lane AT, Drostss (1993) Effects of repeated application of emollient cream to premature neonates' skin. **Pediatrics** 92:415.
715. Rutter N, Hull D (1981) Reduction of skin water loss in the newborn. I. Effect of applying topical agents. **Arch Dis Child** 56:669.
716. Brice JEH, Rutter N, Hull D (1981) Reduction of skin water loss in the newborn. II. Clinical trial of two methods in very low birthweight babies. **Arch Dis Child** 56:673.
717. Vernon HJ, Lane AT, Wischerath LJ et al. (1990) Semipermeable dressings and transepidermal water loss in premature infants. **Pediatrics** 86:357–362.
718. Katz S, McGinley K, Leyden JJ (1986) Semipermeable occlusive dressings. Effects on growth of pathogenic bacteria and reepithelialization of superficial wounds. **Arch Dermatol** 122:58.
719. Harpin VA, Rutter N (1982) Sweating in preterm babies. **J Pediatr** 100:614.
720. Smales ORC, Kime R (1978) Thermoregulation in babies immediately after birth. **Arch Dis Child** 53:58.
721. Keyworth N, Millar MR, Holland KT (1992) Development of cutaneous microflora in premature neonates. **Arch Dis Child** 67:797.
722. Cetta F, Lambert GH, Ross SP (1991) Newborn chemical exposure from over-the-counter skin care products. **Clin Pediatr** 30:286–289.
723. Marzulli FN, Maibach HI (1975) Relevance of animal models: the hexachlorophene story. In: Maibach HI (ed): Animal Models in Dermatology. Churchill Livingstone, Edinburgh, p. 156.

CHAPTER 7

Genodermatoses

Peter H. Itin, Walter H. C. Burgdorf, Rudolf Happle, Amy Paller, Arne König, Adrian Pierini, Patsy Lenane, Bernice Krafchik, Bruce Korf, Seth Orlow, Susan Mallory, Robin Eady and John McGrath

INTRODUCTION

Tremendous progress has been achieved during the past decade in determining the underlying molecular basis of the majority of genetic disorders with cutaneous manifestations, the genodermatoses. This chapter includes contributions about several genodermatoses, including Ectodermal Dysplasias, Neurocutaneous Disorders, Disorders of the Dermis, Disorders of Pigmentation, Immunodeficiencies, Photosensitivity Disorders, Tumor Syndromes, Metabolic Disorders, and Aging syndromes. Mosaic disorders, in which more than one genotype is expressed, and the utility of DNA-based progress in facilitating Prenatal Diagnosis are also reviewed. The reader is referred to other chapters for discussions of Disorders of Cornification, Genetic Disorders of Hair and Nails, and Epidermolysis Bullosa.

ECTODERMAL DYSPLASIA

Peter Itin, Walter C Burgdorf and Rudolf Happle

INTRODUCTION AND HISTORICAL NOTE

Ectodermal dysplasias describe a large and complex group of disorders that involve alterations in multiple structures developing from the primordial external germ layer. Weech in 1929 coined the designation ectodermal dysplasia and recognized heterogeneity.[1] Solomon and Keuer[2] emphasized that the term ectodermal dysplasia has to be limited to those conditions that are congenital, diffusely present, and nonprogressive.

EPIDEMIOLOGY AND CLASSIFICATION

Ectodermal dysplasias are rare diseases with a wide clinical spectrum. Ectodermal dysplasias show anatomic and functional peculiarities in one or more epidermal appendages as a consequence of a developmental defect within the ectoderm. A large and comprehensive classification was initiated by Freire-Maia and Pinheiro on the bases of clinical description.[3] They proposed two main groups specified as A and B. All of the entities belonging to group A have defects in at least two of the classic ectodermal structures such as hair, teeth, nails, and sweat glands. In addition, malformations and other defects may occur. Group B disorders have defects in only one of the four above mentioned structures plus one other ectodermal defect. The diseases belonging to the large group of ectodermal dysplasias are also termed by the number corresponding to the basic affected structure (1, 2, 3, 4 = hair, teeth, nails, and sweat glands, respectively), and by number 5 indicating other ectodermal defects. As a result conditions belonging to this group are labeled 1-5, 2-5, 3-5, or 4-5.

Ectodermal dysplasias may be of unknown etiology but all types of inheritance have been described. The 192 known ectodermal dysplasias are classified into 11 subgroups. The number of ectodermal dysplasias in each subgroup varies from one to 43.[4] The numbers of conditions due to autosomal dominant, autosomal recessive, and X-linked genes are, respectively, 41, 52, and 8. In 53 diseases the cause is not known and in 35 of them some genetic causal suggestions exist (Table 7.1).

A disease that features only ectodermal signs is named a pure ectodermal dysplasia. The combination of ectodermal signs with other anormalies is called an ectodermal dysplasia syndrome.[3] In the classification of Freire-Maia and Pinheiro the above mentioned structures, hair, teeth, nails, and sweat glands, are designated as 1, 2, 3, 4, and several subgropus of group A are called 1-2, 1-3, 1-4, 2-3, 2-4, 3-4, 1-2-3, 1-2-4, 1-3-4, 2-3-4, and 1-2-3-4. An alternative is to mention the affected structures such as tricho–odontic, tricho–onychial, and trichodyshidrotic (Table 7.2).[5]

PRESENTING HISTORY

Children with ectodermal dysplasias may present with different clinical signs and symptoms, depending on the complexity of the ectodermal structures that are functionally and structurally involved. Patients with anhidrosis or hypo–hidrosis often present with hyperthermic crisis. Other children do not develop hair growth in an expected way and this may lead to the diagnosis of an ectodermal dysplasia.

TABLE 7.1 Number of known ectodermal dysplasias from 1971 to 1995

Reference	Year	Number of conditions	Number of subgroups
Freire-Maia	1971	32	8
Freire-Maia	1977	57	10
Freire-Maia and Pinheiro	1984	117	11
Freire-Maia and Pinheiro	1985	131	11
Freire-Maia and Pinheiro	1987	145	11
Pinheiro and Freire-Maia	1994	154	11
Freire-Maia et al.	2001	192	11

1. Weech AA (1929) Hereditary ectodermal dysplasia (congenital ectodermal defect). A report of two cases. Am J Dis Child 37:766–790.
2. Solomon LM, Keuer EJ (1980) The ectodermal dysplasias. Problems of classification and some newer syndromes. Arch Dermatcl 116:1295–1299.
3. Pinheiro M, Freire-Maia N (1994) Ectodermal dysplasias: A clinical classification and a causal review. Am J Med Genet 53:153–162.
4. Priolo M, Laguna C (2001) Ectodermal dysplasias: a new clinical genetic classification. J Med Genet 38:579–585.
5. Stelnicki EJ, Komures LG, Kwong AO et al. (1998) HOX homeobox genes exhibit spatial and temporal changes in expression during human skin development. J Invest Dermatol 110:110–115.

TABLE 7.2 Classification of ectodermal dysplasias

#	1	hair
#	2	teeth
#	3	nail
#	4	sweat glands

Resulting subgroups:

1-2-3-4	Diseases with hair, nail, teeth and sweat gland disorders e.g., incontinentia pigmenti, Bloch–Sulzberger
1-2-3	Diseases with hair, nail and teeth anomalies e.g., Rothmund–Thomson syndrome

PHYSICAL EXAMINATION

Patients may present abnormalities on the skin such as adermatoglyphia, reticular pigmentation, depigmentation, scaling, telangiectases, atrophy, and hyperkeratosis. Often alopecia is a feature of subtypes in ectodermal dysplasias. Hairs sometimes present as brittle and uncombable. Nails can be dystrophic or hyperconvex, or discolored, such as in leukonychia congenita associated with keratoderma and deafness. Enamel defects often occur and lead to severe and early caries. Oral findings include leukoplakia or cheilognathopalathoschisis. In addition, signs of mesodermal and entodermal malformations may be part of an ectodermal dysplasia syndrome.

PATHOPHYSIOLOGY AND HISTOGENESIS

Embryogenesis is regulated by a number of complex signaling cascades, which are critical for normal development. Modern molecular genetics will elucidate the basic defects of the different syndromes and will lead to greater insight into the regulatory mechanisms of embryology. In this way a reclassification of ectodermal dysplasias will be possible. HOX homeobox genes exhibit spatial and temporal changes in expression during human skin development.[5] Recent data underline the complexity of the field, and document that genes related to a family of homeobox-containing transcription factor genes are involved in ectodermal dysplasia because of their crucial role in organ development.[6] McGrath et al.[7] have shown that mutations in the plakophilin 1 gene result in ectodermal dysplasia/skin fragility syndrome and it has been speculated that plakophilin 1 is important in cell–cell adhesion functions and in epidermal morphogenesis. It has been speculated that the gene of hypohidrotic ectodermal dysplasia is an important target for regulatory signals during epithelial morphogenesis that result in the formation of appendages.[8]

The concept of interaction of all germ layers within organ fields during embryogenesis may explain the abnormalities in the mesoderm and endoderm in patients with ectodermal malformations.[9] Complex phenotypes with features of ectodermal dysplasia are progressively explained by molecular causative defects. Causative genes for ectodermal dysplasias can be divided in proteins highly expressed in ectodermal derivatives (EDA1, DL), helicase proteins involved in DNA replication and repair (ERCC2,3), nuclear proteins which act as transcription factors (TRPS1), proteins important for nuclear functions (DKC1) and keratin proteins.[10]

X-LINKED HYPOHIDROTIC ECTODERMAL DYSPLASIA (CHRIST–SIEMENS–TOURAINE SYNDROME)

INTRODUCTION AND HISTORICAL NOTE

X-linked hypohidrotic ectodermal dysplasia was first described by Thurman in 1848 and then by Charles Darwin in 1875.

EPIDEMIOLOGY

X-linked hypohidrotic ectodermal dysplasia (MIM 305100, Freire-Maia A 1-2-3-4) is the most common of the ectodermal dysplasias. However, autosomal dominant[11] and autosomal recessive forms[12] have been described. The clinical features are indistinguishable among the different types of inheritance.

PRESENTING HISTORY AND PHYSICAL EXAMINATION

The disorder is characterized by hypotrichosis with fine, slow-growing scalp and body hair, sparse eyebrows, hypohidrosis, nail anomalies, and hypodontia. Peg-shaped primary and secondary teeth are typical features (Fig. 7.1). Abnormal crown formation and taurodontism are commonly seen radiologically. Decreased sweating leads to heat intolerance and enhances the dryness of the skin (Table 7.3). Sybert and coworkers[13] emphasized that scaling red skin in the neonate might be an important clue to early diagnosis of hypohidrotic ectodermal dysplasia. Affected children characteristically show heat intolerance with episodes of hyperpyrexia, which may result in seizures and neurologic damage. In general, silicone rubber plastic imprints for sweat pore counts, quantitative pilocarpine iontophoresis to determine sweat ability, and skin biopsy for gland structure evaluation are not necessary for establishing the diagnosis, but such methods enable a quantitative assessment of disease activity, the best objective investigations if necessary. Affected persons show a

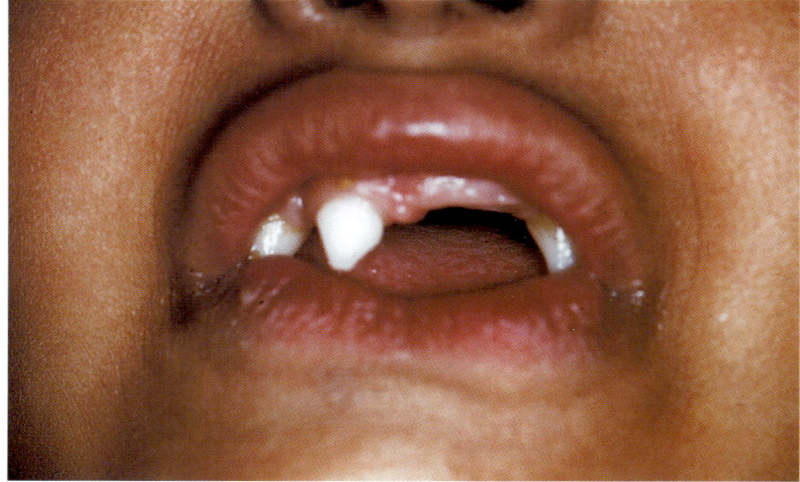

Fig. 7.1 Cone-shaped teeth in a boy with hypohidrotic ectodermal dysplasia.

6. Thesleff I (1996) Two genes for missing teeth. **Nature Genet** 13:379–380.
7. McGrath JA, McMillan JR, Shemanko CS et al. (1997) Mutations in the plakophilin 1 gene result in ectodermal dysplasia/skin fragility syndrome. **Nat Genet** 17:240–244.
8. Kere J, Srivastara AK, Montonen O et al. (1996) X-linked anhidrotic (hypohidrotic) ectodermal dysplasia is caused by mutation in a novel transmembrane protein. **Nat Genet** 13:409–416.
9. De Robertis EM, Larrain J, Oelgeschlager M, Wessely O (2000) The establishment of Spemann's organizer and patterning of the vertebrate embryo. **Nature Rev Genet** 1:171–181.
10. Priolo M, Sclengo M, Lerone M, Ravazzolo R (2000) Ectodermal dysplasias: not only "skin" deep. **Clin Genet** 58:415–430.

11. Ho L, Williams MS, Spritz RA (1999) A gene for autosomal dominant hypohidrotic ectodermal dysplasia (EDA3) maps to chromosome 2q11–q13. **Am J Hum Genet** 62:1102–1106.
12. Munoz F, Lestringant G, Sybert V et al. (1997) Definitive evidence for an autosomal recessive form of hypohidrotic ectodermal dysplasia clinically indistinguishable from more common X-linked disorder. **Am J Hum Genet** 61:94–100.
13. Sybert VP (1989) Scaling skin in the neonate: a clue to the early diagnosis of X-linked hypohidrotic ectodermal dysplasia (Christ-Siemens-Touraine sundrome). **J Pediatr** 114:600–602.

TABLE 7.3 Clinical features in patients with autosomal dominant hypohidrotic ectodermal dysplasia

Smooth, dry skin	78%
Sparse hair	89%
Sparse eyebrows	100%
Sparse body hair	62%
Decreased sweating	85%
Heat intolerance	50%
Onychodysplasia	39%
Dental anomalies	100%

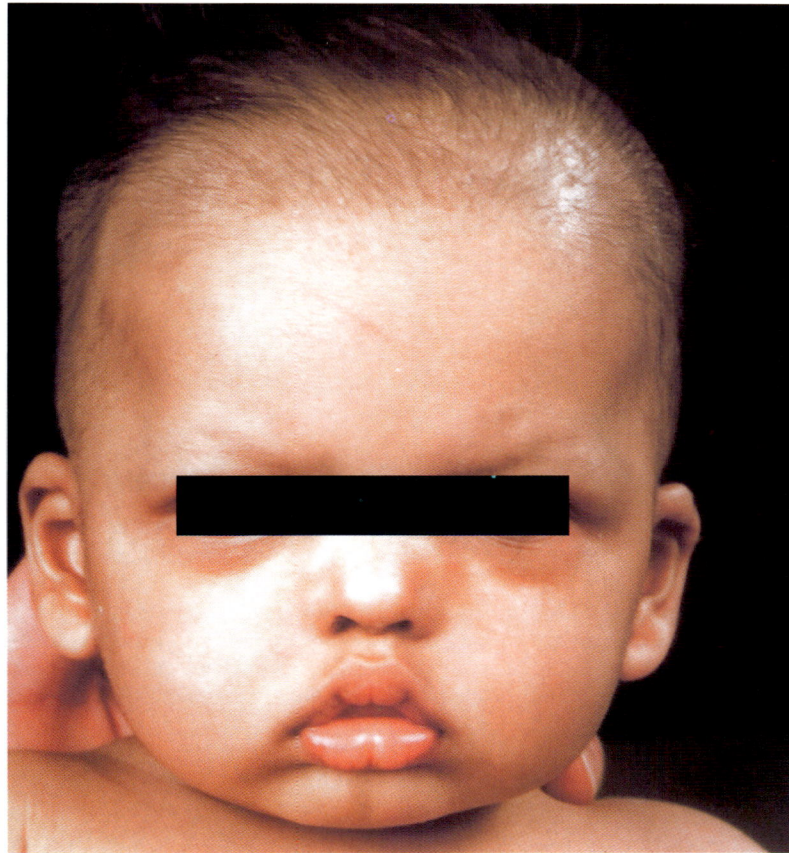

Fig. 7.2 Frontal bossing and large lips in a boy with hypohidrotic ectodermal dysplasia.

distinctive facies with frontal bossing, depressed nasal bridge with a saddle nose and large lower lips (Fig. 7.2). During childhood affected males may have problems with atopic dermatitis, periorbital hyperpigmentation, chronic rhinitis, and frequent respiratory infections. Sometimes extensive sebaceous hyperplasia with multiple papules is noted. Corneal and lenticular opacities and conductive hearing loss are also rare. However, absence of lacrimal puncta is a characteristic finding.

The hair is sparse, dry and lusterless with light color. Rogers[14] suggested that the bar code appearance, which mirrors the microscopic appearance, is often seen in patients with hypohidrotic ectodermal dysplasia. Parallel dark bands of different lengths run across the full width of the shaft. Scanning electron microscopy studies shows follicular distortion, follicular ridging, and distorted bulbs but these findings are nonspecific. Loose anagen hair has been observed.[15] The clinical findings in mosaic carriers of hypohidrotic ectodermal dysplasia have recently been delineated;[16,17] the most impressive finding is the distribution of normal and abnormal skin along Blaschko lines in heterozygous and postzygotic mutation carriers of the X-linked form.

PATHOPHYSIOLOGY AND HISTOGENESIS

Reduced epidermal growth factor receptor number in X-linked hypohidrotic epidermal dysplasia and in the mouse model "Tabby" has been found;[18] but sweat glands are inducible by epidermal growth factor in the murine model of X-linked hypohidrotic ectodermal dysplasia.[19] The human gene maps to Xq12–q13.1 and affects a transmembrane protein which is expressed by keratinocytes, hair follicles and sweat glands. The gene responsible for the autosomal dominant hypohidrotic ectodermal dysplasia has been mapped to chromosome 2q11–q13;[11] clinical findings are shown in Table 7.3. Mutations in the human homolog of mouse downless (dl) gene cause autosomal recessive and dominant hypohidrotic forms of ectodermal dysplasia.[20] The protein has a single transmembrane domain and shows parallels to two separate domains of the tumor necrosis factor receptor (TNFR) family. A novel X-linked disorder of immune deficiency and hypohidrotic ectodermal dysplasia has been described recently and was found to be allelic to incontinentia pigmenti and due to mutations in inhibitory protein of kappaB kinase (IKK)-gamma (nuclear factor–kappaB essential modulator; NEMO).[21] A new subtype of hypohidrotic ectodermal dysplasia with osteopetrosis and lymphoedema results from impaired NF-κB signaling, just as does anhidrotic ectodermal dysplasia and immunodeficiency.[22] The NF-κB transcription factor has an important role in the immune and inflammatory responses, as well as in the control of apoptosis.

TABLE 7.4 Complications of hypohidrotic ectodermal dysplasia

First year	
Mortality	9/43 (21%)
Severe non-fatal illness	14/49 (29%)
Total episodes of severe illness	25/58 (43%)
Years 0–3	
Mortality in years 0–3	12/43 (28%)
Severe non-fatal illness	18/51 (49%)
Total with episodes of severe illness	32/65 (49%)
Other complications in survivors	
Eczema	39/55 (71%)
Asthma or recurring wheezing	35/54 (65%)
Nasal crusting	42/53 (79%)
Recurrent fevers in infancy	27/50 (54%)
Recurrent upper respiratory tract infections in childhood	21/47 (44%)
Feeding problems in infancy	32/47 (68%)
Specific allergies	14/53 (26%)

14. Rogers M (2000) The "bar code phenomenon": a microscopic artifact seen in patients with hypohidrotic ectodermal dysplasia. **Pediatr Dermatol** 17:329–330.
15. Azón-Masoliver A, Ferrando J (1996) Loose anagen hair syndrome in hypohidrotic ectodermal dysplasia. **Pediatr Dermatol** 13:29–32.
16. Happle R, Frosch PJ (1985) Manifestations of the lines of Blaschko in women heterozygous for X-linked hypohidrotic ectodermal dysplasia. **Clin Genet** 27:468–471.
17. Cambiaghi S, Restano L, Paakonen K et al. (2000) Clinical findings in mosaic carriers of hypohidrotic ectodermal dysplasia. **Arch Dermatol** 136:217–224.
18. Vargas GA, Fantino E, George-Nascinento C et al. (1996) Reduced epidermal growth factor receptor expression in hypohidrotic ectodermal dysplasia and Tabby mice. **J Clin Invest** 97:2426–2432.
19. Blecher SR, Kapalanga J, Lalonde D (1990) Induction of sweat glands by epidermal growth factor in murine X-linked anhidrotic ectodermal dysplasia. **Nature** 345:542–544.
20. Monreal AW, Ferguson BM, Headon DJ et al. (1999) Mutations in the human homologue of mouse dl cause autosomal recessive and dominant hypohidrotic ectodermal dysplasia. **Nat Genet** 22:366–369.
21. Zonana J, Elder ME, Schneider LC et al. (2000) A novel X-linked disorder of immune deficiency and hypohidrotic ectodermal dysplasia is allelic to incontinentia pigmenti and due to mutations in IKK-gamma (NEMO). **Am J Hum Genet** 67:1555–1562.
22. Döffinger R, Smahin A, Bessia C et al. (2001) X-linked anhidrotic ectodermal dysplasia with immunodeficiency is caused by impaired NF-kB signaling. **Nature Genet** 27:277–285.

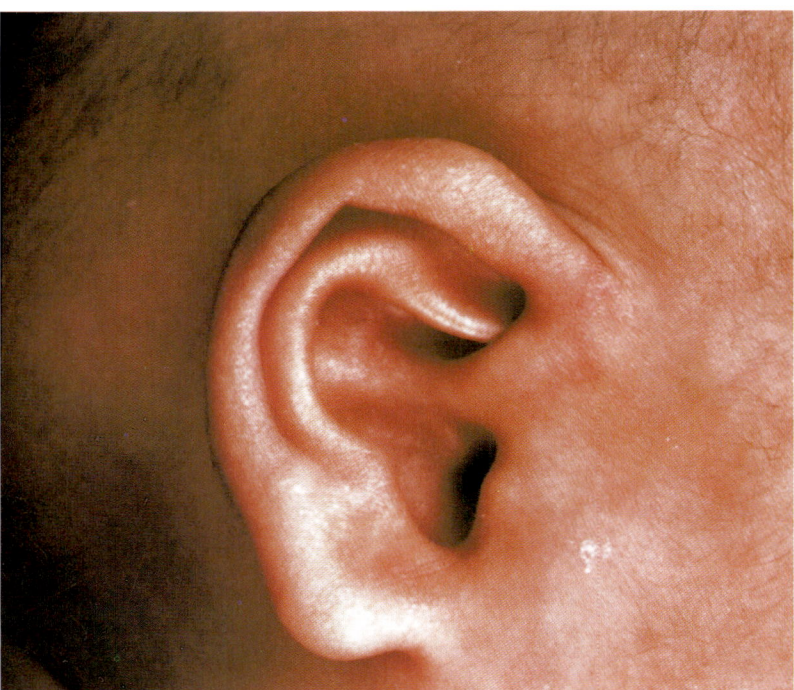

Fig. 7.3   Typical ear deformation in a boy with hypohidrotic extodermal dysplasia.

THERAPEUTICS AND PROGNOSIS

Treatment needs a multidisciplinary approach. Early diagnosis is imperative to avoid life-threatening complications induced by hyperthermia and infections. Zankl *et al.*[23] reported a fatal outcome in a female monozygotic twin with X-linked hypohidrotic ectodermal dysplasia (XLHED) due to a *de novo* t(X;9) translocation with probable disruption of the EDA gene. Autopsy revealed that lack of normal tracheobronchial secretions led to complete tracheal obstruction by mucous debris which was the probable cause of death. Avoiding heat and physical overexertion is the most important prevention and cooling the body with wet clothing, cool drinks and, if available, cooling suits is the only efficient way of treating hyperthermia. Antipyretics are of no effect. Retinoids are not tolerated in patients with hypohidrotic ectodermal dysplasia because of exacerbating dryness and irritation of the skin. Orthodontic intervention with dentures is necessary particularly in those patients for language development, mastication and cosmesis. Meticulous dental hygiene should be taught to the children, as caries develop early. Dental implants have been advocated for older teenagers and adults. Artificial tears and use of moisturizers may add to the patient's comfort. Crusting of the nose is treated by moisturizing nose-creams and intermittent mupirocin topically. Air-conditioned home and school environments are mandatory for these patients. The National Foundation for Ectodermal Dysplasias (NFED) can supply the clinician with excellent reference and patient education materials (see page 9).

HIDROTIC ECTODERMAL DYSPLASIA (CLOUSTON'S SYNDROME)

INTRODUCTION AND HISTORICAL NOTE

Most cases of Clouston's syndrome are also called hidrotic ectodermal dysplasia; initially, most cases were described in French-Canadian families, however, other ethnic groups have also been affected.

EPIDEMIOLOGY

Hidrotic ectodermal dysplasia (MIM 129500, Freire-Maia A, 1-2-3) is a rare autosomal dominant inherited disease defined by generalized hypotrichosis, dystrophic nails and palmoplantar keratoderma.[24]

PRESENTING HISTORY AND PHYSICAL FINDINGS

Reticulated macular or diffuse hyperpigmentation may occur. The skin may be thickened and hyperpigmented over knees, elbows, fingers and knuckles with mild keratoderma (Fig. 7.5). Nails appear thickened and shortened on a bulbous fingertip. Ocular abnormalities include strabismus, pterygium, conjunctivitis, and premature cataracts. The teeth are often normal but caries are rather common. Additional ectodermal abnormalities may be oral leukoplakia, sensorineural hearing loss, polydactyly, syndactyly, and diffuse

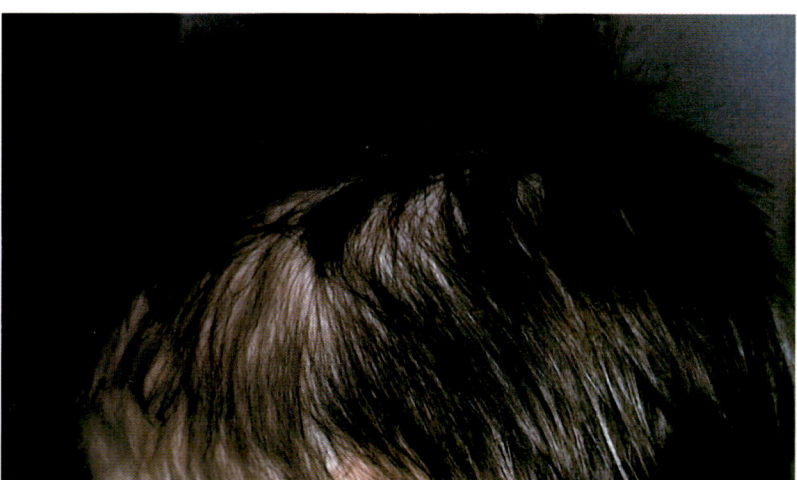

Fig. 7.4   Dry, sparse hair in a boy with hypohidrotic ectodermal dysplasia.

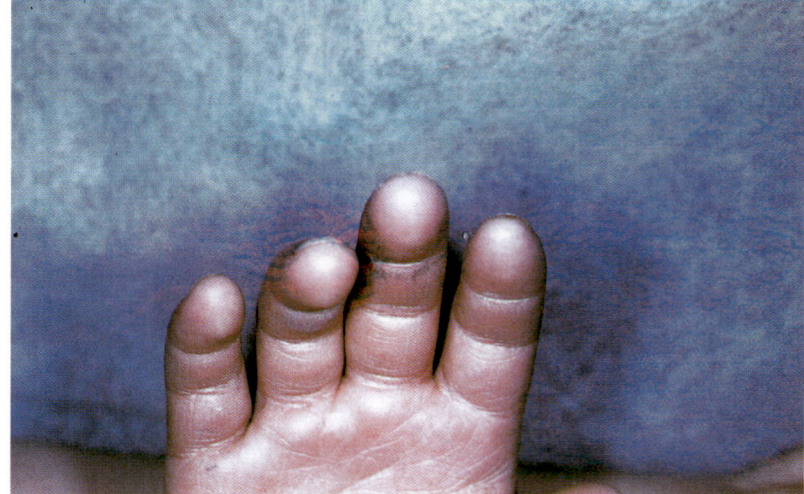

Fig. 7.5   Mild keratoderma in hidrotic ectodermal dysplasia.

23. Zankl A, Addor MC, Cousin P et al. (2001) Fatal outcome in a female monozygotic twin with X-linked hypohidrotic ectodermal dysplasia (XLHED) due to a de novo t(X;9) translocation with probalbe disruption of the EDA gene. **Eur J Pediatr** 160:296–299.

24. Gold RJ, Scriver CR (1972) Properties of hair keratin in an autosomal dominant form of ectodermal dysplasia. **Am J Hum Genet** 24:549–561.

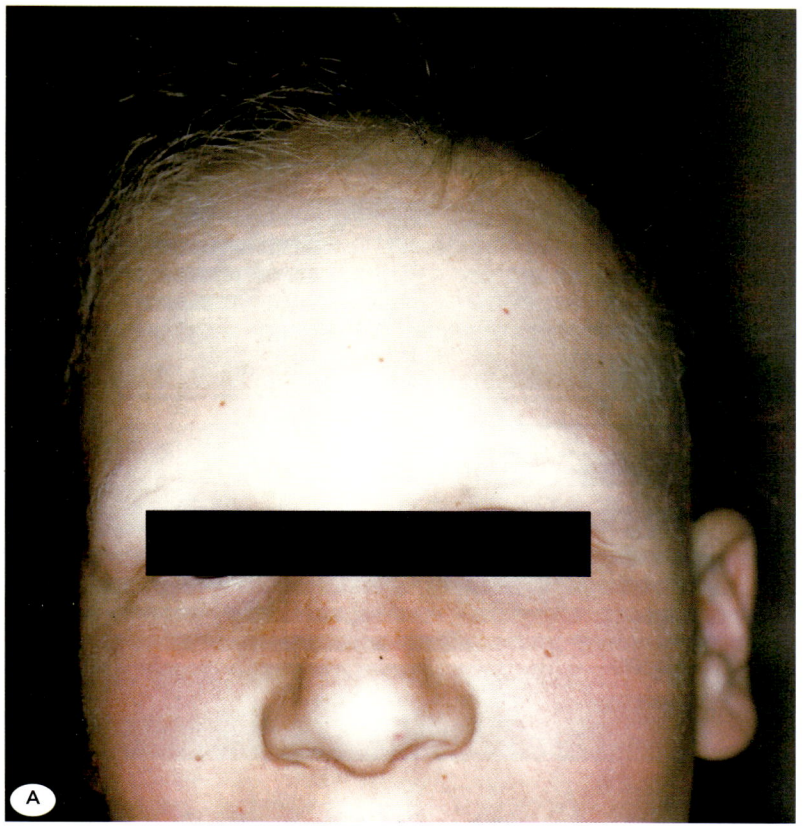
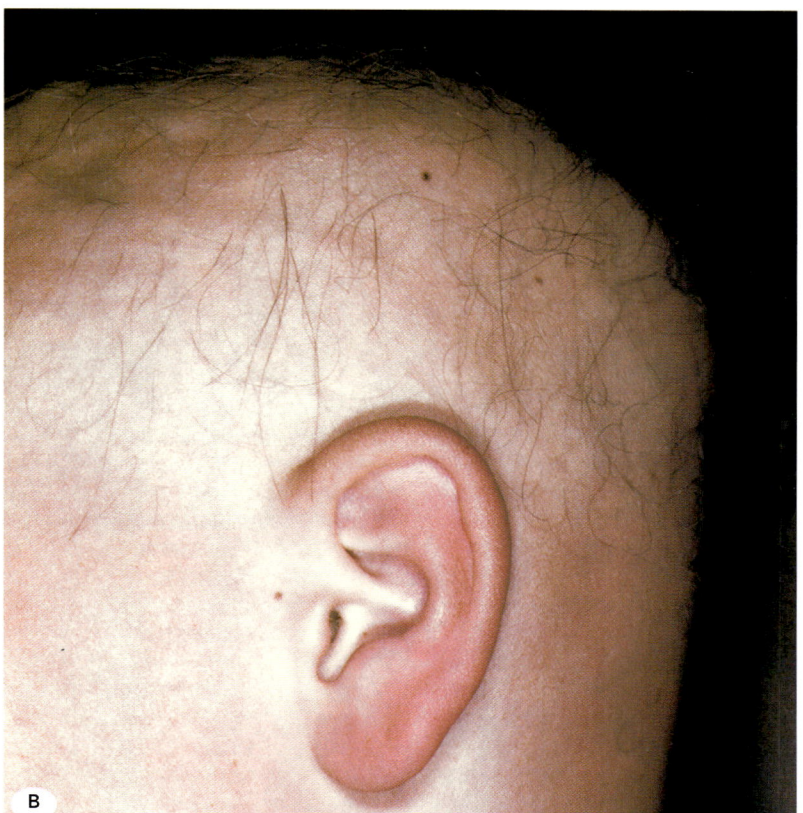

Fig. 7.6   Marked hypotrichosis in a patient with hidrotic ectodermal dysplasia.

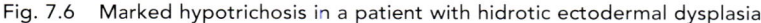

eccrine poromatosis. In contrast to the hypohidrotic form most of the patients have normal sweating and normal function of sebaceous glands. Scalp hair is sparse and brittle with pale color. Hair loss may be progressive and total alopecia can occur. (Fig. 7.6).

PATHOPHYSIOLOGY AND HISTOGENESIS

Ultrastructural investigations of keratoderma show an increased number of desmosomal discs in the thickened stratum corneum, suggesting that hyperkeratosis observed in Clouston's syndrome is due to delayed desquamation. Gold and Scriver[23] described low disulfide-bonded protein content, reduced tensile strength and decreased birefringence when the hair shafts were examined under polarized light. The hair shaft is twisted and grooved as an expression of pilary dysplasia. Eyebrows and eyelashes are thin or absent. The body hair is also sparse. Nail dystrophy is common with short and thickened slow growing and discolored nail plates. Persistent malodorous onychomycosis and squamous cell carcinoma of the nail beds have developed in adults with the syndrome. Lamartine et al.[25] confirmed earlier reports of linkage of Clouston's syndrome to chromosome 13q11–q12.1 and found a mutation in connexin-30.

THERAPEUTICS AND PROGNOSIS

Treatment of plamoplantar keratoderma includes keratolytic agents such as salicylic acid ointment. Systemic retinoids are helpful, but require long-term usage. Careful dental prophylaxis, ocular lubrication and controlling onychomycosis are some of the important aspects in prophylaxis.

ECTRODACTYLY–ECTODERMAL DYSPLASIA–CLEFT LIP/PALATE SYNDROME, EEC SYNDROME

INTRODUCTION AND HISTORICAL NOTE

EEC syndrome was first described by Eckholdt and Matens in 1804 and subsequently further delineated. In 1970 Rüdiger et al.[26] suggested the designation EEC for the syndrome.

EPIDEMIOLOGY

EEC syndrome (MIM 129900 Freire-Maia A, 1-2-3) is an autosomal dominant trait involving ectodermal and mesodermal tissue. About 150 cases have been described.

PRESENTING HISTORY AND PHYSICAL EXAMINATION

The syndrome includes ectrodactyly (split hand or foot deformity, lobster-claw deformity), cleft lip/palate, hypotrichosis, hypodontia, dystrophic nails, eye duct anomalies, and sometimes hypohidrosis[27,28] (Table 7.5). Dental anomalies include microdontia and oligodontia with premature loss of secondary teeth. Caries are often severe. Marked scalp dermatitis may also occur early in the disease process, but occurs more commonly in patients with Rapp–Hodgkin disease or ankyloblepharon–ectodermal dysplasia–clefting;

25. Lamartine J, Munhoz Essenfelder G, Kubarz et al. (2000) Mutations in GJB6 cause hidrotic ectodermal dysplasia. **Nat Genet** 26:142–144.
26. Rüdiger RA, Haase W, Passarge E (1970) Association of ectrodactyly, ectodermal dysplasia and clefting-palate. **Am J Dis Child** 120:160–163.
27. Zlotogora J (1994) Syndactyly, ectodermal dysplasia, and cleft lip/palate. **J Med Genet** 31:957–959.
28. Buss PW, Hughes HE, Clarke A (1995) Twenty-four cases of the EEC syndrome: Clinical presentation and management. **J Med Genet** 32:716–723.

TABLE 7.5   Major and minor criteria for the diagnosis of EEC

Major criteria
Ectodermal dysplasia
Ectrodactyly
Cleft lip/palate
Lacrimal duct anomalies

Minor criteria
Renal anomalies
Deafness
Mental retardation
Choanal atresia

AEC syndrome.[29,30] Scarring folliculitis was observed in a 16-year-old boy by Trüeb *et al.*[31] and in this study reduced hair elasticity was documented, indicating either an abnormal composition or a disordered arrangement of microfibrils with in the apparently normal keratin matrix. Hair is affected in all cases and features light color with a coarse and dry appearance. Axillary and pubic hair may also be sparse.[32] A tendency for increased hair pigmentation with advancing age has been observed. The association with loose anagen hair syndrome has recently been described.[33] Buss *et al.*[28] found skin changes in 78%, particularly dry scaly skin on the extremities. Painful fissuring in interdigital webs and around the finger pads has been reported. Hypohidrosis may occur, but is relatively mild. Nails may be hypoplastic and dystrophic, even on the normal digits.

Ectrodactyly (lobster claw deformity) is a major feature of the disorder and occurs in 80–100%.[34] In more than 75% the anomaly shows tetramelic involvement. The digits most often involved in syndactyly are digits three and four. Radiography of hands and feet deformities reveal absent or hypoplastic metacarpals and metatarsals. Cleft palate with variable lip involvement occurs in 70–100%.[35] In the absence of cleft lip/palate patients have a typical facial morphology with maxillary hypoplasia, short philtrum, and broad nasal tip. Choanal atresia has been observed. Epiphora and recurrent infection with keratitis are commonly induced by nasolacrimal duct obstruction, Meibomian gland dysfunction, and overall reduced tear production. Almost half of the patients have some degree of conductive hearing loss. Mental retardation may occur in up to 5–10%. Genitourinary anomalies are rather common, including glandular hypospadias, ureteric reflux, and hydronephrosis. According to Buss *et al.*[28] the diagnosis of EEC should include ectodermal dysplasia of any variety and two of the additional major features: ectrodactylia, cleft lip/palate, and lacrimal duct abnormalities.

Treatment focuses on surgical correction of the cleft lip/palate, lacrimal duct, limb defects, and genitourinary malformations. In addition, chronic otitis media should be treated and impairment of hearing and speech should be diagnosed early to make intervention possible.

PATHOPHYSIOLOGY AND HISTOGENESIS

Patients with EEC syndrome ("EEC-1") have mutations in the p53 homolog p63 which is critical for maintaining the progenitor-cell populations that are necessary to sustain epithelial development and limb, craniofacial and epithelial morphogenesis.[36,37] A germline missense mutation in the p63 gene

underlying EEC syndrome has also recently been reported.[37] p63 is localized to chromosome 7q11.2–q21.3; other variants of EEC-1, EEC-2, and EEC-3, have been mapped to chromosome 19, and to chromosome 3q27, respectively.

THERAPEUTICS AND PROGNOSIS

Early recognition of EEC may lead to in a more effective intervention. Patients with the EEC syndrome often have ocular and auricular defects that progressively become more severe. These patients are often seen first by cleft palate teams. The patient's dental status requires frequent evaluation after corrective procedures for cleft lip and cleft palate.

HAY–WELLS SYNDROME, AEC SYNDROME, RAPP–HODGKIN SYNDROME

INTRODUCTION AND HISTORICAL NOTE

In 1976, Hay and Wells (MIM 106260, Freire-Maia A, 1-2-3-4) described a syndrome inherited in an autosomal dominant fashion with ankyloblepharon, ectodermal defects, and clefting of the lip and palate.[38] The disorder now is considered identical with Rapp–Hodgkin syndrome (MIM 129400, Freier-Maia 1-2-3-4), which was distinguished previously by lack of ankyloblepharon (Table 7.6).

TABLE 7.6   Clinical features of Rapp–Hodgkin syndrome

Craniofacial anomalies	Midfacial hypoplasia with high forehead, small mouth, narrow nose, short philtrum, short vermillon border of the upper lip
Cleft lip or palate	
Hypoplasia of the uvula	
Poor dentition:	Hypodontia, and conically shaped teeth
Poor hair growth:	Sparseness of eyebrows and eyelashes, pili torti, pili canaliculi
Dystrophic nails: chromonychia	Hypertrophy, brittleness, narrow,
Hypohidrosis	
Hypospadias in boys	
Other clinical features reported	
Erythrodermia and scaling skin at birth	
Short stature	
Low intellectual capacity	
Depapillated tongue	
Conductive hearing loss	
Hypoplastic maxilla	
Atretic ear canal	
Dysplastic eustachian orifices	
Ophthalmological complications:	Bilateral punctal atresia, underdevelopment of lacrimal ducts, corneal scarring

Adapted from Camacho *et al.*[33]

29. Fosko SW, Stenn KS, Bolognia JL (1992) Ectodermal dysplasias associated with clefting: significance of scalp dermatitis. **J Am Acad Dermatol** 27:249–256.
30. Trüeb RM, Bruckner-Tudoman L et al. (1995) Scalp dermatitis, distinctive hair abnormalities and atopic disease in the ectrodactyly-ectodermal dysplasia-clefting syndrome. **Br J Dermatol** 132:621–625.
31. Trüeb RM, Tsambaos D, Spycher MA et al. (1997) Scarring folliculitis in the ectrodactyly-ectodermal dysplasia-clefting syndrome. **Dermatology** 194:191–194.
32. Micali G, Cook B, Blekys I, Soloman LM (1990) Structural hair abnormalities in ectodermal dysplasia. **Pediatr Dermatol** 7:27–32.
33. Camacho F, Ferrando J, Pichardo AR et al. (1993) Rapp–Hodgkin syndrome with pili canaliculi. **Pediatr Dermatol** 10:54–57.

34. Roelfsema NM, Cobben JM (1996) The EEC syndrome: a literature study. **Clin Dysmorph** 5:115–127.
35. Fernandez B, Ruas E, Machado A et al. (2002) Ectrodactyly – ectodermal dysplasia-clefting syndrome (EEC): report of a case with perioral papillomatosis. **Pediatr Dermatol** 19:330–332.
34. Celli J, Duijf P, Hamel BC et al. (1999) Heterozygous germline mutations in the p53 homolog p63 are the cause of EEC syndrome. **Cell** 99:143–153.
36. Mills AA, Zheng B, Wang XJ et al. (1999) p63 is a p53 homologue required for limb and epidermal morphogenesis. **Nature** 398:708–713.
37. Wessagowit V, Mellerio JE Pernbroke AC, McGrath JA (2000) Heterozygous germline missense mutation in the p63 gene underlying EEC syndrome. **Clin Exp Dermatol** 25:441–443.
38. Mancini AJ, Paller AS (1997) What syndrome is this? Ankyloblepharon–ectodermal defects-cleft lip and palate (Hay–Wells) syndrome. **Pediatr Dermatol** 14:403–405.

EPIDEMIOLOGY

AEC/Rapp-Hodgkin syndrome is a rare, autosomal dominant trait with variable expressivity.

PRESENTING HISTORY AND PHYSICAL EXAMINATION

At birth about 90% of patients feature scaling and erythroderma.[40] In one series, 75% of patients had eroded skin at birth and 63% of patients continued to suffer from chronic scalp erosions and recurrent scalp infections.[41] Three of the seven initial patients had scalp infections or folliculitis of the scalp in association with hair loss. The scalp is commonly involved with severe and erosive dermatitis with secondary crusting and superinfection. Scalp hair is sparse, wiry, and often fair. Focal or diffuse scarring alopecia is common, with progression despite quiescence of the erosions and crusting. Patients have rudimentary eyelashes and the eyebrows are often also affected.

Ankyloblepharon or fusion of the eyelids, is an obligatory feature. In its mildest variant, there is a partial thickness fusion of the central portion of the eyelid margins with sparing of the canthi (ankyloblepharon filiforme adnatum). Conjunctivitis and blepharitis may also occur. The original family featured partial or complete hair loss, absent or dystrophic nails, widely spaced teeth and partial anhidrosis. Additional anomalies may include lacrimal duct atresia, supernummary nipples, syndactyly, and auricular deformities.

PATHOPHYSIOLOGY

Scanning electron microscopy shows defective cuticles of hair shaft. Investigation of sweat function reveals patchy loss of sweating. Nails may be hyperconvex and thickened, dystrophic or even absent. CHAND syndrome, with curly hair, ankyloblepharon, and nail disease, is most likely identical with AEC syndrome.[42] McGrath et al.[43] have shown that the syndrome is caused by heterozygous missense mutations in the SAM domain of p63. It appears that p63 gene mutations have highly pleiotropic effects, as the same alterations may also lead to EEC syndrome. Interestingly, in AEC syndrome patients the mutations gave rise to amino acid substitutions in the sterile alpha motif domain. However, in EEC syndrome mutations were found as amino acid substitutions in the DNA-binding domain.

THERAPEUTICS AND PROGNOSIS

Treatment includes ophthalmological correction, application of emollients and scalp care. In addition surgical intervention of cleft lip and palate is necessary. No intervention prevents the progressive cicatricial hair loss, although chronic administration of antistaphyloccocal antibiotics is most helpful.

DYSKERATOSIS CONGENITA (ZINSSER–COLE–ENGMAN SYNDROME)

INTRODUCTION AND HISTORICAL NOTE

Dyskeratosis congenita is a multisystem disease leading to reticulate skin pigmentation, nail dystrophy and leukoplakia with hematological abnormalities. The different aspects were described by Zinsser in 1906, Engman in 1926 and Cole in 1930.

EPIDEMIOLOGY

Dyskeratosis congenita (Freire-Maia A, 1-2-3-4) is a genetically heterogeneous disease. Three different types of inheritance patterns have been documented:[44]

most cases belong to the X-linked forms (MIM 305000) but autosomal recessive (MIM 22430) and autosomal dominant forms (MIM 127550) have also been described. Knight and coworkers[45] have recently summarized the clinical features of 83 patients from 46 families, allowing prevalence data based on physical findings in patients with dyskeratosis congenita.

PRESENTING HISTORY AND PHYSICAL EXAMINATION

Dyskeratosis congenita is a rare genodermatosis with three main cutaneous features: reticulated pigmentation, dystrophy of the nails, and leukoplakia of the mucous membranes (Fig. 7.7). Additional important findings are continuous lacrimation due to atresia of the lacrimal ducts, pancytopenia and in many cases testicular atrophy. The classical findings appear usually between 4 and 10 years of age.

The dermatological findings are the most consistent features (Tables 7.7 and 7.8). Reticulate grayish-brown skin pigmentation with some atrophy and telangiectases most commonly affects the great flexures such as neck, upper

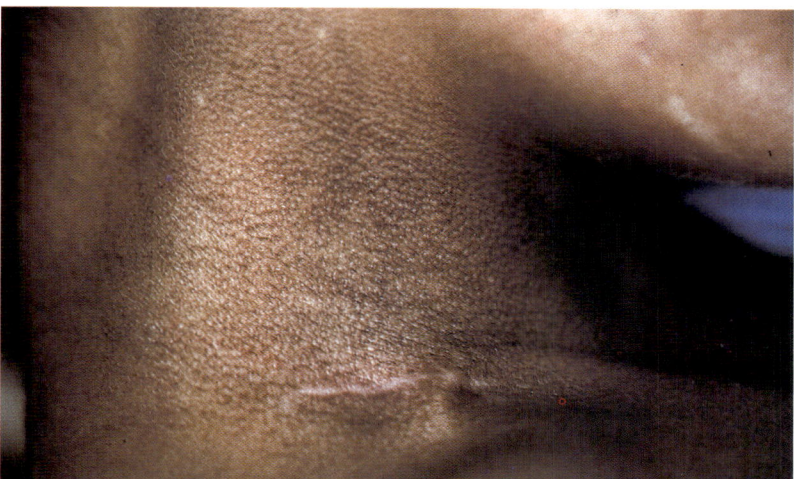

Fig. 7.7 Reticulate pigmentation on the neck in a patient with dyskeratosis congenita.

TABLE 7.7 Somatic abnormalities and complications in families with dyskeratosis congenita with affected males (73 cases)

Somatic abnormality	Number of patients (%)
Pancytopenia	48/61 (79%)
Epiphora	26 (36%)
Learning difficulties/mental retardation	15 (21%)
Pulmonary disease	14 (19%)
Hyperhidrosis	14 (19%)
Extensive caries/dental loss	13 (18%)
Short stature	12 (16%)
Hair loss/grey hair or sparse eyelashes	12 (16%)
Oesophageal stricture	10 (14%)
Hypogonadism/undescended testes	6 (8%)
Urethral strictures/phimoses	5 (7%)
Malignancy	4 (5%)
Liver cirrhosis/adenoma	4 (5%)
Abnormal bone trabeculation/osteoporosis	3 (4%)

Adapted from Knight et al.[45]

39. Fistoral SK, Itin PH (2002) Nail changes in genodermatoses. **Eur J Dermatol** 12:119–128.
40. Drut R, Pollano D, Drut RM (2002) Bilateral nephroblastoma in familial Hay-Wells syndrome associated with familial reticulate pigmentation of the skin. **Am J Med Genet** 10:164–169.
41. Vanderhooft SL, Stephan MJ, Sybert VP (1993) Severe skin erosions and scalp infections in AEC syndrome. **Pediatr Dermatol** 10:334–340.
42. Bertola DR, Kim CA, Sugayama SM et al. (2000) AEC syndrome and CHAND syndrome: further evidence of clinical overlapping in the ectodermal dysplasias. **Pediatr Dermatol** 17:218–221.
43. McGrath JA, Duijf PN, Doetsch V et al. (2001) Hay–Wells syndrome is caused by heterozygous missense mutations in the SAM domain of p63. **Hum Mol Genet** 10:221–229.
44. Drachtman RA, Alter BP (1992) Dyskeratosis congenita: clinical and genetic heterogeneity. Report of a new case and review of the literature. **Am J Pediatr Hematol Oncol** 14:297–304.
45. Knight S Vulliany T, Copplestone A et al. (1998) Dyskeratosis congenita (DC) registry: identification of new features of DC. **Br J Haematol** 103:990–996.

TABLE 7.8   Somatic abnormalities/complications in dyskeratosis congenita families with affected males only (n = 118)

Abnormality	% of patients
Abnormal skin pigmentation	89.0%
Nail dystrophy	88.0%
Bone marrow failure	85.5%
Leukoplakia	78.0%

Adapted from Dokal[83]

TABLE 7.9   Hematological complications in dyskeratosis congenita families with affected males only

Hematological abnormality	% of patients
Pancytopenia	76.3%
Thrombocytopenia only	6.6%
Leukopenia only	2.6%
No cytopenia	14.5%

Adapted from Dokal[83]

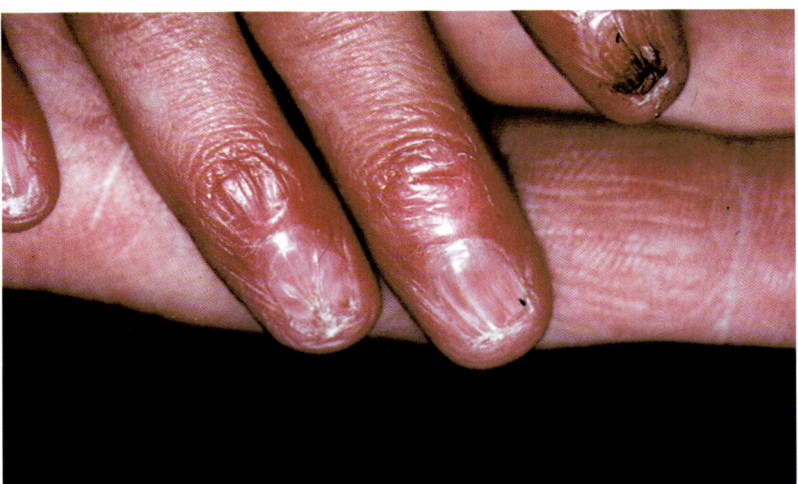

Fig. 7.8   Dystrophic nails in a patient with dyskeratosis congenita.

chest, upper arms.[46] Sometimes interspersed zones of hypopigmentation occur. The cutaneous features occur within the first years of life. Baselga et al.[47] described a patient with typical pigmentation with superimposed linear hyperpigmentation following the lines of Blaschko. This phenomenon was explained by an autosomal dominant inheritance pattern and loss of heterozygosity which occurred in a postzygotic cell giving rise to a population of cells that migrated along these lines during embryogenesis.

Nail dystrophy is found in 98% of patients, usually during the first year of life, and is characterized by longitudinal grooves, thinned nails, or nearly complete atrophy of nails with pterygium formation (Fig 7.8).[39] Loss of dermatoglyphics is characteristic and mirrors the complex ectodermal dysplasia.

Leukokeratosis has been found in about 85% of patients and can occur on the tongue, buccal mucosa, conjunctiva, vagina, rectum, gastrointestinal tract, or genitourinary tract. These lesions usually appear later than the other skin manifestations. Additional dermatologic manifestations include palmoplantar keratoderma, hyperhidrosis of the palms and soles, bullae formation after minor traumas, premature graying of hair, alopecia, and dental anomalies associated with periodontitis. The onset of skin and nail changes in the autosomal dominant form is later and the life expectancy is better.

Epiphora and conjunctivitis with blepharitis as a result of hyperplasia of the epithelial layers occur commonly. Hematological abnormalities occur in 51% of the patients before the age of 10 years and in 34% between 11 and 20 years (Table 7.9). Twelve percent of patients with dyskeratosis congenital develop pancytopenia within 21–30 years and only 2% feature pancytopenia after the age of 30.[45] The earliest sign may be either anemia or thrombocytopenia. Pancytopenia may lead to bleeding and severe infections and death before the age of 40 years. In the study by Knight et al.[45] 93% had peripheral cytopenia and in 71% bone marrow failure was the principal cause of early mortality. Restrictive pulmonary disease rarely develops.

Increased susceptibility to malignancy beginning in the third decade of life is characteristic for almost half of the patients. Squamous cell carcinomas arising from leukoplakia are most common,[48] but Hodgkin's lymphoma are also more prevalent in these patients.[49,50]

PATHOPHYSIOLOGY AND HISTOGENESIS

A gene for dyskeratosis congenita (DKC1) has been assigned to the q28 region of the X chromosome. The gene encodes a 514-amino-acid protein, dyskerin, that is homologous to Saccharomyces cerevisiae Cbf5p and rat Nap57 proteins. Knight and colleagues[51] showed that X-linked dyskeratosis congenita is predominantly caused by missense mutations. Interestingly, incontinentia pigmenti has been mapped to the same locus, but its inheritance pattern, and the mutated gene itself differs, so the conditions are not allelic.[52] The gene has been cloned, showing a nuclear function and a role in the cell cycle.[53] Mitchell and coworkers[54] showed that a telomerase component is defective in dyskeratosis congenita. In addition, impaired DNA repair has been documented in a case of dyskeratosis congenita.[55] Chromosomal instability and T-cell immunodeficiency have also been described, both of which predispose to malignant degeneration. p53 expression seems to be a reliable marker for prediction of premalignant change in the keratoses occurring in dyskeratosis congenita.[56]

THERAPEUTICS AND PROGNOSIS

Treatment should include monitoring of leukoplakias and hematologic counts. Systemically administered retinoids may have a protective effect against neoplasia. Pancytopenia is treated with transfusions and occasionally with androgenic hormones. Granulocyte colony-stimulating factors and bone marrow transplantation have been performed with variable results.[57] As patients have an increased risk for mucosal and cutaneous malignancy, education regarding general risk factors, such as smoking and excessive sun exposure, must be given. Endoscopic screening for possible esophageal or rectal lesions should be initiated in the third decade of life. It should be

46. Itin PH, Lautenschlager S (1998) Genodermatosis with reticulate, patchy and mottled pigmentation of the neck – a clue to rare dermatologic disorders. **Dermatology** 197:281–290.
47. Baselga E, Drolet BA, van Tuinen P et al. (1998) Dyskeratosis congenita with linear areas of severe cutaneous involvement. **Am J Med Genet** 75:492–496.
48. Moretti S, Spallanzani A, Chiarugi A et al. (2000) Oral carcinoma in a young man: a case of dyskeratosis congenita. **J Europ Acad Dermatol Venereol** 14:123–125.
49. Salinas CF, Montes-G GM (1988) Rapp-Hodgkin syndrome: observations on ten cases and characteristic hair changes (pili canaliculi). **Birth Defects** 24:149–168.
50. Baykal C, Bükükbabani N, Kavak A (1998) Dyskeratosis congenita associated with Hodgkin's disease. **Eur J Dermatol** 8:385–387.
51. Knight SW, Heiss NS, Vulliany TJ et al. (1999) X-linked dyskeratosis congenita is predominantly caused by missense mutations in the DKC1 gene. **Am J Hum Genet** 65:50–58.
52. Heiss NS, Poustka A, Knight SW et al. (1999) Mutation analysis of the DKC1 gene in incontinentia pigmenti. **J Med Genet** 36:860–862.
53. Heiss NS, Knight SW, Vulliany TJ et al. (1998) X-linked dyskeratosis congenita is caused by mutations in a highly conserved gene with putative nucleolar functions. **Nature Genet** 19:32–38.
54. Mitchell JR, Wood E, Collins K (1999) A telomerase component is defective in the human disease dyskeratosis congenita. **Nature** 402:551–555.
55. Mazereeuw-Hautier J, Cayrol-Baudouin C, Lachgars et al. (1999) A case of dyskeratosis congenita associated with impaired DNA repair as shown by the comet assay. **Eur J Dermatol** 9:529–532.
56. Ogden GR, Lane DP, Chisholm DM (1993) p53 expression in dyskeratosis congenita: a marker for oral premalignancy? **J Clin Pathol** 46:169–170.

emphasized that irradiation should not be used in the preparative regimen for bone marrow transplantation. Death may result from pancytopenia, malignancy, opportunistic pneumonitis, bronchiolitis obliterans, viral infections, and bleeding in the gut.

Guide to information for families with ectodermal dysplasias

National Foundation for Ectodermal Dysplasia (NFED)
410 East Main, Box 114
Mascoutah, IL 62258-0114
(618) 566 2020
Fax: (618) 566 4718
E-mail: nfed1@aol.com
http://www.nfed.org

INCONTINENTIA PIGMENTI (BLOCH–SULZBERGER)

INTRODUCTION AND HISTORICAL NOTE

Incontinentia pigmenti (IP) (MIM 308310) is characterized by linear cutaneous manifestations following the lines of Blaschko, as well as a variety of systemic problems. The disease was first described by Garrod in 1906 and Bloch further delineated the symptom complex. Subzberger reported Bloch's original patient in greater detail and added the histopathological features. Haber emphasized the multiphasic and multisystemic spectrum of the disease and suggested the eponym Bloch–Sulzberger syndrome.[58,59]

EPIDEMIOLOGY AND GENETICS

By 1987, more than 700 cases had been reported. IP is a genetic disease that segregates as an X-linked dominant disorder and is usually lethal prenatally in males. Therefore 98% of affected patients are female. Several male patients with IP have been described. Four patients had the Kleinfelter genotype. Other boys with limited to more extensive involvement probably had postzygotic mosaicism, although other theories have been proposed.[60]

Linkage analysis in 16 families with IP confirmed the gene locus Xq28.[61] Further studies documented that IP is caused by mutations in the NEMO gene,[62,63] with approximately 70% of mutations involving deletion of the same region. NEMO is required for activation of the transcription factor NF-κB and is therefore central to many immune, inflammatory and apoptotic pathways. A novel X-linked disorder of immune deficiency and hypohidrotic ectodermal dysplasia was found to be allelic to IP and due to mutations elsewhere in NEMO.[21]

PRESENTING HISTORY AND PHYSICAL FINDINGS

IP is a multisystemic disorder that affects tissues and organs derived from embryonic neurectoderm. Eighty percent of patients have systemic manifestations including neurologic, ocular, dental and skeletal abnormalities. Dermatologic findings are specific, diagnostic, and are present in more than 96% of familial cases. Classically the dermatological features are described in four stages. However, not all stages necessarily occur and several stages may overlap.[64] The skin changes are distributed along the lines of Blaschko and the cutaneous lesions in the different stages are characterized as follows:

- Stage 1: erythema, vesicles, and pustules.
- Stage 2: papules, verrucous lesions, and hyperkeratosis.
- Stage 3: hyperpigmentation.
- Stage 4: hypopigmentation, atrophy, and scarring.

In a study of 41 patients, lesions were present at birth in 71.7% and by the second week of life in 87.1%.[65] In this study 90.9% had blisters on an erythematous background and 84.2% developed hyperkeratotic lesions. Hyperpigmentation occurred in 94.8% and hypopigmentation was rarer (9.7%). Secondary skin atrophy on the legs were found in 31%, alopecia of the scalp in 34.2% and nail alteration in 8%. However, in another study, nail changes were found in 40%.[64]

Stage 1 usually occurs within the first few weeks of life and is characterized by blisters or pustules that often occur on an erythematous base. Blisters may be found anywhere on the body, but they usually spare the face. Typically the bullous eruption appears at or soon after birth, often follows the lines of Blaschko, and respects the midline (Fig. 7.9). The blisters clear within weeks and sometimes may be followed by new eruptions. As a rule stage 1 clears by 4 months, although subsequent episodes of vesicobullous eruptions have been reported, even into adulthood.[65,66] During febrile attacks small blisters may recur following lines of Blaschko. The initial inflammatory stage is accompanied by marked infiltration of eosinophils into the epidermis; in the peripheral blood, eosinophils may account for up to 80% of the white cells (A. Paller, personal communication, 2001), sometimes with marked total

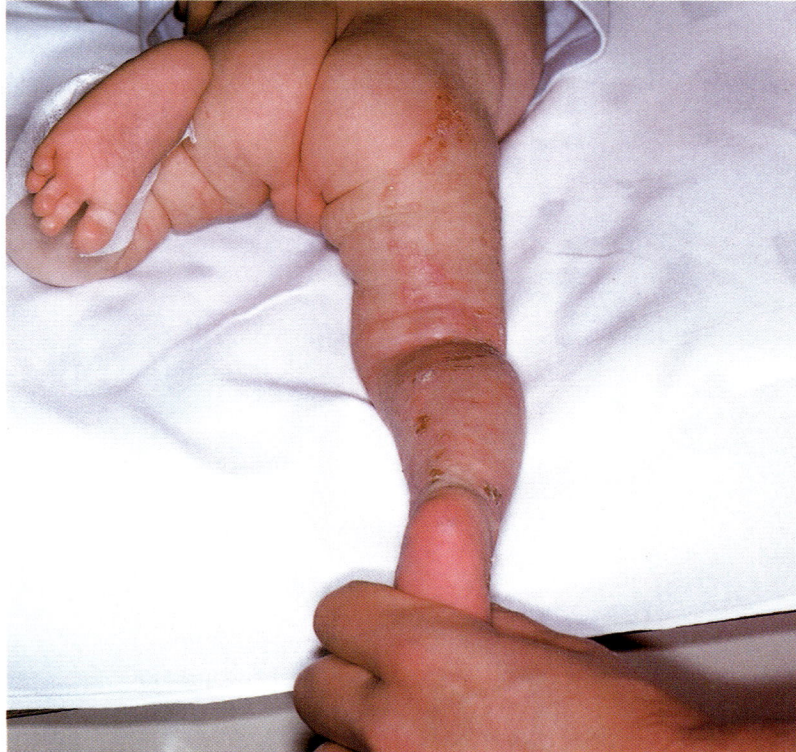

Fig. 7.9   Stage 1: Blistering eruption following the lines of Blaschko in a 4-week-old child.

57. Alter BP, Gardner FH, Hall RE (1997) Treatment of dyskeratosis congenita with granulocyte colony-stimulating factor and erythropoietin. **Br J Haematol** 97:309–311.
58. Carney RG (1976) Incontinentia pigmenti. A world statistical analysis. **Arch Dermatol** 112:535–542.
59. Gorski JI, Burright EN (1993) The molecular genetics of incontinentia pigmenti. **Sem Dermatol** 12:255–265.
60. Vehring KH, Kurleman G, Traupe H et al. (1993) Incontinentia pigmenti bei einem männlichen Säugling. **Hautarzt** 44:726–730.
61. Jouet M, Stewart H, Landy S et al. (1997) Linkage analysis in 16 families with incontinentia pigmenti. **Eur J Hum Genet** 5:168–170.

62. The International Incontinentia Pigmenti Consortium (2000) Genomic rearrangement in NEMO impairs NF-kappaB activation and is a cause of incontinentia pigmenti. **Nature** 405:466–472.
63. Shastry BS (2000) Recent progress in the genetics of incontinentia pigmenti (Bloch-Sulzberger syndrome). **J Hum Genet** 45:323–326.
64. Landy SJ, Donnai D (1993) Incontinentia pigmenti (Bloch–Sulzberger syndrome). **J Med Genet** 30:53–59.
65. Froidevaux D et al. (2000) Incontinentia pigmenti: 41 cas. **Ann Dermatol Venereol** 127 (Suppl.):4S14.
66. Van Leeuwen RL, Wintzen M, Van Praag MCG (2000) Incontinentia pigmenti: an extensive second episode of a "first-stage" vesicobullous eruption. **Pediatr Dermatol** 17:70.

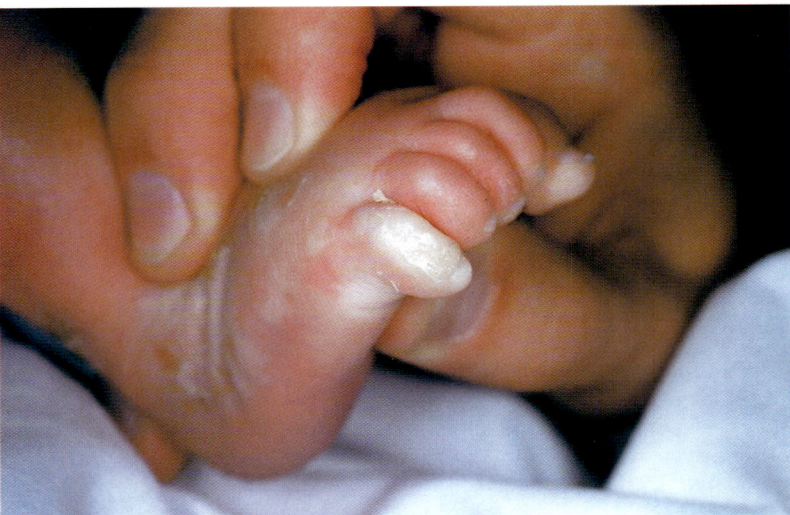

Fig. 7.10   Stage 2: Hyperkeratosis.

leukocytosis. The hyperkeratotic lesions of stage 2 may be present from an early time point (4-week old patient, Fig. 7.10). In general, they appear on the distal limbs, as the blistering starts to heal. The hyperkeratotic lesions clear totally by 6 months in more than 80% of cases.[64] However, Di Landro et al.[67] found warty linear streaks of the palm and sole as a possible late manifestation of IP in an 14-year-old girl and late subungual hyperkeratosis developed in a 10-year-old patient.[68]

Stage 3 is the most typical lesion of IP. Hyperpigmented streaks, especially on the trunk, follow whorls and lines of Blaschko. In some instances they correspond to the blisters and warty lesions; in others, the relationship is not obvious. The timing of appearance of the pigmentary lines varies remarkably.

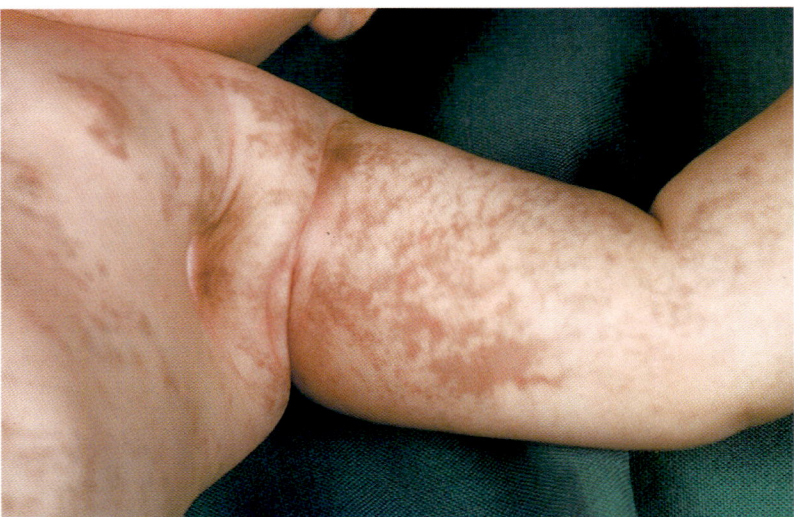

Fig. 7.11   Stage 3: Whorled and linear hyperpigmentations.

The hyperpigmentation fades and disappears by the end of the second decade.

Stage 4 occurs in the minority of patients with IP, with hypopigmented hairless patches or streaks especially on the lower legs.[69] These subtle alterations may be found in mothers of patients with IP not yet known to be affected.[70,71] In addition, focal absence of sweating is a typical hallmark of IP. Nails may show ridging and pitting as well as onychogryphosis-like changes. Subungual hyperkeratotic tumors may develop. Cicatricial alopecia on the vertex is common, and may be found as a residual sign of IP in older patients.

In addition to cutaneous abnormalities, ocular, dental, skeletal and neurological pathologies may occur in patients with IP. Ocular manifestations are often asymmetric and are observed in 20%[65] to 77% of patients.[72] Most characteristic are various retinal alterations that involve both the developing retinal vessels and the underlying pigment epithelium.[72] The following findings may be seen:

- Retinal ischemia
- Retinal neovascularization with bleeding, exudation
- Preretinal gliosis and tractional detachment of dysplastic retina
- Retinal mottling and hypopigmentation with detachment
- Optic atrophy and foveal hypoplasia
- Microphthalmos, cataracts, conjunctival pigmentation
- Corneal changes, iris hypoplasia, uveitis, phthisis
- Iris hypoplasia
- Nystagmus, strabismus, myopia
- Whorl-like epithelial keratitis.

In patients with IP, monthly screening during the first 6–12 months is recommended. Xenon photocoagulation or cryotherapy have been shown to be successful in causing regression of the neovascular changes in IP.

Neurologic features include seizures (often starting in the first week of life), spastic paralysis, mental and motor retardation and microcephaly. Reports of the frequency of neurological abnormalities are variable. Froideveaux et al.[65] found neurologic pathologies in 33.3% and psychomotor retardation in 19.5%. Mental retardation was found in 10.2% and hemiplegia in 5.1%. Landy and Donnai[64] in their series of 111 patients found 14% with seizures and 8% with mental retardation. Disappearance of white matter lesions in incontinentia pigmenti, similar to the fading of skin lesions, has been reported recently by Yoshikawa et al.[73] With high-resolution imaging such as MRI, several central nervous system abnormalities are found.[74]

Dental abnormalities occur in more than 80% of cases. These alterations may help in establishing the definite diagnosis of IP. Dental changes in IP, such as absent teeth, conical teeth with supplemental cups in the posterior teeth, and delayed eruption are typical findings.[75] There is no increased incidence of enamel defects. Cardiovascular anomalies are occasionally reported in IP, including ventricular endomyocardial fibrosis, acyanotic tetralogy of Fallot and tricuspid insufficiency, and abnormal shunt of the right pulmonary vein into the superior vena cava with pulmonary hypertension.[76] In the series of Landy and Donnai[61] breast hypoplasia was found at least 10 times more often than in the general population. Patients with IP and immunologic dysfunctions have also been described.[77] Recently, a novel X-linked disorder of immune deficiency and hypohidrotic ectodermal dysplasia was found to be allelic to IP due to mutations in NEMO, and may provide a clue about the immunologic deficiency in patients with ordinary IP.[21]

67. Di Landro A, Marchesi L, Reseghetti A, Caunelli T (2000) Warty linear streaks of the palm and sole: possible late manifestation of incontinentia pigmenti. Br J Dermatol 143:1102–1103.
68. Abimelec P, Rybojad M, Cambiaghi S et al. (1995) Late, painful, subungual hyperkeratosis in incontinentia pigmenti. Pediatr Dermatol 12:340–342.
69. Moss C, Ince P (1987) Anhidrotic and achromians lesions in incontinentia pigmenti. Br J Dermatol 116:839–849.
70. Dutheil P, Vabres P, Cayla MC, Enjolras O (1995) Incontinentia pigmenti: late sequelae and genotypic diagnosis: a three-generation study of four patients. Pediatr Dermatol 12:107–111.
71. Nazzaro V, Brusasco A, Gelmetti C et al. (1990) Hypochromic reticulated streaks in incontinentia pigmenti: an immunohistochemical and ultrastructural study. Pediatr Dermatol 7:174–178.

72. Holmström G, Thoren K (2000) Ocular manifestations of incontinentia pigmenti. Acta Ophth Scand 78:348–353.
73. Yoshikawa H, Uehara Y, Abe T, Oda Y (2000) Disappearance of a white matter lesion in incontinentia pigmenti. Pediatr Neurol 23:364–367.
74. Mirowski GW, Caldemeyer KS (2000) Incontinentia pigmenti. J Am Acad Dermatol 43:517–518.
75. Macey-Dare L, Goodman JR (1999) Incontinentia pigmenti: seven cases with dental manifestations. Int J Paediatr Dent 9:293–297.
76. Miteva L, Nikolova A (2001) Incontinentia pigmenti: a case associated with cardiovascular anomalies. Pediatr Dermatol 18:54–56.
77. Menni S, Piccino R, Biolchini A, Plebani A (1990) Immunologic investigations in eight patients with incontinentia pigmenti. Pediatr Dermatol 7:275–277.

TABLE 7.10   Histology of skin lesions

Stage 1: Intraepidermal spongiosis and blisters with eosinophils and dyskeratotic cells
Stage 2: Hyperkeratotic lesions with dyskeratosis and still occasional eosinophils
Stage 3: Incontinence of pigment – sometimes large clumps
Stage 4: Scars with no pigment in epidermis, no incontinence, no eosinophils, absent eccrine glands

HISTOLOGY AND PATHOGENESIS

The histopathology depends on the stage of the disorder (Table 7.10). In stage 1 with blistering lesions, intense infiltration of eosinophils into the epidermis with eosinophilic spongiosis is seen. It has been speculated that extracellular deposition of an eosinophil granule major basic protein in lesional tissue plays a role in the pathogenesis of the disease.[78] Light microscopic findings in hyperpigmented areas of IP show dyskeratotic cells in the epidermis and numerous melanin-loaded macrophages in the upper dermis leading to the term of pigment incontinence. Hypopigmented lesions are characterized by round eosinophilic bodies in the upper dermis.[79] In addition, sparse melanocytes and reduced numbers of appendageal structures, epidermal atrophy and thickened dermal collagen are found.[71,80] In hypopigmented lesions no pigment incontinence is seen.

DIFFERENTIAL DIAGNOSIS

Differential diagnosis depends on the clinical stage of IP. Vesicular lesions must be distinguished from herpes simplex, varicella, impetigo, candidiasis, erythema toxicum, pustular melanosis, infantile acropustulosis and miliaria rubra. Verrucous lesions resemble linear epidermal nevus and the hyperpigmented lesions may be confused with Naegeli–Francheschetti–Jadassohn syndrome.[81] Hypomelanosis of Ito, often confused with incontinentia pigmenti, is a description of different patterns of mosaicism and not a diagnosis. In light-skinned children, it may fancifully resemble a mirror image of IP with light swirls on darker normal skin; in darker children, it is clinically hard to separate from IP and other criteria must be employed.

Minor criteria

Dental involvement, alopecia, woolly hair/abnormal teeth, ocular abnormalities may occur.

Major criteria

At least one major criterion is necessary to make a firm diagnosis of sporadic IP. A useful approach to the mothers of children with IP is to check for sweating on their legs. The atrophic, hypohidrotic scars can be identified by starch–iodine.

TREATMENT AND PROGNOSIS

Patient management includes local treatment of blistering lesions to protect them from infection and additional scarring. In the later stages the skin might be dry and moisturizing skin care is important. During the first year of life regular ophthalmologic screening on a monthly basis is recommended. Later, yearly evaluation is justified because of the high incidence of squint and amblyopia. Central nervous involvement often manifests within the first weeks of life. In those patients careful neurologic monitoring is necessary.

TABLE 7.11   Diagnostic criteria for IP (adapted from Landy and Donnai 1993)[64]

Typical neonatal rash with erythema, vesicles and eosinophilia
Typical hyperpigmentations on the trunk following the lines of Blaschko and fading in adolescence
Linear, atrophic, hairless lesions

A source of additional information and support for IP patients and their families is:

National Incontinentia Pigmenti Foundation (NIPF)
30 East 72nd St., 16th Floor
New York, NY 10021 (212) 452–1231
Fax: (212) 452–1406
Email: nipf@pipeline.com
http://imgen.bcm.tmc.edu/nipf

TUBEROUS SCLEROSIS AND NEUROFIBROMATOSIS

Bruce Korf

TUBEROUS SCLEROSIS COMPLEX

Tuberous sclerosis complex is a hereditary disease, also known as Bourneville's disease, epiloia, and hereditary multiple system hamartomatosis. It is characterized by hamartomas involving the skin, eye, CNS, cardiac muscle, lungs, kidneys, and bones. The classical description, first proposed by Vogt in 1908, consists of the triad of adenoma sebaceum, epilepsy, and mental retardation; however, at least 50% of affected persons are not retarded.

HISTORY

Von Recklinghausen in 1862 first described the association of cerebral sclerotic areas and cardiac tumors in an autopsy report of a newborn infant. Bourneville coined the term *sclerose tubereuse* to describe the brain tumors and associate them with epilepsy and mental retardation. In 1885, Balzer and Menetrier described this syndrome's popular facial eruption as "*adenomes sebaces*," without performing histologic studies. Pringle in 1899 correctly classified these facial lesions as angiofibromas. Van der Hoeve in 1920 first reported the presence of retinal lesions, which he termed phakomas. In 1911, Sherlock introduced the term epiloia, combining the words epilepsy and anoia, meaning "minded-less", for the entire syndrome, in which he included convulsions, mental retardation, adenoma sebaceum, and tumors of the brain and other organs.

EPIDEMIOLOGY

This autosomal dominant disease has variable expressivity. Lack of penetrance is relatively uncommon. The disorder is estimated as occurring in 1 in 10 000 and occurs in all ethnic groups.[83] In the past, about one-half to two-thirds of affected patients were thought to represent new mutations, but imaging studies have shown findings compatible with tuberous sclerosis in some asymptomatic parents. The rate of new mutations may therefore be lower

78. Thyresson NH, Goldberg NC, Tye MJ, Leiferman KM (1991) Localization of eosinophil granule major basic protein in incontinentia pigmenti. **Pediatr Dermatol** 8:102–106.
79. Ashley JR, Burgdorf WH (1987) Incontinentia pigmenti: pigmentary changes independent of incontinence. **J Cut Pathol** 14:248–250.
80. Zillikens D, Mahringer A, Lechner W, Burg G (1991) Hypo- and hyperpigmented areas in incontinentia pigmenti. Light and electron microscopic studies. **Am J Dermatopathol** 13:57–62.

81. Itin PH, Lautenschlager S, Meyer R et al. (1993) Natural history of the Naegeli–Francheschetti–Jadassohn syndrome and further delineation of the symptom complex. **J Am Acad Dermatol** 28:942–950.
82. Dokal I (2000) Dyskeratosis congenita in all its forms. **Br J Haematol** 110:768–779.
83. Osborne JP, Fryer A, Webb D (1991) Epidemiology of tuberous sclerosis. **Ann NY Acad Sci** 615:125–127.

than previously believed, and computerized tomography (CT) or magnetic resonance imaging (MRI) of parents and siblings should be done prior to genetic counseling.

CLINICAL MANIFESTATIONS

In infancy and early childhood, presentation is most likely to be prompted by myoclonic generalized or focal seizures. There are no pathognomonic EEG findings in this disease. Developmental delay, mental retardation, autism, and behavioral problems constitute the next most frequent presenting signs. A close correlation has been established between infantile spasms or other generalized seizures and mental retardation; the age of seizure onset and severity of mental retardation are strictly related.

The diagnostic workup is aided by a Wood's light examination of the entire skin surface for hypopigmented macules, reported to be present in 90% of affected patients either at birth or soon afterward. Occasionally, a hypopigmented tuft of scalp or eyelash hair may be present. These white macules can be oval or linear, but the most characteristic lesion are lanceolate (Fig. 7.12), hence the name ash-leaf-spots to describe them. Their size ranges from one millimeter to several centimeters, and the number of lesions varies from a few to more than 75. Histologically, these lesions differ from vitiligo in that they contain hypoactive melanocytes. These lesions are not pathognomonic, but their detection is very helpful in considering the diagnosis of this disease. Specific diagnosis at this age or later is possible if fully dilated indirect ophthalmoscopy or fluorescence angiography reveals retinal hamartomas, or if CT scans or MRI with gadolinium enhancement reveal characteristic features.

Cutaneous angiofibromas, the so-called adenoma sebaceum lesions, usually appear between 2 and 6 years of age, but their appearance has ranged from birth to the mid-20s. They are pathognomonic of tuberous sclerosis, occur in 65 to 90% of reported patients, and consist of 1- to 10-mm pink to red, dome-shaped papules, occurring usually in a symmetric distribution over the nasolabial folds, cheeks (Figs 7.13 and 7.14), and chin, and more rarely over the forehead, eyelids, ears, and scalp. Histologic examination of these lesions demonstrates capillary dilatation and dermal fibrosis with atrophy or downward displacement of sebaceous glands and hair follicles. Clinically, these lesions may be obscured by concomitant acne vulgaris, acne rosacea, or seborrheic dermatitis.

Large fibrotic plaques or nodules can occur on the forehead (Fig. 7.14), cheeks, and scalp and may be present at birth. Histologically, they show connective tissue nevi of the collagen type without vascular dilation. Clinically, they have been reported in persons with mental retardation and in older surviving patients, hence constituting a poor prognostic sign. Shagreen patches, or peau chagrine lesions, are truncal plaques present in 14 to 20% of

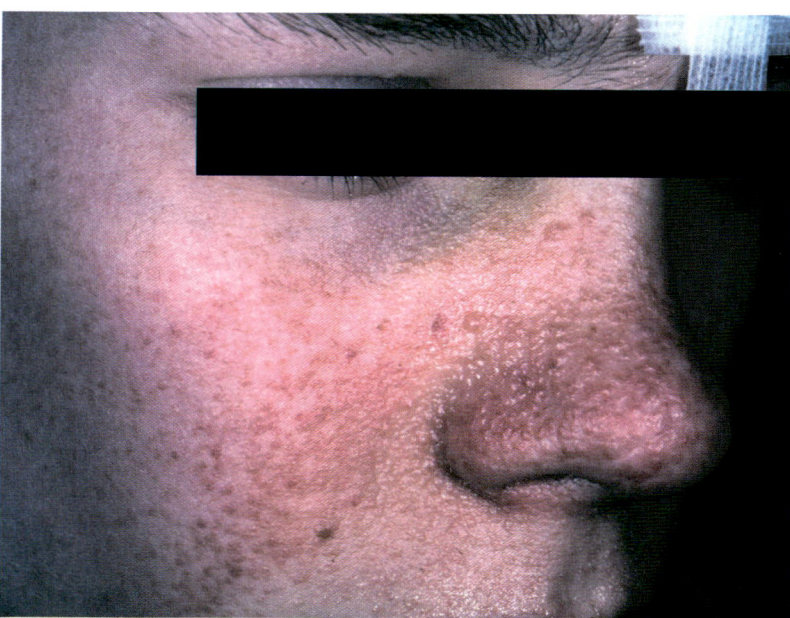

Fig. 7.13 The many angiofibromas called "adenoma sebaceum" on the face of a teenaged boy with tuberous sclerosis who had two white spots, but no neurological abnormalities. (Courtesy Dr. Amy Paller)

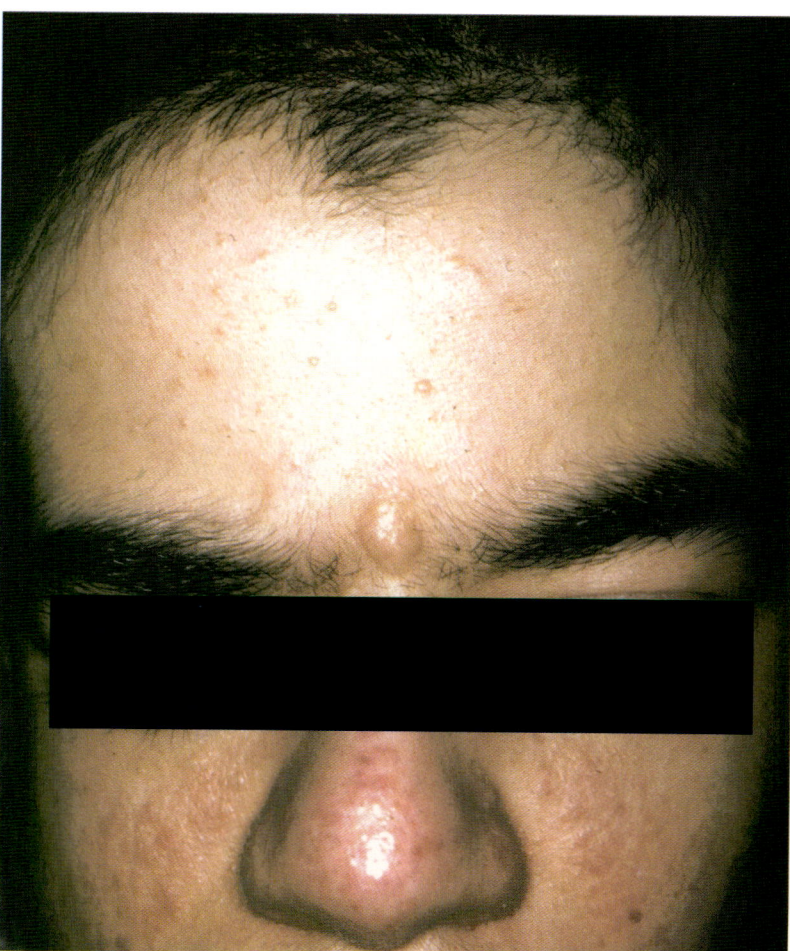

Fig. 7.14 Facial angiofibromas and a congenital fibrous forehead plaque in a boy with seizures and retardation as manifestations of his tuberous sclerosis. (Courtesy Dr. Amy Paller)

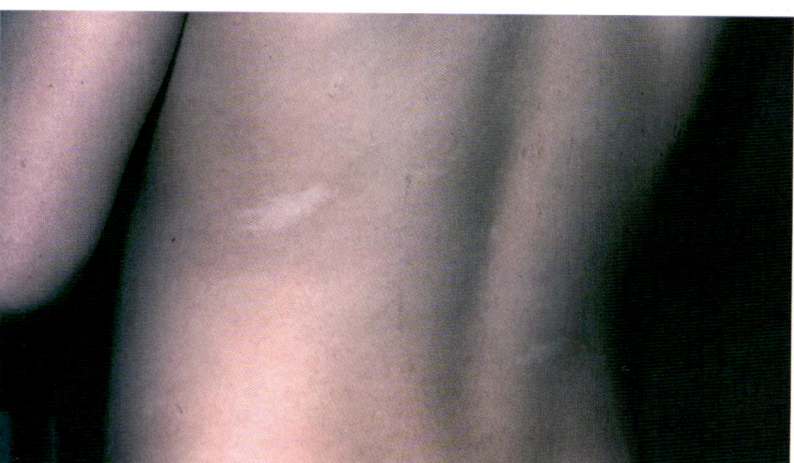

Fig. 7.12 The hypopigmented macules or "white spots" of tuberous sclerosis are often lanceolate and located on the trunk. (Courtesy Dr. Amy Paller)

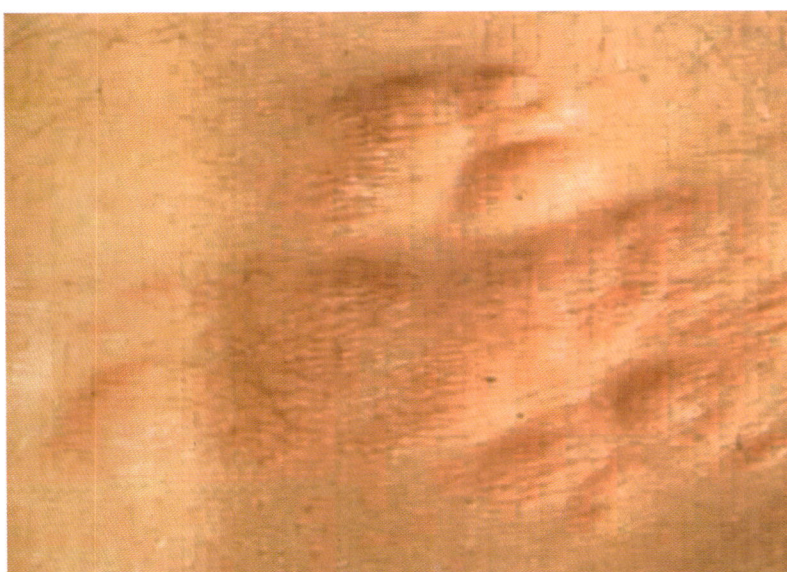

Fig. 7.15   Shagreen patches, such as this one on the lower back, are truncal fibrous plaques.

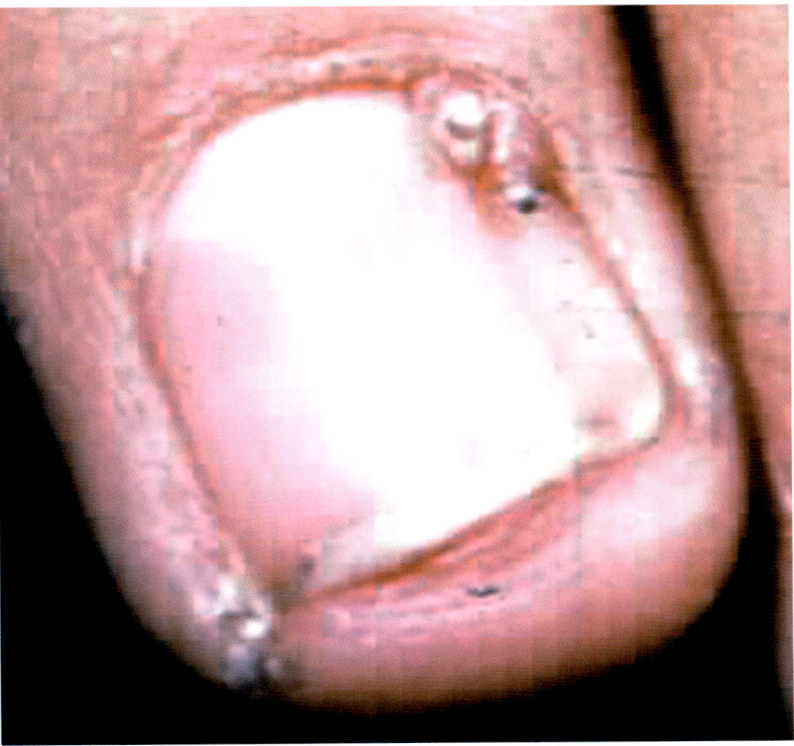

Fig. 7.16   The periungual fibromas can occur on the toes or fingers after the onset of puberty.

patients in an American series and tend to appear at the same time as the angiofibromas. However, in one British report of 18 patients, 15 (83%) had shagreen patches. They are usually found in the lumbosacral region (Fig. 7.15) and may be either solitary or multiple. One woman had a lesion on her left breast as well as the lumbosacral area, and larger lesions frequently have smaller, satellite lesions surrounding them. Lesions vary from being palm-sized to less than 1 cm. They usually appear as slightly raised areas with dimpling at areas of follicular openings and have therefore been described as having a "pigskin," "elephant skin," "orange peel," or "goose flesh" appearance. Histologic examination demonstrates lower dermal sclerosis without vascular proliferation and findings resembling those generally associated with morphea. Many sections show epidermal changes resembling those of acanthosis nigricans.

Subungual and periungual fibromas are pathognomic lesions and are reported in 18–50% of patients; they usually first appear after puberty. Clinically, they consist of 5- to 10-mm firm, smooth, budlike papules growing out of the nail beds (Fig. 7.16). Less common and nonspecific cutaneous lesions include café-au-lait spots, large fibroepithelial polyps, purplish red plaques, diffuse skin bronzing, and mucosal neuromas. Gingival fibromas and small dental enamel pits have been noted.

Retinal hamartomas are pathognomonic of tuberous sclerosis and have been reported in 50–76% of affected patients. These can be seen as two types: (1) a flat gray or yellowish, smooth semitransparent lesion with indistinct borders or (2) an elevated multinodular lesion described as mulberrylike, frog's-egglike, or salmon egglike. Both types have been seen in infants and in adults. The evolution of a flat lesion into a mulberry-type tumor during a 20-year period has been recorded in a single patient. In one series of 44 infants presenting with infantile spasms, rentinal hamartomas were discovered in eight when fully dilated, indirect ophthalmoscopy was done.

Ocular findings also include glial hamartomas of the optic disc, occasionally referred to as giant drusen; white pedunculated tumors of the palpebral conjunctiva; yellow–red thickenings of the bulbar conjunctiva; optic atrophy secondary to papilledema caused by intracranial lesions; retinal angiomas; iris,

lens, choroid, and optic disc colobomatas; and depigmented areas of the iris or retina.

Brain involvement is complex, with pale sclerotic patches or tubers causing broadening or elevations of cerebral gyri. Once calcified, these lesions are visible on skull radiographs as brain stones. When the floors of the lateral ventricles become calcified, they appear as curvilinear opacities on skull films. CT or MRI scanning, both plain and contrast enhanced, permits detection of lesions prior to calcification, by visualizing diagnostic periventricular or subependymal nodules varying in size from less than 1 cm to 2–3 cm. One-third of affected patients show dilation of the lateral ventricles on CT scans. MRI provides sensitive detection of cortical lesions, which may correlate with neurological manifestations of seizures and developmental impairment.[84–86]

Although subependymal nodules are not malignant lesions, some may grow and cause obstructive hydrocephalus, and have the histological appearance of giant cell astrocytoma.[87] Renal hamartomas such as angiomyolipomas and polycystic kidneys occur in about 15% of patients and are never found during the prenatal or neonatal period;[88] abdominal ultrasound or CT scanning is useful in detecting their presence even in asymptomatic patients. Fifty percent of reported cardiac rhabdomyomas have occurred in tuberous sclerosis patients and are usually asymptomic, although they may be a cause of sudden death, usually during the first year of life. Cardiac rhabdomyomas tend to regress spontaneously. Neonatal two-dimensional echocardiography may represent a useful and noninvasive method to identify asymptomatic cardiac rhabdomyomas, especially in newborns.[89,90] Cardiac arrhythmias as well as pulmonary lymphangiomyomatosis and cysts of the liver, pancreas, thyroid, and testes have been noted. About one-half of patients have bony abnormalities visible on hand and skull radiographs.

84. Husain AM, Foley CM, Legido A et al. (2000) Tuberous sclerosis complex and epilepsy: prognostic significance of electroencephalography and magnetic resonance imaging. J Child Neurol 15(2):81–83.
85. Mizuno S, Takahashi Y, Kato Z et al. (2000) Magnetic resonance spectroscopy of tubers in patients with tuberous sclerosis. Acta Neurol Scand 102(3):175–178.
86. Christophe C, Sekhara T, Rypens F et al. (2000) MRI spectrum of cortical malformations in tuberous sclerosis complex. Brain Dev 22(8):487–493.
87. Torres OA, Roach ES, Delgado MR et al. (1998) Early diagnosis of subependymal giant cell astrocytoma in patients with tuberous sclerosis. J Child Neurol 13(4):173–177.
88. Torres VE, Zincke H, King BK, Bjornsson J (1997) Renal manifestations of tuberous sclerosis complex. Contrib Nephrol 122:64–75.
89. Harding CO, Pagon RA (1990) Incidence of tuberous sclerosis in patients with cardiac rhabdomyoma. Am J Med Genet 37:443–446.
90. Watson GH (1991) Cardiac rhabdomyomas in tuberous sclerosis. Ann NY Acad Sci 615:50–57.

PATHOPHYSIOLOGY

Tuberous sclerosis complex is due to mutations in two different genes, TSC1[91] on chromosome 9 and TSC2 on chromosome 16.[92] The two gene products, harmartin and tuberin, respectively, interact with one another in the cell, and appear to function in the regulation of GTPase activity of the Rap1 gene.[93,94] The TSC genes appear to function as tumor suppressors in the pathogenesis of the lesions of TSC.[95,96] A wide variety of mutations occurs in both the *TSC1* and *TSC2* genes; individuals with *TSC1* mutations may have a milder clinical course.[97] Patients with renal cysts have co-deletion of the *TSC2* gene and the *PKD1* gene that leads to polycystic kidney disease, on chromosome 16.[98] Mosaicism has been seen in individuals with TSC.[99]

DIFFERENTIAL DIAGNOSIS

The angiofibromas can be differentiated from trichoepitheliomas, trichilemmomas, milia, xanthomas, and verrucae. Other disease processes associated with intracranial calcifications include Sturge–Weber syndrome, hyalinosis cutis et mucosae, congenital toxoplasmosis, congenital cytomegalic inclusion disease, and basal cell nevus syndrome. Diagnostic criteria for tuberous sclerosis complex have been proposed by an NIH Consensus Development Conference.[100]

THERAPEUTICS

There is some evidence that prevention of seizures, especially in early life, may enhance subsequent mental development. Neurosurgical intervention may be necessary if signs of increased intracranial pressure (e.g., headache, vomiting, visual disturbances, papilledema) develop. Special education or institutional placement may be required if mental retardation is present. Facial angiofibromas can be treated successfully with dermabrasion or laser treatment but slowly recur.

PROGNOSIS

The prognosis varies according to the severity of the disorder, which has varied even in affected monozygotic twins.[101] Some persons have normal intelligence, no seizures, and a normal life span. Severely affected patients in the past had only a 25–50% chance of survival to adulthood, with status epilepticus the cause of death in many of these cases. With improved seizure control, less invasive diagnostic methods such as MRI scanning, and the availability of more precise therapeutic modalities such as microscopic surgery of neoplastic brain lesions, the length and quality of life should improve.

Problems such as cardiac rhabdomyomas can be screened for by echocardiography and arrhythmias by Holter monitoring, but their detection may still not alter an affected patient's prognosis. The most common causes of death, aside from neorologic and cardiac complications, are renal diseases and brain tumors.

NEUROFIBROMATOSIS

"Neurofibromatosis" is a term that encompasses two distinct disorders, NF1 and NF2.[102] Both are characterized by the occurrence of multiple tumors of the nerve sheath and are inherited as autosomal dominant traits. The major distinguishing features are:

1. *NF1*: Classic or von Recklinghausen neurofibromatosis, peripheral neurofibromatosis, is characterized by multiple café-au-lait macules, axillary freckling, numerous neurofibromas, and Lisch nodules or iris hamartomas. It accounts for about 90% of all cases of neurofibromatosis.
2. *NF2*: Bilateral acoustic or "central" neurofibromatosis is characterized by an almost 100% incidence of bilateral vestibular schwannomas. Schwannomas may also occur along other cranial and spinal nerves. Café-au-lait spots tend to be few. Posterior capsular lens opacities are frequent. Lisch nodules are absent. Other tumor types include meningiomas, ependymomas, and gliomas.

HISTORY

The first systemic characterization of neurofibromatosis was made by von Recklinghausen in 1882.[103] Joseph Merrick, also known as the "Elephant Man," was at one time thought to have had neurofibromatosis; the diagnosis is now believed to be Proteus syndrome.[104]

EPIDEMIOLOGY

NF1 is present in 1 in 3000–4000 persons and shows no ethnic or sexual preponderance.[105] The frequency of NF2 is lower, about 1:40 000, but also occurs in both sexes and in populations around the world. Both disorders are characterized by complete penetrance but variable expressivity and exhibit a high rate of new mutation, approximately 50%.

CLINICAL MANIFESTATIONS

Diagnostic criteria for NF1 are the presence of any two of the following: six or more café-au-lait macules measuring 5mm or more before puberty or 15mm or more after puberty; skin-fold freckling; two or more neurofibromas or one plexiform neurofibroma; two or more iris Lisch nodules; optic nerve glioma; characteristic skeletal dysplasia (tibial or orbital dysplasia); affected first-degree relative.

The most common presenting sign is multiple café-au-lait macules (Fig. 7.17A).[106] These may be seen at birth, but often do not appear until several weeks to months of life, and may continue to appear or darken over the first two years. If the diagnostic criterion of six or more café-au-lait macules is met, there is no significance to the overall number, which does not correlate with the severity of the disorder. Also, the location of café-au-lait macules does not predict the future location of neurofibromas. One exception is that large patches of hyperpigmentation, usually with irregular borders and present at birth, may signal the presence of an underlying plexiform

91. Van Slegtenhorst M, De Hoogt R, Hermans C et al. (1997) Identification of the tuberous sclerosis gene TSC1 on chromosome 9q34. **Science** 277(5327):805–808.
92. The European Chromosome 16 Tuberous Sclerosis Consortium. (1993) Identification and characterisation of the tuberous sclerosis gene on chromosome 16. **Cell** 75:1–11.
93. Nellist M, van Slegtenhorst MA, Goedbloed M et al. (1999) Characterization of the cytosolic tuberin-hamartin complex. Tuberin is a cytosolic chaperone for hamartin. **J Biol Chem** 274(50):35647–35652.
94. Wienecke R, Konig A, DeClue JE (1995) Identification of tuberin, the tuberous sclerosis-2 product. Tuberin possesses specific Rap1GAP activity. **J Biol Chem** 270(27):16409–16414.
95. Henske EP, Scheithauer BW, Short MP et al. (1996) Allelic loss is frequent in tuberous sclerosis kidney lesions but rare in brain lesions. **Am J Hum Genet** 59(2):400–406.
96. Henske EP, Wessner LL, Golden J et al. (1997) Loss of tuberin in both subependymal giant cell astrocytomas and angiomyolipomas supports a two-hit model for the pathogenesis of tuberous sclerosis tumors. **Am J Pathol** 151(6):1639–1647.
97. Dabora SL, Jozwiak S, Franz DN et al. (2001) Mutational analysis in a cohort of 224 Tuberous Sclerosis patients indicates increased severity of TSC2, compared with TSC1, disease in multiple organs. **Am J Hum Genet** 68(1):64–80.
98. Brook-Carter PT, Peral B, Ward CJ et al. (1994) Deletion of the *TSC2* and *PKD1* genes associated with severe infantile polycystic kidney disease – A contiguous gene syndrome. **Nat Genet** 8:328–332.
99. Verhoef S, Bakker L, Tempelaars AM et al. (1999) High rate of mosaicism in tuberous sclerosis complex. **Am J Hum Genet** 64(6):1632–1637.
100. Hyman MH, Whittemore VH (2000) National Institutes of Health Consensus Conference: tuberous sclerosis complex. **Arch Neurol** 57(5):662–665.
101. Webb DW, Fryer AE, Osborne JP (1996) Morbidity associated with tuberous sclerosis: a population study. **Dev Med Child Neurol** 38(2):146–155.
102. National Institutes of Health Consensus Development Conference (1988) Neurofibromatosis Conference Statement. **Arch Neurol** 45:575–578.
103. von Recklinghausen FD (1882) Ueber die multiplen Fibrome der Haut und ihre Beiehung zu den multiplen Neuromen. Berlin: Hirschwald.
104. Tibbles JAR, Cohen MM (1986) The Proteus syndrome: The Elephant Man diagnosed. **Br Med J** 293:683–685.
105. Friedman JM (1999) Epidemiology of neurofibromatosis type 1. **Am J Med Genet** 89(1):1–6.
106. Crowe FW, Schull WJ (1953) Diagnostic importance of café-au-lait spot in neurofibromatosis. **Arch Int Med** 91:758–766.

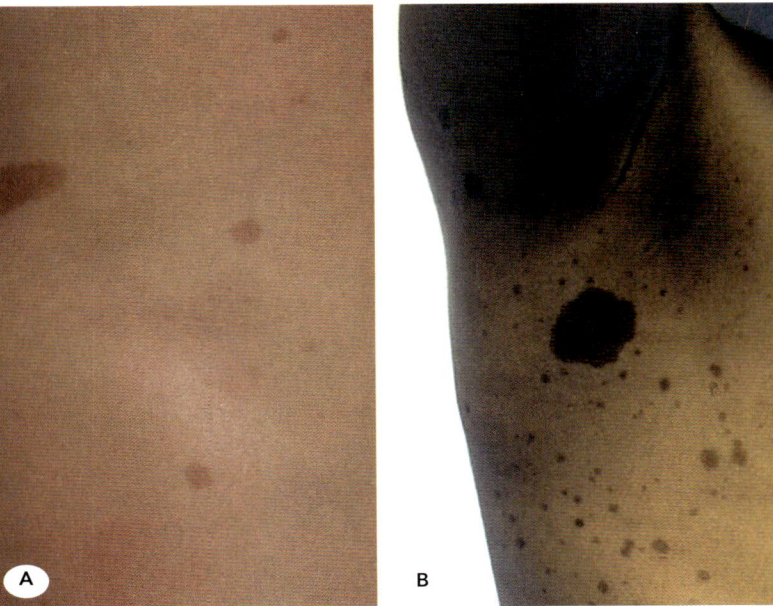

Fig. 7.17   (A) The presence of six or more café-au-lait macules is a major criterion for suspecting the diagnosis in patients with neurofibromatosis, and is usually the only manifestations in children with the disorder. (B) If axillary freckling is present in addition to the multiple café-au-lait macules, the diagnosis of neurofibromatosis may be made with certainty.

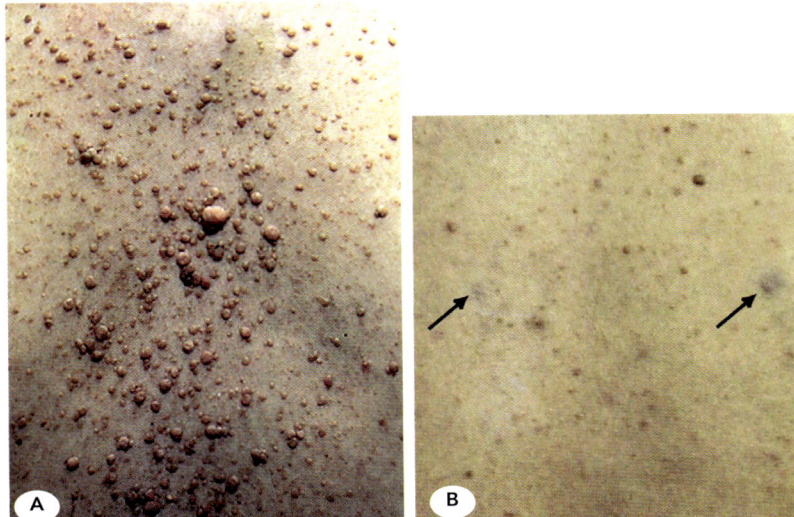

Fig. 7.18   Dermal neurofibromas may present as reddish papules (A) or deeper, more subtle blue nocular lesions (B, arrows). These dermal neurofibromas do not tend to first develop until later in childhood and adolescence.

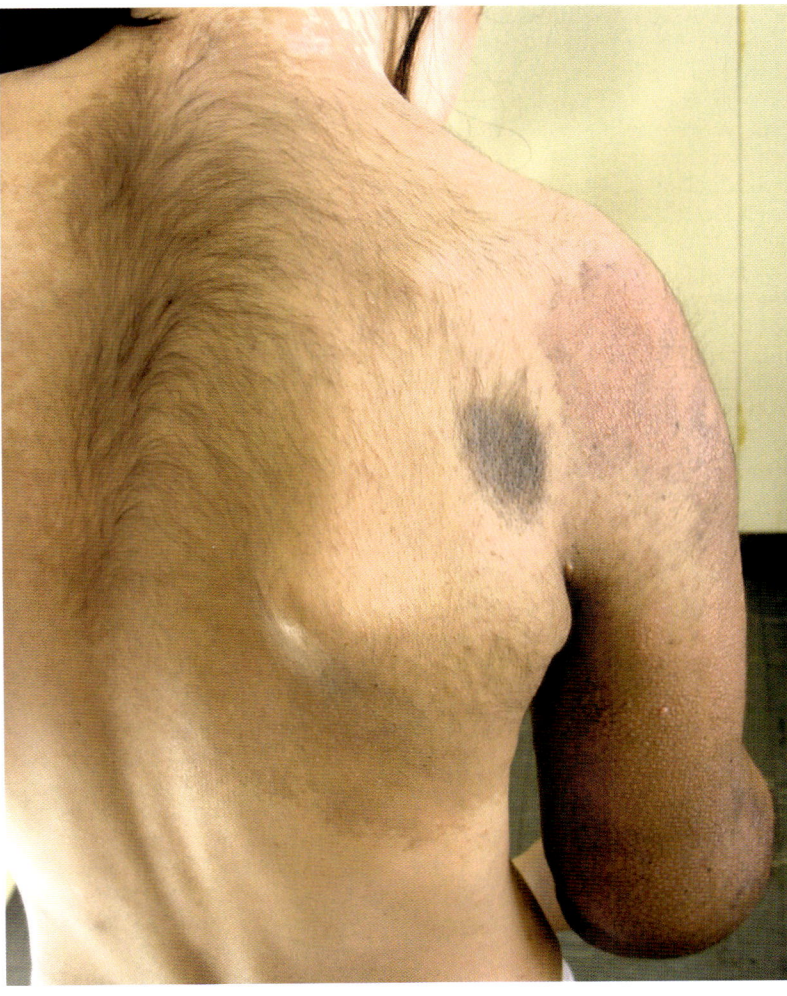

Fig. 7.19   Extensive plexiform neurofibroma involving the back, neck and arm of a patient with neurofibromatosis. Note the overlying hypertrichosis and hyperpigmentation.

neurofibroma.[107] The other major pigmentary feature of NF1, skin–fold freckling (Fig. 7.17B), often confirms a suspected diagnosis, and appears between three and five years of age.[108,109] This sign is highly specific to NF1.

Neurofibromas represent growths of the nerve sheath, including Schwann cells, fibroblasts, and mast cells.[110] They may grow along a single site on a nerve ("discrete neurofibromas") or may extend along the length of a nerve involving multiple fascicles ("plexiform neurofibromas"). Discrete neuro-fibromas occur in the dermis or subdermal layer. These are soft in consistency, range in size from a millimeter to several centimeters, and there may be an associated violaceous discoloration of the skin (Fig. 7.18). Discrete neurofibromas may occur along peripheral nerves deeper in the body, or along nerve roots near the spine. Those that occur along superficial nerves tend to be firm in consistency. Plexiform neurofibromas can occur superficially, including the dermis, the subdermal layers, or deeper in the body (Fig. 7.19).[111] Some are associated with soft tissue and bony overgrowth or bony erosion and can cause local gigantism.

Ocular signs of NF1 include orbital plexiform neurofibroma, Lisch nodules, and optic glioma. The orbital tumors occur rarely, involve the trigeminal nerve, and may cause displacement of the eye and glaucoma.[112] Lisch nodules are melanocytic hamartomas of the iris that do not impair vision, but are useful

107. Riccardi VM (1980) Pathophysiology of neurofibromatosis. V. Dermatologic insights into heterogeneity and pathogenesis. **J Am Acad Dermatol** 3:157–166.
108. Crowe RW (1964) Axillary freckling as a diagnostic aid in neurofibromatosis. **Ann Int Med** 61:1142–1143.
109. Korf BR (1992) Diagnostic outcome in children with multiple café au lait spots. **Pediatrics** 90:924–927.
110. Russell DS, Rubenstein LJ (1989) Pathology of tumors of the nervous system. New York: Williams & Wilkins.
111. Korf BR (1999) Plexiform neurofibromas. **Am J Med Genet** 89(1):31–37.
112. Ferguson VMG, Kyle PM (1993) Orbital plexiform neurofibroma. **Br J Ophthalmol** 77:527–528.

in diagnosis, being present in more than 95% of adults with NF1 and being highly specific to this disorder.[113,114] Optic gliomas occur along the orbital portion of the optic nerve, unilaterially or bilaterally, or may involve the chiasm, or both. They occur in approximately 15% of children with NF1, but fewer than half exhibit progression and cause signs or symptoms of visual impairment or precocious puberty due to hypothalamic involvement.[115–117]

Skeletal manifestations include long bone dysplasias, especially tibial dysplasia, and scoliosis.[118] Tibial dysplasia presents as anteromedial bowing of the tibia, usually visible within the first year of life. There is thinning of the cortex of the bone and sclerosis of the medulla.[119] Fracture may occur at the site of dysplasia, leading in some cases to pseudoarthrosis. There also may be nonossifying cysts in bones, both within areas of long bone dysplasia or elsewhere. The scoliosis in NF1 usually occurs in the thoracic region and is associated with dysplastic changes in the vertebral bodies.[120]

Approximately 50% of children with NF1 exhibit learning disability, including both verbal and nonverbal disabilities as well as attention deficit disorder.[121–123] More severe developmental delay, including "mental retardation", occurs in about 5%, and may be associated with a distinct *NF1* gene mutation consisting of total deletion of the gene.[124,125] Brain MRI reveals areas of enhanced T2 signal intensity in the internal capsule, brainstem, cerebellum, and basal ganglia.[126–128] These tend to disappear with age and may represent areas of abnormal myelination. The number of such foci may correlate with the occurrence of learning disabilities.

Other features of NF1 include macrocephaly, short stature,[129,130] and hypertension. Macrocephaly is common and usually not associated with hydrocephalus, although aqueductal stenosis may occur rarely. Short stature is usually unexplained, with no evidence of neuroendocrine disturbance.[131] Hypertension may be due to renal artery stenosis, or, rarely, pheochromocytoma.[132,133] Some individuals have stenosis of multiple arteries that may cause, in addition to hypertension, strokes or episodes of hemorrhage due to aneurysm.[134]

NF1 is associated with an increased risk of malignancy.[135] Aside from optic gliomas, noted above, other gliomas may occur in the central nervous system. These are usually pilocytic astrocytomas, and tend to be slow-growing lesions. Malignant peripheral nerve sheath tumors may occur, especially along preexisting plexiform neurofibromas. These present with unexplained pain or sudden growth. Other tumors seen in association with NF1 include leukemia (especially nonlymphocytic leukemia), carcinoid, and pheochromocytoma.

The development of multiple small juvenile xanthogranulomas may herald the occurrence of nonlymphocytic leukemia. The lifetime risk of malignancy associated with NF1 is estimated to be around 5%.

The natural history of NF1 includes several epochs of life when particular complications are most likely. Plexiform neurofibromas causing segmental hypertrophy as well as long bone dysplasias tend to be congenital. Optic gliomas and learning disabilities occur during early childhood. Dermal neurofibromas usually begin to appear in late childhood or adolescence, and may continue to appear or grow throughout life. Women often notice an increase in their neurofibromas during pregnancy. Malignant peripheral nerve sheath tumors usually occur after the first decade, peaking in the second and third decades.

Diagnostic criteria of NF2[136,137] require the presence of bilateral vestibular schwannomas, or an affected first-degree relative and unilateral vestibular schwannoma or two characteristic findings (schwannoma, glioma, meningioma, ependymoma, posterior subcapsular cataract). NF2 should also be considered in individuals with unilateral vestibular schwannoma presenting below age 35 and in those with multiple meningiomas.

The cardinal manifestation is the vestibular schwannoma. This presents with tinnitus, hearing loss, and problems with balance.[138,139] Although tumors are almost invariably present bilaterally, onset on one side may precede the other by several years, possibly causing confusion with sporadic unilateral vestibular schwannoma.[140] Vestibular tumors may occur during childhood, but usually do not begin until the second decade, well before most sporadic vestibular schwannomas, however. Schwannomas may affect other cranial nerves, especially the Vth nerve, as well as peripheral and spinal nerves. Schwannomas of cutaneous nerves may present as diffuse plaques, often associated with hair growth. Other tumors associated with NF2 include meningiomas, ependymomas, and gliomas. Multiple meningiomas may cause considerable morbidity. As distinct from NF1, malignant tumors are not seen with increased frequency in NF2. Similarly, more than six café-au-lait macules are not seen regularly in NF2, and learning disabilities are not a feature of this disorder. The only non-tumor manifestation of NF2 is cataract, either presenile posterior subcapsular cataract or cortical wedge opacity.[141]

Both NF1 and NF2 may be associated with mosaic involvement in some individuals. Mosaicism may ameliorate symptoms or segmental involvement of manifestations also may occur.[142,143]

113. Lewis RA, Riccardi VM (1981) Von Recklinghausen neurofibromatosis: Incidence of iris hamartomas. **Ophthalmology** 88:348–354.
114. Lubs M-LE, Bauer MS, Formas ME, Djokic B (1991) Lisch nodules in neurofibromatosis type 1. **N Engl J Med** 324:1264–1266.
115. Listernick R, Charrow J, Greenwald M, Mets M (1994) Natural history of optic pathway tumors in children with neurofibromatosis type 1: A longitudinal study. **J Pediatr** 125:63–66.
116. Listernick R, Darling C, Greenwald M et al. (1995) Optic pathway tumors in children: the effect of neurofibromatosis type 1 on clinical manifestations and natural history. **J Pediatr** 127(5):718–722.
117. Listernick R, Louis DN, Packer RJ, Gutmann DH (1997) Optic pathway gliomas in children with neurofibromatosis 1: consensus statement from the NF1 Optic Pathway Glioma Task Force. **Ann Neurol** 41(2):143–149.
118. Crawford AH, Schorry EK (1999) Neurofibromatosis in children: the role of the orthopaedist. **J Am Acad Orthop Surg** 7(4):217–230.
119. Durrani AA, Crawford AH, Chouhdry SN et al. (2000) Modulation of spinal deformities in patients with neurofibromatosis type 1. **Spine** 25(1):69–75.
120. Ippolito E, Corsi A, Grill F et al. (2000) Pathology of bone lesions associated with congenital pseudarthrosis of the leg. **J Pediatr Orthop B** 9(1):3–10.
121. Cutting LE, Koth CW, Denckla MB (2000) How children with neurofibromatosis type 1 differ from "typical" learning disabled clinic attenders: nonverbal learning disabilities revisited. **Dev Neuropsychol** 17(1):29–47.
122. Moore BD3, Ater JL, Needle MN et al. (1994) Neuropsychological profile of children with neurofibromatosis, brain tumor, or both. **Journal of Child Neurology** 9(4):368–377.
123. North K, Joy P, Yuille D et al. (1994) Specific learning disability in children with neurofibromatosis type 1: Significance of MRI abnormalities. **Neurology** 44:878–883.
124. Kayes LM, Burke W, Riccardi VM et al. (1994) Deletions spanning the neurofibromatosis 1 gene: identification and phenotype of five patients. **Amer J Hum Genet** 54:424–436.
125. Wu BL, Austin MA, Schneider GH et al. (1995) Deletion of the entire *NF1* gene detected by FISH: Four deletion patients associated with severe manifestations. **Am J Med Genet** 59(4):528–535.
126. Es SV, North KN, McHugh K, Silva MD (1996) MRI findings in children with neurofibromatosis type 1: a prospective study. **Pediatric Radiology** 26(7):478–487.
127. Ferner RE, Chaudhuri R, Bingham J et al. (1993) MRI in neurofibromatosis 1. The nature and evolution of increased intensity T2 weighted lesions and their relationship to intellectual impairment. **J Neurol Neurosurg Psychiatry** 56:492–495.
128. Terada H, Barkovich AJ, Edwards MS, Ciricillo SM (1996) Evolution of high-intensity basal ganglia lesions on T1-weighted MR in neurofibromatosis type 1. **Am J Neuroradiol** 17(4):755–760.
129. Clementi M, Milani S, Mammi I et al. (1999) Neurofibromatosis type 1 growth charts. **Am J Med Genet** 87(4):317–323.
130. Szudek J, Birch P, Friedman JM et al. (2000) Growth in North American white children with neurofibromatosis 1 (NF1). **J Med Genet** 37(12):933–938.
131. Carmi D, Shohat M, Metzker A, Dickerman Z (1999) Growth, puberty, and endocrine functions in patients with sporadic or familial neurofibromatosis type 1: a longitudinal study. **Pediatrics** 103(6 Pt 1):1257–1262.
132. Fossali E, Signorini E, Intermite RC et al. (2000) Renovascular disease and hypertension in children with neurofibromatosis. **Pediatr Nephrol** 14(8–9):806–810.
133. Strauss S, Bistritzer T, Azizi E et al. (1993) Renal artery stenosis secondary to neurofibromatosis in children: Detection by Doppler ultrasound. **Pediatr Nephrol** 7:32–34.
134. Hamilton SJ, Friedman JM (2000) Insights into the pathogenesis of neurofibromatosis 1 vasculopathy. **Clin Genet** 58(5):341–344.
135. Korf BR (2000) Malignancy in neurofibromatosis type 1. **Oncologist** 5(6):477–485.
136. Stumpf DA, Alksne JF, Annegers JF et al. (1988) Neurofibromataosis. **Arch Neurol** 45:575–578.
137. Gutmann DH, Aylsworth A, Carey JC et al. (1997) The diagnostic evaluation and multidisciplinary management of neurofibromatosis 1 and neurofibromatosis 2. **JAMA** 278(1):51–57.
138. Kishore A, O'Reilly BF (2000) A clinical study of vestibular schwannomas in type 2 neurofibromatosis. **Clin Otolaryngol** 25(6):561–565.
139. Evans DG (1999) Neurofibromatosis type 2: genetic and clinical features. **Ear Nose Throat J** 78(2):97–100.
140. Evans DG, Lye R, Neary W et al. (1999) Probability of bilateral disease in people presenting with a unilateral vestibular schwannoma. **J Neurol Neurosurg Psychiatry** 66(6):764–767.
141. Pearson-Webb MA, Kaiser-Kupfer MI, Eldridge R (1986) Eye findings in bilateral acoustic (central) neurofibromatosis: Association with presenile lens opacities and cataracts but absence of Lisch nodules. **N Engl J Med** 315:1553–1554.
142. Ruggieri M, Polizzi A (2000) Segmental neurofibromatosis. **J Neurosurg** 93(3):530–532.
143. Evans DG, Wallace AJ, Wu CL et al. (1998) Somatic mosaicism: a common cause of classic disease in tumor-prone syndromes? Lessons from type 2 neurofibromatosis. **Am J Hum Genet** 63(3):727–736.

PATHOPHYSIOLOGY AND HISTOGENESIS

The gene responsible for NF1 is located near the centromere of chromosome 17,[144,145] while the gene responsible for NF2 has been mapped to the long arm of chromosome 22.[146] The *NF1* gene encodes a protein referred to as "neurofibromin",[147,148] the NF2 protein is called "merlin" (or, by some, "schwannomin").[149,150]

Neurofibromas consist of multiple cell types, but it appears that the primary target of the *NF1* gene mutation is the Schwann cell.[151] *NF1* functions as a tumor suppressor gene, so the tumors arise when the wildtype allele undergoes loss or mutation, leaving no functional copy of *NF1*. Some of the Schwann cells within a lesion, and all of the fibroblasts, are not mutated at both loci, but are probably recruited to grow in the lesions by cytokines, perhaps secreted by the abnormal Schwann cells. This tumor suppressor hypothesis is supported by the finding of mutation of both NF1 alleles in neurofibromas,[152] evidence of loss of heterozygosity within neurofibromas,[153] and the fact that chimeric mice that contain *Nf1* −/− cells on a wildtype background develop neurofibromas.

The *NF1* gene product includes a domain with the properties of a GTPase-activating protein (GAP).[154] This domain stimulates the GTPase activity of Ras, causing Ras-GTP to be converted to Ras-GDP, converting this signal transduction molecule from its active to inactive state. It thus appears that the defect in NF1 is related to a failure to regulate Ras, specifically an inability to terminate a signal that may be initiated when the cell is stimulated to divide. It remains unclear whether any of the NF1 phenotype, such as learning disability, may be due to the heterozygous mutation. It is likely that malignant tumors require additional genetic changes besides mutation of both copies of *NF1*.

The spectrum of mutations in the *NF1* gene is broad, although the majority of mutations cause premature termination of translation of the gene product.[155,156] Mutations are widely distributed across the gene, making it difficult to use mutation detection as a diagnostic test. There are no genotype–phenotype correlations, except that deletion of the entire *NF1* gene is associated with a complex phenotype of large numbers of neurofibromas, facial dysmorphism, and severe developmental impairment. These deletions extend for about 1.5Mb, and include flanking genes as well as *NF1*.[157,158]

The *NF2* gene also functions as a tumor suppressor, with mutations of both alleles or loss of heterozygosity occurring in tumors.[159] The *NF2* gene product functions as a cytoskeletal protein,[160] but the mechanism whereby it contributes to tumor formation is unknown. Many of the features of *NF2*

have been reproduced in an animal model, in which a conditional knockout of the *NF2* gene is produced in Schwann cells.[161] *NF2* gene mutations are diverse. Truncating mutations tend to be associated with a more severe phenotype than splicing mutations or amino acid substitutions.[162,163]

DIFFERENTIAL DIAGNOSIS

A distinction has to be made from several other syndromes: multiple mucosal neuroma syndrome, LEOPARD syndrome, Noonan syndrome, Proteus syndrome, McCune–Albright syndrome, multiple lipomatosis, and Klippel–Trenaunay–Weber syndrome. Specific lesions may occur in isolation, such as optic glioma, tibial dysplasia, café-au-lait macules, and neurofibroma. There is an entity of multiple café-au-lait macules without other signs of neurofibromatosis that segregates in families as an autosomal dominant trait.[164–166]

THERAPEUTICS

Although it is hoped that insights into pathogenesis may lead to new methods of treatment, at present the management of individuals with NF1 or NF2 consists of surveillance for treatable complications, anticipatory guidance, and genetic counselling. Those with NF1 should have regular examination by a physician who is familiar with the disorder. Tests such as MRI or X-rays should be done for clinical indications; baseline studies are not recommended.[137] Children should be monitored for learning disabilities and provided cognitive and educational assessments as needed. Regular ophthalmological assessment should be performed during the childhood years to ensure early detection of symptomatic optic glioma. Physical examinations should include measurement of height, weight, head circumference, and blood pressure. There is no treatment available to prevent the growth of neurofibromas. Neurofibromas may be removed by plastic surgical or laser treatments. Plexiform neurofibromas usually cannot be removed entirely,[167] but surgical debulking may be indicated to treat symptoms due to mass effect or to improve cosmesis. Symptomatic and progressive optic gliomas are currently treated with chemotherapy,[168] reserving radiation therapy for older children with tumors that do not respond to chemotherapy. Malignant peripheral nerve sheath tumors are currently best treated by early detection and surgery.

Monitoring of individuals with NF2 is focused on early detection of vestibular schwannomas. This is best accomplished with MRI, although

144. Seizinger RR, Rouleau GA, Ozelius LJ et al. (1987) Genetic linkage of von Recklinghausen neurofibromatosis to the nerve growth factor receptor gene. **Cell** 49:589–594.
145. Barker D, Wright E, Nguyen K et al. (1987) Gene for von Recklinghausen neurofibromatosis is in the pericentromeric region of chromosome 17. **Science** 236:1098–1102.
146. Rouleau GA, Seizinger BR, Wertelecki W et al. (1990) Flanking markers bracket the neurofibromatosis type 2 (NF2) gene on chromosome 22. **Am J Hum Genet** 46:323–328.
147. Wallace MR, Marchuk DA, Andersen LB et al. (1990) Type 1 neurofibromatosis gene: Identification of a large transcript disrupted in three NF1 patients. **Science** 249:181–186.
148. Xu G, O'Connell P, Viskochil D et al. (1990) The neurofibromatosis type 1 gene encodes a protein related to GAP. **Cell** 62:599–608.
149. Trofatter JA, MacCollin MM, Rutter JL et al. (1993) A novel moesin-, ezrin-, radixin-like gene is a candidate for the neurofibromatosis 2 tumor suppressor. **Cell** 72:791–800.
150. Twist EC, Ruttledge MH, Rousseau M et al. (1994) The neurofibromatosis type 2 gene is inactivated in schwannomas. **Hum Mol Genet** 3(1):147–151.

151. Serra E, Rosenbaum T, Winner U et al. (2000) Schwann cells harbor the somatic NF1 mutation in neurofibromas: evidence of two different schwann cell subpopulations. **Hum Mol Genet** 9(20):3055–3064.
152. Rasmussen SA, Overman J, Thomson SA et al. (2000) Chromosome 17 loss-of-heterozygosity studies in benign and malignant tumors in neurofibromatosis type 1. **Genes Chromosomes Cancer** 28(4):425–431.
153. Cichowski K, Shih TS, Schmitt E et al. (1999) Mouse models of tumor development in neurofibromatosis type 1. **Science** 286(5447):2172–2176.
154. Xu G, Lin B, Tanaka K et al. (1990) The catalytic domain of the neurofibromatosis type 1 gene product stimulates ras GTPase and complements ira mutants of S. cerevisiae. **Cell** 63:835–841.
155. Upadhyaya M, Osborn MJ, Maynard J et al. (1997) Mutational and functional analysis of the neurofibromatosis type 1 (NF1) gene. **Hum Genet** 99(1):88–92.
156. Messiaen LM, Callens T, Mortier G et al. (2000) Exhaustive mutation analysis of the NF1 gene allows identification of 95% of mutations and reveals a high frequency of unusual splicing defects. **Hum Mutat** 15(6):541–555.

157. Dorschner MO, Sybert VP, Weaver M et al. (2000) NF1 microdeletion breakpoints are clustered at flanking repetitive sequences. **Hum Mol Genet** 9(1):35–46.
158. Correa CL, Brems H, Lazaro C et al. (2000) Unequal meiotic crossover: A frequent cause of NF1 microdeletions. **Am J Hum Genet** 66(6):1969–1974.
159. Jacoby LB, MacCollin M, Louis DN et al. (1994) Exon scanning for mutation of the NF2 gene in schwannomas. **Hum Mol Genet** 3:413–419.
160. Shaw RJ, McClatchey AI, Jacks T (1998) Localization and functional domains of the neurofibromatosis type II tumor suppressor, merlin. **Cell Growth Differ** 9(4):287–296.
161. Giovannini M, Robanus-Maandag E, van der Valli M et al. (2000) Conditional biallelic Nf2 mutation in the mouse promotes manifestations of human neurofibromatosis type 2. **Genes Dev** 14(13):1617–1630.
162. Parry DM, MacCollin MM, Kaiser-Kupfer MI et al. (1996) Germ-line mutations in the neurofibromatosis 2 gene: Correlations with disease severity and retinal abnormalities. **Am J Hum Genet** 59(3):529–539.
163. Evans DG, Trueman L, Wallace A et al. (1998) Genotype/phenotype correlations in type 2 neurofibromatosis (NF2): evidence for more severe disease associated with truncating mutations. **J Med Genet** 35(6):450–455.
164. Charrow J, Listernick R, Ward K (1993) Autosomal dominant multiple cafe-au-lait spots and neurofibromatosis-1: evidence of non-linkage. **Am J Med Genet** 45:606–608.
165. Arnsmeier SL, Riccardi VM, Paller AS (1994) Familial multiple cafe au lait spots. **Arch Dermatol** 130(11):1425–1426.
166. Abeliovich D, Gelman-Kohan Z, Silverstein S et al. (1995) Familial cafe au lait spots: A variant of neurofibromatosis type. **J Med Genet** 32(12):985–986.
167. Needle MN, Cnaan A, Dattilo J et al. (1997) Prognostic signs in the surgical management of plexiform neurofibroma – The Children's Hospital of Philadelphia experience, 1974–1994. **J Pediatr** 131:678–682.
168. Listernick R, Charrow J, Tomita T, Goldman S (1999) Carboplatin therapy for optic pathway tumors in children with neurofibromatosis type-1. **J Neurooncol** 45(2):185–190.

audiology and auditory brainstem evoked response testing may also be helpful.[169] Treatment of vestibular schwannomas is either by surgery or stereotactic radiation; other schwannomas or meningiomas are treated surgically.[170,171] Auditory brainstem implants may be helpful in partial restoration of hearing.[172]

Individuals with NF1 and NF2 should be provided genetic counselling regarding the 50% recurrence risk. It is not possible to predict severity in the next generation. Prenatal diagnosis may be available in some cases, either by linkage analysis if two or more generations are affected, or by direct mutation analysis in instances where the mutation can be identified. Parents of an apparently sporadically affected child should be examined for signs of neurofibromatosis. If these are not found, their risk of having another affected child is low, based on the rare occurrence of germline mosaicism.

PROGNOSIS

The prognosis of neurofibromatosis is variable, depending on severity of involvement, and development of malignancy. Cosmetic disfigurement from cutaneous and plexiform neurofibromas is progressive and worsens with time. A mild course during childhood and adolescence does not guarantee mild disease in adulthood.

GENETIC DISORDERS OF THE DERMIS

Amy Paller

Many of the heritable disorders of the dermis have significant cosmetic, disabling, or life-threatening complications. It is important for the practitioner to recognize cutaneous clues for the diagnosis of these multisystemic disorders of collagen, elastin, and the microfibrillar system.

PSEUDOXANTHOMA ELASTICUM

This rare entity with progressive calcification of elastic tissue occurs in about 1 in 70 000 to 160 000 persons. Clinically, the most significant changes occur in the skin, eye, and systemic vasculature (e.g., gastrointestinal and coronary vessels).[173]

Four major heritable types of pseudoxanthoma elasticum (PXE) have been recognized, two autosomal dominant and two autosomal recessive.[174,175] Autosomal dominant disease type I has extensive flexural cutaneous elastic tissue involvement with severe retinal and cardiovascular complications, frequently resulting in early blindness and coronary artery disease. Type II autosomal dominant PXE is more benign with primarily skin changes, milder eye findings, and rarely vascular disease. Approximately 50% of these patients also have hyperextensible joints, blue sclerae, and a high arched palate. The type I autosomal recessive variant of PXE is characterized by classic skin findings in flexural areas with moderate retinal disease. These patients occasionally have hypertension, a feature of the vascular degeneration, but have a significant risk (at least 10%) of gastrointestinal bleeding. Type II recessive PXE demonstrates generalized cutaneous elastic tissue destruction with significant skin laxity without systemic involvement, although patients with PXE and severe skin laxity (presumably autosomal recessive type II) have had restrictive lung disease and angioid streaks.[176,177] An autosomal recessive form

in South African Afrikaners has also been described with classical flexural skin changes, severe ophthalmologic abnormalities, and moderate cardiovascular disease.[178] Autosomal recessive PXE type I and autosomal dominant PXE type II are the most common types.

PHYSICAL EXAMINATION

Patients with PXE show marked clinical heterogeneity, with some patients displaying lesions of the skin, eye, and cardiovascular system while others in the same family (presumably the same gene) show only involvement of one

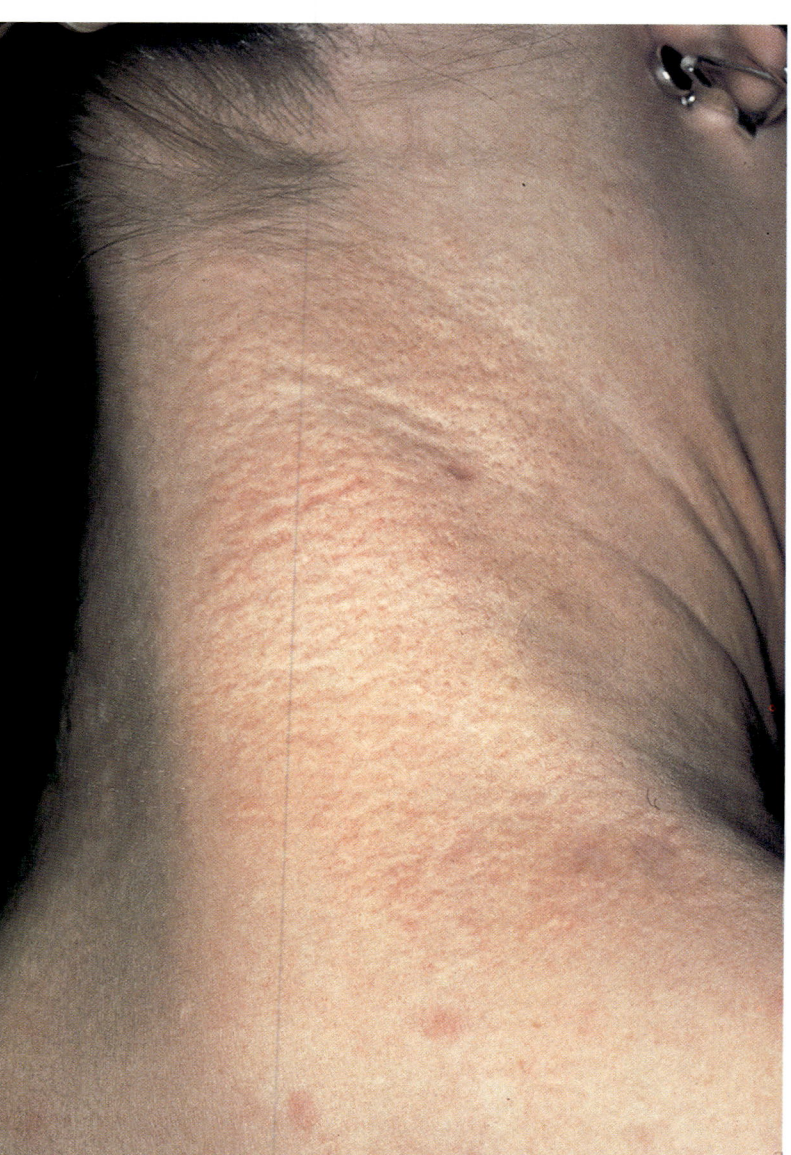

Fig. 7.20   "Plucked chicken skin" on the neck of an adolescent with pseudoxanthoma elasticum.

169. Evans DG, Ramsden R, Huson SM et al. (1993) Type 2 neurofibromatosis: the need for supraregional care? **J Laryngol Otol** 107:401–406.
170. Wiegand DA, Ojemann RG, Fickel V (1996) Surgical treatment of acoustic neuroma (vestibular schwannoma) in the United States: Report from the acoustic neuroma registry. **Laryngoscope** 106(1 PT 1):58–66.
171. Poen JC, Golby AJ, Forster KM et al. (1999) Fractionated stereotactic radiosurgery and preservation of hearing in patients with vestibular schwannoma: a preliminary report. **Neurosurg** 45(6):1299–1305.
172. Seki Y, Umezu H, Usui M et al. (2000) Restoration of hearing with an auditory brainstem implant in a patient with neurofibromatosis type 2 – case report. **Neurol Med Chir** (Tokyo) 40(10):524–527.
173. Lebwohl MG, Neldner K, Pope FM et al. (1994) Classification of pseudoxanthoma elasticum: report of a consensus conference. **J Am Acad Dermatol** 30:103–107.
174. Pope FM (1974) Autosomal dominant pseudoxanthoma elasticum. **J Med Genet** 11:152.
175. Pope FM (1974) Two types of autosomal recessive pseudoxanthoma elasticum. **Arch Dermatol** 110:209.
176. Uenishi T, Uchiyama M, Sugiura H, Danno K (1997) Pseudoxanthoma elasticum with generalized cutaneous laxity. **Arch Dermatol** 133:664–666.
177. Matsuda H, Yoshida H, Nohara N (1979) Pseudoxanthoma elasticum (autosomal recessive type 2). **Jpn J Clin Dermatol** 33:975–981.
178. Viljoen DL, Pope FM, Beighton P (1987) Heterogeneity of pseudoxanthoma elasticum: delineation of a new form? **Clin Genet** 32:100.

of these systems. Typically, the skin in PXE demonstrates yellowish flat-topped discrete and confluent papules in the skin creases of the sides and nape of the neck (Fig. 7.20), perineum, axillae, umbilicus, and flexural folds with skin redundancy that increases with advancing age. These changes are often termed "plucked chicken skin." Calcification of affected skin is common. Multiple comedones have been described in association with the typical skin changes, and may relate to the elastic fiber degeneration as in solar elastosis. Perforating periumbilical PXE has also been described.[179] Oral, anal, and vaginal mucosal lesions may occur, most commonly infiltration of the buccal mucosa of the lip. The dermatologic features generally begin in the second decade but are often subtle and overlooked. More commonly a visual or vascular complication, such as a gastrointestinal tract bleed, prompts the patient to seek medical attention.

The most common ophthalmologic finding is angioid streaks (87% of patients), which are radial extensions of gray, brown, or reddish coloration from the optic disc. The angioid streak is due to visualization of the choroid through tears in the elastic-rich Bruch's membrane. They tend to first appear during the third or fourth decade of life, but the youngest reported patient with angioid streaks was 10 years of age.[180,181] These angioid streaks rarely interfere with visual acuity. Loss of vision in PXE tends to occur later in life and is due to scarring and fibrosis from choroidal neovascularization and retinal hemorrhage. Trauma is probably a precipitating factor in the development of neovascularization and hemorrhagic complications. Characteristic irregular retinal epithelial mottling ("peau d'orange") is also commonly seen and results from degenerated elastic tissue. These pigmentary changes usually precede angioid streaks and are frequently detected in children with PXE. Drusen of the optic nerve have also been associated, and drusen-like lesions of the posterior pole have been reported in a 12-year-old boy with PXE.[181] Calcification of degenerated elastic tissue of the internal lamina of blood vessels with subsequent hemorrhage is a common and potentially serious complication of PXE. The gastrointestinal tract and renal vasculature are sites of early manifestations of this degenerative damage. Both hypertension from resultant renal artery stenosis and gastrointestinal bleeding may occur during adolescence.[182] Late vascular sequelae in PXE include cerebrovascular accidents and intermittent claudication and myocardial infarction.[183] Severe coronary artery disease has been noted in adolescents with PXE; coronary artery bypass surgery may be ameliorative.[184] Physical signs may include diminished peripheral pulses, hypertension, murmurs consistent with mitral valve prolapse and congestive heart failure, and peripheral gangrene. Rectovesical prolapse may also occur.[185]

LABORATORY FINDINGS

The histologic changes on biopsy of lesional skin from patients with PXE are diagnostic, showing distinctive broken curls of basophilic elastic fibers with routine hematoxylin and eosin or Verhoeff–van Gieson staining. Calcium deposition on elastic fibers can be easily detected with von Kossa stain. Soft tissue radiographs of the upper and lower extremities may reveal vessel wall calcification. Dental radiographs may demonstrate early vascular calcification. Ultrasonography shows a characteristic pattern of dotted increased echogenicity of renal arteries.[186] Similar patterns have been described by ultrasound in affected pancreas and spleen.

PATHOPHYSIOLOGY AND HISTOGENESIS

The mutated gene in PXE is ABCC6, a member of the ATP-binding cassette (ABC) transmembrane transporter family that encodes a multidrug resistance protein.[187–189] The reason that mutations in ABCC6 leads to the phenotypic manifestations of PXE is unclear, particularly since it is primarily expressed in the liver and kidney, two sites that are not affected by PXE.

DIFFERENTIAL DIAGNOSIS

The pebbly pattern and yellow discoloration of flexural skin of classical PXE is quite distinctive. The later development of redundancy, particularly in the autosomal recessive type II form may be confused with the sagging skin of cutis laxa. Ten percent of patients with β-thalassemia have both angioid streaks and the skin manifestations of PXE, while 16% have only the skin lesions that are clinically and histopathologically typical of PXE.[190–191] D-Penicillamine may induce an acquired form of PXE, but elastic fibers do not become calcified.[192]

TREATMENT

There is no cure for this genetic alteration of elastic tissue. Plastic surgery may improve the appearance of sagging skin, although extrusion of calcium particles through the surgical wound may result in delayed healing and unsightly scars.[193] Gastrointestinal bleeding can usually be managed conservatively with iced saline lavage and transfusion and rarely requires balloon embolization or surgery for control.[182] All patients should be followed by a retina specialist and instructed in the use of an Amsler Grid. There is no good treatment for the ophthalmologic complications although laser photocoagulation has potential as treatment for the choroidal neovascularization. Although low calcium diets have been advocated, their value has not been tested in trials.

PEDIATRIC ASPECTS

Patients should be advised to protect their eyes from even mild trauma, and about the potential for future visual loss. Because of the potential risk to eyes and calcified vessels when traumatized, contact sports and high-intensity cardiovascular exercise should be prohibited for persons with PXE. This can be quite life-altering for the child or adolescent, who may not fully understand the consequences of the seemingly minor skin changes. Avoidance of high cholesterol foods and smoking, control of blood pressure, and safe aerobic exercises may be recommended by the physician. Two support groups are available: the National Association for Pseudoxanthoma Elasticum (www.napxe.org), and PXE International, Inc. (www.pxe.org).

179. Pruzan D, Rabbin PE, Heilman ER (1992) Periumbilical perforating pseudoxanthoma elasticum. **J Am Acad Dermatol** 26:642.
180. Grand WG, Isserman MJ, Miller CW (1987) Angioid streaks associated with pseudoxanthoma elasticum in a 13-year-old patient. **Ophthalmology** 94:197.   181.   Gills JP Jr, Paton D (1965) Mottled fundus oculi in pseudoxanthoma elasticum: a report on two siblings. **Arch Ophthalmol** 73:792.
182. Cunningham JR, Lippman SM, Renie WA et al. (1980) Pseudoxanthoma elasticum: treatment of gastrointestinal hemorrhage by arterial embolization and observations on autosomal dominant inheritance. **Johns Hopkins Med J** 147:168.
183. Schachner L, Young D (1974) Pseudoxanthoma elasticum with severe cardiovascular disease in a child. **Am J Dis Child** 127:571.
184. Nishida H, Endo M, Koyanagi H et al. (1990) Coronary artery bypass in a 15-year-old girl with pseudoxanthoma elasticum **Ann Thorac Surg** 49:483.
185. Viljoen DL, Beatty S, Beighton P (1987) The obstetric and gynaecological implications of pseudoxanthoma elasticum. **Br J Obstet Gynaecol** 94:1.
186. Suarez MJ, Sarcia JB, Orense M et al. (1991) Sonographic aspects of pseudoxanthoma elasticum. **Pediatr Radiol** 21:538.

187. Ringpfeil F, Lebwohl MG, Christiano AM, Uitto J (2000) Pseudoxanthoma elasticum: mutations in the MRP6 gene encoding a transmembrane ATP-binding cassette (ABC) transporter. **Proc Natl Acad Sci USA** 97:6001–6006.
188. Le Saux O, Urban Z, Tschuch C et al. (2000) Mutations in a gene encoding an ABC transporter cause pseudoxanthoma elasticum. **Nat Genet** 223–227.
189. Bergen AA, Plomp AS, Schuurman EJ et al. (2000) Mutations in ABCC6 cause pseudoxanthoma elasticum. **Nat Genet** 25:228–231.
190. Aessopos A, Savvides P, Stamatelos G et al. (1992) Pseudoxanthoma elasticum-like skin lesions and angioid streaks in β-thalassemia. **Am J Hematol** 41:159.
191. Baccaranni-Contri M, Bacchelli B, Boraldi F et al. (2001) Characterization of pseudoxanthoma elasticum-like lesions in the skin of patients with beta-thalassemia. **J Am Acad Dermatol** 44:33–39.
192. Coatesworth AP, Darnton SJ, Green RM et al. (1998) A case of systemic pseudo-pseudoxanthoma elasticum with diverse symptomology caused by long-term penicillamine use. **J Clin Pathol** 51:169–171.
193. Viljoen DL, Bloch C, Beighton P (1990) Plastic surgery in pseudoxanthoma elasticum: experience in nine patients. **Plast Reconstr Surg** 85:233.

EHLERS–DANLOS SYNDROME

Ehlers–Danlos syndrome (EDS) is a heterogeneous group of disorders of collagen characterized by varying degrees of skin hyperextensibility and fragility, joint hypermobility, and bruisability. A new classification system was proposed in 1997,[194] which consolidates the previous at least 11 subgroups into six subgroups (Table 7.12), including autosomal dominant and autosomal recessive forms. The spectrum of severity ranges from almost imperceptible findings to severe, debilitating disease. The prevalence of EDS, including the mild forms, may be as high as 1 in 5000 individuals. The kyphoscoliosis, arthrochalasia, and dermatosparaxis types are considerably less common than the classical (most common), hypermobile, and arterial types.

PHYSICAL EXAMINATION

In general, patients with EDS share varying degrees of skin and joint hyperextensibility, tissue fragility, and bruising. Skin hyperextensibility should be tested at a site that is not subjected to mechanical forces or scarring, such as the volar surface of the forearm. Joint hypermobility in older children and adolescents can be assessed using a scale derived by Beighton[194,195] that systematically evaluates joints of the hands, elbows, knees and trunk. Mitral valve prolapse is a common manifestation, but aortic root dilatation is uncommon; both can be assessed by echocardiography, CT, or MRI examinations.[196]

Patients with the classical form of EDS have hyperextensible skin that recoils easily to its normal position after stretching (Fig. 7.21). The skin is velvety, thin, and bruises easily (Fig 7.22). Poor wound healing results in atrophic, often widened cigarette paper–like scarring, particularly on pressure points (knees, elbows, forehead, chin), and postoperative wound dehiscence. Calcification and fibrosis of hematomas produces subcutaneous, nodular molluscoid pseudotumors, most frequently found at the elbow and knee areas. Spheroids are small subcutaneous spherical hard nodules, usually on the forearms and shins, that may become calcified and thus detectable radiographically. Blue sclerae may be noted. Joint hypermobility is a frequent feature (Fig. 7.23), often demonstrable at fingers and wrists, and by extension of the tongue to touch the nose (Gorlin's sign). Sprains, dislocations or subluxations, and pes planus occur as complications, and patients complain

TABLE 7.12   Ehlers–Danlos syndrome

Type	Defect	Skin findings	Joint changes	Inheritance	Old classification	Others
Classical	Mutations in COL5A1, COL5A2; rarely, mutations in COL1A1	Hyperextensibility, bruising	Hypermobility	AD	Type I Gravis Type II Mitis	Molluscoid pseudotumors Dislocations Pes planus Hernias Muscle hypotonia
Hypermobility	Unknown	Variable hypertensibility; no atrophic scars	Hypermobility	AD	Type III	Musculoskeletal pain
Vascular	Mutations in COL3A1; abnormal type III collagen secretion, synthesis or structure	Thin, translucent skin; Marked bruising	Minimal hypermobility Limited to digits	AD	Type IV (arterial-ecchymotic)	Acrogeria; clubfoot rupture of bowel, uterus, arteries; family history of sudden death
Kyphoscoliosis	Lysyl hydroxylase deficiency; mutations in PLOD gene	Soft, hyperextensible	Hypermobility	AR	Type VI	Muscle hypotonia, scoliosis; ocular abnormalities
Arthrochalasia	Amino-terminal propeptide cleavage site of COL1A1 type A) or COL1A2 (type B)	Hyperextensible, soft skin with or without abnormal scarring	Marked hypermobility	AD	Type VIIA Type VII B	Congenital hip dislocation; arthrochalasis multiplex congenita; short stature
Dermatosparaxis	Recessive mutations in type I collagen N-peptidase	Severe fragility; sagging, redundant skin; Normal wound Healing	None	AR	Type VIIC	
Other				XL	Type V (X-L)	
				AD	Type VIII (Periodontitis)	
				?	Type X (Fibronectin deficient)	
				AD	Type XI (Familial hypermobility)	
				?	Progeroid EDS	
				–	Unspecified forms	

AD autosomal dominant; AR = recessive.

194. Beighton P, De Paepe A, Steinmann B et al. (1998) Ehlers–Danlos syndromes: revised nosology, Villefranche, 1997. **Am J Med Genet** 77:31–37.
195. Beighton P (1983) The Ehlers–Danlos syndromes. In: Heritable Disorders of Connective Tissue, 5th ed, Beighton P, ed. St. Louis: Mosby, pp. 189–251.
196. Tiller GE, Cassidy SB, Wensel C, Wenstrup RJ (1998) Aortic root dilatation in Ehlers–Danlos syndrome types I, II and III. A report of five cases. **Clin Genet** 53:460–465.

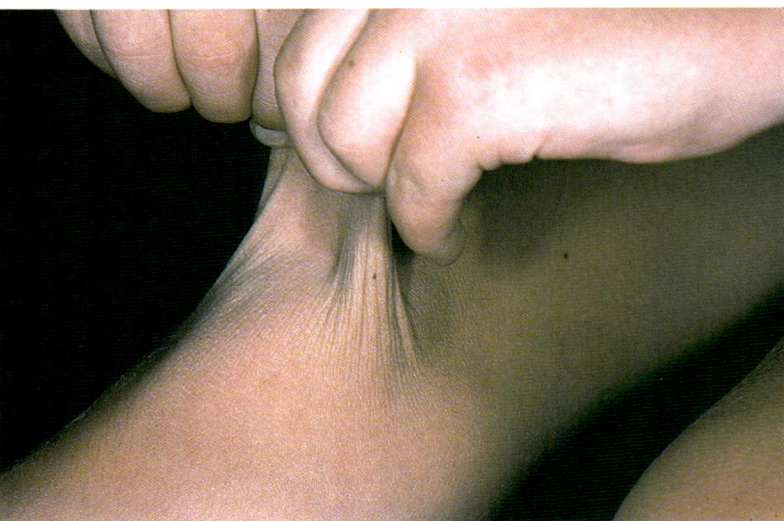

Fig. 7.21   Marked hyperextensibility of the skin in a patient with the classical type of Ehlers–Danlos syndrome.

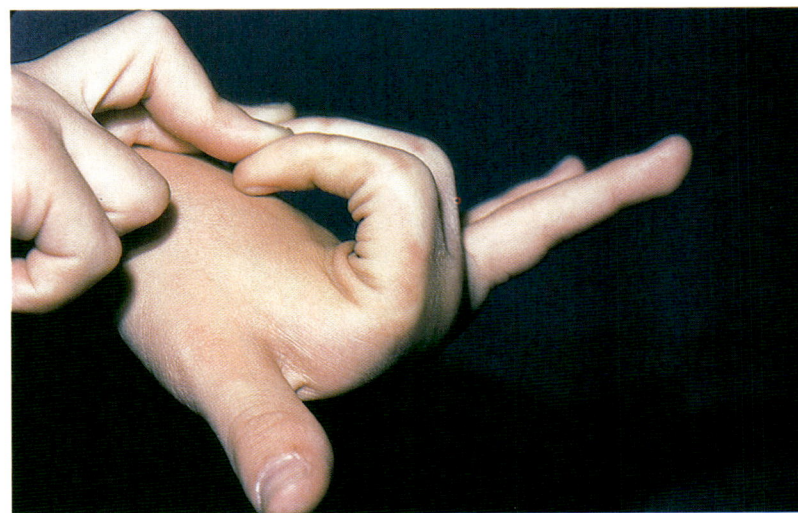

Fig. 7.23   Joint hypermobility in a patient with the classical type of Ehlers–Danlos syndrome.

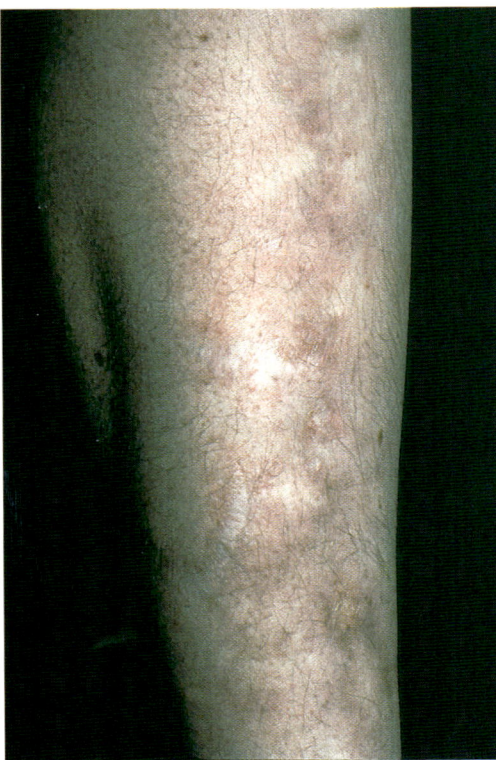

Fig. 7.22   Easy bruisability and persistent discoloration on the legs of a young girl with Ehlers–Danlos syndrome

of chronic joint and limb pain, despite normal skeletal radiographs.[196] Muscle hypotonia and delayed gross motor development have been described. Hiatal hernia, postoperative hernias, and anal prolapse have been noted as manifestations of the tissue hyperextensibility and fragility.[197] Approximately half of affected individuals were born prematurely due to rupture of fetal membranes.

Patients with the hypermobility type show soft, velvety skin with occasional hyperextensibility. If healed wounds are atrophic, the classical type should be diagnosed instead. The joints all tend to be hypermobile, and dislocations of the shoulder, patella and temporomandibular joints are particularly common. Musculoskeletal pain is early in onset, chronic, and sometimes debilitating.

The vascular type of EDS is characterized by thin, translucent skin with prominent venous pattern and extensive bruising.[197] Joint hypermobility is usually limited to the digits. The facial appearance is often typical, and subcutaneous fat is decreased, especially of the face and limbs. Spontaneous rupture of arteries, particularly mid-sized arteries, may occur during childhood, although its peak age of incidence is the third or fourth decade of life. Arterial or intestinal rupture often presents as acute abdominal or flank pain; arterial rupture is the most common cause of death. Pregnancies may be complicated by pre-and postpartum arterial bleeding, and by intrapartum uterine rupture. Vaginal and perineal tears from the delivery heal poorly. The kyphoscoliosis type is characterized by generalized joint laxity with severe muscle hypotonia at birth, which leads to gross motor delay, and congenital scoliosis, which is progressive. By the second or third decade of life, patients tend to lose the ability to ambulate. The skin may be fragile, and heals with atrophic scars. Easy bruisability and arterial rupture have been described. Occasionally, patients show a Marfanoid habitus, osteopenia, and scleral fragility with rupture of the ocular globe. Patients with the arthrochalasia type show generalized joint hypermobility with recurrent subluxations and congenital bilateral hip dislocation. The skin may be hyperextensible, fragile, and easy to bruise. Muscle hypotonia, kyphoscoliosis, and mild osteopenia have been described. Finally, the other established form is the dermatosparaxis form, in which patients have severe skin fragility with sagging, redundant skin;[198] however, wound healing is not impaired and scars are not atrophic. The skin may be soft and doughy in texture, with easy bruisability. Large umbilical and inguinal hernias, and premature rupture of the fetal membranes may be seen. Other types of EDS have been described in single families, or are associated with features that may be serendipitous.

LABORATORY FINDINGS

Routine histopathologic examination of skin from patients with EDS is usually normal, but electron microscopy demonstrates various abnormalities in the appearance of collagen fibrils. Studies of platelet function and coagulation are usually normal, despite a tendency for bruising and increased

197. Pepin M, Schwarze U, Superti-Furga A, Byers PH (2000) Clinical and genetic features of Ehlers–Danlos syndrome type IV, the vascular type. **N Engl J Med** 342:673–680.

198. Petty EM, Seashore MR, Braverman IM et al. (1993) Dermatosparaxis in children. A case report and review of the newly recognized phenotype. **Arch Dermatol** 129:1310–1315.

bleeding, further implicating the defective structural integrity of skin and blood vessels. Although gene diagnosis is possible as a research tool, biochemical tests are available as well. Structurally abnormal collagen type III in cultured fibroblasts has been demonstrated in the vascular form. Measurement of total urinary hydroxylysyl pyridinoline and lysyl pyridinoline crosslinks after hydrolysis using high-performance liquid chromatography is sensitive and specific for diagnosing the kyphoscoliosis type. Electrophoretic demonstration of procollagen $\alpha1(I)$ or $\alpha2(I)$ chains from collagen or cultured fibroblasts is seen with the arthrochalasia and dermatosparaxis forms.

PATHOPHYSIOLOGY AND HISTOGENESIS

The underlying molecular defect for the classical form of EDS is mutations in the $\alpha1$ or $\alpha2$ chain of type V collagen (COL5A1 and COL5A2).[199,200] Haploinsufficiency of the COL5A1 gene probably accounts for approximately one-third of cases.[201] Although uncommon compared to COL5A1 and COL5A2 detects, mutations in COL1A1 have also been associated with the classic form of EDS.[202] The molecular basis for the hypermobility form is currently unknown. The vascular form of EDS has been associated with mutations in type III collagen (COL3A1), resulting in a reduced amount of type III collagen in dermis, vessels, and viscera, as well as decreased production and secretion of type III collagen by cultured fibroblasts.[203] Mutations in the lysyl hydroxylase (PLOD) gene cause the kyphoscoliosis form of EDS. The arthrochalasia and dermatosparaxis forms involve impaired removal of the amino terminal N-propeptides from procollagen. In the arthrochalasia type, mutations lead to deficient processing of the amino terminal end of the pro$\alpha1(I)$ (type A) or pro$\alpha2(I)$ (type B) chains of collagen I. The dermatosparaxis form in both humans and cattle results from mutations in the procollagen I N-proteinase gene.[204] The progeroid variant has been linked to mutations in galactosyltransferase I.[205]

DIFFERENTIAL DIAGNOSIS

EDS must be distinguished clinically and histologically from cutis laxa. In cutis laxa, the hyperelastic skin does not spring back to its usual position after stretching. The joint hypermobility of EDS must also be distinguished from Marfan syndrome, which is characterized by ectopia lentis and characteristic skeletal abnormalities. The nodular pseudomolluscoid tumors on the lower legs may be confused with subcutaneous granuloma annulare. The easy bruisability and poor wound healing may raise the possibility of child abuse. Tenascin-X deficiency, a recessive condition, resembles EDS.[206]

TREATMENT

There is no effective treatment for this syndrome. Wounds should be sutured with tightly spaced sutures and left in place for a prolonged duration. Adhesive tapes or pressure bandages may aid healing, diminish scarring, and lower the risk of pseudotumor formation. Ongoing rheumatologic and orthopedic care may be required to prevent progressive joint disease in certain patients. Low-impact sports are preferable to contact sports and weight training in patients with hypermobility. Ascorbate therapy results in improved wound healing and decreased bleeding tendency in patients with type VI EDS. Prenatal diagnosis is possible by genetic and biochemical analyses.

Unless children are severely affected by their disorder, they generally adjust well to the skin findings and joint hypermobility. Caution must be taken to avoid trauma, and wounds should be repaired by careful suturing and avoidance of infection. The Ehlers–Danlos Foundation is a national support group (www.ednf.org).

MARFAN SYNDROME

Marfan syndrome is an autosomal dominant disorder that primarily affects the skeletal, ocular, and cardiovascular systems.[207,208] About 25% of cases occur sporadically, particularly in patients born of older fathers. Parental germline mosaicism has been described.[209] The overall prevalence of Marfan syndrome is approximately 1 per 10 000 persons.

PHYSICAL EXAMINATION

The characteristic Marfan habitus is a tall, thin person, with the lower body segment longer than the upper segment of the body. Characteristically, the arm span exceeds the person's height. The distal bones are excessively long (arachnodactyly, spider fingers). Kyphoscoliosis may be severe and increases with the adolescent growth spurt.[210] Thoracic cage abnormalities such as pectus excavatum are also commonly seen. The combination of kyphoscoliosis and pectus excavatum rarely compromises cardiopulmonary function. Joint laxity from capsular, ligamentous, and tendinous involvement may cause hyperextensibility and/or dislocation. Patellar dislocation is not uncommon; dislocation of the hip, often detected during the newborn period, may be the first sign of Marfan syndrome. The thumb sign and wrist sign are screening tests for the joint hypermobility of Marfan syndrome.[210] The thumb sign is positive when the thumb extends well beyond the ulnar border of the hand when overlapped by fingers. The wrist sign is positive when the thumb overlaps the fifth finger as they grasp the opposite wrist.

More than one-half of patients have ectopia lentis. Subluxation and complete dislocation of the lens often lead to other secondary ocular abnormalities, including ametropia, myopia, and increased risk of retinal detachment.[208]

Cardiovascular abnormalities occur in approximately 40% of patients with Marfan syndrome by cardiac examination and almost 100% of patients by pathologic examination. Medial necrosis of the aorta is the most common defect and diffuse dilatation of the proximal segment of the ascending aorta with aortic regurgitation often occurs. Death in patients usually occurs in adulthood as a result of cardiovascular sequelae, especially owing to complications related to dilatation of the aortic root.[211,212] Mitral valve prolapse occurs in approximately 25% of affected children and adolescents, and in 86% with associated pectus excavatum.[213]

199. Toriello HV, Glover TW, Takahara K et al. (1996) A translocation interrupts the COL5A1 gene in a patient with Ehlers–Danlos syndrome and hypomelanosis of Ito. **Nat Genet** 13:361–365.
200. Michalickovak K, Susic M, Willing MC et al. (1998) Mutations of the alpha2(V) chain of type V collagen impair matrix assembly and produce Ehlers–Danlos syndrome type I. **Hum Mol Genet** 7:249–255.
201. Wenstrup RJ, Florer JB, Willing MC et al. (2000) COL5A1 haploinsufficiency is a common molecular mechanism underlying the classical form of EDS. **Am J Hum Genet** 66:1766–1776.
202. Nuytinck L, Freund M, Lagae L et al. (2000) Classical Ehlers–Danlos syndrome caused by a mutation in type I collagen. **Am J Hum Genet** 66:1398–1402.
203. Cole WG, Chiodo AA, Lamande SR et al. (1990) A base substitution at a splice site in the COL3A1 gene causes exon skipping and generates abnormal type III procollagen in a patient with Ehlers–Danlos syndrome type IV. **J Biol Chem** 265:17070.
204. Colige A, Sieron AL, Li SW et al. (1999) Human Ehlers–Danlos syndrome type VIIC and bovine dermatosparaxis are caused by mutations in the procollagen I N-proteinase gene. **Am J Hum Genet** 65:308–317.
205. Okajima T, Fukumoto S, Furukawa K, Urano T (1999) Molecular basis for the progeroid variant of Ehlers–Danlos syndrome. Identification and characterization of two mutations in galactosyltransferase I gene. **J Biol Chem** 274:28841–28844.
206. Burch GH, Gong Y, Liu W et al. (1997) Tenascin-X deficiency is associated with Ehlers–Danlos syndrome. **Nat Genet** 17:104–108.
207. Pyeritz RE (2000) The Marfan syndrome. **Annu Rev Med** 51:481–510.
208. Rantamaki T, Kaitila I, Syvanen AC et al. (1999) Recurrence of Marfan syndrome as a result of parental germ-line mosaicism for an FBN1 mutation. **Am J Human Genet** 64:993–1001.
209. Sun QB, Zhang KZ, Cheng TO et al. (1990) Marfan syndrome in China: a collective review of 564 cases among 98 families. **Am Heart J** 120:934.
210. Joseph KN, Kane HA, Milner RS et al. (1992) Orthopedic aspects of the Marfan syndrome. **Clin Orthop** 277:251.
211. Groenink M, Lohuis TA, Tijssen JG et al. (1999) Survival and complication free survival in Marfan's syndrome: implications of current guidelines. **Heart** 82:499–504.
212. Silverman DI, Burton KJ, Gray JR et al. (1995) Life expectancy in the Marfan syndrome. **Am J Cardiol** 75:157–160.
213. Seliem MA, Duffy CE, Gidding SS et al. (1992) Echocardiographic evaluation of the aortic root and mitral valve in children and adolescents with isolated pectus excavatum: comparison with Marfan patients. **Pediatr Cardiol** 13:20.

Lack of subcutaneous fat, and the presence of striae, most prominent on the upper chest, arms, thighs, and abdomen, are the most common cutaneous manifestations of Marfan syndrome. In addition, elastosis perforans serpiginosa occurs with increased frequency in patients with Marfan syndrome.

Infants with the neonatal form of Marfan syndrome have the body disproportion of Marfan syndrome in addition to lax skin, emphysema, ocular abnormalities, joint contractures, kyphoscoliosis, adducted thumbs, crumpled ears, micrognathia, muscle hypoplasia, and deficient subcutaneous fat over joints.[214,215] Severe cardiac valve insufficiency and aortic dilatation result in death during the first 2 years of life.

LABORATORY FINDINGS

The diagnosis of Marfan syndrome is based on a constellation of clinical findings. There is no diagnostic laboratory test or histologic abnormality. Increased urinary hydroxyproline and desmosine are not consistent findings.

PATHOPHYSIOLOGY AND HISTOGENESIS

Marfan syndrome has been shown to result from mutations in the gene for profibrillin 1 on chromosome 15.[216] Fibrillin is a 350kD glycoprotein that is a major component of microfibrils, structural components of the zonular fibers of the lens and associated with elastic fibers in the aorta and skin. Virtually every family's mutation is different, with no hotspots identified, except in cases of neonatal Marfan syndrome.

DIFFERENTIAL DIAGNOSIS

Marfan syndrome is rarely confused with disorders other than homocystinuria. Homocystinuria is an autosomal recessive disorder resulting from deficient cystathionine synthetase with abnormal methionine metabolism and increased levels of urinary homocysteine. Both Marfan syndrome and homocystinuria manifest with dolichostenomelia (long, thin body habitus),

orthopedic abnormalities, and ectopia lentis, but many features differ (Table 7.13) (see Homocystinuria in Hereditary Metabolic Disorders, below). Patients with Weil–Marchesani syndrome also have ectopia lentis, but the orthopedic features are quite different, with short stature, brachydactyly, spherophakia, and stiff joints. Congenital contractural arachnodactyly (Beals syndrome) is a marfanoid syndrome characterized by congenital contractures of the elbows, knees, hips, and fingers, but without ocular or cardiovascular manifestations. A second fibrillin gene on chromosome 5 has been linked to congenital contractural arachnodactyly.

TREATMENT

Management of Marfan syndrome should involve prevention of the disabling and life-threatening potential complications. Early and regular ophthalmologic examinations are required to detect correctable amblyopia and retinal detachment. The ectopia lentis and even complete luxation may be tolerated for decades. Lens extraction may be required to treat diplopia, glaucoma, cataracts, or retinal detachment. Repair of the pectus excavatum is indicated if cardiopulmonary compromise occurs, but should be delayed until skeletal maturation is nearly complete to prevent recurrence and should employ internal stabilization.[217] Scoliosis may be lessened in adolescent girls by estrogen therapy, but this therapy may also produce an overall decrease in height. Bracing, physical therapy, and vertebral fusion may all be necessary to prevent severe scoliosis. Long-term propranolol therapy is being administered to prevent aortic dilatation by decreasing myocardial contractility,[218] but may not affect survival.[219] Aneurysmal and valvular heart defects may require prosthetic replacement, but this should be forestalled as long as possible to avoid recurrent prosthesis replacement, particularly in growing children. Replacement of the aortic root has led to increased life expectancy.

Children should be excused form participation in physical education in order to avoid potentially harmful exertion, contact sports, and isometric exercises, which might lead to aortic rupture or congenital heart failure. This adds to the isolation of a child who may already be concerned about an unusual body image or is socially ostracized because of looking "funny" or being excessively tall. One must keep in mind, however, that not all persons with Marfan syndrome are obviously "different." When the diagnosis in a patient with an atypical presentation is suspected, one must make certain that appropriate studies are performed, so that potentially lethal internal manifestations are not neglected. The web site for the National Marfan Foundation is www.marfan.org.

CUTIS LAXA

Cutis laxa is a heterogeneous group of disorders characterized by widespread laxity of skin and, in some cases, involvement of other organs, due to abnormalities in elastic tissue. The autosomal dominant form of cutis laxa primarily affects the skin. It may present in infancy or often in adulthood and tends to be relatively benign.[220,221] A distinctive facies, inguinal hernia, and bronchiectasis may be associated. An autosomal recessive variety may be very severe with elastic tissue defects occurring in several organs, including fatal cardiopulmonary disease.[220] Other complications include facial dysmorphism with large ears and antimongoloid slanting of the palpebral fissures, diverticula of the gastrointestinal and genitourinary tracts, dislocated hips, osteoporosis, joint hyperextensibility, prolapsed rectal, vaginal or gastric mucosae, hernia, and pectus excavatum.

TABLE 7.13   Comparison of Marfan syndrome and homocystinuria

	Marfan syndrome	Homocystinuria
Defect	Fibrillin-1	Cystathione synthetase
Inheritance	Dominant	Recessive
Eyes	Lens displaced up; myopic	Lens displaced down
Cardiovascular	Aortic aneurysms; mitral regurgitation	Arterial and venous thromboses
Intelligence	Normal	Subnormal
Skin	Striae distensae; elastosis perforanspores; serpiginosa	Malar flush; large facial cutis reticulata; dermatitis
Dolichostenomelia	+	+
Hyperextensibility	−	+
Bones	Marked kyphoscoliosis	Osteoporosis, "codfish" vertebrae

214. Morse RP, Rockenmacher S, Pyeritz RE (1990) Diagnosis and management of infantile Marfan syndrome. **Pediatrics** 86:888.
215. Buntinx IM, Willems PJ, Spitaels SE et al. (1991) Neonatal Marfan syndrome with congenital arachnodactyly, flexion contractures, and severe cardiac valve insufficiency. **J Med Genet** 28:27.
216. Dietz HC, Cutting GR, Pyeritz RE et al. (1991) Marfan syndrome caused by a recurrent de novo missense mutation in the fibrillin gene. **Nature** 352:337–339.
217. Arn PH, Scherer LR, Haller JA Jr, Pyeritz RE (1989) Outcome of pectus excavatum in patients with Marfan syndrome and in the general population. **J Pediatr** 115:954.

218. Shores J, Berger KR, Murphy EA, Pyeritz RE (1994) Progression of aortic dilatation and the benefit of long-term beta-adrenergic blockade in Marfan syndrome. **N Engl J Med** 330:1335–1341.
219. Gray JR, Bridges AB, West RR et al. (1998) Life expectancy in British Marfan syndrome populations. **Clin Genet** 54:124–128.
220. Beighton P (1972) The dominant and recessive forms of cutis laxa. **J Med Genet** 9:216.
221. Damkier A, Brandrup F, Starklint H (1991) Cutis laxa: Autosomal dominant inheritance in five generations. **Clin Genet** 39:321.

PHYSICAL EXAMINATION

The skin in cutis laxa is inelastic and appears pendulous. It is hyperextensible but does not resume its normal shape after stretching, as is seen in EDS. At birth the infant may appear to have unusually soft and loose skin. Joint laxity is not a feature of cutis laxa, in contrast to EDS. Often persons with cutis laxa are described as having a bloodhound-like facial appearance. Young affected children appear aged (Fig. 7.24). In more severe forms of cutis laxa, patients may have gastrointestinal and bladder diverticula, hernias, and pulmonary emphysema. Rarely, severe cardiopulmonary complications of cutis laxa have been reported in young children.

LABORATORY FINDINGS

Special stains for elastic tissue (Verhoeff–van Gieson stain) of skin biopsy specimens demonstrate significantly decreased or absent dermal elastic fibers. Granular degeneration of elastic fibers and increased elastin-associated microfibrils are noted on electron microscopy.

PATHOPHYSIOLOGY AND HISTOGENESIS

Mutations in elastin cause cutis laxa, leading to abnormal elastic fibers in autosomal dominant cases,[222] or absence of elastin, in some cases due to decreased mRNA stability.[223]

DIFFERENTIAL DIAGNOSIS

Cutis laxa has been reported in association with delayed growth and development, ligamentous laxity, widely patent anterior fontanel, and congenital dislocation of hips.[224] This condition has been noted primarily in female patients, but is likely to be autosomal recessive.[225] DeBarsy syndrome is an autosomal recessive condition with cutis laxa in association with progeroid facies, frontal bossing, prominent nose and ears, cutaneous atrophy, hyperextensibility of small joints, short stature, severe mental retardation, and choreoathetoid movements.[226] Cutis laxa, skeletal anomalies, and ambiguous genitalia have been reported in a patient with Lenz–Majewski hyperostotic dwarfism.[227] In addition, two related boys have been described with ambiguous genitalia associated with skeletal abnormalities, cutis laxa, craniostenosis, psychomotor retardation, and facial abnormalities (SCARF syndrome), probably inherited as an X-linked recessive disorder.[228] Cutis laxa-like skin of the hands, feet, and abdomen (when sitting) are characteristic of the wrinkly skin syndrome.[229] Other features include a prominent venous pattern on the chest, hypotonia, mental retardation with microcephaly, and various other musculoskeletal and/or connective tissue findings. A neonate with cutis laxa, emphysema, heart anomalies, a diaphragmatic hernia, and a marfanoid phenotype was found to have a chromosomal break at 7q31.3–7q32 and was found to be deficient in laminin in skin.[230]

Cutis laxa has also been noted with Costello syndrome, thought to be an autosomal dominant disorder.[231] Affected patients have soft, loose skin of the neck, hands and feet, with excessive wrinkling and deep creases. The digits tend to be hyperextensible. Patients show generalized hyperpigmentation with nevi, often on the palms and soles. Other characteristic features are

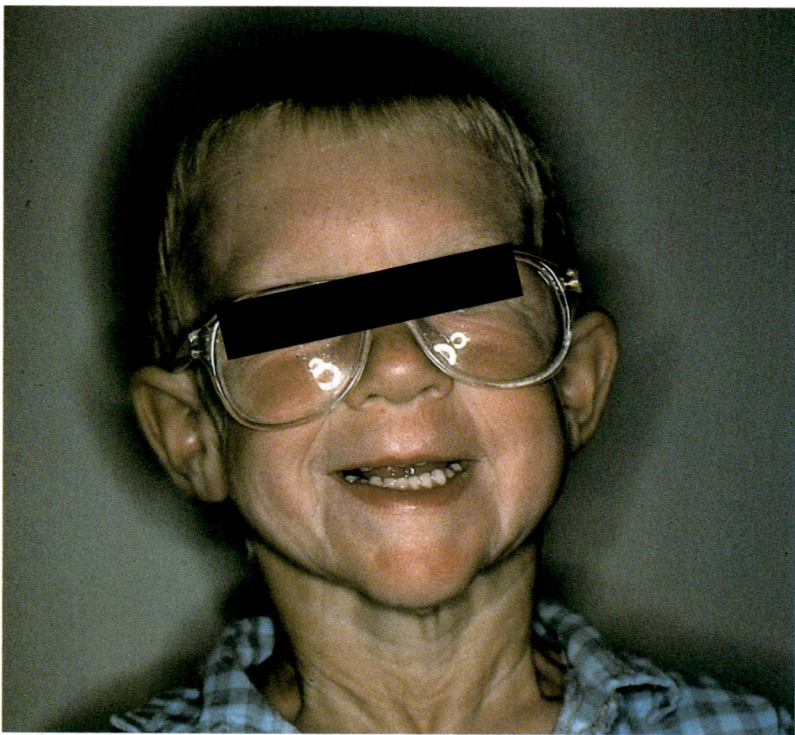

Fig. 7.24   Severe aged appearance in a 10-year-old boy with cutis laxa.

papillomata that develop during childhood around the nares, mouth, and anal areas, and acanthosis nigricans, occasionally in association with abnormal glucose metabolism. Although prenatal overgrowth and polyhydramnios occur, patients tend to have postnatal failure to thrive and a distinctive appearance, with cranofacial findings that resemble those of lysosomal storage disorders. The facies are coarse with thick lips, macroglossia, and relative macrocephaly. Severe short stature, mental retardation, and hypertrophic cardiomyopathy are other associated manifestations. Biopsies show fine, disrupted and loosely constructed elastic fibers in the skin and mucosae, and defects in elastic microfibrils have been proposed.[232]

Acquired forms of generalized and localized cutis laxa occasionally occur.[233] In type I acquired cutis laxa, ill-defined areas of loose skin appear insidiously but progressively. Type I skin lesions involve the face and often progress in a cephalocaudal direction. The development of cutis laxa is often preceded by urticarial eruption. Although type I acquired cutis laxa usually begins in adulthood, children have been described with this condition. Emphysema, aortic aneurysms with subsequent rupture, and gastrointestinal and genitourinary diverticulae have been associated, although most affected children have not had systemic evidence of acquired cutis laxa; aortic dilatation and emphysema, and severe tracheobrachiomegaly have led to the

222. Tassabejhi M, Metcalfe K, Hurst J et al. (1998) An elastic gene mutation producing abnormal tropoelastin and abnormal elastic fibres in a patient with autosomal dominant cutis laxa. **Hum Mol Genet** 7:1012–1018.
223. Zhang MC, Giro M, Quaglino D Jr, Davidson JM (1995) Transforming growth factor-beta reverses a posttranscriptional defect in elastin synthesis in a cutis laxa skin fibroblast strain. **J Clin Invest** 95:986–994.
224. Sakati NO, Nyhan WL, Shear CS et al. (1983) Syndrome of cutis laxa, ligamentous laxity and delayed development. **Pediatrics** 72:850.
225. Allanson J, Austin W, Hecht F (1986) Congenital cutis laxa with retardation of growth and motor development: a recessive disorder of connective tissue with male lethality. **Clin Genet** 29:133.
226. Kunze J, Majewski F, Montgomery P et al. (1985) Debarsy syndrome – an autosomal recessive, progeroid syndrome. **Eur J Pediatr** 144:348.
227. Kaye CI, Fisher DE, Esterly NB (1974) Cutis laxa, skeletal anomalies and ambiguous genitalia. **Am J Dis Child** 127:115.
228. Koppe R, Kaplan P, Hunter A, MacMurray B (1989) Ambiguous genitalia associated with skeletal abnormalities, cutis laxa, craniostenosis, psychomotor retardation, and facial abnormalities (SCARF syndrome). **Am J Med Genet** 34:305.
229. Hurvitz SA, Baumgarten A, Gocdman RM (1990) The wrinkly skin syndrome: a report of a case and review of the literature. **Clin Genet** 38:307.
230. Bonneau D, Huret JL, Godeau G et al. (1991) Recurrent ctb(7)(q31.3) and possible laminin involvement in a neonatal cutis laxa with a Marfan phenotype. **Hum Genet** 87:317.
231. Johnson J, Golabi M, Norton ME et al. (1998) Costello syndrome: phenotype, natural history, differential diagnosis, and possible cause. **J Pediatr** 133:441–448.
232. Mori M, Yamagata T, Mori Y et al. (1996) Elastic fiber degeneration in Costello syndrome. **Am J Med Genet** 61:304–309.
233. Koch SE, Williams ML (1985) Acquired cutis laxa: case report and review of disorders of elastolysis. **Pediatr Dermatol** 2:282.

demise of children with acquired cutis laxa. Children may develop cutis laxa after drug exposure to penicillin, D-penicillamine.[234] or isoniazid. Type II acquired cutis laxa (Marshall syndrome) is a postinflammatory elastolysis characterized by well-demarcated, nonpruritic erythematous plaques that extend peripherally and have a hypopigmented center. They appear in crops during a period of days to weeks, often in association with fever, malaise, and peripheral eosinophilia. Gradually localized, or less commonly generalized, areas of cutis laxa occur at sites of previous inflammation.[235] Systemic involvement is rare, but fatal aortitis has been described.[235,236] Type II cutis laxa occurs in young children. A transient form of neonatal cutis laxa has also been noted in neonates born to mothers who were administered D-penicillamine during pregnancy.[237,238] These babies demonstrate generalized laxity of skin and inguinal hernias, but the loose skin resolves during the first year of life.

Patients with EDS have loose skin that regains a normal appearance when not stretched; other features of the EDS, including joint laxity, increased bruising, and poor wound healing, are not features of cutis laxa. Older patients with PXE may have laxity of skin, especially in flexural areas, but the skin shows a pebbly yellow appearance. Histologic examination of lesional skin further distinguishes these entities.

TREATMENT

Cutis laxa is a progressive disorder that usually worsens with age. The physical appearance can be improved temporarily by plastic surgery, since the vasculature and wound healing capability are normal.[239] However, numerous procedures may be required, so they must be spaced appropriately to lessen the trauma and risk of surgery in the child. Hernia repairs may be necessary. Rarely, cardiopulmonary failure results from pulmonary emphysema, and drug and ventilatory support are required.

PEDIATRIC ASPECTS

Children with cutis laxa are psychologically most traumatized by their aged appearance, which makes them an object of curiosity. Every effort to improve appearance is reasonable and should be customized to the needs of the child, since the clinical spectrum of involvement varies widely.

OSTEOGENESIS IMPERFECTA

Osteogenesis imperfecta (OI) is an inherited disorder of type I collagen that is associated with bone fragility.[240,241] The prevalence of OI in all of its forms is 1:5000 to 1:10 000 individuals.

PHYSICAL EXAMINATION

Clinically, patients with OI have been subdivided into four major types. Patients with type I OI, an autosomal dominant form, tend to have mild to moderate bone fragility with little or no bone deformity, blue sclerae, easy bruisability, hearing loss (50%), and often short stature. A subgroup of patients with type I OI have dentinogenesis imperfecta. Patients with type II OI tend to die in the perinatal period owing to the extreme fragility of bones. The minimal calvarial mineralization, beaded ribs, compressed femora, and marked long bone deformities are common features. Most neonates have intrauterine growth retardation and multiple *in utero* fractures. The inheritance pattern of type II OI may be autosomal dominant (new mutation) or recessive. In type III OI, an autosomal recessive disorder, patients have severe bone fragility with progressive bone deformities and severe osteoporosis. Extreme short stature and scoliosis are associated, but patients tend to have white sclerae, particularly with aging. The fourth type of OI is autosomal dominant, with a greater bone fragility and deformity than in type I OI. Patients have normal sclerae, but moderate short stature and joint hypermobility. One subset of patients with type IV OI have dentinogenesis imperfecta, and hearing loss occasionally occurs.

Not uncommonly, patients have hyperlaxity of ligaments and hypermobility of joints. Many patients have been described with hernias, but joint dislocation does not occur. Bruising is often seen but not hemorrhage. The scleral blueness is due to the thinness of sclera from defects in scleral collagen, permitting scattering of light by normal pigment within the orbit. This often improves with advancing age. Dermatologists may be asked to see children with OI to consider the possibility of child abuse in view of the many fractures and evidence of bruising.[242]

PATHOPHYSIOLOGY AND HISTOGENESIS

Mutations in the two genes that encode the chains of type I collagen have been cited as the molecular cause of different forms of osteogenesis imperfecta.[240] These mutations may reduce the amount of type I collagen synthesized by tissues or alter the structure of the type I collagen. In general those that alter the amount of type I collagen are most mild, whereas the phenotypes of these types with altered structure vary considerably.

DIFFERENTIAL DIAGNOSIS

It is important to remember that blue sclerae are normal in neonates and that this is not a diagnostic criterion in young infants. A variety of other bony disorders need to be considered in the differential diagnosis,[243] but child abuse is also often considered in affected infants.[242]

TREATMENT

The prognosis of patients with OI varies tremendously, depending on the severity. Mild to moderate cases have an excellent chance of ambulation, whereas patients with more severe diseases are usually confined to a wheelchair. Orthopedic intervention involves physical therapy; splints, braces, or casting; and surgical straightening of the bone with intramedually rod placement. Recently, intranasal administration of calcitonin has been shown to decrease the frequency of bone fractures.[244] Since some children with OI and short stature have been shown to have abnormalities of the growth hormone-somatomedin axis, it has been proposed that administration of growth hormone or clonidine may augment growth rates.[245] Prenatal diagnosis has been made by ultrasonic detection of fractures in the affected fetus. Detection of abnormal type I collagen from the skin, chorionic villi, and placental membranes further verified the diagnosis of OI in an affected fetus aborted after detection of bone fractures by ultrasonography.

234. Hill VA, Seymour CA, Mortimer PS (2000) Penicillamine-induced elastosis perforans serpiginosa and cutis laxa in Wilson's disease. **Br J Dermatol** 142:560–561.
235. Muster AJ, Bharati S, Herman JJ et al. (1983) Fatal cardiovascular disease and cutis laxa following acute febrile neutrophilic dermatosis. **J Pediatr** 102:243.
236. Heyl T, Simpson IW, Cronje RE (1971) Post-inflammatory cutis laxa and aortitis (acquired systemic elastolysis). **Br J Dermatol**, 85(suppl. 7):37.
237. Solomon L, Abrams F, Dinner M, Berman L (1977) Neonatal abnormalities associated with D-penicillamine treatment during pregnancy. **N Engl J Med** 296:54.
238. Linares A, Zarranz JJ, Rodriguez-Alarcon J, Diaz-Perez JI (1979) Reversible cutis laxa due to maternal D-penicillamine treatment. **Lancet** 2:43.
239. Nahas FX, Sterman S, Gemperli R, Ferreira MS (1999) The role of plastic surgery in congenital cutis laxa: a 10-year follow-up. **Plast Reconstr Surg** 104:1174–1178.

240. Byers PH, Steiner PH (1992) Osteogenesis imperfecta. **Ann Rev Med** 43:269.
241. Marini JC (1988) Osteogenesis imperfecta: comprehensive management. **Adv Pediatr** 35:391.
242. Gahagen S, Rimsza ME (1991) Child abuse or osteogenesis imperfecta: how can we tell? **Pediatrics** 88:987.
243. Stoltz MR, Dietrich SL, Marshall GJ (1987) Osteogenesis imperfecta: perspectives. **Clin Orthop** 242:120.
244. Nishi Y, Hamamoto K, Kajiyama M et al. (1992) Effect of long-term calcitonin therapy by injection and nasal spray on the incidence of fractures in osteogenesis imperfecta. **J Pediatr** 121:477.
245. Marini JC, Bordenick S, Heavner G et al. (1993) The growth hormone and somatomedin axis in short children with osteogenesis imperfecta. **J Clin Endocrinol Metab** 76:251.

BUSCHKE–OLLENDORFF SYNDROME

Buschke and Ollendorff originally reported the association of connective tissue nevi and osteopoikilosis.[246,247] The disorder is inherited in an autosomal dominant manner with variable expressivity, but usually complete penetrance. The connective tissue nevi appear as collections of 3mm, skin-colored to yellow papules or plaques (dermatofibrosis lenticularis disseminata) that are most commonly located on the buttocks, proximal trunk, and limbs. Many patients begin to develop lesions in early childhood, although later onset and emergence of new lesions while others disappear have also been reported. Histopathologic examination of lesional skin may show increased amounts of elastic tissue (elastoma), although decreased or normal amounts of elastic tissue and abnormalities of collagen have also been described. The bony lesions most frequently appear after 15 years of age. They are discrete spherical areas of increased radiodensity, most frequently noted in the epiphyses and metaphyses of long bone, pelvis, scapulae, carpal and tarsal bones. Although the osteopoikilosis has not been known to cause problems, functional limitation due to decreased mobility of an affected cutaneous area has been described. Other skeletal abnormalities, including short stature, otosclerosis, and supernumerary vertebrae and ribs have been described. Cataracts and peptic ulcer disease have rarely been reported in patients with Buschke–Ollendorff syndrome. Connective tissue nevi without associated bony changes, morphea, and PXE are the most frequent disorders considered in the differential diagnosis. No therapy is available or necessary.

ELASTOSIS PERFORANS SERPIGINOSA

Elastosis perforans serpiginosa (EPS) begins in childhood or adolescence. In approximately one-fourth of patients, EPS is associated with a genetic disorder of connective tissue, particularly Marfan syndrome, PXE, osteogenesis imperfecta, and EDS. EPS has also been found in patients with Rothmund–Thomson syndrome, acrogeria, and particularly in patients with Down syndrome. EPS may be familial, with a suggested autosomal dominant mode of inheritance.[248] Rarely, EPS results from D-pencillamine therapy, and may occur in children treated with this drug for Wilson's disease or juvenile rheumatoid arthritis for as short a duration as 9 months.[234]

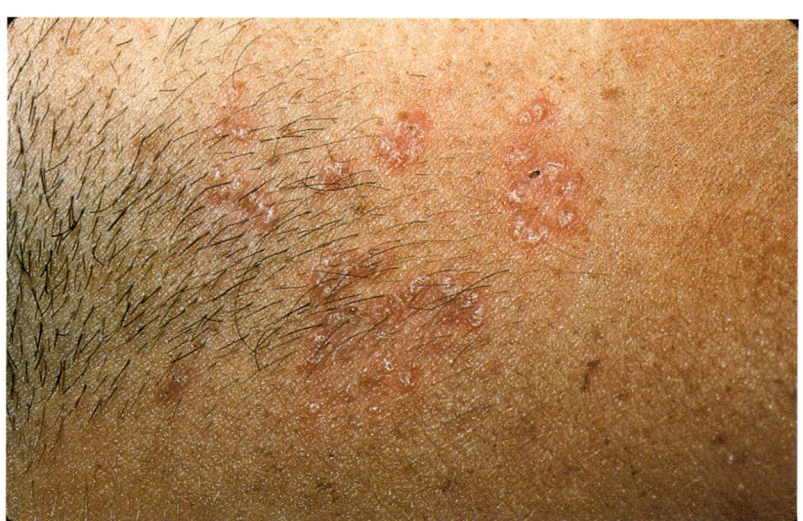

Fig. 7.25   Elastosis perforans serpiginosa in an adolescent.

Reddish to skin-colored hyperkeratotic 1- to 3mm papules with a central keratotic plug occur singly or in arcuate and circinate patterns (Fig. 7.25) The lesions typically appear on the posterior neck and upper extremities but are occasionally seen on the face and trunk. Symmetry of lesions is usually noted, and koebnerization may occur. Lesions are usually asymptomatic and, if few in number, are usually overlooked by the patient; occasionally, irritation, pruritus, or pain may be associated.

LABORATORY FINDINGS

Biopsies of fully developed lesions demonstrate an increase in the number and size of elastic fibers in the papillary dermis associated with a mixed inflammatory infiltrate. The eosinophilic elastic fibers, along with basophilic debris consisting of degenerated epidermal and inflammatory cells, are extruded through narrow winding channels in the acanthotic epidermis. These histopathologic changes are similar to those of Kyrle's disease and perforating folliculitis, but neither of these latter conditions demonstrates an increase in papillary dermal elastic fibers.

PATHOPHYSIOLOGY AND HISTOGENESIS

The etiology of EPS is unknown, but a recent study has shown the expression of the elastin receptor in the epidermis surrounding the eliminated elastic material of EPS. In addition, elastin is known to be a potent inducer of migration and terminal differentiation of keratinocytes. These observations suggest that the elastin receptor is involved in the interaction between keratinocytes and elastin in EPS.[249]

DIFFERENTIAL DIAGNOSIS

Clinically, because of the arcuate array of papules, EPS has been confused with tinea corporis, granuloma annulare, sarcoidosis, and cutaneous larva migrans. The EPS papules may also be mistaken for lichen planus and porokeratosis of Mibelli.

TREATMENT

Therapy is optional, as most lesions resolve spontaneously, although resolution may take 5 to 10 years, and includes Scotch tape stripping for removal of irritating keratotic plugs, various keratolytic agents, liquid nitrogen cryotherapy, and pulsed dye laser.[250]

Most children with EPS are not disturbed by this disorder. The role of the physician is to exclude associated disorders, which can have significant prognostic importance.

GENETIC DISORDERS OF PIGMENTATION

Seth Orlow

INTRODUCTION

In this chapter, genetic disorders causing hypopigmentation and hyperpigmentation will be discussed. The disorders of hypopigmentation have been divided into those causing localized white spotting, various forms of oculocutaneous albinism, and other disorders of diffuse hypopigmentation.

246. Schnur RE, Grace K, Herzberg A (1994) Buschke–Ollendorf syndrome, otoclerosis, and congenital spinal stenosis. **Pediatr Dermatol** 11:31–34.
247. Thieberg MD, Stone MS, Siegfried EC (1993) Buschke–Ollendorff syndrome. **Pediatr Dermatol** 10:85–87.
248. Langeveld-Wildschut EG, Toonstra J et al. (1993) Familial elastosis perforans serpiginosa. **Arch Dermatol** 129:205.
249. Fujimoto N, Tajima S, Ichibashi A (2000) Elastin peptides induce migration and terminal differentiation of cultured keratinocytes via 67 kDa elastin receptor *in vitro*: 67kDa elastin receptor is expressed in the keratinocytes eliminating elastic materials in elastosis perforans serpiginosa. **J Invest Dermatol** 115:633–639.
250. Kaufman AJ (2000) Treatment of elastosis perforans serpiginosa with the flashlamp pulsed dye laser. **Dermatol Surg** 26:1060–1062.

WHITE SPOTTING

A number of genetic disorders are associated with localized areas of absent or diminished pigmentation.

PIEBALDISM

Epidemiology

Piebaldism is a rare autosomal dominant disorder due to mutations in the c-kit proto-oncogene on chromosome 4q12.[251]

Presenting history

The findings of piebaldism are evident at birth.

Physical examination

Clinical findings in piebaldism include patches of depigmentation, often polygonal, especially on the anterior trunk, and areas encircling the mid-portion of the extremities (Fig. 7.26). A white forelock and depigmentation of the central eyebrows is also common. A less well-recognized but also distinctive finding is the presence of melanotic macules both within the border of the depigmented patches as well as on otherwise normal areas of skin. The presence of these brown macules has led to confusion in the literature, as they have been mistaken for the café-au-lait macules of neurofibromatosis type 1 (NF-1). However, patients with piebaldism do not exhibit any of the other stigmata of NF-1.

Pathophysiology and histogenesis

Melanocytes in the skin and hair follicles derive from melanoblasts which themselves arise from the embryonic neural crest, and subsequently migrate to the skin. The c-kit proto-oncogene is thought to play a critical role in melanoblast survival. Dysfunctional copies of the protein bind to normal copies in the cell and prevent them from transducing the signal initiated by the c-kit proto-oncogenes ligand, known as stem cell factor.

Histologic examination of the white areas in piebaldism reveals an absence or marked diminution in the number of identifiable melanocytes.

Differential diagnosis

The lack of associated findings or other dysmorphic features help distinguish piebaldism from Waardenburg syndrome. The congenital nature of the disease as well as its autosomal dominant nature differ from the typically acquired nature of the common disorder of depigmentation, vitiligo.

Therapeutics and prognosis

Although the depigmentation is generally static in nature, both progression of white areas as well as spontaneous repigmentation are well-described phenomena in piebaldism. Efforts at repopulating the skin with melanocytes have included phototherapy, as well as transplantation of autologous skin grafts or melanocytes from normally pigmented areas.

WAARDENBURG SYNDROME

Introduction and historical note

Waardenburg syndrome connotes a group of autosomal dominant disorders in which poliosis and white spotting may be prominent. Although attributed to Waardenburg based upon his 1948 publication, prior descriptions of affected persons are recognized.[252]

Epidemiology

All forms of Waardenburg syndrome are inherited in an autosomal dominant fashion with highly variable expressivity. Each of the types of Waardenburg syndrome is apparently rare. Waardenburg's study from the Netherlands, for example, suggested an incidence of 2–3/100 000.[253] It has been said that 2–5% of all congenitally deaf persons have some form of Waardenburg syndrome.[254]

Presenting history

All forms of Waardenburg syndrome are congenital, and hence presentation in the neonatal period is common. However, if findings are subtle, and especially if there is no preceding family history, presentation may be delayed. Indeed some patients with Waardenburg syndrome may first present to an audiologist due to the associated deafness (see below).

WAARDENBURG SYNDROME TYPES 1 AND 3

Physical examination

The most common skin features in Waardenburg syndrome type 1 are the presence of a white forelock and piebald macules (Fig. 7.27). More than 20% of affected persons will exhibit heterochromia irides or blue-eyed isochromia. Fundal hypopigmentation, if present, is segmental and corresponds to iris hypopigmentation segments. Visual acuity is unaffected by the retinal hypopigmentation.[255] Sensorineural deafness is seen in 10–40%. Hearing loss may be unilateral or bilateral. Additional findings are synophrys (20–70%), as well as dystopia canthorum and a broad nasal root (20–60%). Dystopia canthorum may be assessed by dividing the inner canthal distance by the interpupillary distance; a ratio greater than 0.6 indicates dystopia canthorum. Waardenburg syndrome type 3 is also known as Klein syndrome, and its features are those of Waardenburg syndrome Type 1 accompanied by musculoskeletal anomalies of upper limbs and pectoral areas.

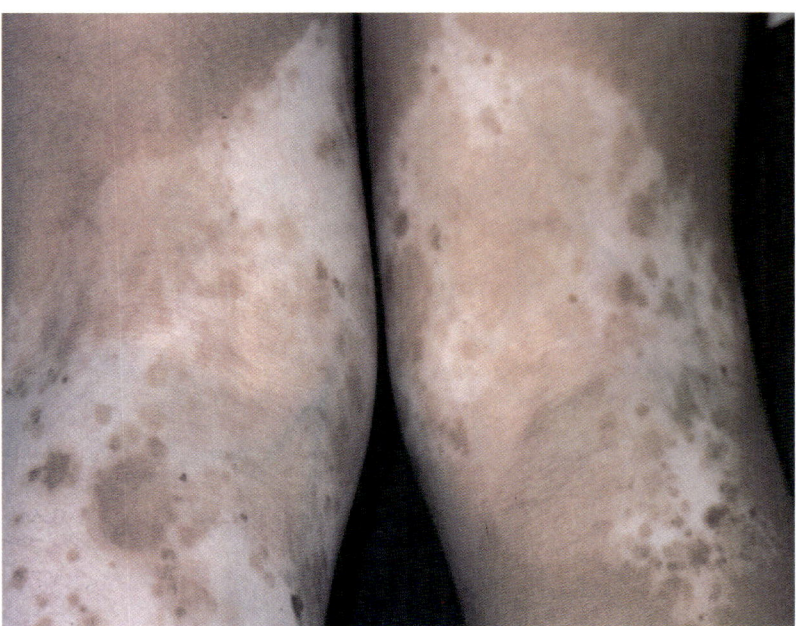

Fig. 7.26   The popliteal areas of this 4-year-old boy with piebaldism show a symmetrical distribution of depigmented patches spotted with macules of normal pigmentation and hyperpigmentation. (Courtesy Dr. Amy Paller)

251. Spritz RA (1997) Piebaldism, Waardenburg syndrome, and related disorders of melanocyte development. **Semin Cutan Med Surg** 16(1):15–23.
252. Gorlin RJ, Cohen MM, Levin LS (1990) Syndromes of the Head and Neck, 3rd edn. New York: Oxford University Press, p. 446–469.
253. Waardenburg PJ (1951) A new syndrome combining developmental anomalies of the eyelids, eyebrows and nose root with congenital deafness. **Am J Hum Genet** 3:195–253.
254. DeSaxe M (1984) Waardenburg's syndrome in South Africa. **S Afr Med J** 66:256–261.
255. Goldberg DJ, Sciales CW (1991) Pyogenic granuloma in children: Treatment with the flashlamp-pumped pulsed dye laser. **J Dermatol Surg Oncol** 17:960–962.

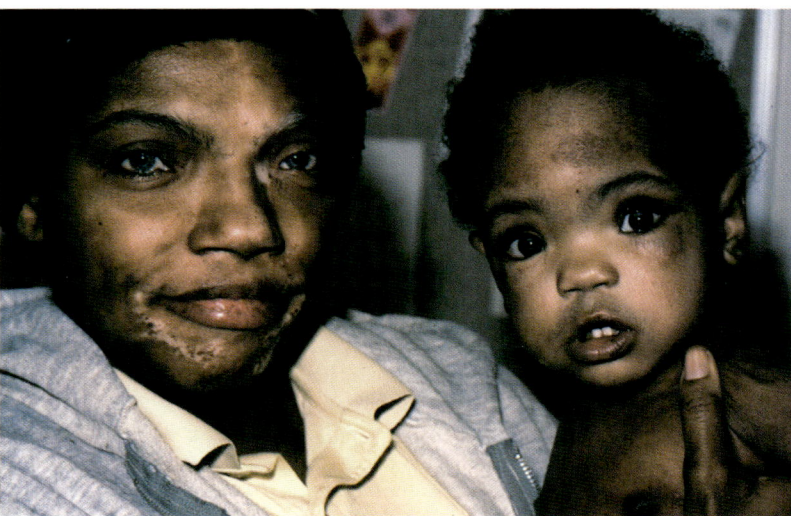

Fig. 7.27 **Mother and son with the autosomal dominant type I Waardenburg syndrome.** Note the dystopia canthorum, synophrys, broad nasal root, and iris heterochromia. Note the loss of pigmentation on the mother's face. The son also has atopic dermatitis. (Courtesy Dr. Amy Paller)

Laboratory findings

Abnormalities upon audiologic testing will depend upon the degree of deafness. The lower and middle ranges of hearing are typically more severely affected.

WAARDENBURG SYNDROME TYPE 2

Physical examination

Dystopia canthorum is absent, but deafness is more common in this type of Waardenburg syndrome than in Waardenburg syndrome type 1.

WAARDENBURG SYNDROME TYPE 4

Waardenburg syndrome type 4, also called Shah–Waardenburg syndrome, is a phenotype in which pigmentary features of Waardenburg syndrome including heterochromia irides, poliosis and white areas of skin are accompanied by aganglisis of the distal bowel resulting in megacolon resembling that seen in Hirschprung disease. Vaginal agenesis has also been noted.[256]

Pathophysiology and histogenesis

Both Waardenburg syndrome types 1 and 3 are caused by mutations in *Pax3*.[257,258] *Pax3* is a key gene in controlling neural crest differentiation by regulating the transcription of a number of other genes including the melanocyte transcription factor MITF (see below). Because the embryonic neural crest gives rise not only to melanocytes but also to the bony and cartilaginous structures of the central face, the dysmorphic features associated with Waardenburg syndrome are not surprising. The hearing loss in Waardenburg syndrome is due to the absence of the Organ of Corti and stria

vascularis, also neural crest drived structures of the ear. Ganglion cells are sparse.[259]

Although few studies have been performed, based upon the known pathophysiology, the number of melanocytes in the white areas of skin or in affected follicles should be markedly diminished. Waardenburg syndrome type 2 is caused by mutations in the gene encoding the MITF transcription factor.[260] *MITF* is downstream of *Pax3*, and *Pax3* controls *MITF*. This hierarchy of effect explains the lesser facial abnormalities in Waardenburg syndrome type 2 and the more restricted pattern of effects compared to the broader abnormalities caused by mutations in the upstream *Pax3*.

Waardenburg syndrome type 4 can be caused by mutations in a number of genes controlling neural crest development, including the genes encoding the Sox10 transcription factor, the signalling molecule endothelin3, and its receptor EDNRB.[261,262]

Differential diagnosis

The distinctive features of Waardenburg syndrome types allow the disorder to be readily differentiated from piebaldism.

Therapeutics and prognosis

The main therapeutic interventions in the different forms of Waardenburg syndrome include the use of devices to augment hearing and surgical correction of megacolon if present. Beyond simple dyeing of the hair, treatment of the pigmentary defects has not been reported upon. In addition to the white areas present at birth, the appearance of new areas of involvement as well as premature graying of the scalp, eyebrow, and eyelash hairs beginning in early adulthood may occur.[252]

OCULOCUTANEOUS ALBINISM (OCA)

Patients with OCA have hypopigmented skin, hair, and eyes. A number of OCA types have been identified, many with varying degrees of severity. Historical classification was based on tyrosinase activity, i.e., tyrosinase-negative or tyrosinase-positive. The identification and mapping of a number of pigment genes has made it possible to reclassify phenotypes based on the locus at which the disease causing mutations occurs.

OCULOCUTANEOUS ALBINISM TYPE I (OCA1)

Introduction and historical note

The biochemical basis of albinism was first speculated on by Garrod in 1908 as an inborn error of metabolism.[263] He correctly theorized, at least for some forms of albinism, that the phenotype was due to the absence of enzyme activity. The enzyme in question has since been identified as tyrosinase.

Epidemiology and genetics

OCA1, also called tyrosinase-related albinism, is an autosomal recessive disorder due to mutations in the gene encoding the key melanogenic enzyme tyrosinase located on chromosome 11q14–21.[264] To date, more than 100 mutations have been described at this locus. OCA1 has been reported throughout the world and occurs with a frequency of about 1 in 40 000 in most populations.[264]

256. Goodman RM, Oelsner G, Berkenstadt M, Admon D (1988) Absence of a vagina and right sided adnexa uteri in the Waardenburg syndrome: a possible clue to the embryological defect. **J Med Genet** 25(5):355–357.
257. Read AP, Newton VE (1997) Waardenburg syndrome. **J Med Genet** 34(8):656–665
258. Hoth CF, Milunsky A, Lipsky N et al. (1993) Mutations in the paired domain of the human PAX3 gene cause Klein–Waardenburg syndrome (WS-III) as well as Waardenburg syndrome type I (WS-I). **Am J Hum Genet** 52(3):455–462.
259. Davis Le RK (1984) Inner ear anomalies in Waardenburg's syndrome with Hirschsprung's disease. **Int Journal of Pediatr** 8:181–189.
260. Nobukuni Y, Watanabe A, Takeda K et al. (1996) Analyses of loss-of-function mutations of the MITF gene suggest that haploinsufficiency is a cause of Waardenburg syndrome type 2A. **Am J Hum Genet** 59(1):76–83.

261. Pignault V, Bondurand N, Lemort N et al. (2001) A heterozygous endothelin 3 mutation in Waardenburg–Hirschsprung disease: is there a dosage effect of EDN3/EDNRB gene mutations on neurocristopathy phenotypes? **J Med Genet** 38(3):205–209.
262. Pingault V, Bondurand N, Kuhlbrodt K et al. (1998) SOX10 mutations in patients with Waardenburg–Hirschsprung disease. **Nat Genet** 18(2):171–173.
263. Garrod AE (1908) Inborn errors of metabolism. Croonian lectues, **Lancet** 2:73.
264. Oetting WS, Brilliant MH, King RA (1996) The clinical spectrum of albinism in humans. **Mol Med Today** 2(8):330–335.

Presenting history

Physical examination

OCA1 presents at birth. There is a range in severity, the most severe phenotype, OCA1A or "tyrosinase-negative albinism," resulting from a complete lack of enzyme activity. Pigment remains completely absent in the skin, hair and eyes throughout life.

The lack of pigmentation is accompanied by a severe ocular phenotype. Irides appear gray to blue, and there is a prominent red reflex as well as foveal hypoplasia. Misrouting of the optic tract leads to a reduction in visual acuity, nystagmus and strabismus. The lack of ocular pigment causes photophobia.

Milder tyrosinase mutations result in production of tyrosinase with some residual enzyme activity and thus result in slightly less severe phenotypes. OCA1B, formerly called yellow albinism, was first described in an inbred Amish population.[265] Affected individuals are born with white skin and hair. With age, the hair develops coloring to varying degrees of yellow–red. Ocular findings are less severe than in OCA1A.

OCA1TS is the human equivalent of the Siamese cat and Himalayan rabbit phenotypes.[266,267] The mutated tyrosinase enzyme has decreased activity at 35–37 °C such that in the cooler regions of the body, including the limbs and head, the enzyme functions normally resulting in pigmentation, while the remainder of the body remains unpigmented.[267]

A fourth tyrosinase-related phenotype, platinum OCA, is also caused by tyrosinase gene mutations. At birth, the phenotype is identical to that of OCA1A. Small amounts of pigment are detectable in the hair and eyes in late childhood, developing into a metallic tinge with age.[268]

Minimal pigment OCA (OCA1MP) is also tyrosinase-related. Individuals are born with the OCA1A phenotype, but accumulate increased ocular pigment with age. The skin remains unpigmented and does not tan.[269]

Laboratory findings/pathophysiology/molecular and biochemical basis/histology

All forms of OCA1 are associated with a decrease in tyrosinase activity. The most severe forms result in a complete loss of activity, while the remainder have varying activity at the low end of the range.

The epidermis, hair follicles and keratinocytes of affected individuals are unaffected with a normal number of melanocytes being present; however there is a significant reduction in melanin content. While the general ultra-structure of the melanocytes also remains unchanged, melanosomes fail to mature and little to no pigment deposition is seen on microscopy.

Differential diagnosis

Definitive diagnoses can only be made by identification of the pathogenic mutations at the tyrosinase locus. Over a hundred mutations have been identified at this locus. It is highly unusual, except in the case of consanguineous marriages, to find the same mutation on both chromosomes. In addition, no one mutation occurs at a significantly increased frequency, thus sequencing of the entire gene is often necessary to identify the pathogenic mutations.

Therapeutics

No treatment is currently available; however, institution of regimens for protection from sun damage are vital. In addition, prescription of corrective eyewear is necessary.

OCULOCUTANEOUS ALBINISM TYPE II (OCA2)
Epidemiology

Genetics

OCA2 results from mutations in the human homolog of the mouse pink-eyed dilution gene, *P*. The gene has been mapped to human chromosome 15q11–12[264,270] and the gene product is predicted to be a transport or channel protein.

Statistics

OCA2 or "tyrosinase-positive albinism" is the most common form of albinism, particulary among non-Caucasian peoples. In Africa it occurs with a preva-lence ranging from 1 in 1100 in the Ibo of Nigeria[271] to 1 in 3900 in southern African populations.[272] Among Caucasian Americans, about 1 in 36 000 people are affected, while among African Americans, 1 in 10 000 will be affected.[264]

Presenting history

Physical examination

Affected individuals are born with some pigmentation and there is a slight increase in pigmentation with age. Hair color ranges from yellow to light brown, while the skin is white. In some kindreds, multiple lentigines develop in sun-exposed areas. Ocular findings are generally less severe than those in OCA1A.

Laboratory findings/pathophysiology/molecular and biochemical basis/histology

This form of albinism was first distinguished from OCA1 in laboratory studies which showed that incubation of anagen hairbulbs in solutions containing high concentrations of tyrosine resulted in pigment formation.[273] Mapping and cloning of the gene has made it possible to definitively diagnose the condition by identification of pathogenic mutations. The gene is, however, large, making the use of general mutation screening unfeasible as a diagnostic tool. In patients of African descent, one mutation has been found to account for a large proportion of pathogenic lesions. The origin of this 2.7kb deletion of exon 7 has been traced back to a founding mutation in central Africa. In parts of Africa, about 80% of OCA2 chromosomes will carry the deletion, making a useful diagnostic marker.

While little data is available on histologic findings in human tissues from OCA2 patients, mouse studies show that melanosomes are smaller in melano-cytes lacking *P*, with the remainder of the dermal tissues remaining unchanged.

BROWN ALBINISM

Introduction and historical note

Brown albinism is a phenotype much milder than OCA1 and OCA2. It was first described in Nigeria.[274] The phenotype was similar to some descriptions of individuals with "xanthism"[275] as well as a condition reported by Burton from west Africa as semi-albinism.[276]

Epidemiology

Genetics/statistics

Brown albinism is inherited in an autosomal recessive fashion.[269,277] One case in the US has been shown to result from mutations in *TYRP1*, a gene with

265. Nance WE, Jackson CE, Witkop CJ (1970) Jr. Amish albinism: a distinctive autosomal recessive phenotype. Am J Hum Genet 22(5):579–586.
266. Giebel LB, Tripathi RK, Strunk KM et al. (1991) Tyrosinase gene mutations associated with type 1B ("yellow") oculocutanecus albinism. Am J Hum Genet 48:1159–1167.
267. King RA, Townsend D, Oetting W et al. (1991) Temperature-sensitive tyrosinase associated with peripheral pigmentation in oculocutaneous albinism. J Clin Invest 87(3):1046–1053.
268. Witkop CJ Jr. (1985) Inherited disorders of pigmentation. Clin Dermatol 3:70–134.
269. King RA, Rich SS (1986) Segregation analysis of brown oculocutaneous albinism. Clin Genet 29(6):496–501.
270. Manga P, Orlow SJ (1999) The pink-eyed dilution gene and the molecular pathogenesis of tyrosinase-positive albinism (OCA2). J Dermatol 26(11):738–747.
271. Okoro AN (1975) Albinism in Nigeria. A clinical and social study. Br J Dermatol 92(5):485–492.

272. Kromberg JG, Jenkins T (1982) Prevalence of albinism in the South African negro. S Afr Med J 61(11):383–386.
273. Kugelman TP, Van Scott EJ (1961) Tyrosinase activity in melanocytes of human albinos. J Invest Dermatol 37:73–76.
274. King RA, Creel D, Cervenka J et al. (1980) Albinism in Nigeria with delineation of new recessive oculocutaneous type. Clin Genet 17(4):259–270.
275. Pearson K, Nettleship E, Usher CH (1911) A monograph on Albinism in Man. London.
276. Burton, Knowles F (1916) Family albinism. Interstate Med J 23:555–559.
277. Manga P, Kromberg J, Turner A et al. (2001) In Southern Africa, brown oculocutaneous albinism (BOCA) maps to the OCA2 locus on chromosome 15q: P-gene mutations identified. Am J Hum Genet 68(3):782–787.

40% identity to that encoding tyrosinase.[278] However, studies in southern Africa show that in the majority of cases on that continent there is linkage to the *P* locus.[277] By contrast, a phenotype seen with some frequency in sub-Saharan Africa, called rufous albinism, is due to mutations in the TYRP1 gene.[279]

Presenting history

Physical examination
Individuals with brown albinism have a cream to light tan skin, beige to light brown hair and blue–green to brown irides with moderate transillumination defects, nystagmus, and reduced retinal pigment.[274] Lentigines, similar to those seen in OCA2, may develop in sun-exposed areas. The reduced severity of the hypopigmentation decreases the risk of developing UV-induced cancerous lesions.

Laboratory findings/pathophysiology/molecular and biochemical basis/histology
The molecular and histological findings in brown OCA are similar to those for OCA2, as would be predicted based on the fact that both conditions are caused by *P* gene mutations. Tyrosinase activity in hairbulbs from affected individuals is above the mean value for brown haired, Caucasian individuals. Melanocyte ultrastructure is normal except for the lack of mature melanosomes.[269]

Differential diagnosis
Differentiation between brown OCA and OCA2 is not always possible. Since both conditions map to the same locus, they can be considered part of a continuum with the more severe OCA2 on one end and brown OCA on the other. `

RUFOUS ALBINISM
Introduction and historical note
The characteristics of the skin and eyes in rufous individuals appear to be distinct from those of brown OCA, although reports in the literature[281] do indicate some difficulty in distinguishing between the two. Historically, the two types were grouped together as xanthism.[280]

Epidemiology

Genetics/statistics
Rufous OCA, at least in patients of African descent, results from autosomal recessive mutations at the tyrosinase-related 1 protein (*TYRP1*) locus. This gene is believed to have evolved from a duplicate copy of the tyrosinase gene. It has retained a high degree of homology with the parent gene. While the precise function of this gene is not known, pigment production is significantly reduced in its absence.

The prevalence of rufous albinism among southern African blacks is at least 1 in 8580, with a carrier rate of approximately 1 in 46,[281] while it is extremely rare in the remainder of the world.

Presenting history

Physical examination
The characteristics of rufous albinism were first described as[282] "mahogany red to deep red" hair, reddish brown skin, occasional presence of pigmented nevi

or freckles, reddish brown to brown eye color, slight transillumination of the iris, fundal pigment, nystagmus, photophobia, and approximately 20/100 visual acuity. Susceptibility to solar damage and skin neoplasia is lower than for OCA2 and BOCA individuals. Affected individuals in a study by Kromberg *et al.*[281] showed no evidence of photoaging, photodamage or carcinomas.

Laboratory findings/pathophysiology/molecular and biochemical basis/histology
To date, two mutations have been shown to account for 90% of the mutated *TYRP1* alleles. Both mutations result in truncation of the protein and there is unlikely to be any residual activity.

Unlike normal black skin, melanocytes in the skin contain both eumelanosomes and phaeomelanosomes at various stages of melanization. Many of the organelles, however, are aberrant "crescent" or racquet shapes and have melanin only at the edges, while the center lacks melanin.[283] Few melanosomes in the hairbulb are completely melanized. There are a normal number of melanosomes in skin keratinocytes, although they are about 30% smaller and packaged as clusters of "rosettes," as seen in normal Caucasoid and Mongoloid skin, instead of singly dispersed as in normal black skin.[283]

Differential diagnosis
The gold–red–brown hair coloring and reddish skin seen in rufous OCA is similar to the cutaneous coloring that results from malnutrition, in particular, kwashiorkor. The distinction can be made based on the presence or absence of visual anomalies. The visual anomalies are, however, extremely mild in some cases of rufous OCA.

Diffuse forms of hypopigmentation with eye involvement are classified under the rubric of oculocutaneous albinism.[264] Patients with albinism are at increased risk of sun-induced skin damage due to the lack of melanin's protective effects, and have a high rate of malignancies, especially squamous cell carcinoma.

OCA1 is also called tyrosinase-related albinism and is an autosomal disorder due to mutations in the gene encoding the key melanogenic enzyme tyrosinase located on chromosome 11q14–21.[264] If the defect is severe, OCA1A ("tyrosinase-negative albinism") ensues. Pigment in skin, hair, and eyes is totally absent for life. Because production of melanin by the retinal pigment epithelium plays a key role during retinal/eye development, photophobia, nystagmus, and hypoplasia of the foveal area of the retina are all found. If at least one allele of tyrosinase carries a milder mutation resulting in some residual enzyme activity, the phenotype is that of OCA1B, formerly called yellow albinism. Here the hair color ranges from yellow to light brown, and skin white to creamy. Ocular findings are less severe than in OCA1A.

The most common form of albinism, especially among non-Caucasian peoples, is OCA2, or "tyrosinase-positive albinism," due to mutations in the *P* (pinkeyed-dilution) locus on chromosome 15q.[264,270] The protein product of this gene is a putative transporter/channel. Hair color ranges from yellow to light brown, and the skin is white. In some kindreds, multiple lentigines develop in sun-exposed areas. Ocular findings are generally less severe than those in OCA1A.

Brown albinism is a phenotype much milder than OCA1 and OCA2. One case in the US was apparently due to mutations in TYRP1, a gene with 40% identity to that encoding tyrosinase,[278] but studies in South Africa suggest that in the majority of cases on that continent there is linkage to the *P* locus.[277] By contrast, a phenotype seen with some frequency in sub-Saharan

278. Boissy RE, Zhao H, Oetting WS et al. (1996) Mutation in the lack of expression of tyrosinase-related protein-1 (TRP-1) in melanocytes from an individual with brown oculocutaneous albinism: a new subtype of albinism classified as "OCA3". **Am J Hum Genet** 58:1145–1156.

279. Manga P, Kromberg JG, Box NF et al. (1997) Rufous oculocutaneous albinism in southern African Blacks is caused by mutations in the TYRP1 gene. **Am J Hum Genet** 61(5):1095–1101.

280. Lowethal L (1944) Partial albinism and nystagmus in Negroes. **Arch Dermatol Syphilol** 50:300–301.

281. Kromberg JG, Castle DJ, Zwane EM et al. (1990) Red or rufous albinism in southern Africa. **Ophthal Paediatr Genet** 11(3):229–235.

282. Witkop CJ, Jr., Quevedo Wc, Jr, Fitzpatrick TB (1983) Albinism and other disorders of pigment metabolism. In: The Metabolic Basis of Inherited Disease, Stanbury J, Wyngerden JB, Fredrickson DS, Goldstein JL, Brown MS, eds. New York: McGraw-Hill p. 301–346.

283. Kidson SH, Richards PD, Rawoot F, Kromberg JG (1993) An ultrastructural study of melanocytes and melanosomes in the skin and hair bulbs of rufous albinos. **Pigment Cell Res** 6(4 Pt 1):209–214.

Africa with reddish hair and albinism-like eye changes, called rufous albinism, is likely due to mutations in the *TYRP1* gene.[279]

HERMANSKY–PUDLAK SYNDROME

Another form of tyrosinase-positive albinism is Hermansky–Pudlak syndrome, a multisystem autosomal recessive disorder.

EPIDEMIOLOGY

The association of oculocutaneous albinism, bleeding diathesis, and the accumulation of a ceroid-like substance in the reticuloendothelial system was first made by Hermansky and Pudlak in 1959.[284] The disorder is prevalent in a number of defined geographic locales, especially the northwestern portion of Puerto Rico, but may occur worldwide.

PHYSICAL EXAMINATION

A broad range of skin findings is possible, with some patients so severely affected as to resemble OCA1 whereas others may be pale tan[285] (Fig. 7.28). Freckling and lentigines may be present and may be accentuated by sun exposure. The extent of ocular findings correlates with the degree of skin pigment dilution. Ocular findings in these patients include nystagmus, photophobia, decreased visual acuity, and iris translucency. Retinal pigmentation may be absent or spotty.[286] Patients with Hermansky–Pudlak syndrome exhibit a bleeding diathesis secondary to an absence of platelet dense granules (Fig. 7.28). Diathesis in these patients may range from easy

bruising to life-threatening bleeding, although epistaxis is the most frequent manifestation. Menometrorrhagia is common in affected adult females. Other disorders occasionally seen in patients with Hermansky–Pudlak syndrome include interstitial pulmonary disease, kidney failure, cardiomyopathy, granulomatous colitis, lupus erythematosus, and frequent bacterial infections.[287,288]

LABORATORY FINDINGS

The hair is usually straw colored, and hair bulbs incubated with L-tyrosine or L-dopa have the ability to synthesize melanin.[289] Bleeding time is prolonged, but platelet number, prothrombin time (PT), partial thromboplastin time (PTT), fibrinogen level, and clotting factors are all normal. Platelets from these patients are deficient in the storage pool of adenosine nucleotides (ADP, ATP) and serotonin. As a result, these platelets lack the normal second stage of aggregation.[290] The accumulation of a ceroid-like pigment in macrophages of the reticuloendothelial system suggests that Hermansky–Pudlak syndrome is a lysosomal storage disorder. The autofluorescent material stored is histochemically similar to that in neuronal ceroid lipofuscinosis. Similar to ceroid lipofuscinosis, patients with Hermansky–Pudlak syndrome show, in the presence of kidney involvement, an increased urinary excretion of dolichols.[291]

PATHOPHYSIOLOGY AND HISTOGENESIS

Many cases of Hermansky–Pudlak syndrome are caused by mutations in the *HPS1* gene, which encodes a protein thought to be involved in the trafficking

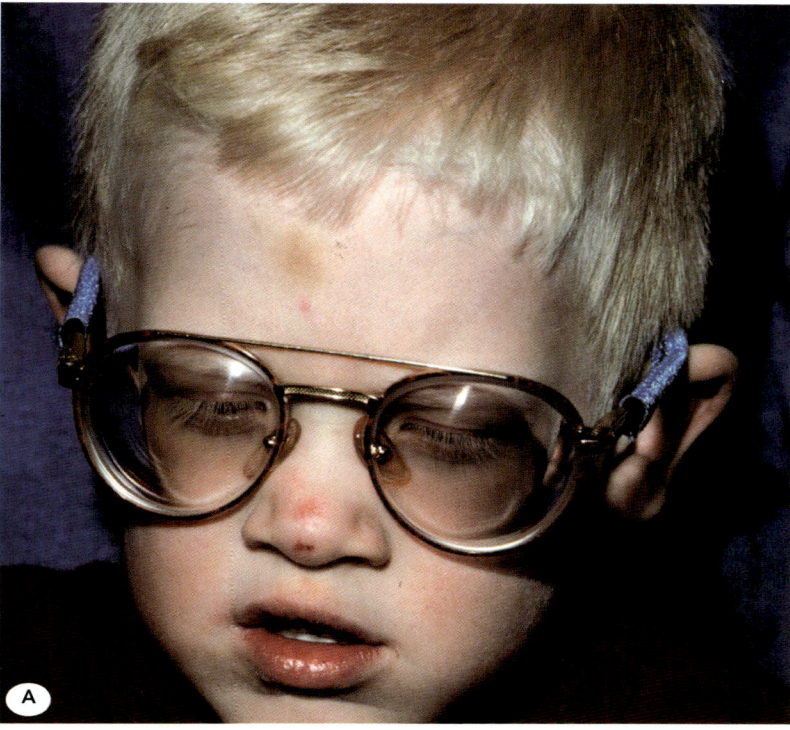

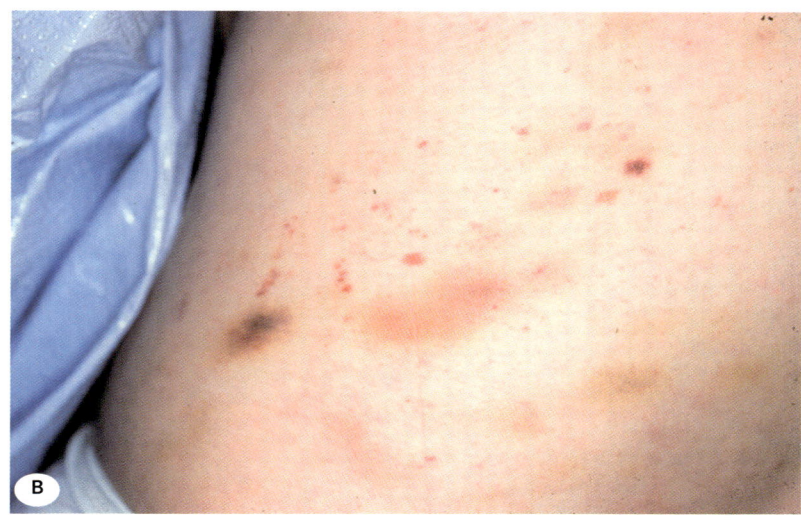

Fig. 7.28   (A) A 3-year-old Puerto Rican boy with Hermansky–Pudlak syndrome. Note the light-colored skin and hair, the need for eyeglasses, and the facial bruising. (B) Multiple ecchymoses and petechiae on the back of a teenaged Puerto Rican girl with Hermansky–Pudlak syndrome. (Courtesy Dr. Amy Paller)

284. Hermansky F, Pudlak P (1959) Albinism associated with hemorrhagic diathesis and unusual pigmented reticular cells in bone marrow: report 2 cases with histochemical studies. **Blood** 14:162.

285. Toro J, Turner M, Gahl WA (1999) Dermatologic manifestations of Hermansky–Pudlak syndrome in patients with and without a 16-base pair duplication in the HPS1 gene. **Arch Dermatol** 135(7):774–780.

286. Summers CG, Knobloch WH, Witkop CJ Jr, King RA (1988) Hermansky–Pudlak syndrome. Ophthalmic findings. **Ophthalmology** 95(4):545–554.

287. White D, Walker-Smith G, Cooper J (1984) Hermansky–Pudlak syndrome and intersitial lung disease: report of a case with lavage findings. **Am Rev Respir Dis** 13:138.

288. Shanahan F, Randolph L, King R et al. (1988) Hermansky–Pudlak syndrome: an immunologic assessment of 15 cases. **Am J Med** 85(6):823–828.

289. Witkop CJ, Jr, White JG, Gerritsen SM et al. (1973) Hermansky–Pudlak syndrome (HPS): a proposed block in glutathione peroxidase. **Oral Surg Oral Med Oral Pathol** 35(6):790–806.

290. Rao GH, Gerrard JM, Witkop CJ, White JG (1981) Platelet aggregation independent of ADP release or prostaglandin synthesis in patients with Hermansky–Pudlak syndrome. **Prostaglandins Med** 6(4):459–472.

291. Witkop C, Jr, Wolfe LS, Cal SX et al. (1987) Elevated urinary dolichol excretion in the Hermansky–Pudlak syndrome. Indicator of lysosomal dysfunction. **Am J Med** 82(3):463–470.

of proteins to lysosome-like organelles including the melanosome.[285] Siblings with a mutation in the beta-3A subunit of AP-3 adaptor also involved in this subcellular pathway have been described as HPS2.[292] Yet a third group of patients has no detectable mutations in either HPS1 or AP3b.

Skin biopsy reveals normal numbers of melanocytes, but there are decreased numbers of melanosomes in both melanocytes and keratinocytes. The melanosomes are incomplete and immature.[293] An occasional macromelanosome has been observed.[294] Pathologic examination of the pulmonary and colonic lesions are both typified by the accumulation of ceroid-like deposits in histiocytic cells.

THERAPEUTICS AND PROGNOSIS

Early identification of patients with this syndrome is critical in achieving several key goals: (1) avoidance of aspirin and other prostaglandin blockers that potentiate hemorrhage; (2) awareness of hemorrhage from minor surgical procedures; (3) avoidance of excessive sun exposure; (4) aggressive treatment of pulmonary infections to minimize fibrosis; and (5) genetic counseling for patients and their parents. For most patients, pulmonary disease is the major cause of premature death.

OTHER DISORDERS OF DIFFUSE HYPOPIGMENTATION

Two other groups of genetic disorders typified by hypopigmentation and multisystem disease deserve mention.

CHÉDIAK–HIGASHI SYNDROME
Epidemiology and Genetics

Chédiak–Higashi syndrome is a very rare autosomal recessive disorder that has been reported in many different populations (see Genetic Disorders of the Immune System, below).

Presenting history

Hypopigmentation and photophobia are generally noted at birth or early in infancy.

Physical examination

Depending upon the ethnic background, the skin is hypopigmented or "muddy" in coloration. Hair color is distinctly unusual, described as silvery to metallic gray. Although photophobia is common, other ocular findings are generally less severe than in OCA.

Laboratory findings

Neutropenia with giant granules within leukocytes is a hallmark of the disease.[295] Neutrophils are deficient in chemotactic and bactericidal activities, being unable to discharge bactericidal enzymes. In addition, a selective profound natural killer (NK) cell function and platelet storage pool deficiencies have been described.[295]

Pathophysiology and histogenesis

Chédiak–Higashi syndrome is caused by mutations the *LYST* (lysosomal trafficking) gene.[296] A number of giant organelle derived granules are seen in blood cells including neutrophils, T cells and natural killer cells, and a variety of tissues.

The cutaneous and hair melanocytes in affected patients consist of a few normal stage IV melanosomes and many giant melanosomes, which are formed by a fusion process similar to the one that is observed among lysosomes. The giant melanosomes occasionally fuse again and then disintegrate. The normal melanosomes are packaged in abnormally large secondary lysosomes instead of being finely dispersed, leading to the hypopigmentation of this syndrome. Thus the pigment dilution is due to defective melanosomal transfer to keratinocytes.

Differential diagnosis

The differential diagnosis might include other forms of diffues hypopigmentation in association with multisystem disease. The presence of giant granules helps readily distinguish Chédiak–Higashi syndrome from Hermansky–Pudlak syndrome and from Griscelli syndrome.

Therapeutics and prognosis

The long-term prognosis is very poor, with death usually occurring in the teenage years or earlier due either to pyogenic infections or the development of an accelerated lymphohistiocytic phase; this frequent complication is characterized by a multivisceral lymphohistiocytic infiltration with hemophagocytosis leading to pancytopenia, a bleeding disorder secondary to low fibrinogen level. Hypertriglyceridemia and hemodilution are also seen. Bone marrow transplantation appears to be the only therapeutic strategy capable of curing the disease.[297]

GRISCELLI SYNDROME

Griscelli syndrome, discussed in greater detail in Genetic Disorders of the Immune System, is caused by mutations in the gene encoding myosin-Va.[298]

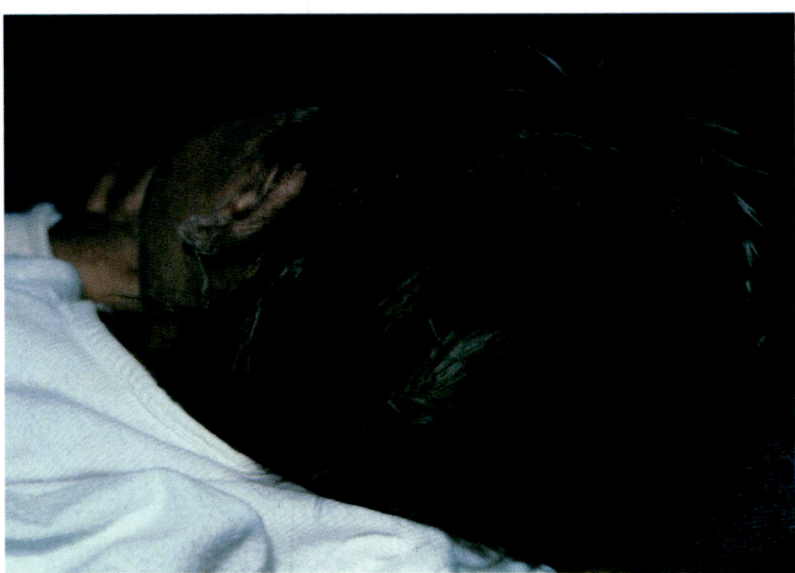

Fig. 7.29 Graying of hair of a baby with Griscelli syndrome who succumbed to hepatic failure (courtesy of Dr Anthony Mancini; reprinted with permission from Mancini AJ, Chan LS, Paller AS (1998)) Partial albinism with immunodeficiency: Griscelli syndrome: Report of a case and review of the literature. J Am Acad Dermatol 38:295–300.

292. Dell'Angelica EC, Shotelersuk V, Aguilar RC et al. (1999) Altered trafficking of lysosomal proteins in Hermansky–Pudlak syndrome due to mutations in the beta 3A subunit of the AP-3 adaptor. **Mol Cell** 3(1):11–21.
293. Schachne JP, Glaser N, Lee SH et al. (1990) Hermansky–Pudlak syndrome: case report and clinicopathologic review. **J Am Acad Dermatol** 22(5 Pt 2):926–932.
294. Frenk E, Lattion F (1982) The melanin pigmentary disorder in a family with Hermansky–Pudlak syndrome. **J Invest Dermatol** 78(2):141–143.
295. Barak Y, Nir E (1987) Chediak–Higashi syndrome. **Am J Pediatr Hematol Oncol** 9(1):42–55.
296. Introne W, Boissy RE, Gahl WA (1999) Clinical, molecular, and cell biological aspects of Chediak–Higashi syndrome. **Mol Genet Metab** 68(2):283–303.
297. Bejaoui M, Veber F, Girault D et al. (1989) [The accelerated phase of Chediak–Higashi syndrome]. **Arch Fr Pediatr** 46(10):733–736.
298. Pastural E, Ersoy F, Yalman N et al. (2000) Two genes are responsible for Griscelli syndrome at the same 15q21 locus. **Genomics** 63(3):299–306.

This specialized myosin controls the ability of melanosomes to attach to actin at tips of dendrites, a necessary prelude to melanosome transfer to keratinocytes in the skin and the nascent hair shaft. Because of this defective transfer, the skin is hypopigmented and the hair silvery gray (Fig. 7.29). Since transfer of melanosomes does not occur in the eye, persons with Griscelli syndrome lack ocular hypopigmentation or other stigmata of OCA. Because of the role of myosin-Va in moving other organelles, additional problems seen in those with Griscelli syndrome include neutropenia, thrombocytopenia and hypogammaglobulinemia. Giant granules, such as those seen in Chédiak–Higashi syndrome, are lacking, but patients have been described with deficient cell-mediated immunity and with an absence of detectable Langerhans cells. A still rarer form of Griscelli syndrome accompanied by a severe reticuloendothelial dysfunction resulting in a hemophagocytic syndrome-type presentation has been found to be caused by mutation in the gene encoding RAB27A, a small protein that has been shown to interact with myosin-Va.[299]

DISORDERS OF HYPERPIGMENTATION

LEOPARD SYNDROME

Introduction and historical note
Moynahan created the acronym LEOPARD to describe the unique constellation of features associated with this syndrome (see below).

Epidemiology and genetics
Although the gene for LEOPARD syndrome has yet to be identified, this rare disorder is thought to be caused by an autosomal dominant mutation with high penetrance. As in many autosomal dominant disorders, however, a majority of cases probably reflect new mutations.[300]

Physical examination
The LEOPARD or multiple lentigines syndrome is characterized by generalized lentigines, sometimes associated with widespread developmental defects. The name LEOPARD syndrome was coined as a description of the skin findings, but it is also an acronym for the developmental defects that may occur: lentigines, ECG abnormalities, ocular hypertelorism, pulmonary stenosis, abnormalities of the genitalia, retardation of growth, and deafness. Lentigines can be present at birth and increase in number until puberty.[307] They are most numerous on the face, neck, and upper trunk (Fig. 7.30). They range in size from pinpoints to 5mm but occasionally may be larger. Numerous café-au-lait macules may also be seen.

Cardiac abnormalities include conduction defects and pulmonary or subaortic stenosis, and several patients have died from obstructive cardiomyopathy. The variably seen genital abnormalities include gonadal hypoplasia, cryptorchidism, delayed puberty, and hypospadia. Ocular hypertelorism, mandibular prognathism, and short stature are the most common skeletal abnormalities. Growth tends to be slowed in affected patients. Sensorineural hearing loss, if present, may be severe and may appear late in life.[302] Additional reported findings include café noir spots, abnormal dermatoglyphics, webbing of the digits, Ehlers–Danlos-like joint hyperextensibility and skin hyperelasticity, and granular cell myoblastomas.[303]

Laboratory findings
Histology of the lentigines shows increased members of melanocytes filled with melanosomes.[303,304] Occasional giant melanosomes can be seen, although this finding is nonspecific of the disease.[305] Electrocardiographic abnormalities are another laboratory hallmark of the disorder.

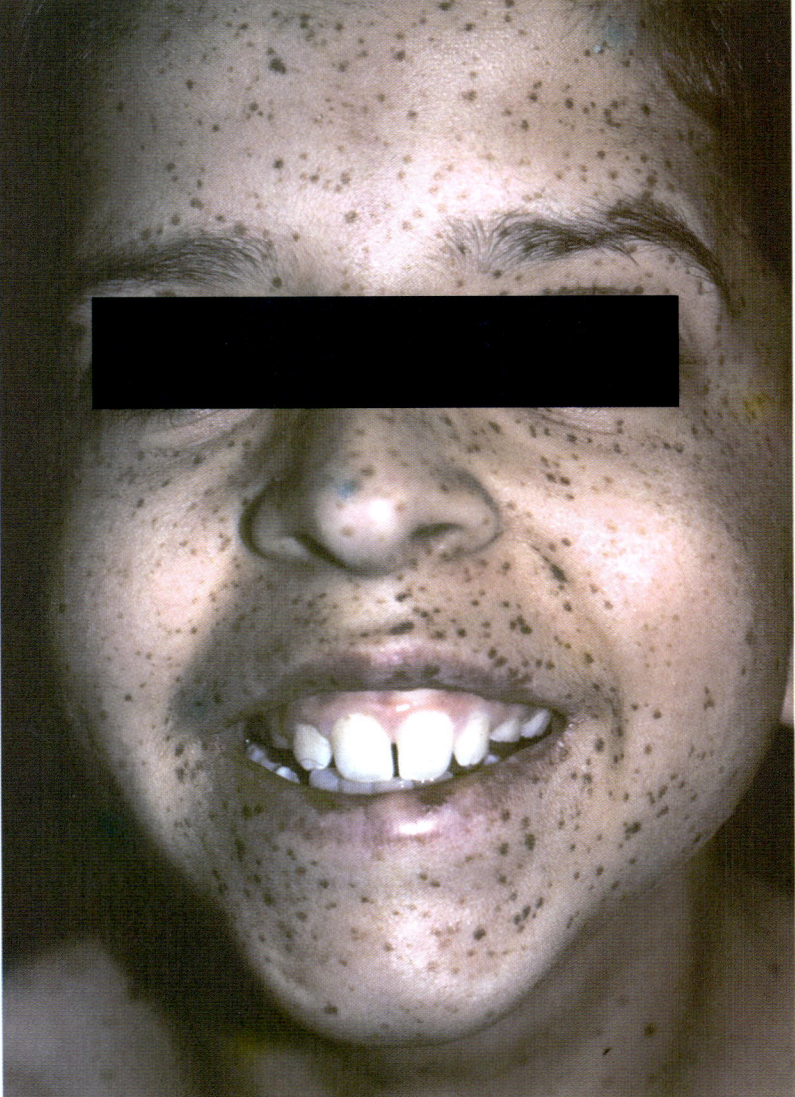

Fig. 7.30 The elongated facies and myriad lentigines on the face of a boy with LEOPARD syndrome (courtesy of Dr Sarah Chamlin).

Prognosis and therapeutics
Although the prognosis in general is good, individual problems may predominate in specific patients. Particular attention must be paid to hearing loss, as its early correction is critical for maximal speech development, and missed hearing loss may result in a child being incorrectly labelled with a learning disability.

Differential diagnosis
LEOPARD syndrome must be differentiated from other disorders characterized by multiple spotty pigmented macules, such as NAME syndrome, LAMB syndrome, and Peutz–Jeghers syndrome. The lack of mucous membrane involvement, the particular facial and body habitus of those with LEOPARD syndrome, and the absence of myxomas help make this distinction.

299. Menasche G, Pastural E, Feldmann J et al. (2000) Mutations in RAB27A cause Griscelli syndrome associated with haemophagocytic syndrome. **Nat Genet** 25(2):173–176.
300. Jozwiak S, Schwartz RA, Janniger CK, Zaremba J (1998) Familial occurrence of the LEOPARD syndrome. **Int J Dermatol** 37(1):48–51.
301. Capute AJ, Rimoin DL, Konigsmark BW et al. (1969) Congenital deafness and multiple lentigines. A report of cases in a mother and daughter. **Arch Dermatol** 100(2):207–213.
302. Voron DA, Hatfield HH, Kalkhoff RK (1976) Multiple lentigines syndrome. Case report and review of the literature. **Am J Med** 60(3):447–456.
303. Nordlund JJ, Lerner AB, Braverman IM, McGuire JS (1973) The multiple lentigines syndrome. **Arch Dermatol** 107(2):259–261.
304. Gorlin RJ, Anderson RC, Blau M (1969) Multiple lentigines syndrome. **Am J Dis Child** 117:652.
305. Weiss LW, Zelickson AS (1977) Giant melanosomes in multiple lentigines syndrome. **Arch Dermatol** 113(4):491–494.

CARNEY COMPLEX

Introduction and historical note

The NAME syndrome (nevi, atrial myxomas, myxoid neurofibromas, and ephelides) was described by Atherton et al.[306] in 1980. The LAMB syndrome (lentigines, atrial myxomas, mucocutaneous myxomas, and blue nevi) was reported by Rhodes et al.[307] in 1984. Endocrine overactivity, hyperplasia, and neoplasias involving various endocrine glands have been described in both syndromes. Carney et al.[308] provided additional details regarding these syndromes, which it now appears represent different aspects of a single disorder (see Chapter 10).

Genetics

It has recently been demonstrated that at least half of all examined cases of Carney complex are the result of mutations in the gene encoding the regulatory subunit Type 1A of protein kinase A (PRKAR1A).[309]

Physical examination

The pigmentary abnormalities described above (Fig. 10.6) may precede the onset of the cutaneous and other tumors associated with the disorder.

Pathophysiology and histogenesis

The activation of cyclic AMP-dependent protein kinase in a number of tissues results in overgrowth of certain cell types as well as endocrine hyperactivity, although the phenotype differs from that in the McCune–Albright syndrome in which the cyclic AMP cascade is activated by mutation in a regulatory subunit of adenylate cyclase.

Prognosis and therapeutics

Endocrine abnormalities require evaluation and management by a knowledgeable endocrinologist. If a myxoma is present in the atrium, surgical removal may be required.

GENETIC DISORDERS OF THE IMMUNE SYSTEM

Amy Paller

Children with genetic immunodeficiency disorders often manifest with skin changes, some of which may be specific for the immune dysfunction and others that share features with a variety of immune and other disorders, such as dermatitis. The dermatologist should work together with the immunologist in determining the correct diagnosis to allow optimal management. The reader is referred to Chapter 1 for more details of the basic science of the immune system.

ACATALASIA

Acatalasia is a heterogeneous group of rare, autosomal recessive disorders characterized by the marked deficiency of catalase, an enzyme present in red blood cells and other tissues.[310] The Japanese variant (Takahara's disease) is the symptomatic form, and pathology is confined to the oral cavity. The enzyme catalase generates oxygen by decomposing hydrogen peroxide and ostensibly protects tissue against oxidizing agents, including the peroxide generated by bacteria such as streptococci and pneumococci. Affected children tend to be normal until the deciduous teeth first erupt. At this time, patients develop deep necrotic periodontal or tonsillar ulcers with surrounding inflammation, dental caries, halitosis, loose teeth, and alveolar bone resorption. Patients rarely manifest for the first time after puberty. The relationship between the function of this enzyme and the resultant ulcerations is unclear. Because of the lack of catalase activity, blood turns brown in contact with hydrogen peroxide and does not generate oxygen (bubbling). Interestingly, there is an associated anomaly in the catabolism of heme, leading to markedly increased urinary excretion of coproporphyrin and bilirubin as well.[311] The differential diagnosis of acatalasia in children is that of the differential diagnosis of oral ulcerations. Entities to be considered as possible causes include agranulocytosis, leukemia, Langerhans cell histocytosis, Chédiak–Higashi syndrome, Papillon–Lefèvre syndrome, and hypophosphatasia. Treatment of this disorder involves surgical debridement of affected areas, extraction of teeth when associated with alveolar bone loss, and scrupulous oral hygiene.

HEREDITARY ANGIOEDEMA

Hereditary angioedema (HAE) is a potentially lethal, dominantly inherited form of angioedema, characterized by nonpruritic swelling of the face, extremities, and gastrointestinal and respiratory tracts without urticaria.[312,313]

EPIDEMIOLOGY

HAE occurs in 1 in 150 000 persons. Decreased antigenic and functional levels of an inhibitor of C1 esterase are found in 85% of affected individuals (Type I HAE). An additional 15% of patients have normal or elevated antigenic levels of a dysfunctional C1 esterase inhibitor (C1 INH) (Type II HAE). The disorder has been reported throughout the world, and involves almost all races and ethnic groups. HAE is almost always inherited as an autosomal dominant disorder with incomplete penetrance, and 75% of patients report a positive family history.

CLINICAL PRESENTATION

The first episode of angioedema tends to occur in early childhood. Since the early episodes most often are manifested as swelling of an extremity following trauma, they are commonly overlooked. The number of attacks usually increases throughout adolescence and young adulthood. The frequency of attacks varies widely among patients; some individuals have only a few attacks over several decades, while others have weekly bouts. No periodicity to the attacks is noted. Although attacks may be spontaneous, approximately 50% of bouts are precipitated by emotional or physical trauma. Dental manipulation and oromaxillofacial surgery of patients with HAE are most likely to trigger life-threatening pharyngeal edema.[314] Female patients commonly report more attacks in association with menses or oral contraceptive use. During the last two trimesters of pregnancy, the frequency of attacks appears to wane and the occurrence of angioedema at delivery is extremely rare.

Patients should be questioned about the occurrence of swelling in other family members, as well as about prodromal signs, including hoarseness, altered taste, difficulty with swallowing, and the presence of abdominal pain. Patients may also report a localized tingling or tightening of the skin prior to the onset

306. Atherton DJ, Pitcher DW, Wells RS, MacDonald DM (1980) A syndrome of various cutaneous pigmented lesions, myxoid neurofibromata and atrial myxoma: the NAME syndrome. Br J Dermatol 103(4):421–429.
307. Rhodes AR, Silverman RA, Harrist TJ, Perez-Atayde AR (1984) Mucocutaneous lentigines, cardiomucocutaneous myxomas, and multiple blue nevi: the "LAMB" syndrome. J Am Acad Dermatol 10(1):72–82.
308. Carney JA, Hruska LS, Beauchamp GD, Gordon H (1986) Dominant inheritance of the complex of myxomas, spotty pigmentation, and endocrine overactivity. Mayo Clin Proc 61(3):165–172.
309. Stratakis CA (2001) Clinical genetics of multiple endocrine neoplasias, Carney complex and related syndromes. J Endocrinol Invest 24(5):370–383.

310. Delgado W, Calderon R (1979) Acatalasia in two Peruvian siblings. J Pathol 8:358–368.
311. Takahara S, Ogata M (1977) Metabolism in Japanese acatalasemia with special reference to superoxide dismutase and glutathione peroxidase. In: Biochemical and Medical Aspects of Active Oxygen, Hayaishi O, Asada K, eds. Baltimore: University Park Press, p. 275.
312. Agostoni A, Cicardi M (1992) Hereditary and acquired C1-inhibitor deficiency: biological and clinical characteristics in 235 patients. Medicine 71:206–215.
313. Frank MM (2000) Complement deficiencies. Pediatr Clin N Am 47:1339–1354.
314. Atkinson JC, Frank MM (1991) Oral manifestations and dental management of patients with hereditary angioedema. J Oral Pathol Med 20:139–142.

of swelling. The attack often begins suddenly without a prodrome. The angioedema progressively increases for several hours, then stabilizes for 1 to 2 days before resolution. The total duration of episodes is typically 48 to 72h, but an attack may last longer. Patients tend to have a refractory period of days or weeks before another episode, in contrast to the often daily occurrence of urticaria. The edema is nonpitting, nonerythematous, and nonpruritic. In about 25% of patients, a transient or erythematous, nonpruritic macular rash resembling erythema marginatum precedes or accompanies the angioedema, but typical urticaria is not a feature of HAE. The most common sites of involvement are the extremities, face, oropharyngeal mucosae, and gastrointestinal tract. Compromise of the airways due to laryngeal angioedema occurs most commonly in adults, and is reported in two-thirds of patients at some time. Often patients are warned of impending obstruction by a voice change or dysphagia. Up to 25% of patients die from airway compromise. Occasionally genitourinary tract edema occurs and results in urinary retention. Rarely the angioedema involves the brain, pleura, or joint space, leading to headaches, seizures, paresis, cough, pleuritic chest pain, or arthralgias. Manifestations in the gastrointestinal tract depend on the location and intensity of the visceral swelling. Jejunal swelling leads to bilious vomiting and crampy abdominal pain; colonic involvement results in watery diarrhea. Rarely the intestinal edema is so extensive that hypotension results. Contrast studies of the intestines during attacks may show edematous mucosae.

A number of patients with HAE demonstrate features of autoimmune disorders as is seen in deficiencies of early complement components of the classical complement pathway. Most of these patients have systemic or discoid lupus erythematosus.[315,316] HAE may also be associated with membranoproliferative glomerulonephritis;[317] patients have also been described with scleroderma or focal lipodystrophy in association with HAE.

LABORATORY FINDINGS

Laboratory confirmation of the diagnosis depends on assays of complement pathway proteins. The best screening tests are levels of C4 and C1 INH. Levels of C4 and C2 are low during attacks, since these complement components are the substrates of C1 esterase. The C4 level tends to be depressed when the patient is asymptomatic as well. Total hemolytic complement (CH50) is often normal, and the C3 level is almost always normal as well. Direct measurement of immunoreactive C1 INH can be done by immunodiffusion assay. When the C1 INH level is normal but the C4 level is low in a patient with possible HAE, an immunodiffusion assay of C1 INH function will identify an antigenically normal but functionally abnormal protein.[318] Serum C1 levels are normal or minimally depressed in HAE. Other normal laboratory values include complete blood count, eosinophil count, sedimentation rate, serum chemistries, rheumatoid factor, antinuclear antibody (ANA), anti-DNA antibody, and immune complex assays.

PATHOPHYSIOLOGY AND HISTOGENESIS

The genetic alterations in HAE affect the structural gene for C1 INH,[319] a serine proteinase inhibitor (serpin). The type I HAE mutations reduced levels of C1 INH to 5–30% of normal, less than the predicted 50% of inhibitor function, suggesting that the mutations may transinhibit porduction of the normal gene or affect its secretion. Although the mutations of type I HAE are quite heterogeneous, the mutations that cause type II HAE are typically found within the active site or in the proximal hinge region of the gene,

which is involved in the proper folding and presentation of the active site. C1 INH modulates clotting, kinin generation, fibrinolysis, and complement pathways. It appears to be produced by hepatocytes, and blocks the generation of C4 and C2 by active C1. The angioedema probably results from uncontrolled activation of the complement pathway. In HAE, C1 becomes activated by proteolytic enzymes, including kallikrein, plasmin, and thrombin, which are produced when Hageman factor is activated by trauma. The mechanism of edema production remains unclear. When purified activated C1 is injected into normal individuals, a wheal develops. In patients with HAE, the injection leads to a typical attack, but patients with homozygous C2 deficiency demonstrate no wheal. This evidence suggests that a polypeptide fragment of C2 with kinin-like activity (C2 kinin) is released, which increases capillary permeability and causes angioedema. The reason for normal C3 levels despite classical complement activation remains unclear, but may relate to the site of C1 activation (in blood rather than on cell surfaces).

DIFFERENTIAL DIAGNOSIS

The diagnosis of HAE is easily made when a patient complains of angioedema with recurrent abdominal pain and reveals a positive family history. However, the clinical diagnosis of HAE in a patient without other affected family members and with a vague history of abdominal discomfort and acral swelling may be difficult. The differential diagnosis includes disorders of painless swelling and recurrent abdominal pain.

The majority of the causes of angioedema involve urticaria and are often pruritic. The causes of angioedema include:

1. Allergic (immediate hypersensitivity): food allergens, drugs, inhalants, parasites.
2. Immune complex disease: serum sickness.
3. C1 INH deficiency: HAE, acquired C1 INH deficiency.
4. Viral infections.
5. Medication-induced histamine release: morphine, codeine, iodinated contrast medium.
6. Physically induced: cold, heat, pressure, solar, aquagenic, vibratory.
7. Syndromes: urticarial vasculitis, urticaria pigmentosa, capillary leak syndrome, carboxypeptidase B deficiency, C3b inactivator deficiency.
8. Idiopathic angioedema.

An acquired deficiency of C1 INH is most commonly associated with lymphomas and cryoglobulinemia. C1 is consumed and levels of C1 are very low, in contrast to normal levels in HAE. Other disorders with facial swelling are the Melkersson–Rosenthal syndrome with facial palsy and a deeply furrowed tongue, patients with lip infiltration from Crohn's disease, and the superior vena cava syndrome associated with cardiovascular manifestations.

The abdominal pain may occur without angioedema involving the skin. If intestinal obstruction or appendicitis is suspected, an exploratory laparotomy may be performed and cause the angioedema to become exacerbated by the increased trauma. Many patients are called "hysterical" and the diagnosis of HAE is not made.

TREATMENT

The mortality of HAE can be reduced significantly by adequate therapy.[320–323] Patients with mild, infrequent attacks do not require long-term prophylaxis, but patients with frequent life-threatening attacks (one to two per month),

315. Massa MC, Connolly SM (1982) An association between C₁ esterase inhibitor deficiency and lupus erythematosus. J Am Acad Dermatol 7:255–264.
316. Pacheco TR, Weston W, Giclas PC et al. (2000) Three generations of patients with lupus erythematosus and hereditary angioedema. Am J Med 109:256–257.
317. Pan CG, Strife CF, Ward MK et al. (1992) Long-term follow-up of non-systemic lupus erythematosus glomerulonephritis in patients with hereditary angioedema: report of four cases. Am J Kidney Dis 19:526–531.
318. Yelvington M, Prograis LJ, Pizzo CJ, Curd JG (1983) Immunodiffusion assay of C₁ inhibitor function in serum: prospective analysis in angioedema-urticaria. Am J Clin Pathol 80:309–313.
319. Brown B, Hawk JJ, Sibunka S et al. (2001) A review of the reported defects in the human C1 esterase inhibitor gene producing hereditary angioedema including four new mutations. Clin Immunol 98:157–163.

320. Webb MD, Hakimeh S, Holly LK (2000) Management of children with hereditary angioedema: a report of two cases. Pediatr Dent 22:141–143.
321. Rosen FS, Beyler A (1980) Hereditary angioneurotic edema and its correction with androgen therapy. Birth Defects: Original Article Series 16:499–507.
322. Cicardi M, Bergamascini L, Cugno M et al. (1991) Long-term treatment of hereditary angioedema with attenuated androgens: a survey of a 13-year experience. J Allergy Clin Immunol 87:768–773.
323. Peltz S, Bateman HE, Reyes R et al. (1996) Hypodermic epinephrine spray and uvular angioedema revisited. J Allergy Clin Immunol 97:717–718.

should receive prophylactic therapy. Long-term treatment includes the use of antifibrinolytic agents, particularly epsilon-aminocaproic acid (EACA), tranexamic acid, and androgens. Danazol, a derivative of ethyltestosterone, is the androgen of choice and has few masculinizing side effects. By inducing mRNA synthesis by hepatocytes, danazol stimulates the synthesis of functional C1 INH. Danazol appears to be effective in elevating C1 INH levels and eliminating attacks in both forms of HAE. In a recent report of use of danazol or stanozolol in 24 patients for more than 5 years, irregular menstruation was the only frequent side effect. However, danazol had to be discontinued in one patient owing to hepatic cell necrosis. Danazol is contraindicated during pregnancy (category X drug). EACA inhibits the C1 and plasmin activation. Side effects include thrombus formation, fatigue, muscle aches, and nausea. Children usually do not need these drugs, but adolescents may have severe attacks.

Children and adolescents should use short-term prophylaxis before elective traumatic procedures, such as dental treatment or surgery, are performed. Antifibrinolytic components, fresh frozen plasma, and C1 INH concentrate (not available in the United States) have been used. Within 15 minutes of administration of C1 INH concentrate, serum levels of C1 INH increase to 50% of normal values and remain elevated for $1\frac{1}{2}$ to 2 days. Fresh frozen plasma or high-dose antifibrinolytic agents (EACA) are the drugs of choice if C1 INH is not available. Occasionally, the administration of fresh frozen plasma may aggravate the attack by renewing early complement components. In the management of acute HAE attacks, antihistamines, epinephrine, corticosteroids, and fresh frozen plasma should be considered.[323] Intubation or tracheostomy is life-saving if medical therapy is not effective. Affected individuals should carry a medical alert card describing the diagnosis and proper therapy. The pain of gastrointestinal edema may be relieved by aspirin or codeine preparations. Swelling of the extremities does not require intervention.

PSYCHOLOGICAL/SOCIAL CONSIDERATIONS

The severity of HAE increases at puberty, and older children may become physically and psychologically debilitated by frequent attacks. The absence from school and careful avoidance of trauma may separate the adolescent patient from peers. Growth and development is not affected. However, first-degree relatives have often suffered fatal or life-threatening episodes, and the risk of such events in a growing child or youth is an ever-present concern. Patients must be encouraged to use common sense in choosing physical activities, and children should not be denied opportunities to play with their peers. In general, noncontact sports, such as swimming, are preferable to contact sports. Traumatic activities, such as dental work, must be undertaken with great caution, with therapy available for ensuing angioedema. There are no medications that are known to induce attacks.

ATAXIA-TELANGIECTASIA

Ataxia-telangiectasia (AT) is a syndrome of progressive cerebellar ataxia beginning in early infancy, progressive oculocutaneous telangiectasia, a tendency to sinopulmonary infections, selective immunodeficiencies, and chromosomal instability with persistent DNA damage after radiation.

EPIDEMIOLOGY

This autosomal recessive disorder has an incidence of approximately 1:100 000 with a carrier rate of 1%.[324] Heterozygote fibroblasts and lymphocytes demonstrate chromosomal breaks after exposure to ionizing radiation. Uninvolved family members have an increased risk of breast cancer and lymphoreticular malignancies, but the risk appears to be function of the specific gene defect, with the highest risk in carriers with dominant negative missense mutations.[325] On average, carriers die 7–8 years earlier than noncarriers.[326] Cancer and ischemic heart disease are the most common cause of the excess numbers of deaths.

CLINICAL PRESENTATION

The initial manifestation is usually ataxia, which typically becomes apparent when the child begins to walk. The syndrome is often not recognized, however, until oculocutaneous features are manifested. In fact, the median age of diagnosis in one study was 78 months of age.[327] The characteristic mucocutaneous telangiectasias are usually first noted at 3 to 6 years of age, but have been described at birth. The telangiectasias first appear at the medial and lateral bulbar conjunctivae, and progress as red, symmetric horizontal streaks on the exposed bulbar conjunctivae. During the next few years, patients begin to develop cutaneous telangiectasias, especially on the ears (Fig. 7.31), eyelids, malar prominences, V of the neck, and antecubital and popliteal fossae. Less commonly, the dorsum of the hands and feet and the hard and soft palate may have telangiectasias. Although the ocular telangiectasias are quite striking, the cutaneous telangiectasias may be subtle and resemble fine petechiae, especially at sites other than the face.

Progeric changes of the skin and hair are noted in almost 90% of patients.[328] Subcutaneous fat is lost early and the facial skin tends to become atrophic and sclerotic. Gray hairs are found in young children and diffuse graying of the hair often occurs by adolescence. Other dermatologic changes that have been described in children with AT include chronic seborrheic dermatitis with blepharitis, poikilodermatous pigmentary changes, eczema, multiple ephelides, hirsutism, pigmentary abnormalities particularly large café-au-lait spots, vitiligo, keratosis pilaris, warts, and acanthosis nigricans. A recently described patient showed ataxia, numerous pigmentary abnormalities, but no mucocutaneous telangiectasia.[329] Two patients developed multiple basal cell carcinomas after 20 years of age. Noninfectious, sometimes ulcerating, cutaneous granulomas have been reported in several patients with AT.[330]

The ataxia is cerebellar, and is characterized by swaying of the head and trunk. Myoclonic jerks, choreoathetosis, oculomotor abnormalities, and dysarthric speech often become prominent in older children. Patients are usually confined to a wheelchair by the time they are 11 years old despite good muscular strength. A characteristic facies develops that is dull, sad, and hypotonic when relaxed. Later, the face becomes mask-like when progeric changes ensue.

Sinopulmonary infections occur in more than 80% of patients in some series. It is the most common cause of death, usually from bronchiectasis and respiratory failure; bronchiolitis obliterans has also been described. Other manifestations of AT include retardation of somatic growth (72%), mental retardation (33%), and endocrine abnormalities, especially ovarian agenesis or hypoplasia and insulin-resistant diabetes. Patients who survive into their late teenage years have an up to 40% risk of developing cancer, with a 70-fold and 200-fold excess of leukemias and lymphomas, respectively.[331] Lymphoid malignancy has been described as the presenting sign of ataxia-telangiectasia in affected infants.[332]

324. Swift M, Morrell D, Massey RB, Chase CL (1991) Incidence of cancer in 161 families affected by ataxia-telangiectasia. **N Engl J Med** 325:1831–1836.
325. Khanna KK (2000) Cancer risk and the ATM gene: a continuing debate. **J Natl Cancer Inst** 92:795.
326. Su Y, Swift M (2000) Mortality rates among carriers of ataxia-telangiectasia mutant alleles. **Ann Intern Med** 133:770–778.
327. Cabana MD, Crawford RO, Winkelstein JA et al. (1998) Consequences of the delayed diagnosis of ataxia telangiectasia. **Pediatrics** 102:98–100.
328. Cohen LE, Tanner DJ, Schaefer HG, Levis WR (1984) Common and uncommon cutaneous findings in patients with ataxia telangiectasia. **J Am Acad Dermatol** 10:431–438.
329. Khumalo NP, Joss DV, Huson SM, Burge S (2001) Pigmentary anomalies in ataxia-telangiectasia: a clue to diagnosis and an example of twin spotting. **Br J Dermatol** 144:369–371.
330. Paller AS, Massey RB, Curtis MA et al. (1991) Cutaneous granulomatous lesions in patients with ataxia-telangiectasia. **J Pediatr** 119:917–922.
331. Morrell D, Cromartie E, Swift M (1986) Mortality and cancer incidence in 263 patients with ataxia-telangiectasia. **J Natl Cancer Inst** 77:89–92.
332. Loeb DM, Lederman HM, Winkelstein JA (2000) Lymphoid malignancy as a presenting sign of ataxia-telangiectasia. **J Pediatr Hematol Oncol** 22:464–467.

infrequently, patients demonstrate increased levels of T-suppressor cells and decreased T-helper cells. Almost all patients with AT tend to have elevated levels of α-fetoprotein and carcinoembryonic antigen, which serves as an easy screening test for diagnosis.

Spontaneous chromosomal abnormalities (fragments, breaks, gaps, and translocations) occur 2 to 18 times more frequently in patients with AT than in normal individuals. Rearrangements of chromosomes 7 and 14, and especially 14:14 translocations, seem to predict the development of lymphoreticular malignancy. Fibroblast DNA is extremely sensitive to ionizing radiation and to radiomimetic agents such as bleomycin; this is probably due to a failure to cease DNA synthesis transiently after radiation exposure, and perhaps also due to defective repair. Heterozygotes for the AT gene are at high risk for neoplasia, especially female breast cancer.[334] Other laboratory abnormalities include mildly elevated liver function tests in 40–50% of patients, and evidence of glucose intolerance with hyperinsulinemia, insulin resistance, and hyperglycemia in greater than 50% of patients.

PATHOPHYSIOLOGY AND HISTOGENESIS

More than 400 mutations have been described in patients with AT, all in the gene ataxia-telangiectasia mutated (ATM), which encodes a protein that is a member of the phosphatidylinositol 3-kinase family.[333,334] The protein is thought to act as an early sensor of DNA damage, particularly by ionizing radiation, and activates by phosphorylation several damage response mechanisms, including a p53-dependent pathway that controls apoptosis and arrest during the cell cycle at G_1/S. ATM also phosphorylates c-abl, another protein kinase implicated in the growth arrest response to DNA damage. Thus, ATM is involved in regulating several cell cycle checkpoints and apoptosis in response to damage to DNA. The neurologic alterations may reflect defective repair of cellular DNA damage in a neurons, a cell population that cannot replicate.

TREATMENT

Patients with AT have progressive ataxia, often leading to the inability to walk without assistance by the early teenage years. The progeric features are also progressive, leading to marked aging by adolescence. Death frequently occurs in late childhood or the early teenage years. The oldest reported patients died at 50 years of age. Fifty-five percent of patients die because of chronic sinopulmonary disease and progressive respiratory insufficiency. The second most common cause of death is malignancy, leading to death in 15% of patients. The remaining 30% of patients tend to die because of sinopulmonary infection and respiratory insufficiency, but show evidence of malignancy on autopsy. Some of the patients who survive into their 30s or 40s show stabilization of the disorder, with improvement in neurologic and immunologic status.

The treatment of patients with AT is supportive. No agent has been demonstrated to control the progressive neurologic and cutaneous changes. The infections must be treated appropriately with antibiotics. Avoidance of sun exposure and use of sunscreens may help to prevent the actinic-like progeric changes. Early physical therapy should be instituted for patients with pulmonary bronchiectasis and physical therapy appropriate for the neurologic dysfunction should be started early to prevent contractures. Patients should be screened aggressively for the development of malignancy. However, when malignancy occurs, radiation and radiomimetic chemotherapeutic agents, especially bleomycin, should be avoided. Standard-dose chemotherapy is more likely to achieve remission and increase survival than reduced-dose chemotherapy.[335] Bleomycin has been shown to accelerate progressive pulmonary fibrosis,[336] which may be controlled by

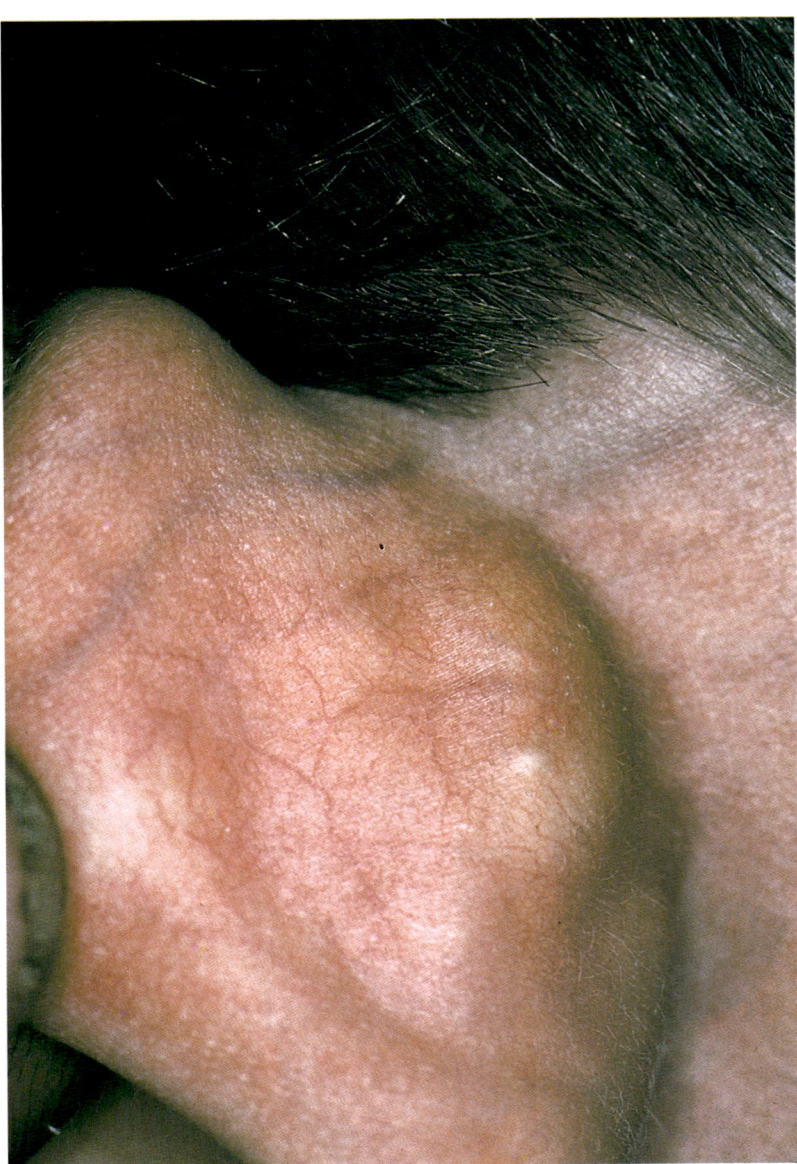

Fig. 7.31   Ataxia telangiectasia. Fine hair-like telangiectasias cover the helix.

LABORATORY FINDINGS

A variety of immunologic defects have been described in patients with AT. Approximately 70% of patients show a deficient or absent level of serum immunoglobulin A (IgA), and many patients demonstrate circulating anti-IgA antibodies. Even if the total serum IgA is normal, patients may demonstrate a specific deficiency of IgA_2. Eighty percent of patients demonstrate deficient to absent levels of IgE. Occasionally, levels, of IgM are increased, and 80% of patients show a low-molecular-weight (8S) serum IgM. Immunoglobulin G is often deficient, especially subgroups IgG_2 and IgG_4. Defective cell-mediated immunity is noted in 70% of patients. Abnormalities include lymphopenia, delayed allograft rejection, impaired self-response to recall antigens, and a deficient response to specific antigens and mitogens. The majority of patients have an absent or abnormally developed thymus. Not

333. Savitsky K, Bar-Shira A, Gilad S et al. (1995) A single ataxia telangiectasia gene with a product similar to PI-3 kinase. Science 268:1749–1753.
334. Spacey SD, Gatti RA, Bebb G (2001) The molecular basis and clinical management of ataxia-telangiectasia. Can J Neurol Sci 27:184–191.0

335. Sandoval C, Swift M (1998) Treatment of lymphoid malignancies in patients with ataxia telangiectasia. Med Pediatr Oncol 31:491–497.
336. Irsfeld H, Korholz D, Janßen G et al. (2000) Fatal outcome of two girls with Hodgkin disease complicating ataxia-telangiectasia (Louis-Bar syndrome) despite favorable response to modified dose chemotherapy. Med Pediatr Oncol 34:62–64.

administration of systemic corticosteroids. AT patients have decreased thresholds for postradiation erythema, tissue necrosis, and radiation-induced cutaneous malignancy. If radiation is necessary, the radiation dose should be restricted to less than 2000 rads, in fractions of less than 100 rads.

Prenatal diagnosis has been successfully performed by molecular techniques to diagnose AT.[337] Bone marrow and fetothymic transplants, transfer factor, and levamisole therapy have not resulted in clinical improvement.

PSYCHOLOGICAL/SOCIAL CONSIDERATIONS

The progressive neurologic deterioration of affected children is often difficult for the family to accept and understand. Despite confinement to a wheelchair by teenage years, two-thirds of children have normal intelligence, and every effort should be made to maintain intellectual stimulation and proper schooling despite the need to accommodate the physical handicaps. Neurologic abnormalities, progressive difficulties with speech and writing, premature aging, and short stature not uncommonly become the basis for teasing by other children. Psychological counseling may be necessary to aid the patient and family in coping with the disease. A national support group, the Ataxia-Telangiectasia Children's Project, is available through www.med.jhu.edu/ataxia and 800-5-HELP-A-T.

CHRONIC MUCOCUTANEOUS CANDIDIASIS

Patients with chronic mucocutaneous candidiasis (CMC) have recurrent, progressive infections of the skin, nails, and mucous membranes most commonly due to *Candida albicans*.[338] The clinical features of CMC may be seen as the manifestations of a variety of immunologic disorders, all characterized by ineffective defense mechanisms against *Candida*. In general, the patients with an earlier onset and greater severity of cutaneous candidal infections tend to have a more severe immunologic alteration.

EPIDEMIOLOGY

Many cases of CMC occur sporadically. The patients with immunodeficiency syndromes and the candidiasis endocrinopathy syndrome (autoimmune poly-endocrinopathy–candidiasis–ectodermal dystrophy syndrome, APECED) often report that other family members are affected. The hereditary pattern is usually autosomal recessive, although the rare association of CMC with chronic keratitis is thought to be autosomal dominant.

CLINICAL PRESENTATION

The extent of involvement is variable, and ranges from recurrent, recalcitrant thrush to mild erythematous scaling plaques with a few dystrophic nails, to severe generalized, crusted granulomatous plaques (Fig. 7.32). The cutaneous plaques tend to occur most commonly in intertriginous and on periorificial sites and on the scalp, but may be more generalized. Scalp infections may lead to scarring and alopecia. The nails are thickened, brittle, and discolored (Fig. 7.33), and the paronychial areas are often erythematous, swollen, and tender. The oral mucosa is the most frequent site of mucosal alteration (thrush with hyperkeratotic plaques), but the esophageal, genital, and laryngeal mucosae may be affected as well by chronic infection with resultant stricture formation. Patients with CMC do not tend to develop systemic candidiasis, but cutaneous dermatophyte infections are not uncommon. Up to 81% of patients have recurrent or severe infections other than candidal, including bacterial septicemia,[339] particularly with disease onset during childhood.

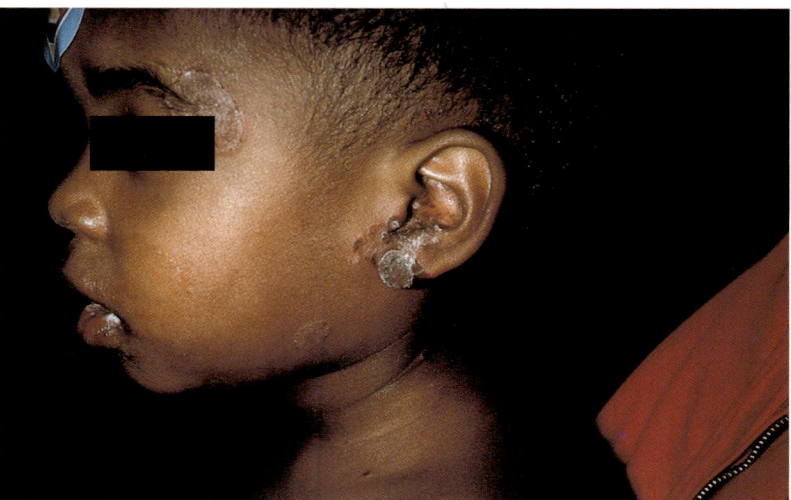

Fig. 7.32   Chronic mucocutaneous candidiasis in a young boy with candidal cheilitis and granulomatous lesions on his face.

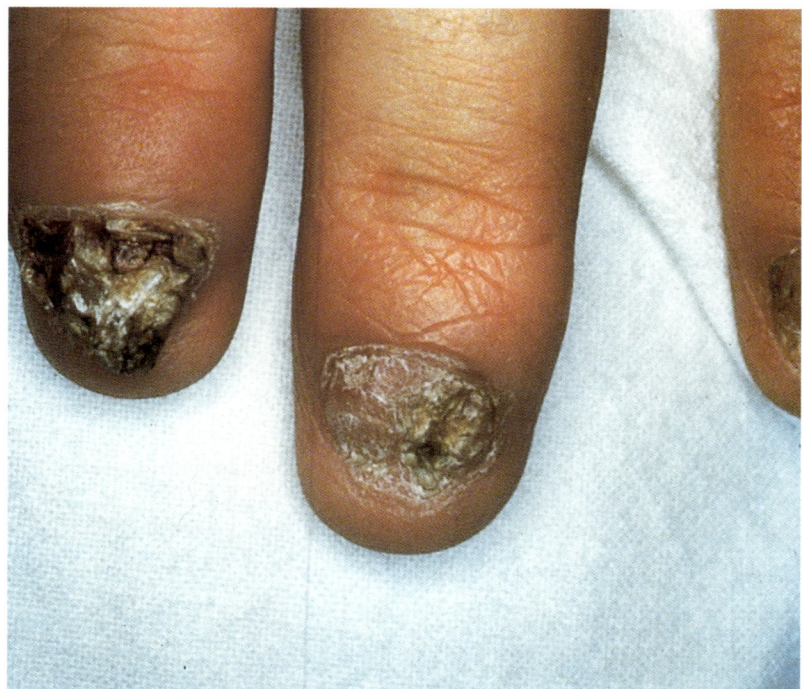

Fig. 7.33   Markedly dystrophic fingernails with paronychial inflammation in chronic mucocutaneous candidiasis.

Pediatric patients with CMC may be classified into the following subgroups:

1. Familial chronic mucocutaneous candidiasis. Oral candidiasis tends to begin by 2 years of age, although cutaneous and ungual candidiasis are less common.[340] No patients develop endocrinopathy. Consanguinity is common.

337. Gatti RA, Peterson KL, Novak J et al. (1993) Prenatal genotyping of ataxia telangiectasia. **Lancet** 342:376.
338. Kirkpatrick CH (2001) Chronic mucocutaneous candidiasis. **Pediatr Infect Dis J** 20:197–206.
339. Herrod HG (1990) Chronic mucocutaneous candidiasis in childhood and complications of non-*Candida* infection: a report of the Pediatric Immunodeficiency Collaborative Study Group. **J Pediatr** 116:377–382.
340. Wells RS, Higgs JM, MacDonald A et al. (1972) Familial chronic mucocutaneous candidiasis. **J Med Genet** 9:302–310.

2. Chronic localized candidiasis ("candidal granuloma"). Most patients with this form show manifestations by 5 years of age. Cutaneous lesions manifest as thick, tightly adherent crusts, most common on the face and scalp. Biopsies of lesional skin show marked hyperkeratosis and acanthosis; the underlying skin is infiltrated with lymphocytes, plasma cells, and sometimes giant cells. Affected patients usually have oral candidiasis as well.

3. Autoimmune polyendocrinopathy–candidiasis–ectodermal displasia (APECED). Most patients with CMC have autoimmune polyendo-crinopathy syndrome.[341] The candidal infections tend to begin by 5 years of age, although the endocrinologic dysfunction may not be apparent until teenage or even adult years. Candidal granulomas, especially of the face and scalp, may be seen. A variety of associated endocrinopathies have been described. Most common are hypoparathyroidism (88%) and hypoad-renocorticism (60%). One-third of patients have candidiasis, hypo-parathyroidism, and defective adrenal function. Other associated endocrinopathies or autoimmune disorders include gonadal insufficiency (45%), alopecia areata (20%), pernicious anemia (16%), thyroid abnor-malities (12%), chronic active hepatitis or juvenile cirrhosis (9%), vitiligo, diabetes mellitus, and hypopituitarism. Chronic diarrhea and malab-sorption have been reported in 25% of patients, and are usually associated with hypoparathyroidism. Affected children may also have pulmonary fibrosis, keratoconjunctivitis, splenic atrophy, and/or dental enamel hypoplasia. The cause of the enamel defects is unknown, as it does not appear to correlate with either periodontal disease or metabolic disorders, including hypoparathyroidism. Patients with APECED often have autoimmune antibodies, including antithyroglobulin, antimicrosomal antibodies, antiadrenal, antimelanocyte antibodies, and rheumatoid factor. Autoantibodies have also been found in patients with CMC who do not have clinical endocrinologic disease.

4. CMC with keratitis. Keratitis can be a feature of APECED, and CMC has been described in keratitis–ichthyosis–deafness syndrome; however, a family with CMC, keratitis and alopecia has also been described. Photophobia developed by 2 years of age, and the alopecia and oral and vaginal candidiasis by 5 years of age.[342] The inheritance pattern in this family was consistent with an autosomal dominant disorder.

5. Late-onset CMC. The candidal infections first develop at the end of the first decade of life or in the early teenage years. Involvement tends to be milder, but otherwise resembles other subgroups of CMC. These patients demonstrate abnormal immunologic responses against *C. albicans*, but the responses may become normal after effective therapy.

6. CMC associated with other immunologic defects. Chronic candidal infections are particularly common in patients with severe combined immunodeficiency, DiGeorge syndrome, and hyper-IgE syndrome.

7. CMC associated with other, predominantly nonimmunologic con-ditions, including the keratitis–icthyosis–deafness syndrome, multiple carboxylase enzyme deficiency, acrodermatitis enteropathica, and the ectodermal–ectrodactyly–clefting syndrome.

Other forms of CMC do not have their onset during childhood. For example, the association of CMC with abnormalities of iron metabolism or with thymoma have only been described in adult patients.

LABORATORY FINDINGS

Scrapings and cultures from cutaneous or mucosal lesions demonstrate candidal organisms. The candidal organisms are confined to the stratum corneum. The majority of patients with CMC demonstrate defective cell-mediated immunity, often restricted to the handling of *C. albicans* although no uniform alteration is found. Twenty-five to 35% of patients with CMC have no demonstrable immunologic defects. The variety of defects include lack of response to candidal antigens in skin testing; reduced lymphocyte blastogenic transformation response to *Candida*; abnormal lymphokine production in response to *Candida*; serum inhibition factors that alter the response to *Candida*; abnormal monocyte/macrophage chemotaxis, phagocytosis, and intracellular killing; and depressed IgA or complement function. The heterogeneity in detected immune disorders results in part from the variety of underlying clinical manifestations. For example, patients with other immune deficiencies such as severe combined immune deficiency or DiGeorge syndrome show lymphopenia, poor mitogenic and cytokine responses to mitogens and *C. albicans*, and anergy to triggers of delayed hypersensitivity. Other patients may have no defects except their altered mitogenic response to *Candida* and anergy. Although the frequent candidal infections are generally assumed to result from the immunologic deficiency, delayed hypersensitivity to candidal antigens has been restored after antifungal therapy in some patients, suggesting that anergy may result from the candidal infection. Recent data suggests that patients with CMC have an excessive response to candidal organisms that is ineffectual, and the resultant inflammatory cytokines trigger overproduction of interleukin-10 and downregulation of Th1 helper cell function[343] although the increase in interleukin-10 (IL-10) has not been demonstrated by other investigators.[344]

PATHOPHYSIOLOGY AND HISTOGENESIS

All patients with CMC have a T-cell deficiency that prevents effective handling of candidal organisms, although verification of T-cell deficits by laboratory tests is not always demonstrable. In some patients, the defect is specific to *Candida*, and in others, the immunologic response to other organisms is defective as well. APECED results from mutations in the gene AIRE (*auto*immune *re*gulator), which encodes a DNA transcription factor.[345] The link between the identified gene defect and the inability to handle candidal infection is unclear.

TREATMENT

In the past, CMC was generally refractory to treatment. The use of gentian violet, flucytosine, amphotericin B, clotrimazole, and miconazole nitrate was limited by side effects or ineffectiveness. Immune enhancement was usually ineffective as well, except for the response to transfer factor of some patients with defective cell-mediated immunity. Bone marrow transplantation, fetal thymus grafts, and leukocyte infusions have been attempted in patients with more severe immunologic deficiencies.

The introduction of the oral imidazole ketoconazole cleared thrush in a week, the skin lesions in 2 months, and the nail dystrophy after 5 to 9 months, although the cutaneous granulomas tended to be less responsive. The rare association of drug-induced hepatitis[346] has led to the preferred administration of alternative azoles, such as itraconazole,[347,348] and fluconazole.[349] Patients should be evaluated at least annually for the possible development of endocrinopathies, and perhaps more frequently if an endocrinopathy has already developed or siblings are affected with APECED syndrome.

341. Okamoto GA, Hall JG, Ochs H et al. (1977) New syndrome of chronic mucocutaneous candidiasis. **Birth Defects Orig Artic Ser** 13:117–125.

342. Ahonen P, Myllärniemi S, Sipilä I, Perheentupa J (1990) Clinical variation of autoimmune polyendocrinopathy-candidiasis-ectodermal dystrophy (APECED) in a series of 68 patients. **N Engl J Med** 322:1829–1836.

343. Lilic D, Gravenor I (2001) Immunology of chronic mucocutaneous candidiasis. **J Clin Pathol** 54:81–83.

344. de Moraes-Vasconcelos D, Orii NM et al. (2001) Characterization of the cellular immune function of patients with chronic mucocutaneous candidiasis. **Clin Exp Immunol** 123:247–253.

345. Finnish-German APECED Consortium (1997) An autoimmune disease, APECED, is caused by mutations in a novel gene featuring two PHD-type zinc-finger domains: autoimmune polyendocrinopathy–candidiasis–ectodermal dystrophy. **Nat Genet** 17:399–403.

346. Macnair AL, Gascoigne E, Heap J et al. (1981) Hepatitis and ketoconazole therapy. **Br Med J** 283:1058.

347. Burke WA (1989) Use of itraconazole in a patient with chronic mucocutaneous candidiasis. **J Am Acad Dermatol** 2 1:1309–1310.

348. Tosti A, Piraccini BM, Vincenzi C, Cameli N (1997) Itraconazole in the treatment of two young brothers with chronic mucocutaneous candidiasis. **Pediatr Dermatol** 14:146–148.

349. Hay RJ (1990) Overview of studies of fluconazole in oropharyngeal candidiasis. **Rev Infect Dis** 12 (Suppl. 3):S334–S337.

PSYCHOLOGICAL/SOCIAL CONSIDERATIONS

Mucocutaneous candidiasis may be extremely disfiguring, and the cosmetic ramifications may represent a tremendous burden, especially to the affected adolescent. Fortunately, the current availability of imidazoles has aided greatly in clearing the mucocutaneous manifestations.

CARTILAGE–HAIR HYPOPLASIA SYNDROME

Cartilage–hair hypoplasia syndrome is an autosomal recessive disorder that is most common in Amish individuals and Finns. Patients have fine, sparse, hypopigmented hair and metaphyseal dysostosis that results in short-limbed dwarfism. Patients may have soft, doughy skin with degenerated elastic tissue.[350] Hypoplastic anemia and neuronal dysplasia of the intestine are other common features, and congenital megacolon (Hirschsprung's disease) has occasionally been described. Patients, but not carriers, have an increased predisposition to non-Hodgkin's lymphoma and basal cell carcinomas.[351] Most patients manifest some degree of defective cell-mediated immunity, often showing particular susceptibility to severe disseminated varicella.[352,353] Thirty-five percent of Finns with this disorder show defective humoral immunity as well,[354] most frequently a deficiency of IgG4. The disorder results from mutations in the RNA component of a ribonucleoprotein endoribonuclease, RNase MRP, which in mitochondria cleaves RNA primers responsible for DNA replication, and in the nucleolus processes pre-rRNA.[355]

CHÉDIAK–HIGASHI SYNDROME

Chédiak–Higashi syndrome is a rare familial disorder characterized by incomplete, decreased and peculiar pigmentation, photophobia, and severe recurrent infections.[356–358]

EPIDEMIOLOGY

The disorder is inherited in an autosomal recessive mode and parental consanguinity is not uncommon.

HISTORY

Patients usually report early severe infections and pigmentary dilution in infancy. Not infrequently, patients are sensitive to sunlight and are very susceptible to sunburn.

PHYSICAL EXAMINATION

Almost all reported patients demonstrate "partial albinism" of the hair, skin, or eyes with pigmentary dilution or slate-gray pigmentation when contrasted with other family members. Hair color is variable, but usually has a silvery sheen. Loss of iris pigmentation results in an increased red reflex and photophobia. Strabismus and nystagmus are common, but visual acuity is usually

normal. Inflammation and ulceration of the oral mucosa, especially of the gingivae, have been described.

Many patients with Chédiak–Higashi syndrome develop progressive neurologic deterioration, particularly with clumsiness, abnormal gait, paresthesias, and dysesthesias. Peripheral and cranial neuropathies and, occasionally, a form of spinocerebellar degeneration may occur.[356] Other findings on physical examination relate to the frequent infections in the accelerated phase of the disease.

Infectious episodes are associated with fever and predominantly involve the skin, lungs, and upper respiratory tract. The most common organisms found are *Staphylococcus aureus*, *Streptococcus pyogenes*, and *S. pneumoniae*. The skin infections are primarily pyodermas, but infections with these organisms that result in deeper ulcerations resembling pyoderma gangrenosum have been reported.

Eighty-five percent of patients undergo an accelerated lymphoproliferative or lymphoma-like phase, characterized by widespread visceral tissue infiltration with lymphoid and histiocytic cells, which are sometimes atypical in appearance. Hepatosplenomegaly, lymphadenopathy, pancytopenia, jaundice, a leukemia-like gingivitis, and pseudomembranous sloughing of the buccal mucosa are associated. The thrombocytopenia and depletion of coagulation factors (decreased hepatic synthesis) may lead to petechiae, bruising, and gingival bleeding. Granulocytopenia and anemia are found in 90% of patients during the accelerated phase.

PATHOPHYSIOLOGY AND HISTOGENESIS

The defective gene in Chédiak–Higashi syndrome is the lysosomal trafficking regulator LYST.[359] This protein appears to regulate the secretory processes of intracellular lysosomal vesicles and melanosomes. Giant abnormal granules are the hallmark of Chédiak–Higashi syndrome, and result from dysregulated fusion of primary lysosomes. They are found in circulating leukocytes, melanocytes, melanosomes of hair, renal tubular epithelial cells, CNS neurons, and other tissues. These giant granules within phagocytic cells of affected children cannot discharge their lysosomal and peroxidative enzymes into phagocytic vacuoles.

Immunologic defects of Chédiak–Higashi syndrome include diminished chemotaxis of polymorphonuclear cells, monocytes, and lymphocytes; decreased antibody-dependent cytotoxicity; and reduced suppressor-cell function. NK cell function is often profoundly decreased, despite a relative increase in the number of γ/δ (immature) T cells. These immune abnormalities have been thought to cause the increased susceptibility to infections and the *lymphoma-like* phase. Deficiency of cathepsin G and elastase has been demonstrated in the neutrophils of patients with Chédiak–Higashi syndrome[360] owing to the presence of excess inhibitors;[361] the inactivation of these enzymes may also contribute to the increased susceptibility to infection. Viral infection, particularly due to Epstein–Barr infection, has been implicated in causing the accelerated lymphomatous phase.[362] The presence of cytotoxic T lymphocyte-associated antigen (CTLA-4 or CD152), which plays a major role in the negative regulation of T cell activation, in enlarged, abnormal vesicles of Chédiak–Higashi syndrome T cells rather than properly

350. Brennan T, Pearson R (1988) Abnormal elastic tissue in cartilage–hair hypoplasia. **Arch Dermatol** 124:1411–1414.
351. Makitie O, Pukkala E, Teppo L, Kaitila I (1999) Increased incidence of cancer in patients with cartilage–hair hypoplasia. **J Pediatr** 134:315–318.
352. Polmar SH, Pierce GF (1986) Cartilage hair hypoplasia: immunological aspects and their clinical implications. **Clin Immunol Immunopathol** 40:87–93.
353. Pierce GF, Polmar SH (1982) Lymphocyte dysfunction in cartilage hair hypoplasia. II. Evidence for a cell cycle specific defect in T cell growth. **Clin Exp Immunol** 50:621–628.
354. Makitie O, Kaitila I, Savilahti E (2000) Deficiency of humoral immunity in cartilage-hair hypoplasia. **J Pediatr** 137:487–492.
355. Ridanpaa M, Van Eenennaam H, Pelin K et al. (2001) Mutations in the RNA component of RNase MRP cause a pleiotropic human disease, cartilage–hair hypoplasia. **Cell** 104:195–203.
356. Blume RS, Wolff SM (1972) The Chédiak–Higashi syndrome: studies in four patients and review of the literature. **Medicine** 51:247–280.

357. Anderson LL, Paller AS, Malpass D et al. (1992) Chédiak–Higashi syndrome in a black child. **Pediatr Dermatol** 9:31–36.
358. Stegmaier OC, Schneider LA (1965) Chédiak–Higashi syndrome: dermatologic manifestations. **Arch Dermatol** 91:31.
359. Barbosa MD, Nyugen QA, Tchernev VT et al. (1996) Identification of the homologous beige and Chédiak–Higashi syndrome genes. **Nature** 382:262–265.
360. Ganz T, Metcalf JA, Gallin JI et al. (1988) Microbicidal/cytotoxic proteins of neutrophils are deficient in two disorders: Chédiak–Higashi syndrome and "specific" granule deficiency. **J Clin Invest** 82:552–556.
361. Takeuchi KH, Swank RT (1989) Inhibitors of elastase and cathepsin G in Chédiak–Higashi (beige) neutrophils. **J Biol Chem** 264:7431–7436.
362. Kinugawa N (1990) Epstein–Barr virus infection in Chédiak–Higashi syndrome mimicking acute lymphocytic leukemia. **Am J Pediatr Hematol/Oncol** 12:182–186.

expressed at the cell surface may lead to the increased risk of lymphoproliferative disease.[363]

DIFFERENTIAL DIAGNOSIS

Chédiak–Higashi syndrome should be differentiated from other "silver hair" syndromes,[320] Griscelli syndrome[364] and Elejalde syndrome.[365,366] The clinical signs of Griscelli syndrome include silver–gray hair and a relatively light skin color, recurrent episodes of fever with or without infection, increasing hepatosplenomegaly due to lymphohistiocytic infiltration, and progressive neurologic deterioration with hypotonia and motor retardation. Blood smears may show pancytopenia, but no leukocyte inclusions. Hypogammaglobulinemia may be an additional feature. Griscelli syndrome results from mutations in myosin-Va or RAB27A, protein thought to participate in membrane transport and organelle trafficking. Elejalde syndrome (neuroectodermal melanolysosomal disease) is another silvery hair syndrome with bronze skin after sun exposure and severe neurologic dysfunction (seizures, severe hypotonia, ocular abnormalities, and mental retardation). While the impairment of the nervous system is more severe in Elejalde syndrome, the defects in cellular or humoral immunity of Chédiak–Higashi and Griscelli syndrome are not seen in Elejalde syndrome. Similar to Griscelli syndrome, no neutrophil giant intracytoplasmic granules are found, although the melanin is distributed in small and large clumps in the hair. It has been postulated that Elejalde syndrome is allelic to Griscelli syndrome. Neutrophilic intracytoplasmic inclusions resembling those of Chédiak–Higashi syndrome have been described in patients with acute leukemia.[367]

TREATMENT

The mean age of death for patients with Chédiak–Higashi syndrome is 6 years. Fatality usually results from overwhelming infection or hemorrhage during the lymphoma-like accelerated phase. Bone marrow transplantation is the treatment of choice for patients with an HLA-matched marrow available. Otherwise, management of the disorder is largely supportive. Antibiotics help to control the recurrent infections. Vincristine and prednisone combination therapy and cyclosporin A have been beneficial in controlling the accelerated lymphoma-like phase, as have high dosages of acyclovir and gammaglobulin injections. Splenectomy has recently been advocated in patients with the accelerated phase unresponsive to other forms of therapy. Ascorbic acid has been administered, and has been found to correct the *in vitro* defect of microtubular function, perhaps through elevation of cAMP. However, when given to patients for weeks to months, it does not appear to decrease the frequency of infections in most cases, nor does it prevent the accelerated phase. Interferon has been demonstrated by some authors to partially restore NK cell function.

The profound NK cell defect and immunodeficiency have been reversed by successful bone marrow transplantation, but the partial albinism is not altered.[368] Bone marrow transplantation has also successfully reversed the relentless deterioration of patients with Griscelli syndrome.[369]

PSYCHOLOGICAL/SOCIAL CONSIDERATIONS

Because of frequent infections, patients with Chédiak–Higashi syndrome miss a great amount of school. They need more calories to balance the requirement of accelerated metabolism. Children affected by neurologic deterioration as well require physical therapy and attention to the special needs of a physical handicap.

COMPLEMENT DEFICIENCY DISORDERS

Isolated complement component deficiencies often result in autoimmune disorders or unusual susceptibility to recurrent infections.[313,370,371]

EPIDEMIOLOGY

All of the complement deficiencies are rare. C2 deficiency is the most common complement component deficiency. The homozygous form of C2 deficiency occurs in 1 in 10 000 to 1 in 40 000 individuals, and the heterozygous form is found in 1–2% of persons. In general, pathology does not occur in the heterozygote state, because enough protein is made to ensure function. Thus, most of the complement defects are inherited as autosomal recessive traits, except for hereditary angioedema (C1 INH deficiency or dysfunction) (see hereditary angioedema).

CLINICAL PRESENTATION

Many patients with complement deficiencies are normal. Only patients with clinical disease or family members of patients come to attention. Deficiencies of the early components of the classical complement pathway (C1, C4, C2) tend to be manifested by lupus erythematosus (LE)-like disorders in childhood. Patients demonstrate photosensitivity and skin changes of systemic or subacute cutaneous lupus erythematosus (SCLE). Most patients have absent or low ANA titers and mild renal disease (Table 7.14). Pyogenic infections, particularly with encapsulated organisms, occur with increased frequency in some patients with deficiencies of components of the classical complement cascade, but are not as frequent as in complement deficiencies involving the alternative pathway or membrane attack complex.

C2 deficiency is the most prevalent of the homozygous deficiencies of the complement components (Table 7.14). It has been reported to be a defect in gene translation (type 1) or a defect in secretion (type 2). Autoimmune disorders occur in almost 50% of persons with the homozygous form and in approximately 10% of those with the heterozygous form of C2 deficiency. Systemic lupus erythematosus (SLE) is more commonly manifested in female patients with homozygous C2 deficiency, 60% of whom show features of SLE. Other disorders have been associated less frequently than lupus with C2 deficiency. They include juvenile rheumatoid arthritis (especially in heterozygous female patients), dermatomyositis, Henoch–Schönlein purpura, glomerulonephritis, vasculitis, atrophoderma, cold urticaria, common variable immunodeficiency, hypogammaglobulinemia, Hodgkin's disease, and inflammatory bowel disease. The time of onset of LE-like manifestations varies, even within affected families. Many patients show characteristics in early childhood; others first have symptoms of autoimmune disease as young adults.

The most typical clinical finding in patients with C2 deficiency is a rash that tends to be exacerbated by exposure to sunlight. The skin lesions are frequently papulosquamous plaques, as in SCLE, but may be more typical of discoid LE or include malar erythema. Skin lesions are often extensive and may be difficult to control. The palmoplantar hyperkeratosis,

363. Barrat FJ, Le Diest F, Benkerrou M et al. (1999) Defective CTLA-4 cycling pathway in Chédiak–Higashi syndrome: A possible mechanism for deregulation of T lymphocyte activation. **Proc Natl Acad Sci USA** 96:8645.
364. Mancini A, Chan L, Paller A (1998) Partial albinism with immunodeficiency: Griscelli syndrome. Report of a case and review of the literature. **J Am Acad Derm** 38:295–300.
365. Ivanovich J, Mallory S, Storer T et al. (2001) 12-year-old male with Elejalde syndrome (neuroecteodermal melanolysosomal disease). **Am J Med Genet** 98:313–316.
366. Duran-McKinster C, Rodriguez-Jurado R, Ridaura C et al. (1999) Elejalde syndrome – a melanolysosomal neuroectodermal syndrome. **Arch Dermatol** 135:182–186.
367. Markovic N (1998) Chédiak–Higashi-like granules in acute promyelocytic leukemia. **Blood** 92:3475.
368. Griscelli C, Virelizier J-L (1983) Bone marrow transplantation in a patient with Chédiak–Higashi syndrome. **Birth Defects** 19:333.
369. Schneider LC, Berman RS, Shea CR et al. (1990) Bone marrow transplantation (BMT) for the syndrome of pigmentary dilution and lymphohistiocytosis (Griscelli's syndrome). **J Clin Immunol** 10:146–153.

TABLE 7.14 Complement deficiency disorders

Complement	Features
Classical pathway	
C1q	SLE, recurrent bacterial and candidal infections, GN
C1r	SLE, infections, GN
C1s	SLE
C1 INH	Hereditary angioedema
C4	SLE with palmoplantar keratoderma and scars, GN, HSP, and urticaria
C2	SLE, DLE, pyogenic infections (see text)
C3 and alternate pathway	
C3	Recurrent infections, SLE, vasculitis, "Leiner's"
Properdin	Fulminant neisserial infections
C3b INH	Recurrent infections, aquagenic urticaria
Membrane attack complex	
C5 dysfunction	"Leiner's," Gram-negative bacterial infections
C5 deficiency	*Neisseria, Pneumococcus*, SLE
C6	*Neisseria, Brucella, Toxoplasma*, GN
C7	*Neisseria*, SLE, CRST syndrome, ankylosing spondylitis
C8	*Neisseria*, SLE, fever with HSM, eosinophilia, hyperglobulinemia
C8 dysfunction	*Neisseria*, SLE
C9	*Neisserial* infections

CRST, calcinosis, Raynaud's phenomenon, sclerodactyly, telangiectasias; DLE, discoid lupus erythematosus; GN, glomerulonephritis; HSM, hepatosplenomegaly; HSP, Henoch–Schönlein purpura; INH, inactivator; SLE, systemic lupus erythematosus.

TABLE 7.15 Features of systemic lupus erythematosus (SLE) in C2 deficiency

Features common to SLE and C2 deficiency	Features more suggestive of C2 deficiency SLE
Photosensitivity	Earlier age of onset
Rash	Extensive cutaneous lesions
Alopecia	Infections
Arthralgias/arthritis	Mild or occult renal disease
Fever	Absent or low titer ANA, anti-DNA
Oral ulcerations	Negative lupus band test
Leukopenia	Less severe
Anti-Ro antibody	
Rheumatoid factor	
Skin histology	

as has been noted in C4 deficiency with LE (Tables 7.14 and 7.15), has not been described in C2-deficient patients. LE-like alopecia is often reported.

Other features of SLE are often present. Arthritis and arthralgias are found in 80% of patients, as are unexplained fevers. Leukopenia and oral ulcerations are noted in almost 50% of patients. Less frequent manifestations include CNS vasculitis, pleuritis, pericarditis, Raynaud's phenomenon, and thrombocytopenia. Renal disease is generally mild or detectable only by biopsy, but occasional patients have severe renal disease.

The most common laboratory abnormality in C2 deficiency is an elevated titer of anti-Ro (SSA) antibodies, found in 75% of patients with SLE and C2 deficiency.[372] The anti-Ro antibody is also found in 60% of patients with SCLE, a subset of LE with prominent papulosquamous plaques, photosensitivity, milder systemic symptoms, and often negative ANA tests. Increased titers of anti-Ro antibodies are not found in homozygous or heterozygous C2 deficiency without LE. Rheumatoid factor is elevated in 40% of patients with C2 deficiency, but ANA and anti-DNA antibodies are usually of low titer or absent. Rarely, elevated levels of Sm and anti-RNP antibodies, circulating immune complexes, and a positive RPR have been found in patients with LE and C2 deficiency.

Patients with C2 deficiency are also susceptible to recurrent infections with pyogenic organisms. Most infections are pulmonary, due to pneumococcus, but other encapsulated bacteria have also been implicated.

Homozygous deficiency of C1q, C1r, C1s, and C4 is extremely rare, but manifests with autoimmune disease more frequently than homozygous C2 deficiency. C4 is unusual in that there are 4 genes that encode this complement, two for C4A and 2 for C4B, each of which have slightly different biologic activity. Interestingly, many individuals are missing one to four alleles of C4, and show reduced functional C4 activity, manifesting as an increased risk of autoimmune disease.

Patients with complement deficiencies involving the alternative and terminal pathways tend to suffer from disseminated infections of Gram-negative diplococci, especially neisseria, as well as from other pyogenic microorganisms.[373,374] Recurrent respiratory tract infections and peritonitis affect patients with deficiencies of C3 and C3 inactivator.[375] Generalized seborrheic erythroderma with failure to thrive, recurrent infections, and diarrhea ("Leiner's phenotype") have been described in patients with C3[376] deficiency and in C5 dysfunction. C3 deficiency has also been associated with partial thoracic or cephalothoracic lipodystrophy, often with mesangioproliferative glomerulonephritis.[377] Patients with deficiencies of components of the membrane attack sequence, C5 to C9, and with properdin deficiency (an X-linked deficiency) have recurrent neisserial infections (gonorrhea, meningococcemia). These neisserial infections tend to begin approximately around the time of puberty, although other infections, especially pneumococcal, often start in earlier childhood. Patients with deficiencies of the membrane attack complex occasionally have autoimmune disorders as well. Patients with C7 deficiency may have features of the calcinosis, Raynaud's, scleroderma, telangiectasia syndrome (see CREST syndrome, Chap. 23).

LABORATORY FINDINGS

The CH50 is markedly decreased or undetectable in complement deficiencies other than hereditary angioneurotic edema (involving C1 INH). The single affected complement component may be shown to be decreased by radioimmunodiffusion assay. All other complement components are within the normal range. An alternative pathway lytic test also exists (AP50), which is a useful screening test for deficiencies of components of the alternate complement pathway, although less sensitive than the CH50.

370. Guenther LC (1983) Inherited disorders of complement. **J Am Acad Dermatol** 9:815–839.
371. Tappeiner G (1982) Disease states in genetic complement deficiencies. **Int J Dermatol** 21:175–191.
372. Provost TT, Arnett FC, Raichlin M (1983) Homozygous C₂ deficiency, lupus erythematosus and anti-Ro (SSA) antibodies. **Arthritis Rheum** 26:1279–1282.
373. Fijen CA, Kuijper EJ, Hannema AJ et al. (1989) Complement deficiencies in patients over ten years old with meningococcal disease due to uncommon serogroups. **Lancet** 2:585–588.
374. Nagata M, Hara T, Aoki T et al. (1989) Inherited deficiency of ninth component of complement: an increased risk of meningococcal meningitis. **J Pediatr** 114:260–264.
375. Borzy MS, Gewurz A, Wolff L et al. (1988) Inherited C3 deficiency with recurrent infections and glomerulonephritis. **Am J Dis Child** 142:79–83.
376. Sonea MJ, Moroz BE, Reece ER (1987) Leiner's disease associated with diminished third component of complement. **Pediatr Dermatol** 4:105–107.
377. Bier DM, O'Donnell JJ, Kaplan SL (1978) Cephalothoracic lipodystrophy with hypocomplementemic renal disease: discordance in identical twin sisters. **J Clin Endocrinol Metab** 46:800–807.

PATHOPHYSIOLOGY AND HISTOGENESIS

Defects involving the early components of the classical complement pathway (C1, C4, C2) tend to resemble autoimmune disorders, especially SLE. These deficiencies do not lead to overwhelming infection because the mannan-binding lectin pathway and the alternative pathway can bypass these proteins to interact with the complement sequence at the level of C3, continuing the complement cascade. The increased risk of autoimmune disorders may be related to the gene location of these complement components as part of the HLA locus. In addition, both alternative and classical complement pathways are required for the solubilization of immune complexes. Ineffective clearance of immune complexes may result in autoimmune disease manifestations. The milder course of SLE in patients with complement deficiency may be explained by the lower or absent titers of anti-DNA antibodies and ANA, and by the inflammatory response that is altered by the complement deficiency. Because skin lesions are common and severe in complement deficiency, other antibodies, such as anti-Ro antibodies, may be more important than complement activation and ANA in the pathogenesis of skin disease.

The variety of recurrent infections associated with complement deficiencies emphasizes the central role of complement components in bacterial clearance. Deficiencies of the early components, especially C2, are associated with infection by encapsulated bacteria, especially *Pneumococcus*. Opsonization of bacteria and fungi may be ineffective in disorders of the classical pathway because of the slow, inadequate formation of C3b. Patients with deficiencies of C5 do not generate chemotactic factors normally and polymorphonuclear leukocyte function may be inadequate. Children with C5 to C9 complement deficiencies tend to develop recurrent neisserial infections in their teenage years because of the importance of the alternative complement pathway for destruction of neisserial organisms.

TREATMENT

Conservative therapy is often effective for patients with autoimmune manifestations of complement deficiency. The use of sunscreens and topical corticosteroids and avoidance of sunlight may be sufficient. Antimalarial drugs, systemic corticosteroids, and other immunosuppressive medications should be employed in more severe cases. The increased risk of infections in patients with complement deficiencies should be recalled in choosing to use immunosuppressive medications. The use of transfusions of plasma to replace the deficient components may activate C3 and C5 and accelerate immune complex deposition in the inflammatory reaction. Vigorous and early use of antibiotics is important in handling the recurrent infections.

CHRONIC GRANULOMATOUS DISEASE OF CHILDHOOD

Chronic granulomatous disease (CGD) is a group of disorders characterized by severe recurrent infections due to an inability of phagocytic leukocytes to kill intracellular bacteria and fungi by generating oxidative metabolites. All of the forms of CGD involve reduced function of the nicotinamide dinucleotide phosphate (NADPH) oxidase complex.

EPIDEMIOLOGY

CGD affects at least 1 in 200 000 live births.[378,379] Ninety percent of patients are male. Of those with known inheritance pattern, 76% have an X-linked transmission, while the remainder show an autosomal recessive form. The most prevalent of the autosomal recessive forms is p47phox (*phagocyte oxidase*) deficiency.

CLINICAL PRESENTATION

The areas of the body that are most involved in chronic granulomatous disease are those that are frequently challenged by bacteria, including the skin, lungs, and perianal tissue. The earliest lesions are usually staphylococcal infections of the skin around the ears and nose, and may be present at birth.[380] The localized pyodermas may progress in infancy to extensive purulent dermatitis with regional lymphadenopathy. Skin abscesses occur in 42% of patients, particularly caused by *S. aureus*; perirectal abscesses occur more commonly with the X-linked form (17% of patients with X-linked vs. 7% with autosomal recessive). Inflammatory reactions, often purulent, tend to develop at sites of minor cutaneous trauma or sites of regional lymph node drainage, which heal slowly with scarring. Cutaneous granulomas occur less frequently than cutaneous infections, and are nodular and often necrotic. Seborrheic dermatitis, scalp folliculitis, perioral ulcers, and intraoral ulcerations, resembling aphthous stomatitis, have also been described. Occasionally, patients may have cutaneous features of systemic or discoid LE.

The extracutaneous organs most frequently involved in CGD are the lymph nodes, lungs, liver, spleen, and gastrointestinal tract (Table 7.16). Suppurative lymphadenitis occurs overall in 53% of patients, and usually affects cervical nodes, with abscess and fistula formation. Axillary, inguinal, mesenteric, and mediastinal lymph nodes are often involved as well (Fig. 7.34). Broncho-pneumonia is the most prevalent infection, occuring in 79% of patients, and often responding inadequately to appropriate antibacterial therapy. Abscess formation, cavitation, and empyema are frequent complications. Hepato-splenomegaly is found in 80–90% of patients. About one-third of patients develop hepatic abscesses, and granulomas of the liver and spleen are common. These granulomas can occlude vital structures, causing gastric outlet obstruction or urinary tract obstruction. Osteomyelitis occurs in 25% of patients, and *Serratia marcescens* is the most common organism. Gastrointestinal abnormalities in CGD are most common, characterized by persistent or recurrent diarrhea and malabsorption, often associated with gastritis, esophagitis, or colitis. In general, the X-linked forms tend to be more severe than the

TABLE 7.16 Signs and symptoms of chronic granulomatous disease

Symptom	% of occurrence
Lymphadenopathy	90
Dermatitis	80
Pneumonitis	80
Hepatomegaly	80
Underweight	75
Splenomegaly	70
Short stature	50
Hepatic/perihepatic abscess	40
Persistent diarrhea	40
Pleuritis/empyema	35
Septicemia or meningitis	35
Osteomyelitis	30
Facial periorificial dermatitis	20
Perianal abscess	15
Lung abscess	15
Conjunctivitis	15
Ulcerative stomatitis	15
Peritonitis	10
Onset by age 1 year	65
Onset with dermatitis	25
Onset with lymphadenitis	25

378. Winkelstein JA, Marino MC, Johnston RB et al. (2000) Chronic granulomatous disease. Report on a national registry of 368 patients. **Medicine** 79:155.
379. Segal BH, Leto TL, Gallin JI et al. (2000) Genetic, biochemical, and clinical features of the chronic granulomatous disease. **Medicine** 79:170.
380. Windhorst DB, Good RA (1971) Dermatologic manifestations of fatal granulomatous disease of childhood. **Arch Dermatol** 103:351–357.

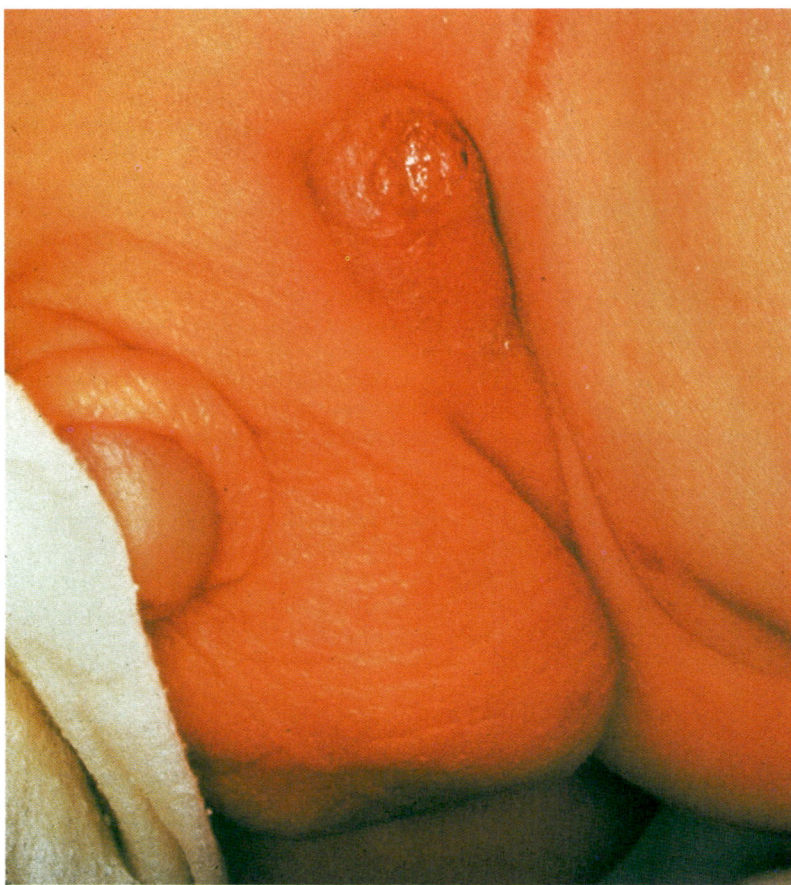

Fig. 7.34 **Infant affected by chronic granulomatous disease.** Draining suppurative inguinal lymph node in an infant with vomiting, failure to thrive, and recurrent staphylococcal pneumonia (courtesy of A. Ammann).

CGD is usually reduced, although the variability in extent reflects the random X-inactivation. Only 5–10% of leukocytes from patients with CGD are able to reduce NBT during phagocytosis. The ferricytochrome C reduction assay and chemiluminescence or fluorescent assays are more accurate and quantitative in reflecting the respiratory burst, and may also be performed to further verify the diagnosis. Immunoblot analysis may demonstrate lack of the gp91[phox] or p22[phox] proteins, which must then be sequenced since mutations leading to absence in either one leads to absense of both. Absence of p47[phox] or p67[phox] by immunoblot analysis is enough to confirm the gene affected.

The organisms associated with CGD are usually *S. aureus* and opportunistic Gram-negative bacteria, including *Klebsiella, Pseudomonas, Escherichia coli,* and *Serratia.* Other organisms involved in the disorder include *Aspergillus, Candida, Cryptococcus,* and *Nocardia.* The generation of oxidative metabolites is necessary for phagocytic leukocytes to kill these microorganisms.

PATHOPHYSIOLOGY AND HISTOGENESIS

For normal bactericidal activity, phagocytotic cells must respond to phagocytosed organisms with a "respiratory burst," producing toxic metabolites of oxygen. The defects in CGD involve four components of phagocyte NADPH oxidase, the membrane-bound glycoprotein gp91[phox] and p22[phox], and the cytoplasmic components p47[phox] and p67[phox]. Patients with CGD have deficient killing because this membrane-associated NADPH oxidase system fails to rapidly generate superoxide anion by transferring electrons from NADPH to molecular O_2 in response to physiologic stimuli, such as phagocytosis. In most X-linked kindreds, cytochrome b_{558} with its 21kDa α subunit (p22[phox]) and 91kDa β subunit (gp91[phox]) components is not detectable, due to mutations in gp91[phox]. Patients with autosomal recessive CGD usually have normal components of cytochrome b, but are deficient in p47[phox] or p67[phox], cytosolic components that are bound in a complex and must be transported together with Rac to the membrane-bound flavocytochrome (with the gp91[phox] and p22[phox] subunits) in order to activate NADPH oxidase. Rarely, patients with autosomal recessive CGD are deficient in cytochrome b_{558} because of mutations in the α-chain (p22[phox]), located on chromosome 16. It is thought that cytochrome b_{558} is the membrane attachment site for the p47 and p67 cytosolic factors that translocate from the cytosol to the plasma membrane and that this assembly of oxidase components, including phosphorylation of p47, allows activation.

The laboratory and clinical abnormalities that are seen in CGD may be explained as compensatory reactions after the failure of phagocytic killing. These include the characteristic classes of microbial organisms involved in producing infections, the intensive humoral reaction reflected by hypergammaglobulinemia, and the brisk cellular reaction characterized by cutaneous inflammation. In addition, granulomas are formed around the invading organisms in an attempt to confine them further, but these granulomas result in visceral impairment. When granulomas involve the skin, a skin biopsy demonstrates histiocytic infiltrates associated with foreign body giant cells, and accumulation of neutrophils with necrosis.

DIFFERENTIAL DIAGNOSIS

CGD should be suspected in children with recurrent cutaneous, nodal, and visceral infections. Laboratory tests (e.g., NBT) allow differentiation of CGD from other disorders with increased susceptibility to bacterial infections, such as hypogammaglobulinemias, myeloperoxidase deficiency, leukocyte adhesion defects, and the hyperimmunoglobulin E syndrome.

autosomal recessive forms, with a higher mean age of onset in the former group (3 years vs. 8 years), and a higher risk of infectious and obstructive complications.[378]

Patients with CGD have an increased risk of inflammatory, noninfectious complications. The clinical manifestations are varied, and include skin ulceration, excessive inflammation leading to dehiscence, pneumonitis, and inflammatory bowel disease, in addition to the autoimmune diseases resembling systemic lupus erythematosus and discoid lupus. Although the mechanisms underlying this inflammatory response are unclear, the tendency for these inflammatory complications to occur may relate to the individual's polymorphisms in genes unrelated to NADPH oxidase.[381]

LABORATORY FINDINGS

The laboratory abnormalities in CGD include leukocytosis, anemia, elevated erythrocyte sedimentation rate, hypergammaglobulinemia, and an abnormal chest radiograph. Skin testing for delayed hypersensitivity is normal, as are phagocytosis and chemotaxis. The screening test for CGD is the nitroblue tetrazolium (NBT) reduction assay. NBT is yellow in its soluble, oxidized form. When reduced, the dye precipitates and becomes blue (formozan precipitate). Approximately 80–90% of normal leukocytes are able to reduce NBT during phagocytosis. The percentage of leukocytes from carriers of

381. Foster CB, Lehrnbecher T, Mol F, et al. (1998) Host defense molecule polymorphisms influence the risk for immune mediated complication in chronic granulomatous disease, *J Clin Invest* 102:2146–2155.

TREATMENT

Cutaneous or nodal infections may be readily apparent. However, small localized areas of inflammation, with or without fever, may be difficult to detect. Vigorous investigation of the lungs, liver, and bones by routine screening X-rays, scans or ultrasound often uncovers an occult focus of inflammation. The use of antibiotics has markedly reduced the morbidity and mortality of CGD. Cultures should be performed to determine the etiologic agent, and appropriate therapy should be initiated. Invasive surgical procedures may be required for adequate cultures. If culture material cannot be obtained or while awaiting culture results, patients should be treated with parenteral antibiotics, including antibiotics effective for staphylococcal infections, for at least 10 to 14 days. A course of oral antibiotics should subsequently be continued for weeks. Long-term prophylactic TMP-SMX therapy decreases the incidence of bacterial infection without increasing the inci-dence of fungal infection.[382] Surgical intervention can be very important for deeper infections and includes debridement, irrigation, and prolonged drainage.

Patients with both X-linked and autosomal recessive CGD have shown clinical improvement after administration of γ-interferon.[383,384] Administration of the interferon likely results in augmentation of oxidant-independent antimicrobial pathways, since superoxide release is not enhanced and levels of cytochrome b are unchanged. The rate of *Aspergillus* infections has been reduced by prophylaxis with itraconazole.[385] Leukocyte transfusions have been used in cases of rapidly progressive, life-threatening infections.[386] Short courses of systemic corticosteroids have been helpful for patients with obstructive visceral granulomas of the bronchopulmonary, gastrointestinal, or genitourinary tracts.[387]

Bone marrow transplantation has been employed successfully in CGD,[388–390] but the morbidity and mortality of transplantation (about 10%) have mitigated against its routine use for CGD. Gene therapy has been performed for patients with the p47phox-deficient form; a single infusion of transduced CD34+ peripheral blood stem cells led to peak levels of corrected granulocytes 3–6 weeks after infusion with persistence at 6 months after infusion in two of the five patients.[391]

The diagnosis of carrier state is important for genetic counseling before pregnancy, including for sisters of the affected male patient. Approximately 50% of women are carriers in families of patients with the X-linked form of CGD,[392] which can be detected by flow cytometric studies showing fewer cells with gp91phox on the surface. Heterozygous carriers have variable proportions of normal and abnormal cells and may demonstrate a partial defect in oxidative metabolism and bacterial killing, but generally do not show increased susceptibility to infections.[393] Many carriers have been described with discoid LE lesions, photosensitivity, severe aphthous stomatitis,[393,394] Jessner's lymphocytic infiltrate, or granulomatous cheilitis.[395] The histopathology of the discoid LE is not typical and immunofluorescence examination is negative.[399] The relation between the development of the lupus-like illness and impaired microbial killing remains unclear. Prenatal diagnosis of X-linked CGD is possible by identifying genetic polymorphisms.[396]

PSYCHOLOGICAL/SOCIAL CONSIDERATIONS

CGD can have devastating effects on the affected child. Patients frequently have an increased metabolic rate requiring increased caloric intake. In addition, gastrointestinal involvement is not unusual, and food may be poorly absorbed. Many of these children are small for their age and grow poorly. The recurrent infections of the skin and other organs lead to frequent absences from school and to considerable psychosocial embarrassment.

DIGEORGE SYNDROME

DiGeorge syndrome is a member of a group of disorders that share a common chromosomal deletion, resulting in monosomy 22q11 (CATCH 22, DiGeorge/Velocardiofacial sydrome). In addition to the thymus abnormality, which results from developmental defects of the third and fourth pharyngeal pouches, conotruncal heart anomalies, dysmorphism, hypoparathyroidism, and cleft palate are prominent features.[397] Although most patients have T-cell defects, some have only mild T-cell abnormalities (partial DiGeorge). T-cell function

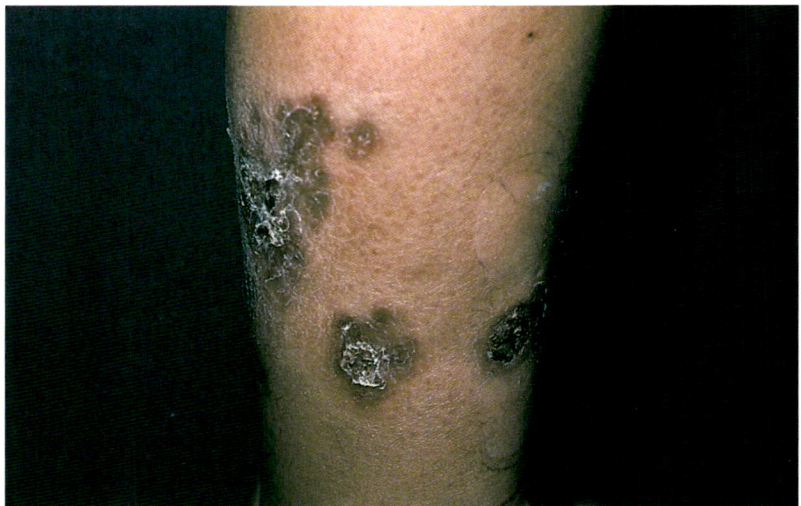

Fig. 7.35   Noninfectious, persistent cutaneous granulomas in a patient with DiGeorge syndrome. The granulomas are indistinguishable clinically from cutaneous granulomas associated with other immunodeficiencies.

382. Margolis DM, Melnick DA, Alling DW, Gallin JI (1990) Trimethoprim-sulfamethoxazole prophylaxis in the management of chronic granulomatous disease. J Infect Dis 162:723–726.
383. International Chronic Granulomatous Disease Cooperative Study Group (1991) A controlled trial of interferon gamma to prevent infection in chronic granulomatous disease. N Engl J Med 324:509.
384. Ahlin A, Elinder G, Palmblad J (1997) Dose-dependent enhancements by interferon-gamma on functional responses of neutrophils from chronic granulomatous disease patients. Blood 89:3396–3401.
385. Mouy R, Veber R, Blanche S, et al. (1994) Long-term itroconazole prophylaxis against Aspergillus infections in thrity-two patients with chronic granulomatous disease. J Pediatr 125:998–1003.
386. Von Planta M, Ozahin H, Schroten H et al. (1997) Greater omentum flaps and granulocyte transfusions as combined therapy of liver abscess in chronic granulomatous disease. Eur J Pediatr Surg 7:234–236.
387. Danziger RN, Goren AT, Becker J et al. (1993) Outpatient management with oral corticosteroid therapy for obstructive conditions in chronic granulomatous disease. J Pediatr 122:303.
388. Ding C, Kume A, Bjorgvinsdottir H, Hawley RG (1996) High-level reconstitution of respiratory burst activity in a human X-linked chronic granulomatous disease (X-CGD). Cell line and correction of murine X-CGD bone marrow cells by retroviral-mediated gene transfer of human gp91 phox. Blood 88:1834–1840.
389. Ho CM, Vowels Mr, Lockwood L, Ziegler JB (1996) Successful bone marrow transplantation in a child with X-linked chronic granulomatous disease. Bone Marrow Transp 18:213–215.

390. Calvino MC, Maldonado MS, Otheo E et al. (1996) Bone marrow transplantation in chronic granulomatous disease. Eur J Pediatr 155:877–879.
391. Malech HL, Mapels PB, Whiting-Theoblad N et al. (1997) Prolonged production of NADPH oxidase-corrected granulocytes after gene therapy of chronic granulomatous disease. Proc Nat Acad Sci USA 94:12133–12138.
392. Crockard AD, Thompson JM, Boyd NA et al. (1997) Diagnosis and carrier detection of chronic granulomatous disease in five families by flow cytometry. Int Arch Allergy Immunol 114:144–152.
393. Sillevis Smitt JH, Weening RS et al. (1990) Discoid lupus erythematosus-like lesions in carriers of X-linked chronic granulomatous disease. Br J Dermatol 122:643–650.
394. Schmitt CP, Scharer K, Waldherr R et al. (1995) Glomerulonephritis associated with chronic granulomatous disease and systemic lupus erythematosus. Nephrol Dial Transplant 10:891–895.
395. Dusi S, Poli G, Berton G et al. (1990) Chronic granulomatous disease in an adult female with granulomatous cheilitis. Evidence for an X-linked pattern of inheritance with extreme lyonization. Acta Haematol 84:49–56.
396. Gorlin JB (1998) Identification of (CA/GT)n polymorphisms within the X-linked chronic granulomatous disease (X-CGD) gene: Utility for prenatal diagnosis. J Pediatr Hematol Oncol 20:112–119.
397. Hong R (1998) The DiGeorge anomaly. (CATCH 22, DiGeorge/velocardiofacial syndrome). Semin Hematol, 35:282–290.

does not tend to improve with advancing age.[398] Humoral immunity is usually normal, and patients with "partial DiGeorge" can mount good antibody responses.[399] The thymic shadow is absent or reduced at birth. Infants often have neonatal tetany with hypocalcemia due to the aplastic parathyroid glands. The cardiac anomalies are most commonly truncus arteriosus, septal defects, and abnormal aortic arch vessels. Characteristic facial features of DiGeorge syndrome include a short philtrum, low-set malformed ears, and hypertelorism.

Many patients have recurrent mucocutaneous candidal infections as neonates, as well as increased susceptibility to viral infections, *Pneumocystic carinii*, and other fungal infections. Graft–versus–host disease may develop in infants that are given nonirradiated blood products. Noninfectious cutaneous granulomas, as in other immunodeficiencies, have been described (Fig. 7.35). Recent studies have shown that the deletion in DiGeorge syndrome results in haploinsufficeincy of Tbx1,[400,401] a member of the T-box transcription factor family that is required for the normal development of the fourth pharyngeal arch arteries; mice heterozygous for a null mutation in Tbx1 have conotruncal defects. HLA-identical bone marrow transplantation or thymic transplantation is recommended for patients with complete DiGeorge syndrome.

HYPERIMMUNOGLOBULIN-E SYNDROME

Hyperimmunoglobulin–E (HIE) recurrent infection syndrome is characterized by repeated cutaneous and sinopulmonary infections and dermatitis from birth or early childhood, associated with extremely elevated immunoglobulin E levels (greater than 2000 IU/ml).[402,403] Job syndrome as a subgroup of HIE, originally described as female patients with fair skin, red hair, and hyperextensible joints in addition to the general features of HIE syndrome.

EPIDEMIOLOGY

The disorder is now considered to be an autosomal dominant disorder with variable expressivity, many of the patients showing only a partial phenotype.

CLINICAL PRESENTATION

Infections usually begin during the first 3 months of life. Cutaneous infections may take the form of excoriated crusted plaques, pustules, furuncles, cellulitis, lymphangitis, or abscesses. Paronychial infections lead to nail dystrophy. The cutaneous abscesses occur most commonly on the neck, scalp, periorbital areas, axillae, and groin, and may be huge. The patient is often afebrile, or has a slight temperature elevation. The abscesses are slightly erythematous and tender, but not nearly to the degree expected for a normal individual ("cold abscesses"). Although the abscesses tend to be staphylococcal, many patients have frequent cutaneous infections from other organisms, particularly *Candida* and *Streptococcus*. In fact, chronic candidiasis of the skin, mucosal and paronychial sites, and of the nails, occurs in 83% of patients, and may precede the pneumonia or skin abscesses in affected infants. Although some patients demonstrate cutaneous manifestations only,[404] patients with HIE syndrome tend to have recurrent bronchitis and pneumonias usually due to *Staph. aureus* and *Haemophilus influenzae*, with resultant empyema, bronchiectasis, and pneumatocele formation. The pneumatoceles tend to persist and become the site of further infections with bacterial or fungal organisms. Rarely, massive hemoptysis ensues. Other common sites of infection include the ears, oral mucosae, sinuses, and eyes. Visceral infections other than pneumonia are unusual.

Affected babies present with a sterile vesiculopustular eruption. However, early cutaneous candidal infections may predinate the eczematous rash is

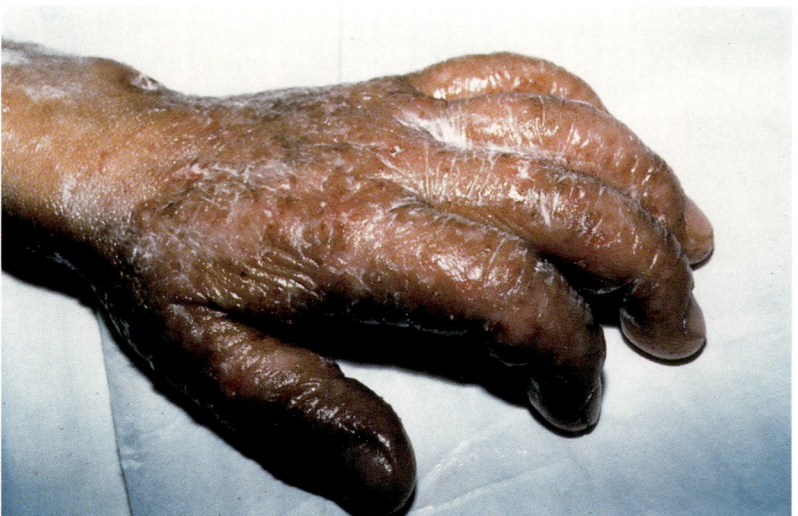

Fig. 7.36 Severe eczema of the hand of a patient with hyper-IgE syndrome.

extremely pruritic and papular with lichenification (Fig. 7.36). Superinfection of the dermatitis with *Staph. aureus* and *Strep. pyogenes* is common. The eczema is always present in infants and young children, but frequently clears by later childhood. Despite the markedly elevated IgE levels and eczematous rash, patients rarely exhibit other signs of atopy, such as a propensity toward hay fever or asthma. Patients with HIE syndrome develop an atypical facial appearance, partially due to severe deforming facial abscesses, with progressive facial coarseness, a broad nasal bridge with a wide, fleshy nasal tip, deep-set eyes, a prominent forehead, and irregularly proportioned cheeks and jaw (Fig. 7.37).

Osteopenia with increased risk of bone fractures has also been described; 57% of patients have had at least three fractures, often due to unrecognized or minor trauma. The long bones, ribs, and pelvis are most frequently affected. Scoliosis occurs in 76% of patients 16 years of age or older, and hyperextensibility of joints has been reported in 68% of patients. A variety of dental abnormalities have been associated with HIE. These include retention of primary teeth, lack of eruption of secondary teeth, and delayed resorption of the roots of primary teeth.

LABORATORY FINDINGS

Extensive studies of complement levels and activities, polymorphonuclear leukocyte phagocytosis and killing, and lymphocyte subgroup distribution have been normal. All patients, by definition, have markedly elevated levels of polyclonal IgE (greater than 2000 IU/ml in adults, although the normal levels of IgE in infants and young children are considerably lower than in adults). IgD levels are also increased in the majority of patients, but other immunoglobulin levels are usually normal. Many patients have eosinophilia of blood and sputum. Abnormal polymorphonuclear leukocyte and monocyte chemotaxis have been noted in a number of patients, but the chemotactic defects have been intermittent and not related to periods of infections. Patients also tend to have positive immediate wheal and flare reactions to a variety of foods and inhalants, as well as to bacteria and fungi, and an impaired anamnestic response to antigens, such as tetanus. Cell–mediated immunity is often abnormal, as manifested by anergy to skin testing,

398. Markert ML, Hummell DS, Rosenblatt HM et al. (1998) Complete DiGeorge syndrome: persistence of profound immunodeficiency. **J Pediatr** 132:15–21.
399. Junker AK, Driscoll DA (1995) Humoral immunity in DiGeorge syndrome. **J Pediatr** 127:231–237.
400. Lindsay EA, Vitelli F, Su H et al. (2001) Tbx1 haploinsufficiency in the DiGeorge syndrome region causes aortic arch defects in mice. **Nature** 410:97–101.
401. Merscher S, Funke B, Epstein JA et al. (2001) TBX1 is responsible for cardiovascular defects in velo-cardiofacial/DiGeorge syndrome. **Cell** 104:619–629.

402. Grimbacher B, Holland SM, Gallin JI et al. (1999) Hyper-IgE syndrome with recurrent infections – an autosomal dominant multisystem disorder. **N Engl J Med** 340:692–702.
403. Borges WG, Hensley T, Carey JC et al. (1998) The face of Job. **J Pediatr** 133:303.
404. Hochreutener H, Wüthrich B, Huwyler T et al. (1991) Variants of hyper-IgE syndrome: the differentiation from atopic dermatitis is important because of treatment and prognosis. **Dermatologica** 182:7.

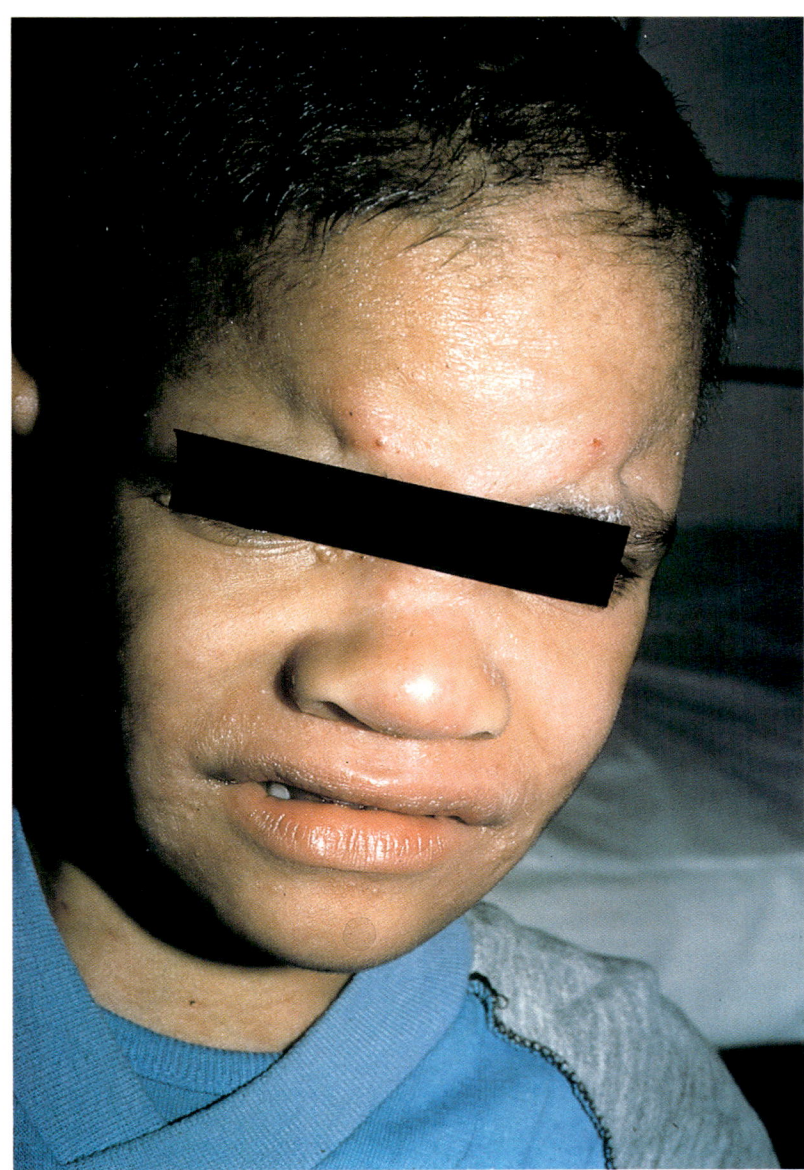

Fig. 7.37   Coarse facial features of a patient with hyper-IgE syndrome. The patient had frequent upper respiratory tract and skin infections, severe eczema, and an IgE level of 56 000IU/ml.

altered responses in mixed leukocyte culture, and impaired blastogenic responses to specific antigens, such as candida and tetanus. In contrast, the blastogenic responses are normal to general mitogens. Patients have high levels of anti-staphylococcal and anti-candidal IgE antibodies.

PATHOPHYSIOLOGY AND HISTOGENESIS

The gene for HIE has been mapped to chromosome 4q,[405] although the identity of the underlying gene is unknown. Although early speculation considered the interleukin-4 receptor to be a candidate gene, its localization on chromosome 16 has excluded its involvement as the primary gene mutated in HIE. The frequency of dermatitis may relate to cytokine abnormalities,

increased levels of IgE, and reactivity against *Staph. aureus*, features shared with atopic dermatitis. IgE of patients with HIE is maximally activated, with high constitutive levels; IL-4 fails to increase further the production of IgE, in contrast to the stimulatory effect of IL-4 on B cells from normal individuals and patients with atopic dermatitis.[406] IFN-γ and IL-12 are able to reduce the excessive IgE (and IgG$_4$) production *in vitro*, while IL-8 and antibodies directed against IL-4, IL-6, and TNF-α completely suppress the IgE and IgG$_4$ production.[407] Patients with HIE have been shown to have deficient T-helper cell type 1 cytokine responses, with decreased interferon (IFN)-γ production after specific antigen stimulation, especially when the patients' cells are activated by staphylococcal antigens.[408] The defect is even more striking when cells are pretreated with IL-12, which should be a strong stimulator of IFN-γ production. This defect in IFN-γ production may be responsible for the high levels in IgE and chemotactic defect, and explains the therapeutic benefit of IFN-γ administration in some patients with HIE.

DIFFERENTIAL DIAGNOSIS

The HIE syndrome must be differentiated from a number of other disorders in which IgE levels may be elevated. Among these are Wiskott–Aldrich syndrome, atopic dermatitis, DiGeorge syndrome, GvHD, Nezelof syndrome, and selected IgA deficiency. Of these, Wiskott–Aldrich and atopic dermatitis, are most easily confused because of the frequent dermatitis with superinfections of *Staph. aureus*. Patients with atopic dermatitis, however, tend to have only superficial pyodermas. Patients with atopic dermatitis often have allergic rhinitis or reactive airway disease as well. Patients with the Wiskott–Aldrich syndrome are almost always male, and have thrombocytopenia, cutaneous petechiae and hemorrhagic episodes. Neither disorder demonstrates the cutaneous abscesses that are so prevalent in HIE syndrome. Bacterial and candidal abscesses may be features of myeloperoxidase deficiency,[407] but the high levels of IgE in HIE syndrome help to distinguish these disorders.

TREATMENT

The mainstay of therapy for HIE syndrome is anti-staphylococcal antibiotics, and incision and drainage of abscesses. When other bacterial or fungal infections develop, the infections must be treated with appropriate antibiotics as well. Recombinant IFN-γ has been shown to increase neutrophil chemotactic responses in patients with HIE and recurrent infections,[408] and administration of gammaglobulin has decreased the atopic dermatitis and level of IgE.[409] A number of other agents have been shown to correct the variable chemotactic defects, including ascorbic acid and cimetidine. However, these agents have not altered the clinical course of the disorder. The cutaneous and pulmonary abscesses often require incision and drainage. The pneumatoceles should be removed surgically, especially if present for longer than 6 months, or the patient is at risk for severe superinfection by bacterial or fungal organisms.

IMMUNOGLOBULIN DEFICIENCIES

IMMUNOGLOBULIN A DEFICIENCY

The most common immunoglobulin deficiency is selective IgA deficiency, found in 1 in 500 persons. Ten to 15% of patients have clinical manifestations. These features usually are sinopulmonary bacterial infections and *Giardia* gastroenteritis. Approximately one-third of patients with clinical disease develop autoimmune disorders, some of which involve the skin. These include SLE, vitiligo, chronic mucocutaneous candidiasis, lipodystrophia centrifugalis

405. Grimbacher B, Schaffer AA, Holland SM et al. (1999) Genetic linkage of hyper-IgE syndrome to chromosome 4. **Am J Hum Genet** 65:735.
406. Claassen JJ, Levine AD, Schiff SE, Buckley RH (1991) Mononuclear cells from patients with the hyper-IgE syndrome produce little IgE when they are stimulated with recombinant human interleukin-4. **J Allergy Clin Immunol** 88:713.
407. Garraud O, Mollis SN, Holland SM et al. (1999) Regulation of immunoglobulin production in hyper-IgE (Job's) syndrome. **J Allerg Clin Immunol** 103:333.
408. Borges WG, Augustine NH, Hill HR (2000) Defective interleukin-12/interferon-γ pathway in patients with hyperimmunoglobulinemia E syndrome. **J Pediatr** 136:176.
409. Parry MF, Root RK, Metcalf JA et al. (1991) Myeloperoxidase deficiency: prevalence and significance. **Ann Intern Med** 95:293.

abdominalis, and idiopathic thrombocytopenic purpura. A number of patients have severe atopic-like dermatitis, asthma, cow's milk allergy, and/or allergic rhinoconjunctivitis. The treatment of IgA deficiency is vigorous treatment with antibiotics. It is imperative that symptomatic patients do not receive immune serum globulin or blood products with IgA-bearing lymphocytes. Almost one-half of patients have serum anti-IgA antibodies, and fatal anaphylactic reactions have occurred from the administration of blood products. Patients with IgA deficiency may develop the immunodeficiency pattern of common variable immunodeficiency; furthermore, 15% of patients with CVI have family members with IgA deficiency.

IMMUNOGLOBULIN M DEFICIENCY

An extremely rare selective immunoglobulin deficiency, IgM deficiency, is apparently due to an inability of T-helper cell function to stimulate IgM production. In addition to recurrent bacterial infections, severe eczema and extensive large warts have been described. Early and vigorous antibiotic use is the only effective therapy.

X-LINKED HYPOGAMMAGLOBULINEMIA WITH HYPER IgM (HIM)

Patients with this X-linked recessive disorder have recurrent infections in association with hepatosplenomegaly, cervical adenitis, recurrent bacterial infections including opportunistic infections, autoimmune disorders (especially thyroiditis and hemolytic anemia), and an increased risk of lymphoma.[410] Cutaneous manifestations include pyodermas, widespread warts (Fig. 7.38), oral ulcerations[411] (Fig 7.39), and ulcerations in the diaper region.[412] Patients tend to have deficiencies of IgA, IgE, and IgG with neutropenia, but increased levels of IgM and isohemagglutinins. The pathomechanism for this form

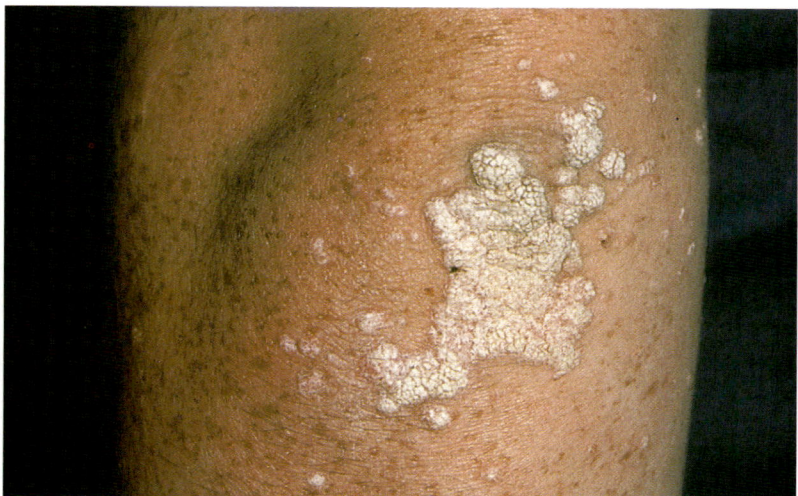

Fig. 7.38   Extensive warts, present for years in a patient with hyper-IgM disorder.

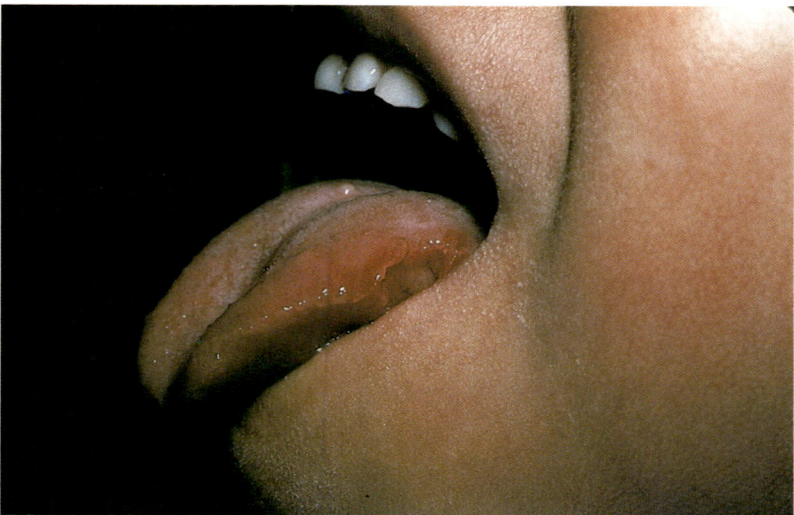

Fig. 7.39   Oral ulceration on the side of the tongue in a patient with hyper-IgM disorder.

of hypogammaglobulinemia involves a T-cell defect, rather than a primary B-cell defect. In the presence of lymphokines, cross-linking of CD40 on B cells induces switching of immunoglobulin classes from IgM to IgG, IgA, or IgE. Mutations in X-linked HIM occur in a transmembrane protein that is the physiologic ligand for CD40, CD40L. B cells from patients with HIM express functional CD40, but the T cells express the defective CD40 ligand and cannot bind CD40.[412–416] Introduction of CD40L by retroviral transfer in a mouse model of X-linked HIM improved immune function, but resulted in T-cell lymphoproliferative disorders in the majority of treated mice.[417] Another form of HIM is autosomal recessive; patients usually present during infancy with bacterial sinopulmonary and gastrointestinal infections; CD40L is normal, but activation-induced cytidine deaminase (AID), which plays an important role in B-cell differentiation and class switch recombination, is mutated.[418] Hyper-IgM production can also be a feature of patients with immunodeficiency ectodermal dysplasia syndrome, resulting from mutations in the NEMO gene.[419]

PAN-HYPOGAMMAGLOBULINEMIA

Hypogammaglobulinemia is found in 1 in 50 000 persons, and is classified into two major subdivisions: Bruton's X-linked hypogammaglobulinemia and common variable immunodeficiency (CVI). Patients with Bruton's X-linked hypogammaglobulinemia develop recurrent bacterial infections after the first several months of life.[420] The organisms most commonly involved are *Staphylococcus*, *Streptococcus*, *Haemophilus*, and *Pneumococcus*. The skin is frequently involved with multiple furuncles and cellulitis. Echthyma gangrenosum may be the presenting sign.[421] Patients have an increased risk of developing eczema, despite the deficiency of IgE. Noninfectious cutaneous granulomas have been described, as has papular dermatitis due to extensive

410. Jeppson JD, Jaffe HS, Hill HR (1991) Use of recombinant human interferon gamma to enhance neutrophil chemotactic responses in Job syndrome of hyperimmunoglobulinemia E and recurrent infections. **J Pediatr** 118:383.
411. Kimata H (1995) High-dose intravenous gamma-globulin treatment for hyperimmunoglobulinemia E syndrome. **J Allergy Clin Immunol** 95:771.
412. Schneider LC (2000) X-linked hyper IgM syndrome. **Clin Rev Allergy Immunol** 19:205.
413. Chang MW, Romero R, Scholl PR, Paller AS (1998) Mucocutaneous manifestations of the hyper-IgM immunodeficiency syndrome. **J Am Acad Dermatol** 38:191.
414. Uguz A, Yilmaz E, Ciftcioglu A, Yegin O (2001) An unusual presentation of immunodeficiency with hyper-IgM. **Pediatr Dermatol** 18:48.
415. DiSanto JP, Bonnefoy JY, Gauchat JF et al. (1993) CD40 ligand mutations in X-linked immunodeficiency with hyper-IgM. **Nature** 361:541.

416. Korthäuser U, Graf D, Mages HW (1993) Defective expression of T-cell CD40 ligand causes X-linked immunodeficiency with hyper-IgM. **Nature** 361:539.
417. Brown MP, Topham DJ, Sangster MY et al. (1998) Thymic lymphoproliferative disease after successful correction of CD40 ligand deficiency by gene transfer in mice. **Nat Med** 4:1253.
418. Revy P, Muto T, Levy Y et al. (2000) Activation-induced cytidine deaminase (AIS) deficiency causes the autosomal recessive form of the hyper-IgM syndrome (HIGM2). **Cell** 102:565.
419. Zonana J, Elder M, Schneider S et al. (2000) A novel X-linked disorder of immune diﬁency and hypohidrotic ectodermal dysplasia is allelic to incontinentia pigmenti and due to mutations in IKK-gamma (NEMO). **Am J Hum Genet** 67:1555–1562.
420. Minegishi Y, Rohrer J, Conley ME (1999) Recent progress in the diagnosis and treatment of patients with defects in early B-cell development. **Curr Opin Pediatr** 11:528.
421. Nussinovitch M, Frydman M, Cohen HA, Varsano I (1991) Congenital agammaglobulinaemia presenting with echthyma gangrenosum. **Acta Paediatr Scand** 80:732.

lymphohistiocytic infiltration of skin.[422] Patients have increased susceptibility to enterovirus infections and hepatitis B. A small percentage of patients develop a dermatomyositis-like disorder, with slowly progressive neurologic involvement, usually related to echovirus meningoencephalitis. Up to 6% of patients develop lymphoreticular malignancies.

In this disorder, pre-B cells are blocked in their conversion in the bone marrow to B cells by interference with early B lineage growth and clonal expansion. X-linked hypogammaglobulinemia is caused by a defect in the gene encoding a tyrosine kinase that regulates B-cell proliferation, differentiation and survival (Btk).[423,424] Female carriers of X-linked hypogammaglobulinemia may be detected through examination of X-inactivation patterns of maternal B cells. Prenatal diagnosis is possible by detecting restriction fragment length polymorphism in regions surrounding the gene or direct gene analysis. An autosomal recessive form that resembles X-linked hypogammaglobulinemia has been described in 10% of affected boys.[425]

Patients with transient hypogammaglobulinemia of infancy often show early failure to thrive, with recurrent sinopulmonary infections and diarrhea, particularly beginning at 6 months of age when maternal antibody levels wane. Affected infants may have recurrent pyodermas and cutaneous abscesses. Immunoglobulin production is delayed, and tends to begin at 18 to 30 months of age.

CVI is a heterogeneous group of disorders.[426] The onset is usually later than the X-linked form (average age 29 years), and the disorder is distributed equally among both sexes. Family members often have evidence of immunodeficiency, including hypogammaglobulinemia and selective IgA deficiency. Patients are especially predisposed to pyogenic upper and lower respiratory tract infections. The infectious agents are similar to those of X-linked hypo-

gammaglobulinemia, but no documented cases of echovirus meningoencephalitis have occurred. *Giardia* infections are more common in CVI than in the X-linked form. Patients frequently have cutaneous pyoderma and eczema. Abnormalities of cell-mediated immunity occur in many patients in addition to the immunoglobulin deficiency and may manifest in the skin as widespread warts and extensive dermatophyte infections. Some patients develop noncaseating granulomas of the lungs, liver, spleen, and/or skin that are not due to microorganisms and may respond to corticosteroids. Patients with CVI have an increased risk of autoimmune diseases,[427] including vasculitis (Fig. 7.40), vitiligo and alopecia areata. The incidence of lymphoreticular malignancy is also increased, with an 8 to 13 times increased risk of cancer overall and a 438-fold increased risk of lymphoma in female patients.[428] Death in patients with CVI usually results from infection, respiratory insufficiency, or neoplasia. The treatment of hypogammaglobulinemia is antibody replacement by intravenous infusions of immune serum globulin and vigorous antibiotic therapy.

X-LINKED LYMPHOPROLIFERATIVE DISEASE

X-linked lymphoproliferative disease (XLP, Duncan's disease) is characterized by an inadequate response to Epstein–Barr virus (EBV) infection.[429] Affected boys are healthy until childhood or adolescence when they develop infectious mononucleosis. Clinical features include fever, pharyngitis, maculopapular rash, lymphadenopathy, hepatosplenomegaly, purpura, and jaundice. Almost 70% of patients die during the disease due to overwhelming B-cell lymphoma stimulated by the virus, often with superimposed bacterial sepsis. Both humoral and cell-mediated immune responses are diminished. Patients cannot adequately produce EBV-specific antibodies or EBV-specific memory T cells. In addition, the affected boys have increased percentages of suppressor T cells, decreased NK cell function, and low antibody-dependent cellular cytotoxicity. Treatment of patients with XLP and acute EBV infection has not been successful; current therapeutic efforts involve prophylaxis with intravenous immunoglobulin. Bone marrow transplantation has been attempted.[430] XLP deficiency results from mutations in SH2D1A, which affects intracellular signaling.[431] Prenatal diagnosis has been achieved by chorionic villus sampling and restriction fragment polymorphic markers,[432] but carrier females show random (normal) X inactivation patterns.[433]

"LEINER'S DISEASE" PHENOTYPE

"Leiner's disease" is characterized by early severe seborrheic dermatitis, diarrhea, failure to thrive, and recurrent Gram-negative and candidal infections during infancy. Although originally reported as a rare, probably autosomal dominant trait due to defective yeast opsonization from dysfunctional C5,[434] the "Leiner's disease" phenotype has been described in infants with a variety of immunodeficiency disorders. These include defective yeast opsonization,[434] C5 deficiency,[376] severe combined immunodeficiency (SCID), hypogammaglobulinemia, and hyperimmunoglobulinemia E.[435]

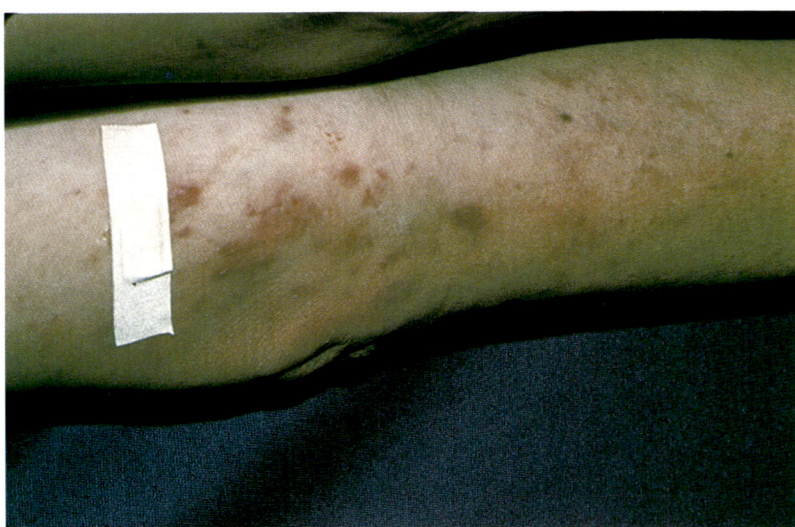

Fig. 7.40   Lower extremity vasculitis in a girl with common variable immunodeficiency.

422. Bentur L, Shear N, Roifman CM (1990) Cutaneous lymphohistiocytic infiltrates in patients with hypogammaglobulinemia. **J Pediatr** 116:68.
423. Vetrie D, Vorechovsky I, Sideras P et al. (1993) The gene involved in X-linked agammaglobulinaemia is a member of the *src* family of protein-tyrosine kinases. **Nature** 361:226.
424. Tsukada S, Saffran DC, Rawlings DJ et al. (1993) Deficient expression of a B cell cytoplasmic tyrosine kinase in human X-linked agammaglobulinemia. **Cell** 72:279.
425. Minegishi Y, Coustan-Smith E, Wang Y-H et al. (1998) Mutations in the human λ5/14.1 gene result in B cell deficiency and agammaglobulinemia. **J Exp Med** 187:71.
426. Cunningham-Rundles C, Bodian C (1999) Common variable immunodeficiency: clinical and immunological features of 248 patients. **Clin Immunol** 92:34–48.
427. Conley ME, Park CL, Douglas SD (1986) Childhood common variable immunodeficiency with autoimmune disease. **J Pediatr** 108:915.
428. Cunningham-Rundles C, Siegal FP, Cunningham-Rundles S, Lieberman P (1987) Incidence of cancer in 98 patients with common varied immunodeficiency. **J Clin Immunol** 7:294.

429. Sullivan JL, Woda BA (1989) X-linked lymphoproliferative syndrome. **Immunodefic Rev** 1:325.
430. Filipovich AH, Blazar BR, Ramsay NK et al. (1986) Allogenic bone marrow transplantation for X-linked lymphoproliferative syndrome. **Transplantation** 42:222.
431. Sylla B, Murphy K, Cahir-McFarland E, Lane WS et al. (2000) The X-linked lymphoproliferative syndrome gene product SH2D1A associated with p62[dok] (Dok1) and activates NF-κB. **Proc Natl Acad Sci USA** 97:7470.
432. Skare J, Madan S, Glaser J et al. (1992) First prenatal diagnosis of X-linked lymphoproliferative disease. **Am J Med Genet** 44:79.
433. Conley ME, Sullivan JL, Neidich JA, Puck JM (1990) X chromosome inactivation patterns in obligate carriers of X-linked lymphoproliferative syndrome. **Clin Immunol Immunopathol** 5:486.
434. Miller ME, Koblenzer PJ (1972) Leiner's disease and C₅ dysfunction. **J Pediatr** 80:879.
435. Glover M, Atherton D, Levinsky R et al. (1988) Syndrome of erythroderma, failure to thrive and diarrhea in infancy: a manifestation of immunodeficiency. **Pediatrics** 81:66.

LEUKOCYTE ADHESION DEFICIENCY

Leukocyte adhesion deficiency (LAD) is a rare autosomal recessive disorder that affects the adherence of neutrophils, cytolytic T lymphocytes, and monocytes[436,437] owing to mutations in the CD18 gene that codes for the β_2 integrin subunit.

CLINICAL PRESENTATION

Patients with LAD have frequent skin infections, mucositis, and otitis. The skin infections often present as necrotic abscesses that resemble pyoderma gangrenosum, but the inflammatory response and production of purulent material are impaired; typically the large ulcerations begin as minor skin wounds that rapidly enlarge (Fig. 7.41). Gingivitis with periodontitis may result in loss of teeth. Moderately affected patients have been noted to have only recurrent skin infections and mild periodontitis or severe gingivitis with only occasional skin infections. Cellulitis of the face and perirectal area is common. Life-threatening severe bacterial or fungal infections may occur. Some patients are susceptible to severe viral infections.[438] Poor would healing leads to paper-thin or dysplastic cutaneous scars. Patients may have delayed separation of the umbilical cord. Cutaneous and visceral granulomas, as described in disorders of ineffective intracellular killing, have not been reported.

LABORATORY FINDINGS

Affected individuals have marked peripheral blood granulocytosis (5 to 20 times normal levels). *In vitro*, leukocytes from patients show defective adhesion-related function, including defective adhesion to endothelial cells and T lymphocytes, with a resultant abnormality in NK-cell-mediated killing,

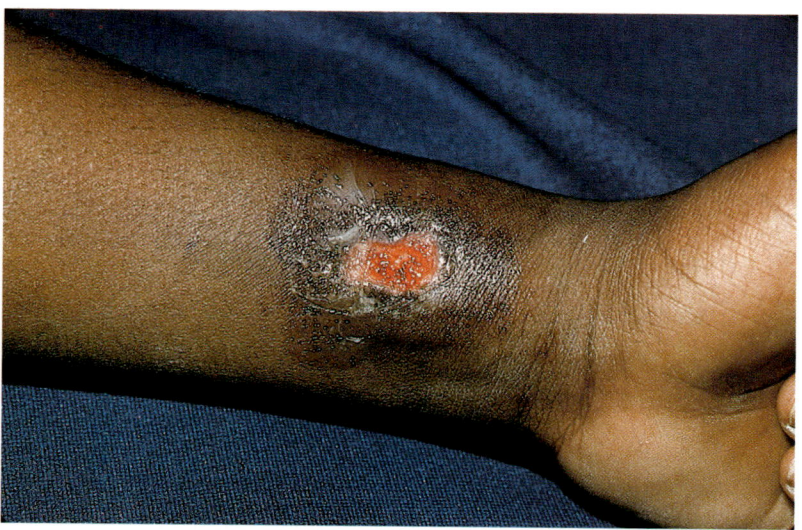

Fig. 7.41 A minor scratch from his sister evolved during the subsequent weeks into a large ulcer on the arm of a boy with leukocyte adhesion disorder.

migration, and antigen presentation. Cultures of soft tissue infections reveal a variety of causative Gram-positive, Gram-negative, or fungal organisms.

PATHOPHYSIOLOGY AND HISTOGENESIS

The infections in both types of LAD result from profound impairment of leukocyte mobilization into extravascular inflammatory sites. Adherence of leukocytes relates in part to a group of cell surface glycoproteins (integrins) that share a common 95-kDa β subunit (CD18) that is encoded on the distal portion of the long arm of chromosome 21 (21q22.3). The β subunit is linked to three distinct α chains to form three different surface glyco-proteins. Because of the deficient or defective β_2 subunit, these glycoproteins, the $iC3_b$ receptor (complement receptor type 3, Mac-1), lymphocyte function associated antigen-1 (LFA-1), and p150,95, are all absent or deficient in affected patients. The principal ligand for these glycoproteins is intercellular adhesion molecule-1 (ICAM-1), which participates actively in the initiation and evolution of localized inflammation in skin and other tissues. As a result, neutrophil and monocyte chemotaxis and phagocytosis are impaired. The degree of glycoprotein deficiency is proportional to the severity of clinical involvement, with "severe" deficiency patients having <0.5% glycoprotein expression and moderate deficiency patients having 3–30% of CD18 detectability. More than 75% of patients with severe disease die by 5 years of age; more than half of the patients with moderate deficiency die between the ages of 10 and 30 years.

DIFFERENTIAL DIAGNOSIS

Type I LAD must be differentiated from type II LAD, which results from a defect in *de novo* GDP-fucose biosynthesis,[439] leading to the absence of the fucosylated ligand for selectins, sialyl–Lewis X, on the surface of neutrophils. In addition to elevated leukocyte counts and recurrent bacterial infections, patients have mental retardation, short stature and a distinctive facies. The value of supplemental fucose administration has been variable.[440,441] Impaired β_2 adhesive functioning has been described in an infant with myelodysplastic syndrome and a "blueberry muffin" rash of dermal erythropoeisis.[442]

TREATMENT

Therapy of the soft tissue infections includes appropriate antimicrobial agents and, in some cases, debridement of wounds. Scrupulous dental hygiene is important in reducing the severity of the periodontitis. In patients with significant LDA, death usually occurs by 2 years of age unless successful bone marrow transplantation or cord blood transplantation is performed.[443] Gene transfer has successfully restored CD18 function in bone marrow progenitor cells.[444]

SEVERE COMBINED IMMUNODEFICIENCY

SCID is a group of heterogeneous disorders that have similar clinical manifestations and functional immunologic capacity, but differ in biochemical and cellular features (Table 7.17).[445–449]

436. Arnaout MA (1990) Leukocyte adhesion molecule deficiency: its structural basis, pathophysiology and implications for modulating the inflammatory response. **Immunol Rev** 114:145.
437. Kishimoto TK, Springer TA (1989) Human leukocyte adhesion deficiency: molecular basis for a defective immune response to infections of the skin. **Curr Probl Dermatol** 18:106.
438. Kohl S, Loo LS, Schmalstieg FS, Anderson DC (1986) The genetic deficiency of leukocyte surface glycoprotein Mac-1, LFA-1, p150,95 in humans is associated with defective antibody-dependent cellular cytotoxicity in vitro and defective protection against herpes simplex virus infection in vivo. **J Immunol** 137:1688.
439. Marquardt T, Brune T, Luhn K et al. (1999) Leukocyte adhesion deficiency II syndrome, a generalized defect in fucose metabolism. **J Pediatr** 134:681.
440. Marquardt T, Luhn K, Srikrishna G et al. (1999) Correction of leukocyte adhesion deficiency type II with oral fucose. **Blood** 94:3976.
441. Etzioni A, Tonetti M (2000) Fucose supplementation in leukocyte adhesion deficiency type II. **Blood** 95:3641.
442. Haris ES, Shigeoka AO, Li W et al. (2001) A novel syndrome of variant leukocyte adhesion deficiency involving defects in adhesion mediated by beta1 and beta2 integrins. **Blood** 97:767.
443. Stary J, Bartunkova J, Kobylka P et al. (1996) Successful HLA-identical sibling cord blood transplantation in a 6-year-old boy with leukocyte ashesion deficiency syndrome. **Bone Marrow Transpl** 18:259.
444. Bauer TR, Schwartz BR, Conrad LW et al. (1998) Retroviral-mediated gene transfer of the leukocyte integrin CD18 into peripheral blood CD34+ cells derived from a patient with leukocyte adhesion deficiency type 1. **Blood** 91:1520.
445. Fischer A (2000) Severe combined immunodeficiencies (SCID). **Clin Exp Immunol** 122:143.
446. Gaspar HB, Gilmour KC, Jones AM (2001) Severe combined immunodeficiency – molecular pathogenesis and diagnosis. **Arch Dis Child** 84:169.
447. Gennery AR, Cant AJ (2001) Diagnosis of severe combined immunodeficiency. **J Clin Pathol** 54:191.
448. Cacalano NA, Johnston JA (1999) Interleukin-2 signaling and inherited immunodeficiency. **Am J Hum Genet** 65:287.
449. DeSandro A, Nagarajan UM, Boss JM (1999) The bare lymphocyte syndrome: molecular clues to the transcriptional regulation of major histocompatibility complex class genes. **Am J Hum Genet** 65:279.

TABLE 7.17 Classification of severe combined immunodeficiency

Disorder	Gene location	Gene	Diagnostic tests	Cells
X-linked SCID	Xq13	Common γ chain	γ_c expression by FACS	T−/B+/NK−
Adenosine deaminase (ADA) deficiency	20q12–13	Adenosine deaminase	Red cell ADA levels and metabolites	T−/B−/NK−
Purine nucleoside phosphorylase (PNP) deficiency	14q11	Purine nucleoside phosphorylase	Red cell PNP levels and metabolites	T−/B−/NK−
Recombinase activating gene (RAG) deficiency, Omenn syndrome	11p13	*RAG1* and *RAG2*	Defects in V(D) J recombination; T&B cell clonal analysis	T−/B−/NK+
T cell receptor deficiencies	11q23	CD3γ/CD3ε	CD3 expression	CD4+ CD8−/B+/NK+
Zap 70 deficiency	2q12	*ZAP-70*	Zap-70 expression	T−/B+/NK−
JAK3 deficiency	19p13	*JAK3*	JAK3 expression/signaling	T−/B+/NK−
IL-7 receptor deficiency	5p13	IL-7 receptor α	IL-7 receptor α expression	T−/B+/NK+
MHC class II deficiency	16p13 19p12 1q21 13q13	*CIITA* *RFX-B* *RFX5* *RFXAP*	HLA-DR expression	T+/B+/NK+ but dysfunctional

EPIDEMIOLOGY

The combined frequency of SCID is 1 in 30 000 to 1 in 100 000 live births. Approximately 42% of patients with SCID have an X-linked recessive form, but most of the forms of SCID are autosomal recessive in their inheritance pattern. Seventy-five percent of affected patients are male. Approximately 20% of cases result from deficiency of adenosine deaminase (ADA); 6% of cases occur because of JAK3 mutations.[448]

CLINICAL PRESENTATION

Patients with SCID usually begin to have recurrent infections, diarrhea, and failure to thrive by 3 to 6 months of age. Among the common early infections are mucocutaneous candidiasis, viral-induced chronic diarrhea with malabsorption, and pneumonia due to bacteria, virus, or *P. carinii*. Patients with SCID lack tonsillar buds and usually lack palpable lymphoid tissue, despite recurrent infections.

The mucocutaneous manifestations of patients with SCID include cutaneous infections, especially due to *C. albicans*, *Staph. aureus*, and *Strep. pyogenes*. The most common rashes are morbilliform or similar to seborrheic dermatitis,[450,451] and the possibility of associated acute graft–versus–host disease (GvHD) must be considered. Thus, lesions may resemble lichen planus, acrodermatitis enteropathica, Langerhans cell histiocytosis, lamellar ichthyosis, or scleroderma, and are manifestations of GvHD in infants with SCID. Skin biopsies of lesional skin may show the histopathologic characteristics of GvHD, which can result from the patient's inability to reject allogeneic cells from unirradiated transfusions or maternal lymphocytes (maternofetal lymphoid engraftment). Extensive eczematous lesions or severe exfoliative erythroderma, often with alopecia, may occur without GvHD in a subgroup of SCID with reticuloendothelial cell proliferation (Omenn syndrome). Lymphadenopathy, hepatomegaly, occasionally splenomegaly, and eosinophilia are associated features of Omenn syndrome; lymph nodes show a typical lymph node architecture with disruption of germinal centers and abundant S-100+ interdigitating reticulum cells.

LABORATORY FINDINGS

Nearly all patients with SCID have a profound deficiency of T lymphocytes and a low absolute lymphocyte count. Patients are then grouped by the results of fluorescent activated cell sorting (FACS) analysis into those with B lymphocytes (T− B+ SCID) and those without B lymphocytes (T− B− SCID). Further subclassification can be made according to the presence or absence of NK cells. For example, X-linked SCID caused by gamma chain deficiency (γ_c) and the autosomal recessive SCID caused by JAK3 deficiency have a characteristic T− B+ NK− profile. The specific laboratory abnormalities of the different types of SCID are noted in Table 7.17. Subtle immunologic abnormalities also characterize particular subgroups; for example, ZAP-70 deficiency infants lack responsiveness to phytohemagglutinin and other T-cell receptor mediated stimuli, while they respond normally to phorbol myristate acetate and ionomycin. Similarly, lymphocytes from patients with IL-2 deficiency only proliferate when exogenous IL-2 is added. Increased levels of deoxy-ATP levels are seen in patients with ADA deficiency, and decreased levels of erythrocyte purine nucleoside phosphorylase (PNP) are noted in patients with PNP deficiency. Certain forms of SCID have diagnostic radiographic features; for example, patients with ADA deficiency show typical cupping and flaring of the costochondral junction on chest X-rays.[452]

Diagnosis now is largely based on direct gene analysis; flow cytometric analysis of peripheral blood mononuclear cells with antibodies directed against specific proteins that are missing from the cell surface, such as JAK3 or γ_c, can help to confirm the diagnosis. Maternal T-lymphocyte engraftment is detected in approximately 50% of patients with SCID.[451] In the majority of cases, the presence of these maternal T cells is asymptomatic; in 30–40% of patients mild changes, such as erythema with skin T-cell infiltration, elevated hepatic transaminases, and eosinophilia have been described. Reports of fatal GvHD resulting from the maternal engraftment are rare, particularly in contrast to the fatal acute GvHD that results from postnatal inoculation of allogenic lymphocytes.

450. Postigo Llorente C, Ivars Amorós J, Ortiz de Frutos FJ et al. (1991) Cutaneous lesions in severe combined immunodeficiency: two case reports and a review of the literature. **Pediatr Dermatol** 8:314.

451. De Raeve L, Song M, Levy J, Mascart-Lemone F et al. (1992) Cutaneous lesions as a clue to severe combined immunodeficiency. **Pediatr Dermatol** 9:49.

452. Hirschhorn R (1983) Genetic deficiencies of adenosine deaminase and purine nucleoside phosphorylase: overview, genetic heterogeneity and therapy. **Birth Defects** 19:73.

PATHOPHYSIOLOGY AND HISTOGENESIS

Several molecular defects lead to the phenotype of SCID.[451–455] Most common is mutations in γ_c, resulting in the absence of T and NK cell development, but normal B-cell numbers. This γ_c chain, together with the IL-2 receptor α and β subunits, generates the high-affinity receptor for IL-2, and plays a major role in signal transduction through activation of its associated tyrosine kinase JAK3. γ_c is also a receptor for IL-4, IL-7, IL-9, and IL-15, thus enabling the function of a variety of cytokines involved in T-cell function. For example, IL-7 is critical for T-cell survival and proliferation of early T-cell progenitors in the thymus, and IL-15 signaling is important for NK cell generation from bone marrow progenitors. ADA belongs to the salvage pathway of purine metabolism, reversibly transforming adenosine to inosine and 2′-deoxyadenosine to 2′-deoxyinosine. The immunodeficiency results from accumulation of adenosine and dAdo substrates that are indirectly toxic to lymphocytes, and especially to immature lymphocytes of the thymus. Mutations in RAG1 or RAG2 are the cause of Omenn syndrome and the immunodeficiency of many patients in the subgroup of SCID with a T⁻ B⁻ NK⁺ phenotype. These RAG (recombination activating gene) proteins mediate the initial DNA double strand break that allows V(D)J (variable/diversity/joining) recombination of genes that encode specific receptor sequences, enabling the diversity of immunoglobulin molecules of the T and B receptors. Major histocompatibility complex (MHC) class II deficiency is an autosomal recessive form of SCID that results from defects in a transacting factor essential for transcription of MHC class II genes. It is characterized by normal numbers of dysfunctional T and B cells (T⁺ B⁺ SCID). All bone marrow cells fail to express MHC class II antigens due to specific defects in the binding of a protein complex, RFX, to the highly conserved X box of the MHC class II promoter. A variety of RFX defects have been shown (RFX5, RFXAP, RFX-B); other patients have mutations in CIITA, an MHC transactivator that is essential for expression of MCH class II genes.[449]

DIFFERENTIAL DIAGNOSIS

SCID must be distinguished from other disorders and immunodeficiency, especially HIV infection. Patients with SCID do not have the HIV virus or anti-HIV antibodies, and usually do not have an inverted CD4/CD8 ratio. Patients with SCID usually have low levels of immunoglobulins.

TREATMENT

The natural outcome of SCID is poor, with most patients dying by 1 year of age without intervention. Early diagnosis of SCID is imperative, if possible before the administration of live vaccines or unirradiated blood products. Infants with SCID should be kept in protective isolation and watched for the presence of infections, which should be vigorously treated. All blood products should be irradiated to prevent GvHD.

Transplantation of infants with SCID is the treatment of choice.[453–455] HLA identical bone marrow transplantation results in rapid reconstitution with the detection of T cells by 3–4 months after transplant. GvHD is virtually absent, and the probability of success is now >90%. In patients without a suitable HLA-identical donor, post-thymic T lymphocytes may be removed with lectins or anti-T-cell antibodies from parental haploidentical marrow. In the absence of GvHD, survival reaches 78% for non-identical transplants. Residual GvHD and especially delay in immune function development (T cells take at least 3–4 months) account for the majority of deaths. *In utero* injection of haploidentical CD34+ cells has been successful in treatment of two fetuses with X-linked SCID.[456,457]

ADA enzyme replacement has been successful in many patients, particularly by injection of polyethylene glycol-conjugated ADA, but does not usually result in complete restoration of immune function. Gene therapy for X-linked SCID has been successfully performed in two affected infants who received retroviral transduced introduction of the normal *gc* gene into bone marrow cells, resulting in normalization of numbers of T cells and NK cells, and freedom from opportunistic infections.[458] Administration of recombinant IL-2 has been used in patients who lack IL-2 production and immunoglobulin synthesis to restore T- and B-cell function.

T and B lymphocytes of female carriers of X-linked SCID exhibit nonrandom X-chromosome inactivation, a feature that in the past allowed proper diagnosis of some boys with "sporadic" SCID as X-linked disease. Prenatal diagnosis of SCID has been performed in families with a previously affected sibling of known phenotype by analysis levels of ADA, examination of maternal X-chromosome inactivation and linkage analysis, and now by direct analysis of fetal DNA obtained by chorionic villus sampling.

TUFTSIN DEFICIENCY

Tuftsin enhances the phagocytic ability of granulocytes. In tuftsin deficiency an abnormal peptide that resembles tuftsin is produced that competitively inhibits tuftsin.[459,460] As a result, granulocyte phagocytosis is defective and there is increased susceptibility to infections. Patients have seborrheic dermatitis-like rashes, enlarged and fluctuant lymph nodes, and respiratory infections; the organisms that most frequently cause infections are *Staph. aureus*, *Pneumococcus*, and *Candida*. Complement levels, immunoglobulin levels, and NBT reduction are normal, but tuftsin activity is deficient. Patients respond to plasma or gammaglobulin injections.

WISKOTT–ALDRICH SYNDROME

Wiskott–Aldrich syndrome (WAS) is a rare disorder consisting of recurrent pyogenic infections, bleeding due to thrombocytopenia and platelet dysfunction, and recalcitrant dermatitis.[461–463]

EPIDEMIOLOGY

The majority of patients are male, with a family history suggesting X-linked recessive transmission. Cases have been described, however, without a familial tendency and in girls.[464] Most patients are Caucasian, and the prevalence in the European population is one in 250 000 individuals; blacks and Orientals are affected in rare cases. The classic association of thrombocytopenia, recurrent otitis media and other infections, and atopic dermatitis is only seen in a proportion of patients, with platelet abnormalities being the most invariable abnormality.[462]

453. Fischer A, Landais P, Friedrich W et al. (1990) European experience of bone-marrow transplantation for severe combined immunodeficiency. **Lancet** 336:850–854.
454. Buckley RH, Schiff SE, Schiff RI et al. (1999) Hematopoietic stem cell transplantation for the treatment of severe combined immunodeficiency. **N Engl J Med** 340:508.
455. Haddad E, Landais P, Friedrich W et al. (1998) Long term immune reconstitution and outcome after HLA-non identical T-cell depleted bone marrow reconstitution for SCI, a European retrospective study of 116 patients. **Blood** 91:3636.
456. Flake AW, Roncarolo MG, Puck JM et al. (1996) Treatment of X-linked severe combined immunodeficiency by in utero transplantation of paternal bone marrow. **N Engl J Med** 335:1806.
457. Wengler GS, Lanfranchi A, Frusca T et al. (1996) In utero transplantation of parental CD34 hematopoietic progenitor cells in a patients with X-linked severe combined immunodeficiency (SCIDXI). **Lancet** 348:1484.
458. Cavazzana-Calvo M, Hacein-Bey S, de Saint Basile G et al. (2000) Gene therapy of human severe combined immundeficiency (SCID)-XI disease. **Science** 288:669.
459. Najjar VA (1975) Defective phagocytosis due to deficiencies involving the tetra-peptide tuftsin. **J Pediatr** 87:1121.
460. Constantopoulos A (1983) Congenital tuftsin deficiency. **Ann NY Acad Sci** 419:214.
461. Ochs HD (1998) The Wiskott–Aldrich syndrome. **Semin Hematol** 35:332–345.
462. Thrasher AJ, Kinnon C (2000) The Wiskott–Aldrich syndrome. **Clin Exp Immunol** 120:2.
463. Sullivan KE, Mullen CA, Blaese RM, Winkelstein JA (1994) A multi-institutional survey of Wiskott–Aldrich syndrome. **J Pediatr** 125:876.
464. Parolini O, Ressman G, Haas OA et al. (1998) X-linked Wiskott–Aldrich syndrome in a girl. **N Engl J Med** 338:291.

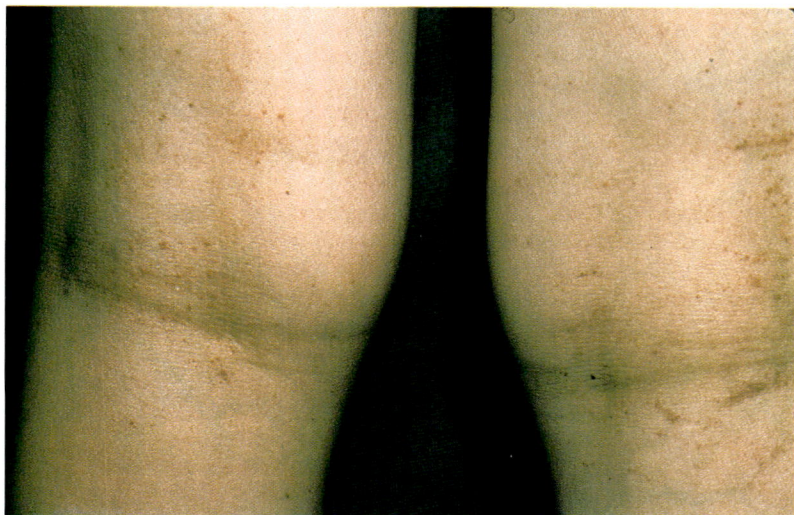

Fig. 7.42   Petechiae and ecchymosis in a young boy with the Wiskott–Aldrich syndrome.

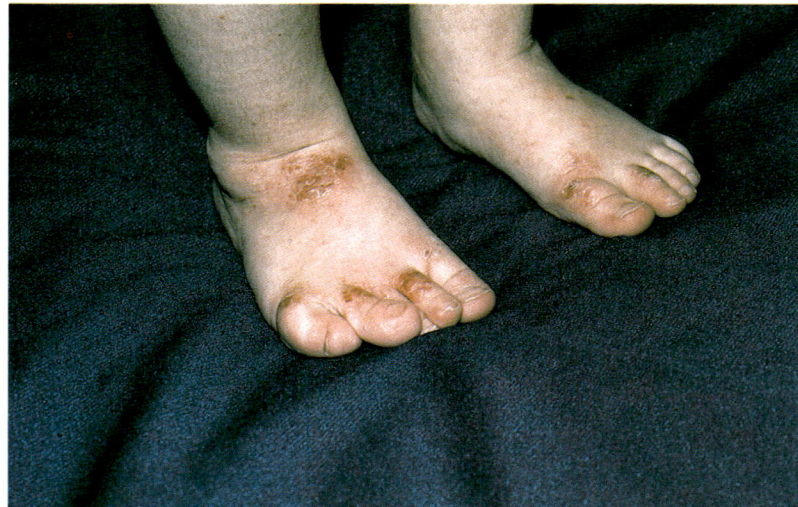

Fig. 7.43   Atopic dermatitis on the feet and lower extremities with serosanguinous drainage in a toddler with Wiskott–Aldrich syndrome.

CLINICAL MANIFESTATIONS

Because thrombocytopenia and platelet dysfunction are often present from birth, the first clinical signs may be petechiae and ecchymoses on the skin (Fig. 7.42) and oral mucosa.[465] Spontaneous bleeding from the oral cavity, cutaneous ecchymoses, epistaxis, hematemesis, melena, and hematuria are common but severity varies. Painful cutaneous vasculitis with purpura and significant edema and induration may also develop, particulary after the first few years.

Dermatitis usually develops during the first few months of life, and fulfills criteria for the definition of atopic dermatitis (Fig. 7.43). The face, scalp, and flexural areas are the most severely involved, although patients commonly have widespread involvement with progressive lichenification. The rash is often more exfoliative than that typical of atopic dermatitis. Excoriated areas frequently have serosanguineous crust and often associated petechiae or purpura. Secondary bacterial infection of eczematous lesions is common, as are eczema herpeticum and molluscum. IgE-mediated allergic problems such as urticaria, food allergies, and asthma are also seen with increased frequency.

Recurrent bacterial infections begin in infancy as placentally transmitted maternal antibody levels diminish and include otitis externa and media, pneumonia, pansinusitis, conjunctivitis, furunculosis, meningitis, and septicemia. Infections with encapsulated bacteria such as *Pneumococcus*, *H. influenzae*, and *Neisseria meningitides* predominate. With advancing age, T-cell function progressively deteriorates and patients become increasingly susceptible to infections due to herpes and other viruses, and to *P. carinii*.

Additional clinical features may be hepatosplenomegaly, lymphadenopathy, and transient arthritis with joint effusions. Lymphoreticular malignancies occur in up to 26% of patients 20 years of age and older, with an increased prevalence in patients with autoimmune disease and WAS. Non-Hodgkin's lymphoma is the most common malignancy, and extranodal and brain involvement predominate. The median survival for WAS patients is now about 15 years. Overall, the usual causes of death (unrelated to transplantation) are infection (44%), bleeding (23%), and malignancy (26%).[463]

LABORATORY FINDINGS

Laboratory studies often demonstrate persistent thrombocytopenia, in the range of 1000 to 80 000 platelets/mm.[3] Platelets tend to be small and aggregation is sometimes defective. Patients may also have Coomb's positive hemolytic anemia, leukopenia, lymphopenia, and eosinophilia. Total serum gammaglobulin is usually normal, but immunoelectrophoresis shows low levels of IgM and sometimes IgM, and IgM antibodies to blood group antigens (isohemagglutinins) are absent. Levels of IgA, IgE, and IgD tend to be elevated. Delayed hypersensitivity skin test reactions are usually absent, and responses to mitogens are often diminished, especially in older patients. The antibody responses to polysaccharide antigens are markedly diminished. Patients with decreased neutrophil or monocyte chemotaxis have been reported. The number of T lymphocytes and response *in vitro* to mitogens may be normal in early life, but often decreases with advancing age.

The expression of WASp protein in mononuclear cells derived from peripheral blood by immunoblot analysis or FACS analysis is a diagnostic screening test in suspected cases prior to mutational analysis.[462] The amount of WASp expressed in circulating cells correlates with the phenotype of affected patients and clinical course.

PATHOPHYSIOLOGY AND HISTOGENESIS

The hemorrhagic diathesis is due to both quantitative and qualitative platelet defects. Platelets from most patients are small, abnormal structurally, and have a reduced half-life without decreased production. No antiplatelet antibodies have been demonstrated. The recurrent infections are secondary to immunodeficiency of both cell-mediated and humoral immune responses because of a primary T-cell defect. The eczema also appears to be related to the T-lymphocyte defect, since it is corrected by T-lymphocyte engraftment; the cause of the high risk of malignancies is poorly understood.

The mutated protein is WASp, which is constitutively expressed in all hematopoietic stem cell–derived lines. WASp controls the assembly of actin filaments required for microvesicle and proplatelet formation; it is critical for T-cell activation and polarization of T cells toward antigen-presenting cells.[466] Mutations in WASp also cause X-linked thrombocytopenia.

DIFFERENTIAL DIAGNOSIS

Several conditions may be confused with WAS. Many of the other immunodeficiencies are characterized by eczema, increased susceptibility to infections, and the development of malignancy. Patients with agammaglobu-

465. Peacocke M, Siminovitch KA (1992) Wiskott–Aldrich syndrome: new molecular and biochemical insights. J Am Acad Dermatol 27:507.

linemias have no bleeding tendency. In the DiGeorge syndrome, facial anomalies, seizures associated with hypoparathyroidism and hypocalcemia, and normal humoral immunity help to distinguish the disorder. Individuals with AT share the eczema and recurrent infections of WAS. However, most patients show decreased levels of IgA and often IgE, and cerebellar ataxia is an early development. Chédiak–Higashi syndrome differs from WAS syndrome by the incomplete albinism, giant granules in leukocytes, and lack of eczema. WAS can also be mistaken for various eczematous processes. The distribution and character of the rash resemble atopic dermatitis. Seborrheic dermatitis, "Leiner's disease," and Langerhans cell histiocytosis may also be confused with WAS. The other clinical findings of hemorrhage, petechiae, and recurrent infections in WAS, and the histopathologic examination of skin for Langerhans cell histiocytosis help to differentiate the conditions.

TREATMENT

Conventional therapy has been directed toward treating the recurrent infections and hemorrhage. Appropriate antibiotics and intravenous infusions of gamma-globulin decrease the risk of fatal infections.[467] Splenectomy has been advocated to ameliorate the bleeding abnormality in patients with recurrent severe hemorrhage; however, splenectomy increases the risk of infection by encapsulated organisms, which is a greater problem in patients with WAS, who cannot mount an immune response from vaccine administration against encapsulated organisms. Platelet transfusions are often given before surgeries and in life-threatening circumstances. Topical corticosteroid preparations and systemic gammaglobulin may improve the dermatitis, and chronic administration of oral acyclovir is appropriate for patients with eczema herpeticum.

Bone marrow transplantation is the treatment of choice for patients with WAS. Full engraftment results in normal platelet numbers and functions, immunologic status, and clearance of the dermatitis (T-lymphocyte engraftment).[468] Survival after allogeneic transplantation below the age of 5 years is 80%; in contrast, survival for patients transplanted when older than 5 years of age is <50%. The survival rate is not significantly different between HLA genetically identical sibling donor recipients and matched HLA unrelated donor recipients if less than 5 years of age; however, older patients have not responded well to unrelated donor transplants.

Genetic counseling is important in families of patients with WAS, including for sisters of involved patients. Female carriers for WAS may be detected by the selective inactivation of the abnormal X chromosome in T and B cells and in platelets.[469] Prenatal diagnosis has been achieved by direct mutational analysis.[470]

PHOTOSENSITIVITY DISORDERS

Adrian Pierini

INTRODUCTION

The sun emits electromagnetic radiation energy comprising mainly the ultraviolet, visible, and infrared spectra. About two-thirds of this energy reaches the earth's surface. Ultraviolet radiation is subdivided into UVA (315–400nm), UVB (280–315nm) and UVC (100–280nm), and recently UVA has been divided into UVAI (340–400nm) and UVAII (320–340nm). The precise

amount of solar UV radiation over a place is determined by a number of different factors, as time of the day, season, latitude, composition of the stratospheric ozone layer, cloudiness, pollution, and altitude.

The cutaneous photobiologic reaction has been well established, and its several steps and consequences can be summarized as follows:[477]

- UVR energy is absorbed by a specific molecule, or chromophore, in the skin;
- this energy may cause either direct photochemical or indirect oxidative damage to biomolecules, such as DNA and proteins;
- DNA damage and repairing is immediately started and the consequence is the release of cytokines and inflammatory mediators;
- these substances modulate the behavior of skin cells, including keratinocytes, Langerhans cells, vascular endothelial cells, fibroblasts, lymphocytes, and melanocytes;
- the skin pigmentation response to solar UVR comprises an immediate pigment darkening and the delayed formation of new melanin;
- UV-induced pyrimidine dimers in DNA can give rise to tumors through the activation of the N-*ras* oncogene;
- the T cells' UV radiation-induced damage leads to some kind of immunosuppression that allows for the rise of cutaneous and organs other than skin malignancies.

Photosensitivity is an abnormal reaction of the skin to ultraviolet or visible light radiation that usually follows exposure to natural sunlight or some artificial sources, such as tanning beds, medical phototherapy lamps, and unshielded fluorescent and tungsten-halogen lamps.[471] Photosensitivity in children is uncommon and encompasses a wide variety of rare diseases, many of which are the result of genetic defects. We must differentiate the skin disorders induced by sun exposure from those aggravated by sun exposure.[472–475]

STUDY OF THE PATIENT WITH PHOTOSENSITIVITY DISORDERS

The child with a suspected photosensitivity disorder must be carefully evaluated on his clinical features, laboratory findings, and phototesting.[472,473]

CLINICAL FEATURES

History is usually the most important issue in diagnosing the photodermatoses. The characteristics of the eruption must be determined, especially duration, distribution over sun-exposed or non-exposed areas, morphology (papules, bullae), seasonal variation, accompanying symptoms (burn, pruritus, pain, swelling), age at onset, systemic and local medications, family history, and effectiveness of sunscreens in prophylaxis.

LABORATORY FINDINGS

All cases of photodermatoses, unless the diagnosis is otherwise certain as in xeroderma pigmentosum, must be evaluated for serum antinuclear factor, anti-SSA (Ro) and anti-SSB (La) antibody titers, and blood, urine and feces porphyrin concentrations. Skin histology may be helpful but is rarely diagnostic. Direct immunofluorescence can be useful in lupus erythematosus patients. DNA excision repair measurements in cultured fibroblasts following UV irradiation is required to diagnose certain genophotodermatoses.

466. Snapper SB, Rosen FS (1999) The Wiskott–Aldrich syndrome protein (WASP): roles in signalling and cytoskeletal organization. **Annu Rev Immunol** 17:905.
467. Litzman J, Jones A, Hann I et al. (1996) Intravenous immunoglobulin, splenectomy, and antibiotic prophylaxis in Wiskott–Aldrich syndrome. **Arch Dis Child** 75:436.
468. Brochstein JA, Gillio AP, Ruggiero M et al. (1991) Marrow transplantation from human leukocyte antigen-identical or haploidentical donors for correction of Wiskott–Aldrich syndrome. **J Pediatr** 119:907.
469. Windelstein JA, Fearon E (1990) Carrier detection of the X-linked primary immunodeficiency diseases using X-chromosome inactivation analysis. **J Allergy Clin Immunol** 85:1090.
470. Giliani S, Fiorini M, Mella P et al. (1999) Prenatal molecular diagnosis of Wiskott–Aldrich syndrome by direct mutation analysis. **Prenat Diagn** 19:36.

471. McGregor JM, Hawk JLM (1999) Acute effects of ultraviolet radiation on the skin. In: Fitzpatrick's Dermatology in General Medicine, 5th edn, Freedberg IM, Eisen AZ, Wolff K et al., eds. New York: McGraw-Hill, pp. 1555–1561.
472. Roelands R (2000) The diagnosis of photosensitivity. **Arch Dermatol** 136:1152–1157.
473. Ramsay CA (1983) Photosensitivity in children. **Pediatr Clin N Am** 30:687–699.
474. Bligard CA, Storer JS (1986) Photosensitivity in infants and children. **Dermatol Clin** 4:311–319.
475. Kahn G (1986) Photosensitivity and photodermatitis in childhood. **Dermatol Clin** 4:107–116.
476. Poh-Fitzpatrick MB (1987) The porphyrias. **Dermatol Clin** 5:55–61.
477. Bonnetblanc JM, Bernard P, Fayol J (1989) Porphyries cutanées. **Encycl Méd Chir (Paris) Dermatologie** 12440 A10, 2-1989.

PHOTOTESTING

The study of the reaction of unaffected skin to solar simulators may be helpful in the diagnosis of some photosensitivity disorders such as actinic prurigo, polymorphous light eruption, hydroa vacciniforme, solar urticaria, and drug-induced photosensitivity. The classification of photosensitivity disorders in children shown in Table 7.18 will allow the dermatologist or pediatrician to consider the most probable diagnoses.

This chapter deals with the genetically determined photosensitivity disorders of infants and children. The other photodermatoses will be treated in separate chapters.

THE PORPHYRIAS

The porphyrias are a group of rare metabolic disorders in which excessive quantities of porphyrins, or their precursors, are produced. They are due to inherited or acquired abnormalities in the metabolic pathway of heme biosynthesis: each type of porphyria results from a specific enzyme defect that leads to the accumulation and excretion of porphyrins (Table 7.19). Since the 2nd edition of this book, important advances has been achieved in the identification of the genes responsible, allowing for the possibility of novel therapeutics of these diseases.

A general summary of the clinical and biochemical features of the porphyrias is presented in Table 7.20, and numerous reviews are available.[476–481]

HISTORICAL ASPECTS

The first descriptions of porphyrins were published by the middle of the 19th century, and the first published case of porphyria is credited to Schultz in 1874.[482,483] The first classification of porphyria was proposed by Günther in 1911.[484] With the advance of biochemistry, the different types of porphyria were identified in the last 50 years: acute intermittent porphyria (Waldenstrom[485] and Goldberg),[486] hereditary coproporphyria (Berger and Goldberg),[487] variegate porphyria (in South Africa),[488] erythropoietic protoporphyria (Magnus *et al.*),[489] erythropoietic coproporphyria (Heilmeyer and Clotten),[490] and hepatoerythropoietic porphyria (Piñol Aguadé *et al.*).[491]

THE BIOCHEMISTRY OF PORPHYRINS AND HEME

Porphyrins are essential biochemical constituents of living beings, controlling oxidation and transporting and exchanging oxygen from the environment to the tissues of the body. The biosynthetic pathway of porphyrins and heme has been almost completely defined[476,478,479] (Table 7.19). Heme, the end product of the pathway, is a tetrapyrrole protoporphyrin chelated with iron. Heme is central to the structure of a number of metabolic proteins such as hemoglobin, myoglobin, catalases, peroxidases, and cytochromes P450.

The starting point of the pathway is the formation of delta-aminolevulinic acid (ALA) from glycine and succinyl-CoA. ALA synthase act as the primary rate-limiting enzyme in the liver, and is regulated by the hepatocellular free heme pool.

In bone marrow, ferrochelatase is the rate-limiting step for heme synthesis. In general, the major porphyrin or porphyrin precursor excreted in a given porphyria is the substrate for the defective enzyme. These intermediates, when present in excess amounts, exert toxic effects on the tissues.[476–479]

MECHANISMS OF PORPHYRIN-INDUCED PHOTOSENSITIVITY

Porphyrins are excited by visible light with a wavelength between 400 and 410nm (Soret's band) and emit an intense red fluorescence. When irradiated with light of the appropriate wavelength in the presence of oxygen, porphyrins will cause photodynamic effects. The energy released reacts with oxygen to produce free radicals and singlet oxygen that damages molecules, cells and tissues.[476,477]

Cell damage results from lysosomal and plasma membrane injury and from complement activation. Beta-carotene exerts its protective activity by quenching both free radicals and singlet oxygen.[492]

Two different phototoxicity patterns can be observed in porphyria patents: (a) the immediate, characterized by erythema, edema, pain, and purpura; and (b) the delayed, which consists of increased fragility of the skin, blistering, and scarring.

Photosensitivity of the skin varies considerably according to the type of porphyria. AIP and ALA-dehydratase deficiency do not present with cutaneous photosensitivity. This variation is likely due to the differing

---

TABLE 7.18   Classification of photosensitivity disorders in children

A. Idiopathic photodermatoses
   Polymorphic light eruption
      Juvenile spring eruption
   Actinic prurigo
      Hereditary PMLE of Native Americans
   Hydroa vacciniforme
   Solar urticaria

B. DNA repair-defective disorders
   Xeroderma pigmentosum
   Cockayne syndrome
   Trichothiodystrophy
   Bloom syndrome
   Rothmund–Thomson and other poikiloderma congenita syndromes
   Ataxia telangiectasia

C. Pigmentary deficiencies
   Albinism
   Phenylketonuria
   Vitiligo

D. Nutritional and metabolic aberrations
   Pellagra
   Hartnup disease

E. Photosensitization by exogenous drugs or exogenous or endogenous chemicals
   Porphyrias
   Acute inflammatory reactions (phototoxicity) to drugs or plants
   Eczematous reactions (photoallergy) to drugs or plants

F. Dermatoses exacerbated by UV irradiation
   Lupus erythematosus
   Dermatomyositis
   Lichen planus actinicus
   Pemphigus
   Psoriasis
   Atopic dermatitis
   Acne

478. Meola T, Lim HW (1993) The porphyrias. **Dermatol Clin** 11:583–596.
479. Paslin D (1998) The porphyrias. **Clin Dermatol** 16:185–307.
480. Jensen JD, Resnick SD (1995) Porphyria in childhood. **Semin Dermatol** 14:33–39.
481. Elder GH (1997) Hepatic porphyrias in children. **J Inherit Metab Dis** 20:237–246.
482. Goldberg A (1985) Porphyria. Introduction – historical background. **Clin Dermatol** 3:3–6.
483. Goldberg A (1998) The porphyrias. Historical background. **Clin Dermatol** 16:189–193.
484. Günther H (1911) Die Haematoporphyrie. **Dtsch Arch Klin Med** 105:89–146.
485. Waldenstrom J (1937) Studien uber Porphyrie. **Acta Med Scand** 92 (suppl):1–254.
486. Goldberg A (1959) Acute intermittent porphyria: A study of 50 cases. **Q J Med (Oxford)** 28:183–209.

487. Berger H, Goldberg A (1955) Hereditary coproporphyria. **Br Med J** 2:85–88.
488. Dean G, Barnes AD (1955) The inheritance of porphyria. **Br Med J** 2:89–91.
489. Magnus IA, Jarret A, Prankerd TAJ et al. (1961) Erythropoietic protoporphyria. A new porphyria syndrome with solar urticaria due to protoporphyrinaemia. **Lancet** 2:448–451.
490. Heilmeyer HP, Clotten R, Kerp I et al. (1963) Porphyria erythropoietica congenita Günther bericht uber Familien mit Erfassung Merkmalsträger. **Dstch Med Wochenschr** 88:2449.
491. Piñol Aguadé J, Castells A, Indacochea A et al. (1969) A case of biochemically unclassificable porphyria. **Br J Dermatol** 81:270–275.
492. Mathews-Roth MM (1998) Treatment of the cutaneous porphyrias. **Clin Dermatol** 16:295–298.

TABLE 7.19   The porphyrin-heme biosynthetic pathway

Porphyria	Normal metabolites	Enzymes
	Glycine + succinyl-CoA	ALA synthase
	↓	
	Delta-aminolevulinic acid (ALA)	
ALA dehydratase	↓	ALA dehydratase deficiency
Acute intermittent porphyria	Porphobilinogen (PBG)	PBG deaminase
	↓	
Congenital erythropoietic porphyria	Hydroxymethylbilane	Uroporphyrinogen III cosynthase
	↓	
	Uroporphyrinogen III	
Porphyria cutanea tarda/HEP	↓	Uroporphyrinogen decarboxylase
	Coproporphyrinogen III	
Hereditary coproporphyria	↓	Coproporphyrinogen oxidase
	Protoporphyrinogen IX	
Variegate porphyria	↓	Protoporphyrinogen oxidase
	Protoporphyrin IX	
Erythropoietic protoporphyria	↓	Ferrochelatase
	Heme	
	↓	
	Hemoglobin Myoglobin Cytochromes	

TABLE 7.20   Clinical and biochemical characterization of porphyrias

Disease	Inheritance	Gene location	Enzyme defect	Photosensitivity	Scarring	Hypertrichosis	Liver	Neurologic	RBC	Plasma	Urine	Feces	Other
CEP	AR	10q25.2	Urogen III S	+++	+++ Mutilating	+	−	−	Uro Copro Proto	Uro Copro	Uro Copro	Uro Copro	Erythrodontia, hemolysis, splenomegaly, bone fragility
EPP	AD	18q22	Ferroc	++	+	+/−	+ to +++	−	Proto	Proto	−	Proto Copro	Cholelithiasis, onycholysis
ECP	?		?	++	+	−	−	−	Copro Proto	−	−	−	Only 3 cases published
PCT	Sporadic AD Type II–III	1p34	Urogen D	++	++ milia	+++	++	−	−	Uro Copro	Uro Copro 7-carboxy	Uro Isocopro Proto Copro	Associated with diabetes, SLE, hepatitis, hematologic
HEP	AD Homozygous PCT	1p34	Urogen D	+++	++	+	+	−	Proto	Uro	Uro 7-carboxy	Copro Isocopro	Erythrodontia, anemia, splenomegaly
VP	AD	1q22 & 6p21.3	Protogen O	+++	++	+	+	+	−	−	ALA, PBG Copro Proto Acute	Proto Copro X-porph	Retarded growth
HCP	AD	3q12	Coprogen O	+	+	+	+	+	−	−	ALA, PBG Copro	Copro	Jaundice, anemia in newborns (hardero-porphyria)
AIP	AD	11q23.3	PBG D	−	−	−	+	++	−	−	ALA, PBG Uro Copro	−	No cutaneous signs

RBC, red blood cell; CEP, congenital erythropoietic porphyria; EPP, erythropotetic protoporphyria; ECP, congenital erythropoietic coproporphyria; PCT, porphyria cutanea tarda; HEP, hepatoerythropoietic porphyria; VP, variegate porphyria; HCP, hereditary coproporphyria; AIP, acute intermittent porphyria; AR, autosomal recessive; AD, autosomal dominant; Uro, uroporphyrin; Copro, coproporphyrin; Proto, protoporphyrin; 7-carboxy, 7-carboxylate porphyrin; ALA, delta-aminolevulinic acid; PBG, porphobilinogen; Isocopro, isocoproporphyrin; X-porph, X-porphyrin; Urogen III S, Uroporphyrinogen III synthase; Ferroc, ferrochelatase; Urogen D, uroporphyrinogen decarboxylase; Protogen O, protoporphyrinogen oxidase; Coprogen O, coproporphyrinogen oxidase; PBGD, porphobilinogen deaminase (also named hydroxymethylbilane synthase).

TABLE 7.21   Classification of porphyrias according to the tissue source of excess porphyrins[476]

Erythropoietic porphyrias
Congenital erythropoietic porphyria (CEP)
Erythropoietic protoporphyria (EPP)
Congenital erythropoietic coproporphyria (ECP)

Hepatic porphyrias
Acute intermittent porphyria (AIP)
Variegate porphyria (VP)
Hereditary coproporphyria (HCP)
Porphyria cutanea tarda (PCT)
ALA-dehydratase porphyria (ALADP)

Hepatic/erythropoietic porphyrias
Hepatoerythropoietic porphyria (HEP)
Harderoporphyria

Classification by mode of transmission
Autosomal dominant
Porphyria cutanea tarda (PCT)
Hereditary coproporphyria (HCP)
Erythropoietic protoporphyria (EPP)
Variegate porphyria (VP)
Acute intermittent porphyria (AIP)
Hepatoerythropoietic porphyria (HEP)

Autosomal recessive
ALA-dehydratase porphyria (ALADP)
Congenital erythropoietic porphyria (CEP)

aqueous and lipid solubility of the various porphyrins (e.g., the intermediates of the first steps are water soluble, and protoporphyrin is lipid soluble).

CLASSIFICATION

There is no completely satisfactory classification of porphyria. The current classification has evolved from Günther's first proposal in 1911,[484] and takes into account the porphyrin pattern in the blood, urine and feces, and the clinical features. The classification in Table 7.21, from Poh-Fitzpatrick,[476] considers the tissue source of excess porphyrins.

CONGENITAL ERYTHROPOIETIC PORPHYRIA

INTRODUCTION AND HISTORICAL NOTE

Also known as Günther's disease, congenital porphyria or congenital hematoporphyria, congenital erythropoietic porphyria (CEP) was first recognized by Günther as "an inborn error of metabolism" but the first case was probably published by Shultz.[483]

EPIDEMIOLOGY

Genetics

Congenital erythropoietic porphyria (CEP, MIM 263700) is inherited as an autosomal recessive trait. The condition is due to mutations in the uroporphyrinogen III synthetase (UROS) gene. A cDNA encoding this enzyme was cloned in 1988[493] and the gene was mapped to 10q25.2–26.3 by the same group.[494]

At least 17 mutations have been described in the UROS gene, explaining the heterogeneous phenotypes of CEP.[495] Patients with severe CEP were noted to be homozygous for a single mutation (C73R).[496–498] The approximately 34kb UROS gene has been isolated and its organization and tissue-specific expression determined. The gene has two promoters, the housekeeping and the erythroid–specific transcripts. The erythroid–specific transcript is present only in erythroid tissues and contains GATA1 and NF-E2 sites.[499] Mutations in these erythroid promoters causes CEP.[500]

CEP is a rare porphyria with a little more than 150 cases in both sexes reported to date. In our hospital, we observed 2 cases in 14 years, from over 80 000 first-visit consultations.

PRESENTING HISTORY

Onset is in infancy or early childhood and has even been reported to be present at birth with the findings of red staining of the diapers from high quantities of porphyrins (uroporphyrinogen I and coproporphyrinogen I) in the urine.[501] The clinical presentation is variable due to the heterogeneous nature of the enzyme defect, being most important in the newborn and infant (Figs 7.44 and 7.45). Rarely, the onset of symptoms occurs in later childhood or even in adult life.

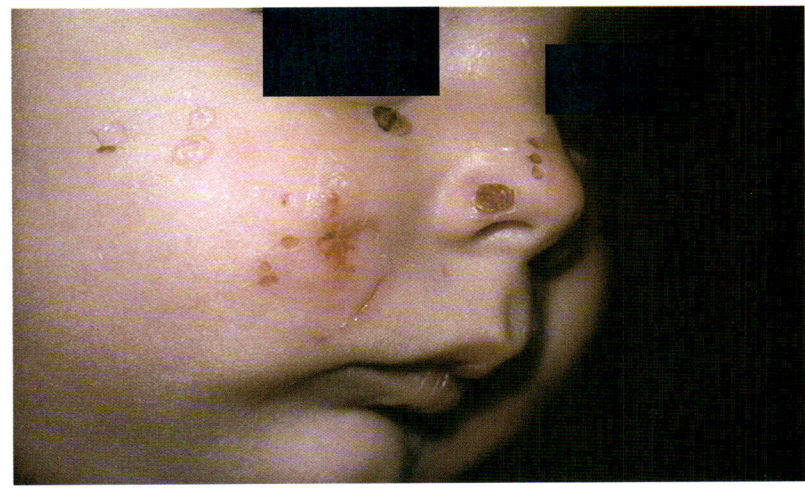

Fig. 7.44   CEP with mild lesions on the cheek and nose of a 1-year-old boy.

493. Tsai SF, Bishop DF, Desnick RJ (1988) Human uroporphyrinogen III synthase: molecular cloning, nucleotide sequence, and expression of a full length cDNA. **Proc Nat Acad Sci USA** 85:7049–7053.
494. Astrin KH, Warner CA, Yoo HW et al. (1991) Regional assignment of the human uroporphyrinogen III synthase (UROS) gene to chromosome 10q25.2–q26.3. **Hum Genet** 87:18–22.
495. Xu W, Astrin KH, Desnick RJ (1996) Molecular basis of congenital erythropoietic porphyria: mutations in the human uroporphyrinogen III synthase gene. **Hum Mutat** 7:187–192.
496. Warner CA, Yoo HW, Roberts AG et al. (1992) Congenital erythropoietic porphyria: identification and expression of exonic mutations in the uroporphyrinogen III synthase gene. **J Clin Invest** 89:693–700.
497. Frank J, Wang X, Lam HM et al. (1998) C73R is a hotspot mutation in the uroporphyrinogen III synthase gene in congenital erythropoietic porphyria. **Ann Hum Genet** 62:225–230.
498. Freesemann AG, Gross U, Bensidhoum M et al. (1998) Immunological, enzymatic and biochemical studies of uroporphyrinogen III-synthase deficiency in 20 patients with congenital erythropoietic porphyria. **Eur J Biochem** 257:149–153.
499. Aizencang G, Solis C, Bishop DF et al. (2000) Human uroporphyrinogen-III synthase: genomic organization, alternative promoters, and erythroid-specific expression. **Genomics** 70:223–231.
500. Solis C, Aizencang GI, Astrin KH et al. (2001) Uroporphyrinogen III synthase erythroid promoter mutations in adjacent GATA1 and CP2 elements cause congenital erythropoietic porphyria. **J Clin Invest** 107:753–762.
501. Poh-Fitzpatrick MB (1998) Clinical features of the porphyrias. **Clin Dermatol** 16:251–264.

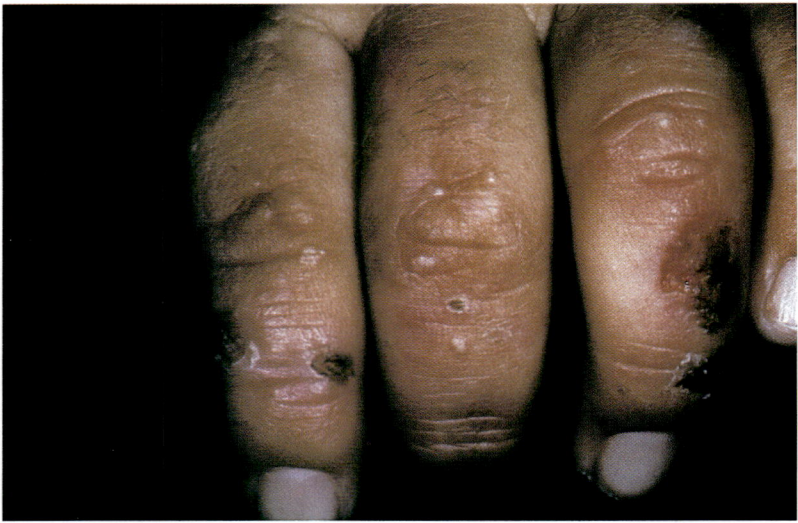

Fig. 7.45   CEP with bullae, crusts, and milia on the hand of the same patient, at age 2.

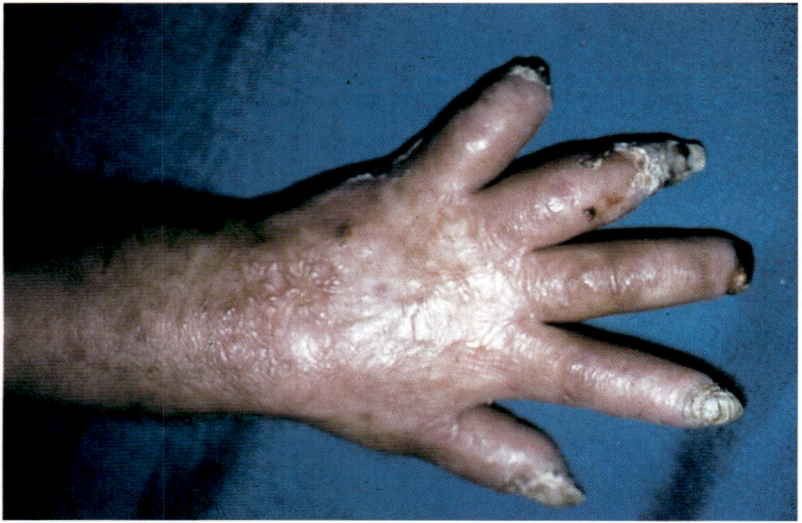

Fig. 7.46   CEP with severe scars and loss of distal phalanges of the digits.

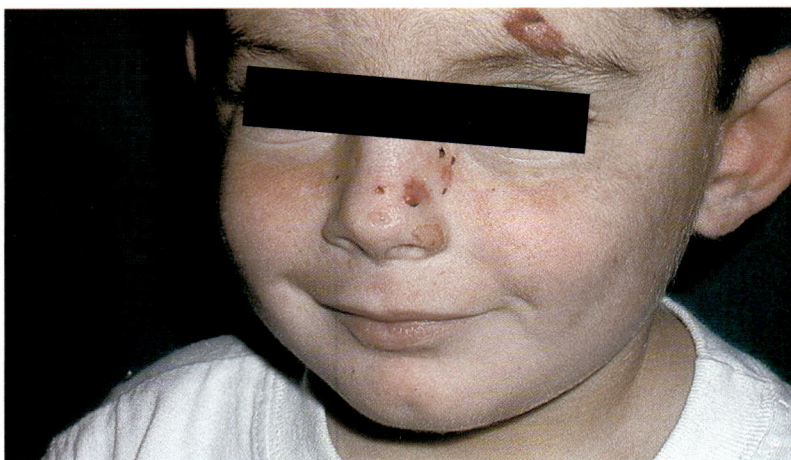

Fig. 7.47   CEP with mild lesions on the cheek and nose at the age of 2 years.

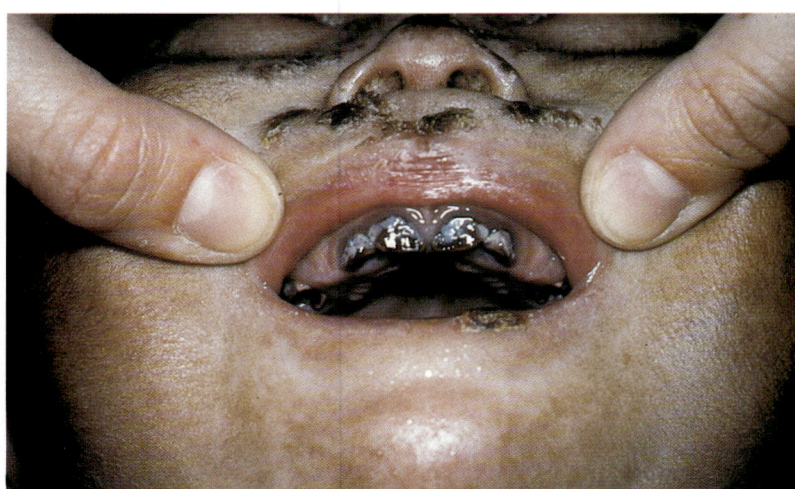

Fig. 7.48   CEP with erythrodontia at age 9 months.

PHYSICAL EXAMINATION

Skin

The cutaneous manifestations of CEP are some of the most dramatic of the porphyrias. There is exquisite photosensitivity with painful vesicles and bullae that are filled with red fluorescent fluid containing free porphyrins. Blisters often become secondarily infected and progress to mutilating scarring (Figs 7.46 and 7.47). The eyelids, nose, ears, and fingers are particularly affected. Most patients develop severe mutilation of the hands and face. Hyperpigmentation and generalized hypertrichosis are seen with the scarring.

Hair, nail, teeth and mucous membranes

A striking pathognomonic feature is erythrodontia (Fig. 7.48), a red to dirty brown staining of the teeth secondary to porphyrin deposition in dentine that is thought to be a result of the affinity of porphyrins for

calcium phosphate. The teeth show characteristic red fluorescence as well. There may be cicatricial alopecia, onycholysis, koilonychia, and nail pigmentation.

Systemic manifestations

Other problems include photophobia, keratoconjunctivitis, ocular ulceration, corneal scarring, ectropion, and cataracts resulting in blindness. There is often intermittent hemolytic anemia, sometimes severe, with associated splenomegaly. Increased bone fragility, due to expansion of the bone marrow or direct toxicity by porphyrins, can lead to fractures and shortened stature.[501–503] Abdominal and neurologic symptoms are absent. In severely affected patients systemic complications can begin *in utero*, with hydrops fetalis, hepatosplenomegaly and anemia. In the newborn with severe CEP, blistering over the entire exposed body surface has been brought on by phototherapy.[504]

LABORATORY FINDINGS

Blood, urine and feces determination of porphyrins allows the biochemical diagnosis of CEP, as shown in Table 7.20. Uroporphyrin I and coproporphyrin I are the main metabolites found to be increased in these patients.

502. Laorr A, Greenspan A (1994) Severe osteopenia in congenital erythropoietic porphyria. **Can Ass Radiol J** 45:307–309.
503. Moore MR (1998) The biochemistry of heme synthesis in porphyria and in the porphyr nurias. **Clin Dermatol** 16:203–223.

504. Huang JL, Zaider E, Roth P et al. (1996) Congenital erythropoietic porphyria: clinical, biochemical, and enzymatic profile of a severely affected infant. **J Am Acad Dermatol** 34:924–927.

Uroporphyrinogen III synthase concentration in erythrocytes can be determined by enzyme-linked immunosorbent assay thanks to a specific antibody. Erythrocyte URO III synthase activities of patients with CEP reduced to 4–33% of the normal controls.[498]

The antenatal diagnosis of CEP is possible by determining increased levels of uroporphyrin I in amniotic fluid and direct detection of the gene mutation in amniotic cells.[505]

PATHOPHYSIOLOGY AND HISTOGENESIS

Molecular, biochemical and immunological basis

The underlying defect is the deficiency of the enzyme uroporphyrinogen III synthetase, the activity of which is reduced to 3–40% of normal in red blood cells. URO synthase is responsible for conversion of the linear tetrapyrrole, hydroxymethylbilane, to the cyclic tetrapyrrole, uroporphyrinogen III, one of the steps of the heme biosynthetic pathway.

Uroporphyrinogen I and coproporphyrinogen I accumulate in the bone marrow, erythrocytes, plasma, bones, and teeth, and their corresponding porphyrins are excreted in the urine and feces. With appropriate UVA light, there is striking red fluorescence of the urine as well.

Histologic findings

Nonspecific changes are observed in CEP. Skin lesions are similar to those observed in other forms of porphyria.

DIFFERENTIAL DIAGNOSIS

Mutilating forms of CEP must be distinguished from other severe deforming diseases, as epidermolysis bullosa, and from HEP by porphyrin determinations. HEP has similar skin manifestations as CEP, but it lacks the erythrodontia, hemolytic anemia and splenomegaly that characterizes the latter.

THERAPEUTICS AND PROGNOSIS

Therapy is aimed at the cutaneous photosensitivity or at the anemia and its complications.

Topical therapy

The patient should be instructed to protect from sunlight (the 400nm wavelength being the most detrimental) by either avoidance, coverings, or topical sunscreens that block visible light.

Systemic management

Beta-carotene may ameliorate some part of the photodamage. Blood transfusions seems to be effective. Splenectomy has been helpful in a few cases with severe hemolytic anemia. Oral superactivated charcoal has given satisfactory results in some patients with CEP, but not in others.[492]

Bone marrow transplantation provided good results in three patients with CEP.[506–509]

Other promising therapeutic approaches include cord blood stem cell transplantation[510] and gene therapy.[511–514]

Prognosis

Despite better therapy for secondary infections in recent years, the ultimate prognosis for a normal life span is poor, and patients succumb in the third or fourth decades. The new therapeutic approaches based on correction of the defective gene (bone marrow transplantation, cord blood stem cell transplantation, and gene therapy) are still in their first steps, but promise a better future for children with CEP.

ERYTHROPOIETIC PROTOPORPHYRIA

INTRODUCTION AND HISTORICAL NOTE

Erythropoietic protoporphyria (EPP) was first defined in 1961 by Magnus,[489] the clinical symptoms having been defined earlier.

Epidemiology

Genetics

Erythropoietic protoporphyria (EPP, MIM 177000) appears to be transmitted as an autosomal dominant trait with variable penetrance. Unlike other dominantly inherited forms of porphyria, enzyme activity levels in EPP are only moderately reduced. The gene for human ferrochelatase (*FECH*) has been assigned to chromosome 18q21.3.[515,516] More than 60 different mutations have been identified in the FECH gene of EPP patients. The carriage of "null allele" mutations seems to be linked with an increased frequency of liver complications.[517,518] The unusual inheritance could be explained by co-inheritance of a "low expression" of the normal *FECH* allele and a mutant allele.[519]

Statistics

Although this was one of the later porphyrias to be described, it represents one of the most common in childhood and puberty.[520] Our Dermatology Service followed 6 cases of EPP between 1987 and 1996, which represents 0.16 per thousand of the total–first visit patients.[521]

505. Ged C, Moreau-Gaudry F, Taine L et al. (1996) Prenatal diagnosis in congenital erythropoietic porphyria by metabolic measurement and DNA mutation analysis. **Prenat Diagn** 16:83–86.
506. Kauffman L, Evans DI, Stevens RF et al. (1991) Bone-marrow transplantation for congenital erythropoietic porphyria. **Lancet** 337:1510–1511.
507. Tezcan I, Xu W, Gurgey A et al. (1998) Congenital erythropoietic porphyria successfully treated by allogeneic bone marrow transplantation. **Blood** 92:4053–4058.
508. Lagarde C, Hamel-Teillac D, De Prost Y et al. (1998) Allogreffe de moelle osseuse dans la porphyrie érythropoïétique congénitale. Maladie de Günther. **Ann Dermatol Venereol** 125:114–117.
509. Harada FA, Shwayder TA, Desnick RJ et al. (2001) Treatment of severe congenital erythropoietic porphyria by bone marrow transplantation. **J Am Acad Dermatol** 45:279–282.
510. Zix-Kieffer I, Langer B, Eyer D et al. (1996) Successful cord blood stem cell transplantation for congenital erythropoietic porphyria (Gunther's disease). **Bone Marrow Transpl** 18:217–220.
511. Moreau-Gaudry F, Mazurier F, Bensidhoum M et al. (1995) Metabolic correction of congenital erythropoietic porphyria by retrovirus-mediated gene transfer into Epstein–Barr virus-transformed B-cell lines. **Blood** 15; 85:1449–1453.
512. Mazurier F, Moreau-Gaudry F, Salesse S et al. (1997) Gene transfer of the uroporphyrinogen III synthase cDNA into haematopoietic progenitor cells in view of a future gene therapy in congenital erythropoietic porphyria. **J Inherit Metab Dis** 20:247–257.
513. Kauppinen R, Glass IA, Aizencang G et al. (1998) Congenital erythropoietic porphyria: prolonged high-level expression and correction of the heme biosynthetic defect by retroviral-mediated gene transfer into porphyric and erythroid cells. **Mol Genet Metab** 65:10–17.
514. Fontanellas A, Mazurier F, Belloc F et al. (1999) Fluorescence-based selection of retrovirally transduced cells in congenital erythropoietic porphyria: direct selection based on the expression of the therapeutic gene. **J Gene Med** 1:322–330.
515. Whitcombe DM, Carter NP, Albertson DG et al. (1991) Assignment of the human ferrochelatase gene (FECH) and a locus for protoporphyria to chromosome 18q22. **Genomics** 11:1152–1154.
516. Brenner DA, Didier JM, Frasier F et al. (1992) A molecular defect in human protoporphyria. **Am J Hum Genet** 50:1203–1210.
517. Schneider-Yin X, Gouya L, Meier-Weinand A et al. (2000) New insights into the pathogenesis of erythropoietic protoporphyria and their impact on patient care. **Eur J Pediatr** 159:719–725.
518. Norris PG, Nunn AV, Hawk JL et al. (1990) Genetic heterogeneity in erythropoietic protoporphyria: a study of the enzymatic defect in nine affected families. **J Invest Dermatol** 95:260–263.
519. Gouya L, Deybach JC, Lamoril J et al. (1996) Modulation of the phenotype in dominant erythropoietic protoporphyria by a low expression of the normal ferrochelatase allele. **Am J Hum Genet** 58:292–299.
520. Baart de la Faille H (1975) Erythropoietic protoporphyria: a photodermatosis. Microscopical and electron microscopical investigations of irradiated skin and a clinical study. Utrecht: Oosthoek, Scheltema & Holkemal.
521. Laffargue JA, Pierini AM, Soliani A et al. (1999) Porfirias en la Infancia. Revisión casuística de 17 niños con porfiria observados en un Servicio de Dermatología Pediátrica. Manifestaciones cutáneas. Evaluación de características hereditarias. Propuesta terapéutica. Revisión de bibliográfica. **Arch Argent Dermatol** 49:49–71.

PRESENTING HISTORY

Onset is in infancy and early childhood with all races and both sexes equally involved. There is a wide spectrum of expression of EPP. The presenting history is usually one of photosensitivity. An infant may cry uncomfortably when exposed to even a few minutes of sunlight, and older children complain of burning, stinging, and itching, and then develop erythema with swelling, urticaria-like plaques, and occasional purpura. Rarely, some patients have vesicles or bullae (Fig. 7.49). In a comprehensive study of 32 patients with the disorder, frequency of symptoms included burning (97%), itching (88%), edema (94%), erythema (69%), scarring (19%), pain (16%), and papulovesicles and petechiae (3%).[522]

PHYSICAL EXAMINATION

Skin

Chronically exposed skin shows thickening with a distinctive waxy, pebbly, superficial, scarred appearance (Figs 7.50 and 7.51). which has been described as "prematurely aged" or "weather-beaten." The bridge of the nose and the knuckles of the hand are most affected. The fine, elliptical, superficial scars of EPP are scattered over the nose, cheeks, chin, or forehead (Figs 7.52 and 7.53). They are quite different from the mutilating scarring seen in CEP. Linear furrowing around the lips is common. (Fig. 7.54).

Hair, nail, teeth and mucous membranes

In severe exposure, nails may be lost (photo-onycholysis). There is no red staining of the urine or the teeth.

Systemic manifestations

Cholelithiasis is common with protoporphyrin-containing gallstones. In some cases there is associated liver disease, including acute fatal hepatic failure or

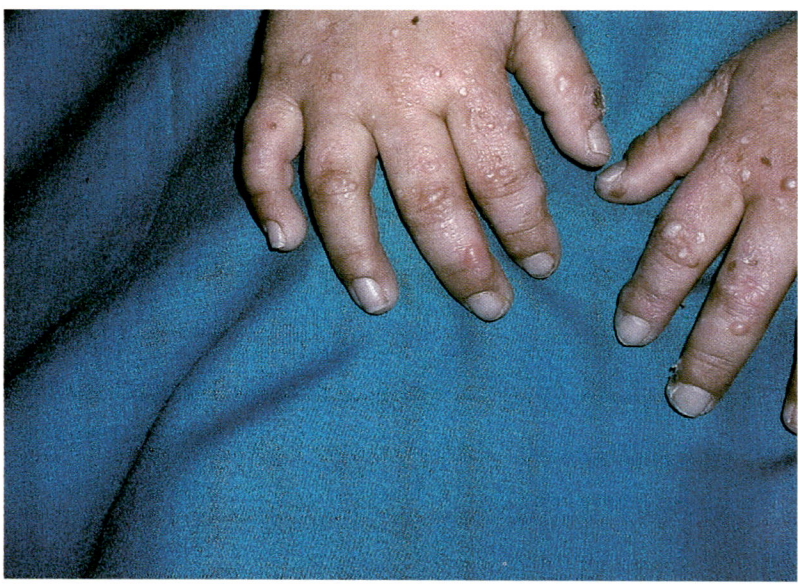

Fig. 7.49   CEP with crusts and milia on the hand of the same patient, at age 2 years.

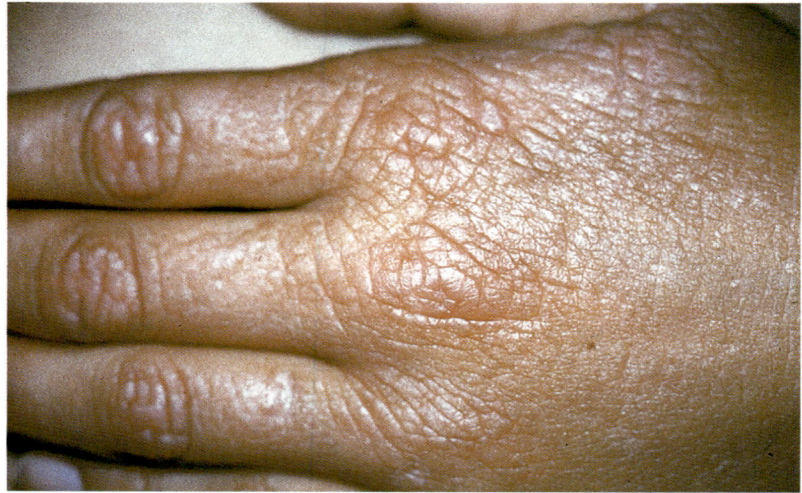

Fig. 7.51   EPP: classic pebbled skin image over the hand of a 7-year-old boy.

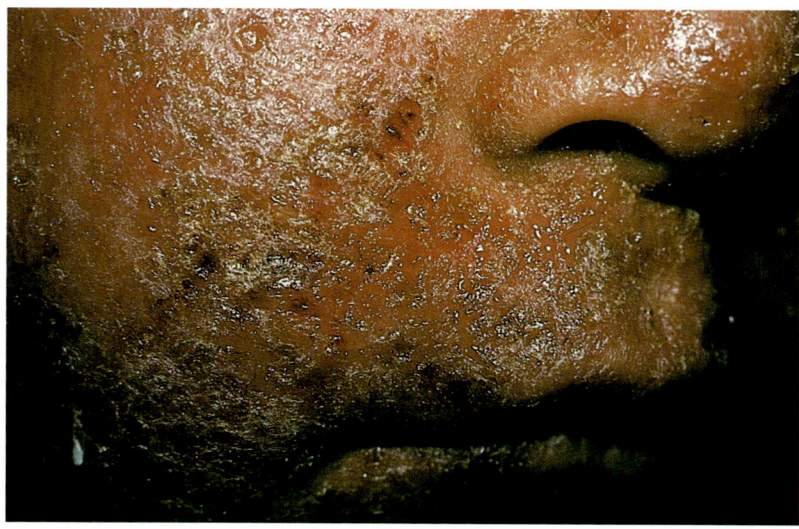

Fig. 7.50   EPP in a 5-year-old girl with acute sunburn reaction, and superimposed bacterial infection.

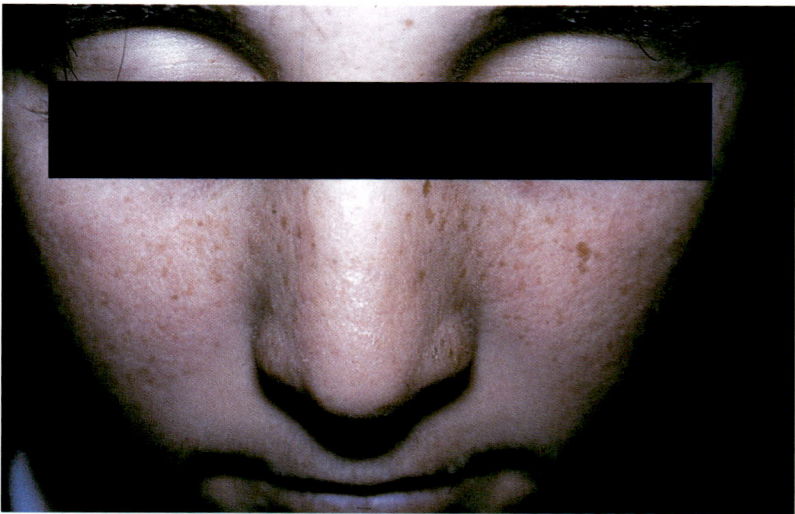

Fig. 7.52   EPP with mild scars over the nose and cheeks in a 17-year-old boy.

522. DeLeo VA, Poh-Fitzpatrick MB, Mathews-Roth M et al. (1976) Erythropoietic protoporphyria. Ten years' experience. Am J Med 60:8–22.

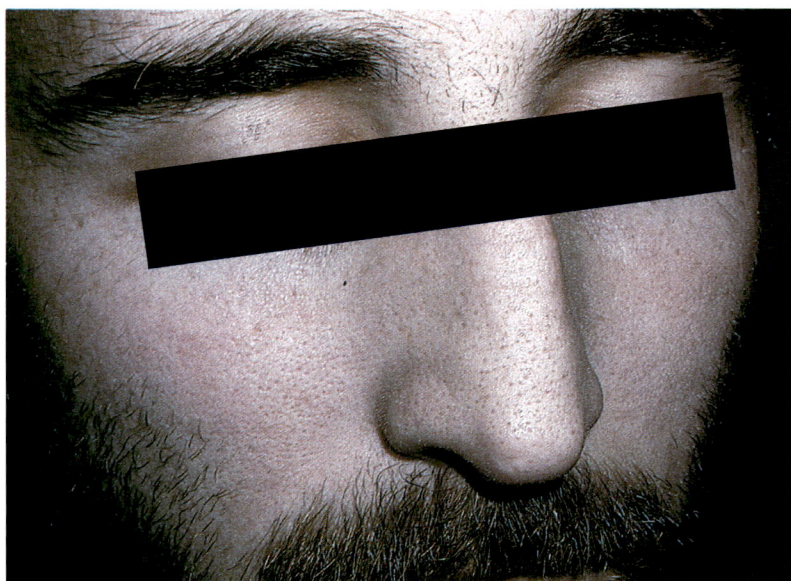

Fig. 7.53   EPP with mild scars over the nose in the same patient as Fig. 7.52 at the age of 21 years.

severe chronic cirrhosis. Approximately one-third of the patients are also anemic.

LABORATORY FINDINGS

Free (not zinc-bound) protoporphyrin is present in massive levels in red blood cells, plasma, and feces. Thus the best test is the free erythrocyte protoporphyrin (FEP) level. However, the more readily available zinc-protoporphyrin assay is usually abnormal as well and, although not reflecting the specific abnormal porphyrin, can be useful if it is elevated. Red blood cells show coral red fluorescence in 5–20% of cells. Liver function tests can be abnormal even in patients without severe hepatic disease. Fluorescence of the hepatic tissue can be positive as the expression of porphyrin's deposition.

PATHOPHYSIOLOGY AND HISTOGENESIS
Molecular, biochemical and immunological basis

The biochemical basis for EPP is a deficiency (10–30% of normal) of ferrochelatase (also known as heme synthetase or heme synthase). This enzyme converts protoporphyrin to heme, and is the final enzyme in the heme synthesis pathway. The defect is in all erythropoietic tissues. EPP is the only porphyria with absent urinary porphyrins since protoporphyrin is not water soluble. It does have high affinity for the liver and bile. Protoporphyrin is activated at 400nm wavelength of light, and generates free radicals that give rise to photodynamic cell injury. The primary event takes place in the endothelial cells of the skin capillaries, but complement activation and mast cell degranulation follow the process.[523]

Histologic findings

Histologic examination of the skin shows perivascular and upper dermal accumulations of periodic acid–Schiff positive, diastase-resistant amorphous material. Immunofluorescence reveals deposits of IgG. There is also cutaneous deposition of complement, neutral glycoproteins, acid glycosaminoglycans, and lipids. Recent studies show photoactivation of complement in this disorder. In cases with hepatic involvement, huge quantities of protoporphyrin are found in bile and hepatic parenchyma.

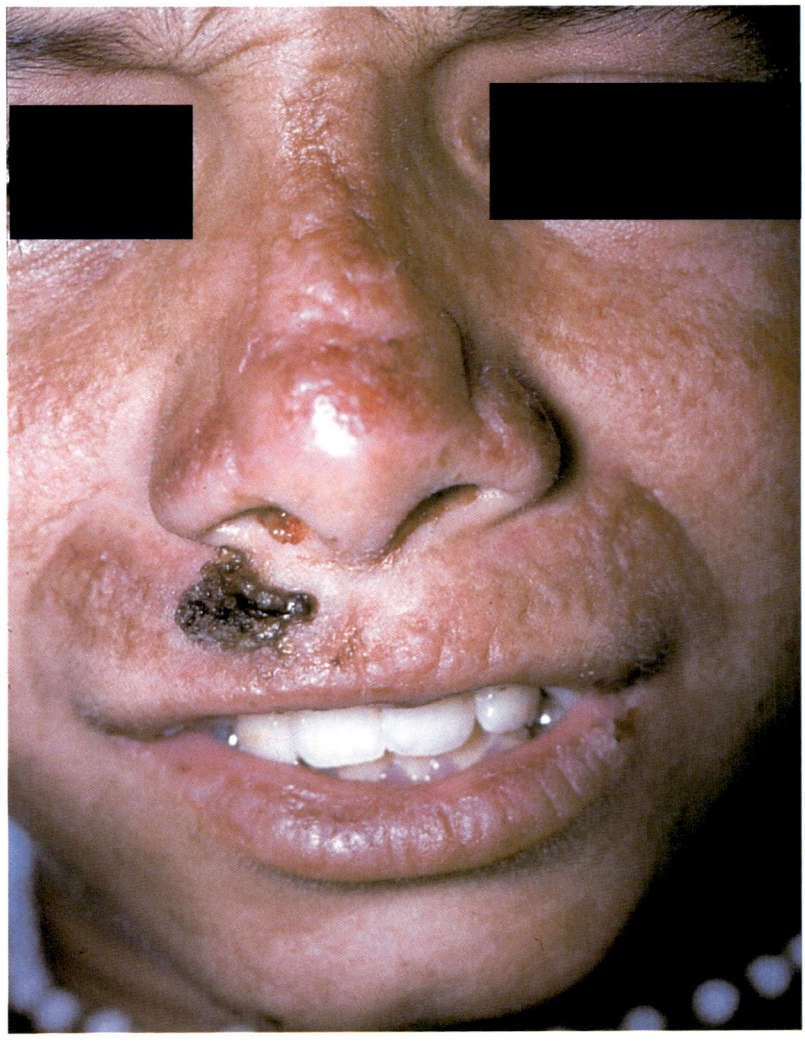

Fig. 7.54   EPP with crusts, scars, and linear furrowing of the lips in a 12-year-old boy.

DIFFERENTIAL DIAGNOSIS

EPP can be distinguished from CEP by the less severe photosensitivity, characteristic linear scarring, and absence of mutilation. Urticaria-like eruptions instead of vesicles are the predominant sign. The hematological picture of red cell protoporphyria can also be seen in iron deficiency anemia and lead intoxication, but in these disorders there are normal fecal porphyrin levels. Other sun-sensitive disorders such as polymorphous light eruption, actinic prurigo, and lupus erythematosus should be considered as well.

THERAPEUTICS AND PROGNOSIS
Topical therapy

Avoidance of sunlight, protective clothing, and sunscreens appropriate for 400nm wavelength of light are adjunctive measures. Common sunscreens protect from sunburn (290–320nm) but not from 400 to 410nm (Soret's band) light. In fact, many patients are condemned to a life in darkness.

523. Thunell S, Harper P, Brun A (2000) Porphyrins, porphyrin metabolism and porphyrias. IV. Pathophysiology of erythropoietic protoporphyria – diagnosis, care and monitoring of the patient. Scand J Clin Lab Invest 60:581–604.

Systemic management

Although only partially successful, beta-carotene (120–300mg/day in adults and 25–150mg/day in children) has been shown to be useful in many cases. Therapy must be given for at least 1 to 3 months, and blood levels of 600–800ng/ml must be achieved. The only side effect appears to be carotenoderma.[524] Terfenadine reduces the photosensitivity in some patients by its H1 receptor antagonism.[525] Cysteine has also been proposed because of its photoprotective effect.[526] Cholestyramine may be of use (4g/day), as well as S-adenosyl-L-methionine, to prevent the hepatic disease.[527] Chenodeoxycholic acid (15mg/kg/day) has been reported to be useful in some cases.[528]

Prognosis

This is a lifelong disorder and the rare occurrence of acute hepatic disease is the most serious potential threat to life. Liver transplantation has been used in such cases.[529]

CONGENITAL ERYTHROPOIETIC COPROPORPHYRIA

Congenital erythropoietic coproporphyria (ECP) is the rarest of all porphyrias, with only three cases published. The clinical picture resembles EPP with photosensitivity presenting in childhood.[490,530,531] All three cases presented elevated red blood cells, coproporphyrins, and protoporphyrins. Neither the enzymatic defect nor the responsible gene has been identified.

PORPHYRIA CUTANEA TARDA

INTRODUCTION AND HISTORICAL NOTE

Porphyria cutanea tarda (PCT) constitutes a heterogeneous group of porphyrias that includes acquired or inherited forms. Type I is a common sporadic disorder that occurs mainly in adults and often is precipitated by ethanol, estrogens, or chemical toxins. Nevertheless, a classic outbreak that occurred in Turkey in 1956, due to contamination of wheat with hexachlorobenzene, affected predominantly children. Type II and Type III (or familial porphyria) are autosomal dominant disorders that have been reported in a few children.

EPIDEMIOLOGY

Genetics

The enzyme defect in PCT is hepatic uroporphyrinogen decarboxylase (also called urogen decarboxylase); its corresponding gene has been identified at chromosome 1p34.[532] The enzyme defect has been found in sporadic and familial cases at the same level. Sporadic cases (PCT type I, MIM 176090) are probably heterozygotes for the gene defect, and manifest under special circumstances of hepatocyte damage by agents as alcohol, hepatitis C virus, iron overload, and estrogens.[533]

Familial cases (PCT type II, MIM 176100) have the deficiency of uroporphyrinogen decarboxylase activity, not only manifesting in their liver, but also in their erythrocytes and other tissues. In these cases it is conceivable that the transmission follows an autosomal dominant pattern. Several mutations have been described.[534–536]

Rare families exist in which PCT identical to the clinical and biochemical presentation of type I occurs, and they constitute type III. It is suggested that type III PCT could be the result of the involvement of other loci.[533] Homozygous cases are known as hepatoerythropoietic porphyria (HEP).[535] An association between PCT and hereditary hemochromatosis has been described, and it is currently accepted that the hemochromatosis gene (HFE) plays a role in the determination of PCT.[537–539]

Statistics

PCT is the most common porphyria observed in adults and children. In our department, it accounts for more than 50% of all porphyria cases.[527] Familial forms of PCT present at any age including the first few years of life, and represent the majority of cases in infancy, but just around 20% of cases in adults.

PRESENTING HISTORY

PCT presents with photosensitivity of the delayed type.[501] Familial forms of PCT appear from early childhood, and sporadic forms usually in middle age. There is a trigger factor in almost all cases of PCT in children, particularly drugs, infections, and malignancies.

PHYSICAL EXAMINATION

Skin

Bullae and vesicles, crusts, ulcerations that healed slowly, and atrophic scars with milia, appear on sun-exposed sites such as the dorsa of the hands, the forearms and the face (Figs 7.55 and 7.56). In distinction from other porphyrias of childhood, skin fragility and milia are prominent signs. Pigmentary changes are common, with hyperpigmentation or a mottled pattern of hypo- and hyperpigmentation over the exposed areas. Sclerodermoid changes and dystrophic calcification are unusual signs in childhood.

Hair, nail, teeth and mucous membranes

There may be striking malar hypertrichosis (Fig. 7.57) and erythrodontia with fluorescence of teeth on Wood's lamp exposure. Scarring alopecia and photo-onycholysis can be observed in adolescents.

524. Mathews-Roth MM (1993) Carotenoids in erythropoietic protoporphyria and other photosensitivity diseases. Ann N Y Acad Sci 691:127–138.

525. Farr PM, Diffey BL, Mathews JNS (1990) Inhibition of photosensitivity in erythropoietic protoporphyria with terfenadine. Br J Dermatol 122:809–815.

526. Mathews-Roth MM, Rosner B, Benfell K et al. (1994) A double-blind study of cysteine photoprotection in erythropoietic protoporphyria. Photodermatol Photoimmunol Photomed 10:244–248.

527. Batlle AM, Stella AM, Melito V et al. (1989) S-adenosil-L-metionina, un posible agente terapéutico anticolestático en las porfirias, con particular referencia a la protoporfiria eritropoyética. Resultados preliminares. Arch Argent Dermatol 39:3–21.

528. Baart de la Faille H, van Hattum J, Rademakers LHPM et al. (1987) Long term effects of chenodeoxycholic acid therapy in erythrohepatic protoporphyria. In: Dermatology in Five Continents, Proceedings 17th World Congress of Dermatology, Orfanos CE, Stadler R, Golnik H, eds. Berlin: Springer Verlag, p. 455.

530. Topi GC, D'Alessandro Gandolfo L, Fazio M et al. (1976) Coproporfiria eritropcyética congénita en 2 hermanos. Med Cutan Ibero Lat Am 4:229–238.

531. Topi GC, D'Alessandro Gandolfo L, Fazio M et al. (1977) Coproporphyrie érythropoïétique congénitale observée chez un frère et une soeur. Forme nouvelle de coproporphyrie érythropoïétique héréditaire. Ann Dermatol Venereol 104:68–70.

532. Dubart A, Mattei MG, Raich N et al. (1986) Assignment of human uroporphyrinogen decarboxylase (URO-D) to the p34 band of chromosome 1. Hum Genet 73:277–279.

533. Elder GH (1998) Genetic defects in the porphyrias: types and significance. Clin Dermatol 16:225–233.

534. Mendez M, Sorkin L, Rossetti MV et al. (1998) Familial porphyria cutanea tarda: characterization of seven novel uroporphyrinogen decarboxylase mutations and frequency of common hemochromatosis alleles. Am J Hum Genet 63:1363–1375.

535. de Verneuil H, Bourgeois F, de Rooij F et al. (1992) Characterization of a new mutation (R292G) and a deletion at the human uroporphyrinogen decarboxylase locus in two patients with hepatoerythropoietic porphyria. Hum Genet 89:548–552.

536. Cappellini MD, Martinez di Montemuros F, Tavazzi D et al. (2001) Seven novel point mutations in the uroporphyrinogen decarboxylase (UROD) gene in patients with familial porphyria cutanea tarda (f-PCT). Hum Mutat 17:350.

537. Santos M, Clevers HC, Marx JJM (1997) Mutations of the hereditary hemochromatosis candidate gene HLA-H in porphyria cutanea tarda. New Engl J Med 336:1327–1328.

538. de Villiers JNP, Hillermann R, Loubser L et al. (1999) Spectrum of mutations in the HFE gene implicated in haemochromatosis and porphyria. Hum Mol Genet 8:1517–1522.

539. Brady JJ, Jackson HA, Roberts AG et al. (2000) Co-inheritance of mutations in the uroporphyrinogen decarboxylase and hemochromatosis genes accelerates the onset of porphyria cutanea tarda. J Invest Dermatol 115:868–874.

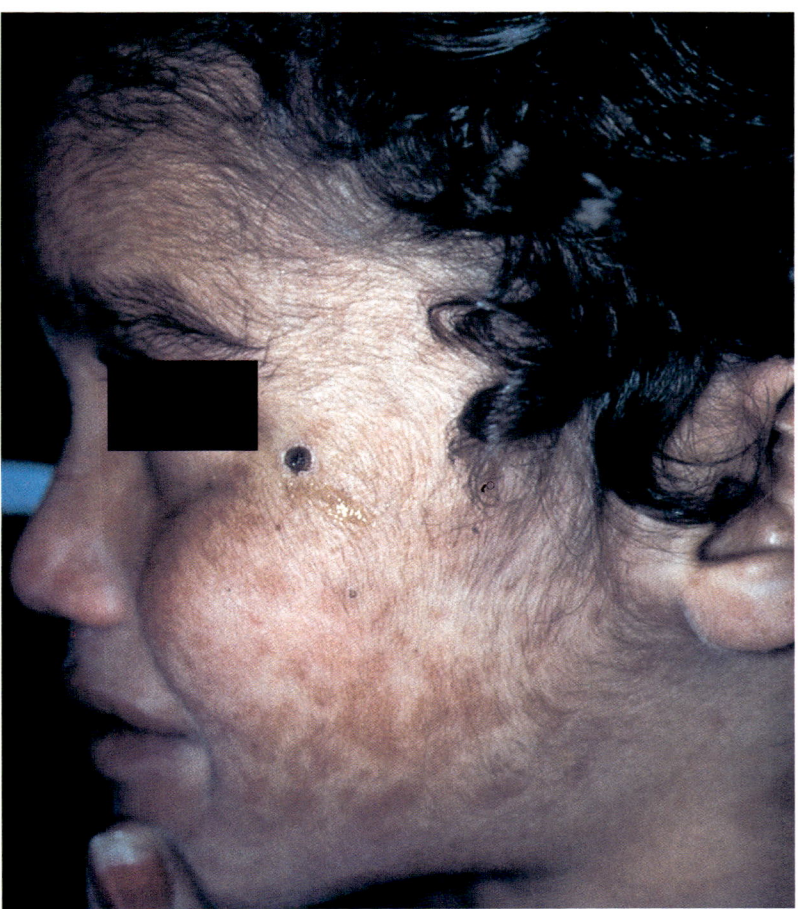

Fig. 7.55   **PCT:** scars, hypertrichosis, and hyperpigmentation on the face.

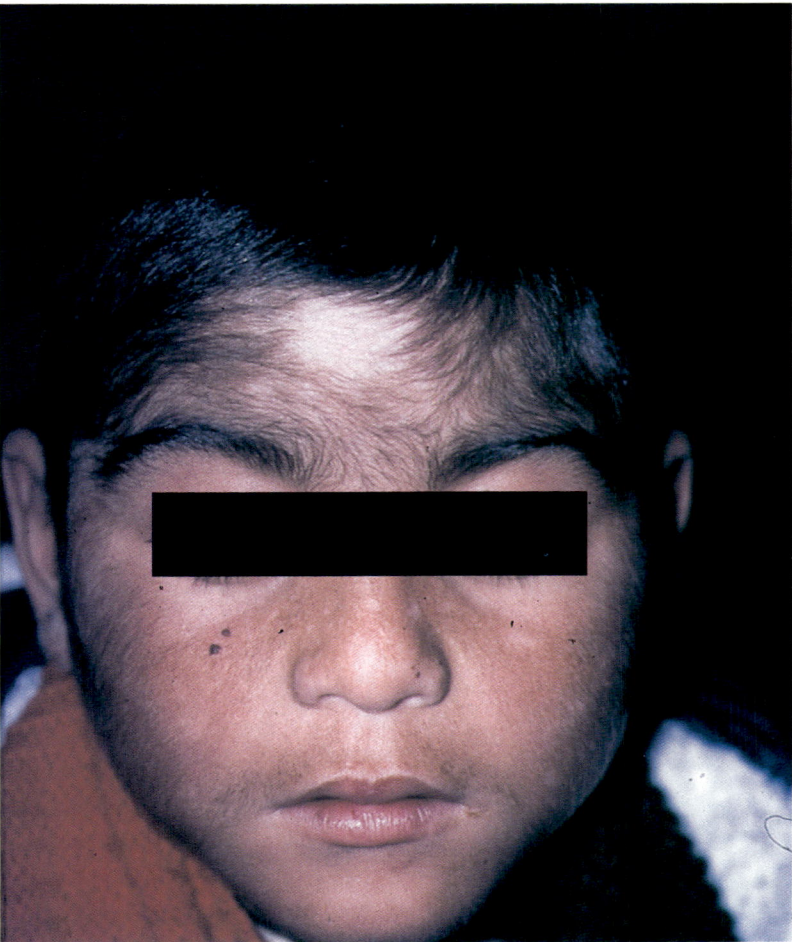

Fig. 7.57   **PCT and leukemia:** striking hypertrichosis and melanosis in an 8-year-old girl.

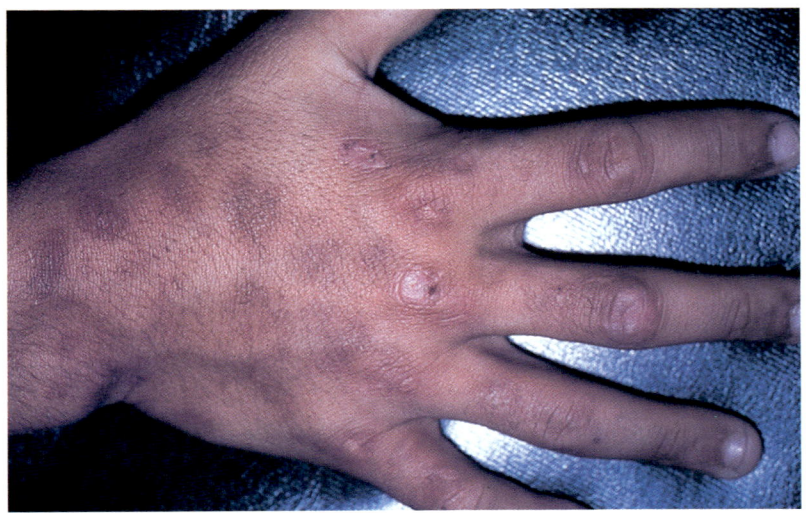

Fig. 7.56   **PCT:** old scars and hyperpigmentation over the hand.

Systemic manifestations

The photodamage to the conjunctiva leads to higher incidence of pinguecula and pterygium than in controls.[540]

There may be hepatomegaly and abnormal liver function tests. PCT has been found in association with diabetes mellitus, systemic lupus erythematosus, type B and type C hepatitis,[541] hematologic disorders (Fig. 7.58),[542] and acquired immune deficiency syndrome (AIDS).[543]

LABORATORY FINDINGS

In PCT there are elevated levels of plasma and urinary uroporphyrins, coproporphyrins, and 7-carboxylate porphyrins. Feces have high levels of isocoproporphyrinogen, sometimes with uro- and coproporphyrins. The examination of urine by Wood's light shows a coral pink fluorescence.

PATHOPHYSIOLOGY AND HISTOGENESIS
Molecular, biochemical and immunological basis

Urogen decarboxylase activity is deficient in PCT, accounting for about 50% of that of normal controls. In sporadic type I PCT there is a decreased

540. Hammer H, Korom I (1992) Photodamage of the conjunctiva in patients with porphyria cutanea tarda. **Br J Ophthalmol** 76:592–593.
541. Sampietro M, Fracanzani AL, Corbetta N et al. (1997) High prevalence of hepatitis C virus type 1b in Italian patients with porphyria cutanea tarda. **Ital J Gastroenterol Hepatol** 29:543–547.
542. Stella A, Melito V, Parera V et al. (1988) Acerca de 2 nuevos casos de porfiria cutanea tardia infantil en una niña con leucemia y en un niño hemodializado en tratamiento con SAMe. Aspectos bioquímicos. **Rev Argent Dermatol** 69:118–124.
543. Cohen PR (1991) Porphyria cutanea tarda in human immunodeficiency virus-seropositive men: case report and literature review. **J Acquir Immune Defic Syndr** 4:1112–1117.

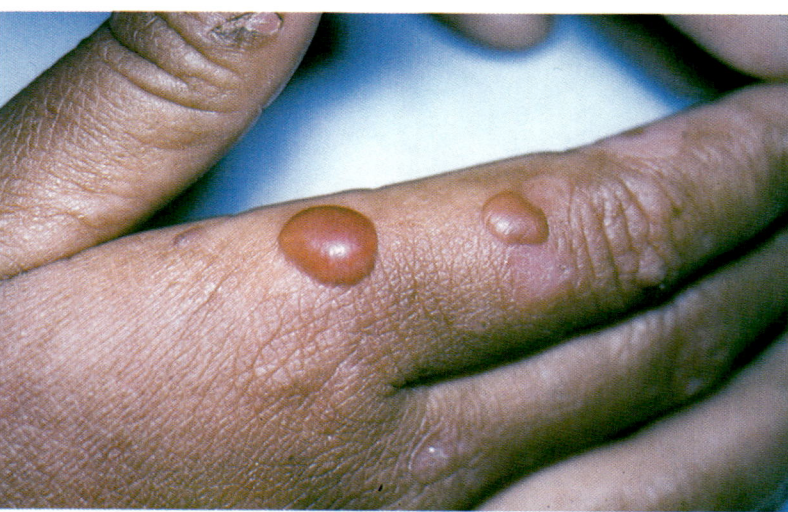

Fig. 7.58 PCT and leukemia: tense hemorrhagic bullae over the hand of the same patient.

enzyme activity in the liver. In familial type II PCT the enzyme activity is decreased both in the liver and the erythrocytes; in the other familial type III PCT, erythrocyte enzyme activity is normal. Iron overload seems to play an important role in the pathophysiology of PCT, through more than one mechanism.[501,544]

Histologic findings

Histologically, all types of PCT show a similar picture of subepidermal bullae with periodic acid–Schiff-positive material in the vessel walls and, less frequently, at the dermoepidermal junction. Immunofluorescence shows these fibrillar deposits to contain IgG and complement. Recently, a distinctive elongated structure ("caterpillar bodies") has been identified in the roof of the bullae.[545]

DIFFERENTIAL DIAGNOSIS

PCT must be differentiated from epidermolysis bullosa in children, because both entities can present with vesicles, skin fragility and milia. However, epidermolysis bullosa has no photosensitivity or hypertrichosis, and no changes in urine color.

Pseudoporphyrias secondary to drug intake or hemodialysis are identified by a careful history. In all cases, porphyrin determination in urine and feces establishes the diagnosis.

THERAPEUTICS AND PROGNOSIS

Topical therapy

Restriction of sun exposure is an essential step in topical prevention.

Systemic management

Therapeutic measures include diet avoidance of hepatotoxic substances and drugs, phlebotomy (150 to 200ml weekly) to remove iron stores and excess porphyrins,[546] low-dose chloroquine (3mg/kg twice a week),[547] S-adenosyl-

L-methionine (200mg/day for 3 weeks),[542] plasmapheresis, and iron chelating agents (deferoxamine).

PROGNOSIS

In contrast to CEP and EPP, there may be spontaneous remission with age. However, a high incidence (5–16%) of hepatocellular carcinoma has been reported in cases of PCT with a long symptomatic period before start of therapy and associated chronic active hepatitis.[548,549]

VARIEGATE PORPHYRIA

INTRODUCTION AND HISTORICAL NOTE

Variegate porphyria (VP, MIM 176200), also called South African porphyria and mixed porphyria, is a rare autosomal dominant disease.[550]

EPIDEMIOLOGY

Only few cases have been described in children. VP is frequent among the Afrikaner population of South Africa, and in Finland.[551]

Genetics

VP is an autosomal dominant disease caused by mutation in the gene for protoporphyrinogen oxidase (*PPOX*) that maps to chromosome lq22.[552]

The association with mutations in the gene for hemochromatosis (*HFE*), mapped to chromosome 6p21.3, has been found in patients with severe forms of variegate porphyria.[538]

Statistics

We mentioned above the rarity of VP in children, with just one case observed in our series.[551,553]

VP is common in South Africa, where an estimated 10 000 to 20 000 descendants from a couple from the Netherlands are affected.[554] Asymptomatic carriers of the gene defect are usually detected by screening of porphyrins.

PRESENTING HISTORY

The first clinical features of VP may include either cutaneous photosensitivity indistinguishable from that of PCT, systemic manifestations that mimic those of AIP, or both. Acute attacks are triggered by exacerbating drug intake and other unknown factors.

PHYSICAL EXAMINATION

Skin

Clinically, VP resembles PCT with excessive skin fragility, sun sensitivity, vesicles, bullae, crusts, and scarring, particularly over face and hands (Figs 7.59 and 7.60). Hyperpigmentation is observed in some cases.

Hair, nail, teeth and mucous membranes

Hypertrichosis is uncommon in children with VP, and onycholysis is associated with chronic skin changes of the hands.

544. Siersema PD, Rademakers LH, Cleton MI et al. (1995) The difference in liver pathology between sporadic and familial forms of porphyria cutanea tarda: the role of iron. **J Hepatol** 23:259–267.
545. Egbert BM, LeBoit PE, McCalmont T et al. (1993) Caterpillar bodies: distinctive, basement membrane-containing structures in blisters of porphyria. **Am J Dermatopathol** 15:199–202.
546. Poh-Fitzpatrick MB, Honig PJ, Kim HC et al. (1992) Childhood-onset familial porphyria cutanea tarda: effects of therapeutic phlebotomy. **J Am Acad Dermatol** 27:896–900.
547. Bruce AJ, Ahmed I (1998) Childhood-onset porphyria cutanea tarda: successful therapy with low-dose hydroxychloroquine (Plaquenil). **J Am Acad Dermatol** 38:810–814.
548. Siersema PD, ten Kate FJ, Mulder PG et al. (1992) Hepatocellular carcinoma in porphyria cutanea tarda: frequency and factors related to its occurrence. **Liver** 12:56–61.
549. Lim HW, Mascaro JM (1995) The porphyrias and hepatocellular carcinoma. **Dermatol Clin** 13:135–142.

550. Dean G (1972) The Porphyrias. A Story of Inheritance and Environment, 2nd edn. Philadelphia: JB Lippincott.
551. Mustajoki P, Tenhunen R, Niemi KM et al. (1987) Homozygous variegate porphyria: a severe skin disease of infancy. **Clin Genet** 32:300–305.
552. Taketani S, Inazawa J, Abe T et al. (1995) The human protoporphyrinogen oxidase gene (PFOX): organization and location to chromosome 1. **Genomics** 29:698–703.
553. Parera V, Alfonso S, Navone N et al. (1984) Porfiria variegata en una niña de 4 años. **Rev Argent Dermatol** 65:68–76.
554. Corrigall AV, Hift RJ, Davids LM et al. (2000) Homozygous variegate porphyria in South Africa: genotypic analysis in two cases. **Mol Genet Metab** 69:323–330.

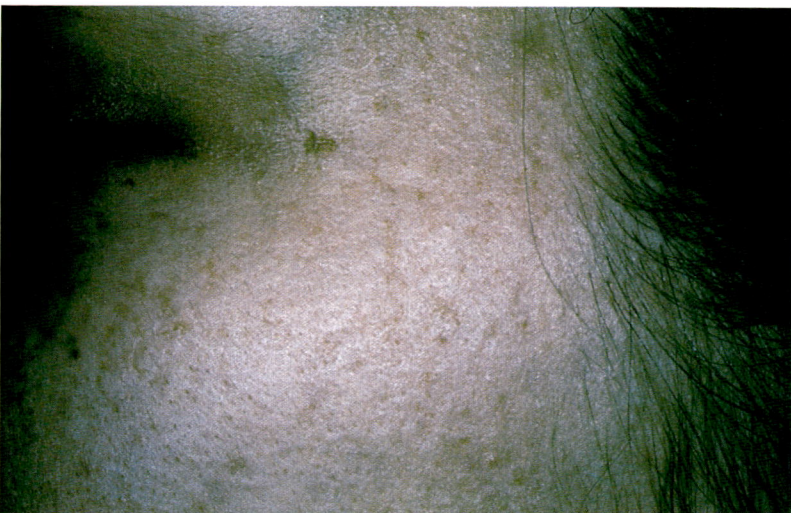

Fig. 7.59   Variegate porphyria with scars over the cheek of a 14-year-old girl.

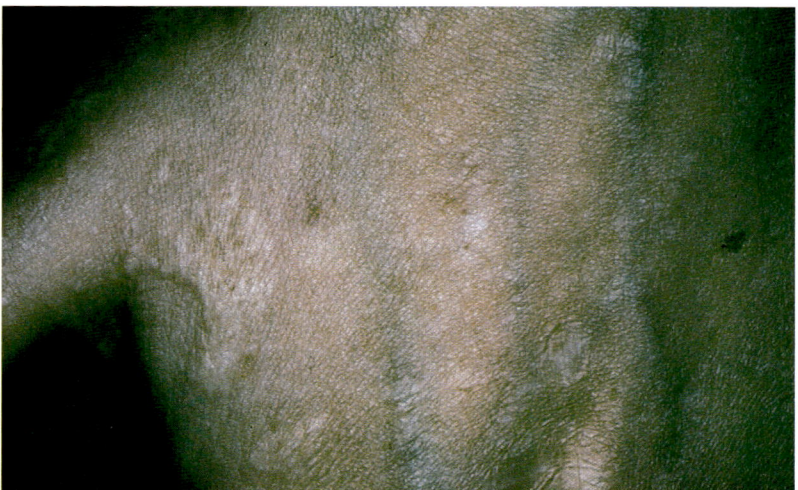

Fig. 7.60   Variegate porphyria with scars over the hand of the same patient.

Systemic manifestations

The acute attack is characterized by neurological symptoms and abdominal pain, similar to those reported in acute intermittent porphyria. The attacks are often induced by drug-intake, and present with constipation, abdominal pain, tachycardia and hypertension, muscular paralysis, and sensory disturbances. Retarded growth has been reported. Seizures, epilepsy, and mental retardation can occur, mainly in homozygous patients. Premature adrenarche has been described in a young girl.[555]

LABORATORY FINDINGS

The enzyme defect in VP is the deficiency of protoporphyrinogen oxidase (PPOX). It leads to the excretion of high amounts of ALA, PBG, coproporphyrinogen and protoporphyrinogen in urine during attacks. Protoporphyrin, and to a lesser extent coproporphyrin as well as X-porphyrins are elevated in feces between attacks and allow the biochemical identification of this porphyria. The plasma has a pathognomonic fluorescence emission pattern at 626nm.

DIFFERENTIAL DIAGNOSIS

Differentiation of VP from PCT is difficult in cases without overt neurologic symptoms, but is essential for the adequate therapeutic approach. Some therapies useful in PCT, such as antimalarials and phlebotomy, are not helpful in VP.[476]

THERAPEUTICS AND PROGNOSIS

Topical therapy and systemic management

Therapy is oriented to suppress the acute symptoms, by the intravenous infusion of glucose and heme analog.[556] Prevention is important, both for the visceral and cutaneous manifestations. Drugs and sun avoidance are imperative, and sunscreens are used. Phlebotomy is ineffective, even though the skin lesions resemble those of PCT. Relatives of patients should be screened to detect the asymptomatic carriers.

Prognosis

No cases of spontaneous remission have been reported. Acute attacks must lead to neurological deterioration. Hepatocellular carcinoma is a rare event that has been described in VP.[549]

HEREDITARY COPROPORPHYRIA

Hereditary coproporphyria (HCP, MIM 121300), first described by Berger and Goldberg in 1955,[487] presents with acute attacks of abdominal pain that resembles AIP but may have photosensitivity (20–30% of cases). It is transmitted by an autosomal dominant gene, located on chromosome 3q12.[557,558]

It is due to a partial deficiency of coproporphyrinogen oxidase, a mitochondrial enzyme that catalyzes the conversion of coproporphyrinogen III to protoporphyrinogen III. As a result of the enzyme deficiency, high quantities of coproporphyrin III are excreted in urine and predominantly in feces. About half of cases are asymptomatic.

It has been described mainly in adults, with hypertrichosis and increased skin pigmentation. The few cases in children have presented as hydroa vacciniforme with vesicles, bullae, burning, and scarring.[559] Acute peripheral neuropathy, a common feature of acute intermittent porphyria, has been described.[560]

Only rare homozygous cases have been reported in the neonatal period with jaundice, hepatosplenomegaly, hemolytic anemia, and photosensitivity. This form, where the activity of coproporphyrinogen oxidase is below 10% of normal levels, is known as harderoporphyria.[561–564] Marked elevation of coproporphyrins or harderoporphyrins in feces is the main finding.[561]

It has been demonstrated that the severity of the phenotype does not correlate with the degree of inactivation of the enzyme, ranging from 1 to 64%.[564]

555. Coakley J, Blake D, Hawkins R et a . (1990) An unusual case of variegate porphyria with possible homozygous inheritance. **Aust N Z J Med** 20:587–589.
556. Kalman DR, Bonkovsky HL (1998) Management of acute attacks in the porphyrias. **Clin Dermatol** 16:299–306.
557. Cacheux V, Martasek P, Fougerousse F et al. (1994) Localization of the human coproporphyrinogen oxidase gene to chromosome band 3q12. **Hum Genet** 94:557–559.
558. Lamoril J, Deybach JC, Puy H et al. (1997) Three novel mutations in the coproporphyrinogen oxidase gene. **Hum Mutat** 9:78–80.
559. Jeanmougin M, Pedreiro J, Manciet JR et al. (1988) Eruption à type d'hydroa vacciniforme, révélatrice d'une coproporphyrie héréditaire. **Ann Dermatol Venereol** 115:1236–1238.
560. Barohn RJ, Sanchez JA, Anderson KE (1994) Acute peripheral neuropathy due to hereditary coproporphyria. **Muscle Nerve** 17:793–799.
561. Nordmann Y, Grandchamp B, de Verneuil H et al. (1983) Harderoporphyria: a variant hereditary coproporphyria. **J Clin Invest** 72:1139–1149.
562. Lamoril J, Martasek P, Deybach JC et al. (1995) A molecular defect in coproporphyrinogen oxidase gene causing harderoporphyria, a variant form of hereditary coproporphyria. **Hum Mol Genet** 4:275–278.
563. Lamoril J, Puy H, Gouya L et al. (1998) Neonatal hemolytic anemia due to inherited harderoporphyria: clinical characteristics and molecular basis. **Blood** 91:1453–1457.
564. Lamoril J, Puy H, Whatley SD et al. (2001) Characterization of mutations in the CPO gene in British patients demonstrates absence of genotype–phenotype correlation and identifies relationship between hereditary coproporphyria and harderoporphyria. **Am J Hum Genet** 68:1130–1138.

HEPATOERYTHROPOIETIC PORPHYRIA

Hepatoerythropoietic porphyria (HEP, MIM 176100.0002), an extremely rare disorder, has been described with onset in the first year of life.[491] Clinically, it mimics CEP, with red teeth, anemia, and hepatosplenic abnormalities. Later on, patients can present with hypertrichosis, skin photosensitivity, and scleroderma-like changes of their hands.[565]

In HEP there is massively elevated erythrocyte protoporphyrin that is not seen in the childhood onset familial form of PCT. Urinary uroporphyrins and 7-carboxylate porphyrins, and fecal isocoproporphyrins and coproporphyrins are increased. This pathway may be related to the extraordinarily elevated levels of abnormal porphyrins found in HEP that suggest overproduction in both the liver and the bone marrow.

The enzyme defect, as in PCT, is hepatic uroporphyrinogen decarboxylase. It is believed that HEP is the homozygous or compound heterozygous form of familial autosomal dominant PCT.[566,567] A specific mutation of the gene at chromosome 1p34 has been found in HEP.[568]

Sun avoidance is essential. Phlebotomy is an ineffective treatment, since plasma iron concentration is normal.

OTHER PORPHYRIAS

Acute intermittent porphyria (AIP, MIM 176000) and ALA-dehydratase porphyria (ALADP, MIM 125270) have no cutaneous manifestations since the porphyrin precursors that accumulate are not photosensitizers. They do not usually occur before puberty.[476,501] Diverse atypical forms of porphyria may be observed. The association of two varieties of porphyria in the same patient or family is called *dual porphyria*.[569]

TABLE 7.22	Drugs that can induce acute attack of porphyria
Alcohol	Hydantoins
Amitriptyline	Hydrochlorothiazide
Amphetamines	Imipramine
Apronalide	Isoniazid
Barbiturates	Mefenamic acid
Busulfan	Meprobamate
Carbamazepine	Methyldopa
Chlorambucil	Methochlorpramide
Chloramphenicol	Metronidazole
Chlordiazepoxide	Nalidixic acid
Chloroquine	Pirazolones
Chlorpromazine	Phenylbutazone
Chlorpropamide	Phenytoin
Colistin	Probenecid
Danazol	Progestogens
Dapsone	Pyrazinamide
Diethyl propionate	Pyrazolone derivatives
Diazepam	Rifampicin
Diclofenac	Sulfonamides
Ergot preparations	Sulfonylureas
Erythromycin	Tetracycline
Estrogens	Theophylline
Flufenamic acid	Valproic acid
Griseofulvin	Xylocaine
Halothane	

Under the name of "pseudoporphyria" are included an array of cutaneous lesions that resemble those of PCT without demonstrable abnormalities of porphyrin metabolism. A PCT-like condition has been described in patients undergoing chronic hemodialysis for renal failure.[542,570,571] The mechanism is unclear, but iron overload could play an important role.

DRUG-INDUCED PORPHYRIA

It is clear that drugs can cause porphyria in the absence of any identifiable genetic predisposition, producing a clinical and biochemical disorder similar to that of other human porphyria (e.g., hexachlorobenzene and PCT in Turkey).[572]

Drugs that have been incriminated in the precipitation of acute attacks of porphyria include anticonvulsants, barbiturates, sex steroid hormones, and griseofulvin (Table 7.22).

PHOTOSENSITIVITY DISORDERS OTHER THAN PORPHYRIAS

XERODERMA PIGMENTOSUM

INTRODUCTION AND HISTORICAL NOTE

The term *xeroderma pigmentosum* was first applied in 1870 by Kaposi[578] to describe a patient with pigmentation accompanying skin atrophy. The first American cases were described in 1878.[573] De Sanctis–Cacchione syndrome, with neurologic deterioration, was first presented in 1883 by Albert Neisser of Germany.[574]

Xeroderma pigmentosum (XP) is now known to be a genetically heterogeneous group of degenerative disorders in which sun sensitivity, oculocutaneous pigmentation, and neoplasia are manifestations of abnormal DNA repair. In some cases, progressive neurologic impairment occurs as well.[573,575]

Intensive research has been performed on XP patients, primarily because it is a model for sun-induced cancer, as well as neurodegenerative disease. Determination of the defective DNA nucleotide excision repair mechanisms in ultraviolet-irradiated skin fibroblasts from xeroderma pigmentosum patients allows the distinction of seven complementation groups (A–G) of the disease.[573] A variant type of xeroderma pigmentosum (XP-V), where unscheduled DNA synthesis is normal but postreplication DNA repair is defective, has been described.[576]

EPIDEMIOLOGY

Genetics

XP is usually inherited as an autosomal recessive trait. Parental consanguinity is common. Autosomal dominant inheritance has been found in few mild cases of XP-B, mainly associated with Cockayne syndrome. Similar phenotypes had different gene defects, most of them having being identified to date (Table 7.23).[577]

Statistics

The frequency in Europe and the United States (1 to 2 per 1 000 000 births) is much lower than in Japan (1 per 40 000).[578,579] All races, including whites, Asians, blacks, and native Americans could be affected. There is no sex preference for XP.[574]

565. Fujimoto A, Brazil JL (1992) Hepatoerythropoietic porphyria in a woman with short stature and deformed hands. **Am J Med Genet** 44:496–499.
566. de Verneuil H, Grandchamp B, Foubert C et al. (1984) Assignment of the gene for uroporphyrinogen decarboxylase to human chromosome 1 by somatic cell hybridization and specific enzyme immunoassay. **Hum Genet** 66:202–205.
567. de Verneuil H, Grandchamp B, Romeo PH et al. (1986) Molecular analysis of urcporphyrinogen decarboxylase deficiency in a family with two cases of hepatoerythropoietic porphyria. **J Clin Invest** 77:431–435.
568. de Verneuil H, Hansen J, Picat C et al. (1988) Prevalence of the 281 (gly-to-glu) mutation in hepatoerythropoietic porphyria and porphyria cutanea tarda. **Hum Genet** 78:101–102.

569. Parera VE, Stella AM, Batlle AM (1988) Porfiria dual: coexistencia de porfiria cutanea tardia y porfiria aguda intermitente en los mismos miembros de una familia. **Rev Argent Dermatol** 69:196–198.
570. Harvey E, Bell CH, Paller AS et al. (1992) Pseudoporphyria cutanea tarda: two case reports on children receiving peritoneal dialysis and erythropoietin therapy. **J Pediatr** 121:749–752.
571. Green JJ, Manders SM (2001) Pseudoporphyria. **J Am Acad Dermatol** 44:100–108.
572. Hebra F, Kaposi M (1874) On Diseases of the Skin, including Exanthemata. London: **The New Sydenham Society** 3:252–258.
573. Lambert WC, Kuo HR, Lambert MW (1995) Xeroderma pigmentosum. **Dermatol Clin** 13:169–209.
574. Kraemer KH, Lee MM, Scotto J (1987) Xeroderma pigmentosum: cutaneous, ocular, and neurologic abnormalities in 830 published cases. **Arch Dermatol** 123:241–250.

TABLE 7.23   Xeroderma pigmentosum complementation groups, genes involved and clinical features

Group	MIM	Gene map locus	Enzyme encoded	Frequency	Skin disease	Skin cancer	Neurologic symptoms	Associations
XP-A	278700	9q22.3	DDB1	Japan +++ US, Europe, Middle East, Tunis	+++	+++	+ to +++ subset with no symptoms, De Sanctis–Cachione	
XP-B	133510	2q21	ERCC3	Extremely rare US, Europe (3 cases)	++ to +++	+++	+++	Cockayne syndrome TTD (one case)
XP-C	278720	3p25	Endonuclease	Commonest worldwide Japan: rare	++ to +++	++ melanoma	rare	
XP-D	278730	19q13.2–13.3	ERCC2	Moderate common: 20% of cases	++	+	absent or moderate late onset	TTD XP–CS complex
XP-E	278740	11p12–p11	DDB2	rare	+	rare	0 or +	
XP-F	278760	16p13.3–p13.13	ERCC4	Moderate rare Japan & Europe	++	few or absent	absent (1 case severe)	
XP-G	278780	13q33	Endonuclease	Extremely rare (5 cases)	+++	few or absent	those of CS	Cockayne syndrome
XP-V	278750	6p21.1–p12	Polymerase eta	1/3 of all cases	++ to +++	late onset ++	++ few cases	

ERCC, Excision-repair cross-complementing genes; DDB, DNA damage-binding protein; 0 = absent; + = mild; ++ = moderate; +++ = severe.
TTD, Trichothiodystrophy; CS, Cockayne syndrome; XP–CS complex, xeroderma pigmentosum–Cockayne syndrome complex.

PRESENTING HISTORY

The following general clinical features are shared to varying degrees by most of patients in different complementation groups. Affected infants present with photophobia and chronic conjunctivitis during the first few months of life. Half of patients with XP have severe sunburn reactions on minimal UV exposure. All patients have some degree of UV reaction on sun-exposed areas of skin. Resolving erythema is then replaced with irregular freckling and mottled hyperpigmentation and hypopigmentation, telangiectasias, dryness, atrophy and scarring that justify the name "xeroderma pigmentosum." The appearance of the skin in children under 2 years of age is similar to that occurring in adults after many years of intense sun exposure, but without dermal elastosis. The tendency to acute sun sensitivity subsides with age.[574]

PHYSICAL EXAMINATION

Skin

Examination of the skin may reveal erythema along with scaling and hyperpigmented macules (Figs 7.61 and 7.62). The facial skin becomes atrophic, with permanent telangiectasias. Blisters, crusts, actinic keratoses, and scars develop at an early age, and with the advent of malignant tumors may cause marked distortion of the nose, eyes, and mouth (Figs 7.63–65). The median age of onset of non–melanoma skin cancer is at about 8 years of age.[573,574,578]

Keratoacanthomas (Fig. 7.66), basal cell carcinomas, squamous cell carcinomas, and malignant melanomas appear, primarily in sun-exposed areas, causing considerable mutilation (Figs 7.65 and 7.66). Lentigo malignant melanoma of the face is the commonest type of such malignancy, with a median age for development of 17.5 years.[580] Multiple primary cutaneous neoplasms commonly occur.[581] It has been estimated that the overall incidence of squamous and basal cell carcinomas is 2500 times greater than that of the general United States population, while that of malignant melanoma is 1000 times greater.[578] Less common skin tumors include sarcomas, fibromas,

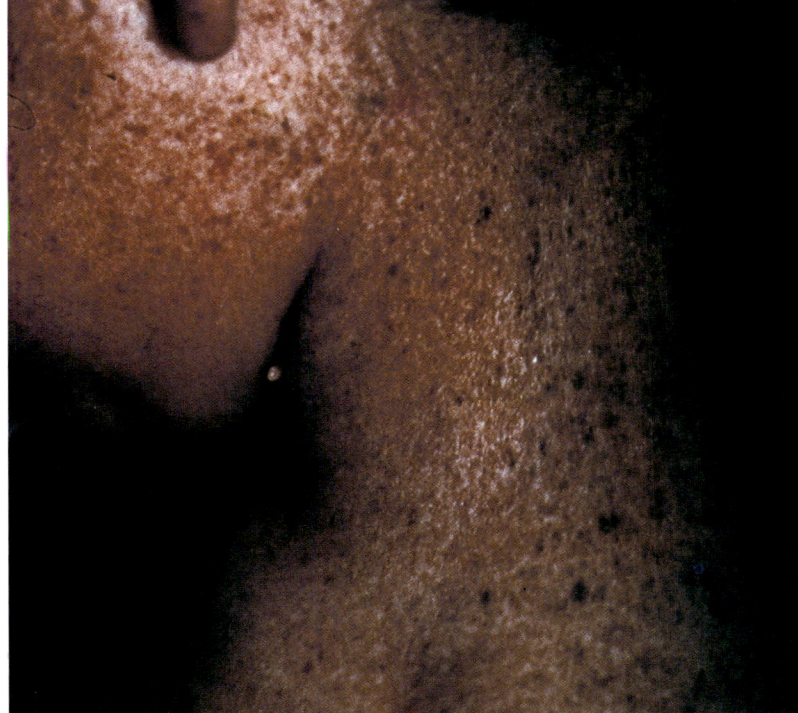

Fig. 7.61   **Xeroderma pigmentosum:** freckling on the neck of a 2-year-old boy.

histiocytomas, and angiomas.[574,580] Variation in occurrence of malignancies in XP appears to be related to the degree of sun exposure and the genetic heterogeneity.[573]

575. Moss C, Savin J (1985) Dermatology and the New Genetics. Oxford: Blackwell, pp. 113–115.
576. Lehmann AR, Kirk-Bell S, Arlett CF et al. (1975) Xeroderma pigmentosum cells with normal levels of excision repair have a defect in DNA synthesis after UV-irradiation. **Proc Nal Acad Sci USA** 72:219–223.
577. McKusick VA (2001) Online Mendelian Inheritance in Man (OMIM). Johns Hopkins University, http://www.ncbi.nlm.nih.gov/omim
578. Kraemer KH (1999) Heritable diseases with increased sensitivity to cellular injury. In: Fitzpatrick's Dermatology in General Medicine, 5th edn, Freedberg IM, Eisen AZ, Wolff K et al., eds. New York: McGraw-Hill, pp. 1848–1862.
579. Takebe H, Nishigori C, Saoth Y (1987) Genetics and skin cancer of xeroderma pigmentosum in Japan. **Jpn J Cancer Res** 78:1135–1143.
580. Bernerd F, Asselineau D, Vioux C et al. (2001) Clues to epidermal cancer proneness revealed by reconstruction of DNA repair-deficient xeroderma pigmentosum skin in vitro. **Proc Natl Acad Sci USA** 98:7817–7822.
581. Fazaa B, Zghal M, Bailly C et al. (2001) Mélanome malin et xeroderma pigmentosum: 12 cas. **Ann Dermatol Venereol** 128:503–506.

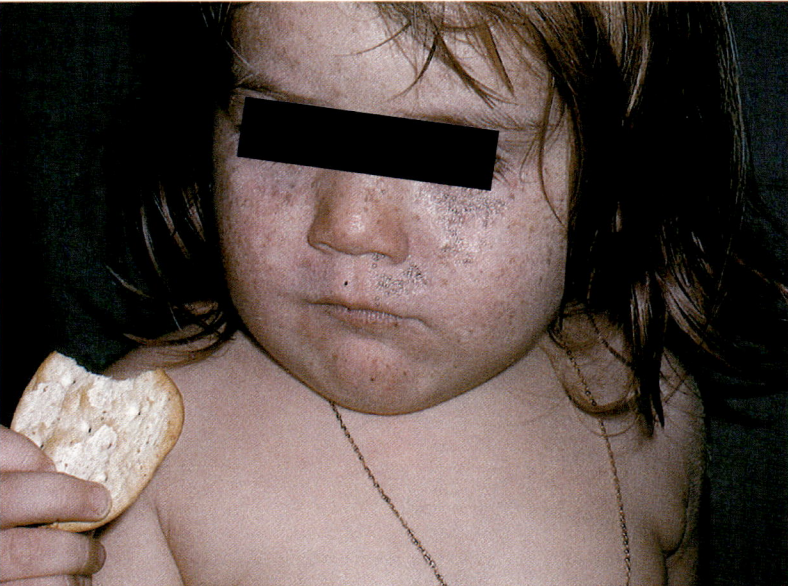

Fig. 7.62   **Xeroderma pigmentosum:** freckling on the face of a 1-year-old girl.

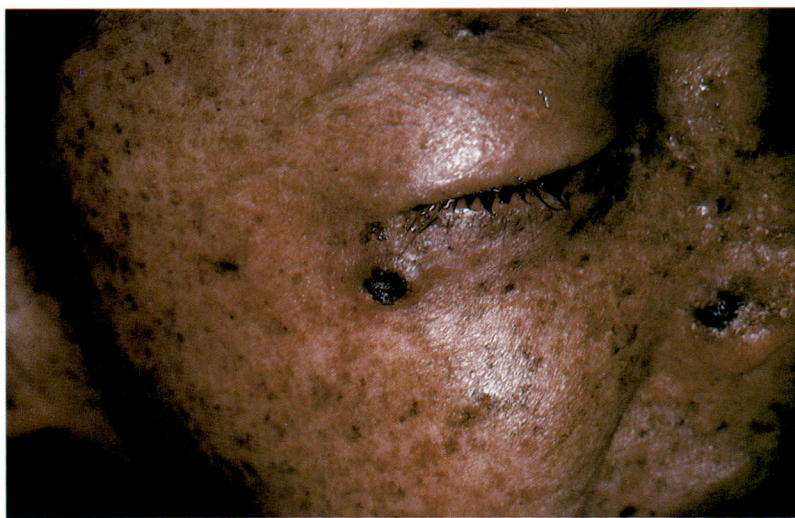

Fig. 7.64   **Xeroderma pigmentosum:** freckling and ulcerated BCC in a 3-year-old boy.

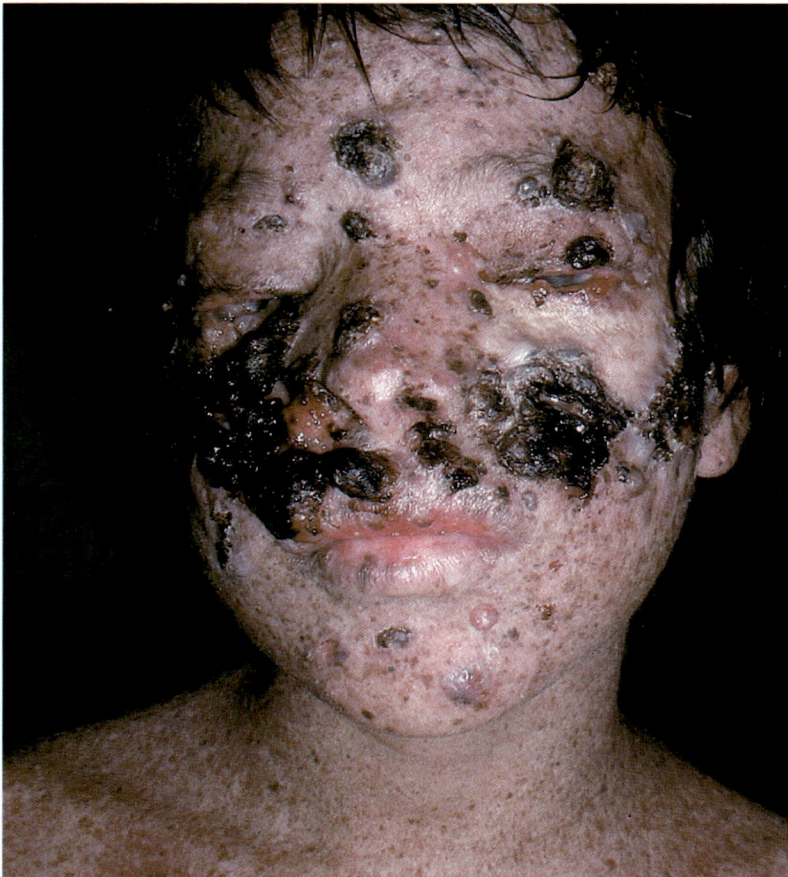

Fig. 7.63   **Xeroderma pigmentosum:** multiple carcinomas on the face of a 9-year-old boy.

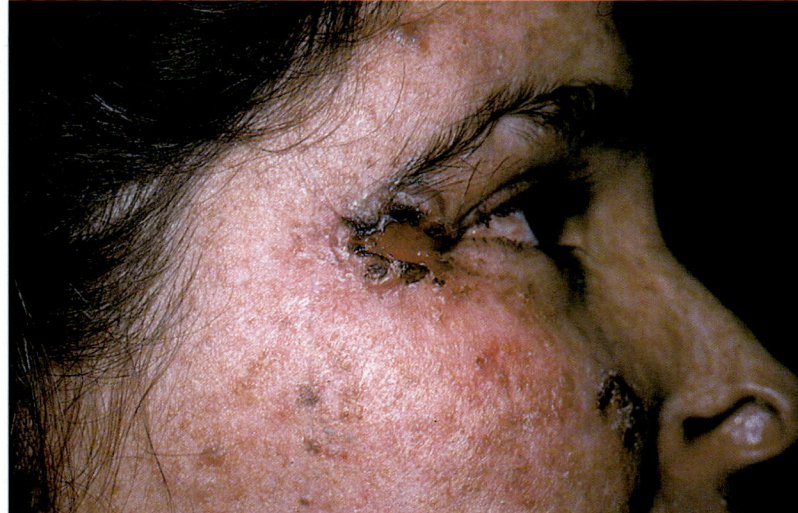

Fig. 7.65   **Xeroderma pigmentosum:** ulcerated basal cell carcinoma in an 18-year-old girl.

Hair, nail, teeth and mucous membranes

Squamous cell carcinomas of the anterior third of the tongue are common, probably because of sun exposure. XP patients younger than 20 years of age have an estimated 1000 times greater frequency of these tumors than expected for their age. Glossal telangiectasias, leukoplakia and other degenerative changes on the tongue and oral cavity may be caused by ultraviolet radiation.[581,582]

Ophthalmologic manifestations

The ophthalmic findings are very important in XP, and almost as common as the cutaneous manifestations.[574,578]

582. Patton LL, Valdex JH (1991) Xeroderma pigmentosum: review and report of a case. **Oral Surg Oral Med Oral Pathol** 71:297–300.

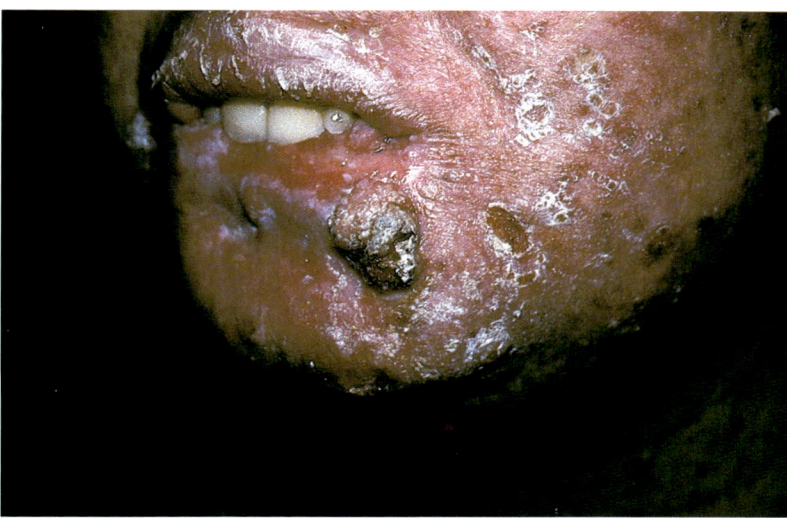

Fig. 7.66   Xeroderma pigmentosum: keratoacanthoma in the same patient as in Fig. 7.65.

Clinical findings are virtually confined to the anterior portion of the eye, exposed to UV radiation, although choroidal melanomas have been seen. Photophobia is usually present since the first months of life, associated with conjunctival injection. Three-quarters of patients aged 6 months to 3 years demonstrate blepharitis, symblepharon, and crusts on palpebral margins.

The lids are often affected with progressive madarosis, scarring, atrophy, entropion or ectropion, trichiasis, lagophthalmos, symblepharon, ankyloblepharon, and even loss of the entire lower lid substance. Basal cell epithelioma, squamous cell carcinoma and melanoma commonly occur on lid margins. Conjunctiva may be involved with hyperemia, xerosis, edema, tenacious mucoid exudates, keratinization, hyperpigmentation, atrophy, pinguecula, pseudopterygiae, or malignancy. The corneas are frequently hypervascularized, opacified, and ulcerated or have nodular neoplasms. The irides may be inflamed, atrophic, or abnormally pigmented or may have synechiae.

Systemic manifestations

The incidence of internal tumors in XP patients is estimated as 10- to 20-fold increased.[574,578,583] Reports of brain (medulloblastoma), central nervous system (astrocytoma), lung, gastric, pancreatic, uterine, breast, renal and testicular tumors account for the higher incidence.[578] Many patients die of neoplastic complications before age 20.

Neurologic involvement has been observed in 30% of patients with XP, mainly in the XP-A group.[573] Mild to severe neurologic abnormalities begin early in infancy or later, up to the second decade (see the section, Xeroderma of De Sanctis and Cacchione).[574] Hyporeflexia, spasticity, seizures, sensorineural deafness, ataxia, and progressive mental retardation have been reported.[584–588] Skeletal and other developmental abnormalities may occur as well.

LABORATORY FINDINGS

Various metabolic and biochemical abnormalities may accompany xeroderma pigmentosum, including renal impairment, aminoaciduria, hypoglycinemia, and adrenal hypofunction.[588] Deficiencies in cellular defenses against oxidative damage, mainly catalase deficiency, have been reported.[573,589–594] Defective adaptive T-cell–mediated immune responses, deficient NK cell function, depressed induction of interferon gamma activity, and immunodeficiencies have been demonstrated.[573,593,595] The quality of immune function may determine the severity of skin neoplasia.

PATHOPHYSIOLOGY AND HISTOGENESIS
Molecular, biochemical and immunological basis
At least seven different genetic defects leading to defective DNA nucleotide excision repair are known.[573,575,577,578] In each form, there is diminished DNA repair in cells exposed to light in the sunburn range (290–310nm). These patients have impaired removal of pyrimidine dimers because of deficient enzyme activity; they may be assigned to one of seven XP complementation groups (A, B, C, D, E, F, or G) based on *in vitro* cell-fusion studies, with DNA repair rates ranging from 0 to 50% of normal.

Each complementation group has its own gene defect, as shown in Table 7.23. These genes regulate the appropriate enzymes in the DNA nucleotide excision repair pathway.[595–597]

Some patients with XP have normal DNA nucleotide excision repair and thus not fall into any of the complementation groups. They have a defect in the postreplication DNA synthesis after ultraviolet irradiation, and constitute the so-called variant type of XP.[598,599]

Studies on gene function and phenotype show a great individual variety.[600–604] The gene mutations in different XP patients have been reviewed by Cleaver *et al.*[605]

583. Mamada A, Miura K, Tsunoda K et al. (1992) Xeroderma pigmentosum variant associated with multiple skin cancers and a lung cancer. **Dermatology** 184:177–181.
584. De Sanctis C, Cacchione A (1932) L'idiozia xerodermica. **Riv Sper Freniatr** 56:269–292.
585. Rapin I, Lindenbaum Y, Dickson DW et al. (2000) Cockayne syndrome and xeroderma pigmentosum. **Neurology** 55:1442–1449.
586. Rolig RL, McKinnon PJ (2000) Linking DNA damage and neurodegeneration. **Trends Neurosci** 23:417–424.
587. Zafeiriou DI, Thorel F, Andreou A et al. (2001) Xeroderma pigmentosum group G with severe neurological involvement and features of Cockayne syndrome in infancy. **Pediatr Res** 49:407–412.
588. Khan SG, Levy HL, Legerski R et al. (1998) Xeroderma pigmentosum group C splice mutation associated with autism and hypoglycinemia. **J Invest Dermatol** 111:791–796.
589. Nishigori C, Miyachi Y, Imamura S et al. (1989) Reduced superoxide dismutase activity in xeroderma pigmentosum fibroblasts. **J Invest Dermatol** 93:506–510.
590. Schallreuter KU, Pittelkow MR, Wood JM (1991) Defects in antioxidant defense and calcium transport in the epidermis of xeroderma pigmentosum patients. **Arch Dermatol Res** 283:449–455.
591. Hoffschir F, Daya-Grosjean L, Petit PX et al. (1998) Low catalase activity in xeroderma pigmentosum fibroblasts and SV40-transformed human cell lines is directly related to decreased intracellular levels of the cofactor, NADPH. **Free Radic Biol Med** 24:809–816.
592. Vuillaume M, Daya-Grosjean L, Vincens P et al. (1992) Striking differences in cellular catalase activity between two DNA repair-deficient diseases: xeroderma pigmentosum and trichothiodystrophy. **Carcinogenesis** 13:321–328.
593. Gennery AR, Cant AJ, Jeggo PA (2000) Immunodeficiency associated with DNA repair defects. **Clin Exp Immunol** 121:1–7.
594. Norris PG, Limb GA, Hamblin AS et al. (1990) Immune function, mutant frequency and cancer risk in the DNA repair defective genodermatoses xeroderma pigmentosum, Cockayne's syndrome and trichothiodystrophy. **J Invest Dermatol** 94:94–100.
595. Moriwaki S, Kraemer KH (2001) Xeroderma pigmentosum – bridging a gap between clinic and laboratory. **Photodermatol Photoimmunol Photomed** 17:47–54.
596. Hanawalt PC (2001) Controlling the efficiency of excision repair. **Mutat Res** 485:3–13.
597. Berneburg M, Lehmann AR (2001) Xeroderma pigmentosum and related disorders: defects in DNA repair and transcription. **Adv Genet** 43:71–102.
598. Yuasa M, Masutani C, Eki T et al. (2000) Genomic structure, chromosomal localization and identification of mutations in the xeroderma pigmentosum variant (XPV) gene. **Oncogene** 19:4721–4728.
599. Itoh T, Linn S, Kamide R et al. (2000) Xeroderma pigmentosum variant heterozygotes show reduced levels of recovery of replicative DNA synthesis in the presence of caffeine after ultraviolet irradiation. **J Invest Dermatol** 115:981–985.
600. Gozukara EM, Khan SG, Metin A et al. (2001) A stop codon in xeroderma pigmentosum group C families in Turkey and Italy: molecular genetic evidence for a common ancestor. **J Invest Dermatol** 117:197–204.
601. Lehmann AR (2001) The xeroderma pigmentosum group D (XPD) gene: one gene, two functions, three diseases. **Genes Dev** 15:15–23.
602. Tomescu D, Kavanagh G, Ha T et al. (2001) Nucleotide excision repair gene XPD polymorphisms and genetic predisposition to melanoma. **Carcinogenesis** 22:403–408.
603. Nag A, Bondar T, Shiv S et al. (2001) The xeroderma pigmentosum group e gene product ddb2 is a specific target of cullin 4a in mammalian cells. **Mol Cell Biol** 21:6738–6747.
604. Emmert S, Schneider TD, Khan SG et al. (2001) The human XPG gene: gene architecture, alternative splicing and single nucleotide polymorphisms. **Nucleic Acids Res** 29:1443–1452.
605. Cleaver JE, Thompson LH, Richardson AS et al. (1999) A summary of mutations in the UV-sensitive disorders: xeroderma pigmentosum, Cockayne syndrome, and trichothiodystrophy. **Hum Mutat** 14:9–22.

Complementation group A is the most common in Japan, and it is also frequently observed in Europe, the United States, and Asia. Complementation group C is the most common worldwide and in particular in Europe and the United States. Complementation groups D and F have intermediate frequency, and the other three (Groups B, E and G) are extremely rare.[573,579]

The variant form of XP accounts for one-third of XP patients worldwide, and it is specially common in Japan.[573] Sister chromatid exchanges are normal in XP patients before irradiation, but are much increased when compared to controlled patients exposed to UV irradiation.[573,578]

Histologic findings

Initially, no specific pathologic findings are present in XP. However, telangiectasias and edema of papillary dermis with chronic lymphocytic infiltration, epidermal atrophy, and hyperkeratosis may be suggestive in a young person. In the pigmented areas, melanin is markedly increased in granular, malpighiian, and basal layers and in the upper dermis. Hyperkeratosis and telangiectasias are pronounced. The atrophic changes resemble chronic radiation dermatitis with epidermal atrophy, absent pigment in areas, collagen degeneration, solar elastosis, and increased vascularity. Malignant proliferations have the same characteristics seen in patients without xeroderma pigmentosum.[573,574]

DIFFERENTIAL DIAGNOSIS

The early sunburn stage of XP may resemble severe sunburn, drug-induced photosensitivity, erythropoietic protoporphyria, polymorphous light eruption, Cockayne syndrome, Rothmund–Thomson syndrome, Bloom syndrome, or Hartnup syndrome. The childhood appearance of basal cell cancers may occur in basal cell nevus syndrome. The pigmentation in xeroderma pigmentosum may mimic radiodermatitis, poikiloderma atrophicans, urticaria pigmentosa, scleroderma, dyskeratosis congenita, arsenic ingestion, or generalized lentigines or ephelides.[578]

XP may be diagnosed by studying the DNA repair or postreplication repair abnormalities in skin fibroblasts following UV radiation exposure. Carriers are clinically normal, although some heterozygotes may have a slight degree of defective DNA repair. Similar findings may be seen in lymphocytes and epidermal cells.

XP can be diagnosed prenatally by showing a decrease in UV-induced damaged DNA repair in cultured amniotic fluid cells, by DNA analysis of trophoblast cells, polymerase chain reaction (PCR), and alkaline comet assay.[606–612]

THERAPEUTICS AND PROGNOSIS

Topical therapy

The treatment of XP should include genetic counseling, and a rigorous program of protection against UV light from infancy with the best sunscreens available, wearing of UV blocking clothing, eyeglasses that block UV radiation, and modification of the patient's lifestyle to minimize UV exposure. Premalignant skin lesions may be treated with cryosurgery or topical antimitotic agents such as 5-fluorouracil (5-FU)[613] and imiquimod. Early removal of neoplasms should be accomplished with excision, chemosurgery, cryosurgery, or intralesional IFN-α.[578]

Dental use of UV light–cured resins such as dental restorative materials, occlusal sealants, and orthodontic bracket adhesives should be avoided in xeroderma pigmentosum patients.[582]

The external use of a prokaryotic DNA repair enzyme has been reported with some success, related to recovery of catalase activity.[614] Pseudocatalase therapy has been reported in one case.[615]

Different surgical approaches, including resurfacing, dermabrasion, and facial full thickness skin grafts can be useful in some patients with extensive carcinomas.[616–621]

Systemic management

In selected XP patients, oral isotretinoin (1mg/kg/day) has been shown to significantly reduce the incidence of skin cancers.[622]

Prognosis

Pigmentation and cutaneous neoplasms in XP patients can rarely be prevented, but early protection from UV irradiation should be attempted. Systemic cancer leads to death at 20 years old in the most severely affected patients.

XERODERMA OF DE SANCTIS AND CACCHIONE

In 1932, De Sanctis and Cacchione[16] described three brothers with XP and microcephaly, delayed motor development, progressive mental deterioration, sensorineural deafness, peripheral neuropathy, dwarfism, and immature sexual development. De Sanctis–Cacchione syndrome is now frequently applied to a subset of patients with xeroderma pigmentosum (20–60% in various series) afflicted with classic cutaneous and ocular manifestations together with a variety of neurologic and developmental abnormalities. According to Lambert[573] the term "De Sanctis–Cacchione syndrome" must be reserved for those severely affected patients, whose signs and symptoms begin in infancy, and have the full syndrome described by those authors. These may include microcephaly with progressive mental retardation, choreoathetosis, cerebellar ataxia, diminished reflexes, spasticity, sensorineural deafness, epilepsy, shortening of the Achilles tendons with the development of quadriparesis, testicular hypoplasia, and dwarfism. When the ability to speak is lost, the term *xerodermic idiocy* has been applied. Less severely afflicted patients may not manifest neurologic abnormalities, such as emotional lability, electroencephalographic (EEG) aberrations, hyporeflexia, deafness, or mental retardation, until adolescence.[573,578]

The most extremely affected individuals with De Sanctis–Cacchione syndrome belong to xeroderma pigmentosum complementation group A, the most common form in Japan. A spectrum of neurologic disease may be seen

606. Ramsay CA, Coltart TM, Blunt S et al. (1974) Prenatal diagnosis of xeroderma pigmentosum. Report of the first successful case. **Lancet** 2(7889):1109–1112.
607. Halley DJ, Keijzer W, Jaspers NG et al. (1979) Prenatal diagnosis of xeroderma pigmentosum (group C) using assays of unscheduled DNA synthesis and postreplication repair. **Clin Genet** 16:137–146.
608. Arase S, Bohnert E, Fischer E et al. (1985) Prenatal exclusion of xeroderma pigmentosum (XP-D) by amniotic cell analysis. **Photodermatol** 2:181–183.
609. Kore-eda S, Tanaka T, Moriwaki S et al. (1992) A case of xeroderma pigmentosum group A diagnosed with a polymerase chain reaction (PCR) technique. Usefulness of PCR in the detection of point mutation in a patient with a hereditary disease. **Arch Dermatol** 128:971–974.
610. Cleaver JE, Volpe JP, Charles WC et al. (1994) Prenatal diagnosis of xeroderma pigmentosum and Cockayne syndrome. **Prenat Diagn** 14:921–928.
611. Matsumoto N, Saito TM, Harada N et al. (1995) DNA-based prenatal carrier detection for group A xeroderma pigmentosum in a chorionic villus sample. **Prenat Diagn** 15:675–677.
612. Alapetite C, Benoit A, Moustacchi E et al. (1997) The comet assay as a repair test for prenatal diagnosis of xeroderma pigmentosum and trichothiodystrophy. **J Invest Dermatol** 108:154–159.
613. Hamouda B, Jamila Z, Najet R et al. (2001) Topical 5-fluorouracil to treat multiple or unresectable facial squamous cell carcinomas in xeroderma pigmentosum. **J Am Acad Dermatol** 44:1054.

614. Quilliet X, Chevallier-Lagente O, Zeng L et al. (1997) Retroviral-mediated correction of DNA repair defect in xeroderma pigmentosum cells is associated with recovery of catalase activity. **Mutat Res** 385:235–242.
615. Schallreuter KU (1999) Pseudocatalase treatment in xeroderma pigmentosum: a case report. **Br J Dermatol** 140:1190–1191.
616. Atabay K, Celebi C, Cenetoglu S et al. (1991) Facial resurfacing in xeroderma pigmentosum with monoblock full-thickness skin graft. **Plast Reconst Surg** 87:1121–1125.
617. Agrawal K, Veliath AJ, Mishra S et al. (1992) Xeroderma pigmentosum: resurfacing versus dermabrasion. **Br J Plast Surg** 45:311–314.
618. Nelson BR, Fader DJ, Gillard M et al. (1995) The role of dermabrasion and chemical peels in the treatment of patients with xeroderma pigmentosum. **J Am Acad Dermatol** 32:623–626.
619. Konig A, Friederich HC, Hoffmann R et al. (1998) Dermabrasion for the treatment of xeroderma pigmentosum. **Arch Dermatol** 134:241–242.
620. Aslan G, Karacal N, Gorgu M (1999) New tumor formation on split-thickness skin grafted areas in xeroderma pigmentosum. **Ann Plast Surg** 43:657–660.
621. Villegas J (1999) Xeroderma pigmentoso en pacientes gemelas. Tratamiento quirúrgico, un aporte a su calidad de vida. **Rev Chil Dermatol** 15:244–246.
622. DiGiovanna JJ (2001) Retinoid chemoprevention in patients at high risk for skin cancer. **Med Pediatr Oncol** 36:564–567.

in patients with group D xeroderma pigmentosum.[601] With computed tomography (CT), patients with De Sanctis–Cacchione syndrome demonstrate ventricular dilatation, cerebrocortical atrophy, and a small brain stem.[573] Commonly seen EEG patterns are diffuse arrhythmia with a poorly developed rhythm and paroxysmal, burst-like slow-wave discharges. Nerve conduction velocities are normal, while electromyography (EMG) and muscle biopsy reveal neuropathic changes. These findings are consistent with chronic lower motor neuron degeneration with attempted reinnervation by adjacent neurons.

The pathologic defect in De Sanctis–Cacchione syndrome is the loss or absence of neurons predominantly in the cerebral cortex and cerebellum without inflammation, abnormal depositions, or changes in the white matter.[573,578]

Attempts to prevent UV radiation exposure or to otherwise alter the environment for these patients have been unsuccessful in preventing the progressive neurologic sequelae.

COCKAYNE SYNDROME

INTRODUCTION AND HISTORICAL NOTE

Cockayne syndrome (CS) is a very rare autosomal recessive disorder with defective repair of cellular injury, characterized by sensitivity to sunlight, dwarfism, precociously senile appearance, pigmentary retinal degeneration, microcephaly, intracranial calcification, hydrocephalus, deafness, and other somatic abnormalities.[573,577,578] Cockayne described the syndrome in 1933,[623] and Nance and Berry reviewed 140 cases of the literature in 1992.[624]

EPIDEMIOLOGY
Genetics
Cockayne syndrome is inherited as an autosomal recessive trait. Two complementation groups have been identified in Cockayne syndrome.[577,625]

CS group A (MIM 216400) gene maps to chromosome 5, and has been identified as ERCC8 (excision-repair cross complementing group 8);[605] and CS group B (MIM 133540) gene (ERCC6) maps to 10q11. CS complementation group C (type III) has been described in one patient, but its identity is under discussion.[626,627]

A XP–CS complex has been described,[573,578] in some patients with features of both XP and CS. They have been identified with XP complementation groups B, D and G, and the gene (ERCC5) maps to 13q33.[587,628,629]

Statistics
Cockayne syndrome is a very rare disorder of worldwide distribution. Sexes are equally affected. Complementation group B, or CS type II, is the most common, accounting for 80% of reported cases. XP–CS complex has been described in only 10 patients to present.[573,577,587,628,629]

PRESENTING HISTORY

Affected infants have a normal appearance at birth, but signs of photosensitivity appear at six months or later, concomitantly with failure of growth and developmental deterioration.[630,631] Late-onset CS complementation group A manifests in childhood or adolescence, by minor photosensitivity in sun-exposed areas of the skin, and neurologic and growth impairment.[577,624,632]

PHYSICAL EXAMINATION
Skin
Frequent acute sun-induced, scaly, erythematous eruptions may resolve, leaving hyperpigmentation and scarring. In some patients, the erythema may be limited to the "butterfly" area of the face, while others manifest severe sun burning similar to that observed in xeroderma pigmentosum. An erythematous papular facial eruption may also be seen several hours after sun exposure.[624]

Patients who have the XP–CS complex are sensitive to UV light but are not predisposed to develop freckling, precancerous skin lesions as solar keratoses, or skin cancer.[573,624]

Progressive periorbital and subcutaneous fat atrophy causes the characteristic prematurely senile birdlike facies and prominent "Mickey Mouse" ears. Sweating may be absent.

Hair, nail, teeth and mucous membranes
Increased incidence of dental caries has been reported as a good indicator for diagnosis.[633,634]

SYSTEMIC MANIFESTATIONS

CS is a multisystem disorder that can be defined by a triad of UV hypersensitivity, retarded growth, and severe progressive neurologic deterioration.

Some patients lack cutaneous manifestations or they appeared very late in their life.

A typical "salt and pepper" pigmentary retinal degeneration was described by Cockayne.[623] Other optical findings are optic atrophy, cataracts, arteriolar narrowing, pupillary unresponsiveness, strabismus, and nystagmus.[635]

Retarded growth can be a striking feature, leading to a "cachectic dwarfism" or progeria-like appearance. Microcephaly, prognathism, kyphosis, disproportionately long limbs, large hands and feet, joint contractures, and skeletal muscle atrophy have been reported.[624] Developmental deterioration can be observed as early as the age of 6 months. Mental retardation can be severe, and accompanied by normal-pressure hydrocephalus, sensorineural deafness, progressive upper motor neuron, cerebellar dysfunction, ataxia, intention tremors, incontinence, and hyperreflexive deep tendon reflexes.[495,636,637]

Accompanying these findings are numerous other defects, including hypertension, nephropathy, adrenal failure,[638–640] hepatomegaly, hyperinsulinemia and growth hormone deficiency.[641]

623. Cockayne EA (1933) Inherited Abnormalities of the Skin and its Appendages. London: Oxford University Press.
624. Nance MA, Berry SA (1992) Cockayne syndrome: review of 140 cases. Am J Med Genet 42:68–84.
625. Lehmann AR (1982) Three complementation groups in Cockayne syndrome. Mutat Res 106:347–356.
626. Cziezel AE, Marchalko M (1995) Cockayne syndrome type III with high intelligence. Clin Genet 48:331–333.
627. Lehmann AR, Bootsma D, Clarkson SG et al. (1994) Nomenclature of human DNA repair genes. Mutat Res 315:41–42.
628. Vermeulen W, Jaeken J, Jaspers NGJ et al. (1993) Xeroderma pigmentosum complementation group G associated with Cockayne syndrome. Am J Hum Genet 53:185–192.
629. Hamel BCJ, Raams A, Schuitema-Djikstra AR et al. (1996) Xeroderma pigmentosum–Cockayne syndrome complex: a further case. J Med Genet 33:607–610.
630. Jaeken J, Klocker H, Schwaiger H et al. (1989) Clinical and biochemical studies in three patients with severe early infantile Cockayne syndrome. Hum Genet 83:339–346.
631. Patton MA, Giannelli F, Francis AJ et al. (1989) Early onset Cockayne's syndrome: case reports with neuropathological and fibroblast studies. J Med Genet 26:154–159.
632. Fryns JP, Bulcke J, Verdu P et al. (1991) Apparent late-onset Cockayne syndrome and interstitial deletion of the long arm of chromosome 10 (del(10)(q11.23q21.2)). Am J Med Genet 40:343–344.

633. Boraz RA (1991) Cockayne's syndrome: literature review and case report. Pediatr Dent 13:227–230.
634. Lehmann AR, Thompson AF, Harcourt SA et al. (1993) Cockayne's syndrome: correlation of clinical features with cellular sensitivity of RNA synthesis to UV irradiation. J Med Genet 30:679–682.
635. Traboulsi EI, De Becker I, Maumenee IH (1992) Ocular findings in Cockayne syndrome. Am J Ophthal 114:579–583.
636. Ozdirim E, Topcu M, Ozon A et al. (1996) Cockayne syndrome: review of 25 cases. Pediatr Neurol 15:312–316.
637. Yamagata T, Momoi MY, Saitoh S et al. (1998) A DNA repair defect in a patient with ataxia, mental retardation, and short stature. Pediatr Neurol 18:358–361.
638. Sato H, Saito T, Kurosawa K et al. (1988) Renal lesions in Cockayne's syndrome. Clin Nephrol 29:206–209.
639. Hirooka M, Hirota M, Kamada M (1988) Renal lesions in Cockayne syndrome. Pediatr Nephrol 2:239–243.
640. Reiss U, Hofweber K, Herterich R et al. (1996) Nephrotic syndrome, hypertension, and adrenal failure in atypical Cockayne syndrome. Pediatr Nephrol 10:602–605.
641. Park SK, Chang SH, Cho SB et al. (1994) Cockayne syndrome: a case with hyperinsulinemia and growth hormone deficiency. J Korean Med Sci 9:74–77.

Death usually occurs by age 30,[578,624] but early death has been reported in severe cases.[630]

LABORATORY FINDINGS

Chidren with CS have an abnormally low or absent thymic hormone level,[642] reminiscent of premature aging. T-cell function may be normal or diminished. Motor nerve conduction velocities are abnormally slow. Sensorineural deafness and neuropathic electromyogram are frequent.[624,636] Epiphyses close prematurely. By CT and MRI examination characteristic calcifications may be seen in the basal ganglia, lateral ventricles, and frontal lobes; atrophy and dysmyelination of cerebrum and cerebellum, and thickening of the meninges and skull bones are other signs.[643]

Decreased levels of 5-hydroxyindole acetic acid in cerebrospinal fluid suggest a primary defect of central serotonin metabolism.[644] Height and weight are usually below the third percentile for the age.[578,624] Prenatal diagnosis is possible on the basis of UV light sensitivity of amniotic fluid cells, and by study of RNA synthesis in cultured aminotic cells.[645,646]

PATHOPHYSIOLOGY AND HISTOGENESIS

Molecular, biochemical and immunological basis

Skin fibroblasts from CS patients exhibit cellular hypersensitivity to sunlight. In contrast to XP patients, who possess high rates of sunlight-induced cancer, CS patients are not cancer prone, and their cells show a normal G_2 response to irradiation with either X-rays or near UV-visible light. However, CS cells show a deficiency in repair of DNA damage inflicted by light during S and G_1 phases of the cell cycle.[573,578] There is a specific defect in the preferential repair of DNA in active genes, resulting in failure of RNA synthesis to recover, and in pronounced hypersensitivity to sunlight and neurodegeneration, even though the bulk of the DNA is repaired at normal rates.[573]

Cell fusion studies have demonstrated two complementation groups in CS based on restoration of a normal rate of recovery of RNA synthesis after exposure of heterokaryons to UV radiation.[578] Cockayne syndrome can be diagnosed by measuring the failure of RNA synthesis to recover in Cockayne syndrome cells after UV irradiation. The human repair gene, ERRC6, has been found to complement Cockayne syndrome group B cells.[647–649]

Histologic findings

Neuropathologic examination reveals diffuse, extensive dysmyelination of the central and peripheral nervous systems, beginning with pericapillary calcification in the cortex and basal ganglia. No inflammation is evident. These findings are consistent with premature aging.

DIFFERENTIAL DIAGNOSIS

CS shares several features with XP, including UV photosensitivity, mental retardation and other complex neurologic abnormalities, and cutaneous dyspigmentation. However, CS may be distinguished clinically by the presence of cachectic dwarfism, pigmentary chorioretinitis, and the absence of skin neoplasia. A few patients have manifestations of both XP and CS.

The premature aging features of CS may resemble those in progeria, but the latter entity lacks the features of photosensitivity, ocular degeneration, or mental retardation. Telangiectasias and dwarfism may be seen in Rothmund–Thomson syndrome and Bloom syndrome; however, patients with these disorders do not regularly manifest premature aging, deafness, mental retardation, or retinal degeneration.

Cerebro-oculofacioskeletal syndrome (COFS, MIM 214150) is caused by a homozygous mutation in the *ERCC6* gene, mapped to 10q11, the same gene that causes CS type B. It comprises microcephaly, hypotonia, failure to thrive, arthrogryposis, eye defects, prominent nose, large ears, overhanging upper lip, micrognathia, widely set nipples, kyphoscoliosis, and osteoporosis.[650,651] Some patients showed photosensitivity and defective DNA repair.[652]

THERAPEUTICS AND PROGNOSIS
Topical therapy
Sunscreens and sun-protecting clothing are useful in patients with photosensitivity.

Systemic management
No evidence of valuable management measures for systemic manifestations of CS exists at present.

Prognosis
Mental retardation and premature aging are the main findings in CS patients, leading to premature death. However, reports of less severe or incomplete cases with isolated cutaneous photosensitivity suggest that the spectrum of CS is larger than previously considered, and prognosis is variable.[653]

TRICHOTHIODYSTROPHY

INTRODUCTION AND HISTORICAL NOTE

The first cases of trichothiodystrophy (TTD) were reported by Pollitt, Jenner and Davies in 1968.[654] They described a family with mental and physical retardation and "trichorrhexis nodosa." Later on, the term trichothiodistrophy was coined by Vera Price.[655]

Currently, TTD refers to a heterogeneous group of autosomal recessive disorders that is characterized by brittle hair and abnormally low sulfur content.[656] At least eight different syndromes have been recognized, and a subset of patients presents with photosensitivity. Crovato *et al.* suggested the acronym PIBIDS (MIM 278730)[657–659] to designate this group. It is characterized by *P*hotosensitivity, *I*chthyosis, *B*rittle hair, *I*ntellectual impairment, *D*ecreased fertility, and *S*hort stature.

This chapter refers to the photosensitivity TTD with DNA nucleotide excision repair defect, which represents about half of the cases reported. The

642. Bensman A, Dardenne M, Bach J-F et al. (1982) Decrease of thymic hormone serum level in Cockayne syndrome. Pediat Res 16:92–94.
643. Demaerel P, Kendall BE, Kingsley D (1992) Cranial CT and MRI in diseases with DNA repair defects. Neuroradiology 34:117–121.
644. Ellaway CJ, Duggins A, Fung VS et al. (2000) Cockayne syndrome associated with low CSF 5-hydroxyindole acetic acid levels. J Med Genet 37:553–557.
645. Lehmann AR, Francis AJ, Giannelli F (1985) Prenatal diagnosis of Cockayne's syndrome. Lancet i:486–488.
646. Sugita T, Ikenaga M, Suehara N et al. (1982) Prenatal diagnosis of Cockayne syndrome using assay of colony-forming ability in ultraviolet light irradiated cells. Clin Genet 22:137–142.
647. Troelstra C, Landsvater RM, Wiegant J et al. (1992) Localization of the nucleotide excision repair gene ERCC6 to human chromosome 10q11–q21. Genomics 12:745–749.
648. Troelstra C, van Gool A, de Wit J et al. (1992) ERCC6, a member of a subfamily of putative helicases, is involved in Cockayne's syndrome and preferential repair of active genes. Cell 71:939–953.
649. Venema J, Mullenders LHF, Natarajan AT et al. (1990) The genetic defect in Cockayne syndrome is associated with a defect in repair of UV-induced DNA damage in transcriptionally active DNA. Proc Nat Acad Sci USA 87:4707–4711.
650. Gershoni-Baruch R, Ludatscher RM, Lichtig C et al. (1991) Cerebro-oculo-facio-skeletal syndrome: further delineation. Am J Med Genet 41:74–77.
651. Del Bigio MR, Greenberg CR, Rorke LB et al. (1997) Neuropathological findings in eight children with cerebro-oculo-facio-skeletal (COFS) syndrome. J Neuropath Exp Neurol 56:1147–1157.
652. Graham JM Jr, Anyane-Yeboa K, Raams A et al. (2001) Cerebro-oculo-facio-skeletal syndrome with a nucleotide excision-repair defect and a mutated XPD gene, with prenatal diagnosis in a triplet pregnancy. Am J Hum Genet 69:291–300.
653. Miyauchi-Hashimoto H, Akaeda T, Maihara T et al. (1998) Cockayne syndrome without typical clinical manifestations including neurologic abnormalities. J Am Acad Dermatol 39:565–570.
654. Pollitt RJ, Jenner FA, Davies M (1968) Sibs with mental and physical retardation and trichorrhexis nodosa with abnormal amino acid composition of the hair. Arch Dis Child 43:211–216.
655. Price VH, Odom RB, Ward WH et al. (1980) Trichothiodystrophy: sulfur-deficient brittle hair as a marker for a neuroectodermal symptom complex. Arch Dermatol 116:1375–1384.
656. Itin PH, Sarasin A, Pittelkow MR (2001) Trichothiodystrophy: update on the sulfur-deficient brittle hair syndromes. J Am Acad Dermatol 44:891–920.
657. Crovato F, Borrone C, Rebora A (1983) Trichothiodystrophy – BIDS, IBIDS and PIBIDS? Br J Dermatol 108:247.
658. Rebora A, Crovato F (1987) PIBI(D)S syndrome – trichothiodystrophy with xeroderma pigmentosum (group D) mutation. J Am Acad Dermatol 16:940–947.
659. Traupe H (1989) The Ichthyoses. A Guide to Clinical Diagnosis, Genetic Counseling, and Therapy. Berlin: Springer, pp. 162–167.

TTD syndromes (MIM 601675) have been the subject of a recent extensive review.[656]

EPIDEMIOLOGY
Genetics
TTD is inherited as an autosomal recessive trait. In patients with TTD and xeroderma pigmentosum group D and B, deletion of two closely linked loci at chromosome 19q13.2–q13.3 has been proposed.[659]

Statistics
The PIBIDS form of TTD is a rare syndrome, with worldwide incidence. Patients have been reported from Italy, Asia, Latin America, and the United States.

PRESENTING HISTORY

Collodion baby and other forms of congenital ichthyosis can be observed in newborns.[656] Congenital alopecia is a characteristic presenting sign.

Forty to fifty percent of patients with TTD present with severe photosensitivity. The clinical spectrum of associated signs is extremely extensive, including cutaneous, neurologic, ocular, skeletal, cardiovascular, pulmonary, urologic, hematologic, and immunologic features.[656]

PHYSICAL EXAMINATION
Skin
Non-bullous ichthyosiform erythroderma or mild, ichthyosis vulgaris–like desquamation are observed at birth or during the first months of life.[656,659]

Sunburn is a common consequence of the extreme photosensitivity that characterizes PIBIDS. This photosensitivity decreases with age, and lacks freckling, telangiectasias, solar keratoses, and other signs of chronic skin actinic damage (Fig. 7.67). Sun sensitivity in these patients does not lead to increased skin cancer incidence.[662]

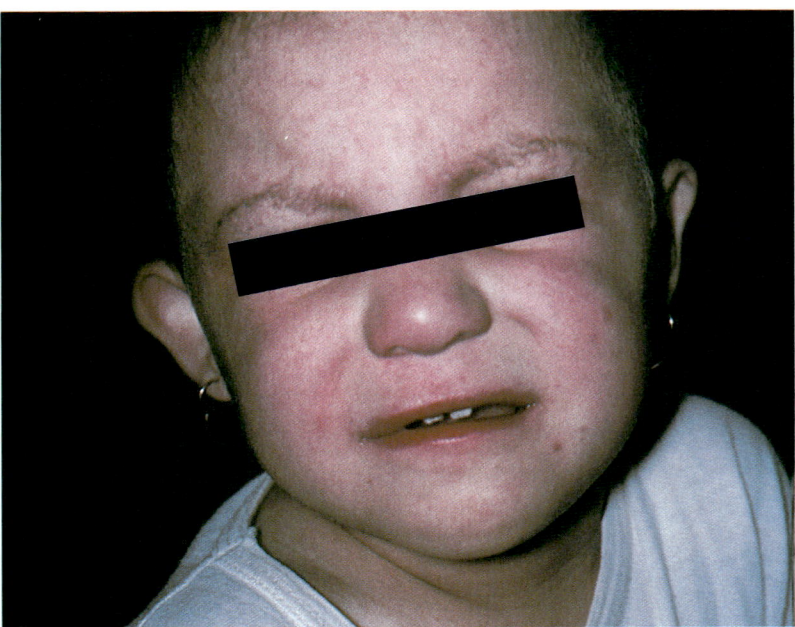

Fig. 7.67 **Trichothiodystrophy.** Photophobia, facial erythema and sparse eyebrows in a 2-year-old girl.

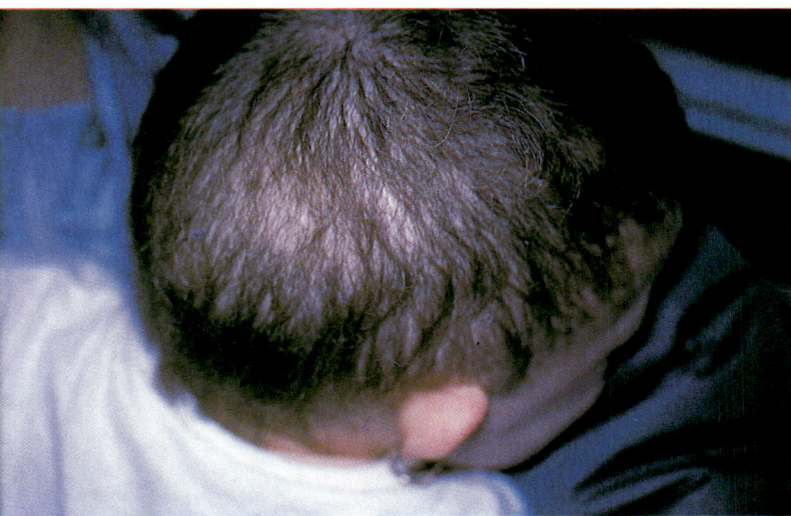

Fig. 7.68 **Trichothiodystrophy.** Alopecia in a 2-year-old girl.

Due to lack of subcutaneous fat, the facies has an aged, progeria-like appearance.

Hair, nail, teeth and mucous membranes
Diffuse alopecia is a common feature in TTD (Fig. 7.68). The hair is dry and sparse, and the hair shaft breaks easily with trauma.[656] Intermittent hair loss, with a cyclic periodicity, has been reported.[660] The biochemical defect also affects eyelashes, eyebrows, body and axillary hair, and otic and nasal hair.

Onychodystrophy accompanies the hair abnormalities: brittle nails, koilonychia, splitting, ridging, onychogryphosis, and yellow discoloration can be present. Dental caries and enamel hypoplasia are observed.

Systemic manifestations
Bilateral congenital cataracts, short stature, impaired mental development, recurrent infections, and premature death have been reported.

LABORATORY FINDINGS

Prenatal diagnosis is based on DNA repair in trophoblasts or amniotic cells.[612,661]

PATHOPHYSIOLOGY AND HISTOGENESIS
Molecular, biochemical and immunological basis
Cells from PIBIDS patients show low levels of unscheduled DNA synthesis following exposure to UV radiation. Some of these cells have similar abnormalities to cells from patients with XP complementation groups D[662] and B,[663] whereas other do not, for at least one independent complementation group referred as TTD-A.[577,656] Normal incidence of skin cancer could be assigned to normal catalase levels and NK cell activity.[656]

Histologic findings
Light microscopy reveals transverse fractures of the hair shafts, and irregular cuticle and diameter. Polarizing microscopy shows the typical "tiger tail" pattern,[656,661] although this may not be present before 3 months of life.[664] Skin biopsy reveals orthokeratotic hyperkeratosis, thin granular layer, moderate acanthosis and papillomatosis, similar to the image of ichthyosis vulgaris.[659]

660. Pollitt RJ, Jenner FA, Davies M (1968) Sibs with mental and physical retardation and trichorrhexis nodosa with abnormal amino acid composition of the hair. **Arch Dis Child** 43:211–216.
661. Sarasin A, Blanchet-Bardon C, Renault G et al. (1992) Prenatal diagnosis in a subset of trichothiodystrophy patients defective in DNA repair. **Br J Dermatol** 127:485–491.
662. Stefanini M, Lagomarsini P, Arlett CF et al. (1986) Xeroderma pigmentosum (complementation group D) mutation is present in patients affected by trichothiodystrophy with photosensitivity. **Hum Genet** 74:107–112.
663. Weeda G, Eveno E, Donker I et al. (1997) A mutation in the XPB/ERCC3 DNA repair transcription gene, associated with trichothiodystrophy. **Am J Hum Genet** 60:320–329.
664. Brusasco A, Restano L (1997) The typical "tiger tail" pattern of the hair shaft in trichothiodystrophy may not be evident at birth. **Arch Dermatol** 133:249.

DIFFERENTIAL DIAGNOSIS

TTD syndromes share a common feature expressed by brittle hair and nails. Extreme photosensitivity is present only in PIBIDS, thus allowing its differentiation from Tay syndrome.[659] XP has striking sun-induced changes and multiple skin cancer of early appearance. CS, another rare DNA nucleotide excision repair deficiency entity, has characteristic neurologic and somatic manifestations.

THERAPEUTICS AND PROGNOSIS

Topical therapy

Sun protection and moisturizers are the main requirements for the skin manifestations of PIBIDS.

Prognosis

Prognosis is a function of the extent and severity of the neurological, immunological, and ectodermal defects of the disease. Early death by severe infections can occur.

BLOOM SYNDROME

INTRODUCTION AND HISTORICAL NOTE

Bloom reported in 1954 a "congenital telangiectatic erythema resembling lupus erythematosus in dwarfs,"[665] thus signaling the importance of the dermatologist in the diagnosis of this rare autosomal recessive syndrome.

The constellation of photosensitivity, facial telangiectasia, dwarfism, immunodeficiency, and a high incidence of malignancy characterizes Bloom syndrome.[578,666]

Increased spontaneous mutation rate in cultured cells may account for the high frequency of internal cancer. German defines Bloom syndrome as the prototype of a group of somatic mutational disorders.[667]

EPIDEMIOLOGY

Genetics

Inheritance is autosomal recessive (MIM 210900), and the gene locus (*BLM*) has been identified in chromosome 15q26.1 as a helicase of the RecQ family.[668,669]

Statistics

This rare, life-limiting disease is most commonly seen among Ashkenazi Jews; this represents one-third of reported cases, with males more frequently affected than females.[666]

PRESENTING HISTORY

Beginning in the first few weeks of life, erythema and telangiectasia appear on the butterfly area of the nose and cheeks, resembling lupus erythematosus. Intrauterine growth retardation, with fairly normal proportions, is present in all patients.[666] Some patients lack the skin photosensitivity, and have short stature and an enormous predisposition to cancer.

PHYSICAL EXAMINATION

Skin

Sun exposure accentuates the lupus-like erythema and telangiectasia of the face (Fig. 7.69), the ears, and the dorsal forearms and hands, and bullae, bleeding, and crusting may appear, even on the lips and eyelids.[578] The eruption worsens in summer sunlight due to UVB exposure.

The intensity of the photosensitivity lesions varies from minimal telangiectasia to severe erythema, but spares the trunk, buttocks, and lower limbs.

Besides erythema, patients with Bloom syndrome have numerous café-au-lait spots and areas of hypopigmentation. These lesions locate specially on the trunk. Less frequently axillary acanthosis nigricans is present.

Hair, nail, teeth and mucous membranes

White hair may be present, but no specific lesions affect the skin appendages.

SYSTEMIC MANIFESTATIONS

Retardation of growth begins *in utero* and continues in the face of normal sexual development. Patients surviving to adulthood are proportionately dwarfed; although mental retardation occasionally occurs, normal intelligence is the rule.

Facies in Bloom syndrome is characterized by a narrow, small cranium with malar hypoplasia, nasal prominence, small mandible, and protuberant ears. The voice is high-pitched and of a coarse timbre. Vomiting and diarrhea are frequent in infancy, often leading to dehydration. Intestinal malabsorption has been observed in some patients. Diabetes mellitus has been diagnosed in 12% of cases of the Bloom's Registry.[666]

Persons with Bloom syndrome have a 150- to 300-fold increased frequency of development of a malignancy, which occurs in 20%. Tissues with high mitotic indices – bone marrow, lymphoid tissues, and gastrointestinal mucosa – are most frequently transformed by neoplasia.[666] Skin, breast, oral cavity, uterine, and lung cancers are also seen, usually at exceptionally early ages. Various types of leukemia develop at a mean age of 16 years. Patients who survive beyond this age develop solid tumors at an average age of 30 years. Striking features of the proneness to neoplasia in Bloom syndrome are the great frequency of benign and malignant tumors, the wide variety of tissues affected, the early age of appearance, and the high frequency of multiple tumors in the same patient.[666] When Bloom syndrome patients develop malignancies, however, their tumors appear exquisitely sensitive to chemotherapy and radiotherapy.[666]

Recurrent respiratory and gastrointestinal infections seen in patients with Bloom syndrome reflect the myriad of immunologic abnormalities that may occur. Chronic lung disease is the second cause of death, after cancer. Men with Bloom syndrome are sterile; women have reduced fertility and a shortened reproductive span.

LABORATORY FINDINGS

A maturational defect in lymphocytes early in their development may account for the deficiencies of immunoglobulin (IgG, IgM, and/or IgA), together with malfunctioning helper-T cells and delayed hypersensitivity reactions.[593,670–672]

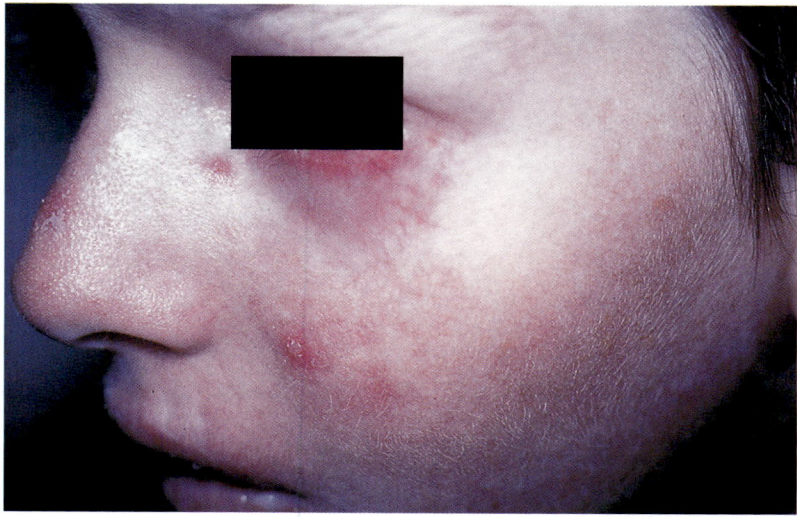

Fig. 7.69   Bloom syndrome. Facial telangiectasia in a 12-year-old boy.

665. Bloom D (1954) Congenital telangiectatic erythema resembling lupus erythematosus in dwarfs. Am J Dis Child 88:754–758.

666. German J (1995) Bloom's syndrome. Dermatol Clin 13:7–18.

Primary hypogonadism affecting the tubular element of the testis leads to azoospermia in men.

PATHOPHYSIOLOGY AND HISTOGENESIS

Molecular, biochemical and immunological basis

The fundamental derangement in Bloom syndrome stems from abnormalities of DNA repair and chromosomal structure. Among these aberrations are a decreased rate of DNA replication, chromatid and isochromatid gaps, breaks and rearrangements, acentric segments, dicentric and abnormal monocentric chromosomes, and a markedly increased (6- to 12-fold) frequency of sister chromatid exchanges with increased triradial and quadriradial configurations.[666,673,674] There is a high spontaneous mutation frequency in both lymphocytes *in vivo* and in cultured fibroblasts.[666]

The *RecQ* gene family, of which *BLM* is a member, is a part of the RecF recombination pathway in which mutations abolish the conjugational recombination proficiency and ultraviolet resistance of a mutant strain. *RecQL* is a human gene isolated from HeLa cells, the product of which possesses DNA-dependent ATPase, DNA helicase, and 3′ 5′ single-stranded DNA translocation activities.[669] Ellis *et al.*[674] have suggested that the absence of the *BLM* gene product probably destabilizes other enzymes that participate in DNA replication and repair, perhaps through direct interaction and through more general responses to DNA damage.

Ellis and German[673] reported that the BLM protein has similarity to two other proteins that are members of the RecQ family of helicases, namely the gene product encoded by the Werner syndrome gene (*WRN*) and the product of the yeast gene *SGS1*.

Histologic findings

Histopathologically, Bloom syndrome manifests epidermal flattening and hydropic degeneration of the basal cell layer with pigmentary incontinence; inflammatory infiltrates may be absent, or perivascular mononuclear cells may be present. Because of the similarities to lupus erythematosus, a direct immunofluorescence examination of the skin may be needed to distinguish Bloom syndrome, in which no dermal-epidermal junction immunoglobulin deposits are seen.

DIFFERENTIAL DIAGNOSIS

The photosensitivity in early childhood can be distinguished from erythropoietic protoporphyria by the absence of red cell protoporphyrins and negative red cell fluorescence. Facial telangiectasias and dwarfism may also be seen in children with Rothmund–Thomson syndrome or CS. Telangiectasias with ataxia-telangiectasia or lupus erythematosus may be distinguished from Bloom syndrome by the accompanying neurologic, rheumatologic, serologic, or other systemic associations. The telangiectasias in hereditary hemorrhagic telangiectasia generally do not appear before the second decade of life.

THERAPEUTICS AND PROGNOSIS

Topical therapy

It is necessary to recommend effective sun protection for affected patients in order to minimize UV damage to the skin and the potential mutagenic stimulation of lymphocytes circulating through the skin.

Systemic management

Early detection of malignancies and its surgical or chemotherapeutic approach are essential steps in the management of Bloom syndrome patients.[666]

Patients and their families need to be educated about the course of the disease, the preventive measures that must be taken, and the early detection of malignant changes. Efforts to avoid other known environmental mutagens are also advisable.

Prognosis

Malignancies of varied cell types and early appearance, as well as recurrent infections, account for death before the age of 50 years in most patients.

ROTHMUND–THOMSON SYNDROME

INTRODUCTION AND HISTORICAL NOTE

Rothmund–Thomson syndrome, also known as congenital poikiloderma, is an extremely rare syndrome characterized by infantile-onset poikiloderma associated with cataracts, photosensitivity, short stature, skeletal abnormalities, and hypogonadism.

Rothmund, a German ophthalmologist, first described in 1868 the association of juvenile cataracts with a peculiar skin degeneration in three patients drawn from interrelated families living in the Klein-Walserthal valley in Austria. Thomson, a British dermatologist, in 1923 and 1936, emphasized the cutaneous findings in naming the same syndrome poikiloderma congenitale.[675]

EPIDEMIOLOGY

Genetics

Autosomal recessive inheritance has been assumed in cases in which marriages were consanguineous. Some cases are caused by mutations in the DNA helicase gene *RecQL4*, which has been mapped to chromosome 8q.24.3 (MIM 268400).[577,676,677]

Statistics

More than 200 cases of Rothmund–Thomson syndrome have been reported worldwide. The disorder has been seen in Indian, Oriental, black, and white children, with a male:female ratio of 2:1.[678]

667. German J (1993) Bloom syndrome: a Mendelian prototype of somatic mutational disease. **Medicine** 72:393–406.
668. German J, Roe AM, Leppert MF et al. (1994) Bloom syndrome: an analysis of consanguineous families assigns the locus mutated to chromosome band 15q26.1. **Proc Natl Acad Sci USA** 91:6669–6673.
669. Mohaghegh P, Hickson ID (2001) DNA helicase deficiencies associated with cancer predisposition and premature aging disorders. **Hum Mol Genet** 10:741–746.
670. Kondo N, Motoyoshi F, Mori S et al. (1992) Long-term study of the immunodeficiency of Bloom's syndrome. **Acta Paediatr** 81:86–90.
671. Weemaes CM, Bakkeren JA. Haraldsson A et al. (1991) Immunological studies in Bloom's syndrome. A follow-up report. **Ann Genet** 34:201–205.
672. Van Kerckhove CW, Ceuppens JL, Vanderschueren-Lodeweyckx M et al. (1988) Bloom's syndrome. Clinical features and immunologic abnormalities of four patients. **Am J Dis Child** 142:1089–1093.

673. Ellis NA, Groden J, Ye T-Z et al. (1995) The Bloom's syndrome gene product is homologous to RecQ helicases. **Cell** 83:655–666.
674. Ellis NA, German J (1996) Molecular genetics of Bloom's syndrome. **Hum Mol Genet** 5:1457–1463.
675. Vennos EM, James WD (1995) Rothmund–Thomson syndrome. **Dermatol Clin** 13:143–150.
676. Kitao S, Shimamoto A, Goto M et al. (1999) Mutations in *RECQL4* cause a subset of cases of Rothmund–Thomson syndrome. **Nat Genet** 22:82–84.
677. Lindor NM, Furuichi Y, Kitao S et al. (2000) Rothmund–Thomson syndrome due to *RECQ4* helicase mutations: report and clinical and molecular comparisons with Bloom syndrome and Werner syndrome. **Am J Med Genet** 90:223–228.
678. Wang LL, Levy ML, Lewis RA et al. (2001) Clinical manifestations in a cohort of 41 Rothmund–Thomson syndrome patients. **Am J Med Genet** 102:11–17.

PRESENTING HISTORY

Affected children develop poikiloderma, usually at 3 to 6 months of age, but varying from birth to 2 years of age. With the knowledge of the gene defect in Rothmund–Thomson syndrome, re-examination of the individuals diagnosed with this disorder showed some patients without poikiloderma.[679]

PHYSICAL EXAMINATION

Skin

The original eruption has been described in various cases as diffuse erythema and edema, reticulate erythema, and in two cases as vesicular. Rarely, this erythematous state is not present. The eruption usually initially involves the face, followed by the buttocks and extremities; however, a reverse order of appearance has been noted in several patients. This stage is followed by a chronic poikilodermatous stage consisting of atrophy, telangiectasia, and patchy or linear hypopigmentation and hyperpigmentation (Fig. 7.70). In most patients, progression of these lesions ceases between 3 and 5 years of age.[675]

Photosensitivity has been reported in 30% of patients and may produce a bullous eruption. However, blistering in patients has been seen without photosensitivity.

After age 2, verrucous hyperkeratoses develop on the hands, feet, knees, and elbows in about one-third of patients. An increased incidence of cutaneous squamous cell carcinoma occurs in adult patients within both hyperkeratotic and atrophic lesions. Actinic keratoses and calcinosis cutis have been documented in few cases.[680]

Hair, nail, teeth and mucous membranes

Scalp and body hair tends to be fine or sparse; loss of vellus hair occurs in sites of the poikilodermatous eruption. This may progress to partial or total alopecia. Occasionally there is an absence of eyebrows or eyelashes (Fig. 7.71). Nail dystrophy occurs in 30% and defective dentition in up to 40% of

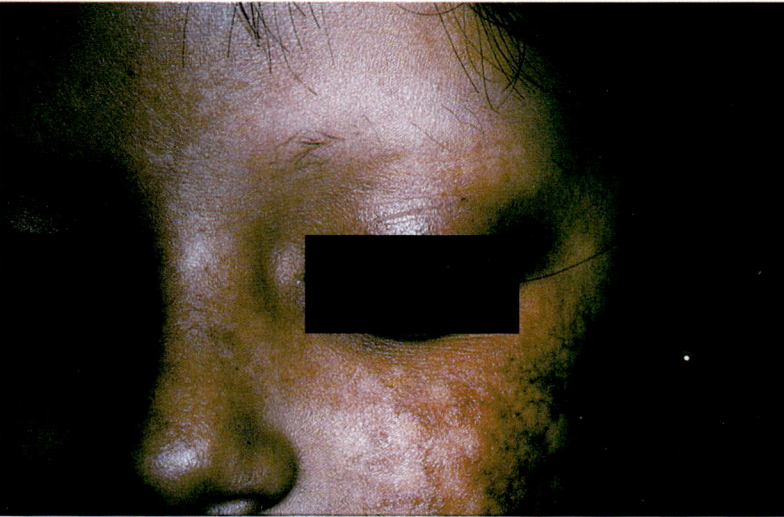

Fig. 7.71   Rothmund–Thomson syndrome. Loss of eyelash and eyebrow hair in a 3-year-old girl.

patients. There is increased incidence of dental caries, and microdontia with conical shape. Anhidrosis has been reported in few patients.[675,681]

SYSTEMIC MANIFESTATIONS

Juvenile cataracts are present in 50% of the patients. These present bilaterally as either posterior or anterior subcapsular opacities that evolve rapidly to total opacity within weeks. They are usually first detected at 3 to 7 years of age but have appeared as early as 4 months or as late as 40 years. Other ocular abnormalities have included keratoconus, colobomata, strabismus, amblyopia with tilted optic discs, microphthalmia with optic atrophy, aneurysmal dilation of retinal veins, exophthalmos, corneal atrophy, corneal scleralization, congenital glaucoma, chorioretinal atrophy, photophobia, hypertelorism, and blue sclerae.[675]

Short stature with small stubby hands and feet has been frequently noted. Low birth weight and length with severe growth failure in childhood are characteristic.

Skeletal abnormalities have been seen in about 68% of patients, and range from minimally to grossly incapacitating. These include a typical facies with frontal bossing, saddle nose and prognathism, absent or rudimentary thumbs, brachymetacarpophalangy, syndactyly, clinodactyly, and fusion or agenesis of carpal and tarsal bones. The radius and ulna may be hypoplastic, absent or bowed. Fibrous dysplasia, osteogenesis imperfecta and soft tissue contractures may be present. An irregular cortical hyperostosis that mimics rickets or chondrodystrophy, a cup-shaped depression of the radial head, and osteoporosis with pathologic fractures have also been reported.[675] Bone age may be lower than chronological age. Hypogonadism has been described in 25% of patients. Mental retardation is rare.

Osteosarcoma has been reported in 32% of cases of Rothmund–Thomson syndrome, suggesting either allelic or genetic heterogeneity.[678,679] Other malignancies reported include squamous cell carcinoma, Bowen's disease, basal cell carcinoma, fibrosarcoma, Hodgkin lymphoma, gastric carcinoma, and acute myelogenous leukemia. Hematological abnormalities include aplastic anemia and myelodysplastic syndrome.[682,683]

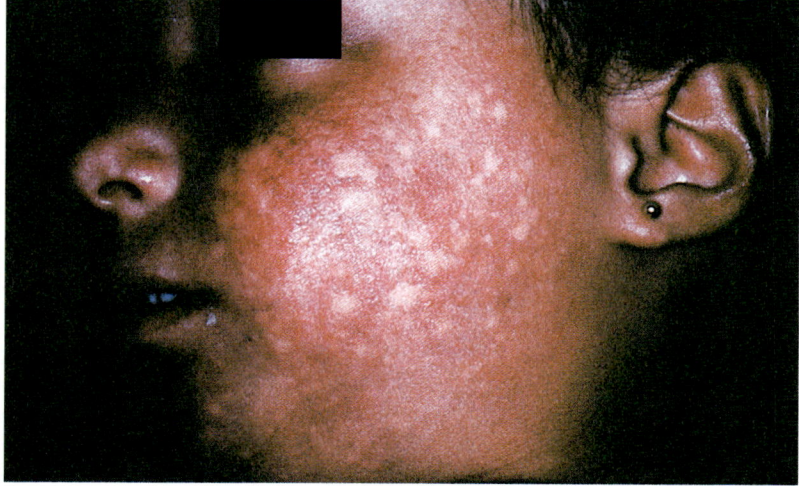

Fig. 7.70   Rothmund–Thomson syndrome. Facial poikiloderma in a 3-year-old girl.

679. Pujol LA, Erickson RP, Heidenreich RA et al. (2000) Variable presentation of Rothmund–Thomson syndrome. **Am J Med Genet** 95:204–207.
680. Aydemir EH, Onsun N, Ozan S et al. (1988) Rothmund–Thomson syndrome with calcincsis universalis. **Int J Dermatol** 27:591–592.
681. Snels DG, Bavinck JN, Muller H et al. (1998) A female patient with the Rothmund–Thomson syndrome associated with anhidrosis and severe infections of the respiratory tract. **Dermatology** 196:260–263.
682. Rizzari C, Bacchiocchi D, Rovelli A et al. (1996) Myelodysplastic syndrome in a child with Rothmund–Thomson syndrome: a case report. **J Pediatr Hematol Oncol** 18:96–97.
683. Knoell KA, Sidhu-Malik NK, Malik RK (1999) Aplastic anemia in a patient with Rothmund–Thomson syndrome. **J Pediatr Hematol Oncol** 21:444–446.

LABORATORY FINDINGS

While most patients have normal immune function, occasional decreases in the relative and absolute numbers of suppressor T cells or in serum IgG_4 levels[684] have been seen.

PATHOPHYSIOLOGY AND HISTOGENESIS

Molecular, biochemical and immunological basis

The basic defect is unknown, since a variety of isolated abnormalities have been noted. Only few studies of fibroblasts demonstrated reduced DNA repair synthesis. It is possible that abnormal DNA repair capacity may account for the susceptibility to cancer in some affected patients.[681]

Normal karyotypes are the rule among patients, though isolated chromosomal abnormalities have been detected. In some cases, mutations in the DNA helicase gene *RecQL4* have been found, similar to those observed in Bloom and Werner syndromes of cancer proneness.[682]

Histologic findings

Poikilodermatous changes are similar in all patients. Direct immunofluorescence studies are usually negative.

DIFFERENTIAL DIAGNOSIS

In childhood, Rothmund–Thomson syndrome must be distinguished from Bloom syndrome, XP, ataxia telangiectasia, CS, acrogeria (Gottron syndrome), Kindler syndrome, acrokeratotic poikiloderma, Mendes da Costa syndrome, sclerosing poikiloderma, dyskeratosis congenita, and progeria. In adulthood, it can be distinguished from Werner's syndrome by early-onset poikiloderma and cataracts and the absence of muscle atrophy and arteriosclerosis.

THERAPEUTICS AND PROGNOSIS

Topical therapy

Treatment consists of avoidance of skin irritants and lubrication in the poikilodermatous state. Facial telangiectasias and poikiloderma have been successfully treated with laser therapy.[685,686] For hyperkeratotic lesions, dermabrasion and keratolytics may be more effective than curettage or topical 5-FU.

Cataract extraction may be necessary and can be successfully performed, although other ocular problems may still interfere with vision.

Photoprotection with the use of lightweight cotton clothing and sun hats along with judicious use of sunscreen agents is advised. Midday sun exposure, especially in summer, should be avoided to the extent possible.

Systemic management

A baseline long bone radiological survey by age 3 is strongly recommended for early detection of osteosarcoma.[675,678] Orthopedic bracing and surgery may be necessary for specific deformities. Genetic counseling for affected families is mandatory.

Prognosis

Cancer proneness shortens life expectancy in some patients. However, many of the original reported patients were still living in their sixth, seventh, and eighth decades, and one was in the ninth decade on follow-up interviews.

TUMOR SYNDROMES

Susan Mallory

GARDNER SYNDROME

INTRODUCTION AND HISTORICAL NOTE

Gardner and Stephens in 1950[687] initially described the syndrome that now bears Gardner's name (MIM 175100). The main features of Gardner syndrome (GS) are premalignant intestinal polyposis, epidermal cysts, osteomas, and desmoid or fibrous tumors of the skin and other organs.[688] It is allelic to familial adenomatous polyposis which does not have other organ involvement.[689]

EPIDEMIOLOGY

The incidence of GS is approximately 1 in 8300 to 1 in 16 000 births.[690] It is inherited as an autosomal dominant trait with a high degree of penetrance and variable expressivity, equally affecting males and females.[691]

PRESENTING HISTORY

Skin lesions and bone abnormalities are often the presenting complaints in early childhood or infancy[689] and frequently occur before polyposis develops

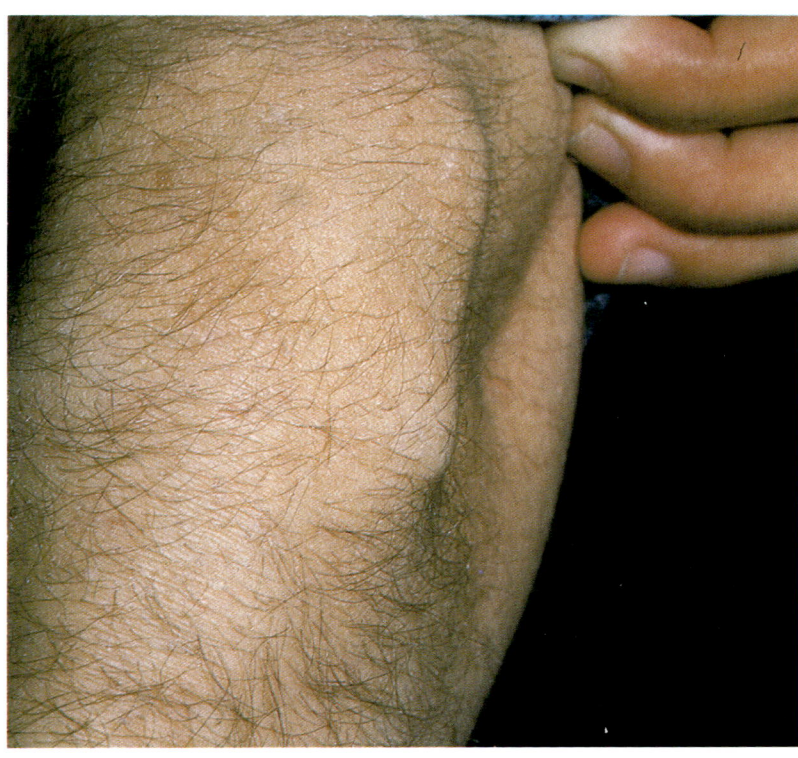

Fig. 7.72   Epidermal cyst in Gardner syndrome.

684. Kubota M, Yasunaga M, Hashimoto H et al. (1993) IgG4 deficiency with Rothmund–Thomson syndrome: a case report. Eur J Pediatr 152:406–408.

685. Potozkin JR, Geronemus RG (1991) Treatment of the poikilodermatous component of the Rothmund–Thomson syndrome with the flashlamp-pumped pulsed dye laser: a case report. **Pediatr Dermatol** 8:162–165.

686. Geronemus RG (1996) Treatment of the cutaneous vascular component of the Rothmund–Thomson syndrome. **Pediatr Dermatol** 13:175.

687. Gardner EJ, Stevens F (1950) Cancer of the lower digestive tract in one family group. **Am J Hum Genet** 2:41–48.

688. Gorlin RJ, Chaudry AP (1960) Multiple osteomatosis, fibromas, lipomas, fibrosarcomas of the skin and mesentry, epidermoid inclusion cysts of the skin, leiomyomas and multiple intestinal polyposis. **N Engl J Med** 263:1141–1158.

689. Ballhausen WG (2000) Genetic testing for familial adenomatous polyposis. **Ann NY Acad Sci** 910:36–47.

690. Sanchez MA, Zali MR, Khalil AA et al. (1979) Be aware of Gardner's syndrome. A review of the literature. **Am J Gastroenterol** 71:68–73.

691. Naylor EW, Lebenthal E (1980) Gardner's syndrome. Recent developments in research and management. **Dig Dis Sci** 25:945–959.

(usually around 25 to 35 years). Malignant transformation of the polyps tends not to occur until 15 to 20 years later.[690]

In adults, diagnosis is commonly made when the patient presents with bleeding secondary to adenomatous polyps. Intussusception, which is common in Peutz–Jeghers syndrome, does not occur in GS.[692]

PHYSICAL EXAMINATION

Epidermal cysts of the skin occur in 35% of cases of GS (Fig. 7.72) These are commonly found on the head and neck, may be present at birth, and tend to increase in size and number and then stabilize.

Osteomas occur in 79% of patients[693] and can appear anywhere on the body but have a predilection for the membranous bones of the face and head, especially the mandible and maxilla. Seen in children as young as 8 years, osteomas may be large enough that they are clinically obvious or they may be picked up only by radiographic survey. Other lesions such as exostoses, endostoses, and cortical thickening of long bones may also be seen. Dental anomalies are seen in 18% of patients with GS[693] and include supernumerary teeth, odontomas, multiple unerupted teeth, and multiple caries.

Desmoid tumors are nonencapsulated, nonmetastasizing, locally aggressive benign tumors that occur in 3.5 to 17.3% of patients with GS, with a marked female preponderance (70 to 85%). They may occur spontaneously or at incision sites, arising from the musculoaponeurotic soft tissues and commonly develop after colectomy. Although benign, desmoid tumors can be invasive and even cause death.

Fibromas may occur in the skin, subcutaneous tissues, mesentery, or retroperitoneal areas.[694] Less commonly seen are lipomas, leiomyomas, trichoepitheliomas, neurofibromas, ovarian cysts[695] and lymphoid hyperplasia of the terminal ileum.

Congenital hypertrophy of the retinal pigment epithelium (CHRPE) is seen in some families with GS and can be a predictive sign of GS.[696,697] Because it is present at birth, it is easily picked up by ophthalmologic screening.

Associated findings that may be found with GS include osteochondromas, papillary carcinoma of the thyroid, hepatoblastoma,[698] adrenal adenomas, skin pigmentation, and transitional cell carcinoma of the urinary bladder.[699]

GASTROINTESTINAL LESIONS

Premalignant adenomatous polyps commonly occur in the colon but can also be seen in the small intestines and stomach in greater than 50%.[655] Polyps are typically less than a centimeter in diameter.[700] Polyps are rarely seen before the age of 10 years; however, they have been recorded as early as age 5 years.[691] By age 20 years, 50% of patients with GS have demonstrable polyps.

Symptoms of polyposis include bleeding and intestinal obstruction. Unlike Peutz–Jeghers polyps, those in GS are adenomatous and have a very high rate of malignancy.

LABORATORY FINDINGS

Skeletal radiographic survey should be performed in all patients with GS and their family members. Skull and facial bones, especially the mandible, may show osteomas or abnormalities of dentition and lead to the diagnosis in an otherwise asymptomatic patient.

PATHOPHYSIOLOGY AND HISTOGENESIS

The gene for GS has been mapped to the adenomatous polyposis coli (*APC*) gene on chromosome 5q21q22, which is a tumor suppressor gene. It is allelic to the familial adenomatous polyposis gene[701,702] and is part of the *ras* family of proto-oncogenes which disrupts signal transduction functions, leading to uninhibited growth.

Histologically, intestinal polyps show focal adenomatous hyperplasia in the colonic mucosa[703] or adenocarcinoma in advanced cases.

Epidermal cysts demonstrate the same microscopic changes as common epidermal cysts, with a typical lining of epithelium, and keratinous debris in the center.[704] Multiple pilomatricomas have also been seen in GS.[705]

Environmental factors may play a role in the timing of the development of carcinoma in those people who have the genetic defect.[691] High dietary fat intake can affect the fecal microflora and ultimately affect the levels of certain fecal bile acids and neutral sterols.[706] These changes, in turn, may affect absorption of carcinogens from the gut and promote tumor formation.[700]

DIFFERENTIAL DIAGNOSIS

GS can be distinguished from familial adenomatous polyposis by the cutaneous findings. In Peutz–Jeghers syndrome one sees hyperpigmented spots on the oral mucosa and periorificial areas. Peutz–Jeghers syndrome polyps in the gastrointestinal tract are hamartomatous and not premalignant. Juvenile polyposis and Cowden syndrome have multiple polyps of the hamartomatous variety.

THERAPEUTICS AND PROGNOSIS

Carcinomatous degeneration occurs in 100% of patients with GS and usually begins between ages 20 and 30 years.[698] Malignant changes have been reported as early as age 9 years.[707] The incidence of cancer in pre–adolescents with polyposis is approximately 5.3–6.6%. Because of the inevitable carcinoma of the bowel, early prophylactic colectomy is recommended.[708] The treatment of choice is colectomy with mucosal proctectomy, followed by ileoanal anastomosis in two stages because of the risk of developing recurrence in the rectum if the rectal mucosa is left after simple colectomy.[700,709] Periodic (semiannual) proctoscopic examination or radiologic examination of the colon and upper GI tract or both is also recommended for affected people,

692. Golitz LE (1980) Heritable cutaneous disorders which affect the gastrointestinal tract. **Med Clin North Am** 64:829–846.
693. Järvinen HJ, Peltokallio P, Landtman M et al. (1982) Gardner's stigmas in patients with familial adenomatosis coli. **Br J Surg** 69:718–721.
694. Michal M (2000) Non-nuchal-type fibroma associated with Gardner's syndrome. **Pathol Res Pract** 196:857–860.
695. Berk T, Friedman LS, Goldstein SD et al. (1985) Relapsing acute pancreatitis as the presenting manifestation of an ampullary neoplasm in a patient with familial polyposis coli. **Am J Gastroenterol** 80:627–629.
696. Shields JA, Shields CL, Shah PG et al. (1992) Lack of association among typical congenital hypertrophy of the retinal pigment epithelium, adenomatous polyposis and Gardner syndrome. **Ophthalmology** 99:1709–1713.
697. Traboulsi EI, Krush AJ, Gardner EJ et al. (1987) Prevalence and importance of pigmented ocular fundus lesions in Gardner's syndrome. **N Engl J Med** 316:661–667.
698. Gruner BA, DeNapoli TS, Andrews W et al. (1998) Hepatocellular carcinoma in children associated with Gardner syndrome or familial adenomatous polyposis. **J Pediatr Hematol Oncol** 20:274–278.
699. Capps WF, Lewis MI, Gazzsaniga DA (1968) Carcinoma of the colon, ampulla of Vater and urinary bladder associated with familial multiple polyposis: A case report. **Dis Colon Rectum** 11:298–305.
700. Rustigi AK (1994) Hereditary gastrointestinal polyposis and nonpolyposis syndromes. **N Engl J Med** 331:1694–1701.
701. Davies DR, Armstrong JG, Thakker N et al. (1995) Severe Gardner syndrome in families with mutations restricted to a specific region of the APC gene. **Am J Hum Genet** 57:1151–1158.
702. Entius MM, Westerman AM, van Velthuysen MLF et al. (1999) Molecular and phenotypic markers of hamartomatous polyposis syndromes in the gastrointestinal tract. **Hepato-Gastroenterol** 46:661–666.
703. Naylor EW, Lebenthal E (1979) Early detection of adenomatous polyposis coli in the Gardner's syndrome. **Pediatrics** 63:222–227.
704. Narisawa Y, Kohda (1995) Cutaneous cyts of Gardner's syndrome are similar to follicular stem cells. **J Cutan Pathol** 22:115–121.
705. Pujol RM, Casanova JM, Egido R et al. (1995) Multiple familial pilomatricomas: a cutaneous marker for Gardner syndrome? **Pediatr Dermatol** 12:331–335.
706. Wynder EL, Reddy BS (1974) Metabolic epidemiology of colorectal cancer. **Cancer** 34:801–806.
707. Reed TE, Neel JV (1955) A genetic study of multiple polyposis of the colon (with an appendix deriving a method of estimating relative fitness). **Am J Hum Genet** 7:236–263.
708. Hampel H, Peltomaki P (2000) Hereditary colorectal cancer: risk assessment and management. **Clin Genet** 58:89–97.
709. Soave F (1964) Hirschsprung's disease: A new surgical technique. **Arch Dis Child** 39:116–124.

with surgical excision of suspicious lesions. Naylor[703] followed four children at risk for GS between the ages of 1½ and 9 years. The youngest patient showed no polyps, but biopsy of "normal" mucosa revealed early adenomatous hyperplasia. He concluded that early mucosal biopsies are mandatory for at-risk children. Endoscopy that includes a thorough view of the duodenum (periampullary area) is also very important because of the high incidence of duodenal cancer.

Carcinoma can arise not only in the intestines but also in the stomach, duodenum, and periampullary areas.[710] The average age of development of periampullary carcinoma is 48 years, but a patient as young as 18 years has been reported.[699] Other malignant tumors, such as papillary carcinoma of the thyroid and hepatoblastomas, should be suspected in symptomatic patients.

Desmoid tumors should be surgically excised; however, there tends to be a high recurrence rate. Tumors can involve the mesentery and thus be difficult to remove. Computed tomographic scan or MRI of the abdomen can demonstrate the origin of the tumors and the extent of involvement of the abdominal structures.

Desmoid tumors are so rare in the general population and so common in GS that any patient with a desmoid tumor should have his or her colon examined for polyps. If wide surgical excision fails, radiotherapy or chemotherapy or a combination can be employed and has met with variable success. Drugs which affect prostaglandin metabolism, such as nonsteroidal anti-inflammatory drugs (NSAID), can reduce the risk of colorectal cancer and desmoids by affecting the enzymatic activity of the cyclo-oxygenases (COX) which are responsible for prostaglandin synthesis.[711,712] IFN-α has been reported to cause regression of a large desmoid tumor in one patient.[713]

Genetic counseling for patients is imperative because of the expected risk that half of the offspring will be affected and develop adenocarcinoma of the bowel. Examination of all family members for extracolonic signs of GS may reveal valuable markers for early detection of asymptomatic family members. Genetic testing can indicate which family members are affected.[689]

Skin lesions can be excised if they are cosmetically or functionally unacceptable.

PEDIATRIC ASPECTS OF THE DISEASE

Gardner syndrome is a genodermatosis associated with carcinoma of the bowel. Genetic testing for all family members, including children, should be performed as early as possible to detect those members who have the disorder.

BROOKE–SPIEGLER SYNDROME

Synonyms: Brooke syndrome, epithelioma adenoides cysticum

INTRODUCTION AND HISTORICAL NOTE

In 1892, Brooke reported an entity which he called epithelioma adenoides cysticum which is now called Brooke tumor or trichoepithelioma. In general, trichoepitheliomas may be solitary or multiple. Brooke–Spiegler syndrome consists of multiple trichoepitheliomas associated with cylindromas inherited in an autosomal dominant fashion[714] (MIM 60541). Other features of the syndrome that are common but not invariably present are eccrine spiradenomas, milia, organoid nevi, and basal cell carcinomas.[715,716]

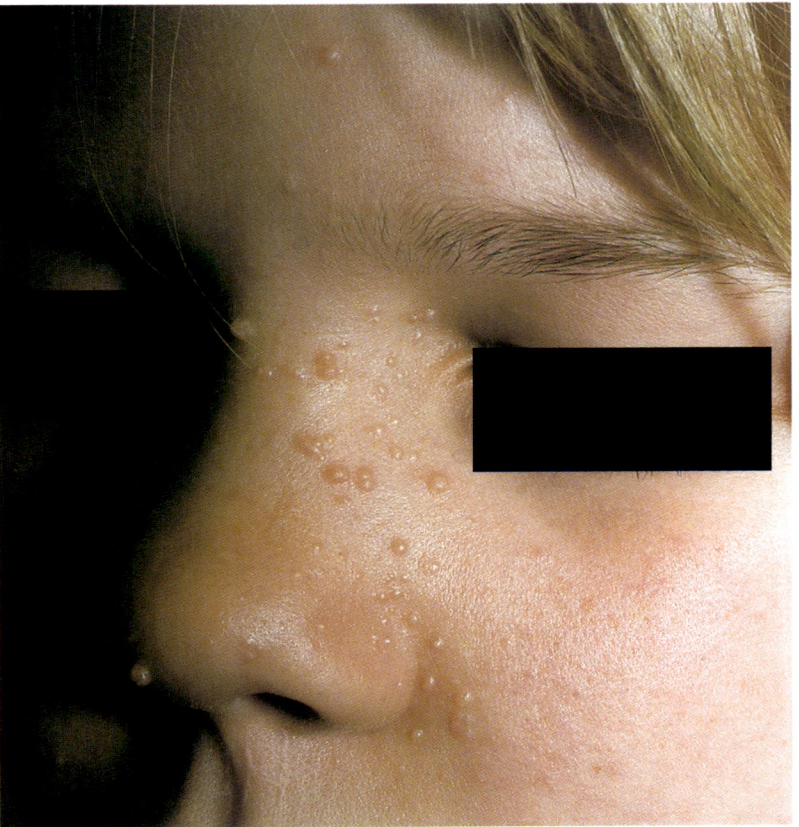

Fig. 7.73 Brooke–Spiegler syndrome, multiple trichoepitheliomas.

PRESENTING HISTORY

Adolescents or children usually present with 1–5mm multiple papules on the face, particularly along the sides of the nose, although these papules can occur anywhere (Fig. 7.73).

PHYSICAL EXAMINATION

Trichoepitheliomas are 1–5mm, skin-colored or white papules with a smooth and sometimes translucent surface which can resemble a basal cell carcinoma.[715] Lesions on the face tend to be smaller, while those occurring in other sites, particularly the scalp, can reach 2–5cm in diameter.[717] They tend to form confluent plaques of tiny papules, especially along the nasolabial folds.

Cylindromas, sometimes called turban tumors, mainly occur in the scalp and behind the ears, more commonly in adults with this syndrome. They are skin-colored or bluish cysts with a smooth surface covered by telangiectasis. They slowly enlarge and can become quite disfiguring.[718] Although rare, malignancy has been reported.[718] A congenital plaque with histological features of both trichoepithelioma and cylindroma has been reported in a patient with Brooke syndrome.[719]

710. Sugihara K, Muto T, Kamiya J et al. (1982) Gardner's syndrome associated with periampullary carcinoma, duodenal and gastric adenomatosis. Report of a case. **Dis Colon Rectum** 25:766–771.

711. Belliveau P, Graham AM (1984) Mesenteric desmoid tumor in Gardner's syndrome treated by sulindac. **Dis Colon Rectum** 27:53–54.

712. Hughes-Fulford M, Boman B (1997) Growth regulation of Gardner's syndrome colorectal cancer cells by NSAIDS. **Adv Exp Med Biol** 407:433–441.

713. Geurs F, Kok TC (1993) Regression of a great abdominal desmoid tumor by interferon alpha. **J Clin Gastroenterol** 16:264–265.

714. Anderson DE, Howell JB (1976) Epithelioma adenoides cysticum: genetic update. **Br J Dermatol** 95:225–232.

715. Puig L, Nadal C, Fernandez-Figueras MT et al. (1998) Brooke–Spiegler syndrome variant: segregation of tumor types with mixed differentiation in two generations. **Am J Dermatolpathol** 20:56–60.

716. Weyers W, Nilles M, Eckert F et al. (1993) Spiradenomas in Brooke–Spiegler syndrome. **Am J Dermatolpath** 15:156–161.

717. Burrows NP, Russell Jones R et al. (1992) The clinicopathological features of familial cylindromas and trichoepitheliomas (Brooke–Spiegler syndrome): a report of two families. **Clin Exp Dermatol** 17:332–336.

718. Pizinger K, Michal M (2000) Malignant cylindroma in Brooke–Spiegler syndrome. **Dermatology** 201:255–257.

719. Schirren CG, Wörle B, Kind P et al. (1995) A nevoid plaque with histological changes of trichoepithelioma and cylindroma in Brooke–Spiegler syndrome. **J Cutan Pathol** 22:563–569.

PATHOPHYSIOLOGY AND HISTOGENESIS

The gene for Brooke syndrome has been mapped to chromosome 16q12–q13, and mutations have been shown in the CYLD gene, a tumor suppressor gene.[720]

Trichoepitheliomas are benign adnexal tumors showing pilar differentiation. However, in contrast to trichofolliculoma, formation of hair shafts is generally not a feature of trichoepithelioma. Microscopically, these tumors are composed of aggregates of basaloid cells within the dermis, without connection to the epidermis.[721] The distinction of typical trichoepithelioma from basal cell carcinoma is sometimes difficult clinically as well as histologically but can be based on the presence of a fibrotic (not myxoid) stroma, and on the lack of retraction of the tumor stroma from the parenchyma. Mitotic figures are rare in trichoepitheliomas but common in basal cell carcinoma.

DIFFERENTIAL DIAGNOSIS

The solitary form of trichoepithelioma can resemble a basal cell carcinoma, and thus a biopsy is indicated. Multiple trichoepitheliomas with the typical appearance and family history is not a diagnostic problem for a child presenting with symptoms. Eruptive syringomas usually occur in a periorbital distribution, not along the nasolabial folds, as in Brooke–Spiegler syndrome.

Multiple trichoepitheliomas may also be part of Rombo syndrome which shows vermiculate atrophoderma, milia, hypotrichosis, basal cell carcinomas and peripheral vasodilatation with cyanosis. Bazex syndrome can also have multiple trichoepitheliomas in addition to follicular atrophoderma and basal cell carcinomas. Basal cell nevus syndrome can feature multiple skin-colored papules, but this can be distinguished by biopsy and clinical features of jaw cysts and palmar pits.

THERAPEUTICS AND PROGNOSIS

Trichoepitheliomas and cylindromas are benign. Most lesions obtain a size no larger than several millimeters. However, some lesions may slowly enlarge to the point of cosmetic disfigurement and may need to be removed.

Individual lesions can be treated by any destructive method such as dermabrasion or shave excision.[717] They may recur if not completely removed, but may be treated by re-excision or electrodesiccation and curettage. Multiple small lesions can be treated by CO_2 laser.[722] Larger lesions will need to be surgically excised.

PEDIATRIC ASPECTS OF THE DISEASE

Multiple trichoepitheliomas begin in childhood and continue to increase in number into early adulthood. Sometimes the lesions remain stable in number and size but occasionally continue to grow in size and number for years. Early detection and removal could potentially aid in cosmesis.

PEUTZ–JEGHERS SYNDROME

INTRODUCTION AND HISTORICAL NOTE

Peutz–Jeghers syndrome (PJS, MIM 175200) is characterized by gastrointestinal polyps and periorificial pigmentation.[723] There is a very high incidence of both gastrointestinal and other malignancies even though the polyps which arise are hamartomatous in origin.[724,725]

In 1896, Hutchinson reported twins with unusual pigmentation of the oral mucosa. One twin died of intussusception, and the other died from carcinoma of the breast. In 1921, Peutz described a family with melanotic spots on the lips and multiple gastrointestinal polyps. Jeghers and colleagues reported the familial pattern and confirmed the association.[726]

EPIDEMIOLOGY

The syndrome is inherited as an autosomal dominant trait, and patients commonly first note the disease in adolescence or adulthood. Males and females are equally affected, and most races and ethnic groups have been affected. The risk of occurrence is approximately 1 in 8300 to 1 in 200 000 live births.

PRESENTING HISTORY

The diagnosis of PJS has been made in infancy, although most patients present later.[727,728] One-third of patients with PJS begin showing signs during the first decade of life,[729] and up to 50–60% show clinical manifestations before age 20 years. The most common gastrointestinal symptoms in children that lead to the diagnosis are abdominal pain (71%), gastrointestinal bleeding (18.5%), anemia (16%), vomiting (6%), and rectal prolapse (7%).[730]

PHYSICAL EXAMINATION

Melanoplakia resembling lentigines is seen in almost all patients, most commonly on the lips (Fig. 7.74), buccal mucosa, and digits, but any mucosal surface can be involved.[731] The pigmentation varies widely in size, shape,

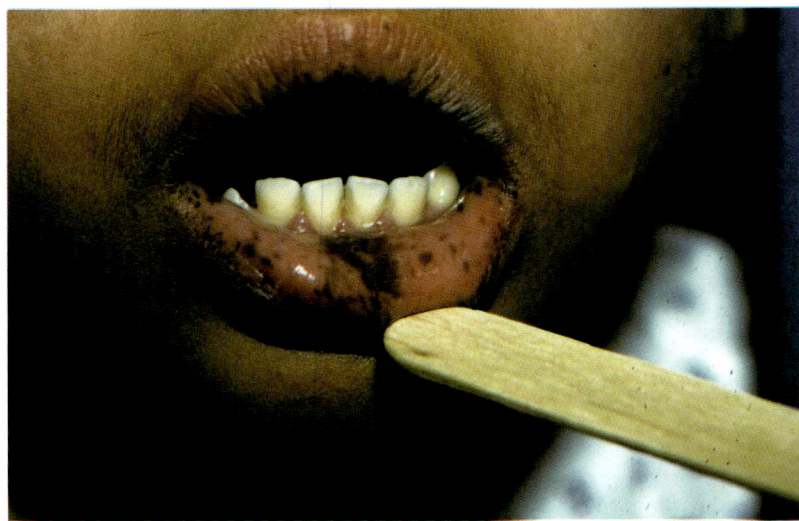

Fig. 7.74 Hyperpigmented macules on lips of a child with Peutz–Jeghers syndrome. The buccal mucosa, fingerpads and toepads also showed hyperpigmented macules.

720. Poblete Guitierrez P, Eggerman T, Holler D et al. (2002) Phenotype diversity in familial cylindromatosis: a frameshift mutation in the tumor suppressor gene CYLD underlies different tumors of skin appendages. **J Invest Dermatol** 119:527–531.
721. Brooke JD, Fitzpatrick JE, Golitz LE (1989) Papillary mesenchymal bodies: a histological finding useful in differentiating trichoepitheliomas from basal cell crcinomas. **J Am Acad Dermatol** 21:523–528.
722. Martins C, Bártolo (2000) Brooke–Spiegler syndrome: treatment of cylindromas with CO_2 laser. **Dermatol Surg** 26:877–882.
723. McGarrity TJ, Kulin HE, Zaino RJ (2000) Peutz–Jeghers syndrome. **Am J Gastroenterol** 95:596–604.
724. Giardiello FM, Brensinger JD, Tersmette AC et al. (2000) Very high risk of cancer in familial Peutz–Jeghers syndrome. **Gastroenterol** 119:1447–1453.
725. Giarcello FM, Welsh SB, Hamilton ST et al. (1987) Increased risk of cancer in Peutz–Jeghers syndrome. **N Engl J Med** 316:1511–1514.
726. Jeghers H, McKusick BA, Katz KH (1949) Generalized intestinal polyposis and melanin spots of the oral mucosa, lips and digits. **N Engl J Med** 241:993–1005, 1031–1036.
727. Howell J, Pringle K, Kirschner B et al. (1981) Peutz–Jeghers polyps causing colocolic intussusception in infancy. **J Pediatr Surg** 16:82–84.
728. Fernandez Seara MJ, Martinez Soto MI, Fernandez Lorenzo JR et al. (1995) Peutz–Jeghers syndrome in a neonate. **J Pediatr** 126:965–967.
729. McKitrick JE, Lewis WM, Doane WA et al. (1971) The Peutz–Jeghers syndrome: Report of two cases, one with 30 year follow-up. **Arch Surg** 103:57–62.
730. Tovar JA, Eizaguirre I, Albert A et al. (1983) Peutz–Jeghers in children: Report of two cases and review of the literature. **J Pediatr Surg** 18:1–6.
731. Agha FP, Nostrant TT, Cohen AR et al. (1985) Giant hamartoma of the colon: Peutz–Jeghers type. **J Clin Gastroenterol** 7:261–265.

and color and may fade in adult years. No obvious features distinguish this pigmentation clinically. Lesions are usually 1–12mm, are regular or irregular in shape, and range in color from brown to black. Pigmentation can either precede or follow the development of polyps. There is no relationship between either the location and distribution of pigmentation or the severity or location of the polyps. Pigmented oral papillomas have also been described.

Gastrointestinal (GI) polyps are characteristically pedunculated, non-neoplastic hamartomas that range from 0.1 to 4cm. They are typically multiple and are most commonly found in the jejunum (70%) and ileum (36%)[730] but have been reported in the stomach (34%), duodenum (27%), and colon (24%). Less commonly, polyps have been found in the nasal passages, bronchi, renal pelvis, ureters,[732] bladder, and gallbladder. PJS polyps can give rise to hemorrhage, intussusception, and obstruction early in life.[733]

LABORATORY FINDINGS

Proctoscopic examination, air-contrast barium enema, ultrasound, and radiographs of the GI tract can all be used to demonstrate polyps.[734]

PATHOPHYSIOLOGY AND HISTOGENESIS

PJS is usually caused by mutations in the serine/threonine kinase LBK1/STK11 gene on chromosome 19p13.3.[702,735] This gene acts as a tumor suppressor gene and alterations in its activity are involved in tumorigenesis.[735] There may be other genetic loci which have similar clinical presentations, as not all families or tumors arising in these patients have this mutation.[737,738]

Histopathologic examination of the oral pigmentation demonstrates an increase in pigment in the basal cell layer, but not an increase in the numbers of melanocytes. Lesions on the hands, however, demonstrate melanosomes that have accumulated within the dendrites of melanocytes, not within the keratinocytes. This implies a disturbance of melanosome transfer. Giant melanosomes are not seen.[739]

PJS polyps are hamartomas with mature, nondividing intestinal epithelial cells organized in arborizing glands surrounded by a delicate, inconspicuous stroma that contains bundles of smooth muscle fibers.[702] They are not adenomatous polyps, which commonly give rise to adenocarcinoma.

DIFFERENTIAL DIAGNOSIS

It is important to distinguish lentigines seen in PJS from freckles, which are never present at birth, are sun-induced, and never occur on the buccal mucosa.[700] LEOPARD syndrome (multiple lentigines syndrome) and Carney complex can be distinguished by other features. Laugier–Hunziker syndrome dermatologically resembles PJS, but even though they may have polyps or gastrointestinal changes, these patients do not have an increased incidence of cancer. Other polyposis syndromes such as Gardner syndrome and Cowden disease are not readily confused with PJS.

THERAPEUTICS AND PROGNOSIS

PJS is frequently misdiagnosed, leading to major consequences. Repeated surgery can cause intestinal crippling in these patients because of extensive adhesion formation and short-bowel syndrome.[733] Endoscopic or surgical removal of large benign lesions may be necessary to prevent hemorrhage and intussusception. It is difficult, however, to differentiate adenomas from hamartomas by either direct visualization or small biopsy specimens. Therefore, complete removal of larger lesions or small-bowel resection may be necessary.

Patients with PJS have a 93% chance of developing cancer from age 15 to 64 years, especially cancer of the esophagus, stomach, small intestine, colon, pancreas, lung, breast, uterus, gallbladder, bile ducts and ovary.[724,725,740] Adenocarcinoma appears to affect younger individuals (less than 40 years of age), and a patient as young as 8 years old developed adenocarcinoma of the duodenum and jejunum.[741]

A distinct type of ovarian tumor, called the sex cord tumor with annular tubules,[742] is found primarily in patients with PJS and is derived from granulosa cells in a pattern more characteristic of Sertoli cells. Precocious puberty can be caused by ovarian tumors in prepubertal children.[743] Sertoli cell testicular tumors with feminizing features can be seen in males.

Cancer surveillance should begin early, looking for breast, gynecological, colorectal, stomach, and pancreatic cancer.[744] Affected individuals should receive a colonoscopy every 1–2 years, starting in adolescence, and upper GI endoscopy and small intestinal double-contrast endoscopy or push enteroscopy every 2 years. Women should have mammography every 2 years beginning at age 25–35 years and annually thereafter. Frequent self-examination of the breast should be encouraged. Routine gynecologic care is of utmost importance starting in the teens.[744]

Treatment of pigmented facial lesions can be accomplished using the ruby laser.[745,746]

PEDIATRIC ASPECTS OF THE DISEASE

Patients with PJS have an increase in the incidence of malignancy, particularly of the gastrointestinal tract, breast, and gonads. Children should be identified as early as possible with genetic testing to watch for signs and symptoms related to these organs.

BASAL CELL NEVUS SYNDROME

INTRODUCTION AND HISTORICAL NOTE

The basal cell nevus syndrome (BCNS), also called nevoid basal cell carcinoma syndrome or Gorlin syndrome (MIM 109400) is an autosomal dominant

732. Sachatello CR, Griffen WO, Jr (1975) Hereditary polypoid disease of the gastrointestinal tract: A working classification. Am J Surg 128:198–203.
733. Mathus-Vliegen EMH, Tytgat GNJ (1985) Peutz–Jeghers syndrome: clinical presentation and new therapeutic strategy. Endoscopy 17:102–104.
734. Navarro O, Dugougeat F, Kornecki A et al. (2000) The impact of imaging in the management of intussusception owing to pathologic lead points in children. Pediatr Radiol 30:594–603.
735. Nakagawa H, Koyama K, Tanaka T et al. (1998) Localization of the gene responsible for Peutz–Jeghers syndrome within a 6-cM region of chromosomes 19p13.3. Hum Genet 102:203–206.
736. Entius MM, Keller JJ, Westerman AM et al. (2001) Molecular genetic alterations in hamartomatous polyps and carcinomas of patients with Peutz–Jeghers syndrome. J Clin Pathol 54:126–131.
737. Boardman LA, Couch FJ, Burgart LJ et al. (2000) Genetic heterogeneity in Peutz–Jeghers syndrome. Hum Mutat 16:23–30.
738. Connolly DC, Katabuchi H, Cliby WA et al. (2000) Somatic mutations in the STK11/LKB1 gene are uncommon in rare gynecological tumor types associated with Peutz–Jegher's syndrome. Am J Pathol 156:339–345.
739. Yamada K, Matsukawa A, Hori Y et al. (1981) Ultrastructural studies on pigmented macules of Peutz–Jeghers syndrome. J Dermatol 8:367–377.
740. Patterson MJ, Kernen JA (1985) Epithelioid leiomyosarcoma originating in a hamartomatous polyp from a patient with Peutz–Jeghers syndrome. Gastroenterology 88:1060–1064.
741. Cordts AE, Chabot JR (1983) Jejunal carcinoma in a child. J Pediatr Surg 18:180–181.
742. Scully RE (1970) Sex cord tumor with annular tubules, a distinctive ovarian tumor of the Peutz–Jeghers syndrome. Cancer 25:1107–1121.
743. Sohl HM, Azoury RS, Najjar SS (1983) Peutz–Jeghers syndrome associated with precocious puberty. J Pediatr 103:593–595.
744. Hampel H, Peltomaki P (2000) Hereditary colorectal cancer: risk assessment and management. Clin Genet 58:89–97.
745. Kato S, Takeyama J, Tanita Y et al. (1998) Ruby laser therapy for labial lentigines in Peutz–Jeghers syndrome. Eur J Pediatr 157:622–624.
746. Ohshiro T, Maruyama Y, Nakajima H et al. (1980) Treatment of pigmentation of the lips and oral mucosa in Peutz–Jeghers syndrome using ruby and argon lasers. Br J Plast Surg 33:346–349.

disorder; its main features are basal cell carcinomas (BCCs), jaw cysts, skeletal anomalies (i.e., bifid ribs, vertebral anomalies, etc.), ectopic calcifications, and palmoplantar pits.[747]

EPIDEMIOLOGY

The prevalence is about 1 per 60 000, but it is more common in northern Europeans than African-Americans or Asians, and has a male to female ratio of one.[748] Causing 0.5% of all the total BCCs, BCNS accounts for 20% of all patients who develop BCCs before the age of 19 years.[749] Blacks develop the syndrome less frequently than whites,[750] although in black patients the syndrome often goes unrecognized because they have fewer BCCs.[751]

PRESENTING HISTORY

Patients may present at any age. In childhood, congenital defects such as jaw cysts,[752] skeletal anomalies, cleft lip or palate,[753] or medulloblastoma may be the presenting complaint.[754] Older children may present with jaw cysts, defective dentition, or skeletal anomalies. Skin manifestations may be present at birth but usually appear in teenage years. Adults are most commonly seen for BCCs or jaw cysts.

PHYSICAL EXAMINATION
Basal cell carcinomas
BCCs usually start between puberty and age 35 years, but they have been reported in newborns.[755] In patients with BCNS, BCCs are seen in half of patients less than 20 years of age, 75–85% of those over 20 years old, and 90–95% of those over 40 years of age.[756,757] Lesions resembling nevi or seborrheic keratoses commonly appear before puberty but behave like benign growths (Fig. 7.75). After puberty, however, the tumors display a greater invasive tendency.[758] Most frequently seen on the face, neck, back, chest, and upper extremities, these 1- to 10-mm hyperpigmented or skin-colored, dome-shaped papules erupt in crops throughout life. If lesions enlarge and are left untreated, secondary changes can occur, such as ulceration, crusting, or bleeding. Patients commonly have 8 to 100 BCCs, and at least one patient has been described who had more than 1000.[759,760]

BCCs of the head and neck in BCNS tend to be more aggressive than sporadic BCCs.[761] The periorbital areas, nose, and central face can show marked invasion with resulting loss of one or both eyes.

Jaw cysts/epidermal cysts
Because jaw cysts cause symptoms (pain, swelling, and drainage), they are commonly the initial complaint in patients with BCNS.[752] Odontogenic keratocysts can appear in childhood, but the average age of presentation is 13 years.[758] They may be single or multiple and vary in size and location, most commonly affecting the molar and premolar regions of the upper maxilla which can cause loosening of the teeth. Patients are frequently edentulous before 30 years of age. Cysts tend to recur after surgical removal, probably because of microcysts or satellite cysts left behind. Squamous cell carcinoma, ameloblastoma,[762] spindle cell carcinoma, and fibrosarcoma have been reported to arise from jaw cysts, but malignant transformation was not

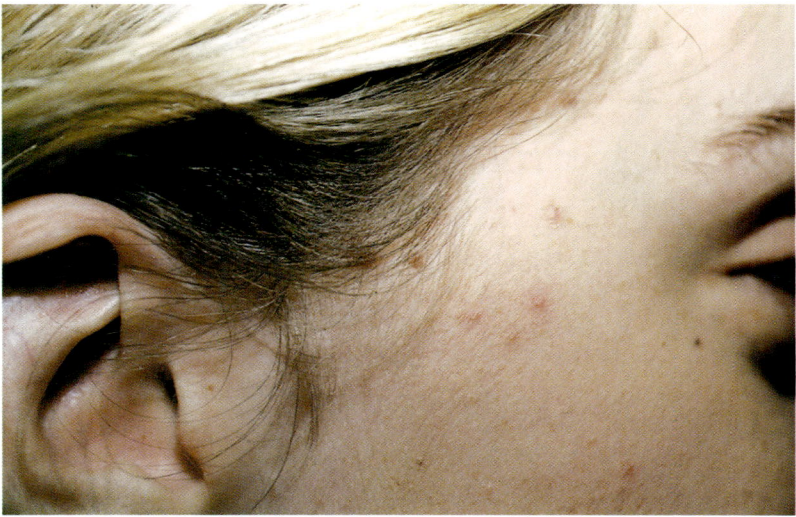

Fig. 7.75 Two brown papules in the hairline which look like benign nevi but which were basal cell carcinomas on biopsy.

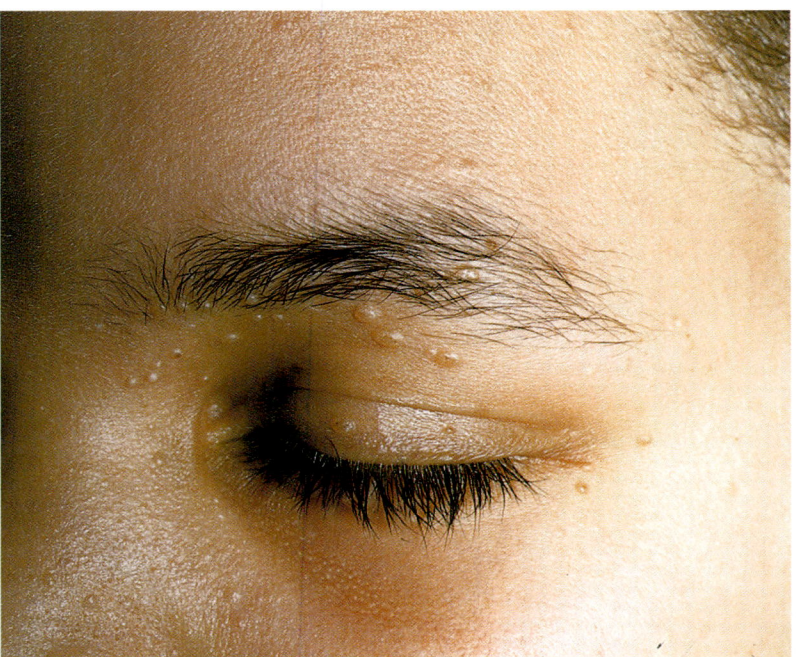

Fig. 7.76 Basal cell nevus syndrome: numerous epidermal cysts around the eyes.

747. Gorlin RJ, Goltz RW (1960) Multiple nevoid basal-cell epithelioma, jaw cysts and bifid rib: a syndrome. **N Engl J Med** 262:908–912.
748. Gorlin RJ (1999) Nevoid basal cell carcinoma (Gorlin) syndrome: unanswered issues. **J Lab Clin Med** 134:551–552.
749. Springate JE (1986) The nevoid basal cell carcinoma syndrome. **J Pediatr Surg** 21:908–910.
750. Johnson AD, Hebert AA, Esterly NB (1986) Nevoid basal cell carcinoma syndrome bilateral ovarian fibromas in a 3½ year old girl. **J Am Acad Dermatol** 14:371–374.
751. Goldstein AM, Pastakia B, DiGiovanna JJ et al. (1994) Clinical findings in two African-American families with the nevoid basal cell carcinoma syndrome. **Am J Med Genet** 50:272–281.
752. Dowling PA, Fleming P, Saunders IDF et al. (2000) Odontogenic keratocysts in a 5-year-old: initial manifestations of nevoid basal cell carcinoma syndrome. **Pediatr Dent** 22:53–55.
753. Lambrecht JT, Kreusch T (1997) Examine your orofacial cleft patients for Gorlin–Goltz syndrome. **Cleft Palate Craniofac J** 34:342–350.
754. Stavrou T, Dubovsky EC, Reaman GH et al. (2000) Intracranial calcifications in childhood medulloblastoma: relation to nevoid basal cell carcinoma syndrome. **AJNR** 21:790–794.
755. Meyvisch K, Andre J, Song M et al. (1993) Basal cell nevus syndrome and congenital hydrocephaly. **Dermatology** 186:311–312.
756. Evans DG, Ladusans EJ, Rimmer S et al. (1993) Complications of the naevoid basal cell carcinoma syndrome: results of a population based study. **J Med Genet** 30:460–464.
757. Shanley S, Ratcliffe J, Hockey A et al. (1994) Nevoid basal cell carcinoma syndrome: review of 118 affected individuals. **Am J Med Genet** 50:282–290.
758. De la Plaza R, Rodriguez E, Castillo E (1983) Two cases of nevoid basal cell carcinoma syndrome. **Plast Reconstr Surg** 71:114–119.
759. Scharnagel IM, Pack GT (1949) Multiple basal cell epitheliomas in a 5 year old child. **Am J Dis Child** 77:647–651.
760. Kimonis VE, Goldstein AM, Pastakia B et al. (1997) Clinical manifestations in 105 persons with nevoid basal cell carcinoma syndrome. **Am J Med Genet** 69:299–308.
761. Howell JB (1984) Nevoid basal cell carcinoma syndrome: profile of genetic and environmental factors in oncogenesis. **J Am Acad Dermatol** 11:98–104.
762. Schultz SM, Twickler DM, Wheeler DE et al. (1987) Ameloblastoma associated with basal cell nevus (Gorlin) syndrome: CT findings. **J Comput Assist Tomogr** 11:901–904.

Musculoskeletal anomalies, which occur in 60 to 75% of patients, are usually congenital. These anomalies include frontal or temporoparietal bossing, prognathism, cleft lip and palate,[756,757] splayed or bifid ribs, kyphoscoliosis, vertebral fusion, spina bifida occulta,[771] marfanoid habitus, pectus excavatum, shortened fourth metacarpals, polydactyly, syndactyly,[747,757,772] and widespread osteolytic lesions in the long bones.[773]

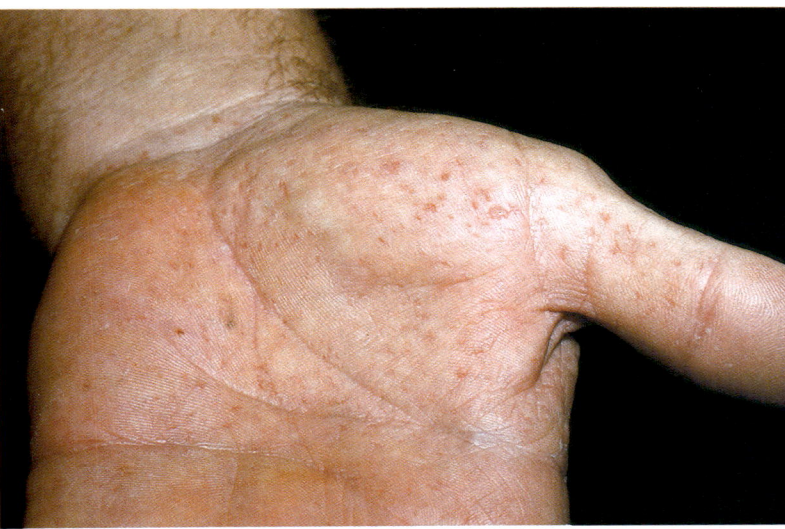

Fig. 7.77   Palmar pits in basal cell nevus syndrome.

reported in two large reviews of 84 and 118 patients.[756,757] The lining of the cysts has an increased number of mitotic figures, suggesting a greater growth potential than in controls. Epidermal cysts are noted in 25% to 55% of patients, mainly on the palms and limbs[763] (Fig. 7.76).

Palmoplantar pits

A hallmark of BCNS is the finding of 2- to 3-mm shallow pits on the palmar or plantar surfaces in 75–90% of patients[756,757] (Fig. 7.77). These pits have an underlying erythema that resembles multiple small red spots on the palms and soles. In blacks, the pits may be hyperpigmented instead. Soaking the hands for 15min accentuates the pits.[757] They usually appear in the second decade of life or later and represent defective keratinization with an altered epidermis.

Ectopic calcifications

Ectopic calcifications of the falx cerebri or dura occur in more than 90% of adults and in some children.[758,764] These calcifications can help in early diagnosis of asymptomatic patients. Calcifications can also be seen in subcutaneous tissue and within the maxillary cysts.

Other systems

Medulloblastoma is the most common malignancy other than BCCs. Its frequency has been estimated to be as high as 5%,[756] and it occurs at an average age of 2 years of age, as compared with the reported onset in control patients after age 7 years.[765]

Seizures can occur even in the absence of brain tumors. Mental retardation,[766] electroencephalographic abnormalities,[767] meningioma,[768] agenesis of the corpus callosum, congenital hydrocephalus,[769] and cerebral gigantism[770] have all been associated with BCNS.

TABLE 7.24   Major findings in basal cell nevus syndrome

Cutaneous
    Basal cell carcinomas
    Palmoplantar pits
    Epithelial cysts
    Milia
    Fibromas
    Lipomas

Skeletal
    Jaw cysts (mandible, maxilla)
    Sellar bridging
    Vertebral anomalies (scoliosis, spina bifida)
    Rib anomalies (bifid, splayed, synostoses, pectus excavatum)
    Cystic changes (long bones, phalanges)
    Brachymetacarpals
    Frontal bossing
    Defective dentition
    Mandibular prognathism
    Cleft lip or palate
    High arched palate

Neurologic
    Ectopic calcification (falx cerebri, tentorium cerebelli)
    Mental retardation
    Electroencephalographic abnormalities
    Medulloblastoma
    Congenital hydrocephalus
    Agenesis of corpus callosum

Ophthalmologic
    Hypertelorism
    Dystopia canthorum
    Strabismus
    Congenital blindness
    Cataract
    Coloboma
    Microphthalmia

Gonads
    Ovarian fibromas
    Hypogonadism (male)
    Adenocarcinoma of the ovary

Miscellaneous
    Cardiac fibroma
    Fibrosarcoma of the jaw
    Squamous cell carcinoma of the jaw
    Lymphomesenteric cysts
    Enterogeneous cysts (bowel)

763. Leppard BJ (1983) Skin cysts in the basal cell naevus syndrome. **Clin Exp Dermatol** 8:603–612.
764. Ratcliffe JF, Shanley S, Ferguson J et al. (1995) The diagnostic implication of falcine calcification on plain skull radiographs of patients with basal cell naevus syndrome and the incidence of falcine calcification in their relatives and two control groups. **Br J Radiol** 68:361–368.
765. Evans DG, Farndon PA, Burnell LD et al. (1991) The incidence of Gorlin syndrome in 173 consecutive cases of medulloblastoma. **Br J Cancer** 64:959–961.
766. Pritchard LJ, Delfino JJ, Ivey DM et al. (1982) Variable expressivity of the multiple nevoid basal cell carcinoma syndrome. **J Oral Surg** 20:261–269.
767. Murphy MJ, Tensor RB (1982) Nevoid basal cell carcinoma syndrome and epilepsy. **Ann Neurol** 11:372–376.

768. Albrecht S, Goodman JC, Rajogopolan S et al. (1994) Malignant meningioma in Gorlin's syndrome: cytogenetic and p53 gene analysis (case report). **J Neurosurg** 81:466–471.
769. Lycka BAS, Chichak VR (1985) Congenital hydrocephalus and the basal cell nevus syndrome. **Can Med Ass J** 132:1037–1038.
770. Cramer H, Niederdellmann H (1983) Cerebral giantism associated with jaw cyst basal cell naevoid syndrome in two families. **Arch Psychiatr Nervenkr** 233:111–124.
771. Barnes DA, Borns P, Pizzutillo PD (1982) Cervical spondylolisthesis associated with the multiple nevoid basal cell carcinoma syndrome. **Clin Orthop** 162:26–30.
772. Gorlin RJ (1995) Nevoid basal cell carcinoma syndrome. **Dermatol Clin** 13:113–125.
773. Blinder B, Barki Y, Pezt M et al. (1994) Widespread osteolytic lesions of the long bones in basal cell nevus syndrome. **Skel Radiol** 12:196–198.

Several patients with BCNS have been reported with ovarian fibromas.[750,774,775] Fibrosarcoma of the ovary can occur[776] and is more common if the patient has undergone radiation therapy. Hypogonadism in men, cryptorchidism, and adrenal cortical adenomas have also been reported.

Ophthalmological abnormalities, including hypertelorism, dystopia canthorum, congenital blindness, cataracts, strabismus, glaucoma, congenital retinal folds, and coloboma of the retina or iris[777] are reported in a third of patients. Epidermal cysts on the palpebral conjunctival surfaces of the upper eyelids are common.[778]

Other neoplasms include Hodgkin lymphoma[779] and non-Hodgkin lymphoma, melanomas,[757] and fetal rhabdomyoma.[772,780]

Cardiac fibromas[781,782] are usually asymptomatic;[783] however, profound bradycardia during general anesthesia can occur and should be considered when undertaking general anesthesia (Table 7.24).

LABORATORY FINDINGS

Histologically, BCCs in this syndrome are indistinguishable from ordinary BCCs. Multiple keratinizing cysts within the tumors occur more commonly than in sporadic BCCs, an interesting fact because of the development of other cystic lesions seen in this syndrome such as odontogenic cysts and epidermal cysts.[784] Osteoid formation may be seen.[785]

Jaw cysts show a keratinizing squamous epithelium with a surrounding fibrous capsule. Commonly, microcysts or daughter cysts are found in the connective tissue stroma.

Palmar pits may show a proliferation of small basaloid cells resembling BCC in situ; however, they rarely form true BCCs.[761] Pits may reveal a thin irregular keratin layer with acanthosis.

Skull X-rays can demonstate intracranial calcifications.[754] Skull radiographs can identify falx calcifications in almost all patients by age 10 years and in some in the first decade of life.[764]

PATHOPHYSIOLOGY AND HISTOGENESIS

BCNS is caused by mutations in PATCHED (*PTC*), a tumor suppressor gene.[786] The malformations found in this syndrome may be caused by a single point mutation in one *PTC* allele.[787] When there is inactivation of both *PTC* alleles, tumors and cysts may arise. The gene defect has been localized to chromosome 9q22.3–3.1. The human *PTC* encodes a transmembrane protein functioning as a receptor for signaling proteins of the hedgehog family.[788] Its role in both organogenesis and carcinogenesis may explain both the birth defects and the cancer predisposition seen in BCNS.[789] This defect in a tumor suppressor gene requires homozygous inactivation ("loss of heterozygosity") to allow BCC growth. One defective copy of the

tumor suppressor gene is inherited. BCCs develop if the other copy is lost, as in nondisjunction, deletion, mitotic recombination, or treatment with ionizing radiation. Whatever the defect causing reduced capacity of DNA repair, tumors may grow following exposure to ultraviolet or ionizing radiation, as evidenced by the development of BCCs in areas irradiated for medulloblastoma.

DIFFERENTIAL DIAGNOSIS

Basal cell carcinomas can resemble benign nevi in childhood or even seborrheic keratoses. A high index of suspicion should be raised if other features of the syndrome are present. Biopsy of a lesion would demonstrate a BCC. Although most BCCs in childhood are associated with this or other syndromes such as XP, Rombo/Bazex syndrome or nevus sebaceus, BCCs have been reported *de novo* in areas of intense sunlight.[790]

Multiple epidermal cysts are also seen in GS.

THERAPEUTICS AND PROGNOSIS

Genetic counseling is important for BCNS patients and their families because of the autosomal dominant transmission. At-risk family members should have skeletal surveys of the skull, mandible, maxilla, ribs, vertebrae, or hands, which may be helpful in identifying affected members, particularly children, before typical BCCs are obvious.

In general, the life span of a patient with BCNS is the same as in the normal population but depends on the location and invasiveness of BCCs and other tumors. Dental radiographs should be performed yearly starting at age 8 years[758,772,791] and cysts should be removed by an experienced surgeon. Neurologic screenings, including magnetic resonance imaging of the head, may be performed yearly until 8 years if warranted clinically.

Patients should use preventative measures such as sun avoidance and sunscreens as well as regular dermatological examinations.

Early BCCs should be surgically removed if growing. Microscopically controlled surgery is the treatment of choice for larger invasive lesions.[792,793] General anesthesia may be necessary to remove numerous lesions at one time, especially in children. Particularly for midface or periorbital BCCS, early detection and treatment are imperative in order to avoid local destruction, metastasis, and even death from invasion of vital structures and hemorrhage.

Topical 5% 5-fluorouracil with 0.1% tretinoin has been used successfully to treat BCCs,[794] but suppression of BCCs requires long-term treatment with both agents. BCCs recur within 6 months of stopping treatment. Topical 5-fluorouracil has also been combined with cryotherapy for treatment.[795]

774. Raggio M, Kaplan AL, Harberg JF (1983) Recurrent ovarian fibromas with basal cell nevus syndrome (Gorlin syndrome). **Obstet Gynecol** 61(suppl):95–96.
775. Fox R, Eckford S, Hirschowitz L et al. (1994) Refractory gestational hypertension due to a renin-secreting ovarian fibrothecoma associated with Gorlin's syndrome. **Br J Obstet Gynaecol** 101:1015–1017.
776. Kraemer BB, Silva EG, Sneige N (1984) Fibrosarcoma of ovary: a new component in the nevoid basal-cell carcinoma syndrome. **Am J Surg Pathol** 8:231–236.
777. Khoubesserian P, Baleriaux D, Toussaint D et al. (1981) Adult form of basal cell naevus syndrome: a family study. **J Neurol** 226:157–168.
778. Levine DJ, Robertson DB, Varma VA (1987) Familial subconjunctival epithelial cysts associated with the nevoid basal cell carcinoma syndrome. **Arch Dermatol** 123:23–24.
779. Potaznik D, Steinherz P (1984) Multiple nevoid basal cell carcinoma syndrome and Hodgkin's disease. **Cancer** 53:2713–2715.
780. DiSanto S, Abt AB, Boal DK et al. (1992) Fetal rhabdomyoma and nevoid basal cell carcinoma syndrome. **Pediatr Pathol** 12:441–447.
781. Coffin CM (1992) Congenital cardiac fibroma associated with Gorlin syndrome. **Pediatr Pathol** 12:255–262.
782. Herman TE, Siegel MJ, McAlister WH (1991) Cardiac tumor in Gorlin syndrome: nevoid basal cell carcinoma syndrome. **Pediatr Radiol** 21:234–235.
783. Cotton JL, Kavey RE, Palmier CE et al. (1991) Cardiac tumors and the nevoid basal cell carcinoma syndrome. **Pediatrics** 87:725–728.
784. Lindeberg H, Jepsen FL (1983) The nevoid basal cell carcinoma syndrome: histopathology of the basal cell tumors. **J Cutan Pathol** 10:68–73.
785. Mason JK, Helwig EB, Graham JH (1965) Pathology of the nevoid basal cell carcinoma syndrome. **Arch Pathol** 79:401–408.

786. Aszterbaum M, Rothman A, Johnson RL et al. (1998) Identification of mutations in the human PATCHED gene in sporadic basal cell carcinomas and in patients with the basal cell nevus syndrome. **J Invest Dermatol** 110:885–888.
787. Cohen MM Jr (1999) Nevoid basal cell carcinoma syndrome: molecular biology and new hypotheses. **Int J Oral Maxillofac Surg** 28:216–223.
788. Ingham PW (1998) The patched gene in development and cancer. **Curr Opin Genet Dev** 8:88–94.
789. Wicking C, Bale AE (1997) Molecular basis of the nevoid basal cell carcinoma syndrome. **Curr Opin Pediatr** 9:630–635.
790. LeSueur BW, Silvis NG, Hansen RC (2000) Basal cell carcinoma in children: report of 3 cases. **Arch Dermatol** 136:370–372.
791. Tokar IP, Fraser MC, Bale SJ (1992) Genodermatoses with profound malignant potential. **Semin Oncol Nursing** 8:272–280.
792. Mohs FE, Jones DL, Koranda FC (1980) Microscopically controlled surgery for carcinomas in patients with nevoid basal cell carcinoma syndrome. **Arch Dermatol** 116:777–779.
793. Krunic AL, Viehman GE, Madani S et al. (1998) Microscopically controlled surgical excision combined with ultrapulse CO$_2$ vaporization in the management of a patient with the nevoid basal cell carcinoma syndrome. **J Dermatol** 25:10–12.
794. Strange PR, Lang PG Jr (1992) Long-term management of basal cell nevus syndrome with topical tretinoin and 5-fluorouracil. **J Am Acad Dermatol** 27:842–845.
795. Tsuji T, Otake N, Nishimura M (1993) Cryosurgery and topical fluorouracil: a treatment method for widespread basal cell epithelioma in basal cell nevus syndrome. **J Dermatol** 20:507–513.

Prophylactic isotretinoin can be used to prevent early BCCs but pregnancy prevention is imperative in women of childbearing age.[796] Photodynamic therapy has been used with some success.[797] A photodynamically active dye (5-aminolevulinic) is preferentially retained by malignant tissues and initiates a cytotoxic reaction when exposed to red light. The major toxic side effect is photosensitivity, which lasts up to 24 hours. The reported recurrence rate with this treatment is only 11%, and as an adjunctive therapy this may be beneficial.[798–800]

Imiquimod 5% has been successful in treating superficial nonfacial BCCs;[801] however, the degree of inflammatory response may affect the tolerability and compliance of the patient.

TABLE 7.25   International Cowden Syndrome Consortium Operational Criteria, 2000[805]

Pathognomonic criteria
Mucocutaneous lesions:
   Trichilemmomas, facial
   Acral keratoses
   Papillomatous lesions
   Mucosal lesions

Major criteria
Breast cancer
Thyroid cancer (nonmedullary) especially follicular type
Macrocephaly
Lhermitte–Duclos disease (LDD)
Endometrial carcinoma

Minor criteria
Other thyroid lesions (e.g., goiter, adenoma)
Mental retardation
GI hamartomas
Fibrocystic disease of the breast
Lipomas
Fibromas
GU tumors (e.g., uterine fibroids, renal cell carcinoma) or malformation

Operational diagnosis in an individual
(1) Mucocutaneous lesions alone if there are:
   (a) ≥6 facial papules, of which ≥3 must be trichilemmoma, or
   (b) cutaneous facial papules and oral mucosal papillomatosis, or
   (c) oral mucosal papillomatosis and acral keratoses, or
   (d) ≥6 palmoplantar keratoses
(2) Two major criteria but 1 must include macrocephaly or LDD
(3) One major and 3 minor criteria
(4) Four minor criteria
Operational diagnosis in a family where 1 individual is diagnostic for CS
(1) Pathognomonic criteria
(2) Any one major criterion ± minor criteria
(3) Two minor criteria

Children with medulloblastoma and BCNS should not receive radiation as a treatment for the medulloblastoma, as it can predispose to multiple BCCs in the site of irradiation.[802]

PEDIATRIC ASPECTS OF THE DISEASE

Basal cell nevus syndrome is a genodermatosis that has a highly variable course. Some family members have minimal disease, whereas others have a highly malignant presentation. It is important to pick up this disease in childhood in order to prevent skin cancers and potentially diagnose medulloblastoma early.

COWDEN SYNDROME (MULTIPLE HAMARTOMA SYNDROME)

INTRODUCTION AND HISTORICAL NOTE

Lloyd and Dennis reported in 1963 a multisystem disorder with characteristic mucocutaneous lesions and abnormalities of the breast, thyroid, and gastrointestinal tract.[803] They named the disorder "Cowden disease" after their first patient.

Cowden syndrome (CS, MIM 158350) is a rare genetic disorder consisting of multiple hamartomatous tumors of ectodermal, mesodermal, and endodermal origin. Mucocutaneous lesions (trichilemmomas, acral keratoses and oral papillomas) are the most constant and characteristic feature.[803,804] Breast lesions including cancer and thyroid abnormalities occur in two-thirds of patients.[805]

EPIDEMIOLOGY

CS is probably more common than is reported because the clinical findings may be very subtle. It is inherited as an autosomal dominant trait with variable expressivity with a strong predominance of female patients.[806] Most of the patients have been Caucasian[807] and it affects 1 in 300 000 individuals.[744]

PRESENTING HISTORY

The International Cowden Syndrome Consortium has developed diagnostic criteria (see Table 7.25).[805] In childhood, macrocephaly may be the presenting sign.[808]

PHYSICAL EXAMINATION

Skin lesions are present in >90% of cases.[803] The age of onset of the characteristic mucocutaneous lesions begins in the second to third decades (average 22 years), but can range from 4 to 75 years.[803]

Frequently presenting before the internal manifestations are the multiple facial trichilemmomas which are skin-colored or yellowish–tan verrucous papules resembling verrucae.[809–811] Other nonspecific cutaneous papules,

796. DiGiovanna JJ (1998) Retinoid chemoprevention in the high-risk patient. J Am Acad Dermatol 39:S82–S85.
797. Wolf P, Kerl H (1995) Photodynamic therapy with 5-aminolevulinic acid: a promising concept for the treatment of cutaneous tumors. Dermatology 190:183–185.
798. Karrer S, Szeimies RM, Hohenleutner U et al. (1995) Unilateral localized basaliomatosis: treatment with topical photodynamic therapy after application of 5-aminolevulinic acid. Dermatology 190:218–222.
799. Tse DT, Kersten RC, Anderson RL (1984) Hematoporphyrin derivative photoradiation therapy in managing nevoid basal-cell carcinoma syndrome: a preliminary report. Arch Ophthalmol 102–990–994.
800. Kopera D, Cerroni L, Fink-Puches R et al. (1996) Different treatment modalities for the management of a patient with the nevoid basal cell carcinoma syndrome. J Am Acad Dermatol 34:937–939.
801. Kagy MK, Amonette R (2000) The use of imiquimod 5% cream for the treatment of superficial basal cell carcinomas in a basal cell nevus syndrome patient. Dermatol Surg 26:577–578.
802. Atahan IL, Yildiz F, Özyar E et al. (1998) Basal cell carcinomas developing in a case of medulloblastoma associated with Gorlin's syndrome. Pediatr Hematol Oncol 15:187–191.

803. Starink TM (1984) Cowden's disease: analysis of fourteen new cases. J Am Acad Dermatol 11:1127–1141.
804. Weary PE, Gorlin RJ, Gentry WC et al. (1972) Multiple hamartoma syndrome (Cowden's disease). Arch Dermatol 106:682–690.
805. Eng C (2000) Will the real Cowden syndrome please stand up: revised diagnositic criteria. J Med Genet 37:828–830.
806. Starink TM, Van Der Veen JPW, Arwert F et al. (1986) The Cowden syndrome: a clinical and genetic study in 21 patients. Clin Genet 29:222–223.
807. Williard W, Borgen P, Bol R et al. (1992) Cowden's disease, a case report with analyses at the molecular level. Cancer 69:2969–2974.
808. Hanssen AMN, Fryns JP (1995) Cowden syndrome. J Med Genet 32:117–119.
809. Takenoshita Y, Kubo S, Takeuchi T et al. (1993) Oral and facial lesions in Cowden's disease: report of two cases and a review of the literature. J Oral Maxillofac Surg 51:682–687.
810. Salem OS, Steck WD (1983) Cowden's disease (multiple hamartoma and neoplasia syndrome). J Am Acad Dermatol 8:686–696.
811. Wade TR, Kopf AW (1978) Cowden's disease: A case report and review of the literature. J Dermatol Surg Oncol 4:459–464.

commonly seen in CS, show a predilection for the face and distal extremities and may be so numerous that they coalesce around facial orifices and ears.

Multiple sclerotic fibromas of the skin have been reported by some authors to be another specific cutaneous marker of this entity.[812–814] These are sharply circumscribed dermal papules with a strikingly uniform storiform pattern staining on histology.

Palmoplantar lesions, present in more than half of the patients,[803] resemble punctate keratoses with central depressions.[811] In addition, keratotic skin-colored papules can be seen on the posterior aspect of the heels, the dorsa of the hands and feet, as well as the extensor surfaces of the forearms and lower legs.[803] Other cutaneous lesions seen with regularity in CS include lipomas, angiolipomas, hemangiomas,[815] and multiple skin tags.

Oral lesions are 1 to 3mm skin-colored papules. Occasionally, lesions cover extensive areas of the oral cavity, including the tongue,[816] and can assume a cobblestone appearance.[811]

The most frequently reported extracutaneous manifestation is thyroid disease, occurring in approximately two-thirds of patients.[803] Both sexes may be affected with a variety of lesions, including goiter, benign adenomas, fetal adenomas, thyroglossal duct cysts, and follicular adenocarcinoma.[803] Patients usually present with an enlarged thyroid. The potential for thyroid carcinoma requires close surveillance.

Fibrocystic disease of the breast and fibroadenomas occur in 76% of female patients. Ductal papillomas and virginal hypertrophy may also be seen.[803] Carcinoma of the breast is the most serious consequence of CS, affecting 25 to 36% of female patients. The onset of breast cancer occurs at the same age as patients without CS.[803,817] Preceding fibrocystic disease or fibroadenomas are often reported in those patients who develop breast carcinoma.[818] Breast cancer has also been reported in male patients.[819]

Multiple hamartomatous polyps may be found anywhere in the gastrointestinal tract including the esophagus, stomach, duodenum, small bowel, colon and anus.[820] They may involve the entire GI tract,[821] but are most common in the colon and usually less than 5mm in size. The degenerative potential of these hamartomas is small, with only a few reported cases of adenocarcinoma of the colon.[700,821]

Benign ovarian cysts and leiomyomas[803,822] of the uterus are commonly seen in affected women. Other less frequent tumors include teratomas, uterine fibroids, endometrial cancer, adenocarcinomas, carcinomas of the urethra or cervix, Gardner duct cysts, vaginal cysts, apocrine hidrocystomas, sebaceous cysts, transitional cell carcinoma of the renal pelvis, renal cell adenocarcinoma, and benign polyps of the urethra. Menstrual irregularities may also be present.

Craniomegaly is the most common skeletal manifestation, occurring in 80% of patients[806] and can be seen in infants.[808] One-third of all patients with CS have other skeletal abnormalities including adenoid facies and high arched palate.[810] Thoracic kyphosis or kyphoscoliosis, bone cysts,[823] pectus excavatum, syndactyly, large hands and feet, and digital abnormalities have been described.[803]

Abnormalities of the eyes have been reported in 13% of patients, including angioid streaks and myopia.

Other organ systems which can be involved include endocrine, central nervous, pulmonary and cardiovascular systems.[803,824]

Several cases of CS have been reported with Lhermitte–Duclos disease, showing a peculiar proliferation of abnormal neuronal cells in the cerebellum, which may represent a hamartoma of neuronal tissue.[825,826] Diagnosis can be made by magnetic resonance imaging and biopsy of the lesions.

LABORATORY FINDINGS

Because multiple facial trichilemmomas are found with such high frequency in CS, this diagnosis should be entertained if a patient presents in this manner. Trichilemmomas show lobular formations of the hair follicle, differentiating toward outer root sheath cells. Some facial lesions may simply show squamous papillomas on biopsy. Oral lesions are usually benign fibromas. Extrafacial lesions and palmoplantar lesions tend to demonstrate hyperkeratotic papillomas.[827]

PATHOPHYSIOLOGY AND HISTOGENESIS

A mutation in the tumor suppressor gene *PTEN* has been found in most cases of CS[828] and has been localized to chromosome 10q22–23. Mutations in this gene can also cause Banayan–Riley–Ruvalcaba syndrome (MIM 153480) and Lhermitte–Duclos syndrome, but these disorders have different clinical manifestations. The significance of the different manifestations of this gene mutation is unknown.

The primary defect in CS is thought to be an abnormality of the regulation of cell proliferation.[805,825] PTEN is a phosphatase that inactivates phosphoinositol-3-kinase; unchecked activity of PI3K promotes cell survival and cycling. Tissues affected mainly include those tissue capable of proliferation, such as the epidermis, the oral and gastrointestinal mucosa, thyroid epithelium, and breast epithelium.

DIFFERENTIAL DIAGNOSIS

Differential diagnosis of papillomatosis of the oral mucosa would include Heck disease, multiple traumatic fibromas, multiple endocrine neoplasia type 2B, tuberous sclerosis, lipoid proteinosis, Darier disease, Goltz syndrome, florid oral papillomatosis, and acanthosis nigricans. These disorders can be differentiated from CS by other characteristic features and histologically.

For multiple skin-colored papules on the face, the differential diagnosis includes tuberous sclerosis (angiofibromas), syringomas, steatocystoma multiplex, multiple trichoepitheliomas (Brooke syndrome), basal cell nevus syndrome, seborrheic keratosis, fibrofolliculomas (Birt–Hogg–Dubé syndrome), neurofibromatosis, epidermodysplasia verruciformis, and verruca vulgaris.

THERAPEUTICS AND PROGNOSIS

Because one-third of all female patients with CS develop breast cancer, periodic (every 6–12 months) mammograms are recommended along with monthly self-examination to detect early lesions. Consideration for bilateral prophylactic mastectomies, particularly in women with other breast lesions

812. Metcalf JS, Maize JC, LeBoit PE (1991) Circumscribed storiform collagenoma (sclerosing fibroma). **Am J Dermatopathol** 13:122–129.

813. Wheeland RG, McGillis ST (1989) Cowden's disease – treatment of cutaneous lesions using carbon dioxide laser vaporization: a comparison of conventional and superpulsed techniques. **J Dermatol Surg Oncol** 15:1055–1059.

814. Requena L, Guiterrez J, Yus ES (1991) Multiple sclerotic fibromas of the skin, a cutaneous marker of Cowden's disease. **J Cutan Pathol** 19:346–351.

815. Barax CN, Lebwohl M, Phelps RG (1987) Multiple hamartoma syndrome. **J Am Acad Dermatol** 17:342–346.

816. Bagan JV, Penarrocha M, Vera-Sempere F (1989) Cowden syndrome. Clinical and pathological considerations in two new cases. **J Oral Maxillofac Surg** 47:291–294.

817. Burgdorf WHC, Koester G (1992) Multiple cutaneous tumors: what do they mean? **J Cutan Pathol** 19:449–457.

818. Brownstein MH, Wolf M, Bikowski JB (1978) Cowden's disease. A cutaneous marker of breast cancer. **Cancer** 41:2393–2398.

819. Fackenthal JD, Marsh DJ, Richardson AL et al. (2001) Male breast cancer in Cowden syndrome patients with germline PTEN mutations. **J Med Genet** 38:159–164.

820. Ortonne JP, Lambert R, Daudet J et al. (1980) Involvement of the digestive tract in Cowden's Disease. **Int J Dermatol** 19:570–576.

821. Chen YM, Ott DJ, Wu WC et al. (1987) Cowden's disease: A case report and literature review. **Gastrointest Radiol** 12:325–329.

822. Burnett JW, Goldner R, Calton GJ (1975) Cowden disease. Report of two additional cases. **Br J Dermatol** 93:329–336.

823. Gentry WC, Reed WB, Siegel JM (1975) Cowden disease. **Birth Defects** 11:137–141.

824. Solli P, Rossi G, Carbognani P et al. (1999) Pulmonary abnormalities in Cowden's disease. **J Cardiovasc Surg** 40:753–755.

825. Albrecht S, Haber RM, Goodman JC et al. (1992) Cowden syndrome and Lhermitte–Duclos disease. **Cancer** 70:869–876.

826. Robinson S, Cohen AR (2000) Cowden disease and Lhermitte–Duclos disease: characterization of a new phakomatosis. **Neurosurgery** 46:371–383.

827. Starink TM, Hausman R (1984) The cutaneous pathology of facial lesions in Cowden's disease. **J Cutan Pathol** 11:331–337.

828. DiCristofano A, Pesce B, Cordon-Cardo C et al. (1998) Pten is essential for embryonic development and tumour suppression. **Nature Genet** 19:348–355.

by the third decade of life, is considered by some authors[807,829] but should not be lightly undertaken.

Facial papules may respond to topical 5-fluorouracil, oral isotretinoin, laser ablation, or surgical excision.[810,813]

Thyroid function tests, thyroid scanning, complete blood count, urinalysis, and chest radiography should be performed as baseline studies in all patients and checked as needed. If abnormalities are detected, fine-needle aspiration biopsy or surgical biopsy for further clarification is indicated.

Work-up of the gastrointestinal tract should be based on symptoms. Screening tests are not generally indicated because hamartomatous polyps often occupy the entire alimentary tract and have little potential for malignant degeneration.[830]

PEDIATRIC ASPECTS OF THE DISEASE

The physician who recognizes a patient with CS in childhood has a unique opportunity to watch for and treat developing carcinomas in both the patient and family members. Findings may be subtle, such as craniomegaly, but further examination of family history may lead to the diagnosis.

CARNEY COMPLEX

Synonyms: LAMB syndrome (*L*entigenes, *A*trial myxoma, *M*ucocutaneous myxoma, *B*lue nevi); NAME syndrome (*N*evi, *A*trial myxoma, *M*yxoid neurofibromata, *E*phelides)

INTRODUCTION AND HISTORICAL NOTE

The Carney complex (CNC, MIM 160980) refers to the association of myxomas (cardiac, cutaneous, breast), spotty mucocutaneous pigmentation, endocrine abnormalities and psammomatous melanotic schwannomas.[831,832]

This syndrome was previously named LAMB syndrome[833] and NAME syndrome.[834] Carney and colleagues describe the clinical characteristics of this disorder in a large series of patients.[831] Endocrine abnormalities include primary pigmented nodular adrenocortical disease causing Cushing syndrome, androgen excess due to Sertoli cell or Leydig cell tumor of the testes and growth hormone-secreting pituitary adenomas.

EPIDEMIOLOGY

Most reported patients have been white, but the disorder occurs worldwide.[835] Both males and females are equally affected. Approximately 50% of the patients have a family history of the disease with an autosomal dominant pattern of inheritance and incomplete penetrance.[836]

PRESENTING HISTORY

The mucocutaneous features of the disease may be the earliest clinical findings and often manifest during infancy and childhood. The patient

TABLE 7.26 Clinical findings in Carney complex[832]

Skin pigmentation	
Lentigines	67%
Blue nevi	19%
Myxomas	
Skin	37%
Cardiac	61%
Breast	20%
Endocrine tumors	
Adrenal	33%
Thyroid	11%
Testicular	30%
Pituitary	11%
Schwannomas	
(GI, skin, sympathetic chain)	11%

might also present to the pediatrician or endocrinologist with Cushing syndrome, acromegaly, male precocious puberty,[837] or an abdominal mass[838] (Table 7.26).

PHYSICAL EXAMINATION

Lentigines vary in number and are usually distributed on the face (periocular, nose, perioral), vermilion borders of the lips, eyelids and ears. Lesions can also be seen on the trunk, limbs, dorsa of the hands, vulva and conjunctiva.[831] The oral mucosa is rarely affected.

Blue nevi, usually 2–10mm in size, have no site predilection and have been seen in children as young as 3 years.[835]

Psammomatous melanotic schwannomas have been seen in patients ages 10–63 years. These present usually as a solitary skin mass in the dermis or subcutis and may have a bluish appearance.[835,839]

Cutaneous myxomas manifest as skin-colored, sessile or pedunculated papules that are usually less than 1cm in diameter. Although they are usually smooth, they may have a papillomatous surface. They are often seen on the eyelid,[840,841] in the external ear canal, on the face, neck, trunk, anogenital area, upper limb and lower limb. The palms and soles are usually spared.

Cardiac myxomas may be single or multiple and may occur in any or all cardiac chambers. Embolic stroke and heart failure may result. Cutaneous signs caused by cardiac myxomas are digital cyanosis, erythematous macules and papules, livedo reticularis, petechiae, splinter hemorrhages or ulcerating lesions.

Thyroid abnormalities include thyroid carcinoma (papillary and follicular), or follicular adenoma, and can be seen in children and adolescents. Ultrasonography can show hypoechoic cystic solid or mixed lesions even with a normal physical examination.[842]

829. Brownstein MH, Mehregan AH, Bikowski JB et al. (1979) The dermatopathology of Cowden's Syndrome. **Br J Dermatol** 100:667–673.

830. Taylor AJ, Dodds WJ, Stewart ET (1989) Alimentary tract lesions in Cowden's disease. **Br J Radiol** 62:890–892.

831. Carney JA, Gordon H, Carpenter PC et al. (1985) The complex of myxomas, spotty pigmentation and endocrine over activity. **Medicine** 64:270–283.

832. Carney JA (1995) The Carney complex (myxomas, spotty pigmentation, endocrine overactivity, and schwannomas). **Dermatol Clin** 13:19–26.

833. Rhodes AR, Silverman RA, Harrist TJ et al. (1984) Mucocutaneous lentigines, cardiomucocutaneous myxomas, and multiple blue nevi: The "LAMB" syndrome. **J Am Acad Dermatol** 10:72–82.

834. Atherton DJ, Pitcher DW, Wells RS et al. (1980) A syndrome of various cutaneous pigmented lesions, myxoid neurofibromata and atrial myxoma: the NAME syndrome. **Br J Dermatol** 103:421–429.

835. Carney JA, Stratakis CA (1998) Epithelioid blue nevus and psammomatous melanotic schwannoma: the unusual pigmented skin tumors of the Carney complex. **Semin Diagn Pathol** 15:216–224.

836. Carney JA, Hruska LS, Beauchamp GD et al. (1986) Dominant inheritance of the complex of myxomas, spotty pigmentation and endocrine over activity. **Mayo Clin Proc** 61:165–172.

837. Malchoff CD (2000) Editorial: Carney complex – clarity and complexity. **J Clin Endocrinol Metab** 85:4010–4012.

838. McCluggage WG, Walsh MY, Thornton CM et al. (2000) Massive abdominal and pelvic myxoma in Carney's syndrome. **J Clin Pathol** 53:558–560.

839. Utiger CA, Headington JT (1993) Psammomatous melanotic schwannoma. **Arch Dermatol** 129:202–204.

840. Carney JA, Headington JT, Su DWP (1986) Cutaneous myxomas. A major component of the complex of myxomas, spotty pigmentation and endocrine over activity. **Arch Dermatol** 122:790–798.

841. Goldstein MM, Casey M, Carney JA et al. (1999) Molecular genetic diagnosis of the familial myxoma syndrome (Carney complex). **Am J Med Genet** 86:62–65.

842. Stratakis CA, Courcoutsakis NA, Abati A et al. (1997) Thyroid gland abnormalities in patients with the syndrome of spotty skin pigmentation, myxomas, endocrine overactivity, and schwannomas (Carney complex). **J Clin Endocrinol Metab** 82:2037–2043.

LABORATORY FINDINGS

Echocardiographic studies can demonstrate tumors in the heart and should be followed by a cardiologist.

PATHOPHYSIOLOGY AND HISTOGENESIS

Mutations in the *PRKAR1A*, which is a protein kinase A type I-α regulatory gene and found on chromosome 17q23–q24, cause CNC in some families and they are referred to as CNC1.[837,843] Another subset, CNC2 (MIM 605244) on chromosome 2p, has yet to be delineated. Histology of the cutaneous myxomas consist of small stellate cells within a myxoid stroma.

Microscopically, blue nevi show spindle or epitheliod cells with light or heavy melanin. Psammomatous melanotic schwannomas are incompletely encapsulated and contain spindle and epithelioid cells, melanin, psammoma bodies and fat in a whirling pattern.[835]

DIFFERENTIAL DIAGNOSIS

Other syndromes which have multiple lentigines include: LEOPARD syndrome, PJS and XP, all of which have different features and presentations.

THERAPEUTICS AND PROGNOSIS

Although most patients live a normal life, death can occur because of cardiac myxoma, metastatic psammomatous melanotic schwannoma, stroke, or sudden death.

Surgical excision of suspicious nodules with microscopic examination will lead one to consider the diagnosis of this multisystem disease.

PEDIATRIC ASPECTS OF THE DISEASE

Patients with CNC can present in childhood with multiple lentigines, multiple blue nevi, cardiac myxoma, cutaneous myxomas, preocious puberty or other endocrine abnormalities. Other possibly affected organ systems should be examined if this diagnosis is made.

HEREDITARY METABOLIC DISORDERS

Peter Itin and Rudolf Happle, Natalie Schaub, Peter Schiller, Jan Izakovic, S.K. Fistarol

AMINOACIDOPATHIES

PHENYLKETONURIA (Fölling disease, hyperphenylalaninemia type I, Phenylalanine hydroxylase deficiency)

Introduction and historical note

Phenylketonuria (phenylpyruvic oligophrenia) is an autosomal recessive disorder (MIM 261600) of amino acid metabolism that leads to mental retardation, diffuse hypopigmentation, seizures, eczematous dermatitis and photosensitivity.[844] Eight subtypes have been described. Pediatric PKU may also result from hyperphenylalaninemia related to maternal phenylketonuria. Without a special diet in the mother, the child is at risk to develop the typical signs and symptoms of phenylketonuria. Genotype-based prediction and classification of the biochemical phenotype is now possible in the majority of newborns with hyperphenylalaninemia. This chapter will be limited to the classical type.

Phenylketonuria was the first inborn error of amino acid metabolism which was clearly defined. Fölling, in 1934, first reported 10 patients with oligophrenia and photodistributed dermatitis, muscle hypotonia and green-colored urine after addition of ferric chloride. In 1937 the condition was named oligophrenia phenylpyruvica. In 1947 Jervis found that the metabolic error is an inability to oxidize phenylalanine and tyrosine, and in 1953 treatment with a phenylalanine-restricted diet was described. Phenylketonuria has been detected by newborn screening programs since the 1960s.

Epidemiology and genetics

The prevalence of phenylketonuria varies markedly in various countries. The highest frequency of phenylketonuria is found in Ireland and Scotland (1:4000), whereas in Finland only 1 in 40 000 births is affected. The overall frequency in northern Europeans is calculated to be about 1:10 000 and in the United States classical phenylketonuria is estimated to occur in about 1:11 000 births within the white population. In the African-American population the frequency is estimated to be only about 1:50 000. In Kuwait there were seven cases among 451 institutionalized mentally retarded persons (1.9%).

The classic form of phenylketonuria is an autosomal recessive disorder that affects both sexes equally. Two of at least three involved enzymes are affected by mutations at different loci, and the phenylalanine hydroxylase apoenzyme locus probably has multiple alleles. There are more than 100 mutations documented. The gene locus for phenylketonuria is on chromosome 12q24.1.

Presenting history and physical examination

Infants appear to be normal at birth and develop manifestations of psychomotor alterations between 4 and 24 months of age. Early symptoms include heavy vomiting. In retrospect, early infantile eczema, indistinguishable from atopic dermatitis, may be one of the first signs of phenylketonuria, which occurs in 20–50% of affected infants during the first year of life. Later on, the incidence may be even higher. A further skin clue is pigment dilution with impressive pale pigmentation, blond hair, and blue eyes, seen in 90% of patients. The pigment dilution is reversible with phenylalanine restriction. The patients develop moderate photosensitivity and, in addition, a sclerodermoid skin change may develop. Edematous scleroderma of the extremities, which spares the hands and feet, is characteristic.[845] Furthermore, resemblance to atrophoderma of Pasini and Pierini has been reported. Typically, a mousy odor induced by phenylacetic acid is noted from urine and sweat. The most important complications are severe mental retardation with irritability, hyperactivity, self-destructive behavior, hypertonicity and seizures. Peculiar gait and increased deep tendon reflexes are noted. Microcephaly, brain calcification, and cataracts are observed.

Laboratory findings

The diagnosis of phenylketonuria is made by documenting elevated levels of phenylalanine in the serum (20mg/dl or higher, 10 to 50 times that of normal). Plasma tyrosine may be normal or elevated. In addition, elevated urinary phenylpyruvic acid can be documented. Additional laboratory abnormalities include phenylalanine hydroxylase deficiency, phenylpyruvic acidemia and increased urinary o-hydroxyphenylacetic acid and phenylacetylglutamine. Increased urinary phenylpyruvic acid can be detected by a typical green coloration of urine after addition of 10% ferric chloride. In numerous countries phenylketonuria screening is performed in the Neonatal Screening Program by either a semiquantitative bacterial inhibition assay method in

843. Kirschner LS, Carney JA, Pack SD et al. (2000) Mutations of the gene encoding the protein kinase A type-I-alpha regulatory subunit in patients with the Carney complex. **Nature Genet** 26:89–92.

844. National Institutes of Health Consensus Development Panel (2001) National Institutes of Health Consensus Conference Statement: phenylketonuria: screening and management. **Pediatrics** 108:972–982.

845. Nova MP, Kaufman M, Halperin A (1992) Scleroderma-like skin indurations in a child with phenylketonuria: a clinicopathologic correlation and review of the literature. **J Am Acad Dermatol** 26:329–333.

which several drops of capillary blood may indicate an elevated level of phenylalanine in a microbiological procedure (Guthrie test) or by a quantitative chemical reaction (Quantase test).[846] In affected babies, serum phenylalanine levels begin to rise on the third or fourth day of life. Prenatal diagnosis is possible by performing amniocentesis or chorionic villus sampling with identification of the gene. In addition, preimplantation genetic diagnosis for phenylketonuria has resulted in phenylketonuria-free children.[847]

Pathophysiology and histology
The classic type of phenylketonuria is induced by a deficiency of phenylalanine hydroxylase or its cofactor tetrahydrobiopterin, and a consequent accumulation of the precursor phenylalanine. The normal phenylalanine to tyrosine ratio is 1:1, whereas in phenylketonuria it is > 3:1. It is widely believed that the pigment dilution is a result of the inhibitory effect of phenylalanine on tyrosinase. Histologic examination shows a normal number of melanocytes but a decrease in mature melanosomes. Histopathology may document dermal thickening in sclerodermoid skin.

Differential diagnosis
Prematurity in infants, defects in biopterin metabolism, use of methotrexate, high protein diets, and liver disease may also elevate plasma levels of phenylalanine.

Treatment and prognosis
With a low phenylalanine diet, which should be continued lifelong, the skin color, photosensitivity, odor and eczema are reversible. In addition, early diet can dramatically reduce mental retardation. If blood levels of phenylalanine are maintained in a reasonable range in early childhood, normal to low-normal intelligence can be expected.[848] Furthermore, no higher risk for psychological disturbance has been found in patients with adequate diet compared with a control population. Late-treated patients with phenylketonuria may mimic Angelman syndrome. It has been shown recently that the individual's blood–brain barrier phenylalanine transport determines the clinical outcome in phenylketonuria and that dietary recommendations might be tailored to the individual.[849] Fish oil supplementation seems to improve visual evoked potentials in patients with phenylketonuria. Although tyrosine supplementation has been recommended, a Cochrane Database Systematic Review did not find clear evidence for efficacy.

Practical guidelines. NIH Consensus Statement on Phenylketonuria. http://consensus.nih.gov

HOMOCYSTINURIA

Homocystinuria is an autosomal recessive trait that maps to 21q22.3. The disorder is caused by a deficiency of cystathionine β-synthase producing increased urinary homocystine and methionine.[850]

Clinical features
The major signs and symptoms involve extracutaneous organs such as the eyes, the central nervous system, the bones and the blood vessels. Infants appear normal at birth but show developmental delay and eventually seizures. Mental capabilities tend to be higher in pyriodoxine responsive patients than in pyridoxine non-responsive patients.[851] Cutaneous features include a distinctive malar flush and livedo reticularis in more that 50% of patients. Children tend to have blond, brittle hair and a thin, fair skin. However, the hallmark of the disease is a downward displacement of the lenses due to disruption of the zonular fiber connecting the lens to the ciliary body. Bone abnormalities include thin habitus, stiff joints and osteoporosis.

A life-threatening problem is the high incidence of thromboembolism of medium- and large-sized blood vessels. Patients typically develop early atherosclerotic cardiovascular disease, strokes, pulmonary emboli, or renovascular hypertension.

Treatment
Some children are responsive to pyridoxine (vitamin B6) in the range of 250–500mg/day. Pyridoxine responsiveness is either present or absent within a particular family. Compound heterozygotes are likely to retain some degree of pyridoxine responsiveness. When initiated neonatally, methionine restriction prevents mental retardation, reduces the rate of lens dislocation, and may reduce the incidence of seizures. Pyridoxine treatment of B6-responsive patients tends to reduce the risk of thromboembolic events. Darkening of newly growing hair has been observed after a pyridoxine administration, giving rise to a clear demarcation between the old, blond and the new, dark hair.[852] The structure of the hair also changes from a coarse to a softer texture.

ORGANIC ACIDURIAS

ALKAPTONURIA (OCHRONOSIS)

Alkaptonuria (McKusick 203500), or homogentisic acid oxidase deficiency, is a rare metabolic disorder inherited in an autosomal recessive pattern. The human gene for alkaptonuria has been mapped to chromosome 3q.[853,854]

History
The earliest verified case of ochronosis is an Egyptian mummy, Harwa, who died in his early 30s, approximately 3500 years ago.[855] In 1584, Scribonius recorded that the urine of an apparently healthy schoolboy became black on standing. In 1859, a chemist named Boedeker[856] correctly concluded that this was not glucose; he introduced the name "alkapton" to emphasize his observation that addition of alkali hastened darkening of alkaptonuric urine. Three decades later, Wolkow and Bauman in 1891 determined the chemical structure of alkapton to be that of 2,5-dihydroxyphenylacetic acid and named it homogentisic acid because of its similarity to gentisic acid.

The name "ochronosis" dates back to Virchow's report in 1866 of gray to blue–black pigmentation in the hip and knee joints found in the postmortem examination of a 67-year-old patient. It was because the microscopic appearance of the pigment was ocher that he named the condition ochronosis.[857] In 1902, Albrecht published the first study tying together alkaptonuria, ochronosis and ochronotic arthritis, and in 1904 Osler published the first account of a diagnosis of ochronosis made during the lifetime of two brothers, noting the

846. Abadie V, Berthelot J, Feillet F et al. (2002) Neonatal screening and long-term follow-up of phenylketonuria: the French database. **Early Hum Dev** 65:149–158.
847. Verlinsky Y, Rechitsky S, Verlinsky O et al. (2001) Preimplantation testing for phenylketonuria. **Fertil Steril** 76:346–349.
848. Lundstedt G, Johansson A, Melin L, Alm J (2001) Adjustment and intelligence among children with phenylketonuria in Sweden. **Acta Pediatr** 90:1147–1152.
349. Weglage J, Wiedermann D, Denecke J et al. (2001) Individual blood-brain barrier phenylalanine transport determines clinical outcome in phenylketonuria. **Ann Neurol** 50:463–467.
850. Sokolova J, Janosikova B, Terwilliger JD (2001) Cystathionine beta-synthase deficiency in Central Europe: discrepancy between biochemical and molecular genetic screening for homocystinuric alleles. **Hum Mutat** 18:548.
851. Yap S, Rushe H, Howard PM, Naughten ER (2001) The intellectual abilities of early-treated individuals with pyridoxine-nonresponsive homocystinuria due to cystathione beta-synthase deficiency. **J Inherit Metab Dis** 24:437.

852. Reish O, Townsend D, Berry SA et al. (1995) Tyrosinase inhibition due to interaction of homocyst(e)ine with copper: The mechanism if reversible hypopigmentation in homocystinuria due to cystathione beta-synthase deficiency. **Am J Hum Genet** 57:127.
853. Janocha S, Wolz W, Srsen S et al. (1994) The human gene for alkaptonuria (AKU) maps to chromosome 3q. **Genomics** 19:5–8.
854. Pollak MR, Chou YHW, Cerda JJ et al. (1993) Homozygosity mapping of the gene for alkaptonuria to chromosome 3q2. **Nat Genet** 5:201–204.
855. Lee SL, Stenn FF (1978) Characterization of mummy bone ochronotic pigment. **JAMA** 240:136–138.
856. Boedeker C (1859) Ueber das Alcapton; ein neuer Beitrag zur Frage: Welche Stoffe des Harns können Kupferreduction biwirken? **Z Rat Med** 7:130.
857. Virchow R (1866) Ein Fall von allgemeiner Ochronose der Knorpel und knorpclähnlicher Theile. **Virchows Arch Pathol Anat Physiol** 37:212–219.

discoloration of their eyes and ears and the presence of spinal arthritis. Alkaptonuria enjoys the historic distinction of being one of the first conditions in which Mendelian recessive inheritance was proposed (in 1902 by Garrod). Garrod[858] believed that the disease resulted from the absence of a hepatic enzyme and that homogentisic acid was produced in the course of a normal tyrosine metabolism. Garrod's idea, however, was not confirmed until 1958, when La Du and associates[859] demonstrated the absence of the enzyme homogentisic acid oxidase in the hepatic tissue of an alkaptonuric patient.

Epidemiology

Inheritance of alkaptonuria is autosomal recessive with a prevalence of 1 in 250 000 or lower in most populations. These estimates are probably low, as very few areas routinely obtain a urine specimen for newborn screening of the disease.[853] A review of reported cases cites a worldwide distribution with an approximately equal incidence in the sexes. Alkaptonuria is unusually frequent in the Dominican Republic.[860] The highest incidence (1 in 19 000 newborns) has been observed in the Slovak Republic.[861] An analysis of the allelic association with intragenic DNA markers and of the geographic origins of the mutated chromosomes suggested that several independent founders had contributed to the gene pool, and that subsequent genetic isolation was probably responsible for the high prevalence of alkaptonuria in Slovakia.[862]

General screening for alkaptonuria is relatively simple and inexpensive: urine alkalinization with 10% sodium hydroxide solution will produce a brownish–black discoloration in the presence of homogentisic acid. The serious disabling arthropathy in adulthood has justified general screening in some countries.[863]

Clinical manifestations

The diagnosis of alkaptonuria depends on awareness of its features and varying presentations at different ages (Table 7.27). The most classic clinical manifestations of alkaptonuria include arthritis with pigment deposition in cartilage and intervertebral disks, homogentisic aciduria with darkening of urine on standing, cortically pigmented renal stones, cutaneous pigmentation and cardiovascular involvement.[864] During the first decade, and as early as the first few days of life, the presenting clinical sign is usually darkening of urine on standing (freshly voided urine is normal colored or slightly gray), generally detected as a brownish discoloration of diapers and bedsheets; washing with soap intensifies stains.[855] However, if the urine is acidic, this sign is not uniformly present. Dark brown or black cerumen may be present in the first decade even in those less than 5 years of age. Axillary skin pigmentation (blue to greenish-blue to greenish-yellow or brownish) has been found as early as 8 to 10 years of age and is regularly present in the teenage years. Brown pigmented spots can be detected in the sweat gland pores of occasional patients. Quaterman et al.[865] described a patient with pigmentary changes confined to sun-exposed areas. A grayish–blue tinge overlying ear cartilage is common in adulthood but is rarely seen before 20 years of age.[866] Ochronotic discoloration is rarely seen in childhood but is common in adulthood and can affect the sclera, cornea, conjunctiva, tarsus and eyelid skin. Scleral involvement is noted in most patients. Extensive ochronosis is uncommon in children. However, it was observed in an 11-year-old boy who died of polycystic renal disease; its early presence was probably secondary to the presence of renal disease.[867] Insidious progression

TABLE 7.27   Clinical features of ochronosis

Skin
Dark pigmentation of axillary skin
Ochronotic discoloration through thin areas of skin overlying pigmented cartilage and tendon

Skeleton
Osteoarthritis
Black ochronotic pigmentation of cartilage

Eyes
Ochronotic discoloration of sclera, cornea, conjunctiva, tarsus and eyelid skin

Genitourinary tract
Cortically pigmented renal stones
Prostatic calculi
Renal failure

Ears and upper respiratory tract
Dark brown to black staining of cerumen
Bluish discoloration of auricular cartilage
Tinnitus and hearing loss
Laryngeal and tracheal cartilage ochronosis

Other manifestations
Cardiovascular involvement
Dura mater involvement
Involvement of other organ systems, including breast, lymph nodes, bone marrow, thyroid, nails and teeth

Laboratory
Homogentisic acid oxidase deficiency
Urine turns dark on standing and alkalinization

of ochronotic arthropathy, which generally begins in the third and fourth decades, is the most disabling manifestation of alkaptonuria. Hip, knee and shoulder limitation are early signs. Ochronotic arthropathy typically involves the spine and larger joints. X-rays show a characteristic appearance of early calcification of the intervertebral disc and later narrowing of the intervertebral spaces, with eventual disc collapse and progressive loss of height. In three siblings with both alkaptonuria and sucrase–solmatase deficiency, arthralgia was present in childhood.[868] Genitourinary tract complications are more common among men than among women, with an increased incidence of renal and prostatic calculi, especially after the age of 50. Zibolen et al.[869] emphasized the increased frequency of urolithiasis in patients younger than 15 years and reported five such patients. The high incidence of prostatic calculi is attributed to the more rapid polymerization of homogentisic acid in the presence of alkaline prostatic secretions, with the resultant pigment serving as a nidus for stone formation. Rarely, renal failure occurs in the late stage of disease.[867]

Although involvement of the ear and upper respiratory tract has not been systematically studied, reports of tinnitus, hearing loss and erosion of cartilage emphasize the need to pay attention to possible hearing difficulties. Laryngeal and tracheal cartilage ochronosis may result in hoarseness and dysphagia.[873]

858. Garrod AE (1908) The Croonian lectures on inborn errors of metabolism, lecture II: alkaptonuria. **Lancet** 2:73–79.

859. La Du BN, Zannoni VG, Laster L et al. (1958) The nature of the defect in tyrosine metabolism in alcaptonuria. **J Biol Chem** 230:251.

860. Milch RA (1960) Studies of alcaptonuria: inheritance of 47 cases in eight highly inter-related Dominican kindreds. **Am J Hum Genet** 12:76–85.

861. Zatkova A, Polakova H, Micutkova L et al. (2000) Novel mutations in the homogentisate-1,2-dioxygenase gene identified in Slovak patients with alkaptonuria. **J Med Genet** 37:539–542.

862. Muller CR, Fregin A, Srsen S et al. (1999) Allelic heterogeneity of alkaptonuria in Central Europe. **Eur J Hum Genet** 7:645–651.

863. Harper PS (1978) Screening for alkaptonuria in the newborn in Wales. **Lancet** 2:576–577.

864. Liu W, Prayson RA (2001) Dura mater involvement in ochronosis (alkaptonuria). **Arch Pathol Lab Med** 125:961–963.

865. Quaterman MJ, Hall JH, Gourdin FW et al. (1992) Photodistributed hereditary ochronosis. **Arch Dermatol** 128:1657–1658.

866. Gutzmer R, Herbst RA, Kiehl P et al. (1997) Alkaptonuric ochronosis: Report of two affected brothers. **J Am Acad Dermatol** 37:305–307.

867. O'Brien WM, La Du BN, Bunim JJ (1963) Biochemical, pathologic and clinical aspects of alcaptonuria, ochronosis and ochronotic arthropathy. **Am J Med** 34:813–838.

868. Garnica AD, Cerda JJ, Maenard D et al. (1981) Alcaptonuria and sucrase-isomaltase deficiency in three offspring of a consanguineous marriage. **Acta Vitaminol Enzymol** 3:157–169.

869. Zibolen M, Srsnova K, Srsen S (2000) Increased urolithiasis in patients with alkaptonuria in childhood. **Clin Genet** 58:79–80.

870. Turiansky GW, Levin SW (2001) Bluish patches on the ears and axillae with dark urine: ochronosis and alkaptonuria. **Int J Dermatol** 40:333–335.

871. McClure J, Smith PS, Gramp AA (1983) Calcium pyrophosphate dihydrate deposition in ochronotic arthropathy. **J Clin Pathol** 36:894.

872. Montagutelli X, Lalouette A, Coude M et al. (1994) AKU, a mutation of the mouse homologous to human alkaptonuria, maps to chromosome 16. **Genomics** 9:9–11.

873. Fernandez-Canon JM, Granadino B, Beltran-Valero de Bernabe D et al. (1996) The molecular basis of alkaptonuria. **Nature Genet** 14:19–24.

Cardiac disease often involves the valves and is associated with calcifications and valvular stenosis.[864] Autopsy involvement of other organ systems, including breast, lymph nodes, bone marrow, thyroid and teeth, has been documented to occur less frequently.[864]

The diagnosis is made by a positive family history, histology and urine testing. Routine histopathology of affected skin demonstrates ochre or yellow–brown pigment within the dermis. The pigment is seen within irregularly shaped degenerated, homogenized and swollen collagen fibers that may display sharp, jagged borders, and within elastic fibers. Fine pigment granules may be seen within macrophages, free within the dermis, in endothelial cells and in the basement membrane and the secretory cells of eccrine glands. Foreign body giant cells may be seen around the granules. The pigment stains black with methylene blue or cresyl violet.[870]

Pathophysiology

Homogentisic acid is an intermediate in the catabolism of the aromatic amino acids phenylalanine and tyrosine. The enzyme homogentisic acid oxidase (homogentisate 1,2-dioxygenase), which cleaves homogentisic acid into its end product maloylacetocetic, normally functions in the liver and kidney; its absence leads to an accumulation of homogentisic acid. As a result, homogentisic acid is excreted in the urine.[870] In patients with alkaptonuria, excess homogentisic acid is oxidized and polymerized by the enzyme homogentisic acid polyphenol oxidase, which catalyzes the oxidation of homogentisic acid into an ochronotic-like pigment, with benzoquinoneacetic acid being one of the known intermediate products in this process. The ochronotic pigment has been found to accumulate irreversibly within collagen fibers, elastic fibers and macrophages.[864] There is some suggestion that in experimental chick embryo models homogentisic metabolites inhibit lysyl hydroxylase activity, which results in poor collagen cross-linking. It also appears that pigment deposition may be enhanced by prior collagen damage.[864] The presence of this pigment in cartilage tissue has been associated with calcium pyrophosphate dihydrate deposition, which in turn may initiate the osteoarthritic process. The relationship between this metabolic defect and the resultant ochronosis and arthritis is not precisely known.[871]

The mutation for alkaptonuria in the mouse was localized to the aku locus[872] and subsequently mapped to the human homologous region on chromosome 3q, AKU, which encodes homogentisic acid oxidase. More than 50 mutations have been described with remarkable allelic heterogeneity,[861,873–875] although a CCC triplet is a mutational hot spot.[876] Most are missense mutations.[861]

Differential diagnosis

Other causes of dark urine, such as the porphyrias, hepatobiliary disease, myoglobinuria, hemoglobinuria and hematuria, can be easily eliminated. Many patients with alkaptonuria are unaware that their urine darkens and, unless directly questioned, staining of undergarments is not revealed in medical history. Ochronosis due to exogenous agents such as phenol, resorcinol or hydroquinone bleaching creams can be differentiated by the absence of homogentisic acid in the urine.[876]

Therapeutics

The course of alkaptonuria is generally slow but irreversible. Despite these features, life expectancy of patients with alkaptonuria is reported to be normal.[866] Treatment is primarily supportive, with close observation for the development of arthropathy, cardiac and urinary tract disease. Appropriate management includes genetic counseling, pain management with non-steroidal anti-inflammatory agents, physical therapy to increase range of motion and regular follow-up visits.[870] Avoidance of high-protein, high-phenylalanine, and high-tyrosine diets was reported to be important.[877] A well-balanced normal diet seems the best approach during childhood. It has been postulated that large amounts of dietary vitamin C may be helpful, since vitamin C protects homogentisic acid against oxidation and thus may prevent the deposition of ochronotic pigment; however, no long-term clinical studies have been undertaken to verify the effectiveness of this approach.[878] Wolff et al.[877] treated two adults and three children with high doses of ascorbic acid and studied the effect on the excretion of homogentisic acid and its derivative benzoquinone acetic acid. The purpose was to determine whether concentrations in body fluids of the latter substance, the putative toxic metabolite in alkaptonuria, would be reduced. Indeed, disappearance of benzoquinone acetic acid from the urine was observed in adults, whereas the level of excretion of homogentisic acid did not change. This could have relevance to the pathogenesis of ochronotic arthritis. In two of the children studied (a 4- and a 5-month-old), ascorbic acid may have doubled the amount of homogentisic acid in the urine, presumably through an effect on the immature p-hydroxyphenylpyruvic acid oxidase. In a 48-year-old man in whom alkaptonuria had been diagnosed during infancy, the effects of four different therapeutic 1-month trials were studied. The authors concluded that supplementation of ascorbic acid in doses of 1g/day represents a simple and rational treatment in patients with alkaptonuria.[879]

In 1999, Suzuki et al.[880] used 2(-2-nitro-4-trifluoromethylbenzoyl)-1,3-cyclohexanedione (NTBC) as a therapeutic agent for alkaptonuria. NTBC is a potent inhibitor of p-hydroxyphenylpyruvate dioxygenase, which catalyzes the formation of homogentisic acid from p-hydroxyphenylpyruvic acid. In a murine model of alkaptonuria they observed a dose-dependent reduction in urinary output of homogentisic acid with administration of NTBC.

ACRODERMATITIS ACIDEMICA

Several types of branched-chain aminoacidopathies may be associated with characteristic cutaneous lesions. Because these features resemble the skin lesions of acrodermatitis enteropathica, yet do not allow distinction among the aminoacidopathies, the term acrodermatitis acidemica has been proposed.[881,882] The branched-chain aminoacidopathies giving rise to acrodermatitis acidemica include methylmalonic acidemia,[883,884] propionic acidemia, glutaric acidemia, biotinidase deficiency,[885] multiple carboxylase deficiency,[886] and maple syrup urine disease[887] (Table 7.28). In general, patients with acrodermatitis acidemica have severe forms of organic acidemias without enzyme activity.[888] These patients tend to be subjected to severe protein restriction which may exacerbate the skin lesions.[889]

874. Beltran-Valero de Bernabe D, Jimenez FJ, Aquaron R et al. (1999) Analysis of alkaptonuria (AKU) mutations and polymorphisms reveals that the CCC sequence motif is a mutational hot spot in the homogentisate 1,2-dioxygenase gene (HGO). Am J Hum Genet 64:1316–1322.
875. Rodriguez JM, Timm DE, Titus GP et al. (2000) Structural and functional analysis of mutations in alkaptonuria. Hum Mol Genet 9:2341–2350.
876. Bory C, Boulieu R, Chantin C et al. (1989) Homogentisic acid determinded in biological fluids by HPLC. Clin Chem 35:321.
877. Wolff JA, Barshop B, Nyhan WL et al. (1989) Effects of ascorbic acid in alkaptonuria: alterations in benzoquinone acetic acid and an ontogenic effect in infancy. Pediatr Res 26:140–144.
878. Lustberg TJ, Schulman JD, Seegmiller JE (1970) Decreased binding of (14)C-homogentistic acid induced by ascorbic acid in connective tissues of rats with experimental alkaptonuria. Nature 228:770–771.
879. Mayatepek E, Kallas K, Anninos A et al. (1998) Effects of ascorbic acid and low-protein diet in alkaptonuria. Eur J Pediatr 157:867–868.
880. Suzuki Y, Oda K, Yoshikawa Y et al. (1999) A novel therapeutic trial of homogentistic aciduria in a murine model of alkaptonuria. J Hum Genet 44:79–84.
881. Happle R (2001) Acrodermatitis acidaemica – ein kutanes Leitsymptom verschiedener Organoazidämien. Z Hautkr 76:205.

882. Happle R (1999) Neurocutaneous diseases. In: Dermatology in General Medicine, Freedberg IM, Eisen AZ, Wolff K et al., eds. New York: McGraw-Hill, pp. 2131–2148.
883. Koopman RJJ, Happle R (1990) Cutaneous manifestations of methylmalonic acidemia. Arch Dermatol Res 282:272.
884. Howard R, Frieden IJ, Crawford D et al. (1997) Methylmalonic acidemia, cobalamin C type, presenting with cutaneous manifestations. Arch Dermatol 133:1563.
885. Wastell HJ, Bartlett K, Dale G, Shein A (1988) Biotinidase deficiency: a survey of 10 cases. Arch Dis Child 63:1244.
886. Williams ML, Packman S, Cowan MJ (1983) Alopecia and periorificial dermatitis in biotin-responsive multiple carboxylase deficiency. J Am Acad Dermatol 9:97.
887. Koch SE, Packman S, Koch TK, Williams MD (1993) Dermatitis in treated maple syrup urine disease. J Am Acad Dermatol 28:289.
888. Bodemer C, De Prost Y, Bachollet B et al. (1994) Cutaneous manifestations of methylmalonic and propionic acidemia: a description based on 38 cases. Br J Dermatol 131:93.
889. Niiyama S, Koelker S, Hoffmann GF et al. (2001) Acrodermatitis acidemica secondary to malnutrition in glutaric aciduria type 1. Eur J Dermatol 11:224

TABLE 7.28   Metabolic disorders giving rise to acrodermatitis acidemica

Disorder	Defective enzyme	Gene locus	MIM numbers	References
Methylmalonic acidemia	Methylmalonyl CoA mutase or its coenzyme adenosylcobalamin	6q21	251000, 251100	Koopman and Happle 1990[883]
Propionic acidemia	Propionyl CoA carboxylase	3q21–q22, 13q32	232000, 232050, 606054	Bodemer et al. 1994[888]
Glutaric acidemia I	Glutaryl-CoA dehydrogenase	19p13.2	231670	Niiyama et al. 2001[889]
Biotinidase deficiency	Biotinidase	3p25	253260	Wastell et al. 1988[885]
Multiple carboxylase deficiency, biotin responsive	Holocarboxylase synthetase	21q22.1	253270	Williams et al. 1983[886]
Maple syrup urine disease, types IA and IB	Branched-chain alpha-keto acid dehydrogenase	19q13.1–q13.2, 6p22–p21	248600, 248611	Assmann et al. 2001[892] Koch et al. 1993[887]
Maple syrup urine disease, type II	Dihydrolipoamide branched-chain transacylase	1p31	248610	

Epidemiology and genetics

All of the metabolic defects leading to acrodermatitis acidemica are autosomal recessive traits. The frequency of glutaric acidemia may be as high as 1:30 000.[890] The incidence of methylmalonic acidemia has been estimated to be about 1:48 000.[891] Neonatal screening for biotinidase deficiency is performed today in many countries.

Clinical features

Branched-chain aminoacidopathies are characterized by acral dermatitis, poor feeding, vomiting, hypotonia, lethargy, and dehydration. These disorders may be associated with progressive neurological symptoms that include a dystonic-dyskinetic movement disorder resulting from encephalopathic crises. In methylmalonic acidemia, hyperammonemia and hyperglycinemia are often present.

The signs of acrodermatitis acidemica include sharply demarcated periorificial and acral erythema and desquamation, reminiscent of acrodermatitis enteropathica. In addition, scaling elsewhere on the face and other body areas may be present. Bodemer et al.[888] described clinical features that may or may not occur simultaneously: (a) superficial scalded skin or superficial desquamation; (b) bilateral and periorificial dermatitis; (c) psoriasiform lesions affecting the trunk and the limbs; characterized by sharply demarcated, erythematosquamous plaques, sometimes with circinate margins; and alopecia associated with fine, dull and brittle hair. Genotypic–phenotypic correlations related to the severity of the acrodermatitis acidemica have not yet been delineated (Figs 7.78 and 7.79).

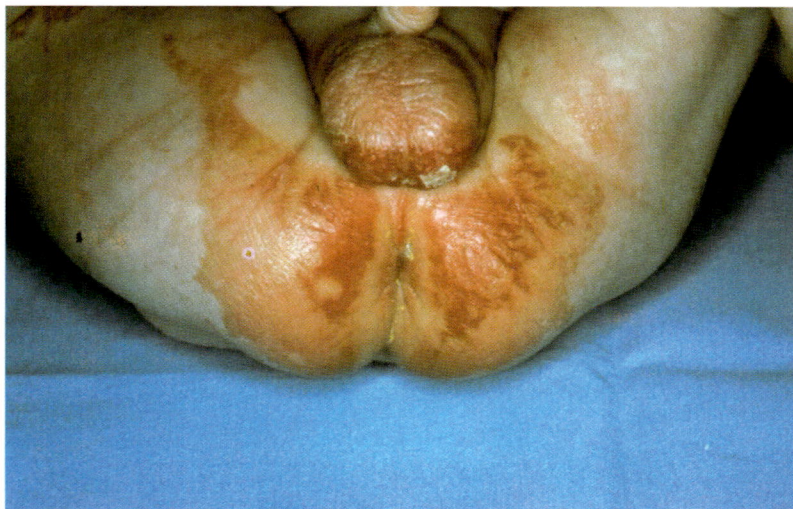

Fig. 7.78   Acrodermatitis acidemica in the diaper area.

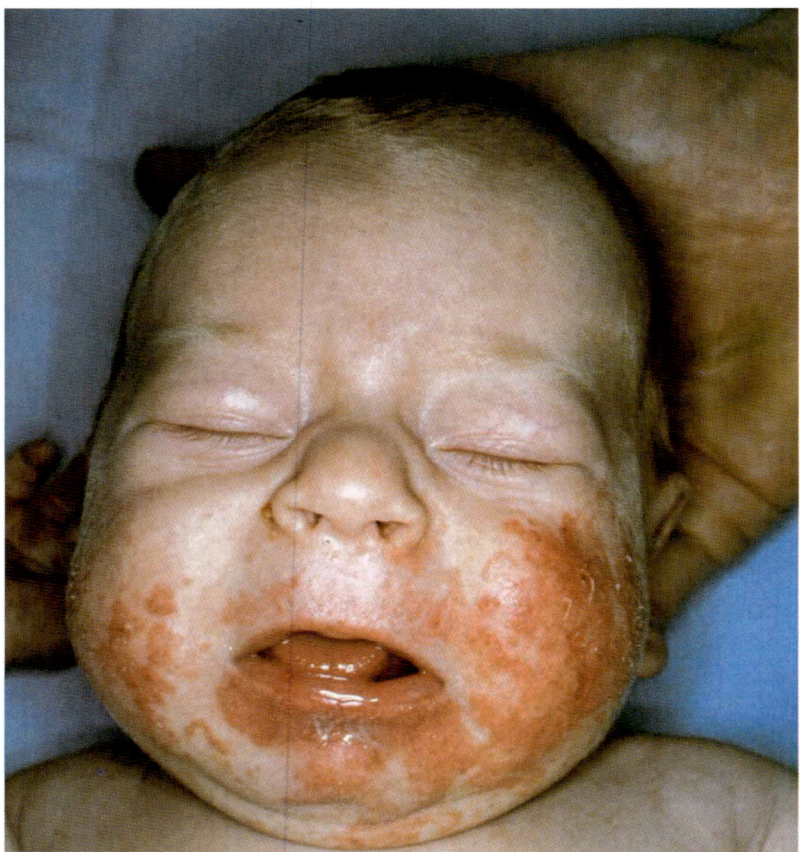

Fig. 7.79   Typical facial appearance of acrodermatitis acidemica.

890. Kyllerman M, Steen G (1980) Glutaric aciduria: a common metabolic disorder? **Arch Fr Pediatr** 37:279.

891. Coulombe JT, Shih VE, Levy HL (1981) Massachusetts Metabolic Disorders Screening Program: II. Methylmalonic aciduria. **Pediatrics** 67:26.

Treatment

The vitamin B_{12}-responsive type of methylmalonic acidemia can be successfully treated with this vitamin. Similarly, the biotin-responsive multiple carboxylase deficiency is treated with biotin. In the other forms of branched-chain aminoacidopathies a protein-restricted diet is necessary but difficult to maintain because manifestations of secondary protein deficiency may occur. Metabolic ketoacidosis should be treated by alkali therapy. In propionic acidemia, oral application of antibiotics may help to reduce propionate production in the gut.[893] In methylmalonic acidemia, tubulointerstitial nephritis with progressive impairment of renal function is a frequent long-term complication, and for this reason a kidney transplant may be a therapeutic choice in children with end-stage renal disease. The low level of enzyme activity present in the transplanted kidney may ensure normal metabolism of organic acids.[894]

TRANSPORT DEFECTS – HARTNUP DISEASE

Hartnup disease is caused by a deficiency of neutral amino acid transport within the kidneys and the small intestine. A typical clinical feature is a pellagra-like rash arranged in a photodistribution. After intensive exposure to sunlight, a severe "sunburn" with blistering may occur. In severe cases, blistering may resemble hydroa vacciniforme. After clearing of the erythema, the skin remains dry and scaly with peripheral depigmentation. Neurological features include cerebellar ataxia and emotional instability. Mild mental retardation may likewise be present. The disease may be genetically heterogeneous because cases with the urinary abnormalities only, without any defect of intestinal transport, have been reported.[895] The diagnosis is established by finding aminoaciduria. The following amino acids are excreted in particularly increased amounts: threonine, tyrosine, histidine, taurine, proline, cystine, and lysine. The disease was found in Massachusetts to have a frequency of 1 in 14 000 live births.[896] The trait has been mapped to chromosome 5p15. Treatment consists of good nutrition and supplementation of nicotinic acid (200–400mg/day). Oral administration of nicotinamide results in clearing of the rash and, possibly, disappearance of the ataxia.

LYSOSOMAL STORAGE DISEASES

FABRY DISEASE (ANGIOKERATOMA CORPORIS DIFFUSUM, α-GALACTOSIDASE A DEFICIENCY)

Introduction and historical note

Fabry disease is a rare storage disorder produced by an inborn error of glycosphingolipid metabolism. The defect in α-galactosidase, a lysosomal enzyme, results in progressive deposition of neutral glycosphingolipids in multiple organs. The first cases were described by Anderson and Fabry in 1898.[897]

Epidemiology and genetics

Fabry disease is a rare pan-ethnic disorder with an estimated prevalence of 1 in 117 000 in Australia and 1 in 42 000 males of the Netherlands.[898,899] The enzymatic defect is transmitted by an X-linked recessive gene, located at Xq21.33–q22, which encodes the gene product α-galactosidase A. Fabry disease may affect both hemizygotes and heterozygotes clinically, although the gene is highly penetrant in the hemizygote.[900] Expressivity in the heterozygote is variable, ranging from completely asymptomatic to the full-blown expression of the disease. The variable disease expression in heterozygous females results from random X-inactivation. At the molecular level several mutations, such as partial deletions, insertions and gene duplication, can lead to classic Fabry disease. However, patients with atypical Fabry disease all have missense mutations that lead to a reduction but not to an absence of α-galactosidase A activity. Residual α-galactosidase A activity was significantly lower in patients with neuropathic pain and in patients with mutations leading to a nonconservative amino acid change.[901] Fluorescence-assisted mismatch analysis (FAMA) has been documented in successful screening of the α-galactosidase A gene and detection of carriers in Fabry disease.[902] Prenatal diagnosis by chorionic villi biopsy at 9 to 10 weeks is possible by the assay of α-galactosidase A activity. The same test can be performed by cultured amniotic cells obtained by amniocentesis in the 15th week of pregnancy.

Presenting history and physical examination

Clinical onset of the disease is variable, occurring usually in childhood but sometimes expression may be delayed until the second or third decade.[903] The first clinical signs and symptoms are periodic crises of severe pain in the extremities (acroparesthesias), appearance of vascular cutaneous lesions (angiokeratomas), edematous upper eyelids, hypohidrosis and characteristic corneal and lenticular opacities. In adulthood, fever, heat collapse and lymphadenopathy combined with abdominal pain occur. Life-threatening complications are renal insufficiency, cardiac failure and cerebrovascular involvement. The clinical manifestations of Fabry disease mainly result from progressive deposition of neutral glycosphingolipids in the lysosomes of the vascular endothelium, although numerous organs and structures are directly affected by the storage of glycosphingolipids.[904]

Damage to vascular endothelial cells in the skin leads to swelling and focal increases in pressure. After sufficient damage has accumulated, telangiectases, angiomas and angiokeratomas develop. Angiokeratomas are vascular lesions which are defined histologically as one or more dilated blood vessel lying directly subepidermal and showing an epidermal proliferative reaction. In the center of pathogenesis is a capillary ectasia in the papillary dermis. The epidermal changes in all forms of angiokeratoma are secondary. Lesions can occur singly and may therefore be overlooked. Often they occur in groups and cover a large area of the body. Predilection sites are thighs, buttocks, groin and lower abdomen together with the genital area. Telangiectases of the labial, buccal, and/or unattached alveolar mucosa and soft palate were seen in 77% of the cases.[905] In addition an increased prevalence of cysts/pseudocysts of the maxillary sinuses and the presence of maxillary prognatism was emphasized. Angiokeratomas may also occur on mucosal surfaces of conjunctiva, airways and gastrointestinal and genitourinary tract. Accumulation of glycosphingolipids in eccrine sweat glands leads to hypohidrosis. Patients are intolerant to heat and exercise. The diagnosis of Fabry disease needs a careful history and clinical examination. Confirmation of the diagnosis is made by a biochemical test (males) or ultrastructure investigation or genetic analysis (females). Variants without the characteristic skin lesions have been observed.

892. Assmann K, Bonsmann G, Werner C, Metze D (2001) Acrodermatitis-enteropathica-ähnliche Hautveränderungen bei Ahornsirupkrankheit. **Z Hautkr** 76:220.

893. Fenton WA, Gravel RA, Rosenblatt DS (2001) Disorders of propionate and methylmalonate metabolism. In: The Metabolic and Molecular Basis of Inherited Disease, 8th edn. Scriver CR, Beandet AL, Sly WS, Valle D, eds. New York: McGraw-Hill, p. 2176.

894. Lubrano R, Scoppi P, Barcotti P et al. (2001) Kidney transplantation in a girl with methylmalonic acidemia and end stage renal failure. **Pediatr Nephrol** 16:848.

895. Sricantia SG, Venkatachalam PS, Reddy V (1964) Clinical and biochemical features of a case of Hartnup disease. **Br Med J** I:228.

896. Levi HL, Magigan PM, Shih VE (1972) Massachusetts metabolic screening program: I. Technique and results of urine screening. **Pediatrics** 49:825.

897. Fabry H (2001) An historical overview of Fabry disease. **J Inherit Metab Dis** 24(Suppl. 2):3–7.

898. Meikle PJ, Hopwood JJ, Clague AE, Carey WF (1999) Prevalence of lysosomal storage disorders. **JAMA** 281:249–254.

899. Poorthuis BJHM, Wevers RA, Kleijer WJ et al. (1999) The frequency of lysosomal storage diseases in The Netherlands. **Hum Genet** 105:151–156.

900. Whybra C, Kampmann C, Willers I et al. (2001) Anderson-Fabry disease: clinical manifestations of disease in female heterozygotes. **J Inherit Metab Dis** 24:715–724.

901. Altarescu GM, Goldfarb LG, Park KY et al. (2001) Identification of fifteen novel mutations and genotype-phenotype relationship in Fabry disease. **Clin Genet** 60:46–51.

902. Germain D, Biasotto M, Tosi M et al. (1996) Fluorescence-assisted mismatch analysis (FAMA) for exhaustive screening of the alpha-galactosidase A gene and detection of carriers in Fabry disease. **Hum Genet** 98:719–726.

903. Beck M, Ries M (2001) Fabry disease. Clinical manifestations, diagnosis and therapy. OOC Europe Ltd, 1–34.

904. MacDermot KD, Holmes A, Miners AH (2001) Anderson–Fabry disease: clinical manifestations and impact of disease in a cohort of 98 hemizygous males. **J Med Genet** 38:750–760.

905. Baccaglini L, Schiffmann R, Brennan MT et al. (2001) Oral and craniofacial findings in Fabry's disease: a report of 13 patients. **Oral Surg Oral Med Oral Pathol Oral Radiol Endod** 92:415–419.

Fig. 7.80 Typical appearance of angiokeratomas in Fabry's disease.

Pathophysiology and histogenesis

The loss of α-galactosidase A leads to increasing accumulation of neutral glycosphingolipids and α-galactosyl breakdown products in affected males and to a smaller percentage in females who are carriers of the disease. The predominant accumulated substance is globotriaosylceramide, which is normally broken down by α-galactosidase A. This accumulation leads to selective damage of endothelial, perithelial and smooth muscle cells of blood vessels and renal glomerular and tubular epithelial cells, myocardial cells and neurons of the dorsal root ganglia and autonomic nervous system.

Histologic examination of the skin lesions show telangiectases or small superficial angiomas in the upper dermis often with overlying epithelial hyperkeratosis. Vascular structures contain pathologic storage. Glycosphingolipids can be stained in frozen sections with lipid soluble dyes. A modified periodic acid–Schiff (PAS) stain is an additional option. Electron microscopic features are typical concentric or lamellar inclusions with alternating light- and dark-staining bands.

Differential diagnosis

Sometimes angiokeratomas are mistaken for melanocytic nevi or malignant melanoma but also for verruca vulgaris, hemangiomas, thrombosed capillary aneurysms and in children for Spitz.

In addition, angiokeratomas may occur in patients without Fabry disease (Fig. 7.78).[906] *Solitary angiokeratoma* is most common and seems to be more frequent in male patients. It present itself as a dark keratotic papule of about 2–10mm in diameter. *Angiokeratoma of Fordyce* is most often situated on the scrotum of patients who have passed the 3rd decade of life. The typical single lesion is a dark red to blue dome-shaped papule 2–4mm in diameter with a very discrete keratotic surface. Typically they are multiple and arranged in line and parallel to the median raphe of the scrotum. *Angiokeratoma circumscriptum naeviforme* is typically present from childhood as a large, mostly linear and unilateral hyperkeratotic plaque, which is composed of confluent keratotic papules. *Angiokeratoma of Mibelli* typically appears in young women on the dorsa of fingers and toes as multiple dark red papules with a slightly verrucous surface one of each measuring about 3–5mm in diameter. In most cases the lesion is preceded by a long history of recurrent perniosis and acrocyanosis. Angiokeratomas not uncommonly occur in patients with vascular malformation, especially nevus flammeus.

Angiokeratomas have been described in several other metabolic disorders. The autosomal recessively inherited *fucosidosis* is caused by a deficiency of α-L-fucosidase with accumulation of fucose containing glycosphingolipids, oligo- and polysaccharides. The main signs are neurologic abnormalities and development disorders. Angiokeratomas tend to be generalized, of earlier onset than in Fabry disease, and are more commonly acral. Progression of the disease is variable and death may occur in preschool years or the disorder is slowly progressive with long-term survival. *Sialidosis* is an inherited storage disease with a primary deficiency of α-neuraminidase with or without accompanying deficiency of β-galactosidase, leading to a cellular accumulation of sialylated oligosaccharides. Angiokeratomas develop very early in infancy and usually the disease is accompanied by multiple organ dysfunction and dysplasias, leading to death before the 2nd year of life. Several cases of angiokeratoma corporis diffusum have been reported without evidence of lysosomal storage disease, and with normal enzyme activities and no relevant family history. Some of these cases were associated with noncutaneous abnormalities, and some appeared to occur in completely healthy individuals. In contrast to the above mentioned entities, these cases had no lysosomal inclusions in their endothelial cells. In addition to these sporadic forms a recent publication describes an autosomal dominant form of diffuse angiokeratomas with arteriovenous fistulas, but no evidence of a metabolic disorder.[907]

Therapeutics and prognosis

Treatment of Fabry disease is symptomatic, and until recently no specific treatment was available. Treatment of neuropathological chronic pain can be tried with membrane stabilizers such as gabapentin, carbamazepine or phenytoin. Antihypertensive drugs are important to slow progressive renal insufficiency. Angiokeratomas of the skin can be treated with laser systems.[908]

Enzyme-replacement therapy for Fabry disease has recently been available and two large randomized studies have been performed.[909] Both studies concluded that enzyme-replacement therapy for Fabry disease is well tolerated and results in significant clearance of the accumulated glycosphingolipids. Adenovirus-mediated gene therapy for Fabry disease has been performed in α-galactosidase-deficient knockout mice with promising results.

MUCOPOLYSACCHARIDOSES

Introduction and historical note

The mucopolysaccharidoses were first described by Hunter in 1917 and labeled as gargoylism in 1936. The mucopolysaccharidoses are a group of heritable disorders caused by deficiency of lysosomal enzymes needed to degrade glycosaminoglycans (Table 7.29) The undegraded or partially degraded glycosaminoglycans are stored in lysosomes of tissues and organs and/or excreted in urine. The storage of incompletely degraded glycosaminoglycans causes marked distortion of many tissues with consequent severe somatic changes and mental retardation. There are at least seven biochemically specified forms of mucopolysaccharidosis with variable subtypes. In some cases evidence has been obtained indicating the existence of additional allelic diseases based on the same enzyme. All forms have an autosomal recessive inheritance with the exception of Hunter syndrome which is an X-linked recessive trait.

Epidemiology and genetics

Estimates of the incidence for numerous types of mucopolysaccharidoses in different populations have shown considerable variation.[910] Sanfilippo syndrome (mucopolysaccharidosis III A-D) is the most common form. However, there are very rare subtypes such as Sly syndrome (mucopolysaccharidosis VII) of which only 40 cases have been described. In the

906. Schiller PI, Itin PH (1996) Angiokeratomas: an update. **Dermatology** 193:275–282.
907. Calzavara-Pinton P, Colombi M, Carlino A et al. (1995) Angiokeratoma corporis diffusum and arteriovenous fistulas with dominant transmission in the absence of metabolic disorders. **Arch Dermatol** 131:57–62.
908. Sommer S, Merchant WJ, Sheehan-Dare RA (2001) Severe predominantly acral variant of angiokeratoma of Mibelli: response to long-pulse Nd:YAG (1064nm) laser treatment. **J Am Acad Dermatol** 45:764–766.
909. Pastores GM, Thadani R (2001) Enzyme-replacement therapy for Anderson–Fabry disease. **Lancet** 358:601–603.
910. Nelson J (1997) Incidence of the mucopolysaccharidoses in Northern Ireland. **Hum Genet** 101:355–358.

TABLE 7.29 Mucopolysaccharidoses

Number/syndrome	Enzyme/biochemical/gene locus	Clinical hallmarks
MPS I/Hurler syndrome	α-L-iduronidase, dermatan sulfate and heparan sulfate in the urine; Chromosome 4p16.3	Severe retardation, corneal clouding, hepatosplenomegaly, chondro-dystrophy, dwarfism, inguinal and umbilical hernia, upper respiratory tract infections, hearing loss, heart disease, hydrocephalus
MPS I/Huler-Scheie syndrome	α-L-iduronidase, dermatan sulfate and heparan sulfate in the urine; Chromosome 4p16.3	Joint stiffness, micrognathism, hearing loss, corneal clouding, less marked mental retardation
MPS I/Scheie syndrome	α-L-iduronidase, dermatan sulfate and heparan sulfate in the urine; Chromosome 4p16.3	Joint stiffness, hearing loss, corneal clouding, less marked or no mental retardation and short stature, excessive body hair, retinitis pigmentosa
MPS IIA/severe Hunter syndrome	Iduronate sulfatase, dermatan sulfate and heparan sulfate in the urine; Chromosome Xq28	Skin papules, hernia, hepatosplenomegaly, short stature, mental retardation, hearing loss, dysostosis multiplex, retinal degeneration, hydrocephalus but no corneal clouding
MPS IIB/mild Hunter syndrome	Iduronate sulfatase, dermatan sulfate and heparan sulfate in the urine; Chromosome Xq28	Skin papules, hearing loss, joint stiffness, heart disease and mild corneal clouding and no mental retardation
MPS III/Sanfilippo syndrome A-D	Heparan-N-sulfatase (A), N-acetyl-alfa-D-glucosaminidase (B), Acetyl CoA: alfa-glucosaminide-N-acetyl transferase (C), N-acetyl-alfa-D-glucosaminide 6-sulfatase (D) Heparan sulfate may be missed due to small amounts; Chromosome 17q25.3 (A) 17q21 (B) 14 (C) 12q14 (D)	Mental retardation, sometimes aggressive behavior, mild hepatosplenomegaly, coarse hair, mild dysostosis multiplex, synophrys as a characteristic feature
MPS IV A/B/Morquio syndrome A-B	Galactosamine 6-sulfate sulfatase (A), beta-Galactosidase (B), keratan sulfate in urine; Chromosome 16q24.3 (A)	Normal intelligence, dwarfism, skeletal abnormalities, corneal clouding
MPS VI/Maroteaux-Lamy syndrome	Arylsulfatase B, dermatan sulfate in the urine; Chromosome 5q11–q13	Marked impairment of vision by corneal clouding, upper respiratory infections, heart disease, hepatosplenomegaly, hearing impairment, dwarfism, hernia, contractures and osseus abnormalities, normal intellect
MPS VII/Sly syndrome	Beta-glucuronidase, dermatan and heparan sulfate in the urine; Chromosome 7q21.11	Hernias, hepatosplenomegaly, orthopedic abnormalities, short stature, upper respiratory infections, mental retardation, hydrocephalus, hearing loss, heart disease, corneal clouding

Netherlands 4.5 patients per 100 000 births have a mucopolysaccharidosis. Extrapolation from the British Columbia data and recent investigations give a total figure for all types of mucopolysaccharidoses of approximately 1:25 000.

Presenting history and physical examination

The characteristic findings usually develop within the first years of life although diagnosis as late as 44 years of age has been reported.[911] Most patients with mucopolysaccharidosis have thickened skin and craniofacial abnormalities resulting in a coarse facial appearance. A thick nose and large tongue with short neck and macrocephaly are typical features. A pebbly skin pattern with ivory–white to skin–colored papules and nodules especially on the back is a diagnostic clue for Hunter's disease and Hurler–Scheie syndrome. Hypertrichosis may also occur. Synophrys is typical for Sanfilippo syndrome. In addition, skeletal abnormalities, mental retardation, corneal clouding and hepatosplenomegaly may be observed. Urinary testing for glycosaminoglycans is the basis for the diagnosis. Enzymatic testing is necessary to confirm the diagnosis.

Mucopolysaccharidosis type I Hurler syndrome (MIM 252800)

It is a progressive disorder with multiple organ involvement that leads to death in childhood. The incidence is estimated to be 1:100 000 with an equal sex distribution. The responsible gene has been located on chromosome 4p16.3. In a recent study of 12 families with Hurler syndrome the most prominent clinical findings were short stature, coarse face with thick lips and enlarged tongue, organomegaly, hernia, cardiac disease, mental retardation and dysostosis. Often the skin is thickened, inelastic and hyperpigmented in exposed areas. Hypertrichosis is often prominent. Gingival hypertrophy is common and dental abnormalities are present. Three patients had no corneal clouding, although this finding was formerly thought to be obligatory. Extensive Mongolian spots have been described in Hurler disease,[912] as well as in GM1 gangliosidosis. Mucopolysaccharidosis type I Scheie syndrome (MIM 252800) is thought to be an allelic variant with milder features than Hurler syndrome.[913]

911. Gösele S, Dithmar S, Holz FG, Völcker HE (2000) Spätdiagnose cincs Morquio-Syndroms. Klinisch-histopathologische Eefunde ciner seltenen Mukopolysaccharidose. **Klin Mbl Augenheilk** 217:114–117.

912. Rybojad M, Moraillon I, de Baulny O et al. (1999) Extensive Mongolian spot related to Hurler disease. **Ann Dermatol Venereol** 126:35–37.

913. Alif N, Hess K, Straczek J et al. (2000) Mucopolysaccharidose de type I au Maroc: manifestations cliniques et profil génétique. **Arch Pédiatr** 7:597–604.

Mucopolysaccharidosis type II Hunter syndrome (MIM 309900)

This may manifest as a severe or mild type, distinguished as types IIA and IIB, respectively. In contrast to Hurler syndrome patients with type IIA mucopolysaccharidoses have a milder phenotype with longer survival. The inheritance is X-linked recessive with an approximate incidence of 1:100 000. The gene is localized to Xq27.3–q28. The skin eruption can be the earliest sign of Hunter syndrome.[914] The skin and hair findings are similar to those of Hurler syndrome. An almost diagnostic feature is pebbly skin, particularly in the scapular area.[915]

Mucopolysaccharidosis type III, Sanfilippo syndrome (MIM 252900, 252920, 252930, 252940)

Mucopolysaccharidosis types III A, B, C, and D are a group of autosomal recessive lysosomal storage diseases caused by mutations in one of four genes which encode enzyme activities required for the lysosomal degradation of heparan sulfate. It is a progressive disorder in which patients have severe central nervous system degeneration together with mild somatic disease.[916] The gene loci are on 17q25.3 (A), 17q21 (B), 14 (C), and 12q14 (D).

Mucopolysaccharidosis type IV, Morquio syndrome (MIM 253000 (A), 253010 (B))

Morquio syndrome is predominantly related to the skeleton. Short trunk, dwarfism, kyphosis and scoliosis are typical skeletal anomalies. The incidence is less than 1:100 000. The gene is located on chromosome 16q24.3.

Mucopolysaccharidosis type VI, Maroteaux–Lamy syndrome (MIM 253200)

Mental development is normal. The somatic involvement in the severe form is similar to that in Hurler syndrome. Severe Maroteaux–Lamy syndrome is usually fatal by early adulthood. This very rare disease is located on 5q11–q13.

Mucopolysaccharidosis type VII, Sly syndrome (MIM 253220)

Sly syndrome, a disease induced by deficiency of β-glucuronidase activity, features the typical signs and symptoms of mucopolysaccharidosis. There is considerable clinical variability among patients with this autosomal recessive disorder. Several laboratories have assigned β-glucuronidase to chromosome 7q21.11.

Pathophysiology and histogenesis

The enzymatic defect leads to accumulation of undegraded glycosaminoglycan molecules such as dermatan sulfate, heparan sulfate and keratan sulfate in numerous tissues. Histology from pebbly lesions of the skin shows extracellular mucopolysaccharides within the lower reticular dermis. Staining with Alcian blue, colloidal iron or Giemsa shows metachromatic granules in fibroblasts.

Differential diagnosis

Mucolipidoses have to be differentiated from mucopolysaccharidoses.

Therapeutics and prognosis

Prenatal diagnosis is possible by enzyme essays of cultured amniotic cells. The natural course of the severe forms is progressive and fatal. However, Scheie syndrome, for example, has a normal life expectancy. Orthopedic, cardiac and ophthalmologic surgery might be necessary and audiologic monitoring is important. Tracheostomy is sometimes requested because of severe sleep apnea. In patients with hydrocephalus, ventriculoatrial shunt might be necessary.

In patients with mucopolysaccharidosis I, treatment with recombinant human alpha-L-iduronidase reduces lysosomal storage in the liver and ameliorates some clinical manifestations of the disease.[917] Neurological correction of lysosomal storage in a mucopolysaccharidosis IIIB mouse model by adeno-associated virus-mediated gene delivery has been reported. Severe Maroteaux–Lamy syndrome (mucopolysaccharidosis type VI) is usually fatal by early adulthood. Bone marrow transplantation is the only form of definitive enzyme replacement therapy available but variable results have been obtained by this method. Enzyme replacement therapy in a feline model of mucopolysaccharidosis VI has been tried successfully. In murine mucopolysaccharidosis type VII syngeneic bone marrow transplantation has prolonged life. In addition, enzyme replacement reduced visceral lysosomal storage. Recently adenovirus-mediated gene therapy for corneal clouding in mice with mucopolysaccharidosis type VII has been performed.[918]

FARBER LIPOGRANULOMATOSIS (DISSEMINATED LIPOGRANULOMATOSIS, CERAMIDASE DEFICIENCY)

Introduction and historical note

Farber disease, or Farber lipogranulomatosis (MIM 228000) is a rare autosomal recessive sphingolipid storage disease due to a deficient activity of lysosomal acid ceramidase, leading to the accumulation of ceramide in cells and tissues such as liver, spleen and lung.[919] Seven different phenetypes can be separated. Type 7 is caused by a deficiency of the sphingolipid activator protein precursor prosaposin. The subtypes differ in age of onset and severity of symptoms. This disorder of lipid metabolism is progressive and involves primarily the skin, the musculoskeletal, respiratory and nervous systems. It manifests during the first year of life.

Epidemiology and genetics

In 1952 Farber *et al.* described a new lipo-glycoprotein storage disease that they called lipogranulomatosis. The responsible gene has been located to chromosome 8p22–p21.3.[920] Koch *et al.*[921] cloned and characterized by full-length complementary DNA encoding human acid ceramidase causing Farber disease.

Presenting history and physical examination

The clinical spectrum of Farber disease includes failure to thrive, subcutaneous brown nodules, painful and progressive deformed and painful swollen joints with restricted mobility, hoarseness, respiratory insufficiency and mental retardation with irritability and seizures.[922]

Hydrops fetalis as a presenting manifestation in Farber disease has been observed.[923] In addition, the typical sites of skin involvement include fingers, elbows, ears and knees. Recurrent infections, hepatosplenomegaly, nephropathy, and macular cherry-red spots may be seen. The diagnosis is confirmed by quantification of ceramide accumulation in tissues or in cultured cells. The degree of tissue accumulation correlates with disease severity. In addition, the diagnosis can be made by determination of residual ceramidase activity *in vitro*. The assay can also be performed using cultured amniotic fluid cells and is a potential tool for detection of carriers of the disease. Radiologic investigations reveal osteopenia, reduced long bone diameters, and underdevelopment of terminal phalanges.

914. Demitsu T, Kakurai M, Okubo Y et al. (1999) Skin eruption as the presenting sign of Hunter syndrome IIB. **Clin Exp Dermatol** 24:179–182.
915. Thappa DM, Singh A, Jaisankar TJ et al. (1998) Pebbling of the skin: a marker of Hunter's syndrome. **Pediatr Dermatol** 15:370–373.
916. Yogalingam G, Hopwood JJ (2001) Molecular genetics of mucopolysaccharidos s type IIIA and IIIB: Diagnostic, clinical, and biological implications. **Hum Mutat** 18:264–281.
917. Kakkis ED, Mucnzer J, Tiller GE et al. (2001) Enzyme-replacement therapy in mucopolysaccharidosis I. **N Engl J Med** 344:182–188.
918. Vogler C, Sands MS, Galvin N et al. (1998) Murine mucopolysaccharidosis type VII: the impact of therapies on the clinical course and pathology in a murine model of lysosomal storage disease. **J Inherit Metab Dis** 21:575–586.

919. Bar J, Linke T, Ferlinz K et al. (2001) Molecular analysis of acid ceramidase deficiency in patients with Farber disease. **Hum Mutat** 17:199–209.
920. Li CM, Park JH, He X et al. (1999) The human acid ceramidase gene (ASAH): structure, chromosomal location, mutation analysis, and expression. **Genomics** 62:223–231.
921. Koch J, Gartner S, Li CM et al. (1996) Molecular cloning and characterization of full-length complementary DNA encoding human acid ceramidase. **J Biol Chem** 271:33110–33115.
922. Kim YJ, Park SJ, Park CK et al. (1998) A case of Farber lipogranulomatosis. **J Korean Med Sci** 13:95–98.
923. Kattner E, Schafer A, Harzer K (1997) Hydrops fetalis: manifestation in lysosomal storage disease including Farber disease. **Eur J Pediatr** 156:292–295.

Differential diagnosis

Juvenile rheumatoid arthritis and juvenile hyaline fibromatosis may mimic Farber disease. Multicentric reticulohistiocytosis has similar findings but does not occur so early in life.

Pathogenesis and histology

Histologic examination of skin lesions shows granulomatous infiltration with lipid-laden macrophages. Light microscopic examination features markedly thickened and hyalinized sclerotic collagen bundles in the reticular dermis and subcutis. Interstitial and perivascular aggregates of foamy histiocytes stain positive for CD68 and form a granulomatous infiltrate. Examination by electron microscopy reveals foamy histiocytes with numerous membrane-bound inclusions that are C-shaped or worm-like. Occasional lipid droplets and rare banana-like bodies may be found.

Therapeutics and prognosis

The types of Farber lipogranulomatosis are severe, intermediate, or mild. Patients with the severe type die before the age of 4 years and those with the intermediate type live more than 4 years and are mentally retarded, but show no visceral involvement. The mild phenotype has a life expectancy of more than 10 years. No treatment is available,[922] although bone marrow transplantation may be an option.

HYPERLIPOPROTEINEMIAS

The term hyperlipoproteinemias (hyperlipidemias) describes a group of metabolic diseases characterized by elevated serum cholesterol levels, elevated triglyceride levels or both. Because plasma lipids are bound to protein, the term hyperlipidemia has been replaced by hyperlipoproteinemia. The plasma level of high-density lipoprotein cholesterol is inversely correlated with coronary heart disease. High-density lipoprotein particles modulate thrombosis, cell adhesion molecule expression, platelet function, and endothelial cell proliferation and apoptosis. The inherited forms of hyperlipoproteinemias are classified into five groups, designated I–V according to Frederickson and Lees, and result from defects of structural components of lipoproteins or receptors that influence production or elimination of lipoproteins. Type I and II are the most common in childhood. With the aid of electrophoresis and ultracentrifugal analysis of lipoproteins the different entities can be identified. Cutaneous markers for hyperlipoproteinemias are xanthomas which may manifest as plane, interdigital, eruptive and tuberous.[924] In addition xanthelasmata are found in type II hyperliporoteinemias. Histopathology shows non-xanthomized histiocytes, foam cells and Touton giant cells. Fat stains such as oil red-O or Sudan red stain are able to document fat storage.

Type I hyperlipoproteinemia (Bürger–Grütz disease, familial lipoprotein lipase deficiency)

In 1939 Holt and coworkers reported the familial occurrence of this disease for the first time (MIM 238600). Havel and Gordon[925] first recognized deficiency of lipoprotein lipase (triacylglycerol acylhydrolase) as the basic defect in type I hyperlipoproteinemia. This rare autosomal recessive disorder is biochemically characterized by marked elevation of chylomicrons and measurable hypertriglyceridemia but normal cholesterol. The responsible gene is located on chromosome 8p22. The type I hyperlipoproteinemia phenotype can also result from deficiency of the activator of lipoprotein lipase, apolipoprotein C-II. Decreased lipoprotein lipase activity leads to defective lipolysis. Apolipoprotein C-II cofactor deficiency secondarily decreases lipoprotein lipase activity and produces a similar phenotype. Cutaneous clues for the diagnosis are eruptive xanthomas, which are papules and nodules that contain lipid. Slight jaundice may occur because of bile duct stenosis and moderate hemolysis may add to this finding. In addition, lipemia retinalis develops in young years. Hepatosplenomegaly and pancreatitis may be associated with abdominal pain and most patients present before 10 years of age with acute abdominal pain. Vomiting and nausea accompany the attacks of abdominal pain. The serum is milky or cloudy with marked elevation of chylomicrons and normal cholesterol levels. Lack of lipoproteinase activity can be measured in adipose tissue biopsies. With lowering of serum triglyceride levels the xanthomas disappear.

Patients with type I hyperlipoproteinemias have no advanced atherosclerosis. A low-fat diet and medium-chain triglycerides can be beneficial. Prevention of recurrent pancreatitis has been reported with high-dose antioxidant therapy.[926]

Type II hyperlipoproteinemia (familial hypercholesterolemia)

This is an autosomal dominant disorder seen in approximately 1:250 to 500 persons in the general population. The responsible mutation of a low-density lipoprotein receptor gene causes the disorder and is located on chromosome 19p13.2. A structural and functional defect of the low-density lipoprotein receptor on cell membrane leads to increase in low-density lipoprotein and cholesterol levels.

This entity is characterized by tendinous, interdigital and tuberous xanthomas and xanthelasmas, corneal arcus, and a high incidence of coronary artery disease.[927] In addition, liver disease with pruritus is common. In homozygous patients serum cholesterol bound to low-density lipoprotein is excessively high and cutaneous xanthomas (tendinous, tuberous, plane and palmar) develop, often within the first years of life. Interdigital xanthomas may be present at birth in the web between the first two digits. In type IIa (MIM 143890) low-density lipoproteins are increased but there is no hypertriglyceridemia whereas in type IIb (MIM 144400) low-density lipoproteins and very low-density lipoproteins are found with increased levels. There is a marked hypertriglyceridemia and IIb type. Dietary regimens combined with modern drugs for lipid lowering are important to prevent early coronary heart disease. Aggressive LDL-cholesterol reduction by atorvastatin results in regression of carotid intima media thickness in patients with familial hypercholesterolemia, whereas conventional LDL lowering does not.[928]

Type III hyperlipoproteinemia (familial hyperbeta- and prebetalipoproteinemia, familial dysbetalipoproteinemia)

This autosomal recessive disease is also called broad-beta disease and is primarily seen in adults and rarely in children (MIM 107741). It occurs in 1:2000–1:10 000 individuals and is more common in males because estrogen has a marked protective potential. A mutation in apolipoprotein E on chromosome 19q13.2 is responsible for this entity.[929] A combination of factors are important, including defective apolipoprotein which impairs receptor-mediated clearance by the liver, elevated levels of apolipoprotein E, which impairs lipolytic processing, and increased levels of apolipoprotein E which stimulates very low-density lipoprotein production.[930] Abnormal glucose tolerance is associated with high levels of triglycerides and cholesterol. The skin may feature plane, tendinous and tuberous xanthomas and patients

924. Maher-Wiese VL, Marmer EL, Grant-Kels JM (1990) Xanthomas and the inherited hyperlipoproteinemias in children and adolescents. **Pediatr Dermatol** 7:166–173.
925. Havel RJ, Gordon RS (1960) Idiopathic hyperlipemia – metabolic studies in an affected family. **J Clin Invest** 39:1777–1790.
926. Heancy AP, Sharer N, Ramch B et al. (1999) Prevention of recurrent pancreatitis in familial lipoprotein lipase deficiency with high-dose antioxidant therapy. **J Clin Endocrinol Metab** 84:1203–1205.
927. Pandhi D, Grover C, Reddy BSN (2001) Type IIa hyperlipoproteinemia manifesting with different types of cutaneous xanthomas. **Indian Pediatr** 38:550–553.
928. Francois J, Lentini F, Hoste P. Rottiers R (1977) Genetic study of hyperlipoproteinemia type IV and V. **Clin Genet** 12:202–207.
929. Eichner JE, Dunn ST, Perveen G et al. (2002) Apolipoprotein E polymorphism and cardiovascular disease: A HuGE review. **Am J Epidemiol** 155:487–495.
930. Mahley RW, Huang Y, Rall SC Jr (1999) Pathogenesis of type III hyperlipoproteinemia (dysbetalipoproteinemia): questions, quandaries, and paradoxes. **J Lipid Res** 40:1933–1949.

develop severe cardiovascular disease. The same treatment approach as in familial hyperlipoproteinemia type II should be planned.

Type IV hyperlipoproteinemia (familial hyperbetalipoproteinemia, familial hypertriglyceridemia)

It is estimated that type IV hyperlipoproteinemia affects 1–10 per 1000 persons. This subclass is inherited in an autosomal dominant manner (MIM 144600). In addition, acquired conditions causing hyperlipoproteinemia IV exist such as uremia, hypopituitarism, contraceptive steroids, and glycogen storage disease I. Urbani and Moneghini.[931] have described the occurrence of palmar spiny keratoderma associated with type IV hyperlipoproteinemia. Type IV hyperlipoproteinemia leads to an elevation of very low-density lipoproteins and to hypertriglyceridemia. Manifestations rarely occur before the age of 20 years. However, in children with renal disease and diabetes clinical signs and symptoms may develop earlier. The clinical findings include eruptive, tuberous and palmar xanthomas, lipemia retinalis, cardiovascular disease and hepatosplenomegaly with abdominal pain. Treatment includes a diet low in carbohydrates, fat and alcohol. In addition, pharmacological treatment with lipid-lowering drugs is necessary.

Type V hyperlipoproteinemia

This disorder is also called familial hyperchylomicronemia with hyper-prebetalipoproteinemia (MIM 144650). The clinical and laboratory features are a mix of type I and type IV disease, with elevated levels of chylomicrons and very low-density lipoproteins. The cholesterol is not as markedly elevated as in type III. The disease is probably transmitted as an autosomal recessive trait. Numerous conditions may cause this phenotype such as insulin-dependent diabetes mellitus, administration of contraceptive hormones, alcohol abuse and glycogen storage disease I. Patients with apolipoprotein C-II deficiency may show a type V pattern. Pancreatitis precipitated by alcohol can produce a major problem. In general, patients are obese and the diagnosis is made in adolescence because of eruptive xanthomas, recurrent abdominal pain, hepatosplenomegaly or lipemia retinalis. Treatment should be performed in the same way as in type IV.

ACRODERMATITIS ENTEROPATHICA

Acrodermatitis enteropathica is an autosomal recessive trait characterized by zinc deficiency resulting in a triad of acral dermatitis, alopecia and diarrhea.[932] The trait has been mapped to 8q24.3.

Pathogenesis

The disorder has traditionally been thought to be caused by the inability of the gut to absorb zinc. However, the impaired uptake of zinc is ubiquitous and not limited to malabsorption within the gastrointestinal tract.

Clinical features

During early infancy, erythema and desquamation appears in the periorificial areas as well as over the bony prominences. Crusting and scaling usually shows a circinate arrangement. Paronychia may result in loss of nails. The scalp hair, eyebrows and eyelashes are brittle and tend to be lost. Blepharitis and conjunctivitis with photophobia frequently occur. Poor wound healing is another feature.

Laboratory findings

Low plasma zinc levels (less than 50μg/dl) are diagnostic. As a secondary phenomenon, low serum lipids and hypobetalipoproteinemia may be noted.

Care must be taken to ensure that blood is drawn into zinc-free tubes to avoid potential contamination. Skin biopsy sections show a nonspecific dermatitis.

Differential diagnosis

Differential diagnosis includes mucocutaneous candidiasis, seborrheic dermatitis, acquired zinc deficiency by malabsorption, and, in particular, acrodermatitis acidemica. In addition, zinc deficiency with the characteristic features of acrodermatitis enteropathica can occur in breast-fed babies of mothers with impaired secretion of zinc into breast milk.

Treatment

Prior to the introduction of oral zinc therapy, acrodermatitis enteropathica usually caused death in early childhood. Surviving patients showed pronounced growth retardation and hypogonadism. Zinc supplementation (2mg/kg/day) has dramatically changed the prognosis. Maintenance therapy is necessary but the disease tends to improve spontaneously with age, often leading to a lower requirement for zinc in the adult patient.

MENKES DISEASE AND OCCIPITAL HORN SYNDROME

HISTORY

Classical Menkes disease (MD, MIM 309400) or Menkes kinky hair syndrome is an X-linked recessive multisystemic disorder that was first described in 1962 by John Menkes and colleagues at Columbia University in New York.[933] According to a recent concept, four types of Menkes disease can be distinguished. The two extreme forms, the severe classical form and the mildest, called occipital horn syndrome (OHS, MIM 304150), comprise more than 90% statistically (Table 7.30); however a moderate and a mild form have also

TABLE 7.30 **The two most characteristic types of Menkes disease (MD) and their main symptoms**

Symptoms	Classical MD	OHS
Neurological		
Mental retardation	++	+/−
Seizures	++	−
Hypothermia	+	+
Feeding difficulties	+	+
Muscle tone changes	+	ND
Connective tissue		
Tortuous vessels	+	+
Skeletal changes	+	++
Bladder diverticula	+	++
Loose skin	+	+
Loose joints	+	+
Other symptoms		
Facial dysmorphism	+	+
Abnormal hair, pili torti	+	+
Hypopigmentation	+	+
Laboratory findings		
Serum copper	↓↓	↓
Serum ceruloplasmin	↓↓	↓
Intracellular copper accumulation	+	+

Adapted from Havel and Gordon 1960.[925]

931. Urbani CE, Moneghini L (1998) Palmar spiny keratoderma associated with type IV hyperlipoproteinemia. **J Eur Acad Dermatol Venereol** 10:262–266.
932. Sehgal VN, Jain S (2000) Acrodermatitis enteropathica. **Clin Dermatol** 18:745.

933. Menkes JH, Alter M, Steigleder GK et al. (1962) A sex-linked recessive disorder with retardation of growth, peculiar hair and focal cerebral and cerebellar degeneration. **Pediatrics** 29:764–779.

been described. In a sense, the latter two most likely represent stages of a seamless clinical transition between MD and OHS than fully independent entities.[934] From all Menkes patients, 5–10% have one of the milder forms.[935]

EPIDEMIOLOGY

The incidence is estimated at a range of 1 per 35 000 live births in Australia to 1 per 300 000 live births in Europe. It usually affects only males although a few females have been reported to express the disease due to genetic defects within the X-chromosome.[934]

PATHOGENESIS

As a disorder affecting copper homeostasis and transport, it is closely related to Wilson disease (ATP7B, > 100 mutations).[936] The importance of copper as an essential trace element lies in its ability to accept and donate electrons. It acts as a cofactor for enzymatic reactions such as oxygenation, dismutation, and hydroxylation. On the other hand, excess copper is toxic by its capability of oxidizing proteins and lipids and promotion of free radical formation. Cells protect themselves against excess copper ions by synthesizing metallothionein.[937] The copper entrapment in intestinal cells after normal uptake from the intestinal lumen leads to copper deficiency and subsequently to a defect of activity of copper-dependent enzymes. Menkes disease has also been termed a disorder of copper maldistribution by some authors.[938]

ATP7A encodes for the copper binding enzyme ATPase which is essential for intracellular copper transport and metabolism. This enzyme is localized in the trans-Golgi membrane and post-Golgi vesicular compartment of cells with the exception of liver and brain where it can be detected only in traces. Reduction, complete absence or functional impairment of this enzyme results in an accumulation of copper in the cytosol and a reduction of its excretion.[939,940] This accumulation may result more from defective copper translocation across an intracellular compartment than defective copper export across the plasma membrane itself.[934]

GENETICS

Menkes disease belongs to a group of disorders that are especially prone to new mutations ("new mutation disorders") and therefore almost every affected family displays a different genetic pattern.[934] More than 160 different mutations of which over 120 are in-gene point mutations, affecting *ATP7A*, also termed Menkes disease gene or *MNK*, have been located on chromosome Xq13.3, close to the centromere region. The center region of this gene seems to be particularly prone to new mutations.[941] The evolutionarily highly conserved Menkes/OHS gene is organized in 23 exons spanning a genomic region of about 165kb. Most of the mutations lead to classical Menkes disease, and only a few to the milder forms such as occipital horn syndrome.[938] The natural course of the disease is severe in more than 90% of the cases and leads to death in early infancy in affected males, usually within the first 3 to 4 years of life.[938] Female carriers of the gene defect are usually phenotypically normal but in 50% of the cases they do have hair shaft anomalies.[942]

CLINICAL FINDINGS

The syndrome is primarily characterized by progressive neurodegeneration, connective tissue abnormalities and abnormal hair.

HAIR

The color of the hair most often is described as white, silver or gray. This unusual color is a result of an explicit reduction of melanin and an associated abundance of tyrosinase, because pigmentation requires copper as a cofactor. The presence of rather short, sparse, coarse, lusterless, twisted and hypo- to depigmented hair is a predominant finding (Fig. 7.81). These typical structural hair changes, namely pili torti and monilethrix, are sometimes trichorrhexis and trichoptilosis, are due to a defect in the copper-enzyme dependent cross-linkage of disulfide bonds in the hair's keratin. This is

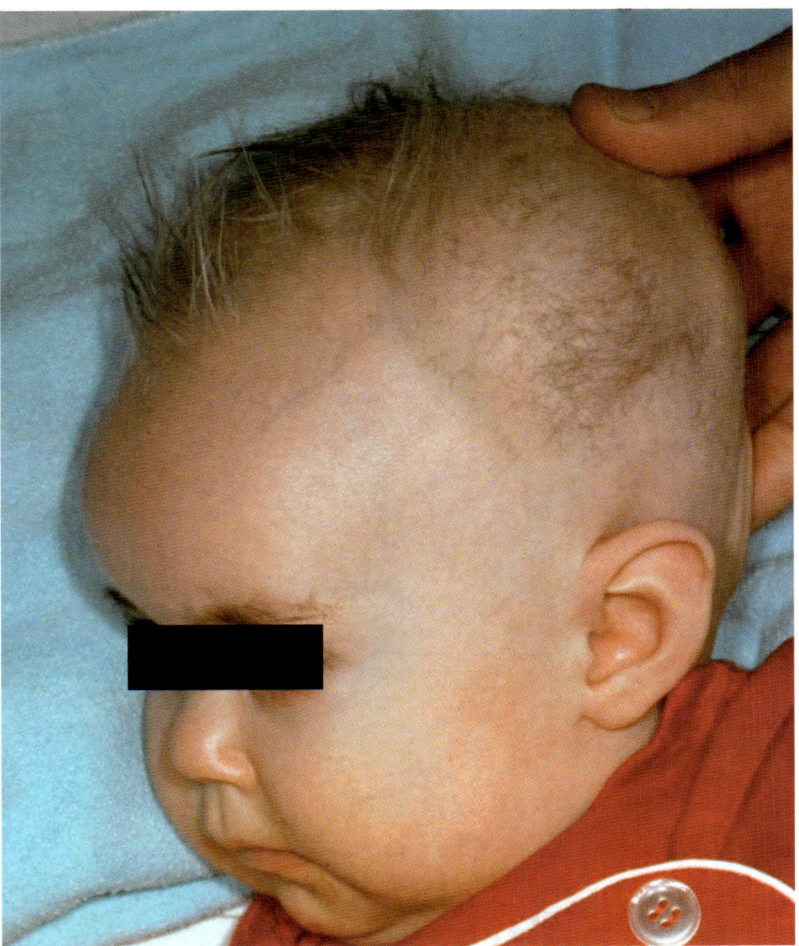

Fig. 7.81 Sparse and dry hair in a patient with Menkes disease. (Courtesy of Dr. Robert J. Gorlin, Minneapolis, Minnesota)

934. Tümer Z, Horn N (1997) Menkes disease: recent advances and new aspects. **J Med Genet** 34:265–274.
935. Møller LB, Tümer Z, Lund C et al. (2000) Similar splice-site mutations of the *ATP7A* gene lead to different phenotypes: classical Menkes disease or occipital horn syndrome. **Am J Hum Genet** 66:1211–1220.
936. Lee J, Prohaska JR, Thiele DJ (2001) Essential role for mammalian copper transporter Ctr1 in copper homeostasis and embryonic development. **Proc Natl Acad Sci USA** 98:6842–6847.
937. Hamer DH (1993) "Kinky hair" disease sheds light on copper metabolism. **Nature Genet** 3:3–4.
938. Dagenais SL, Adam AN, Innis JW, Glover TW (2001) A novel frameshift mutation in exon 23 of *ATP7A* (MNK) results in occipital horn syndrome and not in Menkes disease. **Am J Hum Genet** 69:420–427.

939. Gu YH, Kodama H, Murata Y et al. (2001) *ATP7A* gene mutations in 16 patients with Menkes disease and a patient with occipital horn syndrome. **Am J Med Genet** 99:217–222.
940. Vulpe C, Levinson B, Whitney S et al. (1993) Isolation of a candidate gene for Menkes disease and evidence that it encodes a copper-transporting ATPase. **Nat Genet** 3:7–13.
941. Kaler SG (1998) Metabolic and molecular bases of Menkes disease and occipital horn syndrome. **Pediatr Dev Pathol** 1:85–98.
942. Kapur S, Higgins JV, Delp K, Rogers B (1987) Menkes syndrome in a girl with X-autosome translocation. **Am J Med Genet** 26:503–510.

clinically perceived as coarseness and led to the attribute "kinky" or "steely" to describe the quality of the hair. The eyebrows generally share the features with the scalp hair. Most of the characteristic signs start to become visible at about 3 weeks of age. The clinical picture becomes complete by the age of 3 to 4 months.[933–935,943,944]

CONNECTIVE TISSUE

Many other manifestations are a result of the connective tissue defects due to the impaired function of copper requiring enzymes such as cytochrome oxidase, Zn superoxide dismutase, dopamine β-hydroxylase, lysyl oxidase, and and peptidyl-glycine α-amidating monooxygenase (PAM). These enzymes are involved in hematopoiesis, energy metabolism, cross-linkage of elastin and collagen fibers, pigmentation of the skin and hair, mineralization of bone and formation of myelin.[943,944] In spite of all the connective tissue abnormalities, wound healing does not appear to be impaired.[945] However, bladder diverticula, leading to rupture, peritonitis and death, and inguinal and/or umbilical herniae can develop.[946,947]

SKELETAL SYSTEM

Defects of the skeletal system can manifest as so-called Wormian skull bones, a prominent forehead ("frontal bossing"), metaphyseal spurring of long bones, anterior flaring and fractures of ribs as well as pectus excavatum. Other typical bony changes are the abnormal shape of the upper end of the radius that can lead to luxation, and of the lateral ends of the clavicles and acromion.[948]

BLOOD VESSELS

Arteries, especially in the brain, are tortuous and sometimes aneurysmal, especially in the brain, where collateral vessels can get a "puff of smoke" appearance, a typical pattern otherwise described in Moya-Moya disease.[947] Intra-abdominal arteries can also eventually be affected by tortuosity.[948]

NEURONAL TISSUE

Abnormalities in the central nervous system are best detected by magnetic resonance imaging and include dysmyelination, cerebral and cerebellar atrophy, ventriculomegaly, formation of cystic lesions and subdural fluid accumulation (hygromas).[947] Single cases with associated Dandy-Walker malformation have been described.[949] The most likely culprit for the neurological impairment seems to be the copper-dependent cytochrome oxidase.[948]

SPECIFIC PEDIATRIC ASPECTS

Common features of affected individuals include premature birth with a low birth weight, neonatal jaundice, neonatal temperature instability with tendency to hypothermia, dehydration and low blood pressure (from hypothalamic imbalances), muscular hypotonia with poor head control and a decreased facial expression with noticeable full, sagging cheeks and large-appearing ears. Breathing tends to be sonorous and noisy. Often, affected children suffer from failure to thrive, chronic diarrhea, poor motor and cognitive development and early occurrence of seizures before 1 year of age. Electroencephalograms are moderately to severely abnormal.[941] Regression of cerebral function and visual loss can occur.[945] Cutis laxa and hypopigmented skin become more evident with time. Splenomegaly and hypersplenism as a consequence of a splenic artery aneurysm are another possible complication.[948]

ORAL MANIFESTATIONS

Oral manifestations in Menkes disease are infrequent, and characterized by high-arched palate and usually multiple bluish, fluctuant eruption cysts of the gingivae that contain a sterile serous liquid. Histologically, these cysts are lined with a characteristic nonkeratinizing squamous epithelium.[947,950] Gingival hyperplasia can be severe enough to lead to posterior displacement of the tongue and significant airway obstruction. Unerupted primary teeth and dental malocclusion can also be found.[945,948,951]

MISCELLANEOUS

Normochromic, normocytemic anemia is sometimes observed.[948] Pyloric stenosis, gastrointestinal reflux and gastric polyps are other possible problems.[941]

DIAGNOSIS

Diagnosis is suspected by the clinical features, most notably the typical hair changes. Low serum copper (below 25% of normal range) and low ceruloplasmin levels can be found in blood samples taken shortly after birth and within the first few weeks thereafter. Interpretation of these findings remains difficult for the first 2–3 weeks of life, however, because these levels tend to be low in normal newborns as well. The low levels are more meaningful after the third week of life when levels normally start to increase. On the other hand, cultured fibroblasts from affected individuals show copper accumulation with concentrations up to ten-fold or more of baseline and markedly low lysyl oxidase activity as a result of the defective copper transport and impaired efflux.[952]

PRENATAL DIAGNOSIS

Prenatal diagnosis for Menkes disease in families at risk is possible through amniocentesis, but should be performed before 18 weeks' gestation because of the negative correlation of cell growth and copper accumulation to gestational age. After delivery, the diagnosis can be verified by copper measurements in the placenta.[934] DNA-based prenatal diagnosis of MD is also possible.[953]

Carriers can best and most accurately be identified by direct X-chromosomal mutation analysis. Measuring copper accumulation in cultured fibroblasts is easier and less costly, but also less reliable.[954] The measurement of deoxypyridinoline in urine has recently been proposed as a marker for connective tissue abnormalities, as it reflects the activity of the copper-dependent lysyl oxidase. A low level of deoxypyridinoline (d-Pyr) in urine means a poor lysyl oxidase activity in tissue.[955]

943. Martins C, Gonçalves C, Moreno A et al. (1997) Menkes' kinky hair syndrome: ultrastructural cutaneous alterations of the elastic fibers. **Pediatr Dermatol** 14:347–350.
944. Peterson J, Drolet BA, Esterly NB (1998) What syndrome is this? Menkes' kinky-hair syndrome. **Pediatr Dermatol** 15:137–139.
945. George DH, Casey RE (2001) Menkes disease after copper histidine replacement therapy: case report. **Pediatr Dev Pathol** 4:281–288.
946. Seidel J, Møller LB, Kauf E et al. (2001) Genotype/phenotype correlation in two patients with ATP7A gene mutations leading to classical Menkes disease (MD) and occipital horn syndrome (OHS). **Z Gastroenterol** (abstr) 39:249.
947. Proud VK, Mussell HG, Kaler SG et al. (1996) Distinctive Menkes disease variant with occipital horns: delineation of natural history and clinical phenotype. **Am J Med Genet** 65:44–51.
948. Christodoulou J, Danks DM, Sarkar B et al. (1998) Early treatment of Menkes disease with parenteral copper-histidine: long-term follow-up of four treated patients. **Am J Med Genet** 76:154–164.

949. Bekiesinska-Figatowska M, Rokicki D, Walecki J, Gremida M (2001) Menkes' disease with a Dandy-Walker variant: case report. **Neuroradiology** 43:948–950.
950. Nomura J, Tagawa T, Seki Y et al. (1996) Kinky hair disease with multiple eruption cysts: a case report. **Oral Surg Oral Med Oral Pathol Oral Radiol Endod** 82:537–540.
951. Brownstein JN, Primosch RE (2001) Oral manifestations of Menkes' kinky hair syndrome. **J Clin Pediatr Dent** 25:317–321.
952. Ogawa A, Yamamoto S, Takayanagi M et al. (1999) Identification of three novel mutations in the MNK gene in three unrelated Japanese patients with classical Menkes disease. **J Hum Genet** 44:206–209.
953. Tümer Z, Tønnesen T, Bohmann J et al. (1994) First trimester prenatal diagnosis of Menkes disease by DNA analysis. **J Med Genet** 31:615–617.
954. Tümer Z, Tønnesen T, Horn N (1994) Detection of genetic defects in Menkes disease by direct mutation analysis and its implications in carrier diagnosis. **J Inherit Metab Dis** 17:267–270.
955. Kodama H, Mochizuki D, Kobayashi M et al. (2001) Clinical markers for connective tissue abnormalities in patients with Menkes disease. **Z Gastroenterol** (abstr) 39:248.

TREATMENT

Once the diagnosis is established, early possible copper replacement therapy should be attempted to prevent the deleterious progression of the neurodegenerative features, although not every child with classic Menkes disease will have the same level of benefit. Disabling progressive neurodegeneration can only be stopped or prevented by initiation of treatment before age 2 months.[956,957] Copper-histidine, a copper complex physiologically found in human serum, has proven to be the most effective compound. It is administered subcutaneously in dosages ranging from 500 to 2400µg per day.[948,957,958]

Several well-conducted long-term follow-up studies have repeatedly demonstrated the inability of copper-histidine replacement, even if initiated early, to prevent the persistence or even worsening of connective tissue abnormalities. The duration of the therapy in general must be lifelong, although the first positive effects, e.g., normalization of plasma copper and ceruloplasmin, are only observed after several weeks of administration.[945,948,956,958]

OCCIPITAL HORN SYNDROME

OHS (formerly type IX Ehlers–Danlos, X-linked cutis laxa) represents the mildest variant within the spectrum of Menkes disease. Forty cases of OHS have been reported worldwide.[935,938] Patients with OHS show 2–5% production of correctly spliced *ATP7A*-transcripts,[935,938] perhaps leading to the decreased severity and the more benign course as compared to classical Menkes disease. Only one patient with OHS showed absolutely no normal *ATP7A*, due to a frameshift mutation.[938] It has been hypothesized that the *ATP7A* in OHS is misplaced most likely to the plasma membrane, and not missing. Because lysyl oxidase is more sensitive to copper deficiency than other cuproenzymes[938] the lysyl oxidase activity is particularly affected by this misplacement.

The typical occipital horns are the clinical hallmarks of this mildest variant of the Menkes gene defect,[946,947] and are caused by the exostotic calcification of the tendinous insertions of the trapezius and sternocleidomastoid muscles. Other features include abnormal facies, long neck, narrow thorax (pectus excavatum) and shoulders, deformities of elbows due to luxation of the proximal radius, enlarged lateral ends of the clavicles, abnormal ribs and long bones, cutis laxa, bladder diverticula, kinking of the cerebral and nuchal arteries, and aneurysms of abdominal arteries.

Occasional findings include genu valgum, platyspondyly of parts of the spine, coxa valga, rounded iliac-wing contour, partial scoliosis, broad scapular necks, clavicular handlebar/hammer contour, humeral and femoral diaphyseal wavy contour and bulbous ulnar-coronoid and radial bowing of the forearms.[938] Renal calculus, vesicoureteral reflux, inguinal herniae and neurogenic bladder are additional, infrequently reported features.[938] Affected individuals may have a normal to eventually slightly subnormal intelligence.[945]

HEREDITARY HEMORRHAGIC TELANGIECTASIA (OSLER–RENDU–WEBER DISEASE)

INTRODUCTION AND HISTORICAL NOTE

Hereditary hemorrhagic telangiectasia (HHT, MIM 187300), also known as Osler–Rendu–Weber syndrome, is a group of autosomal dominant inherited disorders characterized by multisystemic vascular dysplasia with recurrent hemorrhage. A century ago Rendu, Osler and Weber first reported families with multiple hereditary telangiectases and epistaxis. HHT may present with a broad clinical spectrum involving skin, mucous membranes, lungs, gastrointestinal tract and brain and may result in serious complications with substantial morbidity and mortality, particularly from brain, pulmonary and hepatic arteriovenous malformations.

EPIDEMIOLOGY AND GENETICS

The overall prevalence of HHT is on the order of 1:10 000.[959,960] It is inherited in an autosomal dominant manner with an age-related penetrance of 97%.[961] Linkage studies have identified two distinct HHT loci. One disease locus, *HHT1* or *ORW1*, has been mapped to chromosome 9q33–34[962–964] and subsequently shown to be the endoglin gene.[965] Endoglin is a homodimeric integral membrane glycoprotein expressed at high levels on human vascular endothelial cells of capillaries, arterioles and venules. On endothelial cells, endoglin is the most abundant transforming growth factor-β (TGF-β) binding protein. TGF-β mediates vascular remodelling through effects on extracellular matrix production by endothelial cells, stromal interstitial cells, smooth muscle cells, and pericytes. Thus endoglin, mediating endothelial–mesenchymal communication, is essential for angiogenesis.[966] A second locus, *HHT2* or *ORW2*, has been assigned to chromosome 12q.[967] The mutated gene on chromosome 12 encodes for activin receptor-like kinase 1 (ALK1).[968] ALK1, a member of the serine–threonine kinase receptor family, is a type I membrane receptor for TGF-β1 and activin A. As endoglin, ALK1 is expressed at high levels in endothelial cells and other highly vascularized tissues as lungs and placenta. The genetic heterogeneity may reflect the heterogeneity of the clinical picture: ORW1 families demonstrate a significantly higher prevalence of pulmonary arteriovenous malformations compared to non-ORW1 families.[969–972] In a large family with an unusual high proportion of liver involvement both disease loci, *ORW1* and *ORW2*, could be excluded, indicating that there might exist at least a third, yet unmapped, HHT locus.[973]

PHYSICAL EXAMINATION

Sixty-three percent of patients with HHT are symptomatic by the age of 16 years, 83% by 26 years and 97% by 35 years.[974] Epistaxis, caused by

956. Sarkar B, Lingertat-Walsh K, Clarke JTR (1993) Copper-histidine therapy for Menkes disease. **J Pediatr** 123:828–830.
957. Ozawa H, Kodama H, Murata Y et al. (2001) Transient temporal lobe changes and a novel mutation in a patient with Menkes disease. **Pediatr Int** 43:437–440.
958. Kirodian BG, Gogtay NJ, Udani VP, Kshirsagar NA (2002) Treatment of Menkes disease with parenteral copper histidine. **Ind Pediatr** 39:183–185.
959. Marchuk DA, Guttmacher AE, Penner JA, Ganguly P (1998) Report on the workshop on hereditary hemorrhagic telangiectasia, July 10–11, 1997. **Am J Med Genet** 76:269.
960. Guttmacher AE, McKinnon WC, Upton MD (1994) Hereditary hemorrhagic telangiectasia: a disorder in search of the genetics community. **Am J Med Genet** 52:252.
961. Plauchu H, de Chadarévian J-P, Bideau A, Robert J-M (1989) Age-related clinical profile of hereditary hemorrhagic telangiectasia in an epidemiologically recruited population. **Am J Med Genet** 32:291.
962. Shovlin CL, Hughes JMB, Tuddenham EGD et al. (1994) A gene for hereditary haemorrhagic telangiectasia maps to chromosome 9q3. **Nat Genet** 6:205.
963. McDonald MT, Papenberg KA, Ghosh S et al. (1994) A disease locus for hereditary haemorrhagic telangiectasia maps to chromosome 9q33–34. **Nat Genet** 6:197.
964. McDonald M, Papenberg K, Ghosh S et al. (1993) Genetic linkage of hereditary hemorrhagic telangiectasia to markers on 9q. **Am J Hum Genet** 53(Suppl):A140.
965. McAllister KA, Grogg KM, Johnson DW et al. (1994) Endoglin, a TGF-β binding protein of endothelial cells, is the gene for hereditary haemorrhagic telangiectasia type 1. **Nature Genet** 8:345.
966. Li DY, Sorensen LK, Brooke BS et al. (1999) Defective angiogenesis in mice lacking endoglin. **Science** 284:1534.
967. Vincent P, Plauchu H, Hazan J et al. (1995) A third locus for hereditary haemorrhagic telangiectasia map to chromosome 12. **Hum Mol Genet** 4:945.
968. Johnson DW, Berg JN, Baldwin MA et al. (1996) Mutations in the activin receptor-like kinase 1 gene in hereditary haemorrhagic telangiectasia type 2. **Nat Genet** 13:189.
969. Berg JN, Guttmacher AE, Marchuk DA, Porteous MEM (1996) Clinical heterogeneity in hereditary hemorrhagic telangiectasia: are pulmonary arteriovenous malformations more common in families linked to endoglin? **J Med Genet** 33:256.
970. Porteous MEM, Curtis A, Williams O et al. (1994) Genetic heterogeneity in hereditary haemorrhagic telangiectasia. **J Med Genet** 31:925.
971. McAllister KA, Lennon F, Bowles-Biesecker B et al. (1994) Genetic heterogeneity in hereditary haemorrhagic telangiectasia: possible correlation with clinical phenotype. **J Med Genet** 31:927.
972. Heutink P, Haitjema T, Breedveld GJ et al. (1994) Linkage of hereditary haemorrhagic telangiectasia to chromosome 9q34 and evidence for locus heterogeneity. **J Med Genet** 31:933.
973. Piantanida M, Buscarini E, Dellavecchia C et al. (1996) Hereditary haemorrhagic telangiectasia with extensive liver involvement is not caused by either HHT1 or HHT2. **J Med Genet** 33:441.
974. Porteous MEM, Burn J, Proctor SJ (1992) Hereditary hemorrhagic telangiectasia: a clinical analysis. **J Med Genet** 29:527.

spontaneous bleeding from telangiectasias of the nasal mucosa, is by far the most frequent and often the presenting symptom (in 90%).[974] Thus, epistaxis is an early marker of the disease with a mean onset age of 12 years (range from 5 to 52 years).[975] The frequency and seriousness often increase in the following years and may be so severe that multiple transfusions and iron supplementation become necessary. Telangiectasias of the skin usually present 5 to 20 years after the epistaxis and become more numerous with age.[974] They typically occur on the face, ears, lips, tongue and palate, palms and soles, tips of the digits and nailbeds. Trunk, arms, legs, and conjunctivae are less often affected. Pulmonary arteriovenous malformations (PAVMs) are discovered in 5 to 15% of persons with HHT.[961,976] Twenty percent of the patients, who present with PAVMs, are under age 20 (range 1–78 years).[961] PAVMs are frequently localized bilaterally with a predilection for the lower lobes. They act as direct right-to-left shunts. They manifest with thoracic murmur, cyanosis, dyspnea, fatigue, and clubbing of fingers. Bleeding may result in hemoptysis and hematothorax. Paradoxical emboli may give rise to ischemic stroke or septic brain abscesses. Standard chest radiographs disclose the PAVMs in 50%.[961] High-resolution computed tomographic scanning seems to be more sensitive.[977,978] For screening patients arterial blood gas measurements are important. Measuring PaO_2 while the patient is breathing 100% O_2 gives information about right-to-left shunting. Pulmonary angiography is required for planning interventional therapy. Gastrointestinal involvement presents usually with recurrent hemorrhage from telangiectasias of stomach and gut. Clinical symptoms are melena, hematemesis, rectal bleeding and chronic anemia. Gastrointestinal bleeding occurs in about 15% of affected persons and usually does not present until the fifth or sixth decade.[961] Rarely, intestinal vascular anomalies may be observed already in childhood.[979] Vascular malformations between the hepatic artery and vein result in left-to-right shunts and thus in high-output heart failure. Shunting from the hepatic artery to the portal vein leads to portal hypertension and esophageal varices. Encephalopathy may result from portal-to-hepatic-vein shunting. In addition, biliary disease has been observed, probably caused by hypoperfusion of the peribiliary plexus due to arteriovenous shunts.[980] The vascular abnormalities in the liver are often associated with fibrosis and atypical cirrhosis.[981] The mean age of patients with hepatic involvement is 65 years.[961] Arteriovenous malformations of the liver can be suspected when there is hepatomegaly or hepatic murmur. Ultrasonography with color and Doppler analysis is a reliable diagnostic tool for liver involvement.[981] Neurologic signs are often secondary to PAVMs and result from embolic complications, which give rise to brain abscesses, transient ischemic attack and ischemic stroke. Cerebral or spinal vascular malformations include telangiectasias, cavernous angiomas, arteriovenous malformations and aneurysms. Cerebral arteriovenous malformations are present in approximately 8% of patients and are described in children as young as 6 years.[974,982] They may be the presenting manifestation of the disease in children, since cutaneous telangiectasias and visceral involvement are unusual before puberty. In HHT typically multiple cerebral arteriovenous shunts are found. In children with multifocal pial arteriovenous fistulas, therefore, HHT should be suspected.[982,983] The cerebral vascular malformations can cause headache, subarachnoid hemorrhage, ischemia, seizure, or paraparesis. In children the most common manifestation is cerebral bleeding.[982] A cranial bruit is often present. Angiography and magnetic resonance imaging are sensitive in detecting cerebral vascular malformations.[984]

PATHOPHYSIOLOGY AND HISTOGENESIS

The earliest morphologic event in the pathogenesis of HHT lesion is a focal dilatation of postcapillary venules, which continue to enlarge and eventually connect with dilated arterioles through capillaries. As the vascular lesion increases in size, the capillary segments disappear and a direct arteriovenous communication is formed. The lesions are associated with a perivascular mononuclear infiltrate of lymphocytes and macrophages.[985]

DIFFERENTIAL DIAGNOSIS

The differential diagnosis from the dermatological point of view includes blue rubber bleb nevus syndrome, scleroderma, and generalized essential telangiectasia. In 2000 Shovlin et al.[986] presented consensus clinical diagnostic criteria. The four criteria for HHT are: epistaxes, telangiectasia, visceral lesions, and an appropriate family history. The HHT diagnosis is definite if three criteria are present. In patients with two criteria the diagnosis of HHT should be recorded as possible and a high clinical suspicion should be maintained. If fewer than two criteria are present a diagnosis of HHT is unlikely.

THERAPEUTICS AND PROGNOSIS

Therapies for epistaxis include cauterization, dermoplasty, laser photocoagulation, estrogen therapy; transcatheter embolotherapy, or ligation of feeding arteries. However, often only a temporary response can be achieved followed by recurrence or even worsening of the symptoms. Laser ablation may be useful for cutaneous telangiectasias if cosmetically disturbing or frequently bleeding. Transcatheter embolotherapy of large pulmonary arteriovenous malformations results in permanent occlusion in the majority of patients and is nowadays the therapy of choice.[987] Most authors prefer to treat asymptomatic lesions as well.[978] Blood loss through gastrointestinal telangiectasias can be reduced by a low-dose combination therapy with progesterone and estrogen. Endoscopic laser or bipolar coagulation may control gastrointestinal bleeding in the short term, but rarely in the long term. Hemodynamically significant hepatic arteriovenous shunts have been treated by catheter embolization of the feeding vessel, but this intervention is associated with a 25% mortality rate.[988] Cerebral arteriovenous malformations have been treated by neurovascular surgery, embolotherapy, and stereotactic radio surgery alone or in combination.

Once the diagnosis of HHT is made, affected patients should be followed carefully. A thorough family history and physical examination with special attention to telangiectasias on the skin, nasal mucosa and oropharynx is essential. Blood cell counts often show anemia caused by epistaxis or gastrointestinal blood loss. Blood chemistry tests may reveal elevated liver enzymes, indicating hepatic involvement. Urine should be examined for hematuria. Examination for pulmonary or brain lesions is of particular importance, because presymptomatic intervention may prevent serious complications.[977] Pulmonary screening for arteriovenous malformations

975. Aassar SO, Friedman CM, White RI Jr (1991) The natural history of epistaxis in Hereditary hemorrhagic telangiectasia. **Laryngoscope** 101:977.

976. Dines DE, Arms RA, Bernatz PE, Gomes MR (1974) Pulmonary arteriovenous fistulas. **Mayo Clinic Proc** 49:460.

977. Guttmacher AE, Marchuk DA, White RI (1995) Hereditary hemorrhagic telangiectaisa. **New Eng J Med** 333:918.

978. Pick A, Deschamps C, Stanson AW (1999) Pulmonary arteriovenous fistula: presentation, diagnosis, and treatment. **World J Surg** 23:1118.

979. Frémond B, Yazbeck S, Dubois J et al. (1997) Intestinal vascular anomalies in children. **J Pediatr Surg** 32:873.

980. Garcia-Tsao G, Korzenik JR, Young L et al. (2000) Liver disease in patients with hereditary hemorrhagic telangiectasia. **N Engl J Med** 343:931.

981. Weik C, Greiner L (1999) The liver in hereditary hemorrhagic telangiectasia (Weber–Rendu–Osler disease). **Scand J Gastroenterol** 34:1241.

982. García-Mónaco R, Taylor W, Rodesch G et al. (1995) Pial arterioevenous fistula in children as presenting manifestation of Rendu–Osler–Weber disease. **Neuroradiology** 37:60.

983. Griffiths PD, Blaser S, Armstrong D et al. (1998) Cerebellar arteriovenous malformations in children. **Neuroradiology** 40:324.

984. Haitjema T, Westerman CJJ, Overtoom TTC et al. (1996) Hereditary hemorrhagic telangiectasia (Osler–Weber–Rendu disease): New insights in pathogenesis, complications, and treatment. **Arch Intern Med** 156:714.

985. Braverman IM, Keh A, Jacobson BS (1990) Ultrastructure and three-dimensional organization of the telangiectases of hereditary hemorrhagic telangiectasia. **J Invest Dermatol** 95:422.

986. Shovlin CL, Guttmacher AE, Buscarini E et al. (2000) Diagnostic criteria for hereditary hemorrhagic telangiectasia (Rendu–Osler–Weber syndrome). **Am J Med Genet** 91:66.

987. Lee DW, White RIJr, Egglin TK et al. (1997) Embolotherapy of large pulmonary arteriovenous malformations: long-term results. **Ann Thorac Surg** 64:930.

988. Allison DJ, Jordan H, Hennessy O (1985) Therapeutic embolization of the hepatic artery: a review of 75 procedures. **Lancet** 1:595.

include chest radiography, arterial blood gas measurements and finger oximetry in the upright position. In case of hypoxemia, a right-to-left shunt can be measured by the 100% O_2 method. Intravenous digital subtraction angiography is performed when the shunt fraction is considered abnormal or if PAVMs are suspected based on the chest radiography.[984,989] Contrast echocardiography demonstrating right-to-left shunting is an effective test to exclude the presence of PAVMs and to monitor the course after therapy.[978] In screening for familial cerebral arteriovenous malformations and aneurysms, magnetic resonance imaging and/or digital subtraction angiography is performed.[984] Capillary microscopy is a simple, noninvasive and unexpensive procedure and can be a useful diagnostic tool in diagnosing HHT, since a high percentage of HHT patients have giant loops between the normal capillaries in the nail fold.[990] Relatives of HHT patients should be encouraged to be screened for presence of the disease and associated PAVMs, since the prevalence of potentially life-threatening vascular lesions in family members is alarmingly high.[989] In the future, more specific screening may be possible, with molecular diagnosis, especially in veiw of evidence that PAVMs are particularly frequent in patients with genetic linkage of the disease to chromosome 9q3.

PEDIATRIC ASPECTS OF THE DISEASE

The age-related penetrance of HHT should always be kept in mind. Children fulfilling only one or two diagnostic criteria who are offspring of affected individuals should be considered at risk to develop the disorder.[986] Because cutaneous telangiectasias are unusual in children, multiple pial arteriovenous fistulas or multiple gastrointestinal vascular malformations or PAVMs may be the only manifestation of the disease and, in these children, HHT should be suspected.[979,982] Examination and screening should be repeated at puberty and again at the end of adolescence.[975,984]

Additional information and support for HHT patients and their families are available from:
Hereditary Hemorrhagic Telangiectasia
HHT Foundation International, Inc. (HHT)
P.O. Box 8087
New Haven, CT 06530
(410) 357-9932
(800) 448-6389
Fax: (419) 357-9932; email: hhtinfo@hht.org
http://www.hht.org

AGING DISORDERS

Patsy Lenane and Bernice Krafchik

Aging is a natural process resulting from deterioration of essential physiological functions. This occurs by a variety of complex biological mechanisms, involving multiple genetic and environmental factors.[991] The protective mechanism of apoptosis (programmed cell death) declines with age, resulting in the failure of the normal destruction of damaged DNA, and the accumulation of carcinogenic genetic material. The end result of aging is cell death and eventual decline of the living organism. This complicated process involves derangement of other biologic pathways, including endocrine failure and the accumulation of free radicals. There is also shortening of normal telomerase function. In human beings this process usually takes 70–80 years. Recognized clinical changes in the skin secondary to aging have been clearly identified. These include dermal atrophy, loss of subcutaneous fat, poikiloderma, alteration in pigmentation and cutaneous sclerosis.[992]

Premature aging syndromes are rare disorders that mimic senescence, in which cell death occurs over a much shorter period of time. Features of premature aging are included in a heterogenous group of genetic disorders ranging from those with true premature aging and early death (Hutchinson–Gilford syndrome) to those with skin atrophy (acrogeria) and skin laxity (Hernandez syndrome), and a normal life span. There are thus many and varied diseases that encompass the group falling under the umbrella of the premature aging conditions (see Table 7.31).

PROGERIA

The Hutchinson–Gilford (HG) syndrome, entitled following its initial description by Hutchinson[993] in 1886 and Gilford[994] in 1897, is a rare entity of premature aging. The term "progeria" was coined by Gilford in 1904[995] from the Greek word "geras" meaning old age. The pattern of inheritance is unclear, with both autosomal dominant and recessive cases having been reported. Most appear to be due to sporadiac mutations. The incidence is one in 8 million but is probably higher, in the order of 1 in 4 million, as not all cases are reported. It is reported almost exclusively in Caucasians and occurs slightly more commonly in males.

Clinical features develop in early infancy with low birth weight and failure to thrive. The cutaneous changes begin within the first year of life and include midfacial cyanosis and prominence of the superficial veins, especially over the scalp and thighs. Sclerodermoid changes are also early findings and are often the first features that precipitate a medical consultation. They generally occur either at or directly after birth and affect the chest, abdomen and thighs. Although diagnostic, they are not always present. Typical facial changes (Fig. 7.82) evolve during the first 2 years and include frontal bossing, development of a glyphic nose, thin lips and micrognathia. Hair changes are a consistent finding ranging from the presence of thin, sparse gray hairs to total alopecia. These affect both the scalp and eyebrows.

Skeletal abnormalities are prominent with joint stiffness and mild knee flexion (Fig. 7.83), both of which result in a characteristic wide-based gait. Acro-osteolysis, osteoporosis and hip dislocation may occur. Nail dystrophy and decreased sweating are frequently seen. Affected individuals have short stature, normal intelligence, lack secondary sexual characteristics and have a high pitched voice.

Severe cardiovascular disease with atherosclerosis and hypertention results in death from myocardial infarction or a cerebrovascular accident. Death usually occurs in the second decade but survival into the 20s has occasionally been reported.

Several laboratory abnormalities have been found in patients with HG although none is diagnostic. These include reduced insulin receptor gene expression in cells[996] and an increase in $\alpha1$ and $\alpha2$ type IV procollagen mRNA in fibroblasts.[997] Elevated levels of urinary hyaluronic acid are consistently found. It has been suggested that an abnormality in hyaluronic acid metabolism may precipitate the clinical features of progeria, as this agent may act as an anti-aging factor.[998] An increased level of hyaluronic acid in conjunction with clinical features is extremely useful in diagnosing this devastating disease.

989. Haitjema T, Disch F, Overtoom TTC et al. (1995) Screening family members of patients with hereditary hemorrhagic telangiectasia. **Am J Med** 99:519.
990. Mager JJ, Westermann CJJ (2000) Value of capillary microscopy in the diagnosis of hereditary hemorrhagic telangiectasia. **Arch Dermatol** 136:732.
991. Makoto KO (2001) Disease models: human aging. **Trends Mol Med** 7(4):179–181.
992. Novice FM, Collison DW, Burgdorf WHC, Esterly NB, eds (1994) Handbook of genetic skin disorders. Philadelphia: WB Saunders Company, pp. 147–161.
993. Hutchinson J (1886) Congenital absence of hair and mammary glands with atrophic condition of the skin and its appendages. **Med Chirur Trans** 69:473–477.

994. Gilford H (1897) On a condition of mixed premature and immature development. **Med Chirur Trans** 80:17–45.
995. Gilford H (1904) Progeria: a form of senilism. **Practitioner** 73:188–217.
996. Briata P, Bellini C, Vignolo M, Gherzi R (1991) Insulin receptor gene expression is reduced in cells from a progeric patient. **Mol cell Endocrinol** 75:9–14.
997. Colige A, Roujeau JC, Lapiere C (1991) Abnormal gene expression in skin fibroblasts from Hutchinson-Gilfords progeria patient. **Lab Invest** 64:799–806.
998. Pesce K, Rothe MJ (1996) The premature aging syndromes. **Clin Dermatol** 14:161–170.

TABLE 7.31   Inherited skin disorders with premature skin aging

Disorder	Mode of Inheritance	Onset	Skin	Skeletal	Systemic	Intellect	Death
Acrogeria	AD, AR	Neonates	Acral atrophy, hyperpigmentation	Short limbs, osteoporosis, acro-osteolysis	None	Normal	Normal life span
Ataxla telangectasia	AR	Infancy	Telangectasia, loss of fat and sclerosis on face	Craniofacial anomalies	Sinopulmonary infections immunodeficiancies Chromosomal instability	Normal	Second decade
Bloom syndrome	AR	Neonatal	Erythema, telangiectasia head, neck, forearms hyper- or hyopigmentation trunk and extremities	None	Cancer predsposition Immunodeficiency – recurrent bacterial infections	Normal but may have some learning disability	Dictated by development of malignancy
Cockayne syndrome	AD	Infancy	Photosensitive eruption Postinflammatory hyperpigmentation	Contractures, kyphosis	Multiple neurological abnormalities	Mental retardation	Second decade
Cutis Laxa	AR, AD Acquired	Neonate childhood	Pendulous skin folds face and body	Joint dislocations	Respiratory, cardiac, GI complications, depending	Normal to severe mental retardation	Unknown
De Barsy syndrome	Unknown	Neonate	Thin skin, loss of fat, wrinkles prominent vasculature	Joint laxity, hands held in listed pattern	Choreoatheosis	Severe mental retardation	Probably normal
Hernandez syndrome	AD ?	Childhood	Ehlers–Danlos like changes	Winged scapulae, pectus excavatum joint hypermobility	Cryptorchidism inguinal herniae	Mild mental retardation	Normal
Hallermann Strieff syndrome	Sporadic	Infancy	Thin, taut facial skin, hypotrichosis telangiactasia	Dyscephaly, severe micrognathia	Ocular, dental abnormalities short stature	Mental retardation in up to 30%	Appears normal
Lee syndrome	AD	Neonate	Premature facial wrinkling	None	Nasolacrimal duct obstruction	Normal	Normal
Lenaert syndrome	AD, X linked dominant	Childhood	Acral atrophy, livedo reticularis	Subluxation interphalangeal joints hyperlaxity large joints	Hypogammaglobulinaemia	Normal	Normal
Mandibuloa-crodysplasia	AR	Childhood	Hyperpigmentation sclerodermoid patches	Bone resorption-clavicles, distal phalanges	Occasional renal disease	Normal	Normal
Metageria	AR ?	Neonates	Limb lipoatrophy	None	Diabetes, atherosclerosis	Normal	Dependent on severity of diabetes/atherosclerosis
Mulvihill–Smith syndrome	Unclear	Childhood	Lack of facial subcutaneous fat, pigmented nevi	Advanced bone age	Sensorineural hearing loss immunodeficiency	Mild–severe mental retardation	Unknown Probably normal
Osteodysplastic geroderma	AR	Neonate	Generalized thin skin, drooping eyelids and cheeks	Osteoporosis, joint laxity	Nil	Normal	Unknown
Progeria	AD, AR	Infancy	Generalized scleroderma-like	Osteoporosis, joint stiffness	Diffuse atherosclerosis	Normal	Second decade
Rothmund–Thompson	AR	Infancy	Poikiloderma, acral keratosis	Skeletal dysplasia	Hypogonadism, osteosarcoma squamous cell carcinoma	Normal	Normal life expectancy
Scleroatrophic syndrome of Huriez	Unclear	Infancy	Scleroatrophy hands	None	Palmar hypohydrosis progressive keratoderma	Normal	Unknown
Werner syndrome	AR	Adult	Generalized scleropoikiloderma	Osteoporosis	Diabetes, hypogonadism cataracts, calcification	Normal	Fifth and sixth decade
Wrinkly skin syndrome	AR	Childhood	Wrinkling skin, hands, feet, abdomen prominent vasculature on chest	Hypermobile joints, kyphosis microcephaly	Potential cardiac complications	Normal or mild mental retardation	Unknown
Wiedemann-Rautenstrauch syndrome	AR	Neonate	Dry, thin skin, generalized lipoatrophy	Skeletal dysplasia	Squamous cell carcinoma	Normal	Unknown
Xeroderma pigmentosum	AR	Infancy	Photosensitivity, photodamage	None	Potential neurological abnormalities, hypogonadism	Normal	Shortened life span

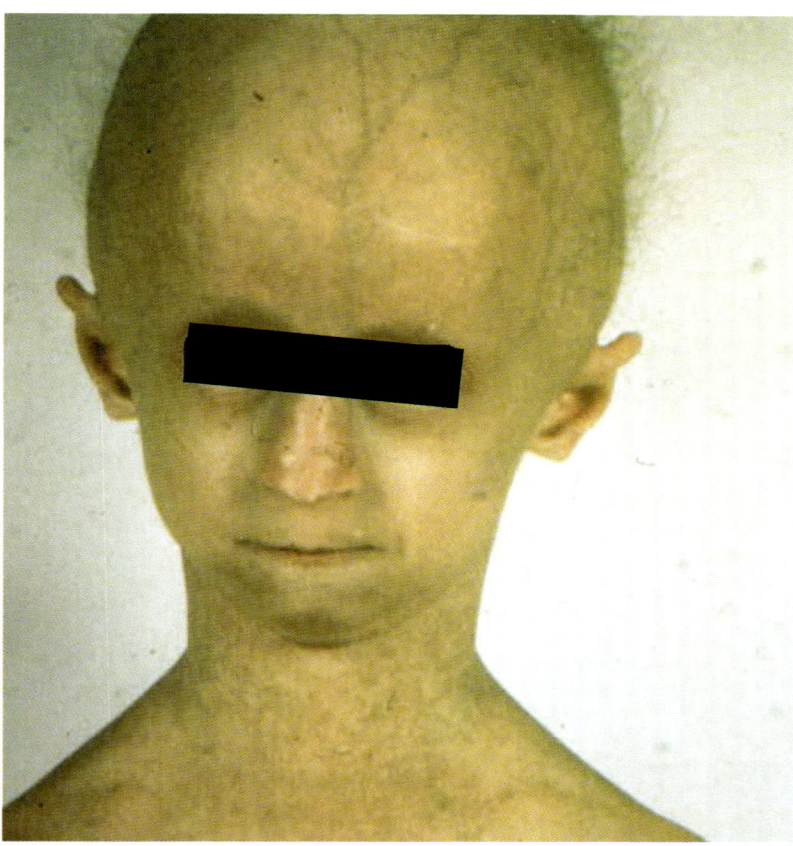

Fig. 7.82   Progeria.

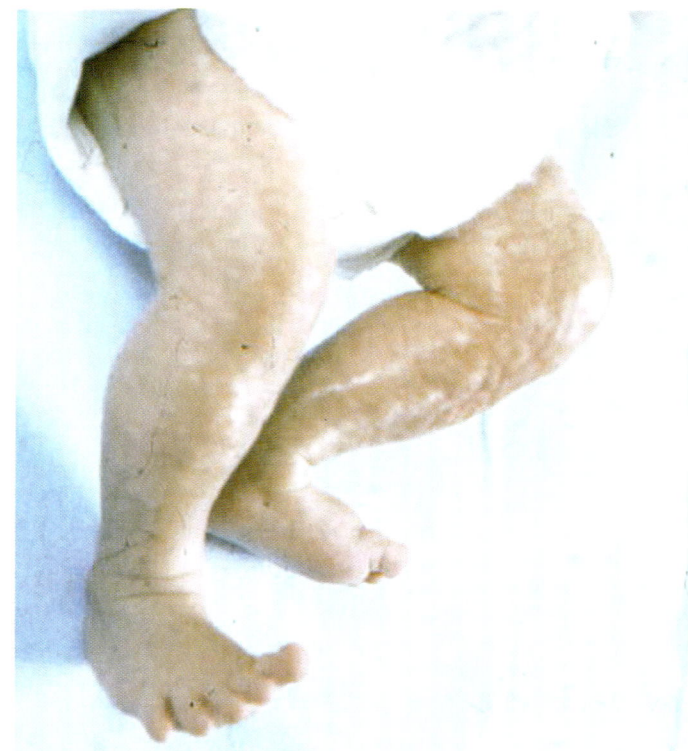

Fig. 7.83   Knee flexion in progeria.

WERNER SYNDROME

Described in 1904 by Werner,[999] this rare autosomal recessive disorder of premature aging is secondary to mutations in the *WRN* gene. The WRN protein is a DNA helicase enzyme. The genetic mutation has been localized to chromosome 8.[1000] The exact molecular deficiency resulting in the clinical phenotype remains to be demonstrated.[1001] Werner syndrome is referred to as progeria of adults; the average age at diagnosis is in the late 30s. Growth retardation is usually the first sign and is generally noticed around puberty. It presents with the unusual combination of short stature, stocky body habitus and thin extremities, the latter resulting from atrophy of the skin, fat and muscle on the limbs. Callus development occurs at the sites of fat loss. Sclerodermoid changes and poikilodermatous hyperpigmentation is noted on the "bird-like" facies, neck and limbs. Premature graying and alopecia are seen in the early 20s. Systemic associations include diabetes, hypogonadism and metastatic calcification. Cataracts and musculoskeletal abnormalities may also occur. Ten percent of patients develop a malignancy, most commonly sarcomas. On the skin, both basal cell epitheliomas and occasional melanomas have been described. Cardiovascular disease and malignancy are the most common cause of death which generally occurs towards the end of the fifth decade.

Urinary hyaluronic acid is raised in patients with Werner syndrome; this is a helpful marker for diagnosis.[1002] Fasting glucose is often elevated as most patients experience mild diabetes. Many chromosomal abnormalities have been identified including increased chromosomal breakage, mosaicism, and sister chromatid exchanges.[1002]

COCKAYNE SYNDROME

Cockayne syndrome was first described in 1936[1003] and since then almost 200 patients have been documented in the literature.[1004] The underlying etiology is related to a delay in recovery of RNA and DNA synthesis following exposure to UV light. This has been demonstrated in lymphocyte cultures from patients[1005] and has allowed the division of the disease into three complement groups, A, B and C. Those in group C have overlapping clinical and biochemical features with XP complement groups B, D and G.[1006] The inability to repair cyclobutane dimers has been recognized in CS patients and may be the most important underlying defect.

The clinical features vary in their expression from mild to severe and in some cases there is an overlap with XP.

999. Werner CWO (1904) Uber Kataract in Verbindung mit Sklerodermie. Thesis, Kiel, Germany, Schmidt and Klauning.

1000. Yu CE, Oshima J, Fu YH et al. (1996) Positional cloning of the Werner's syndrome gene. **Science** 272:258–262.

1001. Bohr VA, Cooper M, Orren D et al. (2000) Werner syndrome protein: biochemical properties and functional interactions. **Exp Geront** 35:695–702.

1002. Salk D (1982) Werner's syndrome: A review of recent research with an analysis of connective tissue metabolism, growth control of cultured cells, and chromosomal aberations. **Hum Genet** 62:1–15.

1003. Cockayne EA (1936) Dwarfism with retinal atrophy an deafness. **Arch Dis Child** 1:11–18.

1004. Nance MA, Berry SA (1992) Cockayne syndrome: review of 140 cases. **Am J Med Gen** 42:68–84.

1005. Venema J, Mullenders LH, Natarajan et al. (1990) The genetic defect in Cockayne syndrome is associated with a defect in repair of UV induced DNA damage in transcriptionally active DNA. **Proc Natl Acad Sci USA** 87:4707–4711.

1006. Rapi I, Lindenbaum Y, Robbins JH et al. (2000) Cockayane syndrome and xeroderma pigmentosa, DNA repair disorders with overlaps and paradoxes. **Neurol** 55:1442–1449.

Cutaneous changes are often the first clinical manifestation of the disease. Exposed areas develop a scaly, erythematous, photosensitive eruption that resolves with hyperpigmentation and occasionally atrophic scarring. Photosensitivity subsides with age. Atrophy of subcutaneous fat on the face occurs in association with microcephaly and prognathism, while on the limbs it results in the appearance of taut, shiny skin. The ears look big and the eyes have a sunken appearance.

Birth weight is generally normal and failure to thrive usually only begins towards the end of the first year of life. Teeth may be hypoplastic or completely absent and hair is generally sparse and occasionally gray. Neurological impairment is an early feature with severely delayed developmental milestones, mental retardation, progressive sensorineural deafness and optic atrophy. The unsteady gait results from both the demyelination of the peripheral and central nervous system, and progressive joint contractures.

Laboratory abnormalities found in patients with Cockyane syndrome depend on the severity of the disease and organ involvement. Ten percent of Cockayne patients have renal disease and should be monitored for abnormal biochemistry. Cerebral imaging is consistently abnormal in all patients with changes that include cerebellar atrophy and calcification of the basal ganglia.

No treatment is available to arrest the pathological process, and management is supportive. Neurological deterioration is progressive with death generally occurring early in the second decade from status epileticus or following a hypertensive crisis.

ACROGERIA AND METAGERIA

First described by Gottron in 1941[1007] these progeria-like diseases are thought to be sporadiac although both autosomal dominant and recessive cases have been reported. The underlying abnormality is unclear. Acrogeria and metageria have been reported in different members of the same family, and features of the two have been described in the same patient. Intellect remains unaffected in both.

The skin and skeleton systems are the main systems involved in acrogeria. At birth or in the neonatal period the changes include atrophy of the cutaneous and subcutaneous tissues of the extremities resulting in prominence of veins. Hyperpigmentation is noted on the trunk and limbs. Easy bruising, hypertrophic scarring and the development of a glyphic nose are the main findings. Skeletal problems may include hypermobile joints, osteoporosis, and short limbs. Life expectancy is normal.

In 1974, Gilkes described metageria, which is associated with more serious complications than acrogeria. Skin abnormalities, which develop in infancy, are more pronounced and include a generalized decrease in subcutaneous fat, affecting the limbs. Similar facial features develop, as are seen in acrogeria. These develop in adolesence in conjunction with mottled hyperpigmentation affecting the limbs and trunk. Systemic complications include the development of early-onset diabetes and premature atherosclerosis. These conditions are the main cause of early death.

No consistent laboratory abnormalities are seen in acrogeria. In metageria elevated fasting glucose levels is usually the only abnormality.

The main premature aging syndrome, HG, has a dismal prognosis. No intervention is available to counteract the relentless destructive process. Management is supportive and symptomatic. The majority of syndromes with progeroid features are less aggressive and in acrogeria the main problem for the patients is cosmetic. The development of the first laboratory animal model, *klotho*, that exhibits a syndrome resembling human aging, occurs from the disruption of the single gene *klotho* and results in the typical aged phenotype. Working with this model it is hoped that a protein may be developed that may act as an anti-aging factor.[1008]

CUTANEOUS MOSAICISM

Rudolf Happle and Arne König

In biology, a mosaic is defined as an organism composed of two or more genetically different populations of cells originating from one genetically homogeneous zygote. Dermatologists are in a privileged situation because the skin reflects the various states of mosaicism in an easily recognizable way.

THE DIFFERENT PATTERNS OF MOSAICISM

In addition to the well known lines of Blaschko, various other mosaic patterns may occur (Fig. 7.84).[1009]

TYPE 1: LINES OF BLASCHKO

Most nevoid skin disorders follow the lines of Blaschko that form a fountain-like pattern on the back, an S-figure on the lateral and ventral aspects of the

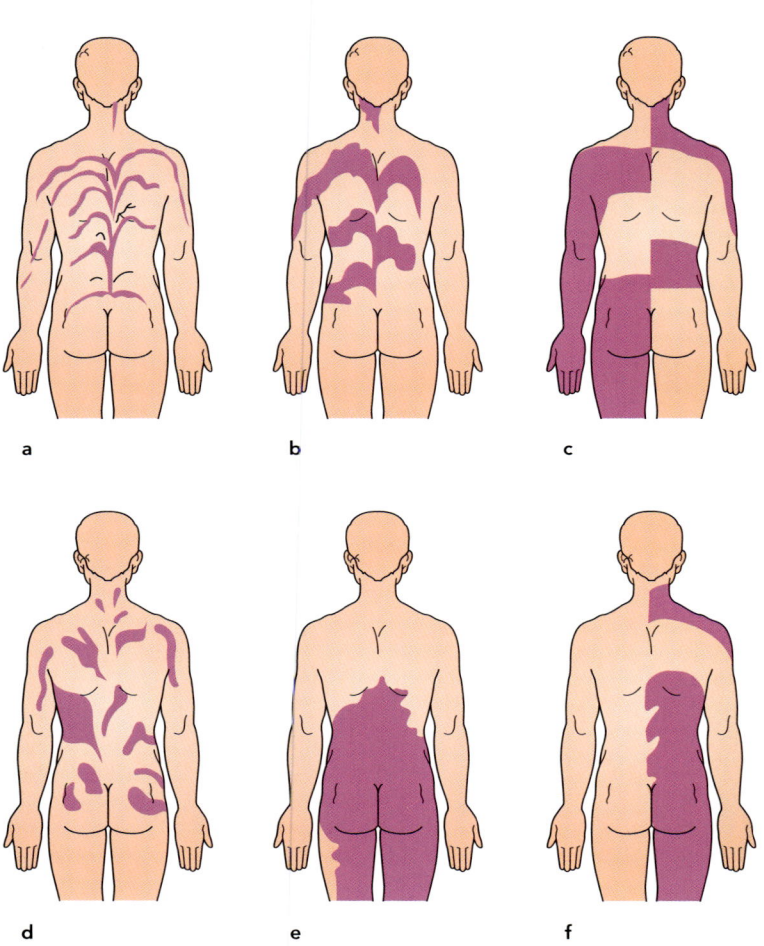

Fig. 7.84 **Patterns of cutaneous mosaicism.** (a) Type 1a: lines of Blaschko, narrow bands; (b) type 1b: lines of Blaschko, broad bands; (c) type 2: checkerboard pattern; (d) type 3: phylloid pattern; (e) type 4: patchy pattern without midline separation; (f) type 5: lateralization.

1007. Gottron H (1941) Familiare akrogerie. **Arch Dermatol Syph** 181:571–583.
1008. Takahashi Y, Kuro-O M, Ishikawa F (2000) Aging mechanisms. **Proc Natl Acad Sci USA** 97:23:1247–1248.

1009. Happle R (1993) Mosaicism in human skin: understanding the patterns and mechanisms. **Arch Dermatol** 129:1460.

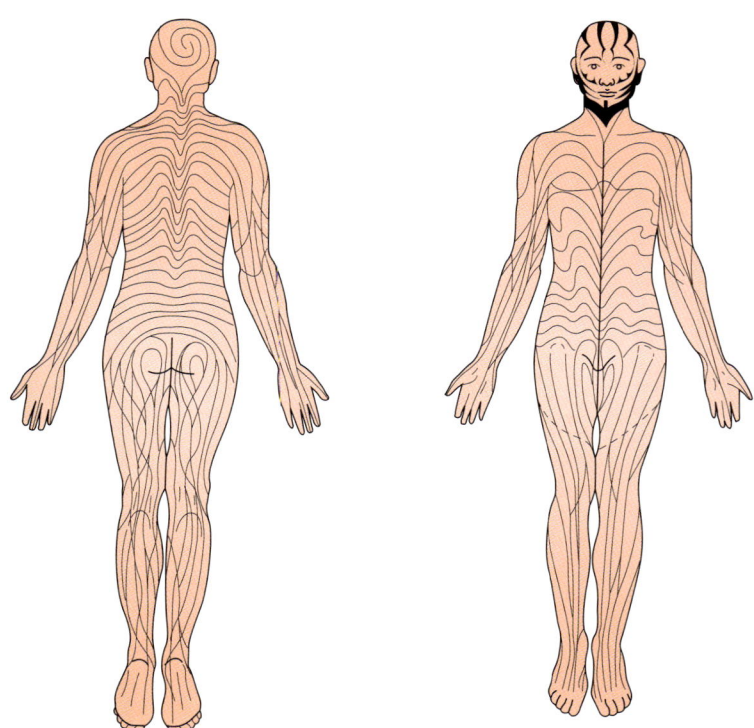

Fig. 7.85   Lines of Blaschko. This is Blaschkos' original diagram, completed on the scalp according to more recent data.[1009]

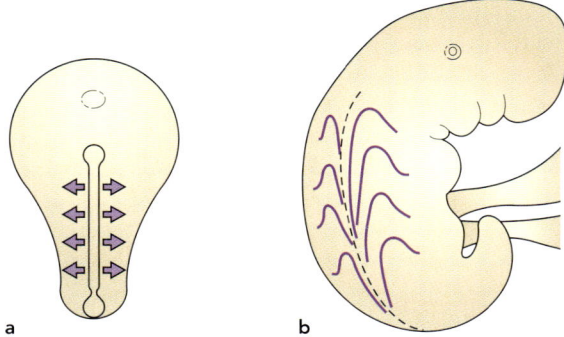

Fig. 7.86   Tentative explanation of the lines of Blaschko. (a) At an early developmental stage precursor cells start from the primitive streak to proliferate in transversal direction in order to form the skin. (b) This transversal clonal proliferation interferes with the longitudinal growth and increasing flexion of the embryo, giving rise to a fountain-like pattern on the back.[1009]

trunk, and a spiral on the scalp (Fig. 7.85). These lines reflect the dorsoventral outgrowth of embryonic cells from the neural crest. Their proliferation interferes with the longitudinal growth and increasing flexion of the embryo, resulting in a characteristic arrangement (Fig. 7.86). On the head and neck, the lines of Blaschko show a rather variable pattern and even tend to intersect at an angle of 90° (Fig. 7.87).[1010] The type 1a is characterized by narrow bands, as observed in incontinentia pigmenti. The type 1b shows the same system in the form of broad bands, as observed in McCune–Albright syndrome. It

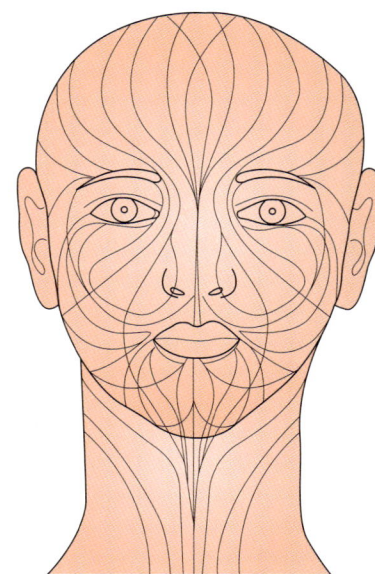

Fig. 7.87   Arrangement of the lines of Blaschko on the head and neck, according to more recent data (reprinted with permission from the Journal of the American Academy of Dermatology).[1010]

should be noted that the distinction of these two subtypes is an oversimplification. Future clinical research may refine this classification.

TYPE 2: CHECKERBOARD PATTERN

This metaphoric term should not be taken literally. The flag-like areas with a sharp midline separation are distributed in a random way and not alternating regularly. Examples are speckled lentiginous nevus, Becker nevus, and the pattern of patchy hairiness as noted in women heterozygous for X-linked hypertrichosis.

TYPE 3: PHYLLOID PATTERN

This type is characterized by peculiar leaf-like patches and oblong macules (Fig. 7.88). Apparently, a midline separation is not always present. The term phylloid hypomelanosis has recently been proposed to denote a new etiologically defined neurocutaneous syndrome. In 5 out of 6 cases in which cytogenetic findings were reported, a mosaic trisomy 13 or translocation trisomy 13 was found.[1011] All patients showed CNS defects with mental retardation. In addition, absence of corpus callosum, conductive hearing loss, choroidal and retinal coloboma, cranio-facial defects as well as brachydactyly, clinodactyly, camptodactyly and other skeletal anomalies were noted. In contrast to so-called "hypomelanosis of Ito" which is associated with many different forms of genetic mosaicism, phylloid hypomelanosis most likely represents a cytogenetically rather uniform neurocutaneous phenotype. On the other hand, a phylloid pattern of hyperpigmentation has likewise been observed.[1012]

TYPE 4: LARGE PATCHES WITHOUT MIDLINE SEPARATION

This arrangement is found in congenital giant melanocytic nevi, with or without neurological involvement. In this disorder the presence of mosaicism

1010. Happle R, Assim A (2001) The lines of Blaschko on the head and neck. **J Am Acad Dermatol** 44:612.
1011. Happle R (2002) Phylloid hypomelanosis is closely related to mosaic trisomy 13. **Eur J Dermatol** 10:511.
1012. Happle R (1993) Pigmentary patterns associated with human mosaicism: a proposed classification. **Eur J Dermatol** 3:170.

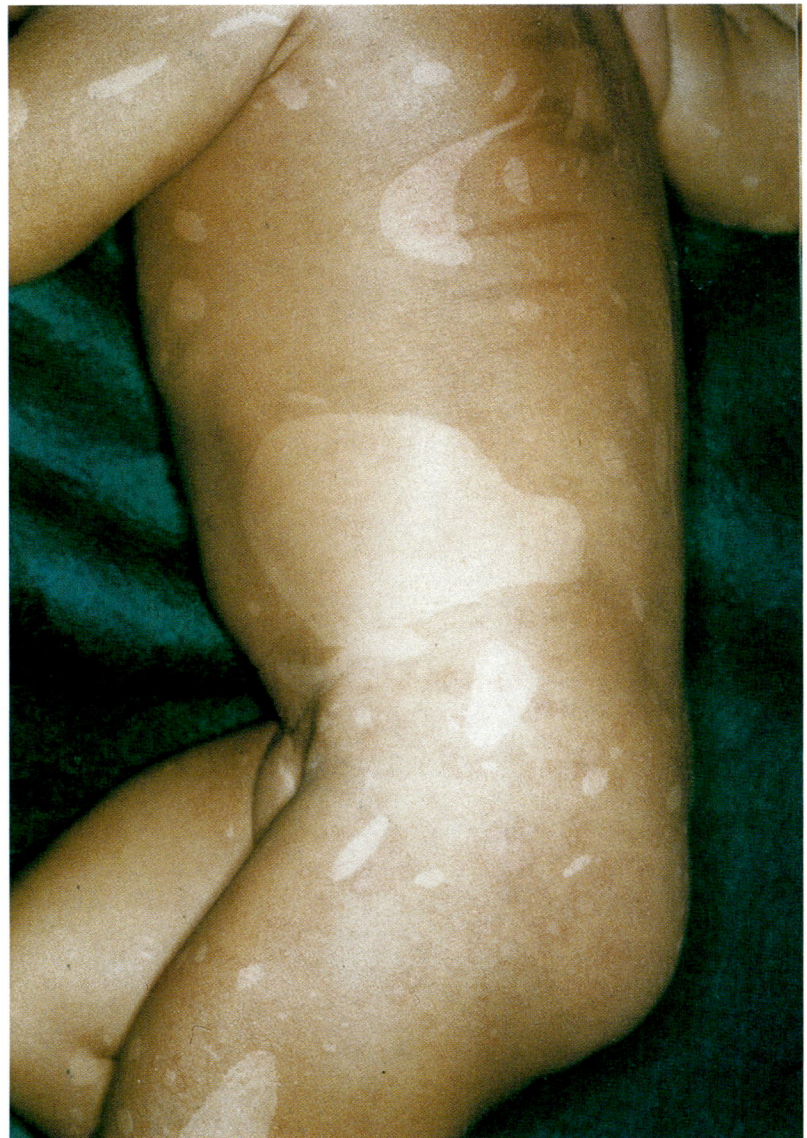

Fig. 7.88   Phylloid hypomelanosis (reprinted with permission from Hautarzt (2001; 52:3–5).

has so far not been proven but is very likely because a clonal origin, and thus a mosaic state, has already been documented in common acquired melanocytic nevi.

TYPE 5: LATERALIZATION PATTERN

A unique lateralization pattern is noted in CHILD syndrome (see Chapter 8). The associated CHILD nevus may diffusely involve one half of the body, with a sharp midline demarcation. In addition, ipsilateral or contralateral lesions following the lines of Blaschko may be present. Because the CHILD syndrome represents an X-linked dominant, male-lethal trait, the lateralization pattern may be explained by the assumption that the event of X-inactivation coincides and interferes with the origin of a clone of organizer cells controlling a large developmental field (Fig. 7.89).[1009]

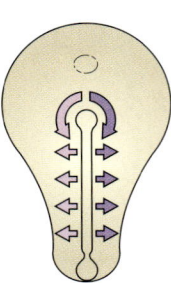
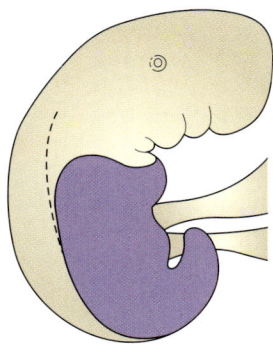

Fig. 7.89   Tentative explanation of the lateralization pattern as found in CHILD syndrome. X-inactivation coincides and interferes with the origin, in the dorsocranial region of the embryo, of a clone of organizer cells controlling a large developmental field. For this reason, the NSDHL mutation results in either intrauterine death or lateralization.

EVIDENCE FOR OTHER CUTANEOUS PATTERNS

In the future, other mosaic patterns will be delineated. For example, it is so far not clear whether lateral vascular nevi show a dermatomal distribution, a checkerboard pattern, or a so far unknown particular mosaic arrangement. The skin lesions of Sturge–Weber syndrome do not correspond well to a trigeminal dermatome, despite the association widely discussed in the dermatologic literature.

A note of caution regarding the term "zosteriform nevi"

The term "zosteriform" is virtually always out of place when applied to a nevoid skin condition.[1013] A zosteriform arrangement corresponds to the system of dermatomes, as noted in a zoster eruption. Virtually all nevi that are described as "zosteriform" are not dermatomal but follow the lines of Blaschko.

LINES THAT DO NOT INVOLVE MOSAICISM

The lines of Voigt are defined as the boundaries of peripheral cutaneous innervation. To date, no skin disorder is known to follow this system of lines. The Matsumoto line[1014] (often called "Futcher's line"[1015]) is a pigment demarcation line on the arms and legs. In traditional Chinese medicine, the well known meridian lines of acupuncture connect the various acupuncture points. Because of the present fad on non-scientific medicine, it seems appropriate to emphasize that this system of "lines" does not exist but represents a speculation for the purpose of magico-religious healing.

GENETIC MECHANISMS GIVING RISE TO MOSAICISM

According to the underlying mechanisms, we can divide the various forms of cutaneous mosaicism into 3 categories: functional X-chromosome mosaicism, genomic mosaicism, and autosomal epigenetic mosaicism.[1009,1016] Mosaic phenotypes reflecting functional X-chromosome mosaicism can be inherited from one generation to the other, and the same is true for epigenetic autosomal mosaicism. By contrast, genomic mosaics usually occur sporadically. Either the underlying mutation is lethal for an embryo,[1009] or it is nonlethal and becomes manifest in a nonmosaic form.[1017] Exceptions are the paradominant traits (see below).[1009]

1013. Happle R (1996) "Zosteriform" lichen planus: Is it zosteriform? **Dermatology** 192:385.
1014. Matzumoto S (1913) Über eine eigentümliche Pigmentverteilung an den Voigtschen Linien. (Beitrag zur Kenntnis der Voigtschen Grenzen). **Arch Dermatol Syph** 118:2157.
1015. Futcher PH (1938) A peculiarity of pigmentation of the upper arm of Negroes. **Science** 88:570.
1016. Happle R (2002) Transposable elements and the lines of Blaschko: a new perspective. **Dermatology** 204:4.
1017. Paller AS, Syder AJ, Chan YM et al. (1994) Genetic and clinical mosaicism in a type of epidermal nevus. **N Engl J Med** 331:1408.

TABLE 7.32   X-linked skin disorders visualizing functional X-chromosome mosaicism

Male-lethal phenotypes
  Incontinentia pigmenti
  Focal dermal hypoplasia
  MIDAS syndrome
  Conradi–Hünermann–Happle syndrome
  Oral–facial–digital syndrome, type 1
  CHILD syndrome
Nonlethal phenotypes
  Hypohidrotic ectodermal dysplasia of Christ–Siemens–Touraine
  Hypohidrotic ectodermal dysplasia with immunodeficiency
  Menkes disease
  Dyskeratosis congenita, X-linked type
  IFAP syndrome
  Partington syndrome
  X-linked hypertrichosis

TABLE 7.33   Autosomal lethal mutations surviving by mosaicism

Pigmentary mosaicism of the Ito type
Phylloid hypomelanosis
Schimmelpenning syndrome
Phacomatosis pigmentokeratotica
Nevus comedonicus syndrome
Phacomatosis pigmentovascularis
McCune–Albright syndrome
Proteus syndrome
Maffucci syndrome
Encephalocraniocutaneous lipomatosis
Delleman syndrome
Sturge–Weber–Klippel–Trenaunay syndrome
Cutis marmorata telangiectatica congenita
Giant congenital melanocytic nevus

TABLE 7.34   Type 1 segmental manifestation of autosomal dominant skin disorders

Neurofibromatosis 1
Epidermolytic hyperkeratosis of Brocq
Gorlin syndrome
Multiple basaloid follicular hamartoma
Multiple syringoma
Tuberous sclerosis
Cutaneous leiomyomatosis
Ehlers–Danlos syndrome
Darier disease
Pachyonychia congenita

FUNCTIONAL X-CHROMOSOME MOSAICISM

Random inactivation of either the paternal or the maternal X-chromosome occurs during the first weeks of gestation, resulting in functional mosaicism. X-linked mutations giving rise to a mosaic skin disorder may be either lethal or non-lethal for a male embryo (Table 7.32). The resulting skin lesions do not always follow the lines of Blaschko but may correspond to a checkerboard pattern, as found in X-linked hypertrichosis, or to a lateralization pattern, as noted in CHILD syndrome. Some less well-known examples of functional X-chromosome mosaicism are MIDAS syndrome (microphthalmia, dermal aplasia and sclerocornea)[1018] as well as carriers with hypohidrotic ectodermal dysplasia with immunodeficiency,[1019] X-linked dyskeratosis congenita and IFAP syndrome (ichthyosis follicularis, atrichia and photophobia).[1020]

MOSAICISM OF LETHAL AUTOSOMAL MUTATIONS

Some autosomal mutations are presumably not compatible with intrauterine life and, therefore, exclusively observed as mosaic phenotypes (Table 7.33).[1009]

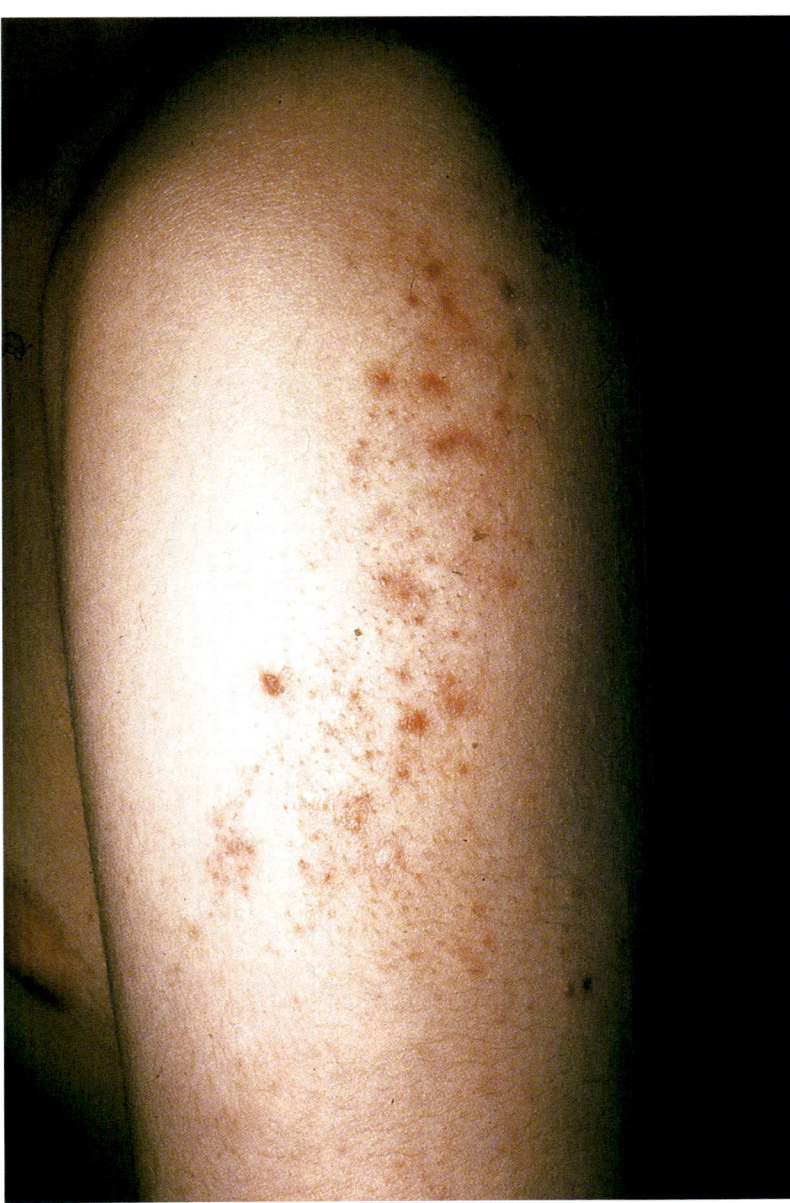

Fig. 7.90 Segmental arrangement of acne on the arm, reflecting mosaicism of the gene of Apert syndrome ("Munro nevus") (reprinted with permission from *Lancet*).[1021]

1018. Happle R, Daniëls O, Koopman RJJ (1993) MIDAS syndrome (microphthalmia, dermal aplasia and sclerocornea): an X-linked phenotype distinct from Goltz syndrome. **Am J Med Genet** 47:710.
1019. Kosaki K, Shimasaki N, Fukushima H et al. (2001) Female patient showing hypohidrotic ectodermal dysplasia and immunodeficiency (HED-ID). **Am J Hum Genet** 69:664.
1020. König A, Happle R (1999) Linear lesions reflecting lyonization in women heterozygous for IFAP syndrome (ichthyosis follicularis with atrichia and photophobia). **Am J Med Genet** 85:365.

MOSAICISM OF NON-LETHAL AUTOSOMAL MUTATIONS

Many autosomal dominant skin disorders have been described in a mosaic arrangement in the form of a type 1 segmental involvement (Table 7.34). In such cases an early postzygotic mutation may likewise involve the gonads, which is why in the next generation the same disorder may involve the entire body. Classical examples are neurofibromatosis 1 and epidermolytic hyperkeratosis of Brocq.[1017] A mosaic manifestation of Apert syndrome has been described in the form of a linear arrangement of acne involving the upper arm (Fig. 7.90), resulting from mutations on fibroblast growth factor receptor 2 (FGFR2).[1021]

GAMETIC HALF-CHROMATID MUTATIONS

If a half-chromatid mutation is present in a gamete and transmitted to a zygote, semiconservative replication will give rise to a chromosome with two chromatids carrying different base pairs. After cleavage, one cell is normal and

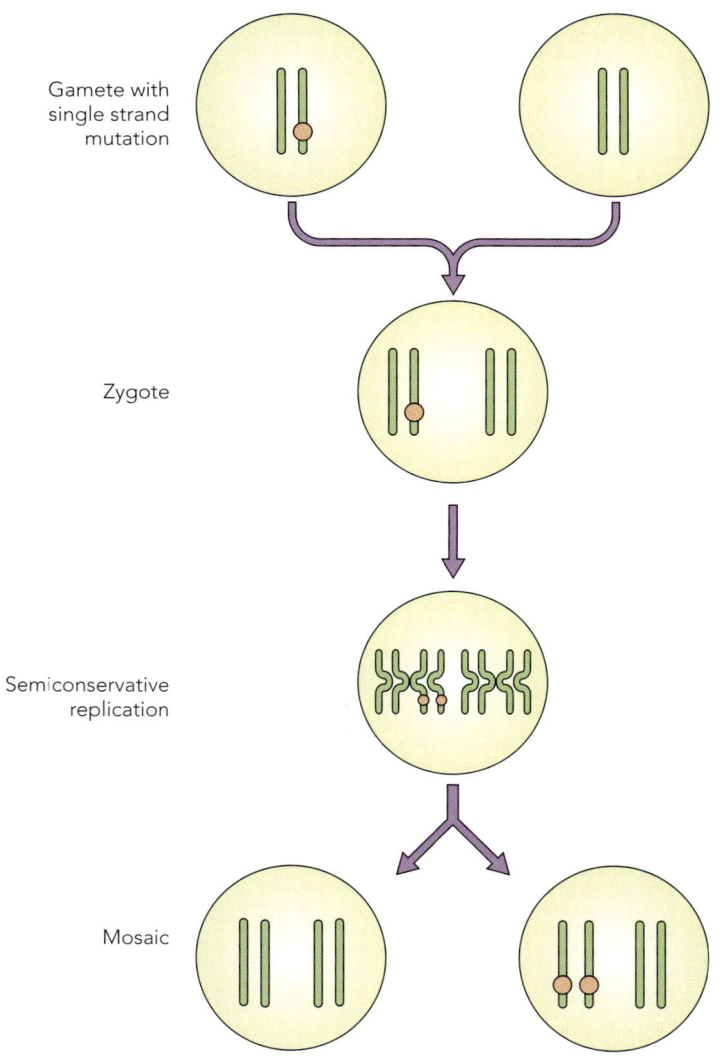

Gamete with single strand mutation

Zygote

Semiconservative replication

Mosaic

Fig. 7.91   Origin of mosaicism from a gametic half-chromatid mutation. If one of the gametes carries a single strand mutation, semiconservative replication within the zygote may give rise, in one of the daughter cells, to a complete point mutation.

the other cell carries a complete mutation. In this way, mosaicism is already present at the two-cell stage (Fig. 7.91).[1009] Nevi or nevoid disorders arranged in a widespread, bilateral form may be tentatively explained by this mechanism although an early postzygotic mutation may result in a similar pattern.

TYPE 2 SEGMENTAL INVOLVEMENT OF AUTOSOMAL DOMINANT SKIN DISORDER

Mosaic forms of autosomal dominant skin diseases have been thought to originate from a postzygotic new mutation. Happle has proposed two types of segmental manifestation (Fig. 7.92),[1022] although the theory awaits molecular confirmation. Type 1 reflects heterozygosity for a postzygotic new mutation, whereas type 2 results from loss of the corresponding wildtype allele occurring in a heterozygous embryo, resulting in either homozygosity or hemizygosity for the underlying mutation. A type 2 manifestation tends to be far more pronounced and usually superimposed on the ordinary non-segmental trait. Possible examples of type 2 segmental involvement have been found in the literature in at least 15 different autosomal dominant skin disorders (Table 7.35). A strikingly high frequency of this proposed type 2 segmental involvement has been documented in cutaneous leiomyomatosis, glomangiomatosis, and disseminated superficial actinic porokeratosis.[1023]

DIDYMOSIS (TWIN SPOTTING)

Didymosis (Greek *didymos* = twin) is a new term proposed by Happle for the mechanism of twin spotting.[1024] Twin spots are paired patches of mutant tissue

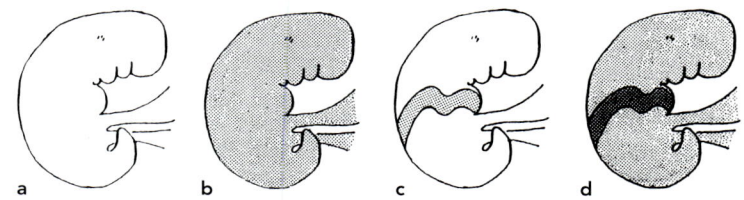

a   b   c   d

Fig. 7.92   Two different types of segmental involvement as observed in autosomal dominant skin disorders. (a) Healthy embryo; (b) heterozygous embryo; (c) type 1 segmental involvement reflecting heterozygosity; (d) type 2 segmental involvement reflecting loss of heterozygosity in a heterozygous embryo.

TABLE 7.35   Type 2 segmental manifestation of autosomal dominant skin disorders

Neurofibromatosis 1
Tuberous sclerosis
Cutaneous leiomyomatosis
Glomangiomatosis
Buschke–Ollendorff syndrome
Multiple syringoma
Multiple trichoepithelioma
Multiple basaloid follicular harmatoma
Nonsyndromic hereditary multiple basal cell carcinoma
Darier disease
Hailey–Hailey disease
Epidermolytic hyperkeratosis of Brocq
KID syndrome
Disseminated superficial actinic porokeratosis
Autosomal dominant dyskeratosis congenita

1021. Munro CS, Wilkie AOM (1998) Epidermal mosaicism producing localised acne: somatic mutation in FGFR2. **Lancet** 352:704.
1022. Happle R (1997) A rule concerning the segmental manifestation of autosomal dominant skin disorders: review of clinical examples providing evidence for dichotomous types of severity. **Arch Dermatol** 133:1509.

1023. Happle R (2001) Segmentale Typ-2-Manifestation autosomal dominanter Hautkrankheiten: Entwicklung eines neuen formalgenetischen Konzeptes. **Hautarzt** 52:283.
1024. Happle R, König A (2001) Didymosis aplasticosebacea: coexistence of aplasia cutis congenita and nevus sebaceus may be explained as a twin spot phenomenon. **Dermatology** 202:246.

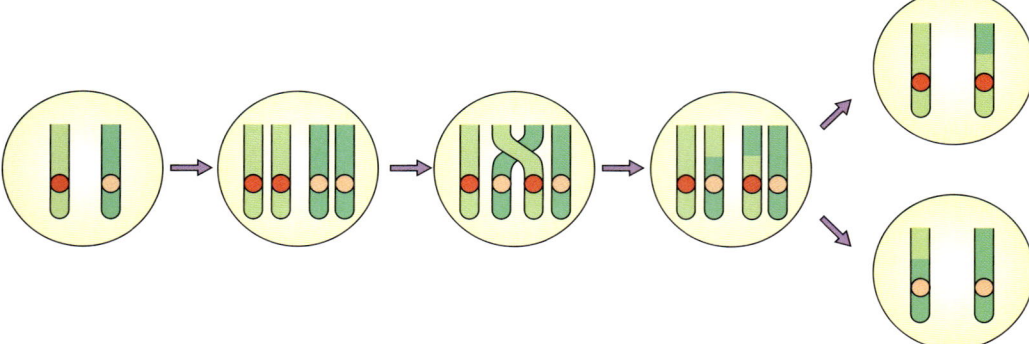

Fig. 7.93   Origin of didymosis (twin spotting). An embryo may show compound heterozygosity, i.e., two different mutations are present at the same locus on either of a pair of homologous chromosomes; or the embryo may be transheterozygous, i.e., two different mutations are present on two different loci on either of a pair of homologous chromosomes. In the first case (as shown in the diagram), somatic recombination may give rise to allelic didymosis, whereas in the second case nonallelic didymosis would occur.

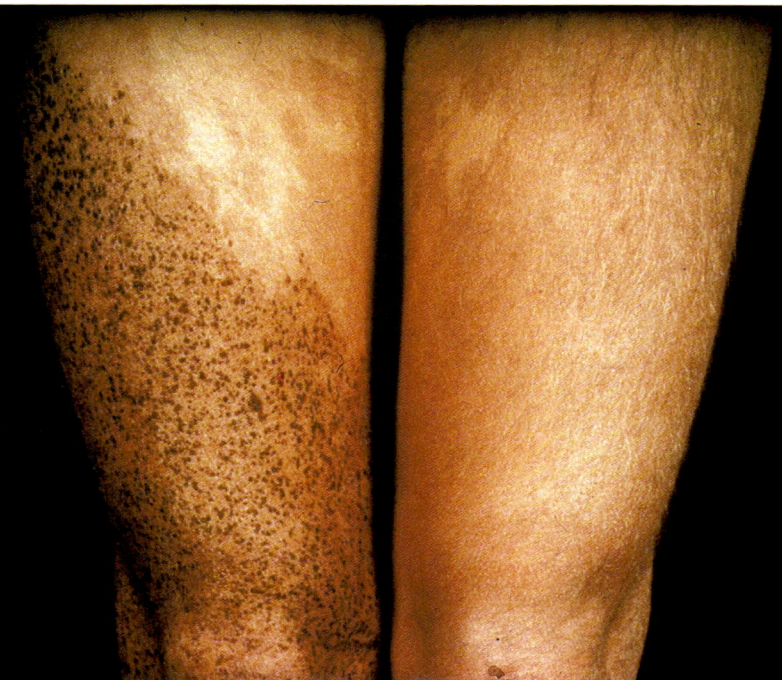

Fig. 7.94 Phacomatosis pigmentovascularis as a possible example of nonallelic didymosis.

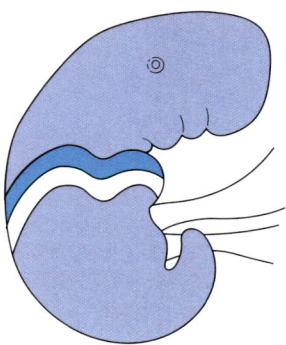

Fig. 7.95 Type 2 segmental involvement with concomitant segment of absent involvement in the form of allelic didymosis, as observed in autosomal dominant skin disorders.

TABLE 7.36   Possible examples of twin spotting

Allelic didymosis
  Vascular twin nevi
  Cutis tricolor
  Hyperplastic and hypoplastic lesions in Proteus syndrome
  Paired segments of either excessive or absent involvement in epidermolytic hyperkeratosis of Brocq
  Paired segments of either excessive or absent involvement in Darier disease
Nonallelic didymosis
  Phacomatosis pigmentovascularis
  Phacomatosis pigmentokeratotica
  Unilateral nevoid telangiectasia associated with Becker nevus
So far unclassifiable
  Didymosis aplasticosebacea

that may differ genetically from each other and from the heterozygous background tissue. An embryo may be doubly heterozygous in a way that two different mutations involve either of a pair of homologous chromosomes. At an early developmental stage, mitotic recombination may give rise to two daughter cells that are homozygous for either mutation (Fig. 7.93), and these would be the stem cells of two different homozygous skin areas that tend to be arranged in close proximity to each other (Figs 7.94 and 7.95).[1025] The underlying mutations may be either allelic on non-allelic. Possible examples are summarized in Table 7.36. The concept of human didymosis has not yet been tested by molecular analysis. Remarkably, in autosomal dominant skin disorders such as Darier disease or epidermolytic hyperkeratosis of Brocq, a type 2 segmental manifestation may occur with a concomitant segment of completely healthy skin in the form of allelic didymosis (Fig. 7.95).[1026,1027]

PARADOMINANT INHERITANCE

Paradominant inheritance is another proposed mechanism to explain mosaic phenotypes that usually occur sporadically but may occasionally affect several members of a family.[1028] Carriers of a paradominant mutation are in general clinically unaffected and, therefore, the mutation can be transmitted

1025. Happle R (1999) Loss of heterozygosity in human skin. **J Am Acad Dermatol** 41:143.
1026. Happle R, König A (1999) Dominant traits may give rise to paired patches of either excessive or absent involvement. **Am J Med Genet** 84:176.
1027. Itin PH, Happle R (2002) Darier disease with paired segmental manifestation of either excessive or absent involvement: A further step in the concept of twin spotting. **Dermatology** 205:344.
1028. Happle R, König A (1999) Familial naevus sebaceus may be explained by paradominant transmission. **Br J Dermatol** 141:350.

TABLE 7.37 Possible examples of paradominant traits

Becker nevus/Becker nevus syndrome
Sebaceous nevus/Schimmelpenning syndrome
Lateral telangiectatic nevus/Sturge–Weber–Klippel–Trenaunay syndrome
Speckled lentiginous nevus/speckled lentiginous nevus syndrome
Nevus anemicus
Unilateral nevoid telangiectasia
Cutis marmorata telangiectatica congenita

undetected through many generations. The trait theoretically only becomes manifest when loss of heterozygosity occurs at an early developmental stage, giving rise to a cell clone in which the wildtype allele has been lost.[1025] Phenotypes that may be explained by the theory of paradominant inheritance are summarized in Table 7.37.

REVERTANT MOSAICISM

In an autosomal recessive trait, a revertant mutation may give rise to a mosaic clone of heterozygous cells that has regained its normal function. A dermatological example has been described in patients with generalized atrophic benign epidermolysis bullosa.[1029,1030] One of these patients showed several patchy areas of unaffected skin, in which a back mutation prevailed.[1029] A more recent case involved a patient with recessive epidermolysis bullosa simplex with gene reversion in one allele.[1031] In this case, however, the clinical phenotype continued to show blistering because the revertant protein did not function. Cases of revertant mosaicism can be taken as examples of a "natural gene therapy." Revertant mosaicism presumably explains patients of normal skin in patients with other autosomal recessive traits such as xeroderma pigmentosum.

AUTOSOMAL EPIGENETIC MOSAICISM

Transposable elements or retrotransposons are particles of retroviral origin that are interspersed in large amounts in the human genome. They may affect the activity of adjacent genes by methylation or demethylation, resulting in silencing or activation of gene expression.[1032] In mice and dogs, certain transposable elements may give rise to a variegated coat pattern reminiscent of the lines of Blaschko. Because the human genome likewise contains large numbers of transposable elements it is conceivable that these particles may cause similar mosaic lesions in human skin.[1016] The inflammatory linear verrucous epidermal nevus as well as cases of pigmentary mosaicism arranged in hypermelanotic or hypomelanotic streaks following the lines of Blaschko, have been proposed by Happle as possible examples of retrotransposon activity in man.[1016] Such phenotypes usually occur sporadically but may occasionally affect several members of a family.

THE GROUP OF EPIDERMAL NEVUS SYNDROMES

In the past, the association of epidermal nevi with exacutaneous defects was considered to represent one clinical entity that was called the epidermal nevus syndrome.[1033] This term is still used in recent articles, although it is today obvious that many different epidermal nevus syndromes exist.[1034] In some of these phenotypes, such as Proteus syndrome or CHILD syndrome, the associated epidermal nevus is of a nonorganoid type, whereas other phenotyes such as nevus sebaceus syndrome or nevus comedonicus syndrome are characterized by organoid epidermal nevi.[1035] Some epidermal nevus syndromes always occur sporadically, whereas other phenotypes such as Schimmelpenning syndrome or Becker nevus syndrome may be paradominant traits, and CHILD syndrome is an X-linked dominant, male-lethal trait.[1034] This section will review 7 well-defined syndromes characterized by epidermal nevi. Several other new epidermal nevus syndromes are presently "in limbo".[1036–1038]

SCHIMMELPENNING SYNDROME

Schimmelpenning syndrome includes sebaceous nevus, cerebral defects and ocular anomalies as well as bone changes.[1039] In addition, developmental delay, seizures, coloboma or lipodermoid of the conjunctiva may be noted.[1040,1041] The cranium is often asymmetrically shaped.

Although isolated sebaceous nevi are sometimes removed before puberty for cosmetic and medical reasons, the incidence of tumors is lower than previously considered.[1042] In children with Schimmelpenning syndrome, with their many other problems, removal of the sebaceous nevus as a prophylactic measure is unnecessary. However, instruction is important so that if basal cell carcinomas develop later in life, they can be easily removed. Histopathological examination of the sebaceous nevus shows hyperplasia of sebaceous glands, but this typical organoid differentiation may be minimal or even absent throughout life in those parts of a sebaceous nevus that involve the trunk or the limbs. In order to establish a correct diagnosis, it is therefore preferable to biopsy a scalp lesion.

The question of whether a child with a large sebaceous nevus should be examined by radiographic techniques for the presence of neurological abnormalities represents a controversial issue, but in general this is not necessary if the child does not show any clinical signs and symptoms of neurological involvement. The Schimmelpenning syndrome tends to occur sporadically.[1043] It is most likely caused by a lethal mutation surviving by mosaicism, and the risk of recurrence is not substantially increased when compared to the general population.

PHACOMATOSIS PIGMENTOKERATOTICA

This type of epidermal nevus syndrome is characterized by a concurrence of sebaceous nevus and speckled lentiginous nevus (Fig. 7.94).[1044] It seems reasonable to distinguish this phenotype from Schimmelpenning syndrome because of the different spectrum of associated neurological defects.

1029. Jonkman MF, Scheffer H, Stulp R et al. (1997) Revertant mosaicism in epidermolysis bullosa caused by mitotic gene conversion. **Cell** 88:543.
1030. Darling TN, Yee C, Hintner H, Yancey KB (1999) Revertant mosaicism: partial correction of a germ-line mosaicism in COL17A1 by a frame-restoring mutation. **J Clin Invest** 103:1371–1377.
1031. Schuilenga-Hut PHL, Scheffer H, Pas HH et al. (2002) Partial revertant mosaicism of keratin 14 in a patient with recessive epidermolysis bullosa simplex. **J Invest Dermatol** 118:626–630.
1032. Whitelaw E, Martin DIK (2001) Retrotransposons as epigenetic mediators of phenotypic variation in mammals. **Nature Genet** 27:361.
1033. Solomon LM, Fretzin DF, Dewald RL (1968) The epidermal nevus syndrome. **Arch Dermatol** 97:273.
1034. Happle R (1995) Epidermal nevus syndromes. **Sem Dermatol** 14:111.
1035. Happle R, Rogers M (2002) Epidermal nevi. **Adv Dermatol** 18:175.
1036. Gobello T, Mazzanti C, Zambruno G, Chinni LM (2000) New type of epidermal nevus syndrome. **Dermatology** 201:51.
1037. Oranje AP, Przyrembel H, Meradji M et al. (1994) Solomon's epidermal nevus syndrome (type: linear nevus sebaceus) and hypophosphatemic vitamin D-resistant rickets. **Arch Dermatol** 130:1167.

1038. Marsch WC, Taube KJ, Käsemann B (1981) Ein Solitärfall von Ichthyosis hystrix gravior unilateralis – Klinische und morphologische Befunde. **Z Hautkr** 56:1073.
1039. Schimmelpenning GW (1957) Klinischer Beitrag zur Symptomatologie der Phakomatosen. **Fortschr Geb Röntgenstrahlen** 87:716.
1040. Feuerstein R, Mims LC (1962) Linear nevus sebaceus with convulsions and mental retardation. **Am J Dis Child** 104:125.
1041. Happle R (1991) How many epidermal nevus syndromes exist? A clinicogenetic classification. **J Am Acad Dermatol** 25:550.
1042. Cribier B, Scrivener Y, Grosshans E (2000) Tumors arising in nevus sebaceus: a study of 596 cases. **J Am Acad Dermatol** 42:263.
1043. Schworm HD, Jedele KB, Holinski E, Hortnagel K et al. (1996) Discordant monozygotic twins with the Schimmelpenning-Feuerstein-Mims syndrome. **Clin Genet** 50:393.
1044. Happle R, Hoffmann R, Restano L et al. (1996) Phacomatosis pigmentokeratotica a melanocytic-epidermal twin nevus syndrome. **Am J Med Genet** 65:363.

Characteristic neurological abnormalities are hemiatrophy with muscular weakness, segmental dysesthesia, and segmental hyperhidrosis.[1045,1046] Remarkably, these abnormalities tend to be ipsilateral with the speckled lentiginous nevus. In addition, mild mental retardation, seizures, deafness, ptosis or strabismus may occur. All cases so far observed have been sporadic. The two different skin lesions may have a common origin in the form of non-allelic didymosis, implying that a sebaceous nevus represents homozygous tissue originating from loss of heterozygosity in a heterozygous embryo, and that a similar mechanism would give rise to speckled lentiginous nevus. Moreover, all of the associated neurological abnormalities would reflect loss of heterozygosity.[1046] As soon as the mutations underlying sebaceous nevus and speckled lentiginous nevus have been elucidated, the concept of non-allelic dydimosis can be tested at the molecular level.

NEVUS COMEDONICUS SYNDROME

This syndrome includes nevus comedonicus, cataract involving mostly the ipsilateral eye, and skeletal defects that are likewise usually ipsilateral.[1035] Cerebral involvement in the form of EEG abnormalities or mental retardation may likewise be noted. Hiernickel et al.[1047] described an ipsilateral corneal erosion. This phenotype likely reflects a mosaic state of a lethal autosomal mutation. The nevus comedonicus that constitutes the hallmark of this syndrome has been misdiagnosed as "atrophoderma vermiculatum."[1048] It should be noted that a nevus comedonicus rather often shows a component of cutaneous hypoplasia or atrophy. On the other hand, rather large sebaceous cysts may also be associated with the nevus comedonicus.[1047] The most frequently associated anomaly is a congenital ipsilateral cataract.[1048–1050] If the nevus comedonicus is distributed in a bilateral systematized pattern, the associated lenticular opacities may likewise be bilateral.

ANGORA HAIR NEVUS SYNDROME

This unusual mosaic phenotype was described by Schauder et al.[1051] A 30-year-old man had systematized bilateral linear lesions covered with long, depigmented hair, involving his entire body. The pattern of distribution corresponded to a mosaic type 1b (lines of Blaschko, broad bands). The white hair was of a smooth, fine structure reminiscent of angora hair. The patient showed short stature, macrocephaly, scoliosis, mild mental retardation, seizures, spastic hemiparesis and hemihypotrophy of the right side of the body, as well as dysdiadochokinesis. The right leg was 2cm shorter than the left one. Facial dysplasia in the form of frontal bossing, macrostomia and malformed ears was noted. MRI revealed asymmetric hemispheres, dilated ventricles and porencephaly of the right hemisphere. Ophthalmological examination showed ectopic pupils, cataract, iridocorneal adhesions, temporal coloboma of the left iris, and membranous thickening over the optic nerve heads.

The associated systematized nevus showed dilated follicular pores and can be categorized as an unusual type of organoid epidermal nevus, hence the inclusion as a distinct epidermal nevus syndrome. The associated epithelial nevus may be best described as "angora hair nevus." The striking similarity of the depigmented hair to that of the angora mutation in animals (FGFR5 mutations) suggests a human homolog (Langenbeck U., personal communication, 2000).

BECKER NEVUS SYNDROME

Becker nevus syndrome is characterized by a pigmented hairy epidermal nevus with hamartomatous augmentation of smooth muscle fibers, in association with other developmental defects. Because this nevus is an androgen-dependent anomaly, the full-blown picture of Becker nevus is in general observed exclusively in adolescent or adult men. In women and pre-pubertal boys the lesion is much less conspicuous because the pigmentation is less intense and hairiness is absent or only mild. Characteristic associated anomalies are unilateral hypoplasia of the breast or the shoulder girdle, hypoplasia of the ipsilateral arm as well as vertebral defects and scoliosis. Other associated anomalies are fused or accessory cervical ribs, pectus carinatum, or bilateral internal tibial torsion. Moreover, extensive patchy hypoplasia of the ipsilateral subcutaneous fat tissue has been noted. The syndrome usually occurs sporadically, but the phenotype may be transmitted as a paradominant trait.[1052–1053]

PROTEUS SYNDROME

Proteus syndrome is characterized by disproportionate overgrowth of multiple tissues in association with various cutaneous and subcutaneous mesodermal harmatomas.[1054,1055] Plantar cerebriform hyperplasia of connective tissue is rather characteristic. The associated epidermal nevus is of a soft, nonorganoid, nonepidermolytic type.[1035] The disorder reflects an autosomal lethal mutation that can only survive in a mosaic state.[1041]

The recognition of a mild manifestation of Proteus syndrome is a difficult task but this problem is inherent in all mosaic phenotypes. Recommendations for diagnostic criteria, differential diagnosis and guidelines for the evaluation of patients have been provided by Biesecker et al.[1056] Mutations in the gene that encodes the PTEN tumor suppressor have been associated with Proteus syndrome,[1057] although the failure to find PTEN mutations in other patients with Proteus syndrome argues against this concept.

A particular variant of Proteus syndrome is Elattoproteus syndrome[1058], which represents an inverse form of the phenotype as originally described by Wiedemann et al.[1054] This disorder is characterized by a mosaic distribution of hypoplastic lesions involving various tissues. Remarkably, patients with Proteus syndrome may show coexisting hyperplastic and hypoplastic lesions which can be best explained as an example of didymosis.[1059,1060] Such patients would carry one allele at the Proteus locus giving rise to overgrowth of tissue (Pleioproteus allele, from Greek pleion = plus), whereas the other allele would cause deficient growth of tissue (Elattoproteus allele, from Greek elatton = minus). At an early developmental stage, postzygotic recombination would give rise to two different clones of cells homozygous for either allele.

1045. Tadini G, Restano L, Gonzáles-Pérez R et al. (1998) Phacomatosis pigmentokeratotica: report of new cases and further delineation of the syndrome. Arch Dermatol 134:333.
1046. Boente C, Pizzi de Parra N, Larralde de Luna M et al. (2000) Phacomatosis pigmentoleratotica: another epidermal nevus syndrome and a distinctive type of twin spotting. Eur J Dermatol 10:190.
1047. Hiernickel H (1982) Naevus comedonicus mit abszedierenden Talgcysten und homolateraler Katarakt. Z Hautkr 57:508.
1048. Hsu S, Nikko A (2000) Unilateral atrophic skin lesion with features of atrophoderma vermiculatum: a variant of the epidermal nevus syndrome? J Am Acad Dermatol 43:310.
1049. Fantini F, Sedona P, Bassi R (1995) Extensive nevus comedonicus, congenital cataract and strabismus. Eur J Dermatol 5:588.
1050. Patrizi A, Neri I, Fiorentini C, Marzaduri S (1998) Nevus comedonicus syndrome: a new pediatric case. Pediatr Dermatol 15:304.
1051. Schauder S, Hanefeld F, Noske UM, Zoll B (2000) Depigmented hypertrichosis following Blaschko's lines associated with cerebral and ocular malformations: a new neurocutaneous, autosomal lethal gene syndrome from the group of epidermal naevus syndromes? Br J Dermatol 142:1204.
1052. Happle R, Koopman RJJ (1996) Becker nevus syndrome. Am J Med Genet 68:357.

1053. Happle R (1992) Paradominant inheritance: a possible explanation for Becker's pigmented hairy nevus. Eur J Dermatol 2:39.
1054. Wiedemann HR, Burgio GR, Aldenhoff P (1983) The proteus syndrome: partial gigantism of the hands and/or feet, nevi, hemihypertrophy, subcutaneous tumors, macrocephaly or other skull anomalies and possible accelerated growth and visceral affections. Eur J Pediatr 140:5.
1055. Cohen MM Jr. (1993) Proteus syndrome: clinical evidence for somatic mosaicism and selective review. Am J Med Genet 47:645.
1056. Biesecker LG, Happle R, Mulliken JB et al. (1999) Proteus syndrome: diagnostic criteria, differential diagnosis, and patient evaluation. Am J Med Genet 84:389.
1057. Zhou X, Hampel H, Thiele H et al.(2001) Association of germline mutations in the PTEN tumor suppressor gene and Proteus and Proteus-like syndromes. Lancet 358:210.
1058. Happle R (19999) Elattoproteus syndrome: delineation of an inverse form of Proteus syndrome. Am J Med Genet 84:25.
1059. Happle R, Steijlen PM, Theile U et al. (1997) Patchy dermal hypoplasia as a characteristic feature of Proteus syndrome. Arch Dermatol 133:77.
1060. Happle R (1995) Lipomatosis and partial lipohypoplasia in Proteus syndrome: a clinical clue for twin spotting? Am J Med Genet 56:332.

CHILD SYNDROME

This is the only epidermal nevus syndrome showing a Mendelian mode of transmission. Moreover, the pattern of lateralization as noted in CHILD syndrome is unique. Within the group of epidermal nevus syndromes, CHILD syndrome is the first entity to be elucidated at the molecular level. The term CHILD syndrome is an acronym for <u>c</u>ongenital <u>h</u>emidysplasia with <u>i</u>chthyosiform erythroderma and <u>l</u>imb <u>d</u>efects.[1061] All except two reported cases have occurred in females and the condition is considered to be inherited as an X-linked dominant trait, and is lethal in males.[1062] The CHILD nevus presents at birth or soon after as an erythematous scaling, sometimes yellow plaque, which shows a striking predominance for one side of the body with a midline cutoff.[1063] Nails are often dystrophic on affected limbs. The skin lesions have an affinity for skin folds, a phenomenon called ptychotropism.[1064] Blaschko-distributed linear areas of spared skin may occur on the side of major involvement and linear areas of affected skin may be found on the opposite side.[1061] The skeletal aplasia or hypoplasia is variable, but often extreme, ipsilateral to the site of maximal skin involvement. Punctate epiphyseal calcification may be seen on X-ray during infancy, but often disappear after the early years of life. Other associated findings in CHILD syndrome include ipsilateral defects of the brain, the lung, the heart or the kidney.[1061,1063] The histologic examination of biopsy sections of lesional skin from patients with the CHILD nevus shows marked hyperkeratosis and parakeratosis with an acanthotic epidermis. The granular layer is variably thickened or absent and ghost granular cells may be seen.[1065] A mixed inflammatory infiltrate occurs in the papillary dermis and may also infiltrate the epidermis. Collections of foam cells in the upper dermis have been noted in several cases producing the changes of verruciform xanthoma.[1066] CHILD syndrome results from mutations in the NSDHL gene located at Xq28,[1067] encoding a 3-beta hydroxysteroid dehydrogenase of the cholesterol biosynthetic pathway.

LESS WELL DEFINED EPIDERMAL NEVUS SYNDROMES

There are several phenotypes that can be taken as epidermal nevus syndromes "in limbo." Further clinical reports may show whether they deserve to be categorized as distinct entities.

GOBELLO SYNDROME

Gobello *et al.*[1036] described an unusual type of epidermal nevus characterized by systematized streaks of nonepidermolytic hyperkeratosis with increased hairiness and follicular hyperkeratosis. The increased hairiness was distinctly different from that observed in the angora hair nevus syndrome.[1051] This skin disorder was associated with hemihypoplasia of limbs, brachydactyly, clinodactyly and onychodystrophy.

HYPHEN SYNDROME (HYPOPHOSPHATEMIA WITH EPIDERMAL NEVUS)

The acronym HYPHEN stands for <u>hyp</u>ophastemia and <u>e</u>pidermal <u>n</u>evus. In several cases of systematized organoid epidermal nevus, rickets with hyperphosphaturia, resistant to vitamin D has been observed.[1068–1070] Sometimes these patients show vascular tumors of the skin or internal organs.[1037,1071,1072] It is so far not clear whether such cases should be categorized within the spectrum of Schimmelpenning syndrome, or whether they represent a distinct phenotype.

NEVADA SYNDROME

The proposed acronym NEVADA stands for <u>n</u>evus <u>e</u>pidermicus <u>v</u>errucosus with <u>a</u>ngio<u>d</u>ysplasia and <u>a</u>neurysms. The associated nevus is always of a nonepidermolytic type and has also been described as "ichthyosis hystrix."[1038,1072] Some authors have mistaken this phenotype as Schimmelpenning syndrome.[1073] In contrast to Schimmelpenning syndrome, it is extremely verrucous and does not show organoid differentiation.[1074,1075] The angiodysplasia with arteriovenous shunts involves the large vessels and may be fatal for the neonate.[1038] Aneurysms, including microaneurysms of the retina, represent another component of this syndrome.[1072]

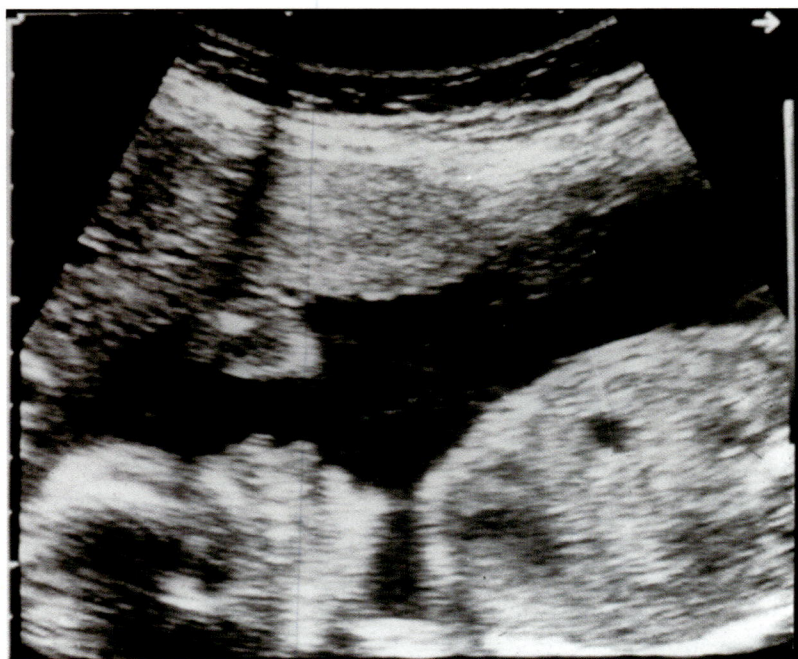

Fig. 7.96 Ultrasound image showing features of a fetus at 18 weeks' gestation (courtesy of Professor K. Nicolaides).

1061. Happle R, Koch H, Lenz W (1980) The CHILD syndrome. Congenital hemidysplasia with ichthyosiform erythroderma and limb defects. Eur J Pediatr 134:27–33.
1062. Happle R, Effendy I, Megahed M et al. (1996) CHILD syndrome in a boy. Am J Med Genet 62:192–194.
1063. Hebert AA, Esterly NB, Holbrook KA et al. (1987) The CHILD syndrome. Arch Dermatol 123:503–509.
1064. Happle R (1990) Ptychotropism as a cutaneous feature of the CHILD syndrome. J Am Acad Dermatol 23:763–766.
1065. Hashimoto K, Topper S, Sharata H, Edwards M (1995) CHILD syndrome: An analysis of abnormal keratinization and ultrastructure. Pediatr Dermatol 12:116–129.
1066. Zamora-Martinez E, Martin-Moreno L, Barat-Cascante A, Castro-Torres A (1990) Another CHILD syndrome with xanthomatous pattern. Dermatologica 180:263–266.
1067. König A, Happle R, Bornholdt D et al. (2000) Mutations in the NSHDL gene, encoding f or 3-beta hydroxysteroid dehydrogenase, cause CHILD syndrome. Am J Med Genet 90:339–346.
1068. Aschinberg LC, Solomon LM, Zeis PM et al. (1977) Vitamin D-resistant rickets associated with epidermal nevus syndrome: demonstration of phosphaturic substance in the dermal lesions. J Pediatr 91:56.
1069. Goldblum JR, Headington JT (1993) Hypophosphatemic vitamin D-resistant rickets and multiple spindle and epitheloid nevi associated with linear nevus sebaceus syndrome. J Am Acad Dermatol 29:109.
1070. O'Neill EM (1993) Linear sebaceous naevus syndrome with oncogenetic rickets and diffuse pulmonary angiomatosis. J Roy Soc Med 86:177.
1071. Stosiek N, Hornstein OP, Hiller D, Peters KP (1994) Extensive linear epidermal with haemangiomas of bones and vitamin D-resistant rickets. Dermatology 189:278.
1072. Burch JV, Leveille AS, Morse PH (1980) Ichthyosis hystrix (epidermal nevus syndrome) and coat's disease. Am J Ophthalmol 89:25.
1073. Mollica F, Pavone L, Nuciforo G (1974) Linear sebaceus nevus syndrome in a newborn. Am J Dis Child 128:868.
1074. Ratzenhofer E, Hohlbrugger H, Gebhart W, Lubec G (1981) Linearer epidermaler Naevus mit multiplen mißbildungen ("epidermal nevus syndrome" Solomon). Klin Pädiatr 193:117.
1075. McAuley DL, Isenberg DA, Gooddy W (1978) Neurological involvement in the epidermal naevus syndrome. J Neurol Neurosurg Psychiatr 41:466.

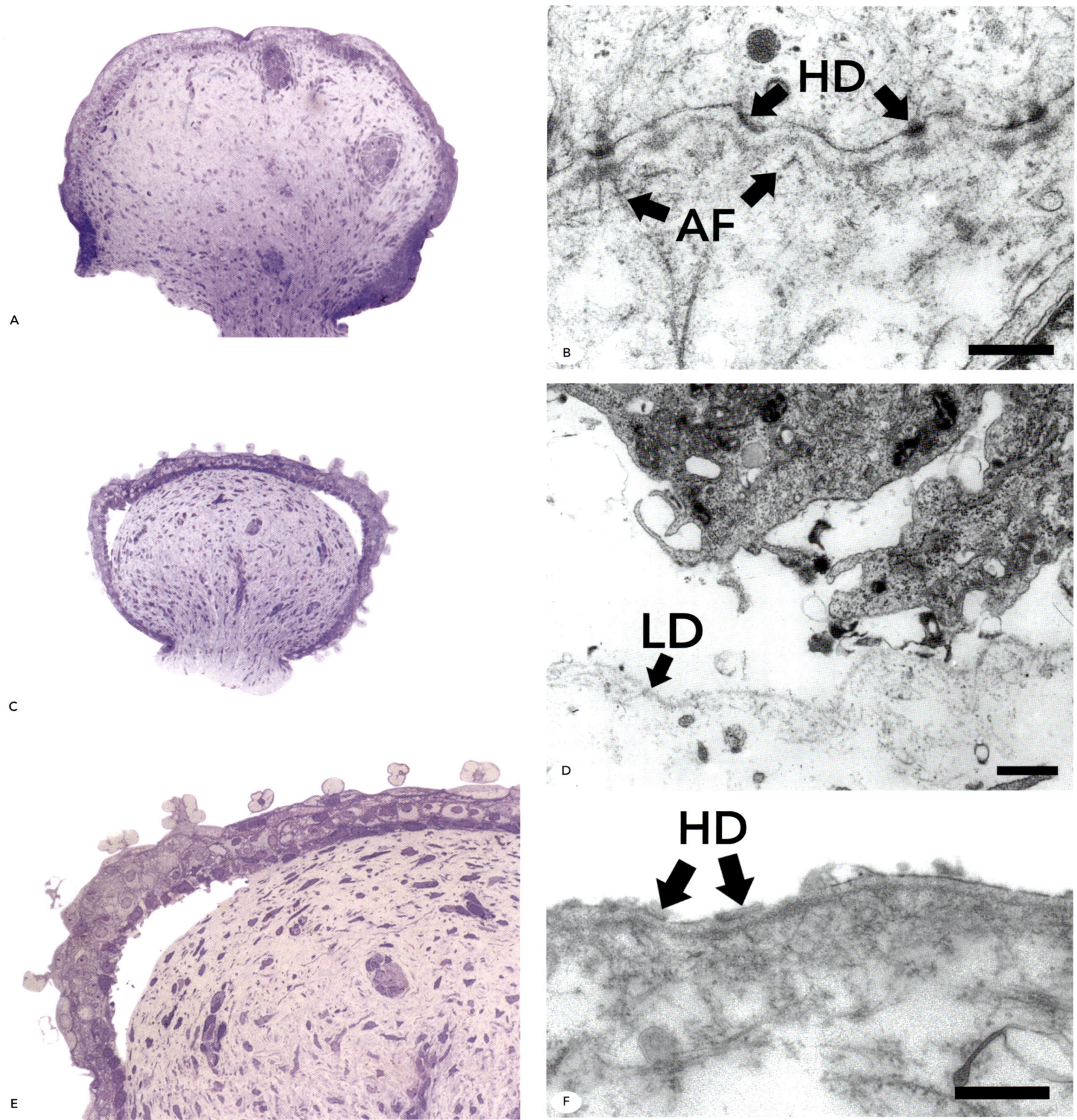

Fig. 7.97   Microscopy of fetal skin biopsies at 18 weeks' gestation. Light micrographs of semithin resin sections (**A, C, E**), and electron micrographs (**B, D, F**). In the normal skin sample (**A, B**) the dermoepidermal junction is intact; and key structures including hemidesmosomes (HD) and anchoring fibrils (AF) are visible. In the sections from a fetus affected with Herlitz junctional EB (**C, D, E**) there is a clear separation through the dermoepidermal junction, at the level of the lamina lucida of the basement membrane, above the lamina densa (LD, in **D**). In a biopsy from a fetus affected with the form of junctional EB associated with pyloric atresia, caused by mutations in the α6 or β4 integrin genes, the split is present at a level immediately above the hemidesmosomes (HD) and associated plasma membrane of a basal keratinocyte. Magnification: (A) 40×, (B) 40×, (E) 100×. Bars: (B, D, F)0.5μm.

PRENATAL DIAGNOSIS OF HEREDITARY SKIN DISORDERS

Robin Eady and John McGrath

FETAL SKIN BIOPSY

A milestone in the recent history of prenatal diagnosis of hereditary skin disorders coincided with the establishment of fetal medicine as a medical specialty in the late 1970s and early 1980s, and a number of centers introduced new methods for sampling fetal tissues, such as cord blood and skin.

The development of the fetoscope,[1076,1077] which allowed direct visualization of the fetus and other uterine contents, including the placenta and umbilical cord, was crucial to the safety and accuracy of the sampling procedure. Initially fetoscopy was accompanied by ultrasound scanning which provided essential monitoring for the precise introduction into the uterine cavity of instruments such as the fetoscope and fine-gauge forceps. Later, the emergence of high-resolution real-time ultrasonography with its ability to produce high-quality images of the fetus and related structures (Fig. 7.96) enabled the fetal skin samples to be safely obtained without the need of the fetoscope. A sound knowledge of the microanatomy of normal fetal skin through graded developmental stages (gestational ages), and particularly during the second half of the mid-trimester, the normal time for performing fetal skin biopsies, is an essential prerequisite for the analysis of the diminutive (about 1mm^3) samples. Light microcopy of semithin resin sections (about 1μm thick) and transmission electron microscopy are essential for the evaluation of the fetal skin samples.[1078–1082] Electron microscopy will reveal the ultrastructural appearances of key components of the fetal dermoepidermal junction (DEJ), such as hemidesmosomes and anchoring fibrils, necessary for the diagnosis of junctional and dystrophic forms of epidermolysis bullosa (Fig. 7.97). Indirect immunofluorescence microscopy used with monoclonal antibodies recognizing normal molecular components of the hemidesmosome-anchoring fibril complex in the DEJ is an alternative method for the diagnosis of junctional and dystrophic forms of epidermolysis bullosa (EB) and for the rapid prenatal diagnosis of these disorders (Fig. 7.98).[1083–1085] This technique has not replaced electron microscopy for the prenatal diagnosis of EB, but is invaluable as a second-line, independent mode of analysis. Key references to the use of fetal skin biopsy in the prenatal diagnosis of a number of hereditary skin disorders are included in Table 7.38.

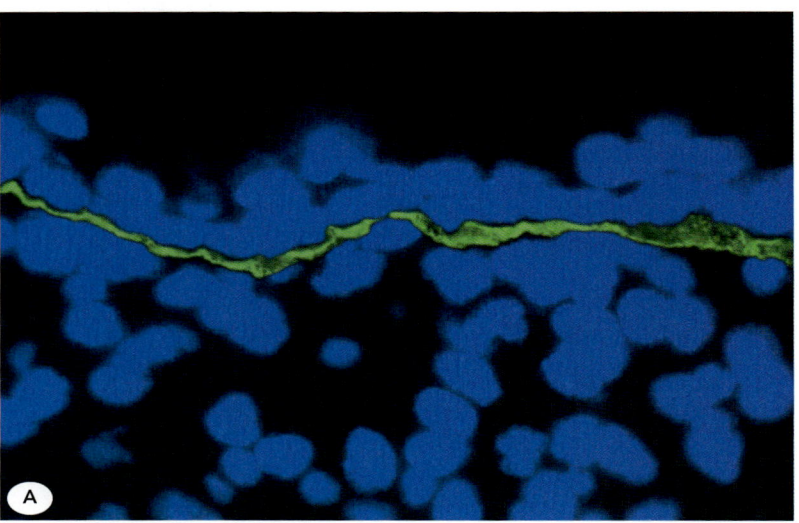

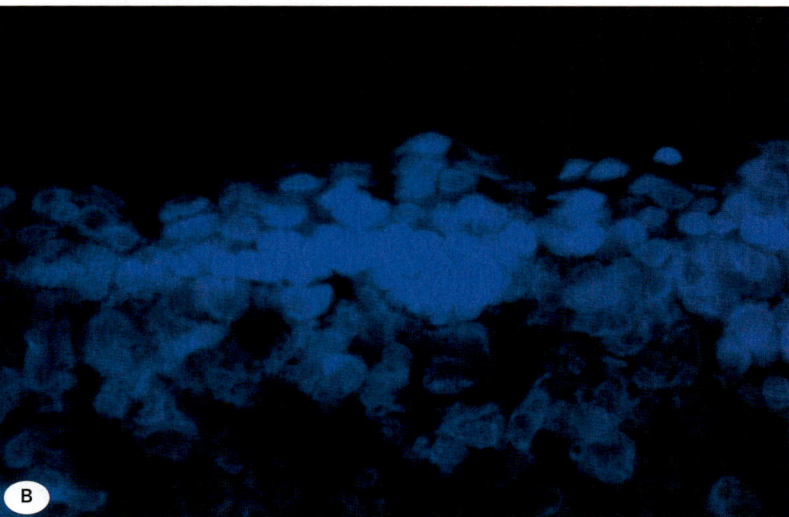

Fig. 7.98 Immunofluorescene microscopy for the prenatal diagnosis of Herlitz junctional EB. (A) Staining with GB3 monoclonal antibody (which recognizes laminin 5) along the dermoepidermal junction in normal fetal skin; (B) GB3 staining is absent in skin from a fetus affected with Herlitz junctional EB. Magnification: A–B 120×. Staining: FITC with Dapi nuclear counterstain.

TABLE 7.38   Prenatal diagnosis using fetal skin biopsies

Disorder	Methods	References
Epidermolysis bullosa		
Junctional EB (Herlitz)	LM, EM, IF	1084, 1085, 1113
Junctional EB with PA	LM, EM, IF	1114, 1115
Recessive dystrophic EB (Hallopeau-Siemens)	LM, EM, IF	1083, 1116
Dominant dystrophic EB	LM, EM	(Eady, unpublished)
EB simplex (Dowling-Meara)	LM, EM	1117
Ichthyosis		
Epidermolytic hyperkeratosis*	LM, EM, AF	1118–1120
Harlequin ichthyosis	LM, EM, AF	1121–1123
Lamellar ichthyosis	LM, EM	1124
Sjögren–Larsson syndrome	LM	1125, 1126
Anhidrotic ectodermal dysplasia	LM, EM	1127
Oculocutaneous albinism	LM, EM, EH	1128,1129

LM, light microscopy; IF, immunofluorescence; EM, electron microscopy; EH, Enjyme histochemistry; AF, Amniotic fluid cells, PA, Pyloric atresia
* Also known as bullous congenital ichthyosiform erythroderma

1076. Rodeck CH, Nicolaides KH (1983) Fetoscopy and fetal tissue sampling. **Br Med Bull** 39:332–337.
1077. Elias S (1987) Use of fetoscopy for the prenatal diagnosis of hereditary skin disorders. In: Prenatal Diagnosis of Heritable Skin Diseases. Current Problems in Dermatology, Gedde-Dahl T, Jr, Wuepper KD, eds. Basel: Karger, 1–13.
1078. Eady RAJ, Gunner DB, Tidman MJ et al. (1984) Rapid processing of fetal skin for prenatal diagnosis by light and electron microscopy. **J Clin Pathol** 37:633–638.
1079. Eady RAJ (1988) Fetoscopy and fetal skin biopsy for prenatal diagnosis of genetic skin disorders. **Semin Dermatol** 7:2–8.
1080. Eady RAJ (1992) Genodermatoses. In: Prenatal Diagnosis and Screening, DJH Brock, CH Rodeck, MA Ferguson-Smith, eds. Edinburgh: Churchill Livingstone, 503–512.

1081. Sybert VP, Holbrook KA, Levy M (1992) Prenatal diagnosis of severe dermatologic diseases. In: Advances in Dermatology, Callen JP, Dahl MV, Golitz LE, Greenway LT, Schachner LA, eds. St Louis: Mosby Yearbook, 179–209.
1082. Holbrook KA, Smith LA, Elias S (1993) Prenatal diagnosis of genetic skin disease using fetal skin biopsy samples. **Arch Dermatol** 129:1437–1454.
1083. Heagerty AHM, Kennedy AR, Gunner DB et al. (1986) Rapid prenatal diagnosis and exclusion of epidermolysis bullosa using novel antibody probes. **J Invest Dermatol** 86:603–605.
1084. Heagerty AHM, Eady RAJ, Kennedy AR et al. (1987) Rapid prenatal diagnosis of epidermolysis bullosa letalis using GB3 monoclonal antibody. **Br J Dermatol** 117:271–275.
1085. Fine JD, Holbrook KA, Elias S et al. (1990) Applicability of 19-DEJ-1 monoclonal antibody for the prenatal diagnosis or exclusion of junctional epidermolysis bullosa. **Prenat Diagn** 10:219–229.

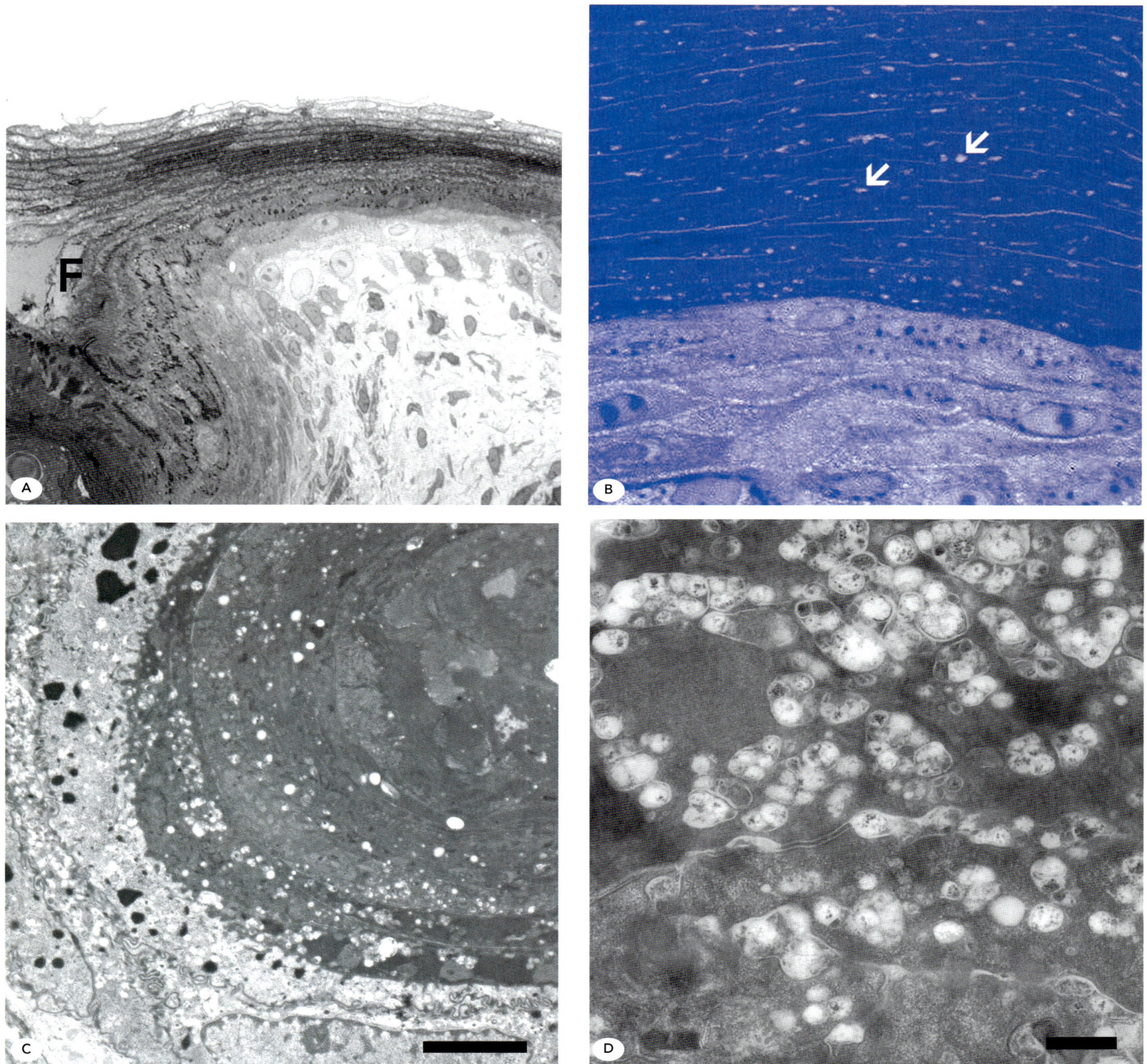

Fig. 7.99   Harlequin ichthyosis. (A, B) Photomicrographs of resin sections from biopsy samples from the scalp of affected fetuses of 22–23 weeks' gestation. **(A)** Note abnormal stacking of newly keratinized cells around the upper part of a hair follicle (F). **(B)** At higher magnification, this section from another fetus shows the abnormal inclusions (arrows) in different layers of newly keratinized follicular epithelial cells. **(C, D)** Electron micrographs showing the same typical inclusions in greater detail. Magnification (A) 160×, (B) 200×. Bars: (C) 2.0μm, (D) 0.5μm.

In 1992 the cumulative world–wide experience of prenatal diagnosis based on fetal skin biopsies indicated the general success of the procedure, especially for junctional and recessive dystrophic forms of EB and for different forms of ichthyosis.[1086] This concurs with our own experience of prenatal diagnosis

1086. Eady RAJ, Holbrook KA, Blanchet-Bardon C et al. (1992) Chair's summary: prenatal diagnosis of skin diseases. In: Dermatology: Progress & Perspectives, The Proceedings of the 18th World Congress of Dermatology, Burgdorf WHC, Katz SI, eds. New York: Parthenon, p. 1159.

in about 170 pregnancies beginning in 1979 (Eady and McGrath, unpublished data). DNA-based techniques, introduced in the early 1990s for the diagnosis and prenatal diagnosis of different genodermatoses, including EB and ichthyosis, have now largely superseded fetal skin biopsy for the prenatal diagnosis of these disorders (see below). However, there is still a role for fetal skin biopsy in the prenatal investigation of at-risk pregnancies, mainly for the following indications:

1. Where the causative gene is unknown but prenatal diagnosis has been shown to be possible in similar cases using fetal skin biopsies. Currently, the main example included in this category is Harlequin ichthyosis. Here, multiple skin samples should be obtained at 21–22 weeks of gestation from the scalp or other sites bearing hair follicles where the pathognomonic ultrastructural changes can be found (Fig. 7.99). Another disorder in this group is a rare autosomal recessive form of ichthyosis in which the newborn is at high risk of asphyxia from aspiration of amniotic fluid with a high content of desquamated skin cells. This little-known skin disorder previously described as "ichthyosis congenita type IV"[1087] is characterized ultrastrucurally by the presence of stacks of (presumably) lipid-rich membrane-type profiles in the cytoplasm of cells of the early keratinizing epidermis of the affected fetus (Fig. 7.100A) and in amniotic fluid cells (Fig. 7.100B). A "snowstorm" type of appearance in the amniotic cavity[1088] may be seen by ultra-

sonography during the second trimester (Mr D Griffin FRCOG, personal communication).

2. Where there is genetic heterogeneity for a particular disorder (e.g., junctional EB) and the pathogenic mutations in an individual case have not been determined.

3. Where the causative gene is known, but informative DNA markers are unavailable, perhaps because an affected offspring or proband had died before appropriate DNA sampling could be achieved.

4. Where the results of DNA-based prenatal diagnosis are equivocal or technically unsatisfactory.

In summary, the use of fetal skin biopsy, combined with electron microscopy and immunofluorescence microscopy for prenatal diagnosis, has a proven track record with a high degree of safety (the fetal loss rate in the more experienced centers is no more than 1–3% above background),[1082] sensitivity and specificity. Major disadvantages of using this method today are that it is moderately invasive and cannot be performed before the middle part of the second trimester, and that only very few centers have the appropriate experience and expertise necessary for the analysis of the fetal skin samples. Diagnostic pitfalls are well recognized.[1089] These methods for the prenatal diagnosis of major genetic skin disorders, including EB and some forms of ichthyosis, have now largely been replaced by DNA-based techniques, which can be used in a wider range of genetic disorders and undertaken at an earlier gestational age.

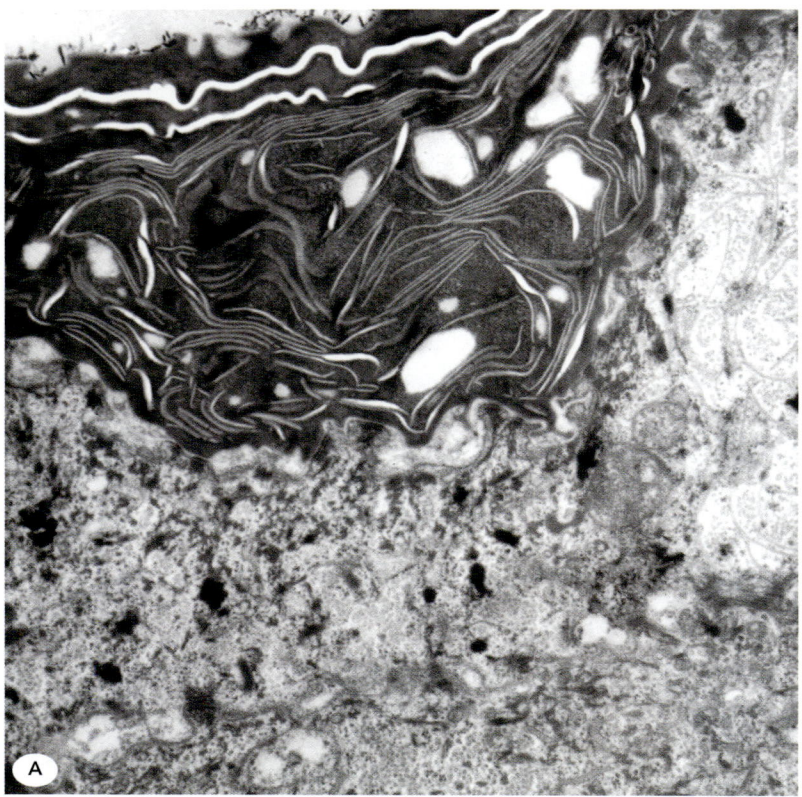
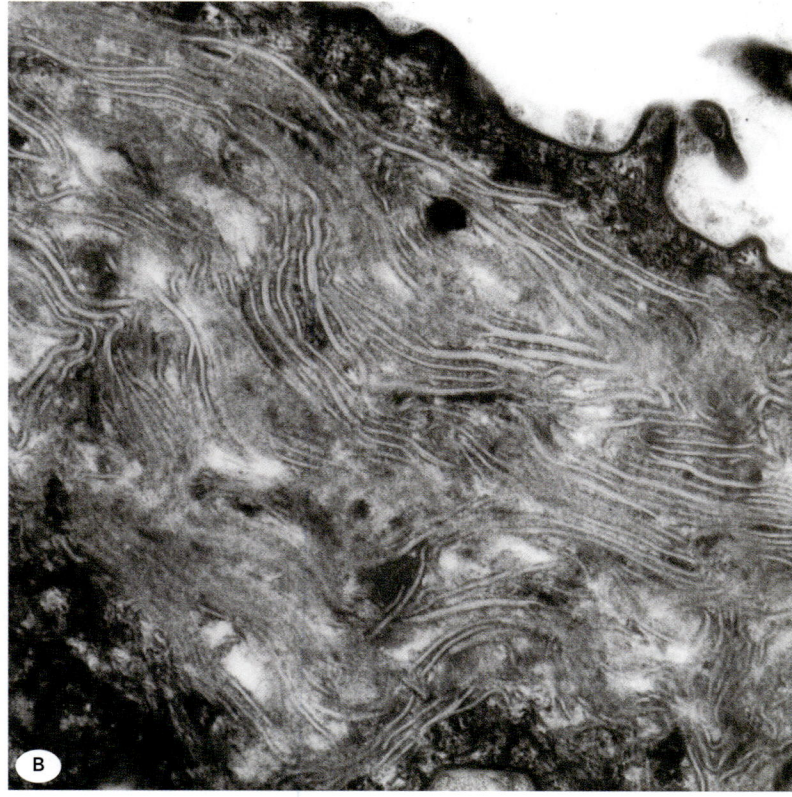

Fig. 7.100   Desquamative ichthyosis. Electron micrographs showing stacks of intracytoplasmic membrane-like profiles in the epidermis (A) and an amniotic fluid cell (B) from an affected fetus of 20 weeks' gestation.

1087. Anton-Lamprecht I (1992) The skin. In: Diagnostic Ultrastructure on Non-Neoplastic Diseases, Papadimitriou JM, Henderson DW, Spagnolo DV, eds. Edinburgh: Churchill Livingstone, pp. 459–550.

1088. Rodeck CH (1990) Prenatal diagnosis of epidermolysis bullosa. In: Epidermolysis Bullosa: A Comprehensive Review of Classification, Management and Laboratory Studies, Priestley JB, Tidman MJ, Weiss JA, Eady RAJ, eds. Crowthorne: DEBRA Publications, pp. 10–12.

1089. Anton-Lamprecht I, Arnold ML, Holbrook KA (1984) Methodology in sampling of fetal skin and pitfalls in the interpretation of fetal biopsy specimens. **Semin Dermatol** 3:203.

DNA-BASED PRENATAL DIAGNOSIS

MOLECULAR BASIS OF INHERITED SKIN DISORDERS

Of the 35 000 or so genes that constitute the human genome, approximately 1500 are known to harbor pathogenic mutations that result in autosomal dominant, autosomal recessive and X-linked single gene disorders.[1090] Of these, over 300 may involve abnormalities of the skin.[1091] A number of these genodermatoses may be associated with a high morbidity or mortality and therefore it may be appropriate to consider molecular prenatal diagnosis in couples at risk for recurrent disease in subsequent pregnancies.[1092] Delineation of specific mutations in several of these disorders has now enabled DNA-based testing to become a feasible option.[1093]

DNA-BASED TESTING

A DNA-based antenatal diagnostic approach requires a source of fetal DNA: this may be derived from early chorionic villus sampling (CVS), early amniocentesis, conventional amniocentesis, placental biopsy (late CVS), as well as fetal blood sampling or endoscopy. However, in most instances, the preferred source of fetal DNA for the diagnosis of single gene or chromosomal disorders is early CVS, usually taken at 10–12 weeks' gestation (Fig. 7.101). Sampling is typically performed either using transcervical or transabdominal forceps techniques. These methods allow for approximately 10–50mg of tissue to be biopsied or aspirated (Fig. 7.102). The risk of fetal loss following CVS (performed after 10 weeks) is approximately 1.7%.[1094] Initially, some reports suggested that CVS might increase the risk of severe limb reduction defects and the hypoglossia/hypodactyly syndrome,[1095] but this has not been borne out in subsequent

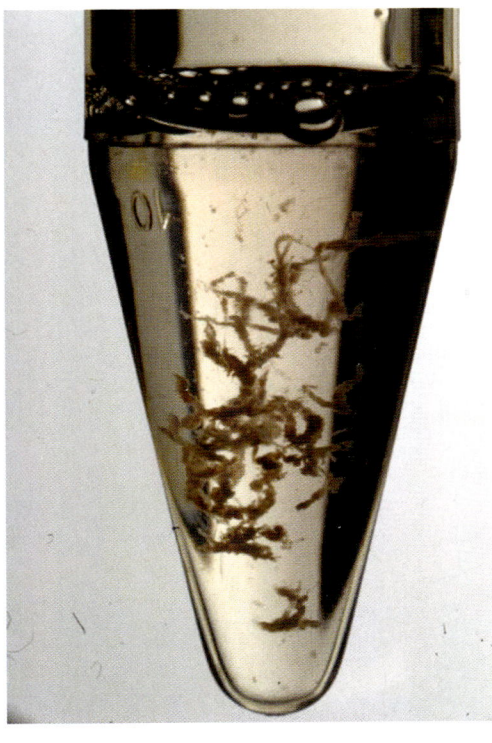

Fig. 7.101   Chorionic villi sampled at 11 weeks' gestation. Maternal decidua has been cleaned from the villi to avoid contamination from maternal DNA when the DNA is analyzed. The villi can now be used for DNA extraction or cultured for further studies.

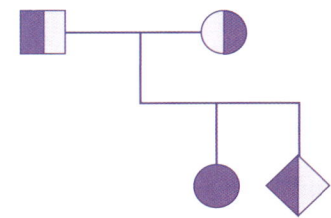

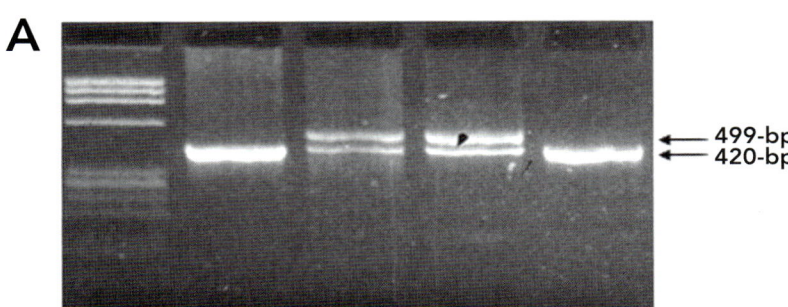

MW

A

← 499-bp
← 420-bp

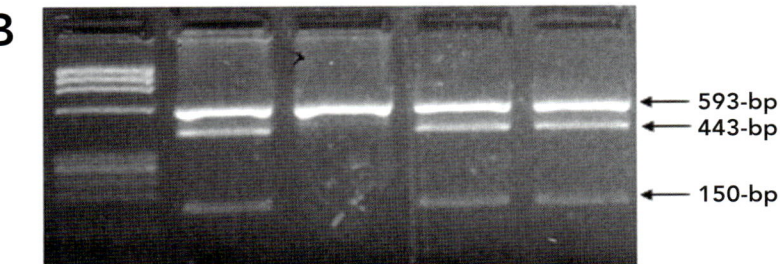

B

← 593-bp
← 443-bp

← 150-bp

Fig. 7.102   DNA-based prenatal exclusion of Herlitz junctional epidermolysis bullosa. The previously affected child is a compound heterozygote for the mutations 957ins77 and R635X in the *LAMB3* gene (encoding the β3 polypeptide chain of laminin 5). (A) Agarose gel electrophoresis of PCR products spanning *LAMB3* exon 10 and flanking introns. In the paternal sample, a single band of 420bp is present. By contrast, in the mother and previously affected child, two bands (420bp and 499bp) are seen consistent with these individuals being heterozygous for the mutation 957ins77. In the fetal amplified DNA only a single band of 420bp is present indicating that the fetus has not inherited the maternal insertion mutation. (B) Restriction endonuclease digestion with *Bgl*II of PCR products spanning exon 14 and flanking introns of *LAMB3*. In the maternal sample, there is a single undigested band of 593bp. However, the mutation R635X introduces a new cut site for *Bgl*II and additional bands of 443bp and 150bp are seen in the digested PCR products from the father, previously affected child and the fetus, consistent with all these individuals being heterozygous for this nonsense mutation. Thus the fetus has inherited the wild-type maternal *LAMB3* allele and the mutated paternal *LAMB3* allele and is therefore predicted to be clinically unaffected with Herlitz junctional epidermolysis bullosa (carrier).

more extensive international studies.[1096] Nevertheless, it is recommended that CVS not be performed before 10 weeks. Tissue obtained from the CVS needs to be cleaned under a dissecting microscope to exclude maternal cells (decidua, blood) that could contaminate polymerase chain reaction (PCR) or biochemical analyses. It is also important that villi are collected in an

1090. Antonarakis SE, McKusick VA (2000) OMIM passes the 1,000-disease-gene mark. **Nat Genet** 25:11.

1091. Uitto L, Pulkkinen L (2000) The genodermatoses: candidate diseases for gene therapy. **Hum Gene Ther** 11:2267–2275.

1092. McGrath JA, Eady RA (2001) Recent advances in the molecular basis of inherited skin diseases. **Adv Genet** 43:1–32.

1093. Ashton GH, Eady RA, McGrath JA (2000) Prenatal diagnosis for inherited skin diseases. **Clin Dermatol** 18:643–648.

1094. Cederholm M, Axelsson O (1997) A prospective study on transabdominal chorionic villus sampling and amniocentesis performed at 10–13 weeks' gestation. **Prenat Diagn** 17:311–317.

1095. Firth HV, Boyd PA, Chamberlain P et al. (1991) Limb abnormalities and chorion villus sampling. **Lancet** ii:51.

1096. Froster UG, Jackson L (1996) Limb defects and chorionic villus sampling: results from an international registry, 1992–4. **Lancet** 347:489–494.

appropriate medium. For example, the presence of heparin in the collection fluid may inhibit the activity of the Taq polymerase enzyme that is fundamental to PCR amplification. Chorionic villi can also be cultured for subsequent diagnostic confirmation of the findings obtained from direct analysis of the villi.

PRACTICAL CONSIDERATIONS IN DNA-BASED PRENATAL TESTING

In contrast to fetal skin biopsy-based diagnoses, in which the diagnostic strategy has to be specific for the disease in question, all DNA-based approaches must be tailored to the precise gene mutations or informative genetic markers relevant to the individual family being tested. In practical terms, this means that DNA-based antenatal tests require optimization before the CVS and ideally before pregnancy is contemplated because of the time needed to establish a robust, family-specific strategy.

For some disorders, such as Hallopeau–Siemens recessive dystrophic EB, analysis can be based on either mutation detection or genetic linkage since there is no genetic heterogeneity in this condition and all cases involve mutations in the type VII collagen gene, *COL7A1*, on 3p21.[1097,1098] However, in disorders such as Herlitz junctional EB there is considerable genetic heterogeneity and DNA-based prenatal diagnosis must be made on the basis of demonstrable mutations in either the *LAMA3*, *LAMB3* or *LAMC2* genes that encode the individual polypeptide chains of laminin 5.[1099] Genetic heterogeneity is also a feature of several other genodermatoses such as lamellar ichthyosis, EB simplex, non-Herlitz junctional epidermolysis bullosa, junctional epidermolysis bullosa associated with pyloric atresia, and bullous congenital ichthyosiform erythroderma/epidermolytic hyperkeratosis.[1092]

Whatever the disorder, in the build-up to DNA-based prenatal testing, it is important to have DNA samples from both parents and the affected individual to determine the pathogenic mutations. Other considerations such as the possibility of *de novo* mutations, nonpaternity, uniparental disomy and germline mosaicism can then all be addressed more fully and the suitability of the prenatal test can be determined.[1093] An illustration of a PCR-based prenatal test is shown in Fig. 7.102 and a list of inherited skin disorders in which antenatal DNA-based mutation analysis has been performed is shown in Table 7.39.

Several further genodermatoses might be added to this list as the repertoire of disease-associated mutations and the feasibility of undertaking such tests expands. Some guidelines for optimal approaches to DNA-based prenatal diagnosis in certain genodermatoses have been published and serve as useful templates for other disorders.[1098,1099]

ETHICAL CONSIDERATIONS IN DNA-BASED PRENATAL TESTING

Before the advent of DNA-based diagnosis, technical limitations meant that fetal skin biopsy testing could only be applied to a small number of genodermatoses. These disorders included conditions such Hallopeau–Siemens recessive dystrophic EB and Herlitz junctional EB, both of which are associated with extensive morbidity and poor prognoses. By contrast, delineation of pathogenic gene mutations in an increasing number of inherited skin disorders now means that, on technical grounds alone, prenatal testing is feasible in a much broader range of conditions, many of which are associated with a relatively less severe phenotype. Consequently, one of the difficult issues that has emerged is trying to define what disorders are appropriate for DNA-based prenatal diagnosis. What clinicians might

---

TABLE 7.39   DNA-based prenatal diagnosis by mutation analysis

Genodermatosis	MIM	Protein (*Gene*)	Gene locus	Reference(s)
Junctional epidermolysis bullosa (Herlitz)	226700	Laminin 5 α3 chain (*LAMA3*) Laminin 5 β3 chain (*LAMB3*) Laminin 5 γ2 chain (*LAMC2*)	18q11.2 1q32 1q25–31	1099, 1130, 1113 1099, 1131, 1114 1099
Junctional epidermolysis bullosa (with pyloric atresia)	226730	Beta-4 integrin (*ITGB4*)	17q11–qter	1132
Dystrophic epidermolysis bullosa (recessive)	226600	Type VII collagen (*COL7A1*)	3p21.3	1099, 1098,1133, 1116
Epidermolysis bullosa simplex (Dowling-Meara)	131760	Keratin 14 (*KRT14*)	17q21–22	1134
Bullous congenital ichthyosiform erythroderma (Epidermolytic hyperkeratosis)	113800	Keratin 10 (*KRT10*)	17q21–22	1135
Netherton syndrome	256500	Serine protease inhibitor (*SPINK5*)	5q32	1136
Oculocutaneous albinism (tyrosinase-negative, OCA1A)	203100	Tyrosinase (*TYR*)	11q14–21	1137, 1138
Lamellar ichthyosis	242300	Transglutaminase 1 (*TGM1*)	14q11	1139, 1140
Sjogren-Larsson syndrome	270200	Fatty aldehyde dehydrogenase (*FALDH*)	17p11	1141
Smith-Lemli-Opitz syndrome	270400	Sterol delta-7-reductase (*DHCR7*)	11q12–q13	1142
Mucopolysaccharidosis: (Hunter, type II)	309900	Iduronate-2-sulphatase (*IDS*)	Xq27.3–q28	1143
Ectrodactyly, ectodermal dysplasia, clefting (EEC) syndrome	129900	TP63 (*p63*)	3q27	1144

1097. Hovnanian A, Hilal L, Blanchet-Bardon C et al. (1995) DNA-based prenatal diagnosis of generalized recessive dystrophic epidermolysis bullosa in six pregnancies at risk for recurrence. **J Invest Dermatol** 104:456–461.

1098. Christiano AM, LaForgia S, Paller AS et al. (1996) Prenatal diagnosis for recessive dystrophic epidermolysis bullosa in 10 families by mutation and haplotype analysis in the type VII collagen gene (*COL7A1*). **Molec Med** 2:59–76.

1099. Christiano AM, Pulkkinen L, McGrath JA, Uitto J (1997) Mutation based prenatal diagnosis of Herlitz junctional epidermolysis bullosa. **Prenat Diagn** 17:343–354.

call "mild, recessive dystrophic epidermolysis bullosa" may be anything but that to the individual or family concerned, who may feel it has only been labeled as such because of the very existence of other cases of dystrophic EB with the Hallopeau–Siemens subtype. Should DNA-based prenatal testing be undertaken in such cases, or considered pro-rata on an individual basis, and who should be involved in making such judgments? Such considerations pose difficult problems and dilemmas for clinicians, geneticists and counselors involved with these families. By comparison, the field of preimplantation genetic diagnosis, which relies on similar DNA-based ascertainment, is underpinned by much more specific legislation and regulation of the actual disorders that are licensed for testing.

PREIMPLANTATION GENETIC DIAGNOSIS

Preimplantation genetic diagnosis (PGD) represents an alternative approach to prenatal diagnosis that combines improved methods of assisted reproduction with single cell genetic analysis. The purpose is to be able to diagnose genetic defects in embryos within days of fertilization, i.e., before the embryo implants and pregnancy is established. The main advantage of PGD is that a couple is able to know that any resulting pregnancy should be normal from the beginning and the possibility of a later termination is therefore avoided.

APPROACHES TO PGD

For preimplantation assessment, approaches to diagnosis may include first polar body analysis, or biopsy at the cleavage or blastocyst stage. Polar body analysis is a preconception diagnosis but has potential diagnostic pitfalls because of frequent crossing-over between non-sister chromatids during first meiotic prophase. Therefore, it is not an optimal consideration in screening for disease mutations and it is mainly used to avoid age-related aneuploidy in women aged 35 years and above undergoing *in vitro* fertilization (IVF) treatment.[1100]

Of more relevance for PGD is cleavage stage biopsy, which involves embryo sampling at the 6–10 cell stage on day 3 postfertilization. Up to 25% of the embryo can be removed at this time without any deleterious effects on the embryo.[1101] To remove blastomeres for analysis, acid Tyrodes solution is used to drill a hole in the zona pellucida and the blastomeres are then aspirated. Individual cells from these embryos are then examined for gene mutations or chromosomal translocations (depending on the disease risk) and then one or more unaffected embryos (which are maintained in culture while the diagnostic tests are being carried out) may be transferred to the uterus and pregnancy established. Worldwide experience reports overall pregnancy rates of around 28%.[1102] Follow-up studies using biochemical, ultrasound and clinical evaluation (including measurements of birth weights and Apgar scores) have not shown any developmental differences in pregnancies obtained from biopsied embryos after preimplantation genetic diagnosis.[1103,1104]

Blastocyst biopsy is performed 5–6 days postfertilization. It has the advantage that a larger number of cells can be removed from the outer trophoectoderm layer without affecting the inner cell mass. However, there is a potential for misdiagnosis using this approach because in at least 1% of all conceptions, evidence of confined placental mosaicism is present, in which the chromosome status of the embryo is different from the placenta. This may reflect a mechanism for preferentially allocating abnormal cells to the trophoectoderm in early development.[1105] A disadvantage further restricting the development of blastocyst biopsies for PGD has been that more than 50% of cleavage stage embryos arrest before the blastocyst stage.

DIAGNOSIS OF SINGLE GENE DISORDERS USING PGD

The first clinical application of PGD was reported in 1992 for couples at risk for transmitting cystic fibrosis.[1106] Subsequently, a number of other disorders including Tay–Sachs disease, Lesch–Nyhan syndrome, β-thalassemia, spinal muscular atrophy, adrenoleukodystrophy, myotonic dystrophy, Huntington's chorea, Charcot–Marie–Tooth 1A, Duchenne muscular dystrophy, and Fragile X syndrome have all been screened for using a similar approach. Applications of this methodology in dermatology have also been reported for Marfan syndrome with a fibrillin-1 gene mutation,[1107] Herlitz junctional EB resulting from mutations in the *LAMB3* gene,[1108] and skin fragility-ectodermal dysplasia syndrome caused by mutations in plakophilin 1.[1109] PGD has also been used for the prenatal diagnosis of incontinentia pigmenti.[1110] In this case, fluorescent *in situ* hybridization labeling for the X and Y chromosome was used to identify male embryos. These embryos were then selectively transferred to the uterus since affected males are lost *in utero* and there is a small risk of females being affected by the condition. However, the gene responsible for most cases of incontinentia pigmenti has now been identified and alternative mutation-based diagnostic testing is feasible.[1111]

The approach to PGD is based on IVF protocols. The IVF cycle commences within a few days of a woman's menstrual period and generally takes 4–6 weeks to embryo transfer. Collected eggs are usually fertilized by single sperm cells using intracytoplasmic sperm injection (ICSI) to avoid contamination by extraneous DNA from other sperm that would interfere with subsequent diagnostic tests (Fig. 7.103A). Most embryo sampling is done at the cleavage stage. For recessive disorders, it is usually technically satisfactory to sample one cell from each embryo to assess the presence or absence of the mutated alleles (Fig. 7.103B). Nevertheless, it is important to establish stringent and robust testing methods on a case-by-case basis. For example, the importance of using specific lysis buffers for the analysis of different genes has recently been recognized.[1112] These findings also highlight a further potential technical problem known as allele dropout, in which single-copy genes are not amplified. This can be due to biopsy of a haploid cell (which may be found in about 15% of embryos) or due to allele-specific amplification failure so that DNA from the gene on one chromosome is not present in the final PCR product. Allele dropout is a particularly relevant issue in PGD for dominant disorders. In such cases, either two cells can be biopsied from each embryo or additional polymorphic markers should be included in the diagnostic test so as to guarantee amplification of both alleles and a reliable PGD test.

1100. Munne S, Dailey T, Sultan KM, et al. (1995) The use of first polar bodies for preimplantation diagnosis of aneuploidy. **Mol Hum Reprod** 1:1014–1020.

1101. Hardy K, Martin KL, Leese HJ et al. (1990) Human preimplantation development in-vitro is not adversely affected by biopsy at the 8-cell stage. **Hum Reprod** 5:708–714.

1102. Harper JC (1996) Preimplantation diagnosis of inherited disease by embryo biopsy. An update of the world figures. **J Assist Reprod Genet** 13:90–94.

1103. Soussis I, Harper JC, Handyside AH, Winston RM (1996) Obstetric outcome of pregnancies resulting from embryos biopsied for preimplantation genetic diagnosis of inherited diseases. **Br J Obstet Gynaecol** 103:784–788.

1104. Soussis I, Harper JC, Kontogianni E et al. (1996) Pregnancies resulting from embryos biopsied for preimplantation genetic diagnosis of genetic disease: biochemical and ultrasonic studies in the first trimester of pregnancy. **J Assist Reprod Genet** 13:254–277.

1105. James RM, West JD (1994) A chimaeric animal model for confined placental mosaicism. **Hum Genet** 93:603–604.

1106. Handyside AH, Lesko JG, Tarin JJ et al. (1992) Birth of a normal girl after in vitro fertilisation and preimplantation diagnostic testing for cystic fibrosis. **N Engl J Med** 327:905–909.

1107. Harton GL, Tsipouras P, Sisson ME et al. (1996) Preimplantation genetic testing for Marfan syndrome. **Mol Hum Reprod** 2:713–715.

1108. Cserhalmi-Friedman PB, Tang Y, Adler A et al. (2000) Preimplantation genetic diagnosis in two families at risk for recurrence of Herlitz junctional epidermolysis bullosa. **Exp Dermatol** 9:290–297.

1109. Thornhill AR, Pickering SJ, Whittock NV et al. (2000) Preimplantation genetic diagnosis of compound heterozygous mutations leading to ablation of plakophilin-1 (PKP1) and resulting in skin fragility ectodermal dysplasia syndrome: a case report. **Prenat Diagn** 20:1055–1062.

1110. McGrath JA, Handyside AH (1998) Preimplantation genetic diagnosis of severe inherited skin diseases. **Exp Dermatol** 7:65–72.

1111. Smahi A, Courtois G, Vabres P et al. (2000) Genomic rearrangement in NEMO impairs NF-kappaB activation and is a cause of incontinentia pigmenti. The International Incontinentia Pigmenti (IP) Consortium. **Nature** 405:466–472.

1112. Thornhill AH, McGrath JA, Eady RA et al. (2001) A comparison of different lysis buffers to assess allele dropout from single cells for preimplantation genetic diagnosis. **Prenat Diagn** 21:490–497.

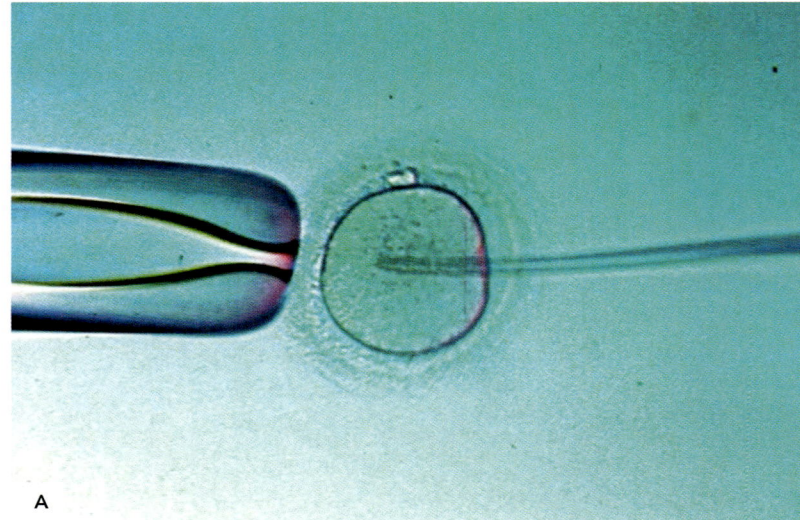

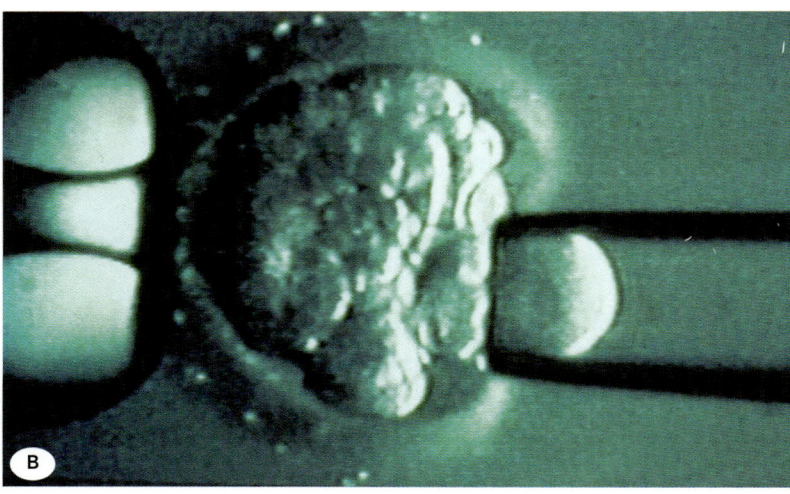

Fig. 7.103 *In vitro* fertilization and preimplantation genetic diagnosis. (**A**) Intracytoplasmic sperm injection (ICSI). A single sperm is injected via the cannula on the right into the egg (note polar body at 12 o'clock position). On the left is the holding pipette used to maintain the position of the egg for the injection procedure. (**B**) Sampling of a single cell from the developing 3-day-old embryo. At this stage, the embryo is about 100μm in diameter. An acidic solution is applied to drill a hole in the zona pellucida. A suction pipette (right) is then used to extract one or more cells from the developing embryo for DNA or chromosomal analyses. (B is courtesy of the Assisted Conception Unit, St Thomas' Hospital, London.)

By January 1997, 29 centers worldwide reported that they had carried out almost 600 PGD cycles, with over 100 pregnancies established and 96 babies born.[1102] Although PGD can be labor-intensive, technically demanding and expensive, its feasibility represents a major advance for certain couples at risk for recurrent inherited disorders. Nevertheless, from a practical standpoint, DNA-based prenatal diagnosis is most likely to remain centered on first trimester CVS-based analyses.

ACKNOWLEDGMENT

We thank Trish Dopping-Hepenstal and Matthew Gratian for help with the preparation of Figs 7.96–7.103.

1113. Rodeck CH, Eady RAJ, Gosden CM (1980) Prenatal diagnosis of epidermolysis bullosa letalis. **Lancet** i:949–952.
1114. Nazzaro V, Nicolini U, DeLuca L et al. (1990) Prenatal diagnosis of junctional epidermolysis bullosa associated with pyloric atresia. **J Med Genet** 27:244–248.
1115. Shimizu H, Suzumori K, Hatton V et al. (1996) Absence of detectable alpha 6 integrin in pyloric atresia – junctional epidermolysis bullosa syndrome. Application for prenatal diagnosis in a family at risk for recurrence. **Arch Dermatol** 132:919–925.
1116. Anton-Lamprecht I, Jovanovic V, Arnold M-L et al. (1981) Prenatal diagnosis of epidermolysis bullosa dystrophica Hallopeau–Siemens with electron microscopy of fetal skin. **Lancet** ii:1077–1079.
1117. Holbrook KA, Wapner R, Jackson L, Zaeri N (1992) Diagnosis and prenatal diagnosis of epidermolysis bullosa herpetiformis (Dowling–Meara) in a mother, two affected children, and an affected fetus. **Prenat Diagn** 12:725–739.
1118. Golbus MS, Sagebiel RW, Filly RA et al. (1980) Prenatal diagnosis of congenital bullous ichthyosiform erythroderma (epidermolytic hyperkeratosis) by fetal skin biopsy. **N Engl J Med** 302:93–95.
1119. Holbrook KA, Dale BA, Sybert VP et al. (1983) Epidermolytic hyperkeratosis: ultrastructure and biochemistry of skin and amniotic fluid cells from two affected fetuses and a newborn infant. **J Invest Dermatol** 80:222–227.
1120. Eady RAJ, Gunner DB, Carbone LDL et al. (1986) Prenatal diagnosis of bullous ichthyosiform erythroderma: detection of tonofilament clumps in fetal epidermal and amniotic fluid cells. **J Med Genet** 23:46–51.
1121. Blanchet-Bardon C, Dumez Y (1984) Prenatal diagnosis of Harlequin fetus. **Semin Dermatol** 3:225–228.
1122. Akiyama K, Holbrook KA (1994) Analysis of skin-derived amniotic fluid cells in the second trimester: detection of severe genodermatoses expressed in the fetal period. **J Invest Dermatol** 103:674.
1123. Akiyama M, Suzumori K, Shimizu H (1999) Prenatal diagnosis of harlequin ichthyosis by the examination of keratinized hair canals and amniotic fluid cells at 19 weeks' estimated gestational age. **Prenat Diagn** 167–171.
1124. Perry TB, Holbrook KA, Hoff MS et al. (1987) Prenatal diagnosis of congenital non-bullous ichthyosiform erythroderma (lamellar ichthyosis). **Prenat Diag** 70:145–155.
1125. Kousseff BG, Matsuoka LY, Stenn KS et al. (1982) Prenatal diagnosis of Sjögren–Larsson syndrome. **J Pediatr** 101:998–1001.
1126. Tabsh K, Rizzo W, Holbrook KA et al. (1993) Sjögren–Larsson syndrome: technique and timing of prenatal diagnosis. **Obstet Gynecol** 82:700.
1127. Arnold ML, Anton-Lamprecht I, Rauskolb R (1984) Prenatal diagnosis of ectodermal dysplasia. **Semin Dermatol** 3:247–252.
1128. Eady RAJ, Gunner DB, Garner A et al. (1983) Prenatal diagnosis of oculocutaneous albinism by electron microscopy of fetal skin. **J Invest Dermatol** 80:210–212.

1129. Shimizu H, Ishiko A, Kikuchi A et al. (1992) Prenatal diagnosis of tyrosinase-negative oculocutaneous albinism. **Lancet** 340:739–740.
1130. McGrath JA, Kivirikko S, Ciatti S et al. A homozygous nonsense mutation in the α3 chain of laminin 5 (LAMA3) in Herlitz junctional epidermolysis bullosa: Prenatal exclusion in a fetus at risk. **Genomics** 1995; 29:282–284.
1131. Vailly J, Pulkkinen L, Miquel C et al. Identification of a homzygous one base-pair deletion in exon 14 of the LAMB3 gene in a patient with Herlitz junctional epidermolysis bullosa and prenatal diagnosis in a family at risk for recurrence. **J Invest Dermatol** 1995; 104:462–466.
1132. Ashton GH, Sorelli P, Mellerio JE et al. α6β4 integrin abnormalities in junctional epidermolysis bullosa with pyloric aresia. **Br J Dermatol** 2001; 144:408–414.
1133. McGrath JA, Dunnill MG, Christiano AM et al. First trimester DNA-based exclusion of recessive dystrophic epidermolysis bullosa from chorionic villus sampling. **Br J Dermatol** 1996; 134:734–739.
1134. Rugg EL, Baty D, Shemanko CS et al. DNA based prenatal testing for the skin blistering disorder epidermolysis bullosa simplex. **Prenat Diagn** 2000; 20:371–377.
1135. Rothnagel JA, Longley NA, Holder RA et al. Prenatal diagnosis of epidermolytic hyperkeratosis by direct gene sequencing. **J Invest Dermatol** 1994; 102:13–16.
1136. Sprecher E, Chavanas S, DiGiovanna JJ et al. The spectrum of pathogenic mutations in SPINK5 in 19 families with Netherton syndrome: implications for mutation detection and first case of prenatal diagnosis. **J Invest Dermatol** 2001; 117:179–187.
1137. Shimuzu H, Niizeki H, Suzumori K et al. Prenatal diagnosis of oculocutaneous albinism by analysis of the fetal tyrosinase gene. **J Invest Dermatol** 1994; 104–106.
1138. Falik-Borenstein TC, Holmes SA, Borochowitz Z et al. DNA-based carrier detection and prenatal diagnosis of tyrosinase-negative oculocutaneous albinism (OCA1A). **Prenat Diagn** 1995; 15:345–349.
1139. Schorderet DF, Huber M, Laurini RN et al. Prenatal diagnosis of lamellar ichthyosis by direct mutational analysis of the keratinocyte transglutaminase gene. **Prenat Diagn** 1997; 17:483–486.
1140. Bichakjian CK, Nair RP, Wu WW et al. Prenatal exclusion of lamellar ichthyosis based on identification of two new mutations in the transglutaminase 1 gene. **J Invest Dermatol** 1998; 110:179–182.
1141. Sillen A, Holmgren G, Wadelius C. First prenatal diagnosis by mutation analysis in a family with Sjogren-Larsson syndrome. **Prenatal Diagn** 1997; 17:1147–1149.
1142. Nowaczyk MJ, Garcia DM, Eng B, Waye JS. Rapid molecular prenatal diagnosis of Smith–Lemli–Opitz syndrome. **Am J Med Genet** 2001; 102:387–388.
1143. Bunge S, Steglich C, Lorenz P et al. Prenatal diagnosis and carrier detection in mucopolysaccharidosis type II by mutation analysis. A 47, XXY male heterozygous for a missense point mutation. **Prenatal Diagn** 1994; 14:777–780.
1144. South AP, Ashton GH, Willoughby C et al. EEC syndrome: heterozygous mutation in the p63 gene and DNA-based antenatal diagnosis. **Br J Dermatol** 2001; in press.

Ichthyosis and Disorders of Cornification

Gabriele Richard, Celia Moss, Heiko Traupe, Mark Pittelkow,
Stephan Lautenschlager, Arne König, Rudolf Happle, Peter Itin

INTRODUCTION

Gabriele Richard

A variety of disorders with abnormal differentiation and desquamation of the epidermis are summarized as disorders of cornification. They are historically separated into several large groups including the ichthyoses, erythrokeratodermas, and palmoplantar keratodermas, comprising at least 24 well-defined entities.[1–3] The descriptive term ichthyosis, derived from the Greek root "ichthys" meaning fish, is used for those disorders sharing generalized scaling of the skin. The group of ichthyoses is both clinically and etiologically extremely heterogeneous resulting in considerable difficulties in their classification. In principle, ichthyoses can be inherited or acquired, presenting at birth or later in life, can be limited to the skin or be an element of a multisystem disorder (Table 8.1). Severity and extent can cover a tremendous range from dry skin in ichthyosis vulgaris to life-threatening harlequin ichthyosis.

It is important to establish an exact diagnosis in a patient or family with ichthyosis because of ramifications for prognosis, therapy, and genetic counseling. Significant diagnostic criteria are: age of onset; quality and distribution of scale; presence or absence of erythroderma, blistering, associated abnormalities of skin adnexae, or other organ systems. Histopathological and ultrastructural features can be helpful to recognize some disorders, as for example epidermolytic hyperkeratosis and ichthyosis hystrix Curth–Macklin, respectively, but can be unrevealing in others. The inheritance pattern of an ichthyosis within a family often assists in establishing a clinical diagnosis. The examination of both parents of a sporadic case may reveal valuable diagnostic hints, such as mosaic presentation (e.g., epidermolytic hyperkeratosis) or minor symptoms in carriers (e.g., X-linked recessive ichthyosis). Although sporadic cases are usually indicative of recessive ichthyoses, in particular when the parents are consanguineous, they may also represent spontaneously occurring new mutations with autosomal dominant inheritance, which has

important implications for genetic counseling. Applying these diagnostic guidelines, several but by far not all types of ichthyoses can be distinguished and reliably diagnosed based on their key features (Table 8.2).

The ichthyoses were first discussed in the dermatological literature in 1808,[4] and they still pose a clinical and diagnostic challenge. One reason is their rarity, which makes it difficult to appreciate the full clinical spectrum of each disorder. Another ensuing problem is the ceaseless development and simultaneous use of different, complex classification systems. The schemes have been based on clinical[5–7] and histopathological features,[8,9] inheritance,[2,3] biochemical, pathophysiological[9–12] and ultrastructural[13–18] criteria, or combinations of them,[1,19] which makes it difficult to correlate them with each other. Moreover, the nosology of ichthyoses is laden with descriptive names, eponyms and synonyms like few other dermatoses, resulting in much confusion and misconception. However, the spectacular advances in cell and molecular biology of the skin over the past decade have provided us with new means for a refined classification based on molecular grounds and a comprehensive understanding of the underlying pathomechanisms of disease (Table 8.3).

PATHOGENESIS OF ICHTHYOSIS AND DISORDERS OF CORNIFICATION

The skin is the barrier to the terrestrial environment. Its uppermost layer, the epidermis, is a highly specialized keratinizing epithelium designed to protect the organism from water loss and physical, chemical, and mechanical insults. In order to establish and constantly maintain this barrier, epidermal keratinocytes undergo a complex, highly organized and tightly controlled process of terminal differentiation, during which they migrate to the surface and form the stratum corneum. Keratin proteins are the major constituents of keratinocytes, representing 85% of the cellular protein.[20] Keratins are a large family of over 20 proteins expressed in tissue and differentiation specific

1. Williams ML, Elias PM (1987) Genetically transmitted, generalized disorders of cornification. The ichthyoses. **Dermatol Clin** 5:pp. 155–178.
2. Siemens HW (1929) Die Vererbung in der Ätiologie der Hautkrankheiten. In: Die Vererbung in der Ätiologie der Hautkrankheiten, Jadassohn J, ed. Berlin: Springer Verlag, pp. 1–165.
3. Wells RS, Kerr CB (1965) Genetic classification of ichthyosis. **Arch Dermatol** 92:1.
4. Willan R (1808) Ichthyosis. In: Ichthyosis. London: Barnard, pp. 197–212.
5. Schnyder UW (1970) Inherited ichthyoses. **Arch Dermatol** 102:240–255.
6. Riecke E (1900) Uber Ichthyosis congenita. **Arch Dermatol Syph (Wien)** 54:289–340.
7. Brocq L (1902) Erythrodermie congénitale ichtyosiforme avec hyperépidermotrophie. **Ann Dermatol Syphiligr (Paris)** 4:1.
8. Lapière S (1932) Epidermolyse ichtyosiforme congénitale. **Ann Dermatol Syph** 3:401–415.
9. Frost P, Van Scott EJ (1966) Ichtyosiform dermatoses. Classification based on anatomic and biometric observations. **Arch Dermatol** 94:113–126.
10. Bergers M, Traupe H, Dunnwald SC et al. (1990) Enzymatic distinction between two subgroups of autosomal recessive lamellar ichthyosis. **J Invest Dermatol** 94:407–412.
11. Hazell M, Marks R (1985) Clinical, histologic, and cell kinetic discriminants between lamellar ichthyosis and nonbullous congenital ichthyosiform erythroderma. **Arch Dermatol** 121:489–493.
12. Williams ML, Elias PM (1985) Heterogeneity in autosomal recessive ichthyosis. Clinical and biochemical differentiation of lamellar ichthyosis and nonbullous congenital ichthyosiform erythroderma. **Arch Dermatol** 121:477–488.
13. Anton-Lamprecht I (1972) [Ultrastructure of inborn errors of keratinization. I. Ichthyosis congenita]. **Arch Dermatol Forsch** 243:88–100.
14. Anton-Lamprecht I (1994) Ultrastructural identification of basic abnormalities as clues to genetic disorders of the epidermis. **J Invest Dermatol** 103:6S–12S.
15. Niemi KM, Kanerva L, Kuokkanen K et al. (1994) Clinical, light and electron microscopic features of recessive congenital ichthyosis type I. **Br J Dermatol** 130:626–633.
16. Niemi KM, Kanerva L, Wahlgren CF et al. (1992) Clinical, light and electron microscopic features of recessive ichthyosis congenita type III. **Arch Dermatol Res** 284:259–265.
17. Niemi KM, Kanerva L, Kuokkanen K (1991) Recessive ichthyosis congenita type II. **Arch Dermatol Res** 283:211–218.
18. Ghadially R, Williams ML, Hou SY et al. (1992) Membrane structural abnormalities in the stratum corneum of the autosomal recessive ichthyoses. **J Invest Dermatol** 99:755–763.
19. Traupe H (1989) The Ichthyoses. A Guide to Clinical Diagnosis, Genetic Counseling, and Therapy. Berlin, Heidelberg, New York: Springer Verlag.
20. Cheng J, Syder AJ, Yu QC et al. (1992) The genetic basis of epidermolytic hyperkeratosis: a disorder of differentiation-specific epidermal keratin genes. **Cell** 70:811–819.

TABLE 8.1   List of the ichthyoses

Types	Synonym
Non-syndromic ichthyoses	
Ichthyosis vulgaris	
X-linked ichthyosis	Steroid sulfatase deficiency
Epidermolytic hyperkeratosis of Brocq (EHK)	Bullous congenital ichthyosiform erythroderma of Brocq; bullous ichthyosis
Mosaic EHK	
Ichthyosis bullosa of Siemens	Exfoliative ichthyosis
Ichthyosis hystrix Curth–Macklin	Epidermal nevus of epidermolytic type
Nonbullous congenital ichthyosiform erythroderma (CIE)	NBCIE, Ichthyosis congenita type 1
Lamellar ichthyosis (LI)	Ichthyosis congenita type 2
CIE/LI intermediate types	
Autosomal dominant lamellar ichthyosis/congenital ichthyosiform erythroderma	
Ichthyosis in confetti	Ichthyosis variegata, congenital reticular ichthyosiform erythroderma
Harlequin fetus	
Peeling skin syndrome Type A	Keratolysis exfoliativa congenita; continual skin peeling
Syndromic ichthyoses	
Netherton syndrome/ichthyosis linearis circumflexa	Comèl–Netherton syndrome
Sjögren–Larsson syndrome	
Neutral lipid storage disease	Chanarin–Dorfman syndrome; triglyceride storage disease with impaired long-chain fatty acid oxidation; ichthyosiform erythroderma with leukocyte vacuolization
Refsum disease	Heredopathia atactica polyneuritiformis
Trichothiodystrophy	Tay syndrome; (P)IBIDS syndrome: Photosensitivity–ichthyosis–brittle hair–impaired intelligence–decreased fertility–short stature syndrome
Infantile Gaucher disease	Gaucher disease type II-GD II; Gaucher disease of the acute neuronopathic type
Neu–Laxova syndrome (NLS)	
Zunich–Kaye syndrome	Zunich neuroectodermal syndrome; CHIME syndrome: ocular colobomas, congenital heart disease, early-onset ichthyosiform dermatosis, mental retardation and ear anomalies (conductive hearing loss), epilepsy
Chondrodysplasia punctata, X-linked dominant	Conradi–Hünermann–Happle syndrome
Rhizomelic chondrodysplasia punctata (RCDP1)	Rhizomelic chondrodysplasia type 1; Chondrodystrophia calcificans punctata, autosomal recessive type
Cardiofaciocutaneous syndrome (CFC)	
Restrictive dermopathy	Tight skin-contracture syndrome, fetal hypokinesia sequence due to restrictive dermopathy
Multiple sulfatase deficiency	
Related disorders	
KID syndrome	Keratitis-ichthyosis-like-deafness syndrome, ichthyosiform erythroderma, corneal involvement, and deafness, autosomal dominant
CHILD syndrome	
Mutilating keratoderma with ichthyosis	Loricrin keratoderma
KLICK syndrome	Keratosis linearis with ichthyosis congenita and sclerosing keratoderma
Keratosis spinulosa delcalvans	
IFAP syndrome	Ichthyosis follicularis, atrichia, and photophobia syndrome
Ichthyosis, follicular atrophoderma, hypotrichosis, and hypohidrosis	
Migratory ichthyosis with diabetes mellitus	
Ichthyosis, hepatosplenomegaly, and cerebellar degeneration	
Ichthyosis–mental retardation syndrome with large keratohyalin granules in the skin	
Desmons syndrome	Ichthyosiform erythroderma, corneal involvement, and deafness; autosomal recessive
Acquired ichthyosis	

patterns. They form keratin intermediate filaments (KIF) and build an elaborate cytoskeleton, which provides structural stability and flexibility for epithelial cells.[21] Keratins are expressed in pairs of acidic (type I) and basic (type II) proteins, the genes of which cluster on chromosomes 17q12–q21 and 12q11–q13. Keratin monomers are organized as a central, alpha-helical rod domain flanked by variable, non-helical head and tail domains. They form obligate heterodimers, which polymerize and assemble into KIF. Short, highly conserved regions at the boundaries of the rod segment, designated helix initiation motif (1A) and helix termination motif (2B), have been recognized as zones of overlap between aligned keratin proteins and are crucial for their

21. McLean WH, Lane EB (1995) Intermediate filaments in disease. **Curr Opin Cell Biol** 7:118–125.

TABLE 8.2   Features of selected ichthyoses

Diagnosis	MIM	Gene	Chromosomal location	Mode of inheritance	Incidence	Onset	Dermatological features	Associated features	Diagnostic
Ichthyosis vulgaris	146700			Autosomal dominant	1:250	Infancy/ childhood	Fine, adherent scale on extremities and trunk with sparing of flexures; larger scale on lower legs; hyperlinear palms/soles, furrowed heels	Keratosis pilaris; atopic diathesis	Clinic; diminished/ absent str. granulosum?
X-linked recessive ichthyosis	308100	STS	Xp22.32		1:2000– 1:6000 males	Infancy	Fine to large, dark, adherent scale on extremities, trunk, neck, and lateral face; occasional palm/sole involvement	Corneal opacities on posterior capsule; increased electrophoretic mobility of beta-lipoproteins; cryptorchism. Female carriers: corneal opacities; prolonged birth with affected child	Lipoprotein electrophoresis; plasma cholesterol sulfate increased; steroid sulfatase activity in leukocytes; molecular testing
Lamellar ichthyosis	242300 LI1 601277 LI2 604777 LI3	TGM1	14q11.2 2q33-q35 19p12–q12	Autosomal recessive	1:300 000	Birth	Frequently collodion membrane at birth; large, thick, plate-like brown scale in generalized distribution; larger scale on lower legs; absent or mild erythroderma	Heat intolerance; scarring alopecia; ectropion; eclabium	Clinic, electron microscopy; in situ transglutaminase-1 expression and activity assay; molecular testing
(Nonbullous) Congenital ichthyosiform erythroderma (CIE)	242100 NCIE1 604780 NCIE2 ALOXE ALOX NCIE3	TGM1	14q11.2 17q 17p13.1 12	Autosomal recessive	1:100 000– 1:200 000	Birth	Frequently collodion membrane at birth; fine, white scale in generalized distribution; variable erythroderma	Heat intolerance; scarring alopecia; rarely ectropion	Clinic, electron microscopy; in situ transglutaminase-1 expression and activity assay; molecular testing
LI/CIE Intermediate types	604781; others are not designated		19p13.2–p13.1;	Autosomal recessive	Rare	Birth	Frequently collodion membrane at birth; fine to large or plate-like scale in generalized distribution; variable color of scale, palm/sole involvement; variable degree of erythroderma	Heat intolerance; scarring alopecia; rarelyectropion	See above
Autosomal dominant lamellar ichthyosis/ congenital ichthyosiform erythroderma	146750			Autosomal dominant	Rare	Birth	Clinically variable; occasionally collodion membrane at birth; either generalized large, dark scale with absent or minimal erythroderma (LI type),or fine, whitish scale with variable erythroderma (CIE type); pruritus	Ectropion possible	Clinic; pedigree analysis

TABLE 8.2   Features of selected ichthyoses—cont'd

Diagnosis	MIM	Gene	Chromosomal location	Mode of inheritance	Incidence	Onset	Dermatological features	Associated features	Diagnostic
Epidermolytic hyperkeratosis of Brocq, EHK (Bullous congenital ichthyosiform erythroderma Brocq, BCIE)	113800 146600	KRT1; KRT10	12q11–q13; 17q12–q21	Autosomal dominant	1:300 000	Birth	At birth erythroderma, blistering and erosions; later clinically heterogeneous; hyperkeratosis with verrucous, cobblestone or ridged pattern most prominent over joints; generalized or localized types; variable degree of erythroderma, palm/sole involvement; and blistering	Frequent skin infections; malodor; gait and posture abnormalities	Clinic, histopathology; molecular testing
Including: Mosaic epidermolytic hyperkeratosis	600648	KRT10	17q12–q21		Rare	Birth/ early infancy	Localized hyperkeratosis with rough, verrucous surface arranged in linear patterns following the lines of Blaschko; unilateral or bilateral		Clinic, histopathology
Ichthyosis bullosa of Siemens, IBS	146800	KRT2e	12q11–q13	Autosomal dominant	Rare	Birth	Erythroderma and blistering at birth; later hyperkeratosis with accentuation of flexures and "molting" of the skin; palms and soles spared		Clinic, histopathology; molecular testing
Ichthyosis Curth–Macklin	146590	KRT1	12q11–q13	Autosomal dominant	Rare	Birth	Variable phenotype: mild to severe, mutilating palmoplantar keratoderma; hyperkeratosis with verrucous, cobblestone or hystrix-like pattern on extremities and trunk	Pseudoainhum, digital contractures	Electron microscopy
Harlequin ichthyosis	242500			Autosomal recessive	Rare	Birth	Very thick, yellow-brown plates of scale that tightly encase the neonate; large, deep, bright red and oozing cracks and fissures; extreme ectropion, eclabium and ear deformities	Premature delivery; demise early postpartum or within days to weeks; sepsis; temperature, fluid and electrolyte imbalance; variable other organ abnormalities	Clinic
Netherton syndrome	256500	SPINK5	5q32	Autosomal recessive	1:300 000– 1:50 000	Birth/ infancy	Occasionally collodion membrane at birth; two principal phenotypes: ichthyosis linearis circumflexa and generalized, CIE-like ichthyosis; pruritus and eczematous plaques are common	Trichorrhexis invaginata and other hair shaft abnormalities; highly elevated serum IgE; neonatal temperature and electrolyte imbalance, failure to thrive; recurrent infections; food and other allergies; often unspecific aminoaciduria	Clinic, psoriasiform histopathology; light microscopic hair shaft analysis; serum IgE; electron microscopy (ruthenium tetroxide); molecular testing

TABLE 8.2   Features of selected ichthyoses—cont'd

Diagnosis	MIM	Gene	Chromosomal location	Mode of inheritance	Incidence	Onset	Dermatological features	Associated features	Diagnostic
Sjögren–Larsson syndrome	270200	*FALDH* (*ALDH10*)	17p11	Autosomal recessive	1:250 000	Birth	Generalized coarse hyperkeratosis with ridged pattern in flexures; pruritus	Spastic di- and tetraplegia; mental retardation; parafoveal glistening white dots; white matter disease of the brain	Fatty aldehyde dehydrogenase activity assay in cultured fibroblasts; molecular testing
Neutral lipid storage disease	275630	CGI-58	3p21	Autosomal recessive	Rare	Birth	Generalized fine, white scale with variable erythema	Lipid-containing vacuoles in leukocytes; cataract; hearing impairment; myopathy; hepatomegaly; developmental delay	Peripheral blood smear to detect lipid vacuoles; (oil stains on frozen skin biopsy material)
Trichothicdystrophy (Tay syndrome, (P)IBIDS)	601675 IBIDS 278730 PIBIDS	*ERCC2*; *ERCC3*	19q13.2–q13.3	Autosomal recessive	Rare	Birth	Occasionally collodion membrane at birth;generalized scaling with absent or minimal erythroderma; flexures may be spared	*Ichthyosis*; *brittle hair and nails*; *intellectual impairment*; *decreased fertility*; short stature; lack of subcutaneous fatty tissue with ensuing progeria-like facies; photosensitivity	Clinic; light microscopic hair shaft analysis under polarizing light
Refsum disease	266500	*PAHX*	10pter–p11.2	Autosomal recessive	Rare	Early childhood/ Ichthyosis in adulthood	Fine, white scale over trunk and extremities resembling ichthyosis vulgaris	Peripheral neuropathy; cranial nerve dysfunction (deafness, anosmia); cerebellar ataxia; retinitis pigmentosa; cardiomyopathy; epiphyseal dysplasia	Plasma level of phytanic acid increased; phytanoyl-CoA hydroxylase activity assay in cultured fibroblasts; molecular testing

proper assembly to KIF.[22,23] In the epidermis, basal keratinocytes predominantly express keratins 5 and 14, while cells in the upper epidermis switch to the expression of the differentiation-specific keratins 1 and 10. Cells of the granular layers also produce keratin 2e, which might assemble with keratin 10. Other site-specific suprabasal keratins include keratin 9, found exclusively in palms and soles, and keratins 6, 16 and 17, which are expressed when the epidermis is stressed. Pathogenic mutations in 19 different keratin genes are responsible for a wide range of genodermatoses affecting skin, mucous membranes, hair, nails, and sebaceous glands. These mutations cluster at mutational "hot spots" at the beginning and end of the central rod domain and disturb KIF assembly, resulting in perinuclear clumping of fragmented KIF and cell fragility, the hallmarks of keratin disorders.

In analogy to a brick wall built from bricks and mortar, the stratum corneum contains two principal elements: protein-rich corneocytes (bricks) and a lipid-enriched extracellular matrix (mortar). The barrier function of the skin is accomplished by formation of the cornified cell envelope, an 8–15nm structure that replaces the plasma membrane in terminally differentiating keratinocytes. It is a highly insoluble and tough polymer of proteins (protein envelope) and lipids (lipid envelope). The protein envelope results from sequential cross-linking of specialized precursor proteins, such as involucrin, small proline-rich proteins, elafin, cystatin A, and loricrin, with KIF and desmosomal proteins facilitated by epidermal transglutaminases.[24] It confers chemical and mechanical resilience as well as water retention of corneocytes. The lipid envelope is formed by a monolayer of long-chain omega-hydroxyceramides, which are covalently attached to the outer surface of the protein envelope by ester bonds, a process which is again mediated by membrane-bound transglutaminase.[25] These protein-linked ceramides coat the corneocytes and intervene with intercellular lipids in a comb-like fashion.

The lipid composition of the stratum corneum is markedly different from the lower epidermis. Instead of phospholipids, the stratum corneum contains large amounts of neutral lipids, such as cholesterol and free fatty acids, as well as polar lipids, such as ceramides and epidermis-specific omega-hydroxy and omega-hydroxyacylceramides. These lipids are synthesized in the spinous layers of the epidermis, where they are stored and transported as stacks of laminar sheets in lamellar bodies. With initiation of formation of

22. Lane EB (1994) Keratin diseases. **Curr Opin Genet Dev** 4:412–418.
23. Fuchs E, Weber K (1994) Intermedite filaments: structure, dynamics, function, and disease. **Annu Rev Biochem** 63:345–382.
24. Steinert PM, Marekov LN (1995) The proteins elafin, filaggrin, keratin intermediate filaments, loricrin, and small proline-rich proteins 1 and 2 are isodipeptide cross-linked components of the human epidermal cornified cell envelope. **J Biol Chem** 270:17702–17711.

25. Nemes Z, Marekov LN, Fesus L et al. (1999) A novel function for transglutaminase 1: attachment of long-chain omega-hydroxyceramides to involucrin by ester bond formation. **Proc Natl Acad Sci USA** 96:8402–8407.

TABLE 8.3   Etiological classification of disorders of cornification

	System	Genes	Disorder	Mechanism
Structural protein defects	Keratin disorders	KRT1; KRT10	Epidermolytic hyperkeratosis of Brocq	
		KRT2e	Ichthyosis bullosa of Siemens	Mutations in epithelial keratin genes predominantly affect the boundaries of the alpha helical rod domain, and dominantly interfere with alignment and assembly of KIF. As a result, the KIF cytoskeleton is weakened and fragile, and may collapse under mechanical stress leading to cytolysis.
		KRT9	Epidermolytic palmoplantar keratoderma	
		KRT10; (KRT1)	Mosaic EHK/Epidermal nevus of the epidermolytic type	
		KRT6a; KRT6b; KRT16; KRT17	Pachyonychia congenita I/II	
		KRT16	Focal non-epidermolytic palmoplantar keratoderma	
		hHb1; hHb6	Monilethrix	
		KRT4; KRT13	White sponge nevus	
		KRT3; KRT12	Meesmann corneal dystrophy	
		KRT1	Diffuse non-epidermolytic palmoplantar keratoderma	Keratin mutations affecting the end domains of keratin-1, dominantly disturbing interaction with KIF associated proteins and cytoplasmic KIF organization.
		KRT1	Ichthyosis hystrix Curth-Macklin	
	Disorders of the cornified cell envelope	LOR	Mutilating keratoderma with ichthyosis (loricrin type)	Frameshift mutations transform the tail domain of loricrin, impair formation of the cornified cell envelope and result in intranuclear accumulation of loricrin.
		LOR	Progressive symmetric erythrokeratoderma (loricrin type)	
	Desmosomal disorders	DSP; DSG1	Striate palmoplantar keratoderma	Dominant mutations in desmoglein-1 and desmoplakin impair desmosomal cell adhesion and interaction with KIF (haploinsufficiency).
		DSP; JUP	Naxos disease	Recessive mutations in plakoglobin disrupt interactions of desmosomal proteins with KIF and weaken desmosomes and adherens junctions, thereby disturbing integrity of cells in skin, hair and myocardium.
Enzyme defects	Disorders of lipid metabolism	TGM1	Lamellar ichthyosis	Recessive transglutaminase-1 mutations result in enzyme deficiency, which severely impairs protein cross-linking and esterification of epidermis-specific ceramides during formation of the protein and lipid envelope of corneocytes, and perturbs the skin barrier function.
		(TGM1)	Congenital ichthyosiform erythroderma (nonbullous)	
		ALOXE3	Congenital ichthyosiform erythroderma (nonbullous)	These 2 ezymes belong to the lipoxigenase family of non-heme, iron-containing dioxygenases and are highly expressed in suprabasal epidermis, trachea, lung, tongue, brain, testis. LOXs catalyze oxygenation of free and esterified polyunsaturated fatty acids, phospholipids and triglycerides, and thus, are involved in etablishing the epidermal lipid barrier.
		ALOX12B	Congenital ichthyosiform erythroderma (nonbullous)	

the cornified cell envelope, lamellar bodies fuse with apical cell membranes in granular cells and extrude their contents into the intracellular space. Hydrolytic enzymes of the lamellar bodies transform glycolipids and phospholipids into free fatty acids and ceramides, respectively. Using the corneocyte lipid envelope as template, discharged lipids reorganize into intercellular lipid lamellae, which form broad double bilayers connecting with each other through intervening lipid monolayers. This arrangement results in the characteristic pattern of alternating electron dense and electron lucent bands visible by transmission electron microscopy with ruthenium tetroxide fixation. Together, lipid envelopes and intercellular lipid lamellae "glue" corneocytes together and impede water loss through the skin. In a normal stratum corneum, 15–20 layers of corneocytes are stacked on top of each other. They are also held together by corneodesmosomes, which are successively degraded by proteolytic lamellar body enzymes to reduce their cohesiveness and allow desquamation of the outermost cells.

Desquamation is a continuous, inconspicuous process by which individual corneocytes or small clumps of them are separated and exfoliated through frictional forces. The human body sheds approximately 2 billion corneocytes

TABLE 8.3   Etiological classification of disorders of cornification—cont'd

System	Genes	Disorder	Mechanism
	FALDH	Sjögren–Larsson syndrome	Recessive mutations inactivate fatty aldehyde dehydrogenase, which catalyzes the oxidation of long-chain aliphatic aldehydes to fatty acids. As a result, the synthesis of epidermal lipids and the catabolism of ether phospholipids and sphingolipids in the brain are impaired.
	STS	X-linked recessive ichthyosis and other sulfatase deficiencies	Steroid sulfatase deficiency results in impaired hydrolysis of cholesterol sulfate leading to accumulation of cholesterol-3 sulfate in the epidermis.
	EPB	X-linked dominant chondrodysplasia punctata	Mutations in delta8-delta7 sterol isomerase (emopamil binding protein) impair postsqualene cholesterol biosynthesis resulting in depletion of cholesterol and accumulation of intermediates. Cholesterol is a major structural element of plasma membranes and a precursor for the synthesis of steroids and bile acids. Sterol toxicity probably interferes with lipid biosynthesis.
	NSDHL	CHILD syndrome	Mutations in NSDHL impair postsqualene biosynthesis upstream to delta8-delta7 sterol isomerase.
	CGI-58	Neutral lipid storage disease	CGI-58 belongs to the subfamily of esterase/lipase/thioesterase enzymes but its function in humans still remains unknown. It is thought that a defect in degradation of endogenously produced diacylgycerols to phospholipids results in widespread tissue deposition of neutral lipids. A defect in degradation of endogenously produced diacylgycerols to phospholipids results in widespread tissue deposition of neutral lipids.
Disorders of protein catabolism	SPINK5	Netherton syndrome	Recessive mutations inactivate the serine proteinase inhibitor KAZAL type 5. Exact pathomechanisms remain to be elucidated.
	CTSC	Papillon–Lefévre syndrome	Allelic disorders caused by deficiency of the lysosomal protease cathepsin C (dipeptidyl aminopeptidase I), which is expressed in skin, gingiva, and a variety of immune cells. Exact pathomechanisms remain to be elucidated.
	CTSC	Haim–Munk syndrome	
Disorders of amino acid metabolism	TAT	Richner–Hanhart syndrome	Tyrosine aminotransferase deficiency results in elevated serum tyrosine and deposition of tyrosine crystals in various tissues and body fluids.
Peroxisomal disorders	PEX7	Rhizomelic chondrodysplasia punctata type 1	Peroxisomal import disorder. Recessive mutations inactivate an import receptor for type 2 peroxisomal targeting sequences (PTS2). Several proteins depending on this pathway fail to be imported from the cytosol into the peroxisomes, resulting in deficient plasmalogen biosynthesis and phytanic acid oxidation, while very long-chain fatty acid oxidation is normal.
	PAHX	Refsum disease	Recessive mutations inactivate the peroxisomal enzyme phytanoyl-CoA hydroxylase and impair degradation of phytanic acid, which subsequently accumulates in tissues and body fluids.

TABLE 8.3   Etiological classification of disorders of cornification—cont'd

	System	Genes	Disorder	Mechanism
Regulatory defects	Disorders of calcium homeostasis			
		ATP2A2	Darier disease	Dominant mutations inactivate intracellular calcium pumps and thereby disturb calcium homeostatsis of the epidermis.
		ATP2C1	Hailey–Hailey disease	
	Connexin disorders	GJB3; GJB4	Erythrokeratodermia variabilis	Dominant mutations in several epidermal connexin genes dominantly interfere with the formation or function of gap junctional intercellular channels implicated in cell-cell signaling.
		GJB2	Diffuse palmoplantar keratoderma associated with hearing impairment	
		GJB2	Vohwinkel syndrome	
	Disorder of nucleotide excision repair			
		ERCC2; ERCC3	Trichothiodystrophy	Recessive mutations inactivate two helicase subunits of the transcription/repair vector TFIIH, thereby impairing excision repair of UV-induced DNA damage.
	?	ARS	Mal de Meleda	Recessive mutations result in deficiency of a secretory protein of the Ly-6/uPAR subfamily, which is closely related to cytotoxins. Expression pattern and pathomechanisms are unknown.

during the course of a day, illustrating the striking magnitude of this imperceptible process. Visible scaling as seen in ichthyosis is produced by exfoliation of clumps of 100–500 or more adherent corneocytes. Under normal conditions, epidermal cell proliferation and desquamation are in a steady-state. Any exogenous or endogenous process that disturbs this homeostasis is bound to impair the barrier function of the skin, eventually resulting in disease. Hyperkeratosis of the stratum corneum can stem from an increased number of cells produced by the epidermis (hyperproliferative ichthyosis), from delayed desquamation (retention hyperkeratosis), or a combination of both mechanisms. The formation of the stratum corneum is controlled by various factors that are not well understood. One of the most important regulators of key metabolic events during epidermal differentiation leading to barrier formation is intracellular calcium, the level of which increases from layer to layer throughout the epidermis.[26] High intracellular calcium concentrations are critical for the expression and processing of differentiation-specific proteins such as keratin-1, keratin-10, profilaggrin, loricrin, involucrin, and others, as well as for the action of transglutaminases. Increased trans-epidermal water loss with ensuing changes in pH and ion concentration, in particular calcium and potassium, is thought to trigger factors for release of cytokines, such as tumor necrosis factor (TNF)-α, interleukin (IL)-8, IL-10, interferon-γ, transforming growth factor (TGF)-α and -β as well as the adhesion molecule intercellular adhesion molecule-1 (ICAM1). These molecules can elicit a host of different homeostatic responses, including secretion of pre-formed lamellar bodies, increase lipid and lamellar body synthesis, stimulation of DNA synthesis to generate more corneocytes and epidermal inflammation.[27,28] Other modulators of terminal differentiation include retinoic acid, vitamin D, protein kinase C, urokinase, and transcription factors, all of which are still under investigation.

In the last decade, genetic tools have been successfully applied to uncover the molecular basis of a large number of heritable disorders of the skin and its appendages, leading to identification of more than 100 disease genes.[29] This knowledge substantially advanced our understanding of the process of cornification itself as well as the pathobiology of disorders of cornification.

It is now possible to categorize ichthyoses and disorders of cornification, at least in part, on the basis of their underlying genetic defects. These may affect (a) structural proteins of the epidermis, including keratins, desmosomal proteins, proteins of the cornified cell envelope, (b) enzymes involved in lipid, protein, and amino acid metabolism as well as (c) regulatory molecules controlling cornification such as calcium and connexins (Table 8.3). Keratin disorders, such as epidermolytic hyperkeratosis, ichthyosis bullosa of Siemens, and epidermolytic palmoplantar keratoderma result from fragility of the KIF network of keratinocytes with ensuing epidermolysis. However, faulty KIF may also directly interfere with the secretory function of lamellar bodies and other differentiation-specific proteins, thus impairing the permeability barrier of the skin. An increasing number of inherited ichthyoses have been associated with defects in the lipid metabolism of the skin, hindering formation of the lipid envelope and intercellular lipid lamellae. Phytanoyl-CoA hydroxylase deficiency in Refsum disease impedes the normal synthesis of ceramides, while fatty aldehyde dehydrogenase deficiency in Sjögren–Larsson syndrome imparis synthesis of fatty acids. Loss of transglutaminase-1 activity in lamellar ichthyosis/congenital ichthyosiform erythroderma has profound effects on the cornified cell envelopes. The dual impairment of protein–protein cross-linkage as well as attachment of ceramides and formation of the lipid envelope leads to severe diminution of the skin barrier and hyperkeratosis. The basic defect in X-linked recessive ichthyosis is steroid sulfatase deficiency causing impaired hydrolysis of cholesterol sulfate and accumulation of cholesterol-3 sulfate in the epidermis. High levels of this metabolite inhibit the normal function of transglutaminase-1 thus explaining the partial overlap between X-linked recessive ichthyosis and lamellar ichthyosis and underscoring the pivotal role of transglutaminase-1 in the cornified envelope formation and normal functioning of the stratum corneum. Disorders of cornification may also arise from genetic defects involving important regulators of epidermal differentiation. In case of Hailey–Hailey disease and Darier disease, a partially reduced function of intracellular calcium pumps negatively affects the calcium homeostasis of the epidermis and response to intercellular signaling. Connexin disorders are thought to arise from impaired gap junctional intercellular com-

26. Menon GK, Elias PM (1991) Ultrastructural localization of calcium in psoriatic and normal human epidermis. **Arch Dermatol** 127:57–63.

27. Elias PM, Feingold KR (1992) Lipids and the epidermal water barrier: metabolism, regulation, and pathophysiology. **Semin Dermatol** 11:176–182.

28. Proksch E, Holleran WM, Menon GK et al. (1993) Barrier function regulates epidermal lipid and DNA synthesis. **Br J Dermatol** 128:473–482.

29. Pulkkinen L, Ringpfeil F, Uitto J (2001) Progress in heritable skin diseases: molecular bases and clinical implications. **J Am Acad Dermatol**, subm.

munication between keratinocytes with ensuing effects on transport of ions such as calcium and cyclic nucleotides.

The etiologic classification of ichthyoses and disorders of cornification based on the underlying genetic defects, though still preliminary and incomplete, is advancing the traditional nosology. Efforts to identify specific mutations and genotype-phenotype correlations advance our ability to diagnose these rare disorders with certainty, allow accurate family counseling, offer the opportunity for reliable and early prenatal testing, and will potentially lead to the development of targeted therapies for these disorders.

ICHTHYOSIS VULGARIS

Heiko Traupe

INCIDENCE

Autosomal dominant ichthyosis vulgaris is a fairly frequent disorder. Many patients are not aware that they are suffering from a skin disease but rather describe their skin as being "a bit dry". Wells and Kerr studied 6061 pupils and found among them 24 children with ichthyosis vulgaris which would correspond to a frequency of 4 in 1000 in the general population.[30]

CLINICAL FEATURES

Ichthyosis vulgaris is not present at birth, but usually develops during the first months of life. Wells and Kerr found demonstrable hyperkeratosis in 40% of their patients at the age of 4 months. The vast majority of cases with ichthyosis vulgaris do not start before the age of 6 months. Typically cutaneous features of ichthyosis vulgaris include light gray scales covering mainly the extensor surfaces of the extremities and the trunk (Fig. 8.1). The groin and the big flexures are always spared. Follicular keratosis projecting above the skin surface is a further characteristic sign of the disease that is present especially in children and young patients. According to Mevorah *et al.*[31] it occurs in 75% of all ichthyosis vulgaris patients compared with 42% of the general population. Accentuated palmoplantar markings are a further hallmark of ichthyosis vulgaris found in 80 to 90% of patients. If the accentuation is marked it may be of considerable diagnostic help (Fig. 8.2), but evaluation of accentuated palmoplantar creases proves rather difficult if this symptom is only mildly expressed. Ichthyosis vulgaris is often associated with atopic dermatitis.[31] Among a patient group of 65 patients attending our department for treatment of autosomal dominant ichthyosis vulgaris, we found concomitant atopic dermatitis in 30% of the patients. Accentuated palmoplantar creases can also be observed in atopic dermatitis and are here often referred to as "hyperlinear palms."

From a clinical point of view it remains difficult to make a clear-cut distinction between X-linked recessive ichthyosis and ichthyosis vulgaris and a recent survey showed that an accurate clinical diagnosis was achieved only in about 50% of the cases.[32] For a definite diagnosis, therefore, a detailed family history and additional diagnostic measures, for example obtaining a histologic examination, or performing biochemical tests to exclude X-linked recessive ichthyosis, for example steroid sulfatase testing or lipoprotein electrophoresis, should be considered.

HISTOLOGIC AND ULTRASTRUCTURAL FEATURES

A reduced granular layer, which may often even be completely lacking in parts of the biopsy, is the most outstanding histologic feature of ichthyosis vulgaris (Fig. 8.3). The stratum corneum usually displays a mild but compact

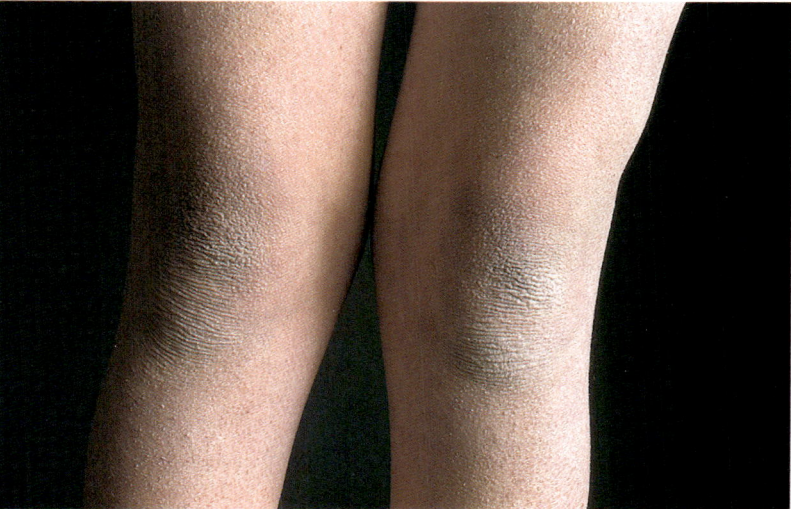

Fig. 8.1 Light gray scales in ichthyosis vulgaris covering the extensor surface of the arms.

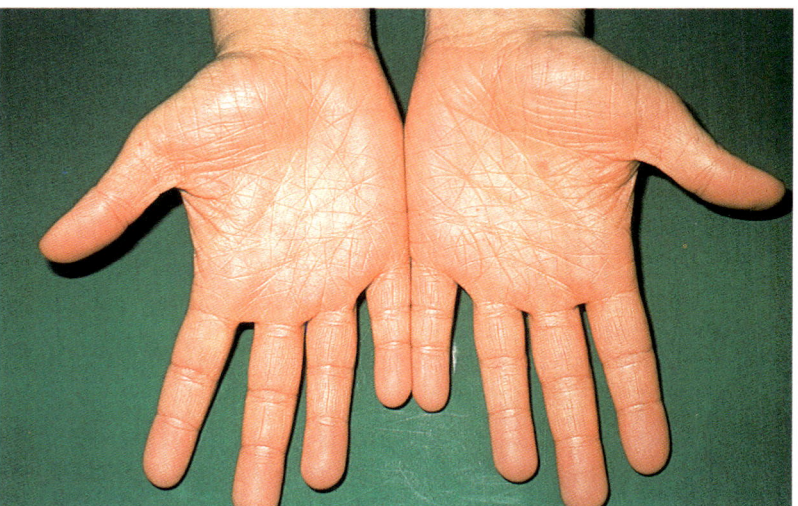

Fig. 8.2 **Accentuated palmoplantar markings in ichthyosis vulgaris.** When present this sign helps to rule out X-linked recessive ichthyosis. Some types of lamellar ichthyosis feature somewhat similar "ichthyosis hands."

orthohyperkeratosis. A reduced rete-papillae pattern, occasional prominent follicular keratosis and reduction in the number of the sebaceous glands are further features of ichthyosis vulgaris.[19] At the ultrastructural level the diminished granular layer is reflected by reduced and abnormal keratohyalin granules which exhibit a crumbly and spongy appearance.[33] It should be noted that it can be difficult on purely histological grounds to exclude the Conradi–Hünermann–Happle syndrome and the Refsum syndrome, which are likewise associated with a reduced granular layer.

BIOCHEMICAL AND GENETIC ASPECTS

It cannot be doubted that ichthyosis vulgaris runs in families and can be transmitted in an autosomal dominant mode of inheritance. Therefore, it is generally considered to be a monogenic skin disease. It is noteworthy,

30. Wells RS, Kerr CB (1966) Clinical features of autosomal dominant and sex-linked ichthyosis in an English population. **Br Med J** 1:947–950.
31. Mevorah B, Marazzi A, Frenk E (1983) The prevalence of accentuated palmoplantar markings and kertosis pilaris in atopic dermatitis, autosomal dominant ichthyosis and control dermatological patients. **Br J Dermatol** 112:679–685.
32. Cuevas-Covarrubias SA, Kofman-Alfaro SH, Palencia AB, Diaz-Zagoya JC (1996) Accuracy of the clinical diagnosis of recessive X-linked ichthyosis vs ichthyosis vulgaris. **J Dermatol** 23:594–597.
33. Anton-Lamprecht I, Jofbauer UC (1972) Ultrastructural distinction of autosomal dominant ichthyosis vulgaris and X-linked recessive ichthyosis. **Hum Genet** 15:261–264.

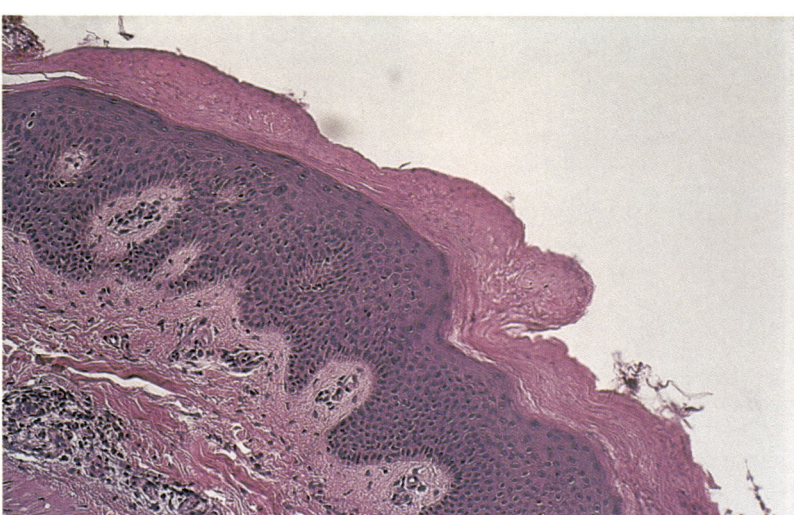

Fig. 8.3   Typical histology of ichthyosis vulgaris. Presence of follicular keratosis and marked reduction or even absence of the granular layer. Refsum disease and the Conradi–Hünermann–Happle syndrome can have a similar histology.

however, that so far all attempts to map or to identify the underlying gene have failed. In our personal experience with many patients it is uncommon to see really large pedigrees and quite often both parents seem to be unaffected. Therefore we now believe that ichthyosis vulgaris actually may be a polygenic disease and has a complex genetics similar to that found in atopic dermatitis with which it may share a predisposing gene.[19] Biochemical studies have demonstrated a decreased profilaggrin expression resulting from a selectively impaired post-transcriptional control. In keratinocytes cultured from the epidermis of affected individuals, profilaggrin was reduced less than 10% of normal controls, while the mRNA level was decreased to 30 to 60% of controls.[34] If this was the primary defect one would expect under an autosomal dominant inheritance pattern an unequal expression of profilaggrin mRNA from both alleles. However, expression of the gene for profilaggrin was biallelic and coequal in both control and affected individuals.[35] Profilaggrin mRNA in ichthyosis vulgaris patients is, however, intrinsically unstable and has a shorter half-life compared with that in normal cells. A labile ribonuclease could act as a stabilizing factor and modulate profilaggrin mRNA steady state level in normal cells while such stabilizing factor could be absent in patients with ichthyosis vulgaris. The autosomal recessive mutation flaky tail (ft) provides an interesting animal model for ichthyosis vulgaris. Biochemical analysis demonstrated that ft/ft mice lacked normal high molecular profilaggrin, and instead expressed a lower molecular weight form of profilaggrin (220kDa) that is not proteolytically processed to profilaggrin intermediates or filaggrin.[36]

THERAPY

Usually ichthyosis vulgaris does not present a major therapeutic problem and responds well to topical ointments containing urea or lactic acid or NaCl. Urea should not be used on large body areas before the age of 1 year, and certainly ichthyosis vulgaris should not be treated by ointments containing

salicylate because this can cause life-threatening poisoning due to percutaneous absorption. Germann *et al.*[37] reported about a 7-year-old boy in whom therapy of ichthyosis vulgaris with ointment containing 10% salicylic acid over large areas of the body surface. After 4 weeks the patient was in a deep somnolent state, apparently caused by hyperventilation following wheezing, vomiting, tinnitus and vertigo. Salicylate intoxication also caused metabolic acidosis, an anion gap and respiratory overcompensation. Therefore, in children total body treatment with salicylic acid should be avoided.[19]

X-LINKED RECESSIVE ICHTHYOSIS

Heiko Traupe

INCIDENCE

X-linked recessive ichthyosis (XRI) is the second most common type of ichthyosis. Population genetics studies disclosed a minimum prevalence in the male population of 1 to 6390 in southern England[30] and 1 in 9855 males in Japan.[38] Routine screening of pregnancies in Denmark showed that the incidence of XRI was 1 in 2000 males.[39]

CLINICAL FEATURES

XRI is the cutaneous manifestation of steroid sulfatase deficiency. Noncutaneous manifestations of this enzyme defect include birth complications, cryptorchidism, and corneal opacities.[40,41]

Prenatal diagnosis of placental sulfatase deficiency has made it possible to follow the course of the disease from birth on. In a Danish study of 21 boys prenatally diagnosed as suffering from placental sulfatase deficiency, 19 displayed a general peeling of the skin with rather large, light and loosely attached scales over the entire integument at the age of 1–3 weeks.[42] During the following weeks this fine scaling was replaced by the typical polygonal dark and firmly attached scales of XRI. The fine scaling in early life is not very striking, however, and usually escapes the attention of parents or nurses. When the patients or their parents are asked with respect to onset of the disease they usually say that it started at the age of 2 to 6 months.

At that time, normally large thick dark-brown to yellow-brown hyperkeratoses cover the trunk, the extremities and the neck (Fig. 8.4). The face is spared except for preauricular scaling, and palms and soles are normal, which is of considerable clinical help in the differential diagnosis from ichthyosis vulgaris. The dark hyperkeratoses are especially prominent over the lateral aspects of the trunk and the back of the neck resulting in "a dirty look" which is a further typical feature of XRI and usually not seen in ichthyosis vulgaris. Axillae and antecubital and popliteal fossae may be involved in some patients and are spared in other patients. This criterion therefore should not be used to separate the disease from ichthyosis vulgaris, which usually spares the antecubital and popliteal fossae completely. From personal experience, about 30% of the patients do not have the classic dark-brown hyperkeratosis, but exhibit large, light-gray hyperkeratoses (Fig. 8.5). This applies in particular also to young boys, and even among two brothers sharing the same mutation one may exhibit the classic yellow–brown hyperkeratoses and the other may show light-gray scaling. These latter patients are often erroneously classified as having ichthyosis vulgaris. Follicular keratosis is absent in XRI – at least from a clinical point of view. It may be seen occasionally in histopathological

34. Nirunsuksiri W, Presland RB, Brumbaugh SG et al. (1995) Decreased profilaggrin expression in ichthyosis vulagris is a result of selectively impaired posttranscriptional control. **J Biol Chem** 270:871–876.

35. Nirunsuksiri W, Zhang SH, Fleckman P (1998) Reduced stability and bi-allelic, coequal expression of profilaggrin mRNA in kekratinocytes cultured from subjects with ichthyosis vulgaris. **J Invest Dermatol** 110:854–861.

36. Presland RB, Boggess D, Lewis SP et al. (2000) Loss of normal profilaggrin and filaggrin in flaky tail (ft/ft) mice: an animal model for the filaggrin-deficient skin disease ichthyosis vulgaris. **J Invest Dermatol** 115:1072–1081.

37. Germann R, Schindera I, Kuch M et al. (1996) Lebensbedrohliche Salizylatintoxikation durch perkutane Resorption bei einer schweren Ichthyosis vulgaris. **Hautarzt** 47:624–627.

38. Sakura N, Nishimura SI, Matsumoto T, Ohsaki M (1998) Frequency of steroid sulfatase deficiency in Hiroshima. **Acta Paediatr Jpn** 40:63–64.

39. Lykkesfeldt G, Hoyer H, Ibsen HH, Brandrup F (19185) Steroid sulfatase deficiency disease. **Clin Genet** 28:231–237.

40. Traupe H, Happle R (1983) Clinical spectrum of steroid sulfatase deficiency: X-linked recessive ichthyosis, birth complications and cryptorchidism. **Eur J Pediatr** 140:19–21.

41. Unamuno P de, Martin C, Fernandez E (1986) X-linked ichthyosis and cryptorchidism. **Dermatologica** 172:3226–3327.

42. Hoyer H, Lykkesfeldt G, Ibsen HH, Brandrup F (1986) Ichthyosis of steroid sulfatase deficiency, clinical study of 76 cases. **Dermatologica** 172:184–190.

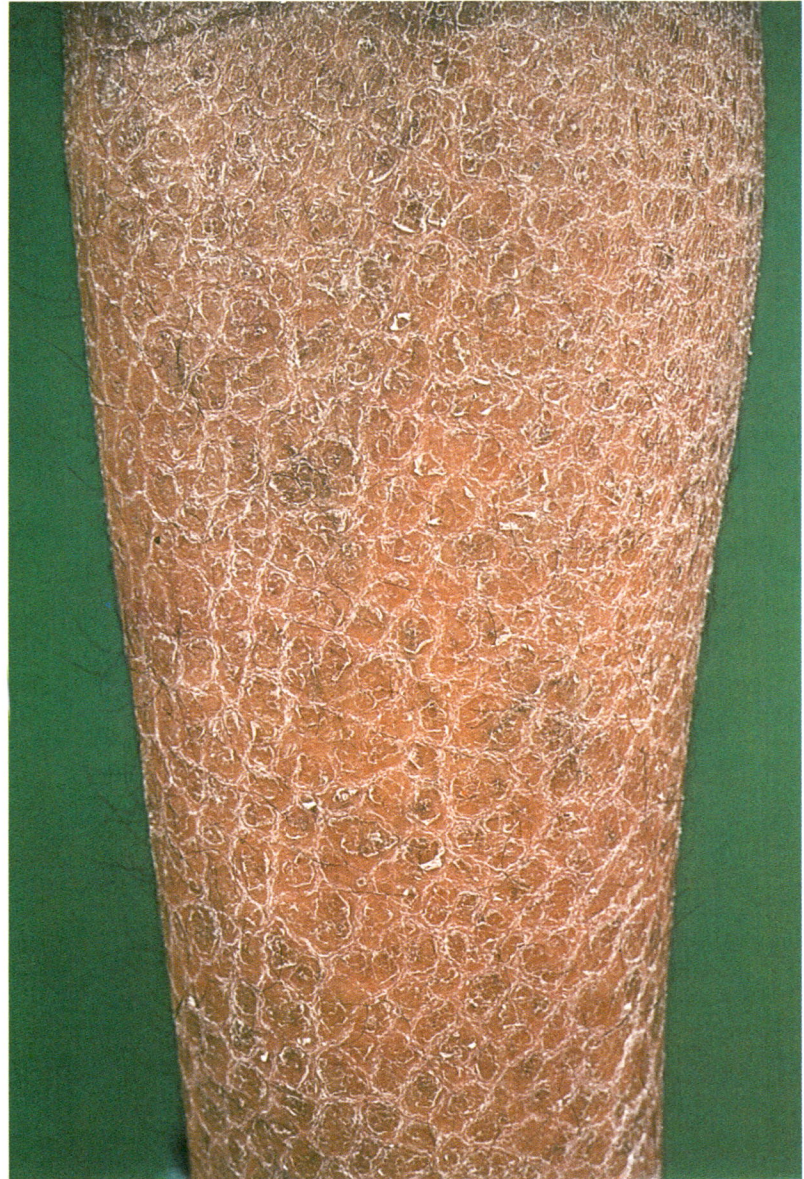

Fig. 8.4   **X-linked recessive ichthyosis.** Typical rhombic yellow–brown hyperkeratosis in older children.

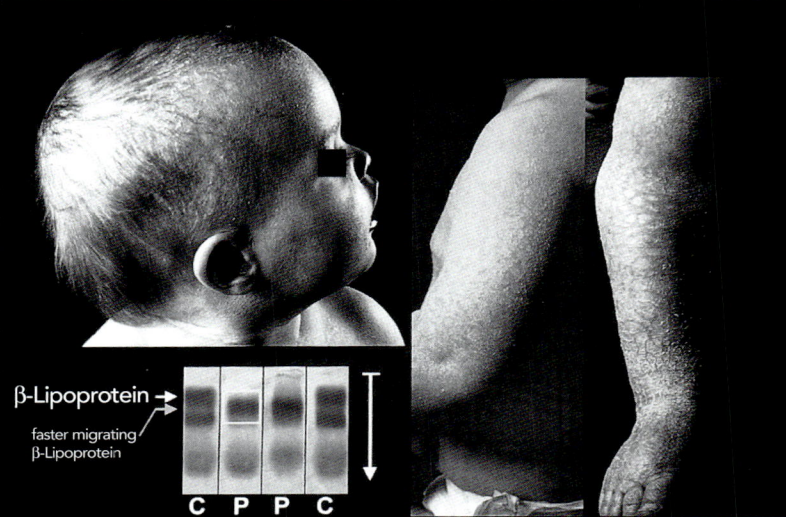

Fig. 8.5   **X-linked recessive ichthyosis.** Clinical aspects in a young boy and increased electrophoretic mobility in the patients (lanes P) contrasting with normal electromobility in the controls (lanes C). Patients with light-gray scaling are often misdiagnosed as having ichthyosis vulgaris.

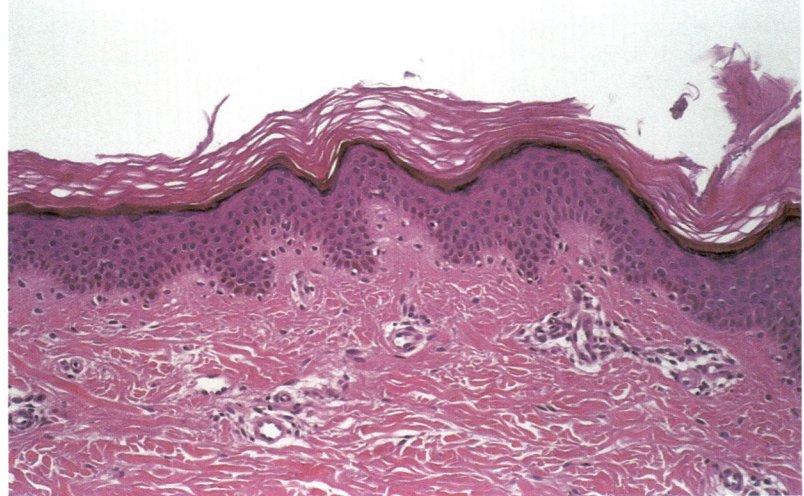

Fig. 8.6   **X-linked recessive ichthyosis.** Typical histology with prominent granular layer and orthohyperkeratosis. It is not possible to exclude mild forms of autosomal recessive lamellar ichthyosis such as transglutaminase-1-deficiency by routine histopathology.

examinations. Female carriers of the disease gene may display a fine, silver-light scaling on the lower legs, especially the calfs.[43]

Obstetric manifestations of steroid sulfatase deficiency include insufficient cervical dilatation which may result in weakness of labor and a prolonged delivery necessitating Cesarean section or forceps delivery. Altogether, a careful medical history reveals that about 30% of boys postnatally diagnosed as having XRI also had a history of clinically manifest birth complications.[33,41] Gonadal abnormalities include cryptorchidism (testicular maldescent), which is seen in about 24% of patients and may be associated with decreased fertility and in extreme cases with hypogenitalism. The rate of testicular cancer may be increased. Risk pregnancies can be detected by prenatal screening of low maternal serum estriol.[44]

HISTOLOGICAL FEATURES

XRI is characterized by a nonspecific epidermal hyperplasia (Fig. 8.6) associated with a usually prominent or broadened granular layer and orthohyperkeratosis.[19,45] If the biopsy has been taken from an area showing maximal scaling then occasionally even a reduced granular layer and an almost atrophic epidermis can be observed. Sebaceous glands are present in XRI and on histologic grounds follicular plugging may sometimes be noted. From a histologic point of view it is usually not possible to exclude mild forms of lamellar ichthyosis.

43. Voss M (1985) Clinical picture of X chromosome recessive ichthyosis. **Dermatol Monatsschr** 171(1):25–37 (in German).

44. Keren DF, Canick JA, Johansen MZ et al. (1995) Low maternal serum unconjugated estriol during prenatal screening as an indication of placental steroid sulfatase deficiency and X-linked ichthyosis. **Am J Clin Pathol** 103:400–403.

45. Feinstein A, Ackermann AB, Ziprkowski L (1970) Histology of autosomal dominant ichthyosis vulgaris and X-linked ichthyosis. **Arch Dermatol** 101:524–527.

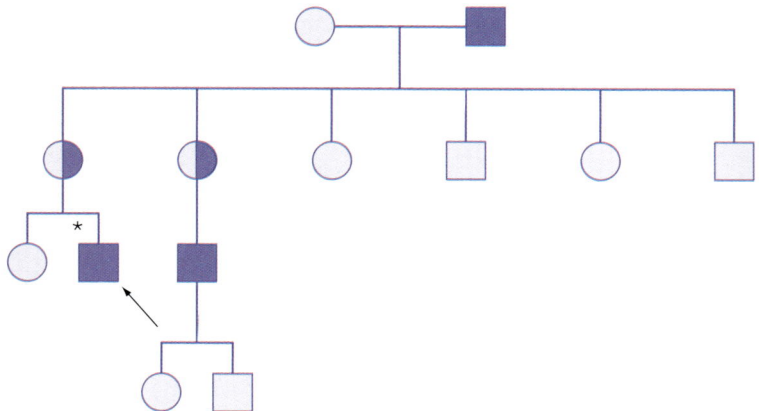

Fig. 8.7   X-linked recessive mode of inheritance visualized by drawing a pedigree. The index patient (arrow) also suffered from severe hypogonadism and cryptorchidism (asterisk). These clinical features of steroid sulfatase deficiency lacked in his likewise affected maternal grandfather and in his maternal cousin who also suffered from XRI. His mother and maternal aunt did not have visible signs of the disease, but were obligate conductors of the mutation.

BIOCHEMICAL AND GENETIC ASPECTS

XRI was one of the first genetic skin diseases that was mapped by classic linkage analysis, namely a close linkage with the Xg-blood group to the X-chromosome.[46] For a clinicogenetic diagnosis it is often extremely helpful to draw a pedigree and then to analyze it. Many clinicians seem to find this difficult at first, but involvement of a maternal grandfather, involvement of further maternally related male relatives and sparing of the female conductor clearly point to an X-linked recessive mode of inheritance and help to make a correct diagnosis (Fig. 8.7).

In 1978 Jöbsis and Shapiro and their coworkers simultaneously discovered that the disease is due to steroid sulfatase deficiency.[47,48] Later on it was established that the gene for steroid sulfatase escapes X-inactivation – which allows biochemical recognition of heterozygous gene carriers by steroid sulfatase testing.[49] Female heterozygous gene carriers have an enzyme activity similar to that of men, while normal women have an enzyme activity that is almost twice as high. The steroid sulfatase gene was cloned and found to be deleted in about 80% of the patients.[50] In those patients who do not have deletion, point mutations have been shown to result in single base pair substitutions causing, for example, a stop codon.[51] The development of ichthyosis is usually attributed to the accumulation of cholesterol sulfate in the stratum corneum. As a consequence of the steroid sulfatase deficiency cholesterol sulfate cannot be cleaved to cholesterol. Another explanation could be that the epidermis actually lacks cholesterol. It is noteworthy that other cholesterol deficiency syndromes such as the CHILD syndrome or the Conradi–Hünermann–Happle syndrome are likewise associated with hyperkeratosis. Somewhat surprisingly, the skin barrier properties in patients with XRI have been shown to be superior to those of normal controls.[52] In particular, the response to sodium lauryl sulfate was less marked when evaluated by transepidermal water loss.

Testing steroid sulfatase activity is of course the ultimate way to make an accurate diagnosis, but the test is quite tedious and performed only in a few laboratories. An increased electromobility of beta-lipoprotein is a convenient way to screen for steroid sulfatase deficiency.[53,54] The reason for the increased electromobility of beta-lipoprotein particles is that cholesterol sulfate is accumulated within this fraction and alters the electric charge and thus the electrophoretic mobility of lipoprotein.

A number of patients with X-linked recessive ichthyosis present with additional clinical features due to a contiguous gene deletion affecting neighboring genes.[55] In particular, Kallmann syndrome and chondrodysplasia punctata caused by mutations in arylsulfatase E are seen in patients with X-linked recessive ichthyosis. Other conditions that can be explained by a contiguous gene deletion effect are hypertrophic pyloric stenosis, unilateral renal aplasia, mental retardation and even hypergonadotropic hypogonadism. In the past such cases have often been erroneously referred to as Rud syndrome. A better designation would be to term such cases as associated steroid sulfatase deficiency.[19]

MULTIPLE SULFATASE DEFICIENCY

Heiko Traupe

INCIDENCE

Multiple sulfatase deficiency was first described in detail by Rampini and coworkers in 1970 and is a very rare and severe neuropediatric disorder. Patients are usually taken care of by neuropediatricians. No reliable data on the incidence can be given.

CLINICAL FEATURES

The signs and symptoms of multiple sulfatase deficiency resemble those of the late infantile form of metachromatic leukodystrophy. Psychomotor retardation usually starts in the second year of life and and an affected child who may already have learned to walk then becomes unsteady and requires support to stand or walk. A flabby weakness and hypotonia of all four limbs develops. During the third year the patient's condition rapidly deteriorates. An obvious mental regression, speech deterioration and severe motor defects are then observed. In the last stage the children are blind, without speech, and must be fed, usually through a nasogastric tube.[56,57] The ichthyosis is rather mild and starts late, often in the third year of life. It develops on the limbs, trunk and scalp. Histopathology reveals orthohyperkeratosis with a normal granular layer.[58] It resembles XRI but is less pronounced. This milder cutaneous involvement reflects some residual activity of steroid sulfatase.

BIOCHEMICAL AND GENETIC ASPECTS

From a biochemical point of view, multiple sulfatase deficiency is a unique autosomal recessive disorder in which all seven known sulfatases are deficient. It is remarkable that the different enzymes are localized in different cellular compartments (lysosomes and microsomes) and that the genes for the various sulfatases are borne on different chromosomes. Certain aspects of the clinical

46. Kerr CB, Wells, Sanger R (1964) X-linked ichthyosis and the Xg groups. **Lancet** 2:1369–1370.
47. Koppe JG, Marinkovic-Ilsen A, Rijken Y et al. (1978) X linked ichthyosis. A sulfatase deficiency. **Arch Dis Child** 53:803–806.
48. Shapiro LJ, Weiss R, Webster D, France JT (1978) X-linked ichthyosis due to steroid sulfatase deficiency. **Lancet** 1:70–72.
49. Müller CR, Migl B, Traupe H, Ropers HH (1980) X-linked steroid sulfatase: evidence for different gene-dosage in males and females. **Hum Genet** 54:201–204.
50. Yen PH, Allen E, Marsh B et al. (1987) Cloning and expression of steroid sulfatase cDNA and frequent occurence of deletions in STS deficiency: implications for X–Y interchange. **Cell** 49:443–454.
51. Oyama N, Satoh M, Iwatsuki K, Kaneko F (2000) Novel point mutations in the steroid sulfatase gene in patients with X-linked ichthyosis: transfection analysis using the mutated genes. **J Invest Dermatol** 114:1195–1199.
52. Johansen JD, Ramsing D, Vejlsgaard G, Agner KTC (1993) Skin barrier properties in patients with recessive X-linked ichthyosis. **Acta Dermatol Venereol** 75:202–204.

53. Traupe H, Kövary PM, Schriewer H (1983) X-linked recessive ichthyosis vulgaris: rapid identification by lipoprotein electrophoresis. **Arch Dermatol Res** 275:63–65.
54. Arndt T, Pelzer M, Nenoff P et al. (2000) Lipoprotein- und Apolipoproteinelektrophorese bei X-chromosomal rezessiver Ichthyose. **Hautarzt** 51:490–495.
55. Paige DG, Emilion GG, Bouloux PM, Harper JI (1994) A clinical and genetic study of X-linked recessive ichthyosis and contiguous gene defects. **Br J Dermatol** 131(5):622–629.
56. Rampini S, Isler W, Baerlocher K et al. (1970) Die Kombination von metachromatischer Leukodystrophie und Mucopolysaccharidose als selbständiges Krankheitsbild (Mukosulfatidose). **Helv Pediatr Acta** 25:436–461.
57. Dulaney JT, Moser HW (1978) Sulfatide lipidosis, metachromatic lipo dystrophy. In: The Metabolic Basis of Inherited Disease, Stanbury J, Wyngaarden B, Frederichson DB, eds. New York: McGraw-Hill, pp. 781–809.
58. Castano-Suarez E, Segurado-Rodrigues A, Guerra-Tapia A et al. (1997) Ichthyosis: the skin manifestation of multiple sulfatase deficiency. **Pediatr Dermatol** 14:369–372.

phenotype can be attributed mainly to deficiency of one specific sulfatase. Patients develop metachromatic leukodystrophy caused by arylsulfatase A deficiency and dysostosis multiplex caused by mucopolysaccharide sulfatase deficiency and ichthyotic skin due to the steroid sulfatase deficiency. As in XRI, low urinary estriol levels can be demonstrated in multiple sulfatase deficiency pregnancies.[59] The deficiency of several sulfatases results from the lack of a post-translational modification that is common to all sulfatases and is required for their catalytic activity. Structural analysis of two catalytically active sulfatases revealed that a cysteine residue that is predicted from the cDNA sequence and conserved among all known sulfatases is replaced by a 2-amino-3-oxopropionic acid residue, while in sulfatases derived from multiple sulfatase deficiency, this cysteine residue is retained.[60] The post-translational conversion of this cysteine residue to 2-amino-3-oxopropionic acid is required for generating a functionally active sulfatase. The oxidation of the cysteine residue to 2-amino-3-oxopropionic acid (C-alpha-formylglycine) occurs in the endoplasmic reticulum at a stage when the nascent polypeptide is not yet folded. The aldehyde alpha-formylglycine is part of the catalytic site of all sulfatases and accepts the sulfatase during sulfate ester clearage. The biochemical elucidation of multiple sulfatase deficiency has enormously contributed to the current understanding of the catalytic mechanisms of sulfatases.[61]

EPIDERMOLYTIC HYPERKERATOSIS (EHK)
Gabriele Richard

Synonyms: Bullous congenital ichthyosiform erythroderma of Brocq (BCIE), Bullous ichthyosis (MIM 113800)

As early as 1897, Nikolski recognized the characteristic histopathology of the bullous form of congenital ichthyosis.[62] Later in 1902, Brocq first differentiated between dry (non-bullous) and wet (bullous) forms of congenital ichthyosiform erythroderma.[7] The term "epidermolytic hyperkeratosis" was coined by Frost and Van Scott in 1965 for the autosomal dominant blistering form of congenital ichthyosis, which is named for the distinctive histopathologic features of vacuolar degeneration and hyperkeratosis of the epidermis.[9] Although these structural abnormalities are not unique to EHK, the name EHK has widely replaced other descriptive terms.

EPIDEMIOLOGY
Genetics
EHK is an autosomal dominant disorder with complete penetrance but extensive clinical variability. It is caused by heterozygous mutations in the genes encoding keratin 1 and keratin 10 (*KRT1, KRT10*), which are expressed in the differentiated layers of the epidermis. Almost half of all cases occur sporadically and represent new mutations. If a spontaneous mutation arises postzygotically during early embryogenesis, it affects somatic cells and may result in a mosaic form of EHK following the lines of Blaschko.[63,64] Extensive, unilateral or bilateral mosaic involvement with massive hyperkeratosis has also been described as ichthyosis hystrix. In the case of epidermal mosaicism, it is possible that the somatic mutation also involves gonadal cells and thereby can be transmitted from the germline to the offspring resulting in generalized disease.[64] Several families have been well documented, in which a parent with a linear, epidermolytic epidermal nevus had offspring with generalized EHK. Based on the autosomal dominant inheritance of EHK, both genders are

affected equally, and an affected person faces in each pregnancy a 50% risk of transmitting the disorder to the offspring. If the parent has mosaic involvement the risk that the offspring will develop full-blown EHK is lower but has to be considered.

Statistics
EHK is a rare disorder with an estimated incidence of 1 in 200 000 to 1 in 300 000 individuals.

PRESENTING HISTORY
EHK usually presents at birth with erosions and widespread areas of denuded skin and erythroderma, which stem from increased epidermal fragility and are provoked by the frictional trauma during passage through the birth canal. Over time, blistering diminishes while hyperkeratosis develops.

PHYSICAL EXAMINATION
Skin
In the neonatal period, infants show erythema, large erosions, peeling, and widespread areas of denuded skin reminiscent of epidermolysis bullosa although focal areas of hyperkeratosis may already be present (Fig. 8.8). Later during infancy and childhood, the bullous component becomes less prominent, while severe hyperkeratosis prevails.

The clinical presentation of EHK is extremely variable, although it tends to be consistent within a family. Based on a survey of 52 patients with histologically confirmed EHK from 21 families, DiGiovanna *et al.*[65] recognized

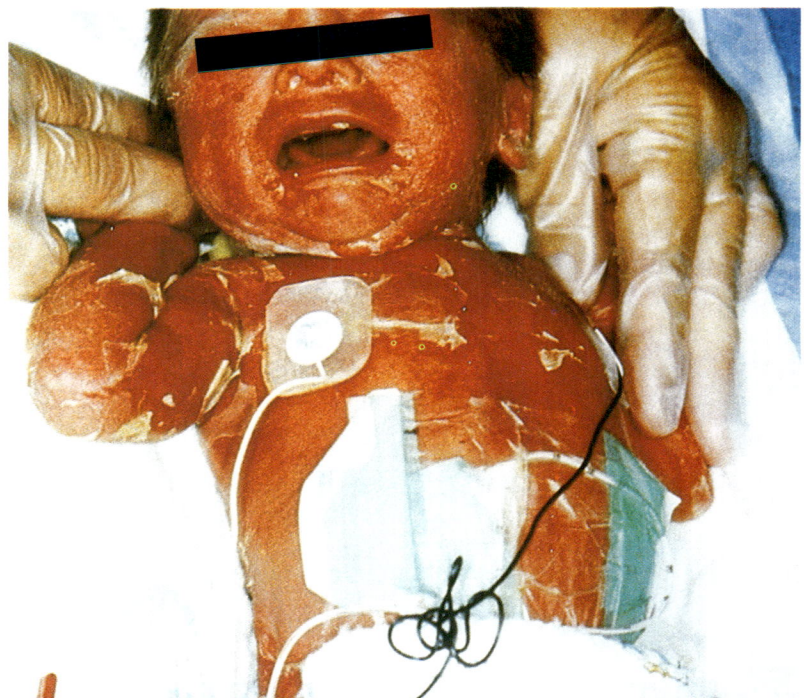

Fig. 8.8 Neonate with epidermolytic hyperkeratosis of Brocq (EHK, bullous congenital ichthyosiform erythroderma). Note erythema and widespread areas of denuded skin. (Courtesy of Dr. M. Williams)

59. Steinmann B, Bieth D, Gitzelmann R (1981) A newly recognized cause of low urinary estriol in pregnancy: multiple sulfatase deficiency of the fetus. **Gynecol Ostet Invest** 12:107–109.
60. Schmidt B, Selmer T, Ingendoh A, von-Figura K (1995) A novel amino acid modification in sulfatases that is defective in multiple sulfatase dificiency. **Cell** 82:271–278.
61. Bond CS, Clements PR, Ashby SJ et al. (1997) Structure of a human lysosomal sulfatase. **Structure** 5:277–289.
62. Nikolski P (1897) Contribution à l'étude des anomalies congénitales de kératinisation. Comptes-Rendus du XII Congres International de Medicine, Moscou, IV, 433–442.
63. Happle R (1990) Acanthokeratolytic epidermal nevus: acanthokeratolysis is hereditary, not the nevus. **Hautarzt** 41:117–118.
64. Paller AS, Syder AJ, Chan YM et al. (1994) Genetic and clinical mosaicism in a type of epidermal nevus. **N Engl J Med** 331:1408–1415.
65. DiGiovanna JJ, Bale SJ (1994) Clinical heterogeneity in epidermolytic hyperkeratosis. **Arch Dermatol** 130:1026–1035.

TABLE 8.4   Clinical subtypes of epidermolytic hyperkeratosis of Brocq

Clinical features	PS-1	PS-2	PS-3	NPS-1	NPS-2	NPS-3
Palmoplantar hyperkeratosis	+	+	+	−	−	−
Surface characteristic	Smooth	Smooth	Ceribriform	Normal	Normal	Hyperlinear
Contractures	−	+	−	−	−	−
Scale	Mild	White scale, peel	Tan	Hystrix	Brown	Fine, white
Distribution	Localized	Generalized	Generalized	Generalized	Generalized	Generalized
Erythroderma	−	+	−	−	−	+
Blistering	Localized	+	Neonatal	+	+	+

PS, epidermolytic hyperkeratosis with severe palmoplantar hyperkeratosis; NPS, epidermolytic hyperkeratosis without severe palmoplantar hyperkeratosis; +, feature present; −, feature absent.
Modified from: DiGiovanna and Bale, Arch Dermatol 130:1026–1035, 1994.

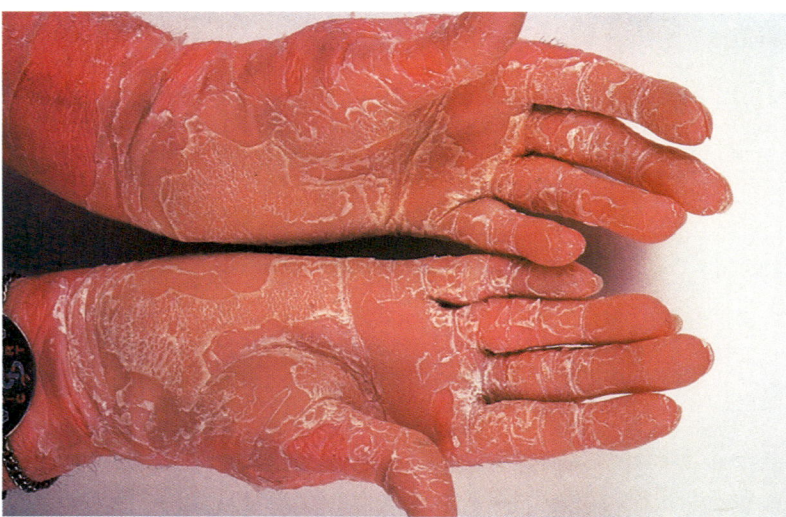

Fig. 8.9   Diffuse palmar hyperkeratosis with flexural contractures, fissures and underlying erythema in a patient with EHK type PS-2. (Courtesy of Dr. J.J. DiGiovanna)

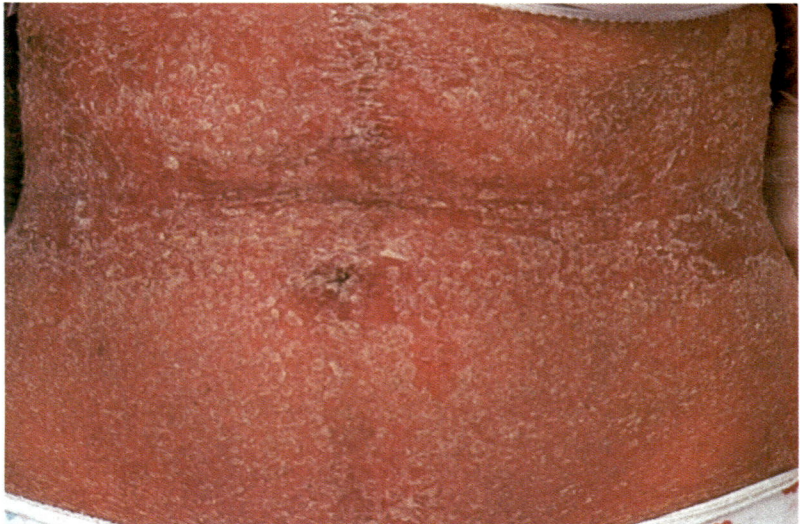

Fig. 8.10   Generalized erythroderma, scaling and peeling. Epidermolytic hyperkeratosis type PS-2. (Courtesy of Dr. J.J. DiGiovanna)

six clinical phenotypes of EHK (Table 8.4). They distinguished between two major subtypes, namely EHK with severe involvement of palms and soles (Palm/Sole types PS1–3) and without (Non-Palm/Sole types NPS1–3). EHK of PS type 1 is characterized by hyperkeratosis predominantly restricted to palms, soles and flexural areas. The palmoplantar keratoderma is diffuse, has a smooth surface and sharply demarcated erythematous border, and often displays areas of peeling. Severe, diffuse palmoplantar keratoderma in PS type 2 leads to fissures and digital contractures, and is associated with generalized, mild to moderate erythroderma as well as hyperkeratosis with a fine, white scale (Fig. 8.9 and 8.10). The rare PS type 3 is characterized by a distinct, cerebriform appearance of palms and soles and generalized hyperkeratosis with ridged or verrucous pattern. In contrast, the generalized, non-erythrodermic hyperkeratosis seen in NPS type 1 almost completely spares the skin of palms and soles. The thickened, yellow to dark brown, dirty-appearing skin has a verrucous surface or sharp, protruding spines, which has been described as ichthyosis hystrix (Fig. 8.11). The extremities over the joints, back, areas around umbilicus and areolae, and the scalp are most severely affected. While the hyperkeratosis usually forms a linear, ridged pattern in flexural areas, it has a cobblestone appearance over the extensor surface of the joints (Fig. 8.12). The face is relatively spared. Patients with NPS type 2 have a similar but much milder disease resembling ichthyosis bullosa of Siemens. NPS type 3 is associated with a generalized mild erythroderma, and a fine white scale.

In general, focal episodes of blistering are common, and often triggered by secondary infections and trauma or friction. Patients shed the thickened, hard superficial epidermis in large plates, most likely due to intraepidermal blistering, thereby revealing a tender, erythematous base or erosions.

Hair, nails, teeth, and mucous membranes
Severe scalp involvement with encasement of the hair shafts is a common feature of EHK. Lips, eyes, mucous membranes and teeth are normal, but linear arrayed hyperkeratosis in the corners of the mouth is not uncommon.

Systemic manifestations
Although EHK affects primarily the skin, there is perinatal morbidity and potential mortality in affected infants due to sepsis, as well as fluid and electrolyte imbalance. Posture and gait abnormalities are not infrequent and might be a result from pain in the skin overlying joints. EHK is accompanied by a very distinct, pungent body odor, which is disturbing to patients and their families and impairs their social life.

LABORATORY FINDINGS
Prenatal diagnosis
EHK is an inherited keratin disorder of the epidermis, which can be detected early during fetal development by electron microscopy of fetal skin or amniotic fluid cells. Diagnostic findings are an abnormal expression pattern of epidermal keratins and cytoplasmic clumping of keratin

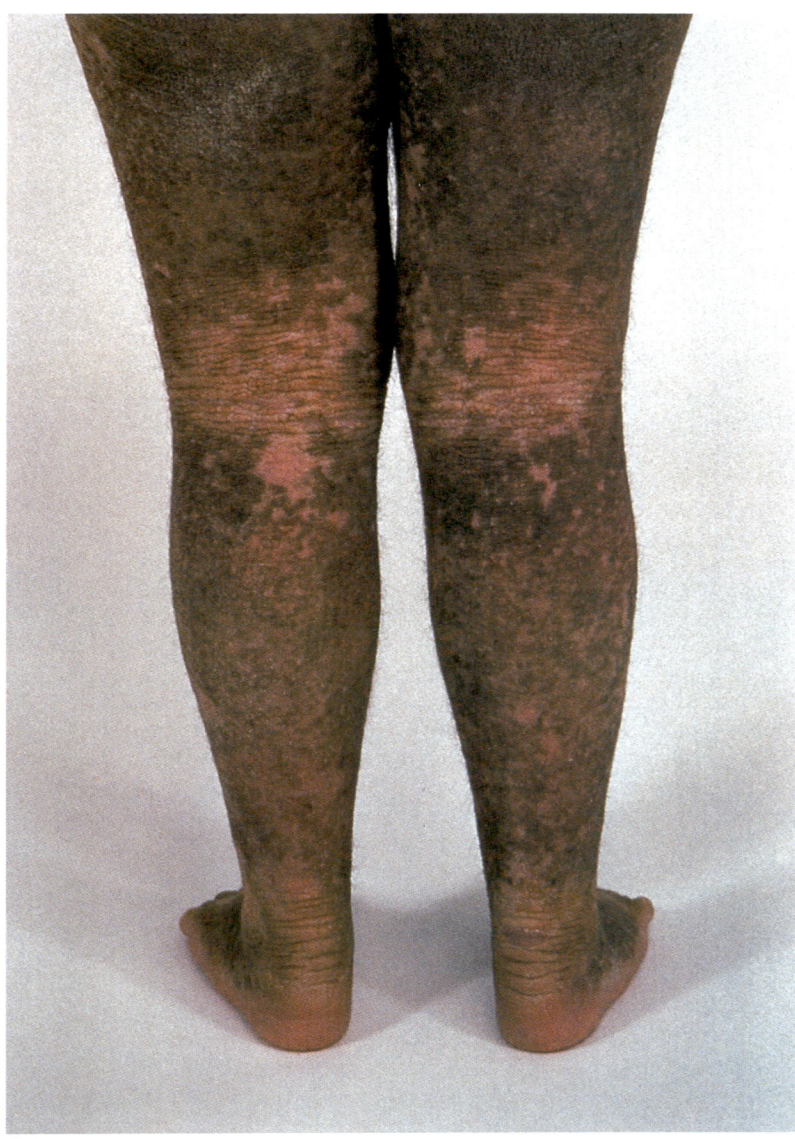

Fig. 8.11   Generalized skin involvement with thick, dark brown, verrucous hyperkeratosis. Note the ridged pattern in the knee folds. Epidermolytic hyperkeratosis type NPS-1. (Courtesy of Dr. J.J. DiGiovanna)

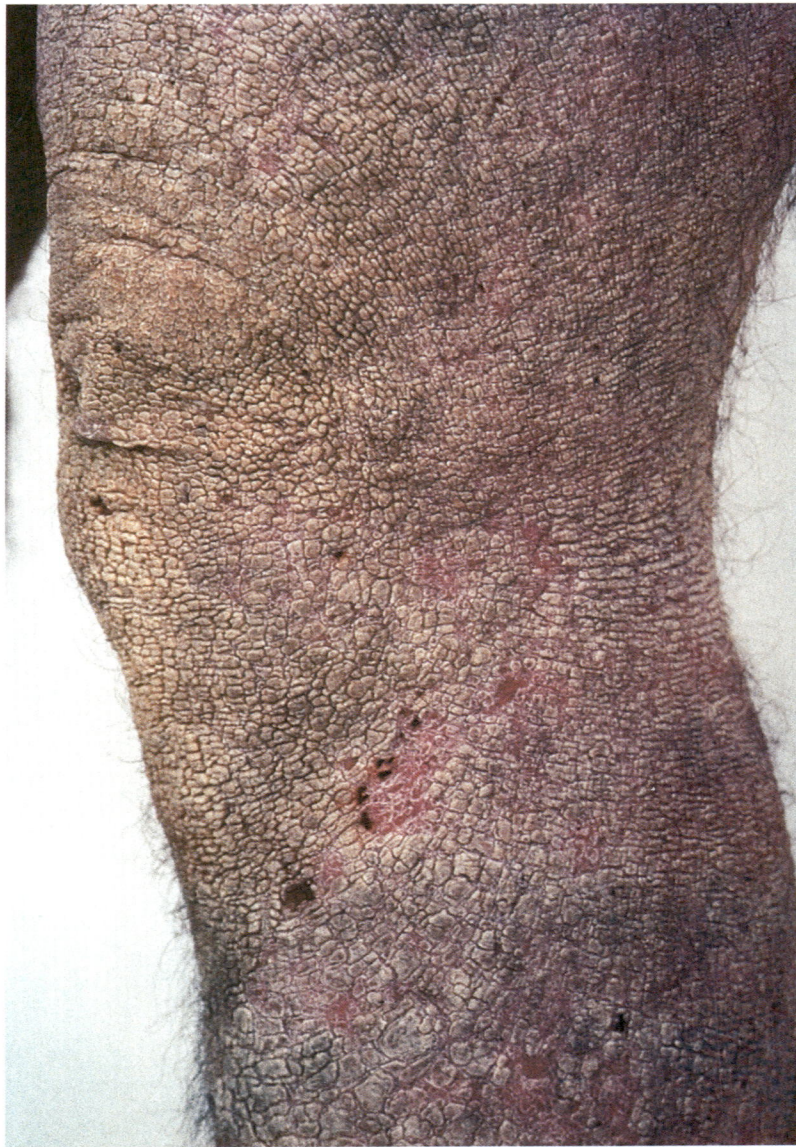

Fig. 8.12   Severe hyperkeratosis with cobblestone surface pattern over the extensor surface of the knee joint and linear arrangement in the knee fold. Note the shedding of large plates of superficial epidermis. Epidermolytic hyperkeratosis type PS-1. (Courtesy of Dr. J.J. DiGiovanna)

intermediate filaments (KIF) in the upper epidermis.[66,67] However, these methods have been widely replaced by molecular testing. In two-thirds of all patients with EHK, disease-causing mutations can be identified in either the keratin 1 or keratin 10 gene (*KRT1*, *KRT10*).[68] Direct DNA sequence analysis or other methods of mutation detection have been successfully performed from CVS or amniotic fluid material, allowing prenatal diagnosis as early as the 10th to 12th week of gestation.[69]

PATHOPHYSIOLOGY AND HISTOGENESIS

Histologic findings

EHK is characterized by distinct structural and ultrastructural abnormalities that separate EHK from other congenital ichthyoses (Fig. 8.13). A strikingly acanthotic epidermis with hypergranulosis is covered by a massive thickened,

dense, orthokeratotic stratum corneum. Keratinocytes of the suprabasal and granular layers exhibit marked intracellular vacuolization and dense clumps of keratin intermediate filaments (KIF). Cytolysis may lead to formation of small intraepidermal blisters with a cleavage plane in the middle or upper spinous layers. Collectively, these histopathological changes are described as "epidermolytic hyperkeratosis." A mild perivascular lymphohistiocytic infiltrate is usually present in the upper dermis.

Molecular and biochemical basis and histogenesis

Ultrastructural analysis in EHK reveals fragmented, clumped KIF in the lower, and perinuclear KIF shells in the upper epidermal layers. The assembly of the

66. Holbrook KA, Dale BA, Sybert VP et al. (1983) Epidermolytic hyperkeratosis: ultrastructure and biochemistry of skin and amniotic fluid cells from two affected fetuses and a newborn infant. **J Invest Dermatol** 80:222–227.
67. Eady RA, Gunner DB, Carbone LD et al. (1986) Prenatal diagnosis of bullous ichthyosiform erythroderma: detection of tonofilament clumps in fetal epidermal and amniotic fluid cells. **J Med Genet** 23:46–51.
68. Bale SJ, Compton JG, DiGiovanna JJ (1993) Epidermolytic hyperkeratosis. **Semin Dermatol** 12:202–209.
69. Rothnagel JA, Lin MT, Longley MA et al. (1998) Prenatal diagnosis for keratin mutations to exclude transmission of epidermolytic hyperkeratosis. **Prenat Diagn** 18:826–830.

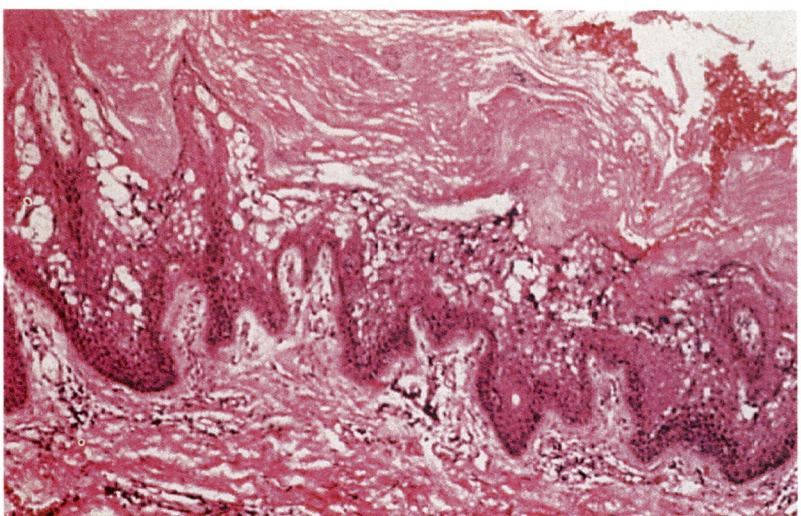

Fig. 8.13   Characteristic histopathologic features of EHK. Massive hyperkeratosis and vacuolar degeneration of the upper spinous layers of the acanthotic and papillomatous epidermis.

cornified cell envelope is altered but keratohyaline granules appear normal. Collapse of the cytoskeleton also impairs association of KIF with desmosomal proteins, thus resulting in cell fragility, acantholysis and cytolysis. Despite the massive hyperkeratosis, the barrier function of the skin is markedly disturbed leading to increased transepidermal water loss[70] and bacterial colonization of the stratum corneum, in particular with *Staphylococcus aureus*. The epidermal proliferation in EHK is markedly increased.[71]

Different approaches including genetic linkage analysis, ultrastructural examination, and mouse models of EHK led almost simultaneously to the discovery of the molecular basis of EHK.[20,72,73] EHK is an inherited disorder of epidermal cell fragility resulting from heterozygous mutations in the genes *KRT1* and *KRT10* localized on chromosomes 17q12–q21 and 12q11–q13. Keratins 1 (type II) and 10 (type I) are the principal, differentiation-specific keratins in the upper epidermis. Their expression pattern correlates with fragility and cytolysis of the superficial epidermis in EHK, while the basal expression of keratins 5 and 14 parallels the site of disease pathology in epidermolysis bullosa simplex.

To date, at least 36 distinct pathogenic mutations have been identified in *KRT1* and *KRT10* in patients with EHK. The mutations are nonrandomly distributed, and more than 80% cluster at the 1A and 2B boundaries of the rod domains representing mutational "hot spots".[21,74,75] The most common mutations, present in more than 30% of all EHK patients, affect the arginine codon 156 in *KRT10*, which contains a methylated and hypermutable CpG dinucleotide.[21] *In vivo* and *in vitro* studies demonstrated that these mutations perturb proper keratin alignment, and thereby oligomerization, filament assembly and integrity. As a result, the KIF network is fragile, disrupted

and less resistant to stress, thus compromising mechanical strength and cell integrity of the epidermis and leading to cytolysis and blistering. Compensatory overexpression of the alternate (hyperproliferative) keratins 6 and 16 in affected skin might contribute to the improvement of skin fragility with age.

The etiology of acanthosis and hyperkeratosis in EHK is not as well understood, and probably includes hyperproliferation of the epidermis combined with decreased desquamation and other factors.[76] The deleterious effect of keratin 1 or 10 mutations on permeability barrier function of the epidermis becomes evident in mice completely deficient in keratin 10, which have an eight-fold increase in transepidermal water loss compared to normal mice, while heterozygous animals exhibit a delay in barrier repair and reduced hydration of the stratum corneum. Although the stratum corneum in EHK appears ultrastructurally normal, its lipid composition is significantly altered with a decreased ratio of ceramides to total lipids due to reduced activity of acid sphingomyelinase.[76,77] Recent biochemical and ultrastructural studies in patients with EHK largely confirmed these observations. In addition, they revealed incomplete lamellar body secretion as evident by decreased delivery of acid lipase to the stratum corneum. This secretion deficiency is likely a direct effect of altered KIF structure and interaction with lamellar bodies (rather than increased fragility of corneocytes or an abnormal cornified cell envelope).[78]

Genotype/phenotype correlations in EHK disclose a tight relationship between the clinical subtype of EHK (PS vs. NPS) and the causative gene. Because KIF formation in suprabasal keratinocytes requires the presence of both keratin 1 and keratin 10, mutations in either gene may produce a similar phenotype. Nevertheless, *KRT1* mutations are usually associated with severe palmoplantar keratoderma whereas mutations in *KRT10* result in EHK with sparing of palms and soles.[65] This difference is explained by the limited expression pattern of *KRT10* that does not include the palmoplantar epidermis. Unusual types of EHK, such as "cyclic ichthyosis with epidermolytic hyperkeratosis" and "annular epidermolytic ichthyosis" have been associated with distinct mutations in the rod domains of *KRT1* and *KRT10*, respectively, but did fall within the helix termination motifs.[79–81] Mutations outside of the helix boundaries are rare and generally associated with a milder phenotype, although the number of mutations identified is still too low to draw definitive conclusions.

The molecular basis of mosaic EHK are somatic mutations in *KRT1* or *KRT10*.[64] Paller *et al.*[64] studied a family in which the parent of a child with generalized EHK had mosaic skin involvement following Blaschko's lines. Mutation analysis in cultured keratinocytes from the affected skin of the parent identified a heterozygous mutation in *KRT10*, which was absent in keratinocytes from normal skin but identical to the mutation of the affected child. A recently developed mouse model for mosaic EHK allowed the temporary activation of a somatic *KRT10* mutation in the murine epidermis, and demonstrated that the lack of selective pressure against this mutation in epidermal stem cells leads to the mosaic phenotype.[82]

DIFFERENTIAL DIAGNOSIS

Widespread blistering and denuded skin in a neonate with EHK are difficult to distinguish clinically from different forms of epidermolysis bullosa, staphy-

70. Frost P, Weinstein GD, Bothwell JW et al. (1968) Ichthyosiform dermatoses. 3. Studies of transepidermal water loss. **Arch Dermatol** 98:230–233.
71. Frost P, Weinstein GD, Van Scott EJ (1966) The ichthyosiform dermatoses. II. Autoradiographic studies of epidermal proliferation. **J Invest Dermatol** 47:561–567.
72. Rothnagel JA, Dominey AM, Dempsey LD et al. (1992) Mutations in the rod domains of keratins 1 and 10 in epidermolytic hyperkeratosis. **Science** 257:1128–1130.
73. Chipev CC, Korge BP, Markova N et al. (1992) A leucine – proline mutation in the H1 subdomain of keratin 1 causes epidermolytic hyperkeratosis. **Cell** 70:821–828.
74. Corden LD, McLean WH (1996) Human keratin diseases: hereditary fragility of specific epithelial tissues. **Exp Dermatol** 5:297–307.
75. Compton JJ (2001) Personal communication.
76. Reichelt J, Doering T, Schnetz E et al. (1999) Normal ultrastructure, but altered stratum corneum lipid and protein composition in a mouse model for epidermolytic hyperkeratosis. **J Invest Dermatol** 113:329–334.

77. Jensen JM, Schutze S, Neumann C et al. (2000) Impaired cutaneous permeability barrier function, skin hydration, and sphingomyelinase activity in keratin 10 deficient mice. **J Invest Dermatol** 115:708–713.
78. Yosipovitch G, Williams ML, Hintner H et al. (2001) Pathogenesis of the permeability barrier abnormality in epidermolytic ichthyosis. **J Invest Dermatol** 116:164.
79. Joh GY, Traupe H, Metze D et al. (1997) A novel dinucleotide mutation in keratin 10 in the annular epidermolytic ichthyosis variant of bullous congenital ichthyosiform erythroderma. **J Invest Dermatol** 108:357–361.
80. Suga Y, Duncan KO, Heald PW et al. (1998) A novel helix termination mutation in keratin 10 in annular epidermolytic ichthyosis, a variant of bullous congenital ichthyosiform erythroderma. **J Invest Dermatol** 111:1220–1223.
81. Sybert VP, Francis JS, Corden LD et al. (1999) Cyclic ichthyosis with epidermolytic hyperkeratosis: A phenotype conferred by mutations in the 2B domain of keratin K1. **Am J Hum Genet** 64:732–738.
82. Arin MJ, Longley MA, Wang XJ et al. (2001) Focal activation of a mutant allele defines the role of stem cells in mosaic skin disorders. **J Cell Biol** 152:645–649.

lococcal scalded skin syndrome, and toxic epidermal necrolysis. Light and electron microscopic examination of frozen skin biopsy material obtained from the margin of a fresh blister and bacterial cultures usually lead to the diagnosis. If epidermolysis bullosa is suspected, immuno-mapping and ultrastructural analysis are necessary to determine the specific subtype. Neonates with AEC syndrome (Hay–Wells syndrome, MIM 106260) may present with erosions and collodion membrane, but have also ankyloblepharon, hair and nail dystrophy, and cleft lip/cleft palate. Incontinentia pigmenti can be discriminated by the nevoid distribution of vesicles and different histopathology. In addition, one should rule out bullous mastocytosis, congenital syphilis, and herpes simplex.

Later during infancy and childhood, EHK is readily distinguished from congenital recessive ichthyoses on account of generalized blistering at birth and occurrence of focal blisters thereafter. These clinical impressions can be confirmed by skin biopsy revealing the distinctive light microscopic features of epidermolytic hyperkeratosis. Similar histologic findings may be also seen in the epidermolytic form of palmoplantar keratoderma (type Vörner, MIM 144200), which is clinically characterized by isolated, diffuse palmoplantar keratoderma with a striking red margin. This autosomal dominant genodermatosis is caused by mutations in the KRT9 gene that is predominantly expressed in the suprabasal epidermis of palms and soles.[74,83]

Ichthyosis bullosa of Siemens can be distinguished from EHK by the absence of erythroderma, the characteristic molting of the outer layer of the epidermis (Mauserung) as well as by the very superficial epidermolysis of the granular cell layers seen on light microscopy. The different site of skin pathology (granular vs. spinous cell layers of the epidermis) is paralleled by the distinct expression pattern of keratin 2e, which is structurally altered due to dominant mutations in the KRT2e gene.[74,84]

Ichthyosis hystrix Curth–Macklin may closely resemble EHK with ridged, verrucous hyperkeratosis over joints and flexures in some patients, while others have only limited hyperkeratosis restricted to palms and soles. In contrast to EHK, there is no clinical or histological evidence for blister formation and epidermolysis. Instead, ultrastructural analysis reveals cytoplasmic shells of fine, tangled KIF in the upper differentiated cell layers of the epidermis associated with perinuclear vacuolization and binucleated cells.[85]

Mosaic EHK may occur unilaterally or bilaterally distributed along the lines of Blaschko. Extensive involvement exhibiting marked hyperkeratosis with verrucous surface or porcupine-like spines has often been described as ichthyosis hystrix. Ichthyosis hystrix is not a disorder per se but a descriptive name for a clinically and genetically heterogeneous group of skin disorders with massive, spiky, or verrucous hyperkeratosis, including EHK, erythrokeratodermia variabilis, ichthyosis hystrix Curth–Macklin, hyperkeratotic epidermal nevi and others.

THERAPEUTICS AND PROGNOSIS
Neonatal period
Infants with erythema, blistering, widespread erosions, and denuded skin require management in a neonatal intensive care nursery. They should be handled gently to avoid further trauma to the skin and blistering, and placed in protective isolation and monitored for development of sepsis. In some patients, treatment with broad-spectrum antibiotics may be necessary. Dehydration and electrolyte imbalances are not uncommon and have to be treated accordingly. Erosions and denuded skin generally heal rapidly, which can be supported by use of lubricants and protective padding.

Topical therapy
The treatment for EHK, like other congenital ichthyoses, is symptomatic and often difficult. It should be tailored to the specific needs of the patient depending on the acute clinical presentation at the time of consultation. Extensive, thick, hard hyperkeratosis requires hydration, lubrication, and keratolytic treatment. Recurrent and long bathing are suitable to moisten the skin and facilitate mechanical abrasion of the thickened stratum corneum (gentle scrubbing with a soft brush, sponges, etc.). Additional use of antiseptics such as antibacterial soaps, chlorhexidine, or iodine may help control bacterial colonization. The use of lubricants and emollients at least twice daily is recommended, but specific agents and formulations may be selected based on individual preferences of the patient. Many commercially available keratolytic creams and lotions containing urea, salicylic acid, alphahydroxy acids, or propylene glycol are effective to diminish and remove scale, and to soften the skin. However, they are often not well tolerated, especially in children, because of burning and stinging when the skin is fissured or denuded. Occlusion may enhance the effect but should be used with care in children or patients with heat intolerance. Widespread topical application of salicylic and lactic acid should be avoided because of the risk of systemic absorption. Topical tretinoin and vitamin D preparations are effective but costly and may cause skin irritation. A therapeutic option is treatment of the exposed skin areas only, rendering the visible parts more acceptable. Bacterial skin infections are common in EHK and often trigger blistering, thus requiring topical treatment with antibiotic ointments or even courses of oral antibiotics.

Systemic management (See also CIE)
Synthetic oral retinoids may be very effective in decreasing hyperkeratosis and frequency of infections in patients with generalized EHK. Nevertheless, these drugs augment the epidermal fragility of EHK and may lead to exacerbation of blistering.[86] It is advisable to start therapy at very low doses with the aim to reach the lowest possible maintenance dose and carefully monitor patients.[87] Methotrexate has limited efficacy in this disorder. Although oral antibiotics are helpful during episodes of blistering and bacterial superinfections, continuous preventive therapy (oral or topical antibiotics) should be avoided because of the risk of development of resistant bacterial strains.

Prognosis
Severe neonatal blistering rapidly improves and most children exhibit only focal blistering in response to trauma or secondary infection. Adult patients may experience little to no blistering. The hyperkeratosis progresses during childhood and persists throughout life but occasionally may improve. Clinical type and course of EHK are relatively consistent within families.

PEDIATRIC ASPECTS OF THE DISEASE

It is important to avoid mechanical trauma to the skin because of the increased skin fragility (e.g., comfortable clothing and shoe wear). The acrid body odor and disfigurement in EHK may pose social problems and can harm the psychosocial development of children and should be addressed. Patient advocacy organizations such as the Foundation for Ichthyosis and Related Skin Types (FIRST) and the National Organization for Rare Disorders (NORD) offer valuable information material, facilitate personal contacts with other affected families, and support patients and their families.

83. Reis A, Hennies HC, Langbein L et al. (1994) Keratin 9 gene mutations in epidermolytic palmoplantar keratoderma (EPPK). Nat Genet 6:174–179.
84. Rothnagel JA, Traupe H, Wojcik S et al. (1994) Mutations in the rod domain of keratin 2e in patients with ichthyosis bullosa of Siemens. Nat Genet 7:485–490.
85. Sprecher E, Ishida-Yamamoto A, Becker OM et al. (2001) Evidence for novel functions of the keratin tail emerging from a mutation causing ichthyosis hystrix. J Invest Dermatol 116:511–519.
86. Happle R, van de Kerkhof PC, Traupe H (1987) Retinoids in disorders of keratinization: their use in adults. Dermatologica 175:107–124.
87. Lacour M, Mehta-Nikhar B, Atherton DJ et al. (1996) An appraisal of acitretin therapy in children with inherited disorders of keratinization. Br J Dermatol 134:1023–1029.

ICHTHYOSIS BULLOSA OF SIEMENS

Gabriele Richard

Synonym: Ichthyosis exfoliativa (MIM 146800)

This autosomal dominant genodermatosis was first recognized as a distinct entity by Siemens in 1937.[88] It has a milder phenotype than EHK and spares palms and soles. Erythroderma and blistering apparent at birth and during early infancy subsequently subside, while hyperkeratosis develops with predilection to flexures, over joints, and on the dorsa of hands and feet. The skin surface may appear ridged, shiny or lichenified. Characteristic are superficially denuded areas with collarette-like borders described as "molting" or "*Mauserung*," which develop due to superficial blistering and shedding of the stratum corneum. The histopathologic abnormalities of orthokeratotic hyperkeratosis, acanthosis, cytolysis, and clumping of tonofilaments are similar to EHK but limited to the granular and uppermost spinous cell layers, which express keratin 2e. Ichthyosis bullosa of Siemens is caused by heterozygous mutations in the *KRT2e* gene, most of which alter glutamic acid codon 493 (E493K) in the helix termination motif.[74]

ICHTHYOSIS HYSTRIX CURTH–MACKLIN

Gabriele Richard

Ichthyosis hystrix Curth–Macklin (MIM 146590) is a rare autosomal dominant disorder of cornification that may clinically mimic EHK but displays no skin fragility. Since the first description in 1954 only two large families and a few sporadic cases of IHCM have been reported. The clinical expression varies not only between but also within families, and ranges from palmoplantar keratoderma, which may be severe and mutilating, to generalized skin involvement. Ichthyosis hystrix Curth–Macklin can be differentiated from

EHK by its peculiar ultrastructural abnormalities of the KIF cytoskeleton in differentiating keratinocytes. KIF are not arranged in thick bundles but instead form a shell–like, interspersed network of tangled filaments often associated with perinuclear vacuolization and formation of binucleated cells. In contrast to EHK, there is no evidence for epidermolysis or keratin clumping. As demonstrated in one family, ichthyosis hystrix Curth–Macklin is also a keratin disorder due to a heterozygous frameshift mutation in *KRT1* affecting the keratin tail domain. Consequently, the mutation results in drastic alteration of the composition, chemical character, structure and properties of the keratin 1 tail, thereby interfering with supramolecular organization of KIF and their interactions with other differentiation-specific proteins such as loricrin.[85]

LAMELLAR ICHTHYOSIS AND CONGENITAL ICHTHYOSIFORM ERYTHRODERMA

Gabriele Richard

The congenital autosomal recessive ichthyoses form a rare, clinically and genetically heterogeneous group of disorders with generalized scaling of the skin from birth. They occur worldwide with an estimated prevalence of 1 in 200 000 persons, but may be more common in inbred populations.[89] Terminology and nosology of these disorders has continuously evolved, resulting in much confusion. More than 100 years ago, the all-comprising group of "ichthyosis congenita" was separated into harlequin ichthyosis, a bullous and a nonbullous form of congenital ichthyosiform erythroderma,[7] or synonymously used, congenital ichthyosiform erythroderma. Frost and Van Scott[9] fortified this distinction and proposed the descriptive terms "lamellar ichthyosis" for all autosomal recessive forms and, based on distinctive histopathological features, "epidermolytic" hyperkeratosis for the autosomal dominant form of congenital ichthyosis. Subsequently, Traupe *et al.*[90] identified also an autosomal dominant form of lamellar ichthyosis with clinical features mainly indistinguishable from the recessive forms.

TABLE 8.5   Differences between congenital ichthyosiform erythroderma (CIE) and lamellar ichthyosis (LI)

	CIE	LI
Clinical	Fine, white scale Bright red erythroderma, but intensity may vary	Thick, dark, plate-like scale Erythroderma absent or mild
Histopathological	SC thickened Parakeratosis to variable extent Prominent mucin or glycosaminoglycans in SC cell membranes	SC massively thickened No parakeratosis No PAS + membranes
Ultrastructural	Abnormal and increased number of lamellar bodies Numerous lipid droplets within cornified cells Extensive bilayer stacks in intercellular spaces of SC Not seen Seen only in few patients	Normal lamellar bodies Not seen Not seen Cholesterol clefts in SC Absent or diminished cornified cell envelope
Molecular	Heterogeneous Mutations in TGM1 in a small subset of patients	Heterogeneous Mutations in TGM1 in about 1/2 of patients
Biochemical	Abnormal intracellular accumulation of TG1 and moderately diminished activity in a small number of patients Butyrase/glucosidase ratio 90 to 100	Absent or strongly diminished TG activity *in vivo* and *in vitro* (≤10% in cultured keratinocytes) in about 1/2 of patients Butyrase/glucosidase ratio <5

CIE, congenital ichthyosiform erythroderma; SC, stratum corneum; TG, transglutaminase-1; *TGM1*, transglutaminase-1 gene (Data from Ghadially et al.[18], Bergers et al.[10], Finlay et al.[461], Laiho et al.[115], Niemi et al.[17], Choate et al.[122], and Hohl et al.[108])

---

88. Siemens HW (1937) Dichtung und Wahrheit ueber die Ichthyosis bullosa, mit Bemerkungen zur Systematik der Epidermolysen. **Derm Syph** 175:590–608.
89. Wells RS (1966) Ichthyosis. **Br Med J** 2:1504–1506.
90. Traupe H, Kolde G, Happle R (1984) Autosomal dominant lamellar ichthyosis: a new skin disorder. **Clin Genet** 26:457–461.

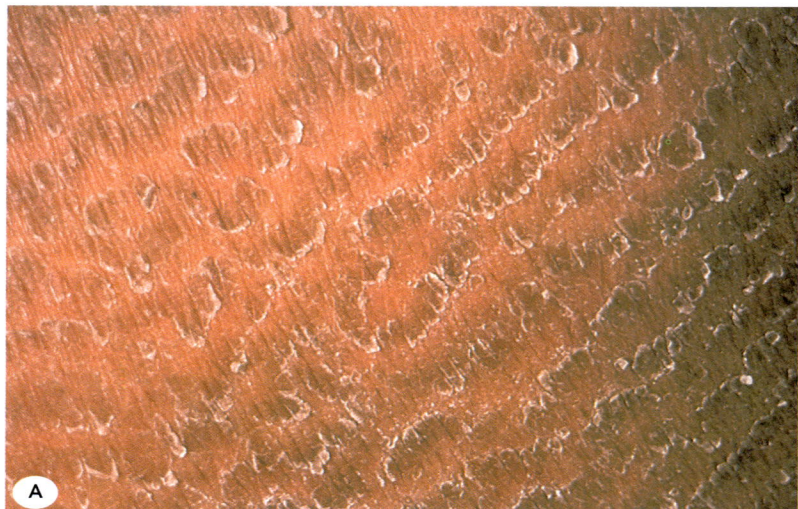

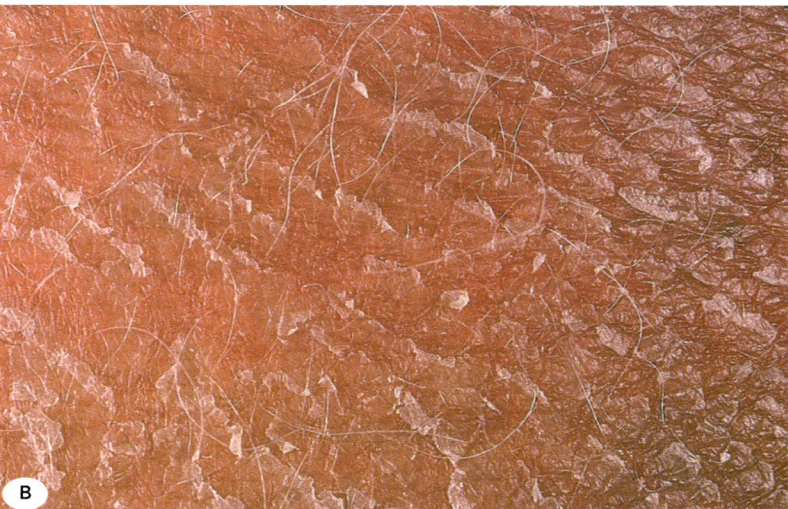

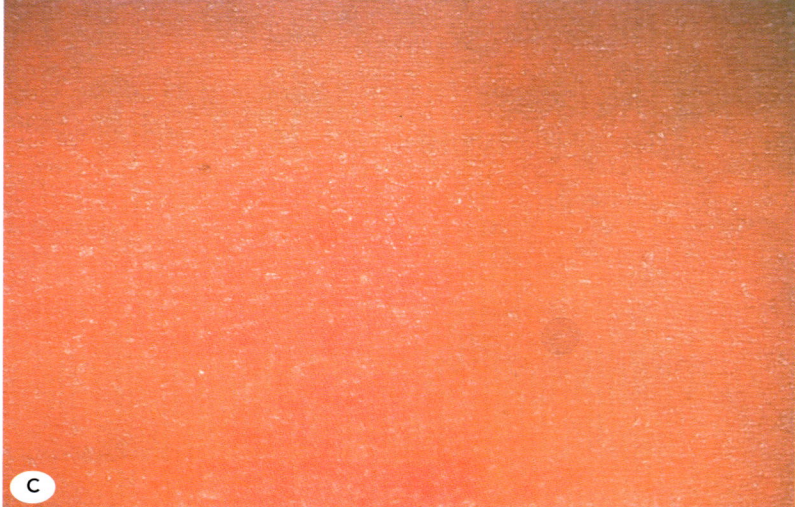

Fig. 8.14   The clinical phenotypes of congenital recessive ichthyoses span a wide range depending on the degree of erythroderma as well as size and quality of scale. On one end of the spectrum lies lamellar ichthyosis with large, dark, plate-like scales, ectropion and without discernible erythroderma (A). The other extreme is represented by congenital ichthyosiform erythroderma, characterized by bright red erythroderma and fine, white scale (C). The intermediate phenotypes fall anywhere between with variable degrees of erythema and scaling (B).

TABLE 8.6   Disorders with collodion membrane presentation

Disorder	Frequency
Lamellar ichthyosis	Common
Congenital ichthyosiform erythroderma	Common
CIE/LI intermediate phenotypes	Common
Autosomal dominant lamellar ichthyosis/congenital ichthyosiform erythroderma	Rare
Self-healing collodion baby	Always
Sjögren–Larsson syndrome	Rare
Trichothiodystrophy	Rare
Infantile Gaucher disease	Rare
Hay–Wells syndrome	Rare

(Data from Larrègue et al.[94], Jagell et al.[484,485], Stone et al.[465], and Frenk et al.[95])

The considerable clinical heterogeneity of autosomal recessive ichthyoses both prompted and limited arduous attempts to further refine their distinction using clinical, histological, biochemical, and ultrastructural markers, which were further hampered by the limited number of patients available for study. Bernhardt and Baden[91] recognized four subtypes predominantly based on severity of disease, while Bergers et al.[10] used discrepancies in the activity of hydrolytic enzymes in the scale of patients to differentiate between an erythrodermic and nonerythrodermic form of autosomal recessive lamellar ichthyosis. Based predominantly on ultrastructural abnormalities of the stratum corneum, Anton-Lamprecht and others identified three major types of congenital autosomal recessive ichthyoses including the accumulation of lipid droplets in type I, formation of "cholesterol" clefts in type II, and lamellated membrane structures in type III.[13,15,17,92] However, these correlate only loosely with the clinical subtypes of ichthyoses. Clinical scrutiny together with the incorporation of up-to-date knowledge on ichthyoses led Traupe[19] to propose a new classification of ichthyoses into 4 major types. He defined lamellar ichthyosis as an isolated congenital ichthyosis, which comprises three forms, the erythrodermic, nonerythrodermic and autosomal dominant lamellar ichthyosis. Using clinical, biochemical, and histologic criteria combined with differences in the epidermal proliferation rate,[11] Williams and Elias[12]

further discriminated the two distinct phenotypes among the recessive forms of nonbullous congenital ichthyoses, distinguishing between lamellar ichthyosis (LI) and (nonbullous) congenital ichthyosiform erythroderma (CIE; Table 8.5). In our current, and certainly preliminary, understanding, the clinical presentation of autosomal recessive ichthyoses encompasses a range of phenotypes with these two entities on each end of the spectrum (Fig. 8.14).[93] Both disorders frequently present at birth with a collodion membrane, which over time develops into lamellar ichthyosis, congenital ichthyosiform erythroderma, other disorders,[94] or may spontaneously resolve (self-healing collodion baby)[95] (Table 8.6). LI in its classic presentation with large, dark, plate-like scales, ectropion without discernible erythroderma can be readily distinguished from classic CIE with generalized redness and fine white scaling. In many patients, however, the skin disorder demonstrates intermediate

91. Bernhardt M, Baden HP (1986) Report of a family with an unusual expression of recessive ichthyosis. Review of 42 cases. **Arch Dermatol** 122:428–433.
92. Arnold ML, Anton-Lamprecht I, Melz-Rothfuss B et al. (1988) Ichthyosis congenita type III. Clinical and ultrastructural characteristics and distinction within the heterogeneous ichthyosis congenita group. **Arch Dermatol Res** 280:268–278.
93. Bale SJ, Russell LJ, Lee ML et al. (1996) Congenital recessive ichthyosis unlinked to loci for epidermal transglutaminases. **J Invest Dermatol** 107:808–811.
94. Larrègue M, Ottavy N, Bressieux JM et al. (1986) [Collodion baby: 32 new case reports]. **Ann Dermatol Venereol** 113:773–785.
95. Frenk E, de Techtermann F (1992) Self-healing collodion baby: evidence for autosomal recessive inheritance. **Pediatr Dermatol** 9:95–97.

phenotypes with variable degrees of erythema and scaling. Since histological, biochemical and ultrastructural features are often not conclusive, there is currently no consensus on a commonly accepted and consistent classification, and further discrimination between LI, CIE, and intermediate phenotypes awaits the discovery of their specific underlying molecular defects.

LAMELLAR ICHTHYOSIS (LI)

Synonym: Ichthyosis congenita type 2, MIM 242300, 601277, 604777, 146750

Lamellar ichthyosis (LI) is a severe disorder of cornification, which usually presents at birth with collodion membrane, and is characterized by generalized skin involvement with large, dark brown scale, ectropion, eclabium, and scarring alopecia (Fig. 8.15). The descriptive name derives from the plate-like, lamellar appearance of the scale.

EPIDEMIOLOGY

Genetics

LI is genetically heterogeneous and in most families inherited as an autosomal recessive trait. Thus families with an affected child face a recurrence risk of 25% for each pregnancy. In as many as 50% of all patients, the disorder is caused by deleterious mutations in the gene encoding transglutaminase-1 (*TGM1*) located on chromosome 14q11.2.[96–98] The *TGM1* gene comprises 14kb including 15 coding exons. Over 49 distinct mutations have been identified so far,[75] most of which are scattered across the gene and either truncate the gene product or impair its function in the epidermis (null alleles). Due to a founder effect, a splice site mutation (2526A to G) resulting in alternative splicing of the *TGM1* message may account for the majority of mutant alleles in patients of northern European descent, and probably originates from a German predecessor.[99,100] However, there is convincing genetic evidence that defects in several other genes may underlie recessive LI. Two loci have been mapped on chromosome 2q33–q35 and 19p12–q12, while others remain to be identified.[101] In addition, exceedingly rare forms of autosomal dominant LI as well as CIE have been reported,[90,94,102] which has important implications for genetic counseling.

Statistics

Although the true incidence is unknown, LI is estimated to occur in 1 in 200 000 to 1 in 300 000 live births. Both genders are affected equally. It has been observed worldwide without ethnic clustering, although it is more common in populations with a high degree of consanguinity.

PRESENTING HISTORY

LI is apparent at birth. Most affected newborns are encased in a tight, shiny, translucent covering called collodion membrane. Over the first weeks of life, this thick horn layer dries, cracks, and is gradually replaced by generalized large scales.

PHYSICAL EXAMINATION

Skin

LI is characterized by dark brown, large and plate-like scales, which form a mosaic or bark-like pattern and involve the entire body surface including the

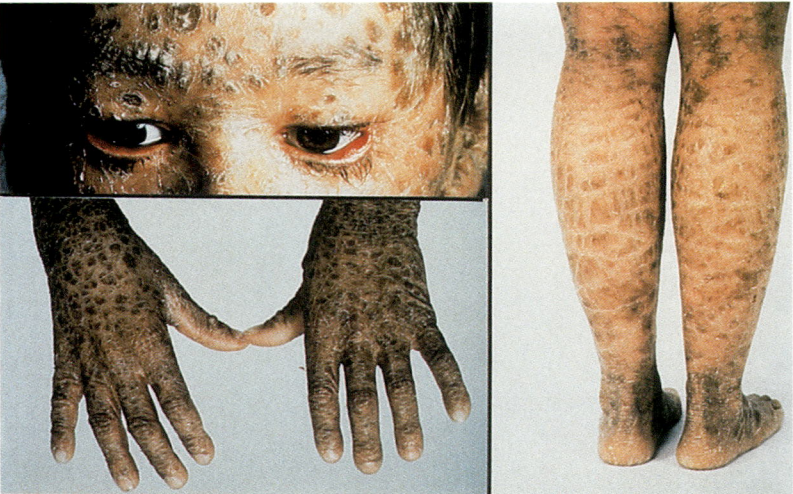

Fig. 8.15 Classical lamellar ichthyosis. Ectropion and madarosis (top left) and large, brown, plate-like scale (bottom left; right). From Russell *et al.*[486] with permission of The University of Chicago Press.

face, flexures and palms and soles (Fig. 8.15). The scales are centrally attached and often have raised borders leading to superficial fissures. Severe tautness of facial skin commonly results in ectropion and eclabium as well as a significant hypoplasia of nasal and auricular cartilage. While an underlying erythroderma can usually be appreciated during infancy, children and adults have minimal to no erythroderma. Palmoplantar keratoderma may vary, ranging from accentuated skin markings to severe thickening with cracking and fissuring.

Hair, nails, teeth, and mucous membranes

Severe scarring alopecia, especially at the periphery of the scalp, is a common feature of LI.[103] Hair shafts emerging from the scalp are encased by the thickened stratum corneum and the taut skin exerts traction and compression. Inflammation of the nail folds may produce secondary nail dystrophy with thickening of the nail plates and ridging. The thickened, firm stratum corneum in LI also constricts the sweat ducts, often resulting in severe heat intolerance. Although lips and mucous membranes tend to be spared, severe ectropion may lead to madarosis, conjunctivitis, and incomplete lid closure with ensuing keratitis.

Systemic manifestations (see also CIE)

LI is not primarily associated with systemic manifestations. Collodion babies have an increased incidence of premature birth with concomitant perinatal morbidity and mortality. They are at increased risk for sepsis, fluid and electrolyte imbalance and particularly hypovolemic hypernatremia.[94]

LABORATORY FINDINGS

Ultrastructural and immunohistochemical studies of skin biopsies in at least half of all LI patients reveal thin or absent cornified cell envelopes.[17,104] Biochemical *in vitro* assays of cultured keratinocytes often demonstrate drastically reduced transglutaminase-1 activity,[105] although it can be normal[106,107] due to genetic

96. Hennies HC, Kuster W, Wiebe V et al. (1998) Genotype/phenotype correlation in autosomal recessive lamellar ichthyosis. **Am J Hum Genet** 62:1052–1061.
97. Huber M, Rettler I, Bernasconi K et al. (1995) Mutations of keratinocyte transglutaminase in lamellar ichthyosis. **Science** 267:525–528.
98. Russell LJ, DiGiovanna JJ, Rogers GR et al. (1995) Mutations in the gene for transglutaminase 1 in autosomal recessive lamellar ichthyosis. **Nat Genet** 9:279–283.
99. Shevchenko YO, Compton JG, Toro JR et al. (2000) Splice-site mutation in TGM1 in congenital recessive ichthyosis in American families: molecular, genetic, genealogic, and clinical studies. **Hum Genet** 106:492–499.
100. Pigg M, Gedde-Dahl T, Jr., Cox D et al. (1998) Strong founder effect for a transglutaminase 1 gene mutation in lamellar ichthyosis and congenital ichthyosiform erythroderma from Norway. **Eur J Hum Genet** 6:589–596.
101. OMIM (2001) Online Mendelian Inheritance in Man. In. http://www3.ncbi.nlm.nih.gov/Omim/.

102. Toribio J, Fernandez Redondo V, Peteiro C et al. (1986) Autosomal dominant lamellar ichthyosis. **Clin Genet** 30:122–126.
103. Traupe H, Happle R (1983) Alopecia ichthyotica. A characteristic feature of congenital ichthyosis. **Dermatologica** 167:225–230.
104. Hohl D, Huber M, Frenk E (1993) Analysis of the cornified cell envelope in lamellar ichthyosis. **Arch Dermatol** 129:618–624.
105. Huber M, Yee VC, Burri N et al. (1997) Consequences of seven novel mutations on the expression and structure of keratinocyte transglutaminase. **J Biol Chem** 272:21018–21026.
106. Lavrijsen AP, Maruyama T (1995) Absent transglutaminase TGK expression in two of three patients with lamellar ichthyosis. **Arch Dermatol** 131:363–364.
107. Huber M, Rettler I, Bernasconi K et al. (1995) Lamellar ichthyosis is genetically heterogeneous – cases with normal keratinocyte transglutaminase. **J Invest Dermatol** 105:653–654.

heterogeneity. Recently, rapid screening procedures were developed to identify patients with transglutaminase-1 abnormalities using *in situ* detection of transglutaminase-1 expression and activity[108,109] and cross-linked cell envelopes.[110] DNA-based molecular studies of the *TGM1* gene are also available for diagnostic and prenatal diagnosis of LI, but are limited by the genetic heterogeneity of the disorder.

Prenatal diagnosis

In families with identifiable *TGM1* mutations or linkage to the *TGM1* locus on 14q11, prenatal diagnosis can be performed by mutation and/or genotype analysis from CVS or amniocentesis material.[111] Although problematic, light and electron microscopic examination of fetal skin samples or amniotic fluid cells obtained by fetoscopy in the second trimester has been successfully performed, predominantly based on the demonstration of marked, early hyperkeratinization of hair follicles.[112,113]

PATHOPHYSIOLOGY AND HISTOGENESIS

Histologic findings

The histological abnormalities in LI are nonspecific and include massive orthokeratotic hyperkeratosis with relatively mild acanthosis, regular papillomatosis, and dilated capillaries in the superficial dermis. In contrast to CIE, the epidermal proliferation rate is normal or only slightly elevated.[11] Elongated cholesterol clefts as well as a variable number of translucent lipid droplets in the stratum corneum and a thin or absent cornified cell envelope have been described as significant ultrastructural abnormalities in LI, although these findings widely overlap with those found in CIE.[17,92,114]

Molecular and biochemical basis and histogenesis

Deleterious mutations of the gene *TGM1* encoding the epidermally expressed enzyme transglutaminase-1 on chromosome 14q11 account for the disorder in many but not all patients exhibiting classical (nonerythrodermic) LI and in some patients with features of CIE (e.g., mild to moderate erythroderma, white or gray, small, sometimes plate-like scales).[96,99,115] The etiology of LI in patients without *TGM1* mutations, however, remains elusive. Transglutaminases are a superfamily of enzymes that catalyze the calcium-dependent cross-linking of proteins through the formation of *N*(epsilon)-(gammaglutamyl)lysine isopeptide bonds widely expressed throughout the body. In the epidermis, *TGM1* (together with *TGM3*) is expressed in the upper, most differentiated keratinocytes of the epidermis, where its gene product transglutaminase-1 serves a dual role during the cornification. The enzyme facilitates the formation of the insoluble protein envelope by cross-linking numerous structural proteins such as involucrin, small proline-rich proteins, loricrin, KIF and desmosomal proteins.[24] In addition, it is paramount for the ester linkage of epidermis-specific omega-hydroxyceramides to the plasma membrane and formation of the lipid envelope.[25] *TGM1* mutations resulting in lack of transglutaminase-1 expression and/or diminished function[104–106] therefore hinder the formation of the protein envelope as well as the lipid envelope and perturb the normal process of cornification and desquamation.[17,18,104,116]

Studies of mice deficient in transglutaminase-1 provided additional insight into the pathophysiology of lamellar ichthyosis.[117] The mice exhibit a phenotype similar to LI, including taut, erythrodermic and scaling skin with impaired barrier function. The faulty cross-linking activity of transglutaminase-1 was shown to result in the complete loss of the cornified cell envelope, disturbed degradation of the nuclei and keratohyaline granules as well as cytoplasmic accumulation of loricrin. The transepidermal water loss and percutaneous absorption rate were tremendously increased, indicative of a severely impaired skin barrier. These results strongly emphasize the essential role of transglutaminase-1 in the development and maturation of the stratum corneum, and in the adaptation of the skin to a dry environment after birth.[117]

LI has become a prototype for therapeutic cutaneous gene delivery. In the human skin/immunodeficient mouse xenograft model, Choate *et al.* succeeded in short-term correction of the molecular, histological and functional abnormalities of LI skin *in vivo*.[118] Transglutaminase-1 deficient primary keratinocytes from LI patients were transduced with a retroviral vector driving the expression of transglutaminase-1, and then grafted onto the skin of nude mice. This bioengineered LI epidermis showed a transient normal expression of the enzyme as well as other differentiation markers and normal barrier function of the skin. However, keratinocytes retained the transglutaminase-1 gene only for a short period of time. Therefore, this and other approaches[119] are not yet practicable for use in human, but demonstrate that *in vivo* functional correction of the primary defect as well as therapeutic gene delivery is feasible.

DIFFERENTIAL DIAGNOSIS (See CIE)

In the neonatal period, there is considerable clinical overlap with other congenital ichthyoses that may manifest as collodion baby, including CIE, Netherton syndrome, Sjögren–Larsson syndrome, and trichothiodystrophy.

THERAPEUTICS AND PROGNOSIS

Therapy
See section on CIE.

Prognosis
Lamellar ichthyosis is a severe disorder persisting unremittingly throughout life.

PEDIATRIC ASPECTS OF THE DISEASE (See also CIE)

Congenital autosomal recessive ichthyoses are characterized by severe impairment of desquamation and barrier function of the skin resulting in substantial loss of water, ions and proteins in the neonatal period. Sufficient dietary protein and fluid intake is required particularly during infancy and childhood. Secondary hypohidrosis due to obstruction of eccrine sweat ducts results in heat intolerance, which is aggravated in a hot climate and may limit physical activity. External cooling by dousing with cool water and the use of air conditioning can ameliorate the symptoms. Accumulation of scale in the external ear canals often leads to occlusion and bacterial colonization with ensuing recurrent ear infections, which may be prevented by periodic scale removal and otologic care. Severe ectropion demands ophthalmologic follow-up and, if necessary, surgical repair to prevent irreversible corneal damage.

Congenital recessive ichthyoses are often severely disfiguring and pose a challenge to the development of a positive body image and hence to normal

108. Hohl D, Aeschlimann D, Huber M (1998) *In vitro* and rapid *in situ* transglutaminase assays for congenital ichthyoses – a comparative study. **J Invest Dermatol** 110:268–271.
109. Raghunath M, Henries HC, Velten F et al. (1998) A novel *in situ* method for the detection of deficient transglutaminase activity in the skin. **Arch Dermatol Res** 290:621–627.
110. Jeon S, Djian P, Green H (1998) Inability of keratinocytes lacking their specific transglutaminase to form cross-linked envelopes: absence of envelopes as a simple diagnostic test for lamellar ichthyosis. **Proc Natl Acad Sci USA** 95:687–690.
111. Schorderet DF, Huber M, Laurini RN et al. (1997) Prenatal diagnosis of lamellar ichthyosis by direct mutational analysis of the keratinocyte transglutaminase gene. **Prenat Diagn** 17:483–486.
112. Akiyama M, Holbrook KA (1994) Analysis of skin-derived amniotic fluid cells in the second trimester; detection of severe genodermatoses expressed in the fetal period. **J Invest Dermatol** 103:674–677.
113. Perry TB, Holbrook KA, Hoff MS et al. (1987) Prenatal diagnosis of congenital non-bullous ichthyosiform erythroderma (lamellar ichthyosis). **Prenat Diagn** 7:145–155.

114. Kanerva L, Lauharanta J, Niemi KM et al. (1983) New observations on the fine structure of lamellar ichthyosis and the effect of treatment with etretinate. **Am J Dermatopathol** 5:555–568.
115. Laiho E, Niemi KM, Ignatius J et al. (1999) Clinical and morphological correlations for transglutaminase 1 gene mutations in autosomal recessive congenital ichthyosis. **Eur J Hum Genet** 7:625–632.
116. Candi E, Melino G, Lahm A et al. (1998) Transglutaminase 1 mutations in lamellar ichthyosis. Loss of activity due to failure of activation by proteolytic processing. **J Biol Chem** 273:13693–13702.
117. Matsuki M, Yamashita F, Ishida-Yamamoto A et al. (1998) Defective stratum corneum and early neonatal death in mice lacking the gene for transglutaminase 1 (keratinocyte transglutaminase). **Proc Natl Acad Sci USA** 95:1044–1049.
118. Choate KA, Medalie DA, Morgan JR et al. (1996) Corrective gene transfer in the human skin disorder lamellar ichthyosis. **Nat Med** 2:1263–1267.
119. Huber M, Limat A, Wagner E et al. (2000) Efficient *in vitro* transfection of human keratinocytes with an adenovirus-enhanced receptor-mediated system. **J Invest Dermatol** 114:661–666.

psychosocial development. Families and patients need continuous support in dealing with psychosocial problems. Patient support organizations such as the Foundation for Ichthyosis and Related Skin Types (FIRST) and the National Organization for Rare Disorders (NORD) have been of tremendous benefit to patients and their families.

CONGENITAL ICHTHYOSIFORM ERYTHRODERMA (CIE)

Synonyms: Nonbullous congenital ichthyosiform erythroderma-NBCIE, Ichthyosis congenita type 1 (MIM 242100, 604781, 604780)

This is another type of congenital autosomal recessive ichthyosis with distinct clinical and biochemical phenotypic features (See Differential Diagnosis below and Table 8.5). It can be clinically distinguished from LI by the presence of marked erythroderma and small, white scale. Nevertheless, there is considerable intra- and interfamilial variability of the phenotype. Many patients may exhibit overlapping features with a variable degree of erythroderma, quality as well as size of scales, and do not fit exactly into one or the other disease category.

EPIDEMIOLOGY
Genetics
In the vast majority of families, CIE is inherited as an autosomal recessive trait, although autosomal dominant inheritance has been occasionally observed.[102,120] In general, parents of an affected child are presumed carriers of a recessive mutation. There is a 25% risk with each pregnancy that both mutant alleles are transmitted to the offspring and the child will be affected. Even more than LI, CIE is clinically and genetically very heterogeneous and its molecular cause remains largely unsolved. A few CIE patients carry pathogenic mutations in the gene *TGM1* encoding the epidermal cross-linking enzyme transglutanminase-1,[96,97,99] whereas most *TGM1* mutations produce a LI phenotype. To date, at least three other genetic loci for CIE phenotypes (3q27–28, 17p) and congenital ichthyosis without erythema (19p13.1–p13.2) have been mapped, while others await identification.[101]

Statistics
CIE might be more common than LI, but its incidence probably does not exceed 1 in 200 000 to 1 in 300 000.

PRESENTING HISTORY

Similar to LI, most infants present at birth with a collodion membrane, which subsequently evolves into generalized scaling and erythroderma.

PHYSICAL EXAMINATION
Skin
The clinical manifestations of CIE are usually milder than in lamellar ichthyosis and demonstrate a greater variability in the intensity of erythema, size and type of scale, even within a family. Generally, scales are white, fine and powdery (Fig. 8.16), although they may become larger, darker or plate-like on the extensor surface of the lower extremities. Severely affected patients show an intense red erythroderma (Fig. 8.16) and develop ectropion and scarring alopecia. Marked hyperkeratosis of palms and soles with cracks and deep fissures often contrasts the fine, translucent scale elsewhere on the body. Patients with milder disease exhibit less or minimal erythroderma but generalized scaling and variable palmoplantar involvement.

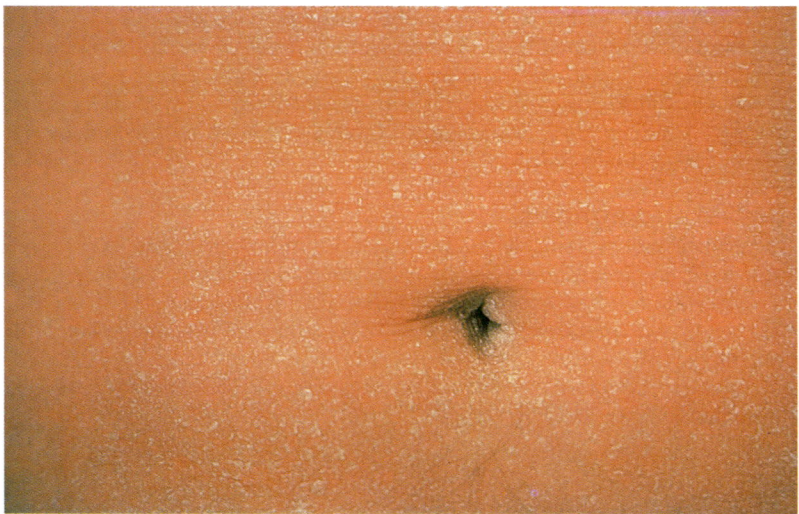

Fig. 8.16 Classical congenital ichthyosiform erythroderma. Intense erythroderma with fine, white scale.

Hair, nails, teeth, and mucous membranes
Scarring alopecia is less common than in patients with LI.[103] The impediment of sweat ducts and pores results in hypohidrosis and heat intolerance. Secondary nail dystrophy (thickened nail plates, ridging) and onychomycosis may develop, while lips, mucous membranes, and teeth tend to be spared.

Systemic manifestations (see also LI)
CIE has no primary systemic manifestations. While most patients with CIE show normal growth and development, severely erythrodermic children may show mild growth retardation.

LABORATORY FINDINGS/PRENATAL DIAGNOSIS

Prenatal diagnosis based on molecular approaches is only available for families carrying known mutations. Fetoscopy and ultrastructural skin examination remain problematic and are not available before the 21st week of gestation.[121]

PATHOPHYSIOLOGY AND HISTOGENESIS
Histologic findings
The histopathological features of CIE are not diagnostic and do not allow a definite distinction from LI. However, they are valuable to exclude epidermolytic hyperkeratosis. Compared to LI, there is pronounced acanthosis of the epidermis with hypergranulosis, mild to moderate hyperkeratosis and focal to extensive parakeratosis. The epidermal cell turnover rate in CIE is markedly increased indicative of epidermal hyperproliferation.[11]

Molecular and biochemical basis and histogenesis
The extensive clinical and genetic heterogeneity of CIE suggests that several different genetic and metabolic defects result in CIE and LI/CIE intermediate phenotypes. The first, and so far only known, disease gene is *TGM1*. A small subset of patients with clinical features of CIE were found to carry inactivating *TGM1* mutations leading to transglutaminase-1 deficiency with ensuing abnormal formation of the cornified cell envelope and perturbed barrier function of the skin.[96,97,99] However, the striking differences in clinical, histological and ultrastructural features in patients with *TGM1* mutations,

120. Rossmann-Ringdahl I, Anton-Lamprecht I, Swanbeck G (1986) A mother and two children with nonbullous congenital ichthyosiform erythroderma. Arch Dermatol 122:559–564.

121. Holbrook KA, Dale BA, Williams ML et al. (1988) The expression of congenital ichthyosiform erythroderma in second trimester fetuses of the same family: morphologic and biochemical studies. J Invest Dermatol 91:521–531.

including classic LI, CIE and overlapping phenotypes, remain unexplained. Thus far, there is no obvious correlation between the specific location and nature of recessive *TGM1* mutations and their phenotypic expression.[96] Nevertheless, abnormal functioning of transglutaminase-1 might be a crucial factor in the pathogenesis of CIE. Choate et al. found in four out of five patients with CIE an aberrant intracellular accumulation of transglutaminase-1 associated with a moderate decrease in enzymatic activity despite normal protein production.[122] These results suggest that CIE may not only stem from a primary transglutaminase-1 deficiency (*TGM1* mutations) but also from a secondary malfunction of the epidermal transglutaminase system (e.g., similar to XRI).[123] Albeit another member of the transglutaminase family is expressed in skin, there is no evidence for the causal involvement of transglutaminase-3 in the pathogenesis of CIE.[93,96]

Ultrastructural and biochemical abnormalities in CIE, although not very well correlated with the clinical phenotypes, are suggestive for abnormalities in the lamellar body secretory system. Electron microscopic examinations reveal abnormal and an increased number of lamellar bodies, many of which appeared to be retained within corneocytes, thereby resulting in accumulation of lipid droplets in the stratum corneum.[13,15,18] Intercellular lipid lamellae of the stratum corneum, which derive from the secretion and reorganization of lamellar body contents, appear highly disorganized in CIE. These structural aberrations are accompanied by differences in the activity of lamellar body enzymes in the stratum corneum,[10] which may play a role in the abnormal persistence of desmosomes.[18] Collectively, these changes might result in a disturbed skin barrier function with increased transepidermal water loss, which in turn has been shown to stimulate epidermal hyperplasia.[27,124] Nevertheless, many ultrastructural features are not specific for CIE and have been observed in other hyperproliferative disorders.[18]

DIFFERENTIAL DIAGNOSIS

Severe forms of CIE and lamellar ichthyosis can be distinguished based on clinical, histological and ultrastructural findings (Table 8.5). CIE is defined by the presence of generalized, bright red erythema and fine white scale. Patients with lamellar ichthyosis have generalized thick, plate-like scale with minimal to no erythroderma. Both disorders may present as collodion baby. Ectropion, eclabium, and scarring alopecia are more commonly seen in lamellar ichthyosis. Keratinocytes in lamellar ichthyosis show a normal granular layer, cell proliferation, and lamellar bodies but massively thickened stratum corneum without parakeratosis.[10,18] The presence of cholesterol clefts in the stratum corneum by electron microscopic examination is suggestive of LI, while a larger number of lipid droplets are more common in CIE.[13,15,17] The mitotic rate in CIE is increased[11] as is the number of lamellar bodies, and the stratum corneum is thickened with focal to complete parakeratosis. The distinction of LI and CIE based on elevated levels of *N*-alkanes in CIE has been refuted because they may originate from exogenous sources.

Other types of ichthyosis can be differentiated from CIE and LI based on specific clinical, histological, and biochemical parameters (Table 8.2). In contrast to ichthyosis vulgaris, skin involvement in LI and CIE is typically generalized, including all flexures, and results in taut facial skin with ensuing ectropion/eclabium and alopecia. However, the distinction between LI/CIE intermediate phenotypes and ichthyosis vulgaris may be difficult. XRI can be excluded by biochemical testing. Chanarin–Dorfman syndrome (neutral lipid storage disease) can be usually identified by examining a peripheral blood smear. Skin findings in Netherton syndrome may closely resemble CIE, but this disorder is often associated with failure to thrive, recurrent or systemic infections, pruritus, highly elevated plasma IgE levels, and hair shaft abnormalities, and has a psoriasiform histopathology. Trichothiodystrophy can be eliminated by light and polarizing microscopy of hair. Finally, epidermolytic hyperkeratosis (See Epidermolytic Hyperkeratosis) can be distinguished clinically based on the occurrence of blisters, flexural accentuation, and absence of ectropion, as well as by its distinctive histopathology.

THERAPEUTICS AND PROGNOSIS

Topical therapy

Topical management of autosomal recessive ichthyosis is a therapeutic cornerstone and complements systemic therapy, although its efficacy is limited by the need for continuous applications. It is aimed to diminish scaling, and to rehydrate and lubricate the skin. Most patients require topical treatment with keratolytic agents such as urea, salicylic acid, alphahydroxy acids (lactic acid, glycolic acid), propylene glycol, or combinations of them. Their use may be limited because of skin irritation and the risk of systemic absorption due to an impaired skin barrier function, especially in children. Topical vitamin D3 derivatives,[125] tazarotene (a receptor-selective retinoid),[126] as well as special formulations of lactic acid and propylene glycol in a lipophilic cream base[127] have been effective in reducing scale in patients with congenital recessive ichthyoses. Adjuvant use of emollients such as petrolatum or lanolin may increase the patient's comfort.

Systemic management

Oral retinoids can have dramatic benefit in the treatment of autosomal recessive ichthyoses. Etretinate as well as acitretin have been shown to effectively alleviate hyperkeratosis and scaling but are less effective to suppress the erythroderma. In a LI patient with transglutaminase-1 deficiency, therapy with etretinate was shown to restore expression of the cross-linking enzyme, possibly due to an upregulation of gene transcription,[128] although it did not have any discernible effect on the ultrastructural abnormalities found in LI.[128,129] Acitretin treatment is usually initiated at a low dose followed by titration to the minimal effective dose, which is dictated by course and severity of disease. In a therapeutic series of nine children with LI and CIE, Lacour et al. observed an excellent to moderate response to acitretin treatment.[87] The therapeutic benefits included improvement of ectropion, avoiding eye complications and reconstructive eyelid surgery. Side effects were related to vitamin A toxicity and included mucocutaneous dryness, skin fragility, fissures, and excessive peeling, the latter especially in LI. Abnormalities of serum lipids and liver function tests were transient and did not necessitate cessation of treatment.[87] Adverse effects of systemic retinoids on the musculoskeletal system occur infrequently, but should be considered before initiating a long-term treatment. Osteoporosis, hyperostoses, calcification of tendons and ligaments, and premature epiphyseal closure were reported in children or adults treated with higher doses of oral etinoids (> 1.0mg/kg/day).[130] In contrast, lower dose treatment over 1 month to 11 years in 42 British children with a series of inherited disorders of cornification did not show evidence for skeletal toxicity or growth retardation.[131] Lacour et al.[87] suggested guidelines for oral acitretin treatment in children. In general, a baseline assessment is recommended, which may

122. Choate KA, Williams ML, Khavari PA (1998) Abnormal transglutaminase 1 expression pattern in a subset of patients with erythrodermic autosomal recessive ichthyosis. J Invest Dermatol 110:8–12.

123. Nemes Z, Demeny M, Marekov LN et al. (2000) Cholesterol 3-sulfate interferes with cornified envelope assembly by diverting transglutaminase 1 activity from the formation of cross-links and esters to the hydrolysis of glutamine. J Biol Chem 275:2636–2646.

124. Williams ML, Elias PM (1993) From basket weave to barrier. Unifying concepts for the pathogenesis of the disorders of cornification. Arch Dermatol 129:626–629.

125. Lucker GP, van de Kerkhof PC, van Dijk MR et al. (1994) Effect of topical calcipotriol on congenital ichthyoses. Br J Dermatol 131:546–550.

126. Hofmann B, Stege H, Ruzicka T et al. (1999) Effect of topical tazarotene in the treatment of congenital ichthyoses. Br J Dermatol 141:642–646.

127. Ganemo A, Virtanen M, Vahlquist A (1999) Improved topical treatment of lamellar ichthyosis: a double-blind study of four different cream formulations. Br J Dermatol 141:1027–1032.

128. Hashimoto K, Gee S, Tanaka K (2000) Lamellar ichthyosis: response to etretinate with transglutaminase 1 recovery. Am J Dermatopathol 22:277–280.

129. Williams ML, Elias PM (1981) Nature of skin fragility in patients receiving retinoids for systemic effect. Arch Dermatol 117:611–619.

130. Peck GL, JDJ (1999) The retinoids. In: The Retinoids, Freedberg IM, Eisen AZ, KW et al. eds. New York: McGraw-Hill, pp. 2810–2820.

131. Paige DG, Judge MR, Shaw DG et al. (1992) Bone changes and their significance in children with ichthyosis on long-term etretinate therapy. Br J Dermatol 127:387–391.

TABLE 8.7   Chronology of pathogenetic aspects in harlequin ichthyosis

Year and author	Biochemical findings	Consequences
1938 Giordano[475]	Abnormal Sudan staining	Concluded that alterations of lipids leads to harlequin ichthyosis
1970 Craig[476]	Normal alpha-helical keratin replaced by a cross-beta pattern	Inborn error of metabolism was suggested
1979 Buxman[477]	Elevated levels of cholesterol and triglyceride in stratum corneum Missing lamellar bodies	Suggests a disorder of lipid metabolism in the skin
1982 Baden[478]	Keratin 51K was found in all 3 cases investigated	
1983 Blanchet-Bardon[479]	Abnormal keratinosomes found in intercellular substance	
1989 Haftek[480]	Increase of lamellar bodies under retinoids; absence of filaggrin	Direct influence of retinoids to the pathogenetically important lamellar bodies
1989 Fleck[481]	Giant lamellar bodies	
1990 Dale[141]	Three different types are recognized; differences between expression of keratin 6/16 and on the ultrastructural level	Keratin staining and ultrastructural investigations are necessary for classification
1997 Sundberg[157]	Mouse model discovered	
1997 Kam[145]	Reduced serine/threonine protein phosphatase activity	Suggested cause of harlequin ichthyosis
1999 Michel[142]	Reduced calcium-activated neutral protease calpain in harlequin ichthyosis	Calcium-signaling is important for normal differentiation
2001 Smith[133]	*De novo* delection on chromosome 18q21.3 documented	

include full blood count, fasting lipids, liver function tests, blood urea, electrolytes, creatinine, and urine analysis as well as a limited skeletal survey (including all four limbs and lateral spine). The follow-up including fasting lipids, liver function tests, and urine analysis is suggested weekly for the first month, then every 3 months thereafter. Periodic radiographic examinations of cervical and thoracic spine and epiphyses might complement the regimen. Overall, systemic retinoids appear to be relatively safe for the long-term treatment of congenital ichthyoses as long as patients are monitored carefully. Because retinoids are potent teratogens, their use in sexually active females requires concomitant use of reliable methods of birth control.

PROGNOSIS

CIE may be severely disfiguring and persists with little change throughout life, although marked improvement was noted in some patients at puberty.

PEDIATRIC ASPECTS OF THE DISEASE (see LI)

The exfoliative erythroderma, especially during infancy, may result in a substantial metabolic stress on the growing child. Therefore, adequate intake of water, calories, protein and iron should be ensured.

HARLEQUIN ICHTHYOSIS

Peter Itin, Mark Pittelkow

INTRODUCTION AND HISTORICAL NOTE

The harlequin ichthyosis represents a serious disorder of cornification in the newborn period. The first description of the condition has been identified in a diary in 1750. The oldest report by a physician was that of from Richter in 1792.

EPIDEMIOLOGY

This extremely rare disease most likely follows an autosomal recessive trait, although dominant mutations with parental mosaicism have been discussed recently.[132] Recently a *de novo* deletion on chromosome 18q in a baby with harlequin syndrome has been documented.[133] The authors speculated that the responsible gene lies distal or at 18q21.3. It is a genetically heterogeneous disorder of cornification with a unique clinical manifestation.

PRESENTING HISTORY AND PHYSICAL EXAMINATION

The newborn, often premature, is encased by a thick plate of stratum corneum showing cracking with deep fissures (Fig. 8.17). The skin has a yellow to gray color and offensive odor. The nose is flat, the ears hypoplastic or absent and the pronounced ectropion and eclabium give the infant a characteristic and grotesque appearance (Fig. 8.17). The limbs remain in rigid semiflexion, hands and feet may have a claw-like appearance and micromelia has been reported.[134] Fingers and toes are often hypoplastic (Fig. 8.18). Strangulation of the digits followed by necrosis may complicate the disease, and constriction of the chest and abdomen interferes with respiration and feeding.[135] Eyelashes and eyebrows may be absent and malformed nails have been noted. Nonspecific alterations in kidney, hypo- or hyperplasia of the thymus, and stenosis of the esophagus were reported, but in many cases no internal abnormalities were found at autopsy. Patients with Neu–Laxova syndrome group III have an appearance similar to the harlequin ichthyosis.[136] Prenatal diagnosis of harlequin ichthyosis is possible by sonographic and structural examination.[137,138] The prognosis is poor because of disturbed thermoregulation, restricted chest movement with respiratory insufficiency, water loss and, in particular, secondary infection with septicemia. However, several reports of long-term survival exist and the treatment with retinoids seems to be promising.[139] Longitudinal studies of harlequin ichthyosis present clinically as non–bullous congenital ichthyosiform erythroderma.

132. Sarkar R, Sharma RC, Sethi S et al. (2000) Three unusual siblings with harlequin ichthyosis in an Indian family. **J Dermatol** 27:609–611.
133. Smith SH, Gaunt L, Moore L et al. (2001) De novo deletion of chromosome 18q in a baby with harlequin ichthyosis. **Am J Med Genet** 102:342–345.
134. Charles A, Moulinasse R, Versailles L (1989) Harlequin fetus and micromelia. **Prenat Diagn** 9:709–713.
135. Rogers M, Scarf C (1989) Harlequin baby treated with etretinate. **Pediatr Dermatol** 6:216–221.

136. Curry CJR (1982) Further comments on the Neu-Laxova syndrome. **Am J Med Genet** 13:441–444.
137. Hashimoto K, De Dobbeleer G, Kanzaki T (1993) Electron microscopic studies of harlequin fetuses. **Pediatr Dermatol** 10:214–223.
138. Bongain A, Benoit B, Ejues L et al. (2002) Harlequin fetus: three-dimensional sonographic findings and new diagnostic approach. **Ultrasound Obstet Gynecol** 20:82–85.
139. Elias PM, Fartasch M, Crumrine D et al. (2000) Origin of the corneocyte lipid envelope (CLE): observations in harlequin ichthyosis and cultured human keratinocytes. **J Invest Dermatol** 115:765–769.

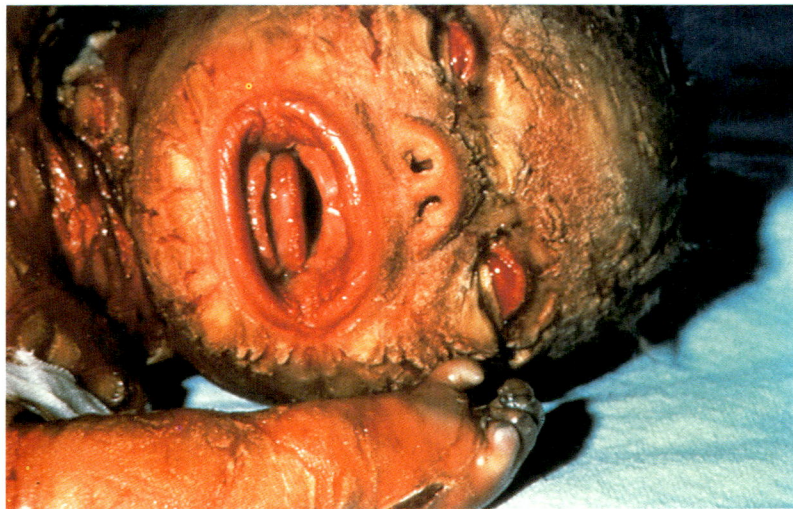

Fig. 8.17   Grotesque hyperkeratosis with eclabion and ectropion.

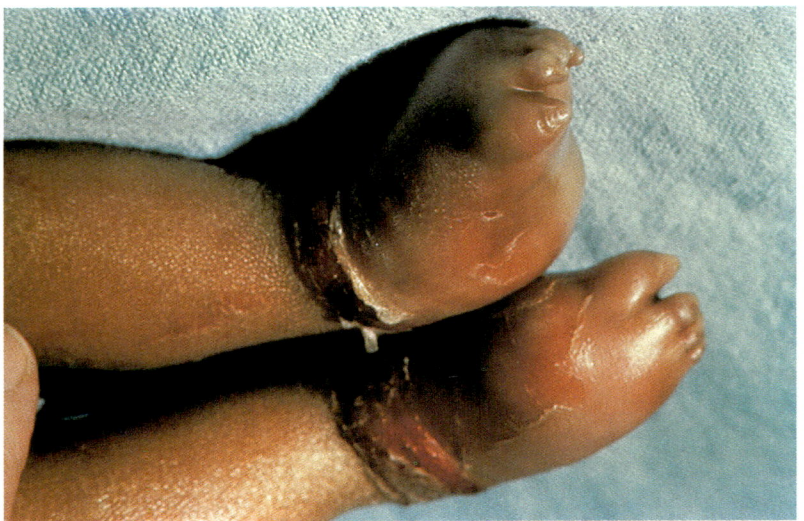

Fig. 8.18   Hypoplastic toes with ischemia.

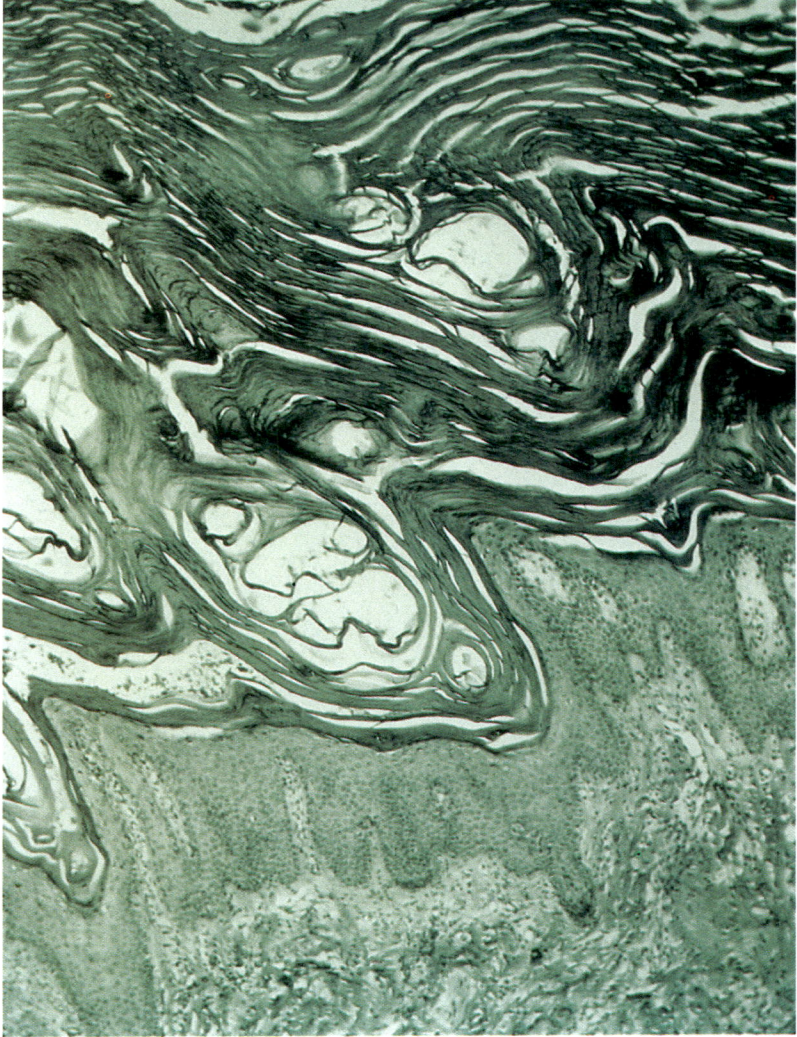

Fig. 8.19   Conventional histology.

Conventional histology is nondiagnostic and variable (Fig. 8.19). An ortho-keratotic or hyperplastic stratum corneum with normal granular layer or thickened granular layer is present but parakeratosis with absence of granular layers may likewise exist. Cultured keratinocytes from harlequin ichthyosis feature excessive hyperkeratosis and failure of desquamation.

The ultrastructural features of the harlequin skin at 17–21 weeks of gestation are the same as those of the newborn.[140] Hashimoto et al.[137] found no lamellar bodies in four harlequin ichthyosis patients. Dale et al.[141] ultra-structurally and biochemically classified harlequin ichthyosis in three different types. They investigated 10 cases. Group I was characterized by absence of keratin pair K6/K16 as well as the presence of profilaggrin in the interfollicular epidermis. Only in this group could keratohylin granules be detected by light microscopy and ultrastructural examination showed large but otherwise normal appearing keratohylin granules. Groups II and III showed positive staining for the keratins 6/16. Presence of profilaggrin in the interfollicular epidermis was found in groups I and II. Profilaggrin

expression was higher than normal in groups I and II because it was not converted to filaggrin. In group III, profilaggrin was reduced and associated with a staining in the intraepidermal sweat ducts. In all cases normal lamellar granules were absent. Group II harlequin ichthyosis patients had tiny, globular keratohyalin granules and group III revealed few or no keratohyalin granules. Analysis of affected siblings showed a clear correlation of the pattern within a given family.[141] Michel et al.[142] showed that calpain (calcium-activated cytoplasmatic proteases) is present throughout the normal epidermis and is expressed from the early stages of development. In harlequin ichthyosis a marked decrease of calpain was found and the authors suggested that calcium-mediated signalling events are important in the alteration of differentiation that occurs in harlequin ichthyosis. Zeeuwan et al. found that cystatin M/E is required for viability of cornified epidermis and they suggested ichg mouse mutation as a model for human type 2 harlequin ichthyosis.[143] A review of the literature suggests that harlequin ichthyosis is a clinical description for a variety of disorders of cornification presenting in the newborn. These entities seem to be the result of altered lipid metabolism or of a defective fibrous polypeptide in the stratum

140. Akiyama M, Kim DK, Main DM et al. (1994) Characteristic morphologic abnormality of harlequin ichthyosis detected in amniotic fluid cells. **J Invest Dermatol** 102:210–213.

141. Dale BA, Holbrook KA, Fleckman P et al. (1990) Heterogeneity in harlequin ichthyosis, an inborn error of epidermal keratinization: variable morphology and structural protein expression and a defect in lamellar granules. **J Invest Dermatol** 94:6–18.

142. Michel M, Fleckman P, Smith LT, Dale BA (1999) The calcium-activated neutral protease calpain I is present in normal foetal skin and is decreased in neonatal harlequin ichthyosis. **Br J Dermatol** 141:1017–1026.

143. Zeeuwan PWM, van Vlijmen-Williams IMSS et al. (2002) A null mutation in the cystatin M/E ichg mice causes lethality and defects in epidermal cornification . **Hum Mol Genet** 11:2867–2875.

corneum. A normal distribution of transglutaminase-1 has been reported.[144,145] Reduced activity of the serine/threonine protein phosphatase in keratinocytes was suggested to be the cause of harlequin ichthyosis.[146] Fleckman et al.[147] showed by culture method that harlequin ichthyosis keratinocytes differentiate poorly by morphologic and biochemical criteria. Their results indicate that both epithelial and mesenchymal structures of the skin are affected in harlequin ichthyosis but that the primary abnormality involves the keratinocytes.

The classification of harlequin ichthyosis among the other types of ichthyoses is difficult, because no objective marker of disease was available until recently. Some authors categorized harlequin ichthyosis within the group of the pronounced forms of nonbullous ichthyosiform erythrodermas, but other see it as a distinct entity or as a genetically heterogeneous group of disorders. Haftek et al.[148] followed for 8 years a patient with harlequin ichthyosis who developed non-bullous congenital erythroderma. However, abnormal lamellar body production and defective filaggrin processing persisted, which is not a feature of the ordinary erythrodermic form of lamellar ichthyosis.

An error in lipid metabolism resulting in abnormal lamellar bodies seems to be involved in this retention-type ichthyosis[139,149] and may also be the reason for frequent lung infections due to abnormal surfactant (Fig. 8.20).

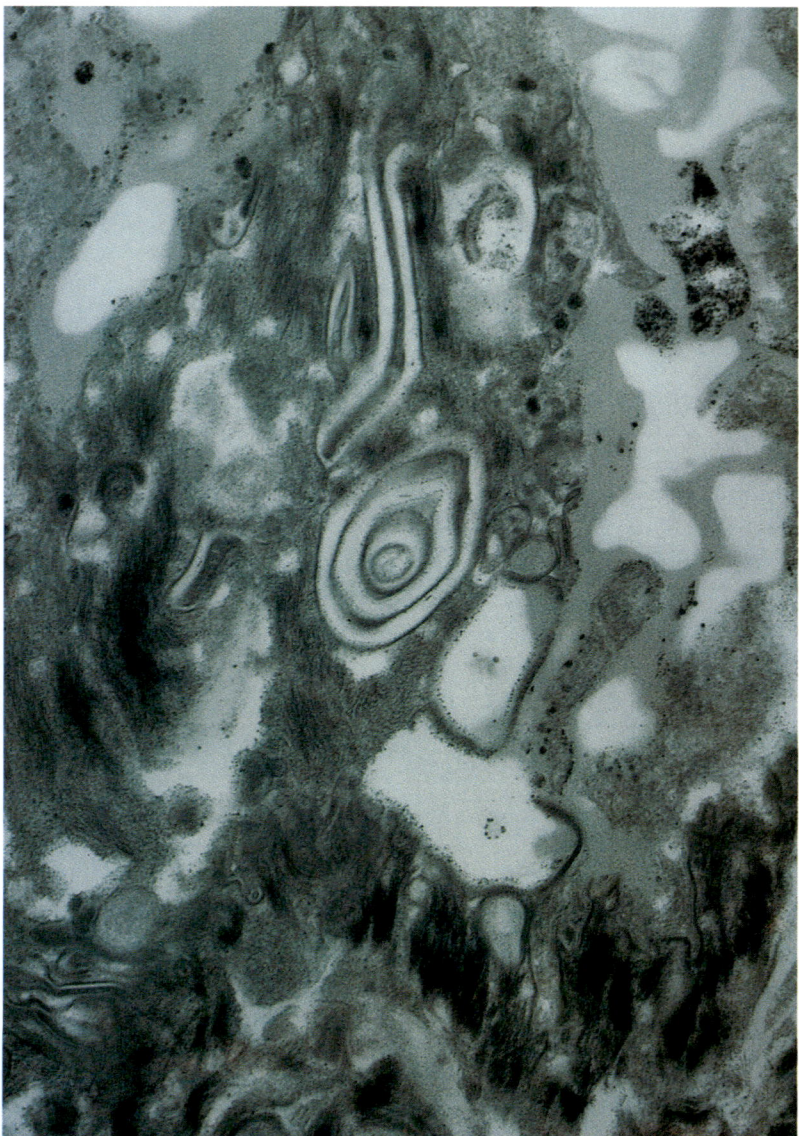

Fig. 8.20 Harlequin ichthyosis: abnormal lamellar bodies under electron microscopy.

THERAPEUTICS AND PROGNOSIS

Intensive nursing and medical care with the use of humidified incubators and fluid replacement may allow prolonged survival. Early use of systemic retinoids and antibiotics seem to contribute to better survival and they accelerate the shedding. The plate-like scales shed within weeks and after severe ichthyosis resembling nonbullous erythrodermic ichthyosis develops. The oldest survivors are now more than 10 years of age. Paraffin-containing emollients are necessary from the beginning, combined with oil baths. Ocular management with topical eye ointment is important because keratitis due to ectropion is rather common and may lead to corneal abscess.[150] Human skin equivalent for repair of cicatrial ectopion in a patient with harlequin ichthyosis was suggested.[151]

Information for families with inherited disorders can be obtained from:
Foundation for Ichthyosis and Related Skin Types (FIRST)
650 N. Cannon Ave., Suite 17
Lansdale, PA 19446
(215) 631 1411
(800) 545 3286
Fax: (215) 631 1413
E-mail: info@scalyskin.org
http://www.scalyskin.org

SJÖGREN–LARSSON SYNDROME

Gabriele Richard

Sjögren–Larsson syndrome (MIM 270200) is an autosomal recessive neurocutaneous disorder characterized by the clinical triad of congenital ichthyosis, di- and tetraplegia, and mental retardation.[152] This rare disorder is most common in Sweden where it has a prevalence of 0.4 in 100 000 persons, but it occurs worldwide.[153] The disorder presents at birth with varying degrees of erythema and ichthyosis, while collodion membrane and ectropion are rarely seen. The type of ichthyosis may vary and range from fine, white scales, larger, plate-like scales to nonscaling hyperkeratosis. Thickening of the skin results in accentuated skin markings (Fig. 8.21) and appearance of lichenification, particularly in flexural areas. Due to the clinical overlap with congenital ichthyosiform erythroderma and other congenital recessive ichthyoses, the diagnosis of Sjögren–Larsson syndrome is often delayed until

144. Choate KA, Williams ML, Elias PM, Khavari PA (1998) Transglutaminase 1 expression in a patient with features of harlequin ichthyosis: case report. **J Am Acad Dermatol** 38:325–329.
145. Akiyama M, Kim SY, Yoneda K, Shimizu H (1997) Expression of transglutaminase 1 (transglutaminase K) in harlequin ichthyosis. **Arch Dermatol Res** 289:116–119.
146. Kam E, Nirunsuksiri W, Hager B et al. (1997) Protein phosphatase activity in human keratinocytes cultured from normal epidermis and epidermis from patients with harlequin ichthyosis. **Br J Dermatol** 137:874–882.
147. Fleckman P, Hager B, Dale BA (1997) Harlequin ichthyosis keratinocytes in liftetd culture differentiate poorly by morphologic and biochemical criteria. **J Invest Dermatol** 109:36–38.
148. Haftek M, Cambazard F, Dhouailly D et al. (1996) longitudinal study of a harlequin infant presenting clinically as non-bullous congenital ichthyosiform erythroderma. 135:448–453.
149. Milner ME, O'Guin WM, Holbrook KA, Dale BA (1992) Abnormal lamellar granules in harlequin ichthyosis. **J Invest Dermatol** 99:824–829.
150. Chua CN, Ainsworth J (2001) Ocular management of harlequin syndrome. **Arch Ophthalmol** 119:454–455.
151. Culican SM, Custer PL (2002) Repair of cicatricial ectopion in an infant with harlequin ichthyosis using engineered human skin. **Am J Ophthalmol** 134:442–443.
152. Sjögren T, Larsson T (1957) Oligophrenia in combination with congenital ichthyosis and spastic disorder. **Acta Psychiatr Neurol Scand** 32:1–113.
153. Liden S, Jagell S (1984) The Sjögren–Larsson syndrome. **Int J Dermatol** 23:247–253.

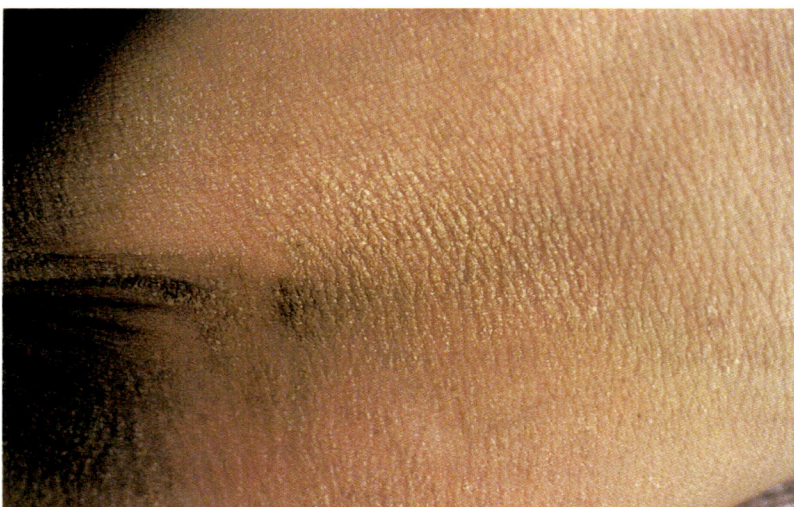

Fig. 8.21   Generalized hyperkeratosis of the skin with accentuated skin markings in the axillary fold. (Courtesy of Dr. W.B. Rizzo)

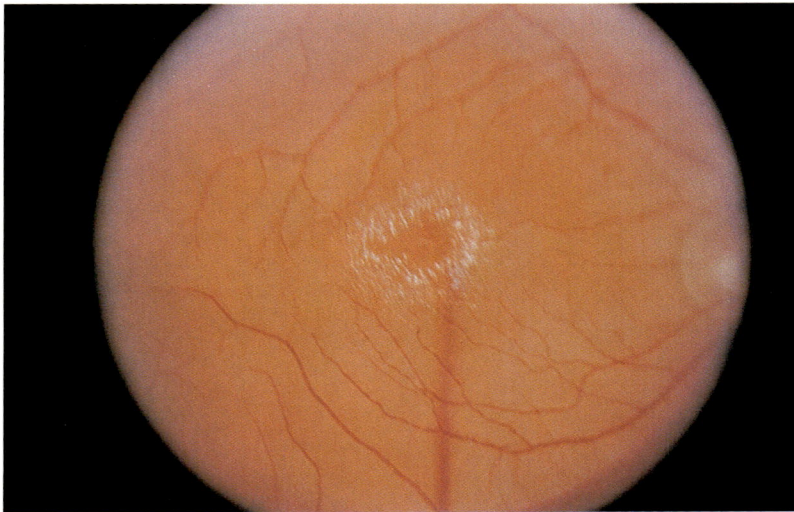

Fig. 8.22   Perifoveal glistening dots of the retina. (Courtesy of Dr. W.B. Rizzo)

the onset of neurological symptoms and/or appearance of perifoveal glistening white dots. After infancy, the erythema tends to fade while hyperkeratosis and scaling become more prominent and darker in color. Predilection sites are the lower abdomen, especially around the umbilicus, the side and nape of the neck, as well as the large flexures. In more than 50% of patients, mild palmoplantar keratoderma is present. In contrast to many other ichthyoses, persistent pruritus is common. The histopathologic features are nonspecific and include hyperkeratosis, papillomatosis, and acanthosis with a well-preserved granular layer. Electron microscopic features are reminiscent of those seen in other congenital recessive ichthyoses.

During the first 2–3 years of life, central nervous system involvement manifests with abnormal gait, pyramidal signs, and di- or tetraplegia. The lower extremities are usually far more severely affected than the arms.[154] Delay in neuromotor development is gradually progressive and accompanied by speech defects, and severe mental retardation. Seizures are present in about one-third of the patients. Neuroimaging studies reveal that most patients have white matter disease with retarded myelination and a variable degree of dysmyelination due to accumulation of free lipids in the periventricular white matter.[155] An almost pathognomonic finding in Sjögren–Larsson syndrome is the presence of perifoveal glistening white dots in the ocular fundus (Fig. 8.22).[156] These develop during the first year of life in many but not all patients, and increase in number over time.[155] Other features of the syndrome reported in some patients are corneal dystrophy, dental and/or osseous dysplasia, and hypertelorism. The combination of congenital ichthyosis with glistening white dots or spasticity is diagnostic for Sjögren–Larsson syndrome.

Sjögren–Larsson syndrome is caused by recessive mutations in the fatty aldehyde dehydrogenase gene *FALDH* on the short arm of chromosome 17, which result in deficient enzyme activity.[156] This enzyme catalyzes the oxidation of long-chain aliphatic aldehydes to fatty acids, a pathway that is important for the synthesis of epidermal lipids as well as the catabolism of ether phospholipids and sphingolipids in the brain.[157,158] The measurement of enzyme activity in cultured fibroblasts or leukocytes is a specific and reliable

diagnostic test that also allows detection of unaffected carriers who exhibit half of normal levels.[157] Another sensitive marker for the enzymatic defect in SLS is the detection of elevated free fatty alcohols in cultured fibroblasts and plasma.[158] In addition, DNA-based molecular testing is possible.[159] Over 50 distinct mutations in the *FALDH* gene have been identified, including mainly frameshift mutations and amino acid substitutions scattered throughout the gene.[159,160] Although the majority of mutations are private, there are a few common mutations with a high allele frequency in the northern European and Middle-Eastern population, which may facilitate DNA-based molecular diagnosis.[159] Prenatal diagnosis is available using enzymatic as well as molecular genetic methods from CVS or amniocentesis material.[157,161,162]

Management of Sjögren–Larsson syndrome patients requires a multidisciplinary approach, including dermatologic, neurologic, ophthalmologic, orthopedic, and social collaboration. Aggressive physiotherapy, followed by appropriate surgical intervention, has been shown to drastically improve the mobility of children.[154] Various forms of a fat-reduced diet have not yet provided consistent and reproducible results, although early dietary intervention during infancy was beneficial in one case.[163] 5-Lipoxygenase inhibitors that block the synthesis of leukotriene B_4 might be a promising class of therapeutics to diminish pruritus, but a beneficial effect on CNS symptoms has not been proven.[164]

NEUTRAL LIPID STORAGE DISEASE WITH ICHTHYOSIS

Heiko Traupe

Synonym: Chanarin–Dorfman syndrome (MIM 275630)

This is a rare autosomal recessive disorder of lipid metabolism with multisystemic accumulation of triglycerides. Most cases have been observed in consanguineous families from the Middle East and from Sicily and Greece,

154. Haddad FS, Lacour M, Harper JI et al. (1999) The orthopaedic presentation and management of Sjögren–Larsson syndrome. **J Pediatr Orthop** 19:617–619.
155. van Domburg PH, Willemsen MA, Rotteveel JJ et al. (1999) Sjögren–Larsson syndrome: clinical and MRI/MRS findings in FALDH-deficient patients. **Neurology** 52:1345–1352.
156. De Laurenzi V, Rogers GR, Hamrock DJ et al. (1996) Sjögren–Larsson syndrome is caused by mutations in the fatty aldehyde dehydrogenase gene. **Nat Genet** 12:52–57.
157. Rizzo WB, Craft DA (1991) Sjögren–Larsson syndrome. Deficient activity of the fatty aldehyde dehydrogenase component of fatty alcohol:NAD+ oxidoreductase in cultured fibroblasts. **J Clin Invest** 88:1643–1648.
158. Rizzo WB, Craft DA (2000) Sjögren–Larsson syndrome: accumulation of free fatty alcohols in cultured fibroblasts and plasma. **J Lipid Res** 41:1077–1081.

159. Rizzo WB, Carney G, Lin Z (1999) The molecular basis of Sjögren–Larsson syndrome: mutation analysis of the fatty aldehyde dehydrogenase gene. **Am J Hum Genet** 65:1547–1560.
160. Sillen A, Anton-Lamprecht I, Braun-Quentin C et al. (1998) Spectrum of mutations and sequence variants in the FALDH gene in patients with Sjögren–Larsson syndrome. **Hum Mutat** 12:377–384.
161. Sillen A, Holmgren G, Wadelius C (1997) First prenatal diagnosis by mutation analysis in a family with Sjögren–Larsson syndrome. **Prenat Diagn** 17:1147–1149.
162. Rizzo WB, Craft DA, Kelson TL et al. (1994) Prenatal diagnosis of Sjögren–Larsson syndrome using enzymatic methods. **Prenat Diagn** 14:577–581.
163. Taube B, Billeaud C, Labreze C et al. (1999) Sjögren–Larsson syndrome: early diagnosis, dietary management and biochemical studies in two cases. **Dermatology** 198:340–345.
164. Willemsen MA, Rotteveel JJ, Steijlen PM et al. (2000) 5-Lipoxygenase inhibition: a new treatment strategy for Sjögren–Larsson syndrome. **Neuropediatrics** 31:1–3.

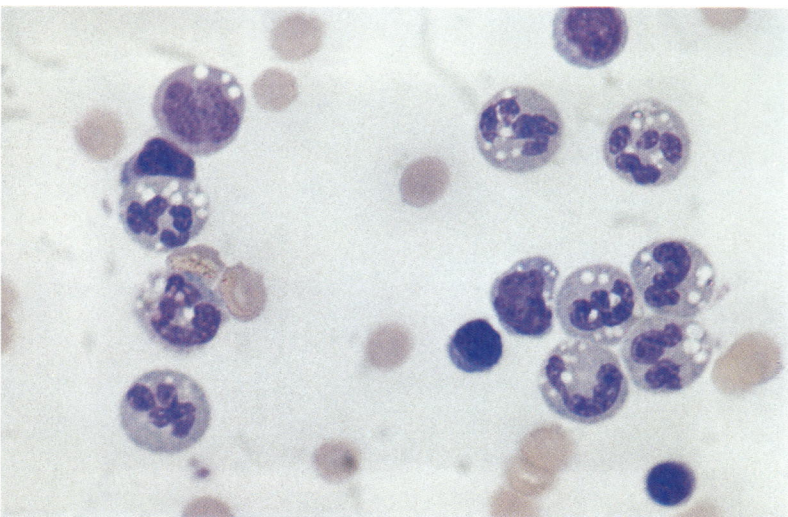

Fig. 8.23 Buffy coat from a patient with neutral lipid storage disease (Wright stain). Note the presence of lipid droplets within granulocytes and monocytes but not lymphocytes or erythrocytes. (Courtesy of Dr. M. Williams)

suggesting a genetic founder effect.[165,166] Clinical characteristics are congenital generalized ichthyosis, vacuolated leukocytes, myopathy, cataracts, and sensorineural deafness.[167–169] The disorder presents at birth with generalized, fine white scaling of the skin and a variable degree of erythema. On the lower extremities and the scalp, the scales may become larger and plate-like with detached borders. Diagnostic are the presence of numerous lipid-containing vacuoles in circulating granulocytes, eosinophils, and monocytes (Fig. 8.23) detectable in a fresh peripheral blood smear.[166] Similar findings to a lesser extent may be seen in heterozygous carriers of the disease.[166] Using lipid stains (oil red-O, Sudan III), cytoplasmic lipid droplets can be also detected in fresh frozen skin sections, in particular in the epithelium of the eccrine sweat glands and ducts, in fibroblasts, basal and sometimes suprabasal keratinocytes.[165,167,170] However, similar findings in basal keratinocytes might be also observed in Refsum disease, a peroxisomal disorder of lipid metabolism.[171] Unique ultrastructural abnormalities of the epidermis include globular electron-lucent inclusions, which disrupt the normal structure of lamellar bodies in cells of the granular layers and change the conformation of intercellular lipid lamellae throughout the stratum corneum.[172] The widespread tissue deposition of neutral lipids results in a wide array of organ manifestations during childhood. Serum liver enzymes and muscle phosphocreatine kinase are usually elevated, although myopathy may be mild and detectable only by neurological examination. Hepatomegaly is common and liver biopsies revealed in all patients severe fatty degeneration and fibrosis of hepatocytes, which might not be reflected in liver function studies.[173,174] Cataract, neurosensory deafness, and developmental delay are common features of the syndrome, while growth retardation, ataxia, microcephaly,

splenomegaly and intestinal malabsorption have been observed only in a subset of patients.[165]

Neutral lipid storage disease has been mapped to 3p21 and inactivating mutations have been identified in the CGI-58 gene. Its gene product belongs to the esterase/lipase/thioesterase family but the specific epidermal biochemical pathways leading to disturbed cornification have not been elucidated. Cytoplasmic accumulation of triglycerides results presumably from a defect in degradation of endogenously produced diacylglycerols. Hydrolyzed fatty acids and the acylated glycerol backbone of triglycerides cannot be properly incorporated into phospholipids, and are instead re-esterified to form triglycerides.[175] Hydrolysis of triglycerides of exogenous origin (serum lipoproteins) via liposomal acid lipase as well as endogenous triglycerides via cytosolic lipase is normal. Nevertheless, the amount and spectrum of produced phospholipids in cultured fibroblasts of affected patients appeared normal.[176] The prognosis of neutral lipid storage disease with ichthyosis mainly depends on the course of liver disease and extent of liver fibrosis. Therapy is symptomatic. Fat-restricted diets were found beneficial in individual cases,[177] and systemic retinoids have been shown to improve ichthyosis.[165]

REFSUM DISEASE

Gabriele Richard

Synonyms: Heredopathia atactica polyneuritiformis, phytanic acid storage disease (MIM 266500)

This is a rare autosomal recessive neurological syndrome characterized by an excessive accumulation of phytanic acid in tissues and body fluids. Due to deficiency of the peroxisomal enzyme phytanoyl-CoA hydroxylase, patients are unable to degrade phytanic acid, a 20-carbon, saturated, branched-chain fatty acid exclusively derived from dietary chlorophyll.[178] The disorder usually leads to insidious neurological symptoms such as muscle weakness, difficulty walking, and failing night vision during childhood. The progressive but undulating course of the disorder with periods of acute exacerbation and remission may delay diagnosis and results in gradual neurological deterioration. Cardinal features of Refsum disease are cerebellar ataxia, atypical retinitis pigmentosa, peripheral polyneuropathy, and elevated protein content in the cerebrospinal fluid. In addition, these may be accompanied by other symptoms, including cranial nerve dysfunction (sensorineural deafness, anosmia), cardiomyopathy, renal tubular dysfunction, and skeletal hyperostosis. Cutaneous symptoms tend to develop in adulthood. The associated ichthyosis is mild to moderate with small white scales covering extremities and trunk often resembling ichthyosis vulgaris. Larger and dark scales or palmoplantar keratoderma have been also reported.[179] Lipid-containing vacuoles in basal keratinocytes may be the only diagnostic finding on histopathologic skin examination.[179] The diagnosis can be established by detecting severely increased phytanic acid levels in the plasma using liquid gas chromatography[180] or severely decreased phytanic acid oxidase activity in cultured fibroblasts.[181] Heterozygous carriers of Refsum disease usually have

165. Judge MR, Atherton DJ, Salvayre R et al. (1994) Neutral lipid storage disease. Case report and lipid studies. **Br J Dermatol** 130:507–510.
166. Williams ML, Koch TK, O'Donnell JJ et al. (1985) Ichthyosis and neutral lipid storage disease. **Am J Med Genet** 20:711–726.
167. Srebrnik A, Brenner S, Ilie B et al. (1998) Dorfman–Chanarin syndrome: morphologic studies and presentation of new cases. **Am J Dermatopathol** 20:79–85.
168. Dorfman ML. Hershko C, Eisenberg S et al. (1974) Ichthyosiform dermatosis with systemic lipidosis. **Arch Dermatol** 110:261–266.
169. Chanarin I, Fatel A, Slavin G et al. (1975) Neutral-lipid storage disease: a new disorder of lipid metabolism. **Br Med J** 1:553–555.
170. Paller AS (1994) Laboratory tests for ichthyosis. **Dermatol Clin** 12:99–107.
171. Dykes PJ, Marks R, Davies MG et al. (1978) Epidermal metabolism in heredopathia atactica polyneuritiformis (Refsum's disease). **J Invest Dermatol** 70:126–129.
172. Elias PM, Williams ML (1985) Neutral lipid storage disease with ichthyosis. Defective lamellar body contents and intracellular dispersion. **Arch Dermatol** 121:1000–1008.
173. Gurakan F, Kaymaz F, Kocak N et al. (1999) A cause of fatty liver: neutral lipid storage disease with ichthyosis – electron microscopic findings. **Dig Dis Sci** 44:2214–2217.

174. Musumeci S, D'Agata A, Romano C et al. (1988) Ichthyosis and neutral lipid storage disease. **Am J Med Genet** 29:377–382.
175. Igal RA, Coleman RA (1996) Acylglycerol recycling from triacylglycerol to phospholipid, not lipase activity, is defective in neutral lipid storage disease fibroblasts. **J Biol Chem** 271:16644–16651.
176. Williams ML, Coleman RA, Placezk D et al. (1991) Neutral lipid storage disease: a possible functional defect in phospholipid-linked triacylglycerol metabolism. **Biochim Biophys Acta** 1096:162–169.
177. Kakourou T, Drogari E, Christomanou H et al. (1997) Neutral lipid storage disease – response to dietary intervention. **Arch Dis Child** 77:184.
178. Wanders RJA, Jacobs C, Skjedal OH (2001) Refsum disease. In: Refsum Disease, Scriver CR, Beaudet AL, Sly WS et al., eds. New York: McGraw-Hill, pp. 3303–3317.
179. Davies MG, Marks R, Dykes PJ et al. (1977) Epidermal abnormalities in Refsum's disease. **Br J Dermatol** 97:401–406.
180. Cingolani L (1987) Rapid gas chromatographic determination of phytanic acid from serum of a patient suffering from Refsum's disease. **J Chromatogr** 419:475–478.
181. Poulos A, Pollard AC, Mitchell JD et al. (1984) Patterns of Refsum's disease. Phytanic acid oxidase deficiency. **Arch Dis Child** 59:222–229.

normal plasma levels of phytanic acid, although the enzyme activity of phytanoyl-CoA hydroxylase is decreased in cultured fibroblasts. Prenatal diagnosis can be performed by measuring phytanic acid oxidation in cultured cells obtained by CVS or amniocentesis.

Abnormalities in catabolism of phytanic acid and its accumulation also occur in other peroxisomal deficiency syndromes including rhizomelic chondrodysplasia punctata, Zellweger syndrome, infantile Refsum disease, and neonatal adrenal lipodystrophy. The combination of neurological symptoms and late-onset ichthyosis, however, is characteristic of Refsum disease.

The disorder is caused by recessive mutations in the *PAHX* gene on the short arm of chromosome 10.[182,183] Missense mutations, insertions, deletions, and splice-site mutations have been observed, many of which inactivate the peroxisomal enzyme phytanoyl-CoA hydroxylase.[183] This enzyme contains a type-2 peroxisomal targeting signal[182] and catalyzes the first step of phytanic acid metabolism by generating pristanic acid. The enzymatic block leads to subsequent accumulation of phytanic acid in plasma and various tissues where it replaces up to 50% of normal fatty acid constituents, thus explaining skin, liver, heart, adipose, and peripheral nervous tissue involvement.[182] In contrast, little phytanic acid is stored in the brain. Preliminary data suggest that a disturbed interaction of *PAHX* with its associated protein number 1 might lead to the development of cranial nerve symptoms.[182]

Restricted dietary intake of phytanic acid of less than 5mg/day may prevent acute attacks and arrest the progression of organ impairment, especially in the peripheral nervous system.[183,184] However, retinal changes are usually irreversible.[185] Therapeutic plasma exchange is recommended for management of acute toxicity as well as in combination with diet for long-term management.[183,184]

CONRADI–HÜNERMANN–HAPPLE SYNDROME
Heiko Traupe

INCIDENCE

The Conradi–Hünermann–Happle syndrome (CHH syndrome) is a rare X-chromosomal dominant skin disease. There are no actual data on its incidence, but it makes up a good proportion of cases of chondrodysplasia punctata and based on our personal experience in Westphalia (about 10 cases in 2 million inhabitants) a prevalence of 1 in 200 000 is realistic.

CLINICAL FEATURES

The CHH syndrome belongs to the group of associated ichthyoses. In other words the CHH syndrome is a multisystem disorder involving skin, bones and eyes. The condition also is often called "X-linked dominant chondrodysplasia punctata."

CUTANEOUS INVOLVEMENT

At birth the skin often exhibits severe erythroderma and the affected girls are born with marked scaling which is arranged in particular on the back in whorls and swirls and follows the lines of Blaschko (Fig. 8.24). Erythroderma and scaling on the trunk usually resolve after the first few months of life leaving follicular atrophoderma, hypo- and hyperpigmentations and circumscribed scarring alopecia on the scalp (Fig. 8.25), whereas ichthyosis on

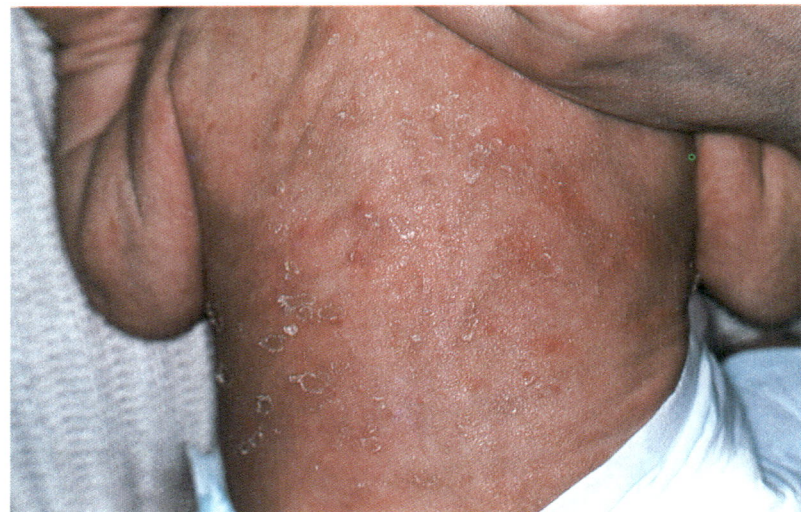

Fig. 8.24   Conradi–Hünermann–Happle syndrome in a neonate. Note arrangement of the hyperkeratoses in whorls and swirls on the back visualizing the lines of Blaschko.

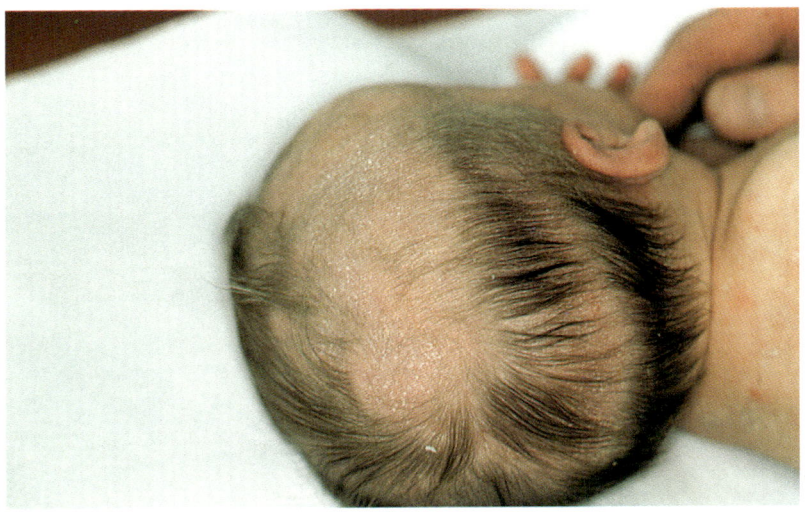

Fig. 8.25   Marked alopecia in a neonate with Conradi–Hünermann–Happle syndrome.

arms and legs often remains present during the entire life (Fig. 8.26). Many patients show minor nail anomalies, for example flattening of the nailplates (platonychia) or splitting into layers (onychochisis).[186,187] In particular in the adult patients patchy areas of cicatricial alopecia are a constant feature and sometimes may even be the only cutaneous manifestation seen in mildly affected female conductors.[188]

NONCUTANEOUS FINDINGS

A further hallmark of the syndrome is the asymmetry of the skeletal involvement. Punctate calcifications of the epiphyseal regions usually result in an asymmetric shortening of the long bones, sometimes in very severe

182. Mihalik SJ, Morrell JC, Kim D et al. (1997) Identification of PAHX, a Refsum disease gene. **Nat Genet** 17:185–189.
183. Jansen GA, Ferdinandusse S, Hogenhout EM et al. (1999) Phytanoyl-CoA hydroxylase deficiency. Enzymological and molecular basis of classical Refsum disease. **Adv Exp Med Biol** 466:371–376.
184. Weinstein R (1999) Phytanic acid storage disease (Refsum's disease): clinical characteristics, pathophysiology and the role of therapeutic apheresis in its management. **J Clin Apheresis** 14:181–184.
185. Claridge KG, Gibberd FB, Sidey MC (1992) Refsum disease: the presentation and ophthalmic aspects of Refsum disease in a series of 23 patients. **Eye** 6:371–375.
186. Goerttier E (1979) Chondrodysplasia punctata Typ Conradi–Hünermann. **Z Hautkr** 54:676–677.
187. Happle R, Kästner H (1979) X-gekoppelt dominante Chondrodysplasia punctata. **Hautarzt** 30:590–594.
188. Manzke H, Christophers E, Wiedemann HR (1980) Dominant sex-linked inherited chondrodysplasia punctata: a distinct type of chondrodysplasia punctata. **Clin Genet** 17:97–107.

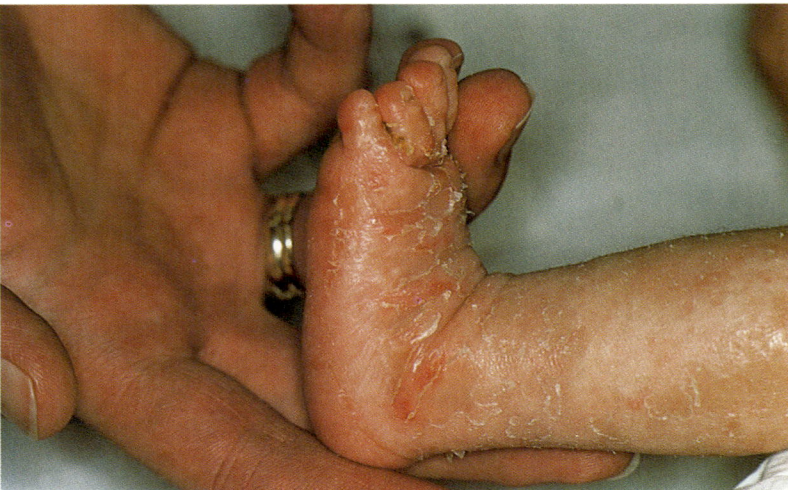

Fig. 8.26 Conradi–Hünermann–Happle syndrome. Hyperkeratoses on the lower leg are often not "linear." Same neonate as in Figs 8.24 and 8.25.

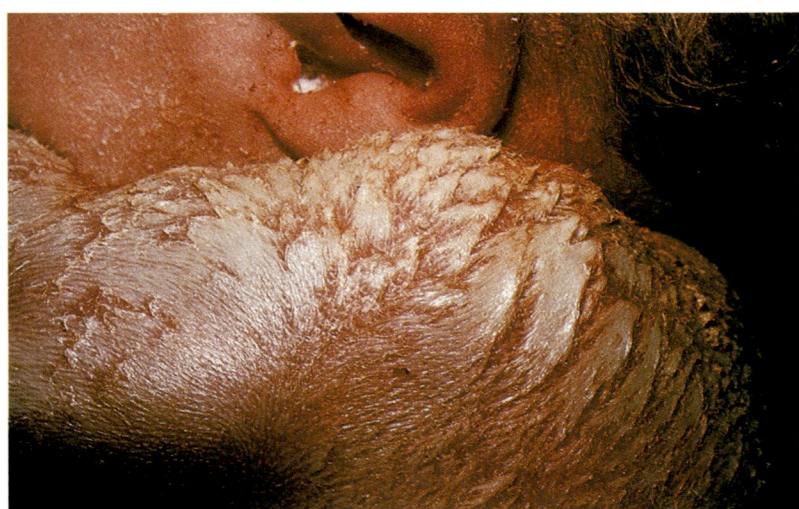

Fig. 8.28 Striking follicular hyperkeratoses in a severely affected neonate with Conradi–Hünermann–Happle syndrome. (Courtesy of Dr. D. Müller, Chemnitz)

kyphoscoliosis, facial dysplasia and congenital hip dislocation.[189,190] Interestingly, one case with a symmetrical shortening of the tubula/bones has also been reported.[191] Skeletal manifestations are not invariably present,[192] and in our personal experience may be clinically inconspicuous at birth but still can become manifest during the first years of life. This applies in particular for kyphoscoliosis. Unilateral and sectorial cataracts (Fig. 8.27) are further typical signs of the disease.[193,194]

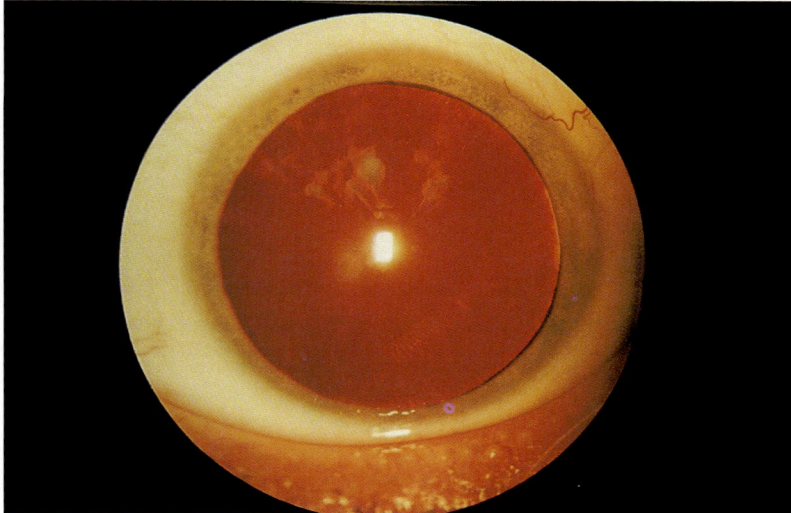

Fig. 8.27 Sectorial cataract as a clinical manifestation of somatic mosaicism in the Conradi–Hünermann–Happle syndrome. We failed to find the mutation in this lady, but her daughter and granddaughter showed clear-cut disease caused by a premature stop codon (Y111X). (Courtesy of Dr. D. Müller, Chemnitz)

HISTOLOGY AND ULTRASTRUCTURAL FEATURES

Histologic features of the CHH syndrome resemble those of autosomal dominant ichthyosis vulgaris. Routine histology discloses a compact ortho-hyperkeratotic stratum corneum, a diminished granular layer, slight epidermal hyperplasia and slight perivascular infiltrates in the upper dermis. In the neonate an extreme follicular hyperkeratosis (Fig. 8.28) can be very striking and at this stage histochemical staining for calcium (von Kossa's stain) reveals calcifications within the epidermis (Fig. 8.29). In older children calcium depositions can often no longer be visualized by histochemistry. Ultrastructural examinations reveal a prominent vacuolization of keratinocytes in the granular layer[195] and cytoplasmic vacuoles containing electron dense stellate bodies in the keratinocytes.[195] Moreover, the number of Langerhans cells is markedly reduced and there is a degeneration of Langerhans cells.[196]

BIOCHEMICAL AND GENETIC ASPECTS

In the years 1977 to 1979 Rudolf Happle delineated the CHH syndrome as a distinct type of chondrodysplasia punctata characterized by a mosaic pattern of skin lesions.[187,197,198] As in incontinentia pigmenti, the disease occurred exclusively in the female sex and the cutaneous changes showed a similar linear distribution pattern with widespread atrophic lesions, pigmentary disturbances and ichthyosis. Based on these peculiar cutaneous findings Happle argued that he was dealing with a further X-linked dominant gene defect that is usually lethal in males, and interpreted the linear cutaneous involvement as an example of X-chromosome inactivation and functional mosaicism.[193,197] A peculiar phenomenon seen in the disease is anticipation of a stepwise increase in disease expression from one generation to the other.[190,199] In part, anticipation may reflect the presence of gonadal and somatic mosaicism in the parent generation.[194]

189. Mueller RF, Crowle PM, Jones RAK, Davison BCC (1985) X-linked dominant chondrodysplasia punctata: a case report and family studies. **Am J Med Genet** 20:137–144.
190. Sutphen R, Amar MJ, Kousseff BG, Toomey KE (1995) XXY male with X-linked dominant chondrodysplasia punctata (Happle syndrome). **Am J Med Genet** 57:489–492.
191. Gobello T, Mazzanti C, Fileccia P et al. (1995) X-linked dominant chondrodysplasia punctata (Happle syndrome) with uncommon symmetrical shortening of the tubular bones. **Dermatology** 191:323–327.
192. Kalter DC, Atherton DI, Clayton PI (1989) X-linked dominant Conradi–Hünermann syndrome presenting as congenital erythroderma. **J Am Acad Dermatol** 21:248–256.
193. Happle R (1981) Cataracts as a marker of genetic heterogeneity in chondrodysplasia punctata. **Clin Genet** 19:64–66.
194. Has C, Bruckner-Tuderman L, Müller D et al. (2000) The Conradi–Hünermann–Happle syndrome (CDPX2) and emopamil binding protein: novel mutations, and somatic and gonadal mosaicism. **Hum Mol Genet** 13:1951–1955.
195. Kolde G, Happle R (1984) Histologic and ultrastructural features of the ichthyotic skin in X-linked dominant chondrodysplasia punctata. **Acta Derm Venereol** 64:389–394.
196. Kolde G, Happle R (1985) Langerhans-cell degeneration in X-linked dominant ichthyosis. A quantitative and ultrastructural study. **Arch Dermatol Res** 277:245–247.
197. Happle R (1979) X-linked dominant chondrodysplasia punctata. Review of literature and report of a case. **Hum Genet** 53:65–73.
198. Happle R (1978) Genetic interpretation of linear skin abnormalities. **Hautzart** 29:357–363.
199. Traupe H, Müller D, Atherton D et al. (1992) Exclusion mapping of the X-linked dominant chondrodysplasia punctata/ichthyosis/cataract/short stature (Happle) syndrome: possible involvement of an unstable pre-mutation. **Hum Genet** 89:659–665.

The hypothesis of an unstable premutation[190] as well as the implication of a primary peroxisomal defect[200,201] proved to be incorrect when recently mutations were identified in the gene that encodes emopamil binding protein (EBP) in several patients.[194,202–204] The EBP gene resides on the short arm of the X-chromosome at Xp11.22–p11.23 and could be shown to be deficient in the mouse mutant *tattered (Td)* as well. The EBP gene has a dual function: on the one hand it serves as a binding protein for the Ca^{2+} antagonist emopamil and thus as a high affinity receptor for several anti-ischemic drugs,[205] and on the other hand it also acts as a delta8-delta7 sterol isomerase which is a key enzyme in the final steps of cholesterol bio-synthesis.[205] Due to the enzymatic block cholesterol precursor molecules such as 8-dehydrocholesterol (8-DHC) and cholest-8(9)-en-3-beta-ol are markedly accumulated, which allows a rapid lipid-biochemical diagnosis of the CHH syndrome by gas chromatography–mass spectrometry (GC–MS) studies.[207] GC–MS analysis of cholesterol precursors demonstrates markedly elevated levels of 8-dehydrocholesterol and of cholest-8(9)-en-3-beta-ol and is a very reliable method that could even help to identify somatic mosaicism in a clinically healthy man.

However, the extent of the metabolic alterations do not correlate well with the molecular genotype nor with the severity of the clinical phenotype. This lack of correlation is probably due to differences in X-inactivation between different tissues of the same patient.

The severe disturbance of cholesterol biosynthesis seen in this disorder is certainly also the metabolic cause for the severe congenital skeletal dysplasia. Other metabolic defects of cholesterol biosynthesis such as the Smith–Lemli–Opitz syndrome or the CHILD syndrome are also associated with congenital skeletal dysplasia and with chondrodysplasia punctata. A lesson that can be learned from the CHH syndrome is that vertebrate embryonic development is dependent on large amounts of cholesterol which is needed for growth and for the synthesis of compounds derived from cho-lesterol, such as steroid hormones. An abnormal cholesterol metabolism obviously impairs the function of "sonic hedgehog" and other related embryonic signaling proteins that help determine the vertebrate body plan during the earliest weeks of embryonic development. It should be noted that the Smith–Lemli–Opitz syndrome which features a related metabolic defect, namely 7-dehydrocholesterol reductase deficiency, has been proposed to be mainly related to deficiency of cholesterol[208] and that in this syndrome the autistic behavior of children can be reduced or even eliminated by treatment with supplementary dietary cholesterol. Whether such a cholesterol supple-mentation is meaningful also in CHH syndrome patients remains to be seen.

CHILD SYNDROME

Arne König

CHILD is an acronym for *c*ongenital *h*emidysplasia with *i*chthyosiform nevus and *l*imb *d*efects. The syndrome was delineated by Happle *et al.* in 1980 as an X-linked dominant trait characterized by the phenomenon of functional X-chromosome mosaicism.[209] In the original publication the "I" stood for "ichthyosiform erythroderma." However, later it became evident that the characteristic cutaneous pathology of this syndrome represents a distinct entity

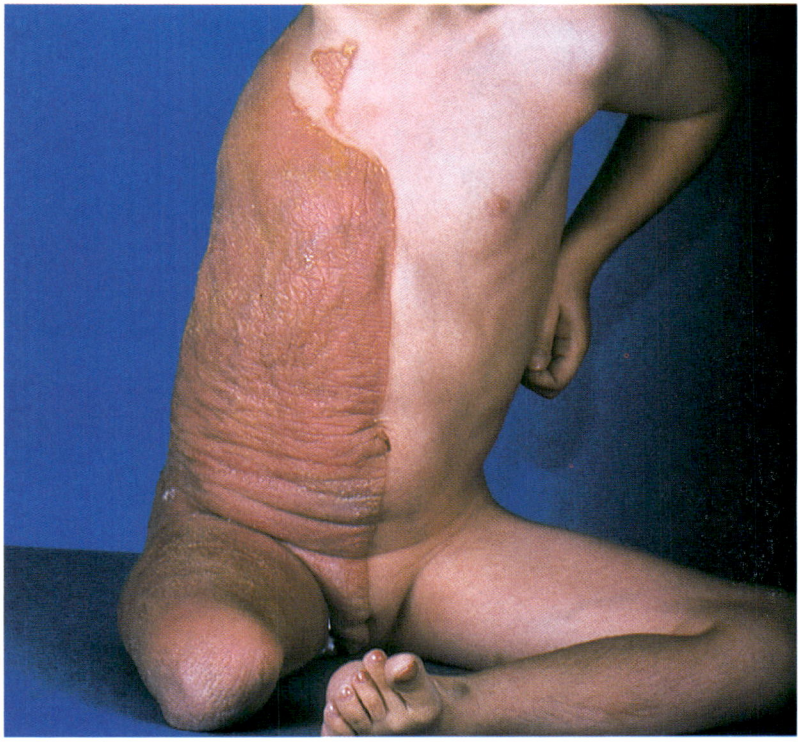

Fig. 8.30 **CHILD syndrome.** Note lateralization of CHILD nevus with strict demarcation as well as ipsilateral absence of arm.

that should be referred to as "CHILD nevus."[210] The X-linked genetic defect represents a lethal factor for male embryos which is why this phenotype is almost exclusively observed in female patients. The most striking feature is an inflammatory nevus with a unique lateralization and strict midline demarcation (Fig. 8.30). In some cases the nevus follows the lines of Blaschko, but there is virtually always a far more pronounced involvement of one side of the body. Ipsilateral hypoplasia of the body may affect all skeletal structures, and shortness or even complete absence of a limb is noted. Development of visceral organs may be impaired on the affected body side; defects of kidney, lung, heart and brain have been reported. The CHILD nevus is characterized by yellowish, wax-like scales that can be removed without bleeding (Fig. 8.31). This nevus may sometimes partially resolve later in life, but usually it shows a pronounced affinity for the body folds, a phenomenon to which the term ptychotropism has been applied.

Histopathological examination shows a psoriasiform dermatitis with acanthosis, zones of parakeratosis and an exocytosis of neutrophils that may form accumulations reminiscent of Munro abscesses. Apart from these epidermal changes, the distinctive feature of verruciform xanthoma may be found in the dermis, especially when the biopsy is obtained from a body fold. The widened dermal papillae abound with foamy histiocytes. Ultra-structurally these cells show intracytoplasmic vacuoles that contain large amounts of so far unidentified lipids.[210] Emami and coworkers have

200. Emami S, Hanley KP, Esterly NB et al. (1994) X-linked dominant ichthyosis with peroxisomal deficiency. An ultrastructural and ultracytochemical study of the Conradi–Hünermann syndrome and its mur ne homologue. **Arch Dermatol** 130:325–336.
201. Wilson CJ, Aftimos S (1998) X-linked dominant chondrodysplasia punctata: a peroxisomal disorder? **Am J Med Genet** 78:300–302.
202. Derry JM, Gormally E, Means GD et al. (1999) Mutation sin a delta 8-delta 7 sterol isomerase in the tettered mouse and chondrodysplasia punctata. **Nat Genet** 22:286–290.
203. Braverman N, Lin P, Mocbius FE et al. (1999) Mutations in the gene encoding 3 beta-hydroxysteroid-delta 8, delta 7-isomerase cause X-linked dominant Conradi–Hünermann syndrome. **Nat Genet** 22:291–294.
204. Ikegawa S, Chashi H, Kogata T et al. (2000) Novel and recurrent EBP mutations in X-linked dominant chondrodysplasia punctata. **Am J Med Genet** 94:300–305.
205. Moebius FF, Sellner KE, Fiechtner B et al. (1999) Histidine 77, glutamic acid81, glutamic acid123, threoninel126, asparagaine194, and tryptophan197 of the human emopamil binding protein are required for in vivo sterol delta 8-delta 7 isomerization. **Biochemistry** 38:1119–1127.
206. Silve S, Dupuy PH, Labit-Lebouteiller C et al. (1996) Emopamil-binding protein, a mammalian protein that binds a series of structurally diverse neuroprotective agents, exhibits delta8delta7 sterol isomerase activity in yeast. **J Biol Chem** 271:22434–22440.
207. Kelley RI, Wilcox WG, Smith M et al. (1999) Abnormal sterol metabolism in patients with Conradi–Hünermann–Happle syndrome and sporadic lethal chondrodysplasia punctata. **Am J Med Genet** 83:213–219.
208. Gaoua W, Wolf C, Chevy F et al. (2000) Cholesterol deficit but not accumulation of aberrant sterols is the major cause of the teratogenic activity in the Smith–Lemli–Opitz syndrome animal model. **J Lipid Res** 41:637–646.
209. Happle R, Koch H, Lenz W (1980) The CHILD syndrome: congenital hemidysplasia with ichthyosiform erythroderma and limb defects. **Eur J Pediatr** 134:27.
210. Happle R, Mittag H, Küster W (1995) The CHILD nevus: a distinct skin disorder. **Dermatology** 191:210.

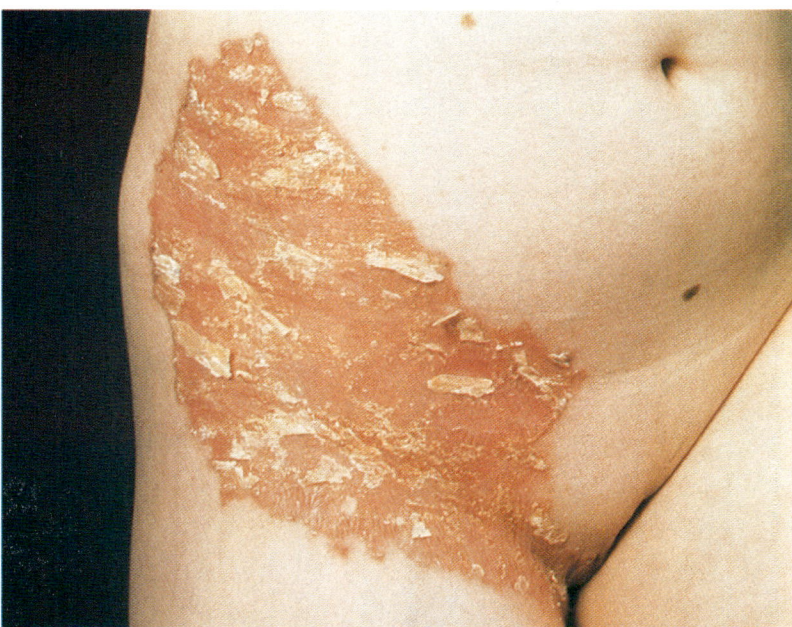

Fig. 8.31   Close-up aspect of CHILD nevus. The typical wax-like scales can be removed without bleeding. A characteristic feature of the CHILD nevus is ptychotropism, i.e., a marked affinity for body folds.

reported a peroxisomal deficiency in lesional skin of CHILD syndrome patients.[211]

The skeletal manifestations include the phenomenon of epiphyseal stippling which can only be seen on X-rays performed in early infancy. Shortening or absence of a limb is the most striking manifestation but many patients also show involvement of the spine or the pelvis. The degree of skeletal involvement may vary considerably and sometimes shortening of a single phalanx may be the only clinical finding. Visceral defects are noted on the side of CHILD nevus and limb malformations. Absence of a kidney, hypoplasia of lung, thyroid or heart have been observed. Involvement of the nervous system includes ipsilateral defects of cranial nerves, pons, medulla, cerebellum, or spinal cord. The electroencephalogram may show ipsilateral abnormalities.

Recently, the underlying molecular defect has been elucidated. Point mutations in the gene *NSDHL* [NAD(P)H steroid dehydrogenase-like protein] at Xq28 were demonstrated in several patients with CHILD syndrome.[212] This gene most likely encodes a novel type of 3β-hydroxysteroid dehydrogenase, similar to that described in the murine *Nsdhl* mutant *bare patches*. The molecular analysis provides a reliable tool for genetic counseling, since mother-to-daughter transmission has sometimes been reported. Moreover, it is possible to confirm the diagnosis in patients with minimal or atypical involvement, for instance in an exceptional case with almost symmetrical manifestation.[213]

Patterned involvement is seen in female carriers of many X-linked genodermatoses such as focal dermal hypoplasia, X-linked dominant chondrodysplasia punctata or incontinentia pigmenti. In most cases the abnormal skin follows the pattern of Blaschko's lines. The concept of functional X-chromosome mosaicism can be applied to these phenotypes. Due to the Lyon effect of X-inactivation two functionally different cell clones develop at an early stage of embryogenesis leading to a patterned involvement of streaks and patches. However, the striking lateralization pattern as seen in CHILD syndrome is unique. Probably the *NSDHL* gene plays an important role in early human embryogenesis and the gene product is likely to be involved in the development of the bilateral body symmetry.

CHILD syndrome has sometimes been confused with X-linked dominant chondrodysplasia punctata (CHH syndrome). Despite some similarities the two syndromes can be clearly distinguished both clinically and at the molecular level without overlapping. The highly characteristic appearance of the CHILD nevus cannot be confused with the atrophodermic skin changes of X-linked dominant chondrodysplasia punctata that usually shows a bilateral asymmetrical pattern of involvement and is caused by mutations in the gene *EBP* at Xp11.22–p11.23.[214,215]

KID SYNDROME

Peter Itin

INTRODUCTION AND HISTORICAL NOTE

In 1915 Burns[216] described a symptom complex consisting of *keratitis*, *ichthyosis* and *deafness*. In 1981 Skinner *et al.*[217] coined the acronym "KID" syndrome. Traupe[218] suggested that the "I" was redefined as ichthyosis-like hyperkeratosis. Nousari *et al.*[219] documented a case of KID syndrome with features of ichthyosis hystrix. There seems to be a second misnomer in the acronym KID, as deafness defines a profound hearing loss.[220] However, in KID syndrome hearing loss is highly variable. Therefore the "D" in the acronym could be replaced by "H" representing hearing loss.

The clinical features are characterized by erythrokeratoderma at birth, which usually fades or disappears after some days. In 1996 a review of all cases was performed by Caceres-Rios *et al.*[221] and these authors realized that patients with KID syndrome have a form of ectodermal dysplasia (Freire-Maia classification 1–2–3–4) and they suggested the name KED for *keratitis*, *ectodermal dysplasia* and *deafness*. Recently, Richard *et al.* and Van Steensel *et al.* reported connexin-26 as the cause of KID syndrome.[222,223]

EPIDEMIOLOGY

KID syndrome is extremely rare and no more than 100 cases have been reported in the literature. Some few inherited cases exist which suggest an autosomal dominant inheritance. However, an inheritance pattern suggestive for autosomal recessive trait has been published. Most cases of KID syndrome occur sporadically due to *de novo* dominant mutations.

211. Emami S, Rizzo WB, Hanley KP et al. (1992) Peroxisomal abnormality in fibroblasts from involved skin of CHILD syndrome: case study and review of peroxisomal disorders in relation to skin disease. **Arch Dermatol** 128:1213.
212. König A, Happle R, Bornholdt D et al. (2000) Mutations in the NSDHL gene, encoding a 3β-hydroxysteroid dehydrogenase, cause CHILD syndrome. **Am J Med Genet** 90:339.
213. König A, Happle R, Fink-Puches R et al. (2002) A novel missense mutation of NSDHL in an unusual case of CHILD syndrome showing bilateral, almost symmetrical involvement. **J Am Acad Dermatol** 46:594–596.
214. Braverman N, Lin P, Moebius FF et al. (1999) Mutations in the gene encoding 3 beta-hydroxysteroid-delta 8, delta 7-isomerase cause X-linked dominant Conradi–Hünermann syndrome. **Nat Genet** 22:291.
215. Derry JM, Gormally E, Means GD et al. (1999) Mutations in a delta 8-delta 7 sterol isomerase in the tattered mouse and X-linked dominant chondrodysplasia punctata. **Nat Genet** 22:286.
216. Burns FS (1915) Generalized congenital keratoderma. A case of generalized congenital keratoderma with unusual involvement of the eyes, ears, and nasal and buccal mucous membranes. **J Cutan Dis** 33:255–260.

217. Skinner BA, Greist MC, Norins AL (1981) The keratitis, ichthyosis, and deafness (KID) syndrome. **Arch Dermatol** 117:285–289.
218. Traupe H (1990) Not an ichthyosis at all: the keratitis, ichthyosis-like hyperkeratosis, and deafness (KID) syndrome. In: The Ichthyoses. A guide to Clinical Diagnosis, Genetic Counseling, and Therapy, Traupe H, ed. Berlin, Heidelberg, New York: Springer-Verlag.
219. Nousari HC, Kimyai-Asadi A, Pinto JL (2000) KID syndrome associated with features of ichthyosis hystrix. **Pediatr Dermatol** 17:115–117.
220. Nowell WA (1988) Keratitis, ichthyosis, and deafness (KID) syndrome: suggested changes in terminology. **Arch Dermatol.** 124:22.
221. Caceres-Rios H, Tamayo-Sanchez L, Duran-Mckinstes C et al. (1996) Keratitis, ichthyosis, and deafness (KID syndrome): review of the literature and proposal of a new terminology. **Pediatr Dermatol** 13:105–113.
222. Richard G, Ronan F, Willoughby CE et al. (2002) Missense mutations in GIB2 encoding connexin-26 cause the ectodermal dysplasia keratitis-ichthyosis-deafness syndrome. **Am J Hum Genet** 10:1341–1348.
223. Van Steensel MA, van Geel M, Nahuys M et al. (2002) A novel connexin-26 mutation in a patient diagnosed with keratitis-ichthyosis-deafness syndrome. **J Invest Dermatol** 118:724–727.

PRESENTING HISTORY AND PHYSICAL EXAMINATION

The skin lesions evolve in hyperkeratotic localized plaques which often underlie erythema and they are best called ichthyosis-like hyperkeratoses (Fig. 8.32). At birth erythroderma often occurs which fades after a few days. Hyperkeratotic plaques with underlying erythema develop and Küster et al.[218] separated two clinical subsets of KID syndrome. One type has a typical facial involvement with bizarre and sharply outlined verrucous hyperkeratotic plaques occurring also on elbows, knees, palms and soles (Fig. 8.33). The other phenotype shows more severe and diffuse involvement

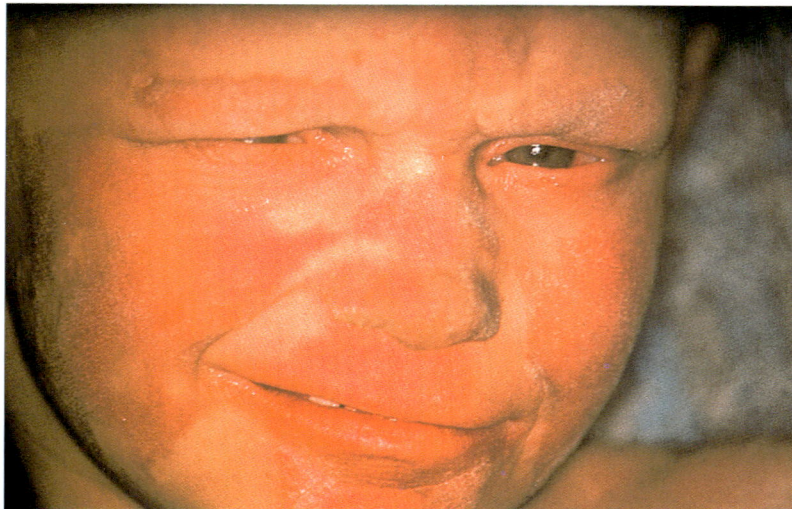

Fig. 8.32   KID syndrome: characteristic facial erythrokeratoderma. (Courtesy of Dr. Robert Gorlin, Minneapolis, MN, USA)

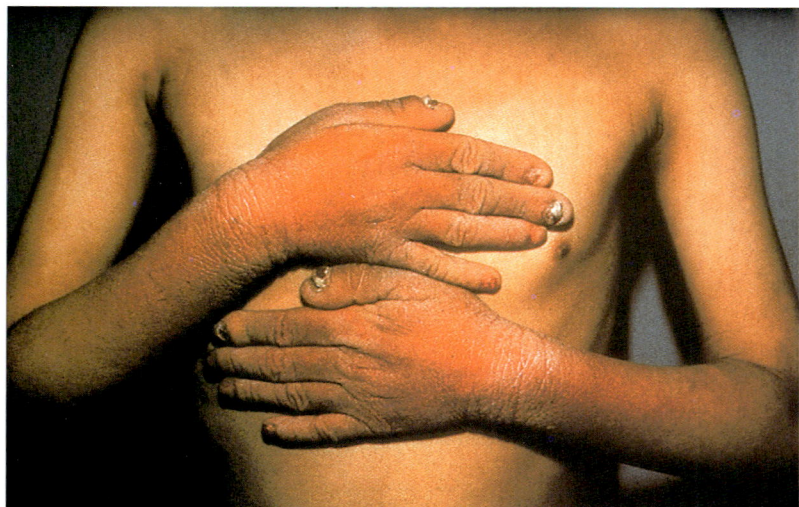

Fig. 8.33   KID syndrome: erythrokeratoderma showing pronounced lichenification. (Courtesy of Dr. Robert Gorlin, Minneapolis, MN, USA)

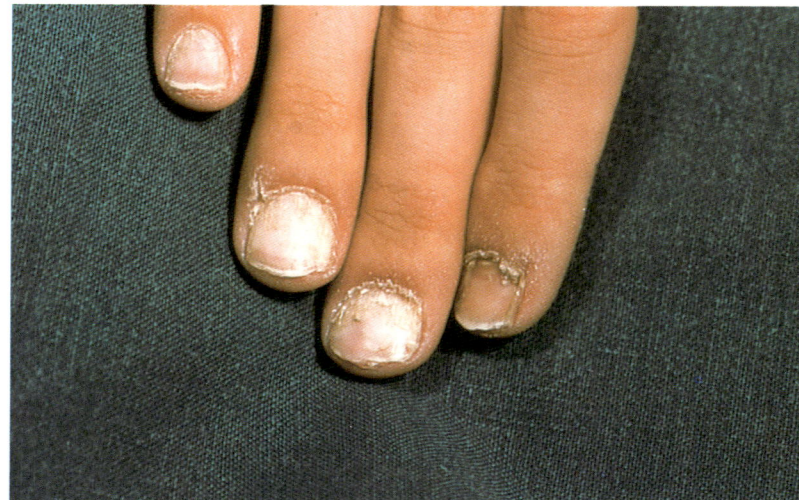

Fig. 8.34   Leukonychia in KID syndrome.

of the skin with severe scarring alopecia. Our review of the literature disclosed that from 70 published patients there are only five documented cases with normal hair. KID syndrome is an ectodermal dysplasia in which hair is often alopecic. All patients show verrucous lesions with rippled hyperkeratosis and a peculiar variant of palmoplantar keratoderma. The nails often show leukonychia and dystrophy (Fig. 8.34). Patients with KID syndrome have a markedly high incidence of squamous cell cancer of the skin. The noncutaneous features include bilateral neurosensory hearing impairment and vascularizing keratitis. Hearing loss is congenital, but vascularizing keratitis develops during the natural course of the disease beginning with photophobia and ending in total blindness. In general physical growth and intellectual development are not affected. There is a large variety of associated signs and symptoms which mirror the ectodermal dysplasia complex.

PATHOPHYSIOLOGY AND HISTOGENESIS

Although patients with KID syndrome often have dry skin, normal sweating and tear production has been documented.[224] Histology of ichthyosis-like skin shows massive expansion of the stratum corneum with basketweave hyperkeratosis, follicular plugging and keratin horns.[225] Immunohistochemical investigation may reveal hyperproliferative changes and malignant development occurs.[226] The constellation of erythrokeratoderma-like skin lesions associated with deafness is extremely suggestive for a mutation in connexin which could produce the disease, but at present no such mutation has been found.

THERAPEUTICS AND PROGNOSIS

Oral fluconazole treatment of fungal candidiasis in KID syndrome has been reported with excellent result. Hazen et al.[227] reported on a possible exacerbation of corneal neovascularization under systemic retinoids in a patient with KID syndrome. Successful topical cyclosporin for progressive vascu-

224. Van Everdingen JJE, Rampen FHJ, Van der Schaar WW (1995) Normal sweating and tear production in congenital ichthyosiform erythroderma with deafness and keratitis. **Acta Derm Venereol (Stockh)** 62:76–78.

225. De Berker D, Branford WA, Soucek S, Michaels L (1993) Fatal keratitis ichthyosis and deafness syndrome (KIDS). Aural, ocular, and cutaneous histopathology. **Am J Dermatopathol** 15:64–69.

226. McGregor J, Markey A, Allen M et al. (1990) Keratitis, ichthyosis and deafness (KID)-syndrome: an histopathological and immunohistochemical study. 28th Annual Meeting of the American Society of Dermatopathology November 28–30, 307. Ref Type: Abstract.

227. Hazen PG, Corney TM, Langston RA, Meister DM (1986) Corneal effect of isotretinoin: possible exacerbation of corneal neovascularization in a patient with the keratitis, ichthyosis, deafness ("KID") syndrome. **J Am Acad Dermatol** 14:141–142.

larizing keratitis has been reported.[228] Local emollients and keratolytics should be applied regularly. The development of squamous cell cancer on skin and tongue is not a rare event. Recently, multiple hair follicle tumors were described in KID syndrome.[229]

NETHERTON SYNDROME

Peter Itin, Stephan Lautenschlager, Rudolf Happle

INTRODUCTION AND HISTORICAL NOTE

In 1949, Comel described a form of ichthyosis called ichthyosis linearis circumflexa, which was characterized by double-edged desquamation at the periphery of erythematous and scaling lesions with a serpiginous pattern. In 1958 Netherton reported a patient with a generalized erythematous ichthyosiform dermatosis associated with bamboo hair abnormalities and allergic asthma.

EPIDEMIOLOGY

Netherton syndrome (MIM 256500) is a rare (< 1 : 100 000) autosomal recessive disease characterized by hair shaft defects, ichthyosis and atopy.

PRESENTING HISTORY AND PHYSICAL FINDINGS

Most children with Netherton syndrome present with a generalized exfoliative dermatitis often combined with atopic diathesis (Fig. 8.35).[230] Newborns with Netherton syndrome may feature erythroderma.[230,231] Eighteen percent of 51 cases with neonatal and infantile erythrodermas were finally diagnosed as Netherton syndrome. Some patients with Netherton syndrome have a distinct form of nonbullous ichthyosis with erythema and

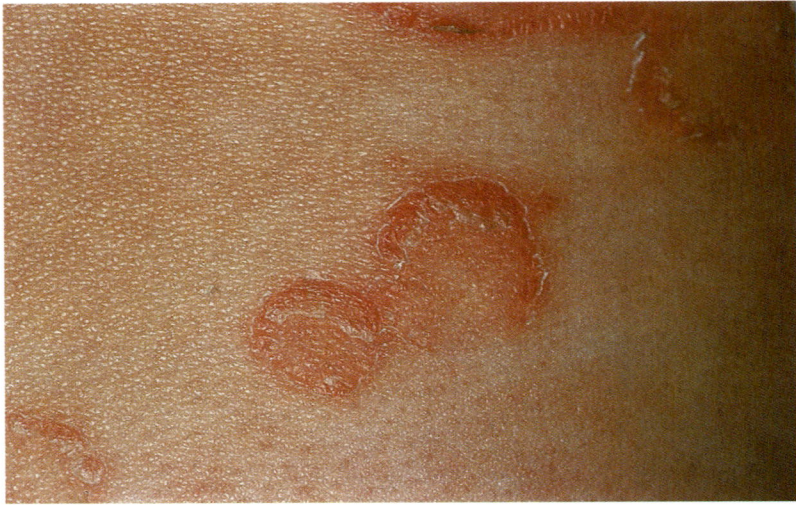

Fig. 8.36   Later, double-edged scaling and crusting developed.

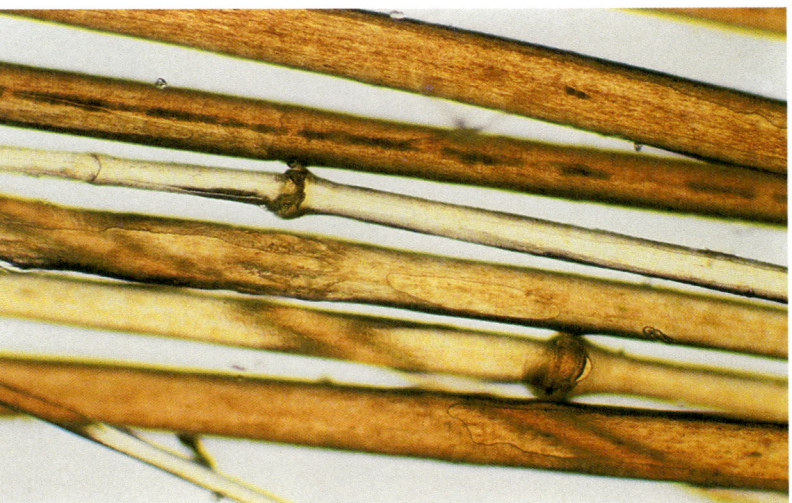

Fig. 8.37   Light microscopy clearly shows trichorrhexis invaginata.

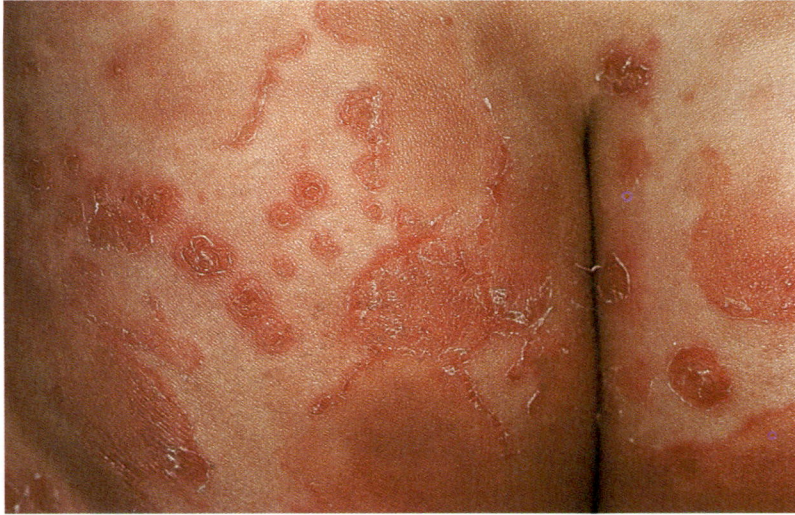

Fig. 8.35   Scaling erythematous lesions resembling atopic eczema.

polycyclic plaques with "double-edged" scale called ichthyosis linearis circumflexa (Fig. 8.36). Out of 43 cases with Netherton syndrome, 30 had ichthyosis linearis circumflexa[232] and congenital erythroderma was the predominant skin disorder in 13 patients. Some patients may present with a congenital psoriasis-like picture (Shwayder and Banerjee 1997).[233]

The main hair abnormality in patients with Netherton syndrome was initially named bamboo hair, and later called trichorrhexis invaginata (Fig. 8.37). Less specific hair abnormalities are torsions, trichorrhexis nodosa, and helical hairs.[234,235] However, in the neonatal period the hair shaft anomaly can still be lacking, which makes an early diagnosis rather difficult.[236] Sometimes the diagnosis of the hair shaft anomaly is easier to perform in the

228. Derse M, Wannke E, Payer H et al. (2002) Ertolgreiche topische Cyclosporin-A-therape bei progredienter vaskularisiere ulzeriernder Keratitis Deim Keratitis-Ichthyosis-Deafness (KID)-Syndrome. **Klin Monals Augenheild** 219:383–386.
229. Kim HH, Kim JS, Piao YJ et al. (2002) Keratitis, ichthyosis and deafness syndrome with development of multiple hair follicle tumours. **Br J Dermatol** 143: 139–143.
230. Hausser I, Anton-Lamprecht I (1996) Severe congenital generalized exfoliative erythroderma in newborns and infants: a possible sign of Netherton syndrome. **Pediatr Dermatol** 13:183–199.
231. Pruszkowski A, Bodemer C, Fraitags et al. (2000) Neonatal and infantile erythrodermas. A retrospective study of 51 patients. **Arch Dermatol** 136:875–880.

232. Greene SL, Muller SA (1985) Netherton's syndrome: report of a case and review of the literature. **J Am Acad Dermatol**. 13:329–337.
233. Shwayder T, Banerjee S (1997) Netherton syndrome presenting as congenital psoriasis. **Pediatr Dermatol** 14:473–476.
234. Lurie R, Garty BZ (1995) Helical hairs: a new hair anomaly in a patient with Netherton's syndrome. **Cutis** 55:349–352.
235. De Berker DA, Paige DG, Ferguson DJ, Dawbes RP (1995) Golf tee hairs in Netherton disease. **Pediatr Dermatol** 12:7–11.
236. Ansai S, Mitsuhashi Y, Sasaki K (1999) Netherton's syndrome in siblings. **Br J Dermatol** 141:1097–1100.

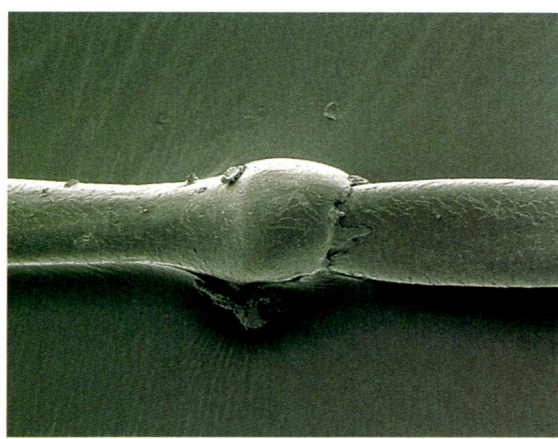

Fig. 8.38 Scanning electron microscopy of trichorrhexis invaginata.

eyebrows than on scalp hair.[237] The typical trichorrhexis invaginata is easily recognized under light microscopy, although scanning electron microscopy gives a better picture (Fig. 8.38). Often, atopy with asthma or increased IgE levels are present. Papillomatous skin lesions induced by papillomavirus often occur.[238] Epidermodysplasia verruciformis-associated HPV-types are often detected, which may lead to numerous skin cancers.[239] Carcinoma of the vulva has been observed repeatedly.[240,241] Selective antibody deficiency to bacterial polysaccharide antigens with recurrent sinopulmonary infections has been reported.[242]

PATHOPHYSIOLOGY AND HISTOGENESIS

Although Netherton syndrome is associated with atopy and high IgE, IgE production is complex and patients are heterogeneous in terms of T helper 2 skewing.[243] In a series of seven cases Fartasch et al.[244] found premature secretion of lamellar body contents. Furthermore, lamellar body-derived extracellular lamellae and stratum corneum lipid membranes were separated extensively by foci of electron-dense material. In addition transformation of lamellar body-derived structures into mature lamellar membranes was altered in patients with Netherton syndrome, which probably leads to an impaired permeability barrier. Chavanas and coworkers[245] mapped the disease to chromosome 5q32 by linkage analysis and homozygosity mapping in 20 families affected with Netherton syndrome. The same group finally found mutations in SPINK5, encoding a serine protease inhibitor which cause Netherton syndrome.[246] SPINK5 may regulate extracellular matrix remodeling, which might have an impact in skin barrier morphogenesis and immunity. Interestingly, SPINK5 mutations show significant association with atopy.[247] Genotype–phenotype correlations suggested in a recent study that

homozygous nucleotide changes resulting in early truncation of LEKT1, a multidomain serine protease inhibitor, are associated with a severe phenotype.[248]

THERAPEUTICS AND PROGNOSIS

Treatment of patients with Netherton syndrome is rather frustrating. Regular moisturing is the basis of a successful therapy. Some patients respond to treatment with 12% ammonium lactate lotion. In addition the patients may benefit from evaluation and treatment of their allergic symptoms. Low-dose systemic treatment with retinoids or phototherapy seems to be an option for some patients. Systemic cyclosporin was not successful in an anecdotal case.[249] Topical tacrolimus led to significant absorption in patients with Netherton syndrome because of skin barrier dysfunction in those patients.[250] Complications in Netherton syndrome include bacterial and viral infections which may lead to severe fluid loss with neonatal hypernatremia and renal vein thrombosis.[251] In addition, malnutrition with growth retardation and allergic manifestations may occur. Widespread multiple skin carcinomas on sunlight-exposed areas have been observed.[239]

OTHER SYNDROMES ASSOCIATED WITH ICHTHYOSIS

Rudolf Happle, Arne König

Many other phenotypes can be categorized within the group of ichthyoses. The interested reader may consider the following 10 existing syndromes as well as one nonexisting phenotype in the form of Rud syndrome.

IFAP SYNDROME

The term IFAP stands for *i*chthyosis *f*ollicularis, *a*trichia and *p*hotophobia. The disorder is inherited as an X-linked "recessive" trait which is why the full-blown picture is observed almost exclusively in boys. They show complete congenital atrichia with absence of eyebrows and lashes (Fig. 8.39). Disseminated filiform follicular hyperkeratoses are highly characteristic and have been likened to a "nutmeg grater" (Fig. 8.40).[252] In addition, mild generalized scaling with underlying erythema may be present. The boys suffer from marked photophobia but the cause is so far not clear. Due to the Lyon effect of X-inactivation, female carriers may show linear areas of follicular hyperkeratosis as well as patchy or linear hairlessness (Fig. 8.41).[253] The disorder should be distinguished from keratosis follicularis spinulosa decalvans in which female carriers may likewise be affected but never show a linear involvement because the responsible gene locus

237. Powell J, Dawber RP, Ferguson DJ, Griffiths WA (1999) Netherton's syndrome: increased likelihood of diagnosis by examining eyebrow hairs, Br J Dermatol 141:544–546.
238. Fölster-Holst R, Swensson O, Stock Fleth E et al. (1999) Comèl-Netherton syndrome complicated by papillomatous skin lesions containing human papillomaviruses 51 and 52 and plane warts containing human papillomavirus 16. Br J Dermatol 140:1139–1143.
239. Weber F, Fuchs PG, Pfister HJ et al. (2001) Human papillomavirus infection in Netherton's syndrome. Br J Dermatol 144:1044–1049.
240. Raykowski S, Küster W, Happle R (1994) Netherton-Syndrom mit Plattenepithelkarzinom der Vulva. ADF – Smposium. Genetik und Dermatologie: Fortschritte der letzten Jahre 29.4–1.5. Marburg, 1994, Ref Type: Abstract.
241. Kubler HC, Kuhn W, Rummel HH et al. (1987) Zur Karzinomentstehung (Vulvakarzinom) beim Netherton-Syndrom (Ichthyosis, Haaranomalien, atopische Diathese). Geburtshilfe Frauenheilkd 47:742–744.
242. Stryk S, Siegfried EC, Knutsen AP (1999) Selective antibody deficiency to bacterial polysaccharide antigens in patients with Netherton syndrome. Pediatr Dermatol. 16:19–22.
243. Van Gysel D, Kaning H, Baest MR et al. (2001) Clinico-immunological heterogeneity in Comèl–Netherton syndrome. Dermatology 202:99–107.
244. Fartasch M, Williams ML, Elias PM (1999) Altered lamellar body secretion and stratum corneum membrane structure in Netherton syndrome. Differentiation from other infantile erythrodermas and pathogenetic implications. Arch Dermatol 135:823–832.

245. Chavanas S, Garner C, Bodemer C et al. (2000) Localization of the Netherton syndrome gene to chromosome 5q32, by linkage analysis and homozygosity mapping. Am J Hum Genet 66:914–921.
246. Chavanas S, Bodemer C, Rochat A et al. (2000) Mutations in SPINK5, encoding a serine protease inhibitor, cause Netherton syndrome. Nature Genet 25:141–142.
247. Walley AJ, Charanas S, Moffatt MS et al. (2001) Gene polymorphism in Netherton and common atopic disease. Nature Genet 29:175–178.
248. Sprecher E, Charanas S, DiGioranna JJ et al. (2001) The spectrum of pathogenic mutations in SPINK5 in 19 families with Netherton syndrome: implications for mutation detection and first case of prenatal diagnosis. J Invest Dermatol 117:179–187.
249. Braun RP, Ramelet AA (1997) Failure of cyclosporine in Netherton's syndrome. Dermatology 195:75.
250. Allen A, Siegfried E, Silverman R et al. (2001) Significant absorption of topical tacrolimus in 3 patients with Netherton syndrome. Arch Dermatol 137:747–750.
251. Pohl M, Zimmerhackl LB, Hausser I et al. (1998) Acute bilateral renal vein thrombosis complicating Netherton syndrome. Eur J Pediatr 157:157–160.
252. Eramo LR, Esterly NB, Zieserl EJ et al. (1985) Ichthyosis follicularis with alopecia and photophobia. Arch Dermatol 121:1167.
253. König A, Happle R (1999) Linear lesions reflecting lyonization in women heterozygous for IFAP syndrome (ichthyosis follicularis with atrichia and photophobia). Am J Med Genet 85:365.

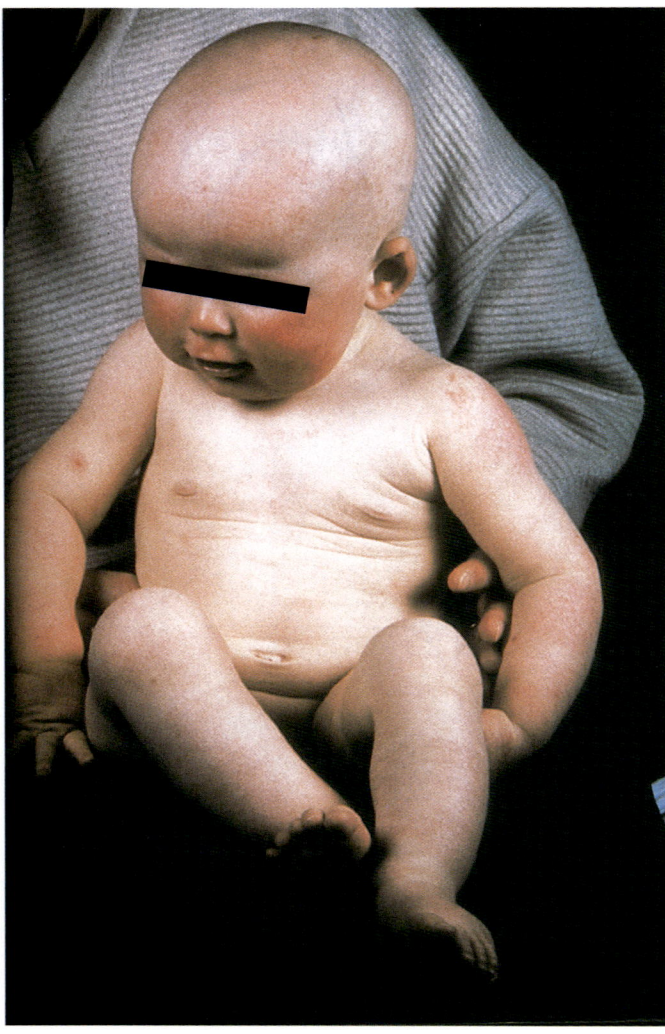

Fig. 8.39 **IFAP syndrome.** Complete atrichia in a boy.

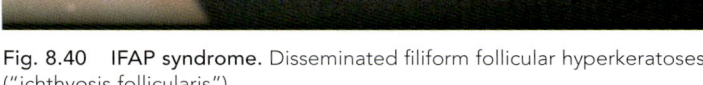

Fig. 8.40 **IFAP syndrome.** Disseminated filiform follicular hyperkeratoses ("ichthyosis follicularis").

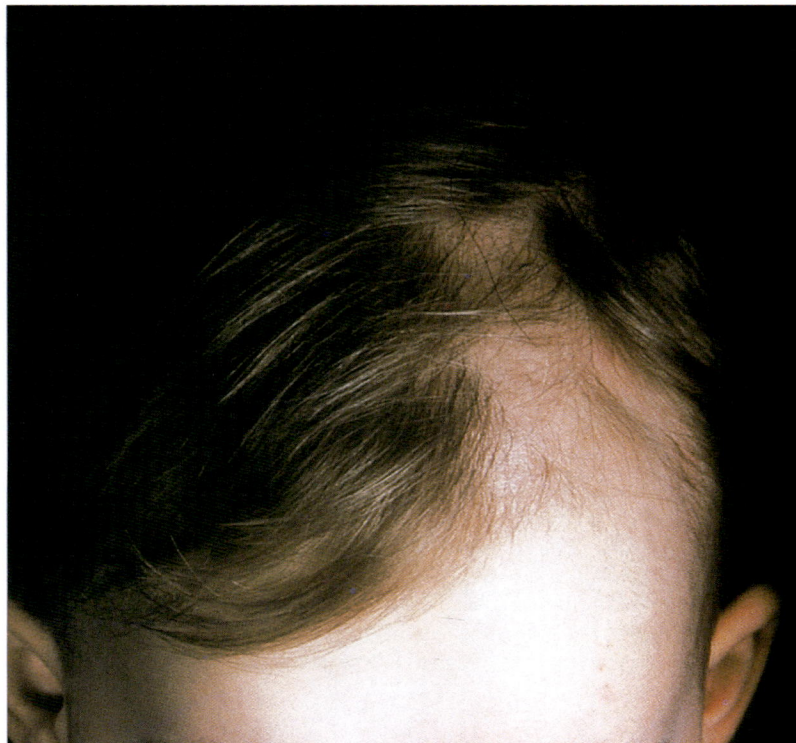

Fig. 8.41 **IFAP syndrome.** Patchy alopecia reflecting functional X-chromosome mosaicism in a heterozygous girl, the sister of the patient shown in Figs 8.39 and 8.40.

apparently escapes the mechanism of X-inactivation.[254] Boente *et al.*[255] reported a case reminiscent of IFAP syndrome but difficult to categorize because of associated seizures, mental retardation and a large inguinal hernia.

ICHTHYOSIS VARIEGATA

This peculiar type of congenital ichthyosis is characterized by disseminated patches of erythematous, hyperkeratotic skin surrounding areas of normal skin in a reticulated pattern.[256] The disorder has also been called "ichthyosis in confetti"[257] but the confetti-like islands are free of ichthyosis and rather surrounded by ichthyotic skin. For this reason the new term ichthyosis variegata was proposed.[258] Remarkably, the variegated hyperkeratotic areas show increased hairiness. In older patients, the ichthyotic skin areas may develop an unusual pattern of hyperpigmentation.[256] Pathognomonic ultrastructural changes consist of perinuclear shells composed of interdigitating filaments. Later in life multiple keratoacanthomas may develop in this genodermatosis.[259] The genetic basis of ichthyosis variegata is unclear. All cases so far reported were sporadic.

YOSIPOVITCH SYNDROME

In a large consanguineous family, Yosipovitch *et al.*[260] described an ichthyosiform skin disorder characterized by migratory hyperkeratotic lesions

254. Happle R (1992) Cutaneous manifestation of X-linked genes escaping inactivation. **Clin Exp Dermatol** 17:69.
255. Boente MC, Bibas-Bonet H, Coronel AN, Asial RA (2000) Atrichia, ichthyosis, follicular hyperkeratosis, chronic candidiasis, keratitis, seizures, mental retardation and inguinal hernia: a severe manifestation of IFAP syndrome? **Eur J Dermatol** 10:90.
256. Brusasco A, Cambiaghi S, Tadini G et al. (1998) Unusual hyperpigmentation developing in congenital reticular ichthyosiform erythroderma (ichthyosis variegata). **Br J Dermatol** 139:893.
257. Camenzind M, Harms M, Chavaz P, Saurat JH (1984) Ichtyose en confettis. **Ann Dermatol Venereol** 111:675.
258. Happle R, Küster W (1997) Ichthyosis variegata: a new name for a neglected entity. **J Am Acad Dermatol** 36:500.
259. Elbaum DJ, Kurz G, MacDuff M (1995) Increased incidence of cutaneous carcinomas in patients with congenital ichthyosis. **J Am Acad Dermatol** 33:884.
260. Yosipovitch G, Mevorah B, David M et al. (1999) Migratory ichthyosiform dermatosis with type 2 diabetes mellitus and insulin resistance. **Arch Dermatol** 135:1237.

involving the trunk and the limbs with onset in early childhood and aggravation during adolescence. Acanthosis nigricans-like lesions involved the flexural areas. This skin disorder was associated with type 2 diabetes mellitus and insulin resistance. The mode of inheritance of this syndrome is so far not clear.

LESTRINGANT SYNDROME

Lestringant et al.[261] described five siblings showing congenital ichthyosis with follicular atrophoderma, hypotrichosis and hypohidrosis. Other phenotypes characterized by follicular atrophoderma such as CHH syndrome or Bazex–Dupré–Christol syndrome were excluded on the basis of clinical evidence. The parents were consanguineous. The authors concluded that this is a new autosomal recessive genodermatosis.

ITIN SYNDROME

Itin and Rufli[262] described a collodion baby with an unusual evolution. The diffuse hyperkeratosis disappeared but the infant developed palmoplantar keratoderma and a peculiar leukokeratosis of the anogenital region. The nails, the oral mucosa and the teeth were normal.

CHIME SYNDROME

The term CHIME stands for coloboma, heart defects, ichthyosiform dermatosis, mental retardation and ear anomalies. This neuroectodermal syndrome was first described by Zunich et al.[263] The congenital ichthyotic erythroderma is characterized by itching and migratory scaling. The upper layer of the stratum corneum is peeling off, reminiscent of a peeling skin syndrome. Follow-up examination shows severe mental retardation, seizures and conductive hearing loss although the general health tends to be good. The syndrome is transmitted as an autosomal dominant trait.

STORMORKEN SYNDROME

Stormorken et al.[264] described a syndrome including thrombocytopenia, muscle fatigue, asplenia, meiosis, migraine, dyslexia and ichthyosis. Traupe[19] discussed the possibility that the associated keratinization disorder may represent autosomal dominant ichthyosis vulgaris. If so, this multisystem birth defect would represent a contiguous gene syndrome, and a candidate locus would be 1q21.

CAMISA–KORGE SYNDROME

Camisa et al.[265] described the association of keratoderma mutilans and ichthyosis affecting six generations of a family. Korge et al.[266] found that this particular type of keratoderma mutilans was caused by a loricrin mutation, whereas Vohwinkel's keratoderma without ichthyosis is caused by mutations in connexin 26. The ichthyosis noted in Camisa–Korge syndrome is rather mild. The disorder is inherited as an autosomal dominant trait.

SHWACHMAN SYNDROME

Shwachman syndrome includes exocrine pancreatic insufficiency, bone marrow hypoplasia and growth retardation.[267] In about one-half of the cases, ichthyosiform skin lesions reminiscent of lamellar ichthyosis are noted.[268] Affected children are particularly prone to infections and may show anomalies of the ribs and the long bones. Children with this autosomal recessive trait are predisposed to hematologic malignancies.

ICHTHYOSIFORM ERYTHRODERMA AND CARDIOMYOPATHY

Hoeger et al.[269] reported two children with ichthyosiform erythroderma who developed dilated cardiomyopathy, which was fatal in one and required heart transplantation in the other. It is likely but so far not certain that this association represents a new genetic syndrome.

A NONEXISTING PHENOTYPE: RUD SYNDROME

The association of ichthyosis with hypogonadism or mental retardation has sometimes been called "Rud syndrome." For two reasons, however, this syndrome does not exist. First, Rud has never described such association because in his first case there was no ichthyosis but some acquired dryness of the skin,[270] whereas in his second case autosomal dominant ichthyosis vulgaris segregated in the family independently from the other symptoms.[271] Second, virtually all cases of so-called Rud syndrome represent X-linked recessive ichthyosis associated with Kallmann syndrome in the form of a contiguous gene syndrome.[19]

PEELING SKIN SYNDROME

Arne König

Peeling skin is a phenomenon that describes generalized and lifelong continual shedding of the corneal layer in sheets. The term "peeling skin syndrome," first coined by Levy and Goldsmith,[272] seemingly comprises at least three different entities. Traupe[19] has pointed out that most cases can be categorized into two major groups, both following an autosomal recessive mode of inheritance. Type A is characterized by a variable onset; the disorder may be congenital or start at 3 to 6 years of age. Patients present with noninflammatory peeling and superficial flaky scaling that includes the face (Fig. 8.42). Histopathologic examination shows orthohyperkeratosis and the splitting is present within or below the stratum corneum, whereas the granular layer is well preserved. Interestingly, ultrastructural studies may reveal an intracellular separation within the corneal layer, i.e., the plasma membrane of the separating cell remains attached to the adjacent underlying cell.[273]

The inflammatory type B is characterized by congenital generalized ichthyosiform erythroderma with gradual improvement. These patients show exfoliative migratory patches that spare the palms and soles. The disorder is accompanied by pruritus and susceptibility to skin infections. Signs of

261. Lestringant GG, Küster W, Frossard PM, Happle R (1998) Congenital ichthyosis, follicular atrophoderma, hypotrichosis, and hypohidrosis: a new genodermatosis? Am J Med Genet 75:186.
262. Itin PH, Rufli T (1994) Collodion baby with evolution to palmoplantar keratoderma and leukokeratosis anogenitalis: a new disease? Eur J Dermatol 4:589.
263. Shashi V, Zunich J, Kelly TE, Fryburg JS (1995) Neuroectodermal (CHIME) syndrome: an additional case with long term follow up of all reported cases. J Med Genet 32:465.
264. Stormorken H, Sjaastad O, Langslet A et al. (1985) A new syndrome: thrombocytopathia, muscle fatigue, asplenia, miosis, migraine, dyslexia and ichthyosis. Clin Genet 28:367.
265. Camisa C, Rossana C (1984) Variant of keratoderma hereditaria (sic) mutilans (Vohwinkel's syndrome): treatment with orally administered isotretinoin. Arch Dermatol 120:1323.
266. Korge BP, Isida-Yamamoto A, Pünter C et al. (1997) Loricrin mutation in Vohwinkel's keratoderma is unique to the variant with ichthyosis. J Invest Dermatol 109:604.
267. Ginzberg H, Shin J, Ellis L et al. (1999) Shwachman syndrome: phenotypic manifestations of sibling sets and isolated cases in a large cohort are similar. J Pediatr 135:81.
268. Goeteyn M, Oranje AP, Vuzevski VD et al. (1991) Ichthyosis, exocrine pancreatic insufficiency, impaired neutrophil chemotaxis, growth retardation, and metaphyseal dysplasia (Shwachman syndrome): report of a case with extensive skin lesions (clinical, histological, and ultrastructural findings). Arch Dermatol 127:225.
269. Hoeger PH, Adwani SS, Whitehead BF et al. (1998) Ichthyosiform erythroderma and cardiomyopathy: report of two cases and review of the literature. Br J Dermatol 139:1055.
270. Rud E (1927) Et tilfælde af infantilisme med tetani, epilepsi, polyneuritis, ichthyosis og anæmi af perniciøs type. Hospitalstidende (Copenhagen) 70:525.
271. Rud E (1929) Et tilfælde af hypogenitalisme (eunuchoidismus femininus) med partiel gigantisme og ichthyosis. Hospitalstidende (Copenhagen) 72:426.
272. Levy SB, Goldsmith LA (1982) The peeling skin syndrome. J Am Acad Dermatol 7:606.
273. Silverman AK, Ellis CN, Beais TF, Woo TY (1986) Continual peeling skin syndrome: an electron-microscopic study. Arch Dermatol 122:71.

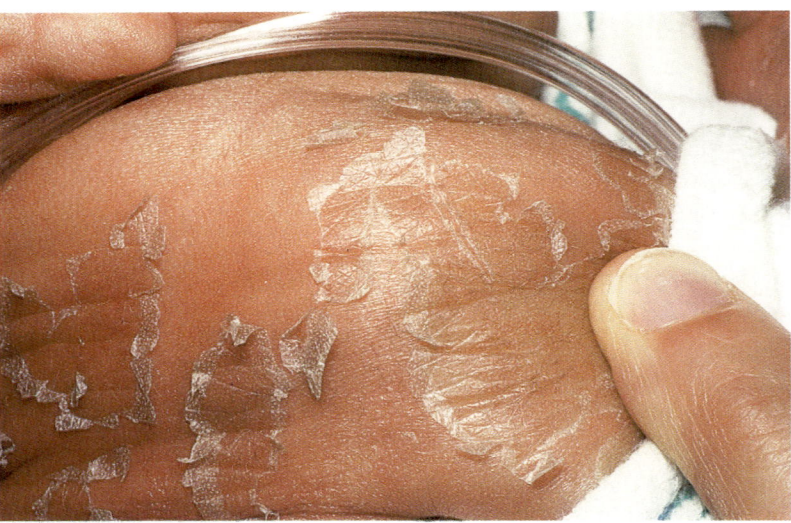

Fig. 8.42   Peeling skin syndrome, Type A. Congenital onset in a premature infant.

THE ERYTHROKERATODERMAS

Peter Itin, Rudolf Happle

INTRODUCTION AND HISTORICAL NOTE

The erythrokeratodermas represent a heterogeneous group of inherited disorders of cornification characterized by the coexistence of transient, figurate erythemas and localized or generalized hyperkeratoses. The group of erythrokeratodermas may be divided in two major subtypes: erythrokeratodermia figurata variabilis of Mendes da Costa (MIM 133200) and progressive symmetric erythrokeratoderma of Darier–Gottron (MIM 602036). In later years additional variants have been described such as erythrokeratoderma with alaxia,[278] progressive partially symmetric erythrokeratoderma with deafness,[279] erythrokeratoderma en cocardes,[280] ichthyosiform erythroderma with changing pattern of annular erythema,[281] erythrokeratoderma annularis migrans,[282,283] and an unusual type of erythrokeratodermia variabilis without mutations in connexin 31.[284] In 1991 MacFarlane *et al.*[285] described two sisters with erythrokeratoderma. One corresponded to erythrokeratodermia figurata variabilis and the other to progressive symmetrical erythrokeratoderma. With this observation it was questioned whether erythrokeratoderma is one disorder.

EPIDEMIOLOGY AND GENETICS

Erythrokeratodermas are very rare genodermatoses inherited as an autosomal dominant trait with marked variability of expression. Van der Schroeff *et al.*[286] documented a large pedigree and found a linkage to the Rhesus blood group system on chromosome 1.

EKV maps to 1p35.1, about 15cM centromeric to the Rh blood group locus – is genetically heterogenous, caused by dominant mutations in the 2 connexin genes encoding cx31 and Cx30.3. Recently, a rare recessive variant has been identified by Gottfried *et al.*[287]

PHYSICAL EXAMINATION

Erythrokeratodermas are characterized by circumscribed migrating and figurate erythematous lesions combined with sharply demarcated, hyperkeratotic, brownish, rather fixed plaques (Fig. 8.43).[288] Subjective complaints include itching and burning sensations. Trigger factors are changes of temperature and emotional stress. Erythema may change within hours but also remain for more than a week.[289] Erythematous lesions may be surrounded by an anemic halo (Fig. 8.44).[289] Often focal hyperkeratotic plaques are present on palms and soles but diffuse keratoderma may occur.[290] Some patients have a characteristic superficial peeling of the palms and soles (Fig. 8.45).[289] Lesions

atopy are characteristic. Short stature and retarded bone age may be present. Laboratory examinations disclose elevated IgE levels. Moreover, aminoaciduria may be present and some authors have described decreased levels of plasma tryptophan. Histopathologic features include psoriasiform dermatitis and cleavage above the stratum granulosum or above the acanthotic epidermis lacking a stratum granulosum. Ultrastructural examination shows that the corneal detachment occurs intercellularly. According to Traupe, type B peeling skin syndrome shares various similarities with the Comèl–Netherton syndrome and thus a genetic relationship might be presumed. Molecular studies should eventually settle this nosological problem.

Mevorah *et al.*[274] described a case of peeling skin syndrome that probably represents a third type of this heterogenous disorder. Congenital generalized ichthyosiform dermatosis with fissured keratosis of the periorificial skin are the key features. Signs of atopy and susceptibility to skin infections are likewise observed. Histologic examination shows lamellar orthohyperkeratosis and cleavage between the granular and corneal layer. Electron microscopic examination reveals that this cleavage occurs at the desmosomal plaque contiguous to the membrane of the corneocyte.

In addition to the above mentioned generalized forms of peeling skin syndrome some cases of localized involvement with onset in early childhood have been published,[275,276] as well as a case report of aquired peeling skin induced by azathioprine in an adult patient.[277]

274. Mevorah B, Salomon D, Siegenthaler G et al. (1996) Ichthyosiform dermatosis with superficial blister formation and peeling: evidence for a desmosomal anomaly and altered epidermal vitamin A metabolism. **J Am Acad Dermatol** 34:379.
275. Hashimoto K, Hamzavi I, Tanaka K, Shwayder T (2000) Acral peeling skin syndrome. **J Am Acad Dermatol** 43:1112.
276. Brusasco A, Veraldi S, Tadini G, Caputo R (1998) Localized peeling skin syndrome: a case report with ultrastructural study. **Br J Dermatol** 139:492.
277. Hermanns-Lê T, Piérard GE (1997) Azathioprine-induced skin peeling syndrome. **Dermatology** 194:175.
278. Giroux JM, Barbeau A (1972) Erythrokeratodermia with ataxia. **Arch Dermatol** 106:133–188.
279. Kiesewetter F, Siemon M, Fartasch M, Geratter M (1993) Progressive partially symmetric erythrokeratodermia with deafness: histological and ultrastructural evidence for a subtype distinct from Schnyder's syndrome. **Dermatology** 186:222–225.
280. Rajagopalan B, Pulimood S, George S, Jacob M (1999) Erythrokeratoderma en cocardes. **Clin Exp Dermatol** 24:173–174.
281. Kelly LJ, Kocsard B, Kocsard E (1970) Congenital ichthyosis with erythema anulare centrifugum. A new form of ichthyosis affecting 12 members of a family of 31 in 5 generations. **Dermatologica** 140:75–83.
282. Vakilzadeh F, Rose I (1991) Erythrokeratodermia anularis migrans – eine neue Genodermatose? **Hautarzt** 42:634–637.

283. Macari F, Landau M, Cousin P et al. (2000) Mutation in the gene for connexin 30.3 in a family with erythrokeratodermia variabilis. **Am J Hum Genet** 67:1296–1301.
284. Ishida-Yamamoto A, Kelsell D, Common J et al. (2000) A case of erythrokeratoderma varibilis without mutations in connexin 31. **Br J Dermatol** 143:1283–1287.
285. MacFarlane AW, Chapman SJ, Verbov JL (1991) Is erythrokeratoderma one disorder? A clinical and ultrastructural study of two siblings. **Br J Dermatol** 124:487–491.
286. Van der Schroeff JG, van Leeuwen-Cornelisse I, van Haeringen A, Went LN (1988) Further evidence for localization of the gene of erythrokeratodermia variabilis. **Hum Genet** 80:97–98.
287. Gotfried I, Landau M, Glaser F et al. (2002) A mutation in GIB3 is associated with recessive erythrokeratoderia variabilis (EKV) and leads to defective trafficking of the connexin 31 protein. **Hum Mol Genet** 11:1311–1316.
288. Knipe RC, Flowers FP, Johnson FR et al. (1995) Erythrokeratodermia variabilis: case report and review of the literature. **Pediatr Dermatol** 12:21–23.
289. Itin P, Levy CA, Sommacal-Schopf D, Schnyder UW (1992) Familienuntersuchung zur Erythrokeratodermia figurata variabilis. **Hautarzt** 43:500–504.
290. Itin PH, Schaub NA (1999) Keratodermies palmoplantaires héréditaires et syndromes associés. In Saurat JH et al. (eds) Dermatologie et maladies sexuellement transmissibles, 3 ed. Paris: Masson.

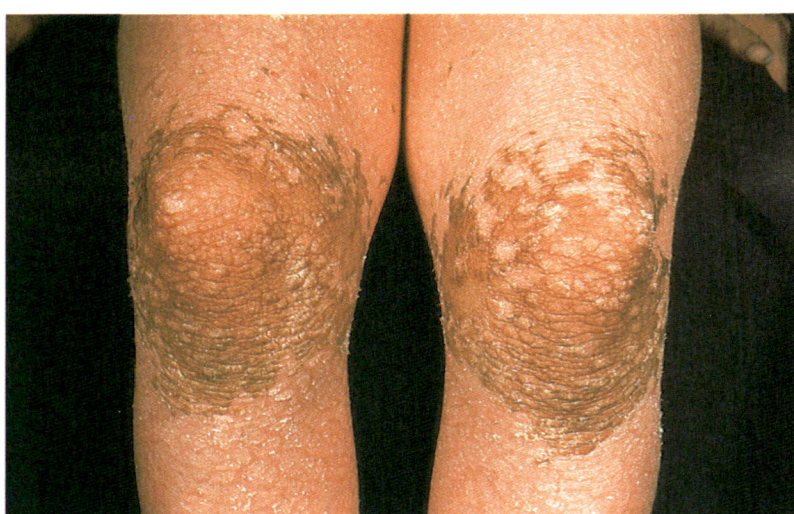

Fig. 8.43   Brownish hyperkeratotic lesions with geographic, sharply demarcated borders. In this patient a mutation in connexin has been documented by Gabriele Richard.

TABLE 8.8   Erythrokeratodermas

Erythrokeratodermia figurata variabilis	connexin-31 and connexin-30.3
Progressive symmetric erythrokertoderma	loricrin
Erythrokeratoderma with ataxia	mutation located at chr. 1p34–1p35.1
Erythrokeratoderma en cocardes	
Erythrokeratodermia with deafness	

irregular acanthosis and papillomatosis psoriasiform aspects. Lipid-like vacuoles are frequently observed within the upper epidermis and a decreased number of lamellar bodies has been found.

Erythkrokeratodermia variabilis of Mendes da Costa

Erythrokeratodermia variabilis (EKV) shows considerable intra- and inter-familial variability.[289] The disorder is characterized by the independent occurrence of two morphologic features: transient irregularly outlined red patches and localized or generalized brownish hyperkeratosis. The brownish hyperkeratotic and well-demarcated plaques are relatively fixed in site and

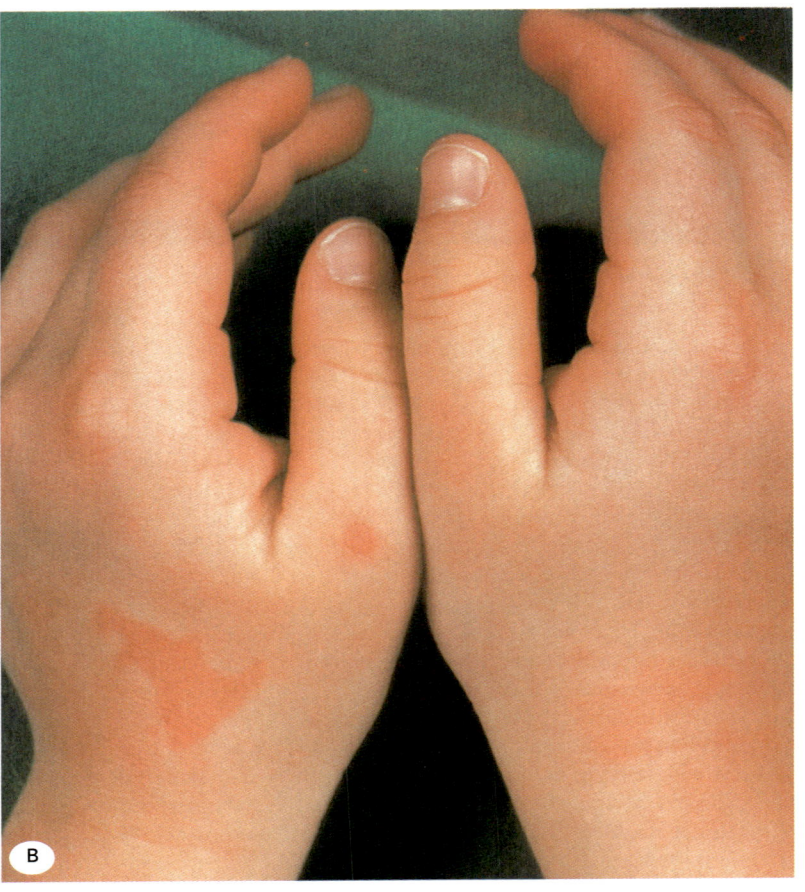

Fig. 8.44   Erythematous, irregularly shaped lesions.

preferentially affect the face, buttocks, and extensor surfaces of the limbs. As this is not an ectodermal dysplasia, teeth, hairs and nails are normal and no associated changes in mucous membranes are found. In our study more than 50% of patients with erythrokeratodermia variabilis had typical erythematous lesions at birth and 100% developed lesions within the first year of life.[289] Patients with the progressive subtype develop lesions later in childhood. The hyperkeratotic lesions appear later than erythemas. Lesions occasionally appear not until late in childhood or adolescence. There is a marked tendency for improvement after puberty. Ishida-Yamamoto et al.[291] emphasized that progressive symmetric erythrokeratodermas have fixed erythemas and not the migratory form as in erythrokderatodermia variabilis and keratoderma is much more pronounced even with pseudoainhum formation. Furthermore, this type of erythrokeratoderma shows a marked improvement in summer.

Histology is nonspecific and shows an orthohyperkeratosis with or without parakeratosis. The stratum granulosum might be thickened and there are

often occur on the extensor surfaces. The hyperkeratotic lesions are rather constant but to some degree extension and regression may occur. Erythemas can easily be provoced by external factors such as trauma to the skin. They change their extent and shapes rather quickly. The skin lesions are often present at birth. It is important to realize that cutaneous lesions in EKV are often dis-

291. Ishida-Yamamoto A, McGrath JA, Lam H et al. (1997) The molecular pathology of progressive symmetric erythrokeratoderma: a frameshift mutation in the loricrin gene and pertubations in

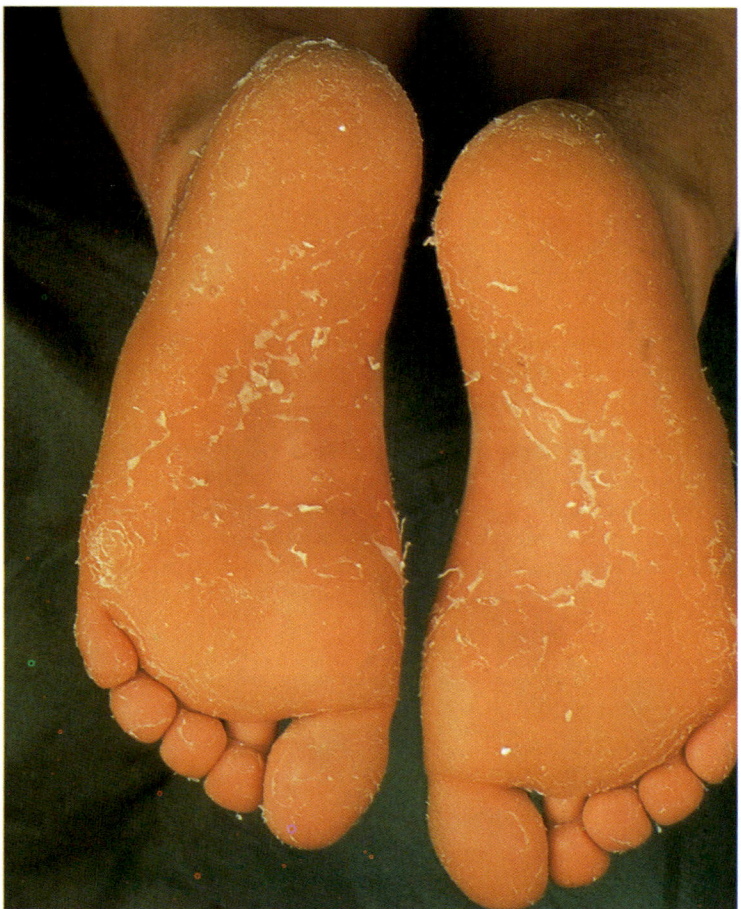

Fig. 8.45   Keratoderma with superficial peeling of palms and soles.

tributed in an asymmetrical way. In 1957, Sommacal and Schnyder reported on a family with 14 affected members. We have re-examined this pedigree, which comprised 77 members with 29 affected persons over five generations (45 females, 31 males).[289] Twenty females and 9 males were affected. In all patients EKV presented in the first year of life, and several mothers noted the erythematous lesions at birth of their children. The hyperkeratotic lesions appeared later. The reddish macules changed within hours or days. The erythematous areas were sharply outlined and sometimes surrounded by an anemic border. Only few members stated that their erythema could persist for more than a week. Clear triggers were emotional stress and changes of temperature. In all but two of the patients erythema was prominent and in the others hyperkeratotic lesions were more severe. Most patients had a burning sensation in their red areas. There was a marked tendency for improvement of EKV after puberty. Five women reported regular superficial skin peeling on hands and feet. The features in these patients were reminiscent of erythrokeratolysis hiemalis. Differential diagnosis includes erythrokeratolysis hiemalis, Netherton syndrome, and some types of ichthyosis. Histopathological features, as in all erythrokeratodermas, are not diagnostic.

Erythrokeratodermia progressiva symmetrica of Darier–Gottron

This group is less homogeneous in the clinical manifestations than in patients with EKV. Patients develop symmetrical erythematous and hyperkeratotic plaques on the extremities and face within the first year of life but the skin is usually normal at birth. Often cheeks, buttocks, and shoulders are affected, as well as wrists and ankles. Itching is only mild or absent. In general progression of the disease with involvement of large parts of the skin occurs. Some regression may start around puberty especially in sporadic cases. Transgenic mice expressing a mutant form of loricrin revealed clinically erythrokeratoderma, and this indicated the molecular basis of some cases of progressive symmetric erythrokeratoderma.[292]

Erythrokeratoderma en cocardes of Degos

Erythrokeratoderma en cocardes are also known as genodermatose en cocardes or Degos' syndrome. The condition is characterized by large round plaques with concentric erythema and scaling. The target-like configuration comes and goes.[280] Lesions are present at birth and superficial scaling on palms and soles may occur resembling erythrokeratolysis hiemalis.

Erythrokeratodermia annularis of Vakilzadeh

In 1991 Vakilzadeh and Rose[282] described this unusual type of erythrokeratoderma in an 11-year-old boy, on the basis of distinguishing clinical criteria such as persisting, slowly migrating, annular lesions, and also by immunohistochemical and ultrastructural findings. A recently described subtype of erythrokeratoderma with erythema gyratum repens-like lesions is most likely the same disease.[283]

MOLECULAR BASIS OF THE GROUP OF ERYTHROKERATODERMAS

Richard et al.[293] documented mutations in the human connexin 31 gene GJB3 as a cause of erythrokeratodermia variabilis. These mutations were predicted to interfere with normal connexin structure and function. Further work revealed that there is a spectrum of mutations in GJB3 in erythrokeratodermas.[294] Connexins form a complex and functionally diverse system of intercellular channels in the skin.[295] In a family with autosomal dominant deafness and palmoplantar kertoderma functional defects of connexin 26 have been found[296] and hidrotic ectodermal dysplasia is also caused by a mutation of connexin 30.[297] Ishida-Yamamoto et al.[292] found a mutation in the loricrin gene and pertubations in the cornified cell envelope of a family with an unusual phenotype of progressive symmetric erythrokeratoderma. Macari et al.[283] found a mutation in the gene of connexin 30.3 in a family with erythrokeratoderma with gyratum repens-like features. In future, disorders of cornification will be reclassified according to detailed clinical aspects and molecular genetic analysis as suggested in a recent editorial.[298]

THERAPEUTICS AND PROGNOSIS

Moisturing agents, topical retinoids and standard keratolytics are of some minor effect. Systemic treatment with retinoids may result in improvement and some patients show a total clearing as long the treatment is performed.[299]

the cornified cell envelope. **Am J Hum Genet** 61:581–589.

292. Suga Y, Janik M, Attar PS et al. (2000) Transgenic mice expressing a mutant form of loricrin reveal the molecular basis of the skin disease, Vohwinkel syndrome and progressive symmetric erythrokeratoderma. **J Cell Biol** 151:401–412.

293. Richard G, Smith LG, Bailey RA et al. (1998) Mutations in the human connexin gene GJB3 cause erythrokeratodermia variabilis. **Nature Genet** 20:366–369.

294. Richard G, Brown N, Smith LE et al. (2000) The spectrum of mutations in erythrokeratodermias – novel and de novo mutations in GJB3. **Hum Genet** 106:321–329.

295. Kelsell DP, Di WL, Houseman MJ (2001) Connexin mutations in skin disease and hearing loss. **Am J Hum Genet** 68:559–568.

296. Richard G, White TW, Smith LE et al. (1998) Functional defects of Cx26 resulting from a heterozygous missense mutation in a family with dominant deaf-mutism and palmoplantar keratoderma. **Hum Genet** 103:393–399.

297. Lamartine J, Munhoz Essenfelder G, Kibar Z et al. (2000) Mutations in GJB6 cause hidrotic ectodermal dysplasia. **Nature Genet** 26:142–144.

298. Hohl D (2000) Towards a better classification of erythrokeratodermias. **Br J Dermatol** 143:1133–1139.

299. Van de Kerkhof PCM, Steijlen PM, van Dooren-Greebe RJ, Happle R (1990) Acitretin in the treatment of erythrokeratodermia variabilis. **Dermatologica** 181:330–333.

PALMOPLANTAR KERATODERMAS

Celia Moss

INTRODUCTION

The skin of the palms and soles is highly specialized. It must resist extreme mechanical forces, and yet remain soft and pliable enough for fine motor and sensory functions. The production and maintenance of palmoplantar skin involves the complex interplay of many genes, and there is a correspondingly large number of disorders caused by mutations in these genes. Many of these disorders manifest as palmoplantar keratoderma (PPK).

During the past few years there have been huge advances in our understanding of PPK.[300–303] Broadly, the known causes of PPK can be classified as disorders of the following aspects of epidermal cells:

- internal structure e.g., keratins[304]
- cornified envelope production, e.g., loricrin, transglutaminase[305]
- cohesion, e.g., desmosomes[306,307]
- intercellular communication, e.g., connexins[308]
- transmembrane signal transduction, e.g., cathepsin C.

There is considerable overlap between ichthyosis and PPK. They often coexist, and most of these pathogenetic mechanisms apply to both. Curiously, ichthyoses caused by abnormalities in lipid metabolism tend to spare the palmar and plantar skin: they include X-linked ichthyosis due to steroid sulfatase deficiency, Sjögren–Larsson syndrome due to fatty alcohol oxidoreductase deficiency, and Refsum syndrome caused by phytanic acid hydroxylase deficiency. This may be related to a lower concentration of lipid in palmoplantar stratum corneum ($2.0 \pm 0.6\%$) compared with abdominal stratum corneum ($6.5 \pm 0.5\%$).[309]

The association of some PPKs with abnormalities beyond the skin also reflects pathogenesis. For example, the association of PPK and cardiac abnormalities in disorders of the desmosomal proteins plakoglobin and desmoplakin reflects the prominence of strong desmosomal junctions in these tissues subjected to high mechanical forces. Sweat glands are a major component of palmoplantar skin, so a link between PPK and ectodermal dysplasia is not surprising. Defects in intercellular cohesion, communication and transmembrane signal transducton may likewise be shared with other organs. Conversely, the genes responsible for keratin and cornified envelop production are expressed only in epidermal cells and therefore disorders due to mutations in these genes affect only the skin.

The information summarized above may provide the basis for a future pathogenetic classification, but while there are still substantial gaps in our knowledge the clinical classification used by Ratnavel and Griffiths is followed here.[301] PPK are divided into diffuse, focal and punctate, and subdivided according to whether or not there are associated extracutaneous features. The abnormality may extend to the dorsal surfaces of the hand and foot, the so-called "transgrediens" pattern (anglicized here to "transgredient") which often also involves extensor surfaces such as knuckles, knees and elbows.

It must be noted, however, that even diffuse PPK may present initially in a focal manner, that walking and manual labor affect the appearance of PPK, and that associated features may appear later than the PPK. Therefore, diagnosis in an infant or child with no affected adult relatives is always difficult.

DIFFUSE PALMOPLANTAR KERATODERMAS

PALMOPLANTAR KERATODERMA: UNNA–THOST AND VÖRNER TYPE

Introduction and historical note

Unna–Thost and Vörner are clinically indistinguishable diffuse types of PPK usually without transgredient spread to the dorsal hand and foot, or involvement of distant sites. Until the early 1990s Vörner's epidermolytic pattern (EPPK) was differentiated histologically from the nonepidermolytic type (NEPPK) described by Unna and Thost. Küster's report of epidermolysis in a descendant of the family described by Thost suggested that they represent the same entity.[310] NEPPK may well be a heterogeneous group with epidermolysis variably present in one type and absent in another.

Epidemiology

Genetics

Unna–Thost and Vörner PPK are inherited as fully penetrant, autosomal dominant traits, affecting males and females equally.

Statistics

These are the commonest of the inherited diffuse PPKs. The incidence of EPPK in Northern Ireland is 1 in 23 000,[311] and of NEPPK in Northern Sweden 3–5.5 in 1000.[312]

Presenting History

The condition may not be apparent at birth but is usually evident by 3 to 12 months. Diffuse thickening of the soles, then palms, is usually the presenting complaint of the parents, who generally will have recognized the familial nature of the condition. Some children develop a habit of removing loose flakes of skin. Unlike bullous ichthyosiform erythroderma, EPPK does not usually blister despite histological epidermolysis. At most there is a decreased threshold to mechanically induced friction blisters, a symptom exacerbated by treatment with oral synthetic retinoids. Some patients complain of painful fissures, or pruritus, maceration and odour due to hyperhidrosis or secondary dermatophyte infection.

Physical examination

The abnormality is largely confined to the hands and feet. Initial involvement may be patchy, but usually by the age of one year there is uniform, dense, white or yellow hyperkeratosis of the palms and soles (Fig. 8.46 and 8.47).

300. Lucker GBH, van de Kerkhof PCM, Steijlen PM (1994) The hereditary palmoplantar keratoses: an updated review and classification. **Br J Dermatol** 131:1–14.
301. Ratnavel RC, Griffiths WA (1997) The inherited palmoplantar keratodermas. **Br J Dermatol** 137:485–490.
302. Paller AS (1999) The molecular bases for the palmoplantar keratodermas. **Pediatr Dermatol** 16:483–486.
303. Kelsell DP, Stevens HP (1999) The palmoplantar keratodermas: much more than palms and soles. **Mol Med Today** Mar; 5(3):107–113. Review.
304. Irvine AD, McLean WHI (1999) Human keratin diseases: the increasing spectrum of disease and subtlety of the phenotype-genotype correlation. **Br J Dermatol** 140:815–828.
305. Christiano AM (1997) Frontiers in keratodermas: pushing the envelope. **Trends Genet** 13:227–233.
306. McGrath JA (1999) Hereditary diseases of desmosomes. **J Dermatol Sci** 20(2):85–91. Review.
307. Green KJ, Gaudry CA (2000) Are desmosomes more than tethers for intermediate filaments? **Nat Rev Mol Cell Biol** 1:206–210.

308. Kelsell DP, Di W-L, Houseman MJ (2001) Connexin mutations in skin disease and hearing loss. **Am J Hum Genet** 68:559–568.
309. Lampe MA, Burlingame AL, Whitney JA et al. (1983) Human stratum corneum lipids: characterization and regional variations. **J Lipid Res** 24:120.
310. Küster W, Becker A (1992) Indication for the identity of palmoplantar keratoderma type Unna–Thost with type Vörner: Thost's family revisited 110 years later. **Acta Derm Venereol (Stockh)** 72:120–122.
311. Covello SP, Irvine AD, McKenna KE et al. (1998) Mutations in keratin K9 in kindreds with epidermolytic palmoplantar keratoderma and epidemiology in Northern Ireland. **J Invest Dermatol** 111:1207–1209.
312. Lind L, Lundstrom A, Hofer PA et al. (1994) The gene for diffuse palmoplantar keratoderma of the type found in Northern Sweden is localised to chromosome 12q11–q13. **Hum Mol Genet** 3:1789–1793.

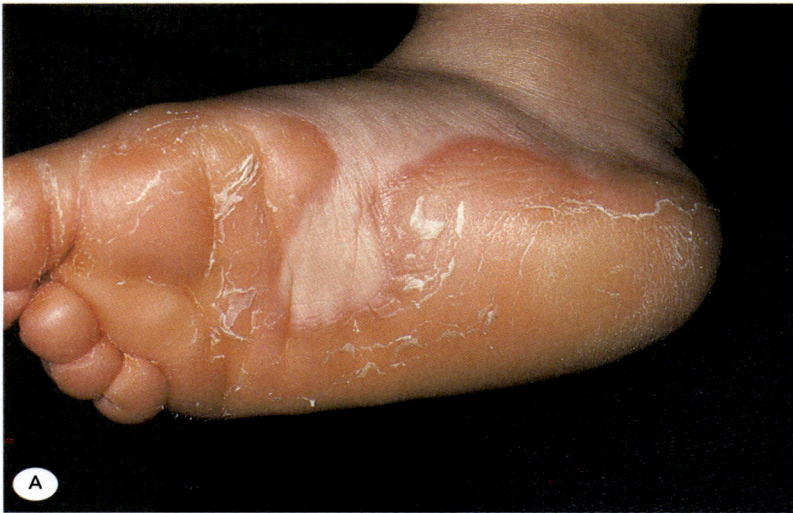

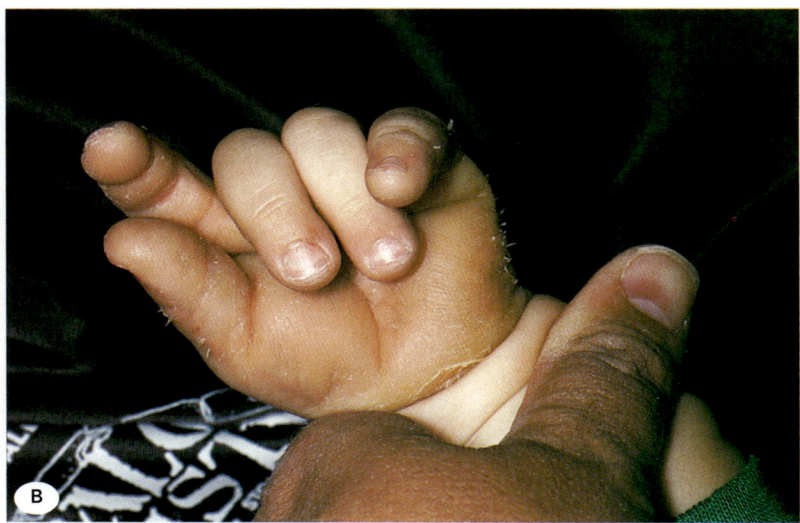

Fig. 8.46   Diffuse EPPK of the soles (**A**) and palms (**B**) in a 2-year-old girl.

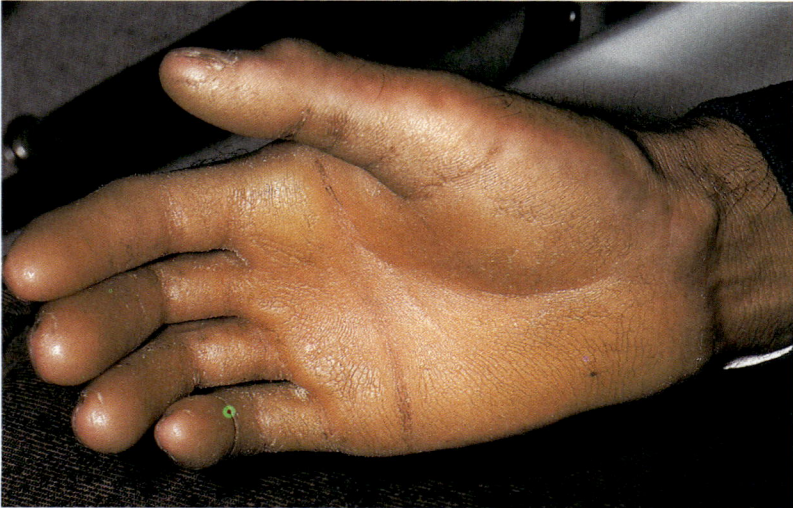

Fig. 8.47   Diffuse NEPPK of the palm in the father of the patient in Fig. 8.46.

Pathophysiology and histogenesis

Molecular basis

The histological similarity of EPPK to bullous ichthyosiform erythroderma (BIE) suggested a keratin abnormality, and the specificity of keratin 9 to palmar and plantar skin made this an obvious candidate gene. Reis *et al.* mapped EPPK to the type I (acidic) keratin gene cluster on 17q, and subsequently identified mutations in the keratin 9 gene (KRT9) in EPPK families.[315] Mutant KRT9 produced disrupted keratin filaments *in vitro* in cell transfection experiments,[316] and *in vivo* when injected into mouse skin.[317] The mutations are heterozygous, so the phenotype is presumably due to a dominant negative effect of the mutant keratin. However, the finding of a *KRT9* stop codon mutation (predicting a markedly truncated and rapidly degraded protein product[318]) makes a dominant negative effect in that family less likely than haploinsufficiency.

Most *KRT9* mutations in EPPK affect amino acid residues 156–171, which correspond to the highly conserved 1A helix initiation region of the alpha-helical domain crucial for keratin filament assembly.[311] The commonest *KRT9* mutation causing EPPK is R162W: this mutation also occurs in *KRT14* in epidermolysis bullosa simplex and in *KTR10* in BIE. Recently, a mutation affecting the *KRT9* 2B helix termination motif (1362ins3) was described in a sporadic case of EPPK.[319]

By analogy with other keratin disorders, the same phenotype should be produced by mutations in the corresponding type II keratin, but the identity of the basic keratin associated with the acidic (type I) KRT9 remains uncertain. Lind *et al.* mapped NEPPK to the type II keratin gene cluster in 1994.[312] KRT1 is a possible candidate, and indeed mutations have now been identified in *KRT1* in both NEPPK[314] and EPPK,[320] further supporting the identity of Unna–Thost and Vörner PPK. The possibility that keratin 1 pairs with keratin 9 in palmoplantar skin, and with keratin 10 elsewhere is consistent with the notion that BIE due to *KRT1* mutations involves the palms and soles while BIE due to *KRT10* mutations does not.[321]

The keratoderma stops abruptly at the lateral margins of hands and feet, often with an erythematous rim. There is no transgredient extension on to the dorsal surface except for occasional thickening of the skin over the proximal interphalangeal joints (knuckle pads) in both EPPK[313] and NEPPK.[314] Hyperkeratosis of umbilicus and areolae, and mild dryness of knees and elbows may occur.[315] The PPK may be complicated by hyperhidrosis, maceration and fissuring. Erythema and fine scaling within the keratoderma may signify a secondary dermatophytosis.

313. Nogita T, Nakagaaawa H, Ishibashi Y (1991) Hereditary epidermolytic palmoplantar keratoderma with knuckle pad-like lesions over the finger joints. **Br J Dermatol** 125:496.

314. Kimonis V, DiGiovanna JJ, Yang J-M et al. (1994) A mutation in the V1 end domain of keratin 1 in non-epidermolytic palmar-plantar keratoderma. **J Invest Dermatol** 103:764–769.

315. Reis A, Hennies H-C, Langbein L et al. (1994) Keratin 9 gene mutations in epidermolytic palmoplantar keratoderma (EPPK). **Nat Genet** 6:174–179.

316. Kobayashi S, Tanaka T, Matsuyoshi N et al. (1996) Keratin 9 point mutation in the pedigree of epidermolytic hereditary palmoplantar keratoderma perturbs keratin intermediate filament formation. **FEBS Lett** 386:149–155.

317. Kobayashi S, Kore-eda S, Tanake T (1999) Demonstration of the pathogenic effect of point mutated keratin 9 in vivo. **FEBS Lett** 447:39–43.

318. Szalai S, Szalai C, Becker K, Torok E (1999) Keratin 9 mutations in the coil 1A region in epidermolytic palmoplantar keratoderma. **Pediatr Dermatol** 16(6):430–435.

319. Coleman CM, Munro CS, Smith FJD et al. (1999) Epidermolytic palmoplantar keratoderma due to a novel type of keratin mutation, a 3-bp insertion in the keratin 9 helix termination motif. **Br J Dermatol** 140:486–490.

320. Hatsell SJ, Eady RA, Wennerstrand L et al. (2001) Novel splice-site mutation in keratin 1 underlies mild epidermolytic palmoplantar keratoderma in three kindreds. **J Invest Dermatol** 116:606–609.

321. Yang JM, Nam K, Kim SW et al. (1999) Arginine in the beginning of the 1A rod domain of the keratin 10 gene is the hot spot for the mutation in epidermolytic hyperkeratosis. **J Dermatol Sci** Feb; 19(2):126–133.

In contrast to the highly disruptive *KRT1* mutations of generalized BIE that affect the important helix boundary motifs, those underlying keratoderma limited to palms and soles involve the central part of the helix in EPPK.[320] In the NEPPK patient, the *KRT1* mutation involved loss of a highly conserved lysine residue within the amino-terminal variable end domain of keratin 1 which normally attaches to the cornified envelope by transglutaminase cross-linking.[314,322]

The *KRT1* EPPK phenotype[320] is milder than that produced by *KRT9* mutations, being confluent with a red border only on weight-bearing areas of the sole, and focal on the palms. It is not transgredient, but callosities develop on the dorsal surfaces of toes and fingers in response to friction.

NEPPK due to *KRT1* mutation is associated with hyperkeratosis of the areola, umbilicus and knuckles.[314]

NEPPK is probably heterogeneous. In three British families NEPPK mapped proximal to the type II keratin gene cluster, excluding *KRT9* and *KRT1* as candidates.[323]

Histologic findings

Histologically, there is acanthosis and dense orthohyperkeratosis. An increased, diminished or absent granular cell layer may be found. There is usually a mild perivascular infiltrate. Vörner-type kindreds exhibit suprabasal epidermolysis with whorls of abnormally aggregated keratin filaments ultrastructurally

---

TABLE 8.9 The inherited primary palmoplantar keratodermas

Disorder	Transgredient?	Extensor keratoses?	Other features?	Gene	Locus	Inheritance
Diffuse palmoplantar keratoderma						
Unna–Thost/Vörner PPK	No	(Knuckle pads)	No	Keratin 9	17q21	Autosomal dominant
				Keratin 1	12q13	
Greither/Sybert	Yes	Yes	No			Autosomal dominant
Norbotten (Gamborg–Nielson)	No	Knuckle pads	Occasional ainhum			Autosomal recessive
Mal de Meleda	Yes	Yes	Occasional ainhum	SLURP 1	8qter	Autosomal recessive
Olmsted	Yes	Yes	Periorificial keratoderma			Sporadic
Vohwinkel	Yes	Yes	Ainhum	Loricrin	1q21	Autosomal dominant
Vohwinkel keratoderma plus deafness	Yes	Yes	Ainhum and deafness	Connexin 26	13q11–12	Autosomal dominant
NEPPK + deafness	No	No	Sensorineural deafness	Mitochondrial	mtDNA	Maternal
Papillon–Lefevre/ Haim–Munk	Yes	Yes	Periodontosis	Cathepsin C	11q14	Autosomal recessive
Naxos (arrhythmogenic right cardiomyopathy + diffuse PPK + wooly hair)	No	No	Abnormal hair and right ventricular cardiomyopathy	Plakoglobin	17q	Autosomal recessive
Huriez sclerotylosis	No	No	Skin cancer		4q23	Autosomal dominant
Focal palmoplantar keratoderma						
Focal PPK (Fuhs/Brunauer/ Siemens/Wachter)	No	No	None	Keratin 16	17q21	Autosomal dominant
Linear (Blaschko) PPK	No	No	None	K16 mosaicism	17q21	Sporadic
Striate PPK (Siemens)	No	No	No	Desmoglein 1	18q12	Autosomal recessive
				Desmoplakin	6p2	Autosomal recessive
Carvajal (arrhythmogenic left cardiomyopathy + striate PPK + wooly hair)	No	No	Abnormal hair and left ventricular cardiomyopathy	Desmoplakin	6p2	Autosomal recessive
Howel–Evans syndrome	No	No	Ca esophagus	TOC	17q	Autosomal dominant
Tyrosinemia type II (Richner–Hanhart)	No	Sometimes	Corneal ulceration, retardation	Tyrosine aminotransferase	16q22	Autosomal recessive
Punctate palmoplantar keratoderma						
Punctate PPK (Buschke, Fischer, Brauer)	No	No	None			Autosomal dominant
Punctate keratoses of palmar creases	No	No	None			Autosomal dominant

---

322. Candi E, Tarcsa E, Digiovanna JJ et al. (1998) A highly conserved lysine residue on the head domain of type II keratins is essential for the attachment of keratin intermediate filaments to the cornified cell envelope through isopeptide crosslinking by transglutaminases. **Proc Natl Acad Sci USA** Mar 3;95(5):2067–2072.

323. Kelsell DP, Stevens HP, Purkis PE et al. (1999) Fine genetic mapping of diffuse non-epidermolytic palmoplantar keratoderma to chromosome 12q11–q13: exclusion of the mapped type II keratins. **Exp Dermatol** 8:388–391.

associated with cellular degeneration in spinous and granular cells.[324] Immunostaining of EPPK[325] showed increased expression of both cornified envelope proteins (transglutaminase-1, loricrin and involucrin) and filaggrin, the protein of the keratohyaline granule.

Even the archetypical nonepidermolytic family of Thost was later found to have epidermolysis.[310] The relative incidence of these two histologic patterns within the clinical group of Unna–Thost PPK is unknown, because biopsy is not usually performed and because the clinical features are often indistinguishable. In general, *KRT9* mutations are associated with epidermolytic histology. However, in a Japanese family with the common R162W mutation, the epidermolysis was very mild, with rounded, dissociated midepidermal cells rather than frank epidermolysis.[326] In *KRT1* EPPK there is minimal cytolysis with tonofilament clumping in occasional cells.[320]

Differential diagnosis

Table 8.9 shows the differentiation from other PPKs. Distinctive features such as transgredient spread, distant keratoses, periodontosis and ainhum are not apparent in infants, and therefore, in the absence of affected relatives, it may be impossible to make a precise diagnosis until later. Hearing should therefore be tested in all infants with PPK because of the occasional association of deafness and keratoderma. Complete skin examination will usually exclude those entities with PPK as a part of a generalized disorder of cornification (Table 8.10).

Therapeutics and prognosis

Topical therapy

The condition is often asymptomatic in young children and treatment must not be more burdensome than the condition itself. Twice daily application of an oily emollient such as emulsifying ointment should be incorporated early on into the child's lifestyle. Older children dislike grease but may accept an oily preparation overnight and a lighter cream during the day. Addition of a keratolytic such as salicylic or lactic acid, or urea, may be required: the appropriate concentration can be found by increasing gradually from 5% and watching for maceration and irritation of adjacent normal skin. Manual paring instantly relieves pain caused by plantar hyperkeratosis[327] and can be carried out by parents who, if affected, usually practice this technique themselves. A chiropodist can advise on equipment and technique. Dermabrasion has also been used successfully.[328] Painful fissures may be sealed with elastoplast or other adhesive tape. Poor gait due to pain on walking can be helped by customized in-soles. Bath PUVA was reportedly successful in an 11-year-old Bosnian girl: used three times weekly for 7 months, then weekly, the condition cleared in a year and stayed in remission a year after stopping the treatment.[329] Calcipotriol is ineffective.[330]

Systemic management

Treatment of secondary fungal infection if present will improve symptoms and signs.[331] Oral retinoids have been used with some success in several of the PPKs: acitretin 20–40mg daily is helpful in many patients, while isotretinoin 30–60mg daily is less effective.[301] Because of their side effects, however, they should only be used for the relief of significant disability. Intermittent therapy, e.g., 4 months "on" and 2 months "off," is sometimes effective. Some patients function better with their hyperkeratotic palm/sole than with a thinned retinoid-treated surface. Oral biotin helped in one family.[332]

Prognosis

Once established, the keratoderma persists.

Pediatric aspects of the disease

Pain from hyperkeratosis with or without fissures may affect motor development, particularly the gait. Likewise, thick palmar keratoderma and hyperhidrosis may impair manual activities. Ideally, treatment is directed at

TABLE 8.10 **Generalized inherited skin disorders featuring palmoplantar keratoderma**

Disorder	Other features?	Gene	Locus	Inheritance
Diffuse palmoplantar keratoderma				
Weber–Cockayne EB Simplex	Palmoplantar blisters	Keratin 5	12q13	Autosomal dominant
		Keratin 14	17q21	
Dowling–Meara EB Simplex	Generalized blisters	Keratin 5	12q13	Autosomal dominant
		Keratin 14	17q21	
Bullous ichthyosiform erythroderma	Generalized epidermolytic hyperkeratosis	Keratin 1	12q13	Autosomal dominant
Clouston hidrotic ectodermal dysplasia	Abnormal hair and nails	Connexin 30	13q12	Autosomal dominant
Naegell–Franceschetti–Jadassohn	Ectodermal dysplasia		17q	Autosomal dominant
Dyskeratosis congenita	Nail dystrophy, oral leukokeratosis, marrow aplasia	Dyskerin	Xq28	X-linked recessive
Rapp–Hodgkin syndrome	Ectodermal dysplasia, clefting			Autosomal dominant
Schöpf–Schultz–Passarge syndrome	Ectodermal dysplasia, eyelid cysts			Autosomal recessive
Weary–Kindler syndrome	Acral blisters and poikiloderma			Autosomal dominant
Focal palmoplantar keratoderma				
Pachyonychia congenita	Oral leucokeratosis, nail dystrophy	Keratin 6a	12q13	Autosomal dominant
		Keratin 16	17q21	
Punctate palmoplantar keratoderma				
Darier disease	Widespread keratotic papules	SERCA2	12q23–24	Autosomal dominant
Cowden syndrome	Cutaneous fibromas, mucosal papillomas, internal malignancies	PTEN	10q23.3	Autosomal dominant

324. Navsaria HA, Swensson O, Ratnavel RC et al. (1995) Ultrastructural changes resulting from keratin-9 gene mutations in two families with epidermolytic palmoplantar keratoderma. **J Invest Dermatol** 104:425–429.

325. Hashimoto K, Mizuguchi R, Tanaka K et al. (2000) Palmoplantar keratoderma (Voerner) with composite keratohyaline granules: studies on keratohyaline parameters and ultrastructures. **J Dermatol** 27:1–9.

326. Mayuzumi N, Shigihara T, Ikeda S et al. (1999) R162W mutation of keratin 9 in a family with autosomal dominant palmoplantar keratoderma with unique histologic features. **J Investig Dermatol Symp Proc** Sep;4(2):150–152.

327. Redmond A, Allen N, Vernon W (1999) Effect of scalpel debridement on the pain associated with plantar hyperkeratosis. **J Am Podiatr Med Assoc** 89:515–519.

328. Daoud MS, Randle HW, Yarborough JM (1995) Dermabrasion of the hyperkeratotic foot. **Dermatol Surg** 21(3):243–244.

329. Kaskel P, Leiter U, Krähn G et al. (2000) PUVA-bath photochemotherapy for congenital palmoplantar keratoderma in an 11-year-old girl. **Br J Dermatol** 143:464–465.

330. Kragballe K, Steijlen PM, Ibsen HH et al. (1995) Efficacy, tolerability, and safety of calcipotriol ointment in disorders of keratinization. Results of a randomized, double-blind, vehicle-controlled, right/left comparative study. **Arch Dermatol** 131(5):556–560.

331. Maruyama R, Katoh T, Nishioka K (1999) A case of Unna–Thost disease accompanied by *Epidermophyton floccosum* infection. **J Dermatol** 26(1):63–66.

332. Menni S, Saleh F, Piccinno R et al. (1992) Palmoplantar keratoderma of Unna–Thost: response to biotin in one family. **Clin Exp Dermatol** 17:337.

relief of functional impairment allowing children to participate fully in all activities. Parents must understand that the condition is lifelong and treatment is not curative.

GREITHER AND SYBERT KERATODERMAS
Introduction and historical note
These diffuse and transgredient NEPPKs may be severe forms of diffuse NEPPK.

Epidemiology
Genetics
Study of a six-generation pedigree in which 10 of 25 family members were affected by Greither PPK suggested autosomal dominant inheritance with variable penetrance.[333] Sybert described one family with clear autosomal dominant inheritance.[334]

Presenting history
This appears in infancy, worsens during childhood, and begins to improve after middle age.

Physical examination
A diffuse, erythematous PPK extends to the dorsum of hands and feet. Plaques also appear on knees and elbows. Older patients in Sybert's family developed ainhum.

Pathophysiology and histogenesis
Molecular basis
Linkage to the erythrokeratodermia variabilis locus on 1p[335] could not be confirmed in a family with both erythrokeratodermia variabilis and Greither syndrome.[336]

Histologic findings
There is acanthosis, hyperkeratosis and hypergranulosis, with prominent and irregular keratohyaline granules.

Differential diagnosis
It can be distinguished from mal de Meleda by the dominant pattern of inheritance, and from NEPPK by the transgredient pattern. See Table 8.9 for differentiation from other PPKs.

Therapeutics and prognosis
Treatment is as for NEPPK. The disease recurred in full-thickness skin grafts in Sybert's patient.

Prognosis
It tends to improve in the fifth decade. Malignant melanoma has been reported in affected skin.[337]

GAMBORG–NIELSEN PPK
This is a severe, mutilating, recessive PPK found in Norbotten, a province of Northern Sweden. It differs from Mal de Meleda only in the absence of distant keratoses. The term Norbotten PPK has, confusingly, been used for both this severe recessive type, and the dominant Unna–Thost NEPPK found in the same area. The two are genetically distinct.[338]

MAL DE MELEDA
Introduction and historical note
For approximately 25 generations, from the late fourteenth to the early nineteenth century, the small island of Mljet (then called Meleda) off the coast of the former Yugoslavia was used to quarantine people with the plague and leprosy. Isolation led to inbreeding and the emergence of recessive traits including this disease from ("mal de") Meleda, in which PPK is associated with keratoses on the extensor surfaces.

Epidemiology
Mal de Meleda has also been seen in northern Europe, North Africa, the Middle East and the Far East.

Genetics
Inheritance is autosomal recessive.

Statistics
The prevalence has been estimated to be 1 in 100 000.[339]

Physical examination
Skin
Keratoderma is not congenital but develops in the first 6 months and progresses during childhood,[340] the other features following later. The PPK is smooth and pink in young children but becomes more rough and sometimes macerated and malodorous by the second decade. Transgredient keratoderma appears by 12 months and increases markedly during the first 4 years. It can encircle the distal phalanges producing a tapering appearance. In children it extends up to the malleoli, with a triangular area on the Achilles tendon and later to the elbows and above the ankles. Lichenoid plaques on the elbows and knees are sharply demarcated and often erythematous with a cobblestone appearance. Knuckle pads, flexion contractures of the hands, digital constricting bands (pseudoainhum), hyperhidrosis and transient perioral erythema may occur.[340,341]

Hair, nails, teeth, and mucous membranes
Nails are usually biconvex but may show koilonychia or subungual hyperkeratosis. Hair and teeth are normal but white plaques on the mucous membranes occur.

Pathophysiology and histogenesis
Molecular basis
Fischer et al. mapped Mal de Meleda to 8qter[339] in two large consanguineous Algerian families. Focussing on the gene encoding SLURP-1 (secreted Ly-6/uPAR related protein 1) at this locus, they identified three different homozygous mutations in 19 affected families of Algerian and Croatian origin.[342] Secreted and receptor proteins of the Ly-6/uPAR superfamily have been implicated in transmembrane signal transduction, cell activation and cell adhesion, but the pathogenesis of the PPK is not yet known.

333. Grilli R, Aguilar A, Escalonilla P et al. (2000) Transgrediens et progrediens palmoplantar keratoderma (Greither's disease) with particular histopathologic findings. **Cutis** Mar; 65(3):141–145.
334. Sybert VP, Dale BA, Holbrook KA (1988) Palmo-plantar keratoderma: a clinical, ultrastructural and biochemical study. **J Am Acad Dermatol** 18:75–86.
335. Gedde-Dahl TJ, Rodge S, Helsing P et al. (1993) Greither's disease and erythrokeratoderma variabilis (EKV) caused by the same mutation on chromosome 1. **Human Genome Mapping Workshop 1** (abstract).
336. Richard G, Whyte YM. Smith L et al. (1996) Linkage studies in erythrokeratodermias: fine mapping, genetic heterogeneity, and analysis of candidate genes. **J Invest Dermatol** 107:481.
337. Seike T, Nakanishi H, Urano Y et al. (1995) Malignant melanoma developing in an area of palmoplantar keratoderma (Greither's disease). **J Dermatol** 22:55–61.
338. Gamborg N (1985) Two different clinical and genetic forms of hereditary palmoplantar keratoderma in the northernmost county of Sweden. **Clin Genet** 28:361–366.
339. Fischer J, Bouadjar B, Heilig R et al. (1998) Genetic linkage of Meleda disease to chromosome 8qter. **Eur J Hum Genet** 6(6):542–547.
340. Lestringant GG, Frossard PM, Adeghate E et al. (1997) Mal de Meleda: a report of four cases from the United Arab Emirates. **Pediatr Dermatol** 14(3):186–191.
341. Bouadjar B, Benmazouzia S, Prud'homme JF et al. (2000) Clinical and genetic studies of 3 large, consanguineous, Algerian families with Mal de Meleda. **Arch Dermatol** 136(10):1247–1252.
342. Fischer J, Bouadjar B, Heilig R et al. (2001) Mutations in the gene encoding SLURP-1 in Mal de Meleda. **Hum Mol Genet** 10(8):875–880.

Histologic findings

Histology from all affected areas shows hyperkeratosis, hypergranulosis, and acanthosis. Electronmicroscopy shows no major abnormalities of keratinization.[343]

Differential diagnosis

See Table 8.9 for differentiation from other PPKs. Mal de Meleda must be distinguished from other recessive and transgrediens forms of PPK, particularly Papillon–Lefevre. After 1 year of age the latter can usually be distinguished by the characteristic periodontosis. Where a single case occurs in a non-consanguineous family, so that recessive inheritance cannot be distinguished from a new case of autosomal dominant disease, Mal de Meleda may be confused with Greither or Vohwinkel PPK, particularly early on before the condition has evolved fully.

Therapeutics and prognosis

The treatment of Mal de Meleda is similar to that for other PPKs (see EPPK). Acitretin or etretinate improves pseudoainhum, keratoderma, lichenoid plaques and contractures, but peeling of the palms limits the dose.[340,341]

Differential diagnosis

See Table 8.9 for differentiation from other PPKs.

OLMSTED SYNDROME

Introduction and historical note

Olmsted syndrome is a rare disorder characterized by diffuse, transgredient, sharply circumscribed, mutilating PPK, and symmetrical periorificial (mouth, nose, genital, and anal) keratoderma.[344]

Epidemiology

Statistics

This condition is exceedingly rare with only 20 cases published in the literature.[345]

Genetics

All cases to date have been sporadic apart from monozygotic twin boys and one case of autosomal dominant transmission.[346]

Presenting history

This condition may present at birth with erythema around the mouth and anogenital area.[347] Progressive, diffuse PPK usually appears in the second year.

Physical examination

The PPK is initially patchy but becomes diffuse, clearly demarcated and transgredient. It appears first on the feet, usually after the child has learned to walk. The grossly thickened skin is later complicated by flexion contractures, constrictions, and autoamputation of digits. The hyperkeratotic periorificial plaques may be detectable at birth as localized erythema which becomes yellow–brown and sharply demarcated. Similar plaques may affect the flexures (axillae, neck, and groins). In addition, these patients may exhibit keratosis pilaris, palmoplantar hyper- or hypohidrosis, oral leukokeratosis, tooth anomalies, nail dystrophy, variable alopecia, joint laxity, and neurosensory deafness.

Pathophysiology and histogenesis

Histologic findings

There is massive acanthosis, parakeratosis, and papillomatosis. The dermis shows increased vascularity and a mononuclear infiltrate in the papillary dermis.[347] Kress *et al.* found suprabasilar staining with a keratin antibody that normally only stains the basal layer.[348]

Differential diagnosis

In infancy, the periorificial keratoses may be mistaken for acrodermatitis enteropathica and, in childhood, the flexor plaques for flexural psoriasis. Later, the mutilating PPK may resemble Vohwinkel and Mal de Meleda. The formation of linear or star-shaped distant keratoses is reminiscent of Vohwinkel's keratoderma. A family with autosomal dominant PPK reported by Rivers as Vohwinkel was clinically more like Olmsted, with periorificial involvement.[349] The other variable features may lead to confusion with ectodermal dysplasia and pachyonychia congenita. See Table 8.9 for differentiation from other PPKs.

Therapeutics and prognosis

Topical therapy

As for EPPK/NEPPK. Full-thickness excision and grafting of the palmar skin may be necessary.[346]

Systemic management

Etretinate 1mg/kg/day was unhelpful in the child reported by Atherton.[346] In the family reported by Rivers as Vohwinkel but clinically resembling Olmsted, the massive hyperkeratosis improved with etretinate.[349]

Prognosis

In some patients the condition is slowly progressive, eventually resulting in mutilating contractures and ainhum of the digits. In others it waxes and wanes in severity.

VOHWINKEL KERATODERMA

Introduction and historical note

Vohwinkel keratoderma, or keratoderma hereditaria mutilans, was first described by Vohwinkel in 1929. More recently two types have been differentiated:[350] Vohwinkel PPK with ichthyosis caused by loricrin mutations, and Vohwinkel with deafness caused by connexin 26 mutations.

Epidemiology

Vohwinkel keratoderma is inherited as a fully penetrant autosomal dominant trait, with occasional sporadic cases presumably representing new mutations.

VOHWINKEL KERATODERMA WITH ICHTHYOSIS (LORICRIN KERATODERMA)

Presenting history

The PPK is evident within a few weeks of birth. The onset of digital constricting bands is variable and is often delayed until adolescence or adulthood.

343. Frenk E, Guggisberg D, Mevorah B, Hohl D. (1996) Meleda disease: report of two cases investigated by electron microscopy. **Dermatology** 193(4):358–361. Review.

344. Poulin Y, Perry HO, Muller SA (1984) Olmstead syndrome – congenital palmoplantar and periorificial keratoderma. **J Am Acad Dermatol** 10:600–610.

345. Larrègue M, Callot V, Kanitakis J et al. (2000) Olmstead syndrome: report of two new cases and literature review. **J Dermatol** 27(9):557–568. Review.

346. Atherton DJ, Sutton C, Jones BM (1990) Mutilating palmoplantar keratoderma with periorificial keratotic palques (Olmsted's syndrome). **Br J Dermatol** 122:245–252.

347. Frias-Iniesta J, Sanchez-Pedreno P, Martinez-Escribano JA et al. (1997) Olmsted syndrome: report of a new case. **Br J Dermatol** 136(6):935–938. Review.

348. Kress DW, Seraly MP, Falo L et al. (1996) Olmsted syndrome. Case report and identification of a keratin abnormality. **Arch Dermatol** 132:797–800.

349. Rivers J, Duke E, Justus D (1985) Etretinate: management of keratoma hereditaria mutilans in four family members. **J Am Acad Dermatol** 13:43–49.

350. Korge BP, Ishida-Yamamoto A, Punter C et al. (1997) Loricrin mutation in Vohwinkel's keratoderma is unique to the variant with ichthyosis. **J Invest Dermatol** 109(4):604–610.

Physical examination

Skin

There is a diffuse PPK with an abrupt margin particularly at the wrist. The PPK is described as "honeycombed," meaning that there is a fine and clearly discernable superficial pattern which completely replaces the normal dermatoglyphs. Starfish-shaped keratoses occur over the elbows and knees and sometimes over the dorsum of hands and feet. Digital constricting bands sometimes lead to autoamputation (ainhum) particularly of the fifth finger. Osteoporotic changes may occur distal to constricting bands. There is a mild, nonerythrodermic generalized ichthyosis with flexural accentuation and linear hyperkeratotic streaks or a more diffuse, verrucous lichenification.

Hair, nails, teeth, and mucous membranes

Alopecia occasionally occurs but nails, teeth, and mucous membranes are normal.

Pathophysiology and histogenesis

Molecular basis

Maestrini et al. mapped Vohwinkel syndrome with ichthyosis to the epidermal differentiation complex (EDC) region at 1q21.[351] Genes that map to the EDC region include loricrin, involucrin, and small proline-rich protein, all of which are associated with formation of the cornified cell envelope. In several families with Vohwinkel syndrome with ichthyosis, mutations have now been identified in the loricrin gene.[350-353] All so far have been single-base insertions producing an extended mutant protein due to a delayed termination codon. Affected individuals are heterozygous for the mutation which has been predicted to disrupt transglutaminase-mediated cross-linking of the peptide to other loricrin molecules and to other components of the cornified envelope in a dominant negative manner.[352]

An identical but recessive phenotype has been reported, also with abnormal intracellular localization of loricrin, but with no loricrin mutation and no linkage to the epidermal differentiation complex.[354]

Histologic findings

Palmoplantar skin shows acanthosis, hypergranulosis, and hyperkeratosis with retention of rounded nuclei. Immunoelectronmicroscopy shows abnormal loricrin distribution, with sparse labeling of the abnormally thin cornified envelopes and strongly labeled intranuclear granules in the granular and cornified layers.[350] Mutant loricrin also localizes to the nuclear granules.[355]

Histogenesis

Ishida-Yamamoto suggests that loricrin mutations disrupt the normal program of apoptosis in the epidermis, leading to the characteristic parakeratotic hyperkeratosis.[355]

Differential diagnosis

Before the development of pseudoainhum this can be differentiated from other forms of PPK by the honeycomb nature of the keratoderma and by abnormal skin on the flexor and extensor aspects of joints. Hearing should be checked because the PPK is identical in Vohwinkel PPK with deafness. See Table 8.9 for differentiation from other PPKs.

Therapeutics and prognosis

Topical therapy

The topical treatment of Vohwinkel PPK is similar to that for other PPKs, but the results are generally unsatisfactory. Constricting bands may require surgical release.[356]

Systemic management

Oral synthetic retinoids may have a role in averting threatened autoamputation, as well as benefiting the keratoderma (see below: Vohwinkel with deafness).

VOHWINKEL KERATODERMA WITH DEAFNESS

Physical examination

The honeycomb PPK, ainhum, and starfish keratoses are common to both types of Vohwinkel keratoderma. Patients with Vohwinkel keratoderma with deafness suffer a moderate to severe sensorineural deafness, and do not have ichthyosis.

Pathophysiology and histogenesis

Following the identification of mutations in a gap-junction protein (GJB2, or connexin 26, CX26) in autosomal recessive nonsyndromic deafness, Richard et al. identified a heterozygous missense mutation (R75W) in a family with autosomal dominant deafness and Vohwinkel PPK.[357] Maestrini et al. found a further missense mutation (D66H) in CX26 in British, Spanish and Italian families with Vohwinkel keratoderma and deafness.[358] Gap junctions are specialized structures on plasma membranes between cells, consisting of cell-to-cell channels. Connexins are proteins extracted from enriched gap junctions. They are tissue specific and designated by their

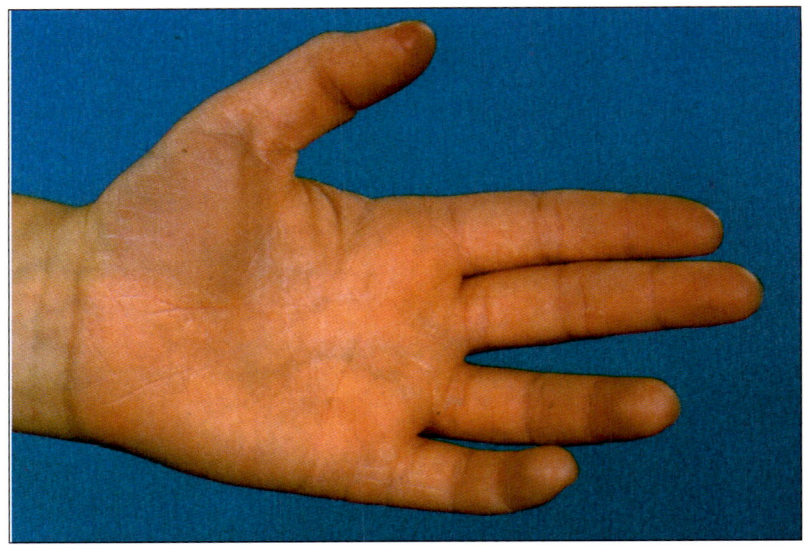

Fig. 8.48   Mild diffuse PPK in a child with congenital sensorineural deafness due to a connexin 26 mutation.

351. Maestrini E, Monaco AP, McGrath JA et al. (1996) A molecular defect in loricrin, the major component of the cornified cell envelope, underlies Vohwinkel's syndrome. **Nat Genet** 13:70–77.

352. Armstrong DKB, McKenna KE, Hughes AE (1998) A novel insertional mutation in loricrin in Vohwinkel's keratoderma. **J Invest Dermatol** 111:702–704.

353. Takahashi H, Ishada-Yamamoto A, Kishi A et al. (1999) Loricrin gene mutation in a Japanese patient of Vohwinkel's syndrome. **J Dermatol Sci** 19:44–47.

354. Akiyama M, Christiano AM, Yoneda K, Shimizu H (1998) Abnormal cornified cell envelope formation in mutilating palmoplantar keratoderma unrelated to epidermal differentiation complex. **J Invest Dermatol** 111(1):133–138.

355. Ishida-Yamamoto A, Kato H, Kiyama H et al. (2000) Mutant loricrin is not cross-linked into the cornified cell envelope but is translocated into the nucleus in loricrin keratoderma. **J Invest Dermatol** 115:1088–1094.

356. Pisoh T, Bhatia A, Oberlin C (1995) Surgical correction of pseudo-ainhum in Vohwinkel syndrome. **J Hand Surg** 20:338–341.

357. Richard G, White TW, Smith LE et al. (1998) Functional defects of Cx26 resulting from a heterozygous missense mutation in a family with dominant deaf-mutism and palmoplantar keratoderma. **Hum Genet** Oct;103(4):393–399.

358. Maestrini E, Korge BP, Ocana-Sierra J et al. (1999) A missense mutation in connexin26, D66H, causes mutilating keratoderma with sensorineural deafness (Vohwinkel's syndrome) in three unrelated families. **Hum Mol Genet** 8:1237–1243.

molecular mass. Connexin subunits assemble as hexamers into connexons. Unlike the loss-of-function mutation that causes autosomal recessive deafness, the *R75W* mutation has a deleterious dominant negative effect on gap channel function *in vitro*. The common *D66H* mutation is located at a highly conserved residue in the first extracellular domain of the CX26 molecule, and interferes with epidermal differentiation as well as inner ear function.[308]

Connexin mutations are responsible not only for deafness and PPK but also Charcot–Marie–Tooth syndrome.[308] PPK has been reported in a family with Charcot–Marie–Tooth syndrome.[359] As more connexin mutations emerge, the PPK + deafness phenotype is proving more variable than originally thought (Fig. 8.48).

Differential diagnosis

Even before the development of pseudoainhum, the honeycomb nature of the keratoderma, and the abnormal skin on the flexor and extensor aspects of joints differentiate Vohwinkel from other types of PPK. This phenotype resembles the maternally inherited sensorineural deafness with NEPPK, associated with a point mutation A7745G in the mitochondrial genome (see below). See Table 8.9 for differentiation from other PPKs.

Therapeutics and prognosis

Oral synthetic retinoids may have a role in averting threatened autoamputation, as well as benefiting the keratoderma.[360]

MATERNALLY INHERITED NEPPK WITH DEAFNESS

Introduction and historical note

Just as for connexin mutations, a mitochondrial mutation was first identified in familial deafness,[361] and then in patients with inherited deafness plus PPK.[362,363] Reassessment of the original deaf patient revealed previously overlooked PPK.[363]

Epidemiology

This has been reported in Scottish, French, New Zealand, and Japanese pedigrees.

Genetics

The condition is transmitted only by females because mitochondria are exclusively inherited from the oocyte. Penetrance is variable, and is higher for hearing loss (60%) than for PPK (37%).[363]

Presenting history

Plantar hyperkeratosis appears during childhood. Palmar involvement develops later and sometimes not at all. Sensorineural deafness starts in infancy or childhood and is slowly progressive, sometimes becoming total.

Physical examination

Skin

The plantar keratoderma is sharply delimited and not transgredient. It predominantly affects the weight-bearing area, but may extend to the instep and Achilles tendon, and keratotic plaques may be found on the dorsum of the foot. Palmar involvement is commoner in manual workers. Pseudoainhum has not been reported.

Hair, nails, teeth, and mucous membranes

These are normal.

Systemic manifestations

The hearing impairment is variable and progressive. High-tone loss predominates.

Pathophysiology and histogenesis

Molecular, biochemical, and immunological basis

There is a mutation designated A7445G in the mitochondrial DNA.[362,363] The mitochondrial genome consists of double-stranded DNA and contains 37 genes that encode 13 respiratory chain polypeptides, two types of ribosomal RNA and 22 transfer RNAs. The A7445G mutation on one DNA strand results in a silent change to the cytochrome oxidase 1 gene, and on the other strand a substitution adjacent to the 3′ end of the serine tRNA gene. The consequences of these rearrangements remain unclear.

Histologic findings

There is acanthosis, hypergranulosis, and ortho- and parakeratosis, but no epidermolysis. Ultrastructurally there are large keratohyaline granules in the granular layer, and perinuclear bundles of tonofilaments.

Differential diagnosis

See Table 8.9 for differentiation from other types of PPK. The late onset of PPK distinguishes it from most other types.

Therapeutics and prognosis

Topical therapy

This is as for other types of NEPPK.

Systemic management

The use of oral synthetic retinoids has not been reported.

Prognosis

Both the PPK and deafness are slowly progressive.

PAPILLON–LEFEVRE/HAIM–MUNK SYNDROME

Introduction and historical note

Papillon–Lefevre syndrome is characterized by PPK associated with rapidly progressive periodontitis. The link between the epidermal and gingival abnormalities has been the subject of much speculation over the years, and is still unclear despite the identification of cathepsin C as the gene responsible.[364]

Epidemiology

Papillon–Lefevre syndrome has been identified throughout the world, while the Haim–Munk variant has been observed only among descendants of an isolated population from Cochin, India.

Genetics

The disorder is inherited as an autosomal recessive trait.

Statistics

The estimated prevalence is 1–4 per million.[364]

Presenting history

The keratoderma may be evident at birth but most commonly begins in the second or third year of life. It is often worse in the winter. Periodontitis with

359. Rabbiosi G, Borroni G, Pinelli P, Cosi V (1980) Palmo plantar keratoderma and Charcot–Marie–Tooth disease. **Arch Dermatol** 116:789–790.
360. Peris K, Salvati EF, Torlone G, Chimenti S (1995) Keratoderma hereditarium mutilans (Vohwinkel's syndrome) associated with congenital deaf-mutism. **Br J Dermatol** Apr;132(4):617–620.
361. Reid FM, Vernham GA, Jacobs HT (1994) A novel mitochondrial point mutation in a maternal pedigree with sensorineural deafness. **Hum Mutat** 3:243–247.
362. Sevior KB, Hatamochi A, Stewart IA et al. (1998) Mitochondrial A7445G mutation in two pedigrees with palmoplantar keratoderma and deafness. **Am J Med Genet** 75(2):179–185.
363. Martin L, Toutain A, Guillen C et al. (2000) Inherited palmoplantar keratoderma and sensorineural deafness associated with A7445G point mutation in the mitochondrial genome. **Br J Dermatol** 143:876–883.
364. Gorlin RJ (2000) Of palms, soles and gums. **J Med Genet** 37:81–82.

premature shedding usually affects both deciduous and permanent teeth, although in a few patients only the permanent teeth are affected. Most patients are edentulous by 15 years. Penetrance is variable, with occasional cases of isolated PPK or isolated periodontosis.[365]

Physical examination
Skin
The severity of the keratoderma is variable, and the soles are usually worse than the palms. The margins are usually well defined and intensely erythematous. Transgredient extension is characteristic. The keratoderma may be punctate or striate rather than diffuse. Hyperhidrosis is often present, and can be malodorous. Hyperkeratotic plaques on the elbows and knees and/or follicular hyperkeratoses may occur. The Haim–Munk variant includes atrophic nail changes.

Teeth
As a rule, the teeth are not carious, and oral inflammation is limited to periodontal tissues but may lead to extensive alveolar bone resorption. Gingival inflammation destroys the periodontal ligaments loosening the teeth and ends in shedding. The deciduous teeth are lost by 4 years, after which the mouth becomes normal until the secondary teeth erupt. The process is repeated with eruption and loss of the permanent teeth by mid teens. The periodontitis and the skin lesions improve after all teeth are shed.

Systemic manifestations
Calcification of the falx cerebri is a characteristic but inconsistent feature of this syndrome. Mental retardation is infrequent. Arachnodactyly occurs in the Haim–Munk variant.

Pathophysiology and histogenesis
Molecular basis
Papillon–Lefevre syndrome was mapped to 11q13–q14 close to the metalloproteinase gene cluster.[366] Toomes et al. narrowed the candidate region, and found mutations in the gene for cathepsin C.[367] A functional assay showed almost total loss of cathepsin C activity in patients and reduced activity in obligate carriers. Hart et al. found several different mutations in an ethnically diverse group of patients, and listed all the mutations to date.[368] The same group identified mutations in cathepsin C in Haim–Munk syndrome, confirming that these two conditions are allelic variants.[369] Most mutations in Papillon–Lefevre syndrome reside within the mature enzyme domain and presumably impair or abolish catalytic activity.[370] Cathepsin C activates serine proteinases expressed in leukocyte granules and implicated in a variety of immune responses, and its deficiency could thus explain the severe periodontitis of Papillon–Lefevre syndrome. The hyperkeratosis is less easy to explain.[364]

Histologic findings
Skin biopsy shows hyperkeratosis with psoriasiform parakeratosis.

Differential diagnosis
The association with periodontosis makes this form of PPK unmistakable. See Table 8.9 for differentiation from other PPKs.

Therapeutic and prognosis
Topical therapy
The dermatological treatment of Papillon–Lefevre syndrome is similar to that for other PPKs (see EPPK). Management of the periodontitis is difficult. Compulsive oral hygiene and vigorous plaque removal may slow disease progression, but this is difficult to achieve in young children. Extractions are frequently required for relief of pain. Early loss of dentition leads to significant distortion of maxillary and mandibular growth but once all teeth have been shed dentures are usually well tolerated.

Systemic management
It has been suggested that early treatment with oral retinoids will preserve dentition and improve keratoderma.[371]

Prognosis
The PPK tends to improve after all the teeth have been lost.

NAXOS DISEASE
Introduction and historical note
Diffuse PPK associated with woolly hair and right ventricular cardiomyopathy was first reported in 1986 in four families on the Greek island of Naxos.[372] Carvajal described a striate PPK with woolly hair and dilated cardiomyopathy (see below).

Epidemiology
PPK with woolly hair and arrhythmogenic cardiomyopathy is an autosomal recessive trait.

Presenting history
PPK and woolly hair are present from infancy. The cardiac condition may be asymptomatic, but can cause arrhythmia, heart failure and sudden death. It is not clinically apparent before the age of 15 years and usually presents first as palpitations and syncope.

Physical examination
Skin
The PPK is indistinguishable from NEPPK.[373]

Hair
The hair is tightly curled, dense, rough and wiry.

Systemic features
The classic cardiac anomalies are right ventricular enlargement and right ventricular band, associated with ventricular arrhythmias. Ebstein anomaly with additional right ventricular myocardial dysplasia has also been reported.

Pathophysiology and histogenesis
Molecular basis
Naxos disease was mapped to 17q21 in 21 patients from nine families in Naxos, and KRT9 was initially the obvious candidate gene.[374] Subsequently,

365. Soskolne WA, Stabholz A, van Dyke TE et al. (1996) Partial expression of the Papillon–Lefevre syndrome in 2 unrelated families. J Clin Periodontol 23(8):764–769.
366. Laass MW, Hennies HC, Preis S et al. (1997) Localisation of a gene for Papillon–Lefevre syndrome to chromosome 11q14–q21 by homozygosity mapping. Hum Genet 101(3):376–382.
367. Toomes C, James J, Wood AJ et al. (1999) Loss-of-function mutations in the cathepsin C gene result in periodontal disease and palmoplantar keratosis. Nat Genet 23:421–424.
368. Hart PS, Zhang Y, Firatli E et al. (2000) Identification of cathepsin C mutations in ethnically diverse Papillon–Lefevre syndrome patients. J Med Genet 37(12):927–932.
369. Hart TC, Hart PS, Michalec MD et al. (2000) Haim–Munk syndrome and Papillon–Lefevre syndrome are allelic mutations in cathepsin C. J Med Genet 37:88–94.
370. Nakano A, Nomura K, Nakano H (2001) Papillon–Lefevre syndrome: mutations and polymorphisms in the cathepsin C gene. J Invest Dermatol 116(2):339–343.
371. Siragusa M, Romano C, Batticane N et al. (2000) A new family with Papillon–Lefevre syndrome: effectiveness of etretinate treatment. Cutis 65:151–155.
372. Protonotarios N, Tsatsopoulou A, Fontaine G (2001) Naxos disease: keratoderma, scalp modifications and cardiomyopathy. J Am Acad Dermatol 44:309–311.
373. Tosti A, Misciali C, Piraccini B et al. (1994) Woolly hair, palmoplantar keratoderma and cardiac abnormalities: report of a family. Arch Dermatol 130:522–524.
374. Coonar AS, Protonotarios N, Tsatsopoulou A et al. (1998) Gene for arrhythmogenic right ventricular cardiomyopathy with diffuse nonepidermolytic palmoplantar keratoderma and woolly hair (Naxos disease) maps to 17q21. Circulation 97(20):2049–2058.

the same group found mutations in the plakoglobin gene at the same locus.[375] Nineteen affected individuals were homozygous, and 29 clinically unaffected family members were heterozygous for a 2bp deletion which caused a frameshift and premature termination of plakoglobin, a key component of desmosomes and adherens junctions in heart and skin.

Histologic findings
The PPK of Naxos disease shows compact hyperkeratosis, hypergranulosis, and acanthosis, as in Unna–Thost PPK.[373]

Differential diagnosis
Naxos disease can be distinguished from NEPPK only by the associated features of woolly hair and cardiomyopathy. Hoeger et al. described an isolated case with diffuse PPK and total anomalous pulmonary venous connection,[376] which seems most likely to be a chance association. See Table 8.9 for differentiation from other PPKs.

Therapeutics and prognosis
These are the same as for NEPPK.

HURIEZ SCLEROTYLOSIS
Introduction and historical note
The cardinal features of this rare and distinctive condition, first reported in 1963, are diffuse scleroatrophy of the hands, ridging or hypoplasia of the nails, mild PPK, and an increased risk of squamous carcinoma of the hands.

Epidemiology
This disorder was first described in two French families. It has since been reported in Germany, Tunisia, India and the UK.

Genetics
Inheritance is autosomal dominant

Presenting history
The hands may be small from birth. The adults studied by Delaporte reported nonerythematous PPK from birth.[377] However, in an infant observed from birth,[378] erythema and peeling developed on the palms and soles at 1 month. At 9 months absence of dermatoglyphics was noted. By age 3 years tapering and flexion contractures of the fingers were apparent. Despite the sclerotic appearance, Raynaud's phenomenon does not occur. Nails become atrophic and may be shed. Focal PPK develops on the soles in adulthood.[379] Squamous cell carcinomas may arise in scleroatrophic skin in middle age.

Physical examination

Skin
This PPK is more marked on palms than soles. The palmar skin is smooth, red and mildly hyperkeratotic, with accentuated palmar creases, absent dermatoglyphics and reduced sweating. Punctate pits sometimes occur over thenar and hypothenar eminences. The keratoderma is not transgredient, but a patchy, reticulate erythema affects the dorsal surfaces of hands and feet, with thickened patches over the knuckles. The digits become tapered and flexed. The soles may show focal PPK over pressure points. Squamous carcinomas develop on the scleroatrophic skin in 10% of patients, appearing in the fourth

or fifth decade. They may be multiple, and fatal metastases have occurred in this condition. Some individuals have poikiloderma-like changes on the nose and lips.[380]

Hair, nails, teeth, and mucous membranes
The nails grow slowly and appear atrophic. They may show beaking, longitudinal ridging, prominence of the lunula, leuconychia or occasionally koilonychia. Hair and teeth are normal.

Systemic manifestations
Carcinomas of the gastrointestinal tract (pharynx and stomach) have been reported, but the risk may not be greater than for the general population.

Pathophysiology and histogenesis
Molecular basis
Linkage to the MN blood group at 4q28–q31, reported in 1967, was subsequently excluded.[377,380] Lee et al. established linkage to 4q23.[381] Because of the association with skin cancer, DNA repair was studied in one patient and was normal.[377]

Histologic findings
Palmar skin shows acanthosis, hyperkeratosis, and hypergranulosis. The upper and mid dermis shows mild fibrosis with an increased vascularity but no inflammation. Eccrine sweat glands are reduced or absent.[379] Ultrastructurally[377] the desmosomes appear normal, tonofilaments are grouped in dense bundles and keratohyalin is abundant and clumped in the granular layer. Langerhans cells were absent in affected palmar skin in one study, suggesting that the tendency to squamous carcinoma on the hands might be due to a defect of immune surveillance involving the presentation of tumor-associated antigens by Langerhans cells.[379]

Differential diagnosis
See Table 8.9 for differentiation from other PPKs. Systemic sclerosis can be excluded by the intact circulation and lack of Raynaud's phenomenon. Progeria and Rothmund–Thomson syndrome show similar changes in the hands, but can be distinguished by their additional features, particularly alopecia and marked cutaneous signs on the face. Acrogeria shows similar skin changes and distribution but less marked nail changes, and is recessively inherited. Acrogeric Ehlers–Danlos syndrome (EDS type 4) shows generalized skin changes.

Therapeutics and prognosis
Topical therapy
Regular emollients reduce cracking and improve mobility.

Systemic management
Oral synthetic retinoids, administered to a patient who had had a squamous carcinoma excised, improved the keratoderma and mobility of the fingers. There were no further malignancies during five years of follow-up.[377]

Prognosis
Patients education and regular surveillance are necessary to minimize the risks of fatal squamous carcinoma.

375. McKoy G, Protonotarios N, Crosby A et al. (2000) Identification of a deletion in plakoglobin in arrhythmogenic right ventricular cardiomyopathy with palmoplantar keratoderma and woolly hair (Naxos disease). Lancet 355(9221):2119–2124.
376. Hoeger PH, Yates RW, Harper JI (1998) Palmoplantar keratoderma associated with congenital heart disease. Br J Dermatol 138:506–509.
377. Delaporte E, N'guyen-Mailfer C, Janin A et al. (1995) Keratoderma with scleroatrophy of the extremities or sclerotylosis (Huriez syndrome): a reappraisal. Br J Dermatol 133(3):409–416.
378. Downs AM, Kennedy CT (1998) Scleroatrophic syndrome of Huriez in an infant. Pediatr Dermatol 15(3):207–209.
379. Hamm H, Traupe H, Brocker EB et al. (1996) The scleroatrophic syndrome of Huriez: a cancer-prone genodermatosis. Br J Dermatol 134(3):512–518.
380. Kavanagh GM, Jardine PE, Peachey RD et al. (1997) The scleroatrophic syndrome of Huriez. Br J Dermatol 137:114–118.
381. Lee Y-A, Stevens HP, Delaporte E et al. (2000) A gene for an autosomal dominant scleroatrophic syndrome predisposing to skin cancer (Huriez syndrome) maps to chromosome 4q23. Am J Hum Genet 66:326–330.

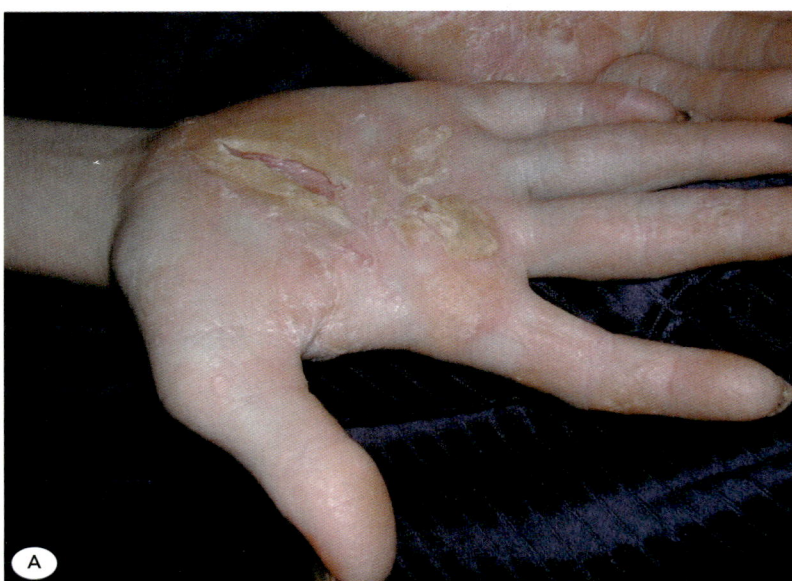

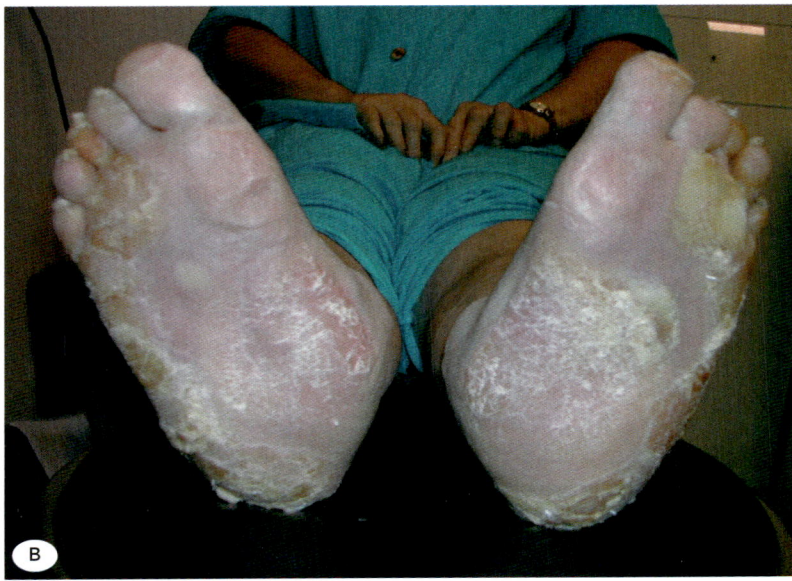

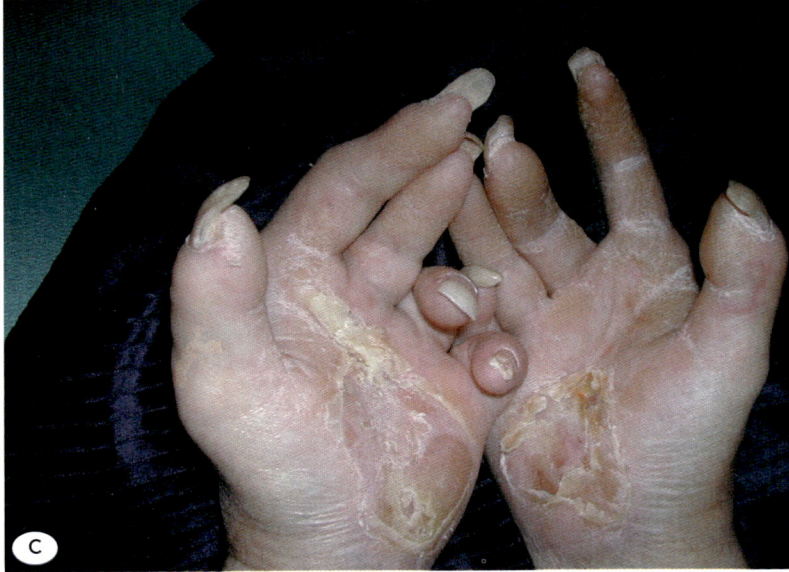

Fig. 8.49   Diffuse PPK with blisters in Dowling–Meara epidermolysis bullosa simplex. (**A**) Palm of mother; (**B**) sole of mother; (**C**) sole of daughter.

GENERALIZED SKIN DISORDERS FEATURING DIFFUSE PPK

Diffuse PPK also occurs in the following generalized disorders (see Table 8.10), which are discussed in more detail elsewhere. Broadly, they can be divided into keratin disorders in which the predominant abnormality is epidermal fragility, and ectodermal dysplasia syndromes in which other ectodermal derivatives are affected.

Epidermolysis bullosa simplex, Weber–Cockayne type

This autosomal dominant keratin 5/14 disorder presents with friction-induced blisters, but in some patients PPK become prominent later, particularly on the soles.

Epidermolysis bullosa simplex, Dowling–Meara type

Severe neonatal blistering characterizes this autosomal dominant keratin 5/14 disorder, but in some families PPK is a serious problem in adult life (Fig. 8.49).

Bullous ichthyosiform erythroderma

Palmoplantar keratoderma is present in some patients with this autosomal dominant keratin 1/10 disorder. In general mutations in keratin 1 are associated with PPK while mutations in keratin 10 are not.

Clouston hypohidrotic ectodermal dysplasia

Clouston syndrome is an autosomal dominant hidrotic ectodermal dysplasia characterized by thickened nails, variable alopecia, and a diffuse PPK. Plantar surfaces are more severely involved, and keratoses may be limited to weight-bearing surfaces. Deafness occasionally occurs. All families so far studied have one of two missense mutations in *GJB6* encoding connexin 30.

Naegeli–Franceschetti–Jadassohn syndrome

Diffuse or punctate PPK may be one of the manifestations of this autosomal dominant ectodermal dysplasia syndrome. Other manifestations include acquired, progressive reticulate pigmentation, and hypohidrosis. Nail abnormalities include onycholysis and subungual hyperkeratosis. Yellow discoloration of tooth enamel occurs.

Dyskeratosis congenita

Atrophic PPK and absent dermatoglyphics are sometimes found in this X-linked recessive degenerative disorder of skin, nails, mucosal epithelium, and bone marrow.

Rapp–Hodgkin syndrome

PPK is an occasional feature of this autosomal dominant ectodermal dysplasia with clefting.

Schöpf–Schultz–Passarge syndrome

Diffuse PPK accompanies cysts of the eyelid margins, nail fragility, hypodontia, and alopecia in this autosomal recessive ectodermal dysplasia.

Weary–Kindler syndrome

Diffuse PPK has been reported in association with congenital poikiloderma and traumatic blister formation (Kindler syndrome). Autosomal recessive inheritance is proposed. A similar syndrome with poikiloderma, PPK, and acrokeratotic papules but no blistering is dominantly inherited (Weary syndrome).

FOCAL PALMOPLANTAR KERATODERMAS

Focal PPKs appear at sites of mechanical pressure. Therefore they are more likely to affect the soles and to develop later than diffuse PPKs. In addition

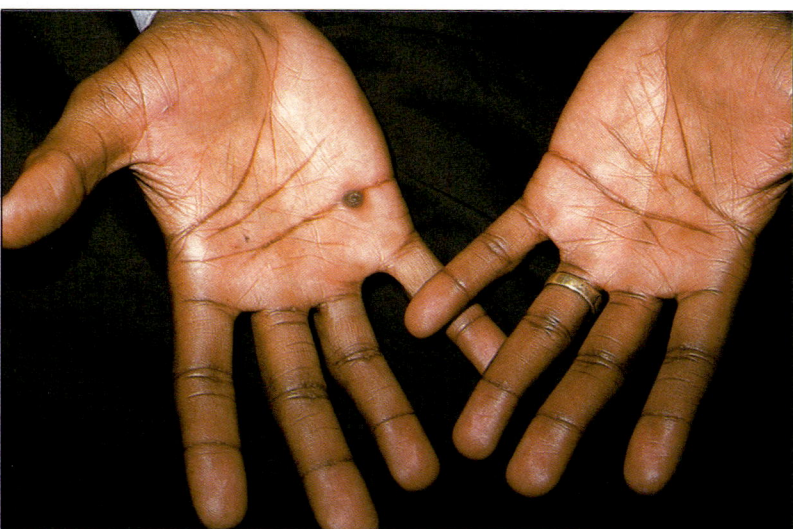

Fig. 8.50   Keratotic pits of the palmar creases in a black teenager.

to the conditions discussed in this section, it should be recalled that disorders classified as diffuse PPK may in some patients present initially with focal involvement, often localized over pressure points.

FOCAL PALMOPLANTAR KERATODERMA (WACHTERS)

Introduction and historical note
Wachter introduced the term "keratosis palmoplantaris varians" for subtypes described by Fuhs, Brunauer and Siemens, reflecting the considerable inter- and intrafamilial variability. This condition is sometimes termed "hereditary painful callosities."

Epidemiology
This is an autosomal dominant trait.

Presenting history
Plantar keratoses become apparent after the child has learned to walk. Palmar keratoses appear only in response to mechanical stress.

Physical examination
Skin
Thick hard yellow hyperkeratoses occur over the pressure points on the sole (Fig. 8.50). The palmar keratoses may be nummular or striate.

Hair, nails, teeth, and mucous membranes
Some individuals have oral mucosal and follicular hyperproliferative lesions similar to those found in pachyonychia congenita type 1. There are no systemic manifestations.

Pathophysiology and histogenesis
Molecular, biochemical, and immunological basis
Keratin 16 mutations have been identified both in pachyonychia congenita type 1, which features focal NEPPK, and in isolated focal NEPPK.[382,383] The

milder phenotype of focal NEPPK is probably due to mutations causing loss of the helix termination motif, rendering this mutant K16 less able to contribute to filament assembly, thereby decreasing any dominant negative effect.[384]

Histologic findings
There is acanthosis, hyperkeratosis, and papillomatosis. Ultrastructurally the keratin filament bundles are condensed, but do not form the dense aggregates seen in some other keratin disorders. Sometimes there is localized epidermolytic hyperkeratosis.

Differential diagnosis
Children with focal NEPPK and their relatives should be examined for other features of pachyonychia congenita type 1 (oral leucokeratosis and nail dystrophy). Focal NEPPK looks like the PPK of Howel–Evans syndrome, but the onset is much earlier in childhood.

Therapeutics and prognosis
Topical therapy
All focal NEPPKs worsen in response to mechanical stress. Suitable insoles should be inserted into footwear. Topical emollients and mechanical relief of pressure are the mainstays of treatment. The patchy distribution makes it difficult to use keratolytics, which may irritate normal skin.

Prognosis
Relief of mechanical pressure and friction leads to improvement.

Pediatric aspects of the disease
Young people should be advised to choose a sedentary, nonmanual job.

LINEAR (BLASCHKO) PPK (EPIDERMAL NEVI)
Linear verrucous epidermal nevus on the palm or sole can be regarded as a form of localized PPK. In general this phenomenon is due to mosaicism for an autosomal dominant gene expressed in palmoplantar epidermis. Terrinoni et al. reported a unilateral palmoplantar verrucous nevus due to a mosaic mutation in keratin 16.[385] The continuous morphology and epidermolytic histology of Terrinoni's mosaic case contrasts interestingly with the focal NEPPK produced by germline keratin 16 mutations. Other genes associated with epidermal nevi include keratin 1, keratin 10, and fibroblast growth factor receptor (FGFR2). None has yet been reported specifically in a palmar or plantar nevus, but keratin 1 is a good candidate.

STRIATE PPK (SIEMENS)
Introduction and historical note
Originally described in the 1920s, this disorder shows considerable inter- and intrafamilial variability, perhaps because mechanical stress is an important provoking and localizing factor.

Epidemiology
Striate PPK is inherited as an autosomal dominant trait.

Presenting history
Onset is often delayed until adolescence or adulthood, and precipitated by mechanical trauma. In one family, a manual laborer had the most prominent clinical features, while those in sedentary occupations had mild or undetectable physical signs.[386]

382. Shamsher MK, Navsaria HA, Stevens HP et al. (1995) Novel mutations in keratin 16 gene underlie focal non-epidermolytic palmoplantar keratoderma (NEPPK) in two families. **Hum Mcl Genet** 4(10):1875–1881.
383. Smith FJD, Steijlen PM, McKenna K et al. (1998) Cloning of multiple K16 genes and genotype-phenotype correlation in pachyonychia congenita type 1 and focal PPK. **J Invest Dermatol** 110:502.

384. Smith FJ, Fisher MP, Healy E et al. (2000) Novel keratin 16 mutations and protein expression studies in pachyonychia congenita type 1 and focal palmoplantar keratoderma. **Exp Dermatol** 9(3):170–177.
385. Terrinoni A, Puddu P, Didona B et al. (2000) A mutation in the VI domain of K16 is responsible for unilateral palmoplantar verrucous nevus. **J Invest Dermatol** 114:1136–1140.
386. Whittock NV, Ashton GH, Dopping-Hepenstal et al. (1999) Striate palmoplantar keratoderma resulting from desmoplakin haploinsufficiency. **J Invest Dermatol** 113(6):940–946.

Physical examination

Skin
Linear keratotic streaks extend in stripes along the flexor aspects of the fingers and onto the palm. Plantar involvement tends to be nummular rather than linear.

Hair, nails, teeth, and mucous membranes
These are usually unaffected. However, striate PPK with islands of thickening at pressure points in association with abnormal teeth, pili torti, sparse hair and eyelashes, hypohidrosis, and sensorineural hearing loss has been reported (Brunauer syndrome.) The onset is usually the second or third decade in both sexes.[387]

Systemic manifestations
Four brothers with striate keratoderma of the palms and diffuse hyperkeratosis of soles with mental retardation, and spastic paraplegia with pes cavus of feet were reported. The mother and sisters were normal.[388]

Pathophysiology and histogenesis

Molecular basis
Hennies et al. excluded linkage to the keratin gene clusters on 12q and 17q, and mapped striate PPK to 18q, in the region of the desmosomal cadherin genes.[389] Rickman et al. identified a mutation in one of these cadherin genes, desmoglein I, in affected members of a three-generation Dutch family,[390] and Hunt found further desmoglein mutations in striate PPK patients.[391] Meanwhile, Armstrong et al. found a mutation in a different desmosomal gene, desmoplakin, 6p21.[392] Both this mutation, and another subsequently identified,[386] resulted in a null allele, suggesting that autosomal dominant striate PPK may be due to haploinsufficiency of desmoplakin in these families. Such a dosage effect might explain the strong influence of mechanical factors, and the variability between family members, and between sites within individuals.

Histologic findings
There is acanthosis, hyperkeratosis, and widening of intercellular spaces throughout the spinous layer. Ultrastructurally, desmosomes are reduced in size and number. Keratin filaments show disruption of their attachment to the plasma membrane, and are compacted in a perinuclear distribution. Keratohyaline granules may show alternating dark and light content characteristic of composite granules.[393]

Differential diagnosis
An association with woolly hair should prompt cardiac evaluation to exclude arrhythmogenic left cardiomyopathy. Occasionally striate PPK can mimic duPuytren's contractures. See Table 8.9 for differentiation from other PPKs.

Therapeutics and prognosis

Topical therapy
Topical emollients and mechanical relief of pressure are the mainstays of treatment. The patchy distribution makes it difficult to use keratolytics which may irritate normal skin. Contractures may develop, requiring surgical release.

Prognosis
Relief of mechanical pressure and friction leads to improvement.

Pediatric aspects of the disease
Young people should be advised to choose a sedentary, nonmanual job.

STRIATE KERATODERMA, WOOLY HAIR AND DILATED CARDIOMYOPATHY (CARVAJAL SYNDROME)

Introduction and historical note
Striate keratoderma with woolly hair and dilated left cardiomyopathy has been described in three families from Ecuador.[394]

Epidemiology
The condition is inherited as an autosomal recessive trait.

Presenting history
Patients are born with wooly hair. PPK develops at around 10 months of age. The first signs of left ventricular dilatation are electrocardiographic and occur in asymptomatic patients. Carvajal-Huerta found ECG abnormalities in children as young as 8 years, and patients can develop heart failure in their teenage years.[394]

Physical examination

Skin
The keratoderma is striate. The hair is tightly curled. Patients also develop striated lichenoid keratoses in major flexures and follicular keratoses on the elbows and knees.

Systemic manifestations
There is dilated left cardiomyopathy.

Pathophysiology and histogenesis

Molecular basis
Affected individuals from three families were homozygous for a deletion in the desmoplakin gene. This produces a premature stop codon leading to a truncated desmoplakin protein missing the C domain of the tail region.[398] Desmoplakin is the most abundant protein in desmosomes, which are particularly prominent in epidermis and cardiac muscle, and may account for the resistance of these tissues to mechanical forces.

Histologic findings
Histologically there is epidermolytic hyperkeratosis with large intercellular spaces. Immunohistochemistry shows perinuclear localization of keratin in suprabasal keratinocytes suggesting a collapsed intermediate filament network.[395]

387. Egelund E, Frentz G (1982) Case of hyperkeratosis palmplantaris striata combined with pili torti, hypohidrosis, hypodontia and hypacusis. Acta Otolaryngol 94:571–573.

388. Fitzsimmons JS, Fitzsimmons EM, McLachkin JI, Gilbert GB (1983) Four brothers with mental retardation, spastic paraplegia and palmoplantar hyperkeratosis. A new syndrome? Clin Genet 23:329–335.

389. Hennies HC, Kuster W, Mischke D et al. (1995) Localization of a locus for the striated form of palmoplantar keratoderma to chromosome 18q near the desmosomal cadherin gene cluster. Hum Mol Genet 4(6) 1015–1020.

390. Rickman L, Simrak D, Stevens HP et al. (1999) N-terminal deletion in a desmosomal cadherin causes the autosomal dominant skin disease striate palmoplantar keratoderma. Hum Mol Genet 8(6):971–976.

391. Hunt DM, Rickman L, Whittock NV et al. (2001) Spectrum of dominant mutations in the desmosomal cadherin desmoglein 1, causing the skin disease striate palmoplantar keratoderma. Eur J Hum Genet 9(3):197–203.

392. Armstrong DK, McKenna KE, Purkis PE et al. (1999) Haploinsufficiency of desmoplakin causes a striate subtype of palmoplantar keratoderma. Hum Mol Genet 8:943.

393. Sidhu GS, Cassai ND, Rico MJ (2000) Composite keratohyaline granules in striate keratoderma. Ultrastruct Pathol 24(6):391–397.

394. Carvajal-Huerta L (1998) Epidermolytic palmoplantar keratoderma with woolly hair and dilated cardiomyopathy. J Am Acad Dermatol 39(3):418–421.

395. Norgett EE, Hatsell SJ, Carvajal-Huerta L et al. (2000) Recessive mutation in desmoplakin disrupts desmoplakin-intermediate filament interactions and causes dilated cardiomyopathy, woolly hair and keratoderma. Hum Mol Genet 9(18):2761–2766.

396. Ellis A, Field JK, Field EA et al. (1994) Tylosis associated with carcinoma of the oesophagus and oral leukoplakia in a large Liverpool family–a review of six generations. Eur J Cancer 30B:102–112.

397. Rogaev EI, Rogaeva EA, Ginter EK et al. (1993) Identification of the genetic locus for keratosis palmaris et plantaris on chromosome 17 near the RARA and keratin type I genes. Nat Genet 5:158–162.

398. Ruhrberg C, Williamson JA, Sheer D et al. (1996) Chromosomal localisation of the human envoplakin gene (EVPL) to the region of the tylosis oesophageal cancer gene (TOCG) on 17q25. Genomics 37(3):381–385.

Differential diagnosis

The wooly hair and cardiac defects distinguish this condition from striate PPK. Carvajal syndrome can be distinguished from Naxos disease[372] both clinically and at the molecular level. See Table 8.9 for differentiation from other PPKs.

Therapeutics and prognosis

These are the same as for NEPPK.

HOWEL–EVANS SYNDROME (TYLOSIS WITH OESOPHAGEAL CANCER)
Introduction and historical note

Howel–Evans syndrome is the association of focal NEPPK with esophageal carcinoma originally described in two kindreds from Liverpool, UK, in 1958. Six generations of the original Liverpool family were reviewed in 1994.[396]

Epidemiology

Further families have been reported from Oxford, UK, the US, and Germany.

Genetics

This is an autosomal dominant trait.

Presenting history

Tylosis is of late onset, between 5 and 15 years, but is always present by puberty. It appears first on the feet.

Physical examination
Skin

Although originally reported as diffuse, the thickened skin is focal, related to physical activity with sparing of the hands, and regresses on bed-rest. There is follicular hyperkeratosis.

Hair, nails, teeth, and mucous membranes

Oral leukoplakia can precede the plantar lesions.

Systemic manifestations

In the original Liverpool family esophageal carcinoma occurred in 18 of 48 tylotic family members and one of 87 nontylotic members. The average age of diagnosis of esophageal carcinoma was 43 years.

Pathophysiology and histogenesis
Molecular basis

Howel–Evans syndrome was mapped in 1993 to 17q, suggesting the keratin type 1 genes and the breast cancer gene *BRCA1* as candidates or contiguous genes.[397] Ruhrberg in 1996 found linkage to the gene for envoplakin, a component of desmosomes expressed in epidermal and esophageal keratinocytes,[398] but the same group later excluded this gene.[399] The Howel–Evans locus, known as *TOC* (tylosis and oesophageal cancer) shows loss of heterozygosity in 69% of sporadic esophageal cancers,[400] and *DMC1* is a specific gene within the *TOC* region that shows loss of expression in a variety of cancers.[401]

Histologic findings

There is acanthosis, hyperkeratosis, and hypergranulosis but no epidermolysis.

Differential diagnosis

The focal nature, clear relationship to weight-bearing, and late onset distinguish this from most other types of PPK. The phenotype is similar to type 1 pachyonychia congenita, with oral leucokeratosis and focal PPK. See Table 8.9 for differentiation from other PPKs.

Therapeutics and prognosis
Topical therapy

As for other forms (see NEPPK).

Systemic management

Patients should be advised to avoid other risk factors for cancer, particularly smoking.[402] Esophageal dysplasia may precede the development of an invasive carcinoma suggesting that endoscopic surveillance and treatment of premalignant lesions might be worthwhile. Oral synthetic retinoids may improve the PPK but do not prevent the development of esophageal dysplasia.[403]

Prognosis

Development of esophageal carcinoma after the third decade is a virtual certainty in family members with PPK, estimated at 95% by age 65. Stevens *et al.* calculated the relative risk as 38.[402]

TYROSINEMIA TYPE II (RICHNER–HANHART SYNDROME)
Introduction and historical note

In 1937 Richner and in 1947 Hanhart described an autosomal recessive syndrome of corneal ulcerations and painful focal keratoses of fingertips and palmar eminences. In 1972, Burns and Goldsmith *et al.* linked the clinical disorder with an inborn error of tyrosine metabolism, called tyrosinemia type II, or Richner–Hanhart syndrome. This disorder is due to mutations in the tyrosine aminotransferase gene on 16q.

Epidemiology

Although cases have been reported from around the world, many patients are of Italian ancestry.

Genetics

Tyrosinemia type II is inherited as an autosomal recessive trait.

Statistics

There are about 100 cases in the literature.

Presenting history

Eye abnormalities usually present during the first months of life with photophobia, redness, and lacrimation. Many patients are erroneously treated for presumed herpes keratitis. The time of onset of PPK is variable, ranging from infancy to the second decade. The palmoplantar keratoses are characteristically painful and may lead to refusal to walk.[403]

Physical examination
Skin

Typically, focal hyperkeratoses are present on the weight-bearing surfaces of the soles, as well as the fingertips and hypothenar, and thenar eminences. The

399. Risk JM, Ruhrberg C, Hennies H (1999) Envoplakin, a possible candidate gene for focal NEPPK/esophageal cancer (TOC): the integration of genetic and physical maps of the TOC region on 17q25. Genomics 59(2):234–242.
400. von Brevern M, Hollstein MC, Risk JM et al. (1998) Loss of heterozygosity in sporadic oesophageal tumors in the tylosis oesophageal cancer (TOC) gene region of chromosome 17q. Oncogene 17(16):2101–2105.
401. Harada H, Nagai H, Tsuneizumi M et al. (2001) Identification of DMC1, a novel gene in the TOC region on 17q25.1 that shows loss of expression in multiple human cancers. J Hum Genet 46(2):90–95.
402. Stevens HP, Kelsell DP, Bryant SP et al. (1996) Linkage of an American pedigree with palmoplantar keratoderma and malignancy (palmoplantar ectodermal dysplasia type III) to 17q24. Literature survey and proposed updated classification of the keratodermas. Arch Dermatol 32(6):640–651.
403. Ashworth MT, Nash JRG, Ellis A et al. (1991) Abnormalities of differentiation and maturation in the oesophageal squamous epithelium of patients with tylosis: morphological features. Histopathology 19:303–310.

keratoses in some patients are sharply circumscribed and in others ill defined. Erythema may or may not be present. The keratoses may blister, ulcerate, and bleed. The keratoderma is episodic, and the clinical characteristics may be quite variable. Increased pain and erythema of lesions during tyrosine loading is reported. Similar keratotic plaques on elbows and knees may occur.

Hair, nails, teeth, and mucous membranes
Hair and nails are unaffected.

Systemic manifestations
Pseudoherpetic keratitis is usually the earliest presenting complaint and, like the keratodermas, may be episodic. Dendritic corneal ulcerations may progress to severe ulcerative keratitis and, left untreated, to neovascularization and blindness. Mental retardation is an inconstant feature but may be severe.

Pathophysiology and histogenesis

Molecular, biochemical, and immunological basis
Tyrosinemia type II is due to deficiency of the hepatic cytosolic enzyme, tyrosine aminotransferase, leading to accumulation of tyrosine in affected tissues. Plasma tyrosine levels and urinary tyrosine metabolites, p-hydroxyphenylacetic acid, N-acetyltyrosine, and p-tyramine, are increased. Several mutations have been identified in the tyrosine aminotransferase gene on 16q.

Histologic findings
Histology of a keratotic papule shows a depressed epidermis surmounted by compact hyperkeratosis. The cytoplasm of spinous cells and Merkel cells is vacuolated due to the presence of minute tyrosine crystals. The corneocytes contain lipid droplets within the cytoplasm.[405] Tyrosine crystals are also deposited in the cornea.[406]

Differential diagnosis
The ocular abnormality is usually diagnosed first as herpetic ulceration.

Therapeutics and prognosis

Topical therapy
As for other PPKs.

Systemic management
A low tyrosine and low phenylalanine diet improves symptoms and may prevent retardation.[407,408] Etretinate therapy has been used.[409]

Prognosis
The condition is lifelong, and the ocular, cutaneous, and neurological changes progress if untreated. Strict dietary treatment can result in complete remission of symptoms.

GENERALIZED SKIN DISORDERS FEATURING FOCAL PPK

Focal PPK also occurs in the following generalized disorder, which is discussed elsewhere (see Table 8.10).

Pachyonychia congenita type 1 (Jadassohn–Lewandowsky)
This autosomal dominant disorder is caused by hetozygous mutations in keratins 6 or 16, and is characterized by thickened, tubular nails, focal PPK, and oral leukokeratosis. Mosaicism for a keratin 16 mutation has been described in a patient with linear (Blaschko) PKK (see above).

Punctate PPK
Confusion abounds in this group because these conditions show considerable variation both within families and within individuals. Onset is usually after the first decade. Only the most clearly defined are mentioned here.

Brauer–Buschke–Fischer punctate PPK
This autosomal dominant disorder is characterized by small, hard keratotic papules which can be picked out leaving a depression.

Keratotic pits of the palmar creases
Punctate hyperkeratoses with a predilection for palmoplantar creases are probably inherited as an autosomal dominant trait. More common in blacks, the disorder affects 2–4% of adults. The keratoses may be painful and may be provoked by manual labor.

GENERALIZED SKIN DISORDERS FEATURING PUNCTATE PPK

These include Darier disease and Cowden syndrome, both of which are discussed elsewhere.

OTHER KERATOSES

Peter Itin, Rudolf Happle

DARIER DISEASE (DARIER–WHITE DISEASE)

INTRODUCTION AND HISTORICAL NOTE

This disorder was described independently by Darier and White more than 100 years ago.[410] Darier first described dyskeratotic features of the epidermis but he incorrectly interpreted these as forms of an epidermal parasite. His term "keratosis follicularis" is a misnomer because the lesions are not follicular. White recognized the genetic nature of the disease. The disease is characterized by altered keratinization of the epidermis which leads clinically to multiple keratotic papules.

EPIDEMIOLOGY

Darier disease (MIM 124200) is an autosomal dominant skin disorder occurring worldwide. The prevalence ranges between 1:30 000 and 1:100 000. It has been shown that *de novo* mutations occur and penetrance is high. It affects males and females equally. Munro noted that in general women show a milder rash than men.[411] Marked intrafamilial clinical heterogeneity is rather common.[412]

404. el-Badramany MH, Fawzy AR, Farag TI (1995) Familial Richner–Hanhart syndrome in Kuwait: twelve-year clinical reassessment by a multidisciplinary approach. **Am J Med Genet** 60(5):353–355.
405. el-Shoura SM, Tallab TM (1997) Richner–Hanhart's syndrome: new ultrastructural observations on skin lesions of two cases. **Ultrastruct Pathol** 21(1):51–56.
406. al-Hemidan AI, al-Hazzaa SA (1995) Richner–Hanhart syndrome (tyrosinemia type II). Case report and literature review. **Ophthal Genet** 16(1):21–26. Review
407. Rabinowitz LG, Williams LR, Anderson CE et al. (1995) Painful keratoderma and photophobia: hallmarks of tyrosinaemia type II. **J Pediatr** 126:266–269.
408. Benoldi D, Orsoni JB, Allegra F (1997) Tyrosinemia type II: a challenge for ophthalmologists and dermatologists. **Pediatr Dermatol** 14(2):110–112.
409. Fraser NG, MacDonald J, Griffiths WAD et al. (1987) Tyrosinaemia type II (Richner–Hanhart syndrome)– report of two cases treated with etretinate. **Clin Exp Dermatol** 12:440–443.
410. Rand R, Baden HP (1983) Commentary: Darier–White disease. **Arch Dermatol** 119:81–83.
411. Munro CS (1992) The phenotype of Darier's disease: penetrance and expressivity in adults and children. **Br J Dermatol** 127:126–130.
412. Tavadia S, Mortimer E, Munro CS (2002) Genetic epidemiology of Darier's disease: a population study in the west of Scotland. **Br J Dermatol** 146:107–109.

PRESENTING HISTORY AND PHYSICAL EXAMINATION

Patients usually present with newly appeared skin-colored or brownish papules in a characteristic distribution. The lesions tend to appear between the ages of 5 and 20.[413] Sometimes the condition is misdiagnosed as acne, seborrheic dermatitis, or genital warts.[414] The primary lesions are firm, rough-textured and greasy, flesh-colored or brown keratotic mostly nonfollicular papules that may be covered by a scaly crust (Fig. 8.51). The clinical spectrum is rather wide. It includes discrete keratotic papules and tumor-like vegetations in intertriginous areas with maceration and malodorous lesions. Rarely, guttate leukodermatous macules and hemorrhagic vesicles in an acral distribution may occur. Coalescence of papules produces plaques that may become papil-

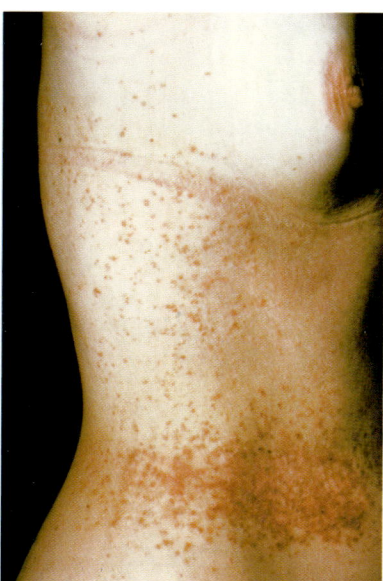

Fig. 8.51 Flesh-colored or brown keratotic, often nonfollicular papules.

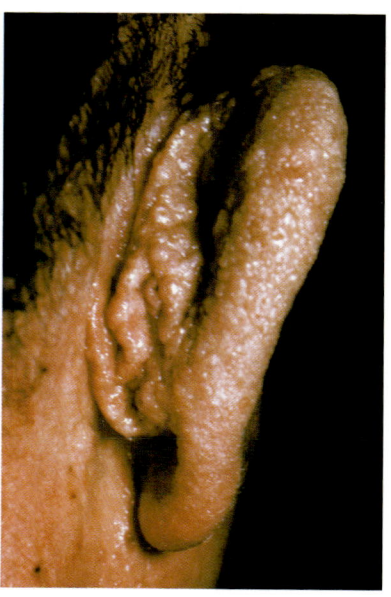

Fig. 8.52 Papillomatous vegetations, especially in intertriginous areas.

lomatous (Fig. 8.52). The disorder is often aggravated by sun, heat, and sweating and therefore the disease manifests often in summer for the first time. In general the distribution is symmetrical. Darier disease may occur anywhere on the body surface but predilection sites are the "seborrheic areas" such as the face, ears, neck, chest, shoulders, and supraclavicular fossae, or the midline of the back. In addition, the flexures such as the anogenital region, the groins, and the gluteal fold are often involved. Often, flat wart-like papules are present on the dorsa of hands and feet. Hand involvement occurs in almost 100% with pits and punctate keratotic plaques (Fig. 8.53). Ten percent of patients develop hyperkeratosis on palms and soles and circumscribed keratoderma may occur.[415] Acrokeratosis verruciformis of Hopf is today considered as an acral variant of Darier disease with wart-like lesions on the dorsum of the hands and feet.[416] Nails are affected in 60% of patients and show diagnostic longitudinal red and white lines (Fig. 8.54).[411] Increased brittleness with fragility, splintering and fissuring associated with V-shaped notches on the distal part of the nail plate are typical findings. Subungual hyperkeratosis may be found. Children may present with nail involvement only. Almost 90% complain of marked itch, and pain was reported in 17% in a large study.[413] Secondary eczematization is often a prominent feature. Papules may coalesce into crusted plaques especially in flexures where hypertrophic and malodorous lesions develop. The odor is mainly due to bacterial overgrowth. Skin fragility and fissuring with painful erosions may occur. Oral involvement occurs in 15–50% of patients and palate, gingiva, buccal mucosa, and the tongue are most commonly affected,[417] often with a cobblestone appearance. In addition, the hypopharyngeal, laryngeal, vaginal, or rectal mucosa may be affected. Duct obstruction due to salivary stones is an uncommon complication. The external auditory canal may be blocked by

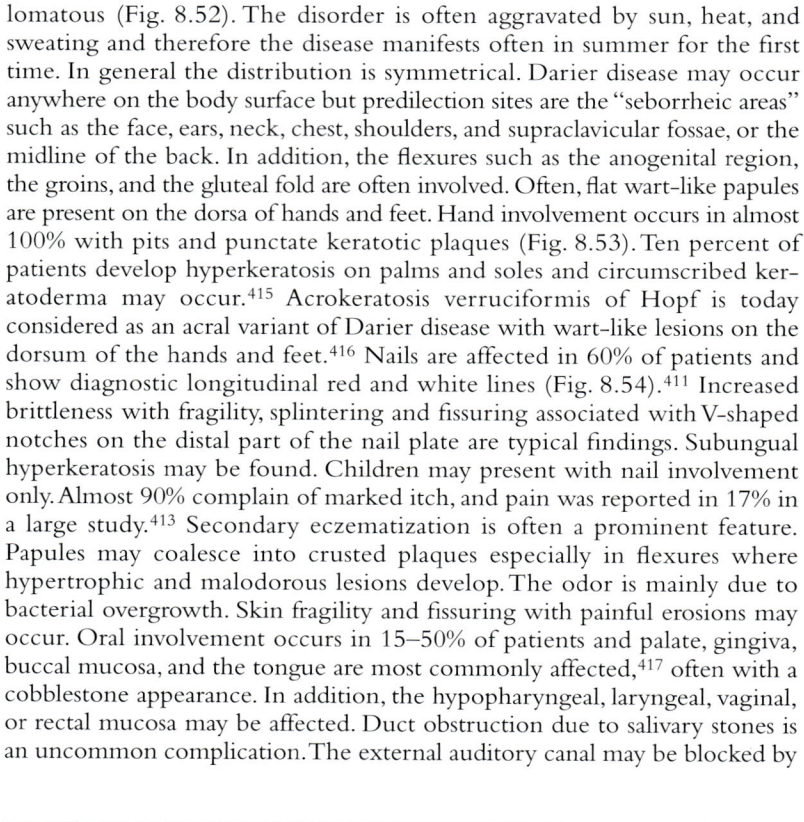

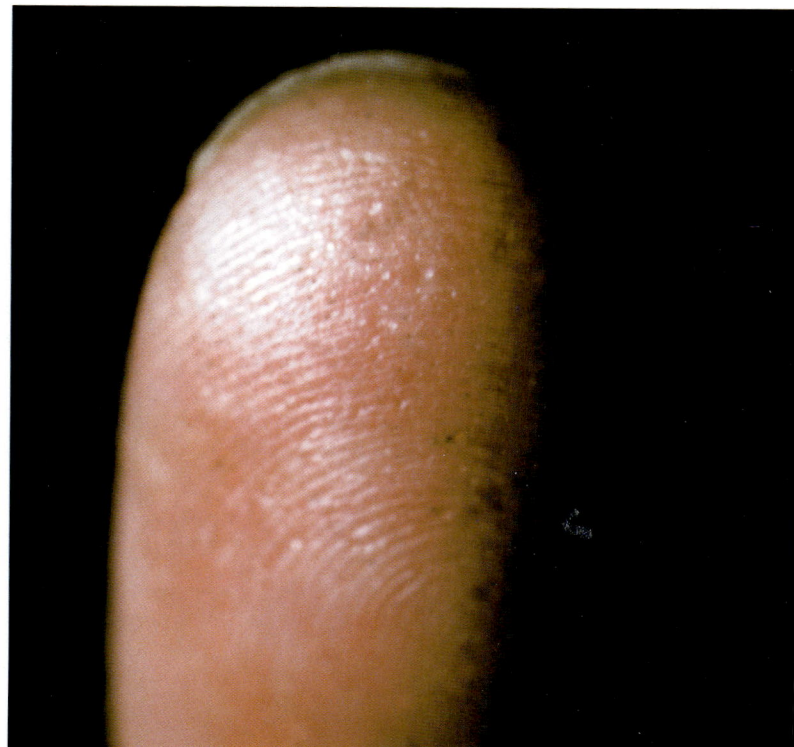

Fig. 8.53 Pits.

413. Burge SM, Wilkinson JD (1992) Darier–White disease: a review of the clinical features in 163 patients. **J Am Acad Dermatol** 27:40–50.
414. Salopek TG, Krol A, Jimbow K (1993) Case report of Darier disease localized to the vulva in a 5-year-old girl. **Pediatr Dermatol** 10:146–148.
415. Thappa DM, Garg BR (1996) Darier's disease with circumscribed plantar keratoderma. **J Dermatol** 23:139–140.
416. MacFarlane CS et al. (2000) Acrokeratosis verruciformis of Hopf is used by mutation in *ATP2A2*, the gene which is defective in Darier's disease. **Br J Dermatol** 143 (Suppl.):47.
417. Tosti A et al. (1996) Oral manifestations of Darier's disease: a clinical and pathological study. **Eur J Dermatol** 6:23–25.

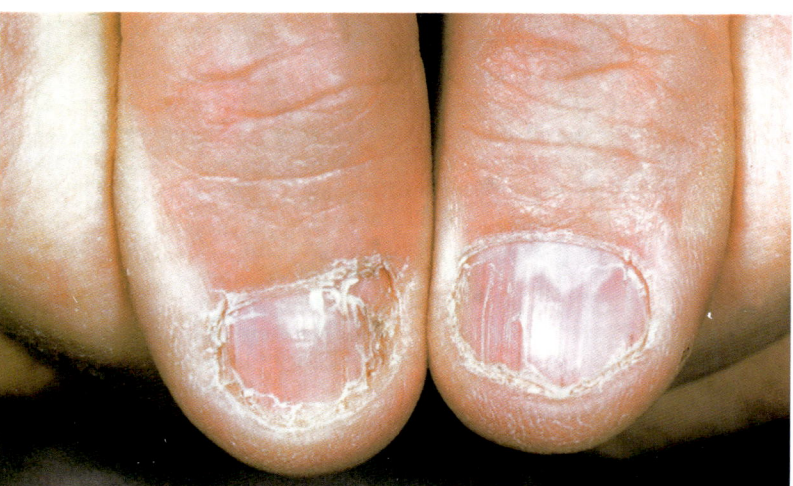

Fig. 8.54   V-shaped notches with longitudinal white and reddish lines.

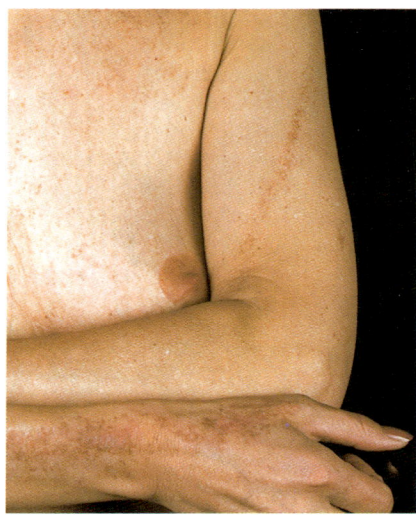

Fig. 8.55   Type 2 segmental Darier disease. Pronounced linear lesions are superimposed on the ordinary phenotype.

accumulated keratotic debris. Retinitis pigmentosa associated with keratosis follicularis has been observed in two affected brothers.[418] Extensive involvement of the scalp has been documented[419] and alopecia may result. Increased susceptibility to bacterial and viral infections are known in such patients but the exact immunologic relationship is not yet clear. A number of researchers believe that it is related to a defect in cell-mediated immunity. The defective skin barrier may increase skin infection rate. Differential diagnoses include Hailey–Hailey disease, seborrheic dermatitis, and keratosis pilaris. Patients with Darier disease are prone to Kaposi's varicelliform eruption due to herpes simplex.[420]

Burge and Wilkinson suggested that Darier disease is associated with mild neuropsychiatric features, including mental handicap, schizophrenia, and bipolar disorder. In neuropsychiatric cases there was a nonrandom clustering of mutations in the 3′ end of the *ATP2A2* gene, and a predominance of the missense type.[421] Ocular involvement leads to focal keratinization of the limbal conjunctiva, a regional increase in conjunctival globlet cells and a diffuse thickening of the basement membrane of the corneal epithelium.[422]

In 1906 Kreibich reported a localized form of Darier disease.[423] Since this time more than 50 cases of localized Darier disease have been reported.[424] Such phenotypes have been called zosteriform, linear, segmental or unilateral. Segmental Darier disease mirrors genetic mosaicism, and in most cases postzygotic mutations very early in the embryogenesis might be responsible for this type.[424–426] Molecular proof of this concept was recently provided.[427] Arin et al.[428] have shown that focal activation of a mutant allele defines the role of stem cells in mosaic skin disorders. The severity of lesions in the circumscribed region commonly corresponds to that observed in the nonmosaic state. The skin outside the segmental manifestation is perfectly normal. This type was designated as type 1 of segmental manifestations of autosomal skin disorders by Happle.[429,430] Type 1 reflects heterozygosity for the underlying postzygotic mutation and shows a severity which corresponds to the expression of the nonsegmental phenotype.[430] Type 1 may also herald gonadal mosaicism which means that the following generation may be affected by the diffuse, nonsegmental form.[431] Rarely, patients may feature a diffuse type of manifestation but, in addition, a segmental form with increased severity of disease may coexist. Happle called this form a type 2 of segmental manifestation of autosomal dominant disorders (Fig. 8.55).[432] He hypothesized that this type 2 reflects loss of heterozygosity for the same allele. The absence of the corresponding wildtype allele results in a marked increase of severity in the linear arrangement as compared with the common phenotype of the disorder. Type 2 originates from an individual with a heterozygous germline mutation and, in addition, a postzygotic mutation occurred, such as mitotic recombination, nondisjunction, or deletion.[432] These mechanisms lead to a population of cells either homozygous or hemizygous for the underlying mutation.[433,434] We recently documented for the first time a case of type 2 segmental Darier disease with concomitant band-like areas of healthy skin similar to a twin spot phenomenon.[435] This case may be taken as a "missing link," thus corroborating the concept of type 2 segmental manifestation of this autosomal dominant skin disorder.

PATHOPHYSIOLOGY AND HISTOGENESIS

Histological hallmarks are focal suprabasal clefting (lacunae) due to acantholysis and subsequent degeneration of keratinocytes (dyskeratosis) with overlying parakeratosis. These dyskeratotic cells are called *grains* and *corps ronds*. Corps ronds are cells showing premature partial keratinization in the spinous

418. Itin P, Büchner SA, Gloor B (1988) Darier's disease and retinitis pigmentosa; is there a pathogenetic relationship? Br J Dermatol 119:397–402.
419. Mailänder W, Stieler W, Stadler R (1991) Ausgedehnte Kopfhautbeteiligung bei Morbus Darier. Akt Dermatol 17:284–286.
420. Pantazi V, Potouridou I, Ratsarou A et al. (2000) Darier's disease complicated by Kaposi's varicelliform eruption due to herpes simplex virus. J Europ Acad Dermatol Venereol 14:209–211.
421. Jacobsen NJ, Lyons I, Hoogendoorn B et al. (1999) ATP2A2 mutations in Darier's disease and their relationship to neuropsychiatric phenotypes. Hum Mol Genet 8:1631–1636.
422. Daicker B (1995) Ocular involvement in keratosis follicularis associated with retinitis pigmentosa. Clinicopathological case report. Ophthalmologica 209:47–51.
423. Kreibich K (1906) Zum Wesen der Psorospermosis Darier. Arch Dermatol Syphilol (Wien) 80:367.
424. O'Malley MP, Haake A, Goldsmith L, Berg D (1997) Localized Darier disease. Implications for genetic studies. Arch Dermatol 133:1134–1138.
425. Plantin P, Le Noac'h E, Leroy JP, Gowcuff H (1994) Maladie de Darier, localisée, récidivante et photo-induite suivant les lignes de Blaschko. Ann Dermatol Venereol 121:393–395.
426. Papadavid E, Dawber RPR (1997) Linear Darier's disease in a patient with recurrent carcinoma of the bladder reflects cutaneous mosaicism. J Europ Acad Dermatol Venereol 9:249–252.
427. Sakuntabhai A, Dhitavat J, Burge S, Horanian A (2000) Mosaicism for ATP2A2 mutations causes segmental Darier's cisease. J Invest Dermatol 115:1144–1147.

428. Arin MJ, Longley MA, Wang XJ, Roop DB (2001) Focal activation of a mutant allele defines the role of stem cells in mosaic skin disorders. J Cell Biol 152:645–649.
429. Happle R (1997) A rule concerning the segmental manifestation of autosomal dominant skin disorders. Review of clinical examples providing evidence for dichotomous types of severity. Arch Dermatol 133:1505–1509.
430. Happle R (2001) Segmentale Typ-2-manifestation autosomal dominanter Hautkrankheiten. Entwicklung eines neuen formalgenetischen Konzeptes. Hautarzt 52:283–287.
431. Paller AS, Syder AJ, Chan YM et al. (1994) Genetic and clinical mosaicism in a type of epidermal nevus. N Engl J Med 331:1408–1415.
432. Itin PH, Buechner SA (1999) Segmental forms of autosomal dominant skin disorders: the puzzle of mosaicism. Am J Med Genet 85:351–354.
433. Happle R, Itin PH, Brun AM (1999) Type 2 segmental Darier disease. Eur J Dermatol 9:449–451.
434. Itin PH, Büchner SA, Happle R (2000) Segmental manifestation of Darier disease. What is the genetic background in type 1 and type 2 mosaic phenotypes? Dermatology 200:254–257.
435. Itin PH, Happle R (2002) Darier disease with paired segmental manifestation of either excessive or absent involvement: A further step in the concept of twin spotting. Dermatology 205:344–247.

layer. They give raise to the grains that are small cells with shrunken cytoplasm in the upper layers of the epidermis. Additional histopathological findings include mild nonspecific perivascular dermal infiltration, dermal villi protruding into the epidermis, hyperkeratosis, and acanthosis.

The causative gene maps to a 2-cM region on chromosome 12q23–24.1.[436–438] Sakuntabai *et al.*[439] described mutations in *ATP2A2*, encoding a calcium pump, which cause Darier disease. This defect of the Ca^{2+}-signaling pathway results in disturbed adhesion of keratinocytes. Recently, in 47 European pedigrees 40 distinct mutations within the *ATP2A2* gene were found.[440] This data documented that classic and variant Darier disease are due to mutations in *ATP2A2*. A striking association was found in families with hemorrhagic variants where all showed a missense mutation, especially N767S substitution in the M5 transmembrane domain.[440]

THERAPEUTICS AND PROGNOSIS

The natural course of Darier disease with waxing and waning makes an evaluation of therapeutic regimens difficult. Keratolytic topicals that contain urea, salicylic acid or retinoid acid are beneficial. Treatment of childhood Darier disease with tazarotene has been described,[441] but irritancy is often limiting, especially in patients with inflammatory disease. In such cases a moderate-potency topical steroid may control inflammation. Observations on

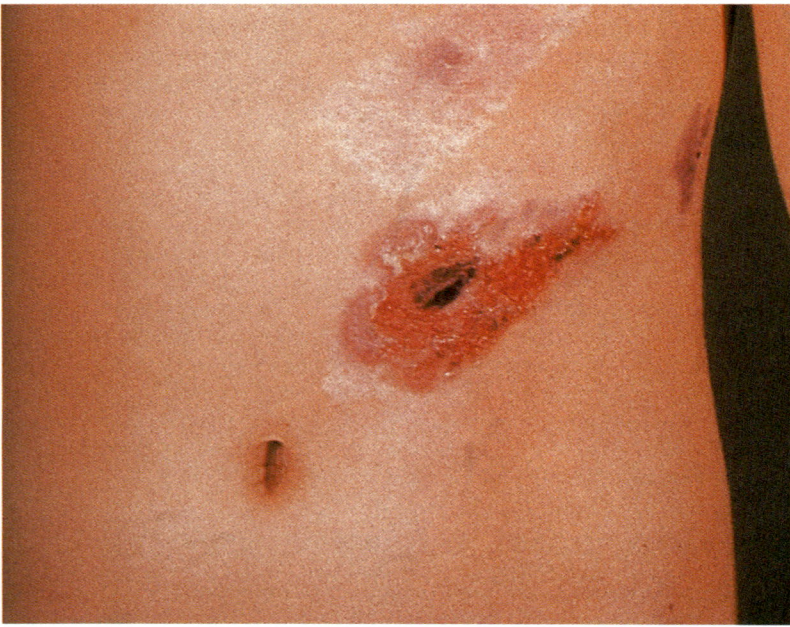

Fig. 8.56   Type 2 segmental manifestation of Hailey–Hailey disease in a 5-year-old girl. Pronounced unilateral lesions characterized by blistering and eczematous changes following the lines of Blaschko. (Courtesy of Dr. F. Vakilzadeh, Hildesheim, Germany.)

successful application of topical vitamin D exist.[442] Some children do profit from systemic retinoids. As this is a long-term treatment monitoring of skeletal and biochemical changes is important. Sometimes the dose can be kept very low and the dose finding has to be performed individually.

Dermabrasion, when done to an adequate depth can be helpful and produce good long-term effects.[443] Carbon dioxide laser vaporization is another alternative for chronic, localized, symptomatic plaques of Darier disease, if medical therapy has been ineffective.

Frequent cleansing with antibacterial soaps is important and intermittent courses of oral antibiotics are sometimes necessary to treat widespread secondary bacterial infections. It has been shown that intracellular persistence of *Staphylococcus aureus* small-colony variants within keratinocytes is a cause for antibiotic treatment failure in a patient with Darier disease.[444] Herpetic infections should be treated by famciclovir or valciclovir systemically. An important preventive regimen is avoidance of direct sun exposure and regular application of sunscreen. Clothing should be cool cotton and not too tight.[445]

Guide to information for families with inherited disorders:
Foundation for Ichthyosis and Related Skin Types (FIRST)
650 N. Cannon Ave., Suite 17
Lansdale, PA 19446
(800) 545 3286
Fax: (215) 631 1413
E-mail: info@scalyskin.org
http://www.scalyskin.org

HAILEY–HAILEY DISEASE

Arne König

Hailey–Hailey disease (familial benign chronic pemphigus) is an autosomal dominant skin disorder characterized by vesicles, erosions, hemorrhagic crusts and eczematous changes that occur predominantly in the body folds. In advanced stages, severe involvement of the axillary or inguinal regions may even lead to immobility of limbs.[446,447] Histopathologically, suprabasal clefting with acantholysis is observed. These changes usually do not affect the hair follicles and sweat glands, and it has been pointed out that these adnexal structures do not express the intrinsic defect of cell adhesion.[448] This explains the beneficial effect of dermabrasion in this disorder. The underlying genetic defect involves the gene *ATP2C1* at 3q21–q24, encoding a calcium pump.[449]

In general, this phenotype cannot be classified as a pediatric condition because it does not become manifest before adulthood. However, Vakilzadeh and Kolde[450] reported on a 5-year-old girl with unilateral manifestation of a "relapsing linear acantholytic dermatosis." A follow-up report of this case revealed that this patient had a family history of Hailey–Hailey disease comprising four generations.[451] Since the age of 3 months the girl had severe lesions of erythema and blistering arranged in a unilateral pattern following the lines of Blaschko (Fig. 8.56). At the age of 24 years additional

436. Craddock N, Dawson E, Burge S et al. (1993) The gene for Darier's disease maps to chromosome 12q23–q24.1. **Hum Mol Genet** 2:1941–1943.
437. Bashir R, Munro CS, Masons et al. (1993) Localisation of a gene for Darier's disease. **Hum Mol Genet** 2:1937–1939.
438. Wakem P, Ikeda S, Haake A et al. (1996) Localization of the Darier disease gene to a 2-cM portion of 12q23–24.1. **J Invest Dermatol** 106:365–367.
439. Sakuntabhai A, Ruiz-Perez VL, Carter S et al. (1999) Mutations in *ATP2A2*, encoding a Ca2+ pump, cause Darier disease. **Nature Genet** 21:271–277.
440. Ruiz-Perez VL, Carter SA, Healey E et al. (1999) ATP2A2 mutations in Darier's disease: variant cutaneous phenotypes are associated with missense mutations, but neuropsychiatric features are independent of mutation class. **Hum Mol Genet** 8:1621–1630.
441. Micali G, Nasca MR (1999) Tazarotene gel in childhood Darier disease. **Pediatr Dermatol** 16:243–244.
442. Kragballe K, Steijlen PM, Ibsen HH et al. (1995) Efficacy, tolerability, and safety of calcipotriol ointment in disorders of keratinization. Results of a randomized, double-blind, vehicle-controlled right/left comparative study. **Arch Dermatol** 131:556–560.
443. Zachariae H (1979) Dermabrasion in Darier's disease. **Acta Derm Venereol (Stockh)** 59:184–186.
444. von Eiff C, Becker K, Metze D et al. (2001) Intracellular persistence of *Staphylococcus aureus* small-colony variants within keratinocytes: a cause for antibiotic treatment failure in a patient with Darier's disease. **Clin Infect Dis** 32:1643–1647.
445. Burge S (1999) Management of Darier's disease. **Clin Exp Dermatol** 24:53–56.
446. Burge SM (1992) Hailey–Hailey disease: the clinical features, response to treatment and prognosis. **Br J Dermatol** 126:275.
447. Michel B (1982) Hailey-Hailey disease: familial benign chronic pemphigus. **Arch Dermatol** 118:781.
448. Metze D, Hamm H, Schorat A, Luger T (1996) Involvement of the adherens junction-actin filament system in acantholytic dyskeratosis of Hailey–Hailey disease: a histological, ultrastructural, and histochemical study of lesional and non-lesional skin. **J Cutan Pathol** 23:211.
449. Hu Z, Bonifas JM, Beech J et al. (2000) Mutations in *ATP2C1*, encoding a calcium pump, cause Hailey–Hailey disease. **Nature Genet** 24:61.
450. Vakilzadeh F, Kolde G (1985) Relapsing linear acantholytic dermatosis. **Br J Dermatol** 112:349.
451. König A, Hörster S, Vakilzadeh F, Happle R (2000) Type 2 segmental manifestation of Hailey–Hailey disease: poor therapeutic response to dermabrasion is due to severe involvement of adnexal structures. **Eur J Dermatol** 10:265.

scattered symmetrical lesions involving the axillary and inguinal folds were noted. This case can be best explained by a recently proposed rule of dichotomy regarding mosaicism in autosomal dominant skin disorders.[452] According to this hypothesis, this patient shows a type 2 segmental manifestation reflecting loss of heterozygosity for the *ATP2C1* mutation. Unlike the ordinary heterozygous phenotype, this mosaic manifestation is characterized by pronounced acantholytic involvement of adnexal structures. This phenomenon apparently reflects the severity of involvement caused by loss of the corresponding wildtype allele within the segmental areas. As a consequence, therapeutic response to dermabrasion was limited in this case.[451]

POROKERATOSIS

Peter Itin, Rudolf Happle

INTRODUCTION AND HISTORICAL NOTE

Porokeratosis is a genetic disorder of keratinization with circular lesions showing central atrophy and a raised horny border that corresponds histopathologically to a column of parakeratotic cells overlying a thinned or absent granular layer, the so-called cornoid lamella.[453] Six clinical variants are recognized (Table 8.11).

EPIDEMIOLOGY AND GENETICS

Porokeratoses are rather common genodermatoses, especially the disseminated actinic type. In general, porokeratoses are inherited as an autosomal dominant trait. A gene locus for disseminated superficial actinic porokeratosis has been mapped on chromosome 12q23.2–24.1.[454] A novel locus for disseminated porokeratosis has been found on chromosome 15q25.1–26.1.[455] Only the recently described syndrome with craniosynostosis, anal anomalies and porokeratosis seems to follow a recessive mode of transmission.

TABLE 8.11   Classification of porokeratosis

Type	Abbreviation	McKusick's catalog
Plaque-type porokeratosis of Mibelli	PM	175800
Disseminated actinic superficial porokeratosis	DSAP	175900
Linear porokeratosis as a mirror of LOH		175900
Porokeratosis palmaris, plantaris et disseminata	PPPD	175850
Porokeratosis punctata palmaris et plantaris	PPPP	175860
Porokeratosis ptychotropica		
Craniosynostosis, anal anomalies, and porokeratosis	CAP-syndrome	603116
Linear porokeratosis*		

* In most, if not all, cases this is a segmental manifestation of DSAP.[483]

PRESENTING HISTORY AND PHYSICAL FINDINGS

Porokeratosis of Mibelli is rare and has an early onset with a male predominance and lesions gradually enlarge centrifugally from a few millimeters to several centimeters with a hyperkeratotic border (Fig. 8.57). Giant lesions rarely occur (Fig. 8.58).[456] Lesions are dry, brownish papules with a very distinct rimmed border. The onset is usually in childhood but later beginning has been observed. The distribution is asymmetric and lesions may be single or numerous. Sites of predilection are the face, trunk, and extremities. In general hair, nails, and mucous membranes are spared. Subtypes associated with reticular erythema exist.

Disseminated actinic superficial porokeratosis is the most common form and occurs symmetrically over sun-exposed areas with often asympto-

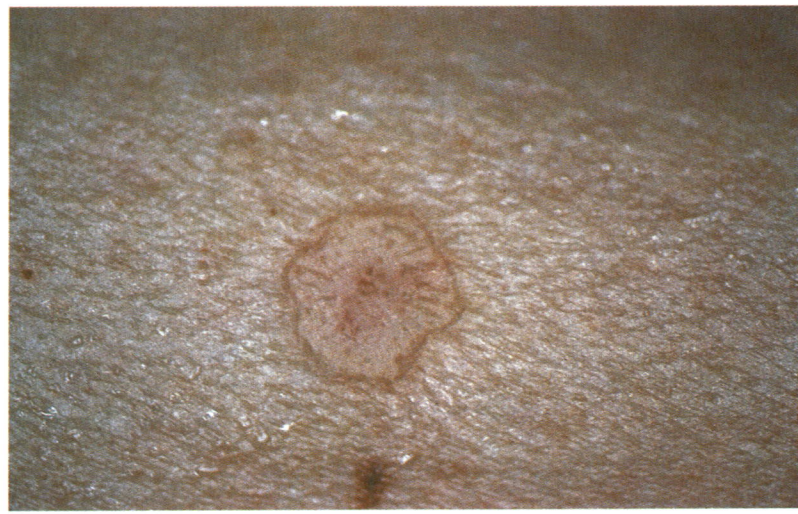

Fig. 8.57   Central atrophic lesion with raised margin on the border.

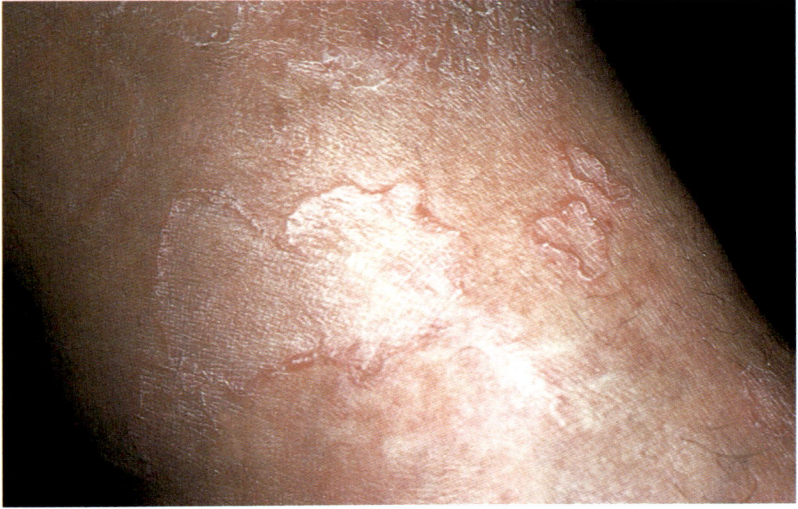

Fig. 8.58   Giant lesion of porokeratosis of Mibelli.

452. Happle R (1999) Loss of heterozygosity in human skin. J Am Acad Dermatol 41:143.
453. Happle R (1997) Cancer proneness of linear porokeratosis may be explained by allelic loss. Dermatology 195:20–25.
454. Xia JH, Yang YF, Deng W et al. (2000) Identification of a locus for disseminated superficial actinic porokeratosis at chromosome 12q23.2–24.1. J Invest Dermatol 114:1071–1074.
455. Xia K, Deng H, Xia JH et al. (2002) A novel locus (DSAP2) for disseminated superficial actinic porokeratosis maps to chromosome 15q25.1–26.1. Br J Dermatol 147:650–654.
456. Thappa DM, Garg BR, Ratnakar C (1995) Giant porokeratosis. J Dermatol 22:964–965.

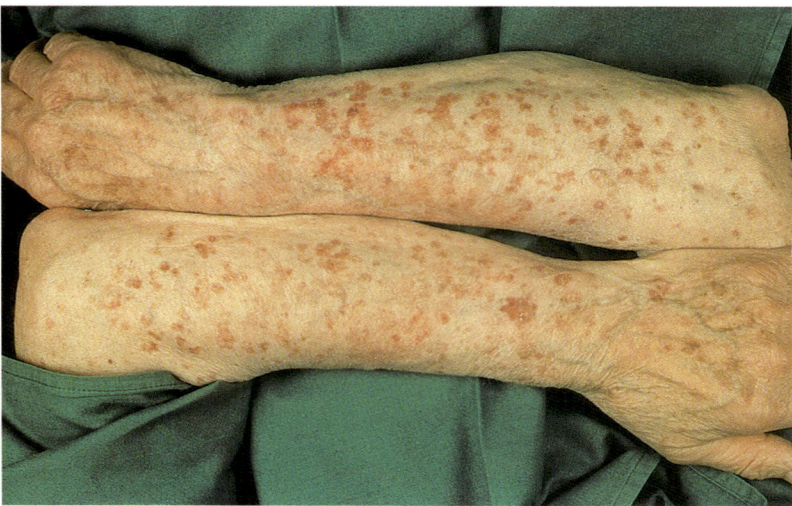

Fig. 8.59 Disseminated actinic superficial porokeratosis occurs symmetrically over sun-exposed areas.

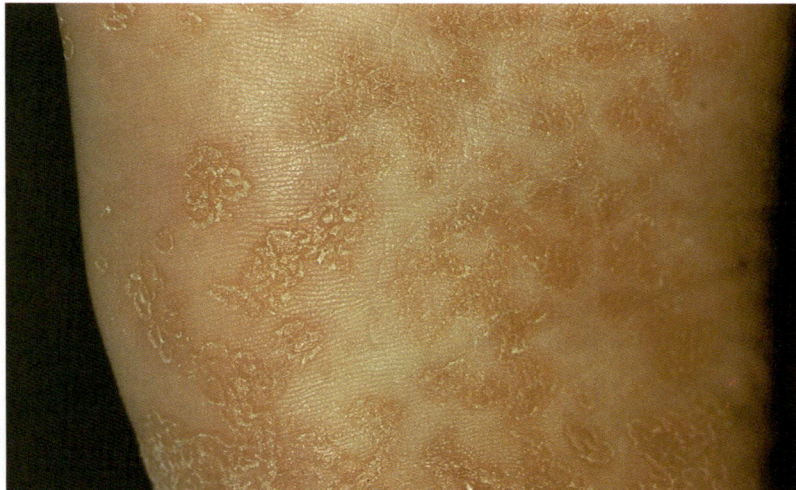

Fig. 8.61 Plantar porokeratotic lesions.

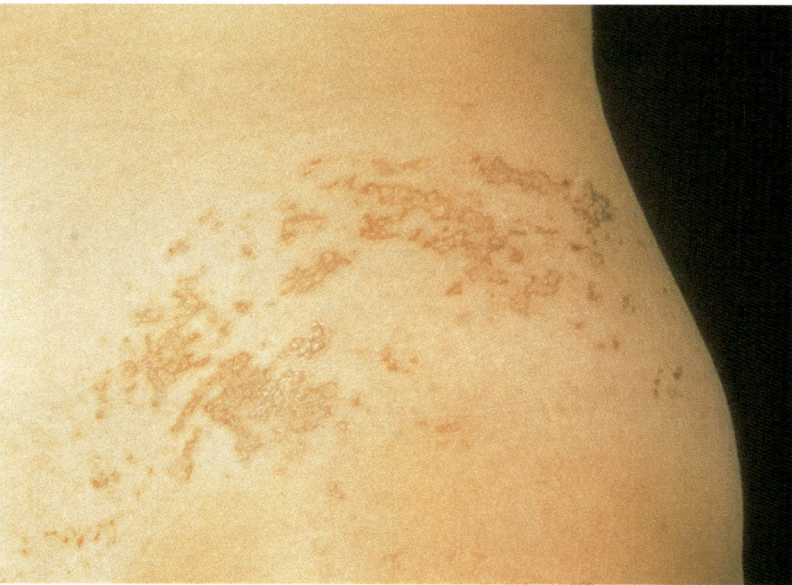

Fig. 8.60 Linear porokeratosis.

matic lesions which may sometimes become rather pruritic (Fig. 8.59).[457] Erosive or bullous variants may occur.[458,459] The dermatosis appears in the third or fourth decade of life. Lesions are smaller than in the Mibelli type and often hundreds are present. The disorder may show amyloid deposition.[462] Malignant degeneration in longstanding lesions may occur.

Linear porokeratosis develops at least in some of the cases, from a loss of heterozygosity and coexistence of linear porokeratosis and disseminated superficial actinic porokeratosis has been documented in a large number of patients (Fig. 8.60).[453,462] This concept is underlined by the recent observation of the coexistence of disseminated superficial actinic porokeratosis in childhood with a congenital linear porokeratosis.[463] It is important to emphasize that linear porokeratosis may occur congenitally whereas disseminated superficial actinic lesions tend to appear in the mid-twenties. Porokeratosis palmaris, plantaris et disseminata is characterized by numerous symmetric lesions with a clearly raised hyperkeratotic margin. The lesions initially erupt on the palms and soles and later sun-exposed and covered body sites may be involved (Fig. 8.61). Oral lesions have been noted. Filiform hyperkeratoses on the trunk and extremities have been observed in this type, and dystrophic nails form porokeratotic lesions may result (Fig. 8.62).[464]

Porokeratosis punctata palmaris et plantaris is a rare variant of porokeratosis with discrete punctate keratotic or spine-like lesions confined to palms and soles.[465] The keratotic papules may be tender and histology shows the columnar parakeratosis.

Flanagan et al.[466] reported the occurrence of coronal craniosynostosis, anal anomalies, and porokeratosis in two male sibs. The pedigree suggested an autosomal or X-linked recessive inheritance.

PATHOPHYSIOLOGY AND HISTOGENESIS

The pathogenesis of porokeratosis is still unclear.[467] Genetic factors are invariably involved in all forms of porokeratosis. In addition, ultraviolet light has at least an impact in disseminated superficial actinic porokeratosis. Remarkably, electron beam radiation seems to be another triggering factor. Trauma such as burning or application of needles for hemodialysis have been suggested to produce a Köbner phenomenon. On a molecular genetic level overexpression of the p53 tumor suppressor protein have been

457. Kanzaki T, Miwa N, Kobayashi T, Ogawas (1992) Eruptive pruritic papular porokeratosis. **J Dermatol** 19:109–112.
458. Watanabe T, Murakami T, Okochi H et al. (1998) Ulcerative porokeratosis. **Dermatology** 196:256–259.
459. Ricci C, Rosset A, Panizzon RG (1999) Bullous and pruritic variant of disseminated superficial actinic porokeratosis: successful treatment with Grenz Rays. **Dermatology** 199:328–331.
460. Yasuda K, Ikeda M, Kodama H (1996) Disseminated superficial porokeratosis with amyloid deposition. **J Dermatol** 23:111–115.
461. Finlay AY (1982) Major autosomal recessive ichthyoses. **Semin Dermatol** 7:26–36.
462. Freyschmidt-Paul P, Holfman R, Konig A, Happle R (1999) Linear porokeratosis superimposed on disseminated superficial actinic porokeratosis: report of two cases exemplifying the concept of

type 2 segmental manifestation of autosomal dominant skin disorders. **J Am Acad Dermatol** 41:644–647.
463. Suh DH, Lee HS, Kim SD et al. (2000) Coexistence of disseminated superficial porokeratosis in childhood with congenital linear porokeratosis. **Pediatr Dermatol** 17:466–468.
464. Itin PH (1995) Porokeratosis plantaris, palmaris et disseminata mit multiplen filiformen Hyperkeratosen und Nageldystrophie. **Hautarzt** 46:869–872.
465. Friedman SJ, Herman PS, Pittelkow MR, Su WP (1988) Punctate porokeratotic keratoderma. **Arch Dermatol** 124:1678–1682.
466. Flanagan N Boyadjiev SA, Harper J et al. (1998) Familial craniosynostosis, anal anomalies, and porokeratosis: CAP syndrome. **J Med Genet** 35:763–766.
467. Kanitakis J, Euvrard S, Fawe M, Claudy A (1998) Porokeratosis and imunosuppression. **Eur J Dermatol** 8:459–465.

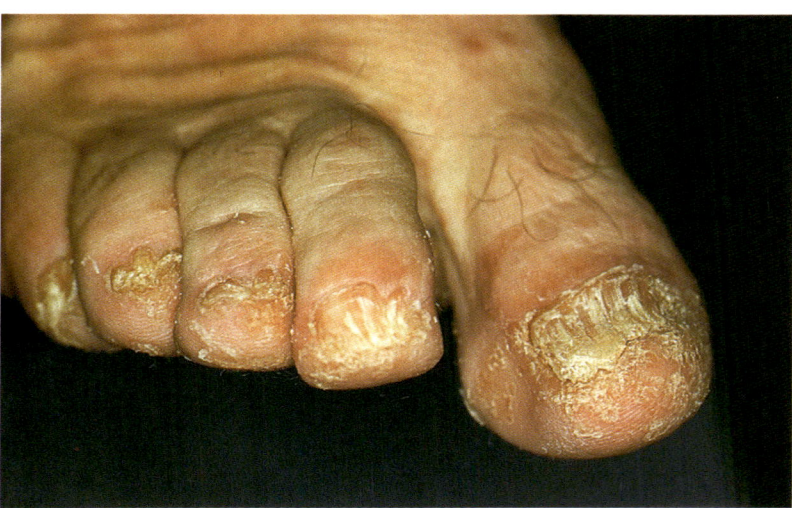

Fig. 8.62 Nail dystrophy induced by porokeratotic lesions.

documented predisposing factor in disseminated porokeratosis. In several cases the course of porokeratosis paralleled the degree of immunosuppression. Immunosuppression seems to reduce the capability of immunosurveillance and facilitates expansion of abnormal keratinocytic clones with possible malignant degeneration. Also, loss of HLA-DR antigen expression by epidermal Langerhans cells in disseminated superficial porokeratosis has been found and it has been interpreted that this has allowed clonal expansion of abnormal lesional keratinocytes.[469] The analysis by Happle[453] showed that among the various forms of porokeratosis, the linear type is particularly susceptible to malignant degeneration. This fact argues for the assumption that the genetic mechanism of allelic loss giving rise to linear porokeratosis may represent an initial step in the development of cancer. A tempting hypothesis for the cancer proneness of linear porokeratosis is the explanation by allelic loss.[453]

Histology shows a parakeratotic columnar keratosis known as cornoid lamella. This is a sharply delineated area of altered keratinization. In addition, a moderate chronic inflammatory infiltrate is present in the dermis consisting mainly of helper T cells intermingled with Langerhans cells.[470]

THERAPEUTICS AND PROGNOSIS

Treatment of porokeratosis is unsatisfactory. Surgical excision has been performed in small lesions. Electrocautery, liquid nitrogen, keratolytics, and intralesional steroids have been tried with variable results. Topical and systemic retinoids may be tried and dermabrasion, CO_2-laser or grenz rays have produced satisfactory results but rapid recurrence may occur.[459,471–473]

The course is chronic and recurrences have been observed.[474]

implicated. Nelson et al.[468] have shown that the p53 tumor suppressor gene product is upregulated together with disregulated cell cycle control in porokeratosis.

It has been suggested that in porokeratosis a mutant clone of epidermal cells expands peripherally. The development of abnormal clones is certainly genetically predisposed but additional factors seem to be important for the clinical manifestations of porokeratoses. Immunosuppression is a well-

468. Nelson C, Cowper S, Morgan M (1999) p53, mdm-2, and p21 waf-1 in the porokeratoses. Am J Dermatopathol 21:420–425.
469. Abe M, Ishikawa O, Miyachi Y (1997) The loss of HLA-DR antigen expression by epidermal Langerhans cell in disseminated superficial porokeratosis. Eur J Dermatol 7:303–304.
470. Jurecka W, Neumann RA, Knobler RM (1991) Porokeratoses: immunohistochemical, light and electron microscopic evaluation. J Am Acad Dermatol 24:96–101.
471. Bhushan M, Craven NM, Beck MN, Chalmers RJ (1999) Linear porokeratosis of Mibelli: successful treatment with cryotherapy. Br J Dermatol 141:389.
472. Liu HT (2000) Treatment of lichen amyloidosis (LA) and disseminated superficial porokeratosis (DSP) with frequency-doubled Q-switched Nd: YAG laser. Dermatol Surg 26:958–962.
473. McCullough TL, Lesher JL Jr (1994) Porokeratosis of Mibelli: rapid recurrence of a large lesion after carbon dioxide laser treatment. Pediatr Dermatol 11:267–270.
474. Adriaans B, Salisbury JR (1991) Recurrent porokeratosis. Br J Dermatol 124:383–386.
475. Giordano A (1938) Contributo allo studio morfologico e patogenetico dell'ittiosi fetale. Giorn It Derm 79:765–789.
476. Craig JM, Goldsmith LA, Baden HP (1970) An abnormality of keratin in the harlequin fetus. Pediatrics 46:437–440.
477. Buxman MM, Goodkin PE, Fahrenbach WH, Dimond RL (1979) Harlequin ichthyosis with epidermal lipid abnormality. Arch Dermatol 115:189–193.
478. Baden HP, Kubilus J, Rosenbaum K, Fletcher A (1982) Keratinization in the harlequin fetus. Arch Dermatol 118:14–18.
479. Blanchet-Bardon C, Dumez Y, Labbe F et al. (1983) Diagnostic prénatal par microscopie électronique d'un foetus arlequin. Ann Pathol 3:321–325.
480. Haftek M, Cambazard F, Réano A et al. (1989) Harlequin foetus: a histological, ultrastructural, and biochemical study of an etretinate-treated patient. Clin Exp Dermatol 14:393.
481. Fleck RM, Barnadas M, Schulz WW, Roberts LJ, Freeman RG (1989) Harlequin ichthyosis: an ultrastructural study. J Am Acad Dermatol 21:999–1006.
482. Sundberg JP, Boggess D, Hogan ME et al. (1997) Harlequin ichthyosis (ichq): a juvenile lethal mouse mutation with ichthyosiform dermatitis. Am J Pathol 151:293–310.
483. Happle R (1991) Somatic recombination may explain linear porokeratosis associated with disseminated superficial actinic porokeratosis. Am J Med Genet 39:237.
484. Jagel S, Liden S (1982) Ichthyosis in Sjören–Larsson syndrome. Clin Genet 21:243–252.
485. Stone DI, Carey WF, Christodolon J et al. (2000) Type 2 Gaudier disease, the collodion baby phenotype revisited. Arch Dis Child Fetal Neonatal Ed 82:F163–F166.
486. Russell JL, Di Giovanna JJ, Haslem N et al. (1994) Linkage of autosomal recessive lamellar ichthyosis to chromosome 14q. Am J Hum Genet 55:1146–1152.

Mucous Membrane Disorders

Adelaide A. Hebert and Eckart Haneke

Disorders of the mucous membranes can occur as isolated findings or may be a reflection of a more generalized process involving the integument or the entire organism. Although lesions of the oropharynx are the most numerous and varied, certain dermatologic problems affect the ocular and anogenital mucous membranes as well. Mucous membrane lesions are grouped for organizational purposes into those that affect the ocular tissues, the anogenital area, and oropharyngeal mucous membranes. More generalized processes regularly involving at least two of these sites are discussed in another section.

Consideration of these conditions as a cohesive group is problematic for a number of reasons. Many of these entities fall within the purview of ophthalmology, gynecology, otolaryngology, dentistry, or infectious disease and are routinely diagnosed and treated by specialists in those areas rather than by dermatologists. Most such disorders have been omitted from this chapter. Certain mucous membrane lesions are a transient or insignificant feature of a more generalized process that also involves the skin; many of these lesions are discussed elsewhere in this book.

DISORDERS OF THE OCULAR MUCOUS MEMBRANES

ANATOMY

See Fig. 9.1.

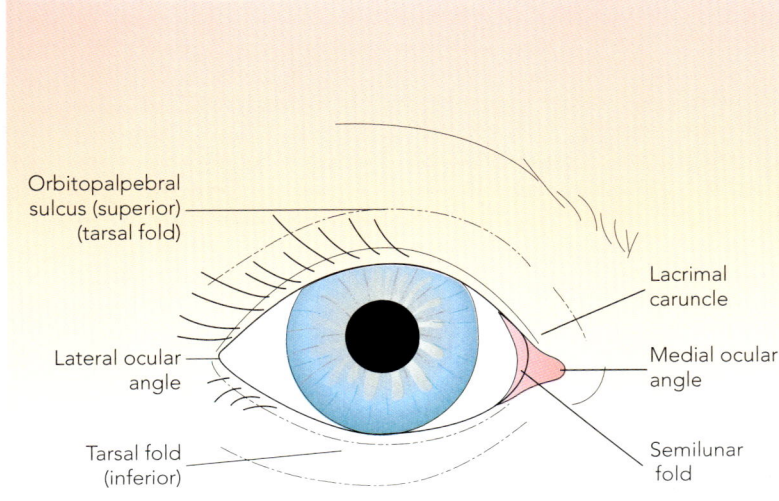

Orbitopalpebral
sulcus (superior)
(tarsal fold)

Lateral ocular
angle

Tarsal fold
(inferior)

Lacrimal
caruncle

Medial ocular
angle

Semilunar
fold

Fig. 9.1 Anatomy of the ocular mucous membranes.

BLEPHARITIS

Blepharitis is an inflammatory condition of the eyelid margins. It is most often chronic and typically begins in childhood. The most common causes are seborrheic dermatitis and infection with *Staphylococcus aureus*, although occasionally secondary infection with other organisms may supervene.[1]

Seborrheic blepharitis usually occurs in association with dermatitis of the scalp and sometimes of the skin of the face and trunk. The lid margins are erythematous and scaly with accumulation of debris at the base of the lashes. The blepharitis seems to fluctuate in severity depending on the extent of the dermatitis. Rarely, with severe involvement, there is an accompanying superficial marginal keratitis. This is most commonly seen in fair-skinned, red-haired children.

Staphylococcal blepharitis is also characterized by erythema and scaling of the lid margins; however, tenacious firm yellow crusts are usually present as well. Removal of the crusts may disclose small ulcers along the lid margin. The contiguous skin of the lids may be eczematized, fissured, and scaly. This type of blepharitis represents a suppurative inflammatory process of the lash follicles and the glands of Zeis and Moll. When acute and severe, conjunctivitis and keratitis may be associated. Ultimately, if the infection becomes chronic and persistent, recurrent styes and chalazions, loss of lashes, and thickening of the lid margins may result. The diagnosis of blepharitis is usually made on clinical grounds. If moist exudate, crusts, or ulcers are present, a bacterial culture for identification of the organism and antibiotic sensitivities should be obtained.

Seborrheic blepharitis can be controlled by mechanical removal of the scales by scrubbing the lid margins with an isotonic shampoo. A soft toothbrush or cotton-tipped applicator is most effective. This procedure should be performed daily until the blepharitis has subsided. A low-potency nonfluorinated corticosteroid (hydrocortisone) ointment can be gently massaged into the lid margin. The use of an ophthalmic preparation (Decadron ointment) will avoid burning and irritation of the conjunctivae.

The crusts of staphylococcal blepharitis can be softened by compressing with tap water or saline or Burow's solution several times daily and ophthalmic petrolatum over night. Once softened, they should be gently removed with a cotton-tipped applicator and an antibiotic ointment (such as bacitracin or erythromycin) massaged into the lash follicles. This treatment should be continued for several weeks, as the condition tends to chronicity.

PEDICULOSIS OF THE EYELASHES (PHTHIRIASIS PALPEBRARUM)

Infestation of the lashes with lice is usually caused by the pubic louse, although in instances of florid scalp involvement, the head louse may populate the eyelashes as well.[2] Signs and symptoms range from simple pruritus of the lid margins to blepharitis with inflammation of the conjunctivae and

1. Nelson LB (1984) Pediatric Ophthalmology. Philadelphia: WB Saunders.

2. Couch JM, Green WR, Hirst LW, DeLaCruz BS (1982) Diagnosis and treating *Phthirus pubis* palpebrum. **Surv Ophthalmol** 26:219.

preauricular lymphadenopathy. Maculae ceruleae and marginal keratitis have been noted in rare instances.[2]

Examination of the lids will disclose small gray or black concretions (nits) attached to the lashes. Reddish-brown granular material (feces) may also be deposited at the base of the lashes. A hand magnifying lens and small tweezers are helpful for discerning nits and capturing live lice for identification.

Discovery of pediculosis of the lashes should prompt a thorough examination of the scalp for head lice and nits. In the adolescent patient, examination of pubic, axillary, and body hair is also mandatory. Identification of public lice in the lashes of prepubertal children raises the possibility of sexual abuse,[3] should be further investigated, and not be lightly dismissed as acquisition by innocent contact with an infested relative.[4]

Treatment consists of eradication of lice and nits by thickly coating the lid margins and lashes with petrolatum four times daily for several days.[5] Probably, the lice suffocate. Physostigmine 0.25 (Eserine) ointment can be used as an alternative agent but must be continued for 14 days to span the entire life cycle of the louse, as it is not effective against nits.[2] Although this drug is a cholinesterase inhibitor, side effects are apparently few. Fluorescein eye drops 20% are also reported to have a toxic effect on lice if applied to the lids and lashes,[6] but staining of the skin is an annoying problem. Yellow oxide of mercury and ammoniated mercury ointments are outmoded therapies, and lindane, pyrethrin, permethrin (Elimite or Acticin), crotamiton, and malathion are too irritating to be used near the eye. Appropriate pediculocidal therapy has to be employed concomitantly for other affected sites. Known human contacts should be examined and treated if evidence of infestation is found. General measures for environmental control must also be instituted.

CONJUNCTIVITIS

Inflammation of the ocular mucous membranes is a common affliction of children and most often represents an infectious process. Although usually a relatively banal rather than a serious problem, certain types of conjunctivitis have the potential to cause significant sequelae. The various types of conjunctivitis are best considered on an age-related basis.

Conjunctivitis in the infant

Chemical conjunctivitis

This type of conjunctivitis is the result of prophylaxis used to prevent gonococcal infection (ophthalmia neonatorum) in the newborn. The most widely employed preparation, in use since its introduction by Credé in 1881, is 1% silver nitrate solution instilled into the conjunctival sac immediately after birth. The resultant mild conjunctivitis, which usually persists for 24 to 36 hours, occurs in up to 100% of newborns so treated.[1,7] Antibiotics, including erythromycin or tetracycline ophthalmic ointment, may be used as a substitute for silver nitrate.

Silver nitrate produces its effect both via its antibacterial activity and by irritation of the conjunctiva, resulting in an influx of neutrophils that directly cause death of the organisms. Saline washes should not be used, because precipitation of the silver by chloride ions reduces the germicidal activity.[7] This type of prophylaxis is ineffective against chlamydial or viral infections.[2] Chemical conjunctivitis from silver nitrate requires no treatment. The rare occurrence of corneal damage due to accidental application of a more concentrated silver nitrate solution is the only deterrent. The topical application of any one of these agents is not useful in treating established gonococcal infections in the neonate, but the smaller inoculum of organisms received during birth is felt to be eliminated.

Bacterial conjunctivitis

This type of conjunctivitis, in contrast to chemical conjunctivitis, occurs after the third day of life and is most often due to infection from staphylococci, streptococci, or pneumococci, although Gram-negative organisms occasionally are implicated. The lids are edematous, with chemosis and a purulent discharge. A Gram stain of the pus will usually disclose the etiologic agent, which can also be identified by culture. Although bacterial conjunctivitis in the newborn is self-limited, local instillation of antibiotics (erythromycin for Gram-positive organisms, gentamicin for Gram-negative organisms) will hasten resolution. When staphylococci are isolated as the causative agent, culture and sensitivity studies are helpful to identify erythromycin-resistant strains.

Gonococcal conjunctivitis

This organism causes the most destructive type of conjunctivitis and can be transmitted during delivery or afterward via the hands of the individuals caring for the infant. Gonococcal infection presents after a 1- to 3-day incubation period as an acute mucopurulent infection with lid edema, chemosis, and copious drainage, at times discolored by hemorrhage. Corneal ulceration and perforation may ensue. Systemic involvement may also complicate the course. Gram-stained smears of pus demonstrating the intracellular Gram-negative diplococci are diagnostic. If the gonococcal infection is localized, ceftriaxone 25–50mg/kg per day should be given intravenously or intramuscularly once daily. Alternatively, cefataxime, 25mg/kg per day, intravenously or intramuscularly, may be given in either two or three daily doses depending on the age of the infant. The duration of therapy is seven days. Ceftriaxone should not be given to hyper-bilirubinemic infants, especially premature infants, as this drug is reversibly bound to plasma proteins and can displace bilirubin from serum albumin.

Aqueous crystalline penicillin G in a dosage of 100 000 units/kg per day in divided doses intravenously every 12 hours and every six hours thereafter for seven days is recommended if the gonococcal isolate is proven susceptible to penicillin. A local antibiotic such as tetracycline, chloramphenicol, or sulfonamide is also advisable until the infection is controlled. (In many European countries, even the use of chloramphenicol in an ointment is banned.)

Chlamydial conjunctivitis

Also known as trachoma inclusion conjunctivitis (TRIC), this type of conjunctivitis has become quite common in the newborn, since approximately 13% of pregnant women shed *Chlamydia* from the cervix during the third trimester.[8] Onset is usually 5–15 days postpartum. The infection is typically mild and evidenced by erythema, chemosis, lid edema, and a mucopurulent exudate. The conjunctivitis is more typically a papillary palpebral one rather than a bulbar type. A Giemsa stain of conjunctival scrapings will demonstrate basophilic intracytoplasmic inclusions in the epithelial cells. Topical prophylaxis is ineffective and prompt culture of the organism is recommended.

Treatment consists of oral erythromycin syrup: 50mg/kg body weight per day in four divided doses for 14 days. If inclusion conjunctivitis recurs after this treatment, erythromycin should be reinstituted for an additional 7–14 days.[9] Conjunctival scarring and pannus formation can complicate the course and mandate precise diagnosis and early treatment.[7] Concomitant infection involving the respiratory tract may occur, requiring systemic therapy with erythromycin.

Conjunctivitis in the child

Viral conjunctivitis

The most common type of conjunctivitis in children is viral in origin and usually occurs in association with a respiratory infection. Erythema, edema,

3. Scott MJ, Esterly NB (1983) Eyelash infestation by *Phthirus pubis* as a manifestation of child abuse, letter. **Pediatr Dermatol** 1:179.
4. Alexander JO (1983) *Phthirus pubis* infestation of the eyelashes. **JAMA** 250:32.
5. Rasmussen JE (1984) Pediculosis and the pediatrician. **Pediatr Dermatol** 2:74.
6. Matthew M, DiSouza P, Mehta DK (1982) A new treatment of phthirus palpebrum. **Ann Ophthalmol** 14:439.

7. Moore RA, Schmitt BD (1979) Conjunctivitis in children. **Clin Pediatr** 18:26.
8. Chandler JW, Alexander ER, Pheiffer TA et al. (1977) Ophthalmia neonatorum associated with maternal chlamydial infections. **Trans Am Acad Ophthalmol Otolaryngol** 83:302.
9. Schachter J, Sweet RL, Grossman M et al. (1986) Experience with the routine use of erythromycin for chlamydial infections in pregnancy. **N Engl J Med** 314:276.

and a watery discharge, as well as preauricular lymphadenopathy, are characteristic. Most commonly adenovirus, echovirus type 11, and coxsackievirus B_2 are the responsible agents.[7] Rubella is no longer considered a common cause of childhood conjunctivitis. Saline compresses are all that is required; antibiotics are to be avoided. TRIC is the exception to this rule and should be treated vigorously with topical sulfonamide or tetracycline. Unlike in the newborn, TRIC in the older child is characterized by marked follicular hypertrophy of the lower eyelids.

Bacterial conjunctivitis

Severe inflammation with lid edema and purulent discharge is highly suggestive of bacterial infection, although a milder presentation can occur. The most common causative agents are *S. aureus*, *Hemophilus* spp., and *Pneumococcus*. A Gram stain or culture of the exudate will confirm the diagnosis and identify the etiologic agent.

Treatment should consist of gentle cleansing and removal of exudates with saline solution and the use of a broad-spectrum topical antibiotic for up to one week. This is effective in most cases of bacterial conjunctivitis because of the extremely high antibiotic concentrations that can be achieved at the ocular surface. Most cases of bacterial conjunctivitis will respond to these ophthalmic preparations even when *in vitro* tests indicate bacterial resistance. Sodium sulfacetamide drops, bacitracin, chlortetracycline, and erythromycin ointments used four times a day are effective. Alternative combination products such as trimethoprim–polymyxin B eye drops, bacitracin–polymyxin B ointment, or gramicidin–neomycin–polymyxin B eye drops can be prescribed. Drops should be instilled in the eyes every two hours initially if the infection is severe. The interval can be extended to every four hours while the patient is awake when the infection is under better control. Ointments may be more useful in younger patients because tearing may rapidly wash away eye drop solutions. Any ointment preparation should be instilled at bedtime as interference with vision is not a contraindication at that time.

Conjunctivitis is a constant symptom of Kawasaki's syndrome, which is characterized by fever of over five days, lymph node enlargement, changes of the oral mucosa, erythema multiforme-like skin alterations, palm and sole lesions, and frequent coronary complications.[10]

Foreign body

Conjunctivitis, particularly when unilateral, may be a manifestation of a foreign body in the eye. Referral to an ophthalmologist is indicated for corneal examination, removal of the material, and appropriate therapy.

Allergic conjunctivitis

Allergic conjunctivitis is usually seen in the setting of other allergic conditions such as allergic rhinitis. It is characterized by watery discharge, conjunctival injection, itching, tearing, swelling of the lids, and chemosis. Smears of the discharge from the conjunctival sac will demonstrate numerous eosinophils. Treatment consists of elimination of the allergen, if possible, as well as cool compresses, oral antihistamines, and a topical corticosteroid.[1]

Vernal conjunctivitis

Vernal conjunctivitis is a recurrent form of allergic conjunctivitis that is more common in children, particularly in boys, and occurs mainly in spring and summer. A family history of atopic disorders is usual. Salient features are itching, tearing, photophobia, a thick ropy discharge, cobblestone papillae observed most easily on the inner aspect of the upper lid, and conjunctival nodules at the corneal limbus. Topical vasoconstrictors and corticosteroids are the treatment of choice.[1,7] Topical cromolyn sodium and lodoxamine 0.1%, have also been used with reasonable success in palliating symptoms.[1]

OCULAR HERPES SIMPLEX INFECTION

Herpes simplex virus (HSV) infection in infants and children may involve the eyelid and ocular tissues rather than the mouth and is almost always due to HSV type 1 (HSV-1). When it develops on the lid or lid margin, the eruption resembles herpes infection elsewhere on the skin and consists of grouped vesicopustules on an erythematous base, usually in a unilateral distribution. These lesions erode, crust, and, if uncomplicated, heal within seven to 10 days without scarring.[1]

Primary ocular HSV infection may also present as an acute follicular conjunctivitis or keratoconjunctivitis with or without lid involvement. Accompanying systemic manifestations include rhinitis, pharyngitis, fever, malaise, and irritability. Ipsilateral preauricular adenitis is found in more than one-half of cases.[11] Ocular infection is most often unilateral but may become bilateral after a unilateral onset. These infections can last for up to five weeks and, in a small percentage of cases, may persist as a chronic blepharoconjunctivitis. Ocular and periocular involvement can develop in patients with atopic dermatitis who become infected with HSV (eczema herpetieum).

Patients with ocular HSV infection most commonly complain of erythema, tearing, itching, irritation, and lid swelling. Pain, photophobia, and blurred vision occur less often. In addition to the characteristic cutaneous lesions, common signs of HSV infection include hyperemia and edema of the conjunctivae, follicular hypertrophy (mainly on the conjunctiva of the lower lid) and, rarely, punctate keratitis, erosions, dendritic ulcers, or stromal keratitis.[11] Because corneal involvement is unusual in a primary childhood HSV infection, the course is generally benign. However, recurrent ocular HSV infection is more often associated with corneal involvement and severe stromal reactions, resulting in scarring and visual loss. About 26% of children with primary ocular HSV infection develop a recurrence within two years of the initial episode. Almost 50% of those with a history of more than one attack will have three or more recurrences within two years.[1,11]

Any child with suspected HSV infection of the eye should have an immediate ophthalmologic consultation. Corneal evaluation by slit lamp or biomicroscopy is critical for optimal care.[1,12] Mild infections are usually treated with topical antiviral agents, such as trifluridine and acyclovir applied two to four times daily.[13,14] However, too long an application of trifluridine has to be avoided.[15] Complicated and severe infections may require debridement and corticosteroid therapy, particularly for stromal keratitis and iridocyclitis. Serious side effects and permanent ocular damage may result from injudicious use of corticosteroids in patients with HSV infection of the eye. In such a setting, steroids should be prescribed only by an ophthalmologist, with careful frequent evaluation of the patient for the development of increased ocular pressure, cataracts, and deterioration of stromal keratitis or iritis.[16]

Newborn infants can also develop ocular HSV infection in association with widespread systemic disease or as a limited infection. Typical cutaneous lesions may develop on the lids; however, corneal involvement may also occur as a primary infection. Recurrent corneal HSV infection may follow. In contrast to older infants and children, neonatal infections are most often contracted during delivery and are therefore due to HSV-2.[17]

10. Blorn US, Zeller B, Perminow KV, Fjærli H-O (2000) Kawasakis syndrome. **Tidsskr Nor Lægeforen** 120:3540–3543.
11. Darougar S, Wishart MS, Viswalingam ND (1985) Epidermiological and clinical features of primary herpes simplex virus ocular infection. **Br J Ophthalmol** 69:2.
12. Dawson CR (1984) Ocular herpes simplex virus infections. **Clin Dermatol** 2:56.
13. Sudesh S, Laibson PR (1999) The impact of the herpetic eye disease studies on the management of herpes simplex virus ocular infections. **Curr Opin Ophthalmol** 10:230–233.
14. Panda A, Das GK, Khokhar S, Rao V (1995) Efficacy of four antiviral agents in the treatment of uncomplicated herpetic keratitis. **Can J Ophthalmol** 30:256–258.
15. Maudgal PC, Van Damme B, Missotten L (1983) Corneal epithelial dysplasia after trifluridine use. **Graefes Arch Clin Exp Ophthalmol** 220:6–12.
16. Wilhelmus KR, Gee L, Hauck WW et al. (1994) Herpetic eye disease study. A controlled trial of topical corticosteroids for herpes simplex stromal keratitis. **Ophthalmology** 101:1883–1895.
17. Nahmias AJ, Visitine AM, Caldwell DR, Wilson LA (1976) Eye infections with herpes simplex virus in neonates. **Surv Ophthalmol** 21:100.

OCULAR VARICELLA-ZOSTER VIRUS INFECTION

Although ocular herpes zoster (HZ) is a well-known entity, eye involvement in varicella is rarely discussed, probably because of its relatively infrequent occurrence as compared with zoster ophthalmicus. In one series of 125 unselected patients with chickenpox, the incidence of ocular lesions was found to be 4%.[18] Common complaints among a group of children referred for ocular involvement included photophobia, redness, soreness, tearing, and lid swelling.[18,19] Physical findings included typical vesicles on the lid margins, conjunctival perilimbal vesicles, palpebral conjunctivitis with prominent follicles, anterior uveitis, and punctate keratitis without frank dendrites that healed without scarring. Complications of ocular varicella noted in the literature include dendritic keratitis, retinopathy, optic neuritis, ophthalmoplegia, oculomotor palsy, cataracts, lacrimal canaliculi obstruction, and optic disk pigmentation.[18,20]

Although HZ occurs less frequently in children than in adults, a comparable percentage of children have involvement of the trigeminal nerve,[21] if one excludes the elderly. Ocular HZ most frequently affects the supraorbital or supratrochlear divisions of the frontal nerve; however, involvement of the nasociliary branch of the ophthalmic nerve has the most significant consequences. Hutchinson's sign, vesicles on the tip of the nose, are an indication of this localization.

All the ocular tissues may be involved in HZ ophthalmicus. Vesicles on the lid may cause ulceration, scarring, hyperpigmentation, trichiasis, permanent anesthesia, lid retraction, and chronic corneal exposure. The conjunctivae may become hyperemic and chemotic, with the occasional appearance of distinct vesicles. Scleritis, punctate uveitis with vesicles and pseudodendrites, serpiginous ulcerations, and severe stromal inflammation may also occur. Uveitis is reflected by photophobia, intense pain, a ciliary flush, pupillary constriction, corneal haziness, and anterior and posterior synechiae. A number of ischemic complications may also occur; however, these problems are relatively rare in children.

Children with ocular HZ should have an immediate, thorough assessment by an ophthalmologist, who should also dictate management. Medications frequently used in the management of ocular herpes zoster include cycloplegics, topical corticosteroids, and, occasionally, systemic corticosteroids. Antiviral agents have to be given very early, if at all. Age, immunocompetence, and general health of the patient must be taken into consideration when formulating individual treatment plans.

DISORDERS OF THE GENITAL MUCOUS MEMBRANES

Sexually transmitted diseases and infectious vaginitis are discussed in Chapter 28.

ANATOMY

For additional information on this topic, see Reference 22.

PRURITUS VULVAE

Because pruritus vulvae is a symptom and not a disease, the etiology reflects the incidence of disorders characterized by itching in the various age groups. In infants and young children, pruritus of the vulval area is most often due to atopic dermatitis, irritant contact dermatitis, allergic contact dermatitis, candidiasis, scabies, and pinworm infestation. In older children, in addition to these conditions, lichen sclerosus et atrophicus, psoriasis, ichthyosis, group A β-hemolytic streptococcal infection, and pubic lice may cause pruritus. Vulval

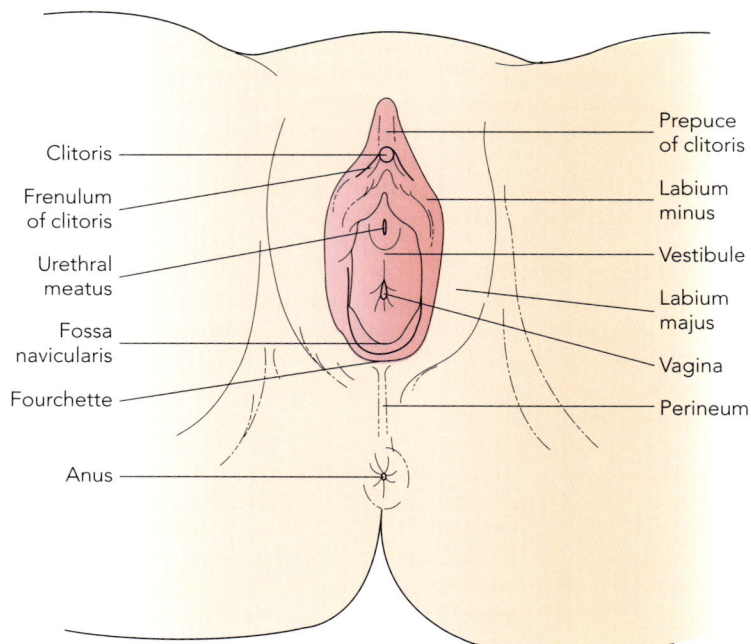

Fig. 9.2 Anatomy of the female genitalia.

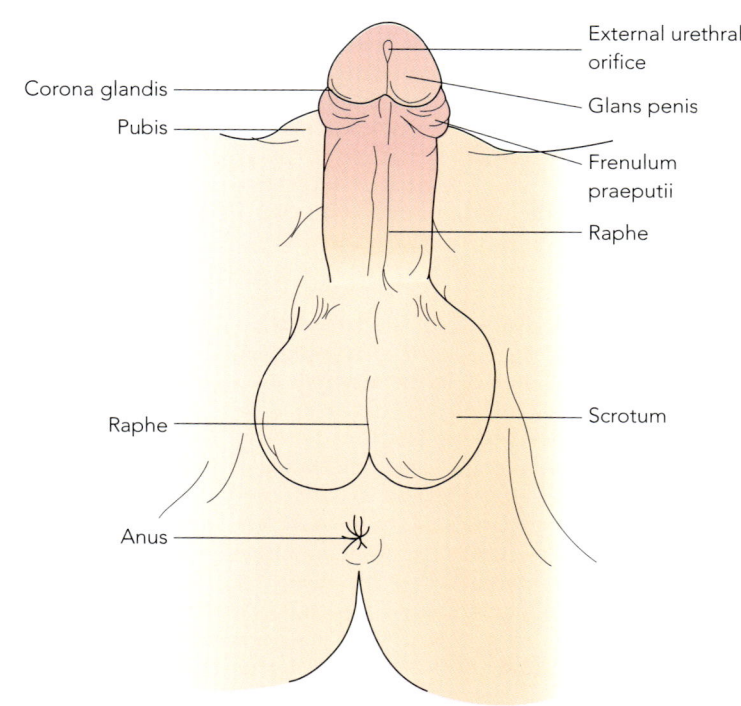

Fig. 9.3 Anatomy of the male genitalia.

itching at any age can result from poor hygiene as well as a bacterial, candidal, trichomonal, or nonspecific vaginitis associated with discharge. Bubble bath dermatitis with *Pseudomonas aeruginosa* superinfection is also a common cause of vulval itching in young girls. However, a specific cause for pruritus vulvae is often not found.[23]

18. Jordan DR, Noel L-P, Clarke WN (1984) Ocular involvement in varicella. **Clin Pediatr** 23:434.
19. de Freitas D, Sato EH, Kelly LD, Pavan-Langston D (1992) Delayed onset of varicella keratitis. **Cornea** 11:471–474.
20. Liesegang TJ (1984) The varicella-zoster virus: systemic and ocular features. **J Am Acad Dermatol** 11:165.
21. Rogers RS III, Tindall JP (1972) Herpes zoster in children. **Arch Dermatol** 106:204.
22. McCann J, Wells R, Simon J, Voris J (1990) Genital findings in prepubertal girls selected for nonabuse: a descriptive study. **Pediatrics** 86:428.
23. Paek SC, Merritt DF, Mallory SB (2001) Pruritus vulvae in prepubertal children. **J Am Acad Dermatol** 44:795–802.

The clinical findings range from little change to florid dermatitis. The most important aspect of the visit will often be to obtain a thorough history, which should include all skin-care products and laundry products used, types of underclothing worn, presence of discharge, or nocturnal itching. Lack of cleanliness as well as overuse of soaps, feminine hygiene products, lubricants, self-prescribed antibiotics or antifungal agents, and contraceptive agents can contribute to or cause pruritus vulvae. Potassium hydroxide (KOH) preparations; cultures for bacteria and fungi; mineral oil scrapings for scabies mites, eggs, and feces; a hand lens examination for pubic lice; and a tape test for pinworm ova may be indicated, depending on the physical findings, the age of the patient, and the historic information provided. Therapy will depend on the cause of the problem as determined by the history, examination, and appropriate laboratory procedures.

PINWORM INFESTATION (ENTEROBIUS VERMICULARIS)

Pinworm infestation is the most common of all the helminth infections and occurs primarily in children. An estimated 20–30% of children are infested with this parasite.[24] Affected children usually experience intense perirectal and vulval itching due to migration of the adult worms over the perineal skin. Because the peak activity of the parasite occurs at night, pruritus often awakens the child and causes nocturnal irritability and restlessness. Occasionally the infestation is reflected by a perianal or vulval eczematous dermatitis, excoriations, or vaginal discharge and inflammation resulting from migration of the worms into the vagina.

Pinworm infestation is acquired by ingestion of eggs transmitted by fomites or via the fingers from the perianal skin or occasionally by inhalation of eggs from the environment. Ingested eggs hatch in the host's duodenum, and the larva mature during their passage through the small intestines. Sexually mature worms copulate in the cecum, following which they migrate to the perianal skin, where the gravid female deposits large numbers of eggs. The eggs become infectious 4–6 hours after deposition on the perianal skin; if the eggs are then swallowed by a human host, the cycle begins again.[24]

The entire life cycle of *Enterobius vermicularis* from ingestion of eggs to maturation of the worms and deposition of fresh eggs takes 4–6 weeks. The child remains well except for the accompanying pruritus and occasional dermatitis. Although mild peripheral eosinophilia has been rarely reported, this hematologic finding should not be attributed to pinworm infection. Likewise, the suggestion that pinworms can cause enuresis, weight loss, and abdominal pain is based on anecdotal information and is regarded as doubtful by most authorities.[24]

The diagnosis of pinworm infection should be suspected in any child with either perirectal or vulval pruritus, or both, and dermatitis. At times the adult worms can be observed on the perineum at night when the distressed child awakens. The diagnosis is most easily made by brief application of a strip of transparent adhesive tape to the perirectal skin and microscopic examination of the tape with low-power objective. *Enterobius vermicularis* eggs are easily identified as thick-walled ovoid structures adherent to the tape. This test is most productive if performed in the early morning before the freshly deposited eggs are dispersed.

Accepted therapy includes pyrantel pamoate in a single dose of 11mg/kg (not to exceed 1g) or mebendazole, 100mg in a single dose. Simultaneous treatment of all household members is recommended. Retreatment in 2–3 weeks is indicated to kill any adult worms that have developed from eggs swallowed at the time of initial therapy because neither drug is effective against

ova. Massive laundering of clothing, bed clothes, and other heroic measures are not required and are generally ineffective. Parents should be made aware of the ubiquity of this parasite and of the likelihood that infection will be reacquired, particularly by preschool children if the napping nits are not treated with a chemotherapeutic active against pinworms, e.g., mebendazole.[25] A nonfluorinated topical corticosteroid can be applied for a few days to clear the dermatitis, if that is necessary.

LICHEN SCLEROSUS ET ATROPHICUS

Although generally regarded as a disease of adulthood, 10–15% of persons with lichen sclerosus et atrophicus (LSA) have onset before the age of 13 years. There is a strong female predominance in all age groups. Seventy-five percent of children with LSA have involvement of the anogenital area and, in most, the disease is confined to those sites.[26] There is a strong association of infantile LSA with DQ 7 pointing at a higher risk of developing other autoimmune diseases.[27]

Anogenital lesions in girls can be asymptomatic or may be associated with irritation, itching, burning, vaginal discharge, pain on urination, and minor bleeding. Cutaneous changes consist of ivory-colored, flattened papules that coalesce into plaques of various sizes, most commonly producing a figure-of-eight or hourglass configuration around the vagina and anus (Fig. 9.4). The skin may feel indurated or become shiny, wrinkled, and parchmentlike; occasionally serous or hemorrhagic bullae, erosions, and fissures develop. The differential diagnosis includes mainly vitiligo and leukoderma but also non-specific vulvitis, vulvitis circumscripta plasmocellularis and perianal dermatitis.[28] The hemorrhagic friable surface of the affected skin is sometimes mistaken for child abuse.

Genital LSA is considered relatively rare in males, and particularly so in boys.[29] Skin lesions are confined to the glans penis (balanitis xerotica obliterans) and prepuce (posthitis xerotica obliterans), sparing the scrotal and perianal skin. The prepuce becomes nonretractable due to a sclerotic ring at the tip of the foreskin, and petechiae may be evident.[30] Less commonly, involvement of the urethral meatus leads to stenosis, dysuria, reduction of the urinary stream, and, potentially, obstructive uropathy. It has been suggested, on the basis of histologic evaluation of foreskins removed because of scarring phimosis, that LSA occurs much more frequently in prepubertal males than has been generally appreciated.[31] Circumcision has been found to have a preventive effect.[32]

Therapy for genital LSA in prepubertal girls is required only if the patient is symptomatic.[33] The disease is usually self-limited involuting spontaneously around the time of menarche in approximately two-thirds of patients. There is little residual skin change. Vulvar LSA in prepubertal children does not predispose to neoplasia and is not an indication for surgical intervention. Reconstructive surgery for severe sequellae is rarely needed.[34]

Topical steroids remain the most commonly used agents to treat childhood LSA and will often suffice to alleviate discomfort. At times, a fluorinated preparation may be required, but the least potent effective preparation should always be prescribed. Progesterone in oil 100mg/30g Aquaphor applied twice daily is also said to be palliative, without side effects, and is well tolerated by children. Progesterone 1% in adequate vehicle applied twice daily for six months resulted in clinical improvement in 10 children (7 girls, 3 boys) after three months with decreased pruritus and recovered skin texture.[33] Estrogen (Premarin) applied once to twice daily for two weeks, then once every other day for 4–6 weeks, provides an alternative approach in prepubertal females. Testosterone propionate, 2% in petrolatum, applied twice daily, has been

24. Hoeprich PD (1983) Infectious Diseases, 3rd ed. Philadelphia: Harper & Row.
25. Sirivichayakul C, Pojjaroen-anant C, Wisetsing P et al. (2000) Prevalence of enterobiasis and its incidence after blanket chemotherapy in a male orphanage. **Southeast Asian J Trop Med Public Health** 31:144–146.
26. Clark JA, Muller SA (1967) Lichen sclerosus et atrophicus in children. A report of 24 cases. **Arch Dermatol** 95:476.
27. Powell J, Wojnarowska F, Winsey S et al. (2000) Lichen sclerosus premenarche: autoimmunity and immunogenetics. **Br J Dermatol** 142:481–484.
28. Albers SE, Taylor G, Huyer D et al. (2000) Vulvitis circumscripta plasmacellularis mimicking child abuse. **J Am Acad Dermatol** 42:1078–1080.
29. Mikat DM, Ackerman HR Jr, Mikat KW (1973) Balanitis xerotica obliterans report of a case on an 11-year-old and review of the literature. **Pediatrics** 52:25.
30. Barton PG, Foyd MJ, Beers BB (1993) Penile purpura as a manifestation of lichen sclerosis et atrophicus. **Pediatr Dermatol** 10:129.
31. Chalmers RJG, Beuton PA, Bennett RF et al. (1984) Lichen sclerosus et atrophicus. A common and distinctive cause of phimosis in boys. **Arch Dermatol** 120:1025.
32. Mallon E, Hawkins D, Dinneen M et al. (2000) Circumcision and genital dermatoses. **Arch Dermatol** 136:350–354.
33. Serrano G, Millan F, Fortea J et al. (1993) Topical progesterone as treatment of choice in lichen sclerosus et atrophicus in children. **Pediatr Dermatol** 10:201.
34. Breech LL, Laufer MR (2000) Surgical in the management of labial and clitoral hood adhesions in adolescents with lichen sclerosus. **J Pediatr Adolesc Gynecol** 13:21–22.

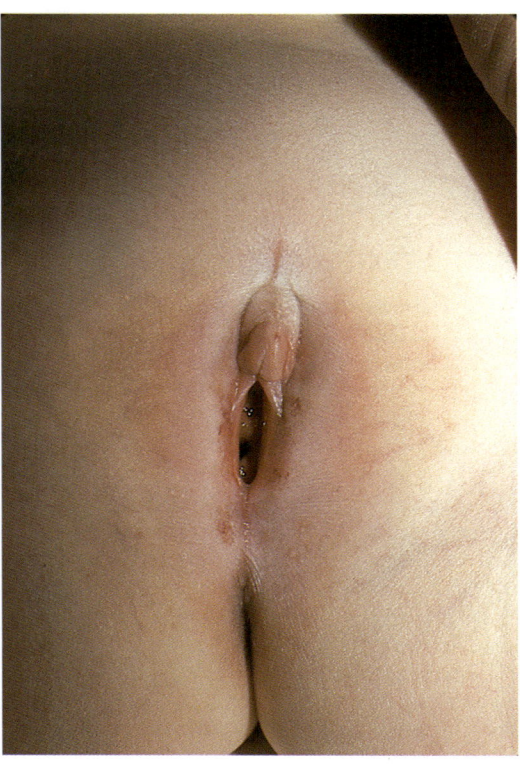

Fig. 9.4 Lichen sclerosus involving the vulvar and perianal skin. Note the hemorrhagic areas.

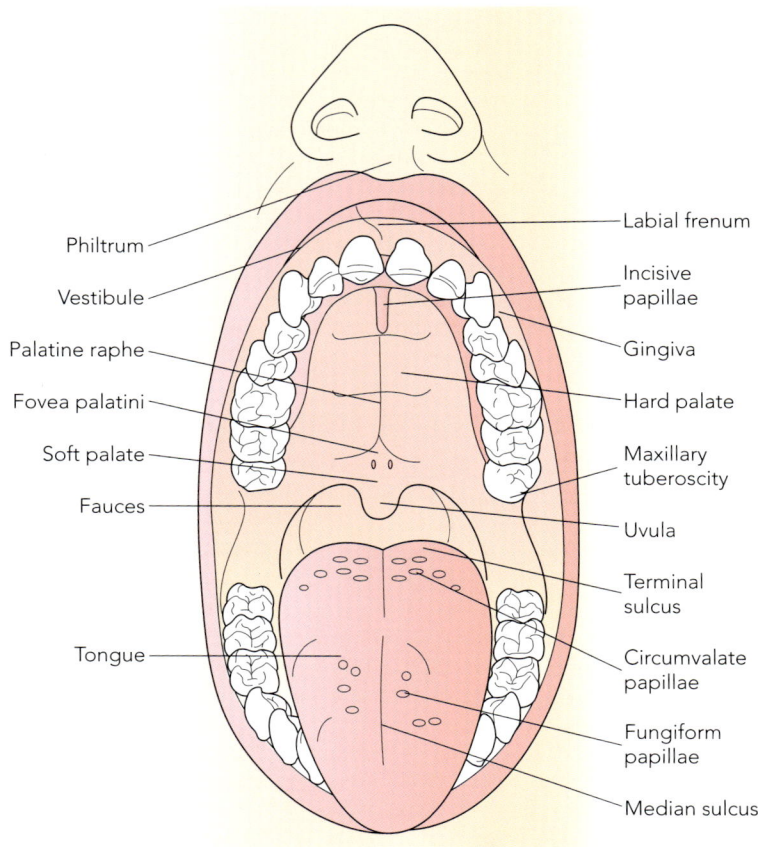

Fig. 9.5 Anatomy of the oral mucous membranes.

effective in severely symptomatic adult patients, but its use in children has been limited. Maintenance dosage is two to three times weekly. Side effects include increased libido and clitoromegaly; however, if used carefully, some of these changes can be avoided.[35]

Studies demonstrating decreased serum levels of dihydrotestosterone and androstenedione in women with LSA lend credence to the postulate that decreased 5α-reductase activity in the tissues may contribute to the development of LSA. Increased levels of androgens coincident with puberty may induce 5α-reductase activity in the vulval skin, thereby accounting for resolution of the dermatosis around the time of menarche.[35]

Although topical corticosteroids and testosterone propionate have been used successfully in affected males, treatment is usually by circumcision. If meatal stenosis is present, meatotomy or meatoplasty may be required.[36]

GENITAL HERPES SIMPLEX

This is usually due to sexual abuse, both in girls and in boys. It presents as a primary herpetic infection with fever, malaise, regional tender lymphadenopathy as well as marked genital edema and disseminated clear vesicles rapidly turning yellow and breaking down to small ulcerations. Healing takes two to three weeks. Recurrences occur earlier and more frequently in HSV-2 than in HSV-1 infections.

Treatment with systemic acyelovir, famciclovir or valacyclovir should be instituted as soon as possible.[37]

DISORDERS OF THE ORAL MUCOUS MEMBRANES

MUCOUS MEMBRANE ANATOMY

Fundamental to the understanding of mucous membrane disorders is the prior understanding of the anatomic and functional relationships of these tissues (Fig. 9.5). A knowledge of which oral mucosal tissues are keratinized and

which are nonkeratinized not only in part explains the function of these tissues (Table 9.1), but also assists in the assessment and distinction of herpetic and aphthous lesions. The above anatomic illustration will enhance the subsequent understanding of pathologic processes involving these same oral mucosal tissues.

TABLE 9.1   The function and keratinization of the oral mucous membranes

Lining mucosa (nonkeratinized/not attached)
    Soft palate
    Buccal and labial mucosa
    Sulcular epithelium
    Ventrum of tongue
    Alveolar mucosae
Masticatory mucosa (orthokeratinized/attached to underlying structures)
    Hard palate
    Gingivae
        Free marginal gingiva
        Attached gingivae
    Dorsum of tongue
    Lip (transitional portion/parakeratinized, skin portion and
        vermilion/orthokeratinized)
Specialized mucosa
    Filiform papillae
    Fungiform papillae
    Circumvallate papillae with taste buds

35. Friedrich EG Jr, Kalra PS (1984) Serum levels of sex hormones in vulvar lichen sclerosus and the effect of topical testosterone. **N Engl J Med** 310:488.
36. Khezri AA, Dovnis A, Dunn M (1979) Balanitis xerotica obliterans. **Br J Urol** 51:229.

37. Leung DT, Sacks SL (2000) Current recommendations for the treatment of genital herpes. **Drugs** 60:1329–1352.

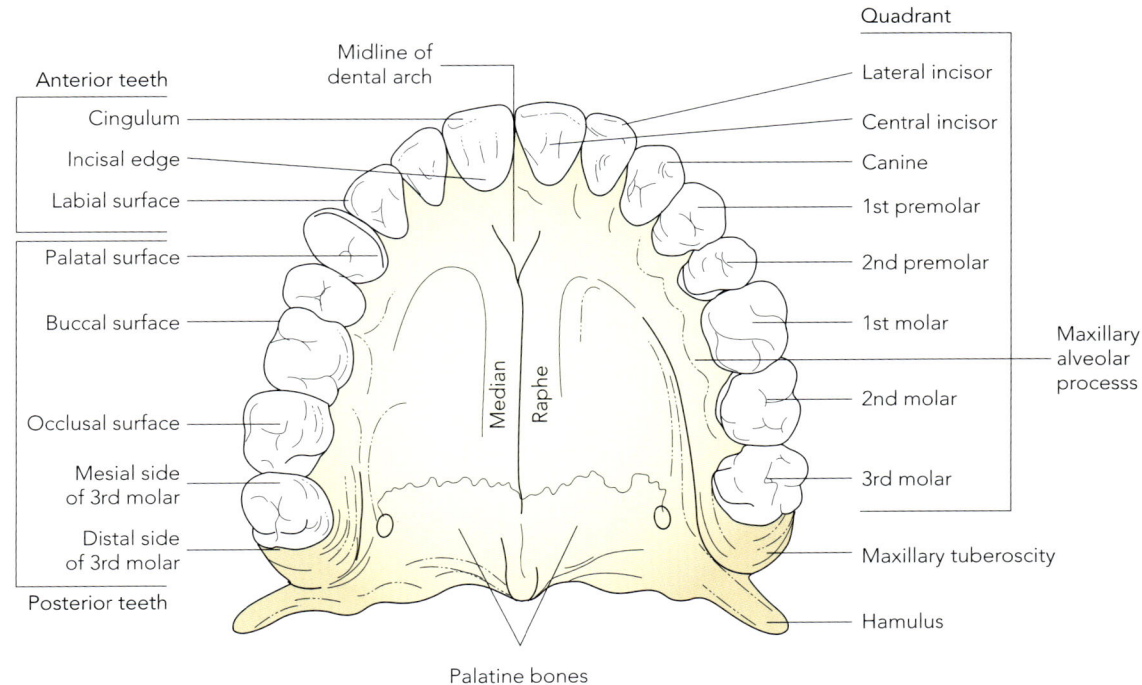

Fig. 9.6   Diagram of the maxillary dental arch and the bones of the hard palate.

TABLE 9.2   Normal chronology of human dentition

Tooth	Hard tissue formation begins	Crown completed	Eruption	Root completed
Deciduous dentition				
Maxillary teeth				
Central incisor	4 mos *in utero*	4 mos	7½ mos	1½ yrs
Lateral incisor	4½ mos *in utero*	5 mos	9 mos	2 yrs
Canine	5 mos *in utero*	9 mos	18 mos	3¼ yrs
First molar	5 mos *in utero*	6 mos	14 mos	2½ yrs
Second molar	6 mos *in utero*	11 mos	24 mos	3 yrs
Mandibular teeth				
Central incisor	4½ mos *in utero*	3½ mos	6 mos	1½ yrs
Lateral incisor	4¼ mos *in utero*	4 mos	7 mos	1½ yrs
Canine	5 mos *in utero*	9 mos	16 mos	3 yrs
First molar	5 mos *in utero*	5½ mos	12 mos	2¼ yrs
Second molar	6 mos *in utero*	10 mos	20 mos	3 yrs
Permanent dentition				
Maxillary teeth				
Central incisor	3–4 mos	4–5 yrs	7–8yrs	10 yrs
Lateral incisor	10–12 mos	4–5 yrs	8–9yrs	11 yrs
Canine	4–5 mos	6–7 yrs	11–12yrs	13–15 yrs
First premolar	1½–1¾ yrs	5–6 yrs	10–11yrs	12–13 yrs
Second premolar	2–2¼ yrs	6–7 yrs	10–12yrs	12–14 yrs
First molar	birth	2½–3 yrs	6–7yrs	9–10 yrs
Second molar	2½–3 yrs	7–8 yrs	12–15yrs	14–16 yrs
Third molar	7–9 yrs	12–16yrs	17–21yrs	18–25 yrs
Mandibular teeth				
Central incisor	3–4 mos	4–5 yrs	6–7 yrs	9 yrs
Lateral incisor	3–4 mos	4–5 yrs	7–8 yrs	10 yrs
Canine	4–5 mos	6–7 yrs	9–10 yrs	12–14 yrs
First premolar	1¾–2 yrs	5–6 yrs	10–12 yrs	12–13 yrs
Second premolar	2¼–2½ yrs	6–7 yrs	11–12 yrs	13–14 yrs
First molar	birth	2½–3 yrs	6–7 yrs	9–10 yrs
Second molar	2½–3 yrs	7–8 yrs	11–13 yrs	14–15 yrs
Third molar	8–10 yrs	12–16 yrs	17–21 yrs	18–25 yrs

From Woelfel[405] with permission.

TABLE 9.3   Syndromes with natal teeth

Syndrome	Associated anomalies	Inheritance/chromosomal abnormality/prevalence
Ellis–van Creveld (chondroectodermal dysplasia)	Bilateral postaxial polydactyly of hands, chondrodysplasia of long bones resulting in cromesolic dwarfism, ectodermal dysplasia affecting nails/teeth, congenital heart malformation	Autosomal-recessive Not known $7/1 \times 10^6$
Hallermann–Streiff	Dyscephaly, hypotrichosis, micro-ophthalmia, cataracts, beaked nose, micrognathia, proportionate short stature	Sporadic Not known 150 cases to date
Pachyonychia congenital (1: Jadassohn–Lewandowsky) (2: Jackson–Lawler)	Dystrophic nails, palmoplantar keratosis, hyperhidrosis, follicular keratosis, oral leukokeratosis, cutaneous cysts	Autosomal-dominant Keratin gene mutations: Type I: 6a/16, type 2: 6b/17 $0.071/1 \times 10^6$ 9:5 male to female
Pallister–Hall (hypothalamic hamartoblastoma)	Hypothalamic hamartoblastoma, craniofacial abnormalities, postaxial polydactyly, cardiac and renal defects	Sporadic Not known 13 cases to date 8:5 male to female
Weidemann–Rautenstrauch	Endocrine dysfunction, aged facies, frontal and biparietal bossing, small facial bones, sparse scalp hair, prominent scalp veins, small beaked nose, low-set ears	Autosomal-recessive Not known 1 case to date
Natal teeth, patent ductus arteriosus, intestinal pseudoobstruction	Dilatation/hypermobility of small bowel, short or micro-colon without obstruction, incomplete rotation of mid gut, patent ductus arteriosus	X-linked recessive Not known 2 cases to date, brothers

DENTAL ANATOMY

Figure 9.6 illustrates the mature maxillary dental arch and bones of the hard palate. Table 9.2 provides the normal chronology of human dentition and Table 9.3 lists syndromes in which natal teeth occur.

ORAL HYGIENE INSTRUCTIONS FOR CHILDREN

Oral hygiene instructions given to parents of infants and young children must be specifically tailored to the individual child. Although there are some general recommendations for cleaning their teeth, the age of the child, their manual dexterity, which is also somewhat dependent on the age, and the emotional and physical stature are significant factors in determining the best mechanism to provide oral hygiene effectively.

The goal of oral hygiene is to remove plaque from the surfaces of the teeth and subgingival areas. Plaque adheres to the enamel surfaces via mechanisms inherent to the plaque bacteria itself. Without an adequate daily regimen, including removal of the plaque, it will accumulate continually until the point of completely covering enamel surfaces. When this occurs, it is easy for the plaque bacteria to cause significant decalcification of mineral surfaces, beneath the area where the plaque resides. Often, children who do not brush their teeth regularly exhibit large white spot areas manifesting decalcified enamel via continual exposure to active acid from plaque bacteria excretions.

Infant positioning

The most effective way of positioning an infant for oral hygiene is the same manner in which the dentist examines the infant. This is referred to as the "knee to knee position," where the child's head is placed on the lap of the individual who is to clean their teeth, and the other individual (typically the other parent) places the legs of the child around their waist. The parent holding the legs around the waist also holds the arms, so that the other parent can have easy access to the mouth. Although this technique may be offensive, and could result in a rebellious response from the child, the enforcement of this technique on a daily basis will soon yield a responsive child who will desire the attention received from cleaning the teeth.

Intention

Cleaning the teeth is not a random event, but a very specific identifiable process. The parent must clearly identify that the bristles of the toothbrush, which must be soft, are cleaning each tooth surface adequately. For this reason, it is essential to clean each tooth surface individually before progressing to the next. Although fluoridated toothpaste can be used as a final topical therapeutic agent for infants in small amounts, it is preferable to brush the infant's teeth without the toothpaste, so that the parent can visualize the tips of the brush cleaning the tooth surfaces. The foaming action of toothpaste will often not allow the parent to visualize the tooth surfaces effectively. Upon complete cleaning of the teeth, a small amount of fluoridated toothpaste, no more than the size of a pea, can be placed on the tooth surfaces to provide a therapeutic effect of fluoride.

School-age children

School-age children can begin to brush their teeth themselves with good confidence and control. Although they may not have complete dexterity to brush all tooth surfaces, and will most likely require the assistance of the parent, they should be encouraged to thoroughly clean their teeth on their own with the approval and support of the parent. It is also a good age to begin teaching dental flossing to the child, so that they can provide the daily removal of plaque from the interproximal surfaces of the teeth, particularly the posterior teeth. Children at this age who gain confidence in their ability to clean their teeth will most likely continue to do so on their own. In school-age children, fluoride supplements may be given not only as adjunctive therapy to replace a fluoride deficiency that might exist in the water supply, but also as a topical agent to aid in the prevention of dental caries, which might be a particular problem for an individual child because of a high caries rate. This situation often requires the recommendation of daily use of over-the-counter flouride rinses (0.05% fluoride) or tooth gels (0.4%) stannous flouride or a weekly dose of a prescription fluoride of 0.2%. The over-the-counter topical fluoride rinse is used daily at bedtime. The stannous flouride gel is used each morning and evening after brushing and flossing. The gel is applied to the teeth for one minute and then spit out. Care must be taken to avoid recommending topical fluoride treatments to children who are not old enough to expectorate.

CONGENITAL FISTULAE OF THE LOWER LIP

Congenital fistulas of the lower lip usually appear as bilateral transverse pits or as symmetric nipple-like projections on the vermilion portion of the lower lip. These pits are typically 1cm apart and equidistant from the midline. The lower lip occasionally appears swollen, thus accentuating the pits.[38]

The fistulas result from failure of closure of embryologic furrows located on the fetal mandibular process at the 7.5–12.5mm stage. This incomplete obliteration of the labial sulcus produces pits that range in depth from a few millimeters to 25mm. The longer fistulas end in a tiny cul-de-sac embedded in the orbicularis oris musculature and, from the opposing open end, a viscous saliva may extrude either spontaneously or during mastication.[39]

The close association with facial clefts makes this minimal deformity quite significant. Nearly 70–80% of persons with paramedian sinuses of the lower lip have either an associated cleft lip or cleft palate, or both (van der Woude syndrome). The trait is transmitted in an autosomal-dominant fashion with a penetrance of almost 100%, but variable expression.[40,41] An affected parent transmits the gene to half of the offspring, whereas a phenotypically normal child may then transmit all or any part of the syndrome (e.g., lip pits with or without clefting) to the subsequent generation. The estimated frequency of lower-lip pits is 1:75 000 to 1:100 000 and that of cleft lip or palate is 1:650. No sex linkage, sex limitation, or sex influence for congenital lip fistulas is recognized, but a slight female predominance has been reported with this anomaly.[42]

Histologically, the labial tubular lumen is lined by a stratified squamous epithelium continuous with that of the vermilion border of the lip. The fistula tapers to a small base, where scattered acini of mucous glands with tubular ducts are present. Occasionally these glands are considerably larger than normal labial glands.

Variations of these labial sulci include single pits of the lower lip, commissural or angular lip pits, and the more rarely described fistulas of the upper lip. Persons with single pits have associated cleft anomalies in roughly the same frequency as for bilateral lip pits.[40] These unilateral or midline fistulas are viewed as an incomplete expression of this trait and not as a distinct entity. Commissural or angular lip pits are thought to be separate entities with a higher incidence and a different embryology. Fistulas of the upper lip are the most rare of these anomalies and have not been shown to be inherited.[40]

Other anomalies associated with lip-pit, cleft-lip syndrome are the van der Woude syndrome and the popliteal web syndrome.[43] Van der Woude syndrome includes missing second premolars with or without lower lip pits, with or without a cleft lip. Popliteal web syndrome is composed of popliteal webs, cleft palate, and lower lip pits.

Congenital lower lip fistulas seldom cause significant deformity or self-harm. Therapy is necessary only to correct the cosmetic deformity or eradicate the aberrant salivation.

DOUBLE LIP

The vermilion in the newborn is divided by a shallow furrow into the anterior pars glabra and posterior pars villosa. This facilitates suckling. When this transverse furrow persists in childhood a double lip forms. Two variants occur: a duplication at the level between the vermilion and mucosa causes the prolabial form, which is permanently visible, whereas a more orally positioned furrow causes a flaccid pouch-like mucosal duplication only visible during speech and smiling. The former is associated with a hyperplasia of the minor labial salivary glands.[44] Most cases are not pronounced and the condition is therefore underdiagnosed.[45]

Treatment is mainly for cosmetic reasons and consists in a transverse wedge excision of the tissue excess.[46,47]

ASCHER SYNDROME

The presence of an acquired double upper lip in association with blepharochalasis and nontoxic thyroid enlargement constitutes Ascher syndrome. An abrupt onset characterizes the changes of the lip and eyelids.[38,48] Although thyroid enlargement may lag several years behind the blepharochalasis, thyroid enlargement develops in a significant number of affected persons during adolescence.[49]

The blepharochalasis may be progressive, with or without antecedent attacks of edema. In addition, hypertrophy of the accessory lacrimal glands may result in pseudoedema of the upper lids. As the upper lip gradually enlarges during infancy or early childhood, discrete areas of soft tissue swelling identifiable by an irregularly lobular mucosal surface become fixed and permanent. The labial enlargement is the result of both hypertrophy and fibrocystic changes within the labial or accessory salivary glands, or both. Inflammation within these glands contributes to the lip distortion.[48,49] Increased salivation is associated with these gland changes.

Therapy is necessary only when speech, mastication, or cosmesis become impaired. Surgical excision of excess tissue is then indicated.[38]

ANGULAR CHEILITIS

This condition, also referred to as perlèche, angular stomatitis, and angular cheilosis, is characterized by inflammation, ulceration, and fissuring at the corners of the mouth. Although it is most common in older persons, particularly denture wearers, angular cheilitis can be attributed to a multiplicity of factors and occurs at any age.[50]

Typically, angular cheilitis presents as erythema and erosions radiating from the labial commissures; edema, scaling, and deep fissures may be associated. The inflammation extends onto the contiguous skin but not onto the buccal mucosa. The involved tissue becomes macerated and crusted, which may produce localized soreness, burning sensations, and pain.

A variety of problems, both local and systemic, may cause or contribute to angular cheilitis (Table 9.4). Many of these factors result in the trapping of excessive moisture at the angles of the mouth, resulting in a constantly wet environment that macerates the skin and facilitates proliferation of certain microorganisms. Persistent or nocturnal drooling associated with mouth breathing, neurologic damage, or orthodontic appliances in the mouth are major contributory factors in some infants and children. The chapping that results from chronic lip licking also predisposes to angular cheilitis in childhood. Unlike adults, poor-fitting dentures are an infrequent cause in the younger age groups.[51] Likewise, loss of vertical dimension, most frequently due to absence of teeth and sagging of the facial musculature, is relatively less common in children.

Contact dermatitis, both irritant dermatitis due to excessive saliva and repetitive lip licking as well as allergic reactions to toothpaste, mouthwash, chewing gum, medications, and cosmetics, is a common etiology in children.

38. Shafer WG, Hine MK, Levy BM (1983) A Textbook of Oral Pathology, 4th ed. Philadelphia: WB Saunders.
39. Goodman RM, Gorlin RJ (1983) The Malformed Infant and Child, An Illustrated Guide. New York: Oxford University Press, p. 234.
40. Cervenka J, Gorlin RJ, Anderson VE (1967) The syndrome of pits of the lower lip and cleft lip and/or palate. Genetic considerations. Am J Hum Genet 19:416.
41. Klausler M, Schinzel A, Gnoinski W et al. (1987) Dominant vererbte Unterlippenfisteln und Gesichtsspalten (Van-der-Woude-Syndrom). Eine Studie an 52 Fällen. Schweiz Med Wochenschr 117:127–134.
42. Lopes MA, Goncalves M, Di Hipolito Junior O, de Almeida OP (1999) Congenital lower lip pits: case report and review of literature. J Clin Pediatr Dent 23:275–277.
43. Smith DW (1982) Recognizable Patterns of Human Malformation, 3rd ed. Philadelphia: WB Saunders.
44. Gorlin TJ (1970) Developmental anomalies of the face and oral structures. In: Thoma's Oral Pathology, 6th ed, Gorlin RJ, Goldman HM, eds. St. Louis: Mosby, pp. 21–95.
45. Witkop jr CJ, Barros L (1963) Oral and genetic studies in Chileans, 1960. I. Oral anomalies. Am J Physiol Anthrop 21:15–24.
46. Greenfield MF, Icochea R, Hoffman C, Gropper C (2000) Double lip: an unusual presentation. Cutis 66:253–256.
47. Reddy KA, Roa AK (1989) Congenital double lip: a review of seven cases. Plast Reconstr Surg 84:420–423.
48. Navas J, Rodriquez P, Chardo A, Camacho F (1991) Ascher syndrome: a case study. Pediatr Dermatol 8:122.
49. Cunliffe WJ (1979) Disorders of connective tissue. In: Textbook of Dermatology, 3rd ed, Rook A, Wilkinson DS, Ebling FJG, eds. Oxford: Blackwell Scientific, p. 1629.
50. Schoenfeld RJ, Schoenfeld FI (1977) Angular cheilitis. Cutis 19:213.
51. Konstantinidis AB, Hatziotis JH (1984) Angular cheilosis: an analysis of 156 cases. J Oral Med 39:199.

TABLE 9.4   Factors related to angular cheilitis

Oral factors
  Drooling, nocturnal or constant
    Orthodontic appliances
    Neurologic deficits
    Persistent mouth breathing
    Macroglossia
  Denture stomatitis: ill-fitting unhygienic dentures
  Lateral lip fistulae
  Xerostomia
Reduced vertical facial dimension
  Sagging of cheeks due to poor tone of facial muscles
  Disturbance of occlusal plane between mandible and maxilla
  Skeletal malformations
  Anodontia, total or partial
Skin disorders
  Dermatologic conditions
    Atopic dermatitis
    Contact dermatitis, allergic or irritant
    Seborrheic dermatitis
    Psoriasis
    Granulomatous cheilitis: Crohn's disease, Melkersson–Rosenthal
      syndrome
    Halogenoderma, pemphigus (vegetans)
    Pachyonychia congenita
  Infections
    Candidiasis
    Herpes simplex infection, viral warts
    Bacterial infection: Streptococci, Staphylococci, secondary syphilis,
      syphilis connata
  Chronic irritation or trauma
General medical disorders
  Deficiencies: Riboflavin (vitamin B$_2$), pyridoxine (vitamin B$_6$), pellagra
    (niacinamide), maple syrup urine disease, kwashiorkor, anorexia
    nervosa, nephrotic syndrome, essential fatty acid deficiency,
    glucogonoma syndrome
  Zinc deficiency syndromes
  Biotin deficiency syndromes
  Anemias
  Gastrointestinal disturbances
  Malnutrition, debilitation

However, atopic dermatitis appears to be the most frequent cause. Other dermatologic conditions, particularly seborrheic dermatitis, psoriasis, and acrodermatitis enteropathica, can also be responsible for skin changes at the angles of the mouth. Although angular cheilitis is commonly attributed to primary or secondary infection with *Candida albicans*,[50] opinions vary as to the prevalence of *Candida* in patients with angular stomatitis.[51,52] *S. aureus* and β–hemolytic streptococci are also commonly cultured from the involved skin.[52]

Systemic disorders account for a minor proportion of patients with angular cheilitis. This easily perceived skin change is a hallmark of riboflavin deficiency but has also been associated with pyridoxine, iron, zinc, biotin deficiencies, and aminoacid metabolism disease. Debilitated patients with gastrointestinal (GI) diseases and malnutrition as well as chronically ill patients receiving systemic corticosteroids, antibiotics, and chemotherapeutic agents may also develop angular cheilitis.[53] In those instances, it is sometimes difficult to isolate the provocative factors.[50]

Therapy consists of correcting underlying disorders or contributory factors, if possible. Institution of measures to ensure good dental hygiene and avoidance of allergens, irritation, and trauma are often helpful. Antifungal agents, preferably in an ointment vehicle, are indicated when *C. albicans* has been identified by KOH preparation or culture. Topical antibacterial ointments (such as mupirocin or bacitracin) should be employed in those patients with a bacterial etiology. Miconazole is favored by some authors because of its broad therapeutic spectrum.[52,54] Protection of the angles of the mouth by application of a thick ointment or bland paste may be palliative in instances where constant drooling or lip licking plays a major role. In patients with an allergic contact dermatitis, patch tests are usually required to identify the causative agent.

CHEILITIS GLANDULARIS

Lip infections originating from, or involving, the minor salivary glands are rare in children.[55] Cheilitis glandularis simplex mainly involves the lower lip and is characterized by lip eversion and protrusion, painless diffuse enlargement and firm nodularity of the affected tissue. It is due to hypertrophy of the labial mucous glands and their ducts, the dilated orifices of which are readily apparent on the labial surface (Fig. 9.7). Pressure exerted on the lip produces a viscid mucous secretion from the ductal openings on the everted hypertrophic lip.[56] Cheilitis glandularis suppurativa exhibits crusting, induration, and incipient ulceration. Cheilitis glandularis apostematosa is a deep suppurative infection resulting in crusting, ulcerations, abscesses and fistulous tracts.[38] Rarely, other minor salivary glands may be involved.[56]

Although the cause is unknown, some cases are familial; others have been attributed to chronic trauma. It has also been suggested that glandular hyperplasia with superimposed long-standing bacterial infection is responsible for the suppurative forms of the disease.[57–59] Squamous cell carcinoma of the lip has been associated in 18% to 35% of cases.[38] Surgical stripping of the involved tissue has been recommended as the treatment of choice.[56]

MELKERSSON–ROSENTHAL SYNDROME AND CHEILITIS GRANULOMATOSA

Melkersson–Rosenthal syndrome (MRS) consists of the classic triad of recurrent or persistent facial swelling, peripheral facial nerve paralysis, and lingua plicata. The *monosymptomatic* and *oligosymptomatic* forms of MRS represent incomplete expression of the disorder. When patients manifest isolated, recurrent, noninflammatory swelling of the lip, the monosymptomatic form is present. These symptoms have also been named Miescher's cheilitis granulomatosa; however, any facial or oral structure may show granulomatous inflammation.[60] When any two features of the classic triad are present, the oligosymptomatic form exists.[61,62]

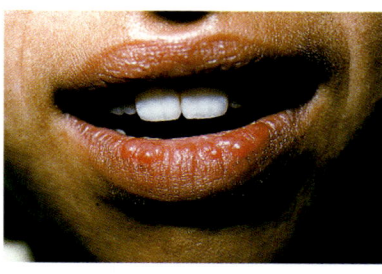

Fig. 9.7   Cheilitis glandularis.

52. Gobetti JP, Colquitt WN (1982) Angular cheilitis—a bacterial infection. **J Mich Dent Assoc** 64:157.
53. Assmann K, Bonsmann G, Werner C, Metze D (2001) Acrodermatitis enteropathica-ähnliche Hautveränderungen bei Ahornsirupkrankheit. **Z Hautkr** 76:220–222.
54. MacFarlane TW, Ferguson MM, MacKenzie D (1978) Sensitivity of miconazole of micro-organisms associated with angular cheilitis. **Br Dent J** 144:199.
55. Yacobi R, Brown DA (1989) Cheilitis glandularis: a pediatric case report. **J Am Dent Assoc** 118:317–318.
56. Rada DC, Koranda FC, Katz FS (1985) Cheilitis glandularis – a disorder of ductal ectasia. **J Dermatol Surg Oncol** 11:372–375.

57. Lederman DA (1994) Suppurative stomatitis glandularis. **Oral Surg Oral Med Oral Pathol** 78:319–322.
58. Doku HC, Shklar G, McCarthy PL (1965) Cheilitis glandularis. **Oral Surg** 20:563.
59. Rogers RS, Bekic M (1997) Diseases of the lips. **Semin Cutan Med Surg** 16:328–336.
60. Hornstein OP (1998) Glossitis granulomatosa—ein ungewöhnlicher Subtyp des Melkersson-Rosenthal-Syndroms. **Mund Kiefer Gesichtschir** 2:14–19.
61. Hornstein OP (1997) Melkersson-Rosenthal syndrome – a challenge for dermatologists to participate in the field of oral medicine. **J Dermatol** 24:281–296.
62. Zimmer WM, Rogers RS III, Reeve CM, Sheridan PJ (1992) Orofacial manifestations of Melkersson–Rosenthal syndrome. **Oral Surg Oral Med Oral Pathol** 74:610.

The earliest literature on MRS is credited to Hübschmann[63] in 1894. Melkersson[64] later reported his collected cases of seventh nerve paralysis and associated facial edema as a syndrome in 1928. Rosenthal[65] added the third feature, plicated tongue, in 1931. Miescher's[66] description in 1945 of several patients with cheilitis granulomatosa suggests to some that the disorder should be named Miescher–Melkersson–Rosenthal syndrome.[62] According to Wadlington,[62] the first report of MRS in the pediatric literature did not appear until 1962, when Ehmann and Stickl described the syndrome in two children aged 22 months and 8 years.

The diagnosis of MRS is based on the clinical findings. The nature of the syndrome is such that dermatologic, oral, or neurologic manifestations may predominate at a given time. Facial swelling, the symptom most frequently reported, occurred in 93% of patients, with the lips being affected in 66%.[60] The edema occurs without prodrome, and signs of acute inflammation are absent. The swelling is usually nonerythematous, painless, nonpruritic, initially soft, and generally asymmetric. The inner aspect of the affected upper lip may enlarge two to three times its normal size (Fig. 9.8). The lip is rolled outward by the edema, exposing the normally moist mucosa to the air, causing secondary chapping and fissuring of the surface.[67]

The edema may persist for one or two days but seldom lasts longer than one week.[60–62] Intervals between attacks range from 1 day to $2\frac{1}{2}$ years, with a median time of $5\frac{1}{2}$ weeks.[60] Following several recurrences, the swelling tends to become persistent, brawny, and deforming. Physiognomic changes resulting from the labial edema include occasional problems with speech and mastication.[68] Despite the fact that the lips may become dry and fissured, xerostomia is not a complicating feature. Excess salivation has occurred in some instances.[68,69]

Lip swelling may be unilateral or bilateral and may involve either the upper or lower lip or both lips. Other oral structures that may become edematous include the tongue, buccal and palatal mucosa, alveolar process, and gingiva.[60] When the gingiva is involved, a distinct, well-demarcated bluish-red swelling is present. The forehead, eyelids, cheek, nose, and chin may become swollen when MRS is present.[60–62]

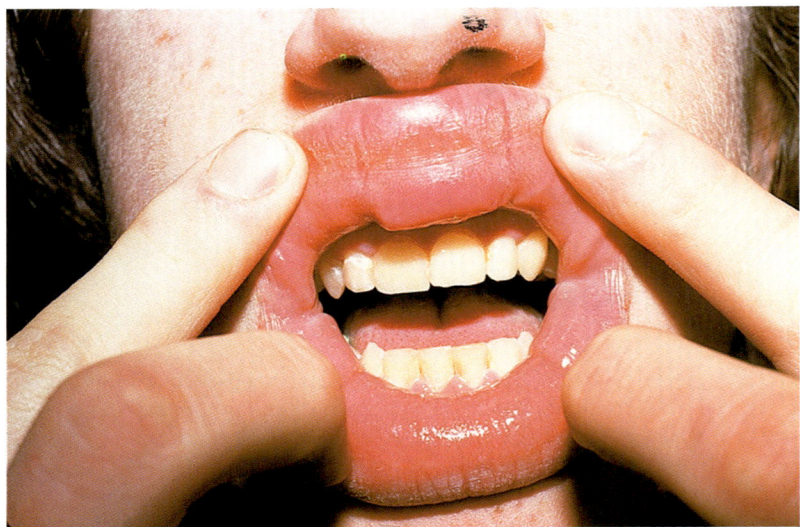

Fig. 9.8 Thickening and fibrosis of the lips in a young man with Melkersson–Rosenthal syndrome. The changes are most pronounced on the middle third of the upper lip.

Most often the facial edema antedates the onset of facial paralysis, but the two may begin simultaneously. Alternatively, the paralysis may even precede the swelling.[61,62] This paralytic component of the clinical triad usually begins suddenly, remains peripheral in nature, and is thus indistinguishable from Bell's palsy. The paralyzed side of the face frequently corresponds to the side that develops swelling but, like the edema, the paralysis is occasionally bilateral.[61,62] During subsequent attacks, the facial palsy may occur on the opposite side of the face from that previously afflicted.[61]

Scrotal tongue is the least frequently reported clinical finding in MRS. When present, as it is in 30% to 50% of cases,[61] it is either present from birth or is a manifestation of granulomatous glossitis. Of 58 cases reported by Alexander,[70] 90% had facial paralysis, 86% had edema of the face, and 77% had lingua plicata. One study found the complete triad in only nine of 23 cases surveyed.[60–62]

Constitutional symptoms occasionally associated with MRS include migraine headaches, hyperpyrexia, hyperhidrosis, chills, loss of taste, and slight visual impairment. Neurologic and ophthalmologic aberrations may be quite severe in certain cases.[61,62] The skin, hair, and nails remain normal, as do laboratory parameters.

MRS seemingly has no racial predilection, and during the first two decades of life the condition occurs more commonly in females.[61,62] Of 58 cases,[70] 45% had onset of their disease by the age of 20. Although the precise incidence is unknown, MRS was seen in 1 of 2100 cases in the dermatology outpatient setting.[69]

Infectious, allergic, and hereditary etiologies have been proposed, but to date no evidence exists to support an infectious or allergic basis for the disorder. It has been suggested that MRS may represent an incomplete autosomal–dominant trait of variable penetrance with the neural deficits and facial edema resulting from abiotrophic changes in the autonomic nervous system. An alternative theory[60,61] attributes the edema of the seventh cranial nerve and oral mucosa to a nonspecific stimulus that triggers vasomotor disturbances in the small arteries, capillaries, and nerves of the subcutaneous tissue.

Histologically, early lesions show only edema below an acanthotic epidermis. Chronically enlarged tissues are due to fibrosis and an increase in connective tissue stroma. Both acute and chronic lesions contain perivascular aggregates of lymphocytes, plasma cells, and histiocytes when specimens are taken from the tongue, check, or buccal mucosa. Noncaseating epithelioid cell granulomas with multinucleated giant cells may be seen in the edematous stroma. These granulomas may bulge into the vascular lumina, causing obstruction.[68] Oral Crohn's disease may exhibit the same clinical and histopathological features.[71]

Included in the differential diagnosis of facial palsy of childhood are Bell's palsy, idiopathic paralysis, otitis media, sarcoid, brain stem tumors, Guillain–Barré syndrome, leukemia or solid tumor malignancies, Ramsay Hunt syndrome, Well syndrome, mycobacterial infections, Hansen's disease, and acoustic neuroma.[69] The differential diagnosis considered in evaluation of facial swelling includes angioneurotic edema, erysipelas, and Ascher syndrome.[60]

Therapeutic measures for controlling the facial edema include systemic and intralesional steroids. Neither has proved curative, however.[60] Intralesional steroids injected every four weeks have provided fair results in some cases of chronic swelling.[62] Antibiotics and antihistamines have failed to alter the course of the disease. Wedge resections of the inner aspect of the lip have yielded good results in some cases, but care must be taken to remove all the underlying glandular tissue and to operate only when the disease is quiescent.[61] Some patients will require more than one surgical procedure to

63. Hübschmann H (1894) Über Recidive und Diplegie bei der sogenannten rheumatischen Facilislähmung. **Neurology** (NY) 13:815.
64. Melkersson E (1928) Ett fall av recidiverande facialispares i samband med angioneurotisk edem. **Hygiea** (Stockh) 90:737.
65. Rosenthal C (1931) Klinisch-erbbiologischer Beitrag zur Konstitutionspathologie. Gemeinsames Auftreten von (rezidivierender familiärer) Facialislähmung, angio-neurotischem Gesichtsödem und Lingua plicata in Arthritismus-Familien. **Z Ges Neurol Psychol** 131:475.
66. Miescher G (1945) Über essentielle granulomatöse Makrocheile (Cheilitis granulomatosa). **Dermatologica** 91:57.
67. Ziem PE, Pfrommer C, Goerdt S et al. (2000) Melkersson–Rosenthal syndrome in childhood: a challenge in differential diagnosis and treatment. **Br J Dermatol** 143:860–863.
68. Worsaae N, Pindborg JJ (1980) Granulomatous gingival manifestations of Melkersson–Rosenthal syndrome. **Oral Surg** 49:131.
69. Roseman B, Mulvihill JJ (1978) Melkersson–Rosenthal syndrome in a 7-year-old girl, **Pediatrics** 61:490.
70. Alexander RW, James RB (1972) Melkersson–Rosenthal syndrome: review of literature and report of case. **J Oral Surg** 30:599.
71. Haneke E (1985) Cheilitis granulomatosa bei Morbus Crohn und Melkersson-Rosenthal-Syndrom. **Dtsch Z Mund-Kiefer- und Gesichtschir** 9:232–234.

bring their disease under control. Clofazimine has been shown to suppress attacks of lip swelling in seven patients, and sustained control of swelling was maintained in the majority subsequent to discontinuation of the drug.[72] Recently, minocycline, both alone and in combination with prednisolone, was found to be effective.[73,74]

The facial paralysis of MRS often undergoes spontaneous resolution. Surgical intervention should be reserved for those patients who fail to recover after two months or in whom spontaneous recovery is incomplete. No recurrences have been noted following such decompression surgery.[60] During the acute stages of facial paralysis, some patients may benefit from ocular lubricants (artificial tears), analgesics, facial massage, and warm compresses. Therapy for lingua plicata is necessary only if trapped food particles inflame the dorsal surface of the tongue. In such instances, enhanced oral hygiene is usually curative. Relapses of MRS and cheilitis granulomatosa may occur many years after seeming recovery; therefore, a conservative approach is best in the management of the orofacial swelling.[61]

CONTACT STOMATITIS AND CHEILITIS

Contact stomatitis and cheilitis are less common than cutaneous dermatitis in all age groups; however, there are no figures for relative incidence in children as compared with adults. Like the skin, the oral mucosa is capable of two types of reactions: irritant contact dermatitis and allergic contact dermatitis. In general, mucosa seems more resistant to primary irritants than does skin and appears to be less easily sensitized, perhaps because the constant dilution by and flushing action of the saliva results in less prolonged contact with the sensitizer. It has also been suggested that the extensive vascularization of the oral mucous membranes aids in the absorption and dispersion of allergens.[75]

Irritant reactions are usually due to heat or chemical injury and most often involve the palate, tongue, and lips. Contact with very hot liquids or foods such as melted cheese may cause intense erythema, vesicles, and bullae, resulting in painful erosions. Chemicals may also cause superficial erosions; a well-known cause is acetylsalicylic acid, particularly when a tablet is held in contact with the buccal mucosa for a lengthy period. Chewing gum containing aspirin can also produce ulcerations of the oral mucosa.[76]

Allergic contact dermatitis can result from a variety of allergens and often involves the lips, angles of the mouth, and perioral skin as well as the oral mucosa (Fig. 9.9). In contrast to the skin, allergic stomatitis is usually characterized by a burning sensation, loss of taste, and numbness rather than itching. The mucosa develops intense erythema, inflammation, and edema, resulting in a smooth, shiny, glazed appearance. Although vesiculation occurs, these lesions are rarely evident because they rupture quickly; rather, erosions and ulcerations may be more prominent. The tongue may become edematous with atrophy of the filiform papillae. Acute allergic cheilitis may present as allergic contact dermatitis, often involving the neighboring skin, particularly when due to so-called herpes remedies, such as tromantadine. At times, there is angular cheilitis, and the lips may be dry, scaly, and fissured; edema and vesiculation of the lips are relatively less common.[38,75] Burning, itching and prickling of the palate and/or tongue may be experienced as so-called pollinosis equivalents, in type I allergy, and several cross-allergies of pollen and food (birch pollen associated with apple and other fruit allergies, artemisia pollen and carrot and celery allergies) are well-known clinical syndromes.[77]

The causative agents of contact stomatitis and cheilitis are numerous and varied. A general classification is provided in Table 9.5; specific ingredients must be sought from specialized publications and manufacturers. Popular brands and

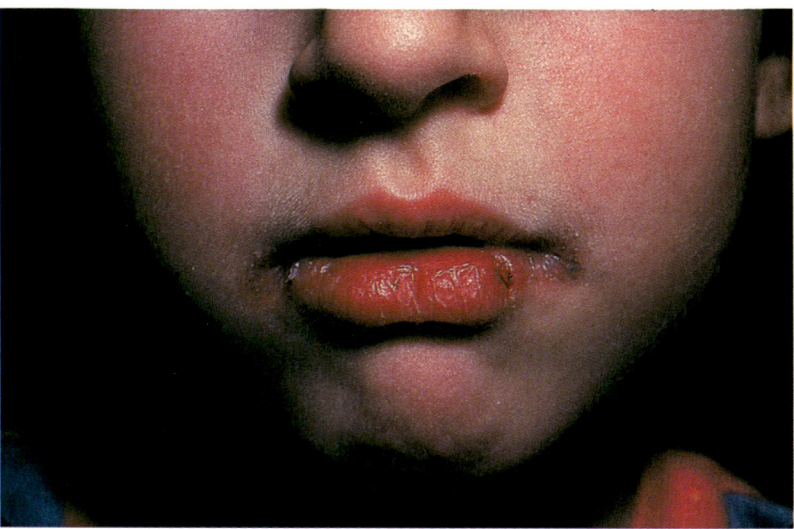

Fig. 9.9 Allergic contact dermatitis involving the lips and angles of the mouth due to toothpaste.

TABLE 9.5 Substances causing contact dermatitis

Dental or cosmetic preparations
  Toothpastes
  Mouthwashes
  Lipstick, chapstick
  Acrylic monomer (also from nail varnish)
  Metal alloy base
  Sunscreen preparations
  Orthodontic elastics
  Dental amalgam
Foods
  Mangoes, oranges, lemons, and other fruits
  Candies, pastries, ice cream, chewing gum
  Selected vegetables
  Beverages: colas, herbal teas
  Fish and seafood, cheese
  Nuts, spices
Therapeutic agents
  Antibiotics, tromantadine
  Procaine
  Alcohol
  Cough drops, lozenges, troches

---

available products change rapidly, and ingredients in a particular product may be altered periodically. Reactions to toothpastes[78] and mouthwashes are often due to flavorings, antiseptics, preservatives such as parabens, or alcohol. Essential oils, such as clove and cinnamon, found in toothpastes, chewing gum, and lipsticks, are commonly incriminated in contact stomatitis. Flavorings may also be responsible for reactions to therapeutic agents, such as antibiotics, lozenges, and troches. A number of plasma-cell gingivitis cases were associated with cinnamon-containing toothpaste and chewing gum.[79] However, most of these cases remained etiologically unclear.[80] A variety of foods are capable of causing

72. Neuhofer J, Fritsch P (1983) Cheilitis granulomatosa (Melkersson Rosenthal-Syndrom): Behandlung mit Clofazimin. **Hautarzt** 35:459.
73. Olivier V, Lacour JP, Castanet J et al. (2000) Cheilitis granulomatosa in a child. **Arch Pediatr** 7:274–277.
74. Stein SL, Mancini AJ (1999) Melkersson–Rosenthal syndrome in childhood: successful management with combination steroid and minocycline therapy. **J Am Acad Dermatol** 41:746–748.
75. Fisher AA (1973) Contact Dermatitis. Philadelphia: Lea & Febiger.
76. Claman HN (1967) Mouth ulcers associated with prolonged chewing of gum containing aspirin. **JAMA** 202:651.
77. Gutschmidt E, Körner E, Haneke E (1979) Saisonales Gaumenbrennen bei Allergie gegen Gräserpollen. **Z Hautkr** 54:817–820.
78. Sainio EL, Kanetra L (1995) Contact allergens in toothpaste and a review of their hypersensitivity. **Contact Dermatitis** 3(2):100–105.
79. Silverman S, Lozada F (1977) An epilogue to plasma-cell gingivostomatitis (allergic gingivostomatitis). **Oral Surg Oral Med Oral Pathol** 43:211–217.
80. Haneke E, Djawari D (1984) Immunoglobulin demonstration in circumorificial plasmocytosis. In: Immunodermatology, DM MacDonald, ed. London: Butterworths, pp. 173–175.

reactions.[81] as well as medicaments and cosmetics. The most common sensitizers in lipsticks are fluorescein stains and eosin indelible dyes, but many of today's products have flavorings as well. Biting of acrylate as well as henna stained nails led to severe allergic mucosal lesions. Piercing the lips or tongue may cause nickel allergy. A thorough history must be obtained; at times, repeated questioning is needed to uncover the offending agent.

Diagnosis can sometimes be made by elimination of the suspected agent. Patch testing is useful to ascertain the specific sensitizer but must be performed in the correct manner by someone knowledgeable in the technique. Direct testing of the oral mucosa is possible but not easily accomplished.[75] Differential diagnosis includes vitamin deficiencies, recurrent aphthous ulcerations, and angular cheilitis due to other causes.

Treatment for acute dermatitis of the lips may include cold wet compresses, applications of petrolatum, and a corticosteroid ointment. When the buccal mucosa is involved, a corticosteroid in Orabase may be helpful. Viscous lidocaine (Xylocaine) may provide relief of discomfort in the event of painful ulceration that interferes with eating, but this therapy should be used with caution in small children due to dose-related toxicity. Most important is identification and discontinuation of contact with the inciting agent.

MACROGLOSSIA

Macroglossia is defined as a resting tongue that protrudes beyond the teeth or alveolar ridge. Enlargement of the tongue may develop as a primary or secondary phenomenon, but it is not itself considered a disease entity.[82] A list of the conditions felt to be responsible for macroglossia is provided in Table 9.6. The tongue may be enlarged at birth or may become so only in adulthood. Macroglossia is not a common finding in the pediatric age group but, when discovered, should alert the clinician that a thorough evaluation is warranted.

In congenital macroglossia, overdevelopment of the musculature occurs with or without associated generalized muscle hypertrophy or hemihypertrophy. The presence of macroglossia due to muscle hypertrophy in an otherwise normal child is rare. Four clinical varieties of muscular macroglossia exist: (1) nodular enlargement not confined to exactly one-half of the tongue; (2) unilateral enlargement associated with localized hypertrophy of the same side of the face or jaw or hemihypertrophy of the body (the most common form); (3) uniform enlargement associated with generalized muscular hypertrophy of the rest of the body; and (4) uniform enlargement with no other ascertainable abnormalities.[83] These as well as other primary forms of macroglossia are less evident clinically than are secondary forms.[84]

Among the many causes of congenital macroglossia, the most frequently encountered is an underlying lymphangioma or hemangiolymphangioma. Enlargement of the tongue may also result from the presence of tumor-like growths of developmental origin (i.e., hamartomas, neurofibromas) or may be due to epithelial inclusion cysts. Although the genesis of these tumors is developmental, they may not become apparent until adolescence or later, when hormonal influences increase. Dermoid cysts are rare in the tongue. The differential diagnosis of newborns with an enlarged tongue must include Down's syndrome, congenital hypothyroidism, and Beckwith–Wiedemann syndrome (exophthalmos-macroglossia–gigantism syndrome with splanchnomegaly and glycolability) (Fig. 9.10).[85] Pseudomacroglossia in which a normal tongue extends beyond the alveolar ridge secondary to a small mouth can be seen in some patients with Down's, Marfan or Robinow syndrome. Many clinical syndromes have an associated macroglossia, particularly those due to inborn errors of metabolism. The lingual hypertrophy in such a setting is caused by excessive deposits of lipid or carbohydrate intermediates. In each case, other abnormalities accompany the macroglossia.

TABLE 9.6   Primary and secondary causes of macroglossia

Primary
  Muscular hypertrophy
Secondary
  Congenital
    Lymphangioma, hemangioma, hemangiomatosis, vascular malformations
  Acute and subacute inflammatory
    Mucosal erysipelas, abscess, actinomycosis, bee and wasp stings, angioedema
  Chronic inflammatory
    Granulomatous glossitis, dissecting glossitis in chronic mucocutaneous candidiasis, glossitis interstitialis luica, lepromatous leprosy
  Chromosome abnormalities
    Trisomy 4p syndrome, triploidy syndrome, trisomy 21 syndrome (Down's syndrome), Panse syndrome
  Dysplastic forms
    Beckwith–Wiedemann syndrome (exophthalmos-macroglossia-gigantism syndrome)
    Bruck–de Lange syndrome
    Fetal face syndrome (Robinow syndrome), maxillo-facial (Peters–Hövels) syndrome
  Metabolic storage disease
    Mucopolysaccharidoses I, II, III, VI
    Generalized gangliosidosis S
    Glycogen storage disease
  Endocrine disorders
    Congenital hypothyroidism
  Tumors
    Granular cell tumor
    Neurofibroma

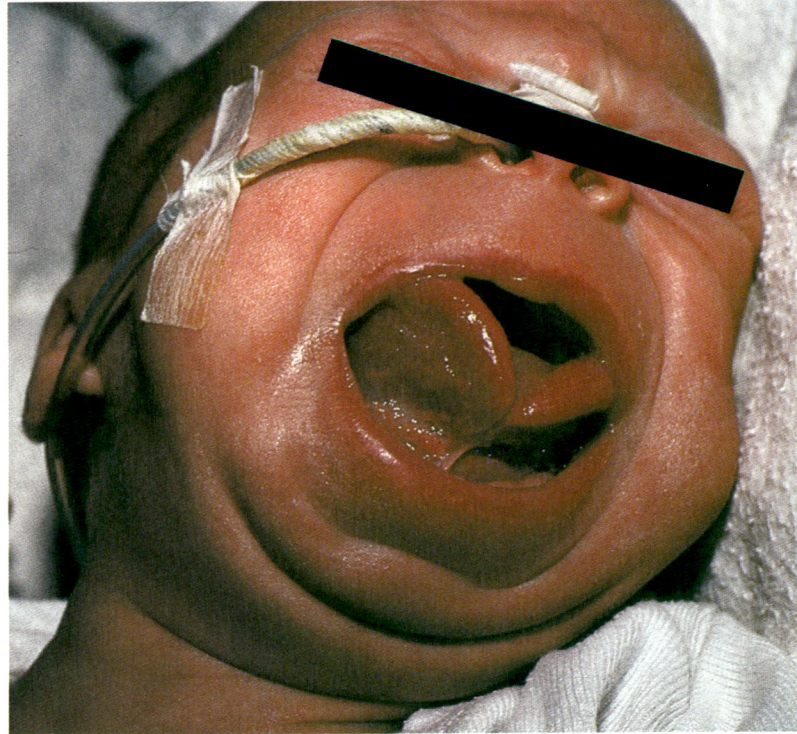

Fig. 9.10   Macroglossia in a child with Beckwith–Wiedemann syndrome.

81. Hausen BM, Hjorth N (1984) Skin reactions to topical food exposure. Dermatol Clin 2:567.
82. Velcek FT, Klotz DH, Hill CH et al. (1979) Tongue lesions in children. J Pediatr Surg 14:238.
83. Bronstein IP, Abelson SM, von Bonin G (1937) Macroglossia in children. Am J Dis Child 54:1328.
84. Shafer AD (1968) Primary macroglossia. Clin Pediatr 7:357.
85. Sotelo-Avila C, Gonzales-Crussi F, Fowler JW (1980) Complete and incomplete forms of Beckwith–Wiedemann syndrome: their oncogenic potential. J Pediatr 96:47.

Macroglossia that develops from either primary or secondary factors may displace the teeth and cause malocclusion because of the strength of the muscles involved and the pressure exerted by the tongue on the teeth. The lateral borders of the tongue may become scalloped or crenated when pushed against the teeth (impressiones dentatae.[38] An enlarged tongue may interfere with respiration, feeding, and speech. Therapy should be aimed at treating the underlying cause, when feasible. Surgery may be necessary to reduce the tissue bulk.[86]

LINGUA PLICATA

Lingua plicata represents the most common developmental anomaly of the tongue. A variety of names have been given to this benign condition including fissured tongue, scrotal tongue, and furrowed tongue. Lingua plicata is an autosomal-dominant trait with variable penetrance. Patterns of fissuring vary from a haphazard arrangement to one of symmetric branching from a central lingual groove that runs anteroposteriorly along the dorsum of the tongue.[87] The fissures may intersect, resulting in a grossly pebbled or cushioned appearance of the surface of the tongue.

These surface changes do not usually affect speech or mastication. The epithelium in the depth of the furrows is thinned with almost no keratinization. If the furrows are deep, they may serve as reservoirs of trapped food debris, permitting bacterial and mycotic proliferation and, ultimately, chronic inflammation. Occasionally painful, this condition responds well to brushing of the tongue with a toothbrush two to four times a day. Alternate therapeutic suggestions include warm (alcohol-free) mouthwash rinses and coating of the tongue with unflavored milk of magnesia.

The overall incidence of fissured tongue increases with age. The prevalence ranges from 3% to 5% in the general population[87] with children between the ages of 5 and 18 years having a prevalence of only 1.08%.[88] No significant race or sexual predominance is recognized. About 20% develop superimposed geographic tongue (Fig. 9.11).[87] Lingua plicata is frequently seen in individuals with Down's syndrome and is also one of the features of MRS.[87]

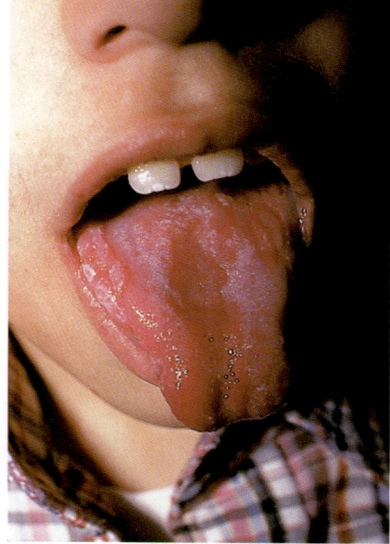

Fig. 9.11 Geographic and fissured tongue.

BLACK HAIRY TONGUE (LINGUA PILOSA NIGRA)

Black hairy tongue is very rare in children. It is a relatively innocuous condition that affects the dorsum of the tongue. The clinical forms of hairy tongue may be divided into two groups. In the first form, true hairy tongue, filiform papillae become elongated with or without discoloration. The second group, pseudohairy tongue, encompasses discoloration of the tongue without associated hypertrophy of the lingual papillae.[87]

The combined effect of elongated, hypertrophic filiform papillae and diminished desquamation results in the development of a thick, matted layer on the mid-dorsal surface of the tongue. Although discoloration may be absent, it may also range from yellowish-white to brown or black.[38] The etiology of this condition remains obscure, but it has been reported in patients on systemic antibiotic therapy and those with colonization of the tongue by *C. albicans* The use of systemic antibiotics may cause a shift in the oral bacterial–mycologic flora, allowing chromogenic bacteria to colonize the tongue and produce a dark pigment.[89] It has also been hypothesized that a lower pH on the surface of the tongue predisposes to the development of black hairy tongue.[90]

Occasionally, the hypertrophied papillae are sufficiently long to cause tickling or gagging as a result of contact with the soft palate or uvula. In pseudohairy tongue, discoloration may result from fruits, other foods, candy, colored or flavored beverages, and medicaments. The tongue coatings are usually removed by salivary flow, speaking, or the ingestion of food.[90] Therefore, debilitated patients receiving no oral feedings or on tube feedings may be rendered particularly susceptible to the development of black hairy tongue. In addition, oral hygiene is typically suboptimal in such a setting.

Therapy should be directed at enhancing the cleanliness of the oral cavity. Brushing the tongue with toothpaste and a toothbrush two to three times daily often remedies the condition within a few day's time.

GEOGRAPHIC TONGUE (ANNULUS MIGRANS, EXFOLIATIO MUCOSAE AREATA)

Annulus migrans or geographic tongue, sometimes also called migratory "glossitis," refers to discrete red patches surrounded by raised white to yellowish polycyclic borders affecting the tongue, buccal mucosa, soft palate, tonsils, or the floor of the mouth. The lateral edges, tip, or undersurface of the tongue may be involved in addition to the dorsal surface. Typically, nonlingual lesions are not seen unless the tongue is also involved.[91] The lesions may already start in early childhood. In 40%, geographic tongue is associated with plicated tongue.

The collarlike polycyclic configurations in the oral cavity change in location and prominence from day to day. The elevated borders range in color from pale gray to bright yellowish-white, and their visibility may span from barely perceptible to florid (Fig. 9.12). The condition may be manifest by a single patch or by multiple areas that are discrete or confluent. The onset of geographic stomatitis is rapid, and persistence is common, with lesions often lasting several months.[92] The circinate lesions may, however, appear and disappear rapidly only to reappear at a later date. They often exacerbate during stress.[93]

The stomatitis usually begins on the lingual surface with loss of the filiform papillae around a fissure and hypertrophy of neighboring papillae. The progression of arcuate borders seemingly occurs in an anterior-medial direction, and changes in configuration can occur as rapidly as within two hours.[94] If only the tongue is involved, the terms of geographic tongue, lingua geographic, annulus migrans, exfoliata areata linguae, lingual dystrophy, and

86. Massengil R, Pickrell K (1978) Surgical correction of macroglossia. **Pediatrics** 61:485.
87. Hornstein OP (1996) Erkrankungen des Mundes. Stuttgart Berlin Köln: Kohlhammer, pp. 138–140.
88. Redman RS (1970) Prevalence of geographic tongue, fissured tongue, median rhomboid glossitis, and hairy tongue among 3,611 Minnesota schoolchildren. **Oral Surg** 30:390.
89. Shklar G, McCarthy PL (1976) The Oral Manifestations of Systemic Disease. Boston: Butterworths.
90. Lynch MA, Brightman VJ, Greenberg MS, eds (1984) Burket's Oral Medicine, 8th ed. Philadelphia: JB Lippincott.
91. Hume WJ (1975) Geographic stomatitis: a critical review. **J Dent** 3:25:80.
92. Barton DH, Spier SK, Crovello TJ (1982) Benign migratory glossitis and allergy. **Pediatr Dent** 4:249.
93. Redman RS, Vancwe FL, Gorlin RJ et al. (1966) Psychological component in the etiology of geographic tongue. **J Dent Res** 45:1403–1408.
94. Zagarelli EV, Kutscher AH, Mercadante JA et al. (1963) Geographic tongue: relation of change in appearance to time. **J South Calif Dent Assoc** 31:11.

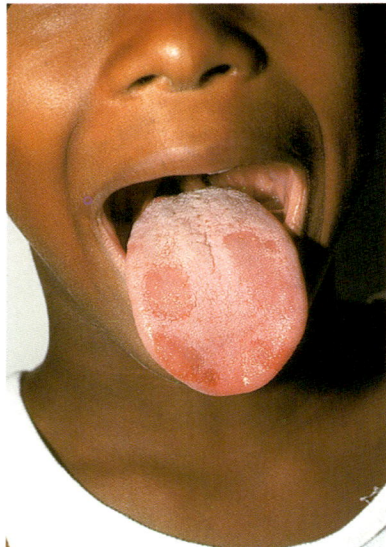

Fig. 9.12   Geographic tongue.

tuberculum impar to retract, allowing interposition of a structure devoid of papillae before the lateral halves of the tongue fuse. The consistently median localization of this condition and an occasional notch in the tip of the tongue favor this theory. It is also suggested that a localized chronic infection, most commonly with *C. albicans*, causes this alteration rather than a developmental defect. The peculiar anatomy of the mid-dorsal surface of the tongue is felt by some[102–104] to permit proliferation of *Candida* in certain predisposed patients. The overgrowth of this organism results in loss of the filiform papillae on the dorsal surface of the tongue.

Wright[104] established the following six diagnostic clinical features: (1) a characteristic location in the median raphe anterior to the circumvallate papillae; (2) a roughly rhomboid shape; (3) a rosy color of the affected area; (4) variable surface changes (smooth to fissured) and absence of papillae, slightly depressed to raised and nodular; (5) slight induration of the tongue; and (6) lack of symptoms. The glossitis becomes evident when the filiform papillae are lost, particularly when the surface of the tongue appears coated or when the papillae are matted.[38] The deeper red or rose color of the anomalous tissue contrasts sharply with the pink color of the normal tongue.[87]

The incidence of median rhomboid glossitis in the general population is approximately 1%.[38,105] Although Baughman[106] detected no cases in a survey of 10 000 schoolchildren, Redman[88] reported three cases in patients under 10 years of age. The condition is without sex or racial predilection.

On histologic examination, there is loss of papillae with varying degrees of parakeratosis, downward proliferation of the spinous layer with elongation of the rete ridges that may branch or anastomose, and a lymphocytic infiltrate within the connective tissue. Numerous blood vessels and lymphatics are apparent. Degeneration and hyalin formation within the underlying muscle are also seen.[104] In two studies 85% and 71% had evidence of candidal hyphae in the parakeratin layer.[104]

The lingual changes are typically asymptomatic. Anticandidal therapy in the form of topical nystatin, clotrimazole troches or even systemically active antifungals may reduce the fungal colonization but will not improve the appearance of the mucosal surface devoid of papillae. No additional specific therapy is warranted, although fastidious oral hygiene may hasten recovery. The differential diagnosis must include a well-developed thyroglossal duct or an aberrant thyroid gland.[90]

GLOSSITIS

Glossitis refers to inflammatory alterations in the normal lingual coating as a result of nutritional deficiency, infection, allergy, or toxic reactions. Glossitis may also be idiopathic. Changes in the inflamed tongue may include erythema, edema, pain, and hypertrophy, or loss of papillae. These changes may occur early in the course of an illness or vitamin deficiency or only after long-standing insult. In most instances, recovery is fairly prompt following institution of appropriate therapy. The various forms of glossitis are detailed under their appropriate etiologies. The discovery of glossitis signals the necessity for a careful history and physical examination (see also Table 9.6).

GLOSSODYNIA AND GLOSSOPYROSIS

Glossodynia and glossopyrosis refer to sensations of pain and burning within the mouth, typically without pathological changes of the mucosa. The typical glossodynia patient is an edentulous postmenopausal woman, and occurrence

transitory benign plaques of the tongue may be applied. The term geographic tongue reflects the resemblances of the oral pattern to land masses and oceans on a map.

The lesions of annulus migrans are typically asymptomatic but affected persons may report mild burning, irritation, or discomfort of the oral mucosal membranes or tongue when exposed to hot, cold, or spicy foods. When the polycyclic borders resolve, healing is complete and no scarring results.

The reported frequency of this entity ranges from 0.28% to 14.4% of the population.[92] Geographic stomatitis occurs more often in children than in adults. One study of 5425 infants up to 2 years of age noted the presence of geographic tongue in 775 (14.29%).[95] Typical oral lesions have been seen as early as 2 to 4 weeks of life.[91] There is no racial predilection, and, although some authorities[96] believe that females are affected more often than males, it is probable that no true sex predominance exists.[91]

The precise etiology of geographic stomatitis remains uncertain. Although an infectious pathogenesis has been suspected, no organism has been isolated, and scrapings of the tongues of affected patients have not provoked disease in disease-free patients following inoculation.[97] Circinate lesions of the tongue have been reported in patients with psoriasis (particularly pustular psoriasis),[98] Reiter syndrome,[99] and atopic dermatitis.[100,101] Other diseases associated with geographic tongue include seborrheic dermatitis, spasmodic bronchitis of childhood, and allergic diathesis.[100] The changes possibly represent a reaction pattern of the tongue to a number of different underlying conditions.

Histologically, the lesions show typical spongiform pustules with necrosis of the superficial epithelium and are thus indistinguishable from those of pustular psoriasis or Reiter syndrome.[99] Therapy of this benign condition is generally unsuccessful and unwarranted.[92]

MEDIAN RHOMBOID GLOSSITIS

Among anomalies of the tongue, median rhomboid glossitis, or central papillary atrophy of the tongue, is the most likely to give rise to diagnostic problems. This abnormality has previously been attributed to failure of the

95. Rahaminoff P, Muhsam HV (1957) Some observations on 1246 cases of geographic tongue. **Am J Dis Child** 93:519.
96. Rowe NH (1986) Diseases of the oral mucosa. In: Clinical Dermatology, Demis DJ, McGuire J eds. vol. 4. Philadelphia: Harper & Row, unit 28–1, p. 1.
97. Redman RS, Shapiro BL, Gorlin RL (1972) Hereditary component in the etiology of benign migratory glossitis. **Am J Hum Genet** 24:124.
98. Hubler WR Jr (1984) Lingual lesions of generalized pustular psoriasis. **J Am Acad Dermatol** 11:1069.
99. O'Keefe E, Braverman IM, Cohen I (1973) Annulus migrans: identical lesions in pustular psoriasis, Reiter's syndrome and geographic tongue. **Arch Dermatol** 107:240.
100. Marks R, Simons MJ (1979) Geographic tongue—a manifestation of atopy. **Br J Dermatol** 101:159.
101. Ullmann W (1981) Korrelation zwischen Exfoliatio areata linguae und Atopie. **Hautarzt** 32:629–631.
102. Cooke BEO (1975) Median rhomboid glossitis, candidiasis and not a developmental anomaly. **Br J Dermatol** 93:399.
103. Farman AG, Nutt G (1975) Oral candida, debilitating disease and atrophic lesions of the tongue. **J Biol Bucc** 4:203.
104. Wright BA (1978) Median rhomboid glossitis: not a misnomer. Review of the literature and histologic study of twenty-eight cases. **Oral Surg** 46:806.
105. Ullmann W, Hoffmann M (1981) Glossitis rhombica mediana. **Hautarzt** 32:571–574.
106. Baughman RA (1971) Median rhomboid glossitis: a developmental anomaly? **Oral Surg** 31:56.

in children is exceedingly rare.[107] These paresthesias most frequently involve the tongue, but the palate, lips, and other sites in the oral cavity may be symptomatic (orolingual paresthesias). The sensations reported include itching, stinging, and a sandy feeling, in addition to pain and burning. Most often, no clinical lesions exist, and thus no physical alterations correlate with the paresthesias.[38,107]

A careful history and physical examination are indicated for patients who complain of glossodynia. The mouth should be examined thoroughly and a culture for *C. albicans* obtained as pain or burning within the oral cavity may herald acute atrophic oral candidiasis. A therapeutic trial of an antiyeast agent such as nystatin is rarely helpful.[108]

Systemic diseases that must be excluded during an evaluation are vitamin B complex deficiency, iron deficiency anemia, diabetes mellitus, and Sjögren syndrome. Local irritation from tongue habits, carious teeth, medicaments, and dentifrices should be considered. Flavoring in chewing gum can produce a painful, burning tongue without observable clinical alteration.[90,107]

Therapy should be directed at correcting whatever systemic or local problems contribute to the oral paresthesias. Even when no etiology is found, chewing gum should be avoided, as the irritating action of the flavoring agents, medicaments, or the slightly abrasive chicle base may worsen pre-existing discomfort. Some benefit maybe derived from chewing unmedicated paraffin, which enhances salivary flow.[90]

XEROSTOMIA

Xerostomia may be divided into subjective and objective. Subjective xerostomia is mainly seen in psychiatrically ill persons who suffer from the sensation of dry mouth but have enough saliva to speak, chew and swallow normally.[107] Objective xerostomia is a clinical manifestation of salivary gland dysfunction and does not of itself comprise a disease entity. Many factors predispose to xerostomia and an outline of these is provided in Table 9.7.[109] The degree of dryness may range from a slight burning sensation with normal-appearing mucous membranes to complete lack of salivary flow with dry atrophic membranes that are pale and translucent.[38] The minor salivary glands of the oral mucosa are mainly responsible for lubrication and oral well-feeling.[107]

In the pediatric age group, xerostomia rarely occurs. Children with agenesis of the salivary glands may have varying degrees of oral dryness. The hypoplastic salivary glands including the intraoral accessory glands predispose those with anhidrotic ectodermal dysplasia to dry mucous membranes. Xerostomia is also a near-constant symptom in chronic graft-versus-host disease,[110] and seen in about one-third of children with AIDS.[111] This is particularly troublesome when dentures are worn, as tenderness and discomfort result from a poorly lubricated interface.

Xerostomia and caries often develop rapidly following initiation of irradiation to the lower face, but also after whole-body irradiation.[112] The caries involve the dentin and cementum exposed at the cervical areas of the teeth and the cusp tips and incisor edges. These alterations are nearly pathognomonic for postirradiation cavities.

Salivary substitutes in the form of sprays or liquids help moisten and lubricate the oral cavity.[113] These agents are formulated to have a viscosity and electrolyte concentration that approximates whole saliva. Flavorings are added to give a pleasant taste, and salivary substitutes may be used, such as the following preparations:

- Rx Sodium carboxymethylcellulose
  0.5% aq.sol. (prepared by your pharmacist)
  Disp: 8-oz bottle
  Rinse as often as needed to moisten and lubricate the mouth.

TABLE 9.7 Etiology of xerostomia

Congenital
  Hypoplasia or aplasia of salivary glands; ectodermal dysplasia
Drug induced
  Anticholinergics
  Sympathomimetics
  Opium and derivatives
  Ergotamine
  Diuretics
Infections
  Mumps
  Tuberculosis
  Syphilis
  Actinomycosis
Neoplasms
  Primary tumors, benign and malignant
  Infiltrative processes, as lymphoma
Collagen vascular
  Systemic lupus erythematosus
  Scleroderma
  Dermatomyositis
  Mixed connective tissue disease
  Sjögren syndrome
Neurologic
  Post-traumatic nerve injury
  Degenerative processes such as multiple sclerosis
Obstructive
  Stone (sialolithiasis)
  Tumor
  Inflammation
  Scar or stricture
Dietary or absorption detect
  Vitamin deficiency (vitamin A, riboflavin, nicotinic acid)
  Pernicious anemia
  Iron deficiency anemia
Endocrine
  Diabetes mellitus
  Hypothyroidism
Postirradiation
Graft-versus-host disease

- Rx Saliv-aid substitute (Copley Pharmaceuticals, Inc.)
  Disp: 2-oz bottle
  Sig: Squeeze 2 to 4 drops into the mouth as often as needed to moisten and lubricate the mouth.
- Rx Salivart saliva substitute (Westport Pharmaceuticals, Inc.)
  Disp: 50-ml spray can
  Sig: Spray into the mouth and throat as needed to moisten and lubricate the mouth.
- Rx Moi-stur (Kingswood Laboratories, Inc.)
  Disp: 120-ml bottle
  Sig: Spray into mouth once or twice to coat all surfaces.
  Use as often as desired.
- Rx Xero-Lube saliva substitute (Scherer Laboratories, Inc.)
  Disp: 6-oz bottle
  Sig: Rinse as often as needed to moisten and lubricate the mouth.

Xero-lube is the only solution containing fluoride, and it is preferable in any patient with dentition. Daily application of stannous fluoride gel, 0.4%

107. Haneke E (1980) Zungen- und Mundschleimhautbrennen. München-Wien: Hanser-Verlag.
108. Zegarelli DJ (1984) Burning mouth, an analysis of 57 patients. **Oral Surg** 58:34.
109. Konzelman JL, Terezhalmy GT (1983) Xerostomia: diagnosis and treatment. **US Navy Med** 74:16.
110. Nicolatou-Galitis O, Kitra V, Van Vliet-Constantinidou C et al. (2001) The oral manifestations of chronic graft-versus-host disease (cGVHD) in paediatric allogeneic bone marrow transplant recipients. **J Oral Pathol Med** 30:148–153.
111. Kozinetz CA, Carter AB, Simon C et al. (2000) Oral manifestations of pediatric vertical HIV infection. **AIDS Patient Care STDS** 14:89–94.
112. Majorana A, Schubert MM, Porta F et al. (2000) Oral complications of pediatric hematopoietic cell transplantation: diagnosis and management. **Support Care Cancer** 8:353–365.
113. Hebert AA, Berg JH (1992) Oral mucous membrane diseases of childhood: I, Mucositis and xerostomia. II. Recurrent aphthous stomatitis. III. Herpetic stomatitis. **Sem Dermatol** 11:80.

5 to 10 drops in a moist carrier for 5 minutes, is recommended to promote remineralization of the tooth enamel in patients with xerostomia.

Comprehensive management objectives for patients with xerostomia[114] include: (1) discovery and treatment of the etiologic factor(s), if possible; (2) implementation of palliative therapy, including local and/or systemic use of various substances that may increase salivary flow; and (3) initiation and implementation of a well-organized preventative dental program to decrease or eliminate the incidence of clinical complications associated with xerostomia.

LYMPHANGIOMA (LYMPHATIC MALFORMATION)
(See also Chapter 20)

Lymphangiomas of the oral cavity are rare in children. When present, the majority are detected at birth or within the first two years of life.[38,115] No sexual predilection or hereditary predisposition has been reported. Lymphangiomas consist of multiple lymphatic vascular channels lined by single or multiple layers of endothelial cells. The surrounding fibrous tissue may be abundant or scanty. Lymphangiomas usually occur as solitary lesions, but bleeding may mimic an association with other vascular malformations such as hemangiomas.

The tongue is the most common location of lymphangiomas within the oral cavity, but the palate, buccal mucosa, gingiva, and lips may also be affected.[38] Lymphangiomas have been noted on the alveolar ridges of neonates.[116] When macroglossia occurs as a result of a lymphangioma, the anterior dorsal two-thirds of the tongue are most often affected (Fig. 9.13). The nasopharynx thus remains patent despite enlargement of the tongue, and respiratory embarrassment is rare.[117] Furthermore, taste is infrequently altered by the presence of a lymphangioma in the tongue.

These intraoral vascular malformations are characterized clinically as spongy compressible masses. The lesions can be unilateral, bilateral, or diffuse. Most often they are bilateral with indistinct lateral margins. Irregular nodularity of the surface of the tongue with gray and pink projections and accompanying macroglossia is pathognomonic of a lingual lymphangioma.[38] The surface of the tongue varies in appearance with the emergence and regression of lymphangiomatous vesicles. Tiny papillomatous residues remain at the sites of resorbed vesicles. These papillomas are painful but, unlike their antecedent counterparts, do not bleed easily following trauma.[118] Included in the differential diagnosis are condylomata acuminata, other oral verrucous lesions, Goltz syndrome, epidermal nevus or neurofibroma of the tongue, and hereditary hemorrhagic telangiectasia.

The lymphangiomatous tongue may grow at a rate equal to or exceeding the growth of the affected child. Following trauma or an upper respiratory infection, the tongue may enlarge within hours and require months to return to its original size. Pain frequently accompanies such swelling. As lymphatic drainage becomes increasingly impaired in the course of repeated trauma or infection, the tongue becomes permanently hypertrophied. Certain foods, particularly salty ones, may trigger some lingual edema and discomfort, but these symptoms are usually temporary.

Lymphangiomas that produce marked enlargement of the tongue tend to cause abnormal bone development, drooling, and difficulties with feeding and speech. During sleep the protuberant tongue dries out, predisposing to both fissuring and bleeding. These clinical complications usually have their onset before 3 years of age. Lymphangiomas causing overgrowth of adjacent structures and destruction of tissues may predispose to mandibular development that is out of proportion to maxillary growth. The associated carious teeth presumably result from lymphangioma-induced alteration of the tooth buds.[118]

Oral lymphatic malformation (Fig. 9.14) may communicate with lymphatic malformations in the neck (cystic hygromas).

Surgery has proved the most efficacious therapeutic modality when such intervention is deemed necessary. Following surgical removal, the lesions have a tendency to recur. This tendency increases with the increasing age of the patient. This is probably due to the fact that intraoral lymphangiomas often extend far beyond their visible border and can often not be removed completely. Electrodesiccation of hemorrhagic lymphangiectasias is followed by edema, pain, and inflammation of the tongue and therefore has little application.

These vascular lesions are more radioresistant and insensitive to sclerosing agents than are hemangiomas (see Chapter 20). Spontaneous regression is rare. Neodymiun:YAG laser therapy, said to be able to "seal off" lymphatic vessels, may prove beneficial for some tongue[119] and other mucous membrane[120] lymphangiomas, but each case must be evaluated carefully before

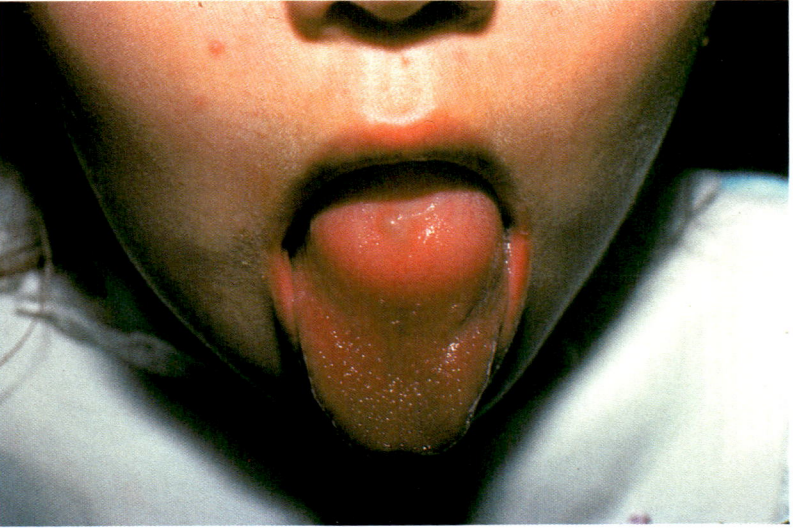

Fig. 9.13   Microcystic lymphatic malformation on the central portion of the tongue.

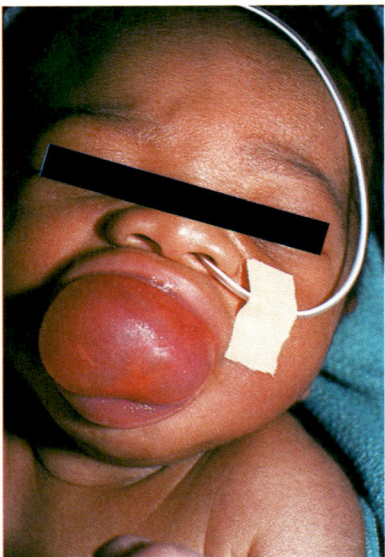

Fig. 9.14   Macrocystic lymphatic malformation of the tongue.

114. Navazesh M, Ship II (1983) Xerostomia: diagnosis and treatment. **Am J Otolaryngol** 4:283.
115. Watson WL, McCarthy WD (1940) Blood and lymph vessel tumors: a report of 1,056 cases. **Surg Gynecol Obstet** 71:569.
116. Levin LS, Jorgenson RJ, Jarvey BA (1976) Lymphangiomas of the alveolar ridges in neonates. **Pediatrics** 58:881.
117. Rice JP, Carson SH (1985) A case report of lingual lymphangioma presenting as recurrent massive tongue enlargement. **Clin Pediatr** 24:47.
118. Koop CE, Moschakis EA (1961) Capillary lymphangioma of the tongue complicated by glossitis. **Pediatrics** 27:800.
119. Dover JS, Arndt KA, Geronemus RG et al. (1990) Neodymium-Yag Lasers. In: Illustrated Cutaneous Laser Surgery. Norwalk, CT: Appleton & Lange, p. 121.
120. Alani HM, Warren RM (1992) Percutaneous photocoagulation of deep vascular lesions using fiberoptic laser wand. **Ann Plast Surg** 29:143.

this modality is employed. Results of therapy with this laser may or may not be acceptable and current literature citing long-term follow-up are lacking.

Systemic steroids may lessen the swelling due to glossitis or postoperative edema but play no role in ongoing management of oral lymphangiomas.

BENIGN PAPULAR LESIONS OF THE TONGUE

In addition to lymphangioma, several other types of benign papular lesions can be localized to the tongue. These lesions differ somewhat in their clinical characteristics and can often be identified by their location, surface configuration, color, and consistency (Table 9.8 and Figs 9.15–9.17). If the diagnosis is not apparent by inspection, histologic examination will usually provide a definitive diagnosis.

MUCOSAL CYSTS

Epstein's pearls and Bohn's nodules are tiny, 1–3mm, circumscribed asymptomatic cysts found in the oral cavity of newborn infants. Epstein's pearls, found at the junction of the hard and soft palate along the midpalatine raphe, represent tiny mucous gland cysts that arise from remnants of salivary gland structures.[78,121] Bohn's nodules develop following entrapment of epithelial remnants during embryologic development of the oral cavity. These inclusion cysts are distributed in a linear fashion along the alveolar ridge (Fig. 9.18).[78,121]

Both varieties of cysts are typically multiple in the newborn, particularly when careful examination is performed within the first 24 hours of life.[121,122] The highest incidence of these cysts occurs in Japanese infants (88.7% to 91.4%), followed by white (76.8% to 85%) and black (63% to

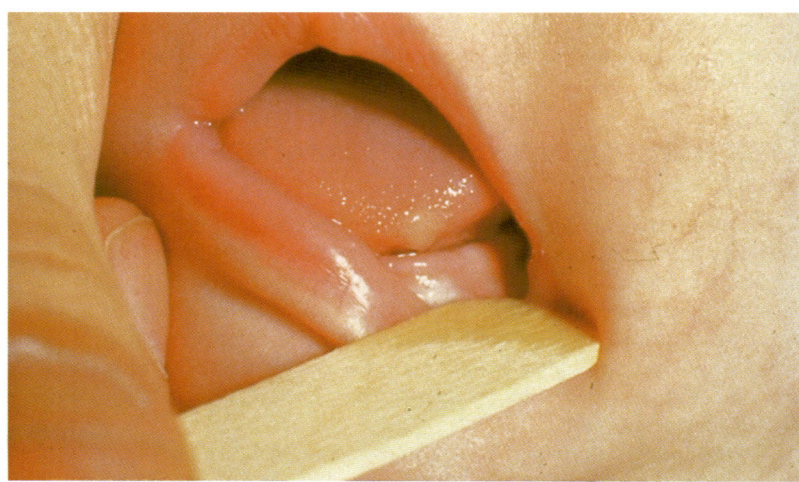

Fig. 9.15   Fibroma on lateral border of the tongue of an infant, congenital.

TABLE 9.8   Benign papular lesions of the tongue/oral mucosa

Lesion	Clinical characteristics	Histologic findings
Fibroma	Smooth, pink or white, firm, sessile or pedunculated; nonpainful; most common on dorsum, tip and and lateral margin (Fig. 9.15)	Dense bundles of collagen, scattered fibrocytes in submucosa; tip may be keratotic
Pseudofibroma (proptosis [diapneusis] linguae, buccalis	Mucosa-colored, soft, flat nodules opposite a missing tooth	Propulsion of normal mucosa, tip may exhibit denser epithelium
Pyogenic granuloma	Deep red, ulcerated, sessile; recurrent bleeding common; rarely painful; usually on dorsum	Localized proliferation of vascular tissue; mixed inflammatory infiltrate; ulcerated mucosa
Traumatic granuloma	Firm, sessile, ulcerated; nonpainful; most common on dorsum	Proliferation of fibroblasts and histocytes into striated muscle of tongue; mixed inflammatory infiltrate including eosinophils
Squamous papilloma	White, pedunculated, painless, digitate surface	Keratinized epithelium; thick connective tissue core; mild inflammation
Verruca (condyloma acuminatum)	Multiple, sessile, or pedunculated, white to pink; painless (Fig. 9.16)	Hyperkeratosis; acanthosis; vacuolated cells in spinous layer, intranuclear viral inclusions
Hemangioma	Red to blue, sessile, blanchable, and compressible; if large, may cause macroglossia; may ulcerate with trauma	Numerous dilated vascular spaces
Lymphangioma	Solitary or multiple; white, pink, or deep red; vesicopapules and nodules; if large, may cause macroglossia	Dilated lymph-filled vessels lined by single layer of endothelial cells
Lipoma	Yellow, compressible, sessile nodules; usually lateral borders	Nodules of fat in fibrovascular stroma
Granular cell tumor	Pink, firm, sessile nodules (Fig. 9.17)	Infiltrate of large oval cells with abundant fine granular cytoplasm within muscle bundles, neural markers positive
Neurofibroma, neurilemmoma	Diffuse or circumscribed pink nodule; lateral border of tongue	Proliferation of neurofibroblasts and collagen within tongue, neural markers positive
Neuroma	Circumscribed sessile pink nodules; usually dorsal surface; traumatic neuromas painful; mucosal neuromas painless	Fibrous connective tissue with intertwining nerve fibers and neurofibroblasts, neural markers including neurofilaments positive
Epidermal nevus	Papillomatous white or pink plaque or linear lesion	Hyperkeratosis, papillomatosis, acanthosis

Adapted from Newland JR[406] with permission.

121. Ikemura K, Kakinoki Y, Nishio K, Suenaga Y (1983) Cysts of the oral mucosa in newborns. A clinical observation. **Sangyo Ika Daigaku Zasshi** 5:163.

122. Flinck A, Paludan A, Matsson L et al. (1994) Oral findings in a group of newborn Swedish children. **Int J Paediatr Dent** 4:67–73.

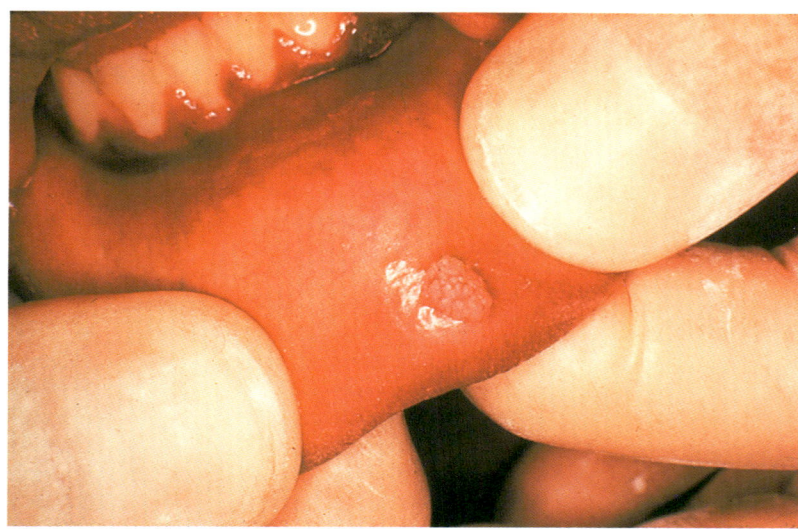

Fig. 9.16   Verrucous papilloma on the lower lip.

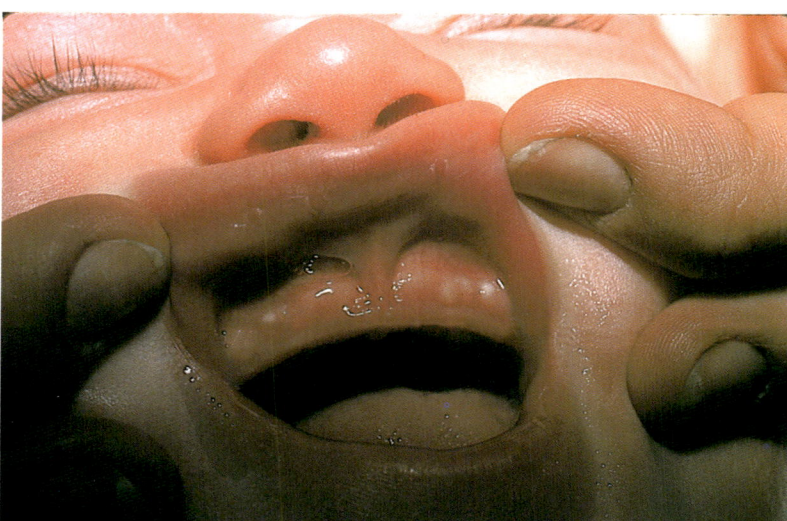

Fig. 9.18   Bohn's nodules along the upper alveolar ridge.

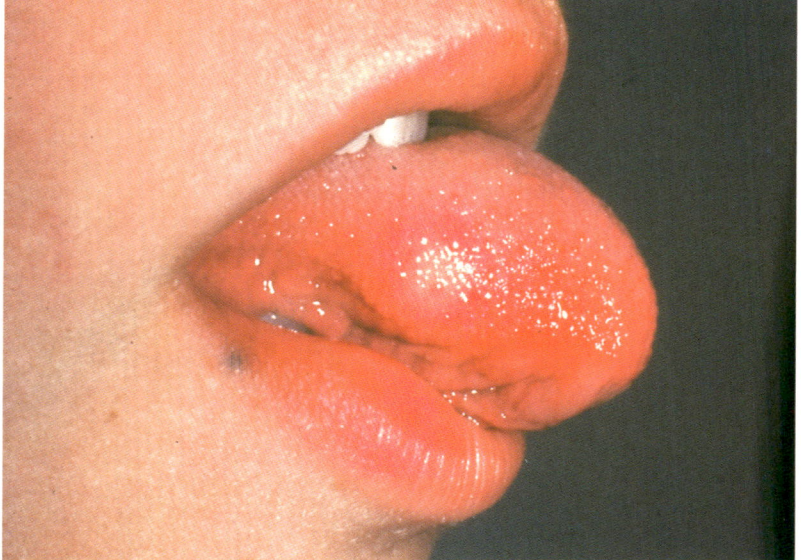

Fig. 9.17   Granular cell myoblastoma on the lateral aspect of the tongue.

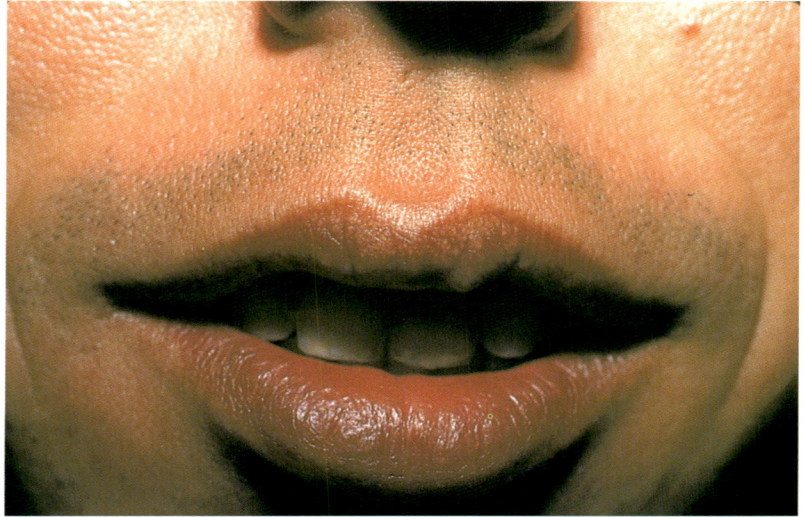

Fig. 9.19   Fordyce spots on the mid-upper lip.

79%) newborns.[121,123] Microscopically, keratin cysts are evident. Within the epithelial lining, the lumen is filled with desquamated keratin. No therapy is indicated, as these cysts are painless, exfoliate spontaneously, and heal without scarring.

The presence of circumscribed, fluctuant swelling over the site of an erupting tooth is called an eruption cyst or eruption hematoma. When the circumcoronal cystic cavity contains blood, the swelling appears purple or deep blue. These lesions are common, occurring in 11% of infants during the eruption of the canines and molars.[38] The cause of eruption cysts is unknown. No therapy is usually warranted, although removing a small portion of tissue overlying the tooth may facilitate its eruption.

FORDYCE SPOTS

Fordyce spots (Fordyce granules) represent normal sebaceous glands within the oral cavity. Ectodermal tissue is included in the early formation of the

maxilla and mandible and explains the unusual location of these structures within the mouth.[38] The primordial ectodermal tissue maintains its ability to differentiate into sebaceous glands during postnatal life.[76]

Clinically, Fordyce spots appear as white to yellow macules and papules visible through the transparent oral epithelium (Fig. 9.19). The well-circumscribed papules measure 1–3mm in size and may occur singly or in great numbers. When many sebaceous glands are present, the papules and macules may coalesce into yellow plaques, projecting slightly above the mucosal surface. The lesions typically appear on the buccal mucosa in a symmetric fashion along the occlusive planes of the teeth. When present on the lips, Fordyce spots are more numerous on the upper lip. Areas less often demonstrating these granular lesions include the retromolar region lateral to the anterior faucial pillar, the tongue, gingiva, frenum, and palate.[38] Affected regions are asymptomatic.

Although Fordyce spots are uncommon in children, the incidence approaches 80% in the adult.[122,124] These sebaceous glands are androgen-dependent and

123. Fromm A (1967) Epstein's pearls, Bohn's nodules and inclusion cysts of the oral cavity. **J Dent Child** 34:275.

124. Halperin V, Kolas S, Jefferis KR et al. (1953) The occurrence of Fordyce spots, benign migratory glossitis, median rhomboid glossitis, and fissured tongue in 2,478 dental patients. **Oral Surg** 54:1072.

therefore often larger in males than in females, but differences in incidence between the sexes or various races do not exist.

Histologically, normal-appearing sebaceous glands are present immediately subjacent to the oral epithelium. The glands may be single or grouped about a short common duct. The glandular structures are rudimentary in young children, enlarge during puberty, and remain large throughout life. No pathologic significance should be attached to Fordyce spots, and no therapy is warranted.

MUCOCELE

The term *mucocele* is applied to several types of lesions characterized by a mucus-filled swelling within the oral cavity. Both the major and minor salivary glands can contribute to the contents of these soft masses.[125] Histologic evaluation of the internal linings surrounding the fluid permits differentiation into true cysts, mucus extravasation cysts, and mucus retention cysts.[90] Of these three types, the least common is the true cyst, which is lined by an epithelium and consists of a small fluid-filled cavity lying within the body of a salivary gland. Mucus extravasation cysts are in fact particular mucus-induced granulomas. They result from trauma to the excretory duct of a minor salivary gland, permitting mucus to flow into the surrounding tissues. Whereas most of the saliva constituents are resorbed, mucins remain in the stroma of the tunica propria attracting macrophages and neutrophils. The latter disappear when the granuloma matures and shows its typical architecture of central mucin lake, inner wall of mucophages, and outer wall of macrophages with fibrous pseudocapsule.[126] The absence of an epithelial lining indicates that the cavity is not a true cyst. The overwhelming majority of these cysts are found on the lower lip (Fig. 9.20), although the floor of the mouth and the upper lip are occasionally affected.[127]

The mucus retention cyst is caused by dilation of a partially obstructed salivary duct, which forms a fluid-filled cystic structure. The cells lining the inner surface are either columnar or pseudostratified squamous epithelium. If the obstruction occurs in the submandibular or sublingual gland, the unilateral lesion formed in the floor of the mouth is called a ranula (Fig. 9.21). These are typically soft, fluctuant, and dark blue in appearance. If the lesion is large, it may interfere with normal oral function.

Clinically, all mucoceles have a bluish translucent appearance if superficially located.[87] When they are deep, the overlying mucosal surface may appear fairly normal. The lesions are smooth, painless, and typically asymptomatic. They may slowly enlarge and rupture spontaneously. Although accidental trauma is occasionally curative, most mucoceles do recur.[87] Similarly, if the mucoid contents are evacuated as a therapeutic measure, the sac fills up after a brief interval. No sexual predilection has been noted, although mucoceles seem to occur more commonly during the first three decades of life when indicated.[38] Therapy should consist of surgical excision, marsupialization or micromarsupialization.[128] Recurrences are common when the associated salivary gland acini are incompletely removed.

EPULIS

The congenital epulis is a rare, benign tumor that presents as a protuberant mass from gum of the newborn. These arise most often in the region of the incisors of the upper jaw. Attachment to the gum can be via a slender stalk or broad pedicle, with the shape of the mass ranging from ovoid to spheroid. Although single tumors are the most common, lobulated and multiple growths have been reported.[129] The maxilla is more often involved than is the mandible, and females are affected far more frequently than males.

The congenital epulis seemingly does not enlarge after birth; thus growth probably ceases at parturition.[130] Spontaneous regression typifies the natural course of this lesion, but simple surgical excision is warranted when there is interference with feeding or respiration. The tumor does not recur postoperatively, and dentition is rarely impaired.[131]

Grossly, the tumor is a firm, moderately pink mass 1–9cm in diameter. Histologically, uniform sheets of closely packed cells with an eosinophilic granular cytoplasm are present. The nuclei are centrally or eccentrically placed. Strands of fine collagenous stroma that are highly vascularized penetrate between the cells. The tumor is nonencapsulated but is separated from the surface epithelium by a zone of normal connective tissue. The surface mucosal epithelium is usually intact.

Although the precise histogenesis remains unclear, congenital epulis can be distinguished from granular cell tumor by the absence of pseudoepitheliomatous hyperplasia and neural elements. Congenital epulis also has both a uniform structure and a prominent vascular component. The typical location in the incisor region of the maxilla or mandible and the almost exclusive incidence in females further distinguish the two lesions.

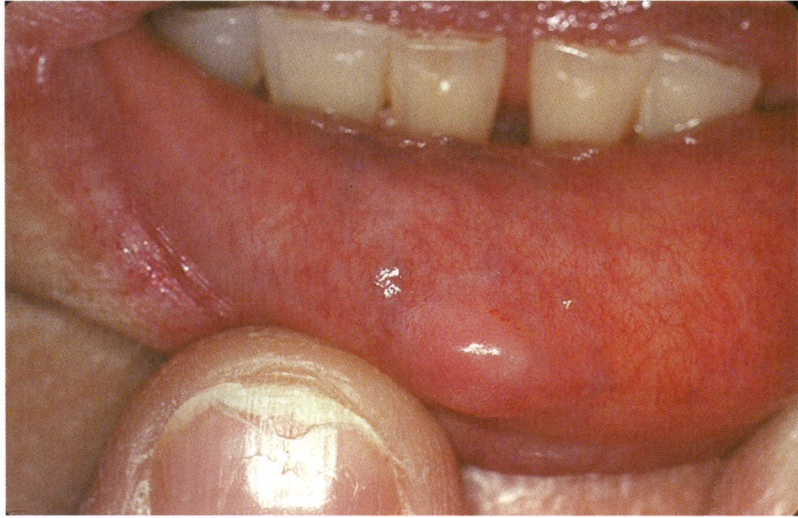

Fig. 9.20   Typical mucocele on the lower lip.

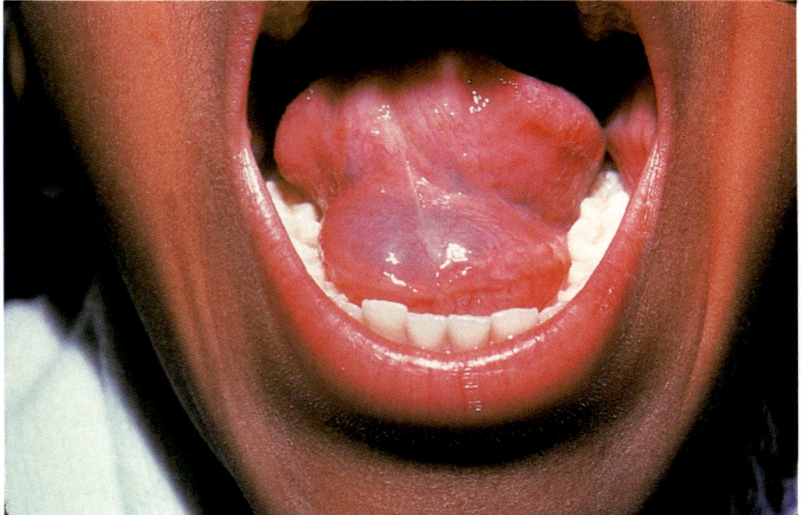

Fig. 9.21   Ranula on the ventral surface of the tongue. (Courtesy T. Laude, MD)

125. Gorlin RJ, Goldman HM (1970) Thomas's Oral Pathology, 6th ed. St. Louis: CV Mosby.
126. Haneke E (1983) Histologie, Elektronenmikroskopie, Enzym- und Immunhistologie des Schleimgranuloms. **Verh Dtsch Ges Pathol** 67, 640.
127. Maia DM, Merly F, Castro WH, Gomez RS (2000) A survey of oral biopsies in Brazilian pediatric patients. **ASDC J Dent Child** 67:128–131.
128. Delbem AC, Cunha RF, Vieira AE, Ribeiro LL (2000) Treatment of mucus retention phenomena in children by the micro-marsupialization technique: case reports. **Pediatr Dent** 22:155–158.
129. Rainey JB, Smith IJ (1984) Congenital epulis of the newborn. **J Pediatr Surg** 19:305.
130. O'Brien FV, Pielou WD (1971) Congenital epulis: its natural history. **Arch Dis Child** 46:559.
131. Sen Gupta SK, Sharma ND (1982) Congenital epulis of the newborn. **Papua New Guinea Med J** 25:53.

FOCAL EPITHELIAL HYPERPLASIA

Focal epithelial hyperplasia (FEH), or Heck's disease, is a benign disorder of the mucous membranes of children. Human papillomavirus (HPV) has been identified as the cause of FEH, and the most frequent, consistent, and disease-specific HPV types are 13 and 32. Less commonly found but previously documented are HPV types 1, 6-related, 11, 13-related, 16, and 18.[132]

A high frequency of FEH occurs in Indian populations from North, Central, and South America; Eskimos from Greenland and North Canada; and blacks from South Africa. However, some cases have also been observed in Europe. Female children are affected more frequently than male children and typical ages of FEH patients range between 3 and 18 years.

The clinical findings include soft, discrete asymptomatic papules that may merge to plaques. They are predominantly located on the lower lip, occasionally also on the buccal mucosa, upper labial mucosa, tongue, and gingivae. Histologically, one sees focal acanthosis of the epithelium with horizontal anastomosis of the elongated and/or clubbed rete ridges. The presence of koilocytes, mitosoid cells (cells demonstrating a mitosis-like nuclear degeneration) and/or cells with ballooning degeneration and more than one distorted nuclei are found. Electron microscopy can be used to demonstrate typical virus particles.[133]

No therapy may be required for FEH as the lesions often involute spontaneously without scarring.[134] Therapeutic modalities with variable efficacy have included cryotherapy, surgical excision, and carbon dioxide laser therapy.

GINGIVOSTOMATITIS

Gingivostomatitis in the child or adolescent is most often due to an infectious etiology but can also be a reflection of one of a number of noninfectious processes. Infectious problems are most often viral; HSV, Coxsackievirus, and varicella-zoster virus are the three most common agents involved. Acute necrotizing ulcerative gingivitis is associated with a proliferation of fusospirochetal organisms, although the disorder is not clearly caused by these agents. Additional conditions that may present as gingivostomatitis include contact stomatitis, erythema multiforme, stomatitis due to chemotherapy agents, recurrent aphthous ulcers, Behçet's disease, pemphigus vulgaris, cicatricial pemphigoid, and lichen planus.

For viral mucosal infections, see also Chapter 25.

HERPANGINA

This common acute infectious illness is caused by several of the Coxsackie viruses, mainly type A16, but also types A5, A9, A10, B2, and B5, as well as Echovirus types 6, 3, 7, 9, and 30. Onset is abrupt with high fever, vomiting, sore throat, anorexia, and dysphagia.[135] Abdominal pain occurs in approximately 25% of cases.[136] Multiple 1–2mm vesicles rapidly breaking down to aphthoid lesions with an erythematous areola are distributed over the fauces, tonsils, uvula, pharynx, and soft palate. These lesions enlarge before forming shallow painful ulcerations. Laboratory findings are generally within normal limits. A similar disease, however, with follicular papules on the soft palate only, is caused by Coxsackievirus A10 and known as acute lymphonodular pharyngitis.

The differential diagnosis includes mainly hand, foot, and mouth disease, herpetic gingivostomatitis, and aphthous ulcers, all of which differ in sites of involvement and accompanying signs and symptoms (Table 9.9). The diagnosis can be confirmed by identification of the viral agent either by inoculation of material obtained from the throat or rectum into a newborn mouse or by demonstration of a rise in antibody titer. The course of the illness is brief, lasting approximately four to six days, and complete recovery without complications is usual. There is no known effective treatment.

HAND, FOOT, AND MOUTH DISEASE

Hand, foot, and mouth disease can usually be attributed to coxsackievirus A16 infection; however, A5, A7, A9, and A10 are also occasionally implicated as etiologic agents.[137] This viral syndrome was first described in 1956 and has been observed to recur in outbreaks since that time.

There is generally a mild prodrome consisting of low-grade fever, malaise, anorexia, and sore mouth. Coryza, cough, diarrhea, vomiting, and lymphadenopathy are less frequent findings. Oral lesions develop 1–2 days later and are typically sparse discrete vesicles, 4–8mm in diameter, on an erythematous base; occasionally these lesions may be as large as 20mm. Most commonly the buccal mucosa, tongue, uvula, and anterior tonsillar pillars are involved. Gingival vesicles are rare. The oral lesions may be the only evidence of infection and, in those instances, may be confused with aphthous stomatitis. The vesicles and ulcers of hand, foot, and mouth disease are larger than those of herpangina; in contrast to herpetic gingivostomatitis, they spare the lips and usually the gingivae.

The cutaneous lesions are much more common in children than in adults and erupt one or two days after the oral lesions. They consist of 3–7mm

---

TABLE 9.9   Common mucosal vesiculoulcerative syndromes

	Musocal lesions	Skin lesions	Associated findings
Herpangina	Pharyngotonsillar	None	High fever, sore throat
Hand, foot, and mouth disease	Sparse lesions; entire oropharynx	Oval vesicles, hand and feet; maculopapular rash, buttocks	Fever, sore mouth
Herpetic gingivostomatitis	Entire mouth involved; lesions rapidly coalesce, gingivae friable and bleeding	Perioral vesicles	Fever, irritability, fetid breath, lymphadenopathy
Varicella	Palate, lips, tongue	Centripetal vesicular eruption	Fever, malaise, headache, anorexia
Aphthous stomatitis	Ulcers, discrete and recurrent, aphthae do not coalesce	None	Prodrome of oral hyperemia, paresthesias
Erythema multiforme	Entire mouth; lips severely involved; gingivae relatively spared	Vesicular, urticarial, target lesions	Fever, malaise, anorexia

132. Cohen PR, Hebert AA, Adler-Storthz K (1993) Focal epithelial hyperplasia: Heck disease. **Pediatr Dermatol** 10:245.
133. Nasemann T, Schaeg G (1985) Der Morbus Heck. **Z Hautkr** 60:1750–1757.
134. Cohen PR, Hebert AA, Adler-Storthz K (1993) Focal epithelial hyperplasia: Heck disease. **Pediatr Dermatol** 10(3):245–251.

135. Cherry JD, Jahn CL (1965) Herpangina: the etiologic spectrum. **Pediatrics** 36:632.
136. Krugman S, Ward R (1973) Infectious Diseases of Children and Adults, 5th ed. St. Louis: CV Mosby.
137. Cherry JD (1983) Viral exanthems. **Curr Probl Pediat** 13:1.

vesicopustules with an erythematous rim and may be sparse or numerous. They are typically oval with their long axis along the dermatoglyphics and are found on the palms, soles, backs of the hands, and around the nails of the fingers and toes. The lesions are nonpruritic and usually resolve without much crusting. A maculopapular eruption is frequently found on the buttocks and occasionally on the arms, legs, or face.[137,138] The disease resolves spontaneously after five to 10 days.

Diagnosis is usually made clinically, although isolation of the virus from vesicle fluid, throat swabs, and feces or documentation of a rise in serum antibody titer to one of the known etiologic agents is confirmatory. Electron microscopy shows typical virus particles.[139] Tzanck smears are always negative for giant cells, balloon cells, and intranuclear inclusions and can be used to distinguish hand, foot, and mouth disease from herpesvirus infections.[140] Treatment is symptomatic only (see also Chapter 25).

HERPETIC GINGIVOSTOMATITIS

The most common form of primary herpes simplex infection is acute gingivostomatitis.[141–144] Infants under 6 months of age usually have a protective maternal antibody; therefore, the infection is usually seen between the ages of 6 months and 5 years.[141] However, only about 1% of the infected children develop this severe infection, 10% get uncharacteristic flu-like symptoms, and probably more 90% will have no symptoms. Following an incubation period of 2–12 days, many patients experience a prodrome consisting of irritability, fever, headache, nausea, and vomiting. The oral eruption consists of small vesicles on an erythematous base scattered over the tongue, buccal mucosa, uvula, soft palate, pharynx, inner aspect of the lips, and floor of the mouth. The vesicles, which are intraepithelial in location, rupture quickly leaving shallow painful ulcers and erosions.[145] The widespread presentation of herpetic lesions on both keratinized and non-keratinized mucosa in primary herpetic gingivostomatitis likely results from a combined bacterial and viral infection. This explains the deviation from the "rule"[146] that herpes lesions occur *only* on keratinized mucosal surfaces. Typically, the gingivae are deeply erythematous and swollen and bleed easily when traumatized. In contrast to aphthous

ulcerations, the lesions soon coalesce to form irregular shallow ulcers. Multiple vesicles may develop on the skin in the perioral area, even at quite a distance from the mouth; thumb suckers may acquire an acute herpetic whitlow on the thumb as well. Because of severe mouth pain, the child may drool excessively and refuse to eat or drink. The breath often has a fetid odor. Although fever is usually low grade, at times it may rise to 105°F. Tender cervical and submental lymphadenopathy is expected.

Children immediately after measles or with immunosuppression may develop a particularly severe form of ulceration known as aphthoid of Pospischill–Feyrter with necrotic lesions around the mouth, perigenitally, and perianally that takes several weeks to heal and is an indication for systemic antiviral therapy.

The diagnosis is usually made clinically but can be confirmed by a positive Tzanck smear, viral culture, or enzyme-linked immunosorbent assay (ELISA). Nearly all primary oral infections are caused by HSV-1. Convalescence coincides with a rise in neutralizing antibody titers that peak at three to four weeks. Differential diagnosis includes herpangina and hand, foot, and mouth disease; aphthous stomatitis; infectious mononucleosis; streptococcal pharyngitis; and Stevens–Johnson syndrome. Evidence for recent contact with someone with an active herpetic infection is helpful in establishing the diagnosis.

In an uncomplicated course, the fever subsides by the fourth day and subsequent healing of lesions occurs over the next 7–10 days. The entire course rarely lasts more than two weeks. Treatment is mainly supportive and consists of antipyretics, topical anesthetics such as dyclonine (Table 9.10). When the manifestations are severe, hospitalization and administration of intravenous fluids may be required to maintain adequate hydration. Measures to improve oral hygiene such as dilute hydrogen peroxide or saline mouthwashes or gargles may reduce bacterial overgrowth and provide some relief from discomfort. Treatment of herpetic gingivostomatitis with acyclovir was shown in one randomized double-blind study to reduce the duration of intra- and extra-oral lesions as well as viral shedding. Those patients treated with acyclovir had earlier resolution of fever and fewer days with difficulty in eating or swallowing.[147] Parents should be educated as to the infectivity of the lesions when acute, in order to prevent spread to others in the immediate environment.[144]

TABLE 9.10   Topical anesthetic agents suitable for use on the oral mucous membranes

Agent	Manufacturer	Anesthetic	Size
Benzo-jel gel (banana flavor)	Schein	20% benzocaine	1-oz jar
Cetacaine	Cetylite	14% benzocaine	
		2% butyl aminobenzoate	
		2% tetracaine HCl	
Liquid (for swab application)			2-oz bottle
Ointment (flavored)			37-g jar
Spray			56g
Gingicaine gingipak (cherry, chocolate milk, piña colada, strawberry)	Schein	20% benzocaine	1-oz jar
Hurricane liquid or gel (original flavor, piña colada)	Beutlich	20% benzocaine	1 oz
Spray			2 oz
Lidocaine ointment 5% (mint flavored)	Schein	5% lidocaine	50g
Topex	Sultan	20% benzocaine	
Gel or liquid (banana, cherry, mint, piña colada)			2 oz
Spray (cherry)	2 oz		
Xylocaine solution topical 4%	Astra	4% lidocaine	50ml
Xylocaine viscous 2%	Astra	2% lidocaine	100ml, 450ml
Dyclone	Astra	0.5% or 1% dyclonine	1 fl oz

138. Richardson HB, Leibovitz A (1965) Hand, foot and mouth disease in children. **J Pediatr** 67:6.
139. Haneke E (1985) Electron microscopic demonstration of virus particles in hand, foot and mouth disease. **Dermatologica** 171:321–326.
140. Cherry JD, Jahn CL (1966) Hand, foot and mouth syndrome. **Pediatrics** 37:637.
141. Wright JM, Taylor PP, Allen EP, Byrd RL (1984) A review of the oral manifestations of infections in pediatric patients. **Pediatr Infect Dis** 3:80.
142. Snavely SR, Liu C (1984) Clinical spectrum of herpes simplex virus infections. **Clin Dermatol** 2:8.
143. McDonald MI, Durach DT (1983) Viral blisters. **Dermatol Clin** 1:281.

144. Blackman JA, Andersen RD, Healy A, Zehrbach R (1985) Management of young children with recurrent herpes simplex lesions in special education programs. **Pediatr Infect Dis** 4:221.
145. Amir J, Harel L, Smetana Z, Varsano I (1999) The natural history of primary herpes simplex type I gingivostomatitis in children. **Pediatr Dermatol** 16(4):259–263.
146. Weathers DR, Griffin JW (1970) Intraoral ulcerations of recurrent herpes simplex and recurrent aphthae: two distinct clinical entities. **J Am Dent Assoc** 81:81.
147. Amir J, Harel L, Smetana Z, Varsano I (1997) Treatment of herpes simplex gingivostomatitis with acyclovir (SIC) in children: a randomized double blind placebo controlled study. **BMJ** 21;314(4097):1800–1803.

VARICELLA-ZOSTER INFECTIONS

Oral mucosal lesions are a common manifestation of varicella and often precede onset of the skin eruption. The vesicles are relatively transient and rapidly progress to small shallow ulcerations on the tongue, lips, palate, and gingiva (Fig. 9.22). They are generally asymptomatic and require no therapy. In herpes zoster infections, oral lesions are typically unilateral in distribution and more painful.

Both types of varicella-zoster virus infections can be confirmed by obtaining a Tzanck smear from an oral vesicle or ulcer and by demonstrating ballooning degeneration of the epithelial cells and multinucleated syncytial giant cells.[148] Topical anesthetics and analgesic agents are palliative (Table 9.10).[141]

ACUTE NECROTIZING ULCERATIVE GINGIVITIS

Acute necrotizing ulcerative gingivitis (ANUG) affects adolescents and young adults and occurs rarely in children. This inflammatory process involves mainly the gingival margins, crest of the gingiva, interdental papillae, and periodontium and is also known as trenchmouth, fusospirochetal gingivitis, and phagedenic gingivitis. When the lesions spread to the cheeks, tongue, soft palate, and pharynx, the term Vincent's stomatitis or angina has been used.[38]

The disorder is characterized by abrupt onset of extremely painful hyperemic gingivae and sharply demarcated ulcerations of the interdental papillae. The eroded papillae and free gingiva bleed easily when touched and become covered by a gray necrotic pseudomembrane. A fetid mouth odor commonly accompanies these findings.

Because of the gingival pain and tendency to bleed easily, the patients find it difficult to eat. Profuse salivation as well as a distinct metallic taste to the saliva are common complaints. The teeth may be extremely sensitive to pressure, are thought to be slightly extruded, and may be slightly movable. Rapid destruction of the dental ligament is observed in acute necrotizing ulcerative periodontitis.[149] Headache, malaise, low-grade fever, as well as regional lymphadenopathy are usual.

Although acute necrotizing ulcerative gingivitis occurs in epidemic patterns as well as sporadically, it is not believed to be a communicable disorder but is rather attributed to a mixed infection superimposed on certain predisposing conditions. Poor oral hygiene is thought to be an important factor as well as inadequate nutrition, heavy smoking, fatigue, and stress. Chronic changes in the oral cavity such as pericoronitis, ill-fitting crowns, inlays and prosthetic appliances, dental caries, impacted food, faulty restorations, and pre-existing

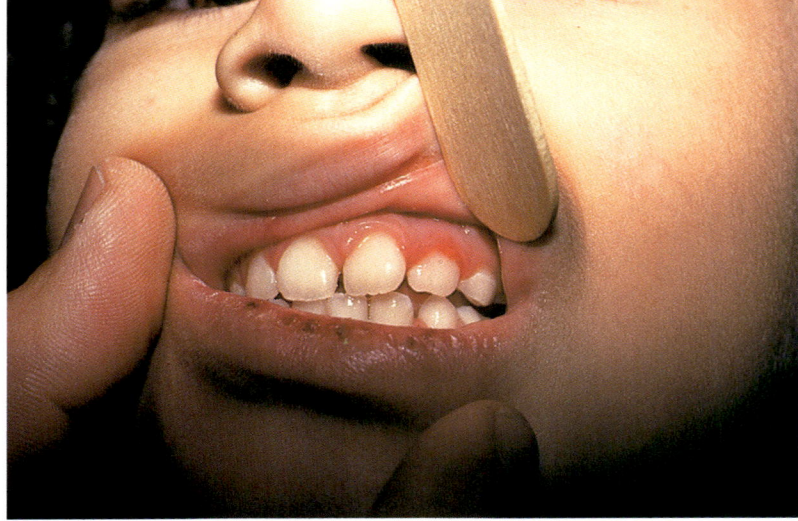

Fig. 9.22   Enanthem of chickenpox.

marginal gingivitis are all considered possible contributory factors.[90,150] Patients with acquired immunodeficiency syndrome, leukemia or blood dyscrasias causing bone marrow depression are also predisposed to this type of gingivitis.

The organisms involved in this condition are the Gram-negative spirochete *Borrelia vincentii* and the fusiform Gram-positive bacillus *Fusobacterium dentium*, which proliferate in the oral cavity and are invariably found in profusion in necrotizing gingivitis. Smears obtained from the gingival surface should demonstrate overwhelming numbers of those two organisms; however, other organisms will be present as well as polymorphonuclear leukocytes. Both *B. vincentii* and *F dentium* require anaerobic conditions for culture. Ultimately, the diagnosis is made on clinical grounds because the organisms present in necrotizing gingivitis can also be found in other types of gingivitis as well as in the normal mouth, although generally in considerably fewer numbers.[38]

Herpetic gingivostomatitis, which is much more common in young children, is most often confused with necrotizing gingivitis. Other conditions to be considered in the differential diagnosis include desquamative gingivitis, chronic gingivitis due to various causes, and mouth ulcerations in patients with blood dyscrasias. Herpetic gingivostomatitis, hand, foot, and mouth disease, aphthous stomatitis, Behçet syndrome, and Stevens–Johnson syndrome may also be confused with necrotizing gingivitis.

Treatment of acute necrotizing gingivitis should be instituted by a dentist after a thorough dental evaluation. Management varies from a conservative approach advocating only superficial cleansing in the acute phase, followed by more thorough scaling and polishing later in the course,[38] to aggressive debridement with irrigation and periodontal curettage early in the disease.[78] Although oxygenating agents and antibiotics are often prescribed, there is no substantive evidence that they hasten resolution of the inflammatory process, which seems to run its course. When extensive involvement of the oral cavity, lymphadenopathy, or systemic signs of disease are present, antibiotic therapy is recommended. Penicillin and/or metronidazole are considered the drugs of choice. All authorities agree that measures to improve oral hygiene, such as gentle brushing and vigorous rinsing several times daily with dilute hydrogen peroxide mixed 1:1 with water, are important aspects of care. The patient should also be educated about the significance of predisposing factors.

Subsequent to recovery from the acute process, a careful periodontal evaluation is appropriate. Recontouring of the gingival papillae by gingivoplasty may be required. Patients with extensive involvement of the oral cavity should be studied for underlying diseases, particularly blood dyscrasias and AIDS. Rarely, serious sequelae, such as gangrenous stomatitis, noma, or septicemia, have resulted from this condition.

ANUG is considered the antecedent lesion of noma (cancrum oris) which is an infectious, but not contagious, disease destroying the oro-facial tissues and other neighboring structures in its fulminating course. Noma affects predominantly children aged 2–16 years in sub-Saharan Africa. The most important risk factors are poverty, malnutrition, poor oral hygiene, deplorable environmental sanitation, close residential proximity to livestock, and infectious diseases, particularly measles. Malnutrition acts synergistically with endemic infections in promoting an immunodeficient state, and noma results from the interaction of general and local factors with a weakened immune system as the common denominator. Recent studies suggest that evolution of ANUG to noma requires infection by a consortium of microorganisms with *Fusobacterium necrophorum* and *Prevotella intermedia* as the suspected key players.[151]

ORAL CANDIDIASIS

The oral mucous membranes constitute the most frequent site of colonization by *Candida* in the pediatric age group. Host factors are responsible for the many different forms of candidiasis. *C. albicans* is the organism usually responsible for the white-gray pseudomembranes (thrush) found on the buccal mucosa, palate, gums, and tongue. These white patches appear curd-like and friable and are easily removed by gentle pressure. Composed

148. Farman AQ (1976) Clinical and cytological features of the oral lesions caused by chicken-pox (varicella). **J Oral Med** 31:94.
149. Navak MJ (1999) Necrotizing ulcerative periodontitis. **Ann Periodontol** 4:74–78.
150. Rowland RW (1999) Necrotizing ulcerative gingivitis. **Ann Periodontol** 4:65–73, 78.
151. Enwonwu CO, Falkler WA, Idigbe EO, Savage KO (1999) Noma (cancrum oris): questions and answers. **Oral Dis** 5:144–149.

of almost pure colonies of *Candida* plus desquamated epithelial cells, inflammatory cells, and fibrin, the yeast is readily identified within such patches by either a KOH preparation or culture on Sabouraud or Mycosel agar, or both. Removal of the white plaques reveals an underlying area of erythema or shallow ulcerations that easily bleeds.

Acute candidiasis

Acute pseudomembranous candidiasis (thrush)

Newborns become colonized with *Candida* as they traverse the maternal vaginal tract. Additional sources of colonization include the hands of the nursery personnel or other infants. When candidal vulvovaginitis develops late in the course of the pregnancy, the infant is at greater risk of developing thrush. Antepartum therapy with intravaginal clotrimazole reduces the risk of neonatal colonization in the birth canal.

The great majority of newborns in whom thrush develops are otherwise healthy. Factors such as sex, season, prematurity, mode of feeding, amount of resuscitation, and use of broad-spectrum antibiotics have not always conclusively influenced occurrence of clinical lesions.[152] Often, candidiasis of the diaper area develops early on in the course of oral thrush. Newborns with thrush warrant treatment with nystatin oral suspension 200 000 units (2ml) on to the tongue four times daily for seven to 10 days. Such therapy usually produces prompt recovery. The solution should be slowly instilled into the mouth to permit adequate contact with affected tissues. Alternatively, a cotton-tipped swab may be employed to apply the medication to infected sites after feeding. Resistant cases may require 400 000 units of nystatin oral solution qid for seven to 10 days or gentian violet 0.5% aqueous solution bid for three days. An alternate method of treatment involves insertion of a 10mg clotrimazole or amphotericin-B troche tightly into a nipple and allowing the child to suck these qid.[153]

Young children are also susceptible to transient episodes of thrush while their oral flora is becoming established. Most often, such infections are unrelated to any known predisposing factors. Immunocompromised children, especially those with AIDS, usually also develop candida esophagitis.[154]

Acute atrophic oral candidiasis

This form of candidiasis is unique in that it is the only form that is consistently painful. Arising from acute pseudomembranous candidiasis or *de novo*, clinical manifestations include red, atrophic, painful, persistent ulcerations. White pseudomembranes are rarely seen.[78]

Acute atrophic oral candidiasis should be suspected if broad-spectrum antibiotics have been prescribed and oral burning, dysgeusia, or a sore throat are reported. Angular cheilitis may be present. KOH preparations from the denuded mucosa reveal budding yeasts and pseudomycelia.

Chronic candidiasis

Chronic hyperplastic candidiasis

This form of candidiasis, mainly seen in middle-aged men, is characterized by firm white plaques on the lips, tongue, or buccal mucosa, which tend to persist.

Candida frequently colonizes oral leukoplakia, although such lesions are exceedingly rare in children.[155] Alternatively, *Candida* does not invade leukedema, lichen planus, squamous papilloma, or carcinoma.

Chronic atrophic candidiasis

Denture sore mouth is synonymous with chronic atrophic candidiasis and is frequently associated with angular cheilitis. Although common in adult denture wearers, it is rare in children even when they wear dentures, such as in the Papillon–Lefèvre syndrome.

Chronic mucocutaneous candidiasis

Typically, this rare condition, which occurs as a result of various genetic defects, is first detected during childhood. *Candida* is one of the opportunistic pathogens that characterize this disease, and evidence of chronic involvement is seen in the skin, scalp, nails, and mucous membranes. Because of such immunodeficiencies as impaired cell-mediated immunity, neutrophil function defects, isolated IgA deficiency, and reduced serum candicidal activity, candidal infections are resistant to common forms of therapy.[38] Ketoconazole, itraconazole and fluconazole therapy has proved effective in most cases.

CHRONIC FAMILIAL MUCOCUTANEOUS CANDIDIASIS

Occurring early in life, this subset is genetically transmitted, probably as an autosomal-recessive trait. Clinical manifestations, including oral lesions, are seen by 5 years of age.

CHRONIC LOCALIZED MUCOCUTANEOUS CANDIDIASIS

In this severe form of candidiasis, which seemingly lacks genetic transmission, granulomatous and horny masses are evident on the face and scalp. Other fungal and bacterial infections commonly occur. The mouth shows typical white pseudomembranes which cannot be easily wiped off, and the nails are often dystrophic by candidal infection.

CANDIDA ENDOCRINOPATHY SYNDROME

The skin, scalp, nails, and mucous membranes are infected with *Candida* as a result of this genetically transmitted entity. Family studies suggest an autosomal-recessive pattern of inheritance. The oral cavity frequently shows candidal lesions in association with hypoadrenalism (Addison's disease), hypoparathyroidism, hypothyroidism, ovarian insufficiency, or diabetes mellitus. The thrush may precede the endocrinopathy by several years.[156]

CHRONIC DIFFUSE MUCOCUTANEOUS CANDIDIASIS

This syndrome usually has its onset during childhood, and patients lack associated endocrinopathies. Affected relatives are uncommon, although eight pedigrees suggest an autosomal-recessive mode of inheritance.[157]

Widespread erythematous serpiginous lesions involving the skin and mucous membranes characterize this condition. Hyperkeratosis is not a prominent feature. The nails are also infected with *Candida*.

A subset of patients with chronic diffuse mucocutaneous candidiasis do not develop their disorder until adolescence. This group often receives multiple antibiotic courses for acne, furunculosis, or urinary tract infections. The antibiotics may alter their cutaneous and oral flora, allowing overgrowth of *C. albicans*. Why progression to chronic diffuse candidiasis occurs remains unclear.[158]

DESQUAMATIVE GINGIVITIS

The term *desquamative gingivitis* is used to describe a specific clinical picture characterized by intense erythema of the gingiva and desquamation of the surface epithelium. Although it occurs primarily in adulthood, children and adolescents may rarely develop this condition as a manifestation of any one of several diseases. Desquamative gingivitis is not a disease *per se* but is in most cases a sign of erosive lichen planus, bullous pemphigoid, or cicatricial pemphigoid whereas pemphigus vulgaris, tuberculosis, histoplasmosis, or blastomycosis are rare.[38,87,159,160] This condition has also been observed as an allergic reaction to tosylamide/formaldehyde resin in a female biting her lacquered nails.[161]

152. Shrand H (1961) Thrush in the newborn. **BMJ** 2:1530.
153. Mansour A, Gelfand EW (1981) A new approach to the use of antifungal agents in infants with persistent oral candidiasis. **J Pediatr** 98:161.
154. Flaitz CM, Hicks MJ (1999) Oral candidiasis in children with immunosuppression: clinical appearance and therapeutic considerations **ASDC J Dent Child** 66:161–166
155. Hornstein OP, Gräßel R, Schirner E, Schell H (1979) Orale Candida-Besiedlung bei Leukoplakie und Karzinomen der Mundhöhle. **Dtsch Med Wschr** 104:1033–1036.
156. de Padova-Elder SM, Ditre CM, Kantor GR, Koblenzer PJ (1994) Candidiasis endocrinopathy syndrome. Treatment with itraconazole. **Arch Dermatol** 130:19–22.

157. Wells RS, Higgs JM, MacDonald A et al. (1972) Familial chronic muco-cutaneous candidiasis. **J Med Genet** 9:302.
158. Kirkpatrick CH (1984) Host factors in defense against fungal infections. **Am J Med** 77:1.
159. Vaillant L, Chauchaix-Barthes S, Huttenberger B et al. (2000) Chronic desquamative gingivitis syndrome: retrospective analysis of 33 cases. **Ann Dermatol Venereol** 127:381–387.
160. Yih WY, Richardson L, Kratochvil FJ et al. (2000) Expression of estrogen receptors in desquamative gingivitis. **J Periodontol** 71:482–487.
161. Staines KS, Felix DH, Forsyth A (1998) Desquamative gingivitis, sole manifestation of tosylamide/formaldehyde resin allergy. **Contact Dermatitis** 39:90.

The clinical picture is one of intense erythema and swelling of the gingiva in a patchy distribution. The involved areas may become hemorrhagic and denuded, and occasionally intact vesicles can be found. The epithelium strips off the gingival surface easily, leaving a raw, sensitive, bleeding base. Oral structures other than the gingiva may also be involved, most frequently the buccal mucosa. There is extreme discomfort from the pain and hemorrhage caused by pressure from toothbrushing, and ingestion of coarse, hard, or spicy foods, or those that are extremely hot or cold.

The precise diagnosis cannot be made without histopathologic evaluation of the involved gingiva. Immunofluorescence preparations and special stains may also be helpful. The disorder is chronic and responsive only to therapy specific for the particular underlying disease process.

ORAL-FACIAL-DIGITAL SYNDROME I (PAPILLON–LÉAGE–PSAUME SYNDROME)

This X-linked dominant syndrome, which represents a lethal factor for males, includes the following facial abnormalities: frontal bossing, pseudocleft of the upper lip, cleft or defect of the hard palate, multiple hyperplastic frenula, cleft tongue with hamartomas between the lobes, ankyloglossia, fibrous bands in upper and lower mucobuccal folds, absent lower lateral incisors, malpositioned and supernumerary teeth, hypoplasia of malar bones, broad nasal root, dystopia canthorum, hypoplasia of the alar cartilages, and milia of the ears and upper face in infancy (Table 9.11).[162]

Additional anomalies are asymmetric shortening of the digits with or without clinodactyly and syndactyly, patchy alopecia, mild mental retardation, unilateral polysyndactyly of the hallux, renal cysts, and pilosebaceous dysplasia.[163–165]

ORAL-FACIAL-DIGITAL SYNDROME II (MOHR SYNDROME)

This autosomal-recessive syndrome includes the following facial features: lobate tongue, nodular hamartomas of the tongue, midline cleft of the upper lip, usually intact but high, arched palate, hypertrophied frenulum, dystopia canthorum with broad nasal root, broad nose with bifid tip, hypoplastic mandible, and variably absent mandibular central incisors. Additional findings include malformed incus and conducive hearing defect, short stature, digital anomalies (syndactyly, brachydactyly, clinodactyly, polydactyly) and bilateral reduplicated hallux, first metatarsal, cuneiform, and cuboid bones.[166]

TRICHO-DENTO-OSSEOUS SYNDROME

This autosomal-dominant syndrome consists of kinky hair that is present at birth but often straightens during childhood, as well as small, pitted, widely spaced teeth and sclerotic bones. The facies is characteristic, with frontal bossing, a square jaw, and dolichocephaly. An additional characteristic finding is brittle, peeling nails.

The teeth become discolored and erode up to the gingival margin due to the defective enamel. Periodontal abscesses are common. Dental radiographs show taurodontia (increase in size of the pulp chamber) in both sets of dentition, lack of contrast between the enamel and dentin, and a moth–eaten appearance of the enamel. By the second or third decade, many affected persons are edentulous.

The sclerotic bones are most readily demonstrable on skull radiographs. Premature closure of the calvarial sutures may be seen. The skeletal findings are not associated with clinical symptoms. An elevation of serum acid phosphatase has been documented in a few affected patients.[167,168]

BÖÖK SYNDROME

A hereditary syndrome involving a kindred of 172 members in which 25 were affected was described by Böök in 1950.[169] Patients with hypodontia of the premolar region (P), hyperhidrosis of the palms and soles (H), and premature whitening of the hair (premature canities) (C) spanned four generations. This constellation of findings is also referred to as PHC syndrome.

The penetrance of this autosomal-dominant gene is nearly complete for the aplasia of the bicuspid region and the premature canities. Expressivity is variable, however, in the number of bicuspids that fail to develop and the age of onset of whitening of the hair (range 6 to 23 years). The loss of hair color occurs in a uniform rather than spotty pattern, with the scalp hair being affected most often. No alteration of skin pigment has been reported. Two-thirds of affected persons with dental and hair changes were found to have detectable hyperfunction of the palmar and plantar sweat glands. Although there is no specific therapy for this disorder, attention should be directed toward providing cosmetic improvement and control of the hyperhidrosis.

PAPILLON–LEFÈVRE SYNDROME

Papillon–Lefèvre syndrome (PLS) is an autosomal-recessive disorder characterized by palmoplantar keratoderma and severe, early onset periodontitis which results from deficiency of cathepsin C activity secondary to mutations in the cathepsin C gene on chromosome 11q14. Different cathepsin C mutations have been reported in PLS patients, 13 of whom are homozygous for a given mutation reflecting consanguinity, and three are compound heterozygotes and inherited as an autosomal-recessive trait.[170–173] This condition has been described in both sexes and all races.[174] Although the skin changes

TABLE 9.11	Differences between OFD I and OFD II syndromes	
	OFD I	OFD II
Genetics	X-linked dominant; females only	Autosomal-recessive; both sexes affected
Skin	Pilosebaceous dysplasia; milia	Normal
Hair	Coarse and sparse	Normal
Alveolar ridge	Thick frenula	Normal or flared
Dentition	Absent lateral mandibular incisors	Normal or absent lateral mandibular incisors
Nose	Alar hypoplasia	Broad bifid tip
Mandible	Hypoplasia of ramus of mandible	Hypoplasia of body of mandible
Digits	Unilateral polysyndactyly of hallux	Bilateral polysyndactyly of halluces
Hearing	Normal	Conductive hearing defect

OFD: oral-facial-digital.

162. Del C, Boente M, Prime N et al. (1999) A mosaic pattern of alopecia in the oral-facial-digital syndrome Type I (Papillon–Leage and Psaume syndrome). Pediatr Dermatol 16:367–370.
163. Solomon LM, Fretzin D, Pruzansky S (1970) Pilosebaceous dysplasia in the oral-facial-digital syndrome. Arch Dermatol 102:598.
164. Rimoin DL, Edgerton MJ (1967) Genetic and clinical heterogeneity in the oro-facial-digital syndromes. J Pediatr 71:94.
165. Goodman RM, Gorlin RJ (1977) Atlas of the Face in Genetic Disorders. St. Louis: CV Mosby.
166. Martinot VL, Manouvrier S, Anastassos Y et al. (1994) Orodigitofacial syndrome type I and II: clinical and surgical studies. Cleft Palate Craniofac J 31:401–408.
167. Wright JT, Kula K, Hall K et al. (1997) Analysis of the tricho-dento-osseous syndrome genotype and phenotype. Am J Med Genet 72:197–204.
168. Lichtenstein J, Warson R, Jorgenson R et al. (1972) The tricho-dentoosseous syndrome (TDO). Am J Hum Genet 24:569.
169. Böök JA (1950) Clinical and genetical studies of hypodontia: premolar aplasia, hyperhidrosis, and canities prematura; a new hereditary syndrome in man. Am J Hum Genet 2:240.
170. Hart TC, Hart PS, Michalec MD et al. (2000) Haim-Munk syndrome and Papillon-Lefevre syndrome are allelic mutations in cathepsin C. J Med Genet 37:88–94.
171. Hart TC, Walker SJ, Bowden DW et al. (2000) An integrated physical and genetic map of the PLS locus interval on chromosome 11q14. Mamm Genome 11:243–246.
172. Nakano A, Nomura K, Nakano H et al. (2001) Papillon-Lefevre syndrome: mutations and polymorphisms in the cathepsin C gene. J Invest Dermatol 116:339–343.
173. Allende L, Garcia-Perez M, Moreno A et al. (2001) Cathepsin C gene: First compound heterozygous patient with Papillon-Lefevre syndrome and a novel symptomless mutation. Hum Mutat 17:152–153.
174. Haneke E (1979) The Papillon-Lefevre syndrome: keratosis palmoplantaris with peridontopathy. Hum Genet 51:1–35.

have been noted in a few affected persons at birth, most experience onset during the first four years of life.

The cutaneous manifestations consist of a diffuse symmetric transgredient keratoderma involving the palms and soles, Achilles area of the heels, and frequently the dorsum of the fingers and toes, volar surfaces of the wrists, dorsal interphalangeal joints of the digits, and the elbows, knees, and lateral malleoli.[174–178] The keratotic areas are sharply demarcated, often displaying an erythematous margin. In some patients the areas of hyperkeratoses fluctuate in severity, even remitting episodically; in others, they persist, causing painful fissures, particularly during the colder months.[131] Several authorities comment that the severity of the keratoderma often parallels the degree of periodontal inflammation. Biopsy of the keratoderma demonstrates hyperkeratosis with parakeratosis and acanthosis.[177]

The deciduous teeth erupt at the expected age and in normal sequence; the teeth are structurally normal. Once the primary dentition is complete, periodontal bone destruction ensues, accompanied by severe purulent gingivitis and fetid mouth odor. The deciduous teeth are shed prematurely in the same sequence in which they erupted and are usually completely exfoliated by the age of 4 to 6 years. Following loss of the teeth, the inflammatory process subsides and the gingivae return to a normal appearance. With the eruption of the permanent dentition, the inflammatory process is renewed and the second set of teeth are also shed, leaving only the third molars intact.[174,175] While the process is active, chewing is painful because of the looseness of the teeth, which tilt and migrate within the gingivae (Fig. 9.23). Radiographic examination will demonstrate the complete resorption of alveolar bone, giving the teeth a "floating-in-air" appearance. Painful regional lymphadenopathy has been observed while the gingivitis is present.[175] Biopsy of the gingivae reveals only the nonspecific changes of acute and chronic inflammation.

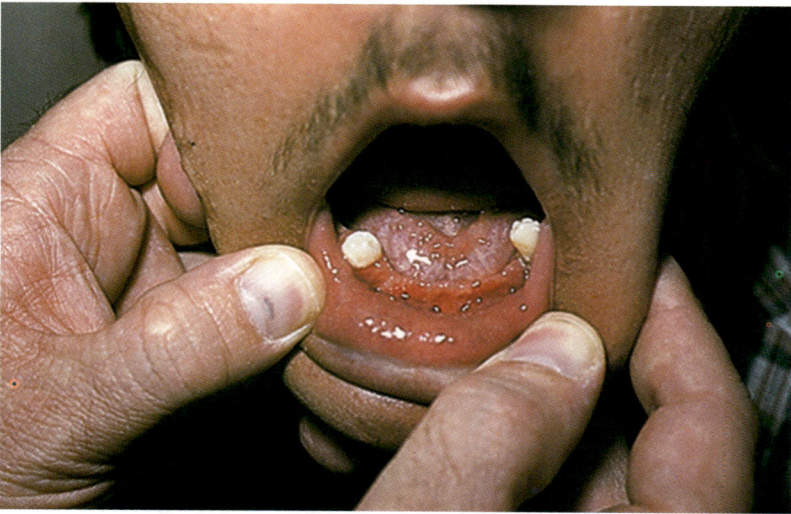

Fig. 9.23 Papillon–Lefèvre syndrome.

Variable findings in this syndrome include calcification of the falx cerebri, increased susceptibility to infection, hyperhidrosis, bromhidrosis, dystrophic nails, as well as scattered additional abnormalities in individual cases.[174,175,179–181]

Keratoderma palmoplantare of Unna–Thost and mal de Meleda must be distinguished from Papillon–Lefèvre syndrome, although neither is associated with dental problems. Conditions associated with gingivitis and causing exfoliation of the teeth include acrodynia, hypophosphatasia, cyclic neutropenia, Ehlers–Danlos type VIII, variable immune defects, and Takahara syndrome.[174,176]

The keratoderma should be treated with emollients and keratolytic agents. Most therapeutic modalities for the gingivitis have been without benefit, but etretinate and acitretin therapy resulted in healing of cutaneous and periodontal lesions within a few months' time in some patients treated thus far.[178,182–184] These patients should be closely followed by a dentist, so that prostheses can be provided at the appropriate time and by a physician due to the potential for life-threatening bacterial infections. Osseointegrated implant appear to be promising.[185]

ACATALASEMIA

Acatalasemia is characterized by the absence of catalase in the blood and tissues, rendering affected persons unable to degrade exogenous or endogenous hydrogen peroxide, which accumulates in the periodontal tissues.[186] The gingivae are thus deprived of oxygen, resulting in ulceration and necrosis of the soft and hard tissues. In more severe cases, inflammation develops into a far advanced gangrene of the maxilla or the soft tissues of the mouth (Takahara's disease).[187]

Numerous pedigrees support an incomplete recessive monogenetic mode of inheritance in this disorder. Acatalasemia cannot be regarded as a single entity but rather as a group of mutations of the catalase gene that result in altered activity levels of a structurally normal enzyme.[188]

The general physical examination of patients with acatalasemia is normal, except for the oral and occasionally the nasal mucosa. No laboratory abnormalities are reported, except for the darkening of blood on exposure to hydrogen peroxide.

Oral ulcerations result from the production of hydrogen peroxide by bacteria proliferating in the crevices of the teeth or tonsillar lacunae. The absence of catalase to metabolize the hydrogen peroxide leads to oxidation of hemoglobin and thus to ulceration or decay of the oral tissues, or both. The early removal of diseased teeth and tonsils and the administration of antibiotics halt the progress of the disease. The healing time for acatalasemics is identical to that of normal persons. Biopsies of ulcerated tissue show chronic inflammation. Immunologically, affected patients are normal, except for their inability to decompose hydrogen peroxide.

Therapy consists of extracting affected teeth and tonsils at an early stage. Systemic antibiotics such as penicillin are necessary to control bacterial proliferation. Meticulous oral hygiene is necessary to prevent recurrence of the ulcerations. The overall prognosis in properly managed cases is good, except for the potential loss of all teeth and some alveolar bone. Topical hydrogen peroxide should be avoided by acatalasemic persons, as it is toxic to them.

175. Schaffer AW, Pearlstein HH (1967) Hyperkeratosis palmoplantaris with periodontosis (Papillon-Lefevre syndrome). **Oral Surg Oral Med Oral Pathol** 24:180.

176. Coccia CT, McDonald RE, Mitchell DF (1966) Papillon-Lefevre syndrome: precocious periodontosis with palmar-plantar hyperkeratosis. **J Periodontol** 37:408.

177. Brownstein MH, Skolnik P (1972) Papillon-Lefevre syndrome. **Arch Dermatol** 106:533.

178. Gelmetti C, Nazzaro V, Cerri D, Fracasso L (1989) Long-term preservation of permanent teeth in a patient with Papillon-Lefevre syndrome treated with etretinate. **Pediatr Dermatol** 6:222.

179. Haneke E, Hornstein OP, Lex C (1975) Increased susceptibility to infections in the Papillon-Lefevre syndrome. **Dermatologica** 150:283–286.

180. Liu R, Cao C, Meng H, Tang Z (2000) Leukocyte functions in 2 cases of Papillon-Lefevre syndrome. **J Clin Periodontol** 27:69–73.

181. Ghaffer KA, Zahran FM, Fahmy HM, Brown RS (1999) Papillon-Lefevre syndrome: neutrophil function in 15 cases from 4 families in Egypt. **Oral Surg Oral Med Oral Pathol Oral Radiol Endod** 88:320–325.

182. Kressin S, Herforth A, Preis S et al. (1995) Papillon-Lefevre syndrome – successful treatment with a combination of retinoid and concurrent systematic periodontal therapy: case reports. **Quintessence Int** 26:795–803.

183. Lundgren T, Crossner CG, Twetman S, Ullbro C (1996) Systemic retinoid medication and periodontal health in patients with Papillon-Lefevre syndrome. **J Clin Periodontol** 23:176–179.

184. Siragusa M, Romano C, Batticane N et al. (2000) A new family with Papillon-Lefevre syndrome: effectiveness of etretinate treatment. **Cutis** 65:151–155.

185. Ullbro C, Crossner CG, Lundgren T et al. (2000) Osseointegrated implants in a patient with Papillon-Lefevre syndrome. A 4 1/2-year follow up. **J Clin Periodontol** 27:951–954.

186. Aebi H, Suter H (1971) Acatalasemia. In: Advances in Human Genetics, vol. 2, Harris H, Hirshckorn K eds. New York: Plenum Press, p. 143.

187. Perner H, Krenkel C, Lackner B et al. (1999) Acatalasemia – Takahara's disease. **Hautarzt** 50:590–592.

ULCERATIVE STOMATITIS WITH NEUTROPENIA

Oral ulcerations may occur as a manifestation of various forms of neutropenia, such as agranulocytosis, cyclic neutropenia, chronic benign neutropenia of childhood, but also of leukemia.[189] The ulcers may be relatively small, localized, and minimally painful or may enlarge gradually to form extensive painful necrotic lesions. A gangrenous stomatitis can develop in patients with severe neutropenia. In addition, necrotizing gingivitis (Vincent's angina) may complicate the clinical picture.[77]

In cyclic neutropenia, the oral ulcers tend to remain small without much peripheral erythema and are randomly distributed throughout the oral cavity.[89–191] The lesions develop during episodes of neutropenia that recur at 3- to 4-week intervals and usually last for five to seven days. A mild gingivitis may also accompany the ulcerations.[89]

Treatment consists of lavage and gentle debridement. Granulocyte-colony stimulating factor has been shown to hasten recovery of neutrophils, reducing the risk of secondary infection.[192]

Drug-induced agranulocytosis may result in necrotizing ulcerations of the oral mucosa, tonsils, and pharynx. The gingiva and palate are the mucosal surfaces most frequently involved in this condition. Shallow ulcers covered by a gray or black membrane are encircled by little or no inflammation. Complications range from severe secondary infection to hemorrhage from the gingiva. Excess salivation is a common finding.

Histologically, denuded areas of mucosa lack polymorphonuclear leukocytes despite the presence of bacteria. Therapy is nonspecific, except for elimination of the drug responsible for the agranulocytosis and administration of appropriate antibiotics. Dental procedures, particularly extractions, are contraindicated in the setting of agranulocytosis. The prognosis in drug-induced agranulocytosis is good if the offending agent can be identified and eliminated and the infection controlled.[38]

Oral mucositis is a common consequence of intensive chemotherapy caused directly by the cytotoxic effect of chemotherapeutic agents and indirectly by sustained neutropenia. This form of mucositis is characterized by edematous erythema, epithelial necrosis, ulcerations with fibrin membranes. It represents an important predisposing factor for life-threatening septic complications during chemotherapy-induced aplasia. A similar clinical picture, however, often associated with severe xerostomia, is also elicited by intraoral radiotherapy.

Topical filgrastim (T-metHuG-CSF) in a viscous mouthrinse alleviated the symptoms.[193]

Another syndrome with cyclic fever is called the periodic fever, aphthous stomatitis, pharyngitis, and cervical adenopathy syndrome (PFAPA). The onset of symptoms is between the age of 3 months and 12 years with a mean age of 5 years. After an initial phase of generalized clinical symptoms such as asthenia, cranial neuritis, dysphagia, and anorexia, high fever suddenly occurs with temperatures over 40°, shivering, multiple aphthous ulcers, pharyngitis and cervical lymphadenitis. Other symptoms may be headache, arthralgia and abdominal pain in about 50% of the cases. Fever recurs every six to nine weeks. During the fever, there is an inflammatory syndrome of hyperleukocytosis, elevated sedimentation rate and increase of C-reactive protein which are not diagnostic.

Differential diagnosis includes familial Mediterranean fever, hyper-IgD syndrome, and cyclic neutropenia.

The prognosis is excellent. No specific cause has yet been identified. The most effective treatment is early administration of corticosteroids.[194–196]

RECURRENT APHTHOUS ULCERATION

Recurrent oral ulcerations, also known as aphthae, aphthous stomatitis, and canker sores, are probably the most common cause of mouth ulcers and are classified as three distinct clinical types. Minor aphthous ulcers were first described by Mikulicz in 1888 and account for the greatest percentage of lesions (more than 80%). Major aphthous ulcers, described by Sutton in 1911, comprise approximately 8% of these lesions. herpetiform ulcers, so named by Cooke in 1960, have a similar frequency, but the latter types are considerably overreported.[197,198] Despite the recommendation of the National Institute of Dental Research Workshop in 1977 that the term *recurrent aphthous stomatitis* be reserved for the major and minor types and that the term *recurrent oral ulcerations* be used to embrace all three clinical types,[199] this suggested alteration in terminology has been applied only occasionally in subsequent publications. The confusion in nomenclature has been further compounded by failure in some publications to distinguish the lesions of recurrent intraoral herpes simplex infection, a totally different entity. Furthermore, even the term "stomatitis" is a misnomer because the aphthae normally appear without a diffuse inflammation of the oral mucosa.

Aphthous stomatitis occurs most frequently during the ages of 10 to 60 years with the highest frequency of onset in the second decade of life.[199] Estimates of prevalence vary from 5% to 60%, but the figure of 20% for the general population is the most widely accepted. A slightly higher prevalence has been observed in females. A positive family history is obtained in up to 40% of affected persons, but a definite mode of transmission has not been established.[200] Children whose two parents are affected are much more likely to have aphthae (67%) than are offspring of affected mothers (53%), affected fathers (34%), or unaffected parents (9%).[201] Twin studies have shown 90% concordance in identical twins as opposed to 57% concordance in fraternal twins.[202]

The signs and symptoms of aphthous stomatitis vary with the particular form of the disorder.[113,203–205]

1. *Minor aphthae*, the most common type of oral ulcerations, begin as erythematous macules that evolve into papules and then into painful yellow necrotic ulcerations surrounded by an erythematous halo. A vesicular stage is absent. Lesions number less than 10, are smaller than 10mm, and develop on the movable nonkeratinized mucosa of the labial, glossal, subglossal, and buccal surfaces and in the mucobuccal folds (Fig. 9.24). Ulcers localized to the hard palate and gingiva are extremely rare. The lesions heal within seven to 10 days without the formation of scars.

2. *Major aphthae* are usually fewer in number (one to five lesions) but do not differ in evolution. They may measure up to 3cm in diameter, are deeper and more painful, and usually persist for longer periods, even up to six weeks. Resolution with scarring is expected.

188. Goth L, Rass P, Madarasi I (2001) A novel catalase mutation detected by polymerase chain reaction-single strand conformation polymorphism, nucleotide sequencing, and western blot analyses is responsible for the type C of Hungarian acatalasemia. **Electrophoresis** 22:49–51.
189. Andrews RG, Benjamin S, Shore N, Canter S (1965) Chronic benign neutropenia of childhood with associated oral manifestations. **Oral Surg** 20:719.
190. Dale DC, Bolyard AA, Hammond WP (1993) Cyclic neutropenia: natural history and effects of long-term treatment with recombinant human granulocyte colony-stimulating factor. **Cancer Invest** 11:219.
191. Rodenas JM, Ortego N, Herranz MT et al. (1992) Cyclic neutropenia: a cause of recurrent aphthous stomatitis not to be missed. **Dermatology** 184:205.
192. Fink-Puches R, Kainz JT, Kahr A et al. (1996) Granulocyte colony-stimulating factor treatment of cyclic neutropenia with recurrent oral aphthae. **Arch Dermatol** 132:1399–1400.
193. Karthaus M, Rosenthal C, Huebner G et al. (1998) Effect of topical oral G-CSF on oral mucositis: a randomised placebo-controlled trial. **Bone Marrow Transplant** 22:781–785.
194. Marshall GS, Edwards KM, Butler J, Lawton AR (1987) Syndrome of periodic fever, pharyngitis, and aphthous stomatitis. **J Pediatr** 110:43–46.

195. Feder HM (2000) Periodic fever, aphthous stomatitis, pharyngitis, adenitis: a clinical review of a new syndrome. **Curr Opin Pediatr** 12:253–256.
196. Ovetchkine P, Bry ML, Reinert P (2000) Syndrome de Marshall: résultats d'une enquête nationale rétrospective. **Arch Pediatr** 7 Suppl 3:578s–582s.
197. Cooke BED (1969) Recurrent oral ulceration. **Br J Dermatol** 81:159.
198. Merchant VA, Molinari J (1984) Recurrent aphthous stomatitis and herpetiform ulcerations. **J Mich Dent Assoc** 66:357.
199. Graykowski EA, Hooks JJ (1978) Summary of workshop on recurrent aphthous stomatitis and Behçet's syndrome. **J Am Dent Assoc** 97:599.
200. Lehner T (1977) Progress report oral ulceration and Behçet's syndrome. **Gut** 18:491.
201. Miller MF, Garfunkel AA, Ram CA, Ship JJ (1980) The inheritance of recurrent aphthous stomatitis. **Oral Surg** 49:409.
202. Miller MF, Garfunkel AA, Ram CA, Ship JJ (1977) Inheritance patterns in recurrent aphthous ulcers: twin and pedigree data. **Oral Surg** 43:886.
203. Rogers RS III (1977) Recurrent aphthous stomatitis: clinical characteristics and evidence for an immunopathogenesis. **J Invest Dermatol** 69:499.

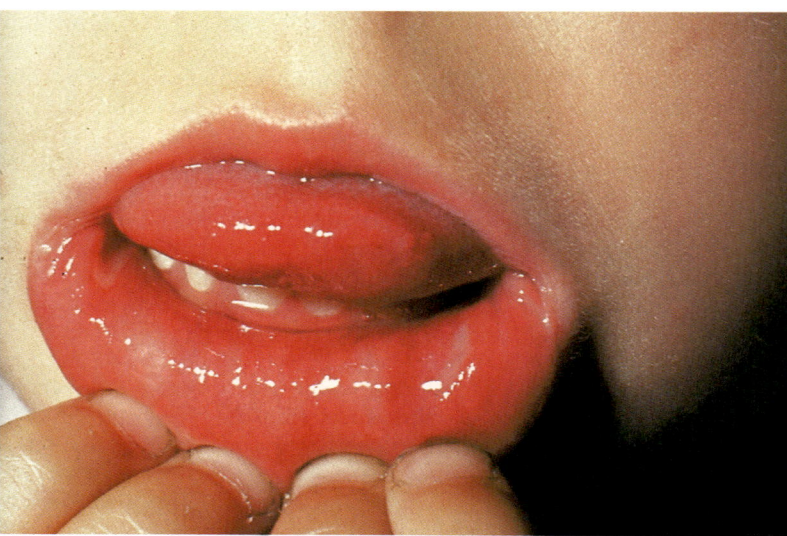

Fig. 9.24 Aphthous stomatitis in a young child.

3. *Herpetiform ulcerations* are profuse in number (up to 100 lesions) but relatively small, measuring only 1–2mm. These ulcers, which have a brief vesicular stage, frequently coalesce to form plaques 5–20mm in diameter and, therefore, have a herpetiform configuration. In contrast to minor and major aphthae, they may develop at any site in the oral cavity. They are intensely painful, persist for approximately seven to 10 days, and heal without scarring.

A premonitory stage is often experienced for all three types for 1–3 days prior to development of these lesions and is characterized by local sensations of tingling, paresthesias, burning pain, and a rough, raw spot on the mucosa. Once the erythema is visible, pain of variable intensity is a prominent feature. Generally, constitutional signs and symptoms such as fever, malaise, and lymphadenopathy are absent, but may occur with the first outbreak. Major aphthous ulcers may cause extreme discomfort and, because of their prolonged course, poor nutrition, and weight loss.

Routine laboratory studies are usually normal. Exceptions occur when systemic disorders such as ulcerative colitis, Crohn's disease, celiac disease, and Behçet syndrome are associated. In the group of patients with nutritional disorders, serum folate, vitamin B_{12}, and iron levels may be altered.

The histopathology of mature aphthae is that of a nonspecific ulcer. There is focal loss of the epithelium with edema and a mixed inflammatory infiltrate limited to the lamina propria. The infiltrate consists predominantly of mononuclear cells, mainly monocytes, macrophages, and blast-forming T lymphocytes.[198,206] Immunofluorescence studies demonstrate immunoglobulins and C3 in submucosal vessel walls.[203]

A definite etiology has not been established for aphthous stomatitis. A number of trigger factors have been implicated in selected individuals including stress, dental trauma, and hormonal changes coincident with the menstrual cycle. Although food hypersensitivity has been considered as an etiologic factor, challenge studies have not substantiated this association.[207] Nutritional deficiencies involving mainly iron, vitamin B_{12} and folate have been documented in approximately 15% of patients.[208] The ulcers in these persons

are not clinically distinctive but are often associated with glossitis and angular cheilitis and respond promptly to restoration of a normal nutritional state.

Attempts to identify an infectious cause have been inconclusive. Adenovirus type 1 has been suspected but not proven as the cause of herpetiform aphthous stomatitis.[199,200] Recovery of L forms of streptococci from patients with aphthae has prompted the suggestion that these organisms stimulate the formation of antibodies that cause cytolysis, a reaction to released antigens from epithelial tissue. Alternatively, an autoimmune reaction might precede direct infection. However, there is no firm evidence to validate the role of streptococci in the production of aphthous ulcerations.

Most investigators favor a cell-mediated immunopathogenic mechanism, although the precise chain of events is still unclear. Circulating antibodies to oral mucous membrane antigens in individuals with aphthae have been identified by several techniques. *In vitro* assays using oral mucosa target cells have demonstrated cytotoxicity of lymphocytes from patients with all three types of aphthous stomatitis.[209]

In children, the differential diagnosis includes acute herpetic gingivostomatitis, herpangina, and hand, foot, and mouth disease, all of which not only differ clinically but are usually associated with constitutional signs and symptoms. Viral cultures and acute and convalescent serum antibody titers will also help distinguish these infections. A positive Tzanck smear and ELISA will establish a diagnosis in herpetic gingivostomatitis and the rare instance of recurrent intraoral herpes simplex infection. Pemphigus vulgaris, Wegener's granulomatosis, and lymphomatoid granulomatosis must be considered but are extremely rare in childhood; immunofluorescence studies and biopsy for histologic changes are diagnostic. Consideration must be given to associated systemic disorders such as inflammatory bowel disease, celiac disease, Behçet syndrome, cyclic neutropenia, and leukemia as well as to drug-related stomatitis. Aphthae occur significantly less frequently in smokers than in nonsmokers.[210] This underlines the observation that benign aphthae predominantly affect nonkeratinized mucosa.

Treatment of aphthous stomatitis is aimed at reducing pain and promoting rapid healing of the ulcers. Treatments can be divided into categories including topical anesthetics, debridement/antiseptic agents, anti-inflammatory agents, and protective products.[211] Topical corticosteroids in an adherent vehicle such as carboxymethylcellulose (Orabase) or applied under a layer of Orabase are often recommended. Hydroxypropylcellulose (Zilactin) forms a more adherent film that outlasts Orabase and offers significant pain relief.[211] Mild oral antiseptics and topical anesthetics such as viscous lidocaine may alleviate discomfort somewhat (see Table 9.10). Antibacterial oral rinse such as chlorhexidine gluconate (Peridex) or tetracycline mouthwash (250mg/5ml water) four times daily diminish secondary bacterial infection and provide symptomatic relief; however, the latter agent should not be used for children because, if swallowed, permanent staining of developing teeth may occur. Five percent amlexanox oral paste (Aphthasol) applied four times daily accelerates healing and pain reduction.[212] Compounded combinations of corticosteroid, diphenhydramine, kaopectate, viscous lidocaine, and tetracycline in various proportions are popular and probably afford some reduction in pain.[113]

Therapy with dyclonine (Dyclone) 0.5% swished or dabbed onto the ulcers may give relief for some patients. Recalcitrant ulcers or large ulcers may require triamcinolone acetonide (10mg/ml) injected in the base for pain control and to promote healing. Cyanoacrylate adhesive provided symptomatic relief within minutes and shortened the healing time in one study.[213] Thalidomide has been successfully used outside the United States to treat aphthous stomatitis in children.[214]

204. Rogers RS (1992) Common lesions of the oral mucosa: a guide to disease of the lips, cheeks, tongue and gingivae. **Postgrad Med J** 91:141.
205. Field EA, Brooks V, Tyldesley WR (1992) Recurrent aphthous ulceration in children: a review. **Int J Paediatr Dent** 2:1–10
206. Weathers DR, Griffin JW (1970) Intraoral ulcerations of recurrent herpes simplex and recurrent aphthae: two distinct clinical entities. **J Am Dent Assoc** 81:81.
207. Eversole LR, Shoppers TP, Chambers DW (1982) Effects of suspected foodstuff challenging agents in the etiology of recurrent aphthous stomatitis. **Oral Surg** 54:33.
208. Wray D, Ferguson MM, Hutcheon AW et al. (1978) Nutritional deficiencies in recurrent aphthae. **J Oral Pathol** 7:418.
209. Rogers RS III, Sams M Jr, Shorter RG (1974) Lymphocytotoxicity in recurrent aphthous stomatitis. **Arch Dermatol** 109:361.
210. Tuzun B, Wolf R, Tuzun Y, Serdaroglu S (2000) Recurrent aphthous stomatitis and smoking. **Int J Dermatol** 39:358–360.
211. Barnes DP, Primosch RE (1990) Therapeutic recommendations for aphthous ulcerations in children. **Comp Contin Educ Dent**, vol XI; no. 5:312–320.
212. Khandwala A (1997) Five percent amelexanox oral paste, a new teatment for recurrent minor aphthous ulcers. **Oral Surg Oral Med Oral Pathol Oral Radiol Endod** 83:222–230.

Although initially thought to be a promising drug, several studies of levamisole therapy in patients with aphthae have failed to prove efficacy, as has thymopentin.[215] Likewise, cromolyn sodium, zinc sulfate, and topical azathioprine have been given without significant response. In patients with severe disease, a short course of oral corticosteroid may be required to induce remission.

Patients with minor aphthae may have recurrences as infrequently as once or twice yearly. Major aphthae and herpetiform ulcerations are likely to recur with greater frequency and may be present almost continuously. The ultimate prognosis is good for most patients, as spontaneous remission in 5–15 years is usual.

PIGMENTED LESIONS OF THE MUCOSAE

Pigmented lesions of the mucous membranes are due to increased production of melanin in the melanocytes, to hyperplasia or neoplastic transformation of the melanocytes, or to deposition of exogenous substances such as heavy metals, iron, and drugs or metabolic products of drugs. In most cases, mainly the oral mucous membranes are affected. The pigmentation may be focal, patchy, or relatively diffuse and, in some entities, has a specific localization and coloration that facilitate diagnosis (Table 9.12).

DIFFUSE MACULAR PIGMENTATION

Racial pigmentation

The most common cause of oral melanosis is racial pigmentation, which occurs in several patterns. Most frequently, a diffuse band of increased pigmentation develops at the junction of the free and attached alveolar mucosa (Fig. 9.25). The band may parallel the line of closure of the teeth or pigment may be distributed in a patchy fashion. The tongue is rarely involved but, when it is, the pigment is characteristically localized to the tips of the filiform or fungiform papillae.[216] Patches of pigment may occasionally be found on the buccal mucosa and the floor of the mouth or along the lips. This type of mucosal pigmentation is common in blacks but can also be found in darker-skinned persons of other races. This finding has been observed at all ages, including infancy, but occurs

with greatest frequency after middle age.[217] The hyperpigmentation has been attributed to increased activity of the melanocytes in affected areas of the mucosa.

Addison's disease

Macular hyperpigmentation of the oral mucosa is an early and prominent manifestation of Addison's disease. The pigment is diffusely distributed in the gingiva, tongue, buccal mucosa, and hard palate; the color varies from blue-black to yellow. In the gingiva, the pigmentation may be spotty or streaked. Although cutaneous pigmentation usually disappears following therapy, mucosal pigmentation persists indefinitely.

Widespread oral mucosal hyperpigmentation

Additional causes of widespread oral mucosal hyperpigmentation are riboflavin (vitamin B_2) deficiency, heavy use of tobacco and snuff, drug-induced pigmentation, and heavy metal deposition.

Familial progressive hyperpigmentation

Familial progressive hyperpigmentation[218] is a very rare cause of hyperpigmentation, described in one family in which it was transmitted in an autosomal-dominant fashion. A family study in China has also been described.[219]

Universal acquired melanosis

Also known as carbon baby,[220] this exceedingly rare condition results in diffuse hyperpigmentation of the entire oral mucosa. The disorder is due to increased melanin and melanosomes in the epithelium of affected areas.

Heavy metal pigmentation

Heavy metal pigmentation is relatively uncommon in infants and children but, when it occurs, can affect the oral and ocular mucous membranes.[221] Mercury, lead, silver, and bismuth can all cause similar slate-gray hyperpigmentation of the gingivae. Mercury-induced pigmentation results from the presence of mercury granules in the dermis as well as increased amounts of melanin in the epithelium and dermal macrophages. Oral pigmentation due to this metal is usually associated with stomatitis and suppurative periodontitis.[222] Bismuth causes conjunctival and oral mucosal hyperpigmentation as well as the blue-black gingival line first seen at the interdermal papillae.

TABLE 9.12   Pigmentation of the oral mucosa in children

Cause	Location
	Diffuse Macular Hyperpigmentation
Racial pigmentation	Gingivae, lips, tongue
Addison's disease	Generalized
Riboflavin deficiency	Generalized or irregular
Heavy use of tobacco and snuff	Generalized
Heavy metal pigmentation (silver, lead, mercury, bismuth)	Generalized, gingival line; conjunctiva (bismuth, silver)
Drug-related (antimalarial agents)	Palatal line
	Focal Hyperpigmentation
Nevocellular nevi	Hard palate; less commonly buccal, labial mucosa, gingiva
Melanotic macules	Lower lips, gingiva, buccal mucosa
Lentigines	Lips; less commonly buccal mucosa, gingiva, hard palate, tongue
Amalgam tattoo	Gingival and alveolar mucosa; buccal mucosa, floor of mouth, mucobuccal fold

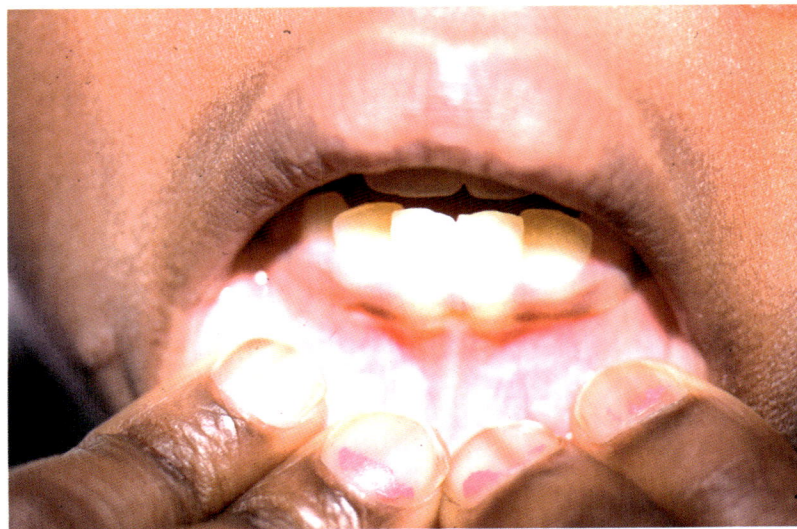

Fig. 9.25   Racial melanosis involving the lower gingiva.

213. Jasmin JR, Muller GM, Jonesco-Benaiche N (1993) Local treatment of minor aphthous ulceration in children. **ASDC J Dent Child** 60:26.

214. Menni S, Imondi D, Brancaleone W, Croci S (1993) Recurrent giant aphthous ulcers in a child: protracted treatment with thalidomide. **Pediatr Dermatol** 10:283.

215. Djawari D, Haneke E (1983) Therapie der rezidivierenden oralen Aphthen mit Thymopoetin-Pentapeptid. **Hautarzt** 34:463–464.

216. Gray RLM (1978) Pigmented lesions of the oral cavity. **J Oral Surg** 36:950.

217. Johnson SAM (1978) The black skin. Norms and abnorms. **Cutis** 22:332.

218. Chernosky ME, Anderson DE, Chang JP et al. (1971) Familial progressive hyperpigmentation. **Arch Dermatol** 103:581.

219. Ling DB, Lo T (1991) Familial progressive hyperpigmentation: a family study in China (letter). **Br J Dermatol** Dec; 125:607.

220. Ruiz-Maldonado R, Tamayo L, Fernandez-Diaz J et al. (1978) Universal acquired melanosis. **Arch Dermatol** 114:775.

Metallic granules are found in the dermal layer on histologic examination. Some authorities believe that the predisposing factors of poor oral hygiene and bacterial interaction with the bismuth compound are required to produce the distinctive gingival line.[172,173] Lead lines in the gingiva indicate chronic poisoning and are due to subepithelial deposits of lead granules that have been converted to lead sulfide. Lead pigmentation is gray and is usually noted a slight distance from the marginal gingiva. Silver is readily absorbed through the mucous membranes as metallic silver or in a relatively insoluble form such as oxide or sulfide.[221] The silver granules are deposited in the subepithelial layer and show a predilection for association with the elastic fibers.

Drug-induced hyperpigmentation

Drug-induced hyperpigmentation in the mucosae is most often seen with administration of antimalarial agents. Antimalarial drugs (quinocrine, chloroquine, hydroxychloroquine) may cause a line of pigmentation, sharply demarcating the soft and hard palates.[221–224] In the skin, hyperpigmentation is presumed to result from deposition of the drug itself, as well as increased melanin and hemosiderin content. Additional drugs that cause dark patches on the oral mucosa are phenolphthalein, phenothiazines, oral contraceptives, and mercurial diuretics in patients with impaired renal function.[216] ACTH and α-methyl dopa can lead to increased mucosal melanin pigmentation.

FOCAL HYPERPIGMENTATION

Nevocellular nevi are much less common in the oral mucosa than in the skin. The site of predilection is the hard palate, but they may also occur on the buccal and labial mucosa, the vermilion border, and the gingiva. They are variously gray, brown, black, or blue, range in size from one to several millimeters, and are most often elevated and sessile, although occasionally they can be flat or pedunculated. Because they are asymptomatic and not easily visualized, age of onset is usually unknown to the patient. Histologically, the most common type of lesion is intramucosal (intradermal), with blue nevi, and compound and junctional types being less frequent in occurrence.[225,226] These lesions can be confused with amalgam tattoo, pigmented neuroectodermal tumor, melanotic macules, or patchy racial or drug-induced pigmentation. The propensity for malignant change is unknown.

The decision to electively remove a pigmented nevus on the oral mucous membranes depends on the overall appearance of the lesion. If the nevus has grown larger, darker, thicker, or become painful or has bled, removal is recommended. Surgical excision should be performed if the edges are irregular or there is extrusion of pigment from the nevus into the surrounding mucosa. Intraoral nevi typically are totally excised rather than sampled due to the technical difficulty in removing these growths in children. Some authorities suggest prophylactic excision of all intraoral pigmented nevi.[227]

Malignant melanoma

Malignant melanoma of the oral cavity is very uncommon in adults and exceedingly rare in children. In several reported series, there have been no cases below the age of 20 years.[228] A single case of a 16-years-old male with dysplastic nevus syndrome did develop a melanoma *in situ* on his hard palate.[229]

The preferred site of involvement is the maxilla; much less commonly, the mandibular alveolus, tongue, buccal mucosa, and lips may be involved. The signs and symptoms are similar to those of melanoma on the skin: development of a mass, changes in pigmentation, pain, ulceration, and bleeding.[227] The presence of a suspicious lesion is an indication for immediate excisional biopsy.

Melanotic macules

Melanotic macules[226,230] are sometimes equated with lentigines or ephelides in the nondermatologic literature, but do not seem to fit into either category clinically or histologically. They are most often solitary, occurring with greatest frequency (30%) on the vermilion borders, almost always on the lower lip. Additional sites of predilection are the gingiva (23%) and buccal mucosa (16%). These pigmented lesions are brown, gray, or blue and range in size from 0.1cm to 2.0cm but are most often 1–3mm. They have been observed in children over 4 years of age, but there are no appreciable data on occurrence in infancy. A slight female predominance has been noted.

Histologically melanotic macules have increased melanin in the basal epidermal layer without increased numbers of melanocytes. In one-half of the lesions, melanin in melanophages is also found in the lamina propria and, in approximately 10%, is found only at this site. Although melanotic macules are benign, clinically they may be confused with lentigines, nevocellular nevi, and malignant melanoma. One authority suggests excision of these lesions on a routine basis because of the confusion they cause diagnostically.[227]

Lentigines

Lentigines are discrete, round-oval, brown, blue or black macules characterized histologically by elongation of the epidermal rete pegs, increased numbers of melanocytes, and increased basal melanin. These lesions develop in the oral mucous membranes in patients with the several syndromes: centrofacial lentiginosis,[231] multiple lentigines with nystagmus and strabismus,[232] lentiginosis with hemangiomas,[233] Carney syndrome (NAME and LAMB syndrome),[234,235] inherited patterned lentiginosis in blacks,[236] Peutz–Jeghers syndrome,[237] and Laugier–Hunziker–Baran syndrome.[238] In patients with centrofacial lentiginosis, multiple lentigines with strabismus, Carney syndrome and inherited patterned lentiginosis in blacks,[235] the hyperpigmentation is limited to the lips, whereas in patients with lentiginosis with hemangiomas, Laugier–Hunziker–Baran syndrome, and Peutz–Jeghers syndrome, the buccal mucosa is affected as well. In the latter syndrome, lesions have also been described on the gums, palate, and tongue.[238,239] The macules in patients with Peutz–Jeghers syndrome are oval or irregular in configuration and most numerous on the lower lip; approximately 98% of affected persons possess these lesions. Onset of pigmentation is usually in early childhood or occasionally in infancy and, unlike the cutaneous lentigines, which may fade during adulthood, mucosal lentigines persist for life.[239,240] Melanonychia is found in about half the cases with Laugier–Hunziker–Baran syndrome.

Amalgam Tattoo

Amalgam tattoo is a relatively common cause of pigmentation of the oral mucous membranes. Although most series include patients from the age of 12 years and up,[241] these lesions occur in children as well. Amalgam tattoos

221. Granstein RD, Sober AJ (1981) Drugs and heavy metal-induced hyperpigmentation. **Arch Dermatol** 5:1.
222. Marlette RH (1975) Generalized melanosis and nonmelanotic pigmentations of the head and neck. **J Am Dent Assoc** 90:141.
223. Kleinegger CL, Hammond HL, Finkelstein MW (2000) Oral mucosal hyperpigmentation secondary to antimalarial drug therapy. **Oral Surg Oral Med Oral Pathol Oral Radiol Endod** Aug; 90:189–194.
224. Ziering CL, Rabinowitz LG, Esterly NB (1993) Antimalarials in children: indications, toxicities, and guidelines. **J Am Acad Dermatol** 28:764.
225. Buchner A, Hansen LS (1979) Pigmented nevi of the oral mucosa: a clinicopathologic study of 32 new cases and review of 75 cases from the literature. **Oral Surg** 48:131.
226. Begleiter A, Moskona D, Gorsky M, Buchner A (1983) Benign solitary pigmented lesions of the oral mucosa. **Dent Digest** 1:9.
227. Batsakis JG, Regezi JA, Solomon AR, Rice DH (1982) The pathology of head and neck tumors: mucosal melanomas, part 13. **Head Neck Surg** 4:404.
228. Liversedge RL (1975) Oral malignant melanoma. **Br J Oral Surg** 13:40.

229. Themblay JF, O'Brien EA, Chauvin PJ (2000) Melanoma in situ of the oral mucosa in an adolescent with dysplastic nevus syndrome. **J Am Acad Dermatol** 42:844–846.
230. Buchner A, Hansen LS (1977) Melanotic macule of the oral mucosa. **Oral Surg** 48:244.
231. Dociu I, Galaction-Nitcelea O, Sirjita N et al. (1976) Centrofacial lentiginosis. **Br J Dermatol** 94:39.
232. Pipkin AC, Pipkin SB (1950) A pedigree of generalized lentigo. **J Hered** 41:79.
233. Bandler M (1960) Hemangiomas of the small intestine associated with mucocutaneous pigmentation. **Gastroenterology** 38:641.
234. Rhodes AR, Silverman RA, Harrist TJ, Perez-Atayde AR (1984) Mucocutaneous lentigines, cardiomucocutaneous myxomas, and multiple blue nevi: the "LAMB" syndrome. **J Am Acad Dermatol** 10:72.
235. Carney JA, Gordon H, Carpenter PC et al. (1985) The complex of myxomas, spotty pigmentation, and endocrine overactivity. **Medicine** 64:270.
236. O'Neill JF, James WD (1989) Inherited patterned lentiginosis in blacks. **Arch Dermatol** 125:1231.
237. Fulk CS (1984) Primary disorders of hyperpigmentation. **J Am Acad Dermatol** 10:1.
238. Haneke E (1991) Laugier–Hunziker–Baran Syndrom. **Hautarzt** 42:512–515.

may be produced in several different ways: (1) by abrasion or laceration of the mucosa by a rotary instrument and inoculation of amalgam particles; (2) by dropping pieces of amalgam into the socket following extraction; (3) by deposition of amalgam fragments into the wound during root canal therapy; and (4) by propelling fine particles through an intact mucosa by a high-speed drill. The embedded amalgam particles consist mainly of silver but also contain a significant amount of tin and smaller quantities of copper and zinc.[242]

Amalgam tattoos are clinically evident as blue or black macules or as slightly elevated lesions having sharp or indistinct margins. They occur most frequently in the gingiva and alveolar mucosa, particularly in the mandibular region; less frequently on the buccal mucosa, floor of the mouth, and mucobuccal fold, and occasionally on the tongue, labial mucosa, and palate.[241,243] They range in size up to 2cm, with most measuring less than 0.5cm. Histologically, the amalgam is detectable in a biopsy specimen as fine dark granules and irregular solid fragments interposed between collagen fibers and around blood vessels and imbibition of elastic fibers is characteristic. There may be no inflammatory reaction or only macrophages or granulomas of the foreign body type with multinucleated cells and Langerhans cells.

Diagnosis is made clinically and can often be confirmed by biopsy. Radiographs may demonstrate opaque particles at the site of the pigmented macule, but often the particles are too small or too diffuse to be visualized. Differential diagnosis includes melanotic macule, heavy metal pigmentation, nevocellular nevus, lentigo, and antimalarial pigmentation. Amalgam tattoos persist indefinitely and sometimes increase in size with time, presumably due to movement of phagocytic cells with ingested particles.[241]

NEVUS OF OTA

This melanotic macular lesion, usually of a gray-blue color, involves the trigeminal area of the face, hence it has also been called nevus fuscocoeruleus ophthalmomaxillaris. Nevus of Ota is most commonly found in Orientals and blacks and has a strong predilection for females. In approximately 60% of affected persons, the nevus is present at birth; in the remainder, the lesion usually develops gradually during the first decade, although in rare instances, it becomes apparent at or after puberty.[244]

Nevus of Ota has a unilateral distribution usually involving the forehead, temple, malar area, and ala nasi, but almost always sparing the nasolabial fold and the upper lip. Mucous membranes of the nose and mouth, the external auditory canal, and tympanic membrane are occasionally involved as well. The size of the patch, which has indistinct margins, usually exceeds 5cm, and the color may vary from a tan-brown to slate blue-black. Although the nevus is usually macular, there may be elevated areas within the patch resembling discrete blue-nevi.[245–247] Two-thirds of patients have blue-gray discoloration of the sclera on the affected side due to melanocytes in the sclera or episclera. The pigment is usually patchy in distribution, most often involving the superior and temporal aspects of the sclera. Rarely, pigmentation may extend to the conjunctiva and other ocular structures, such as the cornea, iris, choroid, and optic disk.[245] Vision is not impaired.

The pigmented patch is due to the presence of melanin-producing melanocytes in the upper and mid-dermis. Depending on the density and distribution of the dermal melanocytes, these nevi may resemble either the blue nevus or the Mongolian spot histologically. Clinically, these lesions are most often confused with Mongolian spots and may be referred to as aberrant Mongolian spots or oculodermal melanocytosis. Café-au-lait spot, ochronosis, contusion, chloasma, and heavy metal pigmentation are additional consid-

erations in the differential diagnosis. When the mucous membranes are involved, Addison's disease, racial melanosis, drug-induced hyperpigmentation, and heavy-metal deposition must also be included. Ocular pigmentation can be confused with scleral defects or pigmented nevi of the conjunctiva.

Nevus of Ota, unlike Mongolian spot, persists indefinitely and has little propensity for malignant change, although melanoma arising in the skin or ocular tissues has been associated in rare instances.[245–247] Q-switched ruby laser therapy has been reported to be an effective and safe method of removing or lightening nevus of Ota pigmentation of the skin.[248–250] The Q-switched alexandrite laser has also been successfully used to treat this condition.[251]

MUCOSAL ALTERATIONS CAUSED BY DRUGS

Phenytoin

Gingival hyperplasia is one of the most frequently recognized sequelae of phenytoin therapy. Nearly one-half of those requiring this anticonvulsant develop painless enlargement of the gingivae. The interdental papillae may reflect changes as early as two weeks following the initiation of therapy, but more often two to three months are required. Maximum hyperplasia occurs following nine to 12 months of phenytoin therapy.

Clinically, the earliest findings include stippling of the interdental papillae and gradual swelling of the gingiva, which acquires a warty, pebbled surface texture. With increasing enlargement, the gingivae begin to encroach on the upper portions of the teeth, obscuring them in some instances. The anterior teeth are more affected than the posterior teeth. The presence of bacterial plaque appears essential for the development of phenytoin-induced gingival hyperplasia.

Therapy consists of meticulous oral hygiene. Surgical excision of excessive tissue is occasionally warranted when the hypertrophy is marked, but recurrences are the rule until the patient reaches middle age. Carbon dioxide laser gingivectomy has been recommended in selected patient populations.[252] Cessation of phenytoin will produce a gradual spontaneous regression over 12 months' time, provided the teeth are kept free of microbial deposits.

Cyclosporine

Cylosporine has many of the same clinical effects on the gingivae as phenytoin. Gingival overgrowth may be seen as early as three months into therapy in predisposed individuals. Patients who develop gingival hyperplasia typically have higher salivary cyclosporine levels than those who are unaffected or have minimal changes.

Gingival overgrowth is seen less frequently in bone marrow transplant recipients than other grafted patients. Both a young age at time of treatment and a high dose of cyclosporine predispose to this adverse effect of the drug. Decreasing the dose of cyclosporine may result in regression of the gingival hyperplasia, but gingivectomy may be required in rare cases.

Other drugs potentially causing gingival hyperplasia are diltiazem, nifedipine, and some antihypertensive agents.

Acetylsalicylic acid (aspirin)

Following the direct application of an aspirin tablet to a painful tooth or aphthous ulcer, a glistening denuded hyperemic erosion may develop on the oral mucosa, occasionally after an initial grayish-white discoloration. These ulcerations occur as a direct effect of the aspirin on the mucosal surface. The

239. Yoskowitz P, Hobson R, Reymann F (1974) Sporadic Peutz–Jeghers syndrome in early childhood. **Am J Dis Child** 128:709.
240. Trovar JA, Eizaquirre J, Albert A, Jimenez J (1983) Peutz–Jeghers syndrome in children: report of two cases and review of the literature. **J Pediatr Surg** 15:1.
241. Buchner A, Hansen LS (1985) Amalgam pigmentation (amalgam tattoo) of the oral mucosa. **Oral Surg** 49:139.
242. Weathers DR, Fine RM (1974) Amalgam tattoo of oral mucosa. **Arch Dermatol** 110:728.
243. Owens BM, Johnson WW, Schuman NJ (1992) Oral amalgam pigmentation (tattoos): a retrospective study. **Quintessence Int** Dec; 23:805–810.
244. Kopf AW, Weidman AJ (1962) Nevus of Ota. **Arch Dermatol** 85:195.

245. Gold DH, Henkind P, Sturner WQ, Baden M (1967) Oculodermal melanocytosis and retinitis pigmentosa. **Am J Ophthalmol** 63:271.
246. Haim T, Meyer E, Kerner H, Zonis S (1982) Oculodermal melanocytosis (nevus of Ota) and orbital malignant melanoma. **Ann Ophthalmol** 14:1132–1136.
247. Kopf AW, Bart RS (1982) Malignant blue (Ota's?) nevus. **J Dermatol Surg Oncol** 8:442.
248. Geronemus RG (1992) Q-switched ruby laser therapy of nevus of Ota. **Arch Dermatol** 128:1618.
249. Ono I, Tateshita T (1998) Efficacy of the ruby laser in treatment of Ota's nevus previously treated using other therapeutic modalities. **Plast Reconstr Surg** Dec; 102:2352–2357.
250. Pfeiffer N (1993) Q-switched ruby laser used to remove pigmented lesions. **J Clin Laser Med Surg** Jun; 11:147–148.

ulcers tend to be painful, although relatively short lived. Recovery occurs within several days and scarring is infrequent. Cotton-roll stomatitis is clinically almost identical.

Silver nitrate

Silver nitrate is occasionally employed to cauterize lesions in the oral cavity, especially in recurrent oral aphthae. Some cases of giant oral ulcers after this treatment have been observed. Injudicious or excessive use result in the development of painful burns. Although long-term sequelae are rare when silver nitrate is used briefly, it is best avoided, when feasible, in the pediatric age group.

Oral ulcerations secondary to cancer chemotherapy

Mucositis and oral ulcerations frequently develop following administration of chemotherapeutic drugs. Commonly implicated chemotherapeutic agents are methotrexate, 5-fluorouracil, actinomycin D, adriamycin, bleomycin, and daunorubicin. Less commonly 6-mercaptopurine, hydroxyurea, vinblastine, and procarbazine are implicated.[78]

Direct and indirect effects of such medicaments on the oral mucosa precipitate the ulceration.[113] The direct effect of methotrexate on cell replication and growth of oral epithelial cells results in interference with nucleic acid and protein synthesis. Thinning is followed by focal ulceration within the oral cavity. Chemotherapeutic agents may have an indirect affect on the mucous membranes by depressing the bone marrow and immune response, ultimately predisposing the patient to invasive infections.

Clinically, the oral ulcerations caused by cancer chemotherapy are deep, large, and necrotic with little inflammation at the base of the ulcer. Virtually all mucosal surfaces may be affected. A history of recent chemotherapy in the presence of these ulcers suggests the diagnosis, but cultures of the ulcers are warranted as Gram-negative sepsis may stem from untreated local infection. When fungal infection is suspected, culture and biopsy are mandatory. Ulcerative herpes simplex and erosive candidiasis must also be ruled out.

When severe oral ulceration occurs, chemotherapy may, of necessity, have to be discontinued or the dosage decreased. These compromises are occasionally impossible. Symptomatic remedies in the form of topical anesthetic mouthwashes (see Table 9.10) and narcotic analgesics where appropriate should be offered to increase patient comfort. Granulocyte-colony stimulating factor may help the patient to recover earlier.

ORAL MANIFESTATIONS OF SYSTEMIC DISEASES

Leukemia

The oral manifestations of leukemia tend to reflect the general status of the patient, the type of leukemia, and the age of the patient.[253–255] Although mucous membrane alterations occur in both acute and chronic forms of leukemia, they occur far more commonly in the acute states and most commonly in monocytic leukemia.[256] In children, the oral manifestations of acute leukemia have been found to be varied rather than pathognomonic.[257,258] Of 292 pediatric patients with leukemia of various types, fewer than 30% had oral findings suggestive of leukemia. Acute lymphocytic leukemia, the most common form of leukemia in childhood, is the least likely to produce oral lesions.[259]

The primary clinical manifestations of leukemia include gingivitis, gingival hyperplasia (Fig. 9.26), hemorrhage, petechiae, and ulcerations of the oral mucosa.[38] Pallor of the mucosa may reflect concomitant anemia. The teeth may become painful and loose, and a sore throat may be

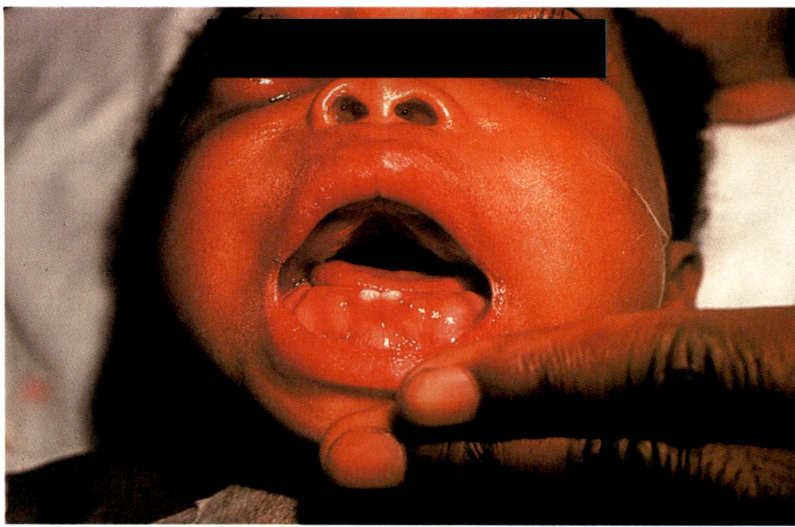

Fig. 9.26 Leukemia: monocytic (infraorbital and gingival infiltrates).

reported.[260] Except for edentulous patients, gingival hyperplasia occurs as an almost constant feature of leukemia. The hyperplasia is typically generalized but varies in intensity. In severe cases, the hypertrophied gums may nearly mask the teeth. Changes in the gingivae include bogginess, edema, and erythema. The surface becomes friable and bleeds readily. The presence of leukemic cell infiltrates in areas of mild chronic irritation contributes to the gingival swelling.

Ulcerations of the sulcus epithelium and necrosis of underlying tissue predispose to gingival hemorrhage. Purpura of the oral mucosa, like cutaneous ecchymoses, occurs as a result of thrombocytopenia. Focal oral ulceration may occur as a consequence of nonfunctioning leukocytes having the same effect as agranulocytosis, or as a direct effect of chemotherapy on mucosal epithelium. Such ulceration typically develops seven days after the onset of antileukemic drug therapy. Bacterial invasion due to severe neutropenia may also contribute to the formation of oral ulcers. These shallow, denuded foci may herald the onset of leukemia and are characteristically large, irregular, and foul smelling. A pale mucosa surrounds these lesions, and an inflammatory response is lacking.

Therapeutic goals for leukemic ulcers should include the prevention of localized infection, minimizing bacteremia, promotion of healing, and the reduction of pain.[78] Local therapy is often effective in managing petechiae, ecchymosis, and minor hemorrhage. Irritants should be removed and direct pressure applied when bleeding occurs. Proper use of adsorbable gelatin sponges with topical thrombin or placement of microfibrillar collagen on packing or splints can reduce the need for platelet transfusions. Oral rinses with antifibrinolytic agents may help in certain cases.[78]

LANGERHANS CELL HISTIOCYTOSIS (HISTIOCYTOSIS X)

Oral and dental manifestations of Langerhans cell histiocytosis (LCH, histiocytosis X) can occur in all three forms of the disorder. The incidence of oral involvement in several series has varied tremendously, ranging from 4.5% to 77%.[261] This variation may be due, in part, to the thoroughness with which the oral cavity was examined in these patients. The presence of jaw swelling or a palpable mass is the most commonly reported finding.[261] Intraosseous

251. Kang W, Lee E, Choi GS (1999) Treatment of Ota's nevus by Q-switched alexandrite laser: therapeutic outcome in relation to clinical and histopathologic findings. **Eur J Dermatol** 9:639–643.
252. Roed-Peterson B (1993) The potential use of CO_2-laser gingivectomy for phenytoin-induced hyperplasia in mentally retarded patients. **J Clin Periodontol** Nov; 20:729–731.
253. Levy-Polack MP, Sebelli P, Polack N (1998) Incidence of oral complications and application of a preventive protocol in children with acute leukemia. **Spec Car Dentist** 18:189–193.
254. Weckx LL, Hidal LB, Marcucci G (1990) Oral manifestations of leukemia. **Ear Nose Throat** 69:341–342.

255. Childrs NK, Stinnett EA, Wheeler P et al. (1993) Oral complications in children with cancer. **Oral Surg Oral Med Oral Pathol** 75:41–47.
256. Burket LW (1944) A histopathologic explanation for the oral lesions in the acute leukemias. **Am J Orthod Oral Surg** 30:516.
257. Michaud M, Bachner RL, Bixler D, Kafrawy AH (1977) Oral manifestations of acute leukemia in children. **J Am Dent Assoc** 95:1145.

lesions predominantly affect the mandible, particularly in the posterior portion. Pain, gingivitis, inflammation, necrosis, and loosening of the teeth are also frequently noted (Fig. 9.27). In small infants, there may be premature eruption of fully or partially formed teeth.

Radiologic studied of the jaw may show a sharply defined lytic lesion with variable loss of alveolar bone. When there is sufficient destruction of bone to permit displacement of teeth, the teeth may appear to the floating in air.[262] Biopsy of gingival ulcerations and lytic bone lesions will demonstrate the characteristic pathology of LCH, thus confirming the diagnosis. The total clinical picture will dictate the type of therapy indicated. Eosinophilic bone granuloma in children is said to heal spontaneously in a high percentage of cases.[262]

WEGENER'S GRANULOMATOSIS

Wegener's granulomatosis is an uncommon disease in adults and is particularly rare in children, with less than 60 pediatric cases currently in the literature.[263–270] Wegener's granulomatosis is a systemic illness characterized by concurrent findings of necrotizing perivascular granulomas and polyvasculitis. Multiple organs, including the skin, are affected by the venous and arteriolar vasculitis.[270] Limited forms have also been described.[265] In such cases, the disease remains localized for prolonged periods before multiorgan system involvement occurs. The necrotizing granulomatous vasculitis typically involves the upper and lower respiratory tract as well as the renal glomeruli. This condition often begins and remains for a long period in the head and neck region.[266] This classic triad of nose, lung, and kidney involvement is less often encountered in children.

If involvement of the lower respiratory tract or kidneys, or both, is evident when oral changes are detected, the prognosis is generally poor. A patient thus affected succumbs to the lungs within a short period of time. If the kidneys and lungs become involved subsequent to the oral lesions, however, survival is prolonged due to the more localized nature of the disease.

As the specific histologic findings of necrotizing, granulomatous inflammation with vasculitis are not always seen and the findings on renal biopsy are almost always nonspecific, other methods to confirm the diagnosis of Wegener's granulomatosis have been developed. Nearly all cases of Wegener's granulomatosis have elevations of the serum autoantibodies to a neutrophilic cytoplasmic antigen (ANCA).[265] Elevation in ANCA titer also heralds disease relapses. However, in children ANCA titers may also be elevated in cystic fibrosis and juvenile rheumatoid arthritis.[271] In adult patients, therapeutic response can be monitored with clinical improvement, a decrease in the erythrocyte sedimentation rate, and ANCA titer levels. Treatment may be discontinued after a disease-free interval of one year. Therapeutic agents used for pediatric patients with Wegener's granulomatosis include cyclophosphamide, prednisone, and methotrexate.[270]

A persistent mucopurulent and sanguineous nasal discharge characterizes this granulomatous process.[266,269] The nasal mucosa may appear swollen, granular, and friable, with rare development of nasal septal perforation.[266] Although involvement of the oral cavity does occur with considerable frequency in Wegener's granulomatosis, oral lesions are seldom the presenting sign.[38] The distinctive hyperplasia of the gingiva that begins in the interdental papillae represents the most common manifestation and represents small vessel vasculitis. The gums become red to purple in color, with numerous petechiae that occasionally extend to the labial and buccal mucosa, eventually involving

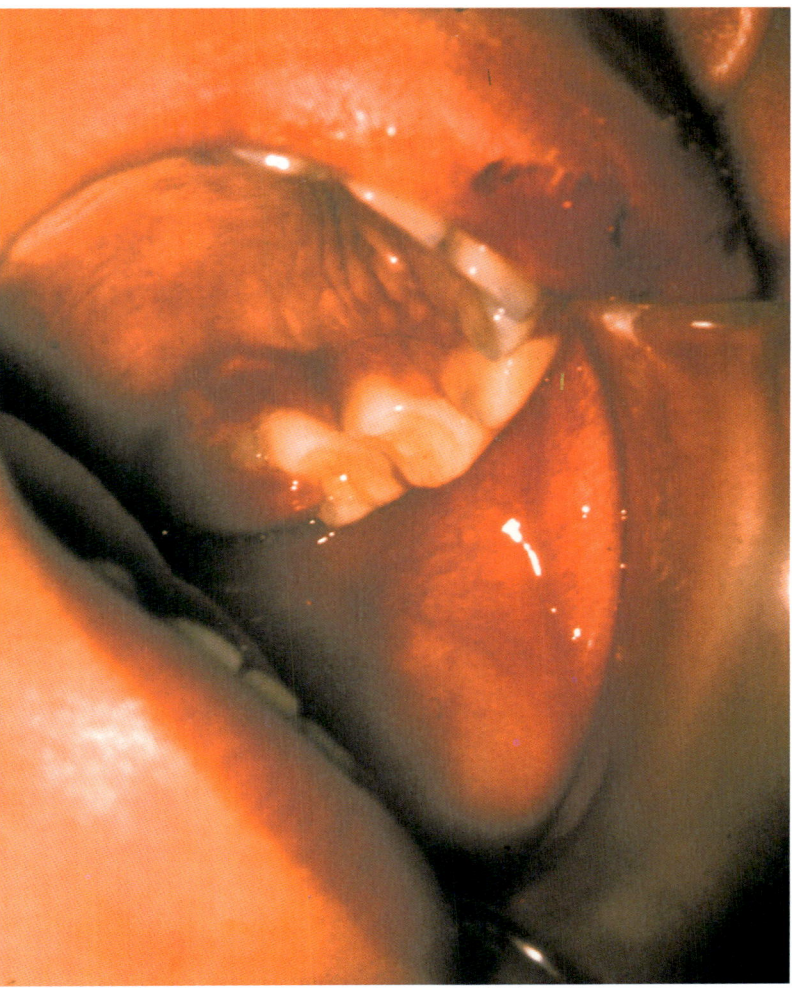

Fig. 9.27   Histiocytosis X (Langerhans cell histiocytosis): periodontal ulceration.

the entire gingiva and periodontium.[265] Other alterations of the gingivae include ulcerations and friable granular growths. The presence of a diffuse ulcerative stomatitis may result in tooth mobility and subsequent spontaneous exfoliation of the teeth. Once these teeth are shed, their extraction sites fail to heal. The hard palate, cheeks and lips may also be involved. Large necrotic ulcers may penetrate the palate to the nose.

Histologically, the gingival lesions demonstrate pseudoepitheliomatous hyperplasia and a nonspecific chronic histiocytic inflammation. Vasculitis of the gingival tissues is uncommon.[265,270] The presence of giant cells is variable and palisading granulomas, although common in classical lesions of Wegener's granulomatosis found in the lung, are rare in gingival biopsy specimens.[272,273] The inflammatory component of the submucosa includes a diffuse infiltrate of epithelioid histiocytes and occasional eosinophils.[265]

The true incidence of Wegener's granulomatosis is unknown.[272] Either sex may be affected, with young adult males showing the greatest propensity for

258. Gruszewska-Lewczuk L (1974) Manifestations of acute leukemia in the oral cavity in children. **Czasopismo Stomatologiczne** 27:887–894.
259. Curtis AB (1971) Childhood leukemias: initial oral manifestations. **J Am Dent Assoc** 83:159.
260. Stawiski MA (1978) Skin manifestations of leukemias and lymphomas. **Cutis** 21:814.
261. Cranin AN, Rockman R (1981) Oral symptoms in histiocytosis X. **J Am Dent Assoc** 103:412.
262. Hartman KS (1980) Histiocytosis X: a review of 114 cases with oral involvement. **Oral Surg** 49:38.
263. Orlowski JP, Clough JD, Dyment PG (1978) Wegener's granulomatosis in the pediatric age group. **Pediatrics** 61:83.
264. Chyu JYH, Hagstrom WJ, Soltani K et al. (1984) Wegener's granulomatosis in childhood: cutaneous manifestations as the presenting signs. **J Am Acad Dermatol** 10:341.

265. Patten SF, Tomecki KJ (1993) Wegener's granulomatosis: cutaneous and oral mucosal disease. **J Am Acad Dermatol** 28:710.
266. Rasmussen N (2001) Management of the ear, nose, and throat manifestations of Wegener granulomatosis: an otorhinolaryngologist's perspective. **Curr Opin Rheumatol** 13:3–11.
267. Hall SL, Miller LC, Duggan E et al. (1985) Wegener granulomatosis in pediatric patients. **J Pediatr** 106:739.
268. Moorthy AV, Chesney RW, Segar WE, Groshong T (1977) Wegener granulomatosis in childhood: prolonged survival following cytotoxic therapy. **J Pediatr** 91:616.
269. Rottem M, Fauci S, Hallahan CW et al. (1993) Wegener's granulomatosis in children and adolescents: clinical presentation and outcome. **J Pediatr** 122:26.

the systemic form. Orlowski *et al.*[263] doubt the authenticity of cases below 10 years of age, stating that the two infants described probably had chronic granulomatous disease of childhood. No genetic predisposition has been determined in Wegener's granulomatosis. The precise etiology remains unclear, but a hypersensitivity reaction to an undefined antigen remains highly suspect. A number of Wegener-like cases have been described.[274]

Current therapy typically includes the use of cyclophosphamide and prednisone. The differential diagnosis of the oral lesions must include eosinophilic granuloma, nonspecific gingivitis, and periodontitis.

GRAFT-VERSUS-HOST DISEASE

Following bone marrow transplantation for leukemia, aplastic anemia, or immunodeficiency, the lymphocytic, hematopoietic, reticuloendothelial, and epithelial cells may undergo an inflammatory reaction mounted by the donor cells against these tissues.[275] Graft-versus-host reaction is said to occur within the specified organ, with the skin, liver, and GI tract being most frequently involved. The host is said to undergo graft-versus-host disease. Mucous membrane alterations are common in the setting of graft-versus-host disease.[276] Furthermore, the manifestations reflected by the oral mucosa indicate successful treatment or progression of a graft-versus-host reaction.[277,278]

Three clinical patterns of acute graft-versus-host disease involve the oral mucosa.[276-278] Each clinical alteration of the oral mucosa may occur as a single distinct finding or as part of a continuum including other mucosal changes. The first clinical variant is one in which numerous tiny papules develop abruptly in the oral cavity. The close proximity of the papules gives an appearance of generalized whiteness. This pattern typically lasts only 2–8 days and may precede the other two recognized forms. The second variant is characterized by the development of a reticular or "lichenoid" pattern on the oral mucosa. Striae-like lesions of interlacing white strands emerge (Fig. 9.28). The third presentation is desquamative. The tiny papules of the first described clinical alteration coalesce. Within 12 to 24 days, these then evolve into irregular plaques of whitened mucosa. The desquamation that follows is asymptomatic with minimal to no surface erosion.

The oral changes seen in acute graft-versus-host disease may gradually evolve into those seen in the chronic graft-versus-host disease. Chronic graft-versus-host disease is characterized by cutaneous and mucosal lesions that mimic lichen planus and scleroderma, both clinically and histologically. Lacy, reticular, keratotic lesions develop on the buccal mucous membranes, cheeks, lips, and gingivae.[78] The salivary and lacrimal gland epithelium may also be involved. Histologically, the patchy and periductal infiltrates of lymphocytes and plasma cells resemble those of Sjögren syndrome.[277,279] The inflammatory cells infiltrate the duct walls and glandular acini, producing fibrosis, ductal dilation with destruction, loss of acini, and replacement by fibrous tissue. Mucus production is markedly diminished in advanced cases.[280]

The combination of xerostomia and desquamation of the oral mucosa predisposes to caries and secondary infection as natural barriers to local tissue invasion are disrupted.[276,277] Greater than three-fourths of patients undergoing bone marrow transplantation have subsequent infection within the oral cavity. *Candida* is a frequent problem, but other opportunistic organisms may also cause morbidity.

Establishing the diagnosis of acute or chronic graft-versus-host disease requires that other factors contributing to mucosal membrane changes be ruled

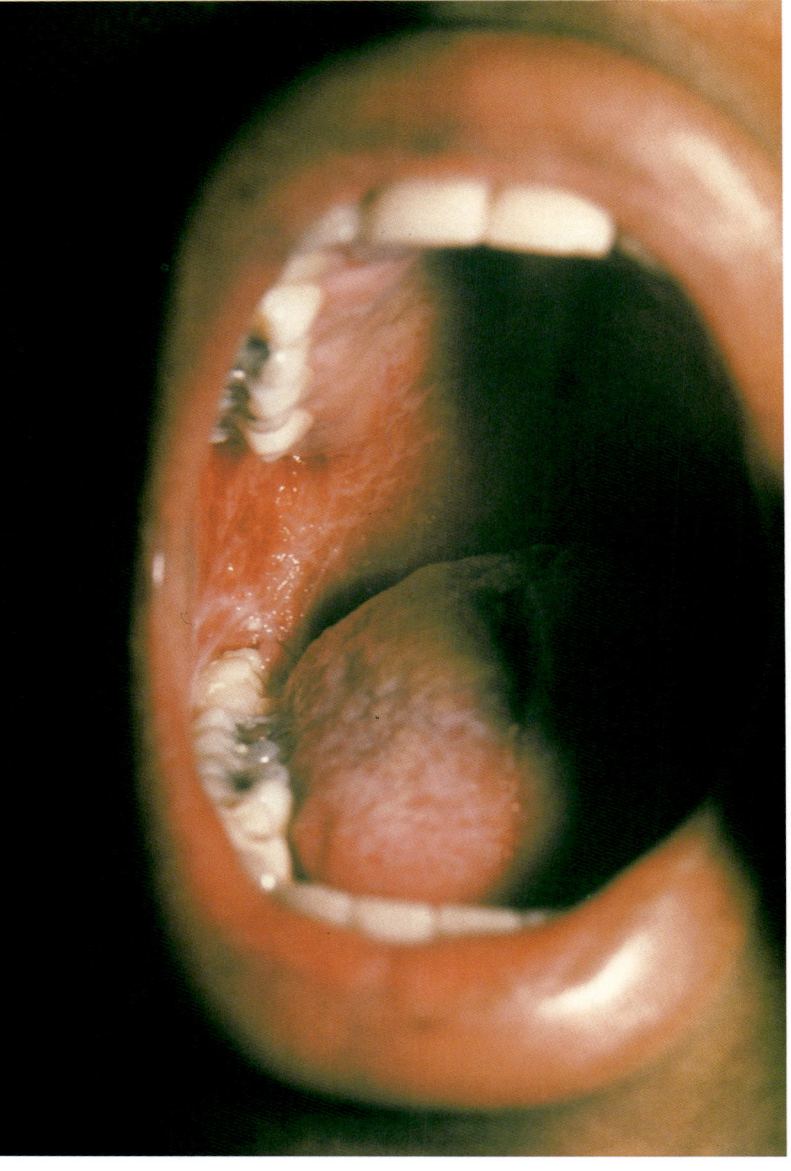

Fig. 9.28 Graft-versus-host disease.

out. Both candidiasis and drug or irradiation-induced mucosal toxicity may simulate or mask the diagnosis.[276-278] Examination of the mucous membranes in those at risk for graft-versus-host disease is crucial, particularly in chronic graft-versus-host disease where changes may predate other manifestations by as much as several weeks.[277]

The treatment of oral GvHD lesions follows the general principles of GvHD therapy. The Sjögren-like symptoms may be improved using pilocarpine.[281] Both intraoral PUVA and selective ultraviolet B irradiation are beneficial.[282-284]

270. Verschuur HP, Struyvenberg PAA, van Benthem PPG et al. (1993) Nasal discharge and obstruction as presenting symptoms of Wegener's granulomatosis in childhood. **Int J Pediatr Otorhinolaryngol** 27:91.

271. Sediva A, Kolarova I, Bartunkova J (1998) Antineutrophil cytoplasmic antibodies in children. **Eur J Pediatr** 157:987–991.

272. Roback SA, Herdman RC, Hoyer J, Good RA (1969) Wegener's granulomatosis in a child. **Am J Dis Child** 118:608.

273. Brooke RI (1969) Wegener's granulomatosis involving the gingivae. **Br Dent J** 127:34.

274. von Vigier RO, Trummler SA, Laux-End R et al. (2000) Pulmonary renal syndrome in childhood: a report of twenty-one cases and a review of the literature. **Pediatr Pulmonol** 29:382–388.

275. Farmer ER, Hood AF (1987) Graft versus host disease. In: Update: Dermatology in General Medicine. 3rd ed, Fitzpatrick TB, Eisen AZ, Wolf K et al., eds. New York: McGraw-Hill, p. 1344.

276. Barret AP, Belous AM (1984) Oral patterns of acute and chronic graft-versus-host disease. **Arch Dermatol** 120:1461.

277. Woo SB, Lee SJ, Schubert MM (1997) Graft-vs-host disease. **Crit Rev Oral Biol Med** 8:201–216.

278. Eisen D, Essell J, Broun ER (1997) Oral cavity complications of bone marrow transplantation. **Semin Cutan Med Surg** 16:265–272.

279. Gratwhol AA (1977) Sjögren-type syndrome after allogenic bone marrow transplantation. **Ann Intern Med** 87:703.

280. Nicolatou-Galitis O, Kitra V, Van Vliet-Constantinidou C et al. (2001) The oral manifestations of chronic graft-versus-host disease (cGVHD) in paediatric allogeneic bone marrow transplant recipients. **J Oral Pathol Med** 30:148–153.

281. Nagler RM, Nagler A (1999) Pilocarpine hydrochloride relieves xerostomia in chronic graft-versus-host disease: a sialometrical study. **Bone Marrow Transplant** 23:1007–1011.

LUPUS ERYTHEMATOSUS

Approximately 25% of patients with lupus erythematosus have oral lesions, most commonly localized to the buccal mucosa, palate, and tongue.[285] These lesions, which occur in both systemic lupus erythematosus (SLE) and discoid lupus erythematosus (DLE), may develop as the initial manifestation or may accompany the onset of the cutaneous lesions. In DLE, the lip lesions consist of small atrophic areas surrounded by a narrow zone of white keratinization, with striae which are net-like or radiate from the margins.[286] Occasionally, there is central ulceration and crusting. When the tongue is involved, deep fissures and atrophy of the papillae are salient features. The oral lesions of SLE are mainly parallel or radiating striae, hyperemia and petechiae. Edema of the involved tissue is more pronounced, and petechiae and ulcerations may be prominent findings. These lesions are most often symptomatic and painful.

The differential diagnosis includes lichen planus, leukoplakia and aphthous stomatitis. Histologic findings on biopsy may be diagnostic, but sometimes even immunofluorescence studies fail to differentiate lupus erythematosus and lichen planus. Immunoglobulins and complement are deposited in a band at the dermo–epidermal junction, as in the skin lesions; this is a consistent finding in patients with SLE and is also noted in most patients with DLE.[287] There is no specific treatment; the oral lesions may improve with therapy instituted for other manifestations of the disease.

KAWASAKI DISEASE

Also known as mucocutaneous lymph node syndrome, this disorder is diagnosed on the basis of the following findings: (1) fever of five or more days; (2) bilateral injection of the bulbar conjunctiva; (3) changes in the oropharyngeal mucous membranes, consisting of dryness, redness, and fissuring of the lips, strawberry tongue, and suffusion of the mucosa; (4) edema and erythema of the feet and hands and periungual desquamation; (5) polymorphous rash; and (6) acute nonpurulent cervical lymphadenopathy.[288] Additional findings include arthalgia and arthritis, diarrhea, sterile pyuria, carditis, pneumonia, aseptic meningitis, hydrops of the gallbladder, aneurysms of the coronary arteries, coronary artery thrombosis, jaundice, and thrombocytosis, as well as other clinical and laboratory abnormalities.[289]

Changes in the ocular and oropharyngeal mucous membranes are considered major criteria for the diagnosis and occur within one to three days following onset of the fever. Ocular conjunctival injection, which is observed in almost all cases,[10,288–293] is always bilateral, and the vascular engorgement is confined to the bulbar conjunctiva, with little change in the palpebral conjunctiva.[290] Most striking is the prominence of individual vessels that may appear tortuous. Mild to moderate conjunctival discharge has been described but is uncommon.[290–292] Also uncommon are the findings of subconjunctival hemorrhage and superficial punctate keratitis. Anterior uveitis has been detected in association with this disease and is usually mild.[291–293]

Marked suffusion of the oropharyngeal mucosa imparts a deep red color to the lips, which are also edematous, dry, and fissured (Fig. 9.29). The tongue is diffusely red with prominent papillae resembling the "strawberry tongue" of streptococcal scarlet fever. Subsequently, the lips may crack and bleed, causing lip soreness, but frank oral ulcerations are rare. The mucous membrane manifestations persist into the second week of the illness and then subside, leaving no sequelae.

An erythematous desquamating perineal eruption has been reported in patients with Kawasaki syndrome. The eruption typically develops in the first six days of the symptoms with a median day of onset on day three. The desquamation of the skin of the perineum occurs earlier than on the

fingertips. No differences in outcome occurred between two groups of patients with or without the perineal rash.[294]

The disorder and treatment are discussed in more detail in Chapter 23.

DISORDERS OF MULTIPLE MUCOUS MEMBRANES

LEUKOPLAKIA

The term *leukoplakia* means "white patch," but it has been used in such a nonspecific fashion as to render it practically meaningless. When applied to oral mucosal lesions, it denotes a white plaque that cannot be removed by rubbing and cannot be ascribed to a diagnosable skin disorder. One cannot make a specific diagnosis with any degree of accuracy from the clinical appearance of the lesion; rather, histopathologic examination is always necessary to establish diagnosis and prognosis.

Oral leukoplakia is a problem of adults, usually of the middle years and beyond, but it is also encountered rarely in adolescents. A preponderance of males has been noted in all series.[78] Etiologic factors include chronic trauma; chemical and thermal irritation, particularly the use of tobacco in any form; neglect of hygiene, and possible nutritional factors.[87,96]

Leukoplakia in the mouth may be limited to a focal area or may be diffuse, involving large areas of the oral mucosa; it is usually painless. Erosions, fissures, and the presence of pain signify malignant change or an erroneous diagnosis. Common sites of involvement are the cheeks near the oral commissure extending posteriorly along the line of closure of the teeth, the tongue, the palate, and the floor of the mouth. When the tongue is involved, the lesion is characterized by absence of papillae, a feature that distinguishes leukoplakia from geographic tongue. In children, disorders likely to be confused with leukoplakia include lichen planus, chronic candidiasis, cheek and lip biting, burns, Heck's disease,[132] and nevoid lesions such as white sponge nevus, epidermal nevus, hereditary benign intraepithelial dyskeratosis, pachyonychia congenita, and

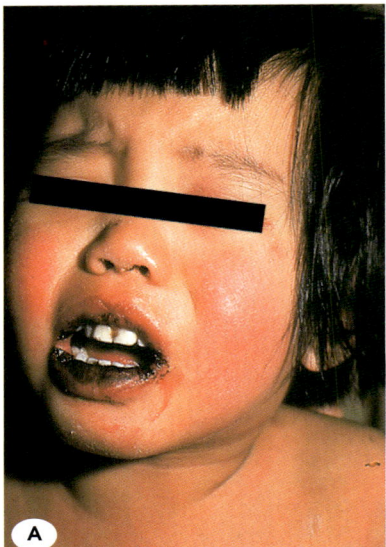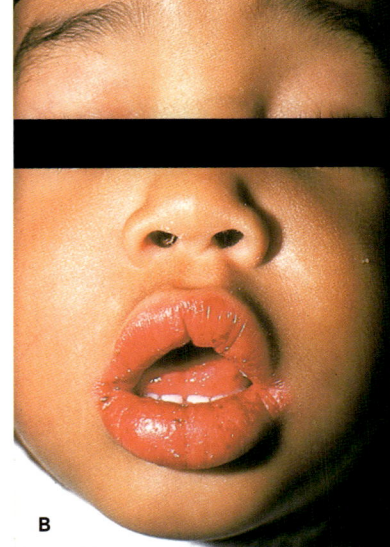

Fig. 9.29   **A, B** Swelling, fissuring, and crusting of the lips in two young children with Kawasaki syndrome.

282. Redding SW, Callander NS, Haveman CW, Leonard DL (1998) Treatment of oral chronic graft-versus-host disease with PUVA therapy: case report and literature review. **Oral Surg Oral Med Oral Pathol Oral Radiol Endod** 86:183–187.

283. Elad S, Garfunkel AA, Enk CD et al. (1999) Ultraviolet B irradiation: a new therapeutic concept for the management of oral manifestations of graft-versus-host disease. **Oral Surg Oral Med Oral Pathol Oral Radiol Endod** 88:444–450.

284. Enk CD, Elad S, Vexler A et al. (1998) Chronic graft-versus-host disease treated with UVB phototherapy. **Bone Marrow Transplant** 22:1179–1183.

285. Schiodt M, Halberg P, Hentzer B (1978) A clinical study of 32 patients with oral discoid lupus erythematosus. **Int J Oral Surg** 7:85.

286. Andreasen JO, Poulsen HE (1964) Oral discoid and systemic lupus erythematosus. **Acta Odontol Scand** 22:295.

287. Schiodt M, Holstrup P, Dabelsteen E, Ullman S (1981) Deposit of immunoglobulins, complement and fibrinogen in oral lupus erythematosus, lichen planus and leukoplakia. **Oral Surg** 51:603.

288. Kawasaki T, Kasaki F, Okawa S et al. (1974) A new infantile acute febrile mucocutaneous lymph node syndrome (MLNS) prevailing in Japan. **Pediatrics** 54:271.

dyskeratosis congenita (Tables 9.13, 9.14).[295] Biopsy must be obtained to distinguish most of these entities. Furthermore, histopathologic examination is required to identify dyskeratotic lesions, although these are rare in children.

Treatment will depend on the cause of the lesion. Chronic irritation from jagged teeth or prosthetic devices should be eliminated. Oral hygiene should be improved and habits such as cheek biting curbed. Dyskeratotic lesions should always be excised because of the predisposition for malignant change. Careful long-term observation of these patients is mandatory.

The term leukoplakia is equally vague when applied to clinical vulval changes. Some modern gynecology tests recommend elimination of the des-

ignation in the classification of gynecologic problems.[296] Others state that vulvar leukoplakia has not been reported in children.[297]

WHITE SPONGE NEVUS OF CANNON

This rare autosomal-dominant nevoid condition most often affects the oral mucosa but can also occur on the labial, nasal, vaginal, and anal mucosa.[298] The mucosal changes have been noted at birth in some affected infants; in others, onset has been noted variably in infancy, childhood, or adolescence.[299] The nevoid change is believed to be fully developed in extent and severity by adolescence. Association with other skin symptoms is rare.[300]

Oral lesions may occur on the buccal mucosa, hard and soft palate, sides of the tongue, gingivae, and floor of the mouth. The involved tissues are spongy and thickened and have a deeply folded or corrugated appearance with an opalescent white tint. In general, the condition is asymptomatic.

Histopathologic specimens show hyperkeratosis with occasional parakeratosis, marked acanthosis of the epithelium with large, swollen vacuolated cells in the granular and prickle cell layers, as well as numerous mitoses. The dermis is remarkable only for increased vascularity of the stroma and absence of inflammatory infiltrates.[298–300] White sponge nevus is a benign disorder requiring no treatment.

HEREDITARY BENIGN INTRAEPITHELIAL DYSKERATOSIS

This congenital disorder has been described in a triracial isolate of white, native American, and black persons in North Carolina and is inherited as an autosomal-dominant trait with a high degree of penetrance.[301] A few more cases have been observed in other populations. A gene duplication at the chromosome locus 4p35 has been found in these patients.[302]

Oral lesions, which are asymptomatic, strongly resemble white sponge nevus clinically. They consist of soft, spongy white folds and plaques of thickened mucosa on the buccal and labial surfaces, at the labial commissures, on the floor of the mouth, on the ventral and lateral surfaces of the tongue, as well as the gingivae, fauces, and palate.[301]

TABLE 9.13   White lesions of the mouth in childhood

Nevoid and hereditary
   Epidermal nevus
   White sponge nevus
   Hereditary benign intraepithelial dyskeratosis
   Hereditary mucoepithelial dysplasia
   Pachyonychia congenita
   Dyskeratosis congenita
Acquired
   Lichen planus
   Candidiasis
   Verrucae
   Heck's disease
   Lichen sclerosus et atrophicans
   Darier's disease
   Pityriasis rubra pilaris
   Lupus erythematosus
   Psoriasis
   Aphthous stomatitis
   Contact dermatitis
   Secondary syphilis
   Focal keratosis secondary to trauma and/or on top of many common lesions

---

TABLE 9.14   Heritable and nevoid white lesions of the mouth

Condition	Inheritance	Anogenital lesions	Ocular lesions	Other	Complications
Epidermal nevus	None	−	−	−	Epidermal nevus syndrome
White sponge nevus	Autosomal-dominant	+	−	−	None
Benign hereditary intraepithelial dyskeratosis	Autosomal-dominant	−	+	−	Blindness
Hereditary mucoepithelial dysplasia	Autosomal-dominant	+	+	Alopecia; hyperkeratotic papules	Fibrocystic-type lung disease; cor pulmonale; severe infections
Pachyonychia congenita	Autosomal-dominant	−	+ (Type III)	Nail dystrophy; keratoderma, bullae palms, and soles	Malignancy, oral mucosa
Dyskeratosis congenita	X-linked recessive; rarely autosomal-dominant	+	+	Nail dystrophy; poikilodermatous skin lesions; keratoderma and hyperhidrosis of the palms and soles; mental deficiency; immunologic abnormalities; alopecia, skeletal anomalies	Blood dyscrasias; pancytopenia; malignancy, oral mucosa

---

289. Wortmann DW (1992) Kawasaki syndrome. **Semin Dermatol** 11:37.
290. Ohno S, Miyajima T, Higuchi M et al. (1982) Ocular manifestations of Kawasaki's disease (mucocutaneous lymph node syndrome). **Am J Ophthalmol** 93:713.
291. Ammerman SD, Rao MS, Shope TC, Rogsdale CG (1985) Diagnostic uncertainty in atypical Kawasaki disease and a new finding: exudative conjunctivitis. **Pediatr Infect Dis** 4:210.
292. Germain BF, Moroney JD, Guggino GS et al. (1980) Anterior uveitis in Kawasaki disease. **J Pediatr** 97:780.
293. Lapointe N, Chael Z, Lacrox J et al. (1982) Kawasaki disease: association with uveitis in seven patients. **Pediatrics** 69:376.
294. Friter BS, Lucky AW (1988) The perineal eruption of Kawasaki syndrome. **Arch Dermatol** 124:1805.
295. Haneke E (1983) Klassifikation und Beurteilung oraler Leukoplakien. **Hautarzt** 34:Suppl VI:53–54.
296. Danforth DN, Dignam WJ, Hendricks CH et al. (1982) Obstetrics and Gynecology, 4th ed. Philadelphia: Harper & Row.
297. Huffman JW, Dewhurst Sir CJ, Capraro VJ (1981) The Gynecology of Childhood and Adolescence. Philadelphia: WB Saunders.
298. Witkop CJ Jr, Gorlin RJ (1961) Four hereditary mucosal syndromes. **Arch Dermatol** 84:762.

Ocular lesions distinguish this condition from others with similar oral lesions. The bulbar conjunctiva becomes hyperemic and foamy gelatinous plaques develop in perilimbal sites both temporally and nasally. Marked photophobia is usual, and temporary blindness can occur from overgrowth of the plaque. The plaques are sloughed spontaneously, usually in summer rather than winter, and vision may be temporarily restored. Permanent blindness may result eventually from vascularization of the cornea.

Oral and conjunctival lesions demonstrate similar histologic features, including an acanthotic epidermis, vacuolization of the prickle-cell layer, and an intraepithelial dyskeratosis characterized by waxy eosinophilic cells and a cell-within-cell pattern. The latter features are also discernible on buccal and conjunctival smears stained with Papanicolaou (Pap) stain and are regarded as diagnostic. There is no known therapy for this condition.

HEREDITARY MUCOEPITHELIAL DYSPLASIA

A rare autosomal-dominant multiepithelial disorder, hereditary mucoepithelial dysplasia, combines dyskeratoses of the oral, nasal, vaginal, urethral, bladder, and conjunctival mucosa with cataracts, follicular keratoses, nonscarring alopecia, lung disease, and premature death.[303,304] Early signs, apparent in infancy, are severe photophobia, tearing and nystagmus, which precede the development of cataracts, corneal vascularization, and keratitis. Intense erythema of the tissues of the mouth and other mucous membranes occurs in infancy and persists throughout life. A generalized eruption of hyperkeratotic pinhead-sized follicular papules may be present as well as diffuse nonscarring alopecia.[305] Additional findings include chronic seborrhea, frequent upper respiratory infections that may progress to pneumonia, diarrhea, melena, pyuria, and hematuria. Spontaneous pneumothorax is common, resulting in fibrocystic-type lung disease and cor pulmonale. HMD should be considered in the differential diagnosis of childhood alopecia, follicular hyperkeratosis, keratoconjunctivitis, juvenile cataracts, gingival hyperemia, restrictive lung disease, and esophageal stenosis or webs.

Biopsy specimens of mucosal epithelium demonstrate thinning, dyscohesion, and dyskeratosis. Mucosal Pap smears show cytoplasmic vacuoles and inclusions, individual cell dyskeratosis, and lack of epithelial maturation. Misinterpretation of these abnormal results could lead to unnecessary hysterectomy being performed on these patients. Ultrastructural studies show sparse desmosomes, cytoplasmic vacuolization, bands and aggregates of filamentous fibers and structures resembling desmosomes and gap junctions, and the absence of keratohyalin granules. It is speculated that the disorder is attributable to a panepithelial cell defect of desmosomal and gap junction structure predominantly affecting mucosal epithelium. Because of the predisposition to severe infections of the eye and respiratory tract, these patients should be carefully cultured and treated promptly with appropriate antibiotics, when infection is evident.[303–305]

PACHYONYCHIA CONGENITA

This relatively rare syndrome is named for the peculiar identifying nail abnormality that may be associated with other multiple defects.[306] Some authorities designate the following three types of the disorder based on the classification proposed by Kumer and Loos:[307]

- Type I   Jadassohn–Lewandowsky (MIM-167200) Pachyonychia, palmoplantar keratoderma, follicular hyperkeratosis biochemically characterized by a mutation of the keratin 6a/16gene.[308,309]
- Type II   Jackson–Lawler (MIM-167210) Pachyonychia, palmoplantar keratoderma, follicular hyperkeratosis, leukokeratosis of the tongue and buccal mucosa characterized by keratin 6b/17 mutations.[310,311]
- Type III   Corneal dyskeratosis or cataracts plus the features of type II.

Additional variable abnormal findings in these patients include hyperhidrosis, palmoplantar blisters, steatocystoma multiplex,[312–314] epidermal cysts, hypertrichosis, thickened tympanic membranes, dental anomalies, including natal teeth, and mental retardation.[315]

The mucous membrane manifestations include white, opaque thickening of the dorsum of the tongue, scalloped tongue, thickening of the tongue along the interdental line, and keratotic changes in the nasal mucosa and larynx.[316,317] These changes are due to hyperkeratosis and parakeratosis of the epithelium rather than to dyskeratosis.[317] The mucosal changes are not apparent at birth; rather, they develop during infancy and childhood. The oral lesions can be confused with other white keratotic lesions of the mouth, but the distinctive nail changes of thickening and wedge-shaped lifting of the nail plates serve to distinguish this disorder from all others.

DYSKERATOSIS CONGENITA

Dyskeratosis congenita (DC) is an inherited bone marrow failure syndrome in which patients undergo premature ageing and have a predisposition to malignancy. X-linked and autosomal (dominant and recessive)[318] forms of the disease are recognized. The gene responsible for X-linked DC (DKC1) encodes a highly conserved protein, dyskerin. This protein is believed to be essential in ribosome biogenesis and involved in telomerase RNP assembly. Peripheral blood cells have dramatically reduced telomere lengths but normal levels of telomerase activity. Also in autosomal DC, patients have significantly shorter telomeres than age-matched normal controls, suggesting that both forms of the disease are associated with rapid telomere shortening in hemopoietic stem cells.[319]

Clinically, DC consists of the classical tetrade of reticulated hyperpigmentation, nail dystrophy, pluriorificial leukoplakia, and immunologic abnormalities.[320] A variety of less common manifestations include keratoderma of the palms and soles, dental dystrophy[321] and caries, obstruction of the lacrimal ducts with blepharitis, mental retardation, small stature, and a predisposition to the development of carcinoma at the sites of leukoplakia. In addition, blood

299. Zegarelli EV. Everett FG, Kutscher AH et al. (1959) Familial white folded dysplasia of the mucous membranes. **Arch Dermatol** 80:97.
300. Haneke E (1988) White sponge nevus and generalized follicular hyperkeratosis. In: Proceeding of the 4th Internat. Congress of Pediatric Dermatology, Urabe H, Kimura M, Yamamoto K, Ogawa H, eds. University of Tokyo Press, 425–427.
301. Witkop CJ Jr, Shank LE, Graham JB et al. (1960) Hereditary benign intraepithelial dyskeratosis. **Arch Pathol Lab Med** 90:696.
302. Allingham RR, Seo B, Rampersaud E et al. (2001) A duplication in chromosome 4q35 is associated with hereditary benign intraepithelial dyskeratosis. **Am J Hum Genet** 68:491–494.
303. Witkop CJ Jr, White JG, King RA et al. (1979) Hereditary mucoepithelial dysplasia; a disease apparently of desmosome and gap junction formation. **Am J Hum Genet** 31:414.
304. Scheman AJ, Ray DJ, Witkop CJ, Dahl MV (1989) Hereditary mucoepithelial dysplasia. **J Am Acad Dermatol** 21:351.
305. Urban MD, Schosser R, Spohn W et al. (1991) New clinical aspects of hereditary mucoepithelial dysplasia. **Am J Med Genet** June; 1:338–341.
306. Su WP, Chun SI, Hammond DE et al. (1990) Pachyonychia congenita: a clinical study of 12 cases and a review of the literature. **Pediatr Dermatol** Mar; 7:33–38.
307. Kumer L, Loos HO (1938) Pachyonychia congenita (Typ Riehl). **Wien Klin Wochenschr** 48:174.
308. Smith FJ, Fisher MP, Healy E et al. (2000) Novel keratin 16 mutations and protein expression studies in pachyonychia congenita type 1 and focal palmoplantar keratoderma. **Exp Dermatol** 9:170–177.

309. Lin MT, Levy ML, Bowden PE et al. (1999) Identification of sporadic mutations in the helix initiation motif of keratin 6 in two pachyonychia congenita patients: further evidence for a mutational hot spot. **Exp Dermatol** 8:115–119.
310. Celebi JT, Tanzi EL, Yao YL et al. (1999) Mutation report: identification of a germline mutation in keratin 17 in a family with pachyonychia congenita type 2. **J Invest Dermatol** 113:848–850.
311. McGowan KM, Coulombe PA (2000) Keratin 17 expression in the hard epithelial context of the hair and nail and its relevance for the pachyonychia congenita phenotype. **J Invest Dermatol** 114:1101–1107.
312. Hodes M, Norins A (1977) Pachyonychia congenita and steatocystoma multiplex. **Clin Genet** 11:359.
313. Covello SP, Smith FJ, Sillevis Smitt JH et al. (1998) Keratin 17 mutations cause either steatocystoma multiplex or pachyonychia congenita type 2. **Br J Dermatol** Sept; 139:475–480.
314. Guistini S, Amorosi B, Canci C et al. (1998) Pachyonychia congenita with steatocystoma multiplex. A report of two cases and a discussion of the classification. **Eur J Dermatol** Apr–May; 8:158–160.
315. Franzot I, Kansky A, Kavicic S (1981) Pachyonychia congenita (Jadassohn-Lewandowsky syndrome). A review of 14 cases in Slovenia. **Dermatologica** 160:462.
316. Stieglitz JB, Centerwall WR (1983) Pachyonychia congenita (Jadassohn-Lewandowsky syndrome): a seventeen-member, four-generation pedigree with unusual respiratory and dental involvement. **Am J Med Genet** 14:21.

dyscrasias, particularly a Fanconi-like pancytopenia, occurs in approximately 50% of affected persons and represents a life-threatening complication.

Both the clinical and genetic aspects of dyskeratosis congenita are heterogeneous, and different patterns of inheritance are associated with distinct clinical manifestations.[322,323] The diagnosis of dyskeratosis congenita should be considered for patients of either sex who have features of the syndrome, as well as patients of any age with aplastic anemia.

The mucous membrane manifestations of dyskeratosis congenita are present in approximately 85–90% of patients.[324] The oral mucosa is involved most frequently (Fig. 9.30). In some persons, the urethra, glans penis, vagina, and rectoanal mucosa have also shown characteristic changes.[324] Atrophy, stenosis, and fissures have been described in the anal, urethral, and vaginal mucosa. Ocular abnormalities, in addition to epithelial hyperplasia of the lacrimal puncta with resultant stenosis, include bullous conjunctivitis, blepharitis, ectropion, and loss of lashes.[325] Gingivitis, periodontitis, dental dysplasia, and early caries may also occur. Squamous cell carcinomas can arise in the buccal, lingual, nasopharyngeal, esophageal, cervicovaginal, and anorectal mucosa, and account for 10–16% of the solid tumors in dyskeratosis congenita patients.[326] Dysphagia as a symptom of esophageal stricture or diverticula has been documented in several cases. Diarrhea has also been noted in association with a friable bleeding rectal mucosa.[327]

Treatment of the mucous membrane manifestations has been difficult. Careful surveillance for the development of carcinoma is all that is currently available. Thymopentin was effective in decreasing the susceptibility to infections.[320] Etretinate or other oral retinoids combined with topical retinoid application might be effective in treating the leukoplakia and merits consideration.[328]

Poikiloderma congenitale may cause similar clinical features with premature cancer development but lacks the typical aplastic anemia.[329]

HYALINOSIS CUTIS ET MUCOSAE

Also known as lipoid proteinosis, lipoglycoproteinosis, and Urbach–Wiethe disease, this rare autosomal-recessive disorder represents a multisystem storage disease with deposition of a hyalin-like material in virtually every organ of the body. The most notable clinical findings are cutaneous waxy nodules coalescing to plaques, vulnerability, crusts, and prolonged wound healing. Scars occur most commonly on the face (Fig. 9.31A). Papules and nodules develop in the mucous membranes, and in the larynx, resulting in striking dysphonia and hoarseness, often since birth, a hallmark of this disease.

The oral manifestations are most frequently noted in the lips, buccal mucosa, posterior tongue, frenulum of the tongue, palate, and posterior pharynx. In very young patients, changes may be limited to the lips and tongue; with increasing age, however, the clinical changes become more widespread.[330] The affected mucosa appears pale and pitted with fissuring of the lips and floor of the mouth. The lower lip is often more severely involved than the upper and may be rigid or sclerotic with multiple infiltrated plaques and nodules.[331] The

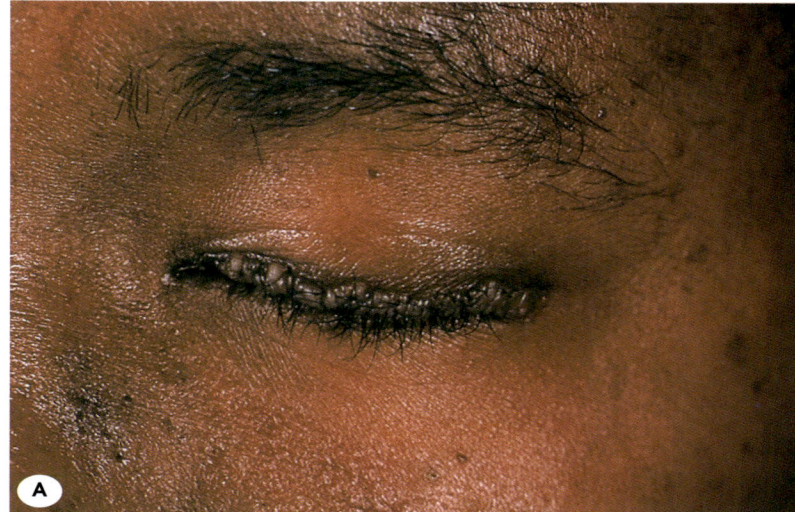

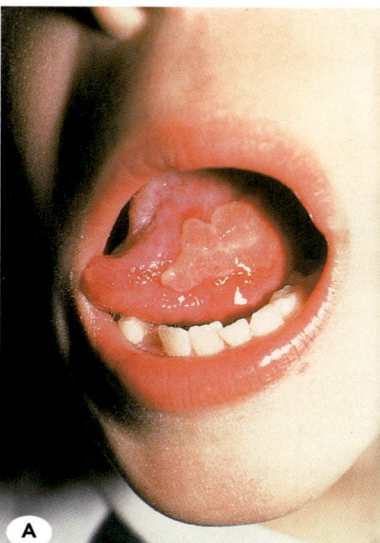
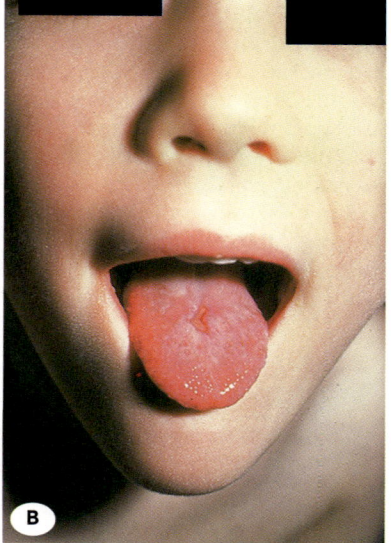

Fig. 9.30   **A, B** Ulcerations and leukoplakia on the tongues of two young boys with dyskeratosis congenita.

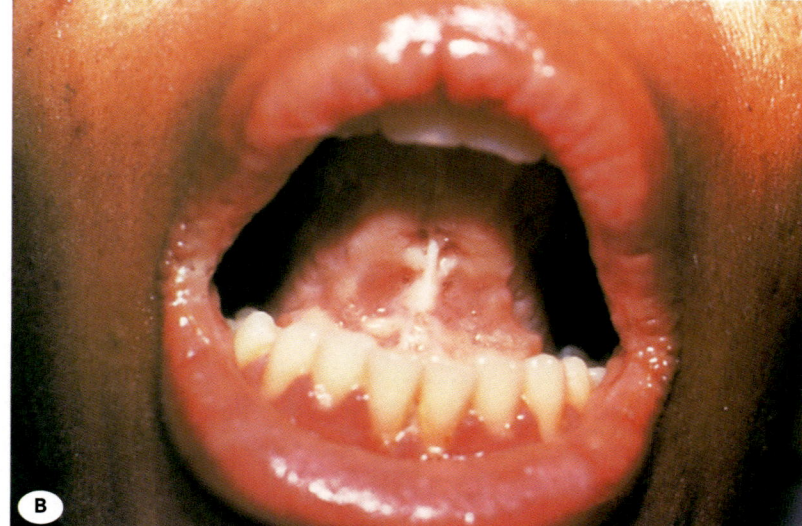

Fig. 9.31   **(A)** Multiple nodules along the lid margin of a child with hyalinosis cutis et mucosae. **(B)** Thickening and induration of the ventral aspect of the tongue in the same patient.

317. Young LL, Lenox JA (1973) Pachyonychia congenita. A long-term evaluation of associated oral and dermatologic lesions. **Oral Surg** 36:663.
318. Elliot AM, Graham GE, Bernstein et al. (1999) Dyskeratosis congenita: An autosomal recessive variant. **Am J Med Genet** 83:178–182.
319. Vulliamy TJ, Knight SW, Mason PJ, Dokal I. (2001) Very short telomeres in the peripheral blood of patients with X-linked and autosomal dyskeratosis congenita. **Blood Cells Mol Dis** 27:353–357.
320. Haneke E, Djawari D, Keller J (1983) Thymopoietin therapy of the susceptibility to infections in dyskeratosis congenita. **Arch Dermatol Res** 275:264–265.
321. Dratchman RA, Alter AP (1995) Dyskeratosis congenita. **Dermatol Clin N Am** Jan; 13:33–39.

322. Solder B, Weiss M, Jager A et al. (1998) Dyskeratosis congenita: multisytemic disorder with special consideration of immunologic aspects. **Clinical Pediatr** 37:521–530.
323. Dokal I (1999) Dyskeratosis congenita: recent advances and future directions. **J Pediatr Hematol Oncol** 21:344–349.
324. Sirinavin C, Trowbridge AA (1975) Dyskeratosis congenita: clinical features and genetic aspects. Report of a family and review of the literature. **J Med Genet** 12:339.
325. Drachman RA, Alter BP (1992) Dyskeratosis congenita: clinical and genetic heterogeneity. Report of a new case and review of the literature. **Am J Pediatr Hematol/Oncol** 14:297.

tongue may be woody and thickened, and induration of the frenulum may limit tongue motion (Fig. 9.31B). The filiform papillae may no longer be detectable by adolescence.[330] The gingivae, alveolar mucosa, hard palate, and uvula are less commonly involved.[331,332] It has been suggested that gingival hypertrophy may be a reflection of periodontal disease or secondary to the administration of anticonvulsants in those patients with seizures.

The larynx is prominently involved, and hoarseness is a common early sign of the disease. Rarely, nodules in this area have caused obstruction necessitating tracheostomy. Nodular lesions in the esophagus have resulted in dysphagia. Recurrent painful swelling of the parotid gland may result from involvement of the buccal mucosa, stenosis of Stensen's duct, and retrograde infection.[331] Rarely, rectal and vaginal lesions have been observed. Asymptomatic infiltrates are also deposited throughout the mucosa of the GI tract, main stem bronchi, and trachea.

There is some dispute as to whether dental abnormalities are characteristic of this disorder.[330] Most frequently noted are hypoplasia or aplasia of the permanent maxillary lateral incisors and premolars.[331] Additional findings include intracranial calcifications and abnormalities of the ocular fundus.

The histopathologic changes in the mucosae are the same as in the skin. Of interest is the finding that even clinically uninvolved tissue such as gingivae show the characteristic pathology.[330] Biopsy specimens demonstrate dermal extracellular deposits of amorphous, eosinophilic, hyaline material and onion-skin proliferation of the adventitia of the small vessels. In the mucosa of the mouth, these deposits may surround the labial, palatal, and laryngeal minor salivary glands. The hyaline material is strongly periodic acid–Schiff (PAS)-positive and resistant to digestion with diastase or amylase. Lipid stains most commonly identify neutral fats. Ultrastructural studies demonstrating marked cytoplasmic vacuolization and increased membranous lamellar material in dermal fibroblasts have led to the hypothesis that hyalinosis cutis et mucosae may be a lysosomal storage disease.[333,334] Nevertheless, the responsible gene or gene-regulation defect for this disorder remains unknown.[335] Differential diagnosis includes primarily erythropoietic protoporphyria, colloid milium, and pseudoxanthoma elasticum. Treatment is ineffective, although carbon dioxide laser surgery of thickened vocal cords has been used successfully to improve hoarseness.[334] (See also Chapter 8.)

MUCOSAL NEUROMA SYNDROME

Also known as multiple mucosal neuroma syndrome, Gorlin–Vickers syndrome, and multiple endocrinopathy syndrome type III or type IIb, this disorder is characterized by multiple mucosal neuromas, medullary carcinoma of the thyroid, and pheochromocytoma. Additional identifying clinical features include a distinctive facies due to thick fleshy lips and a prognathic jaw, a marfanoid habitus, intestinal ganglioneuromatosis, and variable hyperparathyroidism and ophthalmologic abnormalities. Inheritance is consistent with an autosomal-dominant trait, although many instances of incomplete syndrome and many sporadic cases have been documented. The syndrome is due to mutations in the tyrosine kinase domain of the RET proto-oncogene.[336]

The mucosal neuromas occur on the lips, tongue, and eyes, and in the GI tract. In the mouth, they are limited to the anterior third of the tongue and are detectable as pink to white pedunculated or sessile nodules. Similar lesions may develop on the labial commissures. The lips are diffusely infiltrated, causing gen-

eralized enlargement, nodularity, and patulousness. The nasal mucosa and gingivae are less common sites of involvement.[337] Oral lesions may be present at birth or may develop in early childhood. The entire alimentary tract may be involved, causing chronic constipation, diarrhea, vomiting, and cramping abdominal pain. Barium studies demonstrate thickened mucosal folds, diverticuli, and narrowed and dilated segments of the small and large bowel.[338]

Ocular lesions include prominent corneal nerves readily visible at the limbus, medullated retinal nerves, and neuromas of both the bulbar and palpebral conjunctivae. Tumors of the bulbar conjunctiva are smooth and yellow, 1–2mm in diameter, located near the limbus. Lesions of the palpebral conjunctiva measure up to 3mm and develop close to the lid margin, adding to the thickened appearance of the lids. The lids are uniformly thickened or nodular, displacing the cilia toward the cutaneous surface. Eyelid tumors have been noted as early as 4 years and visible corneal nerves by 9 years of age.[339]

Medullary thyroid carcinoma is a neoplasm of the parafollicular C cells responsible for the secretion of calcitonin, the calcium-lowering polypeptide hormone. Elevated calcitonin levels in these patients can be regarded as an indication of the existence of thyroid carcinoma, even though the tumor is as yet clinically undetectable. This marker provides a means for early detection of thyroid malignancy and should be used as a screening test in children with typical facies and mucosal neuromas. Some authors have recommended genetic screening for the RET proto-oncogene with prophylactic thyroidectomy within the first few years of life to obtain an optimum cure rate.[340] Pheochromocytomas and hyperparathyroidism tend to be late manifestations of the syndrome occurring after the second decade.

HEREDITARY HEMORRHAGIC TELANGIECTASIA

Hereditary hemorrhagic telangiectasia (HHT), also known as Osler–Weber–Rendu disease, is a genetic vascular disorder characterized by dilated vessels and arteriovenous malformations. Phenotypic heterogeneity, such as age of onset, severity of disease and organ involvement, is explained in part by two genes being mutated, endoglin (HHT1) on chromosome 9 and ALK-1 (HHT2) on chromosome 12, both members of the TGF-beta receptor family. Haploinsufficiency is the mechanism responsible for HHT.[341,342] The disorder is transmitted as an autosomal–dominant trait with a high degree of penetrance. HHT has a broad spectrum of clinical manifestations that are often inapparent until the third or fourth decade. The characteristic telangiectasias that involve the skin and mucous membranes usually have their onset after puberty.[343] Therefore, symptomatic children, particularly those with a negative family history, may present a diagnostic problem.

The mucosal telangiectasias are found most commonly on the lips, tongue, and buccal surfaces, as well as on the nasal mucosa, consisting of punctate, linear, and spiderlike lesions.[344,345] On the skin, telangiectasias predominate on the head, chest, and limbs, particularly on the palms and soles, on the tips of the digits, and in the subungual and periungual areas.[345] They may also occur in all parts of the GI tract, lungs, brain, retina, liver, and spleen. The most common manifestation of HHT is epistaxis, which usually begins in childhood.[345,346] Chronic GI bleeding resulting in severe anemia is the second most frequent sign but rarely has its onset before the middle adult years.[345] Bleeding may be recurrent and progressively more severe, requiring multiple transfusions and surgical procedures.

326. Steier W, Van Voolen A, Selmanowitz V (1972) Dyskeratosis congenita: relationship to Fanconi's anemia. **Blood** 39:510.
327. Ning Y, Yongshan Y, Pai GS, Gross AJ (1992) Heterozygote detection through bleomycin-induced G₂ chromatid breakage in dyskeratosis congenita families. **Cancer Genet Cytogenet** 60:31.
328. Dodd HJ, Devereux S, Sarkany I (1985) Dyskeratosis congenita with pancytopenia. **Clin Exp Dermatol** 10:73.
329. Haneke E, Gutschmidt E (1979) Premature multiple Bowen's disease in poikiloderma congenitale with warty hyperkeratoses. **Dermatologica** 158:384–388.
330. Hofer P-A, Bergenholtz A (1975) Oral manifestations in Urbach-Wiethe disease (lipoglycoproteinosis; lipoid proteinosis; hyalinosis cutis et mucosae). **Odont Rev** 26:39.
331. Finkelstein MW, Hammond HL, Jones RB (1982) Hyalinosis cutis et mucosae. **Oral Surg** 54:49.
332. Israel H (1992) Gingival lesions in lipoid proteinosis. **J Periodontol** 63:561.
333. Bauer EA, Santa-Cruz DJ, Eisen AZ (1982) Lipoid proteinosis: in vivo and in vitro evidence for a lysosomal storage disease. **J Invest Dermatol** 76:119.

334. Haneke E, Hornstein OP, Meisel-Stosiek M, Steiner U (1984) Hyalinosis cutis et mucosae in siblings. **Hum Genet** 68:342.
335. Hausser I, Biltz S, Rauterberg E et al. (1991) Hyalinosis cutis et mucosae (Morbus Urbach-Wiethe) – ultrastrukturelle und immunologische Merkmale. **Hautarzt** 42:28–33.
336. Iwashita T, Murakami H, Kurokawa K et al. (2000) A two-hit model for development of multiple endocrine neoplasia type 2B by RET mutations. **Biochem Biophys Res Commun** 24;268:804–808.
337. Forsman PJ, Jenkins ME (1973) Medullary carcinoma of the thyroid with Marfan-like body habitus. **Pediatrics** 52:188.
338. Carney JA, Hayles AB (1977) Alimentary tract manifestations of multiple endocrine neoplasia, type 2b. **Mayo Clin Proc** 52:543.
339. Baum JL, Adler ME (1972) Pheochromocytoma, medullary thyroid carcinoma, multiple mucosal neuroma. **Arch Ophthalmol** 87:574.
340. van Heurn LW, Schaap C, Sie G et al. (1999) Predictive DNA testing for multiple endocrine neoplasia 2: a therapeutic challenge of prophylactic thyroidectomy in very young children. **J Pediatr Surg** Apr; 34:568–567.

Pulmonary involvement in the form of arteriovenous (AV) fistulas occurs in approximately one-fifth of affected persons,[345] and, in infants, may cause perplexing cyanosis in the absence of other stigmata of the disease.[346] Standard chest radiographs often demonstrate the vascular abnormality, which may be confirmed by angiography. Liver involvement may cause iron overload, periportal fibrosis, and hepatocellular necrosis.[345] Neurologic manifestations due to leaks from ruptured telangiectasias and vascular malformation include seizures, paresthesias, headaches, visual disturbances, as well as a variety of neurologic deficits.[347] Brain abscess occurs as a result of right-to-left shunting in patients with pulmonary AV fistulas.[347]

The differential diagnosis from the dermatologic standpoint includes blue rubber bleb nevus syndrome, scleroderma (with calcinosis, Raynaud's esophageal dysmotility, sclerodactyly, and telangiectasia), and generalized essential telangiectasia. A characteristic telangiectatic lesion on biopsy consists of dilated blood vessels with a single endothelial layer, classified as venules. On electron microscopy, a defect in the endothelial cell junctions has been identified. These defects have been hypothesized to permit extravasation of blood into the surrounding connective tissue. Repeat episodes of leakage of blood and fibrin, which forms a framework for new endothelial outgrowth, is thought to account for the development of new lesions as the patient ages.[348]

This disorder poses difficult management problems. Surgical measures, including electrocoagulation and laser photocoagulation, have been used with variable success. Transfusions, iron supplementation, and nasal dermoplasty for epistaxis are helpful measures. Enthusiasm for estrogen therapy, which is not without side effects, has not been borne out by clinical trials.[349] (See also Chapters 8 and 21.)

BLUE RUBBER BLEB NEVUS SYNDROME

Delineation of this angiodysplastic syndrome is usually credited to Bean in 1958, although the earliest report dates back to the mid-nineteenth century. The syndrome is characterized by few to many variably-sized vascular malformations in the skin and GI tract. Oral lesions are rare.[350] Three types of lesions have been described: large, disfiguring lesions that may obstruct vital tissues or result in amputation of a portion of a limb; purple-black compressible, rubbery, nipplelike angiomas; and irregular blue-black macules and papules. These angiomas may be spontaneously painful or tender and are occasionally associated with hyperhidrosis of the overlying skin. Lesions may be present at birth, but many patients experience development of new lesions and enlargement of old lesions during the childhood and adult years. Sites of predilection are the upper limbs and trunk, but lesions have been observed on virtually every aspect of the body.

Several reported cases have involved the lips,[351,352] oral cavity,[352,353] and nasopharynx.[354] However, the GI mucosa is the major site of predilection, and hemorrhage from the bowel resulting in severe symptomatic anemia constitutes one of the most serious complications. Gastrointestinal lesions most

often involve the small bowel and may be solitary or multiple and of variable size. Widespread involvement of other organs, including lungs, heart, liver, and brain, may also occur, and hemorrhage from the visceral lesions has resulted in fatalities.[352] Preoperative diagnosis of GI angiomas has been made by barium studies, angiography,[355] and endoscopy.[356]

Some reports suggest familial involvement with autosomal-dominant pattern of transmission,[357,358] but most cases are sporadic. Differential diagnosis includes the Osler–Weber–Rendu (hereditary hemorrhagic telangiectasia) and Maffucci syndromes and, in young infants, miliary hemangiomatosis. Biopsy of the blue rubber bleb nevus demonstrates a variant of cavernous hemangioma; some lesions have also been described as resembling angiokeratoma histologically.

Until recently, therapy has been directed at controlling GI bleeding by excision or cauterization. Surgical excision of small or troublesome cutaneous angiomas has been successful in some instances. Carbon dioxide laser surgery and endoscopic neodymium:YAG laser photocoagulation of colonic vascular lesions proved safe and effective.[359–361] (See also Chapter 21.) Other authors have recommended medical therapy or combinations of lasers and systemic steroids.[362,363]

SJÖGREN SYNDROME

Complaints of recurrent salivary gland enlargement, chronic dry mouth or dry eyes, or a foreign body sensation in the eyes suggests a diagnosis of Sjögren syndrome. This condition is relatively uncommon in the pediatric age group,[364] but is probably underdiagnosed.[365] Sjögren syndrome occurs more often in middle-aged and elderly women. Children with Sjögren syndrome do, however, demonstrate clinical heterogeneity comparable to that seen in adults.[366]

The classic triad of Sjögren syndrome consists of: (1) keratoconjunctivitis sicca or dry eyes with or without lacrimal gland enlargement; (2) xerostomia or dry mouth with or without salivary gland enlargement; and (3) the presence of a connective tissue disease. In children, SLE is the most frequently encountered connective tissue disease, whereas rheumatoid arthritis more often accompanies the adult form. Primary Sjögren syndrome suggests only oral and ocular involvement. When a defined connective tissue disease is associated, Sjögren syndrome is classified as the secondary form. A careful evaluation of children with mixed connective tissue disease and juvenile rheumatoid arthritis for components of Sjögren syndrome is warranted in all instances. This syndrome should also be considered in the differential diagnosis of children with recurrent parotitis, keratoconjunctivitis sicca, or pronounced and early tooth decay associated with xerostomia.[366,367]

Most children with Sjögren syndrome develop parotid involvement but not necessarily early in the course of the disease. Glandular enlargement is usually bilateral, symmetric, and chronic, but occasionally unilateral or intermittent parotid swelling occurs;[368] chronic parotid enlargement may

341. Bourdeau A, Faughnan ME, Letarte M (2000) Endoglin-deficient mice, a unique model to study hereditary hemorrhagic telangiectasia. **Trends Cardiovasc Med** 10:279–285.
342. Kjeldsen A. Brusgaard K, Poulsen L et al. (2001) Mutations in the ALK-1 gene and the phenotype of hereditary hemorrhagic telangiectasia in two large Danish families. **Am J Med Genet** 98:298–302.
343. Garland HG, Anning ST (1950) Hereditary hemorrhagic telangiectasia: a genetic and bibliographical study. **Br J Dermatol** 62:289.
344. Bartolucci EG, Swan RH, Hart WC (1982) Oral manifestations of hereditary hemorrhagic telangiectasia (Osler-Weber-Rendu disease). Review and case reports. **J Periodontol** 53:163.
345. Reilly RJ, Nostrant TT (1984) Clinical manifestations of hereditary hemorrhagic telangiectasia. **Am J Gastroenterol** 79:363.
346. Boynton RC, Morgan BC (1973) Cerebral arteriovenous fistula with possible hereditary telangiectasia. **Am J Dis Child** 125:99.
347. Roman G, Fisher M, Perl DP, Poser CM (1978) Neurological manifestations of hereditary hemorrhagic telangiectasia (Rendu-Osler-Weber disease): report of 2 cases and review of the literature. **Ann Neurol** 4:130.
348. Menefee MG, Flessa HC, Glueck HJ, Hogg SP (1975) Hereditary hemorrhagic telangiectasia (Osler-Weber-Rendu disease). **Arch Otolaryngol** 101:246.
349. Vase P (1981) Estrogen treatment of hereditary hemorrhagic telangiectasia. **Acta Med Scand** 209:303.
350. Langella C, Delaporte E, Beregi JP et al. (1999) Malformation veineuse multifocale majeure à prédominance monomelique. **Ann Dermatol Venereol** 126:817–821.
351. Waybright EA, Selhorst JB, Rosenblum WI et al. (1978) Blue rubber bleb nevus syndrome with CNS involvement and thrombosis of a vein of Galen malformation. **Ann Neurol** 3:364.
352. Belshiem MR, Sullivan SN (1980) Blue rubber bleb nevus syndrome. **Can J Surg** 23:274.
353. Rennie IG, Shortland JR, Mahood JM et al. (1982) Periodic exophthalmos associated with the blue rubber bleb nevus syndrome: a case report. **Br J Ophthalmol** 66:594.
354. Fretzin DF, Potter B (1965) Blue rubber bleb nevus. **Arch Intern Med** 116:924.
355. McCauley RGK, Leonidas JC, Bartoshesky LE (1979) Blue rubber bleb nevus syndrome. **Radiology** 133:375.
356. Baker AL, Kahn PC, Binder SC et al. (1971) Gastrointestinal bleeding due to blue rubber bleb nevus syndrome. **Gastroenterology** 61:530.
357. Walshe MM, Evans CD, Warin RP (1966) Blue rubber bleb naevus. **BMJ** 2:931.
358. Munkvad M (1983) Blue rubber bleb nevus syndrome. **Dermatologica** 167:307.
359. Morris L, Lynch PM, Gleason WA et al. (1992) Blue rubber bleb nevus syndrome: laser photocoagulation of colonic hemangiomas in a child with microcytic anemia. **Pediatr Dermatol** 9:91.
360. Olsen TG, Milroy SK, Goldman L et al. (1979) Laser surgery for blue rubber bleb nevus. **Arch Dermatol** 115:81.
361. Boente MD, Cordisco MR, Frontini MD, Asial RA (1999) Blue rubber bleb nevus (Bean syndrome): evolution of four cases and clinical response to pharmacologic agents. **Pediatr Dermatol** 16:222–227.

cause "chipmunk" facies. Minor salivary glands are also involved in 70% of patients. Both grossly and histologically, the involved glands appear chronically inflamed with ductal ectasia, a lymphoreticular infiltration, acinar destruction, and the presence of epimyoephithelial islands.[369,370]

Evaluation of children suspected of having Sjögren syndrome should include a biopsy of the labial salivary glands, an ophthalmologic examination including evaluation of tear breakup time (performed by slit-lamp examination), staining of the conjunctiva and cornea, and a Schirmer test. Measurement of rheumatoid factor, ANA, Ro and La (anti-SSA and SSB) antibodies, quantitative immunoglobulins, a complete blood count, and urinalysis are indicated. Additional studies that may prove helpful include salivary scintigraphy, and measurement of tear lysozyme levels. All patients with Sjögren syndrome require a complete evaluation to exclude other autoimmune disorders. Certain genetic polymorphisms of the interleukin-10 promoter region appear to be associated with a higher risk of primary Sjögren syndrome.[371]

The goals of therapy are prevention of ocular and oral sequelae and reduction of discomfort caused by symptoms of the disease. Left untreated, keratoconjunctivitis sicca may lead to corneal vascularization, scarring, and ulceration. These complications may be prevented by judicious use of non-sensitizing artifical tears and careful attention to secondary infection. Xerostomia and its attendant caries can be controlled by limiting dietary sucrose, scrupulous oral hygiene and prophylaxis, and topical application of fluoride to the teeth. Xerostomic patients should avoid anticholinergic medications and topical oral preparations (such as commercial mouthwashes) that may contribute to or worsen their symptoms. Careful periodic examination for oral candidiasis is also essential. Therapy must also encompass any associated collagen vascular disease.

Long-term follow-up should include evaluation for extraglandular involvement and other autoimmune diseases. Lymphomas occur with greater frequency in patients with Sjögren syndrome and appear to be associated with lower C4 complement levels, mixed cryoglobulinemia and purpura.[372] These lymphomas are usually of the histiocytic and mixed histiocytic-lymphocytic type. Pseudolymphomas may also occur and are of B-cell origin.

BEHÇET SYNDROME

Behçet syndrome is a chronic multisystem vasculitis involving the ocular, mucocutaneous, skeletal, vascular, GI, and neurologic systems.[373] The classic clinical triad encompasses recurrent oral ulcers, recurrent genital ulcers, and ocular inflammation.[38] The syndrome is rarely seen in children or in the elderly. Most often it afflicts those in their late 20s and early 30s, with men showing three times the predisposition of women.[373,374]

Oral ulceration is the most common initial manifestation of Behçet syndrome, occurring early in greater than 90% of pediatric patients.[375] Oral ulcers often antedate neurologic symptoms by several years.[376,377] The oral lesions, clinically indistinguishable from aphthae, arise in small foci of erythema. The erythema is followed within hours by slight infiltration and, over the course of 24 to 48 hours, shallow, round, to polyhedral ulcerations become evident.[376] Covering these erosions is a white, gray, or yellowish pseudomembrane. The regular, discrete edges of the ulcers help distinguish these lesions from those of Stevens–Johnson syndrome and allergic aphthosis, in which edges remain irregular, and in Reiter syndrome, in which heaped-up borders characterize the mucosal lesions.[378]

The ulcers of Behçet syndrome preferentially form on the gingiva, the mucous membranes of the lips, the buccal mucosa, and the tongue (Fig. 9.32). In contrast to Stevens–Johnson syndrome and Reiter syndrome, the palate, tonsils, and pharynx are rarely involved. The ulcers develop in crops and range in size from several millimeters to 1cm or more in diameter. They persist for several days to a few weeks[379] but typically heal without scarring. The types of oral ulcerations may be minor, major, herpetiform, or combined, but herpetiform aphthae are relatively more frequent.[87] The major factor contributing to morbidity of oral mucosal membrane ulcerations is diminished fluid and caloric intake.[373]

The genital lesions of Behçet syndrome resemble those seen in the oral cavity. In males they occur predominantly on the scrotum and base of the penis and in females on the vulva and vaginal mucosa.[38,373,377] The perianal region and vaginal mucosa may be involved as well. As the genital ulcers are usually deeper than the oral ones, scarring is common. The genital area should be carefully examined for residual scarring when Behçet syndrome is suspected and no active ulcers are evident. Both oral and genital ulcerations tend to remit within 1–2 weeks but often recur.

Ocular manifestations, which range from simple photophobia and irritation to keratoconjunctivitis or uveitis, are less common in pediatric patients with Behçet syndrome.[373,378] In adults, recurrent attacks of anterior and posterior uveitis may ultimately result in blindness. Anterior uveitis may precede hypopyon, a typical but transient clinical sign of Behçet syndrome. Posterior uveitis, hemorrhages, and exudates in the choroid and retina characterize chronic ocular involvement.[374] Gastrointestinal and uncommon lesions are relatively more frequent in children.[380]

Histologically, the oral ulcerations show nonspecific changes similar to those of aphthae. However, the presence of endothelial swelling is characteristic of Behçet's ulcers and helps to differentiate them from aphthae. Vasculitis is another characteristic of some mucocutaneous lesions, and the small vessels, particularly the venules, are filled with immune complex deposits. Neutrophil chemotaxis is enhanced.[38,381]

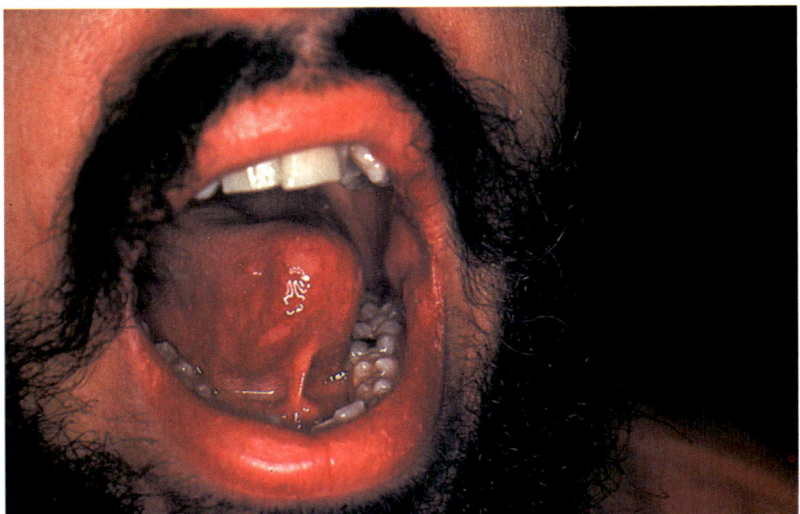

Fig. 9.32 Multiple ulcerations on the tongue of a young man with Behçet syndrome.

362. Kunishige M, Azuma H, Masuda K et al. (1997) Interferon alpha-2a therapy for disseminated intravascular coagulation in a patient with blue rubber bleb nevus syndrome. A case report. **Angiology** Mar; 48(3):273–277.
363. Dieckmann K, Maurage C, Faure N et al. (1994) Combined laser-steroid therapy in blue rubber bleb nevus syndrome: case report and review of the literature. **Eur J Pediatr Surg** 4:372–374.
364. Hearth-Holmes M, Baethge BA, Abreo F, Wolf RE (1993) Autoimmune exocrinopathy presenting as recurrent parotitis of childhood. **Arch Otolaryngol Head Neck Surg** 119:347.
365. Stiller M, Golder W, Doring E, Biedermann T (2000) Primary and secondary Sjögren's syndrome in children – a comparative study. **Clin Oral Investig** 4:176–182.
366. Chudwin DS, Daniels TE, Wara DW et al. (1981) Spectrum of Sjögren's syndrome in children. **J Pediatr** 98 213.

367. Anaya JM, Ogawa N, Talal N (1995) Sjögren's syndrome in childhood. **J Rheumatol** 22:1152–1158.
368. Atheya BH, Norman ME, Myers AR, South MA (1977) Sjögren's syndrome in children. **Pediatrics** 59:931.
369. Rice DH (1984) Salivary gland disease in children. **Cancer Bull** 36:106.
370. Daniels T (1984) Labial salivary gland biopsy in Sjögren's syndrome. Assessment as a diagnostic criteria in 362 suspected cases. **Arthritis Rheum** 27:147.
371. Hulkkonen J, Pertovaara M, Antonen J et al. (2001) Genetic association between interleukin-10 promoter region polymorphisms and primary Sjogren's syndrome. **Arthritis Rheum** 44:176–179.
372. Skopouli FN, Dafni U, Ioannidis JP, Moutsopoulos HM (2000) Clinical evolution, and morbidity and mortality of primary Sjögren's syndrome. **Semin Arthritis Rheum** 29:296–304.

The diagnosis of Behçet syndrome cannot be verified by any reproducible hematologic, immunologic, or infectious studies. Various clinical criteria have therefore been outlined to assist in making the diagnosis.[373–382]

The cause of Behçet syndrome is unknown.[375] Many cases have been shown to be HLA-B 51 positive, and a self-antigenic role for HLA B51 has been postulated. Familial cases are more frequent in childhood Behçet's disease.[380] Etiologies ranging from viral infection, exposure to environmental pollutants, and a variety of immunologic abnormalities have been proposed.[374,381–383] Therapy is not entirely satisfactory. Systemic corticosteroids help control many of the clinical manifestations, but chlorambucil, colchicine, cyclosporine A, levamisole, and azathioprine may be required to maximize therapeutic efficacy. Thalidomide is particularly effective therapy in the mucocutaneous form.

No single form of drug therapy has proven uniformly effective for the treatment of Behçet syndrome. As this disorder has a high prevalence of spontaneous remissions and exacerbations during the course of the disease, the evaluation of the efficacy of any therapeutic regimen is difficult. Combined drug therapy may be more efficacious in some patients than single drug regimens.[383]

REITER SYNDROME

Reiter syndrome is a symptom complex that most frequently consists of the triad of conjunctivitis, urethritis, and arthritis.[384] Asymptomatic mouth ulcers and lesions resembling glossitis/stomatitis geographica are a less common feature, as is the associated cutaneous eruption, keratoderma blennorrhagicum. Although predominantly a disease of the young adult male, this syndrome also occurs in females and has occasionally been recognized in prepubertal children.[385,386] Reiter syndrome is perceived as a reactive response to previous infection and most frequently follows *Chlamydia* urethritis, serotypes D-K, *Salmonella* or *Shigella* dysentery but has also been associated with *Yersinia* gastroenteritis. More than 80% of the patients are HLA-B27 positive, but the reasons for that are unclear.[387]

The mucosal manifestations of the disorder are frequently mild and may be overlooked or forgotten by the patient presenting with arthritis, unless the appropriate history is specifically elicited. In a series of 38 children, 66% had conjunctivitis as the initial finding, 34% had urethritis, and only 24% had arthritis.[388] All three major features are generally detectable during the acute illness.

The conjunctivitis of Reiter syndrome is bilateral and varies considerably in severity from a mild discharge to marked inflammation with edema and erythema of the bulbar and palpebral conjunctivae. Progression to corneal ulceration is uncommon but can occur.[388] An accompanying keratitis[389] or iritis,[390] or both, has also been noted; the latter, if severe and chronic, can result in blindness,[386] an outcome not yet reported in children.

Urethral involvement is most often reflected by dysuria, although the manifestations may range from meatal inflammation only to frank urethral discharge.[388] Pyuria is a common laboratory finding and should always be sought if the diagnosis of Reiter syndrome is under consideration. Balanitis and ulcerations of the labia[390] have been noted in a few patients.

The frequency of oral manifestations in children is unknown. Mouth lesions are nonspecific, consisting of erythema, erosions, and necrotic ulcerations, most commonly involving the buccal mucosa, gingivae, palate, and tongue. The histopathology of these lesions is nondiagnostic.[77] Reiter syndrome and Kawasaki disease have some features in common.[391]

Generally, the mucosal lesions of Reiter syndrome are relatively benign and self-limited; occasionally, however, serious morbidity can result if the inflammatory process becomes chronic. Treatment is largely symptomatic, as no drugs are consistently effective in palliating this disorder.

ERYTHEMA MULTIFORME SPECTRUM

This spectrum of hypersensitivity reactions include erythema multiforme (EM) simplex, bullous EM, Stevens–Johnson syndrome, and toxic epidermal necrolysis (TEN) (Fig. 9.33). In EM simplex, bullous EM, and TEN, the mucous membranes are affected to a variable degree.[38,392,393] By definition,

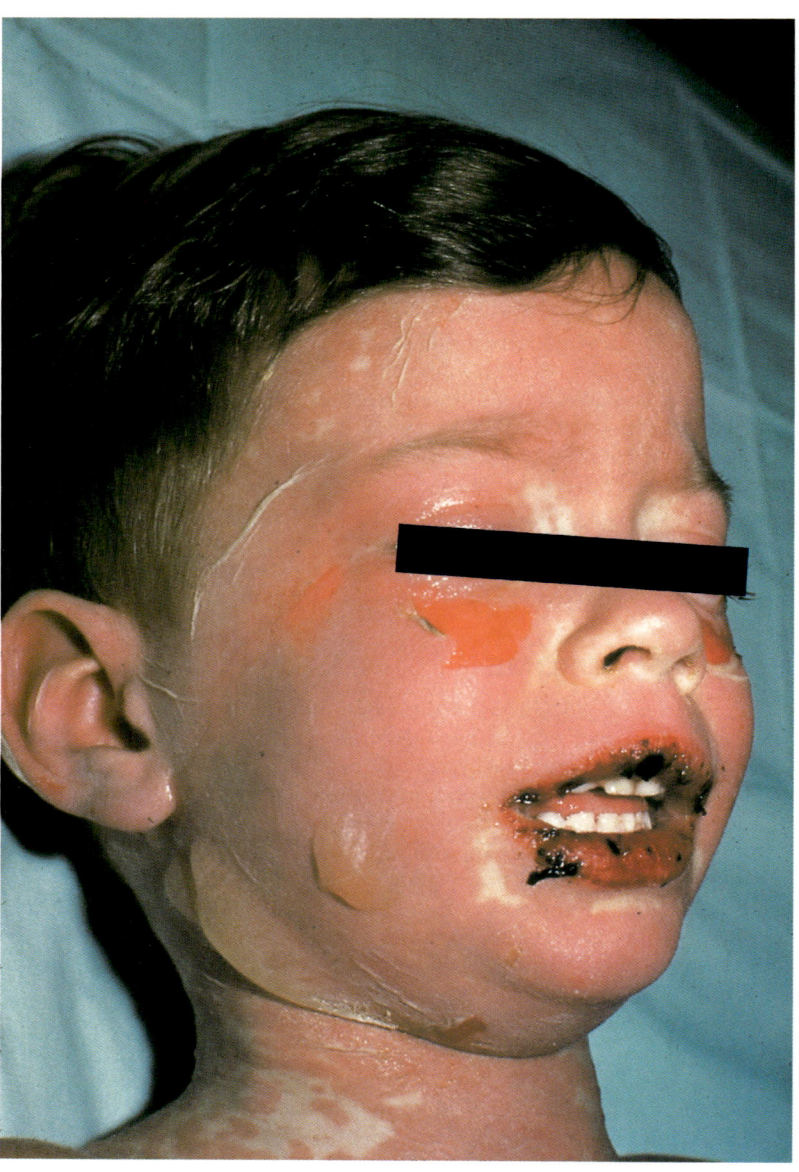

Fig. 9.33 Toxic epidermal necrolysis due to phenytoin.

373. Ammann AJ, Johnson A, Fyfe GA et al. (1985) Behçet's syndrome. **J Pediatr** 107:41.
374. Chajek T, Fainaru M (1975) Behçet's disease: Report of 41 cases and a review of the literature. **Medicine** (Baltimore) 54:179.
375. Yazici H, Yurdakul S, Hamuryudan V (2001) Behçet disease. **Curr Opin Rheumatol** 13:18–22.
376. Haensch R (1974) Behçet's disease (aphthosis). **Cutis** 14:353.
377. Cho MY, Lee S, Bang D et al. (1991) Clinical analysis of 57 cases of Behçet's syndrome in children. In: Behçet's Disease. Basic and Clinical Aspects, O'Duffy JD, Kokmen E, eds. New York: Marcel Dekker, p. 41.
378. Michelson JB, Chisari FV (1982) Behçet's disease. **Surv Ophthalmol** 26:190.
379. Mundy TM, Miller JJ (1978) Behçet's disease presenting as chronic aphthous stomatitis in a child. **Pediatrics** 62:205.
380. Kone-Paut I, Geisler I, Wechsler B et al. (1999) Familial aggregation in Behçet's disease: high frequency in siblings and parents of pediatric probands. **J Pediatr** 135:89–93.
381. Jorizzo JL, Hudson RD, Schmalstieg FC (1984) Behçet's syndrome: immune regulation, circulating immune complexes, neutrophil migration, and colchicine therapy. **J Am Acad Dermatol** 10:205.
382. Haim S, Gilhar A (1980) Clinical and laboratory criteria for the diagnosis of Behçet's disease. **Br J Dermatol** 102:36.
383. O'Duffy JD, Kokmen E, eds. Behçet's Disease, Basic and Clinical Aspects. New York: Marcel Dekker.
384. Calin A (1977) Reiter's syndrome. **Med Clin North Am** 61:365.

Stevens–Johnson syndrome implies activity in at least two mucous membrane sites, most often the conjunctivae and oropharynx, but the nasal mucosa, and urethral, vaginal, and rectal mucosa can also be involved. This form of EM may remain confined to the mucous membranes or may involve the skin as well.

The oral manifestations of this symptom complex are basically similar in all forms of EM but vary in extent and severity.[392,393] The primary lesion is a macular area of erythema that evolves centrally into a thick-walled vesicle or bulla. The duration of the blister is brief and, following rupture, the characteristic irregularly shaped ulcer with indistinct margins and a yellow necrotic base becomes evident. These extremely painful lesions may then become covered with a pseudomembrane prior to healing. The lesions occur in a crop so that, at a given time, lesions in all stages of development may be observed.

Sites of predilection are the lips, where the labial mucosa alone may be affected, or the lesions may extend over the vermilion border to the keratinized skin, the anterior and lateral borders of the tongue, the buccal mucosa, and the palate. The dorsum of the tongue becomes coated but does not ulcerate. The gingivae remain relatively spared, an important clinical finding in differentiating this eruption from acute herpetic gingivostomatitis. As the disease progresses, the ulcers may become confluent on the labial surface so that the entire lip is overlaid with a thick hemorrhagic crust that typifies oral lesions of EM. Erosions of the pharynx occur in severe cases and may extend to cause a necrotizing esophagitis. During the acute stage, swallowing is so painful that ingestion of food and fluids may become impossible. Secondary infection may result in excessive salivation and a fetid mouth odor. Occasionally, ulcerations may also develop in the nasal mucosa and larynx causing bleeding, crusting, and airway obstruction. Healing in all these sites usually occurs without the formation of scars.[394]

Genital involvement in EM causes a urethritis associated with dysuria and purulent discharge. Vulvovaginitis and balanitis accompany the urethral lesions; at times, the rectal mucosa is also inflamed and ulcerated. Genitourinary lesions may be so painful that the child refuses to void, and an indwelling urinary catheter must be placed during the acute phase.

Ocular lesions constitute the most dangerous of the mucous membrane lesions, as they may result in serious sequelae. The early acute phase consists of a mucopurulent conjunctivitis with inflamed swollen papillae in the conjunctiva. Focal ulcerations may lead to the formation of pseudomembranes and synechiae. Secondary complications include symblepharon, entropion, trichiasis, keratitis, corneal pannus, and stricture of the lacrimal puncta. Severe disease may result in profound loss of visual activity or even blindness.[396]

The diagnosis is often made by clinical assessment only but can be confirmed by biopsy of a typical lesion. (See Chapter 20 for a more extensive discussion of the EM spectrum.) Outcome depends on prompt diagnosis and meticulous nursing care for patients with an extensive or severe reaction. Immediate ophthalmologic evaluation is mandatory if the diagnosis of ocular EM is under consideration. Patients with mild disease may need little other than symptomatic therapy. Those with fulminant painful mucosal lesions may require hospitalization and administration of intravenous fluids for correction of dehydration and electrolyte imbalance and maintenance of nutrition. The use of corticosteroids is controversial, since large double-blind multicentered controlled trials have never been carried out.[397,398] High-dose intravenous immunoglobulins have shown dramatic results in Stevens–Johnson syndrome.[399]

TOXIC SHOCK SYNDROME

Toxic shock syndrome (TSS) is an acute febrile illness occurring in both sexes and all age groups, but most frequently in adult women.[400–404] This condition is caused by a toxin elaborated by certain strains of *Staphylococcus aureus* that can be cultured from various body sites. The clinical criteria for diagnosis include: (1) fever of greater than 38.9°C; (2) diffuse macular erythematous rash; (3) desquamation 1–2 weeks after onset of illness; (4) hypotension (less than 90mmHg for an adult or less than the 5th percentile for age for a child; orthostatic hypotension, dizziness, or syncope); (5) involvement of three or more organ systems, including GI (vomiting, diarrhea), muscular (myalgia, elevated CPK), central nervous system (disorientation, altered consciousness), renal (elevated blood urea nitrogen, creatinine, pyuria), hepatic (elevated liver function tests), hematologic (thrombocytopenia), and cardiopulmonary (heart failure, electrocardiogram changes, respiratory distress).[402] Similar signs have also been observed in streptococcal toxic shock syndrome.[405]

Mucous membrane manifestations include hyperemia of the oropharyngeal mucous membranes, occasionally with palatal petechiae.[404] Suffusion of the vaginal mucosa has also been observed.[402] Bulbar conjunctival injection and inflammation sometimes with subconjunctival hemorrhage is a prominent finding[404] mimicking Kawasaki disease. Conjunctival hyperemia is also a salient feature of EM, leptospirosis, certain viral infections such as measles and rubella, and Rocky Mountain spotted fever. (See also Chapter 26.)

385. Lockie GN, Hunder GG (1971) Reiter's syndrome in children. A case report and review. **Arthritis Rheum** 14:767.
386. Cuttica RJ, Scheines EJ, Garay SM et al. (1992) Juvenile onset of Reiter's syndrome. A retrospective study of 26 patients. **Clin Exp Rheumatol** 10:285.
387. Pavlica L, Mitrovic D, Mladenovic V et al. (1997) Reiter's syndrome – analysis of 187 patients. **Vojnosanit Pregl** 54:437–446.
388. Rosenberg AM, Petty RE (1979) Reiter's disease in children. **Am J Dis Child** 133:394.
389. Russell AS (1977) Reiter's syndrome in children following infection with *Yersinia enterocolitica* and *Shigella*. **Arthritis Rheum**, 20 suppl: 471.
390. Iveson JMI, Nanda BS, Hancock JAH et al. (1975) Reiter's disease in three boys. **Ann Rheum Dis** 34:364.
391. Bauman C, Cron RQ, Sherry DD, Francis JS (1996) Reiter syndrome initially misdiagnosed as Kawasaki disease. **J Pediatr** 128:366–369.
392. Shklar G, McCarthy PL (1966) Oral manifestations of erythema multiforme in children. **Oral Surg Oral Med Oral Pathol** 21:713.
393. Giallorenzi AF, Goldstein BH (1975) Acute (toxic) epidermal necrolysis. **Oral Surg** 40:611.
394. Hebert AA, Lopez MD (1997) Oral lesions in pediatric patients. **Adv Dermatol** 12:169–194.
395. Wright P, Collin JRO (1983) The ocular complications of erythema multiforme (Stevens-Johnson syndrome) and their management. **Trans Ophthalmol Soc UK** 103:338.
396. Ginsburg CM (1982) Stevens-Johnson's syndrome in children. **Pediatr Infect Dis** 1:155.
397. Prendiville JS, Hebert AA, Greenwald MJ et al. (1989) Management of Stevens-Johnson syndrome and toxic epidermal necrolysis in children. **J Pediatr** 115:88.
398. Morici MV, Galen WK, Shetty AK et al. (2000) Intravenous immunoglobulin therapy for children with Stevens-Johnson syndrome. **J Rheumatol** 27:2494–2497.
399. Todd J, Fishaut M, Kapral M et al. (1978) Toxic-shock syndrome associated with phage group-I staphylococci. **Lancet** 2:1116.
400. Green SL, LaPeter KS (1982) Evidence for postpartum toxic-shock syndrome in a mother-infant pair. **Am J Med** 72–169.
401. Shands KN, Schmid GP, Dan BB et al. (1980) Toxic shock syndrome in menstruating women. **N Engl J Med** 303:1436.
402. Chesney PJ, Davis JP, Purdy WK et al. (1981) Clinical manifestations of toxic shock syndrome. **JAMA** 246:741.
403. Bach MC (1983) Dermatologic signs in toxic shock syndrome—clues to diagnosis. **J Am Acad Dermatol** 8:343.
404. Huang YC, Hsueh PR, Lin TY et al. (2001) A family cluster of streptococcal toxic shock syndrome in children: clinical implication and epidemiological investigation. **Pediatrics** 107:1181–1183.
405. Woelfel JB (1990) Dental Anatomy: Its Relevance to Dentistry 4th ed. Philadelphia: Lea & Febiger. p. 29.
406. Newland JR (1984) Benign lingual lesions of intrinsic origin. **Postgrad Med J** 75:152.

Pigmentary Abnormalities

Joseph Morelli, Alain Taïeb, Norman Levine and Rafael Falabella

Skin pigmentation is the body's main defence against ultraviolet (UV) light (sunlight). Skin color also is an extremely important social and cultural characteristic that may determine one's station in life. Understandably, parents of children with any deviations from normal pigmentation are concerned about this problem. Even relatively minor pathologic pigmentary changes can cause children to become pariahs in their own communities.

This chapter briefly reviews basic science aspects of pigmentation and then discusses disorders or pigmentation that cause either increased skin color (hyperpigmentation) or decreased cutaneous pigment (hypopigmentation). These pathologic changes may be congenital, as in giant congenital nevi, or acquired, as in vitiligo. They may be localized, as in café-au-lait spots, or generalized, as in oculocutaneous albinism. Emphasis is placed on the clinical features that will usually permit a diagnosis of a given disorder without laboratory testing. In fact, in most pigmentary diseases, physical examination and a detailed history is usually sufficient.

MELANOCYTES AND MELANOGENESIS

Alain Taïeb

Melanocytes are derived from the neural crest and during embryonic development migrate to the skin, eye, and the hairbulbs.[1] These cells are highly specialized dendritic cells that produce a complex polymer, melanin. This is a pigmented substance that has several important functions: (1) it is a potent absorber of ultraviolet radiation and thus protects one from potentially damaging sunlight; (2) it is a scavenger of cytotoxic intermediates; (3) it may be important in the developmental process of the nervous system; and (4) in certain species, the color that it imparts may act as a sexual attractant.[2]

In the skin, melanocytes are present in the basal layer and represent less than 1 percent of the total number of epidermal cells. These cells interact with the immediate environment through a number of cell surface receptors that respond to signaling peptides and hormones, which all may influence the level of melanocytic activity.[2]

Melanin is synthesized in a specialized membrane-bound organelle called a *melanosome*. It begins as a premelanosome after being synthesized on ribosomes and contains a fibrillar network on which melanin will eventually be laid down.

The rate-limiting enzyme for melanin synthesis is tyrosinase, which is produced separately from the melanosome and is then transported and fused to the melanosomal membrane. This enzyme catalyzes two reactions that are critical to melanin synthesis: the hydroxylation of tyrosine to DOPA and the oxidation of DOPA to dopaquinone.[3] Through a series of rearrangements and polymerizations, the final brown-colored compound, *eumelanin*, is produced.

Melanosomes are also capable of producing a melanin of slightly different structure and a different color, *pheomelanin*, which is red or yellow in color and is responsible for the red color of hair and may be partially responsible for the "fair" skin color in individuals who tan poorly and burn easily. Pheomelanins are derived from the interaction of cysteine with dopaquinone.[4] Through a series of nonenzymatic steps, the final product is formed; the exact structure of pheomelanin is unknown. Pheomelanin switch is under the influence of the receptor for alpha-melanocyte stimulating hormone (MSH; the melanocortin 1 receptor or MCR-1). Genetic polymorphisms of the MCR-1 have been associated to hair color, like red hair, and to an increased susceptibility to melanoma.[5,6] The melanin synthetic pathway is schematically represented in Fig. 10.1.[7]

Whatever the phenotype, melanocytes make mixtures of eumelanin and pheomelanin ("mixed melanins"). The ratios of the two compounds differ between individuals and it is not yet known whether this is genetically programmed or is a response to environmental stimuli.

Once melanin is produced, it is transferred to surrounding keratinocytes through a highly efficient system involving the dendrites of the melanocytes;

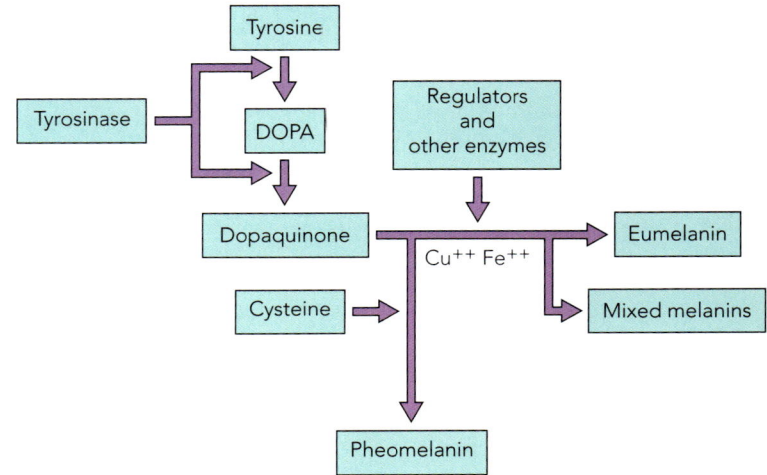

Fig. 10.1 Schematic pathway for eumelanin and pheomelanin synthesis.

1. Quevedo WC Jr, Fleischmann RD (1980) Developmental biology of mammalian melanocytes. **J Invest Dermatol** 75:116.
2. Hearing VJ, King RA (1993) Determinants of skin color: melanocytes and melanization. In: Pigmentation and Pigmentary Abnormalities, Ch. 1, Levine N, ed. Boca Raton, FL: CRC Press.
3. Hearing VJ, Jimenez M (1997) Mammalian tyrosinase – the critical regulatory control point in melanocyte pigmentation. **Int J Biochem** 19:1141.
4. Prota G (1980) Recent advances in the chemistry of melanogenesis in mammals. **J Invest Dermatol** 75:122.
5. Valverde P, Healy E, Jackson I, Rees JL, Thody AJ (1995) Variants of the melanocyte-stimulating hormone receptor gene are associated with red hair and fair skin in humans. **Nat Genet** 11:328–330.
6. Valverde P, Healy E, Sinkkink S et al. (1996) The Asp84Glu variant of the melanocortin 1 receptor (MC1R) is associated with melanoma. **Hum Mol Genet** 5:1663–1666.
7. Carstam R, Edner C, Hansson C et al. (1986) Metabolism of 5-S-gluthathionylDOPA. **Acta Derm Venereol** 126:1.

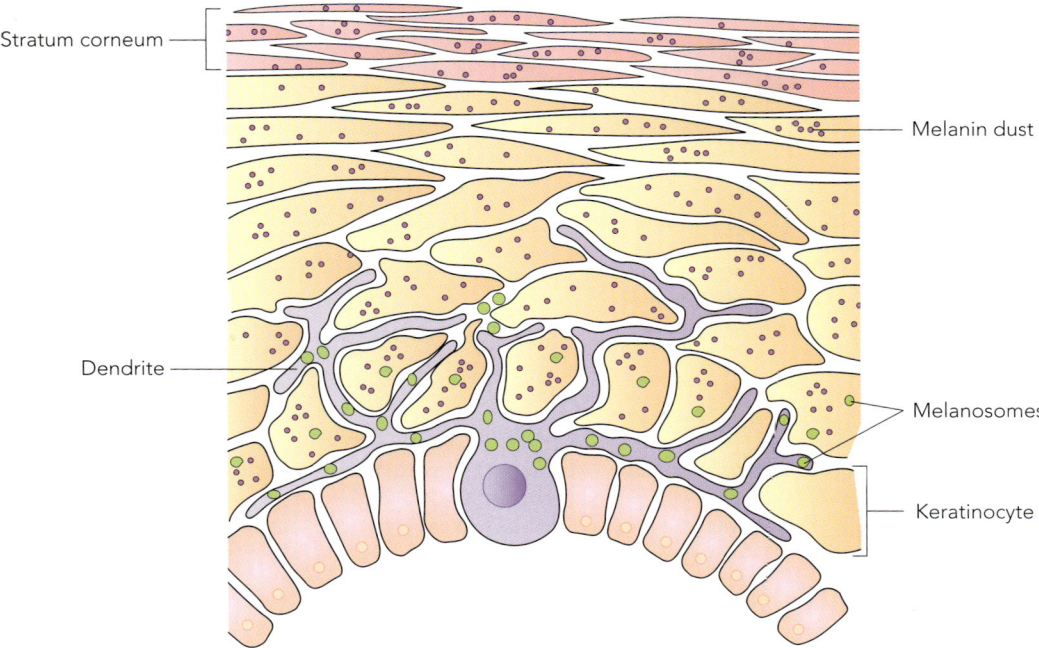

Stratum corneum

Melanin dust

Dendrite

Melanosomes

Keratinocyte

Fig. 10.2   Negroid epidermal melanin unit. One melanocyte supplies melanosomes with melanin to many keratinocytes, which carry it to the stratum corneum layer where it is desquamated. (From Klein and Nordlund,[13] with permission.)

this "epidermal-melanin unit" consists of one melanocyte and about 36 keratinocytes (Fig. 10.2).[8] The type of melanin and melanosomes produced by melanocytes is determining the phototype (i.e., the ability to tan), but keratinocytes are not only passive acceptors of pigment, since they are producing antioxidant enzymes, such as catalase and superoxide dismutase, in a phototype-dependent manner, which act in concert with melanins to limit photodamage.[9] Black skin has more tyrosinase activity and more actively melanizing melanocytes,[10,11] which produce mainly eumelanin. The melanosomes are greater in number, larger, and are dispersed singly throughout the epidermis. Caucasian skin melanocytes have less tyrosinase activity, produce fewer mature melanosomes, distribute melanin granules in clumps that are placed mostly in a suprabasilar location, and may produce more pheomelanin depending on the skin type of the individual.

COMPONENTS OF NORMAL SKIN COLOR

The color that one perceives when viewing the skin is an aggregation of a number of skin constituents. Aside from the constitutive color of the skin, one can increase melanin production after environmental insults. The most obvious example of this is tanning after sunlight exposure. This occurs over a period of days and is called *delayed tanning* (mostly UVB dependent) as opposed to *immediate pigment darkening* (a marker of UVA irradiation), which is a transient phenomenon that does not involve the synthesis of new melanin. If melanin pigment is present in the dermis, the integument takes on a blue-gray hue that looks bluer as the pigment is deposited deeper.

Many vegetables and fruits contain carotenoids, which are yellow polyisoprenoid lipids. These compounds deposit in both the epidermis and dermis and contribute in a minimal way to the yellowish tint of the skin. However, a pronounced yellowing of the integument can be noted in those individuals on high carotenoid diets.

Red and blue hues are the product of oxyhemoglobin and reduced hemoglobin in capillaries, arteries, and veins in the dermis. In areas where the skin is thin such as the lips, red color is a predominant one. On thick skin such as on the palms, one hardly sees red or blue hues.

HYPERPIGMENTARY DISORDERS

Alain Taïeb

Normal skin has essentially all of its melanin in the epidermis. If too much melanin is produced, or if the pigment is distributed in an abnormal fashion (e.g., into the dermis), clinical hyperpigmentation results. Occasionally, foreign materials such as heavy metals deposit in the skin and cause a change in color, but even in these circumstances, pathologic pigmentation is, in part, due to melanin itself. (See also Chapter 7, Pigmentary Disorders.)

PRIMARY CIRCUMSCRIBED EPIDERMAL HYPERMELANOSES

Because the abnormal melanin is close to the surface, these lesions are all tan in color, thus times of onset, distribution pattern, and associated clinical and histopathologic findings are all helpful in differentiating these disorders. Although all the epidermal hypermelanoses discussed below share a similar tan-brown color, they can be differentiated clinically in most instances. Café-au-lait spots are usually larger than lentigines and freckles and are present earlier in life than Becker's nevi or freckles. Lentigines may be indistinguishable from café-au-lait spots but do not vary in color with sunlight as do freckles and do not have coarse hair like Becker's nevi. Histologically, Becker's nevi differ from café-au-lait spots by the downward epidermal proliferation of the rete pegs as well as the presence of increased numbers and activity of melanocytes. Freckles are the only one of these lesions that become substantially darker and coalesce after sun exposure. Becker's nevi occur later in life than café-au-lait spots, are usually much larger than lentigines, and have the unique feature of hypertrichosis.

Café-au-lait spots

Café-au-lait spots present as uniform tan-brown round or oval macules with distinct margins and variable border contour (Fig. 10.3). These lesions tend to enlarge in proportion to general body growth during the first several years of life and then stabilize. They do not regress in later years.

8. Pathak MA, Fanselow DL (1983) Photobiology of melanin pigmentation: dose/response of skin to sunlight and its contents. **J Am Acad Dermatol** 9:724.

9. Bessou S, Picardo M, Maresca V, Surlève-Bazeille JE, Pain C, Taïeb A (1998) Chimeric human epidermal reconstructs to study the role of melanocytes and keratinocytes in pigmentation and photoreception. **J Invest Dermatol** 111:1103–1108.

10. Iozumi K, Hoganson GE, Pennela R et al. (1993) Role of tyrosinase as a determinant of pigmentation in cultured human melanocytes. **J Invest Dermatol** 100:806.

11. Iwata M, Corn Y, Iwata S et al. (1990) The relationship between tyrosinase activity and skin color in human foreskins. **J Invest Dermatol** 95:9.

Histologically, the café-au-lait spots have increased epidermal melanin without melanocytic proliferation. Ultrastructural examination of L-dopa-incubated split-skin preparations reveals giant pigment granules (macromelanosomes) in lesions from patients with neurofibromatosis. At one time this was believed to be specific for this disease,[12] but these granules have subsequently been noted in numerous other pigmented and nonpigmented diseases, including ocular albinism, congenital and acquired melanocytic nevi, and lentigines, as well as in normal skin.[13]

Café-au-lait spots are commonly seen at birth or in early infancy and have also been noted in up to 25% of children, particularly in blacks,[14] but lower figures have been noted. In one study, 1.9% of all infants had café-au-lait spots at birth, but 12% of blacks had at least one lesion at birth, indicating the greatly increased incidence in this racial group.[15] These lower figures may not account for café-au-lait spots that appear after the neonatal period.[16]

Most of the children with café au lait spots have no other associated abnormalities. However, in those with multiple large café-au-lait spots, these may be a sign of one of several multiorgan syndromes (Table 10.1). By far the most common is neurofibromatosis (See also Chapter 7, Neurofibromatosis and tuberous sclerosis). It is generally believed that six or more café-au-lait spots greater than 1.5cm in diameter are pathognomonic of this disease.[17] The importance of this finding was demonstrated in a study that showed that 89% of children with more than six café-au-lait macules with no obvious diseases observed for 3 years eventually developed other changes of neurofibromatosis.[18] Children may have café-au-lait spots as the only manifestation until puberty, when other signs begin to appear. Ninety-five percent of these patients have at least one spot, but other findings such as neurocutaneous neurofibromas, axillary freckling, pigmented hamartomas of the iris (Lisch nodules), skeletal abnormalities, and neurologic changes are necessary to confirm the diagnosis.[19]

Children with McCune–Albright syndrome (polyostotic fibrous dysplasia) usually caused by mosaicism for a mutation in the *GNAS1* gene,[20] also may have multiple café-au-lait spots, but these lesions are characteristically fewer, larger, and darker, and have more jagged margins, supposedly resembling the coast of Maine.[21] Besides the characteristic bony lesions, other findings in this syndrome include endocrinologic abnormalities, especially precocious puberty in females, thyrotoxicosis, pituitary gigantism, and Cushing syndrome.[22]

Watson syndrome is a much rarer disorder in which children have multiple large café-au-lait spots. This is inherited in an autosomal-dominant manner, and is characterized by pulmonary stenosis, low intelligence, axillary freckling, and pigmented patches without neurofibromas.[23] Other conditions in which café-au-lait spots have been described include Russell-Silver dwarfism, ataxia-telangiectasia, tuberous sclerosis, basal cell nevus syndrome, Hunter syndrome, Turner syndrome, and Gaucher's disease, and others (Table 10.2).

There are no medical indications for treating café-au-lait spots. These lesions have no malignant potential and are usually in locations of little cosmetic significance.

Nevus spilus

The nevus spilus is characterized by a light-brown patch stippled with punctuate dark-brown macules or papules (Fig. 10.4), usually present on the trunk or proximal extremities. The nevus spilus has histologic findings that include those of lentigines in the tan patchy areas as well as changes of junctional melanocytic nevi in the darker speckled sites.

Although there have been a few isolated case reports of malignant degeneration in a nevus spilus,[24,25] these should be considered to have little malignant potential; thus, cosmetic considerations alone usually dictate whether these lesions should be surgically removed.

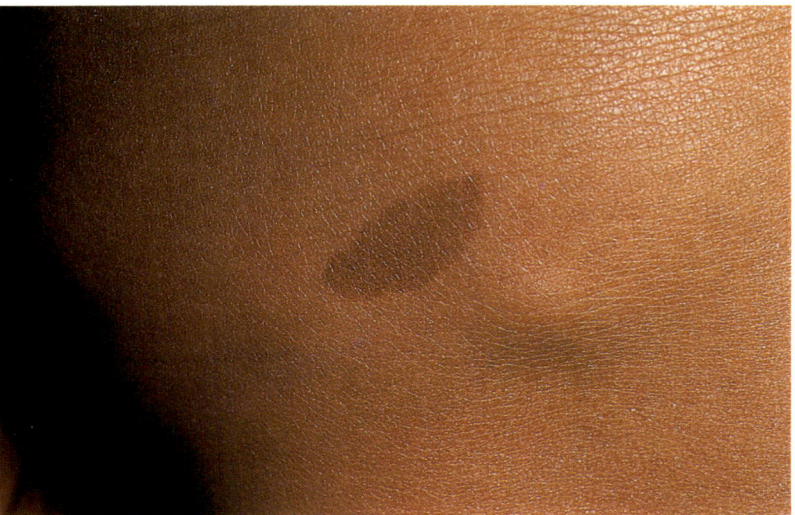

Fig. 10.3   Café au lait macule.

TABLE 10.1   Non café-au-lait spots circumscribed epidermal hypermelanoses

Disease	Clinical findings	Histology
Nevus spilus	Brown patch stippled with brown macules/papules	Lentiginous features plus junctional nests of nevus cells
Peutz–Jeghers syndrome	Multiple lentigines, gastrointestinal hamartomas	Elongated rete pegs, increased number/activity of melanocytes
Carney syndrome	Cardiac/cutaneous myxomas, endocrine overreactivity, testicular tumors, multiple lentigines	Same as Peutz–Jeghers
Nevoid hypermelanosis	Segmental tan patch with brown macules/papules	Same as nevus spilus
Linear whorled nevoid hypermelanosis	Whorled pigment along Blaschko's lines	Basal melanocytic hyperplasia

12. Jimbow K, Szabo G, Fitzpatrick TB (1973) Ultrastructure of giant pigment (macromelanosomes) in the cutaneous pigmented macules of neurofibromatosis. **J Invest Dermatol** 61:300.
13. Klein LG, Nordlund JT (1981) Genetic basis of pigmentation and its disorders. **Int J Dermatol** 20:621.
14. Whitehouse D (1966) Diagnostic value of cafe-au-lait spots in children. **Arch Dis Child** 41:316.
15. Alper J, Holmes LB, Mihm MC Jr (1979) Birthmarks with serious medical significance: nevocellular nevi, sebaceous nevi, and multiple cafe-au-lait spots. **J Pediatr** 95:696.
16. Castella EE, DeGraca DM, Orioli-Parreiras JM (1981) Epidemiology of congenital pigmented nevi, incidence rates and relative frequencies **Br J Dermatol** 104:307.
17. Crowe FW, Schull WJ, Neel JV (1956) A Clinical, Pathological and Genetic Study of Multiple Neurofibromatosis. Springfield, Il: Charles C Thomas.
18. Korf BR (1992) Diagnostic outcome in children with multiple cafe au lait spots. **Pediatrics** 90:924.
19. Riccardi V (1980) Pathophysiology of neurofibromatosis. **J Am Acad Dermatol** 3:157.
20. Weinstein LS, Shenker A, Gejman PV et al. (1991) Activating mutations of the stimulatory G protein in the McCune–Albright syndrome. **N Engl J Med** 325:1688–1695.
21. Benedict PH, Szabo G, Fitzpatrick TB et al. (1968) Melanotic macules in Albright's syndrome and in neurofibromatosis. **JAMA** 205:618.
22. Albright F (1938) Syndrome characterized by osteitis fibrosa disseminata, areas of pigmentation, and a gonadal dysfunction. **Endocrinology** 22:411.
23. Watson GH (1967) Pulmonary stenosis, café-au-lait spots, and dull intelligence. **Arch Dis Child** 42:303.
24. Rhodes AR, Mihm MC Jr (1990) Origin of cutaneous melanoma in a congential dysplastic nevus spilus. **Arch Dermatol** 126:500.
25. Rutten A, Goos M (1990) Nevus spilus with malignant melanoma in a patient with neurofibromatosis. **Arch Dermatol** 126:539.

TABLE 10.2   Diseases associated with multiple café-au-lait spots

Disease	Major features
Ataxia telangiectasia	Progressive ataxia, lymphoreticular malignancy
Bannayan–Riley–Ruvalcaba syndrome	Macrosomia, megalencephaly, lipomas, intestinal polyps
Basal cell nevus syndrome	Multiple basal cell epitheliomas, jaw cysts, skeletal anomalies
Bloom syndrome	Short stature, photosensitivity, chromosome breaks, malignancy
Fanconi's anemia	Limb anomalies, renal anomalies, pancytopenia
Gaucher's disease	Jewish predilection, ataxia, mental retardation
Hunter syndrome	Thickened skin, coarse facies, skin papules, joint contractures
Jaffe–Campanacci syndrome	Fibromas of long bones, hypogonadism, mental retardation, ocular/cardiac anomalies
Maffucci syndrome	Venous malformations, enchondromas
McCune–Albright syndrome	Polyostotic fibrous dysplasia, precocious puberty
Multiple lentigines syndrome	Multiple lentigines, hypertelorism, pulmonic stenosis
Multiple mucosal neuroma syndrome	Mucosal neuromas, thyroid carcinoma, pheochromocytoma, parathyroid adenoma, dysautonomia
Neurofibromatosis	Neurofibromas, central nervous system tumors, iris hamartomas, axillary freckles, skeletal anomalies
Russell–Silver syndrome	Short stature, asymmetry, limb anomalies
Tuberous sclerosis	White macules, multiple hamartomas, central nervous system anomalies
Watson syndrome	Pulmonic stenosis, axillary freckles, low intelligence

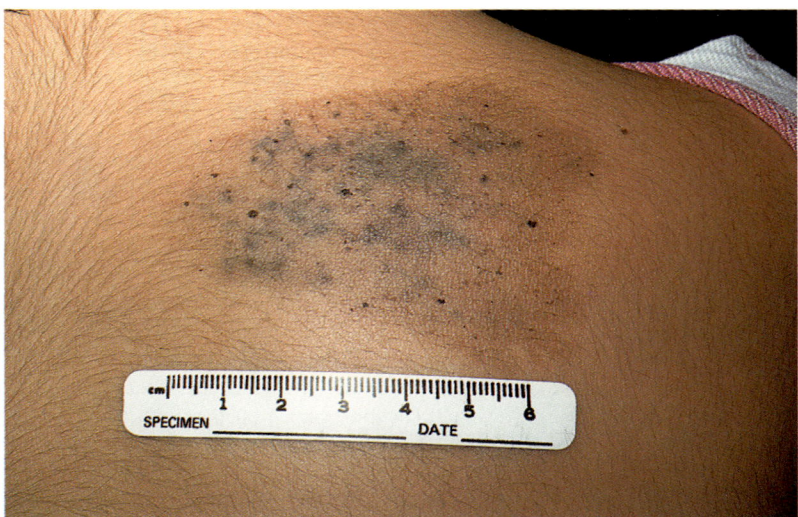

Fig. 10.4   Nevus spilus. Speckled nevus in this case containing a blue nevus component as well.

Non-Blaschkoid and Blaschkoid segmental hypermelanoses

Segmental hypermelanosis is a the expression of a cutaneous mosaicism of the pigmentary system which appears as a hyperpigmented macule in a segmental pattern, and presents early in life.[26] Histologic features are mostly similar to that of lentigines, but foci of junctional clusters of melanocytes may occur on occasional nevus spilus-like areas.

Most cases of segmental hypermelanosis have their onset at birth or in early childhood and may continue to enlarge into adult life. They may appear anywhere on the skin and are typically unilateral with a sharp cutoff at the midline.[27] They often follow a dermatome but may present in a blocklike pattern. In the vast majority of cases, there are no associated dysmorphic features,[28] although there have been a few reported cases of associated neurologic problems.[29] With depigmenting lasers there is the possibility that some of these skin lesions can be lightened.[30]

Another similar but unrelated form of nevoid hypermelanosis is the linear and whorled variety. Within the first few weeks of life, children with this form develop swirls of macular hyperpigmentation along Blaschko's lines (a system of lines on the surface of the skin that certain linear nevi and other dermatoses apparently follow (see Fig. 10.7)). These are not the same as dermatomal lines and thus this condition looks different than zosteriform nevoid hyper-

melanosis. The hyperpigmentation is composed of homogeneous macules that coalesce into reticulated patches. Linear and whorled nevoid hypermelanosis has been associated with serious congenital defects.[31] Differential diagnoses include other Blaschkolinear hyper- and hypomelanoses, such as incontinentia pigmenti and hypomelanosis of Ito.

Lentigines and lentiginoses

A lentigo is an extremely common pigmented lesion that may be present at birth or may appear in early childhood. The typical lentigo (lentigo simplex) is a discrete, small (less than 5mm), tan, brown, or black, oval or circular macule that may occur on any cutaneous surface or on mucous membranes. Exposure to sunlight will not darken it, and it does not disappear spontaneously.

The histologic changes in lentigines are limited to an increased activity of basal epidermal melanocytes, without nesting of melanocytes. These may increase in number well into adult life.[32] Both sexes are equally affected, and a child may have a single lesion or innumerable ones. Lentigines may also be familial.[33] Lentigines should be differentiated from solar lentigines that occurs in exposed areas in older people after significant sun exposure, and comprise an elongation of the rete pegs of the epidermis.

Autosomal-dominant inherited generalized lentigines (lentiginosis profusa) must be differentiated from a multisystem autosomal-dominant disease with progressive lentigines, the multiple lentigines syndrome or LEOPARD syndrome (Fig. 10.5). The acronym LEOPARD identifies the following features:[34] Lentigines, lesions noted most prominently on the face and trunk that increase in number with age; Electrocardiographic abnormalities; Ocular hypertelorism; Pulmonic valve stenosis; Abnormal genitalia, particularly undescended testicles; Retarded growth; and Deafness (sensory).

Another multisystem disease associated with lentigines is Peutz–Jeghers syndrome (PJS), an autosomal-dominant disorder consisting of multiple lentigines, clustered in the perioral area as well as elsewhere, and gastrointestinal hamartomas situated most densely in the jejunum. Unlike other lentiginoses, lesions may remit completely during adolescence.[32] Germline mutations in STK11, a serine/threonine kinase with a wide tissue distribution, probably in conjunction with acquired genetic defects of the second allele in somatic cells, cause the manifestations of PJS.[35] STK11 is a tumor suppressor

26. Simoes GA (1981) Speckled zosteriform lentiginous nevus. **J Am Acad Dermatol** 4:236.
27. Altman DA, Banse L (1992) Zosteriform speckled lentiginous nevus. **J Am Acad Dermatol** 27:106.
28. Ruth WK, Shelburne JD, Jegasothy BJ (1980) Zosteriform lentiginous nevus. **Arch Dermatol** 116:478.
29. Pickering JC (1973) Partial unilateral lentiginosis with associated developmental abnormalities. **Guys Hosp Rep** 122:361.
30. Tan OT, Morelli JG (1989) Lasers in dermatology. **Curr Probl Dermatol** 1:7.
31. Kalter DC, Griffiths WA, Atherton DJ (1988) Linear and whorled nevoid hypermelanosis. **J Am Acad Dermatol** 19:1037.
32. Hurwitz S (1983) Epidermal nevi and tumors of epidermal origin. **Pediatr Clin North Am** 30:482.
33. Fulk CS (1984) Primary disorders of hyperpigmentation. **J Am Acad Dermatol** 10:1.
34. Gorlin RJ, Anderson RC, Blau M (1969) Multiple lentigines syndrome. **Am J Dis Child** 112:652.
35. Jenne DE, Reimann H Nezu J et al. (1998) Peutz–Jeghers syndrome is caused by mutations in a novel serine threonine kinase. **Nat Genet** 18:38–43.

gene that acts as an early gatekeeper regulating the development of hamartomas in PJS which may be pathogenetic precursors of adenocarcinoma. Additional somatic mutation events underlie the progression of hamartomas to adenocarcinomas, and some of these somatic mutations are common to the later stages of tumor progression seen in the majority of colorectal carcinomas.

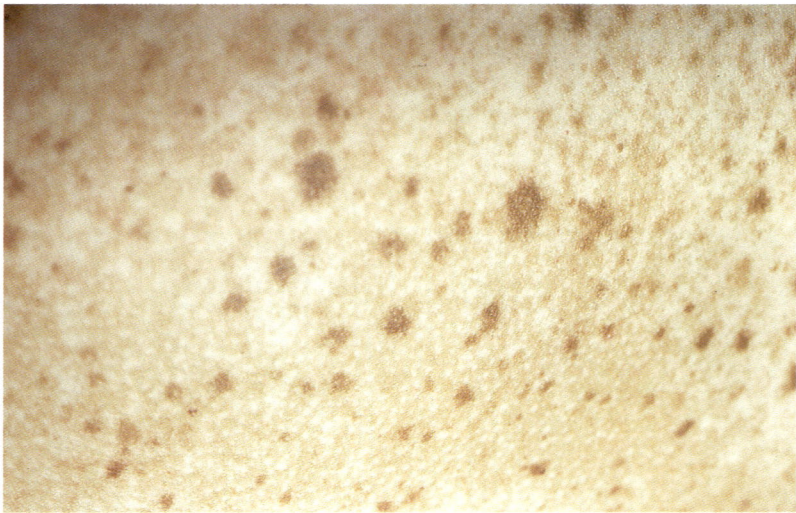

Fig. 10.5 **LEOPARD syndrome.** Diffuse lentiginosis.

A group of patients has been reported that had multiple lentigines but was different from those with other syndromes with these cutaneous findings. Originally given the acronym "NAME" or "LAMB" syndrome, Carney exhaustively reviewed 40 patients with a complex of myxomas, "spotty" pigmentation, and endocrine overactivity,[36] a condition now known as "Carney syndrome" (Fig. 10.6A,B). There appears to be an autosomal–dominant inheritance pattern with variable expressivity[37] and a female predominance. Two genes loci have been associated with this phenotype on chromosomes 2 and 17. The gene situated on chromosome 17 encodes a protein kinase A regulatory subunit.[38] A typical patient with this syndrome has at least two of the following findings: cardiac myxomas; hyperpigmentation of the skin, including lentigines, ephelides, and nevi (although histologically almost all of these lesions are lentigines); cutaneous myxomas; myxoid mammary fibroadenomas; testicular tumors; pigmented nodular adrenocortical disease; and pituitary adenomas with gigantism or acromegaly.[36] The multiple pigmented macules are distributed diffusely but are concentrated most heavily on the central face, including the lips, the neck, and the upper trunk.[39] The skin lesions are present at birth and frequently increase in number at puberty. Multiple subcutaneous myxomas occur in about 50% of cases and usually appear in the periorbital and postauricular areas.[40] Early recognition of this syndrome is important because surgical correction of cardiac myxomas may prevent the potentially fatal complication of embolism of tumor fragments.[41] Endocrinologic studies including cortisol determinations, thyroid function studies, growth hormone levels, and imaging of the sella turcica should be considered if there is a clinical suspicion of endocrine overactivity.

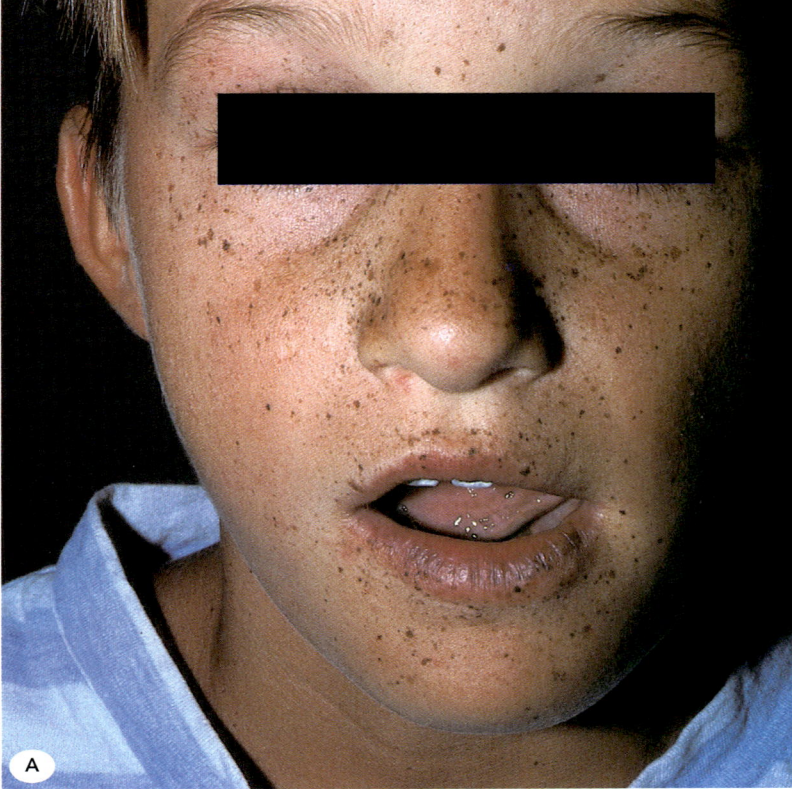

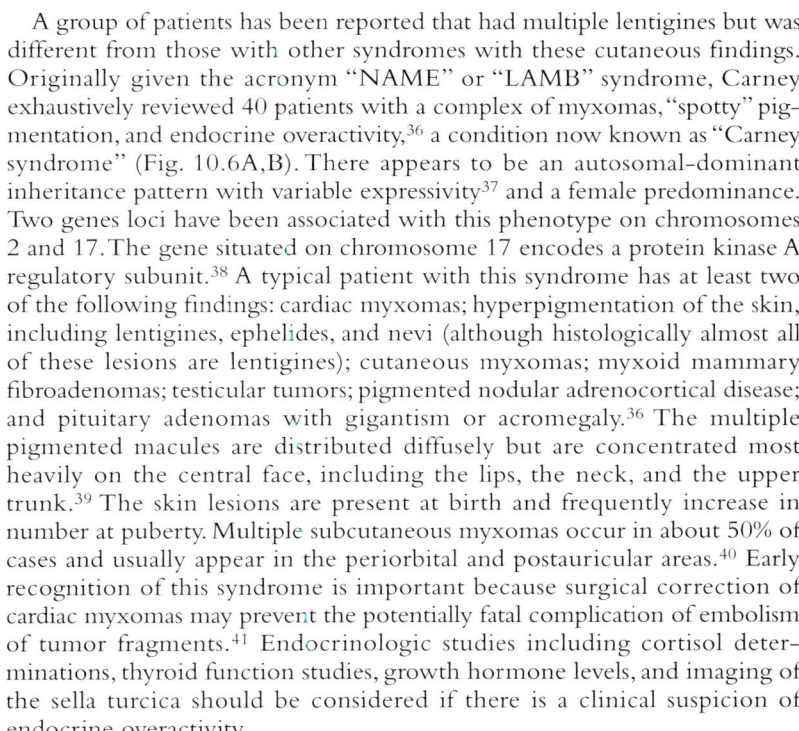

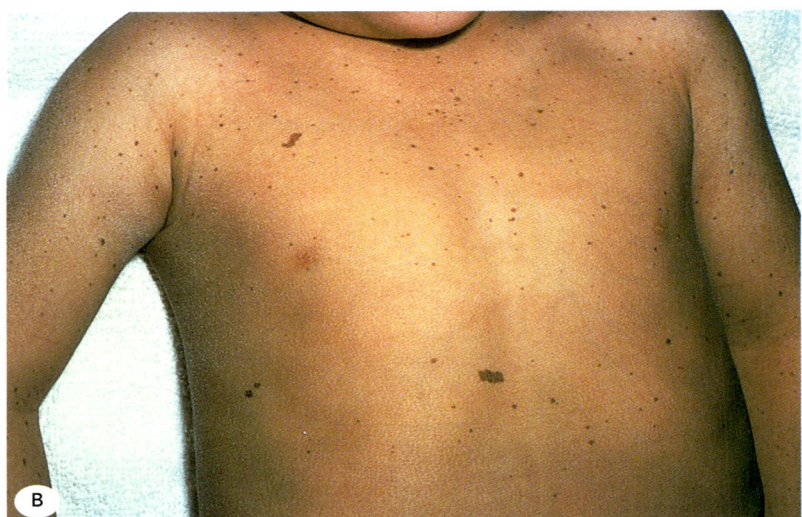

Fig. 10.6 **Carney syndrome.** (A) Central facial and lip lentigines in a 10-year-old boy. (B) Same patient as in (A) as an infant. Multiple truncal lentigines are seen.

36. Carney JA, Gordon H, Carpenter PC (1985) The complex of myxomas, spotty pigmentation, and endocrine overactivity. **Medicine** 64:270.
37. Carney JA, Hruska LS, Beauchamp GD, Gordon H (1986) Dominant inheritance of the complex of myxomas, spotty pigmentation, and endocrine overactivity. **Mayo Clin Proc** 61:165.
38. Kirschner LS, Carney JA, Pack SD et al. (2000) Mutations of the gene encoding the protein kinase A type I-alpha regulatory subunit in patients with the Carney complex. **Nat Genet** 26:89–92.
39. Reed OM, Mellette JR, Fitzpatrick JE (1986) Cutaneous lentiginosis with atrial myxomas. **J Am Acad Dermatol** 15:398.
40. Rhodes AR, Mihm MC (1990) Origin of cutaneous melanoma in a congenital dysplastic nevus spilus. **Arch Dermatol** 126:500.
41. Atherton DJ, Pitcher DW, Wells RS, MacDonald DM (1980) A syndrome of various cutaneous pigmented lesions, myxoid neurofibromata and atrial myxomas: the NAME syndrome. **Br J Dermatol** 103:421.

Ephelides (freckles)

Freckles are extremely common in light-skinned, red-haired people and appear to be inherited as an autosomal-dominant trait.[42] On histologic examination, ephelides show increased melanin in the epidermis without the melanocytic proliferation or epidermal elongation noted in lentigines. They are not present at birth but arise in early childhood (2–4 years), mainly on sun-exposed skin. They darken in summer and tend to fade during the winter months, indicating the necessity of sunlight exposure in their induction. These lesions become less noticeable in adult life. Typically, freckles are well-circumscribed, red-tan macules that occur most commonly on the face (Fig. 10.7), back, and upper shoulders, while sparing the mucous membranes.

Becker's nevus

During the late 1940s, Becker[43] described an acquired localized hyper-melanosis and hypertrichosis in two young men. Subsequently, several hundred cases have been reported in all races and in both sexes, although redheads almost never acquire these lesions. The characteristic presentation is an adolescent boy with a unilateral slightly thickened or pebbly, irregular, hyperpigmented plaque that appears on the upper trunk, although any part of the body may be involved (Fig. 10.8).[44] After a variable period, most of these lesions develop thick, dark hairs. Light microscopic examination of this hyperpigmented lesion reveals an increase in the number of basal melanocytes, along with variable epidermal hyperplasia.[45] There have been cases of Becker's nevus with associated smooth muscle hamartomas where there are dermal

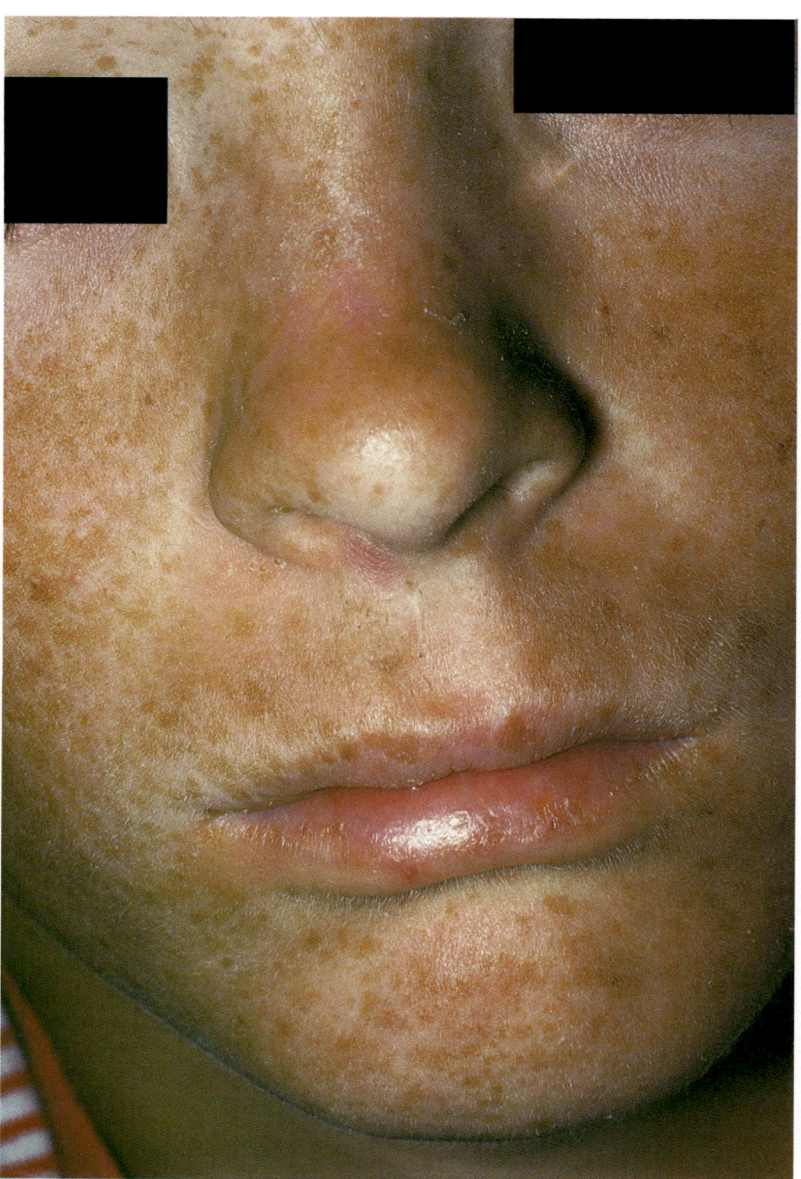

Fig. 10.7   Ephelides. Heavily freckled teenager.

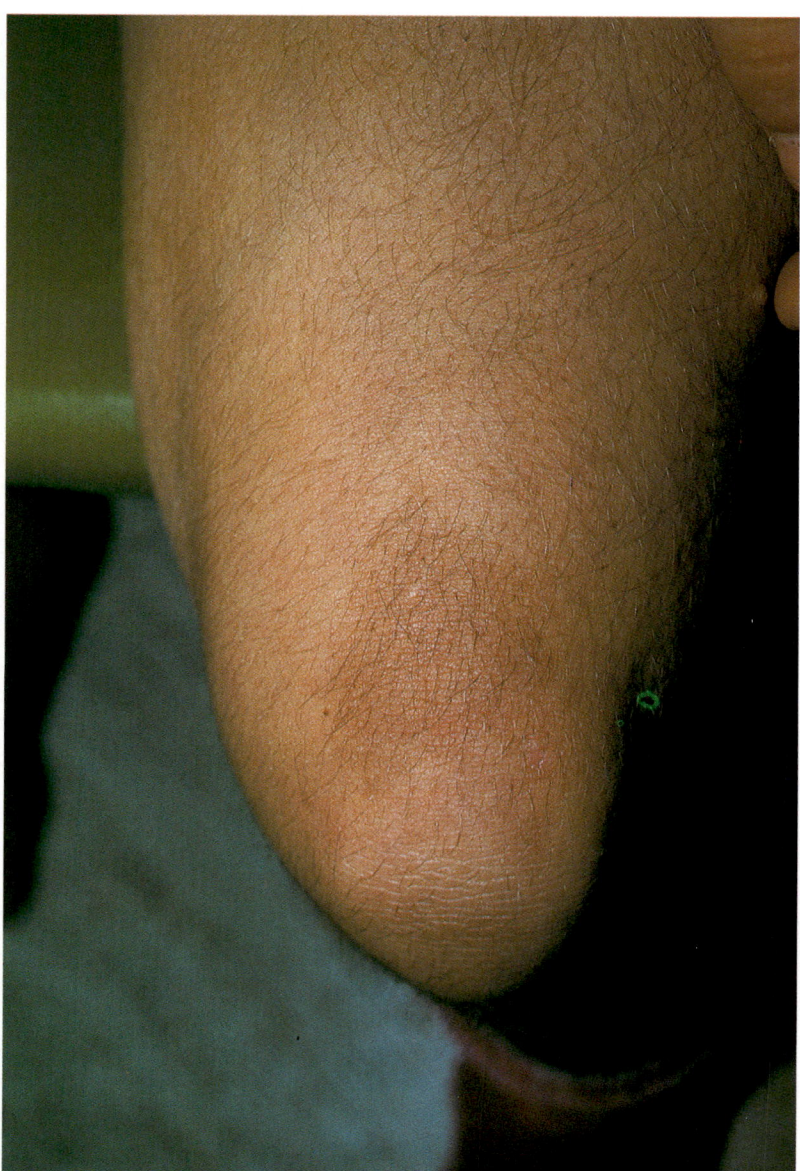

Fig. 10.8   Becker's nevus above knee.

42. Brues AM (1950) Linkage of body build with sex, eye color and freckling. Am J Hum Genet 2:215.
43. Becker SW (1949) Concurrent melanosis and hypertrichosis in distribution of nevus unius lateris. Arch Dermatol 60:155.
44. Tymen R, Forestier JF, Boutel B et al. (1981) Nevus tardef de Becker. Ann Derm Venereol (Stockh) 108:41.
45. Tate PR, Hodge SJ, Owen LG (1980) A quantitative study of melanocytes in Becker's nevus. J Cutan Pathol 7:404.

collections of smooth muscle bundles that connect with the arrector pili muscles.[46] Other hamartomatous proliferations have included sebaceous gland hyperplasia,[47] and in one case, an underlying plexiform neurofibroma.[48] Ultrastructural changes include giant melanosomes in both melanocytes and keratinocytes.[49] The early or even congenital occurrence of lesions similar to classic Becker's nevus suggests a link with smooth muscle hamartomas. Although most of these lesions occur without other pathologic findings, there have been several reports of other abnormalities, particularly in females including unilateral breast hypoplasia,[50] spina bifida, and limb asymmetry.[51] One center reported nine cases of melanoma in patients with Becker's nevi; one of the melanomas arose from the Becker's nevus itself.[52]

The cause of the Becker's nevus is unknown, although the male predominance, onset at the time of puberty, and acquired lesional hypertrichosis suggests androgen-mediated hyperplasia. Two reports of increased lesional androgen receptors indicate that androgen sensitivity and stimulation may play a role in the development of this lesion.[53] Becker's nevus is a benign process and, with rare exceptions aside, without malignant potential. Excision of these lesions is difficult because of the large size and deep-dermal hair follicles and is not recommended in most cases. The most unsightly portion of the lesion is the dark hair, which can be managed by depilatories, hot wax epilation, electrolysis, or shaving. Untreated, these nevi stabilize after several months but do not regress.

DERMAL MELANOCYTOSES

Melanocytes move from the neural crest to the skin during early embryonic life. Failure of complete melanocyte migration into the epidermis before birth with ensuing dermal nesting and melanin production produces characteristic blue patches. Dermal melanin produces a blue color because all but the blue end of the light spectrum penetrates into the deep dermis and is absorbed by dermal melanin. Blue light is reflected from the surface of the skin, producing blue colors in deep dermal melanocytic lesions.[54] Melanocytes are present normally in the dermis in small numbers but do not impart a blue color, since these melanocytes do not synthesize melanin. Prominent dermal melanin synthesis occurs in the Mongolian spot and the nevus of Ota/Ito.

Mongolian spot

The Mongolian spot is a hyperpigmented macule or patch present at birth or shortly thereafter, with a predilection for certain racial groups. Ninety-six percent of black children, 46% of Hispanic infants, and about 10% of white neonates are born with these lesions.[55]

There are two classifications for these lesions based on location and on speed of regression. Mongolian spots are organized as being sacral or extrasacral and are further divided into the common type, which regresses within months to a few years; the extensive type, which regresses more slowly; and the persistent type, which is permanent. This last variety is better considered as a variant of nevus of Ota/Ito. More than 75% of lesions occur in the sacrogluteal region. The shoulder and extensor surface of the upper extremities are other relatively common locations. Mongolian spots uncommonly appear on the abdomen, chest, and rarely on the palms or soles. It has been said that extrasacral lesions may persist longer than those over the sacrogluteal region, but this probably is not the case.[56]

The typical Mongolian spot is noted at birth and presents as a blue-green to blue-gray irregular patch with indefinite margins (Fig. 10.9). It may increase in size for 1 to 2 years and peak in color intensity at 1 year. The lesion may vary in size from a few millimeters to greater than 10cm. During the next 1–4 years, it becomes less noticeable and eventually fades completely. Only 3–4% of lesions remain beyond this time.[57]

Histologic examination of the lesion reveals a deep dermal melanocytic proliferation scattered among the collagen bundles. The pigment is wholly contained within melanosomes and as such is not phagocytosed by melanophages. This is fortunate because pigment within melanophages may remain indefinitely.

There are several intriguing aspects in the pathogenesis of the Mongolian spot. It is reasonable to assume that incomplete migration of melanocytes accounts for the dermal location of these cells, but why does this occur preferentially in certain locations? One theory holds that local hindrance factors prevent melanocytes from entering certain areas and the sacrogluteal area lacks these factors in susceptible individuals.[58] Another interesting question is: Why do these melanocytes disappear early in life and nevocellular nevus cells remain until the sixth or seventh decade? The answer is unknown, but the process of involution does involve the destruction of the melanocytes themselves. In adults, however, dermal melanocytes that are not synthesizing melanin can be detected, so functional alterations of these cells may also be occurring.

The Mongolian spot is so distinctive that when present at birth in the characteristic sacral location, little can be confused with it. Congenital nevi share some similar features but usually have an irregular surface and have shades of brown interespersed with blue and gray colors. Blue nevi are very rare in young children and are smaller and more well defined than Mongolian spots. It is very important that the presence of a Mongolian spot be noted in the newborn medical record, since in cases of suspected child abuse, these lesions can be mistaken for ecchymoses.[58]

Several associated diseases have been described with Mongolian spots but because this is a common anomaly, most are probably coincidental. There is one association that appears to be real, namely multiple Mongolian spots and an abnormality of sphingolipid metabolism, GM1 type gangliosidosis, caused by a deficiency of the enzyme β-galactosidase. These children have severe developmental delay, edema, unusual facies, hepatosplenomegaly, and cherry-red spots

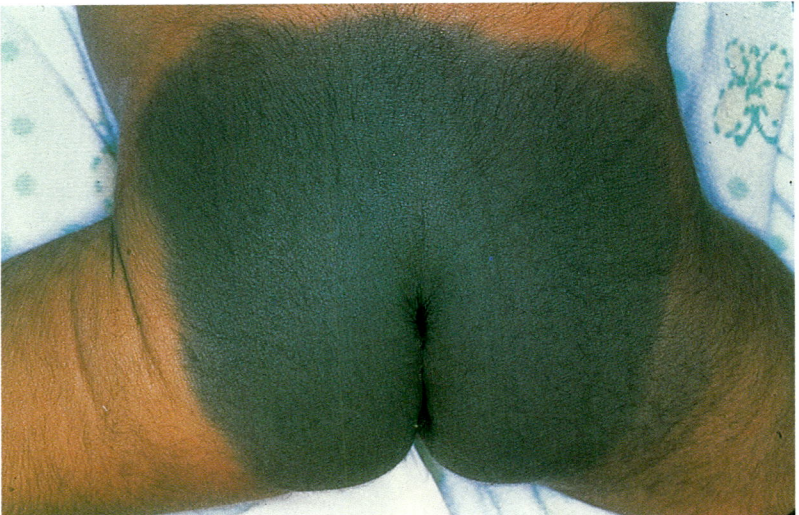

Fig. 10.9 Mongolian spot on the buttocks of a black newborn infant.

46. Urbanek RW, Johnson WC (1978) Smooth muscle hamartoma associated with Becker's nevus. **Arch Dermatol** 114:104.
47. Burgeenk BL, Ackerman AB (1978) Acneform lesions in Becker's nevus. **Cutis** 21:617.
48. Chapel TA, Tavafoghi V, Mehregen A et al. (1981) Becker's melanosis: an organoid hamartoma. **Cutis** 21:405.
49. Bhawan J, Chang WH (1979) Becker's melanosis: an ultrastructural study. **Dermatologica** 159:221.
50. Formigon M, Alsina MM, Mascaro JM et al. (1992) Becker's nevus and ipsilateral breast hypoplasia. **Arch Dermatol** 128:992.
51. Glinick SE, Alper JC, Bogaars H et al. (1983) Becker's melanosis: associated abnormalities. **J Am Acad Dermatol** 9:509.
52. Fehr B, Panizzon RG, Schnyder UW (1991) Becker's naevus and malignant melanoma. **Dermatologica** 182:77.
53. Person JR, Longcope C (1984) Becker's nevus: an androgen-mediated hyperplasia with increased androgen receptors. **J Am Acad Dermatol** 10:235.
54. Rhodes AR (1983) Pigmented birthmarks and precursor melanocytic lesions of cutaneous melanoma identifiable in childhood. **Pediatr Clin North Am** 30:435.
55. Cordova A (1981) The mongolian spot. **Clin Pediatr** 20:714.
56. Hidrano A (1971) Persistent mongolian spot in the adult. **Arch Dermatol** 103:680.
57. Leung AKC (1988) Mongolian spots in Chinese children. **Int J Dermatol** 27:106.
58. Smalek JE (1980) Significance of mongolian spots. **J Pediatr** 97:504.

of the retina. The Mongolian spots range in size from a few millimeters to several centimeters.[59]

Mongolian spots are usually self-limited and of no clinical consequence. Thus, there is no reason to treat these lesions.

Nevus of Ota/Ito

Nevus of Ota was first described in 1939 in Japan but cases have subsequently been recorded from around the world.[60] It most commonly occurs in Asians and blacks, but it is noted in all races. Females account for about 75% of all reported cases. This is usually a sporadic event but rare cases of familial nevus of Ota have been described.[61] Over 50% of lesions are present at birth and 40% appear at puberty, all of which involve the skin over the ophthalmic and/or maxillary division of the fifth cranial nerve. Only rare cases occur after age 21.[62] Four types are described: (1) an orbital type with tan-gray pigment limited to the eyelids or zygomatic region unilaterally (Fig. 10.10); (2) a moderate type with deep slate-gray to brown densely spotted pigment on the eyes, zygomatic region, and base of the nose; (3) an intensive type with deep-blue or purple densely pigmented areas on the side of the scalp and face down to the zygomatic region; and (4) a rare bilateral type. Mucous membrane pigmentation is common with all types, particularly of the ear canal, pharynx, hard palate, and nasal mucosa.[60] An additional clinical feature has been recently described that consists of intralesional or perilesional blue papules resembling blue nevi.[63]

Melanin pigment is deposited in the eye in 46–65% of reported cases. If the eye is affected, the sclera always is pigmented. The iris is involved in 50% of cases, the conjunctiva in 40% of cases, and the optic nerve in 45%.[64] Occasionally, there are melanocytes of the ciliary body of the angle of the anterior chamber that can cause secondary glaucoma. This usually occurs in blacks and Asians and is seen between age 20 and 40.[65]

The nevus of Ito probably represents the same pathologic process as the nevus of Ota, but it is located in a unilateral distribution over the supra-clavicular, deltoid, or scapular regions (Fig. 10.11). This corresponds roughly to the distribution of the posterior supraclavicular and the lateral brachial cutaneous nerves. The lesion is a patch that varies in color from deep blue–purple to light brownish-blue.

The cause of these dermal melanocytic disorders is unknown although an intriguing hypothesis has been proposed. The embryonic environment determines the onset, pattern, and extent of neural crest cell differentiation and these pluripotent cells mature along given phenotypic pathways in response to local factors.[66] The nevus of Ota may occur secondary to alterations in the glycosaminoglycans such that differentiation into melanocytes is favoured.[67] Strong racial differences in incidence suggest that genetic factors are also operative.

Sex hormones may also play a role in the pathogenesis of this hamartoma. The female predominance, the clinical onset at puberty in some children, and the reported variation in the color of the lesion with menstruation provide circumstantial evidence in support of this notion.[60]

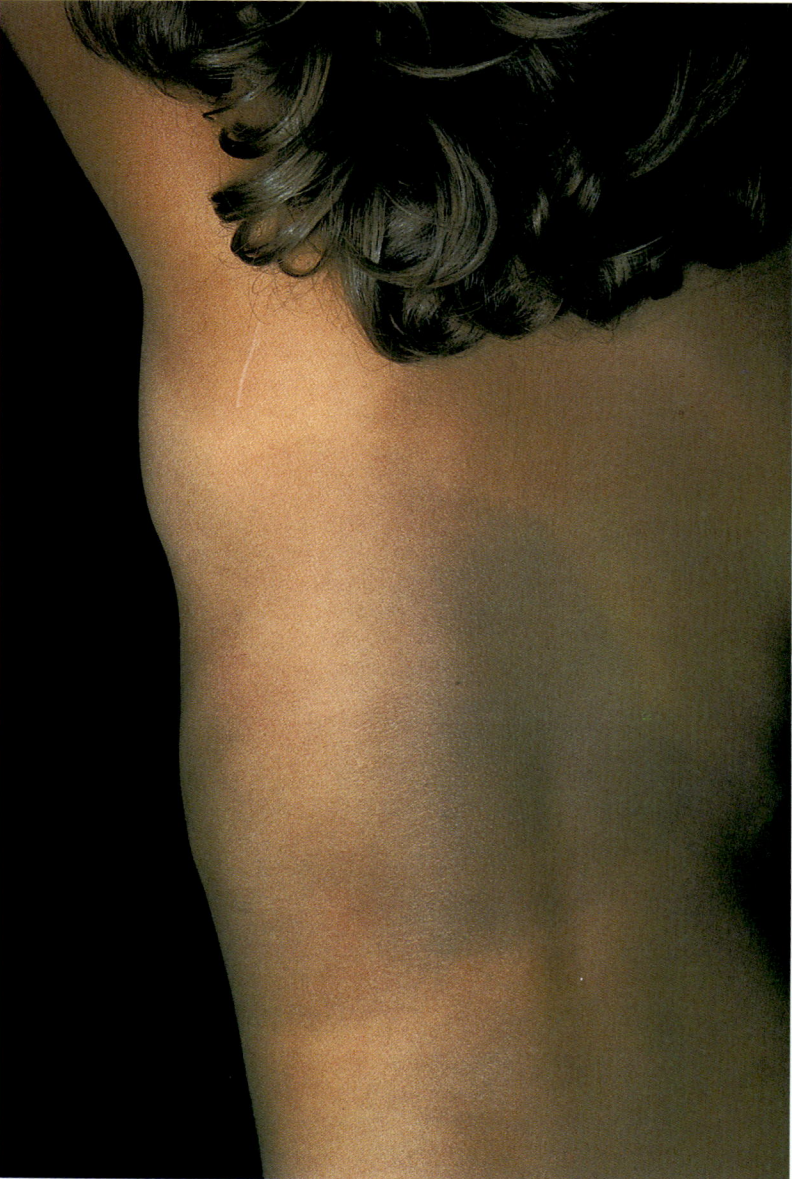

Fig. 10.11   Nevus of Ito.

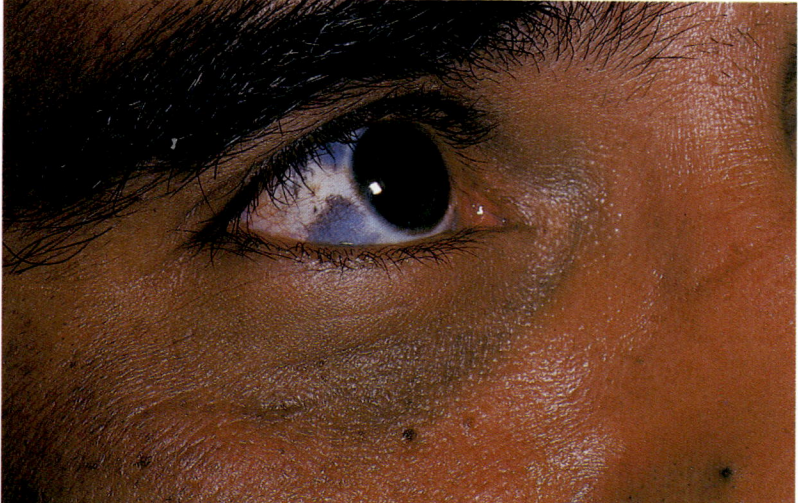

Fig. 10.10   Nevus of Ota.

59. Selsor LC, Lesher JL (1989) Hyperpigmented macules and patches in a patient with GM1 type gangliosidosis. **J Am Acad Dermatol** 20:878.
60. Mishima Y, Mevorah B (1961) Nevus of Ota and nevus of Ito in American Negroes. **J Invest Dermatol** 36:133.
61. Trese MT, Petit TH, Foos RY et al. (1981) Familial nevus of Ota. **Ann Ophthalmol** 13:855.
62. Whitmore SE, Wilson BB, Cooper PH (1991) Late-onset nevus of Ota. **Cutis** 48:213.
63. Hartmann LC, Oliver GF, Winkelmann RK et al. (1989) Blue nevus and nevus of Ota associated with dermal melanoma. **Cancer** 64:182.
64. Haim T, Meyer E, Kerner H et al. (1982) Oculodermal melanocytosis (nevus of Ota) and orbital malignant melanoma. **Ann Ophthalmol** 14:1132.
65. Liu JC, Ball SF (1991) Nevus of Ota with glaucoma: report of three cases. **Ann Ophthalmol** 23:286.
66. LeDorain NM (1975) The neural crest in the neck and other parts of the body. **Birth Defects** 11:19.
67. Benson MT, Rennie IG (1992) Hemi-naevus of Ota: perturbation of neural crest differentiation as a likely mechanism. **Graefes Arch Clin Exp Ophthalmol** 230:226.

Microscopic changes of nevus of Ota/Ito consist of melanocytes scattered in the dermis, most of which are present in the upper corium.[68] This accounts for the browner color than is seen in the Mongolian spot.

The chief differential diagnosis is the Mongolian spot. In those cases of extrasacral lesions, only the passage of time will distinguish these two entities because Mongolian spots usually resolve and the nevus of Ota/Ito is permanent. Several distinguishing features help in making the correct diagnosis: (1) nevus of Ota appears at puberty in 40% of cases, whereas the Mongolian spot always presents in infancy; (2) nevus of Ota has a brownish color with a "powder blast burn" appearance, whereas the Mongolian spot is more uniformly bluish; (3) the characteristic sharp border of nevus of Ota is rarely seen with Mongolian spots; and (4) pigment is commonly present in the mucous membranes and eye in nevus of Ota but is rarely if ever seen in the Mongolian spot. Other differential diagnostic possibilities include melasma, melanoma, postinflammatory hyperpigmentation, exogenous ochronosis, Riel's melanosis, and pigmentation associated with the ingestion of drugs. These subjects will be discussed later in this chapter.

Nevus of Ota is usually a benign dermatosis, but there have been at least 37 cases of associated melanoma reported in the English language literature,[69] almost all of which occurred in white patients. These melanomas have developed in the skin, meninges, frontal brain, choroid, and iris. Ninety-seven percent of these cases have occurred on the ipsilateral side.[69]

Two treatment modalities have recently been touted for the nevus of Ota. The Q-switched ruby laser emits a wavelength of light that is preferentially absorbed by melanin. Selective destruction of upper dermal melanocytes by this method can fade these lesions appreciably.[70,71] A second alternative is a micropeeling procedure where thin strips of tissue are surgically removed from the upper dermis. These presumably contain the abnormally situated melanocytes that produce the brown discoloration.[72] Coverup cosmetics can also be useful in hiding the lesion.

CIRCUMSCRIBED ACQUIRED MELANOSES

There are a number of unrelated conditions that produce a spotty hyperpigmentation, as opposed to a diffuse pattern of hypermelanosis. In some of these dermatoses, such as ashy dermatosis and Riehl's melanosis, there is some inflammatory insult that precedes the increased pigment. Teenagers develop melasma on a hormonal basis in many cases. In all of these diseases, the result is too much melanin being produced and deposited in the skin.

Ashy dermatosis (erythema dyschromicum perstans)

Ashy dermatosis, also known as erythema dyschromicum perstans, is an unusual cutaneous eruption first described in Central America and initially thought to be a disease limited to Latin Americans.[73] Since that time, this condition has been noted in whites, blacks, Native Americans,[74,75] and East Indians,[76] although most cases are in Hispanics. The name originally applied to these patients was *los cenicientos* ("the ash-colored ones"). Others suggested that the name be changed to erythema dyschromicum perstans to relate it to a group of persistent vascular reactions collectively known as erythema perstans. Subsequently, clinical and histologic studies have more closely aligned this disease with inflammatory epidermal and superficial dermal dermatoses,[77,78] hence the descriptive name, ashy dermatosis, has become the preferred term. This condition occurs anywhere from age 5 years through adult life. The sexes are equally affected and there does not appear to be a genetic predisposition.

These patients present with flat to slightly elevated 1- to 2-mm lesions that vary in color from deep blue–gray to gray–brown. The most common locations are on the trunk, face, and arms (Fig. 10.12); the lesions spare the palms, soles, and scalp. Except for occasional minimal pruritus, the involved areas remain asymptomatic. Over weeks to months, the original lesions grow slowly by peripheral extension. Lesions may coalesce to form geometrically shaped patches, and the advancing margins are often slightly raised and erythematous. The evolution of this disorder is insidious and asymptomatic.[79] There are no known internal manifestations.

Histologic changes are characteristic but not specific and include basal layer vacuolization, edema of the dermal papillae, a mild lymphohistiocytic infiltrate, and pigment in dermal macrophages. This latter finding accounts for the blue-gray color of the lesions.

The cause of ashy dermatosis is unknown. The histologic changes are compatible with the notion that the primary disease process occurs in the region of the basal layer.[79] Although there is some similarity to diseases such as lichen planus and cutaneous lupus erythematosus, there are sufficient distinct clinical differences, at least in the Latin American patients, to consider these entities as separate.[80]

In almost all cases of ashy dermatosis in adults, the pigmentation is permanent, although minor degrees of fading may occur over many months. In one study, complete resolution was noted in three of four patients,[75] and spontaneous clearance after years is not frequently noted in children. Numerous treatments including topical or systemic corticosteroids, sunscreens, keratolytic agents, antibiotics, antihistamines, dapsone, antimalarial drugs, and bleaching creams have been tried in ashy dermatosis with almost uniformly disappointing results.[80] This is not surprising, since the cause of the discoloration is melanin in dermal macrophages, which is always resistant to anti-inflammatory or depigmenting strategies. Clofazamine, an agent used in the therapy for leprosy, was given to eight patients with ashy dermatosis for 3 to 8 months. The rationale was that the reddish hue that the drug imparts to the skin would mask the discolored skin spots. In addition, changes in cellular immunity might affect the course of the condition. In seven of the eight individuals, a good or excellent cosmetic result ensued.[80]

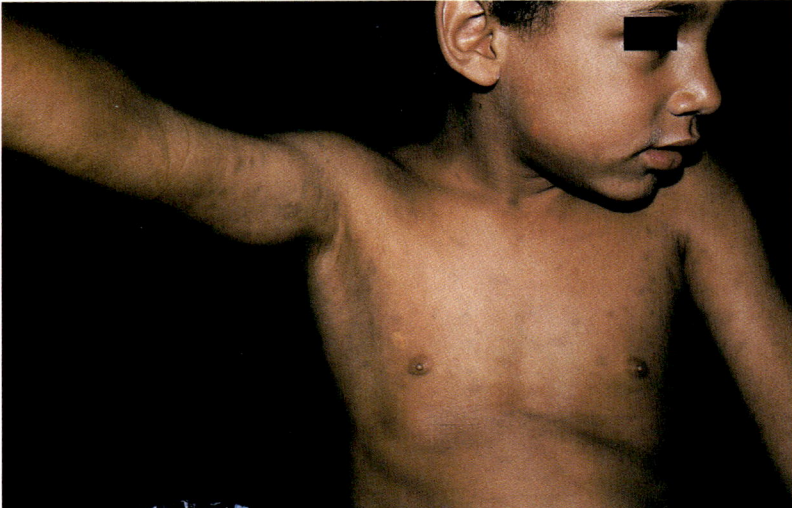

Fig. 10.12   Ashy dermatosis (erythema dischromicum perstans) in a 5-year-old boy.

68. Inoue S (1979) The mongolian spot. **Hifubyoh Shinryoh** 1:104.
69. Shaffer C, Walker K, Weiss GR (1992) Malignant melanoma in a Hispanic male with nevus of Ota. **Dermatology** 1:146.
70. Goldberg DJ, Nychay SG (1992) Q-switched ruby laser treatment of nevus of Ota. **J Dermatol Surg Oncol** 18:817.
71. Geronemus RG (1992) Q-switched ruby laser therapy of nevus of Ota. **Arch Dermatol** 128:1618.
72. Kobayshi T (1991) Microsurgical treatment of nevus of Ota. **J Dermatol Surg Oncol** 17:936.
73. Ramirez CO (1966) Dermatosis cenicienta: estudio epidermologico de 139 casos. **Dermatol Rev Mex** 10:133.
74. Knox JM, Dodge BG, Freeman RG (1968) Erythema dyschromicum perstans. **Arch Dermatol** 97:262.

75. Palatsi R (1977) Erythema dyschromicum perstans. **Dermatologica** 155:40.
76. Bhurani LK, Bedi TR, Pandhi RK et al. (1974) Lichen planus pigmentosus. **Dermatologica** 149:43.
77. Person JR, Rogers RS IV (1981) Ashy dermatosis. **Arch Dermatol** 117:701.
78. Naidorf KF, Cohen SR (1982) Erythema dyschromicum perstans and lichen planus. **Arch Dermatol** 118:683.
79. Vega ME, Waxtein L, Arenas R et al. (1992) Ashy dermatosis versus lichen planus pigmentosus: a controversial matter. **Int J Dermatol** 31:87.
80. Piquero-Martin J, Perez-Alfonzo R, Abrusci V et al. (1989) Clinical trial with clofazamine on treating erythema dyschromicum perstans. **Int J Dermatol** 28:198.

Idiopathic eruptive macular pigmentation

This condition appears to be a distinct clinicopathologic and histologic entity. It is characterized by asymptomatic, pigmented macules involving the neck, trunk, and proximal limbs.[81] Drug intake is not associated with the eruption. The first sign is a pigmented spot without preceding erythematous, papular, or hypopigmented lesions. Histologic study shows enhanced epidermal basal layer pigmentation with pigmentary incontinence, a mild perivascular lymphohistiocytic infiltrate, and many melanophages in the papillary dermis. Electron microscopy shows an increased number of melanosomes in basal and suprabasal keratinocytes as well as clustered melanosomes in dermal melanophages. Differential diagnoses include ashy dermatosis, mastocytosis, and drug reactions. Treatment of this asymptomatic condition is unnecessary because spontaneous resolution of the lesions is to be expected within several months to a few years.

Melasma (chloasma)

Melasma is a very common dermatosis that occurs on the face as patchy tan–brown spots. It may appear in adolescent females and occasionally appears in pubertal boys. Family studies suggest some genetic role, but because this is such a common disorder, an absolute inheritance pattern has not been determined. This occurs in all races but is distinctly more prevalent in individuals of Hispanic origin who live in sunny climates. A typical pediatric-age patient with melasma is a teenaged girl who is either pregnant or who has been taking oral contraceptives. She will relate that the spots darken after sunlight exposure and fade somewhat during the winter months.

Physical examination reveals mottled tan to brown macules that may coalesce into irregular patches. Three clinical patterns of involvement are noted:[82] (1) the most common pattern is one involving the central portion of the face; (2) a malar pattern, limited to the cheeks and nose; and (3) a mandibular type with pigment over the ramus of the mandible.

Two histologic varieties of pigment deposition are seen in melasma.[82] The most common is the epidermal type in which most of the melanin deposition is in epidermis. This superficial pigment imparts a tan color to the skin. Melanin deposition may be mainly in the dermis whereby melanin pigment is engulfed by superficial and deep dermal melanophages. These deeper melanin granules cause a light to dark brown discoloration clinically.

The pathogenesis of melasma is unknown, but the result is an increased number of type-specific melanocytes, which are more active in the synthesis and transfer of melanosomes. A number of etiologic factors have been implicated in the promotion of this melanocyte hyperfunction. Melasma occurs in the context of oral contraceptives[83] and pregnancy,[84] and it rarely occurs before puberty or in old age. Thus it is appealing to consider estrogen and/or progesterone as important etiologic factors. It is difficult to understand why otherwise normal men develop melasma if this is the sole cause of the disease, however. Other hormonal effects involving pituitary melanotropins have also been suggested.[85]

Although sunlight probably does not cause melasma, it is the single most important factor in increasing pigmentation in already darkened areas and in reactivating latent disease.[86] The most likely scenario for the pathogenesis of melasma is that there are sensitive melanocytes that are activated by UV light and are also functionally altered by other factors such as hormones to synthesize and distribute abnormal amounts of melanin.

The differential diagnosis of melasma includes other causes of facial pigmentation. Phytophotocontact (berloque) dermatitis is a patchy hyperpigmentation that occurs in areas in which an applied photosensitive chemical is activated by sun exposure. The most common of these agents are the furo-coumarins (psoralens) contained in perfumes, citrus fruits, and other plants. Although individual patches may be identical to melasma, the limited asymmetric distribution and the history of exposure help confirm this diagnosis. Postinflammatory hyperpigmentation after acne, trauma, and so forth can appear identical to melasma and even the histologic picture may be similar to the dermal type. The asymmetric pattern and association with scarring or other signs of old cutaneous inflammation can be helpful in distinguishing these conditions.

Before embarking on therapy, it is important to ascertain which clinical/histologic type is present. A Wood's light can assist in this determination. Because the light is absorbed by melanin, the epidermal type of melasma will appear darker; in the dermal variety, melanin absorbs this light but there is scattering that produces less visible lesions.[87] In those patients with the epidermal type, prolonged use of hydroquinone-containing agents can cause some improvement. Retinoic acid can also be added to enhance the penetration of the hydroquinone, and, perhaps to bleach the skin on its own.[88] The lesions can also be lightened by the judicious use of physical modalities such as liquid nitrogen cryotherapy, CO_2 laser vaporization, chemical peeling, and superficial dermabrasion. With any of these procedures, the result may not be a perfect color match to the surrounding integument.

If a teenager has the dermal form of the disease, there is little that one can do to bleach the pigment. Because sunlight worsens the condition, broad-spectrum sunscreen protection can minimize the sun's effects at promoting this process.

The prognosis for complete clearing is good in melasma associated with pregnancy or with the use of oral contraceptives, even without therapy. Many of the remaining cases may be present for years with seasonal exacerbation and remission.

Riehl's melanosis (pigmented contact dermatitis)

During World War I, a group of patients of both sexes, children as well as adults, were described with dark-brown pigmentation of the face. Riehl believed that wartime food substitutes were in some way important in the pathogenesis, thus he named this entity *wartime dermatosis*.[89] Since that time, several studies have demonstrated that this is a pigmented variant of contact dermatitis, without the macroscopic evidence of inflammation, to such agents as cosmetic ingredients[90] and optical whiteners.[91]

Darkly pigmented people and Asians are at increased risk for Riehl's melanosis, but what is more important, only certain chemicals are capable of eliciting these changes. Agents that have caused this problem include hydrocarbons, particularly impure mineral oil; coal tar derivatives; aniline dyes in cosmetics; and optical whiteners found in household cleaning products. The typical patient presents with asymptomatic deep-brown macular pigmentation on the face and occasionally on the neck. Certain compounds such as tar derivatives usually have an inflammatory phase preceding the hyperpigmentation. The condition persists as long as the contactant is present.

Histologic changes in Riehl's melanosis include hydropic degeneration of the basal layer, dermal pigment incontinence, and mild dermal inflammation, without the spongiotic changes seen in conventional contact dermatitis.

Melasma is the disease that most resembles Riehl's melanosis. There are subtle differences that can lead one to the correct diagnosis; the lateral cheeks are more commonly involved in Riehl's melanosis and there is less reticulation in the plaques.

The treatment of this and other forms of contact dermatitis is to eliminate the offending agent. Unfortunately, the dermal pigmentation resolves very slowly. Hydroquinones are of little benefit.

81. Sanz de Galdeano C, Leaute-Labreze C, Bioulac-Sage P, Nikolic M, Taieb A (1996) Idiopathic eruptive macular pigmentation: report of five patients. **Pediatr Dermatol** 13:274–277.
82. Sanchez NP, Pathak MA, Sato S et al. (1981) Melasma: a clinical, light microscopic, ultrastructural, and immunofluorescence study. **J Am Acad Dermatol** 4:698.
83. Resnick S (1967) Melasma induced by oral contraceptive drugs. **JAMA** 119:95.
84. Zelenick JS (1967) Endocrine physiology of pregnancy. **Clin Obstet Gynecol** 8:534.
85. Smith AG, Shuster S, Thody AS et al. (1977) Chloasma, oral contraceptives, and plasma immunoreactive beta-melanocyte-stimulating-hormone. **J Invest Dermatol** 68:169.
86. Vasquez M, Sanchez JL (1984) The efficacy of broad-spectrum sunscreen in the treatment of melasma. **Cutis** 32:92.
87. Findlay GH (1970) Blue skin. **Br J Dermatol** 83:127.
88. Pathak MA, Fitzpatrick TB, Kraus EW (1986) Usefulness of retinoic acid in the treatment of melasma. **J Am Acad Dermatol** 15:894.
89. Riehl G (1917) Ueber eine eigenartege melanose. **Wien Klin Wochenschr** 30:780.
90. Nakagawa H, Matsuo S, Kayakawa R et al. (1984) Pigmented contact dermatitis. **Int J Dermatol** 23:299.
91. Osmundsen PE (1970) Pigmented contact dermatitis. **Br J Dermatol** 83:296.

Diffuse acquired hypermelanotic syndromes

Several rare syndromes have been reported in which children become significantly pigmented over large areas of the body. Familial progressive hyperpigmentation has been described in three kindreds.[92,93] This condition is characterized by hyperpigmented patches that are present at birth and that increase in size and number as the infant grows older. Ultimately, most of the skin and mucous membrane surface has increased pigment. Microscopically, the melanin granules are more numerous and larger than normal.

Most infants of dark races are born lighter than they ultimately become, but the nature of hyperpigmentation in these conditions is one of bizarre patterns and uneven darkening. Extensive workup of the members of one of these kindreds has failed to uncover a cause for this pigment abnormality.[92]

Carbon baby

A single case of a striking variant of progressive hyperpigmentation was reported in which a child developed hyperpigmentation at age 3 months and was jet black over his entire body by age 4 years, prompting the investigator to name him "the carbon baby."[94] Histologic examination of the skin revealed heavy melanin deposition of the full thickness of the epidermis with minimal dermal pigmentation. There was no increase in melanocyte number; thus, there was extraordinary melanin production by these normal-appearing melanocytes.

Two children have been described with increased pigmentation limited to the distal extremities. In the first case,[95] a Japanese child developed intensely dark and sharply demarcated areas of hyperpigmentation over the fingers and toes, which rapidly spread proximally. In the second case,[96] jet black patches on all fingers of the right hand developed by age 2 years and did not progress beyond that point over the succeeding 2-year follow-up period. In both cases, there was an increase in the number of melanocytes with increased melanin pigment in the epidermis.

Adrenoleukodystrophy (ALD)

This X-linked acquired generalized hyperpigmentary disorder has been described in association with a slowly progressive disease of the brain and adrenals of affected children. These patients develop uniform macular hyperpigmentation, which spares the palms, soles, and groin areas. ALD is characterized by the accumulation of unbranched saturated fatty acids with a chain length of 24 to 30 carbons, particularly hexacosanoate (C26), in the cholesterol esters of brain white matter and in adrenal cortex and in certain sphingolipids of brain. The encoded gene, designated the adrenoleukodystrophy protein (ALDP), belongs to the ATP-binding superfamily of transporters.[97]

Bronze baby syndrome

This rare acquired generalized pigmentary disorder occurs in neonates. It is characterized by a gray–brown discoloration (see Fig. 6.56, Chapter 6) which occurs only in patients with hepatocellular dysfunction undergoing phototherapy.[98–100] The proposed mechanism for this syndrome is that a porphyrin compound undergoes photodestruction, which results in a brown substance that is deposited in the skin.[101] These children usually have a benign outcome, but deaths have occurred in those with serious hepatic abnormalities.

Miscellaneous acquired hypermelanotic disorders

There are several diseases where reticulate or punctate pigmentation has been described. Many of these cases have been reported in Japanese patients, but they have appeared in other races as well. There has been some debate whether some of these are merely variations of the same disease process.[102] The diseases are presented in tabular form with their characteristic clinical findings in Table 10.3.[103]

Postinflammatory hyperpigmentation

One of the most common causes of acquired hyperpigmentation in children is that associated with inflammatory dermatoses. The intensity and persistence of the increased skin color are greater in pigmented races but occur to some extent in everyone except those incapable of producing melanin (e.g., albinos). The cause of the inflammation is another important determining factor in the degree of hyperpigmentation. Dermatoses that disrupt the basement membrane zone of the epidermis, such as lichen planus and lupus erythematosus, produce significant postinflammatory change, even if the degree of clinical inflammation is relatively modest. Frequently, inflammation can also produce hypomelanosis in the same lesion due to loss of melanocytes. These children usually give a history of some preceding cutaneous insult such as an abrasion, eczema, or infection that heals with irregular brown to gray–blue patches. In the case of exogenous inflammatory stimuli such as infections or burns, the asymmetric pattern of the subsequent pigment is a good clue to the diagnosis. There are several iatrogenic causes of postinflammatory hyperpigmentation. Radiation therapy, even in low dosage, may cause increased skin color with minimal or absent clinical evidence of inflammation. Topical medications such as those used in acne can produce inflammation and postinflammatory pigment changes. There are times, however, when almost inapparent inflammation can result in postinflammatory hyperpigmentation such as in friction melanosis, which was

TABLE 10.3   Punctate and reticulate pigmentation disorders

Disease	Major features
Dowling–Degos disease	Autosomal dominant, progressive symmetric brown macules, comedone-like follicular papules
Reticulate acropigmentation of Kitamura	Autosomal-dominant disorder, reticulated brown atrophic papules of distal extremities, palmar pits and breaks
Haber syndrome	Facial erythema, telangiectases, black keratotic papules of the axilla, neck, torso
Acropigmentation symmetrica of Dohi	Acral hyperpigmentation, hypopigmentation of the face, trunk, extremities
Franceschetti–Jadassohn–Naegli syndrome	Punctate pigment over waist, axilla, neck; hypohydrosis; palmoplantar keratosis; tooth, nail anomalies
Cantu syndrome	Punctate brown macules of the feet, face, forearms; palmoplantar hyperkeratosis
Dermatopathia pigmentosa reticularis	Reticulated pigment of trunk, extremities; loss of nails; hypohydrosis; alopecia; atrophy of skin over elbows, knees
Pigmentatio reticularis faciei et colli with multiple epithelial cysts	Reticulate brown macules of face, neck; folliculitis; cysts; scars on face, trunk

92. Chernosky ME, Anderson DE, Chang JP et al. (1971) Familial progressive hyperpigmentation. Arch Dermatol 103:581.
93. Rebora A, Parodi A (1989) Universal inherited melanodyschromatosis: a case of melanosis universalis hereditaria, letter. Arch Dermatol 125:1442.
94. Ruiz-Maldonaldo R, Tamayo L, Fernandez-Diaz J (1978) Universal acquired melanosis. Arch Dermatol 114:775.
95. Furuya T, Mishima Y (1962) Progressive pigmentary disorder in a Japanese child. Arch Dermatol 86:412.
96. Gonzalez JR, Botet MB (1980) Acromelanosis. J Am Acad Dermatol 2:128.
97. Mosser J, Dcuar A-M, Sarde C-O et al. (1993) Putative X-linked adrenoleukodystrophy gene shares unexpected homology with ABC transporters. Nature 361:726–730.

98. Kopelman A, Brown R, Odell G (1972) The bronze baby syndrome: a complication of phototherapy. J Pediatr 81:466.
99. Ashley JR, Littles CM, Burgdorf WH et al. (1985) Bronze baby syndrome. J Am Acad Dermatol 12:325.
100. Rubatelli FF, Jori G, Reddi E (1983) Bronze baby syndrome: a new porphyrin related disorder. Pediatr Res 17:327.
101. Meisel P, Johrig D, Meisel M (1987) Detection of photobilirubin in urine of jaundiced infants supporting the diagnosis of bronze baby syndrome. Clin Chim Acta 160:61.
102. Kikuchi I (1983) Haber's syndrome or Dowling Degos disease, letter. Arch Dermatol 119:365.
103. Levine N, Hori Y, Kubota K (1993) Acquired hypermelanotic disorders. In: Pigmentation and Pigmentary Disorders, Levine N, ed. Boca Raton, FL: CRC Press, Ch. 8.

first described in Japan in patients who developed brown dyspigmentation after constant use of nylon brushes or coarse towels.[104]

In postinflammatory hyperpigmentation following basal epidermal injury, melanin falls through a damaged basement membrane into the dermis and is phagocytosed by melanophages. Dermal pigment deposition, which acts like a pigment tattoo, is difficult to remove. Thus, the management of post-inflammatory hyperpigmentation can be frustrating, but it is mainly of epidermal origin, the lesions can be expected to fade almost completely within 6 months. Hydroquinone cream and sunscreens as used in melasma may hasten the fading process. In many cases, however, particularly in blacks, it may be permanent.

Hyperpigmentation due to heavy metals and medications

A number of diverse medications and other chemicals can produce changes in cutaneous pigmentation.[105] Some of these agents or their metabolites are deposited directly in the skin and impart a characteristic color. Other compounds stimulate epidermal melanogenesis after being deposited in the dermis. Still others appear to require UV light exposure besides actual deposition to produce increased pigmentation.

Argyria is localized or widespread blue–gray discoloration of the skin caused by the deposition of metallic silver. Although not common in the United States, silver compounds are still used in nose drops and eye drops in many parts of the world. The increased pigmentation may not be noted for months or even years after the use of these agents, and long-time exposure is apparently necessary.[105] These children present with a bluish-gray hue, which is more intense in sun-exposed areas of the skin. Mucous membranes and nail lunulae may also be discolored. Microscopic examination reveals silver granules in the dermis, particularly around sweat glands. Increased epidermal melanin pigment and dermal melanin in macrophages also contribute to the change in color.

Treatment of argyria is unsatisfactory, since the color is usually permanent. Sun avoidance may decrease the intensity of the pigmentation, however.

Children who receive prolonged parenteral gold therapy for rheumatoid arthritis may develop a permanent blue-gray discoloration, most prominently in sun-exposed skin, particularly around the eyes. This must be a rare complication, inasmuch as it was not noted in any of 37 patients treated with gold in a study in which a careful systematic cutaneous toxicity monitoring system was used.[106]

Several medications used in children and young adults can produce either a localized or generalized increase in skin color. Perhaps the most common syndrome is the fixed drug eruption, in which well-circumscribed inflammatory plaques resolve with hyperpigmentation, which recurs locally with reintroduction of the same drug.

Minocycline, a tetracycline derivative commonly used in the treatment of acne, can produce three distinct varieties of pigmentary change.[107,108] Typically, prolonged usage at relatively high dosage precedes the pigment abnormality. Some patients develop blue–gray discoloration in areas of previous inflammation, most notably in old acne scars[107] or rarely, in postacne osteoma cutis.[109] Pigmentation has also been reported in the teeth of young adults.[110] Others develop brown to blue–gray discoloration in noninflamed sites, particularly over the trunk or anterior legs (Fig. 10.13). A third type of pigmentation is the "muddy skin syndrome" where there is generalized gray-

brown discoloration.[111] Although it is stated that these are temporary changes that resolve after discontinuing the medication,[112] this discoloration has persisted for at least 22 months in some patients.[113] Light microscopic examination of hyperpigmented skin reveals pigment-laden macrophages in the papillary and reticular dermis. Electron microscopic studies suggest that this pigment is either a minocycline degradation product[113] or a drug-hemosiderin complex.[112]

Phenothiazines may produce color changes if taken for prolonged periods, especialy on sun-exposed skin. These patients develop a blue–gray or violaceous color that becomes deeper in hue over time and may be exacerbated by UV light exposure. The nail beds may also become blue–gray in color.[114] Histologic examination reveals increased melanin pigment in the epidermis and in dermal melanophages.[115] The pathogenesis of this increase in pigmentation is not known, but phenothiazines do bind to melanin; thus, a drug–melanin complex may in some way appear clinically as a blue–gray pigment in the skin.[116]

Antimalarial agents may be a cause of acquired pigmentation.[117] The most commonly used agent is hydroxychloroquine, which may produce irregular gray plaques over the anterior legs. Other changes noted include subungual and facial pigmentation. Quinacrine causes a diffuse yellowish discoloration that occurs in most patients but is far more obvious in fair-skinned people. Microscopic findings in hydroxychloroquine pigmentation include dermal pigment granules, hemosiderin around capillaries, and melanin in the dermis

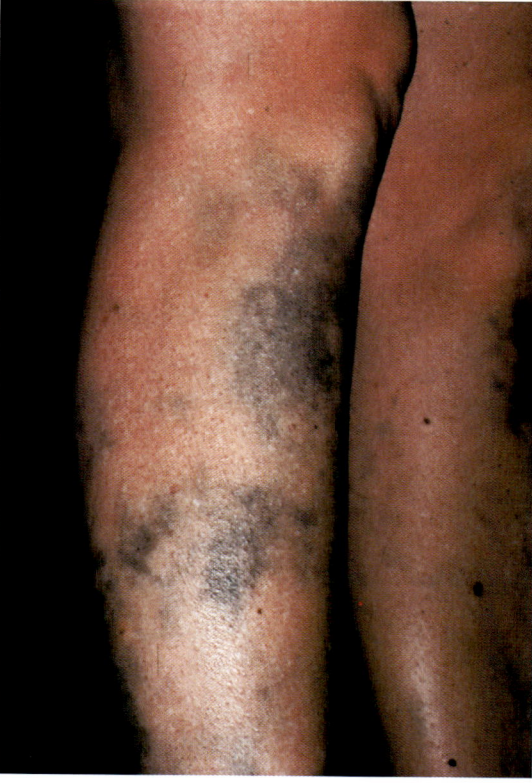

Fig. 10.13 Minocycline pigmentation on the lower legs of a teenage patient.

104. Tanigaki T, Hata S, Kitano Y et al. (1985) Unusual pigmentation on the skin over trunk bones and extremities. **Dermatologica** 170:235.
105. Granstein RD, Sober AJ (1981) Drug and heavy metal induced hyperpigmentation. **J Am Acad Dermatol** 5:1.
106. Pennys NS, Ackerman AB, Gottlieb NL (1974) Gold dermatitis. **Arch Dermatol** 10:372.
107. Basler RSW, Kohnen PW (1978) Localized hemosiderosis as a sequela of acne. **Arch Dermatol** 114:1695.
108. Pepine M, Flowers FP, Ramos-Caro FH (1993) Extensive cutaneous hyperpigmentation caused by minocycline. **J Am Acad Dermatol** 28:292.
109. Moritz DL, Elewski B (1991) Pigmented postacne osteoma cutis in a patient treated with minocycline: report and review of the literature. **Arch Dermatol** 24:851.
110. Poliak SC, DiGiovanna JJ, Gross EG et al. (1993) Minocycline-associated tooth discoloration in young adults. **JAMA** 254:2930.

111. Basler RSW (1985) Minocycline-related hyperpigmentation. **Arch Dermatol** 121:606.
112. Fenski NA, Millns JL (1980) Cutaneous pigmentation due to minocycline hydrochloride. **J Am Acad Dermatol** 3:308.
113. McGrae JD, Zelickson AS (1980) Skin pigmentation secondary to minocycline therapy. **Arch Dermatol** 116:1262.
114. Satanove A (1965) Pigmentation due to phenothiazines in high and prolonged dosage. **JAMA** 191:263.
115. Hashimoto K, Weiner W, Albert J et al. (1966) An electron microscopic study of chlorpromazine pigmentation. **J Invest Dermatol** 47:296.
116. Blois MS (1965) On chlorpromazine binding *in vivo*. **J Invest Dermatol** 45:475.
117. Tuffanelli D, Abraham RK, Dubois EI (1963) Pigmentation from antimalarial therapy. **Arch Dermatol** 88:419.

as well, and these may all contribute to this color change. As with chlorpromazine, chloroquine (and presumably hydroxychloroquine) is known to bind to melanin, and the drug–melanin complex may be deposited in the skin.[118] The yellow color from quinacrine occurs secondary to direct staining of the skin by this pigmented compound. The hyperpigmentation from hydroxychloroquine may fade somewhat after cessation of treatment but does not generally clear completely.[119] The yellow color from quinacrine disappears within a few months of discontinuing the medication.

Children afflicted with human immunodeficiency virus (HIV) disease treated with zidovudine (AZT) can develop pigmentary abnormalities. There have been several reports of nail and mucocutaneous hyperpigmentation with this drug.[120,121] The nail pigmentation often appears as longitudinal bands or a bluish discoloration that involves the entire nail plate of both toes and fingers. Rarely, one can see dark macules at the tips of the digits as well.[121] Histologic examination reveals increased melanin deposition in the basal layer of the epidermis and in dermal melanophages. Ultrastructural studies have failed to demonstrate either drug–melanin complexes or inclusions.[122] The pathogenesis of this pigmentary phenomenon is unknown but other drugs such as 5-fluorouracil and doxorubicin have a similar pattern of pigment deposition, suggesting a common pathogenic mechanism.[123]

In some parts of the world, the normal diet contains such large quantities of carotene-containing food that carotenemia might be considered normal. There are, however, instances in which an infant or small child may ingest large amounts of these compounds and the succeeding yellow–orange color may become disconcerting to the family as well as to the physician caring for the child. An example of this was reported in which a 10-month-old boy became yellow on a diet of junior meats and vegetables that contained a relatively large amount of carrots.[124] Only about one-third of ingested carotene is absorbed in the intestine, but this increases sharply when food is cooked, mashed, or pureed as in infant food. During absorption, some carotene is converted to vitamin A, but most is stored in the tissues, particularly in the keratin of the skin and in the subcutaneous fat. It may also be secreted in sweat and excreted by sebaceous glands.[125] Children with carotenemia appear yellow–orange, most prominently on the palms, soles, forehead, and nasolabial folds.[124] The sclerae of the eyes remain white because carotene does not have a predilection for mucosal surfaces. This helps differentiate this condition from jaundice, for which it may be mistaken. Laboratory testing reveals serum carotene levels greater than 250mg/dl in the face of a normal serum bilirubin. The stool and urine are normal in color.[126] Although the vast majority of children with carotenemia are in good health otherwise, there are several diseases that have been associated with increased serum carotene levels. In hypothyroidism and diabetes mellitus there is thought to be a decreased conversion of carotene into vitamin A secondary to an increase in lipoproteins that carry carotene in the serum.[126] Girls with anorexia nervosa have bizarre eating habits that may lead to carotenemia.[127] There are also rare cases of inborn errors of carotene metabolism that may produce carotenemia.[128] There is no good medical reason to reverse the changes of carotene deposition in the skin. The very slow conversion of the compound to the active vitamin A obviates any threat of hypervitaminosis A syndrome. Most parents are not happy about this color change, however. If the offending foods are eliminated, the skin color will return to normal within 2 to 6 weeks.

HYPERPIGMENTATION IN SYSTEMIC DISEASE

Adrenocortical insufficiency (Addison's disease)

In many instances of the acute type and in more than 90% of the chronic variety of adrenal hypofunction there is generalized hyperpigmentation,[129] which may precede other manifestations of the disease. These children present with a generalized increased skin color which is often a bronze hue in fair-skinned individuals, and is accentuated in skin folds such as occur on the palms (see Fig. 22.7). The mucous membranes, tongue, nipples, and areolae are also pigmented. In the oral mucosa, one may find spotty or speckled blue–brown macules of the gingivae, tongue, palate, and buccal mucosa. In dark-skinned children this increase in color may be mistaken for a suntan, but the mucous membrane and palmar crease color changes should lead to suspicion of adrenal insufficiency in these patients. Histologic examination reveals an increase in epidermal melanin and dermal pigment in macrophages, both of which are nonspecific findings.

The pathogenesis of the hyperpigmentation is not completely clear and there is considerable debate about what role, if any, is played by the pituitary hormones. It is possible that adrenocorticotropic hormone (ACTH), β-lipotropic pituitary hormone (β-LPH), or both have sufficient melanotropic potential that when secreted in excess in Addison's disease they can produce generalized hyperpigmentation. Additional evidence for this hypothesis comes from the fact that in Cushing syndrome there is an increase in ACTH and probably in β-LPH secretion. Many of these patients also develop pigment changes similar to those of adrenocortical insufficiency. Adequate adrenocortical hormone replacement therapy usually results in a decrease in pigmentation in those with Addison's disease. In some younger patients, the skin color may eventually return to normal.

Acromegaly

Acromegaly is a rare disorder, but 17% of patients with this syndrome have the onset of symptoms during adolescence.[130] Both sexes are affected equally. Approximately 45% of these children will develop generalized increased pigmentation along with trophic changes of the skin, sweat glands, sebaceous glands, and hair follicles. Inasmuch as there is no known function of growth hormone in melanin production, there is no satisfactory explanation as to the cause of the hyperpigmentation.

Hemochromatosis

Idiopathic hemochromatosis is rare in children and occurs mainly in men over the age of 40 years. There are reports of symptomatic teenagers, however. The HFE gene maps to 6p21.3, within HLA genes. It is inherited as an autosomal-recessive defect. Heterozygotes may show iron storage abnormalities but usually do not develop clinical disease. The signs of this disease are observed when large amounts of iron are deposited in the liver parenchymal cells. This leads to periportal cell destruction and scarring, which results in cirrhosis. The most dramatic cutaneous finding is a generalized bronze hyperpigmentation that appears in patients with advanced disease. Mucous membranes are pigmented in about 20% of cases.[131] Most of the increased color comes from melanin production rather than from cutaneous iron deposition. A unique experiment in nature demonstrated this fact.[132] In a patient with vitiligo and hemochromatosis,

118. Sams WM, Epstein JH (1965) The affinity of melanin for chloroquine. J Invest Dermatol 45:852.
119. Levantine A, Almeyda J (1973) Drug induced changes in pigmentation. Br J Dermatol 89:105.
120. Furth PA, Kazakis AM (1987) Nail pigmentation changes associated with azidothymidine (zidovudine). Ann Intern Med 107:944.
121. Bendick C, Rasokat H, Steigleder GK (1989) Azidothymidine-induced hyperpigmentation of skin and nails, letter. Arch Dermatol 125:1285.
122. Greenberg RG, Berger TG (1990) Nail and mucocutaneous hyperpigmentation with azidothymidine therapy. J Am Acad Dermatol 22:327.
123. Adrian RM, Hood AT, Skarin AT (1980) Mucocutaneous reactions to antineopolastic agents. CA Cancer J Clin 30:143.
124. Lascari AD (1981) Carotenemia. Clin Pediatr 20:25.
125. Gupta AK, Haberman JF, Pawlowski D et al. (1985) Canthxanthin. Int J Dermatol 24:528.
126. Cohen L (1958) Observations in carotenemia. Ann Intern Med 48:219.
127. Crisp AH, Stonehill E (1967) Hypercarotenemia as a symptom of weight phobia. Postgrad Med J 43:721.
128. McLaren DS, Zekian B ('971) Failure of enzymic cleavage of β-carotene. Am J Dis Child 121:278.
129. Norup J (1974) Addison's disease – clinical studies. A report of 108 cases. Acta Endocrinol 76:127.
130. Gardner LI (ed.) (1975) Endocrine and Genetic Diseases of Childhood and Adolescence. Philadelphia: WB Saunders.
131. Chevrant-Breton J, Simon M, Bourel M et al. (1977) Cutaneous manifestations of idiopathic hemochromatosis. Arch Dermatol 113:161.
132. Perdrup A, Poulsen H (1964) Hemochromatosis and vitiligo. Arch Dermatol 90:34.

bronze hyperpigmentation was seen in unaffected areas of the skin, while the vitiliginous sites remained white. Histologically, the white skin was found to contain deposits of iron.

Childhood cirrhosis

Hepatic fibrosis and cirrhosis in children usually occur secondary to extrahepatic biliary atresia but may also be a consequence of other inherited abnormalities, such as cystic fibrosis, toxins, infections, metabolic disturbances, or autoimmune phenomena. In patients with chronic liver disease, there is usually a diffuse dull-brown hyperpigmentation of the skin. A yellowish hue may also be interposed in those patients with jaundice. In children who are very pruritic, chronic scratching can lead to darker areas of linear hyperpigmentation as a manifestation of postinflammatory change.

Scleroderma

Morphea is the most common variety of scleroderma in children and occasionally produces hyperpigmentation, especially in patches of the Pasini–Pierini variant, when sclerosis is absent. In patients with long-standing extensive sclerosis of the skin, a diffuse increase in pigmentation may occur. This is often interspersed with depigmented macules, giving the skin a confettilike appearance.[133] On the contrary, hypopigmentation is a striking clinical feature of systemic sclerosis in black patients.

Renal failure

Children with chronic renal failure, particularly those on hemodialysis, have been noted to have diffuse hyperpigmentation, caused by changes in the amount of chromogens such as lipochromes, melanins, hemoglobin, and carotenoids.[134] Because many of these patients are pruritic, this increased color is often accentuated in areas that are scratched and traumatized, such as the forearms and legs. Thus, a component of this change in pigment is postinflammatory, as in hemochromatosis. Melanogenesis is increased in the epidermis of these patients. This may be due to the increased serum half-life of β-LPH. The clearance of this hormone in chronic renal failure is markedly prolonged,[135] and there is probably no feedback inhibition once serum levels are elevated.

Pregnancy in adolescence

Although technically not a systemic disease, endocrinologic changes in pregnant adolescent girls cause hyperpigmentation in up to 90% of cases.[136] This pigment change is usually generalized with accentuation in areas that are normally deeply pigmented such as the areolae of the nipples, axillae, and perineal skin. Nevocellular nevi, ephelides, and lentigines may also become darker. A characteristic linear darkening often occurs on the anterior abdomen from the umbilicus to the symphysis pubis (linea nigra).

With the exception of melasma that appears during the latter half of pregnancy, most of the hyperpigmentation appears during the first trimester.[137] In most instances, the color returns to prepregnancy levels but some localized hypermelanotic sites (e.g., nevi) may remain darker indefinitely.

The physiologic mechanism of hyperpigmentation in pregnancy is thought to be due to elevated levels of a compound with MSH activity, but the source and nature of this activity are unknown. One interesting hypothesis is that the melanotropin may be of fetal origin, since the fetal pituitary gland is thought to synthesize α-MSH.

NONGENETIC DISORDERS OF HYPOPIGMENTATION

Rafael Falabella

NEVUS DEPIGMENTOSUS

Nevus depigmentosus (ND), or achromic nevus, is an unusual sporadic leukoderma most commonly present at birth.[138] Males and females are equally affected. These children are born with localized poorly demarcated white patches that tend to be in a dermatomal pattern, which are more common on the trunk and proximal extremities (Fig. 10.14). In a recent study the lesions were mostly found before 3 years of age (92.5%), although some lesions also appeared later in childhood (7.5%); the areas more frequently affected were the back and buttocks, followed by the chest and abdomen, and then the face, neck, and arms; 40 patients in this group (59.7%) had isolated lesions of ND, and 27 others (40.3%) had the segmental type of hypopigmentation.[139] In the majority of patients the lesions are not completely achromic but hypopigmented, and resemble "splashed paint." The individual lesions are permanent and tend to enlarge in proportion to the general body growth. Almost all of these children are otherwise healthy but, as with other pigmentary disorders, exceptional associated neurologic defects have been reported[138] although in a large series of patients with this condition these defects were not found.[139] Among 20 patients reported with the segmental type of ND, 2 of them disclosed associated extracutaneous abnormalities consisting of pes cavus, mental retardation, seizures, and hemihypertrophy.[140] Early in life, hypopigmented lesions as observed in the localized form of the disease, may be indistinguishable from those of tuberous sclerosis and it may not be possible to rule out this potentially serious phakomatosis with certainty, by inspection of the skin alone; furthermore, in the systematized variety, it can be confused with hypomelanosis of Ito, but the presence of whorls and bizarre figures in this condition and multiple organ involvement are helpful for a differential diagnosis.[141]

A recent histopathologic study showed that the staining ability of melanocytes with Fontana–Masson in ND lesions is decreased compared with that of perilesional normal skin, suggesting a functional defect of pigment cells; furthermore, the total number of melanocytes identified as S-100-positive cells in the basal layer were normal, indicating that a pigment cell destruction process does not take place in the pathogenesis of ND and perhaps a functional defect of melanocytes and impaired transfer of melanosomes to keratinocytes may be the possible mechanism originating permanent hypopigmentation.[139]

Electron microscopic examination of affected skin reveals normal melanocytes and normal melanization of melanosomes; however, apparently the melanosomes are not transferred to surrounding keratinocytes appropriately and, instead, aggregate in the melanocyte itself.[142] More recently, a great reduction in the number of melanosomes in melanocytes and some membrane-bound aggregated melanosomes observed in keratinocytes were described.[139]

There are no effective therapies for repigmenting ND and once the clinical picture becomes fully established, the hypopigmented lesions remain unchanged indefinitely. Appropriate sunscreens should be used whenever necessary, mainly to prevent painful sunburns.

133. Krieg T, Meuer M (1988) Systemic scleroderma. **J Am Acad Dermatol** 18:457.
134. Deleixhe-Mauhin F, Krezinski JM, Rorive G et al. (1992) Quantification of skin color in patients undergoing maintenance hemodialysis. **J Am Acad Dermatol** 27:950.
135. Gilkes JJH, Eady RAJ, Rees LH et al. (1975) Plasma immunoreactive melanotrophic hormones in patients on maintenance hemodialysis. **Br Med J** 1:656.
136. Wade TR, Wade SL, Jones HE (1975) Skin changes and diseases associated with pregnancy. **Obstet Gynecol** 52:233.
137. Wong RC, Ellis CN (1984) Physiologic skin changes in pregnancy. **J Am Acad Dermatol** 10:929.
138. Sugarman GI, Reed WB (1969) Two unusual neurocutaneous disorders with facial cutaneous signs. **Arch Neurol** 21:242–247.

139. Lee HS, Chun YS, Hann SK (1999) Nevus depigmentosus: clinical features and histopathologic characteristics in 67 patients. **J Am Acad Dermatol** 40:21–26.
140. Di Lernia V (1999) Segmental nevus depigmentosus: analysis of 20 patients. **Pediatr Dermatol** 16:349–353.
141. Pinto FJ, Bolognia JL (1991) Disorders of hypopigmentation in children. **Pediatr Clin North Am** 38:991–1017.
142. Jimbow K, Fitzpatrick TB, Szabo G, Hori Y (1975) Congenital circumscribed hypomelanosis: a characterization based on electron microscopic study of tuberous sclerosis, nevus depigmentosus, and piebaldism. **J Invest Dermatol** 64:50–62.

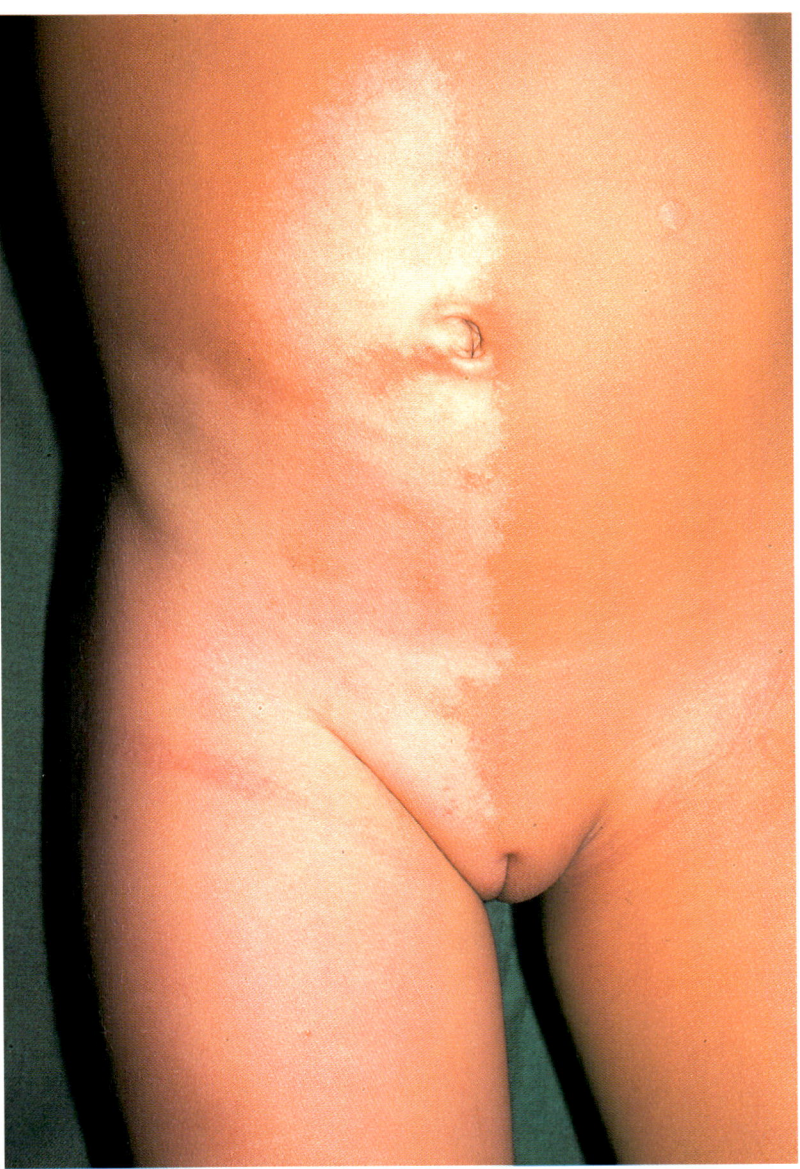

Fig. 10.14   Nevus depigmentosus, segmental type. The hypopigmented areas are unilateral, involving the anterior abdomen with a sharp demarcation at the midline, and the upper part of the right thigh.

HYPOMELANOSIS OF ITO (INCONTINENTIA PIGMENTI ACHROMIANS)

This condition was initially described by Ito in a Japanese woman who presented whorls of hypopigmentation following Blaschko's lines that resembled the pattern of increased pigment seen in incontinentia pigmenti; the condition was named incontinentia pigmenti achromians, but later on it

was renamed hypomelanosis of Ito to avoid the confusion between this entity and a completely unrelated disease, incontinentia pigmenti of Bloch Sulzberger, characterized by linear and bizarre hyperpigmented bands and other lesions. Numerous patients with the classic hypopigmented lesions have been reported worldwide,[143] and females have been observed to outnumber males by a 2.5:1 ratio; in a more recent report from a group of 76 patients, a 1:1 ratio and 57% mental retardation were observed.[144] In a recent work in which 41 new affected individuals are reported, additional literature review disclosed that the term hypomelanosis of Ito was found often misapplied to label nonspecific "patchy depigmentation of the skin" in patients who had several conditions of different etiologies.[145]

The genetic defect, if any, has not yet been determined and has been an issue of controversy for years. In a few instances, it appears to be inherited as an autosomal dominant trait, but in most patients develops sporadically.[146] Some have suggested, however, that the phenotypic changes could be due to gametic half chromatid or somatic gene mosaicism.[147–149]

Many of these children are born with hypopigmented spots, but others develop the lesions in early infancy or later on into childhood. The hypopigmented patches are arranged in broad bands and whorls on the trunk and extremities. Once the lesions become stable and no further depigmentation occurs, the affected areas remain without modification throughout life (Fig. 10.15).

Regarding the coexistence of other anomalies, a case report of three patients with additional review of 70 previously reported patients disclosed that 75% of them had an associated abnormality of the central nervous system, musculoskeletal system, skin, cutaneous appendages, or internal organs,[148,150] although in another group similar anomalies were observed in 16 out of 54 patients (30%).[151] Syndactyly, clinodactyly, abnormalities of the skeleton, asymmetry of the face, ears, body and/or extremities, gynecomastia and asymmetrical breasts, short stature, oral alterations, congenital cardiopathies and genital anomalies have also been occasionally found.[144] The white matter involvement seen at neuroimaging in some patients has been found similar to that reported in well-defined neurocutaneous disorders, particularly central nervous system abnormalities.[145] In another study of brain magnetic resonance imaging, the polymorphism of brain abnormalities in 12 patients was emphasized.[152] On histologic examination melanocytes are present in the hypopigmented skin, but they appear to synthesize less melanin than those of normal skin.

There is no appropriate treatment for the hypopigmented lesions, which remain as a cosmetic alteration; on the other hand, the most important aspects of this condition are the associated anomalies affecting the central nervous system and other organs. The prognosis depends on the severity of involvement of these organs.

ACQUIRED CIRCUMSCRIBED HYPOMELANOSES
Reticulate acropigmentation of Dohi

This is a rare dyschromic disorder that generally has an autosomal-dominant pattern of inheritance; however, recessive[153] and even sporadic cases have been observed. Since reticulate acropigmentation of Dohi was described in Japan, most of the literature has been written in Japanese and dermatologists outside of that country are not familiar with the condition.[154] The clinical manifestations are characterized by the development of a mixture of hyperpigmented

143. Weaver RG Jr, Martin T, Zanolli MD (1991) The ocular changes of incontinentia pigmenti achromians (hypomelanosis of Ito). **J Pediatr Ophtalmol Strabismus** 28:160–163.
144. Pascual-Castroviejo I, Roche C, Martinez-Bermejo A et al. (1998) Hypomelanosis of Ito. A study of 76 infantile cases. **Brain Dev** 20:36–43.
145. Ruggieri M, Pavone L (2000) Hypomelanosis of Ito: clinical syndrome or just phenotype? **J Child Neurol** 15:635–644.
146. Vermittag W, Ensinger C, Raff M (1992) Cytogenetic and dermatoglyphic findings in a familial case of hypomelanosis of Ito (incontinentia pigmenti achromians). **Clin Genet** 41:309–312.
147. Moss C, Burn J (1988) Genetic counselling in hypomelanosis of Ito: case report and review. **Clin Genet** 34:109–115.
148. Chitayat D, Friedman JM, Johnston MM (1990) Hypomelanosis of Ito – a nonspecific marker of somatic mosaicism. **Am J Med Genet** 35:422–424.
149. Kuster W, Konig A (1999) Hypomelanosis of Ito: no entity, but a cutaneous sign of mosaicism. **Am J Med Genet** 85:346–350.
150. Takematsu H, Sato S, Igarashi M et al. (1983) Incontinentia pigmenti achromians (Ito). **Arch Dermatol** 119:391–392.
151. Nehal KS, PeBenito R, Orlow SJ (1996) Analysis of 54 cases of hypopigmentation and hyperpigmentation along the lines of Blaschko. **Arch Dermatol** 132:1167–1170.
152. Steiner J, Adamsbaum C, Desguerres I et al. (1996) Hypomelanosis of Ito and brain abnormalities: MRI findings and literature review. **Pediatr Radiol** 26:763–768.
153. Alfadley A, Al-Ajlan A, Hainau B et al. (2000) Reticulate acropigmentation of Dohi: a case report of autosomal recessive inheritance. **J Am Acad Dermatol** 43:113–117.
154. Oyama M, Shimizu H, Ohata Y et al. (1999) Dyschromatosis symmetrica hereditaria (reticulate acropigmentation of Dohi): report of a Japanese family with the condition and a literature review of 185 cases. **Br J Dermatol** 140:491–496.

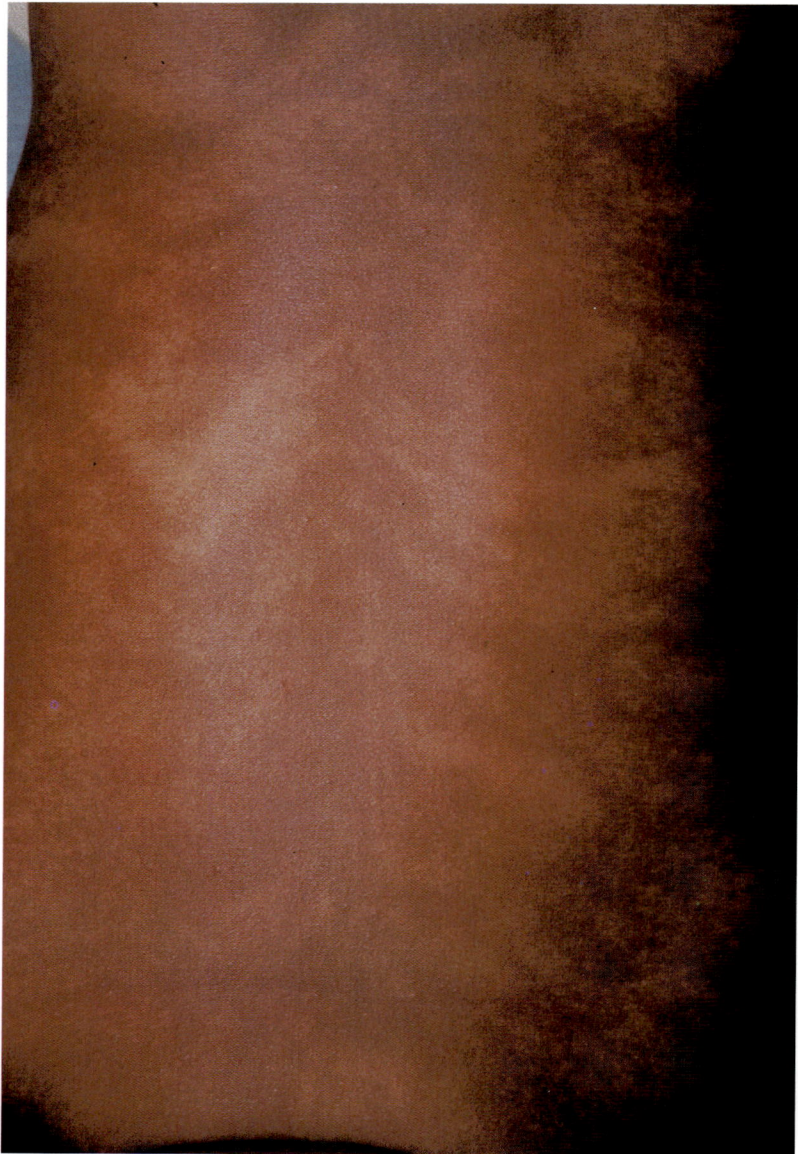

Fig. 10.15   Hypomelanosis of Ito. Several hypopigmented areas in a bizarre bilateral distribution simulating bands and whorls were present at birth in this 14-month-old boy.

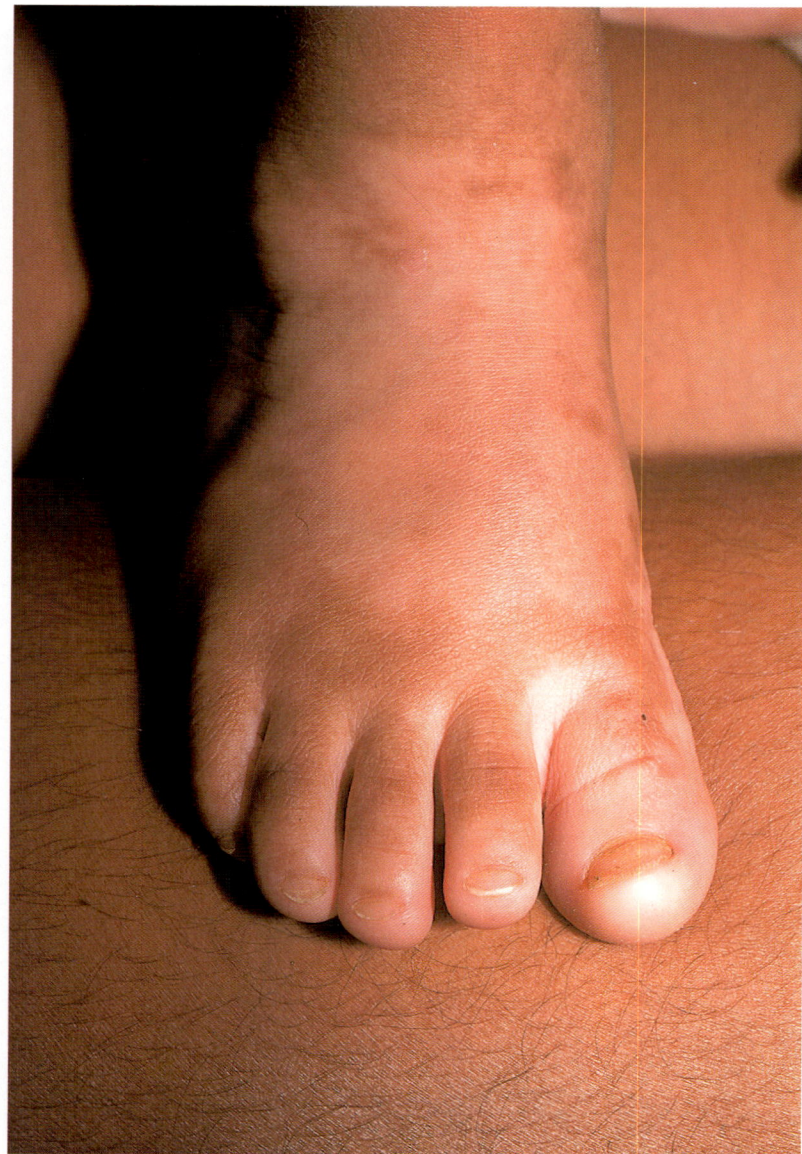

Fig. 10.16   Reticulate acropigmentation of Dohi. Areas of hypopigmentation on the dorsum of the foot that appeared in this infant at age 8 months. Similar bilateral lesions with spotted hyperpigmentation, were present on both feet, hands and neck. (Acknowledgement: Patient kindly referred by Dr. Doralda Castro and published with her permission.)

and hypopigmented macules distributed on the face and the dorsal and acral aspects of the extremities, which appear early in childhood and are limited to these areas (Fig. 10.16). On histologic examination, the hyperpigmented skin discloses increased melanin in all epidermal layers decreasing towards the surface, and on electron microscopy moderate amounts of melanosomes stage III and IV within the cytoplasm of melanocytes have been observed. On the contrary, the hypopigmented macules have a similar pattern but with much less melanin than in normal skin.[153]

Acropigmentation of Dohi should be differentiated from bilateral vitiligo where achromic macules are not restricted to the acral parts of the body since it may progressively spread to other areas; the differential diagnosis should also be made with reticulate acropigmentation of Kitamura, a condition of similar characteristics but with the presence of pits on the dorsa of the distal phalanges of the fingers and toes. This condition has been reported from all over the

world and additional features are being readily recognized, such as widely distributed pits on the palms, palmar aspect and sides of the fingers.[155]

Idiopathic guttate hypomelanosis

Although several authors in the past described similar lesions of this leukodermic defect under different names, this condition has been labelled with its present denomination for many years.[156] As people age, they often develop small hypopigmented macules on the exposed areas of the extremities. The entity is called idiopathic guttate hypomelanosis (IGH) to connote the unknown etiology, the droplike or "guttate" configuration, and the decrease in pigmentation. This occurs in both sexes equally and in all races, although it is more obvious in dark-skinned persons because of the contrast in pigmentation between the lesions and the normal skin. The number of lesions tends to increase with age and after chronic sun exposure.

155. Sharma R, Chandra M (2000) Pigmentation and pits at uncommon sites in a case with reticulate acropigmentation of Kitamura. **Dermatology** 200:57–58.

156. Cummins K, Cottel W (1966) Idiopathic guttate hypomelanosis. **Arch Dermatol** 93:184–186.

Although its etiology is unknown, the chronic actinic exposure and family trend have been implicated as pathogenic factors.[157,158]

Typical lesions are slowly progressive, asymptomatic, porcelain–white macules with sharply defined angular or sometimes "amoeboid-like" borders, 0.5–15mm in diameter, and frequently located over the anterior aspects of the forearms and legs and seldom over unexposed areas. Sometimes, but not so often, a few spots on the face, lower abdomen, trunk or back are observed.[159,160] Slight thinning of some lesions is evident, and some others may present with slight hyperkeratosis. The hypopigmented lesions are asymptomatic, but they are a cause of cosmetic concern to some patients who sometimes confuse IGH with a more serious or progressive leukoderma such as vitiligo.

On light microscopic examination, the most constant features of the hypopigmented spots are flattening of the dermal–epidermal junction, epidermal atrophy and basket weave hyperkeratosis; a moderate to marked focal or patchy reduction of the melanin granules in the basal and prickle cell layers which is more evident with the Fontana–Masson stain is also observed.[159] Studies with the DOPA oxidase reaction reveal a significant reduction in the number of melanocytes, but these cells are never absent even in the clinically depigmented lesions. Ultrastructural studies have demonstrated cytoplasmic vacuolation, scanty and fragmented dendrites, scarce melanosomes and very few mature melanosomes.[161,162]

The differential diagnosis should be made with guttate morphea, lichen sclerosus et atrophicus, monobenzyl ether of hydroquinone toxicity, post-traumatic and postinflammatory hypopigmentation, tinea versicolor, and vitiligo. Size, anatomic location, borders of lesions, and presence of atrophy are important items that may help in defining the diagnosis.

Therapy of IGH may be succesfully accomplished with very superficial dermabrasion done to the affected leukodermic spots, which respond with repigmentation in a good number of patients;[163] liquid nitrogen cryotherapy is another option that may be useful for hypopigmented lesions but it is less effective on the old achromic defects.[162] Once the lesions of IGH become well established, they remain as permanently stable, although with continuing sunlight exposure their number usually increases in time. In children IGH is uncommon but some patients in their teens have been reported,[164] whereas this is a rare disorder in the first decade of life.[158]

Leukoderma punctata

This leukodermic manifestation was described in 1988 in a group of 13 patients, with ages between 7 and 38 years, most of them female children, who developed numerous punctate, hypopigmented and achromic lesions on the sun-exposed areas of the extremities, following oral 8-methoxy psoralens and sunlight exposure (PUVASOL) for treatment of vitiligo; eight of these patients had generalized vitiligo, four others had focal, and the last one had segmental vitiligo; most patients received this therapy on a daily regimen. The small lesions measured 0.5 to 1.5mm and were different from those of idiopathic guttate hypomelanosis because of their small size and the countless number of depigmented spots occurring at an early age in most individuals (Fig. 10.17). The lesions were occasionally observed on the face, gluteal regions and upper aspects of the back and chest areas; in a few patients very few and subtle lesions appeared on the dorsum of the hands. It was notheworthy that no patient developed hypopigmented or achromic lesions on the antecubital fossae, popliteal regions and elbows or knees. None of the patients experienced any signs of acute phototoxicity during PUVASOL therapys.[165]

Histopathologic evaluation of the lesions with Fontana-Masson stain revealed a marked reduction of melanin in five out of six patients. Only one

patient had a slight verruciform hyperkeratosis and no other alterations with hematoxylin and eosin stain were seen. DOPA oxidase stain disclosed a substantial reduction but not complete disappearance of functional melanocytes. Electron microscopic studies of the achromic lesions demonstrated varying degrees of intracellular edema and vacuolar degeneration of the cytoplasm, containing a granular electron-dense material, probably constituted by aggregates of free cytoplasmic ribosomes; these changes were observed in many keratinocytes of achromic and normally pigmented adjacent skin, most of them in a suprabasal location. Some melanocytes showed similar damage with vacuolar degeneration and intracytoplasmic edema. A possible phototoxic effect provoked by natural UVA-UVB and psoralens (PUVASOL) in predisposed individuals with vitiligo, having therapy on a daily schedule, may have been the cause of this hypopigmentation disorder, especially since methoxalen phototoxicity peaks at 48–78h and these patients were treated beyond the two or three doses per week recommended for PUVA or PUVASOL. Avoiding this therapeutic modality in children is strongly recommended. Following this report a few additional patients developing similar but less numerous lesions without PUVASOL therapy have been observed.

The most important differential diagnosis is idiopathic guttate hypomelanosis, a condition that, although very common in adults, is very uncommon in children. The characteristic small size and abundance of lesions also speaks against this dermatosis. A punctate form of vitiligo is a very unlikely presentation that has not been emphasized previously in the many publications on vitiligo. Other leukodermic conditions are not associated with the presence of these minute lesions that often have sharply demarcated borders. No therapy has been described for this condition, and although its course was unmodified in most of the reported patients, in 2 of them a slight reduction of lesions was noted.[165]

Chemical-induced hypomelanosis

A number of chemicals are capable of depigmenting the skin when applied directly onto the cutaneous surface. The primary offending agents are phenols or catechols and benzene derivatives, which are useful as one-step

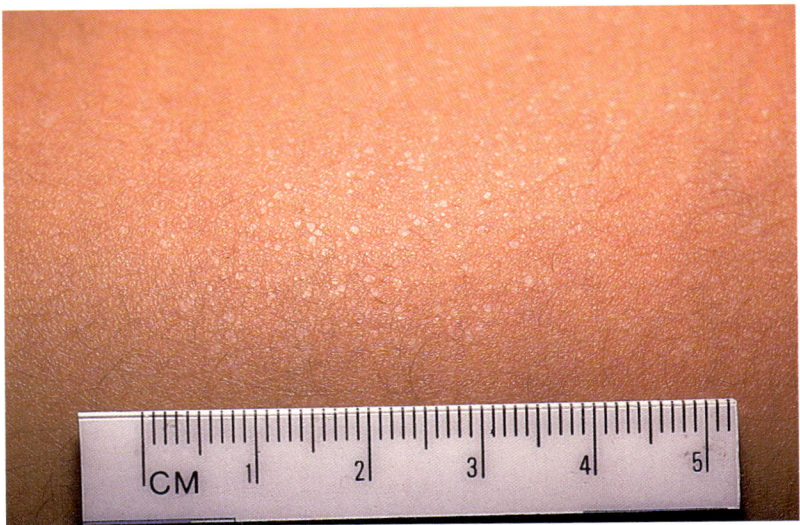

Fig. 10.17 Leucoderma punctata. Numerous, hypopigmented and achromic spots measuring 0.5 to 1.5mm, appeared on the upper extremity in this 10-year-old girl following vitiligo therapy with PUVASOL on a daily regimen.

157. Savall R, Fernandez I, Peyri J (1980) Idiopathic guttate hypomelanosis. Br J Dermatol 103:635–642.
158. Falabella R, Escobar CE, Giraldo N et al. (1987) On the pathogenesis of idiopathic guttate hypomelanosis. J Am Acad Dermatol 16:35–44.
159. Falabella R (1988) Idiopathic guttate hypomelanosis. Dermatol Clin 6:241–247.
160. Wilson PD, Lafker RM, Kligman AM (1982) The nature of idiopathic guttate hypomelanosis. Acta Derm Venereol (Stockh) 62:301–306.
161. Ortonne JP, Perrot H (1980) Idiopathic guttate hypomelanosis. Arch Dermatol 116:664–668.
162. Ploysangam T, Dee-Analap S, Swanprakorn P (1990) Treatment of idiopathic guttate hypomelanosis with liquid nitrogen: light and electron microscopic studies. J Am Acad Dermatol 23:681–684.
163. Hexsel D (1999) Treatment of idiopathic guttate hypomelanosis by localized superficial dermabrasion. Dermatol Surg 25:917–918.
164. Whitehead WJ, Moyer DG, Van der Ploeg DE (1966) Idiopathic guttate hypomelanosis. Arch Dermatol 94:279–281.
165. Falabella R, Escobar C, Carrascal E et al. (1988) Leukoderma punctata. J Am Acad Dermatol 18:485–494.

cleansers and antiseptics, or industrial products used in the rubber industry;[166] sometimes, plants used as topical medications may cause hypopigmentation.[167] Epoxy resins, which are very common household products, have also been reported as a cause of hypopigmentation.[168]

Patients present with localized depigmented patches on the areas exposed to the chemicals, most commonly on the hands. The depigmentation may follow an acute episode of dermatitis or may appear several months after the last exposure without signs of cutaneous irritation. Sites distant from the area of contact may also develop hypopigmentation. Histologic examination of hypopigmented skin reveals only rare melanocytes with few melanosomes and scanty epidermal melanin. Chemical induced hypomelanosis may mimic vitiligo and therefore a history of previous exposure to offending agents may be necessary for diagnosis.

Therapy is often not necessary when the toxic effects of chemicals involved is minimal or transient, since the hypopigmentation may resolve spontaneously. When the hypopigmentation is pronounced and permanent, especially if refractory achromic defects develop, melanocyte grafting may be a therapeutic option for this condition.[169] Since chronic exposure of these agents, such as occurs in occupational dermatitis, is usually necessary to cause hypopigmentation,[170] single exposure of a child to these depigmenting agents usually will not cause cutaneous changes and therefore chemical induced hypopigmentation is not common in children. Nevertheless, this type of depigmentation should always be kept in mind in the differential dignosis when no other explanation for an acquired and localized hypopigmented lesion occurs.

Drug-induced hypomelanosis

It is not uncommon to find hypopigmentation in children around lesions of chronic conditions being treated for prolonged periods of time with potent or even middle strength topical corticosteroids; this can also occur occasionally when the corticosteroid is delivered under occlusion as occurs with an occlusive tape; this can produce transient hypopigmented macules, where the diagnosis is often obvious because the hypopigmented area has a shape that is similar to the shape of the tape strip applied, rather than having the configuration of the dermatosis being treated.[171] Corticosteroids injected intralesionally when indicated for the treatment of hemagiomas,[172] keloids,[173] and for intra-articular use[174] can also produce localized hypopigmentation at the infiltration site. Occasionally, intramuscular injections of long-acting corticosteroids may produce a hypopigmented macule of diffuse borders, measuring 2–4cm^2, often observed with a slight depression at the site of injection that can be confused with a patch of morphea; a retrograde migration of the corticosteroid through the hypodermic needle channel, which may occur immediately after the injection, could explain these findings. Spontaneous resolution of all these pigmentary changes induced by corticosteroids usually occurs in a few months.

Diphenylcyclopropenone, when used for topical immunotherapy of alopecia areata, has also been reported to induce hypopigmentation;[175] from a group of 243 patients treated with this molecule, 4 of them developed localized spotted hypopigmentation on the treated areas ("dyschromia in confetti") which also occurred at distant sites in one patient.[176] The lesions developed several months after treatment was initiated and the hypopigmentation remained unchanged during several months after discontinuation

of therapy. A complete history of previously applied topical medications or other chemicals is important in cutaneous hypopigmentation of recent onset.

Postinflammatory hypopigmentation

In children, many inflammatory dermatoses, burns, minor trauma, eczema and infections may provoke hypopigmentation after healing, which is more evident in the darker skin types; the cutaneous pigmentary changes correspond to the areas of preceding inflammation, and their shape is usually similar to the shape of the previous condition; these two facts are important to establish a correct diagnosis. The underlying mechanisms for developing hypopigmentation are not well understood; an inherited individual predisposition has been proposed as a pathogenic factor.[177]

Postinflammatory hypopigmentation can be confused with tinea versicolor, but the past history of a previous lesion and a negative KOH preparation exclude this diagnosis. It differs from vitiligo by the poor margination and absence of a milk-white color, easily detected under the Wood's light examination.

There is no satisfactory treatment for postinflammatory hypopigmentation, but when residual inflammation remains, low-potency topical corticosteroids may help to solve the pigmentary alteration; however, most hypopigmented macules eventually resolve completely. Nevertheless, there are some patients in whom hypopigmentation remains for prolonged periods of time or indefintely, when more intense or severe damage has been inflicted to the skin. Repigmentation also depends on the age, anatomical location, presence of pigment cell reservoir, a specific response of each individual to inflammation, and other factors.

Lichen sclerosus et atrophicus

This condition is characterized by the onset of whitish papules that gradually coalesce, becoming macular and slightly atrophic. Lesions are frequently observed on the vulvar areas, including clitoris, inner aspect of vestibule, labia majora, and also on the glans penis or prepuce. Sometimes the skin of the abdomen, upper back, or extremities may also become involved and in these areas a shiny surface with some degree of follicular plugging is noticed (Fig. 10.18). Lesions may be pruritic or provoke a marked burning sensation and dysesthesia, although they usually occur without symptoms. The Koebner phenomenon is known to occur, especially around areas of affected skin. The underlying cause is unknown, but genetic susceptibility and possibly autoimmunity seen in the pathogen.[178]

When untreated, marked atrophy may occur, particularly on genital areas. Hypopigmented lesions on the skin or genitalia of recent onset may be difficult to distiguish from vitiligo and a biopsy is required for a definitive diagnosis. On histologic examination epidermal atrophy and vacuolar degeneration of the basal cell layer are seen; in the papillary and upper dermis, edema and homogenization of collagen with an underlying band-like mononuclear infiltrate are observed; a reduction in the number of melanocytes in active lesions has been reported.[179] Tenascin, fibrinogen, and fibronectin are extracellular matrix components that play a significant role in wound repair; their role in the initiation of scarring in lichen sclerosus and the associated increased skin fragility has been recently suggested.[180] In children this condition may occur more commonly in pre-adolescent girls, and in early cases lesions are difficult to differentiate from vitiligo either when present in genital or extragenital areas.

166. O'Malley MA, Mathias CG, Priddy M et al. (1988) Occupational vitiligo due to unsuspected presence of phenolic antioxidant byproducts in commercial bulk rubber. **J Occup Med** 30:512–516.
167. Liao YL, Chiang YC, Tsai TF et al. (1999) Contact leukomelanosis induced by the leaves of *Piper betle* L. (Piperaceae): a clinical and histopathologic survey. **J Am Acad Dermatol** 40:583–589.
168. Kumar A, Freeman S (1999) Leukoderma following occupational allergic contact dermatitis. **Contact dermatitis** 41:94–98.
169. Falabella R (1986) Repigmentation of stable leukoderma by autologous minigrafting. **J Dermatol Surg Oncol** 12:172–179.
170. Kahn G (1970) Depigmentation caused by phenolic detergent germicides. **Arch Dermatol** 102:177–187.
171. Kestel JL Jr (1971) Hypopigmentation following the use of Cordran tape. **Arch Dermatol** 103:460–461.
172. Chowdri NA, Darzi MA, Fazili Z et al. (1994) Intralesional corticosteroid therapy for childhood cutaneous hemangiomas. **Ann Plast Surg** 33:46–51.
173. Friedman SJ, Butler DF, Pittelkow MR (1988) Perilesional linear atrophy and hypopigmentation after intralesional corticosteroid therapy. Report of two cases and review of the literature. **J Am Acad Dermatol** 19:537–541.
174. McCormack PC, Ledesma GN, Vaillant JG (1984) Linear hypopigmentation after intra-articular corticosteroid injection. **Arch Dermatol** 120:708–709.
175. Orecchia G, Stock J (1999) Diphenylcyclopropenone: an important agent known to cause depigmentation. [letter] **Dermatology** 199:277.
176. van der Steen P, Happle R (1992) Dyschromia "in confetti" as a side effect of topical immunotherapy with diphenylcyclopropenone. **Arch Dermatol** 128:518–520.
177. Ruiz-Maldonado R, Orozco-Covarrubias ML (1997) Postinflammatory hypopigmentation and hyperpigmentation. **Semin Cutan Med Surg** 16:36–43.
178. Powell JJ, Wojnarowska F (1999) Lichen sclerosus. **Lancet** 353:1777–1783.
179. Meffert JJ, Davis BM, Grimwood RE (1995) Lichen sclerosus. **J Am Acad Dermatol** 32:393–416.
180. Farrell AM, Dean D, Charnock FM et al. (2000) Alterations in distribution of tenascin, fibronectin and fibrinogen in vulval lichen sclerosus. **Dermatology** 201:223–229.

Because of its peculiar appearance and location on genitalia this disorder may be confused with changes seen in sexual abuse.[178]

Therapy may be accomplished with topical corticosteroids with marked resolution of all changes including hypopigmentation; in nongenital lesions resistant to topical therapy, intralesional corticosteroid may be the treatment of choice and the hypopigmentation may resolve completely. However, care should be taken when administering these medications because of the well-known side effects provoked by corticosteroids, especially atrophy. The prognosis is good but depends on the extent and severity of lesions.

Pitiriasis alba

Pityriasis alba is a very common hypopigmentation disorder that occurs in all races but it is more accentuated in patients with darker skin types; these lesions become more noticeable during the summer months or excessive sunlight exposure, because of the marked contrast between tanned skin and the hypopigmented macules. The characteristic lesion is an ill-defined, pale pink, minimally scaly papule that gradually enlarges as a slightly scaly hypopigmented macule of diffuse borders. Lesions typically measure 1–3cm, although larger lesions are not infrequent. The face is the most commonly affected area, but the neck, trunk, and extremities may develop lesions as well. It is not uncommon to observe a "follicular" variety of pityriasis alba with follicular hyperkeratosis within or around the hypopigmented macules, resembling keratosis pilaris; the hypopigmentation helps in the diagnosis of this condition (Fig. 10.19). These patients have a family or personal history of atopy and the clinical manifestation may last for months and even years with frequent recurrences related to sunlight exposure.

The histopathologic changes are similar to those of a chronic eczema with focal parakeratosis, spongiosis of the epidermis and hair follicle walls, and mild perivascular lymphocytic infiltrates. Electron microscopy studies reveal that the density of functional melanocytes in the affected skin is reduced and melanosomes tend to be fewer and smaller.[181] In a study the alterations found in the horny layer suggested that this condition showed a dermatitic pattern and the resulting hypopigmentation was probably due to postinflammatory mechanisms.[182]

Repigmentation is satisfactorily achieved with a hydrocortisone 1% cream applied daily for several weeks; improvement of lesions is the rule, but avoidance of excessive sunlight and swimming are important general measures for faster improvement; in spite of being long lasting, this condition finally disappears in the postadolescence period.[183]

Macular confluent hypomelanosis of halfcasts ("Creole dyschromia")

This condition, reported in the French West Indies (Martinique), but also observed by many dermatologists in several Latin American countries, is a peculiar macular hypopigmentation occurring more frequently in Mestizo individuals of mixed ethnic origin with dark skin types. Lesions are round or oval shaped, hypopigmented, moderately confluent macules of diffuse borders and different sizes, ranging from 1 to 5cm. Lesions are located in unexposed areas and more often located on the trunk, but more evident on the back; desquamation is generally not observed (Fig. 10.20). From a group of 121 patients, this condition was diagnosed in one-third of the examined

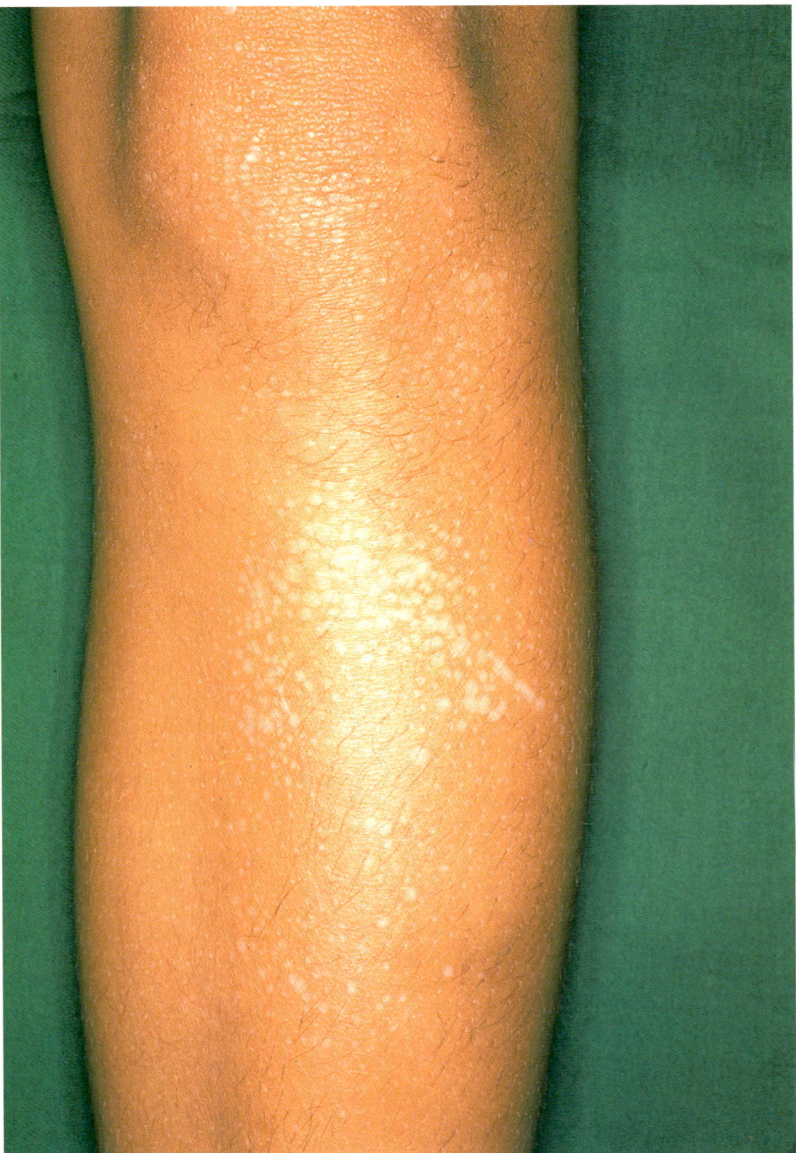

Fig. 10.18   **Lichen sclerosus et atrophicus.** These multiple achromic lesions measuring 0.3–0.5cm show the Koebner phenomenon. This 9-year-old girl was thought to have vitiligo.

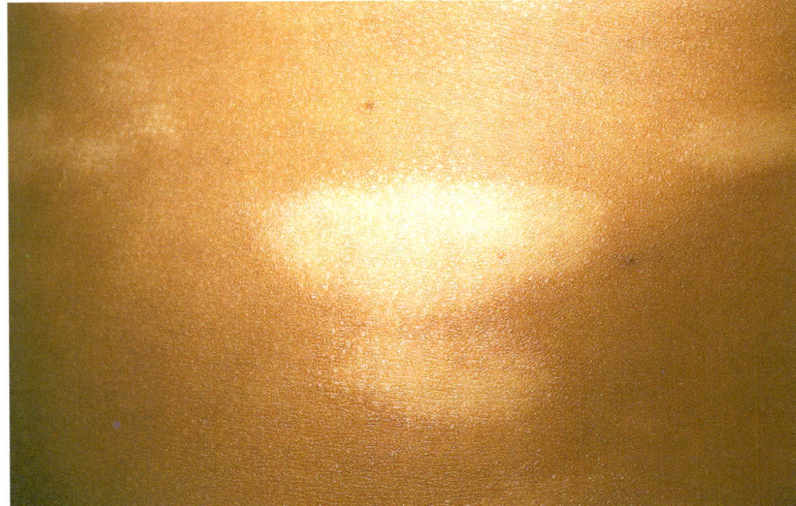

Fig. 10.19   **Pityriasis alba, follicular variety.** Several hypopigmented macules of several centimeters with diffuse borders and peripheral follicular hyperkeratosis are observed.

181. Zaynoun ST, Aftimos BG, Tenekjian KK et al. (1983) Extensive pityriasis alba: a histological histochemical and ultrastructural study. **Br J Dermatol** 108:83–90.
182. Urano-Suehisa S, Tagami H (1985) Functional and morphological analysis of the horny layer of pityriasis alba. **Acta Derm Venereol** 65:164–167.
183. Martin RF, Lugo-Somolinos A, Sanchez JL (1996) Clinicopathologic study on pityriasis alba. **Biol Assoc Med PR** 82:463–465.

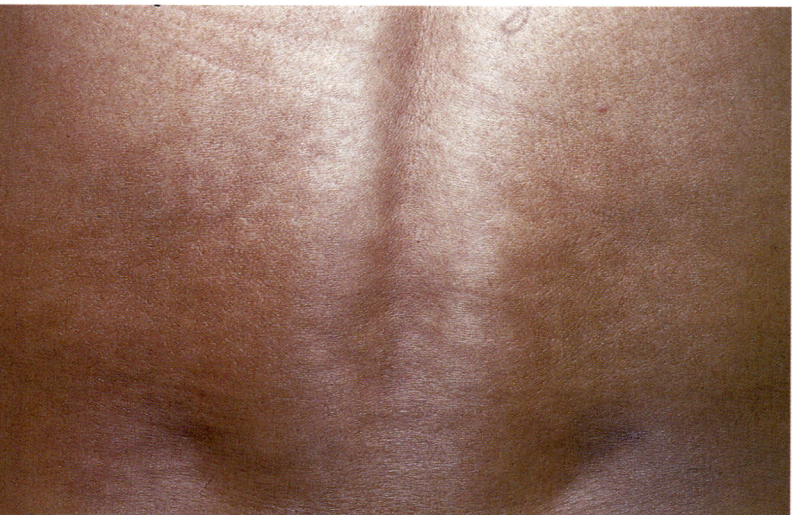

Fig. 10.20   Macular confluent hypomelanosis of halfcasts ("creole dyschromia"). Multiple hypopigmented and characteristic 1–3cm macules of ill-defined borders, on the lower back of a dark skin Mestizo patient.

Fig. 10.21   Tuberous sclerosis. Hypopigmented "ash leaf" macule on the dorsal upper back of a 10-year-old girl with multiple facial angiofibromas. Both features may be observed in this condition.

subjects between the age of 17 and 48 years,[184] but adolescents and older patients may also present with similar findings; more boys than girls are affected.

The pathogenesis of this disorder is unknown but it appears to involve a variation in melanosome size and distribution with decrease in the production of type IV melanosomes.[185] There is no known treatment for this unesthetic hypopigmentation, although sunlight exposure may lead to a partial improvement. A prolonged, indeterminate course is usually expected and the condition may last for many years. This disorder may be misdiagnosed as a fungal disease, extensive pityriasis alba, leprosy, postinflammatory hypopigmentation, or hypopigmented eczema, leading to unnecessary laboratory examinations; however these conditions need to be ruled out. This specific dyschromia deserves to be known and recognized, in particular in those areas of the world with a high population of mixed dark skin types.

HYPOMELANOSIS AND SYSTEMIC DISEASE

Tuberous sclerosis

Children born with tuberous sclerosis (TSC) often develop the characteristic triad of epilepsy, mental retardation, and adenoma sebaceum or typical papular angiofibromas occurring on the face. Although this is an autosomal-dominant disease, the diagnosis may not be evident until later in childhood, when other neurologic or cutaneous manifestations, such as periungual fibromas, become obvious. Two loci for TSC have been clearly identified: one gene is on chromosome 9q34 (*TSC-1*), and the second on chromosome 16p13.3 (*TSC-2*).[186] One of the easily diagnosed manifestations of TSC is the ash-leaf macule, present at birth in at least two-thirds and perhaps as many as 90% of all patients with this disease (Fig. 10.21).[187] These lesions are so named because some of them have the configuration of an ash leaf, consisting of an oval patch with one rounded and one pointed ends. One or many such macules may be distributed over the trunk or extremities. They are usually 1 to 3cm in size and dull white in color.

Occasionally, these children also have poliosis and more extensive hypomelanotic macules may be observed.[188] Wood's light examination in the newborn highlights these light-colored lesions from surrounding normal skin and suggests a diagnosis of TSC without any other clinical findings. However, hypopigmented nevi not associated with this condition occur commonly; thus, the finding of a white macule without other findings of TSC is not diagnostic of the disease.

On histopathologic examination melanocytes have a normal density but there is a decrease in the function of epidermal and follicular pigment cells. Lesions remain unchanged indefinitely.

Mycosis fungoides

Hypopigmented macules may also develop in mycosis fungoides. This pigmentary alteration occurs in adolescents and adults, but is observed more frequently in younger adults; it affects persons with dark skin almost exclusively.[189] In a group of nine patients, this variant occurred in dark-skinned individuals between 30 and 40 years of age who had the condition for several years.[190] The lesions may be small, measuring 1–2cm, or may present as large macules of several centimeters with diffuse hypopigmentation. Lesions may be located on different areas of the cutaneous surface, and facial involvement has also been observed. Lesions are usually nonatrophic, and erythema and slight desquamation may be present.[191] On histopathologic examination lack of epidermal atropy and a moderate to profound epidermotropism with infiltrating mononuclear cells are seen; on electron microscopy decreased numbers of melanocytes and melanosomes within keratinocytes have been reported.[189]

Although infrequent, hypopigmented macules of lymphoma have been reported in childhood and adolescence,[192,193] and must be differentiated from vitiligo; in such cases a biopsy will be necessary to establish the correct diagnosis. Treatment with PUVA[189,190,193] or UVB[190] have been effective with satisfactory repigmentation of affected areas.

184. Lesueur A, Garcia-Granel V, Helenon R et al. (1994) Progressive macular confluent hypomelanosis in mixed ethnic melanodermic subjects: an epidemiologic study of 511 patients. **Ann Dermatol Venereol** 121:880–883.
185. Guillet G, Guillet MH (1997) Creole dyschromia or idiopathic macular hypomelanosis of the melanodermic halfcast of Guillet–Helenon. **Bull Soc Pathol Exot** 90:333–334.
186. Jimbow K (1997) Tuberous sclerosis and guttate leukodermas. **Semin Cutan Med Surg** 16:30–35.
187. Fitzpatrick TB, Szabo G, Hori Y et al. (1968) White leaf-shaped macules – earliest visible sign of tuberous sclerosis. **Arch Dermatol** 98:1–6.
188. Nickel WR, Reed WB (1962) Tuberous sclerosis. **Arch Dermatol** 85:209–212.

189. Lambroza E, Cohen SR, Phelps R et al. (1995) Hypopigmented variant of mycosis fungoides: demography, histopathology, and treatment of seven cases. **J Am Acad Dermatol** 32:987–993.
190. Akaraphanth R, Douglass MC, Lim HW (2000) Hypopigmented mycosis fungoides: treatment and a 6 1/2-year follow-up of 9 patients. **J Am Acad Dermatol** 42:33–39.
191. Goldberg DJ, Schinella RS, Kechijian P (1986) Hypopigmented mycosis fungoides. Speculations about the mechanism of hypopigmentation. **Am J Dermatopathol** 8:326–330.
192. Grunwald MH, Amichai B (1999) Localized hypopigmented mycosis fungoides in a 12-year-old caucasian boy. **J Dermatol** 26:70–71.
193. Neuhaus IM, Ramos-Caro FA, Hassanein AM (2000) Hypopigmented mycosis fungoides in childhood and adolescence. **Pediatr Dermatol** 17:403–406.

Sarcoidosis

Hypopigmentation is a well-known manifestation of sarcoidosis, more frequently and easily observed in patients with dark skin of African ancestry. Lesions are mostly observed as macules without any cutaneous alteration but they may also be associated with the classic lesions of sarcoidosis such as papules, nodules or infiltrated plaques.[194] Sarcoidal granulomas may be present in macular lesions without underlying palpable masses,[194,195] and hypopigmentation has also been reported in systemic sarcoidosis with multiple organ involvement but without cutaneous granulomas and with negative skin biopsies.[196]

On histopathologic examination a reduction of melanin with preservation of melanocytes has been described.[196,197] On electron microscopic studies, dilatation of the endoplasmic reticulum, cytoplasmic vacuolation, edema and reduction of melanosomes have been found.[197] Hypopigmented lesions in sarcoidosis are an uncommon finding but awareness of this type of manifestation is useful for suspecting this condition.

Kwashiorkor

Kwashiorkor is a form of protein-calorie malnutrition that results from a diet poor in protein with an adequate or excessive carbohydrate intake. This condition is more prevalent in developing countries, particularly during times of socio-economical crisis, although it is also the most common form of nutritional deficiency among hospitalized patients in the United States.[198] These children are characteristically well until weaned and then develop erythematous plaques that darken and desquamate, constituting the "flaky paint dermatitis" or "enamel paint sign." This finding is helpful for diagnostic purposes[198] and may even be present in early-onset kwashiorkor.[199] These plaques first appear over pressure points and in the diaper area; in addition, they develop skin pallor that eventually leads to loss of pigment, especially at sites of minor trauma (Fig. 10.22). Hypochromotrichia, presenting as bands of depigmentation, may appear in the hair as well; the breadth of the bands corresponds to the length of time that the child remained malnourished; several of these bands constitute the "flag sign."[198] If kwashiorkor persists for a long time, all the scalp hair becomes pale; in patients of skin type VI, a gray–brown or straw-colored hue may be observed.[200] Mucocutaneous changes such as periorificial glazed erythema represents one of the common, multisystemic clinical manifestations of kwashiorkor.[201] Associated systemic abnormalities include peripheral edema, liver disease, neurologic changes, diarrhea, weight loss, and hypoalbuminemia. Appropriate diet correction eliminates these alterations.

HYPOMELANOSIS AND INFECTIOUS DISEASES

Tinea versicolor (pityriasis versicolor)

A common cause of pigment change is the superficial fungal infection, tinea versicolor. This infection is caused by a lipophilic yeast, *Malassezia furfur* (syn. *Pityrosporum orbiculare*).[202] The taxonomic classification of *Malassezia* yeasts up to the present time describes seven different species based upon molecular, biological, morphological and biochemical parameters. (*M. furfur, M. pachydermatis, M. sympodialis, M. globosa, M. obtusa, M. restricta, M. slooffiae*).[203] Although *M. globosa* may be isolated from uninvolved skin, there is some evidence suggesting that this organism may also be implicated in the pathogenesis of tinea versicolor.[203] This infection is far more common in warm, moist climates, where the incidence may approach 50%.

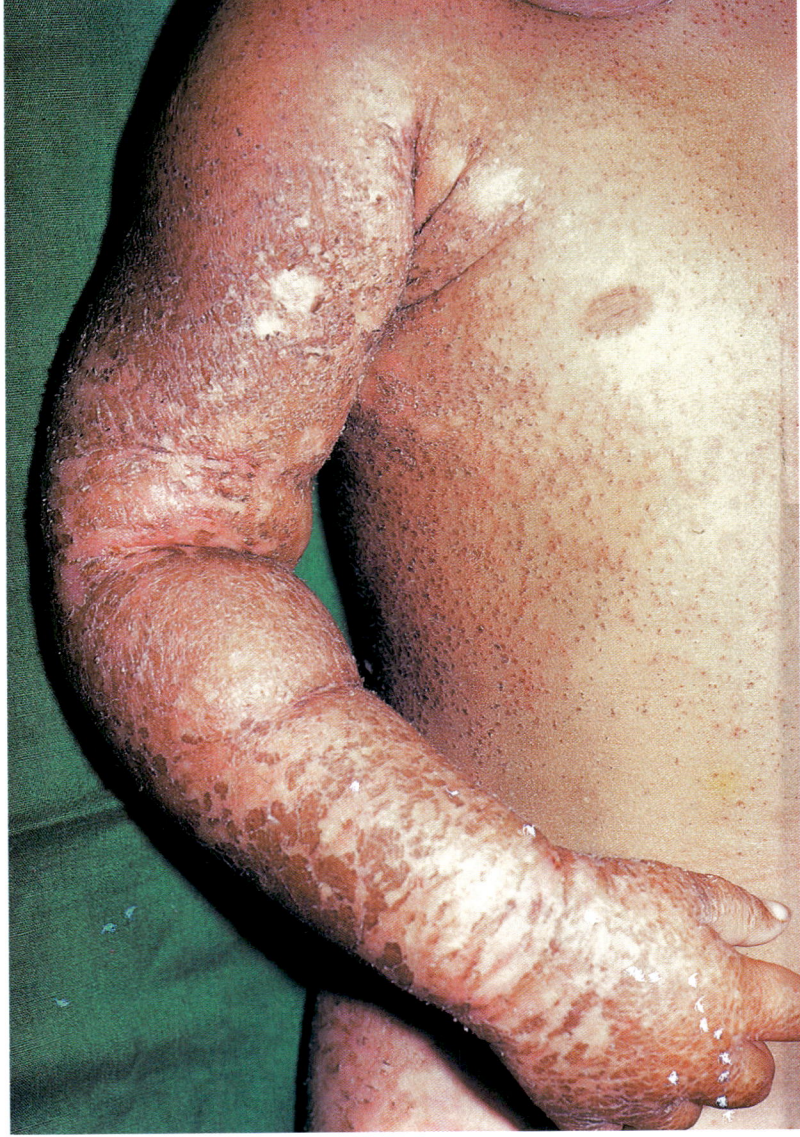

Fig. 10.22 **Kwashiorkor.** Typical areas of dark desquamation and some hypopigmented macules may be observed in this infant ("flaking paint").

The condition is most commonly seen between 28 and 45 years of age[204] but even infants can be affected.[205] These patients present with well-defined, asymptomatic, or slightly pruritic minimally scaly hypopigmented red–brown or brown flat papules, which may coalesce into larger plaques. The lesions are more prominent in the summer months not only because of the warm weather but also because normal skin tans while the affected areas often do not. The lesions are distributed over the upper trunk, neck, and proximal upper extremities; facial lesions are not uncommon on the forehead, as reported in a study of 164 patients.[206] The diagnosis of tinea versicolor is made

194. Hall RS, Floro JF, King LE (1984) Hypopigmented lesions in sarcoidosis. **J Am Acad Dermatol** 11:1163–1164.
195. Cornelius CE, Stein KM, Hanshaw WJ et al. (1973) Hypopigmentation and sarcoidosis. **Arch Dermatol** 108:249–251.
196. Alexis JB (1994) Sarcoidosis presenting as cutaneous hypopigmentation with repeatedly negative skin biopsies. **Int J Dermatol** 33:44–45.
197. Clayton R, Breathnach A, Martin et al. (1977) Hypopigmented sarcoidosis in the negro. Report of eight cases with ultrastructural observations. **Br J Dermatol** 96:119–125.
198. Liu T, Howard RM, Mancini AJ et al. (2001) Kwashiorkor in the United States: fad diets, perceived and true milk allergy, and nutritional ignorance. **Arch Dermatol** 137:630.
199. Buno IJ, Morelli JG, Weston WL (1998) The enamel paint sign in the dermatologic diagnosis of early-onset Kwashiorkor [letter]. **Arch Dermatol** 134:107–108.

200. McLaren DS (1987) Skin in protein energy malnutrition. **Arch Dermatol** 123:1674–1676.
201. Prendiville JS, Manfredi LN (1992) Skin signs of nutritional disorders. **Semin Dermatol** 11:88–97.
202. De Luca C, Picardo M, Breathnach A et al. (1996) Lipoperoxidase activity of *Pityrosporum*: characterisation of by-products and possible role in pityriasis versicolor. **Exp Dermatol** 5:49–56.
203. Weiss R, Raabe P, Mayser P (2000) Yeasts of the genus *Malassezia*: taxonomic classification and significance in (veterinary and) clinical medicine. **Mycoses** 43(Suppl 1):69–72.
204. Faergemann J (1989) Epidemiology and ecology of pityriasis versicolor. **Curr Top Med Mycol** 3:153–167.
205. Wyre HW Jr, Johnson WT (1981) Neonatal pityriasis versicolor. **Arch Dermatol** 117:752–753.
206. Bouassida S, Boudaya S, Ghorbel R et al. (1998) Pityriasis versicolor in children: a retrospective study of 164 cases. **Ann Dermatol Venereol** 125:581–584.

by examination of a KOH preparation of scales from the hypopigmented lesions that shows numerous short hyphae and yeast forms.

The pathogenesis of tinea versicolor involves the morphologic change of *M. furfur* from the yeast to the hyphal form under the influence of various factors including moisture, heat, the degree of host immunity (immuno-suppressed children tend to have more extensive involvement), diabetes mellitus, pregnancy, malnutrition, and inherited predisposition. The organism produces the dicarboxylic acid, azelaic acid, which is a tyrosinase inhibitor and may contribute to the hypopigmentation noted in this infection.[207]

The main differential diagnostic possibilities in tinea versicolor are postinflammatory hypopigmentation and vitiligo. Postinflammatory changes are usually not as well demarcated, but typically show small round macules. If scales are not obvious, tinea versicolor can also be mistaken for vitiligo, but vitiligo lesions are depigmented. The characteristic distribution of bilateral vitiligo differs from tinea versicolor in that it is symmetric, and is commonly found around orifices, bony prominences and distal parts of the extremities; on the contrary, uilateral vitiligo, particularly on light skin types, offers more diagnostic difficulties. Wood's light examination of tinea versicolor exhibits a yellowish color, whereas vitiligo macules are milk white.

Treatment of TV may be accomplished with one of the antiseborrheic shampoos such as selenium sulfide, or ketoconazole, applied as a lotion every other day for 14 days. For limited areas of involvement, one of the topical imidazole antifungal agents such as clotrimazole or miconazole is useful.[208] Oral ketoconazole, and itraconazole or fluconazole[209] in older children may also be effective especially in widespread disease. The hypopigmentation may remain for several months after treatment, even though the pathogenic organism has been eradicated. Sun exposure often evens out the pigmentation changes somewhat more quickly after treatment has been completed. Regardless of what therapy is used, recurrences are common. This hypopigmentation infectious disorder is particularly common in adolescents.

Leprosy

In either the early indeterminate stage or tuberculoid stage, leprosy can present with hypopigmented macules. Because the incubation period for this disease is 2 to 5 years, it is rarely seen in children under the age of 1 year. Children with indeterminate leprosy have one or a few asymptomatic hypopigmented ill-defined macules with normal sensation over the lesion (Fig. 10.23). At this stage, the diagnosis is difficult to confirm, since there is usually no obvious associated palpable nerve enlargement and lesions may be confused with other noninfectious hypopigmented dermatoses; although at this early stage on histological examination no organisms are found, a mononuclear infiltrate of cutaneous nerves observed in the affected dermis or subcutaneous tissue is an important finding to establish a diagnosis. These macules may resolve spontaneously over several months but since they may progress to one of the definite forms of the disease, multidrug therapy is recommended.[210]

Lesions of tuberculoid leprosy are well-defined hypopigmented macules or plaques with elevated papular edges, associated with decreased sweating, pain, and thermoreception sensation within the plaques themselves. Regional cutaneous nerve trunks are often palpably enlarged. The number of melanocytes appear normal in hypopigmented lesions of leprosy.[211]

Tuberculoid leprosy should be treated regardless of the extension of involvement, and in spite of the apparent low-grade infection. Early multi-drug therapy prevents the progression towards a more aggressive clinical form with neural involvement causing severe retractions and functional alterations of the extremities.

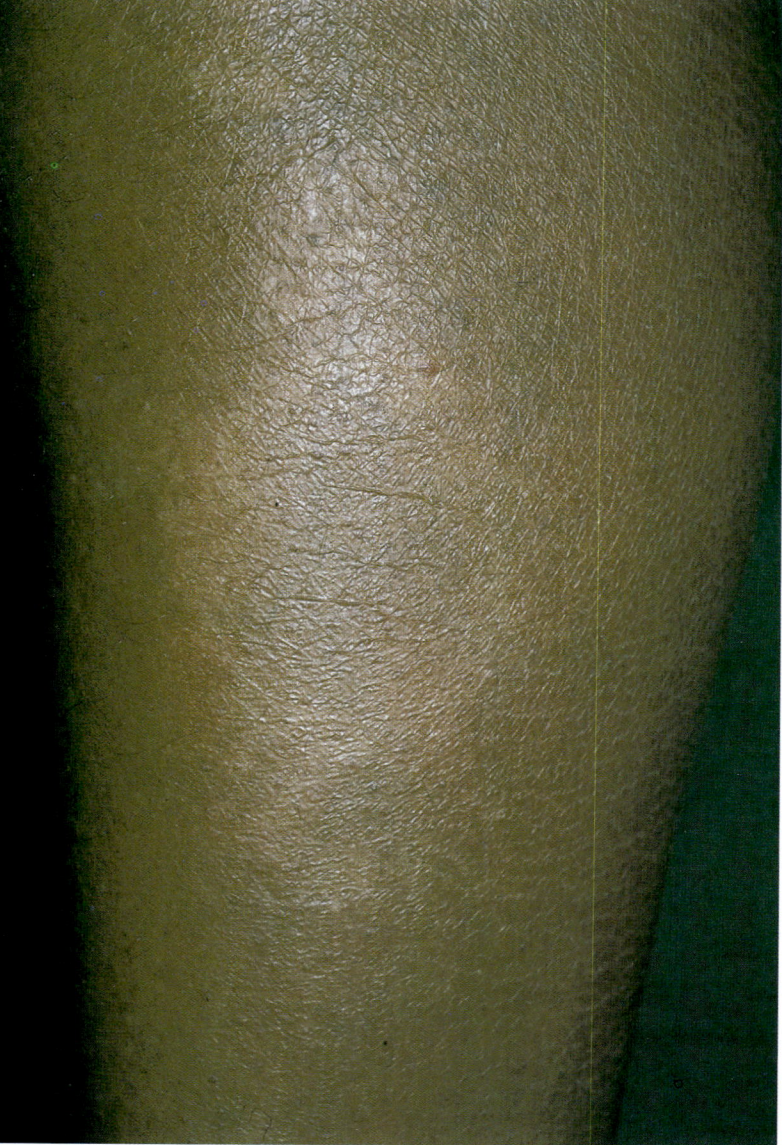

Fig. 10.23 Indeterminate leprosy. A subtle hypopigmented macule of 2 years' duration on the leg of this 11-year-old child. The macule showed normal sensation. (Acknowledgement: Photo is a kind courtesy of Dr. Fabián Sandoval.)

Pinta

Pinta is a chronic treponemal infection caused by *Treponema herrejoni*. Several decades ago many patients in Latin American countries were affected, but after the advent of antibiotics the condition has become limited to remote villages in tropical and subtropical rural areas, affecting socio-economically depressed communities, and certain Indian tribes.[212,213] It is spread by intimate person-to-person contact but is not considered a venereal disease. Pinta rarely occurs in children.[214]

As in other treponemal diseases, there are several evolution stages of pinta. In the initial stage, there are multiple red macules and indurated papules that

207. Jung EG, Bohnert E (1973) Mechanism of depigmentation in pityriasis versicolor. A histochemical and electron microscopic study. **Int J Dermatol** 12:48–52.
208. Strippoli V, Piacentini A, D'Auria FD et al. (1997) Antifungal activity of ketoconazole and other azoles against Malassezia furfur *in vitro* and *in vivo*. **Infection** 25:303–306.
209. Lesher JL Jr (1999) Oral therapy of common superficial fungal infections of the skin. **J Am Acad Dermatol** 40:S31–S34.
210. Kar PK, Jha PK, Snehi PS (1992) Indeterminate leprosy: a therapeutic evaluation. **Ind J Lepr** 64:163–167.
211. Shereef PH, Thomas M (1992) Hypopigmented macules in leprosy, a histopathological and histochemical study of melanocytes. **Ind J Lepr** 64:189–191.
212. Falabella R (1994) Nonvenereal treponematoses: Yaws, endemic syphilis and pinta (Letter to the editor). **J Am Acad Dermatol** 31:1075.
213. Woltsche Kahr I, Schmidt B, Aberer W et al. (1999) Pinta in Austria (or Cuba?): import of an extinct disease? **Arch Dermatol** 135:685–688.
214. Castro LGM (1994) Nonvenereal treponematosis (Letter to the editor). **J Am Acad Dermatol** 31:1075–1076.

may coalesce; in the generalized cutaneous phase, which occurs months or even years after the initial phase, mottled hypo- and hyperpigmented patches sometimes presenting as a bluish discoloration of affected areas. These appear and progress to the late phase, charaterized by extensive pigment mottling and skin atrophy. Histopathologic examination confirms the decrease or absence of epidermal melanocytes in the depigmented skin. Treponemes are occasionally seen in the epidermis.

The treatment of choice in pinta is parenteral penicillin. However, achromic plaques remain almost invariably depigmented in spite of therapy.

Onchocerciasis

This condition, also called "river blindness," is a parasitic infection caused by the filarial nematode, *Onchocerca volvulus*. It infects 18 million people worldwide, most of them in African nations; it is rarely seen in developed countries except in individuals travelling from endemic areas. When patients become affected, one of the most important sequelae is blindness. Onchocerciasis does not only affect the eyes, but can also provoke subcutaneous nodules and a pruritic hypopigmented or hyperpigmented papular dermatitis. Lesions may be observed as hypopigmented macules with slight atrophy.

On histopathologic examination scanty perivascular inflammatory infiltrates with mononuclear cells, eosinophils, and occasional microfilariae in the papillary dermis are observed.[215] Ivermectin is the treatment of choice for onchocerciasis with a high effectiveness and excellent tolerance.[216]

Hypomelanosis in other infectious and parasitic diseases

Hypomelanosis may occur in other treponemal diseases as well. In secondary syphilis, the commonest cutaneous manifestation is the so called "Venus necklace," occurring after the papular rash of secondary lues; discrete hypopigmented lesions appear in previous sites of secondary lesions which disappear spontaneously several months after treatment is completed.[217] Another condition associated with hypomelanosis is post-kala-azar dermal leishmaniasis, an uncommon sequel seen in patients with a previous episode of kala-azar. It is characterized by hypopigmented macules and erythematous eruptions leading to the formation of papules, plaques and nodules.[218] In yaws, the hypopigmented changes may occur in the late stages.

VITILIGO

Joseph Morelli

Vitiligo is macular depigmentation associated with the destruction of melanocytes. The disorder represents a clinical endpoint, may not have a single cause, and may not be a single disease. Vitiligo has been recognized for thousands of years.[219] The social stigma associated with vitiligo arose from its confusion with leprosy and other contagious diseases associated with hypopigmentation. Despite the fact that it is now readily distinguishable from other causes of hypopigmentation or depigmentation these stigma continue in many areas of the world.

GENETICS

Vitiligo is thought to have a genetic component. In one study 42.5% of patients had a first-degree family member with vitiligo and the incidence in either first-, second- or third-degree relatives was 8%,[220] consistent with a polygenic disorder. Vitiligo has been associated with different human leukocyte antigen markers depending on the ethnic groups evaluated.

Vitiligo has been associated with single gene defects,[221] but attempts to identify a single gene that is the cause of vitiligo have so far been unsuccessful.[222,223] The difficulty may be attributed to the likelihood that vitiligo is a heterogeneous condition.

STATISTICS

Vitiligo affects 1–2% of the population worldwide.[224] Both sexes are affected equally. It is unclear whether dark-skinned individuals are more commonly affected, or whether the disease is just more obvious and associated with social stigma in this group, leading patients to seek treatment. Although most people do not think of vitiligo as a childhood disease,[225–227] 50% of patients develop their first lesions before the age of 20 years and 25% before the age of 10 years. Vitiligo has been reported to develop as early in life as 6 months of age.

PRESENTING HISTORY

Generalized vitiligo is the most common type of vitiligo and presents as acral symmetric depigmentation. Many authorities include focal, acral, and acrofacial vitiligo as separate entities from widespread vitiligo, but their shared natural history and response to treatment suggest that they are subsets of generalized vitiligo. In contrast, segmental vitiligo is a less common presentation identified by a more rapid progression of segmental depigmentation. There are minimal data in the literature regarding childhood vitiligo, but there appears to be distinct differences from vitiligo in adults. Although generalized vitiligo are the most common type of vitiligo seen in both children and adults, the percentage of children with segmental vitiligo is significantly greater than in adults.

PHYSICAL EXAMINATION

Skin

The areas of the skin affected by vitiligo are classically devoid of pigmentation and appear as chalk-white macules. They are most common on acral and sun-exposed areas, but may cover the majority of the cutaneous surface (Fig. 10.24). They may be of any size and shape. Developing vitiligo in dark-skinned people may show various shades of color intermediate between the patient's normal skin color and the totally depigmented skin, called trichrome vitiligo. Although most vitiligo strictly undergoes a progressive loss of skin color without inflammation, 5% of patients will exhibit a raised inflammatory border at the edge of the depigmented macules. The Koebner phenomenon may be seen, with new areas of vitiligo developing subsequent to skin injury. Halo nevi may also occur (Fig. 10.25). Segmental vitiligo is localized to one area of skin, (Fig. 10.26), although the

215. Vernick W, Turner SE, Burov E et al. (2000) Onchocerciasis presenting with lower extremity, hypopigmented macules. **Cutis** 65:293–297.
216. Davies JB, Lujan R, Lopez-Martinez LA et al. (1997) Assessment of vector microfilarial uptake as a comparatively non-invasive technique for monitoring onchocerciasis treatment campaigns in the Americas. **Trop Med Int Health** 2:348–355.
217. Fiumara NJ, Kahn T (1982) Leukoderma of secondary syphilis: two case reports. **Sex Transm Dis** 9:140–142.
218. Ramesh V, Singh N (1999) A clinical and histopathological study of macular of post-kala-azar dermal leishmaniasis. **Trop Doct** 29:205–207.
219. Kovacs SO (1998) Vitiligo. **J Am Acad Dermatol** 38:647–666.
220. Kim SM, Chung HS, Hann SK (1998) The genetics of vitiligo in Korean patients. **Int J Dermatol** 37:908–910.
221. Karvonen SL, Haapasaari KM, Kallioinen M et al. (1999) Increased prevalence of vitiligo, but no evidence of premature aging, in the skin of patients with bp3243 mutation in mitochondrial

DNA in the mitochondrial encephalomyopathy, lactic acidosis and stroke-like episodes syndrome (MELAS). **Br J Dermatol** 140:634–639.
222. Bandyopadhyay D, Lawrence E, Majumder PP, Ferrell RE (2000) Vitiligo is not caused by mutations in GTP-cyclohydrolase I gene. **Clin Exp Dermatol** 25:152–153.
223. Tripathi RK, Flanders DJ, Young TL et al. (1999) Microphthalmia-associated transcription factor (MITF) locus lacks linkage to human vitiligo or osteopetrosis: an evaluation. **Pigment Cell Res** 12:187–192.
224. Westerhof W (2000) Vitiligo management update. **Skin Therapy Lett** 5:1–2, 5.
225. Hann SK, Lee HJ (1996) Segmental vitiligo: clinical findings in 208 patients. **J Am Acad Dermatol** 35:671–674.
226. Njoo MD, Das PK, Bos JD, Westerhof W (1999) Association of the Koebner phenomenon with disease activity and therapeutic responsiveness in vitiligo vulgaris. **Arch Dermatol** 135:407–413.
227. Handa S, Kaur I (1999) Vitiligo: clinical findings in 1436 patients. **J Dermatol** 26:653–657.

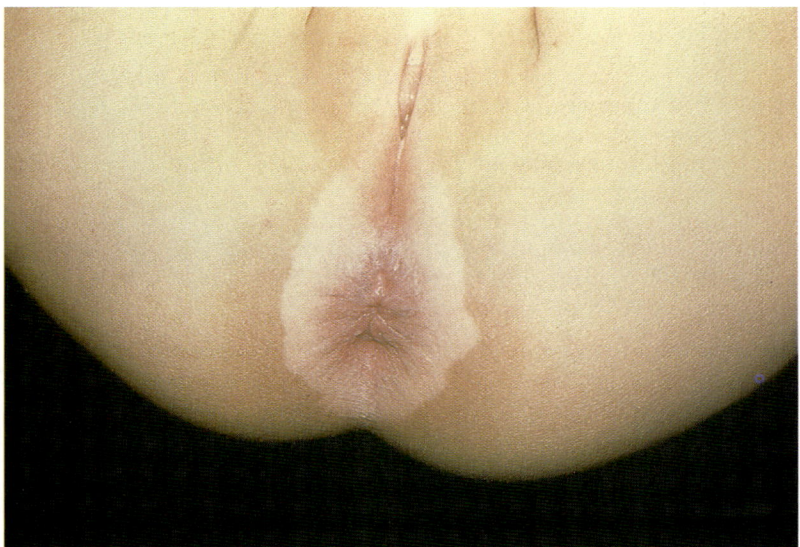

Fig. 10.24   Vitiligo in anogenital region. (Courtesy Dr. Ronald Hansen.)

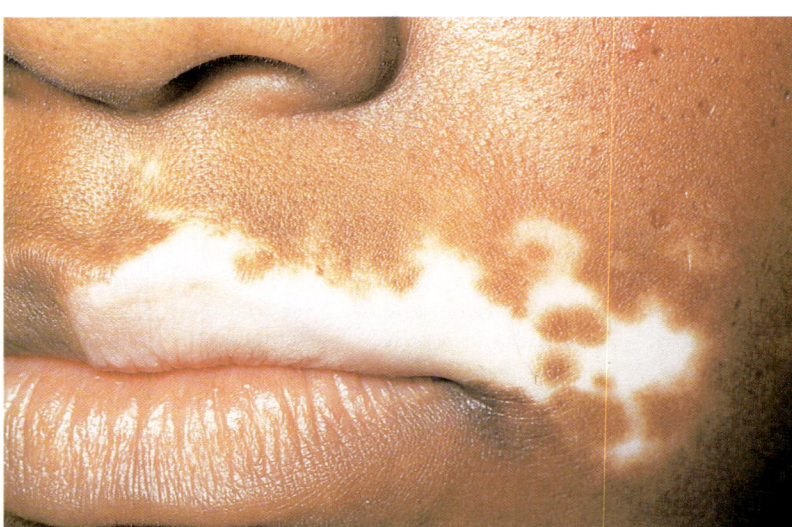

Fig. 10.26   Segmental vitiligo. (Courtesy Dr. Ronald Hansen.)

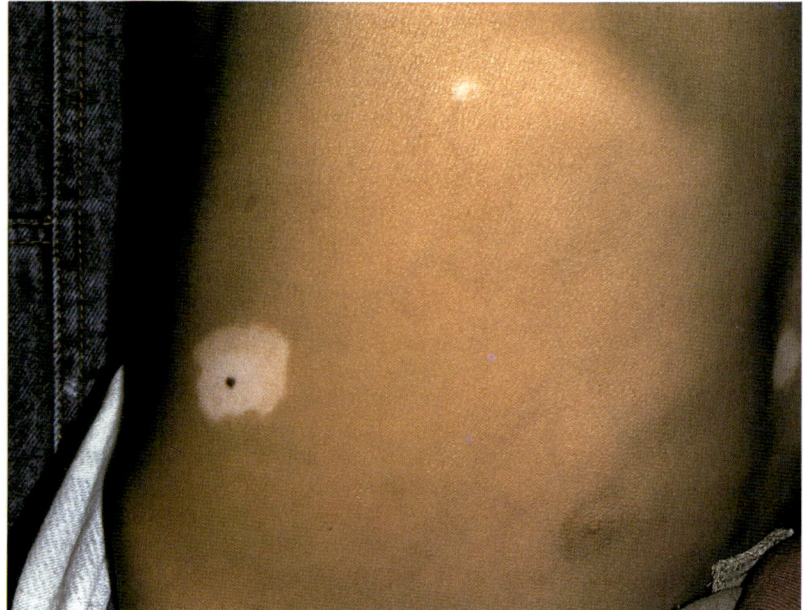

Fig. 10.25   Halo nevi in child with vitiligo. (Courtesy Dr. Ronald Hansen.)

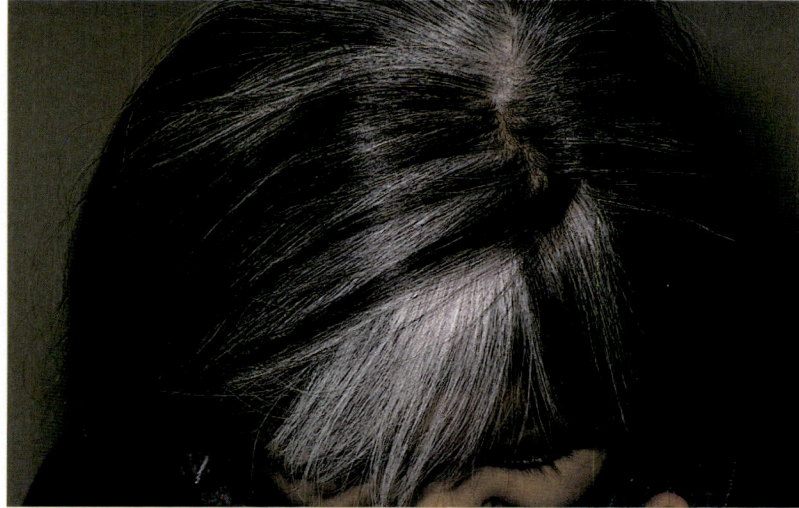

Fig. 10.27   Hair depigmentation (poliosis) with vitiligo. (Courtesy Dr. Ronald Hansen.)

entire segment is not usually involved. The areas of segmental vitiligo do not correspond to dermatomes.

Hair, nails, teeth, and mucous membranes

Areas of hair and mucous membranes may also be depigmented (Fig. 10.27). If the patient has associated alopecia areata, circular areas of hair loss with a normal scalp and nail pits may be seen. The teeth are normal.

SYSTEMIC MANIFESTATIONS

Children with vitiligo are more likely to have an immediate family member with autoimmune disease than are other children, but the familial incidence of autoimmunity is much less than in adults with vitiligo. Children with vitiligo also have a much higher incidence of both nonspecific and organ-specific autoantibodies than other children, but rarely show clinical autoimmune disease. No studies have been performed on the predictive value

of the presence of autoantibodies in childhood and their routine screening is not recommended. Screening for other autoimmune diseases in childhood should only be performed if there is a positive family history or any clinical signs or symptoms of these disorders.

Melanocytes are also found in the retinal pigment epithelium, the choroid of the eye and the scala vestibuli of the inner ear; depigmentation has been described in the retinal pigment epithelium and the choroid. Uveitis may also be seen, but eye color does not change. Mild hearing loss may occur. These changes are extremely rare in childhood and routine screening is not necessary.

LABORATORY FINDINGS

No laboratory tests are routinely performed. Laboratory tests for autoimmune disease should only be checked if personal history, physical examination or family history suggest an increased risk.

PATHOPHYSIOLOGY AND HISTOGENESIS
Molecular, biochemical, and immunologic basis

Several theories have been postulated to explain the cause of vitiligo.[228–232] These include the autoimmune, autocytotoxic, neural and genetic theories. It is likely that vitiligo is a heterogenous disorder with portions of all theories being correct in a given subset of patients.

The autoimmune theory was formulated because of the association of vitiligo with autoimmune disease. Antibodies against melanocyte antigens are present in the serum of patients with vitiligo.[228–231] The extent of vitiligo can be correlated with the incidence and level of these antibodies. Serum from patients with vitiligo is cytotoxic to melanocytes *in vitro*.[232] These antibodies recognize a variety of melanocyte proteins including tyrosinase, tyrosinase-related protein-1 (TRP-1) and Pme1.[229–231] Normal melanocytes are also destroyed in people undergoing antigen-specific immunotherapy for melanoma.[232] It is argued that the antibody formation is not primary, but secondary to antigen release following melanocyte self-destruction.[233]

Many authorities believe that the cause of melanocyte death in vitiligo is a primary cell abnormality. Electron microscopic studies of both skin from patients with vitiligo and melanocytes cultured from patients with vitiligo reveal morphologic abnormalities, including cytoplasmic vacuolization, aggregation of melanosomes, autophagic vacuoles, fatty degeneration, and dilatation of the rough endoplasmic reticulum. Others believe that melanocyte death is related to inherent sensitivity to oxidative stress either in response to toxic intermediates of melanin or abnormal production of and/or lack of protection from hydrogen peroxide and other oxygen radicals.[234,235]

Melanocytes are derived from the neural crest and related to nerve cells. Nerve endings are in direct contact with epidermal melanocytes in depigmented skin. This is the main basis for the neural theory. An excess of catecholamine metabolites may be seen during active depigmentation,[236] although this may be a secondary phenomenon. Although familial vitiligo is definitely seen, the search for a single defect in these patients has so far been unsuccessful.[222,223]

HISTOLOGY

Early lesions of vitiligo show a decreased number of melanocytes. An inflammatory infiltrate containing cutaneous leukocyte-associated antigen T lymphocytes expressing perforin and granzyme-B is seen clustered in the vicinity of disappearing melanocytes.[237]

The classic histology of longstanding vitiligo is the absence of melanocytes.[238] Despite this, it has recently recently been shown that melanocytes may be cultured from the skin of vitiligo that is totally depigmented.[239] Since no clinical pigmentation is seen, any melanocytes remaining are either unable to make melanin, have abnormal interactions with neighboring keratinocytes or are too few to make clinically evident pigmentation. No matter what the pathogenesis, the histogenesis of vitiligo is the destruction of melanocytes. The melanocytes that may be cultured from patches of longstanding vitiligo may either be resistant to destruction or melanocytes that have migrated from the outer root sheath of the hair follicle and are in the process of being destroyed.

DIFFERENTIAL DIAGNOSIS

The differential diagnosis of vitiligo depends on the type of vitiligo and the distribution of the depigmentation.[225] Generalized vitiligo must be distinguished from postinflammatory hypopigmentation, pityriasis alba, tinea versicolor, multiple ash leaf macules, morphea, lichen sclerosis, piebaldism, Waardenburg's syndrome and hypomelanosis of Ito. In a child with segmental disease, one should also consider nevus depigmentosus and nevus anemicus. The two most important factors that aid in distinguishing vitiligo from the other pigmentation disorders are that the lesions must be acquired after birth and that they are totally depigmented. At times, especially in light-skinned children, it is necessary to use a Wood's lamp to determine if the skin is truly depigmented. A small proportion of children will have inflammatory vitiligo, which is characterized by an erythematous raised border, making the differential between vitiligo and postinflammatory hypopigmentation more difficult. Another problem in differential diagnosis arises in dark-skinned children with early vitiligo or with trichrome vitiligo. In early vitiligo some functioning melanocytes may remain and the lesion is not be totally depigmented. In trichrome vitiligo a progression from totally depigmented skin to hypopigmented skin to normal-colored skin is observable.

THERAPEUTICS AND PROGNOSIS
Topical therapy

Not all children with vitiligo want active therapy.[240] This will depend on the age of the patient, location and extent of the vitiliginous lesions and cultural beliefs. Those patients not wishing treatment must be counseled that the areas of vitiligo are totally lacking in pigment and therefore have no intrinsic sun protection. Unless photoprotected they are at risk for the development of the sequelae of acute and chronic sun exposure.[241] Cover-up cosmetics which match the child's skin color may be very beneficial for cosmetically sensitive areas. They are somewhat time-consuming to use; therefore the child must be very motivated. Artificial tanning agents are safe and they do darken the skin, but the color does not match most normal skin colors.

Glucocorticosteroids are the mainstay of topical therapy. There are published studies from many countries using the full range of potency of topical glucocorticosteroids.[240] Using meta analysis of controlled studies of the treatment of localized vitiligo, potent topical steroids had the highest odds ratio for success versus placebo.[242] Interestingly, superpotent topical steroids were less effective and produced greater side effects. In patient series on the treatment of localized vitiligo, potent and superpotent topical steroids were the most effective with 60% of patients achieving 75% clearing (Fig. 10.28). Recently topical tacrolimus has been shown to be effective in treating vitiligo, especially of the face and neck.[243] Segmental vitiligo may respond as well. Superpotent topical steroids produced greater side effects.

228. Norris DA, Horikawa T, Morelli JG (1994) Melanocyte destruction and repopulation in vitiligo. **Pigment Cell Res** 7:193–203.
229. Kemp EH, Waterman EA, Gawkrodger DJ et al. (1999) Identification of epitopes on tyrosinase which are recognized by autoantibodies from patients with vitiligo. **J Invest Dermatol** 113:267–271.
230. Kemp EH, Waterman EA, Gawkrodger DJ et al. (1998) Autoantibodies to tyrosinase-related protein-1 detected in the sera of vitiligo patients using a quantitative radiobinding assay. **Br J Dermatol** 139:798–805.
231. Kemp EH, Gawkrodger DJ, Watson PF, Weetman AP (1998) Autoantibodies to human melanocyte-specfic protein pmel17 in the sera of vitiligo patients: a sensitive and quantitative radioimmunoassay (RIA). **Clin Exp Immunol** 114:333–338.
232. Yee C, Thompson JA, Roche P et al. (2000) Melanocyte destruction after antigen-specific immunotherapy of melanoma: direct evidence of T cell-mediated vitiligo. **J Exp Med** 192:1637–1644.
233. Taeib A (2000) Intrinsic and extrinsic pathomechanism in vitiligo. **Pigment Cell Res** 13(Suppl 8):41–47.
234. Jimbow K, Chen H, Park J, Thomas P (2001) Increased sensitivity of melanocytes to oxidative stress and abnormal expression of tyrosinase-related protein in vitiligo. **Br J Dermatol** 144:55–65.
235. Schallreuter KU, Moore J, Wood JM et al. (1999) In vivo and in vitro evidence for hydrogen peroxide (H_2O_2) accumulation in the epidermis of patients with vitiligo and its successful removal by a UVB-activated catalase. **J Invest Dermatol Symp Proc** 4:91–96.
236. Cucchi ML, Frattini P, Santagostino G, Orecchia G (2000) Higher plasma catecholamine and metabolite levels in the early phase of non segmental vitiligo. **Pigment Cell Res** 13:28–32.
237. Van den Wijngaard R, Wankowicz-Kalinska A, Le Poole C et al. (2000) Local immune response in skin of generalized vitiligo patients. Destruction of melanocytes is associated with the prominent prescence of CLA+ T cells at the perilesional site. **Lab Invest** 80:1299–1309.
238. Le Poole IC, van den Wijngaard RM, Westerhof W, Das PK (1996) Presence of T cells and macrophages in inflammatory vitiligo skin parallels melanocyte disappearance. **Am J Pathol** 148:1219–1228.
239. Tobin DJ, Swanson NN, Pittelkow MR et al. (2000) Melanocytes are not absent in lesional skin of long duration vitiligo. **J Pathol** 191:407–416.
240. Morelli JG (1997) Vitiligo in children: treatment options. **Dermatol Ther** 2:93–97.
241. Akimoto S, Suzuki Y, Ishikawa O (2000) Multiple actinic keratoses and squamous cell carcinomas on the sun-exposed area of widespread vitiligo. **Br J Dermatol** 142:824–825.
242. Njoo MD, Spuls PI, Bos JD et al. (1998) Non surgical repigmentation therapies in vitiligo. Meta-analysis of the literature. **Arch Dermatol** 134:1532–1540.
243. Grimes PE, Soriano T, Dytoc MT (2002) Topical tacrolimus for repigmentation of vitiligo. **J Am Acad Dermatol** 47:789.

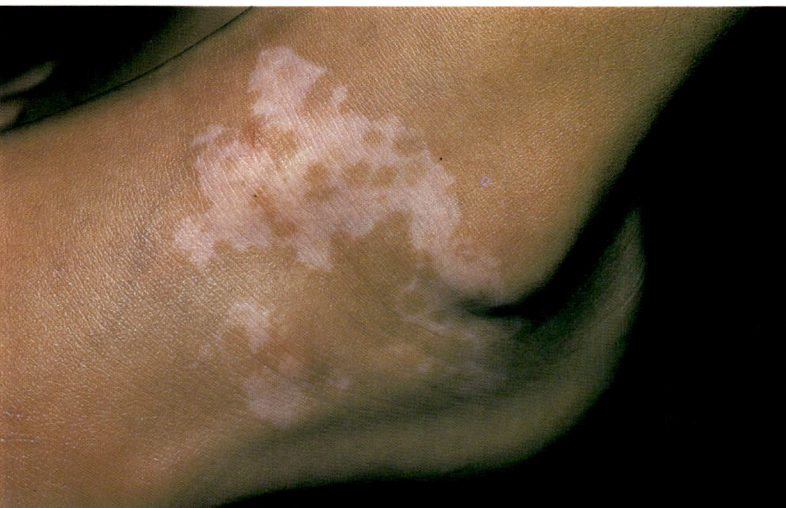

Fig. 10.28   Re-pigmenting vitiligo due to topical corticosteroid therapy. (Courtesy Dr. Ronald Hansen.)

Systemic management

The gold standard for the treatment of vitiligo has been the combination of oral methoxypsoralen and ultraviolet-A radiation (PUVA).[245] There are no studies on PUVA therapy in childhood or adolescents; therefore all recommendations must be drawn from experience in treating adults. It is well accepted that PUVA therapy increases the risk of both nonmelanoma skin cancer and melanoma. Because of the photosensitivity associated with this treatment it has not been recommended for children under the age of 12 years. Natural sunlight and broad-band UVB have also been used. Recently, narrow-band UVB has been advocated as the ultraviolet light treatment of choice. It has been effectively used in children.[244] Since this is a relatively new therapy there are no long-term safety studies. Combination phototherapy with topical calcipotriol or topical steroids may be more effective than phototherapy alone.[245,246] Phenylalanine and natural sunlight has been used in both adults and children, but there is concern about possible neurologic side effects secondary to large doses.[247] For small cosmetically significant areas which have not responded to other therapies, melanocyte transplantation is effective. This may be done either by various methods of direct skin transfer or by using cultured autologous melanocytes.[248] Depigmentation therapy is permanent and should only be considered in children with severe (>75% body surface involvement), stable vitiligo which has been unresponsive to therapy.

PROGNOSIS

Generalized vitiligo is in general a slowly progressive disease. Spontaneous remission may occur, but is rare. In one large study only 5% of the patients had more than 20% of their body surface area covered.[249] It is not known if age at onset of disease correlates with eventual proportion of body surface involved.

Segmental vitiligo usually is rapidly progressive. It then remains stable and is less responsive to treatment than generalized vitiligo. Patients with segmental vitiligo are not expected to develop generalized vitiligo.[250,251]

PEDIATRIC ASPECTS OF THE DISEASE

Very young children with vitiligo are not bothered by the disease and usually do not wish to participate in treatment. It is important in these children to use vigorous methods of sun protection to prevent acute and chronic photodamage.

With advancing age comes an increased knowledge of the differences in skin color, along with an increase in social pressures to be normal. The actual age at which this occurs is quite variable. It is at this time that the child will actively seek treatment. Vitiligo has severe psychosocial effects with two-thirds of vitiligo patients significantly underachieving their potential due to the disfigurement.[252,253]

An excellent support group exists. It is the National Vitiligo Foundation, 611 S. Fleishel Avenue, Tyler, TX 75701. Phone number: 903-531-0074. Fax: 903-525-1234. Website: www.vitiligofoundation.org.

VOGT–KOYANAGI–HARADA SYNDROME

The Vogt–Koyanagi–Harada syndrome is an acute multisystem inflammatory disease that is thought to represent an autoimmune response to pigment cells. The disease usually begins with an acute febrile illness, often accompanied by meningoencephalitis, uveitis and dysacusis. Vitiligo is the cutaneous finding and presents after the other signs. The eye disease can be severe with cataract formation, retinal pigment atrophy, and glaucoma. Treatment with systemic glucocorticosteroids is often required.

Vitiligo vulgaris can affect the eyes and ears as well as the skin. What distinguishes this acute severe disease from the chronic and milder changes in vitiligo vulgaris is unknown. Vogt–Koyanagi–Harada syndrome is primarily a disease of adults, with one series reporting only 3 of 98 patients being younger than 16 years of age. These children had severe ophthalmologic findings.[254]

NEOPLASTIC DISORDERS OF MELANOCYTES

Norman Levine

NEVOCELLULAR NEVUS

A nevocellular nevus (NCN) is defined as a lesion consisting of pigmented or nonpigmented melanocytes with or without the participation of nerve elements. These form a continuum from a hamartomatous growth to very atypical melanocytic proliferation.[255] Nevus cells (melanoblasts) arise from the neural crest and migrate into the skin sometime after the 10th week and before the 6th month of fetal life.[256]

Congenital NCN

Epidemiology

At birth, approximately 4% of children have pigmented lesions, but only about 1% of newborns have NCN. The congenital nevus encompasses a broad group of lesions, both clinically and histologically. Any nevus larger than 1.5 cm which does not have dysplastic features can be considered a congenital nevus, even if it is not evident at birth.[257] Congenital NCN can be divided into three groups, depending on size. *Giant* congenital nevi have been defined variously as those

244. Halder RM, Young CM (2000) New and emerging therapies for vitiligo. **Dermatol Clin** 18:79–89.
245. Yalcin B, Bukulmez G, Karaduman A et al. (2001) Experience with calcipotriol as adjunctive treatment for vitiligo in patients who do not respond to PUVA alone: A preliminary study. **J Am Acad Dermatol** 44:634–637.
246. Westerhof W, Nieweboer-Krobotova L, Mulder PG, Glazenburg EJ (1999) Left–right comparison study of the combination of fluticasone propionate and UV-A vs. either fluticasone propionate or UV-A alone for the long-term treatment of vitiligo. **Arch Dermatol** 135:1061–1066.
247. Burkhart CG, Burkhart CN (1999) Phenylalanine with UVA for the treatment of vitiligo needs more testing for possible side effects. **J Am Acad Dermatol** 40:1015.
248. Yaaar M, Gilchrist BA (2001) Vitiligo: the evolution of cultured epidermal autografts and other surgical treatment modalities. **Arch Dermatol** 137:348–349.
249. Cho S, Kang HC, Hahm JH (2000) Characteristics of vitiligo in Korean children. **Pediatr Dermatol** 17:189–193.
250. Jaisankar TJ, Baruah MC, Garg BR (1992) Vitiligo in children. **Int J Dermatol** 31:621–623.
251. Halder RM, Grimes PE, Cowan CA et al. (1987) Childhood vitiligo. **J Am Acad Dermatol** 16:948–954.
252. Mason PJ (1997) Vitiligo: The psychosocial effects. **Medsurg Nursing** 6:216–218, 232.
253. Nordlund JJ, Halder RM, Grimes P (1993) Management of vitiligo. **Dermatol Clin** 11:27–33.
254. Rathinam SR, Vijayalakshmi P, Namperumalsamy P et al. (1998) Vogt–Koyanagi–Harada syndrome in children. **Ocul Immunol Inflamm** 6:155–161.
255. Banuls J, Climent JM, Sanchez-Paya J et al. (2001) The association between idiopathic scoliosis and the number of acquired melanocytic nevi. **J Am Acad Dermatol** 45:35.
256. Harrison R, Okun M (1960) Divided nevus: a clue to the intrauterine development of melanocytic nevi. **Arch Dermatol** 82:235.
257. Mihm MC, Jr, Barnhill RL, Sober AJ et al. (1992) Precursor lesions of melanoma: do they exist? **Semin Surg Oncol** 8:358.

larger than 20cm,[258] those greater in total area than 120cm², those larger than the palm of the hand at birth (about 6cm),[259] or those that cannot be completely excised with primary suture closure in a single operative procedure.[260] This rare variant occurs in fewer than 1 in 20 000 newborns,[261] but its impact is great because of the considerable cosmetic disfigurement, psychosocial disruption, and the malignant potential of the lesion.

Large congenital nevi are often defined as those greater than 1.5cm but less than 20cm in diameter; these are seen in 0.6% of newborns. *Small* congenital nevi are defined as those less than 1.5cm in diameter and occur in about 1% of newborns.[262]

Physical examination

Giant congenital nevi are often characterized at birth by an uneven verrucous surface with variations in shades of brown and blue throughout the lesion (Fig. 10.29). The margins are usually irregular, and there are often satellite pigmented papules beyond the periphery of the main lesion. As the infant grows, the involved areas acquire more heterogeneous colors, the surface becomes more irregular, and papules, nodules, and coarse dark hairs may appear. These changes are accelerated at the time of puberty.[263]

Giant nevi located in the posterior head and neck region may be associated with leptomeningeal melanocytosis[264,265] and secondary neurologic disorders such as epilepsy. Lesions over the vertebral column may have underlying spinal defects such as meningomyelocele or spina bifida.[260] Melanomas may also occur in these abnormal melanocytic rests.[264]

Small congenital NCN present as light tan-to-brown, uniformly pigmented macules or barely palpable papules, with minimal irregularity of the surface. These lesions tend to be stable over time except for the occasional appearance of coarse dark hair. Large congenital NCN have an initial appearance somewhat between the small and giant NCN with some variations in color

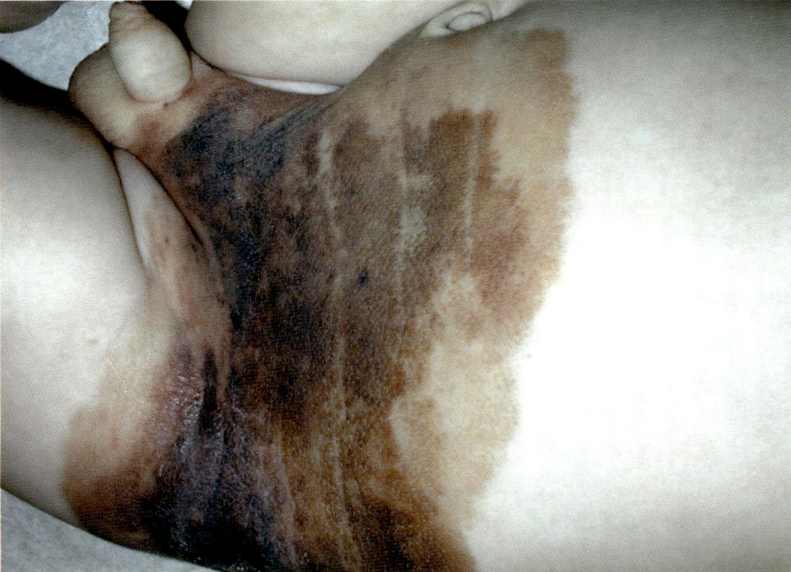

Fig. 10.29   Giant congenital nevus in a newborn child.

and minimal to moderate verrucous changes over the surface and often with subsequent development of dark hair.

Pathophysiology and histogenesis

There is controversy about whether specific histologic changes can differentiate congenital nevi from acquired moles. There are those who contend that most giant congenital nevi and many large congenital nevi have distinguishing histologic features which differentiate them from acquired lesions.[266] These include infiltration of nevus cells between collagen bundles and into nerves, blood vessels, and appendages.[267,268] However, others have noted that only 37% of congenital nevi have deep infiltration of nevus cells and that there are several different patterns noted: patchy or diffuse upper dermal infiltration alone, deep dermal diffuse, or patchy superficial and deep nevus cell infiltration. In many cases, one would be unable to distinguish congenital from acquired nevi by histologic pattern analysis alone.[269] Others have emphasized different microscopic patterns between small and giant congenital nevi. The giant lesions had nevus cells occupying the entire dermis except for a clear upper dermal grenz zone, whereas the small nevi showed a more organized pattern with well-developed nests in the superficial corium, simulating acquired nevi.[258]

Nevus cells are derived from the neural crest and there are reports of differentiation in the deeper portions of the lesions to neurofibroma-like patterns.[270] Thus it appears that congenital NCN are dynamic and can change over the life of the patient.

Differential diagnosis

Several other pigmented lesions that present at birth may be difficult to differentiate from congenital nevi. Café-au-lait spots are more uniformly tan–brown with occasional irregular margins and without any surface change. Mongolian spots are extremely common, particularly in pigmented races and are blue–gray, rather than the brown or tan color of NCN. They are macular, may have either distinct or indistinct margins, and usually disappear by age 5 years.

The nevus of Ota/Ito may be confused with a congenital nevus because of the large surface area that it may cover and because of the persistence of the lesion. However, it is blue–gray in color and is almost always in a dermatomal distribution on the face (Ota) or upper shoulder area (Ito). Epithelial nevi, which are hamartomas of epidermal or dermal structures, may be pigmented, especially if there is a verrucous surface. The margins are very distinct, and the color is usually a variation of a skin tone. The linear shape of the lesion best differentiates it from a congenital nevus.

A lentigo can occasionally be present at birth and may have the identical clinical picture as seen in a small congenital nevus, with sharply marginated borders and a macular surface. Skin biopsy examination is often necessary to distinguish between a lentigo and a nevus. Occasionally, transient neonatal pustular melanosis and acropustulosis of infancy can have brownish discoloration and can be confused with a small congenital nevus. The transient nature of these pigmented lesions easily differentiates them from congenital nevi, lesions that do not fade spontaneously.

Therapeutics and prognosis

The management of the congenital nevus is one of the most unsettled subjects in pediatric dermatology and one in which there are no absolute guidelines

258. Zitelli JA, Grant MG, Abell E et al. (1984) Histologic patterns of congenital nevocytic nevi and implications for treatment. **J Am Acad Dermatol** 11:402.
259. Wyatt AJ, Hansen RC (2000) Pediatric skin tumors. **Pediatr Clin N Am** 47:937.
260. Arons MS, Hurwitz S (1983) Congenital nevocellular nevus: a review of the treatment controversy and a report of 46 cases. **Plast Reconstr Surg** 72:355.
261. Wu SJ, Lambert DR (1997) Melanoma in children and adolescents. **Pediatr Dermatol** 14:87.
262. Rhodes AR, Wood WC, Sober AJ et al. (1981) Nonepidermal origin of malignant melanoma associated with a giant congenital nevocellular nevus. **Plast Reconstr Surg** 67:782.
263. Lefkowitz A, Schwartz RA, Janniger CK (1999) Melanoma precursors in children. **Cutis** 63:321.
264. Bittencourt FV, Marghoob AA, Kopf AW et al. (2000) Large congenital melanocytic nevi and the risk for development of malignant melanoma and neurocutaneous melanocytosis. **Pediatrics** 106:736.

265. Foster RD, Williams ML, Barkovich AJ et al. (2001) Giant congenital melanocytic nevi: the significance of neurocutaneous melanosis in neurologically asymptomatic children. **Plast Reconstr Surg** 107:933.
266. Kanzler MH, Mraz-Gernhard S (2001) Primary cutaneous malignant melanoma and its precursor lesions: diagnostic and therapeutic overview. **J Am Acad Dermatol** 45:260.
267. Mark GJ, Mihm MC, Liteplo MG et al. (1973) Congenital melanocytic nevi of the small and garment type. Clinical, histologic, and ultrastructural studies. **Hum Pathol** 4:395.
268. Bhawan J (1979) Melanocytic nevi. A review. **J Cutan Pathol** 6:153.
269. Stenn KS, Arons M, Hurwitz S (1983) Patterns of congenital nevocellular nevi. A histologic study of thirty-eight cases. **J Am Acad Dermatol** 9:388.
270. Rodriguez H, Ackerman L (1968) Cellular blue nevus. **Cancer** 21:393.

that can be observed. There are two important potential sequelae of these lesions. They can be a major cosmetic disaster and may lead to permanent psychological problems.[271] What is more important, these lesions may undergo neoplastic degeneration, usually into melanomas,[272-278] but also into other spindle cell or neuroectodermal tumors.[279] The precise incidence of these changes has been reported as anywhere from 2 to 31% of cases of giant congenital nevi, the lesion most closely associated with melanoma. In the less worrisome small congenital nevi there are no reliable estimates of melanoma incidence.

Several facts appear to be clear in this debate. The lifetime risk of melanoma in patients with a giant congenital nevus is markedly increased and is probably about 5%.[280-282] Lesions on the trunk most commonly regress into melanoma.[278] Melanoma transformation of extremity lesions is very unusual.[259] There have been numerous cases of malignant transformation of small congenital nevi, but the magnitude of the increased incidence is not yet well established. A review of 52 cases studied in Germany supports an increased incidence. In that study, predominantly superficial spreading types of melanoma were seen, and there were no melanomas that occurred under age 18 in those small congenital nevi.[273]

Most experts agree that if feasible, giant congenital nevi should be excised *in toto*, although there are those who believe that the dangers of the operative procedure may outweigh the risks of melanoma. Since 60% of all melanomas that arise from such lesions do so in the first decade of life, most of which are in the first 5 years of life, early excision is warranted, if feasible. More than 50% of these melanomas have a nonepidermal origin, which makes observation alone a difficult way to follow these lesions (Fig. 10.30).[262,266]

A major debate revolves around the approach to small and medium congenital nevi. Advocates of surgical removal of all congenital nevi present the following line of reasoning:[283,284] (1) an association of small congenital NCN and melanoma is significantly greater than expected based on surface area and the prevalence of small congenital nevi; (2) the relative risk of melanoma as determined by retrospective analysis may be increased; and (3) small lesions are easily excised with minimal morbidity, so that even if only a relatively few melanomas are prevented in children, this preventive measure is justified.

The opponents of wholesale excision of all congenital NCN reason as follows:[272] (1) current data on the incidence of melanoma in small lesions are scanty; (2) the criteria for the histologic diagnosis of congenital nevi are not firmly established, so that retrospective analyses of incidence rates are not valid; and (3) the time and expense of removal of all congenital nevi would make it impractical to excise lesions in about 1% of all newborn infants (about 40 000 nevi per year in the United States). Given the risk of general anesthesia that may be necessary to perform excisional surgery in these young children and the small risk of melanoma occurring in a small congenital nevus before puberty, selected lesions could be removed electively under local anesthesia during the early teenage years. The following additional argument has recently been put forward: since almost all small congenital nevi have only a superficial component and the incidence of melanoma in this histologic variety is extremely low, observation alone is sufficient. If removal is contemplated, it can be postponed until puberty, because these lesions do not undergo malignant degeneration prior to that time.[266]

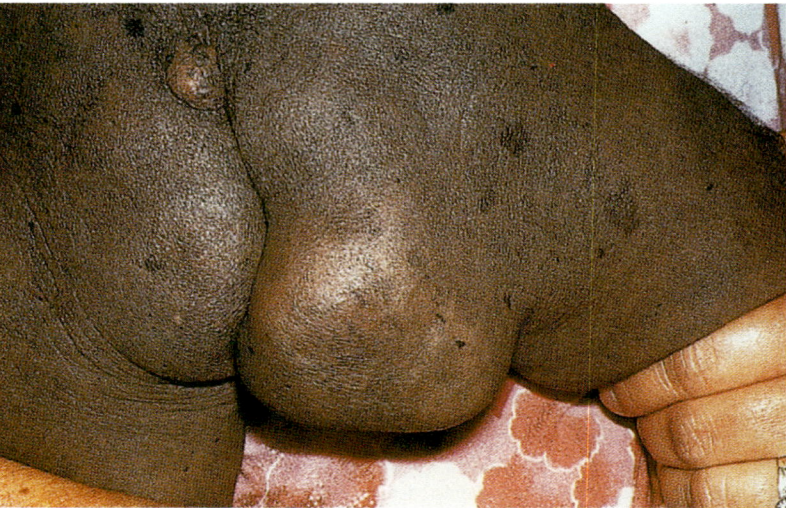

Fig. 10.30 Large malignant melanoma arising medially on the right buttock of a 13-month-old infant. The lesion occurred in the context of a giant congenital nevocellular nevis. It was already metastatic at the time of diagnosis and proved fatal.

After reviewing the data on congenital nevi in 1983, a National Institutes of Health consensus conference concluded that insufficient information is available to recommend prophylactic excision of all congenital nevi. The suggestion is made for periodic examination and biopsy of lesions in which suspicious alteration is noted. There have been no compelling data since that time to alter this recommendation.

Every effort should be made to remove, *in toto*, giant congenital NCN. If possible, surgery should be performed once the child is 6 to 9 months of age,[285] a time when the risks of anesthesia do not outweigh those of the development of melanoma, since melanomas may arise in these lesions even during the first few years of life. The excision must be carried to the deep fascia, because nevus cells may extend to that level. Unfortunately, in some cases, the pigment cells extend deeper into bone, leptomeninges, and other sites, in which case total excision is impractical.[286] There are also instances in which the extent of the melanocytes is so vast that there is insufficient normal skin to cover the defects. Tissue expanders and staged excisions may be the only options in these children. In cases with impossible odds of covering the defect, selective excision of the most abnormal-appearing areas is justified, and careful serial photographic monitoring of untreated areas may be useful. Autologous skin grown in culture may become a feasible alternative for covering large defects after removal of giant lesions.

Many children with a single giant nevus have numerous small pigmented satellite moles. Although there are advocates of surgical removal of all such lesions, there are no reports of any of these nevi regressing to melanoma.

There is no clear consensus as to how to manage large congenital nevi. One suggestion is to perform presurgical diagnostic biopsies to determine

271. Koot HM, de Waard-van der Spek F, Peer CD et al. (2000) Psychosocial sequelae in 29 children with giant congenital melanocytic naevi. **Clin Exp Dermatol** 25:589.
272. Kopf AW, Bart RS, Hennessey P (1979) Congenital nevocytic nevi and malignant melanomas. **J Am Acad Dermatol** 1:123.
273. Illig L, Weidner F, Hundeiker M et al. (1985) Congenital nevi less than or equal to 10cm as precursors to melanoma. 52 cases, a review, and a new conception. **Arch Dermatol** 121:1274.
274. Sharpe RJ, Salasche SJ, Barnhill RL et al. (1990) Nonepidermal origin of cutaneous melanoma in a small congenital nevus. **Arch Dermatol** 126:1559.
275. Paull WH, Polley D, Fitzpatrick JE (1986) Malignant melanoma arising intradermally in a small congenital nevus of an adult. **J Dermatol Surg Oncol** 12:1176.
276. Swerdlow AJ, English JS, Qiao Z (1995) The risk of melanoma in patients with congenital nevi: a cohort study **J Am Acad Dermatol** 32:595.
277. Sahin S, Levin L Kopf AW et al. (1998) Risk of melanoma in medium-sized congenital melanocytic nevi: a follow-up study. **J Am Acad Dermatol** 39:428.
278. Egan CL, Oliveria SA, Elenitsas R et al. (1998) Cutaneous melanoma risk and phenotypic changes in large congenital nevi: a follow-up study of 46 patients. **J Am Acad Dermatol** 39:923.
279. Jerdan MS, Cohen BA, Smith RR et al. (1985) Neuroectodermal neoplasms arising in congenital nevi. **Am J Dermatopathol** 7(Suppl):41.
280. Lorentzen M, Pers M, Bretteville-Jensen G (1977) The incidence of malignant transformation in giant pigmented nevi. **Scand J Plast Reconstr Surg** 11:163.
281. Hendrickson MR, Ross JC (1981) Neoplasms arising in congenital giant nevi: morphologic study of seven cases and a review of the literature. **Am J Surg Pathol** 5:109.
282. Ruiz-Maldonado R, Tamayo L, Laterza AM et al. (1992) Giant pigmented nevi: clinical, histopathologic, and therapeutic considerations. **J Pediatr** 120:906.
283. Rhodes AR, Sober AJ, Day CL et al. (1982) The malignant potential of small congenital nevocellular nevi. An estimate of association based on a histologic study of 234 primary cutaneous melanomas. **J Am Acad Dermatol** 6:230.
284. Solomon LM (1980) The management of congenital melanocytic nevi. **Arch Dermatol** 116:1017.
285. Backman ME, Kopf AW (1986) Iatrogenic effects of general anesthesia in children: considerations in treating large congenital nevocytic nevi. **J Dermatol Surg Oncol** 12:363.
286. Ruiz-Maldonado R, Orozco-Covarrubias ML (1997) Malignant melanoma in children. A review. **Arch Dermatol** 133:363.

the histologic characteristics of the lesion. If the histologic pattern is that of an acquired nevus (superficial variant of congenital nevus), one might consider a plan of watchful waiting rather than surgical excision. If the pattern is one of a dermal tumor, then surgical excision would be indicated.[266]

In those children with extensive scalp or posterior midline nevi, a magnetic resonance imaging (MRI) study should be performed to rule out associated leptomeningeal melanocytosis,[264,265] because the presence of this condition may adversely affect prognosis and may influence subsequent treatment decisions.

Mechanical dermabrasion has been advocated as a method of removing the superficial melanocyte mass and of improving the cosmetic appearance of giant congenital nevi.[287,288] Although improvement in the appearance of the lesion is possible by this method, the bulk of the melanocyte load is deeper in the dermis, hence not affected by this procedure, and the risk of melanoma would still be substantial.

A simple method of partial nevus debulking is the use of curettage alone in the early weeks of life. Apparently, there is a natural cleavage plane in the upper dermis in neonates that makes removal of the superficial melanocytes relatively atraumatic.[289]

Pediatric aspects

The child with a giant congenital nevus presents a challenge to the family and the physician.[271] In certain instances, the parents will reject and even abandon a newborn infant with this condition. Signs of family problems must be detected early to avoid even more emotional trauma in these children. The parents must be given a realistic appraisal of this condition but should be made to understand that most of these children are otherwise completely normal and can live a happy and useful life. Modern plastic surgical techniques can often greatly ameliorate the cosmetic defects in these cases. In addition, the cosmetics industry has developed excellent cover-up make-ups that can hide these lesions fairly well.

The surgical removal of the more common small congenital NCN is usually a routine, single-stage, outpatient procedure and is thus technically feasible in most children. On an individual basis, there is little reason not to suggest removal, if the child or the family is troubled by the lesion. One reasonable approach would be to consider the degree of cosmetic improvement by excision, advise the family of the fact that melanomas have arisen from some lesions, and then make a joint decision based on the degree of concern and wishes of all parties.

Acquired NCN

Most people will develop at least one nevocellular nevus (mole) during the first three decades of life. Reported incidence rates range from 15 to 40 nevi for whites down to two nevi in the average American black person. Nevi have a characteristic natural history. They begin as 2–3-mm tan macules that show a histologic pattern of basal melanocytic proliferation that eventually form nests of nevus cells typical of a darker brown junctional nevus. Nevus cells then migrate into the dermis, which results in a pebbly papule that is a compound nevus with both epidermal and dermal elements. As the nevus ages, the epidermal portion disappears, leaving a intradermal nevus that eventually involutes, usually after age 65. The color may vary from skin-colored to brown or blue–brown to black, depending on the amount and depth of the pigment. Lesional hair may also appear as the moles age.

The number and distribution of NCN may depend on genetic,[290] hormonal,[284] and environmental[291,292] influences. Whites have more moles than Asians or Indo–Pakistanis.[293] Boys tend to have fewer moles than girls and a family history of many nevi is also predictive of an increased number of moles.[294] Hormonal factors have been implicated because the number of moles increases after the onset of puberty and because moles tend to become more prominent during pregnancy. The role of sunlight in NCN appearance is unclear but the number of nevi that a person develops may be strongly influenced by cumulative and/or intermittent intense UV light exposure. For example, nevi do have a predisposition to appear in certain sun-exposed areas such as the lateral arms, as opposed to the sun-protected medial arms.[295] Cancer chemotherapy[296] and immunosuppression after renal allografting[297] have also been associated with an increased number of moles in children.

The characteristic histologic feature of all melanocytic proliferations is the grouping of nevus cells into clusters (thèques), although single cells are also noted. In the deep dermis, spindle-like cells resembling neural elements may be present and may even predominate (neural nevus).

Four special types of NCN are important to recognize and differentiate from cutaneous melanoma. The spindle and epithelioid cell nevus (Spitz nevus, juvenile melanoma) is a benign lesion that usually appears on the extremities or face and may vary in color from brown to red to blue–black. Approximately 60% of Spitz nevi are present before age 14 years, most are less than 1 cm in size, and they almost never ulcerate.[298] These moles are rarely worrisome clinically but may be mistaken for melanoma histologically.[299,300]

Balloon cell nevi appear clinically as ordinary dermal or compound nevi, but are somewhat atypical histologically. Large vesicular cells (balloon cells) predominate in the infiltrate and can be confused with those of a balloon cell melanoma.[301]

Halo nevi usually occur after birth but may appear with congenital lesions in rare cases.[302] Familial cases have been described.[303] The usual history is that of a long-standing pigmented papule that develops a depigmented halo around the margins (Fig. 10.31); the result is often complete regression of the nevus, with only a depigmented macule remaining at the site. Histologic examination of the halo nevus reveals a lymphocytic inflammatory infiltrate that destroys the nevus cells. The halo forms because of the destruction of the normal epidermal melanocytes at the periphery of the lesion.

The pathogenesis of the halo nevus is not completely understood but it is possible that immune mechanisms are involved.[304] These may include antibodies and/or cell-mediated immunity to melanocytes and increased antigen-presenting cells in the depigmented zone. Halo nevi occur relatively commonly in adults with melanomas, again suggesting a host immune response to common antigens in the tumor and the nevus. The halos that appear around melanomas or melanoma metastases differ from benign halo nevi in that the lesion and halo both have irregular margins. Halo nevi also occur commonly in patients with vitiligo, which suggests common pathogenic mechanisms.

287. Chait LA, White B, Skudowitz RB (1981) The treatment of giant hairy naevi by dermabrasion in the first few weeks of life. Case reports. **S Afr Med J** 60:593.
288. Bohn J, Svensson H, Aberg M (2000) Dermabrasion of large congenital melanocytic naevi in neonates. **Scand J Plast Reconstr Surg Hand Surg** 34:321.
289. Moss AL (1987) Congenital "giant" naevus: a preliminary report of a new surgical approach. **Br J Plast Surg** 40:410.
290. Rampen FH, Fleuren BA, de Boo TM et al. (1988) Prevalence of common "acquired" nevocytic nevi and dysplastic nevi is not related to ultraviolet exposure. **J Am Acad Dermatol** 18:679.
291. Kopf AW, Lindsay AC, Rogers GS et al. (1985) Relationship of nevocytic nevi to sun exposure in dysplastic nevus syndrome. **J Am Acad Dermatol** 12:656.
292. Gallagher RP, Rivers JK, Lee TK et al. (2000) Broad-spectrum sunscreen use and the development of new nevi in white children: A randomized controlled trial. **JAMA** 283:2955.
293. Gallagher RP, Rivers JK, Yang CP et al. (1991) Melanocytic nevus density in Asian, Indo-Pakistani, and white children: the Vancouver Mole Study. [see comments]. **J Am Acad Dermatol** 25:507.
294. Green A, Siskind V, Hansen ME et al. (1989) Melanocytic nevi in schoolchildren in Queensland. **J Am Acad Dermatol** 20:1054.
295. Sigg C, Pelloni F (1989) Frequency of acquired melanonevocytic nevi and their relationship to skin complexion in 939 schoolchildren. **Dermatologica** 179:123.
296. Hughes BR, Cunliffe WJ, Bailey CC (1989) Excess benign melanocytic naevi after chemotherapy for malignancy in childhood. **Br Med J** 299:88.
297. Smith CH, McGregor JM, Barker JN et al. (1993) Excess melanocytic nevi in children with renal allografts. **J Am Acad Dermatol** 28:51.
298. Dal Pozzo V, Benelli C, Restano L et al. (1997) Clinical review of 247 case records of Spitz nevus (epithelioid cell and/or spindle cell nevus). **Dermatology** 194:20.
299. Barnhill RL (1998) Childhood melanoma. **Semin Diagn Pathol** 15:189.
300. Orchard DC, Dowling JP, Kelly JW (1997) Spitz naevi misdiagnosed histologically as melanoma: prevalence and clinical profile. **Aust J Dermatol** 38:12.
301. Schrader WA, Helwig EB (1967) Balloon cell nevi. **Cancer** 20:1502.
302. Brownstein MH, Kazam BB, Hashimoto K (1977) Halo congenital nevus. **Arch Dermatol** 113:1572.
303. Herd RM, Hunter JA (1998) Familial halo naevi. **Clin Exp Dermatol** 23:68.
304. Zeff RA, Freitag A, Grin CM et al. (1997) The immune response in halo nevi. **J Am Acad Dermatol** 37:620.

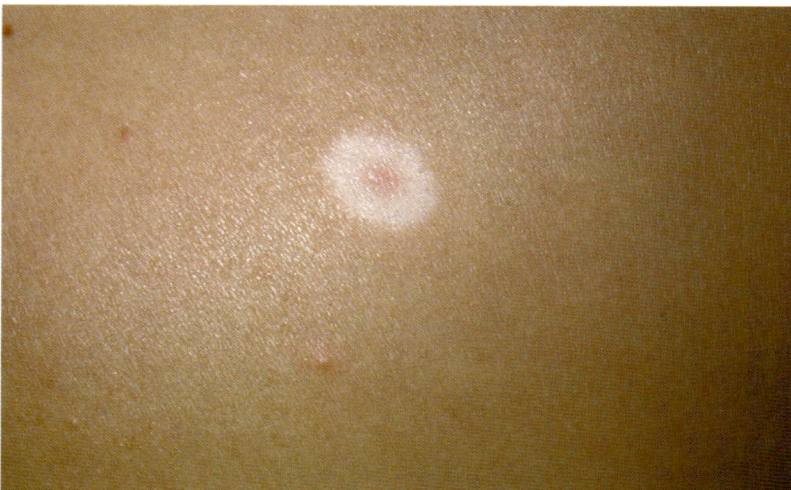

Fig. 10.31   Halo nevus on the upper back. Note the uniform depigmentation around the remnants of the pigmented nevus.

Blue nevi are uncommon in children under age 10 years but can occur later in childhood. They present as discrete blue to blue–gray papules, less than 0.75cm in diameter. Histologically, these lesions are benign infiltrates of dendritic melanocytes, with deep dermal pigment, accounting for the blue color.

Acquired nevi almost always behave in a benign fashion. Although many melanomas arise from preexisting benign moles, the incidence rate is well under 0.1%. Thus, there is little medical justification for the removal of nevi. In those cases in which there are cosmetic considerations or in which there is irritation in a given lesion, excision can be performed. There is no optimum time in childhood to remove these lesions, but a good rule is to wait until the patient is able to give informed consent for the procedure as well as tolerate local anesthesia. Many practitioners prefer to remove nevi by shave excision, which is rapid and almost without morbidity. The only complication of this procedure is that the nevus may recur as a speckled hyperpigmented macule or papule.[305] Complete excision with suture closure is a somewhat more involved procedure but avoids this pitfall and allows for a more certain review of the depth, margins, and histologic characteristics of the lesion. All excised pigmented lesions should be evaluated histologically to rule out melanoma.

Atypical mole (dysplastic nevus)

Dysplastic nevi were described as a clinical entity in 1978[306] but were called other names previously (atypical melanocytic hyperplasia, active junctional nevus). Although initially described as a part of a familial syndrome, the concept has expanded to include sporadic cases with typical clinical and/or histologic features. Although there are those who doubt that this lesion exists,[307] there is general agreement that there is such an entity, which has been renamed *atypical mole* to avoid the controversial issue of dysplasia.[308] The main debates now center on the exact definition, the clinical importance of the lesion, and management of this common problem.

Genetics and epidemiology

The inheritance pattern of the familial atypical mole syndrome (AMS) is autosomal dominant with a high degree of penetrance.[309] There appears to be a linkage of melanoma-prone kindreds to chromosome 9p21 and a correlation between mutations in *CDKN2A*, a gene which encodes p16, and is a cell-cycle inhibitor, with early melanoma in those with atypical moles.[310] The incidence in either sex is approximately equal. Most patients are white, although atypical moles have been seen in other races.

Patients with the familial AMS may also have an underlying hypermutability after injurious stimuli such as UV light, which may be the underlying mechanism that causes benign but atypical moles to regress into melanoma.[311] It has been hypothesized that sun sensitivity deregulates specific genes, which leads to tumor promotion and subsequently to frank melanoma.[312]

During the past 15 years, it has become clear that the vast majority of patients with atypical moles have no obvious familial pattern of inheritance. In fact, at least 5% of Caucasians have at least one clinically diagnosable atypical mole. Depending on the study population and techniques used, it has been estimated that atypical moles occur in 5 to 50% of the white population.[313,314]

History

The clinical and histologic characteristics of both the familial and sporadic types of AMS are similar.[315] The skin of these patients appears normal at birth and during the early years of life. At age 5 to 10 years, small benign-appearing nevi develop, most commonly on the trunk and upper extremities but also on the scalp and buttocks. At the time of puberty, these lesions begin to take on an atypical appearance and new atypical lesions appear *de novo*. One exception to the timing of onset of these lesions is atypical nevi in the scalp that may occur in the first decade in a few children with familial AMS and may be the earliest sign of the emergence of this syndrome in these individuals.[314,316]

Physical examination

Atypical moles have morphologic features of both benign nevi and melanomas. Individual papules are usually 5–15mm in diameter and are round or oval with irregular and indistinct margins. Almost all lesions have a significant macular component, and many have elevation in the center of the mole (Fig. 10.32). The color varies from tan–brown to red–brown with occasional black speckling.[317] The lesions are most common on the posterior trunk and tend to occur in other sun-protected areas of the skin such as over the breasts, on the buttocks, the upper extremities, and on the scalp.[318] The lower extremities are less commonly involved.

Histologic findings

Histopathologic changes are not uniform in all lesions, but at least some of the following findings are present in most atypical moles:[319] (1) features of a benign compound nevus, particularly in the center of the lesion; (2) junctional proliferation of melanocytes with mild to moderate nuclear atypia; (3) lentiginous epithelial proliferation with bridging of adjacent rete pegs; (4) dermal lymphocytic infiltrate; (5) papillary dermal fibroplasia; and

305. Sexton M, Sexton CW (1991) Recurrent pigmented melanocytic nevus. A benign lesion, not to be mistaken for malignant melanoma. **Arch Pathol Lab Med** 115:122.

306. Reimer RR, Clark WH Jr, Greene MH et al. (1978) Precursor lesions in familial melanoma. A new genetic preneoplastic syndrome. **JAMA** 239:744.

307. Ackerman AB (1988) What naevus is dysplastic, a syndrome and the commonest precursor of malignant melanoma? A riddle and an answer. [see comments]. **Histopathology** 13:241.

308. Anonymous (1992) NIH Consensus conference. Diagnosis and treatment of early melanoma. [see comments]. **JAMA** 268:1314.

309. Bale SJ, Chakravarti A, Greene MH (1986) Cutaneous malignant melanoma and familial dysplastic nevi: evidence for autosomal dominance and pleiotropy. **Am J Hum Genet** 38:188.

310. Hashemi J, Linder S, Platz A et al. (1999) Melanoma development in relation to non-functional p16/INK4A protein and dysplastic naevus syndrome in Swedish melanoma kindreds. **Melanoma Res** 9:21.

311. Smith PJ, Greene MH, Devlin DA et al. (1982) Abnormal sensitivity to UV-radiation in cultured skin fibroblasts from patients with hereditary cutaneous malignant melanoma and dysplastic nevus syndrome. **Int J Cancer** 30:39.

312. Holman CD, James IR, Gattey PH et al. (1980) An analysis of trends in mortality from malignant melanoma of the skin in Australia. **Int J Cancer** 26:703.

313. Piepkorn M, Meyer LJ, Goldgar D et al. (1989) The dysplastic melanocytic nevus: a prevalent lesion that correlates poorly with clinical phenotype. **J Am Acad Dermatol** 20:407.

314. Crutcher WA, Sagebiel RW (1984) Prevalence of dysplastic naevi in a community practice. **Lancet** 1:729.

315. Happle R, Traupe H, Vakilzadeh F et al. (1982) Arguments in favor of a polygenic inheritance of precursor nevi. **J Am Acad Dermatol** 6:540.

316. Fernandez M, Raimer SS, Sanchez RL (2001) Dysplastic nevi of the scalp and forehead in children. **Pediatr Dermatol** 18:5.

317. Kim JC, Murphy GF (2000) Dysplastic melanocytic nevi and prognostically indeterminate nevomelanomatoid proliferations. **Clin Lab Med** 20:691.

318. Rhodes AR, Weinstock MA, Fitzpatrick TB et al. (1987) Risk factors for cutaneous melanoma. A practical method of recognizing predisposed individuals. **JAMA** 258:3146.

319. Elder DE, Green MH, Guerry D et al. (1982) The dysplastic nevus syndrome: our definition. **Am J Dermatopathol** 4:455.

(6) dermal telangiectases. There is no invasion of atypical melanocytes into the upper epidermis or into the dermis.

Two recent reports cast doubt on whether there is a real clinicopathologic entity of atypical mole. In both studies, there was a poor correlation between clinical atypia and histologic dysplasia.[320,321] The conclusion of one of the studies was that the atypical mole syndrome should be defined by clinical features alone, because of the poor sensitivity and specificity of the histologic features.[321]

Atypical moles and melanoma

The relationship between familial AMS and melanoma appears to be a close one, and the data supporting the concept of these lesions as melanoma precursors are compelling:[319] (1) atypical moles are found in more than 90% of patients with hereditary melanoma and in up to 13% of sporadic melanoma patients; (2) in families with familial melanoma in which two or more family members have had a melanoma, first-degree relatives with atypical moles have virtually a 100% incidence of melanoma, whereas those family members with no atypical moles do not have excess melanoma risk;[322] (3) atypical moles commonly occur

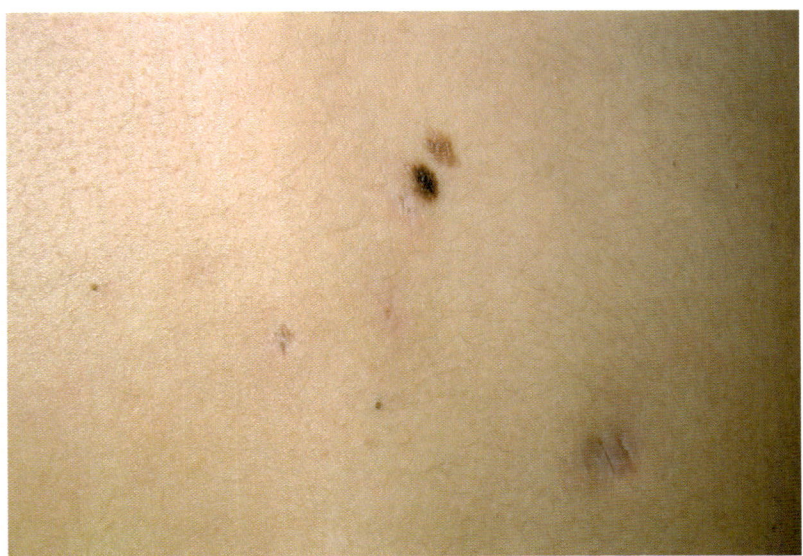

Fig. 10.32 Atypical mole (dysplastic nevus). Note that the lesion is larger than 0.5cm in diameter and has a feathered flat edge.

in contiguity with malignant melanomas;[323] and (4) melanomas have arisen from previously stable atypical moles. This was emphasized in a study where 11 new melanomas arose in 11 patients with atypical moles after an average of only 61 months.[324] A classification of AMS is based on these findings[325] (Table 10.4).

An atypical mole is a common occurrence whereas melanoma is relatively unusual. There appears to be a differential risk of developing this tumor depending on genetic factors. The child with a few atypical moles and no family history may be in no greater jeopardy of a melanoma than one with many normal NCN,[266,326–328] a fair complexion, and a propensity to burn easily. At the other end of the spectrum, the child with atypical moles and two parents who have had a melanoma can expect to suffer this fate sometime in life. Thus atypical moles appear to be both a marker for one at risk for melanoma and a precursor lesion in some cases.

Differential diagnosis

The differential diagnosis of the atypical mole includes two entities, one on the benign end and one on the malignant end of the nevus–melanoma spectrum. Benign acquired nevi are usually smaller (less than 6mm), have very regular borders with sharp margination, and are notably uniform in color as opposed to the irregular margination and hue of atypical moles. Melanomas have a number of common features with atypical moles but often have more grossly irregular margins with geographic shapes and very indistinct borders. They are multicolored and may have shades of red, white, and blue in the same lesion. There are instances where the ABCDs of melanoma fit the description of an atypical nevus perfectly (see below).

Therapeutics

When a child is diagnosed as having AMS it is important to examine all first-degree relatives over age 10 years for evidence of familial involvement. One does this not only to identify other people at risk for melanoma but also to help classify the child as having the familial or sporadic type.

Children with familial AMS should be thoroughly examined by a physician every 6–12 months. Examination for scalp lesions is facilitated by a hair dryer set on the coolest temperature. These children should be encouraged to protect their skin from excess sun exposure and to use sunscreens on a daily basis, since sunlight may promote the growth of these lesions because of possible increased susceptibility to UV-induced cellular damage in these patients.[311]

The responsibility for detecting changing moles should be borne in part by the patient and the family. Self-examination every 1–2 months may uncover early changes in moles that herald the progression to melanoma.

In patients with few atypical moles, surgical excision is easy but not indicated since patients continue to develop new lesions throughout life

TABLE 10.4   Classification of atypical mole syndrome

	Genetics	Incidence	Clinical findings
Group A	Sporadic	High	No melanoma family history, low melanoma rate
Group B	Familial	Moderate	No melanoma family history, melanoma risk fairly low
Group C	Sporadic	Low	Personal history of melanoma, no melanoma family history, moderate melanoma risk
Group D-1	Familial	Very low	One family member with melanoma, high melanoma risk
Group D-2	Familial	Very low	Two or more close family members with melanoma, very high melanoma risk

(Data from Kraemer *et al.*[325])

320. Knoell KA, Hendrix JD, Jr, Patterson JW et al. (1997) Nonpigmented dysplastic melanocytic nevi. **Arch Dermatol** 133:992.
321. Annessi G, Cattaruzza MS, Abeni D et al. (2001) Correlation between clinical atypia and histologic dysplasia in acquired melanocytic nevi. **J Am Acad Dermatol** 45:77.
322. Kraemer KH, Greene MH, Tarone R et al. (1983) Dysplastic naevi and cutaneous melanoma risk. **Lancet** 2:1076.
323. Rhodes AR, Harrist TJ, Day CL et al. (1983) Dysplastic melanocytic nevi in histologic association with 234 primary cutaneous melanomas. **J Am Acad Dermatol** 9:563.
324. Halpern AC, Guerry DT, Elder DE et al. (1993) A cohort study of melanoma in patients with dysplastic nevi. **J Invest Dermatol** 100:346S.
325. Kraemer KH, Tucker M, Tarone R et al. (1986) Risk of cutaneous melanoma in dysplastic nevus syndrome types A and B. **N Engl J Med** 315:1615.
326. Grob JJ, Gouvernet J, Aymar D et al. (1990) Count of benign melanocytic nevi as a major indicator of risk for nonfamilial nodular and superficial spreading melanoma. **Cancer** 66:387.
327. Tucker MA, Halpern A, Holly EA et al. (1997) Clinically recognized dysplastic nevi. A central risk factor for cutaneous melanoma. **JAMA** 277:1439.
328. Schneider JS, Moore DH 2nd, Sagebiel RW (1994) Risk factors for melanoma incidence in prospective follow-up. The importance of atypical (dysplastic) nevi. **Arch Dermatol** 130:1002.

and because the presence of these moles may merely identify children at risk; removal of the moles would not change that situation. In patients with numerous atypical moles, surgical removal is impractical.[308] Serial photographic documentation of the lesions will aid in identifying changes, but in most situations is impractical. Only those lesions that suggest melanoma should be biopsied. There are exceptions to this rule. Atypical moles of the scalp may be removed prophylactically if there is difficulty in monitoring them under a head of hair.

Pediatric aspects

The prognosis in children with even the familial variety of AMS should be very favorable with close follow-up examinations. If lesions progress to melanoma, the vast majority are curable with local excision. Families should be aware of the potential impact of this disease but should not treat these children any differently than unaffected siblings. Cancer phobia is avoidable if the family understands the minimal impact that atypical moles make on the life of the child.

MELANOMA

Epidemiology

Melanoma in childhood is a rare event, representing only 2% of the total melanoma experience,[329,330] and only 3% of the malignant tumors of childhood.[259] In the absence of a congenital nevus or xeroderma pigmentosum it is very rare in the first decade of life.[259,331–333] There are case reports of congnital melanoma resulting from either transplacental spread from maternal melanoma or early malignant degeneration of a congenital nevus.[334] The incidence of melanoma increases somewhat during teenage years and is more common in girls after the onset of puberty.[331,332,335]

Several risk factors influence the development of melanoma.[318,336,337] A very important and easily recognizable one is the number of nevi, either as counted on the arm,[338] or over the entire body.[323,325,339] Other factors noted with increased frequency in children who ultimately develop melanoma include an inability to tan, susceptibility to sunburn, high sun exposure,[337] red hair color,[259] family history of melanoma,[327] the presence of giant congenital nevi, the presence of nevi of the iris, a history of xeroderma pigmentosum, and prolonged immunodeficiency.[259]

History

Children with melanoma usually present with an asymptomatic pigmented lesion that has recently changed. These may occur in any location but are most common in the head and neck region, trunk, and lower extremities, excluding the feet.[340]

Physical examination

Melanoma may present in a number of patterns but there are general guidelines that will help in making the clinical diagnosis (Fig. 10.33). The "ABCD rule" has been devised as a mnemonic in remembering the key features. Although this is not a very sensitive tool, it is a fairly useful guideline for melanoma detection (Table 10.5).

The technique of epiluminescence has been touted as being valuable in clinically differentiating melanoma from its look-alike such as nevus,

seborrheic keratosis, and hemangioma.[341] This is very operator dependent and requires a great deal of experience before one can reliably use this method. Immersion oil is applied to the skin surface and the lesion is then viewed through a magnifying lens. Fairly specific changes can be seen in many melanomas.

Pathophysiology and histogenesis

There are four melanoma clinical subtypes, each having a characteristic biologic behavior. Superficial spreading melanoma is the most common type in children, as in adults. These malignancies have a relatively long phase of radial growth wherein they grow laterally before penetrating deeper into the dermis and assuming the ominous vertical growth phase. When one sees a papule or nodule in a broad melanotic plaque, the nodule represents a focal site of deeper invasion of a previously superficial tumor.

A nodular melanoma has a relatively short radial growth phase before deep invasion (Fig.10.34). Thus, these lesions are usually narrower than superficial spreading tumors but develop nodularity much sooner in the course. Melanomas arising in giant congenital nevi are usually the nodular variety.

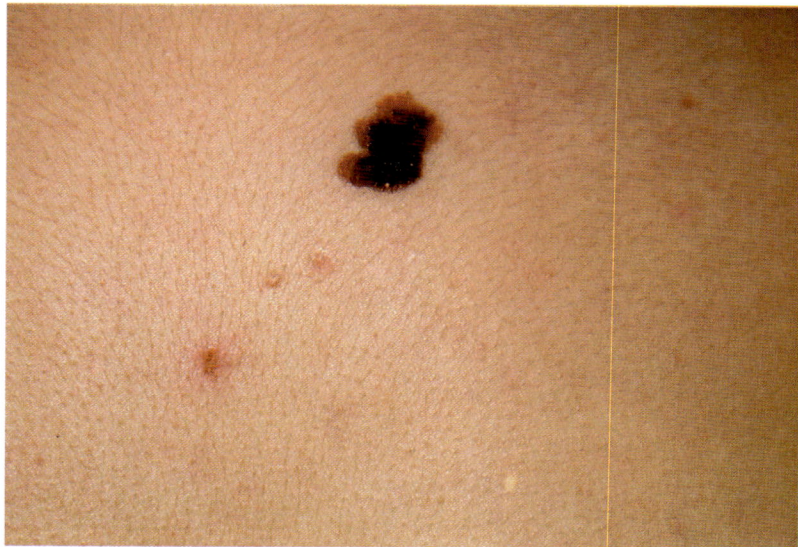

Fig. 10.33 Melanoma of the upper back. There is an irregular border and red and blue hues arranged haphazardly throughout the lesion.

TABLE 10.5   Clinical diagnosis of melanoma

Asymmetry of lesional contour
Border irregularity
Color variation, particularly red, white, and blue
Diameter of lesion that is greater than 0.6cm

329. Bader JL, Li FP, Olmstead PM et al. (1985) Childhood malignant melanoma. Incidence and etiology. **Am J Pediatr Hematol Oncol** 7:341.
330. Whiteman D, Valery P, McWhirter W et al. (1995) Incidence of cutaneous childhood melanoma in Queensland, Australia. **Int J Cancer** 63:765.
331. Temple WJ, Mulloy RH, Alexander F et al. (1991) Childhood melanoma. **J Pediatr Surg** 26:135.
332. Mackie RM, Watt D, Doherty V et al. (1991) Malignant melanoma occurring in those aged under 30 in the west of Scotland 1979–1986: a study of incidence, clinical features, pathological features and survival. **Br J Dermatol** 124:560.
333. Boddie AW, Jr, Smith JL Jr, McBride CM (1978) Malignant melanoma in children and young adults: effect of diagnostic criteria on staging and end results. **South Med J** 71:1074.
334. Baader W, Kropp R, Tapper D (1992) Congenital malignant melanoma. **Plast Reconstr Surg** 90:53.

335. Saenz NC, Saenz-Badillos J, Busam K et al. (1999) Childhood melanoma survival. **Cancer** 85:750.
336. Tucker MA, Fraser MC, Goldstein AM et al. (1993) Risk of melanoma and other cancers in melanoma-prone families. **J Invest Dermatol** 100:350S.
337. Autier P, Dore JF (1998) Influence of sun exposures during childhood and during adulthood on melanoma risk. EPIMEL and EORTC Melanoma Cooperative Group. European Organisation for Research and Treatment of Cancer. **Int J Cancer** 77:533.
338. Elwood JM, Williamson C, Stapleton PJ (1986) Malignant melanoma in relation to moles, pigmentation, and exposure to fluorescent and other lighting sources. **Br J Cancer** 53:65.
339. Holly EA, Kelly JW, Shpall SN et al. (1987) Number of melanocytic nevi as a major risk factor for malignant melanoma. **J Am Acad Dermatol** 17:459.
340. Pratt CB, Palmer MK, Thatcher N et al. (1981) Malignant melanoma in children and adolescents. **Cancer** 47:392.
341. Kenet RO, Kang S, Kenet BJ et al. (1993) Clinical diagnosis of pigmented lesions using digital epiluminescence microscopy. Grading protocol and atlas. **Arch Dermatol** 129:157.

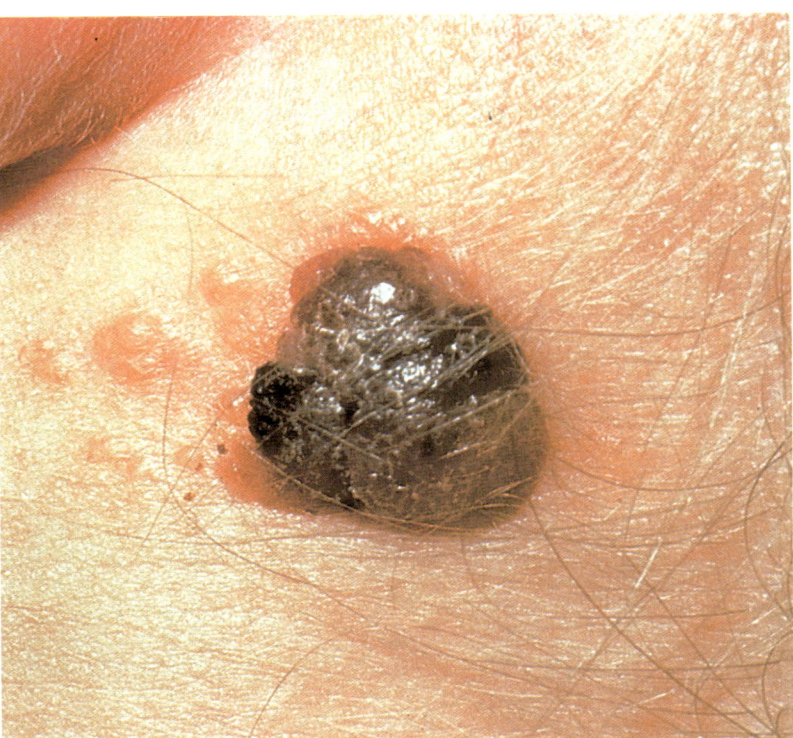

Fig. 10.34 Nodular melanoma arising in mastoid area in a 10-year-old girl. (Reprinted with permission from Wyatt AJ, Hansen RC, Pediatric Skin Tumors. Ped Clin NAM. Philadelphia: Saunders, vol 47, 2000, p. 953.)

Acral lentiginous melanomas are very rare in children but are the most common variety in pigmented races.[342] These aggressive tumors appear on the palms, soles, or mucous membranes, and have a short radial growth phase before vertical extension. The fourth variety of melanoma, lentigo maligna melanoma, does not occur in children. This slow-growing tumor arises in a premalignant lesion, lentigo maligna, which appears on the sun-exposed skin of older people.

The histologic features of all melanoma subtypes have a similar degree of melanocytic cellular atypia. However, the real importance of histologic examination, even in clinically obvious melanomas, is that prognosis is directly related to depth of invasion of the tumor cells. Clark first noted that tumors confined to the papillary dermis have an excellent prognosis, whereas patients having tumors that penetrate deep into the reticular dermis tend to do poorly. He assigned levels I to V to correlate prognosis with invasion.[343] Breslow quantified this relationship by noting that tumors less than 0.76mm in thickness were almost always cured, and melanomas 0.76 to 3.65mm in thickness had an intermediate prognosis, whereas thicker tumors were associated with a very poor outcome.[344]

Subsequently, a number of different prognostic breakpoints have been described associating tumor thickness with the length of survival. A newly proposed system eliminates Clark's level of invasion and changes survival stratification cutoffs to the following: (a) thin melanomas are less than 1mm in thickness, (b) intermediate thickness melanomas are between 1 and 4mm in thickness, and (c) thick melanomas are greater than 4mm in thickness. Ulceration is added as a separate prognostic variable and the number of lymph nodes involved is given more power than the degree of involvement of individual nodes.[345]

Tumor thickness is the most accurate indicator of prognosis. Childhood and adult melanomas appear to behave in a similar way in this regard.[346] Rough averages for survival would be the following: tumors less than 1mm in thickness (90–93% survival rate); melanomas less than 1.5mm in thickness (85% survival rate); tumors that are between 1.5 and 4mm in thickness (70–77% survival rate); melanomas greater than 4mm in thickness (35–40% survival rate). The rates cited here are 5-year survival figures; even very thin tumors can produce recurrences and metastases as long as 15 years after the excision of the primary lesion.[347] Hence, 5-year survival statistics are insufficient to describe adequately melanoma behavior.

Differential diagnosis

The differential diagnosis of melanoma includes other pigmented skin lesions, including acquired nevus, irritated wart or seborrheic keratosis, and traumatic ecchymosis. The irregularity of shape, surface, and color is usually greater in melanomas than in these other processes, but sometimes one cannot make a clinical diagnosis with certainty. If melanoma is in the differential diagnosis, an excisional biopsy should be performed, if possible, so that an assessment of maximal thickness of the lesion can be made. If the lesion cannot be excised *in toto*, a diagnostic punch biopsy of the most nodular area of the tumor should be taken. Shave biopsies of suspected melanomas should be avoided because of the difficulty in determining the thickness of the tumor with this method.

Therapeutics and prognosis

The treatment of primary melanoma is excisional surgery. In the last several years, a definite move toward more conservative procedures has evolved.[348–351] It is evident that thin melanomas have an excellent prognosis even in cases in which only minimal clear surgical margins are taken and that visceral metastases ordinarily reflect subclinical tumor deposits in distant sites at the time of resection of the primary tumor. Most surgeons recommend a 1-cm margin around melanomas thinner than 1mm. This is probably an adequate margin for lesions up to 2mm in thickness. For tumors greater than 2mm in thickness, a 2-cm margin with primary closure if possible is suggested.[266]

The idea of regional lymph node dissection in melanoma is controversial. One large study showed benefit only in those cases with tumors of intermediate thickness,[352] while another study suggested no benefit at all in immediate regional node dissection.[353] Before choosing a course of action, the risks of this procedure[354] must be weighed against the perceived benefit and the patient and the family must be informed of the level of uncertainty that surrounds this issue.

The technology of selective sentinal node biopsy has improved the sensitivity of regional node sampling. The technique involves identifying and biopsying only the first draining node in a given lymph node chain. If the node is free of tumor, it is highly unlikely that other nodes in that chain are

342. Krementz ET, Sutherland CM, Carter RD et al. (1976) Malignant melanoma in the American Black. **Ann Surg** 183:533.
343. Clark WH, Jr, From L, Bernardino EA et al. (1969) The histogenesis and biologic behavior of primary human malignant melanomas of the skin. **Cancer Res** 29:705.
344. Breslow A (1975) Tumor thickness, level of invasion and node dissection in stage I cutaneous melanoma. **Ann Surg** 182:572.
345. Balch CM, Buzaid AC, Soong SJ et al. (2001) Final version of the American Joint Committee on Cancer staging system for cutaneous melanoma. **J Clin Oncol** 19:3635.
346. Gibbs P, Moore A, Robinson W et al. (2000) Pediatric melanoma: are recent advances in the management of adult melanoma relevant to the pediatric population. **J Pediatr Hematol/Oncol** 22:428.
347. Crowley NJ, Seigler HP (1990) Late recurrence of malignant melanoma. Analysis of 168 patients. **Ann Surg** 212:173.
348. Heenan PJ, English DR, Holman CD (1993) The effects of surgical treatment on survival and local recurrence of cutaneous malignant melanoma. **Cancer** 71:3792.

349. Fallowfield ME, Cook MG (1992) Re-excisions of scar in primary cutaneous melanoma: a histopathological study. **Br J Dermatol** 126:47.
350. Balch CM, Soong SJ, Smith T et al. (2001) Long-term results of a prospective surgical trial comparing 2cm vs. 4cm excision margins for 740 patients with 1–4mm melanomas. **Ann Surg Oncol** 8:101.
351. Zitelli JA, Brown CD, Hanusa BH (1997) Surgical margins for excision of primary cutaneous melanoma. **J Am Acad Dermatol** 37:422.
352. Balch CM (1980) Surgical management of regional lymph nodes in cutaneous melanoma. **J Am Acad Dermatol** 3:511.
353. Veronesi U, Adamus J, Bandiera DC et al. (1982) Delayed regional lymph node dissection in stage I melanoma of the skin of the lower extremities. **Cancer** 49:2420.
354. Urist MM, Maddox WA, Kennedy JE et al. (1983) Patient risk factors and surgical morbidity after regional lymphadenectomy in 204 melanoma patients. **Cancer** 51:2152.

positive.[355,356] However, it is still unclear what the therapeutic implications of a positive sentinal node are; thus this procedure should be viewed as a prognostic tool only, until therapeutic interventions based on the sentinal node biopsy result can be shown to be beneficial.[266]

In cases of limited recurrent local disease or a solitary metastasis, surgical excision is sometimes performed. In widespread metastatic disease, there is no curative therapy, although local radiation and chemotherapy, and biologic response modifiers such as cytokines and retinoids occasionally offer short-term palliation.[357,358] Interferon may be useful in select cases,[359,360] but the issue of long-term survival with this modality is still not settled.[266,361]

A potentially exciting development in the therapy for high-risk melanomas is vaccines[362] where the patient is immunized with tumor antigens from one of several different sources. Preliminary reports suggest that some patients do develop delayed-type hypersensitivity to these preparations, and perhaps these people have a more prolonged course.[363] Although there is not yet a clinically effective vaccine available for general use, many competing technologies are under active development.

Pediatric aspects

A diagnosis of melanoma in a child is a devastating development for the whole family. Since melanoma before the age of 15 years is rare, it may be prudent to have the biopsy of a suspected melanoma interpreted by several dermatopathologists before a definitive answer is given. Spitz nevi occur far more commonly in this age group than do melanomas; biopsies of this entity are occasionally very difficult to differentiate from melanoma. The short delay that is entailed in sending the biopsy specimen to several experts is worth the time in equivocal lesions.

Long-term follow-up of children with melanomas is essential for two reasons. Patients with a history of one melanoma are more likely to develop a second primary tumor. In addition, careful observation indefinitely may be necessary for one to be absolutely certain of a clinical cure.

355. Morton DL, Wen DR, Wong JH et al. (1992) Technical details of intraoperative lymphatic mapping for early stage melanoma. **Arch Surg** 127:392.
356. Leong SP, Steinmetz I, Habib FA et al. (1997) Optimal selective sentinel lymph node dissection in primary malignant melanoma. **Arch Surg** 132:666.
357. Mc Clay EF, Mastrangelo MJ (1988) Systemic chemotherapy for metastatic melanoma. **Semin Oncol** 15:569.
358. Rosenberg SA, Lotze MT, Mule JJ (1988) NIH conference. New approaches to the immunotherapy of cancer using interleukin-2. **Ann Intern Med** 108:853.
359. Kirkwood JM, Strawderman MH, Ernstoff MS et al. (1996) Interferon alfa-2b adjuvant therapy of high-risk resected cutaneous melanoma: the Eastern Cooperative Oncology Group Trial EST 1684. **J Clin Oncol** 14:7.
360. Kirkwood JM, Ibrahim JG, Sosman JA et al. (2001) High-dose interferon alfa-2b significantly prolongs relapse-free and overall survival compared with the GM2-KLH/QS-21 vaccine in patients with resected stage IIB–III melanoma: results of intergroup trial E1694/S9512/C509801. **J Clin Oncol** 19:2370.
361. Kirkwood JM, Ibrahim JG, Sondak VK et al. (2000) High- and low-dose interferon alfa-2b in high-risk melanoma: first analysis of intergroup trial E1690/S9111/C9190. **J Clin Oncol** 18:2444.
362. Tartaglia J, Bonnet MC, Berinstein N et al. (2001) Therapeutic vaccines against melanoma and colorectal cancer. **Vaccine** 19:2571.
363. Oratz R, Bystryn JC (1991) Immunotherapy of malignant melanoma. **Dermatol Clin** 9:669.

Hair Disorders

Maureen Rogers and Yong-Kwang Tay

HAIR DISORDERS

Maureen Rogers

Hair is a protein by-product of follicles that are distributed everywhere on the human body surface except the palms, soles, vermilion portion of the lips, glans penis, nail beds, and sides of the fingers and toes. Although hair is of minimal functional benefit to humans and hair disorders are not in themselves dangerous, the cosmetic and associated psychological consequences of hair growth abnormalities are frequently a source of great concern to children and adolescents, and their parents.

Hair follicle anatomy and hair growth are covered in Chapter 1. Neonatal hair patterns, the neonatal hair cycle and postnatal alopecia are covered in Chapter 6.

Although the terms lanugo and vellus are frequently used synonymously, lanugo hairs, except in the rare hereditary syndrome hypertrichosis lanuginosa, are seen only in fetal and neonatal life. They are fine, soft, unmedullated, and poorly pigmented, and they appear as a fine dense growth over the entire cutaneous surface of the fetal infant. Lanugo hair is normally shed *in utero* during the seventh or eighth month of gestation but may cover the entire cutaneous surface of the newborn premature infant. Postnatal hair may be divided into vellus and terminal types. Vellus hairs are the fine, short, non-medullated and lightly pigmented hairs seen on the arms and faces of children and faces of women. Terminal hairs are thicker, longer, pigmented and usually medullated. Terminal hairs occur only in the scalp, eyebrows, and eyelashes in prepubertal children. Post-pubertally vellus follicles convert to terminal follicles in many areas of the body, in particular areas of secondary sexual hair distribution.

CONGENITAL OR EARLY ONSET ALOPECIA

The term alopecia is used here as a general term for sparseness of hair. Alopecia that is present at birth or in the early months of life may be diffuse or localized. Diffuse alopecia may be partial (hypotrichosis) or complete (atrichia). Because of the very variable amount of hair present in neonates the diagnosis of diffuse alopecias may be delayed for some time. In addition there are several conditions, in particular the hair shaft abnormalities, in which there is normal neonatal hair that is replaced by the abnormal fragile hair only after several months.

CONGENITAL DIFFUSE ATRICHIA OR HYPOTRICHOSIS

Diffuse congenital or early-onset hypotrichosis (sparse hair) or atrichia (absence of hair) may occur alone or with other minor cutaneous abnormalities, may be associated with other abnormalities as part of a variety of syndromes, and may occur in some of the genetic hair shaft abnormalities which will be discussed elsewhere in this chapter.

HYPOTRICHOSIS OCCURRING ALONE OR WITH OTHER MINOR ABNORMALITIES

Isolated congenital atrichia or hypotrichosis

There are several distinct genotypes within this group, with recessive, dominant and X-linked inheritance patterns being represented.[1–5] The recessively inherited ones are in general the most severe and are of congenital onset. In some pedigrees there is total absence of hair and no hair follicles are found on biopsy. In others the hair is present but extremely sparse, with biopsy demonstrating a few scattered, miniaturized follicles. Due in part to the persistence of neonatal hair and also to the variability of hair cover in young children the extent of the hypotrichosis may not be evident until the child is several years old.[6] In most cases, the condition involves eyebrow, eyelash and general body hair also. In one family with recessive inheritance, the gene has been mapped to chromosome 8p.[5] In one autosomal dominant form, involving the scalp only, the gene has been mapped to chromosome 6p21.3.[7]

Marie Unna hypotrichosis

This is an autosomal dominant condition in which the hair is usually sparse or absent at birth.[8] In early childhood, characteristic coarse, wiry hair appears, showing irregularly distributed twisting and longitudinal ridging on microscopy. Scalp biopsy demonstrates multiple, small hair follicles budding from the epidermis and from the outer root sheath of the few normal follicles present.[9]

1. Baden HP, Kubilus J (1980) Analysis of hair from alopecia congenita. **J Am Acad Dermatol** 3:623–626.
2. Ahmad M, Abbas H, Haque S (1993) Alopecia universalis as a single abnormality in an inbred Pakistani kindred. **Am J Med Genet** 46:369–371.
3. Pinheiro M, Freire-Maia N (1985) Atrichias and hypotrichoses; a brief review with description of a recessive atrichia in two brothers. **Hum Hered** 35:53–55.
4. Kenue RK, al-Dhafri KS (1994) Isolated congenital atrichia in an Omani kindred. **Dermatology** 188:72–75.
5. Nothen MM, Cichon S, Vogt IR et al. (1998) A gene for congenital alopecia maps to chromosome 8p21–22. **Am J Hum Genet** 62:386–390.
6. De Berker D (1998) Congenital hypotrichosis. **Int J Dermatol** 38(Suppl 1):25–33.
7. Betz RC, Lee Y-A, Bygum A et al. (2000) A gene for hypotrichosis simplex of the scalp maps to chromosome 6p21.3. **Am J Hum Genet** 66:1979–1983.
8. Peachey RDG, Wells RS (1971) Hereditary hypotrichosis (Marie Unna type). **Trans St John's Hosp Dermatol Soc** 57:157–166.
9. Mallon E, Dawber RPR, Dover R et al. (1995) Marie-Unna hypotrichosis – histopathology findings and pathogenesis. **Br J Dermatol** 133(supplement 45):55.

Atrichia with papular lesions

This is a distinctive association of congenital atrichia and small, white papular lesions.[10–12] Scalp atrichia may be present from birth or appear in early childhood. In most cases the normal neonatal hair is shed in the first three months of life and is never replaced;[13] involvement of eyebrows and eyelashes is variable. The papular lesions, which occur diffusely but predominate on the face and scalp, are not present in the neonatal period. A recent histo-pathological study[12] showed the papules to represent keratin-filled follicular cysts. There were tubular epithelial structures devoid of hair bulbs, but demonstrating sebaceous and outer root sheath differentiation, extending from the epidermis to the deep dermis, resembling epidermoid cysts. Recent work has demonstrated molecular homologies between the mutated gene in these patients and the mouse hairless gene.[14,15]

Congenital hypotrichosis and milia

This condition bears some clinical similarity to atrichia with papular lesions. There is hypotrichosis with sparse, coarse hair. Multiple milia are present at birth on the face and sometimes also limbs and trunk. Study of a large pedigree suggests X-linked dominant inheritance.[16]

HYPOTRICHOSIS WITH ECTODERMAL DYSPLASIAS

Hypotrichosis is an important feature in many of the ectodermal dysplasia syndromes but often becomes obvious only after the neonatal period. A selection of conditions in which there may be congenital severe atrichia or hypotrichosis[17–25] is listed in Table 11.1. Ectodermal dysplasias will be discussed in more detail elsewhere.

HYPOTRICHOSIS WITH ICHTHYOSES

Ichthyoses presenting as the "collodion baby" phenotype

The hair is often either absent or shed in the early weeks of life with the membrane in this group of conditions, which includes autosomal recessive and

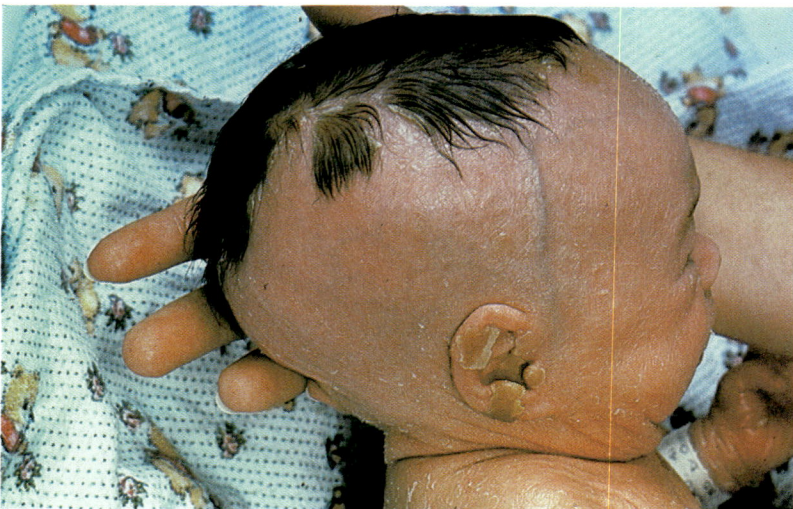

Fig. 11.1   Alopecia in an infant with lamellar ichthyosis; the hair is caught up in the large plates of scale and shed.

autosomal dominant forms of lamellar ichthyosis, congenital ichthyosiform erythroderma, and lamellar ichthyosis of the newborn (self-healing collodion baby).

Lamellar ichthyosis

Alopecia often occurs in this condition as a result of hair being caught up in and shed with the large plates of scale which exfoliate from the scalp. Hair loss may also occur as a result of secondary bacterial infection (Figs 11.1, 11.2).

Ichthyosis follicularis, congenital atrichia and photophobia (IFAP)

From birth these individuals demonstrate atrichia or severe hypotrichosis, keratotic follicular papules and photophobia.[26,27] There are reports in some cases of periorificial erosions and keratotic plaques, nail dystrophy, gingival erythema and recurrent infections suggesting that this condition and hereditary mucoepithelial dysplasia[28] may be the same condition.[29] However, hereditary mucoepithelial dysplasia is believed to be autosomal-dominant whereas the finding of Blaschko-distributed lesions in mothers and sisters of boys with IFAP suggests that this is, in at least some pedigrees, an X-linked trait.[30] In other pedigrees an autosomal-dominant inheritance seems to be operating.[31]

TABLE 11.1   Ectodermal dysplasias in which there is severe neonatal hypotrichosis

- Hidrotic ectodermal dysplasia[17]
- Hypohidrotic ectodermal dysplasia[18,19]
- Ankyloblepharon, ectodermal dysplasia and clefting syndrome (AEC, Hay Wells) and Rapp–Hodgkin syndrome[20–23]
- Bazex–Dupre–Christol syndrome[24]
- Congenital atrichia with nail dystrophy, abnormal facies and retarded psychomotor development[25]

---

10. Lowenthal LJA, Prakken JR (1961) Atrichia with papular lesions. **Dermatologica** 122:85–89.
11. Delprat A, Bonafe JL, Lugardon Y (1994) Atrichie congenitale avec kystes. **Ann Dermatol Venereol** 121:802–804.
12. Misciali C, Tosti A, Fanti PA et al. (1992) Atrichia and papular lesions: Report of a case. **Dermatology** 185:284–288.
13. Miller L, Loffreda M, Lyle S et al. (1998) Atrichia with papules. Presented at the Second Intercontinental Hair Research Societies' Meeting, Washington, DC, November 6, 1998.
14. Ahmad W, Haque M, Brancolini V et al. (1998) Alopecia universalis associated with a mutation in the human hairless gene. **Science** 279:720–724.
15. Sundberg JP, Price VH, King LE (1999) The "hairless" gene in mouse and man. **Arch Dermatol** 135:718–720.
16. Rapelanoro R, Taieb A, Lacombe D (1994) Congenital hypotrichosis and milia: report of a large family suggesting X-linked dominant inheritance. **Am J Med Genet** 52:487–490.
17. McNaughton PZ, Pierson DL, Rodman OG (1976) Hidrotic ectodermal dysplasia in a black mother and daughter. **Arch Dermatol** 112:1448–1450.
18. Rajagopalan K, Tay CH (1997) Hidrotic ectodermal dysplasia: study of a large Chinese pedigree. **Arch Dermatol** 113:481–485.
19. Clarke A, Phillips DIM, Brown R et al. (1987) Clinical aspects of X-linked hypohidrotic ectodermal dysplasia. **Arch Dis Child** 62:989–996.
20. Vanderhooft SL, Stephan MJ, Sybert VP (1993) Severe skin erosions and scalp infections in AEC syndrome. **Pediatr Dermatol** 10:334–340.
21. Felding IB, Bjorklund LJ (1990) Rapp–Hodgkin ectodermal dysplasia. **Pediatr Dermatol** 7:126–131.

22. Camacho F, Ferrando J, Pichardo AR et al. (1993) Rapp–Hodgkin syndrome with pili canaliculi. **Pediatr Dermatol** 10:54–57.
23. Cambiaghi S, Tadini G, Barbareschi M et al. (1994) Rapp–Hodgkin syndrome and AEC syndrome: are they the same entity? **Br J Dermatol** 130:97–101.
24. Goetyn M, Geerts M-L, Kint A et al. (1994) The Bazex–Dupre–Christol syndrome. **Arch Dermatol** 130:337–342.
25. Vogt BR, Traupe H, Hamm H (1988) Congenital atrichia with nail dystrophy, abnormal facies and retarded psychomotor development in two siblings: A new autosomal recessive syndrome? **Pediatr Dermatol** 5:236–242.
26. Keyavani K, Paulus W, Traupe H et al. (1998) Ichthyosis follicularis, alopecia and photophobia (IFAP) syndrome: clinical and neuropathological observations in a 33-year-old man. **Am J Med Genet** 78:371–377.
27. Sato-Matsumara KC, Matsumara T, Kumakiri M et al. (2000) Ichthyosis follicularis with alopecia and photophobia in a mother and daughter. **Br J Dermatol** 142:157–162.
28. Rogers M, Kourt G, Cameron A (1994) Hereditary mucoepithelial dysplasia. **Pediatr Dermatol** 11:133–138.
29. Rothe MJ, Lucky AW (1995) Are ichthyosis follicularis and hereditary mucoepithelial dystrophy related diseases? **Pediatr Dermatol** 12:195.
30. König A, Happle R (1999) Linear lesions reflecting lyonization in women heterozygous for IFAP syndrome (ichthyosis follicularis with atrichia and photophobia). **Am J Med Genet** 85:365–368.
31. Sato-Matsumara KC, Matsumara T, Kumakiri M et al. (2000) Ichthyosis follicularis with alopecia and photophobia in a mother and daughter. **Br J Dermatol** 142:157–162.

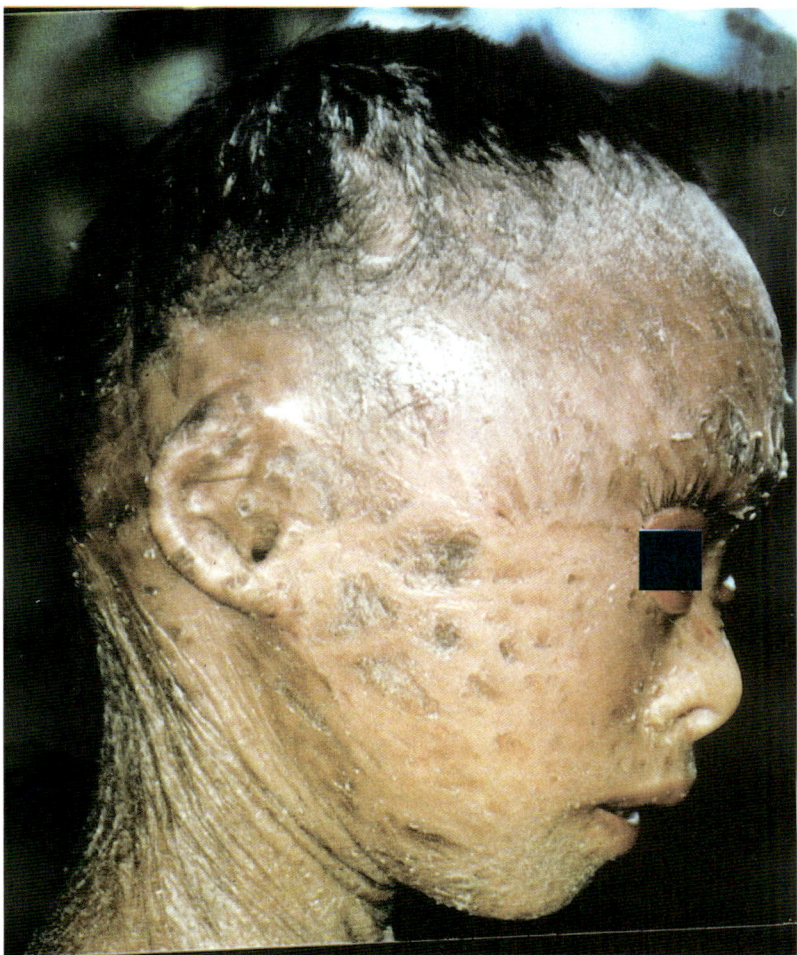

Fig. 11.2 Alopecia in a child with lamellar ichthyosis, subsequent to secondary infection and scarring.

Peeling skin syndrome

There is a single report of a child with the inflammatory variant of the peeling skin syndrome who in addition had hair abnormalities[32] with what were designated trichorrhexis invaginata-like changes, irregular twisting of the hair, and areas of hair shaft narrowing.

Keratitis, ichthyosis and deafness syndrome

Severe hypotrichosis of scalp, eyebrows, and eyelashes may be evident at birth and persists through life. There is also a spiny follicular plugging as well as widespread, thickened erythematous plaques, perioral furrowing, reticulate hyperkeratosis of palms and soles, keratitis and hearing loss.[33]

Congenital ichthyosis, follicular atrophoderma, hypotrichosis and hypohidrosis

This combination of traits has been described as a new autosomal-recessive genodermatosis,[34] and all of the features are present from the neonatal period.

HYPOTRICHOSIS WITH PREMATURE AGING SYNDROMES

While the onset of obvious hypotrichosis is often delayed until several years of age in these conditions, sparse hair is evident in early infancy in some cases of Hutchison–Gilford progeria, Rothmund–Thomson syndrome and Cockayne syndrome. A severe neonatal progeroid syndrome has been described in which sparse anterior scalp hair, thin eyebrows, and absent eyelashes were evident at birth, along with redundant skin, absent subcutaneous fat, and prominent blood vessels.[35]

HYPOTRICHOSIS WITH IMMUNODEFICIENCY SYNDROMES

Alopecia is often a striking feature of a heterogeneous group of congenital immunodeficiency conditions presenting in early infancy with erythroderma, failure to thrive, and diarrhea, which includes severe combined immunodeficiency-associated congenital graft-versus-host disease and Omenn syndrome.[36–38] In cartilage hair hypoplasia syndrome sparsity of scalp, eyebrow, and eyelash hair is often evident in the neonatal period, together with short limbs and prenatal growth failure.[39]

HYPOTRICHOSIS WITH GENETIC DISORDERS OF THE HAIR SHAFT

Increased fragility of hair in many of the genetic disorders of the hair shaft leads to early alopecia. These will be discussed in detail later in this chapter.

CONGENITAL LOCALIZED OR PATCHY ALOPECIA

NEONATAL OCCIPITAL ALOPECIA

A well-defined patch of alopecia commonly develops in the occipital area in the early months of life. This has previously been attributed entirely to rubbing the back of the head on the bedding surface but it is explained more fully by an understanding of the patterns of hair cycle evolution in fetal and early neonatal life, covered in Chapter 6.

SCALP INJURY

Alopecia, which is usually temporary, may occur in areas of scalp damaged by instrumentation such as forceps, vacuum extractor, or scalp monitors and also over cephalhematomas (see Chapter 6).

TEMPORAL TRIANGULAR ALOPECIA

This is a well-circumscribed triangular or lance-shaped area of non-cicatricial hypotrichosis positioned in the fronto-temporal area, with the anterior margin either at the hairline or sometimes separated from it by a small fringe of normal hair (Fig. 11.3).[40] It is unilateral in 80% of cases. Vellus hairs are present in the affected area[40] and occasionally a few terminal hairs are retained.[40,41] Histopathologic examination of transverse sections of a biopsy specimen demonstrates that the majority of follicles are vellus; a normal number of follicles is present but the follicular size is abnormal for the scalp.[40] The

32. Mevorah B, Orion E, de Viragh P et al. (1998) Peeing skin syndrome with hair changes. Dermatology 197:373–376.
33. Harms M, Gilardi S, Levy PM et al. (1984) KID syndrome (keratitis, ichthyosis and deafness) and chronic mucocutaneous candidiasis: case report and review of the literature. Pediatr Dermatol 2:1–7.
34. Lestringant GG, Kuster W, Frossard PM et al. (1998) Congenital ichthyosis, follicular atrophoderma, hypotrichosis and hypohidrosis. Am J Med Genet 75:186–189.
35. Megarbane A, Loiselet J (1997) Clinical manifestations of a severe neonatal progeroid syndrome. Clin Genet 51:200–204.
36. Glover MT, Atherton DJ, Levinsky RJ (1988) Syndrome of erythroderma, failure to thrive and diarrhea in infancy: a manifestation of immunodeficiency. Pediatr 81:66–72.

37. Ricci, G, Patrizi A, Specchia F (1997) Omenn syndrome. Pediatr Dermatol 14:49–52.
38. Farrell A, Scerri L, Stevens A et al. (1995) Acute graft-versus-host disease with unusual cutaneous intracellular vacuolation in an infant with severe combined immunodeficiency. Pediatr Dermatol 12:311–313.
39. Makitie O, Sulisalo T, de la Chapelle A et al. (1995) Cartilage-hair hypoplasia. J Med Genet 32:39–43.
40. Trakimas C, Sperling LC, Skelton HG et al. (1994) Clinical and histologic findings in temporal triangular alopecia. J Am Acad Dermatol 31:205–209.
41. Tosti A (1987) Congenital triangular alopecia. J Am Acad Dermatol 16:991–993.

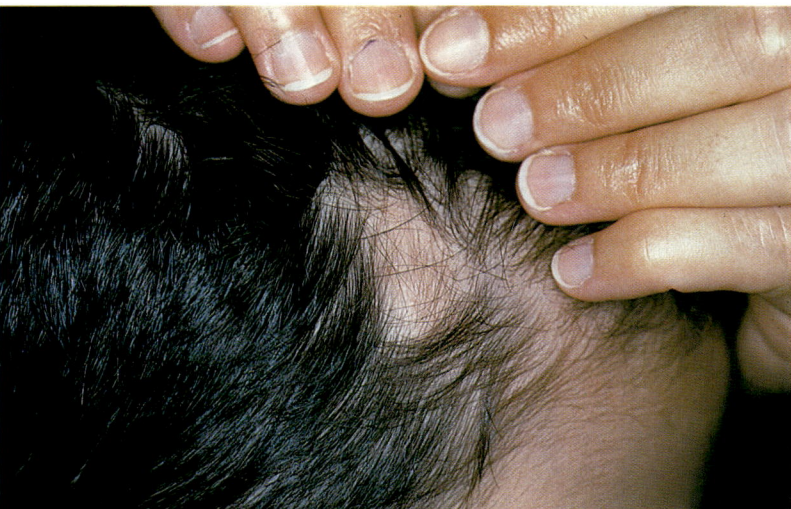

Fig. 11.3   Temporal triangular alopecia.

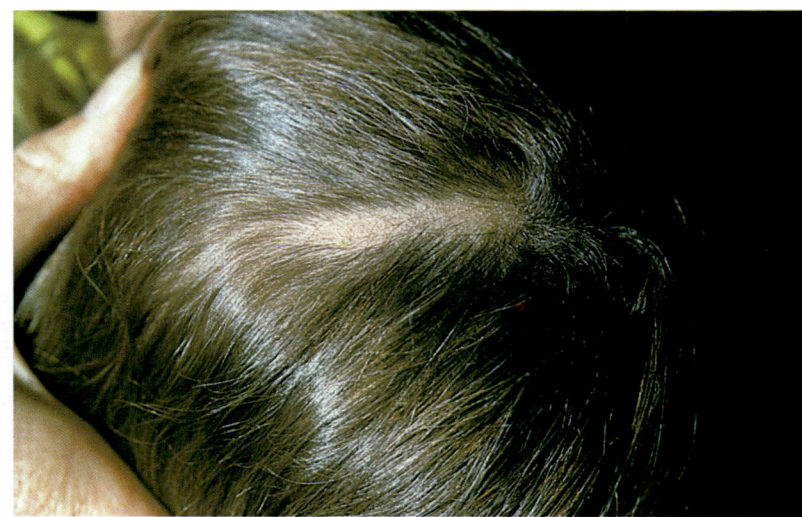

Fig. 11.5   Linear area of alopecia at the site of a very subtle sebaceous nevus.

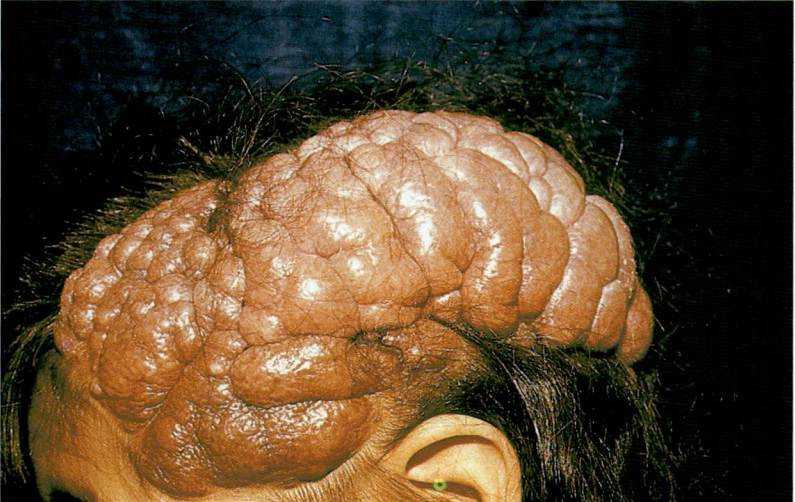

Fig. 11.4   Alopecia over grossly folded congenital melanocytic nevus, with cutis verticis gyrata appearance. (Photograph courtesy of Dr. Marcelo Ruvertoni, British Hospital, Montevideo, Uruguay.)

condition may be congenital and may be noted in the neonatal period in infants with abundant scalp hair, in whom it is often erroneously ascribed to forceps trauma. It is more often first noted in early childhood and adult onset has been reported.[42] A recent report of the condition in a mother and daughter, in both of whom there was also developmental delay and seizures, suggests that in at least some cases the condition may occur as part of a syndrome with autosomal-dominant inheritance.[43]

LOCALIZED ALOPECIA ASSOCIATED WITH OTHER NEVOID CONDITIONS

Congenital melanocytic nevus

These lesions are usually associated with hypertrichosis but large folded lesions on the scalp causing a cutis verticis gyrata appearance may have sparse covering hair or in some extreme cases complete absence of hair (Fig. 11.4).

Sebaceous nevus

These nevi are characteristically hairless. Sometimes the nevus is so flat and subtle that it is only recognized as such later, and the presentation is as a linear or oval-shaped patch of congenital alopecia (Fig. 11.5).

Aplastic nevus (syn. minus nevus)

This is a nevoid condition in which there is a complete absence of skin appendages in an area of otherwise normal skin.[44]

Aplasia cutis

This condition will be dealt with in detail in Chapter 18. Alopecia is a feature of both the common form of aplasia cutis congenita, with an irregularly shaped erosion which eventually heals, often with hypertrophic scarring, and of membranous aplasia cutis where there is an oval or round, hairless area covered by a smooth membrane and occasionally surrounded by a hair collar. The latter condition is probably a form fruste of heterotopic brain tissue.[45] Aplasia cutis producing a localized congenital alopecia may be a feature also of a number of syndromes including Adams–Oliver syndrome (Fig. 11.6)[46] and Toriello oculoectodermal syndrome.[47]

Cranial meningoceles, encephaloceles and heterotopic meningeal or brain tissue

These present characteristically as tumors or cysts which are either hairless or have sparse overlying hair. There is often, however, a surrounding collar of long hair producing the "hair collar sign."

42. Trakimas C, Sperling LC (1999) Temporal triangular alopecia acquired in adulthood. **J Am Acad Dermatol** 40:842–844.
43. Ruggieri M, Rizzo R, Happle R (2000) Temporal triangular alopecia in association with mental retardation and epilepsy in a mother and daughter. **Arch Dermatol** 136:426–427.
44. Schoenfeld RJ, Mehregan AH (1973) Aplastic nevus – the 'minus nevus'. **Cutis** 12:386–389.
45. Drolet B, Prendiville J, Golden J et al. (1995) 'Membranous aplasia cutis' with hair collars. **Arch Dermatol** 131:1427–1431.
46. Mempel M, Abeck D, Lange I et al. (1999) The wide spectrum of clinical expression in the Adams–Oliver syndrome: a report of two cases. **Br J Dermatol** 140:1157–1160.
47. Silengo M, Lerone M, Seri M et al. (2000) New clinical findings in the oculo-ectodermal syndrome. **Clin Dysmorphol** 9:39–41.

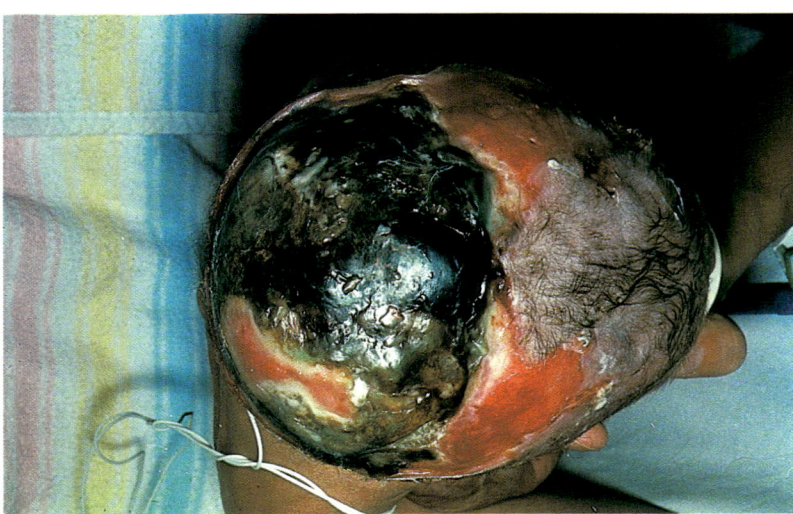

Fig. 11.6 Alopecia in area of aplasia cutis in an infant with Adams–Oliver syndrome.

HYPOTRICHOSIS WITH CONGENITAL FORMS OF CUTIS VERTICIS GYRATA

A marked folding of the scalp associated with sparse hair over the folds can occur at birth with melanocytic nevi, as mentioned above. In addition, it may be a feature of certain syndromes. When it occurs in Turner syndrome it is postulated that the redundant skin results from resolved intrauterine lymphedema.[48,49] In Beare Stevenson syndrome, which is due to a mutation in a fibroblast growth factor receptor gene,[50] it occurs in association with acanthosis nigricans, craniofacial, and anogenital anomalies and developmental delay. In the Michelin-tire baby syndrome[51] there is a generalized folding of the skin due to an excess of various types of connective tissue; while there may be hypertrichosis elsewhere, there may be a marked hypotrichosis of the scalp.[52] Multiple folds of redundant skin, all over the body, due to an accumulation of hyaluronic acid occurs in the so-called Shau Pai dog syndrome,[52] and again there is scalp hypotrichosis. Most other forms of cutis verticis gyrata develop later in life.

LOCALIZED ALOPECIA ASSOCIATED WITH SYNDROMES

Hallermann–Streiff syndrome

The hair may be normal at birth but in some cases the typical alopecia, located in the frontal and parietal areas over the cranial sutures, may be evident in early months, together with atrophic facial skin and multiple craniofacial and ocular abnormalities.[53]

X-linked dominant conditions

Several rare syndromes, caused by X-linked dominant genes which interfere with hair growth, produce a mosaic pattern of alopecia in affected females as a result of functional X-chromosome mosaicism.[54] The hemizygous males with these conditions rarely survive. The conditions include focal dermal hypoplasia (Goltz syndrome),[55] incontinentia pigmenti,[54] oral facial digital syndrome,[56] and X-linked dominant chondrodysplasia punctata.[57] The alopecia in these conditions has a patchy distribution, sometimes obviously linear or spiral as it follows the lines of Blaschko. The pattern of these lines on the scalp has recently been further delineated.[58]

HAIR SHAFT ABNORMALITIES

These conditions have been reviewed in detail by Whiting,[59] Price,[60] and Rogers.[61,62]

MONILETHRIX

This is an autosomal-dominant condition producing a beaded appearance of the hair.[61] On microscopy, spindle shaped "nodes" separated by constricted internodes are seen. The nodes have the diameter of normal hair and may be medullated, whereas the internodes are narrower and usually non-medullated and are the sites of fracture. The abnormality may affect the whole length of the hair or there may be only a few areas of narrowing in an otherwise apparently normal hair (Fig. 11.7).

Recently mutations in the human basic hair keratins hHb1 and hHb6 have been reported.[63,64] However, the failure to demonstrate these mutations in one

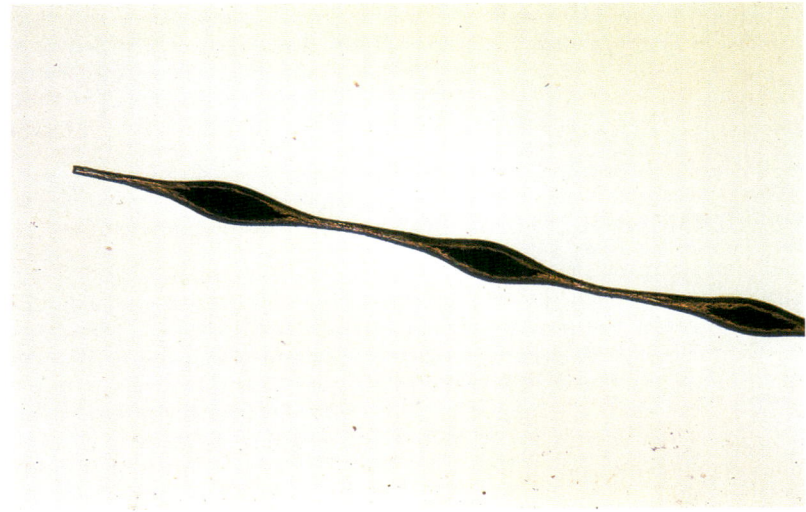

Fig. 11.7 Microscopy of monilethrix demonstrating the beaded appearance.

48. Larralde M, Gardner SS, Torado M et al. (1998) Lymphedema as a postulated cause of cutis verticis gyrata in Turner syndrome. **Pediatr Dermatol** 15:18–22.
49. Marioni LP, Taniguchi K, Giraldi S et al. (1999) Cutis verticis gyrata in a child with Turner syndrome. **Pediatr Dermatol** 16:242–243.
50. Zhang Y, Gorry MC, Post JC et al. (1999) Genomic organization of the human fibroblast growth factor receptor gene (FGFR2) and comparative analysis of the human FGFR gene family. **Gene** 230:69–79.
51. Sato M, Ishikawa O, Miyachi Y et al. (1997) Michelin tyre syndrome: a congenital disorder of elastic tissue. **Br J Dermatol** 136:583–586.
52. Sinclair R, de Berker D (1997) Hereditary and congenital alopecia and hypotrichosis. In: Diseases of the Hair and Scalp, Dawber R, ed. Oxford: Blackwell Science, pp. 151–238.
53. Cohen JJ (1991) Hallermann-Streiff syndrome: a review. **Am J Med Genet** 41:488–489.
54. Traupe H (1999) Functional X-chromosome mosaicism of the skin: Rudolf Happle and the lines of Alfred Blaschko. **Am J Med Genet** 85:324–329.
55. Terashi H, Kurata S, Hashimoto H et al. (1994) A case of Goltz syndrome presenting as congenital incomplete alopecia. **J Dermatol** 21:122–124.

56. Boente M, Primc N, Veliche H et al. (1999) A mosaic pattern of alopecia in the oral-facial-digital syndrome type I (Papillon-League and Psaume syndrome). **Pediatr Dermatol** 16:367–370.
57. Braverman N, Lin P, Moebius FF et al. (1999) Mutations in the gene encoding 3 beta-hydroxysterol-delta 8, delta 7-isomerase cause X-linked dominant Conradi-Hunnermann syndrome. **Nature Genet** 22:291–294.
58. Happle R, Assim A (2001) The lines of Blaschko on the head and neck. **J Am Acad Dermatol** 44:612–615.
59. Whiting D (1987) Structural abnormalities of the hair shaft. **J Am Acad Dermatol** 16:1–25.
60. Price VH (1990) Structural abnormalities of the hair shaft. In: Hair and Hair Diseases. Orfanos C, Happle R, eds. Berlin: Springer Verlag, pp. 363–422.
61. Rogers M (1995) Hair shaft abnormalities: Part I. **Australas J Dermatol** 36:179–186.
62. Rogers M (1996) Hair shaft abnormalities: Part II. **Australas J Dermatol** 37:1–11.
63. Winter H, Clark RD, Tarras-Wahlberg C et al. (1999) Monilethrix: a novel mutation (Glu402Lys) in the helix termination motif of the type II hair keratin hHb6. **J Invest Dermatol** 113:263–266.
64. Horev L, Glaser B, Metzker A et al. (2000) Monilethrix: mutational hotspot in the helix termination motif of the human hair basic keratin 6. **Human Heredity** 50:325–330.

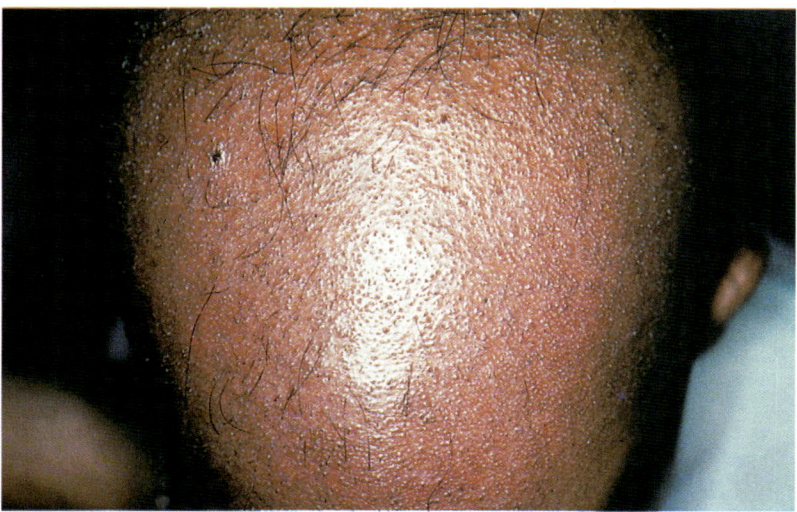

Fig. 11.8   Monilethrix. Most hairs are broken almost flush with the scalp, with some coarse longer hairs and follicular keratosis.

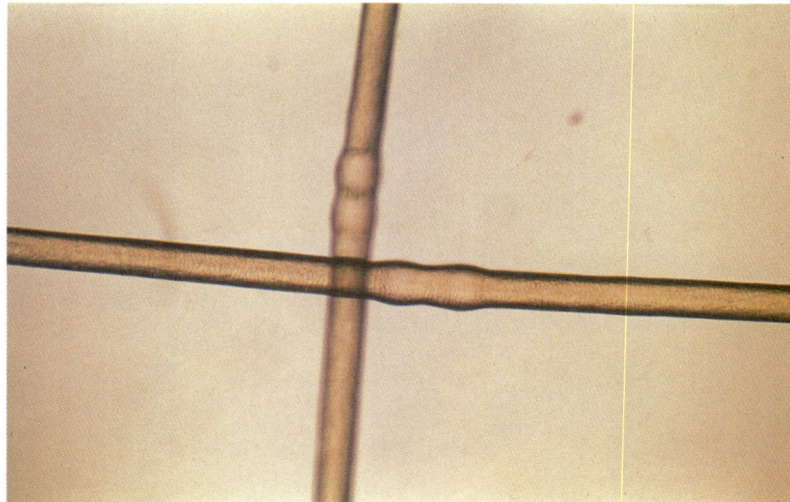

Fig. 11.9   Pseudomonilethrix. Irregularly spaced nodes, wider than the normal shaft, occurring near the site of overlap of the hairs.

family suggests the possibility of genetic heterogeneity.[65] The hair is usually normal at birth but is replaced within weeks by affected hairs which are dry, dull, and brittle, breaking spontaneously to leave a stubble-like appearance. The hairs may break almost flush with the scalp or may attain lengths of 0.5–2.5cm, or occasionally longer (Fig. 11.8). Follicular keratosis is associated in some pedigrees and may involve scalp, face, and limbs. Koilonychia is sometimes found. The condition tends to improve significantly with age, particularly in girls, perhaps in relation to hormonal influences.[66] An acute loss of hair following a fever is a feature of this condition. The hair is lost within days of the fever, and may be of such a severity that it is misdiagnosed as severe alopecia areata. However, the onset of regrowth is immediate. Some residual long hairs may have an unusual coarse texture.

PSEUDOMONILETHRIX

This condition was originally described in 1973 as a developmental defect characterized by fragile hair with irregular nodes along the shaft when seen on microscopy.[67] Autosomal-dominant inheritance with variable penetrance was postulated. Large pedigrees were described in which almost 100% of members demonstrated the abnormality.

The nodes are 0.75–1mm in length, and wider than the normal shaft. The zones between the nodes are of normal thickness. Scanning electron microscopy demonstrates the nodes to be optical illusions, representing indentations of hair with the sides of the depressions protruding beyond the normal diameter of the shaft (Figs 11.9, 11.10). The cuticular pattern is normal over both "nodes" and "internode". In 1986, Zitelli[68] nicely demonstrated that the condition is, in fact, an artifact, caused by the pressure between glass slides of overlapping hairs. He noted that the length of the swelling correlated with the diameter of overlapped hair and the width of the swelling and the depth of the indentation are proportional to the pressure applied. This artifact is seen almost routinely when mounting the fair, fine hair of patients with certain ectodermal dysplasias, if hairs are allowed to overlap. It is often temporary, with the deformation disappearing in a few minutes. Similar deformities are seen in fine hair handled with forceps. It is likely that the early reported pedigrees were examples of ectodermal dysplasias.

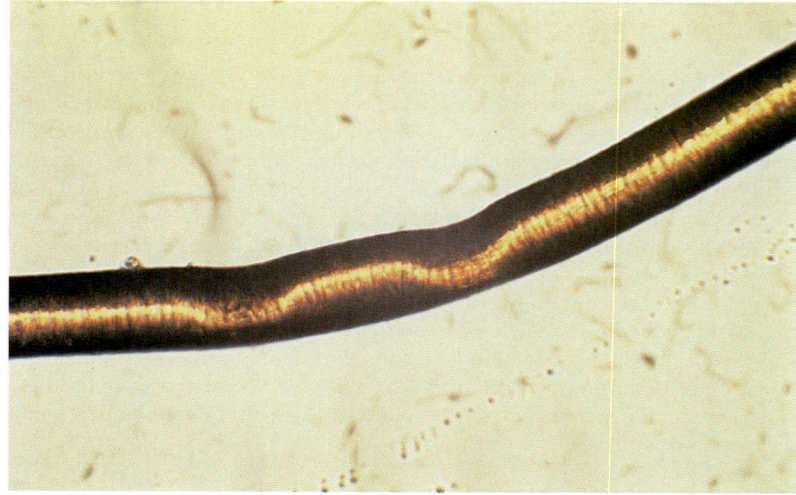

Fig. 11.10   Pseudomonilethrix. Denting of the hair at the site of pressure from an overlapping hair.

PILI TORTI

This is characterized by a twisting of the hair shaft on its own axis.[61] On microscopy, groups of three or four regularly spaced twists, each of 0.4–0.9mm in width, are seen occurring at irregular intervals along the shaft (Figs 11.11, 11.12). Twists are almost always through 180 degrees, although some are through 90 or 360 degrees. The hair shaft is somewhat flattened at the site of the twist.

Pili torti may occur as an inherited, isolated phenomenon with the onset at birth or in the early months of life. The hair is usually fairer than expected and is spangled, dry, and brittle, breaking at different lengths. It may stand out from the scalp and it tends to be short, especially in areas subject to trauma (Fig. 11.13). Both autosomal-dominant and autosomal-recessive pedigrees have been reported.[60]

65. Richard G, Itin P, Lin JP et al. (1996) Evidence for genetic heterogeneity in monilethrix. **J Invest Dermatol** 107:812–814.
66. Gebhart M, Fischer T, Claussen U et al. (1999) Monilethrix – improvement by hormonal influences? **Pediatr Dermatol** 16:297–300.
67. Bentley-Phillips B, Bayles MAH (1973) A previously undescribed hair anomaly (pseudomonilethrix). **Br J Dermatol** 89:159–167.
68. Zitelli JA (1986) Pseudomonilethrix: an artifact. **Arch Dermatol** 122:688.

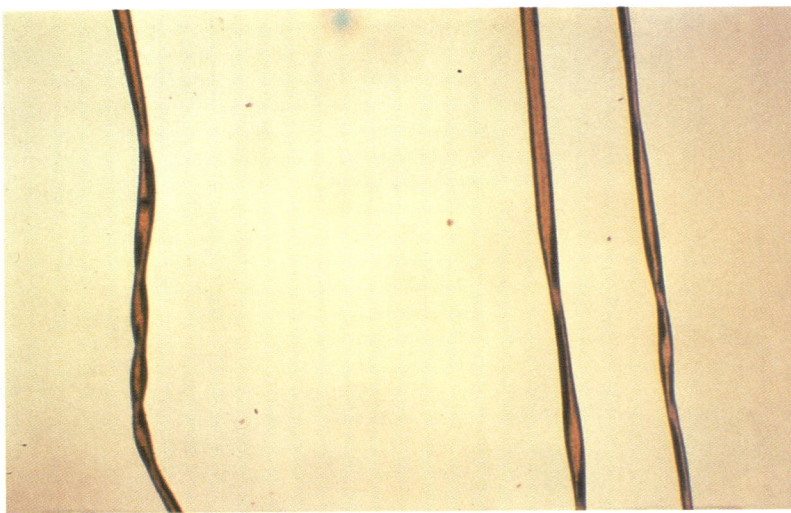

Fig. 11.11   Pili torti. Microscopy showing the series of twists.

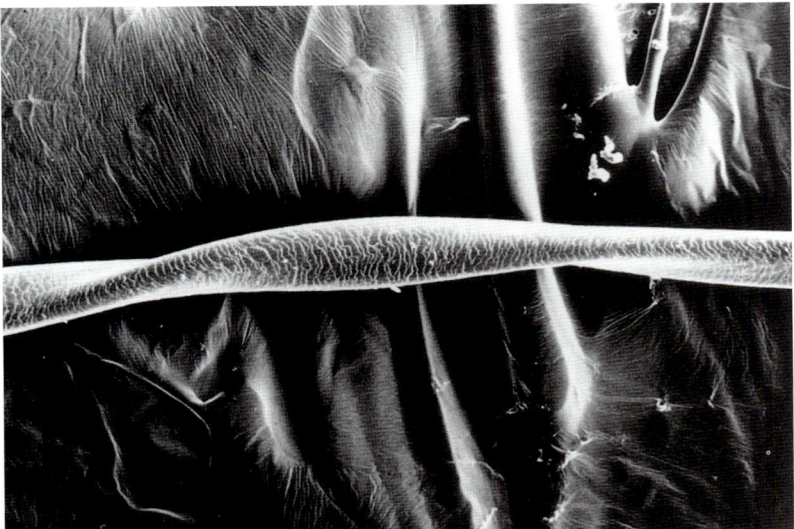

Fig. 11.12   Pili torti. Scanning electron microscopy demonstrating the flattening of the shaft at the site of twisting.

There is a late onset form of pili torti in which alopecia develops after puberty. It is an autosomal-dominant condition in which affected hair is coarse, stiff and jet black. Eyebrow hairs and lashes break off during childhood. After puberty the scalp hair becomes more brittle and a patchy alopecia may develop. Body hair is sparse and may be seen broken off almost flush with the skin surface. Mental retardation has been associated in some pedigrees.[60,61]

Pili torti occurs as a feature of several other defined syndromes.

MENKES SYNDROME

Menkes syndrome is an X-linked recessive condition characterized by progressive neurodegeneration and connective tissue manifestations and is usually

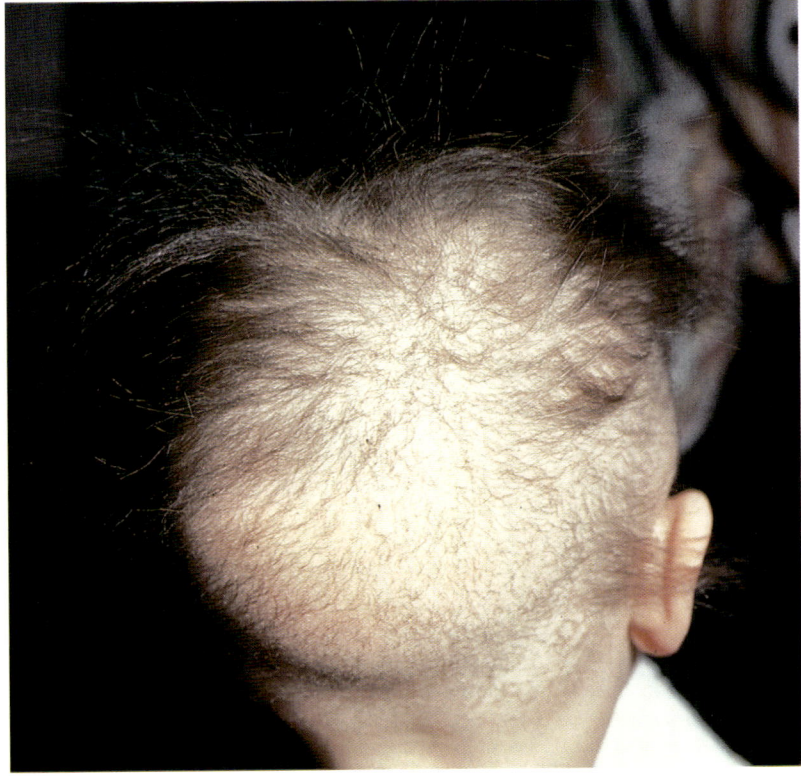

Fig. 11.13   Sparse, spangled hair in pili torti.

lethal in the early years of life. The unusual, twisted hair, demonstrating pili torti on microscopy, has led to the terminology "kinky hair syndrome" or "steely hair syndrome." The basis of the disorder has been found to relate to a defect in copper transport.[69–71]

In 1993, the genes for both Menkes disease[72] and Wilson disease[73] were isolated, and they were found to encode homologous cation copper-transporting P-type ATPase proteins. The Menkes disease protein (ATP7A) is expressed in most tissues except liver, while the Wilson disease protein (ATP7B) is well expressed in the liver, explaining the clinical differences between these two conditions.[74]

The Menkes gene is on chromosome X13.3 and mutations in this gene in patients with Menkes disease show great variety including missense, nonsense, deletion, and insertion mutations.[70] Mutations in the Menkes gene have also been identified in patients with mild Menkes disease, which shows features similar to, but less severe than, classical Menkes disease, and in the occipital horn syndrome (X-linked cutis laxa, Ehlers-Danlos type 9), mainly characterized by connective tissue features, indicating that these conditions represent allelic forms of Menkes disease.[70]

The loss of Menkes protein activity blocks the export of dietary copper from the gastrointestinal tract leading to a decreased bioavailability of copper with resultant functional deficiencies of copper-dependent enzymes.[71,75]

In the classic form, the scalp hair is often sparse at birth and may remain so. It is hypopigmented, sometimes with a silvery sheen, and is twisted or kinked in appearance. It may be rather coarse in texture. It is fragile and breaks easily in areas of trauma, such as the occipital area (Figs 11.14, 11.15). The eyebrows are usually sparse and disordered. Microscopically, pili torti

69. Tumer Z, Horn N (1997) Menkes disease: recent advances and new aspects. **J Med Genet** 34:265–274.
70. Kodama H, Murata Y (1999) Molecular genetics and pathophysiology of Menkes disease. **Pediatrics International** 41:430–435.
71. Kodama H, Murata Y, Kobayashi M (1999) Clinical manifestations and treatment of Menkes disease and its variants. **Pediatrics International** 41:423–429.
72. Vulpe C, Levinson B, Whitney S et al. (1993) Isolation of a candidate gene for Menkes disease and evidence that it encodes a copper-transporting ATPase. **Nat Genet** 3:7–13.
73. Bull PC, Thomas GR, Rommens JM et al. (1993) The Wilson disease gene is a putative copper transporting P-type ATPase similar to the Menkes gene. **Nat Genet** 5:327–337.
74. Suzuki M, Gitlin JD (1999) Intracellular localization of the Menkes and Wilson's disease proteins and their role in intracellular copper transport. **Pediatrics International** 41:436–442.
75. Harrison MD, Dameron CT (1999) Molecular mechanisms of copper metabolism and the role of the Menkes disease protein. **J Biochem Molec Toxicol** 13:93–106.

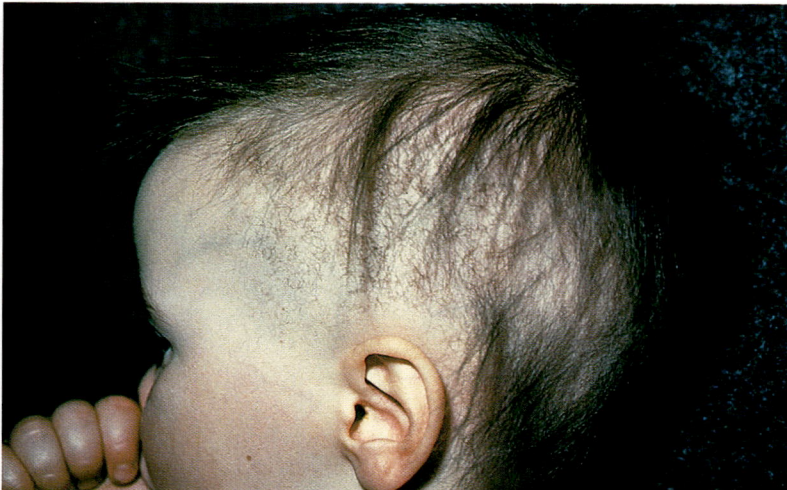

Fig. 11.14   Steely, sparse hair in a patient with Menkes syndrome.

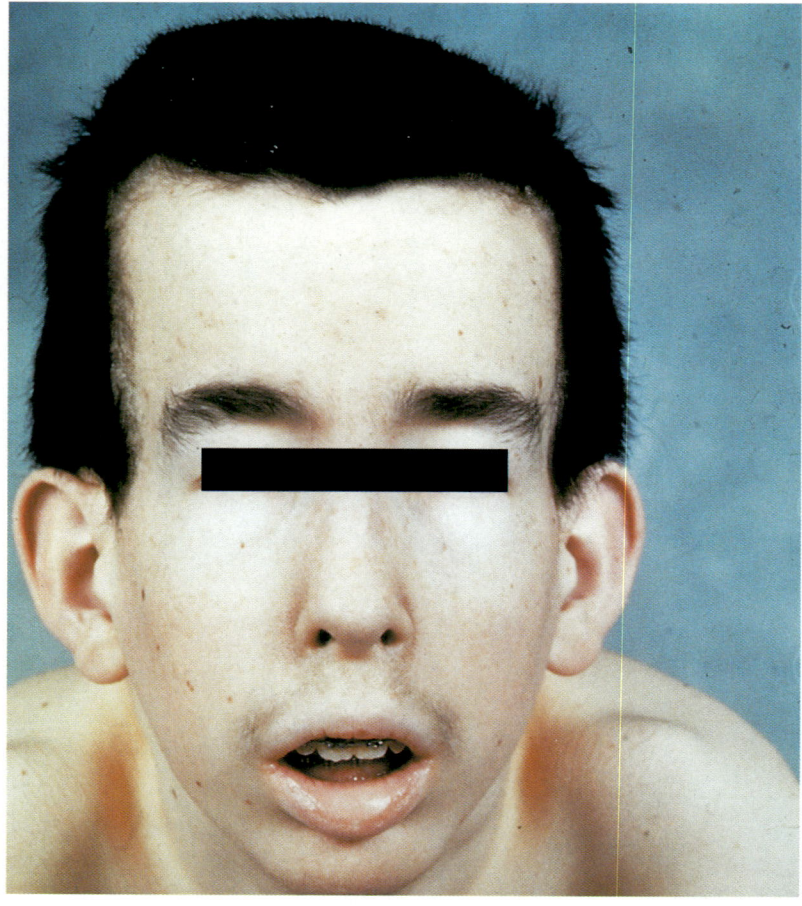

Fig. 11.15   Menkes syndrome. Older survivor with hair remaining fragile and short. (Photograph courtesy of Dr. Agnes Bankier, Royal Children's Hospital, Melbourne, Australia.)

is demonstrated. The skin is pale and lax with a doughy consistency and may be mottled. The hypopigmentation of hair and skin is explained by a deficiency in the copper-dependent enzyme, tyrosinase. Lyonization leads to a Blaschko-distributed hypopigmentation and areas of pili torti noted in some obligate female carriers.[76] These infants are hypotonic and hypothermic and develop early seizures. There is microcephaly and progressive developmental delay. Imaging studies demonstrate osteoporosis, metaphyseal flaring, particularly of ribs and femora, and tortuous blood vessels in the brain and elsewhere. The tortuosity of the vessels results from a defect in elastin crosslinking due to deficiency of another copper-dependent enzyme, lysyl oxidase.

If untreated, most infants die within the first year, but longer-term survivors are now being reported as a result of early treatment.[77,78] Parenteral administration of copper, if commenced in the neonatal period, may prevent neurological deterioration but this advantage is lost after the first 2 months of life and early treatment does not improve the non-neurological features such as connective tissue laxity.[71] Prenatal testing is now available by mutational analysis.

Other syndromes with pili torti

In Bazex syndrome, inherited as an X-linked dominant trait, congenital hypotrichosis with pili torti is associated with follicular atrophoderma, multiple facia milia, and an increased susceptibility to development of basal cell carcinomas.[79] In Bjornstad syndrome, there is an associated sensorineural deafness and in some cases mental retardation.[80,81] In later childhood, normal hair may replace the affected hairs, with considerable improvement in appearance. Mental retardation has been reported in one case.[82] Bjornstad syndrome is autosomal-recessive and has recently been mapped to chromosome 2.[83] In Crandall syndrome, probably inherited as an X-linked recessive trait, congenital hypotrichosis with pili torti is associated with sensorineural deafness and hypopituitarism.[84] Pili torti may occur also in Rapp–Hodgkin syndrome, although pili canaliculi is the more characteristic finding.[85]

TRICHORRHEXIS NODOSA (TN)

This term refers to the light microscopic appearance of a fracture with splaying out and release of individual cortical cells from the main body of the hair shaft producing an appearance suggestive of the ends of two brushes pushed together.[60,61] When the break occurs, the brush-like end is clearly seen (Fig. 11.16). Electron microscopy shows the disrupted cuticle and splaying of cortical cells (Fig. 11.17). The defect renders the hair very fragile and it breaks readily with trauma or sometimes almost spontaneously.

In congenital trichorrhexis nodosa, inherited as an autosomal-dominant trait, the hair is usually normal at birth but is replaced within a few months with abnormal, fragile hair. The condition tends to improve with time.

Acquired trichorrhexis nodosa is a distinctive response of the hair shaft to external injury. In adolescents it may be seen as a result of the use of hot combs, excessively hot hair dryers, hair straightening procedures, and other chemical treatments. In younger children it may be a feature of hair injured

76. Lorette G, Toutain A, Barthes M et al. (1992) Maladie de Menkes. Anomalie particuliare de la pigmentation chez la mere et trois soeurs. **Annales de Pediatrie** 39:453–456.
77. Kaler SG (1998) Diagnosis and therapy of Menkes syndrome, a genetic form of copper deficiency. **Am J Clin Nutrit** 67 (suppl 5):1029S–1034S.
78. Christodoulou J, Danks DM, Sarkar B et al. (1998) Early treatment of Menkes disease with parenteral copper histidine: long term follow up of four treated patients. **Am J Med Genet** 76:154–164.
79. Goetyn M, Geerts M-L, Kint A et al. (1994) The Bazex-Dupre-Christol syndrome. **Arch Dermatol** 130:337–342.
80. Loche F, Bayle-Lebey P, Carriere JP et al. (1999) Pili torti with congenital deafness (Bjornstad syndrome): a case report. **Pediatr Dermatol** 16:220–221.
81. Selvaag E (2000) Pili torti and sensorineural hearing loss. A follow-up of Bjornstad's original patients and a review of the literature. **Eur J Dermatol** 10:91–97.
82. Van Buggenhout G, Trommelen J, Hamel B et al. (1998) Bjornstad syndrome in a patient with mental retardation. **Genetic Counselling** 9:201–204.
83. Lubianca Neto JF, Lu L, Eavey RD et al. (1998) The Bjornstad syndrome (sensorineural hearing loss and pili torti) disease gene maps to chromosome 2q34–36. **Am J Hum Genet** 62:1107–1112.
84. Crandall B, Samec L, Sparkes RS et al. (1973) A familial syndrome of deafness, alopecia and hypogonadism. **J Pediatr** 82:461–465.
85. Camacho F, Ferrando J, Pichardo AR et al. (1993) Rapp–Hodgkin syndrome with pili canaliculi. **Pediatr Dermatol** 10:54–57.

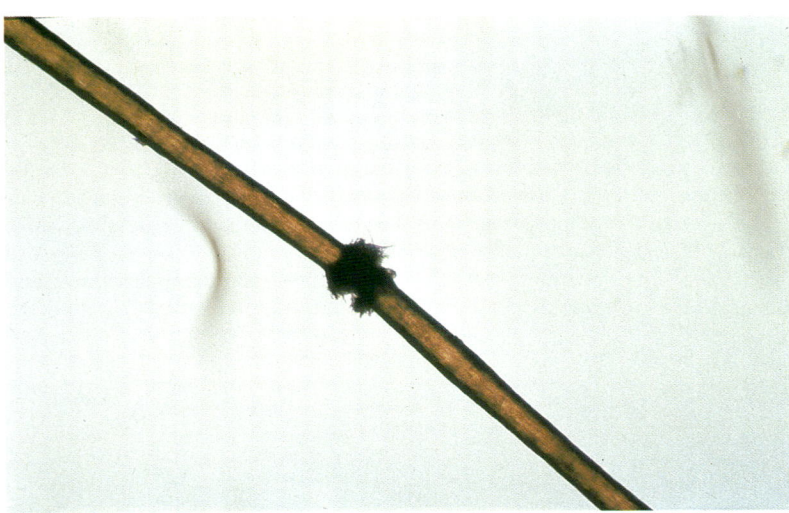

Fig. 11.16   Trichorrhexis nodosa. Microscopy demonstrating the node which appears like two brushes pushed together.

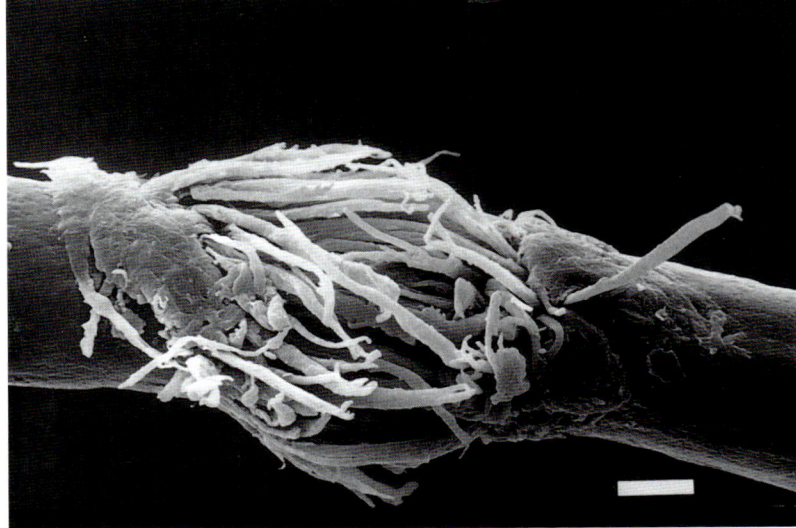

Fig. 11.17   Trichorrhexis nodosa. Scanning electron microscopy of the node demonstrating the disruption of the cuticle and the splaying out of the cortical cells.

by traction, twisting (as in trichotillomania), and rubbing. Trichorrhexis nodosa may occur in hair weakened by other hair shaft abnormalities, in particular monilethrix and trichothiodystrophy.

Trichorrhexis nodosa with arginosuccinicaciduria (ASAU)

There is a neonatal form of ASAU that is fatal in early life and a later-onset form. Most children with late-onset ASAU show trichorrhexis nodosa.[86] The hair may be normal at birth but becomes fragile by 1–2 years. There is a dull, dry, matted appearance especially in the occipital area. The condition reverts to normal with dietary treatment of the metabolic condition but it recurs quickly if the diet is abandoned.

An acquired TN has also been described in association with severe nutritional deficiency.

TRICHOTHIODYSTROPHY

Sulfur-deficient brittle hair is a marker for a neuroectodermal symptom complex occurring in a group of autosomal-recessive genetic disorders.[62,87,88] Named syndromes in this spectrum include Pollitt syndrome, Tay syndrome, Sabinas brittle hair syndrome, and Marinesco–Sjögren syndrome.[89] The words describing the various clinical features of the condition have lead to other mnemonic names, including BIDS, IBIDS, and PIBIDS.[88] The clinical features found in this group of conditions are brittle hair (Fig. 11.18), ichthyosis, short stature, decreased fertility, intellectual impairment, photosensitivity, and osteosclerosis (Fig. 11.19). Mental retardation of varying degree is present in almost all cases but there have been reports of individuals

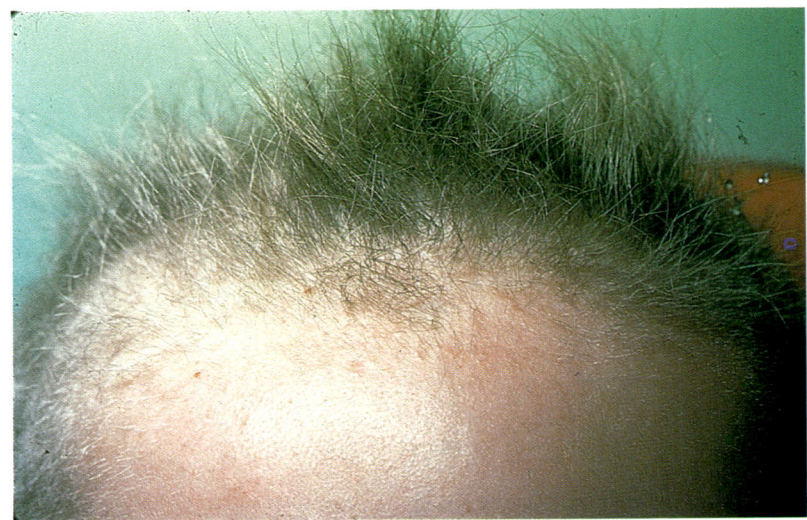

Fig. 11.18   Trichothiodystrophy. Short, disordered sparse hair.

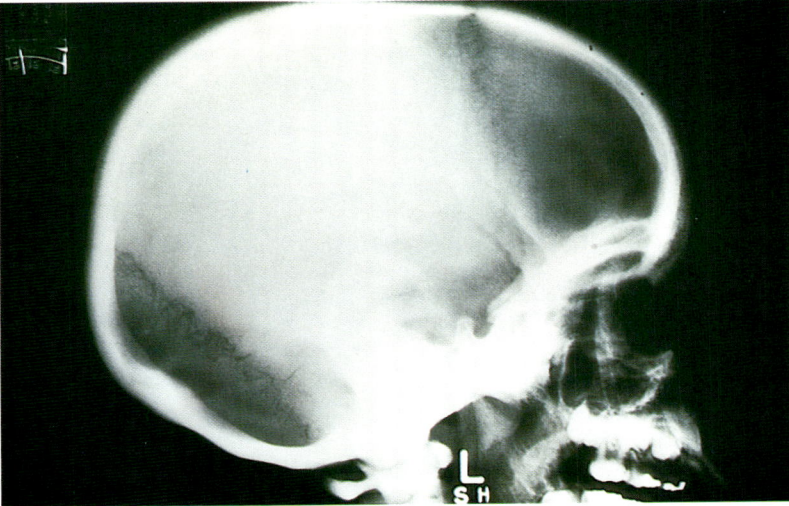

Fig. 11.19   Trichothiodystrophy. X-ray demonstrating osteosclerosis of skull.

86. Potter JL, Timmens GD et al. (1980) Arginosuccinicaciduria: The hair shaft abnormality revisited. **Am J Dis Child** 134:1095–1096.
87. Price VH, Odom RB, Ward WH et al. (1980) Trichothiodystrophy. Sulfur-deficient brittle hair as a marker for neuroectodermal symptom complex. **Arch Dermatol** 116:1375–1384.
88. Itin PH, Pittelkow MR (1990) Trichothiodystrophy: review of sulfur-deficient brittle hair syndromes and association with the ectodermal dysplasias: **J Am Acad Dermatol** 22:705–717.
89. Tolmie JL, de Berker D, Dawber R et al. (1994) Syndromes associated with trichothiodystrophy: **Clin Dysmorphol** 3:1–14.

with typical hair findings and normal development.[90] Photosensitivity is present in about 50% of patients. Photosensitive trichodystrophy, along with xeroderma pigmentosum (XP) and Cockayne syndrome, are explained by mutations in genes involved in nucleotide excision repair. In most patients with photosensitive trichodystrophy the defect is indistinguishable from that of XP complementation type D but two other repair-deficient complementation groups have been described, XP-B and TTD-A.[91,92] Surprisingly, an increased tendency to skin cancer is not a feature in these patients.[93] Individuals with trichothiodystrophy may present with a collodion baby phenotype and intrauterine growth retardation may occur. Other features include facial dysmorphism, congenital cataracts, and nail dystrophy. A rare

variant is reported with severe recurrent infections, failure to thrive, and death in early infancy.[94]

On light microscopy the hair has a wavy, irregular outline and a flattened shaft in which twists like a folded ribbon occur (Figs 11.20, 11.21). Two types of fracture are seen – trichoschisis, a clean, transverse fracture, and an atypical trichorrhexis nodosa with less splaying out of the cortical cells than is usually seen. Using crossed polarizers, bright and dark bands are seen when the hair is aligned in one of the polarizer directions, the so-called tiger-tail appearance (Fig. 11.22). This may be absent at birth and is not fully developed until 3 months of age.[95] Scanning electron microscopy shows irregular ridging and fluting and disordered, reduced, or absent cuticle scale pattern (Fig. 11.23).

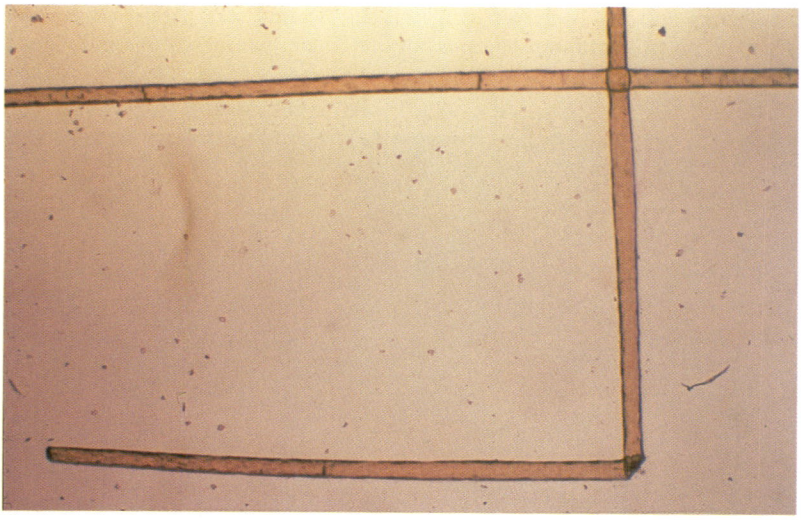

Fig. 11.20 Trichothiodystrophy. Microscopy demonstrating flattened hair shafts twisting like a ribbon. Several areas of trichoschisis.

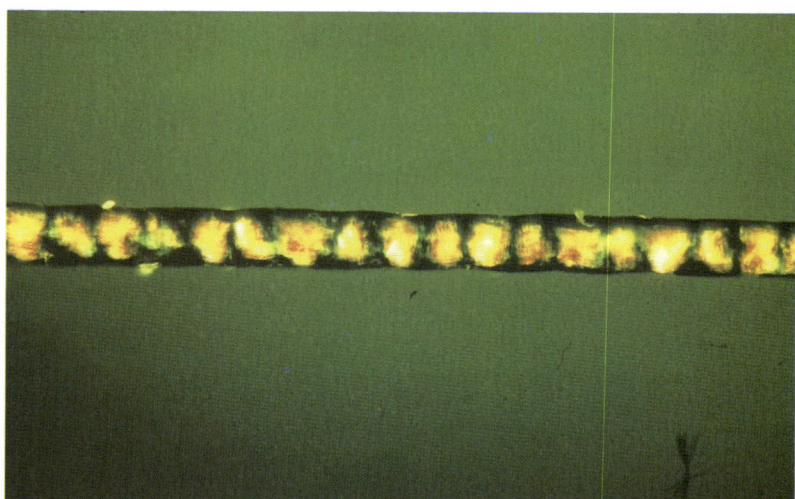

Fig. 11.22 Trichothiodystrophy. Hair viewed microscopically using crossed polarisers, demonstrating the banded "tiger tail" appearance.

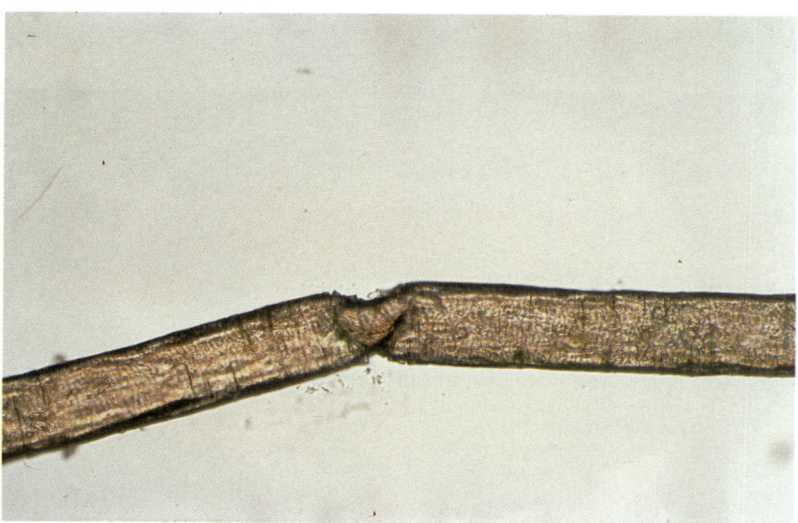

Fig. 11.21 Trichothiodystrophy. Microscopy demonstrating flattened shaft twisted through 360 degrees.

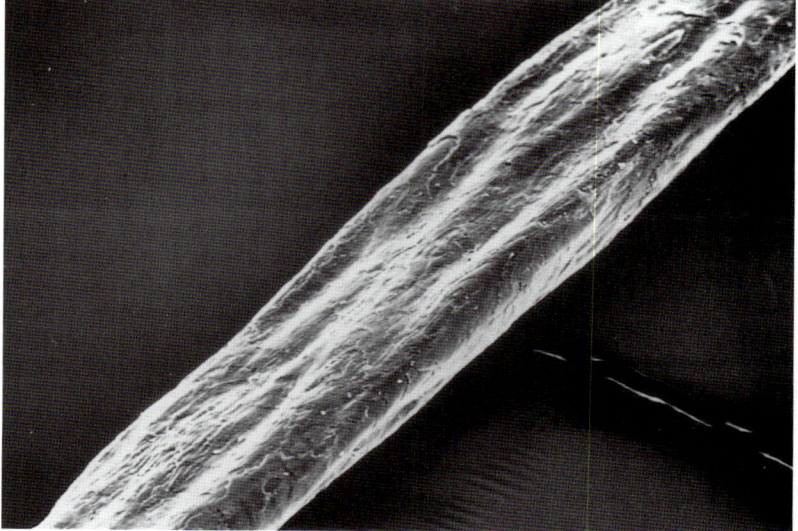

Fig. 11.23 Trichothiodystrophy. Scanning electron microscopy demonstrating the irregular ridging and fluting and disordered cuticle scale pattern.

90. Peter C, Tomczok J, Hoting E et al. (1998) Trichothiodystrophy without associated neuroectodermal defects. **Br J Dermatol** 139:137–140.
91. Taylor EM, Broughton BC, Botta E et al. (1997) Xeroderma pigmentosum and trichothiodystrophy are associated with different mutations in the XPD(ERCC2) repair/transcription gene. **Proc Nat Acad Sci USA** 94:8658–8663.
92. Weeda G, Eveno E, Donker I et al. (1997) A mutation in the XPB/ERCC3 DNA repair transcription gene, associated with trichothiodystrophy. **Am J Hum Genet** 60:320–329.

93. de Boer J, Hoeijmakers JH (2000) Nucleotide excision repair and human syndromes. **Carcinogenesis** 21:453–460.
94. Petrin JH, Meckler KA, Sybert VP (1998) A new variant of trichothiodystrophy with recurrent infections, failure to thrive and death. **Pediatr Dermatol** 15:31–34.
95. Brusasco A (1997) The typical "tiger-tail" pattern of the hair shaft in trichothiodystrophy may not be evident at birth: **Arch Dermatol** 133:249.

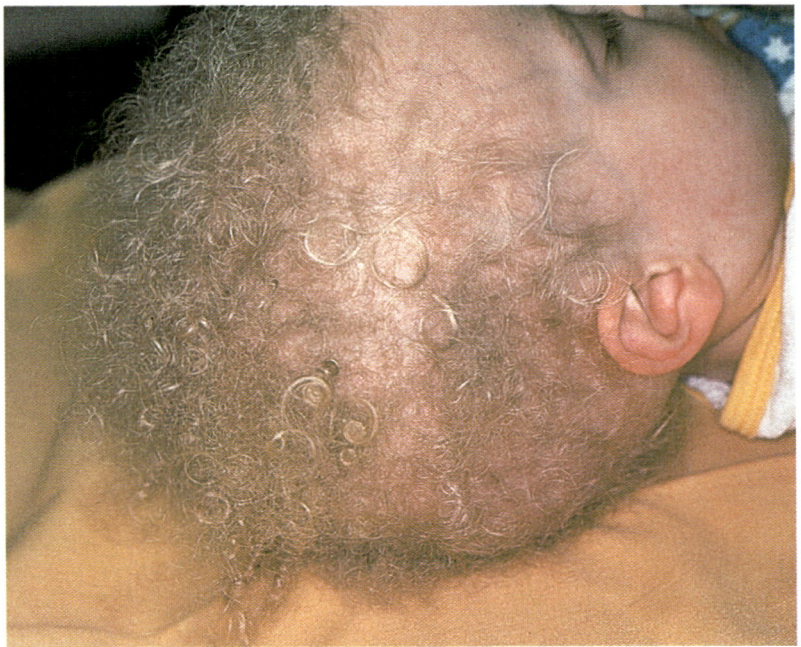

Fig. 11.24   Woolly hair.

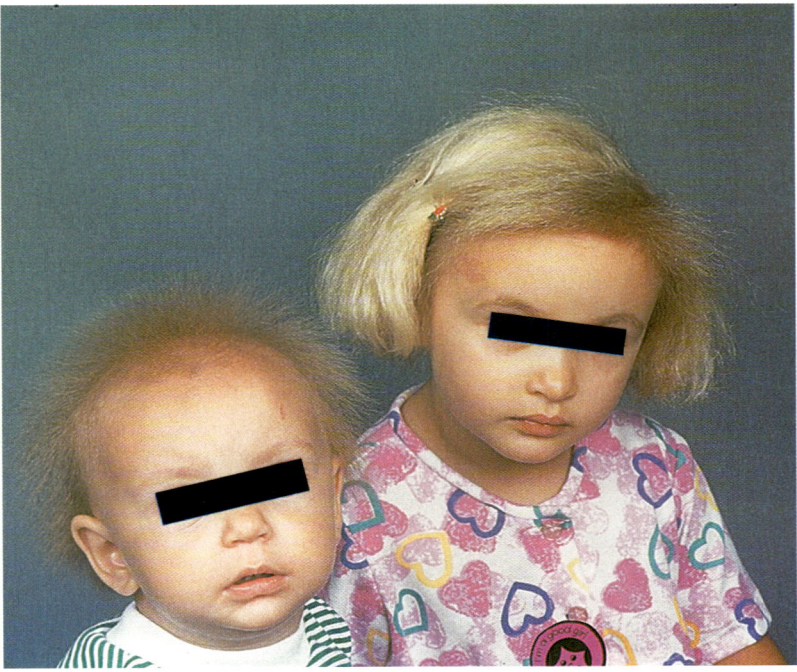

Fig. 11.25   Uncombable hair (pili canaliculi) in two sisters.

WOOLLY HAIR

This is tight, curly hair, which differs considerably from that of other areas of scalp and that of family members (Fig. 11.24).[62] It is usually abnormal from birth. The hair is not fragile in this condition. A wide variety of changes are described in shaft cross-sectional shape, follicle morphology, and cuticular appearance on scanning electron microscopy. The pathogenesis is unclear and may vary from case to case. There are three main groups. Two are diffuse and inherited, one autosomal-recessive and one autosomal-dominant. The other is localized and sporadic, the woolly hair nevus. The condition is important because there are many associations. Diffuse woolly hair has been associated with ocular abnormalities, some present at birth,[96] keratosis pilaris atrophicans,[97] Noonan syndrome,[97] palmoplantar keratoderma and cardiac conduction defects,[98] recently linked with a deletion in the plakoglobin gene,[99] giant axonal neuropathy,[100] and primary osteoma cutis.[101] Woolly hair nevus has been associated with ocular abnormalities[96] and with epidermal nevi, usually away from the site of the woolly hair nevus and sometimes quite extensive.[102]

UNCOMBABLE HAIR (SYNONYMS: SPUN GLASS HAIR, PILI CANALICULI, PILI TRIANGULI ET CANALICULI)

This is a condition defined by its clinical features.[62,103,104] In the classical clinical form the hair is a light silvery-blond, paler than expected. It is frizzy, stands away from the scalp, and cannot be combed flat (Fig. 11.25). It is often glistening or "spangled." It is usually normal in length, quantity, and tensile strength. The onset may be with the first terminal growth or soon after.

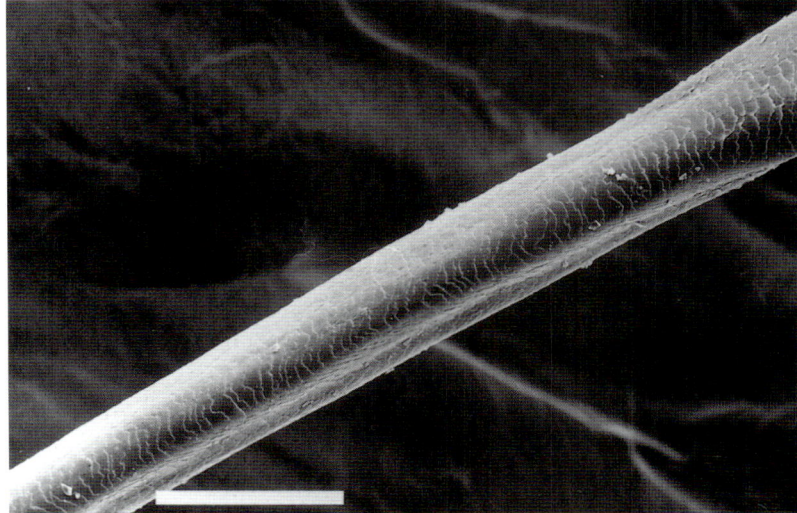

Fig. 11.26   Uncombable hair (pili canaliculi). Scanning electron microscopy demonstrating discontinuous grooving on different faces of the hair shaft.

Eyebrows, lashes, and body hair are normal. There are reports suggesting both dominant and recessive inheritance patterns. Scanning electron microscopy best demonstrates the characteristic shallow grooving or flattening of the surface (Fig. 11.26).[104] These areas are often discontinuous and change orientation many times along the length of the hair, occurring on different faces

96. Taylor A (1990) Hereditary woolly hair with ocular involvement. **Br J Dermatol** 123:523–526.
97. Neild VS, Pegum JS, Wells RS (1984) The association of keratosis pilaris atrophicans and woolly hair, with or without Noonan's syndrome. **Br J Dermatol** 110:357–362.
98. Carvajal-Huerta L (1998) Epidermolytic palmoplantar keratoderma with woolly hair and dilated cardiomyopathy. **J Am Acad Dermatol** 39:418–421.
99. McKoy G, Prontonotarios N, Crosby A et al. (2000) Identification of a deletion in plakoglobin in arrhythmogenic right ventricular cardiomyopathy with palmoplantar keratoderma and woolly hair (Naxos disease). **Lancet** 355:2119–2224.
100. Ouvrier RA (1989) Giant axonal neuropathy. **Brain and Development** 11:207–214.
101. Ruggieri M, Pavone V, Smilari P et al. (1995) Primary osteoma cutis – multiple cafe-au-lait spots and woolly hair abnormality. **Pediatr Radiol** 25:34–36.
102. Wright S, Lemoine NR, Leigh IM (1986) Woolly hair naevi with systematized linear epidermal naevus. **Clin Exp Dermatol** 11:179–182.
103. Ang P, Tay YK (1998) What syndrome is this? Uncombable hair (pili trianguli et canaliculi). **Pediatr Dermatol** 15:475–476.
104. Matis WL, Baden H, Green R et al. (1987) Un-combable hair syndrome. **Pediatr Dermatol** 4:215–219.

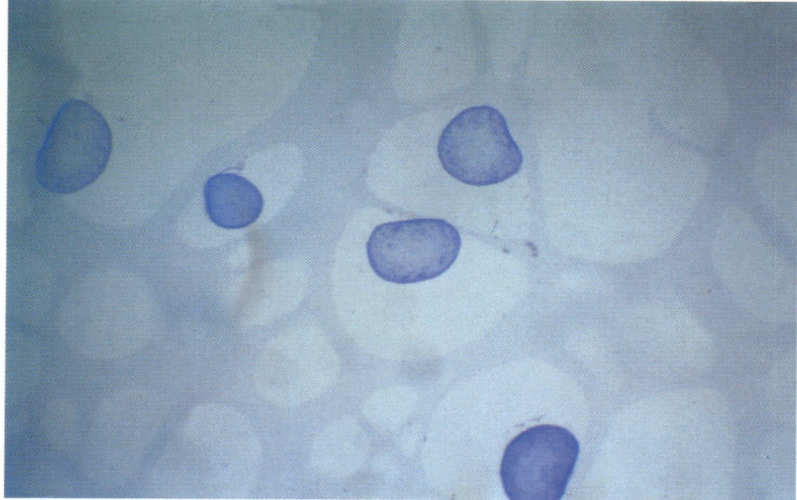

Fig. 11.27 Uncombable hair (pili canaliculi). Cross-sectional microscopy demonstrating reniform and other abnormal shapes.

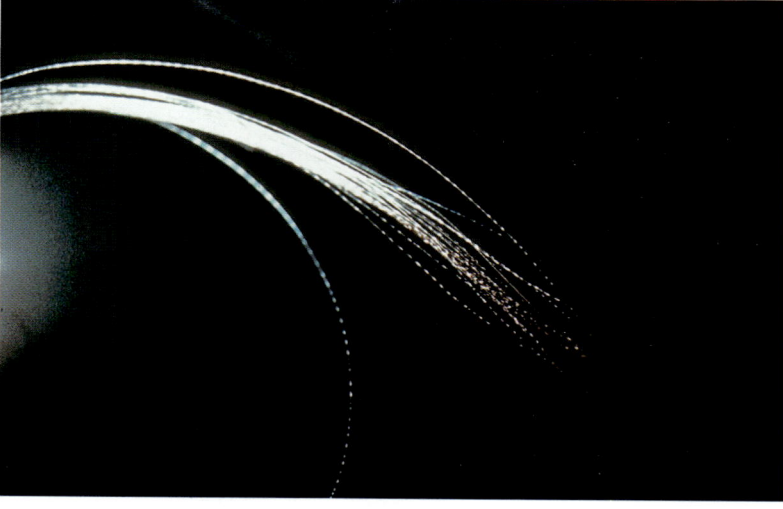

Fig. 11.29 Pili annulati. Banded appearance of hair viewed with reflected light.

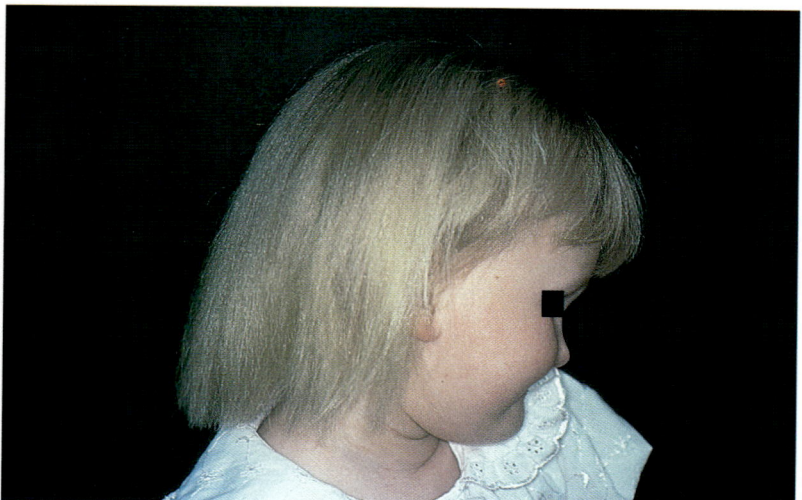

Fig. 11.28 Uncombable hair (pili canaliculi). Spangled hair in a patient with hypohidrotic ectodermal dysplasia.

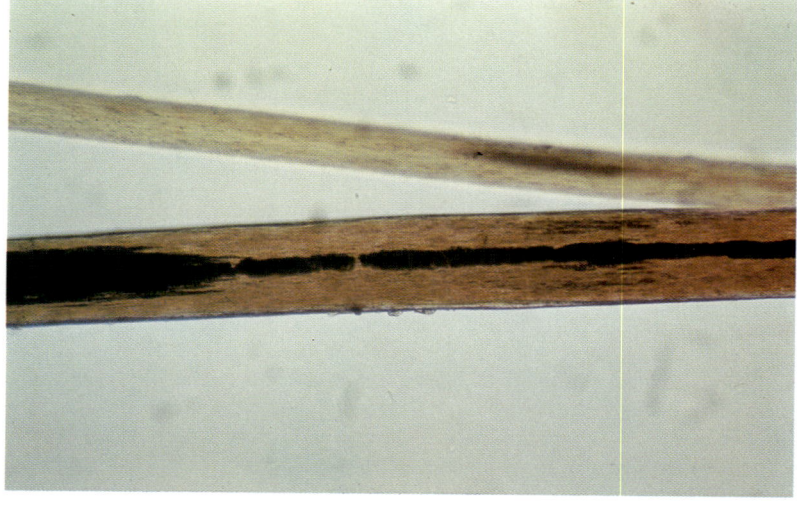

Fig. 11.30 Pili annulati. Microscopy demonstrating air spaces in the cortex of the hair.

of the hair at different points. Cross-sectional microscopy shows triangular, reniform, quadrangular, and other unusual shapes (Fig. 11.27). It is now clear that longitudinal grooving of hair shafts and/or and irregular cross-section is not specific for the clinical entity of uncombable hair. It has been demonstrated in a variety of other syndromes including progeria, Marie Unna hypotrichosis,[8,9] Rapp–Hodgkin syndrome,[80,105–107] oral facial digital syndrome type I,[56] ectrodactyly ectodermal dysplasia and clefting syndrome,[107] hypohidrotic ectodermal dysplasia (Fig. 11.28),[107] and angel-shaped phalango-epiphyseal dysplasia.[108] The classical clinical appearance of spun glass or uncombable hair would seem to depend on a certain proportion of abnormal hairs. The typical spangled appearance as found in the classical patient with no other abnormalities has been seen also in patients with Rapp–Hodgkin syndrome[80] and in hypohidrotic ectodermal dysplasia.[109]

PILI ANNULATI

This hair shaft abnormality, which may be congenital, does not render the hair fragile. The hair looks normally shiny but on close observation alternating bright and dark bands are seen.[62] There are usually no associated abnormalities. The condition may be sporadic or inherited, usually as a dominant characteristic. The bright areas are due to light scattered from clusters of air-filled cavities within the cortex and in a hair mount, viewed with transmitted light, the light areas appear as dark patches (Figs 11.29, 11.30). Scanning electron microscopy shows longitudinal wrinkling and folding in bands corresponding to the abnormal areas, possibly due to the evaporation of air in the spaces when the hair is coated in the vacuum. Transmission electron microscopy demonstrates multiple holes within the cortex.

105. Felding IB, Bjorklund LJ (1990) Rapp–Hodgkin ectodermal dysplasia. **Pediatr Dermatol** 7:126–131.
106. Cambiaghi S, Tadini G, Barbareschi M et al. (1994) Rapp–Hodgkin syndrome and AEC syndrome: are they the same entity? **Br J Dermatol** 130:97–101.
107. Micali GM, Cook B, Blekys I et al. (1990) Structural hair abnormalities in ectodermal dysplasia. **Pediatr Dermatol** 7:27–32.
108. Fritz TM, Trueb RM (2000) Uncombable hair with angel shaped phalango-epiphyseal dysplasia. **Pediatr Dermatol** 17:21–24.
109. Shelley WB, Shelley ED (1985) Uncombable hair syndrome: observations on response to biotin and occurrence in siblings with ectodermal dysplasia. **J Am Acad Dermatol** 13:97–102.

PSEUDOPILI ANNULATI

In this condition, which may simply represent an unusual variant of normal hair, there is a periodic reflection of light along the shaft giving an appearance of light and dark bands with reflected light, as in pili annulati.[60,110,111] The banding is due to superficial optical effects stemming from the geometry of the hair, which is elliptical in cross section and partially twisted in an oscillating fashion along its axis. On examination with transmitted light, the hair appears to vary periodically in thickness. However, the thick and thin segments are not constant and alternate when the hair is rotated, indicating that the appearance is due to twisting. The internal structure of the hair is normal. The banding is seen only when the light strikes the hair at right angles to the hair's long axis and only when the hair is rotated in certain positions about its long axis and not others. The flattened, twisted surfaces of the fiber act as reflective mirrors that preferentially reflect the light at certain angles and not others, and the elliptical hair acts as a variable cylindrical lens to refract and focus the incident light on to the posterior wall of the hair from which it is internally reflected.

TRICHORRHEXIS INVAGINATA

This is the characteristic hair shaft abnormality of Netherton syndrome for which the gene has recently been mapped to chromosome 5.[112] Although the severity varies considerably, the clinical and microscopic findings[62] are present from birth. In the severely affected neonate the hair may be extremely sparse or even absent (Fig. 11.31). What hair is present is fragile, short, and dull (Fig. 11.32). The changes may affect eyebrows, eyelashes, and general body hair also. Sometimes the scalp hair is so minimally affected that the diagnosis cannot be made on sampling from this area but the eyebrows are almost always short and broken and these should be sampled in a suspected case in which the abnormality cannot be demonstrated on scalp hair.

Microscopically, a ball and socket configuration with various patterns is seen. The classical "bamboo hair" occurs when the soft, abnormal hair shaft wraps around a firmer distal shaft, producing the appearance of a shallow invagination of the distal into the proximal shaft (Fig. 11.33). There is a tulip-like form with a deeper invagination and hence longer sides of the "cup" (Fig. 11.34).[60] The

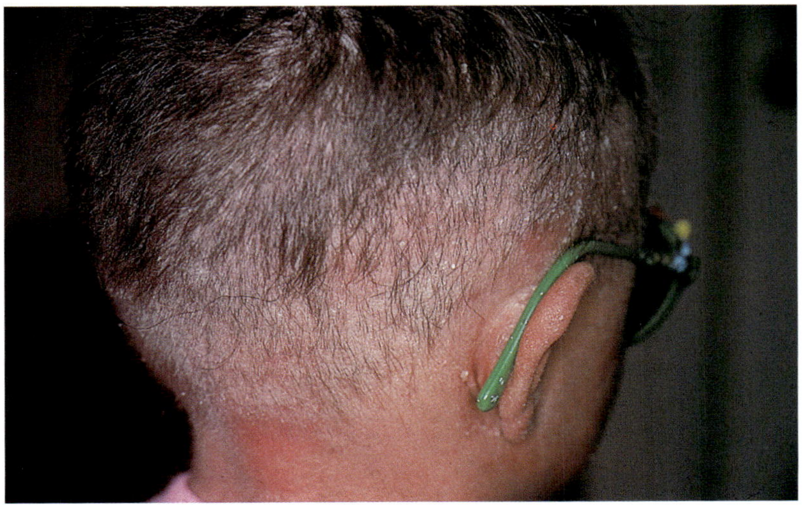

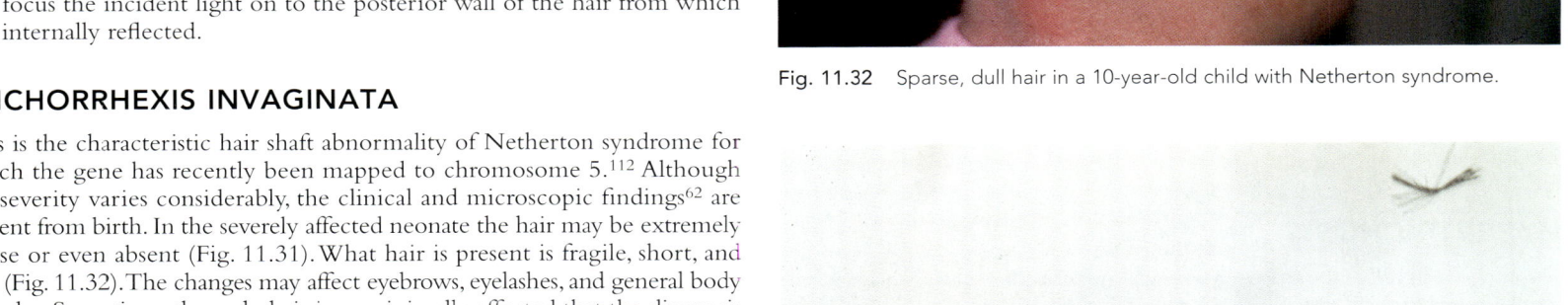

Fig. 11.32   Sparse, dull hair in a 10-year-old child with Netherton syndrome.

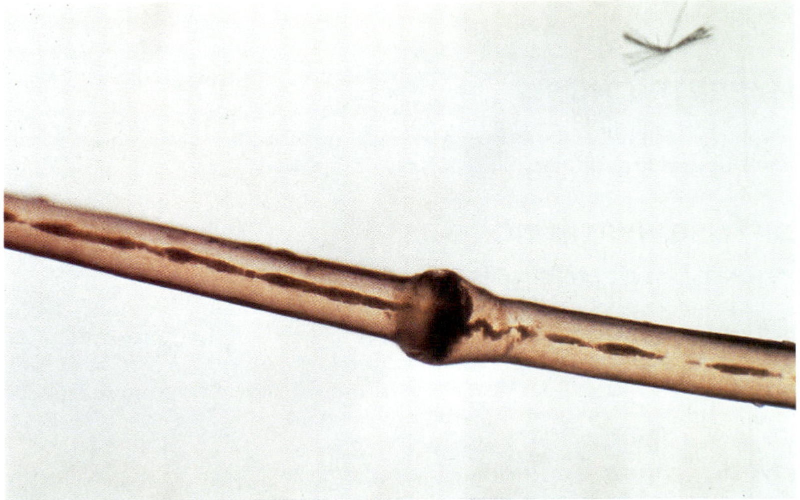

Fig. 11.33   Trichorrhexis invaginata. Microscopy demonstrating the bamboo-like appearance of the invagination.

earliest stage of the invagination may be seen as a circumferential stricture. The term "golf tee hair" has been given to the expanded proximal end of an invaginate node after a break has occurred (Fig. 11.35).[113] Thin vellus hairs may show multiple invaginations, the so-called "canestick hairs."[114] A helical pattern of twisting with obliquely running, parallel invaginations has recently been described[115] and should not be mistaken for pili torti.

ACQUIRED PROGRESSIVE KINKING OF THE HAIR

This condition, in which hair becomes progressively curly, frizzy and dull, usually has its onset in early adult life, involves androgen-dependent scalp hair, leads to hair thinning, and is probably in the spectrum of androgenetic alopecia.[116] However, a reversible form, unassociated with hair thinning, has recently been reported in a prepubertal boy.[117]

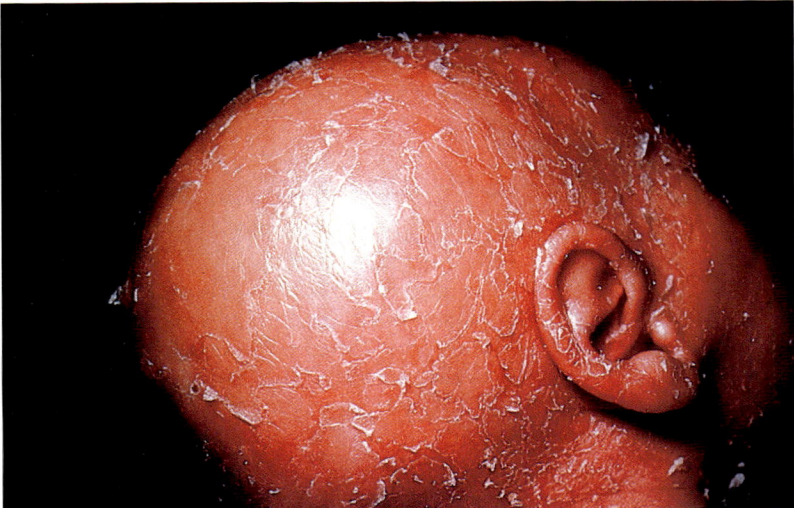

Fig. 11.31   Total alopecia in an infant with Netherton syndrome.

110. Price VH, Thomas RS, Jones FT (1970) Pseudopili annulati: an unusual variant of normal hair. **Arch Dermatol** 102:354–358.
111. Lee S-SJ, Lee Y-S, Giam Y-C (2001) Pseudopili annulati in a dark-haired individual. **Pediatr Dermatol** 18:27–30.
112. Chavanas S, Garner C, Bodemer C et al. (2000) Localization of the Netherton syndrome gene to chromosome q32, by linkage analysis and homozygosity mapping. **Am J Hum Genet** 66:914–921.
113. de Berker D, Paige D, Harper J et al. (1992) Golf tee hairs: a new sign in Netherton syndrome. **Br J Dermatol** 127(suppl 40):30.
114. Menne T, Weisman K (1985) Canestick lesions of vellus hair in Netherton's syndrome. **Arch Dermatol** 121:451.
115. Lurie R, Ben-Zion G (1995) Helical hairs: A new hair anomaly in a patient with Netherton's syndrome. **Cutis** 55:349–352.
116. Tosti A, Piraccini BM, Pazzaglia M et al. (1999) Acquired progressive kinking of the hair. **Arch Dermatol** 135:1223–1226.
117. Rigopoulos D, Katoulis AC, Stavrianeas NG et al. (1997) Acquired progressive kinking of the hair in a prepubertal boy. **Br J Dermatol** 137:832–833.

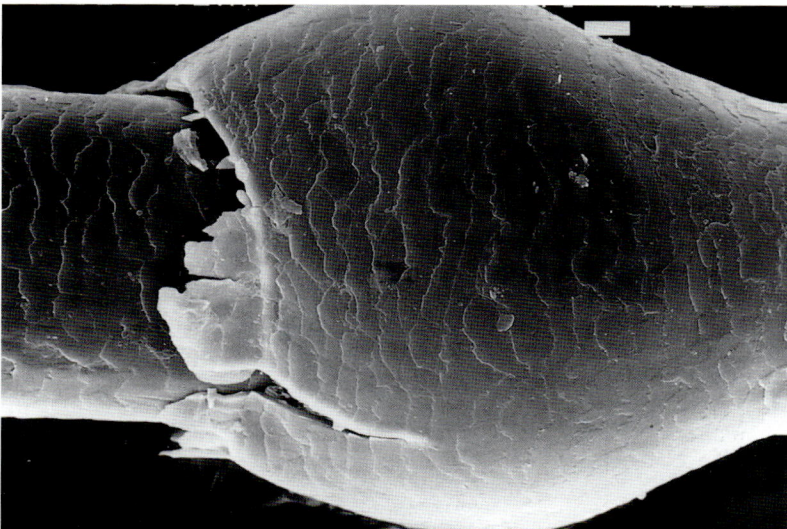

Fig. 11.34 Trichorrhexis invaginata. Scanning electron microscopy demonstrating a tulip-like appearance at the site of invagination.

HYPERTRICHOSIS

Hypertrichosis refers to diffuse or localized patterns of excessive hair growth without evidence of masculinization.

DIFFUSE HYPERTRICHOSIS

Primary hypertrichosis

Because of the wide variety of designations given and the poor clinical descriptions in the early literature there is much confusion surrounding the classification of congenital hypertrichosis occurring alone or with only occasional associations. However, several individual entities can probably be separated out.[118]

Hypertrichosis lanuginosa

This is a very rare condition characterized by retention of lanugo hair. At birth there is a coat of profuse, usually fair, silky, fine hair up to 10cm in length, involving all the usual hair-bearing areas of skin and blending with the hair of scalp and eyebrows.[119–122] There may be accentuation over the spine and on the pinnae and profuse growth in the ear canal may lead to infection and a hearing deficit. Matted hair in the diaper area is particularly troublesome.[123] The prognosis varies, with many authors reporting improvement while others report persistence or even worsening.[122,123] At puberty there may be no conversion to terminal hair in secondary sexual hair areas, with long, fine, lanugo hairs persisting in pubic and axillary areas and in the beard. While about one-third of cases are sporadic, both autosomal-dominant[119,120] and autosomal-recessive inheritance patterns are reported.[121] Most patients have no other abnormalities, but congenital glaucoma[122] and dental abnormalities[120,123] including neonatal teeth[123] have been observed. Management involves cutting or shaving the hair and there is one report of successful removal of hair using a neodymium-YAG laser.[124]

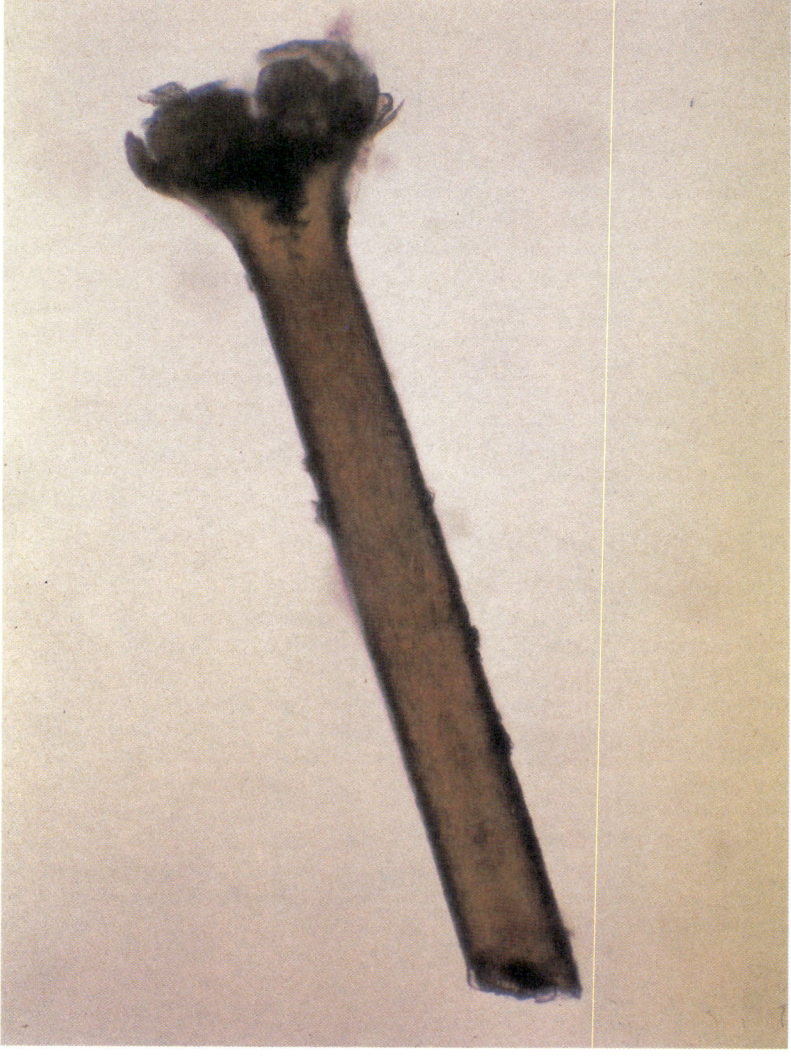

Fig. 11.35 Netherton syndrome. Microscopy demonstrating the "golf tee hair" appearance due to the expanded proximal end of an invaginate node after a break has occurred.

Ambras syndrome

This condition, so designated in reference to the first documented case, has been subsequently reported under a variety of names. It appears to be a unique form of diffuse congenital hypertrichosis in which the hair, which may demonstrate pigmentation and medullation, is said to be vellus rather than lanugo hair.[118,125,126] A balanced structural chromosomal aberration has been reported in a patient with this condition.[125] The hypertrichosis is most marked on face, ears, and shoulders and persists through life. On the face the long hair uniformly covers brow, eyelids, nose, and cheeks. A number of dysmorphic facial features have occurred in these patients.

118. Baumeister FAM, Schwartz HP, Stengel-Rutkowski S (1995) Childhood hypertrichosis: diagnosis and management. **Arch Dis Child** 72:457–459.
119. Felgenhauer WR (1969) Hypertrichosis lanuginosa universalis. **J Genet Hum** 17:1–44.
120. Freire-Maia M, Felizali J, de Figueiredo AC et al. (1976) Hypertrichosis lanuginosa in a mother and son. **Clin Genet** 10:303–306.
121. Janssen TAE, de Lange C (1946) Hypertrichosis (trichostasis) lanuginosa. **Ned Tijdschr Geneesk** 90:198.
122. Judge MR, Rice NSC, Christopher A et al. (1991) Congenital hypertrichosis lanuginosa and congenital glaucoma. **Br J Dermatol** 124:495–497.

123. Partridge JW (1987) Congenital hypertrichosis lanuginosa: neonatal shaving. **Arch Dis Child** 62:623–625.
124. Littler CM (1997) Laser hair removal in a patient with hypertrichosis lanuginosa congenita. **Dermatologic Surg** 23:705–707.
125. Baumeister FAM, Egger J, Schildhaure MT et al. (1993) Ambras syndrome: delineation of a unique hypertrichosis universalis congenita and association with a balanced pericentric inversion (8)(p11.2;q22). **Clin Genet** 44:121–128.
126. Baumeister FAM (2000) Differentiation of Ambras syndrome from hypertrichosis universalis. **Clin Genet** 57:157–158.

X-linked dominant hypertrichosis

A pedigree has been reported with probable X-linked dominant inheritance in which affected individuals had a generalized terminal hair hypertrichosis present at birth and most severe over the face, pubic area, back, and upper chest.[127] (In some cases there was an improvement on the trunk and limbs after puberty.) This condition has recently been mapped to chromosome Xq24–q27.1.[128]

Prepubertal hypertrichosis

A series is reported of children with generalized hypertrichosis present from birth and increasing in severity in early childhood but no other abnormal clinical findings.[129] There is profuse terminal hair growth on the back and proximal limbs and also on the temples, spreading across the brow and merging with bushy eyebrows. The pattern does not resemble hirsutism. There was a patterning of the hair growth on the back with an inverted fir tree distribution centering on the spine. It is not clear whether this condition represents an abnormality or whether it is an extreme form of the normal range of hair growth, as it resembles the patterns of hair growth seen in some racial groups.[129] However, a recent study has demonstrated elevated plasma dihydrotestosterone levels in several patients, suggesting that indeed an endocrine abnormality may be the basis for this condition.[130]

Hypertrichosis as part of other genetically determined disorders

Hypertrichosis, with the onset in the neonatal period or in childhood, is a feature of a number of genetically determined syndromes. A selection of these[131–147] is covered in Table 11.2.

Drug induced hypertrichosis

Neonatal hypertrichosis is an occasional feature of the fetal alcohol syndrome[148] and also can occur due to maternal use of minoxidil.[149] A dose-dependent hypertrichosis of the brow, limbs, and back becomes obvious in the first four weeks of treatment with diazoxide, which is used in neonates with hyperinsulinemia. Other drugs that may be responsible for hypertrichosis in infants and children include cyclosporin, penicillamine, diphenylhydantoin, and minoxidil. An excellent result is reported from the use of a chemical depilatory cream in cyclosporin-induced hypertrichosis in a 6-month-old infant.[150]

Hypertrichosis with systemic diseases

Systemic illnesses in children in which diffuse hypertrichosis may develop include anorexia nervosa[151] and other causes of malnutrition, dermatomyositis[152,153] and primary hypothyroidism.[154]

LOCALIZED HYPERTRICHOSIS

Nevoid hypertrichosis

Several patients have been reported with single or multiple localized patches of terminal hair growing from skin of normal color and texture (Fig. 11.36).[155,156] In one case, underlying lipoatrophy was found in some patches.[155] Additional abnormalities in one patient included areas of lipoatrophy and streaky depigmentation away from the areas of hypertrichosis, developmental delay and seizures, congenital lung cyst, congenital malrotation of the gut, multiple skeletal, dental, and ocular abnormalities.[156] This constellation of findings did not fit into any recognized syndrome. It is likely that these represent mosaic disorders. A case has been recently reported of a definitely Blaschko-distributed pattern of depigmented hypertrichosis in a patient who also had short stature, scoliosis, developmental delay and seizures, structural brain malformations demonstrated on imaging, microphthalmia, eyelid coloboma, and other structural ocular abnormalities.[157] In another case with multiple patches of congenital nevoid hypertrichosis there was an associated epidermal nevus, hypopigmented hairless streaks, and a retinal pigmentary abnormality; surprisingly, the hypertrichosis spontaneously resolved by the age of 2 years.[158]

Familial cervical hypertrichosis with kyphoscoliosis

A family has been reported with congenital localized hypertrichosis of the cervical area overlying a kyphoscoliosis, without other spinal or cutaneous abnormalities.[159] The inheritance pattern was autosomal dominant.

127. Macias-Flores MA, Garcia-Cruz D, Rivera H et al. (1984) A new form of hypertrichosis inherited as an X-linked dominant trait. Hum Genet 66:66–70.
128. Figuera LE, Pardolfo M, Dunne PW et al. (1995) Mapping of the congenital generalized hypertrichosis locus to chromosome Xq24–q27.1. Nature Genet 10:202–207.
129. Barth JH, Wilkinson JD, Dawber RPR (1988) Prepubertal hypertrichosis: normal or abnormal? Arch Dis Child 63:666–668.
130. Balducci R, Toscano V (1990) Bioactive and peripheral androgens in prepubertal simple hypertrichosis. Clin Endocrinol 33:407–414.
131. Lee IJ, Im SB, Kim D-K (1993) Hypertrichosis universalis congenita: a separate entity, or the same disease as gingival fibromatosis? Pediatr Dermatol 10:263–266.
132. Witkop CJ (1971) Heterogeneity in gingival fibromatosis. Birth Defects: Original Article Series VII, 7:210–221.
133. Lacombe D, Biculac-Sage P, Sibout M et al. (1994) Congenital marked hypertrichosis and Laband syndrome in a child: overlap between the gingival fibromatosis-hypertrichosis and Laband syndromes. Genetic Counseling 5:251–256.
134. Chiewchanvit S, Mahanupab P, Vanittanakom P (1998) Congenital erythropoietic porphyria: a case report. J Med Assoc Thailand 81:1023–1027.
135. Parsons JL, Sahn EE, Holden KR et al. (1994) Neurologic disease in a child with hepatoerytropoietic porphyria. Pediatr Dermatol 11:216–221.
136. Garcia-Cruz D, Sanchez-Corona J, Nazara Z et al. (1997) Congenital hypertrichosis, osteochondrodysplasia and cardiomegaly: further delineation of a new genetic syndrome. Am J Med Genet 69:138–151.
137. Robertson SP, Kirk E, Bernier F et al. (1999) Congenital hypertrichosis, osteochondrodysplasia and cardiomegaly: Cantu syndrome. Am J Med Genet 85:395–402.
138. Concolino D, Formicola S, Camera G et al. (2000) Congenital hypertrichosis, cardiomegaly and osteochondrodysplasia (Cantu syndrome): a new case with unusual radiological findings. Am J Med Genet 92:191–194.
139. Lazalde B, Sanchez-Urbina R, Nuno-Arana I et al. (2000) Autosomal dominant inheritance in Cantu syndrome (congenital hypertrichosis, osteochondrodysplasia and cardiomegaly). Am J Med Genet 94:421–427.
140. Ireland M, Burn J (1993) Cornelia de Lange syndrome – photo essay. Clin Dysmorphol 2:151–160.
141. Husain K, Fitzgerald P, Lau G (1994) Cecal volvulus in the Cornelia de Lange syndrome. J Pediatr Surg 29:1245–1247.
142. Levy P, Baraitser M (1991) Coffin-Siris syndrome. J Med Genet 28:338–341.
143. McPherson EW, Laneri G, Clemens MM et al. (1997) Apparently balanced t(1:7)(q21.3;q34) in an infant with Coffin-Siris syndrome. Am J Med Genet 71:430–433.
144. Roth SI, Schedewie HK, Herzberg VK et al. (1981) Cutaneous manifestations of leprechaunism. Arch Dermatol 117:531–535.
145. Santana SM, Alvarez FP, Frias JL et al. (1993) Hypertrichosis, atrophic skin, ectropion and macrostomia (Barber-Say) syndrome: report of a new case. Am J Med Genet 47:20–23.
146. Selmanowitz VJ, Stiller MJ (1981) Rubinstein-Taybi syndrome. Arch Dermatol 117:504–506.
147. Cambiaghi S, Ermacora E, Brusasco A et al. (1994) Multiple pilomatricomas in Rubinstein-Taybi syndrome. Pediatr Dermatol 11:21–25.
148. Hanson JW, Jones KL, Smith DW (1976) Fetal alcohol syndrome: experience with 41 patients. J Am Med Assoc 235:1458–1460.
149. Kaler SG, Patrinos ME, Lambert GH et al. Hypertrichosis and congenital anomalies associated with maternal use of Minoxidil. Pediatrics 79:434–436.
150. Wendelin DS, Mallory GB, Mallory SB (1999) Depilation in a 6-month-old with hypertrichosis: a case report. Pediatr Dermatol 16:311–313.
151. Schultze UM, Pettke-Rank CV, Kreienkamp M et al. (1999) Dermatologic findings in anorexia and bulimia nervosa of childhood and adolescence. Pediatr Dermatol 16:90–94.
152. Pope DN, Strimling RB, Mallory SB (1994) Hypertrichosis in juvenile dermatomyositis. J Am Acad Dermatol 31:383–387.
153. Quecedo E, Febrer I, Serrano G et al. (1996) Partial lipodystrophy associated with juvenile dermatomyositis: report of two cases. Pediatr Dermatol 13:477–482.
154. Stern SR, Kelnar CHJ (1985) Hypertrichosis due to hypothyroidism. Arch Dis Child 60:763–766.
155. Cox NH, McClure JP, Hardie RA (1989) Naevoid hypertrichosis – report of a patient with multiple lesions. Clin Exp Dermatol 14:62–64.
156. Rogers M (1981) Naevoid hypertrichosis. Clin Exp Dermatol 16:74.
157. Schauder S, Hanefeld F, Noske UM et al. (2000) Depigmented hypertrichosis following Blaschko's lines associated with cerebral and ocular malformations; a new neurocutaneous autosomal lethal gene syndrome from the group of epidermal naevus syndromes? 142:1204–1207.
158. Dudding TE, Rogers M, Roddick LG et al. (1998) Nevoid hypertrichosis with multiple patches of hair that underwent almost complete spontaneous resolution. Am J Med Genet 79:195–196.
159. Reed OM, Mellette JR, Fitzpatrick JE (1989) Familial cervical hypertrichosis with underlying kyphoscoliosis. J Am Acad Dermatol 20:1069–1072.

TABLE 11.2 Syndromes featuring hypertrichosis

Syndrome	Hypertrichosis	Other features
Hypertrichosis with gingival fibromatosis There are 3 syndromes which may represent parts of a single spectrum: 1. Gingival fibromatosis[131]	Relatively mild congenital hypertrichosis.	Gingival fibromatosis.
2. Gingival fibromatosis and epilepsy[132]	Severe congenital hypertrichosis. Hair is pigmented. Most severe on face, arms, and lumbosacral area.	Gingival fibromatosis and epilepsy.
3. Laband syndrome[133]	Marked congenital hypertrichosis reported in one patient.	Gingival hyperplasia, dysplasia of the terminal phalanges, hepatosplenomegaly, facial dysmorphism.
Hypertrichosis with hereditary porphyrias 1. Congenital erythropoietic porphyria[134]	Hypertrichosis occurs particularly on light exposed areas.	
2. Familial porphyria cutanea tarda	A marked, diffuse facial hypertrichosis may occur in early childhood; less often limb involvement.	
3. Hepatoerythropoietic porphyria[135]	A variable, sometimes severe hypertrichosis.	
Hypertrichosis with osteochondrodysplasia (Cantu syndrome)[136–139]	Diffuse hypertrichosis.	Congenital macrosomia, coarse facial features, cardiomegaly, narrow thorax, broad ribs, coxa valga, and short phalanges. Recently described megaepiphyses.
Cornelia de Lange syndrome[140,141]	Mild generalized hypertrichosis with low frontal and occipital hairlines, thick eyebrows, synophrys and long, upturned lashes. The hair on the lateral elbows and sacral area may be very long and fine.	Low birth weight congenital livedo, increased susceptibility to infection, growling cry, distinctive facies with hypertelorism, an anti-Mongoloid slant of the palpebral fissures, long philtrum, and thin lips. Rare features are micromelia, phocomelia, gastrointestinal, and urogenital malformations.
Coffin Siris syndrome[142,143]	Hypertrichosis, particularly of face and back. Low frontal hairline, bushy eyebrows, and long eyelashes, but often sparse scalp hair.	Absence or hypoplasia of the nails and distal phalanges of fifth fingers and toes, microcephaly, facial dysmorphism, growth failure, and mental retardation.
Leprechaunism[144]	Coarse curly scalp hair. Extensive body and facial hypertrichosis in 75% of cases.	Low birth weight, wrinkled loose skin with decrease of subcutaneous fat, acanthosis nigricans, periorificial rugosity of skin, thick lips, gingival hypertrophy, large low-set ears, and hypertrophic external genitalia.
Seip–Berardinelli syndrome (congenital generalized lipodystrophy)	Congenital hypertrichosis of face, neck and limbs, increasing with age. Low frontal hairline and thick, curly scalp hair.	Deficient subcutaneous fat, acanthosis nigricans, organomegaly, hypertrophy of genitalia. Insulin resistant diabetes.
Mucopolysaccharidoses: Hunter, Hurler and Sanfilippo forms	Hypertrichosis is an occasional feature of these.	
Barber-Say syndrome[145]	Extensive generalized hypertrichosis, most marked over the back.	Redundant atrophic skin, telecanthus, ectropion, macrostomia, a broad bulbous nose, and abnormal pinnae.
Rubenstein–Taybi syndrome[146,147]	Hypertrichosis of trunk, limbs and face in 2/3 of cases. The eyebrows are highly arched and the eyelashes unusually long.	Capillary vascular malformations, beaked nose, hypertelorism, high arched palate, cryptorchidism and broad thumbs and great toes and sometimes other digits. Pilomatricomas.

Anterior cervical hypertrichosis

A congenital patch of hypertrichosis on the front of the neck has been described as an isolated phenomenon[160] and in association with peripheral sensory and motor neuropathy[161] with or without retinal abnormalities.[162]

Hairy cutaneous malformations of palms and soles

There have been reports of the familial occurrence of hair growth on circumscribed areas of the palms and soles.[163] In one family the skin in the area showed exaggerated skin markings in a geometric pattern. The condition was

160. Braddock SR, Jones KL, Bird LM et al. (1995) Anterior cervical hypertrichosis: a dominantly inherited isolated defect. Am J Med Genet 55:498–499.
161. Trattner A, Hodak E, Sagie-Lerman T et al. (1991) Familial congenital anterior cervical hypertrichosis associated with peripheral sensory and motor neuropathy – A new syndrome? J Am Acad Dermatol 25:767–770.
162. Garty BZ, Snir M, Kremer I et al. (1997) Retinal changes in familial peripheral sensory and motor neuropathy associated with anterior cervical hypertrichosis. J Pediatr Ophthalmol and Strabismus 34:309–312.
163. Jackson CE, Callies QC, Krull EA et al. (1975) Hairy cutaneous malformations of the palms and soles. Arch Dermatol 111:1146–1149.

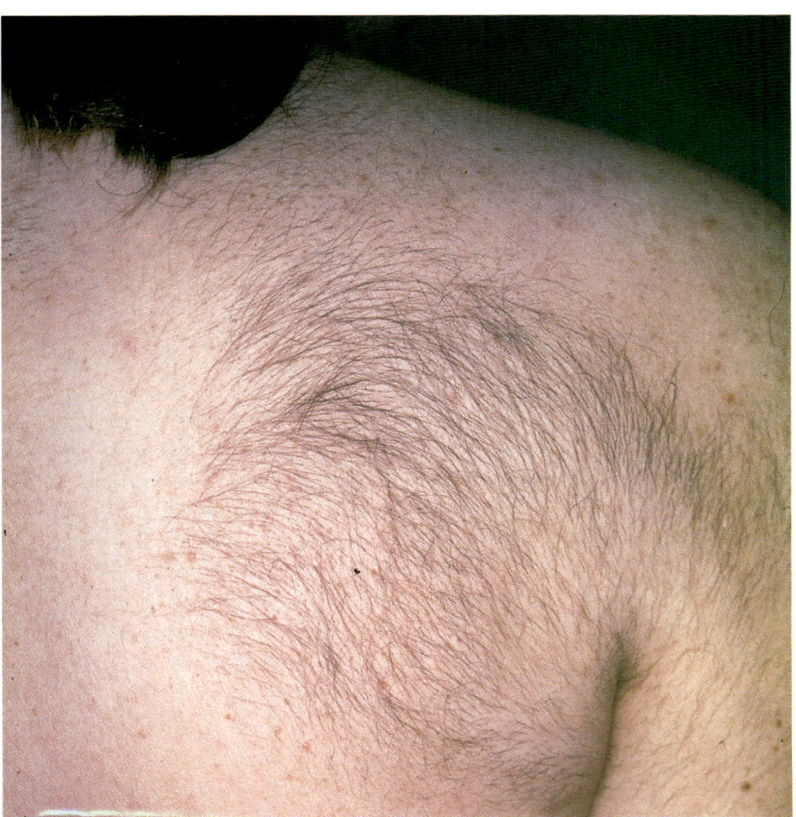

Fig. 11.36 Nevoid hypertrichosis. Swirls of terminal hair on a background of normal skin.

present at birth and persisted through life. Histopathology demonstrated the presence of ectopic hair follicles and some increase in the amount of elastic fibers in the dermis.

Scrotal hair

Several infant boys have been reported to have developed scrotal hair within the first three months of life, in the absence of clinical or biochemical evidence of excessive androgen production.[164,165] The condition was non-progressive and the hair usually disappeared by the age of 18 months.[164]

Hypertrichosis cubiti

This is an uncommon condition in which profuse vellus hair is localized on the extensor aspects of the arms, particularly around the elbow area.[166,167] It is likely that the few associated abnormalities reported represent chance associations. Both dominant and recessive inheritance patterns have been reported but some cases are apparently sporadic. The condition appears in infancy, increases in early childhood and improves spontaneously at puberty.[166]

Hypertrichosis with spinal fusion abnormalities

These occur mainly in the lumbosacral area but can occur elsewhere over the spine. A tuft of long, silky hair often marks the abnormal area, with or without other cutaneous markers such as dimple, sinus tract, aplasia cutis, capillary malformation, hemangioma, lipoma, or pigmented nevus.[168,169] These cutaneous lesions may be found in the presence of clinical spina bifida with myelomenigocele but are particularly helpful as markers for occult spinal dysraphism.

Hypertrichosis with cranial meningoceles, encephaloceles and heterotopic meningeal or brain tissue

They are often marked by a peripheral collar of hair, a tuft of hair nearby or overlying hair (Fig. 11.37).[170–173] Prominent or patulous hair follicle orifices may also be a feature. The membranous form of aplasia cutis, which may also demonstrate a hair collar, is now recognized as a form fruste of a neural tube closure defect.[45] For scalp lesions the hair is longer, thicker, and often darker than the surrounding normal hair. With lesions away from the scalp the presence of hair may be an indication that one is dealing with a neural lesion. A patient has been reported with a congenital patch of hypertrichosis over the lumbar area, well away from the spine, overlying what was demonstrated histologically to be meningeal tissue.[174] The mechanism of this type of case may be displacement of meningeal cells along nerves during embryogenesis rather than the entrapment of meningeal membranes at the time of closure of the neural tube.[175,176]

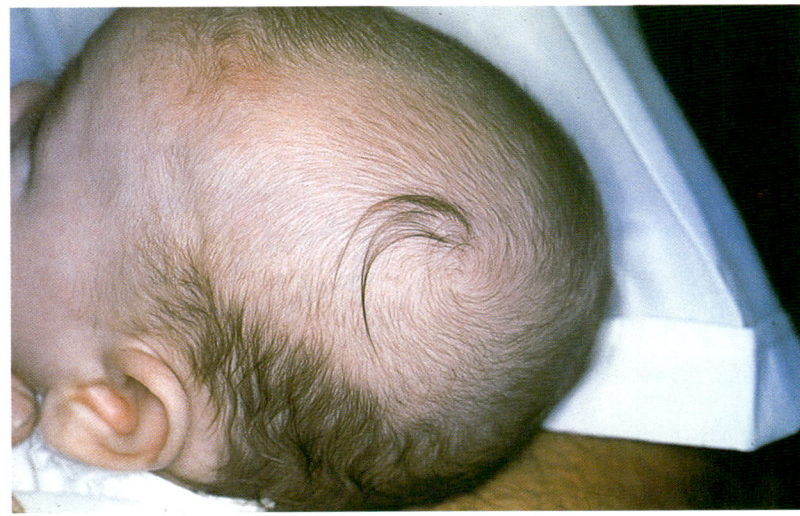

Fig. 11.37 Localized hypertrichosis at the site of a small area of heterotopic brain tissue.

164. Diamond FB, Shulman DI, Root AW (1989) Scrotal hair in infancy. **J Pediatr** 114:999–1001.
165. Slyper AH, Esterly NB (1993) Nonprogressive scrotal hair growth in two infants. **Pediatr Dermatol** 10:34–35.
166. Escallonilla P, Aguilar A, Gallego M et al. (1996) A new case of hairy elbows syndrome (hypertrichois cubiti). **Pediatr Dermatol** 13:303–305.
167. Schwarze HP, Loche F, Kuchta J et al. (1999) A sporadic form of hypertrichosis cubiti. **Clin Exp Dermatol** 24:496–500.
168. Tavafoghi V, Ghandchi A, Hambrick GW et al. (1978) Cutaneous signs of spinal dysraphism. **Arch Dermatol** 114:573–577.
169. Davis DA, Cohen PR, George RE (1994) Cutaneous stigmata of occult spinal dysraphism. **J Am Acad Dermatol** 31:892–896.
170. Commens C, Rogers M (1989) Heterotropic brain tissue presenting as bald cysts with a collar of hypertrophic hair. **Arch Dermatol** 125:1253–1256.

171. Stone MS, Walker PS, Kennard CD (1994) Rudimentary meningocele presenting with a scalp hair tuft. **Arch Dermatol** 130:775–777.
172. Khallouf R, Fetissof F, Machet MC (1994) Sequestrated meningocele of the scalp: diagnostic value of hair abnormalities. **Pediatr Dermatol** 11:315–318.
173. Drolet BA, Clowry L, McTigue K et al. (1995) The hair collar sign: marker for cranial dysraphism. **Pediatrics** 96:309–313.
174. Penas PF, Jones-Caballero M, Amigo A et al. (1994) Cutaneous meningioma underlying congenital localised hypertrichosis. **J Am Acad Dermatol** 30:363–366.
175. Penas PF, Jones-Caballero M, Garcia-Diez A (1995) Cutaneous heterotopic meningeal nodules. **Arch Dermatol** 131:731.
176. Theaker JM, Fletcher CD, Tudway AJ (1990) Cutaneous heterotopic meningeal nodules. **Histopathology** 16:475–479.

Hypertrichosis with focal facial dermal dysplasia

A patient is reported with what is designated as an unusual variant of focal facial dermal dysplasia with symmetrical skin defects at both temples and extending on to the cheeks.[177] These were scar-like, circular, atrophic lesions, each surrounded by a fine rim of hair. These lesions are believed to follow an embryological fusion line. It was suggested that perhaps they would be better described under the broader term of bilateral aplasia cutis.

Hemihypertrophy with hypertrichosis

Hemihypertrophy is a rare congenital disorder in which the whole, or less commonly part, of one side of the body is enlarged. Serious associated malformations include Wilms tumor and tumors of brain and adrenals. The skin is often normal but cutaneous abnormalities reported include pigmentation, telangiectasia, abnormal nail growth, and hypertrichosis, which can be very striking.[178]

Localized hypertrichosis in association with other nevi or tumors

Congenital melanocytic nevus

Congenital melanocytic nevi may be covered at birth with dense, dark terminal hair over part or all of their surface. On the scalp even very flat lesions often have a dense covering of hair which is longer, darker, and coarser than the surrounding scalp hair. In areas other than the scalp the degree of hairiness of the lesion is usually proportional to its degree of elevation.

Congenital smooth muscle hamartoma and Becker's nevus

Congenital smooth muscle hamartomas present most commonly at birth as slightly raised, firm, pebbly plaques, of background skin color or slightly pigmented, with a varying degree of hypertrichosis.[179] They most often occur on the trunk or the proximal limbs but may involve other areas, including the scalp.[180] A transient piloerection or elevation of the lesion after it is rubbed (the pseudo-Darier sign) is a characteristic feature. Extensive hypertrichosis overlying extensive, widespread smooth muscle hamartomas has been reported.[181,182] Becker's nevus usually presents in late childhood or adolescence as a patch of thickened, pigmented, hypertrichotic skin but congenital cases have been reported, although usually lacking hypertrichosis in the neonatal period.[183] An unusual presentation with congenital bilaterally symmetrical lesions, hypertrichotic at birth, has been reported.[184] Controversy remains as to whether Becker's nevus and congenital smooth muscle hamartoma are in the one spectrum[179] or are distinct entities.[185]

Plexiform neurofibroma

There is often hyperpigmentation with irregular outlines over these lesions and hypertrichosis of varying degree may also occur.[186] A prominent paraspinal hair whorl has been reported at the site of a deep mediastinal plexiform neurofibroma[187] and a similar paraspinal whorl has been described in a neurofibromatosis patient with a posterior mediastinal ganglioneuroma.[188]

Sclerosing tufted angioma

A tufted angioma is a rare congenital or acquired vascular proliferation histologically characterized by multiple separated cellular nodules within dermis and subcutaneous fat.[189] Each lobule comprises masses of endothelial cells whorled around a pre-existing vascular plexus, and sometimes bulging into the walls of dilated thin-walled vascular spaces giving a tufted appearance. They usually appear clinically as red to brown plaques or occasionally as nodules.[189] There is a rare clinical variant, preferentially localized to the lower limbs, which progresses to sclerosis.[190] The lesions are present at birth or develop in the first weeks of life as erythematous plaques, which extend and become progressively indurated. On microscopic examination, there is fibrosis in addition to the usual histological features. Several of these lesions demonstrated hypertrichosis and increased sweating.

Linear melorheostotic scleroderma

Melorheostosis is a rare bone dysplasia characterized by eccentric cortical hyperostosis. It has been associated with soft-tissue abnormalities, including vascular lesions and marked dermal thickening, producing a sclerodermoid change.[191] Histologically, the dermis contains excessive normal collagen fibers lacking the hyalinization seen in a true linear scleroderma. There may be significant overlying hypertrichosis. Cases are reported with the cutaneous changes of linear melorheostotic scleroderma but with no skeletal changes demonstrable.[192]

Hypertrichosis due to local heat and cutaneous hyperemia

There are various situations in which hypertrichosis occurs where the likely pathogenesis is related to local heat and cutaneous hyperemia.[193] Examples include sites of PUVA therapy, chickenpox scars, insect bites, at the edges of burns, areas of chronic excoriation, under a plaster cast, and over inflamed joints.

ERUPTIVE VELLUS HAIR CYSTS

Eruptive vellus hair cysts are discrete bluish, pale or skin-colored smooth surfaced, soft papules ranging in diameter from 1 to 4mm, most commonly found on the anterior chest, but also on the upper and lower extremities, the face, neck, posterior trunk and/or buttocks of children and young adults.[194,195] The usual age at onset is between ages 4 and 18 years but presence at birth and adult onset are both reported. The development is usually quite fast and then, following a static period, spontaneous clearing takes place after several years, in some cases.

On histopathology, there is a cystic structure in the mid-dermis lined by four or five layers of squamous epithelium with a discrete granular layer and filled with laminated and amorphous keratinous material as well as fragments of vellus hairs.[195,196] There are no sebaceous glands in the cyst wall as are seen in steatocystoma multiplex. A case has been reported with some umbilicated papules with histological evidence of transepithelial elimination, which may

177. Stone N, Burge S (1998) Focal facial dermal dysplasia with a hair collar. **Br J Dermatol** 139:1111–1137.
178. Hurwitz S, Klaus SN (1971) Congenital hemihypertrophy with hypertrichosis. **Arch Dermatol** 103:98–100.
179. Johnson MD, Jacobs AJ (1989) Congenital smooth muscle hamartoma. **Arch Dermatol** 125:820–822.
180. Knable A, Treadwell P (1996) Pigmented plaque with hypertrichosis on the scalp of an infant. **Pediatr Dermatol** 13:431–433.
181. Glover MT, Malone M, Atherton DJ (1989) Michelin-tire baby syndrome resulting from diffuse smooth muscle hamartoma. **Pediatr Dermatol** 6:329–331.
182. Larregue M, Vabre P, Cavaroc Y et al. (1991) Hamartome diffus des muscles arrecteurs et hypertrichose lanugineuse congenitale. **Ann Dermatol Venereol** 118:796–798.
183. Book SE, Glass AT, Laude TA (1997) Congenital Becker's nevus with a familial association. **Pediatr Dermatol** 14:373–375.
184. Ferreira MJ, Bajanca R, Fiadeiro T (1998) Congenital melanosis and hypertrichosis in a bilateral distribution. **Pediatr Dermatol** 15:290–292.
185. Gagne EJ, Su WPD (1993) Congenital smooth muscle hamartoma of the skin. **Pediatr Dermatol** 10:142–145.
186. Ettl A, Marinkovic M, Koornneef L (1996) Localised hypertrichosis associated with periorbital neurofibroma; clinical findings and differential diagnosis. **Ophthalmol** 103:942–948.

187. Pivnik EK, Lobe TE, Fitch SJ et al. (1997) Hair whorl as an indicator of a mediastinal plexiform neurofibroma. **Pediatr Dermatol** 14:196–198.
188. Flannery DB, Howell CG (1986) Confirmation of the Riccardi sign. **Proc Greenwood Genet Centre** 6:161.
189. Requena L, Sangueza OP (1997) Cutaneous vascular proliferations. Part II. Hyperplasias and benign neoplasms. **J Am Acad Dermatol** 37:887–920.
190. Catteau B, Enjolras O, Delaporte E et al. (1998) Angiome en touffes sclerosant. A propos de 4 observations aux membres inferieurs. **Ann Dermatol Venereol** 125:682–687.
191. Miyachi Y, Horio T, Yamada A et al. (1979) Linear melorheostotic scleroderma with hypertrichosis. **Arch Dermatol** 115:1233–1234.
192. Fimiani M, Rubengi P, de Aloe G et al. (1999) Linear melorheostotic scleroderma with hypertrichosis sine melorheostosis. **Br J Dermatol** 141:747–776.
193. Kara A, Kanra G, Alanay Y (2001) Localised acquired hypertrichosis following cast application. **Pediatr Dermatol** 18:57–59.
194. Esterly NB, Fretzin DF, Pinkus H (1977) Eruptive vellus hair cysts. **Arch Dermatol** 113:500–503.
195. Baums K, Blume-Peytavi U, Dippel E et al. (2000) Guess what: Eruptive vellus hair cysts. **Europ J Dermatol** 10:487–489.
196. Hurlimann AF, Panizzon RG, Burg G (1996) Eruptive vellus hair cyst and steatocystoma multiplex: Hybrid cysts. **Dermatology** 192:64–66.

explain the spontaneous disappearance of lesions.[197] Kindreds with an autosomal–dominant inheritance pattern have been reported.[198] There are reports of families in which milia, eruptive vellus hair cysts, and steatocystoma multiplex all occurred,[199] with some individuals showing more than one type of lesion. Hybrid cysts with features of steatocystoma multiplex in one part and eruptive vellus hair cysts in another have also been reported.[196] This led to the conclusion that these three disorders should be considered as subtypes of multiple pilosebaceous cysts that may all present overlapping histologic features, with the different level of the sebaceous duct from which the cyst originates explaining the different clinical manifestations. However, this concept is challenged by studies reporting the finding of expression of both keratin 10 and keratin 17 in steatocystoma multiplex but only keratin 17 in eruptive vellus hair cysts.[200]

Lesions are usually fairly subtle cosmetically and there is a chance of spontaneous involution. However, successful treatment is reported with needle evacuation[201] and by the use of an erbium:YAG laser.[202]

ABNORMALITIES OF HAIR COLOR
DIFFUSE HYPOPIGMENTATION OF HAIR

This may be primary and present from birth, particularly in certain genetic conditions; it may appear later as premature graying (premature canities) due to autoimmune diseases and certain syndromes and is usually permanent; and it may occur, usually as a result of nutritional deficiencies, as an acquired reversible condition.

Primary diffuse hypopigmentation of the hair

Hair that is hypopigmented from birth is found in a wide range of genetic conditions.[203,204] In some it is simply fairer than expected but in others it may have a silvery aspect. Some of these conditions are listed in Table 11.3.

Premature canities

Canities, or graying of human hair, is caused by a reduction in the activity of melanocytes within hair follicles and is a normal part of the aging process.

TABLE 11.3   Conditions with a primary absence or reduction of color

Condition	Hair color
Tyrosinase negative albinism	Hair has no color
Tyrosinase positive albinism	Hair color is diluted, often yellowish
Chediak–Higashi	Silvery color
Griscelli syndrome	Silvery color
Elejade syndrome	Silvery color
Isolated pili torti	Fairer than expected
Menkes syndrome	Fairer than expected, sometimes silvery
Uncombable hair	Fairer than expected
Phenylketonuria	Alternating light and darker when on and off treatment (flag sign)
Homocystinuria	Probably due to keratinization changes
Oast house disease	Very light, almost white hair

TABLE 11.4   Premature canities

Autoimmune diseases
Generalized vitiligo
Widespread alopecia areata
Pernicious anemia
Addison disease
Hypothyroidism
Hyperthyroidism
Syndromes
Progeria
Werner
Rothmund–Thomson
Dyskeratosis congenita
Down's
Cri du chat
Book

Premature canities refers to a diffuse loss of color, especially of scalp hair, at an age earlier than that generally accepted as physiologic, before the age of 20 in whites and before age 30 in blacks.[203,205] Occasionally, children develop a few gray or white hairs in the apparent absence of any other dermatological or systemic condition but there are some recognized causes of this phenomenon.[203,205] Some of the causes of premature canities are listed in Table 11.4. Canities, once established, is usually permanent.

Acquired reversible diffuse hypopigmentation

Various deficiency states may lead to acquired reversible diffuse hypopigmentation of hair. In protein malnutrition, or kwashiorkor, the hair is lighter than expected. If periods of malnutrition alternate with periods of adequate diet, alternating lighter and darker areas may occur, the so-called flag sign. Lightening of hair is also an occasional feature of severe iron deficiency.[206]

LOCALIZED HYPOPIGMENTATION (POLIOSIS)

Poliosis is defined as a localized patch of white hair due to the absence or deficiency of melanin in a group of neighboring follicles. Some of the causes are covered in Table 11.5.

ALTERATION OF HAIR COLOR DUE TO EXOGENOUS AGENTS

There are various drugs which lead to reversible alterations in hair color, but few of these are regularly used in children. Chloroquine interferes with pheomelanin synthesis and in blonde and red-haired individuals can cause a progressive lightening and silvery coloration.[203,207] A similar change has been noted with alpha-interferon.[207] Lightening of normally dark hair was also been reported during etretinate therapy.[208] There have been no reports of this change with acitretin.

There are various chemicals, usually encountered in an industrial setting, which can cause hair discoloration, but the one most relevant to children is

197. Bovenmeyer DA (1979) Eruptive vellus hair cysts. **Arch Dermatol** 115:338–339.
198. Piepkorn MW, Clark L, Lombardi DI (1981) A kindred with congenital vellus hair cysts. **J Am Acad Dermatol** 5:661–665.
199. Patrizi A, Neri I, Guerrini V et al. (1998) Persistent milia, steatocystoma multiplex and eruptive vellus hair cysts: variable expression of multiple pilosebaceous cysts within an affected family. **Dermatology** 196:392–396.
200. Tomkova H, Fujimoto W, Arata J (1997) Expressions of keratins (K10 and K17) in steatocystoma multiplex, eruptive vellus hair cysts and epidermoid and trichilemmal cysts. **Am J Dermatopathol** 19:250–253.
201. Sardy M, Karpati S (1999) Needle evacuation of eruptive vellus hair cysts. **Br J Dermatol** 141:594–595.
202. Kageyama N, Tope WD (1999) Treatment of multiple eruptive hair cysts with erbium:YAG laser. **Dermatologic Surg** 25:819–822.
203. Dawber RPR, Gummer CL (1997) The colour of hair. In: Diseases of the Hair and Scalp, Dawber R, ed. Oxford: Blackwell Science, pp. 397–417.
204. Duran-McKinster C, Roriguez-Jurado R, Ridaura C et al. (1999) Elejade syndrome – a melanolysosomal neurocutaneous syndrome. **Arch Dermatol** 135:182–186.   205. Tobin D, Cargnello JA. Partial reversal of canities in a 22-year-old normal Chinese male. **Arch Dermatol** 129:789–791.
206. Sato S, Jitsukawa K, Sato H et al. (1989) Segmented heterochromia in black scalp hair associated with iron deficiency anemia. **Arch Dermatol** 125:531–535.
207. Fleming CJ, MacKie RM (1996) Alpha interferon-induced hair discoloration. **Br J Dermatol** 135:337–338.
208. Vesper JL, Fenske NA (1996) Hair darkening and new growth associated with etretinate therapy. **J Am Acad Dermatol** 34:860.

TABLE 11.5   Poliosis

Condition	Symptom
Piebaldism	White forelock
Waardenburg syndrome	White forelock
Tietz syndrome	Multiple white patches
Vitiligo	Patchy
Vogt–Koyanagi–Harada syndrome	Patchy/vitiligo
Alezzandrini syndrome	Patchy/vitiligo
Alopecia areata	Regrowing hair, reversible
Tuberous sclerosis	
Halo nevus	
Halo around neurofibroma	

copper used as an algae retardant in swimming pools. This causes a green discoloration in blonde hair, which may be reversed with a penicillamine shampoo or the application of a 1-hydroxyethyl diphosphonic acid-containing solution.[209,210]

NONSCARRING ALOPECIA

Yong-Kwang Tay

Hair loss disorders can be divided into nonscarring (non-cicatricial) and scarring (cicatricial) alopecia (Table 11.6). Causes of nonscarring alopecia include alteration of the hair growth cycle, structural abnormalities of the hair, and trauma.[211]

TELOGEN EFFLUVIUM

It is calculated that the average human scalp contains 100 000 hairs. The average growth rate of terminal hair is about 2.5mm/week (1cm/month). The human hair follicle has a fairly long phase of growth, the anagen phase,

TABLE 11.6   Classification of hair loss

Nonscarring alopecia	Scarring alopecia
Telogen effluvium	Developmental defects (e.g., Aplasia cutis)
Anagen effluvium	
Alopecia areata	Infections (bacterial, viral, fungal)
Androgenetic alopecia	Trauma (irradiation, thermal or caustic burns)
Hair shaft abnormalities	
Trauma (e.g., traction)	Neoplastic disorders
Infectious disorders (e.g., dermatophyte, syphilis)	Lichen planus (lichen planopilaris), lupus erythematosus, morphea, scleroderma, sarcoidosis
Systemic diseases (e.g., thyroid, systemic lupus erythematosus, iron-deficiency anemia)	Keratosis pilaris atrophicans
	Folliculitis decalvans
	Dissecting cellulitis of the scalp
Intoxications (e.g., vitamin A, Bismuth)	Acne keloidals
	Pseudopelade
Nutritional deficiencies (e.g., zinc, biotin)	Alopecia mucinosa
Medications	

which lasts a period of 2–6 years, average three years. The hairs then undergo a period of involution, the catagen phase lasting about three weeks, followed by a resting telogen or club phase, lasting about three months. At the end of this period, new growth is initiated. In healthy persons, 80–90% of the scalp is in the actively growing, anagen stage; 5% is in the catagen stage; 10–15% is in the resting, telogen stage; and 50 to 100 hairs are shed and simultaneously replaced each day.[212]

During the period of hair growth, the normal cyclic pattern may be interrupted by a variety of different stimuli, resulting in abnormally large numbers of scalp anagen hairs suddenly moving in concert to enter telogen. The resulting increase in hair shedding occurs diffusely over the scalp, usually six weeks to four months after an inciting event (Fig. 11.38). Second in incidence only to androgenetic alopecia in adults, this disorder represents the most common type of alopecia.

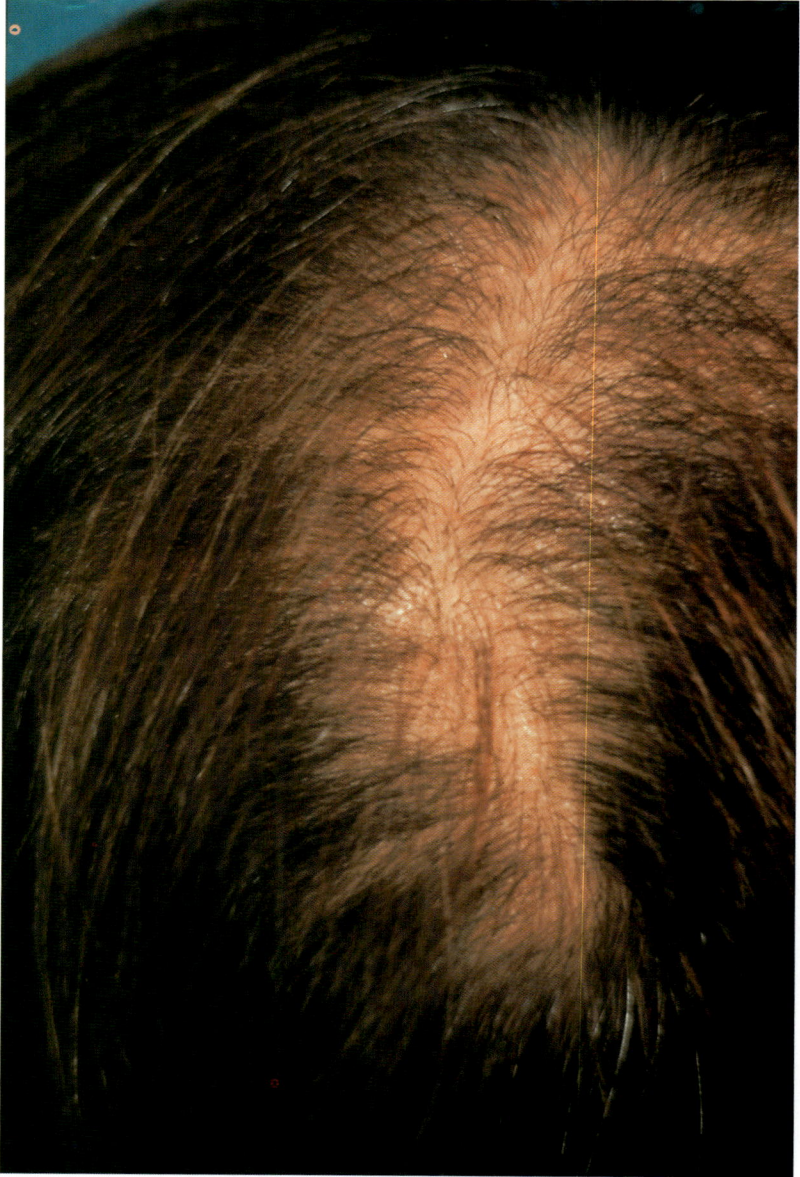

Fig. 11.38   Telogen effluvium. Temporary diffuse alopecia initiated by crash dieting.

209. Goldschmidt H (1979) Green hair. Arch Dermatol 115:1288.
210. Melnik BC, Plewig G, Daldrup T et al. (1986) Green hair: guidelines for diagnosis and therapy. J Am Acad Dermatol 15:1065–1068.
211. Hurwitz S (1993) Clinical Pediatric Dermatology, 2nd ed. Philadelphia: WB Saunders.
212. Kligman AM (1961) Pathologic dynamics of human hair loss: 1, Telogen effluvium. Arch Dermatol 83:175.

TABLE 11.7   Causes of telogen effluvium[213,214]

Physiologic
Physiologic effluvium of the newborn
Postpartum effluvium

Injury or stress
High fever
Severe infection
Severe chronic illness
Major surgery
Hypo- or hyperthyroidism
Crash diets, precipitous decrease of calories or protein (Fig. 11.38)
Iron deficiency
Essential fatty acid deficiency
Biotin deficiency
Drugs (Table 11.8)

TABLE 11.8   Drugs associated with telogen effluvium (including but not limited to)

ACE inhibitors e.g., captopril,[215] enalapril[216]
Albendazole[217]
Amphetamine[218]
Aminosalicylic acid[219]
Anticoagulants e.g., heparin,[220] warfarin[221]
Antiepileptics e.g., carbamazepine,[222] valproic acid[214,220]
Beta blockers e.g., metoprolol,[223] propranolol[224]
Bromocriptine[225]
Cimetidine[226]
Danazol[227]
Interferons[228] e.g., interferon α
Levodapa[229]
Lithium[230]
Oral contraceptive pills – during or after discontinuation[214]
Retinoids e.g., etretinate[231] and excess vitamin A[214]
Pyridostigmine[232]

The diagnosis of telogen effluvium can often be suspected by history alone. Etiologic factors fall into two groups (Tables 11.7, 11.8).[213] In the first group, the effluvium is physiologic in nature and there is no injury to the follicle. Abnormally large numbers of hairs enter telogen because they are programmed to do so. Telogen effluvium of the newborn and postpartum telogen effluvium are examples. The second category of factors resulting in telogen effluvium involves some sort of injury or stress to the follicles, in response to which many hairs prematurely enter catagen and then telogen phases.

The diagnosis of telogen effluvium is suggested by finding a positive hair pull: a lock of hair is grasped between the thumb and forefinger with firm, steady traction applied along the lengths of the hairs. More than six extractable hairs is indicative of active shedding.[213] Loss can be estimated by counting the number of hairs shed each day. Loss of more than 100 hairs per day can be considered excessive. The ratio of resting to growing hairs (the telogen:anagen ration) can be determined by gently plucking approximately 50 hairs from the patient's scalp and examining them under a low-power microscope. This can be done by clamping about 50 hairs about 1cm from the skin surface with a hemostate (the jaws of which have been covered by rubber tubing to prevent trauma to the hair shafts), followed by a gentle but short tug. Anagen hair roots are recognized by the presence of intact outer and inner hair sheaths, with or without a portion of the dermal papilla adherent to the tip of the root. Telogen hair roots have uniform shaft diameters, contain no pigment, and are club shaped. The ratio of telogen to anagen hairs varies from one person to another with an average telogen count of 13%.[212] A telogen count of 25% or more is abnormal. In the typical case of telogen effluvium, the telogen count does not usually exceed 50%.[212] Telogen counts exceeding 70% or 80% do not represent simple telogen effluvium and such cases result from sudden and severe metabolic arrest affecting the actively growing hairs (anagen effluvium).[213]

If a patient is suspected of having a telogen effluvium and a precipitating factor is not evident from the history or physical examination, a search for an occult disease is justified. A complete blood count, chemistry profile, serum iron/ferritin, and thyroid function tests constitute an acceptable screening panel.[213]

There is no effective treatment for telogen effluvium. Spontaneous regrowth occurs and, unless the stressful event is repeated, complete regrowth takes place within six months. Careful explanation of the cause of this disorder and its favorable prognosis with strong psychological support and instructions to avoid manipulation, such as vigorous shampooing, combing, and brushing, until new growth has occurred, is generally all that is required.

ANAGEN EFFLUVIUM

In anagen effluvium, there is marked inhibition of anagen hair-matrix metabolism, such that hair shaft production is greatly diminished.[213] Hair loss is profound since over 80% of scalp hair is normally in anagen at any given time. Causes of anagen effluvium are radiation therapy and chemotherapy. As follicular metabolism ceases under the influence of chemical toxins or ionizing radiation, the hair shaft tapers to a point and is shed.

Chemotherapeutic agents implicated include cyclophosphamide, methotrexate, 6-mercaptopurine, vincristine and doxorubicin.[233–235] Alopecia has also been reported after therapeutic doses of colchicine.[236] Anagen effluvium has been reported after toxic exposure to boric acid,[237] thallium,[238] arsenic, and mercury.[239]

213. Sperling LC (1996) Evaluation of hair loss. **Curr Probl Dermatol** 8:97.
214. Olsen EA (2000) Hair disorders. In: Textbook of Pediatric Dermatology, Harper J, Oranje A, Prose N, eds. Osney Mead (Oxford): Blackwell Science, p. 1463–1490.
215. Leaker B, Withworth JA (1984) Alopecia associated with captopril treatment. **Aust NZ J Med** 14:866.
216. Ahmad S (1991) Enalapril and reversible alopecia. **Arch Intern Med** 151:404.
217. Garcia-Muret MP, Sitjas D, Tuneu L et al. (1990) Telogen effluvium associated with albendazole therapy. **Int J Dermatol** 29:669.
218. Voron DA (1988) Alopecia and amphetamine use. **JAMA** 260:183.
219. Kutty PK, Raman KRK, Hawken K et al. (1982) Hair loss and 5-aminosalicylic acid enemas. **Ann Intern Med** 97:785.
220. Headington JT (1993) Telogen effluvium. New concepts and review. **Arch Dermatol** 129:356.
221. Umlas J, Harken DE (1988) Warfarin induced alopecia. **Cutis** 42:63.
222. Shuper A, Stahl B, Weitz R (1985) Carbamazepine-induced hair loss. **Drug Intell Clin Pharmc** 19:924.
223. Graeber CW, Lapkin RA (1981) Metoprolol and alopecia. **Cutis** 28:633.
224. Scribner MD (1977) Propranolol therapy. **Arch Dermatol** 113:1303.
225. Blum I, Leiba S (1980) Increased hair loss as a side effect of bromocriptine treatment. **N Engl J Med** 303:1418.
226. Kalsha JH, Praham CF, Jones JK (1983) Cimetidine-associated alopecia. **Int J Dermatol** 22:202.
227. Duff P, Mayer AR (1981) Generalized alopecia: an unusual complication of danazol therapy. **Am J Obstet Gynecol** 141:349.
228. Tosti A, Misciali C, Bardazzi F et al. (1992) Telogen effluvium due to recombinant interferon α-2b. **Dermatology** 184:124.
229. Marshall A, Williams MJ (1971) Alopecia and levodopa. **BMJ** 2:47.
230. Dawber R (1982) Hair loss during lithium treatment. **Br J Dermatol** 107:124.
231. Berth-Jones J, Shuttleworth D, Hutchinson PE (1990) A study of etretinate alopecia. **Br J Dermatol** 122:751.
232. Field LM (1980) Toxic alopecia caused by pyridostigmine bromide. **Arch Dermatol** 116:1103.
233. Crounse RG, van Scott EJ (1960) Changes in scalp hair roots as a measure of toxicity from cancer chemotherapeutic drugs. **J Invest Dermatol** 35:83.
234. Brien R, Zelson JH, Schwartz AO et al. (1970) Scalp tourniquet to lessen alopecia after vincristine. **N Engl J Med** 238:1496.
235. Dean JC, Salmon SE, Griffith KS (1974) Prevention of doxorubicine-induced hair loss with scalp hypothermia. **N Engl J Med** 301:1427.
236. Malkinson ED, Lynfield YL (1959) Colchicine alopecia. **J Invest Dermatol** 33:371.
237. Stein KM, Odom RB, Justice GR et al. (1973) Toxic alopecia form ingestion of boric acid. **Arch Dermatol** 108:95.
238. Feldman J, Levisohn DR (1993) Acute alopecia: clue to thallium toxicity. **Pediatr Dermatol** 10:29.
239. Pierard GE (1979) Toxic effects of metals from the environment on hair growth and structure. **J Cutan Pathol** 6:237.

The change in the hair bulb is characteristic and early in the course. A gentle hair pull will yield numerous "pencil-point" dystrophic hairs with proximal tips that taper to a point.[213] As hairs are rapidly shed, fewer and fewer anagen shafts are left in the scalp. A hair pluck performed late in the course of the disease will consist almost exclusively of telogen hairs (which are spared from the metabolic insult). When the telogen count approaches 100%, a form of anagen effluvium is almost certainly the cause.

There is no effective treatment for anagen effluvium. Cessation of the responsible drug or toxin generally results in regrowth of hair. When cytostatic drugs are indicated, the expected hair loss can be minimized to some degree by scalp hypothermia, for example, applying ice packs to the scalp for 30 minutes before the drug is injected.[235] Another approach is to use a specially constructed scalp tourniquet placed around the head just above the ears and inflated to 10mmHg above systolic pressure immediately before injection of the cytostatic drug. This helps to minimize the toxic effects of the drug on the hair follicles.[234] Topical minoxidil has been used to inhibit chemotherapy induced alopecia to some degree.[240]

ALOPECIA AREATA

Alopecia areata is characterized by the sudden appearance of sharply defined round or oval patches of hair loss. It is a common disorder, with an incidence of 17 per 100 000 population per year. About 1% of the population will have had alopecia areata by the age of 50.[241,242] Although the condition occurs at all ages, the first attack usually appears in children, with between 24% to 50% starting before the age of 16.[243,244] There is a history of familial occurrence in 10% to 20% of affected persons.[245] Although there are reports of simultaneous occurrence in identical twins, and autosomal dominance with incomplete penetrance has been suggested, the genetic status of this disorder is unclear.[246]

Clinical features

The typical picture of alopecia areata consists of a sudden appearance of one or more round or oval well-circumscribed patches of hair loss (Fig. 11.39). Patients often report increased hair shedding. The primary patch may appear

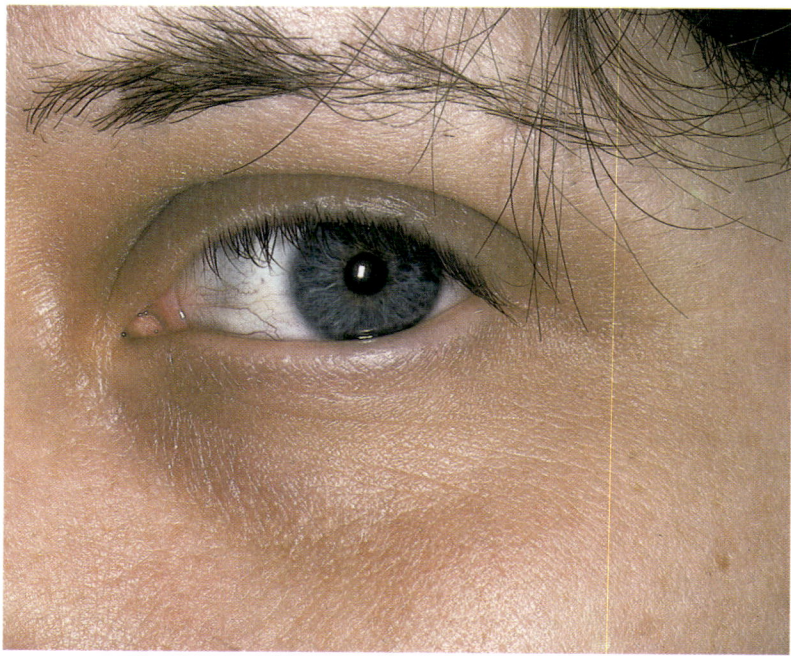

Fig. 11.40 Alopecia areata affecting the eyebrow.

on any hairy cutaneous surface, e.g., eyebrows, beard area (Fig. 11.40), but it usually occurs on the scalp. The skin is smooth, soft, occasionally slightly pink and almost totally devoid of hair. Short hairs that taper as they approach the scalp are called "exclamation-mark hairs" and, if present, are very characteristic of alopecia areata.[213] These loose hairs are easily plucked out of the scalp and when examined under low power, most will be telogen hairs with a frayed distal tip. Hair regrowth in alopecia areata may occur as depigmented hairs which may repigment with time, or may remain white.

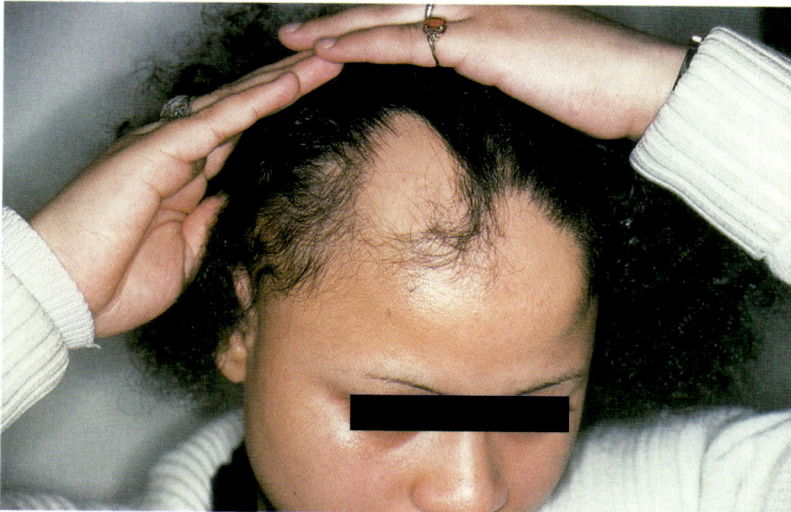

Fig. 11.39 Alopecia areata with a sharply defined oval patch of hair loss.

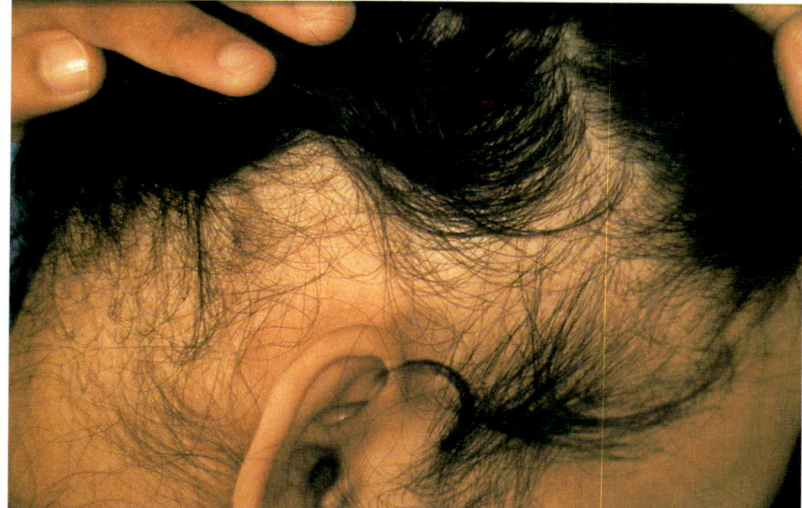

Fig. 11.41 Ophiasis pattern of hair loss in alopecia areata.

240. Duvic M, Lemak NA, Valero V et al. (1996) A randomised trial of minoxidil in chemotherapy-induced alopecia. **J Am Acad Dermatol** 35:74.
241. Price VH (1991) Alopecia areata: Clinical aspects. **J Invest Dermatol** (Suppl) 96:68S.
242. Sahn EE (1995) Alopecia areata in childhood. **Semin Dermatol** 14:9.
243. Sharma VK, Kumar B, Dawn G (1996) A clinical study of childhood alopecia areata in Chandigarh, India. **Pediatr Dermatol** 13:372.
244. DeWaard-Van Der Spek FB, Oranje AP, De Raeymaecker DMJ et al. (1989) Juvenile versus maturity-onset alopecia areata – a comparative retrospective clinical study. **Clin Exp Dermatol** 14:429.
245. Muller SA, Winkelmann RK (1963) Alopecia areata: An evaluation of 736 patients. **Arch Dermatol** 88:290.
246. Scerri L, Pace JL (1992) Identical twins with identical alopecia areata. **J Am Acad Dermatol** 27:766.

Ophiasis, a term derived from the Greek word for serpent, refers to a pattern of alopecia seen mostly in children. It begins as a bald spot on the posterior occiput, extending anteriorly and bilaterally in a 2.5–5cm wide band above the ear and sometimes extending to meet on the anterior aspect of the scalp (Fig. 11.41). This occurs in less than 5% of alopecia areata patients and often progresses to alopecia totalis or universalis.[242] Reticular alopecia areata refers to a very diffuse and somewhat more subtle presentation.

In alopecia totalis, the entire scalp is bald and in the most severe type, alopecia universalis, all body hair is absent, including eyelashes, eyebrows, beard, and pubic hair (Fig. 11.42). Progression to the totalis form occurs more slowly, but more frequently in children than in adults.

Nail changes are seen in 10–44% of cases and more severe nail changes tend to be seen in the more severe types, such as alopecia totalis or universalis.[247] The most characteristic nail abnormality is a fine grid-like stippling, regularly arranged in either horizontal or vertical rows or both, with pits smaller than those seen in psoriasis. Longitudinal ridging and thickening may occur, giving a mycotic appearance.[242] Trachyonychia (rough sandpaper nails) are seen more commonly in children with alopecia areata.[248] Opacity, friability, punctate leukonychia, spotted lunuli, onychomadesis (shedding), and red lunuli have been reported in alopecia areata.[249]

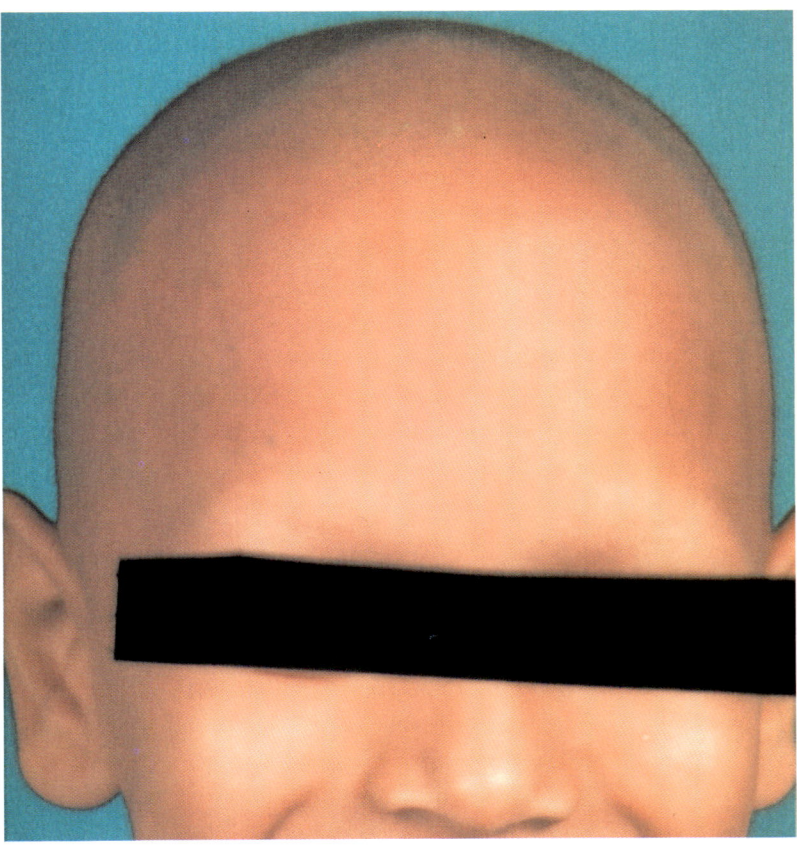

Fig. 11.42 Alopecia universalis with loss of scalp hair and eyebrows.

Diagnosis and differential diagnosis

The diagnosis of alopecia areata is made on the basis of its clinical picture. The sudden appearance and circumscribed nonscarring-patterned nature of hair loss will distinguish it from other disorders of alopecia. Clinically, the differential diagnosis includes telogen effluvium, trichotillomania, androgenetic alopecia, secondary syphilis, and tinea capitis. If regrowth and extension occur simultaneously in one scalp region, the classical round patches of alopecia may not be seen. In children, this may produce either a bizarre pattern, such as that seen in trichotillomania, or a moth-eaten appearance as in secondary syphilis.[242] In trichotillomania, patches of alopecia with twisted and broken hairs of different lengths are seen.

The dearth of signs of inflammation, scaling and lymphadenopathy will help distinguish alopecia areata from that of tinea capitis. Besides its moth-eaten appearance, alopecia due to secondary syphilis may be recognized by its irregular borders, incomplete loss of hair within individual patches and a predilection for the posterior scalp. Patients with androgenetic alopecia usually demonstrate the typical pattern of balding with bitemporal recession of the frontal hair line followed by thinning over the vertex, and shedding is not prominent.

The pull test is usually negative in androgenetic alopecia. Reticular or diffuse alopecia areata resembling telogen effluvium may occasionally be seen and can be difficult to diagnose. When the diagnosis is in doubt, microscopic examination of hairs with potassium hydroxide (KOH), fungal cultures, serologic testing and a 4mm punch biopsy frequently will help establish the proper diagnosis.

A hair pull in newly formed patches of alopecia areata will show an increased number of telogen hairs and dystrophic anagen hairs.[213] Later in the course, most hairs will be in the anagen phase. The most characteristic histopathologic feature of alopecia areata is the presence of a peribulbar lymphocytic infiltrate (swarm of bees) surrounding the hair bulbs. The inflammatory infiltrate is composed mainly of activated T lymphocytes together with macrophages and Langerhans cells.[250] Other histologic features include a reduction in the anagen:telogen ratio, miniaturized dystrophic hairs, fibrous tracts, pigment incontinence, and the presence of eosinophils.[251]

Etiology and pathogenesis

The cause of alopecia areata remains unknown, but is generally believed to be an autoimmune disease. CD4+ T lymphocytes mediate the perifollicular immune attack against a hair follicle antigen by triggering a cascade of events via cytokine production. An aberrant expression of cytokines of the $T_H 1$ type (interferon gamma and IL-2) and IL-1β have been detected in affected areas of the scalp in patients with alopecia areata.[252] Antigen presentation of the responsible epitope that may be in the follicular keratinocyte, melanocyte, or dermal papilla helps drive the condition. Neuropeptides (such as calcitonin gene-related peptide and substance P) as well as increased antibody production to follicular components may also play a significant role.[253]

There is a decrease in calcitonin gene-related peptide and substance P expression in the scalp of patients with alopecia areata.[254] Calcitonin gene-related peptide has potent anti-inflammatory actions[255] and substance P is capable of inducing hair growth.[256]

Alopecia areata is associated with classic autoimmune disorders, mainly thyroid diseases, especially Hashimoto's thyroiditis and vitiligo. The frequency

247. Thiers BH (1989) Alopecia areata. **Clin Dermatol** 2:1.
248. Tosti A, Fanti PA, Morelli R et al. (1991) Trachyonychia associated with alopecia areata: A clinical and pathologic study. **J Am Acad Dermatol** 25:266.
249. Bergner T, Donhauser G, Ruzicka T (1992) Red lunulae in severe alopecia areata. **Acta Derm Venereol** (Stockh) 72:203.
250. Perret C, Wiesner-Menzel L, Happle R (1984) Immunohistochemical analysis of T cell subsets in the peribulbar and intrabulbar infiltrates of alopecia areata. **Acta Derm Venereol** (Stockh) 64:26.
251. Elston DM, McCollough ML, Bergfeld WF et al. (1997) Eosinophils in fibrous tracts and near hair bulbs. A helpful diagnostic feature of alopecia areata. **J Am Acad Dermatol** 37:101.
252. Hoffmann R, Eicheler W, Huth A et al. (1996) Cytokines and growth factors influence hair growth in vitro: possible implications for the pathogenesis and treatment of alopecia areata. **Arch Dermatol Res** 288:153.

253. Madani S, Shapiro J (2000) Alopecia areata update. **J Am Acad Dermatol** 42:549.
254. Hordinsky M, Kennedy W, Wendelschafer-Crabb G et al. (1995) Structure and function of cutaneous nerves in alopecia areata. **J Invest Dermatol** 104 (Suppl):28S.
255. Raud J, Lundeberg T, Brodda-Jansen G et al. (1991) Potent anti-inflammatory action of calcitonin gene-related peptide. **Biochem Biophys Res Commun** 18:1429.
256. Ericson M, Binstock K, Guanche A et al. (1999) Differential expression of substance P in perifollicular scalp blood vessels and nerves after topical therapy with capsaicin 0.075% (Zostrix HP) in controls and patients with extensive alopecia areata. **J Invest Dermatol** 112:653.

of thyroid disease is between 8% to 11.8% in patients with alopecia areata compared with only 2% of the normal population.[245,257] This is further confirmed by an increased prevalence of antithyroid antibodies and thyroid microsomal antibodies in patients with alopecia areata.[258,259] There is also an increased prevalence of gastric parietal cell antibodies, antinuclear and anti-smooth muscle antibodies in sera of patients with alopecia areata.[258,259] Patients with alopecia areata have a fourfold greater incidence of vitiligo.[245] Other associated autoimmune diseases include Addison's disease, pernicious anemia, diabetes, lupus erythematosus, rheumatoid arthritis, myasthenia gravis and Candida endocrinopathy syndrome.[253] An increased incidence has also been noted in patients with Down's syndrome.[260] Atopy is found in 10–22% of cases,[261,262] but this association is unexplained.

Prognosis

The course of alopecia areata is variable and difficult to predict. The natural history includes frequent spontaneous remissions and recurrences. When the process is limited to a few patches, the prognosis is good, with complete regrowth occurring within one year in 95% of children. It is estimated that 7% to 10% of patients can eventually develop the severe chronic form of the condition.[253] Indicators of a poor prognosis are atopy, the presence of other immune diseases, family history of alopecia areata, young age at onset, extensive hair loss, ophiasis, and nail dystrophy.[244]

Therapy

At present, all treatments only control the problem and do not cure the condition. Local treatments may help the treated areas, but do not prevent further spread of the condition. Any mode of treatment may need to be used for long periods because of the chronic nature of alopecia areata. A minimum period of 3–6 months should be tried for any therapy before the treatment can be considered to have failed because of the long period before regrowth. Presently, topical, intralesional and systemic steroids, topical and systemic immunotherapy, arthralin, minoxidil, and photochemotherapy (PUVA) are available for the treatment of alopecia areata.[253]

When first making a diagnosis of alopecia areata, it is important to give psychological support and counselling, with time taken to answer all questions and to provide written material such as pamphlets. Part of psychological support includes addressing cosmetic concerns.[242] A hairstyle change, caps, hats, head bands, and wigs may be required for adequate camouflage. Prescribing no medical therapy is a valid way to manage classical alopecia areata in some children because a high percentage of alopecia areata will spontaneously remit in one year. This option may be the best one in some families.[242]

Topical corticosteroid therapy alone or under occlusion (e.g., under a wig or bathing cap) is used frequently in children with alopecia areata. Mid- to high-potency corticosteroids, applied twice daily to the patch of alopecia will sometimes effect a response in 1–2 months.[263,264] Immunosuppression is the main mechanism of action of the corticosteroids. Intralesional corticosteroids are appropriate only for older children who are highly motivated. Triamcinolone acetonide 2.5–5mg/ml with an upper limit of 10mg/ml is administered with a 0.5-inch-long 30-gauge needle as multiple intradermal

injections of 0.1–0.3ml per site, approximately 1cm apart.[253] A weaker concentration of 2.5mg/ml is used for the beard area and eyebrows. A maximum total of 3ml of triamcinolone acetonide can be used on the scalp in one visit. Treatments can be repeated every four to six weeks.

Children younger than 6 years are not usually treated with intralesional steriods because of pain at the injection sites. Side effects include transient atrophy, telangiectasias, and folliculitis. Atrophy can be prevented by avoiding injections that are too frequent, too great in volume per site, or too superficial (intraepidermal). If there is no response after six months of treatment, intralesional steroids should be discontinued because these patients may lack adequate corticosteroid receptors in the scalp.[265] Patients of all ages may benefit from the use of topical lidocaine (lignocaine) lidocaine pamocaine pre-injection to diminish pain.

Although not recommended for general use, systemic steroids may be considered for selected patients with severe involvement and an associated psychological handicap who do not respond to topical and intralesional steroid therapy. Although frequently effective, the use of systemic steroids is limited because of their side effects, their high relapse rate after dose reduction, and because they may be necessary for long periods of time and may not change the ultimate prognosis.

In such instances, prednisolone in doses of 20–40mg/day with taper of 5mg per week for four to six weeks, followed by alternate-day therapy may be beneficial and cause relatively few significant side effects.[266,267] Pulse therapy with intravenous methylprednisolone (250mg) twice daily for three successive days was found to be effective in controlling the active phase of hair loss in patients with rapidly progressing extensive alopecia areata.[268]

Anthralin is used in the treatment of alopecia areata in concentrations of 0.25% to 1% cream. It may have a nonspecific immunomodulating effect eliciting hair regrowth. Cosmetically acceptable regrowth has been reported to occur in 25% of patients.[269] Anthralin cream may be applied overnight or as short-contact therapy, initially for 30 minutes and gradually to one hour.[270] A mild dermatitis is desired for therapeutic effect. Scalp irritation and staining of the skin and clothing are drawbacks to its use. New hair growth is usually seen within three months and it may take 24 or more weeks for a cosmetically acceptable response. It can be applied simultaneously with twice-daily topical corticosteroid therapy.[242]

Minoxidil is a biologic response modifier that enhances hair growth. Its mode of action in alopecia areata is unknown, but it is known to stimulate follicular DNA synthesis, has a direct effect on the proliferation and differentiation of follicular keratinocytes *in vitro*, and regulates hair physiology independently of blood flow.[271] Cosmetically acceptable hair regrowth in patients with alopecia areata using topical minoxidil solution has been shown to be between 20% to 45%.[272,273] Topical minoxidil is applied twice daily and hair regrowth is usually seen after two months. More successful results are seen in less severe cases and this treatment would not be expected to be effective in patients with alopecia totalis/universalis. Two percent topical minoxidil applied three times daily has been shown to limit hair loss after stopping systemic steroids in patients with alopecia areata.[267] The efficacy of minoxidil solution can be enhanced with anthralin[274] or betamethasone dipropionate.[275] Anthralin is applied two hours after the second minoxidil

257. Shellow WV, Edwards JE, Koo JY (1992) Profile of alopecia areata: a questionnaire analysis of patient and family. **Int J Dermatol** 31:186.
258. Friedmann PS (1981) Alopecia areata and auto-immunity. **Br J Dermatol** 105:153.
259. Milgraum SS, Mitchell AJ, Bacon GE et al. (1987) Alopecia areata, endocrine function and autoantibodies in patients 16 years of age or younger. **J Am Acad Dermatol** 17:57.
260. Wunderlich C, Braun-Falco O (1965) Mongolismus and alopecia areata. **Med Welt** 10:477.
261. Ikeda T (1965) A new classification of alopecia areata. **Dermatologica** 131:421.
262. De Weert J, Temmerman L, Kint A (1984) Alopecia areata: A clinical study. **Dermatologica** 168:224.
263. Gill K, Baxter D (1963) Alopecia totalis: treatment with fluocinolone acetonide. **Arch Dermatol** 87:384.
264. Montes LF (1977) Topical halcinonide in alopecia areata and in alopecia totalis. **J Cutar Pathol** 4:47.
265. Sawaya ME, Hordinsky MK (1995) Glucocorticoid regulation of hair growth in alopecia areata. **J Invest Dermatol** 194 (Suppl 5):30S.
266. Kern F, Hoffman WH, Hambrick GW Jr et al. (1973) Alopecia areata, immunologic studies and treatment with prednisone. **Arch Dermatol** 107:407.
267. Olsen EA, Carson SC, Turney EA (1992) Systemic steroids with or without 2% topical minoxidil in the treatment of alopecia areata. **Arch Dermatol** 128:1467.
268. Perriard-Wolfensberger J, Pasche-Koo F, Mainetti C et al. (1993) Pulse of methylprednisolone in alopecia areata. **Dermatology** 187:282.
269. Fiedler-Weiss VC, Buys CM (1987) Evaluation of anthralin in the treatment of alopecia areata. **Arch Dermatol** 123:1491.
270. Fiedler VC (1992) Alopecia areata. **Arch Dermatol** 128:1519.
271. Buhl AE (1991) Minoxidil's action in hair follicles. **J Invest Dermatol** 96 (Suppl):73S.
272. Weiss VC, West DP, Fu TS et al. (1984) Alopeica areata treated with topical minoxidil. **Arch Dermatol** 120:457.
273. Price VH (1987) Double-blind, placebo-controlled evaluation of topical minoxidil in extensive alopecia areata. **J Am Acad Dermatol** 16:730.
274. Fiedler VC, Wendrow A, Szpunar GJ et al. (1990) Treatment resistant alopecia areata. Response to combination therapy with minoxidil plus arthralin. **Arch Dermatol** 126:756.
275. Fiedler VC (1991) Alopecia areata: current therapy. **J Invest Dermatol** 96 (Suppl):69S.

application. Betamethasone dipropionate cream is applied twice daily, 30 minutes after each use of minoxidil. Side effects of minoxidil are rare. These include local irritation, allergic contact dermatitis, and facial hair growth. Systemic absorption is minimal.[276]

Topical immunotherapy is an accepted therapeutic modality in the treatment of chronic severe alopecia areata.[253] The principle of this type of treatment is to create antigenic competition with putative hair follicle antigens by provoking contact eczema on the scalp.[277] This theory presumes that the generation of T-suppressor cells into the area may exert a nonspecific inhibitory effect on the autoimmune reaction to the hair-associated antigen and thus allow hair to regrow. The first step is sensitization by means of a patch test and then application of increasing concentrations of the allergen after two weeks. The aim is to maintain a low-grade tolerable erythema, scaling and pruritus without causing too much discomfort for the patient.

Three contact sensitizers have been used in alopecia areata: dinitrochlorobenzene (DNCB), squaric acid dibutyl ester (SADBE), and diphenylcyclopropenone (DPCP). DNCB was the first agent used, but was found to be mutagenic in the Ames test and is not frequently used. SADBE is effective in 29% to 87% of patients with alopecia areata.[278–282] Sensitization is achieved with 2% SADBE in acetone applied to a small area on the scalp. Starting doses are low, between 0.0001% to 0.001%, and applications are performed once a week. Doses are increased every month according to individual tolerance. SADBE can be effective for relapses as well. Side effects are minimal and consist of local lymphadenopathy, vesiculation, staining of skin and clothing and skin dryness.

The efficacy of DPCP in alopecia areata ranges from 48% to 85%.[253,283–285] Responses are usually seen after 12 weeks of therapy, with cosmetically acceptable results after 24 weeks.[253] Persistent response was observed in 60% of patients in one study after a mean follow-up of 12 months, suggesting that DPCP may provide prolonged therapeutic benefits.[285] If there is no response by 24 weeks, DPCP is discontinued.[253]

Sensitization is achieved with 2% DPCP solution in acetone to a small area. A starting dose of 0.001% solution is applied to the scalp and left on for 48 hours before being washed off. Concentrations range from 0.001%, 0.01%, 0.025%, 0.05%, 0.1%, 0.25%, 0.5%, and 1%. Applications are performed once a week. The patient must protect the scalp from light because DPCP is degraded when exposed to light.[253]

Side effects of DPCP include eczematous reactions, extension of the contact dermatitis to other body areas, itching, edema of the scalp or face, lymphadenopathy in the cervical and postauricular areas, and postinflammatory hyper- or hypopigmentation.[253] DPCP is contraindicated in pregnancy.

The mechanism of action of PUVA on alopecia areata is believed to be a photoimmunologic action.[286] It may affect T-cell function and antigen presentation and possibly inhibit local immunologic attack against the hair follicle by depleting Langerhans cells. The psoralen is administered either topically or orally and followed two hours later with UVA. Treatments are administered two to three times a week with gradual increase in UVA dosage. There is no difference between oral versus topical psoralens and local versus whole-body irradiation.[287] The response rate varies from 20% to 53%.[287–289] There is a high relapse rate after PUVA is tapered and it is not recommended for use in young (less than age 10) children.

Patients treated with cyclosporine can develop hypertrichosis. Topical cyclosporine was not effective in alopecia areata,[290] but systemic cyclosporine has shown some benefit.[291] Because of their side effect profile, high recurrence rate after discontinuation and long treatment periods, cyclosporine is not practical in alopecia areata.

The National Alopecia Areata Foundation (710 C St, Suite 11, San Rafael, CA 94901-3853) is a valuable support group for patients with alopecia areata and their families.

TRAUMATIC ALOPECIA

Traumatic alopecia results from the forceful extraction of hair or the breaking of hair shafts by friction, traction of other physical trauma. Causes include trichotillomania, and cosmetic practices, such as tight braiding or ponytails; the use of tight curlers, rubber bands; hair straightening practices such as pulling; frequent brushing with nylon bristles and the use of hot combs. Other common causes of traumatic alopecia include pressure, such as seen on the occiput of infants who lie on their backs or who have a habit of head banging, prolonged bed rest in one position in chronically ill persons, thermal or electric burns, a severe blow to the scalp, birth trauma resulting in cephalhematoma, and prolonged pressure over the scalp during surgery.

Most cases of pressure-induced alopecia are associated with surgical operations, especially open-heart surgery or gynecologic surgery and the condition is often referred to as postoperative alopecia (Fig. 11.43). The posterior scalp in the region of the vertex is commonly involved. The cause

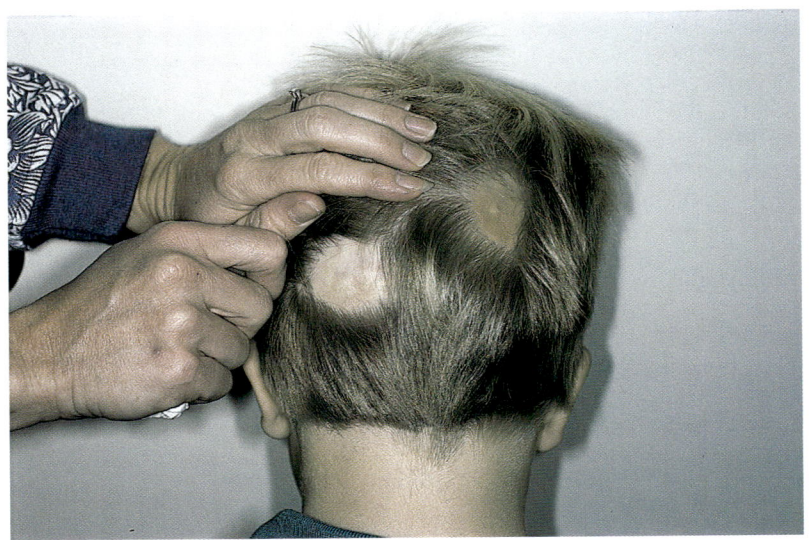

Fig. 11.43   Postoperative alopecia after cardiac surgery.

276. Price VH (1987) Topical minoxidil (3%) in extensive alopecia areata including long-term efficacy. **J Am Acad Dermatol** 16:737.
277. Happle R (1980) Antigenic competition as a therapeutic concept for alopecia areata. **Arch Dermatol Res** 267:109.
278. Happle R, Kalveran K, Buchner U et al. (1980) Contact allergy as therapeutic tool for alopecia areata: application of squaric acid dibutylester. **Dermatologica** 161:289.
279. Flowers F, Slazinski L, Fenske N et al. (1982) Topical squaric acid dibutylester therapy for alopecia areata. **Cutis** 30:733.
280. Gianetti A, Orecchia G (1983) Clinical experience on the treatment of alopecia areata with squaric acid dibutylester. **Dermatologica** 167:280.
281. Orecchia G, Malagoli P, Santagostino L (1994) Treatment of severe alopecia areata with squaric acid dibutylester in pediatric patients. **Pediatr Dermatol** 11:65.
282. Micali G, Licastro-Cicero R, Nasca MR (1996) Treatment of alopecia areata with squaric acid dibutylester. **Int J Dermatol** 35:52.
283. Happle R, Hausen BM, Wierner-Menzel L (1983) Diphencyprone in the treatment of alopecia areata. **Acta Dermatovener** (Stockh) 63:49.
284. Schuttelaar M-La, Hamstra JJ, Plinck EPB et al. (1996) Alopecia areata in children: treatment with diphencyprone. **Br J Dermatol** 135:581.
285. Cotellessa C, Peris K, Caracciolo E et al. (2001) The use of topical diphenylcyclopropenone for the treatment of extensive alopecia areata. **J Am Acad Dermatol** 44:73.
286. Mitchell AJ, Douglass MC (1985) Topical photochemotherapy for alopecia areata. **J Am Acad Dermatol** 12:644.
287. Larko O, Swanbeck G (1983) PUVA treatment of alopecia totalis. **Acta Derm Venereol** (Stockh) 63:546.
288. Claudy AL, Gagnaire D (1983) PUVA treatment of alopecia areata. **Arch Dermatol** 119:975.
289. Healy E, Rogers S (1993) PUVA treatment for alopecia areata – does it work? A retrospective review of 102 cases. **Br J Dermatol** 129:42.
290. Rongioletti F, Guarrera M, Tosti A et al. (1992) Topical cyclosporin A fails to improve alopecia areata: a double blind study. **J Dermatol Treat** 3:13.
291. Gupta A, Ellis C, Cooper K et al. (1990) Oral cyclosporine for the treatment of alopecia areata: a clinical and immunohistochemical analysis. **J Am Acad Dermatol** 22:242.

is a prolonged localized pressure to the scalp during and after operative procedures, which results in focal tissue ischemia.[292] Factors favoring post-operative alopecia include prolonged anesthesia and endotracheal intubation, prolonged head immobilization, and intraoperative Trendelenburg position.[293] The onset of alopecia occurs 3–28 days after surgery and regrowth of hair 28–120 days.[294] Some patients develop a temporary nonscarring alopecia with complete resolution whereas others develop a scarring, permanent alopecia from severe hypoxia. Permanent alopecia was associated with time from anesthesia induction to extubation that exceeded 24 hours, while patients with temporary alopecia averaged 17 hours until extubation.[292]

Initial signs and symptoms that occur within the first postoperative week include local occipitoparietal pain, inflammation and edema followed by crusting and ulceration in severe cases. Over several months, there is partial to complete hair regrowth. Permanent hair loss, if it occurs, is confined to the central portion of the lesion. The histologic findings depend upon when the specimen was obtained. In the immediate postoperative period, there is intravascular thrombosis, edema, early hair follicle necrosis, and perivascular inflammation.[292] Specimens collected later, after alopecia was complete, revealed a moderate to severe obliterative vasculitis in the dermis and fat, with moderate perivascular lymphocytic infiltration, atrophic follicles, and deep dermal fibrosis.[295] Apoptotic cells may be present.[296] Postoperative alopecia can be prevented by frequent repositioning of the head every thirty minutes, both intraoperatively and during recovery until extubation.[292]

TRACTION ALOPECIA

This is common in black females, whose hair is styled by being pulled into tight braids, which are held in place by elastic bands or ribbons. The outermost hairs of the braid are subjected to the most tension and with time a zone of alopecia develops between braids.[213] The margin of the scalp is always most severely affected and the degree of alopecia depends on the vigor with which the braids are tightened.

Traction alopecia can be divided into early and late disease. In early disease, the involved hairs have been subjected to traction for a few months, and if traction is eliminated, the hair will recover. In late disease, patches of alopecia have been present for years, and little regrowth occurs even if traction is discontinued.

In black girls, the alopecia occurs between braids and at the margins of the scalp. In adult black women, hair loss is usually most pronounced in a marginal pattern, especially involving the temporal region, periauricular zone and frontal scalp.[213] Although most terminal hairs are missing from the alopecia area, inspection will reveal numerous fine, vellus hairs. The scalp surface appears normal with no scarring.

Hair loss from hair rollers is usually most conspicuous in the frontocentral area or around the scalp margins. Hot-comb alopecia, seen mainly in black persons who straigthen their hair for cosmetic purposes, usually occurs on the vertex or marginal areas of the scalp. Acute hot-comb injuries may be treated with soaks or topical or systemic steroids with occasional benefit. In severe chronic forms, hot-comb alopecia may affect the entire scalp.

TRICHOTILLOMANIA

Trichotillomania is a self-limiting form of traction alopecia caused by plucking out one's hair and is produced either consciously or subconsciously as a result of habit. It is seen in all age groups, although two-thirds of affected patients

are children, adolescents, and young adults, and is more common in females (76%).[297] It is most commonly seen in children between 4 and 10 years of age although children as young as 2 years can be affected. The scalp is the most common site of involvement, but the eyebrows and eyelashes may also be affected as the patient plucks, twirls or rubs hair-bearing areas, resulting in breakage of hair shafts.

Two types of trichotillomania are recognized: a temporary localized childhood pattern with a good prognosis and a severe adult form, typically occurring in women, in which more widespread areas occur and the prognosis is guarded.[298] The habit is usually practiced in bed before the child falls asleep or when the child is reading, writing, or watching television, and is often associated with a habit of finger or thumb sucking. In many children, trichotillomania occurs in a climate of psychosocial stress in the family (e.g., hospitalization of child or mother, too coercive toilet training, sibling rivalry, inability to focus on activities and play in the younger child, and difficulties at school in the older child).[299] Hair pulling in children may be a mild form of frustration that soon becomes a habitual practice and can be managed by a sympathetic physician and understanding parents. (Older children, teenagers, and adults with this disorder may have deep-rooted psychological problems requiring evaluation and therapy.)

Trichotillomania usually begins insidiously as an irregular linear or rectangular area of partial hair loss. Affected areas are usually single, often frontal, frontotemporal or frontoparietal in location and frequently appear on the contralateral side of right-or left-handed persons. The affected patches have irregularly shaped angular outlines and are never completely bald (Fig. 11.44). The hair is short or stubbly and broken off at varying lengths. Focal perifollicular erythema, hemorrhage or excoriations may be present, but there is no evidence of scarring alopecia. In a variation of this disorder, the alopecia may be noted in the vertex and center of the scalp with a peripheral rim of unaffected hair. Its resemblance to the central shaven crown of the head of a monk has suggested the term "Friar Tuck" alopecia to this variant.[300]

Diagnosis

The diagnosis occasionally can be confirmed by finding wads of hair under the pillow or bed or by observation of the habit by a parent, teacher, or physician. If a circumscribed portion of an affected area is deliberately shaved by the clinician, the window will show increasing density of hair regrowth.[213] The area must be shaved on a weekly basis to keep emerging shafts too short to grasp and pluck. If it becomes clear that the shaved area is improving while other areas are not, the diagnosis of trichotillomania is established. Clinical differentiation from alopecia areata is usually based on the bizarre configuration, irregular outline, and presence of short, stub-like broken hairs, although the concomitant occurrence of trichotillomania and alopecia areata can occur in the same patient.[301] Differentiation from tinea capitis may require Wood's light examination, microscopic examination of plucked hairs with KOH, and fungal culture. The broken hairs of trichotillomania remain firmly rooted in the scalp and the cutaneous surface is normal and stubbled rather than erythematous and scaly as in tinea capitis. Patients with patchy or "moth-eaten" alopecia affecting much or all of the scalp should have syphilis excluded with serologic testing.

If the diagnosis remains in doubt, biopsy of the involved area is often helpful. The histopathologic features of trichotillomania include a marked increase in catagen and telogen hairs, the presence of pigment casts, and trichomalacia.[213,297] Pigment casts are clumps of pigmented hair-matrix cells that become "stranded" in the upper follicle as they are torn out. With time,

292. Lawson NW, Mills NL, Ochsner JL (1976) Occipital alopecia following cardiopulmonary by-pass. **J Thorac Cardiovasc Surg** 71:342.
293. Boyer JD, Vidmar DA (1994) Postoperative alopecia: A case report and literature review. **Cutis** 54:321.
294. Thomson NB Jr, Estrellado R (1962) Occurrence of alopecia after open heart surgery. **Arch Surg** 85:892.
295. Abel R, Lewis G (1960) Postoperative (pressure) alopecia. **Arch Dermatol Syphilol** 81:34.
296. Hanly AJ, Jorda M, Badiavas E et al. (1999) Postoperative pressure-induced alopeica: report of a case and discussion of the role of apoptosis in non-scarring alopecia. **J Cutan Pathol** 26:357.
297. Muller SA (1990) Trichotillomania: A histopathologic study in sixty-six patients. **J Am Acad Dermatol** 23:56.
298. Dawber R (1985) Self-induced hair loss. **Senin Dermatol** 4:53.
299. Oranje AP, Peereboom-Wynia JDR, De Raeymaecker DMJ (1986) Trichotillomania in childhood. **J Am Acad Dermatol** 15:614.
300. Dimmino-Emme L, Camisa C (1991) Trichotillomania associated with the "Friar Tuck" sign and nail-biting. **Cutis** 47:107.
301. Trueb RM, Cavegn B (1996) Trichotillomania in connection with alopecia areata. **Cutis** 58:67.

If patients are reassured, given an opportunity to express their emotional needs, and offered a reasonable therapeutic regimen such as a mild shampoo and scalp lotion (e.g., hydrocortisone in a 1% concentration to relieve pruritus and irritation), the habit will frequently disappear. The hair pulling is usually a "call for help" reflecting an underlying emotional conflict, at least in the older children, and referral to psychologist or psychiatrist for counselling is helpful. For those with persistent or severe obsessive-compulsive or emotional problems, antidepressants such as clomipramine or fluoxetine, and psychiatric consultation should be considered.[302,303]

LOOSE ANAGEN HAIR SYNDROME

Loose anagen hair syndrome is characterized by actively growing anagen hairs that, loosely anchored, can be easily and painlessly pulled from the scalp. The condition is usually sporadic, but may occur in families with an autosomal-dominant mode of inheritance.[304] Although the majority of reported patients were blonde girls 2 to 5 years of age, patients of both sexes, adults, and those with dark hair may also be affected.[305] Parents will complain that their child's hair "won't grow" and seldom requires cutting. Patients are otherwise well, although loose anagen hair has been reported in patients with Noonan syndrome.[306,307] Adults with loose anagen hair usually present during the third or fourth decade of life with a sudden and diffuse hair loss that resembles telogen effluvium.[307]

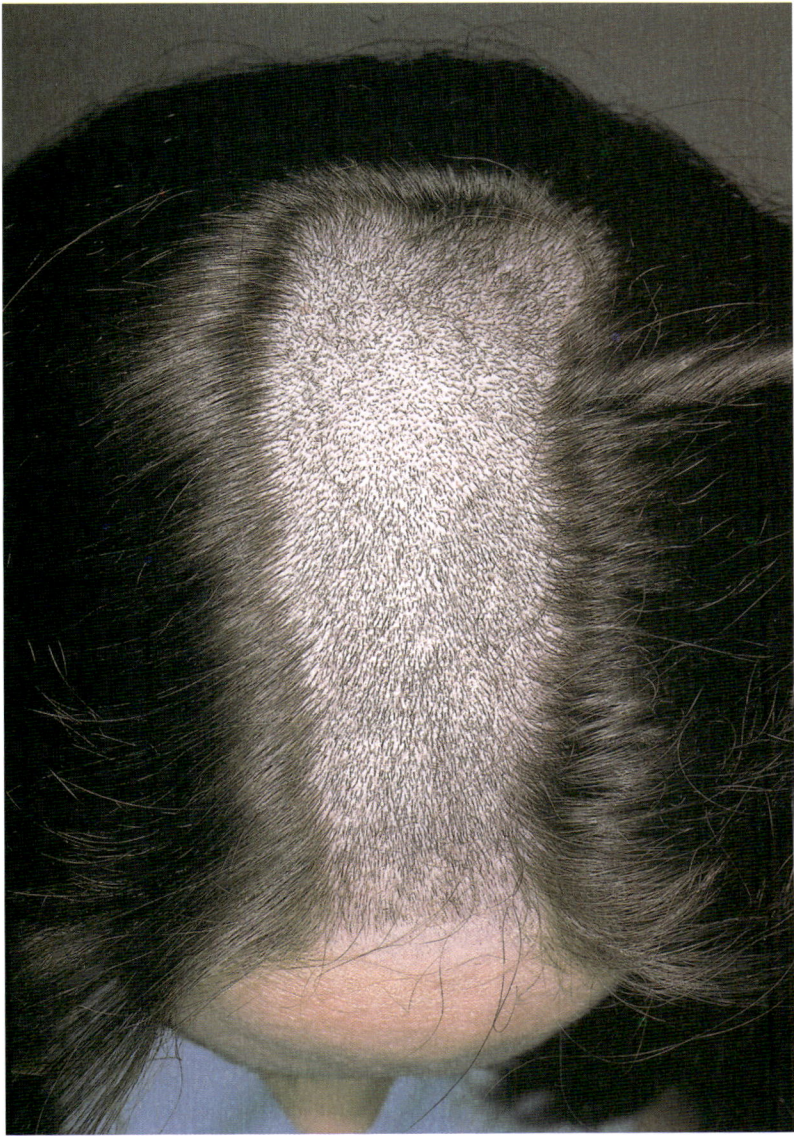

Fig. 11.44 Trichotillomania. Irregular-shaped patch of hair loss with angular outlines.

the casts become compact, black, acellular structures in the interior of a shaftless follicle. Shafts demonstrating trichomalacia are abnormally small, distorted or bizarre in shape, incompletely keratinized, and show irregular pigmentation. Other findings include dilated ostia with soft keratin, empty follicles, traumatized hair bulbs with perifollicular hemorrhage, and absence of bulbar inflammation.[297] In taking biopsy specimens, it is best to select the site of most recent hair loss (less than eight weeks' duration).

Treatment

The management of trichotillomania is often difficult and requires strong physician–patient and physician–parent relationships. Although patients occasionally admit to touching the affected areas, they frequently deny plucking, rubbing, or excessive manipulation. Direct confrontation and accusation frequently are detrimental and rarely helpful.

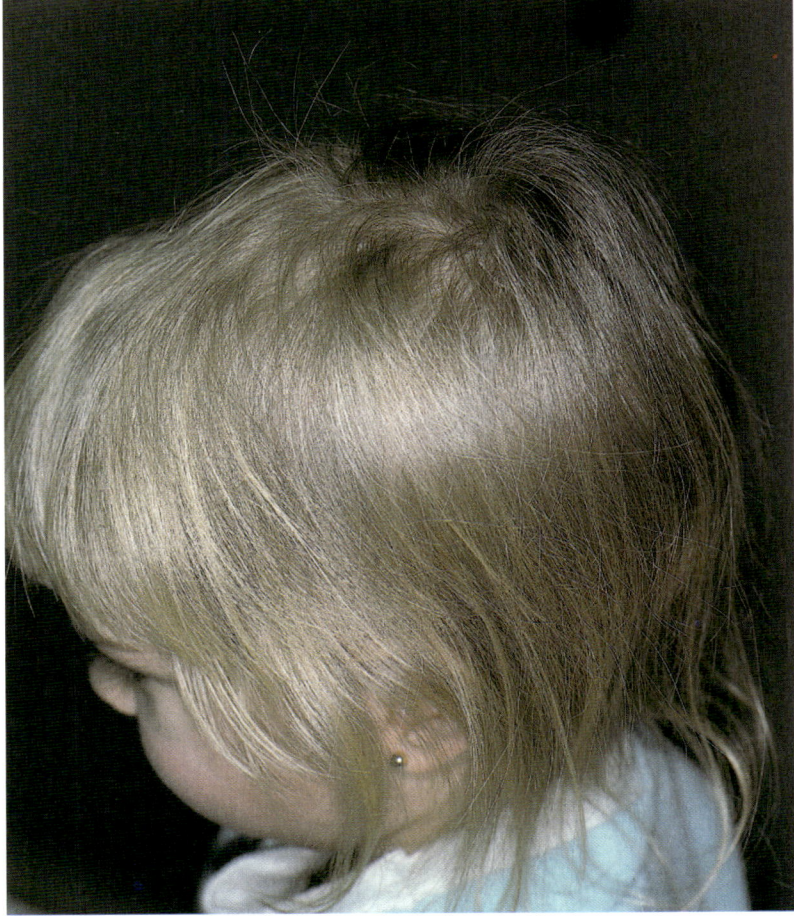

Fig. 11.45 Unruly hair in loose anagen hair of childhood.

302. Swedo S, Leonard H (1989) A double-blind comparison of clomipramine and desipramine in the treatment of trichotillomania. N Engl J Med 321:497.
303. Sheikha SH, Wagner KD, Wagner RF Jr (1993) Fluoxetine treatment of trichotillomania and depression in a prepubertal child. Cutis 51:50.
304. Baden HP, Kvedar JC, Magro CM (1992) Loose anagen hair as a cause of hereditary hair loss in children. Arch Dermatol 128:1349.

305. Price VH, Gummer CL (1989) Loose anagen syndrome. J Am Acad Dermatol 20:249.
306. Tosti A, Misciali C, Borrello P et al. (1991) Loose anagen hair in a child with Noonan's syndrome. Dermatologica 182:247.
307. Tosti A, Peluso AM, Misciali C et al. (1997) Loose anagen hair. Arch Dermatol 133:1089.

On examination, subtle diffuse or patchy thinning is usually present with locks of uneven length (Fig. 11.45). The hair may appear "limp" and a matted, "sticky" feel to the locks has been noted in some cases.[305] Findings from the gentle hair pull test are diagnostic. With each pull, numerous hair shafts (greater than 10 anagen hairs) can be painlessly extracted. A gentle hair pull performed on a normal scalp will yield telogen hairs and the presence of anagen hairs on a gentle hair pull is abnormal.[308] When the bulbs of these shafts are examined microscopically, most or all of the hairs are anagen hairs and the bulbs do not have outer root sheaths, but show a ruffling of the hair shaft.[213] This is because the extracted shafts tear away from their root sheaths at the cuticular zone, where the hair shaft cuticle interlocks with the inner root sheath cuticle.[308] In loose anagen hair syndrome, the normally tenacious bond between the lower hair shaft and the inner root sheath is pathologically weak, allowing trivial amounts of traction to separate the shaft from the sheath.

No treatment is available for loose anagen hair syndrome. It is reassuring for patients and their families to know that the appearance of the hair improves with time, with length and density of the hair gradually increasing with age in both children and adults.[305,307]

ANDROGENETIC ALOPECIA

Androgenetic alopecia, also known as common balding or male-pattern baldness in men and hereditary thinning or female-pattern baldness in women, is the most common cause of hair loss in both men and women. It is characterized by progressive, patterned hair loss from the scalp and is caused by circulating androgens in genetically susceptible men and women. It begins in the teens, 20s, or 30s in both sexes and is usually fully expressed by the 40s.[309] Male-pattern baldness affects up to 70% of all males in later life and female androgenetic alopecia up to 30% of older women.[310] Inheritance of androgenetic alopecia is probably a polygenic trait with heritability from both maternal and paternal sides.[311] Therefore, a history of baldness in grandparents and first-degree relatives on both sides of the family should be obtained.

Dihydrotestosterone is the primary androgen implicated in the pathogenesis of androgenetic alopecia.[312] It is formed by the conversion of testosterone by the enzyme 5α-reductase. Androgens gradually transform large scalp hair follicles to smaller follicles over many cycles resulting in progressively shorter, finer, miniaturized hairs, which ultimately do not cover the scalp effectively.

Most patients with androgenetic alopecia complain of thinning rather than shedding of hair, although early in the course of androgenetic alopecia, hair loss may occur and this has features of a telogen effluvium.[213] This is because the duration of anagen growth shortens and hairs cycle through the telogen phase more frequently. In men, the pattern of androgenetic alopecia varies from accentuation of the bitemporal recession, to frontal and/or vertex thinning, to loss of all hair except hair along the occipital and temporal margins (Fig. 11.46). Women have diffuse thinning, often worse centrally with the central part appearing widened and the scalp becoming visible. In women, there is often retention of hair along the frontal hairline that may be straight or M-shaped. In fact, there is considerable overlap between the sexes, with many women demonstrating a male-pattern of hair loss,[313] and some men showing a female pattern with diffuse crown thinning and retention of the frontal hairline.

On histology, androgenetic alopecia is characterized by a mixture of hairs with various bulb depths and shaft diameters. Below each miniaturized follicle is a "streamer," the collapsed connective tissue sheath that once surrounded

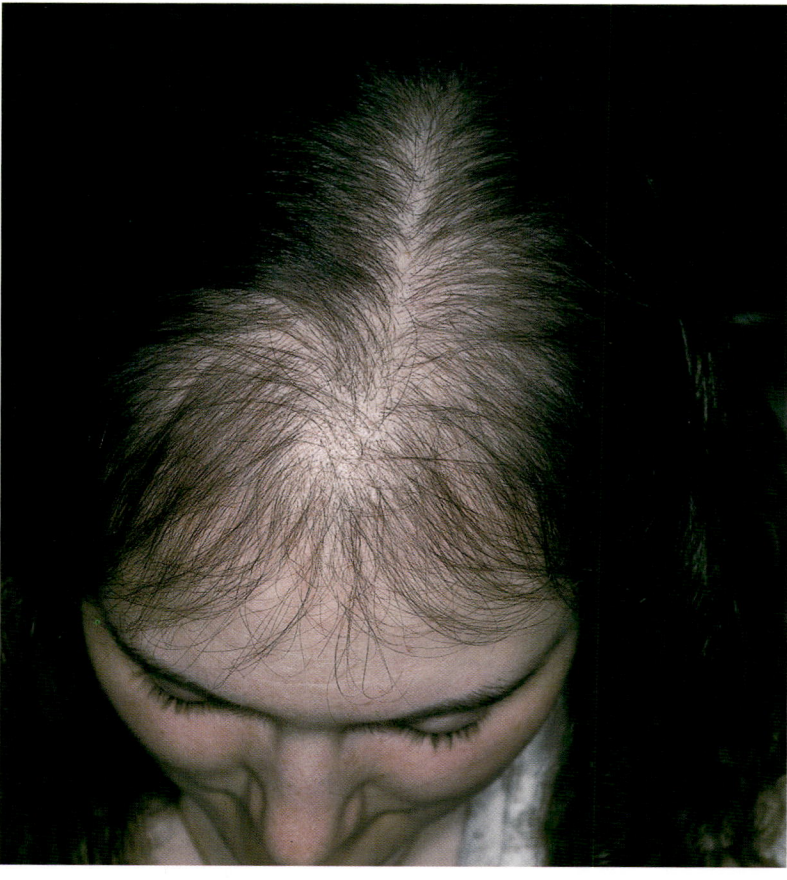

Fig. 11.46   Androgenetic alopecia with vertex thinning and bitemporal recession.

the formerly deep-seated, terminal hair.[314] Miniaturized follicles can be identified on horizontal sections of scalp biopsies. Other features are an increased ratio of telogen to anagen hairs and, in advanced cases, there is an increase in the percentage of vellus and indeterminate hairs compared to terminal hairs. Many biopsy specimens of androgenetic alopecia show mild perifollicular, lymphohistiocytic, upper dermal inflammation. These changes are nonspecific and can be found in a high percentage of normal controls.[314,315]

Men with androgenetic alopecia do not require a laboratory evaluation. In women, hormonal abnormalities are less likely if the patient has no menstrual irregularities, infertility, hirsutism, acne, virilization, or galactorrhea.[316] If one or more of the above symptoms are present, it may be useful to evaluate total and free testosterone, dehydroepiandrosterone sulfate, LH, FSH and prolactin. Referral to an endocrinologist may be indicated.

Without treatment, androgenetic alopecia is progressive.[317] Because of the psychosocial impact of hair loss, it is important to explain to the patient the nature of the condition, assess his or her expectations, stress that response to any therapy may be slow, and emphasize that treatment will need to be used long-term. The aim of treatment is to retard further thinning of the hair and to promote hair regrowth.

Topical minoxidil has been shown to promote hair growth in large controlled clinical studies. The mechanism of action of minoxidil on hair

308. O'Donnell BP, Sperling LC, James WD (1992) Loose anagen hair syndrome. **Int J Dermatol** 31:107.
309. Price VH (1988) Androgenetic alopecia and hair growth promotion state of the art: present and future. **Clin Dermatol** 6:218.
310. Norwood OT (2001) Incidence of female androgenetic alopecia (female pattern alopecia). **Dermatol Surg** 27:53.
311. Ellis JA, Stebbing M, Harrap SB (1998) Genetic analysis of male pattern baldness and the 5α-reductase genes. **J Invest Dermatol** 110:849.
312. Kaufman DK (1996) Androgen metabolism as it affects hair growth in androgenetic alopecia. **Dermatol Clin** 14:697.

313. Venning VA, Dawber RPR (1988) Patterned androgenetic alopecia in women. **J Am Acad Dermatol** 18:1073.
314. Kligman AM (1988) The comparative histopathology of male pattern baldness and senescent baldness. **Clin Dermatol** 6:108.
315. Whiting D (1993) Diagnostic and predictive value of horizontal sections of scalp biopsy specimens in male pattern androgenetic alopecia. **J Am Acad Dermatol** 28:755.
316. Price VH, Baden H, DeVillez RL et al. (1996) Guidelines of care for androgenetic alopecia. **J Am Acad Dermatol** 35:465.
317. Rushton DH, Ramsay ID, Norris MJ et al. (1991) Natural progression of male pattern baldness in young men. **Clin Exp Dermatol** 16:188.

growth promotion is unclear. The hair follicle dermal papilla controls hair growth and minoxidil may be involved in the development of dermal papilla vascularization via stimulation of vascular endothelial growth factor expression.[318]

Two and 5% minoxidil have been studied only in adults, and promote moderate to dense growth in about one-third of subjects.[319–321] Minoxidil works equally well on vertex and frontal scalp thinning.[319,320] Minoxidil is applied directly onto the dry scalp, twice daily. It should be used for at least one year before assessing efficacy.[320] It has to be used indefinitely to maintain its effect; after stopping treatment, the newly regrown hair is shed within six months of drug discontinuation.

Side effects of topical minoxidil include irritation (itching, dryness, erythema) primarily due to propylene glycol and occasionally allergic contact dermatitis. Facial and limb hypertrichosis may occur through local transfer of the drug or via a systemic effect.[322] The hypertrichosis disappears after discontinuing the drug and may occur in 3% to 5% of women, who should be aware of this possibility.[320]

There are two isoforms of the human 5α-reductase enzyme. Type I predominates in the sebaceous glands whereas type II is present in hair follicles and prostate. Oral finasteride, a specific inhibitor of the human type II 5α-reductase, has been shown to reduce both serum and scalp skin dihydrotestosterone levels in balding men.[323,324]

Finasteride is effective in the treatment of men with vertex and frontal male-pattern hair loss in studies up to two years in length.[325,326] A response to finasteride may be seen as early as three months, but patients should be encouraged to continue the treatment for at least 24 months before evaluating it.[326] Continued daily use of 1mg oral finasteride is needed for sustained benefit, otherwise the benefits are lost. The incidence of side effects in the finasteride group was similar to placebo, and the only important side effect was sexual dysfunction in 4.2% of men receiving finasteride versus 2.2% on placebo.[325] This returned to normal in all cases in which the drug was stopped and in many cases with continued treatment. Finasteride is contraindicated in women who are or may potentially be pregnant because of the risk that inhibition of conversion of fetal testosterone to dihydrotestosterone could impair virilization of a male fetus. Finasteride treatment has recently been shown to be ineffective in postmenopausal women with androgenetic alopecia in a one-year, double-blind, placebo-controlled trail.[327] There are no data on the use of finasteride in subjects under age 18.

In certain selected cases, the following treatments may be helpful in women: spironolactone, an aldosterone antagonist, has been used to treat acne, hirsutism, and androgenetic alopecia. Small open trials have shown some benefit in androgenetic alopecia with doses of 50–200mg/day.[328] Cyproterone acetate in doses of 50–100mg/day together with ethinyl estradiol is not available in the USA, but has been successful in preventing progression of hair loss and inducing regrowth.[329]

Excision of bald scalp with or without tissue expansion, scalp flaps and hair transplantation are options in patients with advanced androgenetic alopecia. Hair prostheses are also an option in advanced stages of hair loss.

SCARRING ALOPECIA

Scarring or cicatricial alopecia is the end result of a wide number of inflammatory processes affecting the pilosebaceous units, resulting in destruction of tissue and consequent permanent scarring alopecia of the affected areas. The scarring may be the result of a developmental defect (aplasia cutis), due to infections (e.g., severe bacterial, viral, or fungal infection), physical trauma (e.g., thermal or caustic burns), neoplastic disorders; various dermatoses (e.g., lichen planus, lupus erythematosus, morphea), keratosis pilaris atrophicans, folliculitis decalvans, dissecting cellulitis of the scalp, acne keloidalis, psuedopelade, and alopecia mucinosa.

KERATOSIS PILARIS ATROPHICANS

Keratosis pilaris is a common skin condition characterized by keratinous plugs in the follicular orifices surrounded by a variable degree of erythema over the face, arms and thighs. When rarely atrophy occurs, the condition is called keratosis pilaris atrophicans (KPA). KPA is a group of cutaneous disorders characterized by follicular hyperkeratosis and scarring.[330] There are three distinct clinical entities that show KPA: ulerythema ophryogenes (keratosis pilaris atrophicans faciei), atrophoderma vermiculata, and keratosis follicularis spinulosa decalvans (Table 11.9).[331] Some authors, however, consider atrophoderma vermiculata the final stage of the inflammatory disorders of ulerythema ophryogenes and keratosis follicularis spinulosa decalvans.[332]

Ulerythema ophryogenes is characterized by redness and atrophic scarring of the eyebrows, classically involving the outer half. Occasionally the disorder

---

TABLE 11.9   Classification of keratosis pilaris atrophicans

	Atrophoderma vermiculata	Ulerythema ophryogenes	Keratosis follicularis spinulosa decalvans
Skin lesions	Erythematous papules, follicular plugs, horn cysts, atrophic scars	Follicular papules, plugging, scarring	Milia, thornlike follicular projections, atrophic scars
Sites	Cheeks, neck, limbs	Lateral eyebrows, extending medially	Scalp, eyebrows, eyelashes, cheeks, nose, neck, dorsal hands, fingers
Alopecia	Absent	Minimal eyebrows	Scarring alopecia of the scalp
Photophobia	Absent	Absent	Marked, corneal opacities
Inheritance	Sporadic or autosomal	Sporadic or autosomal dominant	Sporadic or X-linked recessive dominant

---

318. Lachgar S, Charveron M, Gall Y et al. (1998) Minoxidil upregulates the expression of vascular endothelial growth factor in human hair dermal papilla cells. **Br J Dermatol** 138:407.
319. Olsen E (1989) Treatment of androgenetic alopecia with topical minoxidil. **Res Staff Phys** 35:53.
320. Shapiro J, Price VH (1998) Hair regrowth. Therapeutic agents. **Dermatol Clin** 16:341.
321. DeVillez RL, Jacobs JP, Szpunar CA et al. (1994) Androgenetic alopecia in the female. Treatment with 2% topical minoxidil solution. **Arch Dermatol** 130:303.
322. Peluso AM, Misciali C, Vincenzi C et al. (1997) Diffuse hypertrichosis during treatment with 5% topical minoxidil. **Br J Dermatol** 136:118.
323. Waldstreicher J, Fiedler V, Hordinsky M et al. (1994) Effects of finasteride on dihydrotestosterone content of scalp skin in men with male pattern baldness. **J Invest Dermatol** 102:615.
324. Olsen E (1997) Finasteride (1mg) in the treatment of androgenetic alopecia in men (abstract). **Aust J Dermatol** 38:A316.
325. Kaufman KD, Olsen EA, Whiting D et al. (1998) Finasteride in the treatment of men with androgenetic alopecia. **J Am Acad Dermatol** 39:578.

326. Leyden J, Dunlap F, Miller B et al. (1999) Finasteride in the treatment of men with frontal male pattern hair loss. **J Am Acad Dermatol** 40:930.
327. Price VH, Roberts JL, Hordinsky M et al. (2000) Lack of efficacy of finasteride in postmenopausal women with androgenetic alopecia. **J Am Acad Dermatol** 43:768.
328. Burke BM, Cunliffe WJ (1985) Oral spironolactone therapy for female patients with acne, hirsutism or androgenic alopecia. **Br J Dermatol** 112:124.
329. Mortimer CH, Rushton H, James KC (1984) Effective medical treatment for common baldness in women. **Clin Exp Dermatol** 9:342.
330. Baden HP, Byers HR (1994) Clinical findings, cutaneous pathology and response to therapy in 21 patients with keratosis pilaris atrophicans. **Arch Dermatol** 130:469.
331. Bassioukas K, Fragidou M, Nakuci M et al. (1997) Atrophodermia vermiculata. **Cutis** 59:337.
332. Arndt KA, Rand RE (1993) Follicular syndromes with inflammation and atrophy In: Dermatology in General Medicine, 4th ed, Fitzpatrick TB, Eisen AZ, Wolff K et al. eds. New York: McGaw-Hill International, pp. 766.

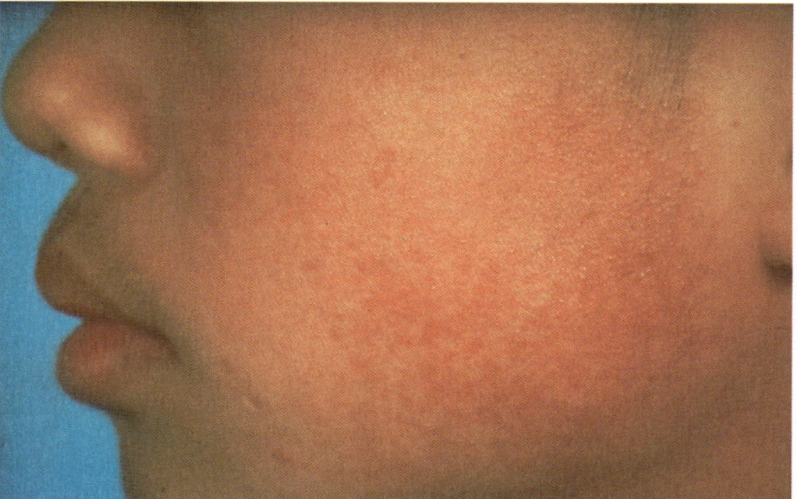

Fig. 11.47 Atrophoderma vermiculata with pit-like scarring.

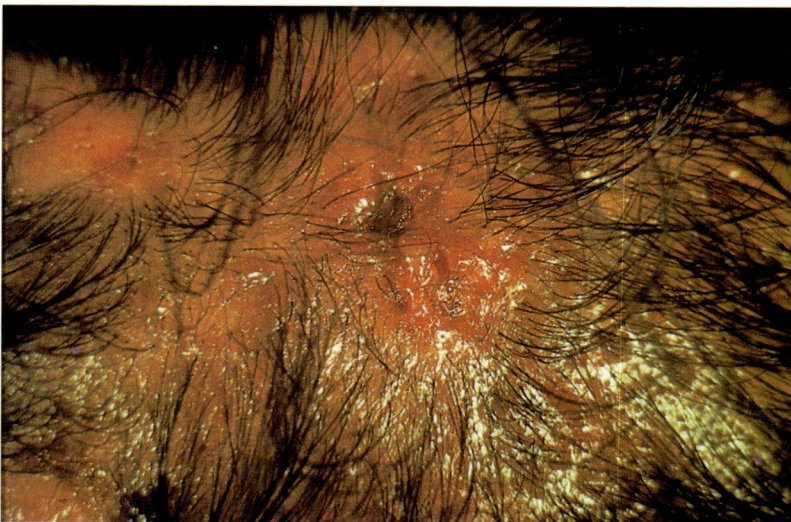

Fig. 11.48 Folliculitis decalvans. Irregular bald atrophic patches with follicular pustules.

extends to include the adjacent skin and scalp. The symptoms present from birth or infancy and inheritance is autosomal dominant. Association of ulerythema ophryogenes with Noonan's syndrome and woolly hair has been described.[333,334]

Atrophoderma vermiculata has its onset between 5 and 12 years of age, occasionally later. It starts with erythema and inflammatory follicular hyperkeratosis on the cheeks leading to pit-like honeycomb scarring.[331] Generally measuring 1–2mm across and 1mm deep, these cribriform lesions with sharp edges are separated by narrow ridges of normal-appearing skin (Fig. 11.47). Other sites of involvement are the neck and the extensor surface of the limbs. It is thought to be of either sporadic or autosomal–dominant inheritance.[331,332]

Keratosis follicularis spinulosa decalvans is characterized by follicular hyperkeratosis of the skin, corneal dystrophy, photophobia, scarring alopecia of the scalp, and absent eyebrows and eyelashes.[335] Other findings are hyperkeratosis of the calcaneal region of the soles and a high cuticle on the nails. Symptoms usually improve spontaneously at puberty. Inheritance of keratosis follicularis spinulosa decalvans is X-linked recessive, and the gene has been localized to Xp21.2–p22.2.[336]

The primary defect of keratosis pilaris atrophicans appears to be abnormal keratinization of the follicular infundibulum, which results in obstruction of the growing hair shaft, producing a chronic inflammatory infiltrate with scarring below that level.[330] It is not surprising that topical therapies are unsuccessful, as the abnormality is present deep in the follicle. Scarring may also limit penetration. Keratolytics and topical corticosteroids are of some help in reducing the keratotic and inflammatory components of keratosis pilaris atrophicans, but the effect is only partial. Other treatments used have included antibiotics, intralesional steroids, tretinoin, and ultraviolet radiation. There has not been any consistent benefit with any of these modalities.[337] In stable atrophoderma vermiculata, dermabrasion and collagen implants have been used to improve the cosmetic appearance. One case report has

demonstrated long-term suppression of atrophoderma vermiculata with oral isotretinoin, provided that it is given during the active inflammatory stage before scarring develops.[338]

FOLLICULITIS DECALVANS

Folliculitis decalvans is a rare form of recurrent, patchy, painful folliculitis of the scalp causing scarring and resultant hair loss. The scalp alone may be involved or it may extend to the axillae, pubic region, and trunk.[339] There are multiple rounded or irregular bald atrophic patches, each surrounded by crops of follicular pustules (Fig. 11.48). Successive crops of pustules, each followed by destruction of the affected follicles, produce slow extension of the alopecia. Folliculitis decalvans affects both sexes, typically affecting women aged 30–60 years and men from adolescence onwards. It rarely occurs in children. Tufted folliculitis is a variant of this entity in which there is progressive folliculitis of the scalp that resolves with irregular areas of scarring alopecia in which numerous hair tufts emerge from dilated follicular openings.[340–342]

The cause of folliculitis decalvans is still uncertain. *Staphylococcus aureus* can nearly always be grown from the pustules and it is possible that folliculitis decalvans may be the result of an abnormal host response to toxins released from *S. aureus*.[341]

Treatment of folliculitis decalvans is difficult. Systemic antibiotics (such as cloxacillin, erythromycin or minocycline) will often prevent extension of the disease; there is rapid relapse after stopping treatment. Oral fusidic acid and oral zinc sulfate together with topical fusidic acid have helped some patients.[343] Rifampicin 600mg daily for 10 weeks led to resolution of the symptoms and no recurrence for a year.[344] Recently, a combination of oral rifampicin 300mg twice daily and oral clindamycin 300mg twice daily, for 10 weeks, produced good results.[341,345] Bacterial culture of pustules in all patients should be done.

333. Pierini DO, Pierini AM (1979) Keratosis pilaris atrophicans faciei (ulerythema ophryogenes): a cutaneous marker n the Noonan syndrome. **Br J Dermatol** 100:409.
334. Neild VS, Pegum JS, Wells RS (1984) The association of keratosis pilaris atrophicans and woolly hair, with and without Noonan's syndrome. **Br J Dermatol** 110:357.
335. Oranje AP, Molewaterplein, Van Osch LDM et al. (1994) Keratosis pilaris atrophicans. **Arch Dermatol** 130:500.
336. Oosterwijk JC, Nelen M, van Zandvoort PM et al. (1992) Linkage analysis of keratosis follicularis spinulosa decalvans and regional assignment to human chromosome Xp21.2-p22.2. **Am J Hum Genet** 50:801.
337. Arreita E, Milgram-Sternberg Y (1988) Honeycomb atrophy on the right cheek. **Arch Dermatol** 124:1101.
338. Weightmann W (1998) A case of atrophoderma vermiculata responding to isotretinoin. **Clin Exp Dermatol** 23:89.

339. Bogg A (1963) Folliculitis decalvans. **Acta Derm Venereol** (Stockh) 43:14.
340. Annessi G (1998) Tufted folliculitis of the scalp: a disinctive clinicohistological variant of folliculitis decalvans. **Br J Dermatol** 138:799.
341. Powell JJ, Dawber RPR, Gatter K (1999) Folliculitis decalvans including tufted folliculitis: Clinical, histological and therapeutic findings. **Br J Dermatol** 140:328.
342. Templeton SF, Solomon AR (1994) Scarring alopecia: A classification based on microscopic criteria. **J Cutan Pathol** 21:97.
343. Abeck D, Korting HC, Braun-Falco O (1992) Folliculitiis decalvans. Long-lasting response to combined therapy with fusidic acid and zinc. **Acta Derm Venereol** (Stockh) 72:143.
344. Brozena SJ, Cohen LE, Fenske NA (1988) Folliculitis decalvans – response to rifampin. **Cutis** 42:512.
345. Brooke RCC, Griffiths CEM (2001) Folliculitis decalvans. **Clin Exp Dermatol** 26:120.

DISSECTING CELLULITIS OF THE SCALP

Dissecting cellulitis of the scalp, also termed perifolliculitis capitis abscedens et suffodiens, is an uncommon, chronic, inflammatory disease of the scalp characterized by painful fluctant nodules and abscesses interconnected by tortuous ridges or deep sinus tracts with scarring alopecia. Pressure applied to one nodule often causes pus to emerge from interconnected nodules and sinuses several centimeters away. The process most commonly begins at the vertex or occiput and may progress to involve the entire scalp. It may be associated with acne conglobata and hidradenitis suppurative to form the follicular occlusion triad.[346]

Dissecting cellulitis is seen primarily in persons between 18 and 40 years of age, although it has been reported in children.[347] The disease occurs in whites and blacks, with a greater frequency in the latter, and men are affected more frequently than women (4:1).[348] Inflammatory tinea capitis (kerion)[349] and folliculotropic mycosis fungoides[350] may mimic dissecting cellulitis. The etiology is not known and both infection and follicular occlusion have been implicated in the pathogenesis. Tissue cultures are usually negative or grow a mixed flora. An immunologic reaction to *Propionibacterium acnes* may also play a role.[351]

In the acute suppurative phase, there is an acniform dilation of the follicular infundibulum with intra- and perifollicular accumulation of neutrophils and subsequent follicular perforation. Later, keratogenous debris incites a granulomatous response with dermal fibrosis surrounding sinus tracts. The abscesses are partially lined with squamous epithelium derived from the overlying epidermis or adjacent follicular epithelium.[342]

The disease follows a chronic relapsing course and is generally considered benign. However, metastasizing squamous cell carcinoma has developed in a long-standing lesion.[352] Treatment options include numerous nonsurgical and surgical modalities or a combination of both. Broad-spectrum systemic antibiotics such as tetracycline or erythromycin are effective in some cases.[353] Topical antibiotics, antibacterial soaps, topical and intralesional corticosteroids, and oral isotretinoin[354] have also been used as adjuncts.

Oral zinc sulfate has been reported to induce complete clearing of lesions by some[355,356] but not all investigators.[357] Surgical interventions include incision and drainage of painful nodules,[347] complete scalp extirpation with skin grafting,[358] and carbon dioxide laser ablation.[359]

Isotretinoin is the systemic drug of choice.[351,357,360,361] Scerri *et al.* consider isotretinoin a first-line treatment, using an initial dose of 1mg/kg per day and a maintenance dose of at least 0.75mg/kg per day after clinical control is achieved. Treatment should be continued for at least four months after the disease appears clinically inactive to reduce recurrence.[357]

ACNE KELOIDALIS

Acne keloidalis (folliculitis keloidalis nuchae) is a chronic scarring folliculitis that begins as small, smooth, firm papules with occasional pustules that occur

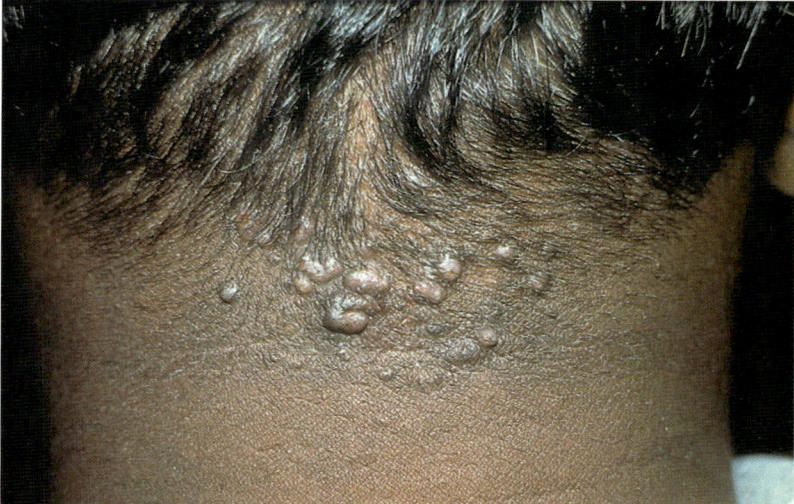

Fig. 11.49   Acne keloidalis. A chronic scarring folliculitis at the nape of the neck.

on the occipital area of the scalp and nape of the neck (Fig. 11.49). With time, the papules coalesce into firm, hairless keloid-like plaques that can be painful and cosmetically disfiguring. Abscesses and sinuses exuding pus may be present in advanced cases.[362] Patients often complain of burning and itching. It is seen most frequently in postpubertal males, especially blacks between the ages of 14 and 25, although it also occurs in white males and black women.

The cause of acne keloidalis remains unclear. Constant irritation by shirt collars, football helmets, low-grade bacterial infection, curved ingrown hairs after a close haircut, chronic scratching, and an autoimmune process have all been suggested as pathogenic mechanisms.[362–366] Recently, it has been proposed that acne keloidalis is a primary form of scarring alopecia with its histology resembling that seen in other forms of cicatricial alopecia, such as the follicular degeneration syndrome.[367]

The histology of early lesions consist of dilatation of the follicular infundibulum similar to that seen in folliculitis decalvans. Intrafollicular neutrophilic inflammation fills the infundibulum and isthmus in inflammatory lesions. Later, there is a chronic, perifollicular lymphocytic and plasmacytic inflammation, most intense at the level of the isthmus and lower infundibulum, with granulomatous inflammation and scarring. Other findings are lamellar fibroplasia, complete disappearance of sebaceous glands, thinning of the follicular epithelium, and total epithelial destruction, with residual "naked" hair fragments.[342,367,368] Herzberg *et al.* proposed the following sequence of inflammatory events.[368] Acute inflammation begins in the sebaceous gland, deep infundibulum, or isthmus. This weakens the follicular wall, which ruptures, releasing hair shafts into the surrounding dermis. The naked hairs

346. Kierland RR (1951) Unusual pyodermas (hidrosadenitis suppurativa, acne conglobata, dissecting cellulitis of the scalp): a review. **Minn Med** 34:319.
347. Ramesh V (1990) Dissecting cellulitis of the scalp in 2 girls. **Dermatologica** 180:48.
348. Jolliffe DS, Sarkany I (1997) Perifolliculitis capitis abscedens et suffodiens (dissecting cellulitis of the scalp). **Clin Exp Dermatol** 2:291.
349. Sperling LC (1991) Inflammatory tinea capitis (kerion) mimicking dissecting cellulitis. **Int J Dermatol** 30:190.
350. Gilliam AC, Lessin SR, Wilson DM et al. (1997) Folliculotropic mycosis fungoides with large-cell transformation presenting as dissecting cellulitis of the scalp. **J Cutan Pathol** 24:169.
351. Stites PC, Boyd AS (2001) Dissecting cellulitis in a white male: A case report and review of the literature. **Cutis** 67:37.
352. Curry SS, Gaither DH, King LE Jr (1981) Squamous cell carcinoma arising in dissecting perifolliculitis of the scalp: a case report and review of secondary squamous cell carcinomas. **J Am Acad Dermatol** 4:673.
353. Moyer DG, Williams RM (1962) Perifolliculitis capitis abscedens et suffodiens: a report of six cases. **Arch Dermatol** 85:378.
354. Shaffer N, Bilick RC, Srolovitz H (1992) Perifolliculitis capitis abscedens et suffodiens: resolution with combination therapy. **Arch Dermatol** 128:1329.
355. Berne B, Venge P Ohman S (1985) Perifolliculitis capitis abscedens et suffodiens (Hoffman): complete healing associated with oral zinc therapy. **Arch Dermatol** 121:1028.
356. Kobayashi H, Aiba S, Tagami H (1999) Successful treatment of dissecting cellulitis and acne conglobata with oral zinc. **Br J Dermatol** 141:1136.

357. Scerri L, Williams HC, Allen BR (1996) Dissecting cellulitis of the scalp; response to isotretinoin. **Br J Dermatol** 134:1105.
358. Moschella SL, Klein MH, Miller RJ (1967) Perifolliculitis capitis abscedens et suffodiens: report of a successful therapeutic scalping. **Arch Dermatol** 96:195.
359. Glass LF, Berman B, Laub D (1989) Treatment of perifolliculitis capitis abscedens et suffodiens with the carbon dioxide laser. **J Dermatol Surg Oncol** 15:673.
360. Schewach-Millet M, Ziv R, Shapira D (1986) Perifolliculitis capitis abscedens et suffodiens treated with isotretinoin (13-cis-retinoic acid). **J Am Acad Dermatol** 15:1291.
361. Bjellerup M, Wallengren J (1990) Familial perifolliculitis capitis abscedens et suffodiens in two brothers successfully treated with isotretinoin. **J Am Acad Dermatol** 23:752.
362. Dinehart SM, Herzberg AJ, Kerns BJ et al. (1989) Acne keloidalis: a review. **J Dermatol Surg Oncol** 15:642.
363. Cosman B, Wolff M (1972) Acne keloidalis. **Plast Reconstr Surg** 50:25.
364. Halder R (1988) Pseudofolliculitis barbae and related disorders. **Dermatol Clin** 6:407.
365. Knable AL, Hanke CW, Gonin R (1997) Prevalence of acne keloidalis nuchae in football players. **J Am Acad Dermatol** 37:570.
366. Burkhart CG, Burkhart CN (1998) Acne keloidalis is lichen simplex chronicus with fibrotic keloidal scarring. **J Am Acad Dermatol** 39:661.
367. Sperling LC, Homoky C, Pratt L et al. (2000) Acne keloidalis is a form of primary scarring alopecia. **Arch Dermatol** 136:479.
368. Herzberg AJ, Dinehart SM, Kerns BJ et al. (1990) Acne keloidalis. Transverse microscopy, immunohistochemistry and electron microscopy. **Am J Dermatopathol** 12:109.

stimulate a foreign body reaction with acute and chronic granulomatous inflammation. The granulomatous inflammation manifests itself clinically as papular lesions. Fibroblasts lay down collagen and scars form in the region of the inflammation. Subsequent fibrosis occurs within the dermis, which may distort and occlude the follicular lumen and consequently lead to hair retention within the deeper follicle and further smoldering granulomatous inflammation and scarring. *Demodex* may play a role in the pathogenesis.

Medical treatment for early papular lesions includes potent topical corticosteroids, intralesional injections of corticosteroids, topical and oral antibiotics such as tetracycline.[362,364,367] Once large keloid-like plaques have developed, the condition is resistant to medical treatment, often requiring surgical removal, e.g., excision or carbon dioxide laser ablation.[369,370] Prophylaxis depends upon avoidance of close "clipper" hair cuts[365] and instructing patients not to scratch affected areas.

PSEUDOPELADE

The term pseudopelade refers to a slowly progressive cicatricial alopecia, without clinically evident folliculitis and no marked inflammation. It may be the end result of several different forms of scarring alopecia such as discoid lupus erythematosus or lichen planopilaris[371,372] although a specific, distinct clinically uninflamed type unrelated to other known forms of scarring alopecia has been recognized.[373] It is generally seen in adults, with an onset between 25 and 45 years of age, although childhood cases have been reported.[374,375] There is a female predominance (3:1).[373] The condition is usually sporadic, although familial cases with an autosomal-dominant pattern have been reported.[376]

Clinically, the alopecia consists of round to irregularly shaped patches of alopecia most commonly located on the vertex or crown. Mild perifollicular erythema may be present, but pseudopelade usually lacks prominent inflammation or follicular hyperkeratosis. Affected areas are shiny, ivory-white with a slightly depressed, atrophic surface giving rise to the classic description of "footprints in the snow."[377] Interspersed between the patches may be a few hair-containing dilated hair follicles.

On histology, early lesions are characterized by perifollicular and perivascular lymphocytic infiltrates without interface changes. As the alopecia develops, the infundibular epithelium becomes atrophic, and in advanced lesions the follicular epithelium is destroyed and only naked hair shafts surrounded by histiocytic and foreign-body giant cell inflammation remain. Characteristic concentric lamellar fibroplasia surrounds inflamed follicles. Sebaceous glands are destroyed and deposits of elastic tissue may occur around these follicular scars.[213,342] Direct immunofluoresence studies are negative or show only IgM.[373]

The condition often worsens in spurts, with periods of activity followed by dormant periods. Pseudopelade is slowly progressive, eventually burning itself out after several years, resulting in permanent hair loss. There is no consistently effective treatment for this disorder. Infiltration of triamcinolone acetonide in a 2.5–5.0 mg/ml concentration into active areas at six to eight weeks intervals may be temporarily beneficial. Other treatments that have been tried include non-steroidal anti-inflammatory and antimalarial drugs.[374,376] If the disfigurement is considerable and no active inflammatory changes are present, autografting of hair from unaffected to scarred scalp may be considered.

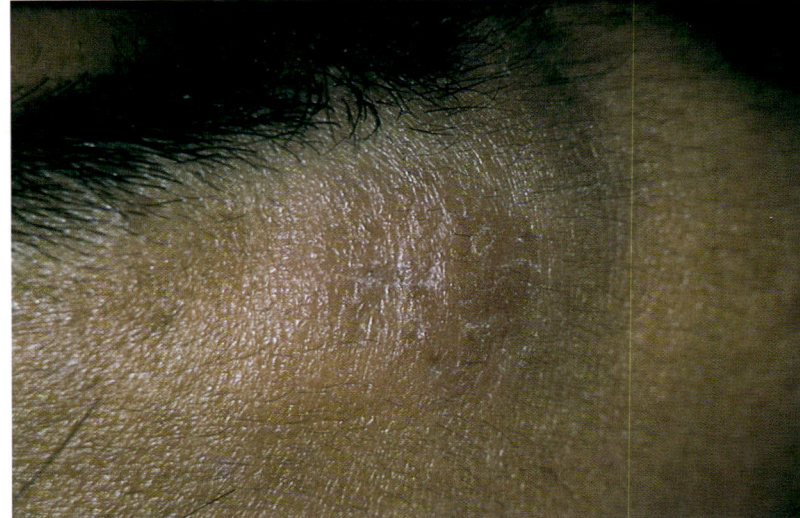

Fig. 11.50 *Alopecia mucinosa. Boggy, erythematous plaque with scaling and loss of hair.*

ALOPECIA MUCINOSA

Alopecia mucinosa or follicular mucinosis is an inflammatory disorder characterized clinically by grouped follicular papules and boggy, erythematous, nodular plaques with scaling and loss of hair (Fig. 11.50) and histologically by the accumulation of mucin (acid mucopolysaccharide) in the sebaceous glands and the outer root sheaths of affected hair follicles.[378] Primary alopecia mucinosa is benign and consists of two forms.[379] The acute form is localized to the head, neck, and shoulders with a few erythematous papules and plaques, prominent follicles, some scaling and shedding of hairs. Spontaneous recovery is usually observed within two years. In the other benign, but more chronic form, the inflammatory plaques with alopecia are more numerous and widespread, involving the trunk and limbs, and may persist for many years without evidence of an associated disorder. Secondary alopecia mucinosa may be associated with cutaneous lymphoma in 9% to 67% of the cases,[380] or rarely with other cutaneous diseases, such as angiolymphoid hyperplasia.[381] Most are T-cell lymphomas of the mycosis fungoides type.[382,383] Less commonly, cutaneous B-cell lymphoma,[380] Hodgkin's disease, or chronic lymphocytic leukemia are associated with follicular mucinosis.[379,383] The cases associated with lymphoma tend to occur more in older patients (above age 30) than the benign ones, although follicular mucinosis with underlying lymphomas have been reported in children.[383]

The temporal relationship between the lymphoma and the follicular mucinosis is variable. The clinical diagnosis is suggested by the presence of papules and plaques that have a soft, gelatinous consistency, the presence of mucin, which can sometimes be squeezed out of affected follicles, and the loss of hair in plaques with prominent follicles that may result in permanent alopecia. Seborrheic dermatitis, pityriasis rosea, tinea capitis, and leprosy may be closely simulated. Biopsy should confirm the diagnosis. The histopathologic picture is characterized by mucin deposition in the outer root sheath and

369. Glenn MJ, Bennett RG, Kelly AP (1995) Acne keloidalis nuchae: Treatment with excision and second-intention healing. **J Am Acad Dermatol** 33:243.
370. Kantor GR, Ratz JL, Wheeland RG (1986) Treatment of acne keloidalis nuchae with carbon dioxide laser. **J Am Acad Dermatol** 14:263.
371. Gay Prieto J (1955) Pseudopelade of Brocq: Its relationship to some forms of cicatricial alopecias and to lichen planus. **J Invest Dermatol** 24:323.
372. Silvers DN, Katz BE, Young AW (1993) Pseudopelade of Brocq is lichen planopilaris: Report of four cases that support this nosology. **Cutis** 51:99.
373. Braun-Falco O, Imai S, Schmoeckel C et al. (1986) Pseudopelade of Brocq. **Dermatologica** 172:18.
374. Bulengo-Ransby SM, Headington JT (1990) Pseudopelade of Brocq in a child. **J Am Acad Dermatol** 23:944.
375. Collier PM, James MP (1994) Pseudopelade of Brocq occurring in two brothers in childhood. **Clin Exp Dermatol** 19:61.
376. Sahl WJ (1996) Pseudopelade: An inherited alopecia. **Int J Dermatol** 35:715.
377. Ronchese F (1960) Pseudopelade. **Arch Dermatol** 82:336.
378. Pinkus H, Macaulay WL, Lund HZ et al. (1957) Alopecia mucinosa. **Arch Dermatol** 76:491.
379. Emmerson RW (1969) Follicular mucinosis: a study of 47 patients. **Br J Dermatol** 81:395.
380. Wolff HH, Kinney J, Ackerman AB (1978) Angiolymphoid hyperplasia with follicular mucinosis. **Arch Dermatol** 114:229.
381. Benchikhi H, Wechsler J, Rethers L et al. (1995) Cutaneous B-cell lymphoma associated with follicular mucinosis. **J Am Acad Dermatol** 33:673.
382. Binnick AN, Wax FD, Clendenning WE (1978) Alopecia mucinosa of the face associated with mycosis fungoides. **Arch Dermatol** 114:791.
383. Gibson LE, Muller SA, Leiferman KM et al. (1989) Follicular mucinosis: clinical and histopathologic study. **J Am Acad Dermatol** 20:441.

sebaceous glands. The keratinocytes of the outer root sheath may appear stellate-shaped and are splayed apart by the mucin. In more advanced lesions, the entire follicular epithelium may be altered with large mucin-filled intrafollicular cystic spaces.[342] Mucin can be demonstrated by the use of colloidal iron and Alcian Blue stains. Variably dense perivascular and perifollicular lymphocytic infiltrates with occasional eosinophils are present in most cases. The presence of large numbers of eosinophils in the inflammatory infiltrate and marked mucinous changes in the follicular epithelium favor a benign form, whereas the presence of a band-like, atypical lymphocytic infiltrate near the dermal-epidermal junction, with significant epidermotropism, favor a lymphoma associated with follicular mucinosis.[384]

Some patients spontaneously improve. Treatment with topical and intralesional steroids, low-dose systemic steroids, superficial radiotherapy,[385] dapsone,[386] interferons,[387] photochemotherapy (PUVA), and retinoids have been reported to be beneficial. Close follow-up of all patients is essential.

LICHEN PLANOPILARIS

Lichen planopilaris, also known as follicular lichen planus, represents lichen planus localized to the follicles. It includes the triad of typical lichen planus, spinous or acuminate follicular papules, and scarring alopecia of the scalp.[388] It is more common in women.

The alopecia of lichen planopilaris is insidious with progressive involvement over several months to years. Patients may be asymptomatic, but mild itching is often present. Early lesions consist of spinous, hyperkeratotic follicular papules with erythema and scaling of the affected scalp. The hair follicles are subsequently destroyed yielding atrophic, irregular, angular-shaped patches of alopecia with similar follicular papules at the periphery (Fig. 11.51). Typical lesions of lichen planus are not usually seen on the scalp. The pattern of scalp hair loss is variable. Most commonly, there are asymmetrical, scattered foci of partial hair loss that may coalesce into larger areas. Occasionally, diffuse hair loss involving the entire scalp may be seen.[389] The end stage may resemble pseudopelade.

Lichenoid interface alteration of the epidermis and follicular epithelium is characteristic of lichen planopilaris.[342] There is disruption of the epithelial-adventitial dermal junction with prominent dyskeratosis and necrotic, basal keratinocytes. A linear lymphocytic infiltrate abuts the follicular infundibular epithelium. Later lesions are characterized by a band-like fibrotic thickening of the papillary dermis accompanied by fibrotic tracts at sites of destroyed follicles.[389] End-stage changes are identical to end-stage pseudopelade and end-stage discoid lupus erythematosus.[342] Direct immunofluoresence shows globular IgM and IgA deposits on cytoid bodies at the dermal-epidermal junction, papillary dermis, along the infundibulum, and isthmus.[390] In addition, patchy deposits of fibrinogen are commonly seen around the hair follicles. It is important to biopsy an early lesion in order to obtain the diagnostic changes.

Treatment consists of high-potency topical steroids, intralesional and/or oral corticosteroids for at least three months, with gradual taper.[390] These agents seem to influence the progression of the alopecia and to provide symptomatic relief, but the effects are temporary and relapse usually occurs within one year after the medication is stopped.

DISCOID LUPUS ERYTHEMATOSUS (DLE)

DLE is a common form of chronic cutaneous lupus erythematosus and is typically found in young to middle-aged adults (mean age 38 years) with a 2:1 female predominance.[391] Lesions are most commonly found on the scalp, face and ears. Between one-third and one-half of the patients with DLE have scalp involvement,[391,392] and have a more chronic course compared to those without scalp involvement. Although chronic discoid lesions may be found in patients with SLE, the majority of patients with DLE do not have systemic disease. Overall, between 6% and 12% of patients with DLE may progress to SLE with time.[391,393]

Lesions consist of scaling, patchy erythema, telangiectases, follicular plugging and central hypopigmentation with peripheral hyperpigmentation within areas of scarring alopecia (Fig. 11.52). Old, burnt-out disease confined to the scalp may be impossible clinically to differentiate from pseudopelade or lichen planopilaris.[213]

Antinuclear antibody (ANA) titers are usually negative in DLE. One study showed positive ANA titers in 22% of cases and this was more common in

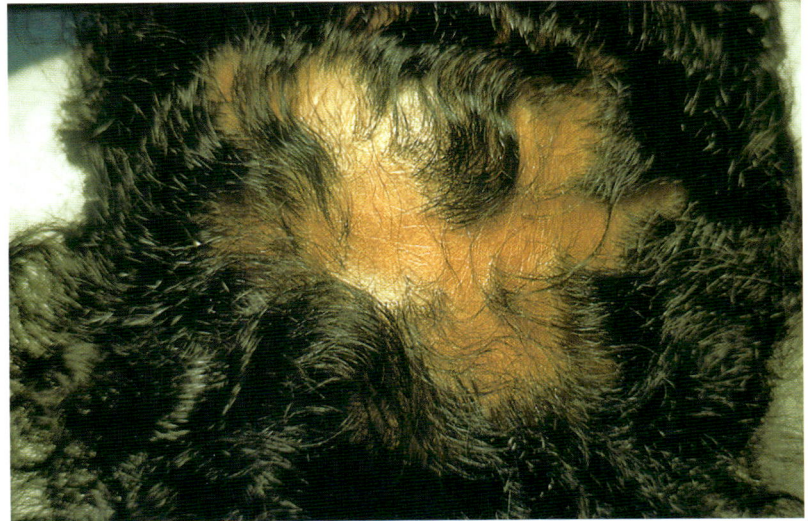

Fig. 11.51 Lichen planopilaris. Irregular patches of scarring alopecia.

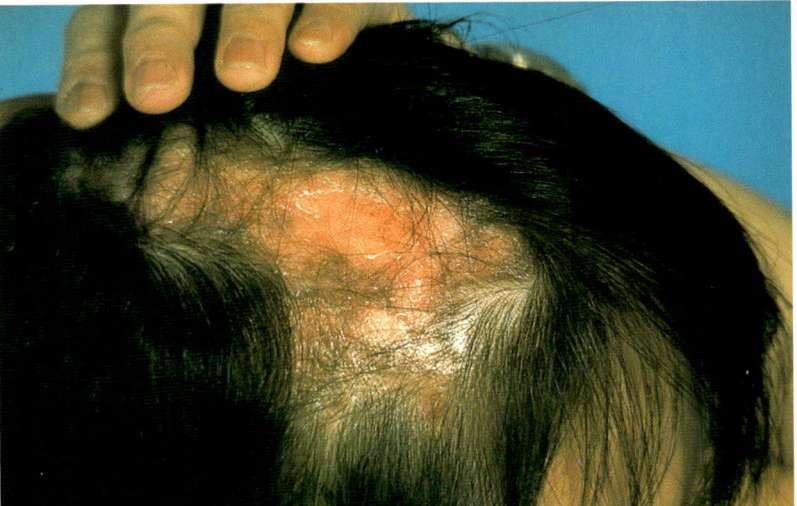

Fig. 11.52 Discoid lupus erythematosus with scaling, erythema and scarring.

384. Logan RA, Headington JT (1988) Follicular mucinosis: a histologic review of 80 cases (abstr). **J Cutan Pathol** 15:324.

385. Coskey RJ, Mehregan AH (1970) Alopecia mucinosa: a follow-up study. **Arch Dermatol** 102:193.

386. Kubba RK, Stewart TW (1974) Follicular mucinosis responding to dapsone. **Br J Dermatol** 91:217.

387. Meissner K, Weyer U, Kowalzick L et al. (1991) Successful treatment of primary progressive follicular mucinosis with interferons. **J Am Acad Dermatol** 24:848.

388. Silver H, Chargin L, Sachs PM (1953) Follicular lichen planus (lichen planopilaris). **Arch Dermatol Syphilol** 67:346.

389. Annessi G, Lombardo G, Gobello T et al. (1999) A clinicopathologic study of scarring alopecia due to lichen planus. **Am J Dermatopathol** 21:324.

390. Mehregan DA, Van Hale HM, Muller SA (1992) Lichen planopilaris: Clinical and pathologic study of forty-five patients. **J Am Acad Dermatol** 27:935.

391. Callen JP (1982) Chronic cutaneous lupus erythematosus. Clinical, laboratory, therapeutic and prognostic examination of 62 patients. **Arch Dermatol** 118:412.

392. Wilson CL, Burge SM, Dean D et al. (1992) Scarring alopecia in discoid lupus erythematosus. **Br J Dermatol** 126:307.

393. Yell JA, Mbuagbaw J, Burge SM (1996) Cutaneous manifestations of systemic lupus erythematosus. **Br J Dermatol** 135:355.

patients with widespread DLE lesions.[391] Histology shows vacuolar interface alteration of the epidermis and follicular epithelium in DLE.[342] Dyskeratotic keratinocytes are occasionally seen and the epidermis ranges from atrophic to acanthotic (hypertrophic DLE). Laminated keratin fills the follicular ostia corresponding to the clinical follicular plugs. Moderate to dense lymphocytic and plasma cell infiltrate occurs in both perivascular and periadnexal locations, and this is most prominent at the level of the follicular infundibulum.

Increased dermal mucin is often present and is helpful in differentiating DLE from lichen planopilaris. Reticular dermal sclerosis is present in advanced disease. Granular deposits of IgG and C3, occasionally IgM or IgA, occurs at the dermoepidermal junction or the junction of the follicular epithelium and dermis.[394]

Treatment consists of topical, intralesional, and systemic corticosteroids. Hydroxychloroquine 200–400mg/day for at least six weeks is effective both in the control of the disease and in the prevention of new lesions.[391]

MORPHEA

Morphea, also termed localized scleroderma, is a disorder of unknown etiology, primarily seen in children and young adults. It is more common in females and is characterized by discrete, circumscribed, nontender sclerotic patches with an ivory-colored center and a violaceous inflammatory border. Lesions may also be guttate, shiny, smooth, hypopigmented or hyper-pigmented, and with time the affected area becomes hairless and anhidrotic.[395] A history of trauma sometimes precedes the onset of morphea.

En coup de sabre (sabre cut) is a form of linear morphea that appears on the face and frontoparietal scalp. In this variant, a linear depressed groove, often with an associated zone of alopecia, occurs on the forehead and fronto-parietal area and may extend downward into the cheek, nose, and upper lip (Fig. 11.53). When the sclerosis is extensive with hypoplasia of facial bones and associated central nervous system abnormalities, such as seizures, hemiparesis and headaches, the condition has been termed Parry Romberg syndrome.[395] Occasionally, bilateral lesions of *en coup de sabre* affecting the frontoparietal area may occur.[396]

On histology, there is epidermal thinning with loss of rete pegs, increased thickness and density of collagen, and adnexal atrophy with an infiltrate of lymphocytes and macrophages around blood vessels and skin appendages.[395]

The management of morphea includes the use of different drugs such as corticosteroids, antibiotics, antimalarials, D-penicillamine, methotrexate, etretinate, gamma-interferon, vitamin E, colchicine, phenytoin, topical cal-cipotriene and oral calcitriol.[397–399] However, no treatment is well established, as evaluation of drug efficacy is difficult and spontaneous remission cannot be excluded. Recently, UVA light has been shown to cause improvement of localized scleroderma.[400]

TINEA CAPITIS

(Please refer to Chapter 26 for complete discussion.)

HIRSUTISM

The perception of hirsutism in women is subjective and there is a wide variation in severity. Both the severity of the hirsutism and the degree of acceptance are dependent on racial, cultural and social factors. In general, hair on the face, chest, or upper back is a good discriminating factor between hirsute women and controls.[397] The incidence of hirsutism in any popula-tion is difficult to assess, since the range of normal is wide. Latin, Jewish and

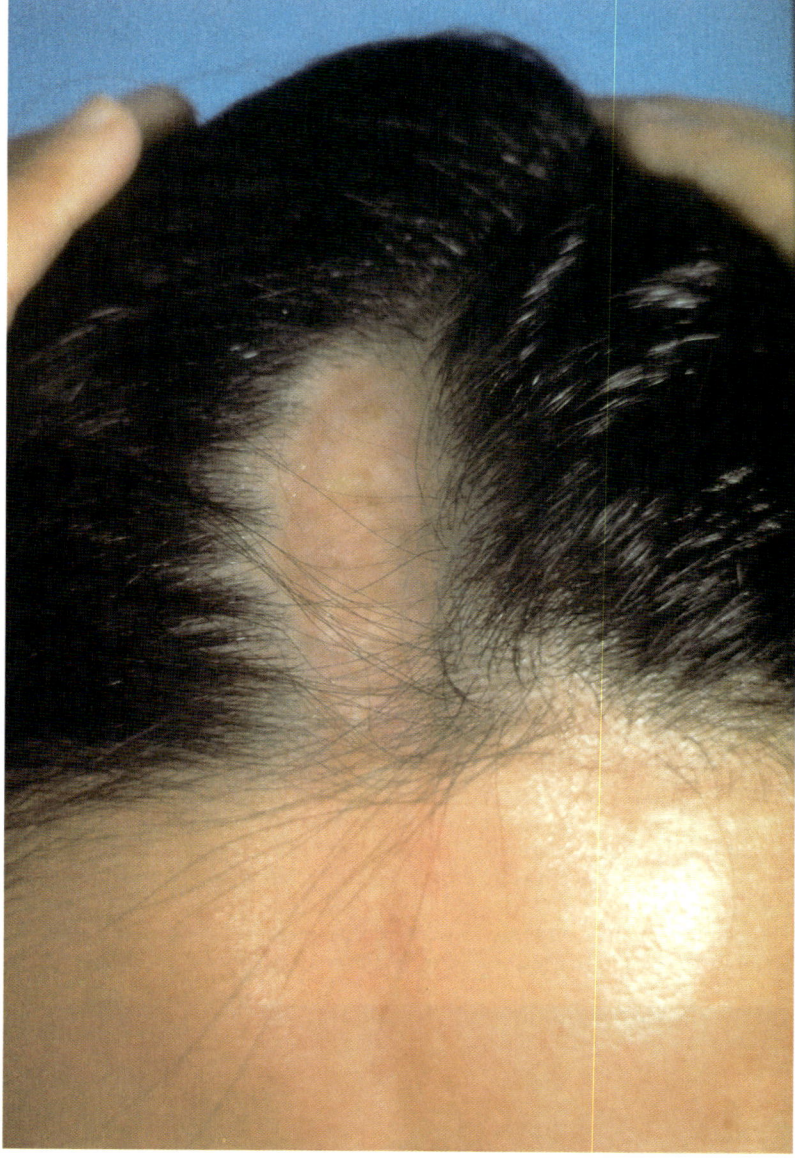

Fig. 11.53 A linear area of morphea with alopecia on the frontal scalp (*en coup de sabre*) extending to the forehead.

Welsh women in general have more hair than their counterparts of northern European and Oriental heritage. There is an increased incidence of hirsu-tism in the female relatives of hirsute woman compared with control populations.[398]

The term idiopathic hirsutism is used to describe the presence in females of excessive body hair in whom no overt underlying endocrine or metabolic disorder can be detected. The pathogenesis of idiopathic hirsutism is assumed to be an increased stimulation of the hair follicles of genetically predisposed females by normal levels of androgenic hormones.

A detailed history and physical examination will help to decide whether a full endocrinologic investigation is indicated. When hirsutism is observed in a

394. Jordan RE (1980) Subtle clues to diagnosis by immunopathology: scarring alopecia. **Am J Dermatopathol** 2:157.
395. Krafchik BR (1992) Localized cutaneous scleroderma. **Semin Dermatol** 11:65.
396. Itin PH, Schiller P (1999) Double-lined frontoparietal scleroderma en coup de sabre. **Dermatology** 199:185.

397. Lunde O, Grottum P (1984) Body hair growth in women; normal or hirsute. **Am J Phys Anthropol** 64:307.
398. Lorenzo EM (1970) Familial study of hirsutism. **J Clin Endocrinol Metab** 31:556.
399. Olsen EA (1999) Methods of hair removal. **J Am Acad Dermatol** 40:143.
400. Richards RN, Uy M, Meharg G (1990) Temporary hair removal in patients with hirsutism: a clinical study. **Cutis** 45:199.

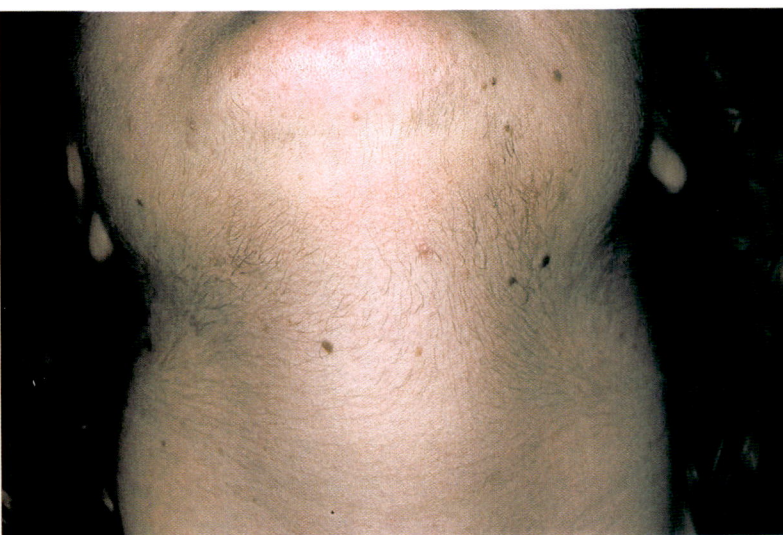

Fig. 11.54 Hirsutism in a woman with polycystic ovary syndrome.

postpubertal female without other signs of virilism (receding hairline, deepening of the voice, menstrual disturbance, increased muscle bulk, clitoromegaly), there is little likelihood of endocrine disease or ovarian tumors. When the disorder does not appear to be physiologic in nature, abnormalities of the pituitary, adrenals, and ovaries must be ruled out. These include polycystic ovary syndrome (Fig. 11.54), congenital adrenal hyperplasia, Cushing's syndrome, hyperprolactinemia, ovarian tumors, and adrenal tumors. These patients should be referred to an endrocrinologist for assessment. Laboratory testing for excessive androgen production should include free plasma testosterone, dehydroepiandrosterone sulfate, and cortisol levels. Other tests that may be useful are urinary 17 ketosteroids, luteinizing hormone and follicle-stimulating hormone ratios, prolactin levels, and pelvic ultrasound to rule out ovarian cysts.

There are several ways in which excessive hair may be removed. These include shaving, epilation, chemical depilatories, electrolysis, and laser hair removal.[399] Shaving with a razor or electric shaver, although occasionally not psychologically acceptable to the patient, is a simple and reasonable method to use and least likely to irritate the skin. Side effects include pseudofolliculitis, irritation, and the need for frequent treatment. Epilation includes plucking, threading, and waxing. Plucking can be done with the use of electronic tweezers or manually. Threading involves using a twisted loop of thread pulled across the skin that catches hairs and either pulls them out or breaks them off.[400] Waxing is performed by the application of a warm wax preparation admixed with resins onto the skin and than stripping off the cooled, stiff wax along with embedded hairs. Waxing is painful and is often complicated by folliculitis. Side effects of plucking include postinflammatory hyperpigmentation, folliculitis, pseudofolliculitis, and even scarring.[400] Chemical depilatories are simple, painless, and can give results that last up to two weeks. The most widely used varieties are substituted mercaptans, 2% to 10% thioglycolates, mixed with 2% to 6% of either NaOH or CaOH.[401] The thioglycolates disrupt disulfide bonds, especially those involving cystine which is found in greater quantities in hair. The alkali is added to increase the pH, and hence the efficacy of the thioglycolate. The depilatory is spread on the area for three to 15 minutes with the resultant dissolution of the hairs into a jellylike mass which is then washed off with soap and water. The main side effect of depilatories is irritant dermatitis (1–5%). Allergic contact dermatitis is rare and may be due either to the thioglycolate or to the fragrance. The above methods of hair removal are acknowledged to be temporary.

Electrolysis is a permanent method of hair removal. A fine electrical wire is introduced down the hair shaft to the papilla which is destroyed by an electrical current. It is a tedious process requiring many treatment sessions over a prolonged period to achieve marked diminution of terminal hair.[402] Erythema and edema are common after treatment, but are temporary. Other side effects of electrolysis include pain, scarring, and postinflammatory dyspigmentation.

Laser hair removal is now widely promoted. None of the presently utilized lasers has been proven to permanently destroy hair. The selective targets identified for hair are either melanin or an exogenous substance topically applied and absorbed down the follicle.[399] Lasers used for hair removal include the ruby laser (694nm),[403] the alexandrite laser (755nm),[404] and the diode laser (800nm), all of which target melanin. Many treatments are required to achieve a lasting reduction in treated hairs. Immediate side effects include edema and erythema, which generally last for a few hours. Postinflammatory hyperpigmentation and hypopigmentation generally clear in months after treatment and usually no scarring occurs. Patients with blond hair do not respond as well as those with dark hair. The Neodymium:Yag laser (1064nm) utilizes a topical preparation of a carbon-based material in mineral oil massaged into the skin.[405] When the carbon particles absorb infrared light, focal photomechanical damage is caused by the short nanosecond pulse. All skin types can be treated, as opposed to lasers that target melanin. Edema and erythema may be present for 24 to 48 hours after treatment and petechiae for up to 5 days. Hormonal therapy of hirsutism is discussed in Chapter 22.

401. Natow AJ (1986) Chemical removal of hair. **Cutis** 38:91.
402. Richards RN, McKenzie MA, Meharg GE (1986) Electroepilation (electrolysis) in hirsutism. **J Am Acad Dermatol** 15:693.
403. Grossman MC, Dierickx C, Farinelli W et al. (1996) Damage to hair follicles by normal-mode ruby laser pulses. **J Am Acad Dermatol** 35:889.
404. Finkel B, Eliezri YD, Waldman A et al. (1997) Pulsed alexandrite laser technology for noninvasive hair removal. **J Clin Laser Med Surg** 15:225.
405. Goldberg DJ (1997) Topical suspension-assisted Q-switched Nd:YAG laser hair removal. **Dermatol Surg** 23:741.

Nail and Appendageal Abnormalities

Robert Silverman and Robert Baran

Epidermal appendages include hair and nails, eccrine, apocrine, and sebaceous glands. These specialized structures form as down-growths of primordial ectoderm in early embryologic development and consist of organized differentiated cell populations with specific functions that together are responsible for many of the diverse properties of human skin. Diseases of the nail unit, and selected disorders of the eccrine and apocrine glands will be discussed. Conditions involving the sebaceous gland, ectodermal dysplasias and appendageal tumors will be addressed elsewhere in this text.

Disorders of epidermal appendages may be global, affecting more than one appendage, as with ectodermal dysplasias, or isolated, affecting only one appendageal type, as in familial leukonychia. Defects may be localized (nevus sebaceous), generalized (steatocystoma multiplex), congenital, or acquired. Such defects may affect the structure or function of an appendage.

The overall prevalence of nail, eccrine, apocrine, and sebaceous gland disorders (except acne) in a general pediatric practice is probably quite small. From 3 to 11% of children in established pediatric dermatology practices were noted to have diseases of the nails or other epidermal appendages.[1,2] Some diseases addressed in this chapter occur almost exclusively in children (e.g., parakeratosis pustulosa); others that occur infrequently are presented so that the reader may become familiar with features that may have prognostic importance during adulthood (e.g., nail-patella syndrome). Infrequently, abnormalities in epidermal appendages may be clues that lead to the diagnosis of a serious underlying illness. For example, capillary loop microscopy of the proximal nail fold may demonstrate changes suggestive of a connective tissue disease (Fig. 12.1).[3,4]

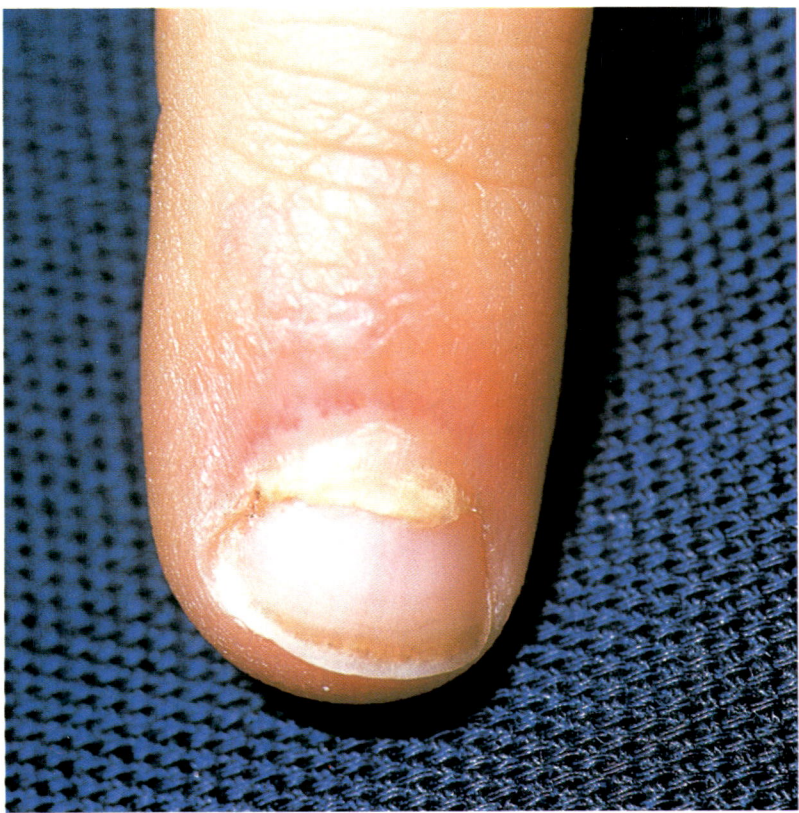

Fig. 12.1 Nail fold capillary loop dilation and cuticular hypertrophy are manifestations of the systemic illness, dermatomyositis.

THE NAIL

Nails are unique to primates that exhibit a high degree of manual dexterity. These hard plate-like structures exert counter-pressure over the digital pulp and make fine-motor grasping more efficient. Nails are used for scratching, and as such, may be defensive weapons or a source of pleasurable sensation.[5] Nails are also the focus of personal satisfaction and social acceptability, especially in young adolescents whose developmental focus is on his or her body image.[6] In Western society, early exposure of children to nail-grooming practices is occurring more frequently. The adornment of children's nails with cosmetics may lead to future sensitization and serve as a source of nail deformity.[7]

NAIL ANATOMY

The nail apparatus consists of a translucent rectangular nail plate with a laterally convex contour (Fig. 12.2).[8] The plate is approximately 0.5mm thick and extends from under the proximal nail fold, which covers about one-quarter of its total length. During infancy, oblique ridges may converge distally to give the plates a "herring bone" appearance.[9] This has also been called "Chevron

1. Schachner L, Ling NS, Press S (1983) A statistical analysis of a pediatric dermatology clinic. **Pediatr Dermatol** 1:157.
2. Iglesias A, Tamayo L, Sosa-de-Martínez C et al. (2001) Prevalence and nature of nail alterations in pediatric patients. **Pediatr Dermatol** 18:107–109.
3. Terreri MT, Andrade Le, Puccinelli ML et al. (1999) Nail fold capillaroscopy: normal findings in children and adolescents. **Sem Arthr rheum** 29:36–42.
4. Spencer-Green G, Schlesinger M, Bove K et al. (1983) Nailfold capillary abnormalities in childhood rheumatic diseases. **J Pediatr** 102:341.
5. Zaias N (1990) The Nail in Health and Disease, 2nd ed. New York: Spectrum.
6. Fotiu E (1982) Modern formulations of coloring agents: face, lips and nails. In: Principles of Cosmetics for the Dermatologist, Frost P, Horwitz SN, eds. St. Louis: CV Mosby, p. 147.
7. Barnett JM, Scher RK (1992) Nail cosmetics. **Int J Dermatol** 31:675.
8. Lewin K (1965) The normal fingernail. **Br J Dermatol** 77:421.
9. Parry EJ, Morley Wn, Dawber RPR (1995) Herringbone nails: an uncommon variant of nail growth in childhood? **Br J Dermatol** 132:1021–1022.

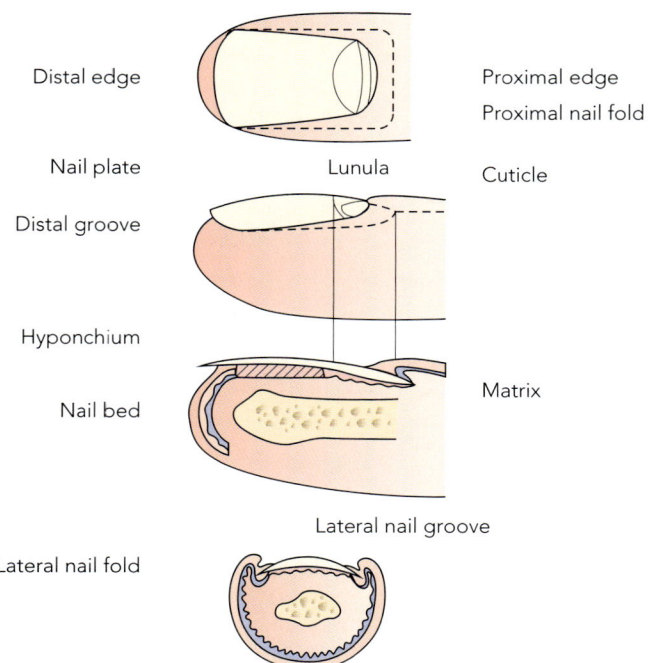

Distal edge

Proximal edge
Proximal nail fold

Nail plate — Lunula

Cuticle

Distal groove

Hyponychium

Nail bed

Matrix

Lateral nail groove

Lateral nail fold

Fig. 12.2 External and cross-sectional anatomy of the nail. (Baran R, Dawber RPR (1984) Disease of the Nail and Their Management. Oxford: Blackwell Scientific.)

nails."[10,11] The cuticle, an acellular extension of the proximal nail fold, is tightly adherent to the dorsal surface of the nail plate and prevents any potentially harmful organisms or chemicals from reaching the underlying matrix. The integrity of the cuticle is particularly important because the matrix in children seems to be very sensitive to any disruptive insult, which may result in permanent deformity. Cuticular hemorrhages occur commonly with trauma. They may also be prominent in patients with collagen vascular disease.[12]

The nail matrix consists of several layers of proliferating epidermal cells. Melanocytes, which may produce melanin pigment and Langerhans cells (antigen-presenting cells of the immune system), are also present.[13,14] The distal portion of the matrix may extend beyond the proximal nail fold. It appears as a pale white crescent under the nail plate called the lunula. Its convex shape parallels the configuration of the distal nail edge. The normal white appearance of the lunula is probably due to the scattering of light from nuclei of the matrix cells.[15] Germinative cells of the lunula give rise to the ventral undersurface of the nail plate, while the proximal matrix (which extends 2–3mm in from the proximal nail fold) forms the exposed or dorsal surface of the nail plate.[16] The nail bed may contribute 20% or more to nail thickness between the lunula and the distal free edge, especially in disease states.[17] However, a sensitive quantitative method of nail production from different regions of the matrix has led to continued controversy about the proliferative potential of the nail bed.[18]

The nail plate is firmly attached to, but grows over, the nail bed, which has a rich supply of nerves, blood, and lymphatic vessels. Numerous glomus bodies (arteriovenous anastomoses), which serve to regulate blood flow, are also present throughout the bed. Sweat glands are absent in this area. The nail bed has regular, closely spaced longitudinal grooves that intercalate with the ventral nail plate. This rugated configuration is responsible for the firm attachment of the plate to the bed and for splinter-shaped hemorrhages when isolated capillary disruption occurs in the nail bed.[19]

Close examination of the distal nail bed reveals a thin red-and-white onychodermal band.[20] This structure is demonstrated most clearly on the third to fifth fingers and is more prominent in young children than in adults. The onychodermal band is thought to be the site of attachment of the fingertip stratum corneum and the nail plate. Its appearance may be exaggerated in acrocyanosis, systemic diseases, Kawasaki disease, or exposure to cytotoxic agents.[21–23]

The lateral borders of the nail plate rest freely in grooves formed from overlying lateral nail folds. Entrapment of foreign material within the grooves may lead to infection or paronychia, while trauma or close clipping may lead to an ingrown nail plate.

The distal border of the nail plate becomes detached from the nail bed at the hyponychium, which then takes on the appearance of normal epidermis beyond its distal groove. This groove may be obliterated by accumulation of subungual debris or by scarring.

NAIL GROWTH

Complete formation of the nail apparatus has occurred by the end of the second trimester of fetal development. A rough estimate of gestational age or a newborn's overall nitrogen balance can be obtained by examining the nails.[24,25] Frequently in premature infants, at less than 32 weeks' gestation, the nail plates will not have grown beyond the distal groove of the hyponychium. Since fetal growth and maturation progress in a cephalocaudal direction, shortened nails are most commonly noted on the toes and may be occasionally observed on term neonates. The nails of post-mature infants are usually long and extend well beyond the hyponychium. This is also true of macrosomic infants of diabetic mothers and other neonates that are large for gestational age.

In adolescents and young adults, nails grow at a rate of about 0.1mm/day.[26,27] Accurate measurements of nail growth in large groups of younger children have not been recorded. It is the author's opinion that nail growth is slow during the first one to three months of life, and then accelerates during infancy and early childhood. Growth rate is determined by the pool of matrix cells actively undergoing cell division, while the size or thickness of the nail plate is determined by other factors, such as the volume of cells present, abnormalities in keratinization, or hypertrophy of the nail bed. Total regeneration of an avulsed fingernail may take four to six months, while toenails can take up to one year to regrow.[28]

Numerous physiologic and pathologic factors may affect nail growth (Table 12.1).[29] Case reports of increased nail growth with dietary supplements of gelatin, dopa (dihydroxyphenylalanine), calcium, and vitamin D have

10. Shuster S (1996) The significance of chevron nails. **Br J Dermatol** 135:144–161.
11. Zaiac MN, Glick BP, Zaias N (1998) Chevron nail. **J Am Acad Dermatol** 38:773.
12. Tosti A (1991) The nail apparatus in collagen disorders. **Semin Dermatol** 10:71.
13. Higashi N (1968) Melanocytes of the nail matrix and nail pigmentation. **Arch Dermatol** 97:570.
14. Hashimoto K (1971) Ultrastructure of the human toenail. I. Proximal nail matrix. **J Invest Dermatol** 56:235.
15. Runne U, Orfanos CE (1981) The human nail. Structure, growth and pathological changes. In: Current Problems in Dermatology, vol 9. Mali JWH, ed. Basel: S Karger, p. 102.
16. Norton LA (1971) Incorporation of thymidine-methyl-H3 and glycine-2-H3 in the nail matrix and bed of humans. **J Invest Dermatol** 56:61.
17. Johnson M, Comaish JS, Shuster S (1991) The nail is produced by the normal nail bed: a controversy resolved. **Br J Dermatol** 125:27.
18. De Berker D, MaWhinney B, Sviland L (1996) Quantification of regional matrix nail production. **Br J Dermatol** 134:1083–1086.
19. Baran R, Dawber RPR (1994) Diseases of the Nails and Their Management, 2nd ed. Oxford: Blackwell Scientific, p. 183.
20. Sonnex TS, Griffith WAD, Nicol WJ (1991) "Onychocorneal band". The nature and significance of the transverse white band of human nails. **Semin Dermatol** 10:12–16.

21. Baran R, Dawber RPR (1994) Diseases of the Nails and Their Management, 2nd ed. Oxford: Blackwell Scientific, pp. 659–660.
22. Lindsley CB (1992) Nail-bed lines in Kawasaki disease. **Am J Dis Child** 146:659.
23. Kowal-Vern A, Eng A (1993) Unusual erythema of the proximal nail fold and onychodermal band. **Cutis** 52:43.
24. Parkin JM, Hey EN, Clowes JS (1976) Rapid assessment of gestational age at birth. **Arch Dis Child** 51:259.
25. Brans YW, Shannon DL (1981) Fingernail nitrogen content in infants of diabetic mothers and macrosomic neonates. **Biol Neonate** 40:237.
26. Hamilton JB, Terada H, Mestler GE (1995) Studies of growth throughout the lifespan of Japanese: growth and size of nails and their relationship to age, sex, heredity and other factors. **J Gerontol** 10:401.
27. Bean WB (1974) Nail growth: 30 years of observation. **Arch Intern Med** 134:497.
28. Runne U, Orfanos CE (1981) The human nail. Structure, growth and pathological changes. In: Current Problems in Dermatology, vol. 9. Mali JWH, ed. Basel: S Karger, p. 107.
29. Orentreich N, Markofsky J, Vogelman JH (1979) The effect of aging on the rate of linear nail growth. **J Invest Dermatol** 73:126.

TABLE 12.1 Factors that alter normal nail growth rate

Slower	Faster
Pysiologic	
Females	Males
Toes	Fingers
First and fifth digits	Third digit
Non-dominant hand	Dominant hand
Winter	Summer
Night	Day
Pathologic	
Severe infections	Psoriasis
Prolonged illness	Erythroderma
Anti-metabolites	Hyperthyroidism
Nerve injury	Pregnancy
Ischemia	AV shunts
Hypothyroidism	Biting
Malnutrition	Typing
Congestive heart failure	Piano playing

appeared in the literature.[30–32] Their usefulness is doubtful, and confirmation of these observations by controlled studies is needed.

Controversy surrounds the formation of the flattened contour and direction of growth of the nail plate. Several investigators believe that the forces that direct nail formation are produced by the restrictive nature of the nail folds. This is supported by transplantation experiments, vertical growth after traumatic matrix disruption, and misdirected growth of ectopic nails.[33–35] However, in one case of congenital absence of the proximal nail folds, nails maintained their normal contour and grew outward.[36] In addition, electron microscopic studies suggest that fetal matrix cells flatten and move in a "centridistal" direction.[37] Dawber and Baran suggested that orientation of the mesenchyme underlying the fetal nail apparatus and interaction between the mesenchyme and epithelium during fetal development probably play a pivotal role in the direction of nail formation.[38] Data supporting this theory are currently being accumulated.[39]

NAIL COMPOSITION

The nail plate is composed of lamellar sheets of tightly adherent, dead corneocytes containing large amounts of protein (78%), smaller amounts of water (18%), and very little lipid (less than 5%).[40] Lamellar dystrophy is a common finding in children. It may result from further reductions in ungual lipid content from prolonged bathing or thumb sucking. The minute amounts of DNA in fingernails can now be amplified for genetic analysis and has become a standard forensic identification technique.[41] Nail rigidity, or hardness, is primarily due to its structural proteins, α–helical keratin, and a cysteine–rich amorphous matrix protein in which the keratin is embedded. The nail unit is composed of numerous distinct types of keratin, some of which are unique to the nail and others of which are constituents of other components of the skin and other organs.[42] The transverse fibril orientation of the former (i.e., arrangement of keratin fibrils at right angles to the direction of nail growth) and the covalent disulfide bonds in the latter combine to give the nail its hard character.[43] The keratin and matrix proteins are confined within the corneocyte plasma membranes, which themselves are supported by a prominent cytoskeleton, the marginal band.[38,44] This envelope is thicker in nails than in other cutaneous structures and is composed of ε-(γ-glutamyl) lysine cross-linked bonds that are also extremely strong.[45] Nail flexibility is related to water content.[46] Soaking nails in water causes the plates to swell and allows for easier trimming.

The mineral content of nails has been thoroughly investigated. Zinc, copper, iron, and magnesium are all present in small quantities.[47] However, calcium and these other metals play little, if any, role in determining nail hardness.[48] Arsenic and lead have been found in nails, and levels of these components in nail clippings have been used as a rough guide of environmental exposure.[49,50] Finally, the element content of nails has been reported to be altered in certain disease states (Table 12.2).[51–54] Techniques for measurement of these elements in nail clippings are generally not available for routine testing.[55]

Measurement of more complex substances in nail clippings has been reported to be useful. For instance, identification of cocaine in nail clippings of newborns by gas chromatography mass spectroscopy can substantiate exposure to the drug during embryogenesis.[56] Also, steroid sulphatase and its substrate, cholesterol sulphate, have been assayed in the nails of patients with X-linked ichthyosis and have been found to be abnormal.[57,58]

TABLE 12.2 Trace elements in nail clippings from patients with systemic diseases

Disease	Element	Level
Cystic fibrosis	Na, Cu	Increased[51]
Wilson's disease	Cu	Increased[52]
Iron-deficiency anemia	Fe	Decreased[53]
Acrodermatitis enteropathica	Zn	Decreased[54]

30. Jank M (1968) Gelatinebehandlung bei onychomykosen. **Wein Med Wochenschr** 118:154.
31. Miller E (1973) Levodopa and nail growth. **N Engl J Med** 788:916.
32. Hogan DB, McNair S, Young J, Crilly RG (1984) Nail growth: calcium and vitamin D. **Ann Intern Med** 101:283.
33. Kligman AM (1961) Why do nails grow out instead of up. **Arch Dermatol** 84:181.
34. Runne U (1980) Nagelveranderungen durch gewohnheits manipulationen, artefackte and trauman. **Hautarzt** 31:344.
35. Kikuchi I, Ogata K, Idemori M (1984) Vertically growing ectopic nail. Nature's experiments on nail growth direction. **J Am Acad Dermatol** 10:114.
36. Baran R (1981) Nail growth direction revisited. **J Am Acad Dermatol** 4:78.
37. Hashimoto K (1971) Ultrastructure of the human toenail: cell migration, keratinization, and formation of the intercellular cement. **Arch Derm Forsch** 240:1.
38. Baran R, Dawber RPR (2001) Diseases of the Nails and Their Management. Oxford: Blackwell Scientific, p. 28–29.
39. Sengel P (1983) Epidermal–dermal interactions during formation of skin and cutaneous appendages. In: Biochemistry and Physiology of the Skin, Goldsmith LA, ed. New York: Oxford University Press, p. 102.
40. Baden HP, Fewkes J (1983) The nail. In: Biochemistry and Physiology of the Skin, Goldsmith LA, ed. New York: Oxford University Press, p. 553.
41. Kaneshinge T, Takagi K, Nakamura S et al. (1992) Genetic analysis using fingernail DNA. **Nucleic Acid Res** 20:5489.
42. Berker DDE, Wojnarowska F, Sviland L et al. (2000) Keratin expression in the normal nail unit: markers of regional differentiation. **Br J Dermatol** 142:89–96.
43. Baden HP (1970) The physical properties of nail. **J Invest Dermatol** 55:115.
44. Forslind B (1970) Biophysical studies of the normal nail. **Acta Derm Venereol** (Stockh) 50:161.
45. Hashimoto K (1971) The marginal band. A demonstration of the thickened cellular envelope of the human nail cell with the aid of Lanthanum staining. **Arch Dermatol** 103:387.

46. Finley AY, Frost P, Keith AD et al. (1980) An assessment of factors influencing flexibility of human fingernails. **Br J Dermatol** 103:357.
47. Alexoiu D, Koutselinis A, Manolidis D et al. (1980) The content of trace elements (Cu, Zn, Fe, Mg) in fingernails of children. **Dermatologica** 160:380.
48. Forslind B, Wroblewski R, Afzelius FA (1976) Calcium and sulfur location in human nail. **J Invest Dermatol** 67:273.
49. Pounds CA, Pearson EF, Turner TD (1979) Arsenic in fingernails. **J Forensic Sci Soc** 19:65.
50. Wilhelm M, Hafner D, Lombeck I, Ohnesorge FK (1991) Monitoring of cadmium, copper, lead and zinc status in young children using toenails: comparison with scalp hair. **Sci Total Environ** 102:199.
51. Kopito L, Mahmoodian A, Townley RRW et al. (1965) Studies in cystic fibrosis. Analysis of nail clippings for sodium and potassium. **N Engl J Med** 272:504.
52. Martin GM (1964) Copper content of hair and nails of normal individuals and of patients with hepatolenticular degeneration. **Nature** (Lond) 202:903.
53. Jacobs A, Jenkins DJ (1960) The iron content of fingernails. **Br J Dermatol** 72:245.
54. Solomons NW (1979) On the assessment of zinc and copper nutrition in men. **Am J Clin Nutr** 32:856.
55. Sirota L, Straussberg R, Fishman P et al. (1988) Xray microanalysis of the fingernails in term and preterm infants. **Pediatr Dermatol** 5:184.
56. Skopp G, Potsch L (1997) A case report on drug screening of nail clippings to detect prenatal drug exposure. **Ther Drug Monit** 19:386–389.
57. Serizawa S, Nagai T, Ito M, Sato Y (1990) Cholesterol sulphate levels in the hair and nails of patients with recessive X-linked ichthyosis. **Clin Exp Dermatol** 15:13–15.
58. Matsumoto T, Sakura N, Ueda K (1990) Steroid sulphatase activity in nails: Screening for X-linked ichthyosis. **Pediatr Dermatol** 7:266–269.

The nail apparatus can be affected by a wide spectrum of acquired, congenital, or familial disorders. Congenital and hereditary nail disorders may be classified by defects in the nail matrix (i.e., size, position, or quality), nail field, nail bed, or ecto-mesodermal interactions.[59] Nails may be damaged by external agents, may be involved with localized or generalized cutaneous disease, or may reflect some underlying systemic abnormality. In each case, the different anatomic parts of the nail apparatus respond in a limited fashion. For instance, the nail folds can become inflamed or scarred; the nail plate can become thickened, thinned, brittle, discolored, or deformed; and the nail plate can separate from the nail bed or become discolored as well.

ALTERATIONS IN THE NAIL PLATE

Beau's lines

Beau's lines are uniform transverse grooves across the nail plate that move distally with nail growth (Fig. 12.3). These depressions are due to an arrest in nail plate formation by systemic illness or toxins. In 1846, Beau first reported these transverse grooves as retrospective indicators of illness,[60] and since that time numerous disease associations have been made (Table 12.3). The depressions may be narrow if the insult is brief, or they may be wide if growth arrest lasts several weeks. In addition, an abrupt leading edge to the groove may indicate an acute onset of disease, while a sloping trailing border may represent a gradual protracted resolution of the illness.[61] In theory, all nails are equally affected, but deformities are most frequently noted on the thumbnails or toenails due to their slower growth rate. In rare cases, patients

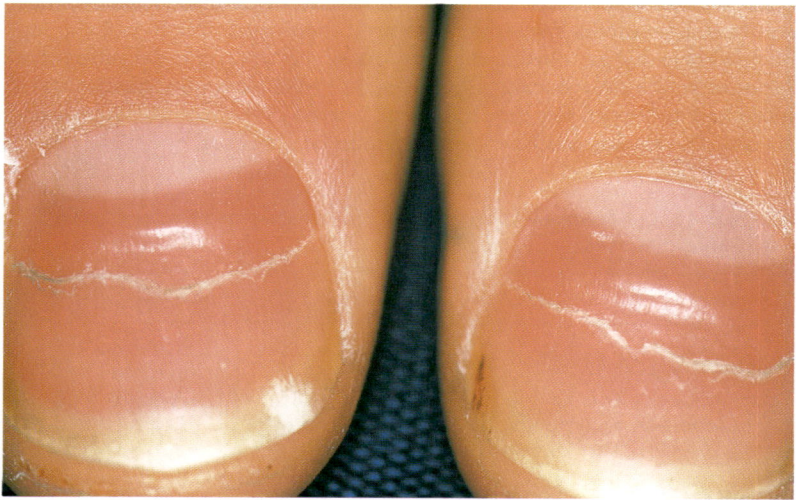

Fig. 12.3 Beau's lines. Uniform transverse grooves following severe illness.

TABLE 12.3 Causes of nail matrix arrest

Insult	Beau's lines	Onychomadesis
High fever (e.g., scarlet fever)	+	+
Local inflammation or trauma	+	+
Kawasaki's disease[67]	+	+
Stevens–Johnson[68] syndrome	+	+
Hand-foot-mouth disease[69] (Coxsackie virus)	+	+
Cytotoxic agents[70]	+	+
Antibiotics[71]	−	+
Retinoids[72]	−	+
Severe bullous eruptions[73,74]	−	+
Radiation therapy[75]	−	+
Acrodermatitis enteropathica[76]	+	+[a]
Hypoparathyroidism[77]	+	+
Amelogenesis imperfecta[78]	−	+
Syphilis[79]	+	+

[a] Schachner L: personal communication.

with Raynaud's phenomenon have Beau's lines localized to the affected digits.[62] Physiologic Beau's lines may be noted in four- to ten-week-old infants as a result of parturition.[63] They may be a reflection of the same process that causes telogen effluvium hair loss, which is commonly observed in newborns and their mothers. Very prominent transverse depressions in all 20 nails were reported in an infant soon after birth and were thought to have resulted from intrauterine distress.[64]

Onychomadesis

Onychomadesis is the complete separation and subsequent shedding of the nail plate, beginning at the proximal nail fold (Fig. 12.4).[65,66] Severe illnesses and many drug toxicities that cause Beau's lines have also been reported to produce onychomadesis (Table 12.3).[67–79] Severe intrauterine distress was theorized as a cause of onychomadesis in one infant.[80] Idiopathic familial onychomadesis has recently been reported.[81] In addition to systemic disease, local inflammatory eruptions of the proximal nail fold, such as eczema or paronychia, and trauma to the nail matrix, as in certain sports injuries, can also result in this deformity. Onychomadesis is a transient phenomenon and new nail plate should grow unless scarring of the nail apparatus occurs.

Washboard nails

Washboard nails may sometimes be confused with Beau's lines. This self-induced deformity of the thumbs is characterized by close, irregularly spaced transverse grooves and ridges that extend only part way across the breadth of

59. Telfer NR (1991) Congenital and hereditary nail disorders. **Semin Dermatol** 10:2.
60. Beau JHS (1846) Note sur certain caracteres des aemaeiologie raetrospectives praesentaes par les ongles. **Arch Gen Med** 11:447.
61. Petrakies NL, Churchill AG (1971) Fingernail furrows (Beau's lines) as a retrospective index of the severity of Asian flu in 1968–69. **Calif Med** 115:77.
62. Samman PD, Strickland B (1962) Abnormalities of the fingernails associated with impaired peripheral blood supply. **Br J Dermatol** 74:165.
63. Turano AF (1968) Transverse nail ridging in early infancy. **Pediatrics** 44:996.
64. Wolf D, Wolf R, Goldberg MD (1982) Beau's lines. A case report. **Cutis** 29:141.
65. Samman PD (1978) The Nails in Disease. London: Heinemann, p. 147.
66. Baran R, Dawber RPR (2001) Diseases of the Nails and Their Management. Oxford: Blackwell Scientific, p. 74–76.
67. Kawasaki T, Kosaki F, Okauwa S (1974) A new infantile acute febrile mucocutaneous lymph node syndrome prevailing in Japan. **Pediatrics** 54:271.
68. Hansen RC (1984) Blindness, anonychia and oral mucosal scarring as sequelae of the Stevens–Johnson syndrome. **Pediatr Dermatol** 1:298.
69. Clementz GC, Mancini AJ (2000) Nail matrix arrest following hand-foot-mouth disease: A report of five children. **Pediatr Dermatol** 17:7–11.
70. Dunagen WG (1982) Clinical toxicology of chemotherapeutic agents. Dermatologic toxicology. **Semin Oncol** 9:14.
71. Eastwood JB, Curtis JR, Smith EKM et al. (1969) Shedding nails apparently induced by the administration of large amounts of cephaloridine and cloxacillin in 2 anephric patients. **Br J Dermatol** 81:750.
72. Ferguson MM, Sampson NB, Hammersley N (1983) Severe dystrophy associated with retinoid therapy. **Lancet** 12:794.
73. Main RA (1973) Periodic shedding of the nails. **Br J Dermatol** 88:497.
74. Parameswara YR, Naik RPC (1981) Onychomadesis associated with pemphigus vulgaris. **Arch Dermatol** 117:759.
75. Adachi I, Haruyama K (1966) Effect of radiation on the nail tissue. **Bull Tokyo Med Dent Univ** 13:369.
76. Weismann K (1977) Beau's lines: possible markers of zinc deficiency. **Acta Derm Venereol (Stockh)** 59:88.
77. Baran R, Dawber RPR (1984) Diseases of the Nails and Their Management. Oxford: Blackwell Scientific, p. 224.
78. Schuppli R (1963) Uber eine mit Paradentose Kombinierte veranderung der Nagel. **Z Haut Gesch** 34:114.
79. Baran R, Dawber RPR (1984) Diseases of the Nails and Their Management. Oxford: Blackwell Scientific, p. 148.
80. Wolf D, Wolf R, Goldberg MD (1982) Beau's lines. A case report. **Cutis** 29:141.
81. Mehra A, Murphy RJ, Wilson BB (2001) Idiopathic familial onychomadesis. **J Am Acad Dermatol** 43:349–350.

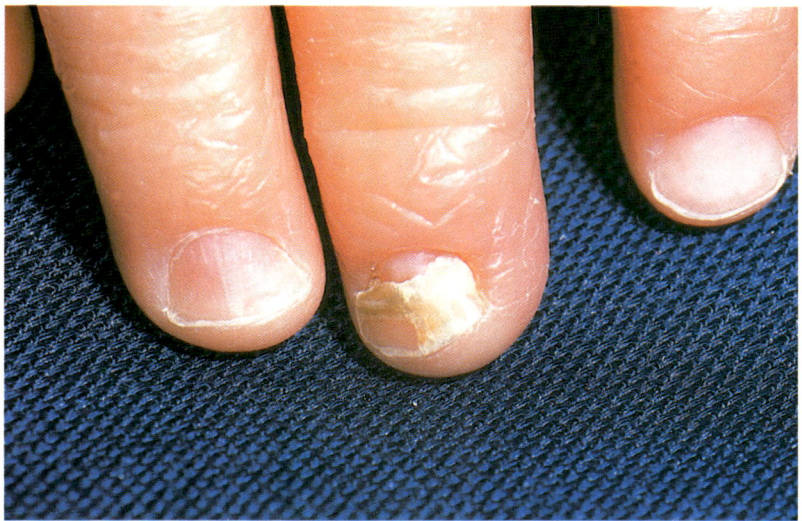

Fig. 12.4   Onychomadesis. Prominal separation of the nail plate from the nail bed.

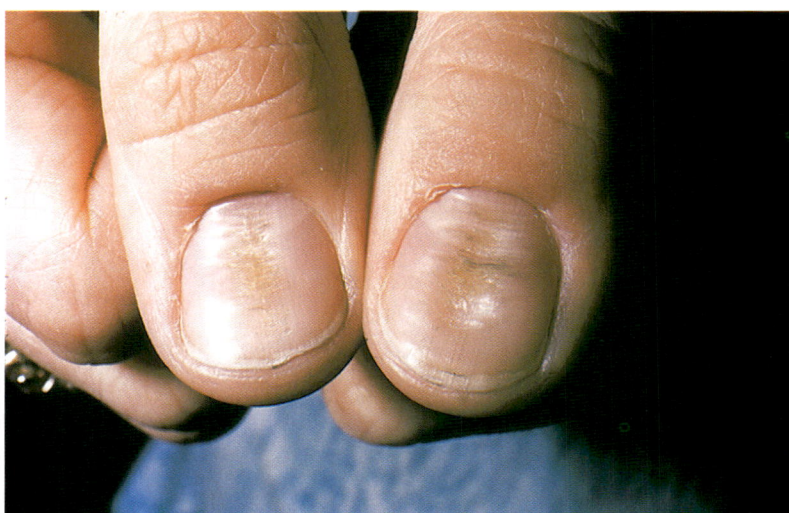

Fig. 12.5   Incomplete transverse grooves and ridges characterize washboard nails.

the nail plate (Fig. 12.5).[82] It is produced by a habit tic of pushing the proximal nail fold back with the index finger. Sometimes the transverse indentations are spaced so closely together that they appear as one large median longitudinal groove. Stopping the behavior allows for healing of the nail fold as well as gradual regrowth of a healthy nail plate.

Koilonychia

The nail plates of children with koilonychia are spoon-shaped. The normally convex contour is replaced by a central concavity surrounded by upturned lateral and distal margins (Fig. 12.6). The plate itself may be thick or thin and longitudinally fissured. Many newborns and young infants demonstrate koilonychia of the great toenails, which spontaneously resolves in several years.[83] In some cases, as in psoriasis or onychomycosis, distal subungual debris

from the hyponychium may alter the direction of nail growth,[84] while in other cases matrix size, shape, or the angle of nail plate exit may cause the deformity.

Isolated koilonychia may be inherited as an autosomal-dominant trait[85] or it may be associated with other syndromes.[86,87] Transient acquired koilonychia is not unusual and may be observed in up to 5% of normal 2-year-olds. It has been associated with iron deficiency anemia.[88] Early observations suggested a causal relationship. However, not all patients with iron deficiency develop spooning.[89] Koilonychia develops when iron deficiency is severe, and the deformity takes months to resolve after iron replacement therapy. Therefore, the sensitivity of koilonychia as an isolated physical sign for the presence of iron deficiency is probably quite low. The mechanism of spooning of the nails in the milieu of low iron remains speculative. Other systemic and local diseases

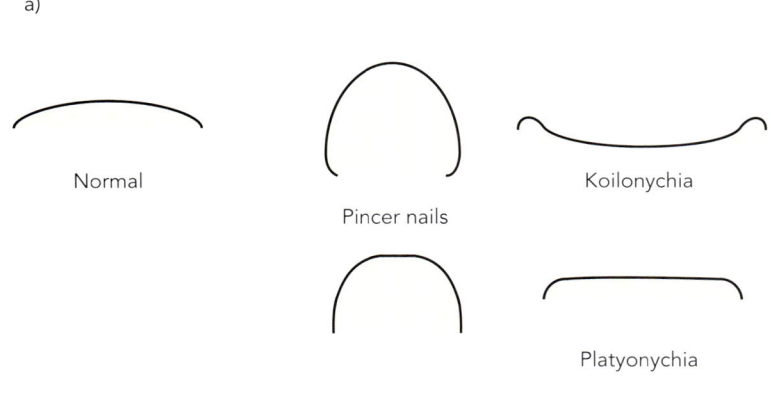

a)

Normal

Pincer nails

Koilonychia

Platyonychia

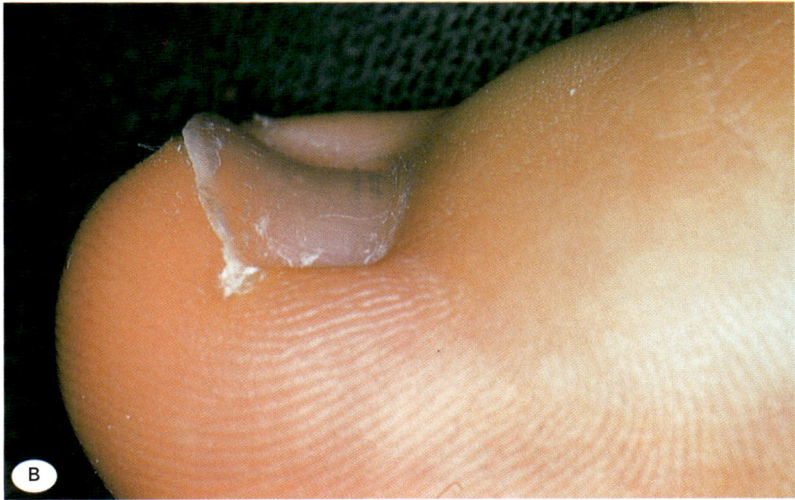

B

Fig. 12.6   (A) Nail shape (contours). (B) Koilonychia, a concave, spoon-shaped deformity.

82. Macauley WL (1966) Transverse ridging of the thumbnails: "washboard thumbnails." **Arch Dermatol** 93:421.
83. Yinnon AM, Matalon A (1988) Koilonychia of the toenails in children. **Int J Dermatol** 27:685–687.
84. Baran R, Dawber RPR (2001) Diseases of the Nails and Their Management. Oxford: Blackwell Scientific, p. 53.
85. Bumpers RD, Bishop ME (1980) Familial koilonychia: a current case history. **Arch Dermatol** 116:845.
86. Baran R, Dawber RPR (1984) Diseases of the Nails and Their Management. Oxford: Blackwell Scientific, p. 310.
87. Keng-Ee T, Sinclair RD (2001) Keratosis pilaris and hereditary koilonychia without monilethrix. **J Am Acad Dermatol** 45:627–629.
88. Hogan GR, Jones G (1970) The relationship of koilonychia and iron deficiency in infants. **J Pediatr** 77:1054.
89. Sato S (1991) Iron deficiency: Structural and microchemical changes in hair, nails, and skin. **Sem Dermatol** 10:313–319.

associated with koilonychia include hemochromatosis, hypothyroidism, lichen planus, and the so-called 20-nail dystrophy of childhood.[90–92]

Platyonychia and pincer nails

Platyonychia (Fig. 12.6A), or flattened nails, should not be confused with koilonychia. In the former, the nail plates are flat, while in the latter the plates are concave. Platyonychia has been described in patients with cirrhosis[93] and has also been observed with a step-like transverse over-curvature of the plates, known as pincer nails.[94]

Pincer nails are characterized by an exaggerated over-curvature of the lateral portions of the nail plate. This is usually a congenital deformity in which the

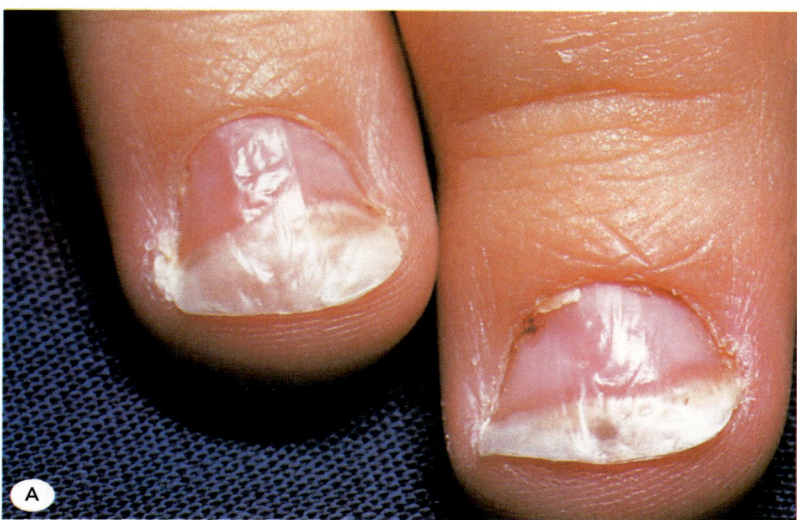

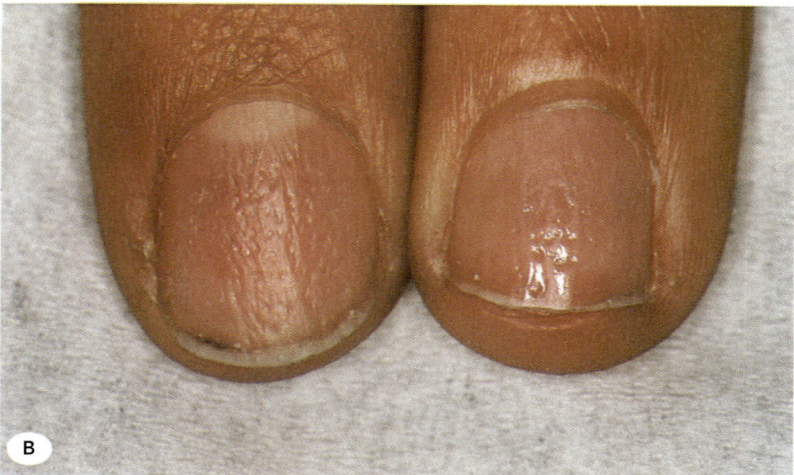

Fig. 12.7 (A) Nail pitting from psoriasis. (B) Nail pitting from alopecia areata.

lateral borders of the nail plate extend down into the lateral nail folds giving them a plicated or ingrown appearance.[95] Acquired pincer nails have been observed in association with distal phalangeal exostosis, epidermoid cysts, and epidermolysis bullosa.[96,97] Transient pincer nails were reported in a 3-month-old girl with Kawasaki's disease.[98] Pincer nails may be quite painful. If they do not resolve on their own, surgical correction may produce a gratifying reduction in symptoms.[99]

Pitting

Pitting of the nail plate surface is a common finding in children with nail disease (Fig. 12.7A). These punctate depressions may be small and shallow or large and deep, involving few or all 20 nails. They are formed by alterations in the proximal matrix.

Theories offered for the formation of pits include pinpoint areas of aberrant keratinization (clusters of dyskeratotic cells or parakeratotic columns), matrix invasion by inflammatory cells (neutrophilic microabscesses, as in psoriasis, or lymphocytic exocytosis, as in pityriasis rosea), or localized spongiosis (intercellular edema formation, as in eczema). In any case, spaces remain in place of loose cellular or acellular material that has been sloughed once the nail plate becomes exposed from under the proximal nail fold.

Pits may be distributed in many ways over the nail plate surface. They may be found in isolated clusters. This is common in normal persons or in those who have suffered localized trauma to the nail matrix. Randomly distributed shallow pits are most frequently observed in inflammatory dermatoses, such as psoriasis. Finally, transverse rows of regularly spaced pits resembling Beau's lines may be observed and are characteristic of alopecia areata (Fig. 12.7B and Table 12.4).[100–110]

Longitudinal markings of the nail plate may take the form of grooves, splitting, striations, or ridges. The nail plates of many normal newborns are longitudinally ridged in a centridistal direction. These ridges flatten with time. Single wide longitudinal grooves are formed by localized disruptions of the

TABLE 12.4   Causes of nail plate pitting

Disease	Relative frequency
Psoriasis[a,b]	7–40%[100,101,102]
Alopecia areata[a]	5–60%[103,104]
Eczema	Common
Normal children	Unusual
Pityriasis rosea	Personal observation[105]
Secondary syphilis	Unusual[106]
Sarcoidosis	Case report[107]
Fluorosis	Case report[108]
Reiter's syndrome	Case report[109]
IgA deficiency	Case report[110]

[a] May be the initial manifestation of the disease.
[b] May be the sole manifestation of the disease.[101]

90. Fairbanks VF, Fairbanks GE (1971) Hemosiderosis and hemochromatosis. In: Clinical Disorders of Iron Metabolism, Beuther E, ed. New York: Grune & Stratton, p. 399.
91. Kiepert JA, Kelley R (1978) Acquired juvenile hypothyroidism presenting with nail changes. **Aust J Dermatol** 19:89.
92. Silverman RA, Rhodes AR (1984) Twenty-nail dystrophy of childhood: a sign of localized lichen planus. **Pediatr Dermatol** 1:207.
93. Kleeberg J (1951) Flat fingernails in cirrhosis of the liver. **Lancet** 2:248.
94. Cornelius CE, Shelly WB (1968) Pincer nail syndrome. **Arch Surg** 96:321.
95. Chapman RS (1973) Overcurvature of the nails. An inherited disorder. **Br J Dermatol** 89:317.
96. Baran R (1974) Pincer and trumpet nails. **Arch Dermatol** 110:639.
97. Kitajima Y, Jokura Y, Yaoita H (1993) Epidermolysis bullosa simplex, Dowling–Meara type: a report of two cases with different types of tonofilament clumping. **Br J Dermatol** 128:79–85.
98. Vanderhooft SL, Vanderhooft JE (1999) Pincer nail deformity after Kawasaki's disease. **J Am Acad Dermatol** 41:341–342.
99. Brown RE, Zook EG, Williams J (2000) Correction of pincer-nail deformity using dermal grafting. **Plast Reconstr Surg** 105:1658–1661.
100. Nyfors A, Lemhold K (1975) Psoriasis in children. A short review and survey of 245 cases. **Br J Dermatol** 92:437.
101. Nanda A, Kaur S, Kaur I, Kumar B (1990) Childhood psoriasis: An epidemiologic survey of 112 patients. **Pediatr Dermatol** 7:19–21.
102. Morris A, Rogers M, Fischer G, Williams K (2001) Childhood psoriasis: A clinical review of 1262 cases. **Pediatr Dermatol** 18:188–198.
103. Tosti A, Morelli R, Bardazzi F, Peluso AM (1994) Prevalence of nail abnormalities in children with alopecia areata. **Pediatr Dermatol** 11:112–115.
104. Horn RT, Odom RB (1980) Twenty nail dystrophy of alopecia areata. **Arch Dermatol** 116:573.
105. Baran R, Dawber RPR (2001) Diseases of the Nails and Their Management. Oxford: Blackwell Scientific, p. 67–68.
106. Baran R, Dawber RPR (2001) Diseases of the Nails and Their Management. Oxford: Blackwell Scientific, p. 211.
107. Patel KB, Sharma OP (1983) Nails in sarcoidosis: response to treatment. **Arch Dermatol** 110:277.
108. Spera L (1943) Mottled nails as an early sign of fluorosis. **J Hyg Camb** 43:69.
109. Lovy MR, Bluhm GB, Morales A (1980) The occurrence of nail pitting in Reiter's syndrome. **J Am Acad Dermatol** 2:66.
110. Leong AB, Gange RW, O'Connor RD (1982) Twenty nail dystrophy (trachonychia) associated with selective IgA deficiency. **J Pediatr** 180:418.

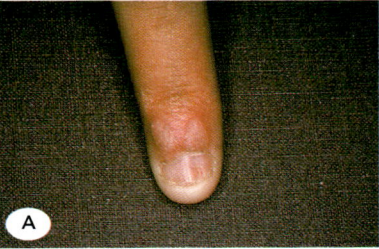 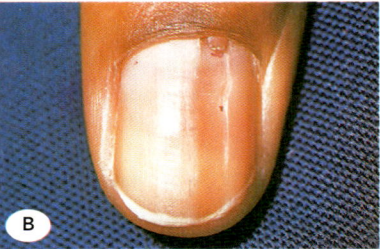

Fig. 12.8 **(A)** Large broad longitudinal groove produced by external pressure on the nail matrix from a wart. **(B)** Longitudinal groove of a Koenen's tumor (periungual fibroma) in tuberous sclerosis.

proximal nail fold that press against the underlying matrix. Periungual warts (Fig. 12.8A), Koenen's tumors of tuberous sclerosis (Fig. 12.8B), myxoid cysts, fibrokeratomas, or other space-occupying lesions may all present in this fashion. Traumatic scars of the nail fold may result in similar deformities.

Multiple longitudinal nail grooves

Multiple longitudinal nail grooves are a prominent finding with thin nail plates of any cause. They may be a reflection of decreased nail matrix volume (atrophy) or of alterations of the normal ridged configuration of the matrix and nailed. Thin grooved nail plates may be found in patients with lichen planus,[111] chronic graft-vs-host disease,[112] psoriasis,[113] alopecia areata,[114] Darier's disease,[115] connective tissue diseases,[116] radiation dermatitis,[117] frostbite, or chilblains.[118]

Onychorrhexis

Onychorrhexis, or longitudinal fissures with splitting and chipping at the free edge, frequently accompanies fragile thin grooved nail plates (Fig. 12.9). Careful close clipping prevents the aggravating and sometimes painful catching of materials that rip the nail plate from the hyponychium when onychorrhexis is present.

Median nail dystrophy

Median nail dystrophy, also called solenonychia or dystrophia mediana canaliformis, is an unusual bilateral defect of the thumbnails characterized by a prominent wide longitudinal midline fissure or a groove flanked by irregularly shaped transverse undulations in the nail plate.[119] This deformity, which has a Christmas tree-like appearance, is occasionally asymmetric or involves other nail plates. Familial cases of this idiopathic deformity have been reported,[120] but some authorities believe it results from repeated pressure on the base of the nail plate. Washboard nails have a similar appearance, but this defect is due to pushing back the cuticle.[121] One case associated with oral administration of isotretinoin (Accutane) has also been documented.[122] Median nail dystrophy may improve spontaneously after several years. Differential diagnosis includes washboard nails, or pterygium (scar) formation.

Trachyonychia

Trachyonychia, or rough nails, occurs when longitudinal grooves and ridges are very superficial and closely spaced (Fig. 12.10).[123] Persons exhibiting this

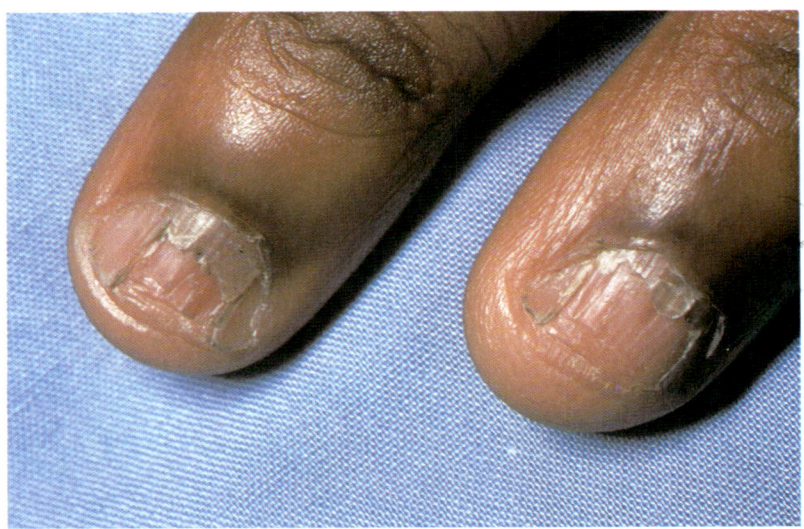

Fig. 12.9 Onychorrhexis. Longitudinal splitting and chipping commonly observed in lichen planus.

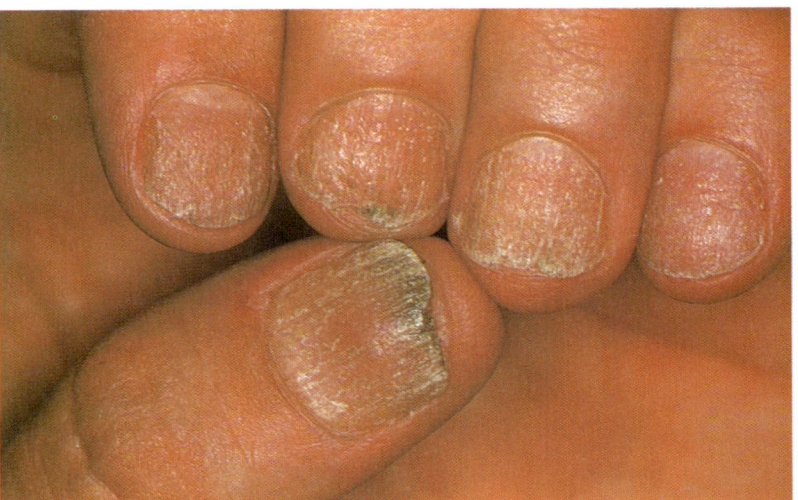

Fig. 12.10 Trachyonychia (rough nails) in idiopathic 20-nail dystrophy of childhood.

physical sign have also been said to have vertical-striated sandpaper nails.[124] Several cutaneous diseases associated with trachyonychia include alopecia areata,[125] lichen planus,[126] psoriasis, atopic dermatitis, and the so-called 20-nail dystrophy of childhood.

20-nail dystrophy

The term 20-nail dystrophy of childhood was popularized in 1977 when Hazelrigg and others described six children who had acquired deformities of

111. Tosti A, Piraccini BM, Cambiaghi S, Jorizzo M (2001) Nail lichen planus in children. Clinical features, response to treatment, and long-term follow-up. **Arch Dermatol** 137:1027–1032.
112. Saurat JH, Gluckman E (1977) Lichen planus-like eruption following bone marrow transplantation: a manifestation of graft-versus-host disease. **Clin Exp Dermatol** 2:355.
113. Kouskoukis CE, Scher RK, Lebovits PE (1983) Psoriasis of the nails. **Cutis** 31:169.
114. Baran R, Dupre A, Aristol B et al. (1978) L'ongle grésé-peladique. **Ann Dermatol Venereol** 105:387.
115. Ronchese F (1965) The nails in Darier's disease. **Arch Dermatol** 91:617.
116. Urowitz MB, Gladman DD, Chalmers A et al. (1978) Nail lesions in systemic lupus erythematosus. **J Rheum** 5:441.
117. Baran R, Dawber RPR (2001) Diseases of the Nails and Their Management. Oxford: Blackwell Scientific, p. 539.
118. Lonsdorf G, Ryckmanns F (1982) Lichen ruber planus beakroucyanose (chilbain-lichen). **Hautarzt** 33:454.

119. Heller J (1928) Dystrophia unguiuna mediana canaliformis. **Dermatol Z** 51:416.
120. Rehtijarvi K (1971) Dystrophia unguis mediana canaliformis (Heller). **Acta Derm Venereol (Stockh)** 51:315.
121. Baran R, Dawber RPR (2001) Diseases of the Nails and Their Management. Oxford: Blackwell Scientific, p. 66.
122. Bottomley WW, Cunliffe WJ (1992) Median nail dystrophy associated with isotretinoin therapy. **Br J Dermatol** 127:447.
123. Samman PD (1979) Trachyonychia (rough nails). **Br J Dermatol** 101:701.
124. Baran R, Dupre A (1977) Vertical striated sandpaper nails. **Arch Dermatol** 13:1613.
125. Tosti A. Fanti PA, Morelli R, Bardazzi F (1991) Trachyonychia associated with alopecia areata. **J Am Acad Dermatol** 25:266.
126. Joshi RK, Abanmi A Ohman S, Haleem A (1993) Lichen planus of the nail presenting as trachyonychia. **Int J Dermatol** 32:54.

all 20 nails.[127] Physical examinations revealed neither mucocutaneous diseases nor ectodermal defects at the time of initial evaluation. Onychomycosis was also absent. Nail plate deformities were characterized by longitudinal grooves, striations, and onychorrhexis with distal chipping and brittleness. Most cases had thin plates with koilonychia, but thick yellowish great toenails were observed as well. Similar nail signs had been described earlier,[128] although the changes listed by Hazelrigg were not purported to be unique. Subsequent reports emphasized the rough sandpaper-like quality of the nail changes (trachyonychia) and the relationship between 20-nail dystrophy and other diseases such as lichen planus and vitiligo.[129–133] Biopsies were performed in several cases; histologic alterations consistent with lichen planus, eczema, and psoriasis were discovered. In addition, congenital, hereditary, and adult-onset cases have been reported.[134–136] Lifelong 20-nail dystrophy in identical twins was described.[137]

It is important to note that trachyonychia may occur months before cutaneous signs of other diseases, as in alopecia areata or dyskeratosis congenita. Therefore, one should observe children with trachyonychia over several months before other diagnoses are excluded. Occasionally, a biopsy of an affected nail might be considered since some diseases such as lichen planus may only affect the nails. Current opinion favors the belief that 20-nail dystrophy of childhood is not a distinct clinical entity but probably a physical sign of some other localized disease (e.g., lichen planus)[138] or malformation. Therefore, the term 20-nail dystrophy of childhood should probably be discarded since it refers to a constellation of physical findings of the nails that may be incompletely expressed and does not refer to a specific disease.

The course of trachyonychia is quite variable. Cases have been reported to improve over periods of time, ranging from six months to 16 years. Daily applications of high-potency topical steroids to the proximal nail fold have proved unsuccessful in the hands of most physicians. Long-term application may result in resorption of the underlying phalanx. Disruption of the proximal nail fold cuticle followed by application of topical steroid solution has been advocated by some clinicians to enhance penetration into the affected matrix. However, this practice may result in paronychia or further matrix injury if not done cautiously. Intralesional steroids have been reported to improve some cases of 20-nail dystrophy, but pain and the necessity for repeated injections make this therapy unsuitable for small children. In the author's experience, topical anesthetics (EMLA-eutectic mixture of lidocaine (lignocaine) and prilocaine) do not reduce the pain of paronychial injections. Years of topical or systemic antifungal medication are also not useful. Treatment with topical PUVA (phototherapy with Psoralen solution soaks followed by localized exposure to ultraviolet A irradiation) was reported to be successful in one case.[139] Oral biotin supplements have also had a positive effect on this condition.[140] Keeping the nails short with frequent careful filing should lessen the incidence of snagging and ripping of the affected nail plates. Clear nail hardeners may be applied if onychorrhexis is a problem. Prolonged exposure to water (habitual washing, long baths or swimming) could, in theory, compound the brittleness associated with the condition.

Onychoschizia

Lamellar splitting of the nail plate at its distal free edge, known as onychoschizia, is most frequently due to repeated trauma (Fig. 12.11A), excessive exposure to nail polish (Fig. 12.11B), or frequent immersion into detergent solutions with subsequent drying.[141] Although onychoschizia occurs most commonly in older women, children are not immune to these exposures. The problem resolves by avoidance of inciting factors.

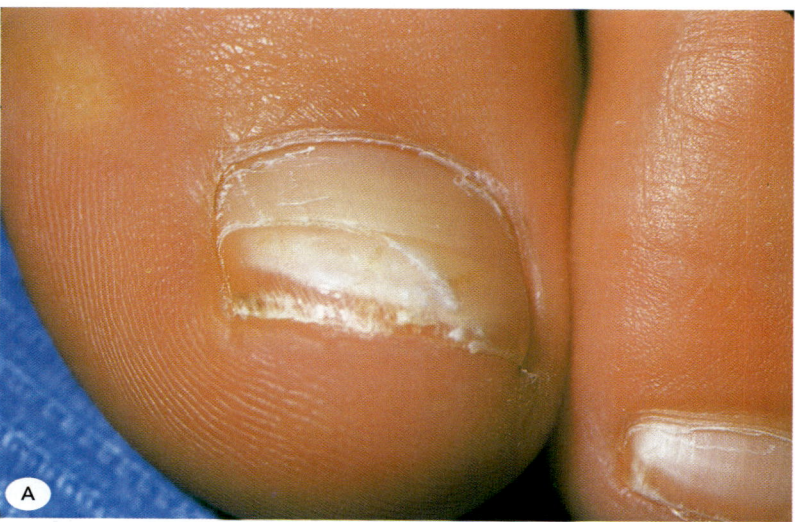

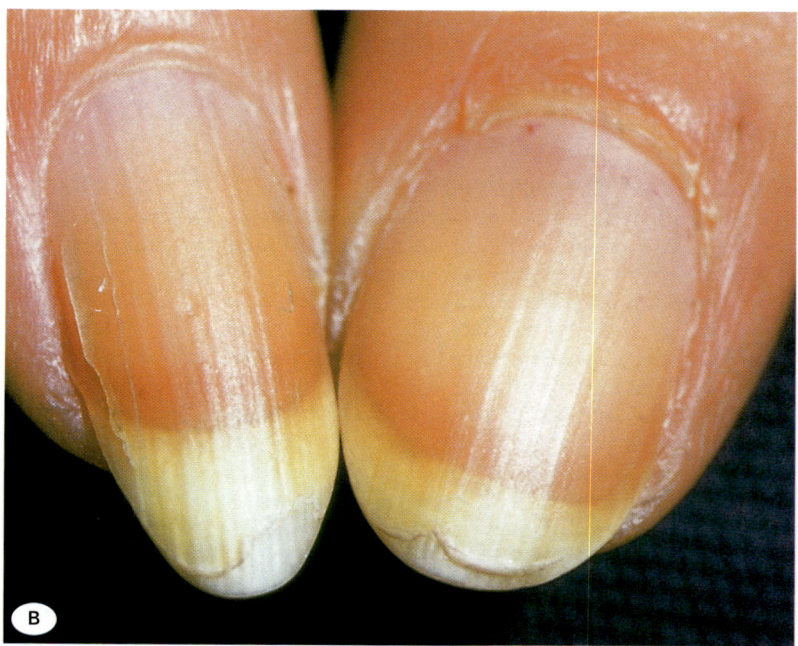

Fig. 12.11 (A) Traumatic onychoschizia. (B) Onychoschizia induced by nail polish.

127. Hazelrigg DE, Duncan C, Jarratt M (1977) Twenty-nail dystrophy of childhood. **Arch Dermatol** 113:73.
128. Samman PD (1965) The Nails in Disease. London: Heinemann, p. 122.
129. Scher RK, Fischbein R, Ackerman AB (1978) Twenty-nail dystrophy. A variant of lichen planus. **Arch Dermatol** 114:612.
130. Wilkinson JD, Dawber RPR, Bowers RP et al. (1979) Twenty-nail dystrophy of childhood. Case report and histopathological findings. **Br J Dermatol** 200:217.
131. James W, Odom RB, Horn RT (1981) Twenty-nail dystrophy and ichthyosis vulgaris. **Arch Dermatol** 117:361.
132. Leong AB, Gange RW, O'Connor RD (1982) Twenty nail dystrophy (trachonychia) associated with selective IgA deficiency. **J Pediatr** 100:418.
133. Barth JH, Telfer NR, Dawber RPR (1988) Nail abnormalities and autoimmunity. **J Am Acad Dermatol** 18:1062–1065.
134. Arias AM, Yung CW, Rendler S et al. (1982) Familial severe twenty-nail dystrophy. **J Am Acad Dermatol** 7:349.
135. Pavone L, Volti SL, Guarneri B et al. (1982) Hereditary twenty-nail dystrophy in a Sicilian family. **J Med Gen** 19:337.
136. Bruynzeel DP, Frankenmolen-Witkiewicz IM (1980) Twenty-nail dystrophy in adults. **Arch Dermatol** 116:862.
137. Commens CA (1988) Twenty nail dystrophy in identical twins. **Pediatr Dermatol** 5:117.
138. Kechijian P (1985) Twenty-nail dystrophy of childhood: a reappraisal. **Cutis** 35:38.
139. Halkier-Sorensen L, Cramers M, Kraballe K (1990) Twenty nail dystrophy treated with topical PUVA. **Acta Dermatol Venereol** (Stockh) 70:510.
140. Möhrenschlager M, Schmidt T, Ring J et al. (1998) Effects of biotin in trachyonychia of childhood. **Ann Dermatol** 125 (suppl1):176.
141. Shelly WB, Shelly ED (1984) Onychoschizia: scanning electron microscopy. **J Am Acad Dermatol** 10:623.

Brittle nails

Hapalonychia and fragilitas unguium are terms used to describe soft or brittle nails.[142] Both onychoschizia (lamellar splitting) and onychorrhexis (longitudinal splitting) may result from softened nails. Irregular chipping of the nail plate surface from repeated applications and removal of nail polish produces hapalonychia of the dorsal surface (Fig. 12.12). Brittleness or friability is also a manifestation of onychomycosis, psoriasis, eczema, lichen planus, iron deficiency anemia, pachyonychia congenita, and trichothiodystrophy.[143] An unusual congenital soft nail dystrophy has been described.[144] No uniformly successful treatment has been found for brittle nails. Outside of adequate nutrition in cases of documented exogenous deficiencies or malnutrition, dietary supplements of gelatin, vitamins, amino acids, or calcium have not proven effective. Two studies of daily biotin supplements (2.5mg per day) improved adults with brittle nails.[145,146] Benefits in children with this condition have not been demonstrated. Nail hardeners may be applied and contact with external agents that worsen the condition avoided.

Onychauxis

Thickening or hypertrophy of the nail plate from any cause is termed onychauxis (Fig. 12.13). Unilateral onychauxis of the fourth toe nail is a distinctive presenting sign of onychomycosis in young children (personal observation, Robert A. Silverman, MD)

Onychogryphosis refers to thickened nails that have a clawlike or curved configuration similar to a ram's horn (Fig. 12.14). This results from uneven rates of matrix growth. The deformity is usually seen on the toes of elderly persons with poor ungual hygiene who have not manicured their nails. Onychogryphosis is rarely a problem in children, although occasionally

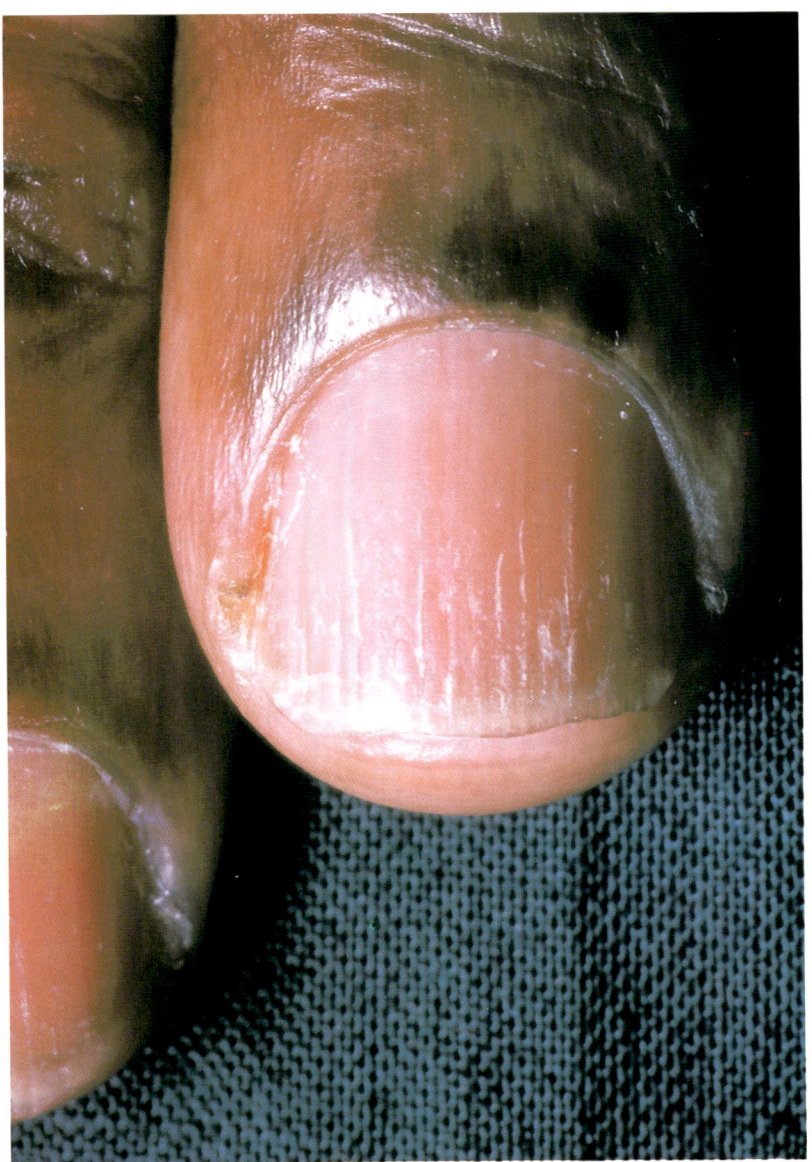

Fig. 12.12 Hapalonychia or fragilitas unguium refer to brittle nails of any cause.

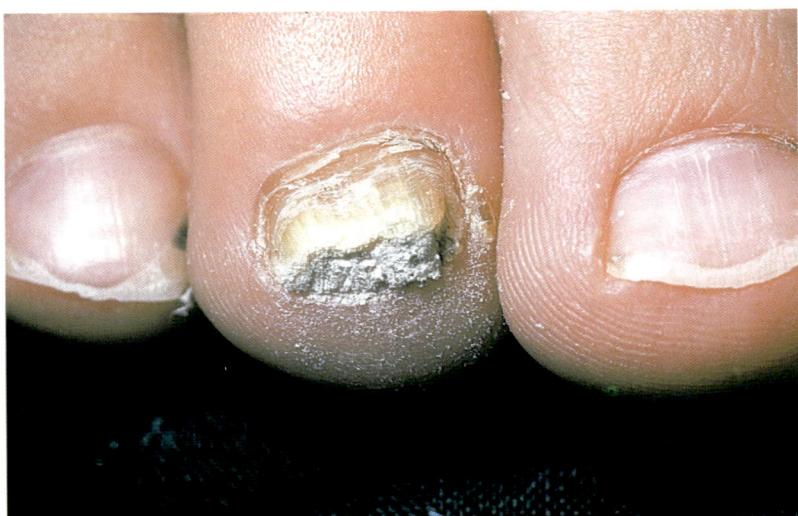

Fig. 12.13 Onychauxis or thickening of the nail may develop from onychomycosis.

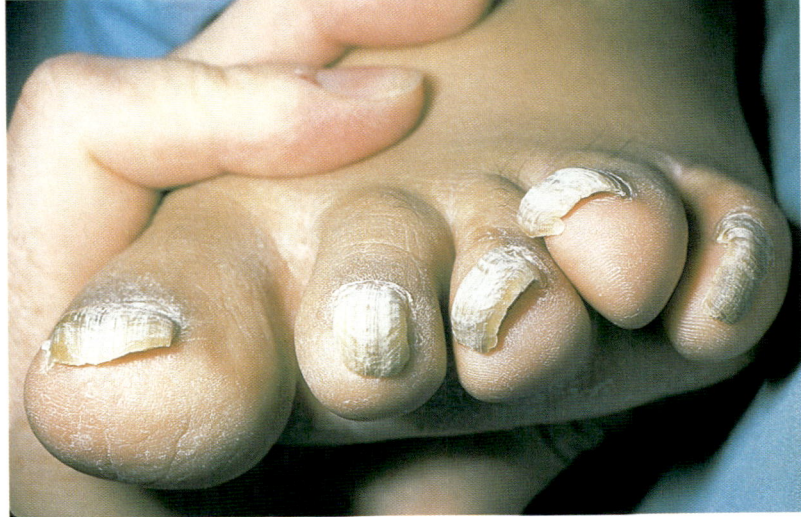

Fig. 12.14 Onychogryphosis is a curved, thickened claw-like deformity.

142. Scher RK, Bodian AB (1991) Brittle nails. Semin Dermatol 10:21.

143. Price VH, Odom RB, Ward WH, Jones FT (1980) Trichothiodystrophy. Arch Dermatol 116:1375.

144. Prandi G, Caccialanza M (1977) An unusual congential nail dystrophy (soft nail disease). Clin Exp Dermatol 2:265.

145. Colombo VE, Gerber F, Bronhofer M, Floersheim GL (1990) Treatment of brittle nails and onychoschizia with biotin: scanning electron microscopy. J Am Acad Dermatol 23:1127.

146. Hochman LG, Scher RK, Meyerson MS (1993) Brittle nails: response to daily biotin supplementation. Cutis 51:303.

ill-fitting shoes and foot deformities may predispose to this abnormality if the toenails are not trimmed. Autosomal-dominant hereditary onychogryphosis has been described.[147] It may be prominent during the first few years of life and should not be confused with congenital malalignment of the great toenail, in which the nail plate is not curved but is deviated laterally.[148]

Pachyonychia congenita

Pachyonychia congenita is a rare hereditary disorder characterized by thickened nails. Cases of these nail changes with keratosis of the palms and soles were mentioned in 17th and 18th century texts and later documented by the English dermatologist, Wilson, in 1905.[149,150] Credit for recognition of the pachyonychia congenita syndrome was given later to Jadassohn and Lewandovsky, who noted the accompanying palmoplantar keratoderma and a variety of additional ectodermal defects.[151]

Pachyonychia congenita syndrome is usually transmitted as an autosomal-dominant trait with a high degree of penetrance.[152] Its variable expressivity may be the basis of reports of sporadic cases. Men seem to be affected more than women. Most persons with the disorder are of Northern European or Jewish extraction, although affected persons with other racial and ethnic backgrounds have been reported.[153]

Patients with pachyonychia congenita may present during the neonatal period with yellowish-brown discoloration of the nails. Within the first few months of life, elevation or thickening of the nail plates occurs from subungual hyperkeratosis (Fig. 12.15). The dorsal surface of the nail plate remains smooth, while the lateral borders curve under in a pincer fashion and the distal free edge angles in an upward direction.[154] Spontaneous nail shedding and regrowth with more severe deformity have been known to occur.[155] Paronychia is a frequent problem and may be due to bacteria or candida organisms.[156]

Other features of pachyonychia congenita in pediatric patients may initially divert attention from nail abnormalities. Though not pathognomonic, the presence of natal teeth may be helpful when the newborn is first examined in the nursery. Affected infants may demonstrate foamy white mucosal plaques that could easily be confused for thrush.[157] Cutaneous examination reveals symmetric thickening of the palms and soles similar to several other keratodermas. Callouses of the soles make ambulation difficult. Palmoplantar hyperhidrosis is not unusual. In toddlers, it may result in painful blister formation, particularly in summer, similar to the Weber–Cockayne form of epidermolysis bullosa. Clusters of rough, dry, grayish spiny papules (follicular hyperkeratosis) develop over the elbows, knees, and other body surfaces, similar to follicular psoriasis.

Pachyonychia congenita has been classified into two variants based on clinical phenotype and recently discovered genetic abnormalities of ungual keratin proteins. Type I cases (PC-1, Jadassohn–Lewandovsky variant [OMIM 167200]) show prominent palmoplantar hyperkeratosis and extensive follicular hyperkeratosis extending onto the trunk, and oral leukokeratosis that may be confused for a white sponge nevus or dyskeratosis congenita. However, malignant degeneration of the leukokeratotic plaques has not been reported, unlike similar lesions in dyskeratosis congenita. Histologic differentiation can also be made between the oral lesions of pachyonychia congenita and Darier's disease, lichen planus, intraepithelial dyskeratosis, and candidiasis. PC-1 patients have mutations in keratins 16 or 6a.[158,159] Prenatal diagnosis of pachyonychia congenita type I has recently been accomplished.[160] Type II patients (PC-2, Jackson–Lawler type [OMIM 167210]) have natal teeth, corneal dystrophy, and cysts that have been described in different reports as epidermoid, cylindromas, or steatocystoma multiplex in addition to the onychodystrophy.[161,162] Leukoplakia is not a prominent feature of this phenotype. Affected members of several kindreds with this variant may also have painful abcesses of hidradenitis suppurativa and myriads of disfiguring facial milia.[163] At least one case of pachyonychia congenita has been observed at birth to present with hundreds of widespread milia (R. Hansen, personal communication, 1993). Mutations in keratin 17 or keratin 6b have been identified in this Jackson–Lawler variant.[164,165]

In 1988, prior to the knowledge of the genetic defects of this disorder, some investigators divided pachyonychia congenita into four clinical subtypes.[166] In addition to PC-1 and PC-2, patients with pachyonychia congenita and very extensive mucosal thickening that extended into the larynx and resulted in hoarseness were observed.[167] Other patients that were thought to be distinctive developed corneal thickening and cataracts. It is now felt that these cases are phenotypic variations of the same keratin gene defects, and for some patients, the distinction between phenotypes is by no means clear.[168] Finally, Paller and other have reported a late-onset variant termed

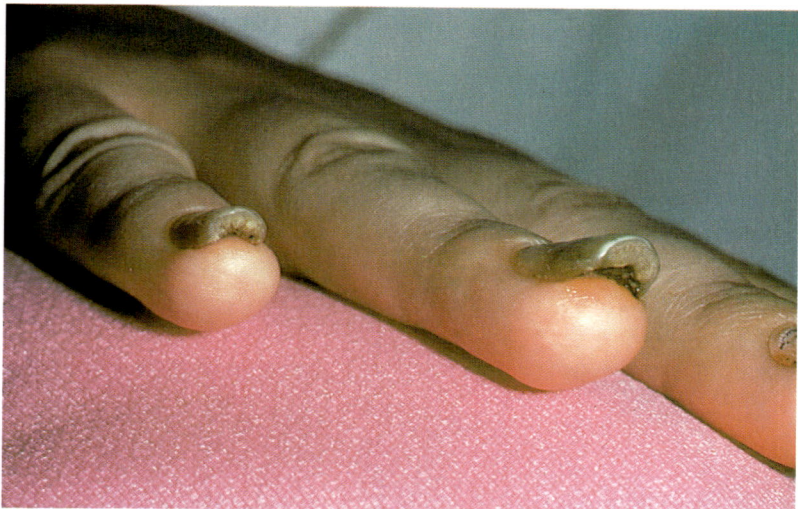

Fig. 12.15   Nail thickening of pachyonychia congenita. (Courtesy of Dr. Craig Elmets.)

147. Lubach D (1982) Erbliche onychogryphoses. **Hautarzt** 33:331.
148. Baran R, Bureau H (1983) Congenital malalignment of the big toenail as a cause of ingrowing toenail in infancy. Pathology and treatment (a study of thirty cases). **Clin Exp Dermatol** 8:619.
149. Bondesson J (1993) Pachyonychia congenita. A historical note. **Am J Dermatolpathol** 15:594.
150. Wilson AG (1905) Three cases of hereditary hyperkeratosis of the nail bed. **Br J Dermatol** 17:13.
151. Jadassohn J, Lewandovsky F (1906) Pachyonychia congenita. **Ikonograph Dermatol** 1:29.
152. Stieglitz JB, Centerwall WR (1983) Pachyonychia congenita (Jadassohn–Lewandovsky syndrome): a seventeen member four generation pedigree with unusual respiratory and dental involvement. **Am J Med Gen** 14:21.
153. Wu WPD, Chun SI, Hammond DE, Gordon H (1990) Pachyonychia congenita: a clinical study of 12 cases and review of the literature. **Pediatr Dermatol** 7:33.
154. Joseph HL (1964) Pachyonychia congenita. **Arch Dermatol** 90:594.
155. Thormann J, Kobayasi T (1977) Pachyonychia congenita. Jadassohn–Lewandowsky: a disorder of keratinization. **Acta Derm Venereol** (Stockh) 57:63.
156. Mawhinney H, Creswell S, Beare JM (1981) Pachyonychia congentia with candidiasis. **Clin Exp Dermatol** 6:145.
157. Anneroth G, Isacsson G, Lagerholm B et al. (1975) Pachyonychia congenita: a clinical, histological and microradiographic study with special reference to oral manifestations. **Acta Derm Venereol** (Stockh) 55:387.
158. McLean WHI, rug EL, Lunny DP et al. (1995) Keratin 16 and keratin 17 mutations cause pachonychia congenita. **Nat Genet** 9:273–276.

159. Bowden PE, Haley JL, Kansky A et al. (1995) Mutation of a type II keratin gene (K6a) in pachyonychia congenita. **Nat Genet** 10:363–365.
160. Smith FJD, McKusick VA, Nielsen K et al. (1999) Cloning of multiple keratin 16 genes facilitates prenatal diagnosis of pachyonychia congenita type 1. **Prenatal Diag** 19:941–946.
161. Soderqvist NA, Reed WB (1968) Pachyonychia congenita with epidermal cysts and other congenital dyskeratoses. **Arch Dermatol** 97:31–33.
162. Hodes Me, Norins AL (1977) Pachyonychia congenita and steatocystoma multiplex. **Clin Genet** 11:359–364.
163. Todd P, Garioch J, Rademaker M et al. (1990) Pachyonychia congenita complicated by hidradenitis suppurativa: a family study. **Br J Dermatol** 123:663.
164. Covello SP, Smith FJD, Sillevis JH et al. (1998) Keratin 17 mutations cause either steatocystoma multiplex or pachyonychia congenita type 2. **Br J Dermatol** 139:475–480.
165. Smith FJD, Jonkman MF, van Goor H et al. (1998) A mutation in human keratin K6b produces a phenocopy of the K17 disorder pachyonychia congenita type 2. **Am J Hum Genet** 7:1143–1148.
166. Feinstein A, Friedman J, Schewach-Millet M (1988) Pachyonychia congenita: **J Am Acad Dermatol** 19:705–711.
167. Cohn AM, McFarlane JF, Knox J (1976) Pachyonychia congenita with involvement of the larynx. **Arch Otolaryngol** 102:233–235.
168. Munro CS (2001) Pachyonychia congenita: mutations and clinical presentations. **Br J Dermatol** 144:929–930.

"pachyonychia congenita tarda." These cases have thickened nails that are not apparent until the teenage years.[169] They may be due to defects in keratin 16, similar to PC-1.[170] Histologic studies of pachyonychia congenita demonstrate abnormal keratin accumulation and occasionally intracellular edema centered around eccrine sweat pores, which may explain the hyperhidrosis from which some patients suffer.[171] Immunologic dyscrasias have been sought in the patients with chronic infections such as paronychia, hidradenitis, and candidiasis, but consistent abnormalities have not been demonstrated.[172]

The differential diagnosis of pachyonychia congenita includes diseases that may have hypertrophied nail plates or subungual hyperkeratosis such as psoriasis, chronic atopic erythroderma, mucocutaneous candidiasis, ichthyosis syndromes,[173,174] distal subungual onychomycosis, pityriasis rubra pilaris, Darier's disease, Norwegian scabies, and pachyonychia with retardation and group-G ring chromosome.[175]

Jadassohn and Lewandovsky used hammers and chisels to reduce nail keratosis in their cases of pachonychia congenita. Treatment with high doses of vitamin A has been disappointing. Partial responses of the oral and follicular keratosis to Accutane™ have been reported.[176] However, nail disease and palmoplantar keratoderma did not respond before serious side effects occurred. The newer retinoid, acitretin, may be safer and more beneficial. Applications of 40% urea in petrolatum followed by careful occlusion and soaking in water softens the nail plates before trimming with professional clippers. Some affected patients have had custom orthotic footwear fabricated to relieve discomfort. Occasionally the nail bed and matrix have to be destroyed, while in other cases amputation of the distal phalanges has been recommended. Once a nail plate is removed, phenol cautery of the nail bed will prevent regrowth of the hypertrophic nail plate, may be repeated, and in most instances is painless. Treatment of the palmoplantar keratoderma with keratolytic agents and emollients has provided only transient relief.[177] One report of a patient with incapacitating blisters that responded to phenytoin has not been substantiated by other investigators.[178]

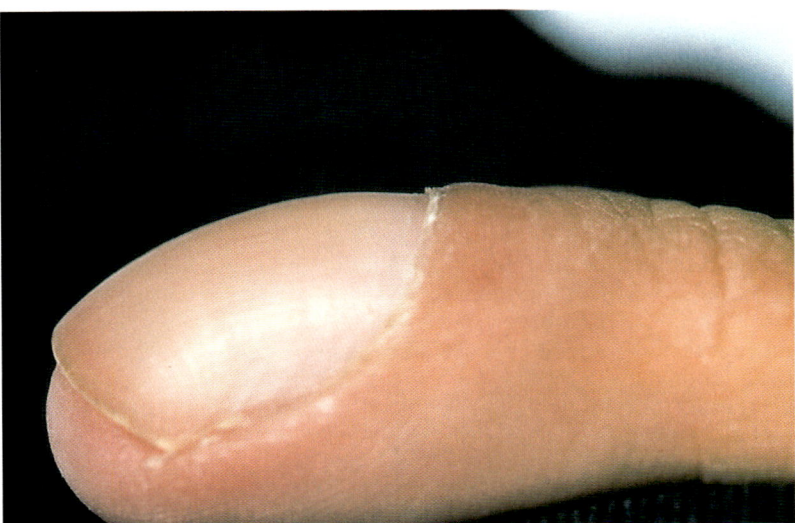

Fig. 12.16   Clubbed (Hippocratic) nails of a patient with cystic fibrosis.

ALTERATIONS IN NAIL SHAPE

Clubbing

Clubbing, or acropachy, was recognized as a reliable sign of internal disease as early as the first century BC. This curved or beak-like deformity, also known as Hippocratic or watch-glass nails, results from hypertrophy and hyperplasia of the fibrovascular support stroma of the distal phalanx (Fig. 12.16).[179] An early sign of clubbing emphasized by Lovibond is increased flexibility of the proximal nail plate due to softened edematous underlying tissues. In addition, the angle formed by the proximal nail fold and nail plate (Lovibond's angle) when viewed from a lateral position exceeds 180 degrees (normally less than 160 degrees).[180]

TABLE 12.5   Clubbing in children[a]

History	System	Disease
Acquired Generalized	Pulmonary	Cystic fibrosis Bronchiectasis Tuberculosis, aspergillosis Asthma complicated by lung infections Sarcoidosis Pulmonary fibrosis Tumors
	Cardiovascular	Cyanotic congenital heart disease Subacute bacterial endocarditis Myxomas
	Gastrointestinal	Inflammatory bowel disease Gardner's syndrome Parasitosis Cirrhosis Chronic active hepatitis
	Endocrine	Diamond's syndrome (myxedema, exophthalomos & clubbing) Hypervitaminosis A Malnutrition
Limited to one or more digits		Aortic/subclavian artery aneurism Brachial plexus injury Trauma Maffucci's syndrome Gout Sarcoidosis Severe herpetic whitlow
Hereditary		Pachydermoperiostosis Familial, isolated[183]
Pseudoclubbing[b]		Apert's syndrome Pfeifer's syndrome Rubinstein–Taybi syndrome

[a] Adapted from Baran R, Dawber RPR (1984) Diseases of the Nails and their Management. Blackwell Scientific: London, p. 29.
[b] Broad distal phalanges with normally shaped nails

169. Paller AS, Moore JA, Scher R (1991) Pachyonychia congenita tarda. Late onset form of pachyonychia congenita. **Arch Dermatol** 127:701.
170. Connors JB, Rahil AK, Smith FJD et al. (2001) Delayed-onset pachyonychia congenita associated with a novel mutation in the central 2B domain of keratin 16. **Br J Dermatol** 144:1058–1062.
171. Schonfeld PHIR (1980) The pachyonychia congenita syndrome. **Acta Derm Venereol** (Stockh) 60:45.
172. Rohold AE, Brandrup F (1990) Pachyonychia congenita: therapeutic and immunologic aspects. **Pediatr Dermatol** 7:307.
173. Harms M, Gilardi S, Levy PM, Saurat JH (1984) KID syndrome (keratitis ichthyosis and deafness) and chronic mucocutaneous candidiasis: case report and review of the literature. **Pediatr Dermatol** 2:1.
174. Jorizzo JL, Crounse RG, Wheeler CE (1980) Lamellar ichthyosis, dwarfism, mental retardation and hair shaft abnormalities: a link between the ichthyosis-associated and BIDS syndromes. **J Am Acad Dermatol** 2:309.
175. Dubowitz V, Cooke P, Colver D, Harris F (1971) Mental retardation, unusual facies, and abnormal nails associated with a group-G ring chromosome. **J Med Gen** 8:195.
176. Thomas DRA, Jorizzo JL, Brysk MM et al. (1984) Pachyonychia congenita. Electron microscopic and epidermal glycoprotein assessment before and during isotretinoin treatment. **Arch Dermatol** 120:1475.
177. Su WPD, Chun SI, Hammond DE, Gordon H (1990) Pachyonychia congenita: a clinical study of twelve cases. **Pediatr Dermatol** 7:33.
178. Blank H (1982) Treatment of pachyonychia congenita with phenytoin. **Br J Dermatol** 106:21.
179. Bigler FC (1958) The morphology of clubbing. **Am J Pathol** 34:237.
180. Lovibond JL (1938) Diagnosis of clubbed fingers. **Lancet** 1:363.

TABLE 12.6   Nail signs as an aid to the diagnosis of congenital heart disease

Nail beds	Nail plates	Diagnosis
Cyanosis of fingers & toes	Normal	Great vessel transposition with preductal coarct and reversed shunt
Cyanosis right & left hand	Normal	Preductal aortic coarctation
Cyanosis of toes & left fingers with pink right fingers	Clubbed toes	Patent ductus with reversed and pulmonary hypertension
Tuft erythema	Normal	Small right to left shunt
Erythematous pulsations (Quincke's)	Normal	Aortic insufficiency or high output state

Clubbing is a sign of many systemic disorders (Table 12.5). It is most commonly recognized in pediatric patients with cyanotic congenital heart disease, cystic fibrosis, and inflammatory bowel disease. In the former instances, right-to-left shunting away from the pulmonary vascular bed occurs, but the precise etiology (hypoxia versus circulating growth factor) is unknown. Localized clubbing may be indicative of specific cardiac defects (Table 12.6).[181] Clubbing associated with malignancy would be distinctly unusual during childhood since primary or metastatic thoracic tumors are uncommon. However, isolated cases of clubbing have been reported with Hodgkin's and non-Hodgkin's lymphomas, both of which may arise during adolescence. Painful clubbing is indicative of the periostitis associated with hypertrophic pulmonary osteoarthropathy, which is characteristic of thoracic malignancy.

Pachydermoperiostosis, an idiopathic sometimes familial form of clubbing, develops around puberty. It is associated with cutis verticis gyrata and eventual spade-like thickening of the hands and feet.[182,183] Thyroid acropachy and acromegaly may both be confused with pachydermoperiostosis.

Shell nails
Shell nails are clinically similar to clubbed nails. They have been reported to form at age 5 years, in a girl with bronchiectasis. However, avulsion of the nail plate revealed atrophy of the nail bed instead of hypertrophy as seen in true clubbing.[184]

Racket nails
Racket nails are broad and shortened and are usually found on the thumb and great toes. They are occasionally confused with clubbed nails because of their stubby appearance (Fig. 12.17). Racket nails reflect an underlying arrest in distal phalangeal formation, which may be dominantly inherited as an isolated trait,[185] or associated with other abnormalities, in which case the more general term brachyonychia can be applied. Brachyonychia has been reported with or without clinical brachydactyly. Disorders associated with brachyonychia include cartilage-hair hypoplasia, acro-osteolysis, Larsen's syndrome, Rubenstein–Taybi syndrome, pyknodysostosis, acrodysostosis, and multiple malignant cylindromas.[186–192] Most syndromes with brachydactyly are manifested as pseudoclubbing with normally proportioned nails.

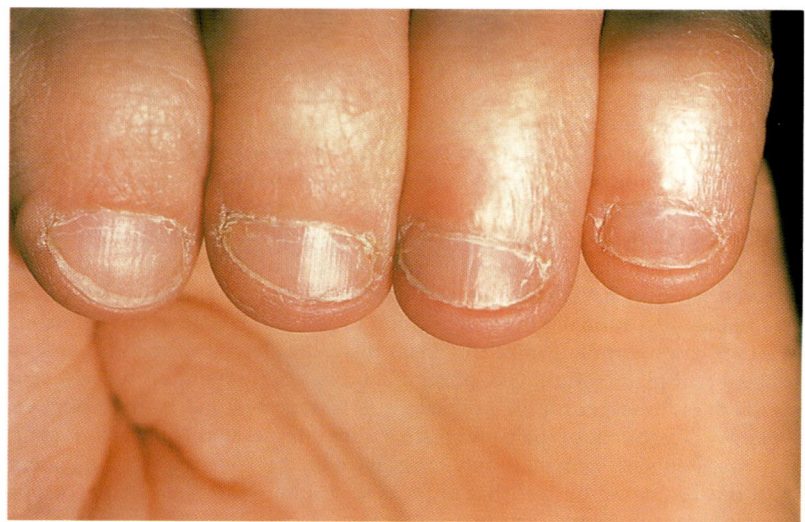

Fig. 12.17   Racket nails in a normal patient.

ALTERATIONS IN NAIL SIZE
Measurements of the dimensions of nails in newborn infants have been recorded.[193] This information may be invaluable to geneticists since about 75% of congenital syndromes are associated with nail abnormalities.[194]

Anonychia
Anonychia refers to the absence of nails. Anonychia is usually accompanied by rudimentary nails on other digits. Congenital anonychia of all nails is rare.[195] It may be an isolated inherited trait or may be a presenting sign of junctional epidermolysis bullosa before blisters develop (Fig. 12.18).[196,197] At birth, anonychia may also be associated with other malformations of ectodermal or mesodermal origin.[198–200] Frequently there are underlying osseous abnormalities that are observed on X-ray.[201,202] Acquired anonychia

181. Silverman ME, Hurst JW (1968) The hand and the heart. **Am J Cardiol** 22:718.
182. Fischer DS, Singer DH, Feldman SM (1964) Clubbing: a review with emphasis on hereditary acropachy. **Medicine** (Baltimore) 43:459.
183. Curth HO, Firschein IL, Alpert M (1961) Familial clubbed fingers. **Arch Dermatol** 83:828.
184. Cornelius CE, Shelly WB (1967) Shell nail syndrome associated with bronchiectasis. **Arch Dermatol** 96:694.
185. Baran R, Dawber RPR (2001) Diseases of the Nails and Their Management. Oxford: Blackwell Scientific, p. 55–56.
186. McKusick VA, Edridge R, Hostetler JA et al. (1965) Dwarfism in the Amish. II. Cartilage-hair hypoplasia. **Bull J Hopkins Hosp** 116:285.
187. Hajdu N, Kaintze R (1948) Cranioskeletal dysplasis. **Br J Radiol** 21:42.
188. Latha RJ, Graham CB, Aase J et al. (1971) Larsen's syndrome: a skeletal dysplasia with multiple joint dislocations and unusual facies. **J Pediatr** 78:291.
189. Dudding BA, Gorlin RJ. Langer LO (1967) The otopalato-digital syndrome. A new symptom complex consisting of deafness, dwarfism, cleft palate, characteristic facies, and generalized bone dysplasia. **Am J Dis Child** 113:214.
190. Schuler SE (1963) Pycnodysostosis: a review. **Arch Dis Child** 38:620.
191. Robinson M, Pfeiffer RA, Gorlin RJ et al. (1971) Acrodysostosis. A syndrome of peripheral dysostosis, nasal hypoplasia and mental retardation. **Am J Dis Child** 121:195.
192. Tsanbaos D, Greither A, Orfanos CE (1979) Multiple malignant Spiegler tumors with brachydactyly and racket nails. **J Cutan Pathol** 6:31.
193. Hudson VK, flannery DB, Karp WB et al. (1988) Finger and nail measurements in newborn infants. **Dysmorph Clin Gen** 1:145–147.
194. Seaborg B, Bordurtha J (1989) Nail size in normal infants. Establishing standards for healthy term infants. **Clin Pediatr** 28:142–145.
195. Solammadevi SV (1981) Simple anonychia. **South Med J** 74:1555–1557.
196. Hopsu-Havu VK, Jansen CT (1973) Anonychia congenita. **Arch Dermatol** 107:752.
197. Parsapour K, Reep MD, Mohammed L et al. (2001) Hurlitz junctional epidermolysis bullosa presenting at birth with anonychia: A case report and review of H-JEB. **Pediatr Dermatol** 18:217–222.
198. Nevin NC, Thomas PS, Calvert J, Reid M (1975) Deafness, onycho-osteodystrophy, mental retardation (DOOR) syndrome. **Am J Med Gen** 13:325.
199. Rahbari H, Heath L, Chapel TA (1975) Anonychia with ectrodactyly. **Arch Dermatol** 111:1482.
200. Verbov J (1975) Anonychia with bizarre flexural pigmentation: An autosomal dominant dermatosis. **Br J Dermatol** 92:169.
201. Baran R, Juhlin L (1986) Bone dependent nail formation. **Br J Dermatol** 114:371.
202. Wood VE (1996) Absence of nails with absent distal phalanges. **J Hand Surg** 3:403.

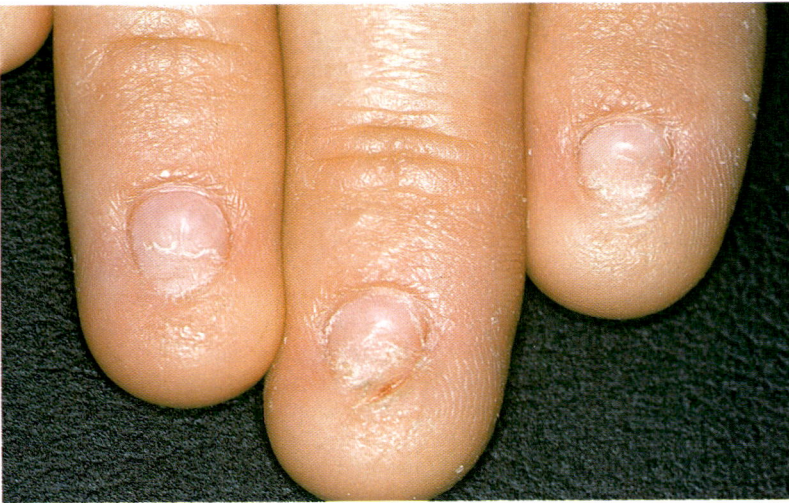

Fig. 12.18   Anonychia, or absent nails, was an isolated ectodermal defect in this child.

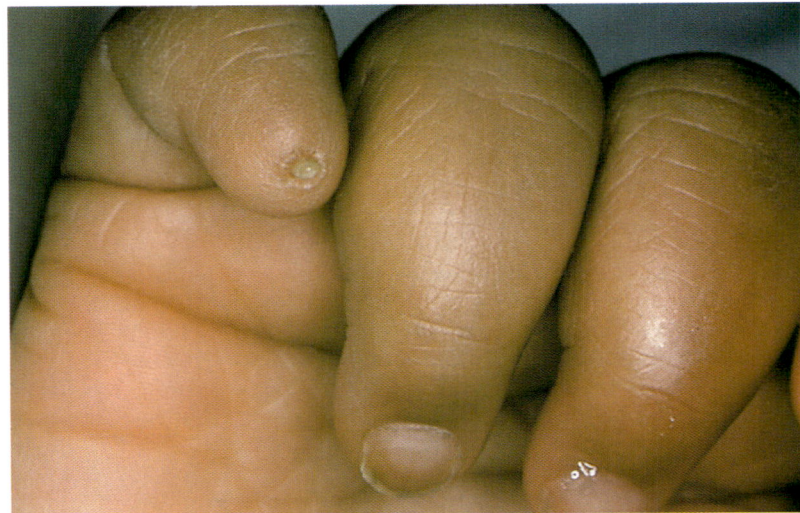

Fig. 12.19   Micronychia of the fifth digit is characteristic of Coffin–Siris syndrome.

TABLE 12.7   Acquired anonychia (absence of nails)

Postinflammatory loss[a]	Stevens–Johnson syndrome
	Severe paronychia
	Epidermolysis bullosa
Pterygium formation	Lichen planus
	Scleroderma
Traumatic[a]	Onychotillomania
	Lesch-Nyhan syndrome

[a] Once scarring occurs, anonychia may be permanent.

may result from severe inflammatory involvement of the nail unit as in Stevens–Johnson syndrome[203] or may gradually occur after progressive scarring called pterygium formation (Table 12.7). Pterygium is a wing-like growth or extension of the proximal nail fold cuticle that develops over a thinned dystrophic nail plate and eventually fuses with the underlying matrix and nail bed. Pterygium may also occur as an extension of the hyponychium onto the ventral surface of the distal nail plate. This pterygium inversum unguis may be idiopathic, inherited, or develop as a consequence of scleroderma.[204] It makes nail trimming unbearable, if not impossible.

Micronychia

Nail hypoplasia is a frequent congenital deformity that may be sporadic, inherited, associated with malformation syndromes, or toxin exposure (Fig. 12.19). *In utero* exposure to dilantin is a well-known cause of micronychia.[205–207] Maternal exposure to polychlorinated biphenyls (PCBs) has also been discovered to cause fetal malformations that include small deformed nails, natal teeth, pigment anomalies, and mucosal changes.[208] The degree of hypoplasia may vary from a minimal reduction in size to complete absence on different digits of the same patient (Table 12.8).[209–214]

TABLE 12.8   Micronychias

Disorder	Other findings
Ectodermal dysplasias	Variable sweating, hair, & tooth abnormalities
Fetal teratogen	
Hydantoins[205–207]	Short stature, retardation hypertelorism depressed nasal bridge, cardiac anomales, dyschromia nail
PCBs[208]	Natal teeth, pigment anomales, mucosal changes
Alcohol[209,210]	Microcephaly, short palpebral fissures, maxillary hypoplasia
Warfarin	Nasal hypoplasia, stippled epiphyses
COIF (**C**ongenital **O**nychodysplasia of **I**ndex **F**ingers)[211–213]	Sporadic inheritance, underlying bone dysplasia, polyonychia
Coffin–Siris syndrome	Hypoplasia of fifth digit, lax joints, blepharoptosis
Dyskeratosis congenita[214]	Hyper- & hypopigmentation, Fanconi-like anemia, blepharitis, leukoplakia
Chromosome abnormalities	
Trisomies	3q, 8, 13, 18
Turner's syndrome	XO, webbed neck, nevi, lymphedema
Noonan's syndrome	male with Turner's phenotype, pulmonic stenosis
Amniotic bands	Hypoplasia of distal phalanx associated with cutis aplasia

203. Wanscher B, Thorman J (1977) Permanent anonychia after Stevens–Johnson syndrome. **Arch Dermatol** 113:970.
204. Nogita T, Yamashita H, Kawashima M, Hidano A (1991) Pterygium inversum unguis. **J Am Acad Dermatol** 5:787–788.
205. Hanson JW, Smith DW (1975) The fetal hydantoin syndrome. **J Pediatr** 87:285.
206. Johnson RB, Goldsmith LA (1981) Dilantin digital effects. **J Am Acad Dermatol** 5:191.
207. D'Souza SW, Robertson IG, Donnai D (1990) Fetal phenytoin exposure, hypoplastic nails and jitteriness. **Arch Dis Child** 65:320.
208. Gladen BC, Taylor JS, Wu Y-C et al. (1990) Dermatological findings in children exposed transplacentally to heat-degraded polychlorinated biphenyls in Taiwan. **Br J Dermatol** 122:799.
209. Crain LS, Fitzmaurice NE, Mondry C (1983) Nail dysplasia and fetal alcohol syndrome. **Am J Dis Child** 137:1069.
210. Clarren SK, Smith DW (1978) The fetal alcohol syndrome. **N Engl J Med** 298:1063.
211. Millman AJ, Stier RP (1982) Congenital onychodysplasia of the index fingers. Report of a family. **J Am Acad Dermatol** 7:57.
212. Kitaejama Y, Tsukata S (1983) Congenital onychodysplasia. Report of 11 cases. **Arch Dermatol** 119:8.
213. Baran R, Stroud JD (1984) Congenital onychodysplasia of the index fingers. Iso and Kikuchi syndrome. **Arch Dermatol** 120:243.
214. Mallory SB (1991) Dyskeratosis congenita. **Pediatr Dermatol** 8:81.

Polyonychia

Polyonychia may accompany any of the micronychias.[215–217] Radiologic evaluation of the digits for underlying bone duplications,[218] chromosomal analysis, and a history of maternal teratogen exposure should be sought. Polyonychia and polydactyly may be inherited as an isolated autosomal-dominant trait, associated with trisomy 13 or Laurence–Moon–Biedl syndrome (obesity, hypogonadism, retinitis pigmentosa).

Nail-patella syndrome (OMIM 161200)

The first reported association between absent or hypoplastic nails and hypoplastic or absent patellae were by Chatelain in 1820 and Little in 1897.[219,220] Recognition of this association, also known as HOOD syndrome (Hereditary Osteo-Onycho-Dysplasia), Turner–Kieser syndrome, or Fong's disease, is important because of potentially debilitating osteoarthritis and renal impairment, which may develop during adulthood.[221] This genodermatosis is an autosomal-dominant disorder with variable expressivity and a high degree of penetrance.[222] Twenty percent of cases are sporadic and due to new mutations. The incidence is 1 in 50 000 and occurs in all ethnic groups throughout the world.

The nail deformities of nail-patella syndrome are recognized at birth and do not progress. However, patients frequently do not come to medical attention until vigorous physical activity leads to knee dislocation, pain, or gait disturbance.[223]

Examination of the nails reveals micronychia, which is most prominent on the thumbs and index fingers, with hemionychia, anonychia, or wide longitudinal fissures occasionally present. These changes decrease toward the 5th finger. Triangular-shaped lunulas with a distal apex may be a clue to the

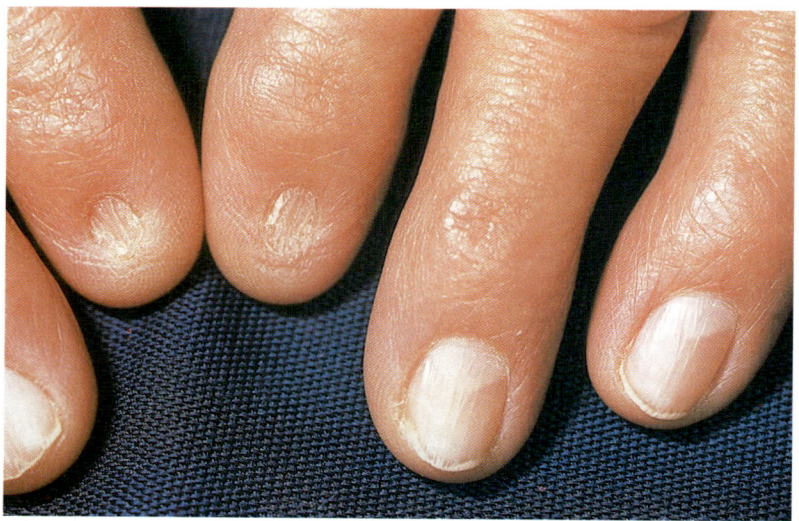

Fig. 12.20   Nail-patella syndrome. Micronychia and triangular lunulas.

presence of nail-patella syndrome (Fig. 12.20).[224] Chipping, splitting, and koilonychia are frequent problems with affected fingernails, but toes are rarely involved. The cutaneous examination is otherwise normal.

Skeletal deformities of nail-patella syndrome include aplastic or luxated patellas in 90% of patients. Knee pain or gait problems after exercise are the most common presenting complaint and result in early osteo-arthritis. Posterior iliac horns are pathognomonic of the disorder. Hypoplasia of the proximal radius and ulna causes frequent subluxations that may result in permanent restrictive deformities. Scoliosis, and thickening of the scapulae may also be present.

Renal disease becomes apparent as asymptomatic proteinuria in adults, although a newborn and a 2-year-old with nail-patella syndrome and nephrosis have been reported.[225,226] It may result in fatal chronic glomerulonephritis. Ultrastructural examinations of renal biopsy specimens have revealed collagen fibril deposition and reduplication of the glomerular basement membrane.[227] Similar findings have been reported at the basement membrane zone of the epidermis and in dermal vascular endothelium.[228] Vasculitis directed at abnormal collagen has also been demonstrated in one case.[229]

Heterochromic irides, colobomas, and other ocular dysplasias are infrequently noted in patients with nail-patella syndrome. Open-angle glaucoma has been reported in these patients. Therefore, regular ophthalmologic examinations are recommended. Mental retardation may be recognized in the school-age child. Organically based psychosis may become a prominent feature as the patient enters adulthood, and significant pain develops from joint deformities and renal disease.

The gene for nail-patella syndrome is linked to the ABO blood group gene and the COL5A1 gene at the 9q34 chromosome locus.[230] Collagen type V is an important component of the glomerular and other basement membrane zones. However, recent evidence suggests that gene which causes nail-patella syndrome codes for a LIM-homeodomain protein Lmx1b at the same site, which plays a central role in dorsal/ventral patterning of the vertebrate limb. The interaction of this gene with others (e.g., COL5A1) probably results in the variation in symptoms that are manifest in these patients.[231]

Differential diagnosis of nail-patella syndrome from other causes of micronychia during childhood may be accomplished by radiologic examination of the pelvis and elbows. Triangular lunulae are distinctive aspects the condition.

Physical activities of patients with nail-patella syndrome should be redirected at an early age in order to prevent trauma-induced osteo-arthritis or joint limitation. Reports of total knee reconstruction are not available; although one would suspect that early intervention when joint degeneration and pain occur would afford an acceptable life-style. All people with nail-patella syndrome should have regular urinalysis to detect renal disease at the earliest possible time. If renal failure supervenes, transplantation may afford a normal survival for these patients.[232]

Information for patients and families with nail-patella syndrome may be obtained from the nail-patella syndrome worldwide support group at www.nailpatella.org.

215. Kikuchi I (1985) Congenital polyonychias. Reduction versus duplication digit malformations. Int J Dermatol 24:211.
216. Miura T, Nakamura R (1990) Congenital onychodysplasia of index fingers. J Hand Surg 15A:793.
217. Kikuchi I (1991) Congenital onychodysplasia of index fingers: a case involving thumb nails. Semin Dermatol 10:7.
218. Cannata GE (1991) Congenital onychodystrophy with hyperplasia and double nail. Clin Exp Dermatol 16:75.
219. Raman D, Haslock I (1983) The nail-patella syndrome–A report of two cases and a literature review. Br J Rheumatol 22:41.
220. Little EM (1897) Congenital absence or delayed development of the patella. Lancet 2:781.
221. Carbonara P, Kane AC, Alpert M (1964) Hereditary osteoonychodysplasia (HOOD). Am J Med Sci 248:139.
222. Lucas GL, Opertz JM (1966) The nail-patella syndrome. Clinical and genetic aspects of 5 kindreds with 38 affected family members. J Pediatr 68:273.
223. Guidera KJ, Satterwhite Y, Ogden JA et al. (1991) Nail-patella syndrome: a review of 44 orthopedic patients. J Pediatr Orthop 11:737.
224. Daniel CR, Osment LS, Noojin RO (1980) Triangular lunulae. A clue to nail-patella syndrome. Arch Dermatol 116:448.

225. Simila S, Vesa L, Wasz-Hockert O (1970) Hereditary onycho-osteodysplasia (the nail-patella syndrome) with nephrosis-like renal disease in a newborn boy. Pediatrics 46:61.
226. Browning MC, Weidner N, Lorentz WB Jr (1988) Renal histopathology of the nail-patella syndrome in a 2 year old boy. Clin Nephrol 29:210.
227. Taguchi T, Takebayashi S, Nishimura M, Tsuru N (1988) Nephropathy of nail-patella syndrome. Ultrastructural Pathology 12:175.
228. Burkhart CG, Bhumbra R, Iannone AM (1980) Nail-patella syndrome. A distinctive clinical and electron microscopic presentation. J Am Acad Dermatol 3:251.
229. Crook AD, Bashar-Kahaleh M, Powerst M (1987) Vasculitis and renal disease in nail-patella syndrome: case report and literature review. Ann Rheum Dis 46:562.
230. Greenspan DS, Byers MG, Eddy RL et al. (1992) Human collagen gene COL5A1 maps to the q34.2'q34.3 region of chromosome 9, near the locus for nail-patella syndrome. Genomics 12:836.
231. Dryer SD, Zhou G, Baldini A et al. (1998) Mutations in LMX1B cause abnormal skeletal patterning and renal dysplasia in nail-patella syndrome. Nat Genet 19:47–50.
232. Chan PC, Chan KW, Cheng IK, Chan MK (1988) Living related renal transplantation in a patient with nail-patella syndrome. Nephron 50:164.

Congenital onychodysplasia of the index fingers (COIF)

The Iso & Kikuchi syndrome, also known as COIF, is a rare but distinctive nail disorder associated with micronychia and underlying skeletal defects.[233] There have been over 70 cases described since the first report by Iso in 1969.[234] Most cases are sporadic, but autosomal–dominant inheritance and cases in identical twins have been reported.[235–237] COIF may be unilateral or bilateral. It may present with anonychia, but asymmetric ulnar micronychia with or without polyonychia is most often present (Fig. 12.21). The nail plates may be thin, have a rolled appearance, or display partial onychogryphosis and malalignment. Rarely, deformities of other fingers are present.[238,239] Radiographs of the underlying boney phalanx disclose a characteristic Y-type bifurcation or a sharpened tip of the distal phalanx.[240]

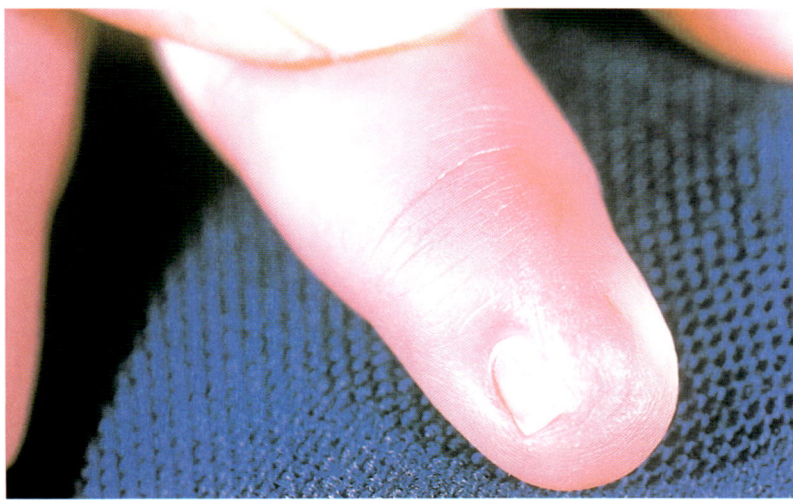

Fig. 12.21 COIF. Asymmetric, ulnar deviated micronychia is characteristic of congenital onychodysplasia of the index fingers.

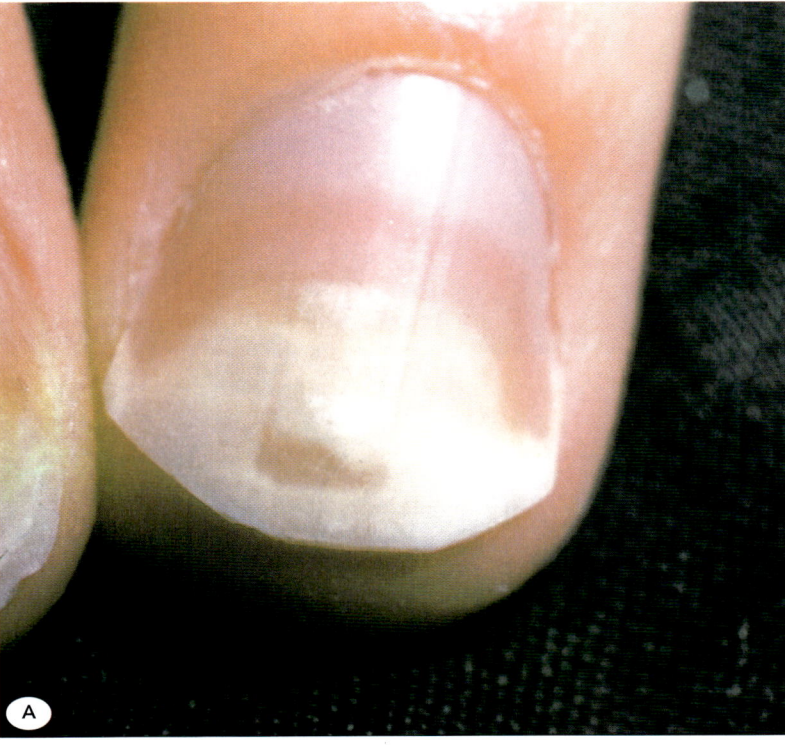

DISEASES OF THE NAIL BED

Numerous diseases may disrupt the normally firm attachment of the nail plate to the nail bed. Distal or lateral separation of these two structures is termed onycholysis (Fig. 12.22).[241] Frequently, onycholysis is accompanied by accumulation of subungual debris. Well-intentioned meticulous attempts at removing foreign matter will occasionally extend the separation. Potential causes of onycholysis in children include the following:

Trauma
    Sportsman's toe
    Compulsive cleaning
Inflammatory disorders
    Psoriasis
    Alopecia areata
    Lichen planus
    Dermatitis (contact or atopic)
Drugs
    Photo-onycholysis (i.e., tetracyclines and thiazides)
    Retinoids (Accutane)
    Antineoplastic agents
    Sodium valproate

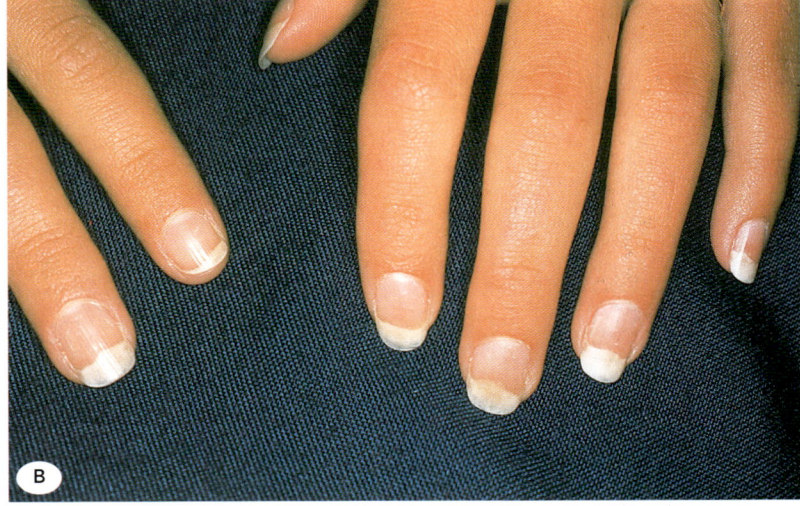

Fig. 12.22 Onycholysis. (A) Separation of the nail plate from the nail bed in a child with candidiasis. (B) Painful photo-onycholysis is a complication of doxycycline therapy for acne.

233. Baran R, Stroud JD (1984) Congenital onychodysplasia of the index fingers–Iso and Kikuchi syndrome. **Arch Dermatol** 120:243.
234. Iso R (1969) Congenital nail defects of the index finger and reconstructive surgery. **Orthop Surg** 20:1383–1384.
235. Millman AJ, Strier RP (1982) Congenital onychodysplasia of the index fingers. Report of a family. **J Am Acad Dermatol** 7:57–65.
236. Harper KJ, Beer WE (1985) Pattern of inheritance in Iso and Kikuchi syndrome. **Clin Exp Dermatol** 10:476–478.
237. Kameyoshi Y, Iwasaki Y, Hide M, Yamamoto S (1998) Congenital onychodysplasia of the index fingers in identical twins. **Br J Dermatol** 139:1120–1122.
238. Kikuchi I (1991) Congenital onychodysplasia of the index fingers: A case involving the thumbnails. **Semin Dermatol** 10:7–11.
239. Koizumi H, Tomoyori T, Ohkawaza A (1998) Congenital onychodysplasia of the index fingers with anomaly of the great toe. **Acta Derm Venereol** 76:322–323.
240. Miura T, Nakamura R (1990) Congenital onychodysplasia of the index fingers. **J Hand Surg** 15:793–797.
241. Daniel CR III (1991) Onycholysis: an overview. **Semin Dermatol** 10:34.

Chemicals
Organic solvents
Alkaline detergents
Cosmetics (formaldehyde)
Depilatories
Nail polish removers
Systemic diseases
Connective tissue diseases
Hypo- or hyperthyroidism
Iron deficiency anemia
Infections
Onychomycosis
Candidiasis
Herpetic whitlow
Warts
Bacterial paronychia

Onycholysis that occurs proximal to the hyponychium has a yellow–brown color and resembles an oil spot. This oil spot sign is nearly pathognomonic for psoriasis but is unusual in children (unlike pitting).

Other disorders of the nail bed present as color changes observed through the transparent nail plate. For instance, a spotted lunula may be observed in patients with alopecia areata.[242] Red lunulas may be observed in a number of diseases, including alopecia areata,[243] cardiac failure,[244] or rheumatoid arthritis.[245] A notched lunula, as seen in Darier–White disease (keratosis follicularis), results in a defect of the distal nail plate margin (Fig. 12.23).[246]

Hemorrhages into the nail bed may appear as small linear punctate discolorations that parallel the microscopic nail bed grooves (splinter hemorrhages) (Fig. 12.24), or as large, painful hematomas (Fig. 12.25). Numerous causes of hemorrhages into the nail bed have been documented (Table 12.9).[247–249] When pain is present in hematomas, it may be alleviated by puncturing the nail plate with a hot sterile paper clip. As hemorrhages age, they move distally, and their coloration changes from red to purple to brown

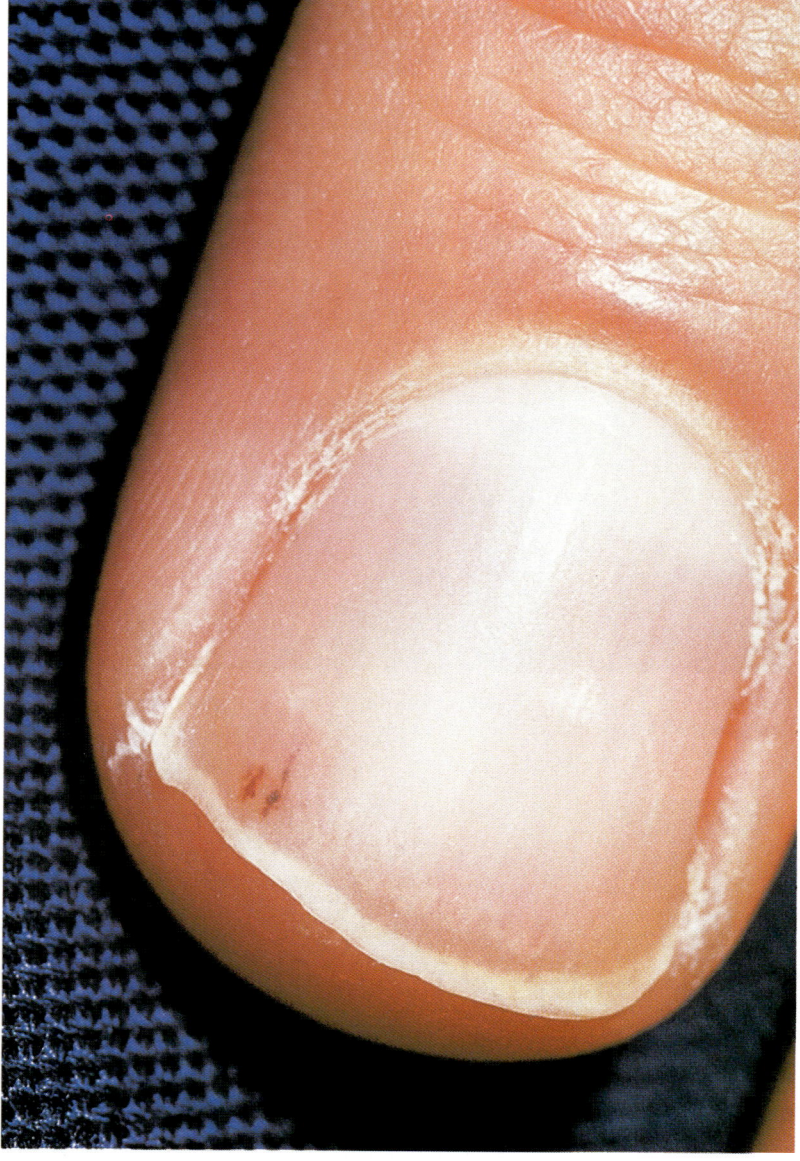

Fig. 12.24   Splinter hemorrhage of the distal nail bed due to trauma.

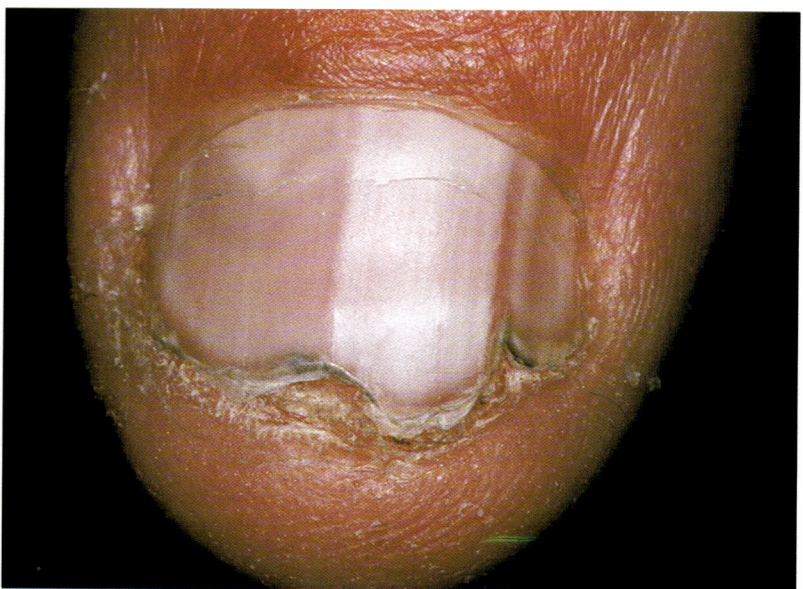

Fig. 12.23   The notched lunula and distal nail plate of Darier–White disease.

or black. Large mature hematomas may be confused with melanocytic nevi or tumors of the nail bed. However, nevi frequently cause longitudinal streaks of pigment across the whole nail plate, while pigmented streaks from hemorrhages usually have an interrupted or incomplete course.

Chromonychia

Chromonychia, or abnormal coloration of the nail apparatus, may be quite striking and is frequently helpful in the diagnosis of various underlying conditions. In general, alterations in color may be due to contact with external agents, systemic medications (antibiotics or anti-neoplastic agents), chronic intoxications, infectious diseases (bacterial or fungal), primary cutaneous

242. Shelly WB (1980) The spotted lunula, a neglected sign associated with alopecia areata. **J Am Acad Dermatol** 2:385.
243. Cohen PR (1992) Red lunulae: case report and literature review. **J Am Acad Dermatol** 26:292.
244. Terry R (1954) Red half-moons in cardiac failure. **Lancet** 2:842.
245. Jorizzo JL, Gonzalez EB, Daniels JC (1983) Red lunulae in a patient with rheumatoid arthritis. **J Am Acad Dermatol** 8:711.
246. Zaias N (1973) The nail in Darier–White disease. **Arch Dermatol** 107:193.

247. Gavin LA, Lanz MJ, Leung DYM, Roesler TA (1997) Chronic subungual hematomas: A presumed immunologic puzzle resolved with a diagnosis of child abuse. **Arch Pediatr Adolesc Med** 151:103–105.
248. Harper JI, Staughton R (1983) Letterer-Siwe disease with nail involvement. **Cutis** 31:493.
249. Timpatanapong P, Hathirat P, Isarangkura P (1984) Nail involvement in histiocytosis-X. A 12 year retrospective study. **Arch Dermatol** 102:1052.

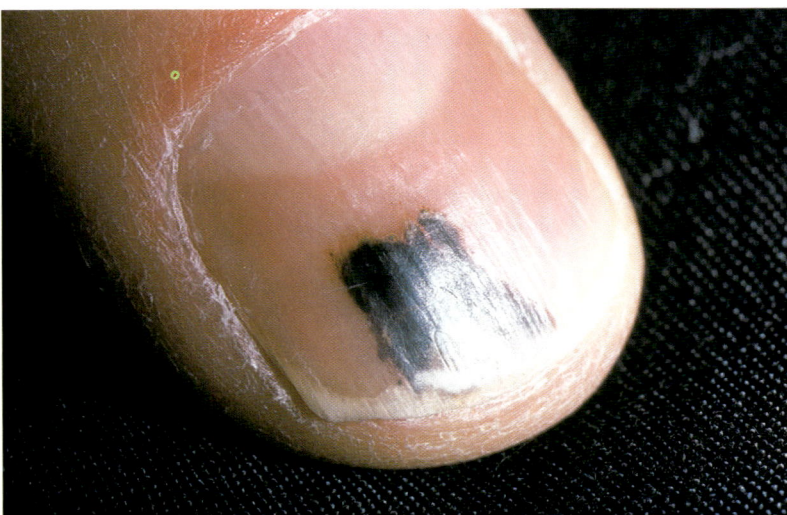

Fig. 12.25 Resolving hematoma of the nail bed in a runner.

TABLE 12.9   Disorders associated with subungual hemorrhage

	Splinter-shaped	Hematomas
Normal variant	+	−
Blood dyscrasias	+	+
Collagen diseases (lupus erythymatosus)	+	+
Trichinosis	+	−
Trauma[a]	+	+
Child abuse[247]		+
Cryoglobulinemia	+	−
Drug eruptions	+	−
Dialysis	+	−
Endocarditis (SBE)	+	−
Emboli	+	+
Histiocytosis-X[248,249]	+	−
Arterial lines or punctures	+	−
Sarcoidosis	+	−
Sepsis	+	−
Thyroid disease	+	−
Vasculitis	+	−
Phototoxicity (tetracyclines)	+	−

[a] Most common.

TABLE 12.10   Leukonychia

History	Configuration	Comments
Hereditary	Total[254]	Associated with duodenal ulcer,[257] Congeni sebaceous cysts & renal calculi,[258] knuckle pads & deafness,[259] LEOPARD syndrome,[260] partial[255]
	Striate[256] Punctate	Congenital candidiasis[261]
Acquired	Striated transversely	Stevens–Johnson syndrome[262] Febrile illness (equivalent to Beau's lines),[263] Mee's lines (arsenic, thallium or lead poisoning intoxication),[264] Muehrcke's paired lines (hypoalbuminemia)[265] Chemotherapy,[266,267] Trauma (e.g., karate),[268] Acrodermatitis enteropathica[269]
	Punctate Partial	Trauma, probable normal variant Lindsey's half & half nails of uremia: proximal white & distal red to brown[270] Terry's nails of cirrhosis or congestive heart failure: proximal white, distal pink to brown[271]
	Total	Vitiligo, sulfonamides
Pseudoleu-konychia		Onychomycoses (especially *candida*) of nail plate or anemia (nail bed pallor)

disorders, systemic disease, trauma, or tumors (Table 12.10).[250–252] Frequently, other nail signs accompany dyschromia.

Leukonychia, or white nails, may present with total (Fig. 12.26) or partial involvement (Fig. 12.27), or striate and punctate configurations.[253] True leukonychia results from opacification of the nail plates by abnormal keratinization, retention of cell nuclei, or formation of air pockets from reabsorbed acellular debris. Apparent leukonychia is seen with onycholysis or when alterations in the nail bed occur (Table 12.11).[254–271]

Yellow nail syndrome

Yellow nail syndrome consists of the triad of thickened yellow nails, lymphedema, and respiratory disease. This association was first emphasized by Samman and White in 1964.[272] Subsequent reports have expanded the list of associations with yellow nails to include thyroid disease, nephrotic syndrome, immunoglobulin A (IgA) deficiency, mental retardation, Milroy's disease, and congenital lymphedema of Meige. An unusual case of fetal hydrops and

250. Baran R, Dawber RPR (2001) Diseases of the Nails and Their Management. Oxford: Blackwell Scientific, p. 85–103.
251. Jeanmougen M, Civatte J (1983) Nail dyschromia. Int J Dermatol 22:279.
252. Daniel CR III, Scher RK (1984) Nail changes secondary to systemic diseases. J Am Acad Dermatol 10:250.
253. Zaun, Hansotto (1991) Leukonychias. Semin Dermatol 10:17.
254. Juhlin L (1963) Hereditary leukonychia. Acta Derm Venereol (Stockh) 43:136.
255. Albright SD, Wheeler CE (1964) Leukonychia: total and partial leukonychia in a single family with a review of the literature. Arch Dermatol 90:392.
256. Higashi N, Sugai T, Yamamoto T (1971) Leukonychia striata longitudinalis. Arch Dermatol 104:192.
257. Ingegno AP, Yatto RP (1982) Hereditary white nails (leukonychia totalis) duodenal ulcer and gallstones. Genetic implications of a syndrome. NY State J Med 82:1797.
258. Bushkell LL, Gorlin RJ (1975) Leukonychia totalis, multiple sebaceous cysts and renal calculi, a syndrome. Arch Dermatol 111:899.
259. Bart RS, Punphyre RE (1967) Knuckle pads, leukonychia and deafness. A dominantly inherited syndrome. N Engl J Med 276:202.
260. Selmanowitz VJ, Orentreich N, Felstein JM (1971) Lentiginosis profusa syndrome (multiple lentigines syndrome). Arch Dermatol 104:393.
261. Arkegast KD, Lamberty LF, Koh JK et al. (1990) Congenital candidiasis limited to the nail plates. Pediatr Dermatol 7:310.
262. Bryer-Ash M, Kennedy C, Ridgway H (1981) A case of leukonychia striata with severe erythema multiforme. Clin Exp Dermatol 6:565.
263. Baran R, Dawber RPR (2001) Diseases of the Nails and Their Management. Oxford: Blackwell Scientific, p. 95.
264. Pounds CA, Pearson EF, Turner TD (1979) Arsenic in fingernails. J Forensic Sci Soc 19:165.
265. Muehrcke RC (1956) The fingernails in chronic hypoalbuminemia. Br Med J 1:1327.
266. James WD, Odom RB (1983) Chemotherapy-induced transverse white lines in the fingernails. Arch Dermatol 119:334.
267. Hogan PA, Krafchik BR, Boxall L (1991) Transverse striate leukonychia associated with cancer chemotherapy. Pediatr Dermatol 8:67.
268. Scher RK (1981) The athletic nail. Dermatology 81:49.
269. Ferrandiz C, Henkes J, Peyri J, Sarmiento J (1981) Acquired zinc deficiency syndrome during total parenteral alimentation. Dermatologica 163:255.
270. Lubach D, Strubbe J, Schmidt J (1982) The "half and half nail" phenomenon in chronic hemodialysis patients. Dermatologica 164:350.
271. Holzberg M, Walker HK (1984) Terry's nails: revised definition and new correlations. Lancet 1:896.
272. Samman PD, White WF (1964) The "yellow nail" syndrome. Br J Dermatol 76:153.

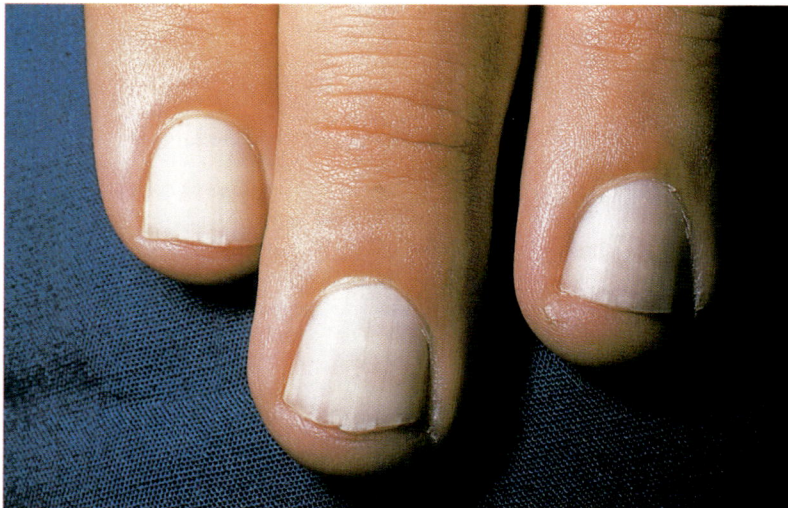

Fig. 12.26   Hereditary total leukonychia.

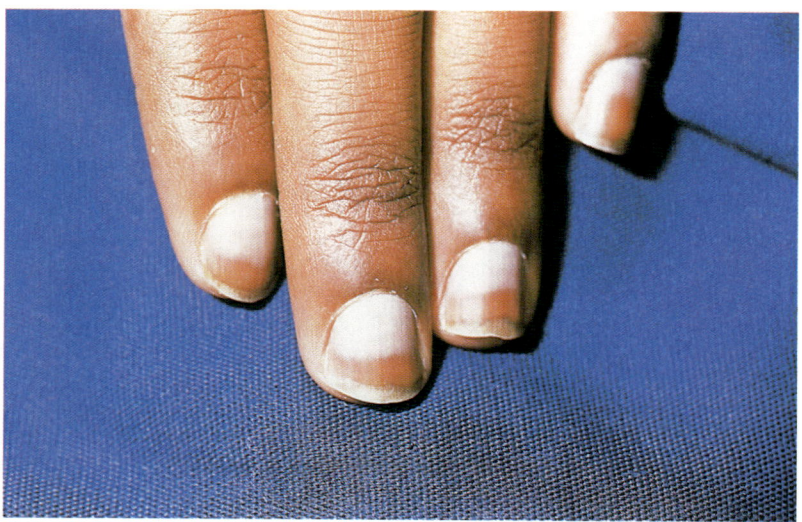

Fig. 12.27   Partial leukonychia similar to that of half-and-half or Lindsey's.

TABLE 12.11	Selected causes of nail dyschromia that may appear in children
Black	Nevocellular nevi or melanoma (long streaks)
	Doxorubicin
	Cyclophosphamide
	Saprophytic onychomycoses
Brown	Anthralin
	Nail enamel and hardeners
	Fetal hydantoin syndrome
	Sulfonamides Actinomycin D (transverse bands)
	Cyclophosphamide
	Doxorubicin
	Adrenal diseases (total or bandlike configuration)
	Nevocellular nevi
	Peutz–Jegher's syndrome
	Ketoconazole
	Normal racial pigmentation
	Pregnancy
Yellow	Nail enamel and hardeners
	Carotene
	Tetracycline (fluorescent)
	Onychomycosis (dermatophytes and others)
	Hyperbilirubinemia
	Penicillamine
	Iodohydroxychloroquin (Vioform)
Blue or blue-gray	Ink
	Minocycline
	Phenophthalein (laxatives)
	Phenothiazines
	Antimalarial agents
	Bleomycin
	Wilson's disease
	Argyria (azure lunulae)
	Congenital pernicious anemia
Green	*Aspergillus*
	Epidermophyton floccosum
	Pseudomonas (fluorescent)
Red/purple	Carbon monoxide
	Glomus tumors (painful)
	Angiomas
	Enchondromas

chylothorax was also reported in association with maternal yellow nail syndrome.[273] The pathogenesis of yellow nail syndrome is unclear, but it is known that nail growth rate in these patients is very slow (less than 0.2mm/week). Yellow nail syndrome persists throughout life, with very few patients reporting spontaneous improvement. There is now increasing clinical evidence that high-dose vitamin E restores the normal growth rate of affected nails and reduces the pigmentation after several months of therapy. The mechanism is unclear, but it is hypothesized that as an antioxidant, vitamin E blocks the production of a lipofuscin pigment deposited in the nail plate.[274] Topical vitamin E is also reportedly beneficial.[275] Yellow nail syndrome has not been described in patients with acrodermatitis enteropathica, but there has been improvement in one case with zinc supplementation.[276] Interestingly, zinc may also act as an antioxidant in some enzyme systems, similar to vitamin E. Itraconazole or fluconazole have been observed to increase the growth rate

of nail plates in yellow nail syndrome, even though onychomycosis was not documented (Baran R., Br J Dermatol, in press).

Longitudinal pigmented bands

Longitudinal pigmented bands may be due to bacterial pigment from Gram-negative organisms, mycotic pigment from Aspergillus, Exophiala, Alternaria or other saprophytic organisms, subungual hematomas, or melanin from melanocytic proliferations of the nail matrix or bed (Fig. 12.28).[277] In Caucasians and less pigmented racial groups, great anxiety develops when a single streak develops because of the concern that it may represent an early subungual melanoma. The likelihood of this in a child is extremely remote, but a few cases have been reported.[278,279]

Longitudinal pigmented bands from melanocytic lesions may be congenital or acquired.[280–282] Isolated lesions occur in 2.5% of black infants and in up

273. Govaert P, Leroy JG, Pauwels R et al. (1992) Perinatal manifestation of maternal yellow nail syndrome. **Pediatr** 89:1016.
274. Norton L (1985) Further observations on the yellow nail syndrome with therapeutic effects of oral alpha-tochopherol. **Cutis** 36:457.
275. Williams HC, Buffham R, DuVivier A (1991) Successful use of topical vitamin E solution in the treatment of nail changes in yellow nail syndrome. **Arch Dermatol** 127:1023.
276. Arroyo JF, Cohen ML (1993) Improvement of yellow nail syndrome with oral zinc supplementation. **Clin Exp Dermatol** 18:62.
277. Haneke E, Baran R (2001) Longitudinal melanonychia. **Dermatol Surg** 27:580–584.
278. Lyall D (1967) Malignant melanoma in infancy. **JAMA** 202:93.
279. Kiryu H (1998) Malignant melanoma in situ arising in the nail unit of a child. **J Dermatol** 25:41–44.
280. Goettmann-Bonvallot S, André J, Bélaïch S (1999) Longitudinal melanonychia in children: A clinical and histopathological study of 40 cases. **J Am Acad Dermatol** 41:17–22.
281. Wong DE, Brodkin R, Rickeert R, McFalls SG (1991) Congenital melanonychia. **Int J Dermatol** 30:278–280.
282. Libow LF, Casey TJ, Varela CD (1995) Congenital subungual nevus in a black infant. **Cutis** 56:154–156.

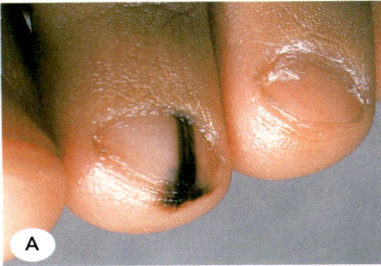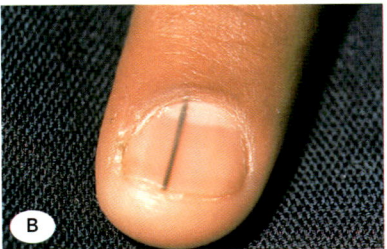

Fig. 12.28   Longitudinal pigmented bands of pigmented nevi. (Courtesy of Dr. Arthur Rhodes.)

to 23% of Oriental infants.[283,284] Their appearance in white patients is very unusual. Benign melanocytic hyperplasias are tan to dark brown in color and may have sharp or ill-defined borders. Measurements from one to several millimeters in width are not uncommon. Interestingly, some benign longitudinal pigmented bands, like common nevi, may regress with time.[285,286] Malignant melanoma of the nail in childhood is very rare.[287,288] The longitudinal streak is black and frequently associated with eczematous paronychia. It should be suspected on a lesion of a single digit when a stable brown streak suddenly becomes darker or wider (greater than 5mm); when the edges become blurred; or if the child has dysplastic nevi and comes from a family with inherited melanoma.[289] In the past, Hutchinson's sign, or "bleeding" of pigment onto the proximal nail fold and cuticle was accepted as pathognomonic of melanoma. However, Hutchinson's sign has been observed with acquired benign and congenital nevocellular nevi and is nonspecific. Many dermatologists believe that any acquired black nail band, especially in a white patient, should be excised for pathologic examination. However, a nail biopsy may lead to significant postoperative deformity and should be performed when there is concordance between several consultants and the lesion is unstable.[290] Multiple pigmented bands are characteristic of Addison's or Cushing's disease, Peutz–Jegher's syndrome, pernicious anemia, or Laugier–Hunziker's syndrome (reported only in adults).[291] They have also been described in patients with AIDS and those HIV-positive individuals taking AZT (zidovudine).[292,293]

Ingrown nails

Ingrown nails are a common problem during infancy and childhood. There are four clinical presentations. Infants may be born with congenital hypertrophic lateral nail folds of the hallux or develop distal embedding with a normally directed nail. The former presents as a firm, red swelling of the lateral nail fold that enlarges progressively.[294] It can resemble recurrent digital fibroma when the lateral soft tissue overgrowth is massive, and tenderness may develop if it persists when the child begins to walk.[295] In general, congenital hypertrophic lateral nail fold of the hallux disappears spontaneously after several months.[296] Congenital hypertrophy of the distal soft tissue of the phalanx may produce a prominent ridge that prevents the free margin of the nail plate from

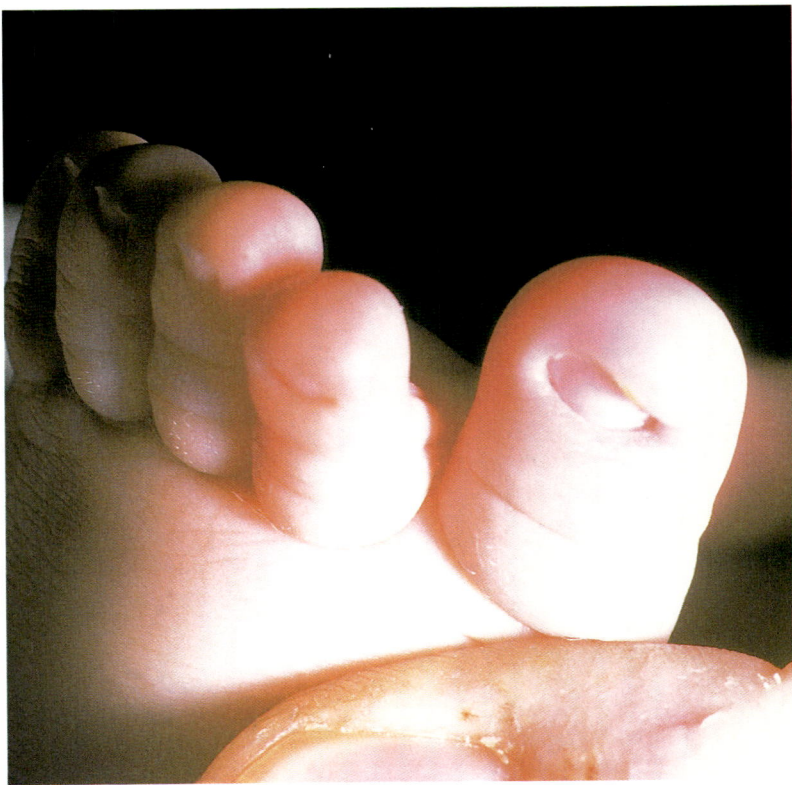

Fig. 12.29   Pseudo ingrown toenail of the newborn.

growing normally. It may be aggravated by bicycling movements when sleeping prone or wearing tight shoes (Fig. 12.29). Severe paronychia has been reported in a few cases.[297] However, some dermatologists believe that this form is a variation of normal development since it, too, has been observed in up to 13% of normal infants and has a tendency towards spontaneous resolution.[298] Distal-lateral nail embedding is a third type of ingrown nail that occurs in toenails and fingernails. It most likely results from uneven cutting or tearing of the nail plate or onychophagia with subsequent growth of the plate into an injured lateral nail fold. Left untreated, ingrown nails can become very painful, as induration and exuberant granulation tissue form around the edge of the embedded plate. Complications of ingrown nails include paronychia (see below) and recurrent blistering dactylitis.[299] Therapy includes silver nitrate cauterization of granulation tissue, adjunctive treatment of inflammation and paronychia with steroid solutions, and oral antibiotics. Surgical removal of entrapped portions of the nail plate or total ungual avulsion may be necessary, but frequently results in a high recurrence rate.[300] Partial nail avulsion to allow phenol cautery of the lateral horn of the nail

283. Higashi N, Saito T (1969) Horizontal distribution of the DOPA positive melanocytes in the nail matrix. **J Invest Dermatol** 53:163.
284. Wong DE, Brodkin RH, Rickert RR, McFalls SG (1991) Congenital melanonychia. **Int J Dermatol** 30:278.
285. Kikuchi I, Inoue S, Sakaguchi E, Ono T (1993) Regressing nevoid nail melanosis in childhood. **Dermatol** 186:88.
286. Tosti A, Baran R, Morelli R et al. (1994) Progressive fading of a longitudinal melanonychia due to a nail matrix melanocytic naevus in a child. **Arch Dermatol** 130:1076–1077.
287. Lyall D (1967) Malignant melanoma in infancy. **J Am Med Assoc** 202:93.
288. Kiryu H (1998) Malignant melanoma in situ arising in the nail unit of a child. **J Dermatol** 25:41–44.
289. Kechijian P (1991) Subungual melanoma in situ presenting as longitudinal melanonychia in a patient with familial dysplastic nevi. **J Am Acad Dermatol** 24:159–161.
290. Léauté-Labrèze C, Bioulac-Sage P, Taïeb A (1996) Longitudinal melanonychia in children. A study of eight cases. **Arch Dermatol** 132:167–169.
291. Baran R (1979) Longitudinal melanotic streaks as a clue to Laugier–Hunziker's syndrome. **Arch Dermatol** 115:1448.

292. Gallais V, Lacour JPh, Perrin C et al. (1992) Acral hyperpigmented macules and longitudinal melanonychia in AIDS patients. **Br J Dermatol** 126:387.
293. Daniel CR, Norton LA, Scher RK (1992) The spectrum of nail disease in patients with human immunodeficiency virus infection. **J Am Acad Dermatol** 27:93.
294. Hammerton MD, Shrank AB (1988) Congenital hypertrophy of the lateral nail folds of the hallux. **Pediatr Dermatol** 5:243–245.
295. Marinet C, Pascal M, Civatte J et al. (1984) Bourrelet latéro-unguéal du gros orteil du nourisson. **Ann dermatol Venereol** 111:731–733.
296. Piraccini BM, Parente GL, Varotti E, Tosti A (2000) Congenital hypertrophy of the lateral nail folds of the hallux: clinical features and follow-up of seven cases. **Pediatr Dermatol** 17:348–351.
297. Bentley-Phillips P, Cole I (1983) Ingrowing toenails of infancy. **Int J Dermatol** 22:115.
298. Honig PJ, Spitzer A, Bernstein R, Leyden JJ (1982) Congenital ingrown toenails. Clinical significance. **Clin Pediatr** 21:424.
299. Telfer NR, Barth JH, Dawber RPR (1989) Recurrent blistering dactylitis of the great toe associated with an ingrown nail. **Clin Exp Dermatol** 14:380.
300. Robb JE (1982) Surgical treatment of ingrowing toenails in infancy and childhood. **Z Kinderchir** 36:63.

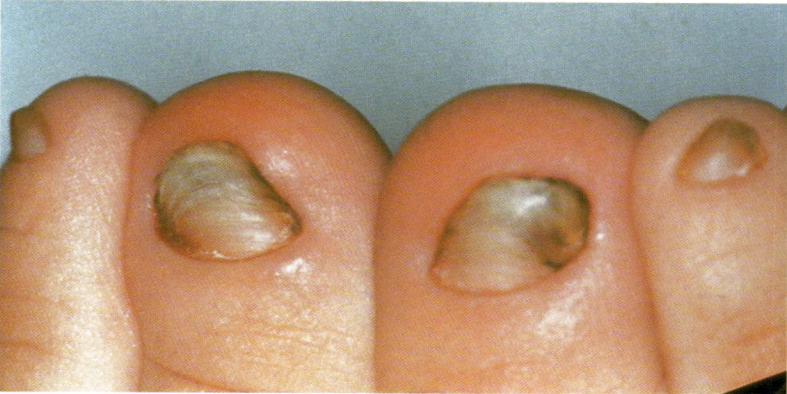

Fig. 12.30 Congenital malalignment of the great toenail is characterized by lateral deviation of the nail plate relative to the axis of the hallux.

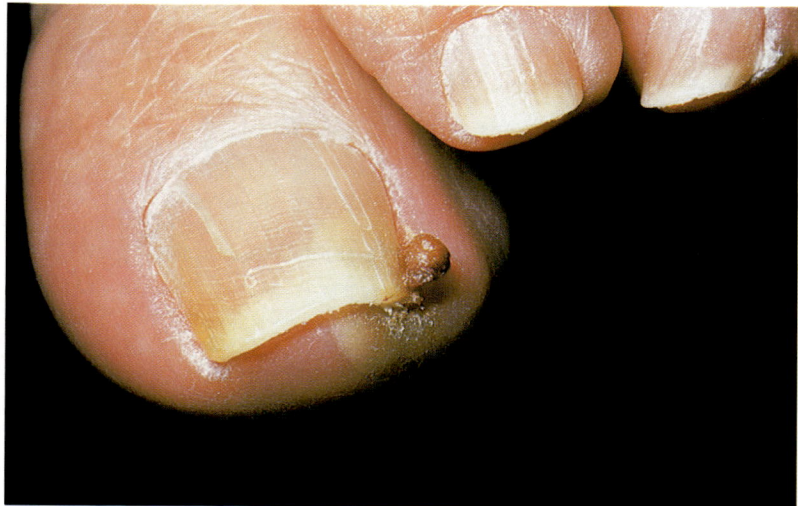

Fig. 12.31 Paronychia secondary to an ingrown nail.

matrix is an effective procedure. Subungual packing of the involved nail fold with a sterile cotton collodion insert may be all that is needed in uncomplicated cases while waiting for growth of the distal free edge of the nail plate to progress beyond the hyponychium.[301,302]

Congenital malalignment of the great toenails was recognized as a distinct clinical entity by Samman in 1978 and popularized by Baran *et al.* in 1979.[303,304] The main characteristic of this condition is lateral deviation of the nail plate with respect to the longitudinal axis of the distal phalanx (Fig. 12.30). Recent evidence suggests that there is traction on the nail unit by a thickened dorsal expansion of the lateral ligament at the distal interphalangeal joint. This may be demonstrated on MRI and results in a bulge in the posterolateral corner of the affected nail. Malalignment predisposes the child to ingrown nails and paronychia.[305,306] One case of a malaligned fingernail has been reported as well.[307] The earliest sign of this condition is transverse ridging that forms regular waves. These represent multiple Beau's lines from recurrent episodes of damage to the matrix. The nail plate may be thickened with gradual tapering towards the distal free edge. It may also take on hues of gray, brown, or green depending on the presence of hemorrhage or colonization with microorganisms. Congenital malalignment of the great toenails is inherited as an autosomal-dominant trait and has been reported in monozygotic twins.[308–310] It may be unilateral or bilateral, and the degree of deformity and disability is quite variable. When severe or recurrent ingrown nails or paronychia supervene, surgical correction should be considered. However, in the absence of marked deviations and complications, one may wait for spontaneous improvement that has been reported in up to 50% of patients before 10 years of age.[311]

Paronychia

Paronychia may follow ingrown nails (Fig. 12.31), but this infection of periungual tissues more commonly results from sucking of the thumb and fingers.[312] Paronychia is characterized by painful erythematous induration of the proximal or lateral nail folds with wet glistening or dry fissured surfaces. The cuticle may be obliterated and nail folds rounded, retracted, and replaced by granulation tissue. Purulent material may be expressed (sterilely) from under the folds, giving relief to the patient. Inflammation of the proximal nail fold may be intense enough to affect the growth of the underlying matrix, resulting in wavy undulation of the nail plate surface. Frequent sucking may also lead to chipping and brittleness of the dystrophic nail plate.

Finger sucking or mouthing objects in general is a normal developmental response.[313] Even at birth, suction blisters measuring up to 1.5cm in diameter may be found on the distal phalanges.[314] These isolated blisters with clear fluid are sterile, but Tzanck and KOH preparations should be performed in order to rule out herpetic or candida infections. Epidemics of inflammatory pustules in the subungual tissues and hyponychium in some nurseries have been attributed to *Veillonella*, small anaerobic, Gram-negative cocci that are nonpathogenic flora of the vaginal vault.[315] Other organisms, including *Fusibacterium*, *Staphylococcus*, *Streptococcus*, and *Candida*, should be expected when paronychia arises from mouthing that occurs regularly during the first months of life.

Toddlers who suck their fingers or thumb almost always have Candida isolated from their nail folds. Trauma to the proximal nail fold disrupts the adherent bond between the cuticle and nail plate. Saliva accumulates in the sulcus, and invading organisms readily proliferate in the moist protected environment (Fig. 12.32).[316] If multiple fingers or digits on both hands and feet are involved, predisposing diseases such as hypoparathyroidism, acrodermatitis enteropathica, biotin-responsive multiple carboxylase deficiency, chronic mucocutaneous candidiasis, or immunodeficiency disorders should be considered. Paronychia from ingrown toenails is frequently due to Pseudomonas or other Gram-negative organisms. Blistering distal dactylitis is a well described common infection with Group A beta-hemolytic streptococcus, or more recently, *Staphylococcus aureus*.[317,318] It too may be associated with paronychia and onychodystrophy. The organism that causes cat scratch disease, *Bartonella henselae*, has also been implicated as a cause of paronychia in one patient who was bitten by a cat.[319]

301. Ilfeld FW (1991) Ingrown toenail treated with cotton collodion insert. **Foot and Ankle** 11:312.
302. Connolly B, Fitzgerald RJ (1988) Pledgets in ingrowing toenails. **Arch Dis Child** 63:71–72.
303. Samman PD (1978) Great toe nail dystrophy. **Clin Exp Dermatol** 3:81–82.
304. Baran R, Bureau H, Sayag J (1979) Congenital malalignment of the big toe nail. **Clin Exp Dermatol** 4:359–360.
305. Baran R, Bureau H (1983) Congenital malalignment of the big toe-nail as a cause of ingrowing toe-nail in infancy. Pathology and treatment (a study of 30 cases). **Clin Exp Dermatol** 8:619–623.
306. Baile FB, Evans DM (1978) Ingrowing toenails in infancy. **Br Med J** 2:737.
307. Murray SC, Dawber RPR, Khumalo N (2001) Congenital malalignment of the left index fingernail. **Br J Dermatol** 144:901–902.
308. Harper KJ, Beer WE (1986) Congenital malalignment of the great toe-nails – an inherited condition. **Clin Exp Dermatol** 11:514–516.
309. Cohen PR (1991) Congenital malalignment of the great toenails: Case report and literature review. **Pediatr Dermatol** 8:43–45.
310. Barth JH, Dawber RPR, Ashton RE et al. (1986) Congenital malalignment of the great toenails in two sets of monozygotic twins. **Arch Dermatol** 122:379–380.
311. Handfields-Jones SE, Harman RRM (1988) Spontaneous improvement of the congenital malalignment of the great toe nails. **Br J Dermatol** 118:305–306.
312. Stone OJ, Mullins JF (1968) Chronic paronychia in children. **Clin Pediatr** 7:104.
313. Brazelton TB (1984) Infant thumb-sucking. (Letter.) **J Am Med Assoc** 252:945.
314. Murphy WF, Langley AL (1963) Common bullous lesions, presumably self-inflicted, occurring in utero in the newborn infant. **Pediatrics** 32:1099.
315. Sinniah D, Sandeford BR, Dugdale AE (1972) Subungual infection in the newborn. An institutional outbreak of unknown etiology, possibly due to Viellonella. **Clin Pediatr** 11:690.
316. Wilson JW (1965) Paronychia and onycholysis, etiology and therapy. **Arch Dermatol** 92:726.
317. McCray MK, Esterly NB (1981) Blistering distal dactylitis. **J Am Acad Dermatol** 5:592–594.
318. Woroszylski A, Durn C, Tamayo L (1996) Staphylococcal blistering dactylitis: report of two patients. **Pediatr Dermatol** 13:292–293.
319. Sander A, Frank B (1997) Paronychia caused by Bartonella henselae. **Lancet** 350:1078.

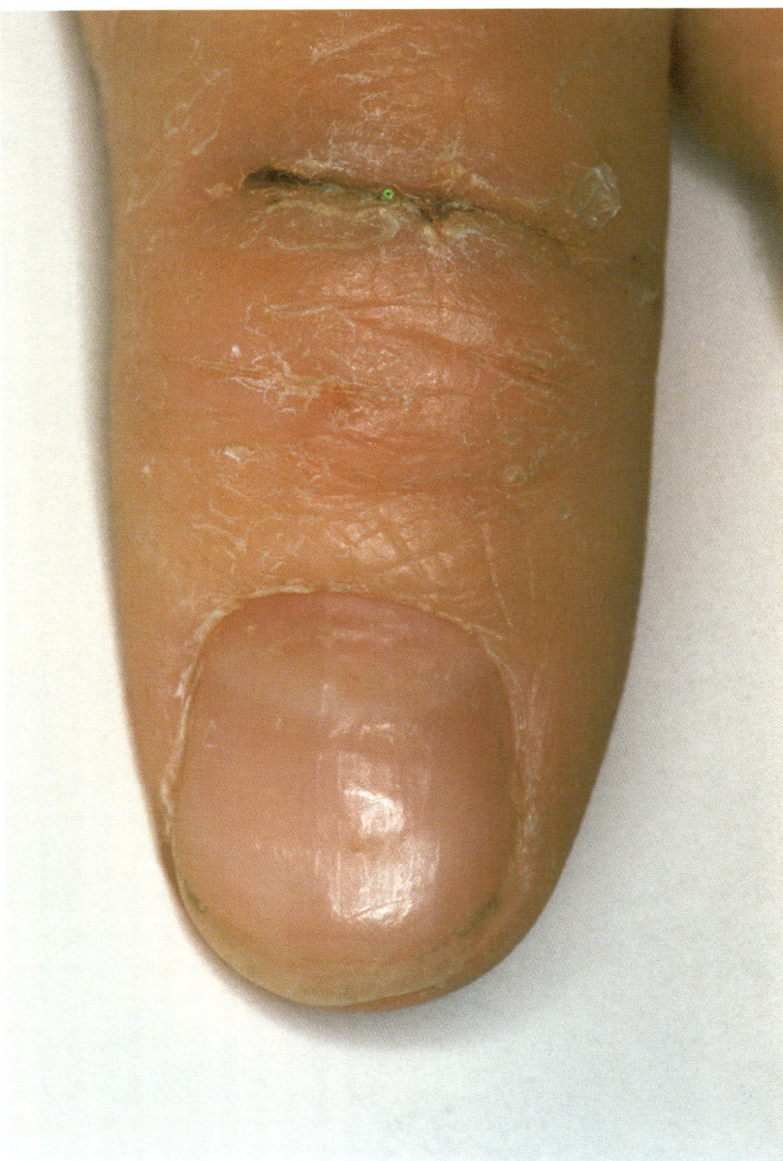

Fig. 12.32 Absence of the cuticle and nail deformity associated with chronic finger sucking.

The treatment of paronychia is difficult as long as predisposing moisture from sucking or mouthing exists. Drops of 4% thymol in chloroform placed in the nail folds will dry out the moist areas. Applications of clotrimazole or sulconizole solution several times daily may be beneficial when Candida is suspected. Successful treatment may be obtained with topical clindamycin solution, too. This acne preparation has a bitter taste that discourages sucking, an alcohol-propylene glycol vehicle that dries out the nail folds, and clindamicin that is active against many secondary bacterial invaders. Side effects from oral absorption of small amounts of these preparations have not been reported, and the comparative efficacy of these therapeutic regimens has not been investigated. Aversive taste treatment of finger and thumb sucking may be beneficial.[320] Reassurance of parents about the transient nature of finger sucking is most important.

Nail biting

It has been estimated that 23% of preschool children bite their nails.[321] In this age group, short periods of onychophagia may be considered to be a normal developmental phase. The incidence of nail biting rises from 28% to 33% of seven- to ten-year-olds.[322] The incidence increases to 45% during adolescence and diminishes thereafter. Frequently, biting is familial. Anxiety and stress from parental disharmony, sibling rivalry, peer rejection, boredom, or overcrowded living conditions accentuate the behavior. Nail biting may also result from poorly manicured nails.

Onychophagia (nail biting) predisposes to ingrown nails and paronychia. It may be a sign of pathology, as in Lesch–Nyhan syndrome, or onychotillomania (a delusional or obsessive-compulsive disorder).[323] In addition, the activity is a means by which warts or other infectious diseases are spread (Fig. 12.33).[324] It is not uncommon that herpetic whitlow begins in this fashion. Dental problems from nail biting are also of concern.[325] Rarely, onychophagia may result in osteomyelitis of the underlying distal phalanx.[326,327]

In older children, application of colored nail polish highlights the damage caused by biting and may serve to heighten awareness of the activity, thus making it consciously unpleasant for the patient to perform. Punishment, ridicule, or nagging are counterproductive and may compound the problem with a more serious psychological disorder. Relaxation-imagery techniques or medications for obsessive-compulsive disorders may also be useful. The approach to young children should be one of distraction from the activity. A hug or compliment for not biting during an anxiety-provoking situation is also preferable. Precipitating stresses should be minimized if possible.

Dactylitis

Dactylitis is an inflammatory condition of the fingers and toes characterized by a bright crimson red color. Unlike simple paronychia, the inflammatory component extends beyond the nail unit. Dactylitis of the distal phalynx may begin as primary nail pathology or result from systemic disease or chemical injury (Table 12.12).[328,329] The former usually presents with involvment of a single digit, while the latter most frequently involves multiple digits.

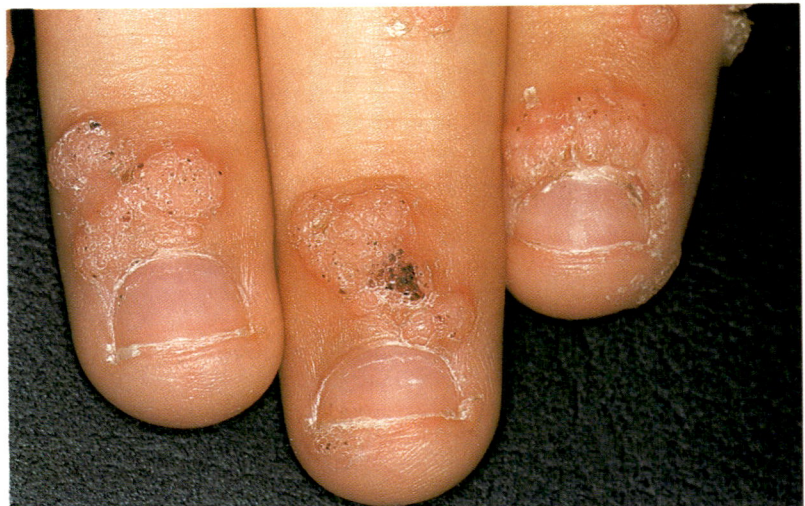

Fig. 12.33 Onychophagia causing periungual; dissemination of wart virus.

320. Friman PC, Barone WJ, Christophersen ER (1986) Aversive taste treatment of finger and thumb sucking. **Pediatr** 78:174.
321. Foster LG (1998) Nervous habits and stereotyped behavior in preschool children. **J Am Acad Child Adolesc Psychiatry** 37:711–717.
322. Leung AKC, Robson WLM (1990) Nailbiting. **Clin Pediatr** 29:690.
323. Colver G (1987) Onychotillomania. **Br J Dermatol** 117:397–402.
324. Tosti A, Piraccini BM (2001) Warts of the nail unit: surgical and nonsurgical approaches. **Dermatol Surg** 27:235–239.
325. Vogel LD (1998) When children put their fingers in their mouths. Should parents and dentists care? **N Y State Dent J** Feb; 64:48–53.
326. Waldman BA, Frieden IJ (1990) Osteomyelitis caused by nailbiting. **Pediatr Dermatol** 7:189.
327. Tosti A, Peluso AM, Bardazzi F et al. (1993) Phalangeal osteomyelitis due to nail biting. **Acta Derm Venerol** 74:206–207.
328. Patrizi A, Bardazzi F, Neri I, Fanti PA (1999) Psoriasiform acral dermatitis: A peculiar clinical presentation of psoriasis in children. **Pediatr Dermatol** 16:439–433.
329. Shaw J, Woolf A (1998) Childhood injuries from artificial nail primer cosmetic products. **Arch Pediatr Adolesc Med** 152:41–46.

TABLE 12.12   Dactylitis of childhood

One digit
   With blisters
      Group A, Beta hemolytic strep
      Herpes simplex (multiple loculations)
      Staphylococcus aureus (atopic dermatitis)
   Without blisters
      Pseudomonas (usually toes)
      Hemophilus influenza (sickle cell disease)
      Mycobacteria tuberculosis
      Parakeratosis pustulosa
Multiple digits
   Primary skin disease
      Psoriasis[330]
      Methacrylic acid burns from nail primers[331]
      Allergic contact dermatitis from nail polish
      Veillonella infection of the newborn
   Systemic diseases
      Acrodermatitis enteropathica
      Systemic candidiasis
      Reiter's syndrome
      Dermatomyositis

Parakeratosis pustulosa

Parakeratosis pustulosa is a distinctive form of distal phalangeal dactylitis that is found almost exclusively in children and young infants (Fig. 12.34). Girls outnumber boys 2.5 to 1.[330] Most of the affected individuals are under 5 years of age. The vast majority of cases involve only one digit, usually a finger. Initially, some parents report a few isolated pustules or vesicles close to the free margin of the nail, but this is rarely observed at the time of initial presentation. No organisms have been consistently identified in cultures taken from these cases. Underlying osteomyelitis or systemic diseases are absent. Shortly after the onset, a confluent bright crimson color covers the skin around the nail unit. Eczematoid changes may be prominent at the free margin of the nail and the phalanx may be densely covered with fine scale. A sharp boundary between the affected and normal skin at the interphalangeal joint is characteristic as is hyperkeratosis beneath the nail tip. When the condition has persisted for many weeks, the nail plate becomes deformed and lifted. Chipping, brittleness, and onycholysis may lead to its eventual destruction. This condition is confused most often with tinea ungum, candida or bacterial paronychia. However, systemic antifungal therapy has no effect on the course of the disease that may go on for several years if left untreated. In addition, unlike these disorders, pain and pruritis, or sucking of the affected digit are not prominent features. Histologic findings of parakeratosis pustulosa are consistent with either psoriasis or eczema.[331] Long-term studies suggest that patients with parakeratosis pustulosa do indeed develop psoriasis, atopic dermatitis, or allergic contact dermatitis.[332] In some instances, treatment with twice-daily applications of fluocinonide and clotrimazole solutions for three or more months is helpful. Once the condition resolves, recurrences are rare. It is the author's opinion that considerable confusion still exists among nail experts regarding the nosology of this condition. Continued confusion will occur in the literature because authors may not have differentiated psoriasis limited to the nails and localized eczema from parakeratosis pustulosa.

Onychomycosis

Fungal infections of the nails may be due to Candida species, saprophytes, or dermatophytes. Although Candida is the most common fungus to be associated with periungual and nail changes in infancy, the nail changes may

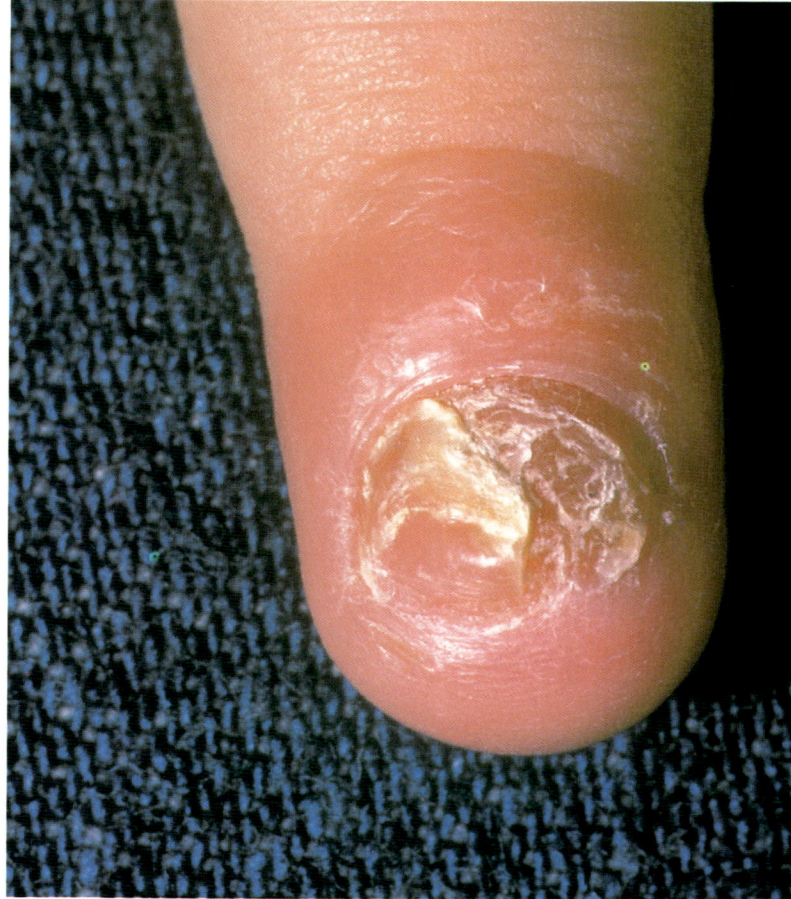

Fig. 12.34   Parakeratosis pustulosa. Well-circumscribed bright erythema and swelling of the distal phalanx associated with destruction of the nail unit.

fail to fulfill the criteria of true nail plate invasion and reproducibility of cultures. In fact, with the exception of Candida paronychia in infancy, onychomycosis is uncommon in childhood. In one North American study of 2500 subjects under the age of 18 visiting a dermatologist for non-fungal disease, the prevalence of onychomycosis was 0.16%. Eleven studies of onychomycosis in children performed in the last 30 years suggest the prevalence of 0.3%.[333] Community rather than office and dermatology-based studies tend to report the lowest figures due to reduced ascertainment bias.[334] Clearly, older children and teenagers are more frequently affected than infants and young children.

Onychomycosis usually presents on the toenails and tends to be associated with concomitant tinea pedis. Adult family members of most children with onychomycosis of the toenails will also have tinea infection.[335] Patients with Down's syndrome, and those with immunodeficiency from chemotherapy, HIV or any cause are also at high risk for onychomycosis. When tinea of the fingernails is present, one should examine the child for tinea capitis.

Onychomycosis has several distinct clinical appearances that can be based on the location of invasion of the nail plate. Distal subungual onychomycosis is the most common and is primarily due to infection with *Trichophyton rubrum* that is acquired from parents. The organisms in these cases will invade under the distal free edge of the nail and will produce onycholysis and subungual debris. Culture or potassium hydroxide examination of the subungual debris collected with a serrated 00 curette will confirm the

330. Hjorth N, Thomsen K (1967) Parakeratosis pustulosa. **Br J Dermatol** 79:527–532.
331. Dulanto F, Armijo-Moreno M, Camacho-Martinez F (1974) Parakeratosis pustulosa: Histological findings. **Acta Dermato-venereol** 54:365–367.
332. Tosti A Peluso AM, Zucchelli V (1998) Clinical features and long term follow-up of 20 cases of parakeratosis pustulosa. **Pediatr Dermatol** 15:259–263.

333. Gupta AK, Chang P, Del Rosso J et al. (1998) Onychomycosis in children: Prevalence and management. **Pediatr Dermatol** 15:464–471.
334. Heikkilä H, Stubb S (1995) The prevalence of onychomycosis in Finland. **Br J Dermatol** 133:699–703.
335. Chang P, Longman H (1994) Onychomycosis in children. **Int J Dermatol** 33:550–551.

diagnosis and differentiate this presentation from ungual psoriasis. White superficial onychomycosis is frequently due to *Trichophyton mentagrophytes* or Candida species, but *Trichophyton rubrum* has also been reported to cause this appearance in children.[336] In these cases, the organisms directly invade the dorsal nail plate. Specimens for diagnosis can be obtained by scraping off the white portions of the nail plate with a #15 blade. The infected nail plate crumbles and is removed easily, unlike punctate leukonychia which enters into the differential diagnosis of this presentation. Proximal subungual onychomycosis occurs when the cuticle of the proximal nail fold is disrupted and organisms invade into the nail plate above the lunula. Although this form of fungal invasion raises a high degree of suspicion for HIV in adults, there has been only one case reported in a child with HIV.[337,338]

Treatment of dermatophyte onychomycosis in childhood is similar to that in adults, although experience with the newer systemic antifungal agents is limited due to licensing restrictions around the world. Consequently, there is a tendency to use topical therapy such as amorolfine, ciclopirox, or topical imidazoles. These topical agents may be appropriate in limited white superficial onychomycosis, but where the nail plate infection is substantial, treatment with bifonozole-urea is the most effective, topically applied preparation.[339] Griseofulvin is still the drug of choice for onychomycosis worldwide. However, one must make sure the infection is a culture-proven dermatophyte since the medication does not affect candida or saprophytes. There is increasing evidence to support the use of terbinafine,[340] itraconazole,[341] or fluconazole[342] but given the lack of licensed indication and relatively little experience, their optimal dosage schedules and safety in young children is difficult to ascertain at this time.

NAIL BIOPSY AND SURGERY

Human beings invest a great deal of emotional energy in their nails to enhance their appearance for social acceptability. An unsightly nail dystrophy may be devastating to an older child or teenager whose behavioral task is the formation of high self-esteem and body image. Because of this, any surgery or biopsy of a nail provokes high levels of anxiety since they are often perceived as mutilating and extremely painful. Parents project these same feelings onto their young infants as well. Therefore, the clinician must spend a significant amount of time preparing the patient and parents for the procedure to be performed. Anesthesia, preoperative sedation, and post-operative analgesia must be optimal. Most importantly, the procedure should be done for the right reasons, perhaps after several opinions have been obtained.

There are two primary reasons to perform a biopsy or undertake surgery of the nail unit: first, to confirm a diagnosis of serious medical importance (i.e., melanoma), or second, to remove a neoplasm or correct a deformity which may be painful or persistent and life-long. One might also consider biopsy of an inflammatory ungual condition if there are serious potential risks of therapy (i.e., corticosteroids or retinoids). X-rays of the distal phalanx should always be obtained prior to surgery in order to rule out underlying osseous pathology.

When nail surgery is performed, preoperative sedation with valium, midozilam, or chloral hydrate is helpful. The topical anesthetic, EMLA (eutectic mixture of lidocaine and prilocaine) may be applied under occlusion to injection sites one hour prior to administration of a local anesthetic. For biopsies of the proximal or lateral nail folds, a wing block of 1% xylocaine without epinephrine (adrenaline) buffered with 1:10 dilution of sodium bicarbonate is recommended. More extensive surgery that may include nail plate avulsion should be preceeded 20 to 30 minutes by digital block with marcaine or bupivicaine or similar long-acting anesthetic in combination with xylocaine (1:1 dilution). Additional xylocaine may be needed at the hyponychium as well.

The location of pathology in the nail unit determines the type of biopsy to be performed. If the matrix is involved, the width of a biopsy should be no more that 2mm in order to minimize the risk of scarring. After reflecting the proximal nail fold, a well-placed punch biopsy is usually adequate, but longitudinal wedge excision after removal of the nail plate may be necessary to completely delineate a problem. If the nail bed is affected, a 4mm punch biopsy through the plate, followed by a 2.5mm biopsy into the bed may alleviate the need for nail plate avulsion. The reader is directed to texts on nail surgery for more complete descriptions of techniques and instrumentation.[343] For best results, surgery of the nail should be undertaken by clinicians who are comfortable with the techniques and have the opportunity to routinely perform them.[344]

DISEASES OF ECCRINE SWEAT GLANDS

Eccrine sweat glands are tubular coiled structures located at the dermal-subcutaneous junction that exit separately onto the surface of the skin. The total complement of fully developed glands (about two to four million) is present in term infants, although complete functional maturation does not occur until after the neonatal period.[345] The major stimulus for sweat production is elevation of core body temperature. Elevations of skin surface temperature or stimulation of the sympathetic cholinergic fibers that enervate the eccrine gland also elicit a sudorific response. Sympathetic adrenergic fibers are present, but play a minor role in sweat production. The neuropeptides, substance P, vasoactive intestinal peptide, and calcitonin-gene related peptide have also been identified around eccrine glands, but their function remains speculative. A new histologic variant of sweat gland in the axilla, called the apoeccrine gland, develops after puberty.[346] Like eccrine glands, apoeccrine glands empty directly onto the skin surface and have similar dual enervation. However, adrenergic and cholinergic stimuli have equivalent responses. Apoeccrine glands are thought to play a major role in axillary hyperhidrosis.

FUNCTIONS OF ECCRINE SWEATING

The major function of sweat is thermoregulatory. Cooling occurs by sweat evaporation off the skin surface. Sweat may also serve as a vehicle for excretion of metabolic byproducts or systemic medications (e.g., griseofulvin). In addition, the relatively large surface area of the eccrine tubular epithelium may be a path for percutaneous absorption of topical medications.[347] Human eccrine sweat has numerous components, including water, electrolytes (Na, K, Cl), urea, lactate, ammonia, immunoglobulins (IgG, IgE), amino acids, epidermal growth factor, and inflammatory mediators (histamine, prostaglandins, and kallikrein), and cytokines (interleukin-1α).[348,349] The participation of organic components of sweat in cutaneous diseases remains speculative. These other components are

336. Ploysangam T, Lucky AW (1997) Childhood white superficial onychomycosis caused by *Trichophyton rubrum*. **J Am Acad Dermatol** 36:29–32.
337. Rongioletti F, Persi A, Tripodi S, Rebora A (1994) Proximal white subungual onychomycosis: a sign of immunodeficiency. **J Am Acad Dermatol** 30:129–130.
338. Pena-Penabad C, Garcia-Silva J, Almagro M et al. (2001) Superficial white onychomycosis in a 3-year-old human immunodeficiency virus-infected child. **J Eur Acad Dermatol Venereol** 15:51–53.
339. Bonifaz A, Ibarra G (2000) Onychomycosis in children: treatment with bifonazole-urea. **Pediatr Dermatol** 17:310–314.
340. Ungpakorn R, Reangchainam S, Kullavanijaya P (1998) Onychomycosis in a 2-year-old child successfully treated with oral terbinafine. **J Am Acad Dermatol** 39:654–655.
341. Huang PH, Paller AS (2000) Itraconazole pulse therapy for dermatophyte onychomycosis in children. **Arch Pediatr Adolesc Med** 154:614–618.
342. Aihara Y, Mor M, Yokota S (1996) Successful treatment of onychomycosis with flucolazole in two patients with hyperimmunoglobulin E syndrome. **Pediatr Dermatol** 13:493–495.
343. Krull EA (2001) Biopsy techniques, In: Nail Surgery, A Text and Atlas, Krull EA, Zook EG, Baran R, Haneke E, eds. Philadelphia: Lippincott Williams & Wilkins, Ch. 3c.
344. Salasche SJ (1990) Surgery. In: Nails: Therapy, Diagnosis, Surgery, Scher RK, Daniel CR, eds. Philadelphia: WB Saunders, p. 258.
345. Green M (1982) Comparison of adult and neonatal eccrine sweating. In: Neonatal Skin Structure and Function, Maibach H, Boisits EK, eds. New York: Marcel Dekker, p. 35.
346. Sato K, Sato F (1987) Sweat secretion by human axillary apocrine sweat gland *in vitro*. **Am J Physiol** 252:R181.
347. Schluplein RJ, Bronaugh RL (1983) Percutaneous absorption. In: Biochemistry and Physiology of the Skin, Goldsmith LA, ed. New York: Oxford University Press, p. 1267.
348. Sato K, Saga KK, Sato KT (1989) Biology of sweat glands and their disorders. I. Normal sweat gland function. **J Am Acad Dermatol** 20:537.
349. Sato K, Sato F (1994) Interleukin-1α in human sweat is functionally active and derived from the eccrine sweat gland. **Am J Physiol** 266:950–959.

implicated in disease states such as atopic dermatitis, xerosis, acanthosis nigricans, and heat stroke. However, elevations of sweat electrolytes (Na and Cl greater than 70mM) measured by pilocarpine iontophoresis are characteristic of cystic fibrosis. This inability of the eccrine duct to reabsorb sodium can result in marked electrolyte loss and heat intolerance in these patients. Thus, the sweat of patients with cystic fibrosis is characteristically salty. Similarly, diabetics in poor control may have sweet sweat from exceeding the tubular reabsorptive capacity for glucose.

ANHIDROSIS

Anhidrosis, the absence of sweating, may result from anatomic defects of the eccrine gland, as in ectodermal dysplasia or scleroderma, and from functional abnormalities that result from insults to the central or peripheral nervous system, such as spinal cord transection, Horner's syndrome, familial sensory neuropathy, and leprosy.[350] The anticholinergic effects of many medications such as antihistamines or tricyclic antidepressants may also produce significant anhidrosis. Air conditioning, cool soaks, light clothing, and a fan may all reduce the likelihood of heat stroke when anhidrosis is present.

HYPERHIDROSIS

Hyperhidrosis, or overreactivity of the eccrine glands, may be generalized or localized to certain body regions.[351] Generalized hyperhidrosis may be associated with emotional outbursts, cocaine abuse, hypoglycemia, shock, pheochromocytoma, thyrotoxicosis, Cushing's syndrome, familial dysautonomia, brain tumors, or defervescence in patients with chronic infections. In these cases, hyperhidrosis is more aptly termed segmental, peripheral, or trunkal. Cases that are related to systemic disease may persist during sleep, unlike those related to emotional stimuli.

Localized hyperhidrosis may be categorized as gustatory, associated with cutaneous disease or idiopathic. Physiologic gustatory hyperhidrosis occurs over the lips, nose and forehead in normal individuals after eating spicy foods. One might speculate that this is related to release of substance P from intraoral exposure to capsaicin. Gustatory sweating associated with underlying pathology is known as Frey's syndrome, and has been reported after salivary gland damage from forceps deliveries, mumps, or other forms of parotitis, and parotid abcess. Sweating in Frey's sydrome is accompanied by flushing in the distribution of the auriculotemporal nerve in response to gustatory and occasionally tactile stimuli. It is frequently misdiagnosed as food allergy, but antihistamines and elimination diets have no effect. Treatment with botulinum toxin A has recently become popular. Some cases will spontaneously resolve.[352] Primary skin disorders associated with localized hyperhidrosis include glomus tumors,[353] blue rubber bleb nevus,[354] POEMS syndrome,[355] pachydermoperiostosis,[356] and eccrine angiomatous hamartoma.[357]

Idiopathic localized hyperhidrosis describes focal areas of sweating that are not associated with underlying abnormalities in other organelles. In some cases there are no histologic differences between the affected area and normal adjacent skin while in others an increased number of eccrine glands is observed. This has also been called nevus sudoriferous or a functional eccrine nevus.[358,359] A starch–iodine test delineates the area of sweat dysfunction. Briefly, iodine solution is applied to the affected area and surrounding normal skin. Starch powder is then sprinkled over the painted surface and blown off. Areas of hyperhidrosis are demonstrated by prominent black dots at the eccrine pores. Treatment of eccrine nevi with topical anticholinergic creams has reportedly been successful. Recently, intralesional botulinum toxin A and topical 0.5% clonazepan have been used to control symptoms, too.[360,361]

Palmoplantar hyperhidrosis, which occurs quite frequently in children, may be so severe that sweat drips from the fingertips or soaks through shoes. Not only is it socially stigmatizing, but it may impede writing, playing musical instruments, driving a car, or have significant occupational repercussions. Hyperhidrosis may be an aggravating factor in juvenile plantar dermatosis or Weber–Cockayne epidermolysis bullosa. The topical anticholinergic agents, formaldehyde, and glutaraldehyde reduce sweating; however, side effects have limited their use. Powders such as cornstarch may be temporarily beneficial. Solutions containing 20% aluminum chloride applied at least two hours after bathing and occluded overnight for two or more consecutive evenings are effective for several days at a time.[362]

The use of oral anticholinergic agents is usually limited by side effects such as drowsiness, flushing, and tachycardia, as well as their contraindication in asthmatic patients. However, low doses of glycopyrrolate, 1–3mg po qd or propantheline bromide, 15mg hs may give some affected individuals adequate relief from symptoms.[363] Small doses of clonazepam may also be useful.[364] Tap water iontophoresis is probably the most effective, noninvasive method for controlling localized palmoplantar hyperhidrosis. A simple, portable, battery-operated delivery system, has been effective after as few as 10 daily 30-minute treatments.[365] Symptomatic relief can be maintained with repeated sessions once every two weeks. It is thought that iontophoresis produces strong acidity from the generation of hydrogen ions within the sweat duct.[366] This results in leakiness of the sweat duct and sweat recycling that results in occlusion and collapse of the sweat pore lumen. Complaints of stinging from this device can be overcome by a thin application of petrolatum. Botulinum toxin blocks the release of acetylcholine from presynaptic terminals of the neuromuscular junction.[367] Injection of small doses of botulinum toxin A into the dermis irreversibly inhibits sympathetic cholinergic production of sweating. Depending on the technique used, injections into the palms, soles or axillae can normalize the hyperhidrotic state for periods of four to nine months.[368–372] Nerve regrowth has been presumed to explain the transient nature of the improvement. Complaints such as localized muscle weakness

350. Sato K, Kang WH, Saga K, Sato KT (1989) Biology of sweat glands and their disorders.II. Disorders of sweat gland function. **J Am Acad Dermatol** 20:713.

351. Sato K, Kang WH, Saga K, Sato KT (1989) Biology of sweat glands and their disorders.II. Disorders of sweat gland function. **J Am Acad Dermatol** 20:713.

352. Rodriguez-Serna M, Marí, Aliaga A (2000) What syndrome is this? Auriculotemporal nerve (Frey's) syndrome. **Pediatr Dermatol** 17:415–416.

353. Cooke SAR (1971) Misleading features in the clinical diagnosis of the peripheral glomus tumors. **Br J Surg** 58:602.

354. Fine RM, Derbes VJ, Clark WH (1961) Blue rubber bleb nevus. **Arch Dermatol** 84:802–805.

355. Kanitakis J, Roger H, Soubrier M et al. (1988) Cutaneous angiomas in POEMS syndrome. **Arch Dermatol** 124:695–698.

356. Sirinavin C, Buist NR, Mokkhaves P (1982) Digital clubbing, hyperhidrosis, acroosteolysis and osteoporosis. A case resembling pachydermoperiostosis. **Clin Genet** 22:83.

357. Morrell DS, Ghali F, Stahr BJ, McCauliff DP (2001) Eccrine angiomatous hamartoma: A report of symmetric and painful lesions of the wrists. **Pediatr Dermatol** 18:117–119.

358. Ghali FE, Fine J-D (2000) Idiopathic localized unilateral hyperhidrosis in a child. **Pediatr Dermatol** 17:25–28.

359. Lorette G, Vaillant L, Grangeponte MC et al. (2000) Localized paroxysmal hyperhidrosis. **Pediatr Dermatol** 17:328–329.

360. Kreyden OP, Schmid-Grendelmeier P, Burg G (2001) Idiopathic localized unilateral hyperhidrosis. Case report of successful treatment with botulinum toxin type A and review of the literature. **Arch Dermatol** 137:1622–1625.

361. Seukeran DC, Highet AS (1998) The use of topical glycopyrrolate in the treatment of hyperhidrosis. **Clin Exp Dermatol** 23:204–205.

362. Sato K, Kang WH, Saga K, Sato KT (1989) Biology of sweat glands and their disorders.II. Disorders of sweat gland function. **J Am Acad Dermatol** 20:713.

363. Shelly WB, Shelly DE (2001) Hyperhidrosis, In: Advanced Dermatologic Therapy II. Philadelphia: WB Saunders, pp. 562–570.

364. Takase Y, Tsushimi K, Yamamato KY (1992) Unilateral localized hyperhidrosis responding to treatment with clonazepam. **Br J Dermatol** 126:416.

365. Arndt K (1983) Manual of Dermatologic Therapeutics with Essentials of Diagnosis, 3rd ed. Boston: Little Brown, p. 286.

366. Sato K, Timm DE, Sato F et al. (1993) Generation and transit pathway of H+ is critical for inhibition of palmar sweating by iontophoresis in water. **J Appl Physiol** 75:2258–2264.

367. Huang W, Foster JA, Rogachefsky AS (2000) Pharmacology of botulinum toxin. **J Am Acad Dermatol** 249–259.

368. Solomon Ba, Hayman R (2000) Botulinum toxin type A therapy for palmar and digital hyperhidrosis. **J Am Acad Dermatol** 42:1026–1029.

369. Naumann M, Hofmann U, Bergmann I et al. (1998) Focal hyperhidrosis. Effective treatment with intracutaneous botulinum toxin. **Arch Dermatol** 134:301–304.

370. Naumann M, Lowe NJ (2000) Botulinum toxin type A in treatment of bilateral primary axillary hyperhidrosis: randomized, parallel group, double blind, placebo controlled trial. **Br Med J** 323:596–599.

371. Schnider P, Moraru E, Kittler H et al. (2001) Treatment of focal hyperhidrosis with botulinum toxin type A: long-term follow-up in 61 patients. **Br J Dermatol** 145:289–293.

372. Swartling C, Naver H, Lindberg M (2001) Botulinum A toxin improves life quality in severe primary focal hyperhidrosis. **Eur J Neurol** 8:247–252.

occur in about 10% of patients when the dose of medication is too high or it is injected too deeply. In addition, the pain of injection has made the procedure difficult to administer without nerve blocks or general anesthesia, especially in children.

Axillary hyperhidrosis may be reduced with surgical curettage of the axillary vaults. Its effects are more long-lasting than injections but there are more reported complications from the procedure.[373] Finally, the most aggressive treatment for palmoplatar hyperhidrosis is transthoracic endoscopic sympathectomy.[374] Under brief general anesthesia administered as an out-patient, the sympathetic chain is bisected at the T_2–T_3 level. Over 90% of patients have satisfactory sweat inhibition. Significant complications are very uncommon and include Horner's syndrome, bradycardia requiring a cardiac pacemaker, and, rarely, postoperative pneumothorax. The most distressing side effect, though, is compensatory perspiration on other areas of the body such as the chest and legs and face, which can occur in over half of patients.[375]

ECCRINE BROMHIDROSIS

Eccrine bromhidrosis is a foul-smelling condition produced when cutaneous microbial flora transform components of excessive stratum corneum softened by sweat to volatile metabolic byproducts. It also may have a metabolic or exogenous basis.[376] The intensity of an odor correlates with population density of bacteria and the types of exoenzymes (proteases or lipases) they produce.[377] Bromhidrosis occurs most frequently in untreated or poorly controlled hyperkeratotic conditions such as exfoliative erythroderma of atopic dermatitis, psoriasis, lamellar icthyosis, hyperkeratosis palmaris et plantaris, or pitted keratolysis. Treatment of bromhidrosis from generalized or localized hyperkeratotic consists of keratolytic agents such as 10% to 40% salicylic acid in petrolatum with overnight occlusion, followed by bacteriostatic washes (chlorhexidine) or topical antibiotics (clindamicin or erythromycin). Topical metronidazol may also be useful for treatment of malodorous ulcers or skin lesions.[378]

Metabolic eccrine bromhidrosis occurs in patients with specific metabolic diseases. For example, fish odor syndrome (trimethylaminuria) is a characteristic metabolic disease that produces a distinctive odor.[379] It is a rare autosomal-recessive disorder that results from a deficiency of trimethylamine oxidase.[380] This enzyme, whose genetic locus is on chromosome 1p, results in the accumulation of a tertiary amine in urine, sweat and breath. When dietary sources of choline (egg yolk, shellfish, liver, fish, soybeans, and peas) or lecithin are ingested by these patients, the distinctive smell of rotten fish develops. Dietary restriction rapidly corrects the malodor. Consequences of this otherwise benign disorder can result in severe psychological problems, and difficulties with socialization and schooling. Similarly, other syndromes with distinctive body odors are due to other volatile substances that may be controlled by diet in most instances.

Acquired exogenous eccrine bromhidrosis could be a sign of ingestion of a toxin. Children with these odors usually present to emergency facilities with other signs and symptoms (i.e., seizures, obtundation, etc.). Occasionally, acquired bromhidrosis may be the sole manifestation of a putrifying foreign body lodged in the nose or other orifice.[381]

MILIARIA

Miliaria is a benign vesicopustular obstructive disorder which is frightening to parents because of its acute onset and widespread nature. Miliaria crystallina (sudamina) presents as asymptomatic, 1–2mm in diameter noninflammatory vesicles. It may be present at birth[382] or form after sunburn, high fevers, or swathing of neonates during summer months. The superficial nature of the eruption is suggested by the ease with which the vesicles are disrupted. Miliaria rubra is characterized by small, nonfollicular, juicy papules found most commonly in the intertriginous or flexor regions of the body. The papules have a narrow red base and may be confused with folliculitis. Tingly sensations are commonplace (prickly heat). Histologic sections reveal periductal intercellular edema of the epidermis (spongiosis) and, on occasion, an amorphous plug and intraluminal bacteria.[383] Mediators from the surrounding inflammatory infiltrate are probably responsible for the symptoms. Miliaria pustulosa is a variant of miliaria rubra. Miliaria profunda occurs after recurrent attacks of miliaria rubra. This symptomatic eruption of deep-seated firm white papules, pustules, or nodules occurs in tropical climates. The lesions may become extremely large.[384] Histologic sections disclose an intradermal location of the eccrine duct disruption.

NEUTROPHILIC ECCRINE HIDRADENITIS

Neutrophilic eccrine hidradenitis is an inflammatory dermatosis of eccrine sweat glands that develops within several weeks of beginning chemotherapy for treatment of a malignancy.[385] First described by Harrist et al. in 1982, this condition appears as numerous erythematous to violaceous papules, plaques, and pustules that may display central necrosis.[386] Lesions are usually located on the trunk or extremities, but unusual sites such as the ears have also been documented.[387] Biopsy reveals degeneration of eccrine epithelial cells and surrounding neutrophilic leukocytoclasia. Culture for pathogens is invariably negative even thought effected individuals may be febrile. The first cases reported were in patients with acute myelocytic leukemia who received cytarabine and doxorubicin. However, subsequent cases have had Hodgkin's disease or have been treated with other antineoplastic agents such as bleomycin, vinblastine or dacarbazine. Immunocompromised patients and several persons on zidovudine for human immunodeficiency virus infection have also contracted the disorder. Children as young as 3 years of age have been affected. Resolution occurs in two to three weeks. Treatment is symptomatic.

GRANULOSIS RUBRA NASI

Granulosis rubra nasi is a rare papular eruption of the cheeks and nasal bridge first described by Jadassohn in 1901.[388] The eruption is preceded by erythema and intermittent localized hyperhidrosis. Patients with this disorder have been infants and children who sometimes have a family history of hyperhidrosis. The differential diagnosis includes rosacea, lupus erythematosus, and lupus vulgaris. Treatment of acute flares has been unsatisfactory, but several reported cases improved by puberty.

373. Rompel R, Scholz S (2001) Subcutaneous curettage vs. injection of botulinum toxin A for treatment of axillary hyperhidrosis. **J Eur Acad Dermatol Venereol** 15:207–211.
374. Lin T-S (1999) Transthoracic endoscopic sympathectomy for palmar hyperhidrosis in children and adolescents: Analysis of 350 cases. **J Laparoendosc Surg** 9:331–334.
375. Johnson JP, Obasi C, Hahn MS, Glatleider P (1999) Endoscopic thoracic sympathectomy. **J Neurosurg** 91:90–97.
376. Senol M, Fireman P (1999) Body odor in dermatology diagnosis. **Cutis** 63:107–111.
377. Marshall J, Holland KT, Grebbone M (1988) A comparative study of the cutaneous microflora of normal feet with low and high levels of odor. **J Appl Bacteriol** 65:61.
378. Rice TT (1992) Metronidazole use in malodorous skin lesions. **Rehab Nursing** 17:244.
379. Rothchild JG, Hansen RC (1985) Fish odor syndrome: trimethylaminuria with milk as chief dietary factor. **Pediatr Dermatol** 3:38–39.
380. Chen H, Aiello F (1993) Trimethylaminuria in a girl with Prader–Willi syndrome and deletion (15) (q11q13). **Am J Med Genet** 45:335.
381. Lucky AW (1991) Acquired bromhidrosis in an 8-year-old boy secondary to a nasal foreign body. **Arch Dermatol** 129:27.
382. Arpey CJ, Nagashima-Walen LS, Chren MM, Zaim T (1992) Congenital miliaria crystallina: case report and literature review. **Pediatr Dermatol** 9:283.
383. Lever WF, Schaumburg–Lever G (1983) Histopathology of the Skin, 6th ed. Philadelphia: JB Lippincott, p. 102.
384. Rogers M, Kan A, Stapleton K, Kemp A (1990) Giant miliaria profunda. **Pediatr Dermatol** 7:140.
385. Bailey DL, Barron D, Lucky AW (1989) Neutrophilic eccrine hidradenitis: a case report and literature review. **Pediatr Dermatol** 6:33.
386. Harrist TJ, Fine JD, Bergman RS et al. (1982) Neutrophilic eccrine hidradenitis. **Arch Dermatol** 118:263.
387. Ostlere LS, Wills J, Stevens HP et al. (1993) Neutrophilic eccrine hidradenitis with an unusual presentation. **Br J Dermatol** 128:696.
388. Aram H, Mohagheghi AP (1972) Granulosis rubra nasi. **Cutis** 10:463.

DISEASES OF APOCRINE GLANDS

Apocrine glands are localized to the axillary and anogenital regions but are not functional until after puberty. Occasionally, clusters of small nonfunctional glands are found on the scalp, face, and abdomen. Unlike eccrine glands, the secretory portions of apocrine glands are embedded in the panniculus, and the duct in most cases enters into the infundibulum of the pilosebaceous apparatus.[389] Apocrine secretion is under adrenergic control. It does not play any role in thermoregulation. They are instead the source of a distinctive personal odor and are closely related to the scent glands of other animal species. Apocrine secretions have no inherent malodor themselves. They are odorless and sterile until they reach the skin surface, where lipophylic diptheroids, staphylococcal, and streptococcal organisms metabolize the milky fluid to form volatile aromatic substances including androgenic steroid aldehydes, alcohols, and ketones. Combinations of these organic compounds produce unique acrid, musky, sweet, or fetid odor.[390]

APOCRINE BROMHIDROSIS

Apocrine bromhidrosis, also known as osmidrosis, is a malodorous condition of the apocrine glands. It develops after puberty, and is more noticeable in the summer months. There may be a racial and genetic component as well. The compound ε-3-methyl-2-hexenoic acid is liberated from nonodorous apocrine secretions by axillary bacteria.[391] Other substances that include short-chain fatty acids and ammonia also add to body odor. Axillary body odor may be controlled by deodorants.[392] These products contain masking fragrances and antibacterial compounds that reduce odor-causing bacteria. Similar results may be obtained by application of topical antibiotics or washing with antiseptic soap solutions, but irritation may limit their use. Unlike deodorants, which do not affect the flow of sweat, antiperspirants literally block sweat secretion. These aluminum halide compounds have been observed to obstruct the intraepidermal portion of the sweat duct.[393] Initial ductal wall necrosis is followed by plug formation and gradual re-epithelialization over a two to four week period.

APOCRINE CHROMHIDROSIS

Apocrine chromhidrosis or pigmented sweat is an embarrassing problem that occurs in up to 10% of darkly pigmented races.[394] Yellow, blue, or green sweat contains lipofucsin and stains skin and clothing. Chromhidrosis is most common in the axillary vaults, but has been reported on the face and on the areolas.[395,396] The pigment accentuates with Wood's light and can increase with emotional, manual, or pharmacologic stimulation. Differential diagnosis should include ochronosis (alkaptonuria), or external pigment from fungi, paint, hair, or clothing dyes. Pseudochromhidrosis may have the same clinical appearance as true apocrine chromhidrosis.[397] The former is due to pigment production by bacteria that may be identified in cultures, while the latter is due to lipofuscin production in apocrine glands that may be observed in skin biopsies. Treatments of axillary apocrine chromhidrosis are generally unsatisfactory. Topical capsaicin that blocks substance P has been beneficial in two non-axillary cases. Pseudochromhidrosis is successfully treated with topical or systemic antibiotics.

APOCRINE MILIARIA

Apocrine miliaria (Fig. 12.35), or Fox–Fordyce disease, is a chronic pruritic papular eruption of the axillary or pubic regions that develops during adolescence and occurs more frequently in women.[398] Apocrine duct obstruction by keratin debris, surrounding spongiosis, and a dermal inflammatory infiltrate are observed on histopathologic examination. Improvement during the last trimester of pregnancy suggests an endocrine

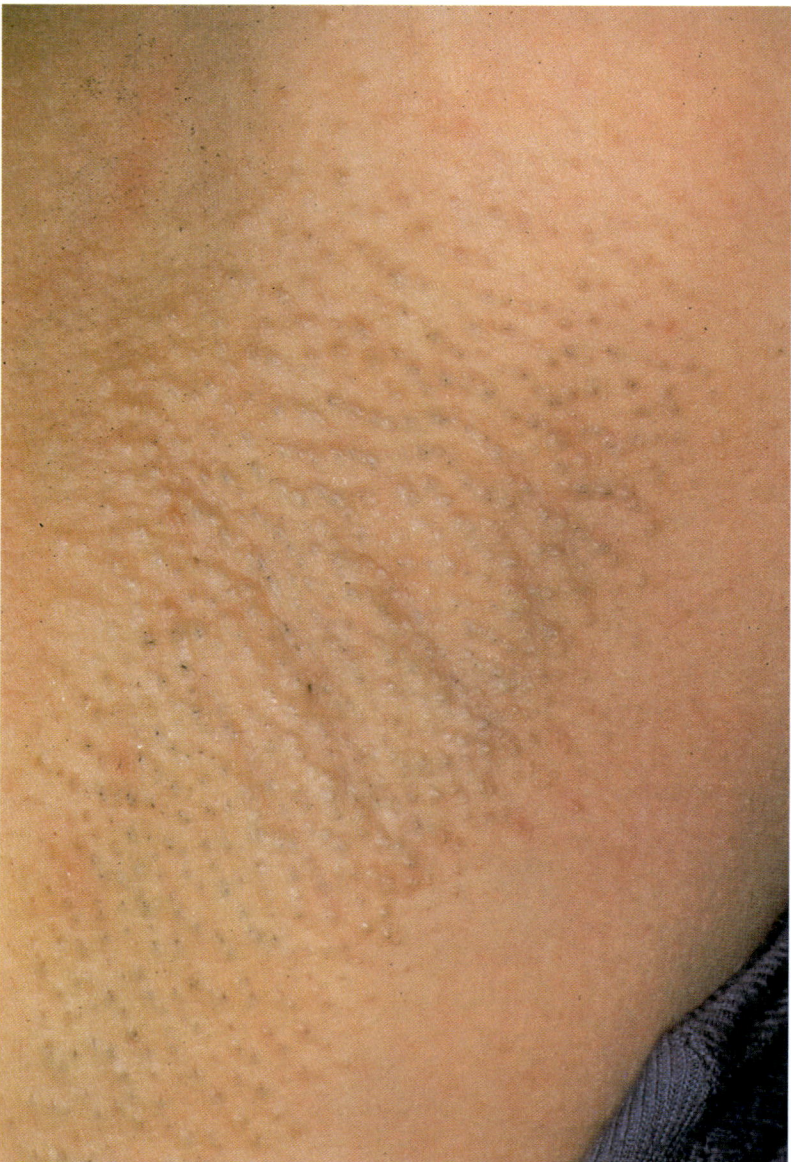

Fig. 12.35 Fox–Fordyce disease.

389. Robertshaw D (1991) Apocrine sweat glands. In: Biochemistry and Molecular Biology of the Skin, 2d ed, vol 1, Goldsmith LA, ed. Oxford, England: Oxford University Press, p. 763.
390. Labows JN, McGinley KJ, Kligman AM (1982) Axillary odor: current status. In: Principles of Cosmetics for the Dermatologist, Frost P, Horowitz SN, eds. St. Louis: CV Mosby, p. 89.
391. Leyden JJ et al. (1981) The microbiology of human axilla and its relationship to axillary odor. **J Invest Dermatol** 77:413.
392. Henkin RI (1995) Body odor. **JAMA** 273:1171–1172.
393. Jass HE (1982) Rationale of formulations of deodorants and antiperspirants. In: Principles of Cosmetics for the Dermatologist, Frost P, Horwitz SN, eds. St. Louis: CV Mosby, p. 98.

394. Shelly WB, Hurley HJ Jr (1954) Localized chromhidrosis: survey. **Arch Dermatol** 69:449.
395. Marks JG, Jr (1989) Treatment of apocrine chromhidrosis with topical capsaicin. **J Am Acad Dermatol** 21:418–420.
396. Saff DM, Owens R, Kahn TA (1995) Apocrine chromhidrosis involving the areola in a 15-year-old amateur figure skater. **Pediatr Dermatol** 12:48–50.
397. Thami GP, Kanwar AJ, Mamta (2000) Red facial pseudochromhidrosis. **Br J Dermatol** 142:1219–1220.
398. Osment LS (1979) Fox–Fordyce disease: self-assessment mini-program. **Int J Dermatol** 18:309.

basis for this condition, but topical and systemic estrogen treatments have not been consistently effective.[399] Judicial use of topical steroids, surgical excision with split-thickness skin grafting, and topical retinoic acid have also been attempted.[400] Oral isotretinoin was only transiently helpful in one case.[401]

399. Shelly WB (1972) Treatment of Fox–Fordyce disease. **J Am Med Assoc** 222:1069.
400. Giaobetti R, Caro WA, Roenigk HH (1979) Fox–Fordyce disease. Control with tretinoin cream. **Arch Dermatol** 115:1365.
401. Effendy I, Ossowski B, Happle R (1994) Fox–Fordyce disease in a male patient–response to oral retinoid treatment. **Clin Exp Dermatol** 19:67–69.

Acne

Carlo C. Gelmetti, Daniel P. Krowchuk and Anne W. Lucky

INTRODUCTION

The term acne encompasses a group of disorders, including acne vulgaris and its variants. Acne vulgaris is a chronic disease that is virtually universal in adolescence and is the most common skin disease treated by physicians.[1] Although often dismissed as trivial, acne may cause emotional distress and physical scarring. For these reasons, clinicians caring for adolescents and young adults must be familiar with the pathogenesis, clinical manifestations, and treatment of acne.

HISTORICAL NOTE

Acne vulgaris has plagued humankind since antiquity. Even King Tut demonstrated acne scars, and his tomb contained medications used by the ancients to treat the disease.[2] The first reference to acne may be the description of *aku-t*, a disorder characterized by "boils, blains, sores, pustules, any inflamed swelling," found in the Ebers Papyrus and elsewhere in Egyptian writing.[3,4] The disorder was recognized by Aristotle and Hippocrates 2500 years ago.[3] Grant suggests that since *ionthoi* meant acne and *ionthus* the first growth of the beard, ancient Greek physicians recognized the association of acne with puberty.[3]

Although the origin of the term acne is uncertain, it first appeared in the works of Atius (AD 542) who was physician to Justinian the Great of Constantinople.[4] The noun sebum is derived from the Latin *sevum*, suet or tallow, and the adjective sebaceous from *sevous*, meaning greasy or full of tallow.[4] Hoefle (1846) observed that blackheads were believed by the laity to represent worms that fed upon the host's nutrients. As a result, the term comedo may be derived from the Latin *comedere*, "to eat up, consume, devour."[4]

During the seventeenth century, the relationship between endocrinologic events and acne was clearly recognized.[3] Riolanus (1638) noted an association between acne and disorders of menstruation, and Jonston (1648) proposed a relationship between virility, repression and acne.[3,4] By the mid-nineteenth century, acne was considered a disease of sebaceous glands or follicles.[2] It was described by Noah Worcester, author of the first American textbook of dermatology, as a "noncontagious eruption characterized by small pustules, upon a chronically inflamed base of greater or less size, usually dull red or livid, though sometimes of natural colors . . ."[2] The importance of *Propionibacterium acnes* in the pathogenesis of acne was recognized by Master (1896), Sabouraud (1897), and Thibierge (1900).[4] The disease was believed to be modified by

"constitutional factors, mode of life, use of cosmetics, affections of the alimentary tract, menstrual abnormalities, and supposedly abnormal sexual behavior."[3]

The belief that acne might represent more than one disease is attributed to Galen who prescribed different treatments for two forms of *ionthoi*.[3] Rosacea was described by Chaucer in the *Canterbury Tales* and by Shakespeare in *King Henry V*.[3] Falcutius (AD 1400) described the permanent blush of rosacea.[3] Willen and Bateman (1813) formally recognized rosacea as a distinct entity, and Fuchs (1840) proposed categorizing various forms of acne as acne vulgaris, acne mentagra, and acne rosacea.[3]

ACNE

EPIDEMIOLOGY

Genetics

Although familial trends are well recognized in patients with acne, an exact pattern of inheritance has not been defined. In addition, because the disease is common and modified by external factors, it is not possible to predict the severity of disease in an individual patient based on family history.[1] Evidence of a role for genetic factors in the expression of acne comes from several sources. Identical twins have similar sebum excretion rates and a high concordance for the presence of acne, although disease severity varies significantly.[5] Persons with the XYY genotype appear more likely than genetically normal individuals to develop nodulocystic acne.[6,7] Finally, the risk of adult acne occurring in a relative of a patient with adult acne is significantly greater than for a relative of an unaffected individual (odds ratio [OR] 3.93, 95% confidence interval [CI] 2.79–5.51, $p<.001$).[8]

Statistics

Acne is the skin disease most commonly treated by physicians.[1] Thirty million Americans have acne,[9] and the prevalence in adolescents aged 15 to 17 years approaches 85%. The incidence is equal in patients of all races.[1] Data from the National Ambulatory Medical Care Survey, an ongoing survey of physician practices in the United States, revealed that in 1998, the most recent year for which data were available, there were an estimated 6.7 million visits to physicians in which the reason for visit or principal diagnosis was acne; women accounted for 65% of these visits.[10] In that same year, there were an estimated 3.5 million visits made by adolescents aged 11 to 20 years.[11] Each year, more than 5 million new and refill oral antibiotic

1. Pochi PE (1990) The pathogenesis and treatment of acne. **Annu Rev Med** 41:187–198.
2. Parish LC, Witdowski JA (1979) History of acne. In: Acne Update for the Practitioner, Frank SB, ed. New York, NY: Yorke Medical Books, p. 7.
3. Grant RNR (1951) The history of acne. **Proc Royal Soc Med** 44:647–652.
4. MacKenna RMB (1957) Acne vulgaris. **Lancet** 1:169–176.
5. Walton S, Wyatt EH, Cunliffe WJ (1988) Genetic control of sebum excretion and acne – A twin study. **Br J Dermatol** 118:393–396.
6. Voorhees JJ, Wilkins JW, Hayes E et al. (1972) Nodulocytic acne as a phenotype feature of the XYY genotype. **Arch Dermatol** 105:913–919.
7. Sosis AC, Panet-Raymond G, Goldberg DM (1973) XYY chromosome complement in a patient with nodulocystic acne. **Dermatologica** 146:222–228.
8. Goulden V, McGeown CH, Cunliffe WJ (1999) The familial risk of adult acne: a comparison between first-degree relatives of affected and unaffected individuals. **Br J Dermatol** 141:297–300.
9. Stern RS (1992) The prevalence of acne on the basis of physical examination. **J Am Acad Dermatol** 26:931–935.
10. Stern RS (2000) Medication and medical service utilization for acne 1995–1998. **J Am Acad Dermatol** 43:1042–1048.
11. National ambulatory medical care survey. URL: ftp://ftp.cdc.gov/pub/Health_Statistics/NCHS/Dataset_Documentation/NAMCS/

prescriptions are dispensed for acne treatment, along with 740 000 for isotretinoin.[10]

Acne often is considered to be a disease of adolescence, but it may be observed in individuals of almost any age. Neonatal acne develops within the first weeks of life and may be more common in males. Lesions typically resolve spontaneously by 1 year of age and rarely persist until age 3 years.[12] A history of acne during infancy appears to be associated with a higher incidence and greater severity of acne during adolescence.[12] Between the ages of 1 and 6 years, acne lesions are unusual and may be a sign of excess androgen production.

Adolescent acne correlates best with pubertal stage; however, acne lesions may precede the physical changes characteristic of puberty.[13] Occasional comedones or small inflammatory papules are common by age 7. Among boys ≥9 years of age who were prepubertal, Lucky et al. found that 57.3% had mild comedonal acne and only 3.5% had no comedones.[14] Inflammatory acne appears to develop later; at pubertal stage 1 (prepuberty), all subjects evaluated by Lucky et al. had fewer than 10 inflammatory lesions and 74% had none.[14] However, by pubertal stage 3, 77% had inflammatory lesions and by stage 4, 94% were affected.[14] Studies in girls demonstrate analogous results; 73.1%, 84.0%, and 90.6% of those in pubic hair stages 1 (prepuberty), 2 and 3, respectively, have some form of acne; comedones are more common than inflammatory lesions.[15] Lucky et al. have shown that girls destined to have severe comedonal or inflammatory acne have significantly more comedonal

and inflammatory lesions, respectively, as early as age 10 years, as well as 2.5 years before menarche.[16] Analogous data do not exist for boys. Early acne occurs in the mid-face (mid-forehead, nose and chin) and later spreads to the lateral cheeks, lower jaw, back, and chest.

By the mid-20s, the incidence of acne in men declines sharply, but about 30% of women in their 30s and 20% of women in their 40s have acne.[13] Worsening or redevelopment of papular or nodular acne is common among women in their 30s.[13] Acne may worsen during menopause but is rarely seen in those who are postmenopausal; less than 3% of men over age 55 have acne.[13]

PRESENTING HISTORY

The patient's concern about the appearance of lesions and their potential impact on interactions with peers may prompt a visit to the clinician when proprietary preparations have failed. Parental pressure also may prompt consultation, either when over-the-counter medications have failed, or in older children or young adolescents with minimal disease when there is a family history of severe acne.

Clinicians should recognize that acne may have a considerable negative impact on quality of life. Studies of adolescents and young adults demonstrate a consistent relationship between the presence and severity of acne and anxiety,[17–20] dissatisfaction with appearance,[17,21–24] self-consciousness,[25] and

TABLE 13.1   Key elements of the history

Question	Rationale
For all patients	
How long has the patient had acne?	Early- or late-onset acne may indicate a hormonal abnormality.
Which medications have been tried?	Which medications have been successful, which have not?
	Were treatment failures the result of improper technique or insufficient duration of use? Did adverse effects occur?
Is the patient using other products to treat acne?	Many nonprescription acne preparations (e.g., abrasive soaps) are irritating and limit the patient's ability to tolerate more effective therapies.
Is the patient receiving other medications?	Topical or oral corticosteroids (including anabolic-androgenic steroids) may induce acne lesions. Lithium, isoniazid, hydantoin and rifampin are among the drugs that may worsen acne.
Does the patient use cosmetics or hair greases?	Cosmetics containing lanolin or oil may cause or worsen acne.
Does the patient have recreational or occupational activities that may worsen acne?	Pressure applied by helmets, chin straps, shoulder pads or tight occlusive garments may worsen acne. Oils or greases inadvertently applied to the skin as part of one's occupation can create obstructive lesions.
Is there a history of other medical problems?	Adolescents with a history of atopic dermatitis or those who report "sensitive" skin may not tolerate topical medications that dry or irritate skin.
For females	
Is the patient menstruating? Are there premenstrual flares?	Premenstrual flares are common in women with acne.
Is there a history of oligomenorrhea or hirsutism?	The presence of oligomenorrhea or hirsutism, coupled with the presence of acne, may suggest androgen excess produced by polycystic ovary syndrome or late-onset congenital adrenal hyperplasia.
Is the patient sexually active? Does she use hormonal contraception?	Patients who are sexually active require effective contraception during treatment with Accutane. Certain hormonal contraceptives may worsen acne (see text). Women using oral contraceptives may require a secondary form of contraception if oral antibiotics are being used to treat acne (see text).

12. Chew EW, Bingham A, Burrows D (1990) Incidence of acne vulgaris in patients with infantile acne. **Clin Exp Dermatol** 15:376–377.
13. Rothman KF, Lucky AW (1993) Acne vulgaris. **Adv Dermatol** 8:347–374.
14. Lucky AW, Biro FM, Huster GA et al. (1991) Acne vulgaris in early adolescent boys. Correlations with pubertal maturation. **Arch Dermatol** 127:210–216.
15. Lucky AW, Biro FM, Huster GA et al. (1994) Acne vulgaris in premenarchal girls. An early sign of puberty associated with rising levels of dehydroepiandrosterone. **Arch Dermatol** 130:308–314.
16. Lucky AW, Biro FM, Simbartl LA et al. (1997) Predictors of acne vulgaris in young adolescent girls: Results of a five-year longitudinal study. **J Pediatr** 130:30–39.
17. Krowchuk DP, Stancin T, Keskinen R et al. (1991) The psychosocial effects of acne on adolescents. **Pediatr Dermatol** 8:332–338.
18. Medansky RS, Handler RM, Medansky DL (1981) Self-evaluation of acne and emotion: A pilot study. **Psychosomatics** 22:379–383.
19. Rubinow DR, Peck GL, Squillace KM et al. (1987) Reduced anxiety and depression in cystic acne patients after successful treatment with oral isotretinoin. **J Am Acad Dermatol** 17:25–32.

20. Wu SF, Kinder BN, Trunnell TN et al. (1988) Role of anxiety and anger in acne patients: A relationship with the severity of the disorder. **J Am Acad Dermatol** 18:325–333.
21. Finlay AY, Khan GK (1994) Dermatology Life Quality Index (DLQI) – a simple practical measure for routine clinical use. **Clin Exp Dermatol** 19:210–216.
22. Gupta MA, Gupta AK, Schork NJ et al. (1990) Psychiatric aspects of the treatment of mild to moderate facial acne. Some preliminary observations. **Int J Dermatol** 29:719–721.
23. Motley RJ, Finlay AY (1989) How much disability is caused by acne? **Clin Exp Dermatol** 14:194–198.
24. Shuster S, Fisher GH, Harris E et al. (1978) The effect of akin disease on self-image. **Br J Dermatol** 99(suppl 16):18–19.
25. Schachter RJ, Pantel ES, Glassman GM et al. (1971) Acne vulgaris and psychologic impact on high school students. **NY State J Med** 24:2886–2890.

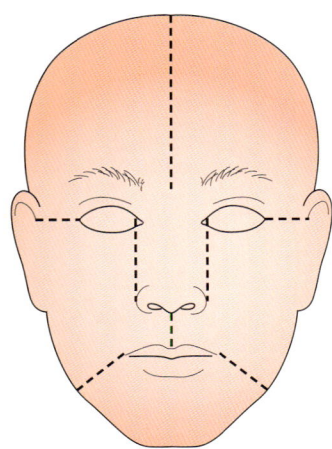

Fig. 13.1 In each region, the physician records the number of open comedones (OC), closed comedones (CC) and inflammatory lesions (IL). (Courtesy of Merck & Co., Rahway, NJ.)

characteristic of these lesions does not represent dirt; rather, it may be the result of oxidation of melanin, interference in transmission of light through compacted epithelial cells, or the presence of certain lipids in sebum.[28–30] Closed comedones are small white papules without surrounding erythema (Figs 13.8, 13.9). They represent follicles that have become dilated with cellular and lipid debris but possess only a microscopic opening to the skin surface.

Inflammatory lesions

Patients with inflammatory forms of acne manifest erythematous papules, pustules or nodules. Papules and pustules are small, measuring <5mm in diameter (Fig. 13.10). Individual papules may become pustules and vice versa. Nodules measure ≥5mm in diameter and often involve more than one follicle. After inflammatory lesions resolve, erythematous or hyperpigmented macules may remain for as long as 12 months and are often mistaken for true scars.

inhibition in social interactions.[17,23,25,26] Importantly, it is the patient's, not the clinician's, impression of acne severity that is most closely associated with dissatisfaction with personal appearance.[17] Successful treatment usually is associated with improved psychological well-being.[17,19,22] For additional information regarding the psychosocial impact of acne, the reader is referred to Chapter 2 of this text.

The first step in patient evaluation is to gather a careful medical history. Helpful questions and their rationale are presented in Table 13.1. Briefly, patients should be questioned about the duration of disease, therapies that have been employed, the use of systemic or topical medications or skin care products (including cosmetics or hair care products), underlying medical conditions and mechanical trauma or friction to affected areas. Females should be questioned about the presence of hirsutism and a menstrual history obtained. Additionally, sensitive and confidential questioning about sexual activity and contraceptive use is vital.

PHYSICAL EXAMINATION

At a minimum the physical examination should include the face, chest and back. Examination of other systems will be dictated by the history. To facilitate later comparison, an approximation of the number and types of lesions may be recorded for each geographic region. For the face, this may be accomplished using a diagram (Fig. 13.1). In each of the five areas in the diagram (excluding the nose), the clinician can document the number of inflammatory lesions and open and closed comedones. For the chest and back, one can also approximate the numbers and types of lesions present. Although this may seem tedious, it can be accomplished quickly and provides the clinician with a valuable, objective assessment. In addition to a "lesion count," it is helpful to make a global assessment of acne severity (e.g., mild, moderate or severe, Figs 13.2–13.4) that represents a synthesis of the number, type, size, and extent of lesions, as well as the presence of scarring.[27] Photographic methods have been employed to assess disease activity and are preferred by some clinicians. Patients with acne may exhibit obstructive (comedonal) or inflammatory lesions, scars, or nodules.

Obstructive (comedonal) lesions

Initially, obstruction within the follicle is microscopic and cannot be perceived clinically; such lesions are termed microcomedones (singular microcomedo) (Fig. 13.5). As comedones enlarge, however, they become apparent as open comedones (blackheads) or closed comedones (whiteheads). Open comedones represent follicles with a widely dilated orifice (Figs 13.6, 13.7). The black color

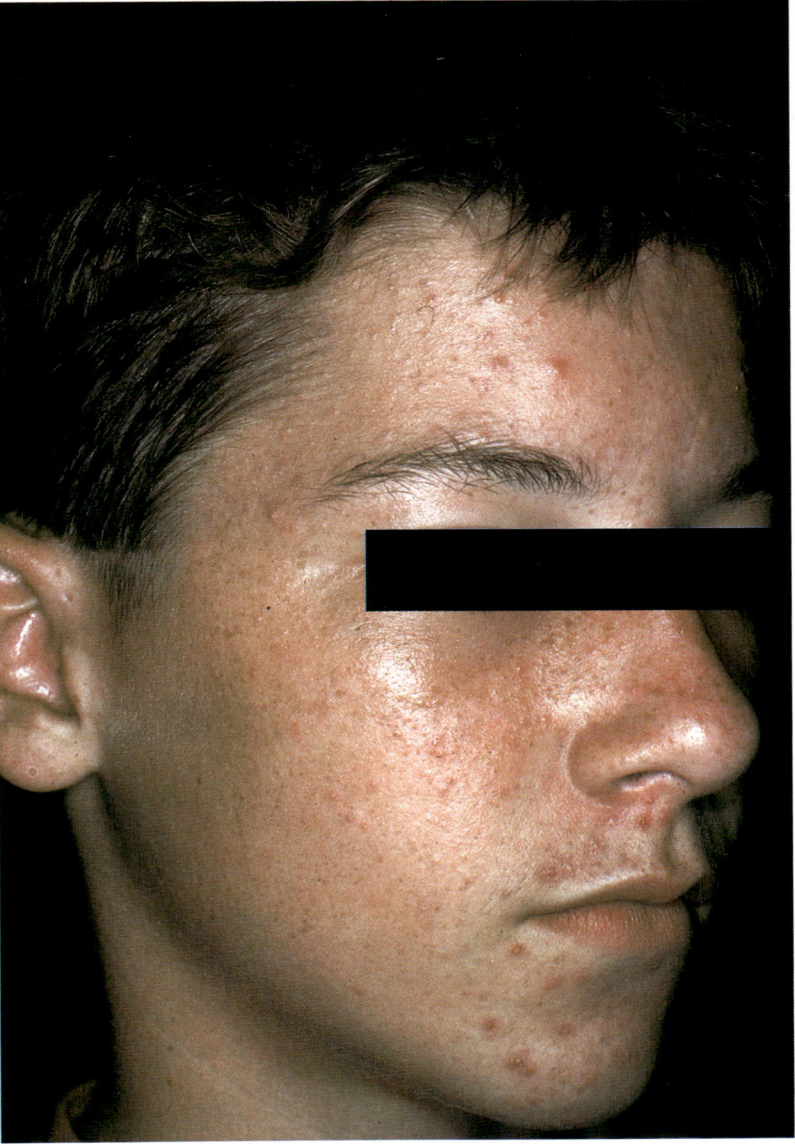

Fig. 13.2 Mild acne: a few small inflammatory lesions are present.

26. Pearl A, Arroll B, Lello J et al. (1998) The impact of acne: A study of adolescents' attitudes, perception and knowledge. **NZ Med J** 111:269–271.
27. Pochi PE, Shalita AR, Strauss JS et al. (1991) Report of the consensus conference on acne classification. **J Am Acad Dermatol** 24:495–500.
28. Blair C, Lewis CA (1970) The pigment of comedones. **Br J Dermatol** 82:572–583.
29. Leyden JJ (1997) Therapy for acne vulgaris. **N Engl J Med** 336:1156–1162.
30. Webster GF (1996) Acne. **Curr Probl Dermatol** 8:237–268.

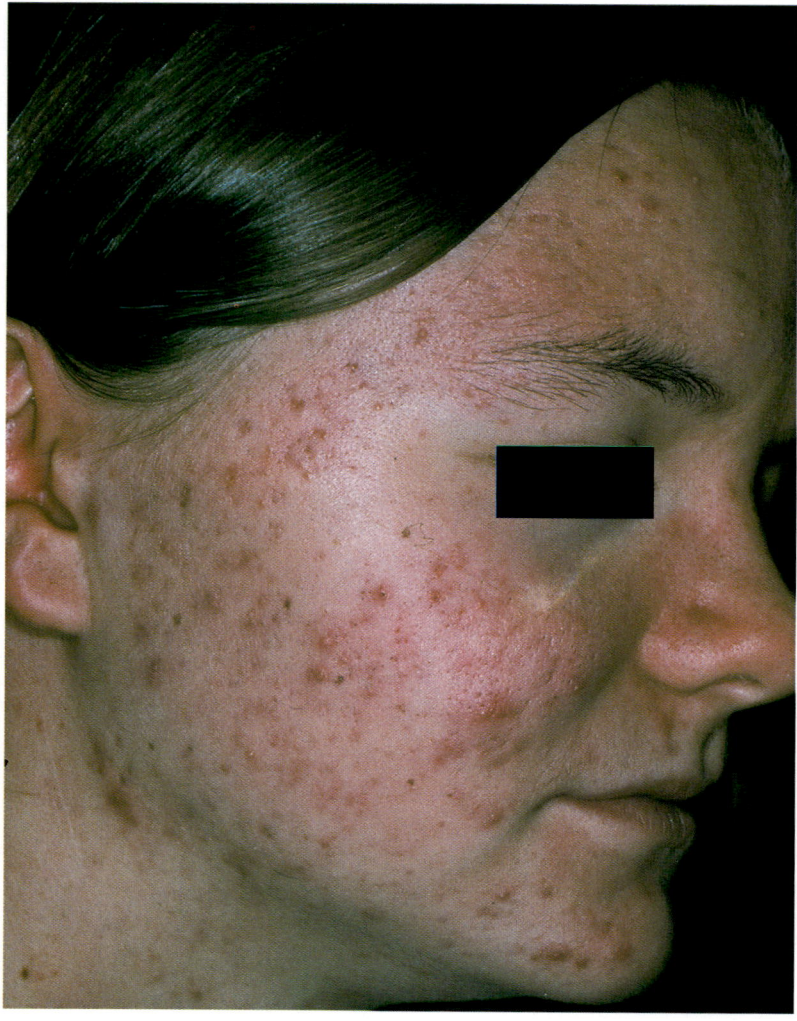

Fig. 13.3   Moderate acne: many inflammatory lesions and early scarring are present.

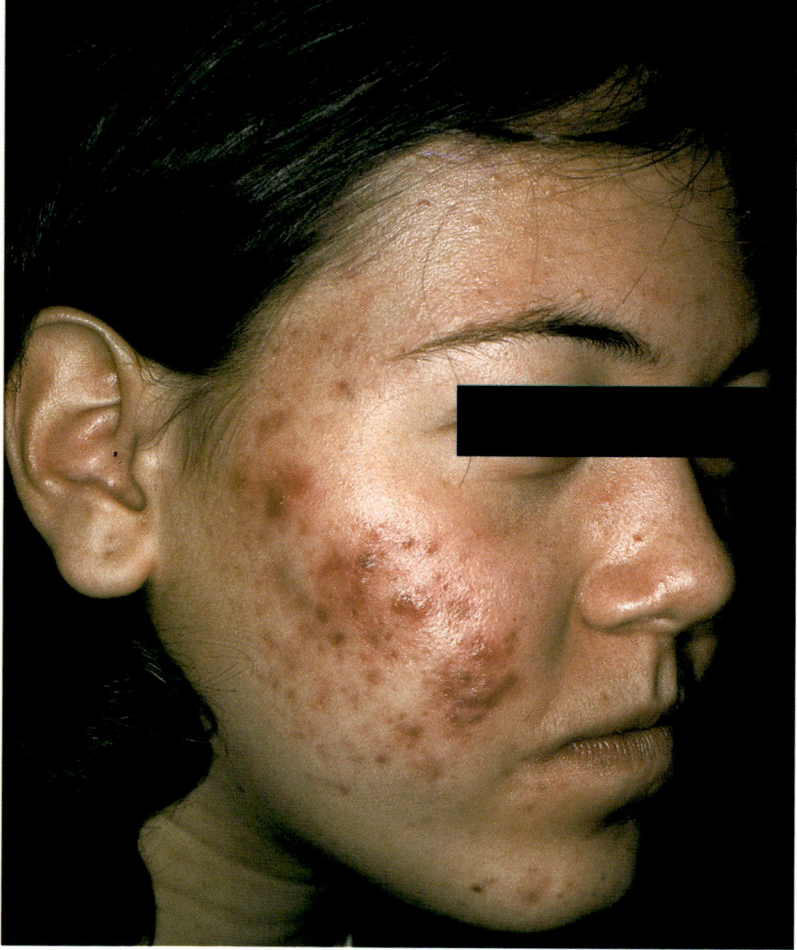

Fig. 13.4   Severe acne: numerous, large inflammatory nodules and scarring are present.

Scars

Some patients with acne develop scars as inflammatory lesions resolve. In general, scarring is most likely in those adolescents with deep papules or nodules.[13] However, even small inflammatory lesions may produce scars. Most often, and particularly on the face, acne scars have the appearance of pits (Fig. 13.11). On the trunk they usually look like small white macules or papules. Rarely, patients develop hypertrophic or keloidal scars. Since scars may be irreversible, their presence should prompt the clinician to be aggressive in the selection of therapeutic agents active against the inflammatory component of the disease. True cysts, compressible nodules that lack overlying inflammation, also may be observed in patients with acne.

LABORATORY FINDINGS

Although serum androgens play an important role in causing acne (see Pathophysiology), most patients have normal hormone levels.[13,31] In females, the picture is more complex; although hormone levels usually are normal, elevations of free testosterone and dehydroepiandrosterone sulfate (DHEAS), and reductions in sex hormone-binding globulin (SHBG) may occur.[13,32–34]

For example, Lucky *et al.* found DHEAS and testosterone levels above the 90th percentile in 29% and 28%, respectively, of girls with severe comedonal acne; only 20% had low SHBG values.[16]

In view of the fact that most patients with acne have normal hormone levels, measurement of androgens should be reserved for those females with acne and other evidence of androgen excess (e.g., irregular menses, hirsutism, alopecia or clitomegaly), or those in whom conventional acne therapy fails.[16,31]

PATHOPHYSIOLOGY AND HISTOGENESIS

Histology

Acne is a disorder of the pilosebaceous unit, comprised of a follicle or pore, sebaceous gland, and rudimentary or vellus hair (Fig. 13.12). These specialized follicles are concentrated on the face, chest, and back. Research on the pathogenesis of acne has focused on the portion of the canal between the surface and the sebaceous ducts known as the infundibulum. The most distal intraepidermal portion of the follicular canal, the acroinfundibulum, merges with the neighboring epidermis. Structurally and functionally, the epithelium lining the acroinfundibulum and epidermis is similar. The epithelium that lines the intradermal region of the infundibulum, the infrainfundibulum, is quite different. Changes occur in a gradient from the well-organized, highly

31. Leyden JJ (1995) New understandings of the pathogenesis of acne. **J Am Acad Dermatol** 32(suppl):S15–S25.
32. Darley CR, Kirby JD, Besser GM et al. (1982) Circulating testosterone, sex hormone binding globulin and prolactin in women with late onset or persistent acne vulgaris. Br J Dermatol 106:517–522.
33. Lucky AW, McGuire J, Rosenfield RL et al. (1983) Plasma androgens in women with acne vulgaris. J Invest Dermatol 81:70–74.
34. Reingold SB, Rosenfield RL (1987) The relationship of mild hirsutism or acne in women to androgens. **Arch Dermatol** 123:209–212.

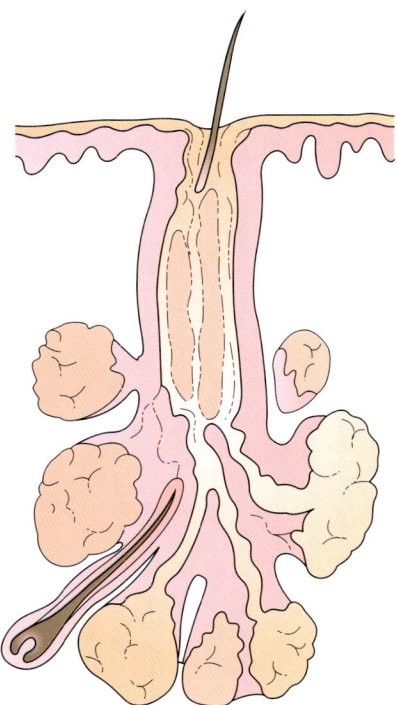

Fig. 13.5   Microcomedo (redrawn from Plewig G, Kligman AM. *Acne and Rosacea*. 2nd ed. Berlin, Germany: Springer-Verlag; 1993).

Microcomedo

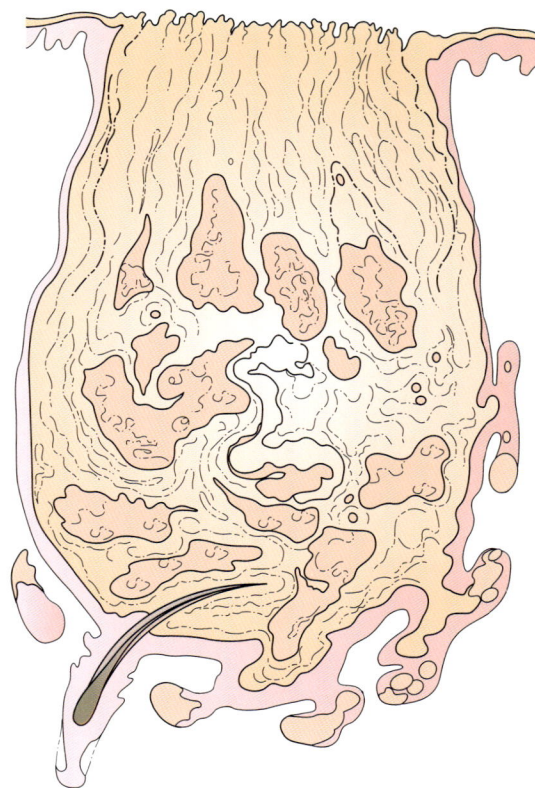

Open comedo

Fig. 13.6   Open comedo (redrawn from Plewig G, Kligman AM. *Acne and Rosacea*. 2nd ed. Berlin, Germany: Springer-Verlag; 1993).

differentiated epithelium near the surface, to the thin, attenuated epithelium near the sebaceous ducts. In the infrainfundibulum, the most striking difference occurs in the stratum corneum, which is markedly thinned. The superficial cells in this layer are readily shed into the lumen, contributing to a loose cellular detritus. Compared with the cells of the granular layer near the surface, those in the infrainfundibulum have fewer tonofilaments and desmosomes and smaller, more discrete keratohyalin granules. Odland bodies (lamellar granules, membrane-coating granules) are prominent in these cells and appear in large clusters in the intercellular space at the junction of the granular and cornified layer.

Pathophysiology
Although the pathogenesis of acne has not been clearly defined, multiple factors contribute, including hormones and sebum production, bacteria and abnormal keratinization.[13,30,31] Well-reasoned therapeutic choices require an understanding of these factors.

Hormones and sebum production
Although it is recognized that androgens play an integral role in causing acne, their exact role remains incompletely understood. A number of studies have been performed to define the relationship between acne and serum and tissue androgen levels.[1,30,31,35] At age 8 or 9 years, prior to the appearance of secondary sexual characteristics, the adrenal glands begin to produce increasing amounts of the androgen DHEAS in a process called adrenarche.[1] Rising levels of DHEAS, perhaps after conversion to more potent androgens

such as testosterone and dihydrotestosterone (DHT), cause sebaceous glands to enlarge and produce more sebum.[36,37] In girls, DHEAS levels correlate with the presence of acne in prepuberty and with the future severity of comedonal acne; analogous data do not exist for boys.[15,16] In both females and males, the prevalence and severity of acne correlate with stage of sexual maturity.[14,15]

Local metabolism of androgens within the sebaceous gland may also play a role in acne. The sebaceous gland possesses the enzymes necessary to convert DHEAS to more potent androgens (Fig. 13.13).[38–40] The final enzyme in this pathway is 5 α-reductase (5 α-R) which converts testosterone to DHT. Two 5 α-R isoenzymes have been identified (types 1 and 2). Thiboutot *et al.* have demonstrated that in adults without acne, 5 α-R activity is concentrated in sebaceous glands, the type 1 isoenzyme predominates and enzyme activity is higher in sebaceous glands from acne-prone areas (e.g., the face) than from non acne-prone regions.[41] Although these investigators have demonstrated that the activities of 5 α-R and 17 β-hydroxysteroid dehydrogenase (the enzyme necessary for conversion of androstenedione to testosterone) in sebaceous glands are higher in men than women, no significant differences in the activity of either enzyme were observed between subjects with or without acne.[38]

Under the stimulation of adrenal and gonadal androgens, sebum secretion peaks during adolescence and begins to decline after age 20.[13,42,43] Patients

35. Pochi PE (1982) Hormones and acne. **Semin Dermatol** 1:265–273.
36. Stewart ME, Downing DT, Cook JS et al. (1992) Sebaceous gland activity and serum dehydroepiandrosterone sulfate levels in boys and girls. **Arch Dermatol** 128:1345–1348.
37. Thiboutot DM (1997) Acne. An overview of clinical research findings. **Dermatol Clin** 15:97–109.
38. Thiboutot D, Gilliland K, Light J et al. (1999) Androgen metabolism in sebaceous glands from subjects with and without acne. **Arch Dermatol** 135:1041–1045.
39. Hay JB, Hodgins MB (1978) Distribution of androgen metabolizing enzymes in isolated tissues of human forehead and axillary skin. **J Endocrinol** 79:29–39.
40. Simpton NB, Cunliffe WJ, Hodgins MB (1983) The relationship between the vitro activity of 3 beta-hydroxysteroid dehydrogenase delta 4-5-isomerase in human sebaceous glands and their secretory activity in vivo. **J Invest Dermatol** 81:139–144.
41. Thiboutot D, Harris G, Iles V et al. (1995) Activity of the type 1 5 alpha-reductase exhibits regional differences in isolated sebaceous glands and whole skin. **J Invest Dermatol** 105:209–214.
42. Pochi PE, Strauss JS (1974) Endocrinologic control of the development and activity of the human sebaceous gland. **J Invest Dermatol** 62:191–201.
43. Pochi PE, Strauss JS (1969) Sebaceous gland response in man to the administration of testosterone, delta-4-androstenedione and dehydroisoandrosterone. **J Invest Dermatol** 52:32–36.

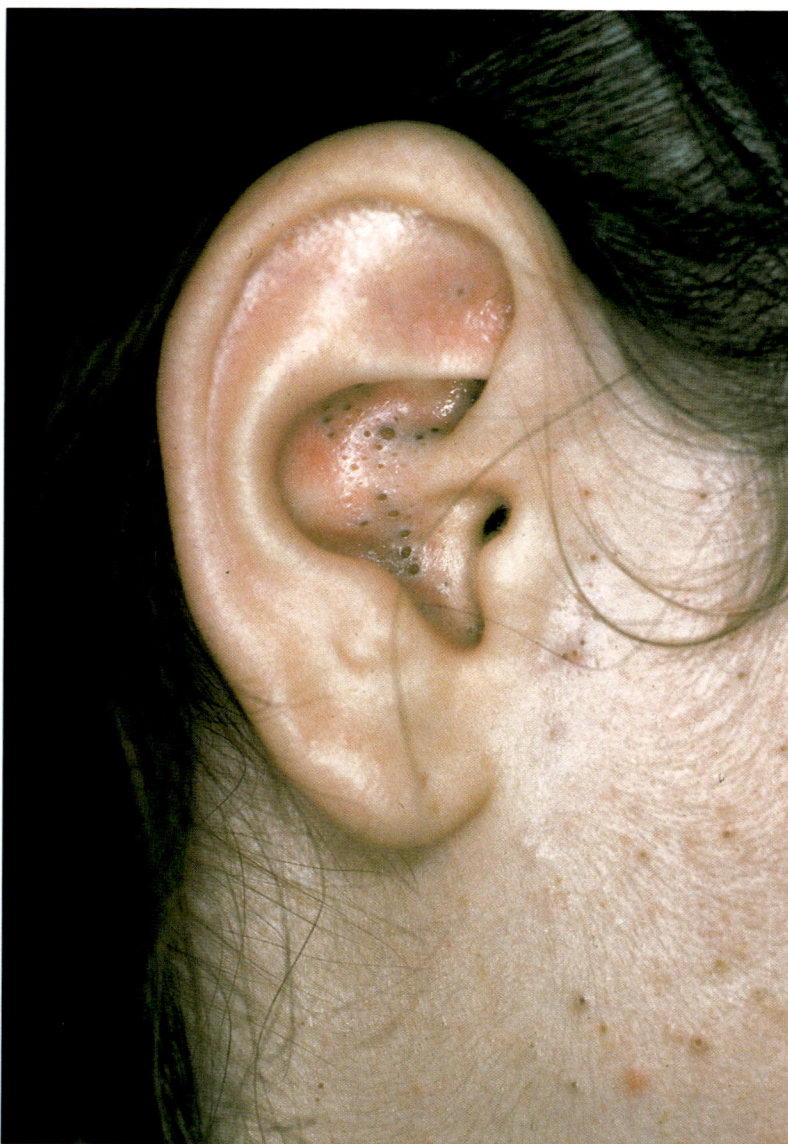

Fig. 13.7 Open comedones in the external ear. (Reprinted with permission from Krowchuk DP, Lucky AW (2001) Managing adolescent acne. *Adolesc Med* 12:355–374.

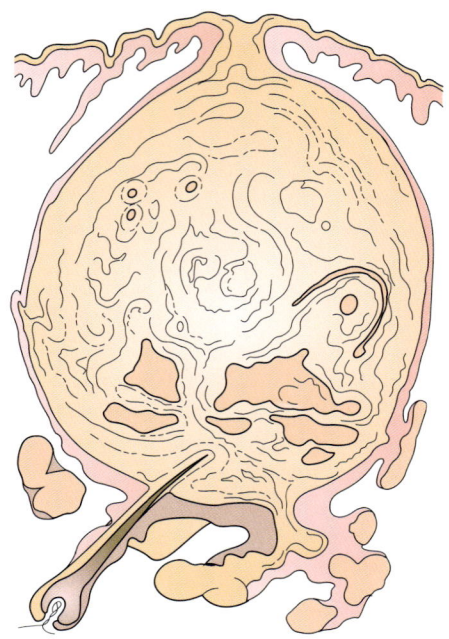

Closed comedo

Fig. 13.8 Closed comedo (redrawn from Plewig G, Kligman AM. *Acne and Rosacea*. 2nd ed. Berlin, Germany: Springer-Verlag; 1993).

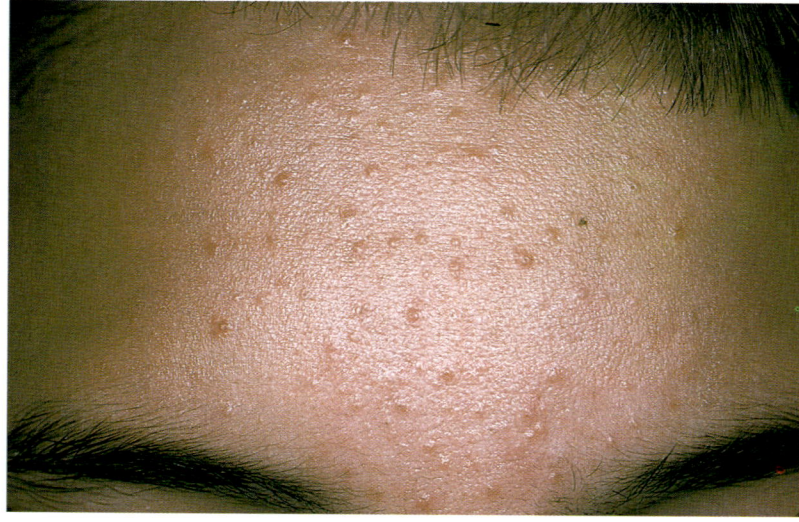

Fig. 13.9 Closed comedones, small white papules without surrounding erythema, located on the forehead.

with acne secrete more sebum than those without disease,[44,45] and, in general, acne severity correlates with rates of sebum secretion.[13,31,46] Sebum from patients with acne is deficient in linoleic acid, a factor that may cause altered follicular epithelial differentiation and obstruction.[13,31,47,48]

Bacteria

Propionibacterium acnes is an anaerobic, Gram-positive diptheroid that begins to colonize pilosebaceous follicles following increases in sebum production that accompany adrenarche.[13,30,49] The organism uses sebum as a nutrient for growth and its numbers correlate with the concentration of triglycerides in sebum.[30,49] Although *P. acnes* is a normal inhabitant of the skin, the number of organisms is higher in patients with acne than in those who are unaffected.[13,50]

44. Pochi PE, Strauss JS (1964) Sebum production, causal sebum level, titratable acidity of sebum, and urinary fractional 17-ketosteroid excretion in males with acne. **J Invest Dermatol** 43:383–388.

45. Harris HH, Downing DT, Stewart ME, Strauss JS (1983) Sustainable rates of sebum secretion in acne patients and matched normal control subjects. **J Am Acad Dermatol** 8:200–203.

46. Burton JL, Shuster S (1971) The relationship between seborrhoea and acne vulgaris. **Br J Dermatol** 84:600–601.

47. Morello AM, Downing DT, Strauss JS (1976) Octadecadienoic acids in the skin surface lipids of acne patients and normal subjects. **J Invest Dermatol** 66:319–323.

48. Wertz PW, Miethke MC, Long SA et al. (1985) The composition of the ceramides from human stratum corneum and from comedones. **J Invest Dermatol** 84:410–412.

49. McGinley KJ, Webster GF, Ruggieri MR et al. (1980) Regional variations in density of cutaneous propionibacteria: Correlation of *Propionibacterium acnes* populations with sebaceous secretion. **J Clin Microbiol** 12:672–675.

50. Leyden JJ, McGinley KJ, Mills OH et al. (1975) Propionibacterium levels in patients with and without acne vulgaris. **J Invest Dermatol** 65:382–384.

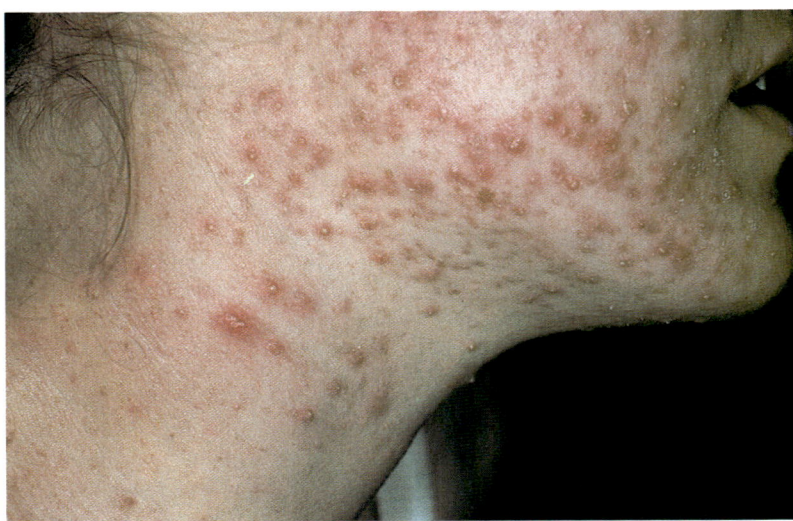

Fig. 13.10 Inflammatory papules and pustules located on the face and neck of a patient with severe acne.

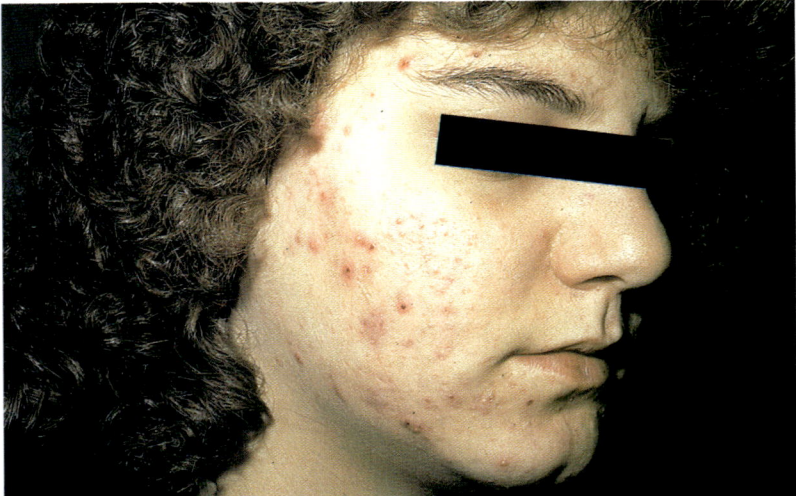

Fig. 13.11 Pitted scars and inflammatory papules and nodules on the face of a girl with severe acne. (Reprinted with permission from Krowchuk DP, Lucky AW (2001) Managing adolescent acne. *Adolesc Med* 12:355–374.

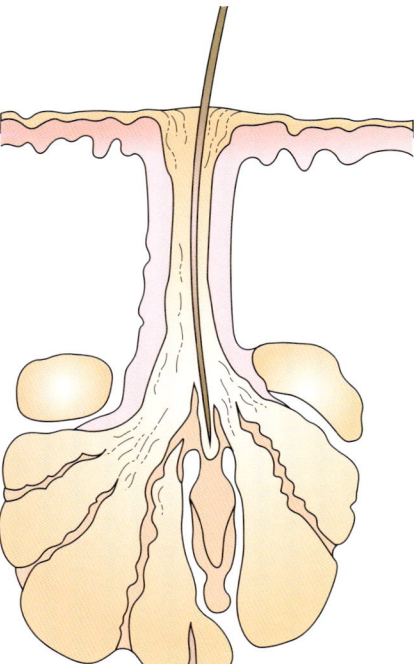

Fig. 13.12 Pilosebaceous follicle (redrawn from Plewig G, Kligman AM. *Acne and Rosacea.* 2nd ed. Berlin, Germany: Springer-Verlag; 1993).

Pilosebaceous follicle

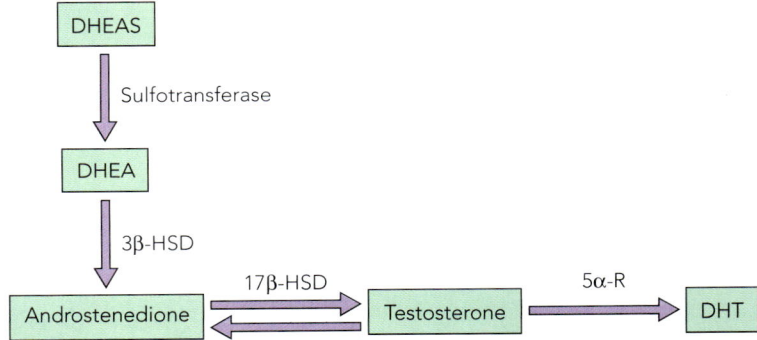

Fig. 13.13 Androgen metabolism in the skin. Dehydroepiandrosterone sulfate (DHEAS) can be converted within the skin to testosterone and dihydrotestosterone (DHT) by means of the following enzymes: sulfotransferase, 3β-hydroxysteroid dehydrogenase (3β-HSD), 17β-hydroxysteroid dehydrogenase (17β-HSD), and 5α-reductase (5α-R). DHEA indicates dehydroepiandrosterone.

P. acnes appears to contribute to the causation of acne in several ways. It produces chemoattractant factors that cause poymorphonuclear neutrophils (PMNs) to enter pilosebaceous follicles.[1,13,30,51,52] As PMNs ingest *P. acnes*, hydrolytic enzymes are released that damage the follicle wall.[1,13,30,53] Follicular contents can then enter the dermis where they incite inflammatory reactions that are manifest clinically as erythematous papules, pustules, or nodules.[13]

P. acnes may induce other immunological reactions.[54] Some patients with acne develop circulating immune complexes and complement fixing antibodies to *P. acnes* that correlate with the severity of inflammation.[54–57] In addition, immediate[58] and delayed[59] hypersensitivity reactions to skin testing with *P. acnes* antigen have been demonstrated in acne patients.[54] *P. acnes* and supernatants from cultures of *P. acnes* can induce significant concentrations of interleukin (IL)–1β, tumor necrosis factor α and IL–8 by human monocytic cell lines and by peripheral blood mononuclear cells from acne patients.[53] These proinflammatory cytokines may result in the expression of vascular and dermal adhesion molecules, attraction of inflammatory cells, and

51. Lee W-L, Shalita AR (1978) Neutrophil chemotaxis and its inhibition by antibiotics. **J Invest Dermatol** 70:219.

52. Puhvel SM, Sakamoto M (1978) The chemoattractant properties of comedonal components. **J Invest Dermatol** 71:324–329.

53. Vowels BR, Yang S, Leyden JJ (1995) Induction of proinflammatory cytokines by a soluble factor of *Propionibacterium acnes*: Implications for chronic inflammatory acne. **Infect Immun** 63:3158–3165.

54. Burkhart CG, Burkhart CN, Lehmann PF (1999) Acne: a review of immunological and microbiologic factors. **Postgrad Med J** 75:328–331.

55. Woolfson H (1987) Acne fulminans with circulating immune complexes and leukaemoid reaction treated with steroids and azothiaprine. **Clin Exp Dermatol** 12:463–466.

56. Kellett JK, Beck MH, Chalmers RJ (1985) Erythema nodosum and circulating immune complexes in acne fulminans after treatment with isotretinoin. **BMJ** 290:820.

57. Puhvel SM, Hoffman IK, Sternberg TH (1966) Corynebacterium acnes. Presence of complement fixing antibodies to *Corynebacterium acnes* in the sera of patients with acne vulgaris. **Arch Dermatol** 93:364–366.

58. Puhvel SM, Hoffman IK, Reisner RM et al. (1967) Dermal hypersensitivity of patients with acne vulgaris to *Corynebacterium acnes*. **J Invest Dermatol** 49:154–158.

59. Kersey P, Sussman M, Dahl M (1980) Delayed skin test reactivity to *Propionibacterium acnes* correlates with severity of inflammation in acne vulgaris. **Br J Dermatol** 103:651–655.

stimulation of other mediators such as prostaglandins and leukotrienes.[53] Finally, within the follicle, *P. acnes* hydrolyzes triglycerides to free fatty acids (FFA), which some believe may contribute to the inflammatory process and increase follicular obstruction.[13]

Abnormal keratinization

Pilosebaceous follicles are lined with squamous epithelium that is contiguous with the skin surface. In persons with acne, keratinization is altered and epithelial cells from the follicle lining are not shed properly and become more cohesive.[30,31] The result is a collection of cells and sebum that become impacted within the follicle. This process, called comedogenesis, is primary in the development of acne lesions.[31] The trigger for comedogenesis has not been identified; current research is focusing on alterations in proliferation or adhesion of keratinocytes, cytokine production, and the effects of androgens.[31,38] Using Ki-67, a monoclonal antibody that reacts with a nuclear antigen expressed by cells in late G1, S, M and G2 phases of the cell cycle, Knaggs *et al.* demonstrated greater cell proliferation in normal follicles from acne-prone skin than in follicles from areas unaffected by acne, and in comedones compared with normal follicles in acne-prone skin.[38,60] Changes in keratin expression[61] or adhesion of keratinocytes due to desmosomal components[62] do not appear to be responsible for these observations. Cytokine production by keratinocytes in pilosebaceous follicles may also contribute to obstruction within follicles. IL-1α is present in high concentrations in open comedones[63] and can induce comedogenesis.[64] Both epidermal growth factor and transforming growth factor-α cause disorganization of infundibular keratinocytes resulting in follicular rupture similar to that seen in acne.[64] A role for androgens in abnormal keratinization is suggested by the observations that the infrainfundibulum and sebaceous gland possess 5 α-R, the enzyme necessary to convert testosterone to DHT[65] and

that the number of comedones is reduced by treatment with ethinyl estradiol and the antiandrogen cyproterone acetate.[66,67]

DIFFERENTIAL DIAGNOSIS

Acne vulgaris occasionally may be confused with other disorders. Unlike acne vulgaris, acne rosacea occurs in older individuals, involves the central face (not the trunk), and lacks comedones. Pityrosporum folliculitis, caused by *P. ovale*, may mimic truncal acne. It presents as erythematous papules or pustules located on the chest, upper back, shoulders and proximal arms. Diagnosis is confirmed by performing a potassium hydroxide preparation that reveals budding yeast. An apparent sudden worsening of acne in patients receiving chronic antibiotic therapy may be the result of Gram-negative folliculitis. In this disorder, infection with *Klebsiella, Enterobacter, Pseudomonas,* or *Proteus* spp. produces pustules, papules and nodules.[13] Other acneiform eruptions, including pomade acne, acne cosmetica and acne medicamentosa may be differentiated from acne vulgaris by the patient history.

THERAPEUTICS AND PROGNOSIS

The successful management of adolescent acne depends on both a solid understanding of the mode of action and possible adverse effects of the various available medications, and an individualized treatment plan based on a thoughtful approach to each patient. No two acne patients are identical in their reaction to their disease, or in the type of care that is optimal for them. For this reason, there can be no standardized treatment plan, only a rational set of guidelines and goals for the control of acne (Table 13.2). The ultimate goal for all acne patients is the avoidance of both the psychological and physical scarring that are so frequently associated with this disease.

TABLE 13.2   Management options for facial acne

Acne severity	Lesion type	Initial treatment	If no response
Mild	Comedonal	Benzoyl peroxide gel 5% once daily, or tretinoin cream 0.025%[1]	If benzoyl peroxide used initially, substitute or combine with tretinoin cream 0.025%[1] once daily
	Inflammatory	Benzoyl peroxide gel 5% once daily	Increase benzoyl peroxide application to twice daily, or substitute oral or topical antibiotic
	Mixed	Benzoyl peroxide gel 5% once daily alone or combined with tretinoin cream 0.025%, or azelaic acid twice daily	If benzoyl peroxide used initially, add tretinoin cream 0.025%[1] once daily (for comedonal component), and/or substitute oral or topical antibiotic (for inflammatory component)
Moderate	Comedonal	Tretinoin cream 0.025% once daily[1]	Increase strength of tretinoin to 0.05% cream
	Inflammatory	Topical antibiotic twice daily, or benzoyl peroxide gel 5% once daily	Oral antibiotic[2,3]
	Mixed	Benzoyl peroxide gel 5% once daily and tretinoin cream 0.025%[1] once daily, or azelaic acid twice daily	Add oral antibiotic[2,3] Continue tretinoin[1]
Severe	Comedonal	Tretinoin cream 0.025%[1] once daily	Increase strength of tretinoin to 0.05% cream
	Inflammatory	Oral antibiotic[2,3]	Consider isotretinoin
	Mixed	Tretinoin cream 0.025%[1] once daily, and oral antibiotic[2,3]	Consider isotretinoin

[1] Or other appropriate topical retinoid (e.g., Retin-A gel micro 0.1%, Differin, avita or tazarotene).

[2] E.g., tetracycline or erythromycin 250–500mg twice daily.

[3] Some experts advise the use benzoyl peroxide in patients treated with oral antibiotics to prevent the emergence of antibiotic resistant *P. acnes.*

60. Knaggs HE, Holland DB, Morris C et al. (1994) Quantification of cellular proliferation in acne using the monoclonal antibody Ki-67. **J Invest Dermatol** 102:89–92.
61. Hughes BR, Morris C, Cunliffe WJ et al. (1996) Keratin expression in pilosebaceous epithelia in truncal skin of acne patients. **Br J Dermatol** 134:247–256.
62. Knaggs HE, Hughes BR, Morris C et al. (1994) Immunohistochemical study of desmosomes in acne vulgaris. **Br J Dermatol** 130:731–737.
63. Ingham E, Eady EA, Goodwin CE et al. (1992) Pro-inflammatory levels of interleukin-1 alpha-like bioactivity are present in the majority of open comedones in acne vulgaris. **J Invest Dermatol** 98:895–901.
64. Guy R, Green MR, Kealey T (1996) Modeling acne in vitro. **J Invest Dermatol** 106:176–182.
65. Thiboutot DM, Knaggs H, Gilliland K et al. (1997) Activity of type 1 5 alpha-reductase is greater in the follicular infundibulum compared with the epidermis. **Br J Dermatol** 136:166–171.
66. Stewart ME, Greenwood R, Cunliffe WJ et al. (1986) Effect of cyproterone acetate-ethinylestradiol treatment on the portions of linoleic and sebaleic acids in various skin lipid classes. **Arch Dermatol Res** 278:481–485.
67. Cunliffe WJ, Holland DB, Clark SM et al. (2000) Comedogenesis: some new aetiological, clinical and therapeutic strategies. **Br J Dermatol** 142:1084–1091.

Patient education

Office visits should allow time to hear the patient's concerns and to provide a simple explanation of the causes, course, and options for treatment of acne. One also should attempt to address and dispel commonly held myths and provide information about those factors and behaviors that may worsen acne. The information contained in Tables 13.1 and 13.3 may be of assistance in guiding this portion of the discussion.

Patients should leave the clinician's office knowing exactly how to use the medications prescribed and any adverse effects to be anticipated. They should be advised that acne treatment is a long-term process, often taking six to eight weeks before any therapeutic benefit is seen, and that when therapy is abandoned prematurely, the acne usually returns. Additionally, once lesions resolve, treatment needs to be continued, even to apparently normal skin, until it is clear that there no longer is a tendency for new lesions to form.

Medications

Medications to treat acne may be separated into topical and systemic preparations.

Topical therapies

Commonly employed topical preparations include benzoyl peroxide, antibiotics, retinoids and salicylic acid.

TABLE 13.3   Elements of patient education

- Acne is not caused by dirt, and frequent washing will not improve the condition. In fact, frequent washing or the use of harsh soaps may irritate the skin and limit a patient's tolerance for topical medications. To control oily skin, patients may wash once or twice daily using a mild, nondrying soap or cleanser of their choice.
- For most adolescents, diet plays no role in acne. Occasionally, a patient may observe an apparent relationship between a particular food and a flare-up. In such instances, common sense would limit the intake of this food.
- Picking at, wearing athletic gear over, or otherwise traumatizing acne lesions may increase inflammation, prolong resolution of lesions, and increase the likelihood of scar formation.
- Cosmetics, sunscreens, and moisturizers, particularly those containing oils, may worsen acne. Advise the adolescent to take care to select cosmetics that are labeled noncomedogenic or nonacnegenic.
- A variant of cosmetic acne, known as pomade acne, may occur when greases used to style hair are inadvertently applied to the skin. Pomade acne is seen almost exclusively in African-Americans and is characterized by the presence of comedones located on the forehead and temporal areas (Fig. 13.14). To prevent such lesions, patients can be advised to avoid placing hair care products on the skin.
- Young women often experience premenstrual flare-ups of acne that may be caused by the androgenic effects of progesterone that is dominant during the second half of the menstrual cycle.[13]
- Environmental factors may exacerbate acne among young people who come into contact with grease at work (e.g., those employed in auto repair shops or fast-food restaurants). Patients may be unwilling or unable, however, to alter their employment status to accommodate concerns about acne.

BENZOYL PEROXIDE

Benzoyl peroxide (BP) primarily has an antibacterial effect and is useful in controlling inflammatory acne.[30,68] BP may also decrease formation of FFA, thereby improving obstructive (comedonal) disease.[30,68] These two actions make it a useful first-line drug in the management of patients with mild inflammatory or mixed (e.g., inflammatory and comedonal) acne.

BP is available with or without a prescription in concentrations ranging from 2.5% to 10%. Over-the-counter products include creams, lotions, washes, or gels. Prescription forms generally employ a gel vehicle, a factor that enhances efficacy. A single daily application of a product containing a 5% concentration is adequate for most patients. Increasing the concentration to 10% does not greatly enhance the therapeutic effect but does increase the likelihood of drying, erythema, and burning.[69]

BP usually is applied once daily, although twice-daily use may be beneficial for some patients. As with all topical medications, BP is applied as a thin coat to all acne-prone areas, not to individual lesions. When the entire face is to be treated, the patient may be instructed to dispense an amount the size of a pea onto a fingertip. To distribute the medication, the finger is touched to each side of the forehead, each cheek, and the chin. The medication is then spread to cover the entire face, avoiding sensitive areas such as the corners of the eyes, the alar folds, and the angles of the mouth. A BP wash that is used during a bath or shower may be used to treat larger areas such as the chest and back, although greater efficacy may be achieved by applying the gel formulation and allowing it to remain in place for several hours.

Adverse reactions resulting from the use of BP include stinging after application and drying, redness, and peeling of the skin. These reactions often can be limited by selecting an emollient or water-based gel, by reducing the concentration of BP, or by reducing the frequency of application.[13] Contact dermatitis is an unusual complication characterized by erythema, small papules, and pruritus. To avoid this, patients using BP for the first time should apply a small amount of medication to the forearm. If there is no reaction after 48 to 72 hours, BP may be used on the face. Those who develop contact dermatitis should avoid BP and use an alternate product (e.g., a topical antibiotic). Patients should be advised that BP may bleach clothing and bedding. BP is considered pregnancy category C by the Food and Drug Administration (e.g., risk to the fetus cannot be ruled out).[70]

TOPICAL ANTIBIOTICS

Topical antibiotics reduce concentrations of *P. acnes*, inflammatory mediators and, possibly, FFA.[30,71] As a result, these agents have been most useful in the management of mild to moderate inflammatory acne. The practical difficulties and cost associated with applying topical antibiotics to large areas limit their use to the treatment of facial acne. In the US, products containing clindamycin or erythromycin are available and have comparable efficacy.[72] Sodium sulfacetamide, with or without sulfur, is also available. Topical antibiotics are available in a variety of vehicles. As with other topical agents, lotions and creams are less drying than solutions or gels.

Products that combine agents enhance the therapeutic effect.[73–76] For example, BP 5% and erythromycin 3% (e.g., Benzamycin) is more effective than either drug alone,[75] and a formulation of erythromycin and zinc is of greater benefit than erythromycin alone.[76] Similarly, a combination of clindamycin and benzoyl peroxide is more effective than individual components.[74] Interestingly, the BP and zinc components of these products

---

68. Cotterill JA (1980) Benzoyl peroxide. **Acta Derm Venereol** (Stockh) 60(suppl 89):57–63.
69. Mills OH Jr., Kligman AM, Pochi P et al. (1986) Comparing 2.5% 5% and 10% benzoyl peroxide on inflammatory acne vulgaris. **Int J Dermatol** 25:664–667.
70. Physicians' Desk Reference. 54th ed. (2000) Montvale, NK: Medical Economics Co., Inc.
71. Gollnick H, Schramm M (1998) Topical drug treatment in acne. **Dermatology** 196:119–125.
72. Eady EA, Cove JH, Joanes DN et al. (1990) Topical antibiotics for the treatment of acne vulgaris: a critical evaluation of the literature on their clinical benefit and comparative efficacy. **J Dermatol Treat** 1:215–226.
73. Chu A, Huber FJ, Plott RT (1997) The comparative efficacy of benzoyl peroxide 5%/erythromycin 3% gel and erythromycin 4%/zinc 1.2% solution in the treatment of acne vulgaris. **Br J Dermatol** 136:235–238.

74. Lookingbill DP, Chalker DK, Lindholm JS et al. (1997) Treatment of acne with a combination of clindamycin/benzoyl peroxide gel compared with clincamycin gel, benzoyl peroxide gel and vehicle gel: Combined results of two double-blind investigations. **J Am Acad Dermatol** 37:590–595.
75. Packman AM, Brown RH, Dunlap FE et al. (1996) Treatment of acne vulgaris: Combination of 3% erythromycin and 5% benzoyl peroxide in a gel compared to clindamycin phosphate lotion. **Int J Dermatol** 35:209–211.
76. Schachner L, Pestana A, Kittles C (1990) A clinical trial comparing the safety and efficacy of a topical erythromycin-zinc formulation with a topical clindamycin formulation. **J Am Acad Dermatol** 22:489–495.

inhibit erythromycin–resistant propionibacteria *in vitro*.[77–79] The disadvantages of combination preparations are cost and the need for refrigeration of some products in order to maintain drug stability.

An area of concern related to the use of topical or systemic antibiotics is the emergence of resistant forms of *P. acnes*. In the United Kingdom, for example, between 1991 and 1996, the percentage of patients attending a dermatology clinic carrying antibiotic-resistant organisms rose from 34.5% to 60%.[78] In 1996, 47%, 41% and 26% of these patients harbored strains of *P. acnes* that were resistant to erythromycin, clindamycin, or tetracycline, respectively.[78] The majority of strains resistant to erythromycin exhibited cross–resistance to clindamycin and other macrolide, lincosamide, and streptogamin antibiotics.[78] Multiple drug resistance was observed in 18% of isolates.[78] Among propionibacteria resistant to tetracyclines, the degree of resistance to tetracycline is greater than that to doxycycline which, in turn, exceeds that to minocycline.[78] Eady and colleagues have demonstrated an association between carriage of erythromycin-resistant propionibacteria and poor clinical response to oral treatment with this agent.[80]

Because multiple factors influence antibiotic efficacy, the exact clinical significance of these data is not known. For example, topical concentrations of an antibiotic surpass those achievable by the oral route and, therefore, may exceed the minimal inhibitory concentration for strains considered resistant by laboratory testing.[78] Nevertheless, these data have led some clinicians to prescribe topical or oral erythromycin only for previously untreated acne patients who are unlikely to harbor resistant organisms,[78,80] and to limit the use of topical antibiotics to prevent the development of drug resistance. Recommendations for antibiotic use to reduce the selection of resistant organisms are presented in Table 13.4.

TABLE 13.4   Recommendations for antibiotic use to reduce the selection of resistant organisms

- Only prescribe antibiotics when necessary
- Treat for as brief a period as possible, recognizing that 3–6 months may be required to achieve a therapeutic effect (resistant strains begin to emerge 12–24 weeks after beginning therapy)
- If antibiotic re-treatment is required, employ the same agent unless there was a previous therapeutic failure
- Use BP for a minimum of 5–7 days between antibiotic courses to eliminate resistant organisms
- Avoid the use of concomitant oral and topical therapy with dissimilar antibiotics

Adapted from Eady EA[78]

TOPICAL RETINOIDS

For patients with significant numbers of comedones, topical retinoids are indicated.[13,30] These drugs normalize the keratinization process within follicles, reducing obstruction and the risk for follicular rupture.[13,81–85] Retinoids exert their effect by activating nuclear receptors (dimers composed of retinoic acid receptors and retinoid X receptors). These dimers bind specific DNA sequences (retinoic acid response elements) in the promoter region thereby regulating transcriptional activity.[86,87] Tretinoin is the best-known topical retinoid and is available in creams (0.025%, 0.05%, 0.1%), gels (0.01%, 0.025%), and a liquid (0.05%). The vehicle has an impact on efficacy; creams are less potent than gels which, in turn, are less potent than the liquid. Newer formulations appear to be as effective but less irritating than traditional varieties.[85,88,89] Tretinoin is also available in generic form.

Many adolescents who use tretinoin experience irritation, redness, or dryness. For persons of color, this inflammation may result in hypo- or hyper-pigmentation that can last several months. To prevent or limit adverse effects, therapy is often begun with a lower-strength preparation (e.g., tretinoin cream 0.025%). Patients are advised to use the medication every third night, progressing as tolerated over two to three weeks to a nightly application. Other adverse effects should be reviewed with the patient. About one-half of individuals experience an apparent temporary worsening of acne two to three weeks after starting tretinoin. Skin irritation may increase sensitivity to sunlight; as a result, a nonacnegenic, noncomedogenic sunscreen should be used. Applying too much tretinoin will worsen the irritant effect.

Because tretinoin is nearly identical in chemical structure to isotretinoin, some have raised concern about potential teratogenicity. However, there have been no reports of malformations occurring in infants born to women who used tretinoin during pregnancy.[13,30,90] Nevertheless, tretinoin is classified as pregnancy category C (e.g., risk to the fetus cannot be ruled out) and, for this reason, its use is avoided during pregnancy.[70] Since BP inactivates tretinoin, the two drugs should not be applied simultaneously. Rather, BP may be applied in the morning and tretinoin at night.

Other retinoids have also become available. Adapalene possesses retinoid-like activity and in a 0.1% gel has been shown to be as effective as tretinoin gel 0.025% but less irritating.[91,92] It is available as a 0.1% alcohol-free gel, cream, solution, or as pledgets. The principles of use and potential adverse effects are the same as those of tretinoin. Like tretinoin, it is classified as pregnancy category C.[70] Tazarotene is formulated in 0.05% and 0.1% gels and creams. Although proven effective in clinical studies, it is much more expensive and may be more irritating than other retinoids and, due to concerns about teratogenicity, is contraindicated in pregnancy.[84,93] For these reasons, it is not widely prescribed for the treatment of acne. Finally, in Europe, topical isotretinoin (0.05%) is available and has been shown to be comparable in efficacy to benzoyl peroxide and tretinoin.[94,95]

77. Bojar RA, Eady EA. Jones CE et al. (1994) Inhibition of erythromycin-resistant propionibacteria on the skin of acne patients by topical erythromycin with and without zinc. Br J Dermatol 130:329–336.
78. Eady EA (1998) Bacterial resistance in acne. Dermatology 196:59–66.
79. Eady EA, Bojar RA, Jones CE et al. (1996) The effects of acne treatment with a combination of benzoyl peroxide and erythromycin on skin carriage of erythromycin-resistant propionibacteria. Br J Dermatol 134:107–113.
80. Eady EA, Cove JH, Holland KT et al. (1989) Erythromycin resistant propionibacteria in antibiotic treated acne patients: Association with therapeutic failure. Br J Dermatol 121:51–57.
81. Bernerd F, Démarchez M, Ortonne J-P et al. (1991) Sequence of morphological events during topical application of retinoic acid on the rhino mouse skin. Br J Dermatol 125:419–425.
82. Kligman LH, Kligman AM (1979) The effect on rhino mouse skin of agents which influence keratinization and exfoliation. J Invest Dermatol 73:354–358.
83. Lavker RM, Leyden JJ, Thorne EG (1992) An ultrastructural study of the effects of topical tretinoin on microcomedones. Clin Ther 14:773–780.
84. Leyden JJ (1998) Topical treatment of acne vulgaris: Retinoids and cutaneous irritation. J Am Acad Dermatol 38(suppl):S1–S4.
85. Webster GF (1998) Topical tretinoin in acne therapy. J Am Acad Dermatol 39(suppl):S38–S44.
86. Chandraratna RAS (1998) Rational design of receptor-selective retinoids. J Am Acad Dermatol 39(suppl):S124–S128.
87. Kang S, Voorhees JJ (1998) Photoaging therapy with topical tretinoin: an evidence-based analysis. J Am Acad Dermatol 39(suppl):S55–S61.
88. Lucky AW, Cullen SI, Funicella T et al. (1998) Double-blind, vehicle-controlled, multicenter comparison of two 0.025% tretinoin creams in patients with acne vulgaris. J Am Acad Dermatol 38(suppl):S24–S30.
89. Lucky AW, Cullen SI, Jarratt MT et al. (1998) Comparative efficacy and safety of two 0.025% tretinoin gels: Results from a multicenter, double-blind, parallel study. J Am Acad Dermatol 38(suppl):S17–S23.
90. Jick SS, Terris BZ, Jick H (1993) First trimester topical tretinoin and congenital disorders. Lancet 341:1181–1182.
91. Cunliffe WJ, Caputo R, Dreno B et al. (1997) Clinical efficacy and safety comparison of adapalene gel and tretinoin gel in the treatment of acne vulgaris: Europe and U.S. multicenter trials. J Am Acad Dermatol 36(suppl):S126–S134.
92. Shalita A, Weiss JS, Chalker DK et al. (1996) A comparison of the efficacy and safety of adapalene gel 0.1% and tretinoin gel 0.025% in the treatment of acne vulgaris: A multicenter trial. J Am Acad Dermatol 34:482–485.
93. Kakita L (2000) Tazarotene versus tretinoin or adapalene in the treatment of acne vulgaris. J Am Acad Dermatol 43(suppl):S51–S54.
94. Hughes BR, Norris JFB, Cunliffe WJ (1992) A double-blind evaluation of isotretinoin 0.05%, benzoyl peroxide 5% gel and placebo in patients with acne. Clin Exp Dermatol 17:165–168.
95. Elbaum KJ (1988) Comparison of the stability of topical isotretinoin and topical tretinoin and their efficacy in acne. J Am Acad Dermatol 19:486–491.

AZELAIC ACID

Azelaic acid 20% is both antibacterial and anticomedonal.[96,97] It is applied twice daily and appears to be well tolerated, although some patients experience pruritus, burning, stinging, tingling, or erythema.[96] No systemic toxicity has been reported. In one controlled trial, azelaic acid was as effective as BP 5%, tretinoin 0.05% or erythromycin 2%.[98] Although it would seem a logical alternative for patients with mild to moderate inflammatory and comedonal acne, or for those with obstructive lesions who are unable to tolerate tretinoin, experience with azelaic acid is limited and, therefore, its exact role in acne treatment remains to be determined.[97]

Systemic therapies

ORAL ANTIBIOTICS

Oral antibiotics possess greater efficacy than topical preparations and, for this reason, are prescribed for patients with more severe or extensive inflammatory acne.[13,30,99] They exert their anti-inflammatory effect by decreasing bacterial colonization and inhibiting neutrophil chemotaxis; however, they also reduce the concentration of FFA in sebum.[13,100–102] Eady et al. have also demonstrated that tetracycline upregulates proinflammatory cytokines, particularly IL-1.[103] Although seemingly paradoxical, since IL-1 is proinflammatory, the authors speculate that enhancement of IL-1 production within follicles accelerates lesion resolution by decreasing the extent and duration of inflammation.[103]

Tetracycline and erythromycin are most often prescribed; both drugs are effective and inexpensive.[30] Depending on disease severity and the patient's weight, each is initiated at a dose of 250–500mg twice daily, although the higher dose is usually favored.[13,30,99] Both are available in liquid form for patients who cannot swallow pills or capsules. The primary adverse effect of erythromycin is gastrointestinal upset that may be avoided by taking the medication with food. Tetracycline, like erythromycin, may cause gastro-intestinal disturbances. To assure absorption, erythromycin should not be taken with milk and should be taken on an empty stomach (e.g., 30 minutes before or two hours after a meal). Tetracycline should not be used during pregnancy or for patients less than 9 years of age due to potential discoloration of teeth. Tetracycline occasionally has caused esophageal ulceration; as a result, patients should be advised to take the medication with a large glass of water and to avoid reclining immediately after ingesting a dose. Other adverse effects include photosensitivity and vulvovaginal candidiasis[13] and, uncommonly, pseudotumor cerebri, hyperpigmentation, and onycholysis.

For those who fail to respond to, or cannot tolerate, tetracycline or erythromycin, doxycycline often is effective.[13] It is begun at a dose of 50–100mg twice daily and can be taken with food.[13,30] Unfortunately, doxycycline is even more likely than tetracycline to induce photosensitivity reactions. An alternative to doxycycline is minocycline.[13] It is the most widely prescribed systemic antibiotic for the management of acne in the US, Canada and the UK.[104,105] Although it is generally considered highly effective, objective data are lacking. In a recent Cochrane Review, only two of 27 randomized controlled trials showed minocycline to be superior to other tetracyclines, and both of these had serious methodological flaws.[106] In clinical practice, however, minocycline may prove more effective than doxycycline or tetracycline when P. acnes resistance is suspected. Among resistant strains of propionibacteria collected from non-responding antibiotic-treated acne patients, Eady et al. found that the mean minimal inhibitory concentrations for tetracycline, doxycycline, and minocycline were $20.61 \pm 4.56\mu g/ml$, $9.70 \pm 2.03\mu g/ml$ and $1.95 \pm 0.35\mu g/ml$, respectively; sensitive strains exhibited MICs $\leq 1\mu g/ml$.[107]

Minocycline is initiated at a dose of 50–100mg bid; the latter dose is recommended when patients are suspected of harboring tetracycline resistant propionibacteria.[106] It is more expensive than other antibiotics and has uncommon but significant adverse effects. Skin pigmentation due to deposition of a melanin-drug complex is well recognized; it may take three forms: blue-black macules that are localized to areas of scarring (type I); localized or diffuse blue-black, brown or slate-gray hyperpigmentation that occurs in normal skin (type II); or a generalized brown pigmentation (type III).[108] Type I pigmentation appears unrelated to the duration of therapy or cumulative dose but types II and III generally occur in patients who have received a cumulative dose exceeding 70–100gm.[108] Types I and II resolve within several months of discontinuing therapy but type III may persist.[108] Minocycline-induced pigmentation has been treated successfully with Q-switched ruby or neodymium: Yag lasers.[107,109] Rarely, pigmentation may affect the teeth, oral mucosa, nails, or eyes.[108]

In recent years, occurrences of autoimmune adverse reactions in patients receiving minocycline have been reported, including a serum sickness-like reaction, a hypersensitivity syndrome, lupus erythematosus, and hepatitis.[105,110] The clinical features of these reactions are summarized in Table 13.5. Although these reactions are uncommon, those receiving minocycline should be counseled appropriately and advised to report unusual symptoms, particularly arthralgias, rash, fever, or jaundice.[105,110]

Other oral antibiotics have been employed in acne management. Trimethoprim-sulfamethoxazole is an alternative for patients who do not respond to other antibiotics, or with Gram-negative folliculitis. However, it should be used with caution due to potential adverse effects, including severe cutaneous allergic reactions. Pulsed azithromycin has proven effective,[111–113] although the emergence of erythromycin-resistant P. acnes may limit its value.

As with other acne therapies, six to eight weeks are required before oral antibiotics produce a significant clinical effect. Once the appearance of new lesions has ceased or been satisfactorily reduced, the dose may be tapered gradually or eventually withdrawn. For example, if an adolescent's inflammatory acne has been controlled with tetracycline 500mg twice daily, the dose may be decreased to 500mg once daily. If control is sustained, the drug could be tapered further or discontinued one to two months later in favor of topical therapy (e.g., benzoyl peroxide or a topical antibiotic). For some adolescents, however, attempts at tapering are unsuccessful and continued oral therapy may be required for months or years.

Concern often is raised that oral antibiotics may diminish oral contraceptive efficacy by decreasing enterohepatic recirculation of contraceptive steroids or by enhancing their hepatic degradation or renal or fecal excretion.[114]

96. Medical Letter, Inc. (1996) Azelaic acid – A new topical drug for acne. **Med Lett Drugs Ther** 38:52–53.
97. Weiss JS (1997) Current options for the topical treatment of acne vulgaris. **Pediatr Dermatol** 14:480–488.
98. Nguyen QH, Bui TP (1995) Azelaic acid: Pharmacokinetic and pharmacodynamic properties and its therapeutic role in hyperpigmentation disorders and acne. **Int J Dermatol** 34:75–84.
99. Leyden JJ (1997) Therapy for acne vulgaris. **N Engl J Med** 336:1156–1162.
100. Esterly NB, Furey NL, Flanagan LE (1978) The effect of antimicrobial agents on leukocyte chemotaxis. **J Invest Dermatol** 70:51–55.
101. Esterly NB, Koransky JS, Furey NL et al. (1984) Neutrophil chemotaxis in patients with acne receiving oral tetracycline therapy. **Arch Dermatol** 120:1308–1313.
102. Freinkel RK, Strauss JS, Yip SY et al. (1965) Effect of tetracycline on the composition of sebum in acne vulgaris. **N Engl J Med** 273:850–854.
103. Eady EA, Ingham E, Walters CE et al. (1993) Modulation of comedonal levels of interleukin-1 in acne patients treated with tetracyclines. **J Invest Dermatol** 101:86–91.
104. Teitelbaum JE, Perez-Atayde AR, Cohen M et al. (1998) Minocycline-related autoimmune hepatitis. Case series and literature review. **Arch Pediatr Adolesc Med** 152:1132–1136.
105. Eichenfield AH (1999) Minocycline and autoimmunity. **Curr Opin Pediatr** 11:447–456.
106. Garner SE, Eady EA, Popescu C et al. (2001) Minocycline for acne vulgaris: efficacy and safety (Cochrane Review). The Cochrane Library, Issue 1. URL: http://www.update-software.com/abstracts/ab002086.htm
107. Eady EA, Jones CE, Gardner KJ et al. (1993) Tetracycline-resistant propionibacteria from acne patients are cross-resistant to doxycycline, but sensitive to minocycline. **Br J Dermatol** 128:556–560.
108. Eisen D, Hakim MD (1998) Minocycline-induced pigmentation. Incidence, prevention and management. **Drug Safety** 18:431–440.
109. Wood B, Munro CS, Bilsland D (1998) Treatment of minocycline-induced pigmentation with the neodymium-Yag laser. **Br J Dermatol** 139:534–562.
110. Elkayam O, Yaron M, Caspi D (1999) Minocycline-induced autoimmune syndromes: An overview. **Semin Arthritis Rheum** 28:392–397.
111. Gruber F, Grubisic-Greblo H, Kastelan M et al. (1998) Azithromycin compared with minocycline in the treatment of acne comedonica and papulo-pustulosa. **J Chemother** 10:469–473.
112. Fernandez-Obregon AC (2000) Azithromycin for the treatment of acne. **Int J Dermatol** 39:45–50.
113. Parsad D, Pandhi R, Nagpal R et al. (2001) Azithromycin monthly pulse vs. daily doxycycline in the treatment of acne vulgaris. **J Dermatol** 28:1–4.
114. Fleischer AB Jr., Resnick SD (1989) The effect of antibiotics on the efficacy of oral contraceptives. A controversy revisited. **Arch Dermatol** 125:1562–1564.

TABLE 13.5   Autoimmune adverse effects associated with minocycline

Features of disease	Serum sickness-like reaction	Hypersensitivity reaction	Lupus-like reaction	Hepatitis
Average duration of treatment before onset (range)	16 days (7–35 days)	17 days	30 months (6–72 months)	19 months (2–120 months)
Clinical features	Rash, often urticaria Fever Arthralgia Lymphadenopathy	Morbilliform rash Fever Pharyngitis Lymphadenopathy Major organ involvement (lungs, liver, brain, kidney)	Polyarthralgia, polyarthritis ANA+ Fever Malaise Anorexia Rash Hepatitis	Arthralgia, arthritis ANA+ Fever Jaundice
Prognosis	Resolves within several days of discontinuing medication	Resoves with discontinuation of minocycline	Generally resolves after drug withdrawal	Generally resolves after withdrawal

Adapted from Eichenfield[105] and Elkayam[110].

Research fails to support this concern for antibiotics used to treat acne.[114–116] However, packaging information provided with some oral contraceptives containing estrogen and progesterone states a "possible" reduction in efficacy during use of ampicillin or tetracyclines.[70] Although "back-up" methods of birth control probably are not warranted, a final resolution of this issue is not likely to be forthcoming.[115] Clinicians should advise patients of this issue; based on this discussion, some may choose to employ a second form of contraception. For adolescents, however, the issue may be moot since clinicians advise those using hormonal contraception to also employ a condom at all sexual encounters to protect against sexually transmitted infections.

ISOTRETINOIN

Isotretinoin (13-cis retinoic acid) is a retinoid used systemically for the treatment of severe, scarring acne.[117–119] Retinoids are derivatives of vitamin A, but in contrast to vitamin A, a fat-soluble vitamin, isotretinoin is excreted and does not accumulate in tissues. Although in the US isotretinoin is indicated for the treatment of severe, scarring nodular acne that has failed conventional therapy, it is widely used for all forms of scarring acne (papular and pustular as well as nodular). Isotretinoin is administered in a dose of 0.5–2.0mg/kg per day; unlike other acne medications, however, it is administered for a finite period, typically 16–20 weeks. The majority of patients treated in this way experience clearing of acne and remain clear, but the dose and duration of therapy must be individualized and repeat courses may be necessary. Initial studies indicated that doses as low a 0.1mg/kg per day could be effective in clearing acne, but that the relapse rate was much higher than in those treated with higher doses.[118] Some dermatologists believe that a treatment course in which the cumulative dose is 120–150mg/kg is associated with success, regardless of the daily dose or duration of therapy. Because some patients experience an initial flare of acne during treatment, half the maintenance dose, or less, may be used during the first month. Clearing may occur at any time during therapy.

Due to potentially serious adverse effects associated with isotretinoin, it should be prescribed only by clinicians experienced in its use.[120] The most serious of these, as with all systemic retinoids, is teratogenicity.[120,121] It is imperative that females of childbearing age be tested to assure that they are not pregnant when they start the drug, and that they begin effective contraception one month in advance of beginning isotretinoin therapy, and maintain this throughout the course of treatment and for at least a month afterwards. Monthly pregnancy tests are mandatory as is regular monitoring of cholesterol, triglyceride, and hepatic function. Other adverse effects include elevations of cholesterol and triglyceride, hepatic dysfunction, mucocutaneous dryness, dryness of the eyes that may preclude the use of contact lenses, headache (with a potential for pseudotumor cerebri), visual changes, and varying degrees of musculoskeletal pain. Although hyperostosis has been found radiographically, there is no evidence that doses used for the treatment of acne cause premature closure of the epiphyses.[122]

It has been postulated that isotretinoin use, through mechanisms unknown, may predispose patients to depression and suicide. The results of a recent study, however, fail to confirm this association. Jick *et al.* compared rates of mental health disorders in more that 7000 acne patients taking isotretinoin with those of more than 13 000 patients taking antibiotics.[123] They also compared rates among isotretinoin users before and during therapy. No statistically significant increase in the risk of depression, psychosis, or suicide among isotretinoin users was observed.[123] Nonetheless, clinicians caring for patients with acne who are receiving isotretinoin should remain alert to the possible presence of mental health disorders, including depression and suicidal ideation.

HORMONAL THERAPY

Oral hormonal contraceptives may affect acne in several ways. Estrogen improves acne by increasing levels of SHBG, which decreases biologically active free testosterone, and by suppressing gonadotropin secretion, thereby reducing ovarian androgen production.[13,124] The inherent androgenic and antiestrogenic potential of the progestin component of an oral or other hormonal contraceptive also may influence acne severity. Thus, oral contraceptives containing progestins with low androgenic potential (e.g., norethindrone or its acetate, ethynodiol diacetate, or newer agents such as norgestimate or desogestrel) often are considered to have the most favorable effects on acne.[13] Among the studies that have examined the impact of oral

115. Helms SE, Bredle DL, Zajic J et al. (1997) Oral contraceptive failure rates and oral antibiotics. **J Am Acad Dermatol** 36:705–710.

116. Miller DM, Helms SE, Brodell RT (1994) A practical approach to antibiotic treatment in women taking oral contraceptives. **J Am Acad Dermatol** 30:1008–1011.

117. Peck GL, Olsen TG, Yoder FW et al. (1979) Prolonged remission of cystic and conglobate acne with 13-cis-retinoic acid. **N Engl J Med** 300:329–333.

118. Shalita AR, Cunningham WJ, Leyden JJ et al. (1983) Isotretinoin treatment of acne and related disorders: an update. **J Am Acad Dermatol** 9:629–638.

119. Goulden V, Layton AM, Cunliffe WJ (1994) Long term safety of isotretinoin as a treatment for acne vulgaris. **Br J Dermatol** 131:360–363.

120. American Academy of Pediatrics Committee on Drugs (1992) Retinoid therapy for severe dermatological disorders. **Pediatrics** 90:119–120.

121. Lammer EJ, Chen DT, Hoar RM et al. (1985) Retionoic acid embryopathy. **N Engl J Med** 313:837–841.

122. Carey BM, Parkin GJ, Cunliffe WJ et al. (1988) Skeletal toxicity with isotretinoin therapy: a clinical-radiological evaluation. **Br J Dermatol** 119:609–614.

123. Jick SS, Kremers HM, Vastlakis-Scaramozza C (2000) Isotretinoin use and risk of depression, psychotic symptoms, suicide, and attempted suicide. **Arch Dermatol** 136:1231–1236.

124. Lucky AW, Henderson TA, Olson WH et al. (1997) Effectiveness of norgestimate and ethinyl estradiol in treating moderate acne vulgaris. **J Am Acad Dermatol** 37:746–754.

contraceptives on acne, however, all appear to demonstrate a benefit, regardless of the progestin component employed.[124–133] Unfortunately, the majority of studies were potentially flawed by the failure to include a placebo control group.[125–130,132,133] Two recent placebo-controlled trials indicate that a combined oral contraceptive containing ethinyl estradiol (35μg) and the progestin norgestimate can improve acne.[124,131] These results notwithstanding, oral contraceptives generally are not viewed as a primary therapy for acne but as adjuncts to standard medications. In Europe, the antiandrogen cyproterone acetate (2mg) combined with ethinyl estradiol (35μg) is employed in the management of patients with recalcitrant disease. Acne is a recognized adverse effect associated with the use of long-acting progestin implants and may occur during the use of depot medroxyprogesterone acetate.[131,134–137]

Adolescents with acne exacerbated by endocrine disorders may require treatment with agents such as spironolactone (an androgen antagonist), low-dose glucocorticoids or gonadotropin-releasing hormone agonists.[13] Patients with these conditions are best managed in consultation with a specialist (e.g., endocrinologist, gynecologist or gynecologic endocrinologist). Clinicians should be aware, however, that acne may be a presenting sign in young women with disorders such as polycystic ovary syndrome or syndrome X (insulin resistance, obesity, hypertension, and dyslipidemia).[137] These women may be at future risk for early-onset Type 2 diabetes mellitus, infertility, obesity, and early cardiovascular disease.

Office therapy

Procedures performed in the office may be an important adjunct to topical and systemic therapy. Comedo extraction is a relatively painless procedure that results in immediate, although often temporary improvement. The resolution of painful nodules may be hastened by the injection of a corticosteroid (e.g., 0.2ml of triamcinolone acetonide 2.5mg/ml) using a 30-gauge needle. There are few data regarding the effectiveness of chemical peels or laser resurfacing in adolescents with active acne.

Complementary and alternative therapies

Although a number of complementary and alternative therapies have been advocated for the treatment of acne, for most, efficacy and safety have not been clearly established. Tea tree oil, derived from *Melaleuca alternifolia*, is a complex mixture of terpenes and related alcohols[138–140] that has antibiotic properties.[135] In a single-blind trial of 124 patients with mild to moderate acne, a 5% water-based gel formulation of tea tree oil was as effective as benzoyl peroxide 5% water-based lotion.[138] Although considered safe when used topically, tea tree oil may cause contact dermatitis[141] and, if applied undiluted, may induce comedogenesis.[142] In young children, inadvertent ingestion of small amounts of tea tree oil has produced confusion, ataxia, and drowsiness.[139,143] The efficacy and safety of other herbal remedies in acne treatment have not been studied. Although uncontrolled trials have demonstrated improvements in acne following accupuncture, controlled trials have not evaluated this or other bioenergetic therapies (e.g., therapeutic touch,

homeopathy, etc.).[141] Similarly, there are no scientific studies demonstrating the benefit of lifestyle (e.g., nutrition, exercise) or biomechanical (e.g., massage, spinal manipulation) therapies.

SYNTHESIS

Deciding which medication(s) should be prescribed for an adolescent with acne is based on a synthesis of several factors, including the types and numbers of lesions present, the clinician's impression of the severity of disease, the extent of acne, and the patient's past experiences with medications and personal preferences. Information contained in Table 13.2 is designed to assist in developing rational treatment plans. Beyond this, however, there is an art to treating acne and two clinicians may differ in their approach to the same patient. Disturbingly, therapeutic choices may be governed by formulary restrictions. In some states in the US, for example, prescription topical acne medications are not approved for Medicaid reimbursement. Thus, clinicians may need to serve as advocates for their patients in order to assure adequate acne care.

FOLLOW-UP

A return visit is typically scheduled for two to three months following the initiation of therapy. However, patients should be encouraged to telephone sooner with questions or concerns regarding possible adverse effects. At the follow-up visit, one can assess compliance, determine the patient's impression

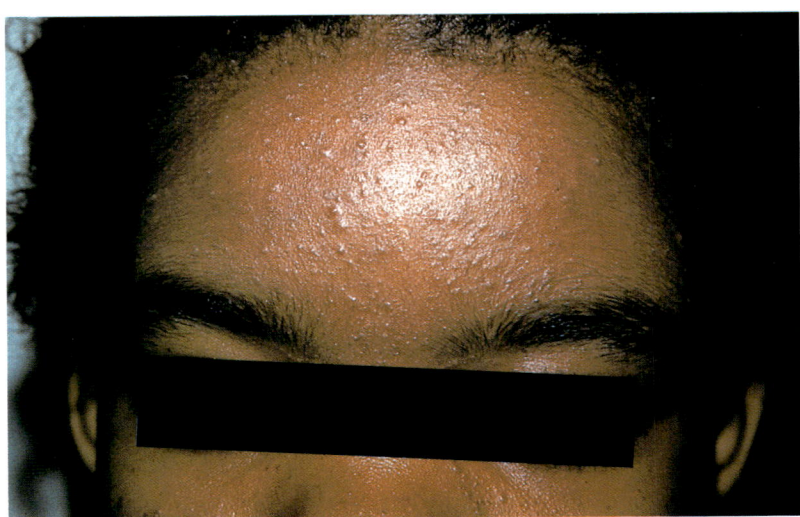

Fig. 13.14 Pomade acne: multiple closed comedones are present on the forehead. (Reprinted with permission from Krowchuk DP, Lucky AW (2001) Managing adolescent acne. *Adolesc Med* 12:355–374.

125. Carlborg L (1996) Cyproterone acetate versus levonorgestrel combined with ethinyl estradiol in the treatment of acne. **Acta Obstet Gynecol Scand** Suppl 134:29–32.
126. Erkkola R, Hirvonen E, Luikku R et al. (1990) Ovulation inhibitors containing cyproterone acetate or desogestrel in the treatment of hyperandrogenic symptoms. **Acta Obstet Gynecol Scand** 69:61–65.
127. Lemay A, Dewailly SD, Grenier R et al. (1990) Attenuation of mild hyperandrogenic activity in postpubertal acne by a triphasic oral contraceptive containing low doses of ethynyl estradiol and d,l-norgestrel. **J Clin Endocrinol Metab** 71:8–14.
128. Mango D, Ricc S, Manna P et al. (1996) Clinical and hormonal effects of ethinyl estradiol combined with gestodene and desogestrel in young women with acne vulgaris. **Contraception** 53:163–170.
129. Miller JA, Wojnarowska FT, Dowd PM et al. (1986) Anti-androgen treatment in women with acne: A controlled trial. **Br J Dermatol** 114:705–716.
130. Palatsi R, Hirvensalo E, Liukko P et al. (1984) Serum total and unbound testosterone and sex hormone binding globulin (SHBG) in female acne patients treated with two different oral contraceptives. **Acta Derm Venereol** (Stockh) 64:517–523.
131. Redmond GP, Olson WH, Lippman JS et al. (1997) Norgestimate and ethinyl estradiol in the treatment of acne vulgaris: A randomized, placebo-controlled trial. **Obstet Gynecol** 89:615–622.
132. Weber-Diehl F, Unger R, Lachnit U (1992) Triphasic combination of ethinyl estradiol and gestodene. Long-term clinical trial. **Contraception** 46:19–27.
133. Wishart JM (1991) An open study of Triphasil and Diane 50 in the treatment of acne. **Australas J Dermatol** 32:51–54.
134. Cullins VE, Garcia FAR (1997) Implantable hormonal and emergency contraception. **Curr Opin Obstet Gynecol** 9:169–174.
135. Darney PD, Klaisle CM, Tanner S et al. (1990) Sustained released contraceptives. **Curr Probl Obstet Gynecol Fertil** 12:30–55.
136. Nelson AL (1996) Counseling issues and management of side effects for women using depot medroxyprogesterone acetate contraception. **J Reprod Med** (Suppl) 41:391–400.
137. DeGroot HE, Friedlander SF (1998) Update on acne. **Curr Opin Pediatr** 10:381–386.
138. Gardiner P, Coles D, Kemper KJ (2001) Herbs and supplements for pediatric dermatology. **Contemp Pediatr** (In Press).
139. Jacobs MR, Hornfeldt CS (1994) Melaleuca oil poisoning. **J Toxicol Clin Toxicol** 32:461–464.
140. Bassett IB, Pannowitz DL, Barnetson RSC (1990) A comparative study of tea-tree oil versus benzoylperoxide in the treatment of acne. **Med J Australia** 153:455–458.
141. Selvaag E, Eriksen B, Thune P (1994) Contact allergy to tea tree oil and cross-sensitization to colophony. **Cont Derm** 31:124–125.
142. Kemper KJ (1996) The Holistic Pediatrician. New York, NY: Harper Perennial, pp. 24–34.
143. Del Beccaro MA (1995) Melaleuca oil poisoning in a 17-month-old. **Vet Human Toxicol** 37:557–558.

of response to treatment, note the occurrence of adverse effects, and make an objective assessment of the effect of therapy. Based on the initial response, the clinician can determine the need to maintain or revise the therapeutic plan.

ACNE VARIANTS

NEONATAL AND INFANTILE ACNE

The appearance of inflammatory papules and pustules and, occasionally, comedones at birth or during the first month of life has been termed neonatal acne (Fig. 13.15). With the recognition of neonatal cephalic pustulosis (see below), however, the frequency and existence of neonatal acne as a distinct entity has been questioned by some. Lesions are located on the cheeks, forehead, and nose. Most infants exhibit few lesions; only a minority have disease severe enough to prompt medical attention.[144–146] Neonatal acne occurs in as many as 20% of newborns; males are more often affected than females (4.5:1).

Acne beginning at 3 to 6 months of age is termed infantile acne (acne infantum). Although less common than neonatal acne, it may be more severe and persistent.[144,145] Open and closed comedones, and inflammatory papules and pustules are present (Fig. 13.16). Lesions usually are confined to the face, typically the cheeks. As in neonatal acne, males are more frequently affected than females.

The mechanisms underlying true neonatal and infantile acne are incompletely understood; however, they likely result from the effects of androgens on sebaceous glands. At birth and for the first 6 to 12 months of life, males produce early pubertal levels of testosterone.[147,148] In both males and females, during the first year of life, the adrenal glands secrete high levels of DHEA and DHEAS; DHEAS has been significantly and specifically associated with the development of acne in young girls.[15,148] That males have an additional testicular androgen component may explain why they are more vulnerable to neonatal and infantile acne.[148] An abnormal sensitivity of pilosebaceous follicles to normal levels of circulating hormones has also been postulated to explain the occurrence of neonatal and infantile acne. The observation that some infants have a family history of severe acne or hyperandrogenism suggests a role for genetic factors.

Neonatal and infantile acne should be differentiated from other disorders, including infantile acne venenata, acneiform reactions due to maternal drug intake during pregnancy (e.g., phenytoin, lithium), candidiasis, and nevus comedonicus.[149] During the first weeks of life, neonatal cephalic pustulosis, pustular miliaria, and neonatal sebaceous gland hyperplasia must be differentiated.[149] Evaluation for hyperandrogenism, such as congenital adrenal hyperplasia, should be reserved for those infants with severe or persistent disease.[149]

Parents must be informed that the disorder may be chronic and that long-term therapy may be required. In addition, they should be advised of the possibility of renewed acne at puberty; one study suggests that those with acne as an infant may be prone to more severe disease during adolescence.[12]

For infants with a few inflammatory lesions, topical benzoyl peroxide or erythromycin may be employed. A low concentration of tretinoin (e.g., 0.025% cream) may be employed to treat comedones. In severe inflammatory disease, oral erythromycin may be considered but tetracycline should not be

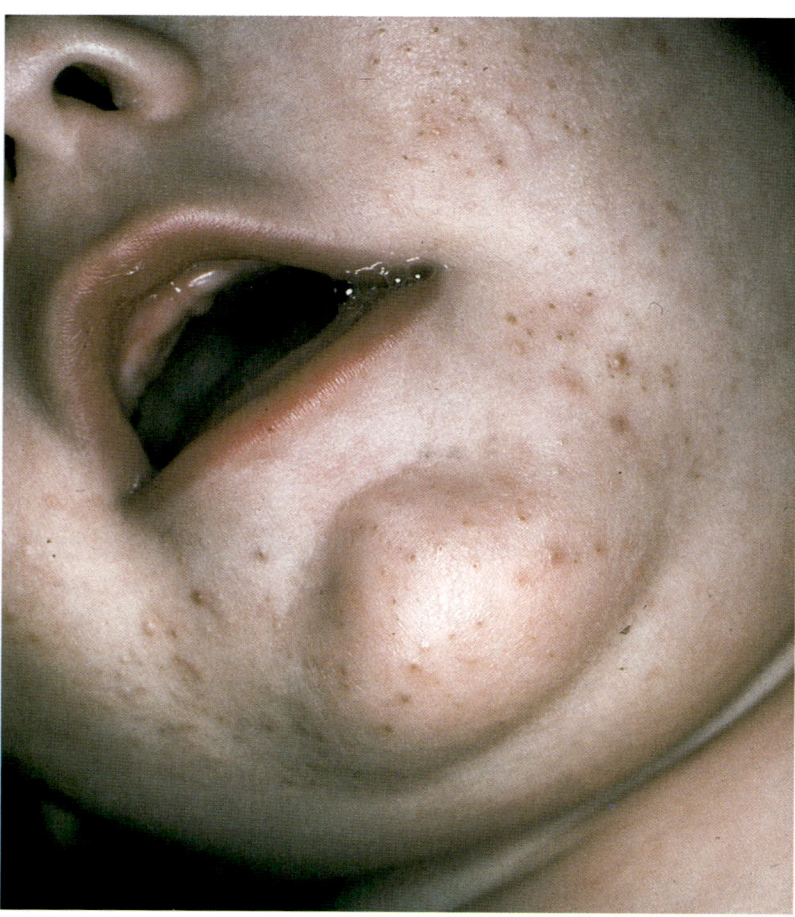

Fig. 13.15 Open comedones and small inflammatory lesions on the chin of an infant with acne.

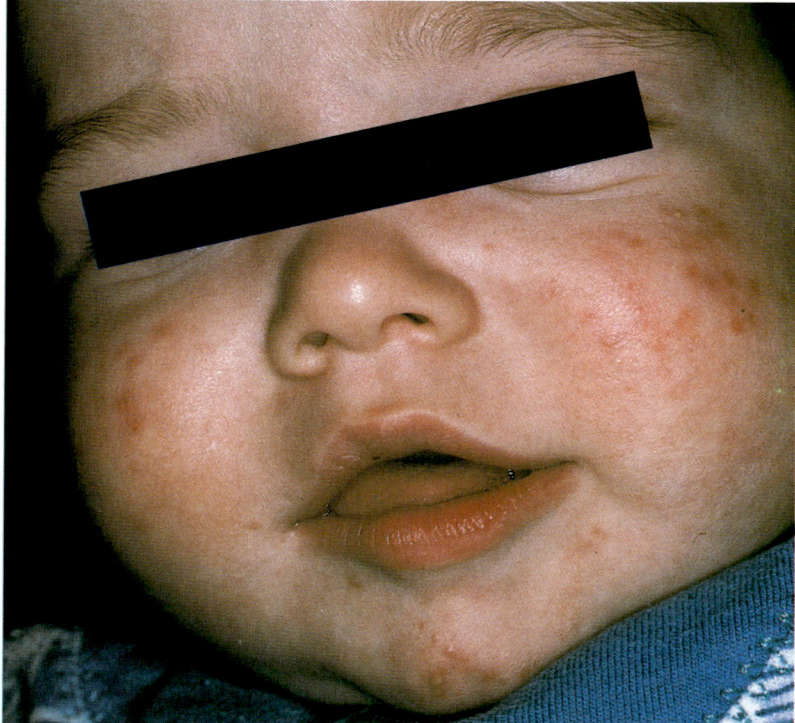

Fig. 13.16 Inflammatory lesions and open comedones on the cheeks and chin of an infant with acne.

144. Jansen T, Burgdorf WHC, Plewig G (1997) Pathogenesis and treatment of acne in childhood. **Pediatr Dermatol** 14:17–21.
145. White GM (1998) Recent findings in the epidemiologic evidence, classification, and subtypes of acne vulgaris. **J Am Acad Dermatol** 39:S34–S37.
146. Giknis F, Hall WK, Tolman MM (1952) Acne neonatorum. **Arch Dermatol Syph** 66:717–721.

147. Bekaert C, Song M, Delvigne A (1998) Acne neonatorum and familial hyperandrogenism. **Dermatology** 196:453–454.
148. Lucky AW (1998) A review of infantile and pediatric acne. **Dermatology** 196:95–97.
149. Katsambas AD, Katoulis AC, Stavropoulos P (1999) Acne neonatorum: a study of 22 cases. **Int J Dermatol** 38:128–130.

on microscopic examination of a potassium hydroxide preparation. It is important to distinguish neonatal cephalic pustulosis from other neonatal disorders characterized by pustules. The absence of comedones, the absence of a follicular distribution, and the monomorphic appearance of lesions distinguish it from neonatal acne. Clinical features also differentiate neonatal cephalic pustulosis from erythema toxicum, transient neonatal pustular melanosis, eosinophilic pustulosis, and acropustulosis of infancy.[155] Treatment with a topical anti-yeast preparation (e.g., ketoconazole or miconazole cream) twice daily for one to two weeks is effective; however, even without treatment the disorder resolves rapidly and spontaneously.[153]

ACNE IN CHILDHOOD

Severe, persistent or therapy-resistant infantile acne, or the appearance of acne between the ages of 1 and 7 years, is rare and should alert the clinician to the possibility of androgen excess due to premature andrenarche, late-onset forms of congenital adrenal hyperplasia, or a gonadal or adrenal tumor.[148] If an endocrine disorder is suspected, measurement of free and total testosterone, DHEA and DHEAS, and the performance of radiographs for bone age should be considered.[151] Treatment of acne in childhood is analogous to that of infantile acne.

SEVERE INFLAMMATORY OR NODULAR ACNE IN CHILDHOOD

Severe inflammatory and nodulocystic acne during childhood (acne conglobata infantum) occurs very rarely.[144] It is characterized by a single or a few large violaceous nodulocystic lesions located on the face. The onset is usually during the second year of life, and males and females may be affected. The cause of the disorder is unknown, but it has been suggested that it reflects an end-organ hypersensitivity to androgens.[157,158] Although reported patients have demonstrated no evidence of androgen excess, clinical and laboratory assessment to investigate this possibility should be performed. The course of nodulocystic acne in children is variable; scarring may occur and patients may experience severe acne during adolescence. Topical or systemic therapy, analogous to that employed in infantile acne, is indicated.[144] Occasionally, children with severe inflammatory acne and scarring require isotretinoin.[144]

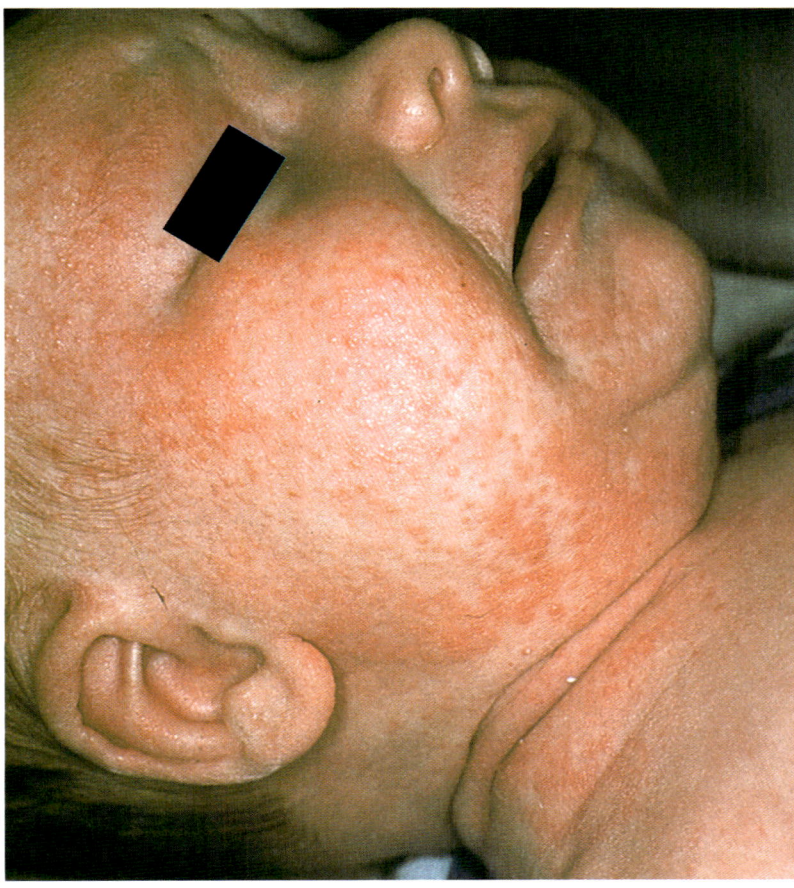

Fig. 13.17 Numerous papules and pustules on the face of an infant with neonatal cephalic pustulosis.

used due to potential discoloration of teeth.[144] The course of infantile acne is variable; often it disappears within one to two years, but it may persist, rarely into puberty. Scarring as a result of inflammation is possible.[150]

NEONATAL CEPHALIC PUSTULOSIS

Neonatal cephalic pustulosis is a recently recognized entity that in the past may have been confused with neonatal acne.[151,152] It appears during the first month of life in both females and males, and is characterized by erythema, pustules, or papules located on the face and neck (Fig. 13.17). Histologic examination reveals a predominance of neutrophils and yeasts of the genus *Malassezia*.[152] This observation has led to speculation that the condition may represent an inflammatory reaction to *Malassezia* spp. Although the role of yeasts has been questioned,[153] and other factors may contribute, the severity of disease correlates with the isolation of *Malassezia* spp. from the skin of affected newborns.[154]

The diagnosis of neonatal cephalic pustulosis is suggested by the age at onset, location of lesions, and absence of comedones. *Malassezia* may be found

ACNE CONGLOBATA

Acne conglobata is a severe variant of nodulocystic acne characterized by cysts, abscesses, and multichanneled draining sinuses that involve the face, neck and trunk (Fig. 13.18).[159] Extensive scarring and keloid formation are common sequelae. *Staphylococcus aureus*, group A β-hemolytic *Streptococcus*, and other bacteria are frequently recovered from lesions and may play a role in disease pathogenesis. Occasionally, patients experience musculoskeletal symptoms, including arthralgia and arthritis.[160] Acne conglobata generally is a chronic progressive disease of adult men; a severe variant has been reported in patients with human immunodeficiency virus infection.[161] Acne conglobata also may occur in association with dissecting cellulitis of the scalp and hidradenitis suppurativa, the so-called "follicular occlusion triad." The development of squamous cell carcinoma in areas of chronic inflammation

150. Janniger CK (1993) Neonatal and infantile acne vulgaris. **Cutis** 52:16.
151. Aractingi S, Cadranel S, Reygagne P et al. (1991) Neonatal pustulosis induced by Malassezia furfur. **Ann Dermatol Venereol** 118:856–858.
152. Rapelanoro R, Mortureux P, Couprie B et al. (1996) Neonatal Malassezia furfur pustulosis. **Arch Dermatol** 132:190–193.
153. Bardazzi F, Patrizi A, Neri I (1997) Transient cephalic neonatal pustulosis. **Arch Dermatol** 133:528–530.
154. Niamba P, Weill FX, Sarlangue J et al. (1998) Is common neonatal cephalic pustulosis (neonatal acne) triggered by Malassezia sympodialis? **Arch Dermatol** 134:995–998.
155. Van Praag MC, Van Rooij RW, Folkers E et al. (1997) Diagnosis and treatment of pustular disorders in the neonate. **Pediatr Dermatol** 14:131–143.
156. De Raeve L, De Schepper J, Smitz J (1995) Prepubertal acne: a cutaneous marker of androgen excess? **J Am Acad Dermatol** 32:181–184.
157. Mengesha YM, Hansen RC (1999) Toddler-age nodulocystic acne. **J Pediatr** 134:644–648.
158. Horne HL, Carmichael AJ (1997) Juvenile nodulocystic acne responding to systemic isotretinoin. **Br J Dermatol** 136:796–797.
159. Berge T, Gundersen J (1967) Acne conglobata. **Acta Derm Venereol** (Stockh) 47:41–45.
160. Olafsson S, Khan MA (1992) Musculoskeletal features of acne, hidradenitis suppurativa, and dissecting folliculitis of the scalp. **Rheum Dis Clin North Am** 18:215–224.
161. Martin AG, Weaver CC, Cockerell CJ et al. (1992) Pityriasis rubra pilaris in the setting of HIV infection: clinical behaviour and association with explosive cystic acne. **Br J Dermatol** 126:617–620.

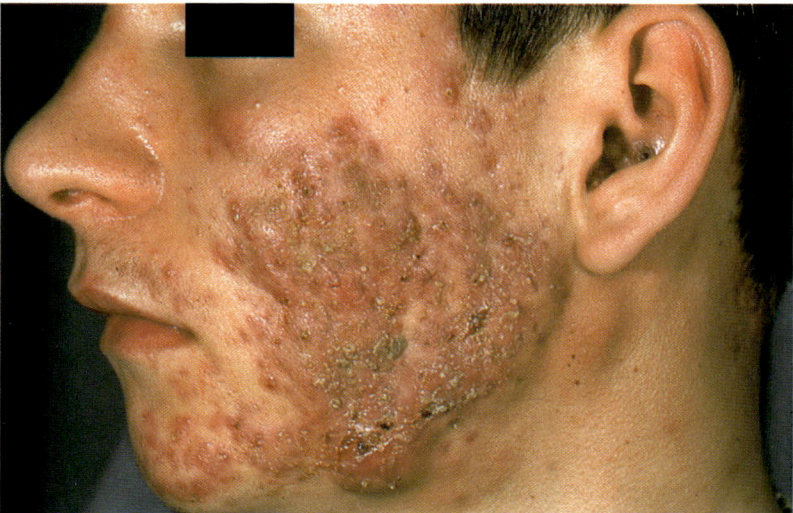

Fig. 13.18   Severe acne conglobata on the cheek of an adolescent boy. (Photo courtesy of John S. Strauss, M.D.)

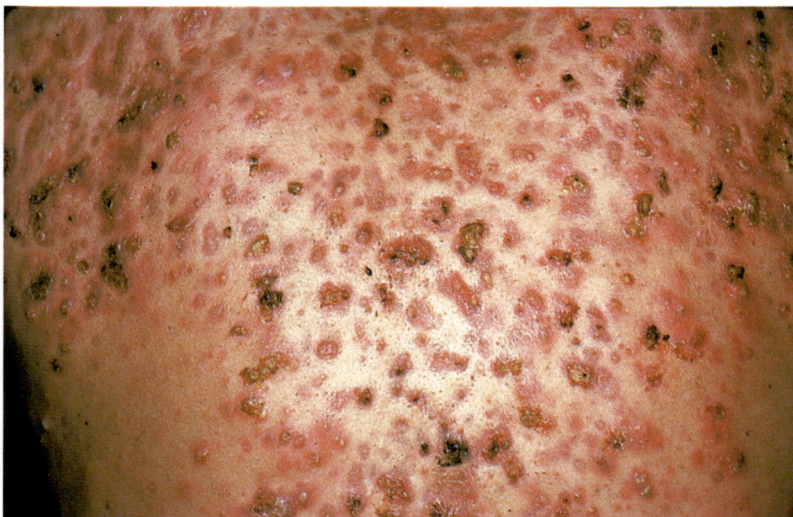

Fig. 13.19   Acne fulminans in a 14-year-old boy. Note the numerous crusted nodules that appeared suddenly and were accompanied by fever and lymphadenopathy.

induced by each of the disorders comprising the follicular occlusion triad has been reported.[162] Acne conglobata must be differentiated mainly from steatocystoma multiplex (sebocystomatosis), a distinct developmental disease of the pilosebaceous unit that is inherited in an autosomal-dominant manner. Pyoderma faciale, a variant of acne conglobata that affects adult women, is distinguished by its abrupt onset, rapid progression, limitation to the face, and lack of systemic symptoms.[163]

The diagnosis of acne conglobata generally is straightforward, although pyoderma and panniculitis may produce similar lesions. Treatment may include a topical or oral antibiotic; however, oral isotretinoin (0.5–1mg/kg per day) is considered the most effective agent. Careful monitoring is required during isotretinoin therapy, but the drug appears to be well tolerated, even in young children.[164,165] A brief course of oral prednisone may be useful to prevent scarring in patients with severe inflammation.

ACNE FULMINANS

Acne fulminans (acute febrile ulcerating acne conglobata, acne maligna) is a devastating disorder of unknown cause usually affecting adolescent males, many of whom are receiving oral antibiotics for the treatment of mild to moderate acne. The onset is marked by the sudden appearance on the back, chest and, occasionally, the face of painful nodulocystic lesions that evolve into hemorrhagic nodules and plaques; these lesions rapidly undergo suppuration and necrotic degeneration (Fig. 13.19).[166] Ulcers may heal slowly with extensive scarring. Patients often experience fever, chills, weight loss, weakness, arthralgia, myalgia, erythema nodosum, or hepatosplenomegaly.[167] Arthritis, primarily involving large joints, the lower back and shoulder girdle, and osteolytic lesions with periosteal reaction suggestive of osteomyelitis, mainly involving the sternum, clavicles, and pelvis, may be present.[168,169] Laboratory abnormalities include leukocytosis, increased erythrocyte

sedimentation rate, and C-reactive protein, anemia, hematuria, hypergammaglobulinemia, and elevation of liver enzymes.

The cause of acne fulminans remains unclear, although bacterial infection, an abnormal immunologic reaction (an altered reaction to *Propionibacterium acnes* has been demonstrated in some patients), or a drug-induced disorder have been hypothesized.[167] Its predominance during adolescence raises the question of whether hormonal factors are important, and reports of familial clustering suggest a genetic susceptibility.[170] A subset of patients with acne of a severity comparable to that of acne fulminans but without characteristic systemic involvement has been reported.[171]

Although acne fulminans may resemble acne conglobata, it occurs in a younger population, is associated with systemic symptoms, and has a more explosive onset. Spontaneous healing occurs but may take years. The response to broad-spectrum antibiotic treatment is usually poor.[172] Antibiotics may be helpful, however, when secondary bacterial infection is suspected. Isotretinoin is often employed to treat acne fulminans, although in some patients, particularly those treated with high doses, the drug actually may precipitate the disorder. The treatment regimen is similar to that used for acne vulgaris (e.g., 0.5–1.0mg/kg daily for 3–5 months). Initially, low doses are used to prevent flaring of the disease, but eventually higher doses (e.g., 1.0–2.0mg/kg daily) may be required. A systemic steroid (e.g., 0.5–1.0mg/kg per day of prednisone) is often recommended as the treatment of choice to control inflammatory skin lesions, reduce fever, and improve musculoskeletal symptoms.[166,167] When used alone, prednisone should be continued for two to four months to avoid relapse. The combination of isotretinoin and prednisone is likely to be the most beneficial approach to the treatment of acne fulminans.[166,167,172,173] Aggressive skin care (e.g., surgical debridement, topical antibiotic application) may be of some value during the active phase of the disease.[167]

162. Camisa C (1984) Squamous cell carcinoma arising in acne conglobata. **Cutis** 33:185–190.
163. Massa MC, Su WPD (1982) Pyoderma faciale: a clinical study of twenty-nine patients. **J Am Acad Dermatol** 6:84–91.
164. Arbegast KD, Braddock SW, Lamberty LF et al. (1991) Treatment of infantile cystic acne with oral isotretinoin: a case report. **Pediatr Dermatol** 2:166–168.
165. Léauté-Labrèze C, Gautier C, Labb L et al. (1998) Infantile acne treated with oral isotretinoin. **Ann Dermatol Venereol** 125:132–134.
166. Karvonen SL (1993) Acne fulminans: report of clinical findings and treatment of twenty-four patients. **J Am Acad Dermatol** 28:572–579.
167. Jansen T, Plewig G (1998) Acne fulminans. **Int J Dermatol** 37:254–257.
168. Erhardt E, Harangi F (1997) Two cases of musculoskeletal syndrome associated with acne. **Pediatr Dermatol** 14:456–459.
169. Gordon PM, Farr PM, Milligan A (1997) Acne fulminans and bone lesions may present to other specialities. **Pediatr Dermatol** 14:446–448.
170. Wong SS, Pritchard MH, Holt PJA (1992) Familial acne fulminans. **Clin Exp Dermatol** 17:351–353.
171. Thomson KF, Cunliffe WJ (2000) Acne fulminans "sine fulminans". **Clin Exp Dermatol** 25:299–301.
172. Seukeran DC, Cunliffe WJ (1999) The treatment of acne fulminans: a review of 25 cases. **Br J Dermatol** 141:307–309.
173. Allison MA, Dunn CL, Person DA (1997) Acne fulminans treated with isotretinoin and "pulse" corticosteroids. **Pediatr Dermatol** 14:39–42.

PYODERMA FACIALE

A condition analogous to acne fulminans may occur in females; it is termed pyoderma faciale or rosacea fulminans. In contrast to acne fulminans, however, the trunk is spared while on the face there appears a rapidly progressive pustular and nodular eruption (Fig. 13.20). Therapy is analogous to that of acne fulminans, with a high dose of a glucocorticosteroid (provided in a long, tapering course) and a gradually increasing dose of isotretinoin.

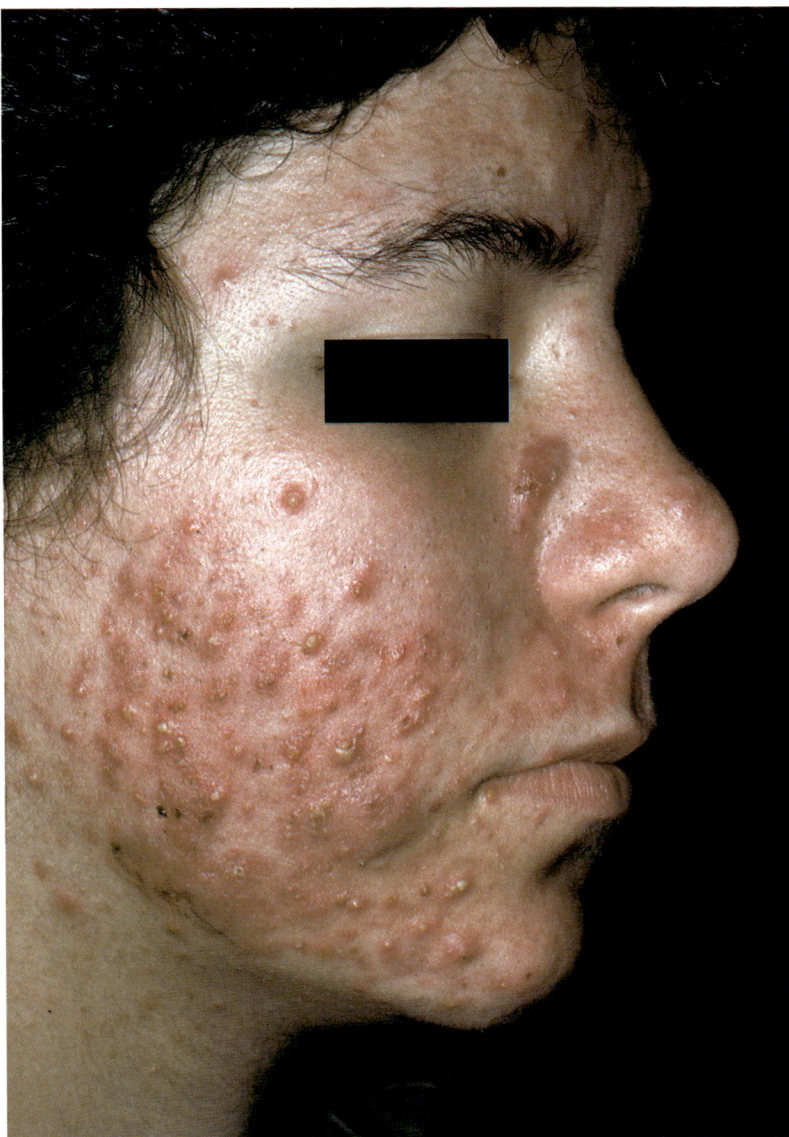

Fig. 13.20 Rapidly progressive pustular and nodular eruption in a patient with pyoderma faciale.

GRAM-NEGATIVE FOLLICULITIS

Gram-negative folliculitis is a cutaneous infection with Gram-negative bacteria that occurs as a complication of long-term, broad-spectrum antibiotic treatment (e.g., tetracycline) for acne.[174,175] More recently, it has been suggested that immunologic factors may play a role in the pathogenesis of the disorder.[176] The face is usually involved and two clinical presentations have been described. In the majority of those affected, pustules and papules are present, often extending outward from the anterior nares. *Escherichia coli*, *Enterobacter* spp. or *Klebsiella* spp. are usually isolated from the pustules. More rarely, the disorder presents with tender, fluctuant, deep-seated nodules of the cheeks produced by *Proteus* spp.

Gram-negative folliculitis should be considered in any acne patient receiving long-term oral antibiotic therapy who experiences a sudden worsening of disease. Because organisms are often scarce, several lesions should be sampled for bacterial culture.[177] The condition may be avoided by withdrawing oral antibiotics whenever possible, and by using oral antibiotics in combination with topical benzoyl peroxide. In established cases, withdrawal of the antibiotic and initiation of isotretinoin (0.5–1.0mg/kg daily for four to five months) usually is effective.[178]

PERSISTENT FACIAL EDEMA

Solid persistent facial edema (Morbihan's disease) is a rare complication of both acne vulgaris[179,180] and rosacea (rosaceous lymphedema).[181,182] It occurs most commonly between the ages of 14 and 20 years and has not been reported prepubertally. Patients develop chronic, inflammatory, and nonpitting swelling of facial skin. The etiology of persistent facial edema is unknown; however, it may be the result of fibrosis and obstruction of lymphatic vessels due to chronic inflammation. A history of antecedent inflammatory acne provides a clue to diagnosis. Persistent facial edema is often resistant to conventional acne treatment; systemic isotretinoin is the preferred therapy, but clofazimine alone and the combination of isotretinoin and ketotifen also have been used successfully.[183]

ACNE EXCORIÉE DES JEUNES FILLES

This form of acne is seen most frequently in adolescent females,[184] but older women and males may be affected.[185] Patients characteristically pick, squeeze, and scratch their real or imagined acne lesions causing crusting, scarring, and linear excoriations. This trauma can prolong the course of the disease, and worsen inflammation and scarring. Most patients do not fulfil diagnostic criteria for psychiatric disease such as obsessive-compulsive or body image disorders;[184] rather, they are believed to be developmentally immature and their skin disease may serve as an appeal for help. When questioned, patients generally admit the self-inflicted nature of their lesions.[186] Acne excoriée is best managed with emotional support and antibiotic therapy to prevent or treat secondary bacterial infection; psychiatric intervention may be helpful in severe cases.

CHILDHOOD ROSACEA AND STEROID ROSACEA

Rosacea is a chronic facial dermatosis that primarily affects women between the ages of 30 and 50 years. It is characterized by a facial eruption composed

174. Leyden JJ, Marples RR, Mills OH et al. (1973) Gram-negative folliculitis – a complication of antibiotic therapy in acne vulgaris. Br J Dermatol 88:533–538.
175. Poli F, Prost C, Revuz J (1988) Gram-negative bacteria folliculitis. Ann Dermatol Venereol 115:797–800.
176. Neubert U, Jansen T, Plewig G (1999) Bacteriologic and immunologic aspects of gram-negative folliculitis: a study of 46 patients. Int J Dermatol 38:270–274.
177. Plewig G, Jansen T (1998) Acneiform dermatoses. Dermatology 196:102–107.
178. James WD, Leyden JJ (1985) Treatment of gram-negative folliculitis with isotretinoin: positive clinical and microbiologic response. J Am Acad Dermatol 12:319–324.
179. Connelly MG, Winkelmann RK (1985) Solid facial edema as a complication of acne vulgaris. Arch Dermatol 121:87–90.
180. Camacho-Martinez F, Winkelmann RK (1990) Solid facial edema as a manifestation of acne. J Am Acad Dermatol 22:129–130.
181. Jansen T, Regele D, Schirren CG et al. (1998) Persistent erythema and edema of the face associated with rosacea and lymph vessel dysplasia. Hautarzt 49:932–935.
182. Harvey DT, Fenske NA, Glass LF (1998) Rosaceous lymphedema: a rare variant of a common disorder. Cutis 61:321–324.
183. Jungfer B, Jansen T, Przybilla B et al. (1993) Solid persistent facial edema of acne: successful treatment with isotretinoin and ketotifen. Dermatology 187:34–37.
184. Bach M, Bach D (1993) Psychiatric and psychometric issues in acne excoriée. Psychother Psychosom 60:207–210.
185. Gupta MA, Gupta AK, Schork NJ (1994) Psychosomatic study of self-excoriative behaviour among male acne patients: preliminary observations. Int J Dermatol 33:846–848.
186. Kent A, Drummond LM (1989) Acne excoriée: a case report of treatment using habit reversal. Clin Exp Dermatol 14:163–164.

of telangiectasias, erythema, edema, flushing, papules, and pustules. Sebaceous hyperplasia and thickening of the skin may result in the development of rhinophyma. Histopathology demonstrates chronic superficial perivascular inflammation surrounding dilated dermal capillaries. Pustules show aggregates of neutrophils and sebaceous glands may be increased in number and size. Noncaseating granulomas may be present in papulonodular lesions.

Rosacea has rarely been reported in children but should be considered in those with a chronic, erythematous, papular, or pustular eruption that involves the cheeks, chin, or nasolabial folds.[187,188] Telangiectasias may be present but rhinophyma and flushing have not been reported in children. Blepharitis, keratoconjunctivitis, and episcleritis are commonly associated and their presence assists in differential diagnosis.[189,190]

Childhood rosacea may be confused with a number of disorders. The absence of comedones and the predominance of the vascular component (e.g., telangiectasias) distinguish it from acne vulgaris. Although folliculitis is characterized by papules and pustules, unlike rosacea it has an acute onset and responds rapidly to appropriate antibiotic treatment. Location of lesions in periorificial areas, lack of telangiectasias, and a paucity of pustules suggest a diagnosis of perioral dermatitis. Excessive or inappropriate cosmetic use may induce comedones (acne venenata) or worsen pre-existing rosacea. Demodicidosis (Demodex folliculitis or demodicosis) has been reported in both immunocompetent and HIV-infected children. The diagnosis is confirmed by recovering abnormal numbers of *Demodex folliculorum* (a common ectoparasite of the human pilosebaceous unit) from pustules.[191]

The persistent or repeated use of topical steroids, particularly potent agents, may cause steroid acne (steroid rosacea).[192] Patients have persistent erythema, telangiectasias, and atrophy, along with papules and pustules (Fig. 13.21). Unlike rosacea, lesions may not be limited to the central face. It has been proposed that affected individuals respond in an unusual manner to the application of topical steroids or are particularly susceptible to rosacea. Supporting this are the observations that all patients in one report had been treated with topical steroids,[188] and that affected children often have a first-degree relative with rosacea.[193]

Sarcoidosis, systemic and discoid lupus erythematosus, papular granuloma annulare, granulosis rubra nasi, and Haber syndrome should also be considered in the differential diagnosis in children with rosacea and steroid rosacea.[168] Haber syndrome, inherited in an autosomal-dominant fashion, is characterized by a childhood rosacea-like eruption that may be exacerbated by sun exposure.[194] Patients may also have pigmented keratotic lesions of the trunk and xerosis. On histological examination, basaloid cells are localized around the hair and sebaceous follicles, or represent true intraepidermal epitheliomas.

Rosacea has a well-known tendency to wax and wane. Children with cutaneous and ocular rosacea respond well to traditional therapies, including systemic or topical antibiotics.[187,188] Topical metronidazole (0.75%) has proven safe and effective for use in children as well as adults. These agents also are effective in the treatment of steroid rosacea, providing that the use of topical steroids is discontinued. Following initiation of treatment, one to four months may be required to clear the eruption.

PERIORAL DERMATITIS IN CHILDHOOD

Perioral dermatitis is a common disorder that typically affects young women but may occur in children or adolescents. Papules and pustules on an erythematous background are distributed around the mouth, sparing a narrow zone around the vermilion border. Although dermatitis in a perioral distribution is common in children, only rarely does it represent the variety seen in adults.[195,196] When the "adult form" of perioral dermatitis occurs in children it often is termed granulomatous perioral dermatitis[197] or childhood granulomatous periorificial dermatitis.[198] These disorders are characterized by small, monomorphous, grouped, skin-colored papules located not only around the mouth (Fig. 13.22) but in the perinasal and periorbital areas (typically the infraorbital area). In view of this distribution, it is clear that the adjective perioral is not entirely accurate. Black children seem to be particularly prone to the granulomatous variant of the disorder[199] and, as a result, the term Facial Afro-Caribbean Childhood Eruption (FACE) has been proposed.[200] In the pediatric age group, perioral dermatitis is seen equally in boys and girls, and affected children are otherwise healthy. Histopathologic examination reveals upper dermal and perifollicular granulomas admixed with lymphocytes. The findings are often nonspecific and similar to those observed in papular or granulomatous manifestations of rosacea.

It has been suggested that granulomatous perioral and periorificial dermatitis represent a granulomatous juvenile variant of classic perioral dermatitis[187] or a juvenile form of rosacea.[201] The etiology of perioral derma-

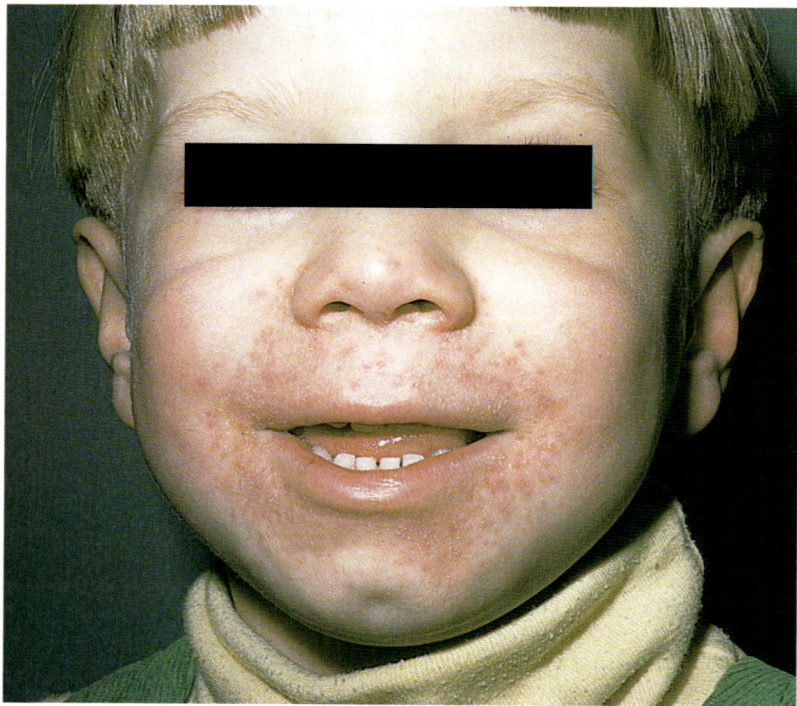

Fig. 13.21 Erythematous papules located around the mouth of a child treated with a mid-potency topical corticosteroid (perioral dermatitis).

187. Howard R, Tsuchiya A (1998) Adult skin disease in the pediatric patient. **Dermatologic Clinics** 16:593–608.
188. Drolet B, Paller AS (1992) Childhood rosacea. **Pediatr Dermatol** 9:22–26.
189. Bourrat E, Rybojad M, Deplus S et al. (1996) Ocular rosacea in a child. **Ann Dermatol Venereol** 123:664–665.
190. Erzurum SA, Feder RS, Greenwald MJ (1993) Acne rosacea with keratitis in childhood. **Arch Ophthalmol** 111:228–230.
191. Patrizi A, Neri I, Chieregato C et al. (1997) Demodicidosis in immunocompetent young children: report of eight cases. **Dermatology** 195:239–242.
192. Martin DL, Turner ML, Williams CM (1989) Recent onset of smooth, shiny, erythematous papules on the face. Steroid rosacea secondary to topical fluorinated steroid therapy. **Arch Dermatol** 125:828–831.
193. Weston WL, Morelli JG (2000) Steroid rosacea in prepubertal children. **Arch Pediatr Adolesc Med** 154:62–64.

194. Kikuchi I, Saita B, Inoue S (1981) Haber's syndrome. Report of a new family. **Arch Dermatol** 117:321–324.
195. Grosieux C, Stalder JF (1997) Perioral dermatitis in children. **Ann Dermatol Venereol** 124:346–350.
196. Manders SM, Lucky AW (1992) Perioral dermatitis in childhood. **J Am Acad Dermatol** 27:688–692.
197. Frieden IJ, Prose NS, Fletcher V et al. (1989) Granulomatous perioral dermatitis in children. **Arch Dermatol** 125:369–373.
198. Knautz MA, Lesher JL (1996) Childhood granulomatous periorificial dermatitis. **Pediatr Dermatol** 13:131–134.
199. Marten RH, Prebury DGC, Adamson JE et al. (1974) An unusual papular and acneiform facial eruption in the negro child. **Br J Dermatol** 91:435–438.
200. Williams HC, Ashworth J, Pembroke AC et al. (1990) FACE – facial Afro-Caribbean childhood eruption. **Clin Exp Dermatol** 15:163–166.
201. Laude TA, Salvemini JN (1999) Perioral dermatitis in children. **Semin Cutan Med Surg** 18:206–209.

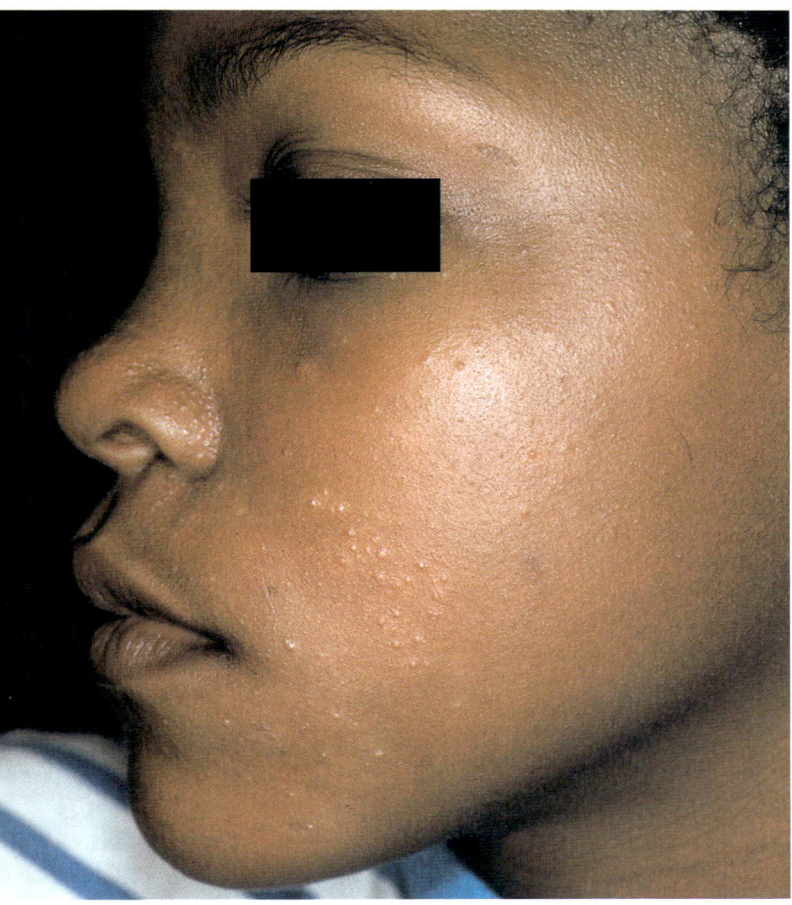

Fig. 13.22 Monomorphous papules located around the mouth of a child with granulomatous perioral dermatitis.

titis is unknown but it may represent a peculiar response to contact with certain substances, most often topical corticosteroids, particularly mid- to high-potency preparations. Other substances implicated include toothpastes,[202] bubble gum, oils, and greases.

A number of disorders may mimic granulomatous perioral dermatitis.[195] Atopic dermatitis, flat warts, folliculitis, allergic contact dermatitis, rosacea, and acrodermatitis enteropathica all may be distributed periorally. However, the most common cause of a perioral eruption in children is an irritant dermatitis caused by salivation, contact with a pacifier, thumb sucking, licking or foods. A skin biopsy may be helpful in differentiating more unusual facial eruptions such as sarcoidosis, lupus miliaris disseminatus faciei, and benign cephalic histicytosis.

The treatment of granulomatous perioral dermatitis is analogous to that of rosacea. Metronidazole 0.75% gel or cream is recommended by most authors.[203,204] Its mechanism of action remains to be elucidated, but it may have an anti-inflammatory or, less likely, antimicrobial effect. In severe cases, a systemic antibiotic (e.g., erythromycin or, depending on the patient's age, tetracycline) may be employed. In those cases resulting from topical steroid use, withdrawal of the steroid may be associated with a temporary worsening of the eruption.

ACNE VENENATA

Acne venenata is the term applied to acne that results from exposure to topical agents that induce comedone formation. It may occur at any age but typically begins beyond the usual age limits for acne vulgaris. Several variants have been described, including acne cosmetica, pomade acne, and occupational acne.

Acne cosmetica

In 1972 Kligman and Mills described a form of acne venenata due to skin care products, which they termed acne cosmetica.[205] It typically affects women in their third decade of life and is rarely observed in infants or children.[144,206,207] Individuals with a history of acne vulgaris have greater susceptibility to acne cosmetica. Numerous cosmetics are comedogenic, as demonstrated in both the rabbit ear model and human subjects.[208,209] Racial differences in follicular reactivity to topical agents have been demonstrated; thus, in blacks the acne cosmetica is predominantly a noninflammatory comedonal disease, while in whites there is a greater inflammatory component.[210] Treatment includes eliminating cosmetics or restricting their use to oil-free, noncomedogenic, nonacnegenic products and the application of a topical retinoid.

Pomade acne

Pomade acne is most often a problem in black patients who use oil-based scalp or hair preparations and inadvertently apply them to facial skin.[211] Densely packed closed comedones occur on the forehead and temples; occasionally, inflammatory papules and pustules may be observed (Fig. 13.14). If the offending agent is applied more widely, large areas of the face may be involved.[212] In infants and young children, a similar eruption may follow long-term application of oily lubricants (acne cosmetica). More elaborate and complex formulations induce pomade acne more frequently and more intensively than simpler preparations, such as petrolatum and mineral oil. Pomade acne often responds to avoidance of contact of hair care products with the skin. A topical retinoid may be helpful in clearing the comedones.

Occupational acne

Occupational acne has been described most often in men beyond the usual age of adolescent acne.[213] Unlike pomades and cosmetics, which are only mildly comedogenic, a number of industrial agents may produce florid acne. Common offending agents include cutting oils, petroleum oil, coal tars, and pitches.[214] Prominent open comedones, papules, pustules, and nodules appear on the face and areas covered by clothing saturated with the offending agent. Treatment consists of the avoidance of industrial comedogenic agents.

Adolescents employed in "fast food" restaurants or automobile repair shops may also develop occupational acne resulting from chronic exposure to cooking oils, greases, or motor oil. This form of acne is primarily comedonal, although inflammatory lesions may develop.

CHLORACNE

Chloracne is a variant of occupational acne caused by exposure to halogenated polycyclic hydrocarbons such as chlorinated dibenzodioxins and dibenzofurans present in paints, varnishes, lacquers, wood preservatives, oils, insecticides, and

202. Ferlito TA (1992) Tartar-control toothpaste and perioral dermatitis. **J Clin Orthod** 26:43–44.
203. Miller SR, Shalita AR (1994) Topical metronidazole gel (0.75%) for the treatment of perioral dermatitis in ch ldren. **J Am Acad Dermatol** 31:847–848.
204. Boeck K, Abeck D, Werfel S et al. (1997) Perioral dermatitis in children – clinical presentation, pathogenesis-related factors and response to topical metronidazole. **Dermatology** 195:235–238.
205. Kligman AM, Mills OH (1972) Acne cosmetica. **Arch Dermatol** 106:843–850.
206. Berlin C (1954) Acne comedo in children due to paraffin oil applied on the head. **Arch Dermatol** 69:683–687.
207. Menni S, Brancaleone W (1992) Cosmetic acne in a child. **Eur J Dermatol** 2:242–243.
208. Fulton JE Jr, Pay SR, Fulton JE III (1984) Comedogenicity of current therapeutic products, cosmetics, and ingredients in the rabbit ear. **J Am Acad Dermatol** 10:96–105.
209. American Academy of Dermatology invitational symposium on comedogenicity (1989) **J Am Acad Dermatol** 20:272–277.
210. Kaidbey KH, Kligman AM (1974) A human model of coal tar acne. **Arch Dermatol** 109:212–215.
211. Fisher AA (1986) Acne venenata in black skin. **Cutis** 37:24–26.
212. Plewig G, Fulton JE, Kligman AM (1970) Pomade acne. **Arch Dermatol** 101:580–584.
213. Plewig G, Kligman AM (1975) Acne Morphogenesis and Treatment. New York: Springer-Verlag.
214. Adams BB, Chetty VB, Mutasim DF (2000) Periorbital comedones and their relationship to pitch tar: a cross-sectional analysis and a review of the literature. **J Am Acad Dermatol** 42:624–627.

herbicides.[215,216] Some dioxins are potent acnegenic agents, both through skin contact and inhalation. In children, chloracne has been reported after accidental exposure to compounds such as 2,3,7,8-tetrachlorodibenzo-p-dioxin.[217] The disorder is probably due to the interference of these chemicals with vitamin A metabolism in the skin, resulting in disturbances of the epithelial tissues of the pilosebaceous follicle.[218] Affected individuals develop large open comedones on the face, particularly on the cheeks and ears, and in the postauricular, axillary and inguinal folds. In patients with prolonged or heavier exposure, keratotic inflammatory papules, pustules, nodules, and cysts appear. Occasionally, the eruption may become generalized, involving the trunk and extremities, particularly the dorsa of the hands. Lesions heal with pitted scars that resemble those of atrophoderma vermiculata.

Beyond the cutaneous effects, exposure to these compounds may cause ophthalmological, neurological (e.g., peripheral neuropathy), hepatic, and lipoprotein abnormalities.[219,220] Although dioxins may be measured in blood lipids, the acneiform eruption remains the most sensitive indicator of systemic poisoning. In fact, chloracne is the most common initial manifestation of halogenated polycyclic hydrocarbon poisoning.[220] Therapy must be individualized, based on the type and severity of lesions; however, the response to treatment may be poor when disease is severe.[221]

ACNEIFORM ERUPTIONS INDUCED BY DRUGS

The term acneiform refers to follicular dermatoses, characterized by papules or pustules, that resemble acne vulgaris but are not thought to be related etiologically.[145,177] These dermatoses are almost always induced by drugs. A generalized acneiform eruption is a well-recognized adverse effect of the chronic administration of systemic corticosteroids or adrenocorticotropic hormone.[222] Steroids act directly on the follicular epithelium, causing focal degeneration and a subsequent inflammatory reaction. This so-called "steroid acne" has clinical similarities to pityrosporum folliculitis and, in fact, high concentrations of *Malassezia furfur* may be found in lesional follicles of most patients with acneiform eruptions associated with systemic steroid therapy.[223] In addition to corticosteroids, acneiform eruptions have been associated with the use of androgens, anabolic steroids,[224] isoniazid, cyclosporin A, lithium carbonate, and other halogenated compounds (e.g., bromide and iodide often present in expectorants and sedatives), vitamin B, and anticonvulsants (e.g., diphenyl-hydantoin, phenobarbital).[177] It should be noted that these agents may cause an acneiform eruption *de novo* or worsen pre-existing acne vulgaris. Newborns may exhibit an acneiform eruption as the result of *in utero* drug exposure as occurs in the fetal hydantoin syndrome.[225]

Acneiform drug eruptions can be differentiated clinically from acne vulgaris. They tend to be uniformly papular or pustular; comedones and cysts rarely occur. Lesions are generally in the same stage of development (e.g., are monomorphous) and often are more widely distributed on the body (e.g., affect large areas of the trunk or the arms). The diagnosis of an acneiform drug eruption is based on the patient's history of exposure to a known causative drug, the clinical findings, and the disappearance of lesions following drug withdrawal.[177]

DISORDERS ASSOCIATED WITH ACNE

In a number of pediatric disorders, acne is an associated clinical manifestation. Apert's syndrome is an autosomal dominantly inherited disorder characterized by craniosynostosis and early epiphyseal closure, causing deformities of the skull, hands and feet.[226,227] Affected individuals have an abnormal sensitivity to normal circulating levels of androgens that predisposes them to the development of severe pustular acne.[228] Conventional therapy is often ineffective, but isotretinoin has been used successfully. As noted previously, acne vulgaris has been reported to be more common and severe in persons with the XYY chromosomal genotype.[6,7,229] This syndrome is characterized by tall stature, mental retardation, and aggressive behavior.[226] Severe acne has also been reported in persons with other chromosomal abnormalities, including Klinefelter syndrome.[230,231]

The acronym SAPHO syndrome (Synovitis, Acne, Pustulosis, Hyperostosis, Osteitis) was coined to emphasize the association between osteoarticular inflammation and neutrophilic skin disorders.[232] Its existence as a unique entity is debated since it shares many features of acne fulminans. SAPHO syndrome occurs rarely in children. Patients have bone and joint involvement that often affects the anterior chest wall; a recurrent multifocal osteomyelitis has been reported. Cutaneous manifestations include severe acne (e.g., acne fulminans or conglobata), a pustular eruption that typically involves the palms and soles, or psoriasis vulgaris.[233] Early recognition of SAPHO syndrome should prevent unnecessary surgery and avoid prolonged and ineffective antibiotic therapy.

215. Coenraads PJ, Olie K, Tang NJ (1999) Blood lipid concentrations of dioxins and dibenzofurans causing chloracne. **Br J Dermatol** 141:694–697.
216. Neuberger M, Kundi M, Jager R (1998) Chloracne and morbidity after dioxin exposure (preliminary results). **Toxicol Lett** 96–97:347–350.
217. Gianotti F (1977) Chloracne due to tetrachloro-2,3,7,8-dibenzo-p-dioxin in children. **Ann Dermatol Venereol** 104:825–829.
218. Coenraads PJ, Brouwer A, Olie K et al. (1994) Chloracne. Some recent issues. **Dermatol Clin** 12:569–576.
219. Rosas Vazquez E, Campos Macias P, Ochoa Tirado JG et al. (1996) Chloracne in the 1990s. **Int J Dermatol** 35:643–645.
220. Mocarelli P, Marocchi A, Brambilla P (1986) Clinical and laboratory manifestations of exposure to dioxin in children. A six-year study of the effects of an environmental disaster near Seveso, Italy. **JAMA** 256:2687–2695.
221. Scerri L, Zaki I, Millard LG (1995) Severe halogen acne due to a trifluoromethylpyrazole derivative and its resistance to isotretinoin. **Br J Dermatol** 132:144–148.
222. Hurwitz RM (1989) Steroid acne. **J Am Acad Dermatol** 21:1179–1181.
223. Yu HJ, Lee SK, Son SJ et al. (1998) Steroid acne vs. pityrosporum folliculitis: the incidence of Pityrosporum ovale and the effect of antifungal drugs in steroid acne. **Int J Dermatol** 37:772–777.
224. Collins P, Cotterill JA (1995) Gymnasium acne. **Clin Exp Dermatol** 20:509.
225. Stankler L, Campbell AGM (1980) Neonatal acne vulgaris: a possible feature of the fetal hydantoin syndrome. **Br J Dermatol** 103:453–455.
226. Downs AM, Condon CA, Tan R (1999) Isotretinoin therapy for antibiotic-refractory acne in Apert's syndrome. **Clin Exp Dermatol** 24:461–463.
227. Parker TL, Roth JG, Esterly NB (1992) Isotretinoin for acne in Apert syndrome. **Pediatr Dermatol** 9:298–300.
228. Henderson CA, Knaggs H, Clark A et al. (1995) Apert's syndrome and androgen receptor staining of the basal cells of sebaceous glands. **Br J Dermatol** 132:139–143.
229. Hook EB (1973) Behavioral implications of the human XYY genotype. **Science** 179:139–150.
230. Funderburk SJ, Landau JW (1976) Acne in retarded boy with autosomal chromosomal abnormality. **Arch Dermatol** 112:859–861.
231. Wollenberg A, Wolff H, Jansen T et al. (1997) Acne conglobata and Klinefelter's syndrome. **Br J Dermatol** 136:421–423.
232. Gmyrek R, Grossman ME, Rudin D et al. (1999) SAPHO syndrome: report of three cases and review of the literature. **Cutis** 64:253–258.
233. Beretta-Piccoli BC, Sauvain MJ, Gal I et al. (2000) Synovitis, acne, pustulosis, hyperostosis, osteitis (SAPHO) syndrome in childhood: a report of ten cases and review of the literature. **Eur J Pediatr** 159:594–601.

Eczematous Dermatitis

Bernice R. Krafchik, Anne Halbert, Kazuya Yamamoto and Rikako Sasaki

Dermatitic eruptions represent a major portion of the skin diseases seen in infancy and childhood. As early as 1992 more than $364 million was spent yearly, in the US, on the care of childhood atopic dermatitis (AD).[1] Annual costs of AD are similar to those of other chronic diseases such as emphysema, psoriasis, and epilepsy.[2] Estimates of costs in the US, including third-party costs, range from $0.9 billion to $3.8 billion annually when projected across the total number of persons younger than 65.[2] Tunnessen reported that one-third of the dermatology cases seen in a pediatric setting were eczematous and that AD was common in both a general pediatric and a special pediatric dermatology clinic.[3] Likewise, Schachner found that 22% of the patients seen in a pediatric dermatology clinic had AD.[4] The referral patterns have changed in recent years; irritant diaper dermatitis is not seen with the same frequency in the Western world owing to the widespread use of disposable diapers, and seborrheic dermatitis is also seen less. There is an increased incidence in AD, which comprises the most common reason for referrals to pediatric dermatology clinics. Although infants and children have the same immunological status as adults, allergic contact dermatitis (ACD), other than nickel, and poison ivy dermatitis in North America, is not commonly seen in the younger age group. The major eczematous eruptions of childhood are atopic dermatitis, seborrheic dermatitis, diaper dermatitis, contact dermatitis, perioral dermatitis and nummular dermatitis. Also of importance are lichen striatus, autosensitization dermatitis, lichen simplex chronicus, prurigo nodularis, papular urticaria, and asteatotic dermatitis.

ATOPIC DERMATITIS

HISTORICAL ASPECTS

AD was described by Besnier[5] as prurigo diasthetique in 1882 and was known in Europe as Besnier's prurigo. In 1923, Coca and Cooke[6] used the term *atopy* (without place or a strange thing) to describe a hypersensitive state in humans characterized by an enhanced capacity to form reagins (now known to be IgE) in response to a variety of antigens. The original description included asthma and hay fever. Later, it was realized that Besnier's prurigo also fell within this category. In 1933, Wise and Sulzberger[7] used the term AD to describe a morphological entity, which was characterized

clinically by Hill and Sulzberger[8] in 1935. Atopic dermatitis is the designation that is now used universally.

DEFINITIONS

The term AD describes a chronic, inherited, relapsing, pruritic skin condition with clinical features of xerosis, inflammation, and lichenification. The disease varies in location according to the age of the patient. Associated with these clinical findings, there is often a family or personal history of AD, asthma, allergic rhinitis, and numerous pharmacological and immunological abnormalities, including a tendency to overproduce IgE in response to common environmental antigens.

Eczema (boiling over) refers both to the infantile form of AD and to the morphology of erythema, scaling, vesicles, and crusts (Fig. 14.1). The term is used loosely by both physicians and the general public. One may find eczematous lesions in conditions other than AD (including scabies, autosensitization reactions, tinea pedis, immunodeficiencies, and ACD). It is a reaction in the skin to a number of different stimuli.

Dermatitis is an all-inclusive term for inflammation of the skin that clinically presents as erythema alone, erythema and scaling, or erythema, scaling, vesicles and crusts The chronic stage of AD is characterized by lichenification, a thickening of the skin with an increase in normal skin markings (Fig. 14.2). This reaction is almost pathognomonic of AD and is caused by rubbing. It may occasionally be seen in chronic ACD.

EPIDEMIOLOGY

Incidence and prevalence

AD is a major cause of morbidity for children in the Western world. The exact incidence and prevalence is difficult to establish, as many of the milder cases are not noted. Atopy (asthma, hay fever, and AD) is common in the general population with a prevalence of 22.5% in 1992.[9] This figure shows a marked increase from the early 1900s, and it is not clear whether there is a real increase[10] or whether the difference is attributable to improved diagnostic and data-collecting procedures.[11] Studies performed prior to

1. Lapidus CS, Schwarz DF, Honig P (1993) Atopic dermatitis in children: Who cares? Who pays? **J Am Acad Dermatol** 28:699–703.
2. Ellis CN, Drake LA, Prendergast MM et al. (2002) Cost of atopic dermatitis and eczema in the United States. **J Am Acad Dermatol** 46:361–370.
3. Tunnessen WW Jr (1984) A survey of skin disorders seen in pediatric general and dermatology clinics. **Pediatr Dermatol** 1:219–222.
4. Schachner L, Ling NS, Press S (1983) A statistical analysis of a pediatric dermatology clinic. **Pediatr Dermatol** 1:157–164.
5. Besnier E (1892) Premiere note et observations preliminaires pour servir d'introduction a l'étude des prurigos diathesiques. **Ann de Dermat et Syph** 3 s iii:634–648.
6. Coca AF, Cooke RA (1923) On the classification of the phenomena of hypersenitiveness. **J Immunol** 8:163–182.
7. Wise F, Sulzberger MB (1933) Editorial remarks. In: Year Book of Dermatology and Syphilogy. Chicago: Year Book Medical Publishers; 59.
8. Hill LW, Sulzberger MB (1935) Evolution of atopic dermatitis. **Arch Derm Syphilol** 32:451–463.
9. Diepgen TL, Fartasch M (1992) Recent epidemiological and genetic studies in atopic dermatitis. **Acta Derm Venereol Suppl** (Stockh) 176:13–18.
10. Carr RD, Berke M, Becker SW (1964) Incidence of atopy in the general population. **Arch Dermatol** 89:27.
11. Wuthrich B (1999) Clinical aspects, epidemiology, and prognosis of atopic dermatitis. **Ann Allergy Asthma Immunol** 83:464–470.

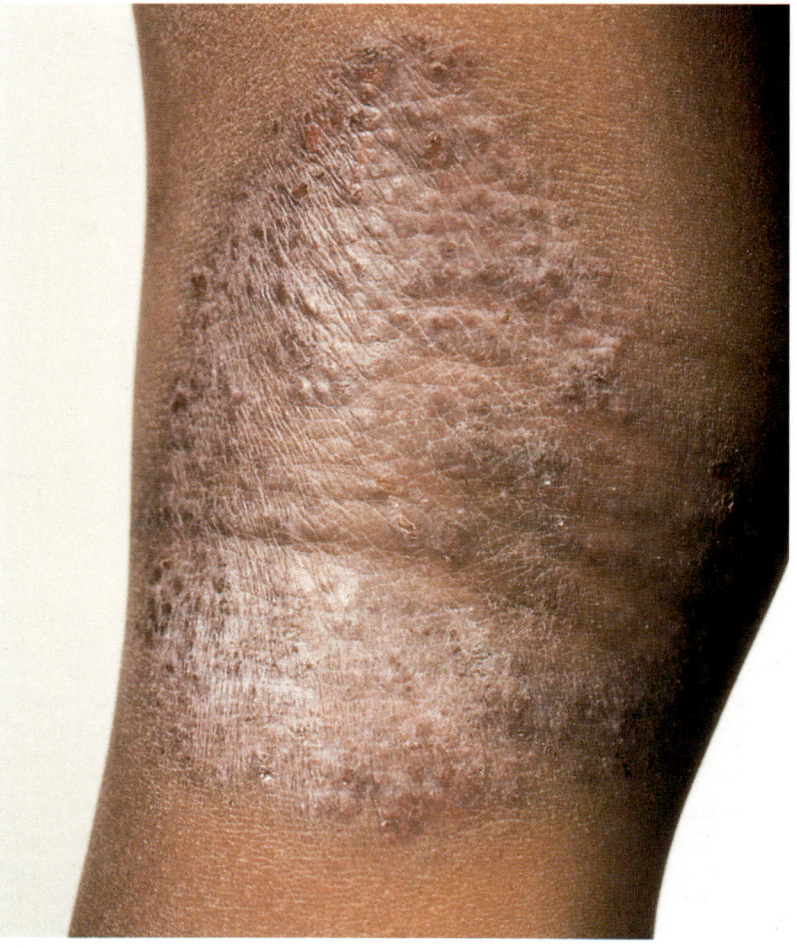

Fig. 14.1 The typical appearance of eczematous plaques in the politieal fossa in an atopic child.

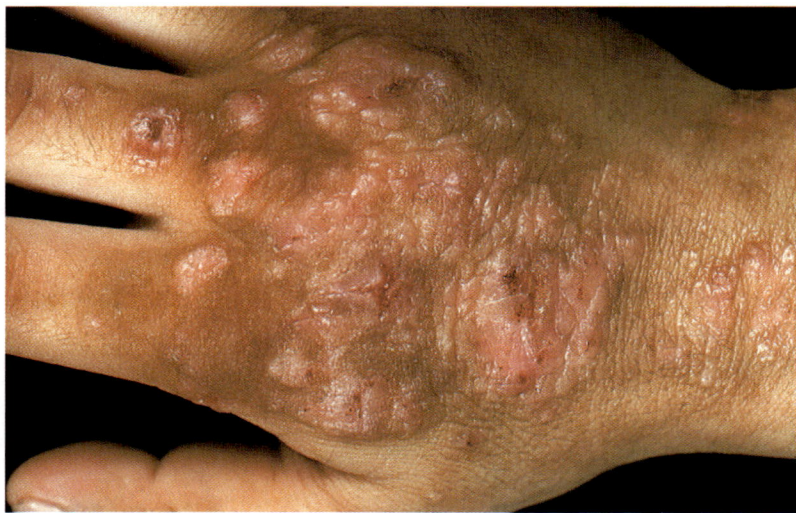

Fig. 14.2 Lichenification manifested as thickened skin with increased skin markings on the back of the hand. Prurigo nodules are also present.

20% in many countries, including Denmark and the US.[22,26–28] These latter studies were performed in children around the age of 7 and in both studies the researchers used standardized questionnaires (albeit slightly differently worded). The consistent rise is not evident in Japan where Sugiura *et al.* found no change in the prevalence of AD compared with figures of 20 years ago reported by Uehara.[29] They found the prevalence of eczema to be 30% in 4-month-old infants and 20% in 3-year-old children. The authors suggested that the discrepancy between their study and other prevalence figures may be due to lack of reporting of mild cases. With the present means of diagnosing AD, there is a large increase in cases in all Western countries, particularly northern Europe.[30,31]

In assessing the prevalence in adults, the figure shifts over a lifetime and is much lower than in children, the highest figure reaching 10% in Norway.[32] This shows a trend toward remission or cure of the disease in adults.

In older children and adults, the disease affects females slightly more than males with an incidence ratio of 1.3:1.[16,33] This has not been consistent in all studies.[34] AD is common in Caucasians.[35] There is an increase in AD in higher social classes.[36,37] The cause is unclear and may be due to increased reporting by mothers in advantaged socio–economic groups, but the trend persists even

1960[12–16] estimated the prevalence of AD to be 1.4–3.1%.[17] From 1960 to 1970, the prevalence of AD increased up to 8%[16,18–21] and after 1970 it rose again to 9–15%.[17,21–25] Recent studies show a prevalence of approximately

12. Service WC (1939) The incidence of major allergic diseases in Colorado Springs. **JAMA** 112:2034–2037.
13. Eriksson-Lihr Z (1955) Special features in allergy in children. **Acta Allergol** 8:289–313.
14. Brereton EM, Carpenter RG, Rook AJ, Tyser PA (1959) The prevalence and prognosis of eczema and asthma in Cambridgeshire schoolchildren. **BMJ** 2:317.
15. Freeman GL, Johnson S (1964) Allergic diseases in adolescents. I. Description of survey; prevalence of allergy. **Am J Dis Child** 107:549.
16. Larsson P-A, Liden S (1980) Prevalence of skin diseases among adolescents 12–16 years of age. **Acta Derm Venereol** 60:415–423.
17. Schultz Larsen F, Hanifin JM (1992) Secular change in the occurrence of atopic dermatitis. **Acta Derm Venereol Suppl** (Stockh) 176:7–12.
18. Arbeiter HI (1967) How prevalent is allergy among United States school children. A survey of findings in the Munster (Indiana) school system. **Clin Pediatr** 6:140–142.
19. Turner KJ, Rosman DL, O'Mahony J (1974) Prevalence and familial association of atopic disease and its relationship to serum IgE levels in 1,061 school children and their families. **Int Arch Allergy Appl Immunol** 47:650–664.
20. Kjellman N-IM (1977) Atopic disease in seven-year-old children. Incidence in relation to family history. **Acta Paediatr Scand** 66:465–471.
21. Engbaek S (1982) The morbidity of school age. Copenhagen: Laegefore-ningens Forlag.
22. Fergusson DM, Horwood LJ, Shannon FT (1982) Risk factors in childhood eczema. **J Epidemiol Community Health** 36:118–122.
23. Taylor B, Wadsworth M, Wadsworth J, Peckham C (1984) Changes in the reported prevalence of childhood eczema since the 1939–45 war. **Lancet** 2:1255–1257.
24. Schultz Larsen F, Holm NV, Henningsen K (1986) Atopic dermatitis. A genetic-epidemiologic study in a population-based twin sample. **J Am Acad Dermatol** 15:487–494.
25. Storm K, Hahr J, Kjellman N-IM, Osterballe O (1986) The occurrence of asthma and allergic rhinitis, atopic dermatitis and urticaria in Danish children born in one year. **Ugeskr Laeg** 148:3295.

26. Laughter D, Istvan JA, Tofte SJ et al. (2000) The prevalence of atopic dermatitis in Oregon schoolchildren. **J Am Acad Dermatol** 43:649–655.
27. Mortz CG, Lauritsen Jm, Bindslev-Jensen C et al. (2001) Prevalence of atopic dermatitis, asthma, allergic rhinitis, hand and contact dermatitis in adolescents: The Odense Adolescent Cohort Study on Atopic Diseases and Dermatitis (TOACS). **Br J Dermatol** 144:523–532.
28. Schultz Larsen F (1993) Atopic dermatitis: A genetic-epidemiologic study in a population-based twin sample. **J Am Acad Dermatol** 28:719–723.
29. Sugiura H, Umemoto N, Deguchi H et al. (1998) Prevalence of childhood and adolescent atopic dermatitis in a Japanese population: Comparison with the disease frequency examined 20 years ago. **Acta Derm Venereol** (Stockh) 78:293–294.
30. Bakke P, Gulsvik A, Eide GE (1990) Hay fever, eczema and utrticaria in southwest Norway. **Allergy** 45:515–522.
31. Schultz Larsen, Diepgen T, Svensson A (1996) The occurrence of atopic eczema in North Europe: an international questionnaire study. **J Am Acad Dermatol** 34:760–764.
32. Smith-Sivertsen T, Dotterud LK, Lund E (1990) Nickel allergy and its relationship with local nickel pollution, ear piercing, and atopic dermatitis: a population-based study from Norway. **J Am Acad Dermatol** 40:726–735.
33. Schultz Larsen F (1993) The epidemiology of atopic dermatitis. In: Epidermiology of Clinical Allergy, Burr ML, ed. Basel, Karger: Monogr Allergy, 31:9–28.
34. Kay J, Gawkrodger DJ, Mortimer MJ et al. (1994) The prevalence of childhood atopic eczema in a general population. **J Am Acad Dermatol** 30:35–39.
35. Rajka G (1984) Some aectiological data on atopic dermatitis. Presented at the Second International Symposium on Atopic Dermatitis, Norway.
36. Williams H, Robertson C, Stewart A et al. (1999) Worldwide variations in the prevalence of symptoms of atopic eczema in the international study of asthma and allergies in childhood. **J Allergy Clin Immunol** 103:125–138.
37. Heinrich J, Popescu Ma, Wjst M et al. (1998) Atopy in children and parental social class. **Am J Public Health** 88:1319–1324.

when detailed examinations are performed.[38] An association between smaller family size and the development of AD has been recognized by numerous authors.[22] It is hypothesized that children with smaller family size are involved in less exposure to infections and an inverse development of AD.[39] Initially thought to adversely influence the incidence of AD, a study by Mills *et al.* has shown that cigarette smoking does not appear to make a difference.[40] This finding was not supported by Schafer *et al.*, who found that maternal smoking during pregnancy or lactation or both might play a role in the development of AD and should be avoided.[41]

Geographical variations

Evidence suggests that there is a difference in prevalence of AD between and within countries.[42] However, there is a great variation in the collection of data, ranging from questionnaires to detailed physical studies. Figures given vary from a low incidence of 2–7.2% in China and 0.7% in Tanzania[43] to a high of 20% in UK, Nigeria, and Hong Kong.[44] The incidence is low in developing countries, outside of fast-growing, densely populated cities[45] and is more common in developed nations.[30,46] These findings were corroborated in Germany where the prevalence was low in East Germany with low industry and high in West Germany with high industrialization.[47]

Numerous studies have shown an increase in AD in children born to immigrants who have moved to more highly industrialized countries;[48] the figures are higher than in the indigenous population of the new country and the country from which they came.[49–51] Leung and Ho in 1994 showed considerable prevalence differences in atopy among three South-east Asian populations (Chinese living in Malaysia, mainland China and Australia) despite similar rates of atopy in the indigenous population.[49] Two studies confirmed that West Indian children living in London had a higher incidence of AD: one study compared similar children living in Kingston, Jamaica, and London;[51] there was a marked increase in AD in the children living in London. Another study showed that AD was present in 16.3% of West Indian children in London and in only 8.7% of whites.[52] A further study showed the incidence of AD in Tokelau (a Polynesian Island) to be 0.1% compared with the incidence in Tokelau children living in Wellington, New Zealand, where the incidence was 8.5%.[53]

Socio-economic, quality of life and occupational factors

Atopic dermatitis is a common condition that creates an enormous financial burden for patients, families, and health care systems around the world. It is a major cause of morbidity in children in the Western world.[54] A report from the US suggests that $364 million is spent on the care of childhood AD yearly.[1] The annual costs are similar to other chronic diseases like asthma and emphysema.[55,56] Studies from the UK divide the burden of cost into individual expenses, those born by the health care system, and society costs.[57] This translated into a cost of £297 million born by families and parents, £125 million born by the health care system, and £43 million born by society. This adds up to £465 million a year,[58] with some individuals spending up to £150 ($240) a month.[57] An Australian study compared the personal cost of looking after patients with AD and asthma, and found the financial burden to the family of AD patients to be higher than asthma, and similar to that needed for caring for a child with diabetes.[59] Studies indicate that 82% of patients with occupational dermatoses are atopic, and these patients are paid proportionally more in lost time.[60–62] Patients with AD are more at risk of developing hand eczema,[63] but it is unclear whether patients avoid certain occupations or change occupations because of their AD.[64]

Atopic dermatitis has profound effects on the lives of adults and children with the disease and has major secondary effects on their families.[65,66] Reports have shown that patients with AD have difficulties with sleep, work, and interpersonal relationships.[67] Efforts have been made to develop a survey instrument, called the Children's Atopic Dermatitis Index (CADI), examining four areas of life style, including physical and emotional health, and physical and social functioning.[68]

Genetic predisposition

In 1916 Cooke and Van de Meer recognized that allergies run in families.[69] There is a strong family history of atopic diseases in families of patients with AD. The mode of inheritance is not entirely clear, but appears to be polygenic.[70] A patient with AD is more likely to have relatives who suffer from AD;[71] similarly, if a patient has respiratory atopy, it is likely that their first-degree relatives will be affected by respiratory atopy, possibly showing

38. Williams HC (1995) Atopic eczema: we should look to the environment. Br Med J 311:1241–1242.
39. Williams HC (1992) Is the prevalence of atopic dermatitis increasing? Clin Exp Dermatol 17:385–391.
40. Mills CM, Srivastava ED, Harvey IM et al. (1994) Cigarette smoking is not a risk factor in atopic dermatitis. Int J Dermatol 33:33–34.
41. Schafer T, Dirschedl P, Kunz B et al. (1997) Maternal smoking during pregnancy and lactation increases the risk for atopic eczema in the offspring. J Am Acad Dermatol 36:550–556.
42. Dotterud LK, Kvammen B, Lund E et al. (1995) Prevalence and some clinical aspects of atopic eczema in the community of Sor-Varanger. Acta Dermatol Venereol (Stockh.) 75:50–53.
43. Henderson CA (1995) The prevalence of atopic eczema in two different villages in rural Tanzania. Br J Dermatol 133 suppl 45:50.
44. The International Study of Asthma and Allergies in Childhood (ISAAC) Steering Committee. Worldwide variation in prevalence of symptoms of asthma, allergic rhinoconjunctivitis, and atopic eczema. (1998) Lancet 351:1225–11232.
45. Falade AG, Olawuyi F, Osinusi K et al. (1998) Prevalence and severity of symptoms of asthma, allergic rhino-conjunctivitis and atopic eczema in secondary school children in Ibadan, Nigeria. East Afr Med J 75:695–698.
46. Paajanen H (1994) Common skin diseases. In: Health and Disease in Developing Countries, Lankinen KS, Bergstrom S, Makela PH et al., eds. London: Macmillan, pp. 271–280.
47. von Mutius E, Fritzsch C, Weiland SK et al. (1992) Prevalence of asthma and allergic disorders among children in united Germany: a descriptive comparison. BMJ 305:1395–1399.
48. The International Study of Asthma and Allergies in Childhood (ISAAC) Steering Committee. Worldwide variation in prevalence of symptoms of asthma, allergic rhinoconjunctivitis, and atopic eczema. (1998) Lancet 351:1225–1232.
49. Leung R, Ho P (1994) Asthma, allergy and atopy in three south-east Asian populations. Thorax 49:1205–1210.
50. McNally NJ, Phillips DR, Williams HC (1998) The problem of atopic eczema: aetiological clues from the environment and lifestyles. Soc Sci Med 46:729–741.
51. Burrell-Morris CE, LaGrenade L, Williams HC et al. (1997) The prevalence of atopic dermatitis in black Caribbean children in London and Kingston, Jamaica. Br J Dermatol 137(suppl 50); 22.
52. Williams HC, Pembroke AC, Forsdyke H et al. (1995) London-born black Caribbean children are at increased risk of atopic dermatitis. J Am Acad Dermatol 32:212–217.
53. Waite DA, Eyles EF, Tonkin SL et al. (1980) Asthma prevalence in Tokelauan children in two environments. Clin Allergy 10:71–75.
54. Lapidus CS (2001) Role of social factors in atopic dermatitis: The US perspective. J Am Acad Dermatol 45:S41–S43.
55. Stevens SR, Drake LA, Prendergast MM et al. (2001) Third-party payer cost of atopic dermatitis and eczema in the United States. Paper presented at the International Symposium on Atopic Dermatitis, National Eczema Association for Science and Education; Portland, Oregon. September 6–9.
56. Ellis CN, Drake LA, Prendergast MM et al. (2002) Cost of atopic dermatitis and eczema in the United States. J Am Acad Dermatol 46:361–370.
57. Herd RM, Tidman MJ, Prescott RJ (1996) The cost of atopic eczema. Br J Dermatol 135:20–23.
58. Herd RM (2002) The morbidity and cost of atopic dermatitis. In: Atopic Dermatitis: The Epidemiology, Causes and Prevention of Atopic Eczema, Williams HC, ed. Cambridge: Cambridge University Press, p. 89.
59. Su JC, Kemp AS, Varigos GA et al. (1997) Atopic eczema: Its impact on the family and financial cost. Arch Dis Child 76:159–162.
60. Shmunes E, Keil JE (1983) Occupational dermatoses in South Carolina: a descriptive analysis of cost variables. J Am Acad Dermatol 9:861–866.
61. Nilsson E (1986) Individual and environmental risk factors for hand eczema in hospital workers. Acta Dermatol Venereol suppl; 128:1–63.
62. Lammintausta K, Kalimo K (1993) Does a patient's occupation influence the course of atopic dermatitis? Acta Dermatol Venereol (Stockh) 73:119–122.
63. Rystedt I (1985) Hand eczema and long term prognosis in atopic dermatitis (thesis). Acta Dermatol Venereol (Stockh) 117:1–59.
64. Coenraads P-J, Diepgen TL (2000) Occupational aspects of atopic dermatitis. In: Atopic Dermatitis: The Epidemiology, Causes and Prevention of Atopic Eczema, Williams HC, ed. Cambridge: Cambridge University Press, pp. 67.
65. Finlay AY (2001) Quality of life in atopic dermatitis. J Am Acad Dermatol 45:S64–S66.
66. Lawson V, Lewis-Jones MS, Finlay AY et al. (1998) The family impact of childhood atopic dermatitis: the Dermatitis Family Impact questionnaire. Br J Dermatol 138:107–113.
67. Lewis Jones MS, Finlay AY (1995) The Children's Dermatology Life Quality Index (CDLQI): initial validation and pratical use. Br J Dermatol 132:942–949.
68. Chamlin SL, Frieden IJ, Williams ML et al. (2001) Quality of life in young American children with atopic dermatitis: instrument development. Paper given at International symposium on atopic dermatitis. National Eczema Association for Science and Education. Portland, Oregon. Sep 6–9.
69. Cooke RA, van der Meer A (1916) Human sensitization. J Immunol 1:201–305.
70. Cookson WOCM (1994) Atopy: a complex genetic disease. Ann Med 26:351–353.
71. Dold S, Wjst M, von Mutius et al. (1992) Genetic risk for asthma, allergic rhinitis, and atopic dermatitis. Arch Dis Child 67:1018–1022.

end-organ sensitivity.[72] A prospective study has shown that AD and asthma are inherited through separate gene pathways although both diseases may be inherited together.[73]

One-third to two-thirds of in-patients with AD have a single or double parental history of atopy and this is even higher when siblings are included.[74] Monozygotic twins are concordant for the disease with an incidence of 75%, whereas in dizygotic twins the concordance is 15%.[75] The incidence in the latter is similar to that occurring in siblings, inferring that genetic susceptibility plays a definite role in AD.[76] An interesting observation that has been replicated a number of times is that children of atopic mothers are more likely to be atopic than children of atopic fathers.[77]

Other indications that AD is inherited come from Cookson et al., suggesting that an atopic gene is present on chromosome 11q13,[78,79] although this site has not been confirmed by other studies.[80,81] Genome-wide screens for AD have identified linkage groups at 3q21, 1q21, 17q25 and 20p,[82,83] and 13q12–14.[84] Several of these identified linkage clusters also correspond to psoriasis susceptibility loci[82] and thus they may represent the end-point of common mediators for cutaneous inflammation. Two studies have shown the transfer of AD by bone marrow transplantation[85,86] and disappearance of AD in a transplanted Wiskott–Aldrich patient.[87] Bradley has suggested that the WAS gene (associated with Wiskott–Aldrich syndrome) may contribute to the severity of the atopic gene phenotype.[88] Until a suitable marker is found for diagnosing AD, it may be impossible to characterize the exact genetic inheritance pattern. AD may be a clinical reaction pattern in the skin representing a number of heterogeneous disorders.

The role of HLA type is controversial. HLA typing has not been useful in elucidating the genetic inheritance pattern of AD;[89] nevertheless, HLA type is known to be important in influencing T-cell expression,[90,91] and there is a presumed link between HLA restriction areas and IgE responsiveness.[92] Studies have not been replicated yet and are too small in number to establish an unequivocal association.

PRESENTING HISTORY

AD is usually the first manifestation of the atopic triad (AD, asthma, and hay fever); it occurs during the first year of life in 60% of patients,[93] generally starting around 3 months of age. In 38% of patients, it develops even earlier.[94,95] More recent studies have estimated the rate of onset to be over 60% by age one.[96] In at least 70–95% of patients, the disease develops by 5 years of age.[93] There has not been a prospective study to establish the exact age of onset of AD; past studies have been retrospective and based on questionnaires.

Hill and Sulzberger characterized three distinct clinical phases of AD, in which both the site and the morphology of the lesions change with age.[97] These phases may overlap or be separated by a period of remission. The sites of predilection have been confirmed by two recent studies.[93,98] The infantile phase occurs up to 2 years of age; the childhood phase from age 2 to puberty; and the adult phase from puberty onward.

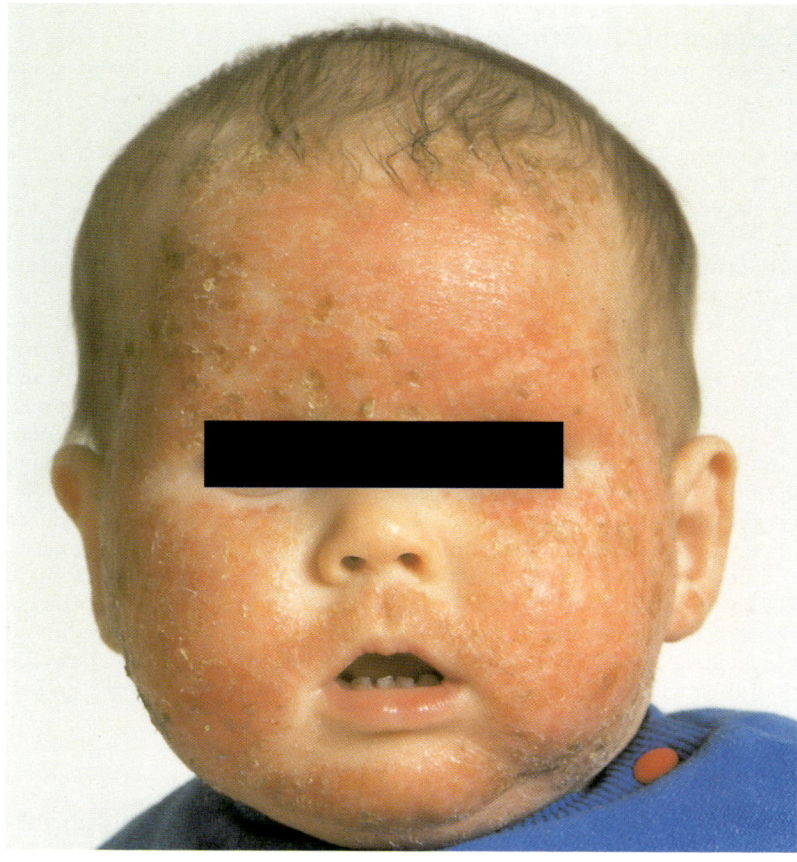

Fig. 14.3 Facial involvement in the infantile form of AD.

72. Dold S, Wjst M, von Mutius E et al. (1992) Genetic risk for asthma, allergic rhinitis, and atopic dermatitis. **Arch Dis Child** 67:1018–1022.
73. Fergusson DM, Horwood LJ, Shannon FT (1983) Parental asthma, parental eczema and asthma and eczema in early childhood. **J Chronic Dis** 36:517–524.
74. Schultz Larsen F (1993) Atopic dermatitis: A genetic-epidemiologic study in a population-based twin sample. **J Am Acad Dermatol** 28:719–723.
75. Schultz Larsen F (1991) Genetic aspects of atopic eczema. In: Handbook of Atopic Eczema, Ruzicka T, Ring J, Przybilla B, eds. Berlin: Springer, pp. 15–26.
76. Luoma R, Koivikko A, Viander M (1983) Development of asthma, allergic rhinitis and atopic dermatitis by age of five years. **Allergy** 38:339–346.
77. Ruiz RGG, Kemeny DM, Price JF (1992) Higher risk of infantile atopic dermatitis from maternal atopy than from paternal atopy. **Clin Exp Allergy** 22:762–766.
78. Cookson WOCM, Sharp PA, Faux JA et al. (1989) Linkage between immunoglobulin E responses underlying asthma and rhinitis and chromosome 11q. **Lancet** Jun 10;1(8650):1292–1295.
79. Fölster-Holst R, Moises HW, Yang L et al. (1998) Linkage between atopy and the IgE high-affinity receptor gene at 11q13 in atopic dermatitis families. **Hum Genet** 102:236–239.
80. Lympany P, Welsh K, MacCochrane G et al. (1992) Genetic analysis using DNA polymorphism of the linkage between chromosome 11q13 and atopy and bronchial hyperresponsiveness to methacholine. **J Allergy Clin Immunol** 89:619–628.
81. Amelung PJ, Panhuysen CIM, Postma DS et al. (1992) Atopy and bronchial hyperresponsiveness: exclusion of linkage to markers on chromosomes 11q and p. **Clin Exp Allergy** 22:1077–1084.
82. Cookson WO, Ubhi B, Lawrence R et al. (2001) Genetic linkage of childhood atopic dermatitis to psoriasis susceptibility loci. **Nat Genet** 27:372–373.
83. Lee Y, Wahn U, Kehrt R et al. (2000) A major susceptibility locus for atopic dermatitis maps to chromosome 3q21. **Nat Genet** 26:470–473.
84. Beyer K, Nickel R, Freidhoff L et al. (2000) Association and linkage of atopic dermatitis with chromosome 13q12–14 and 5q31–33 markers. **J Invest Dermatol** 115(5):906–908.
85. Saarinen UM (1984) Transfer of latent atopy by bone marrow transplantation: a case report. **J Allergy Clin Immunol** 74:196–200.
86. Agosti JM, Sprenger JD, Lum LG et al. (1988) Transfer of allergen specific IgE-mediated hypersensitivity with allogeneic bone marrow transplantation. **N Engl J Med** 319:1623–1628.
87. Saurat JH (1985) Eczema in primary immune-deficiencies. Clue to the pathogenesis of atopic dermatitis with special reference to Wiscott-Aldrich syndrome. **Acta Derm Venereol** (Stockh) Suppl;114:125–128.
88. Bradley M, Soderhall C, Wahlgren C-F et al. (2001) Linkage to the WisKott-Aldrich syndrome gene in Swedish patients with atopic dermatitis. Paper given at International symposium on atopic dermatitis. National Eczema Association for Science and Education. Portland, Oregon. Sep 6–9.
89. Blumenthal MN, Mendel N, Yunis E (1980) Immunogenetics of atopic diseases. **J Allergy Clin Immunol** 65:403–405.
90. Schwartz RH (1989) Acquisition of immunologic self-tolerance. **Cell** 57:1073–1081.
91. Germain RN (1986) The ins and outs of antigen processing and presentation. **Nature** 322:687–689.
92. O Hehir RE, Mach B, Berte C et al. (1990) Direct evidence for a functional role of HLA-DRB3 gene products in the recognition of Dermatophagoides spp by helper T cell clones. **Int Immunol** 2:885–892.
93. Rajka G (1989) Essential aspects of atopic dermatitis. Berlin: Springer-Verlag, pp. 7–16.
94. Kay J, Gawkrodger DJ, Mortimer MJ et al. (1994) The prevalence of childhood atopic eczema in a general population. **J Am Acad Dermatol** 30:35–39.
95. Neame RI, Berth-Jones J, Kurinszuk JJ et al. (1995) Prevalence of atopic dermatitis in Leicester: a study of methodology and examination of possible ethnic variation. **Br J Dermatol** 132:772–777.
96. Williams HC, Wuthrich B (2000) The natural history of atopic dermatitis. In: Atopic Dermatitis: The Epidemiology, Causes and Prevention of Atopic Eczema, Williams HC, ed., Cambridge: Cambridge University Press; p. 43.
97. Hill LW, Sulzberger MB (1935) Evolution of atopic dermatitis. **Arch Derm Syphilol** 32:451–463.
98. Aoki T, Fukuzumi J, Adachi K et al. (1992) Re-evaluation of skin lesion distribution in atopic dermatitis. **Acta Derm Venereol** (Stockh) 176 suppl:19–23.

PHYSICAL EXAMINATION

Infantile phase

The characteristic and most important symptom, and the major cause of morbidity in AD, is pruritus, which may be unbearable and often interferes with normal sleep patterns. Infants will often claw at their skin and rub themselves against hard objects. Some physicians believe there is no primary lesion of AD and that the clinical manifestations are the result of scratching. Jacquet is quoted as saying that AD is "an itch that rashes" as opposed to a rash that itches.[99] However, one frequently sees erythematous lesions with scaling and no excoriations, which makes it unlikely that the eruption is caused by scratching alone. Furthermore, the erythematous eruption may be seen in infants before the "itch-scratch" mechanism develops, which is usually around 3 months of age. This is also the time that parents become concerned about the disease, although many of the features may be present earlier. Prior to the inflammatory phase, the skin may feel rough and dry.

The eruption in infancy characteristically starts on the cheeks (Figs 14.3, 14.4) and scalp, but often involves the lateral aspects of the extensor surfaces of the lower legs[100] and may involve the creases even earlier. Other areas including the trunk may also be involved (Fig. 14.5), but the diaper area is often spared. The lesions are usually symmetric, ill-defined, scaly, erythematous patches

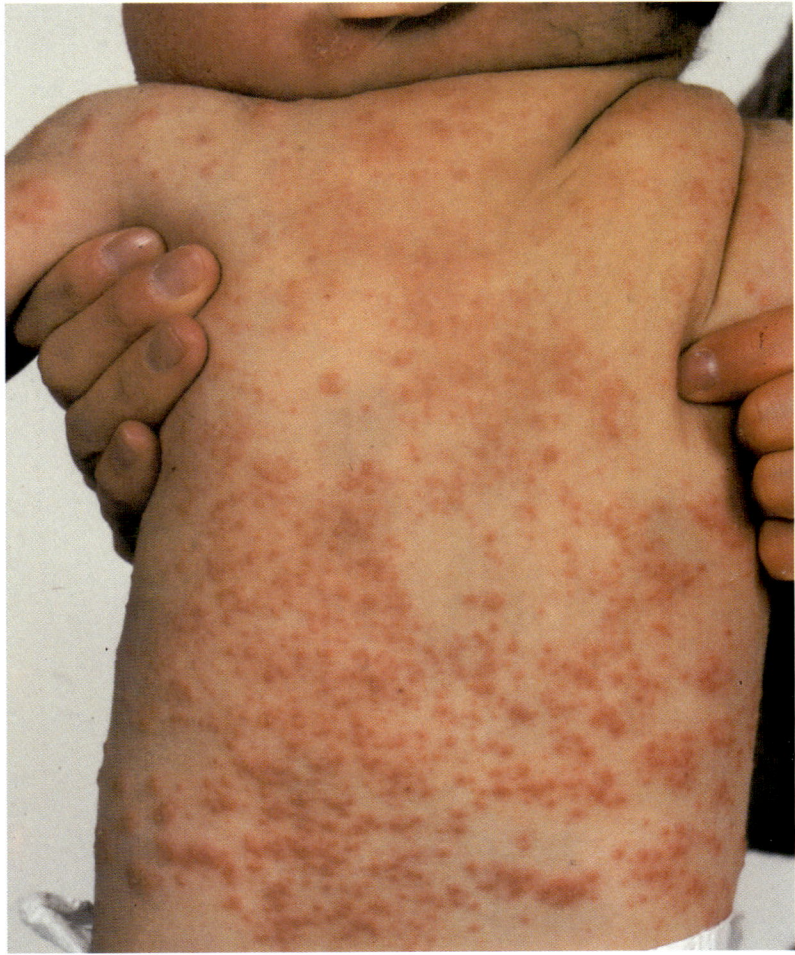

Fig. 14.5 Eczematous lesions on the back of an infant with AD.

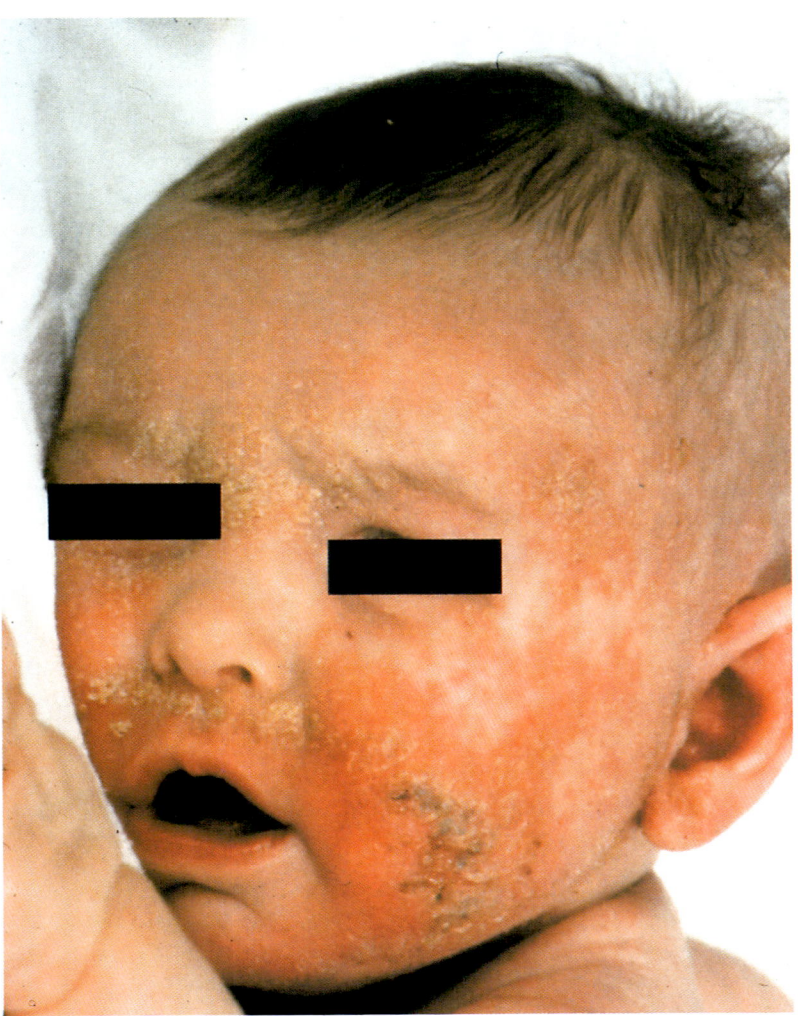

Fig. 14.4 Facial involvement with secondary infection in the infantile form of AD.

with or without small areas of crusting. Generalized xerosis, including dry hair and scalp, is a major feature and is most helpful in establishing the diagnosis. The etiology of this important feature is unknown, but a recent study showed increased water loss and marked skin dehydration compared with controls.[100]

Childhood phase

In the childhood phase, the flexural areas are the sites of predilection. The antecubital and popliteal fossae are most commonly affected, with the neck, flexures of the wrists and ankles, and the buttock/thigh crease also commonly involved (Figs 14.6–14.8). These areas are particularly prone to sweating. The lesions are pruritic, ill-defined, erythematous, scaly patches, often studded with crusts and excoriations. Childhood is the time when lichenification first manifests. It is most evident in the antecubital fossae and around the knees and wrists. Nummular exudative patches may also be seen. The nails may be shiny and buffed from constant rubbing and the eyebrows sparse and broken off. In black children, the lesions of AD are more papular and follicular (Fig. 14.9). Vickers[101] described a variant of AD called the "inverse pattern" that affects the extensor surfaces of the elbows and knees and the dorsa of the hands and wrists. The pattern occurs more commonly in boys and has a poorer prognosis than other forms of AD. Lymphadenopathy is a notable feature often prompting investigation for a lymphoma.

99. Morris M (1912) Prurigo, pruriginous eczema and lichenification. **BMJ** 1:1469–1474.
100. Aoki T, Fukuzumi T, Adach J et al. (1992) Re-evaluation of skin lesion distribution in atopic dermatitis. Analysis of cases 0 to 9 years of age. **Acta Derm Venerol** (Stockholm), suppl 176:19–23.
101. Vickers CFH (1980) The natural history of atopic eczema. Presented at the International Symposium on Atopic Dermatitis 1979. **Arch Dermatol Venereol**, suppl 92:113.

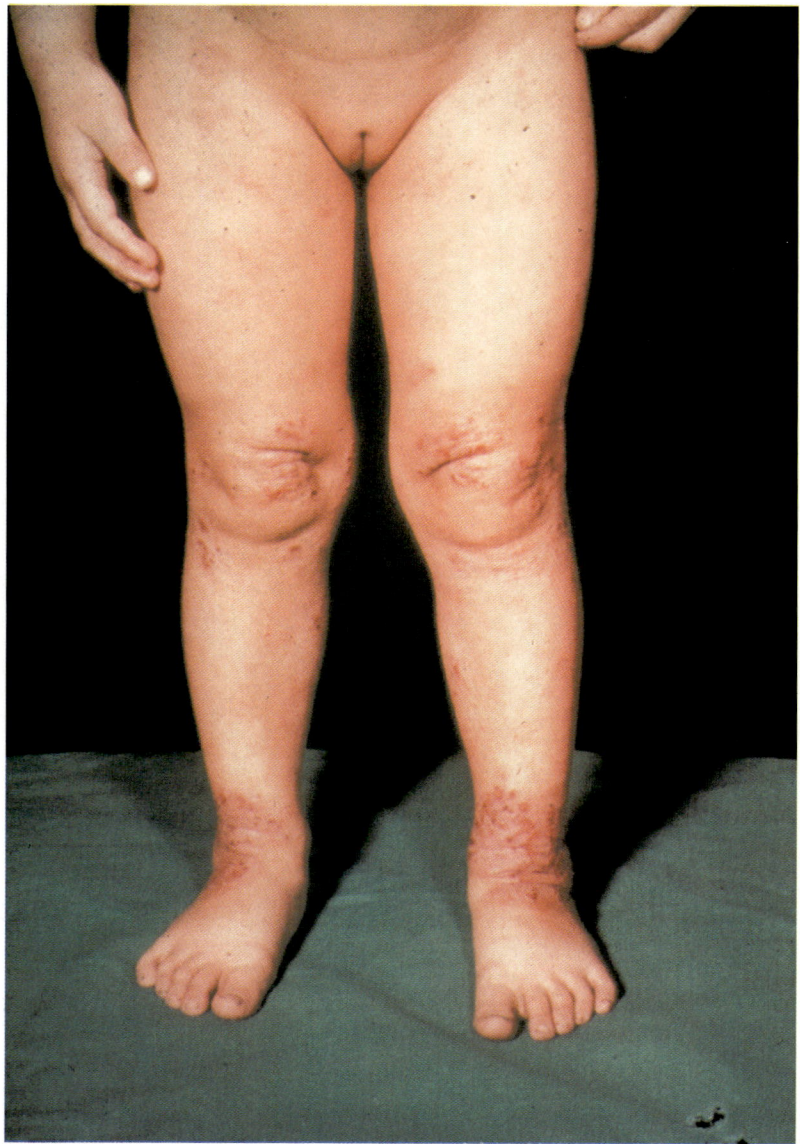

Fig. 14.6   Ankle involvement in childhood AD.

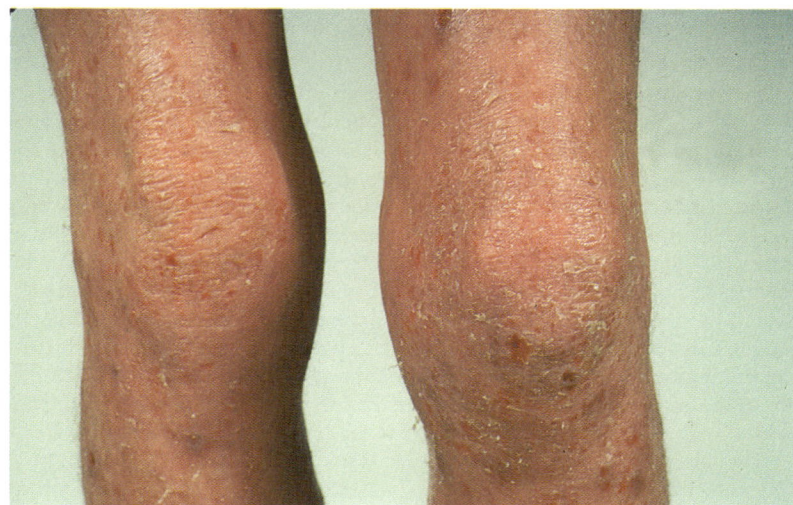

Fig. 14.7   Eczematous lesions on anterior aspects of knees in an older child with AD.

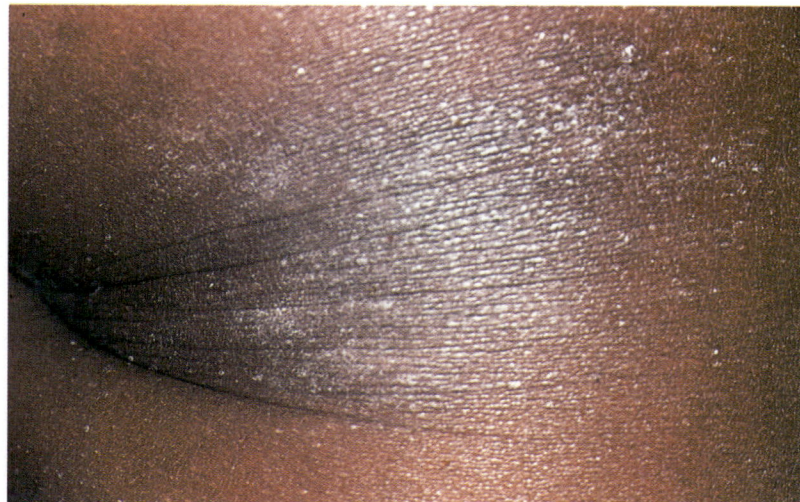

Fig. 14.8   Eczematous lesions at buttocks/thigh crease.

After the child reaches puberty, the clinical features once again involve the face, neck, and body, but more diffusely, with erythema, more scaling, and less exudation. Xerosis and lichenification are still prominent features. The face has a typical central pallor. A distinctive rippled, brown, macular discoloration around the neck has been recognized in adult patients with chronic AD (Fig. 14.10). This is often referred to as the "dirty neck sign." A histologic study of three patients revealed negative Congo red staining, but positive amorphous material on electron microscopy consistent with amyloid.[102]

Children often have postinflammatory hypo- and hyperpigmentation, and parents are very concerned about the possibility of scarring. Atopic dermatitis lesions do not scar unless there is severe secondary infection. The disordered pigmentation disappears weeks to months after the disease becomes quiescent.

Prior to the recognition that AD could begin during the first two weeks of life, the term seboatopic dermatitis was used. Affected children develop their eruption at 2–6 weeks of age and the areas of involvement are primarily the upper part of the body with the scalp and face being the primary targeted areas. The scale is dry, unlike seborrheic dermatitis. These children usually develop other features of AD.

ASSOCIATED FINDINGS

Ichthyosis vulgaris, mainly affecting the lower legs, occurs in 20–37% of patients with AD;[103] hyperlinear palms and soles frequently occur (Fig. 14.11), particularly in those patients with ichthyosis. These findings tend to persist despite improvement in the AD.

The Dennie-Morgan fold is a crease line found under the lower eyelid of patients with AD (Fig. 14.12); it may be present at birth or soon thereafter. Originally thought to be pathognomonic of AD, it may also occur in other acute, inflammatory conditions around the eye. In addition, it was found to be more common in black children living in London than in patients with AD.[104] The fold may last over the lifetime of the affected individual.

102. Humphreys F, Spencer J, McLaren K, Tidman MJ (1996) A histological and ultrastructural study of the "dirty neck" in atopic eczema. **Clin Exp Dermatol** 21:17–19.

103. Uehara M, Hayashi S (1981) Hyperlinear palms. **Arch Dermatol** 117:490–491.

104. Williams HC, Pembroke AC (1996) Infraorbital crease, ethnic group, and atopic dermatitis. **Arch Dermatol** 132:51–54.

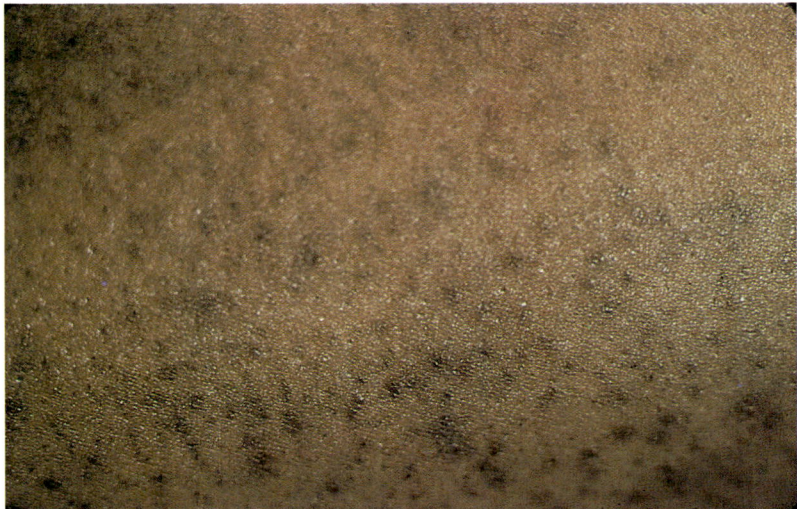

Fig. 14.9   Papular form of atopic dermatitis in the skin of a black child.

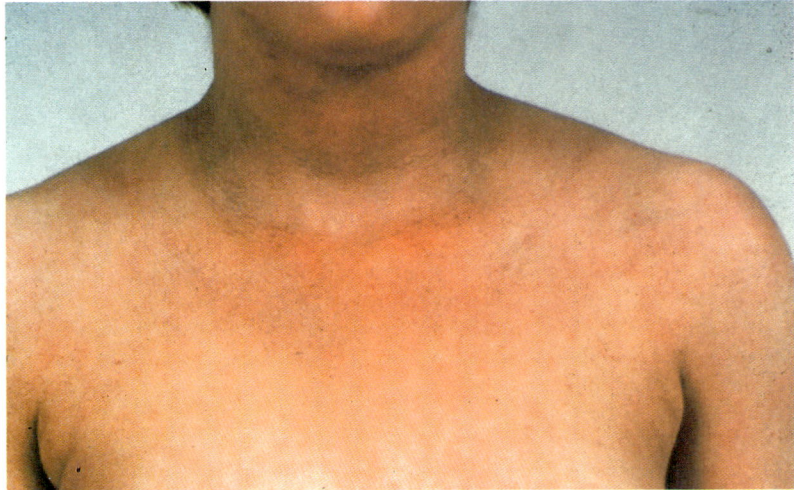

Fig. 14.10   Brown "dirty"-appearing neck and generalized erythema and scale on an adolescent with AD.

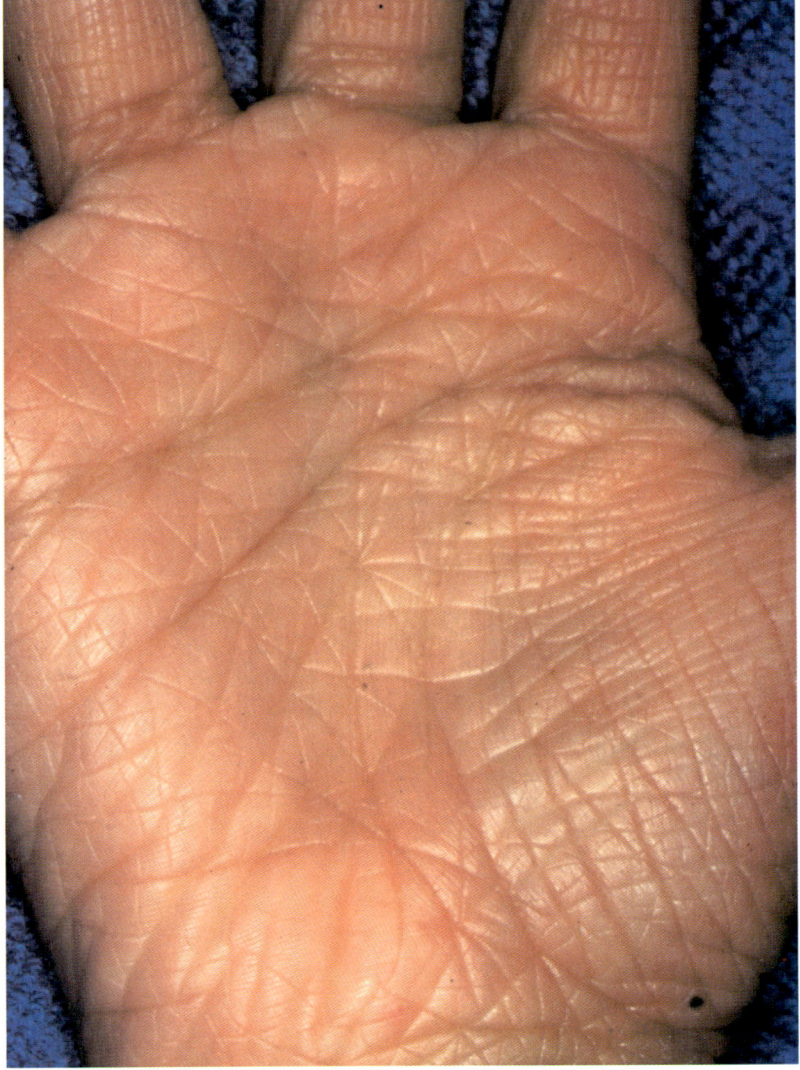

Fig. 14.11   Hyperlinear creases on the palms of a ten-year-old with AD.

Eye findings including keratoconjunctivitis, which may occur in a painful form known as vernal conjunctivitis, and affect 30% of patients with AD.[105] Pruritus and photophobia were the most common findings in the eyes in over 200 patients with AD studied by Gelmetti.[105] Cataracts, which are usually posterior subcapsular, have been described in more severe cases in up to 13% of patients.[106] These usually occur in young adults with AD, but are occasionally seen in children and are usually asymptomatic. Although often ascribed to the use of steroids, this is most unlikely[106] as cataracts were described in children with AD long before the advent of topical corticosteroids. They are thought to be caused by constant rubbing of the eye in response to severe inflammation. Keratoconus (abnormal shaped cornea)

occurs infrequently in very severe cases of AD,[107] and does not occur before adolescence. It was not seen in the study by Gelmetti.[105,108] Retinal changes, including detachment, have also been described in AD patients.[109]

DIAGNOSIS

In 1979, Hanifin and Lobitz[110] and, in 1980, Hanifin and Rajka[111] established for the first time, standardized criteria for the diagnosis of AD (Table 14.1). These criteria have been very useful for epidemiological and drug studies, but many of the features do not occur in children, and the minor criteria have not been validated in a number of studies;[112,113] in fact, they may be present in the normal population, and they may be more evident in certain ethnic types.[114] Many of the tests required to confirm the diagnosis are not readily

105. Gelmetti C (1992) Extracutaneous manifestations of atopic dermatitis. **Pediatr Dermatol** 9:380–382.
106. Garrity JA, Liesegang TJ (1984) Ocular complications of atopic dermatitis. **Can J Ophthalmol** 19:21–24.
107. Oshinskie L, Haine C (1982) Atopic dermatitis and its ophthalmic complications. **J Am Optom Assoc** 53:889–894.
108. Kennedy RH, Bourne WM, Dyer JA (1986) A 48-year clinical and epidemiologic study of keratoconus. **Am J Ophthalmol** 101:267–273.
109. Takashi M, Suzuma K, Inaba I et al. (1996) Retinal detachment associated with atopic dermatitis. **Br J Ophthalmol** 80:54–57.
110. Hanifin JM, Lobitz WC (1977) Newer concepts of atopic dermatology. **Arch Dermatol** 113:663–670.
111. Hanifin JM, Rajka G (1980) Diagnostic features of atopic dermatitis. **Acta Derm Venereol** (Stockh) Suppl 92:44–47.
112. Nagaraja, Kanwar AJ, Dhar S et al. (1996) Frequency and significance of minor clinical features in various age-related subgroups of atopic dermatitis in children. **Pediatr Dermatol** 13(1):10–13.
113. Bohme M, Svensson A, Kull I et al. (2000) Hanifin's and Rajka's minor criteria for atopic dermatitis: Which do 2-year-olds exhibit? **J Am Acad Dermatol** 43:785–792.
114. Lee HJ, Cho SH, Ha SJ et al. (2000) Minor cutaneous features of atopic dermatitis in South Korea. **Int J Dermatol** 39:337–342

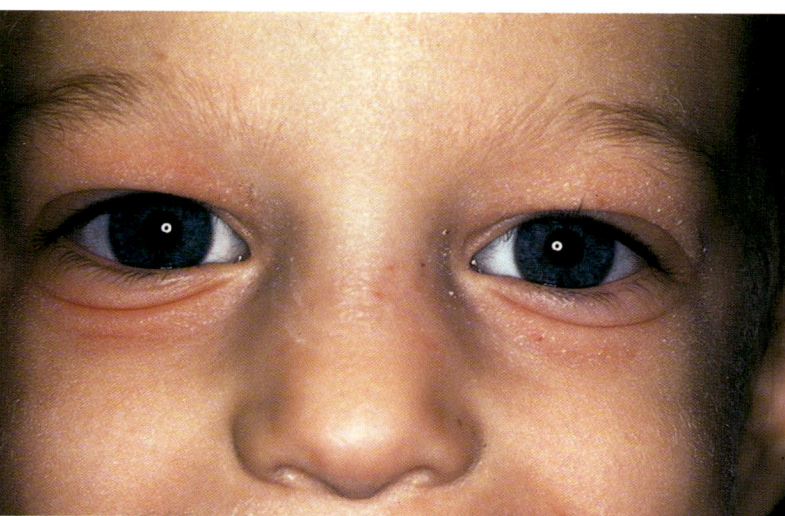

Fig. 14.12   Dennie-Morgan folds and periorbital dermatitis in a child with AD.

TABLE 14.1 **Hanifin and Rajka**[111] **criteria for the diagnosis of atopic dermatitis (1980)**

Must have three or more basic features:
1. Pruritus
2. Typical morphology and distribution:
   flexural lichenification or linearity in adults;
   facial and extensor involvement in infants and children
3. Tendency toward chronic or chronically relapsing dermatitis
4. Personal or family history of atopy (asthma, allergic rhinitis, atopic dermatitis)

Plus three or more of the following:
1. Xerosis
2. Ichthyosis/palmar hyperlinearity/keratosis pilaris
3. Immediate (type 1) skin test reactivity
4. Elevated serum IgE
5. Early age of onset
6. Tendency toward cutaneous infections (esp. *Staphylococcus aureus*) and herpes simplex/impaired cell-mediated immunity
7. Tendency toward nonspecific hand or foot dermatitis
8. Nipple eczema
9. Cheilitis
10. Recurrent conjunctivitis
11. Dennie-Morgan infraorbital fold
12. Keratoconus
13. Anterior subcapsular cataracts
14. Orbital darkening
15. Facial pallor/facial erythema
16. Pityriasis alba
17. Anterior neck folds
18. Itch when sweating
19. Intolerance to wool and lipid solvents
20. Perifollicular accentuation
21. Food intolerance
22. Course influenced by environmental/emotional factors
23. White dermographism/delayed blanch

TABLE 14.2 **Seymour and Hanifin**[115] **diagnostic criteria (1987)**

Major features
   Family history of atopic dermatitis
   Evidence of pruritic dermatitis
   Typical facial or extensor eczematous or lichenified dermatitis

Minor features
   Xerosis/ichthyosis/hyperlinear palms
   Perifollicular accentuation
   Chronic scalp scaling
   Periauricular fissures

TABLE 14.3 **Williams and Burney**[116] **and the UK Working Group to establish diagnostic criteria for the diagnosis of AD (1994)**

For the diagnosis to be made an individual must have:
   An itchy skin eruption or parental report of scratching or rubbing in a child

In conjunction with three of the following:
1. History of flexural involvement (folds of the elbows, behind the knees, front of ankles, around the neck, and the cheeks in children under 10 years of age)
2. Personal history of hayfever or asthma (or a history of atopy in a relative of a child under 10 years of age)
3. A history of generalized dry skin in the last year
4. Visible flexural eczema (or eczema involving the cheeks/forehead and outer limbs in children under 4 years)
5. Onset under the age of 2 years (this is not used if the child is under 4 years of age)

accessible (skin testing, delayed blanch to cholinergic agents), and some findings are extremely rare (keratoconus).

Seymour and Hanifin modified the original criteria as a research tool to aid in assessing AD in infancy (Table 14.2).[115] Williams and Burney, with the UK Working Group, established practical diagnostic criteria for the diagnosis of AD meant to be used mainly in epidemiological studies (Table 14.3).[116] These criteria disregard the inconstant minor findings and the use of serum IgE levels that are not always high. When tested in standardized conditions, these criteria have a sensitivity of 80% and a specificity of 97% in children and are easy to use in everyday practise.[117]

The above definitions of AD do not take into consideration that one may be dealing with a group of different diseases with the same phenotype (atopiform as opposed to true AD). On this premise, Bos has proposed another set of criteria that would more strictly define the basis of true AD. These are known as the Millennium criteria (Table 14.4).[118] In the same vein, the Japanese have created their own criteria which better fit their particular group of patients with AD (Table 14.5).[119] Lastly, Hanifin presented a new set of criteria at the international meeting of AD held in Oregon in September 2001 (Table 14.6).[120]

Most physicians use simple criteria for the diagnosis of AD including xerosis, and a typical eruption in a typical age-related distribution.

Measurement of severity

Studies that were completed prior to 1989 did not have a standardized method of defining improvement or exacerbation of AD and therefore could

115. Seymour JL, Keswick BH, Hanifin JM et al. (1987) Clinical effects of diaper types on the skin of normal infants and infants with atopic dermatitis. **J Am Acad Dermatol** 17:988–997.
116. Williams HC, Burney PGJ, Pembroke AC et al. (1994) The UK working party's diagnostic criteria for atopic dermatitis. III Independent hospital validation. **Br J Dermatol** 131:406–416.
117. Williams HC, Burney PGJ, Pembroke AC et al. (1996) Validation of the UK diagnostic criteria for atopic dermatitis in a population setting. **Br J Dermatol** 135:12–17.
118. Bos JD, Van Leent EJM, Sillevis Smitt JH (1998) The millennium criteria for the diagnosis of atopic dermatitis. **Exp Dermatol** 7:132–138.
119. Japanese Dermatological Association Criteria for the diagnosis of atopic dermatitis. J Dermatol 1997;24:561 cited by Bos JD, Van Leent EJM, Sillevis Smitt JH (1998) The millennium criteria for the diagnosis of atopic dermatitis. **Exp Dermatol** 7:132–138.
120. Hanifin J (2001) Defining AD and assessing its impact: Seeking simplified, inclusive and internationally applicable criteria. Paper presented at the International symposium on Atopic Dermatitis, National Eczema Association for Science and Education. Portland, Oregon. September 6–9.

TABLE 14.4 Millennium criteria for the diagnosis of atopic dermatitis (Bos 1998)[118]

1. Mandatory criterion
   Presence of allergen-specific IgE
     Historical, actual, or expected (in very young children)
     In peripheral blood (RAST, ELISA) or in skin (intracutaneous challenge)
2. Principal criteria (2 of 3 present)
   Typical distribution and morphology of eczema lesions: infant, childhood or adult type
   If distribution is not typical, exclude other entity (dyshidrotic eczema, contact dermatitis, contact urticaria)
   Pruritus
   Chronic or chronically relapsing course

TABLE 14.5 Japanese Dermatological Association (1997)[119]

An atopic diathesis:
  Personal and/or family history of atopic diseases
  and the predisposition to overproduction of IgE antibodies
Must have 3 clinical criteria:
  1) pruritus
  2) typical morphology and distribution
  3) chronic and chronically relapsing course

TABLE 14.6 Hanifin's clinical criteria for the atopic dermatitis complex (2001)[120]

1. Essential features
   (A) Pruritis
   (B) Eczematous changes
     i. Typical and age-specific patterns*
     ii. Chronic or relapsing course
   These features must be present and, if complete, are sufficient for diagnosis.
   *Patterns include: a) facial, neck, and extensor involvement in infants and children; b) current or prior flexural lesions – adults/any age; c) sparing of groin and axillary regions
2. Important features (seen in most cases)
   (A) Early age of onset
   (B) Atopy (IgE reactivity)
   (C) Xerosis
   These features, seen in most cases, add support to the diagnosis
3. Associated features (clinical associations)
   (A) Keratosis pilaris/ichthyosis/palmar hyperlinearity
   (B) Atypical vascular responses
   (C) Perifollicular changes
   (D) Ocular/periorbital changes
   (E) Perioral/periauricular lesions
   These features help in suggesting the diagnosis of AD but are too nonspecific to be used for defining or detecting AD for research and epidemiologic studies
4. Exclusions
   It should be noted that firm diagnosis of AD depends upon excluding conditions such as scabies, allergic contact dermatitis, seborrheic dermatitis, cutaneous lymphoma, ichthyoses, psoriasis, and other primary disease entities

not adequately assess the efficacy of new medications. A plethora of scoring systems has been developed in an attempt to create a useful and practical method to assess changes in clinical features. Many different systems have been proposed, some of which used grid patterns, others severity and extent, and yet others subjective and objective features (Table 14.7). The large number of scoring systems available reflects the requirements of different clinical situations, including natural history and drug investigation.[121,122] Lack of comparative data precludes having a single recognized standard. Some of the scoring methods may obtain a low and positive score while the AD is severe,[123] and with most of the assessments there is a marked intra- and inter-observer variability.

TABLE 14.7 Assessment methods for atopic dermatitis
Severity scoring systems for atopic dermatitis – landmark attempts to produce standardized assessment methods for AD

SSS[124]	1989	Simple Scoring System
		Signs and symptoms, disease extent attributed to Queille-Roussel et al.[125]
The Rajka and Langeland Scoring system[126]	1989	Based on extent, course and intensity of the disease
Hanifin JM[133]	1989	Standardized grading of subjects for clinical research studies in atopic dermatitis; workshop report
ADASI[127]	1991	= atopic dermatitis severity index
	1998	[Based on PASI – Frederiksson and Pettersson 1978 an index for psoriasis]
SCORAD[128]	1993	Uses extent, area of involvement and intensity of six signs
SASSAD[129]	1996	= Six area six sign AD Refinement of SCORAD grading 0–3 (absent, mild, moderate, severe) of six signs – erythema, exudation, excoriation, dryness, cracking and lichenification at six sites – arms, hands, legs, feet, head and neck, and trunk
MRSA[130]	1998	= Modified Rajka and Langeland severity assessment (Nottingham Severity Score)
EASI[131]	1998	= Eczema area and severity index
ADAM[132]	1999	= Assessment Measure for Atopic Dermatitis
TIS[135]	1999	= Three Item Severity score
		Evaluation of erythema, edema/papulation and excoriation on a scale of 0–3.
EASI revision[134]	2001	= Eczema Area and Severity Index Modification of PASI
Quality of life Measures:		
EDI[136]	1990	= Eczema Disability Index developed from the Psoriasis Disability Index
CDLQI[137]	1995	= Children's Dermatology Life Quality Index used to demonstrate the high level of handicap experienced by children with AD
CADI[138]	2001	= Children's Atopic Dermatitis Index

121. Charman C, Williams H (2000) Outcome measure of disease severity in atopic eczema. **Arch Dermatol** 136:763–769.
122. Finlay AY (1996) Measurement of disease activity and outcome in atopic dermatitis. **Br J Dermatol** 135:509–515.
123. Wurtrich B (1991) Minimal forms of atopic eczema. In: Handbook of Atopic Eczema, Ruzicka T, Ring J, Przybilla B, eds. Berlin-Heidelberg: Springer-Verlag, pp. 46–53.

The earliest score of SSS proposed by Costa et al.[124] was based on its simplicity. Attributed to Queille–Roussel et al.,[125] it relies on physician observation plus information from the patient, but severity is assessed at one site only.

Rajka and Langeland[126] developed a scoring system, designed for use at "baseline" for broadly categorizing patients to "mild," "moderate," and "severe" AD groups. It relies on extent, course and intensity of disease.

Scoring systems ADSI and ADASI[127] (Atopic Dermatitis [Area] Severity Index) evolved from more complex attempts to translate PASI, an established and widely accepted system developed for grading psoriasis severity, to suit AD severity scoring. ADASI involves using body charts, color coding for severity, and a grid system.

The European Task Force on AD developed the SCORAD system,[128] which represents an evaluation encompassing the extent of the disease and patient symptomatology. It uses body diagrams to record extent and area of involvement, and records the intensity of six signs (erythema, oedema/papulation, oozing/crusts, excoriation, lichenification, and dryness). Subjective assessment includes pruritus, sleep loss, and "overall skin condition." This system was developed with children in mind.

The SASSAD (Six Area, Six Sign Atopic Dermatitis) severity score[129] is a refinement of SCORAD and allows for quick and easy assessment.[121]

The Nottingham Eczema Severity Score,[130] the Eczema Area and Severity Index (EASI),[131] and the Assessment Measure for Atopic Dermatitis (ADAM)[132] were all refinements of early systems. Hanifin[133,134] and Wolkerstorfer,[135] working on different continents, have published refinements to their severity scores for specific assessment tasks.

For children, their families, and caregivers, AD can profoundly affect their quality of life and indices designed to measure such variables as disturbed sleep, degree of pruritus, and self-esteem have been developed. The EDI (Eczema Disability Index)[136] was developed from the Psoriasis Disability Index; the Children's Dermatology Life Quality Index (CDLQI),[137] designed specifically with children in mind, has been used to demonstrate the high level of handicap experienced by children with AD. The CADI (the Children's Atopic Dermatitis Index)[138] – a 62-question survey instrument – was developed to assess the quality of life of young American children 6 years and younger with AD.

DISEASES THAT MAY BE MORE SEVERE IN AD BUT CAN OCCUR IN UNAFFECTED SUBJECTS

Keratosis pilaris is a condition that is seen mainly on the extensor aspects of the upper arms (Fig. 14.13) and anterior aspects of the thighs. It begins early in life and tends to improve with age. In young children the lateral aspects of the cheeks near the hairline are often involved and may be mistaken for childhood acne (Fig. 14.14). The lesions consist of asymptomatic hyperkeratotic follicular papules, which may have an underlying erythematous telangiectatic background. Keratosis pilaris is an extremely common disorder and is found in many healthy young children, although it may be accentuated by the dryness in AD patients. It is worse in the winter and clears somewhat in the summer. Although the lesions on the cheeks disappear around puberty

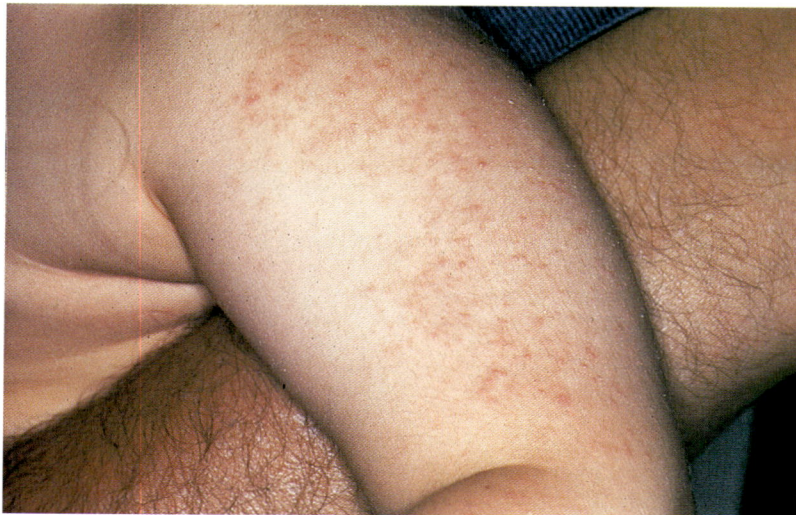

Fig. 14.13 Keratosis pilaris on the upper arm of a child with AD.

or slightly later, keratosis pilaris elsewhere usually persists in a milder form for life and presents no more than a cosmetic problem. Treatment is aimed at hydrating the affected area with oil baths and emollients, including lactic and alpha glycolic acid preparations. In severe cases, treatment with topical retinoids may be helpful.

Pityriasis alba is identified by hypopigmented patches on the cheeks and upper trunk of children mainly 6–12 years, particularly toward the end of summer when the rest of the face is tanned.[139] The lesions are ill-defined, white, at times scaly patches, that are often misdiagnosed as tinea corporis. It is thought to represent a subclinical dermatitis, resulting in postinflammatory hypopigmentation. Lesions of pityriasis alba often recur yearly until puberty, after which time it is unusual to see facial lesions. Histologically, there is acanthosis and mild spongiosis with moderate hyperkeratosis and some parakeratosis. The lesions repigment spontaneously after treatment with low-potency topical corticosteroid preparations (hydrocotisone 1% ointment twice to three times a day) for two to three weeks followed by sun exposure, but they may take several months to resolve and parents should be reassured that complete repigmentation will eventually occur.

Lichen spinulosus is identified by round, occasionally pruritic, follicular plaques on the trunk and extremities with hyperkeratotic follicular accentuation. It is common in black skin and may occur in children with or without AD. At times the lesions are hypopigmented, but their diagnostic feature is the presence of grouped hyperkeratotic follicular spines. They respond well to mild corticosteroid preparations.

Dyshidrotic eczema is a condition that affects the palms, the soles, and the sides of the fingers and toes; it is associated with hyperhidrosis in many cases. The lesions consist of small, pruritic, multiloculated vesicles (Figs 14.15,

124. Costa C, Rilliet A, Nicolet M et al. (1989) Scoring atopic dermatitis: the simpler the better? **Acta Derm Venereol** (Stockh) 69:41–45.
125. Queille-Roussel C, Raynaud F, Saurat J-H (1985) A prospective computerized study of 500 cases of atopic dermatitis in childhood. **Acta Derm Venerol** (Stockh) 114:87–92.
126. Rajka G, Langeland T (1989) Grading of the severity of atopic dermatitis. **Acta Derm Venereol** (Stockh) Suppl 144:13–14.
127. Bahmer FA, Schafer J, Schubert H-J (1991) Quantification of the extent and the severity of atopic dermatitis: the ADASI score. **Arch Dermatol** 127:1239.
128. European Task Force on Atopic Dermatitis (1993) Severity scoring of atopic dermatitis: the SCORAD index. Consensus Report of the European Task Force on Atopic Dermatitis. **Dermatology** 186:23–31.
129. Berth-Jones J (1996) Six area, six sign atopic dermatitis (SASSAD) severity score: a simple system for monitoring disease activity in atopic dermatitis. **Br J Dermatol** 135 (suppl 48):25–30.
130. Emerson RM, Charman CR, Williams HC et al. (1998) Modified Rajka and Langeland severity assessment (MRSA) for atopic dermatitis: a useful tool for epidemiological studies (abstract). **Br J Dermatol** 139 (suppl 51):65.
131. Cherill R, Graeber M, Hanifin J et al. (1998) Eczema area and severity index (EASI): a new tool to evaluate atopic dermatitis (abstract). **J Eur Acad Dermatol Venereol** 11 (suppl 2):48.
132. Charman D, Varigos G, Horne DJ et al. (1999) The development of a practical and reliable assessment measure for atopic dermatitis (ADAM). **J Outcome Meas** 3:21–33.
133. Hanifin JM (1989) Standardised grading of subjects for clinical research studies in atopic dermatitis: workshop report. **Acta Derm Venereol** (Stockh) Suppl 144:28–31.
134. Hanifin JM, Thurston M, Omoto M et al. (2001) The eczema area and severity index (EASI): assessment of reliability in atopic dermatitis. **Exp Dermatol** 10:11–18.
135. Wolkerstorfer A, deWaard van der Spek FB, Glazenburg EJ et al. (1999) Scoring the severity of atopic dermatitis: three item severity score as a rough system for daily practice and as a pre-screening tool for studies. **Acta Derm Venereol** 79:356–359.
136. Eun HC, Finlay AY (1990) Measurement of atopic dermatitis disability. **Ann Dermatol** 2:9–12.
137. Lewis-Jones MS, Findlay AY (1995) The Children's Dermatology Life Quality Index (CSLQI): initial validation and practical use. **Br J Dermatol** 132:942–949.
138. Chamlin SL, Frieden LJ, Williams ML et al. (2001) Quality of life in young American children with atopic dermatitis: instrument development. National Eczema Association International Symposium on Atopic Dermatitis Portland Oregon. [Abstract].
139. Bassaly M (1963) Studies on pityriasis alba. **Arch Dermatol** 88:272–276.

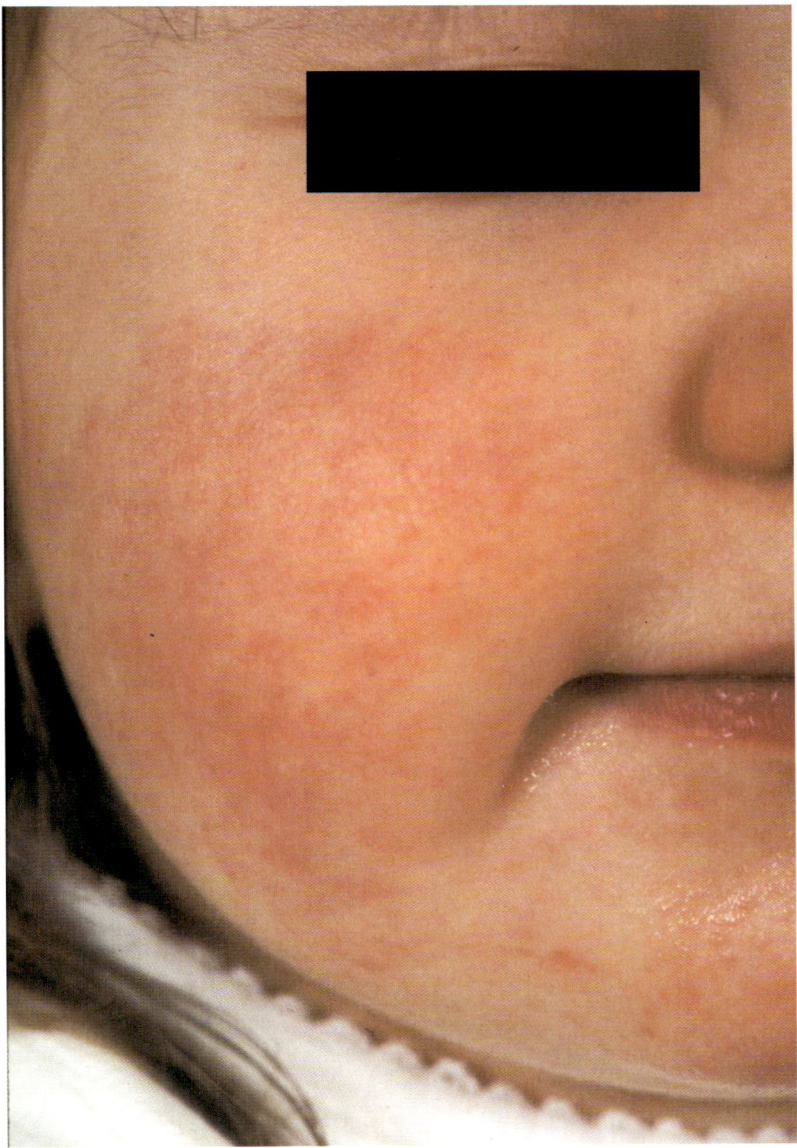

Fig. 14.14   Keratosis pilaris on the lateral aspect of the cheek in a child with AD.

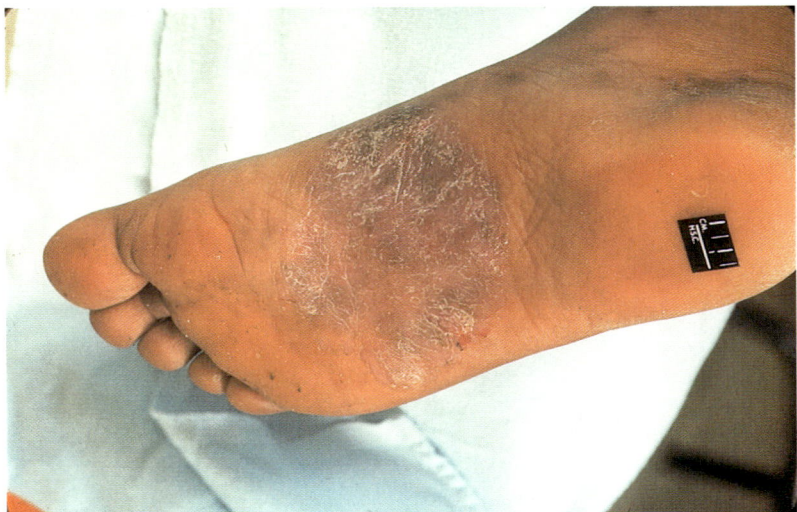

Fig. 14.15   Scaly, hyperkeratotic, fissured plaques in an adolescent with AD.

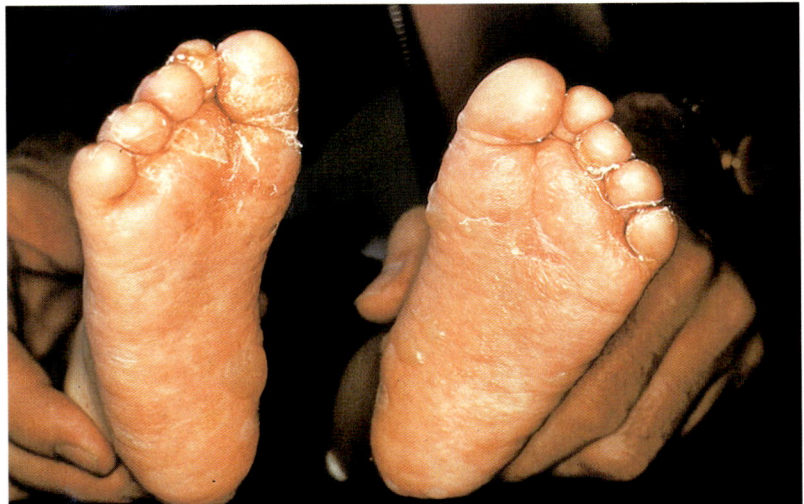

Fig. 14.16   Scaly, hyperkeratotic, fissured plaques in an child with AD.

14.16), resembling "sago grain vesicles." These rupture leaving crusts and scaling with erythema. Occasionally there may be large bullae instead of small vesicles. This condition is difficult to distinguish from an Id reaction or a fungal infection, but the latter tends to be unilateral. Biopsy shows spongiotic vesicles but no occlusion of sweat ducts as previously believed. The pathogenesis of this condition is not understood. Therapy is un–satisfactory. Burow's or saline compresses followed by a medium-strength topical corticosteroid preparation three times a day is helpful. This is both anti-inflammatory and antipruritic. Initially, while the lesions are vesicular, a cream is preferable and later when they become crusted and dry, an ointment should be applied. Recently, topical tacrolimus has been used with good effect in adults.[140]

The term nummular describes coin-shaped lesions. Nummular dermatitis in children differs from that seen in adults; the latter is associated with dry skin, involves the lower legs primarily, and has scaly well-demarcated plaques. In children, the etiology is unknown; lesions begin as exudative and very pruritic follicular papules that coalesce to form plaques anywhere on the body. The disease in adults and children is probably the result of two different path-ogeneses. A refined tar preparation liquor carbonic detergens (LCD) 5% to 10% in a strong corticosteroid ointment used three times a day, with an antibiotic (Cefalexin (Cephalexin) 125mg qid) and antihistamines (hydroxyzine 10–20mg tid) can produce a good therapeutic result. The lesions persist with recurrences until puberty (Fig. 14.17).

Juvenile plantar dermatitis (JPD) presents in childhood with scaling, cracking, and painful fissuring on both feet. The toes (particularly the big toes), anterior third of the soles, and heels are often involved (Fig. 14.18). The problem is much worse when wearing occlusive footwear such as sneakers, and plastic boots, and is thus often worse in the winter. Since fashion now dictates that sneakers are worn both in summer and winter, the condition often persists in the summer months. It is frequently worse in atopics.[141] There is a marked improvement at puberty. Like dyshidrotic eczema, JPD appears to be associated with excessive sweating, which is common in younger children,

140. Hanifin JM, Ling MR, Langley R, Breneman D, Rafal E. (2001) Tacrolimus ointment for the treatment of atopic dermatitis in adult patients: Part I efficacy. **J Am Acad Dermatol** 44(1 suppl): S28–S38.

141. Moorthy TT, Rajan VS (1984) Juvenile plantar dermatosis in Singapore. **Int J Dermatol** 23:476–479.

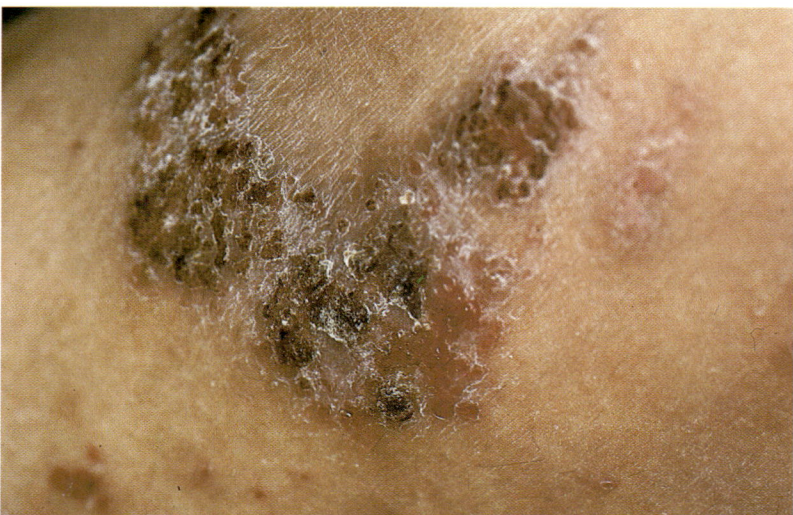

Fig. 14.17   Typical nummular plaques with crusting, oozing and pustules.

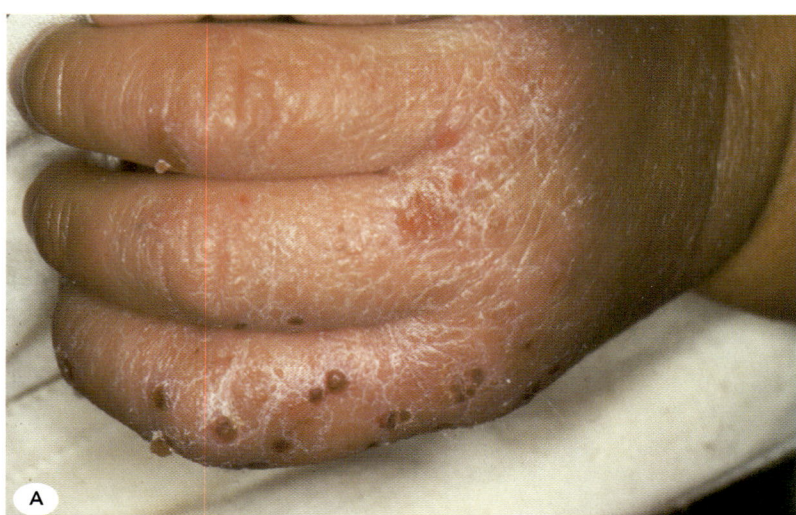

A

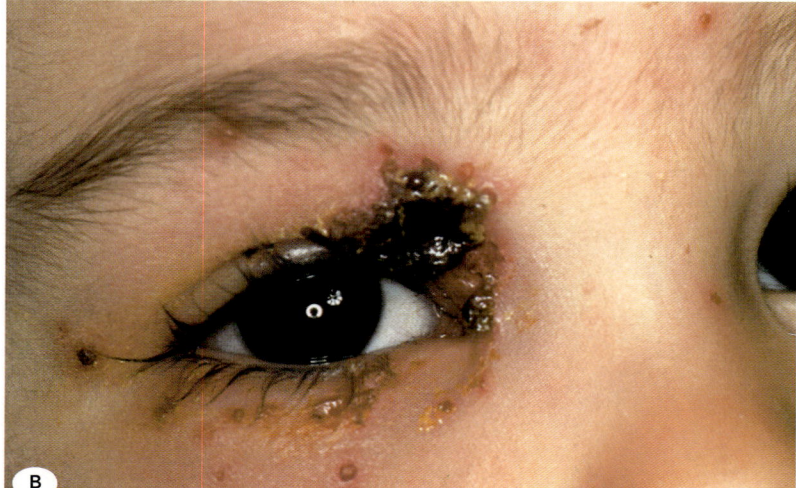

B

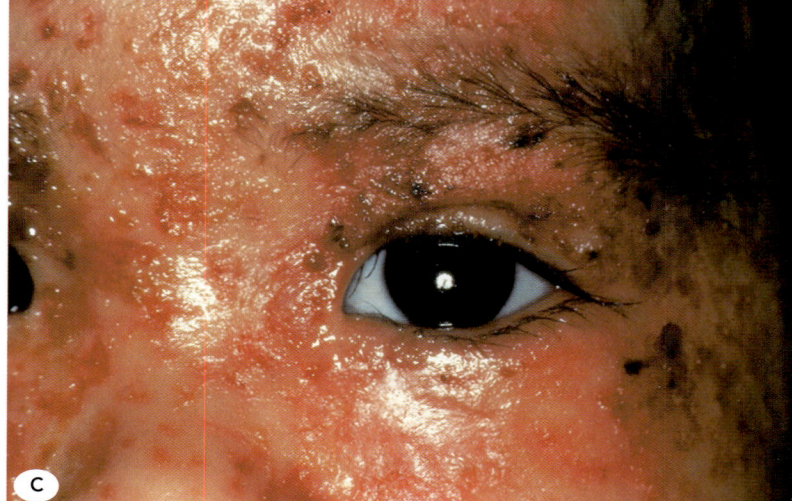

C

Fig. 14.19   (A) Typical vesicular lesions on the hand seen in eczema herpeticum; (B) vesicular lesions around eye in eczema herpeticum; (C) vesicular lesions on face in eczema herpeticum.

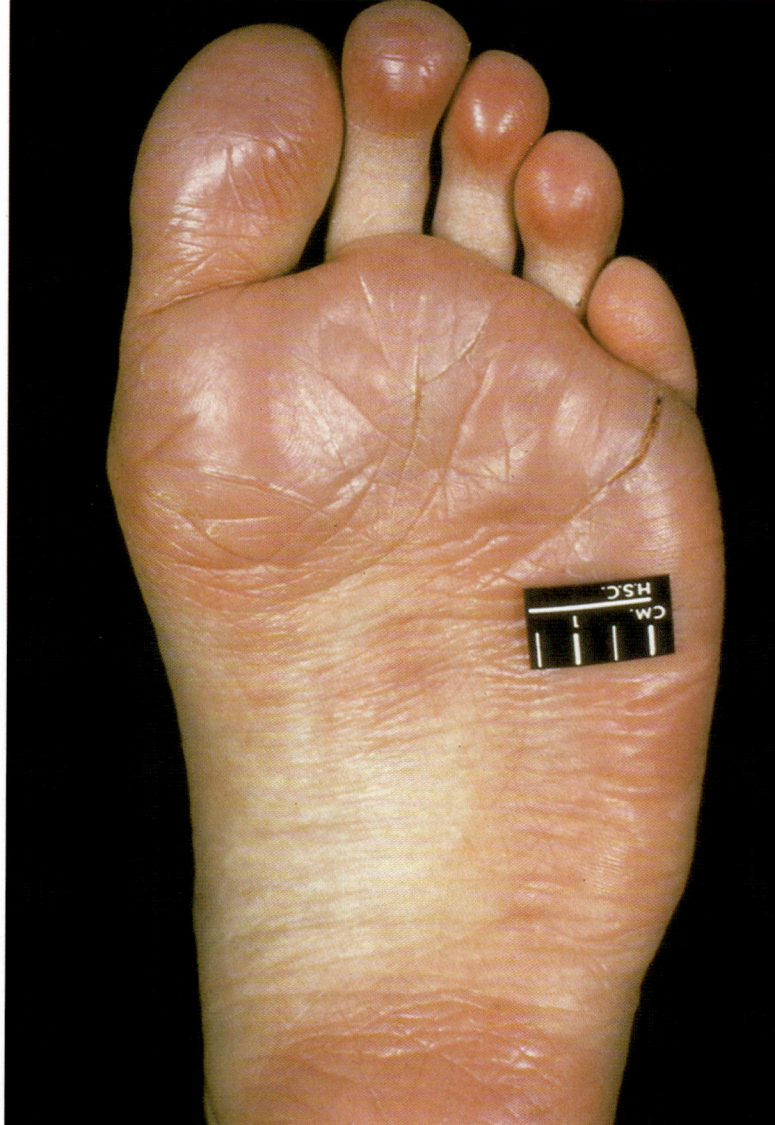

Fig. 14.18   Juvenile plantar dermatosis with fissure on the lateral aspect of the foot of an 11-year-old.

resulting in xerosis as the foot dries. With cotton socks, leather shoes including the soles, and greasy emollients the condition improves. Medium-strength topical corticosteroid ointments three times a day are indicated in more severe cases where fissuring is prominent and pain severe. A colloidal solution of hydrocortisone painted in the fissures three times a day may also be helpful.

COMPLICATIONS OF ATOPIC DERMATITIS

Children with AD have a tendency to develop viral and bacterial skin infections. Eczema vaccinatum occurred when children or their families were vaccinated with the vaccinia virus for the prevention of smallpox, but is no longer seen since vaccination has been discontinued. Herpes simplex virus (HSV) infection is now the main cause of extensive viral infection and is known as eczema herpeticum, or as Kaposi's varicelliform eruption (Figs 14.19, 14.20). The reason that AD patients are susceptible to generalized HSV infection is unknown, but experimentally there have been no demonstrable herpes simplex immune defects found and it is thought that the reduced number of natural killer cells and IL-2 receptors may contribute to the susceptibility of children with AD to cutaneous HSV infections.[142]

Lesions begin soon after a patient with AD has been in close contact with someone who has herpes simplex, most often on the lips. A history of contact with an infected person is not always forthcoming. The eruption is usually associated with a primary infection, although recurrences of eczema herpeticum are not infrequent. In the primary form the child becomes febrile and develops small vesicular lesions in the areas of eczema. The eruption subsequently spreads to normal skin. The vesicular lesions form small erosions which crust over 24 to 48 hours. Prior to the availability of systemic acyclovir and antibiotics, the mortality was high owing to systemic spread of the virus or superinfection with bacteria. Acyclovir should be administered either intravenously 15–30mgs/kg divided into 3 doses or orally in a dose of 30mg/kg per day for seven to 10 days, depending on the severity of the condition. In addition to Acyclovir, saline or Burow's solution compresses may be useful and systemic antibiotics may be warranted.

Verrucae[143] and mollusca contagiosa[144] have been thought to be more common in AD, but this was not corroborated in a report of verrucae and AD in the UK.[145] Mollusca contagiosa tend to be more severe and widespread in children with AD. The associated mollusca dermatitis is also more severe, and the condition persists for a longer period and is more difficult to eliminate. Chickenpox and other viral infections may rarely cause problems in children with AD. Although the incidence of tinea corporis infections is supposedly increased,[146] this has not been reported in children.

Patients with AD have significant *Staphylococcus aureus* (*S. aureus*) colonization on their skin, occurring in 93% of involved skin and 76% of uninvolved skin.[147] In contrast, *S. aureus* colonizes 20% of involved skin in psoriatic patients and less than 10% in the skin in the normal population. David suggests that clinical infection occurs frequently in AD patients (Fig. 14.21).[148] However, despite large areas of excoriated skin and large numbers of staphylococcal organisms, patients seldom develop severe systemic infection. Two studies have found a reduction of *S. aureus* after the use of topical corticosteroids.[149,150]

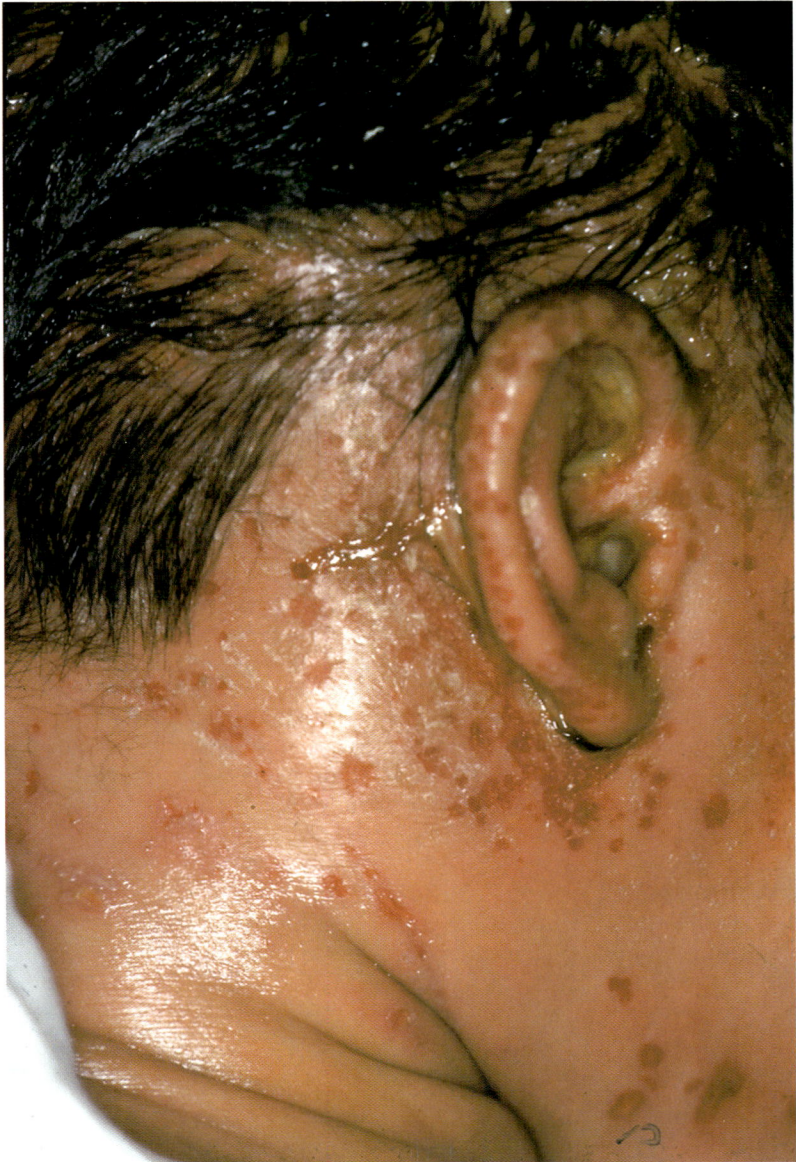

Fig. 14.20 Superficial secondary Staphylococcal infection in patient with eczema herpeticum.

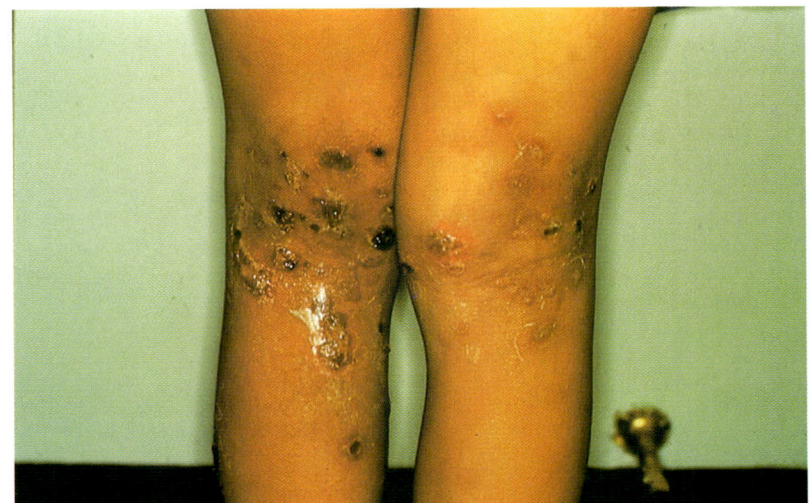

Fig. 14.21 Typical eczematous plaques in the popliteal fossae secondarily infected with *Staphylococcus aureus*.

142. Goodyear HM, McLeish P, Randall S et al. (1996) Immunological studies of herpes simplex virus infection in children with atopic eczema. **Br J Dermatol** 134:85–93.
143. Currie JM, Wright RC, Milelr OG (1971) The frequency of warts in atopic patients. **Cutis** 8:243
144. Solomon LM, Telner P (1966) Eruptive molluscum contagiosum in atopic dermatitis. **Can Med Assoc J** 95:978–979.
145. Williams H, Pottier A, Strachan D (1993) Are viral warts seen more commonly in children with eczema? **Arch Dermatol** 129:717–720.
146. Hanifin JM, Ray LF, Lobitz WC Jr (1974) Immunological reactivity in dermatophytosis. **Br J Dermatol** 90:1–8.
147. Aly R (1980) Bacteriology of atopic dermatitis. **Acta Dermatol Venereol** 1980; suppl. 92:16.
148. David TJ (1989) Infection and prevention: current controversies in childhood atopic enzema: a review. **J R Soc Med** 82:420–422.
149. Stalder JF, Fleury M, Sourisse M et al. (1994) Local steroid therapy and bacterial skin flora in atopic dermatitis. **Br J Dermatol** 131;536–540.
150. Nilsson EJ, Henning CG, Magnusson J (1992) Topical corticosteroids and Staphylococcus aureus in atopic dermatitis. **J Am Acad Dermatol** 27:29–34.

PATHOPHYSIOLOGY AND HISTOGENESIS

Histologic findings

The histologic picture in AD is nonspecific and nondiagnostic. Acute dermatitis is characterized by epidermal intercellular edema (spongiosis). Intra-epidermal vesicles may be permeated by T lymphocytes and neutrophils may be present in the stratum corneum.[151] The stratum corneum is often parakeratotic and contains aggregates of coagulated plasma, forming crusts clinically. The upper dermis shows vascular dilatation, edema, and a perivenular mononuclear cell infiltrate. Eosinophils, basophils, and neutrophils are present in normal numbers in the dermis.

Chronic dermatitis shows epidermal acanthosis with regular elongation of rete ridges, hyperkeratosis, and little spongiosis. There is an increased number of IgE-bearing Langerhans cells (LC) in the epidermis and macrophages dominate the dermal mononuclear cell infiltrate.[152,153] There are increased numbers of mast cells but they are generally fully granulated. Eosinophils may be increased and major basic protein (MBP) is often deposited in large amounts in the superficial dermis.[154] MBP is a cytolytic protein produced by activated eosinophils which, together with other eosinophil-derived cytokines and mediators, contributes to inflammation and tissue injury. Demyelination and fibrosis of cutaneous nerves are seen at all levels of the dermis. The number of capillaries may be increased and their walls thickened.

Histogenesis

The T-cell infiltrate in lesions of acute AD consists of activated memory T cells bearing CD3, CD4 and CD45 RO (indicating previous encounter with antigen),[155] with a CD4:CD8 ratio of 7:1.[156] Infiltrating T cells express high levels of cutaneous lymphocyte antigen (CLA), which functions as a skin homing receptor for T lymphocytes.[157] T-cell activation leads to enhanced adhesiveness of the microvasculature, either directly through lymphokine release or indirectly through the release of mast cell degranulating factors, which in turn leads to enhanced binding and extravasation of leukocytes into lesional skin.[158]

Lesional skin of AD exhibits increased numbers of dermal and epidermal Langerhans cells. Unlike LC from normal skin, these LC are capable of activating autologous resting CD4[+] T lymphocytes in the absence of added antigens.[159] This reactivity may be due to presentation of self-peptides (autoreactivity), presentation of processed foreign antigen, or binding of microbial superantigen.[158] IgE-bearing LC capture selected allergens which are then internalized and processed by the LC for presentation to T lymphocytes, which in turn are of the IL-4 producing Th2 type. Because IL-4 induces IgE synthesis and the expression of receptors for IgE on cells, a positive-feedback loop might be operative. Alterations of LC activity may contribute to depression of delayed-type hypersensitivity (DTH) responses, characteristic of AD. This depression of DTH may be responsible for increased susceptibility to viral and fungal infections in AD and the frequent anergy on intradermal DTH testing.

Cytokines in AD and regulation of IgE synthesis

Total serum IgE is elevated in 43–82% of patients with AD, the highest levels being found in patients with severe skin disease and coexisting respiratory atopy.[160,161] Elevated serum IgE in AD is related to the increased expression of Th2-producing cytokines such as IL-4, IL-5, and IL-13, produced by allergen specific T cells.[162] IL-4 and IL-13 induce germline transcription at the cε exon, promoting isotype switching to IgE.[163] Both cytokines also inhibit production of Th1 cytokines such as interferon-gamma (IFN-γ), upregulate CD23 on monocytes and B cells and stimulate dermal eosinophil infiltration.[164] In addition, peripheral blood mononuclear cells (PBMC) from patients with AD have a reduced capacity to produce interferon-gamma (IFN-γ).[165] IFN-γ inhibits IgE synthesis as well as the proliferation of Th2 cells and expression of the IL-4 receptor on T cells.

Hamid et al.[166] have shown that uninvolved skin of patients with AD has an increased number of cells expressing IL-4 and IL-13 mRNA. Acute skin lesions have a greater number of cells expressing IL-4, -5, -13 and -16 mRNA.[167] IL-4 promotes Th2 cell development and IL-16 may promote the infiltration of CD[+]4 T cells into the skin lesions. In contrast, chronic skin lesions have fewer IL-4 and -13 mRNA expressing cells but increased numbers of IL-5 and IFN-γ expressing cells.[166] There is also overexpression of IL-12 and granulocyte macrophage colony stimulating factor (GM-CSF) in chronic lesions. IL-12, expressed by macrophages and eosinophils, is thought to be responsible for the switch to Th1 cell development, evident in chronic lesions.[168] GM-CSF is likely to enhance cell survival of eosinophils and macrophages.[169]

On a clinical level, the Th2 secretion pattern is associated with IgE-mediated reactions such as exogenous allergic urticaria. Th1 secretion patterns are associated with DTH reactions such as the tuberculin reaction. If Th2-like responses were the only basis of AD, the phenotype of the cutaneous atopic disease would be urticarial lesions. It appears that activation of Th2-type cells initiates AD, but the chronic inflammatory stage is dominated by a Th1-type response resembling a DTH reaction.[170]

Molecular, biochemical and immunological basis

The pathogenesis of AD is not well delineated but appears to be a complex interaction between immune dysregulation, pharmacophysiologic abnormalities, and epidermal barrier dysfunction. AD and the other atopic disorders are most likely to result from multifactorial inheritance with disease expression due to interactions between genetic and environmental factors. The reported development of AD in a previously non-atopic patient after allogeneic bone marrow transplantation suggests bone marrow derived cells play a key role in the formation of AD lesions.[171]

IgE-mediated allergic reactivity

IgE contributes to the inflammatory cell infiltrate in AD by several mechanisms, including a biphasic immediate/late phase reaction, allergen pre-

151. Soter NA (1989) Morphology of atopic eczema. **Allergy** 44Suppl9:16–19.
152. Bruynzeel-Koomen C, van Wichen DF, Toonstra L et al. (1986) The presence of IgE molecules on epidermal Langerhans cells in patients with atopic dermatitis. **Arch Dermatol Res** 278(3):199–205.
153. Barker JNWM, Alegre VA, MacDonald DM (1988) Surface-bound immunoglobulin E on antigen presenting cells in cutaneous tissue of atopic dermatitis. **J Invest Dermatol** 90:117.
154. Cheng JF, Ott NL, Peterson EA (1997) Dermal eosinophils in atopic dermatitis undergo cytolytic degeneration. **J Allergy Clin Immunol** 99:683–692.
155. Leung DYM, Bhan AK, Schneeberger EE et al. (1983) Characterization of the mononuclear cell infiltrate in atopic dermatitis using monoclonal antibodies. **J Allergy Clin Immunol** 71:47–56.
156. Lever R, Turbitt M, Sanderson et al. (1987) Immunophenotyping of the cutaneous infiltrate and of the mononuclear cells in the peripheral blood in patients with atopic dermatitis. **J Invest Dermatol** 89:4–7.
157. Leung DYM (1999) Pathogenesis of atopic dermatitis. **J Allergy Clin Immunol** 104:S99–S108.
158. Cooper KD (1994) Atopic dermatitis: recent trends in pathogenesis and therapy. **J Invest Dermatol** 102:128–137.
159. Taylor RS, Baadsgaard O, Hammerberg C et al. (1991) Hyperstimulatory CD1a+ CD1b+ CD36+ Langerhans cells are responsible for increased autologous T lymphocyte reactivity to lesional epidermal cells of patients with atopic dermatitis. **J Immunol** 147:3794–3802.
160. Johnson E, Irons J, Petterson R et al. (1974) Serum IgE concentrations in atopic dermatitis. **J Allergy Clin Immunol** 54:94–99.
161. Juhlin L, Johansson SGO, Bennich H et al. (1969) Immunoglobulin E in dermatoses. **Arch Dermatol** 100: 12–15.

162. Leung DYM (1995) Atopic dermatitis: the skin as a window into the pathogenesis of chronic allergic diseases. **J Allergy Clin Immunol** 96:302–319.
163. Oettgen HC, Geha RS (1999) IgE in asthma and atopy: cellular and molecular connections. **J Clin Invest** 104:829–835.
164. Nickel R, Beck LA, Stellato C et al. (1999) Chemokines and allergic disease. **J Allergy Clin Immunol** 104:723–742.
165. Jujo K, Renz H, Abe J et al. (1992) Decreased gamma interferon and increased IL-4 production promote IgE synthesis in atopic dermatitis. **J Allergy Clin Immunol** 90:323–331.
166. Hamid Q, Boguniewicz M, Leung DYM (1994) Differential in situ cytokine gene expression in acute versus chronic atopic dermatitis. **J Clin Invest** 94:870–876.
167. Hamid Q, Nareer T, Minshall EM et al. (1996) In vivo expression of IL-12 and IL-13 in atopic dermatitis. **J Allergy Clin Immunol** 98:225–231.
168. Grewe M, Bruijnzeel-Koomen CA, Schopf E et al. (1998) A role for Th1 and Th2 cells in the immunopathogenesis of atopic dermatitis. **Immunol Today** 19:359–361.
169. Bratton DL, Hamid Q, Boguniewicz M et al. (1995) Granulocyte macrophage colony-stimulating factor contributes to enhanced monocyte survival in chronic atopic dermatitis. **J Clin Invest** 95:211–218.
170. Wollenberg A, Bieber T (2000) Atopic dermatitis: from the genes to skin lesions. **Allergy** 55:205–213.
171. Agosti JM, Sprenger JD, Lum Lg et al. (1988) Transfer of allergen specific IgE mediated hypersensitivity with allogeneic bone marrow transplantation. **N Engl J Med** 319:1623–1628.

sentation by IgE-bearing LCs, allergen-induced activation of IgE-bearing macrophages, and IgE autoreactivity to human proteins.[172] However, IgE is not essential to the production of eczematous skin lesions. At least 20% of patients with AD have a normal IgE level and chronic AD has been reported in patients with X-linked agammaglobulinemia in whom IgE was virtually absent.[173] Although IgE has a short half-life of five to seven days, the level does not fluctuate in close association with clinical flares and remissions.[174] When severe AD is treated with systemic steroids, the clinical improvement that ensues is not accompanied by a decrease in the serum IgE level. Patients treated with recombinant IFN-γ improve in the setting of increasing IgE levels.[175] The IgE level returns to normal when patients with a history of severe dermatitis have been free from their disease for at least two years.[174]

Food allergy

The prevalence of IgE-mediated food allergy in patients with AD is increased, although it has been difficult to quantify. Hanifin estimates 10 to 20% of patients with AD have clinically relevant food hypersensitivities.[176] Guillet and Guillet, using an elimination diet followed by open and blind food challenge, could not identify any food allergies in 162 patients with mild to moderate AD, although one or more were detectable in 96% of 88 patients with severe disease.[177] Immediate skin prick tests or radioallergosorbent tests (RASTs) to a range of food allergens yield one or more positive results in 51–85% of patients with AD.[178–180] However, these tests are not useful in predicting clinically relevant reactions. Although negative skin tests virtually exclude IgE-mediated food allergy, only 25–30% of patients with positive skin tests will have a reaction when challenged.[180,181]

Most food reactions develop within minutes to two hours of the food being consumed and last only 30–120 minutes. A pruritic erythematous morbilliform eruption or urticarial lesions are the most common cutaneous reactions and are due to IgE-mediated cutaneous mast cell activation. This is accompanied by a rise in plasma histamine concentration.[182] The IgE-mediated late-phase reaction (LPR) has been proposed as the link between immediate hypersensitivity and the development of atopic eczematous skin, which histologically more closely resembles a type 4 DTH reaction.[183] The LPR begins 3–4 hours after ingestion of antigen. There is a progressive dermal accumulation of eosinophils, neutrophils, and basophils, reaching a maximum concentration at 6–12 hours.[184,185] By 24–48 hours there is a mononuclear cell infiltrate consisting of monocytes and Th2 cells.[186] Although this dermal infiltrate histologically resembles skin lesions of AD, it has been consistently difficult to demonstrate that this IgE-mediated LPR is accompanied by the development of clinically evident eczematous lesions. An alternative mechanism through which foods may aggravate AD is via food allergen-specific T cells, which have been cloned from lesional skin and normal skin of patients with AD.[187] In children with casein aggravated AD, there is significantly increased expression of CLA on casein reactive T cells after *in vitro* stimulation with casein, when compared with *Candida albicans* reactive T cells from the same patients and either casein or *C. albicans* reactive T cells from non-atopic controls.[188] The clinical relevance of these findings needs to be further delineated.

Overall, 90% of children with food allergy react to only one or two foods and only 6 foods are responsible for 90% of all food allergies (egg, peanut, milk, wheat, fish and soy).[178] Avoidance of foods that have produced clinically evident reactions is important to prevent pruritic urticarial exacerbations and anaphylactic reactions. However, despite anecdotal reports in the literature, oral food challenges in a controlled clinical setting are rarely observed to provoke or exacerbate eczematous lesions.[189] Moreover, there is little evidence that more generalized food avoidance with restrictive or elemental diets produces sustained improvement in chronic dermatitis or alters the child's prognosis.[190,191] Many studies have tried to determine if AD can be prevented through maternal (pregnant and breast-feeding) elimination diets, prolonged breast-feeding and the delayed introduction of solids. The results have been variable but overall suggest these measures may delay the development of food allergy and AD but, by 2 years of age, the cumulative incidence of atopic disease is the same as in the control groups.[192–194]

Aeroallergens

Whilst food allergies are most relevant to infants and toddlers, environmental allergens may become a more important aggravating factor for older children and adults. Skin prick test or specific IgE reactions to at least one aeroallergen can be found in the majority of adolescent or adult AD patients with increased total serum IgE.[195] One controlled study has shown that inhalation of house dust mite (HDM) aggravates AD lesions.[196] However, patch testing AD patients with aeroallergens leads to positive DTH reactions in approximately one-third of cases (the results have been variable due to different patch testing techniques utilized).[197–200] Delayed hypersensitivity to aeroallergens is thought to be IgE mediated with the binding of allergen to IgE-bearing epidermal

172. Leung DYM, Soter NA (2001) Cellular and immunologic mechanisms in atopic dermatitis. **J Am Acad Dermatol** 44:S1–S12.
173. Peterson RDA, Page ARP, Good RA (1962) Wheal and erythema allergy in patients with agammaglobulinaemia. **J Allergy** 33:406–411.
174. Johansson SGO, Juhlin L (1970) Immunoglobulin E in healed atopic dermatitis and after treatment with corticosteroids and azathioprine. **Br J Dermatol** 82:10–12.
175. Hanifin JM, Schneider LC, Leung DYM et al. (1993) Recombinant interferon gamma therapy for atopic dermatitis. **J Am Acad Dermatol** 28:189–197.
176. Hanifin JM (1986) Significance of food hypersensitivity in children with atopic dermatitis. **Pediatr Dermatol** 3:161–174.
177. Guillet G, Guillet M (1992) Natural history of sensitizations in atopic dermatitis. **Arch Dermatol** 128:187–192.
178. Sampson HA, McCaskill CC (1985) Food hypersensitivity and atopic dermatitis: evaluation of 113 patients. **J Pediatr** 107:669–675.
179. Burks AW, Mallory SB, Williams LW et al. (1988) Atopic dermatitis: clinical relevance of food hypersensitivity reactions. **J Pediatr** 113:447–451.
180. Sampson HA, Albergo R (1984) Comparison of results of skin tests, RAST and double-blind, placebo controlled food challenges in children with atopic dermatitis. **J Allergy Clin Immunol** 74:26–33.
181. Sampson HA (1983) Role of immediate food hypersensitivity in the pathogenesis of atopic dermatitis. **J Allergy Clin Immunol** 71:473–480.
182. Sampson HA, Jolie PL (1984) Increased plasma histamine concentrations after food challenges in children with atopic dermatitis. **N Engl J Med** 311:372–376.
183. Gleich GJ (1982) The late phase of the immunoglobulin E mediated reaction: A link between anaphylaxis and common allergic diseases. **J Allergy Clin Immunol** 70:160–169.
184. Solley GO, Gleich GJ, Jordan RE et al. (1976) The late phase of the immediate wheal and flare skin reaction. **J Clin Invest** 58:408–420.
185. Leung DYM, Pober JS, Cotran RS (1991) Expression of endothelial leukocyte adhesion molecule-1 in elicited late phase allergic reactions. **J Clin Invest** 87:1805–1809.
186. Kay AM, Ying S, Varney V et al. (1991) Messenger RNA expression of the cytokine gene cluster, IL-3, IL-4, IL-5 and GM-CSF, in allergen induced late phase cutaneous reactions. **J Exp Med** 133:775–778.
187. Van Reijsen FC, Felius A, Wauters EA et al. (1998) T cell reactivity for a peanut derived epitope in the skin of a young infant with atopic dermatitis. **J Allergy Clin Immunol** 101:207–209.
188. Abernathy-Carver KJ, Sampson HA, Picker LJ et al. (1995) Milk-induced eczema is associated with the expansion of T cells expressing cutaneous lymphocyte antigen. **J Clin Invest** 95:913–918.
189. Hanifin JM (1997) Critical evaluation of food and mite allergy in the management of atopic dermatitis. **J Dermatol** 24:495–503.
190. Pike G, Carter CM, Boulton P et al. (1989) Few food diets in the treatment of atopic eczema. **Arch Dis Child** 64:1691–1698.
191. Devlin J, David TJ, Stanton RHJ (1991) Six food diet for childhood atopic dermatitis. **Acta Derm Venereol** (Stockh) 71:20–24.
192. Zeiger RS, Heller S, Mellon MH et al. (1989) Effect of combined maternal and infant food allergen avoidance on development of atopy in early infancy: a randomized study. **J Allergy Clin Immunol** 84:72–89.
193. Arshad SH, Matthews S, Gant C et al. (1992) Effect of allergen avoidance on development of allergic disorders in infancy. **Lancet** 339:1493–1497.
194. Hide DW, Matthews S, Matthews L et al. (1994) Effect of allergen avoidance in infancy on allergic manifestations at age 2 years. **J Allergy Clin Immunol** 93:842–846.
195. Werfel T, Kapp A (1998) Environmental and other provocation factors in atopic dermatitis. **Allergy** 53:731–739.
196. Tupker RA, De Monchy JG, Coenraads PJ et al. (1996) Induction of atopic dermatitis by inhalation of house dust mite. **J Allergy Clin Immunol** 97:1064–1070.
197. Castelain M, Birnbaum J, Castelain P et al. (1993) Patch test reactions to mite antigens: a GERDA multicentre study. **Contact Dermatitis** 29:246–250.
198. Seidenari S, Manzini BM, Danese P et al. (1992) Positive patch tests to whole mite culture and purified mite extracts in patients with atopic dermatitis, asthma and rhinitis. **Ann Allergy** 69:201–206.
199. Clark RAF, Adinoff AD (1989) The relationship between positive aeroallergen patch test reaction and aeroallergen exacerbations of atopic dermatitis. **Clin Immunol Immunopathol** 53(Suppl):S132–S140.
200. Reitamo S, Visa K, Kahonen K et al. (1986) Eczematous reactions in atopic patients caused by epicutaneous testing with inhalant allergens. **Br J Dermatol** 114:303–309.

LCs. Allergen can bind to uncomplexed IgE attached to LC via the high affinity FcεR-I, or preformed IgE-allergen complexes can bind to the low affinity FcεR-II/CD23.[201] Activation of FcεR-I results in the release of proinflammatory mediators from the LCs and activation of both FcεR-I and FcεR-II results in facilitated antigen presentation to CD4+ T lymphocytes in the lesional skin.[202] Many T-cell clones cultured from skin lesions of AD are aeroallergen specific, particularly to *Dermatophagoides pteronyssinus* (house dust mites).[203]

Many studies have attempted to show improvement in AD following aeroallergen avoidance or minimization. Few studies have been well designed and the results have been conflicting. Guillet and Guillet studied 169 patients with moderate to severe AD before and after a two-month period during which relevant aeroallergens were eliminated or reduced.[177] Sensitivity to inhaled allergens was detected and acknowledged as being clinically responsible for respiratory symptoms in 27% of patients, but was believed responsible for skin symptoms in only 4 patients. In a small controlled trial of eradication of HDM with natamycin and vacuum cleaning, Colloff *et al.*[204] found no correlation between clinical improvement and reduced mite numbers. In contrast, Tan *et al.*[205] reported significant improvement in a double-blind controlled trial of HDM avoidance, using Goretex bed covers, benzyltannate spray and a powerful vacuum cleaner. Similarly, there have been conflicting reports on the clinical benefits derived from HDM hyposensitization techniques.[206,207] As yet, no conclusion can be drawn from the small number of studies published.

Autoallergy

Many environmental allergens share structural and immunologic similarities with human proteins. Valenta *et al.*[208] demonstrated that sera from patients with chronic severe AD frequently display IgE reactivity against a broad variety of proteins in histogenetically unrelated human cell types. Patients with strong IgE autoreactivity tend to have more severe forms of AD than those without detectable IgE autoantibodies. These researchers also isolated complementary DNAs coding for autoallergens, mainly intracellular proteins. They postulate that autoallergens may crosslink effector cell-bound IgE autoantibodies and, by release of inflammatory mediators, lead to immediate-type symptoms. Secondly, IgE-mediated presentation of autoallergens may activate autoreactive T cells to release proinflammatory cytokines.

Microbes in AD

Skin colonization with *Staphylococcus aureus* is extremely common in AD. Abeck and Mempel[209] found 90% of children with AD had cutaneous colo-

nization and 71% harbored *Staphylococcus aureus* in their nares. *Staphylococcus aureus* exhibits a greater degree of adherence to corneocytes of patients with AD and may penetrate the epidermis via intercellular spaces.[210] The extracellular lipids of the stratum corneum are altered in AD and this may result in diminished antibacterial activity.[211]

Staphylococci may exacerbate AD in a number of ways. Firstly, up to 57% of patients with AD have anti-staphylococcal IgE antibodies directed toward exotoxins.[212] These specific IgE antibodies may precipitate or aggravate AD by mediating type-1 allergy. Staphylococcal enterotoxin B (SEB)-producing *Staphylococcus aureus* is the most frequently detected strain and anti-SEB IgE levels correlate with disease severity.[213] Secondly, exotoxins such as staphylococcal enterotoxin (SE) A, SEB, SEC, SED, SEE, toxic shock syndrome toxin (TSST-1), and exfoliative toxin A and B may act as superantigens.[214] Superantigens can bind to class II MHC molecules on epidermal LC, macrophages, and monocytes and cause the release of proinflammatory mediators such as IL-1 and tumor necrosis factor-α. In addition, through cross-linking MHC class II molecules on antigen-presenting cells and the variable domain of T-cell receptor-β, T cells can be stimulated to proliferate and secrete a range of inflammatory cytokines.[215] SEB has been shown to induce a Th2 phenotype in lesional T cells, with production of IL-3, -4 and -5.[209] Bunikowski *et al.*[214] have shown that disease severity in children with AD correlates with the presence of toxigenic *Staphylococcus aureus* strains.[215]

Pityrosporum ovale has also been implicated in the pathogenesis of AD, particularly head and neck dermatitis in young adults. In this subgroup, Pityrosporum IgE antibodies are often found and 15–65% have positive skin prick tests to Pityrosporum extracts.[216] However, it is unlikely this organism plays any significant role in childhood dermatitis as it can only be cultured from 5–15% of children younger than 10 years of age[217] and childhood AD does not favor lipophilic areas of skin.

Pharmacophysiologic dysfunction

Leukocytes from atopic patients, particularly monocytes, have reduced cAMP levels due to elevated phosphodiesterase activity.[218,219] This cellular abnormality leads to a higher formation of proinflammatory PGE2 and IL-10.[220,221] Both PGE_2 and IL-10 can inhibit Th1 IFN-γ but not IL-4, tipping the balance of the immune response in favor of a Th2 response. PGE_2 can also act directly on B cells to enhance IgE production.

Epidermal barrier dysfunction

Epidermal barrier function is abnormal in AD, with increased transepidermal water loss.[222] Hara *et al.*[223] have demonstrated reduced ceramide levels in the

201. Bieber T (1992) IgE binding molecules on human Langerhans cells. **Acta Dermatol Venereol** (Stockh) S176:54–57.
202. Van der heijden FL, Joost van Neerven RJ, vanKatwijk M et al. (1993) Serum IgE-facilitated allergen presentation in atopic disease. **J Immunol** 150:3643–3649.
203. Van der Heijden FL, Wierenga EA, Bos JD et al. (1992) High frequency of IL-4 producing CD4+ allergen specific T lymphocytes in atopic dermatitis lesional skin. **J Invest Dermatol** 97:389–394.
204. Colloff MJ, Lever RS, McSharry C (1989) A controlled trial of house dust mite eradication using natamycin in homes of patients with atopic dermatitis: effect on clinical status and mite populations. **Br J Dermatol** 121:199–208.
205. Tan BB, Weald D, Strickland I et al. (1996) Double blind controlled trial effect of house dust mite allergen avoidance in atopic dermatitis. **Lancet** 347:15–18
206. Glover MT, Atherton DJ (1992) A double-blind controlled trial of hyposensitization to Dermatophagoides pteronyssinus in children with atopic eczema. **Clin Exp Allergy** 22:440–446.
207. Leroy BP, Boden G, Lachapelle J-M et al. (1993) A novel therapy for atopic dermatitis with allergen-antibody complexes: a double-blind, placebo-controlled study. **J Am Acad Dermatol** 28:232–239.
208. Valenta R, Seiberler S, Natter S et al. (2000) Autoallergy: A pathogenetic factor in atopic dermatitis? **J Allergy Clin Immunol** 105:432–437.
209. Abeck D, Mempel M (1998) Staphylococcal aureus colonization in atopic dermatitis and therapeutic implications. **Brit J Dermatol** 139:13–16.
210. Morishita Y, Tada J, Sato A et al. (1999) Possible influences of Staphylococcus aureus in atopic dermatitis – the colonizing features and the effects of staphylococcal enterotoxins. **Clin and Exp Allergy** 29:1110–1117.
211. Bibel DJ, Aly R, Shinefield HR (1992) Antimicrobial activity of sphingosines. **J Invest Dermatol** 98:269–273.
212. Leung DYM, Harbeck R, Bina P et al. (1993) Presence of IgE antibodies to staphylococca; exotoxins on the skin of patients with atopic dermatitis. Evidence for a new group of allergens. **J Clin Invest** 92:1374–1380.

213. Nomura I, Tanaka K, Tomita H et al. (1999) Evaluation of the staphylococcal exotoxins and their specific IgE in childhood atopic dermatitis. **J Allergy Clin Immunol** 104:441–446.
214. Bunikowski R, Mielke MEA, Skarabis H et al. (2000) Evidence for a disease promoting effect of Staphylococcus aureus-derived exotoxins in atopic dermatitis. **J Allergy Clin Immunol** 105:814–819.
215. Taskapan MO, Kumar P (2000) Role of staphylococcal superantigens in atopic dermatitis: from colonization to inflammation. **Ann Allergy Asthma Immunol** 84:3–12.
216. Kieffer M, Bergbrant I-M, Faergemann J et al. (1990) Immune reactions to pityrosporum ovale in adult patients with atopic and seborrhoeic dermatitis. **J Am Acad Dermatol** 22:739–742.
217. Broberg AW, Faergemann J, Johansson S et al. (1992) Pityrosporum ovale and atopic dermatitis in children and young adults. **Acta Dermatol Venereol** (Stockh) 72:187–192.
218. Grewe SR, Chan SC, Hanifin JM (1982) Elevated leukocyte cAMP-phosphodiesterase in atopic disease: a possible mechanism for cAMP agonist hyporesponsiveness. **J Allergy Clin Immunol** 70:452–457.
219. Chan SC, Reifsnyder D, Beavo JA et al. (1993) Immunochemical characterization of the distinct monocyte cAMP phosphodiesterase from patients with atopic dermatitis. **J Allergy Clin Immunol** 91:1179–1188.
220. Chan SC, Kim JW, Henderson WR Jn et al. (1993) Altered prostaglandin F_2 regulation of cytokine production in atopic dermatitis. **J Immunol** 151:3345–3352.
221. Ohmen JD, Hanifin JM, Nickoloff BJ et al. (1995) Overexpression of IL-10 in atopic dermatitis. Contrasting cytokine patterns with delayed type hypersensitivity reactions. **J Immunol** 154:1956–1963.
222. Taieb A (1999) Hypothesis: from epidermal barrier dysfunction to atopic disorders. **Contact Dermatitis** 41:177–180.
223. Hara J, Higuchi K, Ohamoto R et al. (2000) High expression of sphingomyelin deacylase is an important determinant of ceramide deficiency leading to barrier disruption in atopic dermatitis. **J Invest Dermatol** 115:406–413.

stratum corneum of lesional and nonlesional skin in patients with AD. This reduced ceramide level appears to be due to upregulation of sphingomyelin deacylase enzyme activity. The defective stratum corneum allows increased penetration of high molecular weight antigens and irritants. Scratching from dryness derived itching may release proinflammatory mediators and cytokines from epidermal cells. It remains unclear whether keratinocytes from AD patients have an intrinsic defect; it is known they produce increased GM-CSF in response to IL-1α.[224] Enhanced production of GM-CSF may contribute to the establishment and chronicity of AD lesions.

Theories of pathogenesis

Hanifin[225] has summarized two pathophysiologic paradigms, one centered on abnormalities of cyclic nucleotide regulation of marrow derived cells, and one centered on allergy.

CAMP PDE hypothesis

The fundamental defect in this hypothesis lies in genetically defined phosphodiesterase isoforms, which lead to reduced cellular cAMP levels. cAMP causes negative modulation of immune and inflammatory reactions, so reduced intracellular levels lead to hyperreactivity to irritants, allergens and microbes.

Allergy hypothesis

This hypothesis proposes that exposure of genetically susceptible individuals to antigens results in proliferation of Th2-dominant T-cell clones which elaborate IL-4, -5, -6, -10 and -13 on re-exposure to antigen. This triggers a vicious circle of spongiotic dermatitis with increased T-lymphocyte activation, hyperstimulatory LC, defective cell-mediated immunity, and B cell IgE overproduction. In this hypothesis, reduced cyclic nucleotide production is secondary to the immunologic abnormalities, but it does not explain the non-immunologic characteristics of AD, such as excess reactivity to irritants. In addition, it does not explain the presence of AD in patients with a normal IgE level and no demonstrable allergies.

DIFFERENTIAL DIAGNOSIS OF ATOPIC DERMATITIS

The differential diagnosis of AD includes other eczematous disorders: scabies, seborrheic dermatitis, contact dermatitis, and psoriasis and other rare causes (Table 14.8).

It is extremely difficult at times to distinguish scabies from AD, particularly in infants. Both diseases are severely pruritic. Xerosis and facial involvement are findings in AD, although in infancy it is not unusual for scabies to affect the face. Recent onset of itching in family members is helpful in the diagnosis of scabies. There are typical burrows and hyperpigmented nodules, which are not features of AD. The eruption of scabies is polymorphous, with papules, nodules, vesicles, eczematous, and urticarial lesions all occurring in the same individual. Palms and soles in infants often have small pustules. If a child presents for the first time with a pruritic eruption at the age of 5, scabies would be more likely than AD.

Seborrheic dermatitis is no longer seen with the same frequency as it was 10 to 15 years ago. It presents in infants around 6 weeks of age and is usually asymptomatic. It is often difficult to distinguish the cradle cap and diffuse scaling on the scalp seen in both AD and SD. Whereas in AD the scale is dry and excoriations are frequent, in SD the scale is yellow and greasy. The intertriginous areas may be affected with erythematous patches in both conditions. In AD the lesions are exudative and in SD are dry. Yates et al. have shown that the differentiation between AD and SD is not always obvious in early infancy, because pruritus may at times be prominent in SD.[226] Vickers included SD as a variant of AD, although the clinical picture and excellent prognosis allow differentiation from AD in retrospect.[101]

Allergy or irritation may result in a contact dermatitis. In infants and young children an ACD is not common; nickel allergy is the most frequently seen. Nickel dermatitis often presents as an eczematous eruption following the pattern of undershirt or sleepwear nickel snaps. There are often other eczematous areas far from the area of contact, particularly in the antecubital fossae making it difficult to distinguish from AD. Children with AD are more prone to develop irritant contact dermatitis from detergents such as bubble baths and harsh soaps.

Psoriasis is increasingly being recognized in infancy and childhood. In infants and young children it is mostly seen in the diaper area and scalp but may be seen anywhere. In children it is most common on the scalp, elbows, and knees, but may occur anywhere. The lesions are asymptomatic or pruritic and consist of scaly erythematous, well-demarcated small plaques. The typical silver scale seen in adults is not common. The main reason for confusion with AD is the lack of recognition of psoriasis in this age group.

Immunodeficiency disorders, including agammaglobulinemia, presenting in the first few months of life, are extremely difficult to distinguish from AD. Pruritus is a feature of all of these diseases. The lack of localization, failure to thrive, and recurrent infections point to an immunodeficiency. There is generally hepatosplenomegaly in Omenn syndrome, which is not a feature of AD. Bleeding with hemorrhagic crusts and dermatitis is typical of Wiscott–Aldridge syndrome.

Other causes of dermatitis may be confused with AD (Table 14.8).

Atopic dermatitis may be so severe that whole-body erythema results. This must be differentiated from other causes of erythroderma in infants and children. These include bullous ichthyosis, Netherton syndrome, psoriasis, pityriasis rubra pilaris, nutritional deficiencies, and drug eruptions.

TABLE 14.8 Rare causes of dermatitic eruptions

1. Acrodermatitis enteropathica
2. Agammaglobulinemia
3. Ataxia telangiectasia
4. Gluten-sensitive enteropathy
6. Langerhans cell histiocytosis
7. Hurler syndrome
8. Leiner's disease
9. Omenn syndrome
10. Phenylketonuria
11. Prolidase deficiency
12. Wiskott–Aldrich syndrome

THERAPEUTICS

Effective management of AD hinges upon establishing good rapport with the affected child and parents. They need to be educated about the nature of the disease, potential aggravating factors to be avoided, and treatment strategies they can implement. Due to the chronic relapsing course of AD, parents have often become disillusioned and skeptical. They are usually subjected to a barrage of information from well-meaning friends, relatives, and health care professionals, much of which may be misleading and conflicting. Having a child with moderate to severe AD has a profound impact on the social, emotional, and financial perspectives of families.[227] Effective treatment not only improves the quality of the child's life but also helps the entire family unit.

224. Pastore S, Fanales-Belasio E, Albanesi C et al. (1997) Granulocyte macrophage colony stimulating factor is overproduced by keratinocytes in atopic dermatitis: implications for sustained dendritic cell activation in the skin. **J Clin Invest** 99:3009–3017.
225. Hanifin JM, Chan S (1999) Biochemical and immunologic mechanisms in atopic dermatitis: new targets for emerging therapies. **J Am Acad Dermatol** 41:72–77.
226. Yates VM, Kerr RE, MacKie RM (1983) Early diagnosis of infantile seborrhoeic dermatitis and atopic dermatitis—clinical features. **Br J Dermatol** 108:633–638.
227. Su JC, Kemp AS, Varigos GA et al. (1997) Atopic eczema: its impact on the family and financial cost. **Arch Dis Child** 76:159–162.

Hydration

Atopic dry skin is characterized by a decrease in skin lipids, an altered water-binding capacity of the stratum corneum, and increased transepidermal water loss.[93] This impaired barrier function leads to increased skin irritability. Bubble baths and excessive exposure to soap, shampoo, and detergents aggravate dryness and should be discouraged. However, bathing is no longer considered to be harmful for atopic dry skin. Indeed, bathing in lukewarm water for 5–15 minutes rehydrates the stratum corneum,[228] although benefits are only seen if an emollient is applied within 2–3 minutes of leaving the water to prevent evaporation.[229] Bathing once or twice daily is soothing during an acute flare, helps reduce bacterial counts, and aids penetration of topical steroids applied after the bath. Showering is not as beneficial, but a short shower is not harmful as long as an emollient is applied immediately after. Moisturizing bath oils help further soften the skin and leave a film after drying. These can be added to the bath or sprayed on to wet skin after showering. A mild, unscented, emollient or moisturizing soap or soap substitute can be used if necessary.

There are many emollients available that are suitable for use on atopic dry skin. In general, creams and ointments are more beneficial than lotions. Urea-based creams are effective for dry skin but cause stinging on areas of inflammation. Some children appear to be very prone to the sensation of stinging and, in this situation, a bland emollient such as petroleum jelly (white petrolatum) or emulsifying ointment is preferable. Compliance deteriorates if treatments produce discomfort. The moisturizer should be applied 2–3 times a day on moist skin but it should be used immediately after the application of a topical steroid, otherwise steroid penetration will be impeded.

Although frequent moisturizing reduces the irritability of atopic skin, it still has a lower itch threshold than normal skin. Irritants to be avoided include woolen clothing, abrasive or occlusive synthetic fabrics, sand and grass, and direct skin contact with irritating foods such as citrus fruits.

Glucocorticoids

Topical glucocorticoids remain the mainstay of treatment for AD. Inflammation should be treated aggressively initially, with the aim of complete or near complete clearance. Treatment regimens vary, but many utilize a medium-potency preparation applied one to three times daily until clearance. Once areas of inflammation have completely cleared, the steroid should be stopped and the skin moisturized regularly. For maintenance, an application of steroid approximately twice weekly is effective.[229] Acute flares should be rapidly aborted by resuming more frequent applications.

Topical steroid ointment preparations are preferable to creams as they penetrate more efficiently, are more moisturizing, and produce less stinging. Their use may need to be substituted in hot, humid weather, where they can be excessively occlusive. Creams are more practical in warm, humid weather and for the scalp; although lotions and gels are more aesthetically acceptable, their alcohol content frequently produces burning discomfort. A 1% hydrocortisone ointment is mostly adequate for thin skin areas such as the face, neck, axillae, and groin, all areas prone to atrophy if more potent preparations are used. For open flexures (wrists, ankles, anticubital, and popliteal fossae) and truncal inflammation, a medium-potency preparation may be used. Potent steroids are not usually required, except for localized areas in longstanding dermatitis where significant lichenification has developed.

Wet dressings are a useful adjunct to topical steroids. The evaporation of water from the skin surface results in vasoconstriction, relief of pruritus, and debridement of crusts from the skin surface.[230] Percutaneous penetration of topical steroids is increased, generally reducing the total quantity of steroid required to settle an acute flare. Some clinicians use total-body wet dressings, which can be done with clothing such as pajamas, cotton tubular dressings or wet towels. After a bath, a low- to medium-potency topical steroid is applied to inflamed areas. A warm, damp layer of clothing or dressing is then applied, followed by a dry layer. These can be left on for as long as eight hours, but are often better tolerated for short periods of 20–30 minutes. The dressings are done two or three times a day for 3–7 days, until the flare settles. Localized wet dressings, such as damp socks for ankles, are useful when there is marked lichenification and slow response to topical steroids alone. An alternative technique for "wet wraps," first described by Goodyear et al.[231] in 1991, involves using cotton tubular dressings impregnated with diluted topical steroid creams.

Failure to respond to topical steroids is usually due to inadequate quantities being applied (poor compliance, fear of adverse effects, or inadequate quantities prescribed) or an inappropriately weak preparation being used. Superinfection or the development of contact allergy to the topical steroid or other topical preparations being applied may also need to be considered. Tachyphylaxis can develop, so periodically changing the topical steroid prescribed may be necessary. A start-stop method of application avoids tachyphylaxis.

When topical steroids are used appropriately, they have a good safety profile and an excellent risk:benefit ratio.[232] It is important to emphasize this to parents, as "corticophobia" is widespread. Hypothalamic-pituitary axis (HPA) suppression can be induced by potent topical steroids used over large areas in children and may transiently develop when diluted steroids are used under wet dressings.[231,233] Ellison et al.[234] recently showed that HPA suppression was rarely found in children or adolescents with moderate to severe AD who used mild- or moderate-potency topical steroids over many years. Growth retardation is another potential systemic complication of topical steroid therapy that has long been a concern. However, it has been difficult to evaluate, as children with AD may have retarded growth due to severe dermatitis per se, nutritional factors, sleep disturbances, and concomitant asthma treated with inhaled or oral steroids. Recently, the knemometer, a lower leg length-measuring device, has been used to assess systemic activity of exogenous glucocorticoids in children. Heuck et al.[235] showed twice-daily application of a potent topical steroid under occlusion did not significantly reduce growth rate, but growth significantly increased after it was discontinued. They hypothesized that, by controlling disease activity, growth potential improves. Patel et al.[236] followed 80 prepubertal children with AD and reported they were not short compared with controls. As they approached teenage years their height velocity decreased and a delay in bone age was noted, features consistent with constitutional growth delay. They did not find that prolonged treatment with moderate-potency topical steroids had any adverse influence on growth.

Local adverse effects include perioral dermatitis (steroid-induced rosacea), persistent facial erythema and telangiectasia, folliculitis, atrophy, striae, local hypertrichosis, and allergic contact dermatitis. Atrophy and striae are the most significant and feared local adverse effects, but are rarely seen with low- to medium-strength preparations, particularly in children under 10 years. These adverse effects may complicate the use of potent and superpotent preparations, particularly when inappropriately used on the face, neck, closed flexures, breasts, and inner thighs in teenagers.

Systemic steroids are rarely appropriate in the management of chronic atopic dermatitis. Although a short course will rapidly settle an acute flare, there is often a rebound flare after discontinuation. Long-term systemic steroids are contraindicated due to the myriad of associated systemic complications.

228. Stender IM, Blichmann C, Serup J (1990) Effects of oil and water baths on the hydration state of the epidermis. **Clin Exp Dermatol** 15:206–209.
229. Hanifin JM, Tofte SJ (1999) Update on therapy for atopic dermatitis. **J Allergy Clin Immunol** 104:S123–S125.
230. Weston WL, Lane AT, Morelli JG (1996) Color Textbook of Pediatric Dermatology. St Louis:Mosby.
231. Goodyear HM, Spowart K, Harper JI (1991) "Wet wrap" dressings for the treatment of atopic dermatitis (Letter). **Br J Dermatol** 125:604.
232. Akers W (1980) Risks of unoccluded topical steroids in clinical trials. **Arch Dermatol** 116:786–788.
233. Wolkerstorfer A, Visser RL, De Waard van der Spek FB et al. (2000) Efficacy and safety of wet wrap dressings in children with severe atopic dermatitis: influence of corticosteroid dilution. **Br J Dermatol** 143:999–1004.
234. Ellison JA, Patel L, Ray DW et al. (2000) Hypothalamic-pituitary-adrenal function and glucocorticoid sensitivity in atopic dermatitis. **Pediatr** 105:794–799.
235. Heuck C, Ternowitz T, Herlin T et al. (1998) Knemometry in children with atopic dermatitis treated with topical glucocorticoids. **Pediatr Dermatol** 15:7–11.
236. Patel L, Clayton PE, Addison GM et al. (1998) Linear growth in prepubertal children with atopic dermatitis. **Arch Dis Child** 79:169–172.

Treatment of infection

With the increasing recognition of the role of *Staphylococcus aureus* as a trigger factor for AD, antibacterial therapy should be considered during acute flares. Widespread golden crusting, follicular pustules, and furuncles suggest staphylococcal infection and this can be readily confirmed with a swab for Gram stain and bacterial culture. Treatment with topical steroids alone reduces the density of staphylococcal organisms on the skin,[237] but clinical outcome is improved if combined with oral antibiotics such as dicloxacillin or cefalexin (cephalexin) (both 40mg/kg per day in four divided doses). Erythromycin (30–50mg/kg daily) is suitable for penicillin allergic patients but increasing staphylococcal resistance should be considered and antibiotic sensitivities checked. For isolated episodes of infection, treatment duration of 10–14 days is usually adequate. For children with severe dermatitis and recurrent infections, more prolonged courses of oral antibiotics may be indicated. In these children, antibiotic sensitivities should be periodically rechecked as resistant strains of *Staphylococcus aureus* may emerge. Nasal swabs taken to determine the presence of chronic nasal staphylococcal carriage are also often useful. If confirmed, intranasal mupirocin twice daily for 10 days is effective, although this may need to be repeated periodically. Moisturizing antibacterial bath oils are now available in many parts of the world and may prove to be useful in reducing staphylococcal colonization and the risk of re-infection.

Antihistamines

Antihistamines have long been used in AD although few randomized, double-blind, placebo-controlled clinical studies have evaluated efficacy. Klein and Clark,[238] in a recent evidence-based review of the efficacy of antihistamines in relieving the pruritus of AD, concluded that the majority of trials (16 studies published between 1966 and 1999) have been flawed in terms of sample size or study design. Anecdotally, sedating antihistamines can be useful in promoting sleep during a flare, but there is no evidence to support or refute the effectiveness of expensive nonsedating agents.

Allergy

Many parents have the simplistic notion that finding the cause of their child's AD through allergy assessment will reduce the need for creams. They should be informed that, even if food or environmental allergies are present, effective treatment for AD still revolves around good skin care and topical therapy. Allergy testing does not need to be routinely ordered but may be considered for children with a history of acute food reactions or those with intractable AD who are not progressing well despite good topical therapy. Any elimination diets instituted should be strictly supervised to ensure they are nutritionally adequate. Reducing exposure to environmental allergens, particularly HDM and animal dander, may also be considered in some cases. It is impossible to completely eradicate HDM from the home environment, but parents can be advised to use protective bed bags, minimize soft furnishings and carpet, and vacuum regularly.[239,240] The value of these measures is still controversial, as is the value of acaricides.[241]

Phototherapy

Phototherapy can reduce both pruritus and inflammation in AD. All forms of ultraviolet radiation have potent inhibitory effects on antigen presentation by LC, and on T-lymphocyte activation, and can modify cytokine production by keratinocytes.[242] Both UVB (280–320) and UVA (320–400) alone have been shown to be effective, but the response rate improves with the combination of UVB and UVA.[243] Treatment regimens usually start with 3–5J of UVA and 30–50mJ of UVB and increase slowly up to 10J UVA and 100mJ UVB.[244] The treatment is best introduced after the stabilization of an acute flare and should be considered an adjunct to topical therapy. Children need to be at least old enough to cooperate with phototherapy and one should be aware of future effects if using ultraviolet light for long periods.

Narrow-band UVB (311nm) is superior to conventional broad-band UVB therapy,[245] as is UVA$_1$ (340–400nm).[246] UVA$_1$ has not yet been studied in children, but is likely to be poorly tolerated as treatment duration is long (30–60 minutes) and, unless the machine is modified,[247] it causes marked overheating and discomfort. The adverse effects of UVA$_1$ are not well delineated.

PUVA therapy (8-methoxypsoralen + UVA) is effective for chronic recalcitrant AD, although potential adverse effects of premature aging and malignancy need to be discussed in detail. Sheehan et al.[248] evaluated 53 children (mean age 11.2 years) with severe AD, unresponsive to other therapy. Twice-weekly treatment resulted in clearance or near clearance of disease in 39 (74%) after a mean of 9 weeks, with a mean cumulative UVA dose of 1118J/cm.[93] Of particular note, 82% of these 39 children were able to maintain remission of disease following gradual withdrawal of treatment.

Immunosuppressive therapy

Tacrolimus

Tacrolimus (FK 506) is a 23-member macrolide produced by *Streptomyces tsukabaensis*. It acts directly on T lymphocytes, particularly CD4$^+$ cells, by binding to immunophilins (FK-binding protein).[249] The tacrolimus-immunophilin complex then binds to, and competitively inhibits, calcineurin, a phosphatase that is active only when bound to calcium and calmodulin. The binding phenomenon inhibits the ability of calcineurin to activate the promotor region of the gene for IL-2, -3, -4, -5, GM-CSF, TNF-α and IFN-γ.[250] It also inhibits the release of mast cell and basophil preformed mediators[251] and downregulates FcεRI on LC.[252] This broad range of inflammatory inhibition mechanisms may downregulate the entire inflammatory cascade leading to clinical disease.

Unlike cyclosporin, tacrolimus is a small molecule with good percutaneous penetration.[252] Some systemic absorption is detectable early in treatment, decreasing as skin barrier function improves.[253] In the largest pediatric study to date involving 351 atopic children, 84% had no detectable blood levels.[254] Increased absorption has been documented in Netherton

237. Nilsson EJ, Henning CG, Magnusson J (1992) Topical corticosteroids and Staphylococcus aureus in atopic dermatitis. J Am Acad Dermatol 27:29–34.
238. Klein PA, Clark RAF (1999) Evidence based review of the efficacy of antihistamines in relieving pruritus in atopic dermatitis. Arch Dermatol 135:1522–1525.
239. Friedmann PS, Tan BB (1998) Mite elimination – clinical effect on eczema. Allergy 53(Suppl 48):97–100.
240. Ricci G, Patrizi A, Specchia F et al. (2000) Effect of house dust mite avoidance measures in children with atopic dermatitis. Br J Dermatol 143:379–384.
241. Cameron MM (1997) Can house dust mite triggered atopic dermatitis be alleviated using acaricides? Br J Dermatol 137:1–8.
242. Cooper KD (1993) New therapeutic approaches in atopic dermatitis. Clin Rev Allergy 11:543–557.
243. Jekler J, Larko O (1990) Combined UVA-UVB versus UVB phototherapy for atopic dermatitis: A paired comparison study. J Am Acad Dermatol 22:49–53.
244. Sidbury R, Hanifin JM (2000) Old, new and emerging therapies for atopic dermatitis. Dermatol Clin 18:1–11.
245. George SA, Bilsland DJ, Johnson BE et al. (1993) Narrowband (TL-O1) UVB airconditioned phototherapy for chronic severe adult atopic dermatitis. Br J Dermatol 128:49–56.
246. Krutmann J, Czech W, Diepgen T et al. (1992) High dose UVA-1 therapy in the treatment of patients with atopic dermatitis. J Am Acad Dermatol 26:225–230.
247. Von Kobyletzki G, Pieck C, Hoffmann K et al. (1999) Medium dose UVA-1 cold-light phototherapy in the treatment of severe atopic dermatitis. J Am Acad Dermatol 41:931–937.
248. Sheehan MP, Atherton DJ, Norris P et al. (1993) Oral psoralen photochemotherapy in severe childhood atopic eczema: an update. Br J Dermatol 129:431–436.
249. Kelly PA, Burckart GL, Venkataramana R (1995) Tacrolimus: a new immunosuppressive agent. Am J Health Syst Pharm 52:1521–1535.
250. Fleischer AB (1999) Treatment of atopic dermatitis: Role of tacrolimus ointment as a topical noncorticosteroid therapy. J Allergy Clin Immunol 104:S126–S130.
251. De Paulis A, Stellato C, Cirillo R et al. (1992) Anti-inflammatory effect of FK-506 on human skin mast cells. J Invest Dermatol 98:800–804.
252. Lawrence ID (1998) Tacrolimus (FK-506): experience in dermatology. Dermatol Ther 5:74–84.
253. Alaiti S, Kang S, Fiedler VC et al. (1998) Tacrolimus (FK-506) ointment for atopic dermatitis: A phase I study in adults and children. J Am Acad Dermatol 38:69–76.
254. Paller A, Eichenfield LF, Leung DY et al. (2001) A 12-week study of tacrolimus ointment for the treatment of dermatitis in pediatric patients. J Am Acad Dermatol 44(Suppl 1):S47–S57.

syndrome, with serum levels reaching the therapeutic range used in organ transplant recipients.[255] Kawashima *et al.*[256] also reported significant blood levels in patients with severe AD who were initially treated with large quantities (10–20g per day) of tacrolimus. However, laboratory results (including serum creatinine) show no changes and no systemic adverse events have been reported. The main adverse effects are stinging and burning on application (10–47%) and erythema (10–12%).[253,254,257–259] It does not block collagen synthesis and therefore does not produce skin atrophy.[260] It is not phototoxic, photosensitizing, or photoallergenic, but avoidance of excessive UV exposure is prudent until long-term effects on photo-carcinogenesis are known.[261]

In 1997, the European Tacrolimus Multicentre AD Study Group showed tacrolimus ointment to be significantly more effective in treating AD than placebo, and there was minimal difference between three concentrations (0.03%, 0.1%, and 0.3%).[257] Boguniewicz[258] showed the safety and efficacy of tacrolimus ointment in 136 pediatric patients (7–16 years) with moderate to severe AD; once again, there was only slight difference between the different concentrations used, with 0.03% not quite as effective as 0.1%. Alait[253] showed 95% of 39 patients (38 children) to have at least good improvement with tacrolimus 0.3% ointment. Paller *et al.*[254] found twice-daily tacrolimus ointment was equally safe for younger (2–6 years) and older (7–15 years) children, with both 0.03% and 0.1% concentrations being safe and significantly more effective than vehicle in the 351 children studies. Sugiura[262] reported reduced efficacy with prolonged use, suggesting tachyphylaxis. There are currently little data directly comparing tacrolimus and topical glucocorticoids, but preliminary evidence suggest it will be comparable to mid-strength glucocorticoids.[261]

At this stage, tacrolimus appears to be a beneficial and a safe alternative to oral immunosuppressants in children with moderate to severe, recalcitrant AD and in those who are recalcitrant to topical glucocorticoids. The long-term safety, especially with respect to future skin malignancy, is not known. It is available in Japan, USA, Canada and Europe but only the 0.03% was approved by the licensing bodies in USA and Canada for children under 12 years of age. A 0.1% ointment has also been marketed for those over 12 years of age. No data are currently available for children under 2 years of age.

Pimecrolimus

Pimecrolimus, also known as SDZ ASM 981, is an ascomycin macrolactam similar to tacrolimus. The configuration of the molecule makes it more lipophilic and thus more specifically targeted to the skin. It produces little, if any, systemic immunosuppression in rat graft vs. host and renal allograft models.[263] It binds to macrophilin 12, the cytosolic macrophilin receptor, and inhibits calcineurin.[263] This downregulates the production of Th1 and Th2 cytokines by T cells and inhibits the proliferation of T cells after antigen specific or nonspecific stimulation. In addition, it inhibits IgE-induced mast cell release of histamine, hexosaminidase, tryptase, leucotriene C4, and TNF-α, as well as basophil production of histamine.[263,264]

Van Leent *et al.*[265] showed that twice-daily application of 1% pimecrolimus cream in 38 adult patients with AD was well tolerated and significantly more effective than placebo. A US multicenter investigator team has recently completed a 26-week trial on 403 patients, aged 1 to 17 years, with AD.[266] The pimecrolimus treatment was more effective than vehicle during the initial six-week double-blind phase, with response to treatment observed as early as day 8. It was well tolerated with stinging and burning in 10–12% of patients, with no significant difference in stinging between vehicle and drug. Studies examining the safety and efficacy of pimecrolimus in infants 3 to 23 months of age have also shown good efficacy with no untoward adverse events[267] and minimal systemic absorption.[268] Harper *et al.*[269] noted consistently low blood levels in children aged 1–4 years, even in those with up to 69% of body surface area treated. As with tacrolimus, cutaneous atrophy does not occur.[270] Similar concerns about long-term risks for cutaneous malignancy apply to pimecrolimus as well as tacrolimus. Pimecrolimus is available as a cream applied twice per day in the United States.

Cyclosporin

Cyclosporin (CyA) is a macrolide immunosuppressive that alters cytokine gene transcription, inhibiting T-cell activation, and modulating the cell mediated immune response.[271] It may work in AD by altering IL-4 transcription and monocyte interleukin-10 production, promoting a Th1 cytokine profile.[272] Since 1987, several studies have confirmed the efficacy of oral CyA in the treatment of AD, in both adults and children. It is mostly used in doses of 2.5–5mg/kg and, because of potential adverse effects, the duration of treatment is kept short (3–6 months). However, Harper *et al.*[273] recently reported 40 patients of 2–16 years who were treated with multiple short courses (12 weeks) or continuous CyA over a 12-month period. Both groups improved significantly (no difference between the groups) and tolerability was considered good or very good in at least 80% of patients. During the course of the study, four patients had a significant rise in creatinine, but in all the creatinine returned to an acceptable level either spontaneously or with dose reduction. No sustained rise in blood pressure was noted in any patient. Prolonged remission occurred in a small group of children, but more commonly AD gradually recurred after CyA cessation.

The use of CyA in childhood AD should be limited to patients with severe disease, poorly controlled with more conservative therapy. Parents must be thoroughly informed of the potential for renal damage, hypertension, cytochrome P_{450} drug interactions and possibly increased malignancy if used long term. Topical preparations of CyA are ineffective.[274]

255. Allen A, Siegfried E, Silverman R et al. (2001) Significant absorption of topical tacrolimus in 3 patients with Netherton syndrome. **Arch Dermatol** 137:747–750.
256. Kawashima M, Nakagawa H, Ohtsuki M et al. (1996) Tacrolimus concentrations in blood during topical treatment of atopic dermatitis. **Lancet** 348:1240–1241.
257. Ruzicka T, Bieber T, Schopf E et al. (1997) A short-term trial of tacrolimus ointment for atopic dermatitis. **New Engl J Med** 337:816–821.
258. Boguniewicz M, Fiedler VC, Raimer S et al. (1998) A randomized, vehicle-controlled trial of tacrolimus ointment for treatment of atopic dermatitis in children. **J Allergy Clin Immunol** 102:637–644.
259. Reitamo S, Wollenberg A, Schopf E et al. (2000) Safety and efficacy of one year of tacrolimus ointment monotherapy in adults with atopic dermatitis. **Arch Dermatol** 136:999–1006.
260. Reitamo S, Rissanen J, Remitz A et al. (1998) Tacrolimus ointment does not affect collagen synthesis: results of a single centre randomized trial. **J Invest Dermatol** 111:396–398.
261. Bekersky I, Fitzsimmons W, Tanase A et al. (2001) Nonclinical and early clinical development of tacrolimus ointment for the treatment of atopic dermatitis. **J Am Acad Dermatol** 44(Supple 1):S58–S64.
262. Sugiura H (2000) Long term efficacy of tacrolimus ointment for recalcitrant facial erythema resistant to topical corticosteroids in adult patients with atopic dermatitis. **Arch Dermatol** 136:1062–1063.
263. Rappersberger K, Meingassner JG, Fialla R et al. (1996) Clearing of psoriasis by a novel immunosuppressive macrolide. **J Invest Dermatol** 106:701–710.
264. Meingassner JG, Grassberger M, Fahrngruber H et al. (1997) A novel anti-inflammatory drug, SDZ ASM 981, to the topical and oral treatment of skin diseases: in vivo phamacology. **Br J Dermatol** 137:568–576.

265. Van Leent EJM, Graber M, Thurston M et al. (1998) Effectiveness of the ascomycin macrolactam SDZ ASM 981 in the topical treatment of atopic dermatitis. **Arch Dermatol** 134:806–809.
266. Eichenfield LF, Lucky AW, Boguniewicz M et al. (2002) Safety and efficacy of pimecrolimus (ASM 981) cream 1% in the treatment of mild and moderate atopic dermatitis in children and adolescents. **J Am Acad Dermatol** 46:495–504.
267. Lakhanpaul M, Allen BR, Wahn U et al. (2001) Pimecrolimus (Elidel® SDZ ASM 981) cream 1%: minimal systemic absorption in infants with extensive atopic eczema. **Poster**.
268. Papp K, Ho V, Halbert A et al. (2001) Pimecrolimus (Elidel® SDZ ASM 981) cream 1% is effective and safe in infants aged 3–23 months with atopic eczema. Poster presented at American Academy of Dermatology 60th Annual Meeting, New Orleans.
269. Harper J, Green A, Scott G et al. (2001) First experience of topical SDZ ASM 981 in children with atopic dermatitis. **Br J Dermatol** 144:781–787.
270. Queille-Roussel C, Paul C, Duteil L et al. (2001) The new topical ascomycin derivative SDZ ASM 981 does not induce skin atrophy when applied to normal skin for 4 weeks: a randomized, double-blind controlled study. **Br J Dermatol** 144:507–513.
271. Liu J (1993) FK 506 and cyclosporin; molecular probes for studying intracellular signal transduction. **Immunol Today** 14:290–295.
272. Campbell DE, Kemp AS (1997) Cyclosporin restores cytokine imbalance in childhood atopic dermatitis. **J Allergy Clin Immunol** 99:857–859.
273. Harper JI, Ahmed I, Barclay G et al. (2000) Cyclosporin for severe childhood atopic dermatitis: short course versus continuous therapy. **Br J Dermatol** 142:52–58.
274. De Prost Y, Bodemer C, Teillac D (1989) Randomised double-blind placebo-controlled trial of local cyclosporin in atopic dermatitis. **Acta Dermatol Venereol** (Stockh) suppl. 144:136–138.

Azathioprine

There have been few studies conducted on the use of azathioprine in AD.[275,276] Despite the paucity of studies, a survey of dermatologists in the United Kingdom reported that 75% used azathioprine to treat adult patients with severe AD and 3% in childhood AD; 89% found it effective.[277] More research is obviously required, but it may be an option for children or adolescents with severe AD unresponsive to other therapies.

Biologic response modifiers

Interferon-gamma

In AD, the Th1 subclass is dominated by an expansion of Th2 cells producing IL-4. The aim of recombinant IFN-γ therapy is to reduce this imbalance, restoring more normal cellular immune responses. Several studies have now shown IFN-γ to produce clinical benefit, with about 45% of patients achieving greater than 50% improvement.[175] Treatment is accompanied by a reduction in circulating eosinophil counts but no decline in serum IgE. It appears to be safe, even when used for as long as 24 months.[278] Adverse effects include flu-like symptoms, leukopenia, and thrombocytopenia. Its cost and the need for subcutaneous administration preclude widespread use.

Thymopentin

Thymopentin is a synthetic pentapeptide derived from the thymic hormone thymopoietin. It promotes the differentiation of mature T lymphocytes and has been proposed to do so preferentially for the Th1 subset.[242] Clinical efficacy has been shown[279,280] but the need for daily subcutaneous injections is a disadvantage.

Other treatments for AD

Tar preparations such as 5–10% liquor carbonis detergens cream can be useful for thick, lichenified plaques of dermatitis. Topical sodium cromoglycate can also be used, with the aim of inhibiting mast cell degranulation. Kita et al.[281] used 1% topical sodium cromoglycate in a water solution and noted benefit; Moore et al.[282] showed anti-inflammatory effect with cromolyn sodium inhalation solution mixed with a water-based emollient cream concentration of 0.21% concentration. These preliminary findings require further follow-up with larger series.

Evening primrose oil contains the n6 series of essential fatty acids. Although a few small studies have shown benefit in AD,[283–285] these have been criticized for methodological flaws. Three large double-blind placebo-controlled parallel group studies have failed to show any benefit.[286–288]

Phosphodiesterase (PDE) inhibitors target the cyclic nucleotide abnormalities characteristic of AD. Potent PDE inhibitors given orally have a high incidence of nausea and vomiting, but Hanifin et al.[289] have identified a type 4 PDE inhibitor (CP-80633) which provided rapid and persistent anti-inflammatory activity when used topically. This is not available for clinical use.

Leukotriene inhibitors (zafirlukast, montelukast and zileuton) are useful in mild to moderate asthma, but their effects in AD are still unknown. Carrucci et al.[290] reported benefit from zafirlukast 20mg twice daily, but only four adult patients were studied.

There are several anecdotal reports of high-dose intravenous immunoglobulin (IVIG) being of therapeutic value in adults and children with AD,[291–293] although Wakim et al. failed to show benefit in one small open label study.[294]

Traditional Chinese herbal medicine has also been used to treat AD. Although benefit has been shown with some concoctions,[295,296] potentially life-threatening adverse events such as hepatotoxicity, cardiomyopathy and renal failure have been reported.[297] A recent analysis of Chinese herbal creams showed eight of 11 samples contained dexamethasone.[298]

Supportive psychotherapy and behavior therapy have also been advocated as adjuncts to other treatment for AD. Recently, Schachner et al.[299] showed benefits from parental massage for 20 minutes each day. The children's affect and activity level improved and parental anxiety decreased.

PROGNOSIS AND COURSE OF THE DISEASE

AD is a disease of exacerbations and remissions. Most patients tend to improve with age. Data from follow-up surveys show variable results due to different patient sampling. In general, the more severe and long lasting the AD, the more likely that it will continue into adult life. One study showed a persistence into adult life in approximately 70% with severe AD and 60% with milder disease.[300] Another study showed that patients with AD in the teenage years persisted into adult life whereas milder cases had a better prognosis.[300–302] Vickers[101] reported that AD cleared by the age of 20 in 90% of patients. However, the inclusion of patients with seborrheic dermatitis, which has an excellent prognosis and clears within weeks, biases his results.

Wuthrich[303] followed 121 patients who had suffered AD from infancy, reviewing them at mean ages of 15 and 23.5 years. In only 11% of patients

275. Buckley DA, Baldwin P, Rogers S (1995) Azathioprine in severe adult atopic eczema. **Br J Dermatol** 133(Suppl 45):18.
276. Lear JT, English JSC, Jones P et al. (1996) A retrospective review of the use of azathioprine in severe adult atopic dermatitis. **J Am Acad Dermatol** 35:642–643.
277. Tan BB, Lear JT, Gawkrodger DJ et al. (1997) Azathioprine in dermatology: A survey of current practice in the UK. **Br J Dermatol** 136:351–355.
278. Stevens SR, Hanifin JM, Hamilton T et al. (1998) Long term effectiveness and safety of recombinant human interferon gamma therapy for atopic dermatitis despite unchanged serum IgE levels. **Arch Dermatol** 134:799–804.
279. Kang K, Cooper KD, Hanifin JM (1983) Thymopentin pentapeptide (TP-5) improves clinical parameters and lymphocyte subpopulations in atopic dermatitis. **J Am Acad Dermatol** 8:372–377.
280. Leung DYM, Hirsch RL, Schneider L et al. (1990) Thymopentin therapy reduces the clinical severity of atopic dermatitis. **J Allergy Clin Immunol** 85:927–933.
281. Kita H, Hiratsuka S (1994) Effect of topical cromoglycate solution on atopic dermatitis: combined treatment of sodium cromoglycate solution with the oral anti-allergic medication, oxatomide. **Eur J Pediatr** 153:66–71.
282. Moore C, Ehlayel MS, Junprasert J et al. (1998) Topical sodium cromoglycate in the treatment of moderate to severe atopic dermatitis. **Ann Allergy Asthma Immunol** 81:452–458.
283. Lovell CR, Burton JL, Horrobin DF (1981) Treatment of atopic eczema with evening primrose oil. **Lancet** 1:278.
284. Wright S, Burton JL (1982) Oral evening primrose seed oil improves atopic eczema. **Lancet** 2:1120–1122.
285. Schalin-Karrila M, Mattila L, Jansen CT et al. (1987) Evening primrose oil in the treatment of atopic eczema: effect on clinical status, plasma phospholipid fatty acids and circulating blood prostaglandins. **Br J Dermatol** 117:11–19.
286. Berth-Jones J, Graham-Brown RAC (1993) Placebo-controlled trial of essential fatty acid supplementation in atopic dermatitis. **Lancet** 341:1557–1560.
287. Bamford JTM, Gibson RW, Renier CM (1985) Atopic eczema unresponsive to evening primrose oil. **J Am Acad Dermatol** 13:959–965.
288. Hederos CA, Berg A (1966) Epogam evening primrose oil treatment in atopic dermatitis and asthma. **Arch Dis Child** 75:494–497.
289. Hanifin JM, Chan SC, Cheng JB et al. (1996) Type 4 phosphodiesterase inhibitors have clinical and in vitro anti-inflammatory effects in atopic dermatitis. **J Invest Dermatol** 107:51–56.
290. Carrucci JA, Washenik K, Weinstein A et al. (1998) The leukotriene antagonist Zafirlukast as a therapeutic agent for atopic dermatitis. **Arch Dermatol** 134:785–786.
291. Kita H (1994) High dose gammaglobulin treatment for atopic dermatitis. **Arch Dis Child** 70:335–336.
292. Gelfand EW, Landwehr LP, Esterl B et al. (1996) Intravenous immune globulin: an alternative therapy in steroid dependent allergic diseases. **Clin Exp Immunol** 104 Suppl 1:61–66.
293. Jolles S, Hughes J, Rustin M (2000) The treatment of atopic dermatitis with adjunctive high dose intravenous immunoglobulin: a report of 3 patients and review of the literature. **Br J Dermatol** 142:551–554.
294. Wakim M, Alazard M, Yajima A et al. (1998) High dose intravenous immunoglobulin in atopic dermatitis and hyper IgE syndrome. **Ann Allergy Asthma Immunol** 81:153–158.
295. Sheehan MP, Atherton DJ (1994) One-year follow up of children treated with Chinese medicinal herbs for atopic eczema. **Br J Dermatol** 140:488–493.
296. Armstrong N, Ernst E (1999) Treatment of eczema with Chinese herbs; a systematic review of randomized clinical trials. **Br J Clin Pharmacol** 48:262–264.
297. Ernst E (2000) Adverse effects of herbal drugs in dermatology. **Br J Dermatol** 143:923–929.
298. Keane FM, Munn SE, du Vivier AWP et al. (1999) Analysis of Chinese herbal creams prescribed for dermatological conditions. **Br Med J** 318:563–567.
299. Schachner L, Field T, Hernandez-Reif M et al. (1998) Atopic dermatitis symptoms decreased in children following massage therapy. **Ped Dermatol** 15:390–395.
300. Roth HL, Kierland RR (1961) The natural history of atopic dermatitis, a 20-year follow-up study. **Arch Dermatol** 89:209.
301. Rajka G (1975) Atopic Dermatitis. London: WB Saunders.
302. Rystedt I (1985) Prognostic factors in atopic dermatitis. **Acta Dermatol Venereol** 65:206–213.
303. Wuthrich B (1999) Clinical aspects, epidemiology and prognosis of atopic dermatitis. **Ann Allergy Asthma Immunol** 83:464–470.

did the dermatitis disappear in childhood; persistence into adult life occurred in 63%, with 32% having a chronic continuous course. During puberty, 25% cleared but reappeared; in another 20% AD reappeared. Prognostically unfavorable factors were delineated as early onset (severe disease within the first 6 months of life), being the eldest or only child, association with respiratory disease, and very high serum IgE levels.

In a large follow-up study from Sweden, Rystedt noted that 50% of adults had persistence of the disease although there were often many years separating recurrences.[302] In this study several risk factors also influenced the eventual prognosis, including severe dermatitis in childhood, family history of AD, associated rhinitis or asthma, and female sex. When many risk factors were present, more than 80% were still affected; when absent less than 15% had persistent disease.

Despite these conflicting results, the majority of patients with AD have periods of complete clearing in teenage and adult life. Those patients with persistent disease are not as severely affected as they were in infancy and have much longer periods of remission between exacerbations of AD.[304]

Asthma develops in approximately 30% of patients with AD.[305,306] A study in a tertiary care centre found 76% of the AD group had wheezing whereas only 12% of the control group had this symptom.[307] Another study of adults found asthma in 10–19% of AD patients.[300] AD tends to develop somewhat earlier than asthma. When asthma occurs in the younger age group, boys are more commonly affected. Allergic rhinitis develops in 25% of AD patients,[305,307] and 15% of patients with AD have both allergic rhinitis and asthma. Roth and Kierland found AD associated with other atopic disease in 55% of their patients.[300] A follow-up survey of patients with AD in Denver showed a 28% incidence of asthma and hay fever in the teenage years but very little AD.[308]

There have been rare reports of AD with Hodgkin's disease,[309] Sézary syndrome,[310] and cutaneous T-cell lymphoma.[311] It is impossible to know if this is a coincidence or not.

Pediatric aspects of the disease

Parents of children with AD are dealing with a chronic condition and usually very uncomfortable children. It is important to discuss the psychological impact of the disease, emphasizing that AD is not caused by stress (as is often believed), but that the condition itself is stressful and may cause problems in family relationships. There is a strong tendency for a child with a chronic pruritic problem to become manipulative.

Patients with AD have extremely dry, sensitive skin. The condition is worse during the dry winter months. A humidifier in the child's room is beneficial. A mild detergent should be used to wash the child's clothes and bleach, and fabric softeners, as well as perfumed products, should be avoided. However, a recent study has not found increased sensitivity in AD children using enzyme detergents.[312]

Clothing is an important factor in controlling itch. Cotton (preferably 100%) should be worn all year and in winter a layering of the cotton provides good insulation. Cotton socks and tights are available. Synthetic fabrics and wool are irritating to the skin of patients with AD.

It is important to allow the child as much freedom as possible. If swimming is part of the school program or a summer activity some clinicians find it helpful to use a barrier of petrolatum after the initial shower and before entering a chlorinated pool. Strenuous activity such as running, soccer, and hockey often make the children hot and sweaty, and their pruritis increases. Nevertheless, for the child's own psychological and physical well-being, it is probably advisable to allow him or her to participate in sports activities.

In the summer months, AD may improve in the sun, but heat exacerbates the pruritus. Thus, a sunny environment with a breeze or access to water (pool or sprinkler) is most helpful. Air conditioning in hot climates is useful in managing the increased sweating. Parents should be warned that extreme fluctuations in temperature as well as fever may produce a flare in the condition. Roth and Kierland reported that most patients found extreme cold also exacerbated their AD.[300]

A clinical observation in many patients with AD is that a change in environment and/or climate (hospitalization or vacation) may improve the clinical condition, particularly when the vacation is taken in warmer climates.[313]

DIAPER DERMATITIS

The term *diaper dermatitis* includes all eruptions that occur in the area covered by the diaper. These conditions are caused directly by the wearing of diapers (irritant contact dermatitis), those that are aggravated by diapers (e.g., psoriasis), and those that occur whether or not diapers are worn (e.g., acrodermatitis enteropathica).[314] In many societies where diapers are not worn, infants escape a condition that is commonly seen in pediatric practice in more industrialized countries.[315]

The first true description of diaper dermatitis was made by Jacquet in 1905,[316] although Parrott described a lesion in the diaper area in 1887.[317] In 1915, Zahorsky described the frequency of diaper eruptions associated with an "ammoniacal" smelling diaper.[318] In Great Britain in the 1970s, diaper dermatitis accounted for 20% of all skin consultations in the 0- to 5-year age group,[319] and in Japan the prevalence varied between 6 and 50% depending on definitions and inclusion criteria.[320–322] Since the advent of newer diapering practices, mainly the introduction of disposable diapers with superabsorbant gel centers, the figure has dropped considerably.[323] Nevertheless, mothers in the US still frequently consult pediatricians for diaper eruptions.[324]

Diapers have only gained widespread acceptance in the Western world during the last 70 years with the appearance of the modern diaper in the 1920s. These have evolved through using pieces of cloth and safety pins, to the 1930s, when diaper services became widely available, and more recently to disposable diapers that have been used extensively in the last 40 years.[315] There are three methods of diapering utilized in most countries. Parents can buy ready-made cloth diapers and launder them at home. With this method there is a residue of chemicals left in the diaper despite numbers of rinses. It is the most common cause of irritant diaper dermatitis (IDD) in infants. Major problems in the past have arisen from antiseptics used in laundering.[325,326] Quaternary ammonium compounds are now the most common chemical

304. Sampson HA (1992) Atopic dermatitis. **Ann Allergy** 69:469–479.
305. Purdy MJ (1953) The long-term prognosis in infantile eczema. **BMJ** 1:1366.
306. Kuster W, Peterson M, Christophers E et al. (1990) A family study of atopic dermatitis: clinical and genetic characteristics of 188 patients and 2,151 family members. **Arch Dermatol Res** 282:98–102.
307. Salob SP, Atherton DJ (1993) Prevalence of respiratory symptoms in children with atopic dermatitis attending pediatric dermatology clinics. **Pediatrics** 91:8–12.
308. Freeman GL, Johnson S (1964) Allergic diseases in adolescents. **Am J Dis Children** 107:549.
309. Winkelmann RK, Rajka G (1983) Atopic dermatitis and Hodgkins disease. **Acta Dermatol Venereol** (Stockh) 63:176.
310. Rajka MD, Winkelmann RK (1984) Atopic dermatitis and Sézary syndrome. **Arch Dermatol** 120:83–84.
311. Lange-Vejlsgaard G, Ralfkiaer E, Larsen JK et al. (1989) Fatal cutaneous T cell lymphoma in a child with atopic dermatitis. **J Am Acad Dermatol** 20:954–958.
312. Belsito DV, Fransway AF, Fowler JF et al. (2002) Allergic contact dermatitis to detergents: a multicenter study to assess prevalence. **J Am Acad Dermatol** 46:200–206.
313. Turner MA, Devlin J, David TJ (1991) Holidays and atopic eczema. **Arch Dis Child** 66:212–215.
314. Koblenzer PJ (1973) Diaper dermatitis: an overview. **Clin Pediatr** 12:386.
315. Levin S (1970) History of medicine-diapers. **S Afr Med J** 44:256–263.

316. Jacquet L (1905) Traitae des maladies de l'enfance. In: Grancher J, Comby J, Marfan AB, eds. Paris: Masson & Co, p. 714.
317. Boisits EK, McCormack JJ (1982) Diaper dermatitis and the role of predisposition. In: Neonatal Skin; Structure and Function, Maibach HI, Boisitis EK, eds. New York: Marcel Dekker, p. 191.
318. Zahorsky J (1915) The ammoniacal diaper in infants and young children. **Am J Dis Child** 10:436.
319. Verbov JL (1976) Skin problems in children. **Practitioner** 217:403–415.
320. Berg RW (1988) Etiology and pathophysiology of diaper dermatitis. **Adv Dermatol** 3:75–90.
321. Jordan WE, Lawson KD, Berg RW et al. (1986) Diaper dermatitis frequency and severity among a general infant population. **Pediatr Dermatol** 3:198–201.
322. Longhi F, Carlucci G, Bellucci R et al. (1992) Diaper dermatitis: a study of contributing factors. **Contact Derm** 26:248–252.
323. Wong DL, Brantly D, Clutter LB et al. (1992) Diapering choices: a critical review of the issues. **Pediatr Nurs** 18:41–54.
324. Krowchuk DP (2000) Characterization of diaper dermatitis in the United States. **Arch Pediatr Adolesc Med** 154:943–946.
325. Brown BW (1970) Fatal phenol poisoning from improperly laundered diapers. **Am J Public Health** 60:901.
326. Jensen JPA (1971) Transcutaneous absorption of boron form a baby ointment used prophylactically against diaper dermatitis. **Nord Med** 86:1425–1429.

used in the laundering of home diapers. Yamamoto, writing in the Japanese literature, found that using cotton diapers with a diagonal weave had a better effect than plain weave diapers for preventing diaper dermatitis.

A diaper service is another method of diapering. Diaper services usually provide their customers with their own new diapers, that are collected weekly or biweekly. They are cycled through as many as eleven hot rinses, the first seven being with detergents. Two or more diapers may be used simultaneously, increasing the absorbency. The diapers are usually covered with a plastic pant.

Disposable diapers were first used in the 1960s and have become increasingly refined. They have changed from paper, to an absorbable cellulose center, to the most modern diapers that have a super-absorbent gel center carrying wetness from the outside to the inside of the diaper and leaving the skin dry. This is achieved by an intricate wicking system preventing back flow and a gel that can hold 80 times its weight. These newer diapers cause the least problem with diaper dermatitis, markedly reducing IDD.[327–331] Even newer changes have employed a slow release of petrolatum,[332] and a breathable outer sheet.[333] Both formulations purport to further reduce the incidence of diaper dermatitis. One study, using diapers with a breathable outer sheet, reports a reduction in candidal diaper dermatitis.[333] An added benefit of disposable diapers has been the development of cuffs that better contain urine and feces, contributing to a reduction in gastroenteritis in day care settings.[334–336]

Numerous studies have compared the incidence of IDD in diapers from a diaper service and disposable diapers, and have reached inconclusive results.[337–339] No studies have compared the newer formulation of disposable diapers with diaper services. The crucial factor in preventing IDD appears to be the number of diaper changes and in this respect both diaper service and disposable diapers are better than home-laundered diapers. One to two percent of non-biodegradable waste in North America is composed of disposable diapers. On the other hand, the eleven or more rinses in boiling water used by diaper services is a drain on natural resources.

Diseases that are most commonly seen in the diaper area are listed and described in Table 14.9.

IRRITANT DIAPER DERMATITIS

In 1921, Cooke[340] described an organism (*Bacterium ammoniagenes*), that was recovered from the feces of infants with IDD. The organism supposedly split urea into ammonia, causing the typical eruption known for many years in the pediatric literature as ammoniacal diaper dermatitis. In 1977, Leyden et al.[341] investigated children who suffered from IDD and found no difference in the ammonia concentration from an early morning diaper of infants with, and without, the diaper dermatitis. In addition, placing various concentrations of ammonia on the buttocks of infants, with occlusion, did not produce a dermatitis and lastly, there was no difference in the number of *B. ammoniagenes*

TABLE 14.9 Causes of diaper dermatitis
1. Chafing, irritant (ammoniacal) dermatitis
2. Candidiasis
3. Psoriasiform dermatitis with Id
4. Nutritional abnormalities
5. Granuloma gluteale infantum
6. Letterer–Siwe disease
7. Bullous impetigo
8. Erosive perianal eruption
9. Seborrheic dermatitis
10. Zinc deficiency
11. Cystic fibrosis
12. Kawasaki's disease

organisms (now shown to be a *Proteus* organism) in children with and without an IDD. They concluded that ammonia was not involved in the etiology of IDD. Nevertheless, children who do suffer from an IDD often have diapers that smell of ammonia.

The etiology and pathogenesis of IDD is only partially understood. Some children seem constitutionally more susceptible, and the ingestion of antibiotics[342] with diarrhea is a risk factor.[343] Occlusion, maceration, and possibly *Candida* and bacteria may all play roles (Fig. 14.22).

Diapers have an impervious plastic covering creating a milieu that is continuously wet from urine and occlusion, resulting in overhydration of the skin. This makes the skin susceptible to friction from movement under the diaper,[317] which does not occur with a dry diaper.[338]

Elevations in the pH of the diaper area from feces mixed with urine[344] activate fecal lipases and proteases; this together with *Candida albicans* causes damage to the epidermis resulting in loss of the barrier function and fostering increased susceptibility to irritation.[344] Fecal bacteria may have a synergistic effect with *Candida* in producing the eruption.[341] *Candida albicans* is capable of penetrating the epidermal barrier by liberating keratinases.

The incidence of IDD is equal between the sexes; it usually begins from 3 to 18 months, peaking between 6 and 9 months. Infants are generally asymptomatic and present with erythema on the convex surface of the inner, upper thigh area and buttock. The creases are spared as is the area over the mons pubis in boys (Fig. 14.23). The eruption subsequently becomes deeply erythematous with a typical glistening or glazed appearance and a wrinkled surface.

Chafing of the diaper area may occur on the convex surfaces and a "tide mark" dermatitis occurs at the margin of the diaper. This is again caused by friction from the diaper and wet skin, and responds well to the use of emollients. A typical contact irritation is seen on the buttock in toddlers

327. Campbell RL, Seymour JL, Stone LC et al. (1987) Clinical studies with disposable diapers containing absorbent gelling materials: evaluation of effects on infant skin condition. **J Am Acad Dermatol** 17:978–987.
328. Lane AT, Rehder PA, Helm K (1990) Evaluations of diapers containing absorbent gelling material with conventional disposable diapers in newborn infants. **Am J Dis Child** 144:315–318.
329. de Prost Y (1987) Results of an efficacy clinical diaper study with superabsorbent panty diaper conducted in French day care centers. In: Diaper Dermatitis: Later Insight into Pathogenesis, Prophylxis, and Therapy, Tronnier H, Schmitt GJ, eds. Munich: Verlag Medical Concepts, pp. 111–114.
330. Oranje AP, Bilo AC, deWaardrd S et al. (1987) In: Diaper Dermatitis: Later Insight into Pathogenesis, Prophylaxis and Therapy, Tronnier H, Schmitt GJ, eds. Munich: Verlag Medical Concepts; pp. 115–122.
331. Tronnier H (1987) Tolerance and efficacy, characteristics of panty diapers with highly absorbent pad. In: Diaper Dermatitis: Later Insight into Pathogenesis, Prophylaxis and Therapy, Tronnier H, Schmitt GJ, eds. Munich: Verlag Medical Concepts, pp. 123–126.
332. Odio MR, O'Connor RJ, Sarbaugh F et al. (2000) Continuous topical administration of a petrolatum formulation by a novel disposable diaper? Effect on skin condition. **Dermatology** 200:238–243.
333. Akin F, Spraker M, Aly R et al. (2001) Effects of breathable disposable diapers: reduced prevalence of candida and common diaper dermatitis. **Pediatr Dermatol** 18:282–290.
334. Van R, Wun CC, Morrow AL et al. (1991) The effect of diaper type and overclothing on fecal contamination in day care centers. **JAMA** 265:1840–1844.
335. Kubinl M, Kressner B, Raynor W et al. (1993) Comparison of stool containment in cloth and single-use diapers using a simulated infant feces. **Pediatrics** 91:632–636.
336. Van R, Morrow AL, Reves RR et al. (1991) Environmental contamination in child daycare centers. **Am J Epidemiol** 133:460–470.
337. Seymour JL, Keswick BH, Hanifin JM et al. (1987) Clinical effects of diaper types on the skin of normal infants and infants with atopic dermatitis. **J Am Acad Dermatol** 17:988–997.
338. Jordan WE, Blaney TL (1982) Factors influencing infant diaper dermatitis. In: Neonatal Skin; Structure and Function, Maibach HI, Boisits EK, eds. New York: Marcel Dekker, p. 205.
339. Stein H (1982) Incidence of diaper rash when using cloth and disposable diapers. **J Pediatr** 101:721–723.
340. Cooke JV (1921) The etiology and treatment of ammonia dermatitis of the gluteal region of infants. **Am J Dis Child** 22:481.
341. Leyden JJ, Katz S, Stewart R, Kligman AM (1977) Urinary ammonia and ammonia-producing microorganisms in infants with and without diaper dermatitis. **Arch Dermatol** 113:1678–1680.
342. Campbell RL, Bartlett AV, Sarbaugh FC (1988) Effects of diaper types on diaper dermatitis associated with diarrhea and antibiotic use in children in day-care centers. **Pediatr Dermatol** 5:83–87.
343. Seymour JL, Keswick BH, Milligan MC et al. (1987) Clinical and microbial effects of cloth, cellulose core, and cellulose core/absorbent gel diapers in atopic dermatitis. **Pediatrician** 149 (suppl 1):39–43.
344. Berg RW (1988) Etiology and pathophysiology of diaper dermatitis. **Adv Dermatol** 3:75–98.

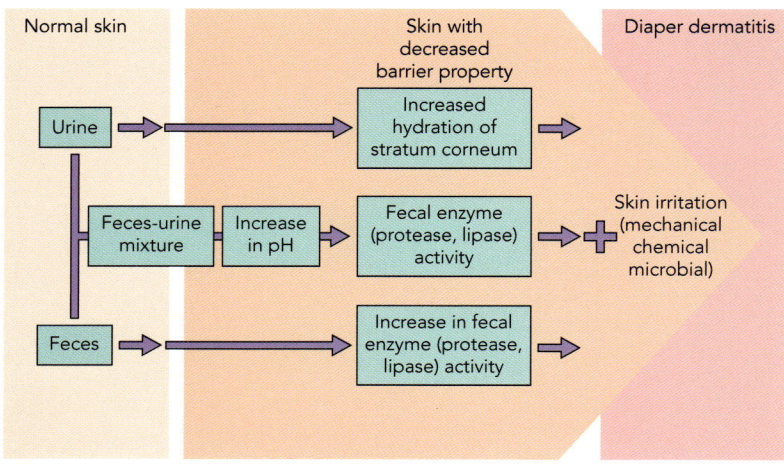

Fig. 14.22   Pathogenesis of irritant diaper dermatitis.

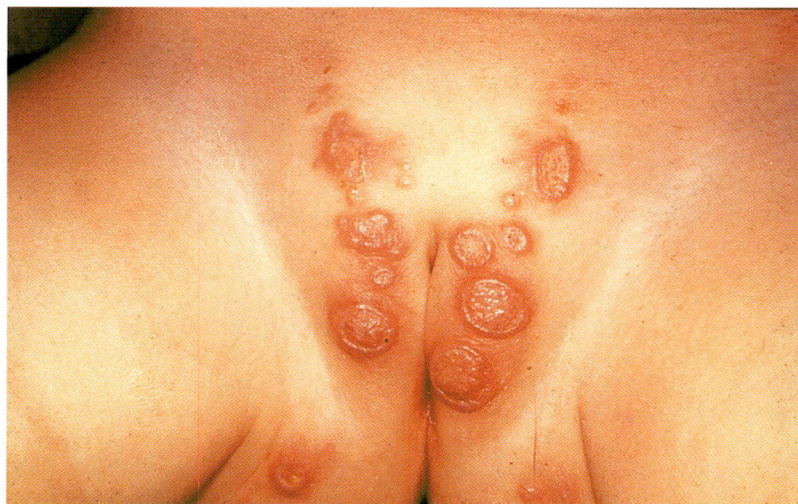

Fig. 14.24   An example of Jacquet's diaper dermatitis with eroded nodules on the labia.

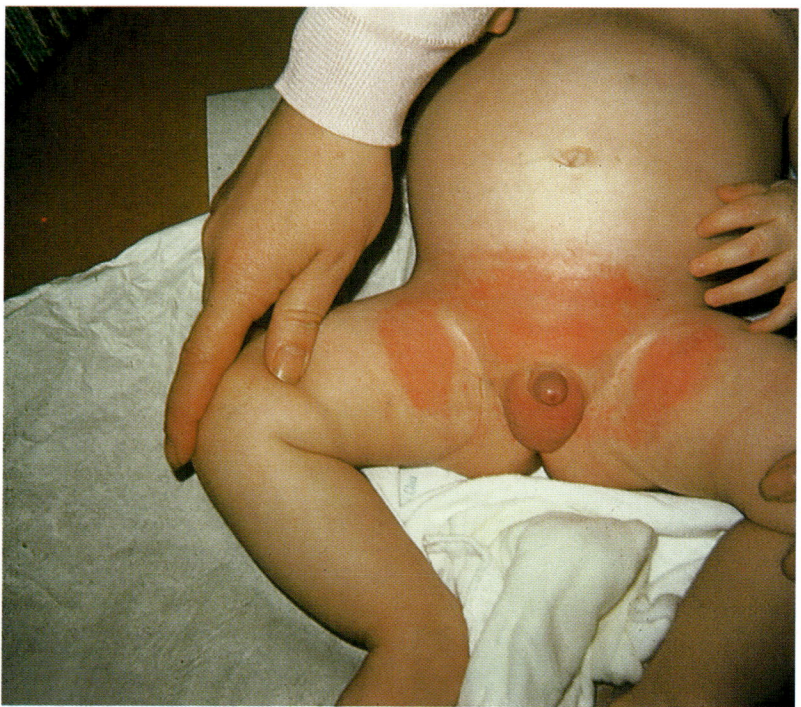

Fig. 14.23   Typical irritant contact dermatitis. The flexures are spared.

wearing pull-up diapers. Erythema on the buttocks may also be seen in infants with cystic fibrosis who are treated with the enzyme cotazyme.

Attempts should be made to prevent all the inciting factors. Diaper changes should be frequent and the often associated diarrhea treated promptly. The diaper area should be gently cleaned at each diaper change. This is best achieved by immersing the area in lukewarm water in a basin (similar to a Sitz bath). Harsh rubbing should be avoided. The area should be gently but completely dried. Treatment employs the use of emollients, particularly zinc oxide preparations and petrolatum. This prevents overhydration of the skin and provides protection from urine and feces. A nonfluorinated corticosteroid (hydrocortisone 1%), covered by the emollient, may be used three times a day if emollients are insufficient to produce improvement. The use of strong cor-

ticosteroid preparations is not recommended in the diaper area as the occlusive effect of the diaper may cause atrophy and striae, and scrotal absorption of corticosteroid is higher than in any other area of the body. Nevertheless, when the eruption is severe a five-day course of a medium-strength steroid often improves a recalcitrant eruption.

When diaper changing is not frequent enough and chemicals are not removed properly in home diapering, a specific eruption occurs on the labia or penis (Fig. 14.24) consisting of well-demarcated punched-out ulcers and erosions. This is known as Jacquet's erosive diaper dermatitis. This responds well to changing to a diaper service or disposable diapers. The fastest cure is to leave the child without any diapers but this is usually not practical. The ulcers heal quickly with a mild corticosteroid preparation, following compresses with Burow's 1/40 solution three times a day, and the use of thick emollients as a barrier. These ulcerations are not seen with the same frequency since the introduction of newer diapering methods. The only instance in which they often occur is in infants who have short bowel syndrome with constant diarrhea.

CANDIDIASIS

As the morphology of lesions in the diaper area has become better recognized, the varied clinical picture of candidiasis has emerged. Infants are particularly prone to candidal infection with 3% of infants affected from the second to the fourth month.[345] Thrush (oral candidiasis) is common in early infancy, presumably through infection from the maternal vaginal canal. Congenital candidiasis is self-limited except in low-weight and ill infants where the prognosis is not good. In this condition the eruption consists of small pustules that occur anywhere, including the palms and soles. The diaper area is not particularly involved.

Candidiasis in the diaper area seems to have become more common, possibly with the more frequent use of oral antibiotics with subsequent diarrhea in infants and children. The clinical picture of candidiasis takes two forms. It may present with a diffuse erythematous patch extending over the genitalia with a peripheral scale (Fig. 14.25) and satellite red pustules; the second presentation is with small pink papules surmounted by a scale, and coalescence in some areas. The anterior perineal and perianal area are either both or separately involved as are the creases, which helps differentiate this from IDD. The more classical picture of a beefy red diaper area with satellite pustules is rarely seen, possibly because of earlier treatment with antifungal and anti-inflammatory agents.

345. Bound JP (1956) Thrush napkin rashes. *Br Med J* 1:782.

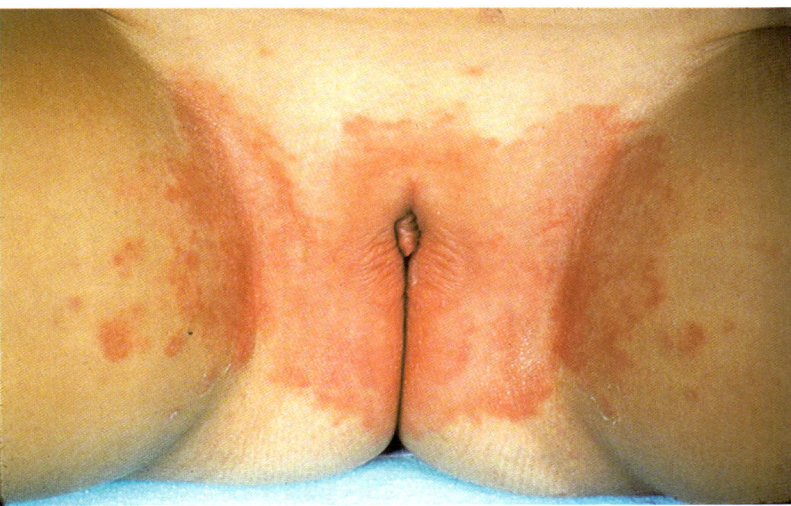

Fig. 14.25   Candidiasis of the diaper area, showing involvement of the creases and a central, red plaque with surrounding satellite papules.

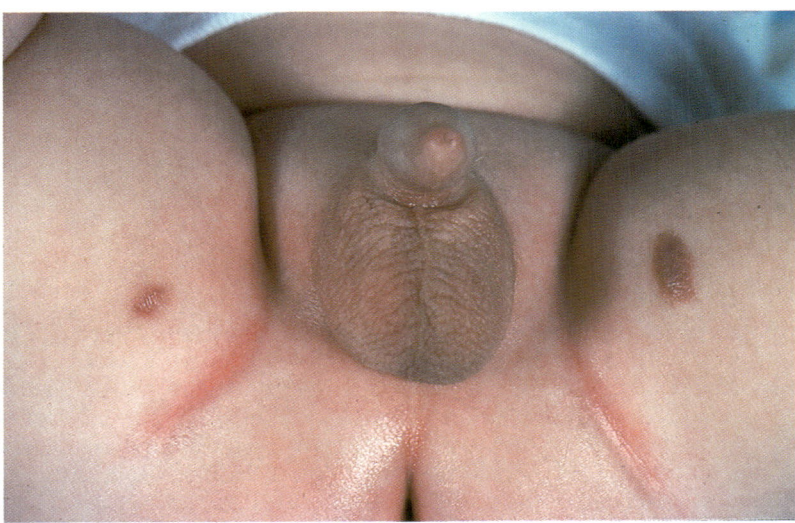

Fig. 14.26   An example of granuloma gluteale infantum.

The significance of recovering *Candida albicans* from the diaper area is at times difficult to interpret as the organism may be recovered in any irritant skin condition in this area after 72 hours,[346] and may even be grown in small amounts from normal skin. The organism appears to have the ability to invade through the epidermal barrier, by liberating keratinases. It is recovered in much larger numbers from the skin and feces when clinical candidiasis occurs.[347,348]

Treatment with topical anticandidal therapy such as nystatin, or one of the imidazoles (e.g., clotrimazole or ketoconazole) two or three times daily produces resolution in under two weeks. Adding hydrocortisone 1% to the above agents may provide an anti-inflammatory effect and promote more rapid healing. Burows or normal saline compresses may also be useful in inflammatory lesions. Potent corticosteroids should be avoided. In a double-blind study, the oral use of nystatin (to eliminate *Candida* from the bowel) in conjunction with topical nystatin did not affect the outcome of the dermatitis more favorably than topical nystatin alone.[349]

CANDIDAL DIAPER DERMATITIS WITH PSORIASIFORM ID

This condition was described in the 1980s and resembles infantile psoriasis.[350] Candidal dermatitis with psoriasiform Id represents a candidal infection in the diaper area[351] followed by an explosive papulosquamous eruption resembling psoriasis on the cheeks and body. The perineal area is often treated with corticosteroids, instead of antifungal preparations. An Id reaction is a generalized and symmetric response to a severe local inflammation.

The condition affects infants between 6 and 24 months. The lesions start in the diaper area as scaly, erythematous patches. Days to weeks later, the trunk and cheeks develop the Id reaction, which consists of well-demarcated psoriasiform plaques.

Lesions on the face are treated with a low-potency corticosteroid cream, those on the body with a mid-potency corticosteroid cream, and those in the diaper area with an antifungal agent, usually a topical imidazole. Cure occurs within two to four weeks and there is no recurrence.

Only certain infants with *Candida* develop this eruption and the question of whether the affected infants have a psoriatic diathesis is not resolved. The eruption is not seen with the same frequency as previously, possibly due to better treatment of candidal diaper dermatitis.

GRANULOMA GLUTEALE INFANTUM

This disorder was first described by Tappeiner and Pfleger in 1971.[352] The condition starts with inflammation in the diaper area that is treated with potent corticosteroids. Subsequently, a variable number of reddish-brown nodules (Fig. 14.26) develop on the inner thighs and perineal area. The buttocks are less often affected.

The histology of the lesions consists of a massive infiltrate of neutrophils, histiocytes, lymphocytes, and eosinophils in the dermis with minimal epidermal changes.

The pathogenesis of this disorder is not well understood. Occlusion from diapers is an important component as is the use of potent topical steroids. Another theory suggests a reaction of the body to the presence of *Candida* treated with strong topical steroids.

The differential diagnosis includes scabetic nodules, urticaria pigmentosa, and xanthogranulomas. It is also important to differentiate this benign process from that of a lymphomatous or histiocytic infiltrate.

Treatment is not necessary, as the condition disappears spontaneously over a period of a few months. Using mild topical or intralesional corticosteroids has not changed the rate of improvement in this condition. Granuloma gluteale infantum has not been seen with the same frequency as in the past.

LANGERHANS CELL HISTIOCYTOSIS (LETTERER–SIWE DISEASE)

Langerhans cell histiocytosis (Letterer–Siwe disease) (see also Chapter 24) is a potentially fatal histiocytic disorder that tends to affect young infants and children under the age of 2 years. The lesions occur anywhere on the body,

346. Beare JM, Cheeseman EA, Mackenzie DWR (1968) The association between Candida albicans and lesions of seborrhoeic eczema. **Br J Dermatol** 80:675–681.
347. Leyden JJ (1978) The role of microorganisms in diaper dermatitis. **Arch Dermatol** 114:56–59.
348. Rebora A, Leyden JJ (1981) Napkin (diaper) dermatitis and gastrointestinal carriage of Candida albicans. **Br J Dermatol** 105:551–555.
349. Munz D, Powell KR, Pai CH (1982) Treatment of candidal diaper dermatitis: a double-blind placebo-controlled comparison of topical nystatin with topical plus oral nystatin. **J Pediatr** 101:1022–1025.

350. Neville EA, Finn OA (1975) Psoriasiform napkin dermatitis: a follow-up study. **Br J Dermatol** 92:279–285.
351. Fergusson AG, Fraser NG, Grant PW (1966) Napkin dermatitis with psoriasiform ide. A review of fifty-two cases. **Br J Dermatol** 78:289–296.
352. Tappeiner J, Pfleger L (1971) Granuloma gluteale infantum. **Hautarzt** 22:383–388.

but tend to be more common in the scalp, retro-auricular, and diaper areas. Individual lesions are erythematous macules and papules, with hemorrhagic crusting being common. Ulceration in the diaper or buttock area may develop as well as on the gingivae and oral mucosa. It is important to differentiate from seborrheic dermatitis and any form of diaper dermatitis. Other features of the disease include anemia, diarrhea, hepatosplenomegaly, lymphadenopathy, and bony involvement. Treatment of systemic disease consists of chemotherapy.

BULLOUS IMPETIGO

Bullous impetigo may occur anywhere, but often affects the diaper area in infants. It usually starts on the second or third day of life. The lesions are caused by *S. aureus* group II and consist of bullae that rapidly rupture, leaving a superficial denuded erythematous base, with a peripheral collarette of scale. Treatment with cloxacillin 50–100mg/kg daily results in rapid resolution within one week. Topical antibiotics, such as fusidic acid or mupirocin, may be a useful adjunct to systemic therapy.

EROSIVE PERIANAL ERUPTION

This condition occurs between 6 weeks and 3 months of age. It consists of small ulcerations around the anal area. The etiology is unknown but is believed to be due to frequent stooling either in breast-fed babies or from short gut syndrome. Frequent diaper changes, thick emollients and the use of a low- or medium-strength topical steroid 3 times per day helps with the ulcers, but the condition may be chronic and meticulous diaper care is needed (Fig. 14.27).

SEBORRHEIC DERMATITIS

First described by Unna in 1887,[353] *seborrhea* means flow of sebum; the name is a misnomer as there is no evidence showing increased sebum production associated with this eruption in children.

Seborrheic dermatitis is a disease of unknown etiology that affects infants from about 3 weeks of age onward with a distinct clinical picture. Many physicians use the term to describe "cradle cap" (retention hyperkeratosis) on the vertex, whereas others imply inflammation with eythema and scaling on the scalp and intertriginous areas. Although the age of occurrence may suggest a role for maternal hormones, there is no evidence that this is the case.[354] The term is also used to describe similar findings in adults. There is no indication

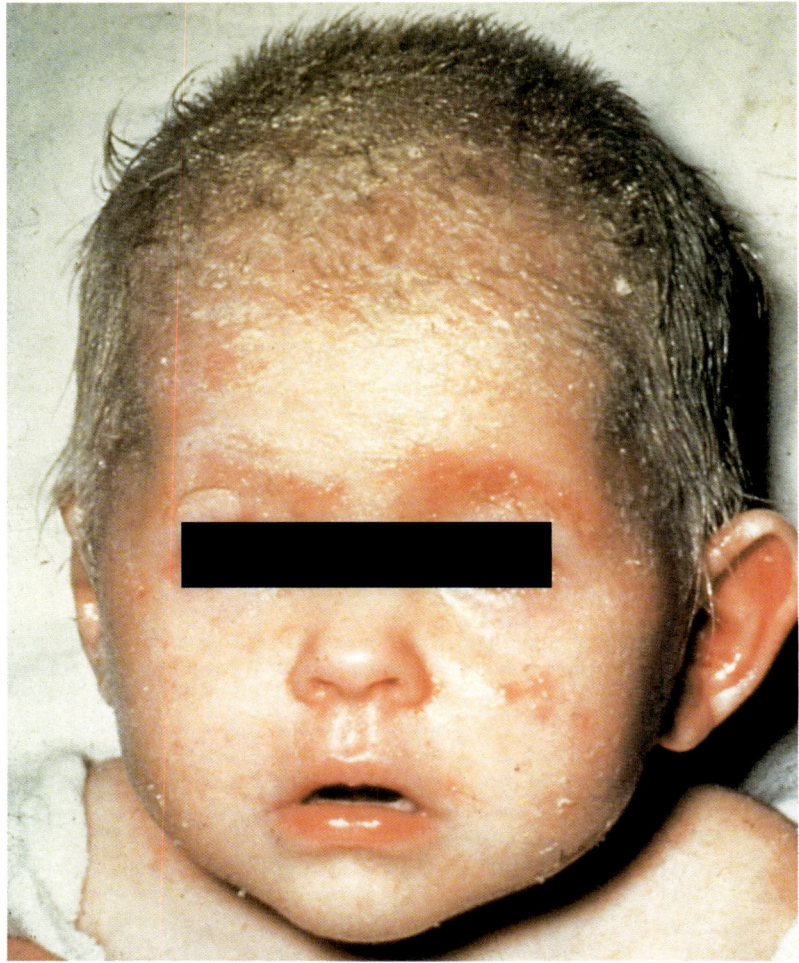

Fig. 14.28 Typical greasy scale of seborrheic dermatitis in the scalp and eyebrows.

that infants with seborrheic dermatitis are more likely to suffer from the adult form of the disease. There is an impression that seborrheic dermatitis is not seen as frequently as in previous years.

The eruption in children begins in infancy, between the ages of 3 and 12 weeks, and is uncommon after 6 months of age. Infants with the disease are usually asymptomatic and it is the parents who are dismayed by the cosmetic appearance. Nevertheless, in a study by Yates, 33% were itchy.[355] On the scalp, which is generally the first area of involvement, the lesions are diffuse greasy yellow or white scales, known as "cradle cap" (Fig. 14.28). Hair loss is not seen and erythema is variable. Lesions may involve the face, particularly the hairline and eyebrow area, where the scale is yellow and greasy overlying erythema. The intertriginous areas are involved in more severe cases, with scaling and linear erythema. In the diaper area well-demarcated erythematous plaques are topped by a thin white scale. The lesions often remain confined to the scalp and diaper areas and then spread to involve other flexural creases, the axillae (Fig. 14.29), retro-auricular area, and neck (Fig. 14.30). These may become macerated, crusted, and superinfected with *Candida albicans*.

The lesions respond quickly to treatment with bathing in soothing oatmeal baths, once or twice a day, and shampooing with a tar shampoo daily, followed by hydrocortisone 1% cream two or three times a day to the affected areas. Shampoos containing salicylic acid should be avoided as they may be irritating and absorption may cause problems with salicylism. Remission is accomplished within 10 days to two weeks, and recurrences are unusual.

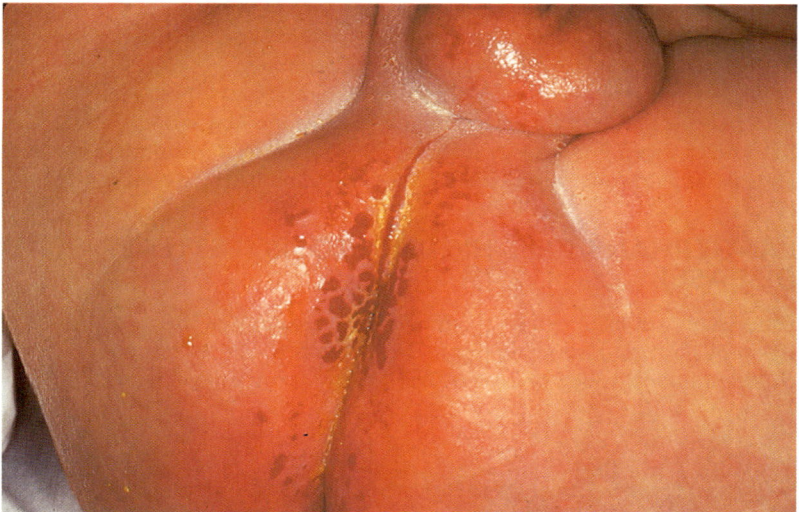

Fig. 14.27 Erosive diaper dermatitis, usually secondary to frequent stooling.

353. Unna PG (1887) Seborrhoeae eczema. **J Cutan Dis** 5:499.
354. Keipert JA (1976) Oral use of biotin in seborrhoeic dermatitis of infancy: a controlled trial. **Med J Aust** 1:584–585.
355. Yates VM, Kerr EI, Frier K et al. (1983) Early diagnosis of infantile seborrhoeic dermatitis and atopic dermatitis total and specific IgE levels. **Br J Dermatol** 108:639–645.

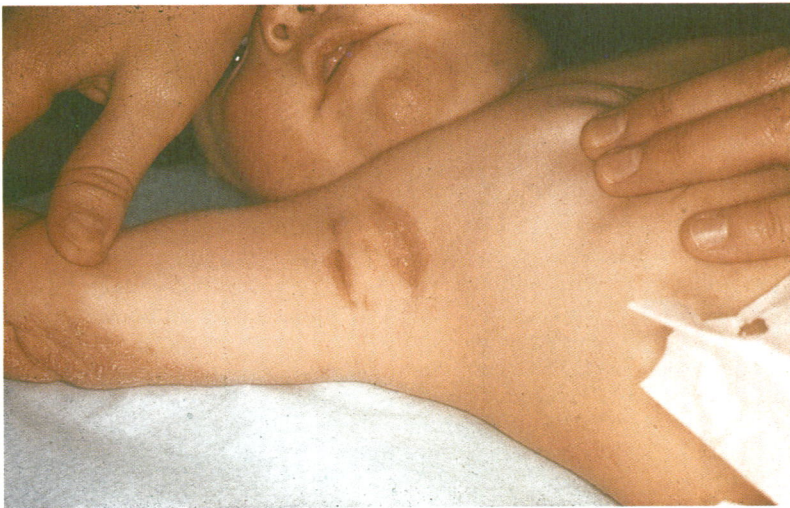

Fig. 14.29 The appearance of typical red axillary plaques in a case of seborrheic dermatitis.

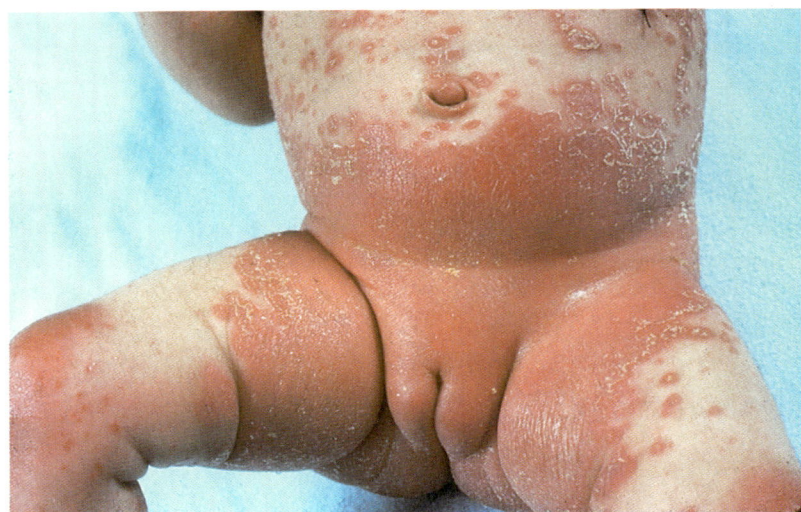

Fig. 14.31 Diaper involvement in psoriasis in an infant.

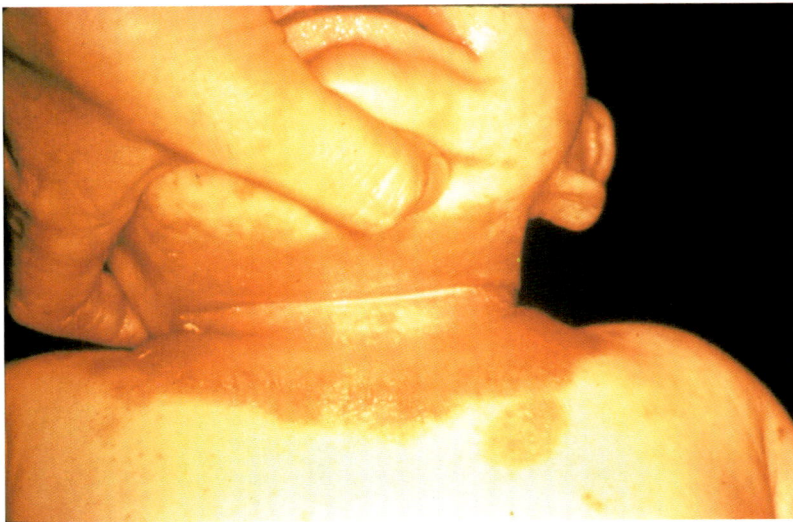

Fig. 14.30 Seborrheic dermatitis of the neck.

The prognosis in seborrheic dermatitis is better than AD, making it important to differentiate between these conditions. In most instances this is quite easy, based on morphology, and the presence or absence of pruritus. However, a study has shown[142] that the two entities may occasionally be difficult to differentiate from one another, with lesions of AD occurring early and those with seborrheic dermatitis manifesting pruritus in one-third of cases.[353] Seborrheic dermatitis is the more likely diagnosis when the axillae are affected and AD when the shins and forearms are involved. In another study, AD patients manifested positive RAST reactions in 80% of patients, whereas in seborrheic dermatitis only 15% were positive.[355]

The pathogenesis of the disease is unknown. Theories of excessive sebaceous gland activity from maternal hormones and nutritional factors, such as biotin deficiency,[354] have not been validated. Recent work has shown that the organism *pityrosporum ovale* (*Malassezia furfur*) is implicated in the etiology

of adult seborrheic dermatitis,[356] but its role in the infantile form of the disease is yet to be proved. Two studies have shown an increased incidence of *P. ovale* in the lesions of infants with seborrheic dermatitis. Broberg[357] isolated the organism in 18 of 20 patients with seborrheic dermatitis and only in four of 20 controls. Ruiz-Maldonado et al.[358] detected *P. ovale* in 73% of patients with infantile seborrheic dermatitis, 33% in AD and other dermatoses, and 53% in normal controls. Treatment of the seborrheic dermatitis group with ketoconazole 2% resulted in clinical cure in 11 of 15 infants in two weeks and mycologic cure in 13 of the 15 infants. *P. ovale* is thought to flourish in areas of increased sebaceous activity, possibly accounting for the prevalence of infantile seborrheic dermatitis in the first 6 months of life. Another study[359] has implicated an abnormality of essential fatty acids in the etiology of infantile seborrheic dermatitis. This work has yet to be corroborated.

Histology of the lesions is not diagnostic and consists of a subacute dermatitis with elongation of the rete ridges.

When considering the differential diagnosis of seborrheic dermatitis, all scaling eruptions should be considered, particularly psoriasis. Napkin psoriasis (Fig. 14.31) and psoriasis in general are more common in infants than was previously recognized. If the disease is persistent, or if crusting and petechial lesions occur, it is important to rule out the possibility of disseminated Langerhans cell histiocytosis (Letterer–Siwe disease).

Follow-up studies of patients with infantile seborrheic dermatitis have produced a variety of findings owing to problems of diagnosis. Vickers, in his study of AD, has classified both AD and seborrheic dermatitis as one disease.[101] Podmore et al.,[360] in a follow-up study after 11 years, concluded that many of the cases of infantile seborrheic dermatitis eventually developed AD. This was also the conclusion of Ruiz-Maldonado et al.[358] These cases were probably AD at the onset. Other studies have shown an increased tendency to develop psoriasis. This is particularly true of napkin psoriasis that was thought to be a variant of seborrheic dermatitis.[350] Since the recognition that psoriasis is not rare in infancy and may occur in the diaper area, the previous diagnosis of seborrheic dermatitis was probably incorrect. Seborrheic dermatitis may well be a reaction pattern in the skin of infants to a variety of different diseases and the term seborrheic dermatitis will eventually be reserved for the lesions that are colonized with *P. ovale*, which respond to anti-yeast therapy.

356. McGinley KJ, Leyden MD, Marples RR et al. (1975) Quantitative microbiology of the scalp in non-dandruff, dandruff, and seborrheic dermatitis. **J Invest Dermatol** 64:401–405.
357. Broberg A, Faergemann J (1988) Infantile seborrheic dermatitis and Pityrosporum ovale. Presented at the 3rd International Symposium on Pediatric Dermatology, Mazara del Vallo, Sicily, September 14–17.
358. Ruiz-Maldonado R, Lopez-Matinez R, Perez Chavariea EL et al. (1989) Pityrosporum ovale in infantile seborrheic dermatitis. **Pediatr Dermatol** 6:16–20.
359. Tollesson A, Frithz A, Berg A, Karlman G (1993) Essential fatty acids in infantile seborrheic dermatitis. **J Am Acad Dermatol** 28:957–961.
360. Podmore O, Burrows D, Eedy DJ et al. (1986) Seborrheic eczema—a disease entity or a clinical variant of atopic eczema? **Br J Dermatol** 115:341–350.

THE RED SCALY BABY

The red scaly baby (which used to be called Leiner's disease) is a rare disorder consisting of lesions similar to those of seborrheic dermatitis but in addition has the associated features of an immunodeficiency with severe exfoliation, failure to thrive, and diarrhea. These patients are susceptible to yeast and Gram-negative bacterial infection. The entity was first described as being due to a quantitative and occasionally a functional C5 deficiency, and has also been described with a C3 dysfunction and other immuno-deficiencies. It is a reaction pattern in the skin to an immune dysfunction. A few patients have benefited from treatment with fresh frozen plasma, or bone marrow transplantation when a specific immune deficiency disorder is identified.

CONTACT DERMATITIS

Contact dermatitis is caused by irritation or an allergic reaction. Whereas the former occurs in all those who are exposed to the irritating substance, depending on the irritancy of the substance and the susceptibility of the person, the latter entity only occurs in a small number of exposed and sensitized individuals.

Irritant contact dermatitis

Irritant contact dermatitis is an inflammatory reaction in the skin resulting from the application of an irritating substance. The reaction depends on the strength of the offending substance and the constitutional composition of the person. Children with AD are more susceptible, and everyone would react to the application of a strong acid. In addition, the barrier function of the patient and percutaneous absorption of the applied agents are very important, and is largely dependent on the structure and thickness of the stratum corneum and on its lipid and water content. Irritant contact dermatitis is commonly seen in the diaper area in infants (IDD), as a result of multiple factors including occlusion, maceration, and friction, all of which influence the function of the stratum corneum. Irritant contact dermatitis is not common in normal infants and children, but is seen with increased frequency in AD.[361]

Allergic contact dermatitis

Allergic contact dermatitis (ACD) is not diagnosed frequently in children under 10 years of age. Even poison ivy dermatitis, a common allergen in North America, is seldom seen in infancy, mainly because of lack of exposure. Nevertheless, children (including infants) mount a normal immunological response and patch test reactions may be positive in 20% of those tested.[362] The risk of developing ACD depends on individual susceptibility, on the sensitizing properties of the substance when applied to the skin, and the amount and concentration per square unit of skin.[363] A substance such as dini-trochlorobenzene (DNCB) induces an allergic response in nearly everyone exposed, and poison ivy dermatitis in approximately 70% of exposed indivi-duals. Most allergies tend to persist, but those not commonly encountered in the environment, such as neomycin, may disappear. In infants the only ACD seen with any frequency is nickel dermatitis; the agents that children react to most commonly include poison ivy, nickel, and rubber, present in shoes. Cosmetics in teenage girls, formaldehyde used to size clothing, flowers, and pollens may all cause allergic reactions, although these are rare in children. Adhesive tape reactions may occur at any age, particularly in hospitalized patients. The lesions usually occur as an acute pruritic dermatitis in the areas of exposure. Id reactions are common.

PHYSICAL EXAMINATION

Poison ivy dermatitis

The most common ACD in children in North America is caused by a plant of the Rhus or Toxicodendron family (poison ivy, oak, or sumac). These family members cross-react. Because the Rhus group belongs to the larger Anacardiaceae family, further cross-reactions may occur with chemicals and nuts from related plants (i.e., skin of the mango or oil from cashew nuts). The actual sensitizing substance is an oleoresin termed urushiol.

The typical lesions occur in the spring, summer, and autumn. The patient may not be aware that exposure has taken place. Sensitization takes five to 25 days and may be followed by the development of an acute pruritic dermatitis. Once sensitized, re-exposure will always result in an eruption within 24 to 48 hours. The lesions do not contain oleoresin and cannot cause an ACD. The initial lesions are usually erythematous vesicular streaks mainly on the lower legs but any area may be involved. A few hours to days later other erythematous patches, papules, and bullae develop (Fig. 14.32). The extent of the eruption is variable. The allergen may be washed off within 20 minutes without causing an eruption, but oleoresin may remain in clothing for months to years, causing a typical dermatitis if contacted by a sensitized individual. It is important for patients to recognize the three-leafed, spiked, green plant with a red stem. The plant develops white berries and the leaves become red, yellow and orange in the autumn. In the western USA poison oak, with smaller leaves, gives a similar reaction.

Two other presentations of poison ivy are well recognized. At the end of the summer when hay is being burnt, it is not uncommon for poison ivy to be mixed with the ash and cause an aeroallergen reaction on the face and neck of those exposed. The eruption is bright erythema over the whole face, often with so much swelling that the eyelids are completely closed. This is often misdiagnosed as a cellulitis and it is not uncommon for these children to be admitted for intravenous antibiotic treatment. The treatment of choice is systemic corticosteroids 1mg/kg per day, reducing the dose over three weeks to avoid a rebound.

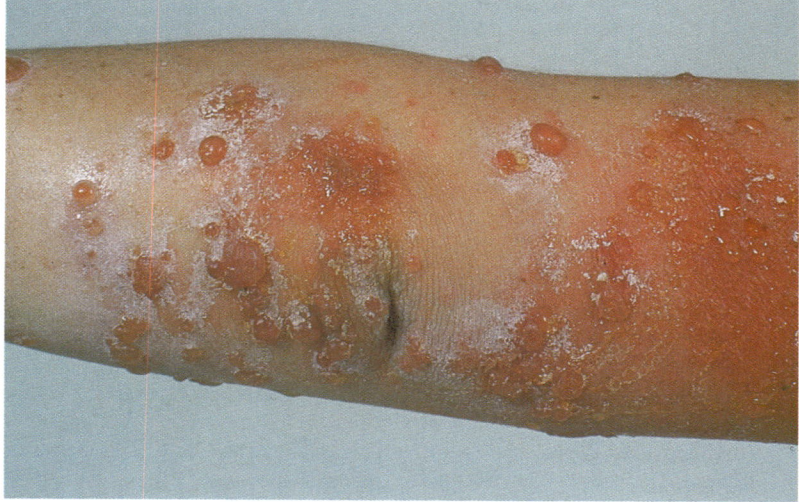

Fig. 14.32 Vesicular eruption seen in poison ivy dermatitis.

361. Manzini BM, Ferdani G, Simonetti V et al. (1998) Contact sensitization in children. **Pediatr Dermatol** 15(1):12–17.
362. Bruckner AL, Weston WL (2001) Beyond poison ivy: understanding allergic contact dermatitis in children. **Pediatr Ann** 30(4):203–206.
363. Mozzanica N (1992) Pathogenetic aspects of allergic and irritant contact dermatitis. **Clin Dermatol** 10:115–121.

Another presentation of poison ivy dermatitis is with black spots. Initially asymptomatic, they subsequently become pruritic. Lesions present as linear black shiny streaks or as black lacquer spots on the skin, sometimes amongst other more typical patches of poison ivy dermatitis. Similar black spots may be found on the clothing. The lesions subsequently erode before healing. A marked concentration of the oleoresin is necessary for this pattern to be seen; that is probably the reason why it is not seen more frequently in typical poison ivy dermatitis reactions.[364]

Nickel allergy

Nickel allergy is the most common allergen seen in infants,[365,366] but it is also particularly common amongst teenagers who wear earrings and necklaces. Earrings have a nickel backing, which results in the typical clinical presentation of bilateral dermatitis (erythema, scaling, vesicles, and crusts) on the back and less often on the front of the earlobes, where the ear has been pierced. Nickel is also widely used in bracelets, necklaces, watches, and rings as a hardening agent for gold. The ACD is seen when larger quantities of nickel are used, such as 9-karat gold jewellery, and seldom seen in 18 and 22 karat gold. Eczematous lesions appear in areas that are exposed.

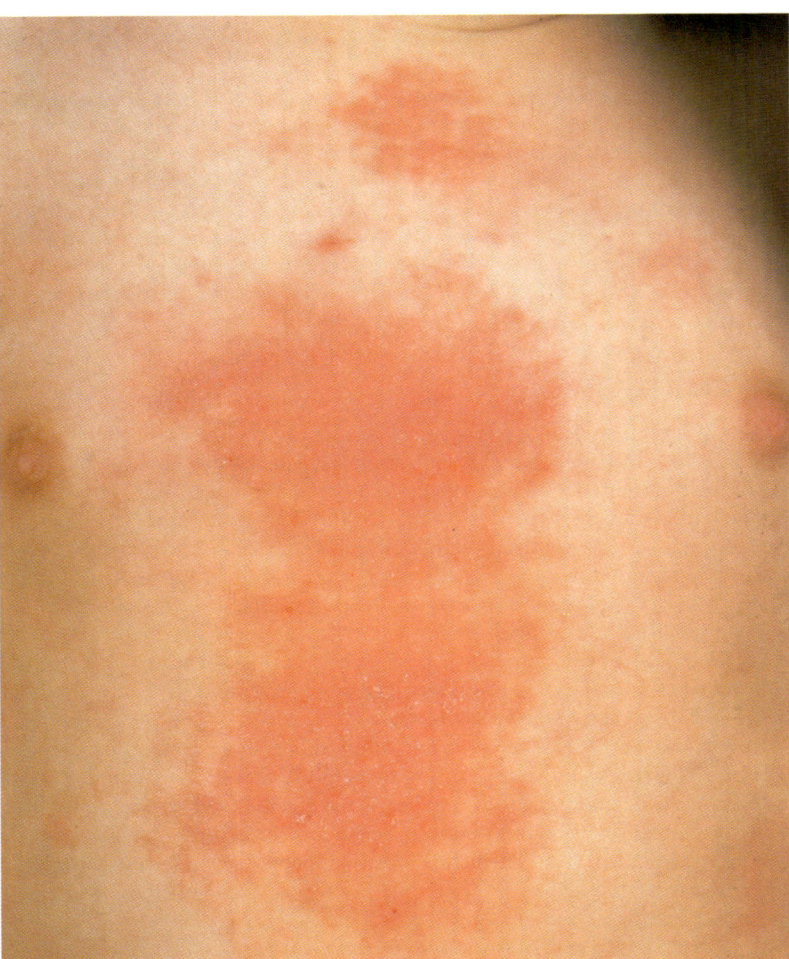

Fig. 14.33 Nickel dermatitis – typical midline involvement on the chest of an infant due to metal snaps on sleeping garments or shirts.

In children, the area immediately below the umbilicus where a nickel snap on blue jeans comes in contact with the skin is commonly involved with a nickel dermatitis. The areas of inflammation may become chronic and the area develops shiny lichenoid papules from constant rubbing. Similarly in infants, the snaps of undershirts (Fig. 14.33) have a large percentage of nickel, resulting in a pruritic eczematous dermatitis that runs along the central chest and onto the abdomen. This is the most common form of ACD seen in infancy and one that is important to differentiate from AD. It may be increasing in frequency. School children, especially girls who wear skirts, may develop nickel contact dermatitis on the backs of the thighs from sitting on metal bolts in school chairs. It is not uncommon in nickel allergic patients to have secondary areas of inflammation away from the areas of contact.

Shoe dermatitis

An acute or subacute dermatitis along the dorsa of the toes with spreading onto the foot is typical of a shoe reaction. The webs of the toes are not involved. The ball and heel are also involved when rubber is the causative agent, although this is a much thicker area and more resistant to sensitization. The most common cause of shoe dermatitis is rubber, but tanning agents including chromates, adhesives, and dyes also cause a shoe ACD. Special trays are available to patch test for shoe sensitivity.

Shoe dermatitis is commonly misdiagnosed as a tinea infection. Tinea normally involves the toe webs whereas ACD involves the surfaces in contact with the shoe. Both conditions are rare in children prior to puberty. More common than shoe dermatitis or tinea pedis is juvenile plantar dermatosis.

Cosmetics

The most common cosmetics causing ACD are deodorants, nail lacquers, lipsticks, and eye make-up. The latter results from the use of mascara, eye shadow, eye liner, and nail hardeners. The eruption usually presents as an acute or subacute dermatitis that varies according to the agent used. Nail lacquers and hardeners often cause an unusual dermatitic reaction around the eyes, favoring one eye over the other. Lipstick allergy causes a rim of erythema around the lips extending beyond the vermilion border. Parabens are frequently added to cosmetics in low concentration to inhibit bacterial growth and may cause ACD. Cosmetics that are advertised as being hypoallergenic do not contain parabens.

Adhesive tape dermatitis

Rubber and colophony are the ingredients that most often cause an allergy to adhesives. The reaction is obvious and occurs as a well-demarcated erythema where the adhesive is applied (Fig. 14.34). Special plastic tapes are available, which may be substituted in allergic individuals. Colophony is also found in the rosin used by violinists and in the powder used by gymnasts.

Corticosteroid allergy

It has recently become well recognized that topical corticosteroids can cause an ACD. This is more common than previously suspected.[367–369] There are four structural corticosteroid classes. Cross-reactions occur more frequently within the classes than between them,[368,369] although a range of corticosteroids should be tested to avoid cross-reaction amongst the various groups. The most common cause is from hydrocortisone sensitivity; tixocortol pivalate is the substance used for testing for an ACD. Parents complain that application of hydrocortisone causes the eruption to become much redder. It is unusual but not impossible to have allergic reactions to betamethasone, which is the least sensitizing of the four groups.

364. Kurlan JG, Lucky AW (2001) Black spot poison ivy: a report of 5 cases and a review of the literature. **J Am Acad Dermatol** 45(2):246–249.
365. Mortz CG, Lauritsen JM, Bindslev-Jensen C et al. (2001) Prevalence of atopic dermatitis, asthma, allergic rhinitis, and hand and contact dermatitis in adolescents. The Odense Adolescence Cohort Study of Atopic Diseases and Dermatitis. **Br J Dermatol** 144:523–532.
366. Smith-Sivertsen T, Dotterud LK, Lund E (1999) Nickel allergy and its relationship with local nickel pollution, ear piercing and atopic dermatitis: a population-based study from Norway. **J Am Acad Dermatol** 20:726–735.
367. Almond-Roesler B, Blume-Peytavi U, Orfanos CE (1995) Kontaktallergien auf kortikosteroide. **Hautarzt** 46:228–233.
368. Dooms-Goossens A (1995) Sensitisation to corticosteroids. **Drug Saf** 13:123–129.
369. Lepoittevin JP, Drieghe J, Dooms-Goossens A (1995) Studies in patients with corticosteroid contact allergy. **Arch Dermatol** 131:31–37.

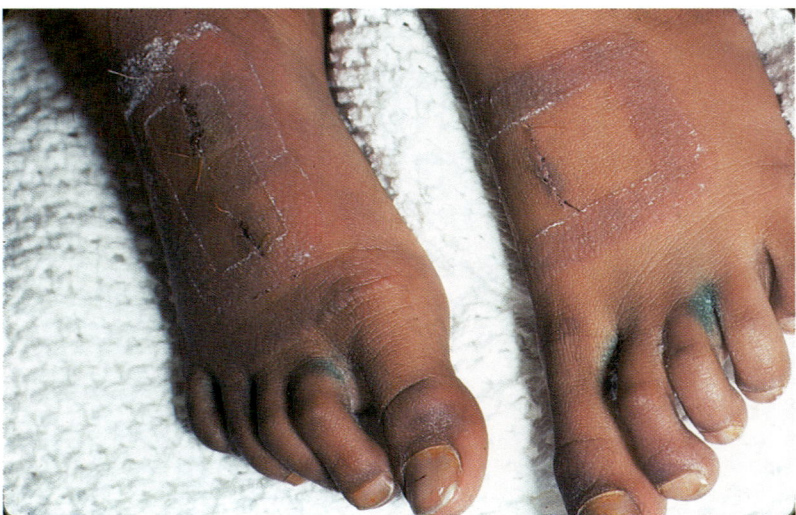

Fig. 14.34 Appearance of adhesive tape dermatitis.

PATHOLOGY

The pathology of ACD is that of an acute, subacute, or chronic dermatitis. Immunohistochemical stains show predominance of helper T cells with some suppressor T cells. Only a small number of the T cells in the infiltrate have specificity for the antigen. The role of the numerous mast cells in the area has not been determined.

PATHOGENESIS

ACD is primarily produced by way of the T-lymphocyte cell-mediated type IV immune response. There are two distinct phases in the development of ACD: the afferent or induction phase and the efferent or elicitation phase.[363] The afferent phase includes the events following first contact with an allergen and is completed when the subject is sensitized and able to produce an elicitation phase. The afferent phase may take five to 25 days whereas the elicitation reaction only requires 24 to 48 hours (see Fig. 14.35).

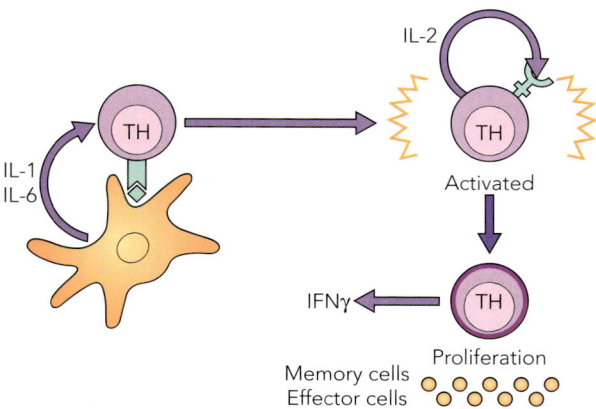

Fig. 14.35 Allergic contact dermatitis (courtesy of Joel DeKoven, MD).

Delayed-type reactions in the skin are produced by foreign materials capable of binding to surface molecules of the Langerhans cell to form new antigens. Most allergens are of low molecular weight and have to penetrate the epidermis where they behave as haptens (bind to skin proteins to form a complete antigen). The carrier protein appears to be a constituent of the Langerhans cell membrane. The bond between the hapten and the carrier protein converts self to nonself against which the immunologic response is directed. The helper T cell is only activated against foreign protein in this context. It is the function of the Langerhans cell to recognize the antigen and present it to the T lymphocytes during the sensitization phase. The Langerhans cells with the environmental haptens leave the epidermis via the lymph vessels and, on arrival in the paracortical areas of the lymph nodes, present antigen to the T cell. In the next phase, the Langerhans cells stimulate naive T cells to differentiate into clones of effector cells directed against foreign antigen. This process involves numerous cytokines and inflammatory cell receptors present on both the Langerhans cell and the T cell. Once this process has taken place and the T lymphocytes are fully activated (a committed, sensitized cell reactive to a specific allergen) they divide and differentiate into clones. These clones consist of both effector T cells of delayed-type hypersensitivity, which possess specific receptors for antigens, whenever they come into contact with them, and also, long-living memory cells that recall sensitivity many years after the initial bout of dermatitis.

Once the induction phase is completed, the elicitation phase begins with the effector cells circulating through the body and into the skin. Re-exposure to the antigen results in an accumulation of delayed-type hypersensitivity effector cells and immune response cells, both of which produce numerous inflammatory cytokines and mediators resulting in a clinical dermatitis limited to the area of contact. Cytokines of importance during the elicitation phase include IFN-γ, tumor necrosis factor-alpha, and granulocyte macrophage colony stimulating factor. The Langerhans cells are not important in the elicitation phase.

PATCH TESTING

When ACD is suspected it is important to identify the causative allergen. This may be clinically easy to identify, but often the cause is not obvious and patch testing is performed.[370] The suspected agent is applied to the skin and the contact site evaluated for a reaction 48 and 72 hours later. The reagents to test against, the method of testing, and the evaluation of tests have been standardized by the North American Contact Dermatitis Group (Table 14.10).[371] There is also a standardized tray in Europe. It is important to have specific trays available as many allergies are only prevalent in specific areas (Table 14.11). At times it is best to test against a battery of common allergens to help identify unknown causative factors. The history is very helpful in delineating suspicious agents.

In a study of ACD, the authors found the disease to be common in children.[372] They found patch testing to be positive in 20% of children with an unknown dermatitis. However, patch testing in children, particularly in those under the age of 8, is known to be inaccurate because the skin is more easily irritated, thus producing false-positive reactions. Patch tests should be interpreted with caution as there are numerous false-positive and false-negative reactions.[373]

A positive patch test presupposes prior sensitization. The percentage of relevant positive patch tests ranges from 25% to 35% in adults who are tested.

The patch test is applied via a closed method fixing the test substances onto the skin, usually the back, with hypoallergenic tape. Occlusion is essential for reliable results. The Finn Chamber has become increasingly popular as it uses more patches with small reaction sites. The patches remain in place for 48 hours, during which the area should be kept dry. The results are read a few

370. Nethercott JR, Cooley JE (1995) Getting the most out of patch testing. **Curr Opin Dermat** 2:10–17.
371. Adams RM (1981) Patch testing: a recapitulation. **J Am Acad Dermatol** 5:629–646.
372. Weston WL (1984) Allergic contact dermatitis in children. **Am J Dis Child** 138:932–936.
373. McAlvany P, Sherertz EF (1994) Contact dermatitis in infants, in children, and adolescents. **Adv Dermatol** 9:205.

TABLE 14.10   The North American standard series (box 81–1) (as presented by Nethercott);[370] the only patch test kit available in the US (Glaxo Wellcome True Test) is similar

1. Benzocaine 5%	13. Epoxy resin 1%
2. Mercaptobenzothiazole 1%	14. Quaternium-15 2%
3. Colophony 20%	15. p-Tert.butyl phenol formaldehyde resin 1%
4. p-Phenylenediamine 1%	16. Mercapto mix 1%
5. Imidazolidinyl Urea 2%	17. Black rubber mix 0.6%
6. Cinnamic aldehyde 1%	18. Potassium dichromate 0.25%
7. Lanolin alcohol 30%	19. Balsam of Peru 25%
8. Carba mix 3%	20. Nickel sulphate 2.5%
9. Neomycin sulfate 20%	21. Cobalt chloride 2%
10. Thiuram mix 1%	22. Fragrance mix 8%
11. Formaldehyde 1%	23. Toluene sulphonamide resin 2%
12. Ethylenediamnine dihydrochloride 1%	

TABLE 14.11   The European standard series

1. Potassium dichromate 0.5%	13. Mercapto mix 1%
2. Neomycin sulfate 20%	14. Epoxy resin 1%
3. Thiuram mix 1%	15. Paraben mix 15%
4. Paraphenylenediamine free base 1%	16. Paratertiarybutyl phenol formaldehyde resin (BPF resin) 1%
5. Cobalt chloride (CoCl₂, 6H₂O) 1%	17. Fragrance mix 8%
6. Benzocaine 5%	18. Quaternium 15 (cis −1-(3-chloroallyl) −3,5,7-triaza-1-azoniaadamanate chloride) 1%
7. Formaldehyde (in water) 1%	19. Nickel sulfate (NiSO₄, 6H₂O) 5%
8. Colophony 20%	20. 5-Chloro-2-methyl-4-isothiazolin 3 – one +2 mthyl-4-isothiazolin 3-one (3:1in water) 0.01%
9. Clioquinoline mix 5%	21. Mercaptobenzothiazole (MBT) 2%
10. Balsam of Peru 25%	22. Sesquiterpene lactone mix 0.1%
11. N-Isopropyl-N-phenyl Paraphenylenediamine 0.1%	23. Primin 0.01%
12. Wool alcohol 5 30%	

hours after the removal of the patches at 48 hours after application and again at 72 hours, when more tests may become positive.

Interpretation of the patch testing is as follows:

0	negative reaction
?	doubtful reaction; faint erythema
+	weak positive reaction; erythema, infiltration, and possibly papules
++	strong (vesicular) positive reaction; erythema, infiltration, papules, and vesicles
+++	extreme positive reaction; bullous reaction

The classical positive patch test consists of erythema, edema, and small closely set vesicles, which extend beyond the border of the patch. Extreme reactions with pustules and bullae rarely occur and almost always represent a severe irritant reaction.

Standard patch test kits are available, as are some additional extra kits for testing special substances, including vehicles commonly used in skin products and those associated with shoe and hair products.

MANAGEMENT

Once the diagnosis of ACD has been made and the causative agent elicited, elimination of the offending substance results in a cure within 2–3 weeks, but during this time patients may be severely incapacitated by the dermatitis, and symptomatic treatment should be initiated as soon as the diagnosis is made.

In an acute generalized dermatitis, oatmeal baths are soothing for the skin but systemic corticosteroid therapy is the treatment of choice; it is given by mouth as prednisone 1mg/kg per day to a maximum dose of 60mg with a gradual reduction over a period of two to three weeks. The prednisone should be cut by 25% every fourth day, but it is important to maintain treatment for a long enough period that a rebound flare does not occur.

In more localized inflammation, topical corticosteroids and antihistamines are moderately helpful and should be used to treat lesions until the inflammation has subsided. The addition of compresses with 1/20 to 1/40 Burow's solution 3–4 times daily is soothing and drying.

PHOTODERMATITIS

Photodermatitis involves a contact dermatitis with sun exposure triggering the reaction. This may be phototoxic (sun plus an irritating agent) or photoallergic (sun plus an ACD). A phototoxic reaction occurs in all individuals who are exposed to the agent and the sun, whereas photoallergic reactions develop only in a small number of those exposed and sensitized to the combination of sun and antigen.

Phytophotodermatitis usually results from handling plants that contain psoralens. Children react particularly to the juice of lime and lemon skin while being sun exposed. Other plants that may cause this are in the celery and parsley family. This reaction is thought to be phototoxic rather than photoallergic. The lesions present as erythema, vesicles, and later streaked hyperpigmentation on the affected areas (Fig. 14.36). Hyperpigmentation is often the predominant feature, with little or no inflammation visible. The most common areas of involvement are the face, chest, hands, and lower legs. In some cases, linear streaks on the child's body may suggest child abuse.[374]

A specific photoreaction known as Berloque dermatitis, takes place from contact with 5-methoxypsoralen contained in oil of bergamot. The substance,

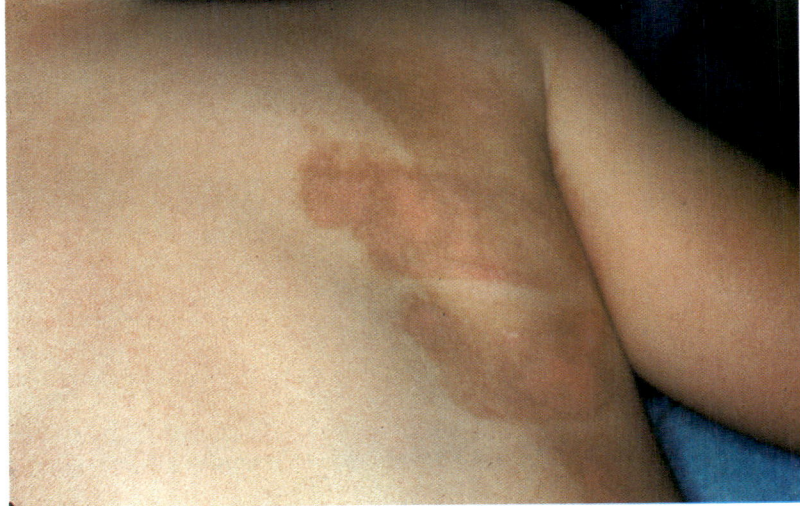

Fig. 14.36 Phytophotodermatitis from lime juice showing hyperpigmented hand marks. This could be mistaken for child abuse.

374. Barradell R, Addo A, McDonagh AJ et al. (1993) Phytophotodermatitis mimicking child abuse. *Eur J Pediatr* 152:291–292.

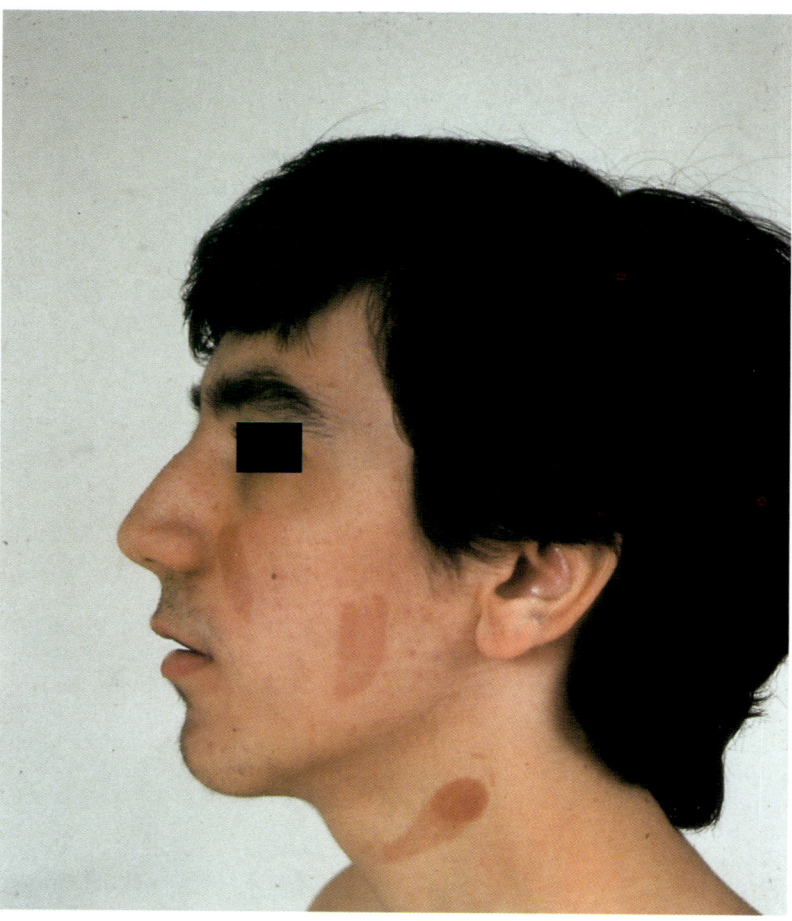

Fig. 14.37   Streaked hyperpigmentation seen in Berloque dermatitis from application of cologne or aftershave.

which is extracted from the peel of ornamental oranges, is used in several perfumes and colognes. The eruption occurs after using the perfume and being exposed to the sun. The clinical picture emerges as streaked hyperpigmentation (Fig. 14.37), commonly seen on the sides of the neck and wrists.

AUTOSENSITIZATION DERMATITIS

The process of autosensitization, which is also known as the Id reaction or the conditioned hyperirritability syndrome, is the rapid spread of an eczematous, papular, or vesicular reaction on the skin surface. The eruption is usually pruritic, symmetric, and widespread over the extremities and trunk. This eczematous response is the result of a severe localized inflammation to an allergic or irritant contact dermatitis, a bacterial or fungal infection, or an inflammatory response as commonly seen in a stasis dermatitis in adults. The most common Id reaction in children is seen following a kerion on the scalp; in this case it affects the upper part of the body and face and consists of symmetrical, small, erythematous papules.

Theories regarding the pathogenesis of autosensitization reactions include antibodies or lymphocytes that are sensitized or committed to react against altered tissue constituents, or that the primary site may release factors that

reduce the skin's threshold to irritation, by diffusing through the epidermis or by being released into the circulation.[375]

Treatment with soothing baths or topical compresses is helpful and the lesions usually disappear when the primary disorder has been adequately treated.

PERIORAL DERMATITIS

This entity was first seen in the 1960s. It is a disease that commonly occurs in young women but is seen with some frequency in children and is more common than previously thought.[376] Many of the patients have used potent corticosteroid preparations to treat an initial eruption, although the eruption may arise *de novo*.

Marks and Black[377] have defined perioral dermatitis as a persistent erythematous eruption composed of tiny papules and papulopustules distributed around the mouth. A small area, close to the vermilion border is usually spared. The eyelids, particularly the lower lids, may develop tiny, erythematous papules (Figs 14.38, 14.39). This may be uni- or bilateral and may accompany the mouth lesions or only affect the eyelid area. The cheeks are spared. The eruption has been described on the vulva, in addition to the mouth and eye.[378] Perioral dermatitis may occur as a granulomatous dermatitis (Fig. 14.40) and on biopsy the histology must be distinguished from sarcoid.[379,380] Histology shows a chronic inflammation with an occasional granulomatous reaction.

Patients seek consultation for the chronic, intermittent eruption that fades when topical steriods are used, flaring one to two days after cessation of their use.[381] This entity may represent a childhood variant of rosacea, but the lesions are usually papules rather than pustules and the vascular component is absent.

In a 12-year follow-up of perioral dermatitis, many of the initially proposed theories of causation, such as the use of fluoride toothpastes and candidal infection, were not substantiated,[382] and potent corticosteroid use was the one exacerbating feature in most cases.

Treatment with tetracycline is effective with tapering dosage over a period of two to three months. Patients should be warned that a marked rebound occurs when the topical steroids are withdrawn and an emollient may be of some benefit as the perioral area usually becomes extremely dry and irritated.

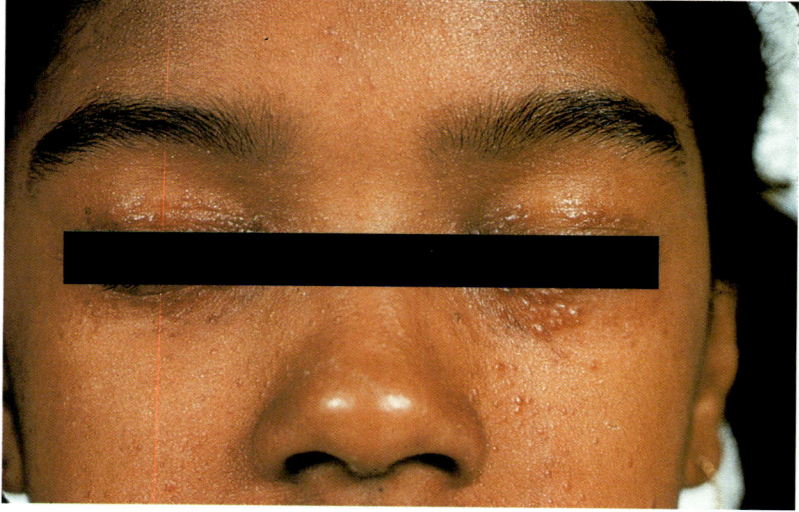

Fig. 14.38   The periorbital component of perioral dermatitis with upper and lower eyelid involvement.

375. Arlette JP, Fritzler MJ (1984) Reduced skin threshold to irritation in the presence of allergic contact dermatitis in the guinea pig. **Contact Dermatitis** 11:31–33.
376. Manders SM, Lucky AW (1992) Perioral dermatitis in childhood. **J Am Acad Dermatol** 27(5 pt 1):688–692.
377. Marks R, Black MM (1971) Perioral dermatitis. A histopathological study of 26 cases. **Br J Dermatol** 84:242–247.
378. Beets-Shay LM (1993) Perioral granulomatous dermatitis with vulvar involvement. Case of the year. Presented at the Society for Pediatric Dermatology Annual Meeting, Snowmass, Colorado.

379. Frieden IJ, Prose NS, Fletcher V, Turner ML (1990) Granulomatous perioral dermatitis or sarcoid? Letter; comment. **Arch Dermatol** 126:1237–1238.
380. Frieden IJ, Prose NS, Flectcher V, Turner ML (1989) Granulomatous perioral dermatitis in children. **Arch Dermatol** 125:369–373.
381. Burry JN (1973) Topical drug addiction: adverse effects of fluorinated corticosteroid creams and ointments. **Med J Aust** 1:393–396.
382. Wilkinson DS, Kirton V, Wilkinson JD (1979) Perioral dermatitis. **Br J Dermatol** 101:245–257.

Tetracycline is contraindicated in patients under 8 years of age, and oral erythromycin can be substituted with few recurrences. The dose is 125mg tid for four weeks and then bid for another six weeks for both medications. The use of topical antibiotics, such as erythromycin 1% or clindamycin 2% in propylene glycol and alcohol, is effective when used bid, but should be covered with an emollient immediately after application, as it is often too irritating to use on already traumatized skin. Some physicians feel there is benefit from using topical metronidazole.

ECZEMA CRACQUELE (ASTEATOTIC ECZEMA, ECZEMA HIEMALIS)

Eczema cracquele (asteatotic eczema) is not often seen in children, but it may, however, occur in association with AD. It is worse in the dry winter months and is also seen in those who shower frequently with subsequent dehydration of the skin. The lesions consist of scaling plaques, mainly on the lower legs. The pattern of the scale is that of a fine cracking or pavement-stone appearance. If the condition worsens, an acute pruritic dermatitis may supervene. Asteatotic eczema may also be seen in cleanliness faddists who wash their hands constantly. A specific dermatitis is seen on the dorsa of the hands associated with erythema, scaling, and a craquele appearance. This is also seen in children who do not wear gloves in winter months and whose hands become dry and chapped.

Patients should be advised to humidify the environment, bathe with an emulsifying oil in lukewarm water, use a mild soap, and follow bathing by leaving a moist film of oil and water on the body and then applying an emollient of petrolatum, or any commercial product preferred by the patient. If a dermatitis occurs, a low- or medium-potency topical corticosteroid (cream or ointment) should be used three times a day until the eruption disappears.

LICHEN STRIATUS

This disease of unknown etiology is most common in children. It has also been described in infants and adults.[383,384] Kennedy and Rogers[385] reviewed 61 patients; in their series there was a 2:1 female to male ratio and the age range in this pediatric population was 9 months to 9 years. Spring and summer was the time of presentation in the majority of patients and the disease seldom affected more than one family member.[385] The most common area of involvement was the lower leg, but any area may be involved in lichen striatus, including the face. At times, multiple sites are involved. The lesions are arranged in a linear pattern, usually on the trunk and extremities (Fig. 14.41), which follow Blaschko's lines.[245] Lesions begin as tiny, asymptomatic, skin-colored or erythematous (Fig. 14.42) lichenoid papules that may coalesce into linear plaques. Lesions persist for one to two years after which the papules flatten out, leaving an area of hypopigmentation that persists for 1–3 years and then disappears. When the lesions involve the area around the nail, grooving of the nail plate may be seen.

The histology is that of a chronic dermatitis. Zang and McNutt found combining features of sweat gland or hair follicle involvement[386] with other histological features including mild spongiosis, a superficial and deep perivascular lymphocytic infiltrate, and exocytosis, hyper- and parakeratosis with a few necrotic keratocytes in the epidermis resulted in a definite diagnosis in 92% of patients.[386] The pathogenesis is poorly understood. The presence of lesions in Blaschko's lines suggests some type of mosaicism, but the initial erythema is suggestive of an infection, possibly a virus.

The disease should be differentiated from other linear conditions, including linear epidermal nevi, verrucae planae, morphea, and linear lichen planus.

As lichen striatus is self-limited, treatment is seldom necessary. Topical corticosteroids may cause more rapid involution of the erythematous lesions. Recurrences seldom occur.[385]

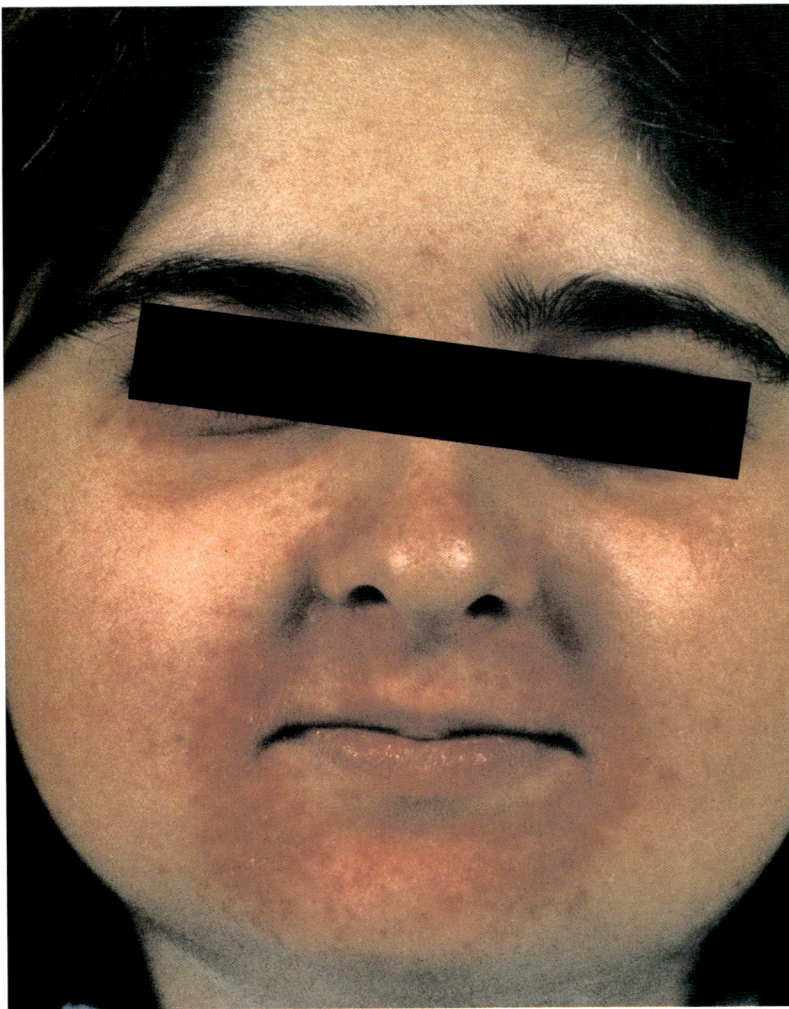

Fig. 14.39   Perioral dermatitis.

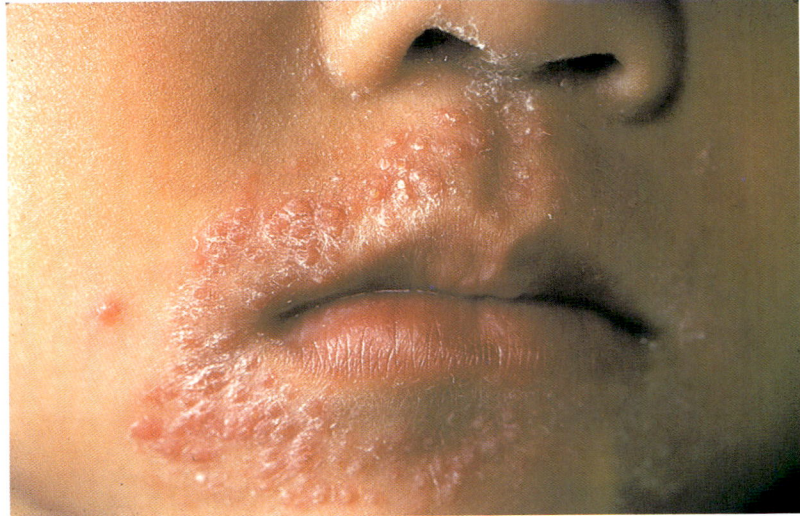

Fig. 14.40   Granulomatous perioral dermatitis in an 8-year-old boy.

383. Kennedy D, Rogers M (1996) Lichen striatus. **Pediatr Dermatol** 13:95.
384. Mitsuhashi Y, Konfo D (1996) Lichen striatus in an adult. **J Dermatol** 23:710.
385. Kennedy D, Rogers M (1996) Lichen striatus. **Ped Dermatol** 13:95–99.
386. Zang Y, McNutt NS (2001) Lichen striatus. **J Cutan Pathol** 28:65–71.

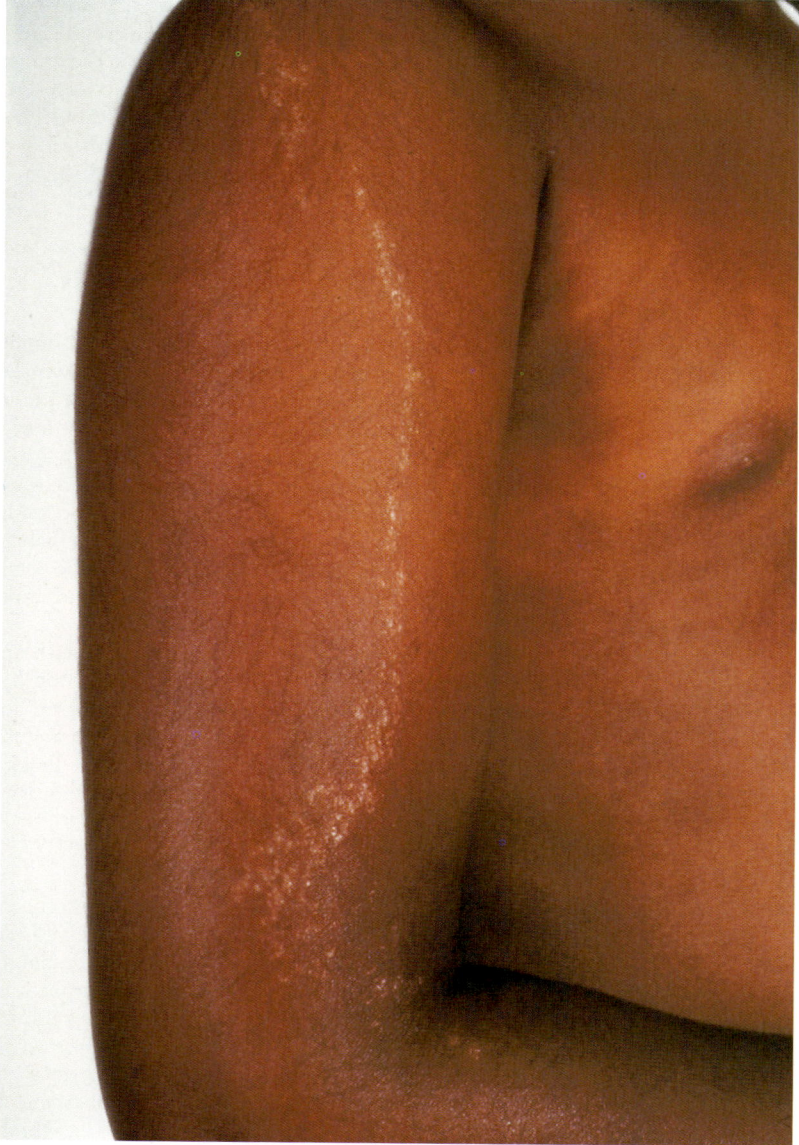

Fig. 14.41 Lichen striatus – typical small lichenoid papules in linear array on the arm in Blaschko's lines.

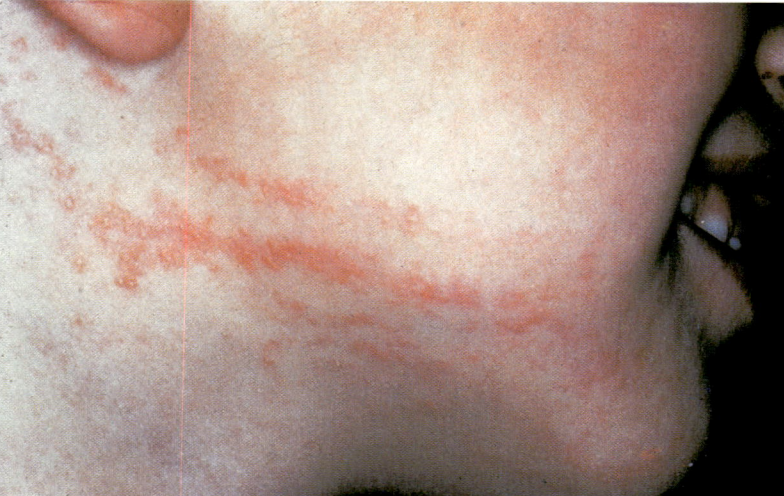

Fig. 14.42 Lichen striatus with inflammation over the face.

continues. In addition to the use of antihistamines, corticosteroid impregnated tape or topical corticosteroids under occlusion or intralesional corticosteroids in recalcitrant cases, may be helpful. The addition of 0.25% methol and 0.25% camphor to the topical steroid may also alleviate the itch. Although lichen simplex chronicus occurs frequently in AD patients, this entity may also occur in patients with no atopic diathesis.

PRURIGO NODULARIS

Prurigo nodularis is common in Asians and is more common in children than lichen simplex chronicus, of which it is probably a variant. The lesions consist of multiple discrete papules and nodules, commonly on the legs and arms, but almost any accessible area may be involved. Crusting and excoriation are common. The etiology is unknown but it is often proceeded by arthropod bites followed by continuous scratching and rubbing. Increased numbers of dermal nerves and Merkel cells have been demonstrated.[387] It is not uncommon for children to have bites in the summer months and to continue to scratch the lesions and pick off the crusts until the late autumn. Histology shows a mixed inflammatory cell infiltrate of chronic dermatitis with some mast cells and eosinophils. It is important to distinguish prurigo nodularis of unknown origin from the pruritus and lesions caused by a lymphoma or liver disease. If there is any question about the association, a full CBC, ESR, chest X-ray, and ultrasound of the abdomen should be performed.[388,389] Treatment is similar to that of lichen simplex chronicus.

LICHEN SIMPLEX CHRONICUS (LOCALIZED NEURODERMATITIS)

Lichen simplex chronicus commonly presents on the nape of the neck, the ankles, and the pretibial areas with single or multiple poorly demarcated circumscribed plaques. The skin becomes thickened, hyperpigmented, and lichenified and at times develops lichenoid papules or excoriated lesions. The pathogenesis of the lesion is unknown, but it is often initiated by a primary pruritic event, such as an insect bite or poison ivy dermatitis followed by continued rubbing in the area. Histology is that of a chronic dermatitis. It is never seen in infants or young children but may occur in older children and teenagers.

Management of lichen simplex chronicus consists of relieving the itch with the use of potent corticosteroid preparations and antihistamines. The patient should be informed that the lesions will not respond if scratching and rubbing

PAPULAR URTICARIA

Children initially do not react to insect bites, and then, when sensitized, with a wheal reaction surrounding a punctum. Typical lesions of urticaria may occur on other body sites. The pathogenesis is unknown but one theory involves an abnormal immune response on the part of the host.

The lesions are extremely pruritic urticarial wheals with a central punctum usually on the lower legs, but in young children, who lie on the ground, any area may be involved including the face and scalp. Bullae may develop. The lesions are often excoriated with a central crust corresponding to the punctum. Within 10 to 14 days they settle down. In those children who are chronic pickers these reactions may last for many months as they meticulously remove the crust and start the itch/scratch cycle all over again. Topical corticosteroids, antihistamines, and time are all helpful.

387. Nahass G, Penneys NS (1994) Merkel cells and prurigo nodularis. **J Am Acad Dermatol** 31:86–89.
388. Jorda E, Zayas AI, Revert A et al. (1991) A lichen striatus-like eruption adopting the morphology of Blaschko lines. **Pediatr Dermatol** 8:120–121.
389. Fina L, Grimalt R, Berti E, Caputo R (1991) Nodular prurigo associated with Hodgkin's disease. **Dermatologica** 182:243–246.

Papulosquamous Disease

Peter A. Hogan

Papulosquamous disorders are common in childhood. They consist of a diverse group of inflammatory conditions of the skin characterized by an eruption that exhibit papule (raised) and squamous (scaling) components. In one large series of pediatric patients, the papulosquamous group accounted for approximately 10% of all cutaneous disorders seen in a busy pediatric dermatology clinic.[1]

PSORIASIS VULGARIS

Robert Willan, an English physician, is given credit for the first description of psoriasis in 1808.[2] Prior to this report, psoriasis was frequently confused with entities such as leprosy and syphilis.

Psoriasis vulgaris is a common papulosquamous disorder; which accounts for 4% of all dermatoses seen in patients under the age of 16 years.[3] It is typically characterized by raised, well-defined, erythematous skin lesions of varying size that are surmounted by a silvery-white scale. Although the scalp, elbows, and knees are the most commonly affected sites, psoriasis can manifest anywhere on the body including the flexural areas and palmoplantar skin. Less common morphologic variants are pustular skin lesions (pustular psoriasis) and widespread erythema with varying degrees of surface scale (erythrodermic psoriasis). Psoriasis of the skin can be accompanied by a variety of nail plate and nail bed changes and inflammatory arthritis (psoriatic arthritis). The nail plate changes are due to involvement of the nail matrix.

EPIDEMIOLOGY

Genetics

Early epidemiologic studies and several twin studies highlighted the role of genetic factors in the pathogenesis of psoriasis. A number of studies have found the incidence of psoriasis to be greater in the relatives of patients with psoriasis compared with the general population.[4-9] The incidence varied from 4.6% in the study by Watson *et al.*[4] to 36% of patients in the study by Farber *et al.*[5] and 91% in the study conducted by Lomholt in the Faroe islands.[6] Swanbeck *et al.* reported the life-time risk of developing psoriasis if no parent, one parent, or both parents were affected was 4%, 28% and 65%, respectively. The risk increased to 24%, 41% and 83%, respectively, if there was an affected sibling as well.[10] The incidence of psoriasis is significantly higher in monozygotic compared with dizygotic twins. The concordance rate was 35–70% in monozygotic twins compared with 12–23% in dizygotic twins.[11-13] When monozygotic twins are concordant for psoriasis, the age of onset, the distribution, severity, and clinical course of the psoriasis is similar in each twin.[11]

Most of the research involving the inheritance of psoriasis has focused on the HLA component of the Major Histocompatibility Complex (MHC) located on chromosome 6p. A strong association exists between psoriasis, particularly early-onset psoriasis, and the HLA-B13,[14-17] HLA-B17(B57),[14-17] HLA-Cw6,[18-21] HLA-DR-7,[22,23] and HLA-DQA1★0201[23] alleles. The association is strongest for the HLA-Cw6 allele in most ethnic groups. Recent studies have identified a psoriasis susceptibility locus within the MHC on chromosome 6 in some families.[24-27] The susceptibility locus has been

1. Schachner L, Ling NS, Press S (1983) A statistical analysis of a pediatric dermatology clinic. **Pediatr Dermatol** 1:157.
2. Farber EM, McClintock RP Jr (1968) A current review of psoriasis. **Calif Med J** 108:440.
3. Beylot C, Puissant A, Bioulac P et al. (1979) Particular clinical features of psoriasis in infants and children. **Acta Derm Venereol** (Stockh), suppl. 87:95.
4. Watson W, Cann HM, Farber EM, Nall ML (1972) The genetics of psoriasis. **Arch Dermatol** 105:197–207.
5. Farber EM, Nall ML (1974) The natural history of psoriasis in 5600 patients. **Dermatologica** 148:1–18.
6. Lomholt G (1963) Psoriasis. Prevalence, spontaneous course and genetics. A census study on the prevalence of skin diseases in the Faroe Islands. Copenhagen: GEC Gad.
7. Hellgren L (1967) Psoriasis: The prevalence in sex, age and occupational groups in total populations in Sweden. Morphology, inheritance and associations with other skin and rheumatic diseases. Stockholm: Almqvist and Wiskell.
8. Farber EM, Bright RD, Nall ML (1968) Psoriasis: a questionnaire survey of 2,144 patients. **Arch Dermatol** 98:248–259.
9. Andreben C, Henseler T (1982) Die Erblichkeit der psoriasis: Eine analyse von 2035 familienanamnesen. **Hautarzt** 33:214–217.
10. Swanbeck G, Inerot A, Martinsson T, Wahlstrom J (1994) A population genetic study of psoriasis. **Br J Dermatol** 131:32–39.
11. Farber EM, Nall L, Watson W (1974) Natural history of psoriasis in 61 twin pairs. **Arch Dermatol** 109:207–211.
12. Brandrup F, Hauge M, Henningsen J, Eriksen B (1978) Psoriasis in an unselected series of twins. **Arch Dermatol** 114:874–878.
13. Duffy DL, Spelman LS, Martin NG (1993) Psoriasis in Australian twins. **J Am Acad Dermatol** 29:428–434.
14. Russell TJ, Schultes LM, Kuban DJ (1972) Histocompatibility (HLA) antigens associated with psoriasis. **N Engl J Med** 287:738–743.
15. White SH, Newcomer VD, Mickey ER et al. (1972) Disturbance of HLA antigen frequency in psoriasis. **N Engl J Med** 287:740.
16. Seignalet J, Clot J, Guilhou JJ et al. (1974) HLA antigens and some immunological parameters in psoriasis. **Tissue Antigens** 4:59.
17. Schunter F, Schieferstein G (1974) HLA Antigene bei Psoriasis vulgaris. **Hautarzt** 25:82.
18. Brenner W, Gschnait F, Mayr WR et al. (1978) HLA B13, B17, B37 and Cw6 in psoriasis vulgaris: association with the age of onset. **Arch Dermatol Res** 262:337–339.
19. Gazit E, Brenner S, Efter T et al. (1978) HLA antigens in patients with psoriasis. **Tissue Antigens** 12:195–199.
20. Tiilikainen A, Lassus A, Karvonen J et al. (1980) Psoriasis and HLA Cw6. **Br J Dermatol** 102:179–184.
21. Henseler T, Christophers E (1985) Psoriasis of early and late onset: characterisation of two types of psoriasis. **J Am Acad Dermatol** 13:450–456.
22. Tiwari JL, Lowe NJ, Abramovits W et al. (1982) Association of psoriasis with HLA-DR7. **Br J Dermatol** 106:227–230.
23. Ikaheimo I, Silvennoinen-Kassinen S, Karvonen J et al. (1996) Immunogenetic profile of psoriasis vulgaris: association with haplotypes A2, B13, Cw6, DR7, DQA1*0201 and A1, B17, Cw6, DR7, DQA1*0201. **Arch Dermatol Res** 288:363–367.
24. Trembath RC, Clough RL, Rosbotham JL et al. (1997) Identification of a major susceptibility locus on chromosome 6p and evidence for further disease loci revealed by a two stage genome wide search in psoriasis. **Hum Mol Genet** 6:813–820.
25. Nair RP, Henseler T, Jenisch S et al. (1997) Evidence for two psoriasis susceptibility loci (HLA and 17q) and two novel candidate regions (16p, 20p) by genome wide scan. **Hum Mol Genet** 6:1349–1356.
26. Burden AD, Javed S, Bailey M et al. (1998) Genetics of psoriasis: paternal inheritance and a locus on chromosome 6p. **J Invest Dermatol** 110:958–960.
27. Oka A, Tamiya G, Ota M et al. (1999) Association analysis using refined microsatellite markers localises a susceptibility locus for psoriasis vulgaris within a 111kb segment telomeric to the HLA-C gene. **Hum Mol Genet** 8:2165–2170.

tentatively narrowed to a few hundred kilobases telomeric to the HLA-C gene region on chromosome 6p.[27,28] Candidate genes currently under investigation include the corneodesmin gene,[29,30] the MICA gene,[31] and the HCR(Pg8) gene.[32] Corneodesmin is a protein expressed within the stratum granulosum and stratum corneum.[33,34] Corneodesmin is translocated to the extracellular part of the desmosome and is believed to play a key role in cornedesmosome formation and/or function.[34,35] A particular allelic form of corneodesmin (allele 5) has been strongly associated with psoriasis.[36] The MICA gene belongs to the MHC class I chain-related (MIC) gene family (MICA, MICB, MICC, MICD, MICE) that have been recently mapped to the region of HLA class I (HLA-A, HLA-B, HLA-C) genes.[37,38] The MICA gene encodes for MICA, which is a MHC-like molecule.[37] Its function is unknown. The HCR (Pg8) gene encodes for the HCR protein, which is overexpressed in psoriatic skin compared with normal skin.[39] A particular allelic variant designated HCR★Arg-Arg was strongly associated with psoriasis in an isolated Finnish population.[40] The physiologic function of the HCR protein is unknown.

In addition to chromosome 6p, linkage analysis has identified other major psoriasis susceptibility loci on chromosome 17q,[25,41] 4q,[42] 1q,[43] and 3q.[44] The candidate genes on 17q, 4q, 1q, and 3q have yet to be identified. The susceptibility loci on 6p, 17q, 4q, 1q, and 3q are now designated ***Psors 1, Psors 2, Psors 3, Psors 4*** and ***Psors 5***, respectively.[45] Minor psoriasis susceptibility loci have been identified on 1p, 2q, 2p, 8q, 16q, 19p, and 20p.[24,25]

Statistics

A recent survey found the incidence of psoriasis ranged from 0% in Samoa to 11.8% in Artic-Kasach'ye. The incidence was 4.6% in the USA, 1.6% in the UK, and approximately 1.5% in Europe.[46] Although females were more commonly affected in the pediatric population[2,47] in two studies, a more recent study found the sex incidence in the pediatric population to be equal.[48] Males and females are equally affected when all age groups are considered.[46] Psoriasis can develop at any age[48] and has been reported at birth (congenital psoriasis).[49] The peak age of onset is 15–25 years,[5,47,50] with a smaller peak between 57–60 years.[47,50] The early-onset group, referred to as Type I, exhibited a strong family history of psoriasis, typical HLA associations, more severe disease, and more nail involvement. In contrast, family history and HLA associations were not features of the late-onset group, referred to as Type II.[47]

PRESENTING HISTORY

Young infants usually present during the first 1–2 years of life with a diaper rash that is not responding to standard diaper dermatitis treatment. Older infants and children usually present with dandruff and/or an asymptomatic erythematous scaling eruption on the face, trunk, and/or limbs.[48] Occasionally, pruritus can be the presenting complaint, particularly with scalp psoriasis. Infants and children can present with guttate psoriasis following a streptococcal infection of the throat[51] or perianal area.[52] It is rare for children to present with nail psoriasis, pustular psoriasis, or erythrodermic psoriasis.[48]

EXAMINATION FINDINGS

Psoriatic diaper rash can develop until the infant is toilet trained. It is characterized by bright red, shiny erythema involving the entire diaper area that responds poorly to conventional diaper dermatitis therapy (Fig. 15.1). Unlike irritant diaper dermatitis, the margins are sharply demarcated and the groin folds are involved. Some of these patients develop an erythematous scaly eruption on the face, scalp, trunk, and limbs within 1–2 weeks of onset of the psoriatic diaper rash (Fig. 15.2). The widespread eruption develops quickly and can be quite alarming to parents. Although the widespread eruption resembles psoriasis, it is still unclear whether it represents true psoriasis or a form fruste of the disease.[48]

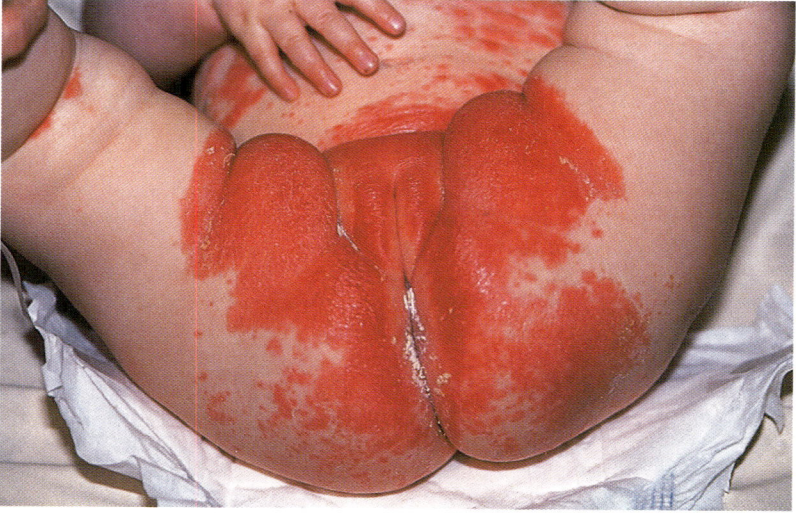

Fig. 15.1 Psoriatic diaper rash.

28. Nair R, Stuart P, Henseler TS et al. (2000) Localisation of psoriasis susceptibility locus PSORS1 to a 60kb interval telomeric to HLA-C. **Am J Hum Genet** 66:1833–1844.
29. Jenisch S, Koch S, Henseler T et al. (1999) Corneodesmin gene polymorphism demonstrates strong linkage disequilibrium with HLA and association with psoriasis vulgaris. **Tissue Antigens** 54:439–449.
30. Ahini RT, Camp NJ, Cork MJ et al. (1999) Novel genetic association between the corneodesmin gene (MHC S) gene and susceptibility to psoriasis. **Hum Mol Genet** 8:1135–1140.
31. Cheng L, Zhang SZ, Xiao CY et al. (2000) The A5.1 allele of the major histocompatibility complex chain-related geneA is associated with psoriasis vulgaris in chinese. **Br J Dermatol** 143:324–329.
32. Asumalahti K, Laitinen T, Itkonen-Vatjus R et al. (2000) A candidate gene for psoriasis near HLA-C, HCR(Pg8), is highly polymorphic with a disease-associated susceptibility allele. **Hum Mol Genet** 9:1533–1542.
33. Zhou Y, Chaplin DD (1993) Identification in the HLA class I region of a gene expressed late in keratinocyte differentiation. **Proc Natl Acad Sci USA** 90:9470–9474.
34. Haftek M, Simon M, Kanitakis J et al. (1997) Expression of corneodesmin in the granular layer and stratum corneum of normal and diseased epidermis. **Br J Dermatol** 137:864–873.
35. Simon M, Montezin M, Guerrin M et al. (1997) Characterisation and purification of human corneodesmin, an epidermal basic glycoprotein associated with corneocyte-specific modified desmosomes. **J Biol Chem** 272:31770–31776.
36. Allen MH, Veal C, Faassen A et al. (1999) A non-HLA gene within the MHC in psoriasis. **Lancet** 353:1589–1590.
37. Baharm S, Bresnahan M, Geraghty DE et al. (1994) A second lineage of mammalian major histocompatibility complex class I gene. **Proc Natl Acad Sci USA** 91:6259–6263.
38. Bahram S, Mizuki N, InokoH et al. (1996) Nucleotide sequence of the human MHC class I MIC gene. **Immunogenetics** 44:80–81.
39. Asumalahti K, Laitinen T, Itkonen-Vatjus R et al. (2000) A candidate gene for psoriasis near HLA-C, HCR(Pg8), is highly polymorphic with a disease-associated susceptibility allele. **Hum Mol Genet** 9:1533–1542.
40. Asumalahti K, Laitinen T, Itkonen-Vatjus R et al. (2000) A candidate gene for psoriasis near HLA-C, HCR (Pg8), is highly polymorphic with a disease-associated susceptibility gene. **Hum Mol Genet** 9:1533–1542.
41. Tomfohrde J, Silverman A, Barnes R et al. (1994) Gene for familial psoriasis susceptibility mapped to the distal end of human chromosome 17q. **Science** 264:1141–1145.
42. Matthews D, Fry L, Powles A et al. (1996) Evidence that a locus for familial psoriasis maps to chromosome 4q. **Nat Genet** 14:231–233.
43. Capon F, Novelli G, Samprini M et al. (1999) Searching for psoriasis susceptibility genes in Italy: genome scan and evidence for a new locus on chromosome 1. **J Invest Dermatol** 112:32–35.
44. Enlund F, Samuelsson L, Enerback C et al. (1999) Psoriasis susceptibility locus in chromosome region 3q21 identified in patients from southwest Sweden. **Eur J Hum Genet** 7:783–790.
45. Burden AD (2000) Identifying a gene for psoriasis on chromosome 6 (Psors 1). **Br J Dermatol** 143:237–241.
46. Farber EM, Nall ML (1998) Epidemiology: Natural history and genetics. In: Psoriasis, 3rd edn, Roenigk HH, Maibach HI, eds. New York: Marcel Dekker, pp. 107–158.
47. Henseler T, Christophers E (1985) Psoriasis of early and late onset: characterisation of two types of psoriasis vulgaris. **J Am Acad Dermatol** 13:450–456.
48. Morris A, Rogers M, Fischer G et al. (2000) Childhood psoriasis: a clinical review of 1262 cases. **Pediatr Dermatol** 18:188–198.
49. Lerner MR, Lerner AB (1972) Congenital psoriasis. **Arch Dermatol** 105:598.
50. Smith AE, Kassab JY, Rowland Payne CME et al. (1993) Bimodality in age of onset of psoriasis in both patients and their relatives. **Dermatology** 186:181–186.
51. Whyte HJ, Baugham RD (1964) Acute guttate psoriasis and streptococcal infection. **Arch Dermatol** 89:350–356.
52. Honig PJ (1988) Guttate psoriasis associated with perianal streptococcal disease. **J Pediatr** 113:1037–1039.

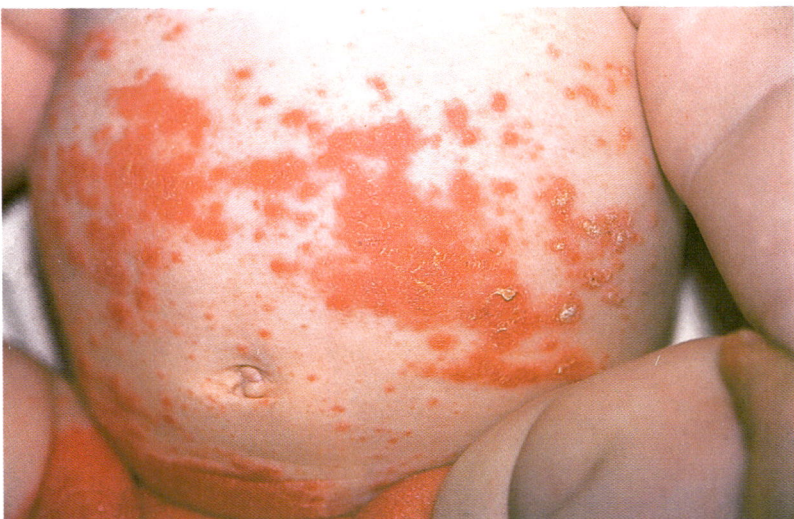

Fig. 15.2   Psoriatic diaper rash with disseminated psoriasiform eruption.

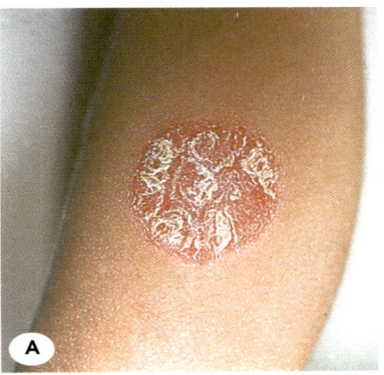
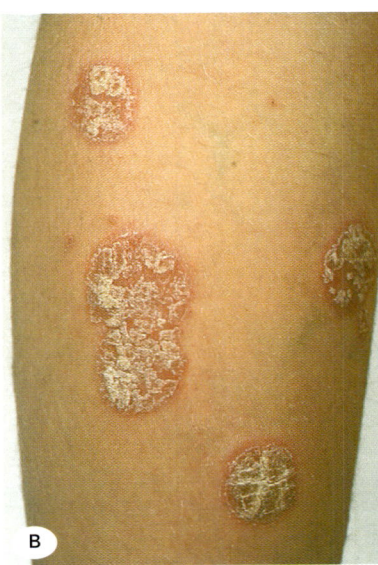

Fig. 15.4   (A) Classic plaque psoriasis.
(B) Typical plaque psoriasis on arm.

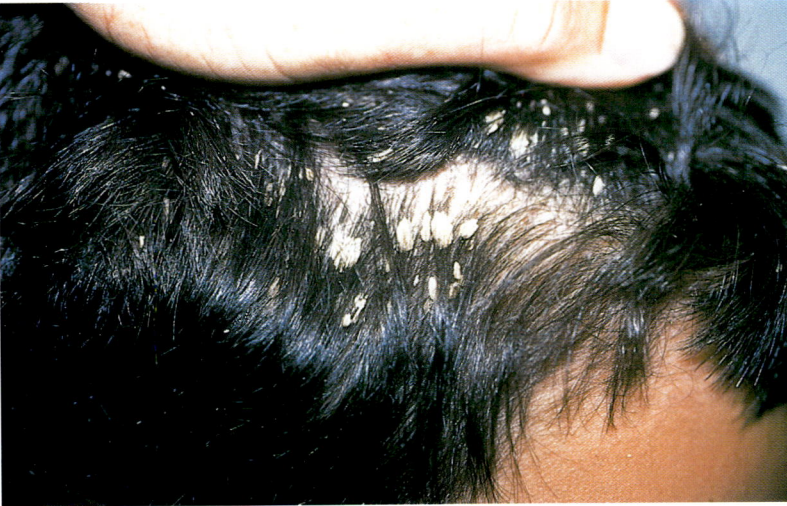

Fig. 15.3   Scalp psoriasis with thick adherent scalp scale (pityriasis amiantacea).

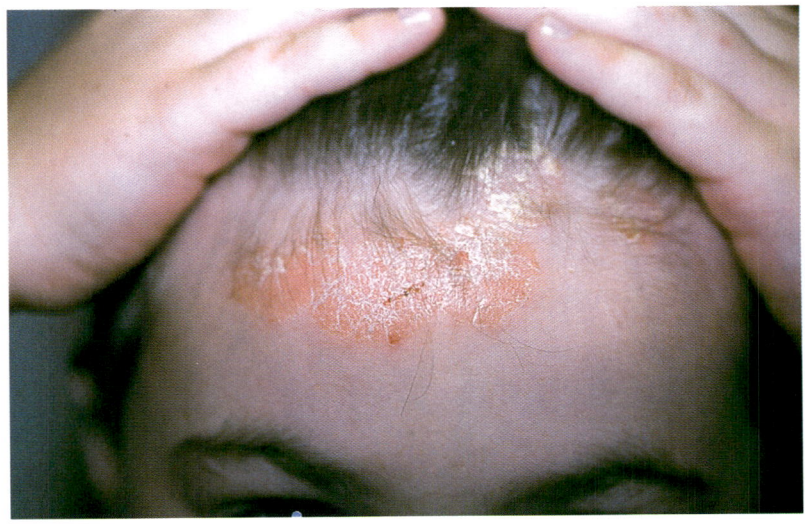

Fig. 15.5   Plaque psoriasis on the face.

Older infants and children usually present with the gradual development of papules or plaques of psoriasis on the scalp and/or body. Although psoriasis is not always pruritic, associated itch can be a feature, particularly with scalp involvement. Psoriasis manifests on the scalp as well-defined, scaly, erythematous papules or plaques or as thick, white scale with very little erythema. The latter presentation, called tinea amiantacea, is associated with matting of the hair and typical scale surrounding the proximal hair shaft at the scalp, resulting in some degree of temporary hair loss when the scale lifts off the scalp surface (Fig. 15.3). Psoriasis on the body manifests as well defined, scaly, erythematous papules or plaques of varying size that are usually, but not always, symmetrically distributed (Fig. 15.4). The plaques can be located on the face, trunk, limbs, hands, feet, genitalia, and/or within flexural areas (retro-auricular folds, axillae, groin folds, guteal cleft, umbilicus) (Figs 15.5, 15.6, 15.7). Flexural and facial involvement is more common compared with adult psoriasis. Surface scale is a prominent feature when plaques are on exposed areas and although classically thick and silvery-white in appearance, many children exhibit plaques with fine surface scale. Bleeding occurs when the scale is lifted. This is known as "Auspitz sign." Surface scale can be minimal or absent on the surface of flexural lesions. The sudden onset of multiple small

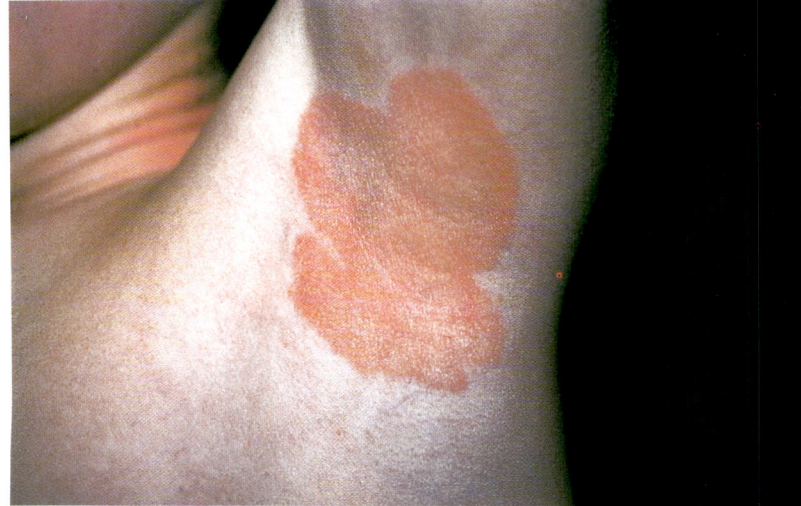

Fig. 15.6   Plaque psoriasis in the axilla.

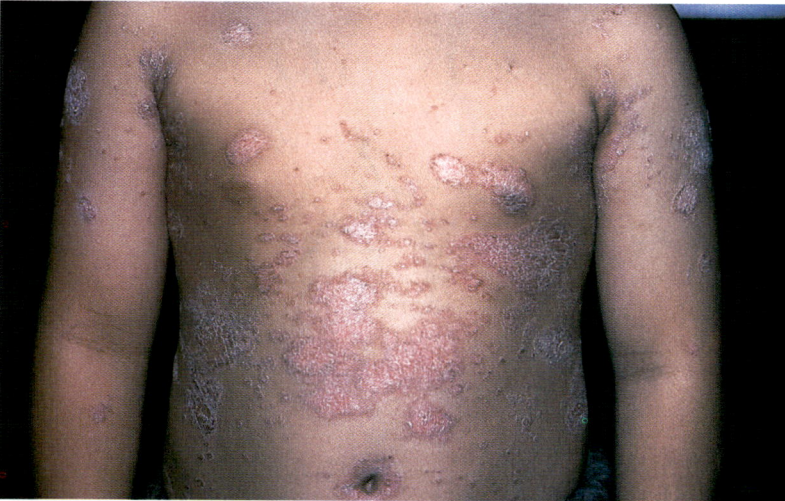

Fig. 15.7 Plaque psoriasis on the trunk.

papules (<1cm) of psoriasis on the trunk, limbs, scalp, and face following strep-tococcal infection is referred to as guttate psoriasis (Fig. 15.8). Morphologic variants of plaque psoriasis on the body in children include grouped follicular papules, annular or figurate lesions (Fig. 15.9), and linear lesions following the lines of Blaschko.[48]

Nail involvement is uncommon in pediatric psoriasis.[48] The most common manifestation is pitting of individual nail plates (Fig. 15.10). Onycholysis and the oil drop sign are uncommon findings. An unusual presentation is the development of marked dystrophy of the nail plate with erythema, scaling, and swelling involving the periungual skin (Fig. 15.11). The nail changes can predate, coincide with, or postdate the diagnosis of psoriasis.

Laboratory findings
No specific laboratory abnormalities are found in patients with plaque psoriasis. Swabs should be collected from the appropriate site (throat, perianal skin) in children with guttate psoriasis to confirm Group A beta haemolytic streptococci as the triggering factor.

PATHOPHYSIOLOGY AND HISTOGENESIS
Pathophysiology
Psoriasis is characterized by proliferation of keratinocytes, abnormal differentiation of keratinocytes, and inflammatory cell infiltration of the dermis and epidermis. Debate has focused on whether the primary defect is located in the skin or immune system. Evidence is mounting that the immune system is the site of the primary defect and is responsible for the hyperproliferation and abnormal differentiation of keratinocytes.

Immune system
The early observation that dermal infiltration with T lymphocytes and macrophages preceded the development of epidermal hyperplasia in early psoriatic lesions suggested a role for the immune system in the pathogenesis of psoriasis.[53] The clearance of psoriasis following an allogeneic bone marrow

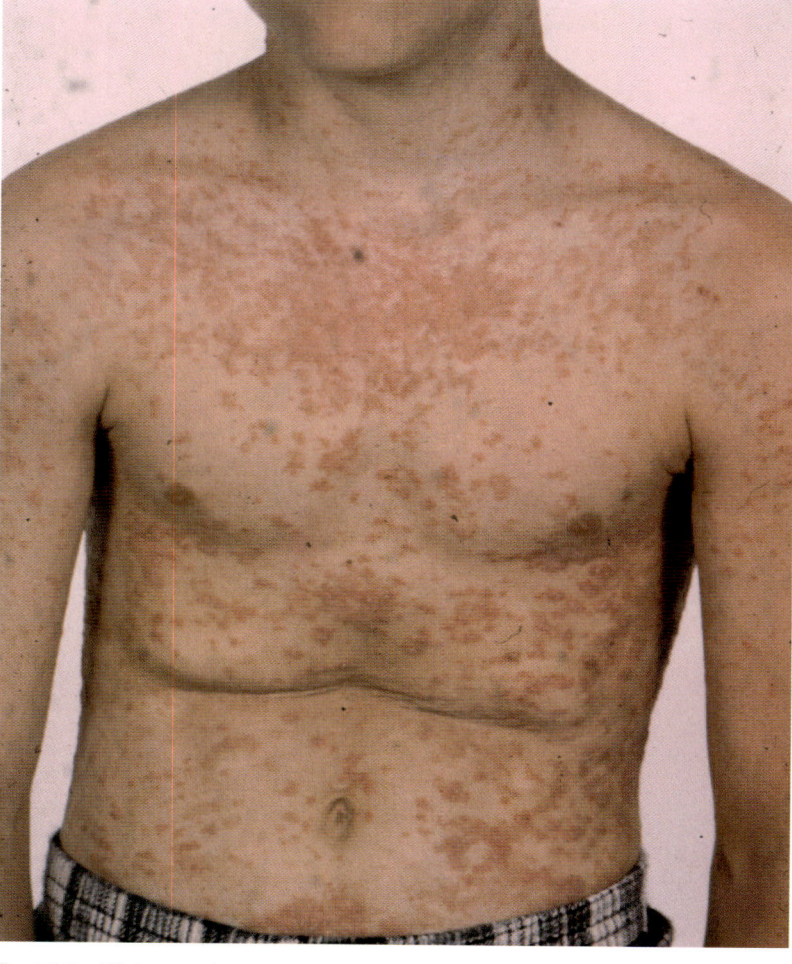

Fig. 15.8 Widespread guttate psoriasis in a seven-year-old child.

transplant[54] and the development of psoriasis in the recipient of a bone marrow transplant collected from a psoriatic patient[55] supported the involvement of immune cells in the development of the disease. The discovery that T lymphocytes, isolated from psoriatic skin, release cytokines that stimulate keratinocyte proliferation *in vitro*[56] and the ability of medications that target T cells, such as cyclosporin A,[57] tacrolimus,[58] anti–CD4 monoclonal antibody,[59] anti–CD3 antibody,[60] and a toxin selective for IL-2 receptor bearing T cells[61] in clearing psoriasis, highlighted the role of activated T lymphocytes in its pathogenesis. A study by Wrone-Smith *et al.*[62] involving severe combined immunodeficient (SCID) mice suggests a primary role for activated CD4+ T lymphocytes in the initiation of the psoriatic process. Unaffected skin from psoriatic patients was grafted onto severe combined immuno-deficient (SCID) mice. Psoriasis developed in the engrafted skin following injection of autologous immunocytes into the dermis of the grafted tissue. The immunocytes required preactivation with IL-2 and staphylotoxin enterotoxin B (SEB). Activated CD4+ T-helper cells rather than activated

53. Baadsgaard O, Fisher G, Voorhees JJ et al. (1990) The role of the immune system in the pathogenesis of psoriasis. **J Invest Dermatol** 95:32S–34S.
54. Eddy DJ, Burrows D, Bridges JM et al. (1990) Clearance of severe psoriasis after allogeneic bone marrow transplantation. **Br Med J** 300:908.
55. Snowden JA, Heaton DC (1997) Development of psoriasis in a syngeneic bone marrow transplant from psoriatic donor: further evidence for adoptive autoimmunity. **Br J Dermatol** 137:130–132.
56. Prinz JC, Grob B, Vollmer S et al. (1994) T cell clones from psoriasis skin lesions can promote keratinocyte proliferation in vitro via secreted products. **Eur J Immunol** 24:593–598.
57. Ellis CN, Gorsulowsky DC, Hamilton TA et al. (1986) Cyclosporin A improves psoriasis in a double-blind study. **JAMA** 256:3110–3116.
58. Jegasothy BV, Ackerman CD, Todo S et al. (1992) Tacrolimus (FK506) – a new therapeutic agent for severe recalcitrant psoriasis. **Arch Dermatol** 128:781–785.
59. Nicholas JF, Chamchick N, Thivolet J et al. (1991) CD4 antibody treatment of severe psoriasis. **Lancet** 338:321.
60. Weinshenker BG, Bass BH, Ebers GC et al. (1989) Remission of psoriatic lesions with muromonab-DC3 (orthoclone OKT3) treatment. **J Am Acad Dermatol** 20:1132–1133.
61. Gottlieb SL, Gilleaudeau P, Johnson R et al. (1995) Response of psoriasis to a lymphocyte-selective toxin (DAB$_{389}$IL2) suggests a primary immune, but not keratinocyte, pathogenesis. **Nature Med** 1:442–447.
62. Wrone-Smith T, Nickoloff BJ (1996) Dermal injection of immunocytes induces psoriasis. **J Clin Invest** 98:1878–1887.

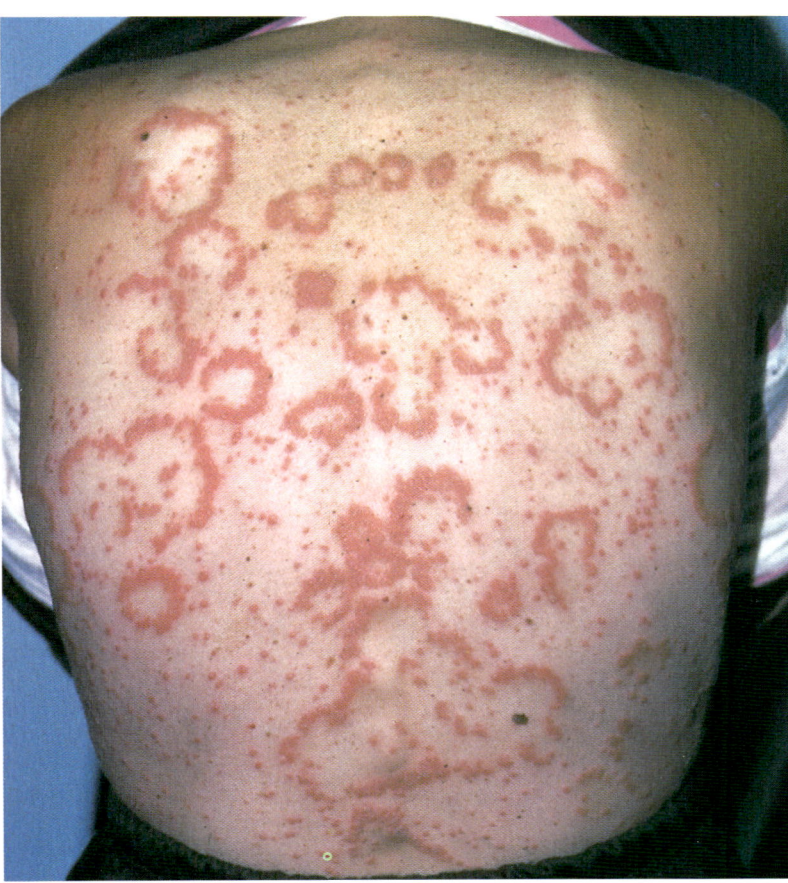

Fig. 15.9   Annular plaque psoriasis.

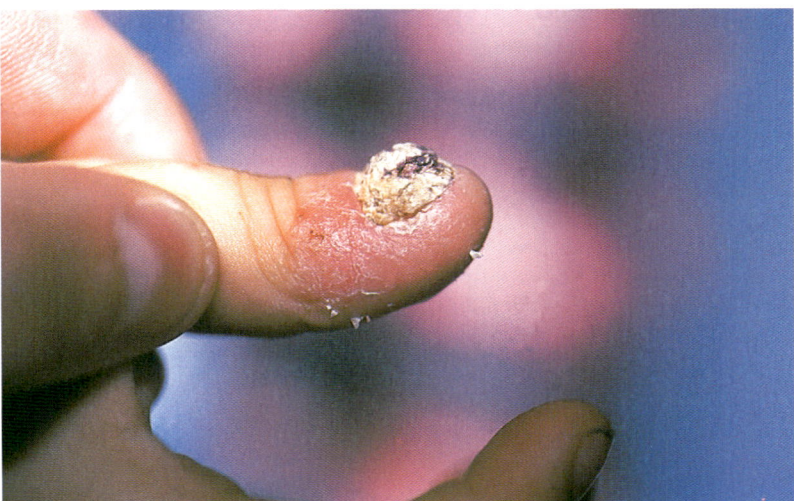

Fig. 15.11   Psoriasis of the fingertip with associated nail dystrophy.

CD8+ T-suppressor cells induced the development of psoriasis when injected into the grafted skin.[63] Although activated CD8+ cells were unable to induce psoriasis when injected into the graft, examination of the engrafted skin

after the injection of CD4+ T cells revealed the presence of activated intraepidermal CD8+ T-cells,[64] a finding that has also been reported in human psoriatic plaques.[65] Activated intraepidermal CD8+ T cells are needed for the establishment and/or maintenance of psoriasis because clinical improvement, following infusion of toxin selective for IL–2 receptor-bearing cells, correlated with the elimination of intraepidermal T cells, which were mainly CD8+.[61] It is not known whether the intraepidermal CD8+ T cells are resident cells that are activated or circulating cells that are recruited to the skin. Recruitment of CD4+ and CD8+ T cells to the skin and their subsequent activation is assumed to be in response to antigen entrapment, processing and presentation by Langerhans cells. Evidence that supports an antigen-driven process is the finding of restricted T-cell receptor expression in psoriatic lesions which reflects clonal expansion of particular T-cell populations.[66,67] The restriction in T-cell receptor expression predominantly involves CD8+ T cells[66] and was constant over long periods of time, in relapsing disease and in skin

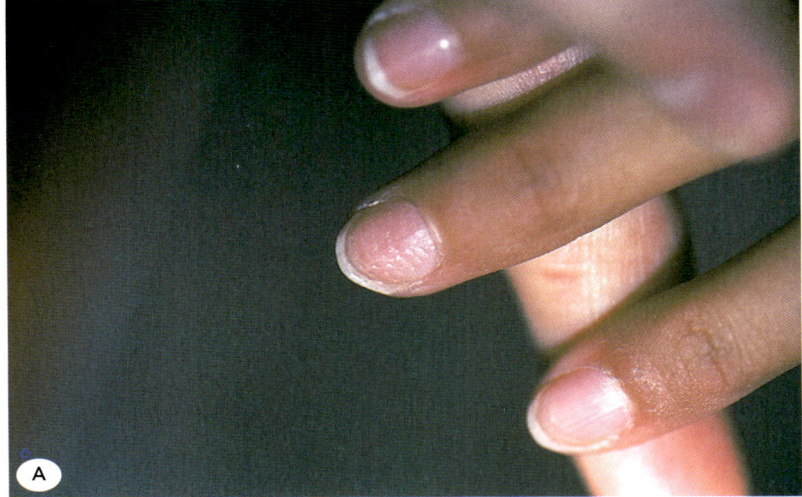

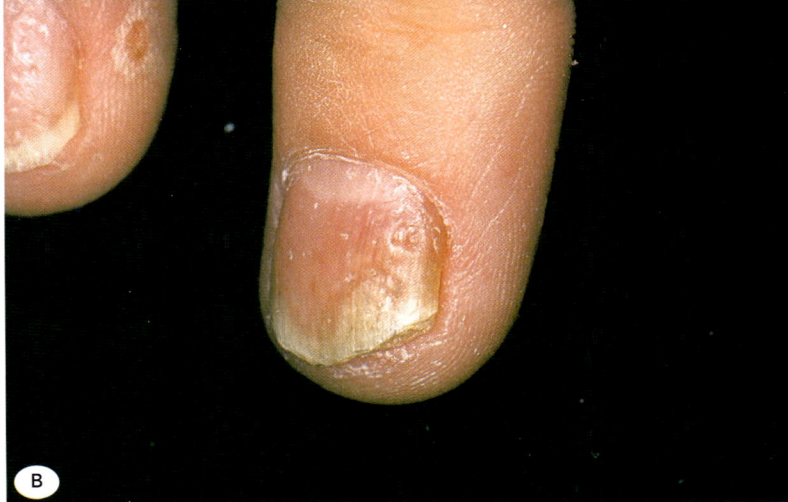

Fig. 15.10   (A) Nail pitting in psoriasis. (B) Typical pitting and oil drop sign of psoriatic nail.

63. Nickoloff BJ, Wrone-Smith T (1999) Injection of pre-psoriatic skin with CD41 T cells induces psoriasis. Am J Pathol 155:145–158.
64. Nickoloff BJ, Wrone-Smith T (1998) Superantigens, autoantigens and pathogenic T cells in psoriasis. J Invest Dermatol 110:459–461.
65. Austin LM, Coven TR, Bhardwaj N et al. (1998) Intraepidermal lymphocytes in psoriatic lesions are GMP-17 (TIA-1)1 CD81 CD31 CTLs as determined by phenotype analysis. J Cutan Pathol 25:79–88.

66. Chang JCC, Smith LR, Froning KJ et al. (1994) CD81 T cells in psoriatic lesions preferentially use T cell receptor Vbeta3 and/or Vbeta13.1 genes. Proc Natl Acad Sci USA 91:9282–9286.
67. Menssen A, Trommler P, Vollmer S et al. (1995) Evidence for an antigen-specific cellular immune response in skin lesions of patients with psoriasis vulgaris. J Immunol 155:4078–4083.

lesions from different sites.[66,67] Identification of a conserved T-cell receptor beta-chain CDR3 motif expression within skin lesions from different patients[68] and identical T-cell receptor expression in skin lesions and synovia of patients with psoriatic arthritis[69] suggest a common antigen is stimulating the immune response in different patients and different tissues affected by psoriasis. Potential antigens include streptococcal superantigens (see below), keratin 14 that cross-reacts with streptococcal M-6 protein (see below), and the L1 capsid protein of human papillomavirus type 5.[70] Keratinocyte proliferation, intraepidermal accumulation of neutrophils, and the production of antimicrobial peptides (beta-defensins)[71] by psoriatic keratinocytes support an infectious antigen as the antigenic stimulus for T-cell activation. Antigen activated CD4+ T cells and CD8+ T cells in psoriatic lesions are of the Th1 phenotype, which produce interferon-gamma, interleukin-2 and tumour necrosis factor-alpha and beta.[72] These cytokines are capable of inducing keratinocyte proliferation.

Skin

Epidermal proliferation in psoriasis is traditionally believed to be due to a reduction in the keratinocyte cell cycle time.[73] Recent studies suggest other factors may contribute to the epidermal hyperplasia.[74,75] The basal layer of the epidermis contains resting and cycling cells; it may be the conversion of resting cells to cycling cells that contributes to an increased growth fraction and epidermal hyperplasia. Attention has also focused on whether epidermal hyperplasia in psoriasis is partly due to reduced apoptosis (cell death). Studies have found increased levels of the anti-apoptotic protein Bcl-x in keratinocytes from psoriatic plaques,[76] which renders the cells more resistant to apoptosis compared with normal skin.[77] Keratinocyte levels of Bcl-x are increased with interferon-gamma, one of the cytokines identified in psoriatic skin.[78] Although current evidence favors epidermal hyperplasia induced by activated T lymphocytes, a study by Carroll et al.[79] highlights the potential for keratinocytes to be the site of the primary defect. The study involved the development of transgenic mice for integrins beta-1, alpha-2, and alpha-5. The beta-1 integrin is only found on basal keratinocytes. When transgenic mice expressed beta-1 alone or in combination with alpha-2 and alpha-5 on suprabasal keratinocytes, skin changes developed that clinically and histologically resembled psoriasis. Notably, the epidermal changes were accompanied by infiltration of the skin with CD4+ and CD8+ T lymphocytes. The skin changes were entirely due to the expression of beta-1 integrin on suprabasal keratinocytes. The expression of beta-1 integrin on suprabasal keratinocytes is erroneously interpreted as a signal for basal cells to proliferate. The altered physiology of the proliferating keratinocytes may lead to the release of cytokines that induce lymphocytic infiltration of the dermis.

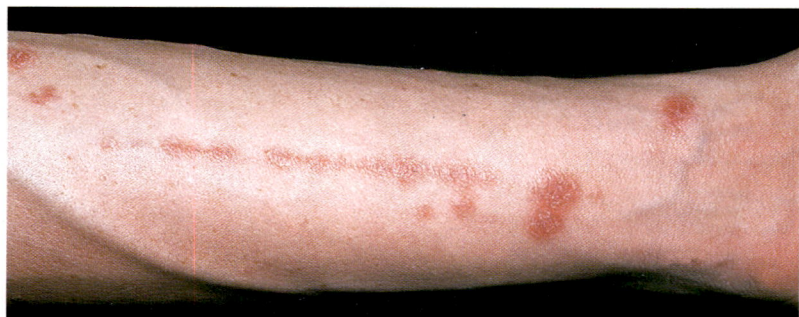

Fig. 15.12 Koebner phenomenon.

Triggering and exacerbating factors

Psoriasis in the pediatric age group can be triggered or exacerbated by trauma, drugs, and certain types of infections. Psoriasis occurring at the site of a physical, chemical, thermal, surgical, or inflammatory insult to the skin is recognized as the Koebner phenomenon (Fig. 15.12).[80] Although psoriasis usually improves during pregnancy, it can flare during pregnancy or the postpartum period.[5,81] Medications that can induce or exacerbate psoriasis in children are antimalarials and rebound experienced after the cessation of oral and potent topical corticosteroid therapy.[82] Exacerbation that occurs with withdrawal of oral and topical steroids may be of the pustular type.[83] Induction and/or exacerbation of psoriasis is a recognized complication of human immunodeficiency infection (HIV).[84,85] It also follows streptococcal infection of the pharynx[51] and perianal skin.[52] Streptococcal infection typically induces the guttate pattern of plaque psoriasis. The development and/or exacerbation of psoriasis with streptococcal infection involves activation of T lymphocytes through two different pathways. The first involves streptococcal proteins functioning as superantigens. Conventional peptide antigens are processed intracellularly by antigen processing cells, placed in the MHC peptide-binding groove and presented to CD4+ T lymphocytes in association with class II MHC molecules. Successful binding between the presented antigen and the T lymphocyte requires antigen recognition by all five variable elements of the T-cell receptor (Vbeta, Dbeta, Jbeta, Valpha, Jalpha).[86,87] In contrast, superantigens directly bind to the outside of the MHC peptide-binding groove on the surface of antigen-presenting cells without prior intracellular processing. Successful binding between the superantigen and CD4+ T lymphocyte only requires recognition of the Vbeta region of the T-cell receptor. In view of the restricted number of Vbeta genes, T-cell response to superantigens far exceeds the response to conventional peptide antigens.[86,87] Leung et al.[88] found a direct link between streptococcal super-

68. Prinz JC, Vollmer S, Boehncke W-H et al. (1999) Selection of conserved TCR-VDJ-rearrangements in chronic psoriatic plaques indicates a common antigen in psoriasis vulgaris. Eur J Immunol 29:3360–3368.
69. Tassiulas I, Duncan SR, Centola M et al. (1999) Clonal characteristics of T cell infiltrates in skin and synovium of patients with psoriatic arthritis. Hum Immunol 60:479–491.
70. Favre M, Orth G, Majewski S et al. (1998) Psoriasis: a possible reservoir for human papillomavirus type 5, the virus associated with skin carcinomas of epidermodysplasia verruciformis. J Invest Dermatol 110:311–317.
71. Harder J, Bartels J, Christophers E et al. (1997) A peptide antibiotic from human skin. Nature 387:861.
72. Austin LM, Ozawa M, Kikuchi T et al. (1999) The majority of epidermal T cells in psoriasis vulgaris lesions can produce type 1 cytokines, interferon-gamma, interleukin-2, and tumour necrosis factor-alpha, defining TC1 (cytotoxic T lymphocyte) and TH1 effector populations: a type 1 differentiation bias is also measured in circulating blood T cells in psoriasis patients. J Invest Dermatol 113:752–759.
73. Weinstein GD, Frost P (1968) Abnormal cell proliferation in psoriasis. J Invest Dermatol 50:254.
74. Van Erp PEJ, Boezeman JBM, Brons PPT (1996) Cell cycle kinetics in normal human skin by in vivo administration of iododeoxyuridine and application of a differentiation marker – implications for cell cycle kinetics in psoriatic skin. Anal Cell Pathol 11:43–54.
75. Van Ruissen F, de Jongh GJ, Van Erp PEJ et al. (1996) Cell kinetic characterisation of cultured human keratinocytes from normal and psoriatic individuals. J Cell Physiol 8:684–694.
   one-Smith T, Nunez G, Johnson T et al. (1995) Discordant expression of Bcl-x and Bcl-2 by atinocytes in vitro and psoriatic keratinocytes in vivo. Am J Pathol 146:1–10.

77. Wrone-Smith T, Mitra RS, Thompson CB et al. (1997) Keratinocytes derived from psoriatic plaques are resistant to apoptosis compared with normal skin. Am J Pathol 151:1321–1329.
78. Uyemura K, Yamamura M, Fivenson DF et al. (1993) The cytokine network in lesional and lesion-free psoriatic skin is characterised by a T-helper type 1 cell-mediated response. J Invest Dermatol 101:701–705.
79. Carroll JM, Romero MR, Watt FM (1995) Suprabasal integrin expression in the epidermis of transgenic mice results in developmental defects and a phenotype resembling psoriasis. Cell 83:957–968.
80. Eyre RW, Krueger GG (1984) The koebner response in psoriasis. In: Psoriasis, Roenigk HH, Maibach HI, eds. New York: Marcel Dekker, pp. 105–116.
81. Dunn SF, Findlay AY (1989) Psoriasis: improvement during and worsening after pregnancy. Br J Dermatol 120:584.
82. Abel EA, DiCicco LM, Orenberg EK et al. (1986) Drugs in exacerbation of psoriasis. J Am Acad Dermatol 15:1007–1022.
83. Boxley JD, Dawber RPR, Summerly R (1975) Generalised pustular psoriasis on withdrawal of clobetasol propionate ointment. Br Med J ii:255–256.
84. Johnson TM, Duvic M, Rapini RP et al. (1985) AIDS exacerbates psoriasis. N Engl J Med 313:1415.
85. Lazar AP, Roenigk HH (1988) Acquired immunodeficiency syndrome (AIDS) can exacerbate psoriasis. J Am Acad Dermatol 18:144.
86. Moller G (1993) Superantigens. Immunol Rev 131:1–200.
87. Kotzin BL, Leung DYM, Kappler J et al. (1993) Superantigens and human disease. Adv Immunol 54:99–166.
88. Leung DYM, Travers JB, Giorno R et al. (1995) Evidence for a streptococcal superantigen driven process in acute guttate psoriasis. J Clin Invest 96:2106–2112.

antigens and the development of guttate psoriasis. Streptococci isolated from the pharynx of guttate psoriasis patients produced the superantigen streptococcal pyrogenic exotoxin C (SPEC), a potent stimulator of T lymphocytes exhibiting the Vbeta2 molecule. All patients had a predominance of Vbeta 2+ CD4+ and CD8+ T lymphocytes in skin biopsies taken from the advancing edge of a new psoriatic lesion. Subsequent cloning of isolated T lymphocytes revealed a polyclonal expansion of the Vbeta 2 type of T-cell receptor. Both findings support SPEC superantigen induced T-lymphocyte activation. An earlier study by Lewis et al.[89] also found a predominance of Vbeta 2+ T lymphocytes in the skin lesions of patients with both guttate and plaque psoriasis compared with matched blood samples. Cloned T lymphocytes collected from the skin lesions were stimulated in vitro by streptococcal proteins. The second pathway of T-lymphocyte activation involves the streptococcal M protein, which forms thread-like projections from the surface of the bacteria.[90] An extensive sequence homology has been identified between streptococcal M protein, which has an alpha-helical coiled structure, and type I keratins.[91] In particular, there is a close sequence homology with keratin 14,[91] which is overexpressed in psoriatic skin compared with normal skin.[92] Valdimarsson et al.[93] found that T lymphocytes isolated from patients with chronic plaque psoriasis were stimulated by M protein and smaller M protein peptides that shared amino acid sequences with type 1 keratins. Stimulation was negligible with T cells from normal patients and not detected with T cells from patients with atopic dermatitis. Stimulation resulted in the production of interferon-gamma,[93] a prominent cytokine in psoriatic skin lesions.[94] After UVB phototherapy, cells collected from psoriatic patients became unresponsive to M-protein and M-protein peptides.[92]

Histogenesis

Current evidence indicates that activation of CD4+ T lymphocytes[62,63] and the subsequent recruitment and activation of CD8+ T cells[61,64,65] is the initial step in the development of psoriasis. The activated CD4+ and CD8+ T cells release a variety of cytokines that promote adhesion molecule formation on keratinocytes[95] and endothelial cells[96] and increased expression of the T-lymphocyte activation molecule CDw60 on keratinocytes.[97] This promotes T-cell infiltration of the epidermis. The ensuing cytokine–induced hyperplasia of the epidermis[56,72] may be due to a shortening of the cell cycle time,[73] an increased growth fraction of basal cells due to recruitment of resting basal cells,[74,75] and/or reduced apoptosis of keratinocytes.[76–78] In guttate psoriasis, CD4+ T-cell activation may be initiated by streptococcal superantigens[88] and perpetuated through the development of M-protein-specific T cells that cross-react with keratin.[93] In chronic plaque psoriasis, the antigen responsible may be streptococcal or an as yet unidentified antigen.

Histologic findings

Established plaque psoriasis is characterized by a number of epidermal changes consisting of (a) acanthosis of the epidermis resulting in club-like elongation of the rete ridges and thinning of the suprapapillary portions of the epidermis, (b) absence of the granular layer with overlying parakeratosis, and (c) collections of neutrophils within the stratum corneum (Munro microabscess). The underlying dermis exhibits elongation of dermal papillae and a mild to moderate lymphohistiocytic infiltrate.[98]

Differential diagnosis

Psoriasis in the diaper area can be distinguished from irritant diaper dermatitis by the confluent nature of the erythema, the involvement of the groin folds, and the shaply delineated edges of the affected area. Zinc deficiency should be considered and excluded if the infant is irritable and has a similar psoriasiform eruption around the mouth. Psoriasis on the scalp can be misdiagnosed as tinea capitis or seborrheic dermatitis. Tinea can be excluded with potassium hydroxide (KOH) microscopy and fungal culture. Seborrheic dermatitis is distinguished by the presence of scaling without plaque formation. Notably, seborrheic dermatitis on the scalp is a postpubertal disorder and any prepubertal child after the age of two with seborrheic dermatitis-like changes on the scalp is most likely to have psoriasis. Psoriatic plaques on exposed areas of the body can be mistaken for chronic discoid eczema (nummular), tinea, or lichen planus. Discoid eczema is very itchy and has an eczematous surface on examination. Tinea can be excluded with KOH microscopy and fungal culture. Lichen planus is distinguished by the violaceous color and the presence of Wickham's striae on the surface. Flexural psoriasis can be distinguished from candidiasis, tinea, and erythrasma with culture and Wood's light examination (erythrasma). The eruptive nature of guttate psoriasis can lead to confusion with pityriasis rosea and syphilis. The history of a herald patch, the Christmas tree-like configuration of lesions on the trunk, and the appearance of the surface scale (collarete) distinguishes pityriasis rosea. Serology will exclude secondary syphilis. All children presenting with psoriatic nail changes should have clippings collected for fungal culture to exclude tinea unguium.

THERAPY AND PROGNOSIS

General principles

During the initial consultation, it is important to discuss the pathogenesis, clinical course, prognosis, and treatment options with the patient and care providers. The two aspects of pathogenesis to highlight with parents are the importance of dealing with triggering factors (eg. streptococcal infection) in susceptible children and the noninfectious nature of psoriasis. The latter point will help parents and patients quickly deal with concerns expressed by other children and adults. Most parents attend the initial consultation unaware that their child has a common condition for which there is no permanent cure and are understandably upset when given the news. Subsequent discussion should focus on the fact that most children have mild psoriasis that is responsive to a variety of treatments. The response can vary from improvement, with maintenance at a cosmetically acceptable level, to complete clearance. The severity of the psoriasis, the site of the psoriasis, and the views of the patient and parents determine the choice of treatment. The treatment options for pediatric psoriasis are listed in Table 15.1. Treatment can be administered as monotherapy or in various combinations. Combination therapy and rotational therapy are gaining support as a way of improving efficacy and reducing the risk of short-, medium- and long-term side effects. Most children can be well controlled with topical therapy. Phototherapy is the preferred option for older children with widespread plaque psoriasis not responding to topical therapy. Systemic therapy is reserved for children with severe disease not responding to topical and phototherapy.

89. Lewis HM, Baker BS, Bokth S et al. (1993) Restricted T-cell receptor VB gene usage in the skin of patients with guttate and chronic plaque psoriasis. Br J Dermatol 129:514–520.

90. Manjula BN, Trus BL, Fischetti VA (1985) Presence of the distinct regions in the coiled-coil structure of the streptococcal PepM5 protein: Relationship to mammalian coiled-coil proteins and implications to its biological properties. Proc Natl Acad Sci 82:1064–1068.

91. McFadden J, Valdimarsson H, Fry L (1991) Cross-reactivity between streptococcal M surface antigen and human skin. Br J Dermatol 125:443–447.

92. Leigh IM, Navsaria H, Purkis PE et al. (1995) Keratinss 16 and 17 as markers of keratinocyte hyperproliferation in psoriasis in vivo and in vitro. Br J Dermatol 133:501–511.

93. Valdimarsson H, Sigmunddottir H, Jonsdottir I (1997) Is psoriasis induced by streptococcal superantigens and maintained by M-protein-specific T cells that cross react with keratin. Clin Exp Immunol 107(Suppl. 1):21–24.

94. Uyemura K, Yamamura M, Fivenson DF et al. (1993) The cytokine network in lesional and lesion-free psoriatic skin is characterised by a T-helper type 1 cell-mediated response. J Invest Dermatol 101:701–705.

95. Dustin ML, Singer KH, Tuck DT et al. (1988) Adhesion of T lymphoblasts to epidermal keratinocytes is regulated by interferon-gamma and is mediated by intercellular adhesion molecule-1 (ICAM-1). J Exp Med 167:1323–1340.

96. Groves RW, Allen MH, Barker JNWN et al. (1991) Endothelial leukocyte adhesion molecule-1 (ELAM-1) expression in cutaneous inflammation. Br J Dermatol 124:117–123.

97. Skov L, Chan LS, Fox DA et al. (1997) Lesional psoriatic T cells contain the capacity to induce a T cell activation molecule CDw60 on normal keratinocytes. Am J Pathol 150:675–683.

98. Lever WF, Schaumburg-Lever G (1975) Histopathology of the skin. 5th ed. Philadelphia: JB Lippincott.

TABLE 15.1 Treatment options for pediatric psoriasis

Topical
    Topical steroids
    Vitamin D analogues
    Coal tar preparations
    Anthralin
    Tazarotene
    Salicylic acid preparations

Phototherapy
    UVB
    Narrow band UVB
    PUVA

Systemic therapy
    Antibiotics
    Acitretin
    Methotrexate
    Cyclosporin

Topical therapy

TOPICAL STEROIDS

Topical corticosteroids are the most commonly prescribed topical therapy for pediatric psoriasis.[99] Their popularity is due to availability, cosmetic acceptability, efficacy, and ease of application. They are particularly useful when pruritus is a problem and for psoriasis on the face, in the flexures, on the genitalia, and around the ears. Creams and ointment preparations are used on the body and lotions and foams are preferred for the scalp. The site of psoriasis determines the strength of the topical steroid. Moderately potent (e.g., betamethasone valerate or triamcinolone acetonide) or potent (e.g., fluocinonide acetonide) steroids are needed for clinical improvement of psoriasis on the scalp, trunk, and limbs. Weaker preparations (e.g., hydrocortisone) are used for psoriasis on sensitive sites such as the face, around the ears, in the flexures, and on the genitalia for safety reasons. The most common side effects of potent topical steroid therapy are atrophy and striae at the site of application following prolonged use. A rare side effect is suppression of the hypothalamic-pituitary-adrenal axis following prolonged, widespread application of a potent topical steroid in infants and young children.[100] The risk of side effects can be minimized by monitoring the amount of steroid used, ensuring the steroid is applied to the correct site, and discouraging continuous use of topical steroids over a long period of time. Strategies to minimize continuous use include intermittent or cyclic therapy, and combination or rotational therapy. Topical steroids have been combined with calcitriol[101–103] and tazarotene[104] in adult patients with greater efficacy, increased duration of remission, and reduction in steroid use. Rotational therapy for mild to moderate psoriasis would involve alternating topical steroids with one of the topical treatments listed in Table 15.1.

CALCIPOTRIOL (VITAMIN D)

Calcipotriol (vitamin D3) is an effective treatment for mild to moderate plaque psoriasis in adults[105,106] and children.[107,108] It is available as a cream, ointment, and lotion. A recent systematic review of the comparative efficacy and tolerability of topical calcipotriol found it to be as effective as potent topical steroids and more effective than tar cream and anthralin in the treatment of mild to moderate plaque psoriasis.[109] Increased efficacy was noted when calcipotriol and potent topical steroids were both applied once a day,[101,102] when calcipotriol was applied twice daily on weekdays with a potent topical steroid applied twice daily on weekends[103] and with twice daily application of calcipotriol with broad band UVB phototherapy.[110,111] The most common side effect is lesional and perilesional irritation, particularly when used on the face, scalp, and flexures; use on these sites should be avoided. To prevent hypercalcemia, the maximum recommended dose of 50g/week per m[2] should not be exceeded during treatment.[108]

COAL TAR PREPARATIONS

Coal tar preparations and shampoos are a useful treatment for mild psoriasis of the skin and scalp.[112] Use in older children and adolescents is limited because of poor compliance related to the smell and staining properties of coal tar. Coal tar preparations can be used on any site and are most effective with plaque psoriasis that has fine rather than thick surface scale. Coal tar is traditionally mixed with salicylic acid in a cream base and applied 2–3 times a day until clear. The strength of the cream is dependent on the age of the patient and the site of the psoriasis. Crude coal tar 2–4% is usually ordered in petrolatum and is applied bid. Because it is so messy, it is usually only used in a hospital setting. Refined tar (liquor carbonis detergens) is often mixed with salicylic acic and a topical steroid. Tar shampoo is used daily as monotherapy or in combination with topical therapy such as tar preparations and steroid lotions. Crude coal tar cream was traditionally combined with UVB therapy (Goeckerman therapy) in a psoriasis day treatment center or hospital for severe widespread plaque psoriasis.[113] A modified Goeckerman treatment can be used at home during the warmer months of the year for school-aged children with the overnight application of tar cream and daily sunlight exposure. The duration of sunlight exposure should be increased slowly to minimize the chances of a phototoxicity reaction between the UVA component of sunlight and the tar cream.

ANTHRALIN

Anthralin is an old and effective treatment for chronic plaque psoriasis.[114] It is traditionally applied as short contact therapy that involves the application of anthralin cream or ointment 0.1–1% to the psoriatic plaques for a short period (10–60 minutes) before wiping and washing off.[115] Clearance is accompanied by temporary staining of perilesional skin. In view of the risk of burning perilesional skin if carelessly applied and permanent staining of any object (e.g., clothing) with which it is in contact, use is restricted to older, cooperative children with large plaque psoriasis. Perilesional staining and irritation can be minimized by the use of a topical spray-on preparation containing triethanolamine (CuraStain) which is sprayed on before and after removing the

99. Stern KS (1996) Utilization of outpatient care for psoriasis. **J Am Acad Dermatol** 35:543–545.
100. McGibbon DH (1979) Infantile pustular psoriasis. **Clin Exp Dermatol** 4:115–118.
101. Lebwohl M, Siskin SB, Epinette W et al. (1996) A multicenter trial of calcipotriene ointment and halobetasol ointment compared with either agent alone for the treatment of psoriasis. **J Am Acad Dermatol** 35:268–269.
102. Kragballe K, Barnes L, Hamberg KJ et al. (1998) Calcipotriol cream with or without concurrent topical corticosteroids in psoriasis: tolerability and efficacy. **Br J Dermatol** 139:649–664.
103. Lebwohl M, Yoles A, Lombardi K et al. (1998) Calcipotriene ointment and halbetasol ointment in the long term treatment of psoriasis: effects on the duration of improvement. **J Am Acad Dermatol** 39:447–450.
104. Lebwohl MG, Breneman DL, Goffe BS et al. (1998) Tazarotene 0.1% gel plus corticosteroid cream in the treatment of plaque psoriasis. **J Am Acad Dermatol** 39:590–596.
105. Highton A, Quell J (1995) Calcipotriene Study Group. Calcipotriene ointment .005% for psoriasis: a safety and efficacy study. **J Am Acad Dermatol** 32:67–72.
106. Harrington CI, Goldin D, Lovell CR et al. (1996) Comparative effects of two different calcipotriol (MC903) formulations versus placebo in psoriasis vulgaris: a randomised, double-blind, placebo controlled, parallel group multicentre study. **J Eur Acad Dermatol Venereol** 6:152–158.
107. Darley CR, Cunliffe WJ, Green CM et al. (1996) Safety and efficacy of calcipotriol ointment (Dovonex) in treating children with psoriasis vulgaris. **Br J Dermatol** 135:390–393.
108. Oranje AP, Marcoux D, Svensson A et al. (1997) Topical calcipotriol in childhood psoriasis. **J Am Acad Dermatol** 36:203–208.
109. Ashcroft DM, Li Wan Po A, Williams HC et al. (2000) Systematic review of comparative efficacy and tolerability of calcipotriol in treating chronic plaque psoriasis. **BMJ** 320:963–967.
110. Kragballe K (1990) Combination of topical calcipotriol (MC903) and UVB radiation for psoriasis vulgaris. **Dermatologica** 181:211–214.
111. Ramsay CA, Schwartz BE, Lowson D et al. (2000) Calcipotriol cream combined with twice weekly broad-band UVB phototherapy: a safe, effective and UVB-sparing antipsoriatic combination treatment. The Canadian Calcipotriol and UVB Study Group. **Dermatology** 200:17–24.
112. Farber EM, Jacobs AH (1977) Infantile psoriasis. **Am J Dis Child** 131:1266–1269.
113. Menter A, Cram DL (1983) The Goeckerman regimen in two psoriasis day care centers. **J Am Acad Dermatol** 9:59–65.
114. Zvulunov A, Anisfeld A, Metzker A (1994) Efficacy of short-contact therapy with dithranol in childhood psoriasis. **Int J Dermatol** 33:808–810.
115. Schaefer H (1985) Short-contact therapy. **Arch Dermatol** 121:1505–1508.

anthralin.[116] The second option involves an anthralin formulation (Micanol) that encapsulates anthralin in a matrix of semicrystalline monoglycerides known as crystalip.[117] The monoglycerides protect the anthralin from oxidation resulting in reduced perilesional staining. The anthralin is only released from the vehicle at a temperature higher than normal skin temperature, which minimizes release on normal skin. The higher temperature is achieved as the cream is rubbed into the psoriatic plaque. The cream is left on for 10–30 minutes before removing with lukewarm water.[118] Anthralin therapy can be combined with other topical therapies and UVB phototherapy.

TAZAROTENE

Tazarotene is the only topical retinoid approved for the treatment of psoriasis vulgaris. It is available as a 0.05% and 0.1% gel and cream. All of the data regarding efficacy and safety relate to adult patients. Although tazarotene monotherapy compares favorably with mid-potency topical steroid therapy,[119] local irritation is a common problem that limits its use. Increased efficacy, reduced local irritation, and longer duration of remission is achieved when tazarotene 0.1% gel is combined with a potent topical steroid.[120] Preliminary data suggest greater efficacy when combined with topical calcipotriol.[121] Tazarotene 0.1% gel therapy also enhances response to broad-band UVB,[122] narrow-band UVB,[123] and PUVA bath phototherapy[124] with the potential benefit of reducing the total dose of ultraviolet light exposure, long-term photodamage, and carcinogenicity.

MISCELLANEOUS

Keratolytic preparations (5–10% salicylic acid in an oil, lotion, cream, or ointment base) are needed when scalp scale is thick and firmly adherent (tinea amiantacea). The keratolytics are used on a daily basis until the thick scale has lifted. This may be used overnight, shampooed out, and then followed by an active ingredient or continued with other agents.

Onycholysis and nail bed hyperkeratosis in children can be treated with steroid lotions, calcipotriol lotion, or a potent topical steroid cream/ointment applied to the nail fold above the matrix. Intralesional steroid injection of the nail matrix is not suitable for pediatric patients.

Phototherapy

Phototherapy is reserved for children with severe widespread plaque psoriasis that is not responding to topical therapy. It can only be used in children mature enough to cope with the confines of the phototherapy cabinet. Informed consent is essential to ensure the patient and family are fully aware of the potential short- (burning) and long-term (photoaging, carcinogenicity) side effects of phototherapy. UVB is the preferred form of phototherapy with narrow-band UVB more effective than broad band.[125] UVB phototherapy is administered three times a week in an outpatient setting until clearance occurs. The efficacy of UVB phototherapy can be enhanced and total dose reduced when combined with tar preparations,[113] short contact anthralin,[126]

topical tazarotene,[123,124] and acitretin.[127–129] PUVA phototherapy is not recommended for pre-adolescent pediatric psoriasis because of the risk of ocular damage during treatment and the long-term risk of skin cancer.[130]

Systemic therapy

Although there is no evidence that antibiotic therapy alters the natural course of streptococcal-induced guttate psoriasis, children with guttate psoriasis and a documented Group A beta-hemolytic infection are often treated with penicillin or erythromycin for 7–10 days. Other systemic therapy is reserved for infants, children, and teenagers with severe plaque psoriasis that has failed to respond to topical and phototherapy and is of sufficiently significant physical and/or cosmetic concern. Informed consent is crucial because of the risk of significant side effects with oral treatment. The three options for oral therapy of pediatric psoriasis are acitretin, methotrexate, and cyclosporin. Acitretin, an aromatic retinoid, is the most commonly used oral medication. It can be used as monotherapy in the treatment of chronic plaque psoriasis, but it is most effective when combined with UVB phototherapy.[127–129] Menstruating females must be informed of the teratogenic potential of acitretin and the need to avoid pregnancy with adequate contraception for a minimum of two years after stopping the medication. After ensuring the patients liver function tests, fasting lipids, and pregnancy test (when appropriate) are normal or negative, the patient is started on a dose of 0.5–0.75mg/kg per day. When given in combination with UVB phototherapy, acitretin is usually begun 2 weeks before the start of light therapy. Acitretin can be started during the course of UVB therapy if needed, provided the dose of UVB is reduced to prevent burning. Routine follow-up investigations (liver function tests, fasting lipids) are needed at regular intervals to monitor for abnormal liver function and elevated serum lipids. When clearance occurs, the UVB and acitretin are stopped. Prolonged acitretin therapy should be avoided because of the risk of premature epiphyseal closure and impaired bone growth.[131]

Methotrexate and cyclosporin are used in children, teenagers, and adult patients with severe psoriasis. Methotrexate is administered once a week as a single dose or divided into two or three doses over a 24 hour period. Patients need regular monitoring because of the potential risk of bone marrow supression and liver dysfunction. Although there are a number of case reports of methotrexate use in children suffering from severe psoriasis,[132–134] there are no studies detailing the efficacy and safety of methotrexate in pediatric psoriasis. Kumar et al.[133] used a dose of 0.2–0.4mg/kg per week to treat seven patients and, apart from nausea and vomiting in three patients, the medication was tolerated and efficacious in all patients. The dose is generally 0.3–0.5mg/kg to a maximum weekly dose of 15–20mg given concurrently with folic acid 1–5mg daily.

Cyclosporin is administered to adult psoriatics with an initial dose of 2.5mg/kg that is increased by 0.5mg–1.0mg/kg every four weeks, if needed, to a maximum dose of 5mg/kg per day. Treatment can be discontinued after remission is achieved and restarted if needed, or the dose

116. Ramsey B, Lawrence CM, Bruce JM et al. (1986) The effect of triethanolamine application on anthralin-induced inflammation and therapeutic effect in psoriasis. **J Am Acad Dermatol** 15:1247–1252.
117. Lindahl A (1992) Embedding of Dithranol in lipid crystals. **Acta Derm Venereol** (Suppl) 172:13–16.
118. Volden G, Bjornberg A, Tegner E et al. (1992) Short contact treatment at home with Micanol. **Acta Derm Venereol** (Suppl) 172:20–22.
119. Lebwohl MG, Ast E, Callen JP et al. (1998) Once-daily tazarotene gel versus twice-daily fluocinonide cream in the treatment of plaque psoriasis. **J Am Acad Dermatol** 38:705–711.
120. Lebwohl MG, Breneman DL, Goffe BS et al. (1998) Tazarotene 0.1% gel plus corticosteroid cream in the treatment of plaque psoriasis. **J Am Acad Dermatol** 39:590–596.
121. Tahnghetti EA (1999) Photographic tracking study of tazarotene treatment alone and in conjunction with mometasone furoate cream or calcipotriene ointment, in mild to moderate plaque psoriasis. Poster presented at the 57th Annual Meeting of the American Academy of Dermatology, March 19–24, New Orleans, LA.
122. Lowe NJ (1999) Ultraviolet B phototherapy plus topical retinoid therapy. **Cutis** 63(3S):6–7.
123. Stege H, Reifenberger J, Bruch-Gerharz D et al. (1998) UVB-311-nm-phototherapie in kombination mit topischer applikation von tazaroten zur behandlung der psoriasis vulgaris. **Z Hautkrank H 1** G 73(10):708–709.
124. Krutmann J (1998) Combination therapy of psoriasis with 311nm UVB phototherapy plus tazarotene. Oral presentation at the Joint Meeting of the 5th European Congress on Psoriasis at the 7th International Psoriasis Symposium. September 3, Milan, Italy.

125. Green C, Ferguson J, Lakshmipathi T et al. (1988) 311 nm UVB phototherapy—an effective treatment for psoriasis. **Br J Dermatol** 119:691–696.
126. Vella-Briffa D, Greaves MW, Warin AP et al. (1981) Relapse rate and long-term management of plaque psoriasis after treatment with photochemotherapy and dithranol. **Br Med J Clin Res Ed** 282:937–940.
127. Ruzicka T, Sommerburg C, Braun-Falco O et al. (1990) Efficiency of acitretin in combination with UV-B in the treatment of psoriasis. **Arch Dermatol** 126:482–486.
128. Lowe N, Prystowsky JH, Bourget T et al. (1991) Acitretin plus UVB therapy for psoriasis: comparisons with placebo plus UVB and acitretin. **J Am Acad Dermatol** 24:591–594.
129. Iest J, Boer J (1989) Combined treatment of psoriasis with acitretin and UVB phototherapy compared with acitretin alone and UVB alone. **Br J Dermatol** 120:665–670.
130. Stern RS, Liebman EJ, Vakeva L et al. (1998) Oral psoralen and ultraviolet-A light (PUVA) treatment of psoriasis and persistent risk of nonmelanoma skin cancer. **J Natl Cancer Inst** 90:1278–1284.
131. Paige DG, Judge MR, Shaw DG et al. (1992) Bone changes and their significance in children with ichthyosis an long-term etretinate therapy. **Br J Dermatol** 127:387–391.
132. Khan SA, Grant Peterkin GA, Mitchell PC (1972) Juvenile generalised pustular-psoriasis. **Arch Derm** 105:67–72.
133. Kumar B, Dhar S, Handa S et al. (1994) Methotrexate in childhood psoriasis. **Pediatr Dermatol** 11:271–273.
134. Juanquin G, Conejomir JS, Ruiz AP et al. (1998) Evaluation of the effectiveness of childhood generalised pustular psoriasis. **Pediatr Dermatol** 15:144–146.

can be gradually reduced by 0.5mg/kg per day every month until the patient is on the lowest dose needed to maintain long-term control. Provided the patient is monitored for side effects, treatment can be continued for up to two years.[135] Although cyclosporin has been studied extensively in pediatric atopic dermatitis,[136] there are no studies examining the efficacy and safety of this therapy for pediatric psoriasis. Most of the case reports of cyclosporin use in pediatric psoriasis involve patients with pustular psoriasis. Cyclosporin was reported to be ineffective in two infants with severe plaque psoriasis.[137] The use of cyclosporin should be reserved for the most severe cases exhibiting significant morbidity and lack of response to alternative therapy.

Prognosis

Most children have mild psoriasis that is responsive to topical therapy. The response varies from improvement with maintenance at a cosmetically acceptable level to complete clearance. Although clearance can be followed by prolonged remission, a chronic relapsing course with intermittent treatment is a feature of most cases. Some children worsen with age, requiring aggressive treatment. Children with guttate psoriasis can clear and have no further problems, redevelop psoriasis only following a streptococcal infection, or gradually develop chronic plaque psoriasis.

PEDIATRIC ASPECTS OF THE DISEASE

Pediatric psoriasis differs from adult psoriasis in terms of morphology, distribution, and approach to management. Plaque psoriasis in children often has finer scale and more commonly manifests on the face, in the flexures, and in a guttate pattern. Nail involvement is less common than with adult patients. Management is more conservative with an emphasis on topical therapy. Phototherapy and systemic therapy are reserved for severe cases. Emotional support of the patient and family is often necessary.

PUSTULAR PSORIASIS

The term pustular psoriasis refers to a group of entities characterized by the development of multiple sterile pustules on an erythematous skin, which can be divided clinically into localized and generalized forms. Localized pustular psoriasis is further subdivided into palmoplantar pustulosis, digital pustulosis (acrodermatitis continua of Hallopeau), and plaque psoriasis that develops surface pustules. Generalized pustular psoriasis is subdivided into acute generalized pustular psoriasis (Von Zumbusch), an annular variant, and impetigo herpetiformis, which refers to acute generalized pustular psoriasis during pregnancy. There is considerable overlap between the acute generalized and annular types and this clinical scenario is often referred to as the mixed variant of generalized pustular psoriasis.[138] Although one study reported digital pustulosis as the most common type of pustular psoriasis in children,[48] the acute generalized and annular forms were the most common types in all other studies.[138–145] A recent review of 39 cases of pustular psoriasis in children by Liao et al.[145] found the annular and mixed forms to be more common than the acute generalized form.

EPIDEMIOLOGY

Genetics

No link has been established between any forms of pustular psoriasis and HLA antigens B13, B17 and Cw6 that are strongly associated with psoriasis vulgaris.[146,147] A link has been found between acute generalized pustular psoriasis and HLA B27.[147] Pustular psoriasis has been reported in siblings,[148] including monozygotic twins[149] and a family history of psoriasis is found in up to 25% of patients.[139]

Statistics

All forms of pustular psoriasis are rare in the pediatric age group.[48,139–140] Only 68 cases were recorded in one series of 1262 pediatric patients with psoriasis[48] and five cases in another series of 479 children with psoriasis.[140] In a series of 104 cases of pustular psoriasis involving patients of all ages, there were only five pediatric patients.[138] Although most reported cases involve the 2–10-year age group, pustular psoriasis can be present at birth[141] or develop at any time during infancy, childhood, or adolescence.[48,138–142] There is a predilection for males, particularly during the first two years of life.[139,141,142]

PRESENTING HISTORY

The acute generalized form of pustular psoriasis presents with the abrupt onset of tender, burning erythema over large areas of the body and increased erythema within pre-existing plaques of psoriasis. Surface pustules develop within 24 hours. The eruption is accompanied by high fever, malaise, and arthralgias.[138–145] The annular form presents with scattered erythematous areas that are plaque-like or annular in appearance with overlying surface pustules towards the periphery of the lesions. Children can be systemically well or have accompanying fever and malaise, which tends to be less severe compared with the acute generalized form.[138–145] Many of the acute generalized, annular, and mixed forms have a preceding history of psoriatic diaper rash as babies or an eruption diagnosed as seborrheic dermatitis.[138,139,143,144] Patients with the palmoplantar and digital forms present with a pustular eruption on acral sites that is not accompanied by a systemic illness. A personal history of plaque psoriasis and/or family history of pustular or plaque psoriasis may be obtained from patients with all types of pustular psoriasis.

PHYSICAL EXAMINATION

In the acute generalized form of pustular psoriasis, the skin is erythematous with superimposed pustules (Fig. 15.13). The extent of skin involvement varies from involvement of large but discrete areas to complete erythroderma. The overlying pustules may remain discrete (1–3mm) or quickly coalesce to produce lakes of pus before drying over a 3–4 day period with pronounced desquamation. Successive waves of pustules develop in severely affected patients over several weeks.[138–145] A linear pattern of pustular psoriasis following the lines of Blaschko has been reported in two adult patients with acute generalized pustular psoriasis.[150,151] The annular form is characterized by scattered, well-delineated, erythematous plaques or annular

135. Lebwohl M, Ellis C, Gottlieb et al. (1998) Cyclosporin concensus conference: with emphasis on the treatment of psoriasis. **J Am Acad Dermatol** 39:464–475.
136. Berth-Jones J, Finlay AY, Zaki I et al. (1996) Cyclosporine in severe childhood atopic dermatitis: a multicentre study. **J Am Acad Dermatol** 34:1016–1021.
137. Mahe E, Bodemer C, Pruszkowski A et al. (2001) Cyclosporine in childhood psoriasis. **Arch Dermatol** 137:1532–1533.
138. Baker H, Ryan TJ (1968) Generalised pustular psoriasis. **Br J Dermatol** 80:771–793.
139. Beylot C, Bioulac P, Grupper C et al. (1977) Generalised pustular psoriasis in infants and children: report of 27 cases. In: Psoriasis, Farber EM, Cox AJ, eds. Proceedings of the 2nd International Symposium New York: Yorke Medical Books, pp. 171–179.
140. Marill FG, Vodov I (1974) Psoriasis pustuleux chez des enfants. Remarques a propos de cinq cas. **Bull Soc Fr Dermatol Syphyiligr** 81:590–592.
141. Beylot C, Puissant A, Bioulac P et al. (1979) Particular clinical features of psoriasis in infants and childre. **Acta Dermatol Venereol** (Stockh) 59 (Suppl 87):95–97.
142. Juanqin G, Zhiqiang C, Zuia H (1998) Evaluation of the effectiveness of childhood generalised pustular psoriasis treatment in 30 cases. **Pediatr Dermatol** 15:144–146.
143. Khan SA, Peterkin GAG, Mitchell PC (1972) Juvenile generalised pustular psoriasis. A report of 5 cases and a review of the literature. **Arch Dermatol** 105:67–72.
144. Zelickson BD, Muller SA (1991) Generalised pustular psoriasis in childhood. **J Am Acad Dermatol** 24:186–194.
145. Liao PB, Rubinson R, Howard R et al. (2002) Annular pustular psoriasis – Most common form of pustular psoriasis in children: Report of three cases and review of the literature. **Pediatr Dermatol** 19:19–25.
146. Zachariae H, Peterson HO, Nielsen FK et al. (1977) The HLA antigens in pustular psoriasis. **Dermatologica** 154:73.
147. Karvonen J, Tiilikainen A, Lassus A (1977) HLA antigens in psoriasis. In: Psoriasis, Farber EM, Cox AJ, Jacobs PH, Nall ML, eds. Proceedings of the 2nd International Symposium. New York: Yorke Medical Books, pp. 405–408.
148. Huber WR (1984) Familial juvenile generalised pustular psoriasis. **Arch Dermatol** 120:1174–1178.
149. Takematsu H, Rokugo M, Takahashi K et al. (1992) Juvenile generalised pustular psoriasis in a pair of monozygotic twins presenting strikingly similar clinical courses. **Acta Dermatol Venereol** 72:443–444.
150. Kanoh H, Ichihashi N, Kamiya H et al. (1998) Linear pustular psoriasis that developed in a patient with generalised pustular psoriasis. **J Am Acad Dermatol** 39:635–637.
151. Ozkaya-Bayazit E, Akasya E, Buyukbabani N et al. (2000) Pustular psoriasis with a striking linear pattern. **J Am Acad Dermatol** 42:329–331.

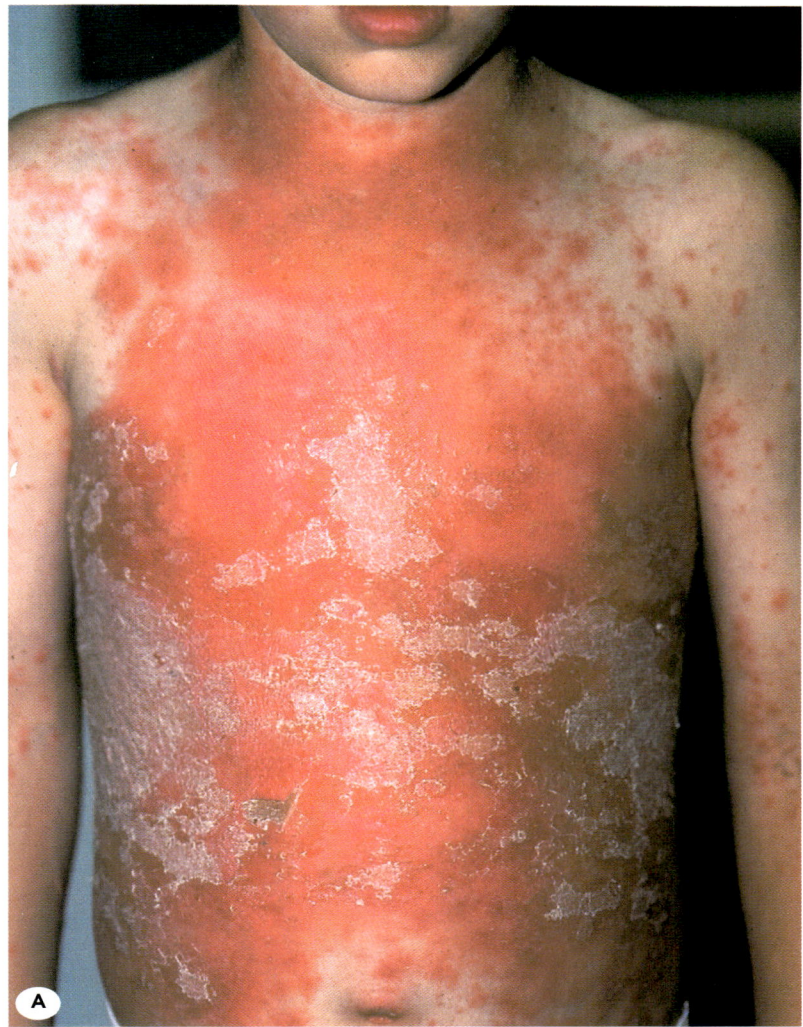

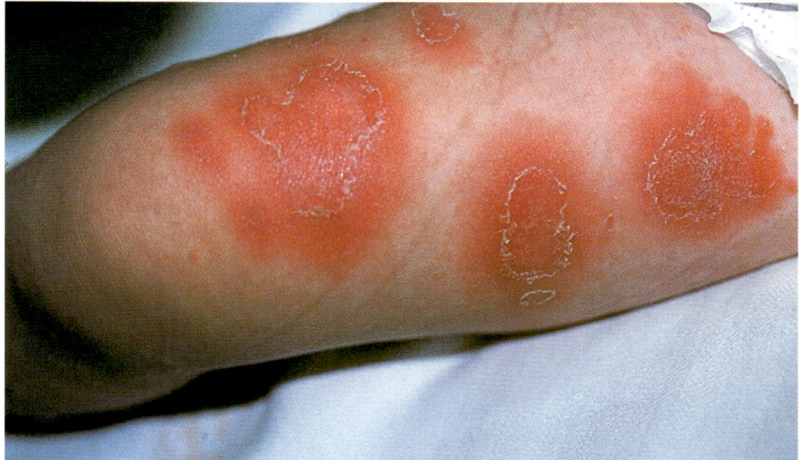

Fig. 15.14   Annular pustular psoriasis.

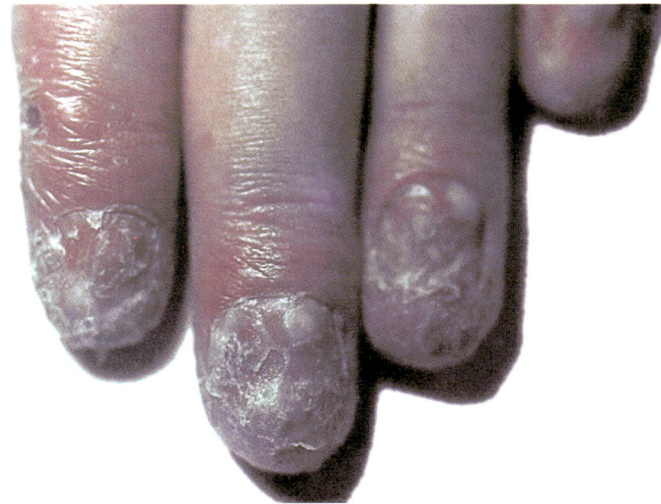

Fig. 15.15   Acropustulosis continua.

lesions with centrifugal enlargement and central clearing (Fig. 15.14). Pustules and desquamation are scattered over the surface of the plaques or along the advancing edge of the annular lesions.[138,139,141–145] The palmoplantar form manifests as pustules on the peripheral and/or central aspects of the palms and soles. As the pustules dry, they develop a characteristic reddish-brown color prior to desquamation. Pruritus is a variable feature.[152] The digital form (acrodermatitis continua of Hallopeau) is characterised by "glazed" erythema, scaling, and pustules on the distal end of a finger and/or toe with dystrophy of the adjacent nail and swelling of the paronychial area (Fig. 15.15).[153] The skin changes are tender and painful rather than pruritic.

Associated findings

Severe cases of acute generalized pustular psoriasis in children may be accompanied by geographic tongue,[142,144] alopecia,[144] nail shedding, nail

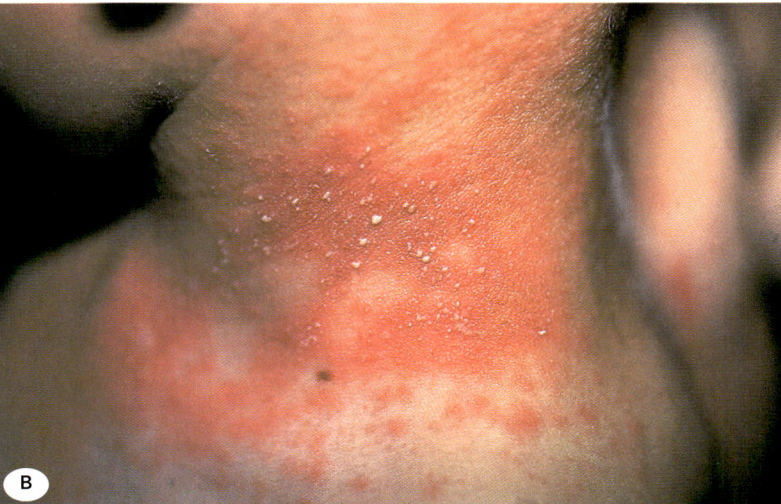

Fig. 15.13   (A) Generalized pustular psoriasis. (B) Generalized pustular psoriasis.

152. Baker H (1984) Pustular psoriasis. *Dermatol Clin* 2:455–470.

153. Mahowald ML, Parrish RM (1982) Severe osteolytic arthritis mutilans in pustular psoriasis. *Arch Dermatol* 118:434–437.

dystrophy,[144] and polyarthritis.[138,144] Rare commplications reported in children are renal failure, cholestatic jaundice,[154] lytic bone lesions,[155] and sterile multifocal osteomyelitis.[156] Rare complications reported in adults with severe acute generalized pustular psoriasis are acute respiratory distress syndrome requiring intubation and ventilation[157] and a number of eye changes which include purulent conjunctivitis, iridocyclitis, corneal ulceration, exfoliation of the cornea,[158] and uveitis.[159] Acute generalized pustular psoriasis was the initial presentation of multiple carboxylase deficiency in a Chinese infant.[160]

Laboratory findings

In severe acute generalized pustular psoriasis, investigations reveal marked leukocytosis with prominent neutrophilia. Some cases have hypoalbuminemia, hypocalcemia and, rarely, impairment of renal and liver function.

PATHOPHYSIOLOGY AND HISTOGENESIS

The development of generalized pustular psoriasis in predisposed children and teenagers can be triggered by the following; an upper respiratory tract infection,[142,144] urinary tract infection,[144] abrupt cessation of oral steroids,[142,144] tar cream therapy,[144] sunburn,[144] calcipotriol therapy,[161] cessation of cyclosporin therapy,[162] vaccination,[142] and pregnancy.[163] Additional triggering factors in adult cases include potent topical steroid therapy,[164] hydroxychloroquine,[165] and recombinant interferon beta injections for multiple sclerosis.[166]

Pustular psoriasis is characterized by massive infiltration of neutrophils into the epidermis resulting in pustule formation. The reasons for the massive infiltration are unknown. One study found the activity of skin derived antileukoproteinase, also known as elafin, significantly reduced in the epidermis of patients with pustular psoriasis patients compared with plaque psoriasis patients.[167] Elafin is an inducible epidermal serine proteinase inhibitor that protects the epidermis against damage caused by elastase and proteinase-3 released by infiltrating neutrophils.[168] Elafin gene expression in plaque psoriasis is greatest around subcorneal microabscesses, which supports a protective or damage-minimization role for elafin.[169] The decreased activity of elafin in pustular psoriasis may theoretically promote neutrophil-induced destruction of the epidermis and pustule formation.

Histologic findings

Pustular psoriasis is characterized by epidermal spongiosis and pronounced neutrophilic infiltration resulting in spongioform pustules (of Kogoj). Significant neutrophil collections are also found in the stratum corneum (Munro microabscesses). The epidermal and dermal features are otherwise those of plaque psoriasis.[98]

Differential diagnosis

Acute generalized pustular psoriasis needs to be distinguished from subcorneal pustular dermatosis, drug induced acute generalized pustular dermatosis (AGEP), and staphylococcal scalded skin syndrome (SSSS). Subcorneal pustular dermatosis is rare in children and does not exhibit spongiform epidermal pustules. This may be a variant of pustular psoriasis. Drug induced AGEP is clinically and histologically similar to acute generalized pustular psoriasis. Distinguishing between the two relies on a history of recent drug ingestion. The tender erythema of SSSS can mimic the very early stages of pustular psoriasis. The absence of pustule formation and the crusted moist eruption around the mouth and in the skin flexures distinguishes SSSS from pustular psoriasis. The main differential diagnosis for the annular form of pustular psoriasis is tinea corporis, erythema annular centrifigum, and Sweet syndrome. Tinea usually manifests as one lesion with positive KOH microscopy and fungal culture. Skin biopsy and routine histology will differentiate erythema annulare centrifigium and Sweet syndrome from pustular psoriasis. Tinea manuum and infected dyshidrotic dermatitis can mimic palmoplantar and digital pustulosis. A KOH microscopy and fungal culture will aid in differentiation. Persistence of pustules after antibiotic therapy and significant associated itch will distinguish infected dyshidrotic dermatitis.

THERAPY AND PROGNOSIS

Localized pustular psoriasis

Localized pustular psoriasis in children is managed adequately in most cases with topical therapy. The choices are potent topical corticosteroids, coal tar preparations, calcipotriol, or dithranol used as monotherapy or in combination. Oral therapy (see below) or PUVA with topically applied psoralen[170] are reserved for children with significant impairment unresponsive to topical therapy.

Generalized pustular psoriasis

The acute generalized type is best managed in the early stages in hospital to ensure adequate fluid intake, urine output, stable blood pressure, and to facilitate monitoring of serum electrolytes, albumin, calcium, liver, and renal function. Removal or treatment of a triggering factor may allow the process to settle with bed rest and the application of a weak topical steroid with or without overlying wet dressings.[144] For most patients, however, repeated waves of pustulation and the associated toxicity necessitates a more aggressive approach with oral therapy. Oral medications that have been used successfully in the treatment of acute generalized pustular psoriasis in children are retinoids,[142,144,171,172] methotrexate,[142,171,172] dapsone,[142,171,173] and cyclosporine.[171,172,174] The choice of oral medication is determined by drug availability, prescribers experience, and the patient's medical status. Particular

154. Li SP-S, Tang WY-M, Lam W-Y et al. (2000) Renal failure and cholestatic jaundice as unusual complications of childhood pustular psoriasis. Br J Dermatol 143:1292–1296.
155. Ivker RA, Grin-Jorgensen CM, Vega VK et al. (1993) Infantile generalised pustular psoriasis associated with lytic lesions of the bone. Pediatr Dermatol 10:277–282.
156. Prose NS, Fahrner L, Miller CR et al. (1994) Pustular psoriasis with chronic recurrent multifocal osteomyelitis and spontaneous fractures. J Am Acad Dermatol 31:376–379.
157. Sadeh JS, Rudikoff D, Gordon ML et al. (1997) Pustular and erythrodermic psoriasis complicated by acute respiratory distress syndrome. Arch Dermatol 133:747–750.
158. Lyons JH (1987) Generalised pustular psoriasis. Int J Dermatol 26:409–418.
159. Yamamoto T, Yokozeki H, Katayama I et al. (1995) Uveitis in patients with generalised pustular psoriasis. Br J Dermatol 132:1023–1024.
160. Law LK, Lau CY, Pang CP et al. (1997) An unusual case of multiple carboxylase deficiency presenting as generalised pustular psoriasis in a Chinese boy. J Inherit Metab Dis 20:106–107.
161. Georgala S, Rigopoulos D, Aroni K et al. (1994) Generalised pustular psoriasis precipitated by topical calcipotriol cream. Int J Dermatol 33:515–516.
162. Georgala S, Koumantaki E, Rallis E et al. (2000) Generalised pustular psoriasis developing during withdrawal of short-term cyclosporin therapy. Br J Dermatol 142:1057–1058.
163. Lee SH, Hunt MJ, Barnetson RS (1995) Pustular psoriasis of pregnancy. Australas J Dermatol 36:199–200.

164. Boxley JD, Dawber RPR, Summerly R (1975) Generalised pustular psoriasis on withdrawal of clobetasol propionate ointment. Br Med J ii:255–256.
165. Vine JE, Hymes SR, Warner NB et al. (1996) Pustular psoriasis induced by hydroxychloroquine: a case report and review of the literature. J Dermatol 23:357–361.
166. Webster GF, Knobler RL, Lublin FD et al. (1996) Cutaneous ulcerations and pustular psoriasis flare caused by recombinant interferon beta injections in patients with multiple sclerosis. J Am Acad Dermatol 34:365–367.
167. Kuijpers AL, Zeeuwen PL, de Jongh GJ et al. (1996) Skin derived antileukoproteinase (SKALP) is decreased in pustular forms of psoriasis. A clue to the pathogenesis of pustule formation. Arch Dermatol Res 288:641–647.
168. Alkemade JA, Molhuizen HO, Ponec M et al. (1994) SKALP/elafin is an inducible proteinase hibitor in human epidermal keratinocytes. J Cell Sci 107:2335–2342.
169. Nonomura K, Yamanishi K, Yasuno H et al. (1994) Up-regulation of elastin/SKALP gene expression in psoriatic epidermis. J Invest Dermatol 103:88–91.
170. Murray D, Warin AP (1979) Photochemotherapy for persistent palmplantar pustulosis (PPP). Br J Dermatol 101(Suppl 17):13–14.
171. Zelickson BD, Muller SA (1991) Generalised pustular psoriasis. Arch Dermatol 127:1339–1345.
172. Ozawa A, Ohkido M, Haruki Y et al. (1999) Treatments of generalised pustular psoriasis: a multicenter study in Japan. J Dermatol 26:141–149.
173. Yu HJ, Park JW, Park JM et al. (2001) A case of childhood generalised pustular psoriasis treated with dapsone. J Dermatol 28:316–319.

care is needed when using retinoids in females of child-bearing age because of its teratogenicity. As a general principle, treatment is initiated at an adequate dose and maintained until clearance occurs. The lowest possible dose required for disease control is determined and continued for as long as needed. Appropriate pretreatment and follow-up investigations are required, particularly during the early stages of the disease when organ dysfunction may be present. Oral corticosteroids are reserved for pregnant patients and non-pregnant patients with evidence of organ dysfunction. One child with cholestatic hepatitis and renal failure required intravenous methylprednisolone therapy to reverse organ dysfunction.[154]

Treatment for the annular and mixed forms of generalized pustular psoriasis is guided by the extent of the eruption and the presence and severity of the associated systemic illness. Topical steroids are sufficient for patients with mild-moderate skin disease and no systemic symptoms.[144,145] Patients with extensive skin disease and any patients with systemic symptoms require oral therapy.[143–145]

Prognosis

The course of generalized pustular psoriasis is variable. It may be a once-only phenomenon, it may recur at intermittent intervals over many years, it may persist indefinitely (annular form), or evolve into localized psoriasis. Morbidity and mortality with the acute generalized form is minimal because of improved medical management and hospital care. Localized pustular psoriasis tends to run a chronic course.

PSORIATIC ARTHRITIS

The first report of a patient with psoriasis and arthritis was made by Alibert in 1818.[175] A formal association between psoriasis and arthritis was reported by Bazin in 1860[176] and Bourdillon in 1888.[177] It was not until the early 1970s, with the implementation of Moll and Wright's classification,[178] that psoriatic arthritis was reliably distinguished from rheumatoid arthritis.

Psoriatic arthritis is an inflammatory arthritis that develops in patients with psoriasis. It is grouped with the other seronegative spondyloarthropathies; Reiter syndrome, ankylosing spondylitis and enteropathic arthritides. It is a heterogenous disease with five clinical subgroups as proposed by Moll and Wright.[178] The subgroups are listed in Table 15.2. There is considerable overlap between the subgroups and patients can evolve from one type to another.

TABLE 15.2   Classification of psoriatic arthritis

Arthritis of the distal interphalangeal joints of the hands and feet
Arthritis mutilans with sacroileitis
Symmetric arthritis indistinguishable from rheumatoid arthritis (negative rheumatoid factor)
Asymmetric pauciarticular arthritis with small joint involvement
Ankylosing spondylitis +/− peripheral arthritis

EPIDEMIOLOGY

Genetics

Studies have identified an association between psoriatic arthritis and HLA alleles Cw6,[179] particularly the Cw*0602 allele,[180] B27,[181] B39,[182] and DR4.[183] HLA-B27 is particularly associated with the sacroileitis variant of psoriatic arthritis. HLA-B39 is linked with poor prognosis and HLA-DR4 is associated with the polyarthritis variant of psoriatic arthritis. Other reported associations with psoriatic arthritis involve a polymorphism at position −238 in the promoter region of the tumour necrosis factor (TNF) gene[184] and a particular allele (MICA-A9) of the MICA gene[185] that encodes for MICA, a major histocompatibility complex-like molecule, whose function remains unknown.[37]

Statistics

Psoriatic arthritis develops in 5–30% of patients with psoriasis; onset is usually between 30 and 50 years of age.[186,187] The prevalence in the general community is 0.33%.[188] Onset of psoriatic arthritis can precede the onset of psoriasis (25%), coincide with development of psoriasis (15%), or succeed the development of psoriasis (60%). The time gap between the development of psoriasis and psoriatic arthritis can be many years.[189] Psoriatic arthritis accounts for 8–20% of cases of childhood arthritis.[190] The peak age of onset is 9–12 years of age with a slight female predominance.[191] With follow-up, 13% remain monoarticular/polyarticular, 10% develop a severe destructive arthropathy, and the remainder become polyarticular.[192]

PRESENTING HISTORY

Patients present to primary care physicians, dermatologists, or rheumatologists with pain involving one or more small or large joints. Many patients will exhibit features of one of the clinical subgroups outlined in Table 15.2. One study found 50% of children will have one joint involved at the time of first presentation.[192] If psoriasis is not clinically evident, a past or family history of psoriasis should be sought.

PHYSICAL EXAMINATION

Joints

The findings of joint examination on first presentation are extremely variable. In mild cases, little may be found apart from mild periarticular tenderness and limitation of movement. More severe cases exhibit varying degrees of tenderness, erythema, swelling, and limitation of joint movement. Sausage-like swelling of the digit is a particularly characteristic feature. Chronicity is associated with progressive reduction in range of movement and variable deformity of affected digits.

Hair, nails, teeth, mucous membranes, and associated findings

Most patients will have evidence of psoriasis vulgaris or pustular psoriasis at the time of initial presentation of the arthritis.[189] There is correlation between the severity of psoriasis and the presence and severity of psoriatic arthritis.[189]

174. Alli N, Gungor E, Karakayali G et al. (1998) The use of cyclosporin in a child with generalised pustular psoriasis. **Br J Dermatol** 139:754–755.
175. Alibert JL (1818) Precis Theorique sur les Malaides de la Peau. Paris: Caille et Ravier.
176. Bazin P (1860) Lecons Theoretiques et Cliniques sur les Affections Cutanees de Nature Arthritique et Arthreux. Paris: Delahaye.
177. Bourdillon C (1888) Psoriasis et arthropathies. MD Thesis, Paris.
178. Moll JM, Wright V (1973) Psoriatic arthritis. **Semin Arthritis Rheum** 3:55–78.
179. Rahman P, Schentag CT, Beaton M et al. (2000) Comparison of clinical and immunogenetic features in familial versus sporadic psoriatic arthritis. **Clin Exp Rheumatol** 18:7–12.
180. Gladman DD, Cheung C, Ng C-M et al. (1999) HLA-C locus alleles in patients with psoriatic arthritis (PsA). **Hum Immunol** 60:259–261.
181. Lambert JR, Wright V, Rajah SM et al. (1976) Histocompatibility antigens in psoriatic arthritis. **Ann Rheumatol Dis** 35:526.
182. Gladman DD, Farewell VT (1995) The role of HLA antigens as indicators of disease progression in psoriatic arthritis. Multivariate relative risk model. **Arthritis Rheum** 38:845–850.
183. Gladman DD, Anhorn KA, Schachter RK et al. (1986) HLA antigens in psoriatic arthritis. **J Rheumatol** 13:586–592.
184. Hamilton ML, Gladman DD, Shore A et al. (1990) Juvenile psoriatic arthritis and HLA antigens. **Ann Rheum Dis** 49:694–697.
185. Gonzalez S, Martinez-Borra J, Torre-Alonso Jc et al. (1999) The MICA-A9 triplet repeat polymorphism in the transmembrane region confers additional susceptibility to the development of psoriatic arthritis and is independent of the association of Cw*0602 in psoriasis. **Arthritis Rheum** 42:1010–1016.
186. Oriente CB, Scarpa R, Pucino A et al. (1989) Psoriasis and psoriatic arthritis: dermatological and rheumatological co-operative clinical report. **Acta Dermatol Venereol** (Stockh) 146(Suppl):69–71.
187. Espinoza LR, Cuellar ML, Silveira LH (1992) Psoriatic arthritis. **Curr Opin Rheumatol** 4:470–478.
188. Kay LJ, Parry-James JE, Walker DJ (1999) The prevalence and impact of psoriasis and psoriatic arthritis in the primary care populations in North East England. **Arthritis Rheum** 42(Suppl):S299.
189. Oriente P, Biondi-Oriente C, Scarpa R (1994) Psoriatic arthritis. Clinical manifestations. (Review). **Baillieres Clin Rheumatol** 8:277–294.
190. Southwood TR, Petty RE, Malleson PN et al. (1989) Psoriatic arthritis in children. **Arthritis Rheum** 32:1007–1013.
191. Shore A, Ansell BM (1982) Juvenile psoriatic arthritis; an analysis of 60 cases. **J Pediatr** 100:529.
192. Wright V (1961) Psoriatic arthritis. **Ann Rheum Dis** 20:123–132.

Psoriatic nail changes are found in 80% of psoriatic patients with arthritis compared with 20–30% of patients with skin disease only.[193] Inflammation of the eye can occur and manifests as conjunctivitis (20% cases), uveitis (10% cases), keratoconjunctivitis (3% cases), and episcleritis (2% cases).[194] Consequently, ophthalmologic assessment is needed if patients complain of eye irritation and/or pain.

Laboratory findings

There is no specific laboratory test to establish the diagnosis of psoriatic arthritis. Nonspecific laboratory findings include mild anemia, elevated erythrocyte sedimentation rate, elevated C–reactive protein, and negative rheumatoid factor.[195] The rheumatoid factor can be mildly positive with the polyarthritis form,[196] which may represent a coincidental finding because a positive rheumatoid factor occurs in 5% of the normal population.[197] Radiologic changes can be indistinguishable from rheumatoid arthritis with local demineralization, narrowing of joint spaces, articular erosions, and periarticular soft tissue swelling.[198] Four characteristic radiologic signs of psoriatic arthropathy noted in one series were; (a) destructive distal interphalangeal arthropathy with bony ankylosis of the interphalangeal joints, (b) destruction of the interphalangeal joints with abnormally wide joint spaces and sharply demarcated adjacent bony surfaces, (c) destruction of the interphalangeal joint of the great toe with bony proliferation of the distal phalanx, and (d) resorption of tufts of the distal phalanges of the hands and feet.[199] Fat suppression magnetic resonance imaging (MRI) has recently identified enthesitis (inflammation at sites of attachment of ligaments, tendons, joint capsule, and fascia to bone) in many patients with psoriatic arthritis.[200]

PATHOPHYSIOLOGY AND HISTOGENESIS

Recent debate has focused on whether the enthesis or synovium is the site of primary pathology in psoriatic arthritis. Fat suppression MRI has identified enthesitis as the initial process in some patients with early psoriatic arthritis.[200] It is proposed that enthesitis triggers the release of inflammatory mediators which induces inflammation of the adjacent synovium.[201] The reason for enthesitis is unknown. Evidence that supports the synovium as the primary site of pathology relates to examination of the T-cell infiltrates in synovial fluid. Studies have found oligoclonal expansion of CD4+ and CD8+ T cells within synovial fluid compared with peripheral blood CD4+ and CD8+ T cells. The clonal expansion is more pronounced with CD8+ T cells, resulting in a significant reduction in the CD4+ : CD8+ ratio.[69,202] This is in contrast with rheumatoid arthritis, which has a high CD4+ : CD8+ ratio due to clonal expansion of CD4+ T cells.[203] The clonal expansion of T cells within the joint suggests stimulation by an unidentified antigen. The finding of common T-cell clonal expansion in the synovium and skin suggests the involvement of a common antigen in the inflammatory process at both sites.[69]

Histologic findings

Histologically, one cannot distinguish psoriatic arthritis from rheumatoid arthritis, and synovial biopsy has no role in the diagnosis and management of psoriatic arthritis.

Differential diagnosis

The diagnosis of psoriatic arthritis is straightforward in patients with definite psoriasis. The polyarthritis form can be difficult to distinguish from rheumatoid arthritis in patients without psoriasis and a negative or weakly positive rheumatoid factor. In this situation, the correct diagnosis will come with time and observation. Distinguishing Reiter disease can be difficult and relies on identification of a triggering illness and the presence or history of urethritis.

THERAPY AND PROGNOSIS

Treatment should be initiated and supervised by a rheumatologist. Mild cases can usually be managed with nonsteroidal anti-inflammatory medication (e.g., naproxen) and intra-articular steroid injections. More severe cases require oral therapy such as methotrexate,[204] salfazalazine (sulphasalazine),[205] retinoids,[206] azathioprine,[207] or cyclosporine.[208] A systematic review of all medications, with the exception of cyclosporin, found that all were better than placebo. Intravenous methotrexate and salazapyrine were the most efficacious.[209] Oral corticosteroids are reserved for severe, fulminant cases with a high risk of irreversible crippling deformities. Physiotherapy is helpful in maintaining full movement in affected joints. Tumor necrosis factor inhibitors, such as etanercept and infliximab may also be efficacious.

Prognosis

The course of childhood psoriatic arthritis is very unpredictable, with numerous remissions and relapses. Severe cases may be rapidly progressive with marked destruction of many joints. In most children, disease activity is intermittent and long-term prognosis is good with minimal joint disease in adult life.[192] Poor prognostic indicators are numerous effusions, peripheral joint involvement, polyarthritis, and elevated erythrocyte sedimentation rate at the time of initial presentation.[210,211]

PEDIATRIC ASPECTS OF THE DISEASE

Education of patients and parents is essential because of the chronic and intermittent nature of psoriatic arthritis in most children. Early assessment by a rheumatologist is important to ensure optimum management.

REITER SYNDROME

In 1916, Hans Reiter reported a case of a young soldier with non-gonococcal urethritis, conjunctivitis, and arthritis following a dysenteric illness.[212] His

193. Eastwood CJ, Wright V (1979) The nail dystrophy of psoriatic arthritis. **Ann Rheumatol Dis** 38:226.
194. Lambert JR, Wright V (1976) Eye inflammation in psoriatic arthritis. **Ann Rheum Dis** 35:354–356.
195. Laurent MR (1985) Psoriatic arthritis. **Clin Rheum Dis** 11:50–55.
196. Roberts MET, Wright V, Hill AGS et al. (1976) Psoriatic arthritis: follow-up study. **Ann Rheum Dis** 35:206–212.
197. Waller M, Toone EC (1968) Normal individuals with positive tests for rheumatoid factor. **Arthritis Rheum** 11:50–55.
198. Lassus A, Mustakallio KK, Laine V (1964) Psoriasis arthropathy and rheumatoid arthritis. **Acta Rheum Scand** 10:62–68.
199. Avila R, Pugh DG, Slocumb Ch et al. (1960) Psoriatic arthritis: a roentgenologic study. **Radiology** 75:691–702.
200. McGonagle D, Gibbon W, O'Connor P et al. (1998) Characteristic magnetic resonance imaging entheseal changes in knee synovitis in spondyloarthropathy. **Arthritis Rheum** 41:694–700.
201. McGonagle D, Conaghan PG, Emery P (1999) Psoriatic arthritis: a unified concept twenty years on. **Arthritis Rheum** 42:1080–1086.
202. Costello P, Bresnihan B, O'Farrelly C et al. (1999) Predominance of CD81 T lymphocytes in psoriatic arthritis. **J Rheumatol** 26:1117–1124.
203. Goronzy JJ, Bartz-Bazzanella P, Hu W et al. (1994) Dominant clonotypes in the repertoire of peripheral CD41 T-cells in rheumatoid arthritis. **J Clin Invest** 94:2068–2076.
204. Willkens RF, Williams HJ, Ward JR et al. (1984) Randomised, double-blind placebo controlled trial of low-dose pulse methotrexate in psoriatic arthritis. **Arthritis Rheum** 27:376–381.
205. Clegg DO, Reda DJ, Mejias E et al. (1996) Comparison of sulphasalazine and placebo in the treatment of psoriatic arthritis: a Department of Veterans Affairs Cooperative Study. **Arthritis Rheum** 39:2013–2020.
206. Hopkins R, Bird HA, Jones H et al. (1985) A double-blind controlled trial of etretinate (Tigason) and ibuprofen in psoriatic arthritis. **Ann Rheum Dis** 44:189–193.
207. Levy J, Paulus HE, Barrett EV et al. (1972) A double-blind controlled evaluation of azathioprine treatment in rheumatoid arthritis and psoriatic arthritis. **Arthritis Rheum** 15:116–117.
208. Mahrle G, Schulze H-J, Brautigam M et al. (1996) Anti-inflammatory efficacy of low-dose cyclosporin A in psoriatic arthritis. A prospective multicentre study. **Br J Dermatol** 135:752–757.
209. Jones G, Crotty M, Brooks P (2000) Interventions for psoriatic arthritis. **Cochrane Database Syst Rev** 3:CD000212.
210. Jones Sm, Armas JM, Cohen MG et al. (1994) Psoriatic arthritis: outcome of disease subsets and relationship of joint disease to nail and skin disease. **Br J Rheumatol** 33:834–839.
211. Gladman DD, Fareqell VT, Nadeau C (1995) Clinical indicators of progression in psoriatic arthritis: multivariate relative risk model. **J Rheumatol** 22:675–679.
212. Reiter H (1916) Ueber eine bisher unerkannte spirochaeteninfektion. **Dtsch Med Wochenschr** 42:1535–1536.

name is now eponymously linked to the syndrome of reactive arthritis associated with urethritis and conjunctivitis.

EPIDEMIOLOGY

Genetics

Most adult[213] and pediatric cases[214–216] of Reiter syndrome are positive for the HLA-B27 antigen. HLA-B51 has also been associated with Reiter syndrome in one Japanese report.[217] Simulataneous occurrence in parents and children[218] and siblings has been reported.[215]

Statistics

In view of the rarity of Reiter syndrome in children, the incidence in this group is unknown. Most of the reported pediatric cases involve males and the age range at the time of presentation is 1.8–16 years.[214–216]

PRESENTING HISTORY

Children with Reiter disease usually present with conjuctivitis and/or asymmetric arthritis involving one or more joints.[214–216] Dysuria and mucocutaneous lesions are uncommon presenting features.[215] The complete triad of arthritis, conjunctivitis, and urethritis is rarely evident on presentation and can take 4–24 days to manifest.[215] Some patients fail to develop the complete triad.[214–216,219] Fever with anorexia, weight loss, and malaise may occur at the time of initial presentation.[215,216] Children and adolescents with Reiter syndrome usually have a history of a preceding gastrointestinal illness.[214–216] Adolescents should be questioned about sexual contacts and the presence of symptoms and/or signs suggestive of chlamydia infection.[215]

PHYSICAL EXAMINATION

Ocular

Conjunctivitis is the most common ocular manifestation of Reiter syndrome. It is bilateral and can vary in severity from mild injection to mucopurulent inflammation of the conjunctiva.[214–216] Infrequent ocular findings in pediatric cases are iritis,[220] keratitis,[221] corneal ulceration,[215] and optic neuritis.[222] Ocular manifestations are self-limited and no long-term sequelae have been reported.[215,216]

Joints

Although large weight-bearing joints (e.g., knee, ankle, hip) are the most commonly affected, any large (e.g., wrist) or small joint (e.g., metatarsophalangeal joint) can be affected.[214–216,220] Most pediatric cases have more than one joint involved in an asymmetric or, less commonly, symmetric distribution.[214–216,220] The affected joints exhibit warmth, tenderness, swelling, and limitation of movement. Unlike adult cases, sacroileitis is uncommon in pediatric cases.[223,224] Many patients will also have enthesitis (inflammation at the site of attachment of tendons and ligaments to bone).[215,219] The enthesitis gives rise to pain and focal tenderness. In most patients, the arthritis and enthesitis is self-limited with resolution occurring within a few months of onset. Occasionally, it lasts for several years as a chronic persistent or chronic recurring problem.[216]

Genitourinary

Most children have asymptomatic urethritis with sterile pyuria as the only evidence of urethral inflammation.[214–216] If there is a history of dysuria, examination may reveal inflammation of the meatus[214,215] and/or urethral discharge.[220]

Mucocutaneous

Circinate balanitis/vulvitis and keratoderma blenorrhagica are the characteristic mucocutaneous findings of Reiter syndrome. Circinate balanitis manifests as shallow, sharply marginated ulcers in females[221] and uncircumcized males.[216] Circumcized males exhibit hyperkeratotic (psoriasiform) patches or plaques.[215,216] Circinate balanitis developed in 15% of pediatric patients in one study[215] and 50% of pediatric patients in another study.[224] In a more recent report, three of four cases were affected.[216] Keratoderma blenorrhagica develops in a minority of children with Reiter's syndrome. It manifests on the palms and soles as yellow, hyperkeratotic papules that can coelesce to form scaly, psoriasiform plaques (Fig. 15.16). Vesicules and/or pustules may be evident in the early stages of development. Psoriasiform changes can develop on the extensor surface of the hands, feet, and limbs.[216,218] Keratoderma blenorrhagica was present in 8% of pediatric patients in one study[215] and 25% of pediatric patients in another study.[224] In another study, two of four pediatric patients were affected.[216] Additional nonspecific mucocutaneous findings include oral ulceration[214,221] and an evanescent erythematous eruption on the trunk and limbs.[215,216]

Other clinical findings

Rare manifestations of Reiter syndrome in children are pleuritis,[215] epistaxis,[215] aortic root dilation,[214] generalized lymphadenopathy,[225] and splenomegaly.[225]

Laboratory findings

Most pediatric patients with Reiter disease are positive for the HLA-B27 antigen.[214–216] Stool cultures and urethral cultures may be positive for the triggering factor if collected at the appropriate time.[215] Nonspecific findings include sterile pyuria, mild anemia, mild leukocytosis, and significantly elevated erythrocyte sedimentation rate.[215] Radiographs of the affected joints

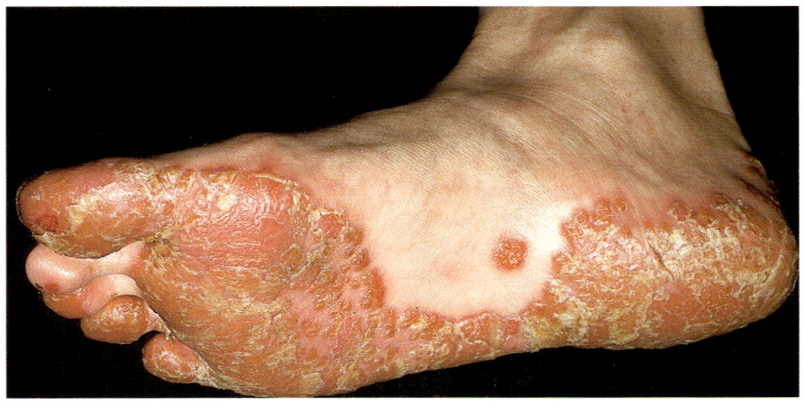

Fig. 15.16 Keratoderma blenorrhagica of Reiter's syndrome.

213. Morris R, Metzger AL, Bluestone R et al. (1974) HLA-B27: A clue to the diagnosis and pathogenesis of Reiter's syndrome. N Engl J Med 290:554.
214. Singsen BH, Bernstein BH, Koster-King KG et al. (1977) Reiter's syndrome in childhood. Arthritis Rheum 20(suppl):402–407.
215. Rosenberg AM, Petty RE (1979) Reiter's disease in children. Am J Dis Child 133:394–398.
216. Zivony D, Nocton J, Wortmann D et al. (1998) Juvenile Reiter's syndrome: a report of four cases. J Am Acad Dermatol 38:32–37.
217. Shimamoto Y, Sugiyama H, Hirohata S (2000) Reiter's syndrome associated with HLA-B51. Intern Med 39:182–184.
218. Gough KR (1962) Reiter's syndrome in father and son. Ann Rheum Dis 21:292–294.
219. Jacobs J, Berdon W, Johnston A (1982) HLA-B27 associated spondyloarthritis and enthesopathy in childhood: clinical, pathologic and radiographic observations in 58 patients. Pediatr 100:521–528.
220. Iveson JMI, Nanda BS, Hancock JAH et al. (1975) Reiter's disease in three boys. Ann Rheum Dis 34:364–368.
221. Russell AS (1977) Reiter's syndrome in children following infection with Yersinia enterocolitica and shigella. Arthritis Rheum 20(Suppl):471–472.
222. Zewi M (1947) Morbut Reiteri. Acta Ophthalmol 25:47–60.
223. Ansell B (1994) Reactive arthritis/Reiter's syndrome in children. Clin Exp Rheumatol 12:581–582.
224. Cuttica R, Scheines E, Garay M et al. (1992) Juvenile onset Reiter's syndrome. A retrospective study of 26 patients. Clin Exp Rheumatol 10:285–288.
225. Lockie GN, Hunder GG (1971) Reiter's syndrome in children. Arthritis Rheum 14:767–772.

are unremarkable in the early stages. Chronicity is associated with periosteal new bone formation secondary to periostitis, heel lucencies, spurs at the attachment of the plantar fascia or Achilles tendon, and demineralization around affected joints.[219]

PATHOPHYSIOLOGY AND HISTOGENESIS

Reiter disease is triggered in predisposed pediatric patients by an infectious illness in the gastrointestinal tract or urethra. Predisposition in most patients is linked to the HLA-B27 antigen. Gastrointestinal infections known to trigger Reiter syndrome in children involve Shigella flexneri,[214,221] Yersinia enterocolitica,[221] and various salmonella species (enteritidis, oranienburg, typhimurium).[214,220,226] Chlamydia has been isolated from the urethra of pediatric patients with post-urethritis Reiter syndrome.[215] Other infectious agents reported as triggering factors in adult patients are human immunodeficiency virus infection[227] mycoplasma pneumonia,[228] streptococcus viridans,[229] cyclospora,[230] and gardinella vaginalis.[231] The link between HLA-B27 antigen, the triggering infection, and development of clinical disease is unknown.

Histologic findings
The early lesions of circinate balanitis and keratoderma blenorrhagica exhibit a spongiform pustule in the upper epidermis similar to psoriasis. The pustule is replaced by nonspecific acanthosis, parakeratosis, and hyperkeratosis in established lesions.[98]

Differential diagnosis
The differential diagnosis includes juvenile rheumatoid arthritis, other seronegative arthropathies (e.g., psoriatic arthritis, inflammatory bowel disease associated arthritis), infectious arthropathies (e.g., lyme disease, post viral, gonococcal), Behçet disease, Kawasaki disease and rheumatic fever. Distinguishing the various conditions will depend on other clinical features (e.g., symptoms of inflammatory bowel disease, criteria for Kawasaki disease), the pattern of joint involvement, serology to exclude particular infections (e.g., lyme disease), serum rheumatoid factor, and HLA-B27 status.

THERAPY AND PROGNOSIS

Therapy is directed at removing the triggering factor and implementing anti-inflammatory therapy to settle the various manifestations of the disease. Antibiotic therapy for the infectious trigger is guided by the results of microbial cultures. Arthritis and enthesitis usually respond to aspirin or a non-steroidal anti-inflammatory medication (e.g. naproxen) given in appropriate doses for as long as needed.[214–216] Occasionally, intra-articular steroids or more aggressive oral therapy is needed. Sulfasalazine has been used sucessfully in combination with aspirin in one child.[216] Methotrexate,[232] acitretin,[233] and cyclosporin[234] have been used successfully in adult patients with difficult-to-control joint disease. The ocular manifestations should be managed with the assistance of an opthalmologist. Circinate balanitis and early keratoderma blenorrhagica may respond to appropriate topical steroid therapy.[216,232] Salicylic acid 10% ointment worked well in one patient with established keratoderma blenorrhagica.[216]

Prognosis
In most children, the disease is self-limiting and clears with no residual sequelae. A small percentage will have persistent or recurring arthritis particularly in the sacroiliac area.[216]

PEDIATRIC ASPECTS OF THE DISEASE

Reiter disease in children is usually triggered by a gastrointestinal infection. Mucocutaneous lesions are not commonly seen. Unlike adults, Reiter syndrome in children is usually self-limited and will respond to simple anti-inflammatory therapy.

GEOGRAPHIC TONGUE

The term geographic tongue (annulus migrans) describes a fluctuating eruption on the anterior two-thirds of the dorsum of the tongue. The eruption conveys the impression of a geographic map. It also known as benign migratory glossitis.

EPIDEMIOLOGY

Genetics
Familial clustering of cases has been reported[235] but the majority of cases are sporadic.

PRESENTING HISTORY

Geographic tongue can manifest at any age. The clinical appearance of the tongue and/or symptoms of burning and tenderness are the usual reasons for presentation. It can also be an incidental finding in patients with pustular psoriasis.[142,144]

PHYSICAL EXAMINATION

Geographic tongue is characterized by flat, smooth, erythematous patches, which contrast with the normal, off-white, furry appearance of the adjacent tongue mucosa (Fig. 15.17). The patches expand and coalesce to produce an appearance that resembles a geographic map. The number of patches, their size, and shape constantly change from day to day, even within hours; this is a typical feature of the disease.[236]

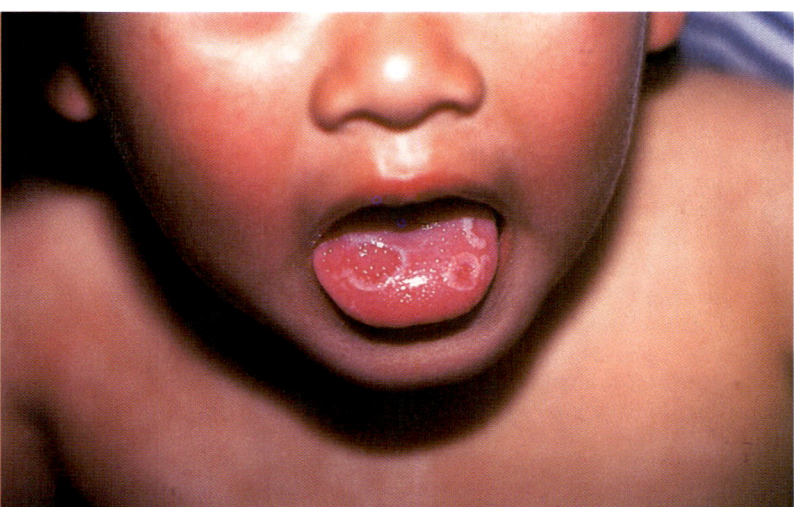

Fig. 15.17 Geographic tongue.

226. Jones RA (1977) Reiter's disease after Salmonella typhimurium enteritis. **Br Med J** 1:1391.
227. Winchester R, Bernstein D, Fischer H et al. (1978) The co-occurrence of Reiter's syndrome and acquired immunodeficiency. **Ann Intern Med** 123:1622–1632.
228. Natarajan UR, Tan TL, Lau R (2001) Reiter's disease following Mycoplasma pneumoniae infection. **Int J STD AIDS** 12:349–350.
229. Huang DF, Tsai CY, Tsai YY et al. (2000) Reiter's syndrome caused by Streptococcus viridans in a patient with HLA-B27 antigen. **Clin Exp Rheumatol** 18:394–396.
230. Sloan VS (2001) Reiter syndrome following protracted symptoms of Cyclospora infection. **Emerg Infect Dis** 7:1070.

231. Toussirot E, Plesiat P, Wendling D (1998) Reiter's syndrome induced by Gardnerella vaginalis. **Scand J Rheumatol** 27:316–317.
232. Rothe M, Kerdel F (1991) Reiter syndrome. **Int J Dermatol** 30:173–180.
233. Blanche P (1999) Acitretin and AIDS-related Reiter's disease. **Clin Exp Rheumatol** 17:105–106.
234. Kiyohara A, Takamori K, Ogawa H (1997) Successful treatment of severe recurrent Reiter's syndrome with cyclosporine. **J Am Acad Dermatol** 36:482–483.
235. Eidelman E, Chosack A, Cohen T et al. (1976) Scrotal tongue and geographic tongue: polygenic and associated traits. **Oral Surg Oral Med Oral Pathol** 42:591.
236. Brooks JK, Balciunas BA (1987) Geographic stomatitis: review of the literature and report of five cases. **J Am Dent Assoc** 115:421–424.

PATHOPHYSIOLOGY AND HISTOGENESIS

The etiology and underlying pathophysiology are unknown. Early reports of a link with atopy or psoriasis have never been substantiated.

Histologic findings

The active, expanding border is characterized by acanthosis with overlying parakeratosis and intraepithelial microabscesses that are indistinguishable from the spongiform pustules of Kogoj seen in pustular psoriasis. The flat smooth center exhibits epithelial thinning.[98]

Differential diagnosis

The geographic appearance and recognition of the changing pattern will distinguish geographic tongue from lichen planus, candidiasis, nutritional deficiency, or the mucus patches seen with secondary syphilis.

THERAPY AND PROGNOSIS

There is no effective treatment for geographic tongue. Most patients only require reassurance and maintenance of good intra-oral hygeine. Symptomatic cases may respond to an intra-oral topical steroid preparation (e.g., Kenalog in Orabase). The clinical course of geographic tongue is variable; it can last from months to years.

SEBORRHEIC DERMATITIS

Seborrheic dermatitis refers to an erythematous, scaly eruption that preferentially involves the scalp, face, and skin folds, which are regarded as the seborrheic areas of the body. An eruption referred to as seborrheic dermatitis may occur during the first year of life (infantile seborrheic dermatitis) or in postpubertal individuals (adolescent or adult seborrheic dermatitis). Whether the two conditions are the same or different is yet to be determined and there is no evidence that an infant with seborrheic dermatitis will develop seborrheic dermatitis as an adolescent or adult.

EPIDEMIOLOGY

Genetics

Although there is no evidence implicating genetic factors in the development of infantile seborrheic dermatitis, patients with adolescent or adult onset seborrheic dermatitis will often give a history of family members with the disease.

Statistics

The incidence of infantile seborrheic dermatitis in the general population is unknown. The incidence of adolescent and adult seborrheic dermatitis in the general population is estimated to be 2–5%. Males appear to be more commonly affected than females.

PRESENTING HISTORY

In infantile seborrheic dermatitis, the eruption develops during the first few months of life with asymptomatic red, scaly lesions in the diaper area, skin folds, and scalp. In adolescent or adult seborrhiec dermatitis, patients present at any time after the onset of puberty with a history of dandruff, scalp pruritus, and/or a facial eruption.

PHYSICAL EXAMINATION

Infantile seborrheic dermatitis usually manifests with erythema on the scalp, in the diaper area, skin folds (retro-auricular folds, neck, axillae, umbilicus, cubital fossae, popliteal fossae) and occasionally the face (Fig. 15.18). The erythema on the scalp, face, and behind the ears is typically covered with greasy, yellow-colored scale. The scaling on the scalp can vary from fine to thick and plate-like. The facial changes are most prominent on the forehead, in the eyebrows, and around the nose. The skin folds are erythematous with mild to moderate scale. Occasionally, the changes extend beyond the flexures, involving the trunk and limbs (Fig. 15.19).

Adolescent seborrheic dermatitis manifests with changes on the scalp that consist of scaling with varying degrees of erythema. Pruritus is a variable feature. Some patients develop changes on the face (Fig. 15.20), presternal area, and skin folds. The facial changes are symmetric and consist of erythema and scaling involving the eyebrows, sides of the nose, the nasolabial folds, the malar area of the face, retro-auricular folds, ears, and external auditory canal. Involvement of the presternal area consists of well-defined, scaly, erythematous patches. Skin fold involvement is characterized by confluent moist erythema. Severe cases can also have blepharitis

Laboratory findings

There are no consistent laboratory abnormalities in either form of seborrheic dermatitis.

PATHOPHYSIOLOGY AND HISTOGENESIS

The link between *Malassezia furfur* (*M. furfur*) and dandruff was first proposed by Malassez in 1874.[237] Thirty years later, Sabouroud suggested a role for the organism in the pathogenesis of adolescent and adult seborrheic dermatitis.[238] *M. furfur* is a normal member of the skin flora of postpubertal individuals. Colonization of the skin begins with the onset of sebaceous gland activity in the early stages of puberty. Although *M. furfur* can be isolated from any part of the skin, its levels are highest in the sebaceous gland-rich areas such as the scalp and face. Clinical improvement that occurs with a reduction in *M. furfur* levels with topical and oral antifungal therapy supports a role for *M. furfur* in the pathogenesis of adolescent and adult seborrheic dermatitis.[239,240] Although total levels of *M. furfur* on the skin surface do not correlate with the presence of seborrheic dermatitis,[241] one study suggests that pathogenicity may be related to the presence of particular *M. furfur* subtypes on the skin surface.[242] The mechanism through which *M. furfur* induces the development of seborrheic dermatitis remains unclear. Immune factors are probably important because of the high incidence of seborrheic dermatitis in patients with human immunodeficiency virus (HIV) infection.[243] There is no evidence of defective humoral and cellular immunity to *M. furfur* in non-HIV patients with seborrheic dermatitis compared with control patients.[244] The immunohistochemistry profile of inflammatory cells and inflammatory mediators in the affected skin of patients with the adult form of seborrheic dermatitis is consistent with an irritant, non-immunogenic stimulation of the immune response.[245] The stimulus may be related to *M. furfur* lipase activity or toxin production.

The etiology of infantile seborrheic dermatitis is unclear. Although there is no quantitative difference in sebum production between infants with infantile seborrheic dermatitis and unaffected controls, one study found a temporary alteration in serum fatty acids in infants with infantile seborrheic

237. Malassez L (1874) Notes sur le champignon de la pilade. **Arch Physiol Norm Pathol** 1:203–212.
238. Sabouroud R (1904) Pityriasis et Alopecies Peliculaire. Les maladies desquamatives. Paris, Massonet, 1st Edition p. 205.
239. Skinner RB Jr, Noah PW, Taylor RM et al. (1985) Double blind treatment of seborrhoeic dermatitis with 2% ketaconazole cream. **J Am Acad Dermatol** 12:852–856.
240. Scaparro E, Quadri G, Virno G (2001) Evaluation of the efficacy and tolerability of oral terbinafine (Daskil) in patients with seborrhoeic dermatitis. A multicentre, randomised, investigator-blinded controlled trial. **Br J Dermatol** 144:854–857.
241. McGinley KJ, Leyden JJ, Marples RR et al. (1975) Quantitive microbiology of the scalp in non-dandruff, dandruff and seborrhoeic dermatitis. **J Invest Dermatol** 64:401–405.

242. Peschere M, Krischer J, Renondat C (1999) Malassezia spp. Carriage in patients with seborrhoeic dermatitis. **J Dermatol** 26:558–561.
243. Smith KJ, Skelton HG, Yeager J et al. (1994) Cutaneous findings in HIV-1-positive patients: a 42-month prospective study. **J Am Acad Dermatol** 31:746–754.
244. Parry ME, Shapre GR (1998) Seborrhoeic dermatitis is not caused by an altered immune response to Malassezia yeast. **Br J Dermatol** 139:254–263.
245. Faergemann J, Bergbrant IM, Dohse M et al. (2001) Seborrhoeic dermatitis and pityrosporum (Malassezia) folliculitis: characterisation of inflammatory cells and mediators in the skin by immunohistochemistry. **Br J Dermatol** 144:549–556.

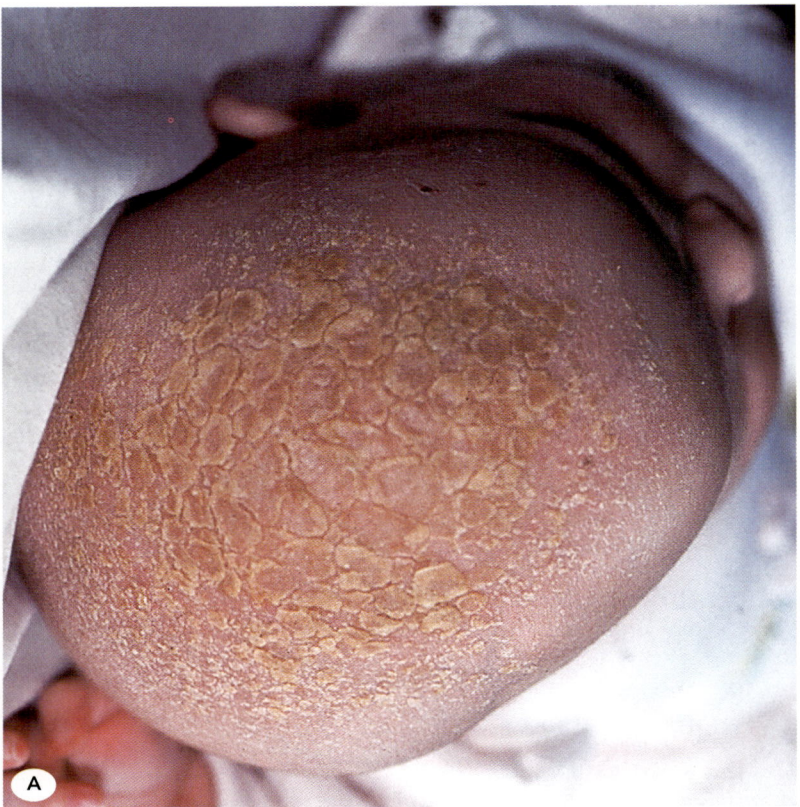

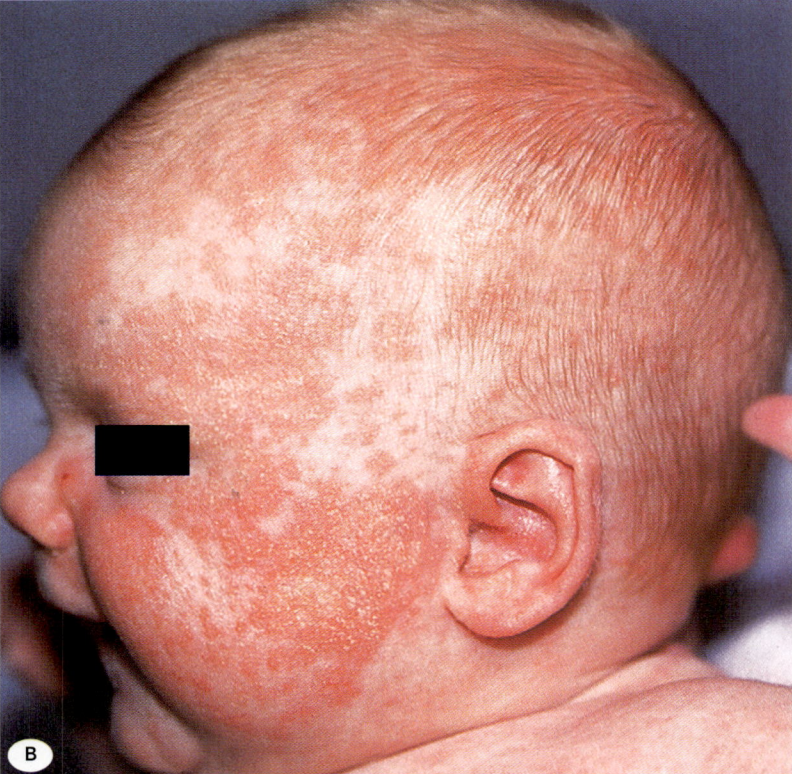

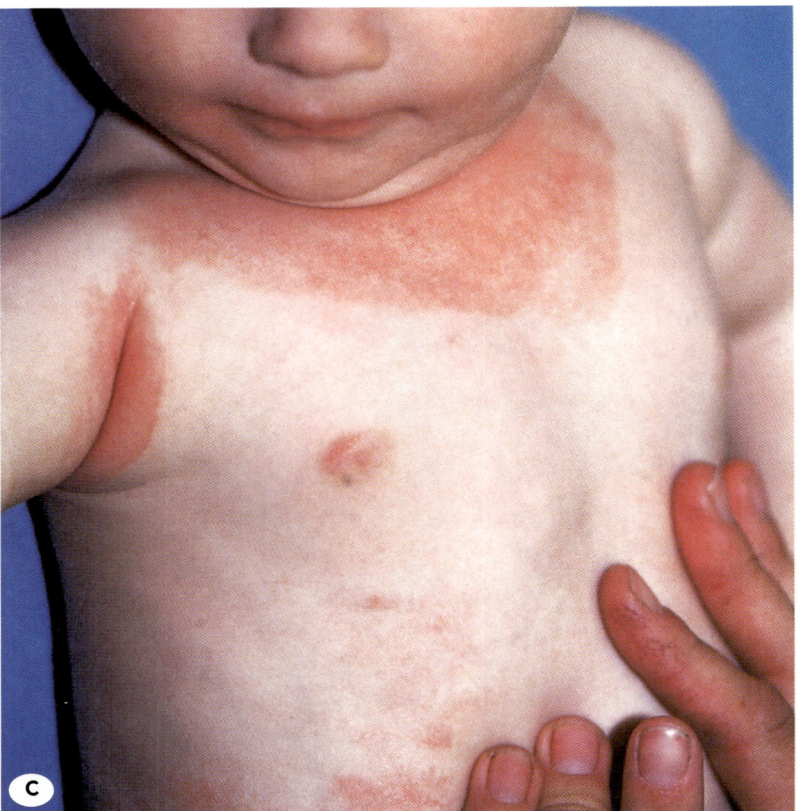

Fig. 15.18 (A) Infantile seborrheic dermatitis on the scalp. (B) Infantile seborrheic dermatitis on the face. (C) Infantile seborrheic dermatitis on his flexures.

dermatitis consistent with transient impaired function of the enzyme delta-6-desaturase.[246] *M. furfur* has been isolated from the skin of infantile seborrheic dermatitis patients at a frequency higher than patients with atopic dermatitis and unaffected controls.[247] Clinical improvement with topical antifungal therapy suggests a pathogenic role for *M. furfur* in infantile seborrheic dermatitis.[247]

Histologic findings

The histopathologic findings in seborrheic dermatitis are nondiagnostic. These consist of focal parakeratosis, moderate acanthosis, and mild to moderate spongiosis with exocytosis of mononuclear cells. A mild superficial perivascular lymphohistiocytic infiltrate is usually present in the dermis.[98]

Differential diagnosis

Conditions to consider in the differential diagnosis of infantile seborrheic are atopic dermatitis, psoriasis, and Langerhans histiocytosis. Atopic dermatitis is readily distinguished by the presence of itch and weepy eczematous lesions outside the skin folds. Psoriasis should be considered in the presence of well-defined scaly plaques on the trunk, limbs, and diaper area. Langerhans histiocytosis must be excluded if purpura, erosions, and/or crusting is evident. The principal differential diagnosis for adolescent seborrheic dermatitis is psoriasis. Distinguishing the two can be difficult when the changes are confined to the scalp and face. A diagnosis of psoriasis is more likely if there are typical plaques on the scalp, plaques on the trunk or limbs, and/or pitting of the nails.

246. Tollesson A, Frithz A, Berg et al. (1993) Essential fatty acids in infantile seborrhoeic dermatitis. J Am Acad Dermatol 22:957–961.

247. Ruiz-Maldonado R, Lopez-Martinez R, Chavarria P et al. (1989) Pityrosporum ovale in infantile seborrhoeic dermatitis. Pediatr Dermatol 6:16–20.

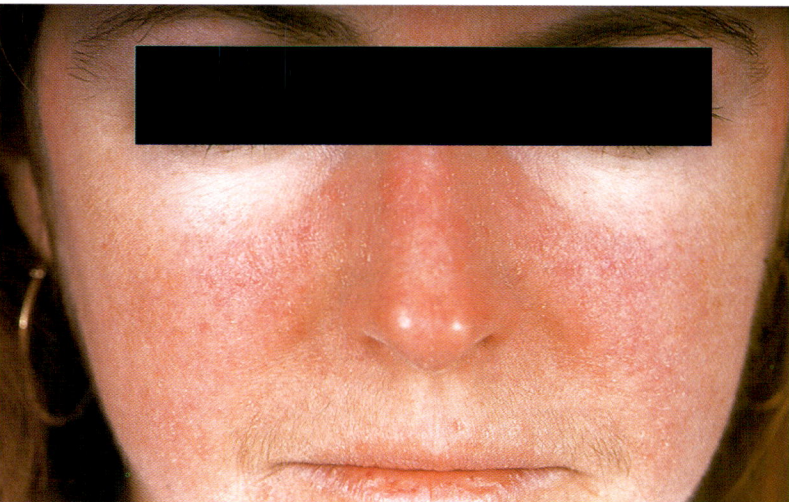

Fig. 15.20   Adolescent seborrheic dermatitis on the face.

Adolescent seborrheic dermatitis of the scalp is usually controlled with the regular use of a medicated shampoo containing zinc pyrithione, selenium sulfide, coal tar, or ketaconazole. If pruritus remains a problem, topical steroid scalp lotions, and foams can be used on an intermittent basis. Patients with severe scaling may benefit from the application of coal tar-salicylic acid preparations.

Prognosis

Infantile seborrheic dermatitis has a good prognosis. Most cases quickly clear with appropriate topical therapy. Adolescent seborrheic dermatitis requires ongoing therapy to maintain disease control. Although no figures are available, there appears to be a marked decrease in the incidence of seborrheic dermatitis in infancy.

SEBOPSORIASIS

Seborrheic psoriasis, also called sebopsoriasis or seborrhiasis, refers to a scaly erythematous eruption on the scalp, face, and skin folds with features that are consistent with both seborrheic dermatitis and psoriasis. A final diagnosis can only be made when typical lesions of psoriasis develop elsewhere on the body. The principles of treatment are identical to those outlined for seborrheic dermatitis and psoriasis. Some suggest that seboatopic dermatitis also exists.

LICHEN PLANUS

Lichen planus (LP) is a distinctive dermatosis aptly summarized by the four Ps; purple, polygonal, pruritic papules. The name lichen planus was first proposed by Wilson in 1869.[248] The reticulate, white lines on the surface of lichen planus papules, eponymously known as Wickham's striae, were first described by Wickham in 1895.[249]

EPIDEMIOLOGY

Genetics

Although LP has been reported in monozygotic twins[250] and families,[251,252] most cases are sporadic. Studies examining links between lichen planus and

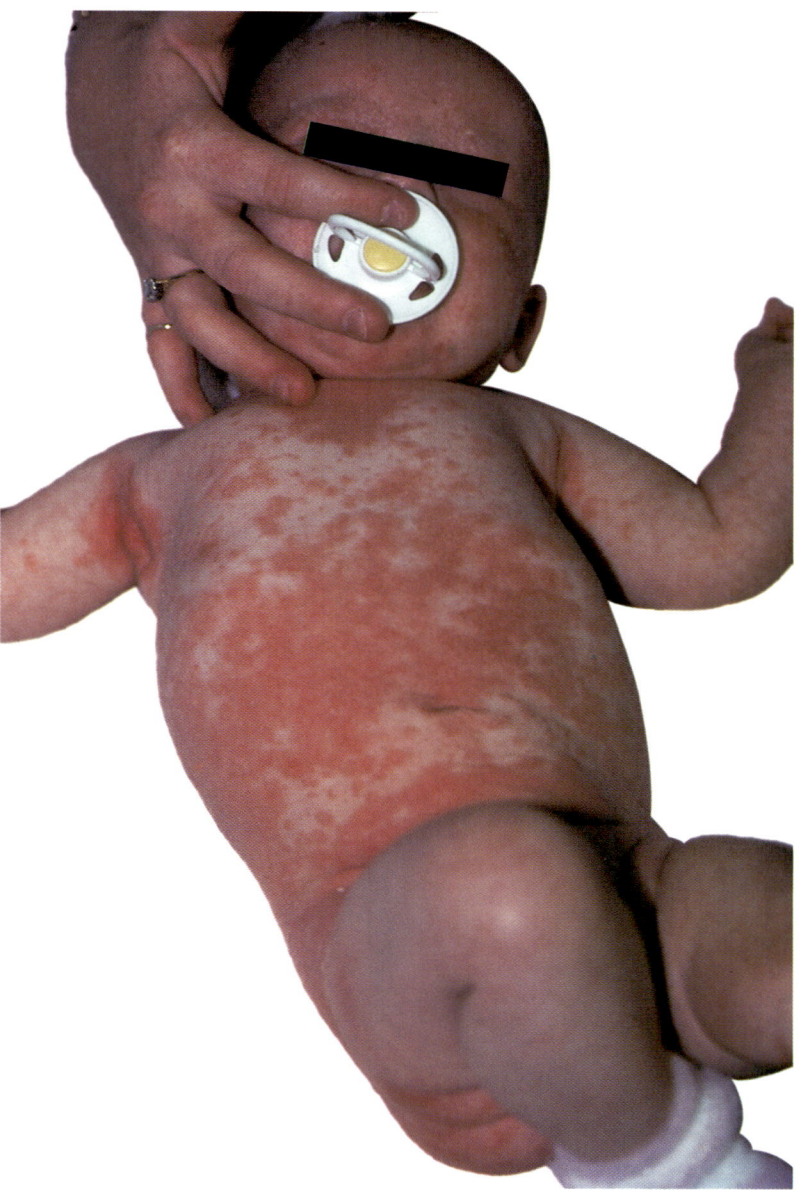

Fig. 15.19   Widespread infantile seborrheic dermatitis.

THERAPY AND PROGNOSIS

Topical

Infantile seborrheic dermatitis responds well to topical therapy. Hydrocortisone 1% is used on the face and skin folds. This may be combined with an antifungal agent for affected skin folds. A mid-potentcy topical steroid (e.g., Betamethasone valerate 0.05%) may be required for the trunk and limbs if hydrocortisone 1% fails to have the desired effect. Scalp scale can be removed after softening with an oil preparation or a weak keratolytic agent. The application of hydrocortisone will prevent the reappearance of erythema and the re-accumulation of scalp scale.

248. Wilson E (1869) On Leichen planus. **J Cutan Med Dis Skin** 3:117–321.
249. Wickham LF (1895) Sur un signe pathognomique de Lichen du Wilson (lichen plan) stries et ponctuations grisatres. **Ann Dermatol Syph** 6:517–520.
250. Gibstine CF, Esterly NB (1984) Lichen planus in monozygotic twins, letter to editor. **Arch Dermatol** 120:580.
251. Mahood JM (1983) Familial lichen planus. A report of nine cases from four families with a brief review of the literature. **Arch Dermatol** 119:292–294.
252. Milligan A, Graham-Brown RAC (1990) Lichen planus in children-a review of six cases. **Clin Exp Dermatol** 15:340–342.

HLA antigens have found an association with a variety of HLA alleles (A3, Bw35, B8, B16, DR1, DQw1), which are of doubtful significance.[253–255]

Statistics

The incidence and prevalence of pediatric LP in the general community is unknown. Several large series of cutaneous LP found the number of pediatric cases to be very small. Little reported 12 pediatric cases in a total of 150 cases,[256] Samman reported two pediatric patients in a total of 200 cases,[257] Singh *et al.* reported 76 cases (10 cases were under 10 yrs; 56 cases were aged 10–18 yrs) in a total of 441 cases,[258] Milligan *et al.* reported six pediatric cases in a total of 154 patients,[252] and Cottoni *et al.* reported five pediatric patients in a total of 234 cases.[259] Only six pediatric cases were identified in one review of 1062 cases of oral lichen planus[260] and five pediatric cases were noted in another series of 723 cases of lichen planus.[261] The four largest series of pediatric cases revealed a predeliction for males.[258,262–264] The age of onset extended from the first year through to adolescence.[258,262–264]

PRESENTING HISTORY

Pediatric patients usually present with a pruritic skin eruption.[258,262–264] Rarely, patients present with the nail[252,262] or oral manifestations[260,261] of LP.

PHYSICAL EXAMINATION

Skin

Classic LP manifests as extremely pruritic, flat-topped, violaceous-colored, polygonal papules which measure 3–15mm in diameter (Fig. 15.21). Wickham's striae are evident on the surface of the papules as a reticulate network of fine white lines (Fig. 15.22). Although lesions are usually symmetrically distributed on the limbs (especially the wrists), lower back, and pretibial areas, any site can be involved, including the face, scalp, and palmoplantar surfaces.[259,262–264] Papules can also develop at sites of trauma, which represents the Koebner phenomenon (Fig. 15.23).[263]

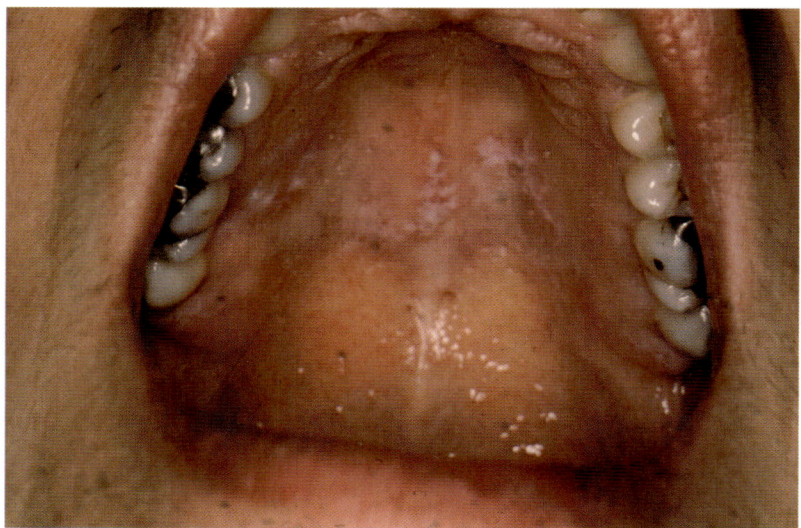

Fig. 15.22 Lichen planus with violaceous color and Wickham's striae.

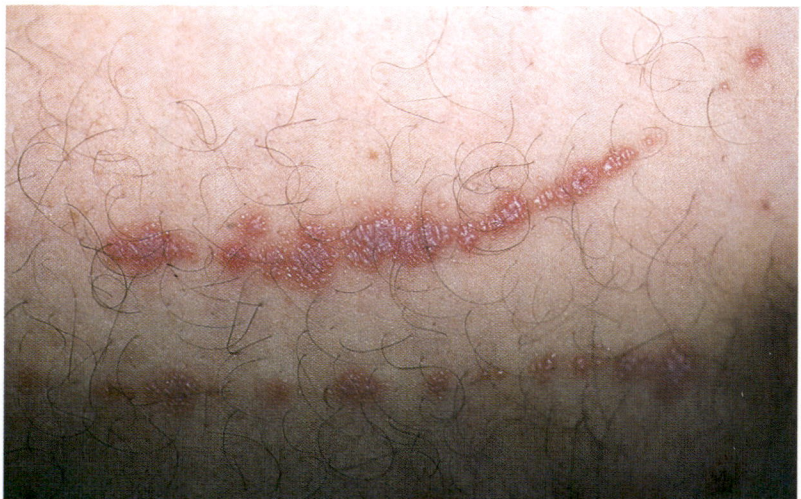

Fig. 15.23 Lichen planus Koebnerising at the site of trauma.

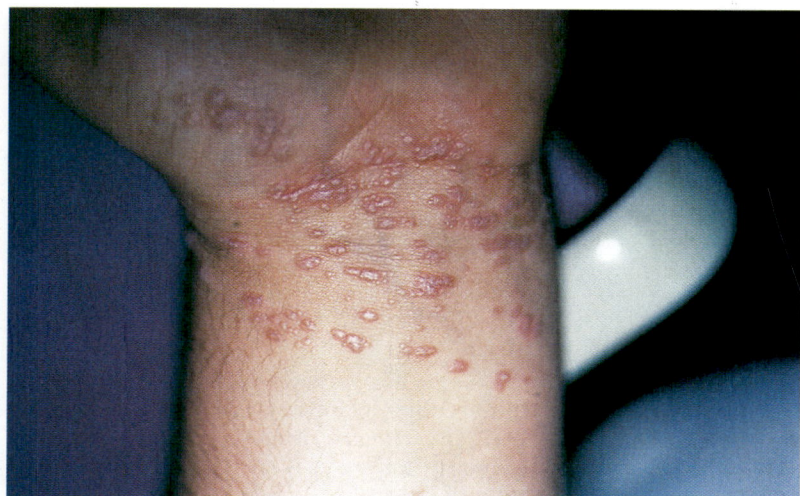

Fig. 15.21 Classic lichen planus; polygonal purple papules.

The morphologic variants of cutaneous LP seen in pediatric patients are linear, hypertrophic, annular, follicular, erosive, actinic, and bullous. Linear LP is is the most common variant seen in children. It is characterized by typical papules arranged in a linear or zosteriform pattern on the limbs and, less commonly, the trunk (Fig. 15.24). It is distinct from linear LP that develops at sites of trauma (Koebner phenomenon).[252,256,262–264] Hypertrophic LP refers to large papules or plaques of LP that develop a verrucous surface (Fig. 15.25). It usually occurs on the pretibial areas and is extremely pruritic.[262–264] Annular LP is characterized by a ring-like cluster of typical papules with a clear or slightly atrophic center (Fig. 15.26). It usually occurs on the penis and

253. Simon M, Djawari D, Schonberger A (1984) HLA antigens associated with lichen planus. **Clin Exp Dermatol** 9:435.
254. Powell FC, Rogers RS, Dickson ER et al. (1986) An association between HLA DR1 and lichen planus. **Br J Dermatol** 114:473–478.
255. Valsecchi R, Bontempelli M, Rossi A et al. (1988) HLA-DR and DQ antigens in lichen planus. **Acta Dermatol Venereol** (Stockh) 68:77–80.
256. Little EG (1919) Lichen planus. **J Cutan Dis** 37:639–670.
257. Samman PD (1961) Lichen planus. An analysis of 200 cases. **Trans St Johns Dermatol Soc** 46:36–38.
258. Singh DVD, Kanwar AJ (1976) Lichen planus in India: an appraisal of 441 cases. **Int J Dermatol** 15:752–756.
259. Cottoni F, Ena P, Tedde G et al. (1993) Lichen planus in children: a case report. **Pediatr Dermatol** 10:132–135.
260. Alam F, Hamburger J (2001) Oral mucosal lichen planus in children. **Int J Paediatr Dent** 11:209–214.
261. Eisen D (2002) The clinical features, malignant potential and systemic associations of oral lichen planus; a study of 723 patients. **J Am Acad Dermatol** 46:207–214.
262. Kanwar AJ, Handa S, Ghosh S et al. (1991) Lichen planus in childhood: a report of 17 patients. **Pediatr Dermatol** 8:288–291.
263. Sharma R, Maheshwari V et al. (1999) Childhood lichen planus: a report of fifty cases. **Pediatr Dermatol** 16:345–348.
264. Nanda A, Al-Ajami HS, Al-Sabah H et al. (2001) Childhood lichen planus: a report of 23 cases. **Pediatr Dermatol** 18:1–4.

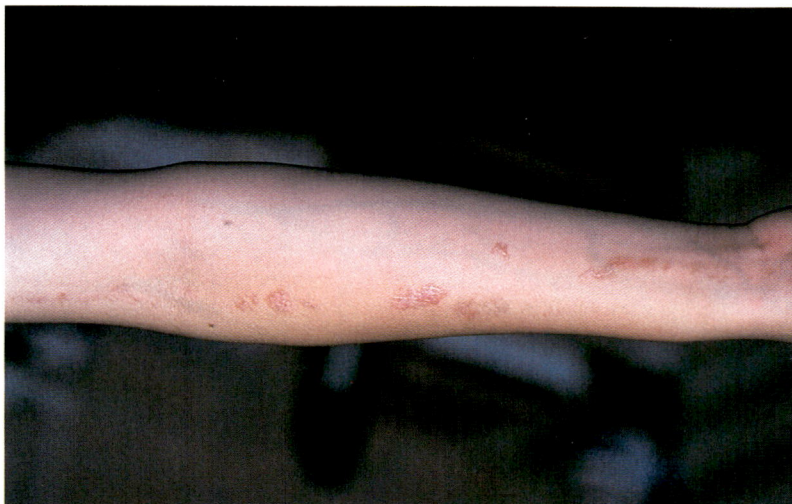

Fig. 15.24   Linear lichen planus.

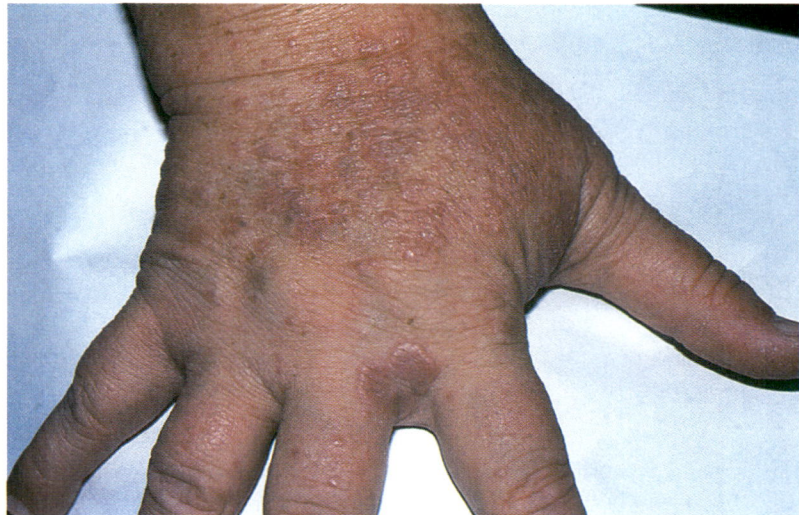

Fig. 15.26   Annular lichen planus and small, typical papules of lichen planus.

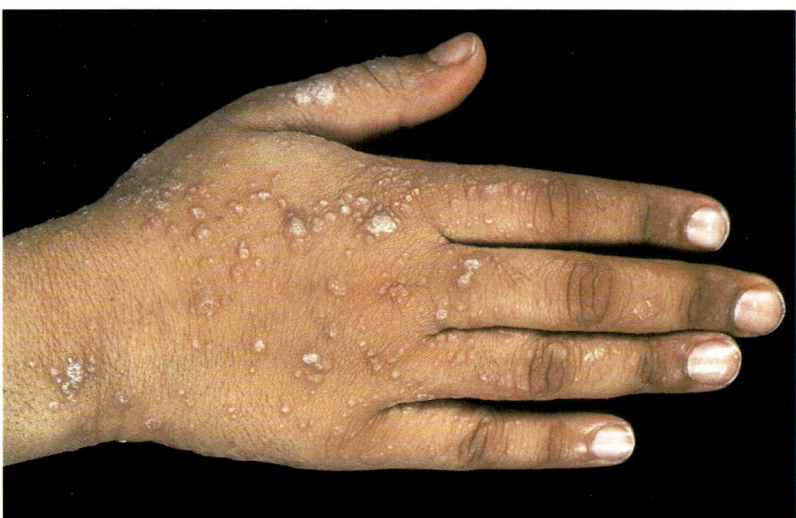

Fig. 15.25   Hypertrophic lichen planus.

trunk.[263] Follicular LP manifests on any hair-bearing area as follicular papules that measure 1–2mm in diameter.[252,262,264] Scalp involvement may be accompanied by scarring alopecia.[262,264] Erosive LP is characterized by the development of erosions on the surface of papular lesions. The palms and soles are the most common site for erosive changes. It has been rarely reported in children.[259] Actinic LP develops on sun-exposed and, to a lesser extent, protected areas, as bluish-brown macules or patches with well-defined borders. Shortly after onset, there is central clearing and induration of the periphery, resulting in an annular lesion with a hyperpigmented center. Most cases have been reported from the Middle East, Italy, India, and Africa.[264,265] This variant of LP accounted for 2% of cases in Sharma et al.'s series of 50 cases.[263] Bullous LP refers to the development of blistering within papules of LP. Blister formation is subepidermal and is due to severe liquefaction and vacuolation

of the basal layer of the epidermis. It is rarely seen in pediatric patients with LP.[259,266] Bullous LP can be confused with LP pemphigoides, which refers to a mixed eruption of LP papules and blisters that develop within the papules and on unaffected skin. Whilst the papules have the histologic features of LP, the blisters have the histologic and immunofluoresence features of bullous pemphigoid.[267] There have been several reported cases in children.[268,269]

Resolution of cutaneous LP is accompanied by the development of postinflammatory hyperpigmentation in all except those with very fair skin. Atrophy may be found following resolution of the hypertrophic and annular variants.

Mucosa

Involvement of the oral mucosa is very uncommon in pediatric patients. Athough Sharma et al.[263] found 30% of their patients with cutaneous LP to have oral manifestations of the disease, only one of Kanwar et al.'s[262] 17 patients and nine of Nanda et al.'s[264] series of 23 patients had oral involvement. In addition, less than 1% of patients presenting with oral LP are in the pediatric age group.[260,261] Oral involvement can predate[260,261] or coincide with the development of skin lesions.[262–264] The most common manifestation is whitish discoloration in the form of papules, plaques, and/or a lacy, reticulate pattern.[260,263,264] Uncommon findings are lichenoid papules on the lips,[262–264] erythematous patches and erosions on the oral mucosa,[260,261] and desquamative gingivitis.[260] The buccal mucosa, lip, and tongue are the most commonly affected sites.[260,261–264] None of the reported cases had evidence of vulval LP.

Nails

Nail involvement is very uncommon in pediatric patients with LP.[262,263] This can predate[262] or coincide with the development of skin disease.[252] Affected nail plates are dull and lusterless with thinning, longtitudinal ridging, and splitting.[252,262] The nails can shed with subsequent fusion of the proximal nail fold with the nail bed, creating an appearance known as pterygium unguis.[252,262] Twenty-nail dystrophy refers to the development of pitting and longtitudinal ridging of all fingernails and toenails. Nail biopsy has revealed this can be an initial manifestation of lichen planus in some patients.[270]

265. Salman SM, Kibbi AG, Zaynoun S (1989) Actinic lichen planus. **J Am Acad Dermatol** 20:226–231.
266. Kavli G (1979) Bullous lichen ruber in a child. **Dermatologica** 159:361–363.
267. Mora RG, Nesbit LT, Brantley JB (1983) Lichen planus pemphigoides: clinical and immunofluorescent findings in four cases. **J Am Acad Dermatol** 8:331–336.
268. Paige DG, Bhogal BS, Black MM et al. (1993) Lichen planus pemphigoides in a child-immunopathological findings. **Clin Exp Dermatol** 18:552–554.
269. Hernando LB, Sebastian F, Sanchez JH et al. (1992) Lichen planus pemphigoides in a 10-year-old girl. **J Am Acad Dermatol** 26:124–125.
270. Peluso AM, Tosti A, Piracinni BM et al. (1993) Lichen planus limited to the nails in childhood. **Pediatr Dermatol** 10:36.

Hair

Untreated follicular LP (lichen planopilaris) on the scalp in children can lead to scarring alopecia.[262,264]

Laboratory findings

There are no specific laboratory findings in any form of lichen planus, although an increased incidence of lichen planus may be seen in hepatitis C infection in adults.

PATHOPHYSIOLOGY AND HISTOGENESIS

The development of a lichenoid skin eruption in mice following intradermal injection of autoreactive T cells directed against murine HLA-DR equivalent antigens[271] and the resolution of LP following transplantation of affected skin onto nude mice,[272] indicates that cell-mediated immune mechanisms are involved in the development of LP. The murine model highlighted the importance of the early interaction between CD4+ T cells and antigen-presenting cells in disease development[273] and the temporal and spatial relationship between autoreactive, cytotoxic T cells and overlying epithelial damage.[274] In humans, the dermal infiltrate of LP consists predominantly of T cells with increased numbers of Langerhans cells and FXIIIa dendritic cells in the epidermis and dermis.[275,276] The T cells are predominantly CD4+ T-helper cells in the early stages[274] and CD8+ T-suppressor cells in the later stages.[277] T-cell infiltration is accompanied by release of a variety of cytokines (IL-1, IL-4, IL-6, IF-gamma, TNF) from T cells, antigen-presenting cells and keratinocytes.[278,279] Tissue damage is mediated by cytoxic T-cell activity and/or released cytokines. Damage involves disruption of anchoring fibrils and the hemidesmosome complex[280] and expression of Fas antigen on keratinocytes.[281]

The reason for the immune response is unknown. The most popular theory involves an infectious agent triggering the immune response with possible amplification via an interaction between CD28+ T cells and a specific ligand (B7/BB1) found on antigen-presenting cells and keratinocytes. This interaction leads to activation of T cells independent of the normal MHC/antigen activation pathway.[282] Evidence that supports an infectious trigger is the demonstration of Mxa protein in LP.[283] Cells produce Mxa protein in response to IFN-alpha/beta that is produced in response to viral infections. Although human papillomavirus DNA has been identified in oral lichen planus,[284] the identity of the infectious trigger is unknown.

Histologic findings

The characteristic histologic features of LP are hyperkeratosis, hypergranulosis, irregular acanthosis that creates a "sawtoothed" appearance, vacuolar damage to the basal cell layer, and a dense band like (lichenoid) infiltrate of lymphocytes and histiocytes that hugs the overlying epidermis. Vacuolar damage of the basal keratinocytes gives rise to globular eosinophilic deposits (Civatte bodies, colloid bodies) at the dermoepidermal junction, the deposition of pigment in the papillary dermis (pigmentary incontinence) and the formation of clefts known as Max Joseph spaces. Wickham's striae correlate with areas of hypergranulosis.

Immunofluorescence may reveal fibrin at the dermoepidermal junction and globular deposits of IgM, IgG, and/or IgA, which correspond to the colloid bodies.[285]

Differential diagnosis

Classic LP should be distinguished from other lichenoid eruptions, such as lichen nitidus, lichen simplex chronicus, and lichenoid drug eruptions, papular granuloma annulare, papular sarcoidosis, a papular viral exanthem, and early guttate psoriasis. The presence of Wickham's striae on the surface of established lesions, a history of drug ingestion, and skin biopsy will distinguish LP from the other conditions. Hypertrophic LP can be hard to distinguish clinically from a viral wart and lichen simplex chronicus. Skin biopsy will readily distinguish the three conditions. Linear LP can be difficult to distinguish from lichen striatus, even with skin biopsy, and relies on the recognition of Wickham's striae and LP elsewhere. Annular LP can resemble granuloma annulare and usually requires skin biopsy for definitive diagnosis. Follicular LP on the trunk and limbs can mimic keratosis pilaris, eruptive vellus hair cysts, lichen nitidus, phrynoderma, and follicular psoriasis. Follicular LP on the scalp with scarring alopecia needs to be distinguished from other causes of scarring alopecia, such as lupus erythematosus. Correctly diagnosing follicular LP, in the absence of classic cutaneous or mucosal LP, ultimately requires skin biopsy. Histology and direct immunfluorescence will distinguish bullous LP from other blistering diseases. Oral LP can be misdiagnosed as candidiasis, bite keratosis, aphthous stomatitis, and herpes simplex infection (desquamative gingivitis). The clinical appearance, microbial studies, and mucosal biopsy will distinguish LP. With the exception of pterygium unguis, LP of the nails can resemble psoriasis, tinea unguium, and 20-nail dystrophy. Fungal culture will distinguish tinea and the presence of LP or psoriasis elsewhere helps lead to the correct diagnosis. If the fungal culture is negative and there is nothing else to find, definitive diagnosis may require nail matrix biopsy.

THERAPY AND PROGNOSIS

Moderately potent or superpotent topical steroids are the treatment of choice for cutaneous LP in pediatric patients.[252,262–264] Overlying occlusion may be needed for hypertrophic lesions. Most patients will clear over a period of several months. Close supervision of potent topical steroid therapy is required to minimize the risk of developing local side effects. Topical steroids can be combined with oral corticosteroids (0.5–1.0mg/kg per day) administered as a tapering dose over a 2–12-week period. This combination is useful for children with widespread involvement or types of cutaneous LP associated with significant morbidity, such as unresponsive hypertrophic LP, follicular LP on the scalp with scarring alopecia, and bullous LP.[262–264] Intralesional triamcinalone 5–10mg/ml is effective for hypertrophic LP in older children and adolescents unresponsive to topical steroid therapy.[262–264]

Topical steroids are also the treatment of choice for symptomatic oral LP. The steroid is applied in an adhesive base several times a day over several months.[286] Kenalog in orabase or a potent topical steroid are helpful when

271. Saito K, Tamura A, Narimatsu H et al. (1986) Cloned auto-Ia-reactive T cells elicit lichen planus-like lesions in the skin of syngeneic mice. **J Immunol** 137:2485–2495.
272. Gilhar A, Pillar T, Winterstein G et al. (1989) The pathogenesis of lichen planus. **Br J Dermatol** 120:541–544.
273. Shiohora T, Moriya N, Nagashima M (1988) The lichenoid tissue reaction. A new concept of pathogenesis. **Int J Dermatol** 27:356–374.
274. Sugerman PB, Savage NW, Walsh LJ et al. (1995) Disease mechanisms in oral lichen planus. A possible role for autoimmunity. **Australas J Dermatol** 34:63–69.
275. Al Fouzan AS, Habib MA, Sallam Th et al. (1996) Detection of T-lymphocytes and T-lymphocyte subsets in lichen planus: in situ and in peripheral blood. **Int J Dermatol** 35:426–429.
276. Akasu R, From L, Kahn HJ (1991) Lymphocyte and macrophage subsets in active and inactive lesions of lichen planus. **Am J Dermatopathol** 15:217–223.
277. Takeuchi Y, Tohnai I, Kaneda T et al. (1988) Immunohistochemical analysis of cells in mucosal lesions of oral lichen planus. **J Oral Pathol** 17:367.
278. Boyd AS, Neldner KH (1991) Lichen planus. **J Am Acad Dermatol** 25:593–619.
279. Yamamoto T, Osaki T, Yoneda K et al. (1994) Cytokine production by keratinocytes and mononuclear infiltrates in oral lichen planus. **J Oral Pathol** 23:309–315.
280. Haaplainen T, Oksala O, Kallioinen M et al. (1995) Destruction of the epithelial anchoring system in lichen planus. **J Invest Dermatol** 105:100–103.
281. Oishi M, Maeda K, Sugiyama S (1994) Distribution of apoptosis-mediating Fas antigen in human skin and effects of anti-Fas monoclonal antibody on human epidermal keratinocyte and squamous cell carcinoma cell lines. **Arch Dermatol Res** 286:396–407.
282. Simon JC, Dietrich A, Mielke V et al. (1994) Expression of the B7/BB1 activation antigen and its ligand CD28 in T-cell mediated skin diseases. **J Invest Dermatol** 103:539–543.
283. Fah J, Pavlovic J, Burg G (1995) Expression of Mxa protein in inflammatory dermatoses. **J Histochem Cytochem** 43:47–52.
284. Miller CS, White DK, Royse DD (1993) In situ hybridization analysis of human papillomavirus in orofacial lesions using a consensus biotinylated probe. **Am J Dermatopathol** 15:256–259.
285. Ragaz A, Ackerman AB (1981) Evolution, maturation and regression of lesions of lichen planus. **Am J Dermatopathol** 3:5–25.
286. Voute AB, Schulten AE, Langendijk PNJ et al. (1993) Fluocinonide in an adhesive base for the treatment of oral lichen planus: a double blind placebo controlled study. **Oral Surg Oral Med Oral Pathol** 75:181–185.

used tid.-qid. There is a risk of systemic absorption of steroid and their use in young children requires close supervision. Topical steroid therapy can be combined with oral corticosteroids (0.5–1.0mg/kg daily) as a tapering dose over 3–6 weeks if the child is very symptomatic, in the early stages of treatment. In addition to anti-inflammatory therapy, adequate intraoral hygeine must be maintained with the assistance of a dentist.

In severe unreponsive cases of cutaneous and/or oral LP, oral retinoids are the preferred option in view of the findings of an evidence-based medicine analysis of treatments for LP.[287] Despite lack of evidence of proven efficacy,[287] cyclosporin,[288] griseofulvin,[289] PUVA phototherapy,[290] dapsone,[263,264,291] and phenytoin[292] have been used with difficult patients not responding to steroids and oral retinoids.

Treatment options for LP of the nail in young children are oral corticosteroids (0.5–1.0mg/kg per day) administered as a tapering dose over 4–12 weeks[252] and oral retinoids.[293] Intralesional triamcinalone injected into the nail matrix is a third option for older patients. Whether treatment is undertaken depends on the severity of nail involvement and the wishes of the patient and their family.

Prognosis

Most pediatric patients with LP respond to treatment with full clearance over 1–6 months.[262–264] Poor response to treatment can be a feature of hypertrophic LP and lichen planopilaris.[252,262–264] Sequelae are rare in pediatric LP and take the form of cutaneous atrophy with resolution of hypertrophic LP, scarring alopecia with uncontrolled lichen planopilaris, and pterygium unguis with chronic nail disease. In published series, recurence rate was very low.[262–264]

PEDIATRIC ASPECTS OF THE DISEASE

The non-infectious nature of the disease should be emphasized to the family. Prolonged topical steroid therapy must be closely supervised to minimize the risk of side effects.

LICHEN PLANUS-LIKE ERUPTIONS
Lichenoid drug eruption

An LP-like eruption can occur with the ingestion of certain medications.[294] The eruption tends to be more eczematous or psoriasiform in appearance with no evidence of Wickham's striae or oral changes of LP. Histologically, a lichenoid drug eruption exhibits focal parakeratosis, spongiosis, and eosinophils in the dermal infiltrate that are features not seen in idiopathic LP.[294,295] The most commonly implicated drugs are the anti-epileptics (e.g., tegretol), antimalarials, anti-arrythmic agents (e.g., quinine, quinidine), antihypertensives (e.g., captopril, beta blockers, thiazide diuretics, methyldopa), nonsteroidal anti-inflammatory drugs, phenothiazines, antibiotics (e.g., sulfonamides, tetracyclines) and gold.[294] When strict criteria are used for the assignment of a drug as a cause of an eruption, of the many drugs regarded as causes of lichenoid drug eruptions, only beta blockers, methyldopa, pencillamine, quinidine, and quinine are definite causes of a lichenoid drug eruption.[296]

Graft-versus-host disease

An LP-like eruption can occur with graft-versus-host disease following bone marrow transplants.[297]

LICHEN NITIDUS

Lichen nitidus was first described by Pincus in 1907.[298] Lichen nitidus, which means shiny papules, is a relatively uncommon, asymptomatic, chronic eruption, consisting of minute sharply demarcated skin-colored papules.

EPIDEMIOLOGY

Genetics

Although familial lichen nitidus has been reported,[299] there is no evidence that genetic factors play a role.

Statistics

Lapins et al. noted a predeliction for males (4:1) in their series of 43 patients. The mean age of onset was 7 years for males and 13 years for females.[300]

PRESENTING HISTORY

Patients present for assessment with an asymptomatic or mildly pruritic eruption. The eruption may be localized to one or more areas or generalized in distribution.[300–302]

PHYSICAL EXAMINATION
Skin

Lichen nitidus is characterized by shiny, skin-colored, flat-topped papules that measure up to 2mm in diameter (Fig. 15.27).[300–302] The papules can rarely be purpuric[303,304] or vesiculobullous.[304] They can develop on any part of the body, including the face, palmoplantar surfaces and genitalia.[300–302,305] The papules can be localized to a particular area or involve most of the body.[300–302] Localization to sites of trauma (Koebner phenomenon) can be a feature in some patients.[300,302] An unusual clinical variant is palmoplanter hyperkeratosis mimicking fissured eczema.[305] All reported patients were adults who had typical lesions of lichen nitidus elsewhere and histologic evidence of lichen nitidus as the cause of the palmplantar hyperkeratosis.

Some patients will have nail changes and lesions on the oral mucosa. The nail changes consist of longtitudinal ridges with a rippled or beaded surface, pitting, and transverse ridging.[300,305,306] The adjacent nail fold may be normal or involved with lichen nitidus.[305] Oral lesions consist of yellowish papules on the gums.[306]

287. Cribier B, Frances C, Chosidow O (1998) Treatment of lichen planus: an evidence based medicine analysis of efficacy. **Arch Dermatol** 134:1521–1530.
288. Ho VC, Gupta AK, Nickoloff BJ et al. (1990) Treatment of severe lichen planus with cyclosporine. **J Am Acad Dermatol** 22:64–68.
289. Sehgal VN, Bikhchandani R, Koranne RV et al. (1980) Histopathological evaluation of griseofulvin therapy in lichen planus. **Dermatologica** 161:22–27.
290. Gonzalez E, Khosrow MT, Freedman S (1984) Bilateral comparison of generalised lichen planus treated with psoralens and ultraviolet A. **J Am Acad Dermatol** 10:958–961.
291. Kumar B, Kaur I, Bhattacharaya M (1994) Dapsone in lichen planus (letter). **Acta Dermatol Venereol** 74:334.
292. Bogaert H, Sanchez E (1990) Lichen planus: treatment of 30 cases with systemic and topical phenytoin. **Int J Dermatol** 29:157–158.
293. Kato N, Ueno H (1993) Isolated lichen planus of the nails treated with etretinate. **J Dermatol** 20:577–580.
294. Halvey S, Shai A (1993) Lichenoid drug eruptions. **J Am Acad Dermatol** 29:249–255.
295. Van den Haute V, Antoine JL, Lachapelle JM (1989) Histopathological discriminant criteria between lichenoid drug eruption and idiopathic lichen planus: retrospective study on selected samples. **Dermatologica** 179:10–13.

296. Thompson DF, Skaehill PA (1994) Drug induced lichen planus. **Pharmacotherapy** 14:561–571.
297. Andrews ML, Robertson I, Weedon D (1997) Cutaneous manifestations of chronic graft-vs-host disease. **Australas J Dermatol** 38:55–64.
298. Pinkus F (1907) Uber eine neue knochtenformige Hauteruption: Lichen nitidus. **Arch Dermatol Syph** (Berlin) 85:11–36.
299. Kato N (1995) Familial lichen nitidus. **Clin Exp Dermatol** 20:336–338.
300. Lapins NA, Willoughby C, Helwig EB (1978) Lichen nitidus: a study of 43 cases. **Cutis** 21:634.
301. Sysa-Jedrzejowska A, Wozniacka A, Robak E et al. (1996) Generalised lichen nitidus: a case report. **Cutis** 58:170–172.
302. Soroush V, Gurevitch AW, Peng S-K (1999) Generalised lichen nitidus: case report and literature review. **Cutis** 64:135–136.
303. Endo M, Baba S, Suzuki H (1998) Purpuric lichen nitidus. **Eur J Dermatol** 8:54–55.
304. Jetton RL, Eby CS, Freeman RG (1972) Vesicular and hemorrhagic lichen nitidus. **Arch Dermatol** 105:430.
305. Munro CS, Cox NH, Marks JM et al. (1993) Lichen nitidus presenting as palmoplantar hyperkeratosis and nail dystrophy. **Clin Exp Dermatol** 18:381–383.
306. Bettoli V, De Padova MP, Corazza M et al. (1997) Generalised lichen nitidus with oral and nail involvement in a child. **Dermatol** 194:367–369.

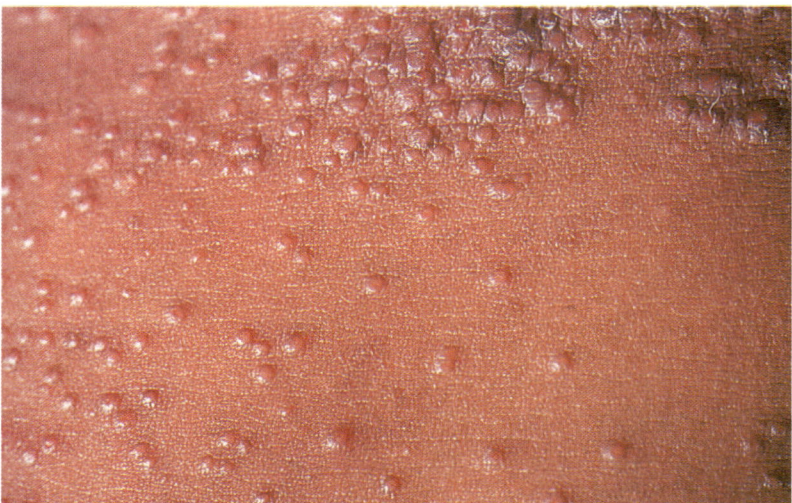

Fig. 15.27   Lichen nitidus on the body.

Laboratory findings

There are no specific laboratory abnormalities in lichen nitidus.

PATHOPHYSIOLOGY AND HISTOGENESIS

The pathophysiology and histogenesis of lichen nitidus is unknown. It was originally believed to be a form of tuberculid and more recently considered to be a variant of lichen planus. Although there is definitely no link with mycobacterial infection, there is still debate regarding the possible link between lichen nitidus and lichen planus.

Histologic findings

Lichen nitidus is characterized by a circumscribed collection of inflammatory cells in the papillary dermis that abuts the overlying epidermis. The inflammatory infiltrate consists of lymphocytes, histiocytes, and multinucleated giant cells. Although the overlying epidermis is flattened with vacuolar degeneration of basal keratinocytes, there is elongation of the rete ridges at the lateral edge of the inflammatory infiltrate, which conveys the appearance of a "claw clutching a ball."[98,300] Rarely, transepidermal elimination channels can be seen.[307]

Differential diagnosis

Lichen nitidus needs to be distinguished from papular eczema, early molluscum contagiosum, small plane warts, keratosis pilaris, eruptive vellus hair cysts, micropapular granuloma annulare, lichen planus, and follicular psoriasis. Papular eczema is pruritic and in addition to lichenoid papules, there is typical eczematous change in adjacent skin. Papules of molluscum contagiosa will exhibit the characteristic central core with magnification. Plane warts tend to be slightly brown in color and have a dull rather than shiny surface. Keratosis pilaris manifests in a symmetric fashion with punctate follicular rather than flat-topped papules. Eruptive vellus hair cysts are dome shaped and vellus hairs can usually be expressed after gently pricking the surface. Micropapular and follicular lichen planus may not have the typical violaceous color and Wickham's striae, which makes it difficult to distinguish from lichen nitidus on clinical grounds. Follicular psoriasis manifests as punctate rather than flat-topped papules and there are usually more typical psoriasis plaques elsewhere. Micropapular granuloma annulare tends to be dome shaped. Skin biopsy will help distinguish lichen nitidus from all these conditions.

THERAPY AND PROGNOSIS

In view of the asymptomatic nature of the eruption, its minimal cosmetic impact, and tendency for spontaneous resolution,[300,306] most cases require no treatment. In Lapins et al.'s series,[300] 69% of patients cleared within 12 months of onset. Symptomatic cases may benefit from moderately potent or potent topical steroid therapy or a short course of oral steroids. There are a number of anecdotal reports of improvement or clearance with extensive sunlight exposure,[301,308] oral astemizole,[309] oral cetirizine-levamisol combination,[310] topical dinitrochlorobenzene,[311] and itraconazole.[312] Oral retinoids have been used successfully in the treatment of palmoplantar lichen nitidus.[305,313]

LICHEN AUREUS

Lichen aureus was first described by Marten in 1958 with the provisional name of lichen purpuricus.[314] In 1960, Calnan proposed the name lichen aureus because of the orange-yellow color exhibited by the eruption.[315] Lichen aureus is defined by its characteristic clinical and histologic features. It belongs to the group of diseases known as the pigmented purpuric dermatoses.

EPIDEMIOLOGY

Genetics

In view of the sporadic nature of reported cases,[316–321] genetic factors are not involved.

Statistics

A review of 104 reported cases by Gelmetti et al.[318] revealed that 17% of cases were in the pediatric age group. This review and a number of other case reports indicate that males and females are affected equally.[316–321] Onset can occur at any age from early infancy onwards.[316–321]

PRESENTING HISTORY

Patients present with an asymptomatic eruption for assessment. Occasionally, slight itch or burning may occur.

PHYSICAL EXAMINATION

Lichen aureus is characterized by macular and/or papular lesions that coalesce to produce discoid lesions of varying size. Established lesions vary from golden-yellow to dark brown in color (Fig. 15.28). Close examination will

307. Itami A, Ando I, Kukita A (1994) Perforating lichen nitidus. **Int J Dermatol** 33:382–384.
308. Arizaga AT, Gaughan MD, Bang RH (2002) Generalised lichen nitidus. **Clin Exp Dermatol** 27:115–117.
309. Vaughn RY, Smith JG (1990) The treatment of lichen nitidus with astemizole. **J Am Acad Dermatol** 23:757–758.
310. Sehgal VN, Jain S, Kumar S et al. (1998) Generalised lichen nitidus in a child's response to cetirizine dihydrochloride/levamisol. **Australas J Dermatol** 39:60.
311. Kano Y, Otake Y, Shiohara T (1998) Improvement of lichen planus after topical dinitrochlorobenzene application. **J Am Acad Dermatol** 39:305–308.
312. Libow LF, Coots NV (1998) Treatment of lichen planus and lichen nitidus with itraconazole: report of six cases. **Cutis** 62:247–248.
313. Lucker GP, Koopman RJ, Steijlen PM et al. (1994) Treatment of palmoplantar lichen nitidus with acitretin. **Br J Dermatol** 130:791–793.

314. Marten R (1958) Case for diagnosis. **Trans St Johns Hosp Dermatol Soc** 40:98.
315. Calnan CD (1960) Lichen aureus. **Br J Dermatol** 72:373.
316. Price ML, Wilson Jones E, Calnan CD et al. (1985) Lichen aureus: a localised persistent form of pigmented purpuric dermatitis. **Br J Dermatol** 112:307–314.
317. Ruiz-Esmenjaud J (1988) Segmental lichen aureus: onset associated with trauma and puberty. **Arch Dermatol** 124:1572–1573.
318. Gelmetti C, Cerri D, Grimalt R (1991) Lichen aureus in children. **Pediatr Dermatol** 8:280–283.
319. Patrizi A, Neri I, Marini R et al. (1996) Lichen aureus with uncommon clinical features in a child. **Pediatr Dermatol** 13:173.
320. Rubio FA, Robayna G, Herranz P et al. (1997) Abdominal lichen aureus in a child. **Pediatr Dermatol** 14:411.
321. Dippel E, Schroder K, Goerdt S (1998) Zosteriform lichen aureus. **Hautzart** 49:135–138.

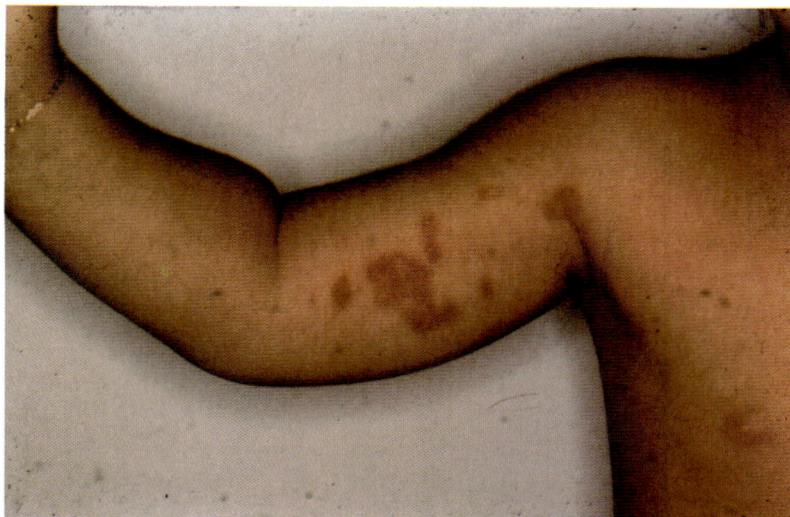

Fig. 15.28   Lichen aureus: burnt orange color with fine petechiae.

often reveal scattered petechiae within the lesion. Although the lower limb is the most commonly affected site, lichen aureus can develop anywhere, including the digits and face. It can manifest as a solitary lesion or as multiple lesions that are distributed in a segmental or zosteriform pattern.[316–321]

Laboratory findings
There are no specific laboratory abnormalities noted in lichen aureus.

PATHOPHYSIOLOGY AND HISTOGENESIS
The etiology and pathophysiology of lichen aureus is unknown.

Histologic findings
The histologic findings in lichen aureus are confined to the superficial dermis. A lymphohistiocytic infiltrate is evident in a perivascular and band-like distribution, with extravasated red blood cells and hemosiderin deposits. The overlying epidermis is unaffected.[316–321]

Differential diagnosis
The two important differential diagnoses are bruising and other pigmented purpuric dermatoses. Lichen aureus can be distinguished from bruising by its persistent nature, the presence of petechiae within the lesion, and histologic findings. The other pigmented purpuric dermatoses (e.g., Schamberg's disease, Majocchi's disease) can be distinguished on the basis of clinical appearance and histology. There is a single case report of Langerhans histiocytosis presenting with a lichen aureus-like eruption in a 13-year-old boy.[322]

THERAPY AND PROGNOSIS
There is no effective topical or oral treatment for lichen aureus. Topical steroids may work but have been ineffective in most reported cases. Resolution in pediatric cases occurs over a period from several months to years.

GIANOTTI-CROSTI SYNDROME

In 1955, Gianotti described a disease characterized by lymphadenopathy, anicteric hepatitis, and an erythematous papular eruption symmetrically distributed on the face, buttocks, and extremities. He believed the disease was virally induced and named it papular acrodermatitis of childhood (PAC).[323] Subsequent reports in the late 1950s used the eponym Gianotti-Crosti syndrome.[324,325] In 1970, Gianotti and an independent group of pediatricians confirmed the infectious etiology of the condition with the identification of Australia antigen (hepatitis B surface antigen) in their patients. They believed PAC was a specific manifestation of hepatitis B virus infection.[326,327] Subsequent reports from various countries highlighted a similar illness unassociated with hepatitis B virus infection. Gianotti considered these cases to be a different disease that was clinically distinguishable from PAC. He coined the term papulovesicular acrolocated syndrome (PALS) for cases not associated with hepatitis B infection.[328] Caputo et al.[329] reviewed 69 cases of PAC and 239 cases of PALS to determine whether the two could be clinically distinguished as proposed by Gianotti. The authors were unable to clinically distinguish cases caused by hepatitis B virus from cases caused by other viruses. They concluded that clinical differences are due to an individual reponse to the virus rather than the type of virus involved. They proposed the terms PAS and PALS be replaced by the term Gianotti-Crosti syndrome, which covers all viral-induced papular or papulovesicular eruptions that are symmetrically distributed on acral sites (face, buttocks, extensor limbs).

EPIDEMIOLOGY
Genetics
There is no evidence for the involvement of genetic factors.

Statistics
Caputo et al.'s review of 308 cases found a slight male predominance and a mean age of onset of 2 years (6 months–14 years). Most cases occurred in the spring and summer months.[329] Adult cases have been reported.[330] Most hepatitis B associated cases have been reported in Italy and Japan.[331,332] Other countries report the involvement of viruses other than hepatitis B.

PRESENTING HISTORY

Patients present with an evolving eruption on the face, buttocks, and limbs. The eruption may be itchy and is preceded or accompanied by symptoms and signs of a viral illness.

PHYSICAL EXAMINATION
Skin
Gianotti-Crosti syndrome is characterized by a monomorphic papular or papulovesicular eruption distributed on the face, buttocks, and limbs (Figs 15.29–15.32). The trunk is typically spared. The individual papules or papulovesicles are firm, dome shaped, and measure 1–5mm in diameter. They can Koebnerize at sites of trauma and coalesce over the elbows and knees to produce plaques of varying size. Although the papules are typically pink or erythematous in color, they can be skin-colored or purpuric (Fig. 15.33) in

322. Megahed M, Schuppe H-C, Holzle E et al. (1991) Langerhans cell histiocytosis masquerading as lichen aureus. **Pediatr Dermatol** 8:213–216.
323. Gianotti F (1955) Rilievi di una particolare casisistica tossinfettiva caratterizzata da eruzione eritemato-infiltrative desquamativa a focolai lenticolari, a sede acroesposta. **G Ital Derm Sif** 96:678–697.
324. Bessone L (1957) Sopra una particolare dermatite eruttiva acroesposta dei bambini (tipo Crosti-Gianotti). **Minerva Dermatol** 32(suppl 12):109.
325. Chapuis H (1958) Acro-erytheme papuleux infantile (syndrome de Gianotti-Crosti). **Rev Med Suisse Romande** 74:136–142.
326. Gianotti F (1970) L'acrodermatite papulosa infantile "malattia". **Gazz Sanitaria** 41:271–274.
327. De Gasperi G, Bardare M, Costantino D (1970) Au antigen in Crosti-Gianotti acrodermatitis [letter]. **Lancet** 1:1116.
328. Gianotti F (1979) Papular acrodermatitis of childhood and other papulovesicular acrorelated syndromes. **Br J Dermatol** 100:49–59.
329. Caputo R, Gelmetti C, Ermacora E et al. (1992) Gianotti-Crosti syndrome: a retrospective analysis of 308 cases. **J Am Acad Dermatol** 26:207–210.
330. Claudy AL, Ortonne JP, Trepo C et al. (1977) Acrodermtite papuleuse de l'adulte. A propose de 3 cas. **Ann Dermatol Venereol** 104:190–194.
331. Ishimaru Y, Ishimaru H, Toda G et al. (1976) An epidemic of infantile papular acrodermatitis (Gianotti's disease) in Japan associated with hepatitis B surface antigen subtype ayw. **Lancet** I:707–709.
332. Gianotti F (1978) HbsAg and papular acrodermatitis of childhood. **N Engl J Med** 298:460.

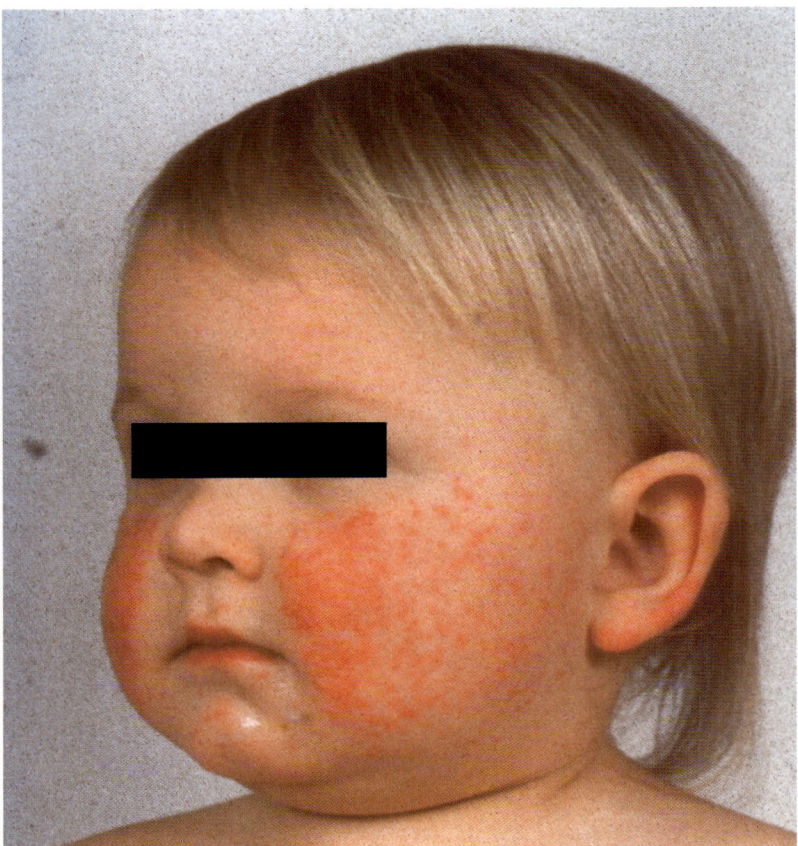

Fig. 15.29   Gianotti-Crosti on face.

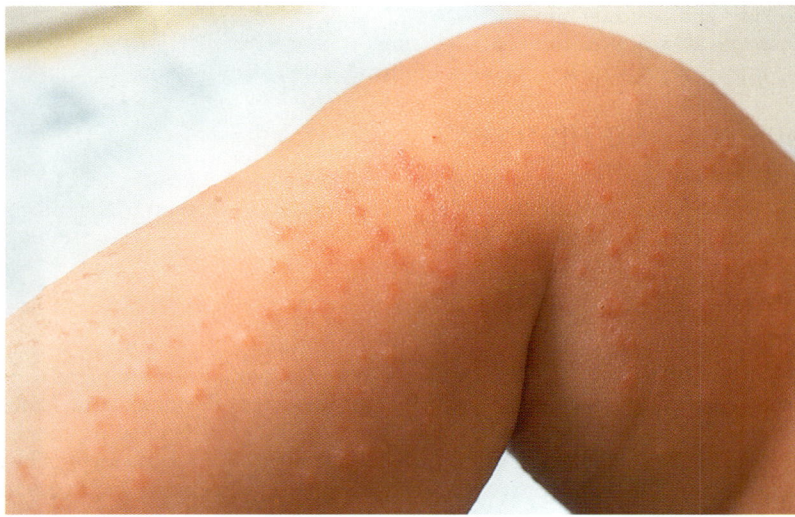

Fig. 15.30   Gianotti-Crosti syndrome on the leg.

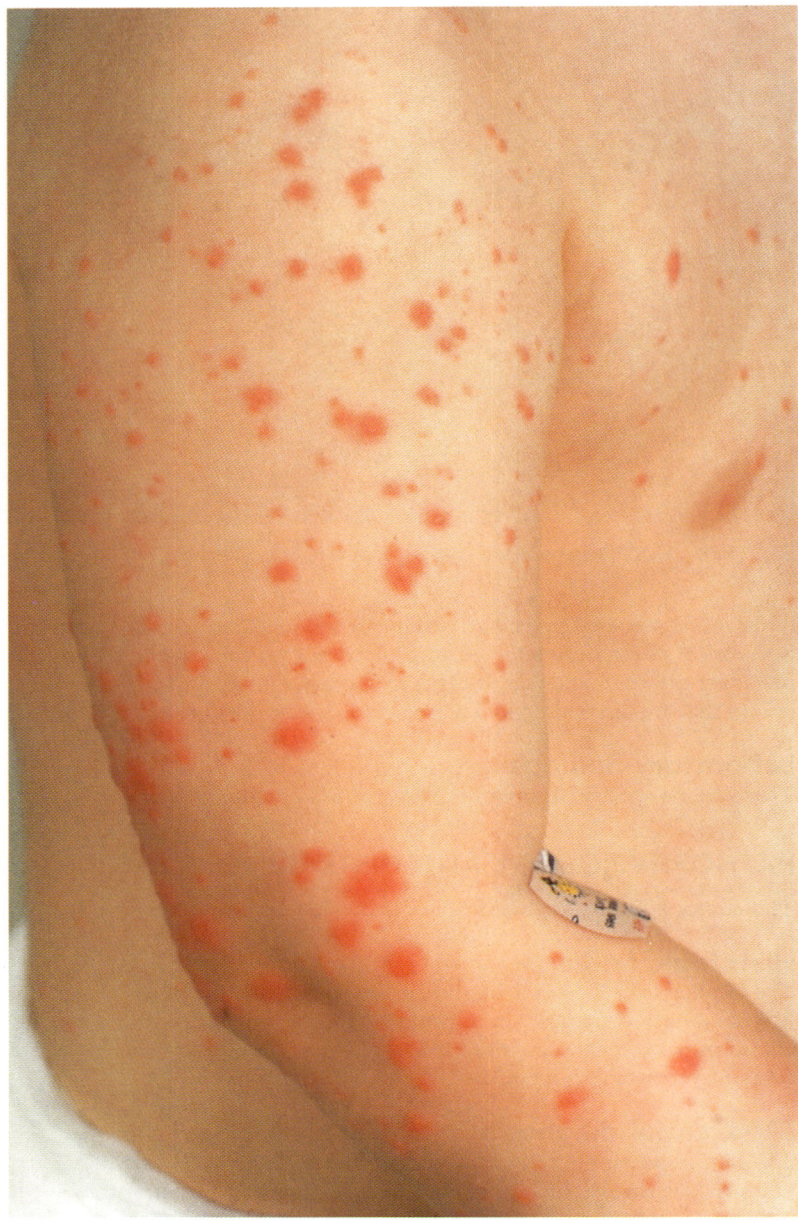

Fig. 15.31   Inflammatory symmetrical lesions of Gianotti-Crosti on arm.

General examination may reveal features of the associated viral infection: fever, lymphadenopathy, hepatosplenomegaly, mouth ulcers, pharyngitis, and respiratory signs. Lymphadenopathy and splenomegaly are not specific for hepatitis B associated cases.[329,333,334]

Laboratory findings

Cases not associated with hepatitis B virus infection usually have no specific laboratory findings apart from virus identification through culture, immunofluorescence, PCR, and/or serology. Lymphopenia or lymphocytosis are often seen as a nonspecific response to the virus infection. Although abnormal liver function tests are a constant feature of hepatitis B associated cases, it can be seen in cases not involving hepatitis B virus (e.g., EBV infection). Most cases of hepatitis B associated Gianotti-Crosti syndrome are caused by the hepatitis B subtype designated ayw.[331,332] Patients with risk

some cases. The eruption can start on the face, buttocks, or limbs, and evolves over a 7-day period to involve the face, buttocks, and limbs. Partial expression is common, with sparing of the face and/or buttocks. The eruption is usually asymptomatic but can be pruritic in come cases. Resolution of the eruption can take 2–8 weeks.[329,333,334]

333. Chuh AAT (2001) Diagnostic criteria for Gianotti-Crosti syndrome: a prospective case-control study for validity assessment. **Cutis** 68:207–213.

334. Hofmann R, Schuppe H-C, Adams O (1997) Gianotti-Crosti syndrome associated with Epstein-Barr virus infection. **Pediatr Dermatol** 14:2733–2777.

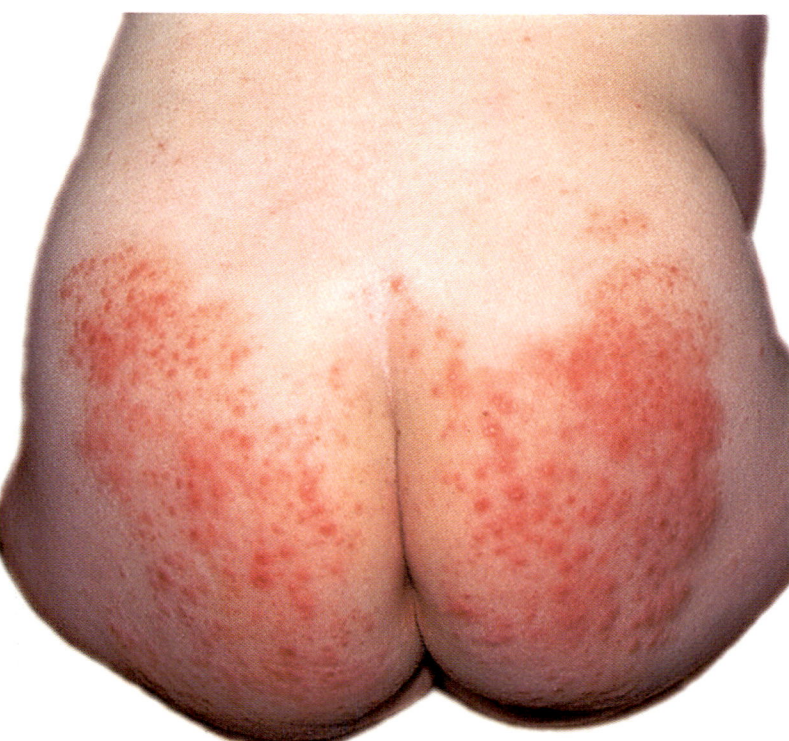

Fig. 15.32 Gianotti-Crosti on buttocks.

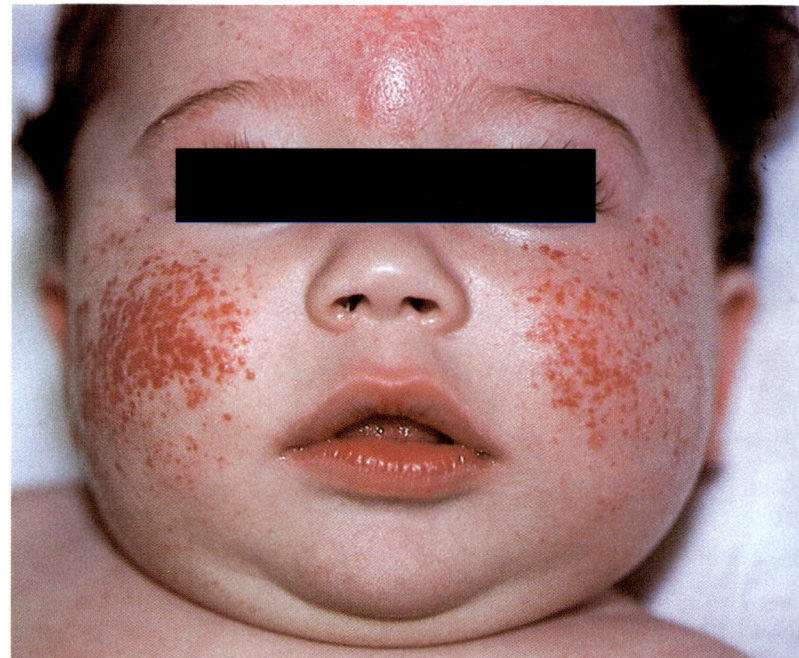

Fig. 15.33 Gianotti-Crosti with purpuric facial lesions.

factors for hepatitis B virus infection should be screened for the virus on initial presentation.

PATHOPHYSIOLOGY AND HISTOGENESIS

Gianotti-Crosti syndrome can develop with the following infections: hepatitis B virus,[326,327,329,331,332] Epstein–Barr virus,[334] cytomegalovirus,[335] rotavirus,[336] parvovirus B-19,[337] coxsackie B virus,[338] coxsackie A-16 virus,[339] respiratory syncytial virus,[340] enterovirus,[341,342] echovirus,[341,342] adenovirus,[341,342] polio virus,[340] rubella virus,[343] parainfluenza virus,[344] human herpesvirus 6,[345] and human immunodeficiency virus infection.[346] Furthermore, the Gianotti-Crosti syndrome has been reported to follow immunization involving diptheria-pertussis,[340] measles-mumps-rubella,[347] influenza,[348] polio,[334,349] diptheria-pertussis-tetanus-oral polio-hemophilus influenzae B combination,[350] hepatitis B,[351] measles-hepatitis B,[352] and bacille Calmette-Guerin (BCG).[353] Like other viral exanthems, the initial step is hematogenous dissemination of the causative virus to the skin. The subsequent immune reponse to the virus generates an inflammatory reaction in cutaneous structures (epidermis, blood vessels) that gives rise to the eruption. It is possible that immune complex deposition in cutaneous vessels may be involved in the development of the eruption in hepatitis B induced cases.

Histologic findings

The histologic features of Gianotti-Crosti syndrome are nonspecific. The epidermis exhibits mild acanthosis, focal parakeratosis, and focal spongiosis. The papillary dermis is mildly edematous with a superficial lymphohistiocytic infiltrate that is usually perivascular, but can be band-like in appearance. Occasionally, lymphocytic vasculitis can be evident with extravasation of red blood cells.[98,344]

Differential diagnosis

Classic Gianotti-Crosti is rarely confused with other skin disease; when purpuric lesions are present they need to be distinguished from septicemia, pityriasis lichenoides, Henoch–Schonlein purpura and, in the presence of lymphadenopathy and hepatosplenomegaly, Langerhans histiocytosis. Skin biopsy and appropriate microbiologic studies will distinguish these entities.

335. Baleviciene G, Maciulevicienen R, Schwartz RA (2001) Papular acrodermatitis of childhood: the Gianotti-Crosti syndrome. **Cutis** 67:291–294.
336. Di Lernia V (1998) Gianotti-Crosti syndrome related to rotavirus infection. **Pediatr Dermatol** 15:485–486.
337. Carrascosa JM, Just M, Ribera M et al. (1998) Papular acrodermatitis of childhood related to poxvirus and parvovirus B-19 infection. **Cutis** 61:265–267.
338. Taieb A, Plantin P, Du Pasquier P et al. (1986) Gianotti-Crosti syndrome; a study of 26 cases. **Br J Dermatol** 115:49–59.
339. James WD, Odom RD, Hatch MH (1982) Gianotti-Crosti-like eruption associated with coxsackie A-16 infection. **J Am Acad Dermatol** 6:862.
340. Draelos ZK, Hansen RC, James WD (1986) Gianotti-Crosti syndrome associated with infections other than hepatitis B. **JAMA** 256:2386–2388.
341. Rogers S, Connolly JH (1974) Gianotti-Crosti syndrome and viral infection. **Br Med J** 3:529.
342. Labbe A, Peyrot J, Goumy P et al. (1982) Syndrome acropapulovesiculeux de l'enfant et maladie de Gianotti-Crosti. **Pediatrie** 37:467.
343. Patrizi A, Di Lemia V, Neri J et al. (1994) An unusual case of recurrent Gianotti-Crosti syndrome. **Pediatr Dermatol** 11:283–284.
344. Spear KL, Winkelmann RK (1984) Gianotti-Crosti syndrome. A review of ten cases not associated with hepatitis B. **Arch Dermatol** 120:891–896.

345. Yasumoto S, Tsujita J, Imayama S et al. (1996) Gianotti-Crosti syndrome associated with human herpesvirus-6 infection. **J Dermatol** 23:499–501.
346. Blauvelt A, Turner M (1994) Gianotti-Crosti syndrome and human immunodeficiency virus infection. **Arch Dermatol** 130:481–483.
347. Velangi SS, Tidman MJ (1998) Gianotti-Crosti syndrome after measles, mumps and rubella vaccination. **Br J Dermatol** 139:1122–1123.
348. Cambiaghi S, Scarabelli G, Pistritto G et al. (1995) Gianotti-Crosti syndrome in an adult after influenza virus vaccination. **Dermatology** 191:340–341.
349. Erkek E, Boztepe Senturk G, Ozkaya O et al. (2001) Gianotti-Crosti syndrome preceded by polio vaccine and followed by varicella infection. **Pediatr Dermatol** 18:516–518.
350. Murphy LA, Buckley C (2000) Gianotti-Crosti syndrome in an infant following immunisation. **Pediatr Dermatol** 17:225–226.
351. Tay YK (2001) Gianotti-Crosti syndrome following immunisation. **Pediatr Dermatol** 18:262.
352. Andiran N, Senturk GB, Bukulmez G (2002) Combined vaccination by measles and hepatitis B vaccines: a new cause of Gianotti-Crosti syndrome. **Dermatology** 204:75–76.
353. Duterque M (1989) Syndrome de Gianotti-Crosti associee a vaccination avec BCG. **Rev Eur Dermatol** 1:198–201.

THERAPY AND PROGNOSIS

There is no specific treatment for the Gianotti-Crosti syndrome.

PITYRIASIS ROSEA

The earliest description of pityriasis rosea was provided by Robert Willan in 1798. He referred to the eruption as roseola annulata.[354] Camille Gibert is credited with the introduction of the name pityriasis rosea,[355] which is derived from the Greek word, pityriasis (fine scale), and the Latin word, rosea (rose-red). Pityriasis rosea is an acute, self-limited, papulosquamous disorder with a highly characteristic morphology and clinical course. It typically begins with a scaly erythematous patch or plaque known as the herald patch, which precedes and heralds the onset of the widespread papulosquamous eruption.

EPIDEMIOLOGY

Genetics

There is no evidence for the involvement of genetic factors.

Statistics

Most cases occur between 10 and 35 years of age with a peak around 20–24 years of age. Males and females are equally affected.[356–359] One series found 45% of cases involved the 0–19 year age group, 14% involved children under 10 years of age and only 4% involved children under 4 years of age.[358] Fewer than 20 cases have been reported in infants less than 2 years of age with the two youngest being 3 and 4 months old.[360,361] Most cases occur in the months of spring and autumn.[356–359]

PRESENTING HISTORY

Patients present either with the initial herald patch, which can be mistaken for tinea, or with the subsequent widespread eruption for assessment. Five percent will give a history of a preceding viral illness.[357]

PHYSICAL EXAMINATION

The clinical findings vary with the stage of the illness (Fig. 15.34, 15.35).[356–359] In 50–80% of cases, the herald patch is usually the only finding in the very early stages of the illness. It usually precedes the onset of the widespread eruption by a period that ranges from several days (the usual presentation) to three months. In a small percentage of cases, its appearance coincides with the onset of the widespread eruption. Any part of the body can be involved, and in 5% of cases more than one herald patch develops. The herald patch begins as a nondescript, smooth erythematous macule or papule, which expands over 1–2 weeks to form an oval shaped patch or plaque. Central clearing may accompany expansion, giving rise to an annular lesion. Desquamation eventually occurs, creating surface scale that is attached at the periphery with the free edge directed toward the center of the lesion. This is referred to as a "collarette of scale" which is characteristic of pityriasis rosea. The widespread eruption evolves bilaterally and symmetrically over 1–3 weeks on the trunk, neck, face, and proximal limbs. The eruption consists of oval shaped, erythematous papules that enlarge to a maximum size of 5–30mm. The lesions are initially smooth but quickly develop the typical

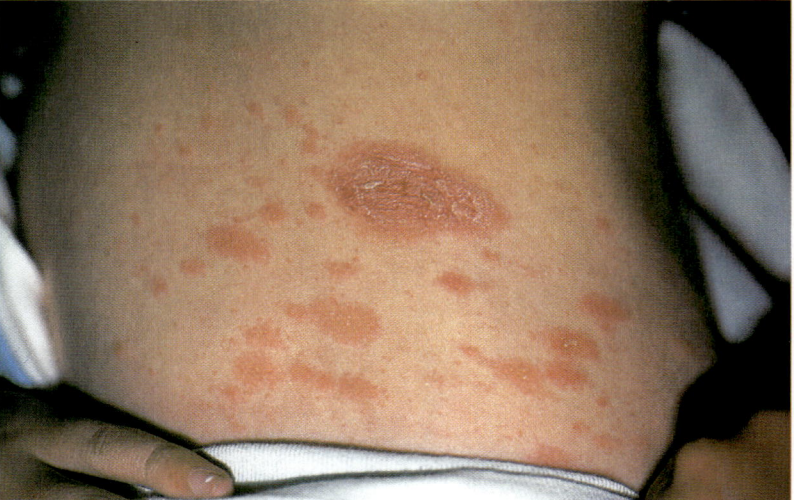

Fig. 15.34 A herald patch and oval lesions of pityriasis rosea.

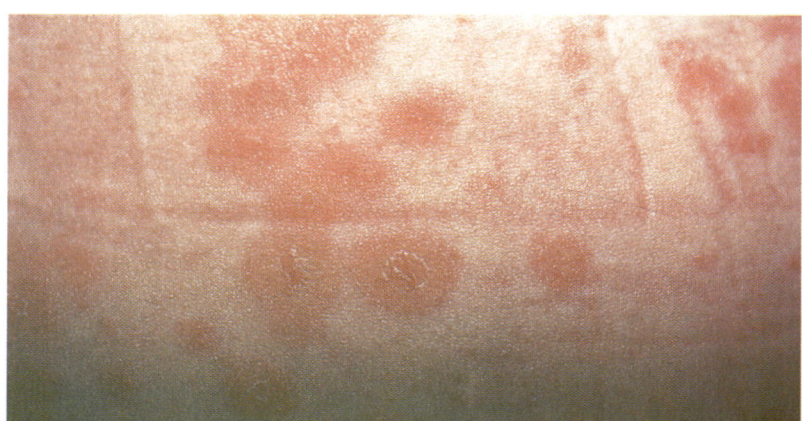

Fig. 15.35 Papules of pityriasis rosea exhibiting a collarette of scale.

collarette of scale on the surface. On the posterior trunk, the long axis of the papules runs parallel to the ribs, giving rise to the highly characteristic Christmas-tree or fir-tree pattern. The eruption is often pruritic in the early stages. Resolution always occurs over over a period of 4–8 weeks. Clearance may be associated with postinflammatory hypopigmentation or hyperpigmentation in patients with dark complexions.

A number of clinical variants have been reported. The eruption can have vesicular,[362] pustular,[363] purpuric,[363,364] or erythema multiforme-like lesions[365] with or instead of the typical papules, and a rare generalized exfoliative erythroderma. The eruption can localize to the face and limbs with sparing of the trunk (inverse pityriasis rosea),[366] localize to the axillae and groin as large plaques (pityriasis circinata et marginata of Vidal),[367] localize to one area of the body[368] or one side of the body.[369] In Black patients, an inverse distribution with facial and acial lesions is called atypical pityriasis rosea.

354. Willan R (1808) On cutaneous diseases. London: J. Johnson, 1796–1808, pp. 189–196.
355. Gibert CM (1860) Traite pratique des maladies de la peau et de la syphilis, 3rd ed. Paris, H. Plon, p. 402.
356. Niles HD, Klumpp MM (1940) Pityriasis rosea: review of the literature and report of two hundred and nineteen cases, in thirty eight of which convalescent serum was used. **Arch Dermatol Syph** 41:265–294.
357. Bjornberg A, Hellgren L (1962) Pityriasis rosea. A statistical, clinical and laboratory investigation of 826 patients and matched healthy controls. **Acta Derm Venereol** (Stockh) 42(suppl 50):1–68.
358. Parsons JM (1986) Pityriasis rosea update: 1986. **J Am Acad Dermatol** 15:159–167.
359. Chuang T, Ilstrup DM, Perry HO et al. (1982) Pityriasis rosea in Rochester, Minnesota, 1969–1978: a 10-year epidemiologic study. **J Am Acad Dermatol** 7:80–89.
360. Hyatt HW (1960) Pityriasis rosea in a 3-month-old infant. **Arch Pediatr** 77:364–368.
361. RuDuskey BM (1963) Pityriasis rosea in a 4-month-old infant. **J Pediatr** 62:159–160.

362. Strauss T, Kuhn A, Steigleder GK (1988) Vesicular pityriasis rosea. **Hautarzt** 39:524–526.
363. Butterworth T (1935) Pityriasis rosea: clinical varieties and etiology. **Penn Med J** 38:400–403.
364. Pierson JC, Dijkstra JWE, Elston DM (1993) Purpuric pityriasis rosea. **J Am Acad Dermatol** 28:1021.
365. Friedman SJ (1987) Pityriasis rosea with erythema multiforme-like lesions. **J Am Acad Dermatol** 17:135–136.
366. Imamura S, Ozaki M, Horiguchi Y et al. (1971) Atypical pityriasis rosea. **Dermatologica** 171:474–477.
367. Sterling JC, Kurtz JC (1998) Viral infections. In: Textbook of Dermatology, 6th edn, Champion RH, Burton JL, Burns DA, Breathnach SM, eds. Oxford: Blackwell Science Publications, pp. 995–1095.
368. Ahmed I, Charles-Holmes R (2000) Localised pityriasis rosea. **Clin Exp Dermatol** 25:624–626.
369. Del Campo DV, Barsky S, Tisocco L et al. (1983) Pityriasis rosea. unilaterlis. **Int J Dermatol** 22:312–313.

Oral lesions may occur during the course of pityriasis rosea. Punctate petechiae, ulceration, erythematous macules, and plaques, vesicles, and bullae have all been reported.[370,371] Oral lesions appear to be more common in children, black patients, and patients with widespread disease.[370] There has been one report of the appearance of nail pitting during the course of pityriasis rosea that evolved into rectangular areas of dystrophy.[372]

Laboratory findings

There are no specific laboratory abnormalities reported with pityriasis rosea.

PATHOPHYSIOLOGY AND HISTOGENESIS

Clinical and epidemiologic data support the long-held belief that an infectious agent is the cause of pityriasis rosea. Pityriasis rosea preferentially develops during autumn and spring.[356–359] There is a viral-like prodromal illness in some patients[356–359] and a history of a preceding upper respiratory tract infection in some cases,[373] as well as clustering of cases within families and institutions.[374] Spontaneous resolution occurs in all patients with a very low incidence of recurrence (<3%).[356–359] CD4+ T cells and Langerhans cells are found in the dermis of early lesions of pityriasis rosea.[375] Recent attention has focused on the role of human herpesvirus 7 (HHV-7) in the pathogenesis. In 1997, Drago et al.[376,377] reported the identification of HHV-7 DNA in cell free plasma, peripheral blood mononuclear cells, and lesional skin of 12 patients with pityriasis rosea. In contrast, HHV-7 DNA was detected in 44% of peripheral blood mononuclear cells but was not isolated from the skin and sera of healthy controls. Serum interferon-alpha was elevated in the pityriasis rosea patients, which was indicative of a viral infection. This implicated HHV-7 as the cause of pityriasis rosea. Other research teams have been unable to confirm HHV-7 as the cause. Kempf et al.[378] were unable to identify HHV-7 in formalin-fixed paraffin-embedded tissues collected from 14 patients with pityriasis rosea. Watanabe et al.[379] detected HHV-7DNA in the sera of only 47% of patients and Kosuge et al.[380] found significant antibody increases in only a minority of patients. Two additional studies from Hong Kong and Taiwan found no DNA or serologic evidence of active HHV-7 infection in patients with pityriasis rosea.[381,382] Like the Gianotti-Crosti syndrome, pityriasis rosea maybe a reaction pattern caused by a variety of viruses.

Histologic findings

The epidermis exhibits focal parakeratosis and spongiosis. In the dermis, there is a perivascular lymphohistiocytic infiltrate with extravasated red blood cells. The extravasated red blood cells may also be found in the epidermis.[358]

Differential diagnosis

The herald patch of pityriasis rosea can be mistaken for tinea corporis. KOH microscopy and fungal culture will distinguish the two. The widespread eruption of pityriasis rosea needs to be distinguished from guttate psoriasis, pityriasis lichenoides, a pityriasis rosea-like drug eruption, and secondary syphilis. Psoriasis and pityriasis lichenoides do not exhibit a collarette of scale or herald patch, and both tend to persist indefinitely without treatment. The presence of psoriasis elsewhere and the recurring crops of lesions with pityriasis lichenoides are additional distinguishing features. Secondary syphilis is a routine consideration in sexually active teenagers and children with symptoms and/or signs of sexual abuse. It is easily excluded with serology. A pityriasis rosea-like drug eruption may occur in patients receiving medications such as gold. If a patient has a persistent pityriasis rosea-like eruption, underlying human immunodeficiency infection should be considered.[383]

THERAPY AND PROGNOSIS

In view of the self-limited nature of the eruption, treatment is only needed for patients suffering from significant pruritus and/or cosmetic impairment. Treatment options are oral erythromycin, UVB phototherapy, topical steroids, and oral steroids. The choice of treatment will be determined by the age of the patient, the availability of phototherapy, and the patient/family's decision. Erythromycin stearate (250mg QID for adults; 25–40mg/kg per day in four divided doses for children) administered over two weeks completely cleared 73% of patients receiving erythromycin compared with no reponse in patients receiving placebo.[384] Daily erythemogenic doses of UVB phototherapy over 5–10 days can significantly improve the eruption with a variable reduction in the degree of pruritus. Despite clinical improvement, the course of the disease is unaffected.[385,386] Potent topical steroids and/or oral steroids may temporarily reduce pruritus without altering the course of the disease. One report highlighted exacerbation of the eruption with oral steroid therapy.[387]

In most cases, cutaneous symptoms resolve in 6–12 weeks, even if left untreated. Reassurance should be given that the disorder is harmless, and that complete spontaneous clearing of symptoms will result.

PEDIATRIC ASPECTS OF THE DISEASE

Parents require reassurance of the benign self-limited nature of the eruption.

PITYRIASIS LICHENOIDES

Pityriasis lichenoides is an inflammatory skin disease with a characteristic clinical and histologic appearance. It was traditionally divided on clinical grounds into acute and chronic forms. Pityriasis lichenoides was first described in 1894 by Neisser[388] and Jadassohn[389] in separate reports. The chronic form was defined by Juliusberg in 1899[390] and given its present name, pityriasis lichenoides chronica (PLC). In 1916, Mucha recognized the acute form of pityriasis lichenoides as a distinct entity.[391] The term pityriasis lichenoides et varioliformis acute (PLEVA) was introduced by

370. Kay MH, Rapini RP, Fritz KA (1985) Oral lesions in pityriasis rosea. **Arch Dermatol** 121:1499–1451.
371. Vidimos AT, Camisa C (1992) Tongue and cheek: oral lesions in pityriasis rosea. **Cutis** 50:276–280.
372. Silvers SH, Glickman FS (1964) Pityriasis rosea followed by nail dystrophy. **Arch Dermatol** 90:31.
373. Chuang T, Perry HO, Ilstrup DM et al. (1983) Recent upper respiratory tract infection and pityriasis rosea: as case control study of 249 matched pairs. **Br J Dermatol** 108:587–591.
374. Messenger AG, Knox EG, Summerly R et al. (1982) Case clustering in pityriasis rosea: support for the role of an infective agent. **Br Med J** 284:371–373.
375. Aiba S, Tagami H (1985) Immunohistologic studies in pityriasis rosea: evidence for cellular immune reaction in the lesional epidermis. **Arch Dermatol** 121:761–765.
376. Drago F, Ranieri E, Malaguti F et al. (1997) Human herpesvirus 7 in patients with pityriasis rosea. Electron microscopy investigations and polymerase chain reaction in mononuclear cells, plasma and skin. **Dermatology** 195:374–378.
377. Drago F, Ranieri E, Malaguti F et al. (1997) Human herpesvirus 7 in pityriasis rosea [letter]. **Lancet** 349:1367–1368.
378. Kempf W, Adams V, Kleinhans M et al. (1999) Pityriasis rosea is not associated with human herpesvirus 7. **ArchDermatol** 135:1070–1072.
379. Watanabe T, Sugaya M, Nakamura K et al. (1999) Human herpesvirus 7 and pityriasis rosea. **J Invest Dermatol** 113:288–289.
380. Kosuge H, Tanaka-Taya K, Miyoshi H et al. (2000) Epidemiological study of human herpesvirus-6 and human herpesvirus-7 in pityriasis rosea. **Br J Dermatol** 143:795–798.

381. Chuh AA, Peiris JS (2001) Lack of evidence of active human herpesvirus 7 (HHV-7) infection on three cases of pityriasis rosea in children. **Pediatr Dermatol** 18:381–383.
382. Wong WR, Tsai CY, Shih SR et al. (2001) Association of pityriasis rosea with human herpesvirus-6 and human herpesvirus-7 in Taipei. **J Formos Med Assoc** 100:478–483.
383. Kaplin MH, Sadick N, McNutt NS et al. (1987) Dermatologic findings and manifestations of acquired immunodeficiency syndrome (AIDS). **J Am Acad Dermatol** 16:485–506.
384. Sharma PK, Yadav TP, Gautam RK et al. (2000) Erythromycin in pityriasis rosea: a double-blind placebo-controlled clinical trial. **J Am Acad Dermatol** 42:241–244.
385. Arndt KA, Paul BS, Stern RS et al. (1983) Treatment of pityriasis rosea with UV radiation. **Arch Dermatol** 119:381–382.
386. Leenutaphong V, Jiamton S (1995) UVB phototherapy for pityriasis rosea: a bilateral comparison study. **J Am Acad Dermatol** 33:996–999.
387. Leonforte JF (1981) Pityriasis rosea: exacerbation with corticosteroid treatment. **Dermatologica** 163:480–481.
388. Neisser A (1894) Zur Frage der lichenoiden eruption. **Verh Dtsch Dermatol Ges** 4:495.
389. Jadassohn J (1894) Ueber ein eigenartiges psoriasiformes und lichenoides exanthem. **Verh Dtsch Dermatol Ges** 4:524–535.
390. Juliusberg F (1899) Ueber die Pityriasis lichenoides chronica (psoriasiform lichenoides exanthem). **A Derm Syph** (Wien) 50:359.
391. Mucha V (1916) Uber einen der Parakeratosis variegata (Unna) bzw. Pityriasis lichenoides chronica (Neisser-Juliusberg) nahestehenden eigentumlichen Fall. **A Derm Syph** (Wien) 123:586.

Habermann in 1925 for the acute form of the disease.[392] The eponym Mucha–Habermann disease is often used for this acute entity. Degos reported the ulceronecrotic and febrile variant of PLEVA in 1966.[393] In view of the common clinical finding of acute and chronic lesions coexisiting at the same time,[394,395] PLEVA and PLC are now regarded as polar ends of a clinicopathologic spectrum rather than two distinct diseases, and the condition is known as pityriasis lichenoides.

EPIDEMIOLOGY

Genetics

Although familial cases have been reported,[396] there is no evidence implicating genetic factors in the disease process.

Statistics

The incidence of pityriasis lichenoides is unknown. Two large series of children with pityriasis lichenoides reported an age of onset that ranged from 8 months to 15 years with peaks around 5 and 10 years of age. Males and females were equally affected.[394,395]

PRESENTING HISTORY

Patients present with an erythematous eruption for assessment. When the eruption is predominantly acute there may be an accompanying fever and malaise.[395]

PHYSICAL EXAMINATION

Skin

The eruption of pityriasis lichenoides can be found on any part of the body. It is usually symmetrically distributed on the trunk with varying degrees of involvement of the neck, face, and limbs.[394,395] Clinical variants include preferential involvement of the limbs[395] and localization to a particular segment of skin.[397] The eruption manifests as recurring crops of lesions, giving rise to a polymorphic appearance with lesions in different stages of evolution (Fig. 15.36A,B). Lesions begin as reddish-brown macules and/or papules that can become purpuric before developing a spectrum of surface change. The acute form develops vesiculation with varying degrees of necrosis, ulceration, and crusting. Healing occurs over 2–6 weeks with postinflammatory hypopigmentation (Fig. 15.36C) or less commonly, hyperpigmentation. Varioliform scarring may follow lesions with significant necrosis and ulceration. The chronic form develops mica-like surface scale before resolving over 2–6 weeks with postinflammatory hypopigmentation or less commonly, hyperpigmentation. Scarring is not a feature of the chronic form.

A rare variant of pityriasis lichenoides is characterized by the sudden onset of high fever and malaise in patients with established pityriasis lichenoides. Skin lesions enlarge before the onset of marked hemorrhagic necrosis and ulceration. The lesions can last for months before healing with residual scarring.[398] This variant is referred to as the febrile ulceronecrotic variant of Mucha–Habermann disease.

Laboratory findings

There are no specific laboratory abnormalities in pityriasis lichenoides. The febrile ulceronecrotic variant will have nonspecific findings consistent with a severe inflammatory process (e.g., elevated ESR, C-reactive protein).

PATHOPHYSIOLOGY AND HISTOGENESIS

The etiology of pityriasis lichenoides is unknown. Recent studies have identified T-cell clonality within skin lesions of the acute and chronic forms of the disease.[399,400] This may represent clonal expansion of T cells in response to an antigenic stimulus provided by an unidentified infectious agent. Alternatively, it may indicate that pityriasis lichenoides is primarily a lymphoproliferative disorder that belongs to the cutaneous T-cell lymphoproliferative spectrum. The benign clinical course exhibited by most patients could be attributed to a vigorous host immune response involving CD8+ T cells, which predominate in the dermal infiltrate of pityriasis lichenoides.[401] Progression of pityriasis lichenoides to cutaneous T-cell lymphoma in children is rare[394,395] but has been reported.[402–404] This may require additional genetic alterations such as those reported for the progression of lymphomatoid papulosis into frank cutaneous T-cell lymphoma.[405]

There has been a report of four children with mycosis fungoides presenting with lesions clinically consistent with the acute and chronic forms of pityriasis lichenoides.[406]

Histologic findings

Pityriasis lichenoides exhibits a spectrum of epidermal and dermal changes. The epidermal changes consist of parakeratosis, exocytosis of lymphocytes, intraepidermal red blood cells, and interface damage that varies from mild vacuolar degeneration of basal keratinocytes through ballooning of keratinocytes to necrosis of individual keratinocytes to confluent necrosis of the epidermis in severe cases. The dermis exhibits a lymphohistiocytic inflammatory infiltrate that varies from superficial to deep involvement. The latter usually has a wedge-shaped appearance. The infiltrate is accompanied by varying degrees of dermal edema and extravasation of red blood cells.[394,395]

Differential diagnosis

The acute form needs to be distinguished from varicella, an insect bite reaction, leucocytoclastic vasculitis, septicemia, vesicular pityriasis rosea, and lymphomatoid papulosis. Varicella is distinguished by the short duration of the eruptive phase, the presence of oral lesions, and laboratory studies (direct immunofluorescence, viral culture). Insect bites will exhibit a central punctum, intense pruritus, and a different histology. Skin biopsy is usually needed to distinguish leukocytoclastic vasculitis and septicaemia. Vesicular pityriasis rosea and the acute form of pityriasis lichenoides share many clinical and histologic features and can be difficult to separate. The absence of recurring crops of lesions and clearance within a short period distinguish the two. Histologic examination is required to definitively differentiate the acute form of pityriasis lichenoides from lymphomatoid papulosis.

The chronic form mimics pityriasis rosea, guttate psoriasis, and lichen planus. The presence of mica-like surface scale and the polymorphic appearance of the eruption distinguishes pityriasis lichenoides from these conditions.

392. Haberman Ch R (1975) Uber die akut vereaufende, nekrotisierende Unterart der Pityriasis Lichenoides (Pityriasis lichenoides et varioliformis acuta). **Dermatol Z** 45:42.
393. Degos R, Duperrat B, Daniel F (1966) Le parapsoriasis ulceronecrotique hyperthermique. **Ann Dermatol Venereol** (Paris) 93:481–496.
394. Gelmetti C, Rigoni C, Alessi E et al. (1990) Pityriasis lichenoides in children: a long-term follow-up of eighty-nine cases. **J Am Acad Dermatol** 23:473–478.
395. Romani J, Puig L, Fernandez-Figueras MT et al. (1998) Pityriasis lichenoides in children: clinicopathologic review of 22 patients. **Pediatr Dermatol** 15:11–16.
396. Dupont C (1995) Pityriasis lichenoides in a family. **Br J Dermatol** 133:338–339.
397. Cliff S, Cook MG, Ostlere LS et al. (1996) Segmental pityriasis lichenoides chronica. **Clin Exp Dermatol** 21:461–462.
398. Luberti AA, Rabinowitz LG, Ververeli KO (1991) Severe febrile Mucha-Habermann's disease in children: case report and review of the literature. **Pediatr Dermatol** 8:51–57.
399. Dereure O, Levi E, Kadin ME (2000) T-cell clonality in pityriasis lichenoides et varioliformis acuta. **Arch Dermatol** 136:1483–1486.

400. Shieh S, Mikkola DL, Wood GS (2001) Differentiation and clonality of lesional lymphocytes in pityriasis lichenoides chronica. **Arch Dermatol** 137:305–308.
401. Varga FJ, Vonderheid EC, Olbricht SM et al. (1990) Immunohistological distinction of lymphomatoid papulosis and pityriasis lichenoides et varioliformic acuta. **Am J Pathol** 136:979–987.
402. Fortson JS, Schroeter AL, Esterly NB (1990) Cutaneous T-cell lymphoma (parapsoriasis en plaque). **Arch Dermatol** 126:1449–1453.
403. Niemczyk UM, Zollner TM, Wolter M et al. (1997) Te transformation of pityriasis lichenoides chronica into parakeratosis variegata in an 11-year-old girl. **Br J Dermatol** 137:983–987.
404. Thomson KF, Whittaker SJ, Russell-Jones R et al. (1999) Childhood cutaneous T-cell lymphoma in association with pityriasis lichenoides chronica. **Br J Dermatol** 141:1146–1148.
405. Knaus P, Lindemann D, DeCoteau JF et al. (1996) A dominant inhibitory mutant of the type II TGF-beta receptor in the malignant progression of a cutaneous T-cell lymphoma. **Mol Cell Biol** 16:3480–3489.
406. Ko J-W, Seong J-Y, Suh K-S et al. (2000) Pityriasis lichenoides-like mycosis fungoides in children. **Br J Dermatol** 142:347–352.

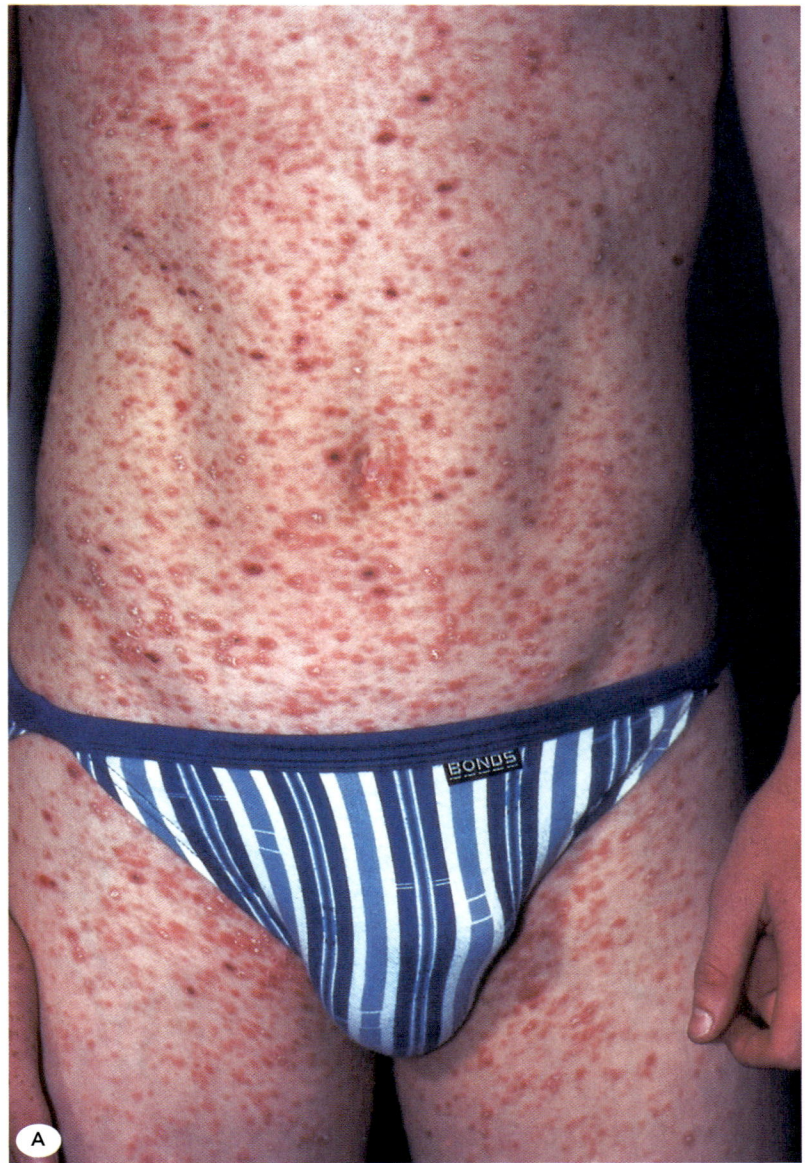

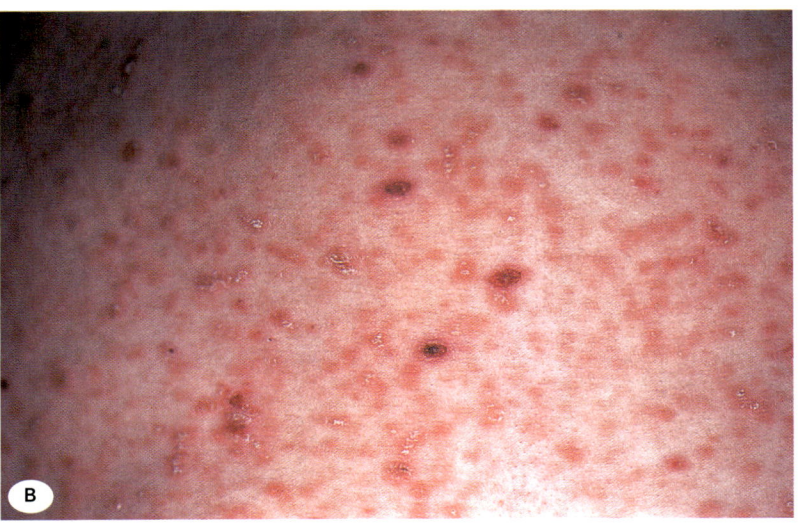

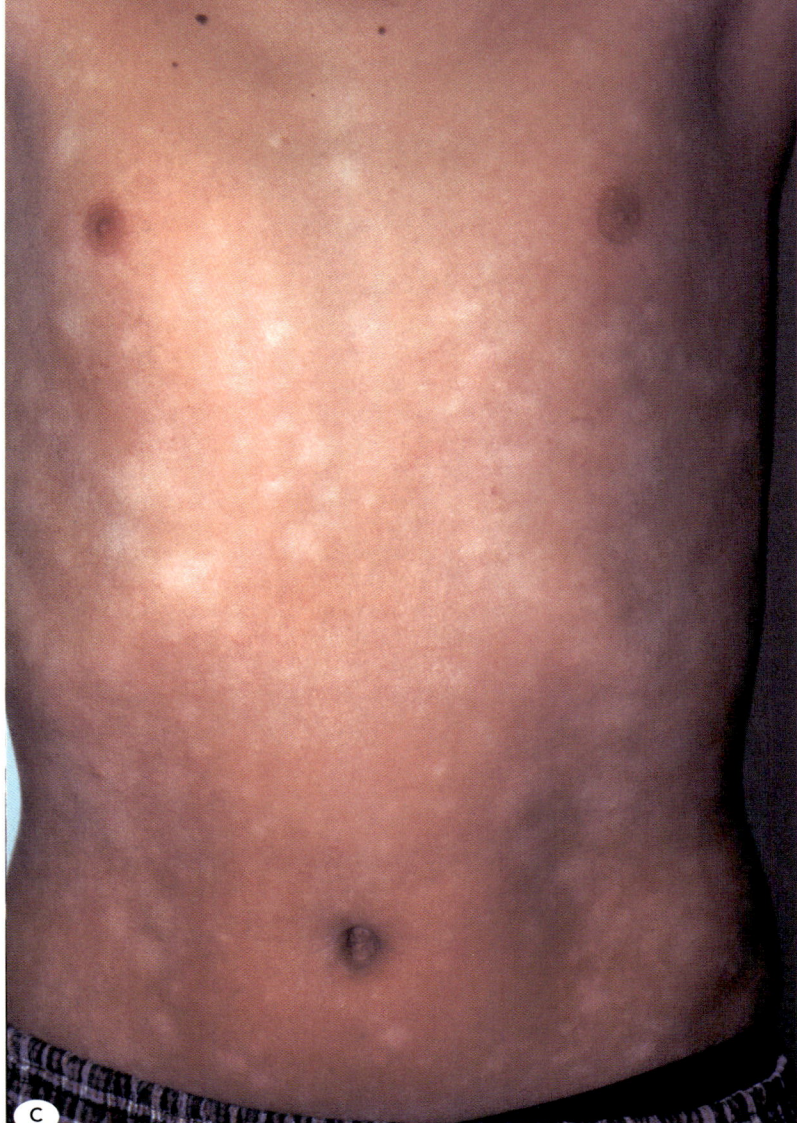

Fig. 15.36 (A) The polymorphic eruption of pityriasis lichenoides; note the mixture of acute (crusted) and chronic (scaly) lesions. (B) Higher power of (A). (C) Postinflammatory hypopigmentation associated with pityriasis lichenoides.

THERAPY AND PROGNOSIS

No treatment is needed for mild cases that are asymptomatic. The treatment options for symptomatic children with pityriasis lichenoides are oral antibiotics and phototherapy. Oral antibiotics are the initial treatment of choice. Both erythromycin (40mg/kg per day in divided doses)[394,395,407] and tetracyline (1–2g/day in divided doses)[408] have been reported to be of benefit. Erythromycin is preferred for children under 10 years of age. Topical steroids and anti histamines may be of some value. Patients not responding to oral antibiotics may benefit from phototherapy administered as natural sunlight exposure, formal UVB phototherapy,[394,395,409] UVA therapy,[409] or PUVA phototherapy.[395,410] Methotrexate has been used for the severe ulceronecrotic form of the disease.[395,411]

407. Truhan AP, Herbert AA, Esterly NB (1986) Pityriasis lichenoides in children: therapeutic response to erythromycin. **J Am Acad Dermatol** 15:66–70.
408. Piamphongsant T (1974) Tetracycline for the treatment of pityriasis lichenoides. **Br J Dermatol** 91:319–322.
409. LeVine MJ (1983) Phototherapy of pityriasis lichenoides. **Arch Dermatol** 119:378–380.
410. Powell FC, Muller SA (1984) Psoralens and ultraviolet A therapy of pityriasis lichenoides. **J Am Acad Dermatol** 10:59–64.
411. Lopez-Estebaranz JL, Vanaclocha F, Gil R et al. (1993) Febrile ulceronecrotic Mucha-Habermann disease. **J Am Acad Dermatol** 29:903–906.

Most patients spontaneously clear but this can take anywhere from several months to several years.[394,395] Approximately 25% of patients will have a chronic relapsing course over many years.[395] It is rare for pityriasis lichenoides in children to evolve into T-cell lymphoma.[402–404]

PEDIATRIC ASPECTS OF THE DISEASE

Families need to be reassured of the noninfectious nature of the condition because of its resemblance to varicella.

LYMPHOMATOID PAPULOSIS

In 1968, Macauley reported a 41-year-old female with a three-year history of a recurrent, asymptomtic, papulonecrotic eruption with the histological features of a lymphoma. The patient had no evidence of lymphoma at the time of presentation.[412] Macauley termed the clinically benign but histologically malignant condition lymphomatoid papulosis. The patient was subsequently monitored over a 25-year period and despite episodic recurrence of the skin eruption, she remained free of lymphoma.[413] Subsequent reports confirmed Macauley's observations, which form the basis for the current definition of lymphomatoid papulosis; a recurring, self-healing, papulonodular eruption with the histological features of a T-cell lympho-proliferative disorder. Although most cases remain clinically benign, 5–20% of cases will eventually develop a malignant lymphoma with mycosis fungoides, Hodgkin's disease, and CD30+ large cell lymphoma accounting for 90% of the malignant lymphomas in patients with lymphomatoid papulosis.[414,415]

EPIDEMIOLOGY
Genetics

There is no evidence for involvement of genetic factors.

Statistics

Lymphomatoid papulosis is rare in children. Cases have been reported from 11 months of age onwards, with a slight male predominance.[416–424]

PRESENTING HISTORY

Patients present with a recurring papulonodular eruption for assessment. The eruption is usually asymptomatic.

PHYSICAL EXAMINATION
Skin

Lymphomatoid papulosis is characterized by recurrent crops of asymptomatic, erythematous papules and nodules that develop at intervals of months

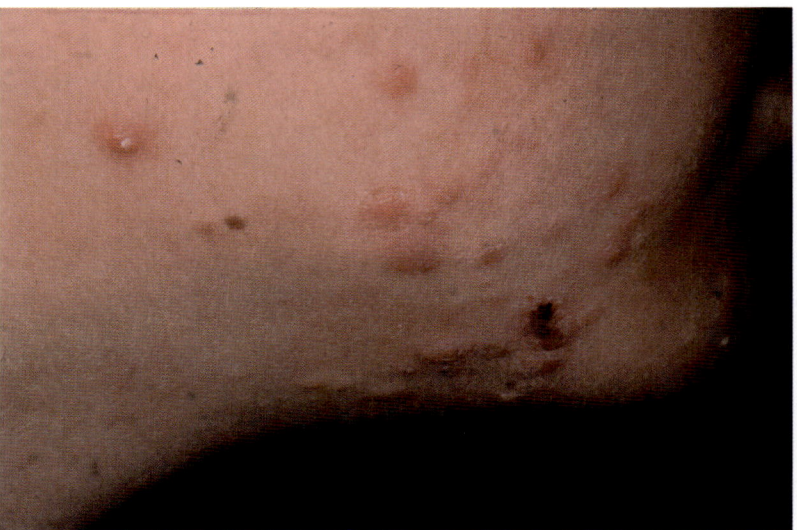

Fig. 15.37 Lymphomatoid papulosis.

to years. Although the papules and nodules are typically scattered over the trunk and limbs, they can develop anywhere and may remain localized to a particular region. Their number can vary from several to more than 100. The papules and nodules may remain smooth or exhibit varying degrees of crusting because of underlying necrosis and ulceration (Fig. 15.37). Lesions last for weeks to months before spontaneous resolution occurs. The affected skin may heal completely or exhibit varying degrees of hypo-pigmentation, hyperpigmentation, or atrophic scarring.[416–422] Morphologic variants include pustular[423] and vesicular lesions that clinically mimic hydroa vacciniforme.[424]

Other sites

Lymphadenopathy and hepatosplenomegaly are not found in pediatric cases.

Laboratory findings

There are no laboratory abnormalities.

PATHOPHYSIOLOGY AND HISTOGENESIS

Lymphomatoid papulosis is a T-cell lymphoproliferative disorder involving CD4+ or, less commonly, CD8+ T cells.[425] A recent report highlighted natural killer cells rather than T cells as the predominant cell type.[426] Studies have identified T-cell clonality within skin lesions of lymphomatoid papulosis.[427,428] The triggering factor for proliferation is unknown. The finding of

412. Macauley WL (1968) Lymphomatoid papulosis: a continuing self-healing eruption, clinically benign histologically malignant. **Arch Dermatol** 97:3–30.
413. Macauley WL (1989) Lymphomatoid papulosis update: a historical perspective. **Arch Dermatol** 125:1387–1389.
414. Harrington DS, Braddock SW, Blocher KS et al. (1989) Lymphomatoid papulosis and progression to T cell lymphoma: an immunophenotypic and genotypic analysis. **J Am Acad Dermatol** 21:951–957.
415. Scheen SR, Doyle JA, Winkelmann RK (1981) Lymphoma-associated papulosis: lymphomatoid papulosis associated with lymphoma. **J Am Acad Dermatol** 4:451–457.
416. Rogers M, De Launey J, Kemp A (1984) Lymphomatoid papulosis in an 11-month-old infant. **Pediatr Dermatol** 2:124–130.
417. Hellman J, Phelps RG, Baral J et al. (1990) Lymphomatosis papulosis with antigen deletion and clonal rearrangement in a 4 year-old boy. **Pediatr Dermatol** 7:42–47.
418. Patrizi A, DiLerna V, Neri I et al. (1991) Long-term follow-up of a patient with lymphomatoid papulosis. **Pediatr Dermatol** 8:93–94.
419. Zirbel GM, Gellis SE, Kadin ME et al. (1995) Lymphomatoid papulosis in children. **J Am Acad Dermatol** 33:741–748.
420. Paul M, Krowchuk DP, Hitchcock MG et al. (1996) Lymphomatoid papulosis: successful weekly pulse superpotent topical steroid corticosteroid therapy in three pediatric patients. **Pediatr Dermatol** 13:501–506.
421. Thomas GJ, Conejo-Mir JS, Ruiz AP et al. (1998) Lymphomatoid papulosis in childhood with exclusive acral involvement. **Pediatr Dermatol** 15:146–147.
422. Van Neer FJMA, Toonstra J, Van Voorst PC et al. (2001) Lymphomatoid papulosis in children: a study of 10 children registered by the Dutch Cutaneous Lymphoma Working Group. **Br J Dermatol** 144:351–354.
423. Barnadas MA, Lopez D, Pujol RM et al. (1992) Pustular lymphomatoid papulosis in childhood. **J Am Acad Dermatol** 27:627–628.
424. Tabata N, Aiba S, Ichonohazama R et al. (1995) Hydroa vacciniforme-like lymphomatoid papulosis in a Japanese child: a new subset. **J Am Acad Dermatol** 32:378–381.
425. Kadin ME (1986) Characteristic immunologic profile of large atypical cells in lymphomatoid papulosis. Possible implications for histogenesis and relationship to other diseases. **Arch Dermatol** 122:1388–1390.
426. Bekkenk MW, Kluin PM, Jansen PM et al. (2001) Lymphomatoid papulosis with a natural killer-cell phenotype. **Br J Dermatol** 145:318–322.
427. Whittaker S, Smith N, Russell-Jones R et al. (1991) Analysis of beta, gamma, and delta T-cell receptor genes in lymphomatoid papulosis: cellular basis of two distinct histologic subsets. **J Invest Dermatol** 96:786–791.
428. Basarab T, Fraser-Andrews EA, Orchard G et al. (1998) Lymphomatoid papulosis in association with mycosis fungoides: a study of 15 cases. **Br J Dermatol** 139:630–638.

paramyxovirus-like particles in skin biopsies from some patients suggests a viral-induced process.[429] The relationship between lymphomatoid papulosis and lymphoma is unclear. The large atypical cells in histologic type A (see below) express the CD30 antigen, which is also seen in Hodgkin's disease and CD30+ anaplastic large cell lymphoma. The smaller atypical cells in histologic type B (see below) resemble the atypical cells seen in mycosis fungoides. Hodgkin's disease, large cell lymphoma and mycosis fungoides can precede, develop with or succeed the onset of lymphomatoid papulosis in adults.[414,415] Several studies have identified the same clone of T cells in the skin lesions of lymphomatoid papulosis and lymphoma arising in the same patient.[428,430] Progression of some cases to lymphoma may involve mutations in the transforming growth factor-beta (TGF-beta) receptor complex, which prevents TGF-beta from regulating growth of lymphocytes.[431]

Histologic findings

Lymphomatoid papulosis is characterized by a superficial and deep, wedge-shaped infiltrate of mononuclear cells with occasional neutrophils and eosinophils. Numerous atypical cells are evident within the infiltrate. Three histologic subtypes (types A, B, and C) have been defined according to the appearance of the atypical cells.[432] Type A is characterized by large cells with vesicular nuclei, prominent nucleolus, and abundant cytoplasm described as lavender-colored on routine H&E examination. Multinucleate forms can be seen and may resemble Reed–Sternberg cells that are seen in Hodgkin's disease. The cells are CD30+ and UCHL-1-negative. Type B is characterized by smaller, cerebriform, mononuclear cells with scant cytoplasm that resemble the atypical cells of mycosis fungoides. The cells are CD3+, UCHL-1-positive and CD30−. Type C is characterized by an abundance of Type A cells that conveys the impression of CD30+ large cell anaplastic lymphoma. Type C can only be distinguished from lymphoma on clinical grounds with spontaneous resolution of Type C skin lesions. A mixture of type A and B can occur.

Differential diagnosis

Lymphomatoid papulosis needs to be distinguished from an insect bite reaction, pityriasis lichenoides, lymphoma, and pseudolymphoma. Insect bites are pruritic and can be differentiated with skin biopsy. The lesions of pityriasis lichenoides are smaller, less indurated and do not have CD30+ cells in the dermal infiltrate. Distinguishing lymphoma from lymphomatoid papulosis can be difficult in view of the clinical and histologic overlap. A final diagnosis relies on evidence of involvement elsewhere (e.g., lymphadenopathy), the clinical behaviour of the eruption, and response to treatment. Histologic findings distinguish lymphomatoid papulosis from pseudolymphoma.

THERAPY AND PROGNOSIS

There are no therapeutic guidelines for the treatment of lymphomatoid papulosis in children. In view of the self-limited nature of the eruption, no treatment is needed for mild cases that spontaneously heal without scarring.[421,422] Treatments that have been used for severe pediatric cases include superpotent topical steroids,[419,420,433] intralesional and oral corti-costeroids,[424,433] oral antibiotics (erythromycin, tetracycline)[417,418,433] UVB phototherapy,[433] and PUVA phototherapy.[434] Methotrexate has been used in adults[435] and remains an option for children with severe disease.

The clinical course of lymphomatoid papulosis in children is variable. In Zirbel et al.'s[419] review of 23 pediatric cases and Van Neer et al.'s[422] review of 10 cases, most patients had a protracted clinical course with recurring crops of lesions over many years. In a minority of patients, the recurrences gradually decreased in severity and frequency until resolution occurred. Scarring can be a problem with severely affected cases. Apart from one recent case of CD30+ anaplastic large cell lymphoma developing in a 16-year-old female with lymphomatoid papulosis,[436] lymphoma is a complication of adult patients. Nevertheless, pediatric patients with lymphomatoid papulosis need regular follow-up as a precautionary measure.

PARAPSORIASIS

In 1902, Brocq created the term parapsoriasis to encompass a number of conditions that clinically resembled psoriasis and seborrheic dermatitis.[437] Brocq divided the patients into three subgroups, termed parapsoriasis en gouttes, parapsoriasis lichenoide, and parapsoriasis en plaques. Parapsoriasis en gouttes was characterized by small papules and papulosquamous lesions that resembled psoriasis or secondary syphyllis. Parapsoriasis lichenoide consisted of a network of pseudopapular lesions with atrophy that exhibited an atrophic appearance. This group included cases referred to as parakeratosis variegata and poikiloderma vascular atrophicans of Jacobi. Parapsoriasis en plaques referred to round or oval-shaped patches with subtle pityriasiform surface scale that measured 2–6cm in size.

The modern classification of parapsoriasis contains only two groups termed large plaque and small plaque parapsoriasis.[438] Large plaque parapsoriasis replaces the parapsoriasis lichenoide group. Small plaque parapsoriasis replaces the parapsoriasis en plaques group and is also referred to as chronic superficial dermatitis or digitate dermatosis. The parapsoriasis en gouttes type has been reclassified as pityriasis lichenoioides.

EPIDEMIOLOGY

Genetics

There is no evidence of involvement of genetic factors.

Statistics

Both types of parapsoriasis are predominantly diseases of adults. Only 5% of small plaque parapsoriasis and 20% of large plaque parapsoriasis cases reported in one large series involved children. Males are more commonly affected than females in both types.[439]

PRESENTING HISTORY

Patients usually present with asymptomatic patches on the skin. The patient is otherwise well.

PHYSICAL EXAMINATION

Small plaque parapsoriasis is characterized by asymptomatic, well-defined, reddish-yellow colored papules and plaques with fine surface scale that imparts a wrinkled appearance. The lesions measure 3–6cm in diameter and are usually

429. Sandbank M, Feuerman EJ (1972) Lymphomatoid papulosis: an electron microscope study of the acute and healing stages with demonstration of paramyxovirus-like particles. Acta Derm Venereol (Stockh) 52:337–345.
430. Chott A, Vonderheid EC, Olbricht S et al. (1996) The same dominant T-cell clone is present in multiple regressing skin lesions and associated T-cell lymphomas of patients with lymphomatoid papulosis. J Invest Dermatol 106:696–700.
431. Kadin ME, Levi E, Kempf W (2001) Progression of lymphomatois papulosis to systemic lymphoma is associated with escape from growth inhibition by transforming growth factor-beta and CD30 ligand. Ann N Y Acad Sci 941:59–68.
432. Willemze R Kerl H, Sterry W et al. (1997) EORTC classification for primary cutaneous lymphomas: a proposal from the Cutaneous Lymphoma Study Group of the European Oranization for Research and Treatment of Cancer. Blood 90:354–371.
433. Ashworth J, Paterson WD, MacKie RM (1987) Lymphomatoid papulosis/pityriasis lichenoides in two children. Pediatr Dermatol 4:238–241.
434. Volkenandt M, Kerscher M, Sander C et al. (1995) PUVA-bath photochemotherapy resulting in rapid clearance of lymphomatoid papulosis in a child. Arch Dermatol 131:1094.
435. Vonderheid EC, Sajjadian A, Kadin ME et al. (1996) Methotrexate is effective therapy of lymphomatoid papulosis and other primary cutaneous CD30-positive lymphoproliferative disorders. J Am Acad Dermatol 34:470–481.
436. Rifkin S, Valderrama E, Lipton JM et al. (2001) Lymphomatoid papulosis and Ki-11 anaplastic large cell lymphoma occurring concurrently in a pediatric patient. J Pediatr Hematol Oncol 23:321–323.
437. Brocq L (1902) Les parapsoriasis. Ann Dermatol Syphilol 3:433–468.
438. Lambert WC, Everett MA (1981) The nosology of parapsoriasis. J Am Acad Dermatol 5:373.
439. Samman PD (1975) Cutaneoud reticuloses. Trans St John's Hosp Derm Soc 61:11.

localized to the trunk and proximal limbs. A digitate pattern resembling fingerprint marks on the sides of the trunk is particularly characteristic of small plaque parapsoriasis.[438,439] Large plaque parapsoriasis manifests as patches or thin plaques that measure more than 5cm in diameter. The lesions can be well defined or blend imperceptibly into the surrounding skin. The bathing trunk area, breasts, and flexures are the most commonly affected sites. The patches or plaques are reddish-brown or salmon pink in color. The surface is slightly scaly and with time develops a wrinkled, atrophic appearance. Atrophic changes are usually accompanied by telangiectasia and mottled pigmentation that is collectively known as poikiloderma. A rare variant is retiform parapsoriasis, which refers to a net-like or zebra-like pattern of scaly macules and papules that eventually becomes poikilodermatous in appearance.[403,438,439]

Laboratory findings

There are no laboratory abnormalities.

PATHOPHYSIOLOGY AND HISTOGENESIS

Both types of parapsoriasis appear to be mediated by CD4+ T cells containing a dominant T-cell clone.[403,440,441] The reason for the T-cell mediated process is unknown. Debate has focused on whether either condition is premalignant or malignant from the outset. Although some authors consider small plaque parapsoriasis to be an early, nonprogressive variant of mycosis fungoides,[442,443] the concensus view is that small plaque parapsoriasis is not a premalignant or malignant condition, based on the findings of several large series of patients.[439,444] In contrast, large plaque parapsoriasis is considered to be a premalignant condition because 10–30% of cases progress to overt mycosis fungoides.[438] The risk is particularly high for patients with the retiform pattern of the disease.

Histologic findings

In small plaque parapsoriasis, the histologic features are nonspecific. The epidermis exhibits mild spongiosis, hyperkeratosis, parakeratosis, and exocytosis. A mild superficial perivascular lymphocytic infiltrate in evident in the dermis. The lymphocytes are not atypical in appearance. In early large plaque parapsoriasis, the epidermis exhibits mild acanthosis, hyperkeratosis, and patchy parakeratosis. The underlying lymphocytic infiltrate is sparse and perivascular in distribution. More advanced lesions have epidermal atrophy, marked exocytosis of lymphocytes, and a band-like infiltrate of lymphocytes in the papillary dermis. The epidermotropic lymphocytes may be scattered singly or grouped together. Additional dermal changes include dilated vessels and melanophages.[403,439,440]

Differential diagnosis

Small plaque parapsoriasis should be distinguished from nummular eczema, tinea corporis, plaque psoriasis, and mycosis fungoides. The presence of pruritus and response to topical steroids distinguishes small plaque parapsoriasis from nummular eczema. Fungal culture helps exclude tinea corporis, and psoriasis will be evident elsewhere. Large plaque parapsoriasis needs to be distinguished from genodermatoses and connective tissue

diseases exhibiting poikiloderma, radiodermatitis, and mycosis fungoides. The genodermatoses, connective tissue diseases, and radiodermatitis can be distinguished by associated clinical findings. Mycosis fungoides can only be excluded with skin biopsy.

THERAPY AND PROGNOSIS

Therapy

Small plaque parapsoriasis usually requires no treatment. If the lesions are itchy or a cosmetic problem, they can be treated with topical corticosteroids or UVB phototherapy.[438,439] Response to treatment is variable and only temporary. Large plaque parapsoriasis can be treated with potent topical steroid therapy, UVB phototherapy, and PUVA phototherapy.[438,439,445] Care needs to be taken if topical steroids are used on lesions with evidence of atrophy. Local radiotherapy can be used if malignant transformation has occurred. Oral treatments are ineffective.

Prognosis

Both forms of parapsoriasis follow a chronic, slowly progressive course over many years. The small plaque type is clinically benign with no risk of progression to lymphoma. In contrast, the large plaque variety will progress to overt mycosis fungoides in 10–30% of cases. Routine follow-up with repeat biopsy is essential for this group of patients.

PITYRIASIS RUBRA PILARIS

Pityriasis rubra pilaris (PRP) was first described by Devergie in 1856, under the title pityriasis pilaris.[446] The full name of pityriasis rubra pilaris was proposed by Besnier in 1889.[447] The term PRP is used to describe a group of conditions that are characterized by a combination of keratotic follicular papules, scaly erythematous patches that coalesce to form plaques or widespread erythroderma, and palmoplantar keratoderma. In view of the unknown etiology and absence of a reliable diagnostic test, PRP has been traditionally classified on clinical grounds into five types (Table 15.3).[448–450] Some authors have proposed a sixth type of PRP that is associated with HIV infection in adults[451–454] and children.[455] Griffith considers these cases to represent a distinct, separate entity unrelated to true PRP and argues against the creation of a sixth type of PRP.[456] The three subtypes of PRP relevant to pediatric dermatology are type III (classic or acute juvenile), type IV (circumscribed or localized juvenile) and type V (atypical juvenile).

TABLE 15.3	Classification of pityriasis rubra pilaris
Type I	Classic type; adult onset
Type II	Atypical type; adult onset
Type III	Classic type; juvenile onset
Type IV	Localized or circumscribed juvenile onset
Type V	Atypical type; juvenile onset

440. Haeffner AC, Smoller BR, Zepter K et al. (1995) Differentiation and clonality of lesional lymphocytes in small plaque parapsoriasis. Arch Dermatol 131:321–324.
441. Wood GS (1994) Detection of clonal T-cell receptor gamma-gene rearrangements in early mycosis fungoides/Sezary syndrome by polymerase chain reaction and denaturing gradient gel electrophoresis (PCR/DGGE). J Invest Dermatol 103:34.
442. King-Ismael D, Ackerman AB (1992) Guttate parapsoriasis/digitate dermatosis (small plaque parapsoriasis) is mycosis fungoides. Am J Dermatopathol 14:518.
443. Ackerman AB (1996) If small plaque (digitate) parapsoriasis is a cutaneous T-cell lymphoma, even an abortive one, it must be mycosis fungoides. Arch Dermatol 132:562.
444. Burg G, Dummer R, Nestle FO et al. (1996) Cutaneous lymphomas consist of a spectrum of nosologically different entities including mycosis fungoides and small plaque parapsoriasis. Arch Dermatol 132:567–572.
445. Laksmitpathi T, Gould PO, Johnson Be et al. (1976) Photochemotherapy: a study of its efficacy in fifty patients suffering from psoriasis and other dermatoses. Br J Dermatol 95(suppl):20.
446. Divergie MGA (1856) Pityriasis pilaris, maladie de la peau non decrite par les dermatologistes. Gazette Hebdomadaire Med Chirug 3:197–201.
447. Besnier A (1889) Observations pour servir a l'histoire clinique du pityriasis rubra pilaire (pityriasis pilaris de Devergie et de Richaaud). Ann Dermatol Syph 10 (series 2):253–287, 398–427, 485–544.

448. Griffiths WA (1975) Pityriasis rubra pilaris-an historical approach. Trans Rep St John's Hosp Dermatol Soc 61:58–69.
449. Griffiths WA (1976) Pityriasis rubra pilaris-an historical approach. 2. Clinical features. Clin Exp Dermatol 1:37–50.
450. Griffith WA (1984) Pityriasis rubra pilaris. J Am Acad Dermatol 10:1086–1088.
451. Blauvelt A, Nahass GT, Pardo RJ et al. (1991) Pityriasis rubra pilaris and HIV infection. J Am Acad Dermatol 24:703–705.
452. Resnick SD, Murrell DF, Woosley JT (1993) Pityriasis rubra pilaris, acne conglobata and elongated follicular spines: A HIV-associated follicular syndrome (letter). J Am Acad Dermatol 29(2 pt 1):283.
453. Auffret N, Quint L, Domart P et al. (1992) Pityriasis rubra pilari in a patient with human immunodeficiency virus infection. J Am Acad Dermatol 27:260–261.
454. Miralles ES, Nunez M, De Las Heras ME et al. (1995) Pityriasis rubra pilaris and human immunodeficiency virus infection. Br J Dermatol 133:990–993.
455. Menni S, Brancaleone W, Grimalt R (1992) Pityriasis rubra pilaris in a child seropositive for the human immunodeficiency virus. J Am Acad Dermatol 27:1009.
456. Griffith W (2000) Pityriasis rubra pilaris. In: Textbook of Pediatric Dermatology, Harper J, Oranje A, Prose N, eds. Oxford: Blackwell Science, p. 667.

EPIDEMIOLOGY

Genetics

Although most cases of PRP are sporadic, familial clustering has been reported in a number of published series.[457–460] In the series published by Griffith,[457] three familes had more than one affected patient, two families had two affected patients each, and the third family had five affected members. The five affected cases in the latter family had the features of type III and fitted an autosomal-recessive pattern of inheritance. Vanderhooft *et al.* reported four cases of PRP affecting three generations with an autosomal-dominant pattern of inheritance.[461] The patients had the features of type V PRP. The genetic abnormality involved in the familial cases is unknown.

Statistics

PRP has been reported around the world with an estimated prevalence of 1 in 500 000.[456] Males and females are equally affected.[457–460,462,463] The percentage of reported cases belonging to type III, type IV, and type V in three reported series are 4–14%, 7–24%, and 4–14%, respectively.[457,459,462] Type III and IV usually manifest in the first decade of life.[457–460,462,463] Type V is usually present at birth or develops in the first few years of life.[448–450,457,459,461,462,464]

PRESENTING HISTORY

PRP presents with erythematous scaly macules, perifollicular erythematous papules with a central scaly plug, and yellow thickening of the palms and soles.[448–450,457–460,462,463] In type III PRP, the erythematous macules and perifollicular papules first appear on the face, neck, and scalp before spreading onto the trunk and limbs. The palmoplantar changes are usually present from the outset.[448–450,457,459,462] In type IV PRP, perifollicular papules appear and coalesce on the elbows and knees to form erythematous plaques with marked follicular prominence.[448–450,457,459,462] Type V presents at birth or the first

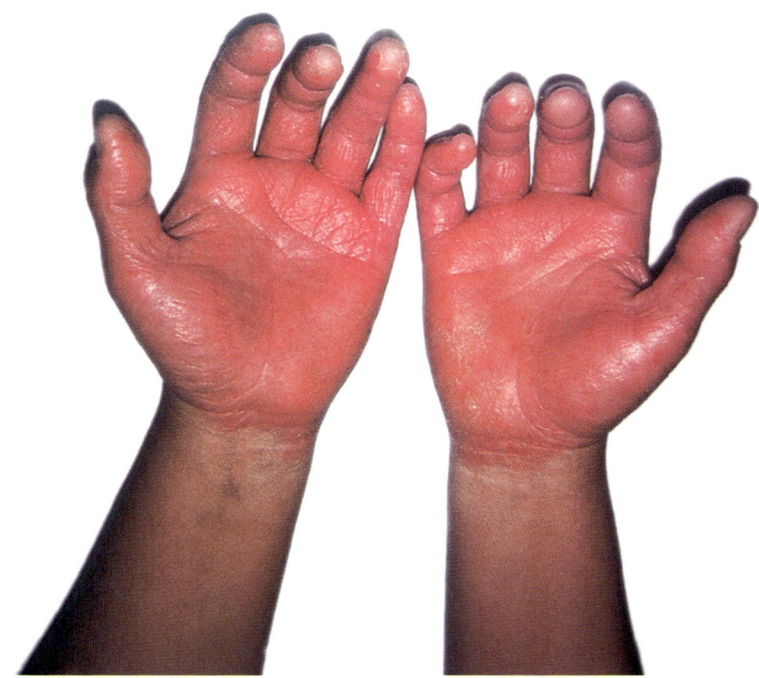

Fig. 15.39   Palmar keratoderma in PRP.

few years of life with widespread erythema and scaling, follicular papules, pronounced keratoderma, and arthritis.[448–450,457,459,461,462,464]

PHYSICAL EXAMINATION

Type III PRP is characterized by scaly, erythematous macules and patches which evolve and coalesce in a cephalo-caudal direction over a period of several weeks to several months. Pruritus can be prominent during the evolving phase. Established cases exhibit erythroderma with patches of unaffected skin ("islands of sparing") scattered within the erythrodermic skin (Fig. 15.38). The facial skin is typically taut with mild ectropion, a common finding. The palms and soles exhibit a uniform, yellow-orange colored keratoderma (Fig. 15.39). Scaling is particularly prominent on the scalp and the nails can thicken with time.[448–450,457–460,462,463] One patient has been reported with an accompanying seronegative arthritis.[465] Type IV is characterized by erythematous plaques on the elbows and knees (Fig. 15.40). The plaques typically exhibit follicular hyperkeratotic plugs. Palmoplantar keratoderma may be present in some patients (Figs 15.13, 15.14).[448–450,457–460,462,463] Type V is characterized by widespread, scaly erythema with prominent follicular papules.[448–450,459,461,462,464] Palmoplantar keratoderma is variable and when present may manifest from mild thickening with fine scaling to pronounced keratoderma resulting in a contracted sclerodermoid appearance.[464,466] Additional features in one reported case included leukonychia, facial dysmorphism, and congenital atrichia.[467]

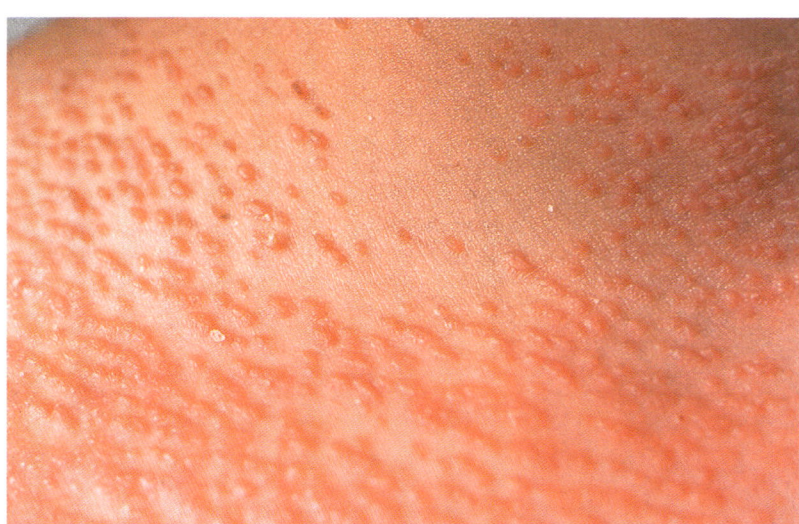

Fig. 15.38   Typical yellow lesions of type III PRP on trunk.

457. Griffith WAD (1980) Pityriasis rubra pilaris. **Clin Exp Dermatol** 5:105–112.
458. Piamphongsant T, Akaraphant R (1994) Pityriasis rubra pilaris: a new proposed classification. **Clin Exp Dermatol** 19:134–138.
459. Sanchez-Regana M, Creus L, Umbert P (1994) Pityriasis rubra pilaris. A long term study of 25 cases. **Eur J Dermatol** 4:593–597.
460. Chuo HF (1985) A clinical analysis of 64 cases of pityriasis rubra pilaris. **Clin J Dermatol** 18:235–236.
461. Vanderhooft SL, Francis JS, Holbrook KA et al. (1995) Familial pityriasis rubra pilaris. **Arch Dermatol** 131:448–453.
462. Lim JT, Tham Sn (1991) Pityriasis rubra pilaris in Singapore. **Clin Exp Dermatol** 16:181–184.

463. Gelmatti C, Schiuma AA, Cerri D et al. (1986) Pityriasis rubra pilaris in childhood: a long term study of 29 cases. **Pediatr Dermatol** 3:446–451.
464. Behr FD, Bangert JL, Hansen RC (2002) Atypical pityriasis rubra pilaris associated with arthropathy and osteoporosis: a cases report with 15-year follow-up. **Pediatr Dermatol** 19:46–51.
465. Lister RK, Perry JD, Cerio R (1997) Pityriasis rubra pilaris and a seronegative polyarthritis. **Br J Dermatol** 137:318–319.
466. Sekkat A, Alami M, Derdabi D et al. (1989) Pityriasis rubra-pilaire sclerodermiforme. **Ann Dermato Venereol** 116:898–900.
467. Sayag J, Koeppel MC, Terrier G et al. (1991) Atrichie congenitale. Ichtyose folliculaire. Keratodermie palmo-plantaire. Leuconychie proximale totale. Dysmorphie faciale. Nouvelle entite? **Ann Dermatol Venereol** 118:771–773.

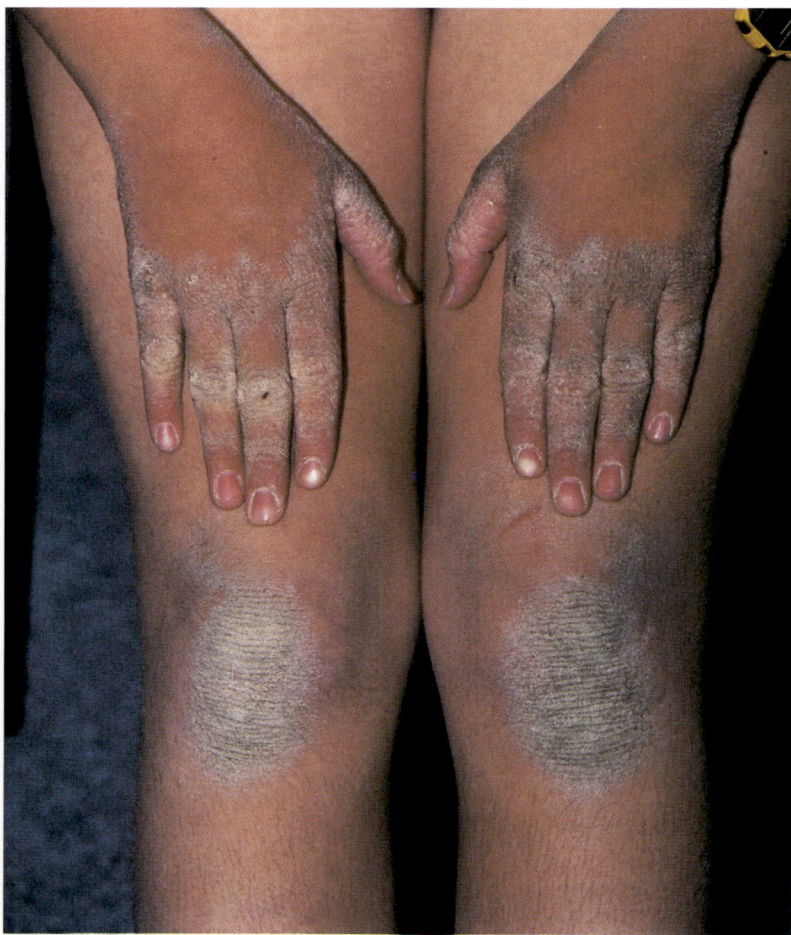

Fig. 15.40 Circumscribed juvenile (type IV) PRP.

Laboratory findings

No consistent laboratory abnormalities are described in PRP.

PATHOPHYSIOLOGY AND HISTOGENESIS

Studies have found the epidermis to be hyperkinetic with a decrease in cell transit time compared with normal skin. Whether this is responsible for the clinical disease is unknown.[468–470] Type III PRP has been reported to follow a febrile illness.[471]

Histologic findings

In established cases, light microscopy reveals epidermal acanthosis with blunting of the rete ridges. Liquefactive degeneration of the basal layer can occur, particularly above the dermal papillae, and perinuclear vacuolation may be seen in suprabasal keratinocytes (poached egg appearance). The granular layer can be thickened or attenuated. There is overlying hyper-keratosis with patchy parakeratosis around the follicular orifice and over the interfollicular epidermis. The follicular orifice is blocked with a keratinous plug. The underlying dermis exhibits vasodilation of dermal vessels with a light superficial perivascular lymphohistiocytic infiltrate.[472] Electron microscopy reveals decreased tonofilaments, enlarged intercellular spaces, parakeratosis with lipid-like vacuoles, and an increased number of keratinosomes.[473]

Differential diagnosis

The principal differential diagnosis for type III and type IV PRP is psoriasis. Distinguishing between the two is often difficult because of shared clinical and histologic features. A final diagnosis requires an assessment of clinical and histologic findings, response to treatment and long-term follow-up. The differential diagnosis for Type V PRP is severe psoriasis, the erythrokeratodermas and non-bullous ichthyosiform erythroderma. The erythrokeratodermas and non-bullous ichthyosiform erythroderma lack follicular papules and prominent palmoplantar keratoderma. Psoriasis can be difficult to distinguish.

THERAPY AND PROGNOSIS

Therapy

Topical therapy is the treatment of choice for patients with mild Type III and Type IV PRP. Emollients are applied regularly to relieve the dryness and tautness of the skin. Calcipotriol may help but should only be used on small areas because of the risk of disturbing calcium metabolism.[474] Retinoic acid 0.05% may improve Type IV, particularly when alternated with topical steroids.[456] Keratolytics can be used to relieve the keratoderma. Systemic therapy is reserved for patients with severe Type III and Type V. Acitretin is the treatment of choice with a daily dose of 0.5–0.75mg/kg per day.[475] Regular monitoring of fasting blood lipids and liver function tests are important. Evidence suggests that acitretin may shorten the duration of the disease.[475] Alternatives to retinoids in the treatment of pediatric PRP are methotrexate[476,477] and cyclosporin.[478]

Prognosis

Spontaneous resolution can occur with Type III and Type IV PRP. Griffith initially reported spontaneous clearance within three years of onset in 16% of Type III patients and 32% of type IV patients.[257] Griffith[456] now believes that spontaneous clearance occurs in approximately 70% of Type III patients, a figure that corresponds with Gelmetti et al.'s[463] series of patients. Type V persists throughout life.[457,461,464]

EXFOLIATIVE ERYTHRODERMA

Exfoliative erythroderma refers to a clinical state of widespread erythema accompanied by marked desquamation of skin. It is a nonspecific reaction pattern that can be induced by a variety of different diseases or medications (Table 15.4).

SUBCORNEAL PUSTULAR DERMATOSIS

Subcorneal pustular dermatosis (SCPD) is a chronic, relapsing vesiculopustular eruption of unknown etiology. It was first described by Sneddon and Wilkinson

468. Ralfs RG, Dawber RPR, Ryan TJ et al. (1981) Pityriasis rubra pilaris: epidermal cell kinetics. **Br J Dermatol** 104:665–667.
469. Griffiths WAD, Pieris S (1982) Pityriasis rubra pilaris – an autoradiographic study. **Br J Dermatol** 107:665–667.
470. Porter D, Shuster S (1968) Epidermal renewal and amino acids in psoriasis and pityriasis rubra pilaris. **Arch Dermatol** 98:339.
471. Larregue M, Champion R, Breissieux JM et al. (1983) Le pityriasis rubra pilaire aigu de l'enfant. A propos de 4 observations. **Ann Dermatol Venereol** 110:221–228.
472. Soeprono FF (1986) Histologic criteria for the diagnosis of pityriasis rubra pilaris. **Am J Dermatopathol** 8:277–283.
473. Kanerva L, Lauharanta J, Niemi KM et al. (1983) Ultrastructure of pityriasis rubra pilaris with observations during retinoid (etretinate) treatment. **Br J Dermatol** 108:653–663.

474. Van de Kerhoff PCM, Steijlen PM (1994) Topical treatment of pityriasis rubra pilaris with calcipotriol. **Br J Dermatol** 130:675–678.
475. Brook M, Lowe NJ (1990) Pityriasis rubra pilaris: further observations of systemic retinoid therapy. **J Am Assoc of Dermatol** 22:792.
476. Dicken CH (1994) Treatment of classic pityriasis rubra pilaris. **J Am Acad Dermatol** 31:997–999.
477. Hanke CW, Steck WD (1983) Childhood onset pityriasis rubra pilaris treated with methotrexate administered intravenously. **Cleve Clin Q** 50:201–203.
478. Rosenbach A, Lowe NJ (1993) Pityriasis rubra pilaris and cyclosporin. **Arch Dermatol** 129:1346–1348.

TABLE 15.4   Classification of exfoliative erythroderma

Diagnosis	Clinical findings	Pathological findings
Neonatal and early infancy		
Atopic dermatitis	Eczematous changes Sparing of diaper area Pruritus (+/− evident in young infants) Family history of atropy Otherwise well	Nonspecific spongiotic dermatitis Elevated serum IgE
Infantile seborrheic dermatitis	Greasy yellow scale on face, scalp, around ears No pruritus Otherwise well	Nonspecific psoriasiform dermatitis

Ichthyosis
  Ichthyosiform erythroderma
  Lamellar ichthyosis
  Bullous ichthyosiform erythroderma
  Keratosis-ichthyosis-deafness
  Sjogren–Larsson syndrome
  Neutral lipid storage disease
  Trichothiodystrophy
  Nethertons syndrome
	Refer to ichthyosis chapter	Refer to ichthyosis chapter

Pustular psoriasis[141]	Recurrent crops of small pustules High fever, toxic appearance	Spongiform pustules Psoriasiform changes
Diffuse cutaneous mastocytosis	Thickening of skin Darier's sign with blister formation	Mast cells with special stains

Infection
  Congenital candidiasis
  Staphylococcal scalded skin
	Multiple small pustules
	Erosions & sloughing face & flexures
	Positive Nikolsky sign
	Fever & toxicity
		KOH microscopy positive for yeast

Immunodeficiency
  Omenn's syndrome
  Hypogammaglobulinemia
  DiGeorge's syndrome
	Refer to immunodeficiency chapter	Refer to immunodeficiency chapter

Graft versus host disease in an infant with primary immunodeficiency	Refer to immunodeficiency chapter	Refer to immunodeficiency chapter
Cutaneous T-cell lymphoma[479]	Lymphadenopathy Splenomegaly Neurologic abnormalities	Atypical mononuclear cells in dermis, epidermis and blood
Metabolic/Nutritional Deficiency Isoleucine deficiency[480]	Periorificial eruption mimicking acrodermatitis enteropathica that evolves into exfoliative erythroderma	Low plasma isoleucine levels
Toxic epidermal necrosis (TEN) associated with klebsiella septicemia[481]	Erythroderma Positive Nikolsky sign Positive blood culture	Epidermal necrosis
Medication	History of recent drug ingestion Widespread erythema Possible TEN picture	Nonspecific perivascular dermatitis with eosinophils Epidermal necrosis with TEN

in 1956.[483] Although all the early cases had negative direct and indirect immunofluorescent studies,[483,484] a number of subsequent case reports have described patients with the clinical and histologic features of subcorneal pustular dermatosis and the presence of intercellular IgA deposition within the epidermis.[485,486] The relationship between these cases, collectively called the intercellular IgA dermatoses, and classic subcorneal pustular dermatosis is unclear. Subcorneal pustular dermatosis has also been reported in association with IgA and IgG gammopathies, pyoderma gangrenosum, inflammatory bowel disease, and rheumatoid arthritis.[486–491]

479. Hendricks GF, Zegers BJ, Van Delden L et al. (1979) Congenital ichthyosis: concurrent immunodeficiency and atypical cells. Int J Dermatol 18:731–740.
480. Spraker MK, Helminski MA, Elsas LJ (1986) Periorificial dermatitis secondary to dietary deficiency of isoleucine in treated infants with maple syrup urine disease. J Invest Dermatol 86:508.
481. Groot de R, Orange AP, Vuzevski VD et al. (1984) Toxic epidermal necrolysis probably due to Klebsiella pneumoniae sepsis. Dermatologica 169:88–90.
482. Meister L, Duarte AM, Davis J et al. (1993) Sezary syndrome in an 11-year-old girl. J Am Acad Dermatol 28:93–95.
483. Sneddon IB, Wilkinson DS (1956) Subcorneal pustular dermatosis. Br J Dermatol 68:385.
484. Sneddon IB (1977) Subkorneale pustulose dermatose. Hautzart 28:63–66.
485. Hashimoto T, Inamoto N, Nakamura K et al. (1987) Intercellular IgA dermatosis with clinical features of subcorneal pustular dermatosis. Arch Dermatol 123:1062–1065.
486. Takata M, Inaoki M, Shodo M et al. (1994) Subcorneal pustular dermatosis associated with IgA myeloma and intraepidermal IgA deposits. Dermatology 189:111–114.
487. Roger H, Thevenet JP, Souteyrand P et al. (1990) Subcorneal pustular dermatosis associated with rheumatoid arthritis and raised IgA: simultaneous remission of skin and joint involvements with dapsone treatment. Ann Rheum Dis 49:190–191.
488. Delaporte E, Colombel JF, Nguyen-Mailfer C et al. (1992) Subcorneal pustular dermatosis in a patient with Crohn's disease. Acta Derm Venereol (Stockh) 72:301–302.
489. Szabo EL, Hamm H (1992) Subkorneale pustulose Sneddon-Wilkinson mit IgG-lamda-paraproteinamie. HG Z Hautkrank 67:792–795, 797.
490. Vaccaro M, Cannavo SP, Guarneri B (1999) Subcorneal pustular dermatosis and IgA lambda myeloma: an uncommon association but probably not coincidental. Eur J Dermatol 9:644–646.
491. Chave TA, Hutchinson PE (2001) Pyoderma gangrenosum, subcorneal pustular dermatosis, IgA paraproteinaemia and IgG antiepithelial antibodies. Br J Dermatol 145:852–854.

TABLE 15.4   Classification of exfoliative erythroderma—cont'd

Diagnosis	Clinical findings	Pathological findings
Older infants, children and adolescents		
Atopic dermatitis	Pruritus Eczematous change Lichenification	Nonspecific spongiotic dermatitis Elevated serum IgE
Psoriasis	Preceding history of plaque psoriasis Nail changes of psoriasis Family history of psoriasis	Acanthosis & parakeratosis Absent granular layer Munro microabscesses
Pustular psoriasis	As above	As above
Pityriasis rubra pilaris	Follicular hyperkeratosis Islands of sparing Palmoplantar keratoderma	Follicular hyperkeratosis Intermittent parakeratosis Acanthosis
Cutaneous T-cell lymphoma[482]	Erythroderma Lymphadenopathy Splenomegaly	Atypical mononuclear cells in the dermis, epidermis (Pautrier microabscess) and blood
Medications	Widespread erythema May have TEN picture with mucosal involvement May have fever, lymphadenopathy & hepatosplenomegaly with drug hypersensitivity syndrome	Nonspecific perivascular dermatitis with eosinophils Epidermal necrosis with TEN
Idiopathic	Nonspecific exfoliative erythroderma with no other clinical clue to diagnosis	Nonspecific perivascular dermatitis

EPIDEMIOLOGY

Statistics

The disease is more common in women, and most cases affect individuals between 40 and 50 years of age. It has been reported in children.[487,488]

PRESENTING HISTORY

Patients present with a vesiculopustular eruption. The eruption is usually pruritic. Children tend to have an associated fever and leukocytosis.[488]

PHYSICAL EXAMINATION

The eruption begins as small, 1–10mm wide vesicles with a slightly erythematous base. The vesicles very quickly evolve into flaccid pustules that rupture and coalesce to produce annular or serpiginous lesions with a scaly edge. The lesions fade over several weeks leaving faint hyperpigmentation. Recurring crops of lesions can occur with a frequency ranging from several days to several weeks. The trunk and limb flexures are the most commonly affected site.[483–493]

Laboratory findings

A Gram stain of the pustular fluid shows numerous polymorphonuclear leukocytes and occasional eosinophils. Bacterial cultures, KOH microscopy, and fungal cultures are all negative.

PATHOPHYSIOLOGY AND HISTOGENESIS

The etiology of subcorneal pustular dermatosis is unknown. Neutrophils migrate through the epidermis to collect on the surface of the epidermis beneath the stratum corneum. The subcorneal collection of neutrophils may be related to overproduction of TNF–alpha.[494]

Histologic findings

Subcorneal pustules filled with neutrophils are the hallmark of the disease. There is no evidence of spongiform pustules, which are a feature of psoriasis. A mild perivascular infiltrate with neutrophils and occasional eosinophils can be seen in the dermis.[98]

Differential diagnosis

The differential diagnosis includes impetigo, dermatophyte infection, pustular psoriasis, immunobullous diseases (dermatitis herpetiformis, pemphigus, linear IgA disease, intercellular IgA diseases), and Hailey-Hailey disease. Microbial studies and response to antimicrobial therapy differentiate impetigo and dermatophyte infection. Pustular psoriasis exhibits spongiform pustules within the epidermis. Histology and immunofluorescence distinguishes the immunobullous group of diseases and Hailey-Hailey disease.

THERAPY AND PROGNOSIS

Dapsone (1–2mg/kg per day) is the treatment of choice. The response is slower compared with the dramatic response seen in dermatitis herpetiformis but most patients respond well and treatment can often be stopped without relapse. Alternative treatments include oral retinoids,[489,490,495] PUVA phototherapy,[495] narrow-band UVB,[496] and colchicine.[497] Some cases may respond to either topical[498] or oral[494] corticosteroids, although their use is generally ineffective. There is a report of resolution of the skin eruption following treatment of the associated paraproteinaemia.[486]

492. Beck AL Jr, Kipping HL, Crissey JT (1961) Subcorneal pustular dermatosis: report of a case. **Arch Dermatol** 83:627.

493. Johnson SAM, Cripps DJ (1974) Subcorneal pustular dermatosis in children. **Arch Dermatol** 73:77.

494. Grob JJ, Mege JL, Capo C et al. (1991) Role of tumor necrosis factor in Sneddon-Wilkinson subcorneal pustular dermatosis: a model of neutrophil priming in vivo. **J Am Acad Dermatol** 25:944–947.

495. Todd DJ, Bingham EA, Walsh M et al. (1991) Subcorneal pustular dermatosis and IgA paraproteinaemia: response to both etretinate and PUVA. **Br J Dermatol** 125:387–389.

496. Cameron H, Dawe RS (1997) Subcorneal pustular dermatosis (Sneddon-Wilkinson disease) treated with narrowband (TL-01) UVB phototherapy. **Br J Dermatol** 137:150–151.

497. Pavithran K (1995) Colchicine in the treatment of subcorneal pustular dermatosis. **Indian J Dermatol Venereol Leprol** 61:56–57.

498. Walkden VM, Roberts A, Wilkinson JD (1994) Two cases of subcorneal pustular dermatosis. Response to use of intermittent clobetasol propionate cream. **Eur J Dermatol** 4:44–46.

The disease follows a chronic relapsing course with a reasonable chance of spontaneous remission. The patients clinical course is influenced by any associated illness or paraproteinemia.

PAPULOSQUAMOUS DRUG REACTIONS

Many medications are capable of producing a papulosquamous eruption that can have an eczematous, psoriasiform, lichenoid, or pityriasis rosea–like appearance.[499,500] The eruption usually begins within several weeks of starting the medication and resolution occurs on cessation of the medication. Consequently, a drug history is essential in the assessment of any patient with a drug eruption.

ACKNOWLEDGMENTS

The author wishes to acknowledge Raymond V. Caputo who authored the chapter on papulosquamous disease in the two previous editions.

499. Litt JZ, Pawlak WA (1997) Drug eruption reference manual 1997, 1st edn. New York: Parthenon.

500. Breathnach SM (1998) Drug eruptions. In: Textbook of Dermatology, 6th edn, Champion RH, Burton JL, Burns DA, Breathnach SM, eds. Oxford: Blackwell Science, p. 3349.

Vesiculobullous Disease

Michael J. Tidman and Maria C. Garzon

INTRODUCTION

The onset of a blistering eruption in a child can be a cause of great concern to parent and physician alike. Not only can the appearance be upsetting and the blisters sore, but also the development of a number of the childhood vesiculobullous disorders may be the harbinger of a life of disability and discomfort and may be potentially fatal.

Bullae may arise as an unusual manifestation of common conditions that are not generally regarded as "blistering disorders," such as acute eczema, cellulitis, and insect bites, where the intensity of the inflammatory process is sufficient to cause the epidermis to separate from the dermis. There are a wide variety of diseases characterized by primary blister formation that in this chapter will be separated into inherited, autoimmune, infectious, reactive and miscellaneous. Virtually all of the acquired vesiculobullous diseases also occur in adults but this chapter will emphasize the clinical features pertaining to children.

INHERITED VESICULOBULLOUS DISEASE

EPIDERMOLYSIS BULLOSA

Introduction

The term epidermolysis bullosa (EB) refers to a heterogeneous group of inherited mechanobullous disorders which are characterized by blistering of the skin, and sometimes the mucous membranes, in response to minor frictional trauma. There are three major forms of EB – simplex, junctional and dystrophic – each with a specific cleavage plane in the region of the epidermal basement membrane; these major forms all have clinical variants. In all types of EB simplex (EBS) blisters form by cytolysis of the infranuclear portion of the basal keratinocytes; in junctional variants (JEB) separation occurs within the lamina lucida of the dermal–epidermal junction; and in the dystrophic forms (DEB) cleavage occurs immediately beneath the lamina densa of the dermal–epidermal junction, in the region normally occupied by the anchoring fibrils. Although the distance spanned by these three planes of cleavage is very small, the major forms of EB are distinct with distinguishing pathophysiology, inheritance and prognosis. The clinical features in older children and adults are fairly distinctive, but it is not usually possible to make a definite clinical diagnosis of the type of EB in the neonatal period and young childhood without undertaking laboratory investigations. Great strides have been made during the last decade in elucidating the pathogenesis of inherited forms of EB and the molecular basis for each of the main types is now understood.

A recent international consensus meeting has clarified the classification and terminology used to describe EB (Table 16.1).[1,2]

Epidermolysis bullosa simplex

Introduction and historical note

Köebner in 1886 described a dominantly inherited seasonal non–scarring mechanobullous disorder, which may be the first record of EBS.[3] Subsequently, a variant localized to acral regions was described independently by Weber in 1926[4] and Cockayne in 1938.[5] It has become customary to use the terms EBS Weber–Cockayne for EBS confined to the palms and soles

TABLE 16.1 Classification of inherited epidermolysis bullosa (major types*)

Epidermolysis bullosa simplex
  Epidermolysis bullosa simplex-Dowling–Meara*
  Epidermolysis bullosa simplex-Koebner*
  Epidermolysis bullosa simplex-Weber–Cockayne*
  Epidermolysis bullosa simplex-muscular dystrophy
  Epidermolysis bullosa simplex-mottled pigmentation
  Epidermolysis bullosa simplex-autosomal recessive
  Epidermolysis bullosa simplex-superficialis

Junctional epidermolysis bullosa
  Junctional epidermolysis bullosa-Herlitz*
  Junctional epidermolysis bullosa-non-Herlitz*
  Junctional epidermolysis bullosa-pyloric atresia*
  Junctional epidermolysis bullosa-Inversa
  Junctional epidermolysis bullosa-late onset

Dystrophic epidermolysis bullosa
  Dominant dystrophic epidermolysis bullosa*
  Dominant dystrophic epidermolysis bullosa-pretibial
  Dominant dystrophic epidermolysis bullosa-transient bullous disease of
    the newborn
  Dominant dystrophic epidermolysis bullosa-pruriginosa
  Recessive dystrophic epidermolysis bullosa-Hallopeau–Siemens*
  Recessive dystrophic epidermolysis bullosa-non-Hallopeau–Siemens*
  Recessive dystrophic epidermolysis bullosa-centripetalis
  Dystrophic epidermolysis bullosa-autosomal dominant/autosomal
    recessive heterozygote

Adapted with permission from Fine JD, Eady RAJ, Bauer EA et al. (2000) **J Am Acad Dermatol** 42:1051–1066.

1. Fine JD, Fady RAJ, Bauer EA et al. (2000) Revised classification system for inherited epidermolysis bullosa: report of the second international consensus meeting on diagnosis and classification of epidermolysis bullosa. **J Am Acad Dermatol** 42:1051–1066.
2. Fine JD (1999) The classification of inherited epidermolysis bullosa. Current approach, pitfalls, unanswered questions and future directions. In: Epidermolyis Bullosa Clinical, Epidemiologic and Laboratory Advances and the Findings of the National Epidermolysis Bullosa Registry. Fine JD,

Bauer EA, McGuire J, Moshell A eds. Baltimore: Johns Hopkins University Press, pp. 20–47.
3. Köebner H (1886) Hereditäre anlage zur Blasenbildung (Epidermolysis bullosa hereditaria). **Deutsch Medicin Wochenschr** 21–22.
4. Weber FP (1926) Recurrent bullous eruption on the feet in a child. **Proc R Soc Med** 19:72.
5. Cockayne EA (1938) Recurrent bullous eruption of the feet. **Br J Dermatol** 50:358–362.

and EBS Köebner for a more widespread involvement which includes blistering at sites of friction. In 1954, Dowling and Meara described a condition, subsequently confirmed to be a form of EBS (EBS Dowling–Meara), presenting with widespread blistering in the neonatal period and progressing to blister formation in characteristic clusters.[6] More recently, other rarer variants of EBS have been described, including EBS associated with mottled pigmentation, EBS with muscular dystrophy and the Ogna variant of EBS. Additionally, a small number of pedigrees with an autosomal recessively inherited form of EBS have been documented.

Genetics and epidemiology

EBS is inherited in an autosomal dominant manner, apart from a small number of pedigrees, all with an element of consanguinity, which have demonstrated a recessive mode of inheritance.[7,8]

The most accurate epidemiological data are derived from Scotland, where the prevalence of EBS in 2001 was determined as 33.2 cases per million of the population and the incidence between 1960 and 1999 was 34.4 per million live births.[9] The equivalent figures from the United States National EB Registry are 4.6 cases per million of the population and 10.75 per million live births.[10] It was probably the capacity of the Scottish study to identify the milder cases of EB that accounts for the quantitative variation in the epidemiological data compared with those from other countries rather than any intrinsic differences.

Clinical features

Within single pedigrees of EBS there are marked differences in the expression of the condition among affected individuals. The Weber–Cockayne and Köebner variants together account for the great majority of EBS cases, with the Dowling–Meara subtype contributing 5%.[11] The remaining subtypes are rare.

Epidermolysis bullosa simplex - Weber–Cockayne

The onset of blistering in EBS Weber–Cockayne may occur at any time between birth and the teenage years. Although there is usually a family history, this is not always the case. Bullae are nonscarring, tense and painful and are virtually confined to the hands and feet, with the soles almost always being affected (Fig. 16.1); occasionally intraoral blistering occurs. Palmoplantar involvement is sometimes associated with hyperkeratosis and hyperhidrosis. The condition is much worse during the summer months and is exacerbated by frictional trauma such as occurs with manual labor and walking, especially with ill-fitting shoes. Thickened, unsightly great toe nails may be present. As a rule, the blistering tendency improves with age, although it may remain troublesome into middle life.

The effect of EBS Weber–Cockayne on the quality of life of a sufferer is often underestimated.[11] The discomfort from bullae on the soles may limit walking to very short distances and some individuals may be confined to wheelchairs during the summer months. Affected children often try to avoid walking and may prefer to crawl or bottom-shuffle when at home. Teenagers may not cope with frequent changes of classroom during their school day, and the less motivated children may have poor school attendance records.

Epidermolysis bullosa simplex - Köebner

EBS Köebner shares many features with EBS Weber–Cockayne, with nonscarring blisters occurring predominantly on the palms and soles but also on other body regions, particularly those that are subject to friction from clothing and jewelry. Some pedigrees with the Köebner variant may show a uniform expression but others may show a mixed picture with some individuals

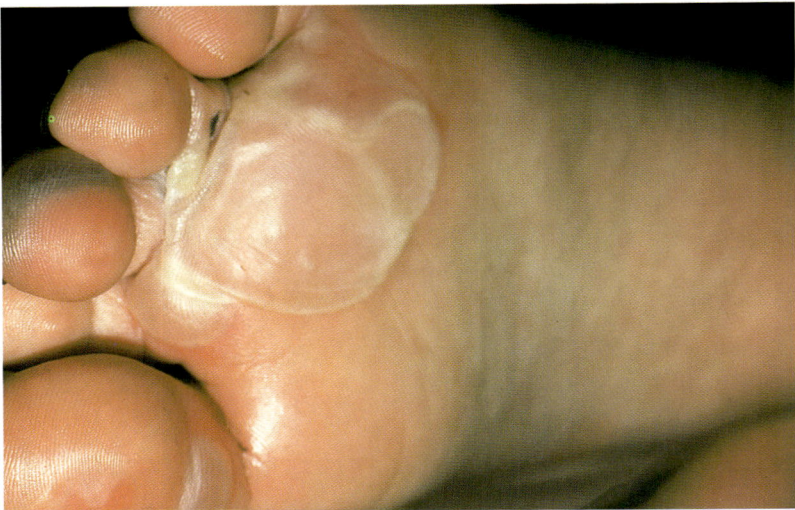

Fig. 16.1   EB simplex-Weber–Cockayne: bullae on forefoot.

demonstrating a Weber–Cockayne phenotype.[11] The Köebner subtype tends towards an earlier onset than EBS Weber–Cockayne but in most respects the two conditions are very similar and differ principally in their degree of severity. Intraoral blistering is more common in the Köebner variant, whereas hyperkeratosis and great toenail dystrophy are similar.[11] Heat is an important predisposing factor to blistering and the warmer months of the year are generally the most troublesome. Improvement tends to occur with age. Both the Köebner and Weber–Cockayne forms may rarely be associated with localized congenital absence of skin ("Bart syndrome"), usually involving a limb, which heals leaving subtle atrophic scarring.[11]

Epidermolysis bullosa simplex - Dowling–Meara

The Dowling–Meara variant of EBS has the most severe blistering tendency of the EBS subtypes. It presents at birth or within the first week of postnatal life with extensive blistering, which may occasionally be life-threatening. There is often no previous family history of the condition, the affected child presenting a *de novo* mutation which subsequently is transmitted in an autosomal dominant fashion. Although EBS Dowling–Meara develops distinctive clinical and pathological features,[12] at the outset it is not possible to distinguish it with certainty from the severe forms of dystrophic and junctional EB on the basis of the clinical features, but ultrastructural examination enables a rapid diagnosis.

After the first few months, bullae tend to assume a clustered, "herpetiform" distribution on the trunk and limbs (Fig. 16.2), hence a former alternative name "EBS herpetiformis." Blisters are nonscarring but often result in postinflammatory hyperpigmentation. Intraoral blistering in infants is very common, and a hoarse cry, the result of laryngeal involvement, may be a prominent feature during the first 2 years. Friction from clothing is an important precipitant of bullae, although they often appear to develop spontaneously, and there is not the same seasonal variation as in the other forms of EBS. The severity of blistering lessens during childhood and adolescence although may still be troublesome in adulthood. A mild degree of palmoplantar hyperkeratosis is common but occasionally it may be florid and be associated with flexion deformities of the digits. Nail involvement is usual and of variable degree. In infants periodic shedding of finger and toe nails

6. Dowling GB, Meara RH (1954) Epidermolysis bullosa resembling juvenile dermatitis herpetiformis. Br J Dermatol 66:139–143.
7. Hovnanian A, Pollack E, Hilal L et al. (1993) A missense mutation in the rod domain of keratin 14 associated with recessive epidermolysis bullosa simplex. Nat Genet 3:327–332.
8. Batta K, Rugg, EL, Wilson N J et al. (2000) A keratin 14 "knockout" mutation in recessive epidermolysis bullosa simplex resulting in less severe disease. Br J Dermatol 143:621–627.
9. Horn HM, Priestley GL, Eady RA, Tidman MJ (1997) The prevalence of epidermolysis bullosa in Scotland. Br J Dermatol 136:560–564.
10. Fine JD, Johnson LB, Suchindran C et al. (1999) The epidemiology of inherited epidermolysis bullosa in: Epidermolysis Bullosa Clinical, Epidemiologic and Laboratory Advances and the Findings of the National Epidermolysis Bullosa Registry, Fine JD, Bauer EA, McGuire J, Moshell A eds. Baltimore: Johns Hopkins University Press, pp. 101–113.
11. Horn HM, Tidman MJ (2000) The clinical spectrum of epidermolysis bullosa simplex. Br J Dermatol 142:468–472.
12. McGrath JA, Ishida-Yamamoto A, Tidman MJ et al. (1992) Epidermolysis bullosa simplex (Dowling–Meara). A clinicopathological review. Br J Dermatol 126:421–430.

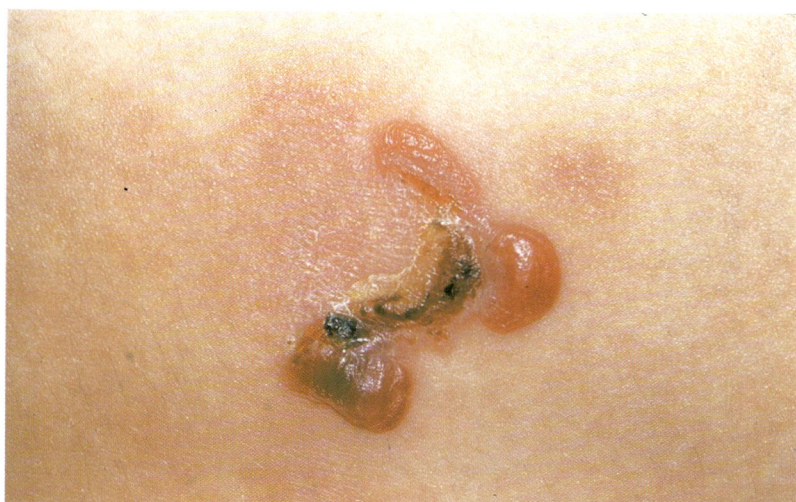

Fig. 16.2 EB simplex-Dowling–Meara: characteristic clustered bullae.

occurs and adults tend to develop thickening of the great toenails. Congenital absence of skin (Bart syndrome) has been recorded.[11]

Epidermolysis bullosa simplex with mottled pigmentation

EBS with mottled pigmentation is a very rare subtype first reported in 1979.[13,14] Patients typically present with acral, nonscarring, seasonal blistering in early childhood and develop a characteristic permanent mottled macular pigmentation on the trunk and limbs. They also develop punctate palmoplantar keratoderma later in life and most have nail abnormalities.

Epidermolysis bullosa simplex with muscular dystrophy

EBS with muscular dystrophy is a very rare autosomal recessive condition with a wide range of clinical severity.[15,16] Generalized blistering is evident at birth or appears shortly thereafter. Blister formation may be seasonal and bullae may leave atrophic scarring. Nail involvement is usual and teeth are often abnormal. The age of onset of muscle weakness ranges widely, from the first year to the fourth decade. There may be associated cerebral and cerebellar atrophy,[17] urethral stricture, scarring alopecia and occasionally respiratory symptoms.[18]

Epidermolysis bullosa simplex - Ogna

The Ogna variant of EBS is inherited in an autosomal dominant fashion and has been described in only two pedigrees.[19,20] Seasonal, nonscarring blistering occurs on the palms and soles in association with generalized nonseasonal skin fragility, resulting in small transient erosions on limbs, face and trunk. Dystrophic great toenails are frequent in this condition.

Epidermolysis bullosa simplex superficialis

EB superficialis is another rare form of EB in which blistering arises just below the stratum corneum.[21] Intact bullae are rarely noted and individuals frequently present with erosions and crusts. Oral erosions, milia formation,

atrophic scarring and dystrophic nails are common. Rarely, conjunctival erosions may occur.

Pathophysiology and histogenesis

It is now well established that the Weber–Cockayne, Köebner, Dowling–Meara and mottled pigmentation variants of EBS are caused by mutations in the genes encoding keratins 5 or 14,[22,23] both of which are expressed by, and constitute, the cytoskeleton of the basal keratinocytes. The degree of impairment of the structural integrity of the keratin molecule is determined by the site and nature of the keratin mutation and this influences the phenotype. The Dowling–Meara subtype is the most severe form of EBS and is characterized by mutations within the highly conserved helix initiation or termination motifs, whereas milder forms of EBS are associated with mutations at other sites in the keratin genes.[24]

The form of EBS associated with muscular dystrophy is caused by mutations of varying disruptive potential in the gene encoding plectin, a hemidesmosomal component.[16,17] The Ogna variant is also caused by a mutation in the plectin gene.[20]

Differential diagnosis

The localized, acral forms of EBS rarely cause diagnostic difficulty, particularly if there is a family history, by virtue of their distinctive clinical features, and usually histological and ultrastructural examination is not necessary. The Dowling–Meara variant of EBS, presenting as it usually does with widespread blistering in the neonatal period, cannot be clinically distinguished from junctional or severe recessive forms of EB. However, ultrastructural examination in Dowling–Meara EBS shows the pathognomonic combination of cytolytic blistering in the lower pole of the basal keratinocytes and clumping of the tonofilaments.

Therapeutics and prognosis

There is no specific treatment for any of the forms of EB and care is essentially preventative and symptomatic. For the localized acral variants of EBS, particularly EBS Weber–Cockayne and EBS Köebner, prevention of blistering is paramount. Keeping the soles and palms cool and dry, especially during the summer months, can be helpful in minimizing the blistering, and if hyperhidrosis is a feature, trying the efficacy of a topical antiperspirant containing 20% aluminium chloride hexahydrate applied last thing at night and gently dried with a hairdryer may be useful. Well-fitting footwear is very important and leather shoes with leather linings, ideally with external seams, are generally recommended. If the leather in new shoes is too stiff, it can be softened by manipulating the shoe. In young children, a boot-type shoe will protect the ankles against knocks. Several pairs of shoes should be worn in rotation to vary the sites of friction and it may be helpful for patient or parent to carry a spare pair of shoes for children to change into partway through the day. During the summer, alternatives to leather shoes are canvas shoes or jelly sandals. Another measure to reduce frictional forces on the soles is to wear two pairs of cotton socks, although this has to be balanced against the possibility of increasing the temperature of the skin. In the worst cases of localized EBS, it may be possible to persuade local authorities to provide transport to and from school. A careful explanation of the nature of EBS to the teaching staff at school will usually ensure that the child is treated sympathetically.

13. Fischer T, Gedde-Dahl T (1979) Epidermolysis bullosa simplex and mottled pigmentation: a new dominant syndrome. Clin Genet 15:228–238.
14. Irvine AD, Rugg EL, Lane EB et al. (2001) Molecular confirmation of the unique phenotype of epidermolysis bullosa simplex with mottled pigmentation. Br J Dermatol 144:40–45.
15. Niemi KM, Sommer H, Kero M et al. (1988) Epidermolysis bullosa simplex associated with muscular dystrophy with recessive inheritance. Arch Dermatol 124:551–554.
16. Shimizu H, Takizawa Y, Pulkkinen L et al. (1999) Epidermolysis bullosa simplex associated with muscular dystrophy: phenotype-genotype correlations and review of the literature. J Am Acad Dermatol 41:950–956.
17. Smith FJ, Eady RA, Leigh IM et al. (1996) Plectin deficiency results in muscular dystrophy with epidermolysis bullosa. Nat Genet 13:450–457.
18. Mellerio JE, Smith FJ, McMillan JR et al. (1997) Recessive epidermolysis bullosa simplex associated with plectin mutations: infantile respiratory complications in two unrelated cases. Br J Dermatol 137:898–906.

19. Gedde-Dahl T (1970) Epidermolysis bullosa. A clinical, genetic and epidemiological study. Universitetsforlaget, Oslo-Bergen-Tromso.
20. Koss-Harnes D, Høyheim B, Anton-Lamprecht I et al. (2002) A site specific plectin mutation causes dominant epidermolysis bullosa simplex Ogna: two identical de novo mutations. J Invest Dermatol 118:87–93.
21. Fine JD, Johnson L, Wright T (1989) Epidermolysis bullosa simplex superficialis. A new variant of epidermolysis bullosa characterized by subcorneal skin cleavage mimicking peeling skin syndrome. Arch Dermatol 125:633–638.
22. Bonifas JM, Rothman AL, Epstein EH (1991) Epidermolysis bullosa simplex: evidence in two families for keratin gene abnormalities. Science 254:1202–1205.
23. Lane EB, Rugg EL, Navsaria H et al. (1992) A mutation in the conserved helix termination peptide of keratin 5 in hereditary skin blistering. Nature (London) 356:244–246.
24. Irvine AD, McLean WHI (1999) Human keratin diseases: the increasing spectrum of disease and subtlety of the phenotype-genotype correlation. Br J Dermatol 140:815–828.

In most cases of localized EBS, discomfort is reduced by puncturing bullae using sterile scissors or needles, and retaining the roof of the bulla which acts as a biological dressing. Antibiotic ointment at the incision site may reduce the risk of secondary infection. Soaking hands and feet in cold water or an antiseptic solution such as potassium permanganate (1:10 000) for 20–30 minutes once or twice each day may be helpful. Some patients prefer the application of a nonadhesive dressing, held in place with a bandage, whereas others find dressings unnecessary.

As with all forms of EB, attention should be paid to adequate pain control, and a nocturnal dose of amitriptyline (0.5mg per kg body weight) is often beneficial.

The Dowling–Meara variant of EBS is managed in the initial weeks in a similar fashion to the severe generalized forms of JEB and DEB. Septicaemia is a particular risk in the early days[25] and management in an intensive care unit may be required. In later years, troublesome palmoplantar hyperkeratosis may respond to low-dose acitretin, although this may increase skin fragility and worsen the tendency to blistering.

JUNCTIONAL EPIDERMOLYSIS BULLOSA

Introduction and historical note

In 1935, Herlitz described a nonscarring variant of EB which was lethal in infancy.[26] Initially, this was considered to be a severe form of dystrophic EB until 1974 when it was demonstrated by ultrastructural examination that the cleavage plane in this condition was within the lamina lucida of the epidermal basement membrane,[27] thereby distinguishing it from DEB. The term junctional EB (JEB) was coined and the lethal form is now known as JEB-Herlitz. However, JEB can be compatable with survival into adulthood and this subtype is designated JEB-non Herlitz. Rarer variants of JEB include a type associated with pyloric atresia (JEB-pyloric atresia), an inverse form (JEB-inversa) and a type manifesting at an older age (JEB-late onset).[1]

Genetics and epidemiology

All the variants of JEB are inherited in an autosomal recessive manner. JEB is the rarest of the three main forms of EB with the Scottish data giving a prevalence of 0.3 cases per million of the population and an incidence of 3.2 new cases per million live births.[9] The equivalent United States figures are 0.44 and 2.04.[10]

Clinical features

Junctional epidermolysis bullosa - Herlitz

JEB-Herlitz presents at birth with tense bullae affecting skin and oral mucous membranes. Occasionally, there may be localized absence of skin on a limb (Bart syndrome). The degree of blistering in the first week or two of postnatal life is no guide to the ultimate prognosis, and the presence of only a few bullae on an otherwise healthy-looking baby can be the harbinger of an ultimately lethal outcome. Provided bullae are not excoriated or infected, they are non-scarring and milia are not a prominent feature. There is no specific pattern of blistering, but involvement of the buttocks (Fig. 16.3) and the pinnae of the ears is quite characteristic in JEB, as is a hoarse cry. Early on, a paronychial inflammation often occurs (Fig. 16.4), followed by nail dystrophy and loss. Dental enamel hypoplasia results in pitting of the tooth surfaces if survival is prolonged until eruption of the secondary dentition (Fig. 16.5). A nonscarring hair loss is common. The gradual development of a distinctive perioral, and occasionally occipital, distribution of granulation tissue occurs in those individuals who survive beyond 6 months of age (Fig. 16.6).

Affected infants fail to thrive, and usually become anaemic despite nutritional supplementation. Death usually occurs within the first few years after a gradual decline, often as the result of septicemia. However, bullae in

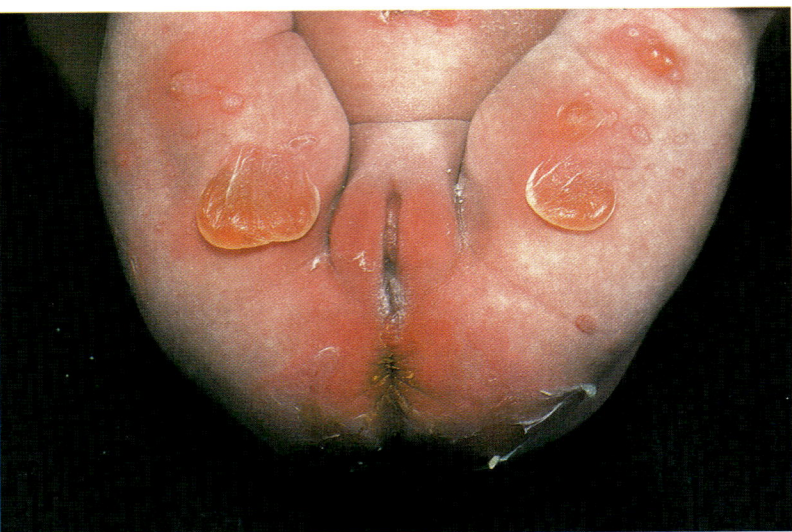

Fig. 16.3 JEB-Herlitz: bullae on the buttocks and thighs.

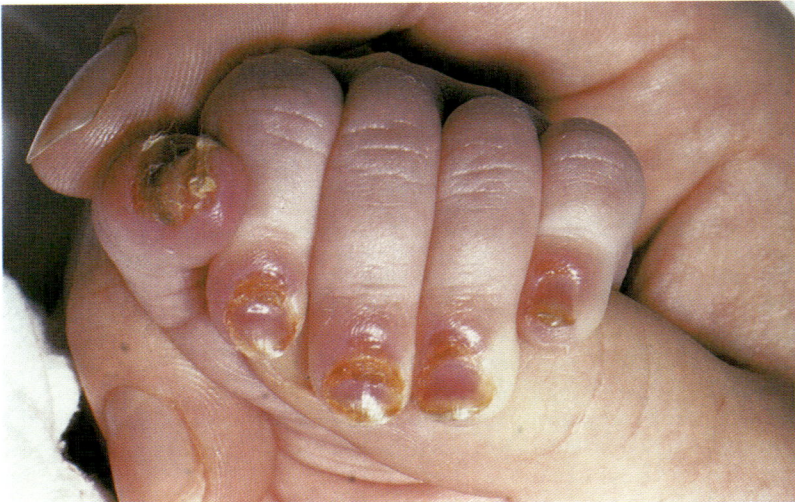

Fig. 16.4 JEB-Herlitz: paronychial inflammation.

the larynx or trachea may cause sudden death. Post-mortem examination often reveals widespread mucous membrane involvement of the upper aerodigestive tract, lower alimentary tract and the urinary tract.

Junctional epidermolysis bullosa - non-Herlitz

This is probably a heterogeneous group of JEB. Some patients with extensive junctional blistering in infancy survive to adulthood, and identification of this subtype in childhood on the basis of the clinical features is not usually possible, although excessive granulation tissue is less of a feature. Another phenotype, originally classified as "generalized atrophic benign EB," is characterized by a normal lifespan and blistering which heals to leave atrophic scarring, which in hair-bearing regions causes alopecia. Pigmentation may occur at sites of previous blisters. Nail dystrophy (Fig. 16.7) and dental enamel hypoplasia are also features. Conjunctival and eyelid involvement may result in scarring or blepharitis. Corneal erosions and scarring with subsequently impaired vision are occasional features of JEB-non-Herlitz. Genitourinary tract abnormalities include urinary retention and urethral meatal stenosis.

25. Denyer J (2000) Management of severe blistering disorders. **Semin Neonatal** 5:321–324.
26. Herlitz O (1935) Kongenitaler nicht syphilitischer Pemphigus. Einc übersicht nebst Beschreibung einer neuen Krankheitsform (Epidermolysis bullosa hereditaria letalis). **Acta Paediatr** 17:315–371.
27. Pcarson RW, Potter B, Strauss F (1974) Epidermolysis bullosa hereditaria letalis. **Arch Dermatol** 109:349–355.

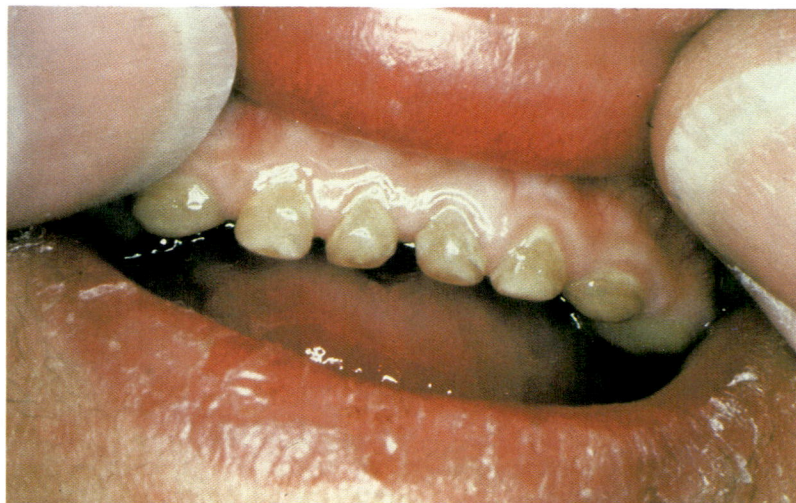

Fig. 16.5   JEB-Herlitz: dental enamel hypoplasia.

There have been descriptions of individuals with clinical features suggestive of DEB who have proved to have junctional blistering. This "cicatricial" form of JEB is now classified as JEB-non-Herlitz.

Junctional epidermolysis bullosa - pyloric atresia

This variant of JEB is characterized by congenital blistering and pyloric atresia. It usually carries a poor prognosis even after surgical correction of the gastrointestinal abnormality. Survivors may develop hydronephrosis and renal failure as the result of strictures within the urogenital tract caused by repeated blistering.

Pathophysiology and histogenesis

JEB is a genetically heterogeneous disorder caused by mutations in several different genes encoding for diverse proteins expressed at the dermal–epidermal junction. JEB-Herlitz is associated with severely disruptive mutations, usually premature termination codons, in both alleles of any of the three genes (*LAMA3, LAMB3* and *LAMC2* encoding respectively the three constituent polypeptide chains (α3, β3 and γ2) of laminin 5,[28] the morphological equivalent of which are the anchoring filaments that cross the lamina lucida. JEB-non Herlitz is usually also the result of laminin 5 mutations, most frequently a premature termination codon on one allele combined with a less disruptive mutation on the paired allele.[28] However, some cases of JEB-non Herlitz, corresponding to the former clinical description of generalized atrophic benign EB, are caused by mutations, usually premature termination codons or missence mutations, in the gene (*COL17A1* or bullous pemphigoid antigen 2 gene) encoding type 17 collagen (the 180kDa bullous pemphigoid antigen),[29] a constituent of hemidesmosomes. Mutations in the genes (*ITGA6* and *ITGB4*) for another hemidesmosome-associated transmembrane protein system, the α6β4 integrin, are responsible for JEB-pyloric atresia.[30]

Differential diagnosis

The diagnosis of EB should be considered for any infant presenting with skin fragility but the differential is quite broad (Table 16.2). JEB cannot usually be distinguished from other severe variants of EB in the neonatal period on the basis of clinical features and early laboratory-based diagnosis is recommended. In the immediate postnatal period, infectious causes of skin blistering (herpes

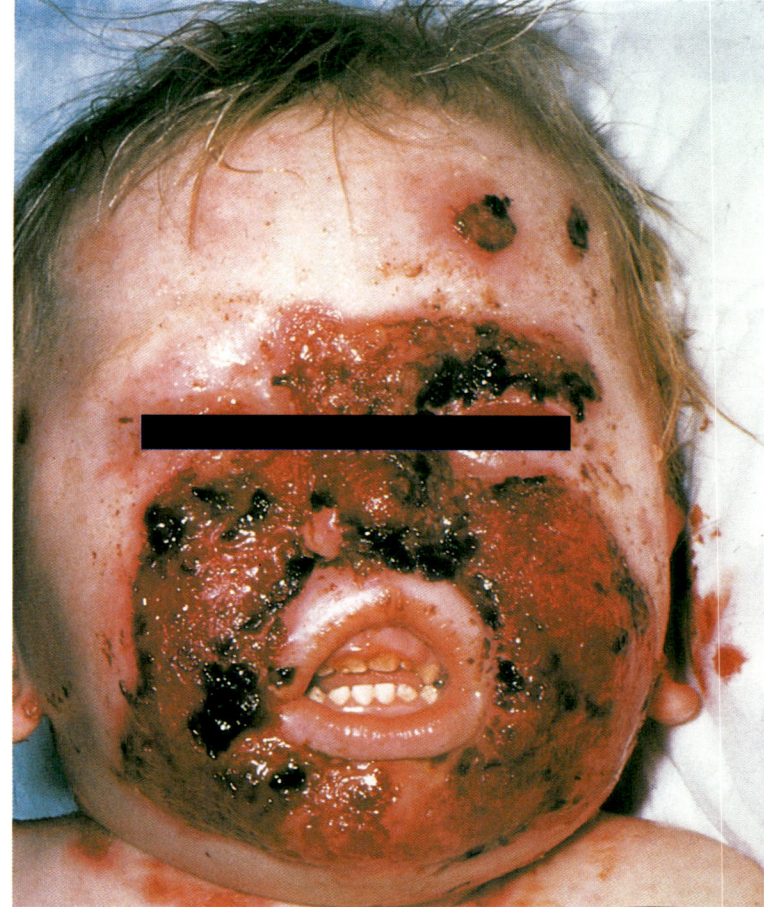

Fig. 16.6   JEB-Herlitz: persistent facial erosions.

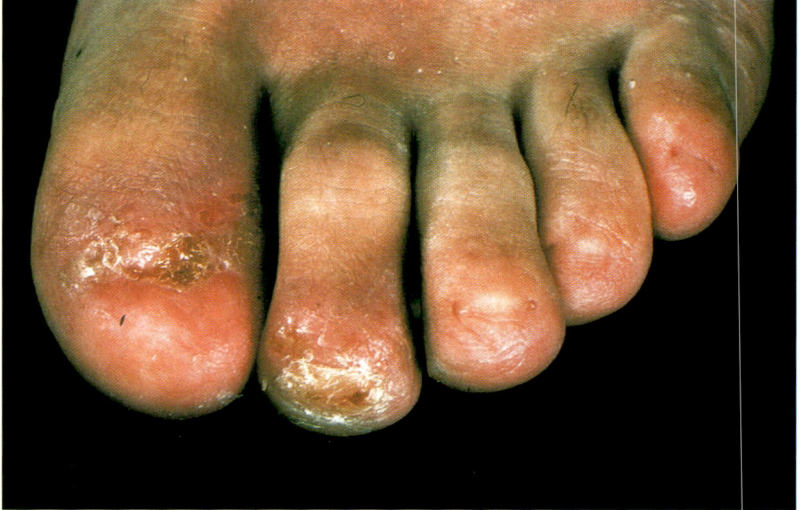

Fig. 16.7   JEB-non-Herlitz: toe nail dystrophy.

simplex, staphylococcal infections, candidiasis, and sepsis related bullae) should be excluded.

28. Nakano A, Chao SC, Pulkkinen L et al. (2002) Laminin 5 mutations in junctional epidermolysis bullosa: molecular basis of Herlitz vs non-Herlitz phenotypes. **Hum Genet** 110:41–51.

29. Pulkkinen L, Marinkovich MP, Tran HT et al. (1999) Compound heterozygosity for novel splice site mutations in the BPAG2/COL17A1 gene underlies generalised atrophic benign epidermolysis bullosa. **J Invest Dermatol** 113:1114–1118.

30. Mellerio JE, Pulkkinen L, McMillan JR et al. (1998) Pyloric atresia-junctional epidermolysis bullosa syndrome: mutations in the β4 gene (ITGB4) in two unrelated patients with mild disease. **Br J Dermatol** 139:862–871.

Therapeutics and prognosis

The treatment of all forms of EB is supportive. The establishment of an appropriate regimen for the immediate care of a neonate with one of the severe generalized forms of EB, which include JEB-Herlitz, EBS-Dowling–Meara and RDEB-Hallopeau–Siemens, will minimize unnecessary damage to the skin and thus help to limit permanent disability. The Dystrophic Epidermolysis Bullosa Research Association (DEBRA) provides invaluable support to parents and nursing staff caring for sufferers of EB and, later in life, to patients themselves. Current treatment strategies are focused on preventing new blisters, preventing and treating infections, enhancing wound healing, providing nutritional support, managing extracutaneous complications, preserving function and providing psychological support to patients and family members.

The essence of caring for the skin of infants and young children with severe EB is careful handling to minimize blister formation and the prevention of infection.[25] Babies should be lifted and moved on a soft pad such as a folded towel inside a pillowcase, trying to avoid applying shearing forces to the skin. Clothing should be soft, and it is helpful to turn them inside out to avoid rubbing of the skin from seams and labels. Cotton mittens may reduce self-inflicted trauma. Nonblistered skin should be kept well moisturized with a greasy emollient such as a 50:50 mixture of white soft paraffin and liquid paraffin. When bathing, the bath should be lined with a thick towel.

A variety of different wound care strategies have been employed to manage EB, but the basic principles are similar.[25] Dressing choices are often determined by parental, and later personal, preference. Probably the best technique of care, to prevent bullae from enlarging, is to puncture them with a sterile needle, leaving the roof intact and allowing it to settle on the floor of the bulla. Dusting the area with cornflour dries up the bullae and limits their spread. A topical antibiotic applied to the ruptured area may be used. Mupirocin ointment is reserved for treatment of small areas for limited periods of time so as not to promote resistance. Systemic antibiotics should be used when significant cutaneous or extracutaneous infection is suspected.

In open exuding wounds, a standard regimen is to apply a nonocclusive hydrocolloid fibre dressing, covered with silicone-based low-adherent dressings, and followed by a simple absorbent secondary dressing; this is secured with a conforming bandage. Care should be taken not to apply tape directly to the skin. Additional protection may be afforded with the use of padding over the secondary dressing. The primary dressing should be changed every 4–7 days in order to minimize the discomfort of the dressing process and to allow the wound to heal undisturbed, although the secondary dressing may be changed daily if required. Care should be taken to give adequate analgesia.[25]

There have been several reports of using tissue-engineered skin (Apligraf) and autologous epidermal grafts for wounds in individuals with inherited EB. In a study of 15 patients with different types of EB and multiple wounds, tissue-engineered skin grafts were effective wound dressings and survived for several months without rejection.[31,32] Limitations of the study include the small number of patients and short follow-up period. Moreover, the cost of treatment may be high. The role of tissue-engineered skin grafts in the routine management of various forms of inherited EB remains to be fully evaluated.

Feeding of the EB patient at any age can be a problem if there is oral involvement. The lips should be protected with vaseline, and if the mouth is ulcerated teething gels may be beneficial. The teat can be moistened prior to feeding to avoid it sticking to ulcerated areas. A Haberman feeder is often helpful if the mouth is very uncomfortable, as this reduces the need for strong sucking and the length of the teat avoids trauma to the nose.[25] Nasogastric tubes are best avoided, but if required a tube suitable for long-term feeding should be used, thereby reducing the need for frequent tube changes. If a pacifier is used it is helpful to avoid those with a plastic ring as this may damage the lips and surrounding skin.

TABLE 16.2   Differential diagnosis of epidermolysis bullosa in infants and children

Genetic conditions
 Bullous congenital ichthyosisform erythroderma (bullae, erosions)
 Ichthyosis bullosa of Siemens (bullae, erosions)
 Porphyrias
  Congenital erythropoeitic porphyria (bullae, erosions)
  Familial porphyria cutanea tarda (bullae, erosions)
 Kindler syndrome (bullae, erosions)
 Mendes da Costa syndrome (bullae, erosions)
 Skin fragility/ectodermal dysplasia syndrome (plakophilin-1 deficiency) (bullae, erosions)
 Pachyonychia congenita (bullae)
 Hailey–Hailey disease (bullae, erosions)
 Hay–Wells syndrome (erosions)
 Laryngo-onychocutaneous syndrome (erosions)
 Incontinentia pigmenti (vesicles, bullae erosions)
 Focal dermal hypoplasia (erosions)
 Microphthalmia and linear skin defects (linear atrophic scars)
 Methylmalonic acidemia (erosions)
 Acrodermatitis enteropathica (erosions)

Infections
 Viral
  Herpes simplex virus (vesicles)
  Varicella zoster virus (vesicles)
  Hand foot and mouth syndrome (Coxsackie A 16) (vesicles, erosions)
 Bacterial
  Staphylococcal pyoderma/bullous impetigo (bullae, erosions)
  Staphylococcal scalded skin syndrome (bullae, erosions)
  Blistering distal dactylitis (bullae)
  Group B streptococcal infection (vesicles, bullae, erosions)
  Congenital syphilis (bullae)
 Yeast
  Candidiasis (pustules, erythroderma, bullae, erosions)
 Parasitic
  Scabies (vesicopustules)

Autoimmune blistering disorders
 Bullous pemphigoid (bullae, erosions)
 Linear IgA disease (chronic bullous disease of childhood)(bullae and erosions)
 Dermatitis herpetiformis (vesicopapules)
 Pemphigus (bullae, erosions)
 Maternal blistering disease (transplacental antibodies, herpes gestationis, pemphigus) (bullae, erosions)
 Epidermolysis bullosa acquisita (bullae, erosions)
 Bullous systemic lupus erythematosus (bullae)

Miscellaneous
 Diffuse cutaneous mastocytosis (bullae, erosions)
 Aplasia cutis congenita (erosions)
 Sucking blisters (bullae, erosions)
 Transient neonatal pustular melanosis (vesicopustules)
 Infantile acropustulosis (vesicopustules)
 Trauma (bullae, erosions)
 Congenital erosive and vesicular dermatosis (vesicles, erosions, reticulate scarring)
 Erythema multiforme (bullae)
 Stevens–Johnson syndrome/toxic epidermal necrolysis (erythema, bullae, erosions)
 Acute contact dermatitis (vesicles, bullae)
 Actinic prurigo (vesicopapules)
 Hydroa vacciniforme (vesicles)
 Miliaria crystallina (vesicles)

Adapted with permission from Fine JD, Eady RAJ, Bauer EA et al. (2000) **J Am Acad Dermatol** 42:1051–1066.

31. Falabella AF, Valencia IC, Eaglstein WH et al. (2000) Tissue-engineered skin (Apligraf) in the healing of patients with epidermolysis bullosa wounds. **Arch Dermatol** 136:1225–1230.

32. Wollina U, Konrad H, Fischer T (2001) Recessive epidermolysis bullosa dystrophicans (Hallopeau–Siemens): improvement of wound healing by autologous epidermal grafts on an esterified hyaluronic acid membrane. J Dermatol 28:217–220.

Genetic counseling is extremely important for affected individuals and their families. DNA-based prenatal diagnosis is available for junctional and dystrophic forms of EB in families in which there is a known history of EB and ideally in whom the mutation has been characterized. It is performed using DNA obtained from chorionic villus sampling or amniocentesis. Future avenues are currently under investigation for early prenatal diagnosis including preimplantation genetics. This technique would permit the genotype to be determined on an embryo produced by *in vitro* fertilization techniques at an eight-cell stage.[33,34]

Gene therapy remains the future hope for treatment of EB. In preliminary work, the laminin 5 β3 gene was transferred to keratinocytes from patients with JEB using a retroviral vector. The transduced JEB cells displayed normal laminin 5 β3 protein activity when used to regenerate skin on severe combined immunodeficient mice. These early studies suggest that gene replacement therapy may prove to be an effective treatment for EB in the future.[35]

There are no accurate clinical or laboratory prognostic features. Cause of death in JEB-Herlitz is not always clear, although infection and laryngeal involvement may contribute.

DYSTROPHIC EPIDERMOLYSIS BULLOSA

Introduction and historical note

Blistering conditions with consequent scarring as a prominent clinical feature were described in the late 19th century by, amongst others, Tilbury Fox (1879)[36] and Hallopeau (1898).[37] Cockayne (1933)[38] and Touraine (1942)[39] both described a dominantly inherited disorder that would now be classified as dominant dystrophic EB (DDEB), and Pasini in 1928 described the same condition that differed principally by the presence of hypopigmented papules on the trunk and limbs that he termed "albopapuloid lesions."[40] For many years DDEB was subdivided into Cockayne–Touraine and Pasini variants but this distinction is now considered spurious. However, in recent years several subtypes of DDEB have become established, including a form centered on the lower legs (DDEB-pretibial), another characterized by a prurigo-like morphology (DDEB-pruriginosa) and one that appears to be expressed only in the early weeks of postnatal life (DDEB-transient bullous disease of the newborn).

In 1921, Siemens described a recessive form of DEB (RDEB) with an aggressively scarring clinical picture,[41] now classified as RDEB-Hallopeau–Siemens. There is a milder variant of RDEB having clinical similarities to DDEB, classified as RDEB-non-Hallopeau–Siemens, and a form of RDEB with predominantly flexural or "inverse" distribution (RDEB-centripetalis). Finally, compound heterozygotes with a mixture of dominant and recessive mutations occur (DEB-autosomal dominant/autosomal recessive heterozygote).

Genetics and epidemiology

DEB may be inherited as autosomal dominant or autosomal recessive conditions. The Scottish prevalence is 24.6 cases per million of the population (compared with 2.4 cases per million of the population in the United States) and the incidence 26.4 new cases per million live births.[9] The majority of these are DDEB (prevalence 17.4 per million of the population).

Clinical features

Bullae in DEB heal with scarring and transient milia, and are usually associated with nail dystrophy of variable degree.

Dominant dystrophic epidermolysis bullosa

DDEB is the most common subtype of DEB and usually presents from birth to 5 years of age. The spectrum of clinical severity is wide even within a particular pedigree and the condition may be expressed by as little as dystrophy of the great toenails. However, characteristically bullae occur over the acral bony prominencies (knuckles, elbows, knees and malleolar regions (Fig. 16.8). Milia develop during the healing process (Fig. 16.9), which eventually leaves atrophic scarring. Thickened, discolored nail plates are common, especially on the toes, although some nails may remain normal (Fig. 16.10). Scarring of the nail bed often results in complete loss of the affected nail. Scarring does not lead to pseudosyndactyly in this type of DEB but occasionally flexion contractures of the fingers may be seen in adults.[42] The presence of albopapuloid lesions, typically over the lower back, is common in, but not specific to, DDEB. Albopapuloid lesions vary from being rather subtle, discrete, hypopigmented, atrophic areas with a finely wrinkled surface to more prominent, ivory–white papules. Their significance is uncertain. Very occasionally, DDEB may be associated with localized congenital absence of skin (Bart syndrome).

Oral bullae are not uncommon in children or adults and may be associated with dental caries.[42] Gastrointestinal tract involvement occurs in about 10–25% of cases of DDEB and includes dysphagia, microstomia, constipation, and anal fissures.[42] Occasionally, esophageal webs at the level of the cricopharyngeus may be a cause of dysphagia, but esophageal strictures are not typical of DDEB. Tracheobronchial and ocular involvement are not characteristic. Anemia occurs in less than one-fourth of patients and growth retardation is an uncommon feature of DDEB.

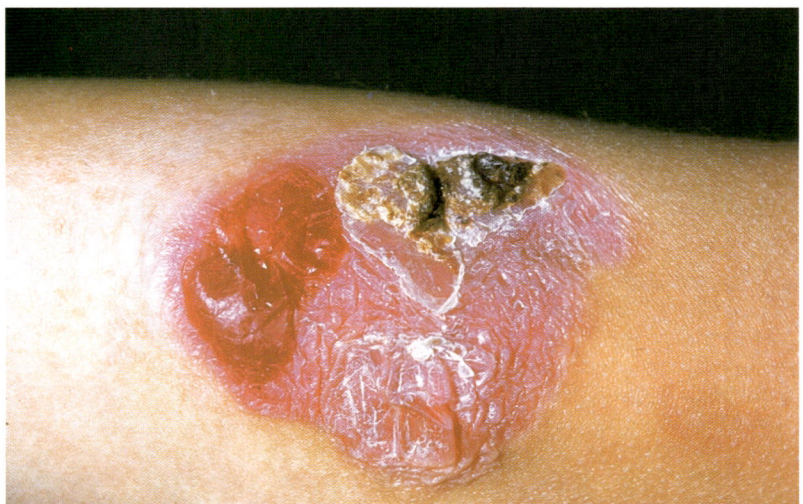

Fig. 16.8 Dominant DEB: bullae and scarring on the knee.

33. Holbrook KA, Christiano AM, Elias S et al. (1999) Prenatal diagnosis of inherited epidermolysis bullosa: ultrastructural, antigenic and molecular approaches. In: Fine JD, Bauer EA, McGuire J, Moshell A eds (1999) Epidermolysis Bullosa: Clinical, Epidemiologic and Laboratory Advances and the Findings of the National Epidermolysis Bullosa Registry. Baltimore: Johns Hopkins University Press, pp. 351–373.

34. Cserhalmi-Friedman PB, Tang Y, Adler A et al. (2000) Preimplantation genetic diagnosis in two families at risk for recurrence of Herlitz junctional epidermolysis bullosa. **Exp Dermatol** 9:290–297.

35. Robbins PB, Lin Q, Goodnough JB et al. (2001) *In vivo* restoration of laminin 5 β3 expression and function in junctional epidermolysis bullosa. **Proc Natl Acad Sci USA** 98:5193–5198.

36. Fox T (1879) Notes on unusual or rare forms of skin disease. **Lancet** 1:766–767.

37. Hallopeau MH (1898) Nouvelle note sur la dermatose bulleuse hereditaire et traumatique. **Ann Dermatol Syph** 9:721–728.

38. Cockayne EA (1933) Inherited abnormalities of the skin and its appendages. Oxford: Oxford University Press.

39. Touraine MA (1942) Classification des épidermolyses bulleuses. **Ann Dermatol Syphiligr** (Paris) 8:141–144.

40. Pasini A (1928) Dystrophie cutanée bulleuse atrophiante et albo-papuloïde. **Ann Dermatol Syph** 9:1044–1066.

41. Siemens HW (1921) Zur klinik, histologie und aetiologie der sog: Epidermolysis bullosa traumatica (Bullosis mechanica) mit klinisch-experimentellen studien über die erzeugung von reibungsblasen. **Arch Dermatol Syph** 134:454.

42. Horn HM, Tidman MJ (2002) The clinical spectrum of epidermolysis bullosa. **Br J Dermatol** 146:267–274.

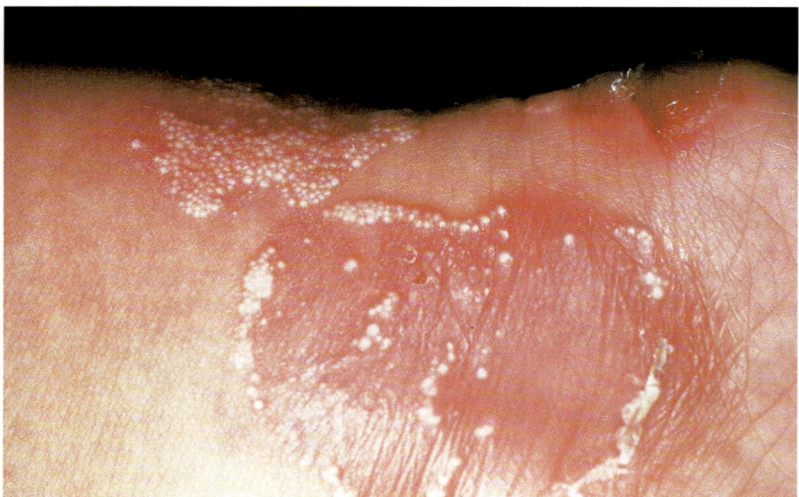

Fig. 16.9   Dominant DEB: milia within scars on ankle.

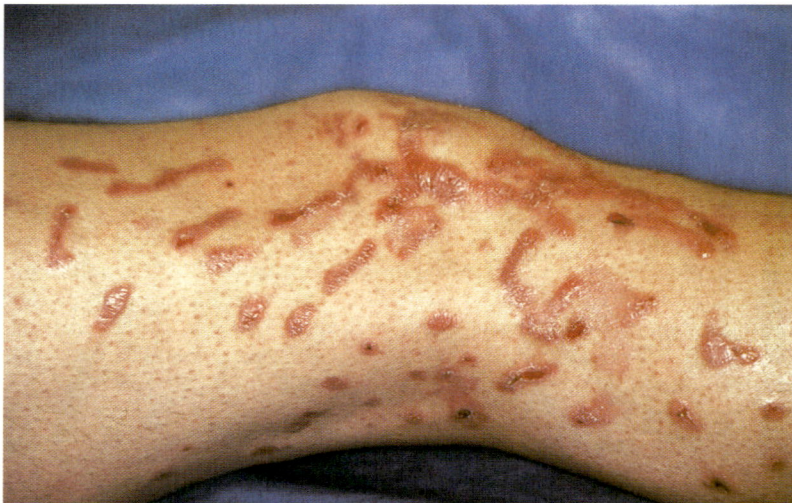

Fig. 16.11   EB pruriginosa: lichenoid lesions on leg.

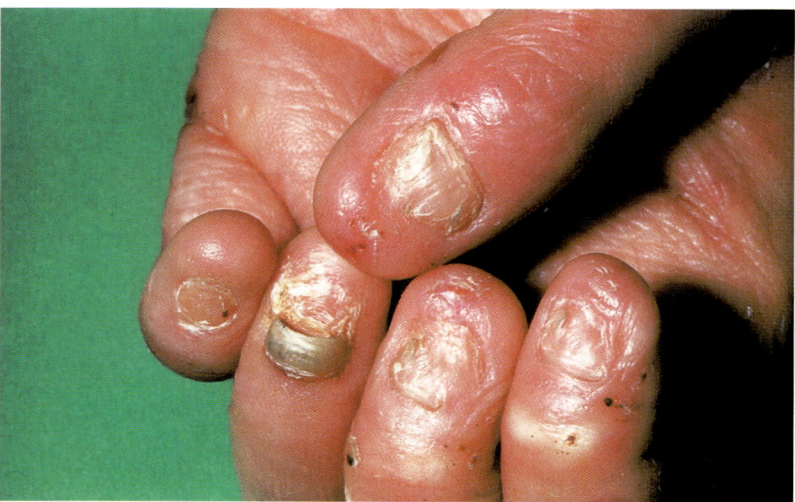

Fig. 16.10   Dominant DEB: fingernail dystrophy.

Data from the United States National EB Registry suggest the incidence of cutaneous malignancies to be increased compared to the general population.[43] The cumulative risk of basal cell carcinoma and malignant melanoma by age 30 in the registry population with DDEB was 0.8% and 0.9%, respectively. Squamous cell carcinomas were reported in older individuals with DDEB.[44]

For the majority, DDEB does not cause serious difficulties and for many the cosmetic consequences of scarring are the most troublesome aspect, resulting in psychological difficulty and social embarrassment rather than physical disability. Most experience improvement of the blistering tendency during early adult life.

Pretibial dominant dystrophic epidermolysis bullosa

Pretibial DEB is rare and is characterized by recurrent blistering, predominantly involving pretibial regions, resulting in milia formation and

scarring, and usually associated with nail dystrophy.[45] Pruritus is a common feature and it may be associated with a prurigo morphology and albopapuloid lesions. Onset may be delayed until the second or third decade. There tends to be significant phenotypic variation even within individual pedigrees. Autosomal dominant transmission is the norm although occasional cases may be the result of recessive mutations. It remains to be determined whether this phenotype is distinct from EB pruriginosa.

Epidermolysis bullosa pruriginosa

EB pruriginosa appears to be a clinically distinctive subset of DEB, which may be inherited in both dominant and recessive manners,[42,46,47] and characterized by intense pruritus associated with the formation of lichenified nodules or plaques. Trauma induced blistering occurs but may not be a prominent feature. Violaceous linear lesions, excoriations, milia, nail dystrophy and occasional albopapuloid lesions are also features. EB pruriginosa may cause clinical confusion with both lichen planus and nodular prurigo (Fig. 16.11).

Transient bullous dermolysis of the newborn

This is a rare subtype of DEB which in the majority of cases is transmitted in an autosomal dominant manner, and is characterized by extensive blistering at birth which resolves or dramatically improves over the succeeding months. Intracytoplasmic retention of type VII collagen within basal and suprabasal keratinocytes typifies this condition during the blistering period.[48]

Recessive dystrophic epidermolysis bullosa

The current recommended classification divides RDEB into two major subtypes, RDEB-Hallopeau–Siemens and RDEB-non-Hallopeau–Siemens.

Recessive dystrophic epidermolysis bullosa of Hallopeau–Siemens subtype

This is a rare form of DEB that presents at birth with generalized blistering. Congenital localized absence of skin may occasionally be a feature (Fig. 16.12). The skin is very fragile and blisters are easily induced by frictional trauma. Milia are usual, although not a prominent feature. It is an aggressively

43. Fine JD, Johnson LB, Suchindran C et al. (1999) Cancer and inherited epidermolysis bullosa. Lifetable analyses of the national epidermolysis bullosa registry study population. In: Epidermolysis Bullosa: Clinical, Epidemiologic and Laboratory Advances and the Findings of the National Epidermolysis Bullosa Registry, Fine JD, Bauer EA, McGuire J, Moshell A eds. Baltimore: Johns Hopkins University Press, pp. 175–192.

44. Schwartz RA, Birnkrant AP, Rubenstein DJ et al. (1981) Squamous cell carcinoma in dominant type epidermolysis bullosa dystrophica. **Cancer** 47:615–620.

45. Lee JY, Chen HC, Lin SJ (1993) Pretibial epidermolysis bullosa: a clinicopathologic study. **J Am Acad Dermatol** 29:974–981.

46. McGrath JA, Schofield OM, Eady RA (1994) Epidermolysis bullosa pruriginosa: dystrophic epidermolysis bullosa with distinctive clinicopathological features. **Br J Dermatol** 130:617–625.

47. Mellerio JE, Ashton GH, Mohammedi R et al. (1999) Allelic heterogeneity of dominant and recessive COL 7A1 mutations underlying epidermolysis bullosa pruriginosa. **J Invest Dermatol** 112:984–987.

48. Fine JD, Johnson LB, Cronce D et al. (1993) Intracytoplasmic retention of type VII collagen and dominant dystrophic epidermolysis bullosa: reversal of defect following cessation of or marked improvement in disease activity. **J Invest Dermatol** 101:232–236.

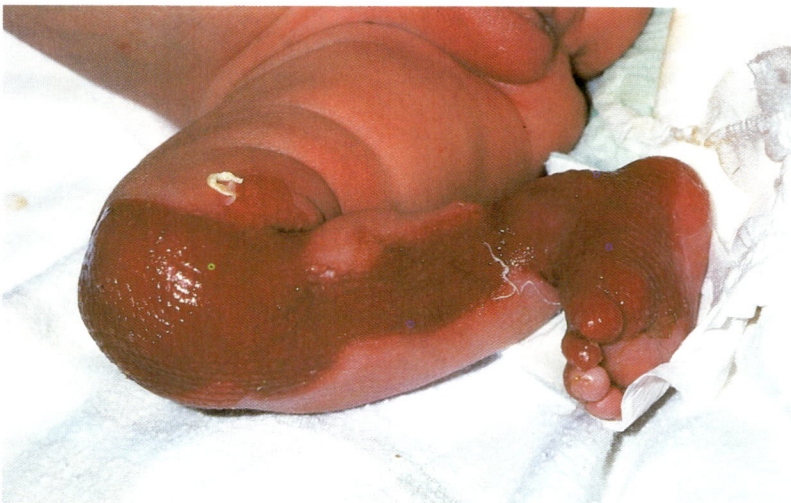

Fig. 16.12   Recessive DEB: congenital absence of skin (Bart syndrome).

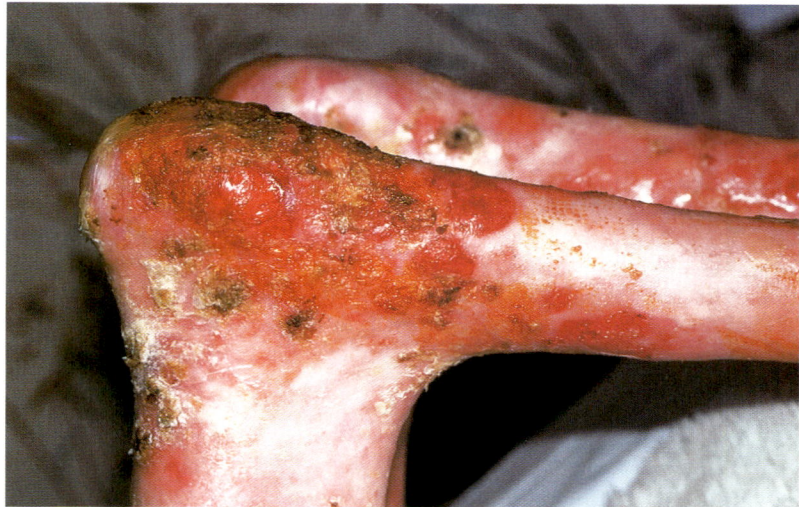

Fig. 16.14   Recessive DEB-Hallopeau–Siemens: fixed flexion deformity at knees.

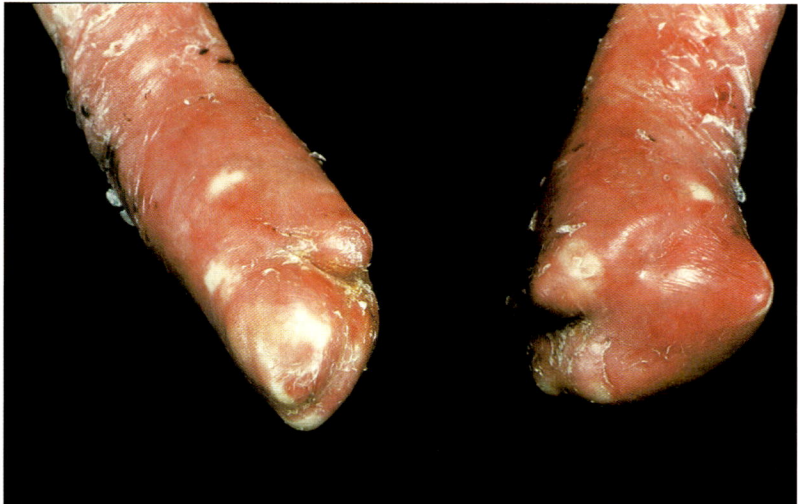

Fig. 16.13   Recessive DEB-Hallopeau–Siemens: pseudosyndactyly of hands.

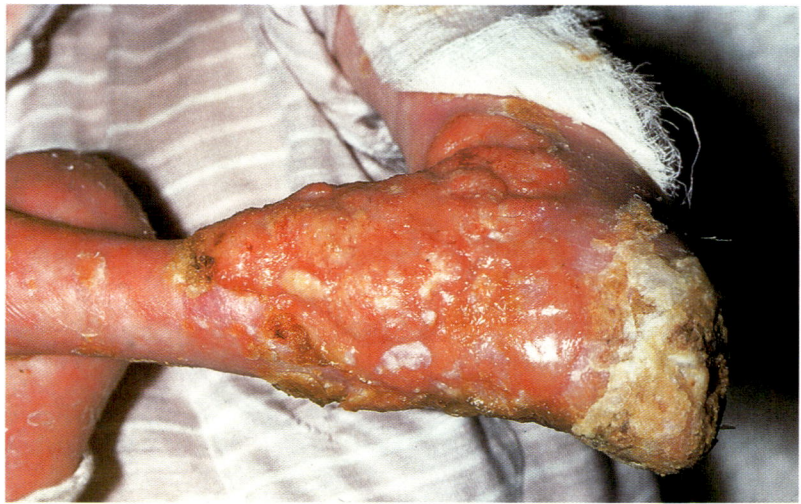

Fig. 16.15   Recessive DEB-Hallopeau–Siemens: squamous cell carcinoma.

scarring condition affecting the skin and gastrointestinal tract. Nail loss is inevitable and early, quickly followed by inexorably progressive flexion contractures of the digits and fusion of the fingers until the hands and feet become encased in a mitten of scar tissue (pseudosyndactyly; Fig. 16.13). Flexion contractures of the limbs contribute to immobility (Fig. 16.14) and sufferers are often confined to a wheelchair by adolescence. Scarring alopecia develops during childhood and scarring of the external ear, corneal erosions, and ectropion may occur.

There is a greatly increased incidence of squamous cell carcinoma (Fig. 16.15) and melanoma in young patients with RDEB-Hallopeau–Siemens and cutaneous malignancy is commonly fatal. The cumulative risk of developing squamous cell carcinoma by age 30 years was 39.6% in the United States National EB Registry and there was a 2.5% cumulative risk of melanoma by age 12 years.[42]

Oral blistering is inevitable and even very gentle brushing of teeth will result in bleeding and erosions. The teeth are normal but dental caries are common and a function of poor oral hygiene and exposure of teeth as a result of intraoral scarring. Microstomia further contributes to the difficulty in maintaining oral hygiene.

Dysphagia is a common symptom and may be due to a combination of ankyloglossia, esophageal dysmotility, and esophageal webs or strictures. Constipation is also common and may also have multifactorial causes, including anal fissuring and inadequate levels of dietary fiber.

Patients with RDEB-Hallopeau–Siemens frequently do not pass through puberty. Anemia, resulting from an inadequate diet, from chronic blood loss from the gastrointestinal tract and the skin, and the consequence of chronic disease, is the rule, and iron deficiency may contribute to esophageal web formation.

Recessive dystrophic epidermolysis bullosa – non-Hallopeau–Siemens

The non-Hallopeau–Siemens variant of RDEB has a phenotype which may be indistinguishable from DDEB, with blisters, transient milia and subsequent atrophic scars localized to acral bony prominences. Nail dystrophy or loss is usual. Congenital absence of skin (Bart syndrome) occasionally occurs. As with DDEB, skin fragility improves in adulthood. A mild degree of flexion contractures of the fingers may be present. Oral blistering, dental caries, and anal fissures may arise, as may a restricted oral aperture and ankyloglossia. Esophageal webs and strictures may cause dysphagia.

Inverse form of recessive dystrophic epidermolysis bullosa

The inverse variant of RDEB is characterized by a combination of flexural and acral bullae and erosions. The inguinal, axillary and, in adulthood, submammary regions are particularly affected. The hands and feet are also involved; the nails are lost and scarring of the hand and feet occur. Flexion contractures of the fingers may result. Dental disease, ankyloglossia, mild microstomia, anal fissures, and esophageal strictures also occur. Other body regions frequently blister and scar although not to the same degree or extent as in RDEB-Hallopeau–Siemens.

Pathophysiology and histogenesis

All variants of DEB are the result of mutations in the gene (*COL7A1*) that encodes type VII collagen, the morphological expression of which is the anchoring fibrils that appear to function in uniting the lamina densa with underlying elements of the papillary dermis. The anchoring fibrils are reduced in number, rudimentary, or absent in DEB. The cleavage plane in DEB coincides with the region normally occupied by anchoring fibrils. The RDEB-Hallopeau–Siemens phenotype is usually associated with premature termination codons on both alleles, either homozygous or compound heterozygous,[49] which results in a grossly defective molecule that cannot assemble anchoring fibrils, which are therefore absent. RDEB-non-Hallopeau–Siemens is associated with missence or frameshift mutations in the collagen VII genes, resulting in somewhat less disruption of the structural integrity and assembly of the collagen VII molecule. DDEB is caused by mutations in *COL7A1* that result in either a glycine substitution or, less frequently, in-frame deletions of 20–30 amino acids,[50] both of which may have a destabilizing effect on the triple helical type VII collagen molecule. However, the presence of a wildtype allele in DDEB allows a small percentage of normal polypeptides to assemble into collagen VII molecules that can form anchoring fibrils. Transient dermolysis of the newborn is caused by a splice site mutation in the gene encoding for collagen VII.[51]

The clinical severity of DEB, as in the other major variants of EB, is determined by the nature of the mutation, its position in the protein molecule and the presence of other mutations that might otherwise be clinically silent.

Differential diagnosis

RDEB-Hallopeau–Siemens is a unique clinical picture and unlikely to be confused with other conditions once the typical consequencies of scarring have developed. In infancy it may be difficult to distinguish from other severe variants of EB, and infections have to be excluded in the affected neonate.

The localized variants of DEB are also quite typical, although in the older child there is the possibility of confusion with conditions such as porphyria cutanea tarda, variegate porphyria, EB acquisita, and pseudoporphyria, all of which can result in very similar appearances of the hands.

Therapeutics and prognosis

The basic skin care of severely blistering DEB is the same as for JEB. The scarring tendency in DEB causes protean problems that demand a multidisciplinary management approach including dermatologists, nurses, plastic surgeons, pediatricians, gastroenterologists, hematologists, ophthalmic surgeons, dentists, dieticians, and physiotherapists. The treatment of systemic complaints, including oral, gastrointestinal, and musculoskeletal manifestations, should be individualized, and a comprehensive discussion of the management of these issues is beyond the scope of this text, but an excellent review of these topics is available from the National EB Registry.[52] Perhaps the single most important aspect of managing DEB, especially the RDEB-Hallopeau–Siemens variant, is the regular monitoring for squamous cell carcinoma, which can be ulcerative or hyperkeratotic. Biopsying of persistent erosions or hyperkeratotic lesions is necessary if there are any unusual features.

Systemic agents such as phenytoin and isotretinoin have been advocated for the treatment of DEB[53–55] but there is insufficient evidence of their efficacy to support their use.[52,56]

DDEB has a normal life expectancy and, in general, the condition improves in adulthood. Nonetheless, patient and physician should be aware of the possibility of squamous cell carcinoma arising on chronically scarred skin. In individuals with RDEB-Hallopeau–Siemens skin fragility and blister formation continue unabated and there is an increased risk of early death from squamous cell carcinoma, sepsis and pneumonia. Squamous cell carcinomas occur at sites of chronic erosions and frequently metastasize.

Laboratory Investigations

If EB is suspected, samples should be taken for ultrastructural confirmation of the cleavage plane and for immunohistochemistry. Routine light microscopy is not helpful for establishing the type of EB, but may exclude other inflammatory blistering disorders. The edge of, or a complete, fresh blister less than 24h old should be biopsied and the perilesional skin used for immunohistochemistry. If a suitable bulla is not available, cleavage may be induced in severe forms of EB by rubbing an unaffected area with a pencil eraser.

Electron microscopy is the gold standard for defining the cleavage plane, but if this is not available immunohistochemical antigen mapping will reveal the level of the split by defining its location relative to proteins that are normally expressed at various levels of the basement membrane zone (e.g., bullous pemphigoid antigen-1, laminin-1, and Type IV collagen). In the case of EBS Dowling–Meara, electron microscopy demonstrates the characteristic tonofilament clumping, and in JEB and DEB abnormalities of the hemidesmosomes and anchoring fibrils, respectively, are present. Immunohistochemistry with antibodies to immunoglobulins should be done routinely to exclude an autoimmune blistering disorder, and immunohistochemistry may also provide information about the presence or absence of particular basement membrane proteins involved in the pathogenesis of EB. Two commercially available antibodies, GB3 (specific for laminin 5) and LH7:2 (specific for type VII collagen), can be used to rapidly confirm or exclude JEB-Herlitz and RDEB-Hallopeau–Siemens, respectively. Patients with JEB-Herlitz will show complete absence of staining with GB3, and RDEB-Hallopeau–Siemens is characterized by totally absent expression of type VII collagen antibody. This type of analysis may be less helpful in milder forms of JEB and DEB.

Gene mutational analysis can now be undertaken for all three main types of EB but at present this is not available routinely outside research departments.

Physician support

The NEBR provides support for physicians evaluating and caring for children with suspected EB. In addition the Dystrophic Epidermolysis Bullosa Research Association (DEBRA), with branches in 15 countries throughout the world, provides valuable support and medical information to physicians, patients and their families.

National Epidermolysis Bullosa Registry
University of North Carolina at Chapel Hill
919-966-2007

49. Pulkkinen L, Uitto J (1999) Mutation analysis and molecular genetics of epidermolysis bullosa. **Matrix Biology** 18:29–42.
50. Christiano AM, Ryynänen M, Uitto J (1994) Dominant dystrophic epidermolysis bullosa: identification of a glycine-to-serine substitution in the triple helical domain of type VII collagen. **Proc Natl Acad Sci USA** 91:3549–3553.
51. Christiano AM, Fine JD, Uitto J (1997) Genetic basis of dominantly inherited transient dermolysis of the newborn: a splice site mutation in the type VII collagen gene. **J Invest Dermatol** 109:811–814.
52. Fine JD, Bauer EA, McGuire J (1999) The treatment of inherited epidermolysis bullosa: nonmolecular approaches. In: Epidermolysis Bullosa Clinical, Epidemiologic and Laboratory

Advances and the Findings of the National Epidermolysis Bullosa Registry, Fine JD, Bauer EA, McGuire J, Moshell A eds. Baltimore: Johns Hopkins University Press, pp. 374–406.
53. Bauer EA, Cooper TW, Tucker DR et al. (1980) Phenytoin therapy of recessive dystrophic epidermolysis bullosa: clinical trial and proposed mechanism of action on collagenase. **N Engl J Med** 303:776–781.
54. Fine JD, Johnson L (1988) Efficacy of systemic phenytoin in the treatment of junctional epidermolysis bullosa. **Arch Dermatol** 124:1402–1406.
55. Andreano JM, Tomecki KJ (1988) Epidermolysis bullosa simplex responding to isotretinoin. **Arch Dermatol** 124:1445–1446.
56. Caldwell-Brown D, Stern RS, Lin AN et al. (1992) Lack of efficacy of phenytoin in recessive dystrophic epidermolysis bullosa. **N Engl J Med** 327:163–167.

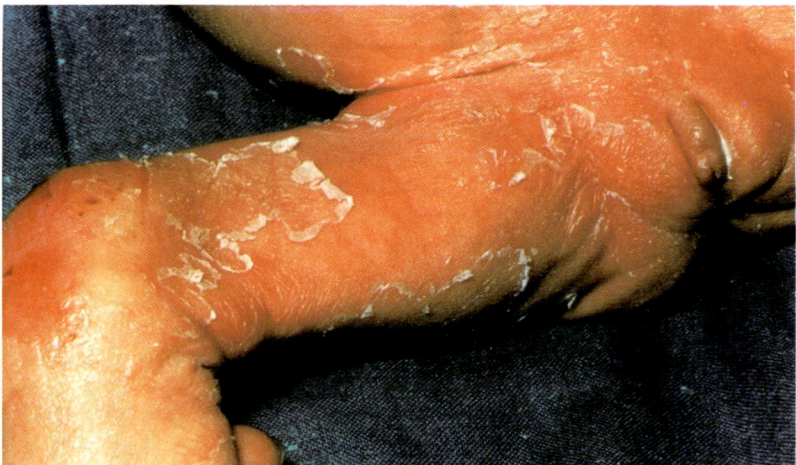

Fig. 16.16   Bullous ichthyosis: blistering in a premature infant.

Dystrophic Epidermolysis Bullosa Research Association of America
www.debra.org
877–88–DEBRA

BULLOUS CONGENITAL ICHTHYOSIFORM ERYTHRODERMA OF BROCQ

Introduction and historical note
Bullous ichthyosis (BI), also known as bullous congenital ichthyosiform erythroderma of Brocq, previously known as epidermolytic hyperkeratosis, is a rare inherited mechanobullous eruption, described by Brocq in 1902,[57] and further defined by Lapière in 1953.[58] A milder variant, BI of Siemens, is recognized (see next section). It is a keratin disorder, with many similarities to EBS, but whereas the latter condition is the result of mutations in the genes encoding the basal keratins 5 and 14, BI is a result of mutations affecting keratins 1 and 10, which are expressed in the suprabasal layers of the epidermis.[59] BI is characterized by blistering and variable erythroderma in early life and the subsequent development of ichthyosis.

Genetics
BI is inherited in an autosomal dominant fashion, but many cases are the result of *de novo* mutations. In an affected parent, the condition may be subtle and localized to the flexures, or rarely the affected parent may have an epidermolytic epidermal nevus; this inheritance pattern is thought to represent mosaicism. Gonadal mosaicism may explain the occurrence of BI in more than one child of unaffected parents.[60]

Clinical features
BI may show pronounced phenotypic variability within a family, possibly related to somatic mosaicism.[61] Blistering and erythroderma are usually present at birth (Fig. 16.16), and the extent of the blistering may resemble the severe forms of EBS or staphylococcal scalded skin syndrome. Mild trauma during normal handling of a baby may induce bullae and erosions. This blistering tendency and the erythema usually subside during the first year, although the bullous element may persist into adult life. Gradually, the skin becomes thickened and hyperkeratotic, and these changes may be widespread or, in mild cases, the hyperkeratosis may be confined to the flexures, producing

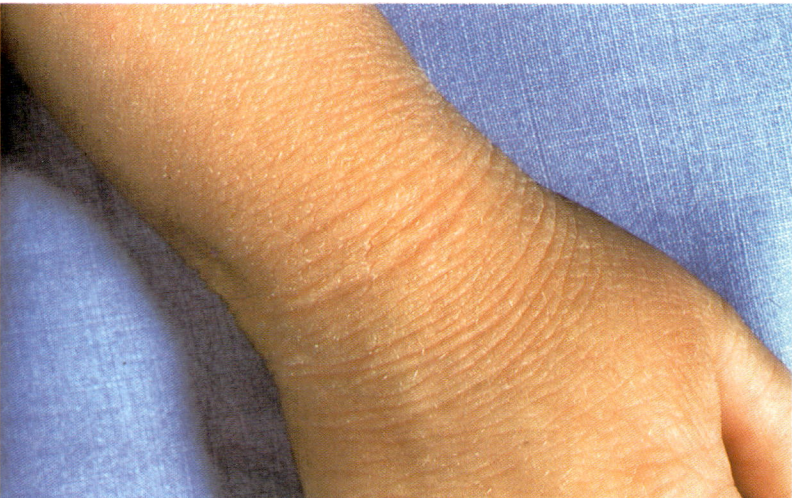

Fig. 16.17   Bullous ichthyosis (same patient as Fig. 16.16, aged 3 years): corrugated hyperkeratosis.

a characteristic corrugated configuration of thickening (Fig. 16.17). The face is not normally involved. There may be severe palmoplantar involvement, associated with flexion contractures of the digits, and such patients usually have mutations of the gene for keratin 1, but occasionally keratin 10 mutations can also produce a similar clinical picture.[62] Severe involvement of the palms and soles may be very disabling and interfere with mobility. Occasionally, widespread cutaneous involvement may be accompanied by developmental delay. The blisters of BI do not leave scarring or atrophy. Widespread hyperkeratosis is sometimes associated with a rather typical musty smell, which is probably the result of overgrowth of yeasts or bacteria within the stratum corneum.

Pathophysiology and histogenesis
BI is the result of mutations in the genes encoding keratins 1 or 10.[59] A number of mutational "hot spots" have been found, and it seems likely that the clinical severity of the condition is related to the location of the mutation and the effect this will have on the integrity of the keratin molecule. The more disrupted the keratin protein is, the weaker the cytoskeleton and the greater the predilection to cytolysis following mild trauma.

Keratins 1 and 10 are expressed by suprabasal epidermal cells, and the lower cell layers of the epidermis are unaffected. The keratinocytes within the upper spinous and granular layers show cytolytic degeneration with cytoplasmic edema and perinuclear vacuolization, clumping of the keratin intermediate filaments and coarse keratohyalin granules. The stratum corneum becomes thick and eukeratotic. These histological features comprise epidermolytic hyperkeratosis, and are similar to the histological and ultrastructural changes seen in the Dowling–Meara variant of epidermolysis bullosa simplex.

Differential diagnosis
In the early stages, BI should be differentiated from severe forms of epidermolysis bullosa and from staphylococcal scalded skin syndrome. As the ichthyotic changes develop, differentiation from other autosomal dominant ichthyoses, such as ichthyosis vulgaris, is necessary.

57. Brocq L (1902) Erythrodermie congénitale ichthyoseforme avec hyperépidermotrophie. **Ann Derm Syph** 3:1–31.
58. Lapière S (1953) Les génodermatoses hyperkératosiques de type bulleux. **Ann Dermatol Venereol** 80:597–614.
59. Ishida-Yamamota A, McGrath JA, Judge MR et al. (1992) Selective involvement of keratins K1 and K10 in the cytoskeletal abnormality of epidermolytic hyperkeratosis (bullous congenital ichthyosiform erythroderma). **J Invest Dermatol** 99:19–26.
60. Paller AS, Syder AJ, Chan YM et al. (1994) Genetic and clinical mosaicism in a type of epidermal naevus. **N Engl J Med** 331:1408–1415.
61. Nomura K, Umeki K, Hatayama I, Kuronuma T (2001) Phenotypic heterogeneity in bullous congenital ichthyosiform erythroderma. **Arch Dermatol** 137:1192–1195.
62. Virtanen M, Gedde-Dahl T, Mörk N-J et al. (2001) Phenotypic/genotypic correlations in patients with epidermolytic hyperkeratosis and the effects of retinoid therapy on keratin expression. **Acta Derm Venerol** 81:163–170.

Therapeutics and prognosis

In the neonatal period the therapeutic considerations are the same as for the severe forms of epidermolysis bullosa, and comprise careful handling and management of blisters. The erythrodermic skin requires careful attention due to increased transepidermal water and heat loss.

With the onset of ichthyosis, standard emollient therapy is required, but in severe cases systemic acitretin therapy appears to be safe and effective.[63] A standard starting dose of acitretin is 0.5mg/kg per day, and the subsequent dose titrated to the response. In BI retinoids can be very effective in treating the hyperkeratosis but an exacerbation of the blistering tendency may limit the dose.[64] Retinoid therapy is thought to be particularly effective in patients with keratin 10 mutations, and less so in those with keratin 1 mutations.[62]

Prenatal diagnosis of BI is possible. Initially, this required a fetal skin biopsy[65] but this has attendant disadvantages and prenatal diagnosis can now be undertaken by direct gene sequencing[66] once the mutation has been identified in the proband. This technique can be done early in pregnancy. The presence of the characteristic tonofilament clumps of BI within amniotic fluid cells raises the possibility of a diagnosis being made by amniocentesis,[67] although there is the potential for a false-negative result.

ICHTHYOSIS BULLOSA OF SIEMENS

Introduction and historical note

Ichthyosis bullosa of Siemens (IBS) was described in 1937,[68] and was resurrected as a unique type of epidermolytic hyperkeratosis in 1986.[69] Whilst it has a number of similarities to BI, there are clinical distinctions, and the demonstration that is caused by mutations in the gene encoding keratin 2e[70] further distinguishes it from BI.

Clinical features

Like BI, it is an autosomal dominant mechanobullous disorder with blisters and erosions caused by minor trauma, although it is a milder condition. It may be present at birth or develop later in infancy, but it is characterized by an absence of erythroderma. Dark hyperkeratotic skin develops mainly on the limbs, with a tendency to spare the trunk except for the periumbilical region. The knees, elbows, dorsa of the hands and feet and the limb flexures are predilection sites. The palms and soles are usually spared. Occasionally, pustulation is a feature. The condition is frequently uncomfortable as a result of skin cracking causing a degree of immobility. Blistering may worsen during the summer, and is exacerbated by sweating. The hyperkeratotic element may improve during the summer months. Like BI, blistering does not result in scarring or atrophy. A particularly distinctive clinical feature is the development of superficially denuded, peeling areas – the so-called "*mauserung* phenomenon" (moulting).

Histological examination reveals a more subtle degree of epidermolytic hyperkeratosis than BI, confined to the granular layer, which is compatible with keratin 2e being expressed only in the upper part of the stratum granulosum.

The clinical features that distinguish ichthyosis bullosa of Seimens from BI are the lack of erythroderma, the typical *mauserung* phenomenon, the confinement of epidermolytic changes to the superficial epidermal layers and the presence of intracorneal blistering.

The differential diagnosis of ichthyosis bullosa of Siemens includes epidermolysis bullosa simplex and other autosomal dominant types of ichthyosis, including ichthyosis vulgaris and BI.

Therapeutics

Treatment should consist of the liberal and frequent application of an emollient, but in troublesome cases the use of an oral retinoid such as acitretin in low dose appears to be very effective.[64] The maintenance dose of retinoid is lower than that for BI and retinoid-induced blistering is not a problem.

HAILEY–HAILEY DISEASE

Introduction and historical note

Hailey-Hailey disease, also known as benign familial pemphigus, was described by two brothers in 1939.[71] It is a rare mechanobullous disease characterized by recurrent small blisters and erosions typically involving the intertriginous sites.

Genetics

Hailey–Hailey disease is inherited as an autosomal dominant trait with the gene located on chromosome 3q21–24.

Clinical features

These have been systematically described by Burge.[72] The onset of Hailey–Hailey disease is rare in the first decade of life and usually presents in the second to fourth decades. It involves intertriginous sites, particularly the axillae, inguinal regions and neck. It occasionally involves the antecubital and popliteal fossae and the scalp may also rarely be involved. Minor trauma results in blisters and erosions, and the condition tends to fluctuate in severity. It tends to be worse during the summer as heat and sweating exacerbate the condition, as does friction of clothing such as collars and underwear. Pruritus and pain are common and the latter can be disabling and limit physical activities, especially when the groin is involved.

The morphology of the lesions is variable. They often take the form of expanding plaques with a peripheral scaly border. Superimposed on the plaques there may be crusts, erosions, vesicles or pustules. Flexural lesions may become hypertrophic. Sometimes the erosions are aligned to resemble the furrows of a plowed field. The lesions of Hailey–Hailey disease are often malodorous and may become secondarily infected with bacteria, dermatophytes, candida, and herpes simplex virus. Nikolski's sign is often positive. The mucous membranes tend not to be involved. Lesions heal without scarring.

Asymptomatic longitudinal white bands on the nails are a common feature of Hailey–Hailey disease.

Pathophysiology and histogenesis

Hailey–Hailey disease is caused by mutations in *ATP2C1*, the gene encoding a novel calcium pump.[73] Intracellular calcium stores seem to be important in regulating epidermal cell–cell adhesion and differentiation, although the precise mechanism whereby defects in the calcium pump cause the clinical phenotype of Hailey–Hailey disease is not clear.

63. Lacour M, Mehta-Nikhar B, Atherton DJ, Harper JI (1996) An appraisal of acitretin therapy in children with inherited disorders of keratinization. **Br J Dermatol** 134:1023–1029.
64. Steijlen PM, van Dooren-Greebe RJ, Happle R, van de Kerkhof PCM (1991) Ichthyosis bullosa of Siemens responds well to low-dosage oral retinoids. **Br J Dermatol** 125:469–471.
65. Golbus MS, Sagebiel RW, Filly RA et al. (1980) Prenatal diagnosis of congenital bullous ichthyosiform erythroderma (epidermolytic hyperkeratosis) by fetal skin biopsy. **N Engl J Med** 302:93–95.
66. Rothnagel JA, Longley MA, Holder RA et al. (1994) Prenatal diagnosis of epidermolytic hyperkeratosis by direct gene sequencing. **J Invest Dermatol** 102:13–16.
67. Eady RAJ, Gunner DB, Carbone LD et al. (1986) Prenatal diagnosis of bullous ichthyosiform erythroderma: detection of tonofilament clumps in fetal epidermal and amniotic fluid cells. **J Med Genet** 23:46–51.

68. Siemens HW (1937) Dichtung und Wahrheit über die Ichthyosis bullosa mit Bemerkungen zur Systematik der Epidermolysen. **Arch Dermatol Syph (Berl)** 175:590–608.
69. Traupe H, Kolde G, Hamm H, Happle R (1986) Ichthyosis bullosa of Siemens: a unique type of epidermolytic hyperkeratosis. **J Am Acad Dermatol** 14:1000–1005.
70. McLean WHI, Morley SM, Lane EB et al. (1994) Ichthyosis bullosa of Siemens – a disease involving keratin 2e. **J Invest Dermatol** 103:277–281.
71. Hailey H, Hailey H (1939) Familial benign chronic pemphigus. **Arch Dermatol Syph** 39:679–685.
72. Burge SM (1992) Hailey–Hailey disease: the clinical features, response to treatment and prognosis. **Br J Dermatol** 126:275–282.
73. Hu Z, Bonifas JM, Beech J et al. (2000) Mutations in ATP2C1, encoding a calcium pump, cause Hailey–Hailey disease. **Nat Genet** 24:61–65.

Histologic findings

Hailey–Hailey disease is characterized by suprabasal acantholysis, associated with mild dyskeratosis. Acanthosis and a mild dermal perivascular infiltrate may be present. Direct and indirect immunofluorescence are negative. Ultrastructural examination demonstrates breakdown of desmosome–keratin filament complexes.

Differential diagnosis

Hailey–Hailey disease is often subtle and may be misdiagnosed as an eczema reaction, fungal infection, impetigo, candidal intertrigo, seborrhoeic dermatitis, or contact dermatitis. Hailey–Hailey disease may be confused with Darier disease.

Therapeutics and prognosis

Hailey–Hailey disease tends to become less troublesome with age and prolonged remissions may occur. There appears to be a small risk of superimposed squamous cell carcinoma.[74,75] Secondary infection with the herpes simplex virus must be considered in cases of severe exacerbation, and eczema herpeticum has been recorded.[76] There is an increased likelihood of allergic contact dermatitis to medicaments in Hailey–Hailey disease.[77]

Both topical corticosteroids and topical antibiotics have proved effective treatments. Topical corticosteroids may abort developing lesions. A combination of a medium potency or potent topical corticosteroid with an antibiotic preparation for a limited time period is a reasonable initial therapeutic option. Oral antibiotics may be helpful and some patients may require oral antibiotics on a long-term, low-dose basis.[72] Topical antiseptic preparations may help to control malodor and emollients are usually helpful.

In recalcitrant cases, a variety of treatments have been used, including Grenz rays, full-thickness excision of affected skin, carbon dioxide laser vaporization, dermabrasion, cryosurgery, dapsone, vitamin E, PUVA, methotrexate, thalidomide, cyclosporin, oral retinoids, and tacalcitol; these are usually employed in adult cases and reports have been anecdotal.

ECTODERMAL DYSPLASIA/SKIN FRAGILITY SYNDROME

Introduction, presenting history and physical examination

Ectodermal dysplasia/skin fragility syndrome is a recently described disorder characterized by features that are reminiscent of ectodermal dysplasia and epidermolysis bullosa. This disorder is caused by a deficiency in plakophilin-1, a structural component of desmosomes.[78]

This rare disorder presents in the newborn period with generalized erythema, bullae, desquamation, and swollen digits. Hair is short and sparse and the nails are thickened and dystrophic. The affected individuals also have perioral erythema and desquamation that persists. The tendency to blister improves over time and becomes more localized. Subsequently, hyperkeratotic plaques develop on the extremities with palmoplantar hyperkeratosis. An inability to sweat normally also characterizes this disorder.[79,80]

Laboratory findings

Skin biopsy reveals acanthosis and widening of intercellular spaces between the keratinocytes of the mid-spinous layer of the epidermis. Immunohistochemical analysis shows absent staining for plakophilin-1 and an altered distribution of desmoplakin.

Pathophysiology and histogenesis

Individuals with ectodermal dysplasia/skin fragility syndrome have mutations in the gene encoding for the desmosmal protein plakophilin-1. The initially reported patients were compound heterozygotes for different combinations of mutations that resulted in a complete absence of plakophilin-1. Plakophilin-1 is an important structural protein involved in cell–cell adhe-sion and also plays an important role in signal transduction pathways and epidermal morphogenesis. An absence of plakophilin 1 leads to abnormal cell–cell adhesion and retraction of the keratin filaments in suprabasal keratinocytes resulting in skin fragility and blistering. The absence of plakophilin-1 probably leads to abnormalities of patterning in embryonic ectodermal development which results in hair, nail and sweating abnormalities.[78]

Prognosis

The prognosis of this rare and newly reported genodermatosis is uncertain. Blister formation improves over time. Management is supportive.

KINDLER SYNDROME

Introduction

Kindler syndrome is a rare distinct genetic disorder characterized by poikiloderma, photosensitivity and skin fragility.[81]

Presenting history and physical examination

Infants often present in the neonatal period with acral blistering although more extensive blistering has been reported. The tendency to develop blisters and photosensitivity improves with maturity, but generalized atrophic scarring and poikiloderma are progressive. Poikiloderma often begins on sun-exposed surfaces and extends to covered areas. Fusion of the digits that resembles recessive dystrophic epidermolysis bullosa is a feature of this disorder (Fig. 16.18). Other less commonly reported findings include palmoplantar hyperkeratosis, esophageal, urethral and anal stenosis, and nail dystrophy. Squamous cell carcinoma of the lip and hard palate and transitional cell carcinoma of the bladder have been reported in Kindler syndrome.[82–84]

Laboratory findings, pathophysiology and histogenesis

Kindler syndrome is a distinct disorder that should be distinguished from dystrophic epidermolysis bullosa. Light microscopy is not specific and shows features of poikiloderma (epidermal atrophy, vacuolization of the basal layer, capillary dilatation, and dermal edema).[83] Electron microscopy of skin biopsy specimens shows duplication of the lamina densa. Cleft formation occurs in the lamina lucida. Beneath areas of clefting the lamina densa is absent or disrupted. The anchoring fibrils and hemidesmosomes are normal. Immunohistochemical analysis demonstrates normal staining with antibodies against hemidesmosomal and anchoring filament proteins. There is no

74. Holst VA, Fair KP, Wilson BB, Patterson JW (2000) Squamous cell carcinoma arising in Hailey–Hailey disease. J Am Acad Dermatol 43:368–371.
75. Cockayne SE, Rassl DM, Thomas SE (2000) Squamous cell carcinoma arising in Hailey–Hailey disease of the vulva. Br J Dermatol 142:540–542.
76. Flint ID, Spencer DM, Wilkin JK (1993) Eczema herpeticum in association with familial benign chronic pemphigus. J Am Acad Dermatol 28:257–259.
77. Reitamo S, Remitz A, Lauerma AI, Förström L (1989) Contact allergies in patients with familial benign chronic pemphigus (Hailey–Hailey disease). J Am Acad Dermatol 21:506–510.
78. McGrath JA, McMillan JR, Shemanko CS et al. (1997) Mutations in the plakophilin 1 gene result in ectodermal dysplasia/skin fragility syndrome. Nat Genet 17:240–244.
79. McGrath JA (1999) A novel genodermatosis caused by mutations in plakophilin 1, a structural component of desmosomes. J Dermatol 26:764–769.
80. McGrath JA, Hoeger PH, Christiano AM et al. (1999) Skin fragility and hypohidrotic ectodermal dysplasia resulting from ablation of plakophilin I. Br J Dermatol 140:297–307.
81. Kindler T (1954) Congenital poikiloderma with traumatic bulla formation and progressive cutaneous atrophy. Br J Dermatol, 66:104–111.
82. Haber RM, Hanna WM (1996) Kindler syndrome clinical and ultrastructural findings. Arch Dermatol 132:1487–1490.
83. Patrizi A, Pauluzzi P, Neri I et al. (1996) Kindler syndrome: report of a case with ultrastructural study and review of the literature. Pediatr Dermatol. 13:397–402.
84. Lotem M, Raben M, Zeltser R et al. (2001) Kindler syndrome complicated by squamous cell carcinoma of the hard palate: successful treatment with high dose radiation therapy and granulocyte–macrophage colony-stimulating factor. Br J Dermatol. 144:1284–1286.

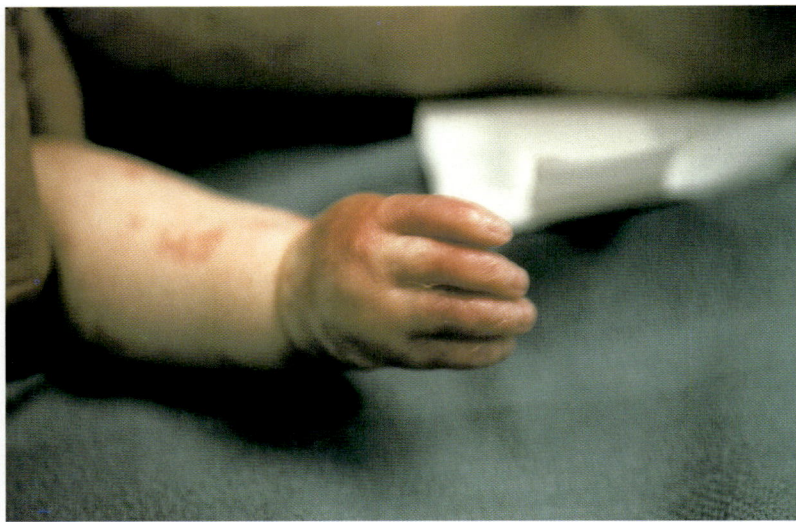

Fig. 16.18   Kindler syndrome.

evidence of mutations in the collagen VII genes.[85] The pathogenesis of Kindler syndrome remains unknown.

Differential diagnosis

The differential diagnosis of Kindler syndrome includes other inherited blistering diseases and the congenital poikilodermas. It may be difficult to distinguish Kindler syndrome from epidermolysis bullosa in the immediate newborn period; however, the development of poikiloderma with age helps to establish the diagnosis. Moreover, a history of blistering and scarring helps to distinguish it from other disorders such as Bloom's syndrome and Rothmund–Thomson syndrome that are also characterized by poikiloderma and photosensitivity.

Therapeutics and prognosis

Individuals with Kindler syndrome often demonstrate improvement of blistering with ageing; however the poikiloderma and atrophy is progressive. There are reports of malignancies arising in individuals with Kindler syndrome.[83]

CONGENITAL EROSIVE AND VESICULAR DERMATOSIS HEALING WITH RETICULATED SUPPLE SCARRING

Introduction

Congenital erosive and vesicular dermatosis with reticulated supple scarring is a very rare disorder that was first reported by Cohen, Esterly, and Nelson in 1985.[86] It may be confused with epidermolysis bullosa in the newborn period. Affected individuals present with crusted erosions and vesicles. The erosions heal relatively rapidly with a reticulate scarring

Epidemiology

Congenital erosive and vesicular dermatosis is a very rare disorder of unknown etiology. There are 11 cases reported in the English language literature.[86–90]

Presenting history and physical examination

Infants with congenital erosive and vesicular dermatosis characteristically present as premature infants in the immediate newborn period. Nine out of the 11 cases in the literature were premature. Erosions, crusts, and vesicles usually appear on the scalp, trunk, and extremities with relative sparing of the palms and soles. Facial involvement is less frequently reported. The lesions heal within the first several weeks to months of life with reticulate or "cobblestoned" scarring. Skin fragility usually resolves relatively soon after the newborn period; however, ongoing mild blistering has been reported.[90] Heat intolerance has been reported and is believed to be secondary to lack of eccrine structures in the areas of scarring.[89] Nail dystrophy, loss of tongue papillae and sparse hair have been seen in some cases.[86,89,90] Chronic recurrent conjunctivitis and nasolacrimal duct scarring was observed in one patient.[90] Neurologic impairment has been reported in some patients but it is unclear whether it is related to the cutaneous disorder or the underlying prematurity.[86]

Laboratory findings

Laboratory findings are nonspecific. In cases in which tests were performed there was no evidence of intrauterine infection. Skin biopsy specimens obtained in the newborn period reveal epidermal erosions with fibrin and neutrophils and a neutrophilic dermal infiltrate. Immunofluorescence and electron microscopy are not diagnostic.[88–90]

Pathophysiology and histogenesis

The etiology of this disorder is unknown. A variety of hypotheses have been considered including intrauterine infection, trauma, vasospastic phenomena and immune complex disease, with little data to support any of these etiologies.[86–90]

Differential diagnosis

The differential diagnosis for this rare disorder includes infectious disease that may present in the immediate newborn period and other disorders characterized by neonatal blistering and erosions. The clinical course and scarring are characteristic and establish the diagnosis.

Therapeutics and prognosis

The treatment of congenital erosive and vesicular dermatosis with reticulated supple scarring is supportive. Local wound care includes application of topical antibiotics and wound dressings until the erosions heal. Physicians following patients should be aware of the potential for future sweating abnormalities.[86–90]

INCONTINENTIA PIGMENTI

Introduction and historical note

Incontinentia pigmenti (IP), or Bloch–Sulzberger syndrome, is a rare multisystem ectodermal disorder characterized by cutaneous, ocular, dental, and neurological features. It is inherited as an X-linked dominant trait which is usually lethal to affected male fetuses *in utero*, but the disease in males is being described with increasing frequency. The clinical features of IP were documented by Bloch[91] and Sulzberger,[92] but IP may have been described 20 years previously in 1906 by Garrod.[93]

85. Shimizu H, Sato M, Ban M et al. (1997) Immunohistochemical, ultrastructural and molecular features of Kindler syndrome distinguish it from dystrophic epidermolysis bullosa. **Arch Dermatol.** 133:1111–1117.
86. Cohen BA, Esterly NB, Nelson PF (1985) Congenital erosive and vesicular dermatosis healing with reticulated supple scarring. **Arch Dermatol** 121:361–367.
87. Plantin P, Delaire P, Guillois B et al. (1990) Congenital erosive and vesicular dermatosis healing with reticulated supple scarring: first neonatal report. **Arch Dermatol** 126:544–546.
88. Sadick NS, Shea CR, Schlessel JS (1995) Congenital erosive and vesicular dermatosis healing with reticulated supple scarring: a neutrophilic dermatosis. **J Am Acad Dermatol** 32:873–877.

89. Sidhu-Malik NK, Resnick SD, Braunstein-Wilson B (1998) Congenital erosive and vesicular dermatosis healing with reticulated supple scarring: report of three new cases and review of the literature. **Pediatr Dermatol** 15:214–218.
90. Stein S, Stone S, Paller AS (2001) Ongoing blistering in a boy with congenital erosive and vesicular dermatosis healing with reticulated supple scarring. **J Am Acad Dermatol** 45:946–948.
91. Bloch B (1926) Eigentumliche, bisher nicht beschriebene Pigmentaffektion (Incontinentia Pigmenti). **Schweiz Med Wochenschr** 7:404–405.
92. Sulzberger MB (1928) Uber eine bisher nicht beschriebene congenitale Pigmentanomalie (IP). **Arch Dermatol Syph (Berl)** 154:19–32.
93. Garrod AE (1906) Peculiar pigmentation of the skin of an infant. **Trans Clin Soc Lond** 39:216.

Epidemiology

Genetics

The mutated gene has been mapped to Xq28,[94] and IP has recently been shown to be caused in most cases by rearrangements in the X-linked gene encoding NF-kappa B essential modulator (NEMO)/I kappa B kinase-gamma (IKK gamma).[95] NEMO/IKK gamma is required for the activation of the transcription factor NF-kappa B (nuclear factor kappa B) and for resistance to tumor necrosis factor (TNF)-induced apoptosis,[96] and is therefore central to many immune, inflammatory and apoptotic pathways.[95]

The mutation is usually a genomic deletion within the NEMO gene and most of the documented mutations cause premature truncation of the protein product of the gene, resulting in absent NF-kappa B activation.[97]

The survival of males with IP can be explained either by somatic mosaicism for the deletational mutation or Klinefelter syndrome, or by the inheritance of less deleterious mutations, which causes diminished rather than absent NF-kappa B activation, and which may also be associated with ectodermal dysplasia or immunodeficiency.[98,99]

Cells expressing the mutated X chromosome are eliminated selectively in females in the perinatal period,[95] resulting in skewed X-inactivation, a hallmark of IP.[100] The precise cause of cell death is not understood, but may relate to a reduced resistance to TNF-induced apoptosis or to NEMO/IKK gamma-deficient cells triggering an inflammatory reaction.[96] The clearing of NEMO-deficient cells results in IP being a self-limited disease, although often leaving permanent and occasionally devastating sequelae.

Clinical features

In affected females, IP causes highly variable abnormalities of the skin, hair, nails, teeth, eyes, breasts, and central nervous system, and is a cause of recurrent miscarriages.

The cutaneous features classically occur in four sequential stages: (1) perinatal inflammatory vesicles; (2) verrucous plaques; (3) a distinctive pattern of hyperpigmentation; and (4) dermal scarring/atrophy and hypopigmentation. It is not necessarily the case that all these stages occur, and they may overlap. In the first stage, small blisters arise in crops, and this usually develops within the first postnatal week, but may take several weeks to become manifest (Fig. 16.19) Bullae may occur anywhere on the body, often orientated along Blaschko's lines, but are frequently seen on the legs in a linear distribution, and usually spare the face. Each crop of blisters settles within about a week, and the vesicular phase does not normally exceed 6 months. The second stage is characterized by warty, short-lived, lesions, which usually appear by 2 months of age and disappear within 3 years. They occur in approximately one-third of patients[101] and predominantly occur in acral regions. They do not always coincide with areas of previous blistering.

The hyperpigmentation that characterizes stage 3, and gives the condition its name, usually appears by 6 months and fades by adolescence. The extent of pigmentation is very variable, from small flecks to extensive hyperpigmentation, which follow Blaschko's lines. A rather bizarre (Chinese figure) pattern may be seen on the trunk. Hyperpigmentation frequently involves the nipples, axillae and groin.

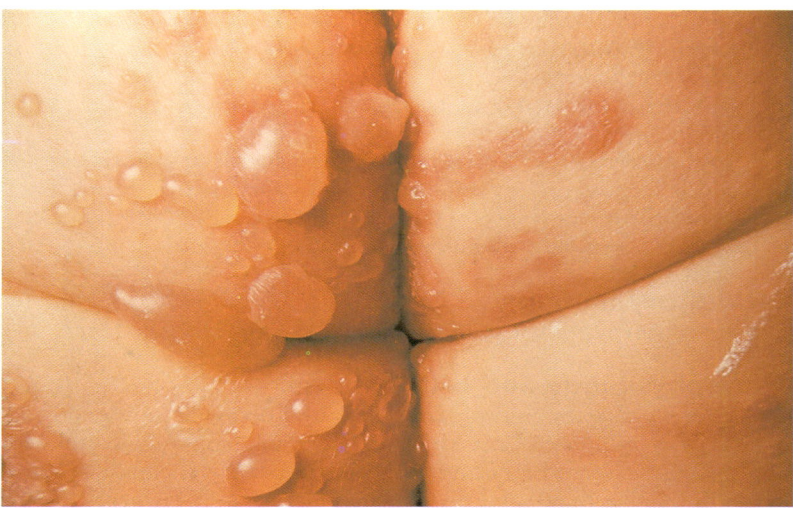

Fig. 16.19   Incontinentia pigmenti: bullae on buttocks.

The fourth stage consists of the development of atrophic or sclerotic, often hypopigmented, streaks, which are usually seen in affected adult females as pale linear lesions, sometimes anhidrotic, and usually on the legs.

The hair is normal, but may be sparse in childhood, and a patch of scarring alopecia may be present from a young age over the vertex of the scalp, usually consequent upon blistering or verrucous lesions at the site. Nail dystrophy is frequent and may affect up to 40% of affected individuals. A wide range of nail abnormalities is seen, from mild ridging to thickened, discolored nail plates; such changes may be transient. Occasionally, painful subungual keratotic tumors develop, usually postpubertally.[102,103]

Dental abnormalities occur in the majority of affected individuals and involve both the deciduous and permanent dentitions. The principal abnormalities are delayed eruption, missing teeth, malformation, and malpositioning of teeth.[104] The incisors may be peg-shaped and there may be retention of the deciduous dentition into adulthood.

Ocular abnormalities occur in approximately 35% of patients, and consist of proliferative vitreoretinopathy, retinal detachment, strabismus, cataracts, microphthalmia, optic nerve atrophy, and iris hyperplasia.[105] Retinal vascular anomalies are the primary cause of severe visual impairment in IP. New vessel proliferation predisposes to bleeding and fibrosis with traction retinal detachment, which may cause blindness. The ocular manifestations are often asymmetrical, with one eye being more affected than the other.[106] These changes occur early in life.[107] and ophthalmological supervision is recommended.

Central nervous system involvement occurs in approximately 25% of cases and is very variable. Seizures are a common symptom, and their onset in early life may be associated with subsequent mental retardation. Small-vessel occlusive central nervous system disease may lead to cerebral infarction, and

94. Sefiani A, Abel L, Heuertz S et al. (1989) The gene for incontinentia pigmenti is assigned to Xq28. **Genomics** 4:427–429.
95. Smahi A, Courtois G, Vabres P et al. (2000) Genomic rearrangement in NEMO impairs NF-kappa B activation and is a cause of incontinentia pigmenti. The International Incontinentia Pigmenti (IP) Consortium. **Nature** 405:466–472.
96. Makris C, Godrey VL, Krahn-Senftleben G et al. (2000) Female mice heterozygous for IKK gamma/NEMO deficiencies develop a dermatopathy similar to the human X-linked disorder incontinentia pigmenti. **Mol Cell** 5:969–979.
97. Aradhya S, Woffendin H, Jakins T et al. (2001) A recurrent deletion in the ubiquitously expressed NEMO (IKK-gamma) gene accounts for the vast majority of incontinentia pigmenti mutations. **Hum Mol Genet** 10:2171–2179.
98. Berlin AL, Paller AS, Chan LS (2002) Incontinentia pigmenti: a review and update on the molecular basis of pathophysiology. **J Am Acad Dermatol** 47:169–187.
99. Kenwick S (2001) Survival of male patients with incontinentia pigmenti carrying a lethal mutation can be explained by somatic mosaicism or Klinefelter syndrome. **Am J Hum Genet** 69:1210–1217.
100. Woffendin H, Jakins T, Jouet M et al. (1999) X-inactivation and marker studies in three families with incontinentia pigmenti: implications for counselling and gene localisation. **Clin Genet** 55:55–60.
101. Landy SJ, Donnai D (1993) Incontinentia pigmenti (Bloch–Sulzberger syndrome). **J Med Genet** 30:53–59.
102. Abimelec P, Rybojad M, Cambiaghi S et al. (1995) Late, painful, subungual hyperkeratosis in incontinentia pigmenti. **Pediatr Dermatol** 12:340–342.
103. Malvehy J, Palou J, Mascaro JM (1998) Painful subungual tumour in incontinentia pigmenti. Response to treatment with etretinate. **Br J Dermatol** 138:554–555.
104. Macey-Dare LV, Goodman JR (1999) Incontinentia pigmenti: seven cases with dental manifestations. **Int J Paediatr Dent** 9:293–297.
105. Nguyen JK, Brady-McCreery KM (2001) Laser photocoagulation in preproliferative retinopathy of incontinentia pigmenti. **J AAPOS** 5:258–259.
106. Holmstrom G, Thoren K (2000) Ocular manifestations of incontinentia pigmenti. **Acta Ophthalmol Scand** 78:348–353.
107. Goldberg MF (1998) Macular vasculopathy and its evolution in incontinentia pigmenti. **Trans Am Ophthalmol Soc** 96:55–65.

the pathology may be similar to the vascular occlusive disease that can occur in the retina.[108] Magnetic resonance imaging may show a variety of central nervous system abnormalities, including hypoplasia of the corpus callosum, enlargement of the lateral ventricles, and periventricular white matter lesions.[109]

Approximately 10% of affected individuals have breast abnormalities,[101] which include aplasia and supernumerary nipples. Occasionally, skeletal abnormalities, usually minor defects of skull and palate, occur and isolated cases of IP have been associated with immunodeficiency.

Laboratory findings
During the vesicular phase of IP, a peripheral eosinophilia is common.

Pathophysiology and histogenesis
Bullae are seen in the midepidermis and are filled with eosinophils; the epidermis is spongiotic and there is a dermal eosinophilic infiltrate. Dyskeratotic cells may be a feature. The verrucous plaques consist of hyperkeratosis, acanthosis, and some degenerate epidermal cells. Pigmented skin in IP is characterized histologically by melanophages within the upper dermis, hence the name of the condition.

Differential diagnosis
The vesicular bullous phase has to be distinguished from other inherited and acquired blistering disorders, but the combination of clinical and histological features is usually distinctive. Neonatal herpes simplex and incontinentia pigmenti have been reported together.[110,111]

Therapeutics and prognosis
There is no specific treatment for IP. Screening for retinal abnormalities in early infancy is recommended. Laser photocoagulation may limit the effects of the ocular vasculopathy.[105,112] Laser treatment for the pigmentation of IP may trigger the reappearance of the vesicular stage.[113] Orthodontic treatment minimizes the cosmetic disability caused by dental anomalies. Systemic corticosteroid therapy for the inflammatory phase of IP is not effective.[114]

PACHYONYCHIA CONGENITA
Introduction
Pachyonychia congenita (PC) is a rare genodermatosis in which combinations of ectodermal defects serve to distinguish two major forms: the Jadassohn–Lewandowsky form (type 1 PC)[115] is characterized by thickened, tented nails, palmoplantar hyperkeratosis, hyperhidrosis, follicular keratoses, leukokeratosis, and a blistering tendency; the Jackson–Lawler form (type 2 PC)[116] is similar, but lacks the oral mucous membrane changes and is associated with natal teeth and steatocystoma multiplex, (see Chapter 12).

Epidemiology
Genetics
PC is usually inherited in an autosomal dominant fashion, but a recessive mode of inheritance has been described.[117]

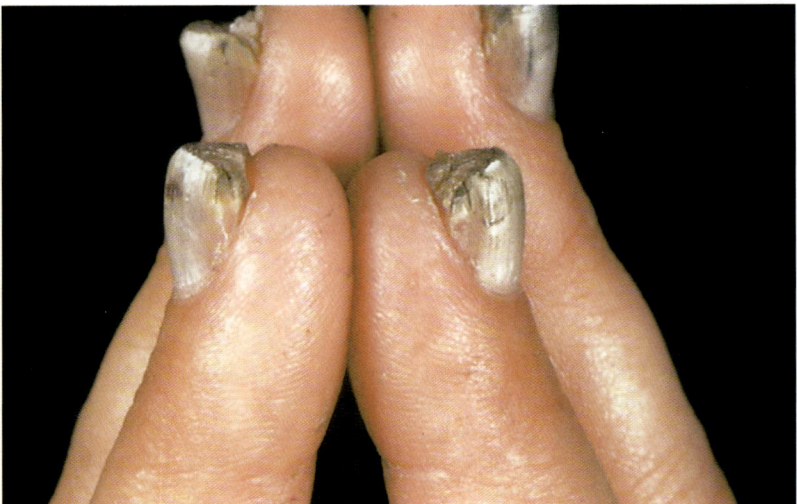

Fig. 16.20 Pachyonychia congenita: tented thickening of fingernails.

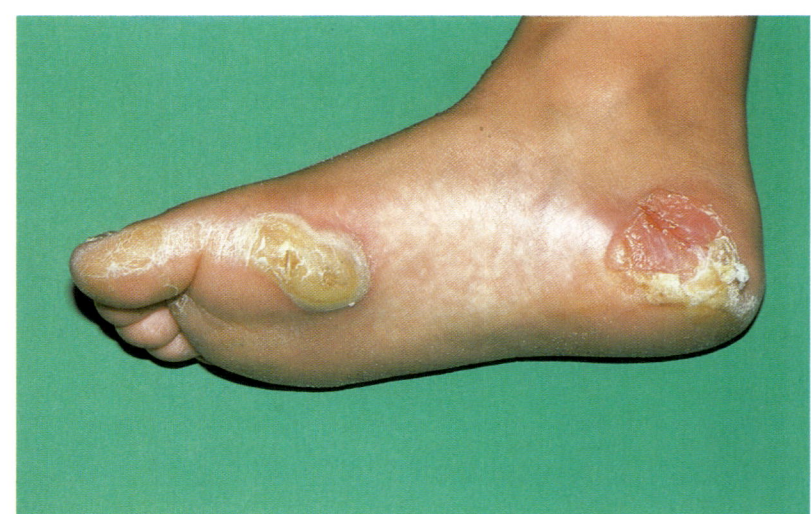

Fig. 16.21 Pachyonychia congenita: plantar bullae.

Clinical features
Patients with the condition usually present in infancy or early childhood with specific nail changes (Fig. 16.20). Palmoplantar bullae in PC, although not a constant or necessarily prominent feature, can be incapacitating (Fig. 16.21). They begin in late childhood or in adulthood. Hyperhidrosis, which is a common feature of PC, increases the blistering. Bullae formation is worse during the summer months.

108. Lee AG, Goldberg MF, Gillard JH et al. (1995) Intracranial assessment of incontinentia pigmenti using magnetic resonance imaging, angiography and spectroscopic imaging. **Arch Pediatr Adolesc Med** 149:573–580.

109. Aydingoz U, Midia M (1998) Central nervous system involvement in incontinentia pigmenti: cranial MRI of two siblings. **Neuroradiology** 40:364–366.

110. Fromer ES, Lynch PJ (2001) Neonatal herpes simplex and incontinentia pigmenti. **Pediatr Dermatol** 18:86–87.

111. Stitt WZ, Scott GA, Caserta M, Goldsmith LA (1998) Coexistence of incontinentia pigmenti and neonatal herpes simplex virus infection. **Pediatr Dermatol** 15:112–115.

112. Shah GK, Summers CG, Walsh AW, Neely KA (1997) Optic nerve neovascularization in incontinentia pigmenti. **Am J Ophthalmol** 124:410–412.

113. Nagase T, Takanashi M, Takada H, Ohmori K (1997) Extensive vesiculobullous eruption following limited ruby laser treatment for incontinentia pigmenti: a case report. **Australas J Dermatol** 38:155–157.

114. Calza AM, Balderrama F, Saurat JH (1994) Systemic steroids for incontinentia pigmenti? **Pediatr Dermatol** 11:83–84.

115. Jadassohn J, Lewandowsky F (1906) Pachyonychia congenita. In: Ikonographia Dermatologica. Berlin: Urban & Schwarzenberg, p. 29.

116. Jackson ADM, Lawler SD (1951) Pachyonychia congenita: report of 6 cases in one family, with note on linkage data. **Ann Eugenics** 16:142–146.

117. Haber RM, Rose TH (1986) Autosomal recessive pachyonychia congenita. **Arch Dermatol** 122:919–923.

Pathophysiology and histogenesis

The Jadassohn–Lewandowsky variant (PC-1) is now known to be the result of mutations in genes coding for keratin 16[118] and keratin 6a.[119] The Jackson–Lawler form (PC-2) is the result of mutations in the keratin 17[118] or keratin 6b[120] genes.

Keratin intermediate filaments constitute the principal stress-bearing cytoskeletal framework within the cytoplasm of epithelial cells, and mutations within the keratin genes may be disruptive to normal filament assembly, which may lead to a weakened keratin molecule less able to withstand stress and strain and thus predisposed to cytolysis.

The bullae in PC arise within the stratum spinosum and are histologically indistinguishable from friction bullae.[121]

Differential diagnosis

The principal differential diagnosis is epidermolysis bullosa simplex, but the wide spectrum of clinical features associated with PC normally allows ready distinction.

Therapeutics and prognosis

The application of 20% aluminum chloride hexahydrate in an alcoholic solution twice daily to the areas of blistering has been shown to reduce the tendency to form bullae.[121] Oral phenytoin has been reported to benefit a patient with PC incapacitated by plantar bullae.[122]

THE PORPHYRIAS

Several of the porphyrias may present in childhood as a bullous eruption including congenital erythropoietic porphyria, porphyria cutanea tarda, and variegate porphyria.[123,124]

Congenital erythropoietic porphyria (Gunther disease) is a rare severe form of porphyria in which the clinical symptoms are initially similar to PCT, with cutaneous hyperfragility, marked photosensitivity and hypertrichosis. Bullae heal with severe scarring which leads to mutilation and scleroderma-like changes. The teeth fluoresce under ultraviolet light. Erythropoietic protoporphyria usually presents at about 2 years of age. Patients develop a severe erythema in a photosensitive distribution which is extremely painful and may result in bullae.

Porphyria cutanea tarda (PCT) may present in childhood. This is a mechanobullous disorder manifesting as hyperfragility of the skin, in which minor trauma results in erosions or blisters that are often hemorrhagic. The dorsa of the hands are usually affected, as is the face and occasionally elsewhere on the limbs. The blisters heal with scarring and milia formation. Hypertrichosis, especially on the forehead, is a feature of familial PCT occurring in 50% of patients. Analysis of plasma, urinary and faecal porphyrins establishes the diagnosis, although a bedside test is the fluorescence under ultraviolet light of a urine specimen. Similar cutaneous manifestations occur in variegate porphyria and hereditary coproporphyria (see Chap. 7).

AUTOIMMUNE VESICULOBULLOUS DISEASE

In children, it is frequently difficult to accurately distinguish between the subepidermal autoimmune blistering disorders on the basis of their clinical, histological, and immunopathological features. The application of sophisticated laboratory techniques such as immunoblotting and immunoelectron microscopy in the subepidermal blistering disorders has enabled the targeted autoantigens to be characterized, but has also demonstrated that there is a great antigenic heterogeneity in what were previously considered to be clearly defined conditions. The boundaries between these diseases are becoming more blurred as knowledge about the target antigens increases.

Immunoblotting and immunoelectron microscopy are not widely available as routine procedures, and information about the plane of blistering can be obtained using salt-split normal human skin as the substrate in the indirect immunofluorescence examination of the patient's serum. Normal skin is cleaved within the lamina lucida of the epidermal basement membrane by 1M NaCl solution, and thus if the circulating antibody involves the epidermal side (roof) of salt-split skin it suggests that the target antigen is either within the upper part of the lamina lucida or associated with the cell membrane or intracytoplasmic stuctures of the basal keratinocyte. If the circulating antibody localizes to the dermal side (floor) of the salt-split skin, the target antigen is beneath the lamina lucida, either within the lamina densa or in the sublamina densa zone. As an example, this simple technique can usually distinguish bullous pemphigoid from epidermolysis bullosa acquisita,[125] although dermal binding of circulating antibody does occasionally occur in bullous pemphigoid.[126] Suction-induced blisters are also characterized by a cleavage plane within the lamina lucida and can be used as the substrate in the same way as salt-split skin.

Another simple technique to establish the cleavage plane in a blistering disorder is to map the dermo–epidermal junction with an antibody to type IV collagen, which is located in the lamina densa of the epidermal basement membrane. In bullous pemphigoid, the blister forms in the lamina lucida and thus type IV collagen will localize to the base of a natural blister, whereas in epidermolysis bullosa acquisita, where the natural blister arises within the sublamina densa zone, type IV collagen antibody will be visualized in the blister roof.[127] Type IV collagen staining can be done on wax-embedded material using a commercially available antibody.

All the autoimmune blistering disorders seen in adults also occur in children, but are very much rarer. Accurate incidence and prevalence data are not available and in the majority the genetic basis for these conditions has yet to be established.

CHRONIC BULLOUS DISEASE OF CHILDHOOD
Introduction and historical note

Chronic bullous disease of childhood (CBDC) is also known as linear IgA disease of childhood; early synonyms included juvenile dermatitis herpetiformis and juvenile pemphigoid. CBDC is an acquired autoimmune subepidermal blistering disorder characterized by the deposition of a linear band of IgA along the dermal–epidermal junction, involving both skin and, less commonly, mucous membranes.

The molecular basis of CBDC has not been clearly defined and it may well represent a heterogeneous disorder. Historically, linear IgA disease (of adults) has been differentiated from CBDC although they probably represent the same entity.[128]

Bowen[129] in 1901 is generally credited with reporting the first cases of CBDC but it was not until immunohistochemistry became a routine diagnostic procedure that CBDC became defined by the presence of a strong

118. McLean WHI, Rugg EL, Lunny DP et al. (1995) Keratin 16 and keratin 17 mutations cause pachyonychia congenita. **Nat Genet** 9:273–276.
119. Bowden PE, Haley JL, Kansky A et al. (1995) Mutation of a type II keratin gene (*K6a*) in pachyonychia congenita. **Nat Genet** 10:363–365.
120. Smith FJ, Jonkman MF, van Goor H et al. (1998) A mutation in human keratin K6b produces a phenocopy of the K17 disorder pachyonychia congenita type 2. **Hum Mol Genet** 7:1143–1148.
121. Tidman MJ, Wells RS (1988) Control of plantar blisters in pachyonychia congenita with topical aluminium chloride. **Br J Dermatol** 118:451–452.
122. Blank H (1982) Treatment of pachyonychia congenita with phenytoin. **Br J Dermatol** 106:123.
123. Meola T, Lim HW (1993) The porphyrias. **Dermatol Clin** 11:583–596.
124. Bickers DR, Pathak MA, Lim HW (1999) The porphyrias. In: Dermatology in General Medicine, 5th edn, Freedberg IM, Eisen AZ, Wolff K et al. eds. New York, McGraw-Hill, pp. 1766–1803.

125. Lacour JP, Bernard P, Rostain G et al. (1995) Childhood acquired epidermolysis bullosa. **Pediatr Dermatol** 12:16–20.
126. Wakelin SH, Allen J, Wojnarowska F (1995) Childhood bullous pemphigoid – report of a case with dermal fluorescence on salt-split skin. **Br J Dermatol** 133:615–618.
127. Nemeth AJ, Klein AD, Gould EW, Schachner LA (1991) Childhood bullous pemphigoid. Clinical and immunologic features, treatment, and prognosis. **Arch Dermatol** 127:378–386.
128. Collier PM, Wojnarowska F, Welsh K et al. (1999) Adult linear IgA disease and chronic bullous disease of childhood: the association with human lymphocyte antigens Cw7, B8, DR3 and tumour necrosis factor influences disease expression. **Br J Dermatol** 141:867–875.
129. Bowen J (1901) Five cases of bullous dermatitis in children following vaccination. **Br J Dermatol** 8:392–394.

linear band of IgA at the epidermal basement membrane, distinguishing it from dermatitis herpetiformis and bullous pemphigoid in childhood.[129–133] CBDC occurs in all ethnic groups and may be more common in developing countries. The annual incidence in the United Kingdom has been estimated at 1 in 500 000 children.[134]

Clinical features

CBDC usually presents in children less than 5 years of age, although it can occur at any time during childhood. There may be a preceding prodromal illness such as upper respiratory tract, urinary tract, or viral infections and there is often a history of preceding treatment with antibiotics or non-steroidal anti–inflammatory agents. The relevance of such prodromal illness remains to be established. Vaccinations have also been implicated as a trigger factor.

There is usually an abrupt onset of tense vesicles or bullae, which may be associated with constitutional symptoms such as fever or anorexia. The lesions often arise on normal-looking skin, but occasionally occur on urticated plaques. The severity of CBDC is variable, and the bullae may be localized or widespread. They can occur in any body region, although the genitalia and perioral regions are commonly involved. In the early stages of the condition, new lesions may arise around the margins of older ones, giving an appearance that has been described as the "string of pearls" rosettes or "cluster of jewels" sign (Fig. 16.22). The central clearing and peripheral blistering may give rise to polycyclic lesions. Pruritus when present is usually not intense, unlike that associated with dermatitis herpetiformis and pemphigoid. Resolved bullae generally do not leave scars but may cause hyper- or hypopigmentation, especially in dark-skinned individuals. Occasionally the lesions are large and hemorrhagic.

Mucous membrane involvement is a common but not invariable feature of CBDC and such involvement may lead to scarring. The oral mucous membranes are most commonly involved with erosions rather than bullae. Conjunctival involvement affects approximately 65% of children[133] causing redness and a gritty discomfort of the eyes, and subsequent conjunctival scarring may lead to entropion and corneal damage. The genital and nasal mucous membranes may also rarely be involved.

Pathophysiology and histogenesis

CBDC is the result of a humoral response to a normal constituent of the epidermal basement membrane zone. However, although the target antigen is known to be present in all human stratified squamous epithelia, it has not yet been defined with certainty. Salt-split skin studies of antibody distribution have been inconclusive and suggest that the ultrastructural localization of the target antigen may be in both the lamina lucida and sublamina densa zones. Immunoelectron microscopy also suggests binding sites for the IgA antibody within the lamina lucida and beneath the lamina densa. Immunoblotting studies have suggested that the IgA autoantibodies appear to recognize different target antigens, most frequently proteins with molecular weights of 97kDa[135] and 285kDa,[136] which are present on the epidermal side of salt-split skin. The 97kDa protein most likely represents a processed form of a recently described 120kDa anchoring filament-associated protein which may correspond to a portion of the extracellular domain of *BP180* or *LAD1*. Some patients have had antibodies against a 290kDa protein corresponding to type VII collagen. These studies show that CBDC is heterogeneous.

Histological examination of fresh lesions is not diagnostic and does not distinguish CBDC from pemphigoid, dermatitis herpetiformis, or EB acquisita. The bullae are subepidermal and associated with a neutrophil or eosinophil-rich inflammatory infiltrate.

The diagnosis of CBDC relies on the immunohistochemical demonstration of a linear band of IgA along the dermal–epidermal junction. This may or may not be associated with weaker bands of IgG, IgM or C3. In the very early stages of the disease, false–negative immunohistochemical results can be obtained and the test may need to be repeated. Immunohistochemical examination requires only a small biopsy of uninvolved, preferably perilesional skin. There may be a regional variation in the intensity of antibody deposition at the dermal–epidermal junction and the forearm is best avoided.[137] A circulating IgA antibody is present in approximately 80% of children with

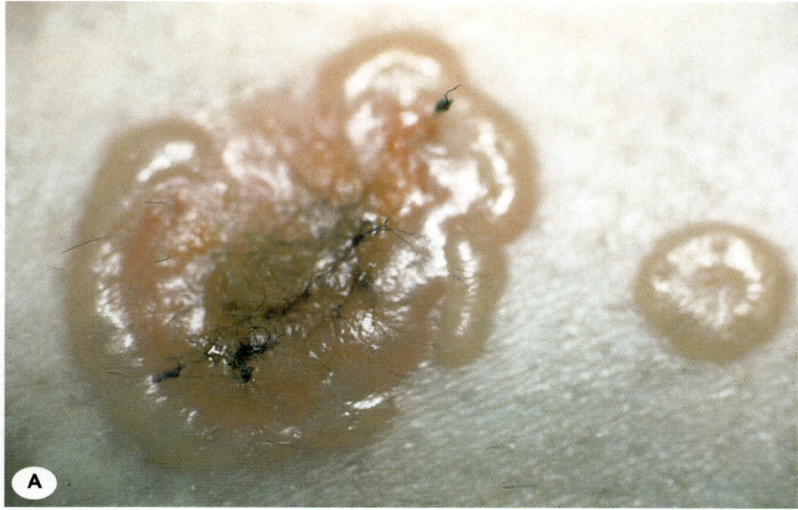
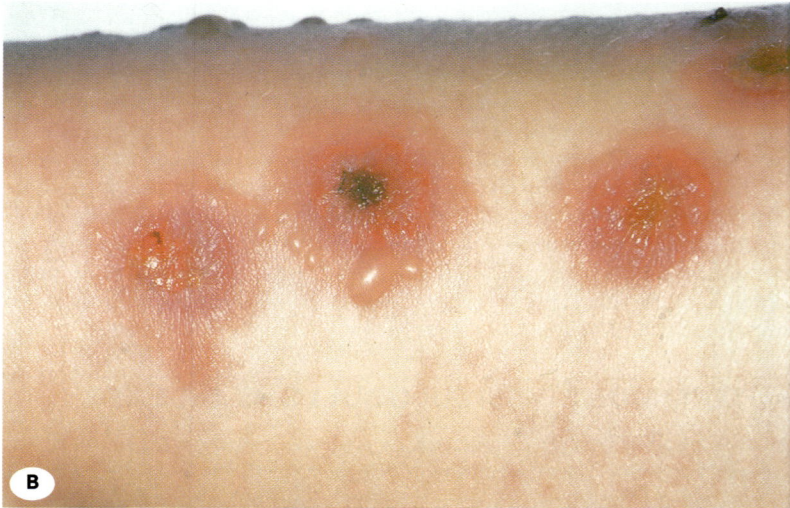

Fig. 16.22   Chronic bullous disease of childhood: new bullae arising around the margins of older lesions.

130. Jablonska S, Chorzelski T, Beutner E, Blaszczyk M (1971) Juvenile dermatitis herpetiformis in the light of immunofluorescence studies. **Br J Dermatol** 85:307–313.
131. Prystowsky S, Gilliam J (1976) Benign chronic bullous disease of childhood. **Arch Dermatol** 112:837–838.
132. Esterly N, Furey N, Kirschner B et al. (1977) Chronic bullous dermatosis of childhood. **Arch Dermatol** 113:42–46.
133. Van der Meer JB, Remme JJ, Nefkens MJ, Baart de la Faille-Kuyper EH (1977) IgA antibasement membrane antibodies in a boy with pemphigoid. **Arch Dermatol** 113:1462.
134. Collier PM, Wojnarowska F (2000) Chronic bullous disease of childhood. In: Textbook of Pediatric Dermatology, Harper J, Oranje A, Prose N, eds. Oxford: Blackwell Scientific, pp. 711–723.

135. Wojnarowska F, Whitehead P, Leigh IM et al. (1991) Identification of the target antigen in chronic bullous disease of childhood and linear IgA disease of adults. **Br J Dermatol** 124:157–162.
136. Zone J, Taylor T, Kadunce D, Meyer L (1990) Identification of the cutaneous basement membrane zone antigen and isolation of antibody in linear immunoglobulin A bullous dermatosis. **J Clin Invest** 85:812–820.
137. Collier PM, Wojnarowska F, Millard PR (1992) Variation in the deposition of the antibodies at different anatomical sites in linear IgA disease of adults and chronic bullous disease of childhood. **Br J Dermatol** 127:482–484.

CBDC, but is often of low titer and not sufficiently sensitive to be useful in monitoring disease activity.

In contrast to dermatitis herpetiformis, CBDC is not associated with gluten-sensitive enteropathy. Although there are anecdotal reports of CBDC and celiac disease coexisting, large series have not confirmed an association.[134]

There may be a genetic susceptibility to CBDC with an increased incidence of HLA-B8, HLA-DR3 and HLA-DQW2.

Differential diagnosis

In the early stages of the disease, localized blistering may be confused with herpes simplex or bullous impetigo, and more generalized blistering may mimic erythema multiforme or Stevens–Johnson syndrome. Without recourse to immunohistochemistry, distinction from bullous pemphigoid and dermatitis herpetiformis may not be possible. When the condition is localized to the genital region, a misdiagnosis of sexual abuse may be made.[138]

Therapy and prognosis

The standard treatments for CBDC, including dapsone, prednisolone, sulfamethoxy pyridazine, and sulfapyridine, all have the potential for significant side effects, and these have to be weighed against the clinical severity of the condition and the fact that natural remission can be expected in the majority of patients within 5 years of onset. A mild blistering tendency may not require systemic treatment, and the judicious short-term application of a moderately potent or potent topical corticosteroid may suffice. If systemic therapy proves necessary, it may be required for only a brief time, although protracted treatment may be required. A gluten-free diet confers no clinical benefit in CBDC.

Dapsone is the most commonly used systemic medication, either as a single agent or in combination with prednisolone. An appropriate starting dose for dapsone is 1mg/kg body weight per day, and this can be increased depending on the response. In our experience, dapsone is well tolerated. It is necessary to monitor the full blood count and reticulocytes on a weekly basis for at least 1 month in case of hemolysis and agranulocytosis, and liver function should also be monitored, as dapsone may cause hepatitis. Thereafter, the frequency of blood tests can gradually be reduced once the condition has been stabilized. It is prudent to screen for glucose-6-phosphate-dehydrogenase deficiency before treatment is started, especially in those racial groups particularly at risk. Dapsone can also cause methemoglobinemia, detectable clinically by blue discoloration of lips and tongue, and the introduction of cimetidine, an inhibitor of the cytochrome P450 family of enzymes, may minimize this. Once blistering is in remission, the dosage of dapsone can gradually be reduced; a convenient way of doing this is to give it on alternate days or less frequently.

If dapsone in acceptable dosage does not control the blistering in CBDC, prednisolone should be introduced, provided there are no contraindications, in a dose of 1mg/kg body weight per day, and the dosage adjusted depending on clinical response. Once blistering is controlled, it is usually possible to taper the dosage of prednisolone and to stop it relatively quickly.

In difficult cases, it may be reasonable to consider the use of sulfapyridine or sulfamethoxy pyridazine. These drugs are associated with potentially serious side effects including bone marrow suppression and, in some countries, are only available on a named patient basis.

There have been anecdotal reports of successful treatment of CBDC with colchicine, azathioprine and cyclosporin, and there has been recent interest in the response of CBDC to antimicrobial agents. Both dicloxacillin[139,140] and erythromycin[141] have been reported to be effective.

Although the majority of cases of CBDC go into natural remission within 5 years of onset, the condition may progress through puberty and into adulthood. There does not appear to be a correlation between severity of blistering and chronicity, and there are no usefully predictive clinical parameters. HLA-B8 positivity may be associated with a more favorable outcome and less risk of ocular disease.[142] Ophthalmic monitoring throughout childhood and beyond is advisable. Possession of the TNF-2 allele is associated with longer disease duration[128] but other major histocompatibility complex associations do not appear to affect the prognosis.

BULLOUS PEMPHIGOID

Introduction

Bullous pemphigoid (BP) is usually a condition of the elderly, but it does, rarely, occur in children, and the major clinical, histopathologic, and immunologic features of childhood BP are the same as in the adult disease. The autoantibodies that occur in childhood BP target the same antigenic epitopes as in the adult condition.[143] BP has been recorded as early as the first few months of postnatal life, but transplacental transmission has not been recorded. The gender incidence is equal.

There have been reports of the onset of childhood BP occurring shortly after vaccination,[144–146] but this may be a chance association. BP in childhood has also been recorded after a second organ transplantation,[147] and in association with chronic renal allograft rejection.[148]

Clinical features

The clinical features of childhood BP are characterized by tense, sometimes hemorrhagic bullae, arising either on normal-appearing or inflamed skin. Urticarial plaques are common, and the inflammation may be in annular or polycyclic patterns. (Fig. 16.23A) The sites of blister predilection are the flexural areas, including the inner thighs, the flexural aspects of the forearms, axillae, the lower abdomen, and groin. Pruritus is variable and lesions tend to heal without scarring or milia formation. There are several subtle distinguishing clinical features from the adult disease. In childhood BP, especially when it involves young children, there is often a marked involvement of the palmar and plantar surfaces (Fig. 16.23B).[149] Facial involvement is more common in childhood BP, and can sometimes be mistaken for impetigo. Involvement of the mucous membranes occurs more frequently in children than in adults, particularly the oral (Fig. 16.23C) and ocular mucous membranes.

138. Coleman H, Shrubb VA (1997) Chronic bullous disease of childhood – another cause for potential misdiagnosis of sexual abuse? Br J Gen Pract 47:507–508.
139. Siegfried EC, Sirawan S (1998) Chronic bullous disease of childhood: successful treatment with dicloxacillin. J Am Acad Dermatol 39:797–800.
140. Skinner RB, Rotondo CK, Schneider MA et al. (1995) Treatment of chronic bullous dermatosis of childhood with oral dicloxacillin. Pediatr Dermatol 12:65–66.
141. Powell J, Kirtschig G, Allen J et al. (2001) Mixed immunobullous disease of childhood: a good response to antimicrobials. Br J Dermatol 144:769–774.
142. Wojnarowska F (1990) Linear IgA disease of adults. In: Management of Blistering Diseases, Wojnarowska F, Briggaman RA, eds. London: Chapman & Hall Medical, pp. 105–118.
143. Chimanovitch I, Hamm H, Georgi M et al. (2000) Bullous pemphigoid of childhood: autoantibodies target the same epitopes within the NC16A domain of BP 180 as autoantibodies in bullous pemphigoid of adulthood. Arch Dermatol 136:527–532.
144. Cambazard F, Thivolet J, Mironneau P (1994) Bullous pemphigoid in a 4-month-old boy. Br J Dermatol 131:449–451.
145. Oranje AP, Vuzevski VD, van Joost T et al. (1991) Bullous pemphigoid in children. Report of three cases with special emphasis on therapy. Int J Dermatol 30:339–342.
146. Baykal C, Okan G, Sarica R (2001) Childhood bullous pemphigoid developed after the first vaccination. J Am Acad Dermatol 44:348–350.
147. Morelli JG, Weston WL (1999) Childhood immunobullous disease following a second organ transplant. Pediatr Dermatol 16:205–207.
148. Yamazaki S, Yokozeki H, Katayama I et al. (1998) Childhood bullous pemphigoid associated with chronic renal allograft rejection. Br J Dermatol 138:547–548.
149. Trueb RM, Didierjean L, Fellas A et al. (1999) Childhood bullous pemphigoid: report of a case with characterization of the targeted antigens. J Am Acad Dermatol 40:338–344.

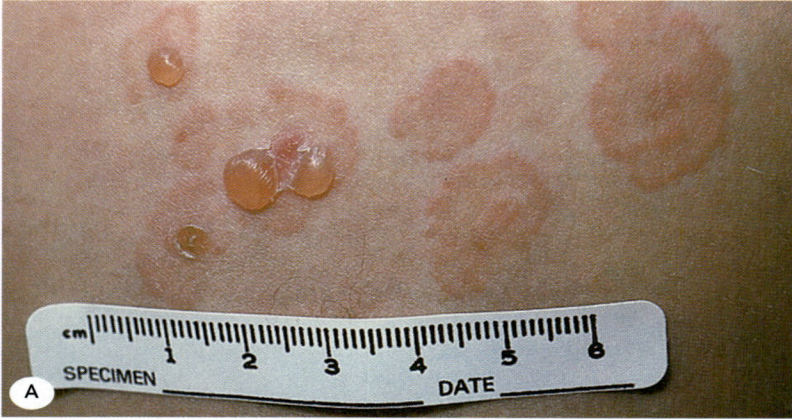

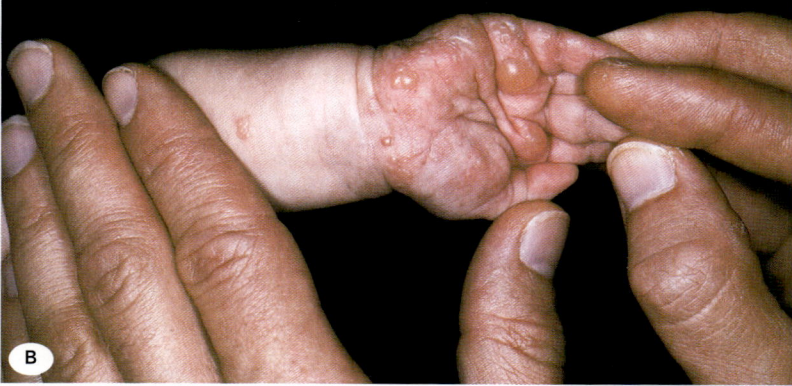

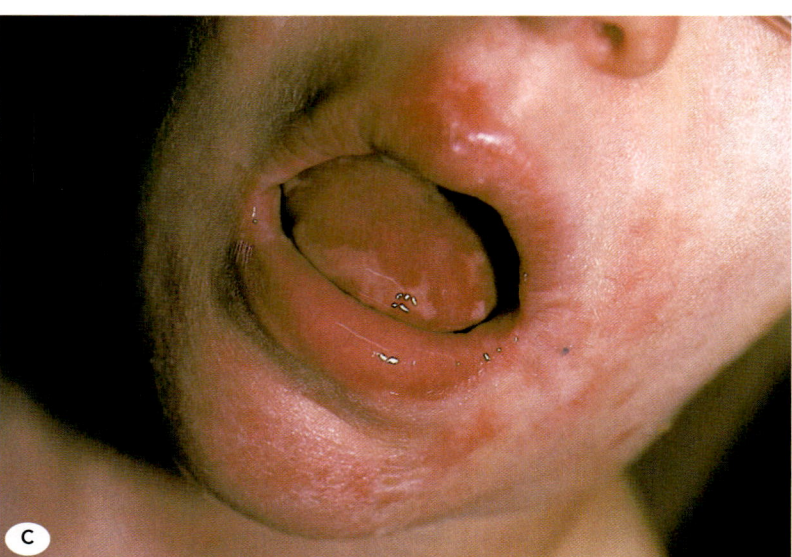

Fig. 16.23 **Bullous pemphigoid.** (A) Polycyclic plaques. (B) Palmar bullae in an infant. (C) Mouth and lip involvement with BP.

Localized vulval pemphigoid is a morphological variant of bullous pemphigoid[150–152] with the target antigens being either BP180 or BP230. It is characterized by localization to the vulval region with recurrent, often hemorrhagic, bullae and painful erosions. Pruritus may be a feature. Painful micturition is usual. Lesions heal without scarring or milia formation, and no other mucous membranes are involved.

Pathophysiology and histogenesis

The targets of the autoantibodies in BP are 2 hemidesmosome-associated proteins, BP230 and/or BP180. BP230 (bullous pemphigoid antigen 1) is an intracellular protein associated with the hemidesmosome attachment plaques. BP180 (bullous pemphigoid antigen 2, Type XVII collagen) is a transmembrane glycoprotein extending from the hemidesmosome into the lamina lucida in association with anchoring filaments.

The histology of bullous pemphigoid is that of a subepidermal blister with an intact overlying epidermis and no necrosis. The inflammatory infiltrate is comprised mainly of eosinophils, with some neutrophils and lymphocytes. Direct immunofluorescence examination usually reveals a linear deposition of IgG and C3, and less frequently IgM and IgA[153] may be found. Indirect immunofluorescence usually, but not always, demonstrates a circulating antibody which is directed against the epidermal side of salt-split normal human skin. However, occasionally dermal binding may be observed, despite Western immunoblotting revealing an epidermal location for the target antigens.[154] The titer of circulating antibody in bullous pemphigoid does not necessarily reflect the disease activity. Antigen mapping with Type IV collagen stains the base of natural blisters, confirming a cleavage plane within

the lamina lucida. Immunoblotting in bullous pemphigoid shows autoantibodies directed against BP230 and/or BP180. Immunoelectron microscopy reveals deposition of autoantibody in the upper portion of the lamina lucida, closely related to the intracellular attachment plaques of the hemidesmosomes.

Differential diagnosis

In the differential diagnosis, epidermolysis bullosa acquisita, chronic bullous disease of childhood, and bullous systemic lupus erythematosus can be difficult to distinguish without resorting to immunoblotting studies. Sexual abuse has to be considered in the localized vulval form, as does bullous lichen sclerosus, bullous impetigo, herpes simplex infection, and a bullous fixed drug eruption.

Therapy and prognosis

The prognosis of childhood BP is good, and most reported cases have had a disease duration of 1 year or less, although the course may occasionally be more protracted. The initial treatment of choice has traditionally been systemic corticosteroids, starting with a dose of prednisolone of 1–2mg/kg/day.[146] Dapsone or sulfapyridine may be used as adjunctive therapy, and a combination of erythromycin and nicotinamide has been suggested as a safe alternative to oral steroids.[154] Increasingly, potent topical corticosteroids are being used in the treatment of adult bullous pemphigoid.[155] and it remains to be seen whether this is as effective in childhood BP. Systemic therapy for localized vulval pemphigoid, with prednisolone or sulfapyridine, may be required, but topical corticosteroid therapy may suffice.[156]

150. Schumann H, Amann U, Tasanen K et al. (1999) A child with localized vulval pemphigoid and IgG autoantibodies targeting the C-terminus of collagen XVII/BP 180. **Br J Dermatol** 140:1133–1138.
151. Saad RW, Domloge-Hultsch N, Yancey KB et al. (1992) Childhood localized vulvar pemphigoid is a true variant of bullous pemphigoid. **Arch Dermatol** 128:807–810.
152. Farrell AM, Kirtschig G, Dalziel KL et al. (1999) Childhood vulval pemphigoid: a clinical and immunopathological study of five patients. **Br J Dermatol** 140:308–312.

153. Arechalde A, Braun RP, Calza AM et al. (1999) Childhood bullous pemphigoid associated with IgA antibodies against BP180 or BP230 antigens. **Br J Dermatol** 140:112–118.
154. Wakelin SH, Allen J, Wojnarowska F (1995) Childhood bullous pemphigoid – report of a case with dermal fluorescence on salt-split skin. **Br J Dermatol** 133:615–618.
155. Joly P, Roujeau J-C, Benichou J et al. (2002) A comparison of oral and topical corticosteroids in patients with bullous pemphigoid. **N Engl J Med** 346:321–327.
156. Guenther LC, Shum D (1990) Localized childhood vulval pemphigoid. **J Am Acad Dermatol** 22:762–764.

MUCOUS MEMBRANE PEMPHIGOID

Introduction

Mucous membrane pemphigoid (MMP), also known as benign cicatricial pemphigoid, is an extremely rare condition in childhood. Clinically, histologically, and immunopathologically, there is an overlap with other autoimmune subepidermal blistering disorders, such as epidermolysis bullosa acquisita and chronic bullous disease of childhood; it has been suggested that cicatricial pemphigoid in childhood may be an unusual and more severe variant of chronic bullous disease of childhood.[157]

Clinical features

MMP occurs at any time in childhood and it may be associated with a generalized eruption involving the face, trunk and limbs, characterized by urticarial or annular, polycyclic or target-like, lesions. The dominant clinical feature is the involvement of mucous membranes. Involvement of the conjunctival mucous membranes may proceed to symblepharon, entropion, and corneal scarring, which may result in blindness. The oral laryngeal, nasal, and genital mucous membranes may also be involved, and scarring is an important feature. MMP may be confined to the oral cavity (oral pemphigoid). It may present in children as a desquamative gingivitis.[158,159] Because of its rarity in childhood, diagnosis may be delayed.[160]

Pathophysiology and histogenesis

MMP is heterogeneous with respect to its target antigens; it is most commonly associated with autoantibodies to BP180,[161] and less frequently to laminin 5 or type VII collagen. A few patients have been described with autoantibodies to the beta 4 subunit of the $\alpha6\beta4$ integrin.[162] The usual target antigen in MMP is BP180, a transmembrane hemidesmosomal glycoprotein. Epitopes on both the extra- and intracellular domains of BP180 are targeted by either IgG or IgA antibodies.

Direct immunofluorescence examination usually reveals IgA and/or IgG deposited in a linear fashion at the dermal–epidermal junction. Circulating antibodies against epithelial basement membrane constituents are detected in approximately 50% of MMP sera by indirect immunofluorescence. Immunoelectron microscopy reveals immunoreactants over the lower part of the lamina lucida or on the lamina densa.

Therapy and prognosis

MMP in childhood may clear completely, but both the cutaneous and mucous membrane involvement may persist and extend into adulthood.

For those rare cases recorded, the usual treatment has consisted of either systemic corticosteroids, dapsone, or sulfapyridine.[157] Topical corticosteroids may give symptomatic relief. Ophthalmological monitoring is mandatory when the conjunctival mucous membranes are involved.

HERPES (PEMPHIGOID) GESTATIONIS

Introduction

Herpes gestationis (HG) is a rare autoimmune disease that develops during pregnancy or in the immediate postpartum period. Its incidence has been estimated at 1:50 000 pregnancies, and cutaneous involvement of the baby on delivery is uncommon, with a reported incidence of 2–10% of neonates at risk.[163,164]

Clinical features

Most of the reported babies with HG have had limited cutaneous involvement, but occasionally the eruption may be widespread. It is characterized by intensely pruritic urticarial plaques with tense bullae. The eruption in the neonate is self-limiting and resolves spontaneously during the weeks after birth, and is rarely evident after 3 months. The gender incidence is equal.

Pathophysiology and histogenesis

HG is the consequence of the formation of an avidly complement-binding autoantibody that usually targets BP180, and occasionally BP230.[165] This IgG-class antibody readily crosses the placenta, and the development of HG in the neonate is due to the transplacental passive transfer of antibody.

The histological features of the eruption are those of subepidermal edema and subepidermal blistering, associated with a moderate dermal infiltrate, composed largely of eosinophils. Direct immunofluorescence examination of perilesional skin usually demonstrates a linear deposition of C3 along the dermal–epidermal basement membrane, with a linear deposition of IgG in 75% of cases. Indirect immunofluorescence examination may reveal a circulating IgG antibody which localizes to the epidermal side of salt-split skin.

Therapy and prognosis

Specific treatment is not normally necessary, although a moderately potent topical corticosteroid may be useful for those infants in whom there is a significant inflammatory element.

The prognosis for infants with cutaneous involvement is not different from that for children without cutaneous lesions born to mothers with HG; they may be small for their gestational age, and there may be a tendency to prematurity. Lesions usually disappear spontaneously in a matter of days.

The possibility of adrenal insufficiency should be considered in neonates born to mothers affected with HG who have received systemic corticosteroids for a prolonged period.

EPIDERMOLYSIS BULLOSA ACQUISITA

Introduction

Epidermolysis bullosa acquisita (EBA) is a chronic subepidermal immunobullous disorder that is rare in adults and particularly rare in childhood. There is no gender or racial predilection to childhood EBA but, like most of the immunobullous disorders, there is probably a genetic susceptibility, and it is known that there is an increased incidence of HLA-DR2 in patients with EBA. The clinical features are variable,[166] and a clinical distinction from bullous pemphigoid and chronic bullous disease of childhood is not usually possible.

Clinical features

EBA may present at any age in childhood, from 3 months onwards, and it can be very variable in its presentation.[167] There are three clinical phenotypes. The first is the classic noninflammatory mechanobullous type presenting with

157. Wojnarowska F, Marsden RA, Bhogal B, Black MM (1988) Chronic bullous disease of childhood, childhood cicatricial pemphigoid, and linear IgA disease of adults. A comparative study demonstrating clinical and immunopathologic overlap. J Am Acad Dermatol 19:792–805.
158. Roche C, Field EA (1997) Benign mucous membrane pemphigoid presenting as desquamative gingivitis in a 14-year-old child. Int J Paediatr Dent 7:31–34.
159. Sklavounou A, Laskaris G (1990) Childhood cicatricial pemphigoid with exclusive gingival involvement. Int J Oral Maxillofac Surg 19:197–199.
160. Cheng YS, Rees TD, Wright JM, Plemons JM (2001) Childhood oral pemphigoid: a case report and review of the literature. J Oral Pathol Med 30:372–377.
161. Schmidt E, Skrobek C, Kromminga A et al. (2001) Cicatricial pemphigoid: IgA and IgG autoantibodies target epitopes on both intra- and extracellular domains of bullous pemphigoid antigen 180. Br J Dermatol 145:778–783.
162. Leverkus M, Bhol K, Hirako Y et al. (2001) Cicatricial pemphigoid with circulating autoantibodies to beta 4 integrin, bullous pemphigoid 180 and bullous pemphigoid 230. Br J Dermatol 145:998–1004.

163. Chen SH, Chopra K, Evans TY et al. (1999) Herpes gestationis in a mother and child. J Am Acad Dermatol 40:847–849.
164. Jenkins RE, Hern S, Black MM (1999) Clinical features and management of 87 patients with pemphigoid gestationis. Clin Exp Dermatol 24:255–259.
165. Ghohestani R, Nicolas JF, Kanitakis J et al. (1996) l'emphigoid gestationis with autoantibodies exclusively directed to the 230-kDa bullous pemphigoid antigen (BP230Ag). Br J Dermatol 134:603–604.
166. Arpey CJ, Elewski BE, Moritz DK, Gammon WR (1991) Childhood epidermolysis bullosa acquisita. Report of three cases and review of the literature. J Am Acad Dermatol 24:706–714.
167. Edwards S, Wakelin SH, Wojnarowska F et al. (1998) Bullous pemphigoid and epidermolysis bullosa acquisita: presentation, prognosis, and immunopathology in 11 children. Pediatr Dermatol 15:184–190.

skin fragility, blisters and erosions at sites of trauma, particularly over acral bony prominences; these heal to leave milia and atrophic scars which, especially in dark-skinned individuals, may be hypo- or hyperpigmented (Fig. 16.24). Occasionally the nails are damaged and may become dystrophic or are shed. The second pattern is an inflammatory type of EBA which mimics other inflammatory bullous disorders, such as bullous pemphigoid and chronic bullous disease of childhood. Pruritic tense bullae, which may become haemorrhagic, arise on normal, erythematous or urticarial skin. These lesions form erosions and crusts, sometimes leaving pigmentary change, but usually without scarring. Involvement of the mucous membranes is frequent and at times may be severe. The oral, genital, conjunctival, and urethral mucous membranes may all be involved. This type may closely mimic chronic bullous disease of childhood when the perioral, periorbital and genital regions develop an annular eruption.[168,169] The third clinical variant is a type resembling cicatricial pemphigoid, defined by predominantly mucous membrane involvement and a pronounced tendency to scarring. The involvement of oral, conjunctival, nasal, esophageal, laryngeal, and genital mucous membranes in children may lead to a variety of complications including malnutrition, symblepharon of the conjunctivae which may progress to blindness,[170] and stenosis of the esophagus, urethra or genital tract. In its clinical course, EBA may progress from a noninflammatory mechanobullous to an inflammatory pattern.

In adults, EBA is associated with a variety of internal disorders, including inflammatory bowel disease, diabetes mellitus, lymphomas, and autoimmune disorders such as rheumatoid arthritis, systemic lupus erythematosus, and thyroiditis. In children such associations have not been recorded.

Pathophysiology and histogenesis

EBA is characterized by the formation of autoantibodies to type VII collagen, the morphological expression of which is the anchoring fibrils in the sublamina densa region of the epidermal basement membrane. Tissue-bound antibody is assumed to activate the complement system which results in the recruitment of inflammatory cells and subsequent separation of the epidermis from the dermis with the cleavage plane immediately beneath the lamina densa of the dermal–epidermal junction. Western immunoblotting of sera from patients with EBA shows the circulating antibody to react with a 290kDa protein (the "EBA antigen") and its breakdown product of 145kDa in a dermal extract of normal human skin.

Histological examination of a fresh lesion reveals a subepidermal bulla with a predominantly neutrophilic inflammatory infiltrate, admixed with eosinophils. Direct immunofluorescence examination of perilesional skin typically reveals a linear deposition of IgG and C3 along the basement membrane zone, and occasionally there is also weak staining for IgA and IgM. Very occasionally, IgA may be the predominant immunoreactant.[170] Indirect immunofluorescence examination is usually positive in EBA and the circulating antibody labels the dermal side of the bulla in salt-split normal human skin.[125]

Direct immunoelectron microscopy reveals IgG deposits under the lamina densa, within the region normally occupied by anchoring fibrils.

Differential diagnosis

The differential diagnosis of EBA is wide and includes other autoimmune blistering disorders such as bullous pemphigoid, chronic bullous disease of childhood, cicatricial pemphigoid, pemphigus vulgaris, and dermatitis herpetiformis. Bullous systemic lupus erythematosus can also present with a similar clinical picture, and the presence of antinuclear antibody will distinguish between the two. Stevens–Johnson syndrome and inherited forms of porphyria should also be considered, as well as infectious disorders such as herpes simplex and bullous impetigo. EBA may develop during infancy[171] and must then be distinguished from dystrophic epidermolysis bullosa.

Therapy and prognosis

The long-term prognosis for EBA in children is much better than in adults, with childhood EBA usually undergoing remission within 1–4 years, although occasionally its course can be more protracted. Whilst EBA in adults tends to be resistant to treatment, the childhood form of EBA is much more responsive.

A combination of prednisolone and dapsone is the best form of therapy for childhood EBA.[172] A reasonable commencing dose of prednisolone is 1mg/kg/day, and for dapsone 2mg/kg/day. Remission is usually quick, within a matter of weeks and, once this is attained, it is standard practice to gradually taper off prednisolone therapy and then to gradually taper the dose of dapsone. Resistant cases may require larger doses of prednisolone, up to 2mg/kg body weight per day, and dapsone, up to 5mg/kg per day. Alternative therapies include the use of sulfapyridine, a combination of nicotinamide and erythromycin, and for localized disease a superpotent topical steroid may suffice.

BULLOUS SYSTEMIC LUPUS ERYTHEMATOSUS

Introduction

Systemic lupus erythematosus has been reported in association with pemphigus vulgaris, bullous pemphigoid, dermatitis herpetiformis, and epidermolysis bullosa acquisita. However, the term bullous systemic lupus erythematosus (BSLE) is used to describe an acquired autoimmune subepidermal blistering disorder in an individual fulfilling the criteria of the American Rheumatism Association for systemic lupus erythematosus. BSLE is likely to be a heterogeneous group of diseases and it may be that in SLE there is a genetic predisposition to form antibodies to constituents of the dermal–epidermal junction that are critical for maintaining epidermal–dermal adhesion.[173] BSLE is an unusual condition, and it has only rarely been reported in children.[174,175]

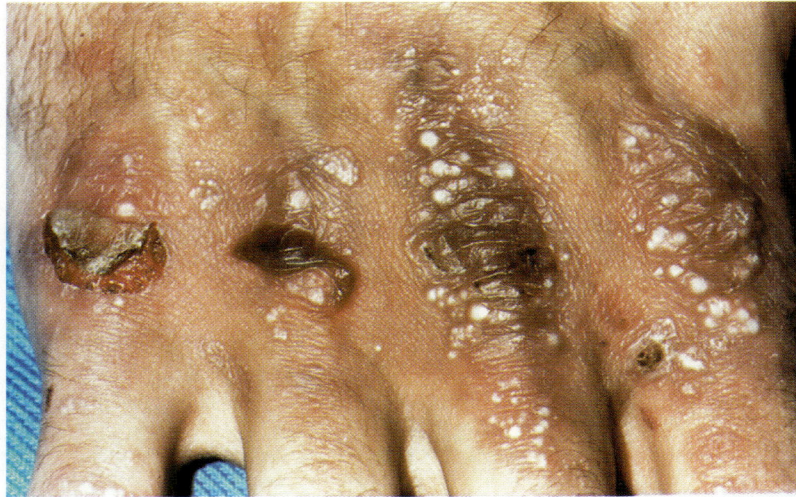

Fig. 16.24 EBA in an adolescent: skin fragility involving knuckles, with subsequent milia and scarring.

168. Inauen P, Hunziker T, Gerber H et al. (1994) Childhood epidermolysis bullosa acquisita. **Br J Dermatol** 131:898–900.
169. Park SB, Cho KH, Youn JL et al. (1997) Epidermolysis bullosa acquisita in childhood – a case mimicking chronic bullous dermatosis of childhood. **Clin Exp Dermatol** 22:220–222.
170. Caux F, Kirtschig G, Lemarchand-Venencie F et al. (1997) IgA-epidermolysis bullosa acquisita in a child resulting in blindness. **Br J Dermatol** 137:270–275.
171. McCuaig CC, Chan LS, Woodley DT et al. (1989) Epidermolysis bullosa acquisita in childhood. Differentiation from hereditary epidermolysis bullosa. **Arch Dermatol** 125:944–949.

172. Callot-Mellot C, Bodemer C, Caux F et al. (1997) Epidermolysis bullosa acquisita in childhood. **Arch Dermatol** 133:1122–1126.
173. Yell JA, Allen J, Wojnarowska F et al. (1995) Bullous systemic lupus erythematosus: revised criteria for diagnosis. **Br J Dermatol** 132:921–928.
174. Kettler AH, Bean SF, Duffy JO, Gammon WR (1988) Systemic lupus erythematosus presenting as a bullous eruption in a child. **Arch Dermatol** 124:1083–1087.
175. Shirahama S, Furukawa F, Yagi H et al. (1998) Bullous systemic lupus erythematosus: detection of antibodies against noncollagenous domain of type VII collagen. **J Am Acad Dermatol** 38:844–848.

Clinical features

BSLE usually presents as a chronic widespread, itchy, nonscarring bullous eruption, with tense blisters arising on normal or urticated skin (Fig. 16.25). The distribution normally includes sun-exposed areas, but nonexposed sites can also be involved. Milia and pigmentary change may or may not be seen, but there is no skin fragility. Mucous membrane involvement, including the oral, nasal, and genital mucous membranes, may occur.

Pathophysiology and histogenesis

The target antigen in BSLE has been shown in a number of cases to be type VII collagen, with Western immunoblotting studies against extracts of human dermis showing that the circulating antibodies bind to the 290kDa and 145kDa dermal proteins that represent the EBA antigens. However, antibodies to type VII collagen are not always present in BSLE patients, and it is possible in some cases that autoantibodies are produced to a variety of other molecules that may be involved in dermal–epidermal adhesion, such as bullous pemphigoid antigen 1 (BP230), laminin 5 and laminin 6.[176] When type VII collagen is the target antigen, the circulating antibody may recognize various epitopes on the noncollagenous domain.

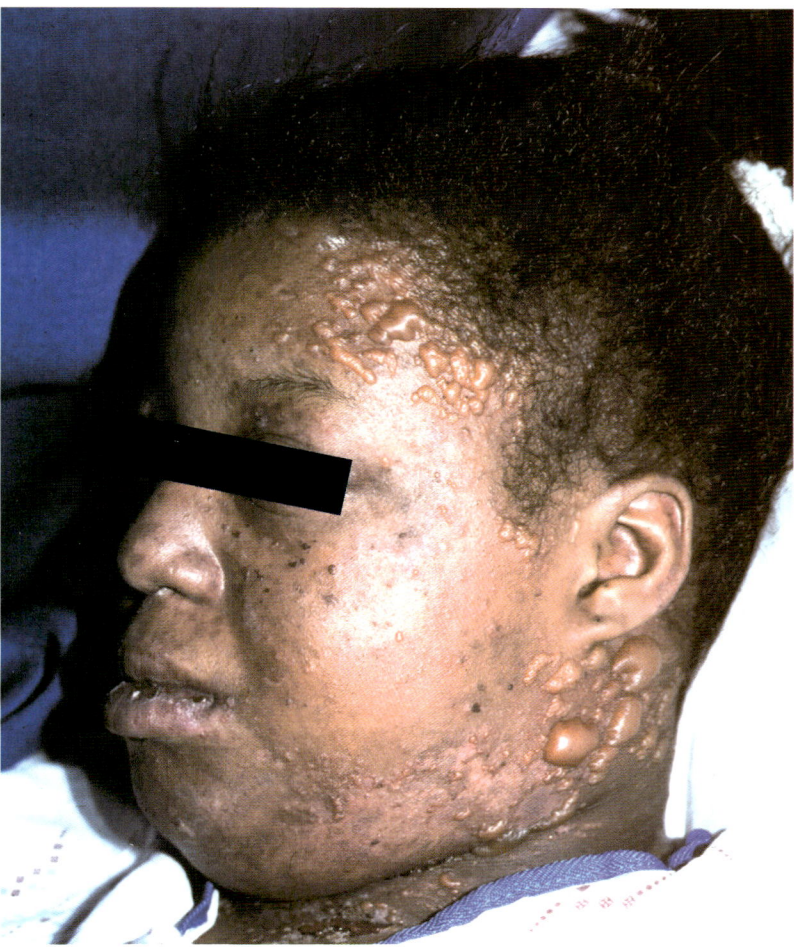

Fig. 16.25   Bullous systemic lupus erythematosus.

BSLE is characterized by a subepidermal blister with a neutrophil-predominant inflammatory infiltrate within the upper dermis. Direct immunofluorescence examination of lesional skin shows IgG and complement deposition along the epidermal basement membrane, with occasional weaker staining with IgA and/or IgM. The immunoreactants along the basement membrane zone may have a granular or linear pattern. Indirect immunofluorescence examination on salt-split skin usually shows antibody localization to the dermal side. Ultrastructural examination shows immune deposits on or beneath the lamina densa of the dermal–epidermal junction.

Therapy and prognosis

The treatment of choice for BSLE is dapsone, and the blistering tendency usually responds quickly. The prognosis is good, and remission the norm. However, the ultimate prognosis depends on the degree of internal organ involvement by the underlying systemic lupus erythematosus.

PEMPHIGUS

Introduction

Pemphigus is a group of autoimmune intraepidermal vesiculobullous diseases, characterized by loss of contact between keratinocytes (acantholysis) as the result of formation of autoantibodies to desmosomal proteins. There are two main forms of pemphigus: the suprabasal type, which includes pemphigus vulgaris (PV) and pemphigus vegetans, and which is usually associated with mucous membrane involvement; and a superficial type, which includes pemphigus foliaceus (PF) and pemphigus erythematosus, in which mucous membrane involvement is not a prominent feature.

Pemphigus is rare in childhood. All the clinical variants that occur in adulthood have been recorded in children, including the paraneoplastic form. The sex incidence is equal, and the mean age of onset of pemphigus in childhood is 12 years.[177] There appears to be a genetic susceptibility, and there are a number of environmental factors which cause the disease to develop. Certain drugs, such as penicillamine, captopril, enalapril and rifampicin, may precipitate pemphigus,[178] and there is a possibility that a number of acantholytic substances, such as thiol-containing molecules, phenols and tannins in plant foodstuffs, may play a role in the initiation and maintenance of pemphigus.[179] In addition, there is a form of superficial pemphigus, fogo selvagem, that is endemic in certain rural developing regions of Brazil. Fogo selvagem occurs mainly in children who live in close proximity to rivers and the distribution of this condition coincides approximately with the habitat of the blackfly, *Simulium nigrimanum*,[180] which may be a vector in disease transmission.

The commonest form of pemphigus in childhood is PV, followed by PF. Pemphigus vegetans[181] and erythematosus[182] are both very rare.

Pemphigus vulgaris

Clinical features

The clinical presentation of pemphigus in children is similar to that in adults. The disintegrating epidermis that characterizes pemphigus cannot withstand a great deal of hydrostatic pressure, and the blisters in PV are usually flaccid and quickly rupture, leaving tender erosions and crusts (Fig. 16.26). Nikolski's sign is positive. Because of the superficial nature of the pathological process, scarring is not usually a feature of PV, but it may occur secondary to infection or excoriation.

176. Chan LS, Lapiere JC, Chen M et al. (1999) Bullous systemic lupus erythematosus with autoantibodies recognizing multiple basement membrane components, bullous pemphigoid antigen I, laminin-5, laminin-6, and type VII collagen. **Arch Dermatol** 135:569–573.
177. Bjarnason B, Flosadottir E (1999) Childhood, neonatal and stillborn pemphigus vulgaris. **Int J Dermatol** 38:680–688.
178. Thami GP, Kaur S, Kanwar AJ (2001) Severe childhood pemphigus vulgaris aggravated by enalapril. **Dermatology** 202:341.
179. Tur E, Brenner S (1998) Diet and pemphigus. In pursuit of exogenous factors in pemphigus and fogo selvagem. **Arch Dermatol** 134:1406–1410.
180. Santi CG, Sotto MN (2001) mmunopathologic characterization of the tissue response in endemic pemphigus foliaceus (fogo selvagem). **J Am Acad Dermatol** 44:446–450.
181. Wananukul S, Pongprasit P (1999) Childhood pemphigus. **Int J Dermatol** 38:29–35.
182. Lyde CB, Cox SE, Cruz PD (1994) Pemphigus erythematosus in a five-year-old child. **J Am Acad Dermatol** 31:906–909.

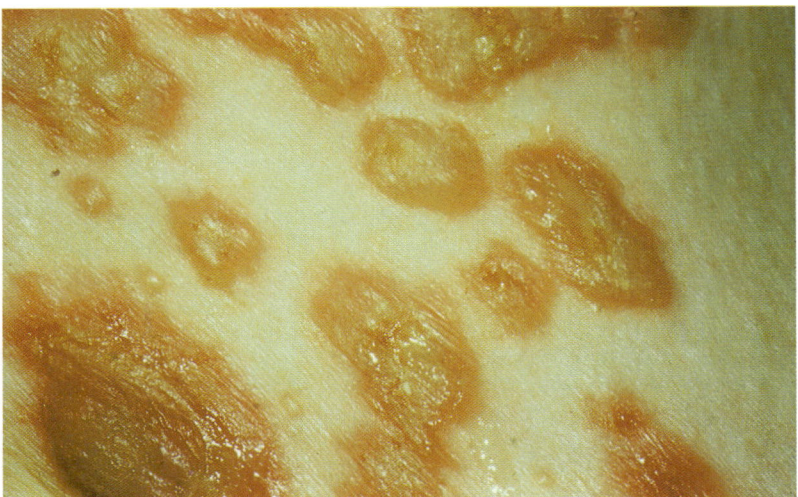

Fig. 16.26 Pemphigus vulgaris: flaccid bullae.

In PV, involvement of the mucous membranes, particularly those of the mouth, is common, and oral involvement may be the presenting feature. Genital and ocular mucous membrane involvement occur less frequently (Fig. 16.27).

Pathophysiology and histogenesis

There is still controversy surrounding the nature of the target antigens in pemphigus, although the evidence points to antidesmoglein antibodies as having a central role in the pathogenesis of both the superficial and suprabasal forms of pemphigus;[183] their circulating titer seems to correlate with the severity of the disease. Desmogleins are structural components of desmosomes and in pemphigus vulgaris, the humoral response is to desmogleins 1 and 3; antibodies to both of these desmosomal constituents seem to be necessary to induce suprabasal acantholysis. However, there may be other autoantibodies, perhaps acting in concert with antidesmoglein antibodies, such as anti-acetylcholine receptor antibodies, that are also important.[184]

In pemphigus vulgaris, the histological changes are those of acantholysis, with individual keratinocytes often seen floating in the suprabasal cleavage plane, and the basal keratinocytes remaining attached to the

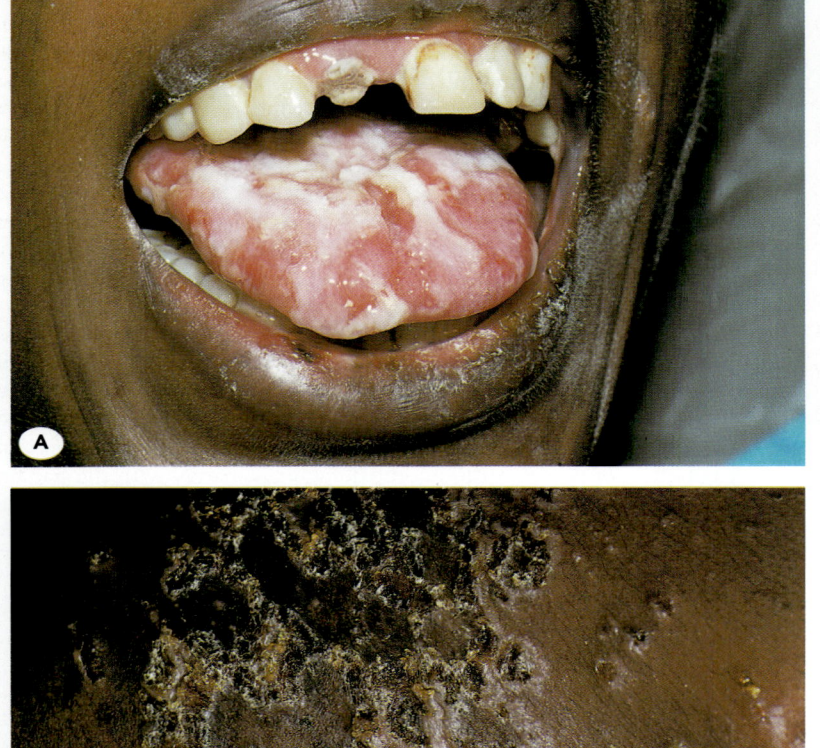

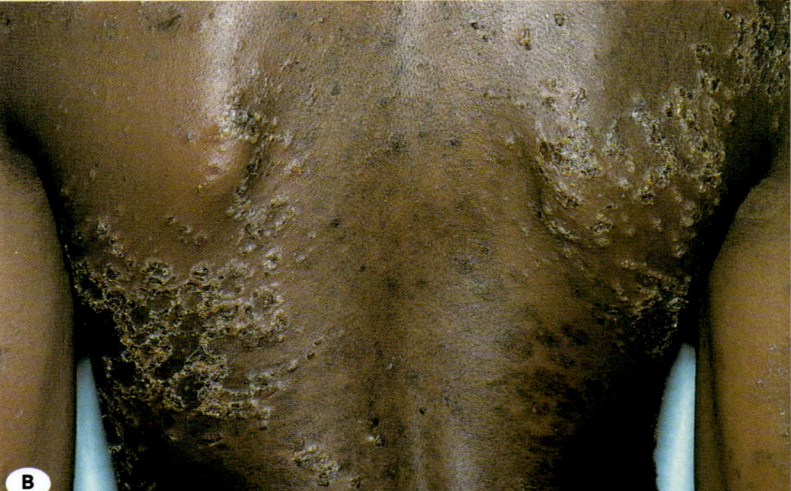

Fig. 16.27 (A) Oral lesions of pemphigus vulgaris. (B) and (C) Pemphigus vulgaris on the back of a child.

183. Stanley JR, Nishikawa T, Diaz LA, Amagai M (2001) Pemphigus, is there another half of the story? **J Invest Dermatol** 116:489–490.

184. Grando SA, Pittelkow MR, Shultz LD et al. (2001) Pemphigus: an unfolding story. **J Invest Dermatol** 117:990–994.

epidermal basement membrane, resembling a "row of tombstones." There is usually a dermal infiltrate consisting of lymphocytes, neutrophils and eosinophils.

Direct immunofluorescence examination of involved or perilesional skin, in both suprabasal and superficial forms of pemphigus, reveals deposition of IgG around keratinocytes, giving a characteristic "chicken wire" or "crazy paving" pattern. C3 may also be present in a pericellular distribution. More than one biopsy may occasionally be necessary to demonstrate the characteristic histology and immunofluorescence.[183]

Indirect immunofluorescence examination of patients' serum usually confirms the presence of circulating antibody, and the titer seems to correlate with clinical severity and can be used to monitor progress during treatment.

Differential diagnosis
The rarity of pemphigus in childhood means that the diagnosis may easily be overlooked. Pemphigus vulgaris may resemble Stevens–Johnson syndrome, and the possibility of a drug eruption should also be considered.

Treatment and prognosis
The prognosis for pemphigus vulgaris in childhood appears to be better than for the adult disease. The mortality is less and it is rarely fatal.[177] The side effects from systemic corticosteroid therapy contribute to morbidity, especially the possibility of infections such as pneumonia and septicemia.

The mainstay of treatment for pemphigus in childhood is systemic corticosteroid therapy, given either orally or as intravenous pulses. A commencing dose of prednisolone of between 1 and 2mg/kg/day is standard, although this may need to be increased depending on response. As the condition comes under control, the dose of prednisolone should be tapered as quickly as possible, and consideration given to an alternating day regimen. The use of potent topical or intralesional corticosteroid preparations should be considered for isolated recalcitrant foci of persistent blistering. Topical corticosteroid therapy may enable reduced systemic doses of corticosteroids.

Dapsone has been advocated as a steroid-sparing measure,[185] and other steroid-sparing drugs that have been used in the treatment of childhood pemphigus include azathioprine,[181] methotrexate,[181] cyclophosphamide,[177] hydroxychloroquine,[186] and intramuscular gold.[177] In cases that are particularly resistant to therapy, the possibility of pulsed intravenous corticosteroid therapy, with or without plasmapheresis should be considered.[177] It remains to be seen whether dietary manipulation, excluding foodstuffs with potentially acantholytic constituents, has a role to play in the control of pemphigus.

Pemphigus foliaceus

Clinical features
The blister roof in the superficial forms of pemphigus is too thin to allow significant fluid accumulation within the cleavage plane and may therefore present as an erythematosquamous condition, perhaps with very superficial erosions, and even as an exfoliative dermatitis, (Fig. 16.28).[181] Arcuate, circinate, or polycyclic lesions, commonly on the head and neck, may be seen in pemphigus foliaceus,[186] and may easily be mistaken for impetigo. Scarring is not a feature.

Pathophysiology and histogenesis
In PF and fogo selvagem the antibody response is to desmoglein 1, a 160kDa constituent of desmosomes at the level of the stratum granulosum, and

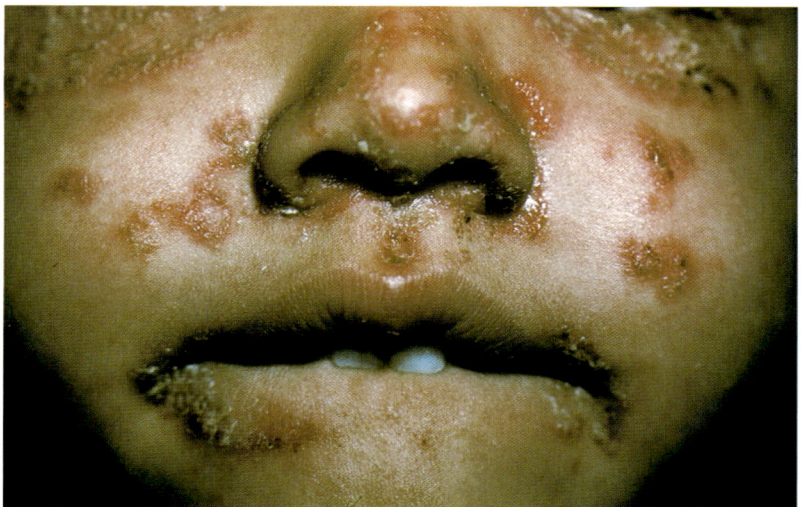

Fig. 16.28   Pemphigus foliaceus: facial lesions. (Courtesy of Annette Wagner.)

desmoglein inactivation at this level is considered to be responsible for the subcorneal cleavage plane in superficial forms of pemphigus. In the superficial forms of pemphigus, the cleavage plane is at the level of the stratum granulosum and the degree of acantholysis may be subtle. In the superficial forms of pemphigus, direct immunofluorescence shows deposition of IgG around keratinocytes. Additionally, in pemphigus erythematosus, there is usually a linear deposition of IgG or IgM at the epidermal basement membrane zone.

Differential diagnosis
PF may present as an exfoliative dermatitis, and impetigo, seborrhoeic dermatitis, psoriasis and staphylococcal scalded skin syndrome may also be mistaken for pemphigus.

Treatment and prognosis
The prognosis for pemphigus foliaceus is good. Treatment is the same as for PV, but PF is a milder condition and topical corticosteroid therapy may suffice.

Neonatal pemphigus
In women with active pemphigus, vulgaris[177] and foliaceus,[187] the possibility of the fetus developing the disease as the result of transplacental passage of circulating maternal antibodies must be considered. Maternal pemphigus is sometimes associated with stillbirth, but the prognosis is excellent for both neonatal pemphigus vulgaris and foliaceus, the bullae resolving spontaneously in neonates within a week or two. A high titer of circulating pemphigus antibody in the maternal circulation prior to delivery may forewarn of neonatal involvement.

Paraneoplastic pemphigus
Paraneoplastic pemphigus associated with Castleman's tumor has been recorded in a child.[188] This case mimicked Stevens–Johnson syndrome and responded to tumor resection and immunosuppressive therapy. Indirect immunofluorescence using rodent bladder epithelium was positive and immunoblotting studies showed the presence of antibodies to epidermal antigens with molecular weights of 190, 210, 230 and 250kDa.

185. Bjarnason B, Skoglund C, Flosadottir E (1998) Childhood pemphigus vulgaris treated with dapsone: a case report. **Pediatr Dermatol** 15:381–383.
186. Metry D, Hebert AA, Jordon RE (2002) Nonendemic pemphigus foliaceus in children. **J Am Acad Dermatol** 46:419–422.
187. Avalos-Diaz E, Olague-Marchan M, Lopez-Swiderski A et al. (2000) Transplacental passage of maternal pemphigus foliaceus autoantibodies induces neonatal pemphigus. **J Am Acad Dermatol** 43:1130–1134.
188. Lemon MA, Weston WL, Huff JC (1997) Childhood paraneoplastic pemphigus associated with Castleman's tumour. **Br J Dermatol** 136:115–117.

DERMATITIS HERPETIFORMIS

Introduction and historical note

Dermatitis herpetiformis (DH) is a chronic autoimmune blistering disorder, the clinical features of which were defined in a seminal description by Duhring in 1884.[189] Its prevalence in childhood has not been established; it is rare although dermatitis herpetiformis may be the most common of the autoimmune blistering disorders in childhood.[190] In children the sex incidence appears equal, whereas in adults it is more common in males. It may be more common in European than in North American children, and it is unusual in children of African and Asian descent. It has been reported as occurring in a child as young as 10 months, but it appears that it can present at any time during childhood, with some sources indicating that its most common presentation is between 2 and 7 years,[181] and others that the mean age is at 14 years.[190]

Clinical features

The cutaneous lesions of DH in childhood resemble those in the adult condition, with intensely pruritic vesicles and erythematous papules, sometimes associated with urticarial plaques, symmetrically involving the extensor surfaces of the limbs, buttocks, shoulders, nape of neck and scalp. Vesicles are excoriated as soon as they develop and blistering may therefore not be evident. Scarring of the skin is not a particular feature, but may occur as a result of excoriation or secondary infection. Mucous membrane involvement is not a feature of DH.

Although DH is a rare condition in childhood, it may be over-diagnosed if only the clinical features are considered[190] and immunofluorescence confirmation is mandatory.

Childhood DH presents with typical features of the adult disease but, in addition, other clinical signs such as the presence of nonpruritic inflammatory papules[191] or the development of pruritic palmar purpuric macules and papules.[192] The latter presentation is associated with extravasated red blood cells, but with the typical histologic and immunofluorescence characteristics of DH.

Gluten-sensitive enteropathy is present in 85–95% of children with DH. If investigated, most of these children will have a degree of villous atrophy of the small intestine, either partial or subtotal. In most instances, the gluten-sensitive enteropathy is asymptomatic at the time of presentation and generally, clinical symptoms if present are relatively mild. Approximately 40% of children with DH have a history of chronic or relapsing diarrhea before a diagnosis of DH is made,[193] and in only 10% is there a diagnosis of celiac disease at presentation.

Pathophysiology and histogenesis

DH is associated with the granular deposition of an IgA antibody within the dermal papillae. The principal target antigen has recently been identified as epidermal transglutaminase.[194]

There is a strong association with gluten-sensitive enteropathy. More than 90% of children with DH have evidence of intestinal abnormality, including partial or subtotal villous atrophy within the small intestine.[193]

The classic histologic picture is that of a subepidermal blister with neutrophilic (and occasionally eosinophilic) microabscesses within the dermal papillae. Fibrin deposition is common. The pathognomonic diagnostic feature is the presence on direct immunofluorescence examination of perilesional skin of a granular deposition of IgA within the dermal papillae, occasionally accompanied by C3. False-negative results can occur if skin at distant sites from the blistering, rather than perilesional skin, is taken for direct immunofluorescence.[190] Circulating IgA autoantibodies to tissue transglutaminase, the target antigen in celiac disease, is found in untreated DH patients and the titer reflects the degree of abnormality in the jejunal mucosa.

Differential diagnosis

DH may be mistaken for a variety of pruritic conditions, including acute or subacute eczema, insect bite reactions, scabies, pityriasis lichenoides et varioliformis acuta, and polymorphic light eruption.

Therapy and prognosis

The mainstays of treating DH are dapsone and a gluten-free diet. A gluten-free diet in isolation causes reversal of the intestinal abnormality in 100% of cases and the disappearance of cutaneous lesions in 82%.[193] Dapsone alone is an effective treatment for the eruption but does not affect the gastrointestinal abnormality. The response to a gluten-free diet tends to be quicker in children than adults. DH may be associated with growth retardation, and a gluten-free diet reverses this.

The standard initial dose of dapsone in childhood is 0.5–2mg/kg/day.[191] In order to minimize the risk of hemolysis at the onset of therapy, it is recommended that the circulating level of glucose-6-phosphate-dehydrogenase be estimated.[193] The main side effects of dapsone are agranulocytosis and hemolysis, and it is recommended that the full blood count and reticulocyte count be checked weekly for 4 weeks after commencing dapsone, and then monthly for the next 5 months. Thereafter, the frequency can be reduced to 3 monthly. Methemoglobinemia may occur with higher dapsone doses, but this rarely requires treatment in childhood. Cimetidine may offer protection. As in the adult disease, the response to dapsone is very quick, but relapse is rapid if the dapsone is stopped.

Once control of the disease has been obtained, the dosage of dapsone should be tapered either by reducing the daily dose, perhaps down to 0.125–0.5mg/kg/day, or increasing the time between doses; control may be possible with as little as a single weekly dosage. If the child is on a gluten-free diet, it may be possible to stop dapsone completely and quickly.

If there are unacceptable side effects with dapsone, such as hepatitis, an alternative is sulfapyridine in a starting dose of 100mg/kg/day,[190] although there may be some cross-reaction with dapsone regarding side effects. The use of superpotent topical corticosteroids for short periods may be considered as a dapsone-sparing measure.

The long-term prognosis for childhood DH is unclear. Short and long remissions are possible, but remission in childhood may be followed by recurrence in adolescence or young adulthood. Until the ideal duration of a gluten-free diet has been established, it should be considered indefinite.

INFECTIONS

A number of cutaneous infections can present with blistering and should be considered in the differential diagnosis of vesiculo-bullous disorders (see Chapter 25).

HERPES SIMPLEX VIRUS (HSV) INFECTION

Primary HSV infection usually presents in childhood as a gingivostomatitis, with vesicles occurring in the mouth and on the perioral region, sometimes associated with malaise and fever. Vesicles on the mucous membranes progress to painful ulcers, usually with regional lymphadenopathy, halitosis, and excessive dribbling. Autoinoculation may result in blistering of the hands and genital regions. Recrudescent HSV infection tends to occur on the lips and adjacent face, although other body regions may be involved. Progression through vesicular, pustular and crusted phases is the rule and healing takes place within 2 weeks.

189. Duhring LA (1884) Dermatitis herpetiformis. **JAMA** 3:225.
190. Weston WL, Morelli JG, Huff JC (1997) Misdiagnosis, treatments and outcomes in the immunobullous diseases in children. **Pediatr Dermatol** 14:264–272.
191. Woollons A, Darley CR, Bhogal BS et al. (1999) Childhood dermatitis herpetiformis: an unusual presentation. **Clin Exp Dermatol** 24:283–285.
192. McGovern TW, Bennion SD (1994) Palmar purpura: an atypical presentation of childhood dermatitis herpetiformis. **Pediatr Dermatol** 11:319–322.
193. Ermacora E, Prampolini L, Tribbia G et al. (1986) Long-term follow-up of dermatitis herpetiformis in children. **J Am Acad Dermatol** 15:24–30.
194. Sardy M, Karpati S, Merkl B et al. (2002) Epidermal transglutaminase (Tgase 3) is the autoantigen of dermatitis herpetiformis. **J Exp Med** 195:747–757.

HSV infection in neonates carries with it the risk of herpes encephalitis, and appropiate early antiviral treatment greatly reduces morbidity and mortality.

CHICKENPOX

Chickenpox is caused by the varicella zoster virus and is a very common childhood exanthem. It is associated with a prodrome of variable severity and characterized by pruritic vesicles, occurring in crops over approximately 1 week, which progress to pustules and then crusts. Secondary bacterial infection is a common complication. Herpes zoster occurs in both immuno-competent and immunocompromised children. If chickenpox is aquired by the mother after the 20th week of pregnancy, there is a risk to the infant of acquiring herpes zoster in the first year of life, and if chickenpox is acquired in the first year of life there is a good chance of the infant developing herpes zoster by 10 years of age.

HAND, FOOT, AND MOUTH DISEASE

Hand, foot, and mouth disease is caused by coxsackie virus A16 and tends to occur in epidemics. Flaccid vesiculopustules arise in the mouth and on the palms and soles, progressing to erosions and ulcers, sometimes associated with a mild prodrome of fever and anorexia. Healing occurs uneventfully. An epidemic of hand, foot, and mouth disease caused by enterovirus 71 resulted in many fatalities from neurological complications and severely handicapped survivors.[195]

CELLULITIS

Bullous changes superimposed on cellulitis is usually associated with *Streptococcus pyogenes* or *Staphylococcus aureus* infection.

BLISTERING DACTYLITIS

Blistering dactylitis is caused by infection with a β hemolytic streptococcus and is characterized by a distinctive blistering of the volar aspects of the fingers and palms. Incision and drainage of tense bullae and a course of oral phe-noxymethyl penicillin or erythromycin is the treatment of choice.

SCABIES

Scabies infestation in young children may be associated with vesiculopustules, chiefly of the hands and feet.

STAPHYLOCOCCAL SCALDED SKIN SYNDROME

Introduction and historical note

Staphylococcal scalded skin syndrome (SSSS) was described more than a century ago by von Rittershain[196] and is sometimes known as Ritter's disease. It is only very recently that a firm understanding of the pathogenesis has developed. SSSS is a toxin-induced epidermolytic bullous disease which usually affects infants and young children and can endanger life, especially when it occurs in the neonatal period. SSSS can also occur, much less commonly, in adults who frequently have a predisposing condition such as immunosuppression, renal impairment or overwhelming sepsis; SSSS has been described in healthy immunocompetent adults. SSSS in adulthood carries a higher mortality rate than in childhood.[197]

Clinical features

The severity of SSSS varies from localized blistering to erythroderma and generalized desquamation. The localized form of SSSS (bullous impetigo) is characterized by the development of fragile flaccid blisters, as the thin roof, comprised only of the stratum corneum and a few cells of the stratum granulosum, cannot withstand significant hydrostatic pressure. These blisters contain a cloudy or frankly purulent fluid, with normal surrounding skin. The child is usually systemically well.

The generalized form of SSSS tends to present with systemic symptoms, including rhinitis, conjunctivitis, fever, irritability, and malaise, and feeding may be affected. This is followed by the development of erythema, which can affect all body regions but with a predilection for the flexures. The next phase of the disease is the development of extensive superficial bullae which become deroofed revealing large areas of raw, red, moist skin, an appearance similar to a hot water scald. Nikolski's sign is positive. The mucous membranes are not usually involved. The primary focus of staphylococcal infection is often not apparent in SSSS. With appropriate treatment, the fever usually subsides rapidly, bullae formation ceases and erythema gradually subsides. In the majority of cases, complete recovery occurs within 2 to 3 weeks, leaving no permanent sequelae.

Pathophysiology and histogenesis

SSSS is the result of the action of staphylococcal exfoliative toxins A and B produced by infection with certain strains of *Staphylococcus aureus*, usually belonging to Phage Group 2.[197] These exfoliative toxins are serine proteases, and recent evidence suggests that the specific substrate for exfoliative toxins A and B is desmoglein 1,[198,199] an important component of desmosomes high in the epidermis in the region of the stratum granulosum. Impaired inter-cellular adhesion is thought to be the consequence of a direct proteolytic attack on desmoglein 1 by the staphylococcal toxins, which reach the skin via the bloodstream. These toxins may[200] or may not[201] act as superantigens although this is still contentious. It is probably not coincidental that desmoglein 1 is also the target antigen of the autoantibody produced in pemphigus foliaceus in which blisters occur at exactly the same level as in SSSS.

The possession of antibodies to staphylococcal exfoliative toxins may, at least partially, explain the epidemiology of SSSS, particularly the fact that it is much less common in adults.[197] Breast-feeding may confer protection against SSSS in neonates as a result of transfer of antibodies in breastmilk.[197] The presence of antibodies may also determine the pattern of infection and may explain why the bullae of bullous impetigo, a localized form of SSSS, contain staphylococcal organisms whereas the contents of the blisters of widespread SSSS are usually sterile.

The diagnosis of SSSS is supported by the characteristic clinical picture, the demonstration of an exfoliative toxin-producing strain of *S. aureus* and the confirmation of a histological cleavage plane at the level of the stratum granulosum. However, in practice, the staphylococcal infection may be covert. Swabs should be taken for bacteriological culture from the nostrils, nasopharynx, and conjunctivae. Blood should be cultured, although it is unusual for bacteremia to occur in SSSS. In generalized SSSS the skin is usually sterile but if there is clinical suspicion of secondary infection swabs for culture from the skin should be taken. Phage typing of the staphylococcus is not considered sufficiently sensitive or specific to be a diagnostic criterion for SSSS.[197] At present the reliable, convenient, and rapid detection of exfoliative toxins is not available.

The most definitive diagnostic test at present is the demonstration of blister formation at the level of the stratum granulosum in the context of a

195. Huang CC, Lin CC, Chang YC et al. (1999) Neurologic complications in children with enterovirus 71 infection. **N Engl J Med** 341:936–942.

196. Ritter von Rittershain G (1878) Die exfoliativa Dermatitis jungerer Sauglinge. **Zentralzeit Kinderheilkd** 2:3–23.

197. Ladhani S, Joannou CL, Lochrie DP et al. (1999) Clinical, microbial, and biochemical aspects of the exfoliative toxins causing staphylococcal scalded-skin syndrome. **Clin Microbiol Rev** 12:224–242.

198. Amagai M, Matsuyoshi N, Wang ZH et al. (2000) Toxin in bullous impetigo and staphylococcal scalded-skin syndrome targets desmoglein I. **Nat Med** 6:1275–1277.

199. Amagai M, Yamaguchi T, Hanakawa Y et al. (2002) Staphylococcal exfoliative toxin B specifically cleaves desmoglein I. **J Invest Dermatol** 118:845–850.

200. Monday SR, Vath GM, Ferens WA et al. (1999) Unique superantigen activity of staphylococcal exfoliative toxins. **J Immunol** 162:4550–4559.

201. Plano LR, Gutman DM, Woischnik M, Collins CM (2000) Recombinant staphylococcus aureus exfoliative toxins are not bacterial superantigens. **Infect Immun** 68:3048–3052.

characteristic clinical picture. It is generally unnecessary to perform a skin biopsy as the diagnosis is usually clinically obvious. If there is doubt, it is simple to obtain a sample by cutting a small piece of the sloughed skin, snap-freezing it in liquid nitrogen and obtaining frozen sections. Not only is the technique entirely atraumatic to everyone involved, as it is painless and does not require local anesthetic, but it enables a rapid result, usually within 1h and very effectively distinguishes SSSS from toxic epidermal necrolysis. In the former condition the exfoliating skin will consist only of stratum corneum and a few cell layers of the stratum granulosum, whereas in the latter condition the roof of the blister will be formed by the entire thickness of a necrotic epidermis (see Fig. 16.29).

Differential diagnosis

The most important differential diagnosis of SSSS is toxic epidermal necrolysis. The clinical picture of a scalded appearance can be very similar although mucosal involvement is very much more likely in toxic epidermal necrolysis. The scalded appearance may raise the possibility of a nonaccidental injury.

Therapy and prognosis

Generalised SSSS requires administration of antibiotics to eradicate the source of the toxin-producing staphylococcus. If the organism has been isolated the choice of antibiotic is guided by the bacteriological sensitivities, otherwise an appropriate choice is flucloxacillin or erythromycin.

Analgesia may be required. Careful attention should be paid to replenishing water loss from greatly increased evaporation through the skin and ensuring electrolyte balance. Body temperature should be maintained

Milder forms of SSSS, including bullous impetigo, are managed with oral antibiotics which should be effective against streptococci as well as staphylococci. As desquamation occurs within a few days into the illness, an emollient should be applied thrice daily.

The more extensive the involvement of the skin in SSSS and the younger the child the worse the outcome, although with appropriate treatment the overall prognosis is good, with a mortality of less than 5%. The superficial exfoliation does not compromise epidermal function as profoundly as the full-thickness epidermal damage encountered in toxic epidermal necrolysis. Nonetheless, fluid loss, temperature dysregulation, and secondary cutaneous infection are all potential complications that have to be strictly addressed.

REACTIVE BLISTERING DISORDERS

ERYTHEMA MULTIFORME

Introduction and historical note

Erythema multiforme (EM) is defined as an acute self-limiting vesiculobullous disorder characterized by the development of erythematous macules and papules, some of which evolve into "target" lesions; it was first described by von Hebra in 1860.[202] Stevens and Johnson described a more severe condition in 1922,[203] subsequently known as Stevens–Johnson syndrome (SJS), which is characterized by severe mucosal, as well as cutaneous disease and, like erythema multiforme, is also associated with epidermal necrosis. For many years EM was classified into minor and major forms, the major variant being synonymous with SJS. However, there is a consensus developing that SJS is best regarded as a distinct entity from EM,[204] despite clinical and histological similarities. The nosological debate continues, and EM is considered

as a separate condition from SJS and toxic epidermal necrolysis (Lyell syndrome).

The list of putative trigger factors for EM and SJS in adults is a long one, but in children it seems that the great majority of cases of EM are the result of a preceding recrudescence of herpes simplex[205,206] even when there is no clinical history of an antecedent herpes infection.[205] SJS in adults is generally drug-induced but in childhood SJS tends to be associated with other infections, particularly with *Mycoplasma pneumoniae*, as well as drugs, often antibiotics and antiseizure medications.[206] EM may occasionally precede varicella zoster virus infection in children.[207]

Clinical features

EM is often preceded by a herpes simplex infection, usually on the face, but occasionally elsewhere. Prodromal symptoms are either absent or mild, consisting of a low-grade fever, cough, and a reluctance to eat. Constitutional symptoms during the course of the eruption may be absent or moderate in degree. Typically, crops of lesions develop over a few days in acral regions, particularly the palms and dorsa of the hands, wrists, feet, extensor aspects of elbow and knees, and occasionally the face. A seasonal clustering in the spring months, presumably the result of sun exposure, is well documented. EM may manifest the Köebner phenomenon.

Individual lesions usually start as dull red macules or maculopapules, which may increase in size up to approximately 3cm in diameter. The lesions are usually asymptomatic but may itch or be uncomfortable. They may develop into target (or iris) lesions, which are a diagnostic feature of EM. The target lesions consist of two or three concentric rings. The central zone represents acute epidermal injury, usually commencing as dusky erythematous or purpuric macules before developing into tense bullae, which often have a lackluster sheen as the result of epidermal damage. The blister contents may be clear or hemorrhagic. There is usually a middle pale zone of edematous skin and finally an outer halo of well-demarcated erythema. As its name suggests, there may be a variable pattern ranging from necrotic macules to an exclusively blistering disorder. Lesions are monomorphous in an individual patient. The lesions tend to fade over a period of 1–2 weeks, without specific treatment.

A mucous membrane is frequently involved in herpes simplex virus-associated EM; this is usually confined to the oral mucosa and tends to be relatively mild, although the lesions quickly become denuded, giving rise to painful erosions which may make eating and drinking difficult. On the lips, identifiable target lesions may form.[208] Rarely, the ocular, genital, pharyngeal, laryngeal, and esophageal mucous membranes are affected.

Cutaneous and mucous membrane lesions heal without scarring, usually with no complications. There is no internal organ involvement. Recurrences of herpes simplex virus-associated EM are common, but recrudescent cold sores do not consistently cause EM.

Pathophysiology and histogenesis

The pathogenesis of EM is unknown. It is considered to be a reaction pattern to a number of different stimuli. It is not a vasculitic process, and it is probably a delayed hypersensitivity immune response, with a cytotoxic immunological attack on keratinocytes expressing foreign antigens such as viruses or drugs. Herpes simplex virus DNA can frequently be demonstrated by polymerase chain reaction amplification of material obtained from the epidermis of EM lesions, whether or not the attack has been preceded by a cold sore.[205] Thus, a high index of suspicion that recrudescent herpes simplex virus has

202. Von Hebra F (1860) Acute exantheme und hautkrankheiten. Handbuch der Speciellen Pathologie und Therapie. Erlangen: Verlag von Ferdinand von Enke, pp. 198–200.
203. Stevens AM, Johnson FC (1922) A new eruptive fever associated with stomatitis and ophthalmia. **Am J Dis Child** 24:526–527.
204. Assier H, Bastuji-Garin S, Revuz J, Roujeau J-C (1995) Erythema multiforme with mucous membrane involvement and Stevens–Johnson syndrome are clinically different disorders with distinct causes. **Arch Dermatol** 131:539–543.
205. Weston WL, Brice SL, Jester JD et al. (1992) Herpes simplex virus in childhood erythema multiforme. **Pediatrics** 89:32–34.
206. Leaute-Labreze C, Lamireau T, Chawki D et al. (2000) Diagnosis, classification and management of erythema multiforme and Stevens–Johnson syndrome. **Arch Dis Child** 83:347–352.
207. Prais D, Grisuru-Soen G, Barzilai A, Amir J (2001) Varicella zoster virus infection associated with erythema multiforme in children. **Infection** 29:37–39.
208. Weston WL, Morelli JG, Rogers M (1997) Target lesions on the lips: childhood herpes simplex associated with erythema multiforme mimics Stevens–Johnson syndrome. **J Am Acad Dermatol** 37:848–850.

precipitated an episode of EM in children should be entertained, even in the absence of obvious preceding herpes infection.[205]

No specific investigations are required. In cases of diagnostic doubt histological examination in mild cases shows a lymphohistiocytic perivascular infiltrate with vacuolar degeneration of the lower epidermis and individual necrotic keratinocytes. In more severe cases, there is necrosis of the entire thickness of the epidermis, and dermal–epidermal separation occurring close to the epidermal basement membrane which tends to lie in the floor of the lesion. There are no specific immunohistochemical changes.

Differential diagnosis

EM in childhood is frequently misdiagnosed[206] and may be mistaken for urticaria, drug reactions, pemphigoid, chronic bullous disease of childhood, and, occasionally, polymorphic light eruption when limited to sun-exposed skin.

Treatment and prognosis

EM in childhood runs a mild course in most cases, and attacks tend to subside within 1–2 weeks, usually without sequelae, apart from occasional pigmentary change. Herpes simplex virus-associated EM in childhood does not progress to SJS.[208] Treatment is symptomatic and oral corticosteroid therapy is not recommended.[208] Herpes simplex virus-associated EM does not usually respond to the topical administration of acyclovir, but prophylactic oral acyclovir, if given early enough, can prevent recurrences.[209] Tense bullae can be ruptured, followed by the topical application of an antibiotic to prevent secondary infection.

STEVENS–JOHNSON SYNDROME/TOXIC EPIDERMAL NECROLYSIS

Introduction

There is now a consensus that Stevens–Johnson syndome (SJS) and toxic epidermal necrolysis (TEN), also known as Lyell syndrome, are similar, if not identical, conditions, and at least part of a single spectrum, differing only in severity. Both are serious conditions, with TEN at the severest end of the spectrum. It has been argued that EM (as described by von Hebra) can reasonably be regarded as a separate entity from SJS-TEN.[204] The particular clinical features said to set SJS-TEN apart from EM are the distribution of the eruption (in EM lesions are acral and in SJS they are centrally located or widespread) and its characteristics (target lesions in EM and either flat atypical target lesions or purpuric macules and bullae in SJS-TEN). The mucous membrane involvement is more severe and extensive in SJS-TEN.[204] This dichotomy is said to correlate well with a principally viral etiology for EM and a drug-induced etiology for SJS-TEN.[204]

SJS-TEN is an episodic condition and recurrences are unusual, in contrast to EM. Drugs are the primary causative factor for SJS-TEN in adults, and appear also to be important in the childhood condition,[210] although this has been challenged.[206] Antibiotics, anticonvulsants, and nonsteroidal anti-inflammatory agents are the classes of drug usually incriminated. A variety of infections may, perhaps less commonly, precipitate SJS-TEN, particularly *Mycoplasma pneumoniae*.[211] Vaccination may rarely be a precipitating factor.[212] At times, the trigger factor cannot be established.

Clinical features

In SJS-TEN there is usually a prodromal illness lasting up to 2 weeks consisting of symptoms such as fever, cough, headache, malaise, arthralgia, myalgia, and gastrointestinal upset. The onset of the rash is sudden and initially takes the form of a macular or morbilliform, tender, dusky erythematous eruption involving the face, trunk and limbs, with at times a suggestion of target lesions. Nikolski's sign is usually positive. The eruption gradually worsens over several days, with coalescence of lesions occurring and the development of flaccid and occasionally hemorrhagic blisters. Depending on the severity of the condition, the epidermis begins to detach as a result of very minor frictional forces and large flaccid blisters, resembling scalds, develop and rupture leaving sheets of necrotic epidermis with a moist erythematous base (Fig. 16.29). In severe cases the nails may be shed. Unusually, SJS-TEN may be associated with subcorneal pustules.[213]

Mucous membrane lesions are common and uncomfortable. Bullae are associated with edema and erythema and break down to form painful erosions. The oral cavity and the vermilion of the lips are almost invariably affected, and the discomfort causes difficulties with eating. The lips are covered with hemorrhagic crusts. The conjunctival and genital mucous membranes are involved, particularly the glans penis in boys and the vulva and vagina in girls, which may lead to dysuria and urinary retention.

SJS-TEN is usually associated with marked constitutional symptoms, particularly fever, arthralgia, and malaise. TEN may affect the respiratory and gastrointestinal tracts. Direct involvement of the respiratory mucosa may lead to respiratory failure.[214] Patchy pulmonary disease also occurs and bronchiolitis obliterans may result. Involvement of the esophagus may cause dysphagia and malnutrition but strictures are unusual.[215] Ileal involvement may lead to abdominal pain and diarrhea, and the colon can also be involved.

Dehydration and electrolyte imbalance may cause the development of hemodynamic shock, coma and seizures, and septicemia and septic shock are potential dangers.

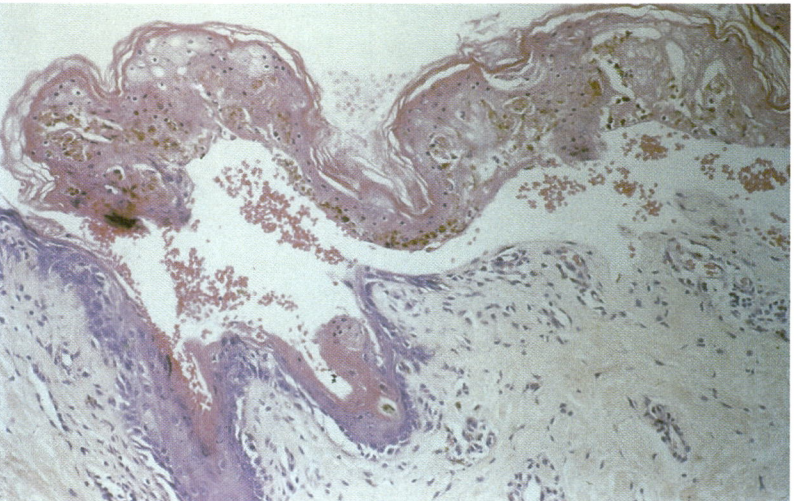

Fig. 16.29   Stevens–Johnson syndrome/toxic epidermal necrolysis: histology showing full thickness necrosis of the epidermis, with a tongue of viable epidermis encroaching onto the blistered area.

209. Weston WL, Morelli JG (1997) Herpes simplex virus-associated erythema multiforme in prepubertal children. **Arch Pediatr Adolesc Med** 151:1014–1016.
210. Sheridan RL, Weber JM, Schultz JT et al. (1999) Management of severe toxic epidermal necrolysis in children. **J Burn Care Rehabil** 20:497–500.
211. Tay YK, Huff JC, Weston WL (1996) Mycoplasma pneumoniae infection is associated with Stevens–Johnson syndrome, not erythema multiforme (von Hebra). **J Am Acad Dermatol** 35:757–760.
212. Ball R, Ball LK, Wise RP et al. (2001) Stevens–Johnson syndrome and toxic epidermal necrolysis after vaccination: reports to the vaccine adverse event reporting system. **Pediatr Infect Dis J** 20:219–223.
213. Reichert-Penetrat S, Barband A, Antunes A et al. (2000) An unusual form of Stevens–Johnson syndrome with subcorneal pustules associated with Mycoplasma pneumoniae infection. **Pediatr Dermatol** 17:202–204.
214. Schamberger MS, Goel J, Braddock SR et al. (1997) Stevens–Johnson syndrome and respiratory failure in a nine-year-old boy. **South Med J** 90:755–757.
215. Lamireau T, Leaute-Labreze C, Le Bail B, Taieb A (2001) Esophageal involvement in Stevens–Johnson syndrome. **Endoscopy** 33:550–553.

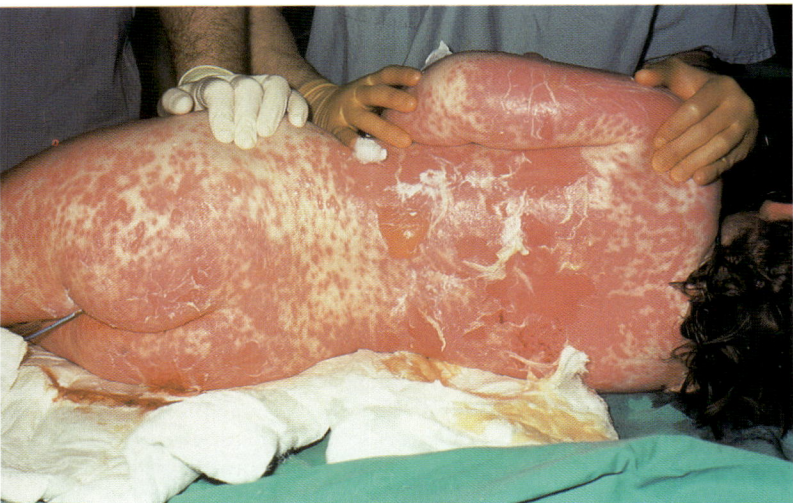

Fig. 16.30 Stevens–Johnson syndrome/toxic epidermal necrolysis: extensive blistering.

Pathophysiology and histogenesis

Like EM, SJS-TEN is probably a cytotoxic immune reaction directed against keratinocytes expressing foreign antigens. However, unlike EM, there is a great over-expression of tumor necrosis factor-alpha (TNF-α) in the epidermis,[216,217] which is thought to play an important role in keratinocyte death, and possibly explains the much greater degree of epidermal necrosis in SJS-TEN than in EM.

Histological examination (Fig. 16.30) of SJS and TEN show a prominent degree of epidermal necrosis occurring on a background of relatively little inflammatory infiltrate. Subepidermal cleavage is usually present. In TEN there is full-thickness epidermal necrosis and widespread dermal–epidermal separation.

Differential diagnosis

Viral exanthems can resemble milder forms of SJS, and burns or scalds have to be considered for the more severe forms of the condition. Staphylococcal scalded skin syndrome can be difficult to distinguish from TEN but histological examination of frozen sections of the blister roof rapidly establish the diagnosis (see Staphylococcal Scalded Skin Syndrome).

Treatment and prognosis

The prognosis of SJS-TEN depends on the severity of the condition and the surface area involved. With appropriate medical treatment, the prognosis in children is good, with a lower mortality than in adults.[210,211] Milder cases can be nursed on a dermatology ward, but more severe cases are probably best managed in a specialized burns unit.[210,218] Initial management should be directed to withdrawing any drugs suspected of causing the reaction, treating any underlying infection, and rectifying any electrolyte and fluid imbalance. In severe cases, a central venous line and urinary catheter may be required, but they should not be used routinely because of the problems of central line

infection and urinary tract infections.[210] Prevention of wound desiccation is desirable and an aerosol emollient is ideal. Regular swabs of the skin should be taken to anticipate secondary infection which should then be treated with appropriate antibiotics; there may be a case to be made for the use of prophylactic antibiotics. Biological wound dressings can be beneficial. General supportive measures include a high-calorie and high-protein diet, and if oral intake is not possible, consideration should be given to parenteral feeding. Close ophthalmic supervision of the eye is important. If severe oropharyngeal involvement prevents a child from guarding the airway, prophylactic intubation should be considered.[210] Gauze or hydrocolloid dressings should be applied to eroded areas and consideration given to the use of a ripple mattress.

The role of systemic corticosteroid therapy is controversial and is considered beneficial by some[219] and detrimental by others.[220] Systemic corticosteroids do increase the risk of infection, but their advocates suggest tapering the dose quickly once disease progression has ceased, and perhaps combining their use with a prophylactic antibiotic. Intravenous immunoglobulin appears to be a safe and effective treatment for TEN in children, and results in a shortening of hospital stay.[221] The dose is 3g/kg in divided doses given over 2–3 days.

Late complications of SJS-TEN include pigmentary change, especially in dark-skinned children, and fingernail loss or deformity.[210] Cutaneous scarring is not usual except when there has been secondary infection, but the mucous membranes are much more likely to scar, especially the conjunctivae, and keratitis sicca is a common cause of long-term morbidity.[210] There are usually no sequelae from involvement of the lips and oral mucosa, but scarring of the genital mucous membranes does occur, causing such problems as phimosis. If bronchiolitis obliterans develops the prognosis is poor.

MISCELLANEOUS BLISTERING DISORDERS

BLISTERING PHOTODERMATOSES

Photosensitivity in childhood may be associated with blister formation. Actinic prurigo is an inflammatory photodermatosis characterized by a pruritic vesiculopustular eruption developing several hours after exposure to sunlight. Hydroa vacciniforme is typified by tender vesicles developing on sun-exposed sites, mainly in boys, that heal with scarring. The distribution of blistering and the temporal relationship to sun exposure usually suggests a photosensitive etiology.

COMA BLISTERS

Blistering in comatose subjects ("coma blisters") has been associated with carbon monoxide exposure, drug overdose, neurological damage, hypoglycemia and diabetic ketoacidosis.[222] Coma blisters usually arise within 24h of the onset of coma and resolve in 10–14 days; they are often associated with ecchymoses. Coma bullae are associated with a rather typical histology, consisting of epidermal necrosis with intraepidermal and subepidermal cleavage and necrosis of the eccrine glands and ducts. There is usually an associated deposition of immunoglobulins or complement, especially around the eccrine apparatus, which is thought to be related nonspecifically to tissue injury. The cause of coma blisters remains unclear but it is assumed that local hypoxia associated with pressure often plays a part, although coma blisters do not necessarily occur at pressure sites.

216. Paquet P, Nikkels A, Arrese JE et al. (1994) Macrophages and tumour necrosis factor alpha in toxic epidermal necrolysis. **Arch Dermatol** 130:605–608.
217. Paquet P, Pierard GE (1997) Erythema multiforme and toxic epidermal necrolysis: a comparative study. **Am J Dermatopathol** 19:127–132.
218. Ringheanu M, Laude TA (2000) Toxic epidermal necrolysis in children – an update. **Clin Pediatr** (Phila) 39:687–694.
219. Kakourou T, Klontza D, Soteropoulou F, Kattamis C (1997) Corticosteroid treatment of erythema multiforme major (Stevens–Johnson syndrome) in children. **Eur J Pediatr** 156:90–93.
220. Prendiville JS, Hebert AA, Greenwald MJ, Esterly NB (1989) Management of Stevens–Johnson syndrome and toxic epidermal necrolysis in children. **J Pediatr** 115:881–887.
221. Morici MV, Galen WK, Shetty AK et al. (2000) Intravenous immunoglobulin therapy for children with Stevens-Johnson syndrome. **J Rheumatol** 27:2494–2497.
222. Mehregan DR, Daoud M, Rogers RS (1992) Coma blisters in a patient with diabetic ketoacidosis. **J Am Acad Dermatol** 27:269–270.

Diseases of the Dermis and Subcutaneous Tissues

CHAPTER 17

Julie S. Prendiville and Alfons L. Krol

NODULAR DISEASES

Swelling or distortion of the skin contours, due to infiltration or expansion of the dermis or the underlying subcutaneous tissues, often presents as a diagnostic problem in infants and children. Most of these skin conditions are rare; a few are common. A diverse group of skin conditions may be considered under this category. To provide the clinician with an organized approach to such conditions, the first part of the chapter is divided into two sections: (1) skin-colored cysts and nodules, and (2) skin nodules with color change of the overlying skin.

The infiltrative diseases of the skin, with the exception of granuloma annulare, are uncommon in children. They are characterized by thickening, swelling, and a firm quality to the dermal tissue on palpation. As in approaching any clinical problem, the clue to the etiology will depend on whether the process is localized or systemic, its degree of infiltration, presence of inflammation, and color changes. Reviewing the various components of the dermis (cellular and supporting structures) allows one to arrive at a correct diagnosis, often aided by histological confirmation.

Cysts and nodules are circumscribed swellings in the skin, whereas infiltrative diseases often result in diffuse thickening and swelling of the skin. Some skin conditions of children that may be included within this classification are discussed in detail in other chapters.

SKIN-COLORED CYSTS AND NODULES

Julie S. Prendiville

Raised lesions with indistinct borders and a palpable deep portion on which the overlying skin is usually of normal color are considered in this category. These include epidermoid cysts, dermoid cysts, bronchogenic cysts, and pilomatricomas.

Epidermoid cysts

Epidermoid cysts (also known as epidermal cysts, epithelial inclusion cysts, sebaceous cysts, and wens) are dermal or subcutaneous nodules in which a keratin-filled cyst is lined by epithelium. Unna credits Schwenninger in 1886 with understanding the experimental production of epidermal inclusion cysts after skin trauma and inversion of the epithelium.[1] Unna recognized that the so-called sebaceous cyst was not lined with sebaceous glands but rather only with epithelium.

EPIDEMIOLOGY

Epidermoid cysts are rare in childhood and occur predominantly in young and middle-aged adults.[2] Epidermoid inclusion cysts on the hands or feet may be induced by trauma. Epidermoid cysts in Gardner syndrome are inherited in an autosomal-dominant pattern and may be present at birth or appear as late as the fourth decade of life.[3] There has been no reported racial or sexual predilection.

PRESENTING HISTORY

Parents will bring a child for medical care because of a lump in the skin. There is sometimes an underlying concern about skin cancer.[4] The cyst may become red and tender from infection, which prompts the parent to seek medical advice. In the circumstance of a sudden appearance of an epidermoid cyst, there may be a history of a preceding puncture wound or other penetrating skin injury.

PHYSICAL EXAMINATION

Epidermoid cysts are firm, spherical nodules that vary in size up to 1–2cm in their greatest diameter. An inflamed cyst is tender on palpation, and the overlying skin is red. Multiple epidermoid cysts in a child should cause one to suspect Gardner syndrome.[3,5] In Gardner syndrome, epidermoid cysts are irregularly distributed over the face, scalp, trunk, and extremities.

In solitary epidermoid cysts, the remainder of the physical examination is normal. In Gardner syndrome, other clinical manifestations may be found.[5] Thick, irregular, firm masses may be observed on the abdominal wall or proximal extremities, which represent a desmoid tumor, a locally invasive fibrous tumor observed in Gardner syndrome. Cutaneous lipomas may also be found. Hard, bony masses on the jaw represent mandibular osteomas.

LABORATORY FINDINGS

Multiple intestinal polyps may be visualized on barium studies or endoscopic examination in Gardner syndrome.[5]

PATHOPHYSIOLOGY AND HISTOGENESIS

Epidermoid cysts have a wall of true epidermis and contain laminated layers of horny material.[6] The wall and contents of the epidermoid cyst are identical

1. Crissey JT, Parish LC (1981) The Dermatology and Syphilology of the Nineteenth Century. New York: Praeger Scientific.
2. Golitz LE, Poomeechaiwong S (1990) Cysts. In: Pathology of the Skin, Farmer ER, Hood AF, eds. Norwalk, CT: Appleton and Lange.
3. Cooper PH, Fechner RE (1983) Pilomatricoma-like changes in the epidermal cells of Gardner's syndrome. J Am Acad Dermatol 8:639–644.
4. Knight PJ, Reiner CB (1983) Superficial lumps in children. What, when, and why. Pediatrics 72:147–153.
5. Gardner EJ, Richards RC (1953) Multiple cutaneous and subcutaneous lesions occurring simultaneously with hereditary polyposis and osteomatosis. Am J Hum Genet 5:139–147.
6. Benharroch D, Sachs MI (1988) Pilomatricoma associated with epidermoid cyst. J Cutan Pathol 16:40–43.

to that of the infundibulum of the pilosebaceous unit, but lack the deeper sebaceous duct and gland. The cyst does not contain sebum. In experimental wounds that invert the epidermis into the skin, epidermoid cysts can be induced. The epidermoid cysts of Gardner syndrome are considered to be developmental and perhaps represent defects in assembly of the skin.[5,6] Inflamed cysts may rupture their keratinous contents through the thin epithelial wall into the dermis, inciting a foreign body immune reaction. Secondary bacterial infection sometimes occurs. Pilomatricoma-like changes, including shadow cells and calcification, have been observed in epidermoid cysts, particularly in cases of Gardner syndrome.[3,6,7]

DIFFERENTIAL DIAGNOSIS

Superficial lymph nodes may be occasionally mistaken for epidermoid cysts because they are also round, firm, skin-colored nodules, which may have a smooth feel on palpation, mimicking the cyst capsule. Superficial lymph nodes in children are frequently found near the skin surface of the neck and groin. Pilomatricomas may be confused with epidermoid cysts but are attached to the overlying epidermis, have a hard, irregular feel, and lack the smooth configuration of epidermoid cysts. Lipomas may also be confused, although they are subcutaneous in location and are softer than true epidermoid cysts. Dermoid cysts may mimic epidermoid cysts, but occur over lines of fusion, and histopathologic differentiation may be required. Epidermal cysts must also be distinguished from congenital developmental cysts on the neck.[8] Thyroglossal cysts occur on the midline of the neck; bronchogenic cysts are found most commonly around the suprasternal notch; branchial cleft cysts occur on the lateral neck area.

THERAPY AND PROGNOSIS

For solitary epidermoid cysts, no therapy is indicated. Parents may wish to have the cyst removed for cosmetic purposes. For red, tender cysts, drainage and oral antibiotics may be required to treat secondary infection before removal.

In Gardner syndrome, large intestinal polyps can occur during adolescence but are more likely to appear during the third decade of life.[5] In at least 50% of patients, colonic cancer develops, in the intestinal polyps, and predictive studies estimate that all affected family members are at risk.[5,9] Careful follow-up by a pediatric gastroenterologist or pediatrician is recommended because malignant transformation in the bowel has been documented in the first decade of life.[9]

Dermoid cysts

Dermoid cysts are epithelium-lined cysts that contain epidermal appendages, including hair follicles, and may contain hair, sebum, keratin, and sometimes associated apocrine glands.[10] They are developmental in origin and are believed to arise as a consequence of displacement of dermal and epidermal cells into and along embryonic lines of fusion.[10] They are usually noted at birth, in infancy, or in early childhood. Sites of predilection are the periorbital region, midline of the nose, scalp, and anterior neck.[11] There is no known racial or sexual predilection, although a slight preponderance of female patients was noted in one study.[10] The exact prevalence of dermoid cysts is not known.

PRESENTING HISTORY

Dermoid cysts present as a nodule on the face, head, or neck. They are usually asymptomatic unless there is infection of the cyst or underlying tissues. An associated sinus tract with intracranial extension may result in recurrent meningitis.[12]

PHYSICAL EXAMINATION

Dermoid cysts appear as round, firm, often slightly compressible, skin-colored nodules on the face or scalp. They are often observed around the eyes (Fig. 17.1), particularly the lateral eyebrow or within the rim of the orbit. Lesions in the nasoglabellar region, and occasionally elsewhere, may have an overlying punctum or sinus opening that contains fine hairs. Extrusion of sebaceous material is sometimes seen.[11] Lesions on the eyelid, although seldom associated with a sinus, may erode underlying bone.

PATHOPHYSIOLOGY AND HISTOGENESIS

Dermoid cysts are the result of sequestration of skin at lines of embryonic closure during skin development.[11] They are differentiated from epidermoid cysts by the presence of hair and sebum within the cystic contents and the presence of sebaceous glands, hair follicle structures, and/or apocrine glands in the epithelial lining of the cyst.[10,11] Dermoid cysts are usually subcutaneous in location. There should be some concern about midline lesions, especially on the nose, because these may have an accompanying sinus tract, sometimes with intracranial extension.[11,12]

DIFFERENTIAL DIAGNOSIS

The differential diagnosis of a dermoid cyst includes nasal glioma, encephalocele, meningocele, ectopic meningeal tissue, epidermoid cyst, and hermangioma. The distinction between epidermoid and dermoid cysts may be difficult clinically. However, except for traumatic epidermoid cysts, which are usually located on the hands and feet, and cysts associated with Gardner syndrome, epidermoid cysts are rare in infants and young children.

THERAPY AND PROGNOSIS

Simple excision is the treatment of choice for lesions on the eyebrow.[11] Midline dermoid cysts may be superficial, may have an accompanying sinus tract that adheres to the underlying periosteum or nasal septum, and may sometimes extend intracranially.[12] A detailed computed tomographic (CT) scan should be obtained before surgery for all midline lesions, lesions with a punctum or sinus opening, and lesions in the orbit with indistinct margins.[11] If present, the CT scan should be followed by a magnetic resonance imaging (MRI) scan to determine whether the sinus tract communicates with the meninges. If there is connection, the sinus tract should be excised at the same time as the dermoid cyst.[11,12] Ophthalmologic evaluation is indicated for lesions within the orbital rim because of possible pressure effects on the globe.[11]

Pilomatricoma

Pilomatricoma (also known as calcifying epithelioma of Malherbe) is a benign adnexal tumor derived from hair matrix cells. It commonly appears in the first or second decade of life and has a slight female preponderance.[13] Familial occurrence is well documented.[7,14] Pilomatricomas have a predilection for the head and neck. They may also occur on the arms and, less commonly, on

7. Pujol RM, Casanova JM, Egido R et al. (1995) Multiple familial pilomatricomas: a cutaneous marker for Gardner syndrome? **Pediatr Dermatol** 12:331–335.
8. Howard R (1998) Congenital midline lesions: pits and protuberances. **Pediatr Ann** 27:150–160.
9. Naylor EW, Lebenthal E (1979) Early detection of adenomatosis polyposis coli in the Gardner's syndrome. **Pediatrics** 63:222–227.
10. Pollard ZF, Robison HD, Calhoun J (1976) Dermoid cysts in children. **Pediatrics** 57:379–382.
11. Bartlett SP, Lin KY, Grossman R et al. (1993) The surgical management of orbitofacial dermoids in the pediatric patient. **Plast Reconstr Surg** 91:1208–1215.
12. Pensler JM (1988) Craniofacial dermoids. **Plast Reconstr Surg** 82:953–958.
13. Moehlenbeck FW (1973) Pilomatricoma (calcifyding epithelioma): a statistical study. **Arch Dermatol** 108:532–534.
14. Demircan M, Balik E (1977) Pilomatricoma in children: a prospective study. **Pediatr Dermatol** 14:430–432.

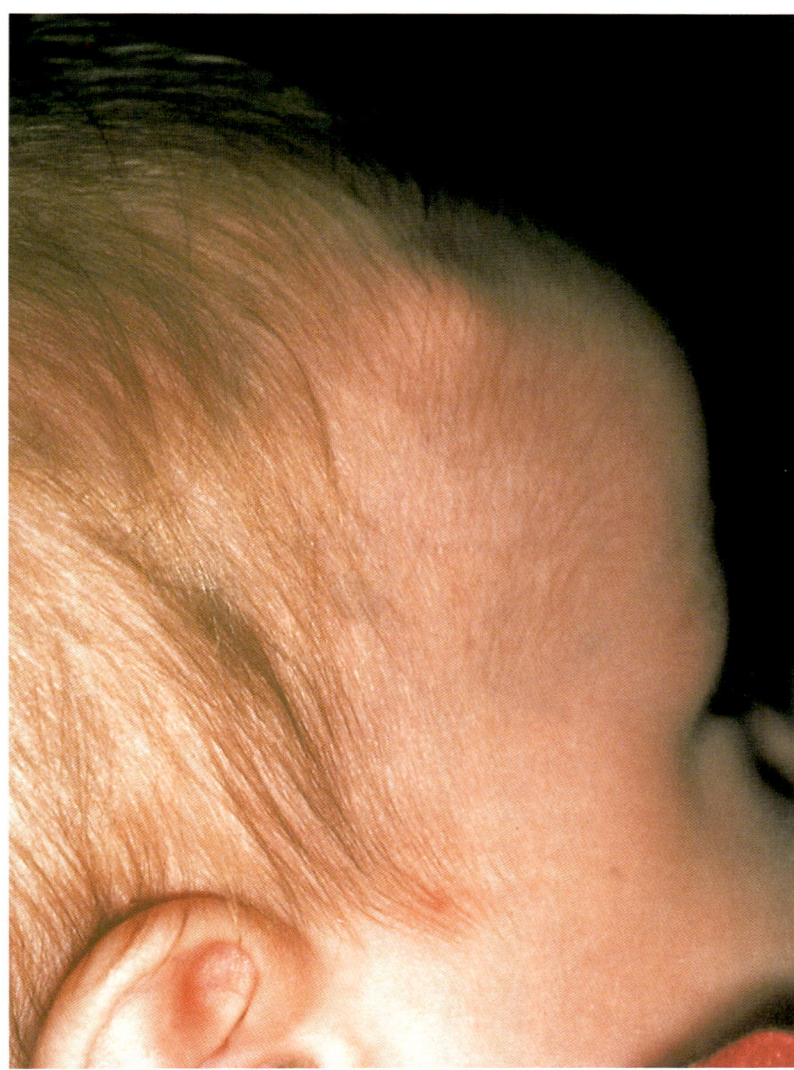

Fig. 17.1   A 10-mm dermoid cyst in the suture line of a toddler.

PATHOPHYSIOLOGY AND HISTOGENESIS

Pilomatricomas have been shown to arise from genetic alterations that influence β-catenin stabilization.[21] A similar genetic defect is found in patients with colon cancer. Ultrastructural and histochemical studies show a keratinization pattern resembling that seen in normal hair cortex. Histopathologically, the pilomatricoma is composed of irregularly shaped islands of epithelial cells located in the deep dermis or subcutaneous fat and surrounded by a capsule of connective tissue. Pilomatricomas are composed of two types of cell: basophilic and shadow. Basophilic cells are seen at the periphery or side of the lesion and have darkly staining round or elongated nuclei and scanty cytoplasm. Shadow

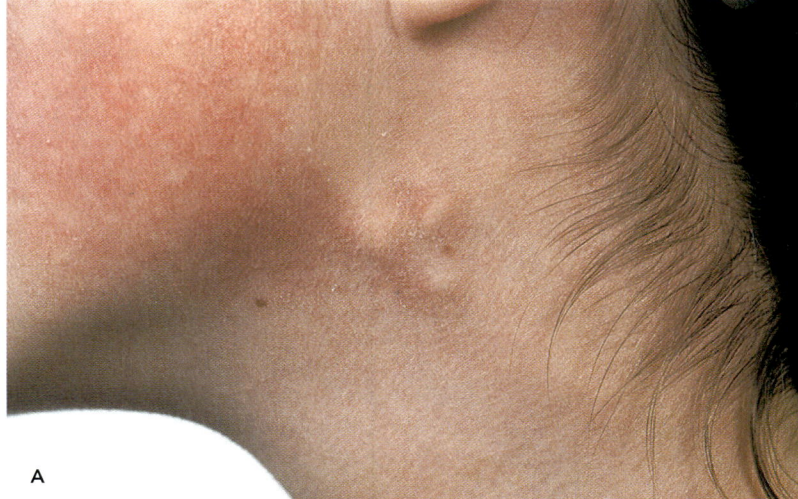

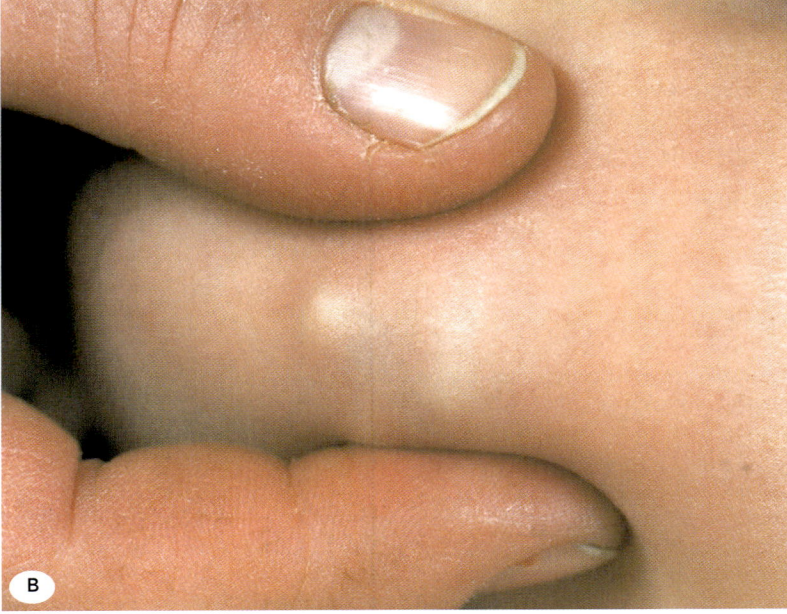

Fig. 17.2   (A) Pilomatricoma in the neck of a teenager. (B) Pilomatricoma on the cheek.

the trunk and lower extremities. Most are solitary nodules, but multiple and eruptive lesions may occur. Multiple pilomatricomas can be associated with myotonic dystrophy,[15,16] and have also been described in Gardner syndrome and Rubenstein–Taybi syndrome.[7,17]

CLINICAL FEATURES

The pilomatricoma presents as a slowly growing, firm to hard, lobulated nodule that is fixed to the epidermis but is freely mobile over underlying structures (Fig. 17.2). The overlying skin is typically skin-colored or white but may show a blue-red discoloration. It can vary in size from 0.5 to 5cm in diameter and, rarely, larger lesions may occur.[6] Anetoderma-like changes of the overlying skin have been described.[18] Rapid enlargement by bleeding into a lesion may occur.[19] Malignant pilomatricoma is very rare, particularly in childhood.[20]

15. Geh JL, Moss AI (1999) Multiple pilomatrixomata and myotonic dystrophy: a familial association. **Br J Dermatol** 52:143–145.
16. Kopeloff I, Orlow SJ, Sanchez MR (1992) Multiple pilomatricomas: report of two cases and review of the association with myotonic dystrophy. **Cutis** 50:290–292.
17. Cambiaghi S, Ermacora E, Brusasco A et al. (1994) Multiple pilomatricomas in Rubenstein-Taybi syndrome: a case report. **Pediatr Dermatol** 11:21–25.
18. Jones CC, Tschen JA (1991) Anetodermic cutaneous changes overlying pilomatricomas. **J Am Acad Dermatol** 25:1072–1076.
19. Julian CG, Bowers PW (1998) A clinical review of 209 pilomatricomas. **J Am Acad Dermatol** 39:191–195.
20. Joshi A, Sah SP, Agrawal CS et al. (1999) Pilomatrix carcinoma in a child. **Acta Derm Venereol** 79:476–477.
21. Chan EF, Gat U, McNiff JM et al. (1999) A common skin tumour is caused by activating mutations in beta-catenin. **Nature Genet** 21:410–413.

cells have a well-defined border and a central unstained area where the nucleus has been lost. Cells in transition between basophilic and shadow cells are also seen. In older lesions, basophilic cells may be few or absent. Areas of keratinization are frequently observed within the tumor, with melanin, melanocytes, and foreign body giant cells. Calcification is a common finding, and ossification occasionally occurs. Pilomatricoma-like histopathologic changes have been described in epidermoid cysts, particularly in patients with Gardner syndrome.[3]

DIFFERENTIAL DIAGNOSIS

The differential diagnosis of pilomatricoma includes epidermoid cysts and other cutaneous adnexal tumors. Ultrasonography has been found to be a useful diagnostic tool, typically showing a mass with an echogenic center and hypoechoic rim at the junction of the dermis and subcutaneous fat.[22]

THERAPY AND PROGNOSIS

Pilomatricomas are benign lesions. Surgical excision is the treatment of choice. Others advocate incision and curettage.[19] It has been suggested that some pilomatricomas regress spontaneously.[23]

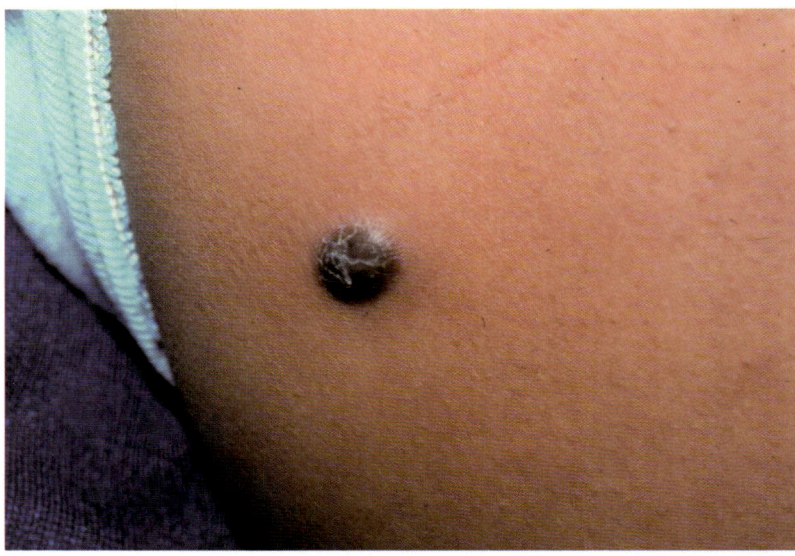

Fig. 17.3   A dermatofibroma.

SKIN NODULES WITH COLOR CHANGE OF THE OVERLYING SKIN

Keloids and hypertrophic scars

These conditions are discussed in Chapter 18.

Dermatofibromas

A dermatofibroma (also known as fibrous histiocytoma, histiocytoma cutis, and sclerosing hemangioma) is a small, benign circumscribed fibrous growth limited to the skin.[24] Unna was credited with first describing dermatofibromas as benign fibrous skin growths.[1] The term *dermatofibroma* was introduced by Schreus in 1930.[25] Some authorities, believing these growths were histiocytic in nature, designated them as histiocytomas or fibrous histiocytomas.[24] In 1943, the term *sclerosing hemangioma* was introduced to describe this tumor. Most authorities, however, prefer the term dermatofibroma.[24]

EPIDEMIOLOGY

The precise prevalence of dermatofibromas is unknown. They are commonly seen in adults. They are not common in young children but may be seen in adolescence.

PRESENTING HISTORY

A dermatofibroma presents as a slowly growing nodule. There are no associated symptoms. There may be concern about skin cancer or cosmesis.

PHYSICAL EXAMINATION

Dermatofibromas are small (1–5mm in diameter), firm, pigmented nodules (Fig. 17.3), usually found on the leg or trunk. Occasionally, they may reach 15mm in diameter but rarely exceed 20mm in size.[24] Multiple lesions may be present, with one to four lesions being the most likely number. Lateral pressure on the lesion produces dimpling of its surface known as the "bullet sign" or "dimple sign." The remainder of the physical examination should be normal.

PATHOPHYSIOLOGY AND HISTOGENESIS

Dermatofibromas contain numerous fibroblasts with excessive deposition of collagen in the dermis accompanied by a proliferation of the overlying epidermis.[24] Often, the acanthotic epidermis has increased melanin present. Histopathologic variants include hemosiderotic dermatofibromas and dermatofibromas with lipidization.[24]

The histogenesis of dermatofibromas has not been clearly established; the cell of origin may be the histiocyte, the fibroblast, or both.[24] Many authorities believe that they represent reactive proliferation of fibroblasts and the overlying epithelium as a result of minor trauma.[24] Because they do not spontaneously regress, some authorities consider them to be neoplasms.[24]

DIFFERENTIAL DIAGNOSIS

Dermatofibromas are pigmented and may be confused with melanoma but, unlike melanomas, dermatofibromas are firm and demonstrate dimpling, "the dimple sign," when the surface of the lesion is pinched or squeezed. The growth rate is slow in dermatofibromas and rapid in melanoma. The overlying epidermis in a dermatofibroma is thickened and firm in contrast to that of a melanoma. Other pigmented nodules, such as intradermal nevi, may be confused with dermatofibromas, and mastocytomas too, which may have overlying pigmentation of the skin. Juvenile xanthogranulomas are usually yellow or orange-brown in color. Pilomatricomas with discoloration of the overlying skin may also be confused. A biopsy may be necessary to distinguish these lesions. It is also important to distinguish the dermatofibroma from other fibrous proliferations of childhood. A dermatofibroma may clinically resemble a keloid scar, a dermatomyofibroma, or dermatofibrosarcoma protuberans. Dermatomyofibroma is a larger plaque-like dermal tumor with distinctive immunohistochemical features.[26] Dermatofibrosarcoma protuberans is also usually larger in size (more than 2cm), more cellular, has a monomorphous infiltrate, and extends deeper into the subcutaneous tissues than the benign dermatofibroma.[24]

22. Hughes J, Lam A, Rogers M (1999) Use of ultrasonography in the diagnosis of childhood pilomatrixoma. **Pediatr Dermatol** 16:341–344.

23. Headington JT (1990) Tumors of hair follicle differentiation. In: Pathology of the Skin, Farmer ER, Hood AF, eds. Norwalk, CT: Appleton and Lange.

24. Sanchez RL (1990) The elusive dermatofibromas. **Arch Dermatol** 126:522–523.

25. Niemi KM (1970) The benign fibrohistiocytic tumors of the skin. **Acta Derm Venereol** (Suppl) 63:1.

26. Rose C, Brocker E-B (1999) Dermatomyofibroma: case report and review. **Pediatr Dermatol** 16:456–459.

THERAPY AND PROGNOSIS

Dermatofibromas tend to persist. They may rarely grow up to 15mm in their maximal diameter. Usually, no treatment is required. If there is concern about the clinical diagnosis, then excisional biopsy is preferred, with complete removal of the lesion. This is easily accomplished because the lesions are usually small.

Digital fibrous tumor of childhood

Digital fibrous tumor of childhood is a benign growth of fibrous tissue found about the distal portion of the fingers or toes.[27,28] Reye[27] is credited with first describing this growth in 1965 and emphasizing its distinction from fibrosarcoma. Although some authorities have called it recurrent digital fibrous tumor of childhood,[27,29] McKenzie et al.[28] correctly determined that its recurrence is related to surgical intervention and that digital fibrous tumor of childhood is a more correct name.

EPIDEMIOLOGY

Digital fibrous tumor of childhood is not inherited and there is no significant sexual or racial predilection. It affects infants. Lesions may be present at birth or may develop up to 12 months of age.[27–29]

PRESENTING HISTORY

A history of a rapidly growing lump about the nail is often given.[27,29] Because these lesions grow rapidly, cancer is often suspected. The lesions are usually asymptomatic but may interfere with nail growth, and a deformed nail is often a secondary component.[27–29] The child may have had a previous biopsy or attempted excision of the lesion followed by rapid regrowth of the fibrous tumor.

PHYSICAL EXAMINATION

A firm nodule occurring around the fingernail or toenail is observed. The nodule is usually asymptomatic, involving one lateral side of the digit, and may cause a deformity within the nail plate. The overlying skin may be red or have a normal color. The lesion is limited usually to a single digit, but a few infants have had two lesions. The remainder of the physical examination is normal.

LABORATORY FINDINGS

There are no associated laboratory abnormalities with digital fibrous tumor of childhood.

PATHOPHYSIOLOGY AND HISTOGENESIS

Reye first observed prominent cytoplasmic inclusions that were not detectable on ordinary histologic stains but were prominently observed on iron hematoxylin stains of the tissue.[27] Initially, it was thought that digital fibrous tumors of childhood were a virus-induced, benign fibroblastic tumor.[29] This idea was based on the eosinophilic inclusions observed within the cytoplasm of proliferating fibroblasts that were accentuated by phosphotungstic acid stains of excised tumors. Electron microscopic studies, however, show that the cytoplasmic inclusions represent degenerated organelles with no evidence of viral particles.[28] Ultrastructural studies have shown the tumor cells to be myofibroblasts.[30]

Nodules of dense proliferating fibroblasts in a collagenous stroma are observed within the dermis and replace most of the normal dermal components. Eosinophilic perinuclear cytoplasmic inclusions surrounded by a clear halo stain pink with trichrome stain. Immunostaining is positive for desmin, actin, vimentin, and keratin.

DIFFERENTIAL DIAGNOSIS

The fibrous thickening overlying a subungual exostosis may exactly mimic fibrous tumor of childhood. A radiograph of the digit should be obtained before attempting a biopsy to rule out a bony exostosis. Thickening of the epidermis, such as in a callous or even a corn, can also sometimes be confused with the deeper thickening of digital fibrous tumor. A calloused pad resulting from vigorous finger sucking by a baby can be occasionally confused. Because of the abrupt onset and rapid growth, a biopsy may be necessary to rule out malignant tumors such as fibrosarcomas.

THERAPY AND PROGNOSIS

Digital fibrous tumor of childhood often involutes spontaneously within a few years. It is recommended to wait for spontaneous resolution.[31] Attempts at surgical excision or other cytodestructive therapies may introduce scarring and should be avoided unless there is functional impairment.

PEDIATRIC ASPECTS OF THE DISEASE

There is no influence of digital fibrous tumor of childhood on the overall growth or development of the child. Larger lesions may cause functional impairment or difficulty with fitting shoes.

Panniculitis

Panniculitis refers to inflammation of the subcutaneous fat. It may arise as a primary idiopathic process or in association with a variety of systemic or cutaneous disorders. Some diseases primarily involve the fat lobules (e.g., cold panniculitis or pancreatic panniculitis), whereas others involve the fibrous septa with extension to adjacent fat lobules (e.g., erythema nodosum and polyarteritis nodosa). However, there is considerable histologic overlap, and a simple classification of septal versus lobular panniculitis can be misleading.[32] No current clinical or histologic classification of panniculitis is entirely satisfactory. The literature is further confused by varied and imprecise terminology. Eponymous terms such as Weber–Christian disease and Rothman–Makai syndrome are no longer considered useful; in the past, these have included cases that would now be classified as lupus panniculitis, erythema nodosum, α_1-antitrypsin deficiency, or factitial panniculitis.[33] To arrive at a satisfactory diagnosis, the clinical history, anatomic location and number of lesions, presence or absence of ulceration or lipoatrophy, and associated systemic disease or symptoms should be evaluated in conjunction with histopathologic examination of an adequately deep skin biopsy.[32]

A classification of panniculitis in childhood is presented in Table 17.1. Erythema nodosum is by far the most common condition in this category.

Erythema nodosum

Erythema nodosum (EN) is characterized by the sudden onset of tender erythematous subcutaneous nodules on the extensor surfaces of the legs. Willan is credited with the introduction of the term *erythema nodosum* in 1798 and he recognized its association with tuberculosis.[1,34] After the incidence of

27. Reye RDK (1965) Recurring digital fibrous tumor of children. **Arch Pathol** 80:228–231.
28. McKenzie AW, Innes ELF, Rack JM et al. (1970) Digital fibrous swellings in children. **Br J Dermatol** 83:446–458.
29. Beckett JH, Jacobs AH (1977) Recurring digital fibromas of childhood: a review. **Pediatrics** 59:401–406.
30. Yun K (1988) Infantile digital fibromatosis. Immunohistocytochemical and ultrastructural observations of cytoplasmic inclusions. **Cancer** 61:500–507.

31. Ishii N, Matsui K, Ichiyama S et al. (1989) A case of infantile digital fibromatosis showing spontaneous regression. **Br J Dermatol** 121:129–133.
32. Peters MS, Su WPD (1992) Panniculitis. **Dermatol Clin** 10:37–57.
33. White JW, Winklemann RK (1998) Weber–Christian panniculitis: a review of 30 cases with this diagnosis. **J Am Acad Dermatol** 39:56–62.
34. Vesey CMR, Wilkinson DS (1959) Erythema nodosum. A study of seventy cases. **Br J Dermatol** 71:139.

tuberculosis waned, other infectious agents such as *Streptococcus, Coccidioides,* and *Histoplasma* became more important in their association with EN.[34–37] Recently , with a resurgence of *Mycobacterium tuberculosis* infection, clinicians may once again be confronted with tuberculosis manifesting with panniculitis, including both EN and erythema induratum of Bazin.

EPIDEMIOLOGY

Erythema nodosum in children has an equal sex ratio, whereas in adults there is a female predominance.[35,36,38] Erythema nodosum is rare before 2 years of age, but a child aged 7 months with EN has been well documented.[35] The peak age in childhood is during adolescence for females and ages 10 to 14 for males.[34] Convincing evidence for a hereditary predisposition is lacking and there is no racial predilection.[35–37]

TABLE 17.1 Classification of panniculitis
Erythema nodosum
Erythema induratum of Bazin   Nodular vasculitis

Physical agents
  Cold, popsicle, or equestrian
  Subcutaneous fat necrosis of the newborn
  Sclerema neonatorum
  Injections, iatrogenic or factitial
  Blunt trauma

Connective tissue disease
  Lupus panniculitis
  Scleroderma, eosinophilic fasciitis, or morphea profunda
  Dermatomyositis
  Juvenile rheumatoid arthritis
  Polyarteritis nodosa

Drug induced
  Poststeroid
  Others

Enzymatic
  α_1-antitrypsin deficiency
  Pancreatic disease[40]

Infections and infestations
  Bacterial, fungal, or mycobacterial[40,130]
  Eosinophilic panniculitis[129]

Subcutaneous noninfectious granulomas
  Subcutaneous granuloma annulare
  Sarcoidosis

Cytophagic histiocytes
  Histiocytic cytophagic panniculitis
  T-cell lymphoma

Idiopathic and lipoatrophic panniculitis[a]
  Connective tissue panniculitis[122]
  Panniculitis associated with autoimmune disorders[123]
  Lipophagic panniculitis of childhood[124]
  Suppressor-cytotoxic T-lymphocyte panniculitis[125]
  Atrophic connective tissue panniculitis of the ankles[126]
  Recurrent lobular panniculitis[127]

[a] Lipoatrophy may also occur in association with lupus panniculitis, dermatomyositis, morphea, juvenile rheumatoid arthritis, injections, and traumatic fat necrosis.

PRESENTING HISTORY

Erythema nodosum presents with an abrupt onset of tender red lesions on the anterior lower legs. Lesions often arise symmetrically but, occasionally, one leg is involved unilaterally for up to 7 days before the other.[35,36] Very painful lesions may cause the child to limp. About 25% of children have a prodrome of sore throat and fever.[34–36] Lymphadenitis occurs in 3% of children, but in contrast to adult cases, joint symptoms are uncommon.[35,36] Cough or other respiratory symptoms may be present in children with associated tuberculosis, coccidioidomycosis, or histoplasmosis.[35–37] Coexisting chronic inflammatory bowel disease may cause bloody diarrhea and weight loss although EN may be the first manifestation of inflammatory bowel disease. In 4% of children, a history of a similar previous episode of EN is obtained.[36]

Tuberculosis was the infectious agent most commonly associated with EN until the mid-twentieth century, but it is now a far less common cause than streptococci.[38] EN is also associated with coccidioidomycosis and histoplasmosis, particularly in endemic areas. Other infectious agents such as mumps and yersinia have been associated.[36,38] Sulfonamides and oral contraceptives are the only drugs convincingly associated with the occurrence of EN in childhood.[34–36] An association with chronic inflammatory bowel disease is also well recognized. EN in adults has been associated with pregnancy,[39] sarcoidosis, blastomycosis, cat-scratch disease, and lymphoreticular malignancies, but such associations in children are not well documented. Many cases of EN are idiopathic.

PHYSICAL EXAMINATION

Erythema nodosum typically presents as a number of erythematous nodules with irregular or indistinct borders on the extensor surfaces of the lower legs (Fig. 17.4).[35,36] Lesions present for more than 4 days appear dull red, and those more than 10 days old have a brown or bruised character.[34] The evolution of lesions is much like that of a bruise. They heal without ulceration or scarring. Lesions have been well described on the trunk, the upper extremities, and the head and neck in adults, and this distribution may occasionally be seen in infancy and childhood.[38] Careful attention should be paid to examination of the respiratory system because of the association of EN with infectious agents of the upper and lower respiratory tract.

LABORATORY FINDINGS

The erythrocyte sedimentation rate is virtually always elevated in children with EN.[35,36] A few children have leukocytosis. A throat culture for streptococci and serologic tests for the presence of streptococcal infection are useful. A chest radiograph should be obtained to rule out pulmonary disease, including sarcoidosis, tuberculosis, coccidioidomycosis, and histoplasmosis. A stool culture and serology for *Yersinia* infection are warranted if symptoms exist.[38] Other laboratory investigations and investigational procedures, such as endoscopy, may be indicated by the history and physical examination.

PATHOPHYSIOLOGY AND HISTOGENESIS

Erythema nodosum is a septal panniculitis without vasculitis.[40] In early lesions, neutrophils and lymphocytes are observed in the fibrous septa, periseptal fat lobules, and around subcutaneous vessels. The overlying dermis often shows a mild, lymphocytic perivascular infiltrate. Abscess formation or fat necrosis are not observed. In lesions more than four days old, neutrophils are absent from the infiltrate, and a lymphocytic infiltrate predominates; this eventually

35. Laurance B, Stone GH, Philpott MG et al. (1961) Aetiology of erythema nodosum in children. **Lancet** 2:14–16.
36. Doxiadis SA (1951) Erythema nodosum in children. **Medicine** (Baltimore) 30:283.
37. Ozols II, Wheat LJ (1981) Erythema nodosum in an epidemic of histoplasmosis in Indianapolis. **Arch Dermatol** 117:709–712.
38. Labbe L, Perel Y, Maleville J et al. (1996) Erythema nodosum in children: a study of 27 patients. **Pediatr Dermatol** 136:447–450.
39. Salvatore MA, Lynch PJ (1980) Erythema nodosum, estrogens, and pregnancy. **Arch Dermatol** 116:557–558.
40. Requena L, Sanchez E (2001) Panniculitis. **J Am Acad Dermatol** 45:163–183.

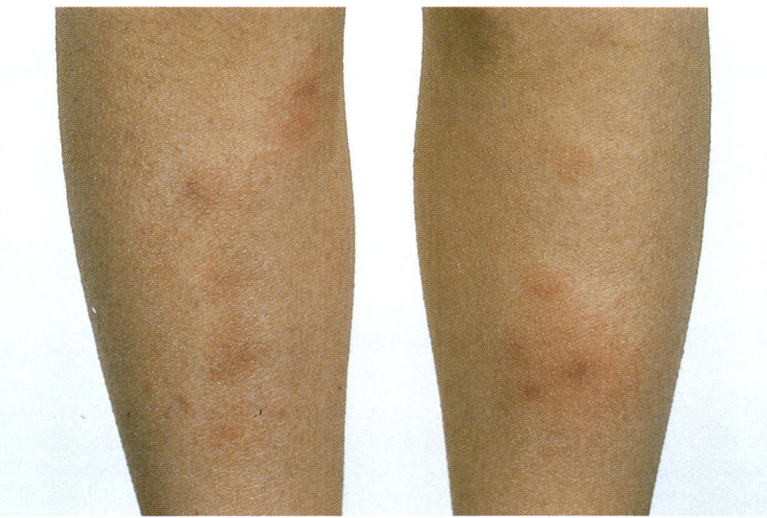

Fig. 17.4 Erythema nodosum: dusky red nodules over the anterior surface of the lower legs.

evolves into granulomatous infiltration with the presence of giant cells. Miescher's radial granulomas are considered a histopathologic hallmark of EN and may be present in evolving or fully developed lesions.[40]

It is believed that EN is a cutaneous reactive response to a variety of possible antigenic stimuli.[40] During epidemics of coccidioidomycosis or histoplasmosis, about 5% of infected children develop EN.[34,37] In addition, the timing of the lesions corresponds to the time it might require to develop a host response to the infectious organism. There is no good explanation for localization of the lesions to the anterior lower legs, but thermal and mechanical factors have been hypothesized.[36]

DIFFERENTIAL DIAGNOSIS

Erythema nodosum may be confused with other processes involving the subcutaneous fat. The location of thrombophlebitis on the flexor rather than the extensor aspect of the leg is a helpful differentiating sign. Early lesions of necrobiosis lipoidica diabeticorum are not tender and have a slow rather than an abrupt onset. Skin lesions of polyarteritis nodosa are associated with a mottled livedo pattern of the surrounding skin and discontinuous livedo in nonlesional sites elsewhere. Factitial panniculitis may also produce red nodules in the skin. Careful inspection for a puncture wound and a period of observation may help establish this diagnosis. Psychogenic purpura (Gardner–Diamond syndrome) should be considered but this is an unusual location and lesions are not tender. Lupus panniculitis (profundus) can mimic EN, although lesions rarely involve the lower legs. Pancreatic fat necrosis, including lupus erythematosus (LE)-induced pancreatic fat necrosis can also mimic EN. Hypersensitivity to biting and stinging insects may produce giant insect bite reactions on the lower legs. The clinical history, presence of pruritus, and observation of a central punctum are helpful in differentiating this condition. Bacterial cellulitis may be confused with EN if lesions are unilateral. Lesions on the soles of the feet that resemble EN are seen in palmar plantar hidradenitis of childhood.[41,42] The cutaneous nodules seen in Behçet syndrome represent a panniculitis that is histologically different from EN and are often associated with vasculitis.[40]

THERAPY AND PROGNOSIS

EN in children is a self-limited disease, usually resolving after 2–4 weeks.[34–37] Rarely, it may have a chronic or recurrent course. In circumstances in which an associated infectious agent can be identified, appropriate antimicrobial therapy should be instituted. If sulfonamides or birth control pills are suspected as precipitating factors, they should be discontinued. A nonsteroidal anti-inflammatory drug such as indomethacin (indometacin) or naproxen may be indicated for analgesia and to reduce inflammation. Indomethacin has been reported to be more efficacious than other nonsteroidal anti-inflammatory drugs in adults.[43] A short, 24- to 48-hour period of bed rest may be most useful. Supportive bandaging may also serve to reduce edema and give symptomatic relief. For chronic, recurrent EN, supersaturated potassium iodide 2–10 drops tid is effective.[44] Systemic corticosteroids are rarely indicated in children with EN.

PEDIATRIC ASPECTS OF THE DISEASE

The limping child has to be restricted in school or physical activities for 10–14 days. The impact of EN is usually limited to this two-week period unless the disorder is recurrent, in which case it can cause more long-term disability. Restrictions imposed by an associated infectious process or inflammatory bowel disease may be limiting.

Erythema induratum of Bazin

Erythema induratum is a lobular granulomatous panniculitis associated with vasculitis. It was first described in association with tuberculosis and is still considered a tuberculid.[45] It presents as nodular lesions, predominantly on the lower legs, that are indistinguishable from idiopathic nodular vasculitis.

EPIDEMIOLOGY

Erythema induratum is most commonly seen on the lower legs of adult women. It is rarely reported in children.[45]

PRESENTING HISTORY

The recurrent tender nodules have a predilection for the posterior lower legs but may occur on the upper limbs and buttocks. There may rarely be an associated fever and/or symptoms of *Mycobacterium tuberculosis* infection. Many patients otherwise appear healthy and have no clinical symptoms of tuberculosis. There may be a history of travel or contact with an individual with active tuberculosis.

PHYSICAL EXAMINATION

Erythematous to violaceous papules and nodules are seen mostly on the calves but occasionally on the upper extremities, face, feet, thighs, and buttocks. The lesions frequently ulcerate. Nodules and ulceration persist for weeks or months before healing, and continue to recur unless treated. The physical examination is often otherwise normal. An intradermal tuberculin test is typically positive.

LABORATORY EXAMINATION

Chest radiography is indicated to look for pulmonary infiltrates or hilar adenopathy. Gastric aspirates and sputum cultures are less helpful in the diagnosis of tuberculosis in children than in adults.[45]

41. Hern AE, Shwayder TA (1992) Unilateral plantar erythema nodosum. **J Am Acad Dermatol** 26:259–260.
42. Naimer SA, Zvulunov A, Ben-Amitai D et al. (2000) Plantar hidradenitis in children induced by exposure to wet footwear. **Pediatr Emerg Care** 16:182–183.
43. Ubogy Z, Persellin RH (1983) Suppression of erythema nodosum by indomethacin. **Acta Derm Venereol** (Stockh) 62:265–267.
44. Sterling JB, Heymann WR (2000) Potassium iodide in dermatology: a 19th century drug for the 21st century – uses, pharmacology, adverse effects, and contraindications. **J Am Acad Dermatol** 43:691–697.
45. Chang MW, Lawrence R, Orlow SL (1999) Erythema induratum of Bazin in an infant. **Pediatrics** 103:498–500.

PATHOPHYSIOLOGY AND HISTOGENESIS

Histopathologic examination of a nodule shows a lobular granulomatous panniculitis with fat necrosis. There is also septal panniculitis and vasculitis with chronic inflammation and fibrosis. Tubercle bacilli are rarely found in the skin lesions either by special stains or tissue culture. In some cases *M. tuberculosis* DNA may be detected by polymerase chain reaction.

A tuberculid is believed to result from a hypersensitivity reaction to antigenic particles of tubercle bacilli that arrive in the skin by hematogenous spread. This theory is supported by the finding of *M. tuberculosis* DNA in skin specimens.[45]

DIFFERENTIAL DIAGNOSIS

Erythema induratum must be distinguished from EN and other forms of panniculitis. Erythema nodosum typically involves the anterior, rather than posterior, lower legs and does not ulcerate. The absence of vasculitis in EN is a further distinguishing feature. Erythema induratum of Bazin may be considered a subset of nodular vasculitis, of which many cases are idiopathic.

THERAPY AND PROGNOSIS

A standard course of antituberculous therapy is curative in patients with clinical evidence of tuberculosis, a strongly positive intradermal tuberculin test, or when *M. tuberculosis* DNA is detected in the skin.

PEDIATRIC ASPECTS OF THE DISEASE

The rarity of erythema induraturn and nodular vasculitis in childhood may cause it to be underrecognized.[45] A high index of suspicion and careful evaluation for underlying disease is essential.

Cold panniculitis

Cold panniculitis (also known as popsicle panniculitis and equestrian panniculitis) is a condition in which cold injury causes erythematous plaques and subcutaneous nodules. It occurs most often in infants and children. It may be more common in black infants.[46] Exposure to frigid air, contact with cold objects such as popsicles, and use of ice packs and cooling blankets before cardiac surgery, or to treat cardiac arrhythmia, have all been implicated as precipitating agents.[46–48] It may also be seen on the thighs and buttocks of young women who ride horseback,[49] or on the inner thighs of hikers walking in cold air wearing light clothing.

PRESENTING HISTORY

The characteristic lesion is a persistent, nontender erythematous nodule. Lesions associated with popsicle injury occur on one or both cheeks. A history of popsicle ingestion, application of cold objects to the skin, or exposure to frigid air should be sought. In young horseback riders, similar lesions may appear on the buttocks or thighs.[49] A recent history of hypothermia induction before cardiac surgery is relevant if subcutaneous fat necrosis develops on the trunk or upper limbs.[48]

PHYSICAL EXAMINATION

The red-purple, indurated nodules on the cheeks of infants and toddlers with popsicle panniculitis have a firm, rubbery consistency and are usually nontender. They may be unilateral or bilateral. The overlying skin is intact,

and there is no epidermal change. The child is usually otherwise healthy. In panniculitis associated with hypothermia related to cardiac surgery, the clinical picture is indistinguishable from that of subcutaneous fat necrosis of the newborn with generalized lesions on the dorsal trunk and limbs.[48]

LABORATORY FINDINGS

No pathologic cold agglutins, cold hemolysins, cryoglobulins, or other laboratory abnormalities are detected in infants or children with localized cold panniculitis.[47]

PATHOPHYSIOLOGY AND HISTOGENESIS

Increased sensitivity of the subcutaneous fat of young infants to cold injury is believed to be due to a higher concentration of saturated fatty acids than is found in later childhood and adult life.[52] Saturated fats have a propensity to solidify at higher temperatures and briefer exposure to cold than unsaturated fats. Application of ice or popsicles may reproduce the lesions.[47] Histologically, cold panniculitis is characterized by fat necrosis; thickening of septa with plump fibroblasts, a few foam cells, neutrophils, and eosinophils.[40]

DIFFERENTIAL DIAGNOSIS

Localized fat necrosis, such as popsicle panniculitis, must be distinguished from bacterial cellulitis, trauma, and frostbite.[47] All of these conditions are associated with pain or tenderness. Facial cellulitis is usually accompanied by fever and systemic symptoms. Epidermal changes, sometimes with vesiculation, are seen in cases of frostbite. Hypothermia-induced lesions that are clinically indistinguishable from subcutaneous fat necrosis may lack the characteristic histopathologic findings of fat crystals and calcium deposition.[48,50]

THERAPY AND PROGNOSIS

Cold panniculitis resolves without sequelae in a few weeks to a few months.[47] No intervention is recommended. In the case of popsicle panniculitis, avoiding the use of popsicles and general cold avoidance strategies should be effective.

Subcutaneous fat necrosis of the newborn

Fat necrosis of the subcutaneous tissues during the first few weeks of life is a disorder of unknown cause.[50] It occurs in full-term or postmature neonates. There is often a history of a difficult delivery or induced hypothermia.[51] The usual age of onset is at 1–6 weeks of age, but it may be seen in the first week.

PRESENTING HISTORY

Firm, red to violaceous, asymptomatic nodules occur in an otherwise healthy newborn. They are not usually present at birth. Sites of predilection are the cheeks, shoulders, back, buttocks, thighs, and legs. There is no limitation of movement even in cases with extensive involvement.

PHYSICAL EXAMINATION

The lesions are often symmetrical, variably circumscribed nodules with a red to violaceous color (Fig. 17.5A,B). Some lesions have a woody hard induration and may develop calcification. The affected areas are freely mobile

46. Ter Poorten JC, Hebert AA, Ilkiw R (1995) Cold panniculitis in a neonate. **J Am Acad Dermatol** 33:383–385.
47. Day S, Klein BL (1992) Popsicle panniculitis. **Pediatr Emerg Care** 8:91–93.
48. Silverman AK, Michels EH, Rasmussen JE (1986) Subcutaneous fat necrosis in an infant, occurring after hypothermic cardiac surgery. Case report and analysis of etiologic factors. **J Am Acad Dermatol** 15:331–336.
49. Beacham BE, Cooper PH, Buchanan CS et al. (1980) Equestrian cold panniculitis in women. **Arch Dermatol** 116:1025–1027.
50. Fretzin DF, Arias AM (1987) Sclerema neonatorum and subcutaneous fat necrosis of the newborn. **Pediatr Dermatol** 4:112–122.
51. Burden AD, Krafchik BR (1999) Subcutaneous fat necrosis of the newborn: a review of 11 cases. **Pediatr Dermatol** 16:384–387.

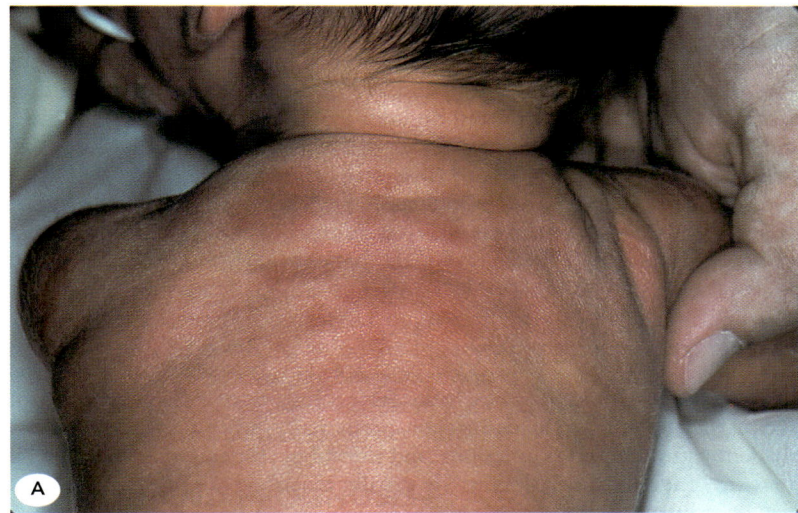

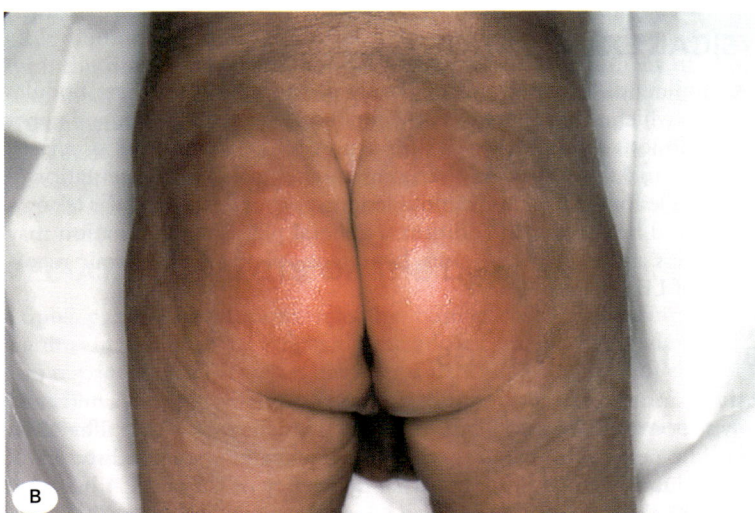

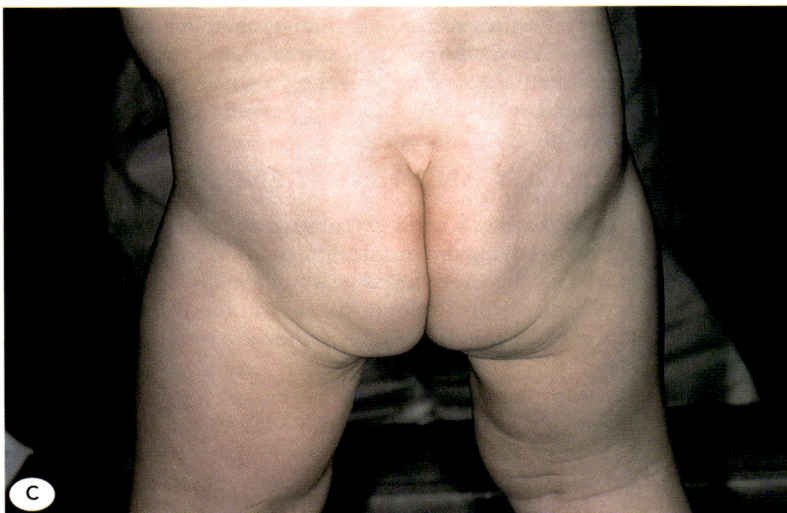

Fig. 17.5   (A) Subcutaneous fat necrosis of the newborn. (B) Subcutaneous fat necrosis, buttocks. (C) Subcutaneous fat necrosis one year later.

over the underlying tissues.[50] Larger nodules may become fluctuant and occasionally ulcerate, discharging an oleaginous material through the skin. Some depression or atrophy of the affected areas may develop (Fig. 17.5C), and a brownish discoloration may replace the original inflammatory appearance. Infants with subcutaneous fat necrosis should be observed for signs and symptoms of hypercalcemia, which can take up to five months to develop.[51,53,56]

LABORATORY INVESTIGATIONS

Fat necrosis of the newborn has been associated with hypercalcemia.[51,53,54] This was fatal in three cases. Serum calcium levels should therefore be monitored in these infants. Radiographic studies may show evidence of calcification in the subcutis.[50] A rare case of calcinosis of the kidneys has been described accompanying hypercalcemia.

PATHOPHYSIOLOGY AND HISTOGENESIS

The subcutaneous tissues show a lobular panniculitis with crystallization of fat.[40,50] Needle-like clefts are surrounded by a granulomatous inflammatory cell infiltrate that extends into the fibrous septa. Deposits of calcium may be seen. The cause and pathogenesis of the subcutaneous fat necrosis are unknown. Obstetric trauma, hypothermia, maternal diabetes mellitus, perinatal respiratory distress or asphyxia, and pre-eclamptic toxemia of pregnancy have been implicated as associated factors.[51] Ten of 11 cases in one study had a cesarian section.[51] Differences in the composition of neonatal adipose tissue resulting in abnormal adaptation to cold exposure have been considered to be a significant predisposing factor. Similar lesions may be induced by hypothermia, although these do not appear to show the characteristic crystallization of fat.[48,52] The association between fat necrosis and hypercalcemia is not well understood.[51]

DIFFERENTIAL DIAGNOSIS

Subcutaneous fat necrosis of the newborn must be distinguished from sclerema neonatorum and other forms of panniculitis. Sclerema neonatorum is associated with diffuse hardening of the skin in an infant who is premature, debilitated, and often moribund. Although needle-like clefts may be seen histologically, sclerema lacks the associated inflammatory response seen in subcutaneous fat necrosis of the newborn.[50] Some authors believe them to be variants of the same disease.[51] Traumatic panniculitis induced by forceps delivery might also be confused.

THERAPY AND PROGNOSIS

Treatment of subcutaneous fat necrosis is usually unnecessary. Most infants have an excellent prognosis with complete resolution of lesions within the first few months of life. Liquefaction and dystrophic calcification of larger lesions may result in more persistent nodules. Subcutaneous atrophy occasionally occurs. Hypercalcemia, if present, may result in a fatal outcome and should be actively treated.[51,52,54] Current treatment includes hydration, furosemide, and corticosteroids.[55] The use of biphosphonates to treat hypercalcemia associated with subcutaneous fat necrosis of the newborn is controversial.[55,56]

Sclerema neonatorum

In the past, there was considerable confusion between sclerema neonatorum and subcutaneous fat necrosis of the newborn. They are presently classified as distinct disorders, although the distinction could be a result of disease severity.[51] They have been observed together in the same infant.[57]

52. Chuang S-D, Chiu H-C, Chang C-C (1995) Subcutaneous fat necrosis of the newborn complicating hypothermic cardiac surgery. Br J Dermatol 132:805–810.
53. Norwood-Galloway A, Lebwohl M, Phelps RG et al. (1987) Subcutaneous fat necrosis of the newborn with hypercalcemia. J Am Acad Dermatol 16:435–439.
54. Fernandez-Lopez E, Garcia-Dorado J, de Unamuno P et al. (1990) Subcutaneous fat necrosis of the newborn and idiopathic hypercalcemia. Dermatologica 180:250.
55. Rice AM, Rivkees SA (1999) Etidronate therapy for hypercalcemia in subcutaneous fat necrosis of the newborn. J Pediatr 134:349–351.
56. Bachrach LK, Lum CK (1999) Etidronate in subcutaneous fat necrosis of the newborn. J Pediatr 135:530.
57. Jardine D, Atherton DJ, Trumpeter RS (1990) Sclerema neonatorum and subcutaneous fat necrosis of the newborn in the same infant. Eur J Paediatr 150:125–126.

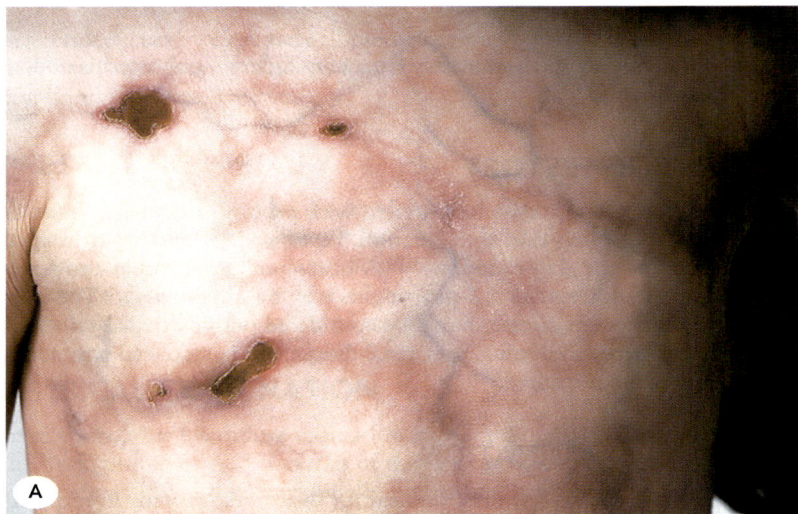
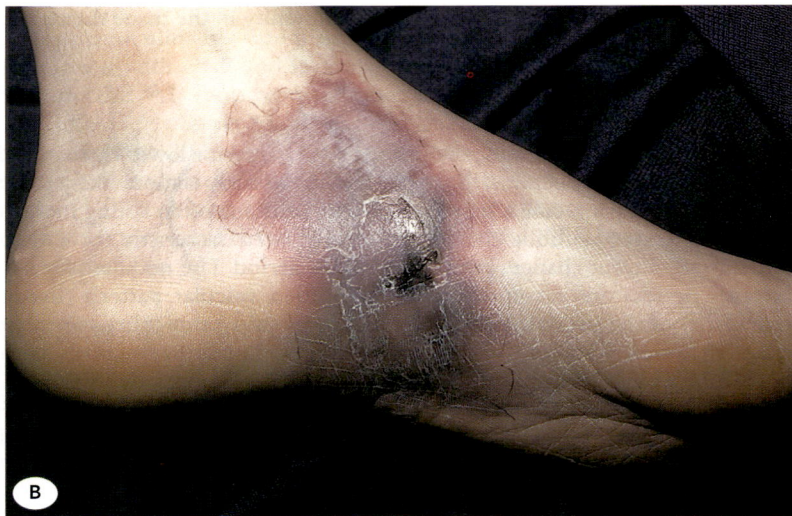

Fig. 17.6   (A) Linear dusky red nodules of cutaneous polyarteritis nodosa on the body of a six-year-old child. (B) Eroded lesion of polyarteritis nodosa.

An infectious agent is suspected as an initiating factor in polyarteritis nodosa. Hepatitis B and C have been implicated in systemic PAN in adults.[80,83] In chronic cutaneous polyarteritis nodosa in children, streptococcal-associated disease has been reported.[77,79] Circulating immune complexes generated as a response to an infectious agent, such as *Streptococcus*, may injure cutaneous vessels, fix complement, and attract neutrophils with subsequent damage to the subcutaneous blood vessels. Other immune mechanisms may modify or amplify the inflammatory response.

DIFFERENTIAL DIAGNOSIS

Erythema nodosum may be confused with the cutaneous findings of polyarteritis nodosa and both can be associated with arthritis. The mottled, purple-red appearance of the skin in polyarteritis nodosa with segmental and linear nodules, rather than the round nodules of EN, is a useful distinguishing feature. In lupus panniculitis, the upper half of the body is involved rather than the lower extremities. Cold panniculitis may also mimic cutaneous polyarteritis nodosa but has a different distribution. Factitial panniculitis can result in linear nodules similar to polyarteritis nodosa, and careful inspection of the nodule surface for a punctum or injection site is mandatory. In factitial panniculitis, usually only one acute lesion is present, whereas many are present simultaneously in polyarteritis nodosa.

THERAPY AND PROGNOSIS

The course of cutaneous polyarteritis nodosa in childhood is often one of relapses, each lasting six weeks to six months, with a chronic course.[70,71] The long-term outlook is uncertain. In adults, the disorder may remain chronic and limited to the skin, only to have systemic involvement appear years later. One should therefore consider cutaneous polyarteritis nodosa as part of the spectrum of systemic polyarteritis nodosa, just as discoid skin lesions may be observed in SLE.

A beneficial response to aspirin alone has been reported in one childhood case of cutaneous disease; another patient required the addition of low-dose alternate-day prednisolone.[70,71] Other nonsteroidal agents may be beneficial. Intravenous immunoglobulin therapy has been found to be effective.[86] If streptococcal infection is identified as an associated factor, prompt treatment of upper respiratory infections with appropriate antibiotics, such as penicillin,

is recommended and these may have to be maintained over a long period. Systemic steroids and/or cyclophosphamide are the treatments of choice for systemic disease. The mortality rate for systemic polyarteritis nodosa in children may be as high as 16%.[67]

PEDIATRIC ASPECTS OF THE DISEASE

The disease may restrict the physical activities of the child because of painful skin nodules or associated systemic disease. One child utilized her disease for school absenteeism as part of a school phobia.[71] The psychological burden of a chronic relapsing disease can have a significant emotional impact on the child.

Factitial panniculitis

Factitial panniculitis is a condition in which red or purple-red nodules result from injection of foreign material into the fat layer.[87–89] Beerman[84] first appreciated that at least some patients with the diagnosis of Weber–Christian panniculitis had factitial panniculitis due to subcutaneous injection. Ackerman *et al.*[87] published the first well-documented case of self-injection producing factitial panniculitis in a child.

EPIDEMIOLOGY

Factitial panniculitis has been recognized most frequently in female patients.[87–90] It is usually seen in adolescence or pre-adolescence rather than in young children. There is no racial predilection.

PRESENTING HISTORY

Frequently, a history of visits to many different doctors is obtained. Invariably, trauma or injection is denied. The history of the present illness is highly variable and often contradictory from visit to visit or from doctor to doctor. The appearance of the lesions varies, as well as their duration.[87–90] Often, the psychosocial history is most revealing, with family separation, death, conflict, or other emotional upsets being events preceding the onset of the skin lesions. Asking the patient, "Do you know the cause of these lumps?" may result in important clues. The lesions are an attention-gaining strategy in a child whose emotional needs are not being met. In small children, factitial lesions should always raise the possibility of Munchausen syndrome by proxy.[91]

86. Uziel Y, Silverman ED (1998) Intravenous immunoglobulin therapy in a child with cutaneous polyarteritis nodosa. **Clin Exp Rheumatol** 16:187–189.
87. Ackermann AB, Mosher DT, Schwamm HA (1966) Factitial Weber-Christian syndrome. **JAMA** 198:731–736.
88. Lyell A (1979) Cutaneous artefactual disease. **J Am Acad Dermatol** 1:391–407.
89. Spraker MK (1983) Cutaneous artefactual disease, an appeal for help. **Pediatr Clin North Am** 30:659–668.
90. Beerman H (1953) Weber-Christian syndrome. **Am J Med** 225:446.
91. Bools CN, Neale BA, Meadow SR (1992) Co-morbidity associated with fabricated illness (Munchausen syndrome by proxy). **Arch Dis Child** 67:77–79.

PHYSICAL EXAMINATION

Red or bruise-like nodules of different ages are noted, usually on the anterior legs. Usually, only one lesion is in the red, acute inflammatory stage, but numerous older lesions may be present. Careful inspection may reveal an injection site, but this can easily be missed, particularly if only older lesions are present. Observation in a hospital situation may be required. Direct observation of injection is the most definitive measure in making the diagnosis. An important clue is the indifferent affect of the patient toward the illness. Some patients may be withdrawn or reclusive. Low-grade fever may follow an injection, but arthralgias and other systemic systems are conspicuously absent.

LABORATORY FINDINGS

All laboratory findings are usually normal, including the erythrocyte sedimentation rate and the white blood cell count.[87–89] Normal laboratory test results in the face of active inflammation should make one suspect factitial disease.

PATHOPHYSIOLOGY AND HISTOGENESIS

The response of the fat layer is inflammatory, and the character of the response is determined by the nature of the injected material. Milk, feces, mineral oil, paraffin, silicone, and pentazocine have all been reported to be injected.[87–90,92]

Focal necrosis of fat and a neutrophilic accumulation may be observed. Hemorrhage, infiltration with lymphocytes, and foreign body giant cells may be present. A biopsy of a late lesion shows considerable fibrosis of the fat layer. In addition, birefringent particles may be present in the fat layer.[40] In every biopsy in which factitial panniculitis is suspected, examination with polarized light is recommended. Occasionally, the material contains pigment, and bizarre pigmented areas are observed in the fat layer. The absence of inflammation of the blood vessels is an important histologic clue to the possibility of factitial panniculitis.

DIFFERENTIAL DIAGNOSIS

Factitial panniculitis may be diagnosed as Weber–Christian panniculitis.[40] Erythema nodosum often has several red nodules present in the same stage, whereas factitial panniculitis usually has only one. The presence of arthritis and an elevated erythrocyte sedimentation rate are suggestive of erythema nodosum. In cutaneous polyarteritis nodosa, a mottled pattern of the skin is helpful. In all circumstances, an excisional biopsy of a nodular lesion is recommended. Biopsy of both an early and a late lesion may be good strategy to help find foreign body giant cells in late lesions and foreign materials in early lesions.

THERAPY AND PROGNOSIS

Therapy is primarily psychiatric. Supportive care for the area of panniculitis includes keeping the weight off the area and rest. Understanding that this represents an emotional problem and being supportive of the child are essential for the clinician. The lesions heal once injections are stopped, but those with severe fat necrosis may heal with atrophy of the fat layer.[87,90,92] Longterm psychiatric care is often required.

PEDIATRIC ASPECTS OF THE DISEASE

The emotional problem leading to factitial panniculitis may also influence school performance, interaction with peers, and physical activities.[88,89] The psychiatric and emotional aspects of this disease predominate over the clinical picture.

Please see Chapter 2 for additional treatment of psychocutaneous disorders.

α_1-Antitrypsin deficiency

α_1-Antitrypsin is a serine protease inhibitor that regulates the action of proteolytic enzymes, including elastase and collagenase.[40] There are more than 33 different alleles for this enzyme, each of which is designated by a letter of the alphabet.[93] In any individual, two of these combine to determine the α_1-antitrypsin phenotype.[94] There is thus a spectrum of enzyme phenotypes from the homozygous MM phenotype, present in most of the population, to the homozygous ZZ variant, which has the lowest plasma levels of α_1-antitrypsin activity.[93] α_1-Antitrypsin deficiency is inherited as an autosomal codominant disorder, with each inherited allele being of equal importance in determining the phenotype. It has been linked principally to emphysema and liver disease. An association with panniculitis was recognized in 1972.[95]

EPIDEMIOLOGY

Most reported cases of panniculitis have occurred in adults,[94–96] but there have been reports of α_1-antitrypsin deficiency presenting as panniculitis in childhood and adolescence.[93,94,97,99] Familial occurrence has been documented.[94]

CLINICAL FEATURES

Lesions are located on the trunk or extremities and present as recurrent painful, ulcerated, subcutaneous nodules that drain an oily serosanguineous fluid. The lesions may be mistaken for bacterial cellulitis. There is often a history of preceding trauma.

PATHOGENESIS AND HISTOGENESIS

The typical histopathologic features are those of an acute lobular panniculitis with numerous neutrophils and necrosis of fat.[40,100] There are often large areas of normal panniculus adjacent to necrotic fat lobules. Hemorrhage and an inflammatory infiltrate may be present at the periphery of the area of panniculitis. Histiocytes and foam cells may be seen. Vasculitis does not occur. Older lesions show lymphocytes, foamy macrophages, and varying degrees of fibrosis.[101]

The mechanisms whereby α_1-antitrypsin deficiency leads to panniculitis are not fully understood. The histopathologic changes of liquefactive necrosis of fat and inflammation may be explained by lack of inhibition of proteolytic enzymes, which results in dissolution of collagen in the dermis and fibrous septa of the subcutis.[93] Lack of neutral proteases that modulate inflammation and chemotaxis may also be implicated.[40]

92. Forstrom L, Winklemann RK (1974) Factitial panniculitis. Arch Dermatol 110:747–750.
93. Edmonds BK, Hodge JA, Rietschel RL (1991) Alpha 1-antitrypsin deficiency-associted panniculitis: case report and review of the literature. Pediatr Dermatol 8:296–299.
94. Breit SN, Clark P, Robinson JP et al. (1983) Familial occurrence of alpha 1-antitrypsin deficiency and Weber-Christian disease. Arch Dermatol 119:198–202.
95. Warter J, Storck D, Grosshans E et al. (1972) Syndrome de Weber-Christian associé a un déficit en alpha 1-antitrypsine. Enquete familiale. Ann Med Interne (Paris) 123:877–882.
96. Smith KC, Su WPD, Pittelkow MR et al. (1989) Clinical and pathologic correlations in 96 patients with panniculitis, including 15 patients with deficient levels of alpha 1-antitrypsin. J Am Acad Dermatol 21:1192–1196.
97. Hendrick SJ, Silverman AK, Solomon AR et al. (1988) Alpha 1-antitrypsin deficiency associated with panniculitis. J Am Acad Dermatol 18:684–692.
98. Smith KC, Pittelkow MR, Su WPD (1987) Panniculitis associated with severe alpha-1 antitrypsin deficiency. Arch Dermatol 123:1655–1661.
99. Chng WJ, Henderson CA (2001) Suppurative panniculitis associated with alpha 1-antitrypsin deficiency (PiSZ phenotype) treated with doxycycline. Br J Dermatol 144:1282–1283.
100. Geller JD, Su WPD (1994) A subtle clue to the histologic diagnosis of early alpha 1-antitrypsin deficiency. J Am Acad Dermatol 31:241–245.
101. Requena L, Sanchez Yus E (2001) Panniculitis. J Am Acad Dermatol 45:325–361.

LABORATORY TESTS

The diagnosis is established by the finding of decreased quantitative serum levels of α_1-antitrypsin. Enzyme phenotyping may also be useful.

DIFFERENTIAL DIAGNOSIS

A combination of panniculitis with ulceration and consistent histopathologic findings should raise the possibility of α_1-antitrypsin deficiency. Factitial panniculitis may be considered in the differential diagnosis because of the presence of ulceration. Ulceration also occurs in pancreatic panniculitis, but the histologic features of this disease are distinctive with fat necrosis, presence of "ghost cells," and saponification. A history of trauma may be misleading and suggest a diagnosis of traumatic fat necrosis or bacterial infection. An infectious cause should always be excluded because α_1-antitrypsin deficiency resembles cellulitis clinically and may have a heavy neutrophilic infiltrate.[40]

TREATMENT

Dapsone is the traditional treatment of choice.[96] Doxycycline and colchicine are also reported to be effective.[99,102] Infusion of proteinase inhibitor concentrate obtained from healthy donors has been used.[98] Corticosteroids and antibiotics are ineffective, and surgical debridement may be detrimental.

Poststeroid panniculitis

Poststeroid panniculitis is a very rare complication of tapering or stopping systemic steroids.[103,104] It has been reported in children receiving long-term, high-dose steroids.

CLINICAL FEATURES

Lesions are tender, erythematous nodules seen during tapering or cessation of systemic steroids. Lesions develop on the cheeks, arms, trunk, or jawline.[103]

PATHOGENESIS AND HISTOGENESIS

The histopathologic features are similar to those of subcutaneous fat necrosis of the newborn.[101] The needle-like clefts are not as numerous as in the newborn disease. The pathogenesis is poorly understood. It is possible that withdrawal of steroids upsets the normal ratio of saturated and unsaturated fat in the panniculus, leading to crystal formation.[103]

THERAPY AND PROGNOSIS

The lesions usually resolve spontaneously with time.[101] A temporary increase in dose and slower tapering of the systemic steroid may be necessary.

Cytophagic histiocytic panniculitis

This entity was first described in 1980 by Winkelmann and Bowie as *histiocytic cytophagic panniculitis*.[104] It is associated with the hemophagocytic syndrome.[105–109] Some cases have been associated with Epstein–Barr virus infection.[109] Although cytophagic histiocytic panniculitis may sometimes follow a benign course, there is convincing evidence that this disorder belongs within the spectrum of malignant T-cell lymphoma.[106,108,109] The term *panniculitis-like subcutaneous T-cell lymphoma with cytophagocytosis* is considered more appropriate by some authors.[109] It is characterized histopathologically by histiocytosis and hemophagocytosis in the skin, subcutaneous fat, and other organs.[40,101] Clinically, it presents as inflammatory subcutaneous nodules associated with fever, serositis, hepatosplenomegaly, lymphadenopathy, and an often fatal hemorrhagic diathesis. Childhood cases have been reported.[107,110–114]

PRESENTING FEATURES

The condition presents with painful, indurated, inflammatory skin nodules associated with fever and malaise. There is often ulceration of the skin overlying the nodules and plaques. The disease may be initially localized to one body area and later become generalized. The initial sites of involvement were the face in two children and the gluteal region and thigh in two others.[110–112] Mucosal ulceration may also occur.

LABORATORY FINDINGS

Anemia, leukopenia, and a coagulopathy are associated laboratory findings. Liver function tests may also be abnormal. The patient should be investigated for Epstein–Barr virus infection. They also have high LDH, ferritin and triglyceride abnormalities.

PATHOPHYSIOLOGY AND HISTOGENESIS

The histology is characterized by a lobular panniculitis consisting of a lymphocytic infiltrate admixed with histiocytes that phagocytose erythrocytes, leukocytes, and platelets.[40,101] These large phagocytic cells are termed "beanbag" histiocytes and have been found in other organs at autopsy. There is evidence that, despite the often apparently benign appearance of the cellular infiltrate, this is a clonal T-cell disorder and, in most cases, represents a variant of cutaneous T-cell lymphoma.[106,108,109]

DIFFERENTIAL DIAGNOSIS

The characteristic histologic findings distinguish this disease from other forms of panniculitis. Immunophenotyping and molecular genetic analysis should be performed to evaluate for T-cell lymphoma.[106]

TREATMENT

The disorder may be associated with a rapidly fatal hemophagocytic syndrome or run a more protracted course. Combination chemotherapy is the treatment of choice for subcutaneous T-cell lymphoma.[110,111,113] Children with more indolent disease have been treated successfully with cyclosporine or prednisone.[107,109] Death may occur despite treatment with systemic steroids and chemotherapy.[111,113]

102. Linnares-Barrios M, Conijo-Mir JS, Artola-Igarza JL et al. (1998) Panniculitis due to α_1-antitrypsin deficiency induced by cryosurgery. **Br J Dermatol** 138:552–553.
103. Reichel M, Diaz Cascajo C (1995) Bilateral jawline nodules in a child with a brain-stem glioma. **Arch Dermatol** 131:1447–1452.
104. Silverman RA, Newman AJ, LeVine MJ (1988) Post-steroid panniculitis: a case report. **Pediatr Dermatol** 5:92–93.
105. Winkelmann RK, Bowie EJW (1980) Hemorrhagic diathesis associated with benign histiocytic, cytophagic panniculitis and systemic histiocytosis. **Arch Intern Med** 140:1460–1463.
106. Hytiroglou P, Phelps RG, Wattenberg DJ et al. (1992) Histiocytic cytophagic panniculitis: molecular evidence for a clonal T-cell disorder. **J Am Acad Dermatol** 27:333–336.
107. Craig AJ, Cualing H, Thomas G et al. (1998) Cytophagic histiocytic panniculitis – a syndrome associated with benign and malignant panniculitis: case comparison and review of the literature. **J Am Acad Dermatol** 39:721–736.
108. Marzano AV, Berti E, Paulli M et al. (2001) Cytophagic histiocytic panniculitis and subcutaneous panniculitis-like T-cell lymphoma. **Arch Dermatol** 136:889–896.
109. Wick MR, Patterson JW (2000) Cytophagic histiocytic panniculitis – a critical reappraisal. **Arch Dermatol** 136:922–924.
110. Hung IJ, Kuo TT, Sun CF (1999) Subcutaneous panniculitic T-cell lymphoma developing in a child with idiopathic myelofibrosis. **J Pediatr Hem Onc** 21:38–41.
111. Chan YF, Lee KC, Llewellyn H (1994) Subcutaneous T-cell lymphoma presenting as panniculitis in children: report of 2 cases. **Pediatr Pathol** 14:595–608.
112. Labeille B, Pautard B, Pare F et al. (1990) Panniculite sévère pseudotumorale de l'enfant: panniculite: histiocytaire cytophagique? **Ann Dermatol Venerol** 117:807–808.
113. Garcia-Consuegra J, Barrio MI, Fonseca E et al. (1991) Histiocytic cytophagic panniculitis: report of a case in a 12-year-old girl. **Eur J Pediatr** 150:468–469.
114. Schuval SJ, Frances A, Valderrama E et al. (1993) Panniculitis and fever in children. **J Pediatr** 122:372–378.

Idiopathic and lipoatrophic panniculitis in childhood

The term *lipoatrophy* refers to loss of subcutaneous fat. It may appear without signs of preceding inflammation or in association with clinical or histologic evidence of panniculitis. This distinction is not always clear-cut.[115] Lipoatrophy is known to occur in lupus panniculitis, in panniculitis associated with morphea, and dermatomyositis,[116–118] and following injections and traumatic fat necrosis.[119] When these and other well-defined entities have been excluded, there remain a number of descriptions in the literature of idiopathic panniculitis, often associated with fever and/or subsequent development of lipoatrophy.[115] Other organ systems may also be involved. Many similar cases have been reported in the past as examples of Weber–Christian disease.[120,121]

Winkelmann[122] used the term "connective tissue panniculitis" to refer to a syndrome of recurrent, progressive, lobular lymphocytic panniculitis with intermittent low-grade fever. The term connective tissue panniculitis was justified by the finding of occasional positive ANA titers in the serum. The lymphoid nodules and hyaline necrosis of lupus panniculitis were not observed. Some lesions healed without sequelae, and others resulted in subcutaneous atrophy and cutaneous hyperpigmentation.

A potential association with autoimmune disease was also postulated by Billings *et al.*[123] who described three children with a lobular panniculitis that resulted in extensive lipoatrophy. Two of these children had associated low-grade fevers during episodes of panniculitis. Two patients had insulin-dependent diabetes mellitus, one child also had Hashimoto's thyroiditis, and in a third patient, juvenile rheumatiod arthritis developed.

There have been a number of cases of lipoatrophy described in the literature with different names. Whether these are variations of the same condition is not known. Winkelmann *et al.*[124] described three children with a lipophagic granulomatous lipoatrophy, which they termed lipophagic panniculitis of childhood. The histologic findings were those of a panlobular panniculitis with lipophagic histiocytes and giant cells. Two children had recurrent fever. One child had an elevated ANA titer. Fourteen similar cases previously reported as Weber–Christian disease were reviewed by these authors. This condition may be the same entity as cytophagic histiocytic panniculitis.

Solomon *et al.*[125] described a case of fever and recurrent lobular panniculitis in a child. The lymphocytic infiltrate in the subcutis consisted predominantly of suppressor-cytotoxic T lymphocytes. Associated lipoatrophy was not described. Roth *et al.*[126] reported panniculitis localized to the ankles with a lobular lymphohistiocytic infiltrate and masses of foam cells. There was associated annular lipoatrophy, and the authors termed this condition "annular atrophic connective tissue panniculitis of the ankles." Randle *et al.*[127] reported four children with idiopathic panniculitis, three of whom had a lobular panniculitis with subsequent lipoatrophy. These patients responded well to systemic corticosteroids. Sorensen *et al.*[121] reported a good response to hydroxychloroquine in a 10-year-old patient with infantile-onset "Weber–Christian" panniculitis and associated recurrent pneumonitis. Martinez *et al.*[128] postulated an association between extensive lipoatrophic panniculitis and a chromosome 10 abnormality in a 3-year-old girl because the human pancreatic lipase gene maps to chromosome 10q24–26.

The pathogenesis of these idiopathic forms of panniculitis and lipoatrophy is poorly understood.

Eosinophilic cellulitis

Eosinophilic cellulitis, or Wells syndrome, is a rare recurrent dermatosis characterized clinically by erythematous, urticarial plaques that resolve slowly with induration and a blue-black discoloration, and histologically by a distinctive pattern of tissue eosinophilia and the presence of flame figures.[129–142]

HISTORICAL ASPECTS

Eosinophilic cellulitis was described first by Wells in 1971 as "recurrent granulomatous dermatitis with eosinophilia." The term eosinophilic cellulitis was introduced by Wells and Smith[131] in 1979. Although these and later authors recognized that a dermal eosinophilic infiltrate with flame figures may be seen in other disorders, the term eosinophilic cellulitis is often used to designate this histologic pattern.[131,135,139] To avoid semantic confusion, some authors prefer the eponym, Wells syndrome, to denote the distinctive dermatosis.

EPIDEMIOLOGY

Eosinophilic cellulitis is a rare disorder. It has been described predominantly in adults but there have been reported cases in children.[134–138] The majority of childhood cases have been male, although there appears to be no sex preponderance in adults.[133,136] There is no known genetic predisposition. Eosinophilic cellulitis has been encountered in association with insect bites, bee stings, onchocerciasis, giardiasis, toxacariasis, varicella, mumps, drug reactions, malignancy, myeloproliferative disorders, atopic dermatitis, and *Trichophyton rubrum* infection.[131–133,136,137,140–142]

CLINICAL FEATURES

The clinical picture of eosinophilic cellulitis evolves through an acute, subacute, and chronic stage before eventual resolution. Lesions may occur on the extremities, face, or trunk. Similar episodes, often at the same anatomic

115. Aronson IK, Zeitz HJ, Variakojis D (1988) Panniculitis in childhood. Pediatr Dermatol 5:216–230.
116. Kavanagh G, Colaco CB, Kennedy CTC (1993) Juvenile dermatomyositis associated with partial lipoatrophy. J Am Acad Dermatol 28:348–351.
117. Commens C, O'Neill P, Walker G (1990) Dermatomyositis associated with multifocal lipoatrophy. J Am Acad Dermatol 22:966–969.
118. Ghali FE, Reed AM, Groben PA et al. (1999) Panniculitis in dermatomyositis. Pediatr Dermatol 16:270–272.
119. Dahl PR, Zalla MJ, Winkelmann RK (1996) Localized involutional lipoatrophy: a clinicopathologic study of 16 patients. J Am Acad Dermatol 35:523–528.
120. Sorensen RU, Abramowsky CR, Stern RC (1986) Ten-year course of early onset Weber-Christian syndrome with recurrent pneumonia: a suggestion for pathogenesis. Pediatrics 78:115–120.
121. Sorensen RU, Abramowsky CR, Stern RC (1990) Corticosteroid-sparing effect of hydroxychloroquine in a patient with early-onset Weber-Christian syndrome. J Am Acad Dermatol 23:1172–1174.
122. Winkelmann RK (1983) Panniculitis in connective tissue disease. Arch Dermatol 119:336–344.
123. Billings JK, Milgraum SS, Gupta AK et al. (1987) Lipoatrophic panniculitis: a possible autoimmune inflammatory disease of fat. Report of three cases. Arch Dermatol 123:1662–1666.
124. Winkelmann RK, McEvoy MT, Peters MS (1989) Lipophagic panniculitis of childhood. J Am Acad Dermatol 21:971–978.
125. Solomon AR, Kantak AG, Ramirez JE et al. (1986) Suppressor-cytotoxic T-lymphocyte panniculitis. Pediatr Dermatol 3:295–299.
126. Roth DE, Schikler KN, Callen JP (1989) Annular atrophic connective tissue panniculitis of the ankles. J Am Acad Dermatol 21:1152–1156.
127. Randle SM, Richter MB, Palmer RG et al. (1991) Panniculitis: report of four cases and literature review. Arch Dis Child 66:1057–1060.
128. Martinez A, Malone M, Hoeger P et al. (2000) Lipoatrophic panniculitis and chromosome 10 abnormality. Br J Dermatol 142:1034–1039.

129. Adame J, Cohen JA (1996) Eosinophilic panniculitis: diagnostic considerations and evaluation. J Am Acad Dermatol 34:229–234.
130. Pao W, Duncan KO, Bolognia JL et al. (1998) Numerous eruptive lesions of panniculitis associated with group A streptococcus bacteremia in an immunocompetent child. Clin Infect Dis 27:430–433.
131. Wells GC, Smith NP (1979) Eosinophilic cellulitis. Br J Dermatol 100:101–109.
132. Schorr WF, Tauscheck AL, Dickson KB et al. (1984) Eosinophilic cellulitis (Well's syndrome): histologic and clinical features in arthropod reactions. J Am Acad Dermatol 11:1043–1049.
133. Melski JW (1990) Wells' syndrome, insect bites, and eosinophils. Dermatol Clin 8:287–293.
134. Lindskov R, Illum N, Weismann K et al. (1988) Eosinophilic cellulitis: five cases. Acta Derm Venereol (Stockh) 68:325–330.
135. Nielsen T, Schmidt H, Sogaard H (1981) Eosinophilic cellulitis (Wells' syndrome) in a child. Arch Dermatol 117:427–429.
136. Reichel M, Isseroff RR, Vogt PJ et al. (1991) Wells' syndrome in children: varicella infection as a precipitating event. Br J Dermatol 124:187–190.
137. Anderson CR, Jenkins D, Tron V et al. (1995) Well's syndrome in childhood: case report and review of the literature. J Am Acad Dermatol 33:857–864.
138. Garty, B-Z, Feinmesser M, David M et al. (1997) Congenital Wells syndrome. Pediatr Dermatol 14:312–315.
139. Aberer W, Konrad K, Wolff K (1988) Wells' syndrome is a distinctive disease entity and not a histologic diagnosis. J Am Acad Dermatol 18:105–114.
140. Prendiville JS, Russell Jones R, Bryceson A (1985) Eosinophilic cellulitis as a manifestation of onchocerciasis. J R Soc Med 78 (Suppl. 11):21–22.
141. Hurni MA, Gerbig AW, Braathen LR et al. (1997) Toxocariasis and Wells' syndrome: a causal relationship? Dermatology 195:325–328.
142. Canonne D, Dubost-Brama A, Segard M et al. (2000) Wells' syndrome associated with recurrent giardiasis. Br J Dermatol 143:425–427.

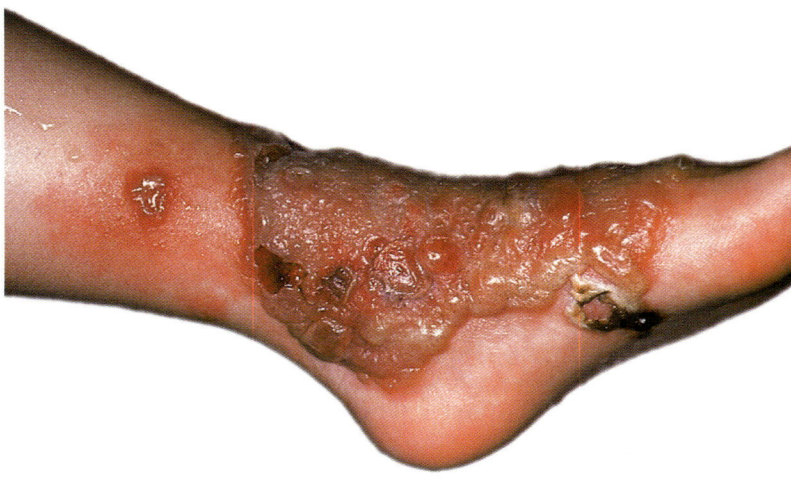

Fig. 17.7 Eosinophilic cellulitis. Acute vesicular bullous stage.

sites, recur over several months or years. The acute stage is characterized by erythematous, urticarial, edematous plaques that resemble bacterial cellulitis but are relatively cool on palpation. There may be a history of prodromal burning or itching. Blisters may develop on the surface and are sometimes hemorrhagic (Fig. 17.7). After several days, the lesions expand with central flattening and develop an indurated consistency resembling morphea, with a bluish or greenish discoloration. This resolves without scarring over a period of several weeks. The patient is usually otherwise healthy. There may be associated fever, malaise, or arthralgia.[133]

LABORATORY INVESTIGATIONS

A peripheral blood eosinophilia is found in at least 50% of cases. The erythrocyte sedimentation rate is occasionally elevated.

HISTOPATHOLOGY

In the acute stage, there is an intense dermal infiltrate, predominantly composed of eosinophils, and dermal edema.[131,133,139] Blisters may be subepidermal or intraepidermal. In the subacute stage, there are multiple histiocytes and eosinophils in addition to the characteristic flame figures. A flame figure consists of granular eosinophilic material that is adherent to collagen and is surrounded by histiocytes and giant cells of the foreign body type. The eosinophilic material has been shown to contain eosinophil major basic protein. As the lesions resolve, the eosinophils disappear, and the phagocytic histiocytes surrounding flame figures remain in the dermis. Vasculitis is not observed.

PATHOGENESIS AND HISTOGENESIS

The cause of eosinophilic cellulitis remains unclear. Some controversy and confusion has arisen because the histologic pattern of eosinophilia and flame figures may be shared by a number of other inflammatory dermatoses, including atopic eczema, prurigo, bullous pemphigoid, and tinea infections.[139] Similar clinical and histologic findings have been observed with insect bite reactions and parasitic diseases such as onchocerciasis.[133,139,140] Some authors

consider eosinophilic cellulitis a histopathologic diagnosis rather than a distinct disease entity, but this has been disputed by others.[139] It is probable that the disorder has more than one etiologic agent in a manner analogous to erythema multiforme or vasculitis.[139] Precipitating agents appear to have in common an ability to induce tissue eosinophilia. The pathogenetic mechanisms whereby an exaggerated and abnormal eosinophilic response occurs in cases of Wells' syndrome are unclear at present. Raised levels of interleukin (IL)-5 and eosinophilic cation protein (ECP) have been found in the peripheral blood and in blister fluid.[143]

DIFFERENTIAL DIAGNOSIS

The diagnosis of eosinophilic cellulitis is based on a combination of the clinical findings, course of the disease, and the characteristic histology. In the acute stage, bacterial cellulitis, erysipelas, parasitic infections, insect bites, and drug reactions must be considered. Other conditions characterized by tissue eosinophilia, such as Churg–Strauss vasculitis or the hypereosinophilia syndrome, can be distinguished by the absence of vasculitis and presence of flame figures in Wells syndrome. Many authors have emphasized that a diagnosis of eosinophilic cellulitis should not be made on the basis of the histologic features alone.[139]

TREATMENT AND PROGNOSIS

Episodes of eosinophilic cellulitis recur over several months or years. Eventual spontaneous remission of the disease without adverse sequelae is the rule. Atrophic scarring of the scalp after secondary bacterial infection has been reported.[135,137] Treatment is not always necessary. Every attempt should be made to rule out and treat any underlying infectious disease. Secondary bacterial infection should be treated with appropriate antibiotic therapy. Systemic steroids may be beneficial.[136–137] There are also reports of benefit from dapsone and phototherapy in adult patients.[143,144]

ACKNOWLEDGMENTS

The editors gratefully acknowledge contributions by Dr William Weston, which were retained from the first edition of *Pediatric Dermatology*.

AMYLOIDOSIS

Alfons L. Krol

Amyloidosis is the name given to a group of distinct syndromes caused by the deposition of an insoluble fibrillar protein in various tissue; this may result in organ dysfunction or failure.[145] Schleiden introduced the term "amyloid" to describe the reactions of plant cellulose to iodine and sulfuric acid.[146] Virchow observed this waxy homogeneous material in human tissue, and used the term "amyloid change" because of the similar characteristics of positive staining with iodine.[147] Konigsstein[147] is credited with the first description of cutaneous amyloidosis, describing a child with this disorder in 1925.

Amyloidosis is classified into two forms based on its distribution; localized and systemic. Each form is further characterized according to the type of amyloid protein within the fibril (amyloid AA, amyloid AL, or keratinocyte derived amyloid, KA)[148,149] (Table 17.2). The amount and site of deposition often determines whether its presence is significant or incidental. Cutaneous

143. Espana A, Sanz ML, Sola J et al. (1999) Wells' syndrome (eosinophilic cellulitis): correlation between clinical activity, eosinophil levels, eosinophil cation protein and interleukin-5. **Br J Dermatol** 140:127–130.
144. Diridl E, Honigsmann H, Tanew A (1997) Wells' syndrome responsive to PUVA therapy. **Br J Dermatol** 137:467–484.
145. Cunnane G (2001) Amyloid precursors and amyloidosis in inflammatory arthritis. **Curr Opin Rheumatol** 13:67–73.

146. Wong C-K (1990) History and modern concepts. **Clin Derm** 8:1–6.
147. Konigsstein H (1925) Uber Amyloidose der Haut. **Arch Dermatol Syph** 148:330.
148. Glenner GG (1980) Amyloid deposits and amyloidosis. The beta-fibrilloses. Part 2. **N Engl J Med** 302:1333–1343.
149. Breathnach SM (1988) Amyloid and amyloidosis. **J Am Acad Dermatol** 18:1–16.

amyloidosis is a rare disease in childhood, usually seen as macular or lichen amyloidosis, which are the most frequent forms of primary localized cutaneous amyloidosis (PLCA).

The most common systemic form of amyloidosis worldwide is that which occurs secondary to chronic inflammation, in which amyloid fibrils are derived from high circulating concentrations of serum amyloid A (SAA).[150] In developed countries rheumatoid arthritis and juvenile rheumatoid arthritis are the most common diseases complicated by secondary amyloidosis,[151] with 50% of the deaths in JRA patients occurring as a result of amyloid-induced renal disease.[152] Renal amyloidosis has also been observed in children with cystic fibrosis and epidermolysis bullosa.[153–155]

The heredofamilial forms of systemic amyloid may be associated with neuropathy beginning in adolescence, with progression to painless ulceration, atrophic scarring, and sclerodermatous skin changes along with hepatic and cardiac involvement occurring in adulthood.[156–158]

TABLE 17.2   Classification of amyloidosis

	Source of Amyloid
Cutaneous Amyloidosis (PLCA)	Keratinocytes
Macular	
Papular (lichenoid)	
Biphasic	
Bullous	
Nodular	Immunoglobin AL protein
Localized organ deposition	
Small deposits in and around tumors and blood vessels in aging	Keratinocytes
Systemic Amyloidosis	
Associated with immune dyscrasias (e.g., myeloma)	Immunoglobin AL protein
Reactive due to chronic inflammatory disease	
(e.g., tuberculosis, juvenile rheumatoid arthritis, or Hodgkin's disease)	SAA protein→ AA protein
Heredofamilial	
Neurotropic	Transthyretin (prealbumin)
Non-neurotropic	SAA protein→ AA protein

Cutaneous lesions occurr in 30% to 40% of cases of systemic amyloidosis; these include macroglossia and periorbital waxy papules and plaques with ecchymosis and pinch purpura. Rarely bullous lesions may be seen.[149,153] The localized cutaneous forms will be the major focus of this section.

EPIDEMIOLOGY

Localized cutaneous amyloidosis usually begins in adolescence. The most common forms seen in children are the macular and lichenoid variants that are often seen in those of Asian, Middle Eastern or Latin American origin.[159–161] Familial variants[162–164] inherited in an autosomal dominant manner have been reported. These often present as a "biphasic" illness with both macular and lichenoid papular lesions present in the same patient.[165–168]

Lichen amyloidosis has been reported with Sipple Syndrome (MEN 2A),[169,170] and in a rare autosomal-dominant disorder associated with poikiloderma, short stature, photosensitivity and blistering.[171] Macular amyloidosis has been reported in association with pachyonychia congenita,[172] epidermolysis bullosa (Weber Cockayne type),[173] dyskeratosis congenita,[174] and the Nageli–Franceshetti–Jadassohn Syndrome.[175] There is no risk of transformation of the sporadic and familial forms of cutaneous amyloidosis to the systemic form.

PRESENTING HISTORY

Cutaneous amyloidosis presents with a history of itching which is at first intermittent and then more intense as the lesions become more fully developed. The most commonly affected areas are the upper back and anterior tibial regions. Hyperpigmentation is often subtle but increases over time.[176–179] A family history of similar skin disorders should be sought in each patient.[164]

PHYSICAL EXAMINATION

Primary localized cutaneous amyloidosis (PLCA) presents as macular or lichenoid lesions. While the lichenoid variety is the most common form seen in adults, it may occur in adolescence. It presents with itchy, closely set, aggregated papules, 1–10mm in size, typically on the anterior tibial or other extensor surfaces. The lesions may vary from skin-colored to varying shades of gray or yellow-brown.

Macular amyloidosis presents with flat hyperpigmented macules, most commonly on the upper back and distal limbs. Close inspection will reveal a

150. Buxbaum J (1998) The amyloidoses. In: Rheumatology, 2nd edn, Klippel JH, Dieppe PA, ed. London: Mosby International 13:615–628.
151. Gertz MA, Kyle RA (1991) Secondary systemic amyloidosis: response and survival in 64 patients. **Medicine** 70:246–256.
152. Savolainen HA, Isomaki HA (1993) Decrease in the number of deaths from secondary amyloidosis in patients with juvenile rheumatoid arthritis. J Rheumatol 20:1201–1203.
153. Rubinow A, Cohen AS (1978) Skin involvement in generalized amyloidosis: a study of clinically involved and uninvolved skin in 50 patients with primary and secondary amyloidosis. **Ann Intern Med** 88:781.
154. Bywaters EGL (1977) Deaths in juvenile chronic polyarthritis. **Arthritis Rheum** 20:256.
155. Cohen AS (1981) An update of clinical, pathologic and biochemical aspects of amyloidosis. Int J Dermatol 20:515.
156. Benson MD (1991) Inherited amyloidos s. **J Med** 28:73–78.
157. Meretoja J (1969) Familial systemic paramyloidosis with lattice dystrophy of the cornea, progressive cranial neuropathy, skin changes and various internal symptoms; a previously unrecognized heritable syndrome. **Ann Clin Res** 1:314–324.
158. Wong C-K, Lin C-S (1988) Friction amyloidosis. Int J Dermatol 27:302–307.
159. Wang W-J (1990) Clinical features of cutaneous amyloidoses. **Clin Derm** 8:13–19.
160. Venkataram MN, Bhushnurmath SR, Muirhead DE et al. (2001) Frictional amyloidosis: A study of ten cases. **Australas J Dermatol** 42(3):176–179.
161. Kyle RA, Bayrd ED (1975) Amyloidosis: review of 236 cases. **Medicine** (Baltimore) 54:271.
162. Newton JA, Jagjivan A, Bhogal B et al. (1985) Familial primary cutaneous amyloidosis. **Br J Dermatol** 112:201.
163. Sagher F, Shanon J (1963) Amyloidosis cutis: familial occurrence in three generations. **Arch Dermatol** 87:171.
164. Toutant DM, San P (1998) Cutaneous deposition disorders. Part 1. **J Am Acad Dermatol** 39:149–171.
165. Rajagopalan K, Tay CH (1972) Familial lichen amyloidosis. Report of 19 cases in four generations of a Chinese family in Malaysia. **Br J Derm** 87:123–129.
166. Ozaka M (1984) Familial lichen amyloidosis. Int J Dermatol 23:190–193.
167. Newton JA, Jagjivan A, Bhogal B et al. (1985) Familial primary cutaneous amyloidosis. **Br J Derm** 112:201–208.
168. De Pietro WP (1981) Primary familial cutaneous amyloidosis: a study of HLA antigens in a Puerto Rican family. **Arch Derm** 117:639–642.
169. Kousseff BG, Espinoza C, Zamore GA (1991) Sipple syndrome with lichen amyloidosis as a paracrinopathy: pleiotropy, heterogeneity, or a contiguous gene? **J Am Acad Dermatol** 25:651–657.
170. Robinson MF, Furst EJ, Nunziata V et al. (1992) Characterization of the clinical features of five families with hereditary primary cutaneous lichen amyloidosis and multiple endocrine neoplasia type 2. **Henry Ford Hosp Med J** 40:249–252.
171. Ogino A, Tanaca S (1977) Poikiloderma-like cutaneous amyloidosis. **Dermatologica** 155:301–309.
172. Tidman MJ, Wells RS, Macdonald DM (1987) Pachyonychia congenita with cutaneous amyloidosis and hyperpigmentation: a distinct variant. **J Am Acad Dermatol** 16:935–940.
173. Kantor GR, Kasick JM, Bergfeld WF et al. (1985) Epidermolysis bullosa of the Weber-Cockayne type with macular amyloidosis. **Cleve Clin Q** 52:425–428.
174. Llistosella E, Moreno A, deMoragas JM (1984) Dyskeratosis congenita with macular cutaneous amyloid deposits. **Arch Dermatol** 120:1381–1382.
175. Frenk E, Mevorah B, Hohl D (1993) The Nageli-Franceschetti-Jadassohn syndrome: a hereditary ectodermal defect leading to colloid-amyloid formation in the dermis. **Dermatology** 187:169–173.
176. MacDonald DM, Fergin PE, Black MM (1980) Localized cutaneous amyloidosis. In: Amyloid and Amyloidosis, Glenner GG, Pinho e Costa P, de Freitas F, eds. Amsterdam: Excerpta Medica. p. 239.
177. Breathnach SM, Black MM (1979) Systemic amyloidosis and the skin. **Clin Exp Dermatol** 4:517.
178. Westermark P (1979) Amyloidosis of the skin: a comparison between localized and systemic amyloidosis. **Acta Derm Venereol** (Stockh) 59:341.
179. Black MM (1976) Primary localized amyloidosis of the skin: clinical variants, histochemistry and ultrastructure. Amyloidosis, In: Wegelius O, Pasternack A, eds. New York: Academic Press, p. 479.

"rippled" or "wavy" pattern on the skin surface which may be accompanied by mild lichenification. The color is brown to grayish brown and itch is usually less than in the lichenoid variety. Friction may play an important role in the evolution of this form of amyloid.[161]

Biphasic amyloidosis is the coexistence of both macular and lichenoid amyloidosis in the same patient.[160] Rubbing, scratching, and friction from brushes or bath sponges may convert the macular form to lichenoid and treatment may reverse the process.[159,160]

Primary systemic or immunocytic amyloidosis is exceedingly rare in childhood,[180] as is secondary systemic amyloidosis.[181,182] Macroglossia, waxy papules (Fig. 17.8) which exhibit "pinch purpura" and sclerodermatous skin changes may occur.[149] Rectal biopsy is usually diagnostic.[149] Amyloid infiltration occurs in the kidneys, liver, heart, and spleen. Skin lesions are rare. Heredofamilial syndromes such as familial Mediterranean fever may culminate in amyloid nephropathy and renal failure in childhood.[183] Muckle–Wells syndrome is an autosomal-dominant disorder characterized by chronic recurrent episodes of urticaria beginning in adolescence followed by progressive deafness and amyloid nephropathy in adult life.[184]

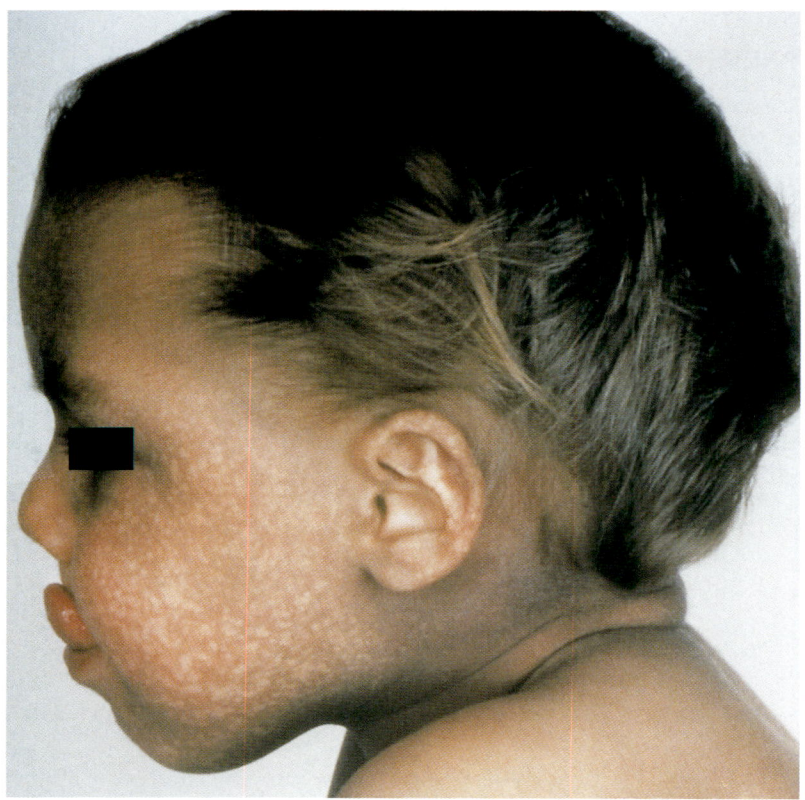

Fig. 17.8 Amyloidosis on the face of a child.

LABORATORY FINDINGS

There are no laboratory abnormalities in the localized cutaneous forms of amyloidosis. In systemic amyloidosis, the type and degree of laboratory abnormalities will vary depending on the extent of the disease and which organ system is involved.[185]

PATHOPHYSIOLOGY AND HISTOGENESIS

Regardless of the source or form of amyloidosis, the histological characteristics are the same.[186] In hematoxylin and eosin-stained sections the lesions appear as a homogeneous, pink deposit that replaces collagen bundles.[176,177] Amyloid stains metachromatically with methyl violet or crystal violet and Congo red stain shows a characteristic apple green birefringence, with yellow-green birefringence when using thioflavin T under fluorescent microscopy.

Ultrastructurally, amyloid appears as straight, non-branching fibrils, 7.5–10nm in diameter. They are configured in an antiparallel (β-pleated) array.[185] Eight sources of amyloid fibrillar proteins have been identified. Plasma cells secrete AL protein derived from IgG lambda light chains, which results in the immunocytic forms of amyloidosis. Serum amyloid A protein (SAA) is the precursor of the AA fibrils. Humans have four types of SAA genes located on the short arm of chromosome 11.

SAA1 and SAA2 are highly homologous and increase sharply in response to inflammation.[187] The main source of SAA is the liver, with other identified sources including endothelial cells, macrophages, and rheumatoid synovium, as well as normal epithelium.[145,188] SAA has significant immunomodulatory effects in upregulating or activation of adhesion molecules, neutrophils, interferon-γ, and metalloproteinases.[145] SAA concentrations are increased by IL-1, TNFα and IL-6.[189]

Damaged and degenerating keratinocytes are the source of keratinocytic amyloid (KA)[190,191] seen in macular and lichenoid amyloidosis.

DIFFERENTIAL DIAGNOSIS

The main differential diagnosis for the papular or lichenoid form is chronic eczema, either lichen simplex chronicus or atopic dermatitis.[162,176,178] Pretibial myxedema, which may be associated with similar epidermal changes of thickening and lichenification, is exceedingly rare in childhood. The macular forms may be confused with tinea versicolor or confluent and reticulated papillomatosis of Gougerot and Carteaud. Biopsy, with special stains to identify amyloid, is required to confirm the diagnosis.

THERAPY AND PROGNOSIS

The main goals of therapy are to alleviate itch and flatten unsightly lesions. This can be achieved through the use of high-potency topical steroids or intralesional steroid injection. Oral antihistamines may be of benefit to alleviate the itch in some patients. Cryosurgery and dermabrasion have been successful in some patients, particularly in the lichenoid or nodular form.[192,193] Actretin has recently been reported to be effective in a case of

180. Pick AI, Versano I, Schreibman S et al. (1977) Agammaglobulinemia, plasma cell dyscrasia, and amyloidosis in a 12-year-old child. **Am J Dis Child** 131:682–686.
181. Woo P (1992) Amyloidosis in pediatric rheumatic diseases. **J Rheum** 19:10–16.
182. Woo P (1994) Amyloidosis in children. **Ballière's Clin Rheumatol** 8:691–697.
183. Gedalia A, Adar A, Gorodischer R (1992) Familial Mediterranean fever in children. **J Rheum** 19:1–9.
184. Muckle TJ (1979) The Muckle-Wells syndrome. **Br. J Dermatol** 100:87–92.
185. Glenner GG (1980) Amyloid deposits and amyloidosis. The beta-fibrilloses. **N Engl J Med** 302:1283.
186. Lever's Histopathology of the Skin, 8th ed. (1997) Philadelphia: Lippincott-Raven.
187. Steel DM, Whitehead AS (1994) The major acute phase reactants: C-reactive protein, serum amyloid P component and serum amyoild A protein. **Immunol Today** 15:81–88.

188. Urieli-Shoval S, Cohen P, Eisenberg S et al. (1998) Widespread expression of serum amyloid A in histologically normal human tissues: predominant localization to the epithelium. **J Histochem Cytochem** 46:1377–1384.
189. Charles P, Elliott MJ, Davis D et al. (1999) Regulation of cytokines, cytokine inhibitors and acute phase proteins following anti-TNF-alpha therapy in rheumatoid arthritis. **J Immunol** 163:1521–1528.
190. Black MM, Heather CJ (1972) The ultrastructure of lichen amyloidosis with special reference to the epidermal change. **Br J Dermatol** 87:117.
191. Husebekk A, Skogen B, Husby G et al. (1985) Transformation of amyloid precursor SAA to protein AA and incorporation in amyloid fibrils in vivo. **Scand J Immunol** 21:283–287.
192. Lien M, Railan D, Nelson B (1997) The efficacy of dermabrasion in the treatment of nodular amyloidosis. **J Am Acad Dermatol** 36:315–316.
193. Wong C-K, Li W-M (1982) Dermabrasion for lichen amyloidosus. **Arch Dermatol** 118:302–304.

biphasic amyloidosis.[194] The long-term prognosis for cutaneous amyloidosis is for persistence or gradual progression of lesions in the skin.

Treatment of systemic amyloid is directed at the underlying disease process. With greater understanding of the mechanisms and control of amyloid production and metabolism, immunomodulatory drug therapy may prove successful in the future.[195]

PEDIATRIC ASPECTS OF THE DISEASE

Growth, development, nutrition, and physical activities are usually unaffected in the localized cutaneous forms of amyloidosis. In systemic forms, organ deposition of amyloid may result in renal, cardiac or hepatic dysfunction.

MYXEDEMA

Myxedema refers to the accumulation of glycosaminoglycans (GAGs) in the form of hyaluronic acid in the skin, giving it a shiny, taut, edematous appearance.[196] Two forms of myxedema are recognized: generalized and localized, or pretibial myxedema. Both forms are related to thyroid abnormalities. Only one report of two pediatric cases with pretibial myxedema have been described.[197] Generalized myxedema is a consequence of congenital hypothyroidism. Sir William Gull is credited with describing myxedema in the skin in 1873, using the term "cretinoid edema."[198] In 1877, Ord suggested the term myxedema after determining that it was due to a deposit of mucinous material.

EPIDEMIOLOGY

Congenital hypothyroidism occurs in approximately 1:4000 births. Females are affected about twice as often as males. Eighty-five percent of cases are sporadic, while 15% are hereditary. The most common sporadic etiology is thyroid dysgenesis, with ectopic glands being more common than aplasia or hypoplasia.[199] The vast majority of infants are now detected through newborn screening programs.[199] The features of congenital hypothyroidism are noted between 1 and 2 months of age. Risk associations with congenital hypothyroidism include birth weight <2000g or greater than 4500g, increased incidence in ethnic groups other than Caucasians, and decreased incidence in African American infants.[200] Congenital hypothyroidism is an important, common, preventable cause of mental retardation. Response to treatment is often dramatic with resumption of growth and skeletal maturation. Early treatment, within the first two to four weeks of life, is important to prevent or minimize neurocognitive deficits in later life.[201]

PRESENTING HISTORY

With the introduction of widespread screening programs in North America, florid congenital hypothroidism with widespread myxedematous skin changes is uncommon. Early signs include a hoarse cry at birth, extensive cutis marmorata that does not respond to warming, and transluscent pallor of the skin with an alabaster hue.[202] Other early signs include prolonged neonatal jaundice, umbilical hernia, prominent fontanelles, bradycardia, and hypotonia.[203,204] Feeding difficulties, lethargy, constipation, thermal instability and hypothermia may be present.[202] Once the disease becomes well established, growth failure and neurodevelopmental delay will be apparent.[205] Acquired hypothyroidism in older children often presents with general symptoms of lethargy, weight gain, constipation, poor school performance, cold intolerance, myalgias and arthralgias, delayed puberty and rarely neuropsychiatric illness.[206–208]

PHYSICAL EXAMINATION

The skin is pale, or sallow in color from accumulation of GAGs as well as the effects of anemia, poor peripheral perfusion, and associated neonatal jaundice or carotenemia. Extensive cutis marmorata is seen. The infant's face may be swollen and the skin of the eyelids, external genitalia, and dorsa of the hands and feet exhibit swelling.[209] With time, macroglossia is noted and the characteristic facial features – thickened facial skin, protruding thick tongue, depressed nasal bridge, and mild hyperteliorism – are seen. The thickened skin does not pit, and has a "doughy" consistency on palpation. The overlying skin surface is dry and cool. The infant is often lethargic, with poor head movement due to hypotonic muscles. The abdomen is large and there is often an umbilical hernia present. Rarely ascites is present. The pulse is slow, and heart murmurs, cardiomegaly and asymptomatic pericardial effusion may be present.[210] If stimulated to cry, there is a delay in the onset of the cry which is hoarse and weak.[209] In older children with acquired myxedema, the cutaneous changes of pale, cool xerotic skin, with puffiness of the face and lips, may be the only features noted, along with poor hair and nail growth, and general symptoms of weight gain.

LABORATORY FINDINGS

Thyroid function studies are abnormal in both congenital and acquired hypothyroidism. A serum thyroxine (T4) level, and TSH, which is more sensitive, should be obtained along with radiographic examination of the hands for bone age. Infants with congenital primary hypothyroidism should undergo radio-isotope scanning to determine the presence and location of thyroid tissue.[199] Elevated serum carotene, cholesterol, and triglyceride levels may be seen. In the neonate, topical iodine containing antiseptics used in nurseries and by surgeons may lead to abnormal results on screening tests and cause transient congenital hypothyroidism, especially in low birthweight infants.[211]

PATHOPHYSIOLOGY AND HISTOGENESIS

Thyroid dysgenesis is the most common cause of congenital hypothyroidism. Mutations in several gene transcription factors, including TTF1, TTF2, and

194. Hernandez-Nunez A, Dauden E. Moreno de Vega MJ et al. (2001) Widespread biphasic amyloidosis: response to acitretin. **Clin Exp Dermatol** 26(3):256–259.
195. Cunnane G (2001) Amyloid proteins in pathogenesis of AA amyloidosis. **Lancet** 358:4–5.
196. Gabrilove JL, Ludwig AW (1957) The histogenesis of myxoedema. **J Clin Endocrinol Metab** 17:925–932.
197. Maldonado Regalado S, Barrio Castellanos R, Alonso Blanco M et al. (1988) Graves' disease in childhood. **An Esp Pediatri** 29(6):440–444.
198. Pusey WA (1932) The History of Dermatology. Springfield, IL: Charles C Thomas.
199. LaFranchi S (1999) Congenital hypothyroidism: etiologies, diagnosis and management. **Thyroid** 9(7):735–740.
200. Waller DK, Anderson JL, Lorey F et al. (2000) Risk factors for congenital hypothyroidism: an investigation of infant's birth weight, ethnicity, and gender in California, 1990–1998. **Teratology** 62(1):36–41.
201. Rovet JF (1999) Congenital hypothyroidism: long-term outcome. **Thyroid** 9(7):741–748.
202. Grant DB, Smith I, Fuggle PW et al. (1992) Congenital hypothyroidism detected by neonatal screening: relationship between biochemical severity and early clinical features. **Arch Dis Child** 67:87–90.
203. Shanker SM, Menon PSN, Karmarker MG et al. (1994) Dysgenesis of the thyroid is the common type of childhood hypothyroidism in environmentally iodine deficient areas of North India. **Acta Paediatr** 83:1047–1051.

204. Tsai WY, Lee JS, Wang TR et al. (1993) Clinical characteristics of congenital hypothyroidism detected by neonatal screening. **J Formos Med Assoc** 92:20–23.
205. Tarim OF, Yordam N (1992) Congenital hypothyroidism in Turkey: a retrospective evaluation of 1000 cases. **Turk J Pediatr** 34:197–202.
206. Callas JS, Foley TP (1990) Hypothyroidism. In: Pediatric Endocrinology: a Clinical Guide, 2nd rev, Lifshitz F, ed. New York: Dekker, pp. 478–493.
207. Keenan GF, Ostrov BE, Goldsmith DP et al. (1993) Rheumatic symptoms associated with hypothyroidism in children. **J Pediatr** 123:586–588.
208. Foley TP, Abbassi V, Copeland KC et al. (1994) Brief report: hypothyroidism caused by chronic autoimmune thyroiditis in very young infants. **N Engl J Med** 330:466–468.
209. Bacon GE, Spencer ML, Hopwood NJ et al. (1983) A Practical Approach to Pediatric Endocrinology, 2nd ed. Chicago: Year Book Medical Publishers.
210. Behrman RE, Kliegman RM, Jensen HB (2000) Nelson Textbook of Pediatrics, 16th ed. WB Saunders Co.
211. Zahidi A, Draoui M, Mestassi M (1999) Iodine status and the use of iodized antiseptics in the mother-newborn pair. **Therapie** 54(5):545–548.

PAX8,[212,213] which play a role in thyroid gland embryogenesis, have been found. Hereditary defects in almost all the steps of thyroid hormone synthesis, secretion, and action have been described, most commonly due to defects in the thyroid peroxidase gene (TPO).[214] Pendred syndrome, an association of congenital hypothroidism and sensorineural deafness results from a mutation in a chloride-iodide transport protein which leads to defective iodine binding to thyroglobulin, and cochlear dysfunction from abnormal endolymph transport in the ear.[215] Rarely, large hemangiomas may produce type 3 iodothyronine deiodinase, which inactivates thyroid hormone, resulting in severe hypothyroidism in affected infants.[216]

The cutaneous changes resulting in myxedema are attributable to low levels of circulating thyroxine, resulting in excess accumulation of GAGs, particularly hyaluronic acid in the dermis. In addition, effects on cutaneous blood flow, diminished sebaceous and eccrine gland activity and reduced hair growth is seen. Histological changes on routine hematoxylin and eosin sections may show little other than swollen collagen bundles. Special stains with Alcian blue or toluidine blue reveal the hyaluronic acid deposits, particularly around blood vessels and appendages.

DIFFERENTIAL DIAGNOSIS

Generalized myxedema must be distinguished from edema, which pits on compression of the surface, while myxedema does not. Accumulation of other mucopolysaccharidoses within the skin may mimic myxedema. Both are accumulations of GAGs. Separation depends on thyroid function tests, analysis of urinary mucopolysaccharides, and the clinical presence of marked hepato-splenomegaly in the mucopolysaccharidoses. Sclerema neonatorum occurs in the immediate newborn period, whereas myxedema takes longer to develop. Infants with lipoid proteinosis will show skin swelling and a hoarse cry, but onset is at 3 to 4 months of age. Trisomy 21 may have lymphedema and Turner syndrome has lymphedema but are easily distinguished by other clinical features including epicanthic folds and transverse palmar creases in Down syndrome, and webbed neck and pedal edema in Turner syndrome, and chromosomal studies which shows XO. Children with Beckwith–Wiedemann syndrome present with macroglossia, but have normal thyroid function and accelerated growth.

THERAPY AND PROGNOSIS

Congenital myxedema is one of the most common preventable causes of mental retardation. There is a firm relationship between when treatment is started and psychometric outcome.[199] Treatment is with levothyroxine (thyroxine). The recommended initial dosae is 10–15μg/kg per day. The goal is to raise the T4 as rapidly as possible into the normal range to minimize the exposure of the neonatal brain to low thyroxine.[199] Complete clearance of the skin lesions occurs within one to two weeks of institution of therapy.[209]

PEDIATRIC ASPECTS OF THE DISEASE

These children show profound neurodevelopmental delay if there is delay in diagnosis. Only 5% are diagnosed by physical examination at birth; the majority are diagnosed through screening programs.[199] In the older child with acquired hypothyroidism, school performance may suddenly drop off, growth rate may flatten, energy is diminished, and delayed onset of puberty may occur. Monitoring of thyroid function on a regular basis throughout infancy and childhood until puberty and growth is complete is recommended for those with the disease.[217] Overtreatment may result in premature closure of the epiphyses and a nervous and jittery child with poor attention span and school performance.

LIPOID PROTEINOSIS

Lipoid proteinosis (hyalinosis cutis et mucosae) is a rare autosomal-recessive disorder, that may present with multiple systemic manifestations involving mucosal deposition of hyaline material. Affected children are hoarse from birth. Gradual development of diffuse papules and nodules on the face, plus thickening of the extremities develop, and the mucosae of the upper aerodigestive tract slowly becomes involved.[218,219] The disorder was first described by Siebenmann in 1908; the first detailed discription was by Urbach and Wiethe in 1929.[220] Urbach proposed the term lipid proteinosis because histochemical investigations showed staining characteristics of both lipid and protein.[220]

EPIDEMIOLOGY

Lipoid proteinosis is a rare disorder with less than 300 cases reported in the literature. A higher prevalence of cases occurs in South Africa and Sweden, with many patients being of Dutch or German ancestry.[221,222] The disorder occurs equally in males and females.

PRESENTING HISTORY

Two-thirds of the patients present with hoarseness in the newborn period. Cutaneous changes usually appear during the first two years of life. Systemic involvement manifests as seizures or neuropsychiatric symptoms. The skin and mucous membrane changes increase with age.

PHYSICAL EXAMINATION

The infant has a poor cry or is hoarse from birth. Initially the lesions are pruritic, subsequently scarring occurs, which is acneiform or varioliform. Numerous papules and nodules and coarse facial features are observed. There is diffuse, firm thickening of the skin of the extremities with hyperkeratosis of the elbows, knees, and dorsa of the hands that may result in decreased joint mobility.

The vermilion border, tongue, gingival and buccal mucosa, and border of the eyelids commonly develop whitish papules which thicken and progress over time.[221,222] The papular infiltration of the margin of the eyelids is associated with dryness and secondary eczematous changes (Figs 17.9, 17.10).

LABORATORY FINDINGS

Calcification of intracranial vessels, particularly in the temporal lobes or hippocampal area, may be seen on skull radiographs or CT scan. These are characteristically "bean shaped."[223] Routine hematology, chemistry, and lipid studies are normal.

212. Krude H, Biebermann H, Schnabel D et al. (2000) Molecular pathogenesis of neonatal hypothyroidism. **Horm Res** 53 Suppl 1:12–18.
213. Macchia PE (2000) Recent advances in understanding the molecular basis of primary congenital hypothyroidism. **Mol Med Today** 6(1):36–42.
214. Ambrugger P, Stoeva I, Bierbermann H et al. (2001) Novel mutations of the thyro d peroxidase gene in patients with permanent congenital hypothyroidism. **Eur J Endocrinol** 145(1):19–24.
215. Scott DA, Wang R, Kreman TM et al. (1999) The Pendred gene encodes a chloride-iodide transport protein. **Nat Genetics** 20:440–443.
216. Huang SA, Tu HM, Harney JW et al. (2000) Severe hypothroidism caused by Type 3 iodothyronine deiodinase in infantile hemanagiomas. **New Eng J Med** 343(3):185–189.
217. Rovet JF, Ehrlich RM (1995) Long-term effects of l-thyroxine therapy for congenital hypothyroidism. **J Pediatr** 126:380–386.

218. Böhme M, Wahlgren CF (1996) Lipoid proteinosis in three children. **Acta Paediatr** 85:1003–1005.
219. Rizzo R, Ruggieri M, Micali G et al. (1997) Lipoid proteincsis: A case report. **Pediatric Dermatol** 14(1):22–25.
220. Urbach E, Wiethe C (1929) Lipoidosis cutis et mucosae. **Virchows Arch Path Anat** 273:285–319.
221. Gorlin RJ, Cohen MM Jr, Levin LS (1990) Hyalinosis cutis et mucosae (lipoid proteinosis, Urbach-Wiethe syndrome). In: Syndromes of the head and neck, 3rd edn, Gorlin RJ, Cohen MM Jr, Levin LS, eds. Oxford Monographs and Medical Genetics no. 19. New York: Oxford University Press, 507–511.
222. Hofer PA (1983) Urbach-Wiethe disease. A review. **Acta Dermatol Venereol** 53 (suppl):1–56.
223. Orlow SJ, Watsky KL, Bolognia JL (1991) Skin and bones I. **J Am Acad Dermatol** 25:205.

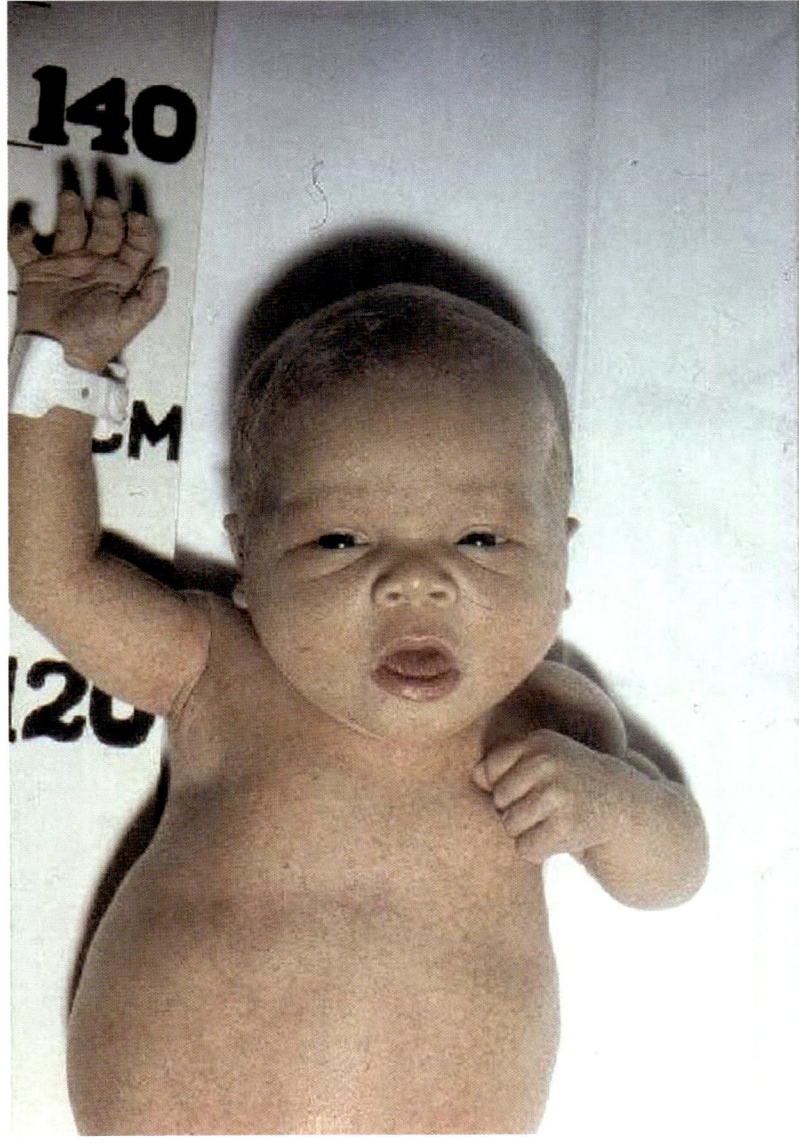

Fig. 17.9   Typical appearance of a child with congenital myxedema. Courtesy of Robert Couch, MD.

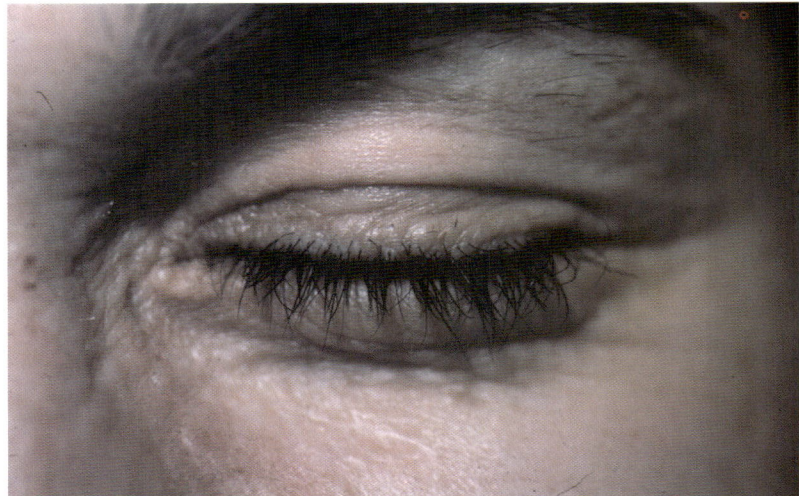

Fig. 17.10   Lipoid proteinosis showing mobiliform beaded papules on the eyelids of a child.

show neutral fat droplets throughout the hyalin material.[186] Cholesterol esters and ceramide may also be found.[225]

Ultrastructurally, reduplication of the basement membrane of vessels and occasionally the dermoepidermal junction is seen.[227] Two separate substances are present in the eosinophilic hyaline material, true hyaline of fibroblastic origin and reduplicated basement membrane produced by multiple cells.[228] One study revealed peculiar cytoplasmic inclusions in lesional fibroblasts and cytoplasmic vacuolization, suggesting the possibility of a lysosomal storage disorder.[229] The inclusions contained granular, electron-dense structures composed of high levels of carbohydrates.[229]

Tissue cultures of cell fibroblasts result in the production of an abnormal glycoprotein, but lipid production is normal. Lipids found within the hyaline materials may result from the affinity of lipids to glycoproteins as this disorder is one of glycoprotein rather than lipid metabolism.[224] Although a reduced proliferative capacity of fibroblasts has been reported,[230] it is doubtful whether the primary underlying defect is an abnormality of collagen metabolism. Hamada *et al.*[231] studied DNA from three siblings with lipoid proteinosis from a consanguinous Saudi Arabian family and mapped the defect to 1q21. Six different homozygous loss of function mutations were found in the extracellular matrix protein 1 gene (ECM1). The precise function of ECM1 is unknown but these findings provide the first indication of its relevence to skin adhesion, differentiation, angiogenesis, wound healing, scarring, and basement membrane physiology.

PATHOPHYSIOLOGY AND HISTOGENESIS

The pathogenesis of lipoid proteinosis is unclear, but some features of a lysosomal storage disorder are present.[224,225] The earliest pathologic change is thickening of dermal capillary walls, with deposition of hyaline material within and around the basement membrane of the vessel.[226] Fully developed skin lesions show papillomatosis and hyperkeratosis of the epidermis, whilst the superficial and deep dermal vessels show a thick, homogeneous, eosinophilic hyaline perivascular deposit. Similar deposits are seen around sweat glands and ducts. The hyalin material stains positive with periodic acid–Schiff (PAS) and Alcian blue stains. Lipid stains such as Sudan IV may

DIFFERENTIAL DIAGNOSIS

Myxedema may mimic lipoid proteinosis. In both conditions, infants present with hoarseness from birth, and have diffuse nonpitting swelling of the skin. Thyroid function tests distinguishes myxedema from lipoid proteinosis. Simple edema will pit. The coarse facies of the infant and the diffusely thickened skin may mimic one of the forms of mucopolysaccharidoses. Analysis for urinary mucopolysaccharides and skin biopsy will help distinguish between the two. Diffuse thickening of sun-exposed areas of skin is observed in erythropoietic protoporphyria.[186] The skin biopsy in erythropoietic protoporphyria may also show perivascular accumulation of PAS-positive material, but in porphyria it

224. Navarro C, Fachal C, Rodriguez C et al. (1999) Lipoid proteinosis. A biochemical and ultrastructural investigation of two new cases. **Br J Dermatol** 141(2):326–331.
225. Konstantionov K, Kabakchiev P, Karche T (1992) Lipoid proteinosis. **J Am Acad Dermatot** 27:293.
226. Caro I (1978) Lipoid proteiniosis. **Int J Dermatol** 17:388.
227. Fleischmajer R, Timpl R, Graves P (1981) Hyalinosis cutis et mucosal: A basal lamina disease, (Abstr). **J Invest Dermatol** 76:314–315.
228. Fleischmajer R, Krieg T, Dziadek M et al. (1984) Ultrastructure and composition of connective tissue in hyalinosis cutis et mucosae skin. **J Invest Dermatol** 82:252–258.
229. Bauer E, Santa Cruz D, Eisen A (1981) Lipoid proteinosis; in vivo and in vitro evidence for a lysosomal storage disease. **J Invest Dermatol** 76:119–125.
230. Moy LD, Moy RL, Matsuoka LY et al. (1987) Lipoid proteinosis: ultrastructural and biochemical studies. **J Am Acad Dermatol** 16:1193–1201.
231. Hamada T, McLean WH, Ramse M et al. (2002) Lipoid proteinosis maps to Iq21 and is caused by mutations in the extra cellular matrix protein 1 gene (ECMI). **Hum Mol Genetics** 11;7:833–840.

is limited to the superficial dermis, whereas in lipoid proteinosis the deposits are also found in the deep dermis and sweat glands. There is hoarseness in lipoid proteinosis but not erythropoietic protoporphyria.

THERAPY AND PROGNOSIS

Effective therapy is not available. Improvement has been reported after dermabrasion of cutaneous lesions,[232,233] and treatment with carbon dioxide laser for eyelid lesions.[234] Oral dimethyl sulfoxide[235] was reported effective in one patient but a long-term trial in three other patients produced no beneficial effects.[236] Oral retinoid was helpful in two patients.[237] The efficacy of these treatments in a disease with a fluctuating course is difficult to evaluate.

The course is chronic, and other than mucocutaneous lesions and hoarseness, the major debility is when neurologic involvement occurs; this is uncommon and may include psychomotor and grand mal seizures, memory loss, rage attacks, and schizophrenic behaviour.[238]

PEDIATRIC ASPECTS OF THE DISEASE

The seizure disorder that some children experience may require control with anticonvulsants.[226] The psychosocial stigma can be severe in the pre-adolescent and adolescent patient.

GRANULOMA ANNULARE

Granuloma annulare (GA) is a common disorder of childhood characterized by grouped dermal papules in an annular or ringed arrangement. The entity was first described by Fox in 1895; the term "granuloma annulare" was introduced by Radcliff-Crocker in 1902.[239] Although the cause is unknown, the common localized form is a benign condition that persists for several years and usually resolves spontaneously.[240] A generalized, disseminated form that presents with widespread, asymptomatic macules, papules and nodules that may coalesce into reticulate patterns is more common in adults.[241]

EPIDEMIOLOGY

GA may occur at any age, but is most common in school-aged children.[242] In a series of 100 cases of generalized GA only eight patients were under the age of 20 years.[243] The generalized form of the disease is more common in adults. Females are affected twice as commonly as males.[240,241] Although familial cases have been reported the disease is usually sporadic. HLA studies are conflicting, with an increased incidence of HLA-Bw35 in Israel,[244] HLA-B8 in Denmark,[245] and HLA-A29, B14, and B15 in Belfast.[246] These findings may reflect the fact that HLA genes are population specific.

PRESENTING HISTORY

Parents usually bring a child for medical care because of asymptomatic ringed papules, often misdiagnosed as tinea corporis and resistant to anti-fungal therapy. Commonly, patients have used numerous topical antifungals or other agents without response. Lesions on the dorsa of the feet may occasionally cause discomfort under sports shoes or skates.

PHYSICAL EXAMINATION

Physical findings in GA are limited to the skin. The most common form of GA is the localized form, which presents as ringed papules on any part of the body, but is most commonly found on the dorsa of the hands and feet and lower extremities (Fig. 17.11). The lesions begin as skin-colored or pale red papules without scale or epidermal change, that slowly expand to form rings with central clearing that has a normal or a violaceous color. The rings vary from one to several centimeters in size. Multiple lesions are common, although 50% of patients have single lesions.[241] A papular umbilicated form of GA limited to the dorsa of the hands and fingers has been described in school-aged children.[247] The generalized form of GA, is characterized by hundreds of small asymptomatic papules forming symmetrical, ringed lesions that usually coalesce into reticulate, circinate patterns or linear bands.[241] The palms, soles, and mucous membranes may be occasionally involved.[242] Patients infected with the human immunodeficiency virus may have the generalized type or extensive localized form of GA.[248]

A subcutaneous form is seen most commonly on the pretibial area of the lower legs in children aged 2 to 5 years.[249-251] Lesions may also be found on the scalp, buttocks, hands, and periorbital regions;[241,252,253] they usually appear as asymptomatic deep dermal or subcutaneous nodules with no overlying epidermal change; they regress spontaneously (Fig. 17.11C). Lesions on the scalp are hard and bound down to the periosteum. Typical ringed lesions are only present in one-fourth of these patients.[254]

Perforating GA is a rare disorder consisting of asymptomatic grouped papules, some of which have a central crust or scale where damaged collagen perforates through the ulcerated epidermis.

LABORATORY FINDINGS

Children with GA are usually healthy.

PATHOPHYSIOLOGY AND HISTOGENESIS

Histologically, GA is characterized by focal degeneration of collagen in the dermis with reactive inflammation and fibrosis[186] and fragmentation of collagen bundles.[255] The epidermis is normal except in perforating GA where

232. Vukas A (1972) Hyalinosis cutis et mucosae: regenerative properties of tissues involved in chronic pathology. **Dermatologica** 144:168–175.
233. Bannerot H, Aubin F, Tropet Y et al. (1998) Lipoid proteinosis: importance of dermabrasion. Apropos of a case. **Ann Chir Plast Esthet** 43(1):78–81.
234. Rosenthal G, Lifshitz T, Monos T et al. (1997) Carbon dioxide laser treatment for lipoid proteinosis (Urbach-Wiethe syndrome) involving the eyelids. **Br J Opthalmol** 81(3):253.
235. Wong C, Lin CS (1988) Remarkable response of lipoid proteinosis to oral dimethyl sulphoxide. **Br J Dermatol** 119:541–544.
236. Ozkaya-Bayazit E, Ozarmagan G, Baykal et al. (1997) Oral DMSO Therapy in three patients with lipoid proteinosis. Results of long-term therapy. **Hautartz** 48(7):477–481.
237. Gruber F, Manestar D, Stasic A et al. (1996) Treatment of lipoid proteinosis with etretinate. **Acta Derm Venereol** 76(2):154–155.
238. Newton FH, Rosenberg RN, Lampert PW, O'Brien JS (1971) Neurologic involvement in Urbach-Wiethe disease (lipoid proteinosis): a clinical, ultrastructural, and chemical study. **Neurology** 21:1205–1213.
239. Radcliff-Crocker H (1902) Granuloma annulare. **Br J Dermatol** 14:1–9.
240. Hurwitz S (1985) The Skin and Systemic Disease in Children, 1st ed. Chicago: Year Book Medical Publishers.
241. Muhlbauer JE (1980) Granuloma annulare. **J Am Acad Dermatol** 3:217.
242. Wells RS, Smith Ma (1963) The natural history of granuloma annulare. **Br J Dermatol** 75:19.
243. Dabski K, Winkelmann RK (1989) Generalized granuloma annulare: clinical and laboratory findings in 100 patients. **J Am Acad Dermatol** 20:232.
244. Friedman-Birnbaum R, Haim S, Gideone O et al. (1978) Histocompatibility antigens in granuloma annulare. **Br J Dermatol** 98:425.

245. Andersen BL, Verdich J (1979) Granuloma annulare and diabetes mellitus. **Clin Exp Dermatol** 4:31–37.
246. Middleston D, Allen GE (1984) HLA antigen frequency in granuloma annulare. **Br J Dermatol** 110:57–59.
247. Lucky AW, Prose NS, Bove K et al. (1992) Papular umbilicated granuloma annulare. **Arch Dermatol** 128:1375.
248. Ghadially R, Sibbald RG, Walter JB et al. (1989) Granuloma annulare in patients with human immunodeficiency virus infections. **J Am Acad Dermatol** 20:232.
249. Grogg KL, Nascimento AG (2001) Subcutaneous granuloma annulare in childhood: clinicopathologic features in 34 cases. **Pediatrics** 107(3):e42.
250. Felner EI, Steinberg JB, Weinberg AG (1997) Subcutaneous granuloma annulare: a review of 47 cases. **Pediatrics** 100:965–967.
251. Evans MJ, Blessing K, Gray ES (1994) Pseudorheumatoid nodule (deep granuloma annulare) of childhood: clinicopathologic features of 20 patients. **Pediatr Dermatol** 11:6–9.
252. Cronquist, SD, Stashower ME, Benson PM (1999) Deep dermal granuloma annulare presenting as a eyelid tumor in a child, with review of pediatric eye id lesions. **Pediatric Dermatol** 16(5):377–380.
253. Hata N, Inamura T, Imayama S et al. (2001) Multiple pallisading granulomas in the scalp of an infant: a case report. **Surg Neurol** 56(6):396–399.
254. Draheim JH, Johnson LC, Helwig EB (1959) A clinicopathologic analysis of "rheumatoid" nodules occurring in 54 children, abstracted. **Am J Pathol** 35:678.
255. Nebesio CL, Lewis C Chuang TY (2002) Lack of an association between granuloma annulare and type 2 diabetes mellitus. **Br J Dermatol** 146:122–124.

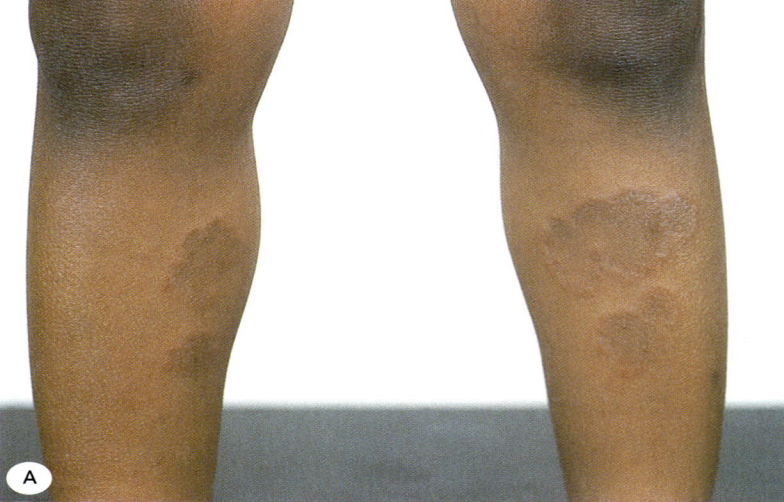

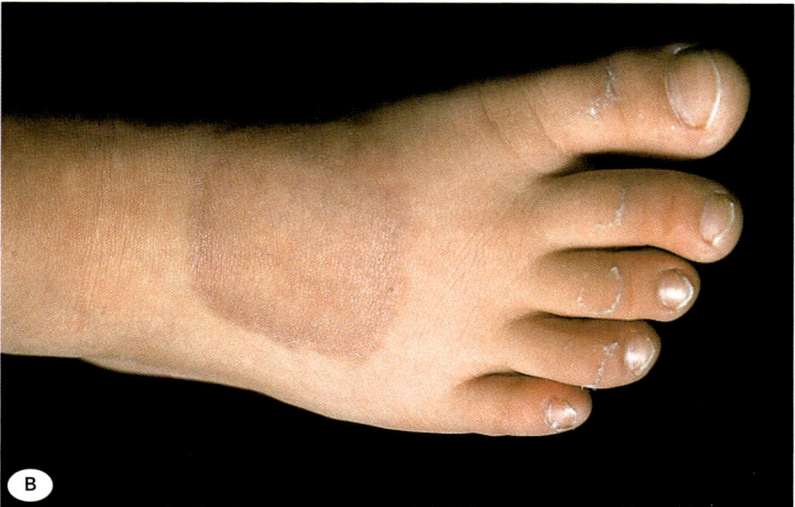

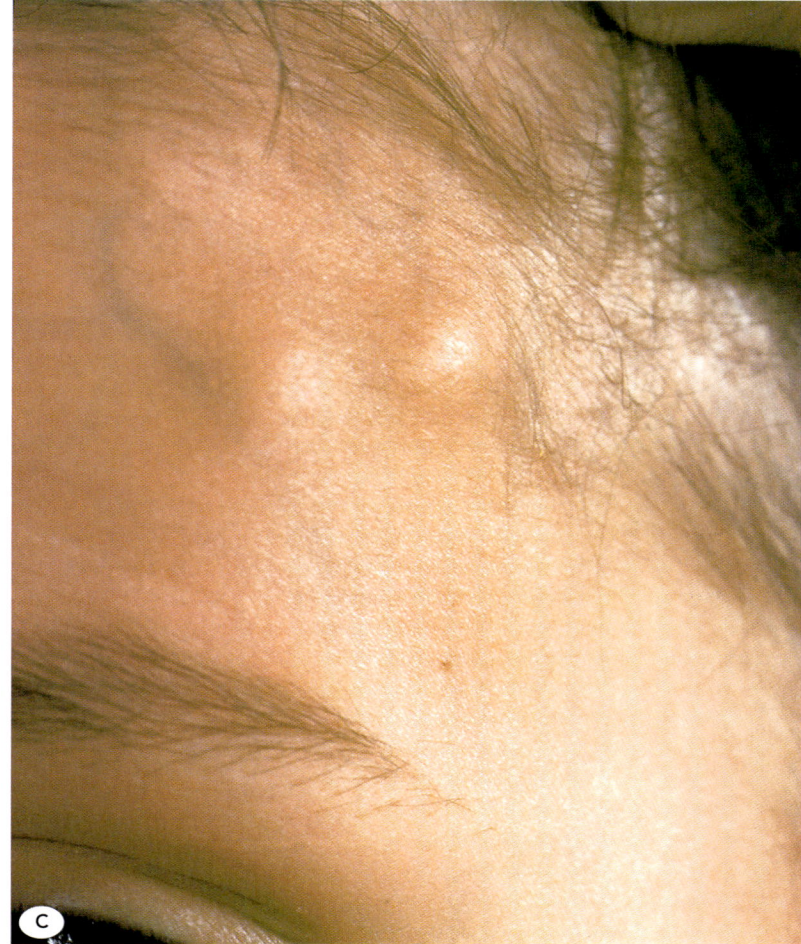

Fig. 17.11   (A) Granuloma annulare on the leg of a child. (B) Granuloma annulare on the foot. (C) Subcutaneous granuloma annulare on forehead and scalp.

degenerated collagen is extruded through the epidermis by transepidermal elimination. In the dermis, there is degeneration of collagen, surrounded by palisading histiocytes with lymphocytes and fibroblasts (the palisading granuloma). In the subcutaneous form, areas of degeneration are located in the subcutaneous layer.

Collagen fibers are separated by mucinous material, some of which is hyaluronic acid, that can be demonstrated on special stains.[241] By immunofluorescent staining, fibrin has also been shown to be a constant feature in the necrobiotic foci.[241,256] IgM, C3, or fibrinogen staining along the dermal-epidermal junction and IgM cytoid bodies have been reported by some authors.[255,257]

Although the cause of GA is unknown, numerous theories have been proposed to account for the degenerated collagen.[257] Dahl et al.[258] found vasculitis on routine biopsy of early lesions, and by direct immunofluorescence, and proposed that the initial event was vascular injury. This has not been substantiated by others.[255] Bergmann et al.,[259] in a study of early lesions, confirmed the presence of neutrophils and nuclear dust, but found evidence of frank vasculitis in only one lesion, and there was no evidence of immune deposits. An underlying defect related to diabetes has been suggested,[260] but the results of glucose tolerance tests and insulin studies are contradictory.[261] Tuberculin skin testing, sarcoidosis,[262,263] insect bites, trauma, herpes zoster,[264] drugs,[265] carcinoma,[266] Hodgkin's disease[267] and other lymphomas,[268] adenovirus,[269]

256. Umbert P, Winkelmann RK (1976) Granuloma annulare. Br J Dermatol 95:487.
257. Dahl MV, Callen JP (1986) Granuloma annulare. In: Pathogenesis of Skin Disease, Thiers BH, Dobson RL, eds. New York: Churchill Livingstone.
258. Dahl MV, Ullman S, Goltz RW (1977) Vasculitis in granuloma annulare. Arch Dermatol 113:463.
259. Bergman R, Pam Z, Lichtig C et al. (1993) Localized granuloma annulare. Am J Dermatopathol 15:544–548.
260. Rhodes EL, Hill DM, Ames AC et al. (1966) Granuloma annulare. Br J Dermatol 78:532.
261. Blohme G, Mobacken H, Waldenstrom J (1974) Early insulin response to glucose injected intravenously in patients with localized granuloma annulare. Acta Derm Venereol (Stockh) 54:259.
262. Ehrich EW, McGuire JL, Kim YH (1992) Association of granuloma annulare with sarcoidosis. Arch Dermatol 128:855.
263. Suite M, Jankey N (1992) Familial granuloma annulare. Int J Dermatol 31:818.

264. Zanolli MD, Powell BL, McCalmont T et al. (1992) Granuloma annulare and disseminated herpes zoster. Int J Dermatol 31:55.
265. Ross EV, Cobb M (1991) Generalized granuloma annulare associated with quinidine therapy. J Assoc Mil Dermatol 17:16.
266. Stewart KA, Cooper PH, Greer KE et al. (1989) Granuloma annulare temporally associated with carcinoma of the breast. J Am Acad Dermatol 21:309.
267. Schwartz RA, Hansen RC, Lynch PJ (1981) Hodgkin's disease and granuloma annulare. Arch Dermatol 117:185–186.
268. Barksdale SK, Perniciaro C, Halling KC et al. (1994) Granuloma annulare in patients with malignant lymphoma: clinicopathologic study of 13 new cases. J Am Acad Dermatol 32:42–48.
269. Coldiron BM, Freeman RG, Beaudoing DL (1988) Isolation of adenovirus from a granuloma annulare like lesion in the acquired immunodeficiency syndrome-related complex. Arch Dermatol 124:654.

and solar radiation have all been reported as possible inciting causes in some patients. The precise antigenic stimulus, whether exogenous or endogenous, is unknown. An inciting event in the center of the lesion may set off a chain reaction of events peripheral to it, eliciting inflammation and causing the characteristic rings.[270]

Buechner et al.[271] and others[272] suggest that the cell-mediated immune response could be the dominant pathogenic event in GA. They demonstrated that most of the mononuclear cell infiltrate was reactive with Leu-1 antibody, which characterizes peripheral and activated T cells. Helper-inducer T cells (identified with Leu-3a) were the major component of the lymphocytic infiltrate; (Leu-2a) suppressor cytotoxic T cells were also found in the area, but to a lesser degree. They concluded that the pathogenesis of this disorder may involve a specific cell-mediated immune response.

Umbert and Winkelmann[273] proposed that sensitized lymphocytes within the dermis, which are consistently found around blood vessels in this condition, release lymphokines including macrophage inhibitory factor, which cause macrophages and histiocytes in the dermis to release lysosomal enzymes that partially degrade connective tissue. The serum lysozyme (muramidase) level has been shown to be elevated in generalized GA.[274] Interferon-β_1, which inhibits maturation of monocytes to macrophages, can cause resolution when injected into a lesion.[275]

The cause of GA remains uncertain. However, with new techniques to explore immunologic characteristics, an immune complex vasculitis or a cell-mediated delayed hypersensitivity reaction may be found resulting from multiple trigger factors.

DIFFERENTIAL DIAGNOSIS

The classic clinical picture in a child is not difficult to recognize, but several other pediatric skin disorders may be confused with GA. Tinea corporis forms ringed lesions but has epidermal changes of scaling or vesiculation. Microscopically, hyphae can be recognized on scrapings. Sarcoidosis may be difficult to distinguish from GA but more commonly affects the face and the typical clinical lesions of GA are not present. Biopsy of a lesion should establish the differences. Rheumatoid nodules may be confused with the subcutaneous form of GA but are usually seen in adults with a high-titer latex fixation test and arthritis. In children, rheumatic fever nodules may mimic the subcutaneous form, but fever, heart murmur, and arthritis are seen in rheumatic fever. Necrobiosis lipoidica is characterized by orange or yellow plaques with atrophy and telangiectasias in the center. This is mainly located on the pretibial areas, and clinically does not resemble GA although the histology may be similar. The flat-topped violaceous plaques of annular lichen planus show Wickham's striae on the surface and occasional scaling. Secondary syphilis can be ruled out with a positive VDRL. Tuberculoid leprosy demonstrates hypopigmentation, decreased sensation, and enlarged nerves. The disseminated or acral papular umbilicated form can mimic lichen nitidus, flat warts, mollusca, or sarcoidosis. Perforating GA can be confused with other perforating disorders such as perforating folliculitis, Kyrle's disease, and elastosis perforans serpiginosa. It can also simulate pitryiasis lichenoides et varioliformis acuta.

PROGNOSIS AND MANAGEMENT

Lesions usually persist for an average of one to four years or may have a more chronic, relapsing course.[243,276] Seventy-three percent of lesions disappear within two years.[242] For this reason, reassurance is usually all that is necessary. Nevertheless, recurrences and/or new lesions are common. The duration of the lesions may last for a few weeks to several decades. Because patients are often concerned about the cosmetic aspect, one may wish to try mid-range topical corticosteroids with or without occlusion. Flurandrenolide tape, an adhesive tape impregnated with corticosteroid, aids penetration and may be helpful. The tape is cut to the size of the lesion and applied for several days at a time. Intralesional steroids, (triamcinolone acetonide 2.5mg/ml) injected directly into the lesion may hasten resolution. Cryotherapy has been used in older children or those with limited areas of involvement. A study of 31 patients showed clearing with cryotherapy in 25; however, due to the pain of the procedure, nitrous oxide anesthesia was required.[277] Occasionaly, biopsy of a lesion is followed by complete involution of the entire lesion. In adults, for cosmetically disfiguring GA, short-term corticosteroid therapy, chlorambucil, etretinate,[278] isotretinoin,[279] dapsone,[280] PUVA,[281] and Cyclosporin A,[282] have been used with some degree of success. Antimalarials were used successfully to clear six children with disseminated GA.[283] Generally, most children do not have disfiguring lesions and do not need such treatments.

Subcutaneous lesions are histologically similar to rheumatoid nodules (pseudorheumatoid nodules).[284] Adults presenting with rheumatoid nodules, histologically identical to subcutaneous GA, are at significant risk for the development of rheumatoid arthritis or other connective tissue disease. Scattered reports of necrobiotic granulomas in children with rheumatoid disease have perpetuated concern about the association of these lesions and connective tissue disorders.[285] Two reviews of 47 and 34 cases of subcutaneous GA have confirmed the self-limited course with no patients developing connective tissue disease after a lengthy follow-up period.[249,250]

In a retrospective study of 557 adult patients, Muhlemann et al.[286] found an association between localized GA and insulin dependent diabetes. The relevance of this study to the common form of childhood GA is unclear. A recent report of 42 children with localized GA followed for three years revealed no increased association with diabetes mellitus.[276]

Whether GA in a child has predictive value regarding development of diabetes mellitus is unknown. A recent case-controlled study of 126 patients found no association between GA and type 2 diabetes, while a previous case-controlled study of 61 patients with GA did show a relationship to type 1 diabetes.[255]

PEDIATRIC ASPECTS OF THE DISEASE

This condition is most commonly seen in the pediatric age group. There is no known influence of GA on nutrition, physical activities, or school performance. It is mainly a cosmetic problem, and whether this entity is associated with insulin-dependent diabetes in childhood requires further investigation. Treatment is limited in children but parental reassurance is usually all that is required.

270. Dahl MV (1986) Is actinic granuloma really granuloma annulare? Arch Dermatol 122:39.
271. Buechner SA, Winkelmann RK, Banks PM (1983) Identification of T-cell subpopulations in granuloma annulare. Arch Dermatol 119:125.
272. Modlin RL, Horwitz DA, Jordan RR et al. (1984) Immunopathologic demonstration of T lymphocyte subpopulations and interleukin 2 in granuloma annulare. Pediatr Dermatol 2:26.
273. Umbert P, Winkelmann RK (1977) Granuloma annulare and sarcoidosis. Br J Dermatol 97:481.
274. Padilla RS, Holguin T, Burgdorf WH, Dahl MV. Serum lysozyme in patients with localized and generalized granuloma annulare. Arch Dermatol 121:624.
275. Baba T, Hoshino M, Uyeno K (1988) Resolution of cutaneous lesions of granuloma annulare by intralesional injection of human fibroblast interferon. Arch Dermatol 124:1015.
276. Martinón-Torres F, Martinón-Sánchez JM, Martinón-Sánchez F (1999) Localized granuloma annulare in children: a review of 42 cases. Eur J Pediatr 158:866–873.
277. Blueme-Peytavi U, Zouboulis CC, Jacobi H et al. (1994) Successful outcome of cryosurgery in patients with granuloma annulare. Br J Dermatol 130:494–497.
278. Botella-Estrada R, Guillen C, Sanmartin O, Aliaga A (1992) Disseminated granuloma annulare: resolution with etretinate therapy. J Am Acad Dermatol 26:777.
279. Schleicher SM, Milstein HJ, Lim SJM (1992) Resolution of disseminated granuloma annulare with isotretinoin. Int J Dermatol 31:371.
280. Steiner A, Pehamberger H, Wolff K (1985) Sulfone treatment of granuloma annulare. J Am Acad Dermatol 13:1004.
281. Kerker BJ, Huang CP, Morison WL (1990) Photochemotherapy of generalized granuloma annulare. Arch Dermatol 126:359–361.
282. Filotico R, Vena GA, Coviello C et al. (1994) Cyclosporine in the treatment of generalized granuloma annulare. J Am Acad Dermatol 30:487–488.
283. Simon M, von den Driesch P (1994) Antimalarials for control of disseminated granuloma annulare in children. J Am Acad Dermatol 31:1064–1065.
284. Patterson JW (1988) Rheumatoid nodule and subcutaneous granuloma annulare. A comparative histologic study. Am J Dermatopathol 10:1.
285. Medlock MD, McComb JG, Raffel C et al. (1994) Subcutaneous palisading granuloma of the scalp in childhood. Pediatr Neurosurg 21:113–116 (Medline).
286. Muhlemann MF, Williams DRR (1984) Localized granuloma annulare is associated with insulin-dependent diabetes mellitus. Br J Dermatol 111:325.

GRANULOMA FACIALE

Granuloma faciale is a rare dermatologic entity characterized by single or multiple, soft, brown-red to violaceous plaques, papules, or nodules that are found most frequently on the face and rarely on other areas. Lever and Leeper[287] and Cobane et al.[288] separated this entity from Langerhans cell histiocytosis, eosinophilic granuloma of the bone, and other nonspecific granulomas of the skin with eosinophilia.[289] It is an uncommon, indolent, benign disorder of unknown cause.[290]

EPIDEMIOLOGY

Granuloma faciale has been reported in children as young as 18 months old[291] but most commonly it occurs in middle-aged adults.[292] Males are affected more commonly than females,[293] and whites more commonly than other races.[294] No genetic predisposition has been demonstrated.

PRESENTING HISTORY

The patient presents with one or more well-circumscribed plaques, most commonly located on the face.[295] Lesions are typically asymptomatic, although some patients report pruritus, burning, and tenderness.[296] The lesions have usually been present for some time before the patient seeks help; a history of resistance to therapy is common.

PHYSICAL EXAMINATION

Lesions are circumscribed, soft, brownish-red macules, plaques, or nodules with a smooth surface.[290] Rarely, they may be seen on other parts of the body.[297,298] The surrounding skin is normal. They vary in size from a few millimeters to several centimeters and do not ulcerate.[293] Hair, nails, and teeth are not affected. A case of intranasal granuloma faciale has been reported.[299] There is no associated internal organ involvement.[292,293]

LABORATORY FINDINGS

Laboratory findings are normal except for an occasional mild blood eosinophilia.[295]

PATHOPHYSIOLOGY AND HISTOGENESIS

Biopsy of the skin shows distinctive changes in the dermis consisting of a dense polymorphous infiltrate of neutrophils and eosinophils.[186] Lymphocytes, histiocytes, plasma cells, and mast cells may be seen. The infiltrate is in the upper dermis, but may extend into the lower dermis, and is separated from the epidermis and pilosebaceous appendages by a Grenz zone of normal collagen.

Immunofluorescent microscopy demonstrates IgG and complement, and less consistently IgA and IgM, along the basement membrane zone and the perivascular areas.[300,301] Fibrin can be demonstrated along the basement membrane zone and blood vessel walls. Indirect immunofluorescence is negative.

Although the cause is obscure,[289] it has been suggested that this is an immunologically mediated disorder, likened to a chronic leukocytoclastic vasculitis.[186] Most current theories suggest that granuloma faciale may be a localized chronic hypersensitivity vasculitis, which involves an antigen-antibody reaction, with deposition of immunoglobulin and complement in the skin.[301] According to this hypothesis, the heavy infiltrate of polymorphonuclear leukocytes perpetuates the inflammatory response by producing chemotactic factors. Smoller and Bortz,[302] demonstrated a predominance of T-helper lymphocytes which costained strongly for antibodies against interleukin and LFA-1, suggesting that the disorder may be mediated by γ-interferon. Electron microscopic studies have shown no evidence of bacterial or viral infection.[303]

DIFFERENTIAL DIAGNOSIS

Clinically, the lesions resemble erythema elevatum diutinum but a biopsy should differentiate erythema elevatum diutinum by demonstrating a leukocytoclastic vasculitis and an absence of both eosinophils and Grenz zone in erythema elevatum diutinum. The histiocytes lack Langerhans granules, which distinguishes this disease from Langerhans cell histiocytosis. Sarcoidosis, lymphocytic infiltrate of Jessner, fixed drug eruption, urticaria pigmentosa, juvenile xanthogranuloma, leprosy, Langerhans cell histiocytosis, and allergic vasculitis can all resemble granuloma faciale clinically. A biopsy helps distinguish among these entities.

THERAPY AND PROGNOSIS

Granuloma faciale is extremely resistant to treatment. The most effective therapies include dapsone,[289,304] or psoralen plus long-wave ultraviolet light (PUVA).[305] Use of the pulsed dye laser has given excellent results.[306,307] Other therapies that have occasionally been effective include cryotherapy,[308] intralesional steroids, dermabrasion, surgical excision, radiation, oral steroids, antimalarials, and the carbon dioxide laser.[309,310] Lesions rarely involute spontaneously.

PEDIATRIC ASPECTS OF THE DISEASE

Granuloma faciale is seen more commonly in middle-aged adults. It has been reported in children and should be considered in a differential diagnosis of persistent plaques on the face. It is primarily a cosmetic problem.

287. Lever WF, Leeper RW (1950) Eosinophilic granuloma of the skin: report of cases representing the two different diseases described as eosinophilic granuloma. Arch Dermatol 62:85.
288. Pinkus H, Straith CL, Cobane JH (1950) Facial granulomas with eosinophilia. Arch Dermatol Syphilol 61:442.
289. Guill MA, Aton JK (1982) Facial granuloma responding to dapsone therapy. Arch Dermatol 118:332.
290. Sears JK, Gitter DG, Stone MS (1991) Extrafacial granuloma faciale. Arch Dermatol 127:742.
291. Pedace FJ, Perry HO (1966) Granuloma Faciale. A clinical and histopathologic review. Arch Dermatol 94:387.
292. Black CI (1977) Granuloma faciale. Cutis 20:66.
293. Fitzpatrick TB (ed) (1999) Dermatology in General Medicine, 5th edn. New York: McGraw-Hill.
294. Sonoda S, Ishikawa Y (1965) A case of granuloma faciale. Excerpta Medica, Sect 13, Derm Venereology 19:554.
295. Johnson WC, Higdon RS, Helwig EB (1959) Granuloma faciale. Arch Dermatol 79:42.
296. Dowlati B, Firooz A, Dowlati Y (1997) Granuloma faciale: successful treatment of nine cases with a combination of cryotherapy and intralesional corticosteroid injection. Int J Dermatol 36:548–551.
297. Roustan G, Sanchez Yus E, Salas C, Simon A (1999) Granuloma faciale with extrafacial lesions. Dermatology 198(1):79–82.
298. Castano E, Segurada A, Iglesias L, Lopez-Rios F et al. (1997) Granuloma faciale entirely in an extrafacial location. Br J Dermatol 136(6):978–979.
299. Holmes DK, Panje WR (1983) Intranasal granuloma faciale. Am J Otolaryngol 4:184.
300. Schroeter AL, Copeman PMN, Jordan RE et al. (1971) Immunofluorescence of cutaneous vasculitis associated with systemic disease. Arch Dermatol 104:254.
301. Nieboer C, Laksbeek GL (1978) Immunofluorescence studies in granuloma eosinophilicum faciale. J Cutan Pathol 5:68.
302. Smoller BR, Bortz J (1993) Immunophentotypic analysis suggests that granuloma faciale is a gamma-interferon-mediated process. J Cutan Pathol 20:442–446.
303. Schnitzler L, Verret JL, Schubert B (1977) Granuloma faciale: ultrastructural study of three cases. J Cutan Pathol 4:123.
304. Goldner R, Sina B (1984) Granuloma faciale; the role of dapsone and prior irradiation on the cause of the disease. Cutis 33:478.
305. Hudson LD (1983) Granuloma faciale: treatment with topical psoralen and UVA. J Am Acad Dermatol 9:559.
306. Hall Welsh J, Schroeder TL, Levy ML (1999) Granuloma faciale in a child successfully treated with the pulsed dye laser. J Am Acad Dermatol 41(2):351–353.
307. Ammirati, CT, Hruza GJ (1999) Treatment of granuloma faciale with the 585-nm. pulsed dye laser. Arch Dermatol 135:903–905.
308. Zacarian SA (1985) Cryosurgery effective for granuloma faciale. J Dermatol Surg Oncol 11:11.
309. Wheeland RG, Ashley JR, Smith DA et al. (1984) Carbon dioxide laser treatment of granuloma faciale. J Dermatol Surg Oncol 10:730.
310. Dinehart SM, Gross DJ, Davis CM et al. (1990) Granuloma faciale. Comparison of different treatment modalities. Arch Otolaryngol Head Neck Surg 116:849.

CUTANEOUS LYMPHOID HYPERPLASIA (PSEUDOLYMPHOMA)

Cutaneous pseudolymphomas are a group of benign diseases that can be difficult to distinguish from true lymphomas. A classification of this group (Table 17.3) has been proposed by Brodell and Santa Cruz.[311]

Cutaneous lymphoid hyperplasia (CLH), also called lymphocytoma cutis or pseudolymphoma of Spiegler–Fendt, is a benign skin disorder that presents as persistent red nodules or plaques. Hyperplasia of the reticuloendothelial tissue in the skin is characteristic, with mature germinal centers resembling the architecture in the cortex of lymph nodes.[312] Cutaneous lymphoid hyperplasia is usually a B-cell predominant or mixed B-cell/T-cell disorder.[313]

EPIDEMIOLOGY

CLH can occur at any age,[314] but it usually occurs in the late teenage years and early adult life.[315] Females are affected more often than males.

PRESENTING HISTORY

The patient usually complains of an asymptomatic nodule or persistent multiple papules on the skin.

PHYSICAL EXAMINATION

There are two forms of skin lesions. The localized form of CLH (circumscribed lymphocytoma cutis) is more commonly seen in infants and children. Lesions are skin-colored, red, or violaceous and often show a follicular arrangement.[312,316] Seventy percent of the lesions occur on the face.[317] Other common sites include the extremities, areola, and genitalia. Lesions slowly enlarge and can grow to a diameter of 3–5cm.(Fig.17.12)

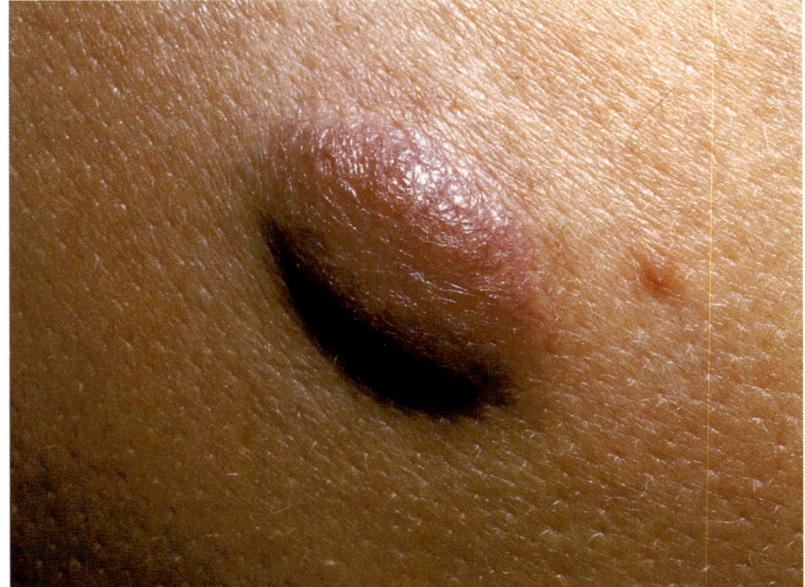

Fig. 17.12 Lymphocytoma cutis on the back of an adolescent.

The disseminated form is rare and is seen mostly in middle-aged adults. Multiple firm papules or small bluish-red nodules are often confined to the face. Sometimes the lesions are large and scattered over the trunk and extremities. Disseminated lesions grow rapidly, tend to recur, and may persist throughout life. There may be temporary loss of hair if the lesions affect a hair-bearing area.[316] There are usually no other associated findings on physical examination, except occasional lymphadenopathy.

LABORATORY FINDINGS

No laboratory abnormalities have been noted with lymphocytoma cutis.[318]

PATHOPHYSIOLOGY AND HISTOGENESIS

Although the cause of lymphocytoma cutis is unknown, the lesions are thought to be a reactive hyperplasia of mature lymphocytes. Some cases have followed insect bites, trauma,[319] gold earring-related dermatitis,[320] contact dermatitis from ophthalmological products,[321] tattooing,[322] herpes zoster,[323] and *Borrelia* infection.[324]

Histologically, a heavy infiltrate of lymphocytes and histiocytes are present in the dermis.[186] Mature lymphoid tissue is seen, which resembles the architecture seen in the cortex of the lymph node, with discrete islands of pale cells surrounded by sheets of dark-staining lymphocytes. A Grenz zone of clear connective tissue between the intense infiltrate and the epidermis, or between the infiltrate and hair follicles, is frequently seen.

Differentiation from true lymphoma (particularly well-differentiated lymphocytic lymphoma) is important but may be difficult. The presence of plasma cells or eosinophils, the lack of extension into the deep dermis and subcutaneous fat, and the absence of mitoses and features of atypia indicate a

TABLE 17.3 Benign and malignant cutaneous lymphoid infiltrates in children

Perivascular lymphocytic infiltrates
  Erythema annulare centrifugum
  Lymphocytic infiltrates with mucinosis
    Lymphocytic infiltrate of Jessner-Kanof

Cutaneous lymphoid hyperplasia (CLH pseudolymphoma)

Arthropod bites, stings, infestations (nodular scabies), Borrelia burgdorferi, vaccinations

"Lymphoproliferative" conditions
  Drug-induced pseudolymphoma
  Lymphomatoid papulosis

Lymphomatoid contact dermatitis

Cutaneous lymphomas
  Primary
    T-cell lymphomas
    B-cell lymphomas
    Histiocytic neoplasms
  Secondary

311. Brodell RT, Santa Cruz DJ (1985) Cutaneous pseudolymphomas. **Dermatol Clin** 3:719.
312. Bafverstedt B (1960) Lymphadenosis benigna cutis (LABC) its nature, course and prognosis. **Acta Derm Venereol** (Stockh) 40:10.
313. Gilliam AC, Wood GS (2000) Cutaneous lymphoid hyperplasias. Cutaneous lymphoid hyperplasias. **Sem Cutan Med Surg** 19(2):133–141.
314. Hurwitz S (1993) Clinical Pediatric Dermatology, 2nd edn. Philadelphia: WB Saunders.
315. Rook A, Wilkinson DS, Ebling FJG, eds. (1998) Textbook of Dermatology, 6th ed. Oxford: Blackwell Scientific.
316. Bafverstedt B (1962) Unusual forms of lymphadenosis benigna cutis. **Acta Derm Venereol** (Stockh) 42:3.
317. Moschella SL, Hurley HJ, eds. Dermatology, 3rd edn. Philadelphia: WB Saunders.
318. Ralfkiaer E, Wantzin GL, Mason DY et al. (1984) Characterization of benign cutaneous infiltrates by monoclonal antibodies. **Br J Dermatol** 111:635.

319. Bafverstedt B (1968) Lymphadenosis benigna cutis. **Acta Derm Venereol** (Stockh) 48:1.
320. Iwatsuki K, Yamada M, Takigawa M et al. (1987) Benign lymphoplasia of the earlobes induced by gold earrings: immunohistologic study on the cellular infiltrates. **J Am Acad Dermatol** 16:83.
321. Braun RP, French LE, Feldmann R et al. (2000) Cutaneous pseudolymphoma, lymphomatoid contact dermatitis type, as an unusual cause of symmetrical upper eyelid nodules. **Br J Dermatol** 143(2):411–414.
322. Blumenthal G, Okun MR, Ponitch JA (1982) Pseudolymphomatous reaction to tattoos. **J Am Acad Dermatol** 6:485.
323. Sanchez JL, Mendez JA, Palacio R (1981) Cutaneous pseudolymphoma at the site of resolving herpes zoster. **Arch Dermatol** 117:377.
324. Albrecht S, Hofstadter S, Artsob H, Chaban O et al. (1991) Lymphadenosis benigna cutis resulting from Borrelia infection (Borrelia lymphocytoma). **J Am Acad Dermatol** 24:621.

benign disease. Using monoclonal antibody staining, the reactive follicles composed of T cells, polytypic B cells, monotypic plasma cells, macrophages, and Langerhans cells have been found.[318,325–327] CLH is generally B-cell rich or a mixed B-cell/T-cell disorder.[326] Occasionally, epidermal involvement, adenexal infiltration, vascular invasion, and deep involvement in the dermis may be seen, features commonly seen in cutaneous lyphoma. Clonality of the infiltrate is suggestive but not diagnostic of cutaneous lymphoma. Gene rearrangement of the T-cell receptor gamma chain gene is present in more than 90% of cutaneous T-cell lymphoma and may be helpful in cases that are not obvious.[327,328] The demonstration of monoclonal immunoglobulin light chain expression in B cells or aberrant antigen expression on B or T cells suggests a malignant process. Patients with clonal populations of B or T cells (clonal cutaneous lymphoid hyperplasia) should be closely observed for emergence of a lymphoma.[313] In the skin, T lymphocytes may have proliferative abilities, as is also seen in lupus profundus, lymphocytic vasculitis, and insect bites.[325] The lymphoid follicles seen in lymphocytoma cutis may be a similar reaction.

DIFFERENTIAL DIAGNOSIS

A clinical differential diagnosis of the solitary form includes histiocytoma, mastocytoma, granuloma faciale, sarcoidosis, DLE, and lymphoma. The disseminated form may resemble polymorphous light eruption, histiocytomas, and lymphocytic infiltrate of Jessner. Histologically, the lesions may resemble insect bites and drug reactions, particularly phenytoin reactions.[329] Malignant lymphoreticular disorders, such as non-Hodgkin's lymphoma, cutaneous T-cell lymphomas, and Langerhans cell histiocytosis, may be difficult to differentiate from lymphocytoma cutis.[330] Direct immunofluorescence, monoclonal antibody studies, T-cell receptor gene rearrangement studies, and a history of photosensitivity may help to separate some of these entities.

THERAPY AND PROGNOSIS

The course is benign, with intermittent spontaneous regression and recurrences. Penicillin,[312] topical and intralesional steroids, cryosurgery,[331] or oral hydroxychloroquine[332] may have some value. The localized form of lymphocytoma cutis responds rapidly to X-ray therapy (500–1500cGy), but this modality should be avoided in children.[314] Use of the argon laser may improve the cosmetic appearance.[333] There have been a few cases reported that have converted to B-cell lymphoma, although these cases usually show clonality of the infiltrate from the outset.[334]

PEDIATRIC ASPECTS OF THE DISEASE

Because this entity tends to involve only the skin, and the general health of the patient is good, only the cosmetic appearance and psychological welfare of the child needs to be assessed.

LYMPHOCYTIC INFILTRATE OF JESSNER

In 1953, Jessner and Kanof[335] described a clinical condition manifested by a lymphocytic infiltrate of the skin with a benign and variable course. The lesions were asymptomatic, erythematous papules or plaques that were associated with spontaneous relapses and recurrences. There is continuing controversy as to whether Jessner's lymphocytic infiltrate represents a distinct clinical entity or is a variant of lupus erythematosus, polymorphic light eruption, or lymphocytoma cutis.[331]

EPIDEMIOLOGY

Lymphocytic infiltrate of Jessner is a sporadic disease affecting people from 4 to 68 years of age.[336,337] Most cases involve young adults.[338] Males are affected more often than females, but female carriers of chronic granulomatous disease may have an eruption similar to lymphocytic infiltrate of Jessner.[339]

PRESENTING HISTORY

Patients present with persistent erythematous discrete papules or plaques. The face, earlobes, and neck are most frequently involved, but lesions may be seen on the upper trunk, extremities, and scrotum. Exacerbations may occur with exposure to sunlight.

PHYSICAL EXAMINATION

The lesions start as asymptomatic, well-defined papules that may expand peripherally and clear in the center as they expand, to form annular lesions. The papules or plaques are pink to reddish-brown and are usually smooth, but occasionally may have an uneven surface. Lesions may be solitary or numerous. Most commonly, they affect the face, but other body areas may also be affected.

The general health of the individual is unaffected and hair, nails, teeth, and mucous membranes are normal. There is no lymphadenopathy or other associated findings on physical examination.

LABORATORY FINDINGS

Lymphocytosis of the peripheral blood has been reported in a minority of patients.[315,335]

PATHOPHYSIOLOGY AND HISTOGENESIS

Histologically, there is a well-circumscribed, intense superficial and deep lymphocytic infiltrate in the dermis, predominantly in the perivascular and periadnexal areas.[186] There are no germinal centers, or significant numbers of reticular or histiocytic elements. A few histiocytes and plasma cells may be found. The epidermis is normal.

325. VanHale HM, Winkelmann RK (1985) Nodular lymphoid disease of the head and neck: lymphocytoma cutis, benign lymphocytic infiltrate of Jessner, and their distinction from malignant lymphoma. **J Am Acad Dermatol** 12:455.
326. Medeiros LJ, Picker LJ, Abel EA et al. (1989) Cutaneous lymphoid hyperplasia. Immunologic characteristics and assessment of criteria recently proposed as diagnostic of malignant lymphoma. **J Am Acad Dermatol** 21:929.
327. Schmid U, Eckert F, Griesser H et al. (1995) Cutaneous follicular lymphoid hyperplasia with monotypic plasma cells. A clinicopathologic study of 18 patients. **Am J Surg Pathol** 19(1):12–20.
328. Flaig MJ, Schuhmann K, Sander CA (2000) Impact of moldecular analysis in the diagnosis of cutaneous lymphoid infiltrates. **Semin Cutan Med Surg** 19(2):87–90.
329. Braddock SW, Harrington D, Vose J (1992) Generalized nodular cutaneous pseudolymphoma associated with phenytoin therapy. **J Am Acad Dermatol** 27:337.
330. Heilman E, Ackerman AB (1980) A histological atlas of pseudomalignant and malignant lymphoreticular disorders of the skin. **J Dermatol Surg Oncol** 6:646.
331. Cerio R, Oliver BF, Jones EW (1990) The heterogenity of Jessner's lymphocytic infiltrate of the skin. **J Am Acad Dermatol** 23:63.

332. Stoll DM (1983) Treatment of cutaneous pseudolymphoma with hydroxychoroquine. **J Am Acad Dermatol** 8:696.
333. Wheeland RG, Kantor GR, Bailin PL et al. (1986) Role of the argon laser in treatment of lymphocytoma cutis. **J Am Acad Dermatol** 14:267.
334. Hammer E, Sangueza O, Suwanjindar P et al. (1993) Immunophenotypic and genotypic analysis in cutaneous lymphoid hyperplasias. **J Am Acad Dermatol** 28:426.
335. Jessner M, Kanof NB (1953) Lymphocytic infiltration of the skin. **Arch Dermatol Syphilol** 68:447.
336. Ralfkiaer E, Lange Wantzin G, Mason DY et al. (1984) Characterization of benign cutaneous lymphocytic infiltrates by monoclonal antibodies. **Br J Dermatol** 111:635.
337. Ashworth J, Morley WN (1988) Jessner and Kanof's lymphocytic infiltration of the skin: a familial variant. **Dermatologica** 177:120.
338. Calnan CD (1957) Lymphocytic infiltration of the skin (Jessner). **Br J Dermatol** 69:169.
339. Nelson CE, Dahl MV, Goltz RW (1977) Arcuate dermal erythema in a carrier of granulomatous disease. **Arch Dermatol** 113:798.

Controversy has surrounded lymphocytic infiltrate of Jessner. Some authors consider it to be a form of lymphocytoma cutis while others classify it as a variant of DLE, polymorphous light eruption, or lymphocytic lymphoma. It may be a heterogeneous group of disorders, but a review of 100 patients classifies it as a single entity.[340] Some of the patients in this study had coexisting polymorphous light eruption suggesting sunlight may play a role in the pathogenesis.[340] Borrelia burgdorferi serology has been reported to be positive by some authors[341] but refuted by others.[342] Lever[186] suggests that the term lymphocytic infiltrate be used as a preliminary term and not a definitive diagnosis because many cases evolve into DLE, polymorphous light eruption, lymphocytoma cutis, or lymphocytic lymphoma at a later time.

Studies using monoclonal antibodies have demonstrated that most of the infiltrating cells are T cells, with a helper/suppressor ratio that is approximately equal.[343,344] B lymphocytes are rare or absent.[345] This distinguishes lymphocytic infiltrate of Jessner from lymphocytoma cutis, which frequently shows a predominance of B cells in the infiltrate. Circulating immune complexes are increased during active disease and decrease when treatment is effective.[346] Natural killer cell function and antibody-dependent cell-mediated cytotoxicity are also decreased, showing that an immune defect may predominate in this disorder. However, T lymphocytes may accumulate from the circulation and not proliferate within the site of inflammation.[347]

Lymphocytic infiltrate of Jessner is most likely a unique benign immuno-reactive process, recognized as a chronic papular lymphocytic dermatosis without associated systemic disease.

DIFFERENTIAL DIAGNOSIS

The major differential diagnoses are with the other lymphocytic infiltrates of the skin such as DLE, polymorphous light eruption, lymphocytoma cutis, lymphoma cutis, and lymphomatoid papulosis. Drug eruptions and sarcoidosis must also be excluded. Direct immunofluorescence and serologic studies may be helpful to rule out LE. Monoclonal antibody studies may also be useful. Cytologic atypia is not seen in lymphocytic infiltrate of Jessner but is seen in lymphoma cutis and lymphomatoid papulosis.[348]

THERAPY AND PROGNOSIS

Therapies for Jessner's lymphocytic infiltrate of the skin include oral antimalarials, intramuscular gold, X-ray therapy, topical steroids, and cryotherapy.[349] Thalidomide given for two months has been reported to be effective.[342] Although many treatments are associated with a clinical response in some patients, this entity tends to be resistant to most modes of therapy. Lesions persist for weeks to years or even as long as 30 years, with an average length of five years. They resolve leaving no residual trace.[350] However, lesions may recur either at the same sites or elsewhere.

PEDIATRIC ASPECTS OF THE DISEASE

This disease has been reported in the pediatric age group; although it is rare, it is important to make the diagnosis, particularly in female carriers of chronic granulomatous disease.

SWEET SYNDROME

Sweet syndrome (acute febrile neutrophilic dermatosis) was first reported by Sweet[351] in 1964. The four cardinal features are: fever; neutrophilic leukocytosis in the peripheral blood; raised painful plaques on the limbs, face, and neck; and histological evidence of a dense dermal infiltrate of neutrophils histologically. Diagnostic criteria are listed in Table 17.4. Although most cases in the original series were preceded by infections, inflammatory diseases of various types, hemoproliferative disorders, and solid carcinomas have been reported with Sweet syndrome.[352–356] Miscellaneous associations include pregnancy, vaccination, POEMS syndrome, and contact with peppers.[352] Patients respond rapidly to systemic corticosteroid therapy.

TABLE 17.4 **Diagnostic criteria for Sweet Syndrome***

Major criteria
1. Abrupt onset of tender or painful erythematous plaques or nodules occasionally with vesicles, pustules, or bullae
2. Predominantly neutrophilic infiltration in the dermis without leukocytoclastic vasculitis

Minor criteria
1. Preceded by nonspecific respiratory or gastrointestinal tract infection or vaccination or associated with:
   ◆ Inflammatory disease such as chronic autoimmune disorders, infections
   ◆ Hemoproliferative disorders or solid malignant tumors
   ◆ Pregnancy
2. Accompanied by periods of general malaise and fever (>38°C)
3. Laboratory values during onset: ESR >20mm; C-reactive protein positive; segmented-nuclear neutrophils and stabs >70% in peripheral blood smear; leukocytosis >8000 (three of four of these values necessary)
4. Excellent response to treatment with systemic corticosteroids or potassium iodide

* Both major and two minor criteria needed for diagnosis.
Initiated by Su and Liu and modified by von den Driesch[352]

340. Toonstra J, Wildschut A, Boer J et al. (1989) Jessner's lymphocytic infiltration of the skin. A clinical study of 100 patients. **Arch Dermatol** 125:1525.
341. Abele DC, Anders KH (1990) The many faces and phases of borreliosis II. **J Am Acad Dermatol** 23:401.
342. Guillaume JC, Moulin G, Dieng Mt et al. Crossover study of thalidomide vs placebo in Jessner's lymphocytic infiltration of the skin. **Arch Dermatol** 131:1032–1035.
343. Willemze R, Dijkstra A, Meijer CJLM (1984) Lymphocytic infiltration of the skin (Jessner): a T-cell lymphoproliferative disease. **Br J Dermatol** 110:523.
344. VanHale HM, Winkelmann RK (1985) Nodular lymphoid disease of the head and neck: lymphocytoma cutis, benign lymphocytic infiltrate of Jessner, and their distinction from malignant lymphoma. **J Am Acad Dermatol** 12:455.
345. Kuo T, Lo SK, Chan HL (1991) Immunohistochemical analysis of mononuclear cell infiltrates in cutaneous lupus erythematosus, polymorphous light eruption, lymphocytic infiltration of Jessner, and cutaneous lymphoid hyperplasia. **J Cutan Pathol** 21:430–436.
346. Braddock SW, Kay HD, Maennle D et al. (1993) Clinical and immunologic studies in reticular erythematous mucinosis and Jessner's lymphocytic infiltrate of skin. **J Am Acad Dermatol** 28:691.
347. Kon Hinen YT, Bergroth V, Johansson E et al. (1987) A long-term clinico-pathologic survey of patients with Jessner's lymphocytic infiltration of the skin. **J Invest Dermatol** 89:205.
348. Mac Donald DM (1982) Histopathological differentiation of benign and malignant cutaneous lymphocytic infiltrates. **Br J Dermatol** 107:715.
349. Gottlieb B, Winkelmann RK (1962) Lymphocytic infiltration of skin. **Arch Dermatol** 86:626.
350. Wantzin GL, Hou-Jensen K, Nielsen M et al. (1982) Cutaneous lymphocytomas: clinical and histological aspects. **Acta Derm Venereol** (Stockh) 62:119.
351. Sweet RD (1964) An acute febrile neutrophilic dermatosis. **Br J Dermatol** 76:349.
352. Von den Driesch P (1994) Sweet's syndrome (acute neutrophilic dermatosis). **J Am Acad Dermatol** 3:535–556.
353. Boatman BW, Taylor RC, Klein LE et al. (1994) Sweet's syndrome in children. **South Med J** 87(2):193–196.
354. Sedel D, Huguet P, Lebbe C et al. (1994) Sweet syndrome as the presenting manifestation of chronic granulomatous disease in an infant. **Pediatr Dermatol** 11(3):237–240.
355. Shimizu T, Yoshida I, Eguchi H et al. (1996) Sweet syndrome in a child with aplastic anemia receiving recombinant granulocyte colony-stimulating factor. **J Pediatr Hematol Oncol** 18(3):282–284.
356. Hassouna L, Nabulsi-Khalil M, Mroueh SM et al. (1996) Multiple erythematous tender papules and nodules in an 11-month-old boy. Sweet syndrome (SS) (acute febrile neutrophilic dermatosis). **Arch Dermatol** 132(12):1507–1510.

EPIDEMIOLOGY

This entity is rare in children, but over 30 childhood cases have been reported.[353–356] Affected children as young as 7 weeks old have been described.[365,366] Nevertheless, Sweet syndrome is most commonly seen in patients aged 30 to 49 years with a female to male ratio of 3.7:1.[352] In children, the sex incidence is equal with peaks of occurrence in the first year of life and between 6 to 12 years of age. In adult cases there is an increased incidence in the spring and autumn. In a review of 176 cases, four broad groups were noted with 71% of patients presenting with classic/idiopathic disease, 16% associated with inflammatory diseases, 11% as a paraneoplastic phenomenon and 2% associated with pregnancy.[352] This contrasts with another review where the rate of paraneoplastic Sweet syndrome was 33%,[367] possibly reflecting the tendancy to publish case reports with associated diseases.

PRESENTING HISTORY

Eighty-five to ninety percent of patients have a high, persistent fever up to 40°C,[368] usually antedating the eruption by several days. Raised, erythematous, painful plaques and nodules appear about one week later.[369] Many of the patients have had a recent infection or other associated illness.

PHYSICAL EXAMINATION

Elevated tender plaques measuring 0.5–4cm are most commonly found on the face, neck, and limbs in an asymmetric distribution. Lesions usually spare the trunk but have been described on the palms and mucous membranes.[370,371] Palmoplantar lesions may mimic palmoplantar pustulosis.[372] Lesions enlarge quickly and develop annular patterns with clearing in the center. The larger plaques have heaped-up mamillated margins and develop vesicles or sterile pustules along their borders (Fig. 17.13); generally, lesions heal without sequelae,[370] except for temporary hyperpigmentation due to hemosiderin deposition. Secondary cutis laxa has been described within the areas of involvement in some children,[373,374] possibly secondary to the intense inflammatory process.

Other associated findings include arthritis and arthralgias in 33–62% of cases, which resolve with treatment.[352,369] Sterile osteomyelitis has been observed in some children.[231] Conjunctivitis and episcleritis have been described in up to 72% of cases;[375] renal involvement including proteinuria, hematuria, and glomerulonephritis may occur.[369] Eleven to thirty-three percent of the cases described in the literature have had an associated malignancy, particularly acute myelogenous leukemia.[267,377,378] This association is mainly in adult males, but has been reported in children.[358] Sterile neutrophilic infiltrates in organs other than skin occur as uncommon manifestations of Sweet syndrome or pyoderma gangrenosum. These infiltrates have been reported in the lungs, bones, joints, central nervous system, liver,

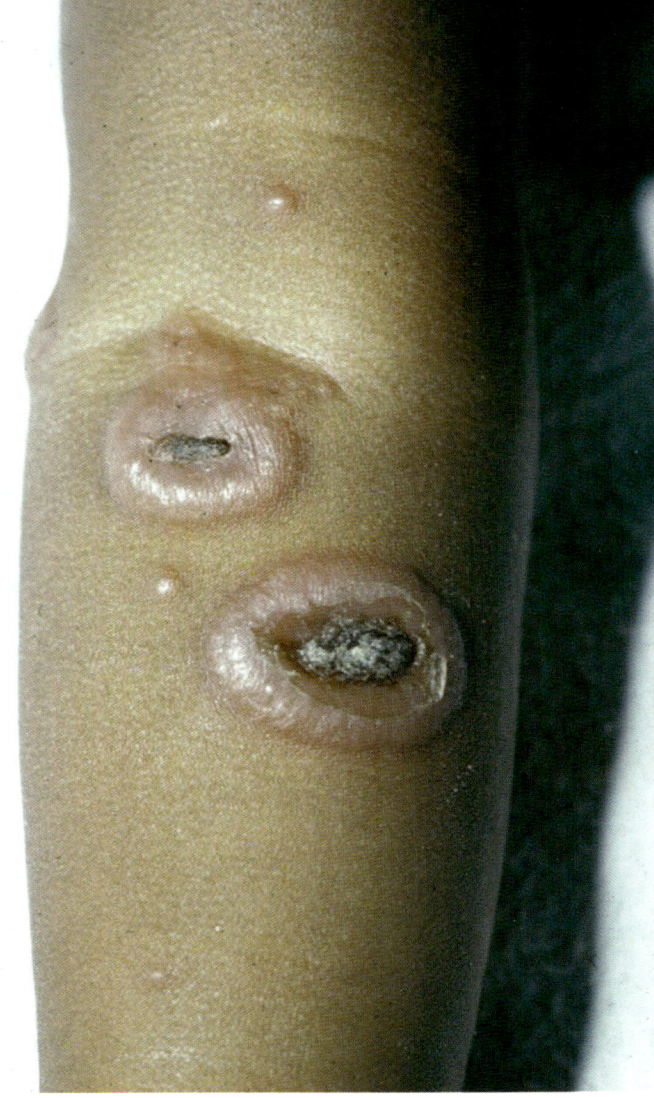

Fig. 17.13 Typical lesions of Sweet syndrome with heaped edges. Courtesy of Nancy Esterly.

gastrointestinal tract, lymph nodes, spleen, cardiovascular system, and eyes.[352,362,379,380] One child, who had cutis laxa-like changes following Sweet

357. Gray LC, Abele DC (1998) Annular erythematous plaques and tibial pain in a child. Sweet syndrome. **Arch Dermatol** 134(5):625–626, 628–629.
358. Schneider DT, Schuppe HC, Schwamborn D et al. (1998) Acute febrile neutrophilic dermatosis (Sweet syndrome) as initial presentation in a child with acute myelogenous leukaemia. **Med Pediatr Oncol** 31(3):178–181.
359. Tuerlinckx D, Bodart E, Despontin K et al. (1999) Sweet's syndrome with arthritis in an 8-month-old boy. **J Rheumatol** 26(2):440–442.
360. Lipp KE, Shenefelt PD, Nelson RP Jr et al. (1999) Persistent Sweet's syndrome occurring in a child with a primary immunodeficiency. **J Am Acad Dermatol** 40(5 Pt 2):838–841.
361. Guia JM, Frias J, Castro FJ et al. (1999) Cardiovascular involvement in a boy with Sweet's syndrome. **Pediatr Cardiol** 20(4):295–297.
362. Nurre LD, Rabalasi GP, Callen JP (1999) Neutrophilic dermatosis-associated sterile chronic multifocal osteomyelitis in pediatric patients: case report and review. **Pediatr Dermatol** 16(3):214–216.
363. Eliott SP, Malloy SB (1999) Sweet syndrome: an unusual presentation of chronic granulomatous disease in a child. **Pediatr Infect Dis J** 18(6):568–570.
364. Sirvent N, Olivier V, Benet L et al. (2000) Sweet syndome in an infant. **Arch Pediatr** 7(5):501–504.
365. Itami S, Nishioka K (1980) Sweet's syndrome in infancy. **Br J Dermatol** 103:449.
366. Dunn TR, Saperstein HW, Biederman A et al. (1992) Sweet syndrome in a neonate with aseptic meningitis. **Pediatr Dermatol** 9:288.
367. Clemmenson OJ, Menne T, Branding F et al. (1989) Acute febrile neutrophilic dermatoses: A marker of malignancy? **Acta Derm Venereol** (Stockh) 69:52–58.
368. Shapiro L, Baraf CS, Richheimer LL (1971) Sweet's syndrome (acute febrile neutrophilic dermatosis). **Arch Dermatol** 103:81.

369. Storer JS, Nesbitt LT, Galen WK, DeLeo VA (1983) Sweet's syndrome. **Int J Dermatol** 22:8.
370. Sweet RD (1979) Acute febrile neutrophilic dermatosis. **Br J Dermatol** 100:93.
371. Spector JI, Zimbler H, Levine R et al. (1980) Sweet's syndrome. **JAMA** 244:1131.
372. Sommer S, Wilkinson SM, Merchant WJ, Goulden V (2000) Sweet's syndrome presenting as palmoplantar pustulosis. **J Am Acad Dermatol** 42(2 Pt 2):332–334.
373. Kibbi AG, Zaynoun ST, Kurban AK, Najjar SS (1985) Acute febrile neutrophilic dermatosis (Sweet's syndrome): case report and review of the literature. **Pediatr Dermatol** 3:40.
374. Levin DL, Esterly NB, Herman JJ, Boxall LBH (1981) The Sweet syndrome in children. **J Pediatr** 99:73.
375. Majeed D, Kalaawi M, Mohanty D et al. (1989) Congenital dyserthropoeitic anemia and chronic recurrent multifocal osteomyelitis in three related children and in association with Sweet's syndrome in two siblings. **J Pediatr** 115:730–734.
376. Gunawardena DA, Gunawardena KA, Ratnayaka RMRS, Vasanthanathan NS (1975) The clinical spectrum of Sweet's syndrome (acute febrile neutrophilic dermatosis): a report of eighteen cases. **Br J Dermatol** 92:363.
377. Klock JC, Oken RL (1976) Febrile neutrophilic dermatosis in acute myelogenous leukemia. **Cancer** 37:992.
378. Cohen PR, Talpaz M, Kurzrock R (1988) Malignancy-associated Sweet's syndrome: review of the world literature. **J Clin Oncol** 6:1887.
379. Lazarus AA, McMillam M, Miramadi A (1986) Pulmonary involvement in Sweet's syndrome (acute febrile neutrophilic dermatosis). Preleukemic and leukemic phases of acute myelogenous leukemia. **Chest** 90:922.
380. Vignon-Pennamen MD, Wallach D (1995) Neutrophilic disease: a review of extra-cutaneous neutrophilic manifestations. **Eur J Dermatol** 5:449–455.

syndrome died suddenly of occlusive coronary artery disease two years after the diagnosis of Sweet syndrome.[381] Two other patients have been described with significant vascular disease of the aorta, coronary and pulmonary vessels without signs of occlusion.[361,382] The phenomenon of pathergy, typical of pyoderma gangrenosum and Behçet syndrome, has been reported in several cases of Sweet syndrome.[383] Sweet syndrome has been associated with embryonal carcinoma of the testicle,[368] ulcerative colitis,[351,384] Crohn's desease,[385] sarcoidosis,[386] Sjögren syndrome,[369] erythema nodosum,[387] chronic granulomatous disease,[363] primary immunodeficiency,[360] arthritis (rheumatoid and sero-negative),[359,388] G–CSF infusion for aplastic anemia,[355] immuno-deficiency,[355,359,360,388] gastrojejunostomy with blind loop syndrome,[389] and HIV infection.[390]

LABORATORY FINDINGS

Leukocytosis ranging from 15 000 to 24 000/mm³ is described in most patients, with 80–90% polymorphonuclear leukocytes.[240] An elevated erythrocyte sedimentation rate is common, often as high as 80mm/h.[374] Thrombocytosis was described in one child who died of occlusive coronary artery disease.[381] Anemia and urinary abnormalities, including red cells and granular casts in the urinary sediment; can occur. Fever and leuko-cytosis may be absent when Sweet syndrome occurs in association with immuno-deficiency.[360] Culture of skin lesions for bacteria and fungi do not grow organisms. Circulating antibodies to neutrophil cytoplasm (ANCA) have been demonstrated in some but not all patients with Sweet syndrome.[391]

PATHOPHYSIOLOGY AND HISTOGENESIS

Sweet syndrome forms part of a spectrum of reactive neutrophilic dermatoses including pyoderma gangrenosum, neutrophilic eccrine hidradenitis, subcorneal pustulosis, pustular vasculitis, erythema elevatum diutinum, rheumatoid neutrophilic dermatosis, and erythema nodosum. Two other entities, chronic recurrent multifocal osteomyelitis (CRMO), and SAPHO syndrome (Synovitis, Acne, Pustulosis, Hyperostosis, Osteitis) also resemble a reactive neutrophilic dermatoses.[362,392] Although the cause of Sweet syndrome remains unclear, studies point to a T-cell dependent cellular immune reaction underlying the disease. CD 25+ activated T cells are noted in the inflammatory infiltrate as well as an increased expression of ICAM-1 and IL-8 immunoreactive cells. IL-1 (α and β) and IFNγ levels are increased in serum of patients with Sweet syndrome.[393] IL-4 levels in the serum are normal, suggesting the disorder is mediated through helper T cell type 1 cytokines. The ensuing cytokine cascade including IL-1, IL-3, IL-6, IL-8, and G-CSF and GM-CSF may explain the local and systemic activation of neutrophils and histiocytes.[352] The trigger to this process may be an antigen or super-antigen,[352] including bacterial or viral infection,[394] an immunologic response to a leukemic or preleukemic state[378] or a drug reaction such as mino-cycline.[395] Because many of the patients have a preceding febrile illness,[242,376]

an immune complex mediated process has been postulated.[352] Two groups found no deposition of immune complexes in 35 patients with Sweet syndrome.[352] Studies of altered function of neutrophils in Sweet syndrome including chemotaxis have given contradictory results and may represent an epiphenomenon.[352]

Histologically, a dense perivascular infiltrate of polymorphonuclear leukocytes with leukocytoclasis is found in the dermis and may extend into the subcutis.[186] Because there are no fibrinoid deposits in the capillaries or extravasated red blood cells, a true vasculitis is not present. The histologic appearance varies with the stage of the process. In the later stages, lymphocytes and histiocytes may predominate. The dermal papillae may be involved with marked edema, which causes subepidermal blisters. Pulmonary infiltrates, on lung biopsies, reveal extensive neutrophilic infiltrates similar to the findings in cutaneous biopsies.[379]

DIFFERENTIAL DIAGNOSIS

Clinically, Sweet syndrome must be separated from other reactive neutrophilic dermatoses. Pyoderma gangrenosum is usually easy to differentiate but the acute disseminated vesiculopustular forms in association with autoimmune bowel disease and hemoproliferative disorders may be more difficult to distinguish. Simultaneous occurrence of both disorders has been reported.[352] Disseminated forms of erythema nodosum may be confusing clinically but histology shows infiltrates predominantly in the septa of the subcutaneous tissue.[186] Bowel bypass syndrome may present with fever, arthralgias and papu-lopustular lesions. The histological changes have been termed "Sweet-like vasculitis."[186] Neutrophilic eccrine hidradenitis is associated with chemo-therapy of malignant disorders. Clinically identical skin lesions may occur accompanied by drug-induced neutropenia.[296] Histology shows dermal infiltration of neutrophils mainly around eccrine sweat glands.[397] The differentiation of this entity from Sweet syndrome may be difficult as both are part of a continuous spectrum of neutrophilic dermatoses.[398]

Idiopathic recurrent palmoplantar hidradenitis (IRPH) is a benign disorder characterized by multiple tender erythematous nodules on the soles and in some cases the palms of otherwise healthy young persons.[399] Fever is usually absent and the disorder clears spontaneously.[399] Mechanical or thermal trauma is thought to lead to rupture of the palmoplantar eccrine glands. The release of eccrine secretions into the surrounding stroma may activate a cytokine cascade including TNFα, IL-8, and G-CSF capable of attracting neutrophils and producing the resultant inflammation. Most cases resolve spontaneously within three weeks without treatment. Pernio (chillblains) may have a similar clinical appearance; however, histology shows a lymphoid infiltrate with endothelial swelling.[186]

An outbreak of "Pseudomonas Hot Foot Syndrome"[400] was reported in 40 children who developed acute inflammatory, painful, plantar nodules after contact with pool water contaminated with *P. aeruginosa*. The floor of the pool had been coated with an abrasive grit to prevent slipping. Culture of skin

381. Muster AJ, Bharati S, Herman JJ et al. (1983) Fatal cardiovascular disease and cutis laxa following acute febrile neutrophilic dermatosis. **J Pediatr** 102:243.
382. Manohar R (1996) Idiopathic dilatation of pulmonary artery. **J Assoc Phys Ind** 44(5):342.
383. Sitjas D, Puig L, Cuatrecasas M et al. (1993) Acute febrile neutrophilic dermatosis (Sweet's syndrome). **Int J Dermatol** 32:261.
384. Benton EC, Rutherford D, Hunter JAA (1985) Sweet's syndrome and pyoderma gangrenosum associated with ulcerative colitis. **Acta Derm Venereol** (Stockh) 65:77.
385. Rappaport A, Shaked M, Landau M, Dolev E (2001) Sweet's syndrome in association with Crohn's disease: report of a case and review of the literature. **Dis Colon Rectum** 44(10):1526–1529.
386. Stuveling EM, Fedder G, Bruns HM et al. (2001) The association of Sweet's syndrome with sarcoidosis. **Neth J Med** 59(1):31–34.
387. Spatz SA (1985) Erythema nodosum in Sweet's syndrome. **Cutis** 35:327.
388. Harary AM (1983) Sweet's syndrome associated with rheumatoid arthritis. **Arch Intern Med** 143:1993.
389. Bechtel MA, Callen JP (1981) Acute febrile neutrophilic dermatosis, Sweet's syndrome. **Arch Dermatol** 117:664.
390. Brady RC, Morris J, Connelly BL, Boiko S (1999) Sweet's syndrome as an initial manifestation of pediatric human immunodeficiency virus infection. **Pediatrics** 104(5 Pt 1):1142–1144.
391. Kemmett D, Harrison DJ, Hunter JAA (1991) Antibodies to neutrophil cytoplasmic antigens: a serologic marker for Sweet's syndrome. **J Am Acad Dermatol** 24:967.
392. Beretta-Piccoli BC, Sauvain MJ, Gal I et al. (2000) Synovitis, acne, pustulosis, hyperostosis, osteitis (SAPHO) syndrome in childhood: a report of ten cases and review of the literature. **Eur J Pediatr** 159(8):594–601.
393. Giasuddin AS, El-Orfi AH, Ziu MM et al. (1998) Sweet's syndrome: Is the pathogenesis mediated by helper T cell type 1 cytokines? **J Am Acad Dermatol** 39(6):940–943.
394. Collins P, Rogers S, Keenan P et al. (1991) Acute febrile neutrophilic dermatosis in childhood (Sweet's syndrome). **Br J Dermatol** 124:203.
395. Thibault M-J, Billick RC, Srolovitz H (1992) Minocycline-induced Sweet's syndrome. **J Am Acad Dermatol** 27:801.
396. Harrist TJ, Fine JD, Berman RS (1982) Neutrophilic eccrine hidradenitis: a distinct type of neutrophilic dermatois. **Arch Dermatol** 118:263–266.
397. Thorisdottir K, Tomecki KJ, Bergfeld WF et al. (1993) Neutrophilic eccrine hidradenitis. **J Am Acad Dermatol** 28:775–777.
398. Gross PR, Margolis D, Starobinski M, Salomon D (1999) Neutrophilic dermatosis versus neutrophilic eccrine hidradenitis. **N Engl J Med** 340:1371.
399. Miklos S, Cremer H, Von den Driesch P (1998) Idiopathic recurrent palmoplantar hidradenitis in children. **Arch Dermatol** 134:76–79.
400. Fiorillo I, Zucker M, Sawyer D et al. (2001) The pseudomonas hot foot syndrome. **N Eng J Med** 345(5):335–338.

lesions grew pseudomonas and biopsy showed a perieccrine neutrophilic infiltrate that extended to the subcutaneous fat. The disorder is self-limited with recovery in 14 days.

Lupus erythematosus, erythema elevatum diutinum, Behçet's disease, granuloma faciale, halogenoderma and other bacterial infections may be excluded by skin biopsy or appropriate cultures.[352]

THERAPY AND PROGNOSIS

Untreated lesions tend to increase in size and persist for one to 12 months, eventually resolving without sequelae. Some children have secondary cutis laxa in the areas of involvement, probably as a result of intense inflammation and degradation of the collagen.[381] One case of Sweet syndrome with fatal cardiac involvement and extensive associated cutis laxa has been described.[381] Milia can also occur.[401]

Lesions respond to oral steroids at a dose of 0.5 to 1.5mg/kg per day given for 10 days and then tapered slowly to prevent recurrences.[352,377] Kemmett[401] in a review of 29 cases reported 21% of patients had more than one episode and another 10% had relapsing disease for at least three years. Alternatives to corticosteroid treatment include potassium iodide, colchicine, dapsone, doxycycline, clofazamine, indomethacin, and interferon-α.[352,402,403] Resistent cases often respond to cyclosporin.[404]

In view of two pediatric patients[358,377] having an associated malignancy, this eruption should be considered a possible cutaneous sign of malignancy, and appropriate investigations should be performed.[374] The prognosis depends on the severity of the systemic disease that accompanies the eruption. In children, the serious complication of occlusive coronary artery or other large vessel disease has been reported in three patients.[361,381,382] As the disorder is considered to be a hypersensitivity reaction, giving aspirin and/or other nonsteroidal anti-inflammatory agents is warranted, particularly if there is thrombocytosis.

PEDIATRIC ASPECTS OF THE DISEASE

Because of a possible relationship to malignancy, this eruption should be thoroughly evaluated with this in mind. If cardiovascular symptoms or signs develop in Sweet syndrome, a thorough investigation of the cardiac status is mandatory to avoid potentially fatal coronary artery disease.[361]

ANGIOLYMPHOID HYPERPLASIA WITH EOSINOPHILIA AND KIMURA DISEASE

The term angiolymphoid hyperplasia with eosinophilia (ALHE) is used for a group of vascular tumor-like lesions of the skin, which have characteristic, nonspecific histiocytoid endothelial cells on histology.[405,406]

In 1969, Wells and Whimster[407] reported their findings on patients with subcutaneous nodules on the head and neck who showed a distinctive vascular proliferation with inflammatory infiltrates containing eosinophils and numerous lymphoid follicles. They termed this disease ALHE, and considered it to be a distinct clinical and pathologic entity that occurred most often in young adults. Kimura disease was originally described by Kim and Szeto in 1937 in a Chinese journal and is exceedingly uncommon in Western countries.[408] It has been reported mainly in the Asian literature and is a similar but distinct entity from ALHE; it occurs more commonly in Asian male children. Many authors consider these entities to be the same disease because of their clinical and pathologic similarities.[407,409] Others contend that the clinical differences and the histiocytoid endothelial cells seen in ALHE are not consistently found in Kimura disease[410] and that they are most likely two separate unrelated disorders.[411–413] A comparison of the two disorders is found in Table 17.5.

EPIDEMIOLOGY

ALHE most commonly occurs sporadically in young adults, with equal sex distribution. Asians, whites, blacks, Native Americans, and Middle Eastern patients all have been reported.[414] Kimura disease occurs most commonly in young Asian boys and men.

PRESENTING HISTORY

The patient usually complains of a growing erythematous nodule, usually in the pre-auricular area, scalp, or forehead. One-third of the patients have pain,[405] and there may be spontaneous bleeding or throbbing in the lesion. Diagnosis before biopsy is unlikely because of the nonspecific morphologic features.

PHYSICAL EXAMINATION

Pruritus is a feature in most, but 21% of patients are totally asymptomatic.[405] Lesions are usually single but may be multiple[405] and appear as dusky, erythematous, or purplish plaques or nodules, measuring 1–2cm in diameter, but may be as large as 10cm.[407] They are occasionally covered with a central crust or scale and occur principally on the head and neck with a predilection for the face and ears. Although many lesions have been reported to be painless,[415] pressure may elicit pain in one-third of patients.[405] In Kimura disease the lesions are bulky subcutaneous masses with normal overlying skin.[416] Oral lesions have been reported.[417,418] Lymphadenopathy is common in Asian children with Kimura disease.[414] Associated conditions include atopic dermatitis[415] and lichen amyloidosis.[419]

LABORATORY FINDINGS

Blood eosinophilia is seen in both diseases and may be as high as 75% in patients with Kimura disease;[419] serum IgE levels may also be elevated.[415]

401. Kemmett D, Hunter JAA (1990) Sweet's syndrome: a clinicopathologic review of twenty-nine cases. J Am Acad Dermatol 23:503.
402. Maillard H, Leclech C, Peria P et al. (1999) Colchicine for Sweet's syndrome. A study of twenty cases. Br J Dermatol 140(3):565–566.
403. Bianchi L, Masi M, Hagman JH et al. (1999) Systemic interferon-alpha treatment for idiopathic Sweet's syndrome. Clin Exp Dermatol 24(6):443–445.
404. Wilson DM, John GR, Callen JP (1999) Peripheral ulcerative keratitis—an extracutaneous neutrophilic disorder: report of a patient with rheumatoid arthritis, pustular vasculitis, pyoderma gangrenosum, and Sweet's syndrome with an excellent response to cyclosporine therapy. J Am Acad Dermatol 40(2 Pt 2):331–334.
405. Olsen TG, Helwig EB (1985) Angiolymphoid hyperplasia with eosinophilia. J Am Acad Dermatol 12:781.
406. Blauvelt A, Cobb MW, Turner ML (2000) Widespread cutaneous vascular papules associated with peripheral blood eosinophilia and prominant inguinal lymphadenopathy. J Am Acad Dermatol 43(4):698–700.
407. Wells GC, Whimster IW (1969) Subcutaneous angiolymphoid hyperplasia with eosinophilia. Br J Dermatol 81:1.
408. Allen PW, Ramakrishna B, MacCormac LB (1992) The histiocytoid hemangiomas and other controversies. Path Annu 2:51.
409. Reed RJ, Terazakis N (1972) Subcutaneous angioblastic lymphoid hyperplasia with eosinophilia (Kimura's disease). Cancer 29:489.
410. Rossai J (1982) Angiolymphoid hyperplasia with eosinophilia of the skin. Am J Dermatopathol 4:175.
411. Helander SD, Peters MS, Kuo TT, Su WP (1995) Kimura's disease and angiolymphoid hyperplasia with eosinophilia: new observations from immunohistochemical studies of lymphocyte markers, endothelial antigens and granulocyte proteins. J Cutan Path 22:319–326.
412. Requena L, Sangueza OP (1997) Cutaneous vascular proliferation. Part II. Hyperplasias and benign neoplasms. J Am Acad Dermatol 37:887–919.
413. Arnold M, Geilen CC, Coupland SE et al. (1999) Unilateral angiolymphoid hyperplasia with eosinophilia involving the left arm and hand. J Cutan Pathol 26:436–440.
414. Henry PG, Burnett JW (1978) Angiolymphoid hyperplasia with eosinophilia. Arch Dermatol 11:1168.
415. Hamrick HJ, Jennette JC, LaForce CF (1984) Kimura's disease: report of a pediatric case in the United States. J Allergy Clin Immunol 73:561.
416. Zhang JZ, Zhang CG, Chen JM (1998) Thirty-five cases of Kimura's disease. Br J Dermatol 139(3):542–543.
417. Buckerfield JB, Edwards MB (1979) Angiolymphoid hyperplasia with eosinophils in oral mucosa. Oral Surg Oral Med Oral Pathol 47:539.
418. Massa MC, Fretzin DF, Chowdhury L et al. (1984) Angiolymphoid hyperplasia demonstrating extensive skin and mucosal lesions controlled with vinblastine therapy. J Am Acad Dermatol 11:333.
419. Danno K, Horio T, Miyachi Y et al. (1982) Coexistence of Kimura's disease and lichen amyloidosis in three patients. Arch Dermatol 118:976.

TABLE 17.5   Comparison of angiolymphoid hyperplasia with eosinophilia and Kimura's disease

	Angiolymphoid hyperplasia with eosinophilia	Kimura's disease
Distribution	Worldwide	Asia
Age	13–67 years	7–50 years
Sex	Males = females	Males > females
Location	Head and neck	Head and neck
Appearance	Superficial papules and nodules usually unilateral	Tumorlike mass with deep soft tissues involved, sometimes bilateral
Size	0.8cm to massive	3–10cm
Lymphadenopathy	No	Yes
Blood findings	Serum IgE normal Blood eosinophilia sometimes	Serum IgE usually elevated Blood eosinophilia usual
Histologic results	Proliferating vessels with histiocytoid endothelial cells, eosinophils, lymphocytes often with follicles, plasma cells Fibrosis absent or minimal	Vessels not prominent Fibrosis prominent surrounding lymphoid follicles, lymphocytes, plasma cells, mast cells with IgE, eosinophils, and eosinophilic microabscesses
	Mast cells commonly increased	Mast cells rarely increased
Nephrotic syndrome	Associated in one case	Associated

PATHOPHYSIOLOGY AND HISTOGENESIS

Histologically, the lesions of ALHE are characterized by vascular proliferations and a lymphocytic infiltration, with eosinophils within the dermis and subcutaneous tissue.[405] Both mature and immature blood vessels are lined by several layers of thick, plump, rounded endothelial cells. The intense infiltrate consists of eosinophils, lymphocytes, mast cells, histiocytes, and lymphoid follicles with germinal centers in many cases. Early lesions show more vascular proliferation than older lesions, which demonstrate more prominent lymphoid tissue with flatter vascular endothelium.[407] Direct immunofluorescence testing demonstrates granular deposits of IgA, IgM, and C3 around small blood vessels in the center of the lesion.[420] Olsen and Helwig[405] showed arterial structures with an internal elastic lamina among the venules and endothelial cell proliferations and suggested that these may be arteriovenous shunts. Renin production by nonendothelial perivascular cells has been demonstrated and may stimulate the vascular proliferation seen in ALHE.

Immunohistochemical markers such as cytokeratins, vimentin, factor VIII-related antigen, collagen type IV, estrogen and progesterone receptors,[421] and adhesion molecule markers have been used to evaluate the pathogenesis of AHLE.[422] The intensity of marker reaction suggests an immunologic activation of proliferating endothelial cells.[422] Gyulai reported the prescence of DNA of Human Herpes Virus type 8 (HHV8) in the lesions of angiolymphoid hyperplasia suggesting a possible infectious cause.[423] However, a more recent study of both Kimura disease and ALHE using heteroduplex PCR showed no evidence of HHV8 in the lesions.[424]

Histologically, Kimura disease shows fibrosis, lymphocytes, plasma cells, eosinophils, mast cells, and eosinophilic microabscesses. Blood vessels are not prominent.

The cause of ALHE is unknown, and opinions are divided on whether the lesions represent a true neoplasm of vascular tissue or a reactive healing process after trauma, infection, or injury.[405] Olsen and Helwig[405] believe that, in a susceptible individual, a traumatic event, immunization[425] or altered estrogen state (such as pregnancy)[421] serves as a stimulus for vascular endothelial proliferation, particularly in exposed areas such as the scalp and ears where the blood supply is abundant. Arteriovenous shunts may result directly from the injury itself or indirectly from release of vasoactive metabolites such as tumor angiogenic factor. Fetsch and Weiss[426] recognized that 63% of cases were associated with an artery or vein, many of which were damaged, and they suggest a reparative, reactive process. The cause of Kimura disease is unknown.

DIFFERENTIAL DIAGNOSIS

Clinically, the lesions do not have a characteristic morphology other than a vascular background. Therefore, diverse lesions such as epidermoid cysts, angiomas, angiosarcomas, Kaposi's sarcoma, bacillary angiomatosis, pseudo-Kaposi's sarcoma, pseudoangiosarcoma, and pyogenic granulomas may be confused with ALHE. Biopsy of the lesion is necessary to rule out these other entities. Histologically, ALHE can resemble angiosarcoma.

THERAPY AND PROGNOSIS

The process is benign, and the general health of the patient is unaffected. Plaques may resolve spontaneously within a few months or may remain active for years with indolent enlargement, persistent eosinophilia, and pruritus.[415] Rarely, lesion can be locally destructive. There are no reports of malignant change.

420. Grimwood R, Swinehart JM, Aeling JL (1979) Angiolymphoid hyperplasia with eosinophilia. **Arch Dermatol** 115:205.
421. Moy RL, Luftman DB, Nguyen QH et al. (1992) Estrogen receptors and the response to sex hormones in angiolymphoid hyperplasia with eosinophilia. **Arch Dermatol** 128:825.
422. von den Driesch P, Gruschwitz M, Schell H et al. (1992) Distribution of adhesion molecules, IgE, and CD23 in a case of angiolymphoid hyperplasia with eosinophilia. **J Am Acad Dermatol** 26:799.
423. Gyulai R, Kemeny L, Adam E et al. (1996) HHV8 DNA in angiolymphoid hyperplasia of the skin. **Lancet** 347:1837.
424. Jang KA, Ahn SJ, Choi JH et al. (2001) Polymerase chain reaction (PCR) for human herpesvirus 8 and heteroduplex PCR for clonality assessment in angiolymphoid hyperplasia with eosinophilia in Kimura's disease. **J Cutan Pathol** 28(7):363–367.
425. Akosa AB, Ali MH, Khoo CTK et al. (1990) Angiolymphoid hyperplasia with eosinophilia associated with tetanus toxoid vaccination. **Histopathology** 16:589.
426. Fetsch JF, Weiss SW (1991) Observations concerning the pathogenesis of epithelioid hemangioma (angiolymphoid hyperplasia). **Modern Pathol** 4:449.

When lesions are few and persistent, excision is the treatment of choice for both AHLE and Kimura disease, but recurrences may still occur.[420,427] Intralesional corticosteroids have been helpful, especially in early lesions,[428,429] oral prednisone may induce regression.[408] Pentoxifylline has been used to treat AHLE and two patients with Kimura disease.[430,431] Withdrawal of birth control pills may be warranted.[421] Vinblastine may be effective for treating the disfiguring lesion of AHLE,[418] as is radiation or carbon dioxide laser therapy. Both pulse dye and copper vapour laser have eradicated lesions of ALHE[432,433] Interferon-α 2a and 2b have both been used sucessfully to treat AHLE in areas not amenable to surgical removal.[434,435]

PEDIATRIC ASPECTS OF THE DISEASE

These entities occur in both children and adults. The general health of the patient is usually unaffected. Large lesions may be cosmetically unsightly, but ALHE and Kimura disease should not interfere with school or physical activities. Kimura disease has been reported with nephrotic syndrome and nephritis however only three of the 14 cases were children.[436] Recently a 13-year-old male with Kimura's disease, coronary spasm, and coronary aneuyrsms has been described.[437] As several children have been reported to develop ALHE after immunization,[425,438] time relationship with vaccination should be considered.

FOREIGN BODY REACTIONS

Foreign body granulomas are caused by a myriad of exogenous materials that have been accidentally implanted or injected into the skin. These sometimes persist indefinitely. Examples of common exogenous materials are vegetable spines, cactus bristles,[439] metals, tick parts, wooden splinters,[440] silk or nylon sutures, paraffin, silicone, silica, starch powder, broken thermometers,[441] acrylic or nylon fibers acquired while walking barefoot on acrylic carpets,[442] and acrylic fibers implanted into the scalp for male-pattern baldness.[443] Rare causes include spurs from rooster attacks,[444] silver,[445] self-sticking bindi disks placed on the glabellar region,[446] and moth cocoon spines.[447] Injections with pentazocine[448] or diphtheria, pertussis, and tetanus vaccine (DPT) secondarily contaminated with aluminum hydroxide have also been reported to cause a foreign body reaction.[449] Erythematous plaques with possible progression to sclerodermatous plaques have been reported with vitamin K injections.[450] Patients with psychiatric illnesses may inject materials into their skin causing foreign body granulomas.[451]

Endogenous materials may also elicit a foreign body reaction. Examples include keratinous material from ruptured epidermal, pilar, or acne cysts, urates (gout), and human hair causing interdigital sinuses on barbers' hands.[452]

EPIDEMIOLOGY

Any age group or sex may be affected. This entity is relatively frequently encountered by dermatologists, pediatricians, family practioners, and internists.

PRESENTING HISTORY

The patient usually complains of a persistent nodule or papule that may be painful. If located on the plantar surface of the foot, the lesion is especially painful during walking. Lesions usually appear weeks to months after the initial inoculation, so that the cause is often not suspected by the patient or the physician.

PHYSICAL EXAMINATION

Lesions appear as firm or fluctuant erythematous papules or nodules, usually on exposed areas. Most often they are single and are localized. Hair, nails, teeth, and mucous membranes are not usually involved. A patient with widespread foreign body granulomas caused by tale application on a chronic generalized dermatitis has been described.[453]

Silica may cause a nonallergic granulomatous reaction in exposed subjects and, years later, a delayed hypersensitivity granulomatous response may take place.[454] Lesions appear in exposed areas, frequently arranged in parallel streaks, and they may be firm or become fluctuant and ulcerate.

Beryllium granulomas result from cuts by fluorescent lamps coated with a beryllium mixture.[455] These lacerations heal incompletely and tend to persist with swelling, induration, tenderness, and ulceration. They often discharge material for months to years.

Zirconium granulomas are often found in the axilla as 1–4mm discrete soft reddish-brown papules.

LABORATORY FINDINGS

Serum angiotensin-converting enzyme levels may be elevated. Studies show that this laboratory test does not differentiate one granulomatous disease from another and thus cannot separate foreign body granulomas from other granulomatous processes such as sarcoidosis.[453] Eosinophilia may occur if lesions are extensive.[453]

427. Bendl BJ, Asano K, Lewis RJ (1977) Nodular angioblastic hyperplasia with eosinophilia and lymphofolliculosis. **Cutis** 19:327.
428. Bonnetblanc JM, Bernard P, Malinvaud G (1985) Treatment of angiolymphoid hyperplasia with eosinophilia. **J Am Acad Dermatol** 13:668.
429. Nelson DA, Jarratt M (1984) Angiolymphoid hyperplasia with eosinophilia. **Pediatr Dermatol** 1:210.
430. Hongcharu W, Baldassano M, Taylor CR (2000) Kimura's disease with oral ulcers: response to pentoxifylline. **J Am Acad Dermatol** 43:905–907.
431. Person J (1994) Angiolymphoid hyperplasia with eosinophilia may respond to pentoxifylline. **J Am Acad Dermatol** 31:117–118.
432. Fosko SW, Glaser DA, Rogers CJ (2001) Eradication of angiolymphoid hyperplasia with eosinophilia by copper vapor laser. **Arch Dermatol** 137(7):863–865.
433. Gupta G, Munro CS (2000) Angiolymphoid hyperplasia with eosinophilia: successful treatment with pulsed dye laser using the double pulse technique. **Br J Dermatol** 143(1):214–215.
434. Rampini P, Semino M, Drago F, Rampini E (2001) Angiolymphoid hyperplasia with eosinophilia: successful treatment with interferon alpha 2b. **Dermatol** 202(4):343.
435. Shenefelt PD, Rinker M, Caradonna S (2000) A case of angiolymphoid hyperplasia with eosinophilia treated with intralesional interferon alfa-2a. **Arch Dermatol** 136(7):837–839.
436. Rajpoot D, Pahl M, Clark J (2000) Nephrotic syndrome associated with Kimura's disease. **Pediatr Nephrol** 14:486–488.
437. Horigome H, Sekijima T, Ohtsuka S, Shibasaki M (2000) Life threatening coronary artery spasm in childhood Kimura's disease. **Heart** 84(2):E5.
438. Hallam LA, Mackinlay GA, Wright AMA (1989) Angiolymphoid hyperplasia with eosinophilia: possible aetiological role for immunization. **J Clin Pathol** 42:944.
439. Synder RA, Schwartz RA (1983) Cactus bristle implantation. **Arch Dermatol** 119:152.
440. Tschen JA, Knox JM, McGavran MH, Duncan WC (1984) Chromomycosis. The association of fungal elements and wood splinters. **Arch Dermatol** 120:107.
441. Sau P, Solivan G, Johnson FB (1991) Cutaneous reaction from a broken thermometer. **J Am Acad Dermatol** 25:915.
442. Pimentel JC (1977) Sarcoid granulomas of the skin produced by acrylic and nylon fibers. **Br J Dermatol** 96:673.
443. Hanke CW, Norins AL, Pantzer JG, Bennett JE (1981) Hair implant complications. **JAMA** 245:1344.
444. Cooler JO, Kleiman MB, West K et al. (1992) Retained spur following a rooster attack. **Pediatrics** 90:106.
445. Rongioletti F, Robert E, Buffa P et al. (1992) Blue nevi-like dotted occupational argyria. **J Am Acad Dermatol** 27:1015.
446. Ramesh V (1991) Foreign-body granuloma of the forehead: reaction to bindi. **Arch Dermatol** 127:424.
447. Shenefelt PD (1991) Moth cocoon dermatitis. **Arch Dermatol** 127:424.
448. Jackson RM, Tucker SB, Abraham JL, Millns JL (1984) Factitial cutaneous ulcers and nodules: the use of electron-probe microanalysis in diagnosis. **J Am Acad Dermatol** 11:1065.
449. Slater DN, Underwood JCE, Durrant TE et al. (1982) Aluminium hydroxide granulomas: light and electron microscopic studies and x-ray microanalysis. **Br J Dermatol** 107:103.
450. Lemlich G, Green M, Phelps R et al. (1993) Cutaneous reactions to vitamin K1 injections. **J Am Acad Dermatol** 28:345.
451. Allen CC, Lund KA, Treadwell PA (1992) Elemental mercury foreign body granulomas. **Int J Dermatol** 31:353.
452. Joseph HL, Gifford H (1954) Barber's interdigital pilonidal sinus. **Arch Dermatol** 70:616.
453. Pucevich MV, Rosenberg EW, Bale GF, Terzakis JA (1983) Widespread foreign-body granulomas and elevated serum angiotension-converting enzyme. **Arch Dermatol** 119:229.
454. Mowry RG, Sams WM, Caulfield JB (1991) Cutaneous silica granuloma. **Arch Dermatol** 127:692.
455. Neave HJ, Frank SB, Tolmach JA (1950) Cutaneous granuloma following laceration by fluorescent light bulbs. **Arch Dermatol Syphilol** 61:401.

PATHOPHYSIOLOGY AND HISTOGENESIS

Two major histological types of foreign body reactions are described by Lever.[186] The first type is the allergic granuloma, which may be caused by zirconium, beryllium, silica, and certain tattoo dyes. It occurs only in sensitized individuals and is a manifestation of a delayed-type hypersensitivity reaction.[456,457] Histologically, epithelioid cells, giant cells, and caseation necrosis are present in varying degrees. There are usually fewer giant cells than are seen in nonallergic granulomas. Phagocytosis of the foreign substance may be slight or even absent. It may be difficult to distinguish these granulomatous reactions from sarcoidosis. The epidermis may show acanthosis with ulceration. Beryllium granulomas often show pronounced caseation necrosis.[455]

Zirconium granulomas used to appear in the axilla when sodium zirconium lactate was commonly found in deodorants.[458] It is still available in underarm deodorants but is thought to be safer in a combined weight of less than 20% in an aluminum salt.[459] Topical lotions for treatment of poison ivy dermatitis may contain zirconium; these are still available over the counter, and may also cause a foreign body reaction in skin damaged by the dermatitis.[460,461]

Silica granulomas can be caused by silicon dioxide found in soil (quartz), talc (magnesium silicate) that are deposited into surgical wounds or used as a dusting powder,[462] asbestos (complex polysilicates), sea urchin spines, and coral polyps.[317] Injection of silicone (polydimethylsiloxane) used for cosmetic purposes (artificial implants), or as prosthetic devices, can result in siliconomas,[462] which are soft tissue masses caused by granulomatous reactions to the silicone. Silicone can migrate in soft tissues and should be considered when evaluating new masses in patients who have received silicone prostheses.

Tattoo granulomas occur most commonly from the red pigment, cinnabar (mercuric sulfide). However, chromium oxide (chrome green),[463] cobalt blue, and cadmium sulfide (yellow) may also be implicated. Such allergic foreign body granulomas may appear years after the acquisition of a tattoo. Tattoo granulomas reveal scattered granules of dye located within macrophages and extracellularly in the dermis.

Zirconium and beryllium particles cannot be detected by polarized light, and thus electron probe X-ray microanalysis must be used to identify beryllium and zirconium within tissue. Some foreign body substances are doubly refractile with a polarizing microscope, and this property can be helpful in localizing and determining the foreign substance.

The second type of foreign body reaction is nonallergic granulomas, caused by silk and nylon sutures, paraffin, wood, talc, surgical glove starch powder,[464] cactus spines, silicone gel, and imbedded hairs. Typically, a nonallergic foreign body reaction shows macrophages and many giant cells surrounding the foreign material.

Paraffinomas are produced when oily substances such as mineral oil (paraffin), cottonseed oil, sesame seed oil, or camphor oil are injected into the skin[465] or applied topically in the nasal cavity.[466] Irregular plaques form and may ulcerate to discharge an oily substance.[186] These may develop years after injection of paraffin.

Paraffinomas cause a "Swiss cheese" appearance in the tissue with numerous ovoid or round cavities that represent spaces occupied by the oil. Macro-phages may have the appearance of foam cells. Multinucleated giant cells are commonly seen. Osmic acid, bromine-silver stains, oil Red-O, and Sudan IV stains may be helpful in distinguishing these exogenous materials from one another.[186] Histologic features of foreign body reactions may be different in patients infected with the human immunodeficiency virus type 1,[467] where abundant macrophages and a lack of giant cells may be seen.

DIFFERENTIAL DIAGNOSIS

Electron probe microanalysis of tissue blocks is very helpful in determining the cause of foreign body reactions when the substance cannot be seen on routine histochemical stains and polarized light.[448,449,468] Talc, silica, zirconium, and aluminum can all be determined by this method, as can the elements from sodium (atomic number 11) to uranium (atomic number 92).

Clinically, lesions can resemble sarcoidosis, pyogenic granuloma, normal granulation tissue, and neurofibromas. Biopsy of such lesions aids in the diagnosis. The Köebner phenomenon may occur at the site of inoculation if the patient has lichen planus, psoriasis, or LE, which may result in further delay of the diagnosis.

THERAPY AND PROGNOSIS

Removal of the foreign body is the treatment of choice. Tweezers, adhesive tape stripping, wax stripping, or glue with gauze may aid in the removal of large quantities of foreign bodies.[469] Topical, intralesional, or systemic steroids inhibit an inflammatory reaction if present. Lesions may persist indefinitely if the foreign material is not removed and may continue to ulcerate and extrude material. With the introduction of foreign material into the body, infection may be introduced, especially bacterial Gram-positive organisms, fungal infections (chromomycosis),[440] syphilis, hepatitis, leprosy, warts, and vaccinia.

PEDIATRIC ASPECTS OF THE DISEASE

Because children more commonly walk with bare feet, they are more likely to pick up foreign material on their exposed parts. Solitary foreign body granuloma on the foot in a child may mimic a solitary wart. DPT immunizations are generally given only to children and produce their intended effect by a foreign body reaction and an allied immune response. A foregn body granuloma of the tissues may occasionally result at the site of the immunization.

HALOGENODERMAS

Halogenodermas are drug eruptions caused by the ingestion or absorption of bromide, iodide, or fluoride, probably representing an idiosyncratic response.[470] The reactions usually occur after a prolonged period of use, but signs may be seen as early as eight days after initial administration. Manifestations include acneiform papules and pustules, vesicles, granulomatous nodules, vegetating plaques, and urticarial lesions. The lesions tend to affect areas of the skin with the highest concentration of sebaceous glands, such as the face, neck, and upper back. Despite the withdrawal of bromide from

456. Hanifin JM, Epstein WL, Cline MJ (1970) In vitro studies of granulomatous hypersensitivity to beryllium. **J Invest Dermatol** 55:284.
457. Henderson WR, Fukuyama K, Epstein WL, Spitler LE (1972) In patients with berylliosis. **J Invest Dermatol** 58:5.
458. Shelley WB, Hurley HJ (1958) The allergic origin of zirconium deodorant granulomas. **Br J Dermatol** 70:75.
459. Lisi DM (1992) Availability of zirconium in topical antiperspirants. **Arch Intern Med** 152:421.
460. Baler GR (1965) Granulomas from topical zirconium in poison ivy dermatitis. **Arch Dermatol** 91:145.
461. LoPresti PJ, Hambrick GW (1965) Zirconium granuloma following treatment of Rhus dermatitis. **Arch Dermatol** 92:188.
462. Travis WD, Balogh K, Abraham JL (1985) Silicone granulomas: report of three cases and review of the literature. **Hum Pathol** 16:19.
463. Epstein WL, Skahen JR, Krasnobrod H (1963) The organized epithelioid cell granuloma: differentiation of allergic (zirconium) from colloidal (silica) types. **Am J Pathol** 43:391.

464. Leonard DD (1973) Starch granulomas. **Arch Dermatol** 107:101.
465. Urbach F, Wine SS, Johnson WC, Davies RE (1971) Generalized paraffinoma (sclerosing lipogranuloma). **Arch Dermatol** 103:277.
466. Feldmann R, Harms M, Chavaz P (1992) Orbital and palpebral paraffinoma. **J Am Acad Dermatol** 26:833.
467. Smith KJ, Skelton HG, Yeager J (1993) Histologic features of foreign body reactions in patients infected with human immunodeficiency virus type 1. **J Am Acad Dermatol** 28:470.
468. Andres TL, Vallyathan NV, Madison JF (1980) Electron-probe microanalysis: aid in the study of skin granulomas. **Arch Dermatol** 116:1272.
469. Martinez TT, Jerome M, Barry RC et al. (1987) Removal of cactus spines from the skin. **Am J Dis Child** 141:1291.
470. Soria C, Allegue F, Espana A et al. (1990) Vegetating iododerma with underlying systemic disease: report of three cases. **J Am Acad Dermatol** 22:418.

prescription medications,[471] these lesions are still occasionally caused by over-the-counter hypnotics such as propantheline bromide.[472,473] Iodides can be found in cough medicines, expectorants, and dyes used in radiography.[474] Iododerma has been described with the use of povidone-iodine.[475] Patients with monoclonal gammopathy or other underlying diseases may be more susceptible to developing these lesions.[470,474]

EPIDEMIOLOGY

Halogenodermas are aquired disorders that can occur at any age, including the neonatal period, from the mother's taking bromides during breast-feeding.[477] Because of an increased incidence of exposure to drugs, they most commonly affect adults. Methyl bromide used in fumigation can cause urticaria and blisters after exposure but not the typical vegetating plaques seen in typical halogenodermas.[478]

PRESENTING HISTORY

Acneiform eruptions occur on the face and upper trunk with the sudden onset of papules and pustules without comedones. Iododermas and bromodermas usually begin as multiple pustules or "boils" that quickly coalesce into vegetating plaques with pustules along the periphery. The lesions may ulcerate and form central crusts. Fluorodermas manifest as scattered papules and nodules no the neck and pre-auricular area.[476]

PHYSICAL EXAMINATION

There are two major types of clinical presentation. The first is with an acute acneiform eruption with papules and pustules, usually on the face, neck, back, and upper extremities. In the second type, a more chronic eruption evolves into vegetating plaques with central ulceration and a pustular border (Fig.17.14). These pustular plaques are seen most commonly on the lower legs. The hair, nails, teeth, and mucous membranes are not usually affected. Fever may accompany the eruption.

LABORATORY FINDINGS

Halogen levels in the blood do not necessarily correlate with clinical findings but may be helpful if elevated.[476] Elevation of the leukocyte count may occur, with eosinophilia as high as 85%.[479] Elevation of the erythrocyte sedimentation rate may also be found. In patients with suspected iododerma, levels of total iodine and inorganic iodine may be elevated. Triiodothyronine and T_4 levels may be low, indicating thyroid dysfunction, compounding the problem. Impaired renal function increases toxicity by decreasing excretion of iodine.[475]

PATHOPHYSIOLOGY AND HISTOGENESIS

The histologic appearance of a lesion is not diagnostic but may be suggestive.[186] The epidermis shows papillomatosis with downward proliferation (pseudoepitheliomatous hyperplasia). Intraepidermal abscesses filled with neutrophils, eosinophils, and keratinocytes are characteristic. Epidermal changes may be more pronounced in bromoderma than iododerma.

The pathogenesis is not well understood. Rosenberg et al.[480] hypothesized a delayed-type hypersensitivity reaction based on lymphocyte transformation

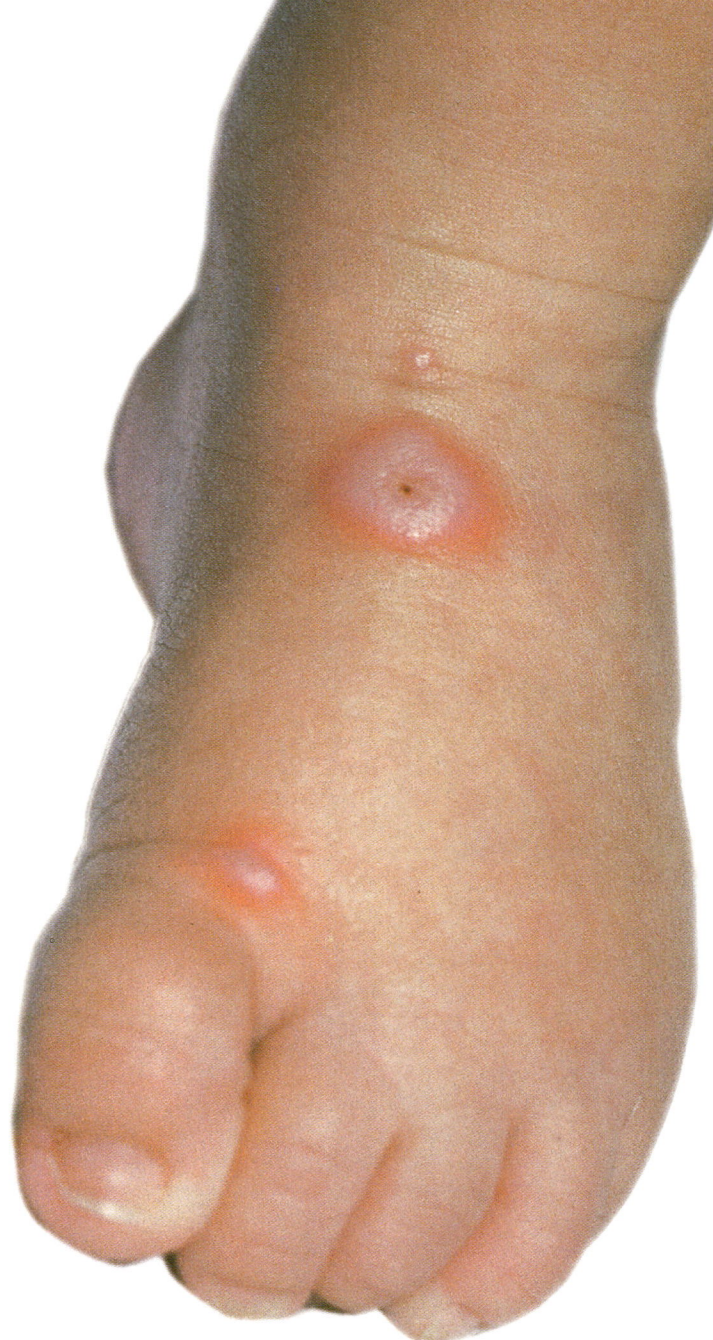

Fig. 17.14   Plaques of bromoderma.

studies. Iodides may act as haptens by combining with serum protein. Once a patient is sensitized, a similar eruption may occur within a few days on readministration of the offending agent.[475,481] Iodides are known to increase movement of polymorphonuclear leukocytes into inflamed tissues.[482]

471. Smith SZ, Scheen SR (1978) Bromoderma. **Arch Dermatol** 114:458.
472. Ewing JA, Grant WJ (1965) The bromide hazard. **South Med J** 58:148.
473. May SB (1972) Ingestion of halogens. **Arch Dermatol** 106:599.
474. Boudoulas O, Siegle RJ, Grimwood RE (1987) Iododerma occurring after orally administered iopanoic acid. **Arch Dermatol** 123:387.
475. Bishop ME, Garcia RL (1978) Iododerma from wound irrigation with providone-iodine. **JAMA** 240:249.
476. Blasic LG, Spencer SK (1979) Fluorocerma. **Arch Dermatol** 115:1134.
477. Yeung GTC (1950) Skin eruption in newborn due to bromism derived from mother's milk. **BMJ** 1:769.
478. Hezemans-Boer M, Toonstra J, Meulenbelt J et al. (1988) Skin lesions due to exposure to methyl bromide. **Arch Dermatol** 124:917.
479. Jacob HS, Sidd JJ, Greenberg BH et al. (1964) Extreme eosinophilia with iodide hypersensitivity. A report of a case with observations on the cellular composition of inflammatory exudates. **N Engl J Med** 271:1138.
480. Rosenberg FR, Einbinder J, Walzer RA, Nelson CT (1972) Vegetating iododerma. **Arch Dermatol** 105:900.
481. Jones LE, Pariser H, Murray PF (1958) Recurrent iododerma. **Arch Dermatol** 78:353.
482. Stone OJ (1985) Proliferative iododerma. **Int J Dermatol** 24:565.

DIFFERENTIAL DIAGNOSIS

Pustular lesions may resemble acne or drug-induced acneiform eruptions. Fungating lesions may resemble deep mycoses, such as blastomycosis. However, fungal elements are not found, and cultures are negative. Folliculitis and other bacterial infections grow organisms on culture. Pemphigus vegetans can be ruled out if there is no acantholysis on biopsy. Mycosis fungoides, syphilis, tuberculosis, anthrax, and pyoderma gangrenosum should be excluded by histologic examination and culture.

THERAPY AND PROGNOSIS

Topical therapy with Burow's solution and topical steroids may be helpful. Once the offending agent is removed, lesions resolve, leaving residual hyperpigmentation. Usually, there is little scarring,[470] but if lesions remain untreated, there may be disfigurement and other serious or fatal sequelae.[483] Corticosteroids may hasten resolution of the lesions.[474]

PEDIATRIC ASPECTS OF THE DISEASE

Chronic iodine ingestion may affect the thyroid gland in children and cause goiter, which should be looked for in children with iododermas. Halogenodermas are mainly a cosmetic problem, and once treated, there should be little cosmetic disfigurement.

CALCINOSIS CUTIS

Calcinosis cutis is the precipitation or deposition of hydroxyapatite, crystals of calcium phosphate, within cutaneous tissues. Normally, calcification occurs only in bone and teeth within the body,[317] but under pathologic circumstances, it may occur in other tissues. Cutaneous calcification may be focal or widespread and symptomatic or asymptomatic. Most forms of calcinosis cutis can be divided into dystrophic, idiopathic, metastatic, and iatrogenic calcinosis.[186,484]

Dystrophic calcinosis cutis

Dystrophic calcinosis cutis, the most common form of cutaneous calcification, is caused by deposition of calcium salts within previously damaged tissues; there are no metabolic abnormalities of the calcium or phosphorus. Internal organ involvement is not found except within the muscles in the rare situation of calcinosis universalis. Localized dystrophic forms of calcinosis cutis arise in inflammatory lesions such as acne, ulcers, foreign body granulomas, traumatic lesions, and subcutaneous fat necrosis of the newborn. Calcinosis has also been noted after heel sticks performed for drawing blood in neonates.[485] Degenerative lesions, such as vascular infarcts and parasitic infections, may also give rise to dystrophic calcinosis cutis. Neoplasms, such as epidermal cysts, lipomas, pilomatricomas, and basal cell carcinomas, can show areas of calcification. Wide-spread calcification (calcinosis universalis) is seen in association with systemic sclerosis, CRST syndrome (calcinosis cutis, Raynaud's phenomenon, sclerodacyly, telangiectasias), dermatomyositis, Werner syndrome,[486] pseudoxanthoma elasticum, Ehlers–Danlos syndrome, DLE[487] and SLE.[488,489]

Calcinosis cutis in dermatomyositis tends to develop two to three years after the onset of disease.[490] Ten to twenty percent of adults and 40–74% of children with dermatomyositis have calcinosis.[491] Deposits may be large and develop slowly accompanied by healing ulcers and draining sinuses; calcium deposits are often extruded from the skin. Increased staphylococcal infections and elevated IgE levels have been associated with the calcinosis in childhood dermatomyositis. The staphylococcal infections can occur before the onset of calcinosis, and an intermittent defect in granulocyte chemotaxis may lead to the areas of calcinosis.[492] Calcinosis universalis, with sheet-like calcified deposits in the intermuscular fascial planes, causing an exoskeleton, forms in a small subgroup of patients with dermatomyositis and portends a poor outcome.[490] These patients tend to have a severe cutaneous vasculitis and the severe calcinosis limits their physical function. Hypercalcemia may occur during resolution.[493]

Calcinosis cutis in scleroderma, on the other hand, usually occurs 10–12 years after the onset of disease, and is rarely seen in childhood.[494] The calcium deposits in scleroderma tend to be smaller than in dermatomyositis, commonly occurring on the fingers and hands but also on the feet, elbows, knees, and hips. Secondary hyperparathyroidism has been reported in patients who had systemic sclerosis and aberrant calcifications, prompting some authors to consider prophylactic treatment with vitamin D to prevent calcinosis.[495]

Idiopathic calcinosis cutis

Idiopathic calcification occurs without evidence of local tissue injury or a systemic metabolic defect. Lesions can be localized (Fig. 17.15) or generalized. One localized form of calcinosis cutis is the subepidermal calcified nodule, which is a solitary, hard lesion or lesions usually seen on the face, particularly the helix of the ear, of infants or small children; it may be congenital (Fig. 17.16)[496] Lesions are usually 3–11mm in size and histologically demonstrate globules of calcified material in the uppermost dermis.[186] The origin of the homogeneous calcified masses is obscure.

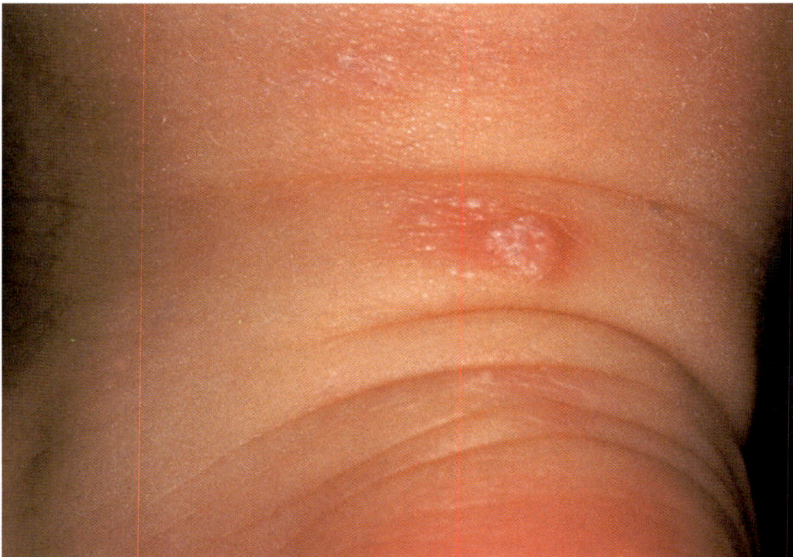

Fig. 17.15   Solitary rock-hard papule of calcinosis cutis on the ankle.

483. Hollander L, Fetterman GH (1936) Fatal iododerma: eleventh case reported in the literature. **Arch Dermatol** 34:228.
484. Orlow SJ, Watsky KL, Bolognia JL (1991) Cutaneous deposition diseases: skin and bone, part 2. **J Am Acad Dermatol** 25:445–462.
485. Sell EJ, Hansen RC, Struck-Pierce S (1980) Calcified nodules on the heel: a complication of neonatal intensive care. **J Pediatr** 96:473.
486. Lucke T, Fallowfield M, McHenry P (1997) Idiopathic calcinosis cutis of the penis. **Br J Dermatol** 137:1011–1013.
487. Ueki H, Takei Y, Nakagawa S (1980) Cutaneous calcinosis in localized discoid lupus erythematosus. **Arch Dermatol** 116:196.
488. Nomura M, Okada N, Okada M et al. (1990) Large subcutaneous calcification in systemic lupus erythematosus. **Arch Dermatol** 126:1057.
489. Carette S, Urowitz MB (1983) Systemic lupus erythematosus and diffuse soft tissue calcifications. **Int J Dermatol** 22:416.
490. Bowyer SL, Blane CE, Sullivan DB, Cassidy JT (1983) Childhood dermatomyositis: factors predicting functional outcome and development of dystrophic calcification. **J Pediatr** 103:882.
491. Muller SA, Winkelmann RK, Brunstig LA (1959) Calcinosis in dermatomyositis: observations on course of disease in children and adults. **Arch Dermatol** 79:669.
492. Moore EC, Cohen F, Douglas SD, Gutta V (1992) Staphylococcal infections in childhood dermatomyositis—association with the development of calcinosis, raised IgE concentrations and granulocyte chemotactic defect. **Ann Rheum Dis** 51:378.
493. Ostrov BE, Goldsmith DP, Eichenfield AH et al. (1991) Hypercalcemia during the resolution of calcinosis universalis in juvenile dermatomyositis. **J Rheumatol** 18:1730.
494. Raimer SS (1985) Calcinosis cutis. **Curr Concepts Skin Disord** 6:9.
495. Serup J, Hagdrup HK (1984) Parathyroid hormone and calcium metabolism in generalized scleroderma. **Arch Dermatol Res** 276:91.
496. Nico MM, Bergonse FN (2001) Subepidermal calcified nodule: report of two cases and review of the literature. **Pediatr Dermatol** 18:227–229.

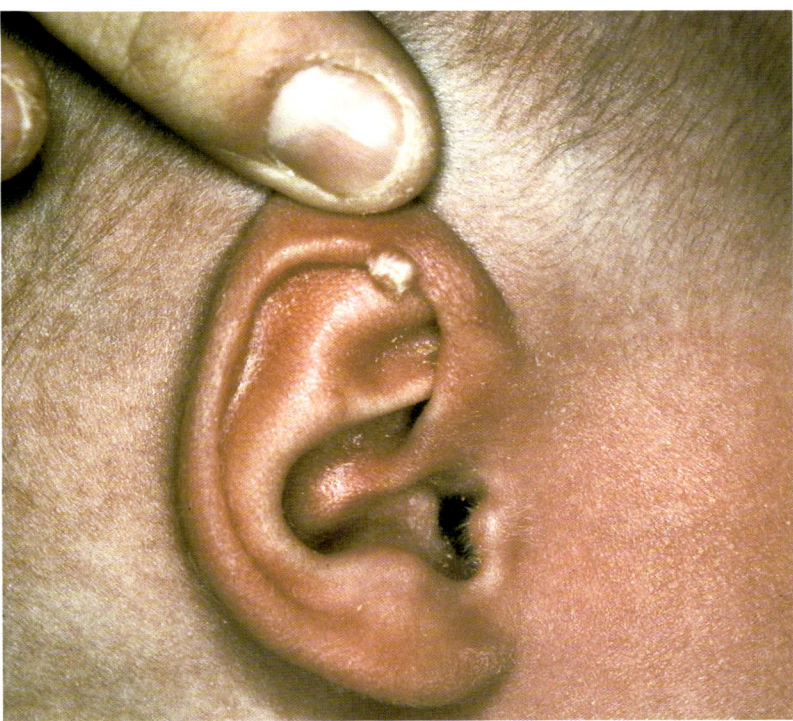

Fig. 17.16   Congenital subepidermal calcified nodule of the ear.

Another localized form is calcinosis of the scrotum, which is characterized by calcified nodules limited to the scrotum or penis.[486,497] Vulvar lesions may occur in females.[498] Lesions begin in childhood or early adult life, increase in size and number, and sometimes break down and discharge chalky material. They are usually asymptomatic, but patients may have itching, tenderness, or a feeling of heaviness of the scrotum. Radiographic examination reveals radio-opaque densities in areas of calcification. Generalized milia-like idiopathic calcinosis cutis has been described in Down syndrome,[499] where in some instances it may represent calcification of syringomas.[500] Rarely the milia-like variety may present as a perforating form with transepidermal elimination.[501]

Metastatic calcinosis cutis

Metastatic calcinosis cutis is caused by the precipitation of calcium salts in undamaged tissue and occurs in disorders associated with abnormal metabolism of calcium and/or phosphorus.[502] Chronic renal failure, vitamin D intoxication, milk-alkali syndrome, sarcoidosis, parathyroid neoplasms, bony destruction from malignant tumors, and tumor-related calcinosis are conditions in which metastatic calcinosis cutis may be seen. In chronic renal failure, decreased renal clearance of phosphate results in supersaturation of the serum with phosphate, causing a compensatory drop in the serum calcium level. This stimulates parathyroid hormone, which in turn mobilizes calcium from bone, with the subsequent release of more phosphorus into the serum. Calcium deposits may occur in various organs including the kidney, lung, gastric mucosa, eyes, and arteries. These deposits are not commonly seen in the skin but, when present, usually occur within the dermis and subcutaneous tissue overlying large joints.

Calciphylaxis, a rare, life-threatening complication of chronic renal failure is manifest by rapidly progressive calcification of small and medium-sized blood vessels.[503] Calciphylaxis presents with livedo reticularis-like changes of the skin which develop overlying subcutaneous plaques. Ultimately, necrosis and deep subcutaneous ulceration develops. Soft tissue calcifications occurr in 60% of children with uremia, but calciphylaxis is extremely rare in children.[503]

Iatrogenic calcinosis cutis

Inadvertent extravasation of intravenous calcium salts into subcutaneous tissue may give rise to dystrophic calcinosis cutis,[504,505] which can break down, causing swelling and induration that may be mistaken for an abscess or cellulitis. Cutaneous lesions develop a few hours to three weeks after injection. Radiographic changes may be seen within five days but become maximal at two weeks.[506] Calcinosis cutis has been reported after electroencephalographic examination and electromyographic examination when there is prolonged contact with calcium-containing electrode paste.[507]

PRESENTING HISTORY

The patient or parent usually complains of firm, stony papules or plaques, which may have an erythematous or purplish border. The lesions may be tender and ulcerate.

PHYSICAL EXAMINATION

The papules and plaques are firm or rock hard and may be located anywhere on the body. They are found most commonly on the extremities, face, or scrotum. The size of the papules ranges from 1 to 30mm. Plaques may ulcerate and discharge a chalky, creamy material or gritty particles that can be demonstrated histologically to be calcium deposits. Secondary infection is common within areas of calcinosis cutis. Metastatic calcinosis cutis occurs more commonly around joints or in areas of increased trauma.

LABORATORY FINDINGS

Radiographs of the skin in calcinosis cutis reveal radio-opaque deposits within the dermis and subcutaneous tissues. Technetium-99m–methylene diphosphonate scans show a high affinity for the surface of hydroxyapatite crystals and are extremely helpful in picking up small asymptomatic nodules.[494] Laboratory abnormalities are not found in the dystrophic and idiopathic forms of calcinosis cutis. In metastatic calcinosis cutis, however, the chronic elevation of either the serum calcium or phosphorus level or both can cause precipitation within tissues.

PATHOPHYSIOLOGY AND HISTOGENESIS

Histologically, calcium deposits may be easily recognized in the dermis or subcutaneous tissues with hematoxylin and eosin stain, which stains calcium a deep blue color.[186] Globules of calcium stain black with von Kossa's stain. Calcified lesions may be present with massive deposits in the subcutaneous

497. Wright S, Navsaria H, Leigh IM (1991) Idiopathic scrotal calcinosis is idiopathic. **J Am Acad Dermatol** 24:727.
498. Jamaleddine FN, Salman SM, Shbaklo Z et al. (1988) Idiopathic vulvar calcinosis: the counterpart of idiopathic scrotal calcinosis. **Cutis** 4:273.
499. Smith ML, Golitz LE, Morelli JG et al. (1989) Milialike idiopathic calcinosis cutis in Down's syndrome. **Arch Dermatol** 125:1586.
500. Kanzaki T, Nakajima M (1991) Milia-like idiopathic calcinosis cutis and syringoma in Down's syndrome. **J Dermatol** 18:616–618.
501. Maroon M, Tyler W, Marks VJ (1990) Calcinosis cutis associated with syringomas: a transepidermal elimination disorder in a patient with Down syndrome. **J Am Acad Dermatol** 23:372–375.

502. Raimer SS, Archer ME, Jorizzo JL (1983) Metastatic calcinosis cutis. **Cutis** 32:463.
503. Zouboulis CC, Blumepeytavi U, Lennert T et al. (1996) Fulminant metastatic calcinosis with cutaneous necrosis in a child with end stage renal disease and tertiary hypoparathyroidism. **Br J Dermatol** 135:617–622.
504. Speer ME, Rudolph AJ (1983) Calcification of superficial scalp veins secondary to intravenous infusion of sodium bicarbonate and calcium chloride. **Cutis** 32:65.
505. Hironaga M, Fujigaki T, Tanaka S (1982) Cutaneous calcinosis in a neonate following extravasation of calcium gluconate. **J Am Acad Dermatol** 6:392.
506. Rodríguez-Cano L, García-Patos V, Creus, M et al. (1996) Childhood calcinosis cutis. **Pediatr Dermatol** 13(2):114–117.
507. Johnson RC, Fitzpatrick JE, Hahn DE (1993) Calcinosis cutis following electromyographic examination. **Cutis** 52:161.

tissue or may form tiny granules with small deposits in the dermis. A foreign body reaction with giant cells, inflammation, and fibrosis may be seen surrounding the area of calcification.

The pathogenesis of calcinosis cutis is unexplained. It tends to occur in areas of damaged tissue or increased trauma,[494] such as the damaged elastic fibers of pseudoxanthoma elasticum.[486,508] In cases of idiopathic calcinosis cutis , there may be unidentified local factors that promote calcification within tissue. Calciphylaxis (soft tissue calcification and necrosis) can be induced experimentally in appropriately sensitized animals and may play a role in human calcinosis cutis.[509] Johnson et al.[510] suggested that sulfated mucopolysaccharides and/or collagen may act as a template for initial crystal formation. Once started, calcification continues unimpeded.

DIFFERENTIAL DIAGNOSIS

Calcinosis cutis is characteristic in forming rock-hard, white nodules in the skin, particularly when seen in areas of dystrophy. Other entities that may be confused with calcinosis cutis include osteoma cutis and myositis ossificans.

THERAPY AND PROGNOSIS

When a metabolic disorder, such as hyperparathyroidism, hypervitaminosis D, chronic renal failure, milk-alkali syndrome, or tumor-related calcinosis occurs, correction of the underlying disorder aids in resolution of the calcinosis. Idiopathic and dystrophic calcinosis cutis may be resistant to therapy and surgical excision for painful deposits may be necessary.[511] Oral phosphate binding agents, such as magnesium hydroxide, or oral aluminum hydroxide antacids, such as aluminum carbonate gel, may decrease the serum phosphate

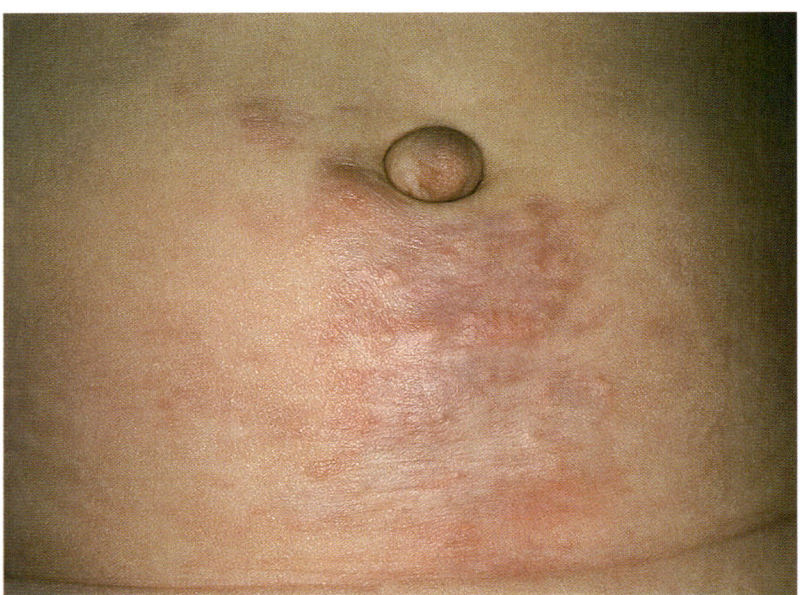

Fig. 17.17   Osteoma cutis in a child with Albright's osteodystrophy.

level and thus decrease deposits of calcinosis. Lowering the dietary calcium intake to 250–300mg/day and decreasing vitamin D intake may also be helpful. Calcium chelating agents, such as edetate trisodium and polyphosphates, have been helpful in treating some patients.[512] Other reported therapies include furosemide, colchicine,[513] diltiazem,[514] monthly injections of intralesional steroid,[515] warfarin,[516] magnesium sulfate, and magnesium lactate.[517] For ulcerations, compresses of 1:40 aluminum acetate, solution may be used to dry the area.

PEDIATRIC ASPECTS OF THE DISEASE

Some forms of calcinosis cutis are seen more commonly in children. These include calcinosis cutis associated with dermatomyositis, subepidermal calcified nodules, solitary congenital calcified nodule of the ear, and calcifications secondary to heel sticks in neonates. With extensive calcinosis, complications of contractures, pain, and suppuration with or without super-infection may occur.

CUTANEOUS OSSIFICATION

Primary dermal ossification is rarely seen in childhood.[518] Osteoma cutis is spontaneous new bone formation within the skin. Calcification, lamellae, lacunae, and bone marrow may all be seen within the dermis or in the sub-cutaneous tissue. Osteoma cutis may be primary, in which there are no preceding cutaneous lesions, or secondary, in which there has been tissue degeneration with secondary bone formation.

Primary osteoma cutis

Primary osteoma cutis is a congenital, benign growth of bone with no invasion of surrounding tissues or tendency to metastasize.[519] There are four types of primary osteoma cutis; Albright hereditary osteodystrophy (AHO), progressive osseous heteroplasia (POH), plate-like osteoma cutis (POC) and a miscellaneous group of other primary osteomas.

Albright hereditary osteodystrophy

Albright hereditary osteodystrophy[520] (AHO), was described in 1952 and includes both pseudohypoparathyroidism and pseudo-pseudohypo-parathyroidism. This is a disorder in which multiple areas of subcutaneous or intracutaneous ossification arises at birth, or in early infancy and early childhood. Lesions may be located anywhere on the body, including the trunk, extremities, and scalp, and range in size from pinpoint to 5cm (Fig. 17.17). Associated abnormalities include short stature, round facies, multiple skeletal abnormalities, short broad nails, basal ganglia calcification, hypothyroidism, mental retardation, defective teeth, and cataracts.[521,522] Skeletal abnormalities seen in AHO include curvature of the radius and shortened metacarpals and metatarsals. A characteristic dimpling sign, particularly over the fourth and fifth metacarpals, results from these shortened bones.[520]

AHO is thought to be inherited as an autosomal-dominant trait.[522] Pseudohypoparathyroidism is characterized by a low serum calcium level, hyper-phosphatemia, and no response to parathyroid hormone (PTH), with no evidence of renal disease, steatorrhea, or generalized osteomalacia. Circulating concentrations of PTH are normal or even increased; there is end-organ

508. Cochran RJ, Wilkin JK (1983) An unusual case of calcinosis cutis. **J Am Acad Dermatol** 8:103.
509. Richens G, Piepkorn MW, Krueger GG (1982) Calcifying panniculitis associated with renal failure. **J Am Acad Dermatol** 6:537.
510. Johnson WC, Forbes PD, Graham JH, Gray HR (1964) Experimental cutaneous calcinosis: a histopathologic and histochemical study. **J Invest Dermatol** 43:453.
511. Shearin JC, Pickrell K (1980) Surgical treatment of subcutaneous calcifications of polymyositis or dermatomyositis. **Ann Plast Surg** 5:381.
512. Rabens SF, Bethune JE (1975) Disodium etidronate therapy for dystrophic cutaneous calcification. **Arch Dermatol** 111:357.
513. Taborn J, Bole GG, Thompson GR (1978) Colchicine suppression of local and systemic inflammation due to calcinosis universalis in chronic dermatomyositis. **Ann Intern Med** 89:648.
514. Palmieri GMA, Sebes JI, Aelion JA et al. (1995) Treatment of calcinosis with diltiazem. **Arthritis Rheum** 38:1646–1654.

515. Hazen PG, Walker AE, Carney JF, Stewart JJ (1982) Cutaneous calcinosis of scleroderma. **Arch Dermatol** 118:366.
516. Martinez-Cordero E, Lopez-Zepeda J, Choza-Tomero F (1990) Calcinosis in childhood dermatomyositis. **Clin Exp Rheumatol** 8:198.
517. Steidl L, Ditmar R (1990) Soft tissue calcification treated with local and oral magnesium therapy. **Magnes Res** 3:113.
518. Roth SI, Stowell RE, Helwig EB (1963) Cutaneous ossification. **Arch Pathol** 76:44.
519. O'Donnell TF, Geller SA (1971) Primary osteoma cutis. **Arch Dermatol** 104:325.
520. Albright F, Forbes AP, Henneman PH (1952) Pseudo-pseudohypoparathyroidism. **Trans Assoc Am Physicians** 65:337.
521. Eyre WG, Reed WB (1971) Albright's hereditary osteodystrophy with cutaneous bone formation. **Arch Dermatol** 104:636.
522. Brook CGD, Valman HB (1971) Osteoma cutis and Albright's hereditary osteodystrophy. **Br J Dermatol** 85:471.

resistance to the action of PTH. Patients with pseudo–pseudohypoparathyroidism have all the other congenital abnormalities of pseudohypoparathyroidism but have normal serum calcium and phosphorus levels. Osteoma cutis is found in both.[521] Thyroid abnormalities frequently occur in these patients.

Progression to pseudohypoparathyroidism with hypocalcemia and seizures has been documented in patients who present in infancy with only osteoma cutis (pseudopseudohypoparathyroidism) and clinical features of AHO; these patients need to be monitored closely.[523] Both types of pseudohypoparathyroidism are recognized as variable expressions of the same disease and may be seen in pedigrees or even in the same individual at different periods.

Most of the actions of PTH are mediated by cyclic adenosine monophosphate. In most patients with AHO the disease is caused by heterozygous mutations in GNASI, a gene on chromosome 20 encoding the α–subunit of the stimulatory G protein of adenyl cyclase ($G_s\alpha$). Patients with AHO have a 50% reduction in the expression or activity of $G_s\alpha$ in multiple cell types. This results in poor coupling of hormone receptors to stimulate adenylate cyclase leading to multiple-organ hormone resistance.[524,525]

Progressive osseous heteroplasia

Progressive osseous heteroplasia, (POH) is an autosomal–dominant disorder characterized by dermal ossification during infancy and progressive herterotopic ossification of cutaneous, subcutaneous, and deep connective tissues during childhood.[526] The disorder is rare with only 29 known cases; sex ratio is equal.[527] The initial lesions appear in the reticular dermis and subcutaneous fat. Over time, the islands of heterotopic bone coalesce into plaques with involvement of the deeper connective tissues including fascia, muscle, tendon and ligaments. Skin lesions appear as small hard papules resembling grains of rice, or larger plaques with a gritty consistency.[528] Extensive ossification eventually results in ankylosis of affected joints and focal growth retardation of affected limbs.[529] The head, face, and extraoccular muscles are characteristically spared. Patients lack the morphological features of AHO and have normal endocrine function.[526] The distribution of lesions is random and asymmetrical, unlike the typical progresive pattern of ossification seen in fibrodysplasia ossificans progressive (myositis ossificans).

Pathology shows ossification. X-ray shows a cocoon-like web of heterotopic bone entangling the soft tissue from the dermis to skeletal muscle and independent of muscle planes.[529] Routine laboratory studies are normal; however, elevated alkaline phosphatase levels may be seen during active phases of osteogenesis. The etiology and pathogenesis remains unknown. A report of a patient with combined features of both POH and AHO and reduced levels of $G_s\alpha$ suggests that POH may be due to GNASI mutations.[527] Treatment is unsatisfactory, with surgical removal often leading to recurrence except when totally removed.[527] The long-term prognosis is uncertain, as only a few patients have been followed beyond adolescence.

Plate-like osteoma cutis

Plate-like osteoma cutis (POC) presents as hard plaques with a gritty consistency one to several centimeters in size. POC is used to describe lesions present at birth or within the first year of life in infants without evidence of abnormal calcium or phosphate metabolism, absence of trauma, and the prescence of at least one bony plate with or without other cutaneous osteomas.[530] The lesions are more common on the scalp and extremities.[531] It is likely that reports of widespread POC represent progressive osseous heteroplasia (POH). A child with severe congenital POC has been reported to have the GNASI mutation identical to a previously described mutation in AHO, but with no evidence of AHO or hormone resistance,[532] suggesting that severe progressive ossification may occur independently of AHO characteristics.[527] Surgical excision is the treatment of choice.

Other forms of primary osteoma cutis

Several forms of primary osteoma cutis are not easily categorized,[533] including single small osteomas that arise later in life and may show transepidermal elimination and multiple miliary osteomas of the face, which are seen in women with or without a history of acne vulgaris.[534] It has been proposed that these miliary lesions represent a hamartoma, where ectopic rests of mesenchymal cells differentiate into osteoclasts for unknown reasons.[535] Primary osteoma cutis has been reported in an adult with unilateral basal cell nevus syndrome with anodontia.[536]

Secondary osteoma cutis

Secondary osteoma cutis, also called metaplastic osteoma cutis, arises in tumors or in areas of inflammation. Tumors that can show osteoma cutis include pilomatricoma (calcifying epithelioma), basal cell carcinoma, nevus sebaceus of Jadassohn, nevus cell nevi, chondroid syringomas, and mixed tumors of the skin. Lesions caused by trauma or injections, acne vulgaris, folliculitis, stasis dermatitis, scars, dermatomyositis, and scleroderma[317] are inflammatory processes that may all have an associated osteoma cutis.

The most common type of secondary osteoma cutis is that seen in patients with acne who have taken tetracycline or minocycline.[537,538] Lesions appear as 1–2mm blue-black papules on the face. Tetracycline is known to form a complex with calcium orthophosphate that is deposited in developing teeth and bone and can cause a characteristic blue-black discoloration within osteoma cutis of acne lesions.[539]

EPIDEMIOLOGY

Cutaneous ossification can occur at any age, even at birth.[540] Albright hereditary osteodystrophy and progressive osseous heteroplasia (POH) are inherited as an autosomal-dominant disease. POC is usually sporadic but familial cases have been reported.[540,541]

PRESENTING HISTORY

The patient or parent usually complains of asymptomatic, solitary or multiple hard, raised 1–5mm nodules with normal or erythematous surrounding skin.

523. Prendiville JS, Lucky AW, Mallory SB et al. (1992) Osteoma cutis as a presenting sign of pseudohypoparathyroidism. **Pediatr Dermatol** 9:11.
524. Izraeli S, Metzker A, Horev G et al. (1992) Albright hereditary osteodystrophy with hypothyroidism, normocalcemia, and normal Gs protein activity: a family presenting with congenital osteoma cutis. **Am J Med Genet** 43:764.
525. Pattern JL, Johns DR, Valle D, Eil C et al. (1990) Mutation in the gene encoding the stimulatory G protein of adenylate cyclase in Albright's hereditary osteodystrophy. **N Engl J Med** 322:1412.
526. Kaplan FS, Craver R, MacEwen GD et al. (1994) Progressive osseous heteroplasia: a distinct developmental disorder of heterotopic ossification. Two new case reports and follow-up of three previously reported cases. **J Bone Joint Surg Am** 76:425–436.
527. Kaplan FS, Shore EM (2000) Progressive osseous heteroplasia. **J of Bone and Mineral Research** 15(11):2084–2092.
528. Miller ES, Esterly NB, Fairley JA (1996) Progressive osseous heteroplasia. **Arch Dermatol** 132:787–791.
529. Urtizberea JA, Testart H, Cartault F et al. (1998) Progressive osseous heteroplasia. Report of a family. **J Bone Joint Surg Br** 80(5):768–771.
530. Worret WI, Burgdorf W (1978) Congenital plaque-like osteoma of the skin in an infant. **Hautarzt** 29:590–596.
531. Sanmartin O, Alegre V, Martinez-Aparicio A et al. (1993) Congenital platelike osteoma cutis: case report and review of the literature. **Pediatr Dermatol** 10:182.

532. Yeh, GL, Mathur S, Wivel A et al. (2000) GNAS1 mutation and Cbfal misexpression in a child with severe congenital plate-like osteoma cutis. **J Bone and Mineral Research** 15(11):2060–2073.
533. Burgdorf W, Naseman T (1977) Cutaneous osteomas: a clinical and histiopathological review. **Arch Dermatol Res** 260:121.
534. Levell NJ, Lawrence CM (1994) Multiple papules on the face. Multiple miliary osteoma cutis. **Arch Dermatol** 130:370–374.
535. Gfeser M, Worret W, Hein R et al. (1998) Multiple primary miliary osteoma cutis. **Arch Dermatol** 134:641–643.
536. Aloi FG, Tomasini CF, Isaia G et al. (1989) Unilateral linear basal cell nevus associated with diffuse osteoma cutis, unilateral anodontia, and abnormal bone mineralization. **J Am Acad Dermatol** 20:973.
537. Basler RS, Taylor WB, Peacor DR (1974) Postacne osteoma cutis, X-ray diffraction analysis. **Arch Dermatol** 110:113.
538. Moritz DL, Elewski B (1991) Pigmented postacne osteoma cutis in a patient treated with minocycline: report and review of the literature. **J Am Acad Dermatol** 24:851.
539. Walter JF, Macknet KD (1979) Pigmentation of osteoma cutis caused by tetracycline. **Arch Dermatol** 115:1087.
540. Peterson WC, Mandel SL (1963) Primary osteomas of the skin. **Arch Dermatol Syphilol** 87:626.
541. Maclean GD, Main RA, Anderson TE et al. (1966) Connective tissue ossification presenting in the skin. **Arch Dermatol** 94:168.

PHYSICAL EXAMINATION

Lesions are common on the trunk or face, particularly the forehead, cheeks, and chin, and tend to be hard, raised, and well defined. The overlying skin may be normal, erythematous, blue pigmented, ulcerated, or atrophic. Superficial lesions sometimes become inflamed and extrude bony particles. When associated with long-standing acne, lesions appear as small blue-gray, hard papules or nodules.[538] The hair, nails, teeth, and mucous membranes are not involved.

LABORATORY FINDINGS

Patients with pseudohypoparathyroidism have decreased serum calcium and high serum phosphorus levels. In other forms of osteoma cutis, levels of calcium, phosphorus, and alkaline phosphatase are normal. In AHO, low thyroid levels may be found.

PATHOPHYSIOLOGY AND HISTOGENESIS

Histologically, there is proliferation of bony tissue with spicules of bone within the dermis and subcutaneous tissue.[186] Osteoblasts, osteocytes, osteoclasts, and mature fat cells are commonly seen within the bone, but only rarely are hematopoietic elements seen. Transepidermal elimination of bone with fragments of bone within channels lined by epidermis leading to the skin surface may be seen. Osteoblasts and osteocytes in primary cutaneous ossification originate from mesenchymal cells[186] and usually form membranous bone but occasionally enchondral bone.[518]

DIFFERENTIAL DIAGNOSIS

Subungual exostosis of the finger or toe may resemble osteoma cutis. These lesions are solitary fibrous nodules on the terminal phalynx, most commonly seen on the great toe, and may develop secondary to trauma, originating from the underlying bone. They commonly project from underneath the nail. Calcification in the skin may be difficult to distinguish from osteoma cutis.

THERAPY AND PROGNOSIS

The treatment of choice for osteoma cutis is surgical excision. Small lesions may not require treatment. Dermabrasion plus excision of individual lesions has been successful for multiple lesions of the face.[542] Isotretinoin may aggravate osteoma formation.[543] Pseudopseudohypoparathyroidism should be closely monitored by a renal or endocrine consultant to prevent severe hypocalcemia and seizures. Vitamin D and calcium supplements are the mainstay of therapy when necessary. Mental retardation may be casually related to hypocalcemia. Patients should be screened periodically for hypothyroidism because of its frequent association with pseudohypoparathyroidism.

PEDIATRIC ASPECTS OF THE DISEASE

Albright hereditary osteodystrophy, progressive osseous heteroplasia, and plate-like osteoma cutis all appear in the pediatric age group, presenting with multiple areas of intracutaneous ossification and/or skeletal abnormalities. Calcifying epithelioma (pilomatricoma) is a disease of childhood.

MYOSITIS OSSIFICANS

Myositis ossificans is a rare, benign, non-neoplastic disorder in which there is formation of true bone, and less frequently cartilage, within muscles.[544] Although uncommon, it has well-described radiologic, pathologic, and clinical features. There are three clinical varieties: traumatic myositis ossificans circumscripta, atraumatic myositis ossificans circumscripta, and myositis ossificans progressiva.

Traumatic myositis ossificans circumscripta

Traumatic myositis ossificans circumscripta develops in a traumatized muscle, often after minor repetitive trauma or an infectious event. It most commonly affects the flexor muscles of the upper arms and thighs,[545] presenting about one month after injury as a solitary 3–6cm localized, well-circumscribed tender soft tissue swelling. The most commonly affected muscle in the head and neck region[544] is the masseter muscle. It has been reported in an infant 5 months of age.[546] Patients usually present with pain or tenderness in subcutaneous tissues, which lasts for two to three weeks, and then progressively becomes indurated, and stony hard to palpation. Diagnostic difficulties may arise in early lesions as the imaging, both ultrasound and radiographic features, may be nonspecific or confusing.[547]

Atraumatic myositis ossificans circumscripta

Atraumatic myositis ossificans circumscripta is a localized lesion that appears without apparent cause and is sometimes referred to as pseudomalignant myositis ossificans. Included in this group is myositis ossificans related to systemic conditions such as paraplegia, poliomyelitis, burns, and hemophilia.[547]

Myositis ossificans progressiva (fibrodysplasia ossificans progressiva or Munchmeyers disease)

Myositis ossificans progressiva is an autosomal-dominant inherited disorder with varied expressivity, the main feature of which is progressive extraskeletal ossification. It is associated with several congenital abnormalities, particularly microdactylia or adactylia of the thumbs and hallux valgus of the great toes. Progressive muscle ossification occurs, usually within the first few years of life. The disease has recently been associated with overexpression of bone morphogenetic protein 4 (BMP-4), which is a member of the TGF-β gene family. The bone morphogenetic proteins appear to induce ossification of cartilage *in vivo*.[548] The disease progresses in a characteristic anatomic pattern—dorsal to ventral, axial to appendicular, cranial to caudal, and proximal to distal.[549] A young child presents with lumps or bruises over the back or nuchal area and in addition may be febrile and irritable. Calcium turnover is elevated, which reflects a large load of extraskeletal bone.[550] Diagnosis is often delayed or erroneously made because the significance of the skeletal abnormalities is not recognized.[551] The prognosis is poor with relentless ossification causing severe incapacitation and eventual death from respiratory failure.[544] Conductive hearing loss appears in 25% of patients.

PHYSICAL EXAMINATION

Clinically, acute lesions of myositis ossificans appear as hard swellings, which can be either localized or generalized. The nodules are warm, red, and painful. There is stiffness and lack of mobility in the areas involved. The

542. Fulton JE (1987) Dermabrasion-Loo-punch-excision technique for the treatment of acne-induced oesteoma cutis. **J Dermatol Surg Oncol** 13:6.
543. Brodkin RH, Abbey AA (1985) Osteoma cutis: a case of probable exacerbation following treatment of severe acne with isotretinoin. **Dermatologica** 170:210.
544. Ferlito A, Barion U, Nicolai P (1983) Myositis ossificans of the head and neck. Review of the literature and report of a case. **Arch Otorhinolaryngol** 237:103.
545. Ackerman LV (1958) Extra-osseous localized non-neoplastic bone and cartilage formation (so-called myositis ossificans): clinical and pathologic confusion with malignant neoplasms. **J Bone Joint Surg [Am]** 40A:279.
546. Heifetz SA, Galliani CA, DeRosa GP (1992) Myositis (fasciitis) ossificans in an infant. **Pediatr Pathol** 12:233.

547. Gindele A, Schwamborn D, Tsironis K et al. (2000) Myositis ossificans traumatica in young children: report of three cases and review of the literature. **Pediatr Radio** 30:451–459.
548. Shafritz AB, Shore EM, Gannon FH et al. (1996) Overexpression of an osteogenic morphogen in fibrodysplasia ossificans progressiva. **N Engl J Med** 335:555–561.
549. Cohen RB, Hahn GV, Tabas JA et al. (1993) The natural history of heterotopic ossification in patients who have fibrodysplasia ossificans progressiva. A study of forty-four patients. **J Bone Joint Surg Am** 75:215–219.
550. Lutwak L (1964) Myositis ossificans progressiva: mineral, metabolic and radioactive calcium studies of the effects of hormones. **Am J Med** 37:269.
551. Kaplan FS (1998) Fibrodysplasia ossificans progressiva. **Clin Orthop** 346:1–140.

acute changes usually subside over a few weeks but intermittent relapses of myositis may occur. This inflammatory stage is followed by fixation of the major joints involved, particularly the hips. Chronic stable lesions may be nontender and manifest as discrete mobile masses. Skeletal muscle involvement is variable.[552]

PATHOPHYSIOLOGY AND HISTOGENESIS

The histological appearance is determined by the age of the lesion. Biopsy may not always show inflammation but this is more likely to occur in early lesions. Traumatic myositis ossificans demonstrates a zonal pattern, which shows a central undifferentiated area surrounded by osteoid material and this is encapsulated by true bone formation.[545] This zone phenomenon helps distinguish myositis ossificans as a benign process, differentiating it from osteogenic sarcoma.

The basic mechanism of ectopic bone formation is unknown. It has been assumed that tissue necrosis, with or without hemorrhage, leads to fibroblastic proliferation and eventual ossification. Once bone matrix is laid down, the area is readily calcified.[553] A metabolic disorder of calcium or phosphorus is not necessary for bone formation, nor is it usually found.

Radiographs of the involved areas show multiple exostoses of bone, and ankylosis, and deformities of the cervical vertebrae. Traumatic myositis ossificans typically shows a soft tissue mass that develops irregular, downy opacities, which as it matures develops a radiolucent center encircled by a well-defined densely calcified periphery.[554] In myositis ossificans progressiva, radiographs show distinct, well-circumscribed areas of deep heterotopic ossification that often correspond to a distinct skeletal muscle.[555] Radiographs of the feet show monophalangic big toes. MRI may be very useful in differentiating these lesions from osteosarcomas because they show characteristic distribution of abnormal signal intensity in the muscles with no abnormality in the adjacent bone marrow or cortex.[556] Calcium and phosphorus levels are usually normal, and there may be a slight elevation of the alkaline phosphatase level[553] and the erythrocyte sedimentation rate. Electromyographic studies suggest a primary myopathy but nerve conduction studies are normal.

DIFFERENTIAL DIAGNOSIS

The differential diagnosis includes nodular fasciitis, traumatic fibrosis, battered child syndrome, the major forms of osteoma cutis, osteomyelitis, osteochondroma, osteogenic sarcoma, subcutaneous fat necrosis, and morphea. Treatment is aimed at alleviating or preventing myositis with systemic steroids.[557]

TREATMENT AND PROGNOSIS

Preventing mineralization by decreasing dietary calcium and using calcium-binding agents (diphosphonates) may reduce ectopic calcification.[553] Surgical excision for painful lesions must be attempted cautiously because of recurrence. The benign nature of the localized form of this non-neoplastic process requires a conservative approach.[554] Acetic acid 2% was administered by iontophoresis into an area of traumatic myositis ossificans on the thigh of a 16-year-old, with 98.9% decrease in the size of the ossified mass after three weeks.[558] In another case, surgery plus isotretinoin at a dose of 2–5mg/kg per day did not prevent ectopic ossification.[559]

MASTOCYTOSIS

Mastocytosis is the broad term used for a group of disorders characterized by the accumulation of mast cells in the skin with or without other organ system involvement[569] (Table 17.6). The most common site of mast cell accumulation is the skin.[561] Nettleship and Tay first described mastocytosis in a 2-year-old girl in 1869.[562] Ehrlich discovered the mast cell in 1877.[563] Mast cells are derived from pleuripotent CD34+ precursors in bone marrow and assume their typical granular morphology after migrating into tissue.[564,565] When bridging of IgE bound to FcεRI receptors on mast cells by specific antigens occurs, mast cells undergo degranulation and release biologically active preformed mediators and newly formed mediators characteristic of stimulated mast cells.

Mast cells are naturally distributed within the dermis, the respiratory system, gastrointestinal tract, genitourinary tract, adjacent to blood and lymphatic vessels, and near peripheral nerves. They act as surveillance cells that can respond to environmental antigens that come in contact with the skin or

---

TABLE 17.6 Classification of mastocytosis

Cutaneous mastocytosis
1. Urticaria pigmentosa
2. Diffuse cutaneous mastocytosis
3. Mastocytoma of the skin
4. TMEP

Systemic mastocytosis (without AHNMD or leukemic mast cell disease)
1. Systemic indolent mastocytosis
2. Systemic smouldering mastocytosis

Systemic mastocytosis with an AHNMD
1. Myeloproliferative syndrome
2. Myelodysplastic syndrome
3. Acute myeloid leukemia
4. Non-Hodgkin's lymphoma

Systemic aggressive mastocytosis
1. Mast cell leukemia
2. Mast cell sarcoma
3. Extracutaneous mastocytoma

Classification adopted from WHO classification (AHNMD **A**ssociated **h**ematological **n**on-**m**ast **c**ell **d**isorder).

Modified from Carter MC, Metcalfe DD (2002) Paediatric mastocytosis. **Arch Dis Child** 86:315–319, with permission.

552. Kaplan FS, Tabas JA, Gannon FH et al. (1993) The histopathology of fibrodysplasia ossifican progressiva. An endochondral process. **J Bone Joint Surg [Am]** 75:220–230.
553. Smith R (1975) Myositis ossificans progressiva: a review of current problems. **Semin Arthritis Rheum** 4:369.
554. Nuovo MA, Norman A, Chumas J, Ackerman LV (1992) Myositis ossificans with a typical clinical, radiographic, and pathologic findings: a review of 23 cases. **Skeletal Radiol** 21:87.
555. Kaplan FS, Strear CM, Zasloff MA (1994) Radiographic and scintigraphic features of modeling and remodelling in the heterotopic skeleton of patients who have fibrodysplasia ossificans progressiva. **Clin Orthop** 304:238–247.
556. Ehara S, Nakasato T, Tamakawa Y et al. (1991) MRI of myositis ossificans circumscripta. **Clin Imaging** 15:130.
557. Illingworth RS (1971) Myositis ossificans progressiva (Munchmeyer's disease). **Arch Dis Child** 46:264.
558. Wieder DL (1992) Treatment of traumatic myositis ossificans with acetic acid iontophoresis. **Phys Ther** 72:133.
559. Crofford LJ, Brahim JS, Zasloff MA, Marini JC (1990) Failure of surgery and isotretinoin to relieve jaw immobilization in fibrodysplasia ossificans progressiva: report of two cases. **J Oral Maxillofac Surg** 48:204.

560. Carter MC, Metcalf DD (2002) Pediatric mastocytosis. **Arch Dis Child** 86:315–319.
561. Soter NA (2000) Mast Cell Disorders. Mastocytosis and the Skin. **Hematology/oncology Clinics North Am:** 14(3):537–555.
562. Nettleship E, Tay W (1869) Rare forms of urticaria. **BMJ** 2:323–324.
563. Ehrlich P (1877) Beiträge zur Kenntnis der Anilinfarbungen und ihrer Verwendurg in der Mikroskopischen Technik. **Arch Mikros Anat** 13:263–277.
564. Kirshenbaum AS, Goff JP, Kessler SW et al. (1991) Demonstration of the origin of human mast cells from CD34+ bone marrow progenitor cells. **J Immunol** 46:1410–1415.
565. Kirshenbaum AS, Goff JP, Kessler SW et al. (1992) Effect of IL-3 and stem cell factor on the appearance of human basophils and mast cells from CD34+ pluripotent progenitor cells. **J Immunol** 148:772–777.
566. Cook J, Stith M, Sahn EE (1996) Bullous mastocytosis in an infant associated with the use of a nonprescription cough suppressant. **Pediatr Dermatol** 13(5):410–414.
567. De Paulis A, Minopoli G, Arbustini E et al. (1999) Stem cell factor is localized in, released from, and cleaved by human mast cells. **J Immunol** 163:2799–2808.
568. Rosbotham JL, Malik NM, Syrris P et al. (1999) Lack of c-kit mutation in familial urticaria pigmentosa. **Br J Dermatol** 140:849–852.
569. Fowler JF, Parsley WM, Cotter PG (1986) Familial urticaria pigmentosa. **Arch Dermatol** 122:80.

mucosal surfaces. Symptoms can be isolated to the organ system involved or may be systemic; they are caused by the release of histamine, cytokines, and other mast-cell mediators such as prostaglandins, leukotrienes, and platelet-activating factor.[566] Recently it has been shown that stimulated mast cells store and release stem cell factor indicating the potential for autocrine growth.[567]

EPIDEMIOLOGY

Reliable data on the incidence of mastocytosis is needed. A recent study from Great Britain estimated two cases annually from a population of 300 000.[568] The disease appears to be sporadic, but there are more than 50 case reports of familial occurrence.[568–570] There is some evidence of an autosomal-dominant pattern in the diffuse cutaneous form.[571] Males and females are affected equally. Most reported patients are white.[572]

Mastocytosis limited to the skin is primarily a disease of children. It can be accompanied by systemic symptoms without systemic infiltration. On the other hand, systemic internal mastocytosis is more common in adults with infiltration of mast cells in other organs. It may be progressive, relenting, debilitating, and fatal. Seventy-five percent of all patients with mastocytosis have lesions in childhood according to one study, usually before 2 years of age.[573] However, the disease may appear at any time from birth to middle age.

PRESENTING HISTORY

In infants, the parent usually seeks attention for a pruritic lesion or multiple lesions that recurrently urticate or blister, usually after a hot bath or rubbing of the lesion (Fig. 17.18). These lesions are commonly mistaken for bullous impetigo. Less commonly, flushing, gastrointestinal complaints such as vomiting, colicky pain, and diarrhea or headaches may be initial problems.

PHYSICAL EXAMINATION

Mastocytosis exhibits a wide spectrum of manifestations. Cutaneous forms include a solitary mastocytoma, urticaria pigmentosa (several lesions), diffuse cutaneous mastocytosis, and telangiectasia macularis eruptiva perstans (TMEP).[561] Systemic forms may or may not be associated with malignancy but rarely occur in childhood.

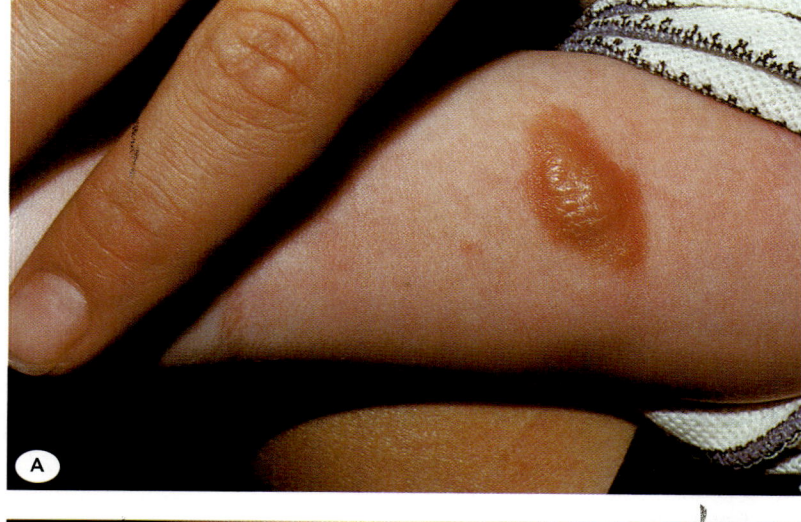

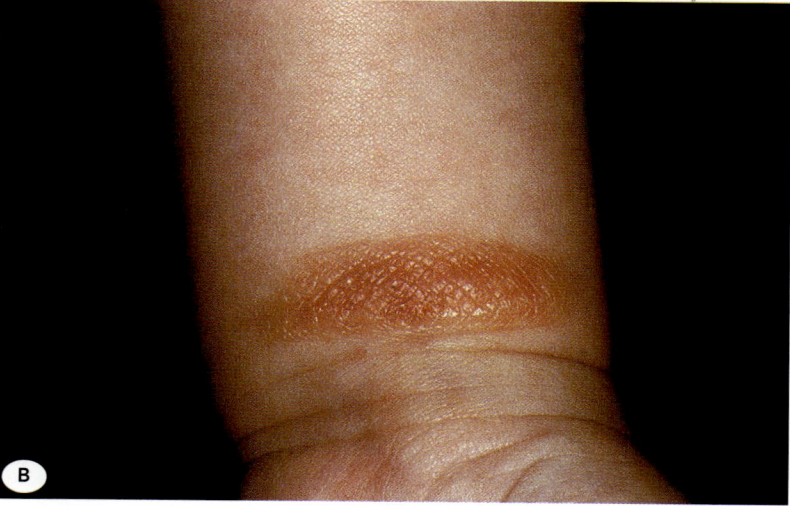

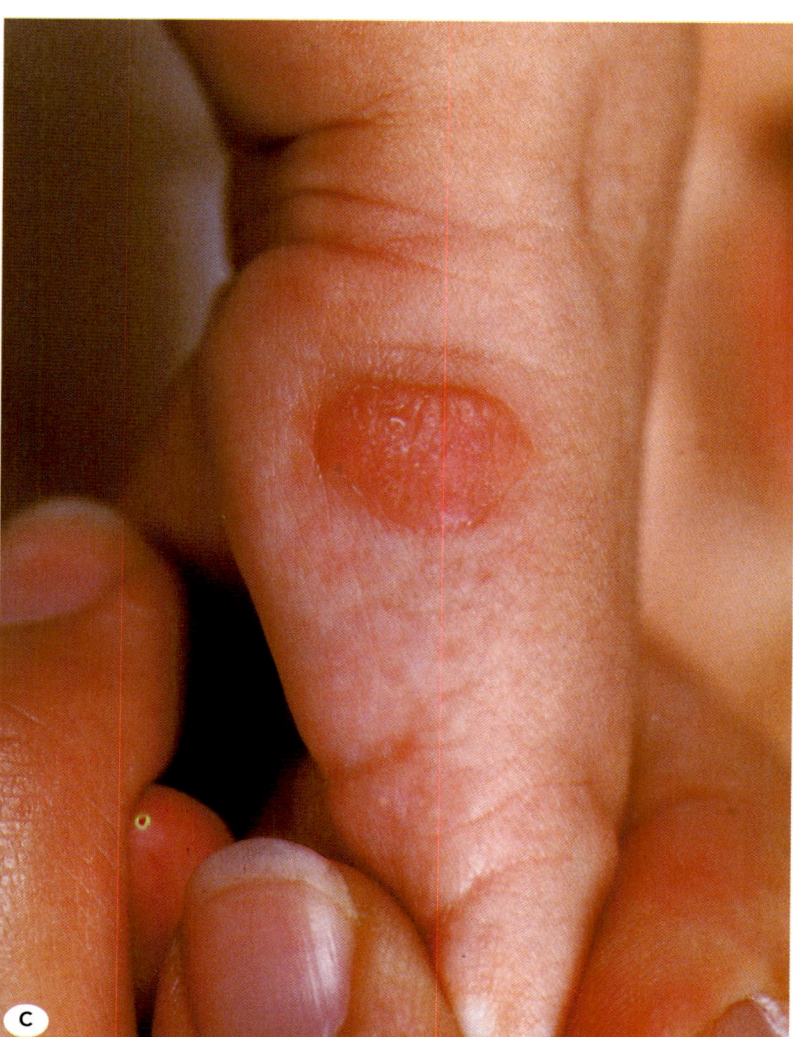

Fig. 17.18   (A) Solitary mastocytoma that has urticated after being rubbed (Darier's sign). (B) Mastocytoma. (C) Mastocytoma.

570. Anstey A, Lowe DG, Kirby JD (1991) Familial mastocytosis: a clinical, immunophenotypic, light and electron microscopic study. **Br J Dermatol** 125:583.
571. Oku T, Hashizume H, Yokote R et al. (1990) The familial occurrence of bullous mastocytosis (diffuse cutaneous mastocytosis). **Arch Dermatol** 126:1478.

572. Fine JD (1980) Mastocytosis. **Int J Dermatol** 19:117.
573. Caplan RM (1963) The natural course of urticaria pigmentosa. **Arch Dermatol** 87:146.

A mastocytoma is a reddish-brown, pink, or yellow nodule that is usually solitary. The surface is usually smooth but may rarely have the appearance of orange peel (peau d'orange). Lesions are round or oval, vary in size from 1 to 5 cm, and may have a thick or rubbery quality. The lesions usually occur at birth or in infancy and account for 10–15% of the cases of cutaneous mastocytosis.[573,574] Symptoms associated with single mastocytomas are usually few, but generalized pruritus, urticaria, and bullae formation over the lesion and systemic symptoms may rarely occur. It is unusual for children who present with a solitary lesion to acquire additional lesions more than two months after the initial lesion.

Urticaria pigmentosa, the commonest form of mastocytosis, usually begins between 3 and 9 months of age.[573] Lesions are usually numerous, red-brown macules, papules, and sometimes nodules and plaques mainly distributed over the trunk (Fig. 17.19). The number of lesions ranges from several to hundreds. Individual lesions are round to oval and vary in size from 1 mm to several centimeters. The numbers of lesions may increase for several years after diagnosis. Urticaria pigmentosa may rarely be associated with systemic involvement, particularly if lesions appear after 10 years of age. Infrequently, hepatosplenomegaly or skeletal lesions may be found that are due to mast cell hyperplasia in these organs.

Diffuse cutaneous mastocytosis is a rare type of mastocytosis that involves skin with an infiltration of mast cells without discrete lesions. The skin is usually thickened, lichenified, and doughy (Figs 17.20, 17.21), with numerous tiny papules, which have a yellowish tint. Initial manifestations often occur at 3 months of age with the sudden appearance of sero-sanguinous bullae (Fig. 17.22). Systemic symptoms including flushing, hemmorrhage, hypotension, diarrhea, dyspnea, or overt shock may occur.[575] When the bullae subside the thickened skin is evident.

TMEP is a term used to describe telangiectatic hyperpigmented macules that are usually extensive and located mainly on the trunk. The lesions do not

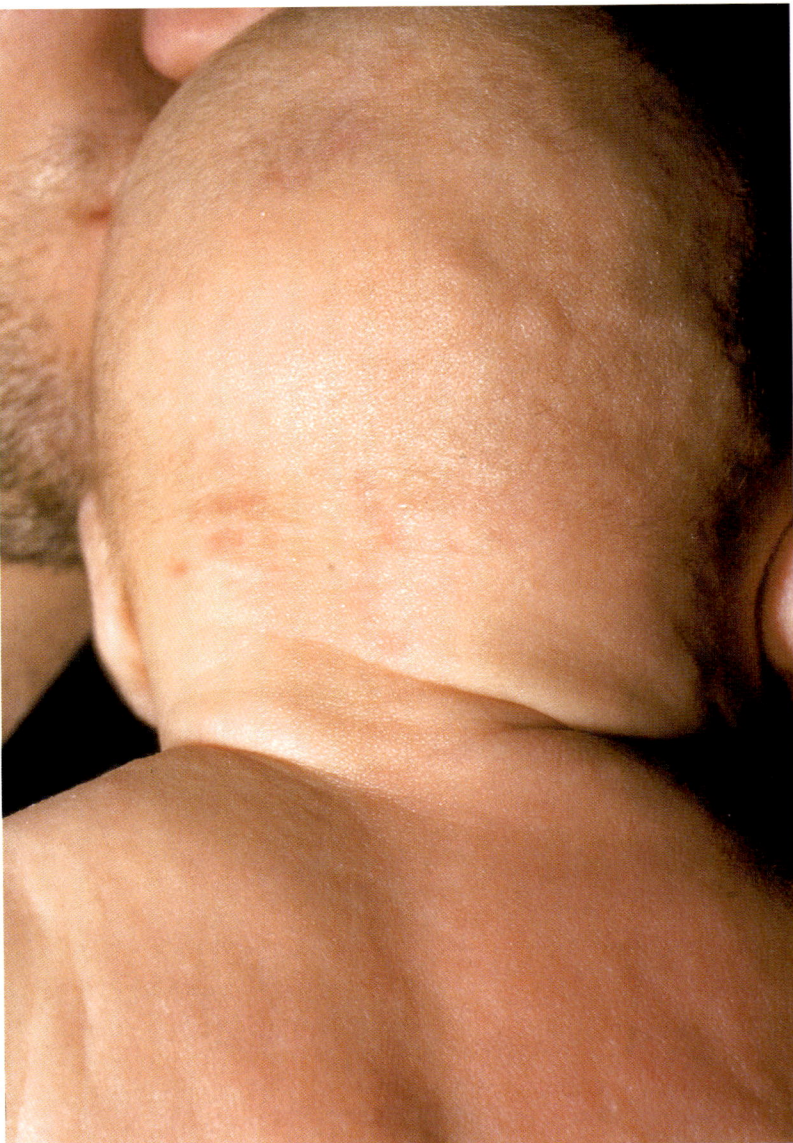

Fig. 17.20   Pebbly changes of diffuse cutaneous mastocytosis in a twelve-month-old infant.

typically urticate when stroked. They are seen more commonly in teenagers and adults and are rarely reported in children.[576]

Systemic infiltration with mastocytosis is more common in adults and older children but has been reported rarely in infants.[577] The gastrointestinal and skeletal systems are most commonly involved, but mast cell infiltration can be found in the lung, kidney, myocardium, pericardium, omentum, and other tissues.

The mastocytosis syndrome results from the massive release of vasodepressor mast cell products with a resultant shock state.[578] It can last from several minutes to several hours. It occurs most commonly in neonates or young children with diffuse cutaneous mastocytosis. Pruritus, headache, bronchospasm, rhinorrhea, flushing, diarrhea, hypotension, tachycardia, dyspnea, and syncope may all result. Occasionally the reaction is so severe that death may result.[575,579]

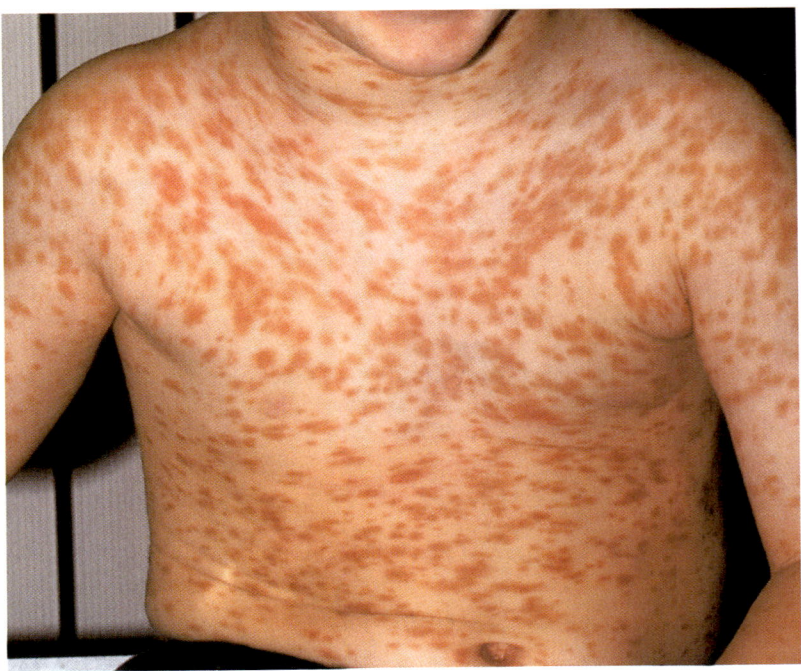

Fig. 17.19   Numerous lesions of urticaria pigmentosa on the abdomen and chest of a child.

574. Johnson WC, Helwig EB (1961) Solitary mastocytosis. **Arch Dermatol** 84:806–815.

575. Golitz LE, Weston WL, Lane AT (1984) Bullous mastocytosis with extensive blisters mimicking scalded skin syndrome or erythema multiforme. **Pediatr Dermatol** 1(4):288–294.

576. Gibbs NF, Friedlander SF, Harpster EF (2000) Telangiectasia macularis eruptive perstans. **Pediatr Dermatol** 17:194–197.

577. Hartmann K, Metcalfe DD (2000) Pediatric mastocytosis. **Hematol/oncol Clinics North Am** 14(3):625–640.

578. Turk J, Oates JA, Roberts LJ (1983) Intervention with epinephrine in hypotension associated with mastocytosis. **J Allergy Clin Immunol** 71:189.

579. Murphy M, Walsh D, Drumm B, Watson R (1999) Bullous mastocytosis: a fatal outcome. **Pediatr Dermatol** 16:452–455.

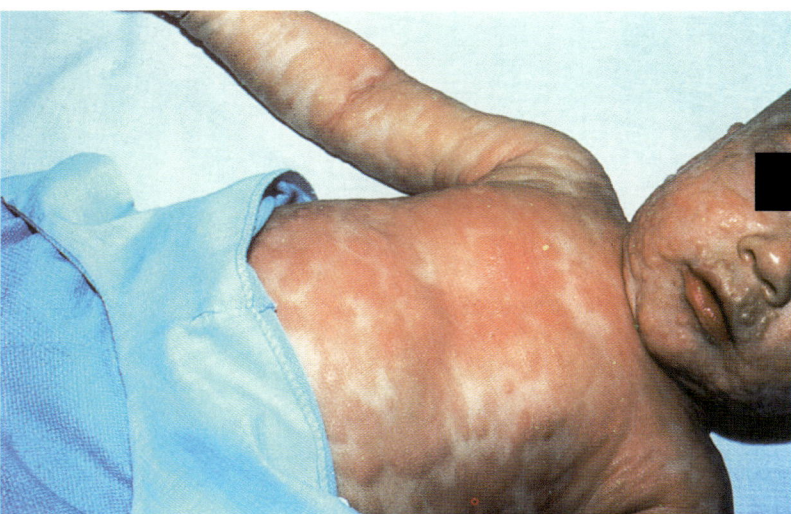

Fig. 17.21 Nodular lesions of mastocytosis.

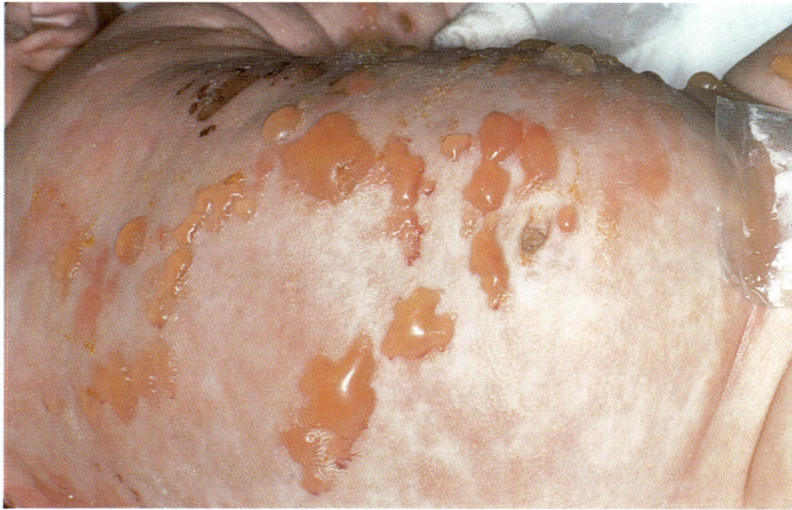

Fig. 17.22 Bullae in a 3-month-old infant with diffuse cutaneous mastocytosis.

In a review of 95 children, 14 showed radiographic bone lesions thought to be related to their mastocytosis.[580] None of these children had an aggressive course, and in three children follow-up radiographs were normal. Skeletal lesions may therefore be transitory and do not correlate with systemic involvement.[581] Obvious radiographic findings include discrete lytic, cystic, or sclerotic lesions and osteoporosis or osteosclerosis; these are most often seen in the axial skeleton.[572] Diffuse bone involvement occurs almost solely in adult-onset disease.[582]

Gastrointestinal symptoms are not common in children[583] but, when present, are usually seen with systemic disease. They may result from direct infiltration of mast cells into the mucosa or from increased tissue levels of histamine, which results in symptoms such as nausea, vomiting, abdominal pain, gastrointestinal hemorrhage, diarrhea, steatorrhea, and malabsorption.[584] Hepatomegaly or splenomegaly occurs in about 12% of cases of urticaria pigmentosa.[585]

The hematopoietic and reticuloendothelial systems are seldom involved in children. Urticaria pigmentosa has been associated with an increased number of hematologic malignancies, including Hodgkin's disease, lymphocytic lymphoma, and leukemia.[586] Diffuse cutaneous mastocytosis has been associated with a myleoproliferative disorder presenting *in utero* or shortly after birth.[587,588]

Darier's sign is a pathognomic sign of mastocytosis. It is defined as the urtication of a lesion after firm stroking. In a young child, the lesion may become bullous. Darier's sign is caused by the release of histamine from degranulation of mast cells secondary to mechanical trauma. The wheal and flare response persists for 30 minutes to several hours and may be intensely pruritic. Other signs of mast cell degranulation include flushing, particularly marked on the upper body and usually lasting 10 to 30 minutes, dermographism on clinically uninvolved skin, and, rarely, telangiectasias (seen in TMEP).

LABORATORY FINDINGS

Elevated urinary or plasma histamine levels may be helpful in making a diagnosis in patients with diffuse involvement, especially with gastrointestinal symptoms.[589] Urinary levels of histamine are metabolized rapidly and the major metabolites (N-methylhistamine and N-methylimidazylacetic acid), when elevated, are a sensitive test for the diagnosis of mastocytosis.[590,591]

Elevation of mast cell secretory products (prostaglandin D_2, α-tryptase, and heparin) can be measured in an attempt to demonstrate systemic mast cell activation.[592–594] Prostaglanding D_2 elevation in the urine suggests that mast cell-derived mediators cause vasodepression and other symptoms.[595] Serum α-tryptase levels when elevated in urine or blood of patients with mastocytosis may be useful in assessing total-body mast cell burden. Levels above 75ng/ml correlate strongly with systemic involvement.[596]

A skeletal radiographic survey or a technetium bone scan is indicated only if the patient has bone pain, hepatosplenomegaly, anemia, or failure to thrive. The usefulness of routine skeletal surveys is doubtful.[597] Examination of the gastrointestinal tract or bone marrow should be reserved for those instances where clinical evidence suggests organ system involvement.

Patients may have hypocholesterolemia secondary to the effects of heparin on lipoprotein metabolism. Hematologic abnormalities, including anemia, thrombocytopenia, and eosinophilia, may also occur with systemic involvement.

580. Lucaya J, Perez-Candela V, Aso C et al. (1979) Mastocytosis with skeletal and gastrointestinal involvement in infancy: two case reports and review of the literature. **Radiology** 131:363.
581. Kettelhut BV, Metcalfe DD (1994) Pediatric mastocytois. **Ann Allergy** 73:197–202.
582. Travis W, Li C-Y, Bergstrahl E et al. (1988) Systemic mast cell disease. **Medicine** 67:345–368.
583. Stein DH (1986) Mastocytosis: a review. **Pediatr Dermatol** 3:365.
584. Lewis RA (1984) Mastocytosis. **J Allergy Clin Immunol** 74:755.
585. Soter NA, Austen KF, Wasserman SI (1979) Oral disodium cromoglycate in the treatment of systemic mastocytosis. **N Engl J Med** 301:465.
586. McElroy EA, Phyliky RL, Li Cy (1998) Systemic mast cell disease associated with the hypereosinophilic syndrome. **Mayo Clin Proc** 73:47–50.
587. Kuint J, Bielorai B, Gilat D et al. (1999) C-kit activating mutation in a neonate with in-utero presentation of systemic mastocytosis associated with myeloproliferative disorder. **Br J Haematol** 106:833–839.
588. Shah PY, Sharma V, Worobec AS et al. (1998) Congenital bullous mastocytosis with myeloproliferative disorder and c-kit mutation. **J Am Acad Dermatol** 39:119–121.
589. Kendall ME, Fields JP, King LE (1984) Cutaneous mastocytosis without clinically obvious skin lesions. **J Am Acad Dermatol** 10:903.

590. Granerus G, Olafasson JH, Roupe G (1983) Studies on histamine metabolism in mastocytosis. **J Invest Dermatol** 80:410–416.
591. Keyzer JJ, deMonchy JGR, van Doormaal JJ et al. (1983) Improved diagnosis of mastocytosis by measurement of urinary histamine metabolites. **N Engl J Med** 309:1603.
592. Roberts LJ, Oates JA (1991) Biochemical diagnosis of systemic mast cell disorders. **J Invest Dermatol** 96:19S.
593. Roberts LJ, Sweetman BJ, Lewis RA et al. (1980) Increased production of prostaglandin D2 in patients with systemic mastocytosis. **N Engl J Med** 303:1400.
594. Morrow J, Guzo C, Lazarus G et al. (1995) Improved diagnosis of mastocytosis by measurement of the major urinary metabolite of prostaglandin D2. **J Invest Dermatol** 104:937–940.
595. Kawai S, Okamoto H (1993) Giant mast cell granules in a solitary mastocytoma. **Pediatr Dermatol** 10:12.
596. Kanthawatana S, Carias K, Arnaout R et al. (1999) The potential clinical utility of serum α-protryptase levels. **J Allergy Clin Immunol** 103:1092–1099.
597. Cooper AJ, Winkelmann RK, Wiltsie JC (1982) Hematologic malignancies occurring in patients with urticaria pigmentosa. **J Am Acad Dermatol** 7:215.

PATHOPHYSIOLOGY AND HISTOGENESIS

Urticaria pigmentosa and mastocytoma lesions have an infiltration of mast cells in the upper third of the dermis with occasional perivascular aggregates.[186] These aggregates may be so extensive that they obliterate all the cutaneous architecture. Mast cells are difficult to demonstrate by routine hematoxylin and eosin staining. Giemsa stain, toluidine blue or Leder's method (napthol AS-D chloracetate esterase) identify the characteristic metachromatic cytoplasmic granules and should be requested if indicated. It is important to choose a biopsy site that has not been recently traumatized. When the lesion has recently been urticated, the mast cells may be degranulated and not evident. Eosinophils, edema, and subepidermal bullae may be seen in some biopsy specimens. TMEP demonstrates a subtle increase in the number of mast cells, usually around capillary venules, along with vascular ectasia. Pigmentation in urticaria pigmentosa is secondary to the presence of increased melanin in the basal cell layer and melanophages in the upper dermis. Electron microscopy demonstrates typical mast cell morphology with rare reports of giant mast cell granules.[595]

The cause of mastocytosis is unknown. Mast cells can be found in the connective tissue of most organs and originate from bone marrow CD34+ precursors. Their granular morphology is only assumed after migrating into tissues. The precursor cells in periperal blood also express the protein kinase KIT (CD117), which is the receptor ligand for stem cell factor (SCF) and FcγRII but not the high-affinity IgE receptors.[598] KIT is the product of the proto-oncogene *c-kit* located on chromosome 4q12 and belongs to the family of tyrosine kinase receptors. It is expressed on numerous cells other than mast cells including melanocytes, primitive hematopoietic stem cells, germ cell lines, and the intestinal cells of Cajal. Abnormalities of the *c-kit* receptor have been described in mastocytosis and piebaldism.[599–601] Alterations in SCF and KIT are seen in mastocytosis patients. The majority of nonfamilial adult mastocytosis cases are associated with a mutation of codon 816 of the *c-kit* proto-oncogene. This results in activation of KIT, which induces cellular proliferation and decreased apoptosis of mast cells.[602] These mutations have not been seen in typical sporadic childhood mastocytosis. Longley[603] investigated *c-kit* auto-activating mutations in 11 adults and 11 children with sporadic mastocytosis. All the adults displayed the codon 816 mutations and all pediatric patients tested negative. Four other pediatric patients with extensive skin involvement, two of whom eventually developed systemic disease, proved positive for the codon 816 mutation.[603] A classification of mastocytosis based on the molecular defect has recently been proposed, as patients who express these mutations regardless of their age appear to have persistent disease with increased risk of systemic involvement and non–mast cell hematologic disorders.[604,605] Increased soluble stem cell factor has been reported in skin lesions of patients with both adult and pediatric mastocytosis and may contribute to mast cell growth and survival as well as to the hyperpigmentation seen clinically.[606–608]

Mast cells are paracrine cells that store products within granules and release them directly into the surrounding tissue fluid. Histamine, a major component of the granules, can alter vascular permeability, increase airway resistance, stimulate cardiac and gastric secretory systems, and mediate T-lymphocyte suppression by acting on specific membrane receptors. Other mediators released include cytokines, TNF-α, IL-4-5-6, and -8. Once stimulated, mast cells may also generate newly formed PGD-2, leukotrienes, platelet activating factor (PAF), and SCF.[567]

Disease results either from the local effects of infiltration of mast cells that interfere with normal organ function or from the pharmacologic effects of chemicals generated by mast cell activation. Immediate type I hypersensitivity reactions may occur secondary to chemical mediators, such as histamine and prostaglandin D_2 which causes injury to tissue, increased vascular permeability, constriction of smooth muscles, enhanced leukocyte migration, and increased platelet activation.

DIFFERENTIAL DIAGNOSIS

A solitary lesion of mastocytosis may be misdiagnosed as bullous impetigo because of the blistering. Other lesions confused with mastocytomas are juvenile xanthogranulomas, nevocellular nevi, connective tissue nevi, bullous insect bites, bullous urticaria, and the nodular lesions of scabies. Darier's sign is helpful in distinguishing these entities. The macular form of mastocytosis may be confused with multiple lentigines, pigmented nevi, eruptive xanthomas, and neurofibromatosis. TMEP may be mistaken for hereditary hemorrhagic telangiectasia. The diffuse or erythrodermic form may be mistaken for Langerhans histiocytosis, bullous erythema multiforme, or other bullous diseases. Biopsy is essential for diagnosis in such cases.

Cutaneous mastocytosis beginning in an older child or adult, or extensive cutaneous lesions associated with symptoms such as episodic flushing, palpitations, or syncope, should alert the physician to evaluate for systemic involvement. Carcinoid syndrome may show similar symptoms, but these patients do not have telangiectasias.

THERAPY AND PROGNOSIS

The patient should avoid precipitating causes for mast cell degranulation (Table 17.7), and a list of medications to avoid should be given to the parent and/or patient. Over-the-counter cough preparations may contain dextromethorphan or codeine which may induce significant histamine release and blistering.[566] If the patient undergoes surgery, the following medications should be avoided: morphine, scopolamine, tubocurarine, gallamine, decamethonium, atropine, procaine, and reserpine.[609] Halothane may prolong the histamine shock state.[572] Propofol, vecuronium, and fentanyl are safe to use in mastocytosis patients undergoing surgery.[610] Intravenously administered lorazepam, a short-acting benzodiazepine, is a safe sedation before diagnostic and investigational procedures.[609]

Various medications have been used to treat mastocytosis. Antihistamines such as hydroxyzine may help alleviate symptoms and are usually given four times a day if symptoms occur. H_1- and H_2-receptor antagonists either alone or together may be of some benefit. Nonsedative H_1 antihistamines such as cetirazine, loratadine, and fexofenadine, have the advantage of not causing drowsiness. Cyproheptadine (0.25mg/kg per day) plus cimetidine (30mg/kg per day) have reduced the bullae in two cases of congenital bullous urticaria pigmentosa.[611] Cromolyn sodium (200–800mg/day) has been effective in

598. Rottem M, Okada T, Goff JP et al. (1994) Mast cells cultured from the peripheral blood of normal donors and patients with mastocytosis originate from CD34+ /Fcε/RI-cell population. **Blood** 84:2489–2496.
599. Lev S, Blechman JM, Givol D et al. (1994) Steel factor and c-kit proto-oncogene: Genetic lessons in signal transduction. **Crit Rev Oncog** 5:141–168.
600. Longley BJ, Tyrell L, Lu SZ et al. (1996) Somatic c-kit activating mutation in urticaria pigmentosa and aggressive mastocytosis: establishment of clonality in a human mast cell neoplasm. **Nat Genet** 12:312–314.
601. Nagata H, Worobec AS, Oh CK et al. (1995) Identification of a point mutation in the catalytic domain of the protooncogene c-Kit in peripheral blood mononuclear cells of patients who have mastocytosis with an associated hematologic disorder. **Proc Natl Acad Sci USA** 92:10560–10564.
602. Boissan M, Fegr F, Guillosson JJ et al. (2000) c-Kit and c-Kit mutation in mastocytosis and other hematological diseases. **J Leukoc Biol** 67:135–148.
603. Longley BJ, Metcalfe DD, Tharp MD et al. (1999) Activating and dominant inactivating c-kit catalytic domain mutations in distinct forms of human mastocytosis. **Proc Natl Acad Sci USA** 96:1609–1614.

604. Tharp M, Longley J (2001) Mastocytosis. **Dermatol Clinics** 19(4):679–696.
605. Longley BJ, Metcalfe D (2000) A proposed classification system of mastocytosis incorporating molecular genetics. **Hematol/oncology Clinics North Am** 14(3):697–701.
606. Longley BJ, Morganroth GS, Tyrrell L et al. (1993) Altered metabolism of mast cell growth factor (c-kit ligand) in cutaneous mastocytosis. **N Engl J Med** 328:1302–1307.
607. Halaban R, Tyrrell L, Longley J et al. (1993) Pigmentation and proliferation of human melanocytes and the effect of melanocyte-stimulating hormone and ultraviolet B light. **Ann NY Acad Sci** 680:290–301.
608. Geissler EN, Ryan MA, Housman DE (1988) The dominant-white spotting (W) locus of the mouse encodes the c-kit proto-oncogene. **Cell** 55:185–192.
609. Greenblatt EP, Chen L (1990) Urticaria pigmentosa: an anesthetic challenge. **J Clin Anesth** 2:108.
610. Borgeat A, Ruetsch YA (1998) Anesthesia in a patient with malignant systemic mastocytosis using a total intravenous anesthetic technique. **Anesth Analg** 86:442–444.
611. Horan RF, Sheffer AL, Austen KF et al. (1990) Cromolyn sodium in the management of systemic mastocytosis. **J Allergy Clin Immunol** 25:852–855.

TABLE 17.7 Nonimmunologic mast cell degranulators
Physical stimuli
Exercise
Skin friction
Hot baths
Cold exposure (especially swimming)
Ingestion of hot beverages, spicy foods, or ethanol
Drugs
Aspirin
Alcohol
Morphine
Codeine
Dextromethorphan
Polymyxin B
Thiamine
Quinine
Tubocuraine
Radiographic dyes
Scopolamine
Procaine
Opiates
Nonsteroidal anti-inflammatory agents
Gallamine
Decamethonium
Beserpine
Reserpine
Other
Intravenous high molecular weight polymers (dextran)
Emotional stress
Bacterial toxins
Snake venoms
Polypeptides released by Ascaris
Jellyfish, crayfish, and lobsters

reducing symptoms of pruritus, dermographism, and blister formation in a number of studies.[612,613] The urinary histamine levels are usually unaffected by cromolyn sodium. Recommendations are 20mg/kg/per day in four divided doses up to age 2 years; for children 2–12 years, 100mg qid can be given. Ketotifen, which has both antihistamine and mast cell stabilizing properties, has been used in both childhood and adult forms of mastocytosis alone or combined with ranitidine.[614,615] One study suggested no advantage over conventional H_1 antihistamines.[614] Dosage of ketotifen is 1–2mg twice daily, and is well tolerated in infants although it may stimulate appetite and weight gain. Aspirin inhibits prostaglandin synthesis[593] but caution should be used in prescribing this, as fatal histamine shock may be precipitated.

Potent topical steroids under occlusion (betamethasone diproprionate 0.05%, clobetasol proprionate 0.05%) may improve the clinical appearance and reduce the number of mast cells in the skin.[616] Occasional prolonged remission of treated areas has been described.[617–620] Intralesional steroids (triamcinolone acetonide 5–10mg/ml) may be used for individual lesions.[618]

Adults with mastocytosis have been reported to have severe anaphylaxis after insect stings.[619] An Epipen or ANA-Kit may be considered for selected children,[579] and a medical alert bracelet may also be suggested.

In the diffuse cutaneous form, PUVA may cause relief of pruritus and symptoms and improve the patient's appearance.[620,621] Caution should be used when starting treatment to prevent massive mast cell degranulation. Bath PUVA was not effective in four patients.[622] The combination of interferon-α 2b and prednisone may be effective in systemic mast cell disease.[623] Symptoms improve but tissue mast cells, particularly bone marrow involvement persists.[624] Interferon has not been adequately studied in pediatric mastocytosis.[561] Oral prednisone is the mainstay of treatment in severe cases of systemic mastocytosis in adults associated with malabsorption.[625,626] In the future, agents which inhibit KIT kinase may be useful in patients with documented activating *c-kit* mutations.[627] Surgical excision of isolated persistent lesions may occasionally be appropriate if other treatments have failed and the lesions produce symptoms.

Episodes of profound hypotension and shock in systemic mastocytosis may require intravenous saline, corticosteroids, pressor agents, epinephrine (adrenaline),[578] and both H_1 and H_2 antihistamines. Treatment of bullae requires local care and prevention of infection. Because many over-the-counter antibiotics contain polymyxin B, a degranulator of mast cells, mupirocin may be a better choice for local wound care. Blisters generally heal without scarring but may leave residual hyperpigmentation.

The course of an isolated mastocytoma is usually spontaneous regression over several years. Childhood urticaria pigmentosa also has a favorable outcome with lesions regressing by puberty.[628] The prognosis in the very young with diffuse cutaneous mastocytosis depends on systemic involvement. Death is usually related to hemorrhage, leukemia, myelofibrosis, or cachexia. Infants who present with bullae are more likely to have systemic involvement. Children whose mastocytosis persists into adulthood typically demonstrate a course similar to adult-onset disease in which 5–10% have systemic involvement.[573] Older children and adults who have serious systemic involvement have a guarded prognosis, as do neonates with massive diffuse cutaneous involvement. Type I allergies may be more severe in mast cell disease than normal because of profound mast cell degranulation.[619]

Rarely, a child may have aggressive mastocytosis with bone marrow and other organ involvement. In these cases, mast cells infiltrate the organs, or circulating mast cells may be seen resembling leukemia. These children have a more guarded prognosis.

612. Frieri M, Alling DW, Metcalfe DD (1985) Comparison of the therapeutic efficacy of cromolyn sodium with that of combined chlorpheniramine and cimetidine in systemic mastocytosis: results of a double-blind clinical trial. **Am J Med** 78:9.
613. Welch EA, Alper JC, Gogaars H et al. (1983) Treatment of bullous mastocystosis with disodium cromoglycate. **J Am Acad Dermatol** 9:349.
614. Czarnetzki BM (1983) A double-blind cross-over study of the effect of ketotifen in urticaria pigmentosa. **Dermatologica** 166:44.
615. Kurosawa M, Amano H, Kanbe N et al. (1997) Heterogeneity of mast cells in mastocytosis and inhibitory effect of ketotifen and ranitidine on indolent systemic mastocytosis. **J Allergy Clin Immunol** 100:S25–S32.
616. Guzzo C, Lavker R, Roberts LJ et al. (1991) Urticaria pigmentosa. Systemic evaluation and successful treatment with topical steroids. **Arch Dermatol** 127:191.
617. Sidhu S, Wakelin SH, Wojnarowska F (1997) Prolonged remission of urticaria pigmentosa following topical steroid therapy under hydrocolloid occlusion. **Clin and Experiment Dermatol** 22:300–304.
618. Barton J, Lavker RM, Schechter NM et al. (1985) Treatment of urticaria pigmentosa with corticosteroids. **Arch Dermatol** 121:1516–1523.
619. Fricker M, Helbling A, Schwartz L et al. (1997) Hymenoptera sting anyphylaxis and urticaria pigmentosa: clinical findings and results of venom immunotherapy in 10 patients. **J Allergy Clin Immunol** 100(1):11–15.

620. Mackey S, Pride HB, Tyler WB (1996) Diffuse cutaneous mastocytosis. **Arch Dermatol** 132:1429–1430.
621. Smith ML, Orton PW, Chu H et al. (1991) Photochemotherapy of dominant, diffuse, cutaneous mastocytosis. **Pediatr Dermatol** 7:251.
622. Godt D, Proksch E, Streit V et al. (1997) Short and long term effectiveness of oral and bath PUVA therapy in urticaria pigmentosa and systemic mastocytosis. **Dermatology** 195:35–39.
623. Kluin-Nelemans HC, Jansen JH, Bruekelman H et al. (1992) Response to interferon alfa-2b in a patient with systemic mastocytosis. **N Engl J Med** 326:619.
624. Worobec A, Kirshenbaum A, Schwartz L et al. (1996) Treatment of three patients with systemic mastocytosis with interferon alpha-2b. **Leuk Lymphoma** 22:501–508.
625. Metcalfe DD (1991) The treatment of mastocytosis: an overview. **J Invest Dermatol** 96:55S–59S.
626. Worobec, AS (2000) Treatment of systemic mast cell disorders. **Hematol/oncol Clinics of North Am** 14:659–687.
627. Longley BJ, Yongsheng M, Carter E et al. (2000) New approaches to therapy for mastocytosis: A case for treatment with kitkinase inhibitors. **Hematology/oncology Clinics of North Am** 14:697–701.
628. Klaus SN, Winkelmann RK (1962) Course of urticaria pigmentosa in children. **Arch Dermatol** 86:116.

TABLE 17.8   Types of xanthomas

Tendinous

Planar
  Xanthelasma palpebrarum
  Corneal arcus
  Xanthoma striatum palmare
  Diffuse infiltrative plaques

Tuberous

Eruptive

Other
  Xanthoma disseminatum
  Cerebrotendinous xanthomatosis
  Phytosterolemia
  Tangier disease

PEDIATRIC ASPECTS OF THE DISEASE

Solitary mastocytomas and urticaria pigmentosa are commonly seen in children and have a favorable outlook. TMEP and diffuse infiltrative mastocytosis are rare in childhood and have a more guarded prognosis. Systemic mastocytosis and mastocytosis with malignancy are very rare in childhood.

HYPERLIPIDEMIAS AND XANTHOMAS

Xanthomas are localized infiltrates of histiocytic foam cells that contain lipid.[629] They are commonly caused by a disturbance of lipoprotein metabolism. In general, five major clinical forms of cutaneous xanthomas exist: tendinous, planar, tuberous, eruptive, and other (Table 17.8).

Xanthomas on the skin may lead to the detection of an associated underlying metabolic lipoprotein abnormality. The number of xanthomas is dependent on the duration and severity of the hyperlipoproteinemia; thus

lesions occur more commonly in adults. When they do occur in children and adolescents, it is an indicator of greater severity. Although a specific diagnosis cannot be made solely on the basis of clinical signs, certain types of xanthomas are more characteristic of specific types of hyperlipidemias. In adults, lipo–protein disturbances may be early clues to other conditions such as diabetes mellitus, thyroid disease, or early atherosclerotic cardiovascular disease. Prompt diagnosis and treatment may help prevent complications such as pancreatitis and early coronary artery disease.[630]

EPIDEMIOLOGY

The epidemiology of xanthomas varies with the lipoprotein abnormality (Table 17.9).

PRESENTING HISTORY

Patients or parents complain of yellow, soft, macular or slightly raised plaques located on charcteristic areas of the body.[631,632]

PHYSICAL EXAMINATION

Tendinous xanthomas arise in tendons, ligaments, and fascia and present as deep smooth, nontender, firm nodules of various sizes that move with the affected tendon. Some are easily seen, but others are detected only by palpation. The lesions are usually 1cm or larger in size and are most frequently located on the Achilles tendons and the extensor tendons of the hands, knees, and elbows. They are seen with other forms of xanthomas and almost always indicate a disturbance of cholesterol metabolism.[631]

Planar xanthomas present as soft yellow macules and slightly elevated papules and plaques located anywhere on the body, with a predilection for surgical or acne scars.[240] There are several subtypes of planar xanthomas. The most common type, xanthelasma palpebrarum, occurs on the eyelids. Most patients with xanthelasmas are normolipemic, but abnormal lipoprotein levels may account for the appearance of these lesions and correspond to an increased tendency to develop atherosclerosis.[633] When these do rarely occur in a child,

TABLE 17.9   Disorders associated with xanthomas

Eruptive (seen with chylomicronemia)	Tuberous	Planar
Lipoprotein lipase deficiency	Familial dysbetalipoproteinemia (type III)	Homozygous familial hypercholesterolemia
Type I glycogen storage disease	Familial hypercholesterolemia	(especially intertriginous)
(von Giercke's disease)	Cerebrotendinous xanthomatosis	Familial dysbetalipoproteinemia (type III)
Familial hyperlipoproteinemia (type V)	β-sitosterolemia	(especially palmar creases)
Diabetes mellitus	Hepatic cholestasis	Severe hepatic cholestasis
Alcohol ingestion	Normocholesterolemic	Dysglobulinemias
Retinoid induced	dysbetalipoproteinemia	Paraproteinemias
Estrogen induced		Leukemia
Familial hypertriglyceridemia (type IV)	Tuberoeruptive	Lymphoma
Hypothyroidism	Familial dysbetalipoproteinemia (type III)	Eosinophilic granulomatosis
Nephrotic syndrome	Hypothyroidism	Rheumatoid arthritis
	Secondary hyperlipoproteinemias	
		Xanthelasmas
	Tendinous (seen with elevated LDL	Familial dysbetalipoproteinemia (type III)
	or altered LDL)	Hypercholesterolemia
	Familial hypercholesterolemia (heterozygous)	Hepatic cholestasis
	Cerebrotendinous xanthomatosis	Cerebrotendinous xanthomatosis
	β-sitosterolemia	β-sitosterolemia
	Hyperapobetalipoproteinemia	Hyperapobetalipoproteinemia
	Familial dysbetalipoproteinemia (type III)	Normolipemic states

Abbreviation: LDL; low-density lipoprotein.

629. Parker F (1985) Xanthomas and hyperlipidemias. **J Am Acad Dermatol** 13:1.
630. Maher-Wiese VL, Marmer EL, Grant-Kels JM (1990) Xanthomas and the inherited hyperlipoproteinemias in children and adolescents. **Pediatr Dermatol** 7:166.
631. Cruz PD, East C, Bergstresser PR (1988) Dermal, subcutaneous, and tendon xanthomas: diagnostic markers for specific lipoprotein disorders. **J Am Acad Dermatol** 19:95.
632. Haber C, Kwiterovich PO (1984) Dyslipoproteinemia and xanthomatosis. **Pediatr Dermatol** 1:261.
633. Douste-Blazy P, Marcel YL, Cohen L et al. (1982) Increased frequency of apo E-ND phenotype and hyperapobetalipoproteinemia in normolipemic subjects with xanthelasmas of the eyelids. **Ann Intern Med** 96:164.

diabetes mellitus, Langerhans cell histiocytosis, multiple myeloma, hepatic disorders, or familial hyperlipidemia should be suspected. Extensive, infiltrative planar xanthomatosis is rare but is usually associated with various paraproteinemias. Diffuse involvement usually involves the face, neck, upper trunk, and arms. Corneal arcus is a translucent yellow infiltrate at the peripheral limbus of the cornea. The lesions begin in the lower or upper cornea and then become circumferential. Deposits consist of cholesterol, triglycerides, and phospholipids. Corneal arcus is associated with an increased incidence of atherosclerosis, especially when seen in patients younger than 50 years of age.[634]

Xanthoma striatum palmare lesions are flat, yellow to orange linear lesions in the creases of the palms and fingers. They are most commonly seen with type III hyperlipidemia, where an increase in cholesterol and triglyceride levels causes the deposition in these specific tissues.

Tuberous xanthomas present as yellow or red nodules located mainly on the extensor surfaces of the extremities, buttocks, and palms (Fig. 17.23). They begin as small, soft papules, which may be confused with eruptive xanthomas; they enlarge and become coalescent and firm, but are not attached to underlying structures like tendinous xanthomas. They indicate an alteration of cholesterol and/or triglyceride metabolism. Atherosclerosis is more common in these patients.

Eruptive xanthomas are small, yellow papules that frequently have an erythematous halo around the base. They range in size from 1 to 4mm and erupt suddenly in crops over the extensor surfaces of the arms, legs, buttocks, and pressure points (Fig. 17.24). They may be associated with the chylomicronemia syndrome, lipemia retinalis (where the fundus appears pale pink secondary to large quantities of light-scattering chylomicrons coursing through the retinal vasculature), recent memory loss, abdominal pain, and occasionally acute pancreatitis.[635] Eruptive xanthomas develop in patients who have markedly elevated triglyceride levels, especially those with uncontrolled diabetes, in patients with type I, III, IV, and V hyperlipidemias, and in patients with the nephrotic syndrome.[636]

Xanthoma disseminatum is rare and usually occurs in adults.[637] Distinctive papulonodular red-yellow lesions appear slowly and develop a dark mahogany

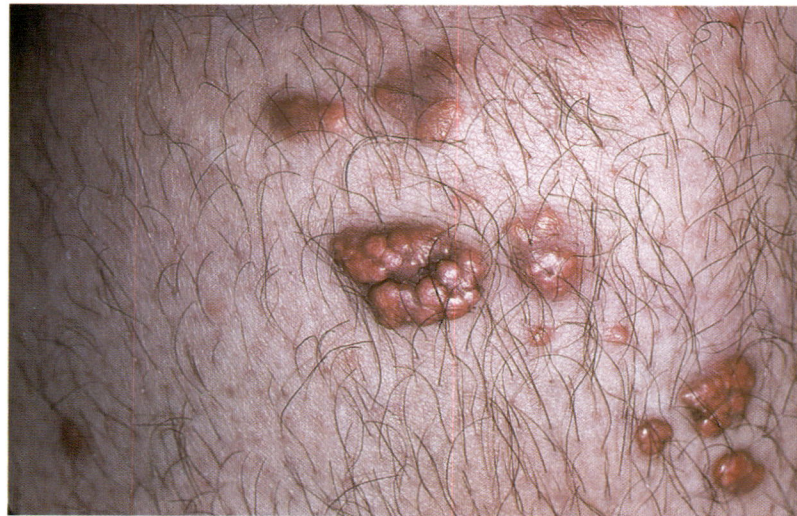

Fig. 17.24 Plaques of xanthomas in a teenager with biliary atresia.

hue with age. There is a predilection for the flexural creases, mucous membranes, central nervous system, corneas, conjunctivae, and occasionally bone. Lesions may be seen in the pharynx, larynx, and the bronchi. They may cause dysphagia, laryngeal obstruction, hoarseness, and dyspnea. When lesions are located in the central nervous system, they can cause diabetes insipidus. Serum lipid concentrations are normal. This disorder is considered part of the spectrum of non-Langerhans cell histiocytosis.

Cerebrotendinous xanthomatosis is a rare autosomal-recessive syndrome consisting of progressive mental retardation, cataracts, and cerebellar ataxia caused by mutations in the sterol-27 hydroxylase gene that results in a disturbance in the lipid storage process of cholestanol.[638,639] The lipid accumulates in the skin, tendons, lungs, and cerebellar white matter. Plasma cholesterol levels are usually normal, but blood cholestanol levels are increased.

Phytosterolemia is a rare disorder in which tissue accumulation of plant sterols (β-sitosterol, campesterol, and stigmasterol) is caused by an increased absorption of plant sterols from the diet.[640,641] It is inherited as an autosomal-recessive trait. Cholesterol levels are either normal or slightly elevated, and tuberous and tendinous xanthomas are seen.

LABORATORY FINDINGS

Cholesterol and triglyceride levels should be measured after having the patient fast for 12–14 hours. Lipoprotein electrophoresis separates lipoproteins according to density; those with the greatest portion of protein have the highest density (e.g., high-density lipoproteins [HDL]). Specific patterns are used to classify the type of hyperlipidemia. To determine whether xanthomas are primary or secondary, ancillary tests for the evaluation of thyroid, liver, renal diseases, and diabetes should be performed.

Plasma lipoproteins are composed of lipids (cholesterol, triglycerides, and phospholipids) and proteins called apolipoproteins. They are divided into five major classes based on physical and chemical properties. Lipoproteins transport fats in the blood by providing emulsifying properties, which help solubilize the hydrophobic lipids. Chylomicrons are the largest, least dense lipoproteins

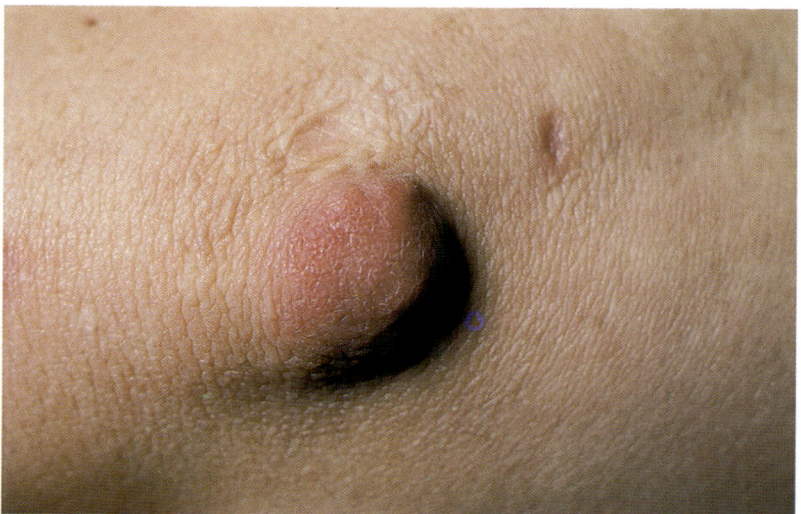

Fig. 17.23 Tuberous xanthomas on the elbow.

634. Rosenman RH, Brand RJ, Sholtz RI et al. (1974) Relation of corneal arcus to cardiovascular risk factors and the incidence of coronary disease. **N Engl J Med** 291:1322.
635. Brunzell JD, Bierman EL (1982) Chylomicronemia syndrome. **Med Clin North Am** 66:455.
636. Teltscher J, Silverman RA, Stork J (1989) Eruptive xanthomas in a child with the nephrotic syndrome. **J Am Acad Dermatol** 21:1147.
637. Mishkel MA, Cockshott P, Nazir DJ et al. (1977) Xanthomas disseminatum. **Arch Dermatol** 113:1094.
638. Philippart M, van Bogaert L (1969) Cholestanolosis (cerebrotendinous xanthomatosis). **Arch Neurol** 21:603.
639. Bel S, Garcia-Patos V, Rodriguez L et al. (2001) Cerebrotendinous xanthomatosis. **J Am Acad Dermatol** 45(2):292–295.
640. Matsuo I, Yoshino K, Ozawa A (1981) Phytosterolemia and type IIa hyperlipoproteinemia with tuberous xanthomas. **J Am Acad Dermatol** 4:47.
641. McArthur RG, Roncari DAK, Little JA et al. (1986) Phytosterolemia and hypercholesterolemia in childhood. **J Pediatr** 108:254.

and contain mostly triglycerides (85%). Very low–density lipoproteins (VLDL), also called pre–β–lipoproteins, are not as dense and carry 30% cholesterol and 50% triglyceride. Intermediate–density lipoproteins (IDL), also called remnant lipoproteins, carry half cholesterol and half triglyceride. Low–density lipoproteins (LDL), also referred to as β–lipoproteins, are the major carriers of cholesterol (50%),[642] and elevated levels of LDL can be correlated with premature development of atherosclerosis. HDL, also called α–lipoproteins, are very dense and contain half apoprotein. They have very little relevance to xanthomas but do play a role in atherosclerosis with increased levels of HDLs protecting against atherosclerosis.

In addition to lipoproteins, 12 apoproteins have been identified in humans, and their deficiencies affect lipoprotein metabolism. Aproproteins not only emulsify lipoproteins and allow them to be transported but also serve as cofactors for enzymes involved in metabolism and act as specific ligands for receptors. Certain apoproteins (B48 and B100) are necessary for the formation of chylomicrons in the enterocyte of the intestine and the formation of VLDL in the hepatocytes.

In many cases, xanthomas are related directly to the degree of elevation in lipoprotein levels and can wax and wane in parallel to fluctuations in serum lipoprotein concentrations. For example, tendinous xanthomas arise when cholesterol levels reach greater than 500mg/dl.[643] Planar xanthomas in obstructive liver disease are seen when plasma cholesterol exceeds 1800mg/dl, and eruptive xanthomas require triglyceride levels to be greater than 1000mg/dl to manifest clinically.

In rare instances, xanthomas can be seen with normal levels of cholesterol,[644] in which case other disorders may be implicated, including the accumulation of plant sterols, cerebrotendinous xanthomatosis, and paraproteinemias or systemic diseases predisposing to the development of lesions, including local factors such as previously inflamed skin in atopic dermatitis or epidermolysis bullosa.

PATHOPHYSIOLOGY AND HISTOGENESIS

The histologic appearance of xanthomas is characterized by macrophages with foamy cytoplasm filled with lipid droplets.[186] Lipoproteins permeate the walls of cutaneous capillaries and are phagocytized by histiocytes, where the lipids accumulate, and result in typical foam cells. Fat stains, such as scarlet red or Sudan red, demonstrate the lipids. Xanthoma cells usually have one nucleus but may have several. Multinucleated xanthoma cells have their nuclei arranged in a wreath-like pattern, or they may look like foreign body giant cells in which the nuclei are randomly scattered. Lymphocytes, histiocytes, and neutrophils may be seen.

Accumulations of lipoproteins in the plasma can result from: (1) excessive endogenous production, (2) defective removal, (3) decreased lipoprotein breakdown, or (4) a combination of these mechanisms.[645,646] Metabolic aberrations in lipoprotein metabolism may be seen as a primary manifestation of a specific genetic disorder, such as lipoprotein lipase deficiency, or as a secondary phenomenon associated with an underlying disease, such as diabetes mellitus, cholestatic liver disease, nephrosis, hypothyroidism, or pancreatitis. In addition, drugs such as estrogens, corticosteroids, isotretinoin, cyclosporine, and protease inhibitors used in HIV may also cause lipoprotein abnormalities.[647] The two sources of lipids from which circulating lipoproteins may be formed are exogenous dietary fats and endogenous fats synthesized by the liver. Reviews of lipid metabolism can be found in the literature and are recommended for in-depth probing into the pathogenesis of lipid disorders.[629,646–649]

Primary hyperlipoproteinemias have been classified into various types, based on specific lipoprotein patterns by paper electrophoretic separation and inheritance (Table 17.10).[629,650] Familial hypercholesterolemia, lipoprotein lipase deficiency, and familial combined hyperlipidemia rarely present in childhood.

Lipoprotein lipase deficiency is a rare recessively inherited disorder. Because of the absence of enzyme activity, there is defective removal of chylomicrons with resultant marked hypertriglyceridemia and either a type I or V pattern on electrophoresis, and hyperchylomicronemia. Clinically it presents before puberty with eruptive xanthomas, hepatosplenomegaly, lipemia retinalis, and pancreatitis.[635,651]

Apoprotein CII deficiency (lipoprotein lipase activator) presents in adolescence with a type I or V pattern. Xanthomas are not usually present. The deficiency results in the inability of lipoprotein lipase recognition, with subsequent nonclearing of chylomicrons from the circulation.

Familial combined hyperlipidemia is responsible for 10% of premature coronary artery disease and reveals patterns of type IIa, IIb, IV, or V. It represents 30% of all genetic lipoproteinemias. Although seldom seen in childhood, it is associated with early coronary atherosclerosis and myocardial infarction and should be screened for in families who have early atherosclerosis.[562]

Childhood xanthomas associated with the Watson–Alagille syndrome are of the planar type and may improve with time.[653] This syndrome consists of a distinctive type of congenital cholestasis with intrahepatic ductular hypoplasia, pruritus, cardiac anomalies, and a characteristic face with a prominent forehead, deep-set eyes, straight nose, and small pointed chin. Vertebral defects, growth retardation, mental retardation, and hypogonadism have been reported.

DIFFERENTIAL DIAGNOSIS

Tendinous xanthomas may be confused with rheumatoid nodules or gouty tophi. Juvenile xanthogranulomas, Langerhans cell histiocytosis, nevus lipomatosis superficialis, and lipoid proteinosis may all have a yellowish nodular appearance, but they may be differentiated by skin biopsy.

Tangier disease (familial HDL deficiency) manifests as enlarged tonsils with distinctive alternating bands of red, orange, yellow, and white striations overlying the normal red mucosa. A maculopapular eruption over the trunk, hepatosplenomegaly, lymphadenopathy, corneal arcus, and alterations of intestinal and rectal mucosa are seen. These patients have an abnormal apolipoprotein AI level, which causes an increased catabolism of HDLs and increased storage of cholesterol esters in body tissues.[654]

THERAPY AND PROGNOSIS

The choice of treatment depends on the underlying lipoprotein abnormality. Treatment is aimed at controlling the associated atherosclerosis, hepatosplenomegaly, abdominal pain, and pancreatitis that may be associated with hyperlipidemias.[655] Medications that elevate lipids should be avoided.[656] In younger patients, early intervention may be helpful in preventing the formation of occlusive vascular lesions in later life. These patients should be referred to a physician specializing in lipid disorders.

642. Valente AM, Newburger JW, Lauer RM (2001) Hyperlipidemia in children and adolescents. Am Heart J 142:433–439.
643. Thiers BH, Dobson RL (1986) Pathogenesis of Skin Disease, 1st edn. New York: Churchill Livingstone.
644. Parker F (1986) Normocholesterolemic xanthomatosis. Arch Dermatol 122:1253
645. Goldstein HL, Kita T, Brown MS (1983) Defective lipoprotein receptors and atherosclerosis. N Engl J Med 309:288.
646. Havel RJ (1992) Role of the liver in hyperlipidemia. Semin Liver Dis 12:356.
647. Knopp RH (1999) Drug treatment cf lipid disorders. N Eng J Med 341:498–511.
648. Brown MS, Goldstein JL (1986) A receptor-mediated pathway for cholesterol homeostasis. Science 232:34.
649. Acton S, Rigott A, Landschulz KT et al. (1996) Identification of scavenger receptor SR-B1 as a high density lipoprotein receptor. Science 271:518–520.
650. Fredrickson DS, Lees RS (1965) A system for phenotyping hyperlipoproteinemia. Circulation 31:321.
651. Eckel RH (1989) Lipoprotein lipase. N Engl J Med 320:1060.
652. Cortner JA, Coates PM, Liacouras CA et al. (1993) Familial combined hyperlipidemia in children: clinical expression, metabolic defects, and management. J Pediatr 123:177.
653. Weston CFM, Burton JL (1987) Xanthomas in the Watson-Alagille syndrome. J Am Acad Dermatol 16:1117.
654. Assman G (1995) Familial high density liporotein deficiency: Tangier disease. In: The Metabolic Basis of Inherited Disease, 7th edn. New York: McGraw-Hill.
655. Gotto AM (1993) Overview of current issues in management of dyslipidemia. Am J Cardiol 71:3B.
656. Stone NJ (1994) Secondary causes of hyperlipidemia. Med Clin North Am 78:117–141.

TABLE 17.10   Primary hyperlipoproteinemias

Disorder	Xanthomas	Major lipoproteins	Metabolic defect	Inheritance	Clinical features	Laboratory features
Lipoprotein lipase deficiency	Eruptive	Chylomicrons	Deficiency of lipoprotein lipase	Autosomal recessive	Hepatosplenomegaly, abdominal pain, pancreatitis, lipemia retinalis usually before puberty and lipemia	Serum: creamy supernatant Plasma TG > 1000mg/dl Electrophoresis: type 1
Apolipoprotein CII	None reported	Chylomicrons with or without VLDL	Absence of apolipoprotein CII	Autosomal recessive	Abdominal pain and pancreatitis	Serum: creamy supernatant, with or without turbid infranatant Plasma TG > 500mg/dl Electrophoresis: type 1 or type 5
Familial combined hyperlipidemia (type IIb and other patterns)	Uncommon	VLDL with or without LDL	Overproduction of VLDL	Autosomal dominant	Premature coronary artery disease with onset in males, in fifth or sixth decade; in females, later; teenagers may show evidence of atherosclerosis	Serum: usually clear Plasma TG > 250mg/dl and chol > 250mg/dl Electrophoresis: type 2a, type 2b, or type 4
Familial hypertri-glyceridemia	Eruptive	VLDL	Probable defect in catabolism of VLDL	Autosomal dominant	Possible premature atherosclerosis, occasional pancreatitis	Serum: may be turbid Plasma TG > 250mg/dl Electrophoresis: type 4 or type 5
Familial hyperlipo-proteinemia (type V)	Eruptive	VLDL and chylomicrons	Overproduction of VLDL and defect in catabolism of VLDL	Probably autosomal dominant	Abdominal pain, pancreatitis, associated with diabetes mellitus, hypertension, hyperuricemia, and polyneuropathy; cardiovascular	Serum: creamy supernatant, turbid infranatant Plasma TG > 500mg/dl Electrophoresis: type 5

contd.

Diet is effective in most primary hyperlipoproteinemias,[657,658] with the exception of familial hypercholesterolemia in which it is rarely helpful. The American Heart Association and the Department of Health and Human Services publish helpful booklets for patient education.[659] Dietary management should be combined with an appropriate exercise program to achieve and maintain a desirable body weight, and elimination of cigarette smoking. Patients with lipoprotein lipase deficiency should restrict fat intake or substitute medium-chain triglycerides that are absorbed without chylomicron formation.

Pharmacologic treatment in children and adolescents should be approached with caution as the long-term benefits and complications of drugs used to lower cholesterol levels have not been established.[642]

Drugs that alter cholesterol and bile salt absorption, such as colestyramine (cholestyramine) and colestipol, are useful in treating hypercholesterolemia.[660] Cholestyramine (8–20g/day) is given in divided doses bid or tid. These medications are not recommended in patients younger than age 6 years and long-term compliance is limited in many patients by undesirable gastrointestinal side effects.[660–662]

657. Polonsky SM, Bellet PS, Sprecher DL (1993) Primary hyperlipidemia in a pediatric population: classification and effect of dietary treatment. **Pediatrics** 91:92.

658. Writing Group for the Dietary Intervention Study in Children (DISC) Collaborative Research Group (1995) Efficacy and safety of lowering dietary intake of fat and cholesterol in children with elevated low-density lipoprotein cholesterol. **JAMA** 273:1429–1435.

659. National Cholesterol Education Program (1992) Report of the expert panel on blood cholesterol levels in children and adolescents. **Pediatrics** 89(suppl):525–584.

660. Mabuchi H, Sakai T, Sakai Y et al. (1983) Reduction of serum cholesterol in heterozygous patients with familial hypercholesterolemia. Additive effects of compactin and cholestyramine. **N Engl J Med** 308:609.

661. McCrindle BW, O'Neill MB, Cullen-Dean G et al. (1997) Acceptability and compliance with two forms of cholestyramine in the treatment of hypercholesterolemia in children: a randomized, crossover trial. **J Pediatr** 130:266–273.

662. Tonstad S, Knudtzon J, Sivertsen M et al. (1996) Efficacy and safety of cholestyramine therapy in peripubertal and prepubertal children with familial hypercholesterolemia. **J Pediatr** 129:42–49.

TABLE 17.10   Primary hyperlipoproteinemias—contd.

Disorder	Xanthomas	Major lipoproteins	Metabolic defect	Inheritance	Clinical features	Laboratory features
Familial dysbetalipo-proteinemia (type III)	Palmar creases, tuberoeruptive, tuberous, xanthelasma	Chylomicrons and VLDL remnants (IDL)	Homozygous apolipoprotein E2 results in decreased remnant clearance; combined with overproduction of VLDL	Autosomal dominant or genetically complex	Premature atherosclerosis, especially peripheral vascular disease	Serum: usually clear Plasma TG > 250mg/dl and chol > 250mg/dl Electrophoresis: type 3
Familial herchole-sterolemia, heterozygous	Tendinous, tuberous, xanthelasma	LDL	50% of LDL receptors nonfunctional	Autosomal dominant	Atherosclerosis; onset in males, fourth or fifth decade, in females, fifth or sixth decade	Serum: clear Plasma chol = 300–500mg/dl Electrophoresis: type 2a
Familial hypercholestero-lemia, (type IIa), homozygous	Intertriginous, tendinous, tuberous, xanthelasma	LDL	No functional LDL receptors	Autosomal dominant	Atherosclerosis; onset in first or second decade	Serum: clear Plasma chol > 600mg/dl Electrophoresis: type 2a

Abbreviations: VLDL, very low-density lipoprotein; LDL, low-density lipoprotein; IDL, intermediate-density lipoprotein; chol, cholesterol; TG, triglyceride.

Drugs that alter lipoprotein synthesis and metabolism, such as clofibrate (0.5 to 1.0g bid), increase the clearance of VLDL and the activity of lipoprotein lipase and are useful in disorders of increased triglyceride production (types IV and V) and increased IDL levels (type III). However, they are less useful in hypercholesterolemia (types IIa and IIb). Nicotinic acid (niacin), given 100mg tid, and gemfibrozil are useful in treating a wide variety of hyperlipidemic disorders, particularly hypertriglyceridemia. They are not recommended for routine use in children because long-term safety and benefit have not been established.[642] Nicotinic acid is the least expensive therapy but requires extensive patient education because of flushing, hypotension, and gastrointestinal side effects. The 3-hydroxy-3-methylglutaryl-coenzyme A (HMG-CoA) reductase inhibitors (statins) are the most potent agents for lowering LDL-cholesterol levels. They include lovastatin, pravastatin, simvastatin, and others. Although several small trials have shown efficacy in children similar to that found in adults, no long-term safety studies on prolonged treatment with statins in children have been published.[642] Because statins are teratogenic, physicians must ascertain this risk in adolescent girls before commencing therapy.

The prognosis depends on the type of hyperlipidemia and the successful management by diet and medication. Eruptive xanthomas tend to respond well to diet and drugs. Tendinous xanthomas and xanthelasmas seldom resolve with treatment. Xanthelasmas may be treated surgically.

PEDIATRIC ASPECTS OF THE DISEASE

Certain genetic disorders of lipid metabolism are more common in children. It is important to identify these patients early to institute management of their disease to prevent premature atherosclerosis and coronary artery disease.

SARCOIDOSIS

Sarcoidosis is characterized by a T-cell-mediated granulomatous response at specific disease sites in the body.[663] It is a common multisystem disorder with the pathologic picture of noncaseating granulomata.[664] Sir Jonathan Hutchinson was probably the first physician to record a case of sarcoidosis in 1892.[664–666] The first article in English was published by Boeck.[667] who described a patient with nodules of the skin and lymphadenopathy in 1899. The histologic appearance of the lesions resembled sarcoma, and thus he named the disease "multiple benign sarkoid." In 1934, at the first international conference on sarcoidosis, the disease was designated a true entity.[668] It primarily affects young adults and presents most frequently with bilateral hilar lymphadenopathy, pulmonary infiltration, and skin or eye lesions. The laboratory criteria for diagnosis should include evidence of noncaseating granulomata with negative stains for organisms or foreign bodies and/or a compatible chemical or radiographic picture.

663. Newman LS, Rose CS, Maier LA (1997) Sarcoidosis. **New Eng J Med** 336:1224–1234.
664. Sharma OP (1990) Sarcoidosis. **Dis Mo** 36:474.
665. Hutchinson J (1892) Recurring ophthalmitis with opacities in the vitreous Mabey's malady. **Arch Surg** (Chicago) 4:361.
666. Hutchinson J (1898) Cases of Mortimer's malady. **Arch Surg** (London) 9:307.
667. Boeck C (1899) Multiple benign sarkoid of the skin. **J Cutan Genitourinary Dis** 17:543.
668. Kerdel FA, Moschella SL (1984) Sarcoidosis. **J Am Acad Dermatol** 11:1.

EPIDEMIOLOGY

Sarcoidosis is found worldwide but is more prevalent in developed countries.[669] A survey of screening chest radiographs in England found an overall prevalence of 20 per 100 000 population.[669]

The greatest incidence is found between ages 20 and 40 years. In children, it is more common in the adolescent age group from 9 to 15 years and is extremely rare in preschool children.[670–672] Women are affected more commonly than men. Although most races are affected, it is more common in Scandinavians and blacks,[669,673] and is seen particularly in the southeastern United States, which is called the "sarcoid belt."[674]

Although sarcoidosis has been described in families[675,676] and in monozygotic twins,[663] there is no consistent mode of inheritance. Patients with class I and II HLA alleles found on chromosome 6 may have increased susceptibility to sarcoidosis including HLA-1, -B8, -DR3, and DRB-1.[677,678] HLA-B13 has been associated with early onset of disease and -DR3 with good outcome. Angiotensin converting enzyme gene polymorphisms may play a role in the susceptibility to sarcoid.[679]

PRESENTING HISTORY

The clinical symptoms of sarcoidosis are often nonspecific and one-third of patients will present with weight loss, fatigue, malaise, anorexia, and fever.[670,680] Any organ system may be affected including skin, lungs, eyes, liver, spleen, lymph nodes, bones, muscles, and central nervous system. Extrathoracic involvement is more common in African-American patients.[681] Twenty-five percent of patients have cutaneous involvement that can occur at any stage of the disease.[673] The lung is the most common organ involved in adults.[680,681] Pulmonary complaints range from a mild, dry cough to significant dyspnea. Pulmonary fibrosis, when it occurs, and upper respiratory tract involvement, tend to correlate with the presence of chronic plaques on the skin, called lupus pernio.[682,683]

The eye is the second most common organ involved, with ocular findings in 30–50% of patients with systemic disease.[684,685] Uveitis (iritis) can range from mild to severe. Conjunctival granulomas can be detected by biopsy in 33–55% of patients with eye involvement.[686] Lacrimal gland involvement is also common.[685] Keratitis, chorioretinitis, and glaucoma may lead to severe disease, resulting in partial or total blindness. Neurologic or central nervous system involvement is seen in about 5–10% of patients.[663,687] Facial nerve paralysis, which is a common neurologic presentation in adults, is rare in children.[672]

Bone involvement is rare and usually affects the distal bones, such as the metacarpals, metatarsals, or phalanges, with asymptomatic small round lytic lesions found on radiographic examination.[669] One-half of patients with osseous sarcoidosis have stiffness and pain.

Generalized lymphadenopathy is common, with nontender, freely movable, slightly enlarged lymph nodes.[663] Hepatic involvement is clinically apparent in one-third of patients, but granulomas can be detected by liver biopsy in 40 to 70% of patients.[663] Splenic involvement occurs in 53% of patients. Patients may be asymptomatic or have massive splenic enlargement.[688] This may be associated with extensive fibrotic changes in other organs and poor outcome.[689] Cardiac sarcoidosis can result from either direct granulomatous infiltration, which can cause arrhythmias, or from congestive cardiac failure secondary to lung involvement. While serious cardiac dysfunction is detected in 5 to 10% of patients, up to 76% of patients will have cardiac involvement at autopsy.[663] Sudden death can occur.[690] Renal involvement is due to overproduction of 1,25-dihydroxyvitamin D leading to increased intestinal absorption of calcium, enhanced bone resorption, and resultant hypercalcuria with or without hypercalcemia.[663] Ultimately, the process may result in nephrocalcinosis and renal failure. Renal involvement with nephrocalcinosis has been reported in children who developed symptoms of chronic erythema nodosum and fever in the first 2 years of life, followed by arthritis, irits, and parotitis years later.[691] Granulomas are found in the kidneys in 15–40% of patients but are thought to be less common in children.

Sjögren syndrome, (keratoconjunctivitis sicca with enlargement of the parotid and lacrimal glands), can be caused by sarcoidosis. Lofgren syndrome,[692] consisting of erythema nodosum, uveitis, fever, and bilateral hilar adenopathy, tends to resolve spontaneously over a few weeks and carries a favorable prognosis.[693] Heerfordt syndrome (uveoparotid fever) is characterized by uveitis, facial nerve palsy, fever, and parotid gland enlargement and may involve the central nervous system.

PHYSICAL EXAMINATION

Approximately 25% of patients with systemic sarcoidosis have cutaneous lesions.[673] Sarcoidosis lesions are both specific, in which granulomas are found, and nonspecific, with no granulomas. Although specific lesions may have characteristic features, no lesion is pathognomonic. The most common presentation is with red to yellowish-brown or violaceous flat-topped papules, nodules, and infiltrated plaques, sometimes in an annular configuration. Diascopy (examination with a glass slide pressed against a lesion) often reveals an apple-jelly color, characteristic of granulomata. Scaly, erythematous patches with palpable infiltrations may also be seen. Although lesions have a predilection for the face, nares, lips, and eyelids, any area of the body may be involved, including the mucous membranes, palms and soles.[673] Granulomata may develop at the sites of old scars[694] and venipuncture sites,[695] and they may resemble keloids.

Subcutaneous nodules, previously called Darier–Roussy sarcoidosis,[696] demonstrate typical sarcoidal granulomas in the subcutaneous tissue on biopsy.

669. James DG (1992) Epidemiology of sarcoidosis. **Sarcoidosis** 9:79–87.
670. Kendig EL, Niitu Y (1980) Sarcoidosis in Japanese and American children. **Chest** 77:514.
671. Rasmussen JE (1981) Sarcoidosis in young children. **J Am Acad Dermatol** 5:566.
672. Shetty AK, Gedalia A (2000) Sarcoidosis in children. **Curr Probl Pediatr** 30:149–176.
673. English JC, Patel PJ, Greer KE (2001) Sarcoidosis. **J Am Acad Dermatol** 44(5):725–743.
674. Abernathy RS (1985) Childhood sarcoidosis in Arkansas. **South Med J** 78:435.
675. Rybicki BA, Harrington D, Major M et al. (1996) Heterogeneity of familial risk in sarcoidosis. **Genet Epidemil** 13:23–33.
676. Rybicki BA, Mallarik MJ, Major M et al. (1998) Epidemiology, demographics and genetics of sarcoidosis. **Semin Respir Infect** 13:166–173.
677. Martinetti M, Tinelli C, Kolek V et al. (1995) The sarcoidosis map: a joint survey of clinical and immunogenetic findings in two European countries. **Am J Respir Crit Care Med** 152:557–564.
678. Ishihara M, Inoko H, Suzuki K et al. (1996) HLA class II genotyping of sarcoidosis patients in Hokkaido by PCR-RFLP. **Jpn J Opthamol** 40:540–543.
679. Furuya K, Yamaguchi E, Itoh A et al. (1996) Delection polymorphism in angiotensin I converting enzyme (ACE) gene as a genetic risk factor for sarcoidosis. **Thorax** 51:777–780.
680. Anonymous (1999) Statement on sarcoidosis: joint statement of the American Thoracic Society (ATS), the European Respiratory Society (ERS) and the World Association of Sarcoidosis and Other Granulomatous Disorders (WASOG) adopted by the ATS board of directors and by the ERS executive committee, Febuary 1999. **Am J Respir Crit Care Med** 160:736–755.
681. Johns CJ, Michelle TM (1999) The clinical management of sarcoidosis: a 50-year experience at the Johns Hopkins Hospital. **Medicine** 78:65–111.
682. Mana J, Marcoval J, Graelis J et al. (1997) Cutaneous involvement in sarcoidosis: relationship to systemic disease. **Arch Dermatol** 133:882–888.
683. Jorizzo JL, Koufman JA, Thompson JN et al. (1990) Sarcoidosis of the upper respiratory tract in patients with nasal rim lesions: a pilot study. **J Am Acad Dermatol** 22:439.
684. Smith JA, Foster CS (1996) Sarcoidosis and its ocular manifestations. **Int Opthalmol Clin** 36:109–125.
685. Ghabrial R, McCluskey FJ, Wakefield D (1997) Spectrum of sarcoidosis involving the eye and brain. **Aust N Z J Ophthalmol** 25:221–224.
686. Nichols CW, Eagle RC, Yanoff M et al. (1980) Conjunctival biopsy as an aid in the evaluation of the patient with suspected sarcoidosis. **Ophthalmology** 87:287.
687. Lower EE, Broderick JP, Brott TG, Baughman RP (1997) Diagnosis and management of neurological sarcoidosis. **Arch Intern Med** 157:1864–1868.
688. Selroos O (1976) Sarcoidosis of the spleen. **Acta Med Scand** 200:337.
689. Salazar A, Mana J, Corbella X et al. (1995) Splenomegaly in sarcoidosis: a report of sixteen cases. **Sarcoidosis** 12:131–134.
690. Shammas RL, Movahed A (1993) Sarcoidosis of the heart. **Clin Cariol** 16:462–472.
691. Nocton JJ, Stork JE, Jacobs G et al. (1992) Sarcoidosis associated with nephrocalcinosis in young children. **J Pediatr** 121:937.
692. Lofgren S (1953) Primary pulmonary sarcoidosis: early signs and symptoms. **Acta Med Scand** 145:424.
693. Liggett PE (1986) Ocular sarcoidosis. **Clin Dermatol** 4:129–135.
694. Manz LA, Rodman OG (1993) Reappearance of quiescent scars: sarcoidosis. **Arch Dermatol** 129:105–108.
695. Burgdorf WHC, Hoxtell EO, Bart BJ (1979) Sarcoid granulomas in venipuncture sites. **Cutis** 24:52.
696. Vainsencher D, Winkelmann RK (1984) Subcutaneous sarcoidosis. **Arch Dermatol** 120:1028.

This variant presents with painful nodules, usually 5–15mm in size on the trunk and legs. Ichthyosiform sarcoid is usually seen on the lower extremities.[697] Erythrodermic forms with erythema and scaling of the entire skin is an uncommon presentation of sarcoidosis. Hypopigmented lesions that may be localized or generalized have been described mainly in black patients.[698,699] Other atypical specific cutaneous presentations of sarcoid include ulcerative, psoriasiform, verrucous, lichenoid and lupus erythematosus–like types.[673]

Nonspecific lesions, including erythema nodosum, may be seen in 17% of patients with systemic sarcoidosis and are considered a manifestation of a hypersensitivity reaction. Erythema nodosum is an important favorable prognostic sign, with subsequent resolution of hilar lymphadenopathy in almost all cases.[700] The combination of hilar lymphadenopathy and erythema nodosum is named Lofgren syndrome. Lupus pernio presents with chronic infiltrated violaceous plaques most commonly seen on the areas of the body exposed to cold, such as the nose, cheeks, and ears. It is associated with chronic upper respiratory tract involvement with sarcoidosis, and rarely resolves spontaneously.[701,702] These lesions can cause marked deformity, with scarring and fibrosis.[683]

Juvenile papular sarcoid

Juvenile papular sarcoid is a subgroup of sarcoidosis presenting in children younger than 4 years of age, with a characteristic triad of skin, joint, and eye disease.[671,703,704] Pulmonary disease is usually absent initially but may develop over time along with cardiac lesions.[704,705] Skin manifestations are often the initial complaint with lesions appearing as typical small red-brown papules (Figs 17.25, 17.26). Frequently the lesions are generalized. The eruption is characterized by exacerbations and remissions and may resolve with scarring. Arthritis affects 60% of patients with nonpainful fusiform swelling of the fingers and wrists with boggy synovial thickening (Fig. 17.27).[705,706] The range of motion of the joints is usually not impaired, as it is in juvenile rheumatoid arthritis. Granulomatous anterior uveitis is common in this entity and may lead to blindness despite therapy.[671] Blau syndrome, a rare autosomal-

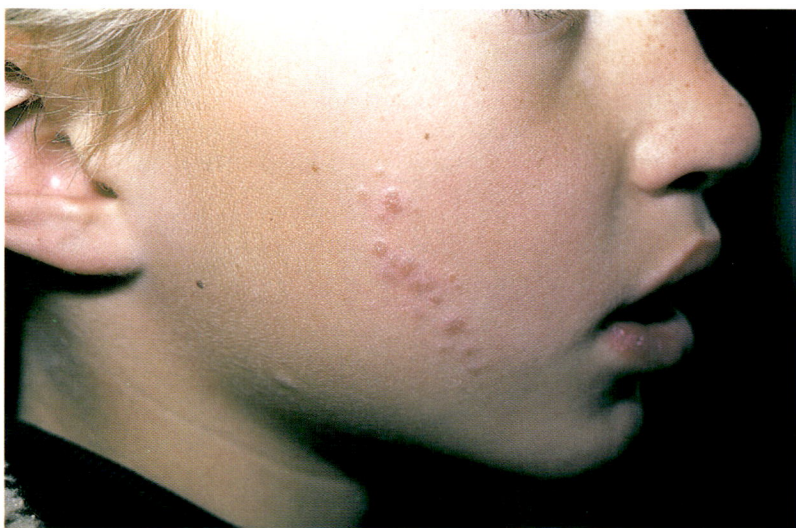

Fig. 17.26 Erythematosus grouped papules of sarcoidosis on the face of a six-year-old boy.

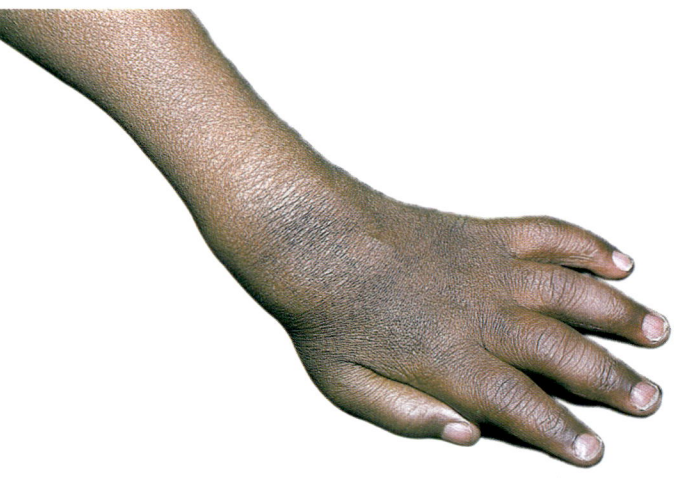

Fig. 17.27 Swollen wrists, synovial thickening and fine papular eruption in a five-year-old with sarcoid.

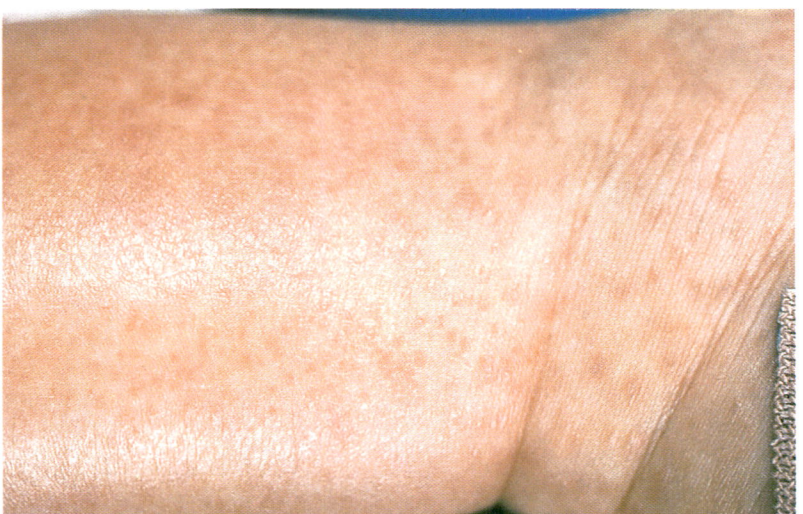

Fig. 17.25 Erythematosus papules of juvenile papular sarcoid on the leg of a preschool child.

dominant disorder characterized by arthritis, uveitis, and skin lesions with noncaseating granulomas, may mimic early-onset sarcoidosis and may be a manifestation of hereditary sarcoid. Pulmonary lesions do not develop and the disorder is linked to chromosome 16.[707]

LABORATORY FINDINGS

There are no pathognomonic laboratory tests to substantiate the diagnosis of sarcoidosis. The most convincing diagnostic procedure is the histologic

697. Cather JC, Cohen PR (1999) Ichthyosiform sarcoidosis. **J Am Acad Dermatol** 40:862–865.
698. Kouh YG, Goody He, Luscombe HA (1978) Ichthyosiform sarcoidosis. **Arch Dermatol** 114:100.
699. Alexis JB (1994) Sarcoidosis presenting as cutaneous hypopigmentation with repeatedly negative skin biopsies. **Int J Dermatol** 33:44–45.
700. Mana J, Salazar A, Manresa F (1994) Clinical factors predicting persistence of activity in sarcoidosis: a multivariate analysis of 193 cases. **Respiration** 61:219–225.
701. Elgart ML (1986) Cutaneous sarcoidosis: definitions and types of lesions. **Clin Dermatol** 4:35–45.
702. Spiteria MA, Matthey F, Gorton T et al. (1985) Lupus pernio: a clinico-radiological study of thirty-five cases. **Br J Dermatol** 112:315–322.

703. Mallory SB, Paller AS, Ginsburg BC et al. (1987) Sarcoidosis in children: differentiation from juvenile rheumatoid arthritis. **Pediatr Dermatol** 4:313.
704. Shetty AK, Gedalia A (1998) Sarcoidosis: a pediatric perspective. **Clin Pediatr** 37:707–717.
705. Hafner R, Vogel P (1993) Sarcoidosis of early onset. A challenge for the pediatric rheumatologist. **Clin Exp Rheumatol** 11:685–691.
706. Hetherington S (1982) Sarcoidosis in young children. **Am J Dis Child** 136:13.
707. Manouvrier-Hanu S, Puech B, Piette F et al. (1998) Blau syndrome of granulomatous arthritis, iritis, and skin rash: a new family and review of the literature. **Am J Med Genet** 76:217–221.

demonstration of noncaseating granulomas in tissue, in association with the clinical picture. Chest radiography reveals bilateral hilar adenopathy in up to 72% of cases and is highly suggestive of sarcoid.[708]

The Kveim-Siltzbach test is of historical interest as a diagnostic test for sarcoidosis with a reliability of up to 80% of patients with active disease.[709] This test is not approved by the Food and Drug Administration and is no longer routinely performed in the United States.[673] A suspension of heat-sterilized human sarcoidal tissue is injected intradermally into the patient. Skin biopsy of a papule formed at the site of injection shows a noncaseating granulomas four to six weeks later.[709]

Transient hypercalcemia can be seen in 7–24% of patients and may be associated with hypercalciuria.[709] If persistent, renal damage may occur. An elevation of angiotension-converting enzyme (ACE) concentration in two-thirds of patients was once once considered to be specific for sarcoidosis.[664] It has since been shown to be elevated in many granulomatous diseases.[673] Although some studies have suggested the degree of enzyme level elevation may reflect disease activity, this may not always be the case.[709,710] ACE levels are generally not a useful guide of disease progression or therapeutic response.[673] Polyclonal hyperglobulinemia with globulin levels above 3.5g/100ml is seen in 22.5–61% of patients, with the highest levels in black patients in the United States.[708]

Cutaneous anergy, demonstrated by decreased delayed-type hypersensitivity and poor reactivity to tuberculin, mumps, and pertussis antigens,[669] is common. Eosinophilia of 6% or greater is found in 50% of children with sarcoidosis.[712]

PATHOPHYSIOLOGY AND HISTOGENESIS

Sarcoidosis has been regarded as a reaction pattern to an unknown infectious agent or allergen. Environmental, infectious, genetic, and immunologic hypotheses have been proposed.[663] Many infectious agents have been implicated but never conclusively demonstrated. Bacterial infections, systemic fungi, mycobacteria, particularly *Mycobacterium tuberculosis*;[711] viruses;[712] and inhaled chemicals or occupational antigens[713,714] have all been studied, but none has been confirmed. Whatever the stimulus, the specific reaction pattern is induced in a genetically or otherwise predisposed host, probably to a persistent, poorly degradable antigen. Sarcoid remains a diagnosis of exclusion.

The development of noncaseating granulomas occurs after local presentation of an antigen by macrophages to T lymphocytes, CD4 helper T cell type 1 (T_H1) phenotype. Once mononuclear inflammatory cells accumulate in the target organ, macrophages aggregate and differentiate into epitheliod and multinucleated giant cells. Abundant CD4 cells are interspersed among these inflammatory cells. Over time CD4 and CD8 lymphocytes, and to a lesser extent B lymphocytes, form a rim around the granuloma. In all but the earliest stages, a dense band of fibroblasts, mast cells, collagen fibres, and proteoglycans begin to encase the ball-like cluster of cells.[663] Once compartmentalized, these CD4 cells produce cytokines including IL-2, interferon-γ, IL-8, and TNF-α along with other immune effector cells including macrophages, mast cells and natural killer cells, that induce

granuloma formation. The granulomas become hyalinized, due to a shift in cytokine profiles to that of T_H2 CD4 T cells, which causes a fibroproliferative response, and ultimate fibrosis.[715] This fibrotic response can produce substantial and often irreversible organ dysfunction and destruction.

Multiple dysfunctions of the immune system have been elucidated,[716] but whether these are primary events or epiphenomena is not known. By biopsy or bronchoalveolar lavage, sarcoidosis in the lung shows an increased ratio of CD4/CD8 cells usually greater than 3.5 to 1.[717] The recruitment of CD4 T cells from the peripheral blood results in the development of anergy, which is seen in two-thirds of patients.[718] Polyclonal hypergammaglobulinemia results from nonspecific induction of B-cell immunoglobulin production activated by the response of localized T cells.[719] The histopathologic findings of the classical chronic cutaneous papules show circumscribed granulomas of epithelioid cells, with little or no caseation necrosis.[186] Similar granulomas are seen in the lungs, bones, eyes, and any organ involved with sarcoidosis. Giant cells and inclusion bodies within the giant cells are frequently observed but are not necessary for the diagnosis.

DIFFERENTIAL DIAGNOSIS

Sarcoidosis is a diagnosis of exclusion; thus every patient with suspected sarcoidosis should have a thorough evaluation. Physical examination, a biochemical panel to measure hepatic and renal function, serum calcium, chest radiograph, ophthalmologic evaluation with slit-lamp examination, electrocardiogram, 24-hour urine calcium determination, serum protein electrophoresis, and histologic tissue confirmation are useful in confirming the diagnosis. A biopsy should be performed on the most accessible involved tissue, whether it is skin, conjunctivae, lymph nodes, minor salivary glands, or lung. Pulmonary function tests should be performed for baseline measurement when indicated. Gallium scans have been shown to reflect the relative degree of inflammation within the parenchyma of the lungs, but lack specificity for sarcoidosis.[663] Angiotensin-converting enzyme (ACE) levels have a false-positive rate of 10% and a false-negative rate of 40%.[720] Cutaneous anergy should be evaluated with common recall antigens if indicated.

Other diseases that can mimic sarcoidosis histologically are tuberculosis, berylliosis,[721] and leprosy. Special stains, cultures, and the use of a polarizing microscope are useful in differentiating amongst these diseases.

THERAPY AND PROGNOSIS

Although there is no specific cure for sarcoidosis, systemic corticosteroids help suppress the acute manifestations.[722] Ideally, patients should be first observed without therapy due to the potential for spontaneous improvement which may occur in 60% of cases.[723] Treatment should be targeted at progressive disease and alleviating symptoms. A trial of corticosteroids is indicated for hypercalcemia, renal insufficiency, neurologic or endocrine disease, myocardial involvement, ocular disease, severe lung disease, and rapidly progressive disfiguring skin lesions.[724–726] Oral prednisone in a dosage of 1mg/kg per day

708. Sitzbach LE, James DG, Neville E et al. (1974) Course and prognosis of sarcoidosis around the world. **Am J Med** 57:847.
709. Siltzbach LE (1976) Qualities and behavior of satisfactory Kevim suspensions. **Ann NY Acad Sci** 278:665.
710. Callen JP, Hanno R (1982) Serum angiotensin-1-converting enzyme level in patients with cutaneous sarcoidal granulomas. **Arch Dermatol** 118:232.
711. Popper HH, Klemen H, Hoefler G, Winter E (1997) Presence of mycobaterial DNA in sarcoidosis. **Hum Pathol** 28:796–800.
712. Di Alberti L, Piattelli A, Artese L et al. (1997) Human herpesvirus 8 in sarcoid tissues. **Lancet** 350:1655–1661.
713. Kon OM, du Bois RM (1997) Mycobateria and sarcoidosis. **Thorax** 52(suppl 3):547–551.
714. Anonymous (1997) Sarcoidosis among US Navy enlisted men 1965–1993. **MMWR Morb Mortal Wkly Rep** 46:539–543.
715. Agostini C, Costabel U, Semenzato G (1998) Sarcoidosis news: immunologic frontiers for new immunosuppressive strategies. **Clin Immunol Immunopathol** 88:199–204.
716. Daniele RP, Dauber JH, Rossman MD (1980) Immunologic abnormalities in sarcoidosis. **Ann Intern Med** 92:406.

717. Winterbauer RH, Lammert J, Selland M et al. (1993) Bronchoalveolar lavage cell populations in the diagnosis of sarcoidosis. **Chest** 104:352–361.
718. Bansal AS, Bruce J, Hogan PG, Allen RK (1997) An assessment of peripheral immunity in patients with sarcoidosis using measurements of serum vitamin D3, cytokines and soluble CD23. **Clin Exp Immunol** 110:92–97.
719. Crystal RG (1998) Sarcoidosis. In: Harrison's Principles of Internal Medicine, Fauci AS, Braunwald E, Isselbacher KJ, Wilson JD, Martin JB, Kasper DL et al, eds. New York: McGraw-Hill, p. 1922–1928.
720. Chesnutt AN (1995) Enigmas in sarcoidosis. **West J Med** 162:519–526.
721. Muller-Quernheim J, Zissel G, Schopf R et al. (1996) Differential diagnosis of berylliosis/sarcoidosis in a dental technician. **Dtsch Med Wochenschr** 121:1462–1466.
722. du Bois RM (1994) Coritcosteroids in sarcoidosis: friend or foe? **Eur Respir J** 7:1203–1209.
723. Gibson GJ, Prescott RJ, Muers MF et al. (1996) British Thoracic Society Sarcoidosis study: effects of long term corticosteroid treatment. **Thorax** 51:238–247.
724. Sharma OP (1993) Pulmonary sarcoidosis and corticosteroids. **Am Rev Respir Dis** 147:1598–1600.
725. Sclroos O (1994) Treatment of sarcoidosis. **Sarcoidosis** 11:80–83.
726. Russo G, Millikan LE (1994) Cutaneous sarcoidosis: diagnosis and treatment. **Compr Ther** 20:418–421.

is given initially[672] and then tapered according to symptoms. The course of treatment is usually 6 months, but this should be modulated by the response and severity of the disease. Most skin lesions heal without scarring.

Topical or intralesional corticosteroids are helpful in the treatment of skin lesions and ophthalmologic steroid preparations are effective in symptomatic eye disease.[705] Other treatments that may control progression include indomethacin or allopurinol for erythema nodosum, cutaneous lesions[727,728] and arthritis; antimalarials for extensive skin lesions,[729] and azathioprine, methotrexate, or chlorambucil[730] as steroid-sparing agents. Thalidomide has been successful in several case reports.[731–734] Isotretinoin may alleviate skin lesions, but does not alter lung disease effectively, and may worsen symptoms of Sjögren syndrome associated with sarcoidosis.[733] Cyclosporin has met with some success in skin and eye lesions but is disappointing in pulmonary disease.[663]

The natural history of sarcoidosis is highly variable in children and adults. The course and prognosis often correlate with the mode of onset.[669,672] Acute forms tend to resolve spontaneously and have a good prognosis.[723] Chronic, progressive sarcoidosis rarely involutes and tends to be more common in older patients with insidious onset. A poorer prognosis is associated with any of the following: black race, chronic cutaneous plaques, lupus pernio, symptoms that last for longer than six months, involvement of more than three organ system,

and later stage pulmonary disease.[735] The disease is chronic and progressive in 10–20% of patients. The mortality rate is reported to be about 1 to 5%.[680]

PEDIATRIC ASPECTS OF THE DISEASE

The degree of involvement affects the amount of physical activity the patient is able to perform. If significant lung involvement is encountered, sports activities may have to be curtailed. If cutaneous lesions are persistent, psychosocial considerations should be addressed. Juvenile papular sarcoidosis is seen exclusively in the pediatric age group and has unique features. Corticosteroid usage in childhood can affect growth and should be managed carefully. Severe eye involvement may lead to partial or total blindness and must be followed closely. Because this is a potentially life-threatening disease and because of both its chronicity and variability, care by a variety of informed specialists such as pulmonologists, immunologists, rheumatologists, ophthalmologists, and dermatologists should be available.

ACKNOWLEDGMENTS

The editors gratefully acknowledge contributions by Dr William Weston, and Dr Susan Mallory that were retained from the first two editions of *Pediatric Dermatology*.

727. Brechtel B, Hass N, Henz BM, Kolde G (1996) Allopurinol: a therapeutic alternative for disseminated cutaneous sarcoidosis. **Br J Dermatol** 135:307–309.
728. Voelter-Mahlknecht S, Benex A, Metzger S et al. (1999) Treatment of subcutaneous sarcoidosis with allopurinol. **Arch Dermatol** 135:1560–1561.
729. Zic JA, Horowitz Dh, Arzubiaga C et al. (1991) Treatment of cutaneous sarcoidosis with chloroquine. Review of the literature. **Arch Dermatol** 127:1034.
730. Baughman RP, Lower EE (1997) Steroid-sparing alternative treatments for sarcoidosis. **Clin Chest Med** 18:853–864.
731. Rousseau L, Beylot-Barry M, Doutre MS, Beylot C (1998) Cutaneous sarcoidosis successfully treated with low doses of thalidomide. **Arch Dermatol** 134:1045–1046.
732. Grasland A, Pouchot J, Chaumaiziere D et al. (1998) Effectiveness of thalidomide treatment during cutaneous sarcoidosis. **Rev Med Interne** 19:208–209.
733. Waldinger TP, Ellis CN, Quint K, Voorhees JJ (1983) Treatment of cutaneous sarcoidosis with isotretinoin. **Arch Dermatol** 119:1003.
734. Lee JB, Koblenzer PS (1998) Disfiguring cutaneous manifestation of sarcoidosis treated with thalidomide: a case report. **J Am Acad Dermatol** 39:835–838.
735. Maná J, Salazar A, Manresa F (1994) Clinical factors predicting persistence of activity in sarcoidosis: a multivariate analysis of 193 cases. **Respiration** 61:219–225.

Sclerosing and Atrophying Conditions

Mary K. Spraker, Edith Garcia-Gonzalez and Lourdes Tamayo Sanchez

This chapter covers a variety of conditions that are characterized by sclerosis and atrophy. The term *sclerosis* means induration or hardening and is taken from the Greek word for hardness, *sclerosis*. Either the subcutaneous tissues and/or the dermis are indurated or sclerotic. Sclerosis is readily detected by palpation. The skin feels taut, unyielding, and thickened.

The term *atrophy* is derived from the Greek and means "wasting away" or "diminution in size." Atrophy refers to changes in the epidermis, the dermis, and subcutaneous fat. In contrast to sclerosis, atrophy is diagnosed with the eye rather than by palpation. The classic morphologic finding of epidermal atrophy is loss of the normal skin markings, which are replaced by fine "cigarette paper wrinkling," best seen when the skin is gently squeezed. The skin may also have a translucent appearance with visible prominence of the underlying vasculature. When the dermis or subcutaneous tissues are atrophic, the skin contour is depressed.

MORPHEA

INTRODUCTION

Morphea is a connective tissue disorder of unknown etiology, characterized by sclerosis of the skin and subcutaneous tissues. Because morphea and scleroderma share the same histology, morphea was previously classified as a subset of scleroderma localized to the skin, and called "localized cutaneous scleroderma." Since systemic involvement almost never occurs in morphea, many clinicians prefer to avoid the term scleroderma completely and instead call the condition "morphea." There are a number of reviews on the subject.[1–4] Progressive systemic sclerosis is discussed in Chapter 23.

EPIDEMIOLOGY

Morphea is an uncommon disease. Schachner's analysis of referrals to a pediatric dermatology clinic estimates that only 3 of 1578 patients (0.19%) seen over a two-year period had morphea.[5] In a report from Mexico City,[6] 68 children were diagnosed with morphea over a thirty-year period (1971–2000). This represents 0.18% of dermatologic patients seen, which is similar to Schachner's estimate. Of the 68 cases, 26 were linear (38.2%), 15 were *en coup de sabre* (22.1%), 14 cases were plaque type (20.6%), nine had generalized morphea (13.2%), and four had the pansclerotic form (5.9%). Girls were more likely to be affected than boys by a ratio of 3:1. A retrospective study from France of seventy children showed similar findings.[7] In a study conducted on thirty patients at the Hospital for Sick Children in Toronto, 18 were female and 12 were male (ratio 1.5:1).[1] Linear morphea affected 87% (including *en coup de sabre*), plaque morphea occurred in 10%, and generalized morphea in one patient (3%).

HISTORY

Children with morphea relate the onset of skin lesions as gradually enlarging plaques that may increase in number. Usually there are no symptoms of skin pain or significant pruritus, but the skin may feel "bound down," especially if the morphea occurs over a joint. In some instances the child or parent may note joint contractures with decreased range of motion and patients may complain of intermittent cramping of the limb. Parents often suggest noticing the lesions after a traumatic event.

PHYSICAL EXAMINATION

There are many clinical variants of morphea that are classified according to the distribution and pattern of the disease. The classic variants are plaque (which includes the rare bullous and keloidal variants), linear, generalized, pansclerotic, and *en coup de sabre*. Parry–Romberg disease, the atrophodermas, the lipoatrophies, and lichen sclerosis are thought by some to be subgroups of morphea. A classification of morphea is shown in Table 18.1.

TABLE 18.1   Classification of morphea

1. Morphea en plaque
   - guttate
   - plaque
   - bullous
   - keloidal
2. Linear morphea
   - linear morphea
   - *en coup de sabre*
   - Parry–Romberg disease (progressive facial hemiatrophy)
3. Generalized
4. Pansclerotic
5. Eosinophilic fasciitis
6. Atrophoderma of Pasini and Pierini
7. Lipoatrophy

---

1. Uziel Y, Krafchik BR, Silverman ED et al. (1994) Localized scleroderma in childhood: a report of 30 cases. **Semin Arthritis Rheum** 23:328–340.
2. Krafchik BR (1992) Localized cutaneous scleroderma. **Semin Dermatol** 11:65–72.
3. Nelson AM (1996) Localized scleroderma including morphea, linear scleroderma, and eosinophilic fasciitis. **Current Problems in Pediatrics** 26:318–324.
4. Albrecht-Nebe H, Harper J (2000) Morphoea. In: Textbook of Pediatric Dermatology, Harper J, Oranje A, Prose N, eds. London: Blackwell Science, pp. 1651–1658.
5. Schachner L, Ling NS, Press S (1983) A statistical analysis of a pediatric dermatology clinic. **Pediatr Dermatol** 1:157.
6. Personal experience. Lourdes Tamayo et al. (2000) Department of Dermatology, National Institute of Pediatrics, Mexico City.
7. Bodemer C, Belon M, Hamel-Teilac D et al. (1999) Scleroderma in children: a retrospective study of 70 cases. **Annales de Dermatologie et de Venereologie** 126:691–694.

There are several clinical patterns of morphea (see above). The plaque type is most common in adults whereas the linear form is most frequently seen in children.[6]

In *plaque morphea*, there is an insidious onset of erythematous, violaceous, indurated plaques, several centimeters in diameter (Fig. 18.1). These lesions are found most commonly on the trunk but may be seen on the extremities, head, and neck. They lose their erythematous color centrally, leaving a violaceous border with a white center. Over weeks to months, the center may become shiny, firm, waxy, and white to yellow-white. Plaques of morphea are devoid of hair, and sweating is absent. Not infrequently there is an associated subcutaneous sclerosis, or at a later stage atrophy, as abnormal collagen fibers replace the subcutaneous fat. When activity ceases a red-brown

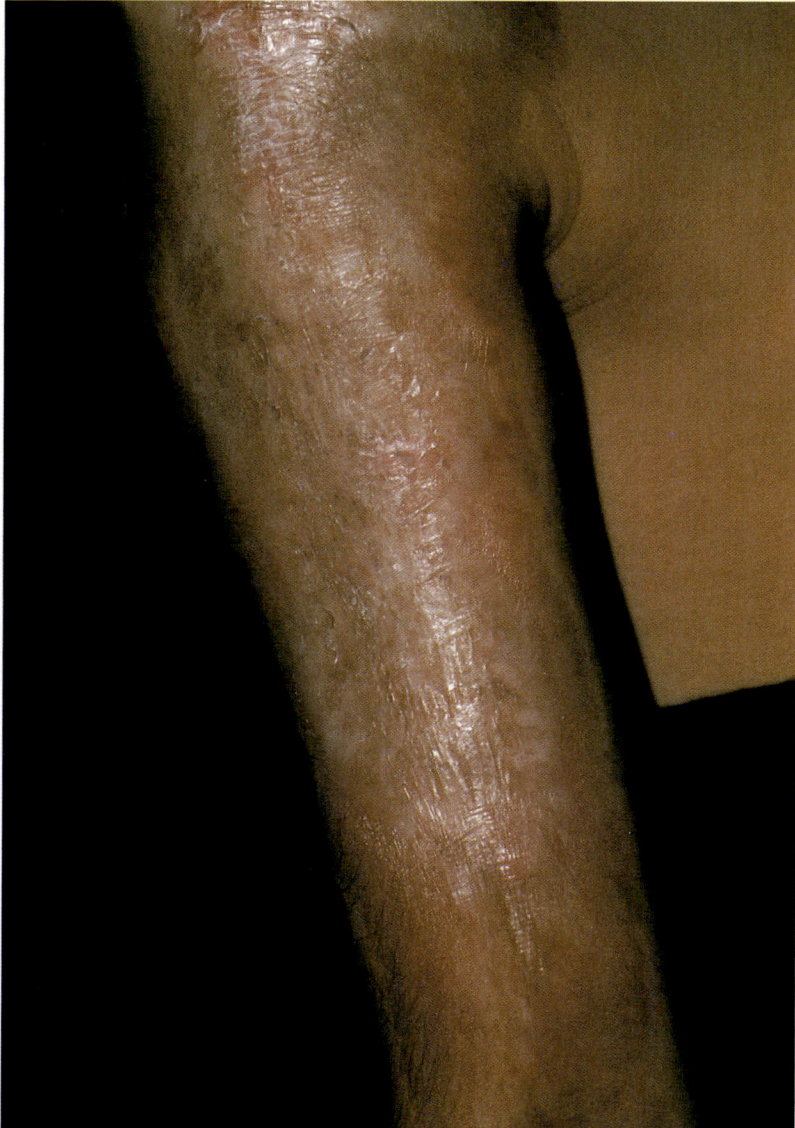

Fig. 18.1 Plaque-like indurated, shiny lesion of linear morphea.

hyperpigmentation develops which may represent postinflammatory changes. When the morphea lesions are small and numerous, they can be called guttate. This usually involves epidermal change and the lesions are white. When large plaques are located in different anatomic locations and numerous lesions are present, the patient is said to have the *generalized* form of morphea. Generalized morphea is rare in children and is mainly seen in adults. If dermal atrophy occurs without sclerosis in localized plaques, the patients may have *atrophoderma of Pasini and Pierini*.

In *linear morphea* (LM), an extremity is usually affected, most commonly a leg followed by an arm (Fig. 18.2 A&B), but lesions may also affect the thorax, abdomen, or buttocks. Occasionally linear and plaque forms are both present in the same patient. Linear lesions are usually unilateral, but occasionally bilateral lesions occur. The condition may involve underlying muscle and occasionally bone. Lesions are initially erythematous or violaceous, and can be mistaken for cellulitis. They gradually lose their pink color centrally, causing the plaques to have a white shiny center with a violaceous edge. The white centers are shiny, and atrophic, or thickened, yellow-white and sclerotic and increased numbers of blood vessels may be seen through the surface of the lesion.

Linear lesions usually extend along the length of an extremity, possibly following the lines of Blaschko (Fig. 18.3).[4] Severe tightening of the skin over a joint may lead to flexion contractures. If the affected leg becomes shortened, compensatory scoliosis occurs.

When LM involves the frontoparietal area, the eponym *en coup de sabre* is given because the condition resembles the scar from a saber cut (Fig. 18.4). An ivory sclerotic plaque with peripheral hyperpigmentation appears on the forehead and may extend into the scalp where it causes a linear area of alopecia. *En coup de sabre* also has a Blaschko line distribution. Sometimes the forehead area alone is involved, but the lesion may extend forward to the nose, cheek, chin, and neck. There are several reports of bilateral *en coup de sabre* morphea.[8] A case report described unilateral eyelid edema preceding the development of *en coup de sabre* by eight months[9] and physicians have noticed a red discoloration preceding the lesions by months. Atrophy of the affected side of the face develops within one year of the onset of the process. *En coup de sabre* can occasionally be associated with central nervous system symptoms and signs, including headaches, seizures, hemiparesis,[10] and eye changes.[11] Some, authors consider *progressive facial hemiatrophy* (Parry–Romberg syndrome) to be a variant of *en coup de sabre* morphea in which atrophy is a more prominent feature than sclerosis and the disease process occurs on the lower face rather than on the upper face. Parry–Romberg syndrome is discussed in the next section of this chapter.

A rare severe form of morphea called *disabling pansclerotic morphea of children*[12] (Fig. 18.5) is occasionally seen. In contrast with the other types that are self-limited, this disease has a relentless disabling course. It usually begins with symmetrical bilateral morphea lesions on the distal extremities that gradually extend longitudinally and circumferentially. Over time, the trunk and neck may also become affected. The disorder differs from other forms of morphea as, in addition to sclerosis of the skin and subcutaneous tissues, the deeper structures including the tendons, fascia, and muscles are involved, producing marked contraction and secondary joint deformity and fixation. Associated hypogammaglobulinemia, lung fibrosis, and esophageal dysmotility have been reported.[12] A progressive cardiomyopathy has been described in a child with large ulcerations within the sclerotic plaques on the legs.[13] Loss of limb function and amputation are sequelae in severe forms. In disabling pansclerotic morphea, Raynaud's phenomenon and other physical signs of systemic sclerosis are absent.

8. Rai R, Handa S, Gupta S, Kumar B (2000) Bilateral en coup de sabre – a rare entity. **Pediatr Dermatol** 17:222–224.

9. Long PR, Miller OF (1982) Linear scleroderma: report of a case presenting as persistent unilateral eyelid edema. **J Am Acad Dermatol** 7:541.

10. Higashi Y, Kanekura T, Fukumaru K, Kanzaki T (2000) Scleroderma *en coup de sabre* with central nervous system involvement. **J Dermatol** 27:486–488.

11. Muchnick RS, Aston SJ, Rees TD (1979) Ocular manifestations and treatment of hemifacial atrophy. **Am J Opththalmol** 88:889–897.

12. Diaz-Perez JL, Connolly SM, Winkelmann RK (1980) Disabling pansclerotic morphea of children. **Arch Dermatol** 116:169.

13. Wollina U, Looks A, Uhlemann C, Wollina K (1999) Pansclerotic morphea of childhood – follow-up over 6 years. **Pediatr Dermatol** 16:245–247.

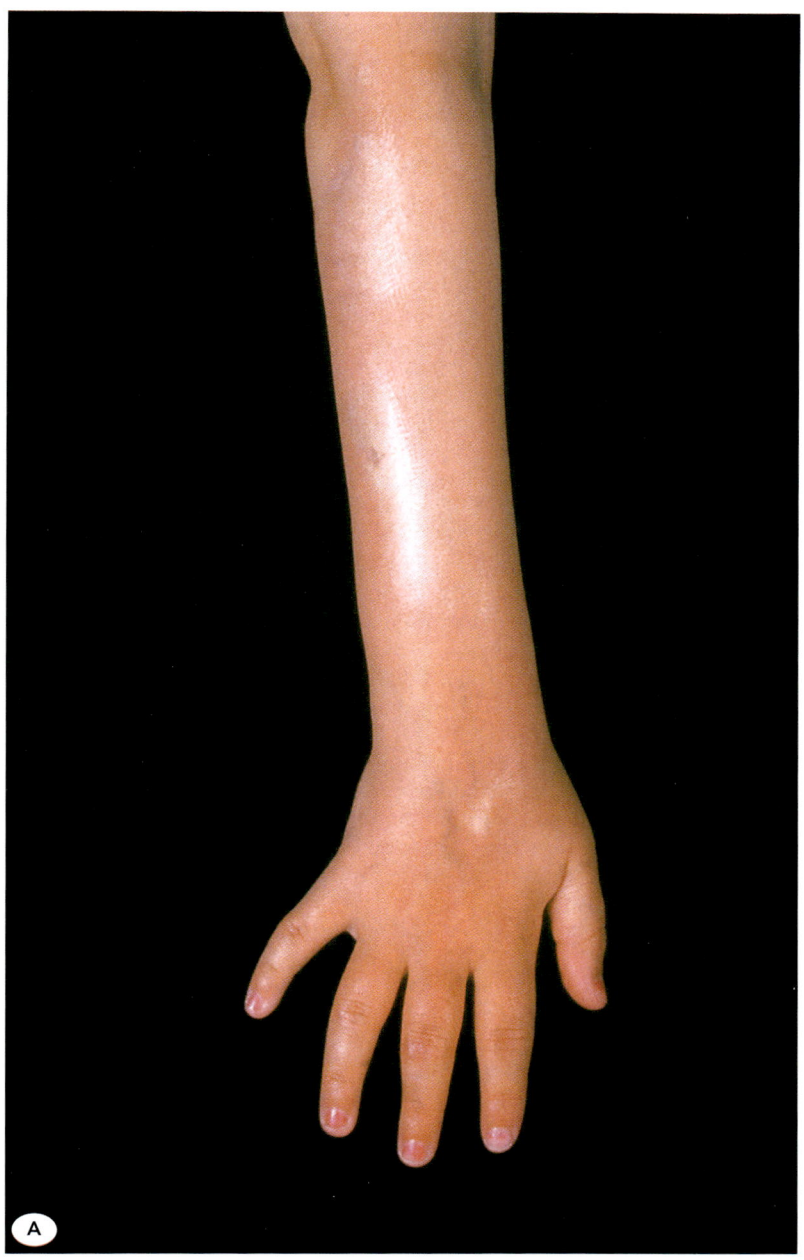

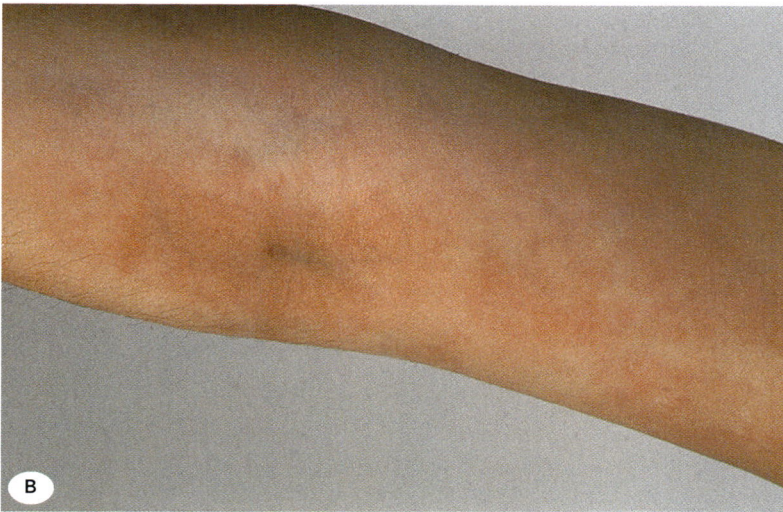

Fig. 18.2 (A) In this child with linear morphea, *white* sclerotic bands extend along the length of the arm. (B) Similar changes, with *dark* sclerotic bands on the arms.

ASSOCIATED FINDINGS

In one series of 68 patients with localized forms of morphea, 32 (47%) had demonstrable anomalies of the vertebral column.[14] Most of these changes occurred in the patients with LM. The most common abnormality was spina bifida occulta. There is one report of elastosis perforans serpiginosa occurring within a plaque of morphea located in the antecubital area of a teenager.[15]

LABORATORY FINDINGS

There are no specific laboratory tests to confirm the clinical diagnosis of morphea, but elevations in serum antinuclear antibodies (ANA) and rheumatoid factor are often present. The frequency of abnormal ANAs varies

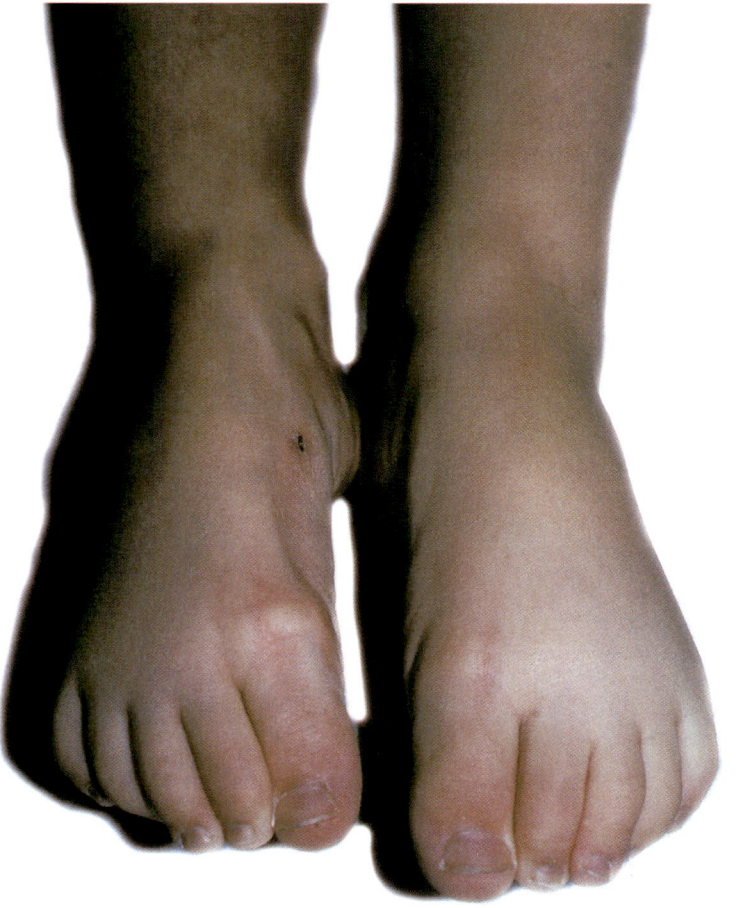

Fig. 18.3 Subcutaneous atrophy may accompany linear morphea.

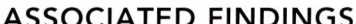

14. Christianson HB, Dorsey CS, O'Leary PA, Kierland RR (1956) Localized scleroderma: a clinical study of 235 cases. **Arch Dermatol** 74:629.

15. Barr RJ, Seigel JM, Graham JH (1980) Elastosis perforans serpiginosa associated with morphea. **J Am Acad Dermatol** 3:19.

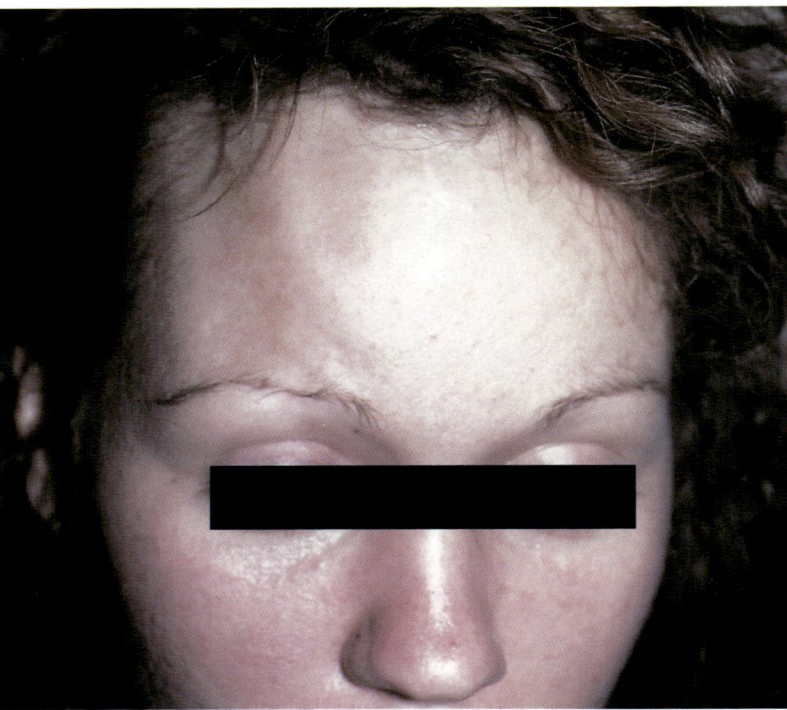

Fig. 18.4 The ivory sclerotic band of *en coup de sabre* morphea results in a vertical depressed linear band on the forehead.

in studies from 25 to 53%, being higher in LM.[16] Patterns of ANA vary, the majority being homogeneous; speckled patterns may also occur.[17] High titers to single-stranded DNA are seen, especially in patients with more extensive cutaneous lesions and prolonged disease duration.[17] Anti-histone antibodies (against histone H1 and H3) have been correlated with the presence of anti-single-stranded-DNA antibodies.[18,19] Anti-topoisomerase I antibodies, a marker for systemic scleroderma, is not detected and if present indicates progressive systemic sclerosis.[3] Anti-Ku antibody (novel DNA-binding protein) was found in one patient with localized morphea.[20] This patient subsequently developed systemic sclerosis and probably had progressive systemic sclerosis at the outset. Autoantibodies to fibrillin I have been found in patients with localized plaque and LM.[21] The serum concentration of pro-collagen type I carboxyterminal propeptide (P1cp) correlates with the number of sclerotic lesions in morphea, as does the anti-single-stranded DNA and anti-histone antibodies.[22] There is no evidence that any of the laboratory markers play a role in the pathogenesis or prognosis of the disease.[4]

Eosinophilia is common in localized morphea.[23] There is an increase in C-reactive protein in childhood morphea, but no similar elevation in other inflammatory markers such as the erythroctye sedimentation rate, immuno-globulins, or complement.[24] In disabling pansclerotic morphea, laboratory abnormalities are frequently present. Eosinophilia and an increased IgG are seen in most pansclerotic patients and some patients have an elevated erythrocyte sedimentation rate and a positive ANA titer.[12]

Magnetic resonance imaging (MRI) and/or computed tomography (CT) imaging abnormalities have been reported in *en coup de sabre* morphea and Parry–Romberg disease.[25] Changes seen include the clinically apparent atrophy of soft tissue and bone, but intracranial calcification and white matter abnormalities in the ipsilateral frontal and parietal lobes are also reported.[25]

PATHOPHYSIOLOGY

The cause of morphea is unknown. It has been postulated that the underlying process involves abnormalities in the metabolism and turnover of collagen, as evidenced by increases in collagen III production.[26] The resemblance and overlap with other collagen vascular disease suggests an autoimmune cause. Factors such as trauma and infection have been suggested as trigger factors in LM.[27]

Some authors consider morphea to be the result of an infection with a *Borrelia organism* because in some cases antibodies to this organism have been found, particularly in European patients.[28] Organisms that are identical or very similar to those seen in Lyme disease have been seen in some skin biopsy samples,[29] and some patients improve with antibiotic therapy.[29] Skin biopsies from patients in western Turkey with morphea tested positive with polymerase chain reaction (PCR) for *Borrelia burgdorferi*.[30] A study of skin biopsies from patients with morphea and lichen sclerosis in the United States, Japan, and Germany were tested for *Borrelia* species with PCR assays; some of the German and Japanese but none of the American samples were positive.[31] Other authors have also found a lack of evidence for *Borrelia* in the US.[32,33] Interpretation of the positive PCR testing results is controversial.

HISTOGENESIS

Jablonska has described the characteristic histologic features in the different variants of morphea.[4] In the early inflammatory stage, there is dermal edema with swelling and degeneration of collagen fibrils and lymphocytic infiltrates around dermal vessels and appendages. This is followed by a progressive increase in dermal thickness with condensation of collagen, loss of appendages, and fragmentation of elastic fibers. There is homogenization of collagen bundles parallel to the skin and hyalinized connective tissue may replace subcutaneous fat. Calcification, myositis, myofibrosis, and IgM and C3 perivascular deposits may be found in LM.[34]

DIFFERENTIAL DIAGNOSIS

The clinical diagnosis is usually not difficult. The indurated lesions of morphea must be distinguished from eosinophilic fasciitis and scleredema of

16. Falanga V (1991) Fibrosing conditions in childhood. **Adv Dermatol** 6:145.
17. Falanga V, Medsger TA Jr, Reichlin M et al. (1986) Linear scleroderma. Clinical spectrum, prognosis, and laboratory abnormalities. **Ann Intern Med** 104:849.
18. Sato S, Ihn H, Soma Y et al. (1993) Antihistone antibodies in patients with localized scleroderma. **Arthritis Rheum** 36:1137–1141.
19. Ruffatti A, Peserico A, Rondinone R et al. (1991) Prevalence and characteristic of anti-single-stranded DNA antibodies in localized scleroderma. **Arch Dermatol** 127:1180–1183.
20. Birdi N, Laxer RM, Thorner P et al. (1993) Localized scleroderma progressing to systemic disease. **Arthritis Rheum** 36:410.
21. Arnett FC, Tan FK, Uziel Y et al. (1999) Autoantibodies to the extracellular matrix microfibrillar protein, fibrillin 1, in patients with localized scleroderma. **Arthritis and Rheumatism** 42:2656–2659.
22. Vuorio T, Kahari VM, Black C, Vuorio E (1991) Expression of osteonectin, decorin and transforming growth factor-beta 1 genes in fibroblasts cultured from patients with systemic sclerosis and morphea. **J Rhematol** 18:247–251.
23. Giardano M, Ara M, Valentini G et al. (1981) Presence of eosinophilia in progressive systemic sclerosis and localized scleroderma. **Arch Dermatol Res** 271:411–417.
24. Vancheeswaran R, Black CM, David J et al. (1996) Childhood-onset scleroderma. **Arthritis Rheum** 39:1041–1049.
25. Liu P, Uziel Y, Chuang S et al. (1994) Localized scleroderma: imaging features. **Pediatr Radiol** 24:207–209.
26. Rahbari H (1989) Histochemical differentiation of localized morphea, scleroderma and lichen sclerosus et atrophicus. **J Cutan Pathol** 16:342.
27. Yamanaka CT, Gibbs NF (1999) Trauma-induced linear scleroderma. **Cutis** 63:29–32.
28. Buechner SA, Winkelmann RK, Lautenschlager S et al. (1993) Localized scleroderma associated with *Borrelia burgdorferi* infection: clinical, histologic, and immunohistochemical observations. **J Am Acad Dermatol** 29:190.
29. Abele DC, Anders KH (1990) The many faces and phases of borreliosis II. **J Am Acad Dermatol** 23(3 Pt 1):401–410.
30. Ozkan S, Atabey N, Fetil E, Erkizan V, Gunes A (2000) Evidence for Borrelia burgdorferi in morphea and lichen sclerosis. **Int J Dermatol** 39:278–283.
31. Fujiwara H, Fujiwara K, Hashimoto K et al. (1997) Detection of Borrelia burgdorferi DNA (B garinii or B afzelii) in morphea and lichen sclerosus et atrophicus tissues of German and Japanese but not of US patients. **Arch Dermatol** 133:41–44.
32. Raguin G, Boisnic S, Souteyrand P et al. (1982) No evidence for spirochaetal origin of localized scleroderma. **Br J Dermatol** 127:218.
33. De Vito J, Merogi A, Vo T et al. (1996) Role of Borrelia burgdorferi in the pathogenesis of morphea/scleroderma and lichen sclerosus et atrophicus: a PCR study of thirty-five cases. **J Cutaneous Pathology** 23:350–358.
34. Vincent F, Prokopetz R, Miller RAW (1989) Plasma cell panniculitis: a unique clinical and pathologic presentation of linear scleroderma. **J Am Acad Dermatol** 21:357–360.

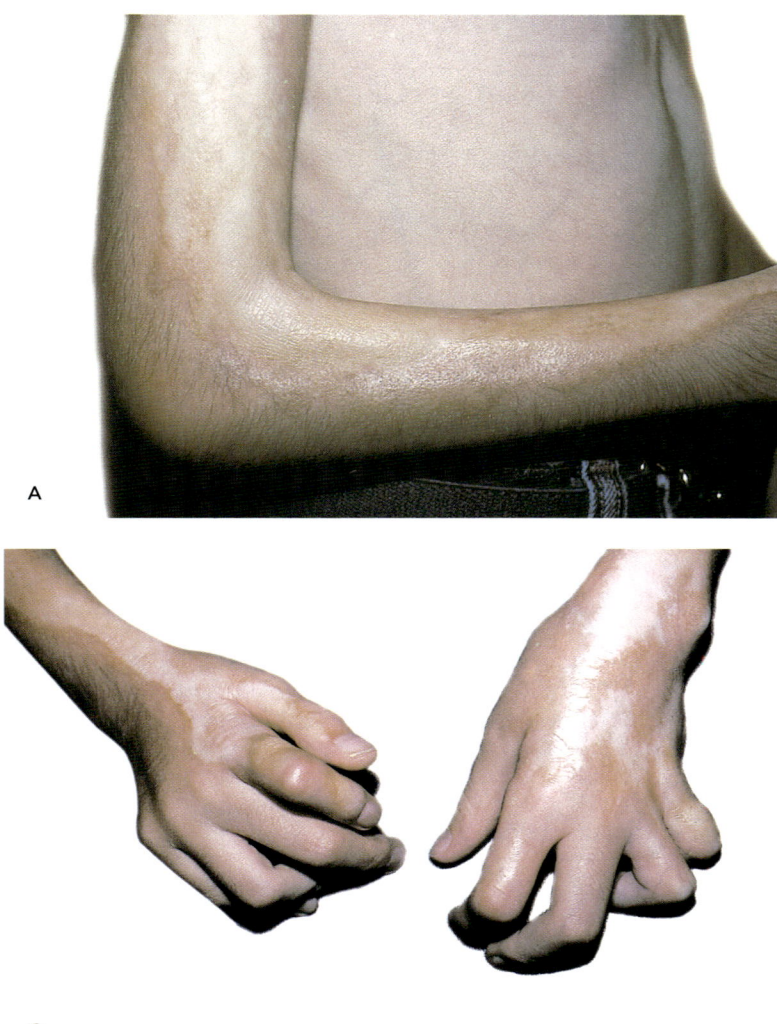

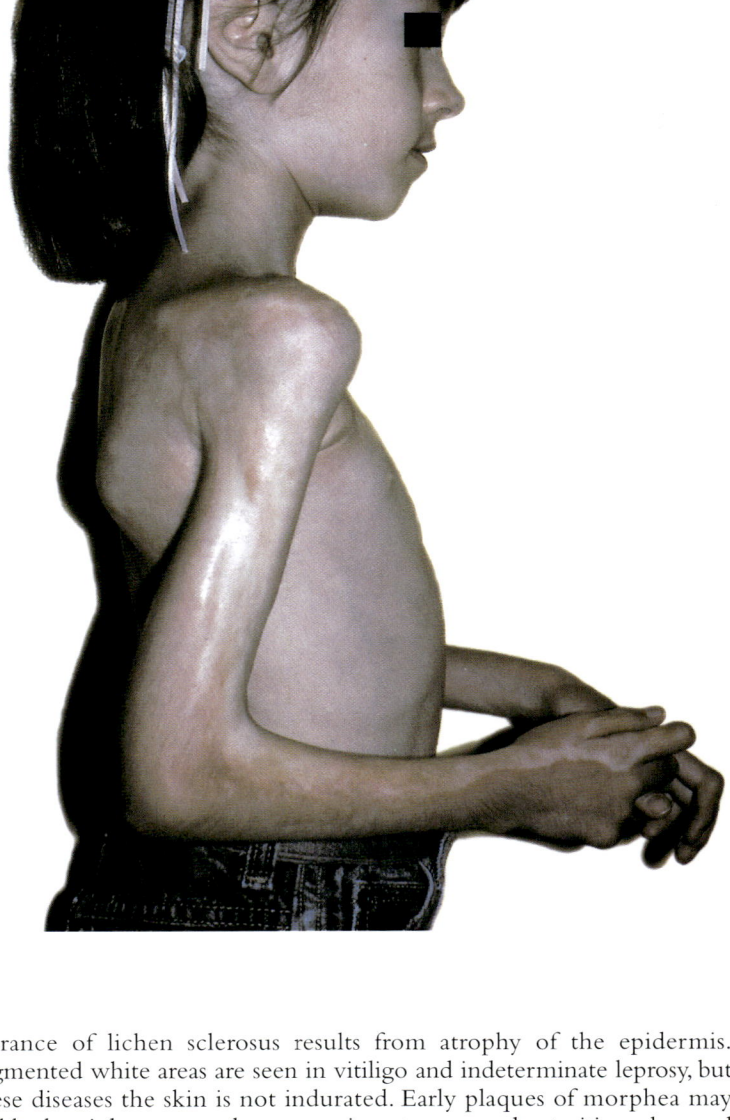

Fig. 18.5 (A) In disabling pansclerotic morphea of children, linear sclerotic bands on the extremities and trunk gradually extend longitudinally and circumferentially. (B) Deep involvement of the muscles, tendons, and fascia produces marked contractions and secondary joint deformities. (C) Involvement of hands in disabling pansclerotic morphea of children.

Buschke. In *eosinophilic fasciitis*, a linear area of erythema, swelling, pain, and induration develops on an extremity, or occasionally on the trunk. There is blood eosinophilia of 30% to 70% in affected patients.[35] A deep skin biopsy that includes fascia shows dermal sclerosis and thickening of the deep fascia from inflammation with plasma cells, histiocytes, and eosinophils. Later, there is fibrosis of the fat and fascia. The condition improves with systemic corticosteroids. Eosinophilic fasciitis may be a morphea variant that differs from classic morphea by the acute onset of erythema and pain, the fascial involvement, and the response to corticosteroids. Eosinophilic fasciitis as well as morphea can be mistakenly diagnosed as *acute cellulitis*. *Scleredema of Buschke* differs from morphea by its location on the back of the neck or face and the presence on biopsy of acid mucopolysaccharides in the dermis rather than sclerosis. Morphea may be morphologically indistinguishable from the lesions of *lichen sclerosus*, and both diseases may coexist in the same patient. The appearance of lichen sclerosus results from atrophy of the epidermis. Depigmented white areas are seen in vitiligo and indeterminate leprosy, but in these diseases the skin is not indurated. Early plaques of morphea may resemble the violaceous erythema seen in cutaneous polyarteritis nodosa and in fixed and gyrate erythemas. Lesions may be identical to the depressed, slightly hyperpigmented lesions of atrophoderma of Pasini and Pierini (see Fig. 18.9); some authors consider the latter to be a form of morphea.[36] The residual hyperpigmentation seen in resolving morphea lesions may be difficult to diagnose from other causes of postinflammatory hyperpigmentation without the history of previous induration.

Other causes of subcutaneous atrophy, such as corticosteroid or vitamin K injection,[37] panniculitis, and lipoatrophy may be confused with morphea. A morphea-like reaction has been reported in patients treated with D-penicillamine.[38] Cutaneous morphea-like lesions in untreated *phenylketonuria*

35. Falanga V, Medsger TA (1987) Frequency levels and significance of blood eosinophilia in systemic sclerosis, localized scleroderma and eosinophilic fasciitis. **J Am Acad Dermatol** 17:648–656.
36. Murphy PK, Hymes SR, Fenske NA (1990) Concomitant unilateral idiopathic atrophoderma of Pasini and Pierini (IAPP) and morphea. Observations supporting IAPP as a variant of morphea. **Int J Dermatol** 29:281.
37. Janin-Mercier A, Mosser C, Souteyrand P, Bourges M (1985) Subcutaneous sclerosis with fasciitis and eosinophilia after phytonadione injections. **Arch Dermatol** 121:1421.
38. Bernstein RM, Hall MA, Gostelow BE (1981) Morphea-like reaction to D-penicillamine therapy. **Ann Rheum Dis** 40:42.

have been reported.[39] In the report, a 10-month-old female infant developed progressive sclerodermatous changes of the legs and upper trunk, with accompanying flexion contractures.[39] Her developmental milestones were delayed, and she was described as irritable. A strongly positive urinary ferric chloride test led to the eventual diagnosis of phenylketonuria.

Progressive facial hemiatrophy (Parry–Romberg syndrome) (PFH) is considered to be another form of morphea. Whereas *en coup de sabre* affects the upper face, PFH affects the cheek and mandible area. In PFH, the subcutaneous tissues, muscle, and bone are initially affected, while the overlying skin may be normal and without pigmentary changes. Many cases begin with a flat erythema resembling a port-wine stain that is followed later by the hemiatrophy. It is questionable whether PFH is a distinct entity different from morphea and *en coup de sabre*. Cases of skin involvement overlying PFH may occur and lesions of typical morphea may be seen in other areas.

The diagnosis of early progressive systemic sclerosis, mixed connective tissue disease, or an overlap syndrome must always be considered in patients with morphea. These systemic conditions are rare in patients with cutaneous morphea, especially in children in whom progressive systemic sclerosis is rare. Progressive systemic sclerosis is associated with Raynaud's phenomenon, nailfold telangiectasias, sclerosis of the face and extremities and usually has evidence of internal organ involvement.

PROGNOSIS

The prognosis depends upon the type of morphea. Most forms of the disease resolve spontaneously, often leaving residual hyperpigmentation and atrophy. Plaque or generalized forms of morphea resolve spontaneously in three to five years. In a series by Torok and Ablonczy, 63 of the 88 children followed for 10 years healed with minimal cosmetic alteration; one case progressed to progressive systemic sclerosis.[40] None of the 82 patients identified in a population study in Olmsted County, Minnesota, diagnosed over a period of 33 years, developed systemic sclerosis.[41] However, some of the patients with LM in this series had severe cosmetic, orthopedic, and psychological sequelae.[41] Fifty percent of patients overall had softening of the skin lesions by 3.8 years in the Olmsted county series.[41] Plaque morphea resolved faster (50% by 2.7 years), compared with deep lesions (50% resolution in 5 years).[41] Linear lesions persist longer than plaque lesions, but resolve spontaneously over time. There may be residual flexion contractures, limb atrophy and occasional calcinosis requiring surgical removal. Children with localized morphea have a normal life expectancy.[2,41] A quality of life survey and self-esteem profile for children with various forms of morphea showed normal self-worth and high quality of life; patients with facial lesions were no more likely to have abnormal scores.[42] The prognosis is not as good in disabling pansclerotic morphea. Of the 14 children reported by Diaz-Perez *et al.*, two died, one of unknown cause and another from bronchopneumonia.[12] The other patients had progression of their disease with loss of function and amputation: two patients improved.[12]

THERAPY

Specific treatment for localized morphea and its variants has not always been tested in a controlled fashion. Aggressive treatments are not usually recommended in children because the disease regresses spontaneously. Patients with mild disease (one or two lesions of plaque morphea) require no therapy other than an emollient to diminish the dryness. Treatment is directed at suppressing the inflammatory and collagen alterations. Local therapy with topical steroids and calcitriol has been used with results that are difficult to evaluate given the nature of the disease. In the localized forms of morphea, a potent topical corticosteroid in an ointment vehicle, or injection with intralesional corticosteroid steroids may be helpful, until the active inflammatory lilac ring has disappeared.[4] A number of reports have discussed the efficacy of topical calcipotriene.[43,44] A small study of pediatric patients treated for three months with topical calcipotriene showed some improvement in lesions[43] although a double-blind study of adults with morphea treated with oral calcitriol showed no more effect than placebo.[45] Systemic therapy with many different drugs has yielded conflicting results. Some cases of morphea in Europe may be associated with *Borreliosis*, and improvement with systemic antibiotics has been reported.[29] A child from Germany with LM and negative serology for *Borrelia* was treated with intravenous penicillin G for 10 days and showed diminished dermal thickness measured by ultrasound.[46] The role of antibiotic therapy is controversial.

Penicillamine, a penicillin breakdown product that decreases collagen synthesis by inhibiting the cross-linking of collagen fibers, has been used to treat morphea.[47–49] Falanga and Medsger's patients with LM improved when treated with penicillamine for one to four years,[47] although this mimics the natural course of the disease. The initial dose used was 3mg/kg per day for two months, which was gradually increased by 2–3mg/kg per day every month up to 10–15mg/kg per day. Improvement began after 3–6 months. Treatment was continued for 6 months after remission was achieved. Disease activity recurred in some patients when the drug was discontinued but remitted on reinitiation of therapy. Significant toxicity with renal disease was seen in half the patients, necessitating the discontinuation of treatment in a third of the patients. The major side effect of penicillamine is proteinuria, but others include bone marrow suppression, allergic reactions, and autoimmune disorders. The authors added prednisone to the penicillamine regimen for the initial three months of therapy to decrease acute inflammation.[47] Moynahan added pyridoxine to a penicillamine regimen.[49] Other clinicians have found the results of penicillamine treatment disappointing.[4] There have been no controlled trials on the use of penicillamine in morphea, and the two deaths in Falanga's series make its use questionable.[47]

Therapy with antimalarials,[4] phenytoin,[50] azathioprine,[4] cyclosporine,[4] colchicine,[51] disodium edetate,[52] intravenous immunoglobulin,[4] and PUVA[4] have also been used. Nineteen children were treated with a combination of topical calcipotriol ointment and low-dose UVA1 photothotherapy with softening and repigmentation.[53] Several studies suggest improvement after UVA1 phototherapy,[54,55] in one there was an associated increase in the number of CD34+ dendritic cells in the dermis.[55]

39. Kornreich HK, Shaw KN, Koch R, Hanson V (1968) Phenylketonuria and scleroderma. J Pediatr 73:571.
40. Torok E, Ablonczy E (1986) Morphea in children. Clin Exp Dermatol 2:607.
41. Peterson LS, Nelson AM, Su WP et al. (1997) The epidemiology of morphea (localized scleroderma) in Olmsted County 1960–1993. J Rheumatology 24:73–80.
42. Uziel Y, Laxer RM, Krafchik BR et al. (2000) Children with morphea have normal self-perception. J Pediatrics 137:727–730.
43. Cunningham BB, Landells ID, Langman C et al. (1998) Topical calcipotriene for morphea/linear scleroderma. J Am Acad Dermatol 39:211–215.
44. Bottomley WW, Jutley J, Wood EJ et al. (1995) The effect of calcipotriol on lesional fibroblasts from patients with active morphea. Acta Derm Venereal 75:364–366.
45. Hulshof MM, Bouwes BJN, Bergman W et al. (2000) Double-blind, placebo-controlled study of oral calcitriol for the treatment of localized and systemic scleroderma. J Am Acad Dermatol 43:1017–1023.
46. Mohrenschlager M, Jung C, Ring J, Abeck D (1999) Effect of penicillin G on corium thickness in linear morphea of childhood: an analysis using ultrasound technique. Pediatric Dermatology 16:314–316.
47. Falanga V, Medsger TA Jr (1990) D-penicillamine in the treatment of localized scleroderma. Arch Dermatol 126:609.

48. Curly RK, MacFarlane AW, Evans S et al. (1987) The treatment of linear morphea with D-penicillamine. Clin Exp Dermatol 12:56.
49. Moynahan EJ (1973) Morphoea (localized cutaneous scleroderma) treated with low-dosage penicillamine (4 cases, including en coup de sabre). Proc R Soc Med 66:1083.
50. Neldner KH (1978) Treatment of localized linear scleroderma with phenytoin. Cutis 22:569–572.
51. Alarcon-Segovia D, Ramos-Niembor F, Ibanez de Kasep G et al. (1979) Long-term evaluation of colchicine in the treatment of scleroderma. J Rheumatol 6:705–712.
52. Neldner KH, Winkelmann RK, Perry HO (1962) Scleroderma: An evaluation of treatment with disodium edetate. Arch Dermatol 86:305–309.
53. Kreuter A, Gambichler T, Avermaete A et al. (2001) Combined treatment with calcipotriol ointment and low dose ultraviolet A1 phototherapy in childhood morphea. Pediatric Dermatology 18:241–245.
54. Gruss CJ, von Kobyletzki G, Behrens-Williams SC et al. (2001) Effects of low dose ultraviolet A-1 phototherapy on morphea. Photodermatology, Photoimmunology and Photomedicine 17:149–155.
55. Camacho NR, Sanchez JE, Martin RF et al. (2001) Medium-dose UVA1 phototherapy in localized scleroderma and its effect in CD34-positive dendritic cells. J Am Acad Dermatol 45:697–699.

Low-dose methotrexate 15mg per week in nine adults with widespread morphea yielded a beneficial effect.[56] One reported protocol for children with severe morphea and/or LM involved the use of monthly pulsed steroid in the dose of 30mg/kg per day for 3 days for 3 months and weekly 0.5–1mg/kg per week methotrexate.[57] Others have also reported the use of intravenous corticosteroids for severe progressive plaque, linear, and *en coup de sabre* forms – intravenous methylprednisolone daily was given for three days and repeated again the following week, and followed by oral prednisolone alone or in combination with once weekly methotrexate.[4]

In patients with disabling pansclerotic morphea, there is no known satisfactory treatment. There was no response to penicillamine, antimalarial agents, or systemic steroids in the series by Diaz-Perez *et al.*[12] There was no response to cytotoxic agents, although two patients in the above series did not develop new lesions while receiving cyclophosphamide (Cytoxan). Large ulcerations within the sclerotic plaques on the legs of a patient with pansclerotic morphea improved with intravenous gammaglobulin, and later with PUVA bath treatments.[13]

The depressed plaques of *en coup de sabre* morphea have been successfully corrected by autologous dermal fat implants.[58] One young adult with cosmetically unacceptable morphea involving the left zygomatic area was treated with local injections of collagen with good cosmetic correction.[59] Surgical excision of localized morphea lesions during the active inflammatory phase of the disease is not recommended because recurrence can result around the scar.[60] Physical therapy is extremely helpful in preventing contractures and an active exercise program with deep massage and splinting improves and possibly prevents the contractures that can complicate LM.[61]

PROGRESSIVE FACIAL HEMIATROPHY

Progressive facial hemiatrophy (Parry–Romberg syndrome) presents with severe atrophy of the soft tissues of half of the face. It may be accompanied by contralateral Jacksonian seizures, trigeminal neuralgia, eye symptoms and signs, hair abnormalities, and malalignment of the jaw causing dental problems.[4,62] The disorder was reported by Romberg in 1846 but had been mentioned as early as 1825 by Parry. There is a long-standing controversy about its relationship to *en coup de sabre* morphea. Most authors think these are variants of the same disease process.[63,64]

EPIDEMIOLOGY

Nearly all cases of PFH are sporadic, but there have been a few cases in families.[65] Males and females are equally affected.

CLINICAL MANIFESTATIONS
Cutaneous
The disease usually begins in the first decade of life[62] but it may rarely begin at any age.[66] Subcutaneous atrophy develops, usually on the cheek. The overlying skin may become hyperpigmented. The process extends to the brow, angle of the mouth, and neck and, occasionally, involves one-half of the body.

Atrophy or growth arrest of the underlying bone and cartilage occurs, probably at the same time as the other changes. The muscles may also be involved but function is maintained. Lesions often extend beyond the hairline causing circumscribed alopecia on the temporoparietal scalp, eyebrow, and eyelashes.[62] The disease progresses slowly for approximately three years and then stabilizes over 3–5 years, often leaving a severe cosmetic defect.[67]

Central nervous system
Trigeminal neuralgia or facial paresthesias occur in some patients and may precede the other changes.[26] Contralateral seizures may occur and are usually Jacksonian in type. Migraine headaches are common. Developmental delay with ipsilateral atrophy of the right hemisphere was documented in one neonate with PFH.[66]

Ocular
The eye is often involved. Loss of periorbital fat results in enophthalmos, and loss of underlying bone may displace the outer canthus downward. Ocular muscle paralysis, ptosis, Horner syndrome, heterochromia iridis, and dilated fixed pupils have been reported.[68] In addition, keratitis, iritis, choroiditis, cataracts, and papillary edema may also occur.

Oral
The tongue and upper lip on the involved side of the face are usually markedly atrophic. The maxilla and mandible do not fully develop, resulting in malocclusion and the teeth may have atrophic roots or be slow to erupt.[62]

LABORATORY FINDINGS

There are no known laboratory abnormalities; there may be many radiological abnormalities. High-resolution ultrasound and magnetic resonance imaging can be used to document dermal and subcutaneous changes.[69]

PATHOPHYSIOLOGY AND HISTOGENESIS

The cause of this disease is not understood. In several patients, a history of trauma has been elucidated, especially following tooth injury or extraction,[67] but the role of injury is controversial. One case report suggests a role for Borrelia infection.[70] In another report, PFH was associated with an intracranial vascular malformation; the authors propose that PFH may be the result of an arrested angiogenic process affecting the central nervous system during growth and development.[71]

DIFFERENTIAL DIAGNOSIS

En coup de sabre and Parry–Romberg disease are difficult to distinguish from one another; there are many who argue that the two conditions are variants of the same disease, rather than two distinct entities.[31] *En coup de sabre* resolves with atrophy of the skin, subcutaneous tissue, and bone that is morphologically identical to hemiatrophy. *En coup de sabre* typically affects the forehead area.[4] During the acute phase of *en coup de sabre*, the skin and deeper

56. Seyger MM, van den Hoogen FH, de Boo T, de Jong EM (1998) Low-dose methotrexate in the treatment of widespread morphea. **J Am Acad Dermatol** 39:220–225.
57. Uziel Y, Feldman BM, Krafchik BR et al. (2000) Methotrexate and corticosteroid therapy for pediatric localized scleroderma. **J Pediatr** 136:91–95.
58. Lapiere JC, Aasi S, Cook B, Montalvo A (2000) Successful correction of depressed scars of the forehead secondary to trauma and morphea en coup de sabre by en bloc autologous dermal fat graft. **Dermatologic Surgery** 26:793–797.
59. Stoner JG, Swanson NA, Siegle RJ (1984) Treatment of localized morphea with Zyderm collagen implant. **J Dermatol Surg Oncol** 8:626.
60. Kamath NV, Usmani A, Pellegrini A (2000) When is surgical treatment not appropriate for morphea? **Annals of Plastic Surgery** 45:199–201.
61. Black CM (1990) Juvenile scleroderma. In: Paediatric Rheumatology Update, Woo P, White PH, Ansell BM, eds. Oxford: Oxford University Press, pp. 194–208.
62. Gorlin RJ, Pindorb JJ, Cohen MM (1976) Syndromes of the Head and Neck. New York: McGraw-Hill.
63. Blaszcyk M, Jablonska S (1999) Linear scleroderma en coup de sabre. Relationship with progressive facial hemiatrophy. **Advances in Experimental Medicine & Biology** 455:101–104.

64. Lehman TJ (1992) The Parry-Romberg syndrome of progressive facial hemiatrophy and linear scleroderma en coup de sabre. Mistaken diagnosis or overlapping conditions? (editorial). **J Rheumatol** 19:844.
65. Lewkonia RM, Lowry RB (1983) Progressive hemifacial atrophy (Parry-Romberg syndrome). Report with review of genetics and nosology. **Am J Med Genet** 14:385.
66. Chang S-E, Huh J, Choi J-H et al. (1999) Parry-Romberg syndrome with ipsilateral cerebral atrophy of neonatal onset. **Pediatr Dermatol** 16:487–488.
67. Crikelear GF, Moss ML, Khuri A (1962) Facial hemiatrophy. **Plast Reconstr Surg** 29:5.
68. Hoang-Xuan T, Foster CS, Jakobiec FA et al. (1991) Romberg's progressive hemifacial atrophy: an association with scleral melting. **Cornea** 10:361.
69. Mauer J, Knollmann FD, Schlecht I et al. (1999) High-resolution magnetic resonance imaging in patients with facial haematrophy. **Acta Dermato-Venereologica** 70:373–375.
70. Abele DC, Dedingfield RB, Chandler FW, Given KS (1990) Progressive facial hemiatrophy (Parry-Romberg syndrome) and borreliosis. **J Am Acad Dermatol** 22:531.
71. Miedziak AI, Stefanyszyn M, Flanagan J, Eagle RC (1998) Parry-Romberg syndrome aosociated with intracranial vascular malformations. **Arch Ophthalmol** 116:1235–1237.

tissues are indurated, whereas in hemiatrophy, they are not. In PFH, it is the deeper tissues rather than the skin that are atrophic. In addition, facial morphea tends to progress over a longer period than the average three years in PFH.

Congenital facial hypoplasia is present at birth and includes diminution in the size of the teeth on the involved side, which may also occur with PFH. Other forms of lipoatrophy are usually not localized to the face. Neuro-muscular paralysis, following polio, can result in secondary atrophy of the face. In the oculo-auriculo vertebral syndrome, the facial bones are not fully developed, and the mandibular ramus is absent. In contrast to hemiatrophy, the ears are not fully formed, and epibulbar dermoids are common.

THERAPY AND PROGNOSIS

The disease tends to progress for three years on average and then becomes stationary. Antibiotic therapy for possible Borreliosis may be attempted. Treatment, as in the more severe forms of morphea, is advocated by some (see discussion of morphea). Serial MRIs may be useful to follow the effect of prednisone and methotrexate therapy.[72] When the disease is no longer progressive, plastic surgical correction can be considered.[73–75]

SCLEREDEMA

Scleredema affects localized areas of the face and back of the neck, which become indurated and tight. It was first recognized as a distinct entity by Buschke in 1900,[76] and has also been called "scleredema adultorum," even though the disease may occur in children.[77–79]

Scleredema is rare, with 223 cases having been reported since 1965.[78] Females are more frequently affected than males. There are occasional reports of familial involvement.[78] In one series, 29% of cases started before the age of 10 years, 22% between the ages of 10 and 20, and the remainder in adulthood.[77] There is one report of neonatal scleredema.[79]

PRESENTING HISTORY

There may be a prodrome of slight fever, malaise, muscle and joint pain, followed by induration, usually on the back and sides of the neck or on the face. Pustules may appear on the skin before the onset of the scleredema.[76] The patient may complain of difficulty in smiling, in wrinkling the forehead, or in opening the mouth. If the tongue and pharynx are involved, there may be difficulty in swallowing. A history of paresthesias and joint stiffness may occur. Later, the shoulders, arms, hands, and upper trunk may become affected. Occasionally, the abdomen is involved. A history of diabetes or precipitation by an infection has been recorded (see Pathogenesis).

PHYSICAL EXAMINATION

The skin is usually skin-colored, markedly thickened and nonpitted and hard. The thickening causes marked limitation in neck movement. The involved skin is not well demarcated from uninvolved skin, as the indurated area gradually fades into normal skin; this contrasts with the well-circumscribed lesions of morphea. The skin feels bound down to the underlying structures. In patients with diabetes, the skin may be erythematous.[76] In one pediatric patient, the scleredema was limited to the upper face and scalp and was initially diagnosed as edema.[80] Temporal tarsorrhaphies were required to prevent exposure keratitis.[80]

The tongue and pharynx are frequently involved, resulting in dysarthria and dysphagia. There is one report of an adult with pharyngeal involvement who developed infiltration of the upper esophagus, with progressive dysphagia, chronic aspiration, pneumonia, and ultimate death from acute aspiration.[81] Pleural and pericardial effusions may occasionally occur, and skeletal and cardiac muscles may be affected.[82] Occasionally, the eyelids and conjunctiva become indurated; the parotid gland may also be affected.

LABORATORY FINDINGS

The streptozyme titer may be raised, especially in children, and the erythrocyte sedimentation rate elevated. Elevation of serum proteins and increased levels of paraproteins have been reported.[83,84] Electrocardiographic abnormalities have been seen in some cases[76] and are thought to be associated with the complications of diabetes.

PATHOPHYSIOLOGY AND HISTOGENESIS

The cause of scleredema is unknown. It was originally thought that most patients had a history of an antecedent infection within a few days to six weeks before the onset of the disease. However, in a 1984 review from the Mayo Clinic, only eight of 33 patients with scleredema and no diabetes had such a history.[76] Although streptococcal infections are the most common precursors, other infections reported include influenza, pharyngitis, measles, mumps, pertussis, impetigo, and cellulitis. A 3-month-old infant reported by Heilbron and Saxe[79] had a fatal cytomegalovirus pneumonia and scleredema. A large number of adult cases have been found in association with long-standing diabetes mellitus and obesity.[85] The diabetes is of late onset and is difficult to control. Monoclonal gammopathy has also been described in association with scleredema.[84,86]

Skin biopsy shows a marked increase in dermal thickness.[85] The epidermis is normal. In the dermis, there are thick, swollen collagen bundles separated by large interfibrous spaces. These fenestrations contain increased levels of acid mucopolysaccharide, probably as a result of an accumulation of hyaluronic acid. The collagen replaces large areas of the subcutaneous tissue. Unlike scleroderma and morphea, the appendageal structures are unchanged. Fibroblast cultures from the involved skin of two patients yielded increased amounts of glycosaminoglycans, especially hyaluronic acid, but only slightly more collagen.[87]

DIFFERENTIAL DIAGNOSIS

The rapid onset makes this condition distinctive. The indurated lesions of morphea are more gradual in onset, ivory-colored, and well circumscribed.

72. Goldberg-Stern H, deGrauw T, Passo M, Ball WS (1997) Parry-Romberg syndrome: follow-up imaging during suppressive therapy. **Neuroradiology** 39:873–876.
73. Inigo F, Rojo P, Ysunza A (1993) Aesthetic treatment of Romberg's disease: experience with 35 cases. **Br J Plast Surg** 46:194.
74. Mordick TG, Larossa D, Whitaker L (1992) Soft-tissue reconstruction of the face: a comparison of dermal-fat grafting and vascularized tissue transfer. **Ann Plast Surg** 29:390.
75. Inigo F, Jimenez-Murat Y, Arroyo O et al. (2000) Restoration of facial contour in Romberg's disease and hemifacial microsomia: experience with 118 cases. **Microsurgery** 20:167–172.
76. Venencie PY, Powell FC, Su WP, Perry HO (1984) Scleredema: a review of thirty-three cases. **J Am Acad Dermatol** 11:128.
77. Greenberg LM, Geppert C, Worthen HG, Good RA (1963) Scleredema "adultorum" in children: report of 3 cases with histochemical study and review of world literature. **Pediatrics** 32:1044.
78. Curtis AC, Shulak BM (1965) Scleredema adultorum. Not always a benign self-limited disease. **Arch Dermatol** 92:526.
79. Heilbron B, Saxe N (1986) Scleredema in an infant. **Arch Dermatol** 122:1417.
80. Burke MJ, Seguin J, Bove KE (1982) Scleredema: an unusual presentation with edema limited to scalp, upper face, and orbits. **J Pediatr** 101:960.
81. Wright RA, Bernie H (1982) Scleredema adultorum of Buschke with upper esophageal involvement. **Am J Gastroenterol** 77:9.
82. Wu EB, Fuller LC, Hughes RA, Chambers JB (2001) Images in cardiovascular medicine: rare cause of cardiomyopathy. **Circulation** 103:2867.
83. Kovary PM, Vakilzadeh F, Macher E et al. (1981) Monoclonal gammopathy in scleredema. Observations in three cases. **Arch Dermatol** 117:536.
84. Ohta A, Uitto J, Oikarinen AI et al. (1987) Paraproteinemia in patients with scleredema. **J Am Acad Dermatol** 16:96.
85. Fleischmajer R, Faludi G, Krol S (1970) Scleredema and diabetes mellitus. **Arch Dermatol** 101:21.
86. Stables GI, Taylor PC, Highet AS (2000) Scleredema associated with paraproteinaemia treated by extracorporeal photopheresis. **Br J Dermatology** 142:781–783.
87. Christy WC, Buckingham RB, Barnes EL, Prince RK (1983) Scleredema adultorum of Buschke: a clinical, pathologic, and cell culture study of 2 patients. **J Rheumatol** 10:595.

Patients with progressive systemic sclerosis usually have Raynaud's phenomenon and other systemic findings. Swelling of the skin can be seen in dermatomyositis, but heliotrope changes and Gottron's papules are helpful differentiating features. Trichinosis can also cause facial edema. Mucinosis, myxedema, scleromyxedema, and mucopolysaccharidosis all cause cutaneous induration but may be distinguished by skin biopsy. Sclerema neonatorum and subcutaneous fat necrosis are diseases of the newborn and differ histologically.

THERAPY AND PROGNOSIS

Twenty-five percent of cases clear in 2 years; some disappear in months[78] but others occasionally persist for many years. It has been suggested that scleredema associated with an acute respiratory tract infection may resolve more rapidly;[76] however, this was true in only three of Venencie et al.'s eight cases.[76]

No effective therapy is known. Therapy with topical and systemic corticosteroids, methotrexate, penicillamine, thyroid hormones, hyaluronidase, estradiol, fibrolysin, pilocarpine, thorium X, and physical therapy have all met with inconsistent results. Scleredema associated with paraproteinemia has been treated successfully with extracorpeal photophoresis.[86]

SCLEREMA NEONATORUM

In this disease, diffuse hardening of the subcutaneous tissues occurs in debilitated preterm to term newborns.[88] The skin is smooth, cold, and stony hard and appears bound down to underlying structures. The face appears mask-like, and the joints are immobile. Induration usually resolves within two weeks, but most patients do not survive this long. Sclerema neonatorum is a nonspecific sign of severe underlying disease. Treatment depends solely on treating the underlying disorder, which can include sepsis, pneumonia, gastroenteritis, and other serious illnesses.

The histologic changes on skin biopsy are minimal. There is some thickening of the fibrous trabeculae in the subcutaneous fat and minimal inflammatory change. The disease must be distinguished from subcutaneous fat necrosis of the newborn (to which it is related), generalized edema, Milroy's disease, and Turner syndrome. See Chapter 6 for further details.

STIFF SKIN SYNDROME

Esterly and McKusick[89] reported four patients with localized areas of stony-hard skin associated with limited joint mobility and mild hirsuitism. The skin was normal in appearance and hard, immovable, and firmly bound to the underlying tissues; it was most severe over the buttocks, thighs, and legs in addition to areas overlying the joints. In the stiff skin syndrome, changes are noted in the neonatal period. Joint stiffness occurs in early childhood with mild limitation of movement. A lordotic stance is present in all patients, preventing full spinal flexion. In Esterly's series, the two most severely affected patients were unable to extend the hips and knees completely. Biopsies of affected skin show abnormal amounts of acid mucopolysaccharide in the dermis, but mucopolysacchariduria is not present. The occurrence in a mother and two children suggested an autosomal-dominant inheritance.[89]

After the initial report, three clinically similar cases were reported from Japan[90] and three from Poland.[91] Skin biopsy shows thickening and homogenization of the connective tissue stroma, with proliferation of connective tissue and an increased number of fibroblasts in the subcutis.[91] Colloidal iron-reactive material is present in the dermis and subcutis and is digestible by hyaluronidase. There are increased numbers of fibroblasts. Jablonska et al.[92] found that the fascia was considerably thickened in their cases, and suggested that their patients had a variant of stiff skin syndrome. They proposed the name *congenital fascial dystrophy* and considered the disorder to be a human counterpart of the tight-skin mouse, a dominant mutant mouse strain characterized by thickened skin firmly bound to the underlying tissues, and excessive collagen accumulation in the dermis and subcutaneous tissue. Jablonska et al. reported four patients with stone-hard indurations of skin and subcutaneous tissue primarily on the buttocks and thighs; the fascia was markedly enlarged.[93] Collagen fibrils were seen in affected fascia on electron microscopy. The authors called this a localized or "abortive" form of congenital fascial dystrophy because it was localized to the buttocks and thighs, not progressive, and involved the fascia only. Affected patients have a nonprogressive and localized disease, aside from joint contractures and occasional modest decreases in pulmonary function if the chest wall is involved.[92]

RESTRICTIVE DERMOPATHY

Restrictive dermopathy is a rare lethal congenital fetal syndrome, which is inherited in an autosomal-recessive manner.[94–96] The skin is abnormal at birth. It is tight, shiny, and taut and may tear or fissure when extended. The erosions can be extensive and mistakenly diagnosed as aplasia cutis congenita. The skin becomes increasingly rigid over time. The facies are distinctive: a small pinched nose with a fixed round open mouth, micrognathia, hypertelorism, and large fontanelles with widened sutures. The extremities have marked flexion contractures. Some patients have natal teeth, skeletal abnormalities, and pulmonary hypoplasia with respiratory insufficiency.

Histologic examination of the skin shows acanthosis, a thin dermis, absent or small elastic fibers, and collagen bundles abnormally oriented in parallel fashion to the epidermis, as seen in a scar or tendon. Keratin filaments and collagen fibrils are abnormal on electron microscopy. In one study, there was no expression of either TGF-alpha or EGFR in the skin at 14, 20 and 34 weeks gestation, whereas these markers were expressed in normal fetuses and in the visceral organs of the affected infant.[97]

Restrictive dermopathy can be readily differentiated from sclerema neonatorum and subcutaneous fat necrosis both clinically by its presence at birth, typical facies, and presence of erosions, and histologically in that there are no abnormalities in fat cells. Stiff skin syndrome and congenital fascial dystrophy are not present at birth, are more localized and usually have a more benign course.[96]

Most affected infants die shortly after birth, but with ventilation and nutritional support, some have survived for several weeks to months. There is a recent report of decreased fetal movement, visualized via ultrasonography in an affected fetus; this occurred at the end of the second trimester, making it less useful for antenatal diagnosis.[98]

KELOIDS AND HYPERTROPHIC SCARS

When skin is wounded, an inflammatory response is triggered, and healing follows. If the wound is deep and extends into the dermis, the resultant wound

88. Fretzin DF, Arias AM (1987) Sclerema neonatorum and subcutaneous fat necrosis of the newborn. **Pediatr Dermatol** 4:112.
89. Esterly NB, McKusick VA (1971) Stiff skin syndrome. **Pediatrics** 47:360.
90. Kikuchi I, Inoue S, Hamada K, Ando H (1985) Stiff skin syndrome. **Pediatr Dermatol** 3:48.
91. Jablonska S, Schubert H, Kikuchi I (1989) Congenital fascial dystrophy: stiff skin syndrome— a human counterpart of the tight-skin mouse. **J Am Acad Dermatol** 21:943.
92. Jablonska S, Groniowski J, Krieg T et al. (1984) Congenital fascial dystrophy—a noninflammatory disease of fascia: the stiff skin syndrome. **Pediatr Dermatol** 2:87.
93. Jablonska S, Blaszczyk M (2000) Scleroderma-like indurations involving fascias: an abortive form of congenital fascial dystrophy (stiff skin syndrome). **Pediatr Dermatol** 17:105–110.
94. Welsh KM, Smoller BR, Holbrook KA, Johnston K (1992) Restrictive dermopathy. Report of two affected siblings and a review of the literature. **Arch Dermatol** 128:228.
95. Graham J, Esterly NB (1999) What syndrome is this? **Pediatr Dermatol** 16:151–153.
96. Nijsten TEC, DeMoor A, Colpaert CG et al. (2002) Restrictive dermopathy: a case report and a critical review of all hypotheses of its origin. **Pediatric Dermatology** 19:67–72.
97. Sergi C, Kahl P, Otto HF (2000) Immunohistochemical localization of transforming growth factor-alpha and epithelial growth factor receptor in human fetal developing skin, psoriasis and restrictive dermopathy. **Pathology Oncology Research** 6:250–255.
98. Mulder EJ, Beemer FA, Stoutenbeek P (2001) Restrictive dermopathy and fetal behaviour. **Prenatal Diagnosis** 21:581–585.

heals with a scar. In some individuals and on some locations of the body, this scar is proliferative, resulting in a thick band of fibrous tissue that is elevated above the surface of the skin. The raised scar is called *hypertrophic* if it remains confined to the site of the injury and resolves in a year; it is called a *keloid* if it extends and invades the surrounding uninjured skin.

Keloids are common. References to their existence have been found in papyrus writings from the Pyramid Age, 3000 to 2500 BC.[99] Oral and sculptural art forms dating from the tenth century AD show that the ancient Yoruba people of western Nigeria practiced ritual facial markings which commonly resulted in keloid formation. They appreciated a familial predisposition to keloids and a time interval between trauma to the skin and keloid formation.[99] Keloids were described in the modern literature by Alibert in the early 1800s. He initially called them *les cancroides* because of their cancer-like extensions and later introduced the term *les cancroides ou keloids*, taken from the Greek *chele*, meaning crab's claw, and referring to the tendency of the lesions to extend laterally into normal tissue. For the next 100 years, there was interest in the rare entity known as "true keloids," keloids that arise spontaneously, and how to differentiate them from "false or cicatricial" keloids, which arise at sites of trauma. This distinction is no longer emphasized.

EPIDEMIOLOGY

Keloids occur equally in males and females.[99] They can occur at any age, but most cases have been reported in patients between the ages of 10 and 30. Prepubescent children and older adults are less commonly affected. Keloids are more common in darkly pigmented individuals.[99] The incidence in random samplings of African populations is approximately 6%. Polynesians are even more susceptible than blacks.[100] There is a familial predilection for keloids, but no genetic predisposition to the development of hypertrophic scars. A pedigree study examining 14 pedigrees with familial keloids found that the pattern of inheritance was autosonal dominant with incomplete clinical penetrance and variable expression.[101] Seven individuals were obligate unaffected carriers, implying environmental factors may also play a role.

PRESENTING HISTORY

Patients note the gradual onset of scar hypertrophy three to six weeks after the inciting trauma to the skin. Common examples of skin injury in the pediatric patient include varicella, ear piercing, lacerations, and surgical incisions. At times, there may be no recollection of prior injury; such "spontaneous keloids" have been reported in the Rubinstein–Taybi syndrome (broad thumbs and broad toes, mental and motor retardation, characteristic facies, and renal and cardiovascular anomalies).[102,103] After several months, a hypertrophic scar stops growing and becomes less red; a keloid, on the other hand, becomes hypersensitive, and sometimes severely pruritic. Even the pressure of clothing may incite irritability. The patient presents either for cosmetic reasons or because of the uncomfortable symptoms.

PHYSICAL EXAMINATION

Hypertrophic scars occur in the area in which trauma occurred, usually at an operation site. After a few months, the erythema abates and the scar flattens.

Keloids may occur anywhere on the body, but are most frequently found over the upper trunk and upper arms, and on ear lobes. The scar is raised and thickened forming a well-defined, firm, red or pink plaque with telangiectatic blood vessels at times coursing through the scar. After 2–3 months, the scar becomes smooth and round and extends beyond the original wound (Fig. 18.6A–C). Over time, the diagnosis of a keloid becomes obvious; it continues to grow, sometimes for years, with the formation of large, irregular, often linear, lesions with crablike projections. The epidermis is thin but does not ulcerate. Lesions may vary in size from 2 to 5mm papules to large pedunculated tumors. In most patients there are one to two lesions, but there may be more.

LABORATORY FINDINGS

There are no known laboratory abnormalities in patients with hypertrophic scars and keloids.

HISTOLOGY

In the early stages, normal wounds, hypertrophic scars, and keloids share similar histologic findings and it is difficult to differentiate amongst them;[99] they show inflammation and early fibroplasia. There are mast cells, plasma cells, and lymphocytes in the inflammatory infiltrate. In a keloid, fibroplasia progresses past the third week of wound healing. Nodular vascular proliferations, heavily cuffed by fibroblasts, enlarge and transform into thickened masses of hyalinized collagen bundles with proteoglycan. In a hypertrophic scar, the number of fibroblasts in capillaries slowly decreases by the fifth week as the collagen bundles organize in a parallel fashion.

Scanning electron microscopy shows that, in normal skin wounds, collagen bundles lie in discrete groups oriented parallel to the skin surface. In keloids, discrete bundles are absent, and collagen fibers are loosely connected and oriented randomly. Electron microscopy of a keloid shows that the lesion is composed entirely of myofibroblasts.[104]

PATHOGENESIS

The bulk of a keloid is composed of extracellular material, proteoglycan, especially chondroitin-4-sulfate, and water.[99] Keloids and hypertrophic scars are more cellular than normal skin wounds, but fibroblasts isolated from keloids appear to have normal growth characteristics.[99] The fibroblasts synthesize increased amounts of collagen, especially types I and III.[105] Keloidal collagen differs from normal dermal collagen in that it is more soluble and has cross-linking similar to that of young skin. There is increased expression of transforming growth factor (TGF)-beta in keloid fibroblasts; and TGF–beta ligands and receptors in keloids may increase collagen production.[106] It is possible that fibrous tissue accumulates in the keloid because collagen is not degraded, but collagenase levels are increased rather than decreased.[99,100] Another theory proposes a balance abnormality between proliferation and apoptotic cell death in keloidal fibroblasts.[107] Keloid fibroblasts may be resistant to apoptosis because they overexpress the insulin–like growth factor receptor I, thereby allowing persistent proliferation and production of excess extracellular matrix.[108] Expression of Gli-1 protein was shown to be strongly elevated in keloids compared with normal scars.[109]

99. Muray JC, Pollack SV, Pinnell SR (1981) Keloids: a review. **J Am Acad Dermatol** 4:461.
100. Nemeth AJ (1993) Keloids and hypertrophic scars. **J Dermatol Surg Oncol** 19:738.
101. Marneros AG, Norris JE, Olsen BR, Reichenberger E (2001) Clinical genetics of familial keloids. **Arch Dermatology** 137:1429–1434.
102. Rubinstein JH (1990) Broad thumb-hallux (Rubinstein-Taybi) syndrome 1957–1988. **Am J Med Genet** Suppl 6:3.
103. Selmanowitz VJ, Stiller MJ (1981) Rubinstein-Taybi syndrome: cutaneous manifestations and colossal keloids. **Arch Dermatol** 117:504.
104. James WD, Besanceney CD, Odom RB (1980) The ultrastructure of a keloid. **J Am Acad Dermatol** 3:50.
105. Low SQ, Moy RL (1992) Scar war strategies: target collagen. **J Dermatol Surg Oncol** 18:981.
106. Chin GS, Liu W, Peled Z et al. (2001) Differential expression of transforming growth factor-beta receptors I and II and activation of Smad 3 in keloid fibroblasts. **Plastic and Reconstructive Surgery** 108:423–429.
107. Luo S, Benathan M, Raffoul W et al. (2001) Abnormal balance between proliferation and apoptotic cell death in fibroblasts derived from keloid lesion. **Plastic and Reconstructive Surgery** 107:87–96.
108. Ishihara H, Yoshimoto H, Fujioka M et al. (2000) Keloid fibroblasts resist ceramide-induced apoptosis by overexpression of insulin-like growth factor I receptor. **J Inv Dermatol** 115:1065–1071.
109. Kim A, DiCarlo J, Cohen C et al. (2001) Are keloids really "gli-oids"?: High-level expression of gli-1 oncogene in keloids. **J Am Acad Dermatol** 45:707–711.

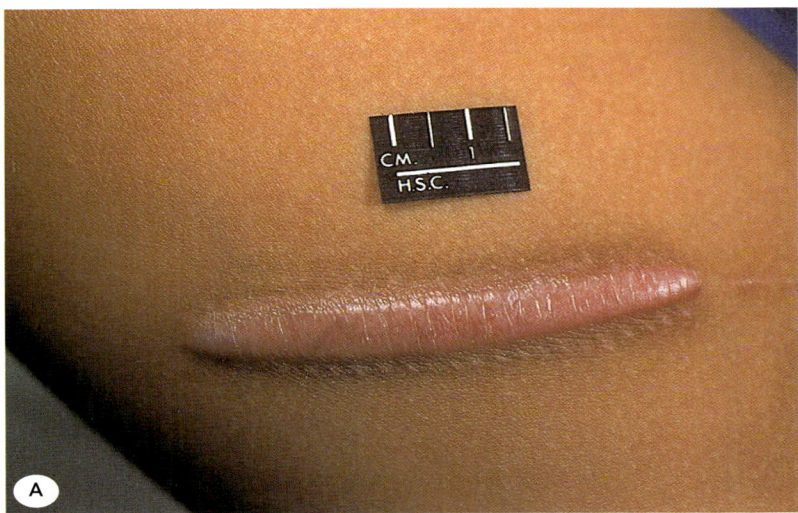

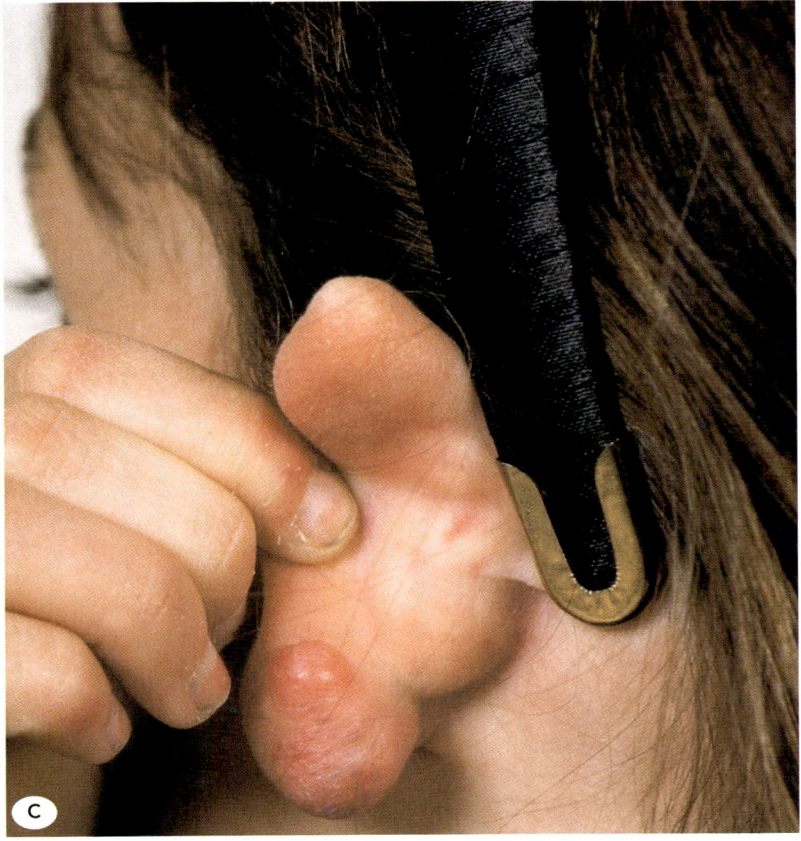

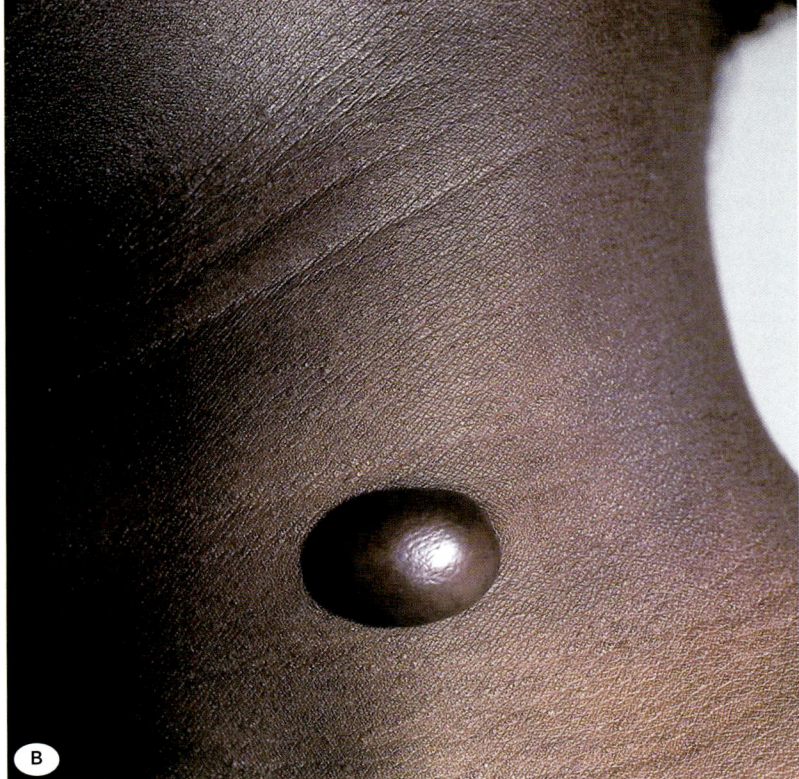

Fig. 18.6   (A) Keloid on chest. (B) Keloid on neck. (C) Keloid on ear.

DIFFERENTIAL DIAGNOSIS

The clinical morphology of a keloid is so distinctive that it is usually easy to diagnose. It should be differentiated from a hypertrophic scar. The keloid's characteristic of extending beyond the original wound is helpful in differentiating the two. Keloids are often hypersensitive or pruritic; hypertrophic scars may or may not be pruritic. Although helpful at times, these distinctions may be blurred enough to be of limited usefulness clinically.

Dermatofibrosarcoma protuberans is a slowly growing, firm, dermal, fibrous mass that at times can look similar to a keloid. These lesions are usually solitary, there is no preceding history of skin trauma, and they can be readily differentiated histologically. Exuberant keloid formation is a feature of Rubinstein–Taybi syndrome[102,103] and should be considered in patients with spontaneous keloids and dysmorphic features.

THERAPY AND PROGNOSIS

Many different treatment modalities have been proposed for the treatment of keloids, most with limited success. Currently, the most utilized treatment, either alone or combined with surgery, is repeated intralesional injections of triamcinolone.[113] Steroids increase the rate of collagen degradation. Murray et al.[99] recommend utilizing test doses of triamcinolone acetonide in concentrations varying from 10 to 40mg/ml injected into various keloid sites to establish a minimum effective dose for each patient; there is considerable variation in patient response. Keloidal tissue is extremely dense and difficult to inject. A Luer-Lok or dental syringe or a Dermajet device can be helpful.

Mast cells are prominent in both keloids and hypertrophic scars, and it has been proposed that histamine causes the pruritus.[99] A higher than normal concentration of neuropeptides has been shown in hypertrophic scars, which may cause the itching and also stimulate growth.[110] There is evidence that histamine in very high concentrations can stimulate fibroblast cell growth *in vitro*.[105] One study showed altered levels of cytokines in patients with keloids.[111] Another showed that keloid fibroblasts are not stimulated by transforming growth factor-β_1, which suggests a modification of regulation of this factor.[112]

110. Crowe R, Parkhouse N, McGrouther DA, Burnstock G (1994) Neuropeptide containing nerves in painful hypertrophic scar tissue. **Br J Dermatol** 130:444–452.
111. McCauley RL, Chopra V, Li YY et al. (1992) Altered cytokine production in black patents with keloids. **J Clin Immunol** 12:300.
112. Babu M, Diegelmann R, Oliver N (1992) Keloid fibroblasts exhibit an altered response to TGF-beta. **J Invest Dermatol** 99:650.
113. Ketchum LD, Cohen ID, Masters FW (1974) Hypertrophic scars and keloids: a collective review. **Plast Reconstr Surg** 53:140.

Cryotherapy with liquid nitrogen has been recommended before injection.[99] The freeze causes the keloid to become edematous and therefore less dense. Injections are repeated on a monthly basis. Care must be taken to infuse the injection into the bulk of the keloid, rather than into the contiguous dermis or epidermis, to minimize steroid-induced perilesional atrophy. Intralesional steroids are frequently used in combination with surgical excision. The wound edges are injected at the time of keloidectomy and at 2–4 week intervals post-operatively, usually with triamcinolone acetonide 10mg/ml. Adverse effects of corticosteroid use include localized atrophy, telangiectasia, depigmentation, necrosis, and ulceration. If systemic absorption is significant, the patient can become Cushingoid. Most of these effects are reversible; if the patient is exquisitely sensitive, the injection itself may incite further keloid formation.

Keloids usually recur after simple excision; thus excision is usually combined with other modalities such as intralesional and oral corticosteroid or pressure therapy. To reduce the probability of recurrence, it is recommended that a minimum amount of suture be used, that hematoma and wound dead space be avoided, and wound tension minimized.[99] To achieve the latter, flaps or Z-plasties are frequently performed. The presence of residual keloid tissue remaining after excision does not enhance recurrence, and it is reported that only the central area of the keloid needs excising.[114] Pressure applied to the area after surgical excision may prevent recurrence. Constant pressure must be maintained for 4–6 months postoperatively, although this is often difficult to achieve. Application to the earlobe with a spring-clip clothespin-like device[115] and to other areas with various types of elastic wraps may be helpful. Some have postulated a roll for topical imiquimod.

Carbon dioxide laser removal of keloids compared with surgical excision does not reduce recurrence. However, when used in combination with intralesional corticosteroids and secondary intention wound healing, results have been good in some patients.[100] Some authors believe that the 585-nm flashlamp-pumped *pulsed dye laser* improves the erythema, height, and pliability of some keloids and hypertrophic scars.[116]

A therapeutic option that is effective in some patients is the topical application of a sheet of *silastic gel*. Initially thought to exert an effect through pressure, new findings suggest the mechanism of action is by hydration and occlusion,[117] or that the surface electrical charge of the skin is altered.[118] Silicone gel and non-silicone gel dressings may be equally effective.[119]

X-ray treatment in the immediate postoperative period is thought to be an effective measure for preventing recurrence X-ray treatment of benign lesions in children is controversial because of the potential long-term hazards of radiation. Protocols that combine surgical excision with radiation, including low-megavoltage single-dose electron beam and roentgen irradiation have been used in adults.[100,120]

Methotrexate,[121] other cytotoxic agents,[67,121] and *topical retinoic acid solution 0.05%* have been recommended.[121] When the latter was applied to 28 patients with keloids and hypertrophic scars, 77% had decreased pruritus and bulk.[121] Some reports advocate the use of *cryotherapy* in keloids less than two years of age.[122,123] The cryogen was delivered intralesionally in one study.[124]

Because expression of Gli-1 protein is strongly elevated in keloids compared with normal scars and a drug called rapamycin inhibits signaling from the gli-1 oncogene, it has been proposed that a clinical trial of topical *tacrolimus* might be helpful, since tacrolimus is chemically similar to rapamycin.[109]

PROGNOSIS

In general, keloids continue to enlarge slowly for some years, then remain dormant and eventually flatten over many years.[125] Hypertrophic scars flatten spontaneously after one to three years.

ACNE KELOIDALIS NUCHAE

Acne keloidalis nuchae (folliculitis keloidalis, sycosis nuchae, or dermatitis papillaris capillitii) is a chronic inflammatory and scarring folliculitis and perifolliculitis that occurs on the nape of the neck and on the occipital scalp, usually in black males. It was first called dermatitis papillaris capillitii by Kaposi in 1869.[126] Basin introduced the term acne keloidalis to describe the later stages of the process.[126] Hebra added the term sycosis frambesiformis, referring to the raspberry-like appearance of the clustered papules.[126]

EPIDEMIOLOGY

The disease can occur occasionally in whites and women, but it is primarily a disease of young black males.[126] It does not occur in young children. In a study of 453 high school, college, and professional football players, acne keloidalis was associated with a family history of similar lesions or a positive personal or family history of keloid formation.[127]

PRESENTING HISTORY

The patient complains of papules in the occipital area that may slowly increase in size and number; they may be pruritic and are often associated with hair loss. Many patients report a short haircut or shaving of the nape of the neck before the onset of the problem.

PHYSICAL EXAMINATION

Firm, dull-pink, 1–3mm rounded, hard, follicular papules develop along the posterior hairline of the scalp (Fig. 18.7). Early papules may show a hair protruding from the center of the lesion, which has been described by Cosmon and Wolff[128] as "trees being engulfed by a moving sand dune." The hair is not embedded or ingrown. Pustules are occasionally present. As the disease progresses, the papules enlarge, coalesce and may form tumors or a thick sclerotic pseudokeloidal band across the occipital area of the scalp; the area is eventually devoid of hair. Draining purulent sinus tracts occasionally develop. There is usually no evidence of acne vulgaris, folliculitis, or keloid formation in other areas. Some patients, however, have or have had acne and hidradenitis.

114. Lee Y, Minn KW, Baik RM, Hong JJ (2001) A new surgical treatment of keloid: keloid core excision. Annals of Plastic Surgery 46:135–140.
115. Russell R, Horlock N, Gault D (2001) Zimmer splintage: a simple effective treatment for keloids following ear-piercing. Br J Plastic Surgery 54:509–510.
116. Manuskiatti W, Fitzpatrick RE, Goldman MP (2001) Energy density and numbers of treatment affect response of keloidal and hypertrophic sternotomy scars to the 585-nm flashlamp-pumped pulsed-dye laser. J Am Acad Dermatol 45:557–565.
117. Sawada Y, Sone K (1992) Hydration and occlusion treatment for hypertrophic scars and keloids. Br J Plast Surg 8:599.
118. Hirshowitz B, Lindenbaum E, Har-Shai Y et al. (1998) Static-electric field induction by a silicone cushion for the treatment of hypertrophic and keloid scars. Plast Reconstr Surg 101:1173–1183.
119. de Oliveira GV, Nunes TA, Magna LA et al. (2001) Silicone versus nonsilicone gel dressings: a controlled trial. Derm Surgery 27:721–726.
120. Ragoowansi R, Cornes PG, Glees JP et al. (2001) Ear-lobe keloids: treatment by a protocol of surgical excision and immediate postoperative adjuvant radiotherapy. Br J Plas Surg 54:504–508.
121. De Limpens J (1980) The local treatment of hypertrophic scars and keloids with topical retinoic acid. Br J Dermatol 103:319.
122. Rusciani L, Rossi G, Bono R (1993) Use of cryotherapy in the treatment of keloids. J Dermatol Surg Oncol 19:529.
123. Zouboulis CC, Blume U, Buttner P, Orfanos C (1993) Outcomes of cryosurgery in keloids and hypertrophic scars. Arch Dermatol 129:1146.
124. Gupta S, Kumar B (2001) Intralesional cryosurgery using lumbar puncture and/or hypodermic needles for large, bulky, recalcitrant keloids. Int J Dermatol 40:349–353.
125. Person communication (2002) BR Krafchik.
126. Dinehart SM, Herzberg AJ, Kerns BJ, Pollack SV (1989) Acne keloidalis: a review. J Dermatol Surg Oncol 15:642.
127. Knable AL Jr, Hanke CW, Gonin R (1997) Prevalence of acne keloidalis nuchae in football players. J Am Acad Dermatol 37:570–574.
128. Cosmon B, Wolff M (1972) Acne keloidalis. Plast Reconstr Surg 50:25.

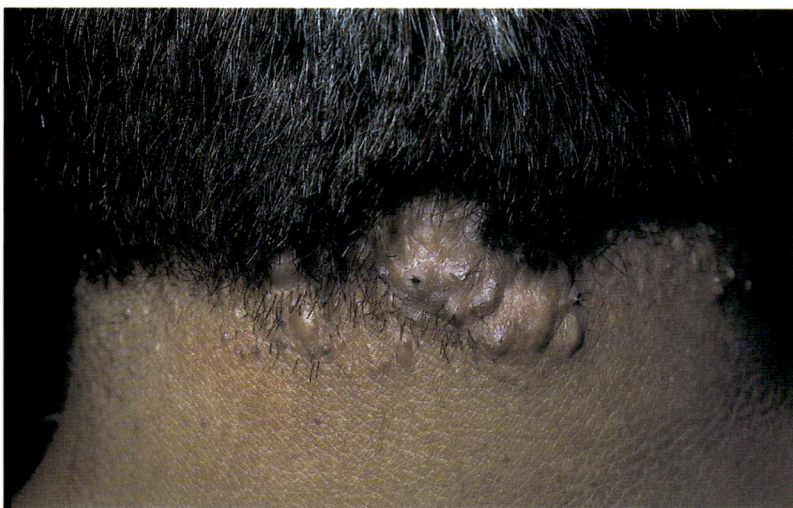

Fig. 18.7 Acne keloidalis in a teenage patient with Down syndrome.

LABORATORY FINDINGS

Staphylococcus aureus is present in intact pustules or from surface cultures in 75% of cases.[126] There are no other known abnormalities.

PATHOPHYSIOLOGY AND HISTOGENESIS

Initially, there is a lymphocytic and neutrophilic folliculitis of the upper third of the hair follicle. This is followed by a perifolliculitis. Later, excessive fibroplasia becomes the dominant feature. Hair follicles disappear or are engulfed by deep collagenous bands that are separated by sheets of plasma cells.

The exact mechanism of scar production is unclear. The lesions are not ingrown hairs, as in pseudofolliculitis barbae. They are also not true keloids, as evidenced by the histologic differences and the absence of keloid formation elsewhere. Almost all patients have used hair pomades, and in many there is a history of trauma from a close haircut or friction from a stiff collar. *S. aureus* is frequently present, but its role in the pathophysiology is probably secondary.

DIFFERENTIAL DIAGNOSIS

Perifolliculitis capitis abscendens et suffodiens (dissecting cellulitis) is also a chronic disease of the scalp that occurs primarily in blacks and causes alopecia. The primary lesions in this disease are nodules containing purulent material that coalesce to form interlacing sinus tracts, in contrast to the fleshy papules and scars of acne keloidalis; often, there is an associated severe acne or hidradenitis suppurativa. In folliculitis decalvans, a pustular dermatitis results in scarring alopecia; there are no raised papules. With a true keloid, there is usually a history of preceding trauma.

THERAPY AND PROGNOSIS

The disease is recalcitrant to therapy. Antiseptics and topical and systemic antibiotics are often used empirically. Some success occurs with the frequent administration of intralesional corticosteroids, in combination with systemic

or topical antibiotics and/or cryotherapy or carbon dioxide laser therapy.[129] Epilation by electrolysis, X-ray, or deep electrodesication has been suggested; healing by second intention is advocated for patients with severe disease. Local excision with primary closure or grafting is an alternative.[130]

AINHUM AND PSEUDO-AINHUM

Ainhum is a condition characterized by the development of constricting bands around a digit that may ultimately lead to spontaneous amputation. The term is derived from an African word meaning "to saw." True ainhum, compared with pseudo-ainhum, is a disease seen mostly in middle-aged black Africans.

Constricting bands can also be found in other situations, and then the term pseudo-ainhum is used. There are several categories of pseudo-ainhum: congenital constricting bands, acquired ainhum-like bands associated with other disease, and constriction due to artifacts.[131]

EPIDEMIOLOGY

True ainhum (dactylolysis spontanea) is primarily a disease of blacks in tropical Africa, who are usually barefoot. In a series by Cole,[132] ainhum was present in 2% of patients admitted for any reason to a university hospital in Nigeria. It has also been reported in all races and in many parts of the world. At least 125 cases have been reported in the United States, most occurring in the South.[133] True ainhum usually occurs in adults, but may occur in children.

The epidemiology of *pseudo-ainhum* is more complex, since it is not a single entity. Congenital constricting bands are usually not inherited, although there have been several familial cases reported.[131] Pseudo-ainhum due to tourniquets from a hair or thread constricting a digit is seen in infants and children and occasionally in the mentally retarded.

PRESENTING HISTORY

In true ainhum, the patient or parent notes the gradual development and widening of a groove at the base of the toe. Edema may develop distally and the underlying bone resorbs. The patient is usually asymptomatic, although there may be intermittent pain. The process slowly progresses over the ensuing 3–10 years, leaving a digit dangling by a piece of soft tissue. Finally, this necrotizes, and autoamputation is complete. In pseudo-ainhum, the patient presents with a band-like constriction; it is acute if due to external forces such as tourniqueting by a hair or thread.

PHYSICAL EXAMINATION
Ainhum

A sulcus or groove occurs at the base of the toe on the plantar surface and gradually deepens and widens circumferentially to finally encircle the toe.[134] The usual site of involvement is the fifth toe; this is usually bilateral but may be unilateral. Edema develops distally, and the underlying bone resorbs.

Amniotic bands (congenital pseudo-ainhum)

In congenital pseudo-ainhum, fibrous bands are found encircling one or more parts of the body, usually the distal portion of an extremity.[131] Any part of the body may be involved, including the trunk. In extreme cases, spontaneous *in utero* amputation may result. Bands vary from shallow depressions to deep constrictions that may extend to and involve bone. They can be single or

129. Kenney J (1965) Management of dermatoses peculiar to Negroes. **Arch Dermatol** 91:126.
130. Cosmon B, Wolff M (1972) Correlation of keloid recurrence with completeness of local excision. **Plast Reconstr Surg** 50:163.
131. Raque CJ, Stein KM, Lane JM, Reese EC (1972) Pseudoainhum constricting bands of the extremities. **Arch Dermatol** 105:434.
132. Cole GJ (1965) Ainhum: an account of 54 patients with special reference to etiology and treatment. **J Bone Joint Surg** [Br] 47:43.
133. Rossiter JW, Anderson PC (1976) Ainhum: treatment with intralesional steroids. **Int J Dermatol** 15:379.
134. Browne SG (1976) Ainhum. **Int J Dermatol** 15:348.

multiple. More than 50% of affected patients have other associated congenital anomalies, most commonly syndactyly and club foot. Occasionally, cleft palate and lip, aplasia cutis, or microdactyly is present.[135] Amniotic bands can occasionally be associated with large body-wall defects causing visceral extravasation of thoracic and/or abdominal organs.[136]

Acquired ainhumlike bands associated with other diseases

Pseudo-ainhum, which is not present at birth, is usually associated with a variety of other diseases.[131] These include conditions that diminish the vascular supply, such as Raynaud's disease, diabetes, and scleroderma, and conditions that diminish sensation, such as leprosy, tertiary lues, syringomyelia, and peripheral neuritis. Constricting bands and digit loss may occur in the verrucous hyperkeratotic plantar lesions of yaws. Vohwinkel syndrome is a hereditary condition, usually seen in females, in which palmar and plantar hyperkeratoses and starfish-shaped and linear keratoses are found on the extremities; constricting bands may develop at puberty.[137,138] Mal de Meleda and other hereditary palmar/plantar keratodermas and the keratoderma associated with pityriasis rubra pilaris and pachyonychia congenita can be associated with pseudo-ainhum. A patient with palmar psoriasis who developed pseudo-ainhum of a digit as a result of a thick epidermal cast has been reported.[139] In this patient, when the cast was removed, the condition resolved. Traumatic scarring from burns and frostbite may also cause constricting scars.

Pseudo-ainhum (tourniquet syndrome)

Threads, hair, or other strands may encircle a body part, such as a digit, nipple, or penis (Fig. 18.8).[140] This results in acute soft tissue swelling that causes the ligating band to be invisible, making the diagnosis difficult. The problem is usually seen in infants and children, but can occur in adults. Five affected infants were analysed by Quinn,[141] who reported fine threads from clothing embedded in the skin of two affected children; the remaining three cases were due to tourniqueting by human hair. Although usually accidental, this problem may be self-induced or may be a manifestation of child abuse.[141]

PATHOPHYSIOLOGY AND HISTOGENESIS

The exact cause of true ainhum is not known, but is probably related to fissuring and infection of the plantar sulcus from walking barefoot. The fissure heals temporarily but breaks down when the toe is extended while walking.[134] This chronic trauma results in the disease process. Four cases reported from India have been associated with *Trichosporon cutaneum* infection.[142] In a series of 83 cases from Nigeria,[134] there were no cases of dermatophyte infection identified. The only constant feature in these patients was chronic fissuring at the site of constriction, often in patients with hyperkeratotic skin. Other theories suggest that ainhum might be due to an abnormal blood supply to the foot, either as a partial blockade of the posterior tibial artery, or to the absence of the plantar arch artery and its branches.[134]

Congenital amniotic bands, on the other hand, are not due to the formation of scar tissue. A skin biopsy obtained after partial surgical excision of a band from an infant's ankle showed deep invagination of the skin in the central portion of the specimen, with thinning of the underlying dermis.[131] Beneath the thin dermis were finger-like strands of connective tissue that projected down deep into the subcutaneous fat. Coarse elastic fibers extended into these connective tissue strands. Sweat glands were present and normal in

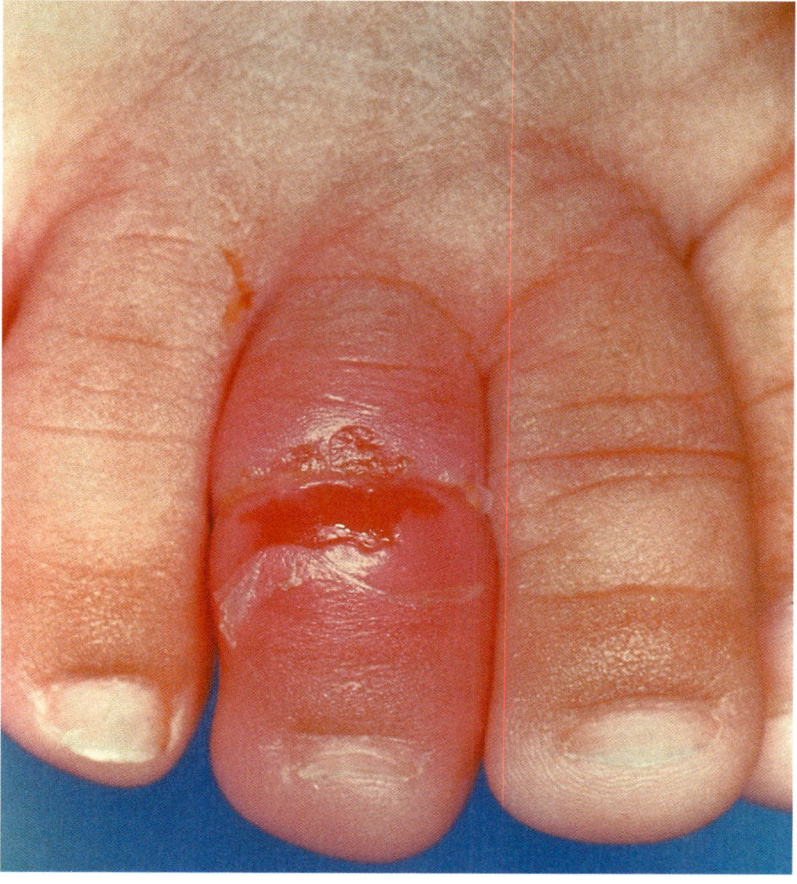

Fig. 18.8   Pseudo-ainhum: constriction of toe from a hair. (Courtesy of Peter Lynch, MD)

appearance. The cause of congenital bands is unknown. It is assumed that there is some developmental abnormality. It has been suggested that the amniotic membrane may adhere to the fetus and, in some way trigger the formation of a constricting band, or that the amniotic membrane itself may encircle the affected part.[143] If this is so, it is difficult to understand why the constrictions seen are always circular instead of spiral.[143] The belief that the umbilical cord encircles the part to cause the constriction is doubtful because the cord is thicker than the digits of the fetus.[143]

It has been assumed that cases of congenital amputation are an extreme form of pseudo-ainhum in which the annular constricting bands are deep enough to constrict the limb during embryonic growth, causing *in utero* amputation. There have been several reports of infants born with the absence of a limb in whom the amputated part is recovered at delivery.[131] Embryologists have thought that limb amputation may be due to a focal degenerative process in the limb itself and not due to extrinsic factors.[131] Moessinger[144] reported cases of congenital constricting bands in which there was a history of amniocentesis. There are rare cases of hereditary congenital pseudo-ainhum, and congenital constricting bands have been associated with Ehlers–Danlos syndrome.[145] It may be that there is a genetic predisposition with involvement of various environmental factors.

135. Izumi AK, Arnold HL (1974) Congenital annular bands (pseudoainhum): association with other congenital abnormalities. **JAMA** 229:1208.
136. Martinez-Frias ML, Bermejo E, Rodriquez-Pinilla E (2000) Body stalk defects, body wall defects, amniotic bands with and without body wall defects, and gastroschisis: comparative epidemiology. **Am J Medical Genetics** 92:13–18.
137. Camisa C, Rossana C (1984) Variant of keratoderma hereditaria mutilans (Vohwinkel's syndrome): treatment with orally administered isotretinoin. **Arch Dermatol** 120:1323.
138. Peris K, Salvati EF, Torlone G, Chimenti S (1995) Keratoderma hereditarium mutilans (Vohwinkel's syndrome) associated with congenital deaf-mutism. **British J Dermatology** 132:617–620.
139. McLaurin CI (1982) Psoriasis presenting with pseudoainhum. **J Am Acad Dermatol** 7:130.
140. Alpert JJ, Filler R, Glaser H (1965) Strangulation of an appendage by hair wrapping. **N Engl J Med** 273:866.
141. Quinn NJ (1971) Toe tourniquet syndrome. **Pediatrics** 48:145.
142. Kamalam A, Thambiah AS (1981) Ainhum, trichosporosis, and Z-plasty. **Dermatologica** 162:372.
143. Neumann A (1953) Pseudoainhum: report of congenital case involving several fingers and left wrist. **Arch Dermatol Syphilol** 68:421.
144. Moessinger AC (1981) Amniotic band syndrome associated with amniocentesis. **Am J Obstet Gynecol** 141:588.
145. Young ID, Lindenbaum RH, Thompson EM et al. (1985) Amniotic bands in connective tissue disorders. **Arch Dis Child** 60:1061.

DIFFERENTIAL DIAGNOSIS

The diagnosis is obvious from the appearance of the affected part. The type of ainhum or pseudo-ainhum is diagnosed according to the presence of the lesion at birth or later, its location, the presence of associated conditions and the finding of constricting material.

TREATMENT AND PROGNOSIS

The acute onset of constriction with erythema and edema of the distal portion of the body part should prompt consideration of the tourniquet syndrome. Patients with severe keratodermas have temporarily improved while receiving treatment with retinoids.[137,138] One patient with pseudo-ainhum from a severe keratoderma was treated surgically by excision of the constriction band and closure with Z-plasties.[146]

True ainhum is a progressive problem that ultimately results in spontaneous amputation. Cole[132] reported reversal of the problem by excision of the groove, followed by single or multiple Z-plasties. Others have reported reversal of the process in a patient treated early in the course of the disease with monthly injections of intralesional triamcinolone acetonide, 5mg/ml, for 10 months.[133] Constrictions caused by congenital bands do not often require intervention, other than for cosmetic reasons, because the bands grow in parallel with the growth of the child. They do persist, however, and can still be seen in the adult.[135] Surgical intervention is not indicated, unless gangrenous changes develop soon after birth.[131]

Pseudo-ainhum associated with keratodermas may respond to plastic surgery repair with Z-plasty.[132] Retinoids administered orally have been helpful in at least two patients with Vohwinkel syndrome.[137]

Treatment of the tourniquet syndrome requires ligation of the offending fiber. Because the area is often edematous, this is not an easy procedure and when the problem has been present for some time, the offending fiber may be buried in scar tissue. If the end of a thread is visible, it can be explored with a fine-tipped forceps, but this may result in incomplete removal. The proximal margin of the constricted area should be explored with a fine-tipped forceps, which can be placed underneath the ligating thread. If the above-mentioned measures do not produce the desired results, a deep longitudinal incision across the constriction is effective.

STRIAE

Striae are linear, white, atrophic bands, commonly called "stretch marks;" other medical synonyms include striae distensae and striae atrophicae.

EPIDEMIOLOGY

Striae occur most frequently during puberty or in women during pregnancy. They are common at puberty and are found in more than 25% of girls and about 10% of boys ages 9 to 16.[147] They do not develop in the elderly.[148] Striae may be found in endocrine disease, especially in Cushing syndrome. They may occur as a side effect of systemic corticosteroids, in some patients after prolonged use of high-potency topical corticosteroids, and/or under occlusion in pubertal children.[149]

PRESENTING HISTORY

The patient notes the appearance of asymptomatic linear lesions that may initially be raised and red but over a period of months to years become white and flat.

PHYSICAL EXAMINATION

Striae are linear lesions, commonly several centimeters long and 1–10mm wide. Their long axis is oriented perpendicular to the direction of skin tension lines. Commonly affected sites include the thighs, buttocks, and breasts in girls and the outer thighs and lumbosacral area in boys. The earliest lesion is usually raised and pink, but soon becomes flat and livid blue-red in color with a fine wrinkled surface. Over time, the lesion becomes white and inconspicuous. Very rarely, severe, extensive striae may ulcerate or tear.[150] Striae of pregnancy occur most commonly on the abdomen and on the breasts. The striae of Cushing syndrome may be larger and more widely distributed. Striae induced by topical steroid use are often found in the inguinal folds[149] but may occur in areas where the steroid is used, particularly if under occlusion.

LABORATORY FINDINGS

There are no known laboratory abnormalities unless the patient has Cushing syndrome, in which case serum and urinary glucocorticoid levels are increased.

PATHOPHYSIOLOGY AND HISTOGENESIS

Striae result from breaks in the connective tissue. Some individuals are more susceptible to the development of striae than others.[151] There is a familial predisposition.[152] It has been hypothesized that striae are caused by stretching of the dermal skin and that physical stress ruptures connective tissue. However, striae almost never develop after the use of tissue expanders,[153] implying factors other than mechanical stresses alone. If skin distension is slow and progressive, there is a lower probability of striae.[148] Striae cannot be produced experimentally, and there is no animal model.

In pregnancy, females with a greater weight gain, primagravidas, and younger pregnant women are more likely to develop striae.[148] Striae are less common in older primagravidas. A history of acne or striae during adolescence is predictive of striae developing during pregnancy.[148]

Obesity is associated with the presence of striae only at puberty[147] or with associated corticosteroid use. Striae are absent in obese pre-adolescents. When striae occur after steroid use, they do not usually develop until adolescence, implying some priming by hormonal factors. On the other hand, striae have also been noted in cachectic states, such as tuberculosis, typhoid fever, and after intense slimming diets.

The striae associated with endogenous or topical corticosteroids are thought to be caused by the epidermal and dermal atrophy that corticosteroids can induce.[154] Atrophy occurs because of epidermal thinning and a reduction in dermal collagen. It has been shown that there is histologic evidence of epidermal atrophy in human skin after one week of daily occlusion with fluocinolone acetonide.[155]

146. Luk KDK, Orth MC, Wu PC, Chow SP (1986) Keratoma hereditaria mutilans: report of a case with successful surgical treatment. **J Hand Surg [Am]** 11A:269.
147. Sisson WR (1954) Colored striae in adolescent children. **J Pediatr** 45:520.
148. Cambazard F, Michel J-L (2000) Striae. In: Textbook of Pediatric Dermatology, Harper J, Orange A, Prose N eds. London: Blackwell, pp. 1847–1852.
149. Barkey WF (1987) Striae and persistent tinea corporis related to prolonged use of betamethasone dipropionate 0.05% cream/clotrimazole 1% cream (Lotrisone cream) (letter). **J Am Acad Dermatol** 17:518.
150. Stroud JD, Van Dersarl JV (1971) Striae. **Arch Dermatol** 103:103.
151. Pottkotter L, Pyeritz RE, Glesby MJ (1989) Striae and systemic abnormalities of connective tissue. **J Am Med Assoc** 262:3132.
152. DiLernia V, Bonci A, Cattania M, Bisighini G (2001) Striae distensae (rubrae) in monozygotic twins. **Pediatric Dermatology** 18:261–262.
153. Marcus J, Horan DB, Robinson JK (1990) Tissue expansion: past, present and future. **J Am Acad Dermatol** 23:813–825.
154. Epstein NN, Epstein WL, Epstein JH (1963) Atrophic striae in patients with inguinal intertrigo. **Arch Dermatol** 87:450.
155. Arndt KA, Clark RA (1979) Principles of topical therapy. In: Dermatology in General Medicine, Fitzpatrick FB, Eisen AZ, Wolff K et al., eds. New York: McGraw-Hill, p. 1753.

The histologic findings are similar to that of a scar. The epidermis overlying striae is flattened and thin. As in scars, appendageal structures are not present. Rare biopsy specimens of striae rubrae show a perivascular inflammatory infiltrate with lymphocytes, monocytes, occasional neutrophils, an increased number of mast cells, and fibroblasts.[156] Sheu *et al*.[157] describes mast cell granulation and elastolysis in the early stage of striae distensae. In mature degranulation and elastolysis, there has been controversy whether the problem is with the elastic fibers or with the collagen fibers. Zheng *et al*.[158] concluded that the elastic fibers in mature striae are normal. They are dense and well developed, on scanning electron microscopy, and may have been previously underestimated with routine staining, because immature fibers contain an insufficient protein matrix and do not stain well. The same authors also showed that the collagen fibers are packed horizontally in bundles and are thin and straight, in contrast to the wavy, thick, randomly arranged collagen fibers seen in normal skin. This horizontal stacking of collagen is identical to the connective tissue arrangement seen in scars. For all these reasons, they concluded that striae are scars. This conclusion is strengthened by the fact that, because of the great tensile strength of collagen fibers, it is not possible in an *in vivo* situation for mechanical stretching to cause parallel alignment of collagen fibers. It is further hypothesized that, in the early stage of striae formation (striae rubrae), there is an inflammatory reaction that destroys collagen and elastin. Healing would then occur, with regeneration of new elastin and collagen and orientation of the collagen fibers in the direction of stress imposed by mechanical forces.[158]

DIFFERENTIAL DIAGNOSIS

The diagnosis is usually obvious because of the distribution and linearity of the lesions, and the lack of preceding trauma, as there is with a scar. The fish-mouthed scars of Ehlers–Danlos syndrome may resemble striae, but occur after mild trauma and are usually located over the knees and elbows. Patients with Ehlers–Danlos syndrome have other stigmata of the disease, including joint hyperextensibility. Endocrine evaluation to exclude the diagnosis of Cushing syndrome is recommended if there is no other obvious cause or if the lesions are severe.

THERAPY AND PROGNOSIS

The patient can be reassured that, over time, the lesions will become less noticeable. If the striae are due to systemic or topical corticosteroids, the medication should be reduced or stopped if possible. Some advocate the topical application of tretinoin, which caused significant improvement in 15 of 16 patients.[159] In our experience the use of topical retinoic acid 0.1% in a cream base once a day during eight weeks improved and even faded pink striae. Breast and hip striae show the best results.[160]

The pulsed dye laser can also be used successfully to improve the appearance of striae, in the inflammatory "rubra" stage.[161] Laser treatment of striae is not recommended in skin types IV, V, or VI because of secondary hyperpigmentation, or lack of effect.[162]

LICHEN SCLEROSUS

Lichen sclerosus (LS) is an uncommon disease of unknown cause in which white, atrophic plaques develop on the body and/or vulva, penis, and perianal areas. The disease is seen most commonly in prepubertal girls and in postmenopausal women. Initially called *lichen sclerosus et atrophicus*, the designation is now LS. Previously, pruritic white lichenified plaques on the vulva were called kraurosis vulvae (kraurosis means "shriveling").[163] It was not appreciated at the time that many but not all patients with kraurosis vulvae actually had LS by histologic examination.[164]

EPIDEMIOLOGY

LS may occur at any age and in either sex. Ten to 15 percent of affected individuals have the onset before the age of 13, and 70% of childhood cases begin before age 7.[165,166] The youngest reported case was several weeks of age.[165] The disease is not inherited, although familial cases have been reported.[167,168] There may also be a family history of autoimmune diseases including vitiligo, morphea, and thyroid disease.[169]

Eighty-five to 90 percent of cases occur in females. Of 130 prepubertal girls reporting to a pediatric dermatology clinic with a vulvar complaint, 18% had LS.[170] Genital LS in males occurs between the ages of 15 and 50, more commonly in young men and, occasionally, in pre-adolescent males. LS is the most common indication for circumcision for phimosis in males.[171] In a prospective study of 100 boys with phimosis, 10% had LS.[172]

PRESENTING HISTORY

The affected patient or parent notices the gradual onset of asymptomatic, ivory-colored plaques. Many patients complain of marked pruritus and discomfort in the vulval area, and perianal involvement may cause painful defecation and bleeding.[173] A vaginal discharge may precede the disease. There is one case report of urinary incontinence from partial obstruction of the urethra due to LS involving the vulva and clitoral head.[174] Extragenital LS is asymptomatic and patients present because of the appearance of the skin lesions.

PHYSICAL EXAMINATION

The characteristic primary lesion of extragenital LS is an asymptomatic small, shiny, ivory-white angular macule or papule several millimeters in diameter. Papules may coalesce into plaques of various sizes that, over time, become atrophic and show fine wrinkling of the epidermis (Figs 18.9 A). Within the plaques, the follicular openings are characteristically dilated and hyperkeratotic (called follicular delling) and appear prominent and plugged. The plaques may occur anywhere, but are often distributed over the clavicles, on the chest and back, around the umbilicus, and on the flexor surfaces of the extremities, neck, and axillae. Occasionally, extensive bullae, telangiectasias, and purpura are found. On resolution, the bullae may heal with milia. The Koebner

156. Ebert MH (1933) Hypertrophic striae distensae. **Arch Dermatol Syphilol** 28:825.
157. Sheu HM, Yu HS, Chang CH (1991) Mast cell degranulation and elastolysis in the early states of striae distensae. **J Cutan Pathol** 18:41.
158. Zheng P, Lavker RM, Kligma AM (1985) Anatomy of striae. **Br J Dermatol** 112:185.
159. Elson ML (1990) Treatment of striae distensae with topical tretinoin. **J Dermatol Surg Oncol** 16:267.
160. Personal communication (2001) Dr Lourdes Tamayo.
161. Alster TS (1997) Laser treatment of hypertrophic scars, keloids, and striae. **Dermatologic Clinics** 15:419–429.
162. Nouri K, Romagosa R, Chartier T et al. (1999) Comparison of the 585nm pulse dye laser and the short pulsed CO2 laser in the treatment of striae distensae in skin types IV and VI. **Dermatologic Surgery** 25:368–370.
163. Personal communication (2002) Dr Marilynne McKay.
164. Ridley CM (1992) Lichen sclerosus. **Dermatologic Clinics** 10:309–323.
165. Chernosky ME, Derbes VJ, Burks JW (1957) Lichen sclerosus et atrophicus in children. **Arch Dermatol** 75:647.
166. Clark JA, Mulb SA (1967) Lichen sclerosus et atrophicus in children. A report of 24 cases. **Arch Dermatol** 95:476.

167. Murphy FR, Lipa M, Haberman HF (1982) Familial vulvar dystrophy of lichen sclerosus type. **Arch Dermatol** 117:329.
168. Sahn EE, Bluestein EL, Oliva S (1994) Familial lichen sclerosus et atrophicus in childhood. **Pediatric Dermatology** 11:160–163.
169. Powell J, Wojnarowska F, Winsey S et al. (2000) Lichen sclerosus premenarche: autoimmunity and immunogenetics. **Br J Dermatology** 142:481–484.
170. Fischer G, Rogers M (2000) Vulvar disease in children: a clinical audit of 130 cases. **Pediatric Dermatology** 17:1–6.
171. Chalmers RJ, Burton PA, Bennett RF et al. (1984) Lichen sclerosus et atrophicus. A common and distinctive cause of phimosis in boys. **Arch Dermatol** 120:1025–1027.
172. Meuli M, Briner J, Hanimann B, Sacher P (1994) Lichen sclerosus et atrophicus causing phimosis in boys: a prospective study with 5-year followup after complete circumcision. **J Urology** 152:987–989.
173. Labandeira J, Pereiro M, Roson E, Toribio J (2001) Rectorrhagia and lichen sclerosus in childhood. **Pediatric Dermatology** 18:543–545.
174. Attaran M, Rome E, Gidwani GP (2000) Unusual presentation of lichen sclerosus in an adolescent. **J Pediatric Adolescent Gynecology** 13:99.

phenomenon has been documented in this disorder, and lesions may occur in surgical scars, vaccination sites, and areas of other trauma or irritation. Lesions of biopsy-proven LS may occur in association with biopsy-proven morphea, and it has been suggested that guttate morphea may be a variant of LS or vice versa. The shiny white changes seen in both disorders are the result of epidermal thinning. Occasionally, blue and white plaques may occur inside the mouth, on the tongue, or on mucosal surfaces. Some patients have associated vitiligo.

Genital LS in females presents with white, atrophic plaques surrounding the vulva and perianal areas in an hourglass or figure-eight configuration (Figs 18.9B,C). Bullae with hemorrhage may occur and small telangiectasias and purpuric areas are common. Because of friction and moisture in the area, the affected skin may break down to form a raw, red, macerated surface. Two patients reported by Loening-Baucke[175] had anal stenosis, and over time atrophy may cause shrinkage of the vulva, particularly of the labia minora and clitoris. There is one case report of infantile pyramidal protrusion as a manifestation of LS.[176] Infantile pyramidal protrusion is a pyramid-shaped red soft tissue swelling that can occur on the perineal median raphe of girls: it is often misdiagnosed as a "skin tag," skin biopsy shows epidermal acanthosis, marked edema of the upper dermis, and mild dermal inflammation.[177] Of the four girls reported in this study with pyramidal protrusion, three had subtle classic LS and the other patient developed LS months later. All four pyramidal papules showed LS histologically.

There is a relationship between vulvar LS, leukoplakia, and malignancy. The histological changes of lichen sclerosus are frequently found in association with vulvar squamous cell carcinoma, seemingly related to the role chronic inflammation can play in oncogenesis. Vulvar intraepithelial neoplasia was found in 9% of adult women with symptomatic LS in one series, and 21% had invasive squamous cell carcinoma.[178] These dysplastic changes have not been found in children. There is no information on the incidence of vulvar carcinoma in LS.

When the disease involves the genital area of males, it is known as balanitis xerotica obliterans. The prepuce becomes sclerotic and cannot be retracted. The glans is blue-white and shiny. Telangiectasias or hemorrhagic bullae may occur, especially when irritated after intercourse. The bullae may cause blood-stained urine if located near the urethral meatus. If the perimeatal mucosa is involved, there may be difficulty in micturition because of phimosis,[172] and back-pressure may affect the urinary tract. Occasionally, the penile shaft is involved, but the scrotum and perianal area are almost always normal. Secondary leukoplakia and carcinoma may occur in males.[179]

LABORATORY FINDINGS

Autoantibodies against thyroid cytoplasm, gastric parietal cells,[180] and against single-stranded DNA may be present.

PATHOPHYSIOLOGY AND HISTOGENESIS

The cause of the disease is unknown. The predominance of the condition in women, frequent onset at menopause, and spontaneous improvement in many patients at puberty all suggest a hormonal factor. Women with LS have low androgen levels.[181] Androgen receptors are diminished in lesional skin[182] and there is local production of 5-alpha reductase.[181] There appears to be a higher incidence of HLA-DQ7 in both children and adults with LS.[169] The

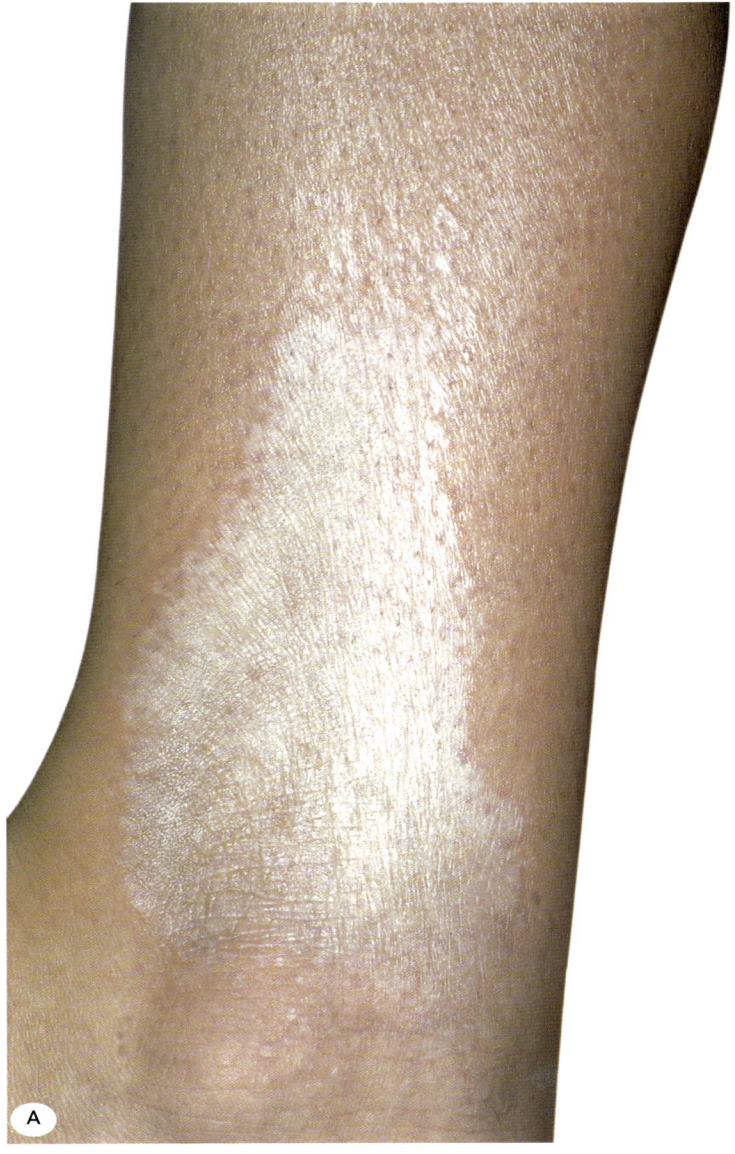

Fig. 18.9   (A) Lichen sclerosis on the leg of a 14-year-old girl.

common history of preceding vaginitis or balanitis suggests that infection may play a role. There is a clinical overlap between LS and localized scleroderma (morphea). *B. burgdorferi* infection has been implicated in some patients with morphea and in two patients with both morphea and extragenital LS in Europe but not in North America.[28]

The histology is distinctive. A skin biopsy shows thinning of the epidermis, vacuolar changes at the dermal-epidermal junction, marked edema of the papillary dermis, and a lymphohistiocytic infiltrate that is bandlike and beneath the edematous zone. Vulvar LS may have histologic variants; the minimal histologic criterion for LS is vacuolar interface changes in

175. Loening-Baucke V (1991) Lichen sclerosus et atrophicus in children. **Am J Dis Child** 145:1058.
176. Cruces MJ, De La Torre C, Losada A et al. (1998) Infantile pyramidal protrusion as a manifestation of lichen sclerosus et atrophicus. **Arch Dermatol** 134:1118–1120.
177. Kayashima K, Kitoh M, Ono T (1996) Infantile perianal pyramidal protrusion. **Arch Dermatol** 132:1481–1484.
178. Carlson JA, Ambros R, Malfetano J et al. (1998) Vulvar lichen sclerosus and squamous cell carcinoma: a cohort, case control, and investigational study with historical perspective; implications for chronic inflammation and sclerosis in the development of neoplasia. **Human Pathology** 29:932–948.

179. Weber P et al. (1987) Verrucous carcinoma in penile lichen sclerosus et atrophicus. **J Dermatol Surg Oncol** 13:529.
180. Goolamali SK, Barnes EW, Irvine WJ, Shuster S (1974) Organ-specific antibodies in patients with lichen sclerosus. **BMJ** 4:78.
181. Friedrich EG Jr, Kalra PS (1984) Serum levels of sex hormones in vulvar lichen sclerosus and the effects of topical testosterone. **N Engl J Med** 310:488.
182. Clifton MM, Garner IB, Kohler S, Smoller BR (1999) Immunohistochemical evaluation of androgen receptors in genital and extragenital lichen sclerosus: evidence for loss of androgen receptors in lesional epidermis. **J Am Acad Dermatol** 41:43–46.

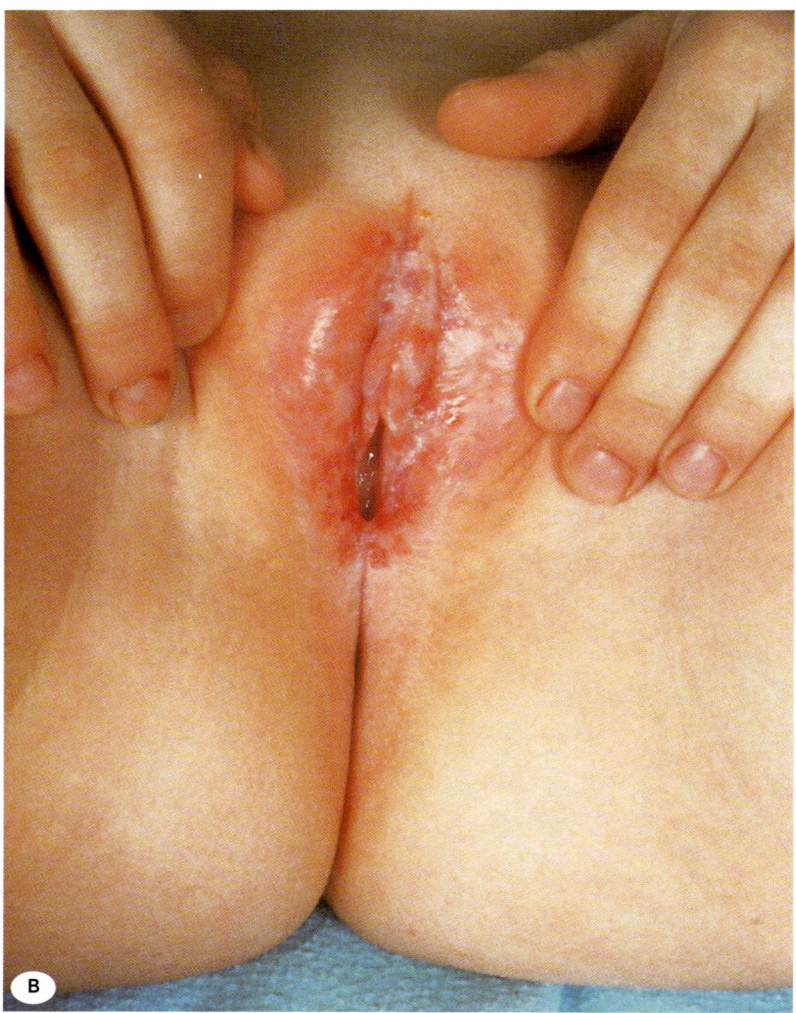

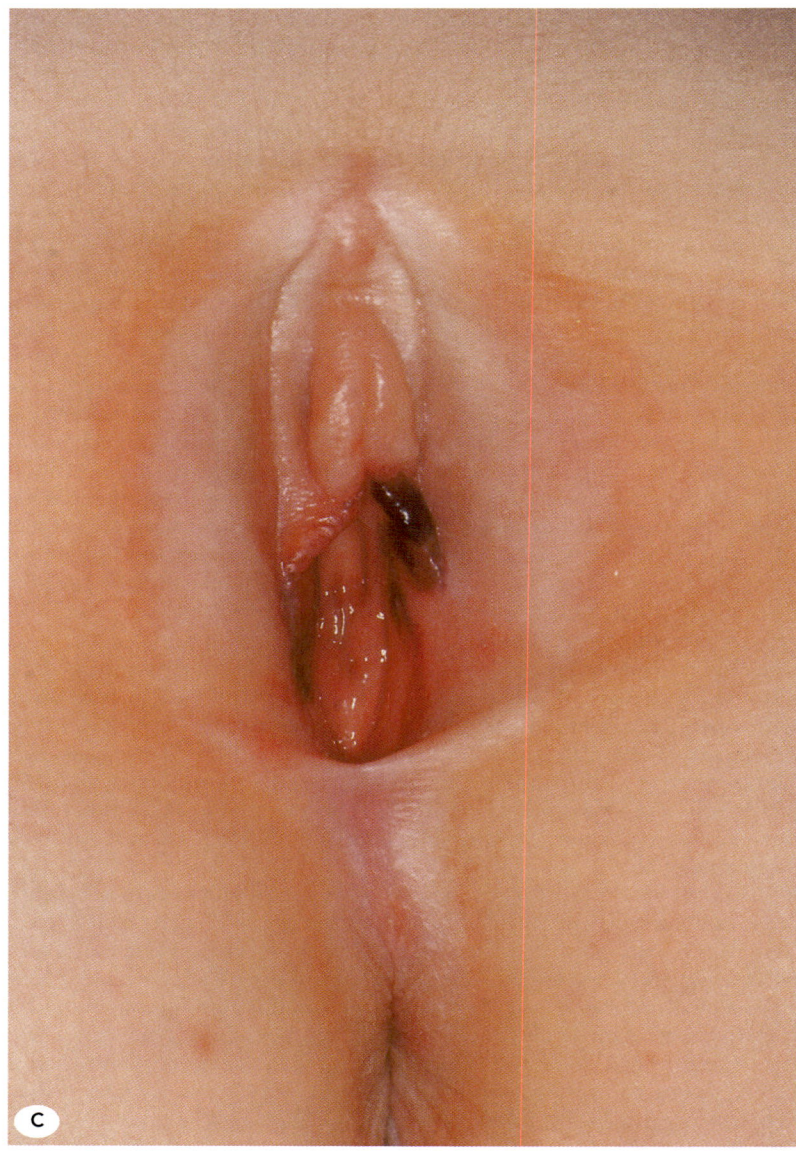

Fig. 18.9 (B) Lichen sclerosis with purpura on labia. (C) Classic hourglass appearance of lichen sclerosis.

conjunction with dermal sclerosis.[183] The distribution of collagen I and III and of elastin and fibrillin are altered, which may contribute to the fragility, scarring, and atrophy seen clinically.[184]

DIFFERENTIAL DIAGNOSIS

The diagnosis is not difficult when typical lesions with follicular plugging are seen or when white plaques involve the anogenital area in an hourglass configuration. Other causes of white plaques should be considered, including morphea, vitiligo, atrophic lichen planus, and annular discoid lupus erythematosus. Lesions in the vulva should be distinguished from candidiasis, bacterial vulvovaginitis, lichen simplex chronicus, pinworm infestations, and psoriasis. The disease may be mistaken for sexual abuse, but the diagnosis of LS should not exclude this possibility because there have been several reported cases of well-documented LS in sexually abused children.[185]

TREATMENT AND PROGNOSIS

There is no known cure for this disease. Therapy is aimed at alleviating symptoms. Because nongenital lesions are usually asymptomatic, therapy is usually not needed but is usually requested by the parents and patients if the lesions are widespread. Genital lesions are often symptomatic and require treatment. A low-potency topical steroid such as 1% hydrocortisone in an ointment base may be effective in alleviating most symptoms in children. Loening-Baucke[175] noted improvement in all children with hydrocortisone 1% ointment bid. If lesions do not respond to a weak steroid, a stronger corticosteroid, either a medium-strength or superpotent steroid, for a short period is very effective. The response to an ultrapotent topical corticosteroid is usually dramatic, and treatment can be altered to once daily and once every other day and then discontinued completely or maintained with a low-potency product.[186,187] Flares of disease activity can be retreated with a short course

183. Carlson JA, Lamb P, Malfetano J et al. (1998) Clinicopathologic comparison of vulvar and extragenital lichen sclerosus: histologic variants, evolving lesion, and etiology of 141 cases. **Modern Pathology** 11:844–854.
184. Farrell AM, Dean D, Millard PR et al. (2001) Alterations in fibrillin as well as collagens I and III and elastin occur in vulval lichen sclerosus. **J European Academy of Dermatology & Venereology** 15:212–217.

185. Harrington CL (1990) Lichen sclerosus (letter). **Arch Dis Child** 65:335.
186. Dalziel KL, Millard PR, Wojnarowska F (1991) The treatment of vulval lichen sclerosus with a very potent topical steroid (clobetasol propionate 0.05%) cream. **Br J Dermatology** 124:461–464.
187. Garzon MC, Paller AS (1999) Ultrapotent topical corticosteroid treatment of childhood genital lichen sclerosus. **Arch Dermatol** 135:525–528.

of a superpotent steroid. In patients who complain of tenderness or maceration, a thick coating of zinc oxide paste may help protect the area and give symptomatic relief, particularly before urinating or defecating. If secondary infection is present, a topical antifungal or antibacterial agent can be added. Topical anesthetics are sometimes useful. Because of the possibility of vulvar carcinoma, all cases that persist beyond puberty or occur in adults should be observed every year. Areas of leukoplakia, nodules, and persistent erosions should be biopsied.

The prognosis of LS with onset in childhood is better than in the adult-onset form of the disease, which tends to be chronic and usually permanent. Fifty percent of childhood cases clear within a period of one to 10 years, within an average of five years. Approximately two-thirds of cases improve or undergo involution before or at the time of puberty, leaving no residual atrophy.[165,166] In Helm et al.'s[188] series of 52 children and young adults, the average age at resolution was 15, which was slightly after menarche. Children may continue to have the disease beyond menarche. In children in whom the disease does not involute, atrophy of the clitoris and labia minora may occur, sometimes with fusion of the latter and stricture of the introitus.[166] A dilating procedure is sometimes indicated. The disease may be reactivated years later in patients who have improved, especially during pregnancy or after the use of oral contraceptives.[189] Males with LS of the glans may require urethral dilation, meatotomy, and circumcision in childhood, adolescence, or adulthood.[190]

ATROPHODERMAS

ATROPHODERMA OF PASINI AND PIERINI

This distinctive form of dermal atrophy resembles the resolved stage of morphea and, in fact, there is speculation that it may be a morphea variant.[191] Atrophic plaques occur primarily on the trunk of young women and, less frequently, young men in their teens and 20s (Fig. 18.10). The plaques are well circumscribed and soft, and have a depressed center with a "cliff-drop" border. They lack the induration typical of morphea.[192] The color ranges from normal, blue-brown or violaceous, unlike the white plaques of morphea that are surrounded by a lilac ring. Lesions vary in size from a few centimeters to twenty or more. They are seen most commonly on the back; the hands, feet, and face tend to be spared. The disease may remain active for 10 to 20 years.

Morphea-like changes may occur within a lesion or develop elsewhere. In a study by Jablonska, 139 patients with atrophoderma of Pasini and Pierini (APP) were followed long-term.[193] Induration resembling morphea appeared within the plaques of atrophoderma in 17% of patients, and in 22%, morphea plaques coexisted outside the atrophic areas; nevertheless, no case evolved into full-blown morphea. Histologically, APP preserves appendageal structures but elastic fibers may be decreased or clumped. Advanced lesions of atrophoderma are indistinguishable from morphea histologically.

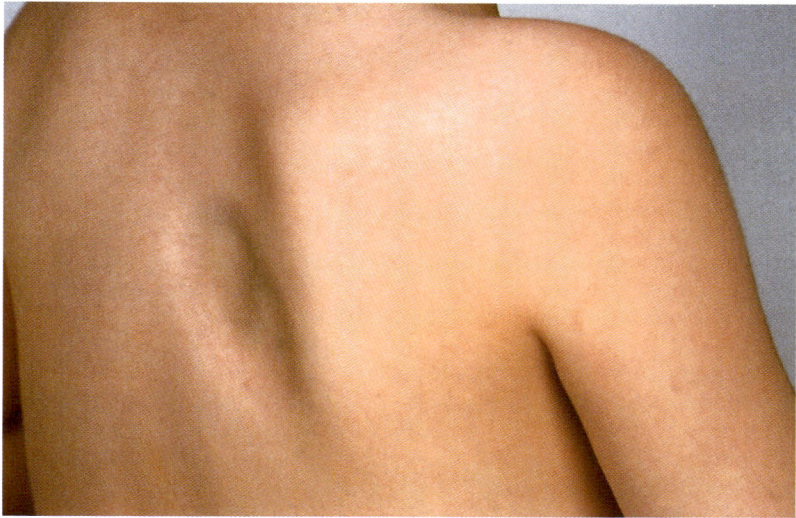

Fig. 18.10   Atrophoderma on back.

In 1992, Moulin reported five patients, reviewed by Wollenberg et al., with a new variant of atrophoderma.[194] The patients had multiple unilateral acquired hyperpigmented depressed linear plaques following Blaschko's lines. The lesions began during the first or second decades and evolved rapidly. They were asymptomatic, with no inflammatory or sclerotic phase. Skin biopsies only showed epidermal hyperpigmentation. One 16-year-old had preceding inflammation.[195] Potaba was helpful in one case;[196] intravenous penicillin had no effect in another case.[197]

The cause of APP is unknown. As in morphea and lichen sclerosis, there have been reports of Borrelia organisms in some patients.[198] Lasser et al.[199] described two siblings with phenylketonuria, one with APP and the other with severe segmental morphea, which suggests a close relationship between these diseases. DeBracco et al.[200] reported on a family with hereditary C2 deficiency in which one sibling had APP and the other had discoid lupus erythematosus.

There is no universally recognized form of treatment. There is one report of lightening of the hyperpigmentation following treatment with the Q-switched alexandrite laser.[201]

FOCAL FACIAL DERMAL DYSPLASIAS

In this group of disorders, congenital atrophic lesions are present on both temples.[202] In some reported families, the inheritance has been autosomal dominant and in others recessive. There may be additional facial features, such as facial clefts and absent or double rows of eyelashes (Seitlis syndrome). Kowalski proposed a classification based on clinical features and mode of inheritance.[203]

188. Helm KF, Gibson LE, Muller SA (1991) Lichen sclerosus et atrophicus in children and young adults. Pediatr Dermatol 8:97.
189. Rook A, Wilkinson DS, Ebling FJ, eds. (1979) Textbook of Dermatology. London: Blackwell Scientific.
190. Barbagli G, Lazzeri M, Palminteri E, Turini D (1999) Lichen sclerosis of male genitalia involving anterior urethra. Lancet 354:429.
191. Murphy PK, Hymes SR, Fenske NA (1990) Concomitant unilateral idiopathic atrophoderma of Pasini and Pierini (IAPP) and morphea. Observations supporting IAPP as a variant of morphea. Int J Dermatol 29:281.
192. Canizares O, Sachs P, Jaimovich L et al. (1958) Idiopathic atrophoderma of Pasini and Pierini. Arch Dermatol 77:42.
193. Kencka, D, Blaszcyk M, Jablonska S (1995) Atrophoderma Pasini-Pierini is a primary atrophic abortive morphea. Dermatology 190:203–206.
194. Wollenberg A, Baumann L, Plewig G (1996) Linear atrophoderma of Moulin: a disease which follows Blaschko's lines. Br J Dermatol 135:277–279.
195. Browne C, Fisher BK (2000) Atrophoderma of Moulin with preceding inflammation. Int J Dermatol 39:850–852.
196. Artola Igarza JL, Sanchez Conejo-Mir J, Corbi Llopis MR et al. (1996) Linear atrophoderma of Moulin: treatment with Potaba. Dermatology 193:345–347.
197. Rompel R, Mischke AL, Langner C, Happle R (2000) Linear atrophoderma of Moulin. Eur J Dermatol 10:611–613.
198. Buechner SA, Rufli T (1994) Atrophoderma of Pasini and Pierini. Clinical and histopathologic findings and antibodies to Borrelia burgdorferi in 34 patients. J Am Acad Dermatol 30:441–446.
199. Lasser AE, Schultz BC, Beaff D et al. (1978) Phenylketonuria and scleroderma. Arch Dermatol 114:1215.
200. DeBracco M, Bianchi C, Bianchi O et al. (1979) Hereditary complement (C2) deficiency with discoid lupus erythematosus and idiopathic atrophoderma. Int J Dermatol 18:713.
201. Arpey CJ, Patel DS, Stone MS et al. (2000) Treatment of atrophoderma of Pasini and Pierini-associated hyperpigmentation with the Q-switched alexandrite laser: a clinical, histologic, and ultrastructural appraisal. Lasers in Surgery & Medicine 27:206–212.
202. Magid M, Prendiville J, Esterly N (1988) Focal facial dermal dysplasia: bitemporal lesions resembling aplasia cutis congenita. J Am Acad Dermatol 18:1203–1207.
203. Kowalski D, Fenske N (1992) The focal facial dermal dysplasias: report of a kindred and a proposed new classification. J Am Acad Dermatol 27:575–582.

FOLLICULAR ATROPHODERMAS

The follicular atrophodermas are a rare group of inflammatory conditions, most of which develop in childhood. They are characterized by the presence of follicular plugging, followed by atrophy, and vary in their distribution and degree of preceding inflammation. Intermediate forms occur. In addition to the conditions described below, follicular atrophoderma can be seen in Conradi–Hunermann syndrome and in keratosis palmaris et plantaris. There is one case report associated with congenital pseudoarthrosis of the tibia,[204] another in a family with diffuse congenital ichthyosis with hypohidiosis and hypotrichosis,[205] and a family with a perioral and pigmented follicular atrophoderma with numerous milia and epidermoid cysts.[206]

Atrophoderma vermiculatum

In classic atrophoderma vermiculatum (folliculitis ulerythematosa reticulata, honeycomb atrophy), there are reticulated atrophic pits on the cheeks bilaterally (Fig. 18.11).[207,208] The condition is occasionally inherited as an autosomal dominant disorder. The disease begins in childhood between the ages of 5 and 12. Erythema and pinhead follicular plugs usually occur first. The plugs are then shed, resulting in reticulate atrophy from widely dilated follicles. Well demarcated atrophic pits 1–2mm across and 1mm deep are

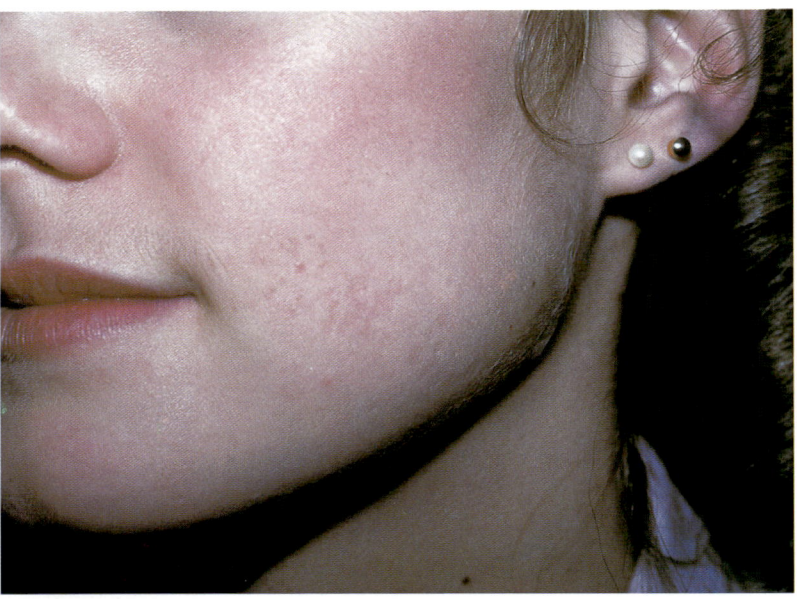

Fig. 18.11 In atrophoderma vermiculatum, reticulated atrophic small and large pits are seen under the cheek.

separated from each other by narrow ridges of normal skin, giving the skin a honeycomb or worm-eaten ("vermiculata") appearance. The cheeks and pre-auricular areas are most commonly involved, although the process can extend to the forehead, chin, and ears. A child with a unilateral form of the disorder has been reported,[209] with the lesions following Blaschko's lines.[210] Another report of unilateral involvement had associated cataracts and seizures.[211] Lesions improve over time, with spontaneous regression in most cases.[212] Dermabrasion and laser therapy[213] have both been utilized. Progression of the disease was halted in one patient after a prolonged course of isotretinoin.[214]

Atrophoderma vermiculatum has been reported in the Rombo syndrome (milia, hypotrichosis, basal cell carcinoma, and peripheral vasodilation with cyanosis).[212,215] Chloracne resulting in atrophoderma vermiculatum was observed in Italian children exposed to dioxin in the Seveso chemical accident.[216]

Keratosis pilaris atrophicans

Keratosis pilaris atrophicans (ulerythema oophyrogenes) is characterized by persistent erythema and small horny follicular papules that classically involve the lateral third of the eyebrows.[208] The process begins in early childhood. The eyebrow follicles are eventually destroyed, resulting in alopecia on the lateral margins of the eyebrows. When the disorder is confined to the lateral eyebrows, is is known as ulerythema ophyrogenes. The same follicular process may begin on the cheeks or temples instead of the eyebrows, or extend there from the eyebrows. The disorder is then called keratosis pilaris atrophicans faciei. The condition is occasionally inherited in an autosomal-dominant fashion and there is an association with Noonan's syndrome.[217] Pulsed dye laser has been successfully utilized to treat the erythema.[218]

Keratosis pilaris decalvans

Keratosis pilaris decalvans (keratosis follicularis spinulosa decalvans, follicular ichthyosis, or Siemen syndrome) begins in early infancy with facial keratosis pilaris.[208,219] The facial keratosis pilaris may be associated with numerous milia in early infancy. Later, follicular plugs develop on the neck and limbs. Shedding of the follicular plugs results in atrophic lesions on the cheeks. A cicatricial alopecia of the scalp and eyebrows develops during early adolescence. The condition is inherited in some patients in a X-linked recessive fashion. There is no known effective therapy. In some cases, corneal opacities, vascularization, and photophobia have been reported, as well as icthyosis vulgaris.[220] A mild palmoplantar keratoderma has been reported in some pedigrees.[221] Alopecia, generalized follicular keratosis, and reduced sweating were reported in one patient.[222]

Bazex syndrome is a *follicular atrophoderma* that occurs on the backs of the hands and feet in infancy.[223] Multiple basal cell carcinomas occur on the face from adolescence onward presenting as lightly pigmented papules. There may be associated hypotrichosis and hypohidrosis. The condition is inherited in

204. Perkins W, Weob DW, White JE (1995) Follicular atrophoderma in association with congenital pseudarthrosis of the tibia. J Roy Soc Med 88:291P–292P.
205. Lestringant GG, Kuster W, Frossard PM, Happle R (1998) Congenital ichthyosis, follicular atrophoderma, hypotrichosis, and hypohidrosis: a new genodermatosis? Am J Medical Genetics 75:186–189.
206. Inoue Y, Ono T, Kayashima K, Johno M (1998) Hereditary perioral pigmented follicular atrophoderma associated with milia and epidermoid custs. Br J Dermatol 139:713–718.
207. Rozyn KT, Mehregan AH, Johnson SA (1972) Folliculitis ulerythematosa reticulata: a case with a unilateral lesion. Arch Dermatol 106:388.
208. In: Andrews' Diseases of the Skin – Clinical Dermatology, Odom RB, James WD, Berger TG, eds. Philadelphia: WB Saunders, pp. 711–713.
209. Nico MM, Valente NY, Sotto MN (1998) Folliculitis ulerythematosa reticulata (atrophoderma vermiculata): early detection of a case with unilateral lesions. Pediatr Dermatol 15:285–286.
210. Cambiaghi S, Restano L, Tadini G (1999) Atrophoderma vermiculata along Blaschko lines (letter). Pediatric Dermatology 16:165.
211. Hsu S, Nikko A (2000) Unilateral atrophic skin lesion with features of atrophoderma vermiculatum: a variant of the epidermal nevus syndrome? J Am Acad Dermatol 43:310–312.
212. Frosch PJ, Brumage MR, Schuster-Pavlovic C, Bersch A (1988) Atrophoderma vermiculatum: case reports and review. J Am Acad Dermatol 18:538.
213. Handrick C, Alster TS (2001) Laser treatment of atrophoderma vermiculata. J Am Acad Dermatol 44:693–695.
214. Weightman W (1998) A case of atrophoderma vermiculatum responding to isotretinoin. Clinical & Experimental Dermatology 23:89–91.
215. van Steensel MA, Jaspers NG, Steijlen PM (2001) A case of Rombo syndrome. Br J Dermatology 114:1215–1218.
216. Pocchiare F et al. (1979) Human health effects from accidental release of TCDD (tetra choloro dibenzo-p-dioxin) at Seveso, Italy. Proc NY Acad Sci 320:300.
217. Snell JA, Mallory SB (1990) Ulerythema ophryogenes in Noonan syndrome. Pediatr Dermatol 7:77–78.
218. Clark SM, Mills, CM, Lanigan SW (2000) Treatment of keratosis pilaris atrophicans with the pulsed tunable dye laser. J Cutaneous Laser Therapy 2:151–156.
219. Maroon M, Tyler WB, Marks VJ (1992) Keratosis pilaris and scarring alopecia. Keratosis follicularis spinulosa decalvans. Arch Dermatol 128:397.
220. Zeligman I, Fleisher TL (1959) Ichthyosis follicularis. Arch Dermatol 80:413.
221. Kuokkanen K (1971) Keratosis follicularis spinulosa decalvans in a family from northern Finland. Acta Derm Venereol (Stockh) 51:146.
222. Morris J, Ackerman AB, Koblenzer PF (1969) Generalized spiny hyperkeratosis, universal alopecia, and deafness. Arch Dermatol 100:692.
223. Viksnins P, Berlin A (1977) Follicular atrophoderma and basal cell carcinomas: the Bazex syndrome. Arch Dermatol 113:948.

PHYSICAL EXAMINATION

Because of the near absence of the dermis, there are circumscribed areas in which the skin is thinned and its surface depressed or pouched out (Fig. 18.13).[257] Fat may herniate through the thinned dermis, causing soft erythematous or tan outpouchings from the skin's surface. Other lesions are telangiectasias on a hypo- or hyperpigmented background. Because of the atrophy and pigmentary changes, the lesions are frequently described as poikilodermatous. Lesions are grouped in a linear pattern. The focal areas of atrophy make the skin appear reticulated and cribriform. At birth, some areas may be ulcerated, as in aplasia cutis congenita; these defects are usually small and heal spontaneously. Bullae and erythematous or urticarial lesions may also be present at birth; histologic studies of one such patient showed a perivascular lymphocytic infiltrate and marked edema of the papillary dermis.[258] There are reports of mild forms of the disease; the patients have linear atrophic telangiectatic scaly macules and patches without fat herniations.[252,259]

Characteristic of focal dermal hypoplasia is the progressive development of raspberry-like papillomas around the lips, anus, genitalia, on the digits and, occasionally, elsewhere on the skin.[260] These are not present at birth but begin to develop within the first few months of life. They can become very large and can erode, ulcerate, and bleed.[258] Papillomas in the larynx can cause stricture, prompting tracheostomy and resection;[261] in the esophagus, they have caused stricture as well.[262]

Other cutaneous changes that have been reported include, urticaria, dermographism, hyperkeratosis of the soles, radial folds that emanate from the corners of the mouth, photosensitivity, sweating abnormalities, and dermatoglyphic changes.[248]

Although several cases have been reported with abnormalities limited to the skin, most patients have extracutaneous findings.[259] The scalp hair may be sparse and brittle, with focal areas of alopecia in areas of severe atrophy or aplasia. The nails may be dystrophic or absent. There are many dental abnormalities associated with Goltz syndrome, including absence of the teeth, enamel defects, and small, defectively formed teeth that erupt slowly. Cleft lip and/or palate may occur.

Skeletal defects are the second most common extracutaneous abnormalities seen in 80% of patients.[246] The most common is fusion or absence of the fingers or toes but other bones may also be absent. Vertebral abnormalities are common and include scoliosis, kyphosis, vertebral body fusions, and spina bifida. Many patients have short stature. One side of the face or body may be underdeveloped.[263] A wide variety of other changes have been reported. Mental retardation is present in some; diffuse cortical and cerebellar atrophy can be seen with magnetic resonance imaging.[264] Eye abnormalities are found in 80% of patients.[246] These include colobomas of the iris, retina, and globe; microphthalmia, anophthalmia, tear duct anomalies, and ocular muscle and corneal abnormalities.[265] The pinnae may be misshapened, and some patients have hearing loss. Cardiac, renal, and central nervous system defects have been described.[248,258] Multiple central giant-cell-like tumors of the maxilla and mandible have occurred in some patients.[266]

LABORATORY FINDINGS
Radiographic findings
Most of the radiographic changes correspond to the clinical skeletal anomalies. However, typical of focal dermal hypoplasia are radiographs of the

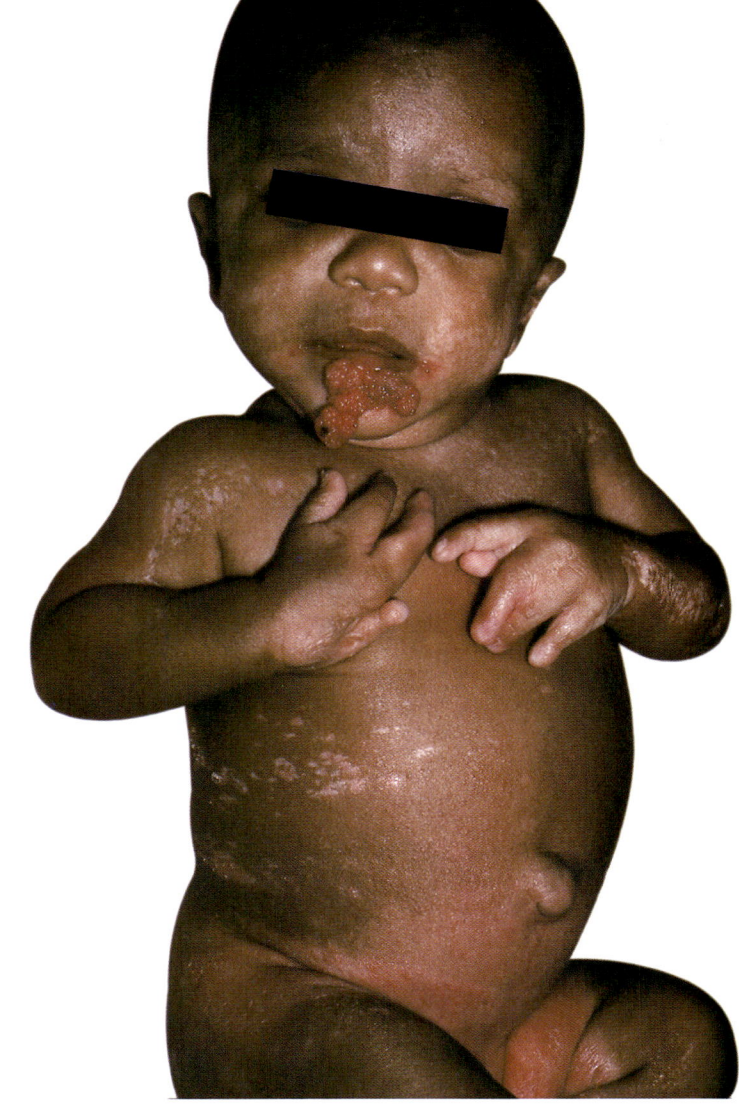

A

Fig. 18.13 (A) Infant with cutaneous, mucosal, and skeletal abnormalities of focal dermal hypoplasia.

long bone that show fine linear striations, called osteopathia striata, at or near the epiphyseal junctions. These occur in many, but not all, patients.[258] Another characteristic change is widening of the symphysis pubis. The bones usually have decreased density, sometimes with cyst formation.[267] Mediastinal dextroposition and intestinal malrotation have been reported.[268]

PATHOPHYSIOLOGY AND HISTOGENESIS

A skin biopsy of an atrophic lesion shows a normal or thinned epidermis overlying a severely hypoplastic dermis, with adipose tissue impinging on the

257. Goltz RW, Henderson RR, Hutch JM, Ott JE (1970) Focal dermal hypoplasia syndrome: a review of the literature and report of two cases. **Arch Dermatol** 101:1.
258. Goltz RW (1992) Focal dermal hypoplasia: an update (editorial review). **Arch Dermatol** 128:1108.
259. Pujol RM, Casanova JM, Perez M et al. (1992) Focal dermal hypoplasia (Goltz syndrome): report of 2 cases with minor cutaneous and extracutaneous manifestations. **Pediatr Dermatol** 9:112.
260. Kore-Eda S, Yoneda K, Ohtani T et al. (1995) Focal dermal hypoplasia (Goltz syndrome) associated with multiple giant papillomas. **Br J Dermatol** 133:997–999.
261. Gordjani N, Herdeg S, Ross UH et al. (1999) Focal dermal hypoplasia (Goltz-Gorlin syndrome) associated with obstructive papillomatosis of the larynx and hypopharynx. **Eur J Dermatol** 9:618–620.
262. Brinson RR, Schuman BM, Mills LR et al. (1987) Multiple squamous papillomas of the esophagus associated with Goltz syndrome. **Am J Gastroenterol** 82:1177–1179.

263. Landa N, Oleaga JM, Raton JA et al. (1993) Focal dermal hypoplasia (Goltz syndrome): an adult case with multisystemic involvement. **J Am Acad Dermatol** 28:86–89.
264. Gunduz K, Gunalp I, Erden I (1997) Focal dermal hypoplasia (Goltz's syndrome). **Ophthalmic Paediatrics & Genetics** 18:143–149.
265. Lueder GT, Steiner RD (1995) Corneal abnormalities in a mother and daughter with focal dermal hypoplasia (Goltz-Gorlin syndrome). **Am J Ophthalmol** 120:256–258.
266. Selzer G, David R, Revach M et al. (1974) Goltz syndrome with multiple giant-cell tumor-like lesions in bones. **Ann Intern Med** 80:714.
267. D'Alise MD, Timmons CF, Swift DM (1996) Focal dermal hypoplasia (Goltz syndrome) with vertebral solid aneurysmal bone cyst variant. A case report. **Pediatr Neurosurg** 24:151–154.
268. Irvine AD, Stewart FJ, Bingham EA et al. (1996) Focal dermal hypoplasia (Goltz syndrome) associated with intestinal malrotation and mediastinal dextroposition. **Am J Med Genet** 62:213–215.

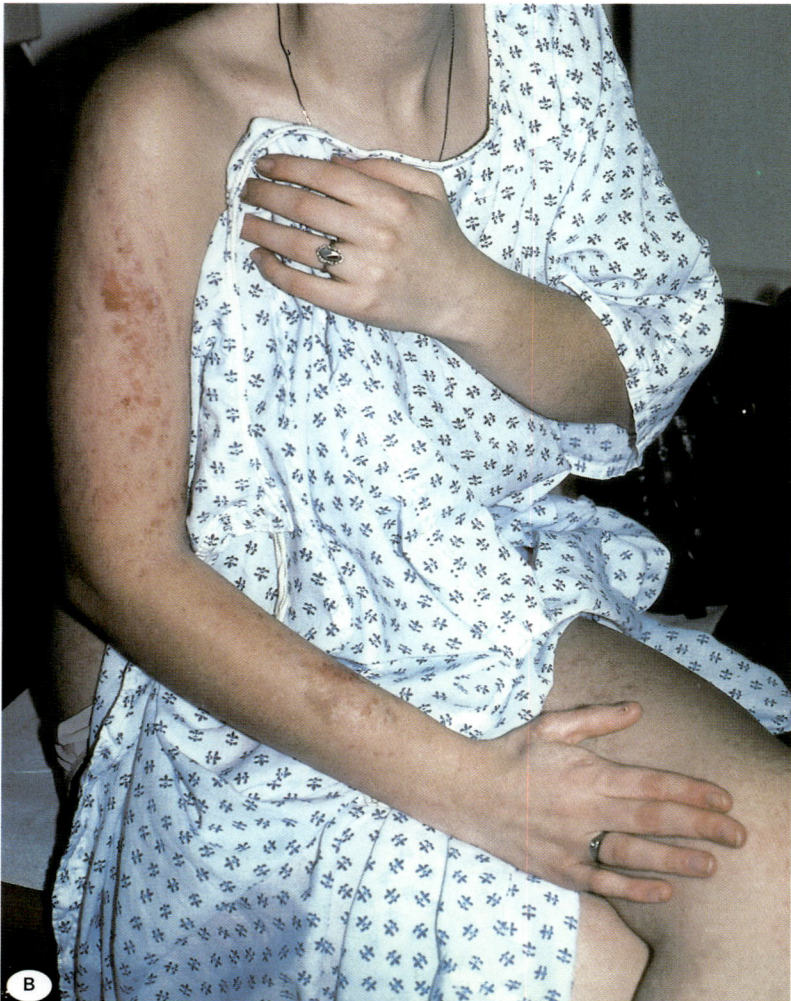

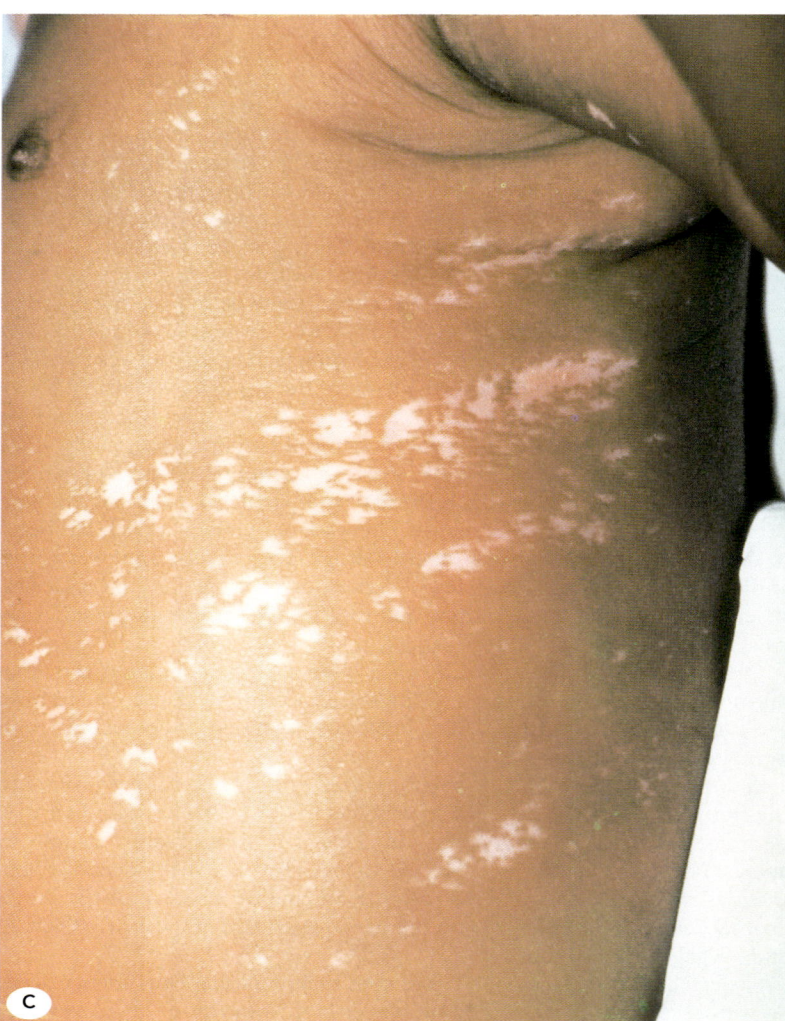

Fig. 18.13   (B) Poikilodermatous grouped linear lesions on the arm of a female adolescent. (C) Linear hypopigmentation on chest wall in a Blaschkoid distribution.

epidermis. A narrow remnant of dermis is usually present along the dermal-epidermal junction and around appendageal structures; in less severely affected areas, there may be remnants of fibrous tissue, especially near the dermal blood vessels. In focal areas where no residual dermis remains, the epidermis cannot survive and ulceration results.[248] The papillomas are fibrovascular structures which, on electron microscopy of an atrophic site, show loose collagen bundles, collagen fibers with loss of regular bands, abnormal fibroblasts, and disruption of the basement membrane zone, suggesting abnormal formation of type IV collagen.[269]

The underlying basic defect is unknown. Happle et al.[249] argue that the linear pattern of the skin lesions conforms to Blaschko's lines and is due to X-chromosomal mosaicism, with X inactivation, according to the Lyon hypothesis. Uitto et al.[270] cultured fibroblasts from a patient with focal dermal hypoplasia and found them to be markedly abnormal. The cells from affected skin had an abnormally long mean doubling time, whereas cells from normal-appearing skin grew normally. The cultured cells also demonstrated unusual cytoplasmic vacuoles although these vacuoles were not seen in a biopsy specimen obtained from another patient and examined

ultrastructurally.[270] The rate of collagen synthesis in the cultured cells, however, was undisturbed and appeared normal. Normal wound healing has been reported in one patient with focal dermal hypoplasia who required a surgical incision through an area of abnormal skin for treatment of a stress fracture of the femur.[271] Tsuji[272] reported multilocular fat cells, which are regarded as young cells, and therefore proposed that the disease is characterized by an overgrowth of adipose tissue and a decreased rate of collagen synthesis. Sato et al. found abnormalities in glycosaminoglycan in cultured fibroblasts.[273]

DIFFERENTIAL DIAGNOSIS

The linear pattern and pigmentary changes are suggestive of incontinentia pigmenti, but can be readily differentiated clinically and histologically. The eosinophilic spongiosis seen in incontinentia pigmenti is not present in focal dermal hypoplasia. Herniations of fat are not seen in incontinentia pigmenti. An epidermal nevus can be linear and associated with underlying skeletal anomalies but is hypertrophic rather than atrophic, and is readily distinguished

269. Lee IJ, Cha MS, Kim SC, Bang D (1996) Electronmicroscopic observation of the basement membrane zone in focal dermal hypoplasia. **Pediatr Dermatol** 13:5–9.
270. Uitto J, Bauer EA, Santa-Cruz DJ et al. (1980) Focal dermal hypoplasia: abnormal growth characteristics of skin fibroblasts in culture. **J Invest Dermatol** 75:170.
271. Burkhart CG (1983) Goltz's syndrome and wound healing (letter). **Arch Dermatol** 119:187.

272. Tsuji T (1982) Focal dermal hypoplasia syndrome. An electron microscopical study of the skin lesions. **J Cutan Pathol** 9:271.
273. Sato M, Ishikawa O, Yokoyam Y et al. (1996) Focal dermal hypoplasia (Goltz syndrome): a decreased accumulation of hyaluronic acid in three-dimensional culture. **Acta Dermato-Venereologica** 76:365–367.

with a biopsy. CHILD syndrome is an acronym for congenital icthyosiform erythroderma with limb defects; there is no dermal hypoplasia and the lesions are unilateral. Areas of epidermal aplasia can be seen in congenital aplasia cutis and in Bart syndrome (local congenital absence of skin associated with epidermolysis bullosa), but these lesions are usually solitary and not associated with the other changes seen in focal dermal hypoplasia. One variant of aplasia cutis, called Adams–Oliver syndrome, has associated limb abnormalities but many of these patients have an associated cutis marmorata. In the Rothmund–Thomson syndrome, the poikiloderma is more severe, and there is an associated photosensitivity and dwarfism. Nevus lipomatosis superficialis is similar to focal dermal hypoplasia histologically but, clinically is composed of raised papules and plaques. Happle et al.[249] reported linear lesions of dermal aplasia in an infant with microphthalmia, sclerocornea, and a congenital heart defect who had a gene defect involving Xp 22.3. The skin lesions differed in that there was no herniation. They called this condition the MIDAS complex and argued that it is distinct from focal dermal hypoplasia. Focal dermal hypoplasia papillomas can be readily differentiated from condyloma acuminatum by skin biopsy.

THERAPY AND PROGNOSIS

There is no known effective treatment for this disease, but patients have a normal life span and can lead normal lives. Surgical correction of skeletal defects should be considered. Families should receive genetic counseling. In some patients, the areas of cutaneous involvement may slowly progress over time. There is one report of a patient with focal dermal hypoplasia in whom a vascular pelvic mass occurred; it was successfully treated with embolization.[274] Cryotherapy effectively controlled giant papillomas on the trunk and extremities in one patient,[260] and pulsed dye laser has been used to treat cutaneous lesions.[275]

APLASIA CUTIS CONGENITA

Aplasia cutis congenita (ACC) is characterized by the absence of localized or widespread areas of skin at birth. The defect is most common on the scalp. It can be associated with other developmental anomalies. More than 500 cases have been reported since Cordon's original article in 1767. Frieden[276] classifies the disorder into nine categories.

EPIDEMIOLOGY

There is no sexual or racial predilection. There have been familial cases reported in Frieden groups 1, 2, 5, 6, 7, and 9.

PRESENTING HISTORY

The clinical findings are present at birth. In some cases, there may be a family history of a similar disorder.

PHYSICAL EXAMINATION
Group 1: scalp without multiple anomalies

The scalp is the most common site of involvement (Fig. 18.14). Scars at birth, especially in the midline area of the scalp, without a history of preceding trauma, are highly suggestive of ACC. A family history of similar lesions is

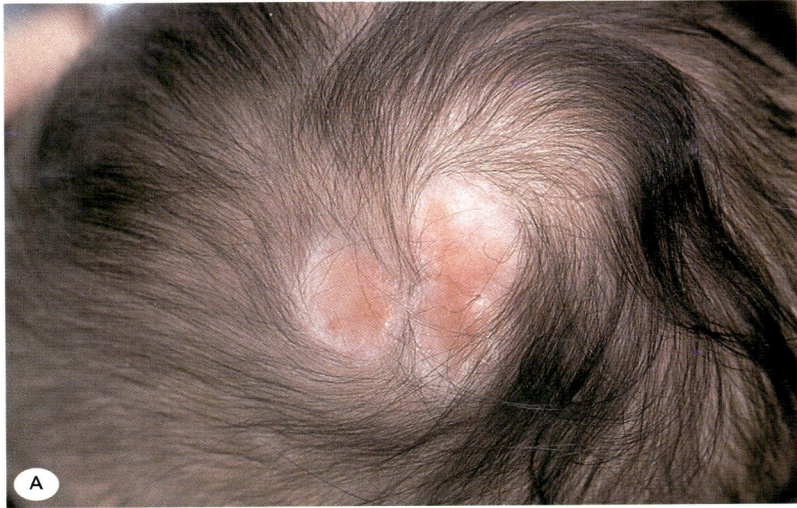

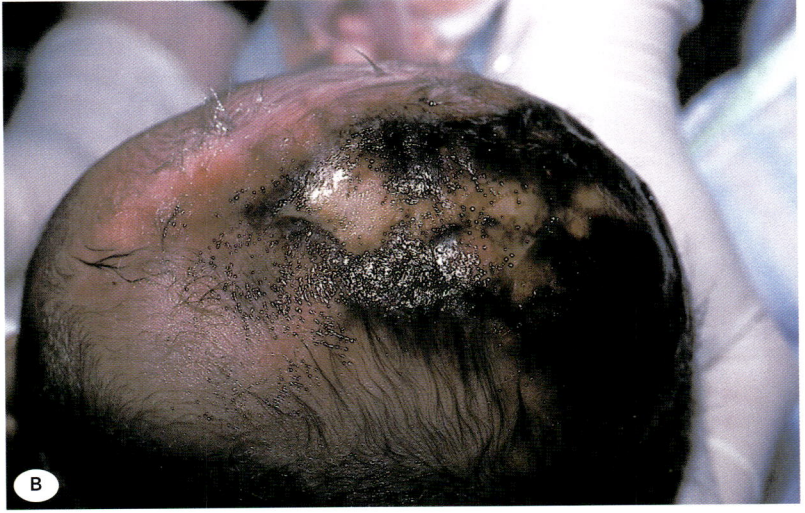

Fig. 18.14   (A) Scar lesions of aplasia cutis congenita at birth. (B) Ulcerated scalp lesion of aplasia cutis congenita.

often obtained. Nearly 86% of all solitary lesions occur on the vertex of the scalp near the parietal hair whorl.[277,278] Seventy to 75% of scalp lesions are single, 20% have two lesions, and 8% have multiple lesions. They range in size from 0.5 to 5.0cm,[276] and may be circular, oval, linear, or stellate. Lesions may be scarred, superficially eroded, or deeply ulcerated, sometimes down to the dura or meninges. There is one report of a scalp lesion covered by a membranous epithelium, looking like a bulla.[279] There are reports of scalp ACC, without other defects, in family members.[280]

Infants do not normally have multiple anomalies, but patients with isolated anomalies are included in this group. Examples are cleft palate, tracheoesophageal fistula, double uterus, congenital heart disease, omphalocele, polycystic kidneys, mental retardation, cutis marmorata telangiectatica congenita, and congenital nystagmus with high myopia[276,281]

274. Lynch RD, Leshner RT, Nicholls PJ, Matthew WE (1971) Focal dermal hypoplasia (Goltz's syndrome) with an expansile iliac lesion. J Bone Joint Surg [Am] 63:470.
275. Alster TS, Wilson F (1995) Focal dermal hypoplasia (Goltz's syndrome). Treatment of cutaneous lesions with the 585-nm flashlamp-pumped pulsed dye laser. Arch Dermatol 131:143–144.
276. Frieden IJ (1986) Aplasia cutis congenita: a clinical review and proposal for classification. J Am Acad Dermatol 14:646.
277. Ingalls NW (1933) Congenital defects of the scalp: studies in the pathology of development. Am J Obstet Gynecol 25:861.
278. Stephan MF, Smith DW, Ponzi JW, Alden ER (1982) Origin of scalp vertex aplasia cutis. J Pediatr 101:850.
279. Yudkin S (1948) Congenital defect of the scalp: an infant with a bullous lesion at birth. Arch Dis Child 23:61.
280. Tan HH, Tay YK (1997) Familial aplasia cutis congenita of the scalp: a case report and review. Annals of the Academy of Medicine, Singapore 26:500–502.
281. Gershoni-Baruch R, Leibo R (1996) Aplasia cutis congenita, high myopia, and cone-rod dysfunction in two sibs: a new autosomal recessive disorder. Am J Med Genet 61:42–42.

Group 2: scalp with limb anomalies (Adams–Oliver syndrome)

In this distinct subtype, distal limb reduction abnormalities are found in association with solitary midline scalp defects (Fig. 18.15). There have been 15 cases reported, usually with an autosomal dominant inheritance pattern, of variable genetic expression.[282] Scalp lesions vary in size but tend to be large and associated with dilated scalp veins and underlying skull defects[283]. The most common limb malformation is hypoplastic or absent distal phalanges, syndactyly, ectrodactyly, club foot, and distal limb absence. Other anomalies include persistent cutis marmorata telangiectatica congenita (Fig. 18.16), hemangiomas, cranial arteriovenous malformation, skin tags, supernumerary nipples, and wooly hair.[276] Intracranial calcifications were seen in one infant,[283] dysplasia of the cerebral cortex in another,[284] and polymicrogyria with psychomotor retardation in two siblings.[285]

Group 3: scalp with epidermal and sebaceous nevi

There have been several cases reported of ACC associated with epidermal or sebaceous nevi involving the scalp, usually adjacent to the ACC.[276] Some patients have also had ophthalmic and neurologic findings similar to those found in the epidermal nevus syndrome, including seizures, mental retardation, corneal opacities, and eyelid colobomas. There have been no familial cases reported to date.

Group 4: overlying embryologic malformations

In various types of major malformations, there may be a congenital absence of skin overlying the deeper defect. Examples include meningomyelocele, gastroschisis, omphalocele, ilial atresia,[286] bilial mid-gut atresia,[287] spinal dysraphism, porencephaly, leptomeningeal angiomatosis, and cranial stenosis. The inheritance pattern in this group depends on the associated underlying condition.

Group 5: associated with fetus papyraceus or placental infarct

Mannino et al.[288] reviewed 17 cases of extensive truncal and limb ACC (Fig. 18.17) associated with the presence of a fetus papyraceus, which is found

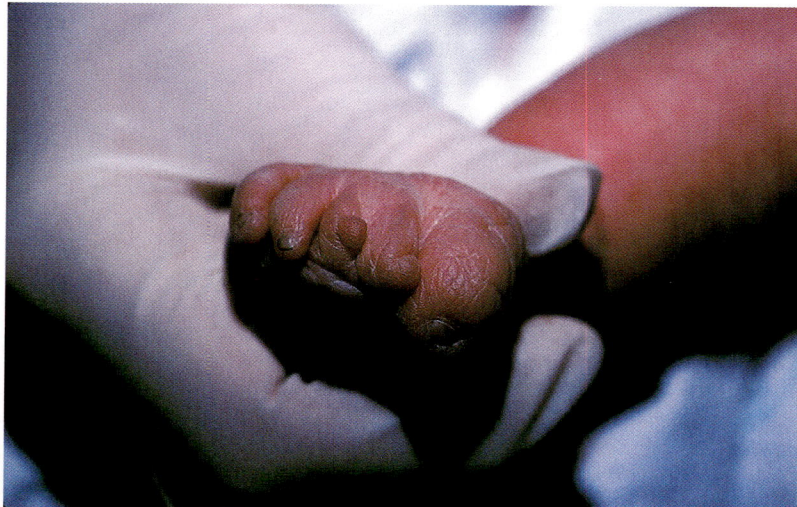

Fig. 18.15   Adams–Oliver with limb shortening.

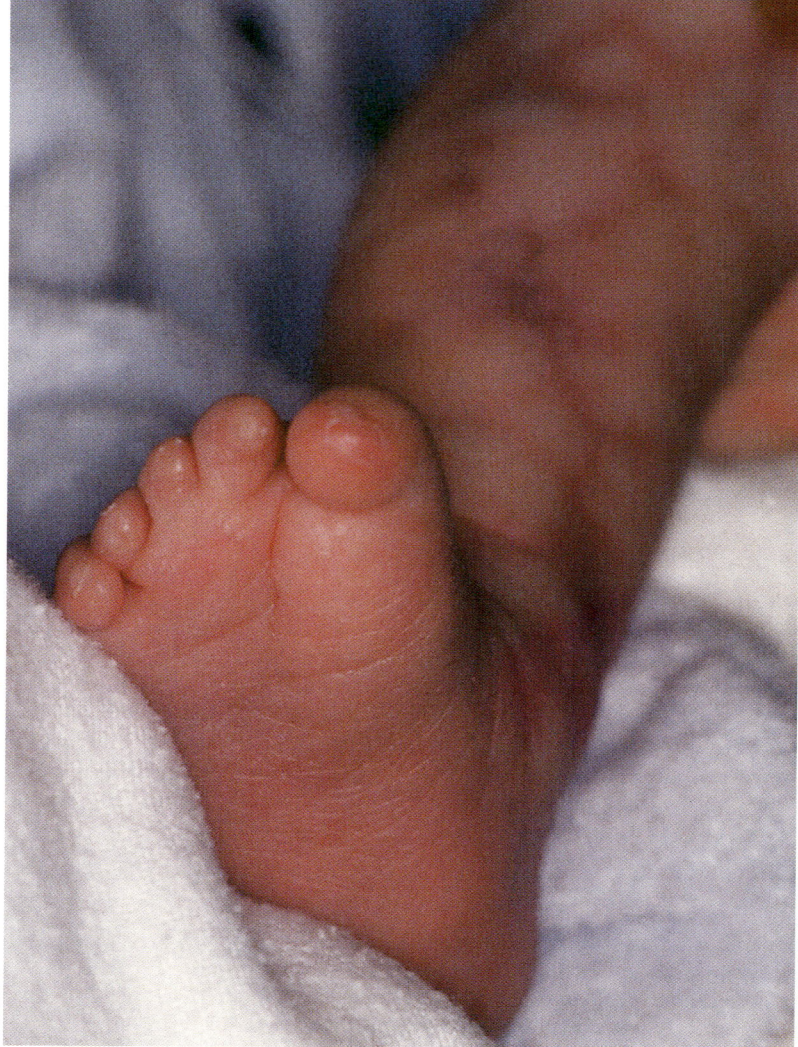

Fig. 18.16   Adams–Oliver with cutis marmorata telangiectatica congenita.

at delivery in the placenta, and is caused by the death of a twin fetus during the second trimester. In a large proportion of twin pregnancies, there are vascular anastomoses or interconnections within the placenta(s).[289] Complications from this shunting can affect one or both fetuses. If one of the co-twins dies, clots or necrotic tissue from the dead twin may enter the circulation of the surviving twin. During the second trimester, vascularization is related to the iliac and umbilical arteries, which explains the frequent distribution of this variant of ACC over the flanks and upper thighs. The surviving twin has ACC, possibly from vascular disruption of the placenta[290] but is usually otherwise normal; there have been associated findings reported, which include constricting bands of tight fibrous tissue on the extremities, psychomotor retardation, hydranencephaly, nail dystrophy, and clubbed hands and feet.[276] No familial cases have been reported. To confirm the diagnosis, a complete pathologic study of the placenta and membranes can be performed to look for the presence of the fetus papyraceus.[290]

282. Wilson WG, Harcus SJ (1982) Variable expressions of a congenital scalp defect/limb malformations syndrome in 3 generations. **Birth Defects** 18:123.
283. Romani J, Puig L, Aznar G et al. (1998) Adams-Oliver syndrome with unusual central nervous system alterations. **Pediatr Dermatol** 15:48–50.
284. Savarirayan R, Thompson EM, Abbott KJ, Moore MH (1999) Cerebral cortical dysplasia and digital constriction rings in Adams-Oliver syndrome. **Am J Med Genet** 86:15–19.
285. Amor DJ, Leventer RJ, Hayllar S, Bankier A (2000) Polymicrogyria associated with scalp and limb defects: variant of Adams-Oliver syndrome. **Am J Med Genet** 93:328–334.
286. Al-Sawan RMZ, Soni AL, Al-Kobrosly AM et al. (1999) Truncal aplasia cutis congenita associated with ileal atresia and mesenteric defect. **Pediatr Dermatol** 16:498–509.
287. Lane W, Zanol K (2000) Duodenal atresia, biliary atresia, and intestinal infarct in truncal aplasia cutis congenita. **Pediatr Dermatol** 17:290–292.
288. Mannino FL, Jones KL, Bernischke K (1977) Congenital skin defects and fetus papyraceus. **J Pediatr** 91:559.
289. Leaute-Labreze, Depaire-Duclos F, Sarlangue J et al. (1998) Congenital cutaneous defects as complications in surviving co-twins: aplasia cutis congenita and neonatal Volkmann ischemic contracture of the forearm. **Arch Dermatol** 134:1121–1124.
290. Cambiaghi S, Schiera A, Tasin L, Gelmetti C (2001) Aplasia cutis congenita in surviving co-twins: four unrelated cases. **Pediatr Dermatol** 18:511–515.

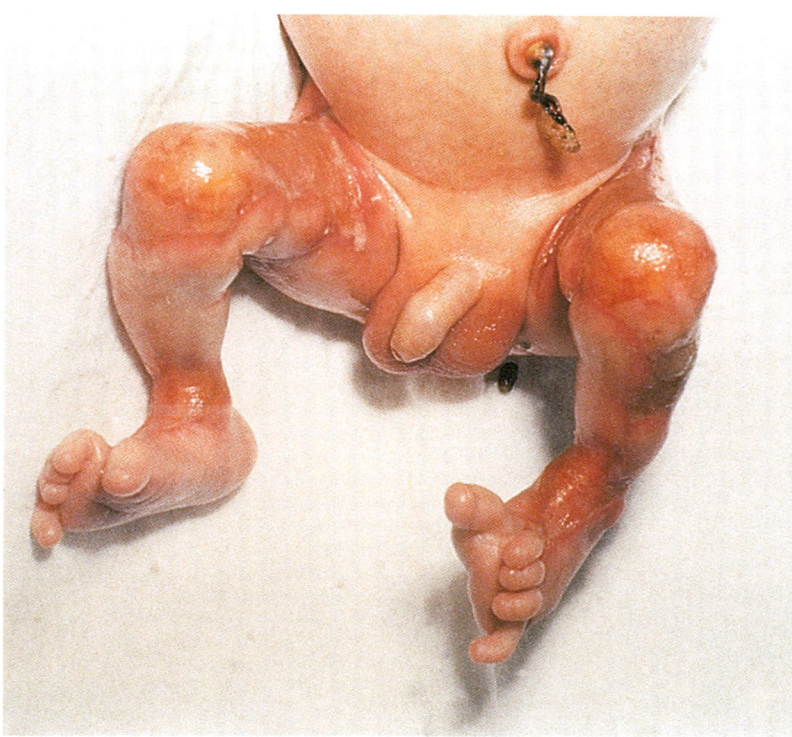

Fig. 18.17   Bilateral aplasia cutis from fetus papyraceous.

Group 6: associated with epidermolysis bullosa

There have been many reports of ACC, usually occurring on the lower extremities, in cases of epidermolysis bullosa (EB). This was thought to represent a distinct entity known as Bart syndrome, but subsequently, it has been shown to represent a specific presentation of EB. At least five types of EB have been reported with ACC: recessive dystrophic EB, dominant dystrophic EB (Cockayne–Touraine variant), Weber–Cockayne EB simplex, EB simplex, and junctional EB. Frieden[276] proposed that the lesions develop on the lower extremities because of mechanical trauma *in utero* due to fetal kicking, which leads to *in utero* blistering and subsequent erosions.

Group 7: extremities without epidermolysis bullosa

There have been at least two families in whom multiple members have had extensive ACC of the lower extremities.[276] Some of these patients have also had affected feet and hands.

Group 8: due to teratogens

There have been a few cases of ACC linked to intrauterine infection with herpes simplex virus or varicella and to the medications valproate and methimazole, which is given during pregnancy for the treatment of thyrotoxicosis.[276]

Group 9: associated with syndromes of malformation

ACC has been reported in association with various syndromes and dysplasias.[276] These include trisomy 134p-syndrome, ectodermal dysplasia, Johanson–Blizzard syndrome, focal dermal hypoplasia (Goltz syndrome), and 46 XY gonadal dysgenesis. In Xp22 deletion syndrome, bilateral linear reticulated defects are found on the malar areas of the face.[291] In the amniotic band syndrome, a ring-like constriction forms that can surround a limb and cause focal aplasia and amputation.[292]

LABORATORY FINDINGS

There are no consistent or specific laboratory abnormalities found in ACC, but there may be abnormalities caused by some of the associated findings.

PATHOPHYSIOLOGY AND HISTOGENESIS

The histology varies according to the depth of the aplasia and its duration. At birth, deeply ulcerated lesions may show complete absence of skin. After healing, the epidermis, if present, is thinned and flattened, and there may be a proliferation of fibroblasts within the connective tissue stroma.

Because ACC is a clinical finding that occurs in more than one disease state, it is very likely that there is more than one mechanism of pathogenesis. The disruption of skin development occurs *in utero*, so genetic factors are one mechanism by which the abnormality may be produced. Other proposed mechanisms include trauma, compromised cutaneous vasculature, and teratogens. Stephan *et al.*[278] noted the proximity of scalp ACC to the scalp hair whorl, which is thought to be the point of maximum tensile force during rapid brain growth. They hypothesized that tension-induced disruption of the overlying skin occurs at 10–18 weeks of gestation, when hair direction, patterning, and rapid brain growth occurs. Early rupture of the amniotic membranes is associated with this disorder in several cases.[276]

DIFFERENTIAL DIAGNOSIS

Diagnostic considerations include an encephalocele or a dermoid cyst. ACC must also be differentiated from the erosions of EB; this can be confusing because patients with EB can also have ACC. Neonatal herpes may present with an eroded plaque, not uncommonly on the scalp. Unlike ACC, neonatal herpes is uncommon at birth. In the first few days of life, congenital erosive and vesicular dermatosis, healing with reticulated supple scarring[293] can look similar to the erythematous erosions or partially healed erosions seen in some infants with ACC. Focal dermal hypoplasia and amniotic band syndrome also needs to be differentiated.

THERAPY AND PROGNOSIS

Treatment is rarely necessary because the erosions and ulcerations almost always heal spontaneously and the prognosis is usually excellent; if the ACC is associated with other syndromes, the prognosis is dependent on the prognosis associated with the syndrome. Genetic counseling is advised for all affected infants. Occasional patients require skin grafting. If the dura is exposed, the defect needs to be covered early with full-thickness skin flaps and/or frequent moist dressings; if an eschar forms over the exposed dura, there is a high risk of infection or life-threatening hemorrhage from laceration of the sagittal sinus.[294–296]

FAT ATROPHY (LIPOATROPHY)

Atrophy of the subcutaneous fat may be a localized problem, as in the localized annular lipodystrophies; it may be more widespread, involving an entire area of the body, as in partial atrophy (lipodystrophy); or rarely, it can affect the entire body, as it does in total lipoatrophy (lipodystrophy).

291. Zvulunov A, Kachko L, Manor E et al. (1998) Reticulolinear aplasia cutis congenita of the face and neck: a distinctive cutaneous manifestation in several syndromes linked to Xp22. **Br J Dermatol** 138:1046–1052.
292. Nagore E, Sanchez-Motilla JM, Febrer MI et al. (1999) Radius hypoplasia, radial palsy and aplasia cutis due to amniotic band syndrome. **Pediatr Dermatol** 16:217–219.
293. Cohen BA, Esterly NB, Nelson PF (1985) Congenital erosive and vesicular dermatosis healing with reticulated supple scarring. **Arch Dermatol** 121:361.
294. Abbott R, Cutting CB, Wisoff JH et al. (1991–1992) Aplasia cutis congenita of the scalp: issues in its management. **Pediatr Neurosurg** 17:182.
295. Kim CS, Tatum SA, Rocziewicz G (2001) Scalp aplasia congenita presenting with sagittal sinus hemorrhage. **Arch Otolaryngol Head Neck Surg** 127:71–74.
296. Simman R, Priebe CJ, Simon M (2000) Reconstruction of aplasia cutis congenita of the trunk in a newborn infant using acellular allogenic dermal graft and cultured epithelial autografts. **Ann Plast Surg** 44:451–454.

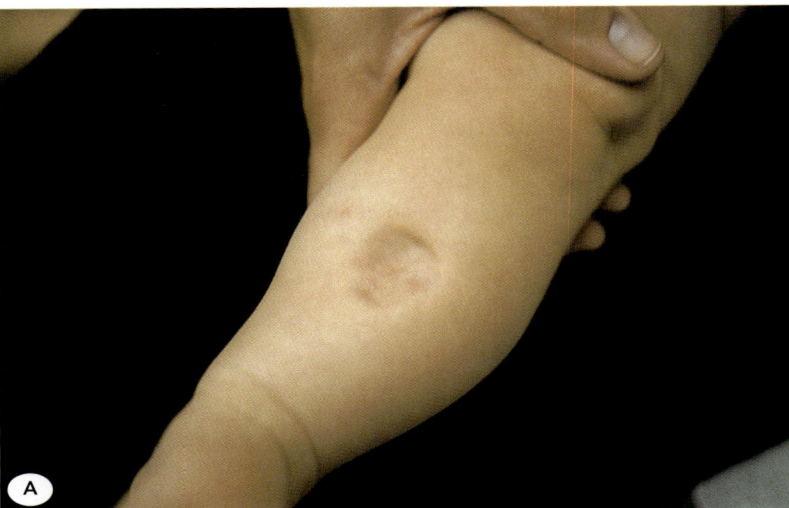

Fig. 18.18 **(A)** Localized annular lipoatrophy on the leg of a child: no antecedent injections or injuries. **(B)** Lipoatrophy of the back.

LOCALIZED ANNULAR LIPOATROPHY

Several clinical forms of localized lipoatrophy are described but are rare. *Lipoatrophia semicircularis* presents with a circular, band-like depression on the extensor surface of the thigh or lateral arms (Fig. 18.18).[297] There is no accompanying epidermal atrophy or color change. The lesions develop rapidly over several weeks. They begin with painless, dusky-red, asymptomatic subcutaneous swelling; arthralgias have been reported in some patients.[297] Histologically, there is degeneration of fat cells. A similar lipoatrophy has been reported that involves the ankles.[298] Nagore detected precipitating trauma in seven cases.[299] Occasionally, the atrophy may completely encircle the arm and cause distal edema; the disease is then called *lipoatrophia annularis (annular lipoatrophy)*. *Panatrophy of Gower* is a localized lipoatrophy associated with autoimmune conditions, such as systemic lupus erythematosis, nephritis, Sjögren syndrome, or diabetes.

Lipodystrophia centrifugalis abdominalis infantilis was originally reported in Japanese children.[300] Most patients are of Asian descent,[301] but it has now been reported in Caucasian children[302] and other racial groups. It usually begins before the age of 3 years. A large depressed area with a slightly erythematous or violaceous and scaling edge is seen on the lower abdomen. The lesion enlarges in a centrifugal fashion. There is no history of preceding trauma. Cases involving areas other than the abdomen have been described.[303,304] Regional lymph node enlargement occurs in about half the cases. Corticosteroid therapy is ineffective. The disease tends to remit spontaneously after puberty. Electron microscopy shows a breakdown in fibrillar collagen[305] and immunohistochemical staining of mononuclear cells shows apoptosis.[306] In a few cases, coexisting morphea has been present.[307]

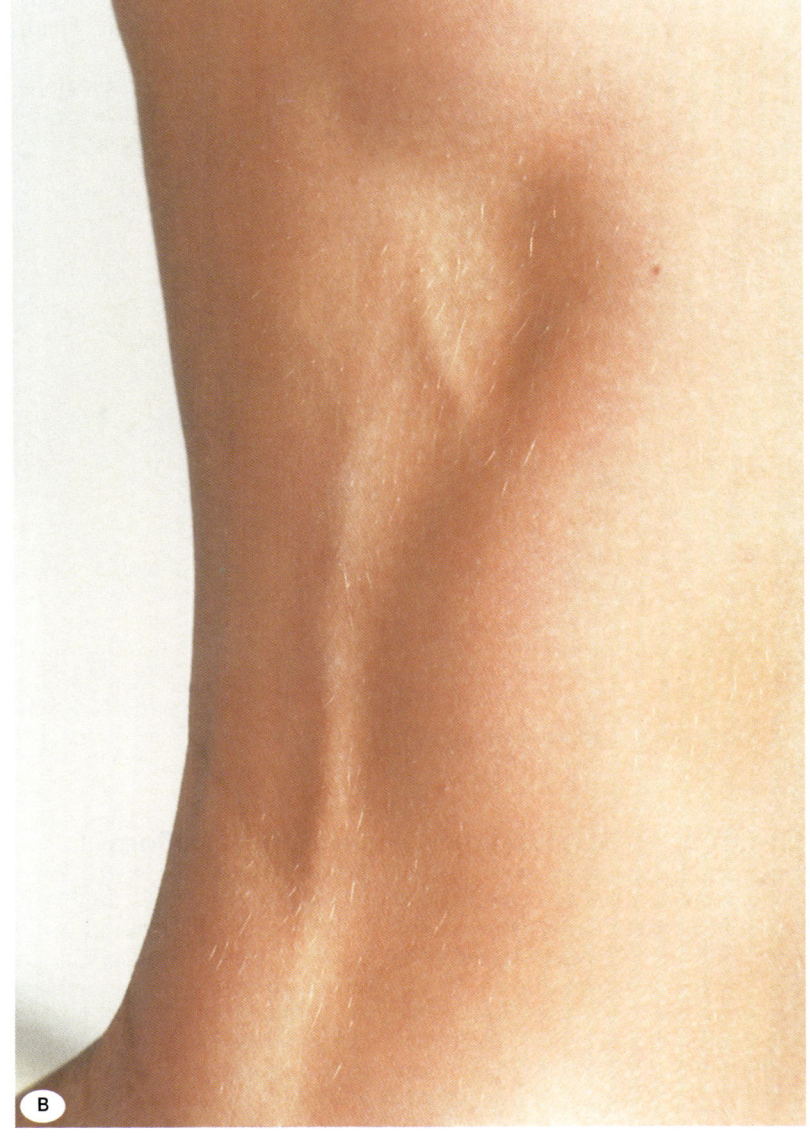

Localized lipoatrophy can occur in the subcutis after the injection of medications.[308] The most common examples are due to injections of corticosteroids particularly common with injections of triamcinolone acetonide in the deltoid area.[309] Insulin and penicillin,[310,311] heparin, dactinomycin, and growth hormone[312] have also been implicated.[298] Parents may not recall the child receiving a local injection in the area. The lipoatrophy usually resolves in several months. Repeated insulin injections at the same site may eventually

297. Jablonska S, Szczeponski A, Gorkiewicz A (1975) Lipoatrophy of the ankles and its relationship to other lipoatrophies. **Acta Derm Venereol** (Stockh) 55:135.
298. Shelley WB, Izumi AK (1970) Annular atrophy of the ankles: a case of partial lipodystrophy. **Arch Dermatol** 102:236.
299. Nagore E, Sanchez-Motilla JM, Rodriguez-Serna M et al. (1998) Lipoatrophia semicircularis – a traumatic panniculitis: report of seven cases and review of the literature. **J Am Acad Dermatol** 39:879–881.
300. Imamura S, Yamada M, Ikeda T (1971) Lipodystrophia centrifugalis abdominalis infantilis. **Arch Dermatol** 104:291.
301. Llistosella E, Puig L, Perez F (1997) Lipodystrophia centrifugalis abdominalis infantilis: a case report. **Pediatr Dermatol** 14:216–218.
302. Muller S, Beissert S, Metze D et al. (1999) Lipodystrophia centrifugalis abdominalis infantilis in a 4-year-old caucasian girl: association with partial IgA deficiency and autoantibodies. **Br J Dermatol** 140:1161–1169.
303. Caputo R (1989) Lipodystrophia centrifugalis sacralis infantilis: a 15-year follow-up observation. **Acta Derm Venereol** (Stockh) 69:442.
304. Hagari Y, Sasaoka R, Nishiura S et al. (1992) Centrifugal lipodystrophy of the face mimicking progressive lipodystrophy. **Br J Dermatol** 127:407–410.
305. Kagoura M, Toyoda M, Matsui C et al. (2001) An ultrastructural study of lipodystrophia centrifugalis abdominalis infantilis, with special reference to fibrous long-spacing collagen. **Pediatr Dermatol** 18:13–16.
306. Okita H, Ohtsuda T, Yamakage A, Yamazaki S (2000) Lipodystrophia centrifugalis abdominalis infantilis – immunohistochemical demonstration of an apoptotic process in the degenerating fatty tissue. **Dermatology** 201:370–372.
307. Ikoma A, Tanaka T, Miyachi Y (1999) A case of lipodystrophia centrifugalis abdominalis infantilis with morphea. **J Dermatol** 26:603–607.
308. Dahl PR, Zalla MJ, Winkelmann RK (1996) Localized involutional lipoatrophy: a clinicopathologic study of 16 patients. **J Am Acad Dermatol** 35:523–528.
309. Fritsch WC (1970) Deep atrophy of the skin of the deltoid area. **Arch Dermatol** 101:585.
310. Kayikcioglu A, Akuyrek M, Erk Y (1996) Semicircular lipoatrophy after intragluteal injection of benzathine penicillin. **J Pediatr** 129:166–167.
311. Kuperman-Beade M, Laude T (2000) Partial lipoatrophy in a child. **Pediatr Dermatol** 17:302–303.
312. Buyukgebiz A, Aydin A, Dundar B, Yorukoglu K (1999) Localized lipoatrophy due to recombinant growth hormone therapy in a child with 6.7 kilobase gene deletion isolated growth hormone deficiency. **J Pediatric Endocrinology** 12:95–97.

result in atrophy, especially in children and women, six months to two years after initiation of insulin therapy.[313] This problem occurs less frequently with recombinant human insulin.

Localized forms of lipoatrophy must be differentiated from partial lipodystrophy, total lipoatrophy, morphea, atrophoderma, Weber–Christian disease, panniculitis, and lupus profundus.

FAMILIAL PARTIAL LIPODYSTROPHY (FPL)

There are at least two phenotypes of x-linked dominant FPL affecting female patients. Progressive loss of subcutaneous fat begins in childhood. It is localized to the limbs in type 1 and involves the limbs and trunk in type 2.[314] Diabetes, hyperlipemia and acanthosis nigricans develop in many patients with type 1 FPL. In type 2, hyperlipoproteinemia and insulin-resistent diabetes can occur, and in some families there is a broad facies. Mutations of the laminin A/C gene have been detected; mapping of heterozygotes indicates plasma lipid abnormalities precede glucose abnormalities.[315]

PROGRESSIVE PARTIAL LIPODYSTROPHY

In the most common variant of this rare disorder, there is complete symmetrical disappearance of the subcutaneous fat from the face that progresses to involve the upper half of the body.[316,317] The loss of facial fat gives these patients a distinctive gaunt appearance. Occasionally, hypertrophy of the subcutaneous fat on the lower part of the body occurs. The disease is much more common in females and primarily affects children between the ages of 5 and 10 years and young adults. It may be preceded by an acute febrile episode, such as measles. The disease is only "progressive" until all the fat is lost, when the process arrests.

Many affected patients eventually have a progressive membranous mesangiocapillary glomerulonephritis, which can be precipitated by pregnancy, oral contraceptive use, and ergot medications. The latter drugs are therefore contraindicated in these patients. The glomerulonephritis is associated with persistently low levels of C3 due to a serum "C3 nephritic" factor that can activate C3 without activating earlier complement components by the alternative pathway.[318] Retinitis pigmentosa occurs in rare patients.

An autosomal-dominant form of partial lipodystrophy in association with the Rieger anomaly (variable eye and tooth abnormalities), midface hypoplasia, short stature, and hypotrichosis has been reported.[319] There is one report of acquired progressive partial lipoatrophy associated with a chromosome 10 abnormality.[320]

The differential diagnosis includes facial hemiatrophy and the generalized wasting that may occur in malnutrition or thyrotoxicosis. There is no known effective therapy for the disorder.

PARTIAL LIPODYSTOPHY IN DERMATOMYOSITIS

There are now multiple reports of lipodystrophy complicating juvenile dermatomysitis (JDM),[321] sometimes years after the initial diagnosis, and at times when the disease is clinically in remission.[322] In a study by Huemer, four of 20 patients with JDM had lipodystrophy and either diabetes or impaired glucose tolerance, and another eight had abnormal glucose and/or lipid studies.[323]

LIPODYSTROPHIC SYNDROME IN HIV-INFECTED CHILDREN

Peripheral lipoatrophy with an increase in central fat is seen in all HIV-infected children treated with highly active antiretroviral therapy (HAART).[324] It may be associated with hypertriglyceridemia and/or insulin resistance.

TOTAL LIPOATROPHY (LIPODYSTROPHY)

These conditions are extremely rare. There are three varieties: leprechaunism, congenital lipodystrophy and adult lipodystrophy. They are all associated with severe insulin resistance and are characterized by diabetes mellitus, acanthosis nigricans, and by hirsuitism and virilization in females.

Leprechaunism

Affected newborns are small due to cessation of growth *in utero*. The facies has a gnome-like appearance and the infant is severely emaciated. Classic cases have hypertrichosis, acanthosis nigricans, and symptomatic hyperglycemia because of insulin resistance. Most die before 1 year of age. Milder variants have been reported.[325] The disease is caused by different mutations in the insulin gene receptor.[326]

Congenital lipoatrophic diabetes (Seip–Bernardinelli syndrome)

Complete loss of subcutaneous fat is noticed at birth or before the age of 2 years.[316] The children are tall (90th percentile) because of an advanced bone age. The muscles appear to be very prominent, in part because of the loss of subcutaneous tissue. The abdomen protrudes and there is hepatomegaly. The skin may be generally hyperpigmented, and acanthosis nigricans may occur. The scalp hair grows luxuriously onto the forehead, almost reaching the eyebrows. Adipose tissue remains in several anatomical sites (orbits, palms, soles),[327] suggesting differences in fat metabolism. The condition is caused by a mutation in chromosome 9q34 and in some pedigrees is autosomal recessive.[328]

Diabetes due to insulin resistance develops by the time the patient reaches adulthood. Younger patients may have glucosuria only after glucose loading, but true hyperglycemia often develops after age 10 years. The hyperglycemia is not associated with significant ketosis, and there is minimal response to insulin; hyperlipidemia from elevated triglycerides also occurs. The disease may be associated with renal abnormalities, cardiomegaly, and disturbances of central nervous system function. Multiple pulmonary artery stenoses have been reported in three patients.[329]

Congenital lipoatrophic diabetes must be differentiated from muscular dystrophy, Cornelia de Lange syndrome, and from leprechaunism. Unlike

313. Huntley AC (1982) The cutaneous manifestations of diabetes mellitus. **J Am Acad Dermatol** 7:427.
314. Kobberling J, Dunnigan MG (1986) Familial partial lipodystrophy: two types of an x-linked dominant syndrome, lethal in the hemizygous state. **J Med Genet** 23:120–127.
315. Hegele RA, Anderson CM, Wang J et al. (2000) Association between nuclear lamin A/C R482Q mutation and partial lipodystrophy with hyperinsulinemia, dyslipidemia, hypertension, and diabetes. **Genome Research** 10:652–658.
316. Senior B, Gellis SS (1964) The syndromes of total lipodystrophy and partial lipodystrophy. **Pediatrics** 33:593.
317. Lenane P, Murphy G (2000) Partial lipodystrophy and renal disease. **Clinical & Experimental Dermatology** 25:605–607.
318. Sissons JG, West RJ, Fallows J et al. (1976) The complement abnormalities of lipodystrophy. **N Engl J Med** 294:461.
319. Aarskoig D, Ose L, Pande H, Eide N (1983) Autosomal dominant partial lipodystrophy associated with Rieger anomaly, short stature, and insulinopenic diabetes. **Am J Med Genet** 15:29.
320. Martinez A, Malone M, Hoeger P et al. (2000) Lipoatrophic panniculitis and chromosome 10 abnormality. **Br J Dermatol** 142:1034–1039.

321. Kavanagh GM, Colaco CB, Kennedy CTC (1993) Juvenile dermatomyositis associated with partial lipoatrophy. **J Am Acad Dermatol** 28:348.
322. Quecedo E, Febrer I, Serrano G et al. (1996) Partial lipodystrophy associated with juvenile dermatomyositis: report of two cases. **Pediatr Dermatol** 13:477–482.
323. Huemer C, Kitson H, Malleson PN et al. (2001) Lipodystrophy in patients with juvenile dermatomyositis – evaluation of clinical and metabolic abnormalities. **J Rheumatol** 28:610–615.
324. Brambilla P, Bricalli D, Sala N et al. (2001) Highly active antiretroviral-treated HIV-infected children show fat distribution changes even in absence of lipodystrophy. **AIDS** 15:2415–2422.
325. al Gazali LI, Khalil M, Devadas K (1993) A syndrome of insulin resistance resembling leprechaunism in five sibs of consanguineous parents. **J Med Genet** 30:470–475.
326. Psiachou H, Mitton S, Alaghband-Zadey J et al. (1993) Leprechaunism and homozygous nonsense mutation in the insulin receptor gene. **Lancet** 342:924.
327. David R, Goodman RM (1981) The Patterson syndrome, leprechaunism and pseudo-leprechaunism. **J Med Genet** 18:294–298.
328. Garg A, Wilson R, Barnes R et al. (1999) A gene for congenital generalized lipodystrophy maps to human chromosome 9q34. **J Clin Endocrinol & Metabolism** 84:3390–3394.
329. Uzun O, Blackburn ME, Gibbs JL (1997) Congenital total lipodystrophy and peripheral pulmonary artery stenosis. **Arch Dis Child** 76:456–457.

leprechaunism, there is no mutation of the insulin receptor gene which makes pregnancy management difficult.[330,331] Treatment consists of good control of the diabetes and hyperlipidemia. Patients usually survive into adulthood.

Acquired lipoatrophic diabetes (adult lipoatrophy)

When the disease has its onset in adulthood, height is normal, and muscularity and abdominal protuberance are not as marked as in childhood lipoatrophy.[332] Adults may have features of acromegaly such as enlargement of the skull, hands, and feet with diabetes. Death occurs from hepatic failure or hematemesis.

Treatment of all forms of lipoatrophy associated with metabolic abnormalities is control of the glucose and lipid abnormalities. An antidiabetic drug troglitazone, which is a ligand for the peroxisome proliferator-activated receptor, is reported to increase insulin sensitivity and promote adipocyte development. It has been used to treat 13 patients with various forms of partial and generalized lipoatrophy.[333] There was improved metabolic control and increased body fat, but the drug has a substantial risk of hepatotoxicity.[333] Therapy with leptin improved glucose and lipid control in nine patients with various forms of generalized and partial lipodystrophy.[334] Intensive plasma exchange therapy dramatically improved triglyceride levels, xanthomata, and hepatomegaly in a 15-year-old with acquired generalized lipoatrophy.[335]

NECROBIOSIS LIPOIDICA

Necrobiosis lipoidica (NL) is a degenerative disease of the dermal connective tissue characterized by atrophic plaques on the anterior legs. Because the first patients seen with the disease were diabetic, it was originally considered to be a complication of diabetes mellitus, but some patients with this condition do not have diabetes, and the disease is uncommon in the diabetic population. NL may begin at any age, but it usually develops in young adults or in midlife. It is unusual in early childhood. The presence of NL may be a marker for greater risk of renal and retinal disease.[336]

In most patients, the disease occurs on the shins (Fig. 18.19). Oval plaques with central atrophy are present, beginning with dull red, asymptomatic, rounded papules that slowly enlarge or coalesce with other lesions. The margin of the lesion is brown-red or violaceous. The center of the lesion atrophies and develops a distinctive yellow waxy hue. Telangiectasias from visible dermal vessels are prominent. Ulceration occurs in 35% of cases,[337] mostly in larger lesions and after minor trauma. It is unusual for the ulcerations to become infected, even in diabetic patients.[337] Occasionally, lesions occur on other areas of the legs and rarely on other body sites, including the arms, trunk, and head.

Sixty-two percent of 171 patients with NL reported in one study were found to have diabetes.[338] In this study, nearly half of the nondiabetic patients

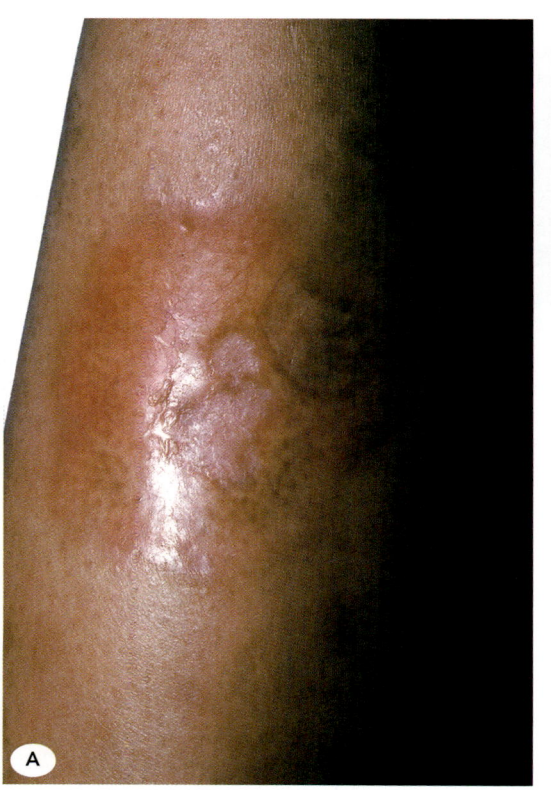
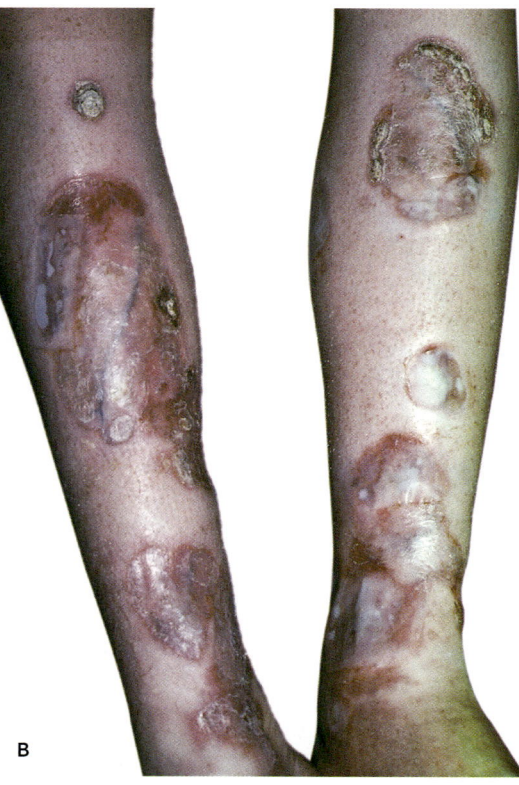

Fig. 18.19 (A) Oval atrophic plaque of necrobiosis lipoidica lesions on a teenager with diabetes mellitus. (B) These lesions of necrobiosis lipoidica have a distinctive yellow waxy appearance.

330. Desbois MC, Magre J, Amselsm S et al. (1995) Lipoatrophic diabetes: genetic exclusion of the insulin receptor gene. **J Clin Endocrinol Metab** 80:314–319.
331. Sturley RH, Stirling C, Reckless JP (1994) Generalised lipodystrophy and pregnancy. **Br J Obstet Gynaecol** 101:719–720.
332. Sasaki T, Ono H, Nakajima H et al. (1992) Lipoatrophic dabetes. **J Dermatol** 19:246–249.
333. Arioglu E, Duncan-Morin J, Sebring N et al. (2000) Efficacy and safety of troglitazone in the treatment of lipodystrophy syndromes. **Ann Intern Med** 133:263–274.
334. Oral EA, Simha V, Ruiz E et al. (2002) Leptin-replacement therapy for lipodystrophy. **N Engl J Med** 346.570–578.
335. Bolan C, Oral EA, Gorden P et al. (2002) Intensive, long-term plasma exchange therapy for severe hypertriglyceridemia in acquired generalized lipoatrophy. **J Clin Endocrinol & Metabolism** 87:380–384.
336. Verrotti A, Chiarelli F, Amerio P, Morgese G (1995) Necrobiosis lipoidica diabeticorum in children and adolescents: a clue for underlying renal and retinal disease. **Pediatr Dermatol** 12:220–223.
337. Lowitt MH, Dover JS (1991) Necrobiosis lipoidica. **J Am Acad Dermatol** 25:735.
338. Muller SA, Winkleman RK (1966) Necrobiosis lipoidica diabeticorum: a clinical and pathological investigation of 171 cases. **Arch Dermatol** 93:272.

had abnormal glucose tolerance tests. All patients with NL should be screened for diabetes.

Skin biopsy initially shows a leukocytoclastic vasculitis followed by collagen degeneration and destruction of adnexal structures.[313] The dermis becomes necrobiotic, then granulomatous, and finally sclerotic.[337] Fatty deposits are present in the upper dermis, which gives the lesions their yellow color clinically.

NL may be a significant cosmetic problem for the affected patient. It is chronic and persistent, with only occasional resolution of the lesions. Control of the hyperglycemia in patients with diabetes does not seem to affect the course of the skin lesions.

Numerous medications have been used to treat this disorder, none with uniform success. Potent topical steroids are occasionally helpful. Intralesional steroids injected into active areas may cause regression but usually do not clear the atrophic centers. A combination of dipyridamole and aspirin was reported to cause marked improvement in several uncontrolled studies, but controlled studies did not show significant differences.[337] Pentoxifylline 400mg bid[339] cleared the condition dramatically in some patients; others showed no response.[339] Petzelbauer et al.[340] advocated the use of a five-week course of systemic corticosteroids (1mg/kg of body weight of methylpred-nisolone for one week, followed by 40mg/day for an additional four weeks) for treating recalcitrant NL in adults. All six patients treated had complete cessation of active disease on the borders of the NL and no recurrence after a follow-up period of seven months. The already atrophic areas were unchanged. Other treatments include high-dose nicotinamide, clofazimine, chloroquine,[341,342] and topical tretinoin.[343] The patient should be instructed to minimize trauma to the lower extremities to prevent ulcerations.

339. Noz KC, Korstanje MJ, Vermeer BJ (1993) Ulcerating necrobiosis lipoidica effectively treated with pentoxifylline. **Clin Exp Dermatol** 18:78.
340. Petzelbauer P, Wolff K, Tappeiner G (1992) Necrobiosis lipoidica: treatment with systemic corticosteroids. **Br J Dermatol** 126:542.
341. Nguyen K, Washenik K, Shupack J (2002) Necrobiosis lipoidica diabeticorum treated with chloroquine. **J Am Acad Dermatol** 46:S34–S36.
342. Ling TC, Thomson KF, Goulden V, Goodfield MJ (2002) PUVA therapy in necrobiosis lipoidica diabeticorum, **J Am Acad Dermatol** 46:319–320.
343. Boyd AS (1999) Tretinoin treatment of necrobiosis lipoidica diabeticorum. **Diabetes Care** 22:1753–1754.

Vascular Reactions

William L. Weston and David Orchard

The diseases considered to be vascular reactions arise as a result of abnormalities either in the blood vessels of the skin or in the blood that flows through them. These abnormalities, which may be functional or structural, give rise to cutaneous lesions that share the clinical characteristics of a smooth surface (nonscaling, noneczematous) and varying degrees of red or white color.

Classification by gross morphology is preferred. With this system, types of vascular reactions can be divided into two major categories based on the presence or absence of purpura. This determination can be made with considerable accuracy through compression of individual lesions. Compression is best accomplished through diascopy, which is the firm application of a clear plastic diascope or, carefully, a glass microscope slide to the surface of the lesion; unfortunately, the application and quick release of finger pressure alone is inadequate. When diascopy is carried out, nonpurpuric lesions blanch completely. On the other hand, the presence of even a modest number of extravasated erythrocytes in purpuric lesions results in the retention of some red or violaceous coloration. Biopsy offers even greater accuracy in separating purpuric from nonpurpuric lesions and is sometimes required for confirmation of a clinical impression or for the evaluation of equivocal lesions such as occur in urticarial vasculitis.

Within the group of nonpurpuric lesions, three subdivisions exist (Table 19.1). The transient erythemas are characterized by the evolution and resolution of individual lesions within a matter of minutes to hours. The persistent erythemas are characterized by greater lesional stability with the resolution of individual lesions over days or weeks. The vasospastic lesions are characterized by the presence of pale white patches, a palpable sense of coolness, or a history of development during cold exposure.

Within the group of purpuric lesions, two subdivisions exist (Table 19.1). The vasculitic or inflammatory purpuras are characterized by the presence of petechiae and, usually, palpable purpuric papules. The noninflammatory purpuras are characterized by the presence of larger lesions of purpura (ecchymoses). Ecchymoses are usually not palpable.

Five major morphologic categories exist within the vascular reactions. It is generally easy for a clinician to assign unrecognized, smooth-surfaced, red lesions to one or another of these categories; for this reason, each of the five categories serves as a section heading within this chapter.

TABLE 19.1   Classification of the vascular reactions

Nonpurpuric lesions
  Transient erythemas
  Persistent erythemas
  Vasospastic reactions
Purpuric lesions
  Vasculitis and inflammatory purpuras
  Noninflammatory purpuras

TABLE 19.2   Transient erythemas

Palpable lesions
  Common urticaria and angioedema
  Anaphylactic reactions
  Serum sickness
  Contact urticaria
  Physical urticarias
  Erythema marginatum
Nonpalpable lesions
  Blushing
  Flushing

TRANSIENT ERYTHEMAS

The diseases in this category, as indicated above, are characterized by the presence of smooth red lesions that evolve individually and resolve within minutes or hours. This degree of transience is possible because inflammatory cells are minimal or absent within the lesions. The redness observed in transient erythemas is due to dilation of upper dermal blood vessels, the size and type of blood vessel involved, and the degree of oxygen saturation of hemoglobin in the circulation. The prototype for the transient erythemas is urticaria.

Transient erythemas can be subdivided into palpable and flat diseases (Table 19.2).

COMMON URTICARIA, ANGIOEDEMA, AND ANAPHYLAXIS

Introduction and historical note

Urticaria is commonly seen in children and the care provider for children should be familiar with the topic. One in five children will have an episode of urticaria before adolescence.[1-3] For many children, the urticarial episode is short lived and simply a nuisance. For a few, urticaria may be a sign of a more serious disorder.

Although the disease now recognized as urticaria was described in antiquity, the term is generally attributed to Johann Peter Frank of Vienna, and in the English literature to William Cullen of Scotland.[1] Angioedema was recognized

1. Warin R, Champion RH (1974) Urticaria. Philadelphia: WB Saunders.
2. Doutre M (1999) Physiopathology of urticaria. **Eur J Dermatol** 9:601–605.
3. Greaves MW (2000) Chronic urticaria in childhood. **Allergy** 55:309–320.

by Donato in the sixteenth century but not named by Strubing until the 1880s.[1] The earliest authors reported urticaria as part of a febrile illness. Robert Willan first associated it with other factors such as foods.[1]

Urticaria represents transient edema within the dermis and epidermis, is initially red throughout, and then clears in the center leaving red borders.[1,2] Most lesions of urticaria are small, less than 10mm, but individual large lesions of 6–10cm may occur, the so-called giant urticaria. Individual urticarial lesions characteristically clear within hours. Angioedema represents subcutaneous extension of edema "deep hives" and frequently is accompanied by urticaria. It is characterized by transient focal deep swellings with indistinct borders. Involvement and swelling of the hands, feet, eyelids, and lips is common.[2]

Epidemiology

Although the precise incidence is not known, urticaria in childhood is believed to be common, and most authorities observe that 15–20% of children have at least one episode of urticaria by adolescence.[1,3–5] Several large studies indicate that 3% of preschool children and about 2% of older children suffer from urticaria.[3–7]

Children who have atopic dermatitis in infancy have an increased incidence of acute urticaria to foods such as peanuts, and reactions to latex.[5] Although urticaria is not believed to be genetic, hereditary angioedema is transmitted as an autosomal-dominant trait, although many individuals may present with new mutations.[7]

Presenting history

A careful history, including a detailed complete review of systems, is the most important aspect of the evaluation of a child with urticaria.[1,3–8] Events that occurred hours or a few days before the onset of urticaria are the most likely associated factors. Specific information should be sought about the most commonly recognized etiologic factors for urticaria and angioedema. These can be remembered by the mnemonic "i-i-i-i-i" (which stand for: infection, ingestion, inhalation, infestation and injection). These categories include the urticaria that may accompany a childhood infection, the ingestion of particular foods or drugs, the inhalation of pollens and other allergens, and the injection of medications or serum products (Table 19.3). Frequently, a history of a preceding infection, particularly respiratory infections, is obtained.[1–7] Less often, a history of a specific ingested product, such as a medication or food, is noted.[3–10] Injections of medications, immunizations, or allergy desensitization treatments might be found. Most uncommonly, an associated infestation is uncovered.

Most patients report the sudden onset of a pruritic eruption, with red raised spots scattered over the body.[1–4,7] Importantly, the history of an individual urticarial lesion is transient. Although the eruption may have been present for days, a history can usually be obtained of new lesions arriving and older lesions fading. The lesions of urticaria are generally accompanied by pruritus, sometimes of extraordinary severity. It is interesting, however, that the quality of this pruritus is different from that which occurs in eczematous disease. Urticarial itching, even when severe, rarely leads to excoriation. Angioedema, on the other hand, is usually not very pruritic and may instead be accompanied by burning or stinging.[7] Angioedema may be associated with dyspnea or dysphagia, but if these symptoms have not occurred within the first few hours of any one urticarial episode, they are not likely to develop during the course of that particular episode.

Physical examination

Uricarial lesions are transient. Individual wheals stay in skin sites for a few hours and are usually completely gone from that area within 24 hours. This

TABLE 19.3   Etiologic agents in urticaria and angioedema: the mnemonic "i-i-i-i-i"

Acute urticaria	Chronic urticaria
Infection	Collagen vascular disease
Bacterial	Lupus erythematosus
Streptococcal	Dermatomyositis
Viral	Juvenile rheumatoid arthritis
Virtually all, especially	Inflammatory bowel disease
enteroviral and adenoviral	Immunobullous skin diseases
infections	Parasitosis
Fungal	"Hidden" infections
Candidiasis	Chronic otitis media
Histoplasmosis	Sinusitis
Coccidioidomycosis	Dental infections
Infestation	Urinary tract infection
Virtually all parasites	Candidiasis of gut or vagina
Ingestion	Malignancies (Hodgkin's
Medications	lymphomas and non-Hodgkin's
Penicillins	lymphomas)
Cephalosporins	
Sulfonamides	
Aspirin	
Nonsteroidals	
Foods	
Nuts	
Shellfish and other	
seafoods	
Chocolate	
Strawberries	
Dairy products	
Grains	
Injections	
Antibiotics	
Immunizations	
Blood products	
Inhalation	
Pollens	
Molds	

rapid change may be dramatized by the placement of ink marks around existing lesions and noting the degree of change a short time later. The initial lesions of urticaria are tense, fluid-filled, flat-topped papules known as wheals. The color is usually pink or light red but may occasionally be bright red, and the wheals are usually 2–10mm in diameter, flat-topped, and have tense edema (Fig. 19.1). The edema can be appreciated by stretching the skin slightly to demonstrate whitish centers. Wheals quickly enlarge to form flat-topped, sharply marginated papules and plaques (Fig. 19.2). In many instances, centrifugal enlargement of closely set lesions leads to the formation of very large urticarial plaques with polycyclic borders, the so-called "giant urticaria." In other instances, the centrifugal expansion is accompanied by central clearing and development of ringed (annular) borders (Fig. 19.3). As urticarial lesions fade, it is not uncommon to leave a dusky purple macule at the site. These lesions can be mistaken for bruises or purpura but are non-tender and often fade in one to two days. Giant urticarial lesions are dramatic and these large polycyclic plaques have no special significance but are often misdiagnosed as erythema multiforme (EM) (Fig. 19.4). The lesions of urticaria may occur

4. Legrain V, Taieb A, Sagi T (1990) Urticaria in infants: a study of forty patients. **Pediatr Dermatol** 7:101–103.
5. Gustafsson D, Sjoberg O, Foucard T (2000) Development of allergies and asthma in infants and young children with atopic dermatitis–a prospective follow-up to seven years of age. **Allergy** 55:240–245.
6. Greaves MW (2000) Chronic urticaria. **J Allergy & Clin Immunology** 105:664–672.
7. Kwong KY, Maalouf N, Jones CA (1998) Urticaria and angioedema: pathophysiology, diagnosis and treatment. **Pediatr Annals** 27:719–724.
8. Janniger CK, Schutzer SE, Schwartz RA (1994) Childhood insect bite reactions to ants, wasps, and bees. **Cutis** 54:14.
9. Knowles S, Shapiro L, Shear NH (1999) Drug eruptions in children. **Advan Dermatol** 14:399–415.
10. Bircher AJ (1999) Drug-induced urticaria and angioedema caused by non-IgE mediated pathomechanisms. **Eur J Dermatol** 9:657–663.

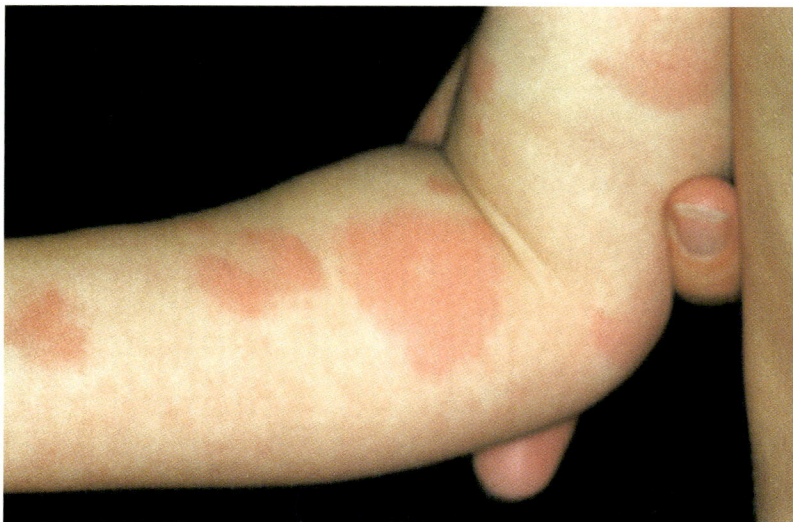

Fig. 19.1   Idiopathic urticaria in a 6-year-old child.

anywhere on the body but are often most prominent at points of pressure, including the belt line and the palms and soles. Exacerbation may occur as a result of vasodilation during body warming. Thus, urticarial lesions may be particularly prominent during exercise, after showering, and under bed coverings at night. These urticarial lesions occur when upper dermal vessels are involved (Table 19.4).

When deep dermal or subcutaneous vessels are affected, the clinical appearance is different. In such situations, light pink to skin-colored, slope-shouldered, large nodules develop. This condition is termed *angioedema* and is a subcutaneous extension of hives or "deep hives."[2,7,10] It is most likely to occur as diffuse swelling of the eyelids, lips, tongue, genitalia, hands, feet, and mucous membranes (Fig. 19.5). Mild angioedema may accompany ordinary urticaria in 10% of infants and children.[2,7,10] The face, hands, and feet are involved in 85% and other areas are involved in 15% of children.

Angioedema of a more severe type occurs in anaphylaxis, serum sickness, and hereditary angioedema. These conditions are considered separately in the section that follows. Anaphylaxis is a medical emergency characterized by the sudden onset of urticaria, angioedema, dyspnea, and hypotension.[7,8,10] The term anaphylaxis came into use more than 75 years ago, when it was recognized that prior exposure to certain agents (e.g., measles virus) offered protection (prophylaxis) against subsequent development of the disease, whereas the reverse was true (anaphylaxis) for other agents such as horse serum. Today, probably because of infrequent use of foreign proteins and better purification steps in pharmaceutical manufacture, anaphylaxis is less commonly encountered but may occur during allergen desensitization strategies.

Patients experiencing anaphylaxis have pruritus within seconds to minutes, followed almost immediately by urticaria and angioedema.[7,8,10] Often, these skin changes appear at the site of antigen entrance (intramuscular injection site, envenomization site, or mouth) but rapidly become more widespread. The rapid shift of fluid from the vessel into the connective tissue results in varying degrees of hypotension and may lead to shock and electrocardiogram abnormalities. Angioedema of the larynx causes difficulty with breathing and speaking. Bronchospasm is often present, and incontinence of the bladder and the bowel sometimes occur. Transient albuminuria has been reported. The diagnosis of anaphylaxis is made on a clinical basis because there are no immediately useful associated laboratory findings.

Mucous membranes of the tongue, soft palate, pharynx, and larynx may rarely be involved, producing acute respiratory distress.[7,8,10] The gastrointestinal mucosa of the stomach and intestines may also rarely be involved, resulting in abdominal cramping, vomiting, or diarrhea. It is not clear whether cerebral edema can cause confusion or coma in these disorders.

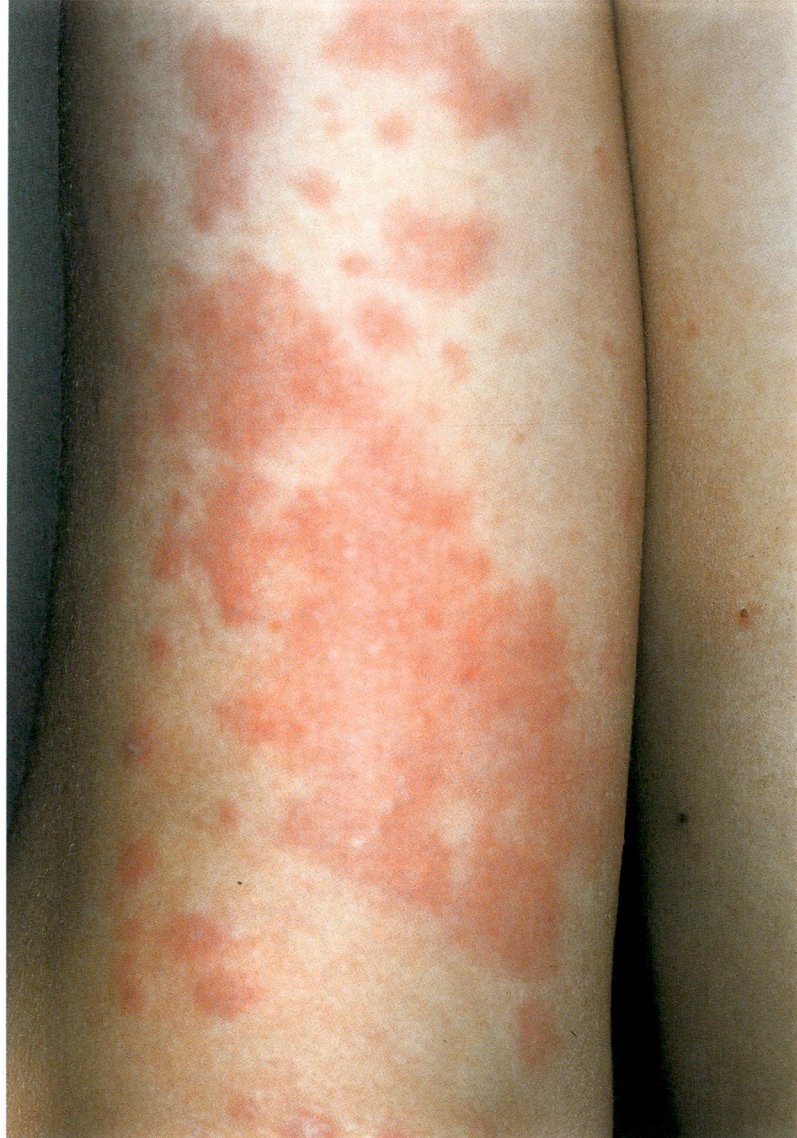

Fig. 19.2   Urticaria with different sized and shaped lesions on arm of 9-year-old.

Laboratory findings

Routine history and physical examination are by far the most useful approaches to the determination of cause. In fact, in children, if this approach does not supply a likely cause, it is safe to say that laboratory testing will seldom be useful. A biopsy is not necessary when the clinician is confronted with typical transient urticaria; when carried out, it does not usually yield significant pathologic changes. However, in instances in which individual lesions persist for many hours or days at a time, biopsy sometimes reveals perivascular lymphocytes or neutrophils.[2]

Pathophysiology and histogenesis

The mechanisms through which urticaria develops can be divided into immunologic and nonimmunologic events. Antigen attachment to, and activation of, specific immunoglobulin [IgE] antibody bound to the membranes of mast cells is the best-studied immunologic event. Only 3% to 5% of children have what can be documented as immunoglobulin E (IgE) mediated allergic urticaria.[2,10] Complement activation through immune complex formation or other non-IgE processes with subsequent C3a-mediated degranulation of mast cells also occurs and may be more frequent than IgE-mediated mechanisms.[2,7,10] IgE mediation is the major mechanism for those urticarias associated with anaphylactic reactions, whereas

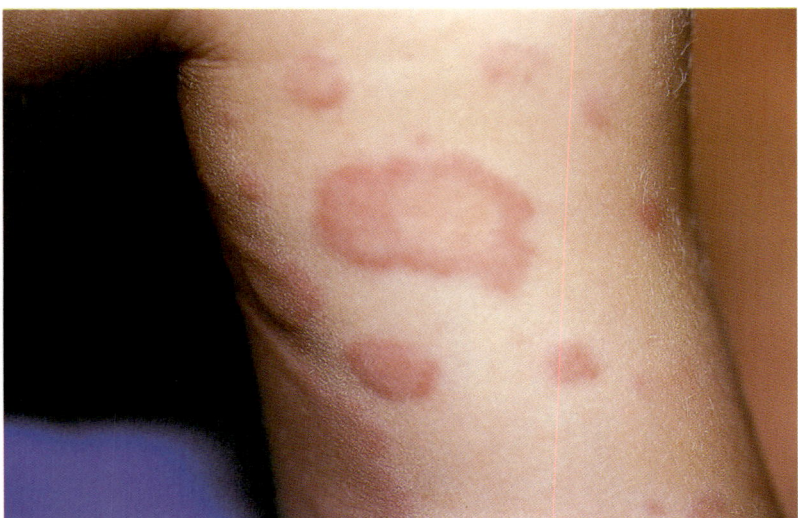

Fig. 19.3   Annular urticarial lesion with clearing in the center.

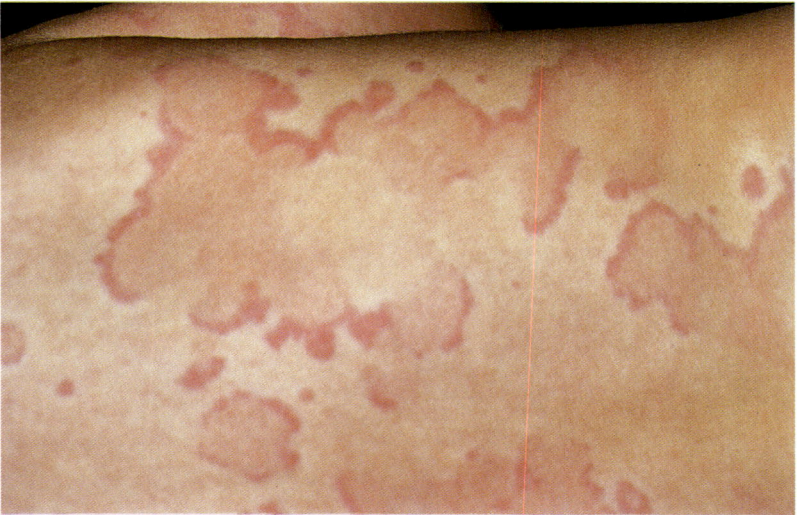

Fig. 19.4   Gyrate polycyclic giant urticarial lesions with dusky centers in a 2-year-old.

TABLE 19.4   The workup of chronic urticaria

Careful detailed history
Erythrocyte sedimentation rate
Antinuclear antibody titer
Examination for parasites

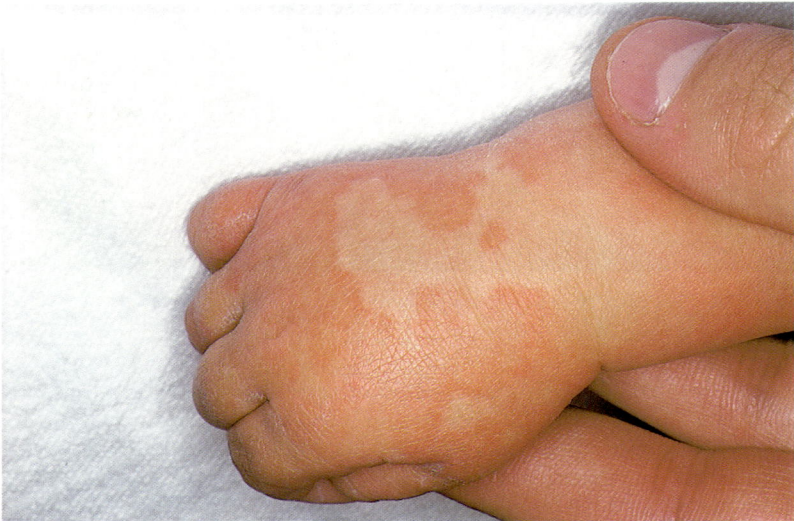

Fig. 19.5   Urticaria with angioedema of the hand in a toddler.

complement activation as a cause of mast cell degranulation occurs in hereditary angioedema, serum sickness reactions, blood transfusion reactions, cryoglobulinemia, and the urticaria-like lesions of dermatitis herpetiformis, bullous pemphigoid, Henoch–Schöenlein purpura and urticarial vasculitis.

Nonimmunologic mechanisms for the development of urticaria include direct pharmacologic degranulation of mast cells and a separate, less well-understood pathway utilized by agents that alter the metabolism of prostaglandins. Both of these nonimmunologic mechanisms can be important in the urticaria and angioedema of anaphylactic reactions.[2,7] The role of non-immunologic mechanisms in chronic urticaria is less certain. However, aspirin and other nonsteroidal anti-inflammatory agents (all of which are antagonists of the prostaglandin cyclooxygenase pathway) worsen chronic urticaria.

Regardless of the specific mechanism through which wheal formation is initiated, the final common pathway is that of mast cell degranulation and release of inflammatory mediators. Histamine is the major chemical mediator of transient urticaria, and the mast cell is central in all forms of transient urticaria and angioedema. Histamine may be nonimmunologically (directly) released from cutaneous mast cells in the case of certain foods or opiate drugs. Specific IgE antibodies bound to IgE receptors on mast cell surfaces "recognize" certain antigens, such as penicillin and other drugs, foods, and venom of certain stinging insects, result in the release of histamine after combining with antigen. In some, the autoantibodies to the epsilon [IgE] receptor on the skin mast cells may be responsible.[1,2,7,10] Individual host factors are probably also important in the pathogenesis of urticaria. Although the role played by the presence of the atopic diathesis remains controversial, those who are genetically atopic readily form IgE antibodies, and it is possible that such individuals are particularly predisposed to wheal formation. The number of mast cells in the skin, a factor that may be genetically determined, may also be important. Although these and other causes should be sought in all patients with urticaria, it must be emphasized that the likelihood of identifying a specific cause is very small in most children with urticaria.[2,3,6–12]

Only the most common causes and underlying illnesses are discussed below. Longer lists of less common or less well-proved etiologic factors can be found in recent review articles.[2–4,6–13] Infections are the most commonly sought cause of urticaria in children.[2,3,6] Acute viral infections, often not specifically identified, are the most frequent offenders, but virtually every infectious agent of childhood has been reported to be associated with urticaria. Among bacterial infections, those caused by streptococci are encountered most often. The fungal infections of histoplasmosis and coccidioidomycosis are well-documented causes in certain areas of the United States. In chronic urticaria, parasitic disease, candidiasis of the gut and vagina, and chronic "hidden" foci of bacterial disease (otitis, sinusitis, dental abscesses, and low-grade urinary tract infection) are somewhat controversial.

11. Jarisch R, Beringer K, Hemmer W (1999) Role of food allergy and food intolerance in recurrent urticaria. **Current Problems in Dermatology** 28:64–73.
12. Heymann WR (1999) Chronic urticaria and angioedema associated with thyroid autoimmunity. Review and therapeutic implications. **J Am Acad Dermatol** 40:229–232.
13. Friedmann PS (1999) Assessment of urticaria and angio-oedema. **Clin & Exper Allergy** 29 Suppl 109–112.

Medications in children are probably second in importance to infection.[2,3,6,7,9,10] Penicillin and its derivatives are by far the medications most likely to cause urticaria. Even when a history of specific penicillin usage cannot be obtained, nonmedical sources of penicillin might be considered because up to 25% of patients with urticaria have demonstrable antibodies to this substance. Cephalosporins (which occasionally cross-react with penicillin), sulfa-derived antibiotics, and anticonvulsants are other well-established offenders. Aspirin and other nonsteroidal anti-inflammatory drugs (NSAIDs) are often associated with worsening of urticaria.[9,10] Infusion or injection of blood products is also commonly associated with the development of urticaria.[2] Rechallenge studies are few, and in suspected urticarial reactions to drugs, only 4% could be reproduced.[10]

Autoimmune disease are commonly associated with urticarial reactions; on occasion, urticaria is an important early diagnostic clue to their presence.[12] Specifically, in patients with urticaria of the chronic type, it is worth considering the possibility of associated lupus erythematosus (LE), juvenile rheumatoid arthritis, dermatomyositis, autoimmune thyroid disease, chronic inflammatory bowel disease, and the immunobullous skin diseases.[1–3,6,7,12]

Food-related products as a cause of urticaria are difficult to evaluate.[2–4,11,13] Certainly some foods, such as nuts, seafood, chocolate, dairy products, grains, and berries, are responsible for episodes of acute urticaria, but the role of foods, food dyes, and food preservatives in chronic urticaria is more controversial. Studies that use provocative double-blind oral food challenges rather than skin tests and radio-allergosorbent tests (RAST) are interpreted to show that food allergy is reproducible in only a few instances.[11]

Factors that are controversial in causing urticaria include having a high frequency of positive skin and RAST test reactions to pollen and molds, and flares of seasonal allergic rhinitis or asthma. Frequently implicated contact factors, such as rubber, have been documented to cause urticaria but others, such as soaps and clothing, are unproven. Psychological stress is believed by some authorities to act as an exacerbating factor, but it is less clear whether it alone can be a true etiologic factor.[1,3] Steps taken to reduce anxiety or improve depression may help, and sometimes completely clear, chronic urticaria.[3] Some antidepressant drugs, such as doxepin, are also strong H_1 blocking agents and may modify the urticarial response.

In anaphylaxis, there must first be a sensitizing exposure, which is ordinarily unaccompanied by a clinical reaction. At the time of the second exposure, the offending antigen bridges adjacent molecules of antigen-specific IgE that have previously attached to the cytoplasmic membrane of mast cells. This bridging attachment triggers mast cell degranulation, allowing mediator release similar to that described for urticaria. These mediators are then responsible for the vasodilation, vasopermeability, smooth muscle contraction, alteration in blood coagulability, and chemotaxis of neutrophils and eosinophils.[7]

A small proportion of individuals who have the signs and symptoms of anaphylaxis do not have identifiable specific IgE antibodies. Such events, not mediated by IgE, are called anaphylactoid reactions. This distinction relates only to pathogenesis; the clinical symptoms and signs are otherwise identical. The mechanism through which these non-IgE reactions occur often involves direct pharmacologic or complement-mediated release of mediators from mast cells. The substances most commonly implicated in the development of urticaria, anaphylaxis, and anaphylactoid reactions are listed in Table 19.3.

Differential diagnosis

Urticaria and angioedema are diagnosed strictly on clinical criteria based on the presence of characteristic wheals, at times accompanied by focal areas of subcutaneous edema, and the transient nature of individual lesions.[1–10] Anaphylaxis is diagnosed based on the presence of acute airway obstruction associated with urticaria.[7,13]

In giant urticaria, the large transient wheals may be misdiagnosed as erythema multiforme.[14] Insect bite reactions, such as papular urticaria, may mimic common urticaria. Rarely, collagen vascular diseases, such as LE or dermatomyositis, may present as urticaria. Photodistributed urticaria and angioedema may be seen in erythropoietic protoporphyria and variegate porphyria. Immunobullous disease, such as dermatitis herpetiformis and bullous pemphigoid, may present with urticaria. Hypocomplementemic vasculitis may also mimic urticaria. Early red papules of guttate psoriasis or pityriasis rosea have also been misdiagnosed as urticaria.

Therapeutics and prognosis

The first therapeutic step is the administration of an H_1-type oral antihistamine.[2,3,6,7] Over-the-counter products, such as chlorphenamine (chlorpheniramine) and diphenhydramine, are less expensive and are often adequate. Prescription products, such as hydroxyzine, cyproheptadine, cetirizine, terfenadine, doxepin, and amitriptyline, may be considered when the over-the-counter antihistamines fail. Ordinarily, one should initiate therapy with a dose that is within the upper level recommended by the manufacturer. This dose can gradually be increased until either improvement occurs or side effects become troublesome. An amount twice the recommended dose should not be exceeded. Sedation is likely to occur even at rather low doses. In infants and toddlers, paradoxical irritability and hyperactivity may occur especially with diphenhydramine. In older children, daytime drowsiness can be minimized by administering most of the entire day's dosage one hour before bedtime. A sedating antihistamine at bedtime and a nonsedating antihistamine in the morning may be useful. Anticholinergic effects secondary to H_1 antihistamine are not usually troublesome in children until high doses are reached. Once the urticaria has been controlled, the antihistamine dosage should be tapered rather than being discontinued abruptly. This approach seems to reduce the risk of immediate exacerbation. However, in the event of recurrences, it is safe and appropriate to carry out longer therapy.

If there is little response after two or more H_1 blockers have been used, an agent such as doxepin can be considered. Alternatively, an H_2 blocker (cimetidine or ranitidine) can be administered. When this is done, the H_1 blocker should be continued because a beneficial synergistic effect occurs.

A small proportion of children with chronic urticaria do not respond even when both H_1- and H_2-blocking agents are used. As an additional step, some authorities recommend the addition of ephedrine or terbutaline, but unacceptable side effects such as night terrors often appear before an effective dose can be achieved. Children may be irritable while receiving these agents. Injected adrenaline (epinephrine) often temporarily clears the urticaria, and is first-line therapy for severe anaphylactic reactions but long-term use is limited. Systemic corticosteroids, given in daily doses of 1mg/kg or greater, sometimes cause resolution of urticaria and angioedema, but concerns about long-term complications should severely restrict the use of these agents. Their use should be restricted to acute urticaria. Long-term use should not be considered. Calcium channel blocking agents, such as nifedipine, have been effective in inhibiting the release of mast cell mediators, but their use for childhood urticaria is not well studied. Oral cromolyn, a mast cell membrane stabilizer, has been advocated, but little of the oral preparation is absorbed, and its efficacy in urticaria has not been established. Non-steroidal, anti-inflammatory drugs given to the child for the urticaria may aggravate and prolong the urticarial episode.[15] Leukotriene antagonists, such as zafirlukast or montelukast, may be useful in treating exacerbations that result from non-steroidal, anti-inflammatory usage.[15]

The second step in the treatment of urticaria involves the identification and removal of any specifically suspected etiologic factors. The parents may have already discontinued the suspected foods or drugs. Removal of the suspected offending agent as a single strategy is rarely successful. Even when the known underlying trigger can be removed, days to weeks are required for urticaria to clear totally.

Therapy for anaphylaxis requires immediate subcutaneous injection of epinephrine in doses up to 0.5ml of a 1:1000 solution. The exact dose is

14. Weston WL (1996) What is erythema multiforme? **Pediatric Annals** 25:106–109.

15. Asero R (2000) Leukotriene receptor antagonists may prevent NSAID-induced exacerbations in patients with chronic urticaria. **Annals of Allergy, Asthma and Immunology** 85:156–157.

0.01ml/kg. The injection can be repeated at 15-minute intervals if necessary. In the event of complete vascular collapse, intravenous or endotracheal administration of a more dilute solution may be required. Venous access for the administration of fluids must be established because, even when the clinical appearance of angioedema suggests the presence of excess fluids, intravascular hypovolemic shock is likely to be present.[7] Intubation is necessary when there is evidence of significant laryngeal edema. Mild degrees of bronchoconstriction can be treated with asthma aerosol inhalers; intravenous aminophylline should be administered if the problem is more severe. Supplemental oxygen can be added as necessary. If the entry site of the offending agent occurred on an extremity, a tourniquet should be placed proximal to it. Antihistamines and corticosteroids may be administered in addition to (but never in lieu of) the steps outlined above.

Anaphylaxis is a frightening event for all concerned. Every attempt should be made to identify the responsible agent and to minimize the chances for subsequent exposure. Appropriate notations of sensitivity should be placed in the patient's medical record, and patients should wear "alert" tags or bracelets. Anaphylaxis kits (bee sting kits) should be prescribed, and both the patient and parents should be instructed regarding injection of the epinephrine contained therein. Occasionally, the fear of subsequent anaphylaxis reaches that of a neurosis. In such instances, psychiatric counseling should be sought.

The outlook for most children with urticaria is excellent.[3,6] If laryngeal edema has not occurred during the first several hours of any given episode, it is very unlikely to occur thereafter. Most children with urticaria experience resolution within 14 days. The remainder experience a more chronic course that can be either intermittent or continuous over a matter of weeks or months. These individuals should be followed with symptomatic treatment. Unfortunately, there is no way of predicting the expected duration of chronic urticaria.

Pediatric aspects of the disease

For most children, urticaria is not a serious problem. The most serious complication is acute airway obstruction from edema, the anaphylactic reaction. Although deaths have been reported, the mortality rate is low. It appears that these fatalities are almost exclusively the result of hereditary angioedema and not ordinary urticaria with anaphylaxis. Most children with urticaria do not have other conditions that require intervention; even with chronic urticaria, the child's growth and development are unaffected. Elimination diets, desensitization strategies, and environmental changes are not indicated and may induce malnutrition or severely disrupt a child's routine. Loss of sleep from itching is rarely a problem for children. It is the child's appearance as a result of the hives that may be a concern.

OTHER TRANSIENT ERYTHEMAS

Serum sickness

Serum sickness is characterized by the development of urticaria, angioedema, arthralgia, myalgia, lymphadenopathy, and fever 7 to 20 days after the administration of animal serum or other foreign proteins.[16,17] Both the likelihood of developing serum sickness and the level of severity when it occurs are dependent on the dose of the antigen and frequency of administration.

The pruritus, urticaria, and angioedema that occur are similar to those observed in anaphylaxis.[16] In fact, anaphylaxis itself occasionally occurs during the course of serum sickness. The development of a serpiginous erythematous and purpuric eruption at the edges of the palms and soles is a useful diagnostic feature of serum sickness. Evidence of systemic involvement is usually confined to joints, muscles, and reticuloendothelial tissues.

The major pathogenetic mechanism in serum sickness involves immune complex deposition at the basement membrane of blood vessels with

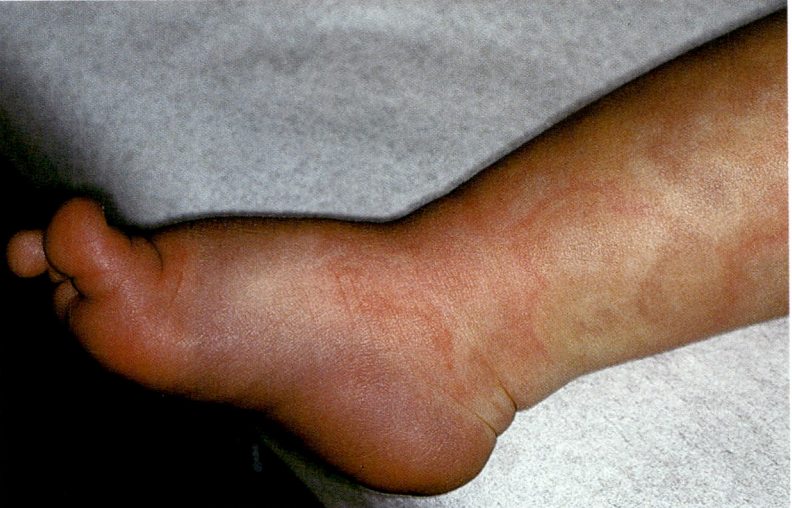

Fig. 19.6 Polycyclic uricarial lesions with angioedema of foot in child with so-called "serum sickness" reaction to Ceclor.

subsequent complement activation. Circulating immune complexes can usually be detected, and serum levels of complement are depressed. Reactions essentially identical to those seen in classical serum sickness are occasionally encountered during the use of medications that do not contain animal serum.[16,17] In these cases, the medication presumably acts as a partial antigen (hapten), which, by attaching to one or more of the patient's own proteins, subsequently forms a complete antigen. This complete antigen may then cause antibody formation and the development of immune complexes.

Serum sickness generally lasts 5 to 30 days and then slowly resolves. Subsequent readministration of the same antigen results in an accelerated reappearance of the original symptoms and signs. The "serum sickness" frequently observed with Ceclor treatment in children more closely resembles urticaria and angioedema than true serum sickness (Fig. 19.6).[16,17]

Antihistamines are only moderately effective in the treatment of serum sickness. For this reason, and because the usual duration of illness is short, systemic corticosteroids are appropriately used in all but the mildest cases. Oral prednisone in doses of 1–1.5mg/kg administered for two to three weeks is usually sufficient.

Hereditary angioedema

Hereditary angioedema accounts for only 0.4% of cases of urticaria, but its specific diagnostic tests and high mortality deserve special mention. It is an autosomal-dominant condition with repeated attacks of swelling of the extremities, face, and throat, accompanied by abdominal pain.[18] The onset usually follows trauma such as surgery, dental manipulation, or accidents. It presents as a diffuse, brawny swelling of the extremities in 75% of patients, abdominal pain in 52%, and swelling of the face and throat in 30%. Its onset is usually in adolescence, with the more severe symptoms associated with the menses. Abdominal pain eventually becomes a major complaint in 93% of patients. They do not have typical urticarial wheals, but 26% have erythema multiforme-like lesions that partially clear in the center.[18] The angioedema seen in the genetically determined hereditary angioedema syndrome is different from that associated with common urticaria, anaphylaxis, and serum sickness, in that it is not triggered by readily identifiable antigens or pharmacologic agents; it is mediated through complement activation and kinin release rather than by an IgE mechanism.[2,18] Individual lesions are of longer duration than common urticaria and pitting of the skin does not occur.

16. Martin-Munoz F, Moreno-Ancillo A, Dominguez-Noche C et al. (1999) Evaluation of drug-related hypersensitivity reactions in children. **J Investigative Allergology & Clinical Immunology** 9:172–177.
17. Hebert AA, Sigman ES, Levy ML (1991) Serum sickness-like reactions from cefaclor in children. **J Am Acad Dermatol** 25:805–806.
18. Laurent J, Guinnepain MT (1999) Angioedema associated with C1 inhibitor deficiency. **Clinical Reviews in Allergy and Immunology** 17:513–523.

Severe airway edema accounts for the mortality of almost 30% in untreated patients. Only 25% of patients give a positive family history. The diagnosis should be suspected if the serum C4 level is persistently low and is confirmed by functional assay of the C1 esterase inhibitor. Mutations in the gene located on chromosome 11 can be either deletions or point mutations. In some children hereditary angioedema is associated with lupus erythematosus or other collagen vascular diseases.[19]

Acute attacks are managed by intravenous fluid replacement, airway maintenance, and intravenous infusion of plasma inhibitor concentrate.[18] Fresh-frozen plasma or ε-aminocaproic acid may be useful before surgical procedures.[18] Unlike other angioedema states, it is not responsive to therapy with steroids, epinephrine, or antihistamines. Good control of the disease is obtained through the use of anabolic steroids, such as danazol or stanozolol. These agents increase the levels of C1 esterase inhibitor.

Contact urticaria

Ordinary urticarial reactions commonly occur by way of mucous membrane exposure to antigens (inhalants or ingestants), but urticaria as a result of skin exposure is also possible.[3,20] In contact urticaria, the lesions are usually confined to the precise site of contact (an important diagnostic clue), but on occasion, satellite or even widespread lesions develop. Systemic reactions in the form of an anaphylaxis have also been rarely observed.[21]

The contactants responsible for these reactions may operate either through pharmacologic or immunologic mechanisms. Some common examples of the former include skin contact to jellyfish, nettles, corals, moths, caterpillars, and certain chemicals.[3,20] Immunologically mediated reactions can occur after exposure to fish, wood dust, rubber chemicals, cosmetics, epoxy resins, parabens, antibiotics, nickel, and certain animal products, such as dander, hair, and saliva. When the pathogenesis involves immunologic reactions, the causative agent may act either as a whole antigen or a partial antigen (hapten). In the latter case, a complete antigen is formed when the hapten binds to specific host proteins. Therapy requires identification and elimination of the contactant together with administration of antihistamines, as described in the section on common urticaria.

Aquagenic urticaria represents a special variant of contact urticaria.[20] In children with this problem, small, uniform urticaria papules develop at the ostia of hair follicles after exposure to water at any temperature. When the reaction is widespread, there are hundreds of these minute lesions. The mechanism through which these lesions develop is unknown. Aquagenic urticaria might be analogous to cholinergic urticaria in which sweat is believed to play a similar inciting role. Antihistamine therapy may be tried but is often only marginally helpful.

Physical urticarias

The physical urticarias are distinguished from other urticarial reactions because the precipitating factors (heat, cold, ultraviolet [UV] light, and pressure) are neither direct antigens nor direct mast cell degranulators.[1,3,20–24] Nevertheless, these agents appear to induce immunologic mechanisms that eventuate in a final common pathway of histamine (and probably other mediator) release from mast cells.

Cold urticaria

There are two distinct forms of cold urticaria: an acquired and a familial type. The former is common and is particularly likely to occur in children. In acquired cold urticaria, symptoms of urticaria and angioedema of conventional type develop during or immediately after exposure to cold. Either of two mechanisms can be responsible for the pathogenesis of acquired cold urticaria. The more common is that of IgE antibody response to an unknown, but presumably cold-induced, antigen. The second is that due to the presence of cryoproteins. These cold-precipitable proteins activate complement with subsequent release of anaphylatoxins and consequent mast cell degranulation, possibly through a mechanism involving immune complex formation. Many of the patients with cryoproteins have or will have symptoms and signs of autoimmune collagen vascular disease. Antihistamines, particularly cyproheptadine and doxepin, may be helpful. Anaphylactic reactions, particularly during swimming, have been reported in those with acquired cold urticaria.

Familial cold urticaria is an autosomal-dominant disease that usually becomes apparent in childhood.[21,22] It has been linked to a gene at chromosome 1q44.[21] In this condition, the development of urticaria is more often caused by cold air than by cold water exposure. The onset of an urticarial episode is usually delayed until several hours after the cold exposure. Burning or stinging is much more prominent than is pruritus. Associated problems include fever, arthralgia, and leukocytosis. The pathogenesis is unknown, but it does not appear to involve an IgE-mediated mechanism. Neutrophils are found in the biopsies.[22] Both types of cold urticaria are covered in greater detail in Chapter 7.

Cholinergic urticaria (heat and exercise urticaria)

This type of urticaria occurs commonly in adolescents.[1,3,23] It is readily identified when numerous, small (2–3mm) red blotches with a tiny (1mm) central urticarial papule occur within a matter of minutes after sweating is induced. The individual papules may be grouped. Headache, faintness, pulmonary distress, and gastrointestinal problems may also develop. Exercise-induced bronchospasm can accompany cholinergic urticaria. There is a refractory period after an attack where another episode cannot be induced for up to 24 hours.

The pathogenesis of cholinergic urticaria is believed to involve heating of the skin surface. Stimulation of sweating by heating the skin surface or with cholinergic-type pharmacologic agents can also induce lesions. The development of lesions may be related to host-determined, heightened reactivity to cholinergic-type chemicals. Attacks can be avoided through rapid cooling. This cooling must, of course, occur before the onset of sweating. One can instruct the child to induce attacks when there is optimal antihistamine coverage. Antihistamines, especially hydroxyzine, can be used to control symptoms. Autosomal-dominant inheritance has been reported but most cases are sporadic.[23]

Solar urticaria

Urticaria as a result of exposure to light occurs occasionally in children.[1,24] Sunlight, which also contains infrared (heat) energy, is the usual source of light exposure. For this reason, cholinergic urticaria (from heat) must also be considered in the differential diagnosis of solar urticaria. Childhood LE, erythropoietic protoporphyria, and polymorphous light eruption may also present with sun-induced urticaria. Children with solar urticaria develop lesions within minutes of light exposure.[24] Pruritic wheals are similar to those found in common urticaria and are occasionally associated with systemic symptoms. Lesions occur most readily on untanned skin.

Appropriate blood tests to rule out LE and erythropoietic protoporphyria should be performed. A clinical diagnosis of solar urticaria can be confirmed with controlled light testing. Most patients with solar urticaria are responsive only to UVB (280–320nm) light; others react to UVA (320–400nm) or visible light. A few respond to UV light across its entire spectrum. Passive transfer experiments are positive in most children with solar urticaria, which suggests that immunoglobulins (probably of the IgE type) are important in the pathogenesis of this disease. Phototesting with a solar simulator or

19. Pacheco T, Weston WL, Collier DH et al. (2000) Three generations of lupus erythematosus and hereditary angioedema. Amer J Med 109:256–257.
20. Wasserman D, Preminger A, Zlotogorski A (1994) Aquagenic urticaria in a child. Pediatr Dermatol 11:29–30.
21. Hoffman HM, Wright FA, Broide DHJ et al. (2000) Identification of a locus on chromosome 1q44 for familial cold urticaria. Am J Hum Genet 66:1693–1698.
22. Toppe Haas N, Henz BM (1998) Neutrophilic urticaria: clinical features, histological changes and possible mechanisms. Br J Dermatol 138:248–253.
23. Onn A, Levo Y, Kivity S (1996) Familial cholinergic urticaria. J Allergy Clin Immunol 98:847–849.
24. Monfrecola G, Masturzo E, Riccardo AM et al. (2000) Solar urticaria: a report on 57 cases. Am J Contact Dermat 11:89–94.

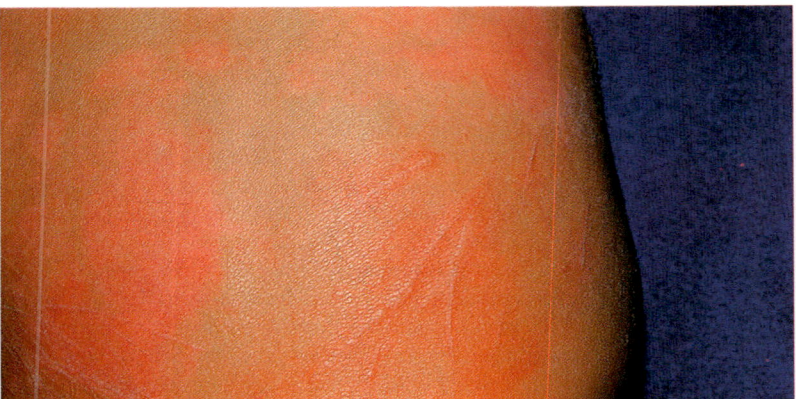

Fig. 19.7 Dermographism in a child.

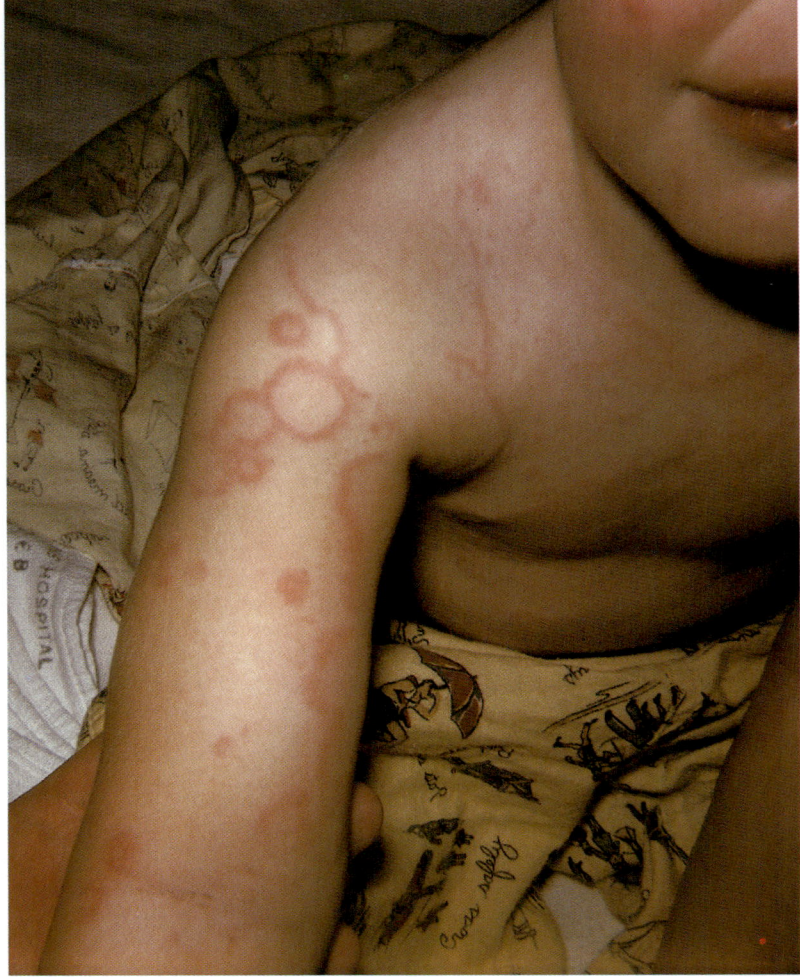

Fig. 19.8 Polycyclic red borders of erythema marginatum in febrile child with acute rheumatic fever.

monochromatic light source can define the action spectrum of light involved. This testing is available in only a few centers.

Therapy depends on the use of sun protection strategies including sun avoidance, clothing, and sunscreens. Unfortunately, the currently available sunscreens, including the newer agents with some UVA protection, are still not very effective for those who are sensitive to UVA or visible light. Systemic administration of β-carotene, antimalarials, or antihistamines may be considered but, in most children, are not often helpful. Attempts to induce "hardening" or "hyposensitization" with UV light therapy may be useful.

Dermographism

In virtually all infants younger than 6 months of age, about one-half of otherwise normal children, 1% of adolescents, and most children that have urticaria, linear stroking of the skin with modest pressure results in (1) the immediate development of a red line at the exact site of stroking, (2) the subsequent replacement of this line with a linear wheal, and (3) development of a surrounding flat red axon flare (Fig. 19.7).[1,3] The wheal reaches maximal size in 6–7 minutes and persists for 10–15 minutes. This phenomenon is known as the triple response of Lewis. In a smaller proportion of patients, the wheal formation is accompanied by significant local or even generalized pruritus. This pruritic reaction, called symptomatic dermographism, may be troublesome enough to warrant medical attention. The wheal is seen in comatose children (e.g., in encephalitis, meningitis, drug overdose) and has been termed tache cerebrale.

Symptomatic dermographism can be passively transferred, which suggests the presence of an immunologic mechanism, presumably IgE in type. Wheals are commonly found around the belt area and may follow widespread insect bites and transient episodes of urticaria. The presence of symptomatic dermographism may be associated with atopic dermatitis, urticaria, or mastocytosis. In infants with autosomal-dominant diffuse cutaneous mastocytosis, dermographism is particularly prominent and may precede the characteristic "Morrocan leather" appearance by several months.

There is no known specific cause for ordinary dermographism, and it is not often a clue to the presence of an underlying systemic disorder. Dermographism may persist for year, but most patients can expect spontaneous regression within two years. Treatment with antihistamines, especially concomitant use of low-dose hydroxyzine and cimetidine, may occasionally be warranted.

Delayed-pressure urticaria is a variant of dermographism. The lesions, however, do not occur until several hours after the pressure has been applied. Moreover, the lesions are painful and deep. No pruritus is present. The palms and soles are involved most commonly. On biopsy, T-helper cells are abundant, which suggests that type IV cell-mediated immune mechanisms may play an important role in the pathogenesis. The response to antihistamine therapy is poor.

Erythema marginatum (erythema circinatum)

Up to 10% of children with rheumatic fever have transient episodic, asymptomatic, annular erythematous lesions.[25] The prevalence of erythema marginatum in rheumatic fever is currently low, but periodic increases in prevalence have been reported in past epidemics. These lesions begin as flat or slightly raised reddened papules that clear in the center and rapidly enlarge in a centrifugal manner. These enlarging lesions appear as thin red lines, forming large annular or polycyclic patterns (Fig. 19.8). These lines and circles appear in successive waves over the trunk and proximal extremities. Each lesion evolves, migrates, and then resolves over one hour or so. They occur most commonly late in the day and usually appear with fever. Inducing cutaneous vasodilation may make the lesions more visible.

The pathogenesis of erythema marginatum is unknown, although it appears to involve the release of vasodilating and permeability-enhancing mediators similar to those responsible for the development of common urticaria.[25] From the lack of itching and the migration of individual lesions one can suggest that the two processes are not identical. A thorough evaluation for acute rheumatic fever is indicated. Erythema marginatum may also be seen following streptococcal infections without evidence of acute rheumatic fever.[25]

25. Report of the Committee on Infectious Disease: Red Book (2000) Elk Grove Village, Il, American Academy of Pediatrics.

Flushing and blushing reactions

The flushing and blushing reactions are characterized by the sudden development of diffuse flat erythema that is most striking over the face and upper trunk.[26] There is no associated increase in vascular permeability during these reactions, and urticaria and angioedema are absent. These reactions may be divided into those related to normal physiologic responses (termed blushing reactions), those related to certain ingestants, and those related to an underlying systemic disease.

Physiologic flushing and blushing

The term *blushing* is usually used for reactions caused by embarrassment and the term *flushing* for those caused by anger or excitement. Little is known about the mechanisms through which these reactions occur. These are most prominent in fair-skinned children.

Flushing may occur during the ingestion of hot or spicy food and beverages and may accompany the ingestion of foods containing sulfites, nitrites, monosodium benzoate, certain "hot" spices, and products containing alcohol.[26] Familial flushing has been linked to inheritance of alcohol dehydrogenase genotypes.[26]

Episodic flushing occurs in some children with mastocytosis and pheochromocytomas. In mastocytosis, the reactions are probably mediated through prostaglandin D_2 mechanisms. In pheochromocytoma, the reactions are believed to be due to catecholamine release.

PERSISTENT ERYTHEMAS

The diseases in this category are characterized by the presence of smooth-surfaced, blanchable red papules and plaques. As such, they are similar to the lesions of the transient erythemas. However, as the name implies, the lesions of the persistent erythemas are considerably more stable and remain at the same skin sites, unchanged in shape or size, for at least one week rather than for minutes or hours.

The stability of the lesion is explained by its histology. All of the diseases in this group are characterized by the presence of mononuclear (primarily lymphocytic) perivascular dermal infiltrates. The deposition and removal of these cells require a much longer time than the simple change in vascular permeability that occurs in the transient erythemas. On the other hand, the persistent erythemas are separated from the purpuras because the lymphocytic infiltrates in the persistent erythemas are non-necrotizing so that the inflammatory infiltrate in the persistent erythemas seldom compromises the integrity of the vascular wall and there is little or no extravasation of red blood cells into the surrounding connective tissue.

The color of the erythema present in the lesions of persistent erythemas is variable, depending on the degree of oxygen saturation, the amount of dermal edema, and the size and type of vessels involved. In general, lesions of the persistent erythemas tend to be duskier in color than are the lesions of the transient erythemas.

There are an extraordinarily large number of diseases that meet the criteria of the persistent erythemas. To enhance their recognition and to simplify discussion, they are subclassified on the basis of shared morphologic features (Table 19.5). The prototype for the persistent erythemas is EM.

ERYTHEMA MULTIFORME
Introduction and historical note

Erythema multiforme (EM) is an acute, self-limited skin condition characterized by the abrupt onset of symmetrical, fixed red papules some of which

TABLE 19.5   Classification of persistent erythemas

Mucocutaneous syndromes 　Erythema multiforme 　Stevens–Johnson syndrome 　Toxic epidermal necrolysis 　Fixed drug eruption Papular erythemas 　Papular urticaria (insect bites) 　Pityriasis lichenoides 　Lymphomatoid papulosis 　Erythema elevatum diutinum Nodular erythemas 　Erythema nodosum 　Subacute nodular migratory panniculitis 　Lobular panniculitis syndromes 　Nodular vasculitis 　Superficial thrombophlebitis Annular and gyrate erythemas 　Erythema chronicum migrans 　Erythema annulare centrifugum 　Erythema gyratum repens Acral erythemas 　Erythromelalgia 　Miscellaneous acral erythemas	Reticulate erythemas 　Livedo reticularis 　Erythema ab igne 　Erythema infectiosum Diffuse and morbilliform erythemas 　Rubeola and atypical measles 　Rubella 　Roseola 　ECHO and Coxsackie viral exanthems 　Erythema infectiosum 　Infectious mononucleosis 　Scarlet fever 　Staphylococcal toxic erythemas

evolve into target lesions.[14,27] A target lesion consists of concentric zones of color change with evidence of damage of the epidermis in the central zone such as bulla formation or crust (Fig. 19.9).[14,27] Early target lesions will have a central dusky zone and a red outer zone, but may evolve to three zones of color change.

The term *erythema multiforme* is attributed to the Viennese dermatologist, Ferdinand von Hebra[28] in 1860.[29] The illness he described was mild, recurrent, and characterized by the evolution of early red papules into "target" lesions. He noted that there was no prodrome and that oral lesions were not present. Since von Hebra's time, the concept of EM has become confused in the literature, possibly because authors interpreted EM to mean many forms of lesions present at one time.[27] This has resulted in many instances of giant urticaria or lesions with polycyclic borders being reported as EM.[14] Further confusion came when Thomas[30] designated the illness described by von Hebra as EM minor and the severe mucocutaneous reaction described by Stevens and Johnson as EM major. This incorrectly linked Stevens–Johnson syndrome (SJS) to EM, and later others linked toxic epidermal necrolysis (TEN) to EM. No author has demonstrated that EM progresses to SJS or TEN.[27,31] Most authorities believe these are distinct conditions.[31]

Epidemiology

The exact incidence of EM is unknown, but it is believed to be very uncommon in childhood, even less common than SJS.[31] Twenty percent of all cases of EM occur in childhood.[27] There is a slight male preponderance but no racial bias. To date, there is no known genetic predisposition. Several small studies of histocompatability antigen (HLA) associations with EM reported differing types, such as HLA-DQw3, –Drw53, and –Aw33.[27]

26. Chen WJ, Chen CC, Cheng AT (1998) Self-reported flushing and genotypes of ALDH2, ADH2 and ADH3 among Taiwanese Han. **Alcohol Clin Exp Res** 22:1048–1052.
27. Brice SL, Huff JC, Weston WL (1990) Erythema multiforme. **Curr Probl Dermatol** II:3–26.
28. von Hebra F (1860) Acute exantheme und hautkrankheiten. Handbuch der Speciellen Pathologie und Therapie. Erlangen: Verlag von Ferdinand von Enke, pp. 198–200.
29. Von Hebra F (1866) On diseases of the skin including the exanthemata. London: New Sydenham Society, p. 285.
30. Thomas, BA (1950) The so-called Stevens–Johnson syndrome. **Brit Med J** 1:1393.
31. Assier H, Bastuji-Garin S, Revuz J, Roujeau J-C (1995) Erythema multiforme with mucous membrane involvement and Stevens–Johnson Syndrome are clinically different disorders with distinct causes. **Arch Dermatol** 131:539–543.

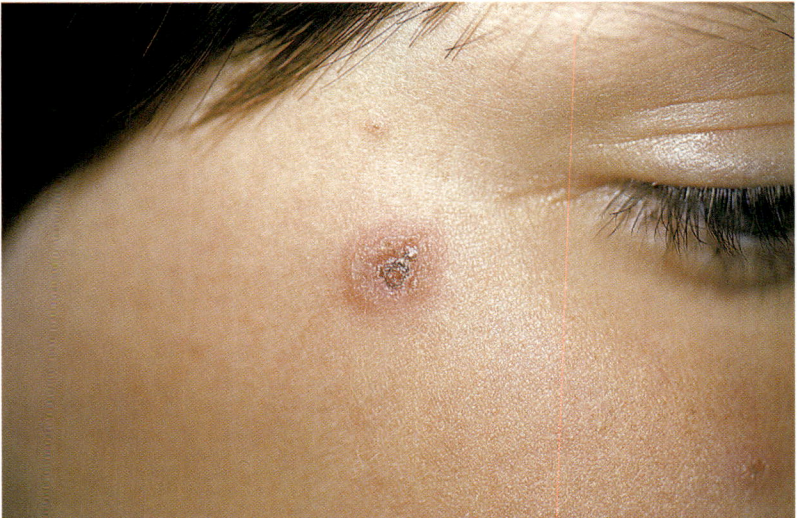

Fig. 19.9 Classic "target lesion" of erythema multiforme with outer red zone and inner zone of epidermal injury with crust and bulla formation. Herpes simplex associated in an 8-year-old boy.

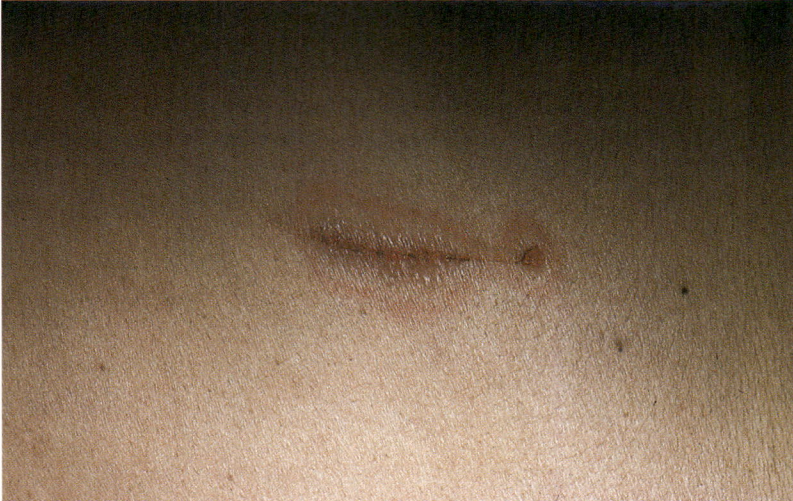

Fig. 19.10 Isomorphic phenomenon in erythema multiforme. Linear target lesions appear within a prior animal scratch on the arm of an 11-year-old child.

Presenting history

There is usually no prodrome.[27] Approximately 50% of children give a history of a preceding herpes labialis or, rarely, herpes progenitalis.[32,33] The preceding herpes simplex virus (HSV) lesion may still be present at the onset of the EM skin lesions but, more often, precedes the onset of EM skin lesions by 3–14 days.[32,33] A history of an abrupt onset of skin lesions is obtained, with almost all the lesions appearing within 24 hours and completely by 72 hours. Itching or burning sensations may be described.

Physical examination

The primary lesion is a round, red papule that remains fixed at the same skin site for seven days or more.[14,27] At least some of the red papules evolve into target lesions. The target lesion is characterized by concentric zones of color change with a central dusky or purple zone and an outer red zone.[14,27,31] Some target lesions develop a blister or crust in the central zone after several days. A few lesions may have three zones of color change with a red border, white inner zone, and dusky center, sometimes referred to as an iris lesion. Whether an individual lesion has two or three concentric zones of color change does not matter (Fig. 19.9). The forearms are the most frequent skin sites, but palms, neck, face, and trunk are also frequently involved.[34,35] Although there is considerable variation from individual to individual, usually over 100 lesions are present.[34] The Köebner phenomenon may be observed, with target lesions appearing within areas of cutaneous injury such as scratches (Fig. 19.10). The injury precedes the onset of the other EM skin lesions and cannot occur once EM lesions are present.[35] EM lesions may also be found within areas of sunburn. Cuticular redness and swelling are observed. Lesions also tend to be grouped, especially around the elbows and knees. The clinical criteria of Brice, Huff and Weston[27] should be strictly observed when diagnosing EM. These include the presence of symmetrical fixed red papules, at least some of which evolve into typical target lesions.[14,27] Oral erosions are present in less than one-half of children with EM and, when present, are few in number and mildly symptomatic.[27,31,34,35] Involvement of the lips, buccal mucosa, and tongue are seen. Occasionally, large bullous target lesions may involve the lips and mimic the crusted lips seen in Stevens–Johnson syndrome (Fig. 19.11).[36,37] Recurrent oral erythema multiforme without skin target lesions has been described but this condition is not universally accepted.[37,39] Recurrent episodes of shallow mouth ulcers mimic aphthous ulcers and these conditions may be impossible to distinguish. Other mucosal sites are not involved. Fever, lymphadenopathy, and organomegaly are absent. Atypical forms of herpes simplex associated-EM have been described.[38] Large, solitary and asymmetrical target lesions are seen on the skin.

Laboratory findings

There are no characteristic laboratory changes in EM.

Pathophysiology and histogenesis

The value of histopathologic examination is to exclude conditions such as LE or vasculitis that may mimic EM. The earliest pathologic change of EM is apoptotic keratinocytes.[40] A perivascular infiltrate of mononuclear leukocytes with exocytosis into the epidermis is seen. Spongiosis and focal liquefaction degeneration of basal keratinocytes are observed with edema of the superficial dermis.[27,31,40] Immunofluorescent findings are nonspecific. Granular deposits of IgM and C3 around superficial blood vessels and at focal areas of the dermal-epidermal junction have been described. Specific HSV antigens have been detected within keratinocytes by immunofluorescence, and HSV genomic DNA has been detected by polymerase chain reaction amplification of skin biopsy samples.[32,33,41,42] By *in situ* hybridization, HSV DNA is located primarily within keratinocytes.[42]

Most childhood EM cases are HSV-associated.[32,33] In some cases, a subclinical HSV lesion may precede the onset of EM.[33] The presence of the entire HSV genome within the skin lesions and the expression of virally encoded

32. Weston WL, Stockert SS, Jester J et al. (1992) Herpes simplex virus in childhood erythema multiforme. **Pediatrics** 89:32–34.
33. Weston WL, Morelli JG (1998) Herpes-associated erythema multiforme in prepubertal children. **Arch Pediatrics & Adolescent Med** 151:1014–1018.
34. Huff JC, Weston WL (1989) Recurrent erythema multiforme. **Medicine** [Baltimore] 68:133–140.
35. Huff JC, Weston WL (1983) Isomorphic phenomenon in erythema multiforme. **Clin Exp Dermatol** 8:409.
36. Weston WL, Morelli JG, Rogers M (1997) Target lesions on the lips: Childhood herpes simplex associated erythema multiforme mimics Stevens–Johnson syndrome. **J Am Acad Dermatol** 37:848–850.
37. Farthing PM, Maragou P, Coates F et al. (1995) Characteristics of the oral lesions in patients with recurrent erythema multiforme. **J Oral Pathol Med** 24:9–11.
38. Weston WL, Brice SL (1998) Atypical forms of herpes-simplex associated erythema multiforme. **J Am Acad Dermatol** 39:124–126.
39. Lozada-Nur F, Gorsky M, Silverman S Jr (1989) Oral erythema multiforme: clinical observations and treatment of 95 patients. **Oral Surg Oral Med Oral Path** 67:36–40.
40. Howland WW, Golitz LE, Huff JC, Weston WL (1984) Erythema multiforme: Clinical, histopathologic and immunologic study. **J Am Acad Derm** 10:438–446.
41. Darragh TM, Egbert BM, Berger TG (1991) Identification of herpes simplex virus DNA in lesions of erythema multiforme by the polymerase chain reaction. **J Am Acad Dermatol** 24:23.
42. Brice SL, Leahy MA, Ong L et al. (1994) Examination of non-involved skin, previously involved skin and peripheral blood for Herpes Simplex Virus DNA in patients with recurrent herpes associated erythema multiforme. **J Cutan Pathol** 21:408–412.

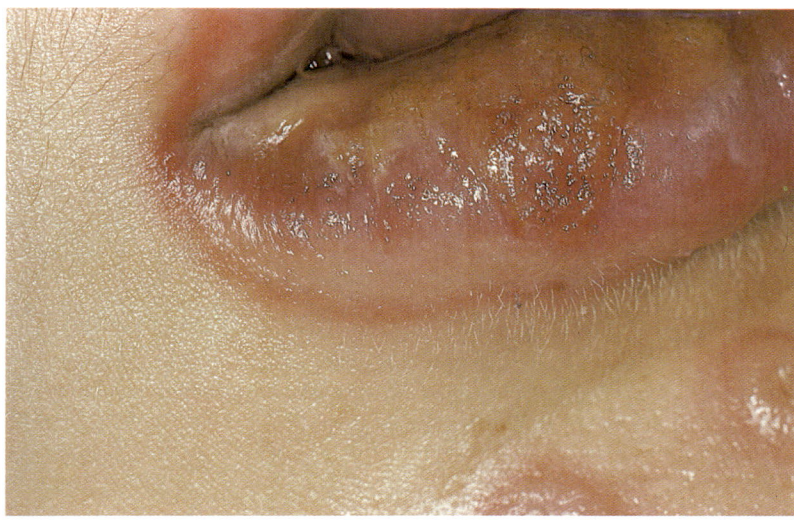

Fig. 19.11 Target lesions of the lips in erythema multiforme. Note outer zone of erythema, inner zone of white edema and central zone of crusting of lips.

antigens on keratinocytes may be interpreted as evidence for replicating HSV within affected skin sites. The inflammation within skin lesions is believed to be a part of the HSV-specific host response.[42] Other infections definitely associated with EM are histoplasmosis and Orf.[27,43,44] Histoplasmosis in endemic areas has occasionally been responsible for EM, especially when both EM and erythema nodosum lesions are present together.[27] Orf is a rare cause of EM.

Differential diagnosis

Giant urticaria is most often confused with EM in pediatric patients.[14] The lesions of urticaria are transient and not persistent; they have a clear central zone, not a dusky one. In children with systemic LE (SLE), individual lesions may mimic true target lesions, but other lesions characteristic of SLE are present. Early lesions of vasculitis, particularly urticarial vasculitis, may mimic target lesions of EM. In the case of both SLE and vasculitis, a skin biopsy, elevated ESR, and low complement level help in the differential diagnosis. Juvenile spring eruption, a form of polymorphous light eruption, may mimic herpes-associated EM.[45]

Therapeutics and prognosis

There are no double-blind or open trials of therapy for the acute episode of EM. For the usual attack of EM, symptomatic treatment will suffice. Oral antihistamines for three or four days reduce the stinging and burning of the skin. Oral antacids may be required for discrete oral ulcers. In children receiving oral steroids, it is advisable to discontinue the steroids, despite the likelihood of an EM flare, as prolonged steroid use may result in more frequent or continuous episodes.[44] There are no trials that support the use of oral steroids in EM. A double-blind, placebo-controlled study in young adults demonstrated efficacy of acyclovir prophylaxis in chronic or frequently recurrent EM.[46] In children with HSV-associated EM with frequent recurrences, 6- to 12-month prophylaxis with oral acyclovir at 10mg/kg per day may be considered. Acyclovir started after symptoms begin is ineffective.[44] A few individuals have attacks precipitated by factors other than reactivation of HSV, and acyclovir will be of no benefit.

All children affected by EM have an uncomplicated course, except when immunosuppressive drugs are used; in these case, secondary infections and more frequent and longer episodes may occur.

For most children with untreated EM, the episode lasts two weeks and heals without sequelae.[32,33] Except for burning and stinging of the skin, the child is usually otherwise healthy. Recurrences are the rule in EM associated with HSV. Most children have one or two recurrences per year, typically each spring and, after two or three years, stop having recurrences.

Pediatric aspects of the disorder

The overall health of the child is unaffected by EM. Growth and development are normal.

STEVENS–JOHNSON SYNDROME
Introduction and historical note

In 1922, two physicians in the United States, Stevens and Johnson,[47] described an acute mucocutaneous syndrome in two young boys. The condition was characterized by severe purulent conjunctivitis, stomatitis with extensive mucosal necrosis, and "EM-like" skin lesions. This became known as SJS and was recognized as a severe mucocutaneous disease with a prolonged course and occasional fatalities.

SJS is usually preceded by a prodrome of a respiratory illness, followed in 1 to 14 days by severe erosions of at least two mucosal surfaces with extensive necrosis of the lips and mouth and a purulent conjunctivitis.[48–50] A varied extent of skin involvement is described, with red macules evolving within hours into bullae and large areas of skin necrosis and denudation rapidly developing. SJS may have mucosal lesions only or both mucosal and skin lesions.[48–50] Fever, lymphadenopathy, and toxicity virtually always accompany the mucocutaneous involvement.

Epidemiology

The exact incidence of SJS is not known, in part because there is considerable confusion over a definition and significant clinical and histologic overlap with other acute epithelial injury states such as toxic epidermal necrolysis (TEN).[48–50] Chan estimated the incidence as 0.8 cases per one million inhabitants.[50] The peak incidence of all cases is in the second decade of life with the majority of patients being pediatric. SJS is more common in childhood than is EM.[48–50] Spring and summer prevalence has been observed for SJS. Recurrences have been described, but are quite unusual. There is no sex or racial predilection.

Presenting history

Most children have a distinct prodrome of an upper respiratory illness with fever, cough, rhinitis, sore throat, headache, vomiting, diarrhea, and malaise.[48–50] During the prodrome, children are often treated with antipyretics or antibiotics or both. After 1 to 14 days, there is an abrupt onset of the skin eruption.

Physical examination

The child with SJS is febrile and appears acutely ill. The lips develop hemorrhagic crusts with denudation of the mucosa, and severe stomatitis ensues (Fig. 19.12). Unlike EM, mucosal involvement is confluent and widespread rather than focal.[36,48] There is a purulent conjunctivitis with photophobia and pseudomembrane formation. The eyelids are adherent to one another. Genital

43. Brice SL, Stockert SS, Ong L et al. (1993) Comparison of the immune response in patients with herpes labialis and those with herpes associated erythema multiforme. **Arch Derm Res** 285:193–195.
44. Schofield JK, Tatnall FM, Leigh IM (1993) Recurrent erythema multiforme: Clinical features and treatment in a large series of patients. **Br J Dermatol** 128:542–545.
45. Wolf P, Soyer HP, Fink-Puches R et al. (1994) Recurrent post-herpetic erythema multiforme mimicking polymorphic light and juvenile spring eruption: two cases in young boys. **Br J Dermatol** 131:364–367.
46. Tatnall FM, Schofield JK, Leigh IM (1995) A double-blind, placebo-controlled trial of continuous acyclovir therapy in recurrent erythema multiforme. **Br J Dermatol** 132:267.

47. Stevens AM, Johnson FC (1922) A new eruptive fever associated with stomatitis and ophthalmia. **Am J Dis Child** 24:526–259.
48. Bastuji-Garin S, Rzany B, Stern RS et al. (1993) Clinical classification of cases of toxic epidermal necrolysis, Stevens–Johnson syndrome, and erythema multiforme. **Arch Dermatol** 129:92.
49. Leaute-Labreze C, Lamireau T, Chawki D et al. (2000) Diagnosis, classification and management of erythema multiforme and Stevens–Johnson syndrome. **Arch Dis Child** 83:347.
50. Chan HL, Stern RS, Arndt KA et al. (1990) The incidence of erythema multiforme, Stevens–Johnson syndrome and toxic epidermal necrolysis: A population based study with particular reference to reactions caused by drugs among outpatients. **Arch Dermatol** 126:43.

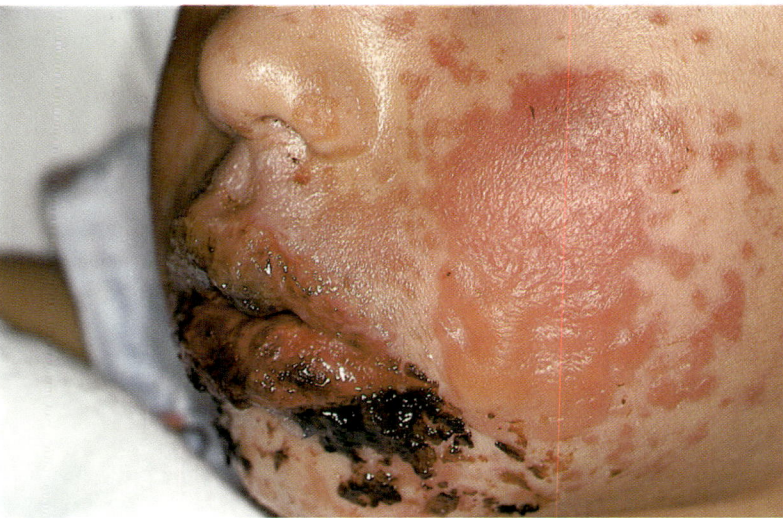

Fig. 19.12 Stevens–Johnson syndrome. Hemorrhagic crusts of lips and red macules on face of two-year-old treated with trimethoprim-sulfonamide combination.

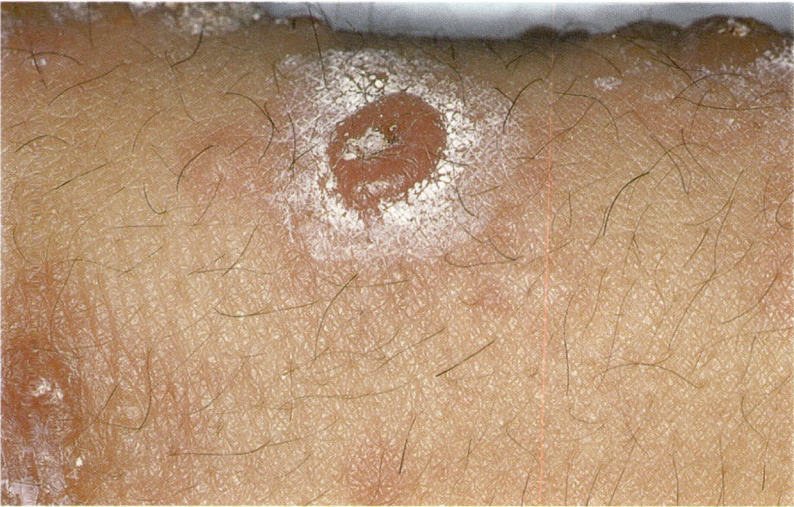

Fig. 19.13 Discrete bullous and crusted lesions of skin in child with SJS.

involvement with pain, redness, and erosions accompanied by bleeding may occur. Anal erosions may be seen; uncommonly, the esophagus, respiratory epithelium, and nasal mucosa are involved. In girls, severe vulvovaginal pain may be observed. The skin eruption consists of symmetrical red macules, which progress to central blister formation and extensive areas of epidermal necrosis. The skin is tender. Involved areas may blister or show central desquamation (Fig. 19.13). All children with SJS have two or more mucosal sites involved; some, in addition, have skin involvement. Skin involvement may be limited or extensive. Some children develop red macules, which rapidly enlarge and may become confluent. Frequently, the child is unable to eat or drink and appears dehydrated at presentation. Generalized lymphadenopathy is usually present, and enlargement of the liver and spleen may

be found. Arthritis and arthralgias are sometimes seen, and hepatitis is common. Myocarditis, pneumothorax, and nephritis are rare associations. Gastrointestinal bleeding can be observed.

The diagnosis of SJS can be made by the characteristic prodrome followed by an abrupt onset of extensive areas of mucocutaneous necrosis with at least two mucosal sites involved.[48–50] Because there may be significant overlap with TEN in those children with SJS and skin involvement, the presence of two or more mucosal sites of injury is a critical diagnostic feature. In SJS the skin involvement is 10–30% of the body surface and, in TEN, over 30%. A biopsy that shows extensive areas of epidermal necrosis is useful.

Laboratory findings

In addition to fluid and electrolyte imbalance, a number of other laboratory abnormalities may be observed. An elevated ESR is found in every child with SJS, with leukocytosis in 60%, eosinophilia in 20%, anemia in 15%, elevated liver enzyme levels in 15%, leukopenia in 10%, and proteinuria and microscopic hematuria in 5%.[48–51]

Pathogenesis

Extensive epidermal necrosis with a paucity of inflammatory cells is characteristic.[48–50] The severity of epidermal necrosis is accompanied by incontinence of melanin pigment, colloid bodies, and subepidermal blister formation. Early lesions sometimes show a prominent neutrophilic dermal infiltrate with nuclear dust; older lesions may be pauci-inflammatory.

Although hundreds of precipitating factors have been implicated in SJS, drugs predominate as the major association.[50–52] Preceding infections with *Mycoplasma pneumoniae* or HSV are uncommonly associated.[52,53] Of the drugs implicated, nonsteroidal anti-inflammatory drugs are the most frequent, followed by sulfonamides, anticonvulsants, penicillins, tetracycline, and doxycycline.[50–52,54–57] Ibuprofen and naprosyn among the NSAIDs and hydantoins and barbiturates among the anticonvulsants are most frequent.[50–52,54–57] NSAIDs, sulfonamides, and anticonvulsants are metabolized by the liver and epithelium through similar mechanisms, including the cytochrome P450 system generated aromatic drug metabolites, which form arene oxides.[54] Shear and Spielberg reported epoxide hydrolases to be deficient in children susceptible to SJS, resulting in accumulation of arene oxides that bind to and inhibit RNA and shut off cell protein synthesis.[55] In drug-associated SJS, the onset of mucosal lesions follows the drug ingestion by 14 to 56 days. Drugs administered a few days prior to the onset of SJS are usually not implicated.[54–57] Rechallenge studies are naturally few unless by oversight, but reproduction of SJS upon rechallenge has been reported.[57]

In *M. pneumoniae*-associated disease and other infectious-related disease, the pathogenesis remains unknown. Recent studies report the detection of autoantibodies to desmoplakin I and II in SJS with binding to the desmosomal plaque of the keratinocytes an important step to keratin cytoskeleton disruption and cell separation.[58] Whether these autoantibodies play an amplifying role or are primarily involved in the pathomechanism is not known.

Differential diagnosis

There are many problems with terminology regarding SJS and TEN.[48–50] It is clear that some children have features of SJS with extensive skin lesions, which mimic those observed in TEN; some have a limited cutaneous involvement; and others have only mucosal involvement. This confusion has resulted in many controversies in the literature. All forms have overlapping features and share in common the presence of large areas of epithelial necrosis,

51. Wong KC, Kennedy PJ, Lee S (1999) Clinical manifestations and outcomes of 17 cases of Stevens–Johnson syndrome and toxic epidermal necrolysis. **Australas J Dermatol** 40:131.

52. Sontheimer R, Garibaldi RA, Krueger GG (1978) Stevens–Johnson syndrome associated with Mycoplasma pneumoniae infection. **Arch Dermatol** 114:241.

53. Tay Y-K, Huff JC, Weston WL (1996) Mycoplasma pneumoniae is associated with Stevens–Johnson syndrome, not erythema multiforme [von Hebra]. **J Am Acad Dermatol** 35:757–760.

54. Rzany B, Correia O, Kelly JP et al. (1999) Risk of Stevens–Johnson syndrome and toxic epidermal necrolysis during the first weeks of antiepileptic therapy. **Lancet** 353:2190.

55. Sullivan JR, Shear NH (2001) The drug hypersensitivity syndrome. What is the pathogenesis? **Arch Dermatol** 137:357–364.

56. Shear H, Spielberg SP (1988) Anticonvulsant hypersensitivity syndrome. **J Clin Invest** 82:1826–1829.

57. Azinge O, Garrick GA (1978) Stevens–Johnson syndrome [erythema multiforme] following ingestion of trimethoprim-sulfamethoxazole on two separate occasions in the same person. **J All Clin Immunol** 62:125–126.

58. Foedinger D, Anhalt GJ, Boecskoer B et al. (1995) Autoantibodies to desmoplakin I and II in erythema multiforme. **J Exp Med** 181:169–179.

and all forms of SJS and TEN may be precipitated by the same factors. If two or more mucosal sites are involved with or without accompanying skin lesions, most authorities consider the condition to be SJS; if large sheets of skin are denuded with no mucosal involvement, TEN is frequently diagnosed. Unfortunately, there are children with overlapping features whose conditions are difficult to classify despite the efforts of the International Cooperative Group.

Kawasaki disease is sometimes confused with SJS in children. In Kawasaki disease, the lips are red and dry and the hemorrhagic crusts and mucosal denudation observed with SJS are absent. The bulbar conjunctivae are red in Kawasaki disease, but there is no exudate as seen in SJS. The skin lesions of Kawasaki disease are transient red macules and bullous lesions or target-like lesions are not seen as would be expected in SJS with the exception of perineal peeling and peeling of the fingertips.

Paraneoplastic pemphigus may also mimic SJS.[59] Although rare, similar severe necrosis of the lips, eyes, and oral mucosa may be observed in paraneoplastic pemphigus. Biopsy will demonstrate epithelial acantholysis and indirect immunofluorescence of serum or immunoblotting will distinguish from SJS. Search for an associated lymphoma or Castleman's tumour is indicated.[59]

Therapeutics and prognosis

The mainstay of management is admission to a burn unit or a pediatric intensive care unit, and the child is managed as if a burn has occurred from the "inside out."[49,51,60–62] If an offending drug is suspected, it should be discontinued.[61] The child should undergo correction of fluid and electrolyte imbalance and monitoring of urinary output and serum osmolality and electrolyte levels; protection from secondary infection; good ophthalmologic care; pulmonary toilet to include postural drainage, sputum cultures, and prompt treatment of pulmonary infections; periodic cultures of the skin, eyes, and mucosal sites; caloric replacement; early skin grafting of large denuded areas or the use of biologic dressings; physical therapy to prevent contractures; use of antacids and mouth rinses; and general skilled nursing care.[49,51,60–62]

The use of systemic steroids has never been demonstrated to be efficacious, and one can suggest from two retrospective studies that systemic steroids may adversely affect morbidity and mortality rates.[63,64] Long-term steroid use should be avoided to reduce the likelihood of infectious complications. Most recently, intravenous immunoglobulin (IVIG) treatment has been championed.[65,66] There is enthusiasm for both IVIG and IV corticosteroid[67] treatments among medical authorities but it is based strictly upon testimonials and not upon comparative trials. Two recently published open, non-blinded, non-placebo-controlled trials have been widely accepted as most promising by clinicians.[65,67] In both, treatments with IVIG or methylprednisolone 4mg/kg per day given iv for four days were employed. Days with fever were reduced by 50% over historical controls but other aspects of the course were not influenced.

SJS is frequently complicated by dehydration; electrolyte imbalance; secondary cutaneous, oral, or pulmonary bacterial infection; and cutaneous scarring and dyspigmentation.[49,51,60] Large areas of denuded skin may scar with contractures if they are over joints. Ocular sequelae are serious and include pseudomembrane formation with immobility of the eyelids, symblepharon, entropion, trichiasis, corneal scarring, and permanent visual impairment.[68] Lacrimal scarring with subsequent excessive tearing, anterior

uveitis, and panophthalmos are complications. Although mouth and lip lesions usually heal without sequelae, esophageal strictures, anal strictures, vaginal stenosis, and urethral meatal stenosis may occur. Severe pneumonitis and pneumothorax may develop.[69] Shedding of the nails may result in permanent anonychia.[51]

SJS often has a protracted course of four to six weeks.[49,51,60]

Pediatric aspects of the disorder

SJS is a severe illness requiring prolonged hospitalization and has significant complications. It may be months before the affected child completely recovers, and permanent sequelae, mostly as the result of scarring, are often observed. Contractures and eye complications are the most common complications.[51] Convalescence for the child is prolonged and requires good physical therapy, a home teacher, and skilled nursing care.

TOXIC EPIDERMAL NECROLYSIS

Introduction and historical note

TEN develops in the form of blistered erythematous patches and plaques, which evolve rapidly to extensive areas of skin necrosis, with loss of sheets of epidermis (Fig. 19.14).[48,50,70] In some, an acute sunburn-like appearance with evolution into extensive epidermal necrosis is seen. Many skin areas denude when the child is handled during the examination. The cutaneous features may be similar to those of SJS, but individual lesions may evolve more rapidly.[48,50,51] Complications and associated cutaneous findings are similar to those of SJS. The precipitating factors appear to be the same for both SJS and TEN.[49,50–54] In one study, TEN was found to be 70% as common as SJS in childhood.[48] Lyell is attributed for the term "toxic epidermal necrolysis" and stated that the condition resembled a "scald."[70] At least one of his initial three patients probably had staphylococcal scalded skin syndrome. Since Lyell's description, the classification of TEN has been confused and the international

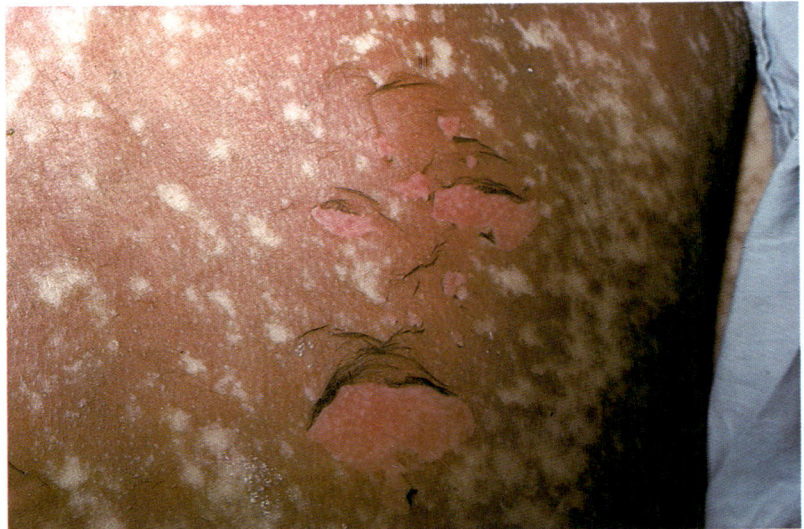

Fig. 19.14   Large sheets of necrotic skin in child with toxic epidermal necrolysis.

59. Lemon A, Huff JC, Weston WL (1977) Childhood paraneoplastic pemphigus associated with Castleman's tumour. Br J Dermatol 136:1`5–117.
60. Prendiville JS, Hebert AA, Greenwald MJ et al. (1989) Management of Stevens–Johnson syndrome and toxic epidermal necrolysis. J Pediatr 115:881–887.
61. Garcia-Doral I, LeCloach L, Bocquet H et al. (2000) Toxic epidermal necrolysis and Stevens–Johnson syndrome: Does early withdrawal of causative drugs decrease the risk of death? Arch Dermatol 136:323–327.
62. Roujeau JC (1999) Treatment of severe drug eruptions. J Dermatol 26:718–724.
63. Rasmussen JE (1976) Erythema multiforme in children: response to treatment with systemic corticosteroids. Br J Dermatol 95:181–186.
64. Renfro L, Grant-Kels J, Feder Jr HM et al. (´989) Controversy: Are systemic steroids indicated in the treatment of erythema multiforme? Pediatr Dermatol 6:43–48.

65. Morici MV, Galen WK, Shetty AK et al. (2000) Intravenous immunoglobulin therapy for children with Stevens–Johnson syndrome. J Rheumatol 27:2494–2497.
66. Brett AS, Phillips D, Lynn AW (2001) Intravenous immunoglobulin therapy for Stevens–Johnson syndrome. South Med J 94:342.
67. Kakourou T, Klontza D, Soteropoulous F, Kattamis C (1997) Corticosteroid treatment of erythema multiforme major [Stevens–Johnson syndrome] in children. Eur J Pediatr 156:90–93.
68. Lehman SS (1999) Long term ocular complcations of Stevens–Johnson syndrome. Clin Pediatr 38:425.
69. Virant FS, Redding GJ, Novack AH (1984) Multiple pulmonary complications in a patient with Stevens–Johnson syndrome. Clin Pediatr 23:412–413.
70. Lyell A (1956) Toxic epidermal necrolysis: an eruption resembling scalding of skin. Br J Dermatol 68:355–361.

group attempting to classify TEN recognizes considerable overlap with SJS.[48–51]

Epidemiology

TEN is less common in children than SJS, although the exact prevalence is unknown.

Differential diagnosis

Differentiation from staphylococcal scalded skin syndrome (SSSS) is necessary. High fever and occurrence in older children favors TEN, whereas evidence of preceding rhinitis and localization to intertriginous areas, acutely tender skin, and occurrence in newborns or infants favors SSSS. Definitive diagnosis depends on the histologic location of the blister. In TEN, it is subepidermal with overlying epidermal necrosis; in SSSS, separation of skin is at the granular portion of the mid-epidermis with a viable overlying epidermis. The histologic location can be rapidly determined microscopically with a shave skin biopsy and frozen-section examination.[48]

Involvement of mucous membranes does not occur with SSSS. The predominance of mucosal lesions over skin lesions generally distinguishes SJS from TEN.[48–51]

Management

Most authorities manage TEN much like a burn, with admission of the child to a burn unit or a pediatric intensive care unit and use a treatment strategy similar to that outlined in the previous section for SJS.[49–51,60–62] The use of intravenous immunoglobulin reduces days of hospitalization and fever.[71]

FIXED DRUG ERUPTION

In children with fixed drug eruptions, the oral ingestion of the causative agent is followed minutes to hours later by the appearance of one (or sometimes several) sharply marginated round or oval patches.[72] A single lesion occurs in half the affected children but those with multiple lesions may have dozens. These smooth, dusky red, or violaceous patches quickly thicken, taking on an edematous appearance (Fig. 19.15). In many instances, the severity of the inflammation is such that blisters arise from within one or more areas of these

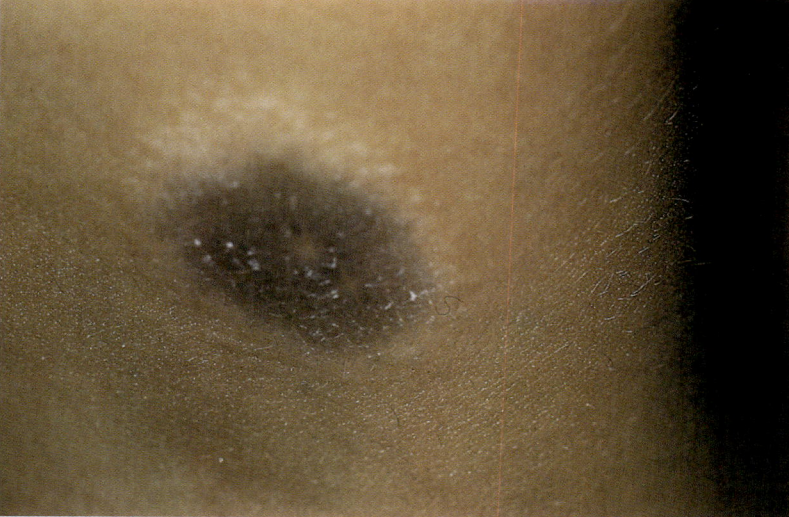

Fig. 19.15 Fixed drug eruption. Edematous, violaceous patch on trunk in 8-year-old with reaction to ibuprofen.

plaques. The lesions may be found anywhere on the skin or mucous membranes, but the most common sites are the lips and genitalia.[72] When more than one lesion develops, clustering is sometimes observed. Itching or burning may be present. In a few instances, associated systemic symptoms and signs have been reported. Several instances of a generalized bullous eruption, intermediate in severity between classical fixed drug eruption and TEN, have been described.[48]

The lesions of fixed drug eruption resolve over 10 to 14 days, leaving a remarkable degree of postinflammatory hperpigmentation. Thereafter, following a refractory period of days to weeks, readministration of the same medication is followed by a recurrent episode.[71] The recurrent episode may be more severe than the first. The fact that these recurrent lesions occur in exactly the same skin sites as the original eruption explains the use of the word "fixed" in the name of the disease.

The pathogenesis of fixed drug eruption is unknown, but the histology mimics that of EM. Many medications have been reported to cause fixed drug eruptions. The most commonly implicated have been trimethaprim-sulfonamide combinations, the paracetamol (acetoaminophen) antipyretics, and ibuprofen anti-inflammatory agents.[72,73] Fixed eruptions have occasionally been reported to have been caused by foods, including strawberries, cheese-flavored snacks, and the food additive tartrazine.[74] A clinical diagnosis can be confirmed by oral rechallenge with the suspected medication, but this is rarely indicated.[72] No efficacious specific therapy is described.

PAPULAR ERYTHEMAS

The individual lesions of papular erythemas share some clinical characteristics with early lesions that occur in EM. In both cases, the papules are red and smooth surfaced. They differ in that the lesions in the papular erythemas tend to be smaller (1cm or less), are dome shaped rather than flat topped, and never progress to form target lesions.

Papular urticaria and insect bites

The cutaneous reaction to bites and stings is frequently that of urticarial papule formation.[75] Generally, this is a short-lived reaction, but in some children these lesions persist for weeks or months. These long-lived reactions presumably occur as a result of allergic sensitization to antigens deposited at the time of the bite. Because sensitization requires repetitive bites over many months, this reaction is generally not seen until after the first year of life. It is most frequent in toddlers.[75] Likewise, long-term re-exposure to the antigen eventually results in hyposensitization. This allows for eventual spontaneous resolution of the problem. It is important to recognize that not all members of a family will become sensitized. Thus, the eruption may appear in a single member of a household, even though others are also bitten. Mites or fleas from dogs or cats are most common, but mites from birds, rats, or mice may also be responsible. A history of pets and birds or rodents around the residence should be sought.

The characteristic lesions of papular urticaria are 5–10mm, dome-shaped, red papules that tend to occur in crops (Fig. 19.16). Occasionally, a punctum, representing the site of the bite, may be observed at the summit of the papule, but usually excoriation has obscured this helpful diagnostic sign.[75] When numerous lesions are present, specific bites may be responsible for only a portion of them. Others may arise as a result of autosensitization. The lesions usually occur on the nonclothed areas of skin.

Therapy (and sometimes proof of causation) depends on the prevention of subsequent bites. Where possible, protective clothing, such as long sleeves and long pants, should be worn. Insect repellents, including those that contain oil of geranium, such as Bite Blocker or N,N-diethyl-m-toluamide (Deet), may be helpful, but removal of the source is preferable. Pets, especially dogs and

71. Viard I, Wehrli P, Bullani R et al. (1998) Inhibition of toxic epidermal necrolysis by blockade of CD95 with human intravenous immunoglobulin. **Science** 282:490–493.
72. Morelli J, Tay YK, Rogers M et al. (1999) Fixed drug eruptions in children. **J Pediatr** 134:365–367.
73. Diaz Jara M, Perez Montero A, Gracia Bara T et al. (2001) Allergic reactions due to ibuprofen in children. **Pediatr Dermatol** 18:66–67.
74. Orchard DC, Varigos GA (1997) Fixed drug eruptions to tartrazine. **Australas J Dermatol** 38:212–214.
75. Howard R, Frieden IJ (1996) Papular urticaria in children. **Pediatr Dermatol** 13:246–249.

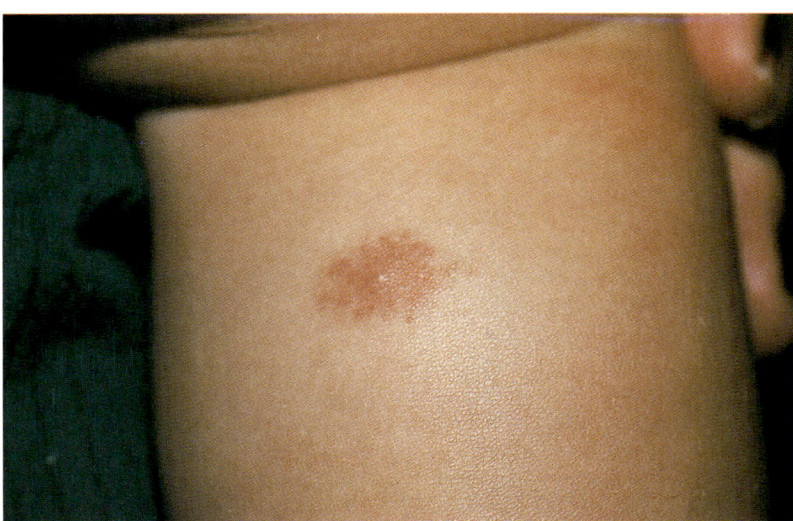

Fig. 19.16 Papular urticaria. Three-millimeter red papule surrounded by red urticarial flare in child with hypersensitivity to dog fleas.

cats, should be examined and should be treated if infested. Individual lesions of papular urticaria may be treated with topical corticosteroids. The oral administration of antihistamines is useful if scratching persists. Other nonspecific treatments of itching may help, such as wet dressings and methol-containing lotions. Antibiotics may be administered if secondary bacterial infection has developed.

Pityriasis lichenoides

Traditionally, both an acute type (Mucha–Habermann disease or acute parapsoriasis) and a chronic type of pityriasis lichenoides (pityriasis lichenoides chronica, chronic parapsoriasis, or digitate dermatosis) have been recognized and are considered under papulosquamous eruptions. It should be remembered that in acute pityriasis lichenoides the characteristic lesions are dome-shaped red papules 3–10mm in diameter and may initially mimic a number of conditions characterized by red papules.[76]

Lymphomatoid papulosis

This disease is considered by many authorities to be a subset of pityriasis lichenoides.[76] The clinical appearance is similar to acute pityriasis lichenoides, although the papules in lymphomatoid papulosis are generally larger and more necrotic. The diagnosis is based on biopsy where, against an inflammatory background similar to that seen in pityriasis lichenoides, marked atypicality of individual lymphocytes is noted. However, in spite of this troublesome histologic appearance, few children eventually develop malignant lymphoma.[76] Lymphomatoid papulosis is extremely rare in children, but it is occasionally encountered in adolescents.

Erythema elevatum diutinum

Clinically, the most prominent skin lesions are nonpurpuric, persistent erythematous papules. The initial papules are small dusky brown-red or even orange-red lesions that gradually enlarge and, through confluent growth, form plaques that are frequently polycyclic in outline. Resolution sometimes occurs in the center of these plaques so that annular lesions are formed. Rarely, bullae develop from the surface of the plaques. These papules and plaques are usually symmetrically located on the dorsal aspects of the hands. The elbows, knees, and buttocks may also be involved. Arthralgia, fever, and malaise often accompany the appearance of the skin lesions. A suspected clinical diagnosis can be confirmed on biopsy by which a vasculitis involving neutrophils (and sometimes eosinophils and mononuclear cells) is found. Leukocytoclasis and fibrinoid deposits are present, but extravasation of erythrocytes is only rarely seen. The course of erythema elevatum diutinum is chronic. Oral treatment with dapsone is the treatment of choice. Unresponsive cases may require prednisone or other immunosuppressive agents.

Another, similar-appearing papular disease, *granuloma faciale*, sometimes develops on the face in children. The histology is similar to that of erythema elevatum diutinum, but the disease is less chronic and is not associated with systemic symptoms and signs.

Miscellaneous papular erythemas

Many other diseases are characterized by the presence of smooth-surfaced small red papules. Most of these are not truly vascular reactions. However, the following should be considered in the clinical differential diagnosis of the vascular papular erythemas: secondary syphilis, pityriasis rosea, miliaria rubra, scabies, papular acrodermatitis (Gianotti–Crosti syndrome), a variety of enteroviral infections, Langerhans cell histiocytosis, and atypical forms of granuloma annulare.

NODULAR ERYTHEMAS

The nodular erythemas are characterized by the presence of one or more smooth-surfaced, slope-shouldered, erythematous nodules 2–10cm in diameter. The deep dermal or subcutaneous location of these lesions generally results in margins that are slope-shouldered and poorly defined. This deep location and large diameter also cause some lesions to appear as flat-topped plaques rather than as nodules. The nodular erythemas are not usually pruritic. They are usually painful and tender on palpation. The presence of lesional pain is unique among the various categories of persistent erythema. The presence of discomfort is due in part to the frequent location of lesions on the lower legs where the skin is tightly stretched, leaving little room for inflammatory distention. Histologic examination of the diseases in this group requires a deep elliptical excision to include the subcutaneous fat; conventional punch biopsies are almost always inadequate. The prototype of nodular erythemas is erythema nodosum. The nodular erythemas are discussed in detail in Chapter 17.

Annular and gyrate erythemas

The conditions considered in this section have in common the presence of erythematous, ringed plaques with prominent central clearing. The adjacent red border of the lesions is narrow (generally less than 1cm in width), but the size of the entire plaque, measured from one border to the other, may be 5–50cm. The centrifugal enlargement that characterizes these lesions occurs over a matter of days or weeks. This relative stability contrasts with the considerably more rapid enlargement of the rings in the annular urticarias and in erythema marginatum. The expanding plaques may be round, but gyrate (polycyclic or serpiginous) forms are often seen. The shape assumed has no particular meaning. The erythematous border of the lesions is slightly raised. Generally, this border has a smooth surface; occasionally, a small amount of fine scale develops as a postinflammatory feature on the trailing edge of the expanding ring. The central clearing left as the border migrates outward contains slightly hyperpigmented but otherwise normal-appearing skin. Pruritus is mild, if present at all.

Biopsy of the lesions in the annular and gyrate erythemas reveals the perivascular lymphocytic infiltrate that is characteristically present in all of the persistent erythemas. The vessels involved are primarily those of the superficial dermis; often in erythema chronicum migrans and sometimes in erythema annulare centrifugum, however, deep dermal vessels are also affected. The overlying epithelium is usually uninvolved, but sometimes mild spongiosis and lymphocytic exocytosis may be noted.

76. Shieh S, Mikkola DL, Wood GS (2001) Differentiation and clonality of lesional lymphocytes in pityriasis lichenoides chronica. **Arch Dermatol** 137:305–308.

The nomenclature of the annular and gyrate erythemas is confusing because of the historical tendency to name every morphologic variant separately. At this time, it seems reasonable to identify two very distinct diseases individually (erythema chronicum migrans and erythema gyratum repens) and to group all of the others under erythema annulare centrifugum, including annular erythema of infancy. All annular erythemas are quite uncommon to rare in children.

Nonvascular diseases that should be considered in the differential diagnosis of the annular and gyrate erythemas include dermatophyte fungal disease (ringworm), subacute cutaneous LE, neonatal LE, ichthyosis linearis circumflexa, granuloma annulare, and sarcoid.

Erythema chronicum migrans

Erythema chronicum migrans is assuming major importance as the frequency with which it is recognized increases.[78,79] It is also the only disease in this group encountered with any frequency by pediatric dermatologists. The initial lesion is a red papule (frequently containing a central punctum) that develops at the site of a tick bite. Over the next several weeks, an erythematous annular ring forms around the papule. The ring can occasionally be vesicular.[78] This ring expands centrifugally to cover an area 30cm or more in diameter (Fig. 19.17). Often the original red papule remains visible in the center of this large ring. In one-half of the affected children, only a single lesion is present, but many smaller, secondary lesions may develop. As the skin lesions evolve, the child develops the insidious onset of fever, malaise, lethargy, arthralgia, and myalgia.[78] Later, if the child remains untreated, arthritis appears, and in some, neurologic or cardiologic complications ensue. In the United States, the combination of erythema chronicum migrans and systemic symptoms and signs is called Lyme disease, after the town in Connecticut where an early epidemic was extensively studied.[79]

Erythema chronicum migrans and the accompanying Lyme disease occur as a result of infection with the spirochete *Borrelia burgdorferi*.[77,78] These spirochetes can be carried by *Ixodes dammini* and related ticks, and they are inoculated at the time of the initial tick bite. The ticks are widely distributed throughout Europe and the United States. The diagnosis of erythema chronicum migrans is generally made on a clinical basis and by serology.[78] The organism can be isolated from the skin lesions by culture.[78] Ten days or more of oral treatment with penicillin V, doxycycline, azithromycin, or cefuroxime is efficacious. Antibiotic treatment in standard doses results in resolution of the skin lesions. The development of the associated internal disease can usually be prevented if these antibiotics are given early in the course of the skin disease. Failure to recognize and treat erythema chronicum migrans may lead to permanent facial palsies and other signs of neuroborreliosis.[79]

Erythema annulare centrifugum

Erythema annulare centrifugum describes a variety of annular and gyrate patterns.[80] Most often, only a few lesions are present; these are usually located on the trunk and proximal extremities. Erythema annulare centrifugum is rare in children. A subset of cases were reported as annular erythemas of infancy.[80] Individual lesions start as dusky red erythematous papules or plaques that expand in a centrifugal pattern (Fig. 19.18). A small amount of fine scale may be present on the trailing portion of the erythematous border. The center of the expanding lesion consists of somewhat hyperpigmented but otherwise normal-appearing skin. Lesions enlarge to a diameter of 10–20cm over a matter of one or two weeks and then gradually fade away. New lesions appear (sometimes as concentric rings within old lesions) as soon as earlier lesions resolve. The entire course of the disease lasts for many months.

If the annular erythema is associated with fever, then one should consider the periodic fever syndromes. Recently, mutations in TNF receptors have been associated with periodic fever syndromes.[81] A specific cause or associated systemic problem is rarely found. Treatment is difficult. Topical steroids are often ineffective. Use of systemic steroids may lead to clearing, but relapse can be expected. Antihistamines decrease any itching that is present but have no direct effect on the lesions.

Gustatory erythema and hyperhidrosis (auriculotemporal nerve syndrome or Frey syndrome)

Gustatory erythema presents in children, during or after eating; a patch of erythema with or without sweating may be seen on one cheek.[82,83] The color

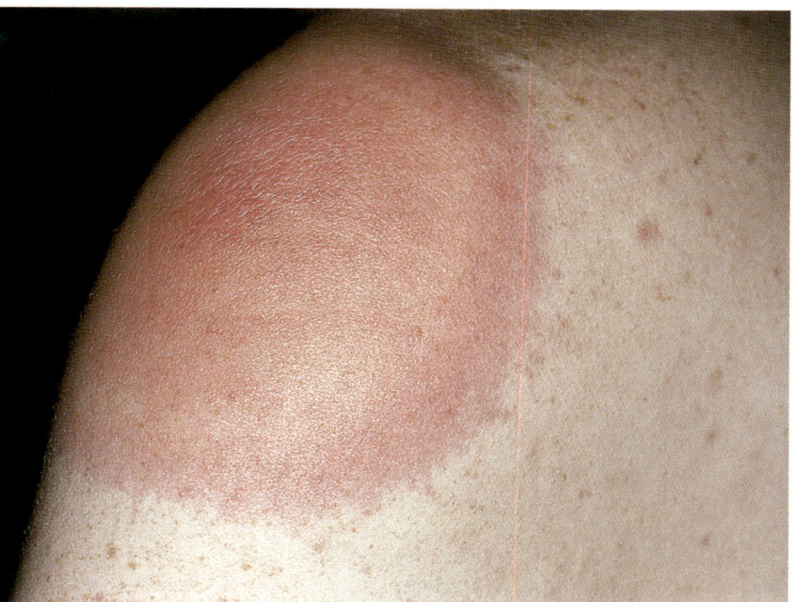

Fig. 19.17 Erythema chronicum migrans. Expanding annular red patch on child's shoulder following tick bite.

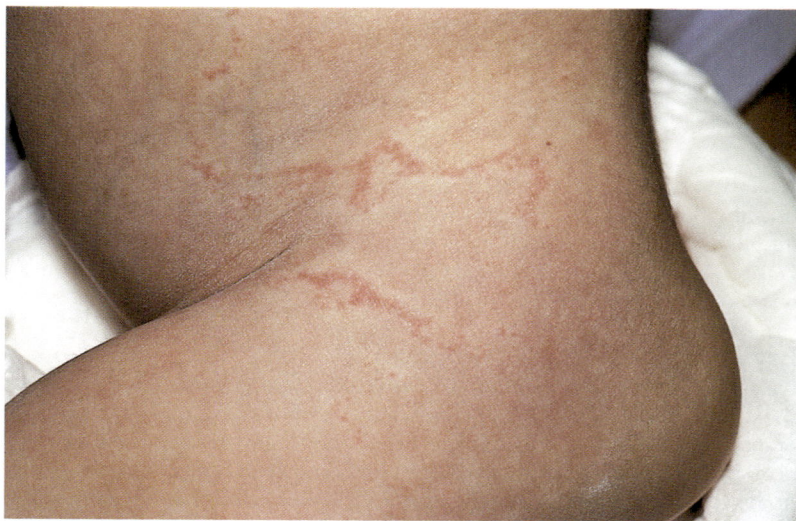

Fig. 19.18 Erythema annulare centrifugum. Large, slowly expanding annular red ring with slight inner scale on a child's hip and abdomen.

77. Gibson LE, al-Azhary RA (2000) Erythema elevatum diutinum. **Clin Dermatol** 18:295–299.
78. Melski JW (1993) Primary and secondary erythema chronicum migrans in Wisconsin. **Arch Dermatol** 129:709–712.
79. Kalish RA, Kaplan RF, Taylor E et al. (2001) Evaluation of study patients with Lyme disease, 10–20 year follow-up. **J Infect Dis** 183:453–460.
80. Tyring SK (1993) Reactive erythemas: Erythema annulare centrifugum and erythema gyratum repens. **Clin Dermatol** 11:135–139.

81. Toro JR, Aksentijevich I, Hull K et al. (2000) Tumor necrosis factor receptor-associated periodic syndrome: a novel syndrome with cutaneous manifestations. **Arch Dermatol** 136:1487–1494.
82. Cliff S, Lever R, Moss AL, Mortimer PS (1998) Frey's syndrome without hyperhidrosis. **J Roy Soc Med** 91:388–389.
83. Dulguerov P, Quinodoz D, Vaezi A et al. (1999) New objective and quantitative tests for gustatory sweating. **Acat Oto-Laryngologica** 119:599–603.

change may persist for several hours. Frequently, the ingested food is implicated as an allergen, but the mechanism is nerve mediated, in which the seventh and eighth cranial nerves have crossed fibers, either as a congenital malformation or as the result of injury to the parotid area.[82,83] Stimulation of the taste buds initiates the sympathetic nervous response of the skin.[83] Intracutaneous injections of botulinum toxin have been reported to reduce the reaction for up to one year in most children.[84,85]

ACRAL ERYTHEMAS

The acral erythemas are characterized by the development of diffuse flat redness over the distal extremities. The diseases in which the acral erythema occurs as a compensatory mechanism after initial vasoconstriction (acrodynia, pernio, and acrocyanosis) are discussed in the section on vasospastic reactions.

Erythromelalgia

This uncommon disease, sometimes known as erythermalgia, consists of episodic reddening and pain of the hands and feet.[86] Primary (idiopathic) and secondary types are recognized. The primary type occurs in children (especially boys) and has recently been found to be hereditary.[86] The secondary type is found almost entirely in adults who have underlying diseases, such as polycythemia vera, thrombocythemia, autoimmune collagen vascular disease, and myeloproliferative malignancy. The clinical appearance of erythromelalgia in the primary and secondary types is identical.

Individual episodes of erythromelalgia may occur spontaneously or, more often, are provoked by heat, exercise, or dependency of the limbs. The child notes the sudden appearance of cyanotic or dusky red color of the hands and feet. The color change is accompanied by local pain and a sensation of warmth. Initially, the episodes may be evanescent; with the passage of time, the attacks last longer. In some cases, they become almost continuous.

The pathogenesis of erythromelalgia is unknown, but it is suspected that the central problem in all types involves microvascular arteriovenous shunting.[87] Some authorities favor abnormalities in platelet aggregation, with contributing factors such as vessel wall damage, changes in patterns of blood flow, and disturbances in prostaglandin metabolism.[88] Therapy is first directed toward reversal of any identified precipitating events. Established attacks are usually treated with the administration of indomethacin 10mg/kg per day in four doses. Aspirin is less helpful. The application of cold packs or immersion in cold water may simply worsen shunting and while providing temporary relief may result in progression of the condition.[89] Anecdotal reports have also suggested the usefulness of vasodilators, vasoconstrictors, and antiplatelet medications.

Reflex sympathetic dystrophy

Reflex sympathetic dystrophy is a regional pain syndrome. After traumatic injury, severe pain, redness, edema, and sweating of the hands or feet occurs.[90,91] The pain begins at the time of injury in one-half of the cases. If there is pain without color change, it is termed causalgia. It occurs rarely in children. In children, associated psychological problems occur in over 80%. Treatment with calcitonin is successful in many, but no analgesic effect was found with sympathetic suppressors, guanethidine, or intravenous regional blocks.[90] Physical therapy may help some children.[91]

Miscellaneous causes of acral erythema

In certain circumstances, children with malignancies who are undergoing systemic chemotherapy have an erythromelalgic-type acral erythema. Redness and swelling of the hands and feet are also prominent components in children with Kawasaki's disease. Redness of the hands and feet without swelling may also be noted in toxic shock syndrome and in streptococcal and staphylococcal scarlatina. In all of these conditions, postinflammatory desquamation is regularly seen. Acrodynia, pernio, and acrocyanosis are discussed in the section on vasospastic disease.

VASOSPASTIC REACTIONS WITH ACRAL ERYTHEMA

The diseases considered in this section (Table 19.6) have an element of vascular constriction as part of their pathogenesis. Whiteness or paleness is an important part of their presentation. This is true in the case of nevus anemicus, but more often cyanosis (as a result of vascular stasis) or redness (as a result of "compensatory" vasodilation) dominates the clinical appearance. Vasospastic changes can be divided into acral and nonacral types.

ACRAL REACTIONS
Raynaud syndrome and related conditions

Raynaud syndrome is characterized by the development of cold- or stress-induced painful vasospastic changes in the digits.[92] Historically, the term Raynaud "disease" was used when these changes were idiopathic, whereas Raynaud "phenomenon" was used when these changes occurred in association with some other underlying disease. The distinction cannot be made with certainty in many patients; for this reason, it seems reasonable to use the term Raynaud syndrome for all patients presenting with this condition.

Raynaud syndrome occurs predominantly in young women; children are not often affected. The fact that this condition frequently occurs in association with collagen vascular disease suggests that at least some of the individuals who develop Raynaud syndrome are genetically predisposed.[92]

The onset of Raynaud syndrome is insidious. Generally, patients first note that their fingers chill more quickly and easily than in the past. Subsequently, they find that considerable discomfort accompanies cold exposure, especially as the fingers start to warm.[92] Patients observe that, with chilling, the fingers first turn white (Fig. 19.19) and that this is followed by the appearance of a blue cyanosis over all but the fingertips. During the warming phase, the hand may redden as a result of reactive hyperemia. These color changes compose the triphasic color response of Raynaud syndrome.[92] The hands alone are

---

TABLE 19.6   Vasospastic reactions

Acral reactions
    Raynaud syndrome
    Acrocyanosis
    Pernio
    Acrodynia

Nonacral reactions
    Cutis marmorata
    Nevus anemicus

84. Laccourreye O, Ake E, Gutierrez-Fonseca et al. (1999) Recurrent gustatory sweating [Frey syndrome] after intracutaneous injection of botulinum toxin type A: incidence, management, outcome. **Arch Otolaryngol Head Neck Surg** 125:283–286.

85. Dulguerov P, Quinodoz D, Cosendai et al. (2000) Frey syndrome treatment with botulinum toxin. **Otolaryngology Head & Neck Surg** 122:821–827.

86. Drenth JP, Finley WH, Breedveld GJ et al. (2001) The primary erythermalgia-susceptibility gene is located on chromosome 2q31–32. **Am J Hum Genet** 68:1277–1282.

87. Mork C, Asker CL, Salerud EG, Kvernebo K (2000) Microvascular arteriovenous shunting is a probable pathogenetic mechanism in erythromelalgia. **J Invest Dermatol** 1114:643–646.

88. Davis MD, Rooke TW, Sandroni P (2000) Mechanisms other than shunting are likely contributing to the pathophysiology of erythromelalgia. **J Invest Dermatol** 115:1166–1167.

89. Cohen JS (2000) Erythromelalgia: new theories and new therapies. **J Am Acad Dermatol** 43:841–847.

90. Perez RS, Kwakke G, Zuurmond WW, deLange JJ (2001) Treatment of reflex sympathetic dystrophy [crps type 1], a research synthesis of 21 randomized clinical trials. **Pain Symptom Manag** 21:511–526.

91. Wesdock KA, Stanton RP, Singsen BH (1991) Reflex sympathetic dystrophy in children. A physical therapy approach. **Arthritis Care Res** 4:32–28.

92. Kahaleh B, Matucci-Cerinic M (1995) Raynaud's phenomenon and scleroderma: dysregulation of neuroendothelial control of vascular tone. **Arthritis Rheum** 38:1–4.

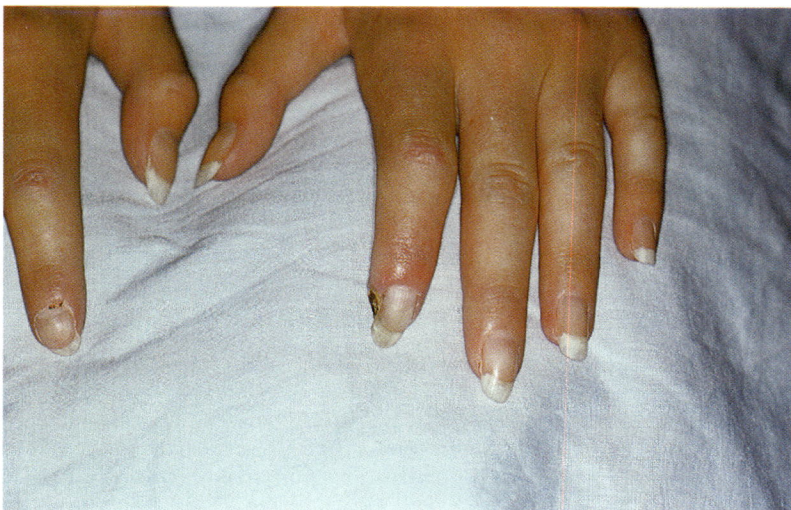

Fig. 19.19 Raynaud phenomenon. Vasoconstrictive (white phase) of characteristic blue, white, then red triphasic color response in a 17-year-old.

TABLE 19.7 Conditions associated with the development of Raynaud syndrome

Autoimmune collagen vascular disease
    Scleroderma
    Lupus erythematosus
    Dermatomyositis
    Rheumatoid arthritis
    Sjögren syndrome
    Various "mixed" and "overlap" syndromes
    Cryoproteins
    Cryoglobulins
    Cold agglutinins
    Cold fibrinogens

Medications
    Ergot derivatives
    Methysergide maleate
    Histamine blockers
    Intra-arterial injection of any drug

Vascular obliterative diseases
    Thromboangiitis obliterans
    Arteriosclerosis obliterans
    Embolus and thrombus formation

Miscellaneous conditions
    Carpal tunnel syndrome
    Thoracic outlet syndromes
    Reflex sympathetic dystrophy
    Postchemotherapy for certain malignancies

affected in about one-half of the patients; both feet and hands are involved in the remainder. Initially, the hands appear normal between attacks, but later, the episodes may be almost continuous as a result of constant triggering by minimal temperature variations or emotional stress. In these later stages, atrophic changes develop on the distal fingers. In such cases, the skin becomes shiny, periungual telangiectasias appear, and often features of sclerodactyly (skin tightness and finger tapering) develop. In the worst circumstances, small infarcts, 1–2 mm in diameter, appear on the fingertips. These heal slowly with eventual development of pitted scarring. Finally, in the most unfortunate individuals, the disease eventuates in considerable gangrenous loss of soft tissue.

The diagnosis of Raynaud syndrome is usually based on historical evidence. The serologic presence of anti-centromere antibodies is considered useful in the diagnosis.[93] Confirmation of the diagnosis can, if necessary, be obtained by provocative cold testing. All patients with Raynaud syndrome should be queried regarding the use of provocative medications and a search should be carried out for evidence of underlying, associated disease (Table 19.7). Particular attention should be paid to signs and symptoms of early scleroderma.[92,93]

The pathophysiology of Raynaud syndrome has not been delineated.[92] Excess sympathetic discharge probably plays an important role; because attacks can be induced after sympathectomy, however, this cannot be the entire explanation. Release of vasoconstricting mediators, such as histamine and serotonin, probably occurs as a result of multiple factors. Females are involved 10 times more frequently than males, suggesting the possibility that hormonal factors may play some role. Moreover, the blood vessels of the fingertips themselves, together with their controlling mechanisms, may be abnormal. Recently, prior infection with parvovirus B19 has been implicated in some children with Raynaud phenomenon.[94] Elimination of provocative factors and induction of cold-protection strategies are the mainstays of therapy for Raynaud syndrome. The softball windup exercise (a whirling motion of the extended arm) may be useful in some. The use of calcium channel-blocking drugs such as nifedipine can be useful in selected children. Topical nitroglycerin paste may help.

Pernio

Prolonged cold exposure, especially associated with dampness, results in the characteristic skin lesions known as pernio or chilblains.[95] Dusky red or violaceous discrete swellings develop on the digits, predominantly the toes (Fig. 19.20). They are remarkable in that, even without further cold exposure, individual lesions may persist for months. Occasionally, diffuse swelling of a digit is observed; rarely, hemorrhagic blister formation or ulceration may ensue. When ulceration of the toes occurs it is called kibes.[95] Cryoproteins, including rheumatoid factor, are found in some children with pernio.[95] Itching or sensory changes occasionally may develop. Protecting the digits from cold, wet conditions will help.

Acrocyanosis

Acrocyanosis presents as cool, sometimes sweaty and dusky red or cyanotic hands and fingers or feet and toes. Acrocyanosis is seen predominantly in adolescent girls but may occasionally be observed in childhood. Rarely, edema of the affected extremity is seen.

The pathogenesis is unknown, although cold sensitivity may be a prominent feature in some. Arterial constriction plus capillary dilation is involved. The progression to skin changes, as described for Raynaud syndrome, is not seen, and the overall prognosis is good.

Acrodynia

Diffuse painful swelling and redness of the digits, hands, and feet characterize acrodynia.[96] The involved areas are palpably cool, presumably as a result of arterial constriction. The overlying redness occurs as a result of the capillary reactive hyperemia that accompanies the deeper vasoconstriction. These changes are accompanied by tachycardia and excess sweating, which suggests that sympathetic stimulation plays a role in the pathogenesis of the disease. This is recognized as the result of chronic mercury exposure and toxicity.[96]

93. Hossny E, Hady HA, Mabrouk R (2000) Anti-centromere antibodies as a marker of Raynaud's phenomenon in pediatric rheumatologic diseases. **Pediatr Allergy Immunol** 11:250–255.
94. Harel L, Straussberg R, Rudich H, Cohen AH, Amir J (2000) Raynaud's phenomenon as a manifestation of parvovirus B19 infection: case reports and review of parvovirus B19 rheumatic and vasculitic syndromes: **Clin Infect Dis** 30:500–503.
95. Weston WL, Morelli JG (2000) Childhood pernio and cryoproteins. **Pediatr Dermatol** 17:97–99.
96. Boyd AS, Seger D, Vanucci S et al. (2000) Mercury exposure and cutaneous disease. **J Am Acad Dermatol** 43:81–90.

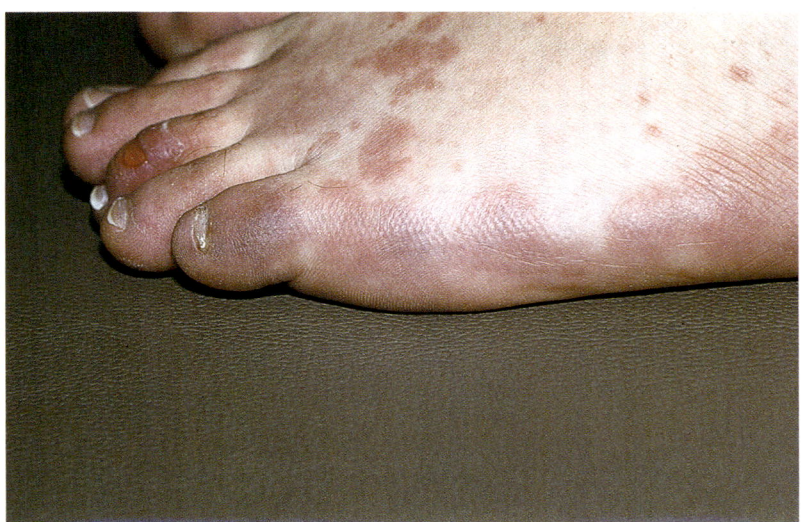

Fig. 19.20   Dusky purple nodules of the toes and side of the foot in an 11-year-old girl with pernio.

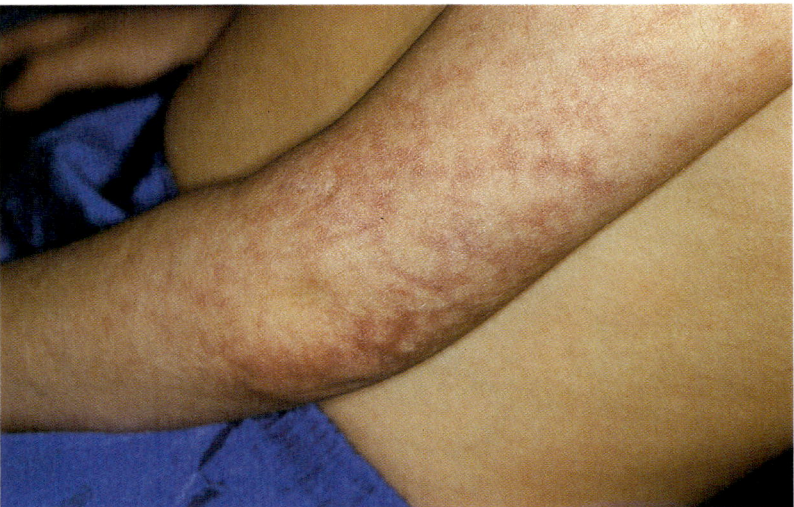

Fig. 19.21   Livedo reticularis. Lacy pattern of red-purple discoloration on the arm of a 9-year-old boy.

Epidemics in children were originally described as "pink disease." Restlessness and irritability, often to a marked degree, are also present. Acrodynia may be mistaken for Kawasaki disease because of redness of plams, soles, and digits. The hypertension may prompt investigation for pheochromocytomas. There is a small but significant mortality rate when the disease remains untreated for prolonged periods. Treatment consists of removing the source of mercury exposure and, in severe cases, the administration of chelating agents.[96]

RETICULATE ERYTHEMAS

The reticulate erythemas are characterized by a flat network of intersecting red lines that enclose small patches of pale or normal-colored skin. The red lines vary in width from several millimeters to as much as 1 cm. These lines are not sharply marginated and instead blend into the adjacent normal skin. This lack of sharp margination gives a mottled or blotchy appearance to the involved areas. The red colors that make up the lines are variable in hue but generally tend toward the dusky end of the spectrum and sometimes even appear violaceous. The lesions have no substance; because there is no scale formation, nothing can be palpated. The conditions considered in this section share nothing in common except their similarity in clinical appearance.

Livedo reticularis

The basic appearance is similar to that described in the paragraph above, but the intersecting lines are generally violaceous (Fig. 19.21). The condition can be widespread, involving most of the body, or it can occur in one or more smaller patches. There is a predilection for distribution on the legs and lower trunk.[97,98] Two forms of livedo reticularis exist. The primary (idiopathic) form is most common in adolescent girls. In this form, the distribution tends to be generalized and symmetrical. The course of the condition, although of long duration, is associated with a good prognosis. The lesions in the secondary form tend to be patchier and are more likely to be associated with ulcerations or nodules. Chronic cutaneous or systemic periarteritis nodosa, LE, and other collagen vascular diseases should come to mind. Embolic disease may occasionally be responsible. The eruption is usually asymptomatic and, although similar to mottling, does not clear when the skin is warmed. Biopsy of secondary forms of livedo lesions often demonstrates vasculitis of small- and large-caliber vessels, most often arteries.[98] Biopsy of a palpable nodule reveals typical changes of periarteritis nodosa.

Cutis marmorata

Cutis marmorata is encountered in virtually all newborns and infants and with considerable frequency in children and adolescent girls. It consists of symmetrical reticular mottling of the skin after exposure to cool or cold temperatures. The color changes are identical in appearance to those found in livedo reticularis, but in contrast, they are variable in intensity from minute to minute and disappear entirely on warming. Generally, cutis marmorata is most prominent on the legs. It is an asymptomatic condition. In infants, cutis marmorata must be distinguished from the congenital vascular malformation known as congenital generalized phebectasia (cutis marmorata congenita). Ordinary mottling clears with rewarming of skin; in the vascular malformation, it does not. In most infants, the mottling response clears by 6 to 12 months. If it persists, congenital hypothyroidism should be considered. In older individuals, it should be differentiated from livedo reticularis.

Anticardiolipin syndrome

This uncommon syndrome is usually described in adult women, but a few cases in adolescent girls have been reported.[97,98] Livedo reticularis is the major cutaneous feature and is associated with major thrombotic episodes, including both venous and arterial thromboses and recurrent ischemic attacks. An additional criterion, that of recurrent pregnancy loss, may be a prominent part of the syndrome. Originally called Sneddon syndrome, this is also known as the lupus anticoagulant syndrome.[97,98]

Autoantibodies against cardiolipin, a phospholipid complex that contains a naturally occurring anticoagulant, are diagnostic of this entity. At least two anticardiolipin antibodies have been detected and are believed to be directed against two separate epitopes of the complex. One is called the lupus anticoagulant and the other, antiphospholipid. It is now appreciated that at least one-half of the affected individuals do not have LE. The exact mechanism of the thrombotic state is not known, but some authorities believe the antibodies may interfere with protein C activity. There may be life-threatening coronary, cerebral, renal, or pulmonary emboli. Cutaneous infarcts and ulcerations sometimes occur. Prophylactic therapy with hydroxychloroquine was believed to be efficaceous.[98] After a thrombotic episode, warfarin is usually given, and antiplatelet therapy such as aspirin is recommended by some. Systemic steroids may predispose to more thromboses. Avoidance of oral contraceptives, smoking and other factors that might promote thrombosis is beneficial.

97. Frances C, Piette JC (2000) The mystery of Sneddon syndrome: relationship with antiphospholipid syndrome and systemic lupus erythematosus. **J Autoimmun** 15:139–143.

98. Lao M, Setty S, Foss C (2001) Antiphospholipid syndrome. A literature review. **Minn Med** 84:42–46.

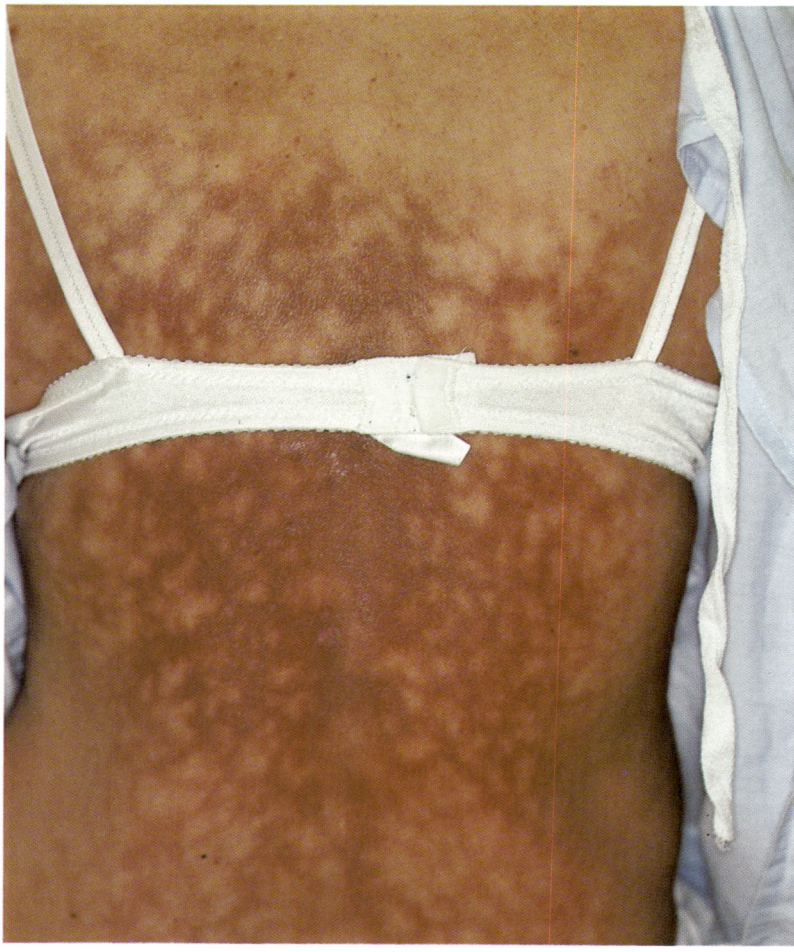

Fig. 19.22 Erythema ab igne. Dusky red-brown pattern involving mid-back of 15-year-old girl using heating pad for back pain.

Erythema ab igne

Children with erythema ab igne have a localized, dusky red, persistent, patchy livedo pattern. Erythema ab igne looks very much like localized livedo reticularis, except that the hues are brown-red rather than violaceous (Fig. 19.22).[99] The lesions are asymptomatic. Erythema ab igne evolves insidiously after repeated exposure of the skin to high (but not burning) temperatures. When encountered today, it usually has developed as a result of habitual heating pad use.

Biopsy shows vasodilation, mild basal layer vacuolization, and incontinent pigment in dermal macrophages.[99] These changes reflect heat-induced toxic damage to both epithelial and vascular structures. In some ways, it may be considered to be a heat analogue to cold-induced pernio (see vasospastic reactions). Discontinuation of heat exposure leads to slow resolution of the red hues, but the reticular postinflammatory hyperpigmentation may persist for years.

Erythema infectiosum (Fifth disease)

Erythema infectiosum occurs primarily in infants and young children. It is characterized by the presence of reticular erythematous patches similar to those described in the introductory paragraph of the reticulate erythemas section. The lesions, however, are distinctly pink, with no violaceous or brown hues present. They may occur anywhere but are most often seen on the lateral arms, lower abdomen, and thighs. The eruption begins after several days of

the infection with human parvovirus B19 and lasts approximately 10 days. Once present, episodes of exacerbation and remission may occur for up to three months. The history of preceding fever, the development of a reticular eruption, and the presence of flat malar erythema (the "slapped cheek" sign) usually allows for easy clinical identification. The slapped cheeks may precede or accompany the onset of other skin lesions. The child usually appears healthy at the time of the rash. The eruption of erythema infectiosum follows the viremic phase and corresponds to the onset of immunity so that the family can be reassured the child is no longer infectious. Erythema infectiosum and other viral exanthems are discussed in detail in Chapter 25.

Miscellaneous reticulate erythemas

Angioma serpiginosum is a nevoid vascular hamartoma in which patches of bright red punctate reticulation may be seen. It primarily affects older children and adolescents and is progressive. Congenital phlebectasia (cutis marmorata congenita) is a reticular vascular hamartoma that is present at birth or develops shortly thereafter. It is often present in segmental patches that are sharply demarcated at the midline. The lesions are similar in appearance to those found in livedo reticularis and cutis marmorata. Mottling (cutis marmorata) is common in infancy and often disappears by 6 months of age. Poikiloderma may sometimes be confused with reticulate erythemas, especially when first presenting in the photosensitive genodermatoses. It is characterized by fine wrinkling of the epidermis, hyper- and hypopigmentation and atrophy.

DIFFUSE AND MORBILLIFORM ERYTHEMAS

Two types of diffuse erythemas can be recognized: morbilliform eruptions and toxic erythemas. Morbilliform eruptions have closely set pink macules or very slightly raised papules that are distributed diffusely over large portions of the body. During the evolution of morbilliform eruptions, areas of coalescence may develop, but on the periphery, discrete individual lesions are always recognizable. On the other hand, in toxic erythemas, there are large areas of flat homogeneous redness, which lack peripheral discrete lesions. As a general rule, morbilliform erythemas occur as a result of drug reaction or viral infection,[100] whereas toxic erythemas occur in bacterial infections secondary to the release of toxins. Additional information about these infections can be found in Chapters 24 and 25.

NONACRAL REACTIONS

Nevus anemicus

Nevus anemicus is an uncommon condition that first presents in infancy or early childhood with one or more flat patches of uniformly pale white skin (Fig. 19.23).[101] The skin, with the exception of this white color, is otherwise normal on inspection and palpation. Most lesions of nevus anemicus are sharply marginated, but sometimes the border is indistinct or "feathered." Generally, the lesions are only several centimeters in diameter, but larger lesions can occur. The trunk is the most common site of involvement. Once present, the patches remain stable indefinitely, in both size and configuration.

Biopsy of affected skin shows a normal histology; the diagnosis is established by two clinical maneuvers instead. First, diascopy of the adjacent normal skin causes a blanching that obliterates the margin between normal and abnormal skin. This indicates that the pale color of the lesion is due to decreased vascularity rather than to the absence of pigment, such as would be seen in vitiligo, Second, firm stroking of the involved skin does not reveal the normally present red axon flare. The absence of the flare indicates that decreased vascularity has occurred as a result of neurally regulated vasoconstriction. There is an association with capillary vascular malformations,[101]

99. Cavallari V, Ciccarello R, Torre V et al. (2001) Chronic heat-induced skin lesions [erythema ab igne]: ultrastructural studies. **Ultrastruct Pathol** 25:93–97.
100. Hogan PA, Morelli JG, Weston WL (1992) Viral exanthems. **Curr Probl Dermatol** 4:35.
101. Katugampola GA, Lanigan SW (1996) The clinical spectrum of naevus anaemicus and its association with portwine stains: report of 15 cases and review of the literature. **Br J Dermatol** 134:292–295.

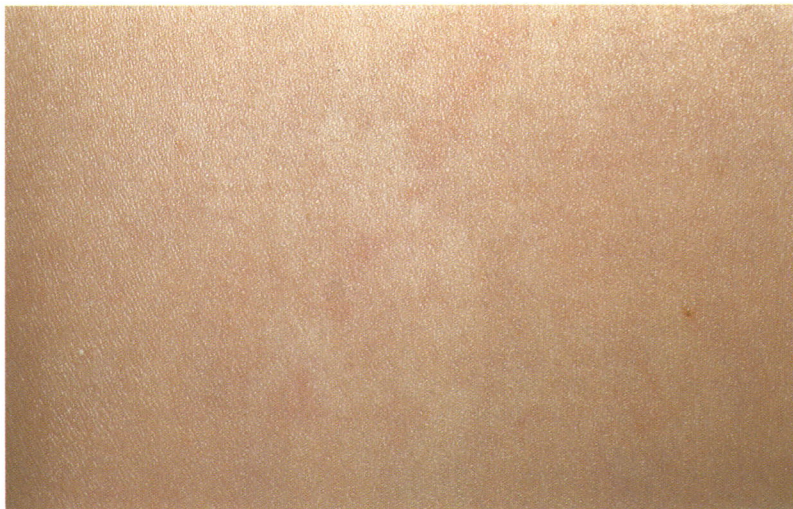

Fig. 19.23 Nevus anemicus in a 2-year-old boy. Permanent patch of pale skin present from birth.

which may be explained by the phenomenon of twin spotting.[102] Cosmetic coverups may be used.

VASCULITIS AND INFLAMMATORY PURPURAS

The diseases considered in this category share in common the presence of nonblanchable purpuric lesions, but, in contrast to the noninflammatory purpuric diseases considered in the next section, the purpuric lesions of the vasculitic group are usually petechial. Ecchymoses and hematomas are rarely encountered. Histologically, the vasculitic purpuras are characterized by the presence of inflammatory infiltrates located within the blood vessel walls. In all instances, these inflammatory reactions cause sufficient disruption of the vascular wall to allow for the extravasation of erythrocytes. It is the extravascular location of these red blood cells that causes the clinically characteristic feature of nonblanchability. When a lesion is blanched by pressure on the skin surface, the red blood cells containing oxyhemoglobin are pushed from superficial vessels into deeper vessels. When the red blood cell is outside the vessel wall, it cannot be pushed into deeper vessels. The diseases in this section are subdivided on the basis of the type and size of vessel involved: capillaritis, venulitis, and arteritis (Table 19.8). The prototype of vasculitis in childhood is Henoch-Shöenlein purpura.

CAPILLARITIS

The diseases in this group are characterized by the presence of nonpalpable petechiae. These petechiae are 1–2mm in diameter, uniform in appearance, and large in number. Histologically, a lymphocytic infiltrate surrounds and infiltrates the walls of those capillaries, which lie within the upper (papillary) dermis. The small size of involved vessels and relative sparsity of inflammatory cells account for the fact that these lesions are not elevated or palpable. Through mechanisms that are not well understood, this lymphocytic vasculitis also produces sufficient vessel wall destruction to result in extravasation of red blood cells. There is no breakup of the inflammatory cell nuclei (leukocytoclasis), and there is little or no fibrinoid deposition. Two types of capillaritis are recognized: a primary (idiopathic) type termed benign pigmented purpura and a secondary type associated with the use of certain medications (Table 19.8).

TABLE 19.8   Vasculitides

Capillaritis (nonpalpable petechiae)
   Benign pigmented purpuras
      Schamberg's progressive pigmented purpura
      Lichen aureus
      Purpura annularis telangiectoides
      Lichenoid pigmented purpura
   Drug-induced inflammatory petechiae
Venulitis (palpable petechiae)
   Leukocytoclastic vasculitis
      Henoch–Schönlein purpura
      Urticarial vasculitis
Arteritis (petechiae, erythematous nodules, and ulcers)
   Polyarteritis nodosa
   Chronic cutaneous polyarteritis nodosa
   Granulomatous vasculitis
   Churg–Strauss vasculitis

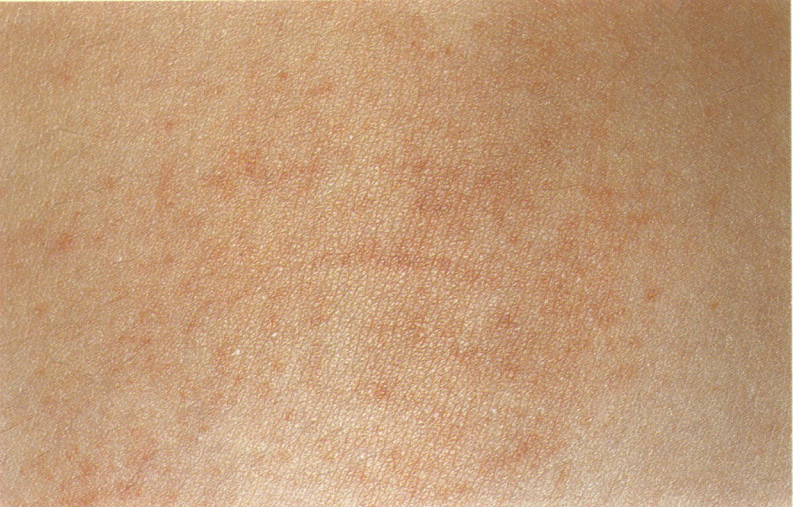

Fig. 19.24 Old (brown) and new (red) petechiae mixed together in a patch on the leg of an adolescent with Schamberg's pigmented purpura.

BENIGN PIGMENTED PURPURAS

This group of closely related conditions is characterized by the appearance of petechiae that are grouped in distinctive patterns. The histology and course of these conditions are similar. They differ in clinical appearance but have in common the presence of both new and old petechiae at the time of examination.

Schamberg's progressive pigmented purpura

This is the most common of these conditions and is one of the most common causes of chronic petechiae in children. Multiple distinct annular patches of closely set, but nonconfluent, petechiae are found on the legs and occasionally elsewhere (Fig. 19.24). Each of the nummular patches is 2–5cm in diameter; clear areas of normal skin separate adjacent patches. Within each patch, the complete life cycle of individual petechiae is demonstrated. That is, some of the petechiae are bright red, others are violaceous, and some have disappeared, leaving brown dots of hemosiderin pigmentation. This latter change accounts

102. Happle R, Koopman R, Mier OD (1990) Hypothesis: vascular twin naevi and somatic recombination in man. **Lancet** 1:376.

for the term "pigmented" in the name of the disease. Individual patches come and go during the months or years in which the process is present. The lesions are asymptomatic and may be asymmetrical or unilateral at the onset, especially in adolescents.[103,104]

Lichen aureus

This differs from Schamberg's purpura in that only one or, at most, a few patches of closely set petechiae are present.[102] Moreover, each patch remains stable in size and location for long periods. In this sense, the patch (or patches) remain "fixed" to one skin site for the entire course of the disease. Within each patch, individual petechiae are continually evolving and resolving. As the name implies, there is often an overall golden background color to the patch. Histologically, lymphocytes are present both in a band-like (lichenoid) and in a perivascular pattern. The individual lesions of lichen aureus are similar to suction-type petechiae, such as those seen in "hickeys" and in suction cup applications. In most cases, the lesions will resolve in two to four years.[104] Children often induce lesions that mimic lichen aureus (in appearance, although not in duration) through oral suction on their own arms.

Purpura annularis telangiectoides of Majocchi

This is similar to Schamberg's purpura, but within each patch there is a predilection for the appearance of telangiectasia. Moreover, individual patches undergo centrifugal spread with central clearing. This results in an annular configuration.

For the most part, the benign pigmented purpuras are asymptomatic, but rarely, an appreciable degree of pruritus is present. In these instances, small lichenoid papules and mild eczematization may occur secondary to chronic rubbing. The term *lichenoid pigmented purpura of Gougerot and Blum* is applied to such lesions. The term *eczematous-like purpura of Ducas and Kapetenakis* is used when eczematous lesions predominate.

The cause and pathogenesis of the benign pigmented purpuras are unknown, with all of them being chronic conditions that generally last for months to years. There is no safe, appropriate therapy. Systemic steroids sometimes result in resolution, but the lesions reappear as soon as the steroids are discontinued.

Drug-induced petechiae

Medications can cause purpuric lesions through at least three different mechanisms: lymphocytic capillaritis, thrombocytopenia, and immune complex venulitis. Lymphocytic capillaritis is the least common of these types and is a reaction generally associated with four classes of medications: barbiturates, sulfa-related medications, carbamate muscle relaxants and anxiolytic agents. Capillaritis has also been associated with interferon-alpha therapy for Hepatitis C.[105] The petechiae in these capillaritic drug reactions are widely and randomly distributed. Moreover, they usually do not occur in well-defined patches. These two features help separate these capillaritic drug reactions from the benign pigmented purpuric eruptions. The pathogenesis of drug-induced lymphocytic capillaritis is unknown.

The differential diagnosis of pigmented purpuric eruption includes pigmented purpuric clothing dermatitis and mycosis fungoides. Mycosis fungoides has been reported to resemble a capillaritis in its early stages on a number of reports.[106,107] It is unclear whether these reports represent a capillaritis evolving to mycosis fungoides or mycosis fungoides clinically resembling capillaritis.

Petechiae with acute infection

During the course of many common acute bacterial and viral infections of childhood, petechiae may appear.[100] These include streptoccocal infections, numerous viral diseases (especially the enteroviruses and herpes-group viruses) and many others. Severe systemic infections due to meningococci and rickettsiae may also result in acute petechiae. The petechiae often appear within a 24-hour period and clear over 5 to 10 days.

A specific clinical entity termed the "papular-purpuric gloves and socks syndrome" has been recently described.[108] It presents as pruritic erythematous papules occurring in a gloves-and-socks distribution associated with oral lesions and fever. The lesions rapidly develop petechial purprua and clear within two weeks, although may be more prolonged in the setting of HIV.[109] Most cases are due to parvovirus B19 with PCR identification of the virus within lesions and serological conversion demonstrated.[110] The histology is not specific and may show a mild interface dermatitis and a superficial lymphocytic vasculitis. Other viruses have been implicated in causing the eruption including rubella,[111] human herpesvirus 6,[112] hepatitis B,[113] cytomegalovirus,[114] and measles.[115]

LEUKOCYTOCLASTIC VASCULITIS (VENULITIS)

Introduction

Petechial diseases in this group are also characterized by the presence of small purpuric lesions. However, these petechiae differ considerably from those described as occurring in capillaritis. They are palpable and are more variable in size, ranging from 2 to 10mm in diameter. They are rather more randomly spread, with little evidence of grouping. Finally, they may be accompanied by other nonpetechial lesions, such as urticarial papules and small hemorrhagic vesicles, infarcts, or ulcers. Venulitis-associated petechiae are microscopically characterized by the presence of a neutrophilic infiltrate in and around the venules of the upper dermis. The vessel walls are visibly damaged, with associated leukocytoclasis, erythrocyte extravasation, and, usually, fibrinoid deposition. Older lesions may contain scattered lymphocytes in the inflammatory infiltrate, but neutrophils still predominate. The pathogenesis for the venulitic type of vasculitis is that of immune complex deposition with consequent complement activation and endothelial injury.

The nomenclature historically applied to the diseases that share these histologic features has been most confusing. All of the following have been used at one time or another to describe essentially similar conditions: leukocytoclastic vasculitis, necrotizing angiitis, hypersensitivity angiitis, allergic vasculitis, immune complex vasculitis, anaphylactoid purpura, and palpable purpura. Because of this confusing nomenclature, many authorities use the term leukocytoclastic vasculitis. The most common form in childhood is Henoch–Schöenlein purpura.

Henoch–Schöenlein purpura

Epidemiology including genetics and statistics

This common condition occurs at all ages and equally in both sexes. Approximately 10% of the cases occur in children.[116] No genetic or infectious predisposing factors are recognized.

103. Mar A, Fergin P, Hogan P (1999) Unilateral pigmented purpuric eruption. **Australas J Dermatol** 40:211–214.
104. Gelmetti C, Cerri D, Grimalt R (1991) Lichen aureus in childhood. **Pediatr Dermatol** 8:280–283.
105. Gupta G, Holmes SC, Spence E, Mills PR (2000) Capillaritis associated with interferon-alpha treatment of chronic hepatitis C infection. **J Am Acad Dermatol** 43:937–938.
106. Barnhill RL, Braverman IM (1988) Progression of pigmented purpura-like eruptions to mycosis fungoides: a report of three cases. **J Am Acad Dermatol** 19:25–31.
107. Georgala S, Katoulis AC, Symeonidou S et al. (2001) Persistent pigmented purpuric eruption associated with mycosis fungoides: a case report and review of the literature. **J Eur Acad Dermatol Venereol** 15:62–64.
108. Harms M, Feldmann R, Saurat JH (1990) Papular-purpuric "gloves and socks" syndrome. **J Am Acad Dermatol** 23:850–854.
109. Ghighiotti G, Mazzarello G, Nigro A et al. (2000) Papular-purpuric gloves and socks syndrome in HIV-positive patients. **J Am Acad Dermatol** 43:916–917.
110. Grilli R, Izquierdo MJ, Farina MC et al. (1999) Papular-purpuric "gloves and socks" syndrome: polymerase chain reaction demonstration of parvovirus B19 DNA in cutaneous lesions and sera. **J Am Acad Dermatol** 41:793–796.
111. Segui N, Zayas A, Fuertes A, Marquina A (2000) Papular-purpuric "Gloves and Socks" syndrome related to rubella virus infection. **Dermatology** 200(1):89.
112. Ruzicka T, Kalka K, Diercks K, Schuppe HC (1998) Papular-purpuric "gloves and socks" syndrome associated with human herpesvirus 6 infection. **Arch Dermatol** 134:242–244.
113. Guibal F, Buffet P, Mouly F et al. (1996) Papular-purpuric gloves and socks syndrome with hepatitis B infection. **Lancet** 347:473.
114. Carrascosa JM, Bielsa I, Ribera M, Ferrandiz C (1995) Papular-purpuric gloves-and-socks syndrome related to cytomegalovirus infection. **Dermatology** 191:269–270.
115. Perez-Ferriols A, Martinez-Aparicio A, Aliaga-Boniche A (1994) Papular-purpuric "gloves and socks" syndrome caused by measles virus. **J Am Acad Dermatol** 30:291–292.
116. Asherson RA, Cruz DD, Stephens CJM et al. (1991) Urticarial vasculitis in connective tissue disease: clinical patterns, presentations and treatment. **Semin Arthritis Rheum** 20:285.

Presenting history

The eruption is frequently preceded by symptoms of fever, malaise, arthralgia, and gastrointestinal upset. The onset in children is usually acute, although may be more insidious on occasion. A detailed history should be sought, looking for symptoms of conditions that may be associated with leukocytoclastic vasculitis, listed in Table 19.9.

Physical examination

The major presentation is that of palpable petechiae. Individual lesions vary in size from 2 to 7mm in diameter, most of them are slightly elevated and palpable. The individual petechiae may be surrounded by a 2–3mm, flat red halo or collar. These petechial lesions may occur anywhere but are most commonly found on the lower legs (Fig. 19.25). Other types of lesions may be intermixed with the petechiae. Dusky red macules and flat-topped papules are the most common lesions, but small hemorrhagic vesicles, infarcts, and ulcers are seen sometimes (Fig. 19.26).[116] The mucous membranes are not often involved. Leukocytoclastic vasculitis should be considered to be a systemic disease involving blood vessels in many organs. Fifty percent of affected children also have involvement of joints, peripheral nervous system, gastrointestinal tract, and lungs.

Laboratory findings

Investigation of leukocytoclastic vasculitis can be subcatagorized into: confirmation of diagnosis; assessment of other organs involved; and investigation for underlying cause. Confirmation of a vasculitic pathogenesis can

TABLE 19.9   Common causes and associated underlying diseases in leukocytoclastic vasculitis

Infections
    Streptococcal and neisserial bacterial infections
    Hepatitis B
    Cytomegalovirus
    Epstein–Barr virus

Medications and related substances
    Sulfa antibiotics
    Thiazides, phenothiazines, sulfonylureas, and other sulfa-related products
    Quinidine
    Phenytoin
    Injected illicit drugs
    Allopurinol
    Radiographic contrast media
    Nonsteroidal anti-inflammatory agents

Autoimmune diseases
    Lupus erythematosus
    Rheumatoid arthritis
    Wegener's granulomatosis
    Giant cell arteritis
    Mixed and overlap collagen vascular diseases
    Sjögren syndrome
    Chronic inflammatory bowel disease

Dysproteinemias
    Cryoglobulinemia
    Monoclonal and polyclonal gammopathies

Malignancies
    Myeloma
    Leukemia
    Lymphoma

Food products
    Food dyes and preservatives

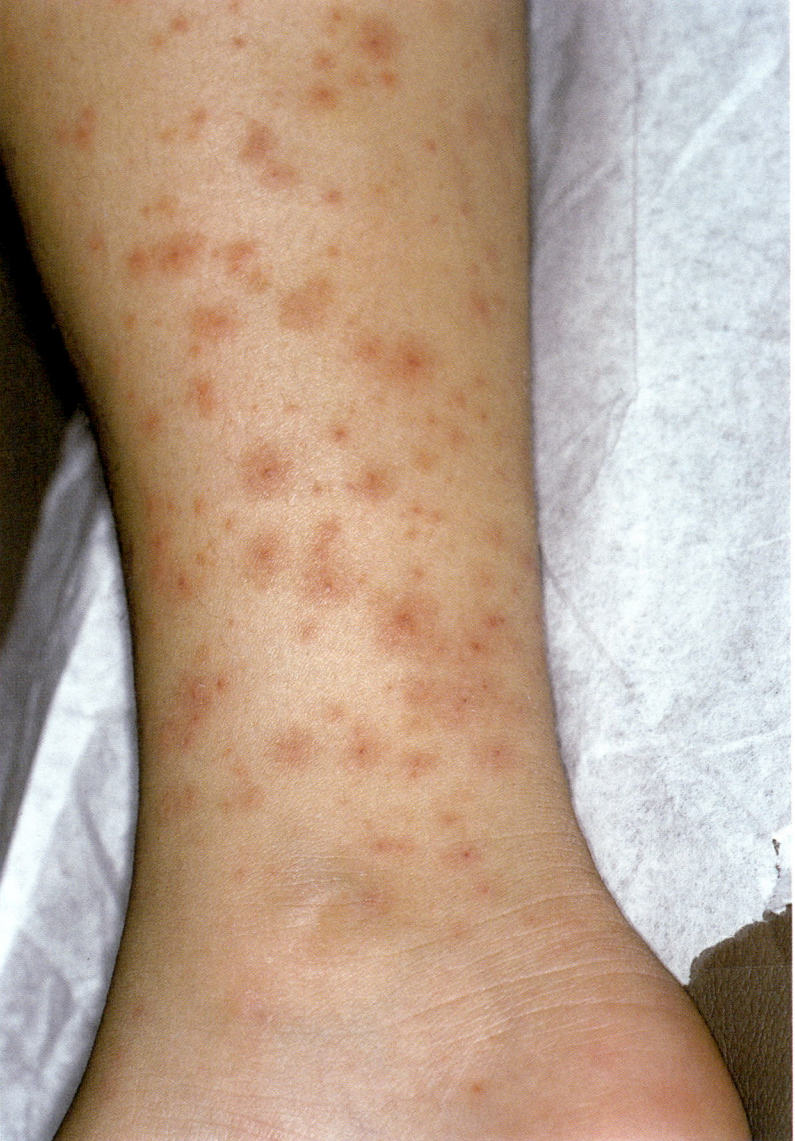

Fig. 19.25   Discrete petechial papules on the leg of an 8-year-old girl with Henoch–Schöenlein purpura.

best be obtained through skin biopsy. The light microscopic changes are essentially those described in the introductory paragraph on venulitis. The severity of the histopathological skin changes is not predictive of internal organ involvement.[117] However, immunofluorescent studies are also often helpful, particularly if IgA deposits are detected around blood vessels, indicating the likelihood of Henoch–Schöenlein purpura. Commonly, IgM, C3, and fibrin are present in and around the blood vessels. IgG rather than IgM is more likely to be present when there is an underlying collagen vascular disease. Decreased serum levels of C3 and C4 complement components are often noted in leukocytoclastic vasculitis.

Testing to exclude internal organ involvement generally includes urinalysis, chest radiograph, stool guaiac, renal function, and liver function studies.

A specific cause or a responsible underlying disease is found in less than 40% of children with leukocytoclastic vasculitis (Table 19.9). Bacterial infection, usually in the form of pharyngitis or other upper respiratory infection, is said to be the single most common cause in childhood vasculitis. However, it is likely that the frequency of associated chronic viral infection

117. Cribier B, Couilliet D, Meyer P, Grosshans E (1999) The severity of the histopathological changes of leukocytoclastic vasculitis is not predictive of extracutaneous involvement. Am J Dermatopathol 21:532–536.

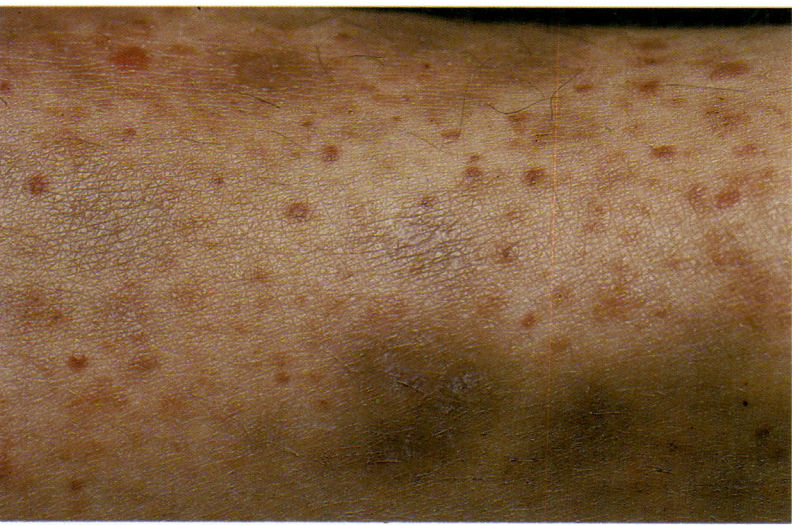

Fig. 19.26 Purpuric papules, ecchymoses and brown old petechiae in a 12-year-old girl with Henoch–Schöenlein purpura.

lysosomal enzymes are released. These proteolytic enzymes then cause basement membrane destruction, leukocytoclasis, and resultant erythrocyte extravasation. This entire chain of events from initial immune complex deposition to removal requires only 24 to 72 hours. After this point, an influx of mononuclear cells signals the initiation of the reparative process.

Differential diagnosis

The most difficult aspect of the diagnosis is the differential between types of vasculitides and their causes rather than differential from other conditions. The most important is the vasculitis associated with meningococcal septicemia due to the serious implications if antibiotic therapy is not immediately instituted.

Papular erythemas such as erythema multiforme and papular urticaria may cause some confusion; however, the lesions are blanchable and do not contain purpura. In the chronic form of pityriasis lichenoides, the child is usually well and the acral areas comparatively spared. Papulonecrotic tuberculid tends to produce monomorphic and scarred lesions with a more insidious onset.

Therapeutics and prognosis

The need for therapy in leukocytoclastic vasculitis depends both on the nature and severity of the organs affected. Children with mild skin involvement only do not require therapy. Those with severe cutaneous disease or with significant systemic involvement may be treated with oral prednisone in a dosage of 1–2mg/kg. In those children unresponsive to steroid therapy, and in those instances in which a steroid-sparing effect is needed, the use of cyclophosphamide can be considered. Nonsteroidal anti-inflammatory drugs such as dapsone, colchicine, and the antimalarials have also been used as safer alternatives to long-term steroid and cytotoxic therapy. Topical therapy is neither necessary nor helpful.

The outcome for children with leukocytoclastic vasculitis is generally good.[116] Cases related to medication usage or infection generally recover completely. When the vasculitis occurs as part of an underlying autoimmune disease, the prognosis is generally that of the associated disease. Idiopathic cases generally resolve spontaneously over several months. Cutaneous scarring does not accompany resolution of the small petechial lesions, but it may occur at the site of infarcts and ulcers.

Pediatric aspects of the disease

The most likely causes of vasculitis in the pediatric population are Henoch–Schöenlein purpura and acute bacterial or viral infections, whereas reactions to medications and connective tissue disease rate higher for adults. Due to the lack of venous stasis in the lower legs, the distribution of lesions in children is more likely to involve the buttocks, arms, and face than with adults.

Acute hemorrhagic edema of infancy

This syndrome in infants and toddlers from 4 to 24 months of age is a vasculitis characterized by an acute onset of purpura in a cockade pattern (Fig. 19.27) accompanied by edema of the hands and feet (Fig. 19.28). It is believed by most authorities to be a variant of Henoch–Schöenlein purpura. The lesions are much larger in size (10–20mm) and more often distributed on the upper extremities. Recurrences are rare and, when present, usually occur shortly after the initial episode.[118] This syndrome usually lacks systemic symptoms. Despite the differences in the size and distribution of lesions, there is leukocytoclastic vasculitis found by skin biopsy, identical to that seen in Henoch–Schöenlein purpura.[119] IgA is usually absent from skin biopsies although is seen on occasion, and the duration of lesions is somewhat shorter than that observed with Henoch–Schöenlein purpura. Importantly, visceral involvement is rare and the prognosis is excellent.[120]

as a cause is underestimated in children. Sometimes it is hard to tell whether an infection or a medication administered for the infection is the true cause of a vasculitic episode. The role played by cryoproteins is also difficult to judge. Small amounts of cryoglobulin may be present in healthy individuals, and thus cryoglobulins sometimes represent a coincidental finding in patients with vasculitis.[117] The situation with food dyes and food preservatives is likewise controversial and unproved. Obviously, most children with vasculitis have been exposed to these agents, but in the absence of challenge testing, an etiologic role usually cannot be proved. Depending on clinical suspicion, investigations that may be performed searching for an underlying cause include throat swab, Anti-Streptolysin O Titer, hepatitis and other viral serology, Tuberculin testing, anti-nuclear antibodies, antineutrophil cytoplasmic antibodies, rheumatoid factor, complement levels, complete blood examination, cryoproteins and protein electrophoresis.[116]

Pathophysiology and histogenesis

The pathogenesis of leukocytoclastic vasculitis is mediated through immune complex formation and deposition. The ability to form circulating immune complexes requires the presence of antigen and antibody in roughly equivalent amounts. Outside of this equivalency ratio, binding sites on either the antigen or antibody are saturated such that interconnecting lattice formation occurs very inefficiently. When circulating immune complexes are formed, they are ordinarily quickly removed by phagocytic cells of the reticuloendothelial system before they can do any harm. However, in leukocytoclastic vasculitis, the reticuloendothelial system is partially blocked or overloaded, and immune complexes are not efficiently removed. These immune complexes do no harm while circulating, but when endothelial cells are separated or the blood vessels are otherwise damaged, they attach to exposed vascular basement membrane. This attachment results in the activation of complement. Complement activation occurs through the classical pathway if the complexes contain IgG or IgM; it occurs through the alternative pathway when they contain IgA. In either case, activation of the complement cascade releases anaphylatoxins (C3a and C5a) that, among other actions, are chemotactic for neutrophils. The neutrophils then accumulate and initiate phagocytosis of the deposited complexes. This removal process is appropriate and desirable, but during phagocytosis, excess neutrophilic

118. Legrain V, Lejean S, Taieb A et al. (1991) Infantile acute hemorrhagic edema of the skin: study of ten cases. **J Am Acad Dermatol** 24:17–22.

119. Saraclar Y, Tinaztepe K, Adalioglu G et al. (1990) Acute hemorrhagic edema of infancy (AHEI): A variant of Henoch–Schonlein purpura or a distinct clinical entity? **J Allergy Clin Immunol** 86:473–483.

120. Gonggryp LA, Todd G (1998) Acute hemorrhagic edema of childhood. **Pediatr Dermatol** 15:91–96.

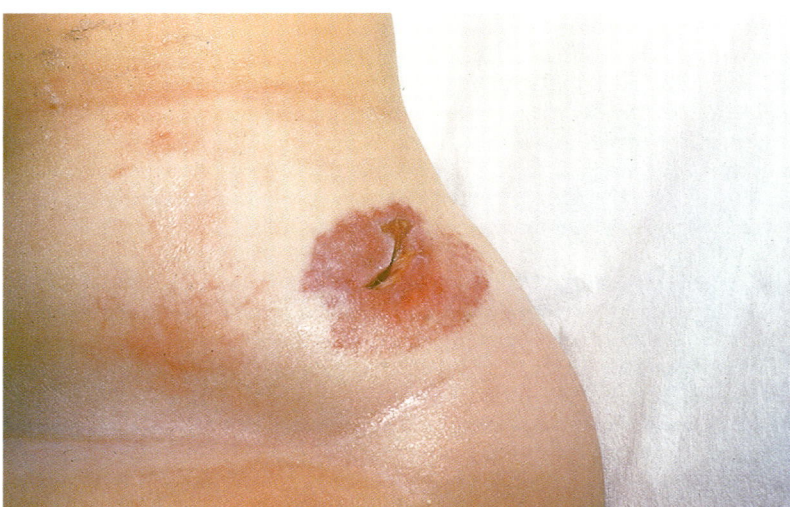

Fig. 19.27 Acute hemorrhagic edema of infancy. Cockade lesion on heel of a 20-month-old.

Urticarial vasculitis (hypocomplementemic vasculitis)

The subtype of leukocytoclastic vasculitis known as urticarial vasculitis occurs rarely in children. It must be kept in mind that many causes of vasculitis, including Henoch–Schöenlein purpura, can produce urticarial wheals and that hypocomplementemia can be seen in the setting of typical palpable purprua. The "hypocomplementemic urticarial vasculitis syndrome" therefore represents a subset of patients with urticarial vasculitis.

The cutaneous lesions in urticarial vasculitis are variable in morphology. They range from typical urticarial papules at one end of the spectrum to petechial lesions at the other. However, most of the lesions are flat-topped, dusky red, and barely palpable, averaging about 1cm in diameter. These lesions are not clinically purpuric, but on diascopy a few petechial dots can sometimes be found within them. The lesions differ from common urticarial wheals in that they remain "fixed" at the same skin site for at least several days rather than hours; they are not associated with itching and leave residual pigmentation when they resolve. Despite the absence of clinical petechiae, biopsy of these lesions usually reveals a typical neutrophilic vasculitis.

Urticarial vasculitis is a chronic process, but it is associated with a good prognosis. It may be associated with cryoglobulins or a monoclonal IgM gammopathy (Schnitzler's syndrome).[121] Hypocomplementemic urticarial vasculitis has a high association with lupus with almost all biopsies showing strong granular immunoreactants along the basement membrane zone, and with the majority of patients suffering from systemic lupus in one series.[122] The pathogenesis and laboratory evaluation are similar to that for conventional leukocytoclastic vasculitis. Therapy similar to that described for leukocytoclastic vasculitis may be required.

ARTERITIS

Conditions in which there is inflammation of cutaneous arteries are uncommon in childhood. The diseases characterized by inflammation of arterial vessels are more polymorphous in appearance than are those of the capillaritis and venulitis groups, and a livedo pattern is often seen. Skin lesions do not always occur in these diseases, although at least a few petechial lesions can generally be found if the search is diligent enough. At other times, however, the petechiae are greatly overshadowed by the presence of more dramatic inflammatory nodules and necrotic ulcers.

Histologically, the arteritis is primarily neutrophilic, but lymphocytes and histiocytes (sometimes to the point of granuloma formation) may be present

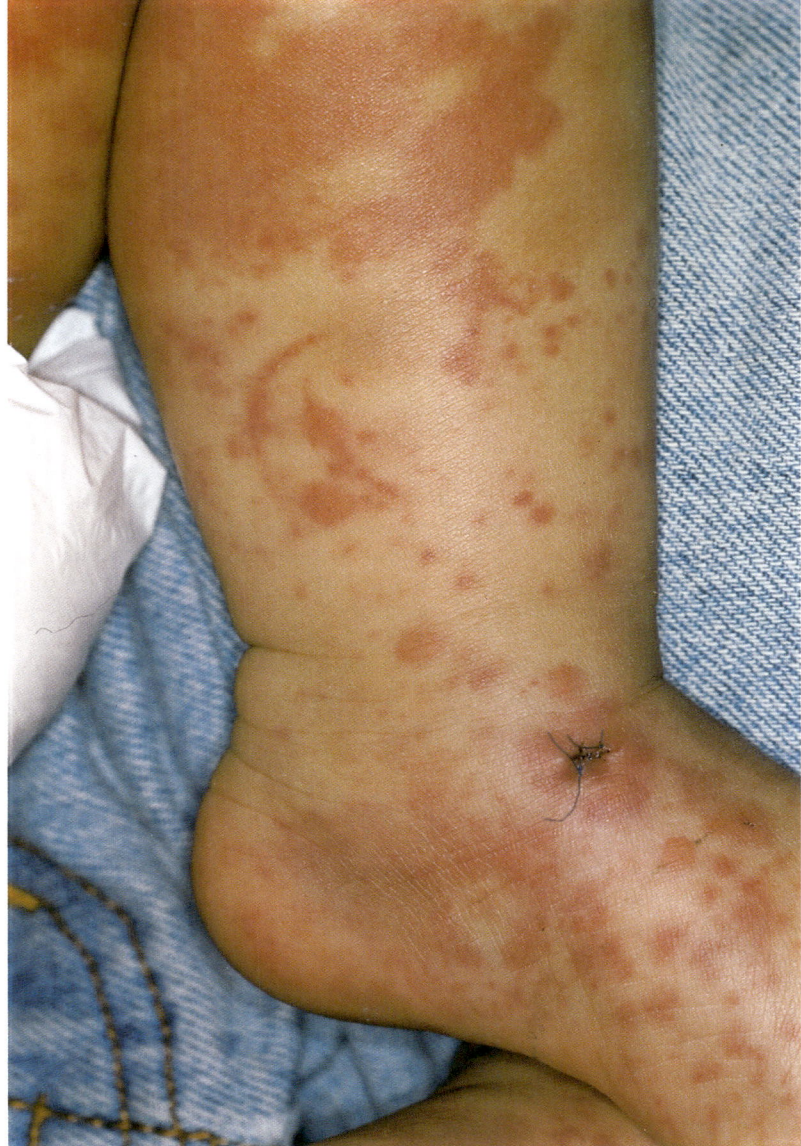

Fig. 19.28 Acute hemorrhagic edema of infancy. Swelling of the leg and foot in an infant with multiple purpuric lesions.

also. Arteries of various size can be involved. Generally, those diseases that involve large arteries demonstrate more severe systemic disease than do those with small-artery involvement. Chronic cutaneous forms may affect only the skin, but most of the diseases considered in this section (Table 19.8) are dominated by systemic symptoms and signs.

Polyarteritis nodosa (periarteritis nodosa)

Introduction and epidemiology

Polyarteritis nodosa is a rare and severe multisystem disease where the primary pathology is due to a necrotizing inflammatory process of small to medium-sized arteries. It has almost certainly been overdiagnosed in the past and the diagnosis should be reserved for conditions where histological evidence of an arteritis is present.

Classical polyarteritis is rare in childhood. Males are said to predominate by a 2:1 ratio.

121. Borradori L, Rybojad M, Puissant A et al. (1990) Urticarial vasculitis associated with monoclonal IgM gammopathy. Schnitzler's syndrome. Br J Dermatol 123:113–318.

122. Davis MD, Daoud MS, Kirby B et al. (1998) Clinicopathologic correlation of hypocomplementemic and normocomplementemic urticarial vasculitis. J Am Acad Dermatol 38:899–905.

Presenting history

Patients with polyarteritis nodosa generally present with fever, weakness, malaise, and hypertension. Multisystem involvement usually occurs early in the disease course.

Physical examination

Skin lesions are found in about one-half of cases. Purpuric papules, similar to those found in leukocytoclastic vasculitis are often present on the lower extremities. They may be accompanied by purpuric infarcts or sharply marginated ulcers. A livedo pattern of the extremities is frequently encountered. In some cases, tender, slope-shouldered, erythematous nodules several centimeters in diameter are intermingled with the other lesions, particularly within an area of livedo. Evidence of internal organ involvement can be found. The joints, nervous system, kidneys, and gastrointestinal tract are the organs affected most frequently.

Laboratory findings

Biopsy of skin lesions reveals a neutrophilic vasculitis of both small and large muscular arteries.[123] The vasculitic lesions, however, are usually segmental and occur most often at points of vessel bifurcation. Because many areas of normal vessels occur between vasculitic lesions, false-negative biopsy findings are obtained with some frequency. The use of elliptical excisions, rather than punch biopsies, helps to minimize this sampling problem. A neutrophilic venulitis may also be found and is especially likely to be present when purpuric lesions undergo biopsy. Appropriate laboratory tests or vascular studies should be carried out for evidence of internal organ involvement.

Pathophysiology and histogenesis

A specific cause for polyarteritis nodosa cannot usually be determined. However, the presence of hepatitis B antigenemia may be found.[124] Hepatitis C is also associated; however, the frequency of the association is uncertain.[124] Polyarteritis has also been found to accompany hairy cell leukemia, Crohn's disease, and certain infections, particularly streptococcal infections.[125] Every case of polyarteritis should be evaluated for the same possibilities of underlying infection, medication reaction, or collagen vascular disease as would be carried out for patients with leukocytoclastic vasculitis. Polyarteritis is likely to be an immune complex disease, based on evidence of the occasional presence of mixed cryoglobulins, rheumatoid factor, antinuclear factor, and depressed levels of complement.

Differential diagnosis

Cutaneous polyarteritis nodosa, discussed below, is separated due to its lack of internal involvement and good prognosis. Microscopic polyarteritis nodosa is the term given to a condition that is associated with the presence of p-ANCA and a segmental necrotizing and crescentic glomerulonephritis.[123] It is a vasculitis that affects venules, capillaries, arterioles and small arteries and therefore is better termed "microscopic polyangiitis."[123] It presents cutaneously primarily as palpable purpura with a leukocytoclastic vasculitis and therefore is better thought as a differential diagnosis in the "venulitis" category.

Therapeutics and prognosis

Systemic polyarteritis nodosa in children is a severe illness with a high mortality rate. Use of systemic corticosteroids in daily dosages of 1.5–2.5mg/kg offers 5-year survival rates of about 50%. Other immunosuppressive agents may be required.

Pediatric aspects of the disease

The condition is less frequent in children. However, essentially the same manifestations are found as with adults.[126] It is reported that there is a higher incidence of convulsions and lymphadenopathy (Infantile polyarteritis nodosa occurs in patients younger than 1 year of age.). It is separated from classical polyarteritis in that the vasculitis is restricted to the coronary arteries almost entirely.[126] The blood vessel changes of infantile polyarteritis are similar to those seen in Kawasaki disease, which is discussed in Chapter 23.

Cutaneous polyarteritis nodosa

Chronic cutaneous polyarteritis nodosa has rarely been described in childhood.[127] The clinical pattern observed is that of livedo reticularis with a few skin nodules (Fig. 19.29). Palpable purpura, cutaneous infarcts, and ulceration generally do not occur with the exception of neonatal cases.[127] Articular, muscular, and neurological manifestations may be present, however, and tend to localize close to the cutaneous lesions.[127] Fever is present in only 30% and other visceral involvement does not occur. Most affected children appear to be cold sensitive and may exhibit serum cryoglobulinemia. The condition tends to be chronic and relapsing but has a much better overall prognosis than does systemic periarteritis.

GRANULOMATOUS VASCULITIS

The diseases considered under this heading are characterized by a combination of neutrophilic vasculitis and associated vascular (or extravascular) necrotizing granulomas. Systemic involvement is prominent; cutaneous lesions are usually incidental features found in only 25–50% of affected children.

Wegener's granulomatosis

Wegener's granulomatosis occurs predominately in mid-adult life, but occasional cases have been recognized in childhood. The onset of Wegener's granulomatosis is usually marked by the development of chronic nasal obstruction and sinusitis.[128] Other prominent early features include otitis, gingivitis, laryngitis, cough, and dyspnea. Skull lesions occur in approximately

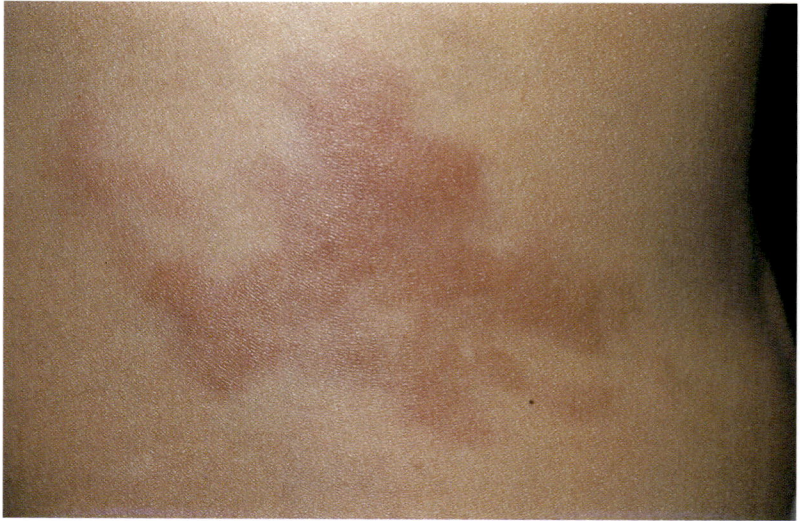

Fig. 19.29 Chronic cutaneous periarteritis nodosa. Palpable linear red nodules within a livedo pattern on the leg of a 6-year-old boy.

123. Jennette JC, Thomas DB, Falk RJ (2001) Microscopic polyangiitis (microscopic polyarteritis). **Semin Diagn Pathol** 18:3–13.
124. Garcia de la Pena Lefebvre P, Mouthon L, Cohen P, Lhote F, Guillevin L (2001) Polyarteritis nodosa and mixed cryoglobulinaemia related to hepatitis B and C virus coinfection. **Ann Rheumatic Dis** 11:1068–1069.
125. Bont L, Brus F, Dijkman-Neerincx RH et al. (1998) The clinical spectrum of post-streptococcal syndromes with arthritis in children. **Clin Exp Rheumatol** 16:750–752.
126. Ozen S, Besbas N, Saatici U, Bakkaloglu A (1992) Diagnostic criteria for polyarteritis nodosa in children. **J Pediatr** 120:206–209.
127. Kumar L, Thapa BR, Sarkar B, Walia BNS (1995) Benign cutaneous polyarteritis nodosa in children below 10 years of age: a clinical experience. **Ann Rheum Dis** 54:134–136.
128. Brazzelli V, Vassallo C, Baldini F et al. (1999) Wegener's granulomatosis in a child: cutaneous findings as the presenting signs. **Pediatr Dermatol** 16:277–280.

50% of children; rarely, chronic skin lesions may precede the development of recognizable systemic involvement. Large, deep, punched-out ulcers, with undermined violaceous borders, are the most characteristic cutaneous lesions. These ulcers are similar in appearance to those of pyoderma gangrenosum. Vesicles, petechial papules, and tender red nodules are found occasionally and there have been two reported cases of pediatric Wegener's granulomatosis with acneiform lesions as the presenting sign.[128] The presence of oral lesions in the form of gingival granulomas (strawberry gums) may be a particularly helpful diagnostic sign.

There is usually prominent clinical evidence of respiratory tract involvement, but the renal impairment, which is also regularly present, may be asymptomatic. The joints, eyes, heart, and nervous system are affected in about 50% of children. Lung disease appears to be significantly less common in children than with adults.[129] A limited form of Wegener's granulomatosis lacking renal involvement is recognized by some authorities. Cutaneous lesions are said to be particularly common in this variant of the classical disease.

Biopsy of lesions from any of the affected organs reveals a necrotizing vasculitis of small to mid-sized arteries and veins. The vasculitis is predominantly neutrophilic, but in older lesions, mononuclear cells become more prominent. The necrotizing granulomas that microscopically characterize the disease may occur as part of the vasculitis or may be located at extravascular sites. Lesions heal with microscopic evidence of fibrotic scar formation. Circulating immune complexes are found in about one-half of patients, but evidence for their deposition in vessel walls is generally lacking. Antineutrophilic cytoplasmic antibody (c-ANCA) is seen in almost all patients and the level is useful in monitoring disease progress.[130] The cause of Wegener's granulomatosis is unknown; development of an immunologic reaction to chronic bacterial infection, viral infection, or inhaled antigens has been suspected.

Children with untreated disease may die within several years. Steroid therapy is only partially effective, but 90% of children respond to cyclophosphamide administered in a daily dosage of 1–2mg/kg with complete remission. A combination of steroids and cytotoxic agents, used concomitantly, is necessary in some.

Churg–Strauss syndrome

Churg–Strauss syndrome is a granulomatous vasculitic syndrome with the primary components being severe asthma, eosinophilia, and vasculitis. It is extremely rare in children. Skin nodules that occasionally ulcerate are the most common cutaneous manifestation, but papules, papulovesicles, livedo reticularis, palpable purpura, necrotic hemorrhagic lesions, and erythema multiforme-like purpuric lesions have been described.[131]

Giant cell arteritis

Temporal arteritis and Takayasu's arteritis, the two major forms of giant cell arteritis, occur infrequently in children and lack skin lesions. For this reason, they are not considered further.

NONINFLAMMATORY PETECHIAL AND ECCHYMOTIC PURPURAS

The diseases considered in this section are characterized by the presence of large areas of purpura. Petechiae are usually present, but ecchymoses dominate the clinical presentation. These ecchymoses, which consist of large, noninflammatory depositions of blood within the skin, usually are not elevated or palpable. Likewise, the petechiae are usually nonpalpable. The noninflammatory petechial and ecchymotic purpuras are subdivided into two groups: intra- and extravascular purpuras (Table 19.10). The intravascular purpuras are so named because they are caused by a disturbance at one or more points in the circulating components of the coagulation cascade. The

TABLE 19.10 Noninflammatory petechial and ecchymotic purpuras

Intravascular purpuras
  Disseminated intravascular coagulation
  Thrombotic thrombocytopenic purpura
  Idiopathic thrombocytopenic purpura
  Thrombocytopenic purpura caused by medications, transfusions, and
  other diseases
  Deficiencies in nonplatelet coagulation factors
  Miscellaneous intravascular purpuras

Extravascular purpuras
  Scurvy
  Ehlers–Danlos syndrome
  Gardner–Diamond syndrome
  Miscellaneous extravascular purpuras

extravascular purpuras, on the other hand, occur because fragility of the vascular wall basement membrane or weakened extravascular connective tissue does not provide adequate structural support for the cutaneous blood vessels.

Clinical differentiation between the intra- and the extravascular purpuras is often possible. Patients with intravascular purpura bleed very easily and cease bleeding only with difficulty. Clinically, this is reflected by "spontaneous" bleeding without a history of specific trauma; oozing from the mucous membranes of the nose, gingiva, and gastrointestinal tract; and cutaneous bleeding brisk enough to form nodular hematomas and flat ecchymoses. In contrast, bleeding in children with extravascular purpura is less troublesome. It usually requires recognizable trauma for initiation, rarely occurs from mucous membranes, and seldom leads to hematoma formation.

DISSEMINATED INTRAVASCULAR COAGULATION

Disseminated intravascular coagulation (DIC) is characterized by the sudden unexpected activation of the coagulation cascade secondary to the presence of one or another underlying disease process. The triggering of this thrombotic process, together with consequent activation of the fibrinolytic process, depletes the blood of platelets and other clotting factors. This depletion then results in the rapid development of a state of hypo- or non-coagulability.

The clinical presentation in DIC is highly variable. In mild cases, only a few cutaneous petechiae and ecchymoses are present. Usually, this is recognized as prolonged bleeding at venipuncture sites and at other sites of skin-piercing trauma. In more severe cases, soft tissue hematomas, hemorrhagic bullae, and skin necrosis are encountered. Moreover, one is likely to find evidence of gastrointestinal, genitourinary, and other types of internal organ bleeding. Almost always, the signs and symptoms of hypocoagulability (bleeding) overshadow those due to the primary hypercoagulability (thromboses).

The diagnosis of DIC usually can be accomplished through the use of screening tests. Specifically, platelet counts are usually (but not always) decreased, and there is prolongation of the prothrombin and partial thromboplastin times. Should a greater degree of diagnostic certainty be required, fibrinogen levels can be obtained (they are decreased), and the presence of fibrin split products can be ascertained. Finally, examination of a blood smear generally reveals the presence of schistocytes from erythrocyte damage caused during passage through partially thrombosed vessels.

DIC may be triggered by a variety of underlying disease processes. Those of importance in pediatric settings include snake bite envenomation, burns, blood transfusions, leukemic malignancies, vascular hamartomas, and, most important of all, various types of infection.[132]

129. Rottem M, Fauci A, Hallahan CW et al. (1993) Wegener granulomatosis in children and adolescents: clinical presentation and outcome. **J Pediatr** 122:26–31.
130. Rao JK, Allen NB, Feussner JR, Weinberger M (1995) A prospective study of antineutrophilic cytoplasmic antibody(c-ANCA) and clinical criteria in diagnosing of Wegener's granulomatosis. **Lancet** 346:926–931.

131. Frayha RA (1982) Churg–Strauss syndrome in a child. **J Rheumatol** 9:807–809.
132. Bick RL, Arun B, Frenkel EP (1999) Disseminated intravascular coagulation: clinical and pathophysiological mechanisms and manifestations. **Haemostasis** 29:111–134.

Treatment of DIC is directed first toward removal or reduction of the triggering process including a thorough investigation for underlying sepsis. The next step involves replacement of depleted clotting factors through administration of fresh-frozen plasma, platelets, or cryoprecipitates containing fibrinogen. Determination of the amount and "mix" of these substances is difficult and requires the assistance of an experienced clinician. Early fears that the addition of these clotting factors would only exacerbate the condition seem unwarranted today.[132] The use of heparin to impede the clotting process and thus decrease consumption of coagulation factors remains controversial. Some authorities would use it in most cases, but most would withhold it until there was evidence that simple replacement of clotting factors was inadequate.[132] The use of heparin seems particularly helpful when fibrinogen levels are found to be extremely low. There is, however, consensus that heparin should not be administered to patients with hypertension, to those with evidence of central nervous system bleeding, and to those in the immediate postoperative period. It has also been suggested that the administration of aminocaproic acid might be helpful because of this product's inhibitory effect on fibrinolysis, but some authorities do not use it because of the risk of thrombosis. The role of other modalities such as antithrombin concentrates, protein C concentrates, and cytokine modifiers may be of value depending on the clinical situation and highlight the need to manage this clinical situation in conjunction with hematological experts.[132] Interferon alfa may also be useful in children with Kasabach–Merritt syndrome, but the response is slow, occurring over weeks to months and reported neurological complications restrict its use.

Purpura fulminans

Purpura fulminans is a variant of DIC that occurs in children during or just after a bacterial (most often meningococcal or streptococcal) or viral (most often varicella) infection.[133] Congenital deficiencies of proteins C and S, in their severe forms, are the most common cause of purpura fulminans in the neonatal period.[133–135] Persons who are heterozygous for protein C deficiency have levels of circulating protein C that are 50% of normal and usually do not have symptoms from thrombosis until early adult life.[134] These persons are also predisposed to coumarin-induced skin necrosis. Persons who are homozygous or doubly heterozygous for the defect have levels of protein C that are less than 1% of normal and purpura fulminans and major thrombotic events usually develop in the neonatal period.[134] Persons homozygous for protein S deficiency usually do not have thromboembolic events in the neonatal period but in early adult life, although neonatal purpura fulminans is reported.[135] A case of neonatal purpura fulminans secondary to activated protein C resistance has been reported.[135–137]

Purpura fulminans is characterized by the sudden onset of tender ecchymoses accompanied by exacerbation of fever and chills. Acral portions of the body are most severely involved. Individual ecchymotic lesions may blister but then rapidly progress to necrosis and gangrene. Shock, coma, and death may ensue. Initial therapy consists of the administration of a source of protein C and S, such as fresh-frozen plasma or prothrombin complex concentrate,[135] with repeated infusions being necessary because of the short half-life of the molecules. Long-term treatment involves careful administration of oral anticoagulants, starting at very low doses and under protective replacement therapy to avoid coumarin-induced skin necrosis. Topically applied nitroglycerin has been helpful for the poorly perfused extremities.

Kasabach–Merritt syndrome

The Kasabach–Merritt syndrome is a variant of DIC in which platelets and clotting factors are locally consumed within a vascular tumor. It has its highest incidence during the first few weeks of life and may be present at birth.[138] It has become apparent that the vascular lesions in this syndrome are kaposiform hemangioendotheliomas[139] or tufted angiomas[140] rather than true hemangiomas. Both sequestration of platelets and consumption coagulopathy are involved in the pathogenesis. Clinically, the onset is manifest by the development of purpura and rapid enlargement of the vascular lesions, which becomes distended and tense. Due to the coagulopathy, evidence of bleeding and bruising at distant sites becomes evident (Fig. 19.22). Both chronic and acute variants of Kasabach–Merritt syndrome exist. Observation without therapy may be sufficient for mild chronic cases, but the acute variants require treatment as indicated above for conventional DIC. In addition, systemic agents, as a treatment for the vascular tumor itself, are usually indicated. These agents include prednisolone, vincristine, interferon alpha, cyclophosphamide, actinomycin D, epsilon aminocaproic acid, compression and embolization, often as multimodal therapy.[141,142]

IDIOPATHIC THROMBOTIC MICROANGIOPATHY

Idiopathic thrombotic microangiopathy includes the two related syndromes thrombotic thrombocytopenic purpura and hemolytic-uremic syndrome. These disorders are due to widespread deposition of intravascular microthrombi consisting mainly of platelets, with subsequent consumption thrombocytopenia, microangiopathic hemolytic anemia, renal abnormalities, and neurologic disturbances.[143]

Thrombotic thrombocytopenic purpura

Thrombotic thrombocytopenic purpura (TTP) is rare in children and may be seen in adolescent girls. Cutaneous lesions consist of petechiae and ecchymoses. Gastrointestinal and genitourinary bleeding are often present but are usually overshadowed by the symptoms and signs of renal and central nervous system disease. Life-threatening acute respiratory distress syndrome can be associated with TTP.[144] Confirmation of a clinical diagnosis requires the demonstration of hyaline-type platelet thrombi in the arterioles and capillaries of involved organs. Biopsy of skin lesions, if present, is usually satisfactory. Gingival biopsy is often recommended, but the false-negative rate is high; only about 40% of such biopsy specimens demonstrate the expected changes.

The pathogenesis of TTP involves a coagulopathic process that is somewhat similar to that which occurs in DIC. There is, however, less evidence of the enhanced fibrinolysis that is characteristically present in classical DIC. Current hypotheses regarding the process through which the coagulopathy develops include both immunologic and nonimmunologic processes. The presence of factors that agglutinate platelets, and the absence of prostaglandin-like factors that, if present, would inhibit platelet agglutination, may also play an important role.

In adults, plasma exchange has improved survival rates from 10% to between 75% and 92%, creating urgency for the initiation of treatment.[145] It has also increased awareness that a chronic, relapsing form of the disease exists. Other forms of therapy sometimes recommended include splenectomy, the admin-

133. Baselga E, Drolet BA, Esterly NA (1997) Purpura in infants and children. 37:673–705.
134. Sills RH, Marlar RA, Montgomery RR et al. (1984) Severe homozygous protein C deficiency. **J Pediatr** 105:409–413.
135. Mahasandana C, Suvatte V, Chuansumrit A et al. (1990) Homozygous protein S deficiency in an infant with purpura fulminans. **J Pediatr** 117:750–753.
136. Pipe SW, Schmaier AH, Nichols WC et al. (1996) Neonatal purpura fulminans in association with factor V R506Q mutation. **J Pediatr** 128:706–709.
137. Sills RH, Marlar RA, Montgomery RR et al. (1984) Severe homozygous protein C deficiency. **J Pediatr** 105:409–413.
138. Esterly NB (1983) Kasabach Merritt syndrome in infants. **J Am Acad Dermatol** 8:504–513.
139. Sarkar M, Mulliken JB, Kosakewich HP et al. (1997) Thrombocytopenic coagulopathy (Kasabach-Merritt phenomenon) is associated with Kaposiform hemangioendothelioma and not with common infantile hemangioma. **Plast Reconstr Surg** 100(6):1377–1386.
140. Enjolras O, Wassef M, Dosquet C et al. (1998) [Kasabach-Merritt syndrome on a congenital tufted angioma]. **Ann Dermatol Venereol** 125:257–260.
141. Blei F, Karp N, Rofsky N et al. (1998) Successful multimodal therapy for kaposiform hemangioendothelioma complicated by Kasabach-Merritt phenomenon: case report and review of the literature. **Pediatr Hematol Oncol** 15:295–305.
142. Hu B, Lachman R, Phillips J et al. (1998) Kasabach-Merritt syndrome-associated kaposiform hemangioendothelioma successfully treated with cyclophosphamide, vincristine, and actinomycin D. **J Pediatr Hematol Oncol** 20:567–569.
143. Sagripanti A, Sarteschi LM, Carpi A (2000) The management of idiopathic thrombotic microangiopathy. Changing trends. **Biomed Pharmacother** 54:423–430.
144. Chang JC, Aly ES (2001) Acute respiratory distress syndrome as a major clinical manifestation of thrombotic thrombocytopenic purpura. **Am J Med Sci** 321:124–128.
145. George JN (2000) How I treat patients with thrombotic thrombocytopenic purpura-hemolytic uremic syndrome. **Blood** 96:1223–1229.

istration of cytotoxic agents, and the use of drugs that inhibit platelet aggregation and activation.

Hemolytic uremic syndrome

Hemolytic uremic syndrome is a disease of infants and young children that, like DIC and TTP, exhibits the presence of microangiopathic anemia and platelet consumption. Hyaline thrombi develop within blood vessels and are especially prominent in the kidneys. Children usually present with acute gastrointestinal problems and evidence of severe renal disease. In contrast to TTP, central nervous system involvement is not prominent. Purpuric skin lesions may be present. Diarrhea-associated hemolytic uremic syndrome develops in about 5 to 10% of children with hemorrhagic colitis due to *Escherichia coli* 0157:H7.[146] Endothelial cell damage, white blood cell activation, and platelet-endothelial cell interactions are important in the pathogenesis. Meticulous supportive care, with attention to nutrition and fluid, and electrolyte balance, is important. Dialysis is necessary in many children Twenty-year follow-up studies report that 75% of children recover without any clinically significant long-term sequelae. Chronic renal failure is reported in about 5% of children.

IDIOPATHIC THROMBOCYTOPENIC PURPURA

Two forms of idiopathic thrombocytopenic purpura (ITP) are recognized. The acute form occurs primarily in children, whereas the chronic form is most often encountered in adolescents. Both types share the features of thrombocytopenia, shortened platelet survival time, and the absence of splenomegaly.

The onset of the acute form of ITP is usually preceded by respiratory infection; 10 to 20 days after this, there is a sudden appearance of cutaneous petechiae and ecchymoses accompanied by gastrointestinal and genitourinary bleeding. Bleeding from the oral cavity is commonly present. In most cases, the disease is self-limited. Mild cases do not require therapy; more severe disease warrants the use of prednisone in doses of 1–2mg/kg. Intravenous administration of γ-globulin has also been recommended. Splenectomy or intravenous anti-D is occasionally necessary in those patients who do not respond to steroids or intravenous γ-globulin.[147]

Chronic ITP, which occurs primarily in adolescent girls, begins more insidiously, with the unexplained development of petechiae, easy bruising, and post-traumatic bleeding. Menorrhagia may be present. The adolescent experiences a long-term, fluctuating course but generally feels reasonably well. In mild cases, therapy may not be necessary. Patients with more severe disease may require prednisone, splenectomy, or the administration of colchicine, danazol, infused γ-globulin, or even cytotoxic drugs.[148]

The pathogenesis of both acute and chronic ITP involves development of IgG antiplatelet antibodies. These antibodies fix to the platelets, which in turn cause their rapid removal by phagocytic cells of the reticuloendothelial system. Not surprisingly, the antibody titer appears to be inversely related to the platelet count.

Patients with autoimmune collagen vascular disease (especially LE), leukemia, or lymphoma and normal individuals during some drug reactions may develop similar antiplatelet antibodies and, thus, a condition similar to that of ITP.

Autoimmune neonatal thrombocytopenia results from placental passage of maternal autoantibodies directed against maternal platelet antigens that are also present in the fetal platelets. This occurs in the course of an autoimmune disease in the mother such as lupus erythematosus, idiopathic thrombocytopenic purpura (ITP), or drug-induced autoimmune thrombocytopenia.[149]

THROMBOCYTOPENIC PURPURA CAUSED BY MEDICATIONS, TRANSFUSIONS, AND OTHER DISEASES

More than 100 different drugs have been identified at one time or another as a cause of thrombocytopenic purpura.[150] The most important of these include the sulfa antibiotics, the thiazides, and quinidine.[148] Children with drug-induced thrombocytopenia present with petechiae and ecchymoses, particularly on dependent areas of the body. The lesions are not palpable, and they have no surrounding erythema. These two factors help differentiate the vasculitic from the thrombocytopenic form of purpuric drug reactions. Fever and malaise are sometimes present. A few of these reactions are due to direct platelet toxicity of the drug or its metabolies, but most reactions are immunologically mediated. The drug or one of its metabolites acts as a hapten, which, after fixing to a carrier protein, becomes a complete antigen. This complete antigen can subsequently induce the formation of antiplatelet antibodies. Laboratory identification of the responsible drug is difficult and is not possible in most clinical settings. A presumptive clinical diagnosis more usually is confirmed by clinical improvement in the subsequent two weeks after withdrawal of the suspected agent.

Immune thrombocytopenia also occurs occasionally in children several days after receiving whole blood transfusions. In these cases, a specific antigen on the transfused platelets stimulates an antibody response in the host. Several systemic diseases are associated with the development of immune thrombocytopenic purpura. The most common of these is LE, including neonatal LE. In LE, an ITP-like immune reaction develops in about 10% of patients.

Thrombocytopenia also occurs frequently in children with leukemia and histiocytosis Langerhans cell. In these conditions, the decrease in platelets is usually due to marrow replacement by tumor, but in some cases, it may be due to ITP-like immune mechanisms. Other conditions less often associated with thrombocytopenic purpura include insect envenomation, rheumatoid arthritis, and various infections. The congenital infections that make up the TORCH (toxoplasmosis, other infections, rubella, cytomegalovirus, and herpes simplex) syndromes are especially likely to be complicated by thrombocytopenic purpura with petechiae, purpura, and, in the clinical form, of the blue-berry muffin lesions. Both thrombocytopenic purpura and infiltrates of extramedullary hematopoiesis play a role in the development of these lesions.[149]

Purpuric lesions are a notable hallmark of the Wiskott–Aldrich syndrome. Fewer than the normal number of platelets and large megakaryocytes are present, and those platelets that remain do not function normally. This disease is discussed in greater detail in Chapter 7.

DEFICIENCIES IN NONPLATELET COAGULATION FACTORS

Genetic absence or functional deficiency of various protein components of the coagulation cascade occur in classical hemophilia, von Willebrand's disease, factor XII deficiency, and other similar conditions.[151] Petechaie and ecchymoses are commonly encountered in these diseases, but these skin lesions are usually overshadowed by other important clinical problems.

Vitamin K is required for active function of factors VII, IX and X and prothrombin. Deficiency of this vitamin results in various hemorrhagic processes, which include petechiae and ecchymoses of the skin. Because vitamin K is not stored in the body, a deficient state can rapidly develop. Vitamin K deficiency of the newborn is commonly accompanied by ecchymoses.[151] Human breast milk (as opposed to cow's milk) contains essentially no vitamin K.[151] Thus, breast milk-fed infants are totally dependent on the production of vitamin K by bacteria in the gut, which is a mechanism that, during the

146. Robson WL (2000) Haemolytic uraemic syndrome. **Paediatr Drugs** 2:243–252.
147. Bussel JB (2000) Overview of idiopathic thrombocytopenic purpura: new approach to refractory patients. **Semin Oncol** 27(6 Suppl 12):91–98.
148. Yang R, Han ZC (2000) Pathogenesis and management of chronic idiopathic thrombocytopenic purpura: an update. **Int J Hematol** 71:18–24.
149. Homans A (1996) Thrombocytopenia in the neonate. **Pediatr Clin North Am** 43:737–756.
150. Litt JZ, Pawlak WA Jr, eds (2001) Drug Eruption Reference Manual (DERM), 5th ed. Cleveland: Wal-Zac Enterprises.
151. Lane PA, Hathaway WE (1985) Vitamin K in infancy. **J Pediatr** 106:351–359.

first few days of life, is very inefficient. Some of these infants, particularly those who are born prematurely, may have hemorrhagic disease with umbilical, gastrointestinal, genitourinary, and central nervous system bleeding.[151] Cutaneous ecchymoses are often prominent. The syndrome can be avoided by prophylactic administration of vitamin K to the mother just before delivery or to the neonate just after delivery.[151]

Late hemorrhagic disease may be due to low vitamin K levels in breast milk in exclusively breast-fed babies, or secondly diseases associated with impaired absorption of vitamin K. These include diarrhea, cystic fibrosis, biliary atresia, α-1 antitrypsin deficiency, hepatitis, abetalipoproteinemia, and celiac disease.[151] Vitamin K is obtained in appropriate dosage through the ingestion of green, leafy vegetables. Dietary deficiency of these vegetables or inadequate absorption as a result of the presence of various malabsorption syndromes can cause purpura and other hemorrhagic problems. Finally, anticoagulants of the coumarin type interfere with the function of vitamin K. The bleeding tendencies and ecchymoses seen with overdosage of these medications can be reversed by administration of vitamin K.

MISCELLANEOUS CAUSES OF INTRAVASCULAR PURPURA

Heparin- and coumarin-related anticoagulants can cause anticoagulant purpura as a result of overdosage, but idiosyncratic ecchymotic reactions unrelated to overdosage are occasionally encountered several days after initiation of therapy. During these idiosyncratic reactions, large ecchymotic areas suddenly appear over areas of plentiful subcutaneous fat. Heparin administration is known to cause thrombocytopenia from heparin-associated antiplatelet antibodies.[152] This syndrome has occurred in neonates in neonatal intensive care units as a result of the administration of low doses of heparin to prevent occlusion of central and peripheral catheters.[150] Minor cutaneous bleeding is seen in one-third of these patients. Aortic thrombosis is the major risk in these babies. Diagnosis can be confirmed by determination of heparin-associated antiplatelet antibodies. Discontinuation of heparin administration leads to rapid recovery of the platelet count in four or five days. Coumarin-induced ecchymosis is usually due to deficiency in the vitamin K-related proteins C and S.

Purpuric lesions are found with some frequency in children with advanced liver and renal disease. The cause of purpura in these settings is multifactorial. Children with primary fibrinolysis can develop purpura through mechanisms that may have some similarity to those found in DIC. On rare occasions, infants with mastocytosis release sufficient amounts of heparin from mast cells to cause purpura. Children with cryoglobulinemia or cryofibrinoginemia may develop purpura as a result of cryoprecipitate damage to vascular endothelium. Those with mixed cryoglobulins may have petechiae secondary to leukocytoclastic vasculitis.

EXTRAVASCULAR PURPURAS

Children with diseases in this category develop cutaneous petechiae and ecchymoses because of connective tissue defects either in the basement membrane of the vessel wall or because of defects in the surrounding, supportive dermal connective tissue. Trauma, which in some cases may be mild, is necessary to provoke the appearance of the purpuric lesions. Hematomas and spontaneous bleeding from mucous membranes usually do not occur.

SCURVY

Vitamin C deficiency, when mild, is reflected by the appearance of petechiae that tend to form around hair follicles. There is an associated keratin plug within the ostia of these follicles, and the hair itself is often twisted in a corkscrew manner. In cases of greater severity, large ecchymoses are found in addition to the petechiae. The ecchymoses are especially likely to be found in dependent areas. Hematoma formation, gingival bleeding, leg edema, and xerosis may also be present.[153] Children with scurvy sometimes develop subperiosteal hemorrhage. The connective tissue defect responsible for the bleeding occurs because of inadequate conversion of proline to hydroxyproline.

EHLERS–DANLOS SYNDROME

The subtypes of Ehlers–Danlos syndrome generally share the problems of abnormal skin extensibility, easy tearing of the skin, poor wound healing, and easy bruisability. Purpuric lesions may occur as a result of both vessel wall fragility, and, particularly in type III disease, easy dissection of extravasated blood through the defectively structured connective tissue of the dermis. Specific biochemical abnormalities in connective tissue synthesis have been identified for several types of Ehlers–Danlos syndrome and are presumably responsible for these changes. Therapy for these defects is not available (See Chapter 23).

GARDNER–DIAMOND SYNDROME AND RELATED CONDITIONS

The conditions considered under the umbrella term Gardner–Diamond syndrome probably have mixed causes. They are considered together here because of the important role that external trauma and psychological disability seem to play in these children. Children with Gardner–Diamond syndrome have in common the development of burning pain in localized cutaneous sites, the appearance of redness and swelling at these sites, and the evolution of these "bruised" areas into ecchymoses.[154] Nearly all of the patients are adolescent girls. Lesions are generally confined to limbs, but they may occur anywhere on the body. Of interest is the fact that the back, an area hard to reach or see, is almost never involved.[155] Adolescents commonly describe an increase in stress at the time the lesions appear, and most patients have readily recognizable depression, anxiety, hysteria, repressed hostility, masochism, or other psychological abnormalities. Characteristically, they are indifferent to the problem.[155] Sometimes, affected individuals have the Munchausen syndrome or suffer Munchausen by proxy syndrome.[156]

All authorities agree that psychological factors are important in the development of these ecchymoses, but it is not clear what proportion are willfully induced, nonwillfully induced, or develop through some psychological effects on coagulation factors.[157] A setting of close observation may be necessary to detect self-induced lesions.

In most cases, significant laboratory abnormalities are not detected, but it is reported that these lesions can be induced by intradermal injection of the individual's own erythrocytes or the erythrocyte stroma. DNA of autologous or calf thymus origin sometimes evoke positive reactions. However, the closer the observation and the greater the use of blinded control injections, the fewer positive results are obtained. A few adolescents have serologic evidence of

152. Spadone D, Clark F, James E et al. (1992) Heparin-induced thrombocytopenia in the newborn. **J Vasc Surg** 15:306–311.
153. Hirschmann JV, Raugi GJ (1999) Adult scurvy. **J Am Acad Dermatol** 41:895–906.
154. Regazzini R, Malagoli PG, Zerbinati N et al. (1998) Diamond-Gardner syndrome: a case report. **Pediatr Dermatol** 15:43–45.
155. Joe EK, Ki VW, Magro CM et al. (1999) Diagnostic clues to dermatitis artefacta. **Cutis** 63:209–214.
156. Archer-Dubon C, Orozco-Topete R, Reyes-Gutierrez E (1998) Two cases of psychogenic purpura. **Rev Invest Clin** 50:145–148.
157. Folks DG, Warnock JK (2001) Psychocutaneous disorders. **Curr Psychiatry** 3:219–225.

other autoimmune phenomena, but it is not clear whether these findings are causally related. Psychological counseling and the use of psychotropic agents such as antidepressants represent the most appropriate approach to therapy.[156]

MISCELLANEOUS CAUSES OF EXTRAVASCULAR PURPURA

Prolonged systemic administration of corticosteroids leads to dermal atrophy and fragility of the dermal connective tissue. As a result, bruising in the form of ecchymoses occurs with even minimal trauma. Most lesions develop on the arms and legs. Recognition of corticosteroid purpura is not difficult based on the history of corticosteroid usage and usual presence of other changes associated with steroid use. Discontinuation of corticosteroids, where possible, allows for resolution of the problem in 6 to 18 months. Similar changes can be encountered after prolonged occlusive application of topical corticosteroids.

Direct trauma of sufficient severity causes ecchymoses in children with entirely normal skin. The appearance of such changes (particularly if linear or angular) in children for whom other causes are not immediately apparent should be considered as suspicious of child abuse. The application of heated coins ("coining") to a child's skin as a remedy is frequent in some Asian cultures and results in round areas of purpura. This should not be considered a marker of child abuse.

ACKNOWLEDGMENTS

The editors gratefully acknowledge contributions by Dr Peter Lynch, which were retained from the first edition of *Pediatric Dermatology* and Dr Peter Hogan, for his contributions from the second edition.

Vascular Birthmarks and Other Abnormalities of Blood Vessels and Lymphatics

Ilona Frieden, Odile Enjolras and Nancy Esterly

THE CLASSIFICATION OF VASCULAR BIRTHMARKS

Vascular lesions are common in infants and children, but their precise classification can be confusing. In 1996, the International Society for the Study of Vascular Anomalies (ISSVA) approved a classification system modified from the schema originally proposed by Mulliken and Glowacki.[1] Their aim was to establish a common language for the many different medical specialists involved in the management of these lesions. Two groups of vascular anomaly are delineated: vascular tumors (of which hemangioma of infancy is the most common) and vascular malformations (Table 20.1).[2] The classification, as

originally conceived, was based on differences in the cellular kinetics and natural history of these lesions. Vascular tumors demonstrate endothelial cell hyperplasia, and the most common of these in children, hemangioma of infancy, spontaneously involutes. In contrast, malformations, such as port-wine stains, have flattened endothelial cells with normal endothelial cell turnover and do not involute spontaneously.

Although there are uncommon examples of either clinical or histologic coexistence of vascular malformations and tumors (Fig. 20.1),[3] this classification has stood the test of time, because of its simplicity and clinical relevance. Most of the entities discussed in this chapter are congenital or arise during infancy; however, some are acquired later in life. During the 1990s, there were exciting new developments in our understanding of angiogenesis, in the appreciation of new clinical associations, and in our therapeutic armamentarium for treating vascular anomalies. Despite this expansion of knowledge, the precise etiology of most of these conditions is not yet known.

TABLE 20.1   Examples of clinically significant vascular tumors and malformations occurring in children

Tumors

Hemangioma of infancy

Lobular capillary hemangioma (pyogenic granuloma)

Rapidly involuting congenital hemangioma (RICH)

Non-involuting congenital hemangioma (NICH)

Tufted angioma (angioblastoma of Nakagawa)

Kaposiform hemangioendothelioma

Congenital eccrine angiomatous hamartoma

Spindle-cell hemangioendothelioma

Malformations

Capillary malformation (port-wine stain)

Venous malformation, including blue rubber bleb nevus (Bean) syndrome

Lymphatic malformation (lymphangioma; cystic hygroma)

Arteriovenous malformation (including Bonnet–Dechaume–Blanc, Wyburn–Mason, and Cobb syndromes)

Capillary–lymphatic–venous malformation (most common type seen in limbs with Klippel–Trenaunay syndrome)

Parkes–Weber syndrome (combined malformation with arteriovenous fistulae)

Cutis marmorata telangiectatica congenita

Glomuvenous malformation (glomangioma–venous malformation, including glomus tumor)

Adapted from International Society for the Study of Vascular Anomalies classification

VASCULAR TUMORS

HEMANGIOMAS OF INFANCY

Hemangiomas of infancy are the most common benign tumors in children and have a distinctive life-cycle, characterized by a proliferative phase in early infancy followed by an involutional phase, leading to complete, spontaneous regression in most patients. A wide variety of vascular anomalies are referred to as "hemangiomas" in the medical literature, so it is preferable to distinguish the specific vascular anomaly being discussed with adjectives and modifiers, i.e., "hemangioma of infancy." For the purposes of this chapter, however, the term hemangioma, unless otherwise

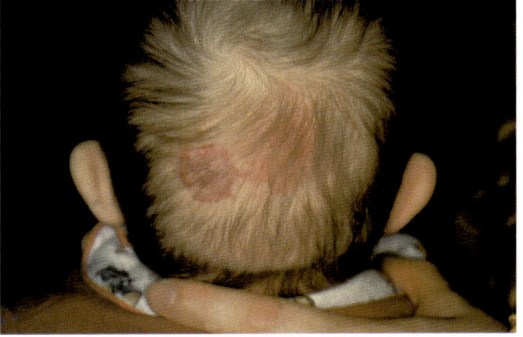

Fig. 20.1 Salmon patch. Coexistence of a salmon patch (nevus simplex) and a hemangioma of infancy on the scalp of this young infant.

1. Mulliken JB, Glowacki J (1982) Hemangiomas and vascular malformations in infants and children. A classification based on endothelial characteristics. **Plast Reconstr Surg** 69:412–422.

2. Enjolras O, Mulliken JB (1997) Vascular tumors and vascular malformations, new issues. **Adv Dermatol** 13:375–423.

3. Garzon MC, Enjolras O, Frieden IJ (2000) Vascular tumors and vascular malformations: evidence for an association. **J Am Acad Dermatol** 42:275–279.

designated, refers specifically to "hemangioma of infancy." Several excellent review articles on vascular anomalies including hemangiomas of infancy have been written.[4–8]

These common vascular tumors occur in approximately 2.5% of all neonates and are seen in up to 5 to 10% of Caucasian infants by 1 year of age. Although hemangiomas appear to be most common in fair-skinned infants, they can occur in any race. Girls are affected three times as often as boys, but the reason for this gender difference remains unclear.[9] It is estimated that 10% of patients have a history of affected family members; however, this feature may be under-reported. Although monozygotic twins do not show consistent concordance nor is there an obvious Mendelian pattern of inheritance in most families, rare families do show an autosomal dominant inheritance pattern for hemangiomas and other vascular anomalies, with a putative localization to 5q.[10] Hemangiomas are also more common in preterm infants weighing less than 1500g, and in infants whose mothers have undergone chorionic villus sampling.[11,12]

Etiology/pathogenesis

Although the precise events leading to the formation of hemangiomas are not known, research in angiogenesis and blood vessel development have provided some clues. During their proliferative phase, hemangiomas are composed of densely packed endothelial cells, forming small sinusoidal channels. Cellular markers of angiogenesis, such as basic fibroblast growth factor, vascular endothelial growth factor (VEGF), proliferating-cell nuclear antigen, and E-selectin, are increased. Immunohistochemical stains confirm blood vessel markers such as CD31 von Willebrand factor and VE-cadherin. Additional studies have shown that hemangiomas of infancy have a unique vascular phenotype which most closely resembles that of placental microvasculature, rather than ordinary cutaneous vasculature, demonstrated by staining markers such as glucose transporter 1 (GLUT-1), merosin, and Lewis Y antigen.[13] Other studies have demonstrated that hemangioma cells cultured *in vitro* behave more like fetal than neonatal endothelial cells, including more readily attaining a spindle-shaped rather than epithelioid morphology, lower levels of expression of platelet–endothelial cell adhesion molecule-1 and von Willebrand factor, and production of interstitial type I collagen rather than epithelium-specific type IV collagen.[14] Clonality has been demonstrated in at least some hemangiomas.[15] Taken together, these observations have led some authors to propose that hemangiomas of infancy represent either placentally derived vasculature or, at the very least, immature vasculature expressing a placental phenotype.[13] In this paradigm, the rapid proliferation of a hemangioma developing in early infancy could be explained by a loss of inhibitors of angiogenesis derived from the placenta or mother. GLUT-1 is present in all phases of hemangiomas. Regression causes histologic changes in hemangiomas with dilatation of vascular lumina, flattening of endothelial cells, and the presence of fibrous tissue. Programmed cell death, also known as apoptosis, is believed to be the mechanism of hemangioma involution. Markers of apoptosis become evident before 1 year of age and reach highest levels by 2 years of age.[16]

Clinical characteristics

Approximately 30 to 50% of hemangiomas are heralded by a premonitory mark, or so-called **precursor lesion**. The varied appearances of precursor lesions include a focal or large area of pallor, often with fine thread-like telangiectases (Fig. 20.2A), a telangiectatic or macular erythematous stain (Fig. 20.2B), a bruise-like area (often erroneously attributed to perinatal

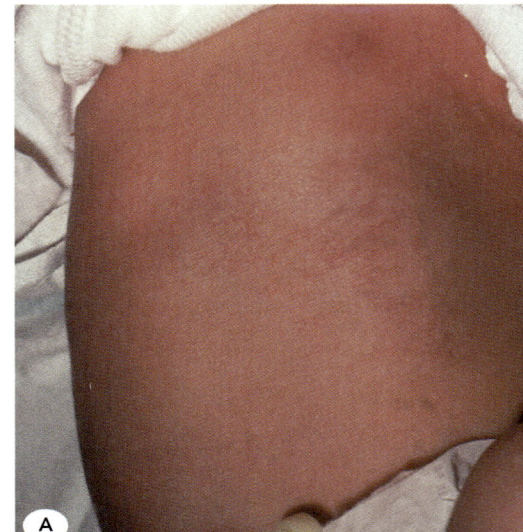
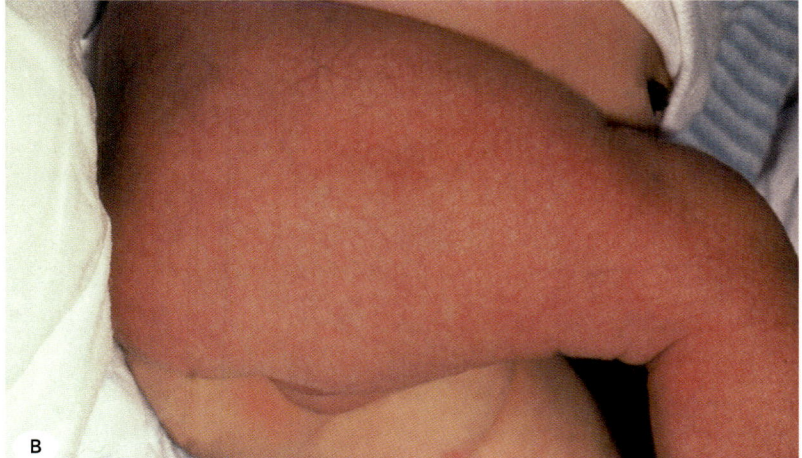
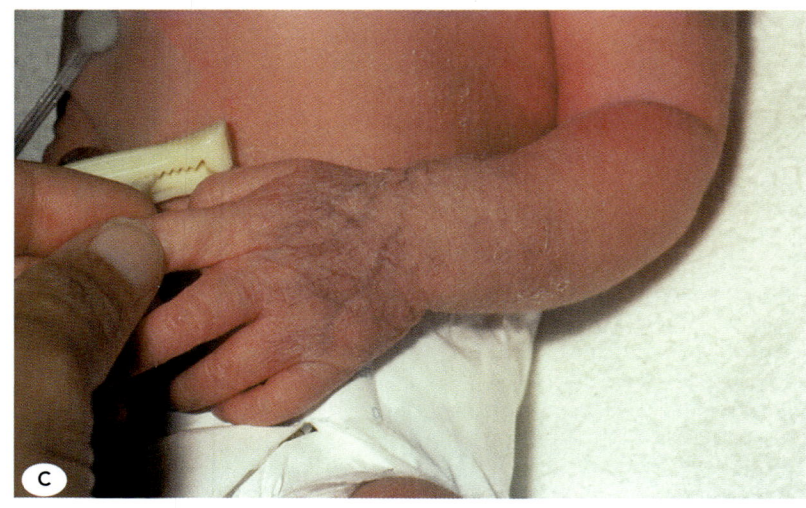

Fig. 20.2 **Hemangioma precursors.** (A) Area of blanching with superimposed telangiectasias. (B) Extensive stain and telangiectasias resembling a port-wine stain. (C) Bruise-like area.

4. Metry DW, Hebert AA (2000) Benign cutaneous vascular tumors of infancy: when to worry, what to do. **Arch Dermatol** 136:905–914.
5. Garzon MC, Frieden IJ (2000) Hemangiomas: when to worry. **Pediatr Ann** 29:58–67.
6. Drolet BA, Esterly NB, Frieden IJ (1999) Hemangiomas in children. **N Engl J Med** 341:173–181.
7. Esterly NB (1995) Cutaneous hemangiomas, vascular stains and malformations, and associated syndromes. **Probl Dermatol** 7:67–108.
8. Mulliken JB, Fishman SJ, Burrows PE (2000) Vascular anomalies. **Curr Probl Surg** 37:519–584.
9. Mulliken JB, Young AE (1988) Vascular Birthmarks: Hemangiomas and Malformations. Philadelphia, PA: WB Saunders.
10. Berg JN, Walter JW, Thisanagayam U et al. (2001) Evidence for loss of heterozygosity of 5q in sporadic haemangiomas: are somatic mutations involved in haemangioma formation? **J Clin Pathol** 54:249–252.
11. Powell TG, West CR, Pharoah PO et al. (1987) Epidemiology of strawberry haemangioma in low birthweight infants. **Br J Dermatol** 116:635–641.
12. Burton BK, Schulz CJ, Angle B et al. (1995) An increased incidence of haemangiomas in infants born following chorionic villus sampling (CVS). **Prenat Diagn** 15:209–214.
13. North PE, Waner M, Mizeracki A et al. (2001) A unique microvascular phenotype shared by juvenile hemangiomas and human placenta. **Arch Dermatol** 137:559–570.
14. Dosanjh A, Chang J, Bresnick S et al. (2000) In vitro characteristics of neonatal hemangioma endothelial cells: similarities and differences between normal neonatal and fetal endothelial cells. **J Cutan Pathol** 27:441–450.
15. Boye E, Yu Y, Paranya G et al. (2001) Clonality and altered behavior of endothelial cells from hemangiomas. **J Clin Invest** 107:745–752.
16. Razon MJ, Kraling BM, Mulliken JB et al. (1998) Increased apoptosis coincides with onset of involution in infantile hemangioma. **Microcirculation** 5:189–195.

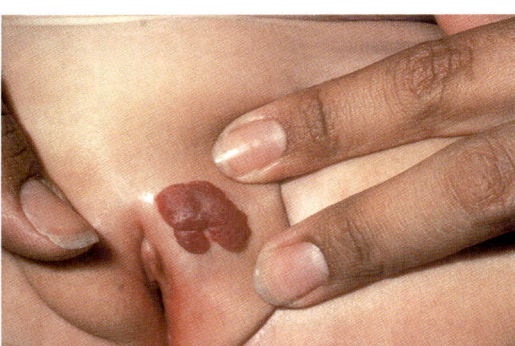

Fig. 20.3 Superficial hemangioma of infancy. Note the resemblance to an upside-down strawberry.

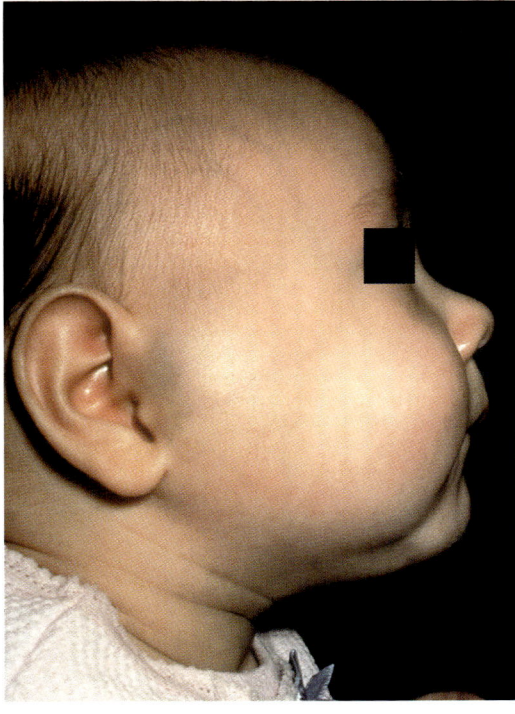

Fig. 20.4 Deep hemangioma. Many deep hemangiomas in the preauricular area involve the parotid gland.

should be avoided since it has been used to refer to several disparate vascular anomalies, rather than one single disease. Superficial and deep hemangiomas are also referred to as "mixed hemangiomas." They involve both the dermis and subcutis and demonstrate clinical features of both the types described above. All hemangiomas of infancy, regardless of their location, are benign neoplasms of capillaries; terms such as combined capillary–cavernous hemangiomas, which imply otherwise, are confusing and should be avoided.[9]

Hemangiomas are rarely painful, unless they have ulcerated. Many, especially large ones, are warm to palpation and occasionally have enough blood flow to produce a bruit. This warmth and high blood flow subsides as the tumor begins to undergo involution. Although rapid growth is a common characteristic during the proliferative phase, some fluctuation of size may be observed even once the tumor growth has ceased; consequently, some parents report a temporary increase in size after the child has a crying episode or an upper respiratory infection.

Specific morphologic patterns of hemangiomas can be recognized, and their clinical implications are now beginning to be appreciated. In addition to marked variations in size and location, some present as discrete papules or nodules whereas others are small or large plaques. Some plaque-type hemangiomas appear as numerous small papules coalescing into a plaque of involvement. Larger plaques may involve broader segments of the skin. The concept of *localized* (Fig. 20.5) and *segmental* (Fig. 20.6) hemangiomas has demonstrable clinical correlates. Large segmental hemangiomas have been associated with structural anomalies, such as Dandy–Walker malformation, arterial anomalies, spinal cord tethering, genitourinary anomalies, as well as subglottic hemangiomas (see discussion below). Large preauricular segmental hemangiomas often have an associated hemangioma within the parotid gland but do not compromise facial nerve function. Based on the known timing of some of their associated structural defects, segmental hemangiomas appear to have their origin as early as 6 to 8 weeks of gestation.[20] Multiple focal hemangiomas have a higher risk of visceral hemangiomas (Fig. 20.7) (see "hemangiomatosis" below). Most hemangiomas are solitary, but a significant percentage of patients (up to 15%) have multiple lesions.

Sites of involvement

Anatomic location plays a critical role in determining whether complications could occur, and if extra concern and vigilance during the growth phase is necessary. Although any area of the body may be affected, approximately 60% occur on the head and neck. Moreover, the distribution of facial hemangiomas does not seem to be random but appears to have a predilection for embryologic fusion lines and facial developmental subunits.[21] Less common anatomic sites include the trunk (25%) and extremities (15%).[7] Hemangiomas can also develop in almost any internal organ. Table 20.2 outlines the risks associated with hemangiomas in several anatomic locations.

Natural history

The natural history of hemangiomas has been well documented.[9,22,23] During the first 6 months, particularly in the first 3 to 4 months, superficial hemangiomas proliferate at a rapid rate. Between 6 and 10 months of age, the lesion may continue to grow, albeit often at a slower rate, usually reaching a maximum size by 9 to 12 months. Despite this generalization, the growth characteristics of a hemangioma in an individual infant are extremely difficult to predict, because some hemangiomas barely proliferate beyond their nascent phase whereas others, particularly large hemangiomas with both a superficial and deep component, continue to grow for longer than expected, occasionally up to 1–2 years.[24,25] Deep hemangiomas are often noted somewhat later than superficial lesions and may also proliferate for somewhat longer periods of time.

trauma) (Fig. 20.2C), or a small "scratch" or ulceration.[17] Most precursor lesions go on to develop fully, but occasionally only a small amount of proliferation occurs at the periphery. Uncommonly, fully formed hemangiomas are present at the time of birth; in rare instances, these are diagnosed *in utero*. These have a different clinical appearance, involute very rapidly, and, recently, their relationship to hemangioma of infancy has been questioned.[18,19] (See the discussion below.)

The appearance of the proliferative phase of cutaneous hemangiomas depends on which level(s) of the skin are affected. **Superficial hemangiomas** (Fig. 20.3) (also called "strawberry" marks) involve the superficial dermis and appear as lobulated, bright red lesions with a thin, delicate surface epithelium. **Deep hemangiomas** (Fig. 20.4) involve the deep dermis and subcutis. In these cases, the epidermis retains its normal thickness and, instead of a superficial red color, the surface of the tumor has a bluish cast or normal skin color. Telangiectases, tortuous vessels, or a few vascular papules may be visible on the surface, and draining veins are noted at the periphery. Deep hemangiomas were formerly called "cavernous hemangiomas," a term that

17. Hidano A, Nakajima S (1972) Earliest features of the strawberry mark in the newborn. **Br J Dermatol** 87:138–144.
18. Boon LM, Enjolras O, Mulliken JB (1996) Congenital hemangioma: evidence of accelerated involution. **J Pediatr** 128:329–335.
19. North PE, Waner M, James CA et al. (2001) Congenital non-progressive hemangioma. A distinct clinicopathologic entity unlike infantile hemangioma. **Arch Dermatol** 137:1607–1620.
20. Hersh JH, Waterfill D, Rutledge J et al. (1985) Sternal malformation/vascular dysplasia association. **Am J Med Genet** 21:177–186, 201–202.
21. Waner M, Waner A, North P et al. (2000) Identification of two distinct types of hemangioma. In: 13th International Workshop on Vascular Anomalies, Montreal, 2000.
22. Jacobs AH (1957) Strawberry hemangiomas. The natural history of the untreated lesion. **Cal Med** 86:8–10.
23. Bivings L (1954) Spontaneous regression of angiomas in children. **J Pediatr** 45:643–647.
24. Blei F, Isakoff M, Deb G (1997) The response of parotid hemangiomas to the use of systemic interferon alfa-2a or corticosteroids. **Arch Otolaryngol Head Neck Surg** 123:841–844.
25. Williams EF, III, Stanislaw P, Dupree M et al. (2000) Hemangiomas in infants and children. An algorithm for intervention. **Arch Facial Plast Surg** 2:103–111.

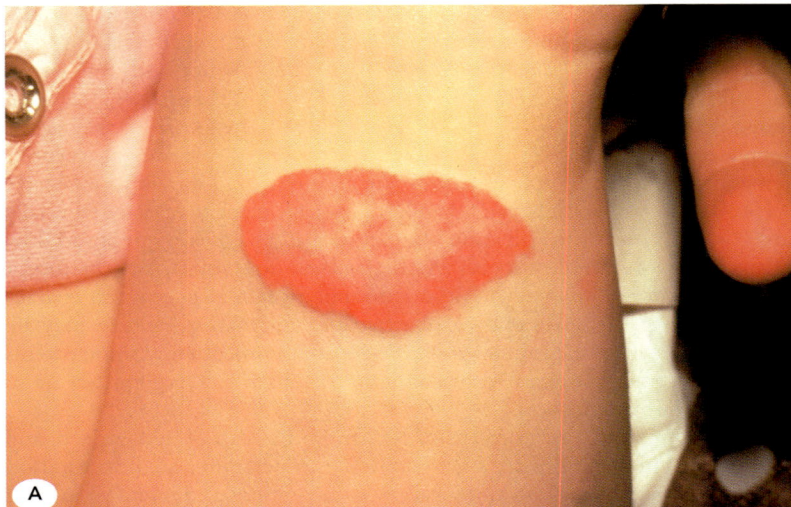

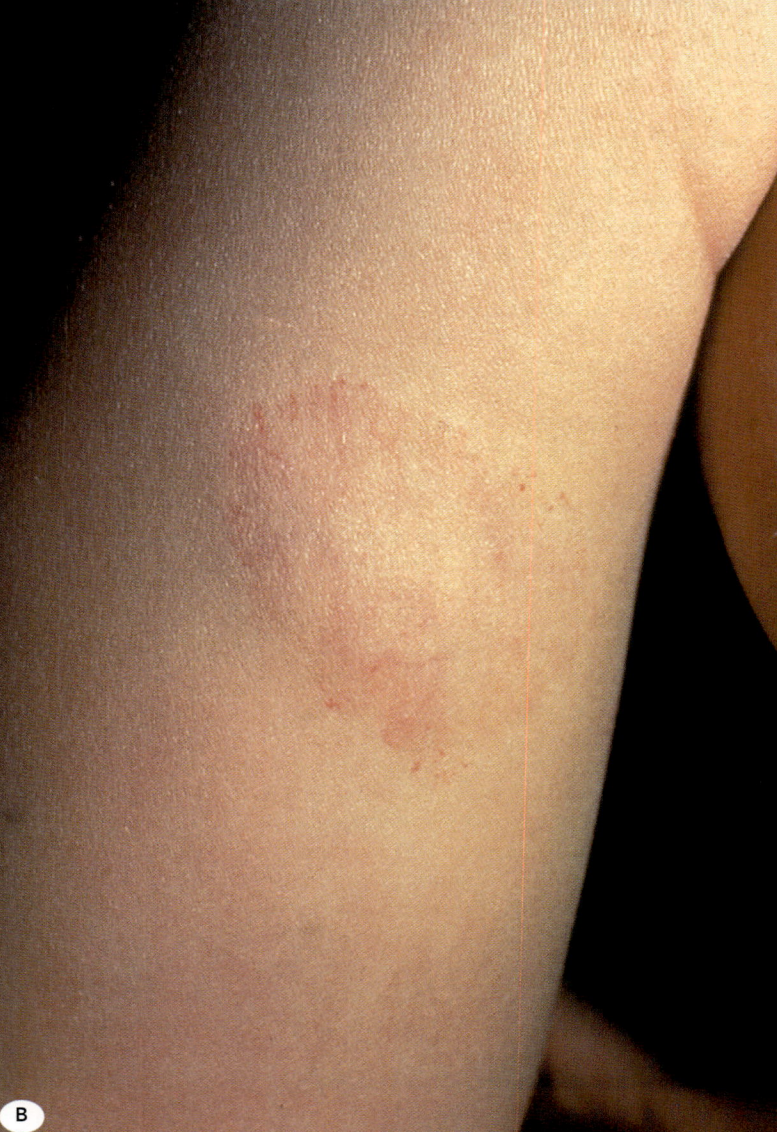

Fig. 20.5 Localized hemangioma. (A) Appearance at 11 months of age. (B) Appearance after spontaneous involution at 2.5 years of age.

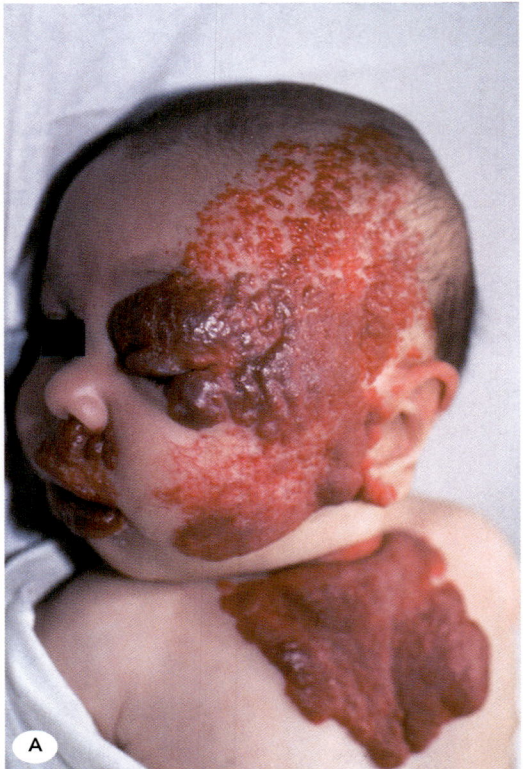

Fig. 20.6 Segmental hemangioma. This hemangioma was extensive (A) and required several modalities of treatment, including prednisolone (which was unsuccessful) and then interferon alfa (which was very effective). The final result at 5 years of age (B), after surgical correction of the eyelid and lip as well as Erbium laser resurfacing was good.

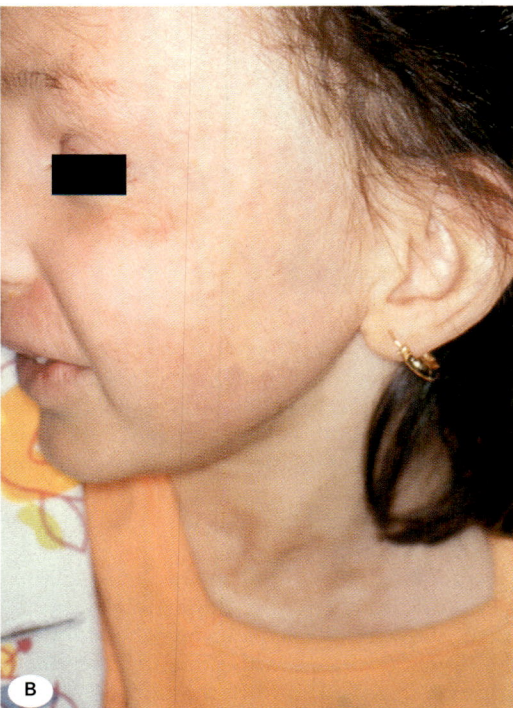

The involution phase of hemangiomas is usually much slower than the proliferation phase. Involution of superficial lesions typically begins by about 1 year of age, occasionally sooner, and its onset is heralded by a color change from bright cherry red to dull red-purple, beginning at the central portion of the tumor and eventually developing a grayish-white color that extends peripherally (Fig. 20.8). In some cases, hemangioma growth actually continues at the margins of the lesion or in deeper components despite signs of

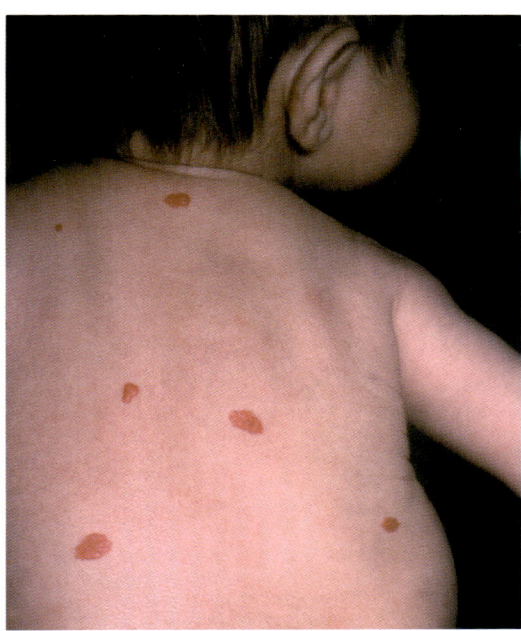

Fig. 20.7 **Multiple disseminated hemangiomas.** These may be associated with visceral involvement, particularly hepatic hemangiomas.

TABLE 20.2 Location and morphology of hemangioma of infancy and associated risks

Anatomic location, morphology	Associated risk
Large segmental facial	PHACE syndrome (see text)
Nasal tip, ear, large facial (especially with prominent dermal component)	Permanent scarring and disfigurement
Periorbital and retrobulbar	Ocular axis occlusion, astigmatism, amblyopia, tear-duct occlusion
Segmental "beard area" and central neck	Airway hemangioma
Perioral, lips	Ulceration, disfigurement
Lumbosacral spine	Tethered spinal cord, genitourinary anomalies
Perianal, axilla, neck	Ulceration
Multiple hemangiomas	Visceral involvement (especially liver, gastrointestinal tract) with high risk of congestive heart failure

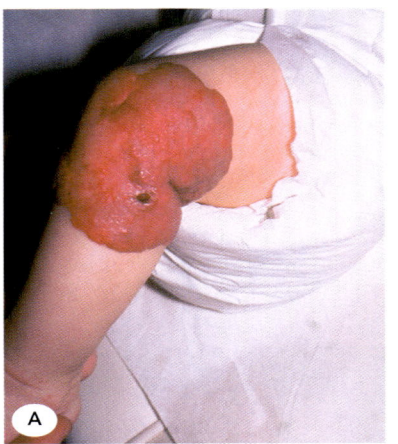
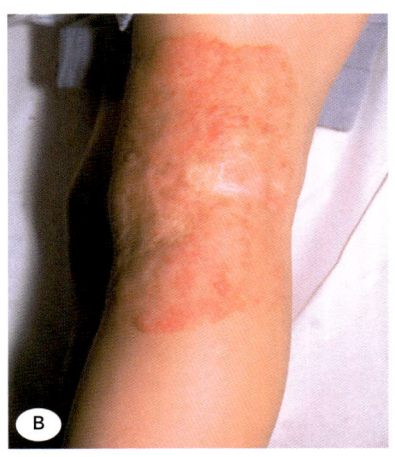
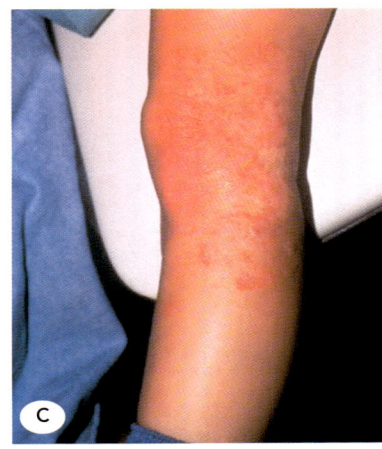

Fig. 20.8 **Plaque-type hemangioma.** Natural involution of a large plaque-type hemangioma of the leg at ages 2 (**A**), 4 (**B**), and 5 (**C**) years. Although some pigmentary and texture remains, the overall result is satisfactory.

regression in the superficial central portions of the hemangioma. As the hemangioma involutes and is replaced by fibrofatty tissue, its volume decreases and it becomes softer and more easily compressible. Similarly, deeper lesions become less blue, softer, and less warm.

Disappearance occurs at a rate of approximately 10% per year, so that approximately 50% have involuted by 5 years of age, 70% by 7 years, and 90% by 9 years.[22,26] Involution, however, should not necessarily be equated with resolution with completely normal skin. Exact estimates of the percentage of hemangiomas that leave significant residual skin changes is a matter of great controversy, with estimates varying widely, from less than 20% to 50%.[8,27] Even when present, the residua in mild cases can be fairly inconspicuous, characterized by focal telangiectases, atrophic wrinkling, slight hypopigmentation, and subtle textural changes. In more severe cases, anetoderma-like scarring or fibrofatty swelling with marked distortion of anatomic structures may be evident. Most small hemangiomas do not result in significant disfigurement, but in certain locations such as the glabella, nose, lips, and ears, the risk of scarring is greater. Large facial hemangiomas, particularly those with a significant superficial dermal component, also have an increased risk of scarring (Fig. 20.9). Ulceration always causes some degree of scarring, with

the severity depending on the size and depth of the antecedent ulcer as well as other prognostic factors such as the location and thickness of the hemangioma itself.[5]

Diagnosis and differential diagnosis

In most cases, the diagnosis of hemangioma is a clinical one, based on appearance and typical growth characteristics. In a small minority of patients, diagnosis is less obvious and ancillary tests are necessary. Deep hemangiomas, in particular, can be difficult to differentiate from other soft-tissue tumors. Table 20.3 lists some of the diagnoses that can resemble hemangioma of infancy. Imaging studies such as magnetic resonance (MR), computed tomography (CT), and ultrasound can be helpful in differentiating hemangiomas from many of these conditions, but biopsy may be necessary in very atypical cases. In the proliferative phase, CT and MR both demonstrate well-circumscribed densely lobulated uniformly enhancing lesions with dilated feeding and draining vessels either at the center or periphery. On MR, the lesions are isointense or hypointense to muscle on T_1-weighted images, and hyperintense on T_2-weighted images. Flow voids are seen within and around the mass. Sonography with Doppler interrogation usually demonstrates a

26. Bowers RE, Graham EA, Tomlinson KM (1960) The natural history of the strawberry nevus. **Arch Dermatol** 82:667–680.

27. Waner M, Suen JY (1999) Hemangiomas and vascular malformations of the head and neck. In: The Natural History of Hemangiomas, Waner M, Suen JY, eds. New York: Wiley-Liss, pp. 13–46.

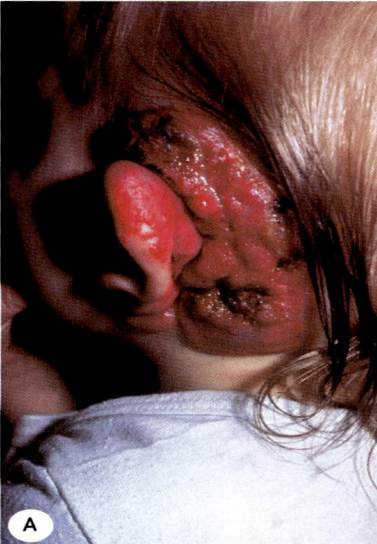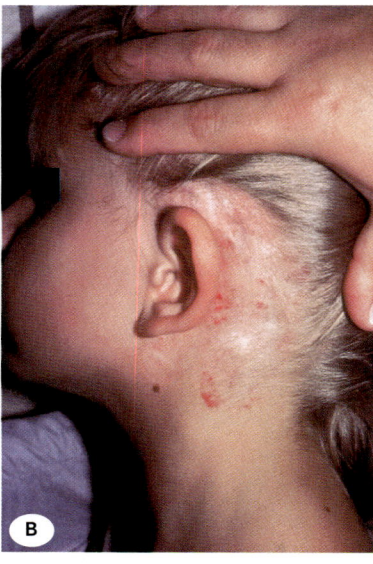

Fig. 20.9 **Large postauricular hemangioma.** The hemangioma is shown at 1 (**A**) and 6 (**B**) years of age. No treatment was given; because the scar is in the postauricular area, it is inconspicuous. In another site (such as the central face) the resultant scar might be much more disfiguring.

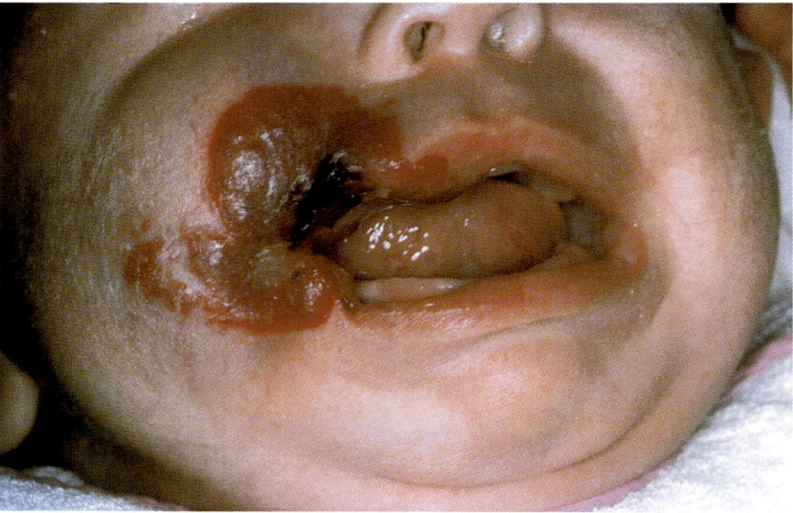

Fig. 20.10 **Ulcerated hemangioma involving the oral commisure.** Pain is a major problem with ulcerations, particularly those in perioral and perianal sites, which are very common locations for ulceration.

TABLE 20.3 Differential diagnoses of hemangioma of infancy
Other vascular anomalies and tumors
capillary malformations
venous malformations
lymphatic malformations
arteriovenous malformations
noninvoluting congenital hemangioma
nonprogressive congenital hemangioma
rapidly involuting hemangioma
lobular capillary hemangioma (pyogenic granuloma)
tufted angioma
spindle cell hemangioendothelioma
Kaposiform hemangioendothelioma
Fibrosarcoma
Rhabdomyosarcoma
Myofibromatosis (including hemangiopericytoma)
Nasal glioma
Lipoblastoma
Dermatofibrosarcoma protuberans (and giant-cell fibroblastoma)
Neurofibroma

well-circumscribed parenchymal mass, often containing anechoic channels.[28] Although true arteriovenous shunting is usually absent (except in hepatic hemangiomas), hemangiomas are fast-flow lesions with numerous high-flow vessels around and within the soft tissue mass; decreased arterial resistance is evident during both the proliferating and the involuting phases.[29] During the proliferative phase, ultrasound demonstrates nonspecific echogenicity and numerous vessels with high Doppler shift (>2kHz) and low resistance.[30]

The histopathology of hemangioma of infancy in the early proliferative phase is characterized by well-defined unencapsulated aggregates of plump endothelial cells with closely associated pericytes. Granulated mast cells are numerous. Normal mitotic figures are often present and may be numerous. Deeper hemangiomas may involve skeletal muscle, salivary gland tissue, and even nerves, not by aggressive invasion but by insinuating themselves between individual cells. When hemangiomas begin to involute, proliferating vessels decrease in number and loose fibrous or fibrofatty tissue begins to separate the vessels.[31] As mentioned above, GLUT-1 is found at all phases in hemangiomas of infancy and can be extremely helpful in their differentiation from other vascular tumors.[13]

Complications

Most complications of hemangiomas of infancy develop during the first 6 months, when growth is most rapid. These complications include ulceration, bleeding, infection, compromise of vital functions, and, in rare instances, congestive heart failure. Cutaneous ulceration is the most common complication, occurring in 5 to 10% (Fig. 20.10). Rarely it may actually precede the development of a hemangioma.[32] If ulceration is mild in degree, it can often be managed with topical therapies, including antibiotics such as metronidazole gel[33] or polymyxin/bacitracin ointment, and covered with an occlusive dressing such as a thin hydrocolloid dressing or petrolatum-impregnated gauze.[33] Pain, which is often a major feature of ulcerated hemangiomas, is usually diminished with the use of occlusive dressings; if the pain is severe, it can be helped by the oral administration of acetaminophen (paracetamol) or acetaminophen with codeine.[33] Flashlamp pumped pulsed dye laser (PDL) can also be helpful in relieving the pain of ulcerated hemangiomas.[34]

28. Paltiel HJ, Burrows PE, Kozakewich HP et al. (2000) Soft-tissue vascular anomalies: utility of US for diagnosis. **Radiology** 214:747–754.
29. Burrows PE, Laor T, Paltiel H et al. (1998) Diagnostic imaging in the evaluation of vascular birthmarks. **Dermatol Clin** 16:455–488.
30. Dubois J, Garel L, Grignon A et al. (1998) Imaging of hemangiomas and vascular malformations in children. **Acad Radiol** 5:390–400.
31. North PE, Mihm MC (1999) The surgical pathology approach to pediatric vascular tumors and anomalies. In: Hemangiomas and Vascular Malformations of the Head and Neck, Waner M, Suen JY, eds. New York: Wiley-Liss, pp. 93–170.
32. Liang MG, Frieden IJ (1997) Perineal and lip ulcerations as the presenting manifestation of hemangioma of infancy. **Pediatrics** 99:256–259.
33. Kim HJ, Colombo M, Frieden IJ (2001) Ulcerated hemangiomas: clinical characteristics and response to therapy. **J Am Acad Dermatol** 44:962–972.
34. Morelli JG, Tan OT, Yohn JJ et al. (1994) Treatment of ulcerated hemangiomas of infancy. **Arch Pediatr Adolesc Med** 148:1104–1105.

SIGNIFICANT BLEEDING

Significant bleeding is a very uncommon complication of hemangiomas. When it does occur, it is virtually always as a sequela of deep ulceration or in scalp lesions. In most cases, local pressure is usually sufficient to control bleeding. In difficult situations, powdered gel-foam or topical thrombin may be used. In recurrent bleeding, an enuresis blanket can be useful, triggering an alarm if bleeding develops during the night. Infection can occur in ulcerated hemangiomas but has probably been overdiagnosed in the past. If infection is suspected, a bacterial culture should be obtained and the patient's antibiotic regimen should be chosen for the organism(s) recovered. Sepsis complicating infected hemangiomas has rarely been reported.[35]

AMBLYOPIA

Amblyopia is a complication of **periocular hemangiomas**. Closure of the eye can lead to occlusion of the visual axis, which will prevent light stimulation and result in loss of vision (amblyopia). However, even if the hemangioma does not completely occlude the eye, the presence of the mass in the periorbital area can cause pressure on the globe and result in astigmatism, which, if uncorrected, can lead to amblyopia. The risk of pressure on the orbit is somewhat greater but not limited to hemangiomas with upper lid involvement. Retro-orbital hemangiomas may cause proptosis.[36] Infants with periocular hemangiomas should have frequent eye examinations during the first few months of life, when most rapid growth is likely to occur.

HEMANGIOMAS OF THE AIRWAY

Hemangiomas of the airway, which are usually subglottic in location, may occur either with or without cutaneous hemangiomas. Large segmental hemangiomas involving the mandibular area and neck have a risk as high as 60% of associated airway hemangiomas, and infants with this anatomic distribution should be followed extremely closely, particularly during the first 12 to 16 weeks of life.[37] These hemangiomas often present with "noisy breathing" or biphasic stridor. Airway involvement can be life threatening; if symptoms are present, direct endoscopic visualization of the airway should be performed. Prompt medical and/or surgical intervention is necessary if symptomatic airway hemangioma is present.[38] Temporary tracheostomy may be necessary to manage rapidly growing airway hemangiomas.

DIFFUSE NEONATAL HEMANGIOMATOSIS

Diffuse neonatal hemangiomatosis is a rare form of hemangioma characterized by multiple cutaneous hemangiomas with visceral involvement. Although some infants with visceral hemangiomatosis have no cutaneous involvement, most have multiple small, cherry-red superficial hemangiomas that are present at birth or develop during the first few weeks of life (Fig. 20.7).[39] An innocuous variant, the so-called **benign neonatal hemangiomatosis,** has identical cutaneous hemangiomas without visceral involvement.[40] The distinction between the two can only be made after careful serial examinations and appropriate investigations (see below). In contrast to other hemangiomas, the hemangiomas in neonatal hemangiomatosis often involute by 2 years of age.

EXTRACUTANEOUS COMPLICATIONS

The most common extracutaneous site of involvement is the liver. Liver hemangiomas are sometimes referred to as hemangioendotheliomas, although the reason for this distinction appears to be based less on true histologic differences than on historical nomenclature. Hepatic hemangiomas can be entirely asymptomatic, but they often lead to hepatomegaly, high-output congestive heart failure, anemia, and, occasionally, thrombocytopenia. Although some authors have defined **diffuse neonatal hemangiomatosis** as occurring in those who have three or more organ systems involved, a more rational approach is to recognize that these infants represent a continuum along a disease spectrum, with tremendous variability. Therefore, thorough evaluation and close follow-up rather than numerical assignation of the absolute number of organ systems involved is central in patient management. After the liver, the most commonly involved organs are the lungs, gastrointestinal tract, and central nervous system (CNS). Complications include hemorrhage, seizures, biliary obstruction with jaundice, and respiratory tract obstruction. Mortality rates in widely disseminated hemangiomatosis are high, reportedly as high as 95%, but a recent review of hepatic hemangiomatosis found a mortality rate of approximately 20% using more current modalities of treatment.[41] Most infants who die from disseminated hemangiomatosis do so because of high-output cardiac failure; however, some have succumbed to CNS or pulmonary complications.[42,43]

Because of the serious consequences of visceral involvement, early diagnostic studies are essential in young infants with multiple (five or more) hemangiomas. Hepatic ultrasound should be performed in all such infants. Other studies should include a complete blood count with platelet count, fibrinogen level, urinalysis, liver function tests (if hepatic involvement is found), and stool examination for blood. Electrocardiogram and chest X-ray should be performed in patients with signs of congestive heart failure. Liver and spleen scans, MR imaging or ultrasonography of the head, ophthalmologic examination, angiography, and gastrointestinal series or endoscopy should be carried out if clinically indicated.[44] Occasionally, asymptomatic small hepatic lesions are detected with imaging studies, and in some cases these hemangiomas will remain small without causing organ dysfunction. Such infants always require close follow-up; while there are no clear guidelines for managing this situation, decision making about whether to treat will depend on evaluating the extent of disease and looking for more subtle signs of organ dysfunction. For example, hepatic hemangio-mas may cause increased hepatic arterial and venous flow (detectable by ultrasound) or cardiomegaly and tachycardia before frank congestive heart failure is evident. In this case, therapy should be initiated as soon as possible.

If symptomatic visceral involvement is present, early aggressive therapy is indicated. Systemic corticosteroids (prednisone 2 to 4mg/kg daily) have been helpful in some patients, with digoxin and diuretics added when indicated for congestive heart failure.[41] The response rate of hepatic hemangiomas to systemic corticosteroids seems to be lower than for cutaneous hemangiomas.[41] Other therapies such as interferon alfa in doses of 3×10^6 IU/m^2 per day or vincristine (standard dosage not established but generally in the range 1–1.5mg/m^2 or 0.05 to 0.65mg/kg intravenously weekly[45] may be helpful if corticosteroid therapy is not effective. When these measures fail to control liver disease, partial hepatectomy, or hepatic artery ligation or embolization, may also be helpful.[44] Liver transplantation has also been used in severe conditions that are unresponsive to other modalities of treatment.[46]

ASSOCIATION WITH HYPOTHYROIDISM

Severe hypothyroidism is a potential complication of hepatic hemangiomatosis and, possibly, hemangiomas in other sites. The mechanism is believed to be tumoral production of type 3 iodothyronine deiodinase, causing peripheral

35. Yagupsky P, Giladi Y (1987) Group A beta-hemolytic streptococcal septicemia complicating infected hemangioma in children. **Pediatr Dermatol** 4:24–26.
36. Haik BG, Karcioglu ZA, Gordon RA et al. (1994) Capillary hemangioma (infantile periocular hemangioma). **Surv Ophthalmol** 38:399–426.
37. Orlow SJ, Isakoff MS, Blei F (1997) Increased risk of symptomatic hemangiomas of the airway in association with cutaneous hemangiomas in a "beard" distribution. **J Pediatr** 131:643–646.
38. Sie KC, Tampakopoulou DA (2000) Hemangiomas and vascular malformations of the airway. **Otolaryngol Clin North Am** 33:209–220.
39. Blei F, Orlow SJ, Geronemus R (1997) Multimodal management of diffuse neonatal hemangiomatosis. **J Am Acad Dermatol** 37:1019–1021.
40. Held JL, Haber RS, Silvers DN et al. (1990) Benign neonatal hemangiomatosis: review and description of a patient with unusually persistent lesions. **Pediatr Dermatol** 7:63–66.

41. Boon LM, Burrows PE, Paltiel HJ et al. (1996) Hepatic vascular anomalies in infancy: a twenty-seven-year experience. **J Pediatr** 129:346–354.
42. Holden KR, Alexander F (1970) Diffuse neonatal hemangiomatosis. **Pediatrics** 46:411–421.
43. Keller L, Bluhm JF, III (1979) Diffuse neonatal hemangiomatosis. A case with heart failure and thrombocytopenia. **Cutis** 23:295–297.
44. Pereyra R, Andrassy RJ, Mahour GH (1982) Management of massive hepatic hemangiomas in infants and children: a review of 13 cases. **Pediatrics** 70:254–258.
45. Moore J, Lee M, Garzon M et al. (2001) Effective therapy of a vascular tumor of infancy with vincristine. **Pediatr Surg** 36:1273–1276.
46. Daller JA, Bueno J, Gutierrez J et al. (1999) Hepatic hemangioendothelioma: clinical experience and management strategy. **J Pediatr Surg** 34:98–105.

inactivation of thyroid hormone.[47] A lingual thryoid, which can lead to hypothyroidism, has also been reported in hemangiomas in association with PHACE (*posterior fossa, hemangioma, arterial anomalies, cardiac defects and coarctation of the aorta, and eye*) syndrome.[48] Although the incidence of hypothyroidism in association with hemangiomas is unknown, some authors recommend performing thyroid function studies (including thyroid-stimulating hormone) in all infants with hepatic and large cutaneous hemangiomas.[47]

Association of hemangiomas with structural malformations

Although most hemangiomas occur without associated anomalies, at least two well-defined hemangioma–malformation complexes have been described. PHACE syndrome describes the association of large segmental hemangiomas with a variety of structural anomalies.[47,48] Affected patients (nearly always girls) usually have one or two of the associated features rather than all components.[49] In the past, PHACE syndrome has sometimes been confused with Sturge–Weber syndrome (SWS), but careful examination reveals more differences than similarities (Table 20.4). In a small number of patients, the neurovascular abnormalities have led to progressive neurologic deterioration.[50]

Patients with large segmental facial hemangiomas should be examined thoroughly for signs and symptoms of PHACE syndrome, including a careful cardiac evaluation, cardiac ultrasound and/or measurement of blood pressure in all four extremities (to exclude coarctation of the aorta), and careful periodic developmental and neurologic assessments. If any neurologic symptoms arise, patients should have MR imaging and angiography of the brain and cranial circulation. In neurologically asymptomatic individuals, recommendations for imaging are less straightforward, but cranial MR imaging and angiography should probably be performed at some point to determine whether aneurysms or other potentially worrisome arterial anomalies are present.[49]

A second constellation of structural malformations is seen in association with hemangiomas overlying the lumbosacral spine (with or without a segmental hemangioma of the lower extremity) (Fig. 20.11). The most common malformation in this setting is a tethered spinal cord, often accompanied by an occult lipomeningocele. Genitourinary anomalies, which are less common, include imperforate anus, abnormal external genitalia, and renal anomalies. Infants with a hemangioma overlying the lumbosacral area and those with perianal hemangioma extending into the gluteal cleft should have MR imaging performed to exclude possible tethered cord.[51,52]

TABLE 20.4   Comparative differences between Sturge–Weber and PHACE syndromes

	Sturge–Weber Syndrome	PHACE syndrome
Gender difference; inheritance	M = F; sporadic	F > M; sporadic
Type, character, and distribution of cutaneous lesion; age of presentation	Port-wine stain (nevus flammeus), V1 ± V2 and V3; usually unilateral but can be bilateral; present at birth; occasionally leptomeningeal and eye findings can occur without cutaneous stain	Hemangioma of the face, with segmental distribution, usually plaque-type morphology (rarely nodular); most commonly involves upper face and forehead but can be any segment of face, unilateral or bilateral; appearance within the first month of life usually with precursor lesion present at birth;
Mucocutaneous complications	May have progressive soft tissue and skeletal hypertrophy beneath the malformation; gingival hypertrophy, epulis, macrochelia (if also involves V2 or V3)	Commonly complicated by ulceration and soft-tissue loss, especially if hemangioma involves the nose and/or lip
Ocular abnormalities	Glaucoma (most common; 42%), increased choroidal vascularity, buphthalmos, homonymous hemianopia, retinal detachment	Increased retinal vascularity, microphthalmia, optic nerve hypoplasia, exophthalmos, choroidal hemangiomas, strabismus, colobomas, congenital cataracts, glaucoma (rare)
Central nervous system (CNS) involvement	Vascular anomaly of the pia mater, often with occipital distribution, over the entire hemisphere or localized to temporal or frontal areas; calcification of the temporal and occipital cortex and/or within or beneath abnormal vessels; cerebral atrophy	Posterior fossa malformations (especially of the Dandy–Walker type) most common; also agenesis of the corpus callosum, cerebellar atrophy, and arachnoid cysts; cervicocranial arterial anomalies also common, may be further complicated by aneurysm development
Association of CNS findings to skin changes	Usually ipsilateral, occasionally contralateral, and may be bilateral (in which bilateral CNS involvement is more likely)	Not directly correlated, although "V1" distribution may have somewhat greater risk of CNS disease
Neurologic findings	Seizures usually begin prior to age 2 but may be delayed until later in childhood; mental retardation and hemiplegia are fairly common; CNS involvement may be progressive, with worsening of seizures and deterioration of intellect; migraine headaches are also common	Structural or cerebrovascular anomalies of the brain may manifest as acute neurologic symptoms (severe headaches and/or seizures) or developmental delay; acute neurologic symptoms, which may be delayed in onset, may be a sign of aneurysm formation within the affected vasculature; many patients are neurologically asymptomatic

---

47. Huang SA, Tu HM, Harney JW et al. (2000) Severe hypothyroidism caused by type 3 iodothyronine deiodinase in infantile hemangiomas. **N Engl J Med** 343:185–189.

48. Frieden IJ, Reese V, Cohen D (1996) PHACE syndrome. The association of posterior fossa brain malformations, hemangiomas, arterial anomalies, coarctation of the aorta and cardiac defects, and eye abnormalities. **Arch Dermatol** 132:317–311.

49. Metry DW, Dowd CF, Barkovich AJ et al. (2001) The many faces of PHACE syndrome. **J Pediatr** 139:117–23.

50. Burrows PE, Robertson RL, Mulliken JB et al. (1998) Cerebral vasculopathy and neurologic sequelae in infants with cervicofacial hemangioma: report of eight patients. **Radiology** 207:601–607.

51. Goldberg NS, Hebert AA, Esterly NB (1986) Sacral hemangiomas and multiple congenital abnormalities. **Arch Dermatol** 122:684–687.

52. Albright AL, Gartner JC, Wiener ES (1989) Lumbar cutaneous hemangiomas as indicators of tethered spinal cords. **Pediatrics** 83:977–980.

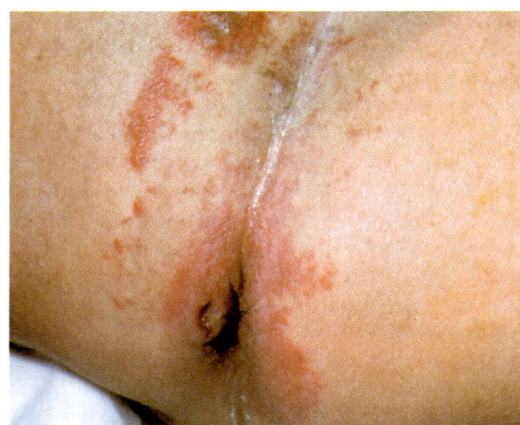

Fig. 20.11 Perianal and lumbosacral hemangioma. This infant had an associated tethered spinal cord.

Management of hemangiomas of infancy

The management of hemangiomas continues to be an area of considerable controversy.[53] Estimates of what percentage of hemangiomas require active treatment and which can be allowed to involute spontaneously without intervention vary widely, at least in part because of ascertainment bias. Hemangiomas are extremely heterogeneous in location, size, and growth characteristics. In the primary care setting, most hemangiomas seen are small and innocuous, and, in many cases, the results of spontaneous involution are superior to those obtained with excisional or laser surgery. For these patients, observation, reassurance, and frequent visits every few weeks during the period of rapid growth are the mainstays of management.[54] Unfortunately, when the hemangioma is in a visible location, families are frequently bombarded with stares, rude comments, accusations of child abuse, and unsolicited advice.[55] The natural history of hemangiomas should be described in detail to the parents, with photographs of other patients (if possible) to illustrate the involutional process. To varying degrees, all families of children with hemangiomas need emotional support and information. For those not receiving a specific treatment, extra support may be needed to bolster the rationale for *not* actively treating, such as photographs and discussions emphasizing that, for some hemangiomas, the final result in an untreated lesion may be superior to that obtained with aggressive therapeutic intervention. A multidisciplinary approach, with dermatologists, surgeons, and other health professionals, may also be helpful.[25]

Even once a decision to treat has been made, the specific treatment(s) used depends on the age of the patient, location and depth of the lesion within the skin (superficial or deep), expertise of the treating physician, and parental preferences. The most commonly used treatments for hemangiomas include corticosteroids (systemic, intralesional, and topical), pulsed dye laser (PDL), interferon alfa, and surgical excision. Other less-common treatment modalities include cryotherapy, other forms of laser surgery, embolization, and chemotherapeutic agents such as vincristine and cyclophosphamide.[56]

SYSTEMIC CORTICOSTEROIDS

Systemic corticosteroids have been a mainstay of therapy of hemangiomas since the 1960s, when their efficacy was first recognized. Their mechanism of action in treating hemangiomas is poorly understood. Prednisolone or prednisone, in doses of 2 to 4mg/kg per day as a single morning dose, is the most common regimen used[57], although some investigators have recommended even higher doses.[58–60] Response is usually seen within 2 to 4 weeks, but often within days of initiating therapy. Once the hemangioma has stabilized, the medication may be tapered, but the duration of treatment needed varies from a few weeks to many months depending on the age of the child, the indications for treatment, and the growth characteristics of the hemangioma being treated. Rapid tapering can lead to rebound growth.[57] Some experts favor switching to alternate-day therapy when the dosage reaches approximately 1mg/kg per day, in order to minimize effects on somatic growth and to help adrenal recovery. In addition, the degree of observed fluctuation of the hemangioma (i.e., whether there is an apparent increase in size on the "off" day) can sometimes be helpful in gauging how quickly to taper the medication.

Corticosteroids are most effective when initiated during the first 6 months of life, when the hemangioma is in its most rapid proliferative stage, but in some cases they can be effective later in infancy. As a corollary, discontinuation is more likely to result in rebound growth in younger patients. A recent meta-analysis of the efficacy of corticosteroids for the treatment of cutaneous hemangiomas found that nearly 90% responded (defined as the cessation of growth and/or shrinkage of the hemangioma) to treatment,[57] and that a daily dosage of 3mg/kg seemed more optimal than 2mg/kg. For unknown reasons, hemangiomas involving the liver and other extracutaneous sites, and those associated with the Kasabach–Merritt phenomenon (KMP; now known to be caused by vascular tumors other than hemangioma of infancy), appear to have a lower rate of response.[41,61]

There are many potential side effects of systemic corticosteroids. The most common are irritability and gastrointestinal upset, which can sometimes be helped by the concomitant administration of a histamine H_2 blocker such as ranitidine. Other reported side effects include hypertension, growth retardation, rapid weight gain, and immunosuppression.[62] Less-commonly reported adverse effects include decreased head growth, delayed motor milestones, hirsutism, and premature thelarche.[63] Despite the risks of administering high doses of corticosteroids to young infants, most treated infants do very well, and catch-up growth nearly always occurs after cessation of therapy.[62]

INTRALESIONAL CORTICOSTEROIDS

Most reports of intralesional corticosteroids were initially seen in the ophthalmologic literature, but this treatment has received growing recognition for well-localized hemangiomas. Paradoxically, the injections have become less popular among ophthalmologists because of the small risk of retinal embolization of particulate matter, which in rare cases has resulted in blindness (either ipsilateral or contralateral). This embolization is likely to be caused by injection pressures exceeding the level of systemic blood pressure.[64] Intralesional corticosteroid usage in other sites can be effective for hemangiomas, especially those that are actively growing and that are small enough to distribute the medication relatively evenly throughout the hemangioma. Doses should not exceed a maximum of 3–5mg/kg triamcinolone per treatment session (to a maximum of 20mg). Several treatments, spaced at monthly intervals, may be necessary, but response rates as high as 85% have been reported.[65] Potential adverse reactions include cutaneous atrophy, anaphylaxis, bleeding, infection, cutaneous necrosis, and adrenal suppression, but the injections are usually well tolerated.

53. Special (1997) Symposia. Management of hemangiomas. **Pediatr Dermatol** 14:57–83.
54. Frieden IJ (1997) Which hemangiomas to treat – and how? **Arch Dermatol** 133:1593–1595.
55. Tanner JL, Dechert MP, Frieden IJ (1998) Growing up with a facial hemangioma: parent and child coping and adaptation. **Pediatrics** 101:446–452.
56. Frieden IJ, Eichenfield LF, Esterly NB et al. (1997) Guidelines of care for hemangiomas of infancy. American Academy of Dermatology Guidelines/Outcomes Committee. **J Am Acad Dermatol** 37:631–637.
57. Bennett ML, Fleischer AB, Chamlin SL et al. (2001) Oral corticosteroids are effective for cutaneous hemangiomas: an evidence-based evaluation. **Arch Dermatol** 137:1208–1213.
58. Akyuz C, Yaris N, Kutluk MT et al. (2001) Management of cutaneous hemangiomas: a retrospective analysis of 1109 cases and comparison of conventional dose prednisolone with high-dose methylprednisolone therapy. **Pediatr Hematol Oncol** 18:47–55.
59. Ozsoylu S (1996) Megadose methylprednisolone therapy for Kasabach–Merritt syndrome. **J Pediatr** 129:947–948.
60. Sadan N, Wolach B (1996) Treatment of hemangiomas of infants with high doses of prednisone. **J Pediatr** 128:141–146.
61. Enjolras O, Riche MC, Merland JJ et al. (1990) Management of alarming hemangiomas in infancy: a review of 25 cases. **Pediatrics** 85:491–498.
62. Boon LM, MacDonald DM, Mulliken JB (1999) Complications of systemic corticosteroid therapy for problematic hemangioma. **Plast Reconstr Surg** 104:1616–1623.
63. Blei F, Chianese J (1999) Corticosteroid toxicity in infants treated for endangering hemangiomas: experience and guidelines for monitoring. **Int Pediatr** 14:146–153.
64. Egbert JE, Paul S, Engel WK et al. (2001) High injection pressure during intralesional injection of corticosteroids into capillary hemangiomas. **Arch Ophthalmol** 119:677–683.
65. Chen MT, Yeong EK, Horng SY (2000) Intralesional corticosteroid therapy in proliferating head and neck hemangiomas: a review of 155 cases. **J Pediatr Surg** 35:420–423.

TOPICAL CORTICOSTEROIDS

Superpotent, topical corticosteroids have anecdotally been reported as being effective in relatively small, superficial hemangiomas.[66,67] They may be considered for treatment of very early hemangiomas that are not causing overt functional impairment and are small and superficial enough to allow adequate percutaneous penetration of the medication. Potential risks of this treatment include cutaneous atrophy and systemic absorption affecting the hypothalamic–pituitary axis.

RECOMBINANT INTERFERON ALFA

Recombinant interferon alfa, an inhibitor of angiogenesis, has been used successfully in the treatment of endangering hemangiomas. Both the 2a and 2b forms have been used with apparently equal success.[68,69] The usual dosage is 3×10^6 IU/m² per day as a subcutaneous injection, although lower dosages at less frequent intervals have also been reported.[70] Interferon alfa often improves severe hemangiomas that have not responded to high doses of corticosteroids, but unfortunately, the discovery of serious neurotoxicity has limited its use. In one report, as many as 20% of infants developed spastic diplegia, which was irreversible in several of those treated.[71] Others have reported less frequent neurotoxicity, but regular monitoring is advised, not only for neurotoxicity but also for the relatively common side effects, which include irritability, neutropenia, and liver enzyme abnormalities.[72] Because of the risk of neurotoxicity, this medication should be used only in severe hemangiomas causing functional impairment or serious soft tissue damage where high-dose corticosteroids have failed or cannot be tolerated.

SURGERY

Indications for surgical removal of hemangiomas can be divided into those appropriate in early infancy and those to be considered later in the course of the hemangioma, usually after 3 or 4 years of age. Early surgical intervention should be considered for sharply demarcated and localized exophytic and pedunculated hemangiomas, which have such a prominent dermal component that they are extremely likely to leave permanent skin changes after involution. Other reasonable indications include those with ulceration and bleeding that are unresponsive to other modalities of treatment and upper eyelid hemangiomas that have not responded to pharmacologic therapy.[8,73]

Surgery can also be considered for children between the ages of 3 and 5 years who continue to have prominent and disfiguring hemangiomas. At this age, enough involution has usually occurred to make the ultimate outcome more predictable (although there are exceptions). Moreover, children at this age are becoming aware of facial differences, and some begin to develop low self-esteem because of their hemangioma. The potential surgical scar must be weighed against the child's emotional distress, as well as the likely outcome if the lesion was left to involute spontaneously. Excision at this age should be seriously considered if resection will be inevitable at some point, if the result of surgery will ultimately be the same whether or not excision is postponed, and in situations where the scar can be easily hidden.[8] In cases with a high degree of uncertainly, it may be best to postpone surgery until later in childhood, in order to allow maximal involution prior to determining how much skin needs to be removed. A multidisciplinary vascular anomalies team may be helpful in decision-making in these cases. Staged resections may be

necessary for larger defects. A purse-string type closure has recently been shown to minimize scar length and give improved results for exophytic focal hemangiomas.[74] Laser surgery (see below) may be helpful for removing residual erythema and superficial telangiectases.

Several kinds of laser have been used to treat hemangiomas. The PDL has been used since the early 1990s and several case series have emphasized its use in the treatment of superficial hemangiomas as well as for residual lesions after involution.[75,76] Treatment of an actively growing hemangioma is typically performed every 2 to 3 weeks until control of proliferation has been achieved. Although this modality has a low risk of scarring when used for treating port-wine stains, there is anecdotal evidence that it may cause ulceration and scarring when used for treating hemangiomas.[77] Paradoxically, PDL has also been used successfully for treating ulcerated hemangiomas, resulting in decreased pain and possibly accelerating reepithelialization.[34] Deep hemangiomas are not effectively treated with PDL because of its limited depth of penetration. Other laser systems including intralesional bare-fiber Nd-YAG (neodymium–yttrium aluminum garnet) have been used for this purpose and appear to be effective, but with some risk of cutaneous ulceration and scarring.[78]

Sclerosing agents and embolization may be helpful in serious, life-threatening hemangiomas. They are not used for routine management. Cryotherapy has been used successfully to treat hemangiomas and is popular in some parts of Europe and South America.[79,80] The risks of scarring, hypopigmentation and epidermal atrophy have limited the popularity of this modality in the USA. Radiation therapy, a treatment option of the past, is no longer considered an acceptable therapeutic modality unless there are life-threatening complications, because of the risk of effects on bone growth and/or late complications such as carcinogenesis.

OTHER VASCULAR TUMORS

Congenital hemangiomas

At least two, possibly three types of fully formed congenital hemangioma have been described; although their relationships to one another are not completely understood, they appear to be distinct entities that are not part of the spectrum of hemangiomas of infancy.

Rapidly involuting congenital hemangiomas

Rapidly involuting congenital hemangiomas, as described by Boon et al.,[18] typically present as raised violaceous tumors with ectatic veins (Fig. 20.12), raised grayish tumors with overlying telangiectasias surrounded by a pale rim of vasoconstriction (Fig. 20.13), or as flat infiltrative tumors with violaceous overlying skin. They vary in size but are often several centimeters in diameter, sometimes even larger. They are frequently warm and occasionally have bruits or even a palpable thrill. In addition to their distinctive appearance, their behavior also differs from hemangiomas of infancy. They do not grow rapidly after birth and many involute extremely rapidly, completing involution by 12–18 months of age.

North et al. have described the pathologic features of fully formed vascular tumors, so-called **congenital nonprogressive hemangiomas**, which share many of the clinical features of rapidly involuting congenital hemangiomas.[19]

66. Elsas FJ, Lewis AR (1994) Topical treatment of periocular capillary hemangioma. J Pediatr Ophthalmol Strabismus 31:153–156.
67. Cruz OA, Zarnegar SR, Myers SE (1995) Treatment of periocular capillary hemangioma with topical clobetasol propionate. Ophthalmology 102:2012–2015.
68. Ezekowitz RA, Mulliken JB, Folkman J (1992) Interferon alfa-2a therapy for life-threatening hemangiomas of infancy. N Engl J Med 326:1456–1463.
69. Chang E, Boyd A, Nelson CC et al. (1997) Successful treatment of infantile hemangiomas with interferon-alpha-2b. J Pediatr Hematol Oncol 19:237–244.
70. Rampini E, Rampini P, Occella C, Bleidl D (2000) Interferon alpha 2b for treatment of complex cutaneous haemangiomas of infancy: a reduced dosage schedule. Br J Dermatol 142:189–191.
71. Barlow CF, Priebe CJ, Mulliken JB et al. (1998) Spastic diplegia as a complication of interferon Alfa-2a treatment of hemangiomas of infancy. J Pediatr 132:527–530.
72. Dubois J, Hershon L, Carmant L et al. (1999) Toxicity profile of interferon alfa-2b in children: A prospective evaluation. J Pediatr 135:782–785.
73. Aldave AJ, Shields CL, Shields JA (1999) Surgical excision of selected amblyogenic periorbital capillary hemangiomas. Ophthalmic Surg Lasers 30:754–757.
74. Mulliken JB, Rogers GF, Marler JJ (2001) Circular excision of hemangioma and purse-string closure - the shortest possible scar. Plast Reconstr Surg in press.
75. Hohenleutner S, Badur-Ganter E, Landthaler M et al. (2001) Long-term results in the treatment of childhood hemangioma with the flashlamp-pumped pulsed dye laser: an evaluation of 617 cases. Lasers Surg Med 28:273–277.
76. Haywood RM, Monk BE, Mahaffey PJ (2000) The treatment of early cutaneous capillary haemangiomata (strawberry naevi) with the tunable dye laser. Br J Plast Surg . 53:302–307.
77. Waner M, Adams D, North P et al. (2000) A rare complication of pulsed dye laser treatment of hemangiomas. In: 13th International Workshop of Vascular Anomalies, Montreal 2000.
78. Achauer BM, Celikoz B, VanderKam VM (1998) Intralesional bare fiber laser treatment of hemangioma of infancy. Plast Reconstr Surg 101:1212–1217.
79. Cremer H (1998) Cryosurgery for hemangiomas. Pediatr Dermatol 15:410–411.
80. Reischle S, Schuller-Petrovic S (2000) Treatment of capillary hemangiomas of early childhood with a new method of cryosurgery. J Am Acad Dermatol 42:809–813.

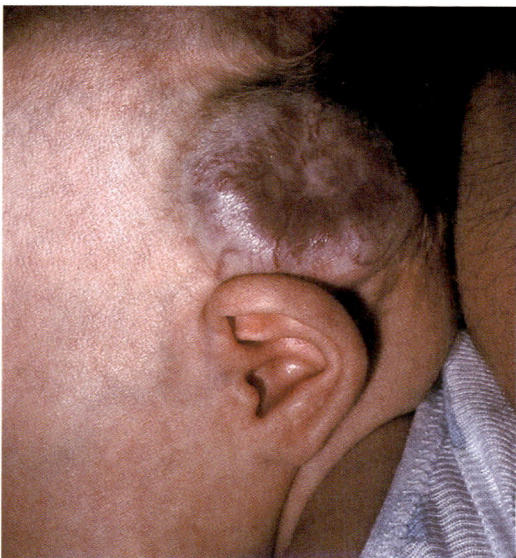

Fig. 20.12 Rapidly involuting congenital hemangioma.

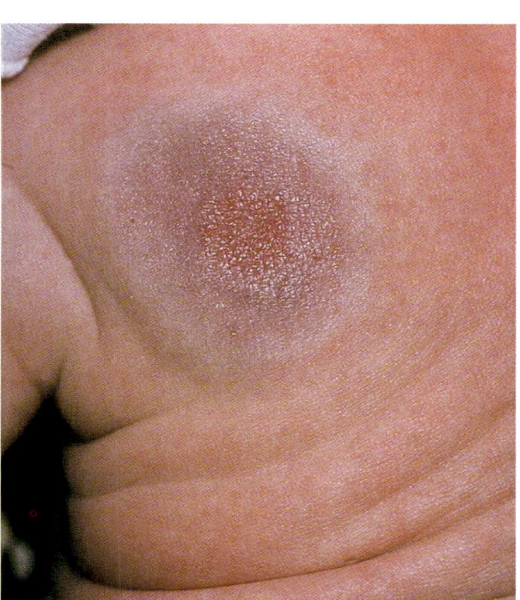

Fig. 20.13 Rapidly involuting congenital hemangioma.

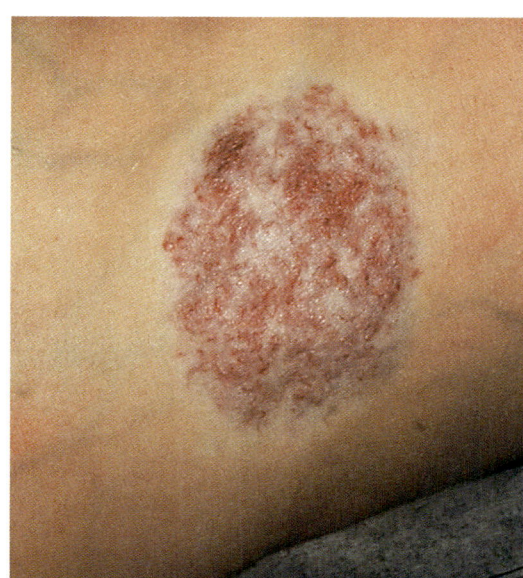

Fig. 20.14 Non-involuting congenital hemangioma.

The pathologic findings of these tumors include cellular lobules with mitotically active capillaries set within a densely fibrotic stroma containing deposits of hemosiderin; focal lobular thrombosis and sclerosis; and frequent association of proliferating lobules with large, thin-walled vessels. The lack of immunoreactivity to GLUT-1 and LeY antigens is also evidence that these tumors are *not* hemangiomas of infancy.

Another recently described tumor is the **noninvoluting congenital hemangioma**.[81] These vascular tumors are also fully formed at birth, occurring slightly more often in male patients, and always appearing as a solitary tumor. Typical lesions are round-to-ovoid in shape, plaque-like or bossed, with central or peripheral pallor as well as coarse, overlying telangiectases (Fig. 20.14). Lesions vary in size, from a few centimeters to 10–15cm, with an average diameter of 5cm. Most have palpable warmth with a component of fast arterial flow that can be demonstrated by Doppler ultrasonography. Pathology typically reveals lobular collections of small, thin-walled vessels with a large, often stellate, central vessel. Interlobular areas contain pre-dominantly dilated, often dysplastic, veins; arteries are also increased in number. Tests for GLUT-1 are negative. These lesions do not involute over time but are usually easily excised without risk of recurrence.

Lobular capillary hemangioma

Lobular capillary hemangioma (pyogenic granuloma) is one of the most common vascular tumors in children, second in frequency to hemangioma of infancy. Lesions can be seen at any age but the majority occur during childhood.[82,83] Pyogenic granulomas may be seen in the early weeks of life though umbilical. Onset during the first year of life is less common but by no means rare, and the tumor is sometimes misdiagnosed at this time as hemangioma of infancy, with false reassurances of spontaneous involution.[84] Pyogenic granulomas may be seen, in the early weeks of life, affecting the umbilicus. Pyogenic granulomas usually present as rapidly growing, bright red papules varying in size from a few millimeters up to 2cm (Fig. 20.15,16). They may have an intact overlying epidermis but frequently become ulcerated. Lesions may be pedunculated and often have a collarette of scale at their periphery. The head and neck are the most common locations, but lesions can occur at any site including mucosal surfaces. While the occurrence of pyogenic granulomas seems to be more frequent in males, females have a much higher frequency of mucosal pyogenic granulomas.[82,83] In contrast to hemangioma of infancy, pyogenic granulomas often bleed repeatedly and profusely, even with very superficial ulceration, prompting this to be called the "Band-Aid disease."[9] In a minority of patients, there is an antecedent history of trauma prior to onset. Pyogenic granulomas usually arise de novo but can develop on the surface of a preexisting vascular malformation. As the revised nomenclature suggests, the pathology of pyogenic granuloma is neither pyogenic nor granulomatous but rather consists of a lobular capillary hemangioma.[82] So-called umbilical granulomas, seen commonly in neonates, are similar in clinical appearance to pyogenic granulomas. Their histology is not well described but their response to silver nitrate treatment suggests that they are probably more similar to granulation tissue rather than a true lobular capillary hemangioma. More persistent "umbilical granulomas" are the result of omphalomesenteric duct cysts and other remnants of the umbilicus.

The management of pyogenic granuloma depends on the location and size. Most small pyogenic granulomas can be removed by shave excision with curettage and light electrodesiccation to the base of the lesion. If the base of the lesion is small, this usually leaves an acceptable scar. PDL has been reported

81. Enjolras O, Mulliken JB, Boon LM et al. (2001) Noninvoluting congenital hemangioma: a rare cutaneous vascular anomaly. **Plast Reconstr Surg** 107:1647–1654.

82. Harris MN, Desai R, Chuang TY et al. (2000) Lobular capillary hemangiomas: An epidemiologic report, with emphasis on cutaneous lesions. **J Am Acad Dermatol** 42:1012–1016.

83. Patrice SJ, Wiss K, Mulliken JB (1991) Pyogenic granuloma (lobular capillary hemangioma): a clinicopathologic study of 178 cases. **Pediatr Dermatol** 8:267–276.

84. Frieden IJ, Esterly NB (1992) Pyogenic granulomas of infancy masquerading as strawberry hemangiomas. **Pediatrics** 90:989–991.

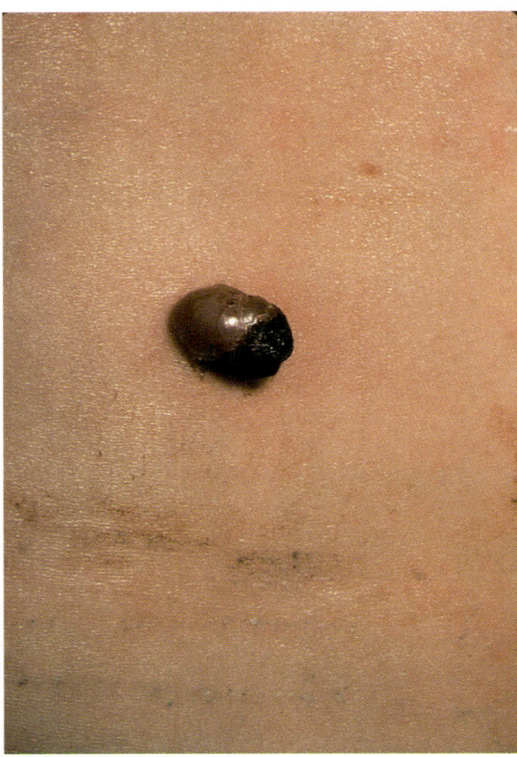

Fig. 20.15 Pyogenic granuloma (lobular capillary hemangioma).

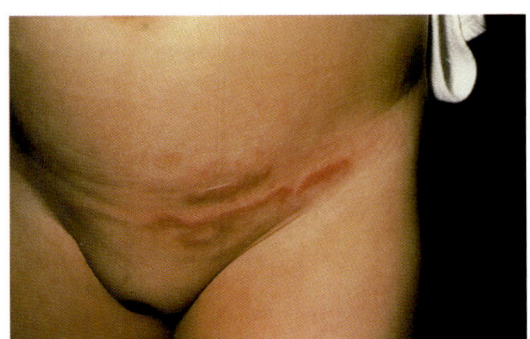

Fig. 20.17 Tufted angioma.

including solitary tumors, large infiltrated plaques (Fig. 20.17), sometimes having increased lanugo hair, and "port-wine stain-like" areas with a cobblestone surface.[87] The characteristic histology is of vascular tufts of tightly packed capillaries dispersed throughout the dermis in a cannonball pattern. Cleft-like lumina are often present at the periphery of the vascular lobules.[88] Some patients with onset of tufted angioma in early infancy develop the Kasabach–Merritt phenomenon (KMP) (see below), and the histology can also be evident in patients with residual tumor following resolution of the KMP. The natural history of tufted angioma is less predictable than that of hemangioma of infancy. Some cases resolve, leaving only minor cutaneous changes whereas others persist and expand over time.

Kaposiform hemangioendothelioma

Kaposiform hemangioendothelioma (KHE) is a rare, distinctive neoplasm that can occur in the skin but has also been reported as a retroperitoneal tumor.[89] It is frequently associated with the KMP (Fig. 20.18). Affected infants have either a congenital tumor or develop a lesion soon after birth and 75% of KHE occurs in early infancy. In rare cases, the tumor arises within a preexisting lymphatic malformation.[89,90] Histologic examination reveals densely infiltrating nodules composed of spindled cells with minimal atypia and infrequent mitoses, as well as slit-like vessels containing hemosiderin.[91] Rare cases of KHE without a consumption coagulopathy have also been reported.[92]

Kasabach–Merritt phenomenon

KMP was first described in 1940. Although originally believed to be a complication of hemangioma of infancy, it is virtually always a complication of other vascular tumors, particularly tufted angioma and KHE.[91,93,94] The clinical features, which can occasionally be present at birth, more commonly appear in the first few months of life, with the development of tenderness, rapid growth, and bruising in a growing soft-tissue tumor (Fig. 20.18A). The central features are a consumption coagulopathy with very low platelet counts and low fibrinogen levels. Other hematologic abnormalities may also be present including elevated D-dimers, prothrombin time and partial thromboplastin time, as well as hemolytic anemia.[95] KMP should *not* be confused with the coagulopathy that may occur in the setting of a large venous or mixed malformation. The coagulopathy associated with malformations usually has a later onset and is characterized by consumption of clotting factors and elevated D-dimers, but the platelet count and fibrinogen level are generally not as low as seen in KMP (Table 20.5).

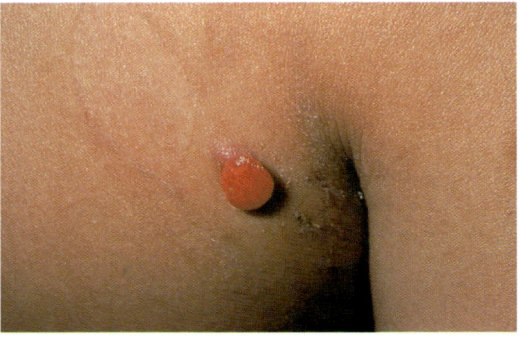

Fig. 20.16 Pyogenic granuloma (lobular capillary hemangioma).

to be effective in many patients,[85] but other authors have found this modality to be disappointing.[83] Excisional surgery, carbon dioxide laser, and cryotherapy have also been used to treat pyogenic granulomas. Estimates of recurrence after removal vary, but recurrence is probably greater with larger lesions. A more worrisome, but rare, complication is the development of multiple satellite lesions after initial removal.

Tufted angioma

Tufted angioma, also known as angioblastoma of Nakagawa, is an uncommon vascular tumor that usually has its onset during infancy or early childhood but rarely can be congenital.[86] Various presentations have been described,

85. Tay YK, Weston WL, Morelli JG (1997) Treatment of pyogenic granuloma in children with the flashlamp-pumped pulsed dye laser. **Pediatrics** 99:368–370.
86. Igarashi M, Oh-i T, Koga M (2000) The relationship between angioblastoma (Nakagawa) and tufted angioma: report of four cases with angioblastoma and a literature-based comparison of the two conditions. **J Dermatol** 27:537–542.
87. Okada E, Tamura A, Ishikawa O et al. (2000) Tufted angioma (angioblastoma): case report and review of 41 cases in the Japanese literature. **Clin Exp Dermatol** 25:627–630.
88. Weiss SW, Goldblum JR (2001) Benign tumors and tumor-like lesions of blood vessels. In: Soft Tissue Tumors, Weiss EA, ed. St Louis: Mosby, pp. 837–890.
89. Zukerberg LR, Nickoloff BJ, Weiss SW (1993) Kaposiform hemangioendothelioma of infancy and childhood. An aggressive neoplasm associated with Kasabach–Merritt syndrome and lymphangiomatosis. **Am J Surg Pathol** 17:321–328.

90. Vin-Christian K, McCalmont TH, Frieden IJ (1997) Kaposiform hemangioendothelioma. An aggressive, locally invasive vascular tumor that can mimic hemangioma of infancy. **Arch Derm** 133:1573–1578.
91. Alvarez-Mendoza A, Lourdes TS, Ridaura-Sanz C et al. (2000) Histopathology of vascular lesions found in Kasabach–Merritt syndrome: review based on 13 cases. **Pediatr Dev Pathol** 3:556–560.
92. Weiss SW, Goldblum JR (2001) Hemangioendothelioma: vascular tumors of intermediate malignancy. In: Soft Tissue Tumors, Weiss EA, ed. St Louis: Mosby, pp. 891–915.
93. Enjolras O, Wassef M, Mazoyer E et al. (1997) Infants with Kasabach–Merritt syndrome do not have "true" hemangiomas. **J Pediatr** 130:631–640.
94. Sarkar M, Mulliken JB, Kozakewich HP et al. (1997) Thrombocytopenic coagulopathy (Kasabach–Merritt phenomenon) is associated with Kaposiform hemangioendothelioma and not with common infantile hemangioma. **Plast Reconstr Surg** 100:1377–1386.
95. Hall GW (2001) Kasabach–Merritt syndrome: pathogenesis and management. **Br J Haematol** 112:851–862.

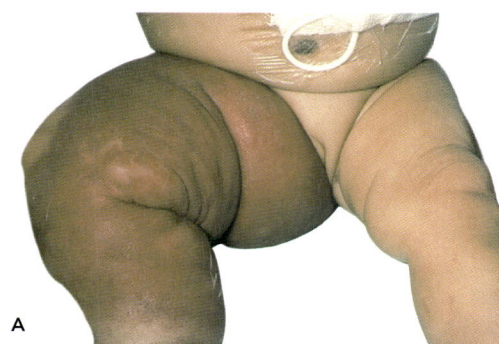

Fig. 20.18 Kaposiform hemangioendothelioma. (A) The hemangioendothelioma with associated Kasabach–Merritt phenomenon. (B) At age 7 residual tumor and lymphedema is still present.

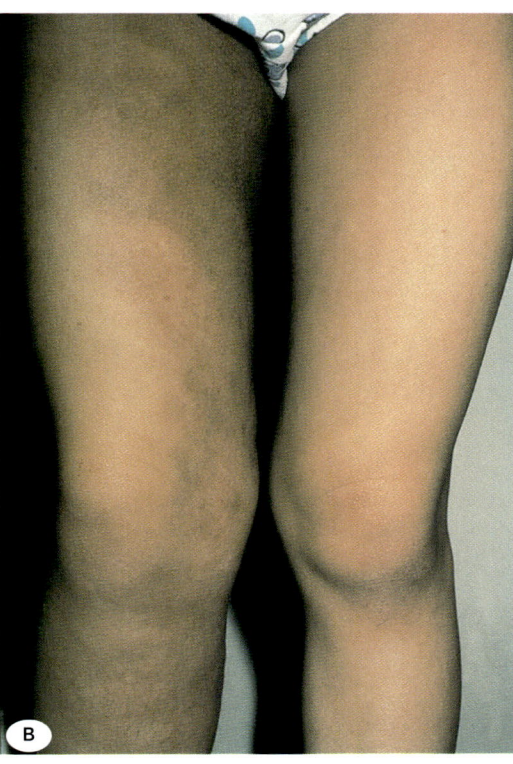

The management of KMP must include a multidisciplinary approach, involving pediatricians, hematologists, dermatologists, and, where appropriate, surgeons and interventional radiologists.[96,97] In contrast to hemangioma of infancy, corticosteroids alone are rarely effective as a sole treatment modality, but they are still often used as a first-line therapy. Surgical excision of the tumor is an effective treatment but is rarely feasible.[98] The addition of interferon alfa has been helpful in some patients, but it is by no means uniformly effective. Recently, vincristine 1–1.5mg/m^2 or 0.05–0.65mg/kg intravenously weekly has been demonstrated to be a highly effective treatment, although relapses may require repeat treatment.[99] Other reportedly effective treatments include aspirin with either ticlopidine or dipyramidole, ε-aminocaproic acid, pentoxifylline (oxpentifylline), and arterial embolization.

X-ray irradiation is reserved for truly life-threatening disease but should be avoided if possible because of its effects on growth and future risk of malignancy.[95,100] Although supportive therapies such as transfusions and infusions of fibrinogen and fresh-frozen plasma may be helpful, platelet transfusions should be avoided except before surgical procedures or if active bleeding is occurring, since the platelets are consumed extremely rapidly and can cause enlargement of the tumor and worsening of the condition.[101] Heparin therapy, which can be helpful in the consumption coagulopathy seen with vascular malformations, is ineffective and can worsen bleeding. Even with current management, the mortality of KMP may be as high as 20%. Residual lesions after resolution of the coagulopathy are relatively common (Fig. 20.18B). They include areas of vascular staining resembling port-wine stains, fibrotic areas of skin, actual tumor mass, or areas of swelling.[102]

Spindle-cell hemangioendothelioma

Spindle-cell hemangioendothelioma is a rare vascular tumor that is most often found on the extremities. It can be associated with Maffucci syndrome[103] (see below) or may arise in conjunction with a preexisting vascular malformation. Although originally believed to be a low-grade angiosarcoma, it is now thought to represent a reactive vascular tumor arising in conjunction with malformed vasculature.[104,105] Surgical excision is the only known effective therapy.

Congenital eccrine angiomatous hamartoma

Congenital eccrine angiomatous hamartoma (sudoriparous angioma) is a rare entity that can present at birth, during infancy, or in early childhood; it is a large, ill-defined vascular plaque, with increased hairs and sweating at the site of the lesion.[106,107] The extremities and abdomen are the usual sites of involvement. Pain may be present. The diagnosis is established by the characteristic histologic findings of closely packed eccrine sweat glands in association with dilated capillaries and venous channels within a dense collagenous matrix.

Infantile hemangiopericytoma is a rare tumor that is now considered to be a form of infantile myofibromatosis rather than a true vascular tumor.

VASCULAR MALFORMATIONS

Vascular malformations are composed of anomalous blood vessels and/or lymphatics lined by a quiescent endothelium without cellular hyperplasia.[2] Although it is believed that all vascular malformations are present at birth, most are evident in infancy. A minority appear in childhood or later, after a dormant phase, as "acquired" vascular anomalies. Depending on their flow characteristics, vascular malformations are defined as either slow flow or fast flow. The slow-flow anomalies include capillary, venous, and lymphatic malformations and combinations thereof. Arterial aneurysms or arteriovenous malformations (AVMs) with arteriovenous shunting are the fast-flow anomalies.[9] Vascular malformations persist lifelong, unchanged, growing proportionate to the child's growth, or, in some cases, worsening and expanding. They never regress spontaneously but only rarely go through a rapid growth phase such as is seen with hemangiomas of infancy. Growth in vascular malformations may be stimulated by trauma, clotting, the effects of hormones during puberty and/or pregnancy, or may occur in the absence of any known triggering factor.

96. Shin HY, Ryu KH, Ahn HS (2000) Stepwise multimodal approach in the treatment of Kasabach–Merritt syndrome. **Pediatr Int** 42:620–624.
97. Blei F, Karp N, Rofsky N et al. (1998) Successful multimodal therapy for kaposiform hemangioendothelioma complicated by Kasabach–Merritt phenomenon: case report and review of the literature. **Pediatr Hematol Oncol** 15:295–305.
98. Drolet BA, Scott LA, Esterly NB et al. (2001) Early surgical intervention in a patient with Kasabach–Merritt phenomenon. **J Pediatr** 138:756–758.
99. Haisley-Royster CA, Enjolras O, Frieden IJ et al. (2002) Kasabach–Merritt phenomenon: a retrospective study of treatment with vincristine. **J Pediatr Hematol Oncol** 24:459–462.
100. Ogino I, Torikai K, Kobayasi S et al. (2001) Radiation therapy for life- or function-threatening infant hemangioma. **Radiology** 218:834–839.
101. Phillips WG, Marsden JR (1993) Kasabach–Merritt syndrome exacerbated by platelet transfusion. **J R Soc Med** 86:231–232.

102. Enjolras O, Mulliken JB, Wassef M et al. (2000) Residual lesions after Kasabach–Merritt phenomenon in 41 patients. **J Am Acad Dermatol** 42:225–235.
103. Pellegrini AE, Drake RD, Qualman SJ (1995) Spindle cell hemangioendothelioma: a neoplasm associated with Maffucci's syndrome. **J Cutan Pathol** 22:173–176.
104. Fletcher CD (1996) Vascular tumors: an update with emphasis on the diagnosis of angiosarcoma and borderline vascular neoplasms. **Monogr Pathol** 38:181–206.
105. Perkins P, Weiss SW (1996) Spindle cell hemangioendothelioma. An analysis of 78 cases with reassessment of its pathogenesis and biologic behavior. **Am J Surg Pathol** 20:1196–1204.
106. Nakatsui C, Schloss E, Krol A et al. (1999) Eccrine angiomatous hamartoma: report of a case and literature review. **J Am Acad Dermatol** 41:109–111.
107. Requena L, Sangueza OP (1997) Cutaneous vascular anomalies. Part I. Hamartomas, malformations, and dilation of preexisting vessels. **J Am Acad Dermatol** 37:523–549.

TABLE 20.5   Differences between Kasabach–Merritt syndrome and coagulopathy associated with vascular malformations (usually venous malformation or lymphatic–venous malformation)

Differences	Kasabach–Merritt syndrome	Vascular malformations-associated local or disseminated intravascular coagulation
Ages	Birth and infancy: growth of the tumor; onset of coagulopathy; childhood: cure of coagulopathy, residual tumor	Lifelong biologic process of localized intravascular coagulopathy (LIC) with flares and risk of disseminated intravascular coagulopathy (DIC)
Clinical features	Congenital or early-onset plaque or tumor followed by a distinctive ecchymotic, inflammatory, painful mass; purpura, bruises; visceral hemorrhages are rare	Occurs mainly with extensive limb or trunk venous malformations and, very rarely, with head-and-neck venous malformations; plaques, patches, masses of blue vascular anomalies, soft, compressible; swelling when dependent, pain; normal temperature; phleboliths
Hematology	Severe thrombocytopenia (often < 5000 × 10^6 cells/l); low fibrinogen, elevated D-dimers	Mild thrombocytopenia (> 80 000 × 10^6 cells/l); very high D-dimers; low fibrinogen; von Willebrand deficiency in some patients
Course	Acute, sudden; involution of the tumor occurs subsequently	Vascular malformation persists and slowly worsens lifelong; coagulopathy may also worsen
Pathology	Vascular tumor: either kaposiform hemangioendothelioma or tufted angioma (occasionally associated with lymphatic malformation)	Vascular malformation: usually venous malformation (sometimes lymphatic and venous malformation)
Radiodiagnostic	Doppler: high-flow; MRI: parenchymal tumoral signal and flow voids	Doppler: slow-flow; MRI: hypersignal on T2-weighted image; radiograph: phleboliths
Treatment	Heparin ineffective; a number of drugs have been useful including: corticosteroids, interferon alfa, vincristine and ticlopidine plus aspirin (see text)	The most effective treatment is low-molecular-weight heparin; compressive stockings for extremity lesions

Pathogenesis

Although some progress in the understanding of the pathogenesis of vascular malformations has been made, the precise origin of most is not known. They are presumed to be errors in blood vessel development most likely caused by localized dysfunction in pathways regulating vascular embryogenesis, especially the molecular events responsible for vascular remodeling.[108] The study of rare families with Mendelian inheritance of their vascular malformations has enhanced our understanding of molecular genetics in this field.[109] Mutant genes responsible for familial venous malformations, glomangiomas, lymphedema, cerebral cavernomas, hereditary hemorrhagic telangiectasia (HHT), and ataxia-telangiectasia have been identified. The functions of these mutations, and how they affect signaling pathways between endothelial cells and other mural cells, are currently being investigated. It is hoped that a better understanding of pathogenesis as well as new treatment modalities may arise from such research.

Cutaneous AVMs usually present as a faint stain in childhood, expanding at or after puberty. Hormonal changes and trauma are known to trigger growth. Many head and neck AVMs are located at so-called "choke zones," representing the anastomotic junction of two arterial blood supplies. It has been hypothesized that their occurrence in these areas as well as their growth in response to trauma may be a consequence of their vulnerability to oxidative stress.[110] The cells cultured from skin AVMs differ from normal endothelial cells in culture, demonstrating higher rates of proliferation with lack of inhibition by known angiogenic inhibitors, such as interleukin 1β, tumor necrosis factor α, interferon-γ, and transforming growth factor β, and a lack of expression of leukocyte adhesion molecules; they also express the proto-oncogene c-ets-1.[111] Brain AVMs have been studied more extensively. Cerebral AVMs express basic fibroblast growth factor in the endothelium and subendothelium, as well as in the brain tissue intermingled within the AVM.[112] Capsase-3 immunoreactivity has been detected in the endothelium, media, and perivascular tissue of CNS AVMs, indicating that apoptosis and vascular remodeling play a role in their development.[113] Childhood cerebral AVMs that recur after surgery have a high degree of endothelial expression of VEGF in the primary vascular lesion, while nonrecurring lesions have low expression of VEGF.[114] Upregulation of VEGF mRNA has been observed in the parenchyma adjacent to brain AVMs, with elevated levels of *Tie* endothelial cell-specific receptor tyrosine kinase in the AVM vessels and VEGF protein in the AVM endothelia compared with those in normal brain tissue and vasculature.[115] The applicability of these findings to cutaneous AVMs remains controversial as no comparable experimental data exist for them, but the expression of angiogenic cytokines in the AVM environment could explain their propensity to recur and recruit new vessels when the overlying stained skin is left in place after embolization and excision of the AVM nidus.

CAPILLARY MALFORMATIONS

Capillary malformations are the most common vascular malformations. They involve vessels of the capillary network in skin and mucous membranes. Capillary malformations may be isolated and innocuous, may cause disfigurement and stigmatization, and, in some cases, may herald the presence of an extracutaneous disease.

108. Chiller KG, Arbiser J, Frieden IJ (2001) Vasculogenesis and Angiogenesis in the Development of Cutaneous Vascular Birthmarks. Submitted.
109. Vikkula M, Boon LM, Mulliken JB (1998) Molecular basis of vascular anomalies. **Trends Cardiovasc Med** 8:281–292.
110. Mitchell EL, Taylor GI, Houseman ND et al. (2001) The angiosome concept applied to arteriovenous malformations of the head and neck. **Plast Reconstr Surg** 107:633–646.
111. Wautier MP, Boval B, Chappey O et al. (1999) Cultured endothelial cells from human arteriovenous malformations have a defective growth regulation. **Blood** 94:2020–2028.
112. Kilic T, Pamir MN, Kullu S et al. (2000) Expression of structural proteins and angiogenic factors in cerebrovascular anomalies. **Neurosurgery** 46:1179–1191.
113. Takagi Y, Hattori I, Nozaki K et al. (2000) DNA fragmentation in central nervous system vascular malformations. **Acta Neurochir (Wien)** 142:987–994.
114. Sonstein WJ, Kader A, Michelsen WJ et al. (1996) Expression of vascular endothelial growth factor in pediatric and adult cerebral arteriovenous malformations. **J Neurosurg** 85:838–845.
115. Hatva E, Jaaskelainen J, Hirvonen H et al. (1996) Tie endothelial cell-specific receptor tyrosine kinase is upregulated in the vasculature of arteriovenous malformations. **J Neuropathol Exp Neurol** 55:1124–1133.

Salmon patches

The most common vascular lesion in infancy is the salmon patch, also known as nevus simplex, erythema nuchae, angel's kiss, and stork bite. The term nevus flammeus is synonymous with port-wine stain and should *not* be used to describe a salmon patch. The latter lesion is best classified as a superficial vascular malformation, although its course is typically different from that of the port-wine stain. Salmon patches consist of ectatic capillaries that have been thought to represent the persistence of fetal circulatory patterns in the skin. Their disappearance may be based on maturation of the autonomic innervation of these vessels in early infancy, but this is hypothetical, not proven.

The salmon patch is present at birth in about 40% of infants and appears as a pink to red macule on the nape, glabella, forehead, upper eyelids, nasolabial region, and occasionally on the parietal and occipital scalp and overlying the thoracic or lumbosacral spine (Fig. 20.19) In contrast to the port-wine stain, the salmon patch tends to be located in the central portion of the face and does not follow a dermatomal distribution. Occasionally, however, port-wine stains occur in this more medial location (so-called "medial telangiectatic nevus"); at times, these can be difficult to differentiate from salmon patches. Many infants have salmon patches in several locations. Of those infants born with salmon patches, 81% have lesions at the nape, 45% on the eyelids, and 33% on the glabella.[116,117]

A variant of the salmon patch termed the **butterfly-shaped mark**, a red-violet rhomboid-shaped macule, can occur in the sacral region. These lesions are less common than salmon patches at other sites and tend to disappear more slowly. Although some authors have concluded that radiographic studies of the lumbosacral area are not indicated when the butterfly-shaped mark is present, this premise remains controversial and many physicians continue to suggest routine imaging studies of the lumbar spine in patients with a midline cutaneous vascular malformation, because it can be a marker of occult spinal dysraphism.[118,119] Salmon patches of the face are, in rare instances, a manifestation of other diseases. Prominent and persistent salmon patch (often referred to as a midline facial nevus flammeus) has been described in the Beckwith–Weidemann syndrome, a condition that has several other features including omphalocele, macroglossia, dysmorphic facies, hemihypertrophy, and neonatal hypoglycemia, as well as a risk of Wilm's tumor and other malignancies.[120,121] In Nova syndrome, glabellar salmon patches are reported as an autosomal dominant trait in association with posterior fossa brain malformations.[122]

Usually no treatment of salmon patches is necessary, as most of those on the face fade by 1 to 2 years of age.[116] The nuchal lesions tend to be more persistent and are present in many adults. If salmon patches do not fade completely, they can be effectively treated with a PDL. Nuchal salmon patches may occur in association with a hemangioma, as an overlap between vascular malformation and vascular tumor.[3] (Fig. 20.1) Predisposed infants may develop a superimposed eczematous dermatitis.

Port-wine stains

The port-wine stain, or nevus flammeus, occurs in 0.3% of all newborns and has an equal sex distribution.[117] Port-wine stains are present at birth and do not undergo spontaneous resolution. These well-demarcated vascular stains grow in proportion to the growth of the child. They are usually unilateral and segmental, generally (but not always) respecting the midline, although occasionally there is a contralateral component in the same or adjacent dermatome. The stain may appear on any area of the body. In a review of 310 patients with port-wine stains, 85% were unilateral, 15% were bilateral, and 68% had more than one dermatome involved. In this group, 8% of port-wine stains involving the V1 dermatome were associated with ocular or CNS involvement, but this increased to 25% if there was bilateral V1 or complete involvement of all three trigeminal dermatomes (Figs 20.20 and 20.21).[123]

Port-wine stains are usually pink or red during infancy. They sometimes appear to lighten somewhat in the first 1–6 months of life, probably because of the marked drop in circulating blood hemoglobin concentration during this time period. This lightening should not be interpreted as an indication

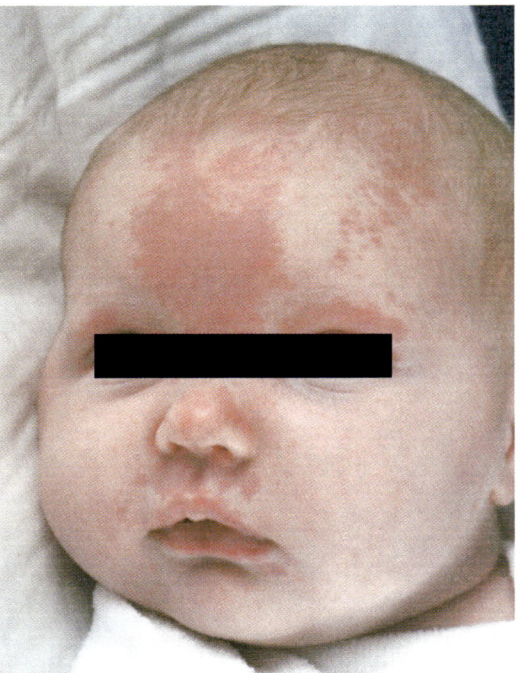

Fig. 20.19 Salmon patch (nevus simplex). Note that in addition to the glabella and upper eyelids – the most common sites of involvement – the nose and upper lip are often affected (Courtesy of Howard Pride.)

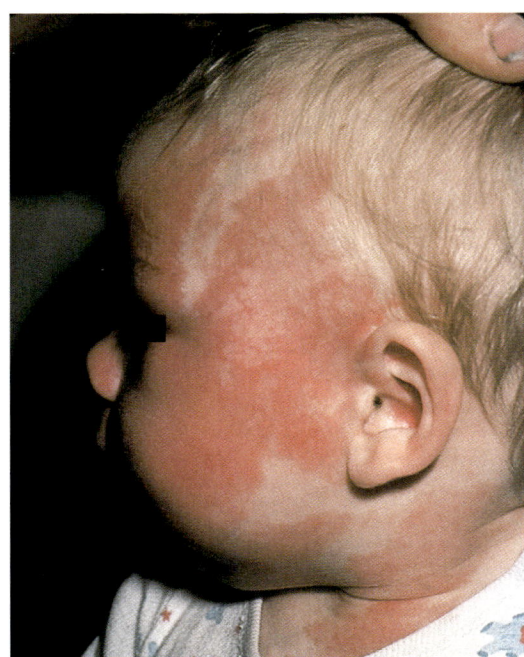

Fig. 20.20 Port-wine stain involving both V1 and V2 dermatomes. This infant had Sturge–Weber syndrome.

116. Leung AK, Telmesani AM (1989) Salmon patches in Caucasian children. **Pediatr Dermatol** 6:185–187.
117. Jacobs AH, Walton RG (1976) The incidence of birthmarks in the neonate. **Pediatrics** 58:218–222.
118. Metzker A, Shamir R (1990) Butterfly-shaped mark: a variant form of nevus flammeus simplex. **Pediatrics** 85:1069–1071.
119. Ben-Amitai D, Davidson S, Schwartz M et al. (2000) Sacral nevus flammeus simplex: the role of imaging. **Pediatr Dermatol** 17:469–471.
120. Jonas R, Kimonis V (2001) Chest wall hamartoma with Wiedemann–Beckwith syndrome: clinical report and brief review of chromosome 11p15.5-related tumors. **Am J Med Genet** 101:221–225.
121. Lam W, Hatada I, Ohishi S et al. (1999) Analysis of germline CDKN1C (p57-KIP2) mutations in familial and sporadic Beckwith–Wiedemann syndrome (BWS) provides a novel genotype-phenotype correlation. **J Med Genet** 36:518–523.
122. Nova H (1979) Familial communicating hydrocephalus, posterior cerebellar agenesis, mega cisterna magna, and port-wine nevi. Report on five members of one family. **J Neurosurg** 51:862–865.
123. Tallman B, Tan OT, Morelli JG et al. (1991) Location of port-wine stains and likelihood of ophthalmic and or central nervous system complications. **Pediatrics** 87:323–327.

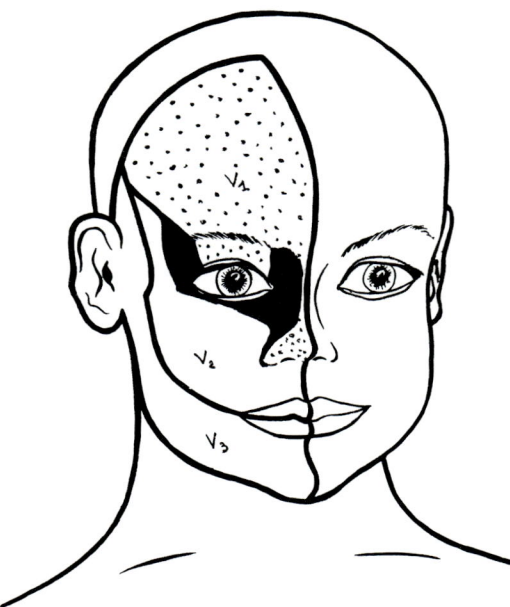

Fig. 20.21 Anatomic drawing of trigeminal dermatomes. Note the blackened area – the so-called V1–V2 watershed area, which can be ennervated by either V1 or V2. (Reprinted with permission Irom Enjolras O, Garzon MC (2001) Vascular stains, malformations, and tumors. In Textbook of Neenatal Dermatology, Eichenfield LF, Frieden IJ, Esterly NB, eds. Philadelphia, PA: WB Saunders, p. 332.)

of spontaneous resolution as this rarely if ever occurs. Port–wine stains often darken to a dull erythrocyanotic or purple hue with advancing age. Although most are initially macular, the surface may become irregular, thickened, and nodular during adulthood. This feature is frequent in facial port–wine stains but is less commonly observed in those located on the trunk and limbs.[124] Bony and soft tissue hypertrophy can be associated with overlying port–wine stains, particularly in the V2 facial distribution. Progressive ectasias manifest by thickening and nodularity of the port–wine stains may develop over time. In addition, pyogenic granulomas may arise within port–wine stains, presenting as small papules or nodules.[3]

Histologically, the port–wine stain is composed of normal numbers of ectatic mature capillaries in the superficial dermis with no evidence of cellular proliferation. These vessels become more dilated over time and are found in the deep dermis and subcutaneous tissue when the clinical lesion is raised or nodular.[9] Loosely arranged collagen fibers surround the ectatic vessels.[125] Studies have demonstrated a decrease in the number of nerves surrounding the abnormal blood vessels. Progressive vascular dilatation is thought to be a result of impairment of neural control of the vascular elements.[126] Additional studies have documented impaired neural regulation of blood flow in port–wine stains.[127]

Although almost all port–wine stains are present at birth, rare instances of later onset have been documented. These "acquired" port–wine stains sometimes develop after injury to the skin or in association with the use of oral contraceptives. Perhaps **acquired telangiectatic nevus** would be a more accurate term for these puzzling lesions.[128–130] Differential diagnosis includes mastocytosis (the telangiectasia macularis eruptiva perstans type) and telangiectasias occurring in aluminum workers.[131]

Port–wine stains can occur as isolated cutaneous lesions or in association with other abnormalities. Although a midline port–wine stain alone, without other associated hallmarks (e.g., fatty mass, dimple, tuft of hair), is very rarely associated with dysraphism,[132] some physicians still recommend the evaluation of these areas with ultrasound (very early in infancy) or MR imaging. Neurogenic bladder and accompanying voiding dysfunction may be the initial symptom of tethered spinal cord and once established may be irreversible.

Sturge–Weber (SWS) and Klippel–Trenaunay (KT) and Proteus syndromes typically feature port–wine stains as a clinical manifestation. Rarely, lesions resembling port–wine stains occur overlying AVMs or in rare disorders such as Cobb, Bonnet–Dechaume–Blanc, or Wyburn–Mason syndromes, but in these cases it is not understood whether the port–wine stain is an associated capillary malformation or if it is a true component of the AVM. In some patients, it is the only indication of a dormant AVM for many years.

The development of lasers that selectively ablate vascular lesions has greatly advanced our ability to treat these congenital anomalies, and the rationale for treatment, including psychosocial and ethical issues have been well documented.[133] Port–wine stain, especially when located on visible skin such as the face, can invoke teasing and stigmatization, causing significant emotional distress in affected children. A British study examining psychological disabilities among patients with port–wine stains found a high level of psychological morbidity, resulting from a feeling of stigmatization, but these morbidities were not evident in casual social interactions or with standard psychological tests.[134] Troilus,[135] after quantifying the psychological disabilities associated with port–wine stains, stressed the considerable emotional turmoil encountered in 259 patients and their families and advised early treatment with the aim of finishing prior to beginning school. Although as yet unproven, treatment in childhood could potentially prevent the thickening and vascular nodules that develop over time in many port–wine stains. The mainstay of treatment of port–wine stains in children is the PDL with wavelengths between 585 and 595nm and a pulse duration between 450 and 1500ms. The latter duration is usually used together with a cooling device to minimize thermal damage. Newer lasers using even longer pulse durations (up to 10ms) have recently been introduced. PDLs have been used in children and adults for more than 10 years and have a low risk of scarring and high percentage of clinical response (Fig. 20.22). Although initial reports emphasized complete

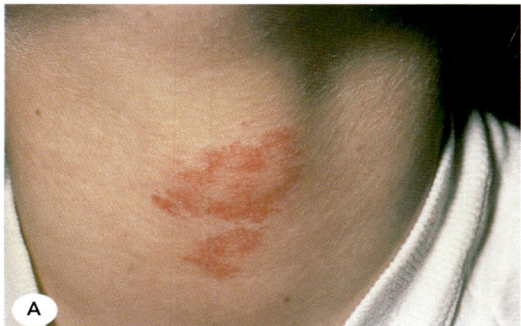

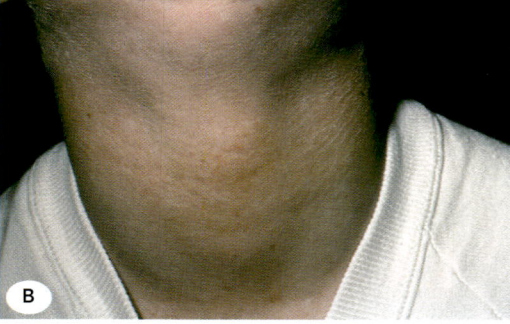

Fig. 20.22 Telangiectactic port–wine stain. (A) Before laser treatment. (B) Complete resolution after three laser treatments.

124. Klapman MH, Yao F (2001) Thickening and nodules in port-wine stains. **J Am Acad Dermatol** 44:300–302.
125. Lever W, Schaumburg-Lever G (1990) Histopathology of the Skin, 7th edn. Philadelphia, PA Lippincott.
126. Smoller B, Rosen S (1986) Port wine stains. A disease of altered neural modulation of blood vessels? **Arch Dermatol** 122:177–179.
127. Gaylarde PM, Dodd HJ, Sarkany I (1987) Port wine stains. **Arch Dermatol** 123:861.
128. Colver GB, Ryan TJ (1986) Acquired port wine stains. **Arch Dermatol** 122:1415–1416.
129. Goldman L (1970) Oral contraceptives and vascular anomalies. **Lancet** ii:108–109.
130. Tsuji T, Sawabe M (1988) A new type of telangiectasia following trauma. **J Cutan Pathol** 15:22.

131. Theriault G, Cordier S, Harvey R (1980) Skin telangiectases in workers at an aluminum plant. **N Eng J Med** 303:1278–1281.
132. Tavafoghi V, Ghandehi A, Hambrick G et al. (1978) Cutaneous signs of spinal dysraphism. **Arch Dermatol** 114:573–577.
133. Strauss RP, Resnick SD (1993) Pulsed dye laser therapy for port wine stains in children: psychosocial and ethical issues. **J Pediatr** 122:504–510.
134. Lanigan SW, Cotterill JA (1989) Psychological disabilities amongst patients with port wine stains. **Br J Dermatol** 121:209–215.
135. Troilus A, Wrangsjö B, Ljunggren B (1998) Potential psychological benefits from early treatment of port-wine stains in children. **Br J Dermatol** 139:59–65.

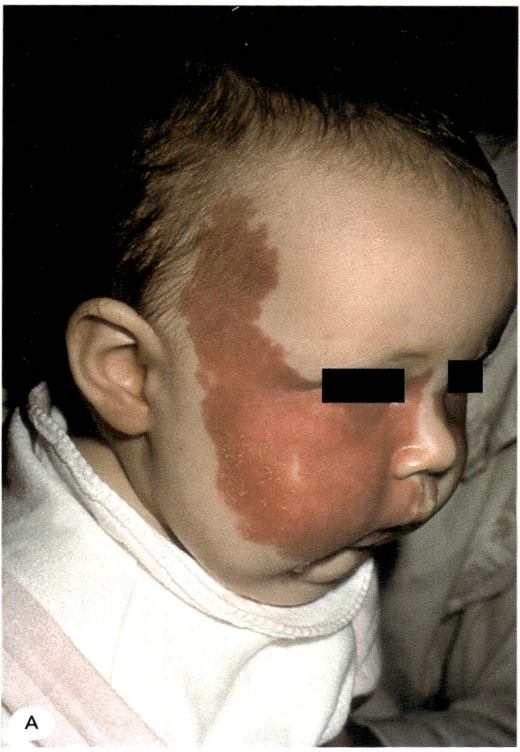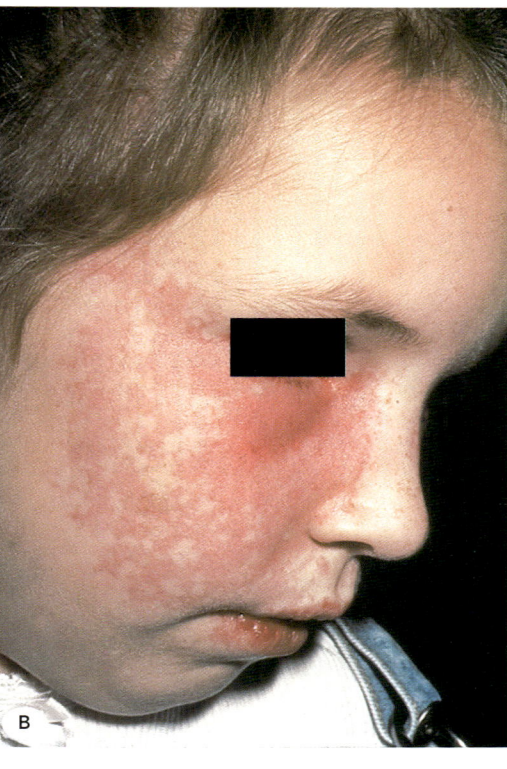

Fig. 20.23 Port wine stain V2 dermatome. (A) Before laser treatment. (B) After eight laser treatments the lesion is considerably lighter but still persists.

clearing,[136] more recent studies have emphasized that this is the exception, with most patients achieving lightening but not complete clearance. The response to treatment is based on a number of factors including the size and location of the port-wine stain. Very large port-wine stains and those located in a V2 distribution or those involving the extremities do respond, but less well than lesions in other sites (Fig. 20.23). Stains over bony prominences require fewer treatments. Scarring is rare, but transient pigmentary changes are sometimes seen. Although many authors have reported that earlier treatment results in better clearance[137,138] others disagree.[139] Recurrences of port-wine stains after completion of treatment can occur, but the incidence of recurrence is uncertain. Michel *et al.*[140] reported no recurrences in children treated before 10 years of age, which might hint at a lower recurrence frequency with early treatment. Laser treatments are typically performed every 2 to 3 months, allowing for maximal lightening of the lesion prior to subsequent treatment. The type of anesthesia or sedation necessary for treatment with PDL is controversial. With the introduction of EMLA (eutectic mixture of local anesthesia) cream in 1993, many older children and those with small, well-localized port-wine stain can be treated without general anesthesia or sedation. The cream consists of a combination of prilocaine and lidocaine. Its efficacy depends on the amount of cream applied, duration of contact, and proper use of an occlusive covering. The cream should be applied thickly, and the site must be completely occluded with a nonpermeable, airtight patch. Duration of contact should be at least 1 hour, preferably 2. The maximum action time is between 1.5 and 3 hours. The recommended maximum application of EMLA to children weighing 5–10kg is 20cm². There have been reports of methemoglobinemia induced by topical application of EMLA, particularly when used in infants less than 6 months of age.

Sturge–Weber syndrome

SWS, also known as encephalotrigeminal angiomatosis, is the triad of a facial port-wine stain in a V1 distribution (Fig. 20.20), an ipsilateral leptomeningeal vascular malformation, and a choroidal vascular malformation of the eye, which can lead to ipsilateral glaucoma and buphthalmos. There is no clear evidence of a genetic predisposition, and the etiology remains unknown. The three tissues involved are all derivatives of the so-called mesoectoderm. Theoretical causes of this disorder include an error of morphogenesis within the cephalic neural crest and lethal genes surviving by mosaicism.[141,142]

Port-wine stains in SWS follow the distribution of the first branch of the trigeminal nerve. Consequently, the stain typically involves the forehead and upper eyelid. The distribution of V1 varies somewhat, so V1 can involve the skin below the eye and on the nose in some patients; however port-wine stains that spare the upper face and eyelids are almost never associated with an intracranial vascular malformation (Fig. 20.21).[141] Approximately 10% of patients with a port-wine stain in the V1 distribution have SWS. Extensive and bilateral involvement including other trigeminal dermatomes may also occur, but the midline is respected in most cases. Even in infants with bilateral involvement of the V1 areas, often in association with other stains on face and body, only one side of the brain and eye is usually affected. Bilateral brain lesions, observed in about 15% of patients (including some patients with hemifacial port-wine stains) carries a greater risk of neurologic impairment.[142]

Patients may have partial forms of SWS, including port-wine stain with only eye or only CNS involvement. In addition, individuals with typical CNS or eye findings of SWS without a facial port-wine stain have also been reported.[143] Common neurologic abnormalities include contralateral seizures, episodes of contralateral hemiparesis or hemiplegia, headaches, and intellectual impairment. Seizures are usually of the focal motor or generalized tonic–

136. Tan OT, Sherwood K, Gilchrest BA (1989) Treatment of children with port wine stains using the flashlamp-pulsed tunable dye laser. **N Engl J Med** 320:416–421.
137. Ashinoff R, Geronemus RG (1991) Flashlamp-pumped pulsed dye laser for port wine stains in infancy: earlier versus later treatment. **J Am Acad Dermatol** 24:467–472.
138. Nguyen CM, Yohn JJ, Huff C et al. (1998) Facial port-wine stains in childhood: prediction of rate of improvement as a function of the age of the patient, size and location of the port-wine stain, and the number of treatments with the pulsed dye (585 nm) laser. **Br J Dermatol** 138:821–825.
139. van der Horst CM, Koster PH, de Borgie CA et al. (1998) Effect of the timing of treatment of port-wine stains with the flashlamp pumped pulsed dye laser. **N Eng J Med** 338:1028–1033

140. Michel S, Landthaler M, Hohenleutner U (2000) Recurrence of port-wine stains after treatment with the flash-lamp pumped pulsed dye laser. **Br J Dermatol** 143:1230–1234.
141. Enjolras O, Riche MC, Merland JJ (1985) Facial port wine stains and Sturge–Weber syndrome. **Pediatrics** 76:48–51.
142. Happle R (1987) Lethal genes surviving by mosaicism: a possible explanation for sporadic birth defects involving the skin. **J Am Acad Dermatol** 16:899–906.
143. Martinez-Bermejo A, Tendero A, Lopez-Martin V et al. (2000) Angiomatosis leptomeningea sin angioma facial. Debe considerarse como variante del syndrome de Sturge Weber? **Rev Neurol** 30:837–841.

clonic types initially. They usually have their onset before two years of age. Developmental delay in motor and cognitive skills is seen in about half of affected children. Continued seizures predispose the child to severe mental impairment. Extensive brain lesions contribute to poor intellectual development, behavioral abnormalities, and learning disabilities. The reason for the developmental delay is not known but it may be because of the seizures or atrophy of the affected areas of the brain.

Ocular abnormalities are included in the classic triad of SWS but need not be present in order to make a definitive diagnosis. Glaucoma develops in approximately half of patients whose port-wine stain is adjacent to the eye and occurs independent of neurologic involvement. The precise cause of elevated intraocular pressure is a matter of debate, and more than one mechanism is probably responsible. Hyperemia of the ciliary body, anomalies of the anterior chamber angle structures, and abnormal arteriovenous communications in the episcleral vascular plexus may all play a role in the pathogenesis of glaucoma in SWS.[144] Ophthalmologic examination at regular intervals (every six to 12 months) should be performed in all those affected, as glaucoma can develop early and should be tested for as soon as possible. Long-term follow-up is important because glaucoma can develop later in life. Early detection of increased intraocular pressure is important in order to prevent progressive disease. For 60% of patients with SWS and glaucoma, onset is in infancy, when the eye may stretch because of the increased intraocular pressure; these infants have an enlarged cornea, buphthalmos (bull eye – large eye), and myopia. For the other 40%, glaucoma begins in childhood or adulthood and there is no eye enlargement.[145]

Because most affected children are initially normal, neuroimaging studies can be helpful in detecting brain involvement. Radiographic examination of the brain in patients over 2 years of age reveals characteristic calcifications in two-thirds of patients, but this finding has only rarely been detected in the neonate.[146] Calcifications follow the convolutions of the cerebral cortex and are characterized by sinusoidal parallel lines simulating "railroad tracks," most often in the occipital region of the brain adjacent to the leptomeningeal vascular lesions. They are best demonstrated by CT scan and are usually evident by 1 year of age. MR imaging with gadolinium enhancement is the most useful study for even earlier detection of SWS, because it provides clear identification of increased blood vessels as well as any accompanying cortical atrophy. MR occasionally fails initially to detect small areas of vascular malformation in infants less than 6 months of age, but advanced myelination or an enlarged choroid plexus may be seen in the involved hemisphere.[146,147] The use of functional cerebral imaging such as positron emission tomography (evaluating the glucose metabolism in the brain) or single photon emission computed tomography (SPECT: studying the regional cerebral blood flow) may indicate increased metabolism and increased cerebral blood flow in the abnormal hemisphere early in infancy. After the development of seizures, however, rapid cerebral impairment with hypometabolism and hemispheric hypoperfusion develops.[148–150]

The management of SWS depends on the clinical manifestations. Seizures require anticonvulsant medications;[151] in those with severe, intractable seizures, surgical intervention, such as localized resection of the involved brain tissue or hemispherectomy, is necessary.[152] Glaucoma, when present, can be treated medically but most cases of congenital glaucoma require surgery. Argon laser photocoagulation of prominent conjunctival and episcleral vessels in SWS has been reported to be successful and is accompanied by no apparent vision-threatening complications. Laser treatment of the port-wine stains is

not contraindicated and can begin as soon as seizures are controlled by anticonvulsants. Gum hypertrophy, which is particularly common in patients receiving phenytoin, can be resected with a photocoagulator. Because the malformation is a low-flow one, there is no need for preoperative embolization. Children with a V2 port-wine stain, in association with V1 location, frequently develop an enlarged maxilla. This bony hypertrophy creates an occlusion deformity and crossbite and requires orthodontic evaluation and follow-up. A team approach is very important in managing these patients, because many children need the expertise of neurologists, ophthalmologists, pediatricians, neurosurgeons, dermatologists, plastic surgeons, ear, nose, and throat surgeons, and neuroradiologists.

Klippel–Trenaunay syndrome

KT syndrome (angio-osteohypertrophy) is characterized by a triad of port-wine stain, varicose veins (venous malformation), and bony and/or soft tissue hypertrophy. The cutaneous stains are the earliest sign and are typically limited to a single extremity, although multiple extremities can be involved. A lymphatic component is common, evidenced either by lymphedema or by lymphatic vesicles, usually intermingled with the port-wine stain in the lateral or anterior aspect of the thigh and knee (Fig. 20.24). Osteohypertrophy is rarely present at birth. Overgrowth of the affected limb appears either at birth or within the first few months or years of life. In a review of 144 patients with KT syndrome, 95% had a cutaneous vascular malformation, 93% had soft tissue or bony hypertrophy, 76% had varicosities, and 71% had involvement limited to one leg.[153] The etiology of KT syndrome is unknown. Although it has been suggested that this syndrome may be inherited in a

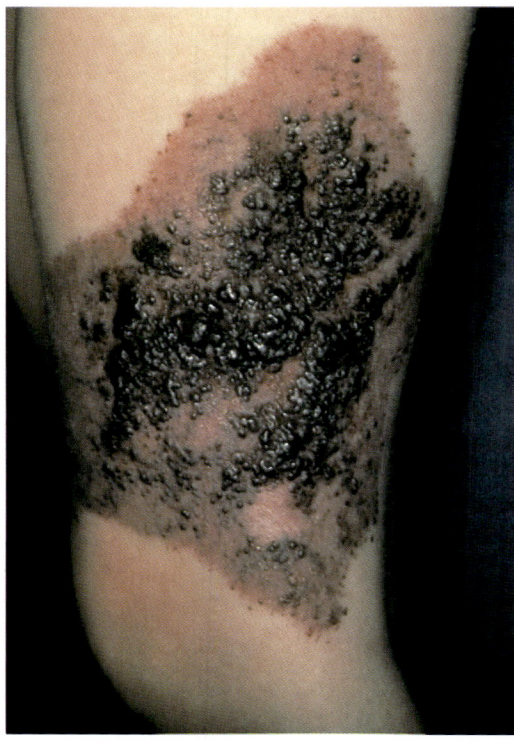

Fig. 20.24 Klippel–Trenaunay syndrome in association with a capillary–lymphatic–venous malformation. The geographic stain and multiple eclasias are common when a lymphatic component is present.

144. Celebi S, Alagoz G, Aykan U (2000) Ocular findings in Sturge–Weber syndrome. Eur J Ophthalmol 10:239–243.
145. Cheng KP (1999) Ophthalmologic manifestations of Sturge–Weber syndrome. In Sturge–Weber Syndrome, Bodensteiner JB, Roach ES, eds. Mt Freedom: Sturge–Weber Foundation, pp. 17–26.
146. Griffiths PD (1996) Sturge–Weber syndrome revisited: the role of neuroradiology. Neuropediatrics 27:284–294.
147. Adamsbaum C, Pinton F, Rolland Y et al. (1996) Accelerated myelination in early Sturge–Weber syndrome: MR–SPECT correlations. Pediatr Radiol 26:759–762.
148. Maria BL, Hoang K, Robertson RL et al. (1999) Imaging brain structure and function in Sturge–Weber syndrome. In Sturge–Weber Syndrome, Bodensteiner JB, Roach ES, eds. Mt Freedom: Sturge–Weber Foundation, pp. 43–69.
149. Pinton F, Chiron C, Enjolras O et al. (1997) Early single photon emission computed tomography in Sturge–Weber syndrome. J Neurol Neurosurg Psychiatry 63:616–621.
150. Maria BL, Neufeld JA, Rosainz LC et al. (1998) Central nervous system structure and function in Sturge–Weber syndrome: evidence of neurologic and radiologic progression. J Child Neurol 13:606–618.
151. Kramer U, Kahana E, Shorer Z et al. (2000) Outcome of infants with unilateral Sturge–Weber syndrome and early onset seizures. Dev Med Child Neurol 42:756–759.
152. Bruce DA (1999) Neurosurgical aspects of Sturge–Weber syndrome. In Sturge^=Weber Syndrome, Bodensteiner JB, Roach ES, eds. Mt Freedom: Sturge–Weber Foundation, pp. 39–42.
153. Gloviczki P, Stanson AW, Stickler GB et al. (1991) Klippel–Trenaunay syndrome: the risks and benefits of vascular interventions. Surgery 110:469.

multifactorial fashion, it is generally a sporadic disorder.[154] It affects males more often than females.

There is no known cure for KT syndrome. Management includes regular visits, with clinical and radiographic measurements of affected limbs at regular intervals. Scanograms should be obtained to evaluate limb length discrepancy more accurately in any children with more than 1–2 cm difference in limb length. Those with significant differences in length should be referred for orthopedic evaluation. Non-invasive arterial/venous evaluation with ultrasonography/Doppler is preferred to conventional contrast angiography and contrast venography during childhood. MR imaging[155] is the single best method for evaluation and delineation of the extent of the disorder. In addition, MR angiography and venography will demonstrate the anomalous vessels, located in the skin and subcutis, and indicate whether muscle involvement is present, although, in contrast to venous malformations, muscle involvement is actually very uncommon. MR lymphography, a new non-invasive tool, is useful for differentiating veins from lymphatics as enlarged axial and extra-axial lymphatic channels may be seen in children with KT syndrome.[155] Pelvic, intestinal, and/or bladder vascular anomalies may be associated.

Treatment of this condition is usually aimed at controlling specific symptoms and is, in general, conservative.[156,157] Compression stockings are a mainstay of treatment, but accurate fitting for these stockings is not usually practical until the child is 2 or 3 years of age. Compressive wraps may be used in younger infants with significant venous congestion. Intermittent pneumatic compression devices can reduce limb size and control varicosities. This modality can be combined with use of elastic garments to provide continuous compression. Surgical correction of varicose veins is controversial. Some feel it is contraindicated and others feel it may be beneficial as long as the deep venous system is intact.[153] Most patients do relatively well with compression alone. Debulking of soft tissue may be indicated to restore function of the affected extremities; however, it carries a high risk of long-term complications (severe scarring, fibrosis, pedal edema). Orthopedic management is mandatory during childhood to decide if epiphysiodesis will be necessary at early puberty, as a means of equalizing the limbs if discrepancy in length is significant.

Other abnormalities have been described in association with KT syndrome, including the association with SWS, ocular anomalies, glaucoma, and retinal exudative vascular masses. Lymphatic obstruction, lymphatic involvement of the lungs,[158] nonimmune hydrops fetalis, severe menorrhagia,[159] cerebral aneurysm, gastrointestinal hemorrhage,[160] and pulmonary embolism[161] have also been reported. Many orthopedic abnormalities have been noted to occur in these patients, including frequent polydactyly and syndactyly that may also suggest possible Proteus syndrome. Patients frequently have a low-grade coagulopathy similar to that seen with venous malformations (see discussion below).

The differential diagnosis of KT syndrome includes extensive pure venous malformations of the extremities,[162] and the Parkes–Weber, and Maffucci syndromes. Features of typical KT syndrome may also occur in Proteus syndrome.

Phakomatosis pigmentovascularis

Phakomatosis pigmentovascularis consists of an extensive port-wine stain accompanied by either melanocytic or epidermal lesions. The melanocytic

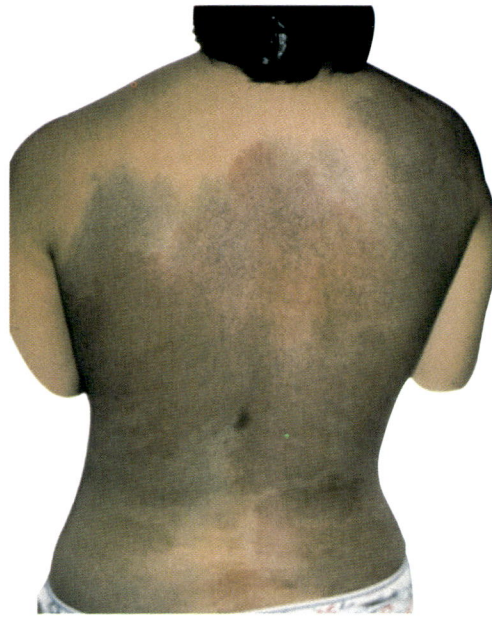

Fig. 20.25 Phakomatosis pigmentovascularis type IIB. This patient also had facial involvement and glaucoma.

lesions may be persistent dermal melanocytosis (Fig. 20.25) or a speckled lentiginous nevus.[163,164] The macules of dermal melanocytosis resembles Mongolian spots and are often present at sites other than the lumbosacral region. In most cases, these lesions are extensive. Four distinct types of phakomatosis pigmentovascularis, all characterized by a port–wine stain and either a pigmented or an epidermal nevus, have been described. Type I has an associated epidermal nevus; type II has dermal melanocytosis (ectopic Mongolian spots) with or without nevus anemicus; type III has a speckled lentiginous nevus with or without nevus anemicus; and type IV has dermal melanocytosis and a speckled lentiginous nevus with or without nevus anemicus. Additional subtypes further classify the disorder as to the absence (type a) or presence (type b) of systemic manifestations. Happle has proposed that phakomatosis pigmentovascularis is caused by so–called "twin spotting."[165]

TELANGIECTASIA

Telangiectasias are dilated small vessels that may or may not blanch on diascopy. They appear on the skin and mucous membranes as small, red, linear, stellate or punctate markings. There are many causes of secondary telangiectasia, such as rosacea, actinic or radiologic damage; various connective tissue diseases; mastocytosis; poikiloderma; prolonged application of topical corticosteroids; and miscellaneous genodermatoses. Primary telangiectases include spider angioma, angioma serpiginosum, HHT, ataxia telangiectasia, generalized essential telangiectasia, hereditary benign telangiectasia, unilateral nevoid telangiectasia, and cutis marmorata telangiectatica congenita.

Spider angioma

The spider angioma (nevus araneus) is the most common of the telangiectases. In adults, spider angiomas frequently develop in large numbers during pregnancy and are also characteristically associated with liver disease. In

154. Aelvoet GE, Jorens PG, Roelen LM (1992) Genetic aspects of the Klippel–Trenaunay syndrome. **Br J Dermatol** 126:603–607.
155. Laor T, Hoffer FA, Burrows PE et al. (1998) MR lymphangiography in infants, children and adults. **Am J Roentgenol** 171:1111–1117.
156. Rogalski R, Hensinger R, Loder R (1993) Vascular abnormalities of the extremities: clinical findings and management. **J Pediatr Orthopaed** 13:9–14.
157. Berry SA, Peterson C, Mize W et al. (1998) Klippel Trenaunay syndrome. **Am J Med Genet** 79:319–326.
158. Joshi M, Cole S, Knibbs D et al. (1992) Pulmonary abnormalities in Klippel–Trenaunay syndrome. **Chest** 102:1274.
159. Markos AR (1987) Klippel–Trenaunay syndrome-a rare cause of severe menorrhagia. **Br J Obstet Gynaecol** 94:1105.
160. Azizkhan RG (1991) Life-threatening hematochezia from a rectosigmoid vascular malformation in Klippel–Trenaunay syndrome: long term palliation using an argon laser. **J Pediatr Surg** 26:1125.
161. Gianlupi A, Harper R, Dwyre D et al. (1999) Recurrent pulmonary embolism associated with Klippel–Trenaunay-Weber syndrome. **Chest** 115:1199–1201.
162. Enjolras O, Ciabrini D, Mazoyer E et al. (1997) Extensive pure venous malformations in the upper or lower limb, a review of 27 cases. **J Am Acad Dermatol** 36:219–225.
163. Ruiz-Maldonado R, Tamayo L, Laterza AM et al. (1987) Phakomatosis pigmentovascularis: a new syndrome? Report of 4 cases. **Pediatr Dermatol** 4:189–196.
164. Guiglia MC, Prendiville JS (1991) Multiple granular cell tumors associated with giant speckled lentiginous nevus and nevus flammeus in a child. **J Am Acad Dermatol** 24:359–362.
165. Happle R (1991) Allelic somatic mutations may explain vascular twin nevi. **Hum Genet** 86:321–322.

childhood, however, these lesions are commonly found in the absence of systemic disorders.

The spider angioma is composed of small telangiectases radiating from a central point in fine hair-like branches. The central point or punctum is an arteriole from which the superficial blood vessels radiate peripherally. Because the central vessel is an arteriole and blood flow is centrifugal, gradually increasing pressure over the central vessel will cause blanching of the lesion in a centripetal fashion. This phenomenon will help to differentiate the spider angioma from other telangiectases.

In childhood, spider angiomas appear most commonly on the face (malar areas), upper trunk, arms, and hands. They are never present at birth but are often detectable after 2 years of age, reaching a frequency of 30% of normal children by age 4 and 40% by age 8. The prevalence figures start to decline in the early teens to approximately 10–15% in the adult population.[166] From these data, it is clear that more than 50% of spider nevi disappear by adult life.

Therapy for the spider nevus, when desired for cosmetic reasons, consists of gentle electrodesiccation of the central vessel or ablation of the lesion by the PDL. Almost immediately after coagulating the central vessel, all the branches disappear.

Angioma serpiginosum

Angioma serpiginosum is a distinctive rare entity involving the capillaries of the dermis. The onset of this condition is usually in childhood, and 90% of the reported cases have been in females.[167]

The primary lesion consists of an asymptomatic vascular ectasia that appears clinically as a minute, partly compressible, red-to-purple punctum, which may require slight magnification for visualization. These small puncta appear in groups that fuse into patches and spread by forming new satellite puncta at the periphery. This extension results in the formation of annular or serpiginous patterns. Because of the confluence of capillary ectasias, there may be an erythematous background. Angioma serpiginosum usually develops on the lower extremities and the buttocks, but occasionally lesions occur elsewhere. Although the lesions extend gradually, widespread cutaneous involvement is infrequent. The condition is progressive despite periods of relative stability; although areas of fading and involution are evident, complete spontaneous resolution does not occur.

Angioma serpiginosum can be confused with the various pigmented purpuric eruptions; however, it is not a capillaritis but rather a nevoid telangiectatic condition. There is no evidence of variegated pigmentation, scaling, atrophy, or lichenification in angioma serpiginosum. These lesions must also be distinguished from other localized telangiectases.

Histopathologically, the fundamental lesion is a dilatation of the capillaries of papillary and subpapillary regions of the dermis. The vessel walls may be slightly thickened. Other dermal structures are normal. An inflammatory infiltrate is not a significant feature, and no red cell diapedesis or hemosiderin pigment is present.

Obliteration of angioma serpiginosum is probably best accomplished by laser therapy.

Hereditary hemorrhagic telangiectasia (Osler-Weber-Rendu disease)

This autosomal-dominant mucocutaneous and visceral vascular malformation is characterized by the triad of telangiectasia, recurrent epistaxis, and a positive family history of the disorder. Completely normal carriers are rare, but about 20% of patients are unaware of other affected family members. HHT is heterogeneous in terms of age of onset and clinical expression. In a given family, symptoms and severity may vary considerably even in individuals with the same mutation.[168] Recurrent epistaxis from telangiectases over the nasal septum and inferior turbinates is the presenting sign in over 50% of individuals and occurs in approximately 80% of patients at some time during their course.[169,170] This manifestation is usually seen by puberty, in contrast to hemorrhage from other sites such as the gastrointestinal and genitourinary tracts, which occur later in life. Epistaxis may become severe, requiring transfusions. Anemia is a common complication.

The mucocutaneous lesions are not commonly observed in childhood but generally become evident during the third or fourth decade, occasionally somewhat earlier. These vascular lesions develop primarily on the face, lips, nasal mucosa, tongue, palms, and palate, but they can also be found in the nail beds, on the soles of the feet, and even on the tympanic membrane. They are dark red and tend to be slightly elevated, with an ill-defined border and one or more legs radiating from an eccentrically placed punctum.

Gastrointestinal hemorrhage is the second most common complication, occurring in about 40% of affected individuals; however, unlike epistaxis, onset of this complication is rare before midlife. Bleeding may occur from lesions in the upper and lower bowel, but despite careful evaluation by endoscopy and radiologic studies, the bleeding site may remain undetermined. The bleeding pattern is one of chronicity and recurrence and tends to be progressive as new telangiectases appear.

Some patients have pulmonary AVMs, and one-third have multiple pulmonary lesions. Patients may be asymptomatic or may exhibit dyspnea, cyanosis, fingernail clubbing, and polycythemia; both ischemic and septic neurologic complications may ensue as a result of these lesions.[168–170] In addition, a small number of affected individuals have cerebral telangiectases, aneurysms, and AVMs of the brain and spinal cord, giving rise to focal and generalized neurologic deficits. Hepatic AVMs can cause liver enlargement and portal hypertension. Liver disease in HHT is rare but severe, combining vascular anomalies, fibrosis, and cirrhosis;[171] these patients may develop a severe coagulopathic disorder as a result of the cirrhosis, complicating any surgical procedure on their vascular lesions.

HHT involves capillaries, arteries, veins and arteriovenous fistulae, and the combinations of vessels vary in different individuals. Cutaneous telangiectases are composed of a subepidermal tortuous mass of dilated capillaries and post-capillary venules with markedly thinned walls comprising a single layer of endothelium. Hemorrhage is thought to result from malformation of the vessel walls or possibly defects in the surrounding perivascular tissue. No specific hematologic defects have been consistently identified.

New advances in molecular genetics have helped to explain the previously obscure heterogeneity of HHT. It is now clear that there are various phenotypes and genotypes. Identification of two genes *endoglin* (for HHT type 1) and *ALK-1* (for HHT type 2), both of which can be affected by differing intragenic mutations, have brought new insights in the pathogenesis of HHT, as well as the hope of new treatments.[172] Genotype–phenotype correlations are not yet completely defined; however, pulmonary AVMs seem more common in HHT1 than in HHT2, and hepatic AVMs are more common in HHT2.[168] Other genes may be involved, as demonstrated by a family with HHT and pulmonary AVMs[173] when no genetic abnormality could be established.

The vast majority of patients survive the disease and die of some other cause, although frequent treatment for hemorrhages and anemia is a lifelong necessity. Therapy is primarily directed at the control of hemorrhage and blood replacement. The local therapy of the bleeding nasal telangiectases with chemical cautery or electrocoagulation has temporary value, as does tamponade. For severe recurrent epistaxis, laser coagulation, sclerotherapy by means of direct puncture of the telangiectases, or septal dermoplasty are the

166. Wenzl JR, Burgert EO (1964) The spider nevus in infancy and childhood. **Pediatrics** 33:227–232.
167. Stevenson JR, Lincoln CS (1967) Angioma serpiginosum. **Arch Dermatol** 95:16–22.
168. Mc Donald JE, Miller FJ, Hallam SE et al. (2000) Clinical manifestations in a large hereditary hemorrhagic telangiectasia (HHT) type 2 kindred. **Am J Med Genet** 93:320–327.
169. Porteous MEM, Burn J, Proctor SJ (1992) Hereditary hemorrhagic telangiectasia: a clinical analysis. **J Med Genet** 29:527.
170. Reilly PJ, Nostrant TT (1984) Clinical manifestations of hereditary hemorrhagic telangiectasia. **Am J Gastroenterol** 79:363.
171. Weik C, Johanns W, Janssen J et al. (2000) The liver and hereditary hemorrhagic telangiectasia. **Gastroenterology** 38:31–37.
172. Azuma H (2000) Genetic and molecular pathogenesis of hereditary hemorrhagic telangiectasia. **J Med Invest** 47:81–90.
173. Wallace GM, Shovlin CL (2000) A hereditary hemorrhagic telangiectasia family with pulmonary involvement is unlinked to the known *HHT* genes, endoglin and ALK-1. **Thorax** 5:685–690.

treatments of choice. Resection or, if possible, embolization of pulmonary AVMs is mandatory in order to prevent the occurrence of pulmonary insufficiency, high-output heart failure, or brain abscess (owing to loss of pulmonary filtration of bacteria). Treatment of AVMs in other locations depends on accessibility. Genetic counseling should be offered to all affected individuals, and if both partners are affected, they should be warned that the homozygous state might be lethal in childhood.

Generalized essential telangiectasia

This uncommon disorder might more appropriately be called **essential progressive telangiectasia**, because it does not become generalized until many years after its onset. The condition occurs more frequently in females and most commonly develops in late childhood or early adult life. It is not familial. It usually begins on the legs and slowly spreads to involve the thighs, lower abdomen, occasionally the arms, and rarely the face. The telangiectases are macular, retiform, and linear and may coalesce to form confluent sheets over large areas. Occasionally, patients experience sensations of numbness, tingling, and burning in an involved limb.[174]

Essential telangiectasia must be differentiated from relangiectasia secondary to underlying disease as well as from HHT. For some patients, it represents a serious cosmetic problem, and lasers offer the best option for successful treatment.

Hereditary benign telangiectasia

Hereditary benign telangiectasia has been described in several kindreds. Affected persons were noted to have widespread asymptomatic telangiectases unassociated with systemic disease.[175,176] It is inherited as an autosomal dominant trait. The telangiectases are not present at birth or during the first year of life but begin to appear between 2 and 12 years of age. Predominantly affected areas are the face, arms, and upper trunk, but lesions have been noted on the vermilion border of the lips and palate in some individuals. Typical lesions are macular, punctate or plaque-like, radiating, arborizing, or merely a diffuse blush; they often have a halo of pallor. Capillary microscopy reveals that the main feature is dilatation of the horizontal subpapillary venous plexus. This is accompanied by loss of the more superficial capillaries that normally stain with alkaline phosphatase and supply the papillae. The disorder is slowly progressive, but in old age it becomes less obvious because of the normal skin changes of aging.

Hereditary benign telangiectasia must be differentiated from other primary telangiectases, the most important of which is HHT. Intervention is unnecessary except for cosmetic reasons; as with other benign telangiectasias, laser therapy or electrocautery may help to improve the lesions.

Unilateral nevoid telangiectasia

Unilateral nevoid telangiectasia (also known as unilateral dermatomal superficial telangiectasia) is a relatively rare condition that occurs in both a congenital and an acquired form. The acquired type has occurred mainly in females, either at puberty or during pregnancy, and is thought to be estrogen related; this disorder has also occurred in male alcoholics suffering from cirrhosis of the liver.[177] Some authors have proposed that this entity represents a localized form of generalized essential telangiectasia.[177]

Congenital unilateral nevoid telangiectasia has been documented only rarely and reportedly affects males predominantly.[178] None of the children reported have had evidence of endocrine abnormalities.[178]

Lesions occur unilaterally on the face, neck, chest, and arms (trigeminal, C3 and C4 or adjacent dermatomes) and only rarely elsewhere. They are evident as macular telangiectatic mats, although elevated puncta and even pulsatile spider angiomas may be found in some cases. Lesions fade on pressure. Blanching or vasoconstriction surrounding individual lesions is common and represents "vascular steal." In the congenital type, the telangiectasia is permanent; the acquired form of the disorder (e.g., onset during pregnancy) may resolve spontaneously in some patients. Lasers with selectivity for cutaneous vascular structures are the best treatment for areas causing disfigurement.

Cutis marmorata telangiectatica congenita

Cutis marmorata telangiectatica congenita (CMTC), also known as **congenital generalized phlebectasia**, is an unusual, clinically distinctive cutaneous vascular anomaly. The variable presence of cutaneous atrophy and/or coexistent port-wine stains are frequent. The condition is said to be rare. However, one report of 13 cases, 10 of them seen by one physician in a 10-year period,[179] and another of 22 patients seen by a single physician in an 8-year period,[180] suggest that many instances of CMTC remain undiagnosed. The etiology is unclear, and there is no evidence of genetic origin. It is usually stated that CMTC occurs predominantly in females, but in four large series the male to female ratios were 7:6, 9:13, 5:5, and 5:3, respectively.[179–182]

This disorder, which is present at birth, mimics the physiologic vascular marbling effect (cutis marmorata) commonly seen in young infants,

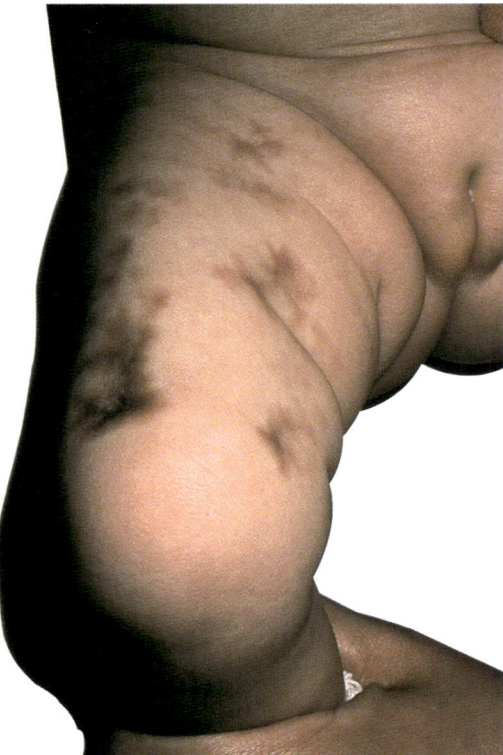

Fig. 20.26 Cutis marmorata telangiectatica congenita.

174. Abrahamian LM, Rothe MJ, Grant-Kels JM (1992) Primary telangiectasia of childhood. Int J Dermatol 31:307.

175. Ryan TJ, Wells RS (1971) Hereditary benign telangiectasia. St Johns Hosp Dermatol Soc Trans 57:148–156.

176. Gold MH, Eramo L, Prendiville JS (1989) Hereditary benign telangiectasia. Pediatr Dermatol 6:194–197.

177. Colver GB, Shrank AB, Ryan TJ (1985) Unilateral dermatomal superficial telangiectasia. Clin Exp Dermatol 10:455.

178. Wilkin JK, Smith JG, Jr., Cullison DA et al. (1983) Unilateral dermatomal superficial telangiectasia: 9 new cases and a review of unilateral dermatomal superficial telangiectasia. J Am Acad Dermatol 8:468–77.

179. South DA, Jacobs AH (1993) Cutis marmorata telangiectatica congenita (congenital generalized phlebectasia). J Pediatr 93:944–949.

180. Picascia DD, Esterly NB (1989) Cutis marmorata telangiectatica congenital; report of 22 cases. J Am Acad Dermatol 20:1098–1104.

181. Kennedy C, Oranje AP, Keizer K et al. (1992) Cutis marmorata telangiectatica congenita. Int J Dermatol 31:249–252.

182. Pehr K, Moroz B (1993) Cutis marmorata telangiectatica congenita: long-term follow-up, review of the literature, and report of a case in conjunction with congenital hypothyroidism. Pediatr Dermatol 10:6–11.

particularly when they are chilled or exposed to low environmental temperatures. However, the pattern of CMTC is more vivid and darker in color, with a coarser pattern of mottling (Fig. 20.26). Although it is always discernible at rest, it can be accentuated by cold exposure, vigorous movement, or crying. The reticulated mottling of the skin is accompanied by varying degrees of telangiectasia, phlebectasia, ulcerations with crusts, and atrophy.[179,183] The pattern of CMTC may be either generalized or localized, often with a segmental distribution and a sharp midline demarcation. The extremities are most commonly affected, followed by the torso, and only rarely the face, palms, soles, and mucous membranes.

Most patients with CMTC experience definite improvement of their mottled vascular pattern, with the most dramatic change occurring in the first year and tapering thereafter. It has been theorized that this improvement may be a result of the normal maturation process with thickening of the epidermis and dermis. However persistence of a purple vascular reticulated network is a common finding.[184]

Associated abnormalities occur in up to 50% of patients but may be overstated through ascertainment bias.[184] The following have been reported: subcutaneous atrophy, deep ulceration, port-wine stain, body asymmetry (both hemiatrophy and hemihypertrophy), dystrophic teeth, glaucoma, patent ductus arteriosus, pulmonary hypertension, mental retardation, SWS, macrocephaly, varicosities, hemangiomas, syndactyly, hypothyroidism, and delayed psychomotor development. CMTC has been described as an associated finding in a large number of patients with the Adams–Oliver syndrome, which is characterized by distal transverse limb defects and aplasia cutis congenita.[185] Decrease in the size of an affected limb is probably the most common finding associated with CMTC,[186] especially those with involvement of the lower limb.[187] A decrease in girth, rather than length, is obvious in some infants with a single affected limb. Clinically, CMTC must be differentiated from physiologic cutis marmorata and from genuine diffuse phlebectasia of Bockenheimer. The latter is a deep venous malformation that begins in childhood rather than being present at birth, with the gradual development of multiple large venous sinusoids. It may be difficult to distinguish CMTC from a reticulated port-wine stain. Persistent livedo and telangiectases resembling CMTC have been described in neonates with Down syndrome, Cornelia de Lange syndrome, homocystinuria, neonatal lupus erythematosus, and other genetic, neurologic, and metabolic conditions. A distinct syndrome (or phenotype?) of macrocephaly and cutis marmorata, reminiscent of CMTC, includes a high risk of growth disturbances and cardiac and neurologic complications.[188]

The microscopic findings in CMTC are not specific, and diagnosis is best made on the basis of clinical criteria. The histologic appearance usually consists of an increased number of dermal thin-walled dilated capillaries, occasionally with venous lakes and large dilated veins in all layers of the dermis and subcutaneous tissue. Cutaneous atrophy, ulceration, and microthromboses may also be evident histopathologically.

The management of CMTC involves careful examination for associated disorders. Laser therapy may help those components with true capillary malformation. Occasionally, ulcerations may be severe enough to require specific ulcer wound care regimens. They may also become secondarily infected and may require topical or systemic antibiotics.

ANGIOKERATOMAS

The term angiokeratoma is applied to a group of disorders characterized by ectasia of the superficial dermal vessels (capillaries) and compact hyperkeratosis of the overlying epidermis.[107] All present as asymptomatic, firm, dark-red to black papules, with varying degrees of secondary hyperkeratosis, increasing with time. Classically, four types of localized angiokeratoma are described, all of which are probably related but vary in size, depth, and location. They are solitary papular angiokeratoma, angiokeratoma circumscriptum, angiokeratoma of Mibelli, and angiokeratoma of the scrotum and vulva. Angiokeratoma corporis diffusum represents a distinctive fifth group. In addition, angiokeratomas may occur in the setting of KT syndrome.

Papular angiokeratoma

Papular angiokeratomas represent a response to trauma and can occur at any age and at any site, although the legs are the favored location. They can be solitary or multiple and consist of blue-black warty papules 2–10mm in diameter. A single angiokeratoma may be mistaken for a viral wart, nevus, or malignant melanoma, but it can be differentiated on the basis of histopathologic examination or dematoscopy. Microscopic features include grouped dilated papillary blood vessels, acanthosis and hyperkeratosis of the epidermis, and elongation of the rete ridges, which tend to enclose the underlying capillary spaces. Treatment of a solitary angiokeratoma for cosmetic reasons or because of undue anxiety can be accomplished by local excision, electrodesiccation, or by laser ablation.

Angiokeratoma circumscriptum

Angiokeratoma circumscriptum is a rare disorder typically appearing as a large, solitary, hyperkeratotic plaque on a lower extremity. The most common sites of involvement are the extremities. These vascular malformations may be present at birth or develop during infancy or childhood. They extend during adolescence. The aggregates of warty, keratotic, deep-red to blue-black papules and nodules are often distributed in a band-like configuration. These angiokeratomas may enlarge to form a plaque several centimeters in size; there are reports of lesions as large as one-quarter of the body.

Microscopically, these lesions consist of dilated capillaries, some of which may be thrombosed, in the papillary dermis. The closely approximated epidermis is papillomatous, acanthotic, and hyperkeratotic.

Angiokeratoma circumscriptum may be confused with the so-called **verrucous hemangioma**; however, in the latter, the abnormal vascular structures extend into the deep dermis and subcutaneous tissue. Verrucous "hemangioma" is a misnomer[107] for a vascular malformation with hyperkeratosis and involvement of capillaries, veins, and, in some cases, lymphatics.

Distinctive hyperkeratotic, cutaneous capillary–venous malformations resembling angiokeratomas have been described in a small group of patients with **cerebral capillary malformations** (also known as **familial cerebral cavernomas**). These patients may present with headaches and life-threatening cerebral hemorrhages.[189] In some families, the skin lesion represented a hallmark for risk of brain involvement.[190] The first mutated gene, *CCM1*, detected is located on 7q21-22 and encodes the protein KRIT-1.

Angiokeratoma circumscriptum has also been confused with lymphangioma circumscriptum, both clinically and histologically. Thrombosis within a solitary angiokeratoma may cause changes in size and color simulating melanoma.[191] Small lesions can be removed by electrodesiccation and curettage, cryosurgery or laser ablation; for larger lesions surgical excision is the treatment of choice.

183. Gerritsen MJ, Steijlen PM, Brunner HG et al. (2000) Cutis Marmorata telangiectatica congenita. **Br J Dermatol** 142:366–369.

184. Enjolras O (2001) Cutis Marmorata telangiectatica congenita. **Ann Dermatol Venereol** 128:161–166.

185. Dyall-Smith D, Ramsden A, Laurie S (1994) Adams Oliver syndrome: aplasia cutis congenital, terminal transverse limb defects and cutis marmorata telangiectatica congenital. **Australas J Dermatol** 35:19–22.

186. Devillers ACA, de Waard-van der Spek FB, Oranje AP (1999) Cutis marmorata telangiectatica congenita. Clinical features in 35 cases. **Arch Dermatol** 135:34–38.

187. Ben Amitai A, Fichman S, Merlob P et al. (2000) Cutis marmorata telangiectatica congenital: clinical findings in 85 patients. **Pediatr Dermatol** 17:100–104.

188. Yano S, Watanabe Y (2001) Association of arrhythmia and sudden death in macrocephaly-cutis marmorata telangiectatica congenita syndrome. **Am J Med Genet** 102:149–152.

189. Labauge P, Enjolras O, Bonerandi JJ et al. (1999) An association between autosomal dominant cerebral cavernomas and a distinctive hyperkeratotic capillaro-venous cutaneous vascular malformation in 4 families. **Ann Neurol** 45:250–254.

190. Eerola I, Plate KH, Spiegel R et al. (2000) KRIT 1 is mutated in hyperkeratotic cutaneous capillaro-venous malformation associated with cerebral capillary malformation. **Hum Mol Genet** 9:1351–1355.

191. Goldman L, Gibson SH, Richfield DF (1981) Thrombotic angiokeratoma circumscriptum simulating melanoma. **Arch Dermatol** 117:138.

Angiokeratoma of Mibelli

Angiokeratoma of Mibelli is a rare condition that occurs primarily in female children and adolescents. It has been seen in siblings and in children with an affected parent, suggesting a dominant mode of inheritance with variable penetrance.[192]

The frequent association of lesions with acrocyanosis, chilblains, and frostbite suggests that cold sensitivity is the precipitating factor of this disorder. The lesions are most often seen on the dorsal and lateral aspects of the toes and fingers, and the knees and elbows. Less frequently, they arise on the knuckles, malleoli, palms, soles, and ears. Early lesions are minute bright-red macules that fade somewhat on diascopic pressure. They slowly increase in size and become elevated, warty, and darker in color, attaining a diameter of 5–10 mm. The papules are asymptomatic but bleed easily. There is no tendency for spontaneous involution, although occasionally involution may occur following trauma.

Microscopically, there are ectatic vessels in the papillary dermis. The epidermis is hyperkeratotic and often acanthotic, with elongated rete ridges that enclose the vascular lacunae. There may be some cellular infiltrates, which are predominantly lymphocytic. Clinically these lesions may resemble those of **acral pseudolymphomatous angiokeratoma of children (APACHE)**. However, pseudolymphomatous angiokeratoma is usually unilateral, unassociated with cold exposure, and has histologic features of a pseudolymphoma rather than true angiokeratoma.[193,194] Treatment of angiokeratoma of Mibelli consists of cryosurgery, electrodesiccation, or laser ablation.

Angiokeratoma of the scrotum and vulva (Fordyce)

Although relatively common, angiokeratomas of the scrotum and vulva are primarily a phenomenon of aging. The lesions usually appear in middle to later adult life and arise as multiple, small, bright-red vascular papules that subsequently become keratotic. They are distributed along the superficial veins of the scrotum and rarely over the penis, inguinal area, and upper thighs in men and on the labia majora in women. With increasing age, they may become quite numerous. On occasion, these angiokeratomas become bothersome and may itch or bleed when traumatized.

The diagnosis of angiokeratoma corporis diffusum must be considered in any patient with these lesions, particularly if onset is early in life. Symptomatic lesions can be removed with cryotherapy, electrodesiccation, or laser ablation.

Angiokeratoma corporis diffusum

In the past, angiokeratoma corporis diffusum has been used synonymously with Fabry syndrome, but, currently, it can only be used as a descriptive term because the characteristic clinical findings can be seen in patients with several metabolic diseases as well as in some metabolically normal individuals.[195]

Anderson-Fabry disease (Fabry disease; angiokeratoma corporis diffusum)

Fabry disease is a rare X-linked recessive lysosomal storage disorder caused by an error in glycosphingolipid catabolism. The defect in α-galactosidase A results in intracellular accumulation of globotriaosylceramide (ceramide trihexoside), which is responsible for the multisystemic involvement. Various mutations have been described in the gene for α-galactosidase A.[196] The disorder exhibits complete penetrance but variable clinical expressivity in hemizygous males. Heterozygous females generally have α-galactosidase A activity and plasma globotriaosylceramide levels intermediate to that of hemizygous males and normal individuals. Among female carriers, 15% have

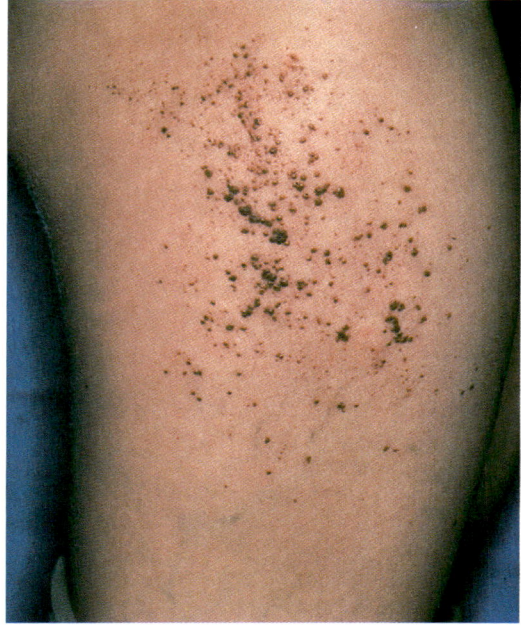

Fig. 20.27 Fabry disease with multiple angiokeratomas in a mother of an affected male.

similar clinical findings in one or more organs, and approximately 70% show evidence of the distinctive whorl-like corneal dystrophy.[197]

The first sign of Fabry syndrome is the onset of cutaneous vascular lesions, usually between 5 and 10 years of age, although occasionally as late as age 20. The lesions are small macules and papules, red, purple, or dark blue, usually 1–2mm in size (Fig. 20.27). They develop on the trunk predominantly, particularly on the periumbilical skin, genitalia, inguinal folds, upper thighs, buttocks, and lumbosacral area, seldom occurring on the hands, feet, or face. They are distributed symmetrically and do not blanch with pressure. These angiokeratomas gradually increase in size and number with age and persist indefinitely. The overlying hyperkeratosis is of a very mild degree.

The oral (and occasionally nasal) mucosa is involved in most of the patients with Fabry disease. Typical lesions are small discrete blue papules, which on the vermilion border of the lower lip resemble petechiae. These lesions have also been identified in the gastrointestinal, genitourinary, and respiratory mucosae.

A decrease in sweating is often noted by the time puberty begins. Sweating may be entirely absent by the third decade, with the exception of the face where sweating may be normal or increased. Bouts of severe, often excruciating, pain occur in association with fever of unknown origin and paresthesias in the hands and feet. The pain, caused by vasomotor disturbances, usually occurs subsequent to changes in temperature, but it also may be spontaneous or elicited by exertion or emotional stress. Pedal and ankle edema is usually present and may result in stasis ulcers. These findings are believed to be caused by impaired autonomic reflexes resulting from glycolipid deposits in the autonomic and sensory ganglia.[198]

Involvement of the ocular tissues occurs early in the disease. The conjunctiva, cornea, lens, and retina can all be affected. Deposits of glycosphingolipid in the corneal epithelium produce a corneal opacity with a characteristic whorled vortex configuration (corneal verticillata) that is asymptomatic and visible only on slit-lamp examination. The opacities are usually present during childhood and are found in all affected males as well

192. Smith RBW, Prior IAM, Park RG (1968) Angiokeratoma of Mibelli: a family with nodular lesions of the legs. **Aust J Dermatol** 9:329.
193. Ramsay B, Dahl MCG, Malcolm AJ et al. (1990) Acral pseudolymphomatous angiokeratoma of children. **Arch Dermatol** 126:1524.
194. Hara M, Matsunaga J, Tagami H (1991) Acral pseudolymphomatous angiokeratoma of children (APACHE): a case report and immunohistological study. **Br J Dermatol** 124:387.
195. Gasparini G, Sarchi G, Cavicchini S, Bertagnolio B (1992) Angiokeratoma corporis diffusum in a patient with normal enzyme activities and Turner's syndrome. **Clin Exp Dermatol** 17:56.
196. Ashton-Prolla P, Tong B, Shabbeer J et al. (2000) Fabry disease: twenty-two novel mutations in the alpha-galactosidase A gene and genotype/phenotype correlations in severely and mildly affected hemizygotes and heterozygotes. **J Invest Med** 48:227–235.
197. Burda CD, Winder PR (1967) Angiokeratoma corporis diffusum universale in female subjects. **Am J Med** 42:293.
198. Brady RO, Schiffmann R (2000) Clinical features and recent advances in therapy for Fabry disease. **J Am Med Assoc** 284:2771–2775.

as almost all female carriers and are thus highly diagnostic of the disease. A pathognomonic posterior cortical cataract with narrow wavy spokes also develops in the lens of about 50% of the hemizygotes but not in the heterozygous females. Ectasia and tortuosity of the conjunctival and retinal vessels are another early finding.

The onset of renal involvement during early adult life is indicated by abnormal findings on urinalysis or renal biopsy. Renal failure, the most common cause of death, usually ensues. Hypertension, angina pectoris, and congestive heart failure are also frequent findings. Myocardial infarction may occur as early as age 29, and cerebrovascular disease also may be evident in early adult life. Death usually occurs by age 40 as a result of renal, cardiac, or cerebrovascular disease.

The diagnosis of Fabry disease should be suspected in any individual with the characteristic clinical findings, a positive family history, and a marked decrease in activity of α-galactosidase A in white blood cells or cultured fibroblasts. Early in the course of the disease, casts, red cells, fat-laden epithelial cells (mulberry cells), and lipid inclusions with characteristic birefringent "Maltese crosses" appear in the urinary sediment. Biopsy of the skin or kidney is confirmatory if intracellular birefringent lipoid deposits can be demonstrated. Skin biopsy specimens contain deposits of glycosphingolipid in the walls of the blood vessels, which stain positively with Sudan black and periodic acid–Schiff reagent. Analysis of genomic DNA, isolated from patients and related family members, allows the accurate detection of heterozygous carriers, so that effective genetic counseling can be provided.[196] Prenatal diagnosis in a pregnant female carrier is possible by demonstration of deficient α-galactosidase activity in cultured cells obtained by amniocentesis or biopsies of chorionic villi, or by detecting mutations in the gene.[197]

Treatment of Fabry disease has traditionally been supportive, but recently recombinant human α-galactosidase replacement therapy has been shown to clear microvascular endothelial deposits of globotriaosylceramide from the kidney, heart and skin in patients with Fabry's disease, offering hope of a specific biologic treatment.[199] Protection from extremes of temperature is advised. Phenytoin and carbamazepine have been found to provide relief from the severe pain crises of Fabry syndrome, although the latter drug may exacerbate autonomic dysfunction in some patients. Hemodialysis is indicated for chronic renal failure; renal transplantation has restored renal function and provided a source of functional enzyme in some individuals.

Fucosidosis

Disseminated angiokeratomas may also be seen in patients with fucosidosis,[200] an autosomal-recessive lysosomal storage disorder, caused by deficient $α_1$-fucosidase activity in all tissues. This very rare disorder is manifest by accumulation of fucose-containing glycolipids and glycoproteins in the skin and other organs; various kinds of mutation of the gene *FUCA 1* lead to nearly absent enzyme function.[201] Phenotypically, there is a spectrum of severity of the disease. Patients dying at an early age usually lack the angiokeratomas that develop later in the course.

Common clinical manifestations include progressive mental and motor deterioration, coarse facies, growth retardation, recurrent infections, dysostosis multiplex, visceromegaly, and seizures. Angiokeratoma corporis diffusum is seen in more than 50% of patients. The skin lesions appear in the groin and on the genitalia, rarely as early as 6 months of age but more often later in life, and gradually spread over the trunk and limbs. Mats of telangiectases develop on the palms and soles and occasionally on the trunk as well. The gingivae may also be the site of vascular ectasia, and there is dilatation and tortuosity of the conjunctival vessels in almost all affected individuals. Sweating abnormalities, both hypo- and hyperhidrosis, have been recorded in a number of patients.

Clinical differences[202] distinguish fucosidosis from other metabolic disorders characterized by angiokeratomas. The diagnosis is firmly established by biochemical assay of fucosidase enzyme activity in fibroblasts or peripheral leukocytes. The gene *FUCA* has been localized to chromosome 1. Fucosidase assays of amniocytes and direct detection of the mutation by DNA analysis should permit prenatal diagnosis.

Miscellaneous disorders with angiokeratomas

Several other rare metabolic disorders are associated with angiokeratomas. These include β-galactosidase deficiency (GM1 gangliosidosis), sialidosis with combined deficiency of β-galactosidase and neuraminidase, aspartyl glycosaminuria, mannosidosis, partial combined deficiency of fucosidase and α-galactosidase, and α-*N*-acetylgalactosaminidase deficiency.[202] Several well-studied patients with angiokeratoma corporis diffusum with and without systemic abnormalities but without demonstrable enzyme defects have also been reported.

VENOUS MALFORMATIONS

Venous malformations are usually evident at birth and may occur either as localized or segmental lesions with no associated abnormalities or as a part of a complex syndrome. Lesions comprise anomalous dilated veins with irregularly thickened walls, which often have focal regions lacking smooth muscle cells.[9,107,109] There are slit-like or open lumens. Interconnected channels dissect through normal tissues. Thromboses give rise to calcifications, which can become progressively more evident over time as phleboliths.

The clinical expression, sequelae, and management of venous malformation differ, depending on the age of the patient, the severity, and the anatomic location, but they share some common features. Venous malformations give a blue hue to the involved skin and mucous membranes. They can be small and well localized (Fig. 20.28) or large, crossing several anatomic planes (Fig. 20.29). They swell and enlarge when dependent and with exertion or activities (such as Valsalva maneuver or crying) that increase venous pressure. Skin temperature is normal or minimally warm; neither thrill nor bruit is present. Pain is variable but fairly common. Slow enlargement is commonly observed over time. Radiologic imaging is helpful in delineating the extent

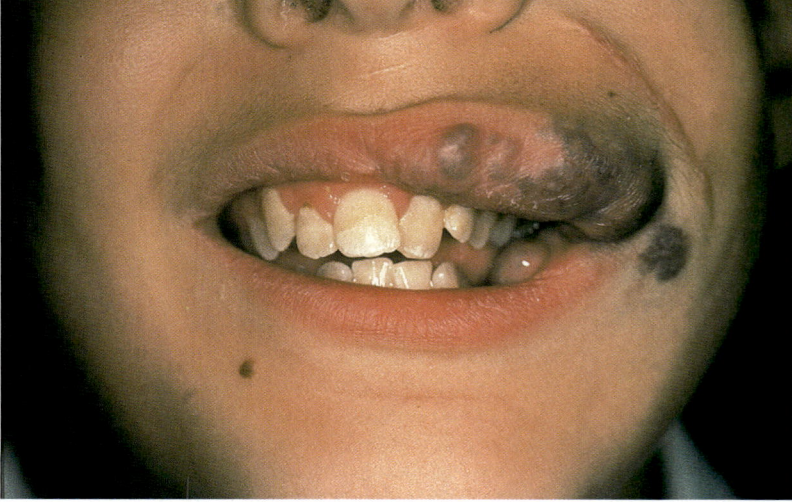

Fig. 20.28 Venous malformation of the lip and oral mucosa, resulting in an openbite.

199. Eng CM, Guffon N, Wilcox WR et al. (2001) Safety and efficacy of recombinant human α-Galactosidase A replacement therapy in Fabry's disease. **N Engl J Med** 345:9–16.
200. Willems PJ, Seo HC, Coucke P et al. (1999) Spectrum of mutations in fucosidosis. **Eur J Med Genet** 7:60–67.
201. Fleming C, Rennie A, Fallowfield M et al. (1997) Cutaneous manifestations of fucosidosis. **Br J Dermatol.** 136:594–597.
202. Kodama K, Kobayashi R, Abe A et al. (2001) A new case of *N*-acetylgalactosaminidase deficiency with angiokeratoma corporis diffusum, with Menière's syndrome and without mental retardation. **Br J Dermatol.** 144:363–368.

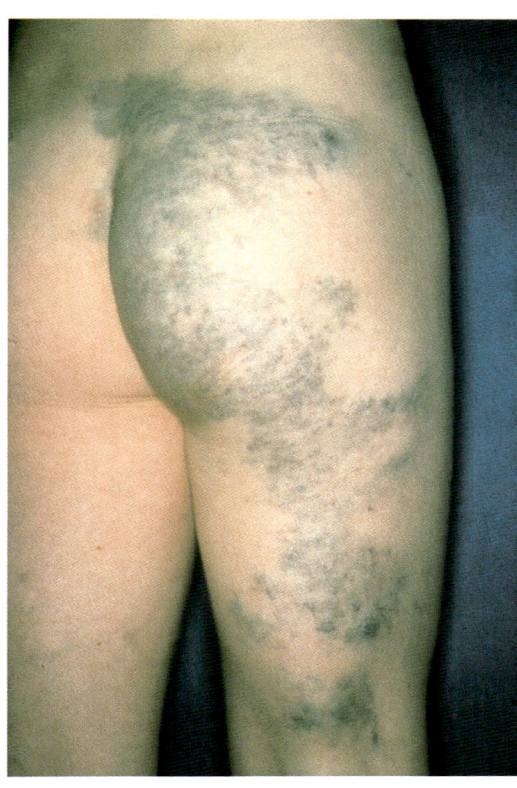

Fig. 20.29 Venous malformation of the leg involving the skin and musculature.

of involvement and in differentiating venous malformations from other vascular anomalies and soft tissue tumors. MR imaging is the best single imaging modality: it gives a bright hypersignal on T_2-weighed spin-echo sequences, because of slow flow, and this clearly indicates the extent of the lesions throughout the involved tissues.[29] There is rarely a need for CT scans to look for associated bony defects. Doppler ultrasound is a useful study for limb venous malformations: as it is a rapid and easy method of portraying the vascularization and low-flow velocity.[203] Arteriography and venography are usually not necessary.[29]

Cephalic venous malformations create a blue discoloration of the skin and mouth, distortion of facial features, and pain when swelling occurs in dependent positions or with straining. Involvement of the cheek and tongue can cause dental malocclusion, crossbite and/or openbite deformity through a mass effect on the developing jaws during childhood (Fig. 20.28). Deep mucous membranes lesions, involving the palate, pharyngeal and laryngeal areas, can cause snoring, progressive sleep apnea and respiratory difficulties. Orbital involvement, in communication with cheek and infratemporal venous malformations through the sphenomaxillary fissure, can cause enophthalmos when standing, and exophthalmos when supine; dark-blue veins may be visible on the inner surface of the conjunctiva or sclera. Usually there is no visual impairment. Management of cephalic venous malformations combines percutaneous sclerotherapy and staged excisions. A multistep approach, through multiple procedures over the years, will give the best results. In many patients, "cure" is impossible; treatment will aim at improving appearance, maintaining facial symmetry and muscle dynamics, and restoring lip competence. Soft tissue venous lesions and bone deformities can be treated in parallel.[204,205]

Venous malformations of the limb can be well localized or diffuse. Deeper venous malformations often involve the musculature and in some cases the

synovium of the joints may also be affected.[162,206] In rare cases, the muscle is affected without overlying skin involvement. Genitalia are commonly affected in association with a lower extremity venous malformation. Limb length discrepancy is uncommon and generally mild. If there is synovial involvement, the symptoms often manifest before 10 years of age and include pain, swelling, and functional impairment, owing to effusion or hemarthrosis. Permanent joint damage and severe muscle pain may follow. Chronic localized intravascular coagulopathy is common in patients with severe, extensive, or bulky lesions. This coagulopathy causes pain, thromboses, and phlebolith formation and may result in severe bleeding during surgical procedures. Low fibrinogen and elevated D-dimers are the hallmarks of this disorder. This venous malformation-associated local and disseminatred intravascular coagulation is often mislabeled in the literature as Kassabach–Merritt (KM) syndrome, but it is not the same condition (see discussion of KMP and Table 20.5).[162] The platelet count may be slightly low, but not to the degree seen in the KMP. Treatment with low-molecular-weight heparin is indicated in severe disease. Conservative management with elastic stockings is always recommended, and for localized lesions percutaneous sclerotherapy may be helpful.[206] Excision may be considered in some patients with symptomatic lesions.[207] Staged excisions are usually necessary and, in contrast to AVMs, this does not trigger the growth of the residual venous malformation. Knee joint venous malformation embedded in the synovial membrane that causes repeated episodes of hemarthrosis is an indication for resection to prevent joint degeneration, similar to that observed in hemophiliacs.

The glomuvenous malformations: glomus tumors (glomangiomas) and glomangiomatosis

Glomus tumors (glomangiomas) are relatively uncommon hamartomas of the glomus body, a special temperature-regulating arteriovenous shunt that bypasses the usual capillary bed of the dermis. Solitary tumors are more likely to occur in adults, whereas multiple lesions, more commonly have their onset in childhood. Although some cases are sporadic, rather than familial, a recent study carefully searching for small lesions in family members found familial occurrence in more than 75% (LM Boon, personal communication 2001). Although very rare in infancy, congenital glomus tumors have been reported.[208] In a review of 731 cases of glomus tumors occurring in children, six were congenital and one of those was also multiple.[209]

Solitary glomus tumors usually occur on the upper extremities, particularly in the nail beds, although occasionally they are found on the lower extremities, head, neck, or genitalia. These extremely tender purple nodules vary in size from 1mm to several centimeters. In addition to marked tenderness, there may be paroxysms of pain, either spontaneously or evoked by trauma. The solitary tumors are not genetically transmitted. Multiple glomus tumors are transmitted in an autosomal dominant fashion. In a given family, some affected members have small lesions, sometimes only a solitary lesion, whereas others have widely scattered (disseminated) lesions and still others have grouped lesions, often in a segmental distribution (Fig. 20.30). These large plaque-like lesions are usually congenital. They may be pink and macular at birth, becoming thicker and more nodular during childhood or may already be thick at the time of birth. Diagnosis can be particularly difficult in deeply pigmented skin. The lesions are usually dark blue and multinodular; although they resemble venous malformations superficially, they are firmer, less compressible and show less change with dependency or exercise.[210]

Familial glomangiomas have been linked to chromosome 1p21-22.[211] The gene VMGLOM is currently a poorly understood regulator of vasculogenesis or angiogenesis.[212]

203. Trop I, Dubois J, Guibaud L et al. (1999) Soft-tissue venous malformations in pediatric and young adult patients: diagnosis with Doppler. US Radiology. 212:841–845.
204. Enjolras O, Deffrennes D, Borsik M et al. (1998) Les "tumeurs vasculaires" et les règles de prise en charge chirurgicale. Ann Chir Plast Esthet. 4:455–490.
205. Berenguer B, Burrows PE, Zurakowski D et al. (1999) Sclerotherapy of craniofacial venous malformations. Plast Reconstr Surg. 104:1–15.
206. Yakes WF (1994) Extremity venous malformations. Semin Intervent Radiol. 11:322–329.
207. Upton J, Coombs CJ, Mulliken JB et al. (1999) Vascular malformations of the upper limb: a review of 270 patients. J Hand Surg (US). 24:1019–1035.

208. Landthaler M, Braun-Falco O, Eckert F et al. (1990) Congenital multiple plaquelike glomus tumors. Arch Dermatol 126:1203–1207.
209. Kohout E, Stout AP (1961) The glomus tumor in children. Cancer 14:555–566.
210. Mounayer C, Enjolras O, Wassef M et al. (2001) Facial glomangiomas masquerading as venous malformations. J Am Acad Dermatol in press.
211. Boon LM, Brouillard P, Irrthum A et al. (1999) A gene for inherited cutaneous venous anomalies ("glomangiomas") localizes to chromosome 1p21-22. Am J Hum Genet 65:125–133.
212. Irrhum A, Brouillard P, Enjolras O et al. (2001) Linkage disequilibrium narrows locus for venous malformations with glomus cells (VMGLOM) to a single 1.48 Mbp YAC. Eur J Hum Genet 9:34–38.

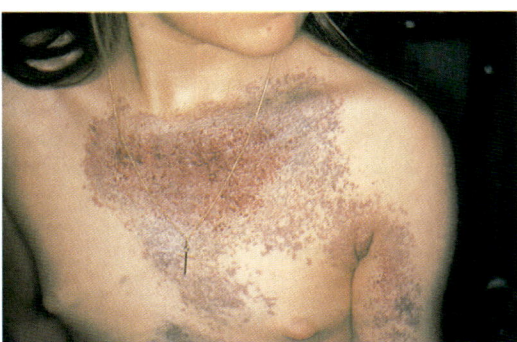

Fig. 20.30 Glomangiomatosis. Family history was positive in this case.

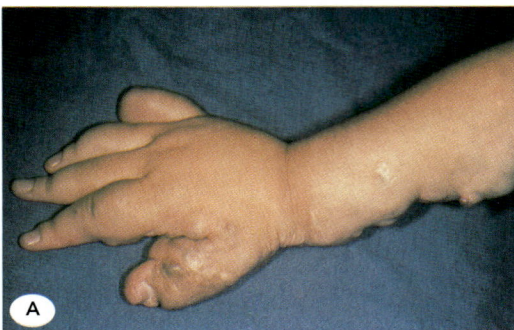

Fig. 20.31 Maffucci syndrome with radiographic evidence of bony involvement.

On histopathologic examination, the large tortuous dysplastic venous channels are reminiscent of a capillary–venous malformation. However in many vessels, the walls contain one or several rows of poorly differentiated cubical cells with eosinophilic or pale cytoplasm and a round nucleus; these cells stain with stains specific for vimentin, and smooth-muscle cell α- actin, a pattern consistent with glomus cells.[210] The pattern has features of both a vascular malformation and a tumor. Therefore the names **venous malformation with glomus cells** or **glomuvenous malformation** have been proposed as more appropriate names than glomangioma.

Complete surgical excision is the only reliable treatment for these tumors, although percutaneous sclerotherapy may improve some.

Maffucci syndrome

Maffucci syndrome is a rare congenital disorder with no recognized genetic basis. It is characterized by dyschondroplasia of one or more limbs, multiple enchondromas, and vascular malformations that are often large and located in the subcutaneous tissues. The lesions appear early in life, often in infancy. There is no racial or sex predilection. The vascular malformations are blue or purple, soft, compressible, and occasionally tender. Cutaneous lesions exhibit clinical (blue color of the nodules), radiological (presence of phleboliths and vascular tufts on the late phase of the angiogram), and pathologic features of venous malformations (Fig. 20.31). However, on pathologic specimens there is coexistence of anomalous venous channels and of a vascular tumor, the spindle cell hemangioendothelioma.[107,213] Although the vascular lesions may develop anywhere on the body surface, the hands and feet are involved most frequently. Localized forms involving a single extremity are observed. The site of the vascular malformation does not necessarily correlate with that of skeletal lesions, and lesions in bones may appear before the skin lesions.[214]

Skeletal changes consist of multiple enchondromas, exostoses, and recurrent fractures. Bone lesions are usually bilateral but asymmetric (Fig. 20.31B). Radiographic findings include oval defects in association with expansion and thinning of the cortex of involved bones. Limb deformity and leg lengthening, as well as scoliosis, occur in approximately one-third of patients.

The diagnosis of Maffucci syndrome is usually based on clinical findings. The differential diagnosis of the skeletal changes includes Ollier and Gorham syndromes. The skin changes often resemble multiple venous malformations clinically.

The most serious complications of Maffucci syndrome, aside from multiple fractures in childhood, are the neurologic deficits, resulting from encroachment of cranial enchondromas on the cerebral cortex, and the development of malignant tumors. Chondrosarcomas are the most common malignancy and are estimated to occur in 15% of patients. Other malignancies such as angiosarcomas, fibrosarcomas, lymphangiosarcomas, and intracranial tumors,[215] have also been reported.

Treatment involves surgical extirpation of skeletal and vascular lesions where possible. Diagnostic biopsy is mandatory to exclude malignancy in any bony or soft tissue tumor that enlarges rapidly or becomes painful. Radiation is of no therapeutic value.

Blue rubber bleb nevus syndrome

The blue rubber bleb nevus syndrome consists of multiple venous malformations in the skin and gastrointestinal tract associated with massive or occult intestinal hemorrhage and anemia. This disorder is rare, without known sexual predilection. Most cases are sporadic; some are inherited in an autosomal dominant fashion. The etiology is unknown. The syndrome usually is manifest at birth or during early childhood, but adult onset has been reported.[216]

The cutaneous malformations may be solitary or may number in the hundreds and can occur anywhere on the skin surface. The trunk and upper extremities are involved most often. Oral mucosal lesions may be evident as well. Skin lesions range in size from 1–2mm to several centimeters, vary in color from purplish-red to blue or black, and may be flat or elevated. According to the original description by Bean, they have "the feel and look of rubber nipples, are compressible and refill fairly promptly from their rumpled compressed state." In some cases, they may contain thrombi and phleboliths. These patients may also develop large combined venous and lymphatic vascular malformations with blue nodules on their surface. The vascular lesions tend to increase in size and number with age; spontaneous involution does not occur.

Histologically, the cutaneous venous malformations have certain distinctive features. In some areas, the vascular spaces, which are separated by a smooth muscle or fibrous stroma, are lined by cuboidal cells and intimately associated with sweat glands.

Gastrointestinal involvement can easily be detected by endoscopic examination. The gastrointestinal vascular malformations are usually multiple and submucosal, involving the small intestine and distal colon.[217] The lesions can be macular, polypoid, or, rarely, tumor-like masses. Each nodule has an overlying central blue or purple cap.[218] They vary in size and number, but there is no correlation with extent of cutaneous involvement. MR imaging is a useful noninvasive modality to detect gastrointestinal lesions. Selective

213. Hisaoka M, Aoki T, Kouho H et al. (1997) Maffucci's syndrome associated with spindle cell hemangioendothelioma. **Skeletal Radiol** 26:191–194.

214. Enjolras O, Wassef M, Merland JJ (1998) Syndrome de Maffucci; une fausse malformation veineuse? Un cas avec hémangioendothéliome à cellules fusiformes. **Ann Dermatol Venereol** 125:512–515.

215. Balcer LJ, Galetta SL, Cornblath WT et al. (1999) Neuro-ophthalmologic manifestations of Maffucci's syndrome and Ollier's disease. **J Neuroophthalmol** 19:62–66.

216. Oranje AP (1996) Blue rubber bleb nevus syndrome. **Pediatr Dermatol** 3:304–310.

217. Goraya JS, Marwaha RK, Vatve M et al. (1998) Blue rubber bleb nevus syndrome. **Pediatr Hematol** 15:261–264.

218. Gallo S, McClave S (1992) Blue rubber bleb nevus syndrome: gastrointestinal involvement and its endoscopic presentation. **Gastrointest Endosc** 38:72–76.

abdominal angiography performed during bleeding episodes can demonstrate location and extent of vascular lesions. These vascular malformations can also arise in other organs, including the liver, lung, pleura, urinary tract, brain and muscle.

Management is directed toward control of chronic gastrointestinal bleeding and correction of the resultant iron-deficiency anemia. Endoscopic electrocautery or surgical removal may be indicated if bleeding is severe.[219] Cutaneous lesions do not need to be removed unless they are disabling or disfiguring. The prognosis of this condition cannot be predicted.

Blue rubber bleb nevus syndrome, with its malformations of the venous network, can easily be differentiated from Osler–Weber–Rendu syndrome, which has malformations of the capillaries and arterioles.

ARTERIOVENOUS MALFORMATIONS

AVMs are fast-flow vascular malformations with direct arteriovenous shunts without an intervening capillary bed. They are among the most dangerous of the vascular anomalies. There is no gender predominance. AVMs are noted at birth in 40% of patients. Progression during childhood occurs in a majority. Known trigger factors include puberty, pregnancy (25% in a group of 102 women),[219] and trauma, including iatrogenic causes such as subtotal surgical resection, proximal artery ligation, or arterial embolization that is too proximal. AVMs can be classified according to the ISSVA–Schobinger staging[2] into four clinical stages: 1, dormancy; 2, expansion; 3, destruction; and 4, destruction plus congestive cardiac failure. In stage 1, AVMs mimic a port-wine stain or an involuting hemangioma, or they create a small pulsatile mass under normal skin (Fig. 20.32). In stage 2, the expansion creates plaques or masses, which are red and warm, with local tenderness, pulsations, bruits, and enlarged tortuous veins. In stage 3, skin necrosis, torpid ulcers, bleeding and hemorrhage become evident and lytic bone lesions may develop. Stage 4 is rare, occurring in approximately 2.5% and consists of increasing congestive cardiac failure from increased arterial pressure.[220,221]

Once a diagnosis of AVM is considered, certain investigations are necessary. Ultrasound/Doppler studies can help to confirm the high-flow nature of the condition and will provide measurements of the comparative output between arteries on the affected and unaffected sides of the body. This helps in serial reevaluation. If the output is markedly increased on the affected side, cardiac evaluation and follow-up become mandatory. MR imaging and arteriography plus conventional arteriography are all helpful in characterizing the angioarchitecture and extent of the AVM. Effects on the bone are best evaluated with CT scan, which can identify complications such as draining veins penetrating the skull and draining into an intracranial sinus.

Management

Treatment is often fraught with difficulty and no one treatment can be guaranteed to provide total cure. Embolization alone may initially appear to be successful, but good long-term results are rare, particularly for lesions on the extremities or facial AVMs.[220] Combining embolization and resection of the AVM nidus and overlying skin may give good results for small AVMs,[221] but the need for systematic excision of small AVMs (stage 1 or 2) in order to prevent further extension is controversial. For larger lesions (stage 2 and 3), embolization and excision are also performed, but covering the surgical wound is not easy; in addition, the therapeutic outcome is uncertain. In patients with pain, ulcers, and hemorrhages, particularly those with extensive AVMs in limbs, distal amputation may be required, even years after a technically and clinically effective embolization.[222] In some distal extremity AVMs with local complications, one may stabilize the disease by covering the region with a vascularized, anastomosed cutaneous and muscular flap transfer, after wide excision or localized amputation.[223] Similar flap transfer is used for severe

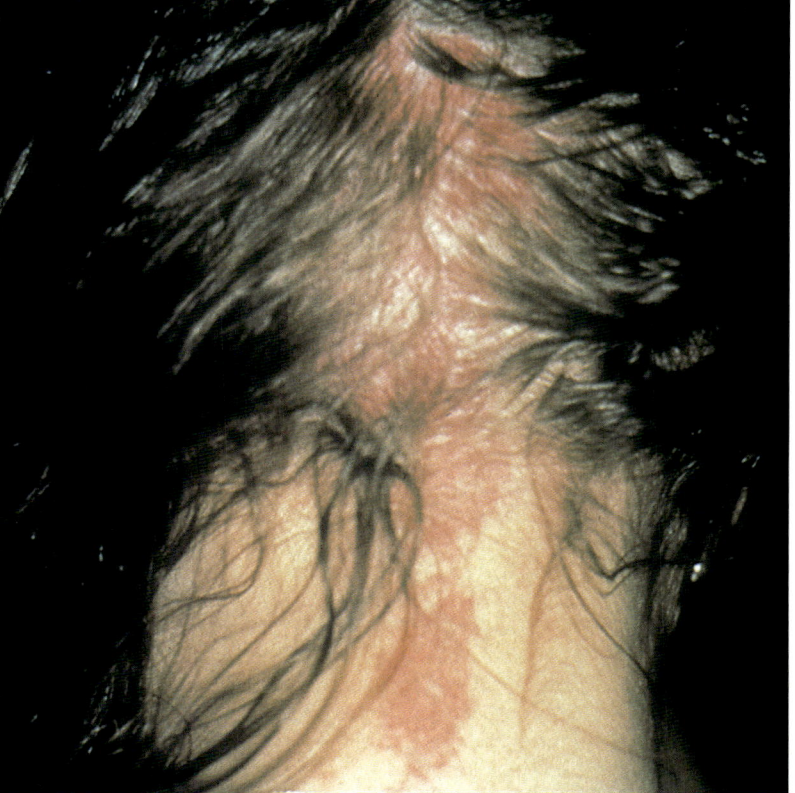

Fig. 20.32   Scalp arteriovenous malformation mimicking a port-wine stain.

facial AVMs in adolescents and adults, and this may also cure the lesion or stabilize the progress of a residual AVM; nevertheless, the results are cosmetically poor.[204] Therapies that are known to be trigger factors of AVMs, such as arterial ligation, partial excision, proximal or incomplete embolization, PDL for the red staining of the skin overlying the arteriovenous nidus, and cryosurgery, should be avoided whenever possible.

Parkes–Weber syndrome

The presence of arteriovenous fistulae distinguishes Parkes–Weber syndrome from KT syndrome.[9] Other features of Parkes–Weber syndrome include warmth and tenderness overlying the malformation, dilated veins with a thrill on palpation, lengthening of the affected limb, and hypertrophy in girth owing to both lipomatosis and lymphatic hyperplasia. Patients with Parkes–Weber syndrome may develop high-output congestive heart failure secondary to the arteriovenous fistulae. The prognosis is not as good as in KT syndrome, because there may be progressive worsening with pain and worsening functional outcome.

Treatment of Parkes–Weber syndrome should not be aggressive. Conservative management (such as compression stockings) is recommended. Surgical orthopedic management is necessary when leg length discrepancy is prominent. Epiphysiodesis may be considered, to achieve symmetric lower extremities; in many patients, this surgical procedure in the knee area, where arteriovenous fistulae are commonly located, induces worsening of the fast-flow malformation. Embolization is usually unsatisfactory because of multiple arteriovenous shunts along the limb. Surgical resection of the shunts usually fails, as new vessels are recruited and complicate the anomalous vascular network. Overaggressive surgical management can precipitate local

219. Ertem D, Acar Y, Kotoliglu E et al. (2001) Blue rubber bleb nevus syndrome. **Pediatrics** 107:418–420.

220. Enjolras O, Logeart I, Gelbert F et al. (2000) Malformations artérioveineuses. Etude de 200 cas. **Ann Dermatol Venereol** 127:17–22.

221. Kohout MP, Hansen M, Pribaz JJ et al. (1998) Arteriovenous malformations of the head and neck: natural history and management. **Plast Reconstr Surg** 102:643–654.

222. White RI, Pollack J, Persing J et al. (2000) Long-term outcome of embolotherapy and surgery for high-flow extremity vascular malformations. **J Vasc Interv Radiol** 11:1285–1295.

223. Toh S, Tsubo K, Arai H et al. (2000) Vascularized free-flaps for reconstruction after resection of congenital arteriovenous malformations of the hand. **J Reconstr Microsurg** 16:511–517.

complications, including pigmentary changes in skin, pseudo-Kaposi sarcoma skin alterations, pain, ulcers, hemorrhage, and ischemic distal changes in toes or digits necessitating amputation. These patients are evaluated initially with Doppler studies, MR arteriography, and conventional arteriography. Isotopic lymphography should be performed if lymphatic involvement is suspected. Many patients with Parkes–Weber syndrome have been grouped with those with KT syndrome under the rubric Klippel–Trenaumay–Weber syndrome, as the distinction between the two entities has not always been clear.

Cobb syndrome

Cutaneomeningospinal angiomatosis (Cobb syndrome) consists of a capillary stain or a fast-flow skin mass on the posterior thorax (and sometimes on the limb) in association with a contiguous or nearly contiguous fast-flow vascular malformation of the spinal cord.[224] A vertebral body is sometimes involved. The location of the spinal cord lesion corresponds within a segment or two with the involved dermatome of the skin lesion. The syndrome is very rare, much rarer than isolated intraspinal AVMs.[225]

The neurologic problems, which usually develop during adolescence or young adulthood, are the result of cord compression by the AVM or of spinal subarachnoid hemorrhages (occurring in one-third of patients). They vary with the level of spinal cord involvement and are thought to result from physical cord compression and/or anoxia. The spinal AVM is intramedullary in most patients; it may also be medullary and meningeal, or perimedullary. The patient becomes symptomatic as the spinal AVM increases in size. The onset of neurologic signs and symptoms can be gradual, episodic and progressive, or sudden and acute. They include pain in the areas supplied by the involved segment of the spinal cord, radiculopathy, weakness and atrophy of the limb muscles, loss of sensation, monoplegia, paraparesis and paraplegia. Scoliosis is present in 20% of reported cases.

The diagnosis of Cobb syndrome is suggested by the presence of a posterior thoracic vascular lesion in association with neural deficit. The vascular lesion either mimics a port-wine stain or is evident as an AVM with a thrill and bruit (with or without stained overlying skin); it is accompanied by neurologic evidence of a vascular abnormality of the spinal cord. MR imaging and angiography[226] and spinal angiography will demonstrate the vascular fast-flow lesion and pinpoint its precise location. Patients are generally not considered at risk for Cobb metameric syndrome if the cutaneous vascular malformation is venous, capillary–lymphatic–venous, or purely capillary, although on rare occasions quiescent AVMs may appear as a macular "pseudo-port-wine stain," making this a relative, rather than absolute, rule.

Endovascular embolization of spinal AVM has greatly improved the neurologic prognosis of Cobb syndrome; however, results may be temporary. If there is also a symptomatic vertebral vascular lesion, it can be treated by means of intralesional injections of ethanol or glue under CT guidance. Intramedullary lesions can be resected in some patients when embolization is impossible or too dangerous.[227]

Bonnet–Dechaume–Blanc and Wyburn–Mason syndromes

Bonnet-Dechaume-Blanc syndrome is the association of a pseudo-port-wine vascular anomaly of the skin (which is actually an AVM in a quiescent stage) with retinal and brain AVMs. Lesions tend to worsen progressively or become evident during childhood in all three locations. The cutaneous lesion is either hemifacial, involving the eyelids and cheek, or located in the central portion of the face (nose, forehead and, upper lip). It worsens over many years, particularly when incomplete resection is performed. The intracranial lesions occur predominantly around the thalamus and mesencephalon and are clinically manifest after hemorrhage; vascular accidents may occur in childhood or early adult life.

Wyburn–Mason syndrome is similar, combining a facial cutaneous AVM, midbrain AVM and unilateral congenital anomalies of the retinal vessels.

Treatment of these unusual but severe syndromic neuro-ophthalmologic and cutaneous AVMs is daunting; it is rarely possible to excise the whole facial lesion, using either free-flap transfer or cutaneous expansion to cover the large wound created, and arterial embolization is a palliative therapy that is usually unable to change a frequently bad prognosis.

LYMPHATIC MALFORMATIONS

Lymphatic malformations, or so-called **lymphangiomas**, are disorders of the lymphatic system and of the circulation of lymphatic fluid. Several subcategories appear in the medical literature based on clinical features (e.g., lymphangioma simplex, lymphangioma circumscriptum, cavernous lymphangioma, cystic hygroma, acquired progressive lymphangioma, benign lymphangioendothelioma); there are also several severe diffuse, often lethal, visceral types known as **diffuse visceral lymphangiectasia** or **visceral lymphangiomatosis**. It is probably more helpful to think of lymphatic malformations as microcystic (corresponding to lymphangioma circumscriptum and cavernous lymphangioma) and macrocystic (previously called cystic hygroma). Combined micro- and macrocystic types are common, particularly in the head and neck area, as well as in other sites (Fig. 20.33). In a review of 186 patients, lymphatic malformations involved the head and neck in 48%, the trunk and extremities in 42%, and were internal and visceral in 10%.[228] Common complications of lymphatic malformations include disfigurement, infection, and bleeding (superficial vesicles become hemorrhagic or there is a sudden hemorrhage in a large cyst). Recurrent inflammation with swelling can be particularly dangerous in some locations. For example, in orbital locations it can cause proptosis and may impair vision. In the mouth and perioral area it can create deformity of the maxilla and mandible; it may then cause crossbite, openbite, and speech impairment. The diagnosis is often clinical but is best confirmed with MR imaging, which often demonstrates fluid levels to suggest cystic components and shows the extent of the malformation. The stagnant lymphatic lesions show a bright hypersignal on T_2-weighed sequences.

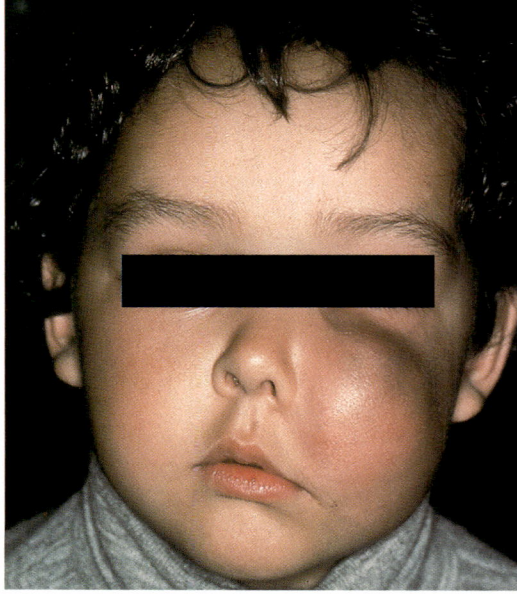

Fig. 20.33 Lymphatic malformation of the cheek.

224. de Vera C, Peiro R, Gort. A et al. (1996) Cobb syndrome. **Rev Neurol** 24:720.
225. Aminoff MJ, Logue V (1974) Clinical features of spinal vascular malformations. **Brain** 97:197–210.
226. Binkert CA, Kollias SS, Valavanis A (1999) Spinal cord vascular disease: characterization with fast three-dimensional contrast-enhanced MR angiography. **Am J Neuroradiol** 20:1785–1793.
227. Huffmann BC, Spetzger U, Reinges M et al. (1998) Treatment strategies and results in spinal vascular malformations. **Neurol Med Chir (Tokyo)** 38:231–237.
228. Alqahtani A, Nguyen LT, Flageole H et al. (1999) 25 years' experience with lymphangiomas in children. **J Pediat Surg** 34:1164–1168.

Macrocystic lymphatic malformations

Macrocystic lymphatic malformations are uncommon lesions that most often occur in the neck, axilla, groin, or chest wall. They are large, single or multiple cysts that are usually present at birth or by the age of 2 years. Rare documented cases of sudden development in an adolescent or an adult have been described. Large congenital forms are documented by ultrasound as early as the fourth month of pregnancy; in some of these fetuses a chromosomal abnormality is present (Down or Turner syndrome). In all cases, there is an increase of amniotic fluid α-fetoprotein level.[229] Usually macrocystic lymphatic malformations persist unchanged, if not treated, or they expand; however, there are instances of spontaneous regression, usually after infection of the cysts. Some lymphatic malformations of the neck extend into the mediastinum; others involve the tongue and floor of the mouth. Infection and hemorrhage into the lesion or close to it may lead to rapid enlargement, with resultant respiratory compromise, dysphagia, infection, and death. Radiologic assessment of the upper airway is essential for proper management of patients with neck lesions, as acute obstruction may supervene at any time.

Management

Recommendations for the management of macrocystic lymphatic malformations have varied from early total excision to waiting for spontaneous regression for several years. However, as resection often has considerable morbidity, techniques of percutaneous sclerotherapy have been developed, using a number of sclerosants with high irritant capabilities: the most widely used have been killed bacteria, known as OK-432[230] or Picibanil[231,232] and Ethibloc, a mixture of a corn protein and ethanol.[233] Other sclerosants that have been used include sodium morrhuate, dextrose, bleomycin, cyclophosphamide, and doxycycline.[234] Shrinkage of the lesions after single or multiple procedures is the result of the intense inflammatory reaction and subsequent fibrosis. It occurs in more than 50% of patients and the technique is now considered a first-line effective treatment.

Microcystic lymphatic malformations

Microcystic lymphatic malformations are more common than macrocystic lymphatic malformations. The lesions are sometimes present at birth or appear in childhood. They may develop anywhere on the body surface, but the most common sites are the axillary folds, shoulders, neck, proximal limbs, perineum, tongue, and floor of the mouth, where they may encroach on parapharyngeal spaces and the larynx, and create bony overgrowth.[235,236] The lesions consist of grouped small papules and translucent thin-walled vesicles resembling frog spawn, occasionally with superimposed hyperkeratosis. Some of the vesicles may contain varying amounts of blood, giving them a pink-red cast; coagulation of blood will produce a purple to black color.[237] Microcystic lymphatic malformations range in size from small (1 cm) plaques of vesicles to exceedingly large lesions covering extensive areas. A deeper component is almost always present and may be detectable as diffuse swelling or thickening and a bluish hue of the underlying tissues. Massive lymphatic malformations, deeply invading the dermis, subcutis, and underlying muscles, may involve an entire limb and appear as spongy subcutaneous masses without overlying color change or as multiple dark red vesicles, often with a hyperkeratotic or even verrucous surface (sometimes labeled angiokeratomas).[237] Very often, clusters of vesicles develop in the vicinity of the scar from a previously excised

lymphatic malformation. Leakage of lymphatic fluid may occur. Recurrent cellulitis is common and can cause worsening lymphedema.

Management

The treatment of microcystic and combined micro-macrocystic lymphatic malformations is exceedingly difficult. If therapy is indicated, deep and extensive surgery is necessary. If possible, this should be performed after tissue expansion of adjacent normal skin to take a larger area and avoid recurrences. A number of patients with extensive lesions of the head and neck undergo multiple resections with a high rate of recurrence and persistent disease, and poor cosmetic and functional results.[236,238] Patients with jaw involvement and overgrowth need orthodontic and orthognathic procedures after completion of skeletal growth, but overgrowth may recur and is difficult to repair. Carbon dioxide, diode and Nd–YAG lasers have been used successfully to obliterate the vesicular component in some lymphatic malformations, while the PDLs usually give only a temporary improvement after multiple procedures.

Acquired progressive lymphangioma

Acquired progressive lymphangioma (benign lymphangioendothelioma) is a rare but distinctive form of lymphatic malformation that develops gradually over a period of years.[239] It may occur at any age but is often seen in young individuals and takes the form of a well-defined solitary erythematous macule or plaque that is usually asymptomatic. These lesions may become quite large, in some instances measuring more than 30 cm. The histologic findings of anastomosing, often widely dilated, channels lined by a single flat layer of endothelial cells dissecting through the collagen fibers in the dermis and occasionally the fat make it difficult to distinguish from a well-differentiated angiosarcoma or patch-stage Kaposi's sarcoma. Excision is the treatment of choice.

Lymphedema

Lymphedema is the result of inadequate lymphatic drainage. Lymphatic obstruction from any cause produces a similar sequence of events. The protein content of the extravascular tissue rises and, because of its osmotic effect, additional water is retained. The newly established equilibrium permits the lymphatics to remove a smaller volume of lymph that is richer in protein. Unfortunately, an excess of extravascular protein often leads to proliferation of fibroblasts and organization of the edema fluid. This gives rise to the characteristic firm, nonpitting, and largely irreversible swelling of chronic lymphedema. For this reason, it is important to institute treatment early. Advances in diagnostic imaging studies and the development of improved lymphotropic contrast agents allow more accurate assessment of lymphatic function and lymphatic vascular morphology. Molecular genetic studies are delineating the origins of congenital lymphedema.[240]

Lymphedema is divided into primary and secondary forms. Secondary lymphedema is caused by lymphatic obstruction following surgery, by recurrent lymphangitis or cellulitis, by an extralymphatic process (such as compression by neoplastic invasion of lymphatics), or by fibrosis resulting from radiation therapy or scar formation. Secondary lymphedema is rare in childhood.

Patients with primary lymphedema are usually subdivided into clinical groups according to the age of onset. In congenital lymphedema, the swelling

229. Musone R, Bonafiglia R, Menditto A et al. (2000) Fetuses with cystic hygroma. A retrospective study. Panminerva Med 42:39–43.

230. Ogita S, Tsuto T, Deguchi et al. (1991) OK-432 therapy for unresectable lymphangiomas in children. J Pediatr Surg 26:263–270.

231. Brewis C, Pracy JP, Albert DM (2000) Treatment of lymphangiomas of the head and neck in children by intralesional injection of OK-432 (Picibanil). Clin Otolaryngol 25:130–135.

232. Luzzato C, Midrio P, Tchaprassian Z et al. (2000) Sclerosing treatment of lymphangiomas with OK-6432. Arch Dis Child 82:316–318.

233. Brevière GM, Bonnevalle M, Pruvo JP et al. (1993) Use of Ethibloc in the treatment of cystic and venous angiomas in children. Eur J Pediatr 3:166–170.

234. Molitch HI, Unger EC, White CL et al. (1995) Percutaneous sclerotherapy of lymphangiomas. Radiology 194:343–347.

235. Padwa BL, Hayward PG, Ferraro NF et al. (1995) Cervicofacial lymphatic malformation: clinical course, surgical intervention, and pathogenesis of skeletal hypertrophy. Plast Reconstr Surg 95:951–960.

236. Hartl DM, Roger C, Denoyelle F et al. (2000) Extensive lymphangioma presenting with upper airway obstruction. Arch Otolaryngol Head Neck Surg 126:1378–1382.

237. Davies D, Rogers M (2000) Morphology of lymphatic malformations, a pictorial review. Australas J Dermatol 41:1–7.

238. Orvidas LJ, Kasperbauer JL (2000) Pediatric lymphangiomas of the head and neck. Ann Otol Laryngol 109:411–421.

239. Guillou L, Fletcher CD (2000) Benign lymphangioendothelioma (acquired progressive lymphangioma): a lesion not to be confused with well-differentiated angiosarcoma and patch-stage Kaposi's sarcoma) clinicopathologic analysis of a series. Am J Surg Pathol 24:1047–1057.

240. Irrthum A, Karkkainen MJ, Devriendt K et al. (2000) Congenital hereditary lymphedema caused by a mutation that inactivates VEGFR3 tyrosine kinase. Am J Hum Genet 67:295–301.

is firm and is characterized by pitting on pressure. In lymphedema praecox, females are primarily affected, and the swelling appears spontaneously, generally between the ages of 9 and 25 years. It is common to see patients with one extremity involved for years and later have a second one become affected. It is evident, using isotopic lymphography in patients with one limb involved, that the lymphatic network of these patients is bilaterally impaired; however, the clinical manifestations may occur at different periods of life.

About 20% of primary lymphedema is familial. Lymphedema occurring distally and present at birth is referred to as **Milroy disease; Meige disease** describes later onset. In these autosomal dominant disorders, the edema is almost always confined to the legs and feet. The edema is at first pitting and disappears completely with elevation. Subsequently, with the development of fibrosis, the swelling becomes harder and more or less nonpitting. The epidermis may become hyperkeratotic and warty (so-called pseudoverrucous hyperplasia) and the skin is often chronically thickened. Fissures and secondary infection often occur. Changes of elephantiasis, similar to that caused by parasitic infection in the tropics, occurs in severe cases. Another familial form is **Hennekam disease**, combining limb lymphedema, facial anomalies (flat face, flat nasal bridge, tooth and ear anomalies), intestinal lymphangiectasia with protein-losing enteropathy, mental retardation, and cerebral anomalies; most reported patients were born from consanguineous parents.[241,242]

Several other syndromes have been described that combine congenital primary lymphedema with various associated anomalies. Many are genetic and of varied inheritance. Lymphedema has been associated with Turner and Noonan syndromes. Opitz has proposed that the presence of generalized congenital lymphedema can contribute to certain facial dysmorphisms as well as minor abnormalities of the ears, hair patterns, nails, and palmar prints.[243]

Management

Treatment of advanced lymphedema is very unsatisfactory, but early treatment can often prevent further deterioration. This includes external pressure by elastic stockings or bandages, active muscle exercises, and centripetal massage. Diuretics may also be helpful. Systemic antibiotics may be necessary for the recurrent inflammatory episodes and infections. Sequential pneumatic compression devices have been efficacious in many instances in preventing progression of the lymphedema. Operations to restore the damaged or absent lymphatics are generally unsatisfactory, with only transient improvement. Surgery, to remove the grossly thickened tissues, and liposuction are sometimes performed. Lymphaticovenous shunts have given some improvement in visceral forms with massive effusions. Visceral lymphangiomatosis in the thoracic or abdominal area, or both, is a life-threatening situation in childhood, often occurring in association with intravascular coagulopathy and leading to severe visceral hemorrhages.

GORHAM SYNDROME (GORHAM–STOUT SYNDROME)

Gorham syndrome (Gorham's massive osteolysis, disappearing bone disease, phantom bone disease) is an extremely rare sporadic disorder. It is characterized by massive osteolysis and partial or complete replacement of bone by fibrous tissue. The translucent "phantom" bones develop in any part of the skeleton. Bone loss may stop after a few years of progression but may create local complications. When the spine is affected, neurologic deficits may develop. Thoracic involvement may cause chylothorax. The associated vascular lesions are usually venous, lymphatic, or capillary. Areas of osteolysis are probably the result of intense osteoclastic activity.[244] Similar lesions have been observed in patients with an antecedent history of KMP in infancy and in patients with AVMs, so they are not entirely specific to low-flow vascular malformations. In addition, lesions have rarely been described in areas of the skeleton remote from a cutaneous vascular anomaly. Rare cases are lethal: in most patients, Gorham's osteolysis is considered a benign, self-limited condition. Multiple pathologic poorly healing fractures occur and require orthopedic care. Because of increased osteoclastic activity, it has been suggested that bisphosphonates and calcitonin be given to these patients. Implants of bone in the osteolytic areas are usually absorbed in a few months; therefore, artificial devices like titanium implants should be utilized to stabilize the lesions or to replace the bone after curettage of the vascular lesion.[245] Amputation may rarely be necessary.

BANNAYAN–RILEY–RUVALCABA SYNDROME

Three autosomal dominant disorders, Riley–Smith syndrome, Bannayan–Zonana syndrome and Ruvalcaba–Myrhe syndrome, have been demonstrated to have clinical overlap and are now considered a part of the same disease spectrum named Bannayan–Riley–Ruvalcaba syndrome (BRRS). Interestingly, families with BRRS share mutations of the same tumor suppressor gene, *PTEN*, as families with Cowden syndrome.[246,247] Mutations in *PTEN* have also been seen in patients with features of Proteus syndrome. Symptoms in BRRS include macrocephaly without hydrocephalus, lipomas, capillary and/or venous malformations, lymphatic anomalies, pigmented macules of the genitalia, intestinal polyps, macrodactyly, pseudopapilledema and Hashimoto thyroiditis.[248] There is normal CNS function and, therefore, awareness of the benign nature of the macrocephaly should help to avoid unnecessary intervention.

241. Hennekam RC, Geerdink RA, Hamel BC et al. (1989) Autosomal recessive intestinal lymphangiectasia and lymphedema, with facial anomalies and mental retardation. Am J Med Genet 34:593–600.
242. Huppke P, Christen HJ, Sattler B et al. (2000) Two brothers with Hennekam syndrome and cerebral abnormalities. Clin Dysmorphol 9:21–24.
243. Opitz J (1986) On congenital lymphedema. Am J Med Genet 24:127–129.
244. Moller G, Priemel M, Amling M et al. (1999) A report of six cases with histopathological findings. J Bone Joint Surg Br 81:501–506.
245. Sato K, Sugiura H, Yamamura S et al. (1997) Gorham massive osteolysis. Arch Orthop Trauma Surg 116:510–513.
246. Tok Celebi J, Chen FF, Zhang H et al. (1999) Identification of PTEN mutations in five families with Bannayan–Zonana syndrome. Exp Dermatol 8:134–139.
247. Lowichik A, White FV, Timmons CF et al. (2000) Bannayan–Riley–Ruvalcaba syndrome: spectrum of intestinal pathology including juvenile polyps. Pediatr Dev Pathol 3:155–161.
248. Gorlin RJ, Cohen MM, Condon LM et al. (1992) Bannayan–Riley–Ruvalcaba syndrome. Am J Med Genet 44:307–314.

Benign and Malignant Tumors

Walter H.C. Burgdorf and Ramón Ruiz-Maldonado

INTRODUCTION

The spectrum of tumors in the skin of children is vast.[1] A broad range of lesions ranging from congenital malformations to hamartomas to epithelial and mesenchymal neoplasms to cutaneous infiltrates by hematopoietic cells may all present with papules, plaques, or nodules. While most are harmless, life-threatening soft tissue sarcomas, leukemias, and lymphomas must be promptly recognized. Many other childhood tumors are discussed elsewhere in this text, such as cysts (Ch. 17), melanocytic nevi and malignant melanoma (Ch. 10), nodular and infiltrative conditions (Ch. 17), and vascular neoplasms (Ch. 20).

CLINICAL APPROACH

The unexpected finding of a new growth in an infant or child causes great anxiety for the parents and grandparents and usually results in a prompt visit to either the pediatrician or dermatologist. Five clinical danger signs suggest the possibility of a malignant tumor.[2]

- Onset in the neonatal period
- A history of rapid growth
- A firm mass > 3cm in diameter
- Skin ulceration
- Fixation to deep tissues or location below the fascia

Before attempting to apply these criteria, one should exclude a hemangioma, since these common benign lesions of infancy often fulfill several of the points. If an exact clinical diagnosis is not obvious and one or more of these signs is present, a biopsy should be undertaken. If none is present, the lesion usually can be observed, depending on the clinical judgment of the physician. When evaluating melanocytic lesions, the clinical ABCD criteria (Ch. 3) should also be kept in mind. In many instances a tumor will be removed for cosmetic purposes. Using this approach, only a small number (~3/1000) of malignant tumors will be missed on the first assessment.

CONGENITAL TUMORS

Congenital lesions are those present at birth or appearing within the first 30 days of life. They are even a bit more distressing to the parents as they are noticed at a time when emotions are high. Counseling done at this time should always be repeated later to be sure the desired information is conveyed.

Dermatologists take congenital tumors somewhat for granted since both melanocytic nevi and hemangiomas are frequently present at birth. Estimates of the prevalence of either a vascular or melanocytic tumor at birth range

from 5 to 15%. Included among the malignant tumors that may present at birth are leukemia, neuroblastoma and sarcomas (usually rhabdomyosarcoma), as well as Langerhans cell disease.

The classification of congenital tumors is confusing because there are overlaps among the following:

1. Hamartoma – an overgrowth or disarray of tissues at their usual anatomic site. Many hamartomas are present at birth or in early infancy, but this is not a prerequisite. Hamartoma has been used to describe so many unrelated processes that it has lost specificity.
2. Nevus – often used as a synonym for a hamartoma, such as a connective tissue nevus. Nevus is also employed to describe benign melanocytic lesions, such as compound nevus or Spitz nevus. When used without qualification, the term nevus generally implies a melanocytic process.
3. Choristoma or heterotopia – an overgrowth or disarray of tissues at the wrong site.
4. Teratoma – a germ cell neoplasm involving two or more of the primitive germ layers: ectoderm, mesoderm, and endoderm.
5. Malformation – a morphological defect resulting from aberrant developmental process. All the overlaps between the above terms cause more confusion than clarity. Thus, we have avoided such classification.

MOSAICISM

As first espoused by Happle and discussed by him in detail (Ch. 7), mosaicism is responsible for a wide range of lesions which are sometimes interpreted as tumors. The underlying principle is that if a mutation occurs early in embryonic life, cutaneous lesions may be segmental following Blaschko lines, such as in an epidermal nevus. If the same mutations occur in later life, solitary tumors develop. A simple example is that of epidermolytic hyperkeratosis – a distinctive histologic pattern caused by specific keratin mutations that may produce a widespread ichthyosis if a germline mutation, an epidermal nevus if an early somatic mutation, and focal acanthomas if a late sporadic mutation. Happle has refined his concepts regarding the segmental lesions, dividing them into two types:[3]

Type 1 segmental lesions arise from a post-zygotic new mutation as outlined above.

Type 2 lesions result from a loss of heterozygosity in a patient who already has a germ line mutation. For example, a patient with multiple leiomyomas may have a segment of skin with many more leiomyomas than the background of the rest of the body. In another instance, someone with neurofibromatosis 1 may have an area following Blaschko lines where there is an extremely high number of neurofibromas and café-au-lait macules.

1. Ruiz-Maldonado R, Orozco-Covarrubias M de la L (1999) Skin tumors in children. In: Malignant Tumors of the Skin, Chu AC, Edelson RL eds. London: Arnold, pp. 314–342.
2. Knight PJ, Reiner CB (1983) Superficial bumps in children: what, when and why? *Pediatrics* 72(2):147–153.
3. Happle R (2001) Segmentale Typ-2-Manifestation autosomal dominanter Hautkrankheiten. *Hautarzt* 52(2):283–287.

The clinical relevance of this phenomenon is that even after identifying an apparent segmental mutation, one must examine the entire patient carefully to exclude this Type 2 phenomenon, for such patients are capable of transmitting their disease to their offspring in 50% of cases.

SOLITARY VERSUS MULTIPLE

Another good general rule of childhood tumors is that while a solitary lesion, be it epithelial or adnexal, is likely to be sporadic; just as in adults, multiple cutaneous tumors should suggest autosomal-dominant inheritance and an underlying syndrome. Often the cutaneous changes may be a marker for underlying systemic changes or even for potential tumors, which may be expected to appear later in life, as discussed later under cancer-associated genodermatoses.[4]

BENIGN VERSUS MALIGNANT

The terms tumor and neoplasm are used interchangeably in this chapter, connoting a palpable swelling of tissue in which growth may be relatively uncontrolled and progressive. Benign tumors usually show a lesser degree of histologic atypia and lack the properties of invasion and metastasis. Several studies exist on the prevalence of skin tumors in childhood. One analysis of 775 superficial lumps of childhood gives an indication of the prevalence of various tumors. Pilomatricomas, epidermoid cysts, and hemangiomas (three tumors not covered in this chapter) make up about 75% of all lesions.[2] Only 1–2% of lesions are malignant, which is reassuring. In some childhood tumors, the microscopic appearance correlates poorly with the clinical course. Some bland tumors with little atypia (e.g., desmoid tumors) can behave aggressively, while on the other hand, some microscopically worrisome tumors have a good prognosis (Spitz nevi).

SOFT TISSUE TUMORS

Childhood tumors are often puzzling to the dermatologist used to dealing with primarily epithelial tumors. Because there are so few basal cell carcinomas and squamous cell carcinomas in childhood, the entire spectrum is shifted a bit, placing increased emphasis on mesenchymal and hematopoietic tumors. The classification of soft tissue tumors remains in flux. We have followed the standard WHO classification, but also attempted to include the alternative terms more familiar to many clinicians.[5,6]

Sarcomas are malignant soft tissue tumors of mesodermal origin. They account for about 7% of pediatric cancers; the incidence is about eight per million. Rhabdomyosarcomas and undifferentiated sarcomas account for over half of this group, while fibrosarcomas, synovial sarcomas, and malignant peripheral nerve sheath tumors account for most of the rest. There are striking differences between infants and older children.[7] The vast majority of tumors in infancy are benign, usually vascular or fibroblastic-myofibroblastic in nature. Most sarcomas present as ill-defined, often large masses, in the deep soft tissues of extremities, retroperitoneum, or head and neck. Sarcomas of the extremities are often fixed to underlying fascia and muscle. Deep incisional biopsy with expert pathologic diagnosis is often required for these tumors. Superficial punch biopsies can be helpful when dealing with smaller or more superficial lesions but may suffer from sampling defects. Needle biopsies or similar approaches to possible sarcomas may also not be desirable because biopsy tract seeding may be a cause of disease recurrence.

In most instances, the sarcoma can be classified as to its "cell of origin" or "direction of differentiation," and even subclassified with significant therapeutic implications. The mainstays of diagnosis are expert light microscopic evaluation, coupled with immunohistochemical stains. The latter usually enable the pathologist to identify the tissue of origin or direction of differentiation of the sarcoma, although poorly differentiated tumors may often lack expected markers (Table 21.1). This is a highly simplified table and ignores the complex determinations needed to study hematological tumors. A wide range of relatively specific chromosomal abnormalities have been recognized in both benign and malignant soft tissue tumors; today the diagnosis of sarcoma is rarely made without specific cytogenetic analysis.[8]

The mainstay of treatment of all sarcomas is meticulous surgical excision with particular attention paid to spread along fascial lines followed by exact histologic control of margins. True soft tissue sarcomas are thus usually resectable; the problems arise when the tumor involves skeletal, neurovascular,

---

TABLE 21.1   Common immunohistochemical stains

Antigen	Normal structures identified	Most common tumors
Actin	Smooth muscle cells, pericytes, myofibroblasts, myoepithelial cells	Leiomyoma, leiomyosarcoma, some dermatomyofibromas
CD1a	T cells, Langerhans cells	Langerhans cell disease
CD 34	Stem cells, endothelial cells, others	Dermatofibrosarcoma protuberans
Desmin	Myogenous cells	All muscular tumors
Factor VIII	Endothelial cells	Vascular tumors
Factor XIII	Dermal dendrocytes	Dermatofibromas, fibrous papule
Keratins	Keratinocytes	Epidermal tumors
Many	Macrophages	Xanthogranuloma family (not Langerhans cell disease)
Neurofilaments	Neurons, nerve fibers	Neural tumors
S100	Melanocytes, Langerhans cells, neural cells	Malignant melanoma, Langerhans cell disease
Ulex europeaus I	Endothelial cells	Vascular tumors
Vimentin	Endothelial cells, fibroblasts, many others	All mesenchymal tumors

4. Burgdorf WH, Koester G (1992) Multiple cutaneous tumors: what do they mean? **J Cutan Pathol** 19(6):449–457.
5. Weiss SW (1994) Histological Typing of Soft Tissue Tumors, 2nd edn. Berlin: Springer.
6. Weiss SW, Goldblum JR (2001) Enzinger and Weiss' Soft Tissue Tumors, 4th edn. St. Louis: Mosby.
7. Coffin CM, Dehner LP (1990) Soft tissue tumors in the first year of life: a report of 190 cases. **Pediatr Pathol** 10(4):509–526.
8. Singer S, Demetri GD, Baldini EH et al. (2000) Management of soft-tissue sarcomas: an overview and update. **Lancet Oncology** 1:75–85.

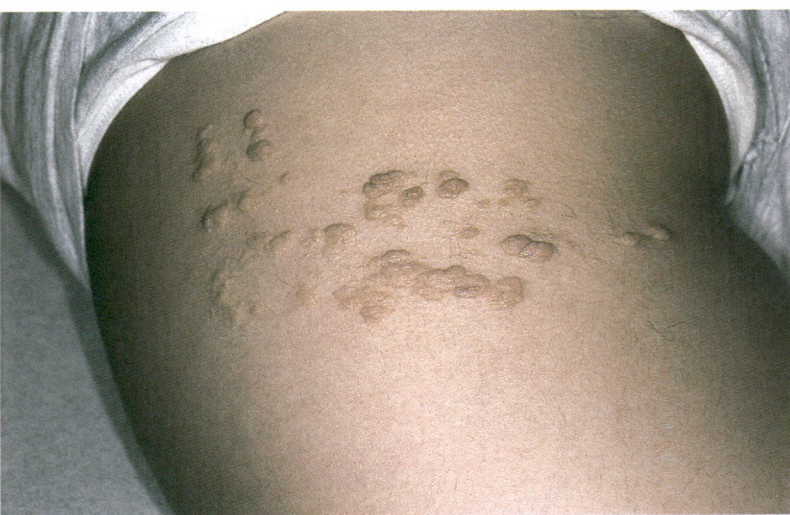

Fig. 21.1   Nevus lipomatosus with herniations of fat.

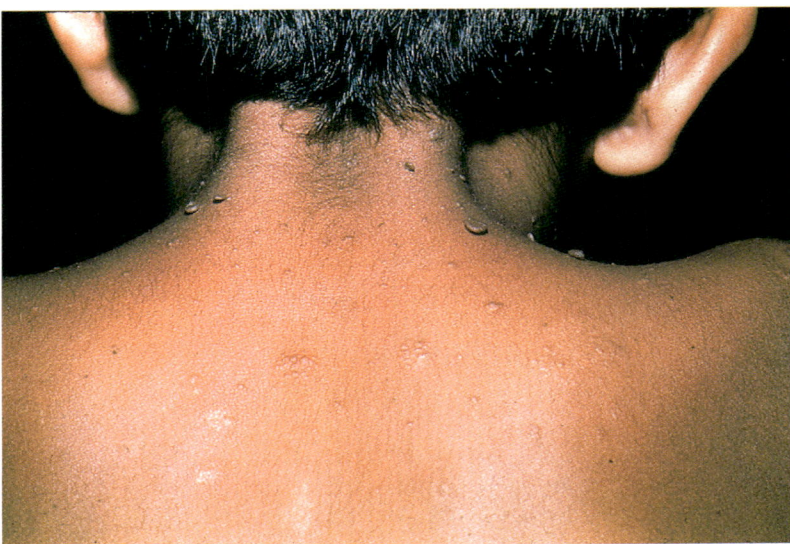

Fig. 21.2   Multiple tiny skin tags in a patient with tuberous sclerosis.

or internal organ structures. The number of amputations done for sarcomas of limbs has dropped markedly. In adult sarcomas, both radiation therapy and chemotherapy are employed both for prophylaxis after an apparently successful excision and to control recurrences and metastases. The exact indications vary widely from tumor to tumor and center to center. In childhood sarcomas, there are more chemotherapy-sensitive tumors and thus this approach plays a far greater role.

BENIGN TUMORS AND TUMOR-LIKE LESIONS OF SUBCUTANEOUS FAT

NEVUS LIPOMATOSUS

Nevus lipomatosus presents at birth or in childhood as a plaque or linear lesion composed of coalescing soft, polypoid, skin-colored, slightly yellow or red papules (Fig. 21.1).[9] The individual papules are similar to a skin tag. These nevi most often occur in the pelvic or lumbosacral region. They may be large and cosmetically disfiguring,[10] but are usually not associated with other developmental abnormalities. Larger pedunculated lesions have been described as pedunculated lipofibromas.[11] Histopathologically, there is mature fat in the superficial dermis. Skin tags can be microscopically identical. Focal dermal hypoplasia (Goltz syndrome) (Ch. 7) is also characterized by high dermal fat, so it too may enter into the histologic differential diagnosis, but can usually be readily excluded by clinical evaluation. Smaller lesions can be excised if desired; larger lesions are a surgical challenge, but fortunately are almost never on exposed sites.

SKIN TAG

Skin tags, acrochordons, or soft fibromas are soft, fleshy, polypoid, and pedunculated lesions commonly found in the folds of the axillae and neck in adults. Occasionally, adolescents also acquire skin tags in these areas. More commonly, childhood acrochordons are solitary, often congenital, and larger than acquired skin tags in adults. They occur most commonly over the trunk, lumbosacral, groin, and perineal areas. Skin tags of the neck are common in tuberous sclerosis (Fig. 21.2). Histologic examination reveals a polypoid tumor with an epidermis that may range from atrophic to acanthotic, and a dermis

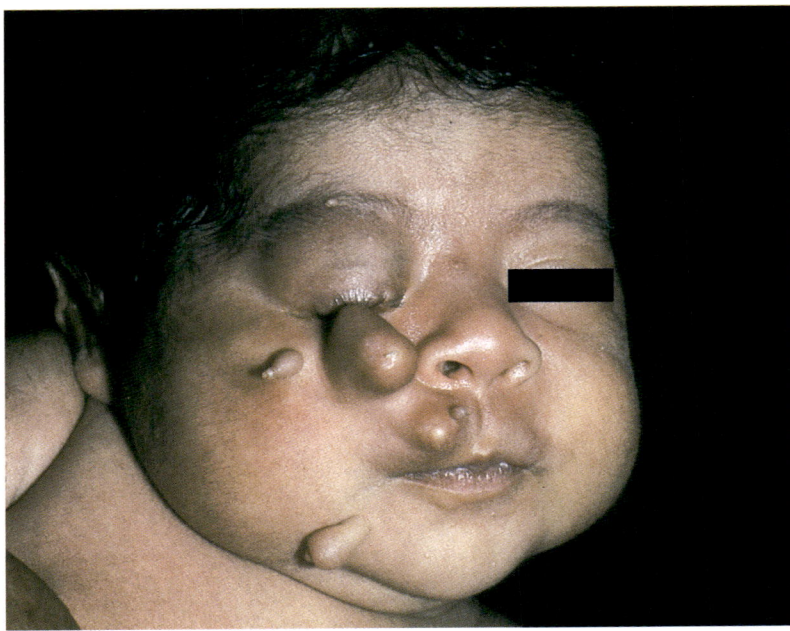

Fig. 21.3   Oculocerebrocutaneous syndrome with multiple skin tags and orbital cysts.

that lacks appendages and is composed of loose connective tissue, fat, and telangiectatic vessels. Oculocerebrocutaneous syndrome (Delleman syndrome) presents with periorbital or facial skin tags, orbital cysts, cerebral malformations, and focal cutaneous hypoplasia (Fig. 21.3).[12,13] Moving skin tags suggest a striated muscle hamartoma. Congenital "skin tags" in the preauricular area usually turn out to be accessory tragi or branchial cleft remnants. Smaller lesions can be simply removed by scissors or shave excision; larger ones can be excised. On occasion, deeper sinus tracts are present complicating the surgery. In addition, patients should be screened for hearing loss.

9. Wilson-Jones E, Marks R, Pongsehirun D (1975) Naevus superficialis lipomatosus. A clinicopathological report of 20 cases. **Br J Dermatol** 93(2):121–133.
10. Bergonse FN, Cymbalista NC, Nico MM et al. (2000) Giant nevus lipomatosus cutaneus superficialis: case report and review of the literature. **J Dermatol** 27(1):16–19.
11. Ozturkcan S. Terzioglu A, Akyol M et al. (2000) Pedunculated lipofibroma. **J Dermatol** 27(4):288–290.
12. Delleman JW, Oorthuys JW (1981) Orbital cyst in addition to congenital cerebral and focal dermal malformations: a new entity? **Clin Genet** 19(3):191–198.
13. Moog U, de Die-Smulders C, Systermans JM et al. (1997) Oculocerebrocutaneous syndrome: report of three additional cases and etiological considerations. **Clin Genet** 52(4):219–225.

GENERALIZED FOLDED SKIN WITH UNDERLYING LIPOMATOUS NEVUS

Symmetric ringed creases associated with thickened subcutaneous tissue in a newborn has been referred to as the "Michelin tire baby syndrome" (Fig. 21.4). This is a very rare condition with fewer than 20 case reports. The folds may be caused by an underlying lipomatous nevus,[14] smooth muscle hamartoma,[15,16] constriction bands,[17] or fibrosis.[18] Chromosomal abnormalities, familial occurrence, cleft palate, and other developmental abnormalities have been reported. Michelin tire baby syndrome is most probably not a single syndrome, but a clinical finding seen in unrelated disorders.

LIPOMAS AND RELATED TUMORS

Solitary lipoma

Ordinary lipomas are uncommon in children but are encountered so frequently in adults that they are the most common mesenchymal neoplasm. The wide histological spectrum of lipomas seen in adults is of little significance in children. Lipomas are most often found on the trunk (Fig. 21.5) and proximal extremities. On palpation, they tend to be multilobular, slightly compressible, subcutaneous masses with smooth margins.

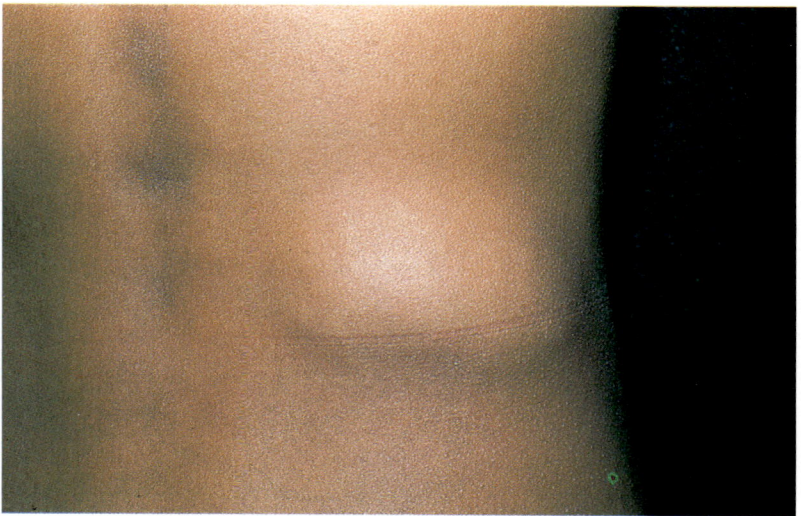

Fig. 21.5   Large lipoma on trunk of young child.

Several variants are of clinical interest in young adults. The subgaleal lipoma is a firm forehead nodule, often misdiagnosed as an osteoma. It presents a surgical challenge to the unwary because of its deep location.[19] The mobile encapsulated lipoma is typically on the forearm and is freely mobile, much like a subcutaneous marble.[20] Angiolipomas tend to be painful. Sclerotic lipomas are more common in young adults and can be mistaken for the sclerotic fibromas of Cowden syndrome.[21] Lipomas can be easily excised, but they can almost always be identified clinically with certainty and the patient reassured.

Lumbosacral lipoma

A lumbosacral lipoma is a rare congenital developmental anomaly with mature fat forming a lobular mass in the lumbosacral region (Fig. 21.6).[22] Superficially, there may be associated hypertrichosis, skin tags, nevus lipomatosus, hemangioma, or a cutaneous dimple or pit. There is almost invariably a laminar defect in the underlying spine. Mature fat may extend through this defect as an intradural or extradural lipoma. Slow progressive enlargement with compression or tethering of the spinal cord and compressive symptoms such as spasticity, anesthesia, and incontinence may result. Recognition of the neurologic features may be delayed until early childhood or later. Suspicion of a lumbosacral lipoma should prompt imaging studies (MRI) and neurologic evaluation. Early surgical intervention is generally the treatment of choice, although there is not always reversal of neurologic symptoms. Spinal cord lipomas have also been described in association with the vertebral defects in the VATER association (**V**ertebral defects, **A**nal atresia, **T**racheo**E**sophageal fistula with atresia, and **R**adial dysplasia).[23]

Hibernoma

A hibernoma is a tumor of brown fat, a tissue normally found only in children (and, of course, hibernating mammals); surprisingly it occurs most often not in children but in young adults, usually in the mediastinum or interscapular region. The lesions are typically slow growing soft tissue tumors that attract no attention clinically but are assumed to be large lipomas. The mutation seen in multiple endocrine neoplasia (MEN) 1 syndrome involving a growth control protein known as menin has also been found in hibernomas, so

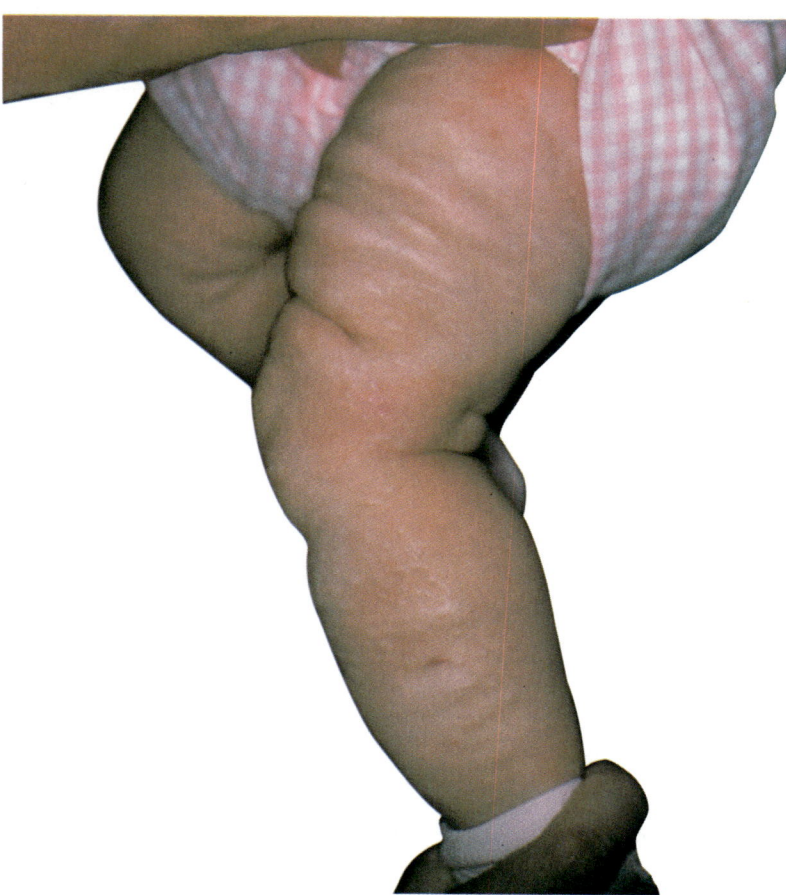

Fig. 21.4   Michelin tire baby with excessive skin folds.

14. Ross CM (1969) Generalized folded skin with an underlying lipomatous nevus: "The Michelin Tire baby". **Arch Dermatol** 100(3):320–323.
15. Glover MT, Malone M, Atherton DJ (1989) Michelin-tire baby syndrome resulting from diffuse smooth muscle hamartoma. **Pediatr Dermatol** 6(4):329–331.
16. Schnur RE, Herzberg AJ, Spinner N et al. (1993) Variability in the Michelin tire syndrome. A child with multiple anomalies, smooth muscle hamartoma and familial paracentric inversion of chromosome 7q. **J Am Acad Dermatol** 28(2):364–370.
17. Bass HN, Caldwell S, Brooks BS (1993) Michelin tire baby syndrome: familial constriction bands during infancy and early childhood in four generations. **Am J Med Genet** 45(3):370–372.
18. Burgdorf WH, Doran CK, Worret WI (1982) Folded skin with scarring: Michelin tire baby syndrome? **J Am Acad Dermatol** 7(1):90–93.

19. Wörle B, Kunte C, Schaller M et al. (2000) Das Lipom der Stirn. **Hautarzt** 51(9):661–665.
20. Sahl WJ Jr (1978) Mobile encapsulated lipomas. Formerly called encapsulated angiolipomas. **Arch Dermatol** 114(11):1684–1686.
21. Zelger BG, Zelger B, Steiner H et al. (1997) Sclerotic lipoma: lipomas simulating sclerotic fibroma. **Histopathology** 31(2):174–181.
22. Xenos C, Sgourcs S, Walsh R et al. (2000) Spinal lipomas in children. **Pediatr Neurosurg** 32(6):295–307.
23. Chesnut R, James HE, Jones KL (1992) The Vater association and spinal dysraphia. **Pediatr Neurosurg** 18(3):144–148.

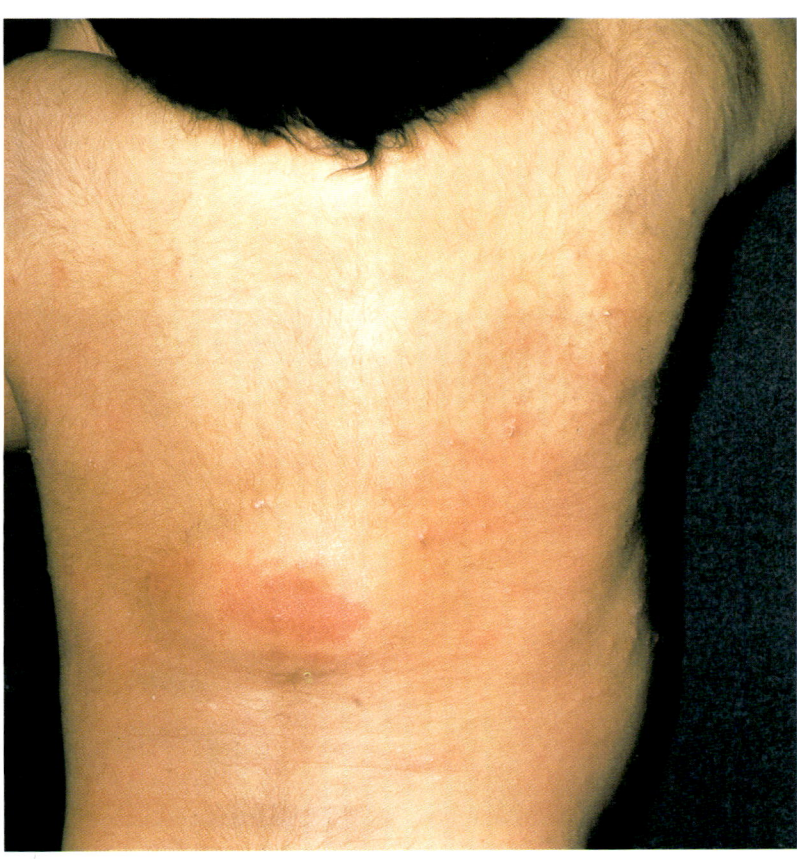

Fig. 21.6   Lumbosacral lipoma in child with underlying spinal defect.

perhaps younger patients with MEN 1 syndrome are at risk for this rare tumor.[24]

LIPOMATOSES

There are a number of rare syndromes in which multiple or diffuse lipomas may be identified.

Encephalocraniocutaneous lipomatosis

The syndrome is either a variant of Proteus syndrome (Chapter 7) or a closely related form of mosaicism.[25,26] It is also known as Fishman syndrome, and may clinically overlap with oculocerebrocutaneous syndrome. Patients present at birth with a unilateral fatty nevus of the scalp associated with alopecia, as well as facial skin tags, usually periocular. The scalp lesion has been described as nevus psiloliparus,[27] differing from nevus lipomatosus because of the presence of numerous arrector pili muscles. In addition, the patients have ipsilateral ocular choristomas and intracranial lipomas which lead to both epilepsy and mental retardation.

Infiltrating lipomatosis

Infiltrating, diffuse, or congenital lipomatosis usually presents in the first two years of life as a soft, poorly circumscribed, enlarging mass. Histologically, mature fat without hypercellularity or pleomorphism is present in increased quantities in the subcutis and extending into muscle. Recurrence often follows surgical resection. There is often underlying hypertrophy of bone and clinical hemihypertrophy or macrodactyly.[28]

Fibrolipoma

A fibrolipomatous hamartoma of nerve consists of a proliferation of mature fat and fibrous tissue surrounding peripheral nerves of an extremity. Eighty percent of cases involve the median nerve and thus the hand. Some patients present with macrodactyly. The tumor is palpable as a sausage-shaped mass and there is no muscle infiltration.[29]

Lipofibromatosis

This rare neoplasm combines features of a fibrous proliferation with a lipoma. Most lesions involve the extremities and may be present at birth. Typically, there is mature fat tissue with fibroblastic proliferation involving the fat septa and adjacent muscle fascia. Nerves are frequently entrapped. The tumors often persist or recur following surgery, but do not metastasize.[30]

Multiple familial lipomas

Also known as familial lipomatosis, this condition is inherited in an autosomal-dominant pattern. Patients develop multiple otherwise ordinary lipomas, most often in adult life, frequently with a rapid onset. Other pedigrees show multiple angiolipomas. Touraine–Renault syndrome refers to the same condition in a segmental pattern, suggesting somatic mosaicism. Despite the genetic background, lesions in children appear to be uncommon. A number of other genodermatoses (Ch. 7) may also feature multiple lipomas. They include Gardner syndrome, Cowden syndrome, the closely related Bannayan–Riley–Ruvalcaba syndrome, and Proteus syndrome.

Visceral lipomatosis

Visceral lipomas are uncommon but one variant is of particular interest. Epidural lipomatosis has been described several times following high-dose corticosteroid therapy. Patients who develop localized neurological symptoms and signs while receiving such therapy should be examined with available imaging techniques.[31]

LIPOBLASTOMA AND LIPOBLASTOMATOSIS

Lipoblastoma and lipoblastomatosis occur most frequently in children less than 3 years of age and most often involve the extremities.[32] In lipoblastoma, the tumor is clinically discrete and lobular; solitary acral lesions have been described.[33] In lipoblastomatosis, the tumor often infiltrates the subcutis and muscle diffusely.[34] Histopathologically, these tumors are characterized by the presence of lipoblasts. These are immature fat cells in a mucinous stroma, often admixed with mature fat. Lipoblastomas are benign but may be confused clinically and histopathologically with liposarcoma, a very rare tumor in childhood. A lobular tumor with fibrous septae and without marked pleomorphism, hyperchromatic nuclei, or atypical mitoses favors the diagnosis of lipoblastoma. Often there is a deletion of chromosome 8q. Complete excision is recommended; local recurrence is occasionally seen. The tumors tend to contain more mature fat in older children and may recur as lipomas.

Liposarcomas

Liposarcomas are extremely uncommon in childhood. Myxoid liposarcomas almost always have a t(12;16) karyotype, which should be sought before making the diagnosis of malignancy in a childhood fatty tumor.

24. Chen DY, Wang CM, Chan HL (1998) Hibernoma. Case report and literature review. **Dermatol Surg** 24(3):393–395.
25. Nosti-Martinez D, del Castillo V, Duran-McKinster C et al. (1995) Encephalocraniocutaneous lipomatosis: an uncommon neurocutaneous syndrome. **J Am Acad Dermatol** 32(2):387–389.
26. Ciatti S, Del Monaco M, Hyde P et al. (1998) Encephalocraniocutaneous lipomatosis: a rare neurocutaneous syndrome. **J Am Acad Dermatol** 38(1):102–104.
27. Happle R, Küster W (1998) Nevus psiloliparus. **Dermatology** 197(1):6–10.
28. Gorken C, Alper M, Bilkay U et al. (1999) Congenital infiltrating lipomatosis of the face. **J Craniofac Surg** 10(4):365–368.
29. Silverman TA, Enzinger FM (1985) Fibrolipomatous hamartoma of nerve. A clinicopathologic analysis of 26 cases. **Am J Surg Pathol** 9(1):7–14.
30. Fetsch JF, Miettinen M, Laskin WB et al. (2000) A clinicopathologic study of 45 soft tissue tumors with an admixture of adipose tissue and fibroblastic elements and a proposal for classification as lipofibromatosis. **Am J Surg Pathol** 24(11):1491–1500.
31. Berking C, Przybilla B (1997) Epidurale Lipomatose als Komplikation der Glukokortikoidbehandlung. **Hautarzt** 48(11):787–790.
32. Collins MH, Chatten J (1997) Lipoblastoma/lipoblastomatosis: a clinicopathologic study of 25 tumors. **Am J Surg Pathol** 21(10):1131–1137.
33. Young RJ 3rd, Warschaw KE, Elston DM et al. (2000) Acral lipoblastoma. **Cutis** 65(4):243–245.
34. Calobrisi SD, Garland JS, Esterly NB (1998) Congenital lipoblastomatosis of the lower extremity in a neonate. **Pediatr Dermatol** 15(3):210–213.

FIBROBLASTIC AND MYOFIBROBLASTIC TUMORS

Fibrous proliferations in infancy are a particularly befuddling area. Nomenclature has changed many times over the years, but no consensus has been reached. After many attempts at devising a new, dermatologist- and pediatrician-friendly classification of this wide array of lesions, we have chosen to follow the approach of Weiss and Goldblum[6] with only minor modifications. We have not attempted to distinguish between fibroblastic, myofibroblastic, and fibrohistiocytic lesions, as the overlaps far exceed the clean borders.

The cellular machinery of the fibroblast is normally geared toward production of collagen, elastin, and ground substance. Fibroblasts both in culture and in a variety of proliferative disorders may assume some features of smooth muscle cells and have thus been designated myofibroblasts. Myofibroblasts always express vimentin but may also display alpha-smooth muscle actin and/or desmin. They are normally present in early granulation tissue and play an important role in wound contraction. Thus the interaction between fibroblasts and myoblasts is seen in diverse processes ranging from ordinary scar formation, to hypertrophic scars and keloids, to a variety of tumor-like proliferations. Not surprisingly, in many instances, there is a tendency for spontaneous improvement, but frankly malignant lesions do arise.

FIBROUS LESIONS OF INFANCY

Coffin and Dehner analyzed over 100 fibroblastic or myofibroblastic tumors in children.[35] Three-quarters were benign, most appeared early in life, and the extremities were the favored site. Infantile myofibromatosis was the most common diagnosis. In a companion paper, the same authors looked at 190 soft tissue tumors in infancy. Once again, most were fibrous and benign.[7] The fibroblastic and myofibroblastic disorders that are most commonly seen at birth or in infancy are shown in Table 21.2 and are first to be considered.[36]

Connective tissue nevus

Connective tissue nevi are benign, often congenital lesions presenting as firm, asymptomatic, skin-colored plaques composed of closely grouped papules (Fig. 21.7) with a surface texture described as "peau d'orange," pigskin (as seen in an American football), or cobblestone (the German term *Pflastersteinnaevus*).[37,38] The plaques are most often solitary, although they may occasionally be multiple, with a symmetric distribution over the back, buttocks, arms, and thighs. Occasionally, they present in a segmental pattern. Unusual clinical forms including exophytic lesions have been described.[39]

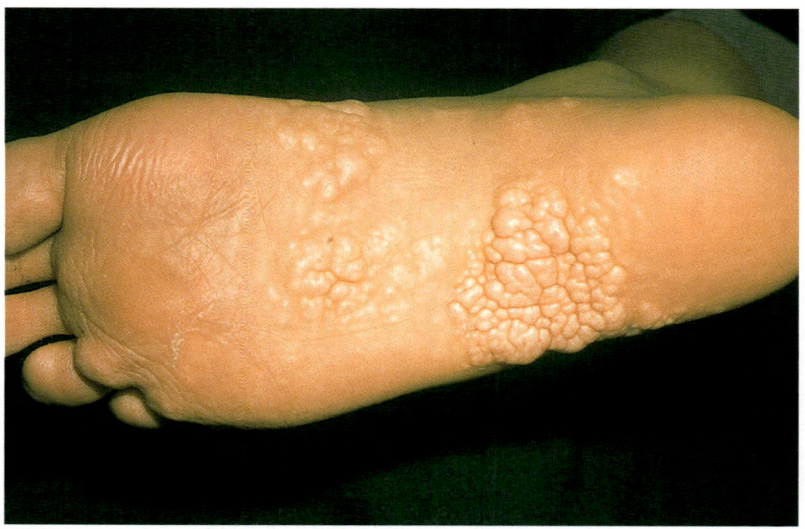

Fig. 21.7   Connective tissue nevus with multiple firm papules and nodules on sole. While this patient did not have Proteus syndrome, the possibility should be considered with plantar connective tissue nevi.

TABLE 21.2   **Fibroblastic and myofibroblastic disorders**

Diagnosis	Age	Location	Solitary	Multiple	Recur
Fibrous hamartoma	B-2	Flexural regions	±	– –	Rare
Myofibroma/ myofibromatosis	B-2	Soft tissue, bones, viscera	±	±	Rare
Fibromatosis colli	B-2	Sternocleidomastoid muscle	±	BIL	Rare
Digital fibromatosis	B-2	Fingers and toes	±	±	Common
Infantile desmoid-type fibromatosis	B-5	Musculature	±	– –	Common
Calcifying aponeurotic fibroma	2-A	Hands and feet	±	– –	Common
Hyaline fibromatosis	2-A	Dermis, soft tissue	– –	±	Common
Gingival fibromatosis	B-A	Gingiva	– –	±	Common

B – birth
A – adult life
BIL – bilateral

35. Coffin CM, Dehner LP (1991) Fibroblastic-myofibroblastic tumors in children and adolescents: a clinicopathologic study of 108 examples in 103 patients. **Pediatr Pathol** 11(4):569–588.
36. Cooper PH (1992) Fibrous proliferations of infancy and childhood. **J Cutan Pathol** 19(4):257–267.
37. Uitto J, Santa Cruz DJ, Eisen AZ (1980) Connective tissue nevi of the skin. Clinical, genetic, and histopathologic classification of hamartomas of the collagen, elastin and proteoglycan type. **J Am Acad Dermatol** 3(5):441–461.
38. Pierard GE, Lapiere CM (1985) Nevi of connective tissue. **Am J Dermatopathol** 7(4):325–333.
39. Fork HE, Sanchez RL, Wagner RF Jr et al. (1991) A new type of connective tissue nevus: isolated exophytic elastoma. **J Cutan Pathol** 18(6):457–463.

Multiple connective tissue nevi may be familiar, as an isolated event, or more often as part of a syndrome. Both the shagreen patch and the facial plaque in tuberous sclerosis are connective tissue nevi, so a search for other stigmata of tuberous sclerosis is essential when an apparently isolated connective tissue nevus is identified. Similar changes are seen in MEN 1 syndrome.[40] Connective tissue nevi in association with a hereditary bony dysplasia called osteopoikilosis are seen in dermatofibrosis lenticularis disseminata or Buschke–Ollendorff syndrome (Ch. 7). The cerebriform thickenings of the feet and occasionally other areas in Proteus syndrome represent excess collagen, so they too can be viewed as connective tissue nevi. Some cases of Michelin tire baby have also shown excessive dermal connective tissue.[18]

Often, the diagnosis can be made clinically. If a skin biopsy is performed, we prefer a small ellipse, sectioned longitudinally, extending from normal skin into the nevus. Alternatively, two small punch biopsies can be taken, one from the lesion and one from contralateral normal skin. Connective tissue nevi are histologically heterogeneous, showing an excessive accumulation and/or degeneration or fragmentation of collagen, elastin, or dermal ground substance. Changes in collagen are difficult to assess, even when one finds a thickened dermis, as collagen stains are usually disappointing. If elastin is increased, comparison of elastin stains in suspected and normal tissue is rapid and dramatic. In such a situation, the diagnosis of elastoma may be justified. There is a marked variation in the patterns of elastin and collagen excess and deficiency in clinically distinct connective tissue nevi and one must remain flexible. We do not usually attempt to distinguish between collagenoma and elastoma.

The clinical differential diagnosis includes a smooth muscle hamartoma. These lesions look similar but may change on palpation or with a drop in temperature as their muscular components contract. The histology is decisive. Connective tissue nevi have no malignant potential and require no treatment. They rarely lend themselves to a simple surgical approach.

Fibrous hamartoma of infancy

This relatively common tumor of infancy is typically a single nodule of the axilla, nape, thigh, or buttocks (Fig. 21.8).[41–43] It may be congenital. Boys are affected far more often than girls. There may be overlying hypertrichosis. The histologic pattern is almost pathognomonic; there is mature fat, fibrous tracts or strands and nests of small blue immature mesenchymal cells in a myxoid stroma. Both the fibrous tracts and the less-differentiated cellular areas consist of myofibroblasts. In most instances, the lesions regress spontaneously. Excision is curative.

Myofibroma and myofibromatosis

These lesions may be solitary (myofibroma) or multiple (myofibromatosis).[44,45] They were formerly known as congenital fibrosarcomas but this is a most misleading designation and should not be employed. The histologic picture is distinctive with a relatively well-circumscribed lesion containing fascicles of plump or elongated spindle cells. The fascicles are surrounded by collagen. There may be vascular spaces, so that a myofibroma is one of the tumors with a hemangiopericytoma pattern. The cells are positive for vimentin and alpha-smooth muscle actin, usually negative for desmin, and always S-100 negative.

About 80% are solitary and over half of these involve the head and neck region. About half are in the deep soft tissues but the rest are subcutaneous. In such a case, a firm subcutaneous mass is noted at birth or early in life, most often in a boy. The mass may be erythematous or lack overlying surface changes. Once the diagnosis has been confirmed on biopsy, there is no need to excise the entire lesion unless it fails to regress over a period of months.

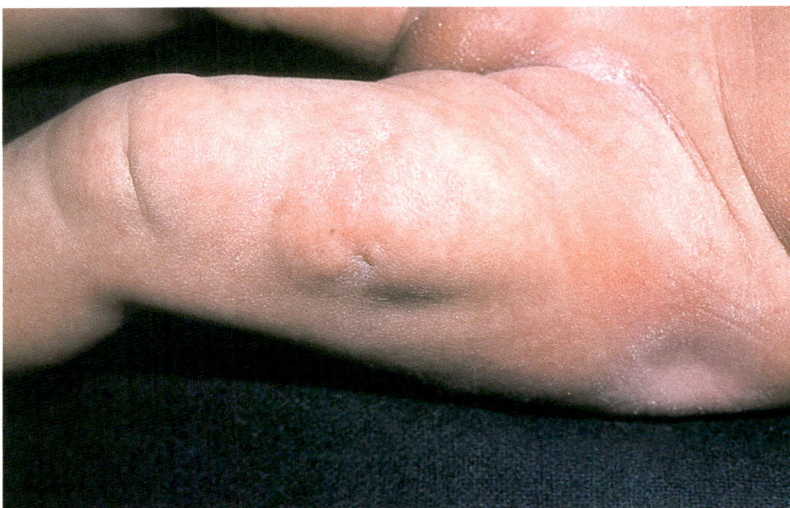

Fig. 21.8 Fibrous hamartoma of infancy.

Almost all do regress spontaneously so the outlook is excellent. They often resolve with atrophy; some may present as atrophic patches.

Multiple lesions are a slightly different story. They are more common in girls and may be familial.[46,47] The myofibromas involve not only the subcutaneous tissues, but also the skeleton and a variety of solid viscera. Those restricted to the soft tissues and bones do well, but visceral involvement can end fatally. The individual lesions do not expand aggressively or metastasize, but as space-occupying lesions they interfere with vital functions, especially in the gastrointestinal tract and lungs. Clinical features which indicate the likelihood of recurrence include age > 5 years and location on an extremity, while worrisome pathological features include incomplete resection, high mitotic count, and areas of necrosis within the tumor.[48] Treatment is obviously more difficult, as surgery is often impossible, and the luxury of waiting for regression not available.

Fibromatosis colli

Fibromatosis colli or congenital torticollis (wryneck) is a peculiar but common congenital fibromatosis of the sternocleidomastoid muscle. It is presumably secondary to trauma. Patients present either with a mass at the base of the muscle or with a distorted neck. The mass usually resolves spontaneously but the muscle may be permanently deformed, requiring surgical correction after the lesion has regressed.

Infantile digital fibromatosis

This relatively common disorder was first described by Reye. It almost always occurs at birth or in the first year of life and is far more common on the fingers than the toes (3:1) but spares the thumbs and great toes. It presents as a firm, usually red-brown mass (Fig. 21.9). Some lesions occur away from the digits.[49] The tumor consists of plump spindle cells interlaced with collagen bundles. The spindle cells are myofibroblasts with characteristic perinuclear cytoplasmic inclusions. The trichrome stain is useful for highlighting these particles, which consist primarily of actin. Following surgical removal, recurrence occurs in more than 50% of cases while the other lesions eventually involute over time, sometimes leaving residual deformities.[50] Not surprisingly, the role of surgical intervention is controversial.

40. Darling TN, Skarulis MC, Steinberg SM et al. (1997) Multiple facial angiofibromas and collagenomas in patients with multiple endocrine neoplasia type 1. **Arch Dermatol** 133(7):853–857.
41. Paller AS, Gonzalez-Crussi F, Sherman JO (1989) Fibrous hamartoma of infancy. Eight additional cases and review of the literature. **Arch Dermatol** 125(1):88–91.
42. Scott DM, Pena JR, Omura EF (1999) Fibrous hamartoma of infancy. **J Am Acad Dermatol** 41(5):857–859.
43. Dickey GE, Sotelo-Avila C (1999) Fibrous hamartoma of infancy: current review. **Pediatr Dev Pathol** 2(3):236–243.
44. Chung EB, Enzinger FM (1981) Infantile myofibromatosis. **Cancer** 48(8):1807–1818.
45. Stanford D, Rogers M (2000) Dermatological presentations of infantile myofibromatosis: a review of 27 cases. **Australas J Dermatol** 41(3):156–161.
46. Parker RK, Mallory SB, Baker GF (1991) Infantile myofibromatosis. **Pediatr Dermatol** 8(2):129–132.
47. Bracko M, Cindro L, Golouh R (1992) Familial occurrence of infantile myofibromatosis. **Cancer** 69(5):1294–1299.
48. Baerg J, Murphy JJ, Magee JF (1999) Fibromatoses: clinical and pathological features suggestive of recurrence. **J Pediatr Surg** 34(7):1112–1114.
49. Purdy LJ, Colby TV (1984) Infantile digital fibromatosis occurring outside the digit. **Am J Surg Pathol** 8(10):787–790.
50. Ishii N, Matsui K, Ichiyama S et al. (1989) A case of infantile digital fibromatosis showing spontaneous regression. **Br J Dermatol** 121(1):129–133.

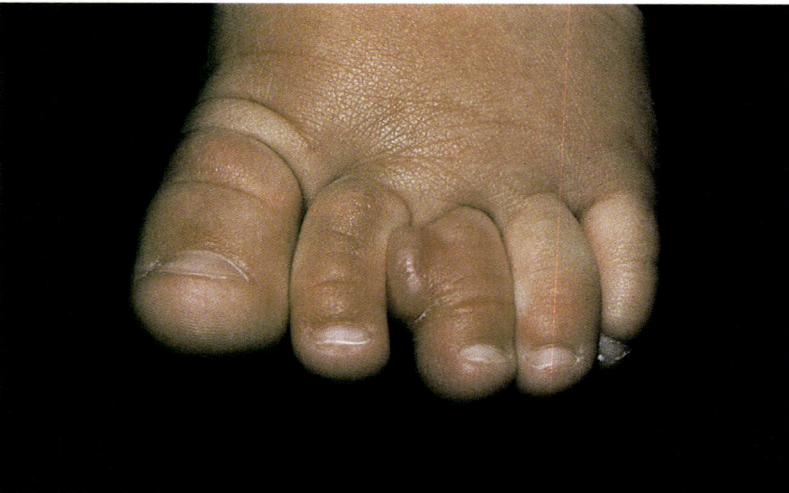

Fig. 21.9   Infantile digital fibroma between the 2nd and 3rd toes.

Gingival fibromatosis

Hyperplasia of the gums, or gingival fibromatosis (Fig. 21.10), is a well-known clinical picture because it is a frequent medication side effect, especially with phenytoin usage. It also occurs spontaneously, either as an isolated finding or as part of a variety of syndromes including juvenile hyaline fibromatosis and Winchester syndrome. When isolated, it is usually sporadic although familial forms have been described. In older children with poor dental care, it may reflect a reactive process. Periodontal surgery can produce dramatic improvements but unless there is an addressable underlying cause, the proliferations invariably recur.[51]

Calcifying aponeurotic fibroma

First described by Keasbey as juvenile aponeurotic fibroma, this tumor typically develops on the palms or soles of teenagers. The mass is usually fixed to the overlying skin but not often painful. The microscopic picture shows a fibrous proliferation often with palisading fibroblasts and foci of calcification and cartilage. Surgery may be necessary but spontaneous improvement often occurs.[52]

Juvenile hyaline fibromatosis

Hyaline is not a specific substance but simply refers to amorphous eosinophilic material that appears to be altered collagen. There are several diseases which fall under this rubric. The most common of a list of rare disorders is juvenile hyaline fibromatosis, characterized by the triad of fibroblastic tumors of the head, neck and extremities, gingival hyperplasia, and flexion contractures (Fig. 21.11).[53] In addition to the large fibrous tumors, there may also be small white papules primarily on the face, as well as perianal papules. It starts in infancy and is relentlessly progressive. Adolescent patients are usually disfigured and bedridden with their contractures. The metabolic defect is unknown, although inheritance shows an autosomal-recessive pattern. The soft tissue lesions show large strands of hyalinized or glassy collagen admixed with few fibroblasts, and occasional chondroid areas. No treatment has been devised.

Clinically related diseases include:

- Infantile systemic hyalinosis (Landing syndrome) is clinically similar to juvenile hyaline fibromatosis but far more severe. Infants are affected at birth and rarely live past two years of age. This disorder is most likely an extreme variant of the juvenile disease.[54]

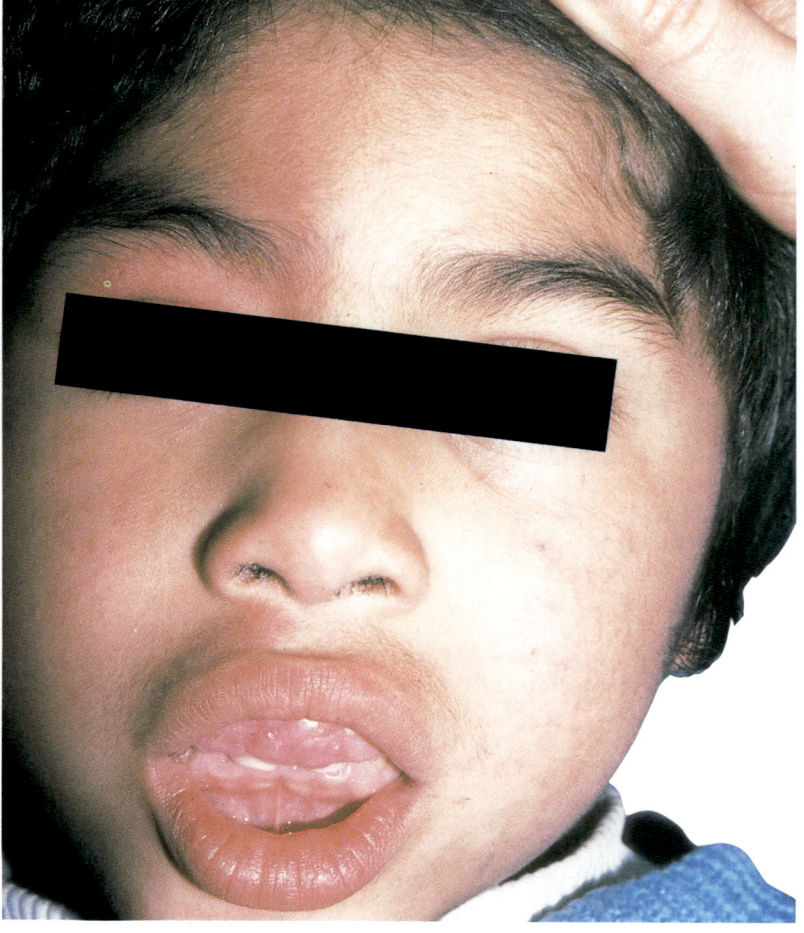

Fig. 21.10   Gingival fibromatosis.

- Winchester syndrome features gingival hyperplasia and joint contractures, but has ocular abnormalities and lacks the cutaneous nodules.
- Francois syndrome (dermo-chondro-corneal dystrophy) is inherited in an autosomal-recessive pattern. Patients have deforming arthritis, corneal dystrophy, and firm fibrous dermal nodules.[55]
- Hyalinosis cutis et mucosae (lipoid proteinosis, Urbach–Wiethe disease) (Chs 7, 9) is similar in name only. This disorder is inherited in an autosomal-recessive pattern, often found in isolated European or South African populations, and features papules on face, neck, and hands. The most striking clinical sign is hoarseness, because of similar lesions on the vocal cords. Histology shows deposits of amorphous hyaline material in the dermis, especially around the blood vessels.

Infantile desmoid-type fibromatosis

Fibromatoses in general are considered below; they represent an interface between a reactive process and a neoplastic one, as they are frequently locally aggressive but do not metastasize. The infantile desmoid-type fibromatosis typically presents as a rapidly expanding solitary mass involving skeletal muscle, fascia, or aponeurosis. Favorite sites are the head and neck region, shoulder girdle, and thighs. These tumors generally appear in the first five years of life. The histologic appearance is variable, perhaps reflecting the stages of fibroblast differentiation. In younger patients, the lesions can be quite cellular with plump fibroblasts in a myxoid stroma. Later the lesions are more

51. Bittencourt LP, Campos V, Moliterno LF et al. (2000) Hereditary gingival fibromatosis: review of the literature and a case report. **Quintessence Int** 31(6):415–418.
52. Fetsch JF, Miettinen M (1998) Calcifying aponeurotic fibroma: a clinicopathologic study of 22 cases arising in uncommon sites. **Hum Pathol** 29(12):1504–1510.
53. Mancini GM, Stojanov L, Willemsen R et al. (1999) Juvenile hyaline fibromatosis: clinical heterogeneity in three patients. **Dermatology** 198(1):18–25.
54. Glover MT, Lake BD, Atherton DH (1992) Clinical, histological, and ultrastructural findings in two cases of infantile systemic hyalinosis. **Pediatr Dermatol** 9(3):255–258.
55. Ruiz-Maldonado R, Tamayo L, Velazquez E (1977) Dystrophie dermo-chondro-cornéenne familiale (syndrome de François). **Ann Dermatol Venereol** 104(6–7):475–478.

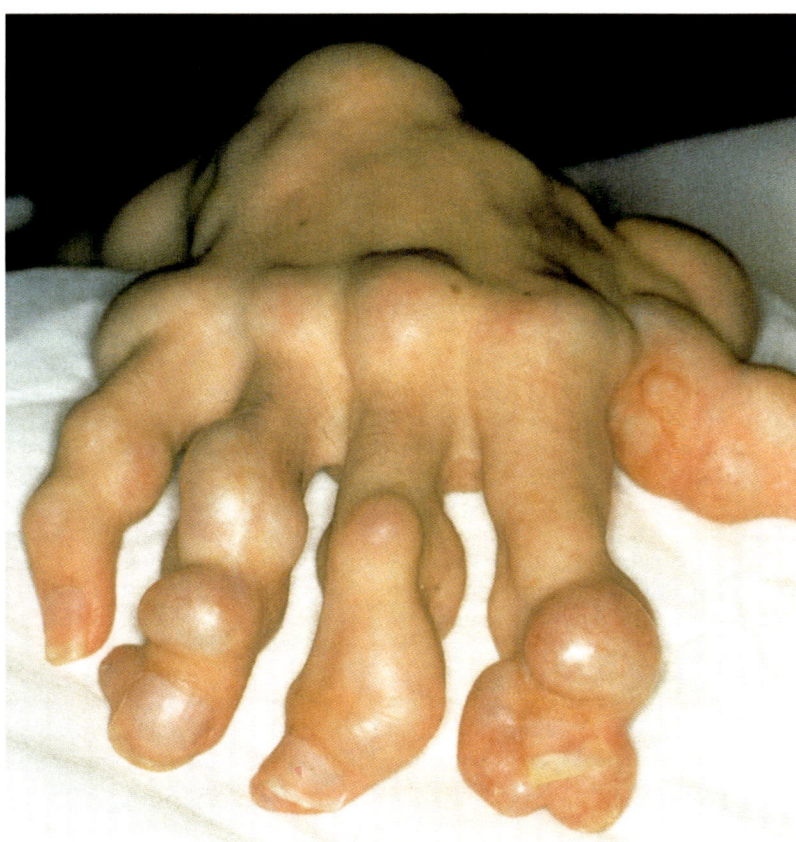

Fig. 21.11 Juvenile hyaline fibromatosis with multiple disfiguring nodules (Courtesy of Peter Kind MD, Frankfurt, Germany).

acellular and fibrous. The cells are usually bland and mitoses are uncommon. The histologic dilemma arises when the fibroblasts are quite cellular and atypical. These lesions have been diagnosed as aggressive fibromatosis, differentiated fibrosarcoma, or fibrosarcoma-like fibromatosis. The essential distinction between a desmoid-type fibromatosis with a significant risk of local recurrence and an infantile fibrosarcoma that has a small but real risk of metastasis requires expert pathological consultation. Treatment consists of complete excision, which often may be extensive or compromised by involvement of vital structures. At least half of the lesions recur and subsequent therapy is difficult. Features pointing towards recurrence include not only extension to the surgical margin, but also onset at more than 5 years of age and location on an extremity. Anti-estrogens, such as tamoxifen, are the usual resort, as with other desmoids.[48,56]

BENIGN FIBROUS LESIONS
Hypertrophic scar and keloid

These common problems are seen on a daily basis (Ch. 18). A hypertrophic scar is a thickened scar within the confines of the original insult, while a keloid is a scar that has proliferated beyond the expected margins and may continue to grow. The classic example of a keloid is a large nodule that occurs on the ear lobe after piercing. There is clearly a racial predisposition, as keloids are far more common in blacks, as well as a site predilection, with favored areas being the sternum, ankles, shoulders, and other areas of tension. Keloids are also a feature of the Rubenstein–Taybi syndrome (Ch. 18). A hypertrophic scar is usually perceived by the patient as a scar that has healed poorly, often being reddened or raised. It may improve spontaneously, while a keloid rarely does. Both processes are myofibroblastic proliferations.

Dermatofibroma

Dermatofibromas (Ch. 17) are common dermal tumors that may occur at any age, including childhood. In some countries they are called histiocytomas. A dermatofibroma often presents as a small (less than 1cm) firm but movable nodule with a predilection for the extremities. The overlying skin may dimple when the lesion is pinched. Dermatofibromas may appear yellow to blue to brown because of hemosiderin within the tumor. They are most likely reactive processes, often triggered by an insect bite or folliculitis, which occasionally flatten or regress. Multiple dermatofibromas are a possible marker for systemic lupus erythematosus, especially in young black women. Microscopically, they show an admixture of collagen, fibroblasts and macrophages, as well as vessels and hemosiderin. Many histological variants have been described but they are of little clinical significance. The aneurysmal fibrous histiocytoma is a variant with large vascular spaces associated with hemorrhage; its name is often confused with angiomatoid fibrous histiocytoma, a more aggressive tumor discussed below.[57] The best treatment is probably no treatment, as excision often leads to unacceptable scarring.

Sclerotic fibroma

Sclerotic fibromas are small waxy papules with a peculiar hyalinized stroma, resembling a cut onion. They may also contain mucin and are sharply demarcated from the adjacent dermis. Although sclerotic fibromas were first described in patients with Cowden syndrome, they also occur sporadically and are best viewed as dermatofibroma variants. If desired, excision is curative.[58]

Pleomorphic fibroma

Pleomorphic fibromas are usually pedunculated lesions resembling a skin tag, although some resemble dermatofibromas. Although they are clinically indistinct, histologically they show striking atypia of spindle-shaped cells that stain with myofibroblastic markers. Excision is curative.[59]

Dermatomyofibroma

Dermatomyofibroma is a plaque-like proliferation of both fibroblasts and myofibroblasts.[60,61] It tends to occur around the shoulder girdle or neck of young women. Occasional childhood lesions have been reported.[62] Histologically, it is a bland lesion consisting of spindle-shaped cells often arranged parallel to the epidermis and separated by collagen fibers. Elastin fibers are also present. Immunochemistry reveals positive staining for vimentin and alpha-smooth muscle actin. No treatment is required, but smaller lesions can be conveniently excised.

Angiofibroma

A number of clinically quite different lesions have been grouped together as cutaneous angiofibromas. The unifying feature is that they feature fibrosis of the papillary and periadnexal dermis associated with prominent vessels. The stellate fibroblast-like cells are most often positive for Factor XIIIa, a marker for dermal dendritic cells, but the significance of this variation is unclear. Included in the group are:

56. Keltz M, DiCostanzo D, Desai P et al. (1995) Infantile (desmoid-type) fibromatosis. **Pediatr Dermatol** 12(2):149–151.
57. Calonje E, Fletcher CD (1995) Aneurysmal benign fibrous histiocytoma. Clinicopathological analysis of 40 cases of a tumour frequently misdiagnosed as a vascular neoplasm. **Histopathology** 26(4):323–331.
58. Chang SN, Chun SI, Moon TK et al. (2000) Solitary sclerotic fibroma of the skin: degenerated sclerotic change of inflammatory conditions, especially folliculitis. A **J Dermatopathol** 22(1):22–25.
59. Garcia-Doval I, Casas L, Toribio J (1998) Pleomorphic fibroma of the skin, a form of sclerotic fibroma: an immunohistochemical study. **Clin Exp Dermatol** 23(1):22–24.
60. Hügel H (1991) Die plaqueförmige dermale Fibromatose. **Hautarzt** 42(4)223–226.
61. Kamino H, Reddy VB, Gero M et al. (1992) Dermatomyofibroma. A benign cutaneous plaque-like proliferation of fibroblasts and myofibroblasts in young adults. **J Cutan Pathol** 19(2):85–93.
62. Rose C, Bröcker EB (1999) Dermatomyofibroma: case report and review. **Pediatr Dermatol** 16(6):456–459.

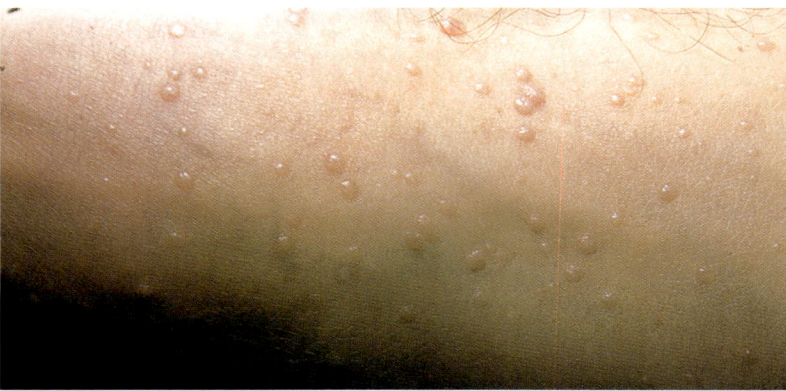

Fig. 21.12 Many tiny pale to red papules, which on biopsy were angiofibromas. The patient had other family members with the same lesions.

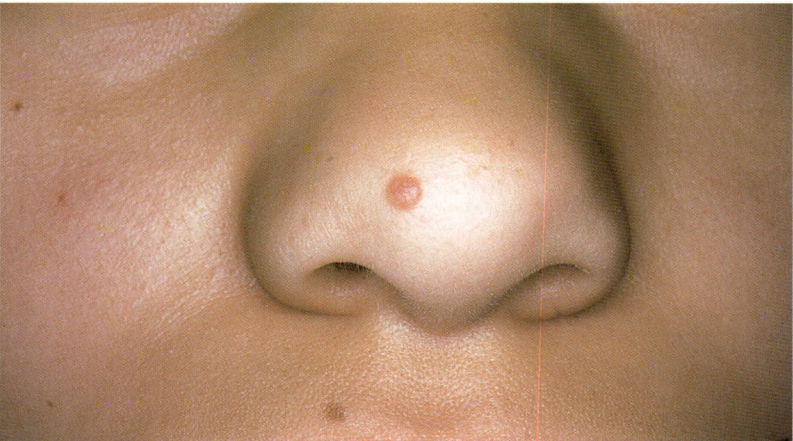

Fig. 21.13 Fibrous papule of the nose.

- Facial lesions in tuberous sclerosis (Ch. 18). The usual designation of adenoma sebaceum is a misnomer; the lesions are not sebaceous gland proliferations. Genital angiofibromas may also be seen.[63] In addition, segmental distribution of angiofibromas occurs.[64] Finally, patients with MEN 1 syndrome also have facial angiofibromas.[40]
- Multiple angiofibromas can occasionally be seen in patients with no other disease stigmata (Fig. 21.12). Our guess is that such individuals carry mutations for tuberous sclerosis of MEN 1 but only with partial expression of the phenotype.
- Fibrous papule of the nose (and face) is a skin-colored papule, common in adults, but rarely seen in children (Fig. 21.13). Its etiology is unclear; some lesions are regressing melanocytic nevi but this is unlikely to be the case in children. Often a shave excision is the best approach to minimize scarring on the nose.
- Pearly penile papules are multiple white papules along the corona of the glans. They are usually misdiagnosed as warts, but quite common, present in at least 10% of young men. The same lesions in females surround the vaginal orifice and may be elongated; they are known as hirsuties papillaris vulva or vestibular papillae of the vulva. Both are harmless and require no therapy.

- Acral fibrokeratoma is an acquired digital tumor usually misdiagnosed as a therapy-refractory wart. There is typically a collarette of scale about a firm papule, usually arising in the nail fold. The periungual Koenen tumors of tuberous sclerosis are clinically quite similar, but usually occur on more than one digit. Microscopically, there is prominent hyperkeratosis, often with a sharp lateral invagination at the border. In the dermis are numerous vessels, stellate fibroblasts and thickened collagen.

Nodular fasciitis and related diseases

Nodular fasciitis is a benign, reactive myofibroblastic growth that may appear alarming under the microscope, prompting the former disturbing designation of pseudosarcomatous fasciitis. It presents as a rapidly growing firm subcutaneous nodule, several centimeters in size, occasionally adherent to underlying muscle fascia. It occurs most commonly on the arm, thigh, or chest wall. Histologically, these lesions show a variety of patterns, with a predominance of myxoid, cellular, or fibrous elements. Intradermal variants have been described.[65] While it can be difficult to separate the cellular variants from sarcomas, nodular fasciitis is usually well circumscribed and lacks atypical mitoses. Local surgical excision is adequate treatment, with recurrence a rare event, highlighting the benign nature of this clinical entity. When recurrence does occur, careful reconsideration of the original diagnosis is essential.[66]

There are several closely related forms of fasciitis, all rare and unlikely to be encountered by dermatologists. One is proliferative fasciitis, which is characterized by both spindle cells and bizarre ganglion-like cells in a myxoid and collagenous matrix. Although it is primarily an adult disease, some cases have been described in childhood.[67] Cranial fasciitis occurs almost exclusively in the first year of life, involving the scalp and underlying skull. It, too, grows rapidly, may be related to trauma, and often causes alarm as it can erode the skull.[68] Similarly, intravascular fasciitis appears as multiple nodules in both veins and arteries. Over 50% of cases occur in children.[69] The differential diagnosis includes reactive intravascular processes, such as intravascular pyogenic granuloma and Masson phenomenon (papillary endothelial hyperplasia).

Fibroma of tendon sheath

The exact nature of this tumor is unclear. It may represent a late collagenous phase of an inflammatory traumatic response such as nodular fasciitis. It presents as a solitary rubbery mass attached at the tendon sheath (Fig. 21.14), most often of the hands in young adults. There is a male predominance.[70] In the original series, about 20% occurred in children or adolescents.[71] Histologic examination reveals a lobular arrangement of dense fibrous and collagenous areas with large clefts and focal cellular portions. Surgery is usually curative; 25% recur but can be retreated and permanent sequelae are rare.

Giant cell tumor of tendon sheath

This tumor probably represents a different stage of fibroma of tendon sheath.[72] It typically involves the dorsal aspects of the hands, especially about the distal intraphalangeal joints, usually affects adults, and is more likely to be multiple. Microscopically, it shows a large of number of multinucleate giant cells admixed with a fibrous stroma. Individual lesions can be excised if they are painful or disfiguring.

FIBROMATOSES

A fibromatosis is defined in the WHO classification as "a differentiated fibroblastic tumor with a biologic behavior intermediate between benign

63. Nico MM, Ito LM, Valente NY (1999) Genital angiofibromas in tuberous sclerosis: two cases. J Dermatol 26(2):111–114.
64. Silvestre JF, Banuls J, Ramon R et al. (2000) Unilateral multiple facial angiofibromas: a mosaic form of tuberous sclerosis. J Am Acad Dermatol 43(1):127–129.
65. Goodlad JR, Fletcher CD (1990) Intradermal variant of nodular "fasciitis". Histopathology 17(6):569–571.
66. Sarangarajan R, Dehner LP (1999) Cranial and extracranial fasciitis of childhood: a clinicopathologic and immunohistochemical study. Hum Pathol 30(1):87–92.
67. Meis JM, Enzinger FM (1992) Proliferative fasciitis and myositis of childhood. Am J Surg Pathol 16(4):364–372.

68. Sajben FP, Eichenfeld LE, O'Grady TC et al. (1999) Cranial fasciitis of childhood. Pediatr Dermatol 16(3):232–234.
69. Patchefsky AS, Enzinger FM (1981) Intravascular fasciitis: a report of 17 cases. Am J Surg Pathol 5(1):29–36.
70. Pulitzer DR, Martin PC, Reed RJ (1989) Fibroma of tendon sheath. A clinicopathologic study of 32 cases. Am J Surg Pathol 13(6):472–479.
71. Chung EB, Enzinger FM (1979) Fibroma of tendon sheath. Cancer 44(5):1945–1954.
72. Maluf HM, De Young BR, Swanson PE et al. (1995) Fibroma and giant cell tumor of tendon sheath: a comparative histological and immunohistological study. Mod Pathol 8(2):155–159.

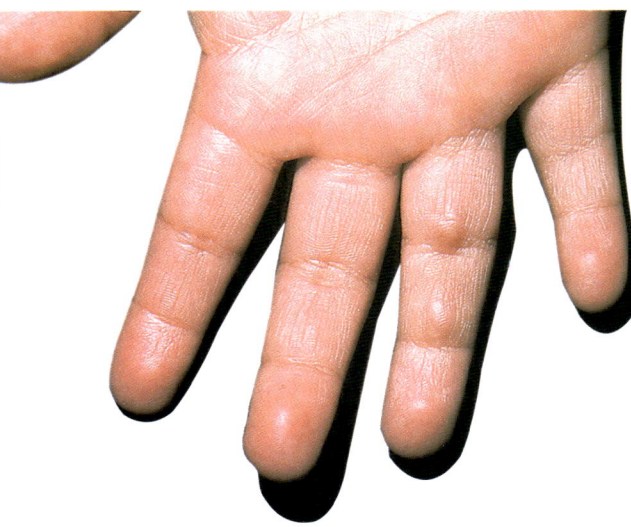

Fig. 21.14   Fibroma of tendon sheath with multiple nodules over the flexor tendon of the 4th digit.

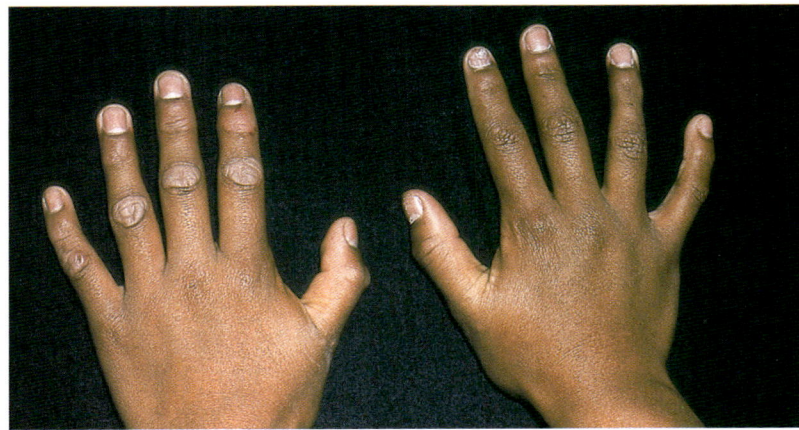

Fig. 21.15   Knuckle pads.

fibroblastic tumors and fibrosarcoma, having the capacity to recur locally but not to metastasize."[5] The most troublesome fibromatosis is the infantile-desmoid type fibromatosis, considered above under infantile tumors.

Superficial fibromatoses

The two most common lesions in this group primarily involve the elderly; they are palmar fibromatosis or Dupuytren contracture and penile fibromatosis or Peyronie disease. The other less common members may be seen in children.

- Plantar fibromatosis (Ledderhose disease) presents as a firm nodule, usually on the mid-plantar surface. Contractures are uncommon in contrast to Dupuytren disease, but the lesions are usually excised because of discomfort.
- Precalcaneal congenital fibrolipomatous hamartoma is a rare lesion which may be confused with Ledderhose disease.[73,74] It presents as a nodule just anterior-medial to the heel on the plantar surface, usually present at birth. When excised, there is an admixture of fibrous and fatty tissue, reflecting the usual mix on the sole.
- Knuckle pads are asymptomatic fibrous plaques over the knuckles (Fig. 21.15).[75,76] In children, a solitary knuckle thickening is usually from trauma, such as sucking or rubbing, or cracking the joints.[77] Multiple lesions, especially those present in infancy, are more likely to reflect inherited connective tissue abnormalities, such as Bart–Pumphrey syndrome.[78] In adolescents and adults, occupational trauma sometimes plays a role, placing knuckle pads in the same category as calluses. Biopsies are rarely done, but reveal thickened dermal collagen. No treatment is effective.
- Pachydermodactyly represents a more widespread form of reactive digital fibromatosis, almost always seen in individuals who interlock their fingers, exert pressure, and attempt to pull against the pressure.[79] They develop thickened digits, sometimes with discrete lesions on the medial and lateral aspects of the fingers.

Deep or musculoaponeurotic fibromatoses

While these disorders rarely come to the attention of a dermatologist, they are of considerable significance. They feature a striking contrast between a bland histologic appearance and the ability to grow rapidly, attain great size, and interfere with vital functions.[80] Extra-abdominal desmoids involve the muscles and aponeuroses of the shoulder girdle and pelvic muscles of young adults, whereas abdominal desmoids arise typically in the muscle sheath of the abdomen in young females after pregnancy or abdominal surgery. Extra-abdominal desmoids have been described in association with idiopathic multicentric osteolysis or disappearing bone disease.[81]

Intra-abdominal fibromatosis is usually a complication of familial adenomatous polyposis (Gardner syndrome) (Ch. 17). Almost every Gardner syndrome patient has a colectomy for prophylactic removal of their premalignant colonic polyps. A major complication of this surgery is the development of desmoid tumors in the mesentery and retroperitoneum, as well as in the abdominal scar, usually within a few years of the surgery. Another common trigger is a cesarean section. Familial desmoids involve a mutation in the APC gene, just as Gardner syndrome, but in a slightly different region so only the fibroblastic response is abnormal. Other patients may develop sporadic desmoids which may reflect sporadic mutations in the APC gene.

SARCOMAS OF FIBROBLASTIC ORIGIN

Dermatofibrosarcoma protuberans

Dermatofibrosarcoma protuberans (DFSP) is a slowly progressive fibrous tumor usually occurring on the shoulder girdle of young adults (Fig. 21.16). In one series, 8 of 136 (5.9%) of DFSP tumors presented before 13 years of age.[82] Lesions at birth and in infancy have been reported.[83–85] Early lesions are often flat, or even atrophic.[86] Later lesions are nodular or claw-like and often characterized as a bumpy "scar" in an area where no trauma has occurred. Bednar tumor is a pigmented DFSP and also may occur in children.[87] The differential diagnosis is limited, once a true scar has been excluded. Dermatomyofibroma and morphea profunda may be similar clinically but have different histology. Under the microscope the hallmark is the infiltration of the dermis and subcutaneous fat septae by slender uniform

73. Ortega-Monzó C, Molina-Gallardo I, Monteagudo-Castro C et al. (2000) Precalcaneal congenital fibrolipomatous hamartoma: a report of four cases. Pediatr Dermatol 17(6):429–431.
74. Jacob CI, Kumm RC (2000) Benign anteriomedial plantar nodules of childhood: a distinct form of plantar fibromatosis. Pediatr Dermatol 17(6):472–474.
75. Paller AS, Hebert AA (1986) Knuckle pads in children. Am J Dis Child 140(9):915–917.
76. Guberman D, Lichtenstein DA, Vardy DA (1996) Knuckle pads – a forgotten skin condition: report of a case and review of the literature. Cutis 57(4):241–242.
77. Peterson CM, Barnes CJ, Davis LS (2000) Knuckle pads: does knuckle cracking play an etiologic role? Pediatr Dermatol 17(6):450–452.
78. Ramer JC, Vasily DB, Ladda RL (1994) Familial leuconychia, knuckle pads, hearing loss, and palmoplantar hyperkeratosis: an additional family with Bart-Pumphrey syndrome. J Med Genet 31(1):68–71.
79. Kopera D, Soyer HP, Kerl H (1995) An update on pachydermodactyly and a report of three additional cases. Br J Dermatol 133(3):433–437.
80. Mendez-Fernandez MA, Gard DA (1991) The desmoid tumor: "benign" neoplasm, not a benign disease. Plast Reconstr Surg 87(5):956–960.

81. Sahn EE, Cook WJ, Gross RH et al. (1993) Musculoaponeurotic fibromatosis (extraabdominal desmoid tumor) in a child with idiopathic multicentric osteolysis. Pediatr Dermatol 10(1):49–53.
82. McKee PH, Fletcher CD (1991) Dermatofibrosarcoma protuberans presenting in infancy and childhood. J Cutan Pathol 18(4):241–246.
83. Bouyssou-Gauthier ML, Labrousse F, Longis B et al. (1997) Dermatofibrosarcoma protuberans in childhood. Pediatr Dermatol 14(6):463–465.
84. Checketts SR, Hamilton TK, Baughman RD (2000) Congenital and childhood dermatofibrosarcoma protuberans: a case report and review of the literature. J Am Acad Dermatol 42(5):907–913.
85. Patrizi A, Vespignani F, Fraternali GO et al. (2000) A pediatric case of dermatofibrosarcoma protuberans: an immunohistochemical study. Pediatr Dermatol 17(1):29–33.
86. Martin L, Combemale P, Dupin M et al. (1998) The atrophic variant of dermatofibrosarcoma protuberans in childhood: a report of six cases. Br J Dermatol 139(4):719–725.
87. Marcus JR, Few JW, Senger C et al. (1998) Dermatofibrosarcoma protuberans and the Bednar tumor: treatment in the pediatric population. J Pediatr Surg 33(12):1811–1814.

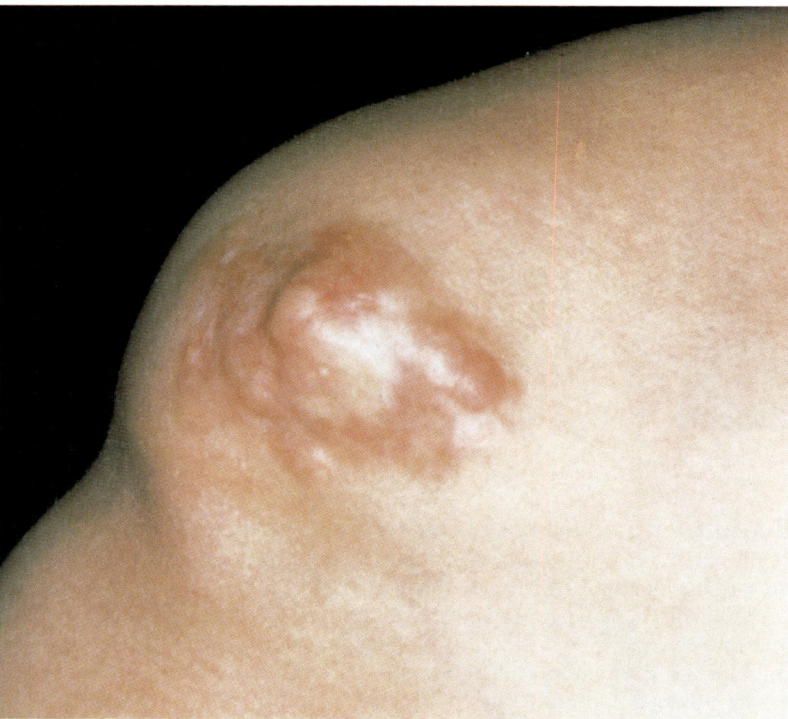

Fig. 21.16 Dermatofibrosarcoma protuberans in typical location on shoulder with irregular finger-like projections.

spindle cells arranged in a cartwheel or storiform pattern, almost invariably CD34 positive. The typical cytogenic change is a t(17;22)(q22;q13) translocation fusing the collagen 1 gene (COL1A1) with a growth control gene. Fibrosarcomatous degeneration can occur, in which case the histologic features more closely resemble a fibrosarcoma and the prognosis is worse.[88] Initial surgery should be generous; at least 3cm margins appear judicious. Micrographic surgery has been recommended.[89] When the initial surgery is inadequate, recurrences are common but metastases rare.

Giant cell fibroblastoma

Giant cell fibroblastoma presents as a solitary dermal nodule in young children, typically involving the thigh, groin or, less often, trunk.[90,91] Histologically, it is characterized by sinusoidal spaces lined by giant cells as well as pleomorphic spindle cells in a myxoid matrix. Similar areas can be identified in DFSP and the same lesion may show both patterns at different times. The same cytogenetic changes are also seen. Thus, it is best viewed as a variant of DFSP. Recurrences are common but metastases extremely rare.

Plexiform fibrohistiocytic tumor

This tumor presents as a solitary deep nodule, usually in the upper arm, in teenagers or young adults.[92] Microscopically, there are plexiform fibrous bundles admixed with fibrohistiocytic nodules, often with giant cells. The

histologic differential diagnosis is vast, including neural, fibrous, smooth muscle, and histiocytic tumors.[93,94] About 70% are cured by initial excision but the tumors can be locally aggressive or even metastasize.

Malignant fibrous histiocytoma

As soft tissue tumors have been reclassified over the past two decades, malignant fibrous histiocytoma (MFH) has gone from being an unknown to becoming the most common adult sarcoma to once again having its existence questioned. The histogenesis of this sarcoma remains unclear; it is hard to reconcile the fibrous and histiocytic features with a single cell of origin. Fewer than 5% of MFH occur before the age of 20. The superficial variant of MFH is known as an atypical fibroxanthoma.[95] It may be seen in severely sun-damaged skin, in xeroderma pigmentosum in children,[96] or rarely as a papule or nodule on the trunk or extremities in non-sun-damaged skin in young adults.[97] Local excision is usually curative for the superficial lesions; deeper lesions must be approached like any other sarcoma.

Angiomatoid fibrous histiocytoma

This tumor was for years classified at the least aggressive end of the malignant fibrous histiocytoma spectrum.[98] Most cases appear in children and young adults, usually involving subcutaneous or deeper soft tissues, but occasionally extending to the dermis. A small percentage of cases behave aggressively and may even rarely present with lymph node involvement.[99] There are no reliable microscopic criteria to identify the lesions more likely to behave aggressively. Because of the confusing biology, the initial excision should be generous.

Fibrosarcoma

Fibrosarcomas have become less common in recent years, probably because of increased diagnostic precision. Although rare, they are the second most common childhood sarcoma involving the skin, following rhabdomyosarcoma. Both congenital and infantile lesions are identified; almost all appear before 5 years of age. The tumors are rapidly growing, usually subcutaneous masses tending to involve the extremities, pelvis, and head and neck region.

Histologically, the prototypic infantile fibrosarcoma has sheets of spindle-shaped cells with abundant mitoses. Often there is a herring bone pattern, with tumor fascicles running at angles to each other. The characteristic translocation is t(12;15)(p13;q25). The chief diagnostic difficulty lies in distinguishing between an infantile desmoid-type fibromatosis and an infantile fibrosarcoma. In one large series, 50% of fibrosarcomas in children over 10 years of age (which can be viewed as adult fibrosarcomas) metastasized. In patients less than 5 years old, the metastatic rate was only 7%, but local recurrences appeared in over 40% of cases.[100] This suggests that whatever name is applied, infants with histologically worrisome fibrous tumors do much better than their older counterparts. Surgery is the treatment of choice, with radiation and chemotherapy reserved for postsurgical prophylaxis or treatment of recurrences and metastases.

Two rare variants of fibrosarcoma which primarily affect young adults are:

- Fibromyxoid sarcoma is often labeled as a low-grade tumor, although 50% of patients develop metastases. It arises primarily in the deep soft tissues of young adults. Microscopically, there are spindle cells, often quite bland, admixed with a myxoid stroma.

88. Mentzel T, Beham A, Katenkamp et al. (1998) Fibrosarcomatous ("high-grade") dermatofibrosarcoma protuberans: clinicopathologic and immunohistochemical study of a series of 41 cases with emphasis on prognostic significance. **Am J Surg Pathol** 22(5):576–587.
89. Goldberg DJ, Maso M (1990) Dermatofibrosarcoma protuberans in a 9-year-old child: treatment by MOHS micrographic surgery. **Pediatr Dermatol** 7(1):57–59.
90. Shmookler BM, Enzinger FM, Weiss SW (1989) Giant cell fibroblastoma. A juvenile form of dermatofibrosarcoma protuberans. **Cancer** 64(10):2154–2161.
91. Diaz-Cascajo C, Borrego L, Bastida-Inarrea J et al. (1996) Giant cell fibroblastoma. New histological observations. **Am J Dermatopathol** 18(4):403–408.
92. Enzinger FM, Zhang RY (1988) Plexiform fibrohistiocytic tumor presenting in children and young adults. An analysis of 65 cases. **Am J Surg Pathol** 12(11):818–826.
93. Zelger B, Weinlich G, Steiner H et al. (1997) Dermal and subcutaneous variants of plexiform fibrohistiocytic tumor. **Am J Surg Pathol** 21(2):235–241.

94. Remstein ED, Arndt DA, Nascimento AG (1999) Plexiform fibrohistiocytic tumor: clinicopathologic analysis of 22 cases. **Am J Surg Pathol** 23(6):662–670.
95. Fretzin DF, Helwig EB (1973) Atypical fibroxanthoma of the skin. A clinicopathologic study of 140 cases. **Cancer** 31(6):1541–1552.
96. Dilek FH, Akpolat N, Metin A et al. (2000) Atypical fibroxanthoma of the skin and the lower lip in xeroderma pigmentosum. **Br J Dermatol** 143(3):618–620.
97. Rothman AE, Lowitt MH, Pfau RG (2000) Pediatric cutaneous malignant fibrous histiocytoma. **J Am Acad Dermatol** 42(2):371–373.
98. Enzinger FM (1979) Angiomatoid malignant fibrous histiocytoma: a distinct fibrohistiocytic tumor of children and young adults simulating a vascular neoplasm. **Cancer** 44(6):2147–2157.
99. Costa MJ, Weiss SW (1990) Angiomatoid malignant fibrous histiocytoma. A follow-up study of 108 cases with evaluation of possible histologic predictors of outcome. **Am J Surg Pathol** 14(12):1126–1132.
100. Soule EH, Pritcharc DJ (1977) Fibrosarcoma in infants and children: a review of 110 cases. **Cancer** 40(4):1711–1721.

- Inflammatory fibrosarcoma is a tumor of the mesentery and retroperitoneum which may represent a myofibroblastic tumor of less malignant potential than a fibrosarcoma.

NEURAL TUMORS

BENIGN NEURAL TUMORS

There are a wide variety of benign neural tumors, several of which are markers for a series of genodermatoses. In each case, conservative local excision is curative, except for the plexiform or diffuse neurofibromas of NF1 in which an excision can lead into therapeutic quagmires.

Neurofibroma

Solitary neurofibromas occur most commonly in adults as soft compressible pedunculated papules or nodules. While a single neurofibroma in an adult is almost never associated with neurofibromatosis, a solitary superficial neurofibroma in childhood should prompt a search for other clinical features of neurofibromatosis type1 (NF1) and various other neurofibromatosis subtypes. A frequently misdiagnosed solitary neurofibroma in children is the subungual variant which is usually not associated with NF1.[101] Multiple neurofibromas may also occur in a linear or segmental distribution unaccompanied by the systemic features of NF1, suggesting somatic mosaicism.[102] Histologically, neurofibromas are well circumscribed without a distinct capsule. Tumor cells are spindled with thin, wavy nuclei and the tumor stroma is delicate and often contains mucin and mast cells. The neurofibromas of neurofibromatosis cannot be distinguished from solitary neurofibromas by histologic criteria. If treatment is desired, shave excisions should be avoided as they often produce gaping scars. Simple excision and closure is preferable. Children with NF1 may also develop deep-seated or plexiform neurofibromas, appearing as worm-like masses involving major nerves. This tumor has approximately a 5% chance of malignant degeneration; the resulting sarcoma is confusingly called malignant peripheral nerve sheath tumor, neurofibrosarcoma, or malignant schwannoma. Diffuse neurofibroma is another rare variant seen sporadically and in NF1 patients. It presents most commonly as a firm, large plaque with indistinct borders on the head and neck. Histologically, there is diffuse infiltration of surrounding fat and dermis with spindled cells. Malignant degeneration is most rare, in contrast to plexiform neurofibroma. Both plexiform and diffuse neurofibromas present an extreme therapeutic challenge because of their size and association with deeper structures. Surgery is usually delayed unless there is suspicion of malignant change or involvement of vital structures.

Neurilemmoma

Neurilemmomas, also known as schwannomas, occur most commonly as small, painful, solitary nodules on the head, neck, and proximal extremities in adults. Solitary neurilemmomas are rare in childhood. While some patients with typical NF1 with typical café-au-lait macules and neurofibromas also have neurilemmomas, they are far more strongly associated with NF2 and acoustic neuromas. Neurilemmomatosis or schwannomatosis is the diagnosis applied to patients with multiple neurilemmomas and no other stigmata for NF2 (Fig. 21.17).[103,104] Such patients also have a mutation in the NF2 gene. In some instances, the neural tumors are present at birth or in early infancy. The patients should be carefully followed for the development of acoustic neuromas. In the Gorlin–Koutlas syndrome, there are multiple neurilemmomas, multiple vaginal leiomyomas, and multiple melanocytic nevi; the gene has not been identified.[105]

Histologically, neurilemmomas are well circumscribed and often have a fibrous capsule. The tumor has a distinctive biphasic pattern, as cellular areas with palisaded nuclei (Antoni A) tend to alternate with loose, unorganized,

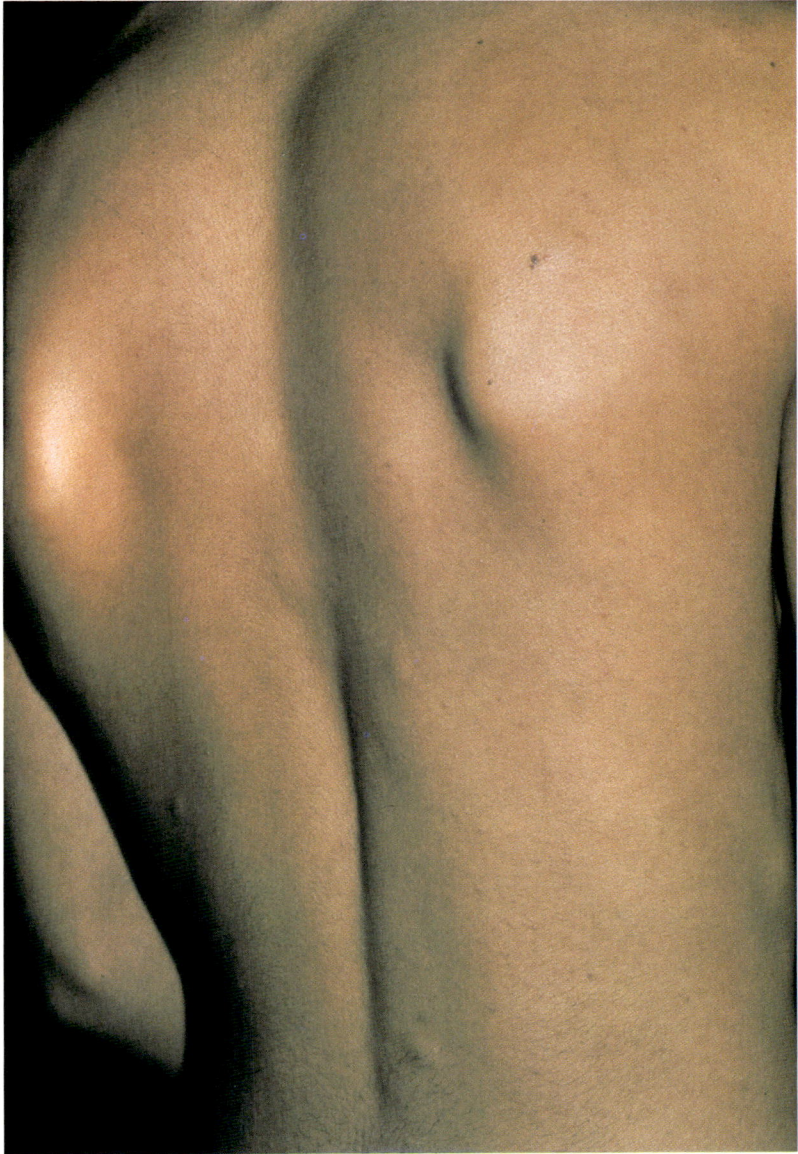

Fig. 21.17   Neurilemmomatosis with multiple subcutaneous nodules.

relatively acellular areas (Antoni B). Excision is usually simple, as the lesions shell out nicely but may be attached to a nerve.

Neuroma

Neuromas are usually the result of disorganized overgrowth of a nerve following surgery or trauma. They are often painful. The most common painful tumors are listed using the mnemonic BENGAL:

Blue rubber bleb nevus
Eccrine tumors
Neural tumors
Glomus tumor
Angiolipoma
Leiomyoma

In children, neuromas occasionally form at the base of a supernumerary digit, which presents as a congenital papule on the ulnar portion of the hand near

101. Niizuma K, Iijima KN (1991) Solitary neurofibroma: a case of subungual neurofibroma on the right third finger. **Arch Dermatol Res** 283(1):13–15.
102. Tinschert S, Naumann I, Stegmann E et al. (2000) Segmental neurofibromatosis is caused by somatic mutation of the neurofibromatosis type 1 (NF1) gene. **Eur J Hum Genet** 8(6):455–459.
103. Murata Y, Kumano K, Ugai K et al. (1991) Neurilemmomatosis. **Br J Dermatol** 125(5):466–468.
104. Iyengar V, Golomb CA, Schachner L (1998) Neurilemmomatosis, NF2 and juvenile xanthogranuloma. **J Am Acad Dermatol** 39(5):831–834.
105. Gorlin RJ, Koutlas IG (1998) Multiple schwannomas, multiple nevi, and multiple vaginal leiomyomas: a new dominant syndrome. **Am J Med Genet** 78(1):76–81.

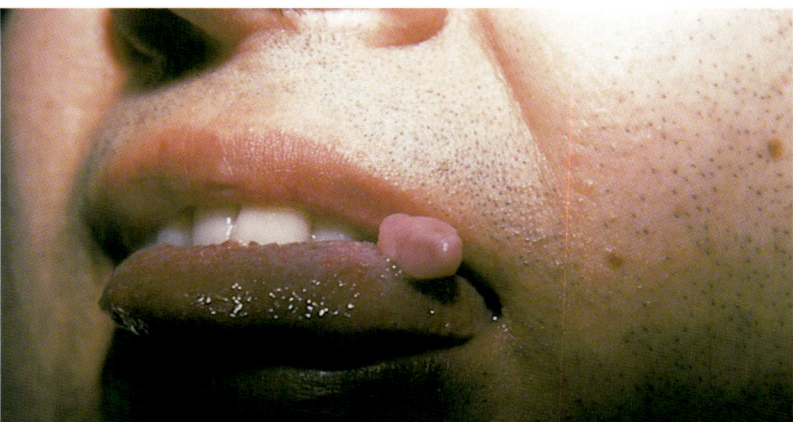

Fig. 21.18   Granular cell tumor on lip.

the fifth finger. Mucosal neuromas are a feature of the MEN 2B syndrome (Ch. 22) along with medullary carcinoma of the thyroid and pheochromocytomas. Ocular conjunctival neuromas in these patients may result in a permanently everted eyelid – another Gorlin sign. The mucosal neuromas usually precede the other tumors, appearing in childhood.

Granular cell tumor

Granular cell tumors occur most commonly as solitary dermal or subcutaneous nodules on the tongue (Fig. 21.18) or trunk of middle-aged people. While solitary tumors are rare in children, multiple granular cell tumors have been reported occasionally, sometimes in association with NF1.[106–108] Malignant granular cell tumors have not been reported in childhood and adolescence. Histologically, the tumors are poorly circumscribed and composed of distinctive round cells with coarsely granular cytoplasm. The overlying epithelium often has pseudoepitheliomatous hyperplasia, which may be confused with squamous cell carcinoma. The congenital epulis or congenital granular cell tumor is a rare gingival tumor occurring in infancy that often regresses spontaneously. The exact nature of granular tumors is still unclear, with conflicting evidence for neural, pericytic and smooth muscle origin. They may well represent a reaction pattern rather than a highly specific tumor. Excision is generally curative.

Neurothekeoma

Neurothekeomas or nerve sheath myxomas are relatively uncommon, small, superficial soft tissue tumors.[109,110] These tumors of nerve sheath origin occur most frequently between 10 and 30 years of age as small, painless nodules on the face, neck, or shoulder. Histologically, the tumor has two variants. A myxoid variant is composed of mucinous fascicles with a few spindled cells. A cellular variant is composed of fascicles of more epithelioid cells with pink or pale-staining cytoplasm and scant mucin. Since clinical identification is almost impossible, the usual approach is an excisional biopsy.

Meningoceles and meningiomas

A baffling number of names have been given to ectopic meningeal tissue which results from abnormal neural tube closure.[111] A true or classic meningocele is the result of an outbulging or malformation of the meninges and by definition is connected to the underlying neural structures and often associated with a skeletal defect. Classic meningoceles tend to be present at birth or an early age. They are a neurosurgical problem.

Rudimentary meningocele refers to remnants of meningothelial elements in the skin and soft tissue.[112,113] These tumors may clinically mimic an epidermoid cyst or skin tag on the forehead, scalp, or paravertebral areas of a newborn. While in most cases there is no underlying bony defect or connection to the meninges, imaging studies should be performed prior to any surgical intervention. Rudimentary meningoceles have also been called meningothelial hamartomas. In contrast, meningiomas are usually solitary tumors felt to result from the growth of meningeal cells displaced along cutaneous nerves or as a sequel to skull trauma when presumably fragments of the meninges are trapped and then grow in an ectopic fashion. Both are usually excised. Primary cutaneous meningiomas have also been described in NF1.[114]

Nasal glioma

A nasal glioma is a rare developmental anomaly in which an encephalocele or herniation of both brain tissue and meninges is separated from the underlying frontal lobes by closure of the cranial sutures. The most common presentation is a congenital gray or red–gray nodule on the bridge of the nose. In contrast to meningioma, the likelihood of an underlying connection is greater and brain tissue is seen on the biopsy.

Ganglioneuroma

This rare lesion usually develops after birth, but may be congenital.[115] Typical neural ganglion cells are aggregated in the dermis or soft tissue. The differential diagnosis includes a well-differentiated metastasis of neuroblastoma, so the patient should be evaluated with this in mind. Rarely, neurofibromas in patients with NF1 may entrap ganglion cells. If the lesion is solitary, local excision is curative.

MALIGNANT NEURAL TUMORS

Malignant peripheral nerve sheath tumor, formerly known as neurofibrosarcoma or malignant schwannoma, is a rare complication in children with neurofibromatosis. It presents as a changing, tender subcutaneous mass in a plexiform neurofibroma but may extend to the dermis. Sporadic peripheral malignant nerve sheath tumors are extremely uncommon in children (Fig. 21.19). Treatment is generous resection; often it is necessary to sacrifice a major nerve. If the resection achieves free margins, the outlook is promising. Otherwise the chances are dismal.[116]

SMOOTH MUSCLE TUMORS

BENIGN SMOOTH MUSCLE TUMORS

Congenital smooth muscle hamartoma

This lesion is present at birth or early infancy. Typically it is a slightly pigmented plaque which has increased vellus or terminal hairs (Fig. 21.20), and becomes firmer or shows goose bumps when the infant becomes colder or the lesion is rubbed.[117,118] Some lesions are atrophic. The trunk, buttock,

106. Martin RW 3rd, Neldner KH, Boyd AS et al. (1990) Multiple cutaneous granular cell tumors and neurofibromatosis in childhood. A case report and review of the literature. **Arch Dermatol** 126(8):1051–1056.
107. Sahn EE, Dunlavey ES, Parsons JL (1997) Multiple cutaneous granular cell tumors in a child with possible neurofibromatosis. **J Am Acad Dermatol** 36(2)327–330.
108. Dorta S, Sanchez R, Garcia-Bustinduy M et al. (2000) Multiple granular tumours in a teenager. **Br J Dermatol** 143(4):906–907.
109. Gallager RL, Helwig EB (1980) Neurothekeoma – a benign cutaneous tumor of neural origin. **Am J Clin Pathol** 74(6):759–764.
110. Pepine M, Flowers F, Ramos-Caro FA (1992) Neurothekeoma in a 15-year-old boy: case report. **Pediatr Dermatol** 9(3):272–274.
111. Marrogi AJ, Swanson PE, Kyriakos M et al. (1991) Rudimentary meningocele of the skin. Clinicopathologic features and differential diagnosis. **J Cutan Pathol** 18(3):178–188.

112. Chan HH, Fung JW, Lam WM et al. (1998) The clinical spectrum of rudimentary meningocele. **Pediatr Dermatol** 15(5):388–389.
113. El Shabrawi-Caelen L, White WL, Soyer HP et al. (2001) Rudimentary meningocele: remnant of a neural tube defect. **Arch Dermatol** 137(1):45–50.
114. Argenyi ZB, Thieberg MD, Hayes CM et al. (1994) Primary cutaneous meningioma associated with von Recklinghausen's disease. **J Cutan Pathol** 21(6):549–556.
115. Gambini C, Rongioletti F (1996) Primary congenital cutaneous ganglioneuroma. **J Am Acad Dermatol** 35(2):353–354.
116. deCou JM, Rao BN, Parham DM et al. (1995) Malignant peripheral nerve sheath tumors: the St. Jude Children's Research Hospital experience. **Ann Surg Oncol** 2(6):524–529.
117. Gagne EJ, Su WP (1993) Congenital smooth muscle hamartoma of the skin. **Pediatr Dermatol** 10(2):142–145.
118. Grau-Massanes M, Raimer S, Colome-Grimmer M et al. (1996) Congenital smooth muscle hamartoma presenting as a linear atrophic plaque: case report and review of the literature. **Pediatr Dermatol** 13(3):222–225.

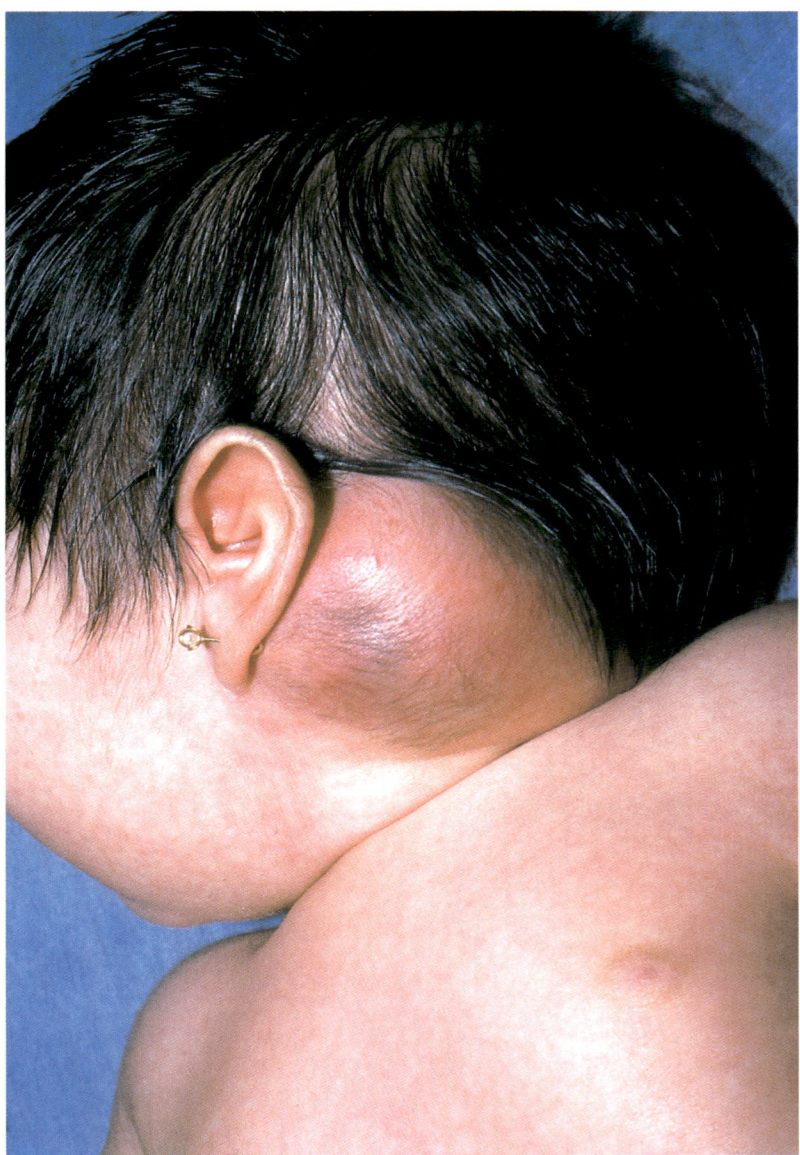

Fig. 21.19 Malignant peripheral nerve sheath tumor presenting as rapidly expanding mass behind the ear in child without neurofibromatosis.

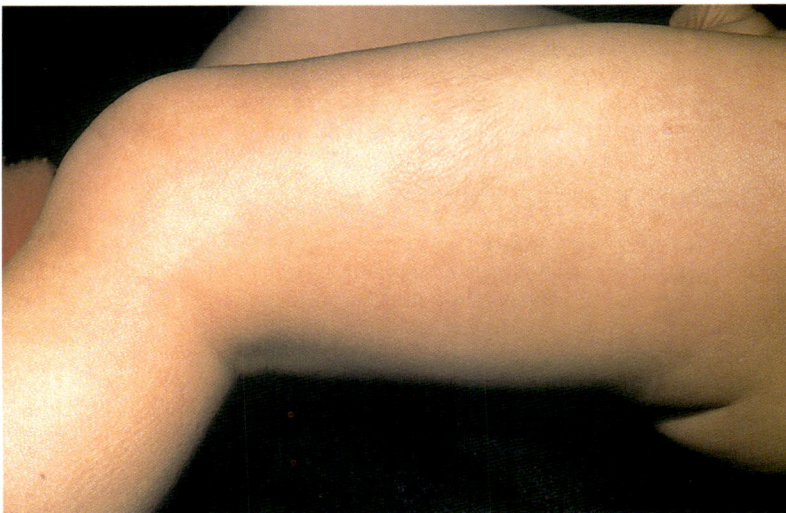

Fig. 21.20 Subtle smooth muscle hamartoma on thigh with slight hypertrichosis. These tumors are very difficult to identify and frequently overlooked unless the patient points out that they may have increased goose bumps in the area following cold exposure or rubbing.

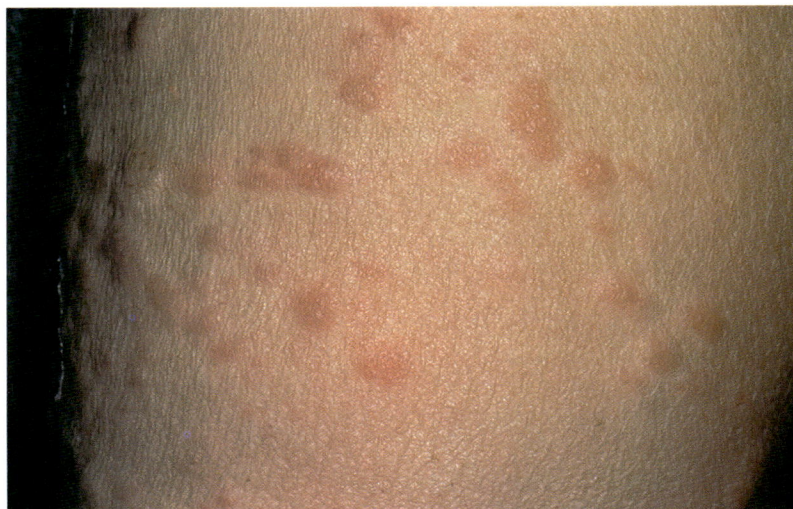

Fig. 21.21 Multiple leiomyomas with typical red-brown color and grouped pattern. These lesions were painful to touch.

or proximal portions of the extremities are the most common sites. A biopsy shows bundles of smooth muscle throughout the dermis. Smooth muscle hamartomas have many similarities with Becker nevus (Ch. 10), when a Becker nevus is biopsied, an increase in smooth muscle tissue may be found, suggesting the two conditions overlap. An accessory scrotum typically is a congenital perineal mass containing both smooth muscle fibers and excess fat.[119] Michelin tire babies have also been described with an underlying smooth muscle hamartoma.[15,16] Congenital smooth muscle hamartomas need not be excised.

Leiomyoma

Leiomyomas may arise anywhere smooth muscle is found. Typical cutaneous variants appear to involve the arrector pili muscles of hair follicles, the dartos muscle of the scrotum and labia majora, and the erectile muscle of the nipple. A unifying feature of leiomyomas is that they tend to be painful, especially

when rubbed or otherwise stimulated so that their muscle bundles contract. Arrector pili leiomyomas are most common. They are red-brown papules or nodules most common on the arms and usually multiple (Fig. 21.21). They may occur in childhood and have been described at birth.[120-122] The nipple and genital lesions are usually solitary. With multiple leiomyomas, there is often a positive family history and autosomal-dominant inheritance is found. In such families, there is also an increase in uterine leiomyomas. Multiple leiomyomas may also be seen in Cowden syndrome.

Angioleiomyoma

Angioleiomyomas are deep, painful, subcutaneous or deep dermal nodules without distinguishing clinical features. On microscopic examination, bundles of spindled fibers are seen. They often are arranged in an intersecting pattern surrounding a central vessel. Although the benign nature of the lesion is

119. Amann G, Berger A, Rokitansky A (1996) Accessory scrotum or perineal collision-hamartoma. A case report to illustrate a misnomer. **Pathol Res Pract** 192(10):1039–1043.
120. Lupton GP, Naik DG, Rodman OG (1986) An unusual congenital leiomyoma. **Pediatr Dermatol** 3(2):158–160.
121. Henderson CA, Ruban E, Porter DI (1997) Multiple leiomyomata presenting in a child. **Pediatr Dermatol** 14(4):287–289.
122. Raj S, Calonje E, Kraus M et al. (1997) Cutaneous pilar leiomyoma: clinicopathologic analysis of 53 lesions in 45 patients. **Am J Dermatopathol** 19(1):2–9.

apparent, on occasion neural, fibrous, and smooth muscle cells can appear so similar that the exact diagnosis may be difficult. A helpful clue for smooth muscle cells is nuclei that are cigar-shaped with perinuclear halos. Immuno-histochemistry greatly facilitates the identification of the cell of origin, as staining with alpha-smooth muscle actin is positive.

MALIGNANT SMOOTH MUSCLE TUMORS

Cutaneous leiomyosarcomas can be seen in children, but are uncommon.[123,124] A variety of patterns may be seen, including an epithelioid variant which has been described in infancy.[125] Systemic leiomyomas and leiomyosarcomas occur in children with HIV/AIDS.[126,127] It is felt that these tumors are caused by infection of the smooth muscle cells by EBV; they are the second most common malignancy in children with AIDS.

SKELETAL MUSCLE TUMORS

BENIGN SKELETAL MUSCLE TUMORS

Striated muscle hamartoma

Just as with smooth muscle, hamartomas of striated muscle have been described. The term striated muscle hamartoma was proposed for two infants with papillomatous tumors rich in striated muscle as well as appendageal structures.[128,129] In an even more unusual case, an infant had multiple periocular skin tags similar to the oculocerebrocutaneous syndrome, but with skeletal muscle cores, resulting in spontaneously moving tags.[130] Rhabdomyomatous hamartomas are also often rich in fat; they appear to be most common on the chin, where superficial skeletal muscle is normally found. The lesions can be excised easily if they are pedunculated.[131]

Rhabdomyoma

Rhabdomyomas or benign skeletal muscle tumors are rare, outnumbered 50:1 by their malignant counterparts. There is an infantile form, presenting as a head and neck tumor, usually before the age of 4.[132] Because this is also the clinical setting for rhabdomyosarcoma, caution must be used and expert pathologic consultation sought. In one instance, a rhabdomyoma was described in association with nevoid basal cell carcinoma syndrome.[133] Cases have been described that appeared to be a typical rhabdomyoma initially, but recur and then behave like a rhabdomyosarcoma. For this reason, complete excision with careful margin control is recommended.

MALIGNANT STRIATED MUSCLE TUMORS

Rhabdomyosarcoma

Rhabdomyosarcoma is the most common childhood sarcoma with an incidence of 4–7 per million. There are four histologic subtypes of rhabdomyosarcoma – embryonal, alveolar, botryoid, and pleomorphic. The embryonal is most common in children; the botryoid presents as protuberant nodules (botryoid comes from the Greek for grapes) in a mucosal cavity such as the vagina or nasopharynx (Fig. 21.22). The tumors are positive for

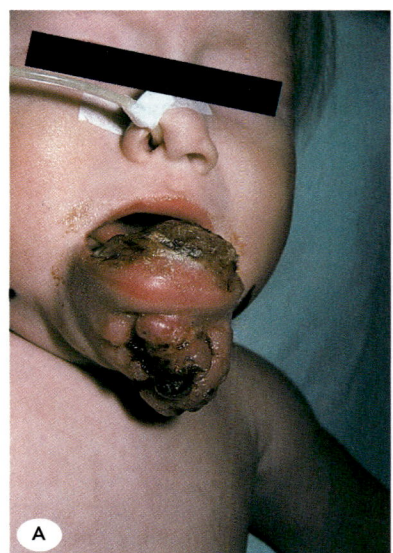

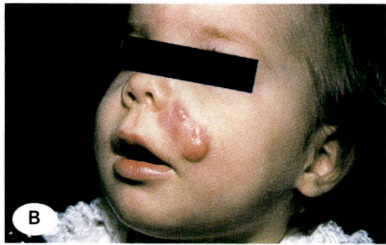

Fig. 21.22 Rhabdomyosarcomas. (A) Botryoid rhabdomyosarcoma protruding from mouth with clustered nodules. (B) Rhabdomyosarcoma of the cheek in an infant girl (photo courtesy of Sharon Raimer MD).

actin, myoglobin, desmin, and vimentin to varying degrees. Alveolar rhabdomyosarcoma typically has either a t(2;13)(q35;q14) or a t(1;13)(p36;q14) translocation involving the FKHR gene and a PAX control gene. Pleomorphic rhabdomyosarcoma must be differentiated from other small, blue-cell cutaneous malignancies in childhood such as lymphoma, neuroblastoma, or extraskeletal Ewing sarcoma.

Less than 1% of rhabdomyosarcomas involve the skin, either primarily or as metastases.[134] The alveolar is most likely to present with metastases and thus involve the skin. Around 50% of cases occur in children less than 5 years of age, with 2% present at birth,[135] sometimes with blueberry muffin lesions.[136] Congenital alveolar rhabdomyosarcoma is a rare uniformly fatal tumor in which more than half of infants present with multiple cutaneous metastases.[137] Although arising in the soft tissue, the tumor may extend into the dermis and present as a papule or plaque on the face of a child. Rhabdomyosarcoma with this presentation may be misdiagnosed as a cyst, hemangioma, or an inflammatory process.[138,139] Unfortunately, when the diagnosis is delayed, the tumor may grow rapidly and become widely destructive, fulfilling the deservedly bad reputation of sarcomas.

123. Yanguas I, Goday J, Gonzalez-Guemes M et al. (1997) Cutaneous leiomyosarcoma in a child. Pediatr Dermatol 14(4):281–283.
124. de Saint Aubain Somerhausen N, Fletcher CD (1999) Leiomyosarcoma of soft tissue in children: clinicopathologic analysis of 20 cases. Am J Surg Pathol 23(7):755–763.
125. Kato K, Arai K, Tanaka Y et al. (2000) Epithelioid leiomyosarcoma in a non-immunocompromised infant: additional differential diagnosis of pediatric "round cell tumors". Mod Pathol 13(10):1156–1160.
126. Chadwick EG, Connor EJ, Hanson IC et al. (1990) Tumors of smooth-muscle origin in HIV-infected children. JAMA 263(23):3182–3184.
127. Jenson HB, Leach CT, McClain KL et al. (1997) Benign and malignant smooth muscle tumors containing Epstein-Barr virus in children with AIDS. Leuk Lymphoma 27(3–4):303–314.
128. Hendrick SJ, Ranchez RL, Blackwell SJ et al. (1986) Striated muscle hamartoma: description of two cases. Pediatr Dermatol 3(2):153–157.
129. Scrivener Y, Petiau P, Rodier-Bruant C et al. (1998) Perianal striated muscle hamartoma associated with hemangioma. Pediatric Dermatol 15(4):274–276.
130. Sahn EE, Garen PD, Pai GS et al. (1990) Multiple rhabdomyomatous mesenchymal hamartomas of skin. Am J Dermatopathol 12(5):485–491.
131. Ashfaq R, Timmons CF (1992) Rhabdomyomatous mesenchymal hamartoma of the skin. Pediatr Pathol 12(5):731–735.
132. Crotty PL, Nakhleh RE, Dehner LP (1993) Juvenile rhabdomyoma. An intermediate form of skeletal muscle tumor in children. Arch Pathol Lab Med 117(1):43–47.
133. Dahl I, Angervall L, Save-Soderbergh J (1976) Foetal rhabdomyoma. Case report of patient with two tumours. Acta Pathol Microbiol Scand [A] 84(1):107–112.
134. Schmidt D, Fletcher CD, Harms D (1993) Rhabdomyosarcomas with primary presentation in the skin. Pathol Res Fract 189(4):422–427.
135. Ahmed OA, Hussain A, King DJ et al. (1999) Congenital rhabdomyosarcoma. Br J Plast Surg 52(4):304–307.
136. Godambe SV, Rawal J (2000) Blueberry muffin rash as presentation of alveolar cell rhabdomyosarcoma in a neonate. Acta Pediatr 89(1):115–117.
137. Grundy R, Anderson J, Gaze M et al. (2001) Congenital alveolar rhabdomyosarcoma: clinical and molecular distinction from alveolar rhabdomyosarcoma in older children. Cancer 91(3):606–612.
138. Chang Y, Dehner LP, Egbert B (1990) Primary cutaneous rhabdomyosarcoma. Am J Surg Pathol 14(10):977–982.
139. Wiss K, Solomon AR, Raimer SS et al. (1988) Rhabdomyosarcoma presenting as a cutaneous nodule. Arch Dermatol 124(11):1687–1690.

OTHER SARCOMAS

Epithelioid sarcoma

Epithelioid sarcoma typically presents as a subcutaneous nodule on the arm or hand of a young man (Fig. 21.23). About 30% of patients are less than 20 years old. Histopathologically, the tumor has zonal necrosis that may mimic the appearance of a rheumatoid nodule or granuloma annulare at scanning magnification. There are nodular aggregates of spindle and epithelioid neoplastic cells that stain with antibodies against vimentin and various keratins, as well as muscle-specific actin and CD34 in about half of the cases. Thus, the cell of origin remains unclear. Local recurrences and lymph node or hematogenous metastases may occur with a long-term mortality rate of about 30%.[140–142]

EPIDERMAL TUMORS

The vast number of epidermal tumors in adults, squamous cell carcinomas and basal cell carcinomas, are caused by actinic exposure. In children this is not true, so one must approach the problem differently, searching for other predisposing factors as shown in Table 21.3 Actinic damage is considered both here and under photosensitivity (Ch. 29). The other predisposing factors can be combined into several groups – syndromes in which basal cell carcinoma is a feature, immunodeficiency or immunosuppression, human papilloma virus infections (especially when combined with immunosuppression), chronic trauma (especially that associated with dystrophic epidermolysis bullosa) and other environmental factors. In sharp contrast to the situation in adults, malignant melanoma is the most common skin cancer of childhood.[143]

ACTINIC DAMAGE

The role of sunlight in the induction of premalignant and malignant skin neoplasms has been well accepted for almost a century. Ultraviolet (UV) light, especially UVB (290–320nm), causes sunburns and is a proven risk factor for actinic keratosis, squamous cell carcinoma, basal cell carcinoma, and malignant melanoma. Clearly it is not the only risk factor, as all these tumors except

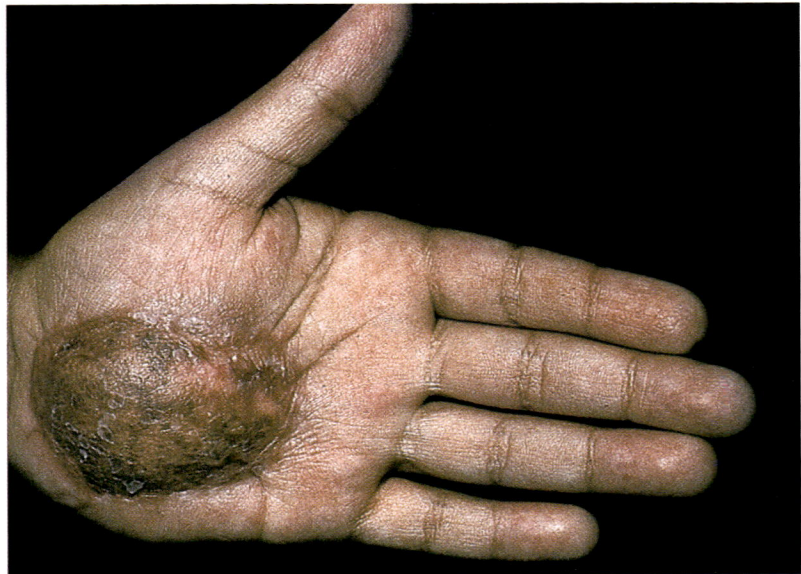

Fig. 21.23   Epithelioid sarcoma in typical location on palm.

TABLE 21.3   Predisposing factors for basal and squamous cell carcinomas

Condition	BCC	SCC
Sunlight	X	X
Nevoid basal cell carcinoma syndrome	X	
Bazex–Dupre–Christol syndrome	X	
Xeroderma pigmentosum	X	X
Rothmund–Thomsen syndrome	X	
Epidermolysis bullosa dystrophica		X
Hidrotic ectodermal dysplasia		X
Albinism	X	X
Fanconi anemia		X
Dyskeratosis congenita		X
Erythropoietic porphyria		X
Congenital/acquired immunodeficiency	X	X
Immunosuppression	X	X
Epidermodysplasia verruciformis		X
Other human papilloma virus infections		X
Burn scars		X
Tuberculosis sinus tracts		X
Osteomyelitis sinus tracts		X
Chemotherapy	X	X
Ionizing radiation	X	X
Arsenic exposure	X	X
Nevus sebaceus	X	

for actinic keratosis can be seen in sunlight-shielded areas. The carcinogenic effects of sunlight have been attributed to UV-induced DNA damage within epidermal cells and melanocytes, as well as to reduced immune surveillance by Langerhans cells. The risk for developing actinic keratoses and skin cancer is highest in fair-skinned people, often from a northern European or Celtic background, with blond or red hair, blue or hazel eyes, who freckle and sunburn easily, and tan with great difficulty. Table 21.4 shows the usual classification of skin phototypes based on Fitzpatrick's work.[144] Basal cell carcinoma and squamous cell carcinoma tend to occur on sun-exposed skin after high cumulative lifetime exposure to UV light. Malignant melanoma may occur at any age and correlates better with infrequent high intensity exposure, such as sunburn in childhood. About 80% of the lifetime UV exposure is estimated to occur before 20 years of age.

Malignant melanoma and nonmelanoma skin cancer should be considered as preventable tumors. The regular use of sunscreens beginning in childhood has been estimated to reduce the risk of developing skin cancer by as much as 75%. Current recommendations for fair-skinned children include avoiding sun exposure during midday when UVB exposure is highest and the regular use of sunscreen and clothing as a barrier. Sunscreens are standardized by sun protection factor (SPF), but current recommendations are in flux because of lack of agreement on UVA protection (broad spectrum sunscreens) and increasing information that the degree of protection in actual usage is almost always less than in laboratory testing. Sun avoidance is probably the best approach in the newborn period and infancy. Since most UV damage occurs in childhood, the active insistence on sunscreens by pediatricians is of inestimable value in helping prevent both tumors and other stigmata of actinic damage.

ACTINIC KERATOSIS

Actinic keratoses are very rare in childhood and adolescence but may be seen in pale children with intense sun exposure (Fig. 21.24). As rare as xeroderma

140. Miettinen M, Fanburg-Smith JC, Virolainen M et al. (1999) Epithelioid sarcoma: an immunohistochemical analysis of 112 classical and variant cases and a discussion of the differential diagnosis. Hum Pathol 30(8):934–942.
141. Billings SD, Hood AF (2000) Epithelioid sarcoma arising on the nose of a child: a case report and review of the literature. J Cutan Pathol 27(4):186–190.
142. Theunis A, Andre J, Larsimont D et al. (2000) Epithelioid sarcoma: a puzzling soft tissue neoplasm in a child. Dermatology 200(2):179–180.
143. Ruiz-Maldonado R, Orozco-Covarrubias M de la L (1997) Malignant melanoma in children. Arch Dermatol 133(3):363–371.
144. Fitzpatrick TB (1975) Soleil et peau. J Med Esthet 2(1):33–34.

TABLE 21.4   Skin phototypes

Skin type	Color of unexposed skin	History – Burn	History – Tan	Skin cancer risk
I	White	Always	Never	High
II	White	Easily	Poorly	High
III	White	Moderate	Moderate	Moderate
IV	Beige, light tan	Minimal	Easily	Low
V	Brown	Rarely	Deeply	Almost none
VI	Dark brown or black	Never	Deeply	Almost none

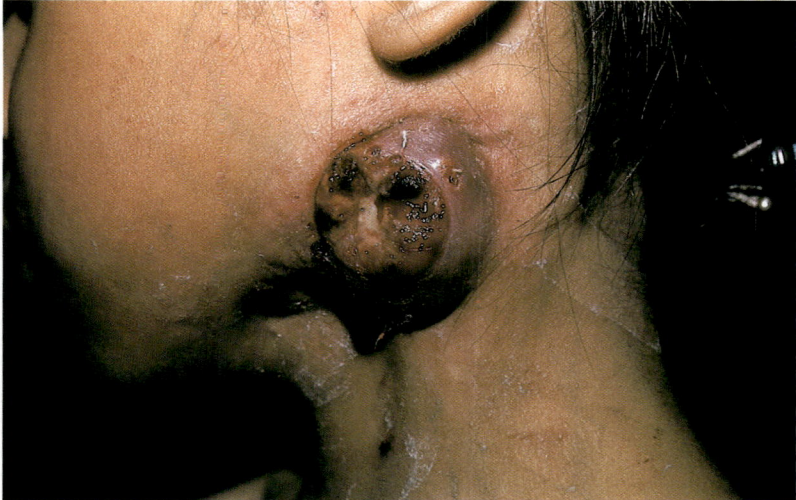

Fig. 21.25   Squamous cell carcinoma on neck in 8-year-old girl following radiation therapy.

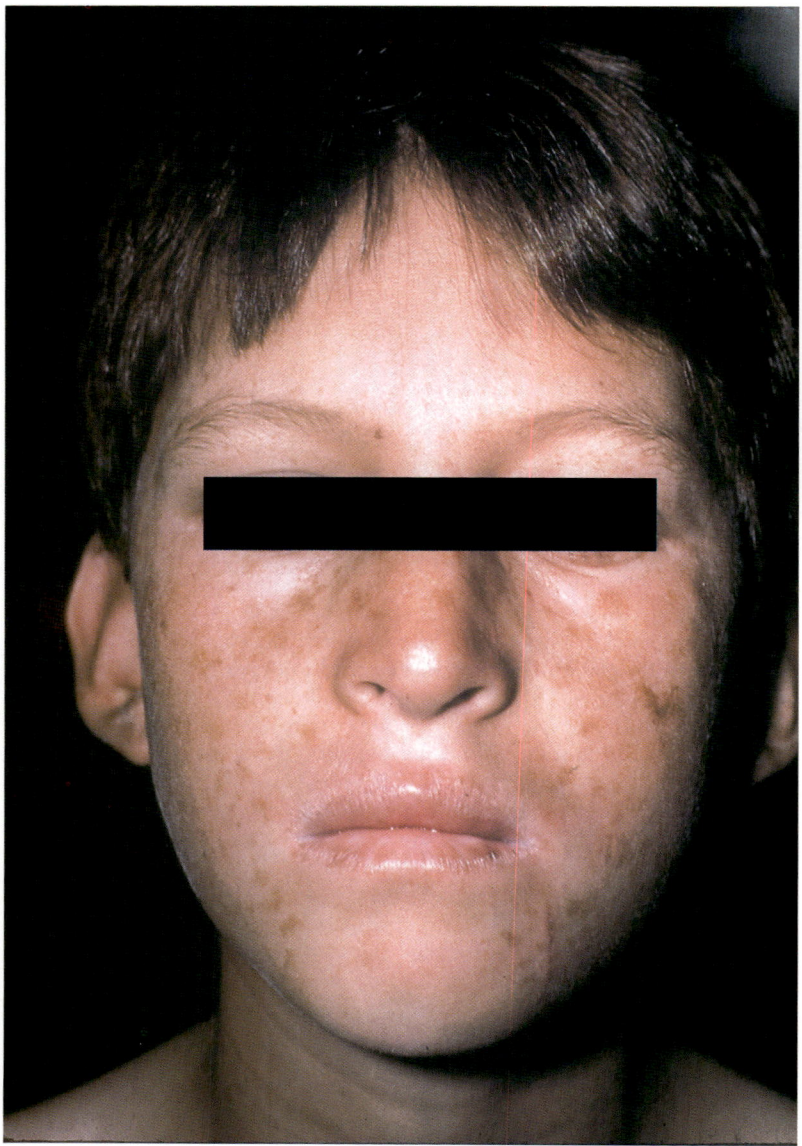

Fig. 21.24   Multiple actinic keratoses in 14 year-old without known predisposing factors other than fair skin.

pigmentosum is, if one encounters a child with actinic keratoses, this geno-dermatosis (Ch. 7) should be excluded. The individual actinic keratoses are indistinct, scaly, small, erythematous, pink or brown, macules appearing on a background of solar lentigines, solar elastosis, and other evidence of sun damage.

Histologically, there is epidermal keratinocyte atypia without dermal invasion. The likelihood of any one lesion turning in squamous cell carcinoma in a given time period is small. Actinic keratoses respond well to liquid nitrogen therapy. Actinic keratoses that are indurated, painful, or therapy-resistant should be biopsied to exclude squamous cell carcinoma. Actinic cheilitis can be observed on the lips of heavily sun-exposed teenagers; it is the mucosal equivalent of actinic keratosis.

SQUAMOUS CELL CARCINOMA

Squamous cell carcinoma usually presents as a scaly or crusted indurated papule on sun-exposed skin. The average age of presentation is in the 60s. In children, it comprises less than 0.10% of all childhood malignancies and at most 5% of childhood cutaneous malignancies. In addition to UV radiation and xeroderma pigmentosum,[145] other significant risk factors are ionizing radiation (Fig. 21.25) and human papillomavirus (HPV) infection. Squamous cell carcinoma may develop from the interaction of HPV, UV light, and immunosuppression in patients with epidermodysplasia verruciformis, or after solid organ transplantation, or chemotherapy with immunosuppression. The median age for the first squamous cell carcinoma in patients with epidermodysplasia verruciformis is in the 20s.[146] Although warts are common in children with solid organ transplantation, squamous cell carcinoma is rare.

Bowenoid papulosis, which histologically is squamous cell carcinoma in situ, presents as multiple hyperpigmented, warty plaques in the genital region. Human papillomavirus 16 and 18, which have been associated with invasive cervical cancer, are also found in bowenoid papulosis. Progression to squamous cell cancer occurs rarely in adults. Several cases of bowenoid papulosis have

145. Hadi U, Tohmeh H, Maalouf R (2000) Squamous cell carcinoma of the lower lid in a 19-month-old girl with xeroderma pigmentosum. **Eur Arch Otorhinolaryngol** 257(2):77–79.

146. Kaspar TA, Wagner RF Jr, Jablonska S et al. (1991) Prognosis and treatment of advanced squamous cell carcinoma secondary to epidermodysplasia verruciformis: worldwide analysis of 11 patients. **J Dermatol Surg Oncol** 17(3):237–240.

been reported in children.[147] In these few cases, clinical resolution of the lesions occurred spontaneously or with liquid nitrogen therapy.

Scars from dystrophic epidermolysis bullosa may be associated with squamous cell carcinoma. Although the average age of onset of squamous cell carcinoma in these patients is 40, the tumor may occasionally present in childhood.[148,149] Children with burn scars must also be monitored for the development of squamous cell carcinoma.[150] Complete excision is the treatment of choice for cutaneous squamous cell carcinoma.

BASAL CELL CARCINOMA

Most, if not all, basal cell carcinomas are more closely related to hair follicle structures than to the epidermal basal cells, so their name and classification are both misnomers.[151] Basal cell carcinoma usually presents as a pearly, translucent papule with telangiectases and often a central dell or crusted erosion (Fig. 21.26). In a large experience in Mexico City, basal cell carcinoma accounted for 0.24% of all tumors in children and for 13% of cutaneous malignancies. Children less than 3 years of age have been diagnosed with basal cell carcinoma, and even congenital forms have been seen. Often, the diagnosis is delayed in children because the index of suspicion is low. In fair-skinned adolescents, basal cell carcinoma in sun-exposed skin can be viewed as similar to the lesions seen in adults. It may be locally aggressive with resultant significant morbidity.[152,153] A history of ionizing radiation exposure should be sought.[154] A solitary nonulcerated facial papule with a basaloid histologic pattern in a young adult is often a benign adnexal tumor of hair follicle origin, which may be misidentified as a basal cell carcinoma.

In younger children, one must search for a pre-existing cause. The most common answer is nevoid basal cell carcinoma syndrome (Ch. 7). Often the lesions do not resemble the stereotypical basal cell carcinoma, but instead present as skin tags (the so-called nevoid form) or innocent papules. One should take a family history and check for other stigmata, including palmoplantar pits, acral epidermoid cysts, and dysmorphic features. The other syndromes with basal cell carcinomas are all extremely uncommon; they include Rombo,[155] Bazex,[156] and Oley[157] syndromes. The latter two are probably phenotypic variants of the same disorder. Families with only multiple

basal cell carcinomas and no other stigmata have been described.[158] Basal cell carcinoma only rarely occurs with nevus sebaceus, as discussed below.

Excision is the treatment of choice although electrodesiccation and curettage, as well as cryotherapy, are also effective for superficial or small lesions. Radiation therapy must be avoided, especially in patients with nevoid basal cell carcinoma syndrome, because it leads to the induction of hundreds of new tumors. We prefer to avoid this modality entirely in treating childhood skin tumors. Regular follow-up is indicated because of the risk of local recurrence or subsequent primary tumors. Regular use of sun screens should be emphasized.

ADNEXAL TUMORS

Tumors of the skin adnexal structures or appendages have follicular, sebaceous, or sweat gland differentiation. In childhood, these tumors present most commonly as nodules in the head and neck region.[159] All may be occasionally seen as multiple tumors, then inherited in an autosomal-dominant fashion and in a localized or linear pattern, following Blaschko lines as a reflection of mosaicism. Definitive diagnosis of adnexal tumors requires microscopic evaluation; usually an excisional biopsy provides a diagnosis and treatment simultaneously. Malignant adnexal tumors are so rare in younger patients that we will ignore them. We describe only those tumors with unique clinical features; the histologic details should be sought in a dermatopathology text such as that of Weedon.[160]

TUMORS WITH FOLLICULAR DIFFERENTIATION

Pilomatricomas and cysts

Pilomatricoma is far and away the most common adnexal tumor in childhood, accounting for 75% of the group. The next most common tumors are epidermoid and trichilemmal cysts – despite their name, both are also follicular tumors. All of these common lesions are considered under nodular diseases (Ch. 17).

Trichoblastomas and trichoepitheliomas

Trichoepitheliomas, or superficial trichoblastomas, are most often seen as a single, small, skin-colored nodule on the face of an older child. Deeper lesions, often on the scalp, are today designated trichoblastomas. Multiple trichoepitheliomas are usually inherited in an autosomal-dominant pattern (Brooke syndrome), most often associated with cylindromas (Spiegler syndrome). The association of milia with the above mentioned adnexal tumors is known as Rasmussen syndrome.[161] Multiple trichoepitheliomas present as many small skin-colored nodules (Fig. 21.27), often clustered around the central face and nose. They may be confused with multiple angiofibromas in tuberous sclerosis or multiple basal cell carcinomas in the nevoid basal cell carcinoma syndrome. Nevoid plaques with both trichoepitheliomas and cylindromas have been described in a patient with Brooke–Spiegler syndrome, supporting the concept of Type 2 mosaicism and the overlap between the two tumors.[162] Desmoplastic trichoepitheliomas tend to be flatter tumors clinically and have a more fibrous stroma; they, too, may be familial.[163]

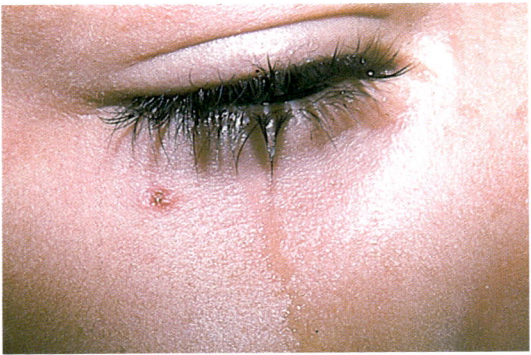

Fig. 21.26 Tiny basal cell carcinoma under eye in 7-year-old boy.

147. Weitzner JM, Fields KW, Robinson MJ (1989) Pediatric bowenoid papulosis: risks and management. **Pediatr Dermatol** 6(4):303–305.
148. McGrath JA, Schofield OM, Mayou BJ et al. (1992) Epidermolysis bullosa complicated by squamous cell carcinoma: report of 10 cases. **J Cutan Pathol** 19(2):116–123.
149. Bosch RJ, Gallardo MA, Ruiz del Portal G et al. (1999) Squamous cell carcinoma secondary to recessive dystrophic epidermolysis bullosa: report of eight tumours in four patients. **J Eur Acad Dermatol Venereol** 13(3):198–204.
150. Love RL, Breidahl AF (2000) Acute squamous cell carcinoma arising within a recent burn scar in a 14-year-old boy. **Plast Reconstr Surg** 106(5):1069–1071.
151. Schirren CG, Rütten A, Kaudewitz P et al. (1997) Trichoblastoma and basal cell carcinoma are neoplasms with follicular differentiation sharing the same profile of cytokeratin intermediate filaments. **Am J Dermatopathol** 19(4):341–350.
152. Comstock J, Hansen RC, Korc A (1990) Basal cell carcinoma in a 12-year-old boy. **Pediatrics** 86(3):460–463.
153. LeSueur BW, Silvis NG, Hansen RC (2000) Basal cell carcinoma in children: report of 3 cases. **Arch Dermatol** 136(3):370–372.
154. Garcia-Silva J, Velasco-Benito JA, Pena-Penabad C et al. (1996) Basal cell carcinoma in a girl after cobalt irradiation to the cranium for acute lymphoblastic leukemia: case report and literature review. **Pediatr Dermatol** 13(1):54–57.
155. Van Steensel MA, Jaspers NG, Steijlen PM (2001) A case of Rombo syndrome. **Br J Dermatol** 144(6):1215–1218.
156. Goeteyn M, Geerts ML, Kint A et al. (1994) The Bazex-Dupre-Christol syndrome. **Arch Dermatol** 130(3):337–342.
157. Oley CA, Sharpe H, Chenevix-Trench G (1992) Basal cell carcinomas, coarse sparse hair and milia. **Am J Med Genet** 43(5):799–804.
158. Guarneri B, Borgoia F, Cannavo SP et al. (2000) Multiple familial basal cell carcinomas including a case of segmental manifestation. **Dermatology** 200(4):299–302.
159. Marrogi AJ, Wick MR, Dehner LP (1991) Benign cutaneous adnexal tumors in childhood and young adults, excluding pilomatrixoma: review of 28 cases and the literature. **J Cutan Pathol** 18(1):20–27.
160. Weedon D (2002) Skin Pathology, 2nd edn. Edinburgh: Churchill Livingstone.
161. Rasmussen JE (1975) A syndrome of trichoepitheliomas, milia, and cylindromas. **Arch Dermatol** 111(5)610–614.
162. Schirren CG, Wörle B, Kind P et al. (1995) A nevoid plaque with histological changes of trichoepithelioma and cylindroma in Brooke-Spiegler syndrome. An immunohistochemical study with cytokeratins. **J Cutan Pathol** 22(6):563–569.
163. Shapiro PE, Kopf AW (1991) Familial multiple desmoplastic trichoepitheliomas. **Arch Dermatol** 127(1):83–87.

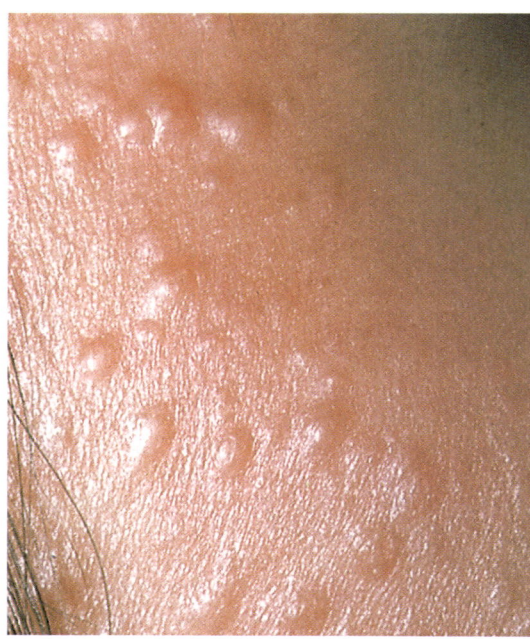

Fig. 21.27 Multiple trichoepitheliomas.

Microscopic evaluation reveals a basaloid tumor with hair germs or other unequivocal signs of hair follicle differentiation. Such lesions can be viewed as the benign equivalent of a basal cell carcinoma,[151] explaining why they cannot always be separated with certainty and why on rare occasions basal cell carcinomas are seen in Brooke–Spiegler syndrome. Conservative excision is the treatment of choice for solitary trichoepitheliomas. Treatment of multiple trichoepitheliomas for cosmetic reasons is problematic. Destruction of these dermal tumors results in scarring, which may or may not be cosmetically superior to no therapy at all.

Cylindroma

Cylindroma has long been an interesting tumor. It is almost invariably benign, usually multiple, and favors the scalp (Fig. 21.28). Patients with multiple large cylindromas were initially described as wearing a turban, so it has become well-known as the "turban tumor." Despite its affinity for the scalp, the cylindroma has long been identified as a sweat gland tumor, although modern evidence supports the more logical association with hair follicle differentiation. Molecular genetics has clarified much of the confusion. The CYLD tumor suppressor gene has been identified on chromosome 16q12-q13 in patients with documented familial cylindromatosis inherited in an autosomal-dominant fashion.[164] This same mutation has been found in patients with multiple trichoepitheliomas, multiple eccrine spiradenomas, and all the variants thereof. Histologically, a cylindroma features islands of small blue cells, often arranged in rosettes and surrounded by a dense PAS-positive membrane, resembling the outer root sheath. Any single lesion can be easily excised, but multiple lesions challenge the most skilled cosmetic surgeon.

Trichofolliculoma

Trichofolliculoma presents as a solitary, skin-colored papule on the face, scalp, or neck. Characteristically, a tuft of whitish hair protrudes from a pore in the center of the papule, often allowing clinical diagnosis. In one series, 25% of trichofolliculomas were present during childhood.[165] Trichofolliculoma has been reported as a congenital lesion. Histologically, well-differentiated secondary hair follicles radiate from a primary cystic follicle, which often contains multiple hairs. Excision is curative.

Trichilemmoma

Trichilemmomas may present as a solitary lesion on the face or as multiple papules in Cowden syndrome (Ch. 7). The multiple facial trichilemmomas of Cowden syndrome may be seen in childhood, but solitary trichilemmomas are unusual before 20 years of age. The lesions may be smooth papules but are more often verrucous. There is increasing evidence that human papillomavirus is associated with the solitary lesions and perhaps even with those seen in Cowden syndrome. Histologically, a trichilemmoma is a sharply demarcated epithelial tumor within the epidermis, composed of clear cells with a prominent, hyalinized basement membrane zone. Solitary lesions can be easily excised.

Fibrofolliculomas/trichodiscomas

These tumors, when multiple, suggest Birt–Hogg–Dubé syndrome, but may also present as a solitary lesion. They involve varying degrees of perifollicular fibrosis and later follicular involution. Clinically, they appear as white or pale perifollicular papules, often resembling acne scarring.

TUMORS WITH SWEAT GLAND DIFFERENTIATION

To the dismay of purists, it remains very difficult to distinguish between apocrine and eccrine tumors. There are few immunohistochemical markers. Decapitation secretion is the only reliable marker for apocrine differentiation, while eccrine tumors tend to have an admixture of basaloid and clear cells and are often vascular. Since the apocrine-eccrine issue plays almost no clinical role, we will avoid it. One peculiarity is that eccrine tumors are occasionally stimulated to become pruritic or tender when the patient sweats.

Syringomas

Syringomas are the most common tumors with sweat gland differentiation in children. These tumors present most often as multiple, small, skin-colored nodules around the eyes and nose (Fig. 21.29). A particularly distinctive association is the presence of syringomas and milia-like calcinosis cutis in Down syndrome.[166] Syringomas may also present as solitary lesions or in an eruptive form occurring in crops over the abdomen and chest. Another variant is the presence of multiple vulvar lesions, often appearing around

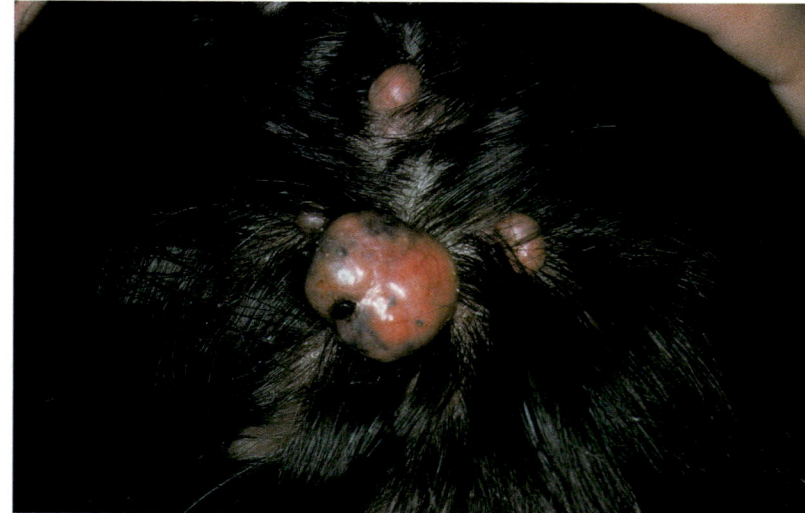

Fig. 21.28 Cylindromas on scalp in teenager who also had multiple spiradenomas.

164. Takahashi M, Rapley E, Biggs PJ et al. (2000) Linkage and LOH studies in 19 cylindromatosis families show no evidence of genetic heterogeneity and refine the CYLD locus on chromosome 16q12–q13. **Hum Genet** 106(1):58–65.

165. Ishii N, Kawaguchi H, Takahashi K et al. (1992) A case of congenital trichofolliculoma. **J Dermatol** 19(3):195–196.

166. Schepis C, Siragusa M, Palazzo R et al. (1994) Perforating milia-like idiopathic calcinosis cutis and periorbital syringomas in a girl with Down syndrome. **Pediatr Dermatol** 11(3):258–260.

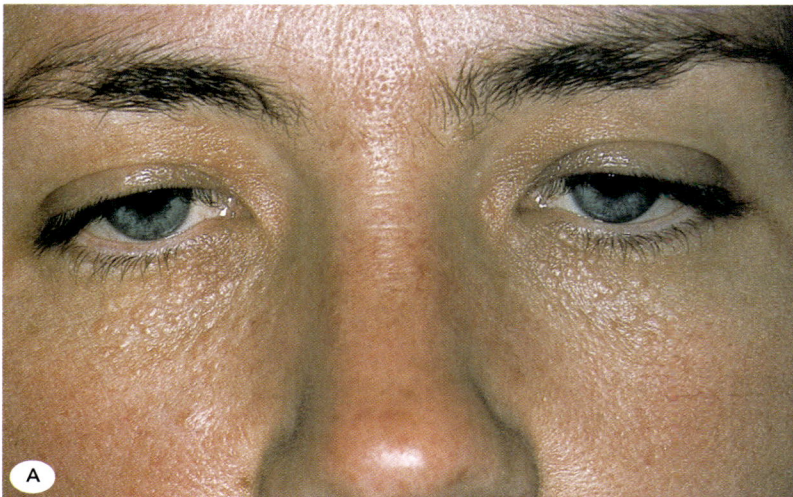

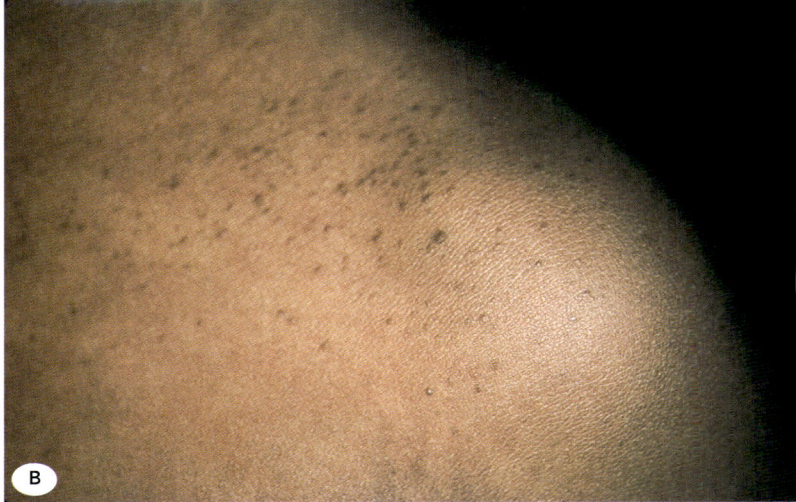

Fig. 21.29   Syringomas. (A) Multiple syringomas in classic location about the eyes (Courtesy of Gerd Plewig MD, Munich, Germany). (B) Multiple syringomas on the shoulder of a girl with Down Syndrome. (Courtesy of Anne W. Lucky MD).

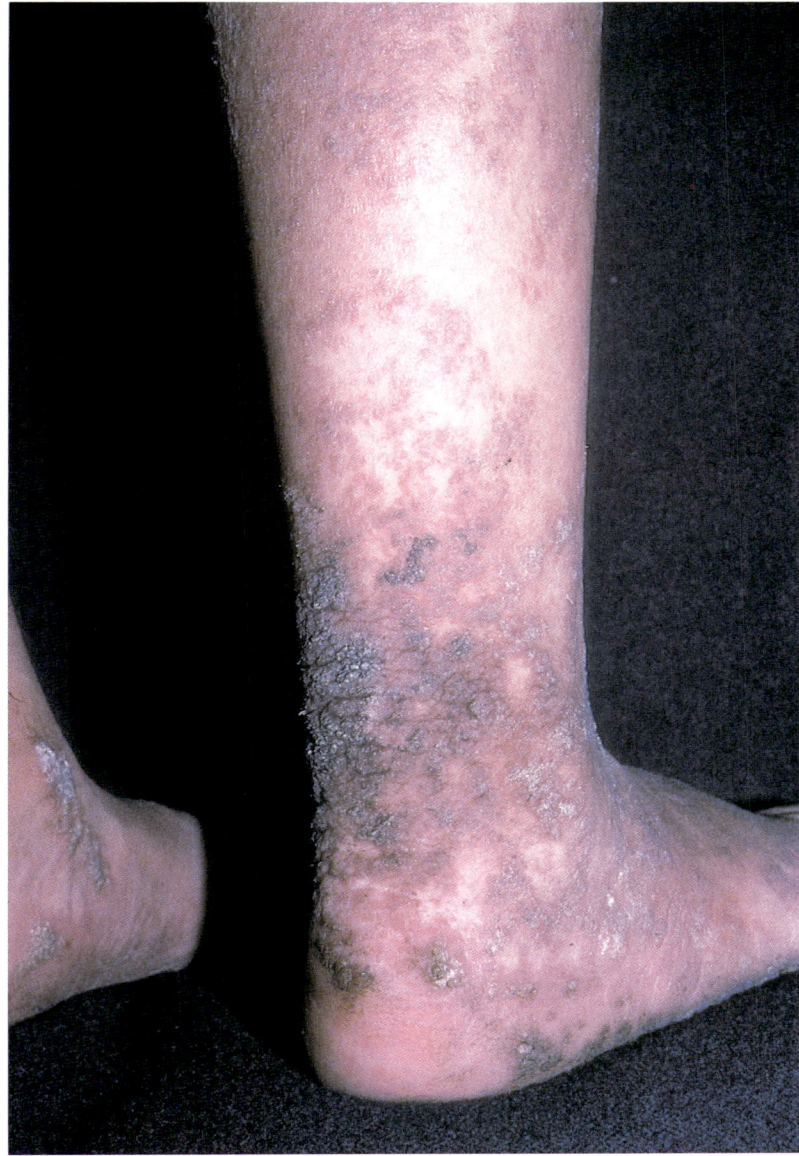

Fig. 21.30   Porokeratotic eccrine ostial and dermal duct nevus.

puberty. Histologically, eccrine duct-like structures with a tadpole shape are present within a fibrous stroma, which may be difficult to distinguish from the surrounding dermis. The differential diagnosis of facial lesions includes plane warts and xanthomas, while the disseminated lesions can be confused with granuloma annulare and eruptive vellus hair cysts. Treatment of multiple syringomas is difficult, as the destruction of each lesion can result in a scar.

Eccrine nevus

An eccrine nevus is a localized accumulation of excessive numbers of entirely normal eccrine glands, usually following the distribution of the lines of Blaschko and reflecting mosaicism. Typically, the lesions are difficult to see, but hyperhidrotic. There are two relatively distinct variants of the ordinary eccrine nevus. Porokeratotic eccrine ostial and dermal duct nevus tends to present at birth as multiple keratotic pits on the palms or soles (Fig. 21.30).[167,168] Histologically, acral epidermal invaginations with parakeratosis plug underlying dilated eccrine ducts. Because of the size and location, excision is usually difficult. Eccrine angiomatous hamartoma also

presents congenitally or in childhood. It is usually not considered a tumor by the patient or parents, because it is typically a hyperhidrotic, sometimes hypertrichotic plaque or nodule on the leg.[169,170] The lesion is usually linear and may be painful. Multiple tumors are occasionally seen; they have been reported in association with knuckle pads.[171] Histologically, eccrine angiomatous hamartoma is a proliferation of sweat glands and blood vessels, often with increased hair follicles.

Eccrine poroma

Eccrine poromas are typically red, often friable nodules on the scalp (Fig. 21.31) or feet; they may be mistaken for a hemangiomas or warts and occasionally are seen in adolescents. They are often painful, probably because anything on the sole can hurt. For this reason, excision is usually recommended.

167. Valks R, Abajo P, Fraga J et al. (1996) Porokeratotic eccrine ostial and dermal duct nevus of late onset: more frequent than previously suggested. **Dermatology** 193(2):138–140.
168. Sassmannshausen J, Bogomilsky J, Chaffins M (2000) Porokeratotic eccrine ostial and dermal duct nevus: a case report and review of the literature. **J Am Acad Dermatol** 43(2):364–367.
169. Sanmartin O, Botella R, Alegre V et al. (1992) Congenital eccrine angiomatous hamartoma. **Am J Dermatopathol** 14(2):161–164.
170. Nakatsui TC, Schloss E, Krol A et al. (1999) Eccrine angiomatous hamartoma: report of a case and literature review. **J Am Acad Dermatol** 41(1):109–111.
171. Morrell DS; Ghali FE, Stahr BJ et al. (2001) Eccrine angiomatous hamartoma: a report of symmetric and painful lesions of the wrists. **Pediatr Dermatol** 18(2):117–119.

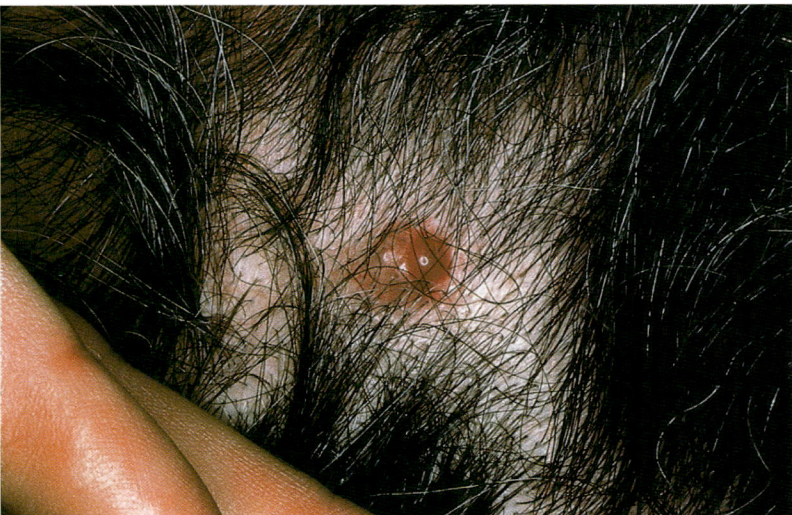

Fig. 21.31   Eccrine poroma in typical scalp location and resembling a vascular tumor.

Eccrine spiradenoma

These tumors are typically painful or tender slowly growing dermal nodules in children and young adults. Multiple lesions may be seen in children, often in association with cylindromas or other adnexal neoplasma and inherited in an autosomal-dominant fashion. Lesions distributed along the lines of Blaschko may also be seen. While we have seen the development of an eccrine carcinoma in such a lesion, the malignant potential is vanishingly small and excision should be viewed as elective.

Hidrocystomas

Hidrocystomas are clear cystic lesions typically located on the eyelid or in the mid-facial region. They may be of apocrine or eccrine origin, but the classification is unreliable. Sometimes the lesions are blue or even darker and mistaken for a melanocytic nevus or even malignant melanoma. Multiple lesions resemble syringomas and are seen in focal dermal hypoplasia (Goltz syndrome) (Ch. 18) and in some ectodermal dysplasia syndromes. Some lesions may become pruritic or swollen when the patient is stimulated to sweat. Solitary lesions can be excised; multiple lesions are often treated with systemic or topical anticholinergic agents, but this approach is not very helpful.

Syringocystadenoma papilliferum

This tongue-twister of a name refers to a relatively common tumor that in childhood is most often seen in association with nevus sebaceus. In one large series, about 45% were present at birth and another 20% identified during childhood or adolescence. Typically, the lesion is verrucous or eroded and microscopically complex folded glandular structures are seen with a surface connection. Linear lesions may also be seen.[172] Hidradenoma papilliferum is a microscopically similar tumor but without surface connection and usually found in the vulvar or perianal regions.

Other tumors

Other solitary eccrine tumors are very rare in childhood. One case of a clear cell hidradenoma (eccrine acrospiroma) has been reported in a 3-year-old.[173]

Apocrine nevi have also been described, but are even more uncommon than their eccrine counterparts. Apocrine tumors tend to have an associated fibrous stroma and are most common in the perianal region.

TUMOR OF SEBACEOUS GLANDS

Nevus sebaceus

Nevus sebaceus is a complex appendageal hamartoma that was first described by Jadassohn in 1895, when he distinguished this excess of epidermal and glandular skin structures from a melanocytic nevus. It is the prototype of an organoid nevus, representing another example of somatic mosaicism. Nevus sebaceus was long considered a fertile ground for basal cell carcinoma, as well as for a variety of other adnexal tumors including syringocystadenoma papilliferum. Today it is well accepted that most of the basaloid tumors arising in nevus sebaceus are trichoblastomas.[174,175] In rare instances, clinically aggressive neoplasms do develop, but their classification remains a point of argument. Aggressive or metastasizing lesions are not seen in childhood. Excision of nevus sebaceus should no longer be thought of as tumor prophylaxis, although it is still appropriate for cosmetic reasons. Usually these lesions can be easily excised under local anesthesia in the pre-teen years before they start to become more verrucous at puberty.

Steatocystoma multiplex

Steatocystomas are true sebaceous cysts, in contrast to epidermoid cysts, which are often so designated by non-dermatologists. They are more likely to be multiple than single, usually involve the chest, head, and neck and become clinically apparent in teenagers. The individual cysts are small and flaccid, containing a cloudy or milky fluid (Fig. 21.32). Hundreds of lesions may be present; they are often misidentified as acne cysts and scars. Steatocystoma multiplex is one of the hallmark features of pachyonychia congenita type 2; mutations in keratin 17 have been associated with both disorders.[176] The other major clinical differential diagnosis is eruptive vellus hair cysts. Some feel that the two conditions are identical or at least overlap frequently. Individual lesions can be excised. Systemic retinoids produce improvement when surgery is impractical, but it is rarely long-lasting.

Other tumors

Large cystic sebaceous tumors should suggest Muir–Torre syndrome (Ch. 7), but they are uncommon in children. Folliculosebaceous cystic hamartoma is a rare lesion, most often seen on the mid-face of children and young adults. Under the microscope, it features an overlap of sebaceous and follicular elements. Excision is curative.[177] Rarely, sebaceous hyperplasia is seen in adolescents; in such instances it may be familial, inherited in an autosomal-dominant fashion.[178] Treatment with isotretinoin is often helpful in such children. In addition, renal transplant recipients, even when young, are likely to have sebaceous hyperplasia.

CANCER-ASSOCIATED GENODERMATOSES

There is a long list of genetic disorders associated with cancer. Of special interest to pediatric dermatologists are a group of autosomal-dominantly inherited disorders in which cutaneous neoplasms are a marker and often the first clue to the diagnosis of an underlying genodermatosis. Some have a considerable lifetime risk of developing an internal malignancy (Table 21.5). More details on these disorders is contained in Chapter 7.

172. Patterson JW, Straka BF, Wick MR (2001) Linear syringocystadenoma papilliferum of the thigh. **J Am Acad Dermatol** 45(1):139–141.

173. Faulhaber D, Wörle B, Trautner B et al. (2000) Clear cell hidradenoma in a young girl. **J Am Acad Dermatol** 42(4):693–695.

174. Kaddu S, Schaeppi H, Kerl H et al. (2000) Basaloid neoplasms in nevus sebaceus. **J Cutan Pathol** 27(7):327–337.

175. Cribier B, Scrivener Y, Grosshans E (2000) Tumors arising in nevus sebaceus: A study of 596 cases. **J Am Acad Dermatology** 42(2):263–268.

176. Covello SP, Smith FJ, Sillevis Smitt JH et al. (1998) Keratin 17 mutations cause either steatocystoma multiplex or pachyonychia congenita type 2. **Br J Dermatol** 139(3):475–480.

177. Templeton SF (1996) Folliculosebaceous cystic hamartoma: a clinical pathologic study. **J Am Acad Dermatol** 34(1):77–81.

178. Weisshaar E, Schramm M, Gollnick H (1999) Familial nevoid sebaceous hyperplasia affecting three generations of a family. **Eur J Dermatol** 9(8):621–623.

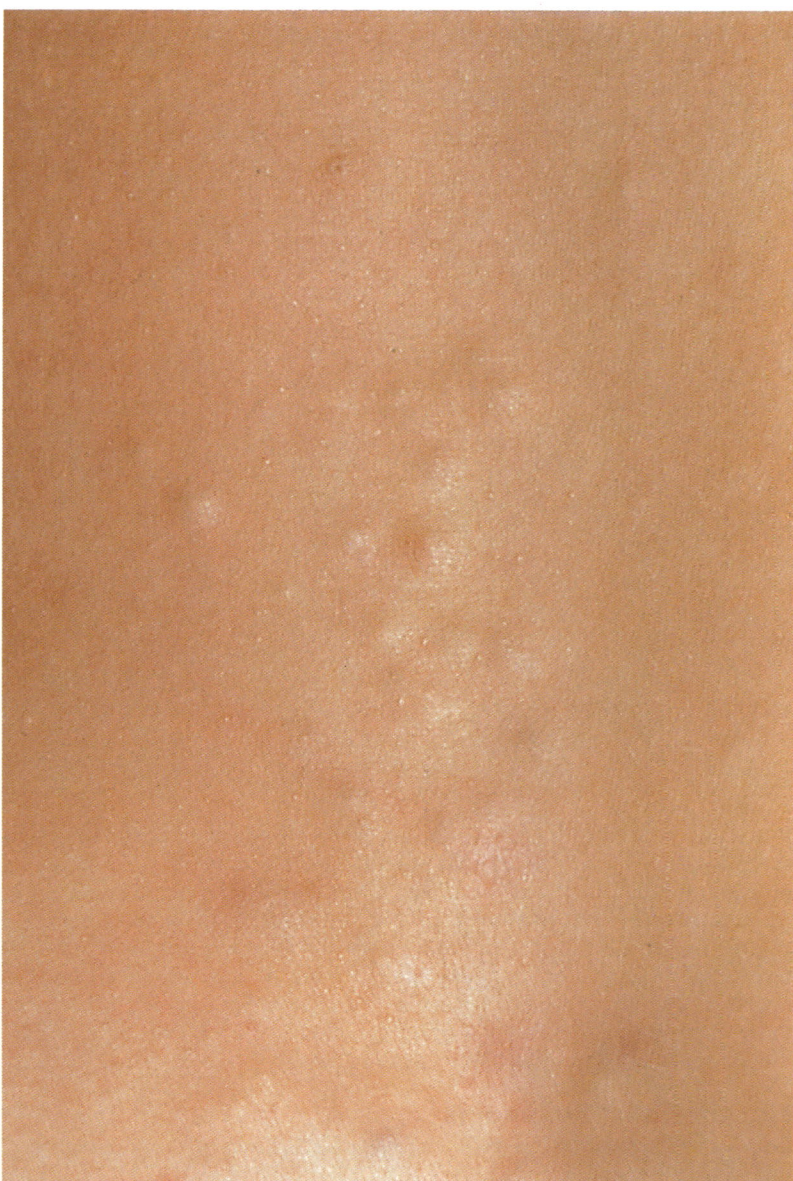

Fig. 21.32 Steatocystoma multiplex with many flaccid cysts on chest.

LYMPHOCYTIC INFILTRATES

The distinction between benign and malignant cutaneous lymphocytic infiltrates has been highly technical and refined in recent years.[179] No longer are routine light microscopic criteria of much utility; their employment, even by highly skilled individuals, led to mistaken diagnoses in the past. The mainstays of diagnosis are the use of monoclonal antibodies against various CD (cluster determination) antigens expressed in different stages of development of T and B cells. These steps are refined by a search for kappa or lambda chains to identify B cell clonality, and by evaluation of the T-cell gamma receptor to identify the same feature in T-cell proliferations. Many lymphomas are also characterized by typical cytogenetic changes, usually involving a translocation placing a growth control or oncogene under the influence of a immunoglobulin or other structural protein coding domain,

leading to uninhibited cell proliferation or impaired apoptosis. In MALT (*m*ucosa-*a*ssociated *l*ymphoid *t*issue) lymphomas of the gastrointestinal tract, infection with *Helicobacter pylori* plays an important role and some such proliferations can be arrested with antibiotic treatment directed against the bacteria. The same scenario has not been so cleanly identified in the skin.

BENIGN LYMPHOCYTIC INFILTRATES

The term pseudolymphoma is imprecise, but it has won acceptance in recent years to describe reactive or benign lymphocytic infiltrates. At the same time, it has become clear that many lesions formerly identified as benign are low-grade lymphomas. Pseudolymphomas are typically red–brown nodules that on histology show a benign lymphocytic infiltrate, often with germinal centers, and are without immunohistochemical or cytogenetic evidence for lymphoma. In Europe, the most common cause is infection with *Borrelia burgdorferi*. Patients tend to develop nodules of lymphocytes involving the ear lobe and nipple, although any body part can be affected. In areas where *B. burgdorferi* is common, a history of a tick bite should be ascertained and serological studies obtained (Ch. 24). Borrelial pseudolymphomas are uncommon in the USA, perhaps suggesting that they are not caused by *B. burgdorferi sensu stricto*, the prevailing subspecies in North America. The organism can often be found in the cutaneous lesion with PCR techniques. The infiltrate is a polyclonal B-cell type. The lesions respond well to appropriate anti-borrelial antibiotics.

Other causes of pseudolymphoma in the pediatric age group include the inflammatory response associated with mollusca contagiosa,[180] persistent arthropod bite reaction, and the closely related nodular scabies. All are usually predominated by T cells with a generous admixture of eosinophils. A most uncommon pediatric lymphoma is acral pseudolymphomatous angiokeratoma or APACHE, in which multiple red–violet papules develop, usually on the hands. The infiltrate is primarily T cell and there is an admixture of superficial vessels. These lesions may simply be a variant of a persistent arthropod bite reaction.[181] In addition, lupus erythematosus can occasionally present with pseudolymphomas; this form is known as lupus tumidus and is uncommon in children. Typically there are symmetrical papules and plaques; biopsy shows a lymphocytic infiltrate usually accompanied by mucin without the expected epidermal changes of lupus erythematosus.[182]

LYMPHOMAS

Lymphomas are the third most frequent malignancy in childhood, after leukemias and central nervous system tumors, appearing at a rate of about 13 cases per million children per year. The separation into Hodgkin lymphoma and non-Hodgkin lymphomas of B- and T-cell types is well agreed upon, but beyond that the classification is difficult.

Hodgkin lymphoma

Hodgkin lymphoma (HL), formerly called Hodgkin disease, occurs most commonly in adolescence and rarely before age 5. It accounts for about 40% of childhood lymphomas. There is a bimodal distribution of HL in the USA with a peak in young adulthood and then in later life. HL is very rare in children less than 5 years of age; in older children, about one-third of USA cases and the majority of those in developing lands are associated with EBV.[183] Recent studies have shown that the Reed–Sternberg cell, the cellular hallmark of HL, is a germinal B cell. Thus HL is a B-cell lymphoma. HL is classified based on the histological appearance of the lymph nodes into five classes – lymphocyte predominance, nodular sclerosis, mixed cellularity, lymphocyte depletion, and unclassified. Lymphocyte predominance HL usually presents with localized disease and may be curable with less aggressive regimens.

179. Cerroni L, Kerl H, Gatter K (1998) An Illustrated Guide to Skin Lymphoma. Oxford: Blackwell.
180. de Diego J, Berridi D, Saracibar N et al. (1998) Cutaneous pseudolymphoma in association with molluscum contagiosum. **Am J Dermatopathol** 20(5):518–521.
181. Kaddu S, Cerroni L, Pilatti A et al. (1994) Acral pseudolymphomatous angiokeratoma. A variant of the cutaneous pseudolymphomas. **Am J Dermatopathol** 16(2):130–133.
182. Kuhn A, Richter-Hintz D, Oslislo C et al. (2000) Lupus erythematosus tumidus – a neglected subset of cutaneous lupus erythematosus: report of 40 cases. **Arch Dermatol** 136(8):1033–1041.
183. Stiller CA (1998) What causes Hodgkin's disease in children? **Eur J Cancer** 34(4):523–528.

TABLE 21.5   Cancer-associated genodermatoses

Syndrome	Skin findings	Internal malignancies
Birt–Hogg–Dubé	Fibrofolliculomas/trichodiscomas	Renal
Carney	Multiple lentigines and blue nevi, myxomas	Testes, breast, cardiac myxomas
Cowden	Trichilemmomas, sclerotic fibromas, oral papules	Breast, thyroid, GI
Gardner	Multiple epidermoid cysts	GI, hepatoblastoma, desmoids
Howel–Evans	Palmoplantar keratoderma, buccal leukoplakia	Esophagus
MEN 1	Facial angiofibromas, connective tissue nevi	Pituitary, parathyroid and islet cell tumors
MEN 2B	Mucosal neuromas	Medullary thyroid carcinoma, pheochromocytoma
Muir–Torre	Sebaceous neoplasms (especially cystic sebaceous tumors), keratoacanthomas	Varied; mainly GI, GU, lung
Nevoid basal cell carcinoma	Multiple basal cell carcinomas, palmoplantar pits, acral epidermoid cysts	Medulloblastoma, ovarian tumors (occasionally carcinomas)
Peutz–Jeghers	Labial, acral pigmented macules	GI, ovarian, testicular

Mixed cellularity subtypes are more likely to be associated with EBV. In general the histologic subtype does not influence the outcome with effective chemotherapy.

Boys are affected more frequently than girls. Clinical presentation is most often painless, firm, enlarging, lymphadenopathy in the neck. The lymphoma is staged based on degree of spread and presence or absence of weight loss, unexplained fever, and night sweats. Over 90% of patients are cured by combined chemotherapy and radiation therapy, so cutaneous lesions have become even more uncommon.[184] The risk of developing a second malignancy later in life is considerable for survivors of childhood HL.[185] This phenomenon has been responsible for a delicate adjustment of treatment regimens, seeking to balance cures versus lower incidence of second tumors. Chemotherapy regimens are associated with secondary leukemias, while both breast and thyroid cancers are associated with radiation therapy.

Specific skin lesions with infiltrating malignant cells are uncommon (<1%) in adult HL and even rarer in children. Papules, tumors, ulcerative lesions, and diffuse dermal infiltrates can be seen by direct extension from lymph nodes or in advanced disease that has often failed chemotherapy and radiation. A diagnosis of HL should not be made on skin biopsy alone but requires confirmation by biopsies from lymph nodes or other tissues. The monoclonal antibody CD30 marks Reed–Sternberg and other HL lymphocytes, as well as the large lymphocytes in lymphomatoid papulosis and anaplastic large cell lymphoma. These diseases may be histologically indistinguishable from cutaneous HL and probably are responsible for many of the earlier diagnoses of cutaneous HL. Follicular mucinosis is also occasionally associated with HL although it is more often seen with T-cell lymphomas.[186]

Several secondary skin findings may be presenting features of HL and should prompt lymph node examination in these children. Skin findings, except for the rare specific infiltrates, do not alter the classification or staging of HL. They include pruritus, prurigo nodules, and acquired ichthyosis. The pruritus associated with HL is severe and responds poorly to treatment; excoriations are common. As a result of the repeated scratching and rubbing, prurigo nodules may appear. Acquired ichthyosis of HL presents with thick, often dark scales most prominent on the lower extremities. This uncommon change overlaps clinically with extremely dry skin, which is common and often seen in hospitalized patients. Herpes zoster is uncommon in children, but seen in almost every HL patient. It is rarely a presenting sign, but may be more extensive, hemorrhagic, or pustular. Finally, HL patients tend to have therapy-resistant warts and mollusca contagiosa.

Non-Hodgkin lymphoma

Non-Hodgkin lymphomas (NHL) account for 60% of childhood lymphoma, with about 800 new cases yearly in the USA.[187] In contrast to HL, there is a lifelong gradual increase in the incidence of NHL. There has also been a marked increase in childhood NHL of about 30% over the past three decades. Over 90% of these tumors are classified as high grade and fall into the categories of Burkitt lymphoma, lymphoblastic lymphoma, and anaplastic large cell lymphoma. In addition to their high grade, NHL in childhood are frequently extranodal. Boys are 2–3 times more frequently affected than girls, and white children are about twice as frequently affected as blacks. NHL is the most frequent malignancy associated with HIV/AIDS in childhood; it may occur before 4 years of age. HIV screening is a reasonable measure in all children with NHL. EBV play a role in AIDS-associated NHL as well as in Burkitt lymphoma.

The paradox of lymphomas is that the high-grade tumors respond better to therapy, so that with aggressive chemotherapy, the survival rate is over 75%, varying with histologic subtype and degree of involvement. The risk of a second malignancy does not appear to be as great as with HL. Skin involvement is so vanishingly rare that it is not mentioned in most reviews of childhood NHL. We will concentrate on those lymphomas that occur both

184. Schellong G (1998) Pediatric Hodgkin's disease: treatment in the late 1990s. Ann Oncol 9 (Suppl 5):115–119.
185. Bhatia S, Robison LL, Oberlin O et al. (1996) Breast cancer and other second neoplasms after childhood Hodgkin's disease. N Engl J Med 334(12):745–751.
186. Ramon D, Jorda E, Molina I et al. (1992) Follicular mucinosis and Hodgkin's disease. Int J Dermatol 31(11):791–792.
187. Sandlund JT, Downing JR, Crist WM (1996) Non-Hodgkin's lymphoma in childhood. N Engl J Med 334(19):1238–1248.

in childhood and in the skin, considering first mycosis fungoides and then the various other T- and B-cell lymphomas.[188]

Cutaneous T-cell lymphoma (mycosis fungoides)

Cutaneous T-cell lymphoma (CTCL), also known as mycosis fungoides, is an indolent T-helper cell lymphoma that affects the skin primarily with late spread to lymph nodes, bone marrow, and viscera. It is traditionally thought of as a disease of older adults, but has been reported in recent years with increasing frequency in children.[189,190] CTCL usually begins as large scaly or atrophic patches on the lower trunk and buttocks (Fig. 21.33), also known as

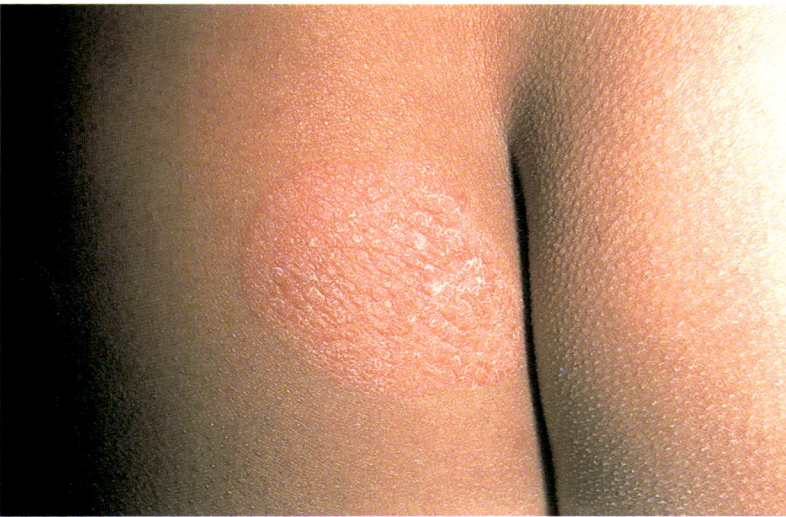

Fig. 21.33 Solitary lesion of cutaneous T-cell lymphoma (CTCL) (mycosis fungoides) with erythema and discrete border.

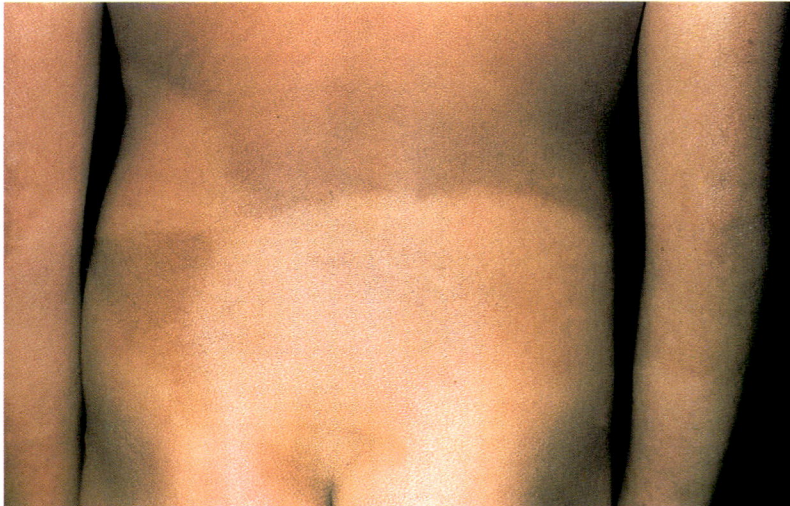

Fig. 21.34 Widespread hypopigmented cutaneous T-cell lymphoma, CTCL (mycosis fungoides).

large patch parapsoriasis (Ch. 15), which is almost certainly lymphoma. CTCL may also present as one or more hypopigmented macules Fig. 21.34).[191] This feature has been diagnosed more often in darker-skinned children, but probably because it is easier to see in this group. The discoloration is caused by postinflammatory hypopigmentation. Some cases clinically diagnosed in children as pityriasis lichenoides turn out under the microscope to be mycosis fungoides.[192] Solitary lesions may also be seen in children.[193] The diagnosis is often delayed, particularly in patients less than 20 years old, because the disease has the appearance of a chronic, unresponsive dermatitis and the index of suspicion is low. Nonetheless young patients with more advanced plaque or tumor stage disease are uncommon.

Biopsy reveals an infiltrate of helper T cells with large cerebriform nuclei that have an affinity for the epidermis and form loosely cohesive microabscesses within the epidermis. Lichenoid, spongiotic, and psoriasiform patterns may be seen. Usually the cells are positive for CD2, CD3, CD4 and CD5, but negative for CD8. T-cell receptor rearrangement indicating clonality is found in the later stages of the disease, but is often not present in early cases. Several biopsies often months or years apart may be required to produce diagnostic histopathology. Definitive histologic diagnosis is difficult and controversial and may vary between dermatopathologists.

Sézary syndrome is either a very unusual variant of mycosis fungoides or a closely related disease. The condition is characterized by erythroderma, lymphadenopathy, and circulating atypical cerebriform lymphocytes. Generally, more than 10% of the circulating lymphocytes must be Sézary cells for the diagnosis to be considered. This is particularly important in the pediatric population where severe atopic dermatitis patients frequently have some atypical circulating cells. Although the Sézary syndrome is extremely rare in children, it should be considered in the differential diagnosis of childhood erythroderma.

Follicular mucinosis presents as localized indurated or edematous plaques. If follicular mucinosis involves the scalp or eyebrows, hair loss is a prominent feature and the term alopecia mucinosa may be employed. In adults, follicular mucinosis may occasionally precede or even follow the development of cutaneous T-cell lymphoma. Although most follicular mucinosis in children is self-limited, it may progress to mycosis fungoides.[194] Those with more widespread disease are clearly at greater risk of lymphoma. Since most childhood lesions are solitary, this is another reassuring feature.

Treatment of childhood mycosis fungoides is difficult, because many of the measures recommended in adults are difficult to justify to parents because of long-term problems.[195] Many cases are kept well in check with high-potency topical corticosteroids. In older patients, PUVA, especially bath PUVA, and even topical nitrogen mustard, may be considered. The systemic retinoid bexarotene (Targretin) may be useful for refractory or persistent early-stage disease, although experience is limited and the expense is enormous.[196] Both localized and even total body electron beam therapy also appears efficacious but in our experience is rarely needed for children. Cures of mycosis fungoides are rare and controversial; control is the most reasonable treatment goal, although in children complete remissions are occasionally seen.

Other non-Hodgkin lymphomas

None of the other NHL frequently have skin involvement in children. Only 2% have skin involvement at the time of diagnosis, and most cutaneous disease occurs late in the disease course. Typically, there are papules, nodules and plaques (Figs 21.35, 21.36). Skin involvement is a poor prognostic sign with rare exception.

188. Sander CA, Kind P, Kaudewitz P et al. (1997) The Revised European-American classification of lymphoid neoplasms (REAL): a new perspective for the classification of cutaneous lymphomas. **J Cutan Pathol** 24(6):329–341.

189. Peters MS, Thibodeau SN, White JW Jr et al. (1990) Mycosis fungoides in children and adolescents. **J Am Acad Dermatol** 22(6):1011–1018.

190. Garzon MC (1999) Cutaneous T cell lymphoma in children. **Semin Cutan Med Surg** 18(3):226–232.

191. Neuhaus IM, Ramos-Caro FA, Hassanein AM (2000) Hypopigmented mycosis fungoides in childhood and adolescence. **Pediatr Dermatol** 17(5):403–406.

192. Ko JW, Seong JY, Suh KS (2000) Pityriasis lichenoides-like mycosis fungoides in children. **Br J Dermatol** 142(2):347–352.

193. Hodak E, Phenig E, Amichai B et al. (2000) Unilesional mycosis fungoides: a seven of seven cases. **Dermatology** 201(4):300–306.

194. Gibson LE, Muller SA, Peters MS (1988) Follicular mucinosis of childhood and adolescence. **Pediatr Dermatol** 5(4):231–235.

195. Zackheim HS (1999) Cutaneous T cell lymphoma: update of treatment. **Dermatology** 199(2):102–105.

196. Duvic M, Martin AG, Kim Y et al. (2001) Phase 2 and 3 clinical trial of oral bexarotene (Targretin capsules) for the treatment of refractory or persistent early-stage cutaneous T-cell lymphoma. **Arch Dermatol** 137(5):581–593.

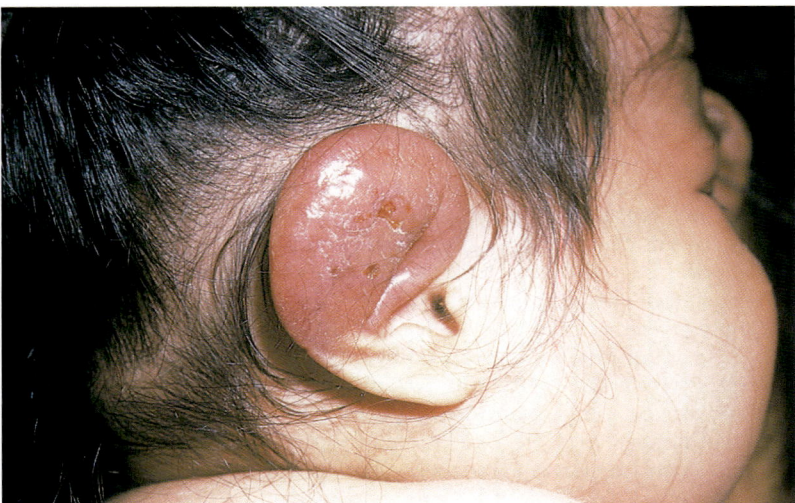

Fig. 21.35 Non-Hodgkin lymphoma in 11-month-old infant. The location suggests a pseudolymphoma but the child had lymph node involvement and the histology was that of lymphoma.

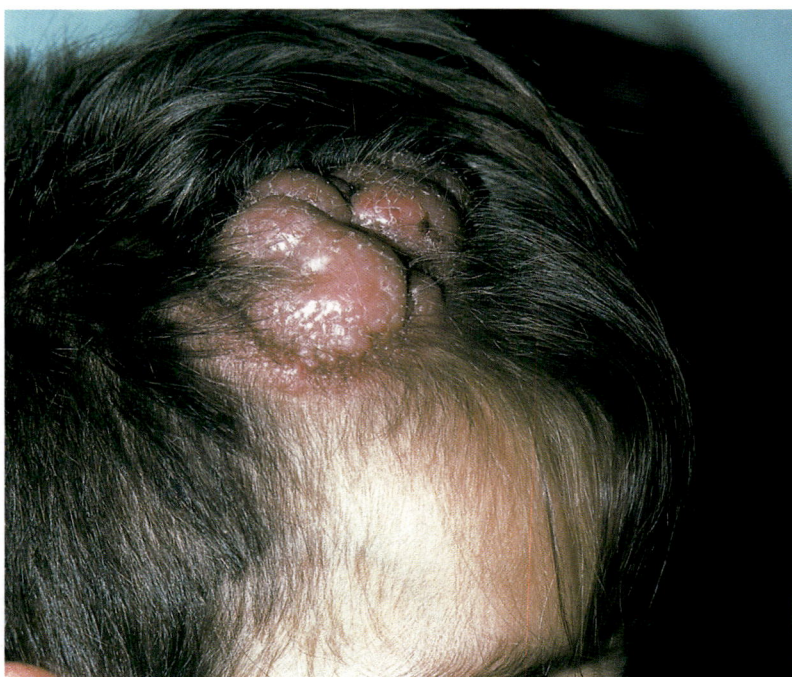

Fig. 21.36 Non-Hodgkin lymphoma in a 5-year-old boy with a prominent scalp nodule.

PRECURSOR B-CELL LYMPHOBLASTIC LYMPHOMA

This precursor B-cell neoplasm most commonly affects children and adolescents. About 80% of cases present with leukemia but the remainder are identified with solid tumors. In one series, the skin was a more common presenting site than the lymph nodes.[197] We have seen a scant number of patients whose first manifestation was a skin nodule or infiltrate. Microscopically, the lesions are very similar to T-lymphoblastic leukemia/ lymphoma, which also involves young adults, but typically presents in the mediastinum or lymph nodes and rarely involves the skin. The microscopic pictures are similar and the diagnosis is made with immunophenotyping. While the disease is highly aggressive, it is frequently curable. Those patients presenting with lymph node or skin involvement do better than those with leukemia.

MARGINAL ZONE LYMPHOMA

Marginal zone lymphomas are of particular interest as the prototypic MALT lymphoma in the gastrointestinal tract is associated with *Helicobacter pylori*. As a logical step, the cutaneous equivalent of this B-cell lymphoma has been linked to inflammatory processes but with less convincing results. A few cases have presented in the skin of adolescents. Those involving the skin are indolent tumors, but not presently curable.

BURKITT LYMPHOMA

Burkitt lymphoma is the most common childhood tumor in Africa and accounts for about 30% of non-African pediatric lymphomas. Most cases have a characteristic translocation of c-myc to the Ig heavy chain [t(8;14)] or light chain, so there is distorted B-cell growth and function. In Africans and immunosuppressed patients, Epstein–Barr virus is also often identified in the tumor cells. The most typical presentations involve the jaws, other facial bones, and cervical lymph nodes. Skin involvement is common but almost always secondary to direct spread. Burkitt lymphoma in non-immunosuppressed hosts responds well to chemotherapy.

PITYRIASIS LICHENOIDES ET VARIOLIFORMIS ACUTA

Pityriasis lichenoides et varioliformis acuta (PLEVA or Mucha–Habermann disease (Ch. 15) is a relatively common papulosquamous disorder of childhood. While it is usually self-limited, in some cases it may persist and is then known as pityriasis lichenoides chronica (PLC). Histologically it features a lymphocytic vasculitis but the infiltrate may contain atypical cells, CD30-positive cells and even cells with a monoclonal rearrangement of the T-cell receptor gene.[198–200] In rare cases, documented PLEVA or PLC has over years evolved into lymphoma.[201] Cases which clinically represent PLEVA but have cytological atypia and/or CD30-positive cells are classified by some as lymphomatoid papulosis. In other instances, CTCL may present with papules and macules, as may some NK/T-cell lymphomas.

LYMPHOMATOID PAPULOSIS

Lymphomatoid papulosis is a rare T cell disease which presents with multiple self-healing papules and nodules that may be eroded, ulcerated, or crusted (Fig. 21.37). It most often affects young adults, although children[202] and even infants[203] may be involved. Many clinical patterns are possible; some patients present with widespread disease with many papules, while others have localized or regional disease which may latter generalize.[204] Other children may have "dwindling outbreaks" with a reduction in frequency of attacks and number of lesions. Other patterns include large solitary tumors, acral lesions,[205] pustular lesions,[206] and even hydroa vacciniforme–like lesions.[207] In any case, the lesions heal spontaneously, often as new tumors are developing.

197. Lin P, Jones D, Dorfman DM et al. (2000) Precursor B-cell lymphoblastic lymphoma: a predominantly extranodal tumor with low propensity for leukemic involvement. **Am J Surg Pathol** 24(11):1480–1490.
198. Romani J, Puig L, Fernandez-Figueras MT et al. (1998) Pityriasis lichenoides in children: clinicopathologic review of 22 patients. **Pediatr Dermatol** 15(1):1–6.
199. Dereure O, Levi E, Kadin ME (2000) T-cell clonality in pityriasis lichenoides et varioliformis acuta: a heteroduplex analysis of 20 cases. **Arch Dermatol** 136(12):1483–1486.
200. Shieh S, Mikkola DL, Wood GS (2001) Differentiation and clonality of lesional lymphocytes in pityriasis lichenoides chronica. **Arch Dermatol** 137(3):305–308.
201. Niemczyk UM, Zollner TM, Wolter M et al. (1997) The transformation of pityriasis lichenoides chronica into parakeratosis variegata in an 11-year-old girl. **Br J Dermatol** 137(6):983–987.

202. Zirbel GM, Gellis SE, Kadin ME et al. (1995) Lymphomatoid papulosis in children. **J Am Acad Dermatol** 33(5):741–748.
203. Rogers M, de Launey J, Kemp A et al. (1984) Lymphomatoid papulosis in an 11-month-old infant. **Pediatr Dermatol** 2(2):124–130.
204. Scarisbrick JJ, Evans AV, Woolford AJ et al. (1999) Regional lymphomatoid papulosis: a report of four cases. **Br J Dermatol** 141(6):1125–1128.
205. Thomas GJ, Conejo-Mir JS, Ruiz AP et al. (1998) Lymphomatoid papulosis in childhood with exclusive acral involvement. **Pediatr Dermatol** 15(2):146–147.
206. Barnadas MA, Lopez D, Pujol RM et al. (1992) Pustular lymphomatoid papulosis in childhood. **J Am Acad Dermatol** 27(4):627–628.
207. Tabata N, Aiba S, Chinohazama R et al. (1995) Hydroa vacciniforme-like lymphomatoid papulosis in a Japanese child: a new subset. **J Am Acad Dermatol** 32(2):378–381.

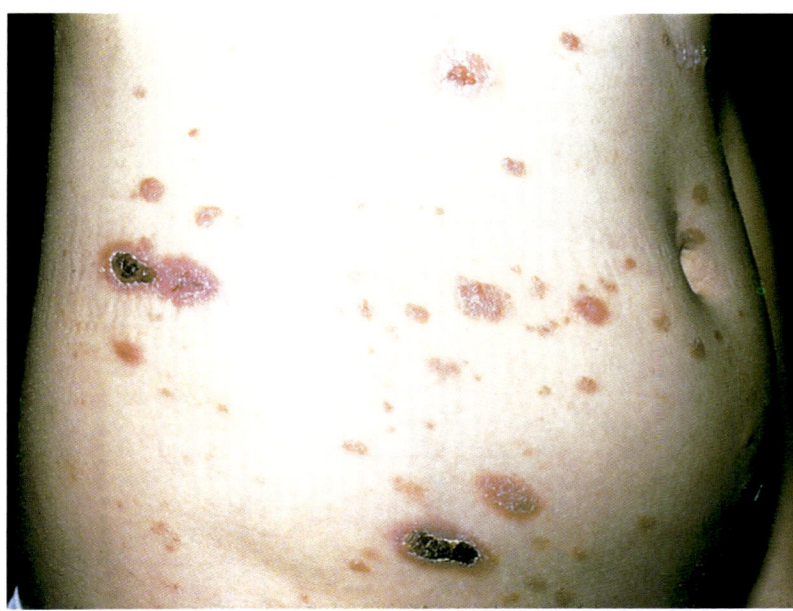

Fig. 21.37 Lymphomatoid papulosis in a 10-year-old girl with multiple lesions at various stages.

Histologically, several patterns can be seen but in all cases the cells are large atypical T cells, usually positive for CD 30. In most cases, analysis of the T-cell receptor gene shows evidence for clonality. Treatment with high-potency topical corticosteroids,[208] PUVA, or more recently bath PUVA appears efficacious.[209] Extremely low-dose oral methotrexate is also effective, but usually not employed in children. About 10–20% of patients advance to lymphoma, usually Hodgkin lymphoma or large cell anaplastic lymphoma but also CTCL. Those with the hydroa-vacciniforme variant appear at highest risk.

ANAPLASTIC LARGE CELL LYMPHOMA

Sometimes referred to as CD30-positive lymphoma, the anaplastic large cell lymphoma (ALCL) was initially identified on the basis of its striking cell morphology with large T cells with pleomorphic appearance, often containing multinucleate cells.[210,211] There are two forms of ALCL. In the more common systemic variant, the lymphoma presents in the lymph nodes and often the skin, with about 25% of patients under 20 years of age. The primary cutaneous form primarily involves adults, is indolent, and may be part of a continuum with lymphomatoid papulosis. ALCL may also arise in association with either Hodgkin lymphoma or CTCL. We have seen several teenagers who first came to the dermatologist with cutaneous infiltrates that microscopically were ALCL; in all such cases, the odds are that the systemic disease is present and one should search aggressively. Nonetheless, there are primary cutaneous cases in children, which tend to be indolent and locally recur without going on to systemic involvement.[212] Primary cutaneous ALCL in children often shows the same t(2;5) translocation seen in systemic cases in adults, but not usually seen in primary cutaneous cases in adults.[213] The systemic form is more therapy-responsive than the indolent localized form.[214]

HTLV-1-ASSOCIATED LYMPHOMA

Adult T-cell leukemia/lymphoma is associated with the HTLV-1 virus and is most common in parts of Japan and the Caribbean. Infected children have a weeping severe dermatitis known as infective dermatitis.[215] In rare instances, children infected with the virus may present with cutaneous infiltrates and other signs of lymphoma.[216,217] The histology may be confusing, resembling mycosis fungoides or even its granulomatous variant, but study of the lymph nodes and a search for the HTLV-1 virus should establish the diagnosis. There is a long latency period after infection, explaining the infrequent appearance of lymphomas in childhood, but once the disease is full-blown, survival is limited.

CYTOTOXIC NATURAL KILLER/T-CELL LYMPHOMA

The classic form of this disease is the aggressive nasal lymphoma associated with Epstein–Barr virus and seen primarily in Asia. Such tumors can also present in the skin. The cutaneous infiltrate consists of large monomorphous T cells, often extending into the subcutaneous fat, and positive for CD56. In rare cases, the infiltrate is also positive for CD30 and that may suggest a better prognosis.[213] Two closely related conditions are:

- so-called hypersensitivity to mosquito bites with an intense local reaction and high fever, previously reported in Japan as a precursor to "malignant histiocytosis," appears to involve an NK lymphoma with Epstein–Barr virus;[218]
- some forms of lymphomatoid granulomatosis, an angiodestructive lymphocytic process usually involving the lungs and upper airways, but occasionally the skin.[219]

PANNICULITIC LYMPHOMA

Panniculitic or subcutaneous lymphomas are very rare in children. They are generally suppressor T cell in type although they may also have a helper T-cell or NK phenotype. In the past, they were also designated as cytophagic histiocytic panniculitis, as erythrophagocytosis may occur. In contrast to more common types of panniculitis, such lymphomas are more likely to involve areas other than the legs and may present with unusual features, such as facial swelling or even acneiform lesions.[220]

EDEMATOUS SCARRING VASCULITIC PANNICULITIS

This clinically distinct variant of a lymphocytic panniculitis has also been described as hydroa vacciniforme-like lymphoma or lymphomatoid papulosis, primarily by Japanese authors.[221] We prefer the original term, which was applied to the disorder in Mexican children.[222] Hydroa vacciniforme is an uncommon photodermatosis (Ch. 29) that features superficial vesicles that leave behind mild varicelliform scars. Edema is uncommon, and there is no

208. Paul MA, Krowchuk DP, Hitchcock MG et al. (1996) Lymphomatoid papulosis: successful weekly pulse superpotent topical corticosteroid therapy in three pediatric patients. **Pediatr Dermatol** 13(6):501–506.
209. Volkenandt M, Kerscher M, Sander C et al. (1995) PUVA-bath photochemotherapy resulting in rapid clearance of lymphomatoid papulosis in a child. **Arch Dermatol** 131(9):1094.
210. Willemze R, Beljaards RC (1993) Spectrum of cutaneous CD30 (Ki-1)-positive lymphoproliferative disorders. A proposal for classification and guidelines for management and treatment. **J Am Acad Dermatol** 28(6):973–980.
211. LeBoit PE (1996) Lymphomatoid papulosis and cutaneous CD30+ lymphoma. **Am J Dermatopathol** 18(3):221–235.
212. Tomaszewski MM, Moad JC, Lupton GP (1999) Primary cutaneous Ki-1(CD 30) positive anaplastic large cell lymphoma in childhood. **J Am Acad Dermatol** 40(5):857–861.
213. Gould JW, Eppes RB, Gilliam AC et al. (2000) Solitary primary cutaneous CD30+ large cell lymphoma of natural killer cell phenotype bearing the t(2;5)(p23;q35) translocation and presenting in a child. **Am J Dermatopathol** 22(5):422–428.
214. Bekkenk MW, Geelen FA, van Voorst Vader PC et al. (2000) Primary and secondary cutaneous CD30+ lymphoproliferative disorders: a report from the Dutch Cutaneous Lymphoma Group on the long-term follow-up data of 219 patients and guidelines for diagnosis and treatment. **Blood** 95(12):3653–3661.
215. LaGrenade L, Hanchard B, Fletcher V et al. (1990) Infective dermatitis of Jamaican children: a marker for HTLV-I infection. **Lancet** 336(8736):308–309.
216. Lin BT, Musset M, Szekely AM et al. (1997) Human T-cell lymphotropic virus-1-positive T-cell leukemia/lymphoma in a child. Report of a case and review of the literature. **Arch Pathol Lab Med** 121(12):1282–1286.
217. Lewis JM, Vasef MA, Stone MS (2001) HTLV-I-associated granulomatous T-cell lymphoma in a child. **J Am Acad Dermatol** 44(3):525–529.
218. Ishihara S, Yabuta R, Tokura Y et al. (2000) Hypersensitivity to mosquito bites is not an allergic disease, but an Epstein-Barr virus-associated lymphoproliferative disease. **Int J Hematol** 72(2):223–228.
219. LeSueur BW, Ellsworth L, Bangert JL et al. (2000) Lymphomatoid granulomatosis in a 4-year-old boy. **Pediatr Dermatol** 17(5):369–372.
220. Chan YF, Lee KC, Llewellyn H (1994) Subcutaneous T-cell lymphoma presenting as panniculitis in children: report of two cases. **Pediatr Pathol** 14(4):595–608.
221. Iwatsuki K, Xu Z, Takata M et al. (1999) The association of latent Epstein-Barr virus infection with hydroa vacciniforme. **Br J Dermatol** 140(4):715–721.
222. Ruiz-Maldonado R, Parilla FM, Orozco-Covarrubias M de la L (1995) Edematous, scarring vasculitic panniculitis: a new multisystemic disease with malignant potential. **J Am Acad Dermatol** 32(1):37–44.

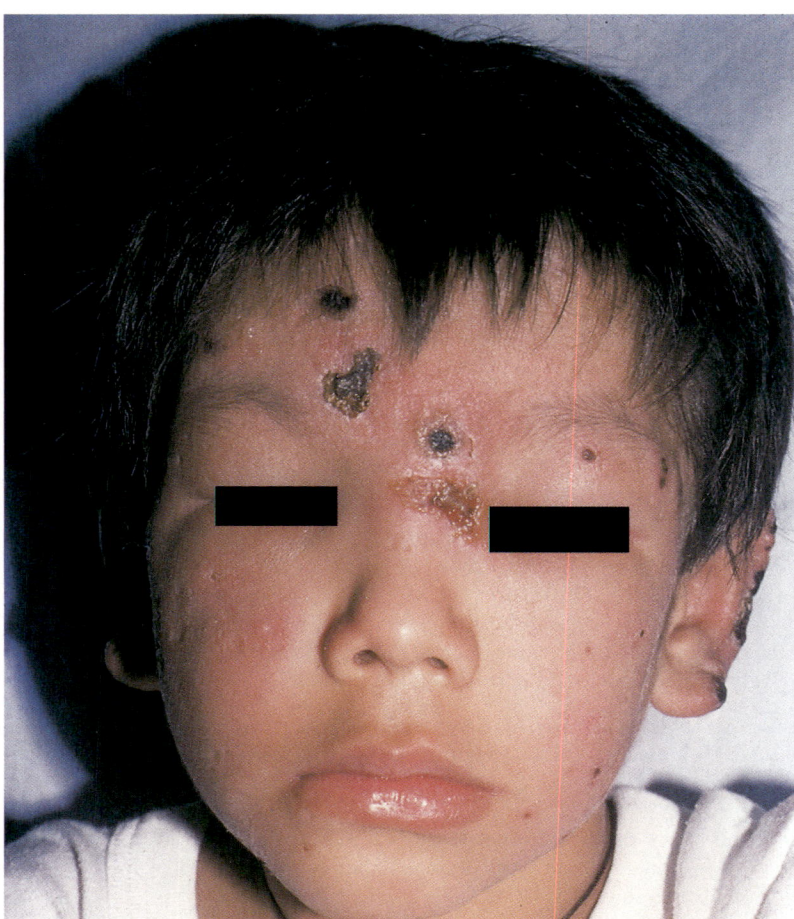

Fig. 21.38 Edematous scarring panniculocytic T-cell lymphoma with typical hydroa-like scars and facial edema.

panniculitis. Spontaneous healing during adolescence is the rule and there is no association with lymphoma. In contrast, in this disorder, while the vesicles and scarring are similar (Fig. 21.38), there is deeper involvement, the patients are often systemically ill, and a significant percentage advance to lymphoma.[223] The role of Epstein–Barr virus is confusing; it has been identified in some Japanese cases but the molecular biology and type of lymphoma remain unclear.

LEUKEMIAS

Leukemia is the most common malignancy of childhood, with an inci-dence of 40 per million, thus accounting for 25–40% of all childhood malignancies. Leukemia is somewhat more common in males and in whites. The peak incidence is 3–5 years of age. Just as with lymphomas, leukemias are classified with increasingly refined immunologic and genetic methods. Often the exact mutation can be identified, explaining the aberrant cell growth pattern and allowing highly targeted therapy to be employed. In our experience, leukemic infiltrates are the fourth most common cutaneous malignancy and the most common cause of cutaneous metastases. Cutaneous findings in leukemia include both primary leukemic infiltrates as well as a host of secondary lesions.

While only about 1% of children with leukemia have leukemic infiltrates, a much higher percentage have secondary involvement including such common problems as petechiae and hemorrhage.[224]

ACUTE LYMPHOBLASTIC LEUKEMIA

Acute lymphoblastic leukemia (ALL) is the most common form of childhood leukemia, accounting for 80% of all leukemia diagnoses and 25% of all cancer diagnoses. ALL occurs most frequently in early childhood with a peak incidence at 2–3 years of age.[225] About 2500 cases are diagnosed yearly in the USA. White children are three times as likely to be affected.

The best-established risk factors are either prenatal or postnatal exposure to ionizing radiation. Genetic disorders associated with ALL include NF-1, Bloom syndrome, and ataxia telangiectasia. About 80% of ALL is of B-cell lineage; the rest is T cell. Almost all children go into remission with aggressive chemotherapy and CNS preventive therapy (intrathecal chemotherapy and/or CNS irradiation). The five year survival is 75–80%. Second tumors are not as common as in Hodgkin lymphoma but include AML and CNS tumors. Prognosis depends on clinical presentation and subtype of acute ALL. With chemotherapy, more than 90% of patients will achieve remission and more than 50% are cured.

Leukemia cutis is rarely a presenting feature of ALL, but may signal late extramedullary relapse following chemotherapy. In such a setting, it is obviously a poor prognostic sign. Aleukemic leukemia cutis refers to the rare presentation of this type of leukemia in the skin.[226] Petechiae of the skin or mucous membranes are present at the time of diagnosis in close to 50% of patients.

ACUTE MYELOID LEUKEMIA

AML, also known as acute nonlymphocytic leukemia (ANLL), is responsible for 20% of childhood leukemias. Here, the leukemic cells have myelocytic or monocytic differentiation.[227] AML is responsible for most congenital leukemia. In Down syndrome patients, AML is quite common in the first three years of life, while later ALL is also seen. Such patients have a spectrum of leukemoid reactions, sometimes associated with vesiculopustular erutions.[228] Patients with a variety of hematological disorders (especially myelodysplastic syndrome), as well as a number of other syndromes, such as Fanconi anemia, Bloom syndrome, Wiskott–Aldrich syndrome, and ataxia telangiectasia, are also at risk. Those with ALL or other malignancies treated with alkylating agents or topoisomerase II inhibitors (epipodophyllotoxins) are also at risk for AML. Once again, 75–85% achieve complete remission with aggressive chemotherapy with CNS treatment or prophylaxis. Then either bone marrow transplantation or further aggressive chemotherapy is required, as bone marrow control in AML is considerably poorer than in ALL. The long-term outlook is slightly worse than ALL, with an event-free 5-year survival around 40%.

Leukemia cutis is more frequent in AML than in ALL, with its prevalence approaching 50% in congenital cases.[229] In this setting, the many nodules are often purpuric and referred to as "blueberry muffin lesions." These leukemic infiltrates must be differentiated by biopsy from clinically identical lesions of dermal erythropoiesis caused by intrauterine infections (toxoplasma, rubella, cytomegalovirus, herpes simplex virus, syphilis) or severe intrauterine anemia (hemolytic disease of the newborn, hereditary spherocytosis, or twin transfusion syndrome), as well as from other tumors, such as neuroblastoma, rhabdomyosarcoma, and mastocytoma.[230]

223. Magana M, Sangueza P, Gil-Beristain J et al. (1998) Angiocentric cutaneous T-cell lymphoma of childhood (hydroa-like lymphoma): a distinctive type of cutaneous T-cell lymphoma. **J Am Acad Dermatol** 38(4):574–579.

224. Su WP, Buechner SA, Li CY (1984) Clinicopathologic correlations in leukemia cutis. **J Am Acad Dermatol** 11(1):121–128.

225. Pui CH, Evans WE (1998) Acute lymphoblastic leukemia. **N Engl J Med** 339(9):605–615.

226. Taniguchi S, Hamada T, Kutsuna H et al. (1996) Lymphocytic aleukemic leukemia cutis. **J Am Acad Dermatol** 35(5):849–850.

227. Lowenberg B, Downing JR, Burnett A (1999) Acute myeloid leukemia. **N Engl J Med** 341(14):1051–1062.

228. Nijhawan A, Baselga E, Golzalez-Ensenat MA et al. (2001) Vesiculopustular eruptions in Down syndrome neonates with myeloproliferative disorders. **Arch Dermatol** 137(6):760–763.

229. Francis JS, Sybert VF, Benjamin DR (1989) Congenital monocytic leukemia: report of a case with cutaneous involvement, and review of the literature. **Pediatr Dermatol** 6(4):306–311.

230. Meuleman V, Degreef H (1995) Acute myelomonocytic leukemia with skin localizations. **Dermatology** 190(4) 346–348.

Rarely, AML may present as a soft tissue mass prior to bone marrow or hematological involvement. This lesion is known as a chloroma (because the cut surface acquires a greenish hue from myeloperoxidase granules) or granulocytic sarcoma.[231] The most common location is the deep soft tissues of the head and neck, especially the orbit, but skin involvement has been described. Two-thirds of the chloroma associated with AML occur in children less than 15 years of age. Other presenting manifestations of AML include purpura,[232] calcinosis cutis,[233] and gingival infiltrates. The presence of extramedullary infiltrates has no prognostic significance in children.[234]

CHRONIC LEUKEMIAS

Chronic lymphocytic leukemia is extremely rare in childhood and has no special dermatological features. Chronic myeloid leukemia is also uncommon in children, accounting for less than 5% of leukemia diagnoses. There are two forms: the adult form, which occurs in older children with cells that are usually Philadelphia chromosome positive; and the juvenile form, which occurs in children less than 2 years old and is Philadelphia chromosome negative.[235] Both may occasionally have cutaneous infiltrates.[236] Juvenile chronic myeloid leukemia is sometimes associated with café au lait spots, juvenile xanthogranulomas, and a family history of NF1.[237]

TYPES OF LESIONS

Primary lesions

Leukemic infiltrates or leukemia cutis appear as multiple brown-red to violaceous papules and nodules (Fig. 21.39). A biopsy from one of these indurated papules or nodules will often reveal a diffuse infiltrate of leukemic cells around blood vessels and between collagen bundles. It is not reasonable to differentiate the type of leukemia from skin biopsy specimens; examination of the blood smear and bone marrow is required. Other rare clinical presentations of leukemic infiltrates include bullae, ulcerations (Fig. 21.40), diffuse dermal infiltration, and erythroderma.

Secondary lesions

The most common secondary lesions in childhood leukemia are listed below and discussed throughout the book:

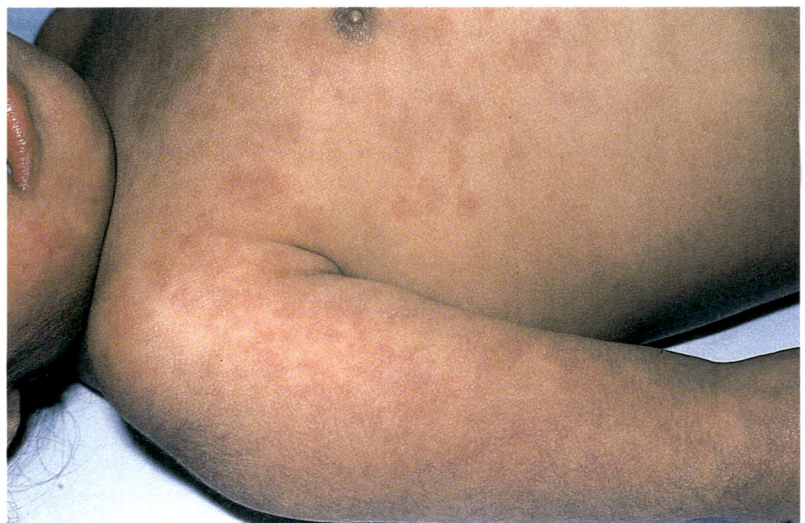

Fig. 21.39 Leukemia cutis in exanthem pattern.

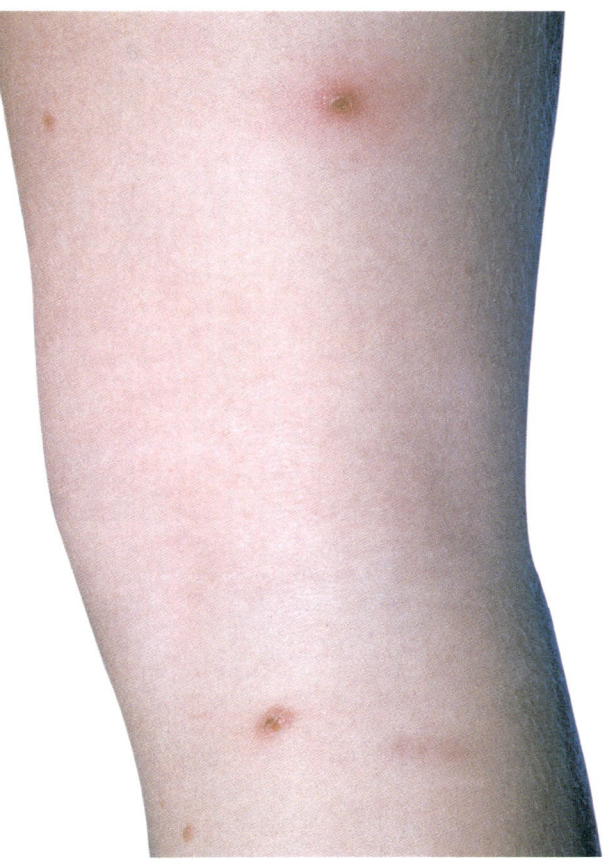

Fig. 21.40 Leukemia cutis with occasional ulcerated nodules, initially mistaken for insect bites.

- Pyoderma gangrenosum
- Sweet syndrome
- Thrombocytopenia with petechiae, hemorrhage
- Opportunistic infections, often more severe (e.g., herpes simplex, varicella-zoster)
- Alopecia, mucosal lesions secondary to chemotherapy
- Other drug reactions

NEUROBLASTOMA

Neuroblastoma is the second most common solid malignancy of childhood, following CNS tumors. It accounts for about 7–10% of childhood malignancies but 15% of childhood cancer deaths. Neuroblastoma has an incidence of around 10 per million. Boys and girls are equally affected, although boys are more likely to have metastatic disease and girls tend to have localized tumors. Race and environment also play a role as this disease is extraordinarily rare in African black children. It is also the most common congenital tumor, as 25% are present at birth, 50% before 2 years of age and over 90% before 5 years of age. Neuroblastoma is most often sporadic, although familial occurrence with autosomal-dominant inheritance can also be seen. This tumor of primitive neural crest cells of the sympathetic nervous system has many clinical presentations and may regress or differentiate spontaneously into mature neural ganglion cells. Autopsies on children who have died of other causes often show asymptomatic neuroblastomas, which would have presumably regressed.

231. Sun NC, Ellis R (1980) Granulocytic sarcoma of the skin. **Arch Dermatol** 116(7):800–802.
232. Rybojad M, Bredoux H, Vignon-Pennamen M-D et al. (1999) Leucémie monoblastique néonatale révélée par des lésions cutanées spécifiques transitoires. **Ann Dermatol Venerol** 126(2):157–159.
233. Lestringant GG, Masouye I, El-Hayek M et al. (2000) Diffuse calcinosis cutis in a patient with congenital leukemia and leukemia cutis. **Dermatology** 200(2):147–150.
234. Bisschop MM, Revesz T, Bierings M et al. (2001) Extramedullary infiltrates at diagnosis have no prognostic significance in children with acute myeloid leukemia. **Leukemia** 15(1):46–49.
235. Sawyers CL (1999) Chronic myeloid leukemia. **N Engl J Med** 340(17):1330–1340.
236. Buescher L, Anderson PC (1990) Circinate plaques heralding juvenile chronic myelogenous leukemia. **Pediatr Dermatol** 7(2):122–125.
237. Zvulunov A, Barak Y, Metzker A (1995) Juvenile xanthogranuloma, neurofibromatosis, and juvenile chronic myelogenous leukemia. World statistical analysis. **Arch Dermatol** 131(8):904–908.

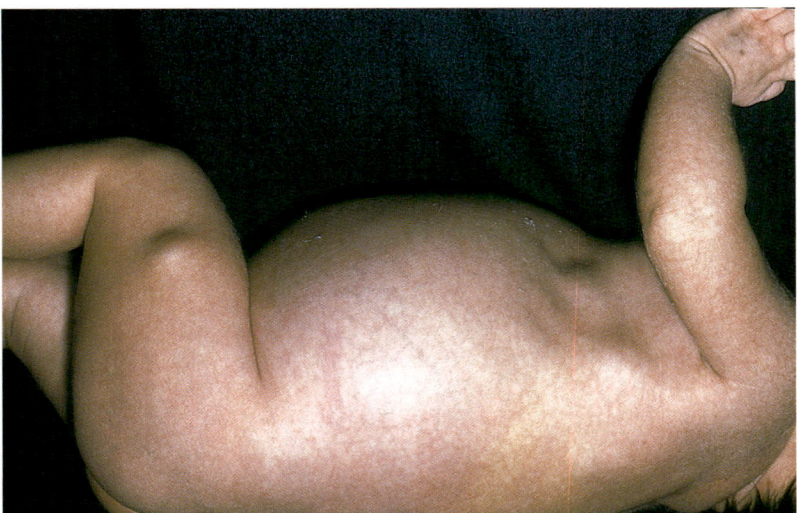

Fig. 21.41 Neuroblastoma with multiple subcutaneous nodules of metastatic disease.

Primary neuroblastomas may occur anywhere neural crest cells migrate. The neural crest cells are responsible for both the adrenal medulla and the sympathetic ganglia. Thus in simplistic terms one can expect a spectrum from pure medullary cells (classic neuroblastoma) to admixtures of ganglia elements to well-differentiated ganglioneuromas, which are benign and mentioned under neural tumors. The most common presentation is an enlarging mass within the upper abdomen with the tumor located within the adrenal gland or in the retroperitoneum. Two-thirds of patients with neuroblastoma have metastatic disease at the time of diagnosis.

Although cutaneous metastases are seen in only approximately 2% of all children with neuroblastoma, about 30% of newborns with metastatic disease have skin lesions as an initial sign of the disease. On physical examination, cutaneous metastases appear as multiple, 2mm to several centimeter, firm, skin-colored to blue papules and nodules over the trunk and extremities (Fig. 21.41). These lesions may give a baby a "blueberry muffin" appearance. Occasionally, the papules will blanch within two to three minutes when stroked.[238,239] This may be from localized release of catecholamines. Another unusual dermatologic finding in neuroblastoma is "raccoon eyes" (periorbital ecchymoses from orbital metastases).

Microscopic examination of cutaneous neuroblastoma reveals a dermal or subcutaneous infiltrate of small blue cells with round, heterochromatic nuclei and scant cytoplasm. There may be scattered mitoses and hemorrhage. More differentiated lesions will have a more diagnostic appearance with pseudo-rosettes, a mucinous stroma, and a few, more mature, ganglion cells. The differential diagnosis of cutaneous lesions in children with small blue cells includes other undifferentiated tumors such as lymphoma, leukemia, Ewing tumors and embryonal rhabdomyosarcoma. Neuroblastoma contains neuron-specific enolase and neurofilaments, both of which may be identified by immunoperoxidase stain. Increased urinary catecholamines are found in 90% of patients. Ferritin levels may be increased in some patients from tumor production of carcinofetal isoferritin.

The therapy and prognosis of this disease vary widely, depending on the age of the child and the stage of the disease. Surgery for localized disease results in a 95% cure rate. Children with widespread disease have a far less favorable outlook, despite surgery, chemotherapy, irradiation, and even bone marrow transplantation. Thirteen-*cis*-retinoic acid (isotretinoin) has been added to most chemotherapy regimens, as it seems to favorably influence differentiation of the neuroblastoma cells. Children under 1 year of age at the time of diagnosis achieve a survival rate of approximately 90% at two years. Older children and children with widespread metastatic neuroblastoma have a poor prognosis with 20–40% two-year survival. An unusual stage of neuroblastoma with a good prognosis is stage IV-S, which features widespread metastases involving liver, skin, or bone marrow with a small primary tumor and no radiographic evidence of skeletal involvement in a neonate. These patients are likely to have a "blueberry muffin" appearance. Spontaneous differentiation and regression occur in more than 75% without treatment.[240] Differentiation to neural ganglion cells has been documented by serial biopsies of regressing cutaneous metastases.

EWING FAMILY OF TUMORS

There is a large, confusing family of childhood tumors that only rarely involve the skin.[241] Members of the group include:

- Ewing tumor of bone (Ewing sarcoma)
- Extraosseous Ewing tumor
- Primitive neuroectodermal tumor (PNET) or peripheral neuroepithelioma
- Askin tumor (PNET of the chest wall).

All these tumors seem to arise from the same primordial stem cell, have a consistent alteration of the EWS gene on chromosome 22 q12 and express the MIC2 gene product CD99 on their surface. How a primitive neural cell can so often involve the bone remains a mystery; for years, Ewing tumor of bone was classified as a tumor of unknown origin. They are all small round blue-cell tumors under the microscope with varying degrees of rosette formation in PNET. The Ewing family of tumors arise most commonly in the second decade of life and account for 4% of childhood tumors. Those with localized disease do well with surgery; up to 20–30% have metastases at the time of diagnosis, typically in involving lung, bone, or bone marrow, sparing lymph nodes and CNS. Skin involvement results either by direct extension from bone or from tumors arising in the soft tissues.[242,243]

METASTASES

The most common childhood cancers are also the most likely to have cutaneous metastases. Leukemia, lymphoma, and neuroblastoma may present primarily as skin lesions or skin lesions may be a late finding in disease that is unresponsive to therapy. Wilms tumor of the kidney and central nervous system tumors, although relatively common during childhood, rarely have cutaneous metastases. Sarcomas may present in the skin from direct extension from underlying tumor or rarely from cutaneous metastases. Malignant melanoma may rarely metastasize from mother to fetus, presenting as congenital metastases. Choriocarcinoma may arise in the placenta and spread to both the mother and infant; in addition, childhood choriocarcinomas can metastasize to the skin.[244]

HISTIOCYTIC DISORDERS

The histiocytic disorders remain a confusing area. Most confusing of all is the concept of a histiocyte – a cell not recognized by modern biology. While the term "histiocytoses" is firmly entrenched in the literature, we prefer to speak of diseases of dendritic cells (antigen-processing cells) or of macrophages.[245]

238. Lucky AW, McGuire J, Komp DM (1982) Infantile neuroblastoma presenting with cutaneous blanching nodules. **J Am Acad Dermatol** 6(3):389–391.

239. Maher-Wiese VL, Wenner NP, Grant-Kels JM (1992) Metastatic cutaneous lesions in children and adolescents with a case report of metastatic neuroblastoma. **J Am Acad Dermatol** 26(4):620–628.

240. DuBois SG, Kalika Y, Lukens JN et al. (1999) Metastatic sites in stage IV and IVS neuroblastoma correlate with age, tumor biology, and survival. **J Pediatr Hematol Oncol** 21(3):181–189.

241. Delattre O, Zucman J, Melot T et al. (1994) The Ewing family of tumors – a subgroup of small-round-cell tumors defined by specific chimeric transcripts. **N Engl J Med** 331(5):294–299.

242. Suster S, Ronnen M, Huszar M (1988) Extraskeletal Ewing's sarcoma of the scalp. **Pediatr Dermatol** 5(2):123–126.

243. Ahmad R, Mayol BR, Davis M et al. (1999) Extraskeletal Ewing's sarcoma. **Cancer** 85(3):725–731.

244. Wesche WA, Khare VK, Chesney TM et al. (2000) Non-hematopoietic cutaneous metastases in children and adolescents: thirty years experience at St. Jude Children's Research Hospital. **J Cutan Pathol** 27(10):485–492.

245. Caputo R (1998) Text Atlas of Histiocytic Syndromes. St. Louis: Mosby.

CELLS

Dendritic cells

The dendritic cells are also bone marrow-derived cells that are generically described as antigen-presenting cells. Members of the group include the following:

- Langerhans cells: the main epidermal antigen-presenting cell present as a clear cell in the epidermis, staining with S-100, CD1a, and containing highly specific intracellular Birbeck granules. Langerhans cells (LC) migrate to regional lymph nodes after contact with an epidermal antigen and there present antigen to T cells. The veiled cell may be an LC in transit.
- Indeterminate cells are found primarily in the epidermis; they are identical to LC but lack Birbeck granules. They may represent a stage in LC development or a closely related dermal dendritic cell.
- Interdigitating dendritic cells are found in T-cell-rich, paracortical regions of lymph nodes and help present foreign antigens to T cells. They are S-100 and CD45 positive.
- Follicular dendritic cells are larger than interdigitating cells and are present in B-cell-rich germinal follicles where they capture antigen-antibody complexes and activate memory B cells. They have some macrophage and B-cell markers as well as a specific antigen identified by monoclonal antibodies R4/23 and Ki-M4.
- Dermal dendrocytes are mesenchymal cells that are S-100 negative and Factor XIII positive and have been identified in the normal dermis, as well as in a variety of fibrous tumors including dermatofibromas and fibrous papules of the nose. Their relationship to the bone-marrow derived dendritic cells is unclear.

Macrophages

Tissue macrophages derive from bone marrow progenitors that develop into circulating monocytes and then migrate to various tissues such as bone marrow, spleen, lymph nodes (medullary sinuses), liver (Kupffer cells), lung (alveolar macrophages), brain (microglial cells), bone (osteoclasts) and skin. Their individual characteristics in each tissue seem to be dependent on that specialized biochemical milieu and on activation by antigenic stimulation, soluble mediators, and other factors. When appropriately stimulated, macrophages enlarge, proliferate their intracytoplasmic organelles, and form epithelioid and multinucleated giant cells. They have a broad range of immunologic activities including chemotaxis, phagocytosis, ingestion, and killing. Macrophages have phagolysosomes on electron microscopy and contain phagocytic enzymes such as lysozyme, α1-antitrypsin and α1-antichymotrypsin. A variety of monoclonal antibodies such as Ki-1Mp are usually used to identify macrophages.

CLASSIFICATION OF HISTIOCYTIC DISORDERS

Table 21.6 shows a simplified classification of the cutaneous histiocytoses. The entire concept is more one of convention than of logic. Infectious diseases such as tuberculosis or leprosy, xanthomas, sarcoidosis, necrobiotic disorders, and many lysosomal disorders all clearly involve macrophages. None is referred to as a histiocytosis.

LANGERHANS CELL DISEASE

Introduction

There are several disorders in which Langerhans cells are the predominant infiltrative cell in the skin; the most common is Langerhans cell disease (LCD), also known as Langerhans cell histiocytosis or histiocytosis X [246] In addition, we view self-healing reticulohistiocytosis or Hashimoto–Pritzker disease as a variant of LCD.

TABLE 21.6 The cutaneous histiocytoses

Disease	S-100	CD1a	Birbeck granules	Macrophage markers
Langerhans cell diseases	+	+	+	−
Indeterminate cell diseases	+	+	−	+/−
Sinus histiocytosis with massive lymphadenopathy	+	−	−	+/−
Macrophage diseases (xanthogranulomas)	−	−	−	+

TABLE 21.7 Histiocyte Society classification of Langerhans cell disease

Traditional name	Histiocyte Society name
Letterer–Siwe disease	Acute disseminated LCD
Hand–Schüller–Christian disease	Chronic multifocal LCD
Eosinophilic granuloma	Chronic focal LCD
Congenital self-healing reticulohistiocytosis (Hashimoto–Pritzker)	Not recognized

Histiocytosis X was suggested by Lichtenstein as a unifying term for a group of related disorders including the following: (1) Letterer–Siwe disease: infants with a seborrheic distribution of the rash and most often multiorgan involvement; (2) Hand–Schüller–Christian disease: a classical triad of lytic skull lesions, exophthalmos, and diabetes insipidus; (3) eosinophilic granuloma: children or adults with one or several lytic bone defects.

All of these disorders are unified at the microscopic level, as the causative cell is a foamy mononuclear cell with a kidney-shaped nucleus having the same markers as an LC. The Histiocyte Society has suggested a classification, shown in comparison to the traditional terminology in Table 21.7.[247,248] Neither system addresses the main problems, which are marked overlaps between categories and the puzzling phenomena associated with neonatal disease.

The argument has longed raged over whether LCD is a malignancy or a reactive process. The clonality of the involved dendritic cells has been conclusively shown. Nonetheless, there are many clonal proliferations which are clearly benign, such as warts. In LCD, regression is common and there are frequently periods of waxing and waning. In addition, there is also evidence for immunosuppression. This uncertainty has led to confusion in both classification and, more importantly, therapy. The main need is to distinguish the more aggressive infantile forms from the less threatening disease in older children.

Presenting history

The presentation varies greatly depending on the stage of the disease but typical complaints include a refractory cradle cap or diaper rash, a weeping dermatitis, cutaneous nodules, and diabetes insipidus.

Physical examination

Infants usually have widespread cutaneous disease, presenting with a seborrheic rash, often with petechiae, involving the scalp (Fig. 21.42) and

246. Maarten Egeler R, D'Angio GJ, eds (1998) Langerhans Cell Histiocytosis. Hematol/Oncol Clinic North America 12(2):213–482.
247. Writing Group of the Histiocyte Society (1987) Histiocytosis syndromes in children. **Lancet** 1(8526):209–209.
248. Favara BE, Feller AC, Pauli M et al. (1997) Contemporary classification of histiocytic disorders. The WHO committee on histiocytic/reticulum cell proliferations. **Med Pediatr Oncol** 29(3):157–166.

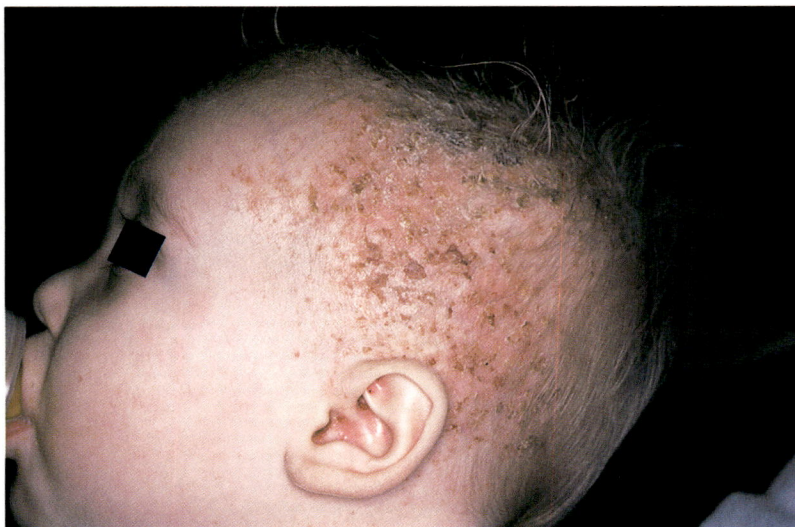

Fig. 21.42 Langerhans cell disease with prominent scaling and erythema of scalp.

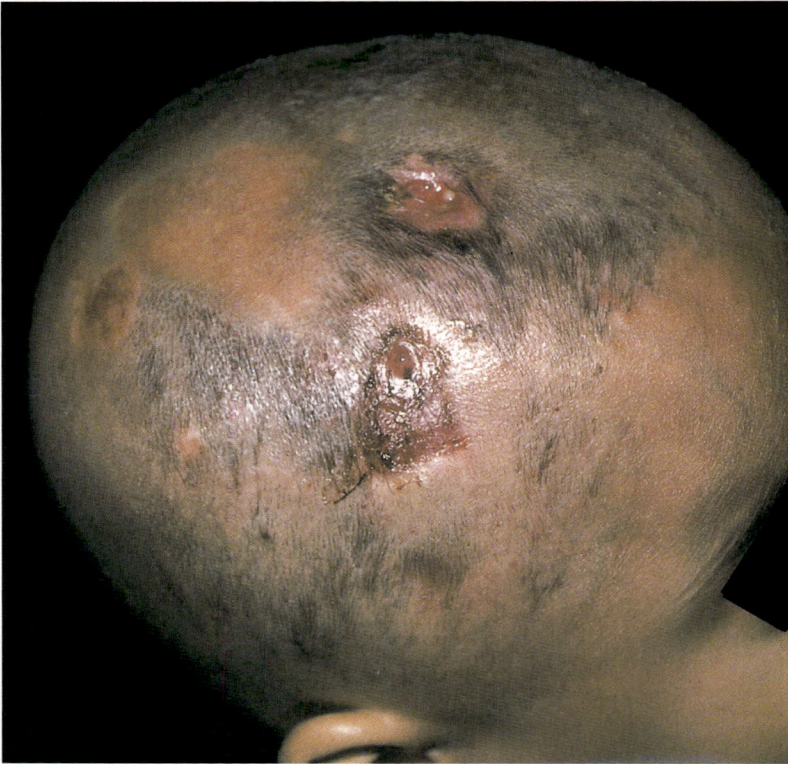

Fig. 21.44 Langerhans cell disease with ulcerated scalp nodules.

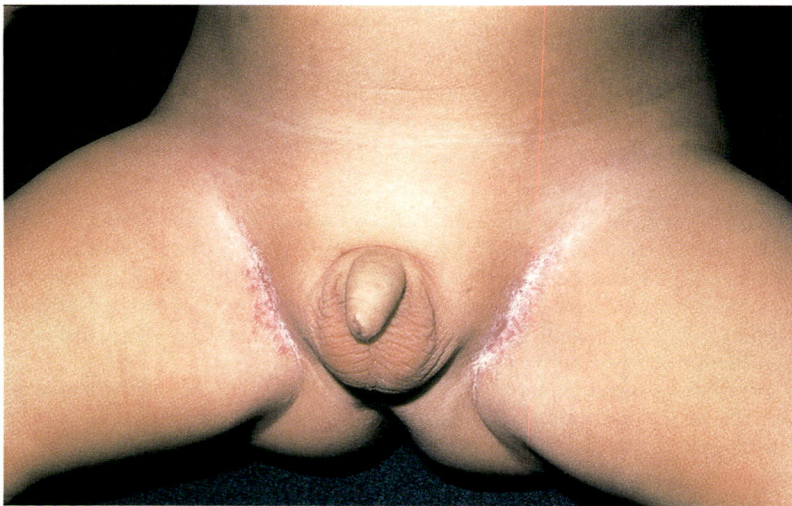

Fig. 21.43 Langerhans cell disease mistaken for refractory diaper dermatitis in the inguinal folds.

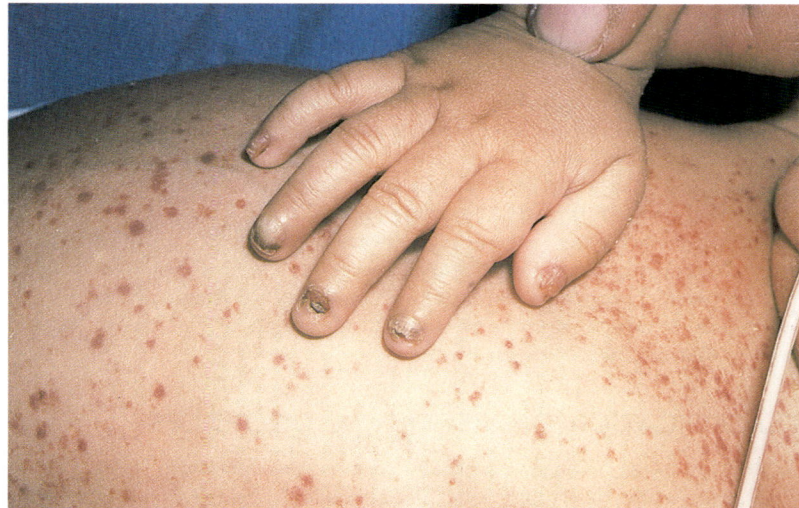

Fig. 21.45 Langerhans cell disease with petechiae and nail involvement.

flexural areas (Fig. 21.43). Ulcerations in the groin are common. Less often they may have one or more nodules, often ulcerated. Occasionally, very early in life there may be a vesiculopustular eruption. In dark-skinned children, the macules and papules tend to be hypopigmented. Older children are more likely to have ulcerated nodules (Fig. 21.44), once again most often in flexural areas. Many other unusual presentations of LCD have been described. The small papules are frequently hemorrhagic, mimicking pigmented purpura (Fig. 21.45)[249] or angiomas.[250] Groin and perianal lesions may be mistaken for condylomata.[251] Involvement of the palms and soles is common and may be mistaken for dermatitis or a dermatophyte infection (Fig. 21.46). Nail involvement is frequently overlooked or blamed on nail sucking or chewing (Fig. 21.45). Sometimes there are sufficient accompanying mast cells to produce urticaria, thus mimicking mastocytosis.[252] The disease may be limited to the skin; this favorable situation has been designated pure cutaneous LCD, but should be taken with a grain of salt as such individuals may progress to

systemic disease. Extracutaneous manifestations are common and their identification is essential toward adequately staging the disease. One should search for hepatomegaly, bone marrow involvement, lymphadenopathy, and bone lesions. Central nervous system involvement occurs more often in older children. Parapituitary infiltrates may lead to diabetes insipidus. Orbital infiltrates may produce exophthalmos. Oral involvement is common with gingival or palatal ulceration (Fig. 21.47). An eosinophilic granuloma is a common cause for a loose or floating tooth in a young adult.

249. Megahed M, Schuppe HC, Hölzle E et al. (1991) Langerhans cell histiocytosis masquerading as lichen aureus. **Pediatr Dermatol** 8(3):213–216.
250. Messenger GG, Kamei R, Honig PJ (1985) Histiocytosis X resembling cherry angiomas. **Pediatr Dermatol** 3(1):75–78.
251. Cavender PA, Bennett RG (1988) Perianal eosinophilic granuloma resembling condyloma lata. **Pediatr Dermatol** 5(1):50–55.
252. Butler DF, Ranatunge BD, Rapini RP (2001) Urticating Hashimoto-Pritzker Langerhans cell histiocytosis. **Pediatr Dermatol** 18(1):41–44.

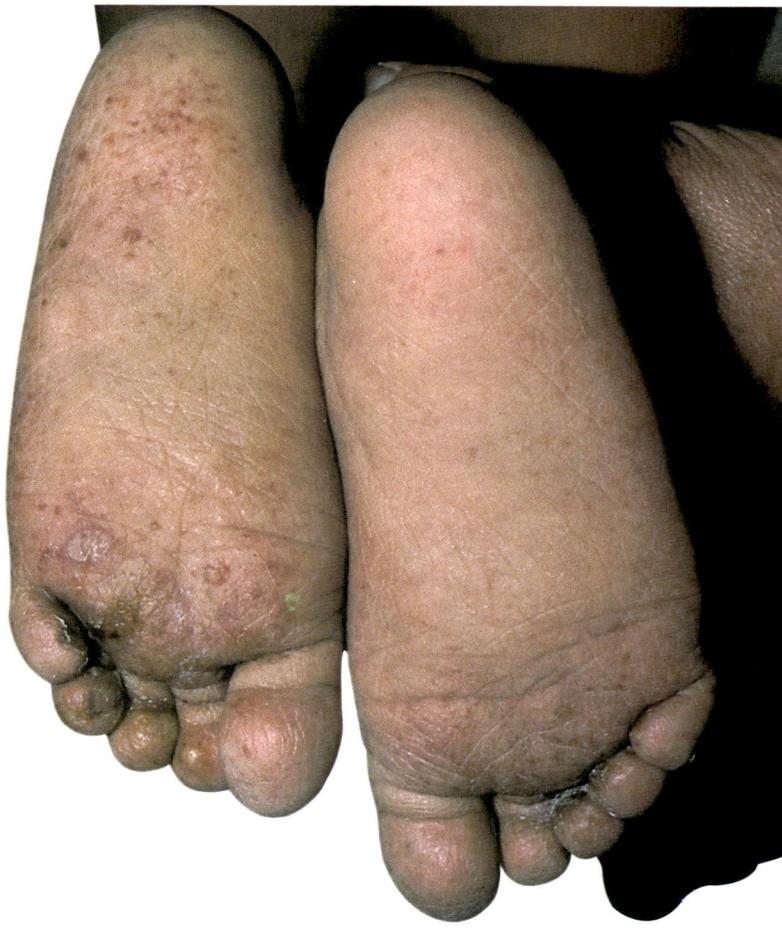

Fig. 21.46   Langerhans cell disease with hemorrhagic scaly plantar lesions.

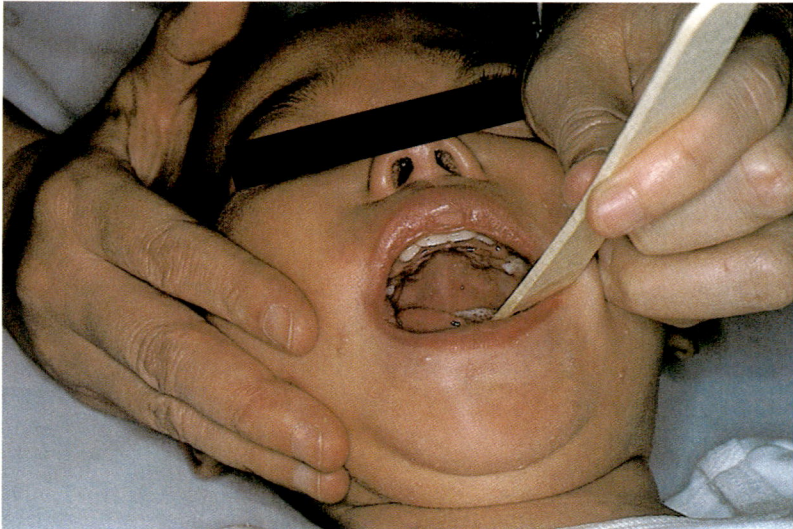

Fig. 21.47   Langerhans cell disease with gingival and palatal erosions.

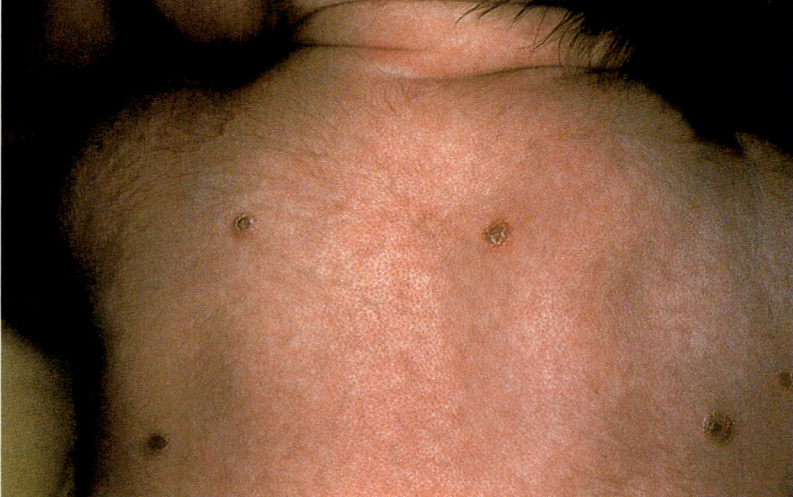

Fig. 21.48   Congenital self-healing reticulohistiocytosis in a 1-week-old child, whose lesions resolved over two weeks.

The congenital variant of LCD has been designated congenital self-healing reticulohistiocytosis (Hashimoto–Pritzker disease) and is considered a separate entity by some groups.[253] In these newborns, there are typically one or more papules or nodules which usually become crusted or ulcerated and then regress spontaneously (Fig. 21.48).[254,255] In rare instances, there may be associated systemic involvement, which also tends to resolve rapidly.[256] Despite this pristine description, congenital self-healing histiocytosis is not a unique disease but part of the spectrum of LCD. In any large collection of patients with LCD, there are some children with disease present at birth, and others who present in infancy with nodules. Furthermore, patients with typical congenital self-healing histiocytosis may see their lesions resolve, only to recur with straightforward LCD.[257] Thus such children need to be followed closely for many years.

Histologic findings

The diagnosis is made by histologically identifying LC in one or more organs, using the already discussed criteria of S-100 and CD1a positivity, and in many cases the ultrastructural presence of Birbeck granules. In the appropriate clinicopathologic setting the presence of S-100- and CD1a-positive cells allows a presumptive diagnosis of LCD, whereas demonstration of Birbeck granules is confirmatory. Other stains recommended in the original criteria of the Histiocyte Society are rarely used today. Typically, the large oval cells with a kidney-shaped nucleus are accompanied by other histiocyte, lymphocytes, eosinophils, and on occasion giant cells. In the skin, the cells are usually epidermotropic, producing the clinically noted petechiae and erosions. On other occasions, there may be a band-like infiltrate, corresponding to the lichenoid papules, or even a nodule or tumor similar to the granulomas seen in bone. There is no reliable way to distinguish between ordinary LCD and congenital self-healing reticulohistiocytosis microscopically, despite the original contention that fewer Birbeck granules were suggestive of the latter diagnosis.

Other diagnostic methods

Radiological examination is extremely useful in LCD.[258] Lytic scalp lesions, pituitary saddle changes, floating teeth, and a variety of other changes can be identified.

253. Hashimoto K, Pritzker MS (1973) Electron microscopic study of reticulohistiocytoma. An unusual case of congenital, self-healing reticulohistiocytosis. **Arch Dermatol** 107(2):263–270.
254. Alexis JB, Poppiti RJ, Turbat-Herrara E et al. (1991) Congenital self-healing reticulohistiocytosis. Report of a case with 7-year follow-up and a review of the literature. **Am J Dermatopathol** 13(2):189–194.
255. Berger TG, Lane AT, Headington JT et al. (1986) A solitary variant of congenital self-healing reticulohistiocytosis: solitary Hashimoto-Pritzker disease. **Pediatr Dermatol** 3(3):230–236.
256. Zaenglein AL, Steele MA, Kamino H et al. (2001) Congenital self-healing reticulohistiocytosis with eye involvement. **Pediatr Dermatol** 18(2):135–137.
257. Longaker MA, Frieden IJ, LeBoit PE et al. (1994) Congenital "self-healing" Langerhans cell histiocytosis: the need for long-term follow-up. **J Am Acad Dermatol** 31(5):910–916.
258. Caldemeyer KS, Parks ET, Mirowski GW (2001) Radiologic images in dermatology: Langerhans cell histiocytosis. **J Am Acad Dermatol** 44(3):509–511.

In newborns, leukemic infiltrates can be similar clinically and histologically, so a bone marrow biopsy may on occasion be required.

Differential diagnosis

There are several issues in the differential diagnosis. They include the following:

- Any infant with what appears to be refractory or purpuric seborrheic dermatitis must be biopsied to rule out LCD. Similarly, any ulcerated nodule, especially in the flexures, must be biopsied, especially if scabies is not a consideration.
- In the newborn, LCD falls into the blueberry muffin syndrome differential.

Therapeutics and prognosis

Treatment of histiocytosis X is a prototype of the concept of "do no harm."[246] Initially aggressive chemotherapy regimens have proved disastrous. Instead, the therapy should be tailored to meet the degree of involvement and be limited. For example, solitary lesions, such as in bone, respond well to local destruction, such as curettage. The skin lesions often need no treatment although they do respond well to topical corticosteroids or nitrogen mustard.[259] Systemic treatment is indicated only when there is dysfunction of a vital organ; the skin does not usually qualify for this designation. Most studies have used systemic corticosteroids and vinblastine, although etoposide and cladribine have also shown promise. Patients requiring systemic therapy should be treated by oncologists with access to investigative protocols. The following four clinical variables seem most important:[260–262]

- Age – young patients do worse than older ones, if one excludes patients with congenital lesions (who do better).
- Number of organs involved – more sites means a worse outlook.
- Rate of progression – rapid changing of a clinical sign (such as rapid decrease in liver function) is a poor sign.
- Organ dysfunction – the extent of dysfunction of the liver, lungs, spleen, and hematopoietic system is the mainstay of most staging systems. The cutaneous histology is not helpful in staging the disease.[263] Children less than 2 years of age with disseminated disease have a mortality over 50%; in other settings, there may be significant morbidity but death is uncommon. Another problem is the not uncommon association of LCD with a second malignancy; the explanation for this phenomenon remains speculative. Our approach to newborns or small infants with nodules of LCD is to be very cautious in making any prognostic statements. If there is no hepatosplenomegaly or lymphadenopathy on physical examination and complete blood count, liver function tests, chest X-ray, and skeletal survey are normal, most children do well, but a minority will progress to systemic involvement.

Indeterminate cell histiocytosis

In contrast to all the other histiocytoses, this disorder does not have a distinct clinical picture. Patients have ranged from a newborn to an octogenarian, and the lesion morphology varies from single nodules to disseminated disease.[264–266] The only unifying factors are the immunohistochemical evidence of both LC and macrophage markers and the lack of Birbeck granules on electron microscopy.[267] In some instances, indeterminate cell histiocytosis may be reactive. The lesions of nodular scabies may contain such cells,[268] and we have recently seen a case in which pityriasis rosea evolved into a papulonodular infiltrate rich in the same cells. In other instances, indeterminate cell histiocytosis has developed in patients with B-cell lymphoma.[269] Until basic scientists define a role for the indeterminate cell and more reproducible criteria, we view this diagnosis with a bit of healthy skepticism.

SINUS HISTIOCYTOSIS WITH MASSIVE LYMPHADENOPATHY

Also known as Rosai–Dorfman disease, sinus histiocytosis with massive lymphadenopathy (SHML) is a poorly understood, presumably reactive proliferation of sinus histiocytes, macrophages in the sinuses of lymph nodes.[270] The nature of the precursor cell remains elusive since there are no normal cells which are S-100 positive, CD1a negative, and express macrophage markers. While both Epstein–Barr virus and HHV-6 have been postulated as triggers, the evidence is underwhelming.

SHML is very much a pediatric disease. The typical patient is a young child with striking lymphadenopathy, especially cervical. About 10% of these patients have cutaneous disease, but it is the least of their problems.[271] Typically, there are widespread small red-brown papules or nodules. Pustular lesions have also been described.[272] The skin is a frequent extranodal site; along with soft tissue, it is the most common location for solitary SHML, in which there are no distinguishing features, just a lump in an otherwise healthy child.[273] Such solitary lesions can be excised; the systemic disease has no well-established therapy but the overwhelming percentage of cases resolve spontaneously.

MACROPHAGE DISORDERS: XANTHOGRANULOMA FAMILY

We group a series of related disease together as members of the xanthogranuloma family or macrophage disorders:

- Juvenile xanthogranuloma
- Multicentric reticulohistiocytosis
- Reticulohistiocytoma
- Progressive nodular histiocytosis
- Benign cephalic histiocytosis
- Generalized eruptive histiocytosis
- Xanthoma disseminatum
- Papular xanthoma.

In the past, terms such as non-X histiocytosis or non-LCD were employed for this group. Zelger has convincingly shown that all have histological features of xanthogranuloma, sharing a variety of morphological variants of macrophages, including vacuolated, foamy, oncocytic, spindle-shaped, and scalloped forms. This approach makes it easier to interpret the histological features but

259. Hoeger PH, Nanduri VR, Harper JI et al. (2000) Long term follow up of topical mustine treatment for cutaneous Langerhans cell histiocytosis. **Arch Dis Child** 82(6):483–487.
260. Esterly NB, Maurer HS, Gonzalez-Crussi F (1985) Histiocytosis X: a seven-year experience at a children's hospital. **J Am Acad Dermatol** 13(3):481–496.
261. Rivera-Luna R, Martinez-Guerra G, Altamirano-Alvarez E et al. (1988) Langerhans cell histiocytosis: clinical experience with 124 patients. **Pediatr Dermatol** 5(3):145–150.
262. Braier J, Chantada G, Rosso D et al. (1999) Langerhans cell histiocytosis: retrospective evaluation of 123 patients at a single institution. **Pediatr Hematol Oncol** 16(5):377–385.
263. Risdall RJ, Dehner LP, Duray P et al. (1983) Histiocytosis X (Langerhans' cell histiocytosis). Prognostic role of histopathology. **Arch Pathol Lab Med** 107(2):59–63.
264. Wood GS, Hu CH, Beckstead JH et al. (1985) The indeterminate cell proliferative disorder: report of a case manifesting as an unusual cutaneous histiocytosis. **J Dermatol Surg Oncol** 11(11):1111–1119.
265. Levisohn D, Seidel D, Phelps A et al. (1993) Solitary congenital indeterminate cell histiocytoma. **Arch Dermatol** 129(1):81–85.
266. Flores-Stadler EM, Gonzalez-Crussi F, Greene M et al. (1999) Indeterminate-cell histiocytosis: immunophenotypic and cytogenetic findings in an infant. **Med Pediatr Oncol** 32(4):250–254.
267. Sidoroff A, Zelger B, Steiner H et al. (1996) Indeterminate cell histiocytosis – a clinicopathological entity with features of both X- and non-X histiocytosis. **Br J Dermatol** 134(3):525–532.
268. Hashimoto K, Fujiwara K, Punwaney J et al. (2000) Post-scabetic nodules: a lymphohistiocytic reaction rich in indeterminate cells. **J Dermatol** 27(3):181–194.
269. Vasef MA, Zaatari GS, Chan WC et al. (1995) Dendritic cell tumors associated with low-grade B-cell malignancies. Report of three cases. **Am J Clin Pathol** 104(6):696–701.
270. Foucar E, Rosai J, Dorfman R (1990) Sinus histiocytosis with massive lymphadenopathy (Rosai-Dorfman disease): review of the entity. **Semin Diagn Pathol** 7(1):19–73.
271. Thawerani H, Sanchez RL, Rosai J et al. (1978) The cutaneous manifestations of sinus histiocytosis with massive lymphadenopathy. **Arch Dermatol** 114(2):191–197.
272. Ang P, Tan SH, Ong BH (1999) Cutaneous Rosai-Dorfman disease presenting as pustular and acneiform lesions. **J Am Acad Dermatol** 41(2):335–337.
273. Lazar AP, Esterly NB, Gonzalez-Crussi F (1987) Sinus histiocytosis clinically limited to the skin. **Pediatr Dermatol** 4(3):247–253.

also explains why so often there are clinical overlaps or even progression from one type of macrophage disorder to another.[274,275]

Juvenile xanthogranuloma

Juvenile xanthogranuloma (JXG) is one of the more common pediatric tumors and the only member of this family which every reader can expect to see at least once. The name is a misnomer and xanthogranuloma is preferable, but for a pediatric dermatology text we have retained the traditional designation. JXG can be highly variable in clinical appearance. The typical patient has one to several yellow to red-brown papules or nodules often with overlying telangiectases (Fig. 21.49). The most common sites are the flexural areas and scalp. Most patients are young children, but the lesions may be congenital and there is no upper age limit. Many different clinical variations can be seen.[276] Deeper subcutaneous nodules do not have any surfaces changes or are simply erythematous and may thus be difficult to diagnose clinically.[277] Macular, lichenoid, and plaque variants are also seen. The Cyrano form refers to disfiguring nasal lesions, but JXG at other sites can also be destructive (Fig. 21.50). Most lesions resolve spontaneously but with atrophic scars.

Xanthogranulomas are not limited to the skin.[278] Erdheim–Chester disease is probably the best-established example of cutaneous and systemic xanthogranulomas, with bone involvement most common.[279] The soft tissue is the second most common site affected by xanthogranulomas, but the possibility of ocular involvement attracts the most attention. Some have emphasized the micronodular cutaneous variant with many small lesions and an increased risk of eye involvement, as compared to the macronodular form with fewer larger lesions and a greater risk of internal involvement. This distinction is difficult in practice. Typical eye findings include bleeding into the anterior chamber and conjunctival or bulbar tumors. Many patients require ophthalmologic consultation. The current recommendations include targeting screening to patients under 2 years of age with multiple skin lesions and a newly made diagnosis.[280] We tend to have almost every patient examined by

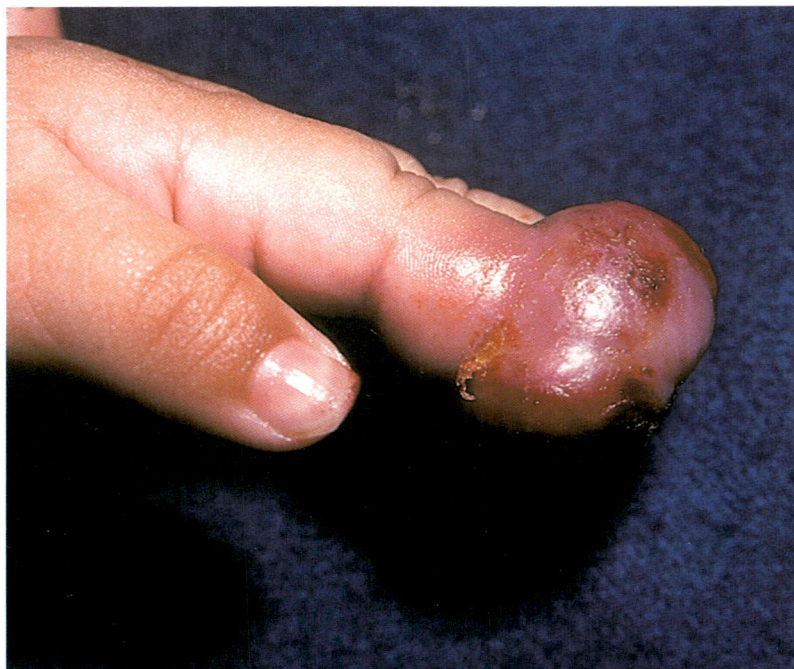

Fig. 21.50 Disfiguring juvenile xanthogranuloma of the digit in a 8-month-old infant.

an ophthalmologist. We search further for other systemic involvement based only on signs and symptoms. The relationship of JXG, NF1, and juvenile chronic myeloid leukemia is well-established but surely rare.[237] NF2 has also been associated with xanthogranulomas but not simultaneously with leukemia.[104]

All of the macrophage forms mentioned above can be identified in ordinary JXG with a bit of careful searching and luck. Typically, there is a dense dermal infiltrate of vacuolated cells, along with wreath-like giant cells (Touton cells) and eosinophils. The plasmacytoid monocyte may be the normal counterpart of the predominant cells in a xanthogranuloma.[281] Some lesions, especially early ones, lack Touton cells and the inexperienced may then shy away from the correct diagnosis.[282] The change from an early lesions with only vacuolated macrophages to a more classic picture with Touton cells can be very rapid.[283]

If the diagnosis is clinically straightforward, no therapy is necessary. After the usual spontaneous regression, a slightly depressed, often hyper- or hypopigmented macule or patch remains. If treatment is desired, excision can be performed.

Multicentric reticulohistiocytosis

Multicentric reticulohistiocytosis is a systemic disorder which is extremely rare in children, involving the skin, skeletal system, and a variety of internal organs.[284,285] Patients typically develop a disfiguring arthritis and multiple nodules, especially over the involved joints. In addition, multicentric reticulohistiocytosis is associated with a variety of autoimmune diseases and is a paraneoplastic marker. The skin and joint lesions are rich in macrophages and

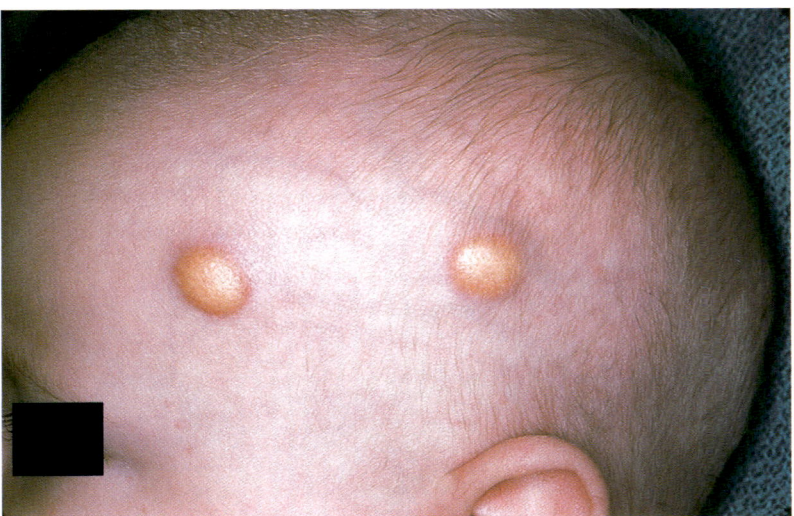

Fig. 21.49 Juvenile xanthogranulomas on the scalp.

274. Zelger BW, Sidoroff A, Orchard G et al. (1996) Non-Langerhans cell histiocytoses. A new unifying concept. **Am J Dermatopathol** 18(5):490–504.
275. Burgdorf WH, Zelger B (1996) The non-Langerhans' cell histiocytoses in childhood. **Cutis** 58(3):201–207.
276. Cohen BA, Hood A (1989) Xanthogranuloma: report on clinical and histologic findings in 64 patients. **Pediatr Dermatol** 6(4):262–266.
277. Janney CG, Hurt MA, Santa Cruz DJ (1991) Deep juvenile xanthogranuloma. Subcutaneous and intramuscular forms. **Am J Surg Pathol** 15(2):150–159.
278. Freyer DR, Kennedy R, Bostrom BC et al. (1996) Juvenile xanthogranuloma: forms of systemic disease and their clinical implications. **J Pediatr** 129(2):227–237.
279. Shamburek RD, Brewer HB Jr, Gochuico BR (2001) Erdheim-Chester disease: a rare multisystem histiocytic disorder associated with interstitial lung disease. **Am J Med Sci** 321(1):66–75.
280. Chang MW, Frieden IJ, Good W (1996) The risk of intraocular juvenile xanthogranuloma: survey of current practices and assessment of risk. **J Am Acad Dermatol** 34(3):445–449.
281. Kraus MD, Haley JC, Ruiz R et al. (2001) "Juvenile" xanthogranuloma: an immunophenotypic study with a reappraisal of histogenesis. **Am J Dermatopathol** 23(2):104–111.
282. Shapiro PE, Silvers DN, Treiber RK et al. (1991) Juvenile xanthogranulomas with inconspicuous or absent foam cells and giant cells. **J Am Acad Dermatol** 24(6):1005–1009.
283. Kubota Y, Kiryu H, Nakayma J et al. (2001) Histopathologic maturation of juvenile xanthogranuloma in a short period. **Pediatr Dermatol** 18(2):127–130.
284. Caputo R, Ermacora E, Gelmetti C (1988) Diffuse cutaneous reticulohistiocytosis in a child with tuberous sclerosis. **Arch Dermatol** 124(4):567–570.
285. Raphael SA, Cowdery SL, Faerber EN et al. (1989) Multicentric reticulohistiocytosis in a child. **J Pediatr** 114(2):266–269.

giant cells with a ground-glass cytoplasm. There is no effective systemic treatment. Familial histiocytic dermatoarthritis appears to be a variant.[286,287] The same changes can be seen in solitary lesions which are then termed reticulohistiocytoma and represent simply a variant of xanthogranuloma.

Progressive nodular histiocytosis

This rare disorder has been described in children[288] as well as adults.[289] The clinical key is the presence of two types of lesions – superficial xanthomatous papules and deeper nodules rich in spindle-shaped macrophages. The latter lesions may become hemorrhagic or necrotic and thus painful. Resolution of lesions does occur, but is the exception, not the rule. Systemic findings have been reported, but their relationship to the macrophage disorder are unclear.[290] The solitary equivalent is a xanthogranuloma rich in spindle-shaped cells, sometimes even showing immunoreactivity against smooth muscle actin.[291] It is usually mistaken for a dermatofibroma although it lacks the overlying epidermal changes. Hereditary mucinous histiocytosis is clinically similar, but only females are affected and the dermal nodules are rich in mucin.[292,293]

Benign cephalic histiocytosis

This form of xanthogranuloma is both clinically distinct and almost limited to children.[294–296] The young patients typically have multiple small yellow to red-brown papules primarily on their cheeks and forehead (Fig. 21.51). Systemic involvement in the form of diabetes insipidus has been reported, but is extremely uncommon.[297] In some instances, the lesions may evolve into juvenile xanthogranuloma. In one case, varicella-zoster virus infection seemed to trigger this change.[298] Other body sites can be involved, but if facial lesions do not predominate, we prefer to diagnose generalized eruptive histiocytosis. Histologically the lesions show monomorphous vacuolated macrophages. In the past, such patients were confused with LCD, but today special stains settle the issue. In older children one may also consider syringomas and flat warts. Resolution is spontaneous over months to years.

Generalized eruptive histiocytosis

By definition, patients with generalized eruptive histiocytosis have multiple papules and nodules which appear rapidly and often may wax and wane.[299] We have seen both spontaneous resolution and long persistence of lesions. These patients may also evolve into other forms of xanthogranuloma.[300] Cases have been described at birth and in childhood.[301] Histology shows primarily vacuolated macrophages. In adults, generalized eruptive histiocytosis may be a paraneoplastic marker.

Xanthoma disseminatum

Xanthoma disseminatum (Montgomery syndrome) is an unusual chronic type of xanthogranulomatosis. Patients present with extensive yellow to red-brown papules, often coalescing into plaques, involving the flexural areas. (Fig. 21.52) Onset is usually in childhood or young adult life. Additional features include

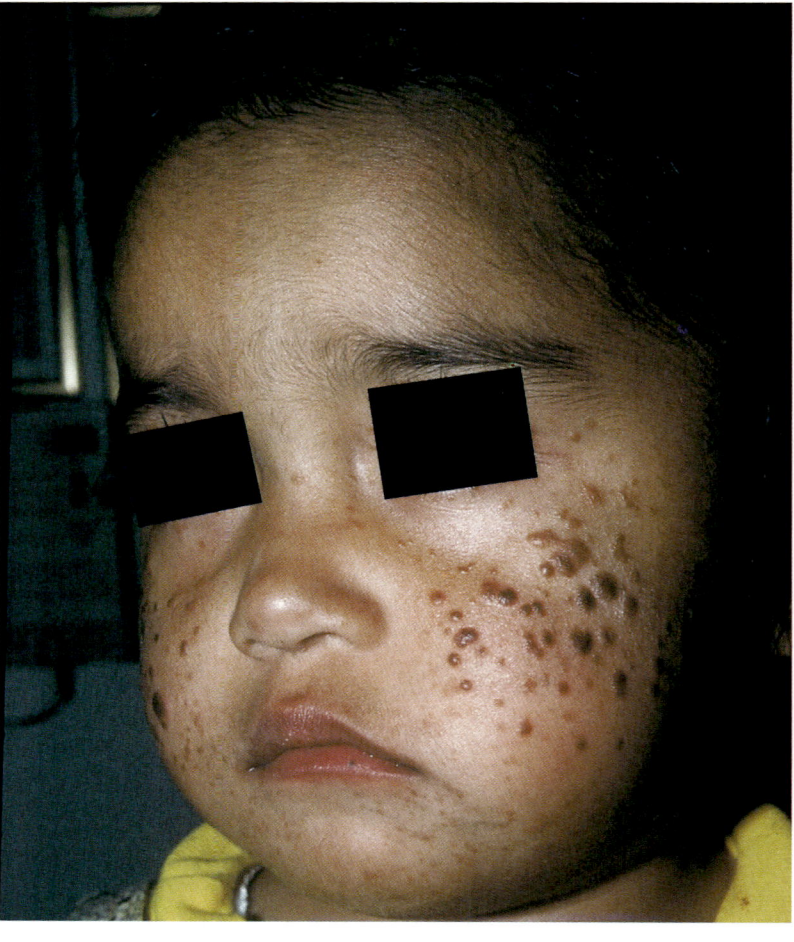

Fig. 21.51   Benign cephalic histiocytosis.

mucosal lesions, diabetes insipidus, and elevated cholesterol or triglycerides.[302] Initially, under the microscope one may find the intriguing scalloped macrophages, but in later stages the lesions are very foamy and indistinguishable from an ordinary xanthoma.[303] Most patients follow a chronic course, although some show spontaneous improvement. There is no satisfactory treatment.

Papular xanthoma

Papular xanthoma is the solitary equivalent of xanthoma disseminatum. It has been described in infants, children, and adults as one or several clinically

286. Zayid I, Farraj S (1973) Familial histiocytic dermatoarthritis. A new syndrome. **Am J Med** 54(6):793–800.

287. Valente M, Parenti A, Cipriani R et al. (1987) Familial histiocytic dermatoarthritis. Histologic and ultrastructural findings in two cases. **Am J Dermatopathol** 9(6):491–496.

288. Taunton OD, Yeshurun D, Jarratt M (1978) Progressive nodular histiocytoma. **Arch Dermatol** 114(10):1505–1508.

289. Burgdorf WH, Kusch SL, Nix TE Jr et al. (1981) Progressive nodular histiocytoma. **Arch Dermatol** 117(10):644–649.

290. Gonzalez Ruiz A, Bernal Ruiz AI, Aragoneses Fraile H et al. (2000) Progressive nodular histiocytosis accompanied by systemic disorders. **Br J Dermatol** 143(3):628–631.

291. Zelger BW, Staudacher C, Orchard G et al. (1995) Solitary and generalized variants of spindle cell xanthogranuloma (progressive nodular histiocytosis). **Histopathology** 27(1):11–19.

292. Bork K, Hoede N (1988) Hereditary progressive mucinous histiocytosis in women. Report of three members in a family. **Arch Dermatol** 124(8):1225–1229.

293. Antoni-Bach N, Pfister R, Grosshans E et al. (2000) Histiocytose mucineuse héréditaire progressive. **Ann Dermatol Venereol** 127(4):400–404.

294. Laralda de Luna M, Glikin I, Golberg J et al. (1989) Benign cephalic histiocytosis: report of four cases. **Pediatric Dermatol** 6(3):198–201.

295. Gianotti R, Alessi E, Caputo R (1993) Benign cephalic histiocytosis: a distinct entity or part of a wide spectrum of histiocytic proliferative disorders of children? A histopathological study. **Am J Dermatopathol** 15(4):315–319.

296. Pena-Penabad C, Unamuno P, Garcia-Silva J et al. (1994) Benign cephalic histiocytosis: case report and literature review. **Pediatr Dermatol** 11(2):164–167.

297. Weston WL, Travers SH, Mierau GW et al. (2000) Benign cephalic histiocytosis with diabetes insipidus. **Pediatr Dermatol** 17(4):296–298.

298. Rodriquez-Jurado R, Duran-McKinster C, Ruiz-Maldonado R (2000) Benign cephalic histiocytosis progressing into juvenile xanthogranuloma: a non-Langerhans histiocytosis transforming under the influence of a virus. **Am J Dermatopathol** 22(1):70–74.

299. Winkelmann RK, Kossard S, Fraga S (1980) Eruptive histiocytoma of childhood. **Arch Dermatol** 116(5):565–570.

300. Repiso T, Roca-Miralles M, Kanitakis J et al. (1995) Generalized eruptive histiocytoma evolving into xanthoma disseminatum in a 4-year-old boy. **Br J Dermatol** 132(6):978–982.

301. Wee SH, Kim HS, Chang SN et al. (2000) Generalized eruptive histiocytoma: a pediatric case. **Pediatr Dermatol** 17(6):453–455.

302. Caputo R, Veraldi S, Grimalt R et al. (1995) The various clinical patterns of xanthoma disseminatum. Considerations on seven cases and review of the literature. **Dermatology** 190(1):19–24.

303. Zelger B, Cerio R, Orchard G et al. (1992) Histologic and immunohistochemical study comparing xanthoma disseminatum and histiocytosis X. **Arch Dermatol** 128(9):1207–1212.

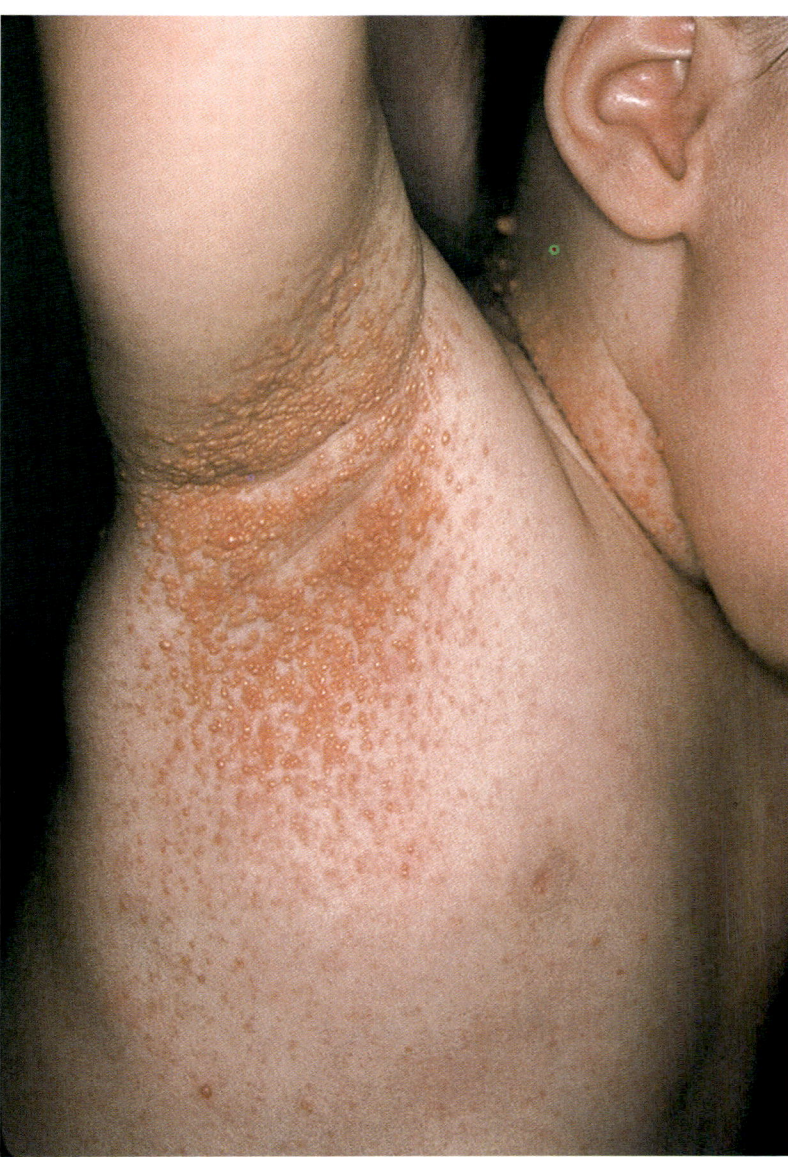

Fig. 21.52 Xanthoma disseminatum in a three-year-old girl showing coalescent yellow papules in the axilla and around the neck (Photo courtesy of Anne W. Lucky MD).

indistinct papules that on histology contain foamy macrophages.[304–306] While the first consideration in children with such lesions should be true xanthomas, associated with genetic disorders of cholesterol or triglyceride metabolism or liver disease, these patients have normal blood lipid studies. In children, the following disorders should be considered as causes of normolipemic xanthomas:

- Non-cholesterol sterol deposits – cerebrotendinous xanthomatosis and phytosterolemia both may present with large xanthomas in childhood, often about tendons.
- Verruciform xanthoma is usually a solitary oral lesion, but can be seen on the genitalia, in inflamed skin and especially in CHILD syndrome.
- Postinflammatory xanthomas have been described in children with severe atopic dermatitis.

MALIGNANT HISTIOCYTOSIS

Malignant histiocytosis is a disease that has become decidedly more rare as modern immunologic techniques have reclassified many, but not all, cases as T-cell lymphomas. Robb-Smith first described the disease as histiocytic medullary reticulosis, but this term is rarely used today. Patients typically are seriously ill with fever, hepatosplenomegaly, lymphadenopathy, and bone marrow involvement. About 20% have been reported to have skin involvement, usually in the form of purpura but also with infiltrative nodules. Only a few cases of true histiocytic lymphoma starting in nodes and true malignant histiocytosis starting as a multisystem disease in which the cells show only histiocytic markers have been reported. The main differential diagnosis in children includes familial hemophagocytic lymphohistiocytosis, X-linked lymphoproliferative syndrome, and infection-associated hemophagocytic syndrome. All of the latter have similar histologic findings and none shows distinctive cutaneous features.[307]

ACKNOWLEDGMENTS

The authors gratefully acknowledge contributions to this chapter in previous editions–
1st Edition – Drs Jerry Bangert, Libby Edwards, Gerald Goldberg and Ronald Hansen
2nd Edition – Dr Carl Bigler
They also thank Dr Anne Lucky for editorial guidance and advice.

304. Caputo R, Gianni E, Imondi D et al. (1990) Papular xanthoma in children. **J Am Acad Dermatol** 22(6):1052–1056.

305. Horiuchi Y, Ito A (1991) Normolipemic papuloeruptive xanthomatosis in an infant. **J Dermatol** 18(4):235–239.

306. Fonseca E, Contreras F, Cuevas J (1993) Papular xanthoma in children: report and immunohistochemical study. **Pediatr Dermatol** 10(2):139–141.

307. Woda BA, Sullivan JL (1993) Reactive histiocytic disorders. **Am J Clin Pathol** 99(4):459–463.

Cutaneous Manifestations of Endocrine, Metabolic, and Nutritional Disorders

Anne W. Lucky and Julie Powell

THYROID DISORDERS

Anne W. Lucky

Hypothyroidism and hyperthyroidism both can have distinctive cutaneous manifestations.

HYPOTHYROIDISM

Severe congenital hypothyroidism has been documented for centuries in illustrations and sculptures of goitrous retarded individuals. The obsolete term *cretin* has been used in the past but is no longer applicable.[1] Nongoitrous and acquired hypothyroidism in childhood were appreciated later. The absence of thyroid hormone may be congenital or acquired, and either form may be associated with an enlarged thyroid gland (goitrous hypothyroidism) or an absent or atrophic gland (nongoitrous hypothyroidism). More rarely, hypothyroidism can be caused by pituitary failure or by end-organ insensitivity to thyroid hormones.

Epidemiology

Congenital hypothyroidism is usually sporadic, except in rare cases of inborn errors of thyroid metabolism. Congenital hypothyroidism is not uncommon: it occurred in 1 in 4300 births of 1 million infants screened in North America and in 1 in 3600 of more than 3 million newborns screened in Europe.[2–4] Secondary hypothyroidism due to congenital pituitary failure is much more rare, occurring in 1 in 68 200 births.[2] Congenital hypothyroidism occurs equally in both sexes. Acquired hypothyroidism in later childhood is sporadic and is most often associated with Hashimoto's thyroiditis. There is a predilection for females, and a positive family history for thyroid disease or other autoimmune diseases can often be found.

Presenting history

In congenital hypothyroidism, symptoms are subtle; prior to mandatory newborn screening programs, diagnosis was often made in retrospect. The insidious symptoms include docility (these are described as "good" babies), thermal instability with hypothermia, lethargy, poor feeding, constipation, hoarse cry, and poor linear growth after the newborn period. At birth, these infants do not have short length. Slow development and profound mental retardation are the ultimate consequences. Acquired hypothyroidism is also subtle and the most reliable sign is a decrease in linear growth rate. Children tend to be docile and well-behaved, and consequently have above average grades in school. Subtle change in facies due to myxedema, dry skin, or change in bowel habits may be presenting findings.

Physical examination

In congenital hypothyroidism, the physical examination is distinctive once the metabolic changes are florid[5] (Fig. 22.1). Unfortunately, few signs are present at birth.

The skin is cool, dry, and vasoconstricted and often shows a pattern of cutis marmorata, even at average room temperature. A distinctive yellow-tinged translucent pallor (described as alabaster) results from a combination of abnormalities: anemia, prolonged jaundice, carotenemia, and nonpitting dermal infiltration with glycosaminoglycans (acid mucopolysaccharides), primarily hyaluronic acid and chondroitin sulfate. These myxedematous deposits of glycosaminoglycans are most prominent perioribitally and in the lips and tongue, causing macroglossia. There is puffiness of the dorsa of the hands and feet and supraclavicular fossae. General laxity of tissues results in umbilical and occasionally inguinal hernias. The hair is lusterless and brittle and may be relatively hypopigmented or reddish. Nails grow slowly. Tooth eruption is delayed, with possible enamel hypoplasia.

Skeletal abnormalities include normal length at birth but dramatic failure of linear growth with rapid downward crossing of growth percentiles. The distal femoral epiphyses, usually present in full-term neonates, are absent. Long bones show proximal shortening and infantile body proportions with an elevated ratio of upper to lower segment. Maldevelopment of facial bones results in a depressed nasal bridge. All fontanels are large, including a patent metopic suture in the midforehead, and there is delayed closure of

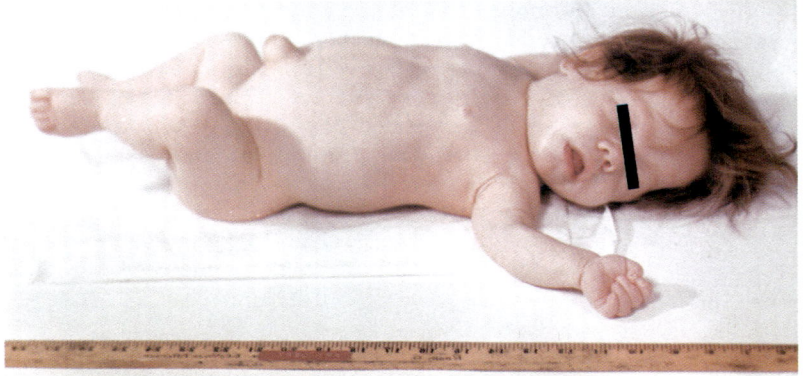

Fig. 22.1 An 8-month-old girl with profound signs and symptoms of congenital hypothyroidism, including short stature, proximal shortening of the extremities, umbilical hernia, macroglossia, depressed nasal bridge, dry lusterless hair, alabaster pallor, and hypotonia. (From Lucky,[1] with permission.)

1. Lucky AW (1985) Congenital hypothyroidism. In: Clinical Dermatology, vol. 2, unit 12–32, Demis DJ, Dobson RL, McGuire J, eds. Hagerstown, MD: Harper & Row, p. 1.
2. Fisher DA, Dussault JH, Foley TP Jr et al. (1979) Screening for congenital hypothyroidism: results of screening one million North American infants. J Pediatr 94:700.
3. Delange F, Illig R, Rochiccioli P, Brock-Jacobsen B (1981) Progress report 1980 on neonatal thyroid screening in Europe. Acta Paediatr Scand 70:1.
4. Burrow GN, Dussault JH (1992) Neonatal Thyroid Screening. New York: Raven Press.
5. Heymann WR (1992) Cutaneous manifestations of thyroid disease. J Am Acad Dermatol 26:885–902.

fontanelles. Head circumference fails to enlarge normally, reflecting poor brain growth.

Gastrointestinal (GI) signs include prolonged jaundice as well as early and often severe carotenemia. Both signs presumably reflect hepatic immaturity. Poor feeding and constipation are progressive and constant symptoms. Cardiovascular features include poor peripheral circulation, bradycardia, and, ultimately, congestive heart failure (CHF), often with pericardial effusion. The neurologic sequelae of congenital hypothyroidism are the most devastating, with profound mental retardation being the ultimate outcome for untreated cases. Prior to screening programs, it was believed that treatment delayed beyond 3 months of age would result in irreversible retardation. Early intervention with thyroid screening has prevented severe developmental delay. However, long-term neuropsychological sequelae in adolescence, such as declines in IQ and poor performance in a variety of skills at school, indicated that pre- and perinatal influences of hypothyroidism may persist.[6] Other neurologic signs include hypotonia, hyporeflexia, and profound delay in the relaxation phase of deep tendon reflexes.

The physical examination of children with acquired hypothyroidism is more subtle. The skin may be cool and dry but rarely shows the ichthyosis-like changes seen in the elderly. Sweating and sebum production are reduced with myxedematous infiltrate of the appendages. There is a yellow pallor due to carotenemia as well as a nonpitting dermal infiltrate with glycosaminoglycans, causing gradual alteration of facial appearance. Prominent features include macroglossia, thickening of the lips, puffy eyes, and general coarsening of features. An enlarged symmetric thyroid gland may be present.

Scalp hair may become sparse, lusterless, and brittle. A distinctive finding is acquired hypertrichosis with coarse dark terminal hairs appearing on the back and upper arms (Fig. 22.2).[7,8] This is not hirsutism, because the hair is not in a secondary sexual distribution. Such hypertrichosis is reversible with treatment. Other findings include profound failure of linear growth with downward crossing of growth percentiles and delayed bone age. Constipation may occur. Obesity is rarely seen in the hypothyroid child, although many obese children are brought to physicians to be evaluated for hypothyroidism. By contrast, obese children tend to be tall, with accelerated growth and bone age.

Other rare syndromes have been reported in association with acquired hypothyroidism in childhood. The Kocher–Debré–Semelaigne syndrome[9,10] consists of muscular pseudohypertrophy of the calves and testicular enlargement. Muscle weakness and tenderness with elevated creatine kinase (CPK) may mimic dermatomyositis.[11] The Van Wyck–Grumbach syndrome[12] represents pseudoprecocious puberty, which is probably a result of simultaneous overproduction of prolaction and gonadotropins as well as thyroid-stimulating hormone (TSH) in profound primary hypothyroidism. The resultant hypersecretion of these pituitary hormones results in precocious thelarche (breast development) associated with galactorrhea and early onset of menses in girls. Hypothyroidism as a result of resistance to TSH is common in pseudohypoparathyroidism (see pseudohypoparathyroidism below). Finally, there has been a single case report of acanthosis nigricans in a 15-year-old obese boy, associated with insulin resistance. Both the insulin resistance and the acanthosis nigricans resolved with thyroid hormone treatment, although there was no significant change in weight.[13] Hypothyroidism can be induced in adults and children by chronic use of povidone-iodine as a topical disinfectant.[14]

Laboratory findings

The diagnosis of primary hypothyroidism is based on low levels of serum thyroxine (T_4) accompanied by high levels of circulating TSH. Low T_4 and/or

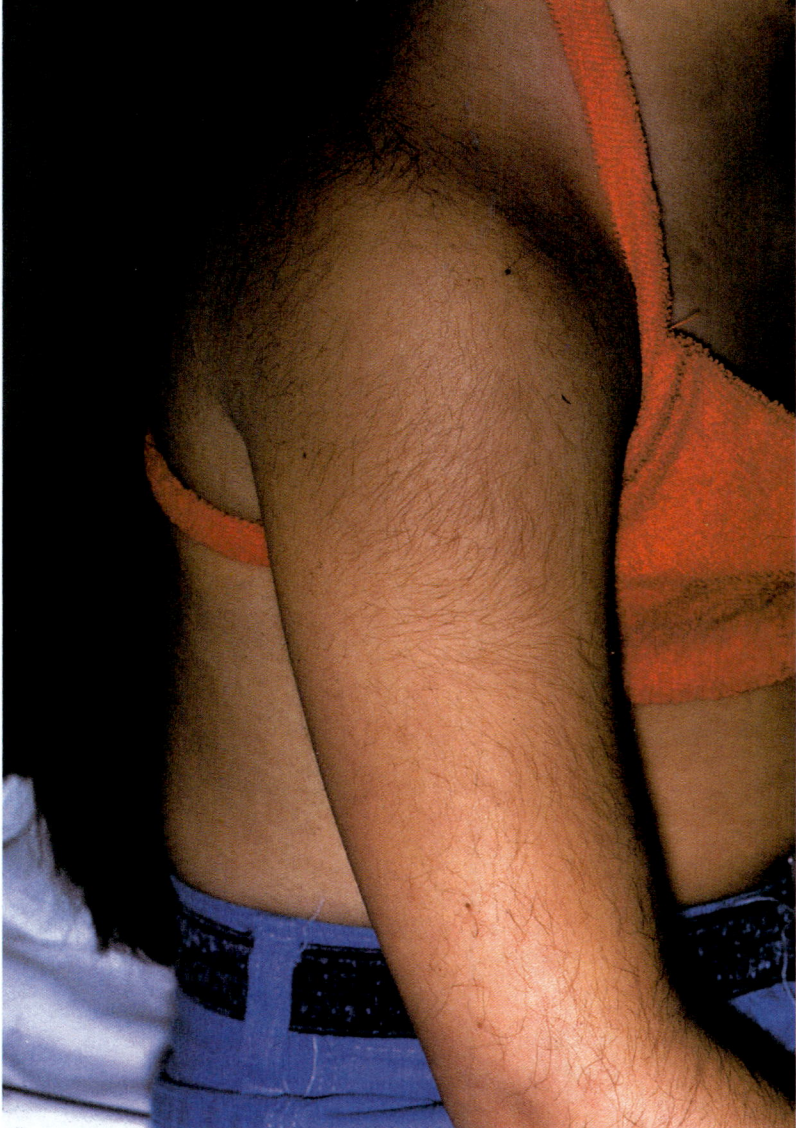

Fig. 22.2 The shoulders of a child with acquired hypothyroidism demonstrating typical acquired hypertrichosis. This hair pattern reverts to normal with therapy.

high TSH can be measured from a few drops of blood collected from a heel stick onto filter paper and eluted for radioimmunoassay (RIA). This is the basis for the newborn screening of congenital hypothyroidism. Because T_4 circulates bound to a large protein, thyroid-binding globulin (TBG), variations in TBG may give false impressions about the functional state of thyroid hormone. For example, in congenital TBG deficiency there will be a low level of total T_4 in a euthyroid state. If available, a measurement of the biologically active free T_4 is preferable. An approximation of this can be provided by measurement of a triiodothyronine (T_3) resin uptake, which measures the available binding sizes on TBG. Direct measurement of T_3 by RIA is not useful in the diagnosis of hypothyroidism. Radionucleotide scans can detect the presence or absence of thyroid tissue. Associated laboratory findings may

6. Rovet, JF (1999) Long-term neuropsychological sequelae of early-treated congenital hypothyroidism: effect in adolescence. **Acta Paediatr Suppl** (432):88–95.
7. Perloff WH (1955) Hirsutism – a manifestation of juvenile hypothyroidism. **JAMA** 157:651.
8. Nishi Y, Hamamoto K, Kajiyama M et al. (1989) Pituitary enlargement, hypertrichosis and blunted growth hormone secretion in primary hypothyroidism. **Acta Paediatr Scand** 78:136.
9. Najjar SS (1974) Muscular hypertrophy in hypothyroid children: the Kocher-Debré-Semelaigne syndrome. A review of 23 cases. **J Pediatr** 85:236.
10. Hopwood NJ, Lockhart LH, Bryan GT (1974) Acquired hypothyroidism with muscular hypertrophy and precocious testicular enlargement. **J Pediatr** 85:233.
11. Newman AJ, Lee C (1980) Hypothyroidism simulating dermatomyositis. **J Pediatr** 97:772.
12. Van Wyck JJ, Grumbach MM (1960) Syndrome of precocious menstruation and galactorrhea in juvenile hypothyroicism: an example of hormonal overlap in pituitary feedback. **J Pediatr** 57:416.
13. Ober KP (1985) Acanthosis nigricans and insulin resistance associated with hypothyroidism. **Arch Dermatol** 121:229.
14. Nobukuni K, Hayakawa N, Namba R et al. (1997) The influence of long-term treatment of povidone-iodine or thyroid function. **Dermatol** 195 (suppl 2):69–72.

include a normochromic normocytic anemia, carotenemia, hypercholesterolemia, triglyceridemia, and prolonged hyperbilirubinemia in the newborn.

Secondary hypothyroidism due to pituitary failure will show a depressed T_4 but normal or low baseline TSH levels. Failure of TSH to respond to thyrotropin-releasing hormone (TRH) may be helpful but is not a constant diagnostic finding.

Pathophysiology and histogenesis

Congenital hypothyroidism occurs most commonly as a sporadic event with thyroid hypoplasia or aplasia (35%), or ectopic (43%) placement such as on the base of the tongue (lingual) or as goitrous hypothyroidism (22%) due to inborn errors of thyroid biosynthesis. Biochemical defects in most of the steps of thyroid hormone biosynthesis and degradation have been described. These inherited inborn errors of thyroid biosynthesis are usually autosomal-recessive. Exogenous causes of hypothyroidism in the newborn also include maternal use of antithyroid drugs such as methimazole (Tapazole) and propylthiouracil (PTU) taken during pregnancy,[15] but this occurs very rarely. In a few mountainous regions isolated from sources of iodine, endemic iodine deficiency goiters and hypothyroidism may still exist. Paradoxically, iodine toxicity due to cutaneous absorption of iodine from skin scrubs has caused goiter and hypothyroidism in newborn infants in intensive care units.[14,16] Peripheral unresponsiveness to TSH or to T_3 and T_4 can also occur. Infiltration of the thyroid gland causing hypothyroidism in some metabolic disorders such as cystinosis[17] and Langerhans cell histiocytosis[18] has been reported. A variety of congenital and acquired hypothalamic and/or pituitary disorders can result in secondary hypothyroidism. Acquired hypothyroidism is usually an end result of autoimmune Hashimoto's thyroiditis or, rarely, Graves' disease.

The most distinctive histologic finding in the skin of patients with hypothyroidism is diffuse infiltration of acid mucopolysaccharides, primarily hyaluronic acid, throughout the dermis and occasionally extending into the subcutaneous fat. There is a predilection for accumulation around appendages such as hair, eccrine, and pilosebaceous units. Specific mucin stains such as toluidine blue, Alcian blue, or colloidal iron are essential for diagnosis of myxedema.[19]

Differential diagnosis

Infants with trisomy 21 (Down syndrome) are also hypotonic with growth retardation and delayed milestones, but they lack the characteristic myxedema and manifestations of low basal metabolism. Older children with trisomy 21 do, however, have a high incidence of Hashimoto's thyroiditis and acquired hypothyroidism, which may be overlooked. Newborns with gonadal dysgenesis (XO Turner syndrome) have short stature and puffy hands and feet due to lymphedema rather than to myxedema. They also have a higher than normal incidence of thyroiditis in later life. Patients with mucopolysaccharidoses, such as Hunter and Hurler syndromes, also have coarse facies and retarded growth and development, but they are distinguished by hepatosplenomegaly and normal thyroid hormone levels. The Weideman–Beckwith syndrome also has profound macroglossia and coarse facies, but these children are large with accelerated rather than retarded growth. They have true omphaloceles rather than simple umbilical hernias. Achondroplasia, hypochondroplasia, and other forms of rhizomelic dwarfism with short proximal extremities may mimic the skeletal features of congenital hypothyroidism, but the laboratory studies of thyroid hormone function are normal.

Therapy

Treatment of hypothyroidism requires adequate replacement with thyroid hormone, preferably synthetic L-thyroxine. Fortunately, in the United States, newborn screening for hypothyroidism has virtually eliminated undiagnosed disease in that country. However, in many parts of the world congenital hypothyroidism is still a problem. Newborns with profound hypothyroidism may need to be hospitalized. Under an endocrinologist's care, dosage can be adjusted to achieve normal T_4, TSH, and proper growth rate. All secondary manifestations of hypothyroidism respond to thyroid hormone replacement. If treatment is prescribed early, prevention of profound mental retardation may be achieved. However, more subtle neuropsychologic disorders may persist.[6] Treatment should begin slowly to avoid high-output cardiovascular failure. Gross overtreatment may cause rapid advancement of linear growth with early epiphyseal fusion, CHF, and craniosynostosis in infancy. However, lack of adequate T_4 levels in the upper range of normal may cause intellectual impairment.

Pediatric aspects

Children with acquired hypothyroidism tend to be docile and well-mannered and consequently achieve excellent grades in school. Parents should be forewarned that with replacement therapy their children will become more appropriately active for their ages and consequently may have a decline in their apparent school performance. This is not a reflection of intellectual ability but rather of the way in which school grades are often given.

HYPERTHYROIDISM

Hyperthyroidism or in its advanced state, thyrotoxicosis, is most often caused by autoimmune thyroid disease, either chronic lymphocytic thyroiditis (Hashimoto's thyroiditis) or Graves' disease. Females are affected significantly more often than males, in a 5:1 ratio. All ages can be affected, including newborns who may receive transplacentally transmitted antibodies from a thyrotoxic mother with Graves' disease. There are familial clusters of autoimmune thyroid disease in association with such disorders as Addison's disease, diabetes, pernicious anemia, alopecia areata, and vitiligo (see Autoimmune polyglandular disease section). Multinodular goiter with hyperthyroidism may also be found in McCune–Albright Syndrome.[19,20]

Presenting history

Early signs of hyperthyroidism are subtle; in retrospect, it is often behavioral changes with poor school performance due to a short attention span, insomnia, emotional lability, and nervousness that are first noted. Heat intolerance, increased appetite with weight loss, diarrhea or a change in bowel habits, and tremor are frequent symptoms.

Physical examination

An enlarged thyroid gland (goiter) is present in almost all cases.[5] General cutaneous features of thyrotoxicosis include warmth, increased sweating, flushing, and a very smooth velvety texture to the skin. Heat will radiate from the outstretched palms and can be felt without touching the patient. A few case reports have documented diffuse brown hyperpigmentation of unknown etiology, but this is rare. Patients may complain of generalized pruritus, and urticaria has been reported. Three specific findings are characteristic of Graves' disease: ophthalmopathy, pretibial myxedema (PTM), and thyroid acropachy. All three may occur when the patient is hyper-, hypo-, or euthyroid.

Thyroid ophthalmopathy is milder and rarer in children than in adults, occurring in 0.1 in 100 000 young children and 3.0 in 100 000 adolescents.[21] It is a result of infiltration of glycosaminoglycans and lymphocytes in the orbit and extraocular muscles. Infiltration of extraocular muscles results in ocular paralysis, especially inward gaze. Unilateral or bilateral proptosis results from

15. Refetoff S, Ochi Y, Selenkow HA, Rosenfield RL (1975) Neonatal hypothyroidism and goiter in one infant in each of two sets of twins due to maternal therapy with anti-thyroid drugs. **J Pediatr** 87:958.

16. Chabrolle JP, Rossier A (1978) Goitre and hypothyroidism in the newborn after cutaneous absorption of iodine. **Arch Dis Child** 53:495.

17. Lucky AW, Howley PM, Megyesi K et al. (1977) Endocrine studies in cystinosis: compensated primary hypothyroidism. **J Pediatr** 91:204.

18. Braunstein GD, Kohler PD (1981) Endocrine manifestations of histiocytosis. **Am J Pediatr Hematol Oncol** 3:67.

19. Heymann WR (1997) Advances in the cutaneous manifestations of thyroid disease. **Inter J Dermatol** 36:641–645.

20. Isotani H, Sanda K, Kameoka K, Takamatsu J (2000) McCune-Albright syndrome associated with non-autoimmune type of hyperthyroidism with development of thyrotoxic crisis. **Horm Res** 53:256–259.

21. Gruters A (1999) Ocular manifestations in children and adolescents with thyrotoxicisis. **Exp Clin Endocrinol Diabetes** 107 (Suppl) 15:S172–S174.

accumulations of glycosaminoglycans within the orbit and can be threatening to eyesight. Lid lag results from tonic spasm of the upper lid and can also be seen with chemical hyperthyroidism as well as Graves' disease.

PTM is a localized accumulation of acid mycopolysaccharides, specifically hyaluronic acid, usually on the anterior tibia.[19] Rarely, lesions have been reported on the back of the lower legs, arms, and trunk. PTM is rare in children but may be seen in adolescents. Lesions are small localized nodules or diffuse plaques that are cool, nontender, nonpitting, and sometimes pruritic. Borders are well defined. The surface has dilated follicular orifices with coarse hairs and has been described as peau d'orange (orange peel) in appearance. The color may vary from brown to red to waxy yellow. A rare hypertrophic form of PTM in which the skin is folded exuberantly and extends out to the dorsa of the feet has also been reported.

The last of the triad, thyroid acropachy,[5] is rarely reported in a child. Distal extremities are thickened and soft tissues as well as bone become enlarged. There is associated clubbing of the nails. Radiographic findings of lacy periosteal new bone formation are characteristic.

Hair characteristically becomes fine, limp, oily, and unable to hold a curl in hyperthyroidism. There may be diffuse scalp hair thinning. Nails characteristically show distal onycholysis, especially of the fourth finger (Plummer's nail). Other physical findings include tachycardia, tendency to arrhythmia such as atrial fibrillation, mitral valve prolapse, and high-output CHF.[22] Diarrhea may be significant. Neurologic findings include hyperactivity of the sympathetic nervous system with tremor, accentuated deep tendon reflexes, and emotional lability with unpredictable behavior.

Laboratory findings

Elevated levels of free T_4 are diagnostic. False elevations of total T_4 may be seen with states of excess TBG such as are induced with oral contraceptives. Free T_4, if available, is a better measurement. If T_4 is normal in the face of suspected hyperthyroidism, T_3 may be elevated in so-called T_3 toxicosis. TSH is low or undetectable and fails to respond to TRH stimulation or exogenous T_3 suppression. Iodine-131 radionucleotide scans will reveal either a diffusely enlarged thyroid gland or a single overactive nodule.

Pathophysiology and pathogenesis

Graves' disease has been associated with the presence of anti-thyroid antibodies which have a stimulatory effect on thyroid membranes in inducing adenylate cyclase. Histologically, there is lymphocytic infiltration of the thyroid gland and, ultimately, destruction of thyroid tissue. Chronic lymphocytic thyroiditis (Hashimoto's disease) is very similar and many authors consider it on the same spectrum as Graves' disease. The most prominent cutaneous feature of Graves' disease, PTM, represents localized accumulation of hyaluronic acid in the dermis of the anterior lower legs. Similar pathophysiology involves hyaluronic acid deposits around the orbit in thyroid ophthalmopathy. Histologically, PTM shows hyaluronic acid deposits primarily in the mid-dermis without atrophy of the appendages, in contrast to the infiltrative myxedema of hypothyroidism. The exact mechanism of induction of PTM with its propensity for the shins has been studied but is not well understood. The general manifestations of thyrotoxicosis, such as warmth, smoothness of skin, tremor, and sweating, are independent of immune status and reflect the thyrotoxic state, which could also be induced by exogenous thyroid hormone.

Differential diagnosis

The thyrotoxic child may be thought to have a psychiatric or emotional disturbance. PTM could be confused with cellulitis or erythema nodosum although the lack of tenderness and heat and infiltrative appearance are quite distinctive. Lichen myxedematosis (scleromyxedema) and lichen amyloidosis can also present with pretibial plaques, but these characteristically occur in older persons. Thyroid acropachy may be mistaken for acromegaly or clubbing from pulmonary etiology. Graves' disease is seen in frequent association with such disorders as diabetes mellitus, systemic lupus erythematosus (SLE), rheumatoid arthritis, myasthenia gravis, idiopathic thrombocytopenic purpura, pernicious anemia, Addison's disease, vitiligo, and alopecia areata. It is also more common in Down syndrome and Turner syndrome.

Therapy and prognosis

Graves' disease in childhood has been recently reviewed.[23] Thyrotoxicosis secondary to Graves' disease usually responds to the antithyroid drugs methimazole (Tapazole) and propylthiouracil (PTU). Agranulocytosis is the most severe potential adverse reaction to PTU. Cutaneous adverse reactions to these drugs, especially PTU, are quite common and include both a diffuse papular urticarial eruption as well as leukocytoclastic vasculitis. Iodine has been used to block the thyrotoxic gland prior to subtotal thyroidectomy. Its side effects include a diffuse pruritic papular eruption and a classical pustular iododerma. β-blockers are useful prior to surgery but have their own adverse effects on the skin, such as maculopapular rash and reversible alopecia. Although thyrotoxicosis can usually be brought under control medically, surgery is often considered the treatment of choice because of problems with compliance with long-term medication. Postoperatively, patients may remain hyperthyroid or become hypothyroid or euthyroid. The use of radioactive iodine in children is becoming more accepted.[23] With any form of therapy for Graves' disease, the patient may be left with lifelong problems, including possible hypothyroidism, recurrent hyperthyroidism, PTM, ophthalmopathy, or acropachy.

There is no good specific therapy for PTM, although systemic steroids, adrenocorticotropic hormone (ACTH), intralesional steroids, and high-potency topical steroids have been tried.[24] Skin grafting and excision of lesions is not successful.[25] Plasmapheresis has been tried in severe cases of crippling ophthalmopathy and PTM in experimental circumstances.[26]

Pediatric aspects

One of the primary manifestations of hyperthyroidism is a change in personality, including poor school performance due to short attention span, emotional lability, and unpredictable behavior. Gradually, this will improve with return to the euthyroid state.

GROWTH HORMONE DISORDERS

GROWTH HORMONE DEFICIENCY

Primary pituitary insufficiency of growth hormone (idiopathic hypopituitarism) is rare, occurring in approximately 1 in 60 000 births.[27] Infants may present with hypoglycemia and, after the second year of life, growth failure. The cutaneous manifestations of growth hormone deficiency are subtle and include fine smooth skin. The dermis is thinner, stiffer, and less elastic.[28] There is infantile fat distribution. Hair is spare and fine, and nails grow slowly. Sebum production is low. An unusual defect reflecting the midline origin of the pituitary gland is the presence of a single central upper incisor[29] in association with growth hormone deficiency (Fig. 22.3). Micropenis probably due to concomitant gonadotropin deficiency is common in males.

Although primary idiopathic hypopituitarism is the most common cause of growth hormone deficiency, other disorders, such as tumors (especially craniopharyngioma), Hand–Schüller–Christian variant of Langerhans cell

22. Lester LA, Sodt PC, Rich BH et al. (1982) Cardiac abnormalities in children with hyperthyroidism. **Pediatr Cardiol** 2:213.
23. Kraiem Z (2001) Graves' disease in childhood. **J Pediatr Endocrinol Metab** 14(3):229–243.
24. Lang PG, Sisson JC, Lynch PJ (1975) Intralesional triamcinolone therapy for pretibial myxedema. **Arch Dermatol** 111:197.
25. Kucer KA, Luscombe HA, Kauh YC (1980) Pretibial myxedema: recurrence after skin grafting. **Arch Dermatol** 116:1076.
26. Dandona P, Marshall NJ, Bidey SP et al. (1979) Successful treatment of exophthalmos and pretibial myxedema with plasmapheresis. **BMJ** 1:374.
27. Kaplan SA (1982) Growth and growth hormone: disorders of the anterior pituitary. In: Clinical Pediatric and Adolescent Endocrinology, Kaplan SA, ed. Philadelphia: WB Saunders, p. 1.
28. Conte F, Diridollou S, Jouret B et al. (2000) Evaluation of cutaneous modifications in seventy-seven growth hormone-deficient children. **Horm Res** 54:92–97.
29. Rappaport EB, Ulstrom RA, Gorlin RJ et al. (1977) Solitary maxillary central incisor and short stature. **J Pediatr** 91:924.

After epiphyseal closure, the bony, soft tissue, and metabolic changes of acromegaly predominate. There is no hereditary pattern associated with growth hormone excess in childhood. The major manifestation of growth hormone excess before epiphyseal closure is rapid linear growth without concomitant advancement in bone age. Hands and feet enlarge, and facial features coarsen. Puffiness of the eyelids has been reported. Shifts in teeth require dental therapy. Children may complain of headache and visual disturbances, or exhibit change in behavior. The changes of acromegaly are insidious and are more apparent in adulthood than in childhood. There is profound overgrowth of soft tissues of the hands, feet, face, and the tip of the nose. Shoe and glove size slowly increase. Although the acromegalic individual may be tall and heavy, he or she may manifest incoordination, muscle weakness, and joint disturbance. The mandible and supraorbital ridges become prominent. Redundant skin on the scalp and forehead result in cutis verticis gyrata. There may be marked hypertrichosis and hyperpigmentation sometimes accompanied by acanthosis nigricans.

Laboratory diagnosis is made by elevated levels of circulating growth hormone and abnormal response of growth hormone to glucose tolerance tests and other provocative tests. Pituitary eosinophilic or chromophobe adenomas are the cause of growth hormone excess and the preferred therapy is surgical ablation via a transsphenoidal hypophysectomy. In recalcitrant cases, bromergocryptine may be useful as a medical therapy.

GONADAL DYSGENESIS

In 1938, Turner[40] described seven girls with short stature, absent secondary sexual characteristics, and a distinctive body habitus and physical features. These girls were eventually found to have primary ovarian failure and possessed only fibrous streaks instead of gonads. Ullrich had previously described a similar case.[41] Now a variety of chromosomal abnormalities involving an absent or aberrant X chromosome have been described as gonadal dysgenesis, Turner syndrome, or Ullrich–Turner syndrome.

Epidemiology
Patients with gonadal dysgenesis are phenotypic females with either a missing X chromosome (45 XO) or some abnormality of one of the X chromosomes. The occurrence is sporadic and believed to be secondary to nondisjunction during fertilization. Gonadal dysgenesis is estimated to occur in 1 in 2000 to 1 in 5000 live births, but it is believed that more than 99% of conceptuses with this karyotype are spontaneously aborted.[42] There is no increased risk to a family for a recurrence.

Presenting history
Gonadal dysgenesis becomes apparent in two stages of life. First, in the newborn period, an astute clinician will pick up physical findings including lymphedema of the extremities and webbed neck with redundant skin (pterygium colli) and will be suspicious of the disorder. Most cases, however, are discovered around puberty because of short stature, delayed secondary sexual development, and primary amenorrhea.

Physical examination
In the newborn child with gonadal dysgenesis, there is distinctive, transient, nonpitting lymphedema of the dorsa of the hands and feet. Deep folds of skin on the scalp and forehead resembling cutis verticis gyrata may be a result of

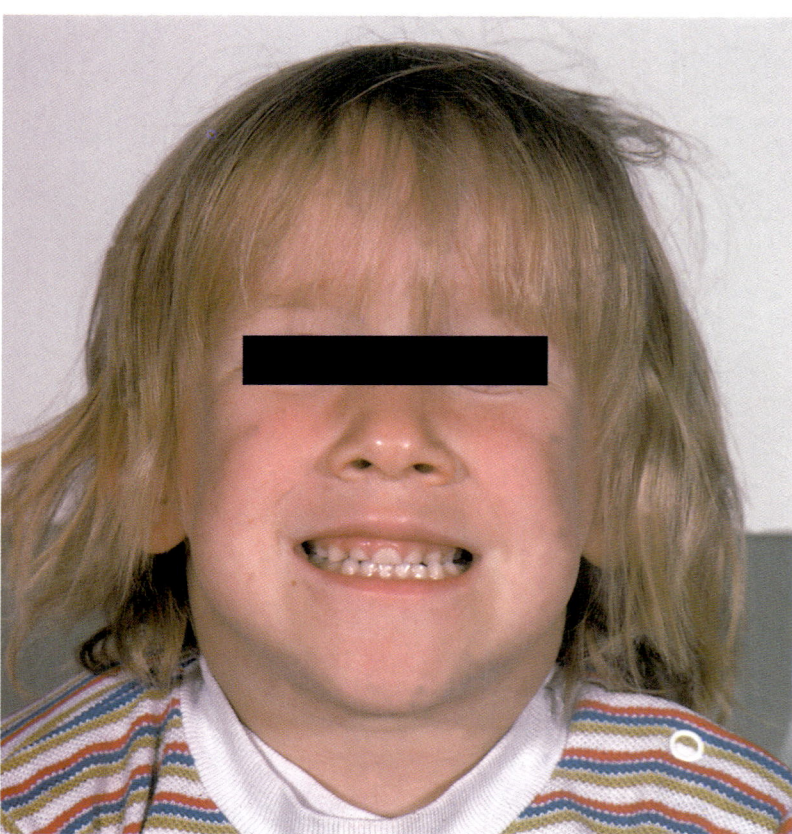

Fig. 22.3 A single, central upper incisor in a body with growth hormone deficiency reflects a basic midline defect affecting the pituitary as well as embryonal tooth development.

histiocytosis, vascular malformations, trauma, and, rarely, inflammatory diseases such as sarcoidosis and histoplasmosis, can cause later-onset growth hormone deficiency. A rare syndrome of peripheral resistance to growth hormone has also been reported.[30]

Therapy with human growth hormone (HGH) has been the treatment of choice. However, the occurrence of Creutzfeldt–Jakob disease in recipients of HGH[31–33] has made synthetic growth hormone, manufactured using recombinant DNA techniques, the only treatment available today.[34] Therapy with recombinant human growth hormone (RHG) has been shown to improve the thickness of the dermis, but not the stiffness or inelasticity.[28] However, concern for a stimulatory effect of growth hormone on the size of melanocytic nevi and the production of nonmalignant atypical changes has been raised.[35] Other investigators[36,37] have found no change in nevus counts or density in large longitudinal studies of HGH-treated patients.

GROWTH HORMONE EXCESS (GIGANTISM AND ACROMEGALY)

Growth hormone excess is rare in childhood.[38,39] When it occurs before epiphyseal closure, there is excessive linear growth, producing gigantism.[39]

30. Laron Z (1974) Syndrome of familial dwarfism and high plasma immunoreactive growth hormone. Isr J Med Sci 10:1247.
31. Brown P, Gajdusek DC, Gibbs CJ, Asher DM (1985) Potential epidemic of Creutzfeldt-Jakob disease from human growth hormone therapy. N Engl J Med 313:728.
32. Koch TK, Berg BO, DeArmond SJ, Gravina RF (1985) Creutzfeldt-Jakob disease in a young adult with idiopathic hypopituitarism. N Engl J Med 313:731.
33. Gibbs CJ, Joy A, Heffner R et al. (1985) Clinical and pathological features and laboratory confirmation of Creutzfeldt-Jakob disease in a recipient of pituitary-derived human growth hormone. N Engl J Med 313:734.
34. Saenger P (2000) A lifetime of growth hormone deficiency: a US pediatric perspective. J Pediatr Endocrinol Metab 13 (Suppl 6):1337–1342.
35. Pierard GE, Pierard-Franchimont C, Nikkels A et al. (1996) Naevocyte triggering by recombinant human growth hormone. J Pathol 180:74–79.
36. Zvulunov A, Wyatt DT, Laud PW, Esterly NB (1997) Lack of effect of growth hormone therapy on the count and density of melanocytic naevi in children. Br J Dermatol 137:545–548.
37. Wyatt D (1999) Melanocytic nevi in children treated with growth hormone. Pediatrics 104(4):1045–1050.
38. Eugster EA, Pescovitz OH (1999) Gigantism. J Clin Endocrinol Metab 84(12):4379–4384.
39. Cohen MM Jr (1999) Overgrowth syndromes: an update. Adv Pediatr 46:441–491.
40. Turner HH (1938) A syndrome of infantilism, congenital webbed neck and cubitus valgus. Endocrinol 23:566.
41. Ullrich O (1949) Turner's syndrome and status Bonneville-Ullrich. Am J Hum Genet 1:179.
42. Lippe BM (1982) Primary ovarian failure. In: Clinical Pediatrics and Adolescent Endocrinology, Kaplan SA, ed. Philadelphia: WB Saunders, p. 269.

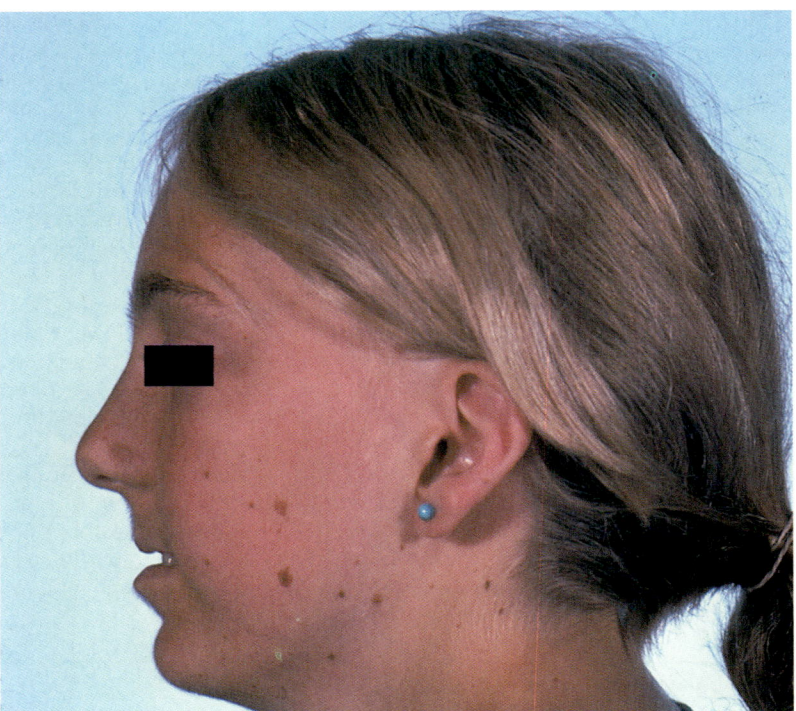

Fig. 22.4 Low-set hairline typical of gonadal dysgenesis.

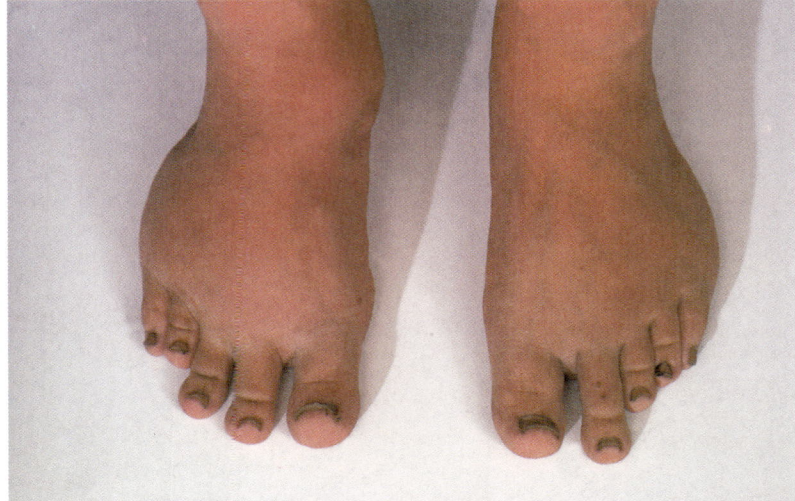

Fig. 22.5 Hypoplastic hyperconvex toenails and hypoplasia of the fourth and fifth metatarsals in a girl with gonadal dysgenesis.

in utero lymphedema in these locations.[43,44] Severe nail hypoplasia may be pathognomonic in the neonate. A few cases have been reported with hemangiomas as well.[45] There may be a webbed neck or perhaps only redundant skin at the nape of the neck which, in fetal life, represented a large lymphangioma.[46,47] Children with Turner syndrome have a distinctive triangular-shaped face with micrognathia. There is an antimongoloid slant to the eyes and ptosis. There is a low-set W-shaped hairline (Fig. 22.4), a downward turned mouth, and a narrow, high-arched ogival (omega-shaped) palate with broad ridges of gum. Eyelashes tend to be quite thick and appear to be in a double row. The nails have a distinctive shape and are nearly pathognomonic of gonadal dysgenesis, being thin but markedly hyperconvex (Fig. 22.5). There may be nail hypoplasia in association with bony hypoplasia of the fourth and sometimes fifth metacarpals and metatarsals.

In later childhood, all patients exhibit short stature with ultimate height rarely reaching 5 feet. At puberty, recurrent problems with peripheral lymphedema and occasional intestinal lymphangiectasia may occur. Patients appear to have a high tendency to keloidal scar formation. Although estrogen is low because of absence of functioning ovarian tissue, adrenal androgens are present and pubic and axillary hair may be present in the absence of other manifestations of normal pubertal development. Thus there is usually primary amenorrhea with failure to develop full secondary sexual characteristics. Psoriasis (17 vs 1.6%), blue sclerae (29 vs 1.4%) vitiligo (6 vs 0.3%) and alopecia areata (3 vs 0.3%) were found in greater frequency in 35 girls with gonadal dysgenesis compared to controls.[48]

Other abnormalities include skeletal deformities, left-sided heart disease (especially coarctation of the aorta, which may result in overdevelopment of the upper trunk in comparison to the lower extremities), reduced femoral pulses, and structural renal abnormalities such as horseshoe kidney.

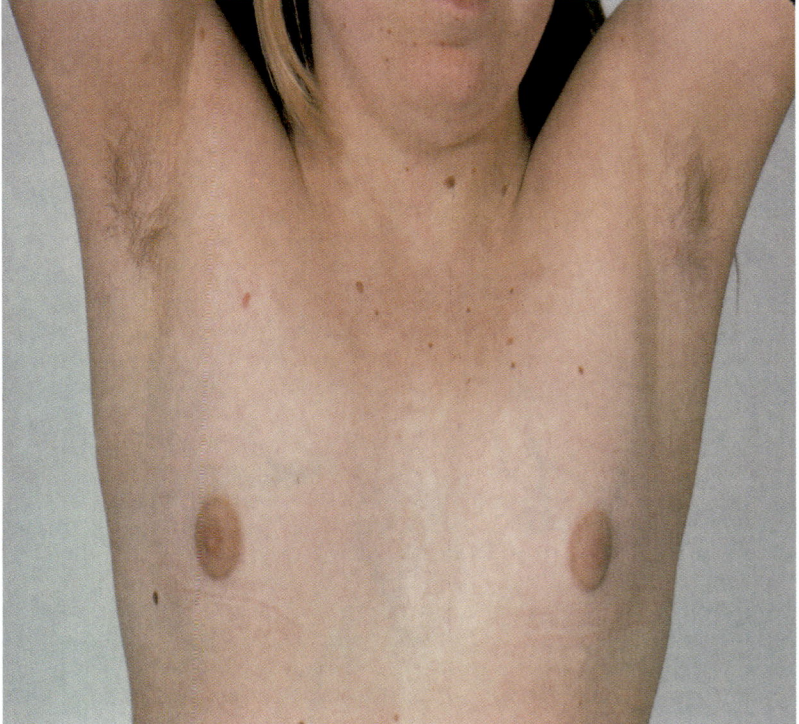

Fig. 22.6 Multiple acquired nevi in a girl with gonadal dysgenesis.

A large number of dark brown nevi are seen compared to the general population (Fig. 22.6 and Table 22.1). Interestingly, there are fewer than expected reported cases of melanoma, considering the larger number of nevi ($50/m^2$ vs $24/m^2$) in this population.[49–51]

43. Marinoni LP, Tangiguchi K, Giraldi S et al. (1999) Cutis verticis gyrata in a child with Turner syndrome. **Pediatr Dermatol** 16:242–243.
44. Larralde M, Gardner SS, Torrado M et al. (1998) Lymphedema as a postulated cause of cutis verticis gyrata in Turner syndrome. **Pediatr Dermatol** 15:18–22.
45. Paller AS, Esterly NB, Charrow J, Cahan FM (1983) Pedal hemangiomas in Turner's syndrome. **J Pediatr** 103:87.
46. Singh RF, Carr DH (1966) The anatomy and histology of XO human embryos and fetuses. **Anat Rec** 115:369.
47. Van der Putte SCJ (1977) Lymphatic malformation in human fetuses. A study of fetuses with Turner's syndrome or status Bonneville-Ullrich. **Virchows Arch** 376:233.
48. Dacou-Voutetakis C, Kakourou T (1996) Psoriasis and blue sclerae in girls with Turner syndrome. **J Am Acad Dermatol** 35(6):1002–1004.
49. Becker B, Jospe N, Goldsmith LA (1994) Melanocytic nevi in Turner syndrome. **Pediatr Dermatol** 11(2):120–124.
50. Zvulunov A, Wyatt DT, Laud PW, Esterly NB (1998) Influence of genetic and environmental factors on melanocytic nevi: a lesson from Turner's syndrome. **Br J Dermatol** 138:993–997.
51. Gibbs P, Brady B, Gonzalez R, Robinson A (2001) Nevi and melanoma: Lessons from Turner's Syndrome. **Dermatol** 202:1–3.

TABLE 22.1 Physical findings in gonadal dysgenesis

Lymphatic malformation of nape of neck *in utero*
Pterygium colli (webbed nack)
Triangular-shaped face
Rotated ears
Antimongoloid slant of eyes
Ptosis
Double row of eyelashes
High-arched (ogival) palate
W-shaped low-set posterior hairline
Puffy hands and feet
Wide carrying angle of arms
Hyperconvex, hypoplastic nails
Hypoplasia of fourth and fifth metacarpals and metatarsals
Keloids
Multiple nevocellular nevi
Shield-shaped chest
Short stature
Delayed puberty with primary amenorrhea

Laboratory findings

Diagnosis can be made on a chromosomal determination showing a missing X chromosome (45 XO) or one of a variety of X chromosome mosaicisms. The occasional presence of a Y chromosome should alert the clinician to look for a higher risk of malignant transformation of the gonadal tissue. A buccal smear is not a reliable test in the neonatal period. In infancy, up to 1 year of age, and again at puberty, there is a characteristic highly elevated level of follicle-stimulating hormone (FSH), reflecting the absence of gonadal development.

Pathophysiology and histogenesis

The absence or malfunction of an X chromosome has innumerable profound effects on normal development. From a cutaneous perspective, there is a failure of normal lymphatic development and, thus, the resulting webbed neck or pterygium colli in infancy and postpubertal lymphedema.[44,45]

Differential diagnosis

The most difficult differential diagnosis is between gonadal dysgenesis and Noonan syndrome.[48] Patients with Noonan syndrome have an identical phenotype to those with gonadal dysgenesis but have normal female (XX) or male (XY) karyotype. Noonan syndrome may be inherited as an autosomal–dominant trait and a mutation has been located.[49] Many of the cutaneous features, including facial shape, nails, nevi, and lymphedema, are identical to those seen in gonadal dysgenesis, although short stature and infertility are not constant features. Interestingly, cardiac disease in these children tends to be pulmonic stenosis rather than the coarctation of the aorta seen in gonadal dysgenesis. In the newborn period, infants with Down syndrome and congenital hypothyroidism may appear somewhat similar to those with gonadal dysgenesis. Slow growth rate may raise the question of growth hormone deficiency or pituitary dysfunction in later childhood. All short girls with primary amenorrhea should be suspected of having gonadal dysgenesis.

Therapy and prognosis

Female hormone (estrogen) replacement therapy at an appropriate age during adolescence is essential for normal maturation. However, because these children have extreme short stature, a variety of treatments, including low-dose estrogen, low-dose androgen, and, most recently, growth hormone, have been tried to maximize linear growth since, untreated, most of these children do not achieve 5 feet in stature.

There is a high incidence of Hashimoto's thyroiditis associated with gonadal dysgenesis. Because these patients are already short, growth failure may not be picked up as readily. Periodic examination of the thyroid gland and blood studies of thyroid hormone, TSH, and/or thyroid antibodies may be indicated.

Pediatric aspects

Girls with gonadal dysgenesis need counseling about their absent secondary sexual characteristics, hormone replacement therapy, and infertility. Although they are not mentally retarded, these children are often socially immature. Some psychologists believe there are specific visuomotor learning disabilities unique to gonadal dysgenesis.

ADRENAL DISORDERS

The adrenal cortex produces three major classes of hormones: glucocorticoids, mineralocorticoids, and androgens. Excesses or deficiencies of glucocorticoids and androgens may have profound cutaneous manifestations. Adrenal steroid hormone biosynthesis is under the control of pituitary ACTH, which in turn is controlled by hypothalamic corticotropin-releasing hormone (CRH). In order to evaluate the impact of the adrenal on the skin, primary adrenocortical insufficiency, adrenocortical excess, and adrenal androgen excess are discussed separately.

ADRENOCORTICAL INSUFFICIENCY

Adrenocortical insufficiency, also known as hypoadrenalism or Addison's disease, is rare but does occur in children and adolescents.[51] It is often undiagnosed for long periods of time.

Epidemiology

Primary Addison's disease is seen in Western countries at a rate of approximately 120 per million.[52] Both sexes are affected equally. Addison's disease may appear at any age.

Presenting history

Insidious onset of weakness, lethargy, and apathy, which may be interpreted as psychiatric or emotional disturbance, is the earliest sign of primary adreno-cortical insufficiency. Patients often deny feeling ill and may not note how poorly they are feeling until after therapy has been initiated. Abdominal pain is common in children with Addison's disease. Vomiting, diarrhea, salt craving, headache, sweating, and behavior changes occur later. Eventually, most patients note gradually increasing hyperpigmentation or failure to lose a summer suntan. They often do not seek medical attention unless they present in acute hypocortisolemic crisis.

Physical examination

The skin of the patient with primary adrenal insufficiency shows diffuse brown hyperpigmentation as the hallmark of this disease (Fig. 22.7). There is prominent darkening of the areolae, scrotum, labia, pre-existent nevi, palmar and plantar creases, and scars. Pigmentation of the linea alba (changing it to a linea nigra) may appear on the lower abdomen. Ironically, in the face of generalized hyperpigmentation, there is also a strong association of vitiligo with Addison's disease.

In postpubertal patients, public and axillary hair becomes sparse. Some patients will also complain of loss of scalp hair. Hyperpigmented, longitudinal streaks may appear on the nails (Fig. 22.8). Blue–black pigment deposits can be seen in the gums, along the tooth margins, and on the hard palate. Associated findings include a wan and weak appearance and a narrow cardiac silhouette on chest radiography. Blood pressure tends to be quite low.

52. Ten S, New M, Maclaren N (2001) Clinical Review 130: Addison's disease 2001. J Clin Endocrinol Metab 86(7):2909–2922.

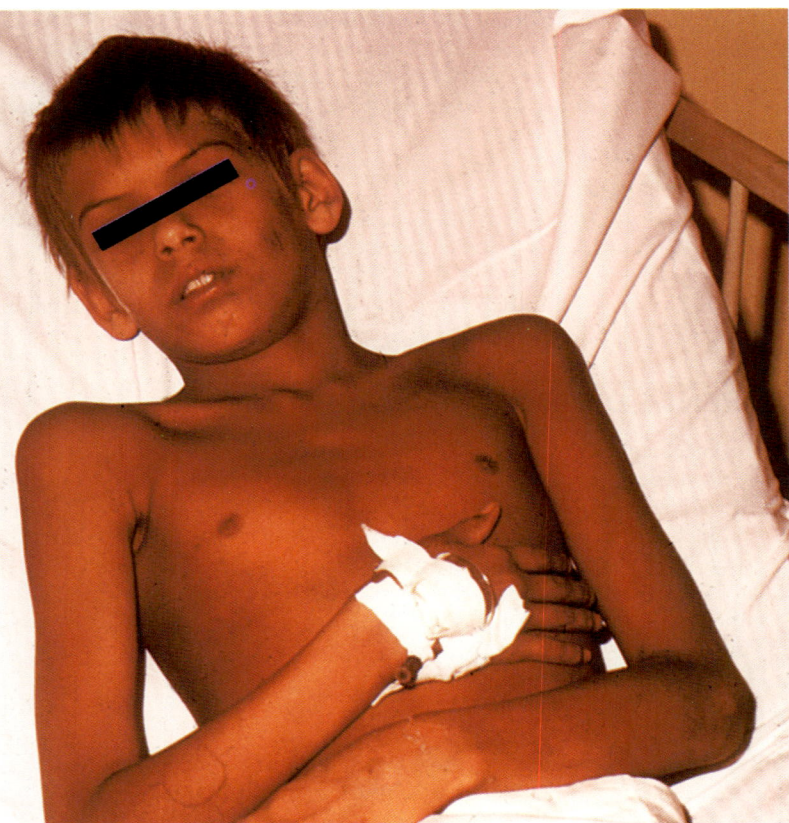

Fig. 22.7 Diffuse hyperpigmentation, which persisted into autumn months, in a 11-year-old boy with Addison's disease.

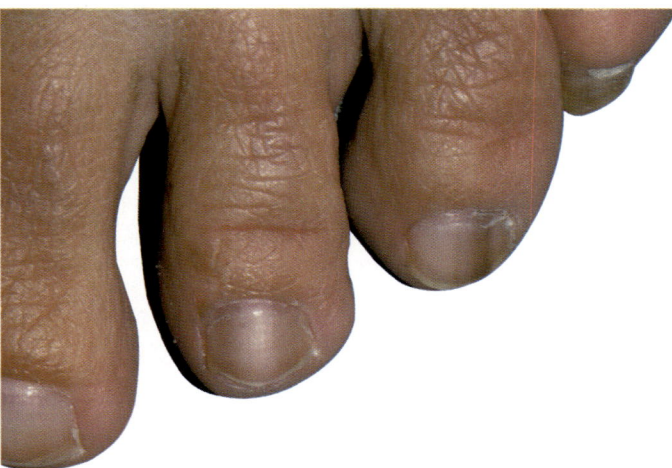

Fig. 22.8 Pigmented linear streaks appeared on the nails of this young lady with primary idiopathic adrenal failure. She sought medical attention for her darkening complexion.

Laboratory findings

Low or absent cortisol can be diagnosed by plasma samples or by 24-hour collections of urine for 17-hydroxysteroids or urinary-free cortisol. The best diagnostic test for primary adrenal insufficiency is the failure of adrenal cortisol levels to rise in response to im or iv ACTH stimulation. If available, direct RIA of ACTH will reveal high levels. Metabolic abnormalities include low sodium and high potassium with hypoglycemia. Secondary pituitary hypothalamic ACTH insufficiency can be diagnosed by failure of the adrenal to produce 11-deoxycortisol (compound S) during a metyrapone test. Such patients retain normal mineralocorticoid function and do not have pigmentary abnormalities.

Pathophysiology and histogenesis

The causes of adrenocorticoid hypofunction have recently been summarized (Table 22.2).[52] In those disorders in which there is primary destruction or unresponsiveness of the adrenal gland, there will be consequent high levels of ACTH to produce cutaneous hyperpigmentation. It remains unclear whether this hyperpigmentation is secondary to an effect of the elevated levels of ACTH or to simultaneous overproduction of melanocyte-stimulating hormone (MSH). It is also possible that there is elevation of another peptide derived from prepro-opiomelanocortin, the large precursor hormone for many of the neuroactive peptides, including ACTH and MSH.

Differential diagnosis

In childhood, presenting complaints may most closely mimic inflammatory bowel disease. Likewise, emotional and/or psychiatric disorders may be suspected in the patient with Addison's disease until adrenal crisis occurs. The diffuse and progressive hyperpigmentation, however, should distinguish Addison's disease.

Therapy

With replacement of physiologic levels of glucocorticosteroids, there is rapid reversal of all symptoms, including hyperpigmentation. Prognosis is excellent if appropriate therapy is maintained and increased to cover periods of stress, such as surgery or major illness (Table 22.3).[53,54] Patients diagnosed with adrenal insufficiency with positive anti-adrenal antibodies should be followed prospectively for the detection and treatment of other manifestations of polyglandular immune syndromes.

ADRENOCORTICAL EXCESS

The term Cushing disease is applied to endogenous overproduction of adrenocortical glucocorticoids, specifically cortisol, in reaction to stimulation from

TABLE 22.2 Causes of hypoadrenalism
Adrenal dysgenesis/hypoplasia
Mutations in nuclear hormone receptor genes
Congenital adrenal hypoplasia
Familial glucocorticoid deficiency (unresponsiveness to ACTH)
Adrenal destruction
Autoimmune Addison's disease (APS-1 and APS-2)
Adrenal leukodystrophy (males)
Infections (TB, histoplasmosis, coccidiomycosis)
Adrenal hemorrhage
Meningococcus (Waterhouse–Fredrickson)
Neonatal sepsis (pseudomonas)
Impaired steroidogenesis
Cholesterol biosynthesis
A betalipoproteinemia
Smith–Lemli–Opitz syndrome
Steroid Biosynthesis
Congenital adrenal hyperplasias
Mitochondrial disorders
Drugs

Modified from Ten et al.[52]

53. Lucky AW (1984) Principles of the use of glucocorticosteroids in the growing child. **Pediatr Dermatol** 1:226.

54. Axelrod L (1976) Glucocorticoid therapy. **Medicine** (Baltimore) 55:39.

TABLE 22.3   Stress doses of glucocorticoids

Moderate stress or illness
    Double or triple oral maintenance
    Prednisone 10–15mg/m²/day
    Hydrocortisone 50–75mg/m²/day

If unable to take oral medication
    Hydrocortisone 75mg/m² im and cortisone acetate 75mg/m² im at least
      every other day

Severe stress or shock
    Hydrocortisone 50mg/m² im or iv STAT and then every 6 hours

From Lucky,[53] with permission.

TABLE 22.4   Skin manifestations of Cushing disease in children and adolescents*

Striae	77.7%
Acne	58.3%
Hirsutism	63.7%**
Acanthosis nigricans	27.7%
Ecchymoses	27.7%
Hyperpigmentation	16.6%
Fungal infections	11.1%

* From Stratakis et al.[55] based on 36 patients with pituitary Cushing Syndrome
** of 22 girls

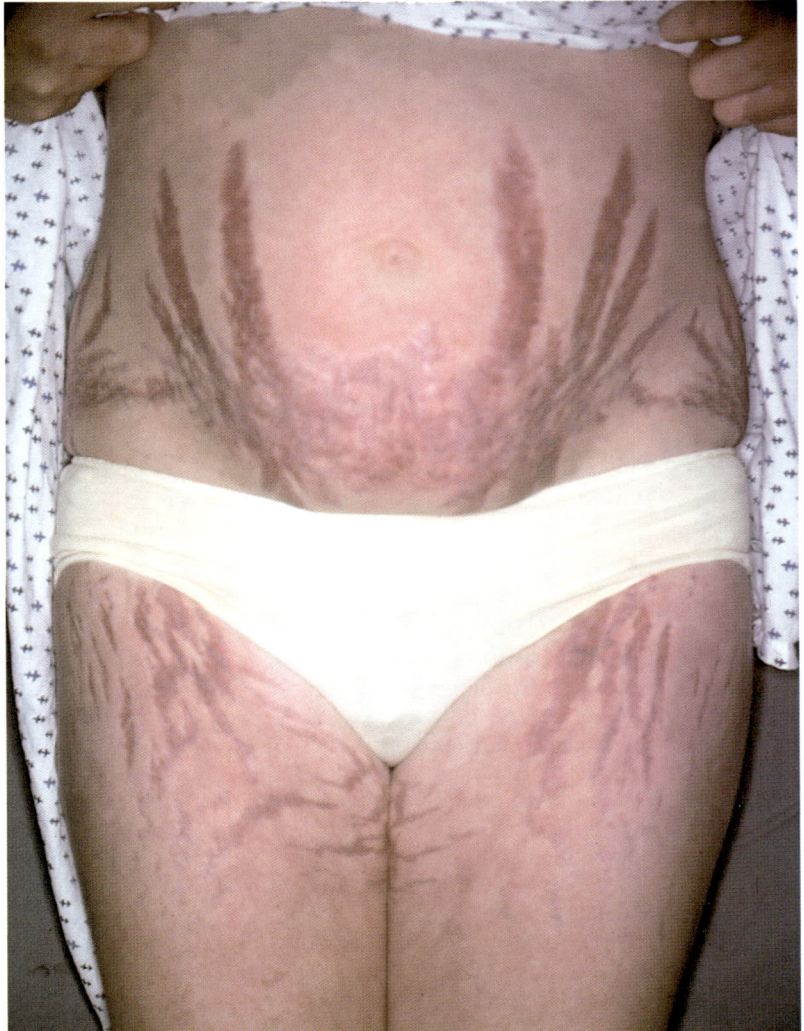

Fig. 22.9 Striking number and distribution of deep, red striae in a young woman with Cushing syndrome.

pituitary and/or hypothalamic hormones. Cushing syndrome, however, is a phenotypic copy due to the effects of excessive glucocorticosteroids from causes other than pituitary hypothalamic overstimulation. Cushing syndrome is most commonly produced from the iatrogenic overuse of steroids, usually systemic but rarely also topical. All causes of Cushing syndrome except exogenous steroid hormone administration may manifest signs of combined glucocorticoid and androgen excess. By contrast, congenital adrenal hyperplasia (CAH) is a disorder of underproduction of glucocorticoids due to specific enzymatic defects in the biosynthesis of cortisol and resulting overproduction of androgens. (CAH is described separately under Disorders of androgen excess.)

Presenting history

The most consistent finding in the prepubertal child with Cushing syndrome is growth failure with markedly delayed skeletal osseous maturation (bone age). Linear bone growth is exquisitely sensitive to glucocorticosteroids. In addition, there may be weight gain with a redistribution of normal fat to the trunk. Children may also present with insomnia, emotional lability, and headaches associated with hypertension. There may be menstrual irregularities in the postmenarchal female. New onset or exacerbation of acne and/or hirsutism may also be presenting complaints.

Physical examination

The most common skin conditions noted in 36 children with pituitary Cushing syndrome are listed in Table 22.4.[55] Except for striae, all findings resolved within one year of therapy (Fig. 22.9). Striae are due to glucocorticoid stimulation and represent both epidermal thinning and dermal atrophy and appear to occur in areas of skin tension. Large subcutaneous vessels can be seen under wrinkled, atrophic, transparent epithelial covering. Rupture of striae with slow healing may be a severe cutaneous complication

of Cushing syndrome. Hyperpigmentation of striae is associated with generalized hyperpigmentation (such as that seen in Addison's disease) and is due to overproduction of ACTH and/or MSH. Excessive glucocorticoids also cause redistribution of subcutaneous fat to produce roundness of the cheeks (moon facies), accumulation in the upper back (buffalo hump), and deposits in the buttocks and abdomen, with striking sparing of the extremities. In some cases of Cushing syndrome, there may be secondary plethora, telangiectasia, and flushing of the face. Because of androgen excess, there may be typical acne vulgaris. Acne in childhood may be the presenting sign of an adrenal tumor. However, glucocorticoids alone produce distinct perifollicular pustules on the back, upper arms, chest, and face that are all in the same stages of development. This is called "steroid acne" and is more of a folliculitis. Initially, comedones are not present. With a prolonged course, these primary follicular pustules may develop abnormal keratinization and secondary comedones, a pathophysiology quite different from that seen in acne vulgaris. Acanthosis nigricans can also be a feature of Cushing syndrome and will be discussed later in this chapter. Glucocorticoids promote fine, long, downy hair, especially on the sides of the face (Fig. 22.10), but androgens cause true hirsutism in secondary sex locations such as upper lip, chin, mid chest and abdomen, and around the areolae.

55. Stratakis C, Mastorakos G, Mitsiades NS et al. (1998) Skin manifestations of Cushing disease in children and adolescents before and after the resolution of hypercortisolemia. **Pediatr Dermatol** 15(4):253–258.

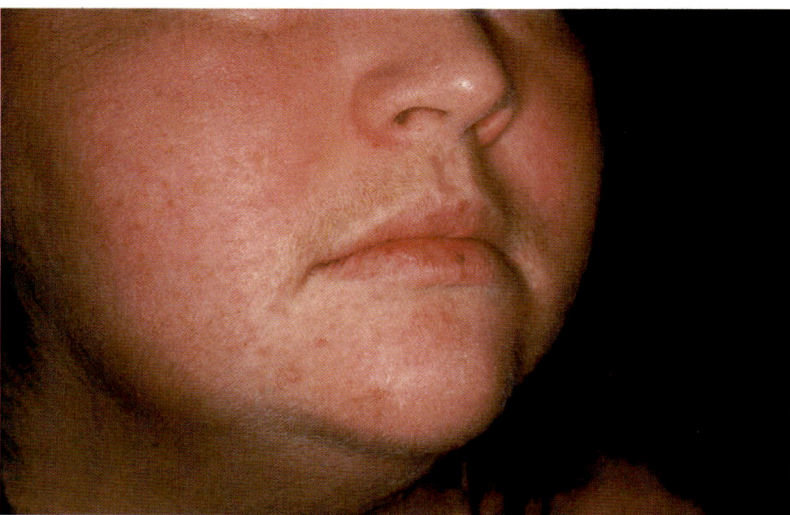

Fig. 22.10 Fine downy hair on the cheeks of a young woman with Cushing syndrome. She also had new onset of acne, oral and nail candidiasis, and redistribution of body fat.

Secondary cutaneous features associated with glucocorticoid excess are primarily due to superinfection with organisms whose normal colonization becomes pathologic in the milieu of excessive glucocorticoids. Tinea versicolor (due to superficial colonization of *Pityrosporum ovale*) may appear prepubertally and may be refractory to standard therapy. Candidiasis can occur on the oral mucosa (thrush), vaginal mucosa (vaginitis), nail plate and bed (onychomycosis) and surrounding tissues (paronychia), interdigital webs (blastomycetes interdigitalis erosio), the corners of the mouth (perleche), and intertriginous folds such as neck, axillae, and under the breast and groin (intertrigo).

Bacterial infections, especially with *Staphylococcus aureus*, can cause diffuse folliculitis, furunculosis, and large carbuncles and abscesses in glucocorticoid excess. Other features of adrenocortical excess include hypertension, glucose intolerance or frank diabetes mellitus, altered mental status, emotional lability, and menstrual disturbances.

Laboratory findings
The most reliable diagnostic tools to diagnose glucocorticoid excess are serum ACTH levels, a 24-hour urine level of free cortisol, and plasma cortisol levels showing absence of normal diurnal variation. Normally, plasma cortisol is highest in the early morning and reaches a low level after noon. Failure to reach the low afternoon levels is suggestive of Cushing syndrome.

Dexamethasone suppression tests and diagnostic imaging studies such as ultrasound, computed tomography (CT) and magnetic resonance imaging are essential to differentiate pituitary ACTH excess from primary adrenal tumors.

Pathophysiology
Glucocorticoid excess can be a result of excessive stimulation of the adrenal gland from ACTH or of primary adrenal hypersecretion. ACTH overproduction includes disorders of the pituitary and/or hypothalamus as well as rare cases of ectopic ACTH production from neural crest tumors arising in pancreas, thymus, or ovary. These rare tumors have been described primarily in adults. Primary nodular adrenal hyperplasia (now also reported in McCune–Albright syndrome[56]), benign adenomas,[57] or malignant carcinomas[57,58] will result in suppressed ACTH, as will exogenous excess of glucocorticosteroids therapeutically.[59] In all of the disorders except exogenous treatment, there may be concurrent adrenal androgen hyperproduction.

Iatrogenic Cushing syndrome may occur when prolonged use of systemic steroids is prescribed for a variety of skin and other disorders. Rarely, signs of glucocorticoid excess result from intralesional or topical steroid therapy.

Differential diagnosis
The usual diagnostic dilemma is to distinguish between Cushing syndrome and exogenous obesity. In addition, patients with polycystic ovary syndrome, who tend to be obese with irregular menses as well as acne and hirsutism, may also be thought to have Cushing syndrome. Children presenting with precocious puberty or pseudoprecocious puberty (i.e., partial precocious development without true puberty) should be evaluated for adrenal tumors. Differential diagnosis also includes diabetes mellitus and obesity with multiple secondary infections.

Therapy and prognosis
Cushing syndrome is now treated primarily by transsphenoidal hypopophysectomy of pituitary adenomas[55] Adrenal nodular hyperplasia and adrenal tumors must be surgically removed.[57,58] Malignant adrenal tumors have a very poor prognosis[57,58] despite surgical excision and chemotherapy.

The various potencies of systemic glucocorticoids are illustrated in Table 22.5.[53] Although there are studies of average plasma and tissue half-life and hypothalamic pituitary suppression, each individual has a different metabolic clearance rate and thus treatment must be individualized. In general, therapy with the shortest acting, least potent steroid for the shortest period of time that will give therapeutic benefit is most highly recommended. Guidelines for what duration of treatment will require careful tapering rather than immediate discontinuation of steroids are not established. Certainly, therapy beyond two to three weeks has been shown to have prolonged suppressive effects on the hypothalamic pituitary-adrenal axis. In fact,

TABLE 22.5 Potencies of glucocorticoids

Compound	Plasma half-life (min)	Tissue duration (h)	HPA suppression (h)	Glucocorticoid potency	Dose equivalents (mg)	Mineralocorticoid activity
Cortisol (hydrocortisone)	60–115	4–8	24–36	1	20	+
Cortisone acetate	30–90	6 (po, iv) 72 (im)	24–36	0.8	25	+
Prednisone	60	6–8	24–36	4	5	+
Dexamethasone	110–300+	8–12	48	25–40	0.5–0.75	−

From Lucky,[53] with permission.

56. Kirk JMW, Brain CE, Carson DJ et al. (1999) Cushing's syndrome caused by nodular adrenal hyperplasia in children with McCune-Albright syndrome. **J Pediatr** 134:789–792.
57. Ciftci AO, Senocak ME, Tanyel FC, Buyukpamukcu N (2001) Adrenocortical tumors in children. **J Pediatr Surg** 36(4):549–554.
58. Liou LS, Kay R (2000) Adrenocortical carcinoma in children. Review and recent innovations. **Urol Clin North Am** 27(3):403–421.
59. Curtis JA, Cormode E, Laski B et al. (1982) Endocrine complications of topical and intralesional corticosteroid therapy. **Arch Dis Child** 57:204.

suppression is achieved with doses as low as 30mg prednisone for five days or 20mg prednisone for seven days in adults.[53] Response to a 30-minute im or iv bolus of ACTH (or Cortrosyn® may provide useful information about adrenal recovery in patients treated for long periods of time. Doses can be tapered gradually to a physiologic level and then switched to an alternate-day regimen, which allows for more recovery of the pituitary-adrenal axis. Alternately, some physicians prefer gradually reducing an alternate-day dose until one day's dosage is eliminated and then reducing the other alternate dosage. The recurrence of primary disease or appearance of withdrawal symptoms are guidelines for this kind of taper. For intercurrent illnesses or major stress, such as surgery or trauma, guidelines are available for replacement (Table 22.3).[52] Excessive use of intralesional and even topical steroids, especially high-potency steroids, can lead to iatrogenic Cushing syndrome with growth retardation and many of the major side effect , including extraordinary local atrophy.[57] For this reason, children on long-term topical steroids should, if possible, be treated with the smallest amount of low-potency steroids needed for therapeutic effect.

DISORDERS OF ANDROGEN EXCESS

Excessive amounts of circulating androgens can contribute to cutaneous disorders including acne, hirsutism, and alopecia. Since manifestations of androgen excess are quite variable from individual to individual, a high index of suspicion is required for diagnosis of an underlying hyperandrogenic disorder. The causes of androgen excess are varied: these include tumors as well as functional overproduction of androgens from the ovary and/or adrenal gland (Table 22.6) and exogenous use of anabolic steroids by athletes. The importance of insulin resistance in the pathogenesis of polycystic ovary syndrome (PCOS) has been recently recognized and is discussed below.

Epidemiology

Onset of androgen excess may occur at any age and can affect both sexes. Depending on the disorder, there may be a genetic predisposition.

Clinical features

Prepubertal children with androgen excess may present with precocious sexual development as a primary complaint. Such development would be sex appropriate in males and inappropriate in females. Besides rapid linear growth and development of axillary and pubic hair, there s increased maturation of genitalia in boys and clitoromegaly in girls. Acne vulgaris and hirsutism may be early signs of an androgen abnormality. One of the earliest

signs of androgen excess is the appearance of adult-type underarm odor. Postpubertally, diagnosis may be more difficult because acne is so common, but hirsutism, alopecia of the scalp, amenorrhea, irregular menses, and infertility are more reliable indicators of androgen excess.

Physical examination

The main clinical features of androgen excess – acne, hirsutism and androgenetic alopecia[60–62] – have been covered in Chapters 13 (Acne) and 11 (Hair). Acne may be the first sign of androgen excess and, in normal puberty, is associated with rising levels of DHEAS.[63,64] In older adolescents and adults, acne is also associated with higher levels of free testosterone.[65] Hirsutism is defined as excessive terminal hair in androgen-dependent locations. Although normal amounts of terminal hair have been established for women over age 18,[66] only recently have standards for adolescent girls been established that demonstrated that smaller amounts of upper lip hair are abnormal in girls ages 10–19 than in adult women.[67] Androgenetic alopecia in females is usually confined to the crown of the scalp (Fig. 22.11); in males there is bi-frontal as well as vertex thinning.

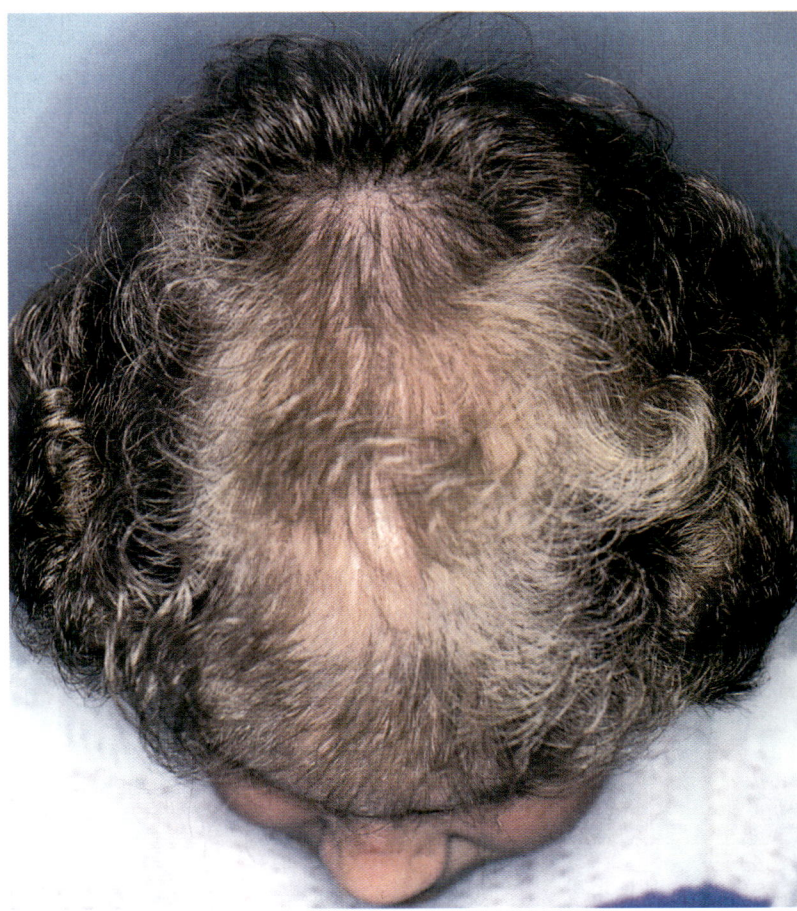

Fig. 22.11   Typical thinning hair on the crown of the scalp in a 13-year-old girl. Onset was early, just prior to menarche. Her mother had had a similar pattern of female pattern hair loss (androgenic alopecia).

TABLE 22.6   Causes of androgen excess
Ovarian or testicular
Benign or malignant tumors
Polycystic ovarian disease
Adrenal
Benign or malignant tumors
Congenital adrenal hyperplasia
Functional adrenal androgen overproduction (premature or exaggerated adrenarche)

60. Rosenfield RL, Lucky AW (1993) Acne, hirsutism, and alopecia in adolescent females. Endocrin Metab Clin North Am 22:507–532.
61. Sperling LC, Heimer WL II (1993) Androgen biology as a basis for the diagnosis and treatment of androgenic disorders in women. I. J Am Acad Dermatol 28:669.
62. Sperling LC, Heimer WL II (1993) Androgen biology as a basis for the diagnosis and treatment of androgenic disorders in women. II. J Am Acad Dermatol 28:901.
63. Lucky AW, Biro FM, Huster GA et al. (1991) Acne vulgaris in early adolescent boys. Correlations with pubertal maturation and age. Arch Dermatol 127(2):210–216.
64. Lucky AW, Biro FM, Huster GA et al. (1994) Acne vulgaris in premenarchal girls. An early sign of puberty associated with rising levels of dehydroepiandrosterone. Arch Dermatol 130(3):308–314.
65. Lucky AW, Biro FM, Simbartl LA et al. (1997) Predictors of severity of acne vulgaris in young adolescent girls: Results of a five-year longitudinal study. J Pediatr 130(1):30–39.
66. Ferriman D, Gallwey JD (1961) Clinical assessment of body hair growth in women. J Clin Endocrinol Metab 21:1440–1447.
67. Lucky AW, Biro FM, Daniels SR et al. (2001) The prevalence of upper lip hair in black and white girls during puberty: A new standard. J Pediatr 138:134–136.

Laboratory findings

Accelerating growth with upward crossing of percentiles is indicative of androgen excess. Advancement of the bone age (derived from standards of radiographs of the bones of the left hand and wrist[68]) is also indicative. Elevated plasma free testosterone (T) and dehydroepiandrosterone (DHEAS) are two common findings in androgen excess. Testosterone circulates bound to a carrier protein, testosterone estrogen-binding globulin (TEBG), also known as sex hormone-binding globulin (SHBG). A small fraction of T is also bound to albumin. The small, free fraction of T is biologically active. Assays of total T measure both T and TEBG; thus changes in TEBG may misleadingly affect the total T value without biologic significance. For example, estrogen increase TEBG production and elevates total T, but in fact the increased availability of binding sites actually lowers biologically active free T. By contrast, androgens depress TEBG; thus, total T values appear relatively lower in precisely those patients who have functionally high free T. Free T is a much more reliable measurement than total T. One problem with measurements of T is that there are fluctuations in circulating levels over minutes, hours, and days. The ideal way to overcome this problem is by multiple sampling, such as three consecutive hourly samples. But this plan has economic limitations. The origin of T is approximately equal from the ovary and the adrenal gland and thus measurement of T or free T cannot distinguish ovarian from adrenal sources.

DHEA and its sulfate, DHEAS, have been found to be elevated in about one-half of female acne patients.[60–62] These hormones are more than 95% adrenal in origin and serve as markers for adrenal overproduction of androgen.

Other hormones may be elevated in special circumstances. Delta$_4$-androstenedione (A) is produced by both the ovary and the adrenal gland and provides about one-half the plasma T via peripheral conversion. It is very rapidly metabolized and thus an unreliable marker for elevated androgens. 17-α-Hydroxyprogesterone (17-Prog) is a specific marker for 21-hydroxylase deficiency, and 11-deoxycortisol (compound S) is a specific marker for 11-β-hydroxylase deficiency, the two most common forms of congenital adrenal hyperplasia. In milder forms of this disease, baseline levels of these hormones may not be elevated, and diagnostic stimulation with ACTH is necessary to diagnose such enzymatic defects definitively.[69] Baseline levels of 17-Prog should be measured in the follicular phase of the menstrual cycle because in the luteal phase there is a large ovarian contribution of 17-Prog. The gonadotropins luteinizing hormone (LH) and follicle stimulating hormone (FSH) demonstrate a ratio of LH/FSH elevated above 3:1 in a majority of patients with polycystic ovarian (PCO) disease. ACTH stimulation and dexamethasone suppression tests may define specific enzymatic defects and diagnose nonsuppressible adrenal tumors. From a practical point of view, plasma free T, DHEAS, LH, and FSH seem to be reasonable tests to screen patients in whom hyperandrogenemia is suspected.

Pathophysiology

There are three sources of androgenic steroid hormones: the gonads (ovary or testes), the adrenal gland, and a variety of peripheral organs including the skin, which can convert less potent precursors to highly potent androgens. Interactions between these are abundant and often frustrate our attempts to neatly categorize the cause of androgen excess.

The ovary

Ovarian tumors may be virilizing and can be benign or malignant. Usually there is rapid onset of symptoms and the timing is not necessarily associated with puberty. Testosterone is often very high (i.e., greater than 200ng/dl).

Ovarian tumors can be diagnosed by pelvic examination, ultrasound, magnetic resonance imaging (MRI) scan, laparoscopy, or laparotomy.

Polycystic ovary syndrome (PCOS)[70,71] is the most common ovarian abnormality encountered in association with hyperandrogenemia and will be discussed in detail below. The ovary is relatively quiescent in childhood until puberty when the production of LH and FSH increases. This phenomenon begins as early as age 7 or 8 years, with nighttime spikes of LH that may be detected with 24-hour urinary assays. LH stimulates the thecal cells of the ovarian follicle to produce T and, most abundantly, A, which are converted by the enzyme aromatase to the estrogens, estrone (E$_1$) or estradiol (E$_2$), respectively. These androgens are the primary product of the ovary. Androstenedione can be converted to T inside or outside the ovary, and ovarian production accounts for approximately 50% of circulating T. Aromatase is present in granulosa cells and is catalyzed by FSH. As granulosa cells multiply in a dominant, growing follicle cyclically each month before ovulation, that follicle produces a surge of estrogen that helps induce ovulation. After ovulation, the granulosa cells transform to luteal cells and primarily produce progesterone (Prog) and 17-Prog. If instead of a cyclic production of estrogen there is tonic, continuous output, especially of E$_1$, a paradoxical positive feedback of LH occurs.[72] Thus, if there is overproduction of A, it can be converted to E$_1$, which will stimulate high levels of LH, perpetuate further increase in androgen, and further disrupt normal cyclic ovulation. The result of elevated androgens, from any source including the adrenal gland, may be to raise the ratio of LH/FSH by the tonic production of estrogen and the process becomes self-perpetuating. Thus, follicles that might have become dominant and ovulated become the androgen-producing cysts of polycystic ovaries instead.

In summary, the ovary produces about 50% of the circulating T, much of which is derived from A. E$_1$ and E$_2$ are derived from A and T, respectively, in a cyclic manner during normal ovulation, but when follicular maturation is interrupted, there may be androgen-producing cysts associated with increased ratio of LH/FSH. The rationale for treatment of PCOS is primarily to interrupt tonic LH stimulation, and this is most easily accomplished with estrogen-containing oral contraceptives.

The adrenal gland

Adrenal tumors, including adenomas and carcinomas as well as pituitary-hypothalamic ACTH-producing tumors (Cushing syndrome), can all be rare causes of virilization in children and adults. Usually, onset is abrupt and signs of androgen excess severe. Diagnosis is made by imaging techniques or exploratory surgery. More common adrenal abnormalities causing hyperandrogenemia are biochemical disorders: congenital adrenal hyperplasia and functional overproduction of androgens in response to ACTH.

The primary secretory product of the adrenal is cortisol (Fig. 22.12). In order to produce cortisol from the basic precursor cholesterol, a series of enzymatic steps produce intermediates that have androgenic potential. ACTH stimulates the adrenal and responds only to cortisol (or very similar compounds such as prednisone or dexamethasone) for negative feedback control.

Similar to the ovary, the androgen-predominant cells of the inner zona reticularis of the adrenal cortex are quiescent in childhood from about ages 1 to 7 but are quite active in the perinatal months and pubertal years.[73,74] The inner fetal adrenal zone of the newborn adrenal gland (which is analogous to the zona reticularis, both histologically and biochemically) disappears in the first year of life and a well-defined zona reticularis first appears in late childhood between the ages of 5 and 8.[75] The presence of these zones is

68. Greulich WW, Pyle, SI (1959) Radiographic Atlas of Skeletal Development of the Hand and Writst, 2nd ed. Stanford: Stanford University Press.
69. Levine LS, Dupont B, Lorenzen F et al. (1980) Cryptic 21-hydroxylase deficiency in families of patients with classical congenital adrenal hyperplasia. **J Clin Endocrinol Metab** 51:1316.
70. Kahn JA, Gordon CM (1999) Polycystic ovary syndrome. **Adolescent Medicine** 10(2):321–336.
71. Dunaif A, Thomas A (2001) Current concepts in the polycystic ovary syndrome. **Ann Rev Med** 52:401–419.
72. Yen SSC (1980) The polycystic ovary syndrome. **Clin Endocrinol** 12:177.

73. De Peretti E, Forest MG (1978) Pattern of plasma dehydroepiandrosterone sulfate levels in humans from birth to adulthood: evidence for testicular production. **J Clin Endocrinol Metab** 47:572.
74. Winter JSD, Hughes IA, Reyes FI, Faiman C (1976) Pituitary-gonadal relations in infancy. 2. Patterns of serum gonadal steroid concentrations in man from birth to two years of age. **J Clin Endocrinol Metab** 42:679.
75. Dhom G (1973) The prepubertal and pubertal growth of the adrenal (adrenarche). **Beitr Path Bd** 150:357.

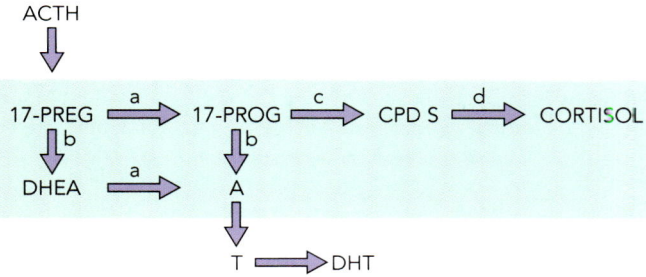

(a) 3β-Hydroxysteroid Dehydrogenase
(b) C$_{17-20}$-Lyase
(c) 21-Hydroxylase
(d) 11β-Hydroxylase

Fig. 22.12 Simplified diagram of adrenal steroid biosynthesis. Any interruption in the production of cortisol will lead to excessive ACTH production and consequent androgen excess. 17 Preg, 17-hydroxypregnenolone; 17 Prog, 17α-hydroxyprogesterone; Cpd S, 11-deoxycortisol; DHEA, dehydroepiandrosterone; A, Δ^{4-} androstenedione; T, testosterone, DHT, dihydrotestosterone.

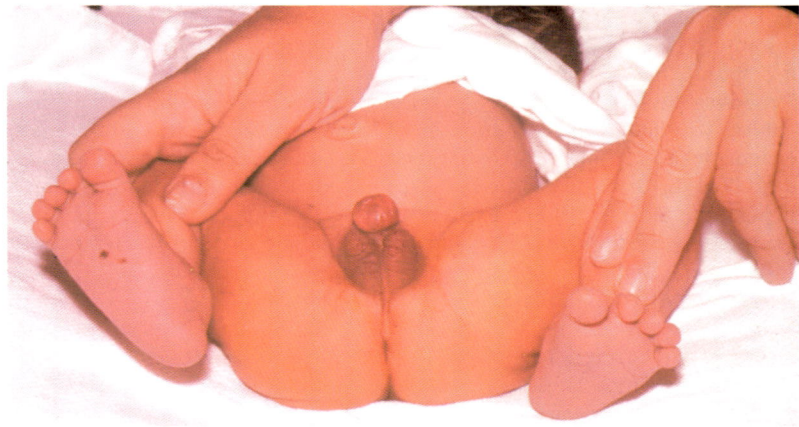

Fig. 22.13 Ambiguous genitalia (intersex) in a female 46XX infant with congenital adrenal hyperplasia due to severe 21-hydroxylase deficiency. Note hyperpigmentation of the fused labia, clitoral hypertrophy, and a phallic urethra.

associated with a biochemical synthetic pathway that favors the production of androgens and androgen precursors, notably DHEA and its sulfate DHEAS.

Premature adrenarche

The process of adrenal maturation is termed adrenarche, and it appears to be independent of gonadal development. The specific changes noted in adrenarche are a relatively decreased efficiency of the enzyme 3β-hydroxysteroid dehydrogenase (3β–HSD) and increased efficiency of C17–20 lyase, resulting in elevated levels of 17-α-hydroxypregnenolone (17-PREG), DHEA, and A.[76,77] Premature adrenarche (PA) is the early (before age 8) reappearance of adrenal androgens (adrenarche) and stimules growth of public and axillary hair (pubarche). It is much more common in girls. Although considered "benign" for many years, there is growing evidence that PA may be the first sign of hormonal imbalance: many of these girls will go on to develop insulin resistance, NIDDM, and/or PCOS.[78–80] Girls with PA and acanthosis nigricans or elevated insulin/glucose ratios may be particularly at risk.[81] Some girls with premature adrenarche actually have late-onset congenital adrenal hyperplasia.[82,83]

The mature adrenal gland contributes approximately one-half of the circulating plasma T, primarily via conversion of A to T. The adrenal is also the source of more than 95% of the circulating DHEA and DHEAS, which can serve as markers of adrenal androgen production. DHEAS is present in 1000-fold higher quantities than DHEA. Although DHEA itself is not a strong androgen, it can be metabolized peripherally in tissues, including skin, to more potent androgens and thus has androgenic potential.

Congenital adrenal hyperplasia

If there is a deficient or inefficient enzyme in any step along the pathway to cortisol biosynthesis, which results in lowered cortisol, there will be a compensatory increase in ACTH via negative feedback control. The resulting accumulation of androgens or androgenic precursors will produce

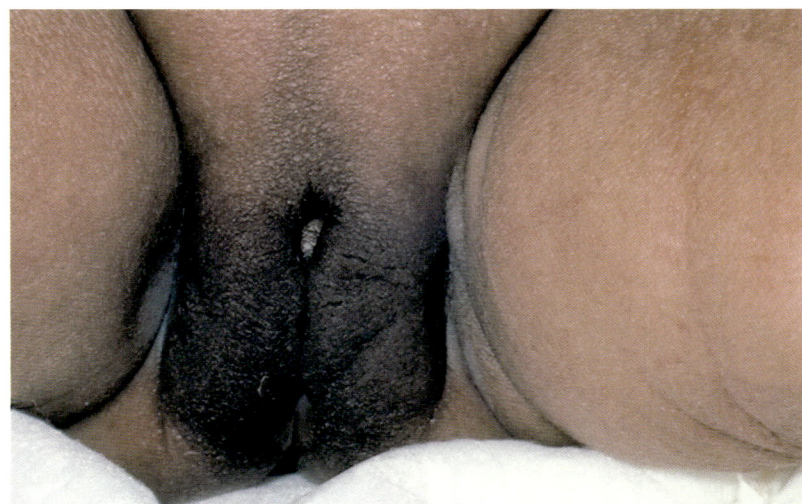

Fig. 22.14 Normal black newborn girl with hyperpigmentation of the labia.

clinical signs of androgen excess. In the classical form of congenital adrenal hyperplasia (CAH) where the enzyme block has been severe *in utero*, infants are born with ambiguous genitalia and shock from lack of cortisol. The primary skin manifestation seen is hyperpigmentation of the genitalia (Fig. 22.13). It can be confused with the normal hyperpigmentation seen in dark-skinned neonates (Fig. 22.14). However, of interest to dermatologists are the milder enzymatic defects, which may not manifest with signs of androgen excess until puberty. Among the young women who present with acne and/or hirsutism, ACTH stimulation tests can detect some specific enzyme defects (i.e., mild- or late-onset CAH).[84,85] The most common form of CAH is 21-hydroxylase deficiency.[86,87] It is an autosomal-recessive disorder and the heterozygote carrier state occurs as frequently as 1 in 35 to 1 in

76. Rich BH, Rosenfield RL, Lucky AW et al. (1981) Adrenarche: changing adrenal response to adrenocorticotropin. J Clin Endocrinol Metab 52:1129.

77. Dickerman Z, Grant DR, Faiman C, Winter JSD (1984) Intraadrenal steroid concentrations in man: zonal differences and developmental changes. J Clin Endocrinol Metab 59:1031.

78. Ibanez L, Potau N, Zampolli M et al. (1996) Hyperinsulinemia in postpubertal girls with a history of premature pubarche and functional ovarian hyperandrogenism. J Clin Endocrinol Metab 81(3):1237–1243.

79. Ibanez L, Potau N, Marcos MV, de Zegher F (2000) Adrenal hyperandrogenism in adolescent girls with a history of low birthweight and precocious pubarche. Clin Endocrinol 53:523–527.

80. DiMartino-Nardi J (2000) Pre- and postpubertal findings in premature adrenarche. J Pediatr Endocrinol Metab 13:1265–1269.

81. Vuguin P, Saenger P, DiMartino-Nardi J (2001) Fasting glucose insulin ratio: A useful measure of insulin resistance in girls with premature adrenarche. J Clin Endocrinol Metab 86:4618–4621.

82. Siegel SF, Finegold DN, Urban MD et al. (1992) Premature pubarche: etiological heterogeneity. J Clin Endocrinol Metab 74:239.

83. Hawkins LA, Chasalow PI, Blethen SL (1992) The role of adrenocorticotropin testing in evaluating girls with premature adrenarche and hirsutism/oligomenorrhea. J Clin Endocrinol Metab 74:428.

84. Siegel SF, Finegold DN et al. (1990) ACTH stimulation tests and plasma dehydroepiandrosterone sulfate levels in women with hirsutism. N Engl J Med 323:845.

85. Eldar-Geva T, Hurwitz A, Vecsei P et al. (1990) Secondary biosynthetic defects in women with late-onset congenital adrenal hyperplasia. N Engl J Med 323:855.

86. Lobo RA, Geobelsmann U (1980) Adult manifestation of congenital adrenal hyperplasia due to incomplete 21-hydroxylase deficiency mimicking polycystic ovarian disease. Am J Obstet Gynecol 138:720.

87. Migeon CJ, Rosenwaks Z, Lee PA et al. (1980) The attenuated form of congenital adrenal hyperplasia as an allelic form of 21-hydroxylase deficiency. J Clin Endocrinol Metab 51:647.

50 individuals. Elevated 17-OH-Prog response to ACTH is a marker for this disorder. 11-β-Hydroxylase deficiency (with high 11-deoxycortisol or Cpd S response to ACTH) and 3β-HSD (with high 17 PREG and DHEA response to ACTH)[88] are other forms of CAH found in young adult women.

Not all adrenal overproduction of androgen neatly fits into specific enzymatic defects. There also exist functional abnormalities of adrenal response to ACTH that have been called exaggerated adrenarche, or functional adrenal hyperandrogenism.[89,90] The existence of such a functional state might help explain how stress, via ACTH, could cause flares of androgen-dependent acne.

Peripheral metabolism of androgens

Many tissues, including skin, hair, and sebaceous glands, have androgen receptors and enzymes to further metabolize steroid hormones.[91] Androgens are taken up into the cytoplasm, attach to cytosol receptors, and are translocated to nuclear receptors where their effect is mediated via RNA synthesis. Testosterone is converted to the more potent dihydrotestosterone (DHT) by 5-α-reductase in the skin as well as other tissues. Skin has the ability to metabolize less potent androgenic precursors such as DHEA into potent androgens such as T and DHT. Inactive steroid end products such as 5-α-androstanediol glucuronide, a reduced metabolite of DHT, may serve as a marker for cutaneous androgen metabolism.[92]

Therapy and prognosis

Primary treatment of acne is discussed at length in Chapter 13. Hormonal therapy should be reserved for specific patients not responsive to conventional therapy or who have a well-documented ovarian or adrenal disorder. Most patients with acne do not have androgen excess. By contrast, significant hirsutism and androgenetic alopecia are very likely due to androgen excess. Non-hormonal therapy for hirsutism includes bleaching, plucking, waxing, shaving, chemical depilatories, topical eflornithine, electrolysis, and laser therapy (see Chapter 11). Topical minoxidil is the only non-hormonal therapy for androgenetic alopecia to be shown clinically superior to placebo, despite many claims that other over-the-counter products stimulate hair growth (see Chapter 11).

Hormonal therapy for acne, hirsutism, and androgenetic alopecia includes oral contraceptives, low-dose steroids, and antiandrogens. Oral contraceptives have been shown to be effective for acne.[93,94] Oral contraceptives act by elevating TEBG and thus decreasing available free T as well as by interfering with the normal gonadotropin feedback mechanism and essentially eliminating ovarian hormone production. GnRH analogs, alone or in combination with estrogens,[95,96] may be useful in some situations. Progestagen-only contraceptives, given orally, intramuscularly, or via implantation, are not useful for acne and actually exacerbate it because of the androgenic activity of some progestins.[97]

Low-dose corticosteroids act by suppressing adrenal production of androgens via ACTH suppression.[98] Doses such as 2.5–5mg prednisone or 0.25–0.5mg dexamethasone, given at night to suppress the late night diurnal surge of ACTH, may be effective. However, patients need to be carefully monitored for adrenocortical suppression, especially with dexamethasone, which could be life threatening.

Antiandrogens are drugs which interfere with the effect of androgens on the end organ, either as competitive inhibitors of the androgen receptor or as blockers of 5-α-reductase.[99] Spironolactone, a competitive inhibitor of the androgen receptor, is the most widely used antiandrogen in the United States, although blockage of androgen excess is an off-label use of this medication.[100–102] It is given as 50–200mg per day in two doses with meals. Polymenorrhea, increased urination, breast tenderness, and fatigue are the most common side effects. Hyperkalemia is rare, especially at the lower doses. Spironolactone seems to be especially useful in older adolescents and women with acne flares related to the menstrual cycle. It is not used in males. Cyproterone acetate, another inhibitor of the androgen receptor,[96] combined with ethinyl estradiol, is successfully used in many countries for hyperandrogenemia but is not available in the USA. Flutamide, a non-steroidal competitive inhibitor of the androgen receptor,[103] has also been recommended for hirsutism, even in adolescents, but with its potential for hepatotoxicity, it is less popular. Finasteride inhibits the Type 2, 5-alpha reductase found in hair follicles and thus is useful in hirsutism and androgenetic alopecia.[104] However, the Type 1 enzyme predominates in sebaceous glands[91] and it is not useful in acne. Extreme caution needs to be exercised when using antiandrogens in

---

TABLE 22.7 Endocrine and metabolic disorders associated with acanthosis nigricans

Metabolic disorders

Obesity
  Insulin-resistance syndromes
    Leprechaunism (Donohue syndrome)
    Rabson–Mendenhall syndrome
    Generalized lipodystrophies
      Congenital (Berardinelli–Seip)
      Acquired (Seip–Lawrence)
    Partial lipodystrophies
      Cephalothoracic
      Face-sparing (Dunnigan–Koeberling)
    Polycystic ovary syndrome (PCOS)

Other endocrine disorders
  Hyperandrogenic states
  Acromegaly, gigantism
  Cushing disease, pituitary basophilism
  Glucocorticoid therapy
  Diethylstillbestrol, oral contraceptives
  Hypogonadal syndromes with insulin resistance
    Prader–Willii
    Alstrom and other familial hypogonadal syndromes
  Addison's disease
  Hypothyroidism
  Hormone production by malignant neoplasms?
  Crouzon syndrome
  Ataxia telangiestasia

88. Rosenfield RL, Rich BH, Wolfsdorf JI et al. (1980) Pubertal presentation of congenital delta5-3β-hydroxysteroid dehydrogenase deficiency. J Clin Endocrinol Metab 51:345.

89. Lucky AW, Rosenfield RL, McGuire J et al. (1986) Adrenal androgen hyperresponsiveness to adrenocorticotropin in women with acne and/or hirsutism: adrenal enzyme defects and exaggerated adrenarche. J Clin Endocrinol Metab 62:840.

90. Rosenfield RL (1996) Evidence that idiopathic functional adrenal hyperandrogenism is caused by dysregulation of adrenal steroidogenesis and that hyperinsulinemia may be involved. J Clin Endocrinol Metab 81(3):878–880.

91. Thiboutot D, Bayne E, Thorne J et al. (2000) Immunolocalization of 5 alpha-reductase isozynes in acne lesions and normal skin. Arch Dermatol 136(9):1125–1129.

92. Lookingbill DP, Horton R, Demers LM et al. (1985) Tissue production of androgens in women with acne. J Am Acad Dermatol 12:481.

93. Lucky AW, Henderson TA, Olson WH et al. (1997) Effectiveness of norgestimate and ethinyl estradiol in treating moderate acne vulgaris. J Am Acad Dermatol 37(5 pt 1):746–754.

94. Thiboutot D, Archer DF, Lemay A et al. (2001) A randomized, controlled trial of a low dose contraceptive containing 20 microg of ethinyl estradiol and 100 microg of levonorgestrel for acne treatment. Fertil Steril 76(3):461–468.

95. Vegetti W, Testa G, Maggiono P et al. (1996) An open randomized comparative study of an oral contraceptive containing ethinyl estradiol and cyproterone acetate with and without the GnRH analogue goserelin in the long-term treatment of hirsutism. Gynecol Obstet Invest 41:260–268.

96. Carmina E, Lobo RA (1997) Gonadotrophin-releasing hormone agonist therapy for hirsutism is as effective as high dose cyproterone acetate but results in a longer remission. Human Reproduction 12(4):663–666.

97. Darney PD (1998) The androgenicity of progestins. Am J Med 98(1A):104S–110S.

98. Carmina E, Lobo RA (1998) The addition of dexamethasone to antiandrogen therapy for hirsutism prolongs the duration of remission. Fertil Steril 69(6):1075–1079.

99. Schmidt JB (1998) Other antiandrogens. Dermatology 196:153–157.

100. Cumming DC, Yang JC, Rebar RW, Yen SSC (1982) Treatment of hirsutism with spironolactone. JAMA 247:1295.

101. Moghetti P, Castello R, Zamberlan N et al. (1999) Spironolactone, but not flutamide, administration prevents bone loss in hyperandrogenic women treated with gonadotropin-releasing hormone agonist. J Clin Endocrinol Metab 84(4):1250–1254.

102. Sprtizer PM, Lisboa KO, Mattiello S, Lhullier F (2000) Spironolactone as a single agent for long-term therapy of hirsute patients. Clin Endocrinol 52:587–594.

103. Ibanez L, Potau N, Marcos MV, de Zegher F (2000) Treatment of hirsutism, hyperandrogenism, oligomenorrhea, dyslipidemia and hyperinsulinism in nonobese, adolescent girls: Effect of flutamide. J Clin Endocrinol Metab 85(9):3251–3255.

104. Moghetti P, Tosi F, Tosti A et al. (2000) Comparison of sprinolocatone, flutamide and finasteride efficacy in the treatment of hirsutism: A randomized, double blind, placebo-controlled trial. J Clin Endocrinol Metab 85(1):89–94.

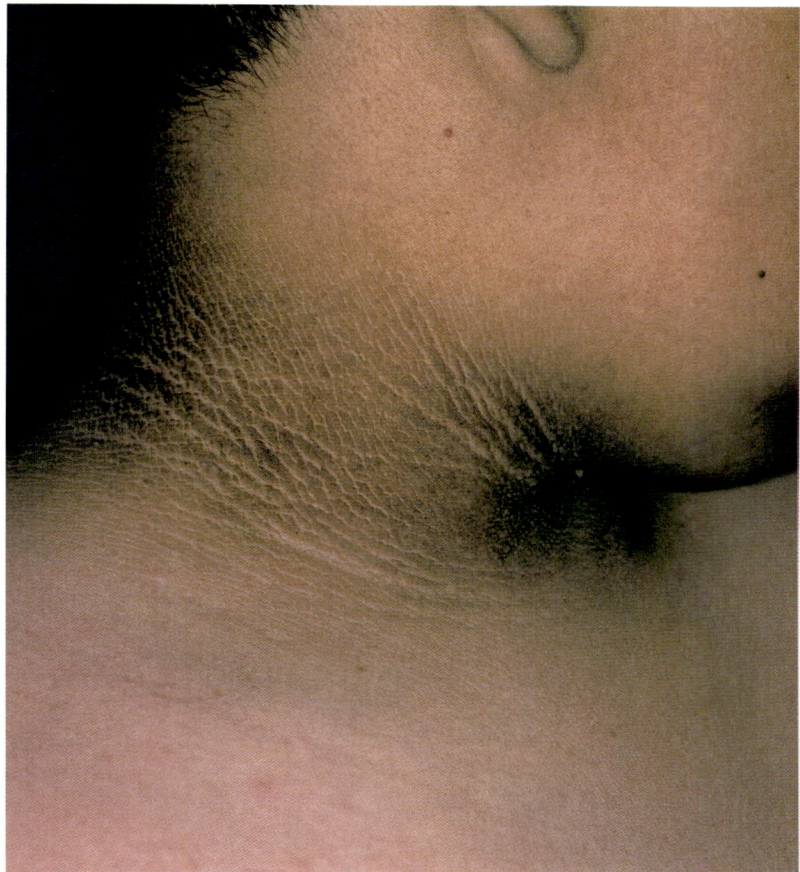

Fig. 22.15   Acanthosis nigricans of the neck in an obese adolescent boy with Down syndrome and hypothyroidism.

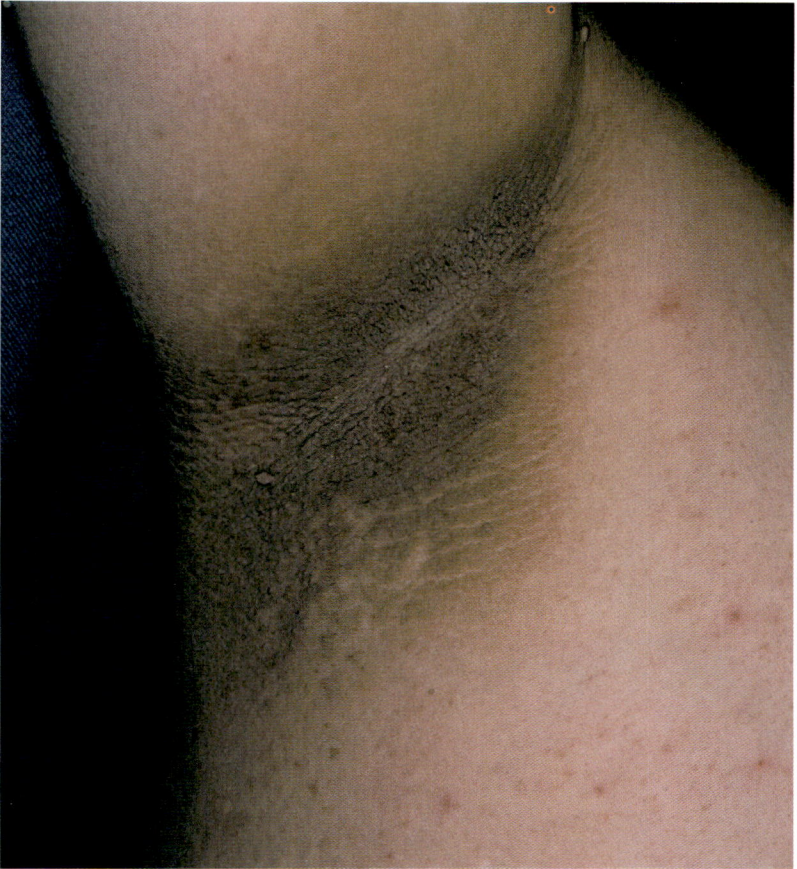

Fig. 22.16   Acanthosis nigricans of the axilla in the same patient shown in Fig. 22.15.

reproductive-aged women to avoid potential teratogenicity to development of male genitalia.

DISORDERS OF INSULIN RESISTANCE

Introduction

The concept of insulin resistance has unified a group of seemingly unrelated disorders, many of which are familiar to dermatologists. Insulin resistance is the inability of insulin to exert its metabolic effects.[105,106] It can result from a variety of mechanisms including primary and secondary disorders of the insulin receptor post-receptor defects, antibodies to the insulin receptor, and other abnormalities of gluconeogenesis. Obesity is one of the primary causes of insulin resistance. No matter what the cause, the end result is hyperinsulinemia. High circulating levels of insulin are important in the pathogenesis of a variety of disorders which will be discussed below.

ACANTHOSIS NIGRICANS

The association of acanthosis nigricans (AN) with tumors, endocrine disorders, and obesity has been noted in the literature for decades. The correlation of insulin resistance with AN has been recognized with the landmark work of Kahn *et al.* in 1976,[107] and has been reviewed more recently.[108] The old classification of "malignant" and "benign" AN should now

be discarded in favor of a more etiologic classification. There are diverse causes of insulin resistance and AN (Table 22.7); for that reason, the genetic inheritance and epidemiology of this disease cannot be discussed as such. However, the clinical findings and various pathophysiologic mechanisms for this group of syndromes are discussed below. Because AN is common, occuring in 0.5% of adolescents of European ancestry, 6% of Hispanics, 13% of African-Americans and up to 40% of native Americans,[109] dermatologists need to be aware of the associated findings.

Physical examination

Acanthosis nigricans refers to a complex of skin findings usually localized to flexural areas of the body such as the neck, axilla, groin, and under the breasts (Figs 22.15, 22.16). There is hyperpigmented, velvety, rugated hypertrophy of the overlying skin. Parents complain that their children's skin is dirty and cannot be scrubbed clean. Often there are associated papillomatous overgrowths, which appear to be skin tags. In addition to these changes in the flexural areas, one also finds firm, verrucous, hyperpigmented plaques with pebbly surfaces located over bony prominences such as elbows, knees, and knuckles (Fig. 22.17). The buccal mucosa can also develop a pebbly surface.

Laboratory findings

Laboratory findings vary with the etiology of the AN in each individual. Hyperinsulinemia seems to be present in most, if not all, cases.

105. Krook A, O'Rahilly S (1996) Mutant insulin receptors in syndromes of insulin resistance. **Bailliere's Clin Endocrinol Metab** 10(1):97–122.

106. Nakae J, Accili D (1999) The mechanism of insulin action. **J Pediatr Endocrinol Metab** 12:721–731.

107. Kahn CR, Flier JS, Bar RS et al. (1976) The syndromes of insulin resistance and acanthosis nigricans. **N Engl J Med** 294:739.

108. Schwartz RA (1994) Continuing Medical Education. Acanthosis nigricans. **J Am Acad Dermatol** 31:1–19.

109. Stuart CA, Gilkison CR, Smith MM et al. (1998) Acanthosis nigricans as a risk factor for non-insulin dependent diabetes mellitus. **Clin Pediatr** 37:73–80.

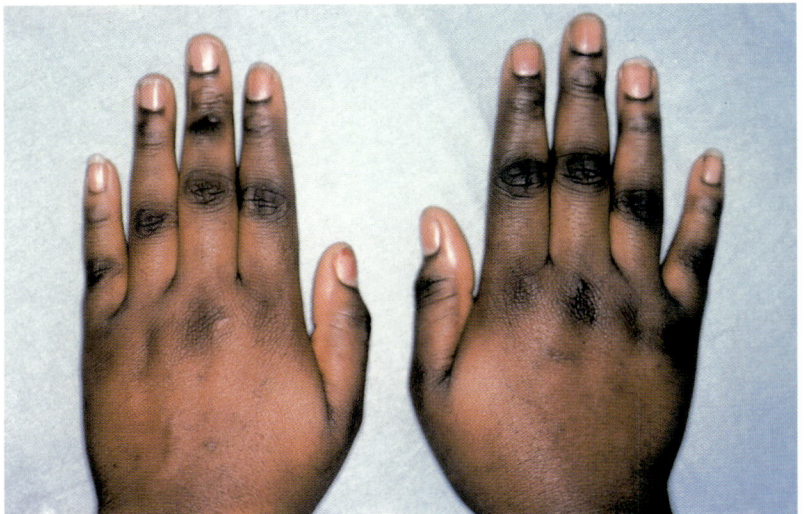

Fig. 22.17 Hyperpigmentation and skin thickening over the knuckles of a patient with acanthosis nigricans.

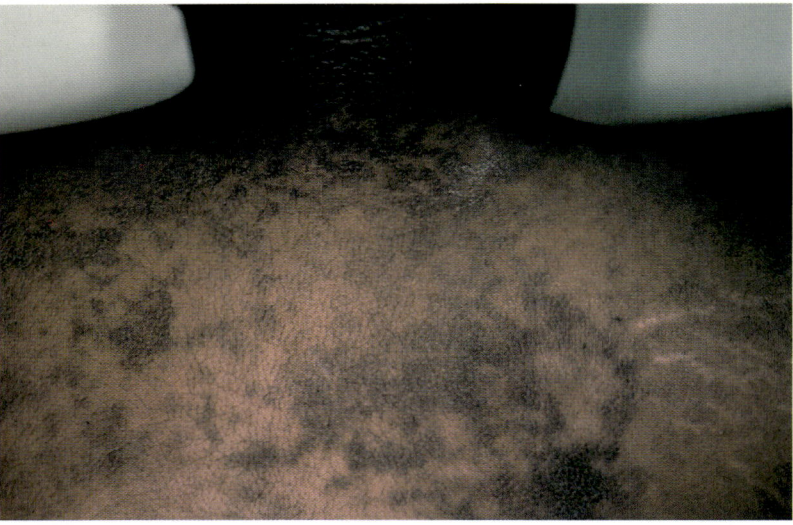

Fig. 22.18 An adolescent girl with confluent and reticulate papillomatosis of Gougerot and Carteaud on her back. This responded to therapy with minocycline.

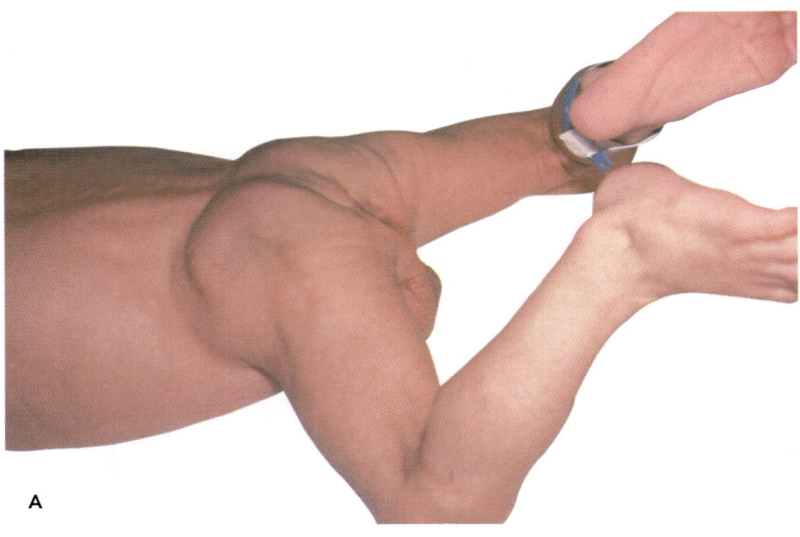

A

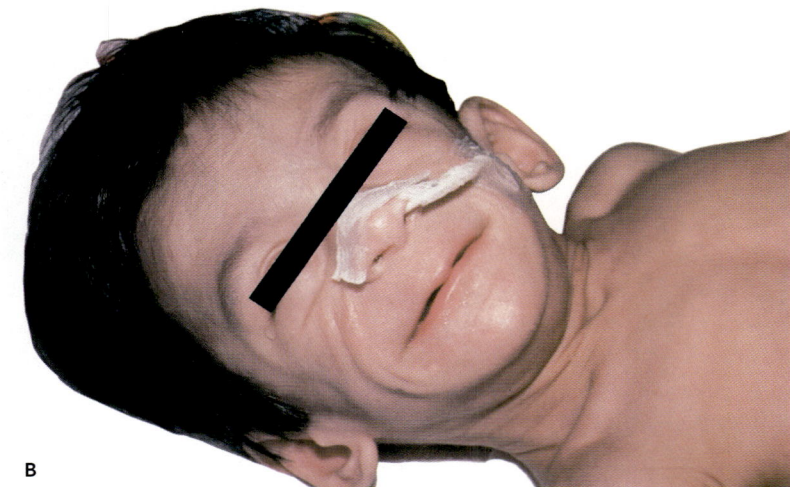

B

Fig. 22.19 An infant with leprechaunism showing lipoatrophy of the buttocks (**A**) and a typical "elfin" facies (**B**). (Photo courtesy of Dr Nancy Esterly.)

Table 22.7 summarizes many of the conditions associated with AN.

Pathophysiology and histogenesis

The term acanthosis nigricans is really a misnomer, as skin biopsy exhibits neither acanthosis nor hyperpigmentation. The primary abnormality is papillomatosis of the epidermis with orthokeratotic scale and no apparent abnormality of pigmentation. It is believed that high levels of circulating insulin directly stimulate epidermal growth, but a specific mechanism of action has not been elucidated.[109] Obesity is the most common cause of AN.

Differential diagnosis

The primary conditions simulating AN are retained keratin and confluent and reticulate papillomatosis of Gougerot and Carteaud (CARP) (Fig. 22.18). Retained keratin can be found in areas such as the supraclavicular notch, behind the ears, and on the neck, and is easily removed with alcohol, but not with soap and water. CARP is histologically identical to AN but occurs on the trunk in a reticulate pattern. Oddly, it responds to the tetracycline class of of antibiotics.[110]

Therapy and prognosis

The therapeutic options for AN itself are dismal, as it does not respond well to keratolytics or bleaching agents. Therapy of the underlying disorder, presumably thus lowering levels of circulating insulin or other peptides that are stimulating the skin, may be helpful.

Pediatric aspects of the disease

When AN is found in routine cutaneous examination, physicians should be aware of the variety of underlying associated problems and initiate appropriate diagnostic measures, especially if obesity is not present.

INSULIN RESISTANCE SYNDROMES

Leprechaunism

Patients with leprechaunism, or Donahue's disease,[111,112] have absent subcutaneous fat, acanthosis nigricans, hyperpigmentation, and hypertrichosis.

110. Fuller LC, Hay RJ (1994) Confluent and reticulate papillomatosis of Gougerot and Carteaud clearing with minocycline. **Clin Exp Dermatol** 19(4):343–345.
111. Roth SI, Schedewie HK, Herzberg VK et al. (1981) Cutaneous manifestations of leprechaunism. **Arch Dermatol** 117:531.
112. Taylor SI, Hedo JA, Underhill LH et al. (1982) Extreme insulin resistance in association with abnormally high binding affinity of insulin receptors from a patient with leprechaunism: evidence for a defect intrinsic to the receptor. **J Clin Endocrinol Metab** 55:1108.

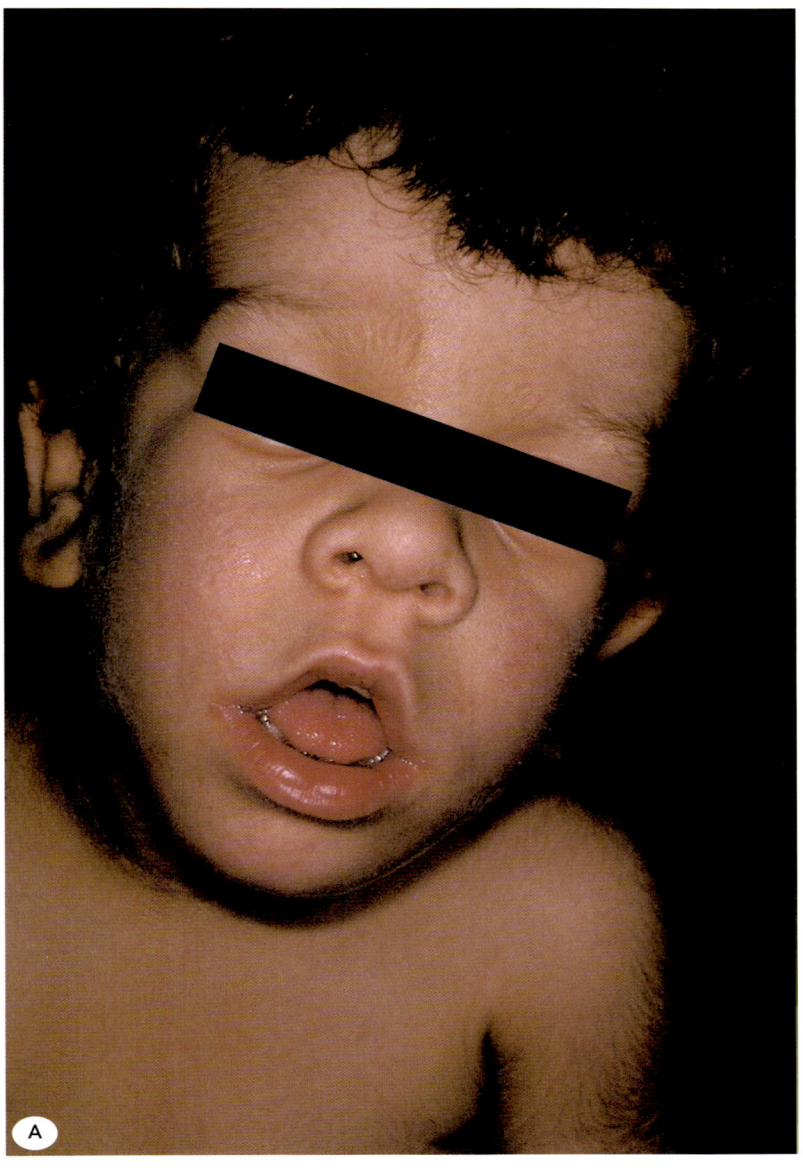

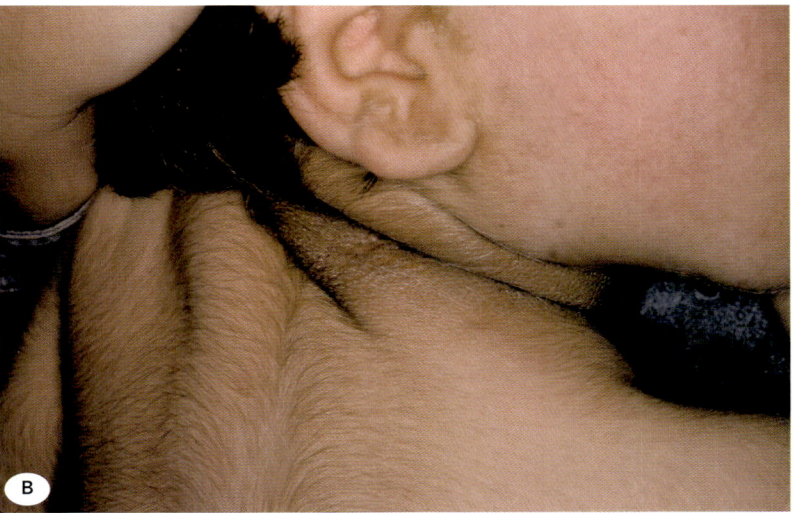

Fig. 22.20 A 3-year-old boy with Rabson–Mendenhall syndrome with coarse facial features and a "cupid's bow" mouth (A) also had hypertrichosis, low-set, large ears and acanthosis nigricans (B).

They also have distinctive features of wrinkled skin and thick lips with gingival hypertrophy leading to a so-called "elfin" facies (Fig. 22.19A,B). There is rugation of periorificial skin. In addition, patients have visceromegaly and large genitalia, and some reportedly show a yellow discoloration of the palms and soles with hyperkeratotic nodules of unknown etiology. Café-au-lait spots, coarse curly scalp hair, and low frontal hairline are associated. Some cases have been reported with dysplastic, small, hyperconvex, thin nails. Because many of these children die early and suddenly in infancy, not all have had acanthosis nigricans reported, as this is a later manifestation. In some cases, mutations in the insulin receptor gene have been identified.[105]

Rabson–Mendenhall syndrome

Children with this rare syndrome have severe disorders of glucose metabolism with hypo- and hyperglycemia at different stages of life. They have acanthosis nigricans, unusual coarse facies (Fig. 22.20A,B), and may exhibit pineal hypertrophy and sexual precocity. Mutations in the insulin receptor gene have been found in some cases.[113,114]

The lipodystrophies

Generalized lipodystrophies

The congenital, autosomal-dominant, Beradinelli–Seip type is characterized by acanthosis nigricans, hyperhidrosis, thick hair, and muscular hypertrophy (Fig. 22.21). The patients have a high anabolic rate, precocious growth and development, and, unfortunately, cardiomyopathy that can lead to early death. It is due to a post-receptor glucose transport defect. The acquired, autosomal-recessive or post-viral Seip–Lawrence type has similar features, but they are milder. There are associated xanthomas and autoimmune disorders.[115,116]

Partial lipodystrophies

The autosomal-recessive or sporadic cephalothoracic type exhibits loss of fat in the face and upper thorax. Mainly females are affected. These women are at risk for C3 deficiency and glomerulonephritis.[115] The autosomal-dominant or X-linked face-sparing Dunnigan–Koeberling type is characterized by excess fat on the face and neck with lipoatrophy on the limbs. Most patients

113. Longo N, Wang Y, Pasquali M (1999) Progressive decline in insulin levels in Rabson-Mendenhall syndrome. **J Clin Endocrinol Metab** 84(8):2623–2629.
114. Takahashi Y, Kadowaki H, Ando A et al. (1998) Two aberrant splicings caused by mutations in the insulin receptor gene in cultured lymphocytes from a patient with Rabson-Mendenhall's syndrome. **J Clin Invest** 101:588–594.
115. Seip M, Trygstad O (1996) Generalized lipodystrophy, congenital and acquired (lipoatrophy). **Acta Paediatr** Suppl 413:2–28.
116. Sovik O, Vestergaard H, Trygstad O, Pedersen O (1996) Studies of insulin resistance in congenital generalized lipodystrophy. **Acta Paediatr** Suppl 413:29–38.

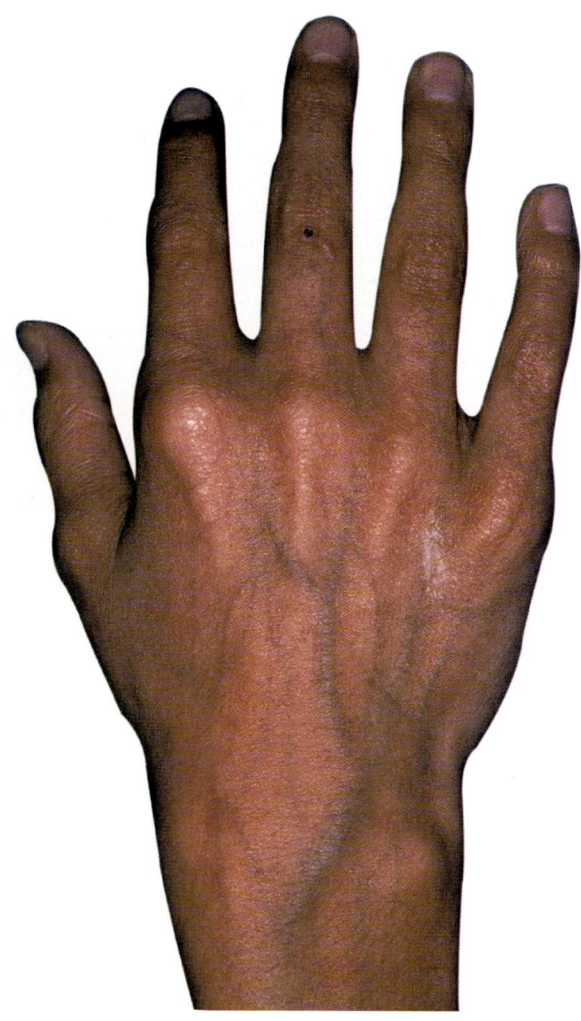

Fig. 22.21   The hand of a 7-year-old girl with congenital, generalized lipoatrophy.

are female. They exhibit acanthosis nigricans, xanthomas, and a high metabolic rate.[115,117]

Polycystic ovary syndrome (PCOS)

PCOS may be the most common endocrinopathy in women, affecting 4–12% of reproductive-aged females.[71,118] It has been described by a variety of names including Stein–Leventhal syndrome, HAIR-AN syndrome, Syndrome X, and SAPHO syndrome: all of these reports are describing the same group of patients. Earlier diagnoses are being made in pubertal and even prepubertal girls. There is some evidence that PCOS may be genetic.[70,71] Dermatologists and pediatricians are likely to see these patients because of cutaneous manifestations such as acne, hirsutism, and androgenetic alopecia. However, irregular or absent menstrual periods, obesity, ovarian cysts, and infertility can be presenting complaints.

The physical examination of these patients is similar to that described above for women with androgen excess. Not all patients are obese. Acanthosis nigricans, especially in the thin patient, may be a clue of underlying insulin resistance. The specific android body habitus with a high waist:hip ratio of greater than 0.85 is also characteristic.

Laboratory findings

Laboratory findings are similar to those found in other hyper-androgenic disorders with elevations in DHEAS, free testosterone, and a ratio of LH:FSH of > 3:1. However, many patients with PCOS will have normal laboratory studies, perhaps because a single blood test only reflects one moment in time and is not an indication of integrated hormone levels. Because of the risks for more serious metabolic disorders in PCOS (discussed below), other studies should be obtained in patients suspected of having PCOS: fasting blood glucose and insulin levels may reveal elevated insulin levels and/or NIDDM; a fasting lipid profile may show hypertriglyceridemia with elevated VLDL and LDL cholesterol and low HDL cholesterol.

Pathophysiology

The pathophysiology of PCOS is complex, but appears to be related to insulin resistance. Anovulation with the physical findings noted above usually make the diagnosis. Not all patients need to have ovarian cysts, and conversely not all patients with ovarian cysts have PCOS. Similarly, not all patients have demonstrably high insulin levels, especially the younger girls. Four categories of medical consequences of insulin resistance and PCOS are important (Table 22.8): (1) Hyperandrogenism;[70,71] the primary origin of elevated androgen in PCOS is the ovary and insulin stimulation of ovarian cells as well stimulate the ovary to promote steroidogenesis has been demonstrated *in vitro*,[119] and this propensity may be genetic and intrinsic to ovarian cells from women with PCOS. The adrenal gland also responds to hyperinsulinemia with high output of DHEA. (2) Obesity;[70,91] insulin resistance is directly related to obesity of any cause. In turn, it is difficult for women with PCOS to lose weight, and therapy with insulin-lowering agents may reverse this. (3) Early onset NIDDM;[70,71,120] women with PCOS are more likely to develop NIDDM and the earliest signs are elevated fasting plasma insulin levels or slight elevations of fasting glucose. Oral glucose tolerance tests may be helpful in borderline cases. (4) Early cardiovascular disease; patients with PCOS have a variety of risks including early macrovascular coronary artery disease, such as angina, myocardial infarction, stroke, dyslipidemias, hypercoagulability, hypertension and early death.[121]

Therapy and prognosis

Therapy for PCOS needs to be individualized for the specific concerns of each particular patient (i.e., acne, hirsutism, alopecia, infertility etc.). Weight reduction and exercise are simple measures that can lower insulin resistance and reduce risks. The standard therapy for acne, hirsutism, and androgenetic alopecia is noted above. However, the recent availability of drugs for NIDDM

TABLE 22.8	**Medical consequences of insulin resistance**
Hyperandrogenism	
Acne	
Hirsutism	
Androgenetic alopecia	
Non-insulin dependent diabetes mellitus	
Obesity	
Cardiovascular disease	
Coronary artery disease	
Dyslipidemia	
Hypercoagulability	
Hypertension	

117. Jackson SNJ, Howlett TA, McNally PG et al. (1997) Dunnigan-Kobberling syndrome: An autosomal dominant form of partial lipodystrophy. Q J Med 90:27–36.
118. Knochenhauer ES, Key TJ, Kahsar-Miller M et al. (1998) Prevalence of the polycystic ovary syndrome in unselected black and white women of the Southeastern United States: a prospective study. J Clin Endocrinol Metab 83(9):3078–3082.
119. Franks S, Gilling-Smith C, Watson H, Willis D (1999) Insulin action in the normal and polycystic ovary. Endocrinol Metab Clin North Am 28(2):361–378.
120. Legro RS, Kunselman AR, Dodson WC, Dunaif A (1999) Prevalence and predictors of risk for Type 2 diabetes mellitus and impaired glucose tolerance in polycystic ovary syndrome: A prospective, controlled study in 254 affected women. J Clin Endocrinol Metab 85(1):165–169.
121. Amowitz LL, Sobel BE (1999) Cardiovascular consequences of polycystic ovary syndrome. Endocrinol Metab Clin North Am 28(2):439–458.

that lower insulin levels may enhance the dermatologists' therapeutic armamentarium. Metformin, a bioguanide that improves insulin resistance probably via enhanced gluconeogenesis, has been noted to reduce obesity, lower serum lipids, improve fibrinolysis and induce ovulation in infertile women with PCOS.[122,123] The thiazolidinediones (the "glitazones") including troglitazone, roziglitazone, and pioglitazone reduce insulin resistance through activation of PPAR λ.[124,125] Troglitazone has been removed from the US market because of hepatotoxicity. Although none of these agents has been studied for specific effects on acne, hirsutism, or androgenetic alopecia, they may turn out to be useful. Because many patients with PCOS may be treated with insulin-lowering agents, dermatologists should be familiar with them.

Pediatric aspects of the disease

PCOS may present in prepubertal girls with acanthosis nigricans, premature adrenarche, or very early acne. Recognition of these high-risk factors, especially in light of a positive family history of PCOS, should allow early diagnosis, but the classic hallmarks of PCOS may not be apparent for several years. Careful follow-up of girls suspected to have PCOS, with repeat monitoring of laboratory studies, may lead to early diagnosis and prevent some of the severe medical consequences of PCOS.

TABLE 22.9   Cutaneous changes in diabetes mellitus

Skin disorders associated primarily with diabetes mellitus
    Limited joint mobility syndrome
    Waxy skin syndrome
    Finger pebbles
    Pigmented pretibial patches
    Necrobiosis lipoidica diabeticorum
    Disseminated granuloma annulare[a]
    Bullosis diabeticorum[a]
    Scleredema of Buschke[a]
    Kyrle's disease[a]

Skin disorders secondary to complications of diabetes mellitus
    Eruptive xanthomas
    Lipoatrophy/lipohypertrophy at injection site
    Infections
        Candidiasis
        Severe, recurrent staphylococcal infections
        Malignant otitis externa (*Pseudomonas*)

Associated cutaneous manifestations of diabetes mellitus
    Vitiligo
    Acanthosis nigricans
    Hemochromatosis
    Lipodystrophy

[a] Rarely reported in childhood.

DIABETES MELLITUS

Cutaneous findings in diabetes mellitus can be related primarily to the disease process, associated with the diabetic state, secondary to infection, manifestations of related diseases, or a response to therapy (Table 22.9).[126,127]

Type I is insulin-dependent diabetes mellitus (IDDM), which used to be called juvenile, ketosis-prone, or brittle diabetes. Type II is non-insulin-dependent diabetes mellitus (NIDDM), which was formerly called the adult-onset form. Because both types may occur in either childhood or adult life, the designations Types I and II are preferable. Most children have IDDM. Diabetes mellitus can also occur secondary to disorders that destroy the pancreatic islet cells, such as hemochromatosis or cystic fibrosis, or may occur in one of the insulin-resistance syndromes.

Epidemiology

About 5% of the world population has diabetes,[128] and about half of these patients have cutaneous manifestations.[128,129]

A prevalence rate of 0.9 in 1000 schoolchildren has been reported.[130] Male-to-female ratios appear equal. Blacks develop IDDM only 20–30% as often as whites.

Presenting history

Type I diabetes mellitus in childhood presents with a relatively short history, usually less than one month, of polyuria, polydypsia, polyphagia, and weight loss. Less often, there is frank diabetic ketoacidosis as an initial symptom with Kussmaul breathing, prostration, coma, and shock. Some skin manifestations of diabetes mellitus, notably necrobiosis lipoidica diabeticorum (NLD), may precede the onset of Type I diabetes mellitus.

Physical examination

The cutaneous changes associated with diabetes mellitus are summarised in Table 22.9

Primary skin disease associated with diabetes mellitus

Limited joint-mobility syndrome, waxy skin, and finger pebbles

These changes occur in up to 30% of Type I diabetics in the first two decades.[131–134] The limited joint-mobility syndrome consists of diffuse, although sometimes subtle, joint contractures of the hands with inability to fully extend the fingers (Fig. 22.22). There is thickened waxy skin, especially on the dorsa of the hands, and there may be stiffness of the large joints. There may be a pebbly appearance to the skin, but these finger pebbles are more common in adults with NIDDM.[135] Limited joint mobility is seen in patients with poor growth and short stature. It has been associated with duration but not with severity of disease. The contractures are analogous to Dupuytren's contractures in adults and appear to affect the fourth and fifth fingers most commonly. Histologically, the thick waxy skin shows increased dermal collagen. Although the changes may be described as scleroderma-like,[136] there have been no reports of atrophy or pigmentary alterations. It has been

122. Pugeat M, Ducluzeau PH (1999) Insulin resistance, polycystic ovary syndrome and metformin. **Drugs** 58(Suppl) 1:41–46.
123. Moghetti P, Castello R, Negri C et al. (1985) Metformin effects on clinical features, endocrine and metabolic profiles and insulin sensitivity in polycystic ovary syndrome: a randomized, double-blind placebo-controlled 6-month trial, followed by open, long-term clinical evaluation. **J Clin Endocrinol Metab** 85(1):139–146.
124. Balfour JA, Plosker G (1999) Rosiglitazone. **Drugs** 57(6):921–930.
125. Horikoshi H, Hashimoto t, Fujiwara T (2000) Troglitazone and emerging glitazones: new avenues for potential therapeutic benefits beyond glycemic control. **Prog Drug Res** 54:191–212.
126. Edidin DV (1985) Cutaneous manifestations of diabetes mellitus in children. **Pediatr Dermatol** 2:161.
127. Perez MI, Kohn SR (1994) Cutaneous manifestations of diabetes mellitus. **J Am Acad Dermatol** 30(4):519–531.
128. Paron NG, Lambert PW (2000) Cutaneous manifestations of diabetes mellitus. **Dermatology** 27(2):371–383.
129. Romano G, Moretti G, Di Benedetto A et al. (1998) Skin lesions in diabetes mellitus: prevalence and clinical correlations. **Diabetes Research and Clinical Practice** 39:101–106.
130. Sperling MA (1982) Diabetes mellitus. In: Clinical Pediatric and Adolescent Endocrinology, Kaplan SA, ed. Philadelphia: WB Saunders, p. 131.
131. Grgic A, Rosenbloom AL, Weber FT et al. (1976) Joint contracture – common manifestation of childhood diabetes mellitus. **J Pediatr** 88:584.
132. Rosenbloom AL, Silverstein JH, Lezotte DC et al. (1981) Limited joint mobility in childhood diabetes mellitus indicates increased risk for microvascular disease. **N Engl J Med** 305:191.
133. Seibold JR (1982) Digital sclerosis in children with insulin-dependent diabetes mellitus. **Arthritis Rheum** 25:1357.
134. Rosenbloom AL, Silverstein JH, Lezotte DC et al. (1982) Limited joint mobility in diabetes mellitus of childhood: natural history and relationship to growth impairment. **J Pediatr** 101:874.
135. Huntley AC (1986) Finger pebbles: A common finding in diabetes mellitus. **J Am Acad Dermatol** 14:612–617.
136. Buckingham BA, Uitto J, Sandborg C et al. (1984) Scleroderma-like changes in insulin-dependent diabetes mellitus: clinical and biochemical studies. **Diabetes Care** 7:163.

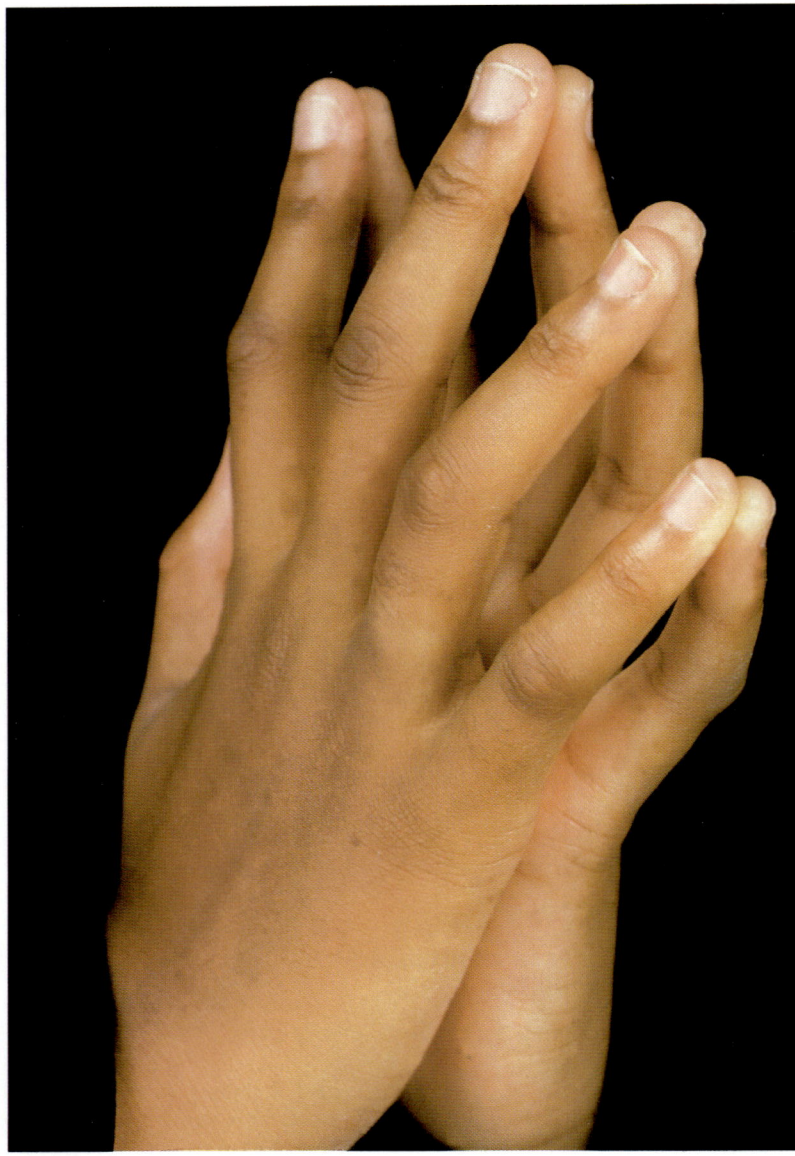

Fig. 22.22 Contractures of the fingers with inability to fully extend the digits and approximate the palms is the hallmark of the limited joint-mobility syndrome seen in type I diabetes. There is also a waxy thickening of the skin on the dorsa of the hands. (From Rosenbloom et al.,[123] with permission.)

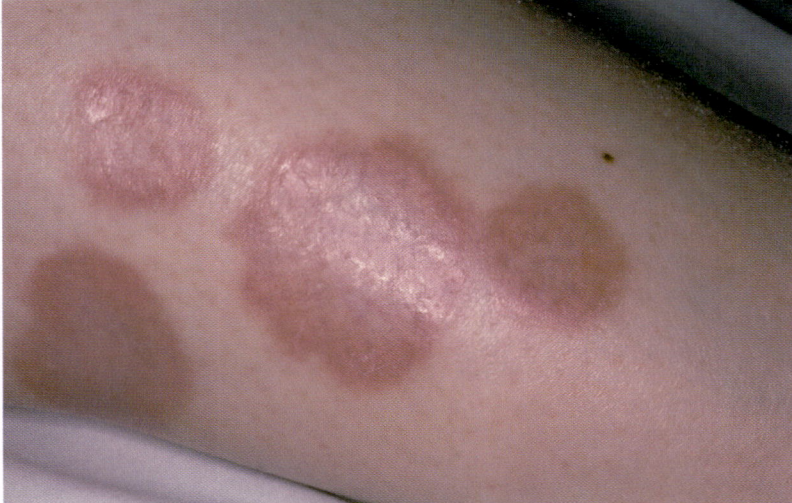

Fig. 22.23 Necrobiosis lipoidica diabeticorum (NLD) on the anterior tibia of a 14-year-old girl. These lesions preceded the onset of her insulin-dependent diabetes mellitus.

deposits of acid mucopolysaccharides have been noted. The lesions of diabetic dermopathy do not evolve into NLD. They may resolve and often leave brown hyperpigmentation.

Necrobiosis lipoidica diabeticorum

NLD lesions also characteristically appear on the anterior tibiae (Fig. 22.23) but may be found on the upper extremities and on the trunk on rare occasions.[127] The skin lesions may precede the onset of diabetes mellitus. The primary lesions are oval plaques that expand up to several centimeters in size from their origins as small erythematous papules. The borders are usually sharply demarcated, somewhat raised, and more erythematous than the center of the lesion. There is rarely some scale at the borders. Centrally, there may be a waxy, translucent, atrophic epidermis with colors ranging from red to brown to a characteristic yellow. Often, the atrophy is so prominent that large subcutaneous vessels are easily visible coursing under the surface of the plaque. There is a tendency to ulceration with slow healing. Histologically, there is necrobiosis of collagen and infiltration of collagen bundles with pallisading histiocytes and accumulations of mucin. This histology closely resembles granuloma annulare as well as rheumatoid nodule.

High-potency topical corticosteroids under occlusion and intralesional steroids have been tried for NLD with minimal success. In some cases, grafting has improved cosmetic appearance.[139] Aspirin and dipyridamole were not successful treatments.[140]

Granuloma annulare

The common childhood form of localized granuloma annulare (GA), consisting of discrete rings with raised papular borders that occur in countable numbers, does not correlate well with the presence of diabetes mellitus. Such patients with typical GA need not be studied for the presence of diabetes or glucose intolerance. In addition, because most children develop IDDM of rapid, rather than insidious, onset, a prospective glucose tolerance test (GTT) is not indicated in GA (Fig. 22.24). It is not clear whether the disseminated form of GA, especially in elderly patients, is associated with diabetes; estimates of 12–15% have been published,[141,142] but one study of subcutaneous GA in

postulated that accumulations of glycosylated proteins in the collagen matrix or increased fibroblast proliferation are responsible.

Diabetic dermopathy

Pigmented pretibial patches or shin spots are seen in up to 50% of adult diabetics; they are rare, but do occur in childhood.[137,138] Lesions begin as small pretibial papules and evolve into 1–2cm patches that have a brownish-red to yellow color and may be depressed. There is no waxy alteration of the epidermis such as seen in NLD. Histopathology is similar to the progressive pigmented purpuras with extravasated red blood cells (RBCs), hemosiderin, and mild perivascular lymphohistiocytic infiltrate. Increased

137. Danowski TS, Sabeh G, Sarver ME et al. (1966) Shin spots and diabetes mellitus. **Am J Med Sci** 106:104.
138. Bauer MF, Levan NE, Frankel A, Bach J (1966) Pigmented pretibial patches. **Arch Dermatol** 93:282.
139. Marr TJ, Traisman HS, Griffith BH, Schafer MA (1977) Necrobiosis lipoidica diabeticorum in a juvenile diabetic. **Cutis** 19:348.
140. Statham B, Finlay AY, Marks R (1980) A randomized double blind comparison of an aspirin dipyridamole combination versus a placebo in the treatment of necrobiosis lipoidica. **Acta Derm Venereol** (Stockh) 61:270.
141. Studer EM, Calza AM, Saurat JH (1996) Precipitating factors and associated diseases in 84 patients with granuloma annulare: a retrospective study. **Dermatology** 193(4):364–368.
142. Tan HH, Goh CL (2000) Granuloma annulare: A review of 41 cases at the National Skin Centre. **Ann Acad Med Singapore** 29(6):714–718.

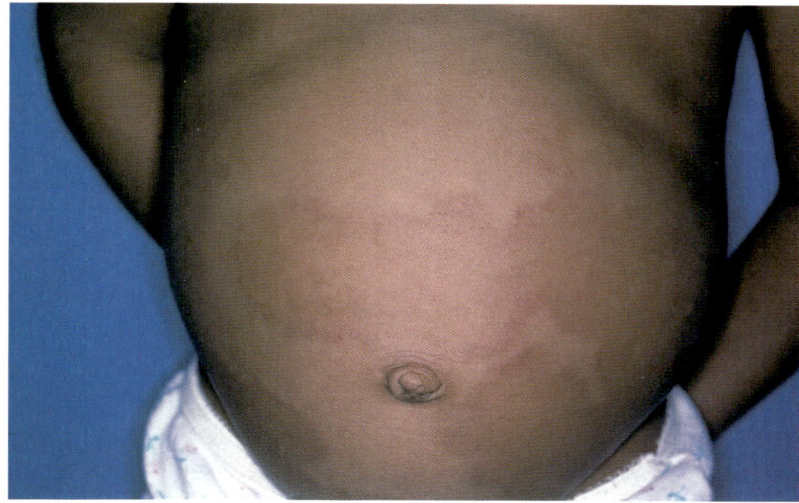

Fig. 22.24   Large plaques of granuloma annulare on the abdomen of a toddler who had developed IDDM at age 1 year.

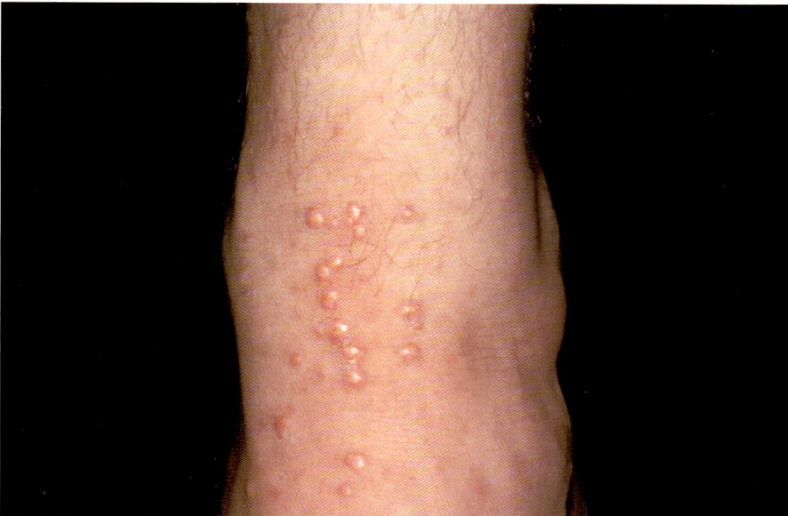

Fig. 22.25   Pink-yellow firm papules, here in linear array, on the ankle of a type I diabetic patient in poor control. He had massively elevated triglycerides as the basis of his eruptive xanthomas.

children under age 10 years revealed diabetes in 6% (2/34) [143] Lesions resembling GA have been noted on the anterior tibiae in proximity to, or in association with, typical lesions of NLD; rarely, these two disorders have been reported to coexist.[144] It may be a matter of semantics whether such pretibial lesions are distinctly NLD and/or GA. GA may be long-standing but eventually resolves without scarring.

Diabetic skin changes primarily found in adults

Bullosis diabeticorum
Tense bullae on the distal portions of the extremities that appear without preceding trauma and usually resolve without scarring have been reported in adults with long-standing diabetes mellitus.[145]

Scleredema
In scleredema adultorum of Buschke, broad areas of woody, hard nonpitting edema with erythema typically appearing on the upper back have been noted in long-standing, poorly controlled adult diabetics who have many microangiopathic complications.

Perforating disorders
Disorders such as Kyrle's disease (hyperkeratosis follicularis et parafollicularis in cutem penetrans) and/or reactive perforating collagenosis have been described in adults with DM, often when they are in renal failure and receiving dialysis.

Diabetic ulcers
In long-standing IDDM, ulcerations of the distal lower extremities with eventual gangrene can occur on the basis of poor peripheral perfusion and secondary trauma if there is severe neuropathy. Diabetic ulcers are rare in childhood.

Skin disorders secondary to metabolic changes in diabetes mellitus

Eruptive xanthomas
In IDDM that is poorly controlled, there may be massive hypertriglyceridemia. In such cases, there may be sudden appearance of diffuse xan-

thomatosis. Lesions consist of firm, 1–3mm red to yellow papules that may coalesce (Fig. 22.25) or appear in linear array in lesions of previous trauma to the skin (Köbner's phenomenon). With control of the hyperlipidemia, the lesions resolve.

Local lipodystrophy at injection sites
Paradoxically, both lipoatrophy and/or lipohypertrophy may occur at sites of insulin injection. Hypertrophic lesions are composed of collagen mixed with adipose tissue and are often anesthetic and preferred by juvenile diabetics for injection sites. However, absorption from these sites is erratic.

Local reactions to insulin
Local cutaneous reactions at the site of injection of insulin used to occur in 15–55% of patients.[146] These are rare with the use of human recombinant insulin.

Infections associated with diabetes mellitus

It is not established whether cutaneous fungal and bacterial infections are more common in diabetics or simply more severe when they occur. *Candida* can be found in many locations: oral mucosa (thrush), vaginal mucosa (vaginitis), on the nail (onychomycosis), or surrounding soft tissues (paronychia), in the toe and the finger webs (blastomycosis erosio interdigitalis), or on moist flexural surfaces (intertrigo). Topical anticandidal therapy usually is effective. Recurrent staphylococcal furunculosis is common in diabetics. Patients may be intranasal *Staphylococcus* carriers or may have recurrent insignificant staphylococcal folliculitis, which then develops into more serious lesions. Chronic or intermittent systemic antibiotics, antibacterial cleansers, and intranasal antibiotic ointment may be helpful. Mucormycosis of the nasal cavity can cause perforation in poorly controlled disease, usually in elderly diabetics, and is usually fatal. Malignant otitis externa due to *Pseudomonas aeruginosa* has been reported as a complication of diabetes in elderly patients. Although a few cases of this destructive infection have been reported in childhood,[147] only one has been associated with diabetes.[148]

143. Grogg KL, Nascimento AG (2001) Subcutaneous granuloma annulare in childhood: clinicopathologic features in 34 cases. **Pediatrics** 107(3):E42.
144. Schwartz ME (1982) Necrobiosis lipoidica and granuloma annulare. **Arch Dermatol** 118:192.
145. Paltzik RL (1980) Bullous eruption of diabetes mellitus. Bullosis diabeticorum. **Arch Dermatol** 116:475.
146. Kahn CR, Rosenthal AS (1979) Immunologic reactions to insulin: insulin allergy, insulin resistance, and the autoimmune insulin syndrome. **Diabetes Care** 2:283.
147. Joachims HZ (1976) Malignant external otitis in children. **Arch Otolaryngol** 102:236.
148. Merritt WT, Bass JW, Bruhn FW (1980) Malignant external otitis in an adolescent with diabetes. **J Pediatr** 96:872.

Other disorders associated with diabetes mellitus

Vitiligo, psoriasis, and eczema

These disorders were found in nearly 10% of a series of 64 patients with IDDM[129] suggesting a possible autoimmune link between these disorders.

Lipodystrophies

Congenital, acquired, partial, or total, lipodystrophies have been associated with diabetes mellitus, and underlying insulin resistance (see above).

Hemochromatosis

Either primary or secondary, excessive iron deposition can lead to destruction of pancreatic islet cells and produce so-called bronze diabetes, which is insulin dependent. Such patients have diffuse, deep hyperpigmentation, due not only to deposits of iron but to hypermelanization as well. Hemochromatosis can be primary or secondary to multiple transfusion therapy for diseases such as thalassemia.

Pathophysiology and histogenesis

There is a distinct familial predisposition to development of IDDM with preponderance of HLADR3, and HLADR4.[127] However, clear-cut evidence for autosomal-recessive or dominant inheritance is lacking.

Environmental triggers such as viral infections and autoimmune mechanisms also appear to play a role. A major debate remains as to whether chronic hyperglycemia plays a role in the secondary complications of diabetes mellitus. There is evidence that non-enzymatic glycosylation of many proteins, including dermal collagen, may play an etiologic role in the ultimate degeneration and destruction of tissues.[149–151] Glycosylated hemoglobin A₁C is used as a marker of diabetic control. Several studies on glycosylation of collagen in patients with diabetes have indicated that diabetic collagen is less acid soluble, less susceptible to collagenase, and more susceptible to increased cross-linking than collagen from normal controls. This structural alteration in the collagen protein resembles accelerated aging in many ways and may explain some of the cutaneous manifestations of diabetes mellitus. Similarly, glycosylation of basement membrane proteins around endothelial cells may explain the widespread capillary microangiopathy characteristic of diabetes mellitus. Another theory involves sorbitol accumulation in tissues with secondary edema.

Therapy

The only treatment for Type I diabetes mellitus at this time is parenteral administration of human recombinant insulin. Current therapeutics[152] are leaning toward more stringent control of hyperglycemia with either multiple daily injections or computer-controlled insulin pumps maintaining normal blood glucose levels. On the horizon is an intranasal preparation of insulin which may be a useful new method for delivery.

DISORDERS OF G PROTEIN SIGNAL TRANSDUCTION

Introduction

Several endocrine disorders have been attributed to mutations in G (guanine nucleotide) stimulating protein signal transduction. G proteins couple receptors for many hormones to effectors that regulate second messenger metabolism.[153–155] Mutations in G proteins or their receptors may result in loss or gain of function. Loss-of-function mutations create hormone resistance. Gain-of-function mutations create hormone hypersecretion. Relevant to dermatology are two syndromes caused by mutations in the GNAS1 gene which codes for G$_s$-α: pseudohypoparathyroidism (Albright's hereditary osteodystrophy) which results from a loss-of-function mutation causing resistance to Parathyroid Hormone (PTH); and polyostotic fibrous dysplasia with multiple endocrine abnormalities and café au lait spots (McCune–Albright syndrome) which results from a gain-of-function mutation causing excessive endocrine function, especially precocious puberty.

PSEUDOHYPOPARATHYROIDISM

Pseudohypoparathyroidism (PHP1a), also known as Albright's hereditary osteodystrophy, is an autosomal-dominant disorder which has a distinctive phenotype.[156] Patients present with typical facies and body habitus and may exhibit signs of hypocalcemia. Typically, they have a round face with a broad, flat nasal bridge, short stature with brachydactyly (broad, short digits) and short fourth and sometimes fifth metacarpals and metatarsals causing dimpling of the knuckles, especially of the fourth and fifth fingers (Figs 22.26A, B, C). Patients have ectopic calcifications in the basal ganglia, calcinosis cutis, and, most diagnostically, osteoma cutis (Fig. 22.27). Osteoma cutis can present at birth or in the early years of life and may be an important first sign of PHP.[156–160] Mental retardation was initially considered to be part of the syndrome. However, children treated early and aggressively with calcium and 25-hydroxy vitamin D appear to develop normally, suggesting that prolonged hypocalcemia was the cause of the delayed development.[161] Concurrent hypothyroidism is usually found, although its onset may be delayed. This is not surprising because resistance to thyroid stimulating hormone (TSH) is also a result of the loss-of-function mutation.[162]

Laboratory findings include hypocalcemia, hyperphosphatemia, and elevated serum levels of PTH. There is an absent urinary cyclic AMP response to PTH stimulation. Those with hypothyroidism have elevated levels of TSH. Radiographs of the hands reveal short fourth and fifth metacarpals.

As noted above, the underlying causes are loss-of-function mutations of the gene that encodes G$_s$-α (GNAS1) located on chromosome 20q13.3.[153,155,162] Therapy consists of prospective monitoring for development of hypocalcemia, hyperphosphatemia, and rising levels of serum PTH and TSH. These changes may occur in infancy or later in childhood, and require replacement with appropriate doses of calcium, Vitamin D, and thyroid hormone.

Pseudo-pseudohypoparathyroidism (PPHP) is the cumbersome term used to denote a phenotype identical to pseudohypoparathyroidism but without the hypocalcemia. It has been postulated, but not proven, that the difference between PHP and PPHP may be due to paternal imprinting:[162–164] if only the allele from the mother is expressed and the mother is the source of the mutant gene, the full phenotype (PHP) will be expressed. If the father's allele is the affected one, progressive osseous heteroplasia (POH), a disorder with osteoma cutis without the PPH phenotype occurs.[165] However, infants with normocalcemia who have congenital osteoma cutis or a primary relative with pseudohypoparathyroidism need to be prospectively and closely followed

149. Chang K, Uitto J, Rowold EA et al. (1980) Increased collagen cross-linkages in experimental diabetes. Reversal by β-aminopropionitrile and D-penicillamine. **Diabetes** 29:778.
150. Kohn RR, Schnider SL (1982) Glucosylation of human collagen. **Diabetes** 31(suppl) 3:47.
151. Kirschenbaum DM (1984) Glycosylation of proteins: its implications in diabetic control and complications. **Pediatr Clin North Am** 31:611.
152. Santiago JV (1993) Insulin therapy in the last decade. **Diabetes Care** 16(suppl) 3:143.
153. Aldred MA, Trembath RC (2000) Activating and inactivating mutations in the human GNAS1 Gene. **Hum Mutat** 16:183–189.
154. Bastepe M, Juppner H (2000) Pseudohypoparathyroidism: New insights into an old disease. **Endocrinol Metab Clinics N Amer** 29:569–589.
155. Spiegel A (2000) Protein defects in signal transduction. **Horm Res** 53(suppl 3):17–22.
156. Prendiville JS, Lucky AW, Mallory SB et al. (1992) Osteoma cutis as a presenting sign of pseudohypoparathyroidism. **Pediatr Dermatol** 9:11.
157. Izraeli S, Metzker A, Horev G et al. (1992) Albright hereditary osteodystrophy with hypothyroidism, normocalcemia, and normal Gs protein activity: a family presenting with congenital osteoma cutis. **Am J Med Genet** 43:764.
158. Lucky AW, Tsang R (1997) Clinical vignette pseudopseudohypoparathyroidism, presenting with osteoma cutis. **Bone Mineral Res** 12:995.
159. Kappy M, Kummer M, Tyson RW et al. (1999) Pathological case of the month. Osteoma cutis/pseudohypoparathyroidism **Arch Pediatr Adolesc Med** 153:427–428.
160. Goeteyn V, De Potter, CR, Naeyaert JM (1999) Osteoma cutis in pseudohypoparathyroidism. **Dermatology** 198:209–211.
161. Patten JL, Johns DR, Valle D et al. (1990) Mutation in the gene encoding the stimulatory G protein of adenylate cyclase in Albright's hereditary osteodystrophy. **N Engl J Med** 322:1412.
162. Spiegel AM (1999) Hormone resistance caused by mutations in G proteins and G protein-coupled receptors. **J Pediatr Endocrinol Metab** 12:303–309.
163. Nakamoto JM, Sandstrom AT, Brickman AS et al. (1998) Pseudohypoparathyroidism type Ia from maternal but not paternal transmission of a G$_s$α gene mutation. **Am J of Med Genetics** 77:261–267.
164. Lui J, Litman D, Rosenberg MJ et al. (2000) A GNAS1 imprinting defect in pseudohypoparathyroidism type IB. **J Clin Invest** 106:1167–1174.
165. Shore EM, Ahn J, Jan de Beurs S et al. (2002) Paternally inherited inactivating mutations of the GNAS1 gene in progressive osseous heteroplasia. **N Engl J Med** 346:99–106.

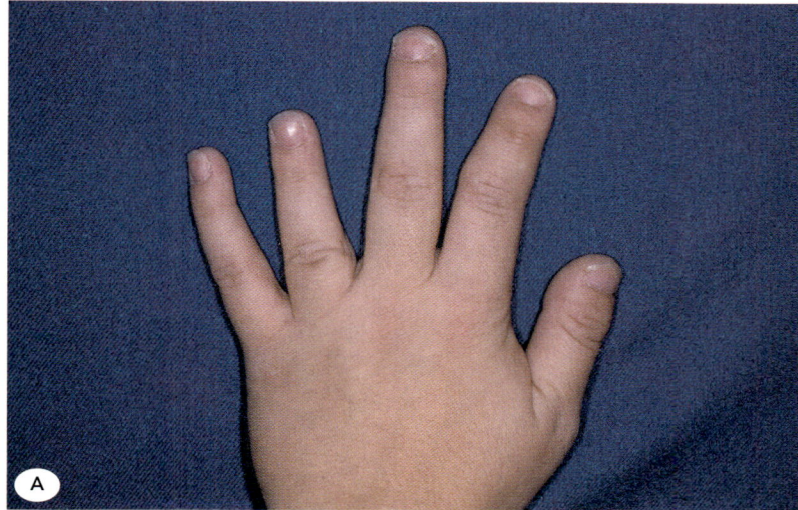

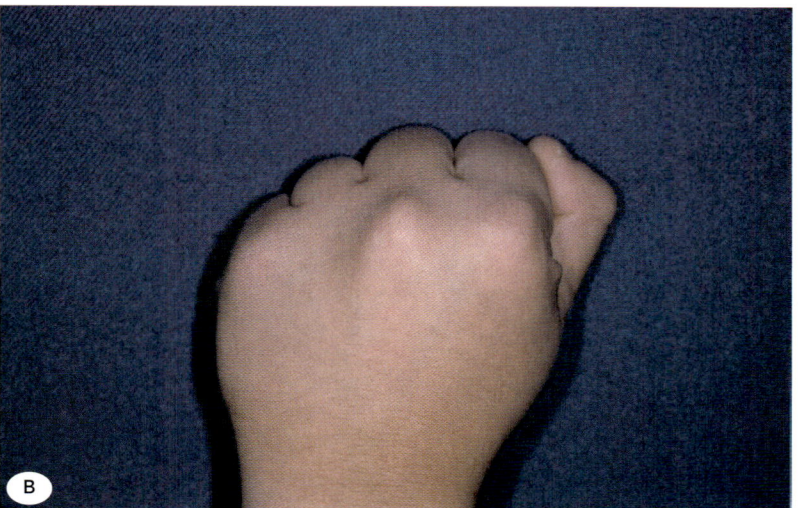

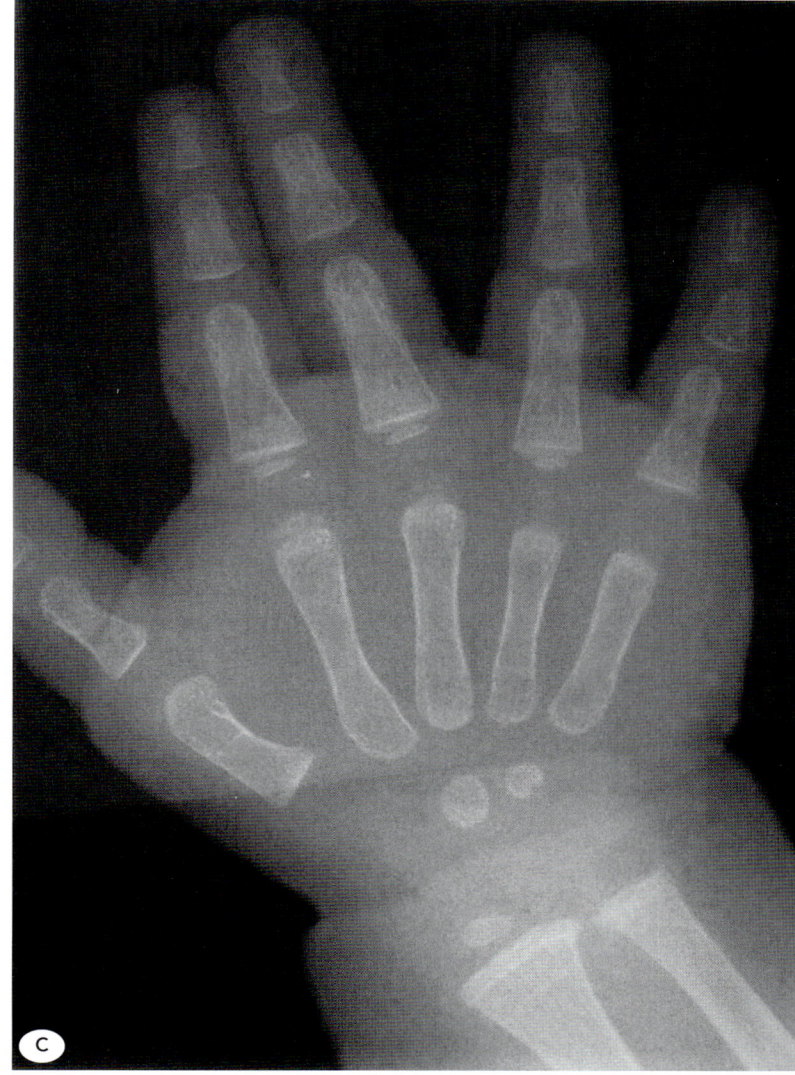

Fig. 22.26   Brachdactyly in a girl with pseudohypoparathyroidism with short 4th and 5th metacarpals (**A**) and the "knuckle, knuckle, dimple, dimple" sign when she makes a fist (**B**). Radiograph of the hand of an infant girl born with osteoma cutis showing short 4th and 5th metacarpals. She had pseudo-pseudohypoparathyroidism (**C**).

for development of hypocalcemia and hypothyroidism. Another form of the disorder, PHP1b, expresses only the renal metabolic defect and has none of the clinical or dermatologic features of PHP1a.

POLYOSTOTIC FIBROUS DYSPLASIA WITH MULTIPLE ENDOCRINE ABNORMALITIES AND CAFÉ-AU-LAIT SPOTS (McCUNE–ALBRIGHT SYNDROME)

McCune–Albright syndrome (MAS) is a sporadic disorder characterized by polyostotic fibrous dysplasia, café-au-lait spots, and endocrine hyperfunction.[166,167] The cutaneous manifestations are primarily café au lait spots that tend to be large with irregular borders (like the "coast of Maine") and segmental (Fig. 22.28). They often follow Blaschko's lines and tend not to cross the midline. They usually appear on the same side as the skeletal abnormalities. The typical bone lesions of polystotic fibrous dysplasia are usually multiple. Endocrine abnormalities consist of autonomous and excessive functioning of endocrine organs with nodular overgrowth and hormone elevation with low levels of stimulating hormones. Precocious puberty is the

most common clinical manifestation, but excessive growth hormone, prolactin, thyroid hormone, and nodular adrenal hyperplasia with Cushing syndrome are reported. Abnormal radiographs and specific hormone tests can be useful but must be tailored to each clinical situation.

These patients do not have the genetic abnormality in all of their tissues and are thus mosaic for mutations of the GNAS1 gene. This disorder thus represents postzygotic rather than germline mutation. The gain–of-function mutation causes elevation of cyclic AMP levels, but specific clinical manifestations may appear at different times of life. One study showed increased c-AMP mediated expression of tyrosinase in melanocytes isolated from a pigmented patch in one patient.[168] Therapy is directed towards specific hormonal abnormalities as they become manifest, with careful attention to early pubertal development.

AUTOIMMUNE POLYGLANDULAR SYNDROMES

The autoimmune polyglandular syndromes, also known as polyendo-crinopathy-candidiasis-ectodermal dystrophy (APECED) syndromes, have

166. Levine MA (1999) Clinical implications of genetic defects in G proteins: Oncogenic mutations in Gα$_s$ as the molecular basis for the McCune-Albright syndrome. **Arch Med Res** 30:522–531.

167. de Sanctis C, Lala R, Matarazzo P et al. (1999) McCune-Albright syndrome: A longitudinal clinical study of 32 patients. **J Pediatr Endocrinol Metab** 12(6):817–826.

168. Kim IS, Kim ER, Nam HJ et al. (1999) Activating mutation of GSα in McCune-Albright syndrome causes skin pigmentation by tyrosinase gene activation on affected melanocytes. **Horm Res** 52:235–240.

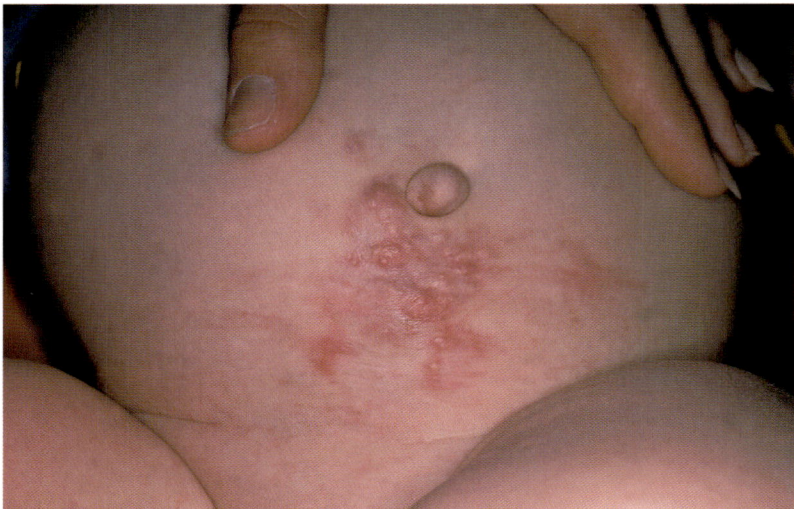

Fig. 22.27 A large plaque of osteoma cutis in an infant boy who had pseudohypoparathyroidism.

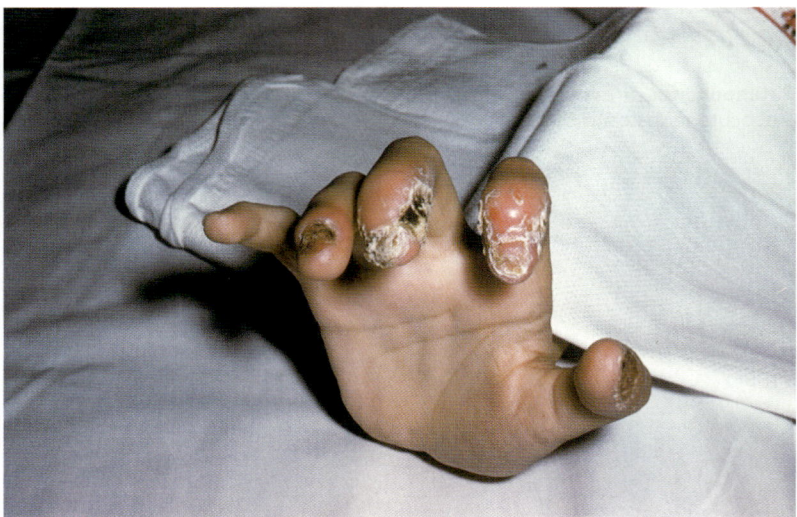

Fig. 22.29 Severe nail candidiasis in a teenage girl with autoimmune polyglandular syndrome Type I (APS-1).

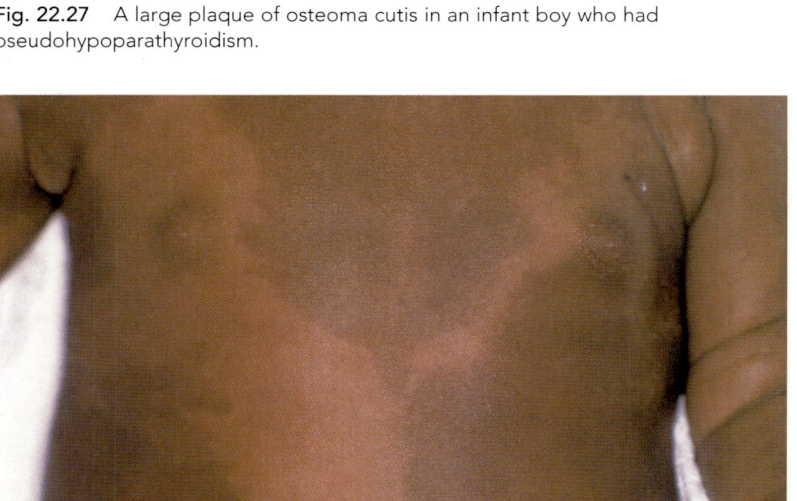

Fig. 22.28 Large, segmental café-au-lait macules with a "coast of Maine" border in an infant with McCune–Albright syndrome. (Photo courtesy of Philippe Backelijauw, Cincinnati Children's Hospital.)

been subdivided into two types.[169] Type 1 (APS-1)[170–172] occurs in childhood as an autosomal-recessive disorder that has been localized to mutations of the autuoimmune regulator gene AIRE located at 21q22.3. Type 2[171,173] occurs later in midlife. The prevalence is high in Iranian Jews (1:9000), Finns (1:25 000) and Sardinians.[172] There is wide variation of expression within and between families.[169] Associated cutaneous signs of APS-1 include vitiligo, alopecia areata, and nail dystrophy. Severe mucocutaneous candidiasis of nails (Fig. 22.29) and mucous membranes (Fig. 22.30) is the hallmark of the disorder and is often refractory to conventional topical antifungal therapy and requires chronic oral imidazole treatment. Enamel hypoplasia may also occur.[174] Other features are listed in Table 22.10. Specific endocrine disorders associated with both Types 1 and 2 include hypoparathyroidism, adrenal insufficiency, gonadal failure in females, and insulin dependent diabetes mellitus (IDDM).

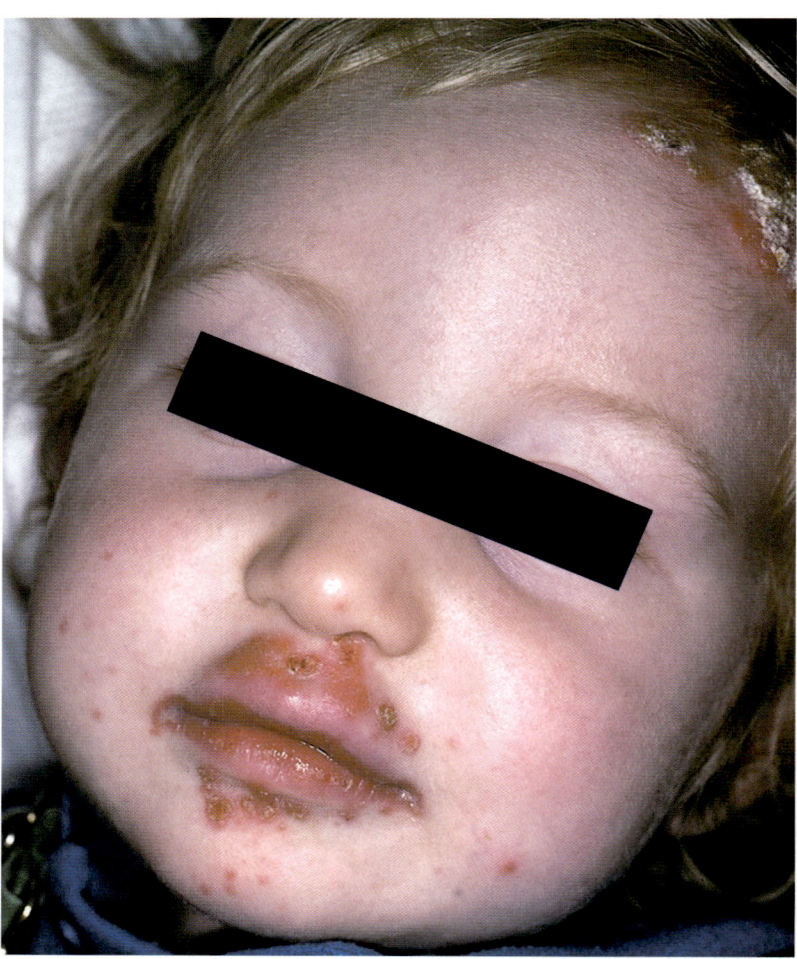

Fig. 22.30 Mucous membrane and lip involvement with chronic candida in a child with APS-1.

169. Ahonen P, Myllarniemi S et al. (1990) Clinical variation of autoimmune polyendocrinopathy-candidiasis-ectodermal dystrophy (APECED) in a series of 68 patients. **N Engl J Med** 332:1829.

170. Obermayer-Straub P, Strassburg CP, Manns MP (2000) Autoimmune polyglandular syndrome Type I. **Clin Rev Allergy and Immunol** 18:167–183.

171. Obermayer-Straub P, Manns MP (1998) Autoimmune polyglandular syndromes. **Bailliere's Clinical Gastroenterology** 12(2):293–315.

172. Winer KK, Merke DP (2000) Picture of the month. Autoimmune polyglandular syndrome Type I. **Arch Pediatr Adolesc Med** 154:745–746.

173. Betterle C, Volpato M, Greggio AN, Presotto F (1996) Type 2 polyglandular autoimmune disease (Schmidt's syndrome). **J Pediatr Endocrinol Metab** 9(1):113–123.

174. Porter SR, Haria S et al. (1992) Chronic candidiasis, enamel hypoplasia, and pigmentary anomalies. **Oral Surg Oral Med Oral Pathol** 74:312.

TABLE 22.10   Autoimmune polyglandular syndrome-1 (APS-1)

Cutaneous features

Mucocutaneous candidiasis	73–100%
Alopecia	29–37%
Vitiligo	8–15%
Nail dystrophy (pitting)	52%
Enamel hypoplasia	77%

Endocrine features

Hypoparathyroidism	76–93%
Adrenal failure	72–100%
Gonadal failure	7–50%
Parietal cell atrophy	13–15%
Insulin dependent diabetes mellitus	2–12%
Autoimmune thyroid disease	2–11%

Other features

Keratoconjunctivitis	12–35%
Chronic hepatitis	12–20%
Intestinal malabsorption	77%

TABLE 22.11   Autoimmune polyglandular syndrome-2 (APS-2)

Cutaneous features
Vitiligo (rare)
Alopecia (rare)

Endocrine features
Adrenal failure
Autoimmune thyroid disease
Insulin dependent diabetes mellitus
Gonadal failure

Other features
Myesthenia gravis
Celiac disease
Pernicious anemia

In APS-2, (Schmidt's syndrome),[173] Addison's disease, thyroid autoimmune disease, and insulin-dependent diabetes mellitus are the endocrine hallmarks. Cutaneous features such as vitiligo and alopecia are rare. Other features are listed in Table 22.11.

MULTIPLE ENDOCRINE NEOPLASIA (MEN) SYNDROMES

The multiple endocrine neoplasia (MEN) syndromes are a group of autosomal-dominantly inherited disorders in which there are multiple tumors in a variety of endocrine organs. Most are associated with specific cutaneous findings.[175–177] The major cutaneous and endocrine features are summarized in Table 22.12.

MEN-1[178–180] occurs in 0.01–2.5:100 000 in the population and has been attributed to a loss-of-function mutation of the tumor suppressor gene MEN-1 (which produces the protein menin) located on chromosome 11q13. It

TABLE 22.12   Multiple endocrine neoplasia (MEN) syndromes

MEN 1

Cutaneous features	Endocrine features
Angiofibromas	Parathyroid hyperplasia and
Collagenomas	adenomas
Leiomyomas	Gastroenteropancreatic tumors
Lipomas	Pituitary adenomas
Collagenomas	Adrenocortical tumors
Confetti-like hypopigmented	
macules	
Café-au-lait macules	
Gingival papules	
Melanoma	

MEN-2A (Sipple syndrome)

Cutaneous features	Endocrine features
Lichen amyloidosis	Medullary carcinoma of the thyroid
	Pheochromocytoma
	Parathyroid hyperplasia

MEN-2B

Cutaneous features	Endocrine features
Mucosal neuromas	Medullary carcinoma of the thyroid
Marfanoid habitus	Pheochromocytoma
Elongated facies	
Café-au-lait macules	

rarely presents in childhood. Endocrine features include primary hyperparathyroidism with parathyroid hyperplasia or adenomas, gastroenterohepatic tumors, especially those producing gastrin or insulin, pituitary adenomas, particularly prolactinomas, and more rarely adrenocortical tumors.

Cutaneous manifestations of MEN-1[178–180] include angiofibromas, which occur in more than 90% of patients. These are smaller and less numerous than in tuberous sclerosis (TS) and are often located around the upper lip. Other skin signs such as collagenomas and confetti-like hypopigmentation also overlap with TS. Leiomyomas, lipomas, gingival papules and café-au-lait macules have been reported. Melanomas may occur more frequently.[181] Allelic deletions of the MEN-1 gene have been demonstrated within several cutaneous tumors.[182]

The MEN-2 disorders result from activation mutations in the proto-oncogene RET, which encodes a tyrosine kinase receptor in neural crest-derived tisues.[183] MEN-2A is characterized by medullary carcinoma of the thyroid (MCT), pheochromocytoma, and parathyroid hyperplasia. The cutaneous hallmark is lichen amyloidosis.[178,184] Hirschprung's disease has also been associated. The gene defect is a gain-of-function mutation in the RET extracellular domain.

MEN-2B[178] patients also have MCT and pheochromocytomas as well as a Marfanoid habitus and multiple mucosal, cutaneous, and gastrointestinal ganglioneuromas (Fig. 22.31). Patients are tall, thin, and have elongated faces with thickened lips. Mucosal neuromas are usually present by age 3 and may be visible at birth. Such patients also have multiple café-au-lait macules and

175. Brandi ML, Gagal RF, Angeli A et al. (2001) CONSENSUS: Guidelines for diagnosis and therapy of MEN Type 1 and Type 2. **J Clin Endocrinol Metab** 86:5658–5671.

176. Gorlin RJ, Sedano HO, Vickers RA, Cerbenka J (1968) Multiple mucosal neuromas, pheochromocytoma and medullary carcinoma of the thyroid – a syndrome. **Cancer** 22:293.

177. Brown RS, Colle E, Tashijian AH (1975) The syndrome of multiple mucosal neuromas and medullary thyroid carcinoma in childhood. Importance of recognition of the phenotype for the early detection of malignancy. **J Pediatr** 86:77.

178. Stratakis CA, Ball DW (2000) A concise genetic and clinical guide to multiple endocrine neoplasias and related syndromes. **J Pediatr Endocrinol Metab** 13:457–465.

179. Darling TN, Skarulis MC, Steinberg SM et al. (1997) Multiple facial angiofibromas and collagenomas in patients with multiple endocrine neoplasia Type I. **Arch Dermatol** 133:853–857.

180. Schussheim DH, Skarulis MC, Agarwal SK et al. (2001) Multiple endocrine neoplasia type 1: New clinical and basic findings. **Trends in Endocrinol and Metab** 12(4):173–178.

181. Nord B, Platz A, Smoczynski K et al. (2000) Malignant melanoma in patients with multiple endocrine neoplasia Type I and involvement of the MEN1 gene in sporadic melanoma. **Int J Cancer** 87:463–467.

182. Pack S, Turner ML, Zhuang Z et al. (1998) Cutaneous tumors in patients with multiple endocrine neoplasia type I show allelic deletion of the MEN1 gene. **J Invest Dermatol** 110:438–440.

183. Hansford JR, Mulligan LM (2000) Multiple endocrine neoplasia Type 2 and RET: from neoplasia to neurogenesis. **J Med Genet** 37:817–827.

184. Kousseff, BG (1995) Multiple endocrine neoplasia 2 (MEN2)/MEN 2A (Sipple syndrome). **Dermatol Clin** 13(1):91–97.

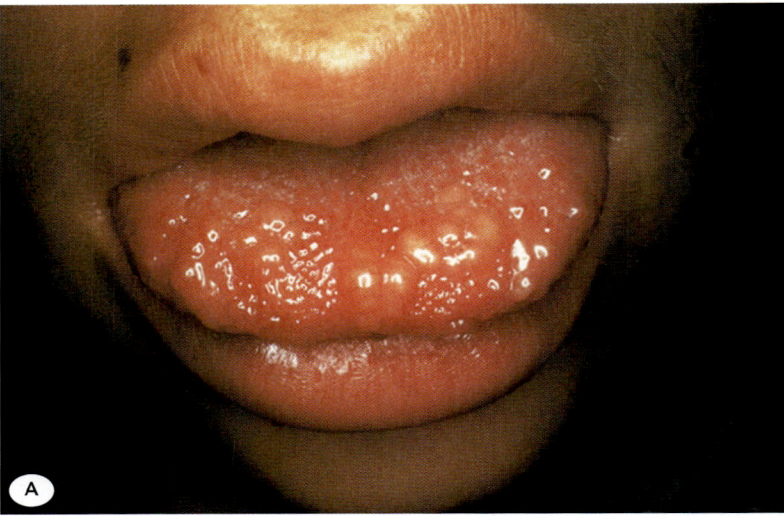

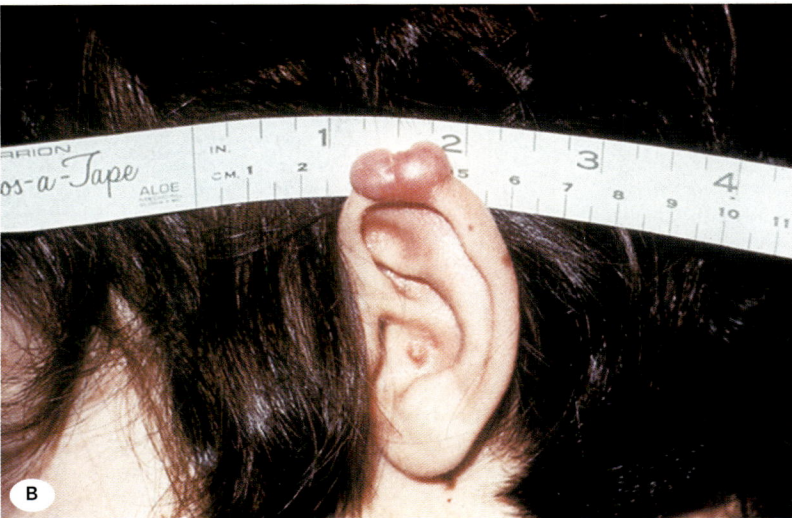

Fig. 22.31 Patient with Type 2B multiple endocrine neoplasia (MEN 2B) syndrome showing (A) characteristic thick lips and mucosal neuromas on the tongue and (B) a cutaneous neuroma on the pinna.

TABLE 22.13 Carney complex	
Cutaneous features Lentigines (spotty skin pigmentation)* Cutaneous and mucosal myxomas* Multiple epithelioid blue nevi* Conjunctival pigmentation Combined nevi Small café-au-lait macules Depigmented macules Multiple skin tags Lipomas Pigmented schwannomas Pilonidal sinus	**Endocrine features** Adrenal tumors (PPNAD) with Cushing syndrome* Pituitary tumors with gigantism or acromegaly Precocious puberty* Testicular tumors (LCCSCT)* Thyroid nodules and carcinomas* **Other features** Cardiac myxomas* Breast myxomas* Breast ductal adenomas* Psammomatous melanotic schwannomas*

* Diagnostic criteria
PPNAD = Primary pigmented nodular adrenocortical disease
LCCSCT = Large-cell calcifying Sertoli cell tumors

CC is inherited as a rare autosomal–dominant trait; only 338 cases have been reported as of 2001.[186] More than half of the cases are familial. Of these, more are from affected mothers than fathers.

CC has been diagnosed as early as at birth, but the mean age of diagnosis is 20 years. Lentigines are often the first sign, unless one of the endocrinopathies such as Cushing disease, precocious puberty or gigantism arises first. The main clinical findings are listed in Table 22.13. The lentigines are the "dark spots" originally described and occurr in about three-quarters of the patients, although nevocellular nevi and café-au-lait macules occur as well. The lentigines characteristically occur in the midface, the borders of the lips (Fig. 22.32) and in the genital skin of females. Buccal mucosal involvement is rarer (5–10%). Pigmentation of the conjunctivae is characteristic, in particular the lacrimal caruncle and the semilunar fold. Multiple epithelioid blue nevi are found on the face, trunk, and singly on the extremities.[187] Depigmented macules also occur. Myxomas are small, flesh-colored papules seen on the eyelids, external ear canals, mucosae, and elsewhere on the skin in one-third of the cases. Pigmented schwannomas of the skin are rare, but can metastasize and be fatal.[187]

The most common endocrine findings are in the adrenal, pituitary, gonads and thyroid.[186,188,189] Primary pigmented nodular adrenocortical disease (PPNAD) is the hallmark of CC and often manifests as Cushing disease. Growth hormone producing tumors of the pituitary can cause gigantism or acromegaly. Large-cell calcifying Sertoli cell tumors (LCCSCT) are also characteristic of CC and are rarely found in other settings: ultrasound of the testes may reveal calcifications even in infancy. Testicular adrenocortical rests and Leydig cell tumors also occur. Thyroid nodules and carcinoma have been recently added to the list of endocrine tumors. Non-endocrine tumors include cardiac myxomas, occuring in half of the cases and possibly life-threatening breast myxomas and ductal adenomas, as well as psammomatous melanotic schwannomas of the upper GI tract and sympathetic chain, which may become malignant.

Laboratory findings are myriad and reflect the particular manifestations of each patient. However, regular adrenal and testicular screening are recommended for identified patients. The genetics of CC have been extensively studied and two loci have been identified: 2p16 and 17q22-24. The latter locus involves a tumor suppressor gene (PRKARIA) which produces an

lentigines. MEN–2B is also an autosomal-dominant trait, but it has onset in early childhood. Screening of first-degree relatives for MCT should begin by age 1 year. These manifestations can be seen in early childhood. The genetic defect is a gain-of-function mutation in the RET intracellular domain. Early screening for the gene defect has superceded pentagastrin-calcitonin stimulation tests. Prophylactic thyroidectomy by age 5 is recommended. Finally, the familial MCT syndrome[178] has no endocrine or cutaneous manifestations and is also due to a mutation in the RET extracellular domain.

CARNEY COMPLEX

Carney complex (CC) was first described as such in 1985 as a syndrome consisting of "spotty skin pigmentation, myxomas, endocrine overactivity and schwannomas."[185] It is closely related to other multiple lentigines syndromes (see Chapter 10) as well as the MEN syndromes. Patients previously described as having LAMB and NAME syndromes undoubedly had CC.

185. Carney JA, Gordon H, Carpenter PC et al. (1985) The complex of myxomas, spotty pigmentation and endocrine overactivity. **Medicine** (Baltimore) 64:270–283.
186. Stratakis CA, Kirschner LS, Carney JA (2001) Genetics of Endocrine Disease. Clinical and molecular features of the Carney complex: Diagnostic criteria and recommendations for patient evaluation. **J Clin Endocrinol Metab** 86:4041–4046.
187. Carney JA, Stratakis CA (1998) Epithelioid blue nevus and psammomatous melanotic schwannoma: The unusual pigmented skin tumors of the Carney complex. **Semin Diagnost Pathol** 15:216–224.
188. Stratakis CA (2000) Genetics of Carney complex and related familial lentiginoses and other multiple tumor syndromes. **Frontiers in Bioscience** 5:353–366.
189. Carney JA (1995) The Carney complex (myxomas, spotty pigmentation, endocrine overactivity and schwannomas). **Dermatologic Clinics** 13:19–26.

This paradoxically high level of vitamin D is related to peripheral resistance to hormonal action. The inheritance appears to be autosomal recessive. Patients may have hair at birth but, usually over a six- to seven-month period of time in association with onset of rachitic bone changes, striking hair loss progresses to total alopecia. Patients tend to be irritable and to have growth failure. In those few patients who have had scalp biopsies, no lymphocytic infiltrate was noted about the hair bulbs (such as seen in alopecia areata). Clinical response of the rickets to pharmacologic doses of vitamin D3, 25-hydroxy D3, 1,25-dihydroxy D3, or 1-α-hydroxy D3 was variable, suggesting more than one mechanism of action. In one case in which the rickets was documented to respond to therapy, no regrowth of hair occurred. Although all of these children can be classified as having vitamin D resistance, distinct biochemical defects have been documented in nuclear uptake and binding[192,193] or in postreceptor events, including decreased receptor affinity for vitamin D.[195] The mechanisms by which such vitamin D receptor defects produce alopecia is unclear. Vitamin D resistance should be added to the list of disorders that cause alopecia in infancy.

ANOREXIA AND BULIMIA NERVOSA

Anorexia nervosa (AN) is a generalized disorder that almost exclusively affects 1–3% of prepubertal and pubertal females (20:1) and may persist into the third and fourth decades. It often coexists with bulimia nervosa (BN), which is binge eating and forced vomiting or laxative abuse. Anorexic patients develop an abhorrence of food intake, and often participate in excessive physical exercise. Cutaneous manifestations primarily reflect malnutrition (Fig. 22.33),[198,199] but repetitive self-induced vomiting in patients with bulimia and concomitant self-inflicted injury in some patients can also produce characteristic skin findings. Cutaneous manifestations of AN and BN have been studied in several series of patients under psychiatric treatment,[200–202] and those findings noted on examination are listed in Table 22.14. The prevalence of each of these conditions varies with the stage (early, late, recovery) and duration of the illness, accounting for discrepancies between studies. Cutaneous xerosis, carotenodermia, and acral changes including coldness, cyanosis, and erythema are common. Hair changes of note are generalized hypertrichosis, telogen effluvium, dry scalp hair, and pili torti.[203] Oral manifestations include cheilitis, perleche, aphthae, gum recession and erosion, enamel erosion, and dental caries. Salivary glands are enlarged. Nails become brittle and dystrophic. Self-inflicted injuries are common, but calluses on the backs of the hands from repetitive forced vomiting (Russell's sign) is most characteristic. Most of the changes are reversible with weight regain. It has been proposed that a Body Mass Index (BMI) of <16kg/m^2 is the critical value when most skin manifestations become apparent.

DISORDERS OF PREGNANCY

Julie Powell

The disorders of pregnancy are considered in a textbook of pediatric dermatology because of the associated fetal morbidity and mortality and because of the high incidence of adolescent pregnancies. The literature is

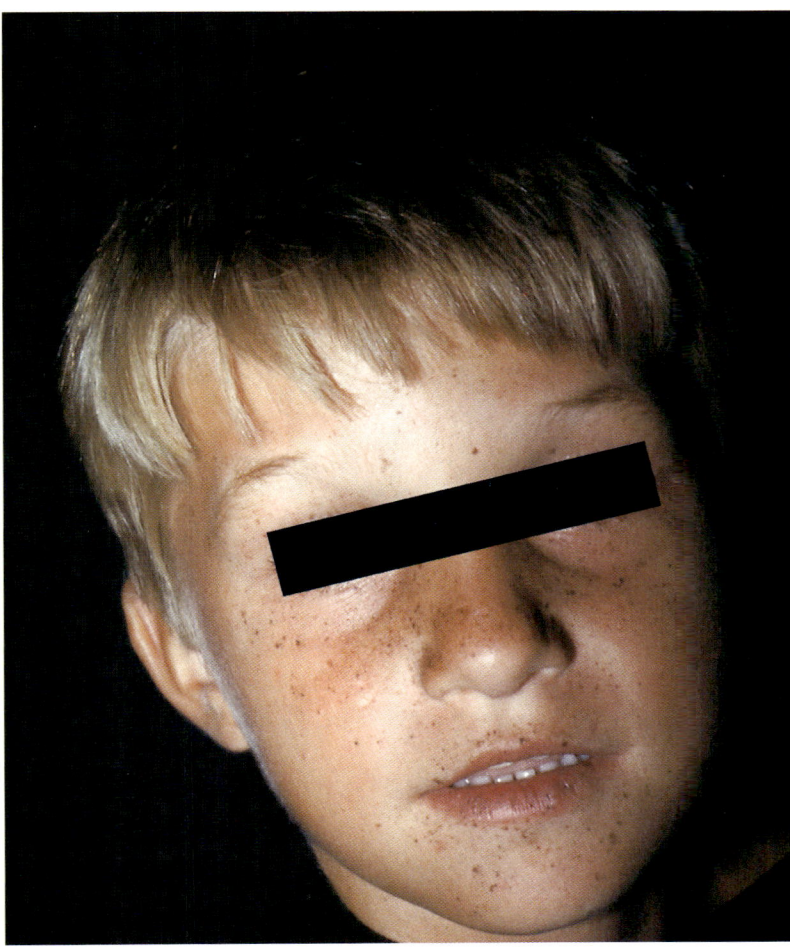

Fig. 22.32   Carney complex. Facial and lip lentigines.

effector molecule important in many endocrine signaling pathways.[186,188] The differential diagnosis includes the other familial lentigines syndromes such as Peutz–Jehgers, LEOPARD, Cowden, Ruvalcaba–Myhre–Smith (Bannayan–Zonana), Multiple endocrine neoplasia and Laugier–Hunziker syndromes.[188] Therapy is directed to specific manifestations of CC as they appear. All 1st degree relatives should be screened. Pediatricians and dermatologists are in a unique position to recognize the cutaneous findings of this probably underdiagnosed condition.

VITAMIN D RESISTANCE AND ALOPECIA

Of interest to dermatologists are the reports of several kindreds with clinical syndromes of vitamin D-dependent rickets (VDDR) and alopecia.[190–197] Affected individuals have rickets associated with elevated rather than decreased circulating levels of 1,25-dihydroxy vitamin D, the active form of vitamin D.

190. Rosen JF, Fleischman AR, Finberg L et al. (1979) Rickets with alopecia: an inborn error of vitamin D metabolism. J Pediatr 94:729.
191. Liberman UA, Halabe A, Samuel R et al. (1980) End-organ resistance to 1,25-dihydroxycholecalciferol. Lancet 1:504.
192. Tsuchiya Y, Matsuo N, Cho H et al. (1980) An unusual form of vitamin D-dependent rickets in a child: alopecia and marked end-organ hyposensitivity to biologially active vitamin D. J Clin Endocrinol Metab 51:685.
193. Beer S, Tieder M, Kohelet D et al. (1981) Vitamin D resistant rickets with alopecia: a form of end organ resistance to 1,25-dihydroxy vitamin D. Clin Endocrinol (Oxford) 14:395.
194. Balsan S, Garabedian M, Liberman UA et al. (1983) Rickets and alopecia with resistance to 1,25-dihydroxyvitamin D: two different clinical courses with two different cellular defects. J Clin Endocrinol Metab 57:803.
195. Hochberg Z, Benderli A, Levy J et al. (1984) 1,25-dihydroxyvitamin D resistance, rickets, and alopecia. Am J Med 77:805.
196. Hochberg Z, Gilhar A, Haim S et al. (1985) Calcitriol-resistant rickets with alopecia. Arch Dermatol 121:646.
197. Hewison M, O'Riordan JL (1994) Hormone – nuclear receptor interactions in health and disease. Vitamin D Resistance. Baillieres Clin Endocrinol Metab 8:305–315.
198. Rapaport MJ (1985) Pellagra in a patient with anorexia nervosa. Arch Dermatol 121:255.
199. Van Voorhees AS, Riba M (1992) Acquired zinc deficiency in association with anorexia nervosa: case report and review of the literature. Pediatr Dermatol 9:268.
200. Schulze, UME, Pettke-Rank CV, Kreienkamp M et al. (1999) Dermatologic findings in anorexia and bulimia nervosa of childhood and adolescence. Pediatr Dermatol 16:90–94.
201. Glorio R, Allevato M, De Pablo A et al. (2000) Prevalence of cutaneous manifestations in 200 patients with eating disorders. Int J Dermatol 39:348–353.
202. Hediger C, Rost B, Itin P (2000) Cutaneous manifestations in anorexia nervosa. Schweiz Med Wochenschr 130:565–575.
203. Lurie R, Danziger Y, Kaplan Y et al. (1996) Acquired pili torti – a structural hair shaft defect in anorexia nervosa. Cutis 57:151–156.

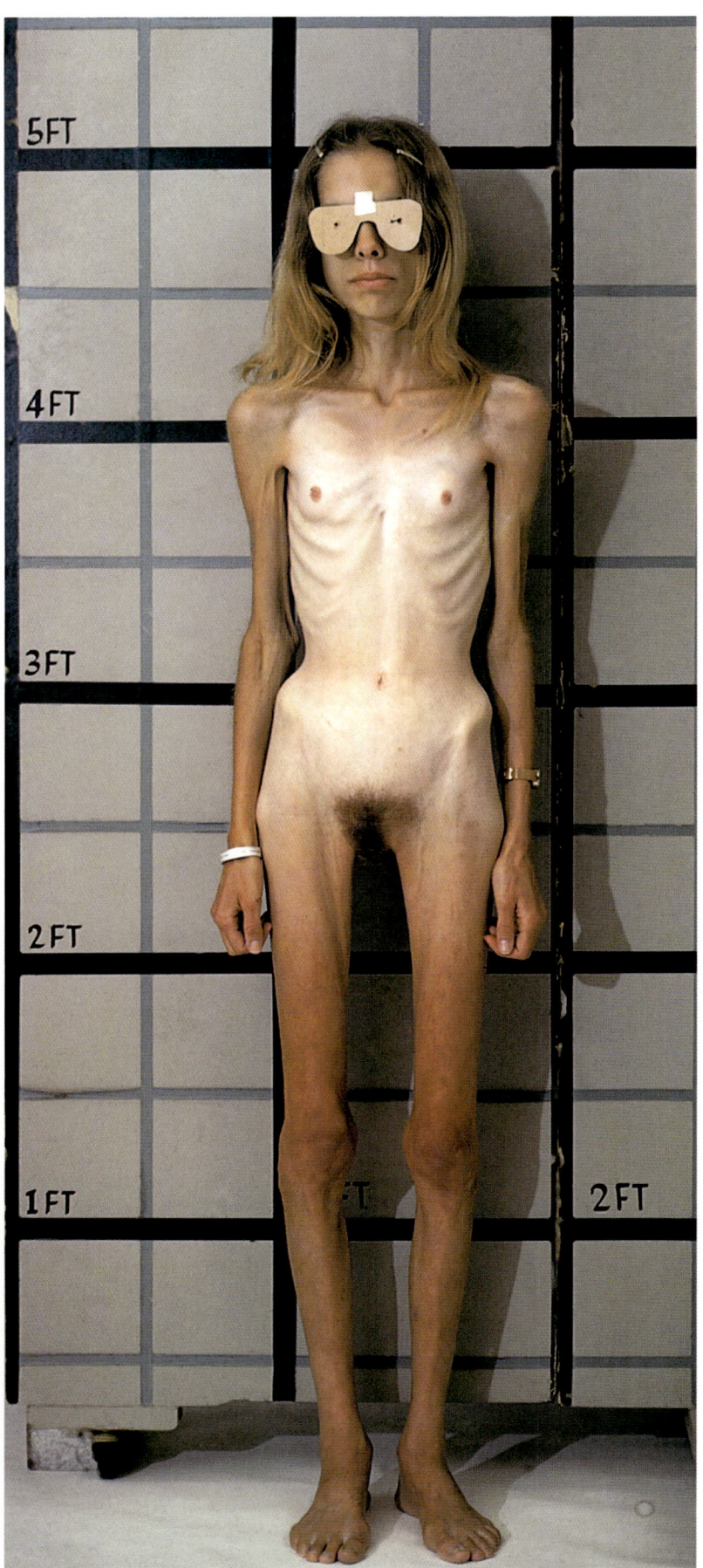

TABLE 22.14   Cutaneous manifestations of anorexia nervosa and bulimia nervosa*

	Prevalence on examination
Xerosis	71–97%
Carotenodermia	24%
Acral changes	
Acral coldness	38%
Acrocyanosis	24–40%
Periungual erythema	48%
Hair changes	
Hypertrichosis	36–77%
Telogen effluvium	37–86%
Dry scalp hair	20–48%
Pili torti	82%*
Oral changes	
Cheilitis and perleche	15–76%
Aphthae	9–18%
Gum recession, erosion**	37%
Enamel erosion**	5–12%
Dental caries**	5–47%
Brittle/dystrophic nails	30%
Calluses on dorsum of hand (Russell's sign)**	23%–30%
Other self-inflicted injuries	12%
Sialadenosis (enlarged parotid and salivary glands)**	5–13%

* from Lurie, *et al.*
** in patients with BN
from Schilze *et al.*, Hediger *et al.*, and Glorio *et al.*

replete with discrepancies and controversies over nomenclature and classification of the disorders of pregnancy. There have recently been several excellent reviews.[204–207] This section discusses the major disorders likely to be seen and affect the fetus. Cutaneous findings during pregnancy can be classified as (1) physiologic changes, (2) specific disorders seen only in pregnancy, and (3) effects of pregnancy on cutaneous disorders previously present.

Physiologic skin changes[207] that occur with pregnancy are listed in Table 22.15. These include disorders of pigmentation such as hyperpigmentation of pre-existing pigmented lesions (i.e., nevi, lentigines, linea nigra), melasma (which is also known as chloasma), and jaundice (which is a result of cholestasis of pregnancy). Cholestasis is also responsible for the common pruritus gravidarum that occurs in nearly 20% of normal pregnancies. Vascular changes are also common during pregnancy and include growth in number and size of spider telangiectasia, varicosities (both large deep-vessel varicosities and stellate varicosities of the lower extremities), and palmar erythema. Pyogenic granulomas are commonly seen during pregnancy, as well as edema and hyperemia of the gingivae. Abdominal striae distensae develop in up to 90% of women during the sixth and seventh months of pregnancy.[206] Hair changes during pregnancy include prolonged anagen cycle of the hair with consequent thickening and less loss of hair during gestation followed by a predictable telogen effluvium three months postpartum. This telogen effluvium is seen in the newborn at approximately the same time. There is increased eccrine hyperhidrosis and heat intolerance associated with pregnancy, increased sebaceous activity, and decreased apocrine activity. Finally, besides pyogenic granulomas, other cutaneous tumors seem to be stimulated

◀ **Fig. 22.33**   A teenage girl with severe emaciation characteristic of anorexia nervosa.

204. Shornick JK (1998) Dermatoses of pregnancy. **Semin Cutan Med Surg** 17:172–181.
205. Vaughn Jones SA, Black MM (1999) Pregnancy dermatoses. **J Am Acad Dermatol** 40:233–241.
206. Kroumpouzos G, Cohen LM (2001) Dermatoses of pregnancy. **J Am Acad Dermatol** 45:1–19.
207. Elling SV, Powell FC (1997) Physiological changes in the skin during pregnancy. **Clin Dermatol** 15:35–43.

TABLE 22.15   Cutaneous changes observed during pregnancy

Physiologic
Pigmentary
  Hyperpigmentation
  Melasma (chloasma)

Vascular
  Spider telangiectasia
  Venous varicosities
  Palmar erythema
  Vasomotor instability
  Gingival hypertrophy
  Hemorrhoids

Hair
  Prolonged anagen cycle
  Telogen effluvium (3 months postpartum)
  Hirsutism

Cholestasis
  Jaundice
  Pruritus gravidarum

Striae distensae

Glandular
  Increased eccrine gland activity
  Decreased apocrine function
  Increased sebaceous function

Nail
  Transverse ridging
  Brittleness
  Distal onycholysis

Tumors
  Skin tags (molluscum fibrosum gravidarum, fibroma molle)
  Dermatofibroma
  Neurofibromas
  Melanocytic nevi
  Keloids
  Leiomyoma

Specific disorders of pregnancy
  Herpes gestationis (pemphigoid gestationis)[a]
  PUPPP (also known as polymorphic eruption of pregnancy, toxic erythema of pregnancy, toxemic rash of pregnancy, and late-onset prurigo of pregnancy)
  Prurigo of pregnancy
  Pruritic folliculitis of pregnancy
  Impetigo herpetiformis (pustular psoriasis of pregnancy)[a]
  Autoimmune progesterone dermatitis

Cutaneous disorders aggravated by pregnancy
  Autoimmune
    SLE, systemic sclerosis
    Dermatomyositis/polymyositis
    Pemphigus vulgaris, vegetans, foliaceous

  Metabolic
    Porphyria cutanea tarda
    Acrodermatitis enteropathica

  Infectious
    Condyloma accuminata
    Fungal (Candida, Pityrosporum)
    AIDS

  Miscellaneous
    Neurofibromatosis
    Tuberous sclerosis
    Erythema nodosum

[a] Associated with either fetal morbidity or mortality, or both.

by pregnancy, including skin tags or larger similar lesions called molluscum fibrosum gravidarum or fibroma molle, dermatofibromas, keloids, leiomyoma, neurofibromas, and nevi.

The specific skin disorders of pregnancy are listed in Table 22.15. Although classified in various ways, the following classification highlights the major features of the most common conditions.

HERPES GESTATIONIS (PEMPHIGOID GESTATIONIS)

This disorder closely resembles bullous pemphigoid (BP) and has been estimated to occur in 1 in 50 000 births, an incidence much lower than reported earlier. It has been recently reviewed,[208–210] and the term pemphigoid gestationis is proposed to avoid any confusion with a herpesvirus infection. It has been reported to occur as early as 9 weeks of gestation and as late as 6 days postpartum, but it usually occurs in mid-trimester (mean onset, 21 weeks). There may be earlier onset in subsequent pregnancies. Individual lesions begin as urticarial papules and plaques that develop into polycyclic wheals, target-like lesions, and ultimately vesicles and bullae that crust over.

Rarely, they are pustular.[211] The lesions begin around the umbilicus and rapidly progress to become generalized, usually sparing the face, mucous membranes, palms and soles. Patients may be quite ill. Earlier reports suggested a higher than expected infant mortality and prematurity rate,[212] but this has been disputed.[209,210] Infants born to affected mothers may have transient papulovesicular eruptions lasting several weeks[213–215] and herpes gestationis factor (HG factor), an IgG, can be found in cord blood.

Histologically, lesions of herpes gestationis are subepidermal bullae with a mixed perivascular inflammatory cell infiltrate[216] and a predominance of C3 localized to the lamina lucida of the basement membrane zone. IgG can also be found but in only about 25% to 30% of patients.[206,210] Thus, although there may be many features of herpes gestationis that resemble bullous pemphigoid, one major difference is the rarity of IgG compared with C3. A circulating complement-fixing IgG called HG factor is not easily detected by routine indirect immunofluorescence (IF) but can be demonstrated in the majority of cases by using indirect complement-added IF.[210] This antibody belongs to the IgG1 subclass and the antigen is a 180-kd protein similar to the bullous pemphigoid antigen (bullous pemphigoid antigen 2, BPAG2). This can cross

208. Yancey KB (1990) Herpes gestationis. Dermatol Clin 8:727.
209. Jenkins RE, Hern S, Black MM (1999) Clinical features and management of 87 patients with pemphigoid gestationis. Clin Exp Dermatol 24:255–259.
210. Engineer L, Bhol K, Ahmed AR (2000) Pemphigoid gestationis: a review. Am J Obst Gynecol 183:483–491.
211. Bercovitch L, Bogaars HA, Murray DO (1983) Pustular herpes gestationis. Arch Dermatol 119:91.
212. Lawley TJ, Stingl G, Katz SI (1978) Fetal and maternal risk factors in herpes gestationis. Arch Dermatol 114:552.
213. Chorzelski TP, Jablonska S, Beutner EH et al. (1976) Herpes gestations with identical lesions in the newborn. Passive transfer of the disease? Arch Dermatol 112:1129.
214. Karna P, Broecker AH (1991) Neonatal herpes gestationis. Pediatrics 119:299.
215. Chen SH, Chopra K, Evans TY et al. (1999) Herpes gestationis in a mother and child. J Am Acad Dermatol 40:847–849.
216. Hertz KC, Katz SI, Maize J, Ackerman AB (1976) Herpes gestationis. A clinicopathologic study. Arch Dermatol 112:1543.

the placenta, has been found in cord blood, and probably accounts for the transient symptoms reported in some infants. Immunogenetic studies have shown a marked increase in the HLA antigens DR3 and DR4 in patients with HG; the most striking observation is the simultaneous presence of both DR3 and DR4 in about 45% of patients compared with only 3% in the general population.[206,210] These observations suggest that both genetic (HLA type) and environmental (pregnancy) factors are involved in the pathogenesis of HG.

Therapy for herpes gestationis is quite successful with systemic glucocorticosteroids. Such treatment may be responsible for the recent apparent decline in infant morbidity and mortality with this disease. Mild cases may respond to topical corticosteroids and oral antihistamines.

There is no maternal risk in HG other than pruritus and discomfort. An increased association with Graves' disease and other autoimmune disorders has been reported.[206,210] Neonatal HG can occur in up to 10% of cases, but is mild and self-limited. There has been considerable controversy regarding the increase in fetal mortality and morbidity with HG. Most studies show a tendency for complications associated with low-grade placental insufficiency, such as prematurity and small-for-gestational-age infants; this does not seem to be altered by systemic corticosteroids. However, recent studies show no additional increase in fetal mortatility and morbidity. A few cases of HG progression to bullous pemphigoid have been reported.[217]

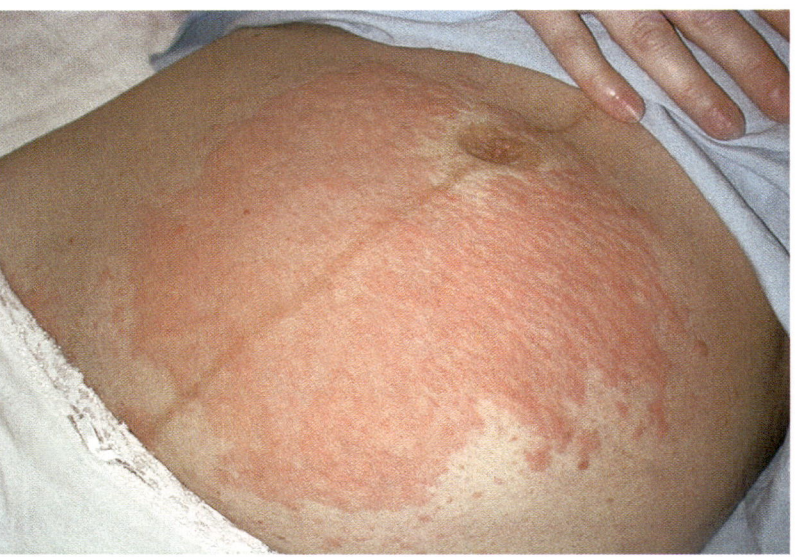

Fig. 22.34 Pruritic urticarial papules and papules of pregnancy: periumbilical striae involved.

PRURITIC URTICARIAL PAPULES AND PLAQUES OF PREGNANCY

Pruritic urticarial papules and plaques of pregnancy (PUPPP) was described as such in 1979 by Lawley, followed by massive confusion in the literature concerning the inclusion or exclusion of previously described but less well-documented disorders.[218–224] PUPPP still seems to be the preferred acronym in the United States at this time but the name polymorphic eruption of pregnancy (PEP) is also widely used;[205] these incorporate toxic erythema of pregnancy, toxemic rash of pregnancy, and late-onset prurigo of pregnancy. This pruritic disorder tends to occur in the last trimester of pregnancy, usually in a primigravida. In contrast to herpes gestationis, it does not recur with subsequent pregnancies. The incidence is estimated to be as frequent as 1 in 120 to 1 in 240 pregnancies, and its common occurrence in mild forms probably accounts for the lack of reported cases.

Lesions begin as pruritic urticarial papules, primarily within abdominal striae around the umbilicus (Fig. 22.34). The papules progress to plaques, polycyclic wheals, and target-like lesions. Rarely, tiny vesicles are seen. The abdomen and proximal portions of the extremities are most often affected. In contrast to herpes gestationis, these do not develop large vesicles or bullae. Although there has been one report of an infant with papular lesions born to a mother with PUPPP,[225] the diagnosis of PUPPP in the infant was not well substantiated; the neonate is usually not affected. There appears to be no increased infant morbidity or mortality.

Histologically, lesions show upper dermal and epidermal spongiosis with a mixed perivascular infiltrate including prominent eosinophils. In contrast to herpes gestationis, there is no evidence for an immune etiology and direct and indirect immunofluorescence are negative. Lesions often respond nicely to high-potency topical steroids and oral antihistamines, and rarely are systemic steroids needed for relief of pruritus.

PRURIGO OF PREGNANCY

This is the current term used to describe a heterogeneous group of disorders including Besnier's prurigo gestationis, Spangler's papular dermatitis of pregnancy[226,228] and Nurse's early onset prurigo[227] because of extensive clinical overlap between these conditions.[206] Its incidence is approximately 1 in 300 pregnancies. It is similar to nodular prurigo in non-pregnant individuals and typically presents as an intensely pruritic papular disorder on the extensor surfaces of the limbs and on the abdomen. Lesions are 0.5–1.0cm in size, with or without a central crust. Histopathologic features are nonspecific, showing a chronic upper dermal infiltration with occasional epidermal involvement and negative direct and indirect IF. Spangler described an association with a higher than expected level of urinary human chorionic gonadotropin (HCG) and low levels of urinary cortisol and estriol, but this has not been further substantiated.[204–206] Prurigo of pregnancy is now thought to be a result of physiologic pruritus in patients with an atopic tendency. Liver function tests should be performed to exclude cholestasis. There are no adverse effects to mother or infant. The disease may last for weeks to months and resolves postpartum. Recurrence in subsequent pregnancies is variable. Treatment is usually satisfactory with mid-potency topical corticosteroids and oral antihistamines.

PRURITIC FOLLICULITIS OF PREGNANCY

This disorder, which presents as its name describes, with pruritic follicular inflammation, is the most recent addition to the specific disorders of pregnancy; described in 1981 by Zoberman and Farmer.[229] It presents as widespread erythematous, follicular papules occurring in the fourth to ninth month of gestation and carries no fetal risk. Histologically, there is an acute

217. Jenkins RE, Vaughan Jones SA, Black MM (1996) Conversion of pemphigoid gestationis to bullous pemphigoid – two refractory cases highlighting this association. Br J Dermatol 1996;595–598.
218. Lawley TJ, Hertz HC, Wade TR et al. (1979) Pruritic urticarial papules and plaques of pregnancy. JAMA 241:1696–1699.
219. Callen JP, Hanno R (1981) Pruritic urticarial papules and plaques of pregnancy (PUPPP). J Am Acad Dermatol 5:401–405.
220. Ahmed AR, Kaplan R (1981) Pruritic urticarial papules and plaques of pregnancy. J Am Acad Dermatol 4:679.
221. Schwartz RA, Hansen RC, Lynch PJ (1981) Pruritic urticarial papules and plaques of pregnancy. Cutis 27:425–427.
222. Faber WR, Van Joost TH, Hausman R, Weenink GH (1982) Late prurigo of pregnancy. Br J Dermatol 1982; 511–516.
223. Noguera J, Moreno A, Moragas JM (1983) Pruritic urticarial papules and plaques of pregnancy (PUPPP). Acta Derm Venereol (Stockh) 63:35–38.
224. Aronson IK, Bond S, Fiedler VC et al. (1998) Pruritic urticarial papules and plaques of pregnancy: clinical and immunopathologic observations in 57 patients. J Am Acad Dermatol 39:933–939.
225. Uhlin SR (1981) Pruritic urticarial papules and plaques of pregnancy. Involvement in mother and infant. Arch Dermatol 117:238.
226. Spangler AS, Reddy W, Bardawil WA et al. (1962) Papular dermatitis of pregnancy. A new clinical entity? JAMA 181:577–581.
227. Nurse DS (1968) Prurigo of pregnancy. Aust J Dermatol 9:258–267.
228. Michaud RM, Jacobson D, Dahl MV (1982) Papular dermatitis of pregnancy. Arch Dermatol 118:1003.
229. Zoberman E, Farmer ER (1981) Pruritic folliculitis of pregnancy. Arch Dermatol 117:20–22.

sterile folliculitis with negative immunofluorescence, and cultures are negative. It bears some resemblance to steroid acne; increased levels of androgens were reported in one case. Some authors think that this condition should be included in the PUPPP or polymorphic eruption of pregnancy category.[230] Therapy with 1% hydrocortisone, 10% benzoyl peroxide, or UVB has been effective.

IMPETIGO HERPETIFORMIS

This generalized pustular disorder represents pustular psoriasis of Von Zumbusch exacerbated by pregnancy.[204–206] It can occur in any trimester and often in patients without a prior family or personal history of psoriasis. Patients may become extremely ill with fever, chills, nausea, vomiting, diarrhea, and hypocalcemic tetany. Indeed, hypocalcemia has become a hallmark of acute exacerbations of this disease. Individual lesions are millimeter-size pustules that coalesce into large lakes of pus, desquamate, and recur in crops. The lesions often begin in flexural areas, spreading centrifugally; the face, hands, and feet are spared. Postinflammatory hyperpigmentation is common. Histopathologic features are the same as pustular psoriasis and direct immunofluorescence is negative. There is some response to systemic steroids, usually at doses of 15–30mg per day of prednisone. Serum calcium and albumin levels should be monitored closely as risks to the mother include tetany, seizures, and delirium. Stillbirth and placental insufficiency are still frequently seen even if the disease appears well controlled with corticosteroids. Remission occurs postpartum but recurrence in further pregnancies is common.

AUTOIMMUNE PROGESTERONE DERMATITIS OF PREGNANCY

Although in the minds of some scholars this entity does not exist, there have been a series of reports of cyclic cutaneous eruptions occurring during the luteal phase of the menstrual cycle, with some oral contraceptives, and exacerbated by pregnancy.[231,232] Patients may have positive skin tests to intradermal progesterone. Most of the patients reported have had prior exposure to synthetic progestins. Manifestations of the disease range from urticaria to erythema multiforme-like lesions to dermatitis to frank anaphylaxis. Intradermal challenge with progesterone not only produces a wheal and flare but often reproduces the original symptoms. Treatment is successful with agents that decrease endogenous progesterone production; often an oral contraceptive may be useful if the progestin in the pill does not itself produce the symptoms. In one report, postpartum treatment with luteinizing hormone-releasing hormone analogue (LHRHa), followed by oophorectomy, was curative in a patient who had severe anaphylaxis every 3–7 days during pregnancy.[231]

SYSTEMIC DISORDERS EXACERBATED BY PREGNANCY

There is a group of disorders that seem to be aggravated by pregnancy (Table 22.15), which include porphyria cutanea tarda,[233,234] SLE, the renal manifestations of systemic sclerosis, polymyositis/dermatomyositis, acrodermatitis enteropathica,[235] Ehlers–Danlos syndrome, pseudoxanthoma elasticum, condyloma acuminata, neurofibromatosis,[236] tuberous sclerosis, erythema nodosum, and pemphigus vulgaris and foliaceus. Some other conditions, such as atopic dermatitis, psoriasis, acne vulgaris, hidradenitis suppurativa, rheumatoid arthritis and sarcoidosis, may either improve or deteriorate during pregnancy.[206]

DISORDERS OF MINERALS AND CO-FACTORS

ZINC

Epidemiology

Human clinical zinc deficiency states have been recognized only relatively recently. Three types of zinc deficiency have been described: (1) a rare autosomal-recessive disorder, acrodermatitis enteropathica; (2) nutritional zinc deficiency, found sporadically in premature and full-term infants and endemically in adolescents in some Middle Eastern countries; and (3) iatrogenic zinc deficiency associated with total parenteral nutrition (TPN). This last cause is now rare because of heightened awareness of necessary zinc supplementation in TPN. Although clinical descriptions of acrodermatitis enteropathica have appeared in the literature for decades, Moynahan[237] was the first to associate zinc deficiency with the clinical syndrome. Subsequently, the more subtle forms of zinc deficiency that are not genetically inherited have been recognized. Several excellent reviews are available.[238–245]

Presenting history

Infants with acrodermatitis enteropathica present with a classic triad of diarrhea, skin rash with alopecia, and extreme irritability and depression. Onset is approximately one to two weeks after weaning or four to 10 weeks of age in bottle-fed infants. Left untreated, severe failure to thrive and death may ensue. Frequent secondary bacterial and fungal infections are not uncommon. Acquired nutritional zinc deficiency has been reported in both bottle- and breast-fed premature infants[246–249] and in full-term infants as well.[250,251] These children present with cutaneous eruptions, alopecia, irritability, and failure to thrive. Adolescents, primarily in the Middle East, have been noted to have growth failure and delayed pubertal maturation.[252] In the past, premature infants receiving TPN[253] appeared with symptoms similar to nutritionally deprived children. In some adults and children, disturbances in taste appear secondary to zinc deficiency. Two children have been reported

230. Kroumpouzos G, Cohen L (2000) Pruritic folliculitis of pregnancy. J Am Acad Derm 43:132–134.
231. Bierman SM (1973) Autoimmune progesterone dermatitis of pregnancy. Arch Dermatol 107:896–901.
232. Meggs WJ, Pescovitz OH, Metcalfe D et al. (1984) Progesterone sensitivity as a cause of recurrent anaphylaxis. N Engl J Med 311:1236.
233. Goerz G, Hammer G (1983) Porphyria cutanea tarda and pregnancy. Dermatologica 166:316.
234. Baxi L, Rubeo TJ, Katz B, Harber LC (1983) Porphyria cutanea tarda and pregnancy. Am J Obstet Gynecol 146:333.
235. Bronson DM, Barksy R, Barsky S (1983) Acrodermatitis enteropathica. Recognition at long last during a recurrence in pregnancy. J Am Acad Dermatol 9:140–144.
236. Swapp GH, Main RA (1973) Neurofibromatosis in pregnancy. Br J Dermatol 88:431–435.
237. Moynahan EJ (1974) Acrodermatitis enteropathica: a lethal inherited human zinc deficiency disorder. Lancet 2:399–400.
238. Sehgal VN, Jain S (2000) Acrodermatitis enteropathica. Clin Dermatol 18:745–748.
239. Prasad AS (1995) Zinc: An overview. Nutrition 11:93–99.
240. Gordon EF, Gordon RC, Passal DB (1981) Zinc metabolism: basic, clinical, and behavioral aspects. J Pediatr 99:341.
241. Hambidge KM (1981) Zinc deficiency in man: its origins and effects. Phil Trans R Soc Lond 294:129.
242. Kay RG (1981) Zinc and copper in human nutrition. J Hum Nutr 35:25.
243. Aggett PJ (1983) Acrodermatitis enteropathica. J Inher Metab Dis 6(suppl) 1:39.
244. Di Silvestro RA, Cousins RJ (1983) Physiological ligands for copper and zinc. Annu Rev Nutr 3:261.
245. Van Wouwe JP (1989) Clinical and laboratory diagnosis of acrodermatitis enteropathica. Eur J Pediatr 149:2.
246. Zimmerman AW, Hambidge KM, Lepow ML et al. (1982) Acrodermatitis in breast-fed premature infants: evidence for a defect of mammary zinc secretion. Pediatrics 69:176.
247. Heinen F, Mathern D, Pringsheim N et al. (1995) Zinc deficiency in an exclusively breast-fed preterm infant. Eur J Pediatr 154:71–75.
248. Stevens J, Lubitz C (1998) Symptomatic zinc deficiency in breast-fed term and premature infants. J Paediatr Child Health 34:97–100.
249. Moore MEC, Moran JR, Green HL (1984) Zinc supplementation in lactating women: evidence for mammary control of zinc secretion. J Pediatr 105:600.
250. Krieger I, Evans GW (1980) Acrodermatitis enteropathica without hypozincemia: therapeutic effect of a pancreatic enzyme preparation due to a zinc-binding ligand. J Pediatr 96:32.
251. Bye AME, Goodfellow A, Atherton DJ (1985) Transient zinc deficiency in a full-term breast-fed infant of normal birth weight. Pediatr Dermatol 2:308.
252. Prasad AS, Halsted JA, Nadimi M (1961) Syndrome of iron deficiency, anemia, hepatosplenomegaly, dwarfism, hypogonadism and geophagia. Am J Med 31:532.
253. Arlette JP, Johnston MM (1981) Zinc deficiency dermatosis in premature infants receiving prolonged parenteral alimentation. J Am Acad Dermatol 5:37.

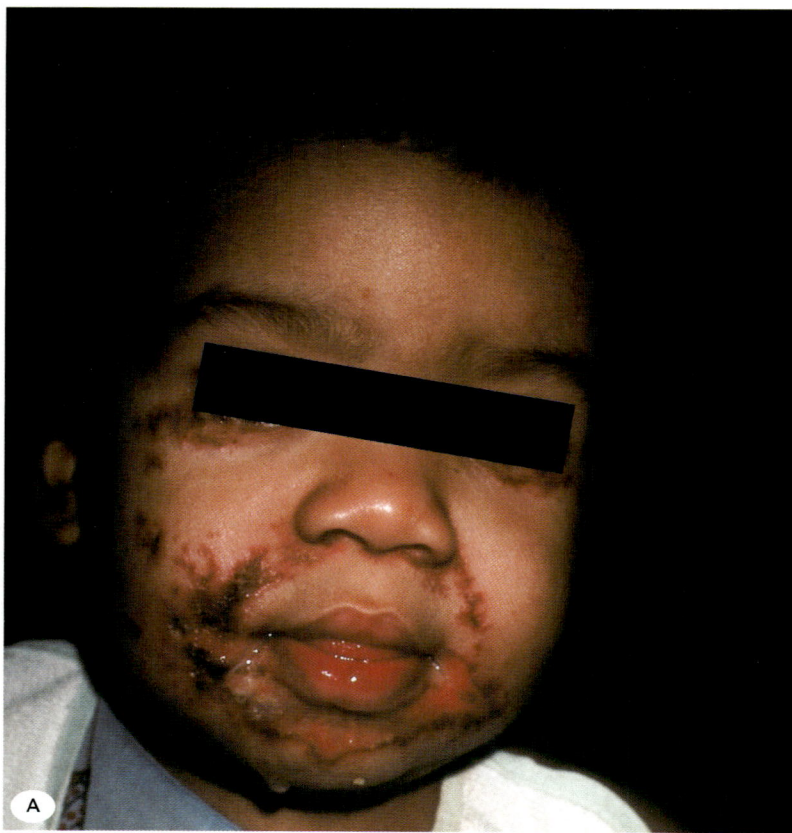

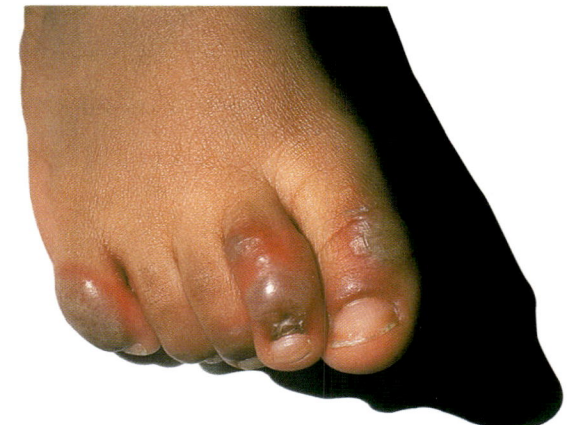

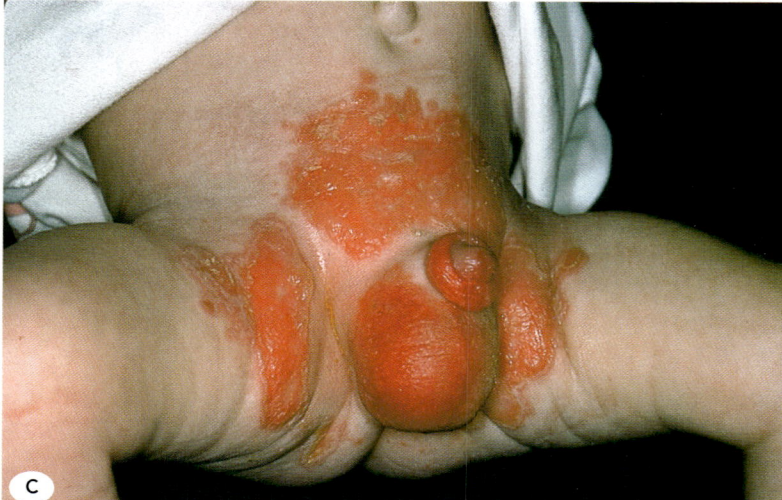

Fig. 22.35 Acrodermatitis enteropathica. (A) Periorificial erosions (Courtesy of Dr Ilona Frieden); (B) acral vesiculobullous lesions (Courtesy of Dr Ilona Frieden); (C) recalcitrant diaper dermatitis.

who had alopecia, trichorrhexis nodosa, and dry, scaly skin who responded to zinc supplementation despite normal serum zinc levels, adding further confusion to the clinical diagnosis of zinc deficiency.[254]

Physical examination

Infants with acrodermatitis enteropathica have a classical erythematous, scaly, psoriasiform, and sometimes vesiculoerosive eruption located periorifically (Fig. 22.35A) (i.e., around the mouth, eyes, and genital area). Similar lesions may occur on the distal portions of the extremities (Fig. 22.35B), but these are not always present in infancy. In premature infants, scaly, red, macerated plaques in the neck folds are characteristic. Refractory diaper dermatitis may be the presenting complaint (Fig. 22.35C). Nail changes consisting of paronychia as well as dystrophy of the nail plate may occur. Secondary staphylococcal and candidal superinfections are very common, and *Candida* may not respond to topical therapy unless the zinc deficiency is corrected. If the disorder is left untreated, the skin rash appears first and, followed by a period of several weeks, near-total alopecia develops. In addition, there is usually photophobia, blepharitis, conjunctivitis, and corneal opacity. Diarrhea may present before or after the cutaneous changes. The affected child is typically irritable with failure to thrive. The Middle Eastern adolescents who have been reported have similar acral and periorificial cutaneous findings, but they also have short stature and delayed puberty.[252]

Laboratory findings

Low levels of plasma zinc are pathognomonic of acrodermatitis enteropathica. Zinc levels must be carefully collected in special acid–washed or plastic tubes, so that exogenous zinc present on ordinary glassware will not contaminate the specimen. In milder forms of zinc deficiency, plasma levels may be misleadingly normal,[250] although there would be a clinically favorable response to zinc.

Another useful associated laboratory finding is low serum alkaline phosphatase, a zinc-dependent metalloenzyme.[255] Investigational testing of immune function has revealed anergy, hypogammaglobulinemia,[254] abnormal cell-mediated immunity,[256,257] as well as monocyte and neutrophil chemotaxis defects.[258,259]

Pathophysiology and histogenesis

The clinical signs and symptoms of all the zinc deficiency states correct dramatically upon replacement with zinc.[239–243] In acrodermatitis enteropathica, the actual metabolic error has not yet been defined, but it is clearly a problem with intestinal absorption and/or transport of zinc. One hypothesis suggests a primary disorder of tryptophan metabolism based on finding high levels of kynurenine, a tryptophan metabolite, in affected patients. Picolinic acid, which enhances the intestinal absorption of zinc, is a tryptophan metabolite.[260] The observation that acrodermatitis enteropathica does not usually occur during

254. Slonim AE, Sadick N et al. (1992) Clinical response of alopecia, trichorrhexis nodosa, and dry, scaly skin to zinc supplementation. **J Pediatr** 121:890.
255. Weismann K, Hyer H (1978) Serum alkaline phosphatase activity in acrodermatitis enteropathica: an index of the serum zinc level. **Acta Derm Venereol** (Stockh); 59:89.
256. Oleske JM, Westphal ML, Shore S et al. (1979) Zinc therapy of depressed cellular immunity in acrodermatitis enteropathica. Its correction. **Am J Dis Child** 133:915.
257. Chandra RK (1980) Acrodermatitis enteropathica: zinc levels and cell-mediated immunity. **Pediatrics** 66:789.

258. Businco L, Menghi AM, Rossi P et al. (1980) Zinc-dependent chemotactic defect in an infant with acrodermatitis. **Arch Dis Child** 55:996.
259. Weston WL, Huff JC, Humbert JR et al. (1977) Zinc correction of defective chemotaxis in acrodermatitis enteropathica. **Arch Dermatol** 113:422.
260. Krieger I, Cash R, Evans GW (1984) Picolinic acid in acrodermatitis enteropathica: evidence for a disorder of tryptophan metabolism. **J Pediatr Gastroenterol Nutr** 3:62.

breast-feeding but one to two weeks after weaning and the fact that breast milk seems more beneficial than cow's milk in this disorder has led to extensive studies of zinc metabolism in human milk.[246,249] Although the zinc content of human milk is not significantly greater than that of cow's milk, human milk contains higher amounts of picolinic acid. Control of zinc levels in human milk is independent of maternal plasma zinc, as shown by the failure to increase milk zinc levels by maternal ingestion of zinc.[246,249] Individual abnormalities in breast milk zinc excretion have resulted in the development of zinc deficiency states in premature and full-term breast-fed infants.[246–251] Conversely, it is believed that the Middle Eastern adolescents with symptomatic zinc deficiency develop it on the basis of concurrent ingestion of high amounts of a zinc-binding ligand, phytate, present in high quantities in these areas and perhaps in the local clay, which is often ingested. Phytate binds the zinc and renders it unavailable for absorption. Finally, in TPN-associated zinc deficiency and in sick premature infants, the zinc deficiency state occurs because of a combination of factors. These include inadequate intake as well as enhanced losses and need for zinc in severe illness and/or stress, as plummeting plasma zinc levels are associated with such stressful events as sepsis.

Absorption of zinc is in the duodenum and proximal small intestine and excretion is primarily intestinal with a small component being excreted in sweat. Thirty percent of ingested zinc is absorbed. In blood, 80% of zinc is in RBCs in carbonic anhydrase. Zinc is an essential mineral that has been found to be present in at least 100 metalloenzymes. Notable enzymes include carbonic anhydrase, carboxypeptidases A and B, alkaline phosphatase, alcohol dehydrogenase, retinene reductase, lactate dehydrogenase, glutamate dehydrogenase, glyceraldehyde 3-phosphate dehydrogenase, and superoxide dismutase. Thus, zinc deficiency has profound widespread metabolic effects. The specific cutaneous manifestations of zinc deficiency may be in part due to zinc interaction with vitamin A metabolism.[261] The interaction of zinc and vitamin A may be mediated via the enzyme retinol alcohol dehydrogenase, which converts photoactively inert retinol to the active retinaldehyde[241] or by impairing synthesis of retinol-binding protein.[241] Zinc also may interact with essential fatty acid metabolism mediated via prostaglandins.[262,263] Zinc

also seems to play an important role in wound healing. The histopathology of zinc deficiency is not specific.[264] It shows a chronic dermatitis with possible neutrophilic infiltration of the epidermis and intraepidermal vesicle formation.

Differential diagnosis

Zinc deficiency in infants resembles severe seborrheic dermatitis as well as essential fatty acid and biotin deficiencies. Secondary candidal infection may be mistakenly thought to be the primary disorder. An acrodermatitis enteropathica-like eruption has been reported as a presenting sign of cystic fibrosis,[265,266] acquired immune deficiency syndrome, and organic aciduria.[267]

Therapy and prognosis

Left untreated, acrodermatitis enteropathica can progress to a fatal outcome. Before the discovery of zinc deficiency, 8-hydroxyquinoline (diodoquin) was found empirically to provide partially successful therapy. It is now speculated that the mechanism of action of diodoquin is to enhance intestinal zinc absorption. Zinc supplementation has a rapid and dramatic effect that reverses all cutaneous, GI, and neurologic manifestations of the disease. In acrodermatitis enteropathica, zinc may need to be supplemented for a lifetime, or at least during times of metabolic stress such as pregnancy. In transient zinc deficiency associated with prematurity or TPN, there is gradual lessening of the need for zinc supplementation as the underlying medical problems are resolved. There is no evidence that zinc supplementation will enhance growth or intellectual function or improve hair growth in children with normal levels of plasma zinc. The daily dietary requirements for zinc and suggested replacements in deficiency states are listed in Table 22.16.

COPPER

Two disorders of copper metabolism are of interest to pediatric dermatologists: Wilson's disease and Menkes' steely hair disease (kinky hair syndrome).[268] They are discussed separately.

TABLE 22.16 Elemental zinc requirements and replacement[a]

Clinical state	PO (mg/day)	IV (μg/kg/day)	Reference
<1 year	3–5	–	253
1–10 years	10	–	253
11–51 years	15	–	253
Pregnant female	20	–	253
Lactating female	25	–	253
Premature, sick, on TPN	–	40–200	255, 266
Premature, not sick	13–30	–	259–262
Full-term infant, not sick	20–45 (3mg/kg/day)		263, 264
Acrodermatitis enteropathica	1–2mg/kg/day	–	253
Adult on TPN	–	20	253

[a] 200mg zinc sulfate = 55mg elemental zinc.

2.8mg zinc acetate = 1mg elemental zinc.

---

261. Solomons NW, Russell RM (1980) The interaction of vitamin A and zinc: implications for human nutrition. Am J Clin Nutr 33:2031.

262. Horrobin DF, Cunnane SC (1980) Interactions between zinc, essential fatty acids and prostaglandins: relevance to acrodermatitis enteropathica, total parenteral nutrition, the glucagonoma syndrome, diabetes, anorexia nervosa and sickle cell anaemia. Med Hypoth 6:277.

263. Cunnane SC (1982) Maternal essential fatty acid supplementation increases zinc absorption in neonatal rats: relevance to the defect in zinc absorption in acrodermatitis enteropathica. Pediatr Res 16:599.

264. Gonzalez JR, Botet MV, Sanchez JL (1982) The histopathology of acrodermatitis enteropathica. Am J Dermatopathol 4:303.

265. Hansen RC, Lemen R, Revsin B (1983) Cystic fibrosis manifesting with acrodermatitis enteropathica-like eruption. Arch Dermatol 119:51.

266. Schmidt CP, Tunnessen W (1991) Cystic fibrosis presenting with periorificial dermatitis. J Am Acad Dermatol 25:896.

267. De Raeve, De Meirieir L, Ramet J et al. (1994) Acrodermatitis enteropathica-like cutaneous lesions in organic aciduria. J Pediatr 124:416–420.

268. Culotta VC, Gitlin JD (2001) Disorders of copper transport, In: The Metabolic and Molecular Basis of Inherited Disease, 8th ed, Scriver CR, Beaudet AL, Sly WS et al. eds. New York: McGraw Hill, pp. 3105–3118.

Wilson's disease (hepatolenticular degeneration)

This disorder[268,279] was first described in 1912 as an autosomal-recessive trait distinguished by toxic copper accumulation in several organ systems. It occurs in approximately 1 in 100 000 births. Chronic liver disease, occasionally progressing to rapid massive hepatic failure, is the presenting sign in the first decade of life. Later, in the second and third decades, CNS copper accumulation, especially in the basal ganglia, causes symptoms including dysarthria and loss of control of voluntary movements. Eventually the disease progresses to deterioration of intellectual function. Hemolytic anemia, joint symptoms, renal stones, and renal tubular acidosis are less common findings. The visible sign in Wilson's disease is the Kayser–Fleischer ring, a brownish-green pigmentation of copper deposition in Descemet's membrane of the cornea. It first appears at the upper and lower poles. Early on, it is visible only with a slit lamp. By the time CNS manifestations are present, it is usually visible. Blue lunulae may also be seen in the nails.

Laboratory studies reveal low plasma ceruloplasmin with high plasma and urinary levels of copper. Liver biopsy specimens also show an accumulation of copper. Radioactive copper studies show failure of normal copper incorporation into ceruloplasmin. The Wilson's disease gene has been mapped to chromosome 13q14.3. The basic defects are thought to be abnormal biliary copper excretion and failure of normal copper incorporation into ceruloplasmin in the liver.[268,269]

Therapy may be successful with the chelating agent, penicillamine. Cutaneous complications of this treatment include elastosis perforans serpiginosa and pemphigus foliaceous and/or vulgaris as well as cutaneous adverse drug reactions. Nephrotic syndrome is also a possible complication. Other treatment options include ammonium tetrathiomolybdate, triethylene tetramine dihydrochloride, and zinc acetate.

Menkes' kinky hair disease

This disorder,[268] also known as steely hair disease, trichopoliodystrophy, X-linked copper malabsorption, and X-linked copper deficiency, was first described clinically as an X-linked disease in 1962 by Menkes et al.[270] but its relationship to copper deficiency was not noted until a decade later by Danks et al.[271] The incidence has been estimated in Australia as 1 in 35 000 births,[272] but in Northern Europe the incidence was found to be only 1 in 298 000 live births.[273] The clinical features of this disorder of copper storage, which result in systemic copper deficiency for many vital tissues, illustrates the ubiquity and importance of copper. The Menkes' disease gene has been located on chromosome Xq13.3 and codes for an intracellular copper binding P-type ATPase similar to that in Wilson's disease.[268,274]

Affected infants, often born prematurely, may have normal appearance and development for the first 2 to 3 months of life. In retrospect, hypothermia and prolonged jaundice are common. Gradually, there is loss of normal psychomotor development, severe hypotonia, and seizures. Cutaneous findings include a striking appearance of the hair, resembling steel wool (Fig. 11.17). The hair is usually light, almost depigmented, with a spangled appearance (Fig. 11.16). Under the microscope, the main finding is pili torti (Fig. 11.15). Trichorrhexis nodosa, brushlike breaks along the hair shaft, may be found also. In careful studies of obligate female heterozygotes, variable levels of pili torti have also been found. The face is characteristically pudgy, with a cupid's bow upper lip and horizontal fuzzy eyebrows. There is generalized marked pigment dilution, with the patient having fairer skin, hair, and eye color than in first-degree relatives. In addition to kinky hair, there are kinky tortuous

TABLE 22.17   Some important copper-containing enzymes

Enzyme	Function
Cytochrome oxidase	Mitochondrial electron transport
δ-Amino levulinate dehydrase	Hemoglobin synthesis
Ceruloplasmin	Catecholamine metabolism
Tyrosinase	Melanin formation
Superoxide dismutase	Protection from free radicals
Monoamine oxidases	Catecholamine metabolism
Lysyl oxidase	Collagen and elastin production
Dopamine β-hydroxylase	Catecholamine metabolism
Peptidylglycine α-amidating monooxygenase	Neuropeptide and peptide hormone processing

blood vessels due to abnormalities of the internal elastic lamina of large and small arteries. Bones are fragile, and fractures, often resembling those seen in child abuse, may be present.[275] Inguinal hernias are common. Infants rarely survive beyond the first decade and invariably show progressive deterioration before death.

Most patients are males because this is an X-linked recessive disease. However, several female patients have now been reported, presumably clinically affected because of unfortunate random inactivation of a large percentage of their normal X chromosomes.[276]

Laboratory findings include low levels of serum copper and ceruloplasmin, although incorporation of copper into ceruloplasmin appears normal.[268,272,274,277] Anemia is common. Intestinal biopsies show high levels of copper in the brush border of the intestinal mucosa. The abnormalities in this disorder reflect the numerous enzymes that are dependent on copper (Table 22.17).[277–279] Thus the anemia, connective tissue and bone abnormalities, and pigment dilution are readily understood as direct abnormalities of δ-amino levulinate dehydrase, lysyl oxidase, and tyrosinase, respectively. It is believed that the poor CNS development may be a result of abnormal catecholamine metabolism in the brain. Arterial abnormalities are due to abnormal elastin tissue on the internal elastic lamina of arteries. There also is an abnormality of cross-linking of free sulfhydryl groups in hair, which may account for the pili torti.

Although Menkes' disease was initially thought to be a simple disorder of copper deficiency due to malabsorption of copper, the high levels of copper found in intestinal mucosal cells as well as in the kidney put it more in the category of a copper storage disease. Indeed, cultured fibroblasts from affected individuals accumulate copper in vitro, providing a basis for possible prenatal diagnosis.[280,281] In a mouse model, the mottled (or brindled) mutants have served as a good source of study.[268] Prenatal screening is possible by demonstrating accumulation of copper in chorionic villus sampling in the first trimester or in cultured amniotic fluid cells in the second.

Ultrastructural studies of the skin have shown abnormal elastin fibrils with deficiency of mature elastin but normal-appearing collagen.[282] Recent biochemical studies of collagen biosynthesis in cultured fibroblasts showed not only copper accumulation, but low lysyl oxidase activity, similar to the abnormality found in Ehlers–Danlos syndrome type IX.[281]

Treatment with both oral and parenteral replacement of copper has unfortunately been uniformly unsuccessful. This may be because CNS damage is

269. Menkes JH (1999) Menkes disease and Wilson disease: two sides of the same copper coin. PartII: Wilson disease. **Eur J Paediatr Neurol** 3:245–253.
270. Menkes HJ, Alter M, Steigleder GK et al. (1962) A sex-linked recessive disorder with retardation of growth, peculiar hair, and focal cerebral and cerebellar degeneration. **Pediatrics** 29:764.
271. Danks DM, Campbell PE, Stevens BJ et al. (1972) Menkes' kinky hair syndrome. An inherited defect in copper absorption with widespread effects. **Pediatrics** 50:188.
272. Hart DB (1983) Menkes' syndrome: an updated review. **J Am Acad Dermatol** 9:145.
273. Tonnesen T, Kleijer WJ, Horn N (1991) Incidence of Menkes disease. **Hum Genet** 86:408.
274. Menkes JH (1999) Menkes disease and Wilson disease: two sides of the same coin. Part I: Menkes disease. **Eur J Paediatr Neurol** 3:147–158.
275. Adams PC, Strand RO, Bresnan MJ, Lucky AW (1974) Kinky hair syndrome: serial study of the radiological findings with emphasis on the similarity to the battered child syndrome. **Radiology** 112:401.

276. Gerdes AM, Tonnesen T, Horn N et al. (1990) Clinical expression of Menkes syndrome in females. **Clin Genet** 38:452.
277. Lucky AW, Hsia YE (1979) Distribution of ingested and injected radiocopper in two patients with Menkes' kinky hair disease. **Pediatr Res** 13:1280.
278. Kay RG (1981) Zinc and copper in human nutrition. **J Hum Nutr** 35:25.
279. Waggoner DJ, Barthikas TB, Gitlin JD (1999) The role of copper in neurodegenerative disease. **Neurobiol Dis** 6:221–230.
280. Kivirikko KI, Peltonen L (1982) Abnormalities in copper metabolism and disturbances in the synthesis of collagen and elastin. **Med Biol** 60:45.
281. Peltonen L, Kuivaniemi H, Palotie A et al. (1983) Alterations in copper and collagen metabolism in the Menkes syndrome and a new subtype of the Ehlers-Danlos syndrome. **Biochemistry** 22:6156.
282. Oakes BW, Danks DM, Campbell PE (1976) Human copper deficiency: ultrastructural studies of the aorta and skin in a child with Menkes' syndrome. **Exp Mol Pathol** 25:82.

irreversible prenatally. The prognosis is poor for survival beyond the first few years of life. Early administration of copper–histidine may be benificial in less severe cases.[268]

Biotin deficiency and multiple carboxylase deficiencies

Skin disorders secondary to biotin deficiency were first reported in the 1940s when diets high in raw eggs were popular.[283] Avidin, a component of egg white, binds biotin and renders it biologically unavailable. More recently, several inborn errors of metabolism, the multiple carboxylase deficiencies, have also been identified as causing biotin-dependent skin and neurologic disease.

Epidemiology

Biotin deficiency can occur as an acquired or dietary deficiency in children and adults, or as an inborn error of metabolism. The two major metabolic syndromes associated with multiple carboxylase deficiency are inherited autosomal recessively: neonatal (early-onset) multiple carboxylase deficiency (OMIM 253270) presents in the first weeks of life and is associated with a deficiency of the enzyme holocarboxylase synthetase; the juvenile (late infantile) form (OMIM 253260) occurs after the second or third month of life and is caused by biotinidase deficiency, an enzyme necessary for the recycling of endogenous biotin. There is no sex predilection.

Presenting history

Acquired dietary biotin deficiency has been produced experimentally in adult volunteers.[283] After the fifth week of a biotin-free diet, symptoms included depression, lassitude, somnolence, hallucination, muscle pains, hyperesthesia, anorexia, and nausea.

In the inherited neonatal and juvenile forms of multiple carboxylase deficiency, vomiting, seizures, developmental delay or regression, hypotonia, and later ataxia are prominent symptoms.[284–289] Similar neurologic findings can also be found in the acquired form secondary to total parenteral alimentation.[290–293]

Physical findings

In the neonatal form of multiple carboxylase deficiency, the earliest signs in the first weeks of life are a sharply marginated seborrheic rash in the scalp, eyebrows, and eyelashes that can spread to perioral, perianal, and other flexural areas.[288] There is associated crusting and erosion, but there are no pustules or vesicles. Over several months, hair thinning can progress to total and even universal alopecia. Prominent fissures on the feet, in the perianal area, and on the cheeks have been reported. There has been associated blepharitis and keratoconjunctivitis with photophobia. Severe cutaneous manifestations may not appear before an early demise. The juvenile (or late infantile) onset and the acquired forms of biotin deficiency secondary to TPN have similar signs but they present at later ages (i.e., over 2 to 3 months in the juvenile form and at the time of TPN). In one family,[289] three affected children developed neurologic and cutaneous signs at 2 to 3 months of age. These children had distinctive, sharply marginated, brightly erythematous periorificial scaly plaques with secondary *Candida* infection as well as severe alopecia. Of note, there are reported cases of well-documented multiple carboxylase deficiency without mention of cutaneous findings. In addition, secondary candidiasis is a frequent complication and is often difficult to treat despite topical antifungal medication until biotin therapy is instituted.

Laboratory findings

Metabolic acidosis, often lactic acidosis, ketosis, and hyperammonemia are all reported. Specific elevations of the urinary organic acids β-methylcrotonyl glycine, β-hydroxyisovaleric acid, and tiglyglycine can aid in diagnosis. Plasma levels of biotin are unreliable indicators of this disorder, unless they are diagnostically low. Holocarboxylase synthetase deficiency can be demonstrated in cultured fibroblasts of affected children. The diagnosis of biotinidase deficiency is made by measuring the enzyme activity in serum.

Etiology and pathogenesis

There are at least three different mechanisms whereby a patient may be biotin deficient (Table 22.18). First, dietary deficiency of biotin coupled with binding of available biotin with avidin can occur.[283,290] One such case was reported in an 11-year-old retarded boy who subsisted on formula supplemented with raw eggs.[294] Second, there may be biotin deficiency due to inadequate replacement during total parenteral nutrition.[291,292] In such cases, the etiology is clear, although there may be individual variation of response to standard biotin supplementation in TPN fluids. Differentiation from essential fatty acid and zinc deficiencies can be extremely difficult clinically. In fact, since one of the key enzymes in long-chain fatty acid synthesis, acetyl CoA carboxylase, contains biotin, there may be a common mechanism.[289] Of note, some children who have responded well to biotin therapy (after failure on zinc and essential fatty acid supplementation) had normal plasma biotin levels, making diagnosis of this deficiency difficult.

The third and most important etiology of biotin responsive disease is the group of multiple carboxylase deficiencies.[284–289] These involve poor activity of any or all of four carboxylases: 3-methylcrotonyl CoA carboxylase (MCC), propionyl CoA carboxylase (PCC), pyruvate carboxylase (PC), and acetyl CoA carboxylase (ACC). These four enzymes are biotin dependent, biotin acting as an obligatory cofactor.[284,294] In the neonatal form, diagnosis of a deficient holocarboxylase synthetase can be made in cultured skin fibroblasts with defects localized to at least four loci. Holcarboxylase synthetase is necessary for biotinylation or attachment of biotin to the other carboxylase enzymes. Enzyme activity can be restored *in vitro*.[295] In the juvenile (late infantile) form, total and partial deficiencies of the enzyme biotinidase have been found.[296–300] These are both inherited as autosomal–recessive disorders occurring as frequently as 1 in 40 000 births.[300]

TABLE 22.18   Biotin deficiency states

Dietary deficiency =/− avidin binding
Total parenteral nutrition
Multiple carboxylase deficiencies
    Neonatal (holocarboxylase synthetase deficiency)
    Juvenile (biotinidase deficiency)

---

283. Sydenstricker VP, Singal SA, Briggs AP et al. (1942) Observations on the "egg white injury" in man. JAMA 118:1199.
284. Wolf B (2001) Disorders of biotin metabolism. In: The Metabolic and Molecular Basis of Inherited Disease, 8th ed, Scriver CR, Beaudet AL, Sly WS et a . eds. New York: McGraw-Hill, ch. 156, p. 3935.
285. Cowan MJ, Wara DW, Packman S et al. (1979) Multiple biotin-dependent carboxylase deficiencies associated with defects in T-cell and B-cell immunity. Lancet 2:115.
286. Charles BM, Hosking G, Green A et al. (1979) Biotin-responsive alopecia and developmental regression. Lancet 2:118.
287. Thoene J, Baker H, Hoshino M, Sweetman L (1981) Biotin-responsive carboxylase deficiency associated with subnormal plasma and urinary biotin. N Engl J Med 304:817.
288. Mock DM (1991) Skin manifestations of biotin deficiency. Semin Dermatol 10:296–302.
289. Williams ML, Packman S, Cowan MJ (1983) Alopecia and periorificial dermatitis in biotin-responsive multiple carboxylase deficiency. J Am Acad Dermatol 9:97.
290. Sweetman L, Surh L, Baker H et al. (1981) Clinical and metabolic abnormalities in a boy with dietary deficiency of biotin. Pediatrics 68:553.
291. Mock DM, DeLorimer AA, Liebman WM et al. (1981) Biotin deficiency; an unusual complication of parenteral alimentation. N Engl J Med 304:820.
292. Mock Dm, Baswell DL, Baker H et al. (1985) Biotin deficiency complicating parenteral alimentation: diagnosis, metabolic repercussions, and treatment. J Pediatr 106:762.
293. Navarro PC, Guerra A, Alvarez JG (2000) Cutaneous and neurologic manifestations of biotinidase deficiency. Int J Dermatol 39:363–365.
294. Gompertz D, Bartlett K, Blair D, Stern CMM (1973) Child with a defect in leucine metabolism associated with β-hydroxyisovaleric aciduria and β-methylcrotonylglycinuria. Arch Dis Child 48:975.
295. Burri BJ, Sweetman L, Nyhan W (1985) Heterogeneity of holocarboxylase synthetase in patients with biotin-responsive multiple carboxylase deficiency. Am J Hum Genet 37:326.
296. Wolf B, Brier RE, Parker WD Jr et al. (1983) Deficient biotinidase activity in late-onset multiple carboxylase deficiency. N Engl J Med 208:161.
297. Wolf B, Grier RE, Allen RJ et al. (1983) Phenotypic variation in biotinidase deficiency. J Pediatr 103:233.
298. Wolf B, Grier RE, Allen RJ et al. (1983) Biotinidase deficiency: the enzymatic defect in late-onset multiple carboxylase deficiency. Clin Chim Acta 131:273.
299. Wolf BW, Heard GS (1991) Biotinidase deficiency. Adv Pediatr 38:1.
300. Heard GS, Wolf B, Jefferson LG et al. (1986) Neonatal screening for biotinidase deficiency: results of a 1-year pilot study. J Pediatr 108:40.

Therapy

All cutaneous findings, including the alopecia, are rapidly responsive to biotin therapy. Pharmacologic doses of biotin of 5–20mg/day in infants and children have been employed in most cases, although some authors believe that 100μg/day supplementation may be adequate.

Differential diagnosis

The clinical findings of biotin deficiency are nearly indistinguishable from essential fatty acid and zinc deficiencies, including location and appearance of the skin manifestations as well as secondary refractory candidiasis.

Hypoxanthine-guanine phosphoribosyltransferase deficiency

This X-linked recessive disorder of purine metabolism, known also as Lesch–Nyhan syndrome, is characterized by the total absence of hypoxanthine-guanine phosphoribosyltransferase (HPRT).[301] The HPRT gene has been mapped to chromosome Xq26-Q27 and over 200 mutations have been characterized. The condition occurs only in males, the female carriers being unaffected, and can present anywhere from early infancy to later life with some degree of genetic heterogeneity. Besides mental retardation, choreoathetosis, and dysarthria, the striking manifestation of this disorder is compulsive, uncontrollable self-mutilation, primarily of the lips, mucous membranes, and hands. This behavior is unwanted by the patient but appears to be uncontrollable, and the patients are often grateful for external restraints. There is no absence of pain, and it is one of the few, if not the only, disorder in which there is massive destruction of tissue rather than callous formation or chronic dermatitis from biting or compulsive picking of the skin. Biochemically, the disorder is characterized by massive elevation of uric acid and, in later life, renal stones and gouty tophi can be present. Of interest, a milder defect of the same enzyme produces no neurologic signs, but early and severe renal disorders and gout.

Therapy toward reducing the uric acid is advised but has no effect on the neurologic manifestations; unfortunately, there is no significant curative treatment for this disorder.

ESSENTIAL FATTY ACID DEFICIENCY

Essential fatty acid (EFA) deficiency does not occur naturally in humans. It has been observed secondary to nutritional deficiencies that are induced either by abnormal diets or severe malabsorption in individuals who have had large portions of their intestine resected and require low-fat diets to prevent severe diarrhea. It has also been observed in individuals who were treated with TPN before the need for replacement of EFAs was recognized. The two major EFAs are linoleic and linolenic acids, and, although arachidonic acid has also been considered essential, it can be metabolized from linoleic acid. Hopefully, with increased awareness of EFA deficiency in the situations noted above, this will become a rare if not extinct disorder. EFA deficiency may be one of the factors responsible for the malnutrition-associated rash of cystic fibrosis.[302]

Pathophysiology and histogenesis

Descriptions of EFA deficiency are sparse, but our major clinical understanding of the disorder comes from studies in the late 1950s and early 1960s[303,304] in which over 400 infants were fed diets with graded deficiencies of linoleic acid for six to 12 months. Skin changes were noted to be most striking in infants with the lowest levels of linoleic acid and were most easily seen in black infants, but were present in all races. After several weeks of either fat-free or low linoleic acid diets, the skin became dry, leathery, and scaly with underlying erythema. The intertriginous areas became exudative. Although there was no increase in bacterial infections in the linoleic acid-deficient group, the children who did develop infections seemed to tolerate them less well. In one instance, a child with full-blown clinical symptoms reversed these after two weeks of oral supplementation of linoleic acid. However, after the supplement was discontinued, she relapsed within six weeks to the previous clinical state. Histologic differences were not apparent in the skin between linoleic acid-deficient and normal children. In most other scattered case reports, the skin is referred to as "dry," "flaky," or "scaly." Other manifestations of EFA deficiency include growth failure, alopecia, poor wound healing, and, at least in animal studies, impaired reproduction, abnormal liver and kidney function, capillary fragility, and increased susceptibility to infection.[305]

Laboratory findings

Laboratory findings in EFA deficiency include decreased levels of plasma linoleic acid, linolenic acid, and arachidonic acid. There is also the presence of 5, 8, 11 eicosatrienoic acid, a lipid not usually found in measurable levels in the circulation, and elevated levels of palmitoleic and oleic acids. The trienoic/tetraenoic ratio is greater than 0.4[306,307] Essential fatty acids are C18, C20, or C22 fatty acids with two to six methylene interrupted unsaturated bonds.[308] The two major EFAs are linoleic and linolenic acids. These cannot be synthesized *de novo* in humans, and can be obtained only through the diet. Arachidonic acid can be metabolized from linoleic acid and is important as a precursor to the prostaglandins, leukotrienes, and thromboxane. Major functions of the EFAs are thought to be multiple because they provide a structural role for fluidity in phospholipid membranes, they serve as energy stores or sebum precursors in triglycerides, and they are also found in sterol esters in the skin. It has been argued that their most important role is as a precursor to prostaglandins. Clinical studies have indicated that reversal of abnormalities noted in EFA deficiency, such as dry, flaking skin, and increased transepidermal water loss, can be improved with oral, parenteral, or even topical applications of linoleic acid. For example, in one study (in adults) topical application of sunflower seed oil to one arm provided increased epidermal linoleic acid, decreased transepidermal water loss, and reversed the scaliness of the skin. This was seen in contrast to the contralateral arm treated with olive oil.[309] However, controlled studies on premature neonates showed no effect of topical application of safflower oil.[310] Animal studies[311] have shown that topical linoleic acid directly corrected skin signs of EFA deficiency (scaling, dryness, dandruff) even when prostaglandin synthesis was blocked with indomethacin; this suggests that the linoleic acid effect was a direct one not mediated via prostaglandins. Such studies have not yet been confirmed in humans. It should be noted that there are many well-documented cases of biochemical EFA deficiency where there are no cutaneous manifestations.

Differential diagnosis

Differential diagnosis will include other nutritional deficiencies and indeed there may be coexistence of multiple deficiencies in individuals with poor diet (i.e., protein calorie malnutrition syndromes) or specific malnutrition due to illness. Therapy involves replacing linoleic acid orally, parenterally, or topically, but most important is the awareness of potential EFA deficiency in situations of poor nutrition.

301. Jinnah HA, Friedemann T (2001) Lesch-Nyhan disease and its variants. In: The Metabolic and Molecular Basis of Inherited Disease, 8th ed, Scriver CR, Beaudet AL, Sly WS et al. eds. New York: McGraw-Hill, ch. 107, p. 2537.
302. Darmstadt GL, McGuire J, Ziboh VA (2000) Malnutrition-associated rash of cystic fibrosis. **Pediatr Dermatol** 17:337–347.
303. Hansen AE, Haggard ME, Boelsche AN et al. (1958) Essential Fatty acids in infant nutrition. III. Clinical manifestations of linoleic acid deficiency. **J Nutr** 66:565.
304. Hansen AE, Wiese HF, Boelsche AN et al. (1963) Role of linoleic acid in infant nutrition. Clinical and chemical study of 428 infants fed on milk mixtures varying in kind and amount of fat. **Pediatrics** 31:171.
305. Paulsrud JR, Pensler L, Whitten CF et al. (1972) Essential fatty acid deficiency in infants induced by fat-free intravenous feeding. **Am J Clin Nutr** 25:897.

306. Caldwell MD, Jonsson HT, Othersen HB Jr (1972) Essential fatty acid deficiency in an infant receiving prolonged parenteral alimentation. **J Pediatr** 81:894.
307. Friedman Z, Danon A, Stahlman MT, Oates JA (1976) Rapid onset of essential fatty acid deficiency in the newborn. **Pediatrics** 58:640.
308. Horrobin DF (1989) Essential fatty acids in clinical dermatology. **J Am Acad Dermatol** 20:1045–1053.
309. Prottey C, Hartop PJ, Press M (1975) Correction of the cutaneous manifestations of essential fatty acid deficiency in man by application of sunflower-seed oil to the skin. **J Invest Dermatol** 64:288.
310. Lee EJ, Gibson RA, Simmer K (1993) Transcutaneous application of oil and prevention of essential fatty acid deficiency in preterm infants. **Arch Dis Child** 68:27.
311. Elias PM, Brown BE, Ziboh VA (1980) The permeability barrier in essential fatty acid deficiency: Evidence for a direct role for linoleic acid in barrier function. **J Invest Dermatol** 74:230.

PROTEIN ENERGY MALNUTRITION

The term *protein energy malnutrition* refers in a general sense to a variety of nutritional disorders due to either limited intake, malabsorption, or an excessive catabolic state. The two best-known syndromes include kwashiorkor and marasmus, which, although uncommon in the United States, are endemic worldwide. Other causes of exogenous starvation include anorexia nervosa and iatrogenic causes when inadequate replacement is given during TPN for a variety of disorders. Malabsorption syndromes including cystic fibrosis, celiac sprue, liver disease, and intractable diarrhea can cause loss of protein, fat-soluble vitamins, and a variety of minerals. Catabolic states such as malignancies, or renal and hepatic failure, can also cause negative nitrogen balance that leads to starvation. In developed countries, protein energy malnutrition is rarely encountered in the absence of chronic disease but has been described occasionally with food faddism or nutritional ignorance. The clinical features of kwashiorkor and marasmus are discussed below. Specific features of vitamin deficiencies are discussed separately.

KWASHIORKOR

Kwashiorkor is a form of protein energy malnutrition in which there is a specific protein intake deficiency with normal caloric intake. This usually occurs in impoverished areas in children in the first 5 years of life at or after the time of weaning when breast milk, the only source of protein, is removed. Such children are usually fed on a diet of carbohydrate staples such as maize. To date, the best clinical descriptions of kwashiorkor remain those of Cicely Williams, put forth in 1933.[312] Williams described children in the Gold Coast of Africa who, after weaning, went onto a diet consisting nearly entirely of maize. Classic symptoms include irritability, diarrhea, and edema of the hands and feet. After one week to 10 days, cutaneous findings become apparent. There is generalized hyperpigmentation from "dark glossy brown" to "dull reddish muddy" color, and occasional depigmentation is also seen. Specific signs include the appearance of small black patches over pressure points on the extensor surfaces of the ankles, knees, and above the wrists and elbows that gradually spread to the legs, forearms, knees, and elbows in a "crazy pavement of thickened epidermis." As the older patches mature, they strip off very readily leaving a pink raw surface exposed underneath; this is called the "enamel paint," "flaky paint," or "peeling paint" appearance (Fig. 22.36A). There is also desquamation at the corners of the mouth and eyes with photophobia. The mucous membranes begin to erode. The thickened black patches of desquamating skin appear first in areas of pressure. In addition, erosions in intertriginous areas with fissuring also occur. Most striking in these children is extreme irritability, apathy, and dejection. Edema can be massive and appear as anasarca. The edema contributes to a large protruding abdomen (Fig. 22.36B), which is also due to hepatomegaly secondary to fatty infiltration of the liver. Edema also accounts for the puffy cheeks and moon-faced appearance.

The hair becomes dry, hypopigmented, and sparse. When children are treated following a bout of kwashiorkor, there is repigmentation of the hair

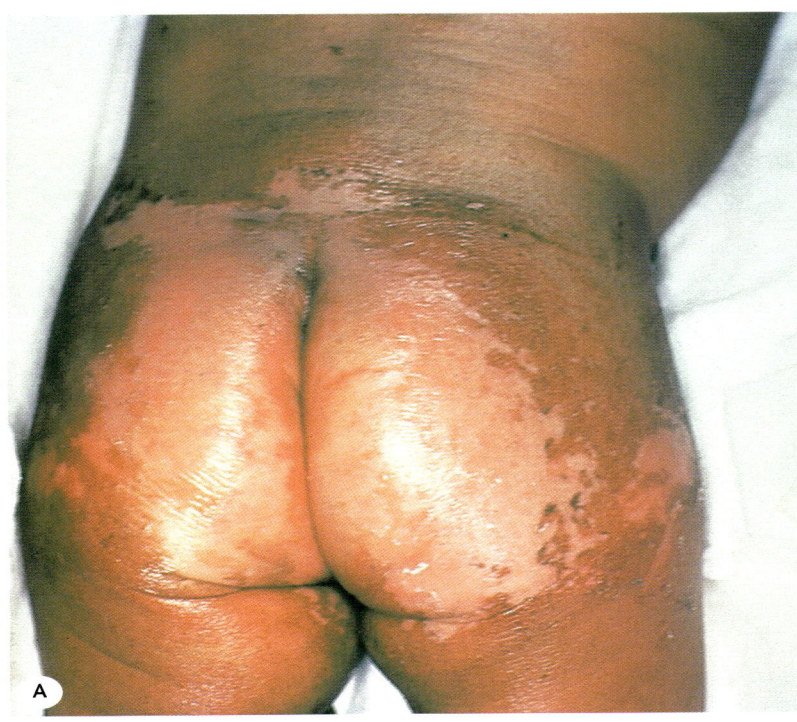

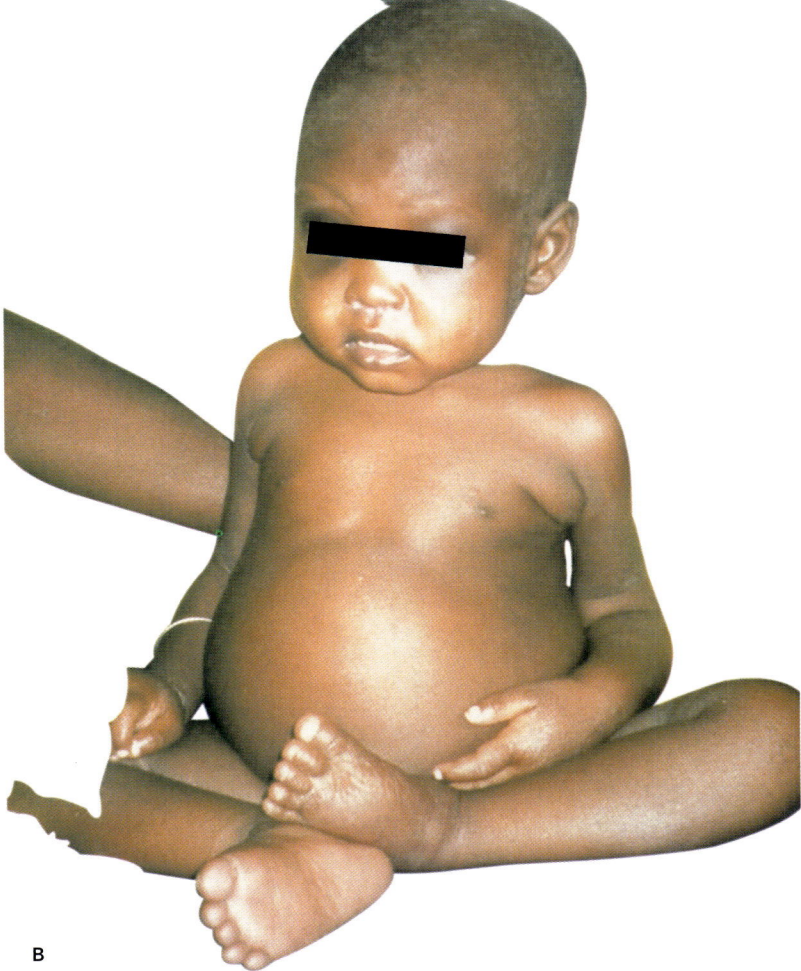

Fig. 22.36 Kwashiorkor: **(A)** classical flaky paint desquamation (Courtesy of Amy Paller); **(B)** bronze color, edema, protuberant abdomen (Courtesy of Hélène Decaluwe MD, Sainte-Justine Hospital, Montreal).

312. Williams CD (1933) A nutritional disease of childhood associated with a maize diet. **Arch Dis Child** 8:423.

shaft leading to the classical "flag sign." A band of depigmented hair along the hair shaft marks the span of time during which there was relative protein malnutrition. Other hair findings include a change in the character of the hair to a softer, finer, and sometimes, straight shaft in normally curly or kinky hair. Ultrastructural studies of such hair has revealed oval shafts with asymmetric loss of the cuticle at the ends of the oval. This weathering of the cuticle is apparently responsible for the dull lusterless look of the hair. No abnormalities in distribution or relative amounts of sulfur-containing amino acids have been found.[313] Copper and zinc levels in hair of children with kwashiorkor have been apparently normal.[314] Nails were thin and soft. The cutaneous findings in kwashiorkor are quite striking and specific and are all reversible with therapy.[315]

Protein energy malnutrition in developed countries occurs predominantly in chronically ill patients such as those with cystic fibrosis. However, several recent cases have been reported in North America in infants without chronic disease intentionally on unorthodox diets because of suspected milk allergy or intolerance, food faddism, nutritional ignorance, or food aversion.[316–318] The most common diagnostic sign is the characteristic skin eruption. The diagnosis of kwashiorkor in these children was often missed initially because of their chubby appearance, due to the edema.

The histopathology is distinctive but not pathognomonic, being similar in other nutritional deficiencies: it shows superficial perivascular lymphocytic infiltrate, pallor of keratinocytes in a band across the upper epidermis, and confluent parakeratosis. A psoriasiform pattern can also be seen.

Pathophysiological features are still not precisely defined. Increased lipid peroxidation seems to play an important role.[319] The differential diagnosis includes other nutritional deficiencies (with which it often coexists) such as zinc, essential free fatty acid, or multiple carboxylase deficiency; immunodeficiencies; metabolic disorders; and Langerhans cell histiocytosis.

MARASMUS

In contrast to kwashiorkor, marasmus represents total calorie starvation and is often seen in younger children under 1 year of age. These children are emaciated with extensive loss of subcutaneous fat and muscle (Fig. 22.37), but they remain alert as opposed to those with kwashiorkor, who are more irritable and apathetic. Rare cutaneous findings may include thin, dry, and elastic skin. However, striking desquamation, hair changes, pigmentary changes, and edema are absent.

VITAMINS

VITAMIN A

Vitamin A (retinol) is a fat-soluble vitamin found in green leafy vegetables, animal fats, milk, and liver. Although the infant's liver stores are quite low at birth, vitamin A derived from colostrum, breast milk, and cow's milk rapidly saturates this primary reservoir. Ultimately, a supply is established that provides enough vitamin A for the body's needs for a 12-month period.

In the setting of a well-balanced diet, vitamin A deficiency is not encountered. If, however, intake of retinol is inadequate, symptoms may develop as early as 2 to 3 years of age. In infants and young children, in whom the pilosebaceous follicles are immature, very dry cracked skin is found. Follicular hyperkeratosis (phrynoderma) may develop, particularly on the shoulders, buttocks, and the extensor surface of the extremities. Acneiform eruptions have been described in adolescents, involving the anterolateral

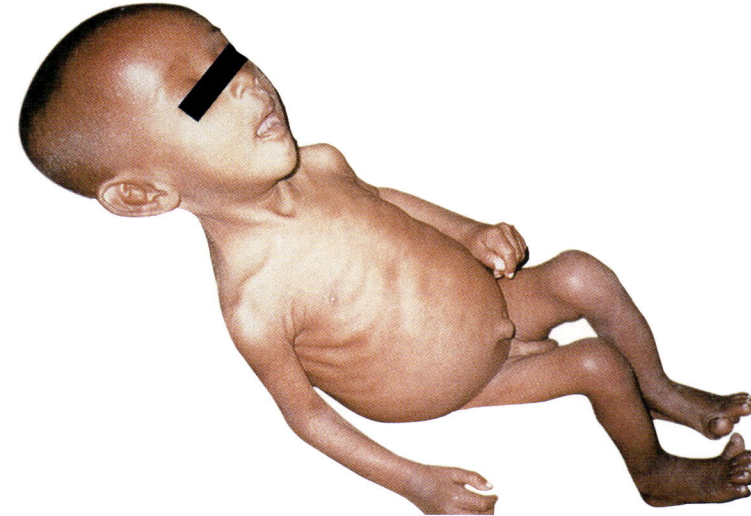

Fig. 22.37 Marasmus (Courtesy of Hélène Decaluwe MD, Sainte-Justine Hospital, Montreal).

surfaces of the arms and back, sparing the face and abdomen. Enhanced keratinization of mucosal surfaces transforms nonkeratinized mucosa into hyperkeratotic white patches. Associated findings may include metaplasia of the salivary ductal epithelium and xerostomia.

Ocular changes are among the earliest manifestations of vitamin A deficiency. Initial changes include impairment of dark adaptation and night blindness. Later, conjunctival and corneal dryness develop as a result of keratinizing metaplasia. Keratomalacia (wrinkling and clouding of the cornea) and Bitot spots (dry, silver-gray plaques on the bulbar conjunctiva) may accompany photophobia.

Vitamin A deficiency may produce both mental and physical retardation and apathy. Vitamin A is also essential for normal immune functions.[320] Anemia with or without hepatosplenomegaly is usually present. Increased intracranial pressure and hydrocephalus may occur. Normal values of vitamin A are age related: from 0 to 6 months, serum levels should exceed 20mg/dl, and from 6 months to adulthood they should fall within the range of 30 to 80mg/dl. Infants require at least 500 international units (iu)/day, whereas older children and adults require 600 to 1500iu/day of either vitamin A or carotene.

Both vitamin A and carotene (which is broken down to vitamin A following ingestion) are absorbed with fats. Absorption may be grossly diminished when fat maldigestion or malabsorption occurs as a result of GI disease or surgery.[321] Celiac disease, hepatic and pancreatic diseases, iron deficiency anemia, chronic infectious diseases, or chronic ingestion of mineral oil impair vitamin A absorption. Premature infants also absorb vitamin A and fat less efficiently than do full-term infants. Low dietary intake of fat also minimizes vitamin A absorption.

Diagnosis is based on dietary history and dark adaptation tests; ophthalmologic examination for conjunctival xerosis is helpful. Treatment is based on the severity of the ophthalmologic impairment and ranges from 5000 to 25 000iu vitamin A in oral or intramuscular forms. In the setting of xerophthalmia, 5000iu/kg per 24 hours orally for 5 days should be followed by daily intramuscular injections of 25 000iu vitamin A in oil until recovery. Keratomalacia requires that doses between 50 000 and 100 000iu be given

313. Gummer CL, Dawber RPR, Harman RRM, King IS (1982) Kwashiorkor: an electron histochemical study of the hair shaft. **Br J Dermatol** 106:407.

314. Bradfield RB, SooHoo T, Baertl JM (1980) Effect of hypochromotrichia on hair copper and zinc during kwashiorkor. **Am J Clin Nutr** 33:1315.

315. Latham MC (1991) The dermatosis of kwashiorkor in young children. **Semin Dermatol** 10:270–272.

316. Buno IJ, Mordei JG, Weston WL (1998) The enamel paint sign in the dermatologic diagnosis of early-onset kwashiorkor. **Arch Dermatol** 134:107–108.

317. Eastlack JP, Grande KK, Levy ML et al. (1999) Dermatosis in a child with kwashiorkor secondary to food aversion. **Pediatr Dermatol** 16:95–102.

318. Liu T, Howard RM, Mancini AJ et al. (2001) Kwashiorkor in the United States. Fad diets, perceived and true milk allergy, and nutritional ignorance. **Arch Dermatol** 137:630–636.

319. Lenhartz H, Ndasi R, Annikos A et al. (1998) The clinical manifestation of the Kwashiorkor syndrome is related to increased lipid peroxidation. **J Pediatr** 132:879–881.

320. Stephensen CB (2001) Vitamin A, infection, and immune function. **Annu Rev Nutr** 21:167–192.

321. Schwartz KB (1996) Vitamins. In: Nutrition in Pediatrics: Basic Science and Clinical Application, 2nd ed, Walter A, Watkins JM, eds. London: BC Decker, Hamilton, ch. 8, pp. 115–135.

parenterally. Children with malabsorption syndrome, celiac disease, or cystic fibrosis should be given supplements of 2000iu in a water-miscible preparation of vitamin A per day (i.e., 1iu vitamin A = 0.3 units of retinol).

Vitamins A excess can be seen in children chronically receiving high doses of vitamins. Manifestations of hypervitaminosis A include lethargy and anorexia. The skin becomes dry and itchy, with follicular keratosis; cheilitis and hair loss are also observed. These mucocutaneous changes are similar to those encountered with isotretinoin therapy. No treatment is necessary other than discontinuation of the vitamin supplement.

Infants should not receive more than 20 000iu/day, as vitamin A toxicity may occur. Toxicity has been reported with intakes as low as 18 000iu/day over a period of a few weeks and from a single dose of 300 000iu.[320] Supplements of vitamin A (400 000iu) are effective in decreasing morbidity and mortality due to measles.

THIAMINE (B₁)

Deficiency of vitamin B₁ (thiamine) leads to beriberi. This water-soluble vitamin plays an important role in pyruvate metabolism; in the setting of poor vitamin intake, both lactate and pyruvate accumulate. These by-products interfere with carbohydrate metabolism, and a high carbohydrate diet accentuates the pre-existing vitamin deficiency state.[322]

Thiamine is present in many foods, including breast and cow's milk, pork, vegetables, cereals, fruits, eggs, yeast, and unmilled cereal grains. It is absent in oils, fats, and refined sugars. Both heat and alkalinity destroy the vitamin, and loss into the water used for boiling is high. When GI or liver disease is present, absorption of thiamine is often poor. Minimum daily requirements are elevated with fever, stress, surgery, dialysis, use of diuretics, and folate deficiency.

Nonspecific systemic indications of thiamine deficiency include fatigue, apathy, irritability, depression, drowsiness, poor concentration, anorexia, nausea, and abdominal discomfort. Characteristic developments that appear later are polyneuritis, muscular weakness, cardiac failure, mental changes, and growth retardation. Neurologic sequelae of beriberi include decreased tendon reflexes, loss of vibratory sense, ptosis, hoarseness, ataxia, and loss of coordination and deep sensation. Prolonged deprivation of thiamine may induce signs of increased intracranial pressure, meningismus, and coma.[323]

A plump, pale child who appears flabby, listless, and dyspneic characterizes the "dry" form of beriberi. These children have a rapid heart rate and hepatomegaly. When "wet" beriberi occurs, peripheral edema develops secondary to high-output biventricular cardiac failure. Skin breakdown may ensue. These children appear undernourished, pale, edematous, and dyspneic. Vomiting and tachycardia are associated features. The skin is waxy and may develop changes as a consequence of peripheral neuropathy. Although no pathognomonic oral changes are seen in beriberi, glossodynia has been reported.

The diagnosis is based on the characteristic clinical findings. Lowered erythrocyte transketolase activity and clinical improvement in response to thiamine help confirm the diagnosis. Prevention is possible if the daily diet includes 0.5mg thiamine for infants and 0.7 to 1.5mg for older children. When hyperalimentation is required, up to 3mg/day may be necessary. A high carbohydrate intake should be avoided when thiamine deficiency is present.[324]

Therapy should be directed at correcting dietary inadequacies. Thiamine supplementation should include both mother and child when the infant is being breast-fed. Oral administration of 10mg thiamine daily will correct beriberi provided absorption is not diminished by GI disturbance. Intramuscular or intravenous thiamine is indicated when cardiac failure is present. Fortunately, the cardiac changes are reversible. Infants suffering from beriberi often have other vitamin deficiencies and the entire B complex should be provided.

RIBOFLAVIN (B₂)

Riboflavin (vitamin B₂) is the coenzyme of flavin mononucleotide and flavin-adenine dinucleotide and essential for redox reactions. Deficiency (oculo-orogenital syndrome) is rarely encountered without concomitant deficiencies of the other B vitamins. Poor dietary intake accounts for most cases of ariboflavinosis, but riboflavin status is not dependent exclusively on dietary intake of the vitamin.[325] Certain non-dietary factors can modify riboflavin status. Respiratory infection, certain diseases, drugs and hormones can influence riboflavin metabolism, and poor absorption may play a role in the setting of biliary atresia or hepatitis. Minimum daily requirements are higher during increased physical activity and in patients with GI disease, hyperthyroidism, fever, and in patients receiving probenecid, tricyclic antidepressants or phenothiazine, or the antagonist galactoflavin.[323] Riboflavin levels are lowered during phototherapy for neonatal hyperbilirubinemia and during psoralen and ultraviolet A light (PUVA) therapy for psoriasis. Although destruction of riboflavin is accelerated in the presence of light, patients receiving phototherapy do not show clinical evidence of vitamin deficiency.

Diets high in carbohydrates accentuate ariboflavinosis, but foods such as liver, kidney, brewer's yeast, milk, cheese, eggs, and green leafy vegetables contain large amounts of riboflavin. Cow's milk provides five times as much of the vitamin as does breast milk.

None of the oral, ocular, or cutaneous sequelae of ariboflavinosis are pathognomonic. When several of the clinical stigmata appear simultaneously, they suggest the deficiency. Among the earliest and most frequently encountered clinical signs is angular cheilitis, which begins with painless gray papules at the corners of the mouth. As the papules enlarge, they ulcerate and become indolent fissures. Similar lesions may develop at the ocular canthi and nasolabial folds.

During the early stages of ariboflavinosis, the fungiform papillae become flattened and swollen, giving the dorsal surface of the tongue a pebbly or granular appearance. With ongoing vitamin deficiency, a progressive papillary atrophy develops and an irregular denudation of the papillae occurs. Rarely, the edema at the bases of the papillae modifies the color of the tongue to a deep purple-red, hence the name magenta cobblestone tongue.

Ocular features of riboflavin deficiency include superficial keratitis, conjunctival edema, lacrimation, blepharospasm, disturbances of vision, changes in iris pigment, and photophobia. Fine, greasy scale mimicking seborrheic dermatitis (dyssebacea) is found on the nasal ala, nasal vestibule, nasolabial and nasomaxillary folds, cheeks, and chin. A normochromic, normocytic anemia with an associated bone marrow hypoplasia represents the hematologic aberration. The erythrocyte glutathione reductase activation test confirms the diagnosis. Oculo-orogenital syndrome is thought to result from riboflavin deficiency. It has been described in adult prisoners of war but not in children.

Measurement of riboflavin stores is possible by determining the erythrocyte glutathione reductase activity. Urinary excretion of riboflavin below 30mg/24 hours is considered low.[323] Ariboflavinosis is preventable if the daily intake for infants is 0.6mg and for older children and adults, 1–2mg.[323] A balanced diet is important to ensure adequate intake. If vitamin deficiency is detected, 3–10mg riboflavin can be given daily by mouth. If no alteration in clinical status occurs within a few days, 2mg should be given intramuscularly three times a day.[323]

PYRIDOXINE (B₆ GROUP)

The three forms of vitamin B₆ are pyridoxol, pyridoxal, and pyridoxamine. Pyridoxine is a cofactor for numerous enzymes of the amino acid metabolism (transaminases, hydroxylases, synthetases) and the transformation of linolic acid to arachidonic acid. Pyridoxol is present in plant foods, the remaining two in animal products.[322] As pyridoxine is widely distributed in

322. Ferguson MM, Dagg JH (1980) Nutritional disorders. In: Oral Manifestations of Systemic Disease, Jones JH, Mason DK, eds. Philadelphia: WB Saunders, p. 211.

323. Curran JS, Barness LA (2000) Vitamin Deficiencies and Excesses. In: Textbook of Pediatrics, 16th ed, Behrman RE, Kliegman RM, Jenson HB. Philadelphia: WB Saunders.

324. Vidal S, Andrianjatovo JJ, Dubau B et al. (2001) Postoperative encephalopathies: thiamine deficiency, an unrecognized etiology. **Ann Fr Anesth Reanim** 20:40–43.

325. Lakshmi AV (1998) Riboflavin metabolism – relevance to human nutrition. **Indian J Med Res** 108:182–190.

nature, deficiency does not occur in the presence of a balanced diet. Malabsorption states, as in celiac disease, may play a role in the development of B_6 deficiency. Riboflavin deficiency can cause conditioned deficiency of vitamin B_6 and the mucocutaneous lesions observed in these two vitamins deficiencies could be due to impaired skin collagen maturity. The metabolic antagonists of pyridoxine (desoxypyridoxine, and isonicotinic acid hydrazide [isoniazid]), as well as oral contraceptives, hydralazine, and penicillamine may induce a vitamin deficiency state.

Clinical findings that develop when vitamin B_6 levels are inadequate include dermatitis, glossitis, and neurologic and GI disturbances. A scaly eruption mimicking seborrhea develops around the eyes, nose, and mouth. The onset of glossitis is heralded by a scalding sensation in the mouth, followed by reddening and hypertrophy of the filiform papillae at the tip and on the margins and dorsum of the tongue. Pain and edema are associated features. Angular cheilitis and a generalized stomatitis may also be present.[322] Additional clinical aberrations include peripheral neuropathy, dizziness, weakness, seizures, nausea, and vomiting.

Although the anemia of pyridoxine deficiency is uncommon in infants, it is of a microcytic, hypochromic nature when present. The determination of vitamin B_6 levels is based on erythrocyte pyridoxal phosphate concentrations or erythrocyte aspartate transaminase levels. Provided the infant's diet contains 0.5–1.5mg, intake is adequate to prevent vitamin deficiency. Adults require 1.5–2.0mg/day.[323] Intake must be supplemented when drug use induces the deficiency state. Among the pyridoxine-responsive inherited disorders are seizures from B_6 dependency, B_6-dependent anemia, homocystinuria, xanthinuric aciduria cystathionuria, and pyridoxine-responsive chronic anemia.

PANTOTHENIC ACID

Pantothenic acid, like biotin, is synthesized by the bacterial flora within the gut. The vitamin is required for the synthesis of coenzyme A, and this plays an essential role in metabolism. Deficiency states occur when nutrition is poor, as with protein-energy malnutrition. Manifestations of inadequate pantothenic acid include fatigue, muscle cramps, headaches, incoordination, paresthesias, vomiting, and diarrhea. No characteristic skin or mucous membrane changes are attributable to a deficiency of this vitamin.

NIACIN (B₃)

Niacin, one component of the vitamin B complex, is unlike other vitamins in that humans are capable of synthesizing it from tryptophan, an essential amino acid. Liver, lean pork, salmon, poultry, and red meat are good sources of niacin. Pellagra is a deficiency disease caused by inadequate intake of niacin (nicotinic acid). Pellagra (*pelle* for "skin" and *agra* for "rough") is limited primarily to populations whose major dietary intake is maize (which is low in tryptophan) and millet (which may interfere with tryptophan metabolism due to its high leucine content) or who suffer from malnutrition due to psychic alterations.[326] Some drugs may cause pellagroid skin and mucosal reactions.[327]

The earliest symptoms of pellagra include lassitude, anorexia, numbness, dizziness, and paresthesias.[322] The tongue is often the focus of clinical changes, with both edema and glossitis noted as prominent features. The swollen papillae at the tip and lateral margins gradually atrophy and disappear, leaving a slick red dorsal surface. The entire tongue gradually becomes enlarged, painful, and erythematous. The lateral surfaces may become deeply ulcerated, and superinfection is common. The buccal and vaginal mucosa are also susceptible to deep ulceration and secondary infection.

The classical triad of dermatitis, diarrhea, and dementia develops only after months of niacin or tryptophan deficiency. Tissue stores of niacin are generally large and the symptom complex of pellagra is often not well developed in infants and children.[323] The dermatitis may develop suddenly or insidiously following exposure to an irritant or to bright sunlight. Areas exposed to heat, friction, or pressure are also susceptible to the development of pellagrous dermatitis. Early lesions are pruritic and burning and have sharp margination. A symmetric distribution of erythematous patches with or without vesicles develops. The underlying skin may be slightly edematous. The facial lesions, which are often large and thick, can become pustular. Well-demarcated lesions around the neck, called Casal's necklace, are rarely present in the absence of dermatitis elsewhere. Dermatitic skin becomes rough, hard, brittle, cracked, and dark reddish-brown to black. Areas that have healed may remain hyperpigmented. Painful fissures occasionally develop on the digits and palms.[328]

Children infested with parasites or suffering from other chronic diseases demonstrate more severe effects as a result of niacin deficiency. GI manifestations include vomiting and diarrhea or diarrhea alternating with constipation. Other dietary deficiencies as well as anemia may exist simultaneously.

Changes in the nervous system occur late in the course of the illness and are associated with irritability, anxiety, and apathy.[323] The posterior and lateral columns are demyelinated when niacin deficiency is prolonged.

The diagnosis of pellagra is suspected in the clinical setting of glossitis, GI problems, and a symmetric dermatitis. Clinical response to niacin remains an important diagnostic parameter. *N*-Methylnicotinamide, a normal metabolite of niacin, is nearly absent in the urine of pellagrous patients. Included in the differential diagnosis of pellagrous dermatitis are carcinoid syndrome, Hartnup's disease, and isoniazid-induced alteration of tryptophan metabolism.

Prevention of pellagra is possible if 8mg niacin is provided in the daily diet of infants and 9–20mg/day for older children. The addition of 50–300mg niacin daily brings about rapid reversal of pellagra. If the vitamin deficiency is severe or GI absorption poor, 100mg niacin may be given by the intravenous route. Within 30 minutes, flushing and a sensation of increased local heat may be noted. These side effects are not present when nicotinamide (niacinamide) is used, but with large doses of that medication, cholestatic jaundice and hepatotoxicity may supervene.[323]

VITAMIN B₁₂

Vitamin B_{12} is ubiquitous in foods, and most cases of deficiency are due to failure of absorption. Inadequate intake does result, however, from diets lacking in milk, eggs, and animal products as in strict vegetarianism (vegans), or the breast milk of mothers with pernicious anemia. Infants with kwashiorkor or marasmus are not usually B_{12} deficient.

Juvenile pernicious anemia, a rare condition, differs from the adult form in that gastric acid secretion is normal. The ability to secrete gastric intrinsic factor is lost, possibly as a result of genetic influences, as parental consanguinity is common in such cases. Symptoms of juvenile pernicious anemia may appear between 9 months and 3 years of age. Congenital transcobalamine deficiency predisposes of vitamin B_{12} deficiency in older children. Intestinal causes of poor absorption of vitamin B_{12} include surgical resection of the terminal ileum for regional enteritis or tuberculosis, overgrowth of intestinal bacteria in diverticula or blind loops of bowel, and infestation with the fish tapeworm *Diphylobothrium latum* in the upper small intestine.

Glossopyrosis antedates swelling and pallor of the tongue when vitamin B_{12} levels are inadequate. The filiform and fungiform papillae are lost, in either a focal or diffuse pattern, leaving a smooth, red, painful dorsal surface (Hunter's or Moeller's glossitis). These oral changes may precede significant anemia. Neurologic sequelae include ataxia, paresthesias, hyporeflexia, clonus, Babinski responses, and even coma.[323] A symmetric but patchy hyperpigmentation may develop over the joints of the hands and feet.

Diagnosis of vitamin B_{12} deficiency is based on characteristic changes in the peripheral blood smear and bone marrow. Radioassay of vitamin B_{12} levels

326. Ballmer-Weber BK, Braathen LR, Ballmer PE (1999) Erythem nach Fehlernährung und Sonnenexposition. **Schweiz Med Wochenschr** 129:1492–1495.

327. Heyer G, Simon M, Schell H (1998) Dosisabhängige pellagroide Hautreaktion durch Carbamazepin. **Hautarzt** 49:123–125.

328. Yoshikawa K (1999) Vitamin and dermatology. **Nippon Rinsho** 57:2385–2389.

in the serum may also be employed. Therapy should include oral therapy only if poor oral intake is causing the deficiency, as most cases result from malabsorption of the vitamin. Intramuscular injection of hydroxycobalamin, which is retained more efficiently than cyanocobalamin, effects a prompt clinical response and rapidly replenishes body stores. If chronic replacement is required, $1000\mu g$ injected every two months provides a wide margin of safety.[321,323] The liver stores vitamin B_{12}; if gastric absorption ceases, and stores are generally adequate for 6 to 10 years. Daily metabolic requirements may be as little as $2-5\mu g$ of vitamin B_{12}.

VITAMIN C (ASCORBIC ACID)

Vitamin C (ascorbic acid) is a hydrosoluble vitamin that is not synthesized in the human body. Dietary intake is essential and recommended daily allowance is 40–50mg/day for children and 60mg/day for adults. Its main sources are fresh fruit and vegetables. Vitamin C is important in collagen formation and various enzymatic processes as well as an antioxidant.

Inadequate dietary intake of vitamin C results in the metabolic deviations and clinical manifestations known as scurvy. Deficient ascorbic acid leads to the production of functionally defective collagen as a result of failure of hydroxylation of procollagen, proline, and lysine. Abnormal collagen is responsible for widespread changes affecting principally the bones, teeth, and supporting tissues of blood vessels.

Scurvy is rare in the United States and Europe, but most cases in the pediatric age group occur between the ages of 6 and 24 months.[329] At birth, scurvy is extremely rare, and breast-fed infants usually receive adequate vitamin C. Infants fed with formula may require additional supplementation. Deficiency may occur with peculiar dietary habits, food fads, or parental ignorance.[330,332] The need for vitamin C increases with febrile illnesses, particularly those of an infectious nature or accompanied by diarrhea. Exposure to cold, iron deficiency, and protein depletion also increases metabolic demands for ascorbate.[323]

Mucous membrane changes in scurvy are most noticeable after the teeth have erupted. Patients under 6 months of age and those who have become edentulous often lack the mucosal changes entirely. Redness, swelling, and tiny hemorrhages become evident at the tips of the interdental papillae. The gums may become bluish-purple and spongy, swelling to the point of concealing the upper incisors. Gradual loss of periodontal bone may follow with loosening and, ultimately, loss of the teeth.[329,331]

Follicular hyperkeratosis with broken corkscrew hairs represents one of the most distinctive and earliest signs of scurvy.[329,330] The enlarged follicles are reddened by the congestion and proliferation of the surrounding blood vessels. The anterior forearms, abdomen, and lower extremities show the most marked follicular hyperkeratosis, with the follicles of the lower extremities having the greatest tendency to become hemorrhagic. These petechiae are prominent in hair-bearing areas due to defective collagen within the supporting tissue of the blood vessels.

Bone pathology as a result of scurvy includes fractures of the cartilaginous matrix, decreased osteoid formation, and large subperiosteal or marrow hemorrhages. Epiphyseal separation may result. The femur and tibia are the long bones most often affected. Generalized tenderness and increasing irritability frequently accompany the bony alterations. The legs may assume a "frog position," with semiflexion at the hips and knees and the feet rotating outwardly. Overall growth is impeded. Vitamin C deficiency in infants, known as Möller–Barlow disease, shows particularly pronounced petechiae and hemorrhages in the gastrointestinal and urinary tracts.

Systemic features of scurvy include low-grade fever, anemia, lethargy, and poor wound healing. When scurvy is severe, cardiac hypertrophy, bone marrow depression, adrenal atrophy, and degeneration of skeletal muscles may occur.[332]

The diagnosis of scurvy is based on a history of poor ascorbate intake in the setting of characteristic clinical changes. Laboratory evaluation of serum or leukocyte vitamin C levels can be employed to confirm the diagnosis. The differential diagnosis includes leukemia, meningococcemia, thrombocytopenic purpura, suppurative arthritis, osteomyelitis, and other vitamin deficiencies. Therapy consists of a daily oral intake of 100–200mg ascorbic acid. Recovery is generally rapid.

VITAMIN K

Vitamins K_1 and K_2 are naphthaquinone derivatives that participate in oxidative phosphorylation and hepatic synthesis of coagulation factors II (prothrombin), V, VII, IX, and X. Protein C, protein S, and osteocalcin are also vitamin-K dependant. The production of these coagulation components is dependent both on normal hepatic function and on adequate dietary intake of vitamin K_1. This naturally occurring fat-soluble form of vitamin K is found in varying concentrations in hog's liver, soybeans, alfalfa, spinach, and tomatoes. The intestinal bacteria synthesize vitamin K_2, but alteration of the gut flora by antibiotics may hinder its manufacture, with resultant diminution of prothrombin production.

Low levels of vitamin K are frequently encountered in newborn infants, particularly those of low birth weight, as a result of inadequate intake and an uncolonized GI tract. Breast milk serves as a less valuable source of the vitamin than does cow's milk. Infants with diarrhea, particularly if breast-fed, are susceptible to the development of a deficiency state. Other GI diseases predisposing to inadequate levels of vitamin K are biliary obstruction, fistulas, sprue, and other malabsorption diseases. By acting as competitive antagonists of vitamin K, drugs such as coumarin, salicylates, isoniazid and cholestyramine produce thrombocytopenia.[333]

The clinical stigmata of thromcytopenia due to inadequate vitamin K include ecchymoses of the skin and bleeding from the gums. The ecchymoses may become confluent at sites of pressure or trauma. The gums are not friable despite their tendency to be hemorrhagic.

Diagnosis of vitamin K deficiency is based on these clinical changes and a prolonged prothombin time. Mild cases in infants are amenable to oral administration of 1–2mg vitamin K daily. When the hemorrhagic state is severe, a daily dose of 5mg vitamin K_1 should be given parenterally.

Use of large doses of synthetic vitamin K analogue (but not vitamin K_1) can produce hyperbilirubinemia and kernicterus in the glucose-6-phosphate-dehydrogenase-deficient newborn as well as the premature infant.[323] If liver damage is the source of hypothrombinemia, both vitamin K_1 and whole blood are often required to correct the deficiency.

ACKNOWLEDGMENT

The section on vitamin deficiency is courtesy of Dr Adelaide Hebert.

329. Ellis CN, Vanderveen EE, Rasmussen JE (1984) Scurvy: a case caused by peculiar dietary habits. **Arch Dermatol** 120:1212–1214.
330. Levin NA, Greer KE (2000) Scurvy in an unrepentant carnivore. **Cutis** 66:39–44.
331. Fuchs J (1994) Vitamine und Haut. **Ther Umsch** 51:489–495.
332. McLaren DS (1979) Cutaneous changes in nutritional deficiencies. In: Dermatology in General Medicine, 2nd ed, Fitzpatrick TB, Eisen AZ, Wolff K et al. eds. New York: McGraw-Hill, p. 1024.
333. Bor O, Akgün N, Yakut A et al. (2000) Late hemorrhagic disease of the newborn. **Pediatr Int** 42:64–66.

Collagen Vascular, Connective Tissue Diseases, and Selected Systemic Diseases with Skin Manifestations

Nancy K. Barnett, Dowain A. Wright, Tomisaku Kawasaki and Patricia A. Treadwell

CONNECTIVE TISSUE DISEASES AND ARTHRITIDES

Nancy K. Barnett and Dowain A. Wright

LUPUS ERYTHEMATOSUS

Lupus erythematosus (LE) is a chronic inflammatory disorder of unknown origin involving multiple organ systems. The clinical signs and symptoms, primarily the result of small vessel vasculopathy, can be protean and episodic. Advances in serologic technology, as well as the establishment[1] and revision[2,3] (first in 1977 and again in 1999) by the American College of Rheumatology (ACR) of criteria for the diagnosis of systemic lupus erythematosus (SLE), have provided clinicians with clinical and laboratory guidelines for the early diagnosis of SLE (Table 23.1). Four of these criteria must be present to establish a diagnosis of SLE.

These laboratory and clinical guidelines, together with aggressive treatment, have improved the prognosis of childhood SLE. During the late 1950s and early 1960s, childhood SLE was viewed as a usually fatal disease. Now early diagnosis and the use of steroid and immunosuppressive therapy have dramatically improved the survival of childhood SLE patients, although it is still frequently more severe than its adult counterpart.[4,5]

EPIDEMIOLOGY

Approximately 25% of SLE begins during the first two decades of life.[6] The peak incidence of the occurrence of SLE in childhood is early adolescence.[7] Another study has demonstrated that 60% of childhood SLE occurs between the ages of 11 and 15 years, 35% begins between 5 and 10 years of age, and 5% of cases occur before the age of 5.[4] SLE is rare under 1 year of age.[5]

The frequency of SLE among white male and female children appears to be about 3:4 until puberty, at which time a striking increased predominance in female to male involvement occurs (9:1).[8]

The exact incidence and prevalence of childhood SLE are unknown because no central registry exists. The prevalence of childhood SLE has been estimated at 5 to 10 per 100 000 but racial differences in the frequency of childhood SLE appear to exist. Black, Hispanic, and Asian children may have at least a two- to threefold increased frequency of SLE compared with whites.[9–12] Tucker[8] reports an incidence of 9.4 per 100 000 in white females compared to almost 20 per 100 000 in black females before age 10 and the frequency of SLE at puberty appears to rise at a disproportionately greater level among black, Asian, and Hispanic females than white females.[9] There is some evidence to suggest that the disease process may also be more severe among black and Hispanic children. For example, black and Hispanic children with lupus nephritis appear to have a slightly earlier age of onset (approximately 10 years) and a higher mortality and morbidity than their white counterparts.[13]

TABLE 23.1   1982 Revised criteria for the classification of SLE

1. Malar rash
2. Discoid rash
3. Photosensitivity
4. Oral ulcers
5. Arthritis: peripheral nonerosive arthritis involving two or more joints
6. Serositis: pleuritis or pericarditis
7. Renal disorder: proteinuria or cellular casts
8. Neurologic disorder: seizures or psychosis*
9. Hematologic disorder: hemolytic anemia or leukopenia $<4000/mm^3$ or lymphopenia $<1500/mm^3 \times 2$ or thrombocytopenia $<100\,000/mm^3$ without offending drugs
10. Immunologic disorder: positive LE preparation or anti-DNA or anti-Sm or false-positive serologic test for syphilis for 6 mos (using the *Treponema pallidum* immobilization or fluorescent treponemal antibody absorption test)**
11. ANA: in the absence of drugs known to be associated with "drug-induced lupus" syndrome

(From Tan et al.[1] with permission.)

* Item 8 revised in 1999 to include 19 central and peripheral nervous system syndromes.[3]

** Item 10 revised in 1997 to delete positive LE preparation and add positive finding of antiphospholipid antibodies based on (1) an abnormal serum level of IgG or IgM anticardiolipin antibodies, (2) a positive test result for lupus anticoagulant using a standard method, or (3) a false positive serologic test for syphilis known to be positive for at least 6 months and confirmed by treponema pallidum immobilization or fluorescent treponemal antibody absorption test.[2]

---

1. Tan EM, Cohen AS, Fries JF et al. (1982) The 1982 revised criteria for the classification of systemic lupus erythematosus. **Arthritis Rheum** 25:1271.
2. Hochberg MC (1997) Updating the American College of Rheumatology Revised Criteria for the Classification of Systemic Lupus Erythematosus. **Arthritis Rheum** 40 (9):1725.
3. ACR Ad Hoc Committee on Neuropsychiatric Lupus Nomenclature (1999) The American College of Rheumatology Nomenclature and Case Definitions for Neuropsychiatric Lupus Syndromes. **Arthritis Rheum** 42(4):599.
4. Kornreich HK, Hanson V (1974) The rheumatic diseases of childhood. **Curr Probl Pediatr** 4:3.
5. Dale RC, Tang SP, Heckmatt JZ, Tatnall FM (2000) Familial systemic lupus erythematosus and congenital infection-like syndrome. **Neuropediatrics** 31(3):155.
6. Fish AJ, Blau EB, Westberg NG et al. (1977) Systemic lupus erythematosus within the first two decades of life. **Am J Med** 62:99.
7. Lo JT, Tsai MJ, Wang LH et al. (1999) Sex differences in pediatric systemic lupus erythematosus: a retrospective analysis of 135 cases. **J Microbiol Immunol Infect** 32(3):173.
8. Tucker LB (1998) Caring for the adolescent with systemic lupus erythematosus. **Adolesc Med** 9(1):59.
9. Lehman TJA (1993) Systemic lupus erythematosus in childhood and adolescence. In: Dubois Lupus Erythematosus, 4th edn, Wallace DJ, Hahn BH, eds. Philadelphia: Lea & Febiger, p. 431.
10. Siegel M, Lee SL (1973) The epidemiology of systemic lupus erythematosus. **Semin Arthritis Rheum** 3:1.
11. Lehman TJA, McCurdy D, Spencer C et al. (1990) Prognostic value of antibodies to Ro/SSA, La/SSB, and RNP in children with systemic lupus erythematosus. **Arthritis Rheum** 33:S154.
12. Schaller J (1982) Lupus in childhood. **Clin Rheum Dis** 8:219.
13. Tejani A, Nicastri AD, Chen CK et al. (1983) Lupus nephritis in black and hispanic children. **Am J Dis Child** 137:481.

SLE appears to be the most common form of LE among children. Benign cutaneous lupus (discoid, i.e., cutaneous lupus with no clinical or serologic evidence of systemic disease), is relatively unusual in children, whereas renal disease and central nervous system disease are prominent in childhood LE.[4,6,12,14,15] It is likely that less severe forms of SLE in childhood go underreported.

ETIOLOGY

The etiology of SLE at the present time is unknown. However, the etiology appears to be multifactorial, with evidence being accumulated for the roles of viral, hormonal, environmental, and immunogenetic factors. Recent studies have demonstrated a more compelling role for immunogenetic factors. Several studies demonstrate an aggregation of autoimmune diseases and autoimmune phenomena among first-degree relatives of patients with LE.[16] In addition, studies of the occurrence of LE in monozygotic and dizygotic twins present the most striking evidence of a genetic association with LE. In one study, the concordance in monozygotic twins for SLE was approximately 70% and in another study approximately 25%.[17,18] The concordance among dizygotic twins ranges between 2 and 9%. It has also been observed that when identical twins develop SLE, the age of onset of the disease is closer and the occurrence is at a younger age compared with siblings who develop SLE.

SLE is associated with an increased frequency of the HLA-DR2 and DR3 phenotypes. The relative risks of developing SLE associated with the presence of these phenotypes are small (2 to 3). More recent studies indicate that the anti-Ro(SSA) antibody response is associated with the HLA-DR2 and DR3 phenotypes. If one subtracts the anti-Ro(SSA) antibody positive patients from the total lupus cohorts, the association of lupus erythematosus with the HLA-DR2 and DR3 phenotypes disappears. This suggests that the anti-Ro(SSA) antibody response and not the clinical presentation of lupus erythematosus is associated with these HLA phenotypes. Furthermore, in a study of 34 families with children with SLE, Lehman, *et al.* demonstrated that anti-Ro(SSA) antibodies were detected more frequently in daughters of anti-Ro(SSA) antibody positive mothers than among daughters of anti-Ro(SSA) negative mothers.[19] Work by Reveille *et al.* has demonstrated that the anti-Ro(SSA) antibody response is under genetic control by alleles at the DQ locus. Virtually all anti-Ro(SSA) and La(SS-B) antibody-positive patients have glutamine at position 34 on the outer domain of the β-chain of the DQ molecule, and a leucine residue at position 26 on the α-chain of the DQ molecule.[20]

Other studies have demonstrated a very close immunogenetic relationship between some anti-Ro(SSA) positive females presenting with primary Sjögren syndrome or presenting with subacute cutaneous LE, and those female patients presenting with the Sjögren syndrome/lupus erythematosus overlap syndrome. These patients all share an increased frequency of the HLA-B8, DR3, DQ2, and DRw52 phenotypes.[21,23] All of these women are at risk of giving birth to a child with the neonatal lupus syndrome (see below).

Further evidence demonstrating the strong genetic relationship with LE have come from a study of patients with hereditary deficiencies of various components of the complement system.[22] Those patients possessing homozygous deficiencies of the early complement components (i.e., C1q, C1r, C1s, C4, C2) have an increased frequency LE (many beginning in childhood)[23] when compared with those patients with homozygous complement deficiencies of the late complement components (i.e., C3, C5, C6, C7, and C8). It should be noted that C2 and C4 are encoded for by class III alleles located in the major histocompatibility complex of chromosome 6. Furthermore, the lupus-like disease process that homozygous C2 and C4 patients develop is characterized by the frequent presence of anti-Ro(SSA) antibodies.[24] The most common complement deficiency associated with the development of LE is null alleles for the fourth component of complement, most commonly C4AQ0.[25]

As noted above, gender differences emerge strikingly in adolescence, becoming more common in the female by 5:1. Studies have suggested that there may be an effect of sex hormones with estrogen or lower testosterone predisposing to the development of SLE.[25]

Thus, although the pathogenesis of LE is multifactorial, these recent studies demonstrate that immunogenetic factors most likely play a substantial role in the pathogenesis of LE in some patients. Positional candidate genes have been suggested on chromosome 1[26] and a genetic mutation of T-cell regulation may allow apoptosis with impaired regulation of B-cell clones producing autoantibodies in susceptible individuals.[27]

PHYSICAL EXAMINATION

It is important to emphasize that the true frequency of occurrence of various manifestations in childhood LE is difficult to obtain. It is very conceivable that children with milder forms of LE (i.e., lacking cerebral and renal disease) are underreported. Furthermore, the early recognition of LE and the institution of aggressive therapy with corticosteroids, etc. have undoubtedly modified the frequency of occurrence of manifestations.

Classical discoid lupus erythematosus (DLE) lesions are the most common cutaneous manifestation in childhood SLE.[28] The term *discoid* is employed as a morphologic descriptive term meaning coin-shaped. Unfortunately, this term has been used to mean benign cutaneous lupus as opposed to SLE and this misuse of the term discoid has created a great deal of confusion. It is important to realize that DLE lesions can be seen in the total absence of serologic and clinical data of systemic involvement (Fig. 23.1A), and can also be seen as cutaneous manifestations in patients with classic SLE (Fig. 23.1B).

In the largest report of eight cases of childhood benign cutaneous lupus (DLE), George and Tunnessen indicate that although benign cutaneous lupus (DLE) is similar to its adult counterpart in presentation and chronicity, there may be some significant differences. These authors note a lack of female predominance, a low incidence of photosensitivity, and an increased risk of progression to SLE.[28] There is increasing evidence that these cases in children are seldom reported[29] as is lupus erythematosus tumidus (LET).[30] LET consists of erythematous, edematous, non-scarring plaques in sun-exposed areas without systemic disease.

14. Yancy CL, Doughty RA, Athreya BH (1981) Central nervous system involvement in childhood systemic lupus erythematosus. **Arthritis Rheum** 24:1389.
15. Cameron JS (1994) Lupus nephritis in childhood and adolescence. **Pediatr Nephrol** 8(2)230.
16. Arnett FC, Reveille JD, Wilson RW et al. (1984) Systemic lupus erythematosus: current state of the genetic hypothesis. **Arthritis Rheum** 14:24.
17. Block SR, Lockshin MD, Winfield JB et al. (1976) Immunologic observations on 9 sets of twins either concordant or discordant for SLE. **Arthritis Rheum** 19:545.
18. Deapen DM, Escalante A, Weinrib L et al. (1992) A revised estimate of twin concordance in systemic lupus erythematosus. **Arthritis Rheum** 35:311.
19. Lehman TJA, Reichlin M, Harley JB (1990) Familial concordance for antibodies to Ro/SSA among female relatives of children with systemic lupus erythematosus: evidence for a supergene hypothesis. **Arthritis Rheum** 33:125A.
20. Reveille JD, MacLeod MJ, Whithington K, Arnett FC (1991) Specific amino acid residues in the second hypervariable region of HLA-DQA1 and DQBI chain genes promote the Ro(SSA)/La(SSB) autoantibody responses. **J Immunol** 146:3871.
21. Provost TT, Watson R (1993) Anti-Ro(SSA) HLA-DR3 positive women: the interrelationship between some ANA negative, SS, SCLE and NLE mothers and SS/LE overlap female patients. **J Invest Dermatol** 100:14s.
22. Arnett F (1992) Genetics of systemic lupus erythematosus. **Rheum Dis Clin North Am** 18:865.
23. Stone NM, William A, Wilkinson JD et al. (2000) Systemic lupus erythematosus with C1q deficiency. **Br J Dermatol** 142:521.
24. Provost TT, Arnett F, Reichlin M (1983) C2 deficiency, lupus erythematosus, an anti-cytoplasmic antibodies. **Arthritis Rheum** 26:1279.
25. Petty RE (1998) Etiology and pathogenesis of rheumatic disease of adolescence. **Adol Med** 9(1):11.
26. Tsao BP (2000) Lupus susceptibility genes on human chromosome 1. **Int Rev Immunol** 19:319.
27. Andrade F, Casciola-Rosen L, Rosen A (2000) Apoptosis in systemic lupus erythematosus. **Rheum Dis Clin North Am** 26:215.
28. George P, Tunnessen WW Jr (1993) Childhood discoid lupus erythematosus. **Arch Dermatol** 129:613.
29. Magana M, Vazquez R (2000) Discoid lupus erythematosus in childhood. **Pediatr Dermatol** 17(3):241.
30. Kuhn A, Richter-Hintz D, Osliislo C et al. (2000) Lupus erythematosus tumidus-a neglected subset of cutaneous lupus erythematosus: a report of 40 cases. **Arch Dermatol** 136(8):1033.

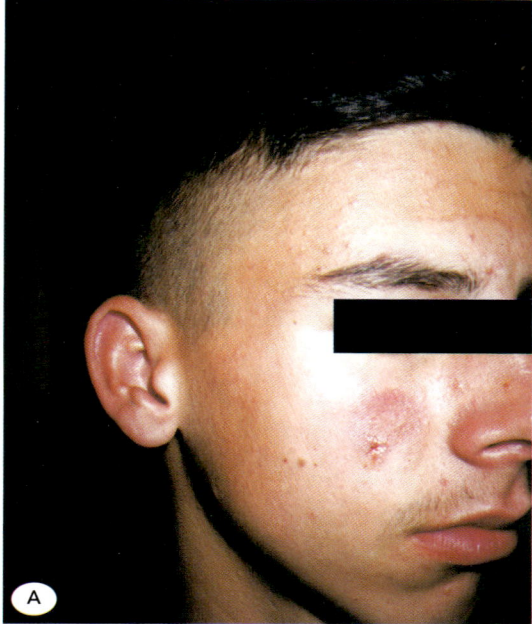
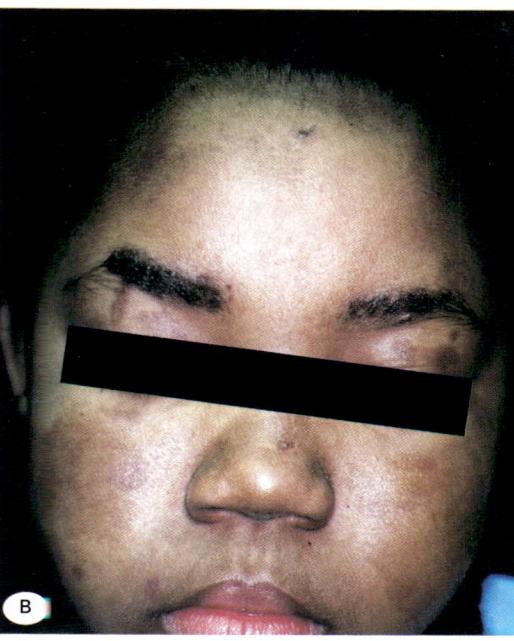

Fig. 23.1   (A) Erythematous discoid lupus erythematosus lesion on the cheek in an adolescent male with no systemic disease. (B) Discoid lesions, hyperpigmentation and alopecia in a 12-year-old female with SLE cushingoid from steroid therapy.

The DLE lesions are characterized as erythematous, sharply demarcated, round lesions demonstrating adherent scale formation, follicular plugging, telangiectasia, and scarring. These lesions are also most prominent in the light-exposed areas occurring most frequently on the face and scalp. In 55% the DLE lesions can involve the malar eminence producing a classical butterfly dermatitis in which the involvement of the malar eminences are the wings of the butterfly and involvement of the nose is the body of the butterfly (Fig. 23.1B).

In addition to the classic DLE and rare LET lesions, childhood SLE patients may have an urticaria-like or a papulosquamous malar dermatitis in which there is little, if any, scaling, telangiectasia, follicular plugging, or scar formation. This type of lesion occurs primarily on sun-exposed surfaces and is known as subacute cutaneous lupus erythematosus (SCLE). Patients with SCLE have few systemic disease manifestations and often are anti-Ro positive.

SLE patients may also have both nasal and oral ulcerations, as well as scarring or nonscarring alopecia (25%). Petechiae or purpuric lesions, nail fold telangiectasia, or small digital ice pick infarcts (Fig. 23.2) may be manifestations of an underlying vasculopathy accompanying the lupus disease process. Urticaria-like vasculitic lesions can also occur, as well as livedo reticularis, and rarely blister formation. Erythema nodosum and lupus panniculitis are also skin manifestations that may be seen in SLE.

Fever and arthralgias/arthritis are common presenting features in childhood SLE. The arthritis is a nondeforming polyarthritis that can affect all joints. In addition, weight loss, lymphadenopathy (50%), fatigue, abdominal pain, night sweats, proximal muscle weakness (20%) and Raynaud phenomenon (20%) have also been described.

Raynaud phenomenon is characterized by a triphasic reaction triggered by cold exposure or emotional distress. An initial blanching of the digits is followed by cyanosis and painful reactive hyperemia upon rewarming. Small ice pick-like scars representing infarcts may occur on the fingertips (Fig. 23.2) and distal toes.

Pulmonary involvement such as pleuritis has also been commonly detected in childhood SLE, occurring in as many as two-thirds of patients.[31] Cardiac disorders may occur in as many as 50% of childhood SLE patients.[32] These

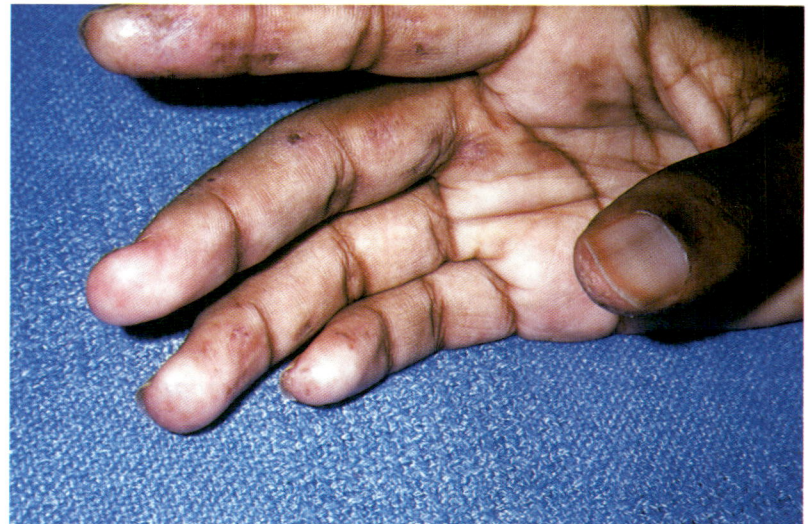

Fig. 23.2   Digital infarcts in SLE.

include pericarditis, myocarditis, and vasculitis affecting the coronary arteries. In addition, Libman–Sachs endocarditis has also been reported.

It has been reported that as many as 50% of childhood SLE patients may have central nervous system involvement[14] now known as neuropsychiatric SLE (NPSLE). The ACR has now defined nineteen neuropsychiatric manifestations of the central and peripheral nervous systems including seizures, alteration in mental status, psychosis, and peripheral neuropathy.[33]

As many as 60 to 80% of childhood SLE patients may develop clinical renal disease.[12,15,34] This is usually detected at the onset of the disease or within the first 2 years. It is important to note that in some patients, especially with anti-dsDNA antibodies and hypocomplementemia, direct immunofluorescence examination of the kidney may demonstrate a significant immunologic insult

31. Delgado EA, Malleson PN, Pirie GE, Petty RE (1990) Pulmonary manifestations of childhood onset systemic lupus erythematosus. **Semin Arthritis Rheum** 29:285.

32. England JA, Lucas RV Jr (1983) Cardiac implications in children with systemic lupus erythematosus. **Pediatrics** 72:724.

33. ACR Ad Hoc Committee on Neuropsychiatric Lupus Nomenclature (1999) The American College of Rheumatology nomenclature and definitions for neuropsychiatric lupus syndromes. **Arthritis Rheum** 42(4):599.

34. Morris MC, Carmeron JS, Chantler C et al. (1981) Systemic lupus erythematosus with nephritis. **Arch Dis Child** 56:779.

in the absence of hematuria or proteinuria. It appears that nephritis occurs more frequently in childhood SLE than in adult SLE and can be a devastating complication of childhood LE.

The prognosis of childhood lupus nephritis has improved with early recognition and aggressive steroid and/or immunosuppressive treatment and only about 5% of patients currently progress to renal failure. Like adult LE patients, the survival rates for childhood lupus nephritis have dramatically improved during the past 20 years.[34,35]

LABORATORY FINDINGS

Serologic examination is the most important laboratory evaluation of children suspected of having LE.[36] As in adult LE, the following laboratory tests have played a significant role in the early detection of SLE.

The antinuclear antibody (ANA) determination is almost always positive in SLE when human substrates derived from tissue culture (Hep-2, Kb, etc.) cells are employed to detect the ANA. If, however, heterologous tissues (e.g., rat kidney, mouse liver) are employed as ANA substrates, approximately 5 to 10% of SLE patients may fail to demonstrate a significant ANA titer. The human tissue culture or tumor cell lines provide a much more sensitive substrate for the detection of the ANA. Recent studies indicate that anti-Ro antibodies, unlike autoantibodies against Sm, U_1RNP, or La(SS-B), are directed against epitopes unique to human-derived Ro(SSA) macromolecules. These antibodies show variable or occasionally no cross-reactivity with nonhuman sources of the Ro(SSA) macromolecule.[37] This fact, in all probability, explains the high frequency of anti-Ro(SSA) antibody positivity in lupus patients previously found to have insignificant ANAs ("ANA-negative SLE") when heterologous substrates were employed in the detection of ANAs.

Five distinct patterns have been associated with ANAs. These are the speckled pattern, the most nonspecific; a homogeneous pattern, associated with antinucleoprotein antibodies; a shaggy or peripheral pattern, associated with the presence of anti-nDNA antibodies; a centromere pattern predominantly associated with CREST (calcinosis, Raynaud, esophageal dysmotility, sclerodactyly, and telangiectases) syndrome; and a nucleolar pattern, commonly detected in patients with progressive systemic sclerosis. Because patients with lupus erythematosus make autoantibodies against many different nuclear autoantigens, less significance is now placed on the pattern of the ANA. However, if a shaggy or peripheral pattern is detected, a specific test to determine the presence or absence of native DNA antibodies should be performed.

It is important to emphasize that the ANA determination is a screening test. It is not specific for LE. ANAs can be detected in various connective tissue diseases and in approximately 5 to 10% of the general population. It was previously held that the magnitude of a titer has no relationship to the presence of LE, but a recent study in children suggests that an ANA of > or = 1:160 correlates with autoimmune disease.[38] When one detects a significant ANA titer especially > 1:640, other ANA profile serologic tests should be performed and definite clinical and historic features should be detected before a possible diagnosis of SLE is made. The diagnosis of SLE evokes a tremendous amount of anxiety in the patient and family.

Children suspected of having SLE should be examined for the presence of antinative [double stranded (ds)] DNA antibodies. These antibodies are highly specific for SLE and are found in approximately 50% of SLE patients. Lupus patients with anti-dsDNA antibodies have a guarded prognosis and a high frequency of renal disease. The presence of anti-dsDNA antibodies and

hypocomplementemia, even in the absence of hematuria and proteinuria, almost always indicates a significant immunologic insult occurring in the kidney. It has been the early detection of these patients with anti-dsDNA antibodies that has played a major role in the reduction of the mortality that has previously been associated with this group of patients.

Anti-single-stranded DNA (ssDNA) antibodies are found in approximately 70% of patients with LE. These antibodies, unlike anti-dsDNA antibodies, are not specific for LE and can be seen in a variety of other conditions. However, complement-fixing single-stranded DNA antibodies in the absence of anti-dsDNA antibodies have been associated with the presence of renal disease.

In addition to anti-DNA antibodies, SLE patients frequently make autoantibodies directed against small nuclear ribonuclear proteins (snRNPs). The first of these antibodies against ribonuclear proteins to be described were anti-Sm antibodies. These antibodies, like anti-dsDNA antibodies, are specific for SLE and occur in approximately 20% of SLE patients. These anti-Sm antibodies rarely occur alone and are almost always seen in the presence of anti-nRNP (U_1RNP) antibodies.

Unlike anti-Sm antibodies, anti-nRNP antibodies can occur alone. They have been seen in a lupus disease process in which there is an increased frequency of sclerodactyly, esophageal dysmotility, pulmonary disease, and Raynaud phenomenon. In addition, a small percentage (approximately 5%) of scleroderma and dermatomyositis/polymyositis patients possess these antibodies. Some patients possessing this antibody system have been described previously as having the mixed connective tissue disease syndrome. A follow-up study of patients with the mixed connective tissue disease syndrome has indicated that over a 10-year period, most of these patients evolved into a classical scleroderma or, more likely, LE disease process.

A third antibody directed against ribonuclear proteins is the anti-Ro(SSA) antibody. These antibodies are found in approximately 30% of SLE patients and approximately 40 to 45% of Sjögren syndrome patients as detected by gel double diffusion. LE patients with anti-Ro(SSA) antibodies generally have a disease process that is characterized by intense photosensitive cutaneous LE lesions. It has been estimated that approximately 90% of these patients are photosensitive.[39] Frequently they give a history of burning through window glass, indicating that low-energy, long-wave ultraviolet light is capable of activating or aggravating their disease process. Approximately 40% of these patients develop either papulosquamous or widespread annular polycyclic lesions. Of these patients, approximately 30 to 50% have features that will satisfy the minor criteria of the American College of Rheumatology for the diagnosis of SLE.[40,41] These patients have been described under the term SCLE. In addition, as noted above, some of these patients previously were reported under the rubric of "antinuclear antibody negative" SLE patients.

The anti-La(SS-B) antibody is found in approximately 10% of patients with SLE. The La(SS-B) antibody is very often found in association with anti-Ro(SSA) antibodies.

In adult lupus patients, antiphospholipid antibodies (anticardiolipin lupus anticoagulant) occur frequently (30–50%).[42] These antibodies may also occur in the absence of LE (primary antiphospholipid syndrome). These autoantibodies are associated with an increased frequency of arterial and venous thrombosis involving all organs including the brain and heart. Cutaneous manifestations include acrocyanosis and livedo reticularis with and without ulceration. In addition, these patients have an increased frequency of thrombocytopenia, Libman–Sachs endocarditis, and central nervous system disease.

Laboratory tests involving direct immunofluorescence, gel double diffusion, and enzyme-linked immunosorbent assay (ELISA) technologies have proved

35. Abeles M, Urman JD, Weinstein A et al. (1980) Systemic lupus erythematosus in the younger patient: survival studies. **J Rheumatol** 7:515.
36. Tan EM (1989) Antinuclear antibodies: diagnostic markers for autoimmune diseases and probes for cell biology. **Adv Immunol** 44:93.
37. Reichlin M, Reichlin MW (1989) Autoantibodies to the Ro(SSA) particle react preferentially with the human antigen. In: Second International Symposium on Sjögren's Syndrome, Talal N, ed. Academic Press, London, p. 51.
38. Perilloux BC, Shetty AK, Leiva LE, Gedalia A (2000) Antinuclear antibody (ANA) and ANA profile tests in children with autoimmune disorders: a retrospective study. **Clin Rheumatol** 19(3):200.

39. Mond CB, Peterson MGE, Rothfield N (1989) Correlation of anti-Ro antibody with photosensitivity rash in systemic lupus erythematosus patients. **Arthritis Rheum** 32:202.
40. Sontheimer RD, Maddison PJ, Reichlin M et al. (1982) Serologic and HLA associations of subacute cutaneous lupus erythematosus: a clinical subset of lupus erythematosus. **Ann Intern Med** 97:664.
41. Watson RM, Talwar P, Alexander E et al. (1991) Subacute cutaneous lupus erythematosus—immunogenetic associations. **J Autoimmun** 4:73.
42. Asherson RA, Cervera R (1993) Antiphospholipid syndrome. **J Invest Dermatol** 100:21s.

invaluable in the early diagnosis of children suspected of having LE. Lehman *et al.* have reported that there may be an increased prevalence of single-stranded DNA, nRNP, and Sm in adult, as compared with childhood, SLE populations.[43,44] The authors have found that the prevalence of these autoantibodies in childhood SLE (under 18 years of age) is roughly the same as it is in adult SLE in a small population (Table 23.2). Serologic profiles for children under the age of 1 are not yet available in sufficient numbers to detect the prevalence of these autoantibodies.

Monitoring of SLE activity is best performed by frequent physical examination and determination of serum complement (C3/C4) levels.[45] The clinical onset of disease activity, especially renal disease, is frequently heralded by the gradual development of hypocomplementemia. Studies from one institution have demonstrated that therapeutic attempts to normalize complement levels are associated with a much better prognosis than treatment designed to treat only symptoms.[46] Total complement activity is measured by a functional hemolytic assay (CH_{50}). In addition, complement can also be measured using single radioimmunodiffusion techniques examining for C3 and C4. It should be noted that frequently C4 levels are depressed when C3 levels are normal. The most likely explanation for this dichotomy is the presence of one or more null alleles for C4 rather than low-grade complement consumption.

Other laboratory procedures are of value in monitoring childhood SLE patients. The erythrocyte sedimentation rate (ESR) usually increases with disease activity, although there are exceptions. In addition, thrombocytopenia, coagulation abnormalities (secondary to circulating anticoagulants), a Coomb's positive hemolytic anemia, and leukopenia are also seen alone or in combination in as many as 90% of active childhood SLE patients.[45]

Routine urinalysis, serial complement determinations, anti-dsDNA antibody levels, and a renal biopsy are important procedures in monitoring childhood lupus patients suspected of having renal disease. Frequent blood pressure determinations are also indicated in childhood SLE patients with active renal disease to detect the onset of a complicating hypertension. Renal biopsies have proven to be of immense value in the management of children with lupus nephritis. Four pathologic types of nephritis have been detected. These include mesangial lupus nephritis, membranous lupus nephropathy, focal glomerulonephritis, and diffuse proliferative glomerulonephritis. The diffuse proliferative glomerulonephritis carries the worst prognosis. Unfortunately this type of nephritis appears to be a common type of nephritis seen in childhood SLE. The indications for renal biopsy in childhood SLE can be found in the review by Garrin *et al.*[47]

Newer imaging techniques such as MRI and CT may help to delineate disease processes in SLE.[48] Bosma *et al.*[49] detected brain parenchyma abnormalities in adolescents with NPSLE with magnetization transfer imaging

(MTI). Chest X-rays have not been particularly helpful in discriminating LE from infectious causes in children.[50]

PATHOGENESIS

The pathogenesis of various features of LE is now becoming clarified and are reviewed by Petty.[25] The best evidence at present indicates that the glomerulonephritis is the result of immune complex formation with complement activation. In the past, circulating immune complexes have been thought to play the primary role. There is evidence to suggest, however, that both double-stranded, as well as single-stranded DNA, but not various ribonuclear proteins [Sm, nRNP (U_1RNP), Ro(SSA), and La(SS-B)] may preferentially bind to the collagen molecules along the glomerular basement membrane.[51] Once having bound to the collagen molecules, the anti-DNA antibodies can bind to these various forms of DNA (*in situ* immune complex formation). This observation could be one explanation for the increased frequency of renal disease associated with anti-DNA antibodies compared with the frequency of renal disease in lupus patients possessing antibodies against Sm, nRNP (U_1RNP), Ro(SSA), and La(SS-B).

Another reason for the increased frequency of renal disease associated with anti-dsDNA antibodies compared with the frequency of renal disease associated with anti-U_1RNP and Ro(SSA) antibodies may be related to the fact that lupus patients generally produce small quantities of anti-dsDNA antibodies. Thus, immune complexes involving anti-dsDNA tend to be formed in antigen excess. These immune complexes are small and soluble and escape clearance by the reticuloendothelial system.

Antibodies directed against various riboprotein macromolecules, however, generally are present in large quantities. Thus, these immune complexes, in contradistinction to DNA immune complexes, are formed in antibody excess. These complexes generally are large and insoluble, and are easily removed by the reticuloendothelial system.

In addition to anti-DNA and anti-RNP antibodies, lupus patients make antibodies against a variety of cell surface markers on platelets, neutrophils, and red blood cells. It is conceivable that these autoantibodies play a direct role in the development of cytopenias seen in LE. However, Petty indicates enhanced phagocytosis by the reticuloendothelial system as the cause of low platelets and leukopenia, with the antibodies being serologic markers.[25]

Cutaneous lupus lesions (DLE and SCLE) demonstrate an inflammatory mononuclear infiltrate characterized by the predominance of activated T cells (CD4 and CD8).[52] Because the scarring discoid lesions most commonly occur in the total absence of autoantibodies, it is very conceivable that this inflammatory lesion is the result of this T-cell inflammatory infiltrate. The deposition of immunoglobulin and complement has been shown to develop after the cutaneous lupus lesion is formed. At times, heavy deposition of

TABLE 23.2   Prevalence of autoantibodies in 23 untreated SLE patients with disease onset prior to age 18

	Autoantibodies				
	nDNA	Sm	nRNP	Ro(SSA)	La(SS-B)
No. of patients (total, 23)	11	8	7	5	3
Percentage	48	35	30	22	13

Barnett N, Sills E, and Provost TT, unpublished observations.

43. Lehman TJA, Hanson V, Singsin BH et al. (1980) The role of antibodies directed against double stranded DNA in the manifestations of systemic lupus erythematosus in childhood. J Pediatr 96:657.

44. Lehman TJA, Hanson V, Zvaifler N et al. (1984) Antibodies to non-histone nuclear antigens and anti-lymphocyte antibodies among children and adults with systemic lupus erythematosus and their relatives. J Rheumatol 11:644.

45. Schaller JG (1998) Diagnosis and management of rheumatic diseases in adolescence. Adolesc Med 9(1):1.

46. Laitman RS, Glichklich D, Sablay LB et al. (1989) Effective long term normalization of serum complement levels on the course of lupus nephritis. Am J Med 87:132.

47. Garrin EH, Shulman ST, Donnelly WH et al. (1981) Systemic lupus erythematosus glomerulonephritis in children. Paediatrica 10:351.

48. Hanlon R, King S (2000) Overview of the radiology of connective tissue disorders in children. Eur J Radiol 33(2):174.

49. Bosma GP, Rood MJ, Zwinderman AH et al. (2000) Evidence of central nervous system damage in patients with neuropsychiatric systemic lupus erythematosus demonstrated by magnetization transfer imaging. Arthritis Rheum 43(1):48.

50. Chantarojanasiri T, Sittirath A, Preutthipan A et al. (1999) Pulmonary involvement in childhood systemic lupus erythematosus. J Med Assoc Thai 82(Suppl) 1:S144.

51. Izui S, Lambert PH, Miescher PA (1976) In vitro demonstration of a particular affinity of glomerular basement membrane and collagen for DNA. J Exp Med 144:428.

52. Synkowski DR, Provost TT (1983) Characterization of the inflammatory infiltrate in lupus erythematosus lesions using monoclonal antibodies. J Rheumatol 19:920.

immunoglobulin and complement at the dermal–epidermal junction can be seen in the total absence of clinical as well as histologic evidence of inflammation or an inflammatory cell infiltration. This implies that immune complex formation at the dermal–epidermal junction does not play a primary role in the pathogenesis of the cutaneous lupus lesions.

Studies of the neonatal lupus syndrome have provided a good deal of evidence to suggest that the lesions of SCLE are antibody mediated, perhaps by antibody-dependent cellular cytotoxicity. These studies have demonstrated that the inflammatory infiltrate in SCLE contains T cells. UV light may stimulate DNA to increase expression of Ro and recruit T cells (see below).[25] Furthermore, since this type of cutaneous lupus lesion can occur in infants born of anti-Ro(SSA) antibody-positive mothers, it is hypothesized that the maternal anti-Ro(SSA) antibody passes to the infant via the placenta and recruits the infant's T cells to participate in this inflammatory lesion (see below).

The vasculitic lesions, including palpable purpura, urticarial-like, livedo reticularis with ulceration, as well as nodular vasculitis are thought to be primarily the result of immune-complex mediated mechanisms. Indeed, immunoglobulin and complement deposition can be seen in and about affected blood vessels. Evidence exists that another mechanism could also be potentially involved. Studies indicate that some patients with SLE make autoantibodies reactive against non-HLA-derived endothelial cell surface markers.[53] Thus, it is conceivable that a Gell and Coomb's type II antibody-mediated complement-dependent (cytotoxic) immunologic mechanism in addition to type III (immune complex) type of immunologic mechanism may be involved in some of the vasculopathies seen in SLE.

The alopecia that is seen in patients with SLE appears to arise from at least three different mechanisms. The most obvious mechanism is the presence of a scarring DLE lesion in the scalp resulting in destruction of the hair follicles. A second possible mechanism frequently seen in children with the acute onset of SLE is a diffuse alopecia most likely the result of a telogen effluvium secondary to the catabolic effects of the acute lupus disease process. A third type of alopecia, so-called lupus hair, is probably related to the catabolic effects of the lupus disease process. In this case, the patient develops characteristic thinning of the hair, especially around the periphery of the scalp, and most commonly observed at the temple and forehead area. The alopecia is characterized by thin, short hairs that easily fragment. It is likely that this type of alopecia, which is seen in patients with acute onset of SLE or recurrence of the SLE, is the result of catabolic effects on the normal growth of the hair, producing weakened hairs that easily break resulting in shortened broken hairs.

Bullous lesions, which are rare in SLE, can also arise via three potential mechanisms.[54] Blisters can arise from widespread dissolution of the dermal–epidermal junction caused by liquefaction degeneration even to the point of mimicking toxic epidermal necrolysis. This has been seen in anti-Ro(SSA) positive patients following intense ultraviolet light or sunlight exposure. The second form of bullous disease associated with lupus erythematosus most probably results from a low-grade vasculopathy involving the blood vessels high in the papillary portion of the dermis resulting in neutrophilic papillary dermal microabscesses resembling dermatitis herpetiformis. These blisters have been reported to be responsive to dapsone therapy. The third form of bullous formation in lupus erythematosus was described by Gammon et al.[55] These investigators have determined that some lupus patients make an autoantibody against type VII collagen in the anchoring fibrils. This autoantibody results in destruction of the normal integrity of the dermal–epidermal junction

producing subepidermal blister formation. This type of bullous formation in lupus erythematosus can be very recalcitrant to therapy.

The role of ultraviolet light in the pathogenesis of the cutaneous lupus lesions has intrigued investigators for many years. Data by Lehmann et al. indicate that both short-wave ultraviolet light (UVB), as well as long-wave (UVA) are capable of activating or aggravating lupus lesions.[56] Their studies have confirmed that patients with SCLE appear to be the most photosensitive. The exact mechanism of how ultraviolet light induces formation of a cutaneous lupus lesion is unknown. However, recent evidence suggests that ultraviolet light plays a very significant role in the generation of potential autoantigens to which the patient is sensitized. For example, work by Natali and Tan has demonstrated that ultraviolet light is capable of denaturing DNA in epidermal cells producing thymidine dimers.[57] This denatured DNA is excreted from the keratinocyte and crosses the dermal–epidermal junction. In experimental animals sensitized to the denatured DNA, immunoglobulin deposits then form along the dermal–epidermal junction. Additional studies by LeFeber et al. have demonstrated that ultraviolet light is capable of inducing the de novo synthesis of the Ro and other RNP macromolecules in the nucleus and cytoplasm.[58] With time, the Ro(SSA) macromolecule and other small nuclear ribonuclear proteins may be expressed on the plasma membrane. In this location, it is conceivable that these autoantigens are exposed to host-sensitized T cells or autoantibodies. These data provide evidence that ultraviolet light may generate specific autoantigens in the pathogenesis of photosensitive cutaneous lesions. There is no evidence that ultraviolet light induces a de novo induction of an autoimmune response.

The anticardiolipin antibody is found as a serologic marker in SLE and gave the old false positive VDRL test in LE. It causes primary antiphospholipid antibody syndrome[59] and has an unknown substrate, but does bind to beta 2 glycoprotein 1.[59,60] This results in intravascular coagulation and vessel endothelium adhesion causing thromboses.[25]

Inflammatory mediators affect pleuropericardial disease in SLE but no specific serologic markers have been identified.[25]

DIFFERENTIAL DIAGNOSIS

Childhood SLE is often misdiagnosed as juvenile rheumatoid arthritis (JRA) (see under Juvenile Rheumatoid Arthritis below for distinguishing features). In addition, infections such as infectious mononucleosis and other viral infections plus rheumatic fever, which can usually be distinguished by the documentation of the Jones' criteria, as well as a history of a recent streptococcal infection, are in the differential. Bacterial endocarditis must also be considered and can be distinguished from LE by clinical evidence of embolic phenomena, as well as positive blood cultures. Septicemia with arthritis must also be considered in the diagnosis, especially septicemia secondary to a gonococcal or a meningococcal infection. The purpuric dermatosis plus positive blood cultures help distinguish these two entities from lupus erythematosus.[8,61]

A serum sickness-like drug reaction can also be confused with LE. In this case, a careful drug history plus discontinuation of the suspected offending drug should reveal the appropriate diagnosis. Of special consideration are the drug-induced lupus-like states associated with isoniazid, hydralazine, and procainamide drugs. These lupus-like states are associated with a polyserositis, but generally no skin or renal disease.[62] High-titer antihistone antibodies (directed predominantly against H2A/H2B histones) are present and ANA

53. Cines DB, Lyss AP, Reeber M et al. (1984) Presence of complement fixing anti-endothelial cell antibodies in systemic lupus erythematosus. **J Clin Invest** 73:611.
54. Gammon WR, Briggaman RA (1993) Bullous SLE: a phenotypically distinctive but immunologically heterogeneous bullous disorder. **J Invest Dermatol** 100:28s.
55. Gammon WR, Briggaman RA, Inman AO III et al. (1983) Evidence supporting a role for immune complex mediated inflammation in the pathogenesis of bullous lesions of systemic lupus erythematosus. **J Invest Dermatol** 81:320.
56. Lehmann P, Hölze E, Kind P et al. (1990) Experimental reproduction of skin lesions in lupus erythematosus by UV-A and UV-B radiation. **J Am Acad Dermatol** 22:181.
57. Natali PG, Tan EM (1973) Experimental skin lesions in mice resembling systemic lupus erythematosus. **Arthritis Rheum** 16:579.
58. LeFeber WP, Norris DA, Ryan SS (1984) Ultraviolet light induces expression of selected nuclear antigens on cultured human keratinocytes. **J Clin Invest** 74:1545.
59. Gattornd M, Buoncampagni A, Molinari AC et al. (1995) Antiphospholipid antibodies in paediatric lupus erythematosus, juvenile chronic arthritis and overlap syndromes: SLE patients with both lupus anticoagulant and high-titre anticardiolipin antibodies are at risk for clinical manifestations related to the antiphospholipid syndrome. **Br J Rheumatol** 34:873.
60. McNeil HP, Simpson RJ, Chesterman CN, Krilis SR (1990) Antiphospholipid antibodies are directed against a complex antigen that includes a lipid-binding inhibitor of coagulation beta 2 glycoprotein 1 (apolipoprotein). **Proc Natl Acad Sci USA** 87:44129.
61. Ansell BM (2000) Rheumatic disease mimics in childhood. **Curr Opin Rheumatol** 12(5):445.
62. Cush JJ, Goldings EA (1985) Drug induced lupus: clinical spectrum and pathogenesis. **Am J Med Sci** 290:36.

may be directed toward single-stranded DNA as opposed to the double-stranded DNA of true SLE. However, a lupus-like state, including skin disease, renal disease, and anti-dsDNA antibodies, can occur in patients receiving D-penicillamine. Complement levels are usually normal in drug-induced SLE. In the last decade a lupus-like syndrome has been increasingly reported in adolescents on minocycline for acne.[63]

Occasionally the early onset of juvenile dermatomyositis in which the myositis is not a prominent feature (amyopathic dermatomyositis) can be confused with LE. Unfortunately, the dermatitis can be photosensitive and histologically indistinguishable from that LE. Serologically, the presence of lupus-specific autoantibodies such as anti-dsDNA and anti-Sm are of great help in establishing a diagnosis of lupus. On the other hand, myositis-specific antibodies, if present, or elevated muscle enzymes (see below under Dermatomyositis) help to establish the diagnosis of dermatomyositis.

It is also conceivable that with the increased prevalence of syphilis, secondary syphilis characterized by arthralgias, fever, lymphadenopathy, and a papulosquamous disease process may be confused with lupus erythematosus. In this case, the diagnosis would be established by the demonstration of a positive Venereal Disease Research Laboratory (VDRL) test and confirmation by a fluorescent treponemal antibody (FTA) determination. It should be pointed out that in lupus erythematosus, it is possible to have the speckled positive FTA that represents staining of the nuclei of the treponema. This speckled pattern of staining is in reality a positive ANA determination. The staining pattern on the FTA for syphilis is a homogeneous staining of the treponema.

THERAPY

Corticosteroids have assumed the major therapeutic role in the treatment of childhood SLE. High doses of corticosteroids are employed until the anti-dsDNA antibodies and complement levels are normalized with improvement in clinical state. Prednisone is usually preferred. A tuberculosis skin test is advised before therapy is begun. Then, the corticosteroids are very slowly tapered to the lowest dose capable of controlling lupus disease process symptoms and maintaining normalized complement levels. Both alternate day and single morning dose corticosteroids have been shown to be therapeutically effective in treating lupus and minimizing the side effects of infection, aseptic necrosis, cushingoid features, and osteoporosis. High dose pulse corticosteroids have also been shown to be effective in providing rapid control of acutely ill SLE patients.

Immunosuppressive agents such as azathioprine (Imuran) and cyclophosphamide are generally reserved for individuals with severe renal disease or severe systemic involvement of other vital organs, especially the central nervous system. Steroids plus immunosuppressive agents have been shown to be more effective than steroids alone in the treatment of lupus nephritis.[15] The combination of steroids and immunosuppressive agents permits lower doses of steroids to be used. While steroid exposure may risk growth failure, severe infections and avascular necrosis, these immunosuppressive agents also have significant potential side effects such as sterility and hemorrhagic cystitis (cyclophosphamide), chemical hepatitis (azathioprine), and proneness to infection and aplastic anemia and malignancy (azathioprine and cyclophosphamide). They should be employed only in the most severe cases and with great caution, and treatment should be individualized by histologic class as discussed by Niaudet.[64] Pulse intravenous cyclophosphamide (Cytoxan) has been especially effective and relatively non-toxic in the treatment of diffuse proliferative lupus glomerulonephritis.[65,66] Other immunosuppressive drugs such as methotrexate, chlorambucil and mycophenolate mofetil

(Cellcept) have also been employed in the management of childhood lupus and can be tried to achieve control if the above regimen has been unsuccessful.

Renal transplant is a reasonable therapeutic choice for progressive end-stage lupus nephritis unresponsive to therapy. Lupus nephritis rarely recurs in the new organ[64] and dialysis poses the risk of predisposing to sepsis. Of course, for lesser renal disease standard antihypertensive and renal medical management is appropriate.

Cutaneous lesions in childhood LE can be treated with topical steroid preparations. Less often employed, but also effective, is the intralesional injection of steroids. Complications such as atrophy, telangiectasia, and striae can result from local repetitive use of potent topical steroid therapy to treat cutaneous lupus lesions. Clofazimine has been employed in adult patients with cutaneous lupus lesions; however, skin pigmentation complications must be considered. Also, retinoids and tazarotene have been employed with success in adults to control recalcitrant cutaneous lupus lesions. Thalidomide has been shown to be effective in treating cutaneous lupus.[67] This drug is now available in the United States. Imiquimod off-label is being tried by some sparked by the observation that thalidomide helps.

In addition to topical steroids, oral hydroxychloroquine, an antimalarial, has been shown to be effective in treating photosensitive cutaneous lesions. Patients treated with hydroxychloroquine have less recurrence of minor flares including cutaneous, as well as joint disease. If antimalarials are used, the patient must have an ophthalmologic examination every 6 months to assess for possible macular degeneration. In addition, care should be observed in prescribing antimalarials to glucose-6-phosphate-dehydrogenase deficient (G6PD) patients. Blood counts, liver functions, and electrolytes were previously recommended to be monitored every 2 months but this frequency is no longer recommended by the ACR as alterations of significance in these are so extremely rares.[68]

Aspirin and nonsteroidal anti-inflammatory drugs (NSAIDs) may be beneficial in treating myalgias and arthralgias. Care must be taken to avoid excessive gastrointestinal irritation and the potential of a bleeding ulcer. Chronic ibuprofen use is contraindicated in lupus patients because it can rarely cause creatinine elevation in some individuals and is also associated with aseptic meningitis. In the presence of thrombocytopenia, aspirin should *not* be used but in lupus patients with the lupus anticoagulant (anticardiolipin antibody), 1mg/kg/day of aspirin may help prevent platelet aggregation.

Because of the potential deleterious effects of excessive sunlight exposure, patients and their families should be cautioned about excessive sun exposure. Protective clothing and the judicious use of sunscreens (with a sun protective factor #30 rating or above) should be stressed.

Children with SLE should not receive live viral immunizations and may benefit from vaccines to help prevent infection such as DTaP, Varivax, Pneumovax and meningococcal vaccines.

PROGNOSIS

The prognosis of childhood SLE, like that of adult lupus erythematosus, has markedly improved during the past quarter century. Children with the worst prognosis appear to be those with diffuse proliferative glomerulonephritis in whom hypertension develops within 6 months of diagnosis. The 5-year survival, however, from the time of diagnosis is at least 80%. In all probability, this spectacular improvement in survival is due to earlier diagnosis, aggressive steroid and antibiotic treatment, and, most recently, the judicious use of pulse corticosteroids and iv cyclophosphamide. Infection is the cause of most

63. Akins E, Miller LE, Tucker LB, Schaller JG (1997) Minocycline related lupus-like syndrome: Possible association with anti-neutrophil cytoplasmic antibodies [abstract]. Arthritis Rheum 40:A962.

64. Niaudet P (2000) Treatment of lupus nephritis in children. Pediatr Nephrol 14(2):158.

65. Lehman TJA, Onel K (2000) Intermittent intravenous cyclophosphamide arrests progression of the renal chronicity index in childhood systemic lupus erythematosus. J Pediatr 136(2):245.

66. Lehman TJA, Sherry DD, Wagner-Weiner L et al. (1989) Intermittent intravenous cyclophosphamide therapy for lupus nephritis. J Pediatr 114:1055.

67. Ordi-Ros J, Cortes F, Cucurull E et al. (2000) Thalidomide in the treatment of cutaneous lupus refractory to conventional therapy. J Rheumatol 27(6):1429.

68. Sontheimer RD (2000) Questions answered and a $1 million question raised concerning lupus erythematosus tumidus. Is routine laboratory surveillance testing during treatment with hydroxychloroquine for skin disease really necessary? Arch Dermatol 136:1044.

deaths in children with SLE, especially those on chronic daily steroids, so vigilance for evidence of infection is mandatory in caring for these patients.

Unfortunately, children with SLE are at risk of developing additional autoimmune disorders over time.[69] Ultrasound has been documented in carotid wall thickening in severe renal lupus nephritis with nephrotic range proteinuria, suggesting that these patients are also at risk of early atherosclerosis.[70]

PEDIATRIC ASPECTS

With the improved prognosis, patients with childhood SLE who do not have diffuse proliferative glomerulonephritis will have a normal life expectancy, but they must be closely monitored. Every means should be employed to minimize the disruption of the normal socialization of the child and adolescent.[71] Once the disease is under control, physical activities such as play and physical education should be reinstituted as promptly as possible. Compliance with medication is essential for good control of disease and often becomes difficult to manage in the adolescent years as independence, which must be respected, is asserted by the patient.[8] Development of neuropsychiatric lupus confounds the situation beyond the stress of a chronic disease and may impact greatly on cognitive function, school performance and peer and family interaction. Support groups and psychiatric medications help coping mechanisms in some patients.

Cutaneous lupus lesions in exposed areas should be treated as aggressively as possible to attempt to minimize their disfiguring nature. In order to minimize any misunderstanding regarding the possible contagious nature of the patient's disease, school staff, playmates, and playmates' parents may be educated as to the nature of the patient's illness with their consent. The cushingoid features and growth abnormalities of corticosteroid therapy have an especially detrimental effect on the child's self-image. Modified disease therapy effects and psychosocial factors have been documented to improve quality of life for SLE patients.[72]

NEONATAL LUPUS ERYTHEMATOSUS

The neonatal lupus erythematosus (NLE) syndrome is primarily characterized by the development in newborn infants of lupus skin lesions and/or isolated congenital heart block.[73–76] The overwhelming majority of these infants are females[77] born of anti-Ro(52kDa and 60kDa SSA) antibody and/or anti-La (48Kda SS-B)positive mothers,[78] although occasionally they have been born to anti-nRNP (U$_1$RNP) positive mothers.[79] In addition to the cutaneous lesions and the isolated congenital heart block, neonatal lupus syndrome (NLS) infants have also demonstrated thrombocytopenia,[80,81] transient hepatic involvement,[80] aplastic anemia, and neurologic symptoms secondary to central nervous system vasculopathy.[82]

The mothers of these infants may or may not show features of connective tissue disease at the time of birth of the affected infant. Approximately 60% will demonstrate features of Sjögren syndrome, LE,[75,78] or rheumatoid arthritis.[83,84] Most of the asymptomatic mothers will with time either develop features of Sjögren syndrome or LE. At times, this may not occur for several decades after the birth of the affected child. Rarely, the mothers remain asymptomatic. We are aware of one instance in which a 43-year-old male was admitted for a cardiac transplant for intractable congestive failure secondary to complete heart block that began in infancy. His 77-year-old mother was totally asymptomatic, although she possessed in her serum anti-Ro(SSA) and anti-La(SS-B) antibodies.

It has been estimated that an infant born of an anti-Ro(SSA) antibody positive mother has a 1 in 20 chance of developing NLE syndrome. In an excellent review, Kitridou and Mintz detected 21 children with NLE in 292 live births of anti-Ro(SSA) positive Sjögren syndrome and lupus erythematosus mothers, giving an overall prevalence of 7.2%.[85] Isolated congenital heart block (CHB) is estimated to occur once in 15 000–20 000 live births.[86] It is rare even in anti-Ro antibody positive mothers with SLE with one report of six instances of CHB in 79 births.[87] Buyon et al.[88] report in a retrospective study of anti-SSA/Ro and anti-SSB/La positive antibody mothers who have had a child with CHB and NLE syndrome that the probability of a subsequent child with manifestation of NLE is 22%

Immunogenetic studies indicate that anti-Ro(SSA) antibody positive mothers of NLE infants have a strikingly increased frequency of the HLA-DR3 phenotype.[75,78,89]

Congenital heart block in the NLE syndrome is complete in approximately 90% of patients. In addition, 2:1 atrioventricular (AV) and transient AV block, as well as a right bundle branch block and sinus bradycardia have also been reported. Since the 1980s isolated congenital heart block has been detected, generally before 30 weeks' gestation and often between 20 and 24 weeks.[88]

Associated congenital heart abnormalities have been detected in approximately 30% of affected infants. These congenital defects include patent ductus arteriosus, ventricular septal defect, transposition of the great vessels, atrial septal defect, patent foramen ovale, coarctation of the aorta, tetralogy of Fallot, hypoplastic right ventricle, dysplastic pulmonic valve, anomalous pulmonary venous drainage, pulmonary regurgitation, tricuspid insufficiency, and mitral insufficiency. Whether or not these associated cardiac abnormalities are part of the cardiac manifestations of the neonatal lupus syndrome is unclear. At Johns Hopkins Hospital the examination of 50 children born with various cardiac abnormalities in the absence of isolated congenital heart block failed to detect in their mothers any evidence of connective tissue disease or the presence of autoantibodies associated with lupus including anti-Ro(SSA) antibodies.

The mortality associated with isolated congenital heart block is significant (approximately 14–20%) especially in the first 3 months of life. Pacemakers

69. McDonagh JE, Isenberg DA (2000) Development of additional autoimmune diseases in a population of patients with systemic lupus erythematosus. **Ann Rheum Dis** 59(3):230.
70. Falaschi F, Ravelli A, Martignoni A et al. (2000) Nephrotic-range proteinuria, the major risk factor for early atherosclerosis in juvenile-onset systemic lupus erythematosus. **Arthritis Rheum** 43(6):1405.
71. White PH (1998) Psychosocial aspects of rheumatic disease in childhood and adolescence. **Adolesc Med** 9(1):171.
72. Thumboo J, Fong KY, Chan SP et al. (2000) A prospective study of factors affecting quality of life in systemic lupus erythematosus. **J Rheumatol** 27(6):1414.
73. Franco HL, Weston WL, Peebles C et al. (1981) Autoantibodies directed against sicca syndrome antigens in the neonatal lupus syndrome. **J Am Acad Dermatol** 4:67.
74. Kephardt D, Hood AF, Provost TT (1981) Neonatal lupus erythematosus: new serologic findings. **J Invest Dermatol** 77:331.
75. Watson RM, Lane AT, Barnett AK et al. (1984) Neonatal lupus erythematosus: a clinical, serological and immunogenetic study with review of the literature. **Medicine** 63:362.
76. Scott JS, Maddison PJ, Taylor PV et al. (1983) Connective tissue disease, autoantibodies to ribonuclear protein an congenital heart block. **N Engl J Med** 309:209.
77. Weston WL, Morelli JG, Lee LA (1999) The clinical spectrum of anti-Ro-positive cutaneous neonatal lupus erythematosus. **J Am Acad Dermatol** 40:675.
78. Petri M, Watson RM, Hochberg MC (1989) Anti-Ro antibodies and neonatal lupus. **Rheum Dis Clin North Am** 15:335.
79. Provost TT, Watson RM, Gammon WR et al. (1987) The neonatal lupus syndrome associated with U$_1$RNP (nRNP) antibodies. **N Engl J Med** 316:1135.
80. Watson RM, Kang JE, May M et al. (1988) Thrombocytopenia in the neonatal lupus syndrome. **Arch Dermatol** 124:560.
81. Laxer RM, Roberts EA, Grass KR et al. (1990) Liver disease in neonatal lupus erythematosus. **J Pediatr** 116:238.
82. Cabanas F, Pelliter A, Valverde E et al. (1996) Central nervous system vasculopathy in neonatal lupus erythematosus. **Pediatr Neurol** 15(2):124.
83. Neiman AR, Lee LA, Weston WL, Buyon JP (2000) Cutaneous manifestations of neonatal lupus without heart block: Characteristics of mothers and children enrolled in a national registry. **J Pediatr** 137(5):647.
84. Askanase AD, Neiman A, Lee LA, Buyon JP (1999) Clinical parameters of mothers whose children have permanent and transient manifestations of neonatal lupus and risk of crossover in siblings. **Arthritis Rheum** 42(Suppl.):55225.
85. Kitridou R, Mintz G (1992) The neonatal lupus syndrome. In: Dubois Lupus Erythematosus, Wallace DJ, Hahan BH, eds. Philadelphia: Lea & Febiger, p. 516.
86. Michaelsson M, Engle MA (1972) Congenital complete heart block: an international study of the natural history. **Cardiovasc Clin** 4:85.
87. Ramsey-Goldman R, Hom D, Deng J-S et al. (1988) Anti-SSA antibodies and fetal outcome in maternal systemic lupus erythematosus. **Arthritis Rheum** 31:697.
88. Buyon JP, Hiebert R, Copel J et al. (1998) Autoimmune-associated congenital heart block: demographics, mortality, morbidity and recurrence rates obtained from a national neonatal lupus registry. **J Am Coll Cardiol** 31:1658.
89. Lee LA, Bias WB, Arnett FC et al. (1983) Immunogenetics of the neonatal lupus syndrome. **Ann Intern Med** 99:592.

are needed in approximately two-thirds of infants with isolated congenital heart block.[88]

Autopsies of affected infants with isolated congenital heart block demonstrate dense connective tissue replacing the entire conduction system, including the sinoatrial and AV nodes, as well as the bundle of His. Endocardial fibroelastosis is also a common finding.

PRESENTING HISTORY AND PHYSICAL EXAMINATION

The prenatal care and examination of mothers at risk for giving birth to a child with the NLE syndrome is discussed in the excellent review by Kitridou and Mintz previously cited.[85]

The cutaneous lesions in the NLE syndrome generally occur within the first few days of birth, but may be seen at birth. The lesions are multiple and are characterized as erythematous, nonscaling, sharply demarcated lesions that may occur on all parts of the body including the scalp (Fig. 23.3A). There is a special predilection for involvement around the eyes giving a very peculiar, but characteristic "owl-like" appearance. The skin changes frequently demonstrate the annular polycyclic type of lesions seen in subacute cutaneous lupus erythematosus (SCLE). These lesions may expand peripherally leaving a central ecchymotic area. The lesions generally heal without any evidence of scar formation. A transient postinflammatory hyperpigmentation or hypopigmentation may occur and residual telangiectasia may occur at the sites of previous involvement (Fig. 24.3B). Telangiectasias have lasted at least eight years.[77]

A recent retrospective study of eighteen antiRo positive patients with cutaneous NLE noted crusted plaques more often in male infants who also had thrombocytopenia, cholestatic jaundice and cardiac disease.[77]

There is evidence that ultraviolet light may precipitate these lesions. Historically, mothers have related the onset of cutaneous lupus lesions in their infants following sunlight exposure but Weston et al.[77] report three infants with lesions at birth so sun exposure is not a prerequisite. There is also a report of the development of cutaneous lupus lesions in the neonate following the use of bilirubin lights for the treatment of jaundice. The skin lesions generally disappear by the seventh month of age, which corresponds to the disappearance of the maternal IgG antibodies from the infant's serum, but rarely last months longer.

The NLE skin lesion must be differentiated from infantile atopic eczema, erythema multiforme, tinea faciei, seborrheic dermatitis, and psoriasis. The photosensitive genodermatoses, Rothmund–Thomson, Cockayne, and Bloom syndromes, must also be considered in the differential diagnosis.

EPIDEMIOLOGY

The expression of the manifestations of the NLE syndrome is variable. For example, there is an approximately equal distribution of cutaneous lesions and isolated congenital heart block. However, only 10% or less of the infants demonstrate both the heart and skin manifestations.[78,85] Initial studies of family pedigrees in which there was more than one NLE infant indicated that if the initial neonatal lupus infant had cutaneous disease, then subsequent infants generally had cutaneous disease. If the initial affected infant had isolated congenital heart block, the subsequent children born to that mother generally had isolated congenital heart block.[78] However, more recent data from the Research Registry for Neonatal Lupus reports three families where the first child with NLS had CHB and the subsequent child had only cutaneous manifestations[88] so the former observation may not hold up over time. Recent studies have shown a threefold risk of CHB recurrence in anti-SSA/Ro and SSB/La antibody-positive mothers in subsequent pregnancies compared to women without affected children.[84,88] These studies support echocardiographic monitoring of infants in subsequent pregnancies from 18 weeks of gestation onward.

Seventy-six percent of the mothers of children with NLS with CHB are white.[88] Immunogenetic studies have shown that there is a strikingly increased frequency of the HLA-DR3 phenotype in mothers of infants with NLE. Further studies have indicated a much closer relationship between these NLE mothers and female patients with primary Sjögren syndrome, female patients with SCLE, and female patients with Sjögren syndrome/lupus erythematosus overlap syndrome. It has been reported that all of these anti-Ro(SSA) antibody positive lupus subsets possess an increased frequency of the HLA-B8, DR3,

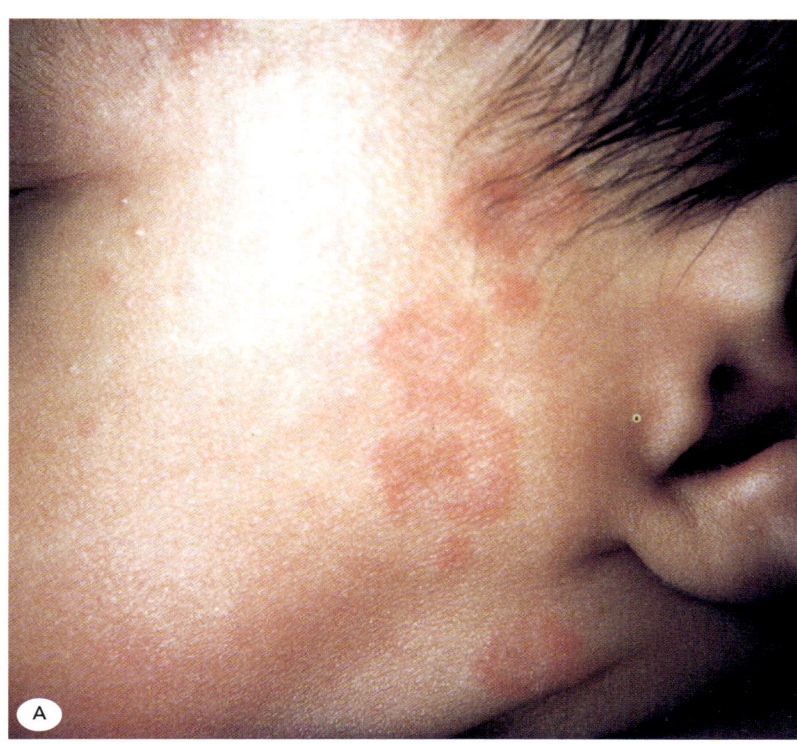

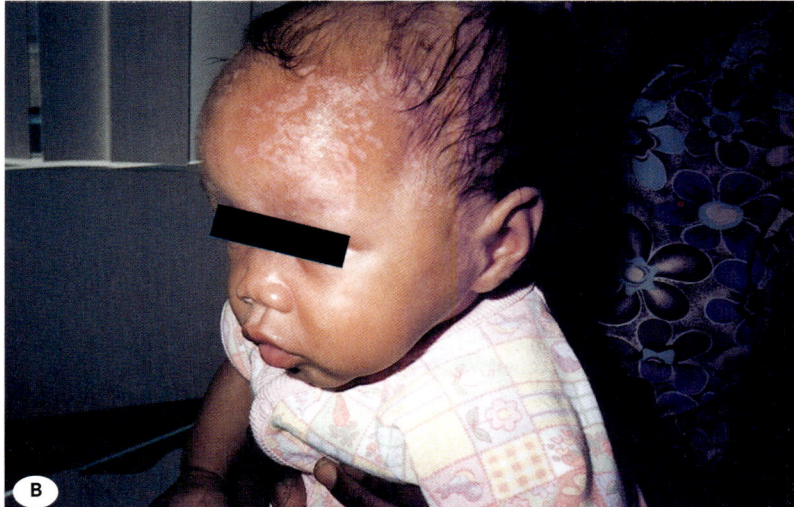

Fig. 23.3   (A) Red, annular targetoid lesions of neonatal lupus erythematosus (NLE). (B) Atrophic hypopigmented sequelae of NLE.

DQ2, and DRw52 phenotypes.[90,91] but whether this will remain true as more cases of NLE syndrome are reported and registered remains to be seen. Clinical studies indicate that all of these anti-Ro(SSA) positive females, whether or not there is overt maternal LE, are at risk of giving birth to children with the NLE syndrome. Studies indicate that the NLE mothers have a disease process that frequently extends for three to four decades associated with a variable degree of morbidity and a low mortality. At times, these patients are totally asymptomatic or may show exquisite photosensitivity. They may develop a photosensitive cutaneous lupus disease process, and then later lose the photosensitivity and the cutaneous manifestations. Some develop features of Sjögren syndrome, sometimes demonstrating extraglandular manifestations such as cutaneous vasculopathy and peripheral and central nervous system disease.[90]

Studies by Reveille *et al.*, employing molecular genetic techniques such as site-specific oligonucleotides, polymerase chain reaction, and DNA sequencing, demonstrate that all anti-Ro and La antibody–positive patients (these patients are almost always HLA-DR3-positive) possess one or more alleles at the DQ locus that encode for the presence of glutamine in position 34 and leucine in position 26 of the α-chain of the HLA-DQ encoded cell surface molecule.[92] These studies collectively indicate that there is a much closer relationship between these various anti-Ro(SSA) antibody positive subsets of LE and primary Sjögren syndrome than has previously been appreciated.

PATHOGENESIS

The study of the NLE syndrome has provided the best evidence for a direct role of anti-Ro(SSA) and/or anti-La (SS-B) antibodies in the pathogenesis of some of the clinical features of lupus erythematosus. Studies have demonstrated the presence of the Ro(SSA) macromolecule in the keratinocytes and in the fetal heart conduction system and myocardium at the sites of pathology.[93] Furthermore, the work of Norris's group indicates that ultraviolet light is capable of inducing the synthesis of Ro(SSA) and other small nuclear ribonuclear proteins and that with time there was a translocation of these small nuclear ribonuclear proteins including the Ro(SSA) macromolecule to the plasma membrane of the keratinocyte.[94]

At the present time, the best evidence is that the IgG autoantibodies (anti-Ro and anti-La) are produced in the mother and passed to the fetus via the placenta. These autoantibodies then can bind to fetal Ro and La autoantigens and induce, via antibody-dependent cellular cytotoxicity mechanisms, an inflammatory infiltrate in the skin or heart resulting in either the cutaneous lesions of LE or the isolated congenital heart block.[95] This hypothesis is supported by the demonstration that T cells are the predominant inflammatory cell in anti-Ro(SSA) positive lupus lesions. In addition, epidermal direct immunofluorescence has demonstrated the presence of anti-Ro IgG and complement deposits in lupus lesions and in the heart of an infant dying of isolated congenital heart block.[77]

THERAPY

Neonatal lupus dermatitis usually responds to low-potency topical steroids, but treatment is discretionary. Because of the history of exacerbation of

induction of these lesions in some infants following sunlight exposure, avoidance of ultraviolet light exposure is recommended. The skin lesions usually heal with no residua, although in some cases, telangiectasia and/or color change in the sites of previous involvement is detected. Rarely, increasingly potent topical steroids or even oral steroids may be necessary to prevent scarring from diffuse and significant neonatal lupus cutaneous lesions.

Isolated complete congenital heart block is permanent and is associated with a significant morbidity and mortality.[88] If an anti-Ro(SSA) positive pregnant woman is detected by M-mode echocardiography to have a fetus with a conduction defect, all attempts should be made to have the mother carry the infant to term. Long-term oral dexamethasone has been given to the mother in an attempt to treat the inflammatory infiltrate occurring in the infant's heart. This therapeutic approach is based on the fact that dexamethasone, unlike prednisone, passes across the placenta. Use of this treatment has resulted in improvement of conduction defects in infants with incomplete block.[96,97] For infants born with isolated congenital heart block, pacemaker implantation and revision is frequently required.

PROGNOSIS

The prognosis for infants born with isolated congenital heart block is guarded with a 14% mortality rate by three months of age.[88] The neonatal cutaneous lesions are transient, leaving little if any residua. There are now several NLE infants who subsequently have developed SLE as adolescents or adults.[85] One of these patients was the original case report by McCuiston and Schoch in 1956.[98]

The recurrence rate of CHB is two- to threefold for antiSSA/Ro and antiSSB/La antibody positive mothers so subsequent pregnancies should have echocardiographic monitoring. Infants with neonatal lupus syndrome need serial EKGs as intrauterine cardiac damage may be progressive.[88]

PROGRESSIVE SYSTEMIC SCLEROSIS (PSS, SCLERODERMA)

Progressive systemic sclerosis is rare in childhood.[99–101] The first case report of PSS was in a 17-year-old girl reported by Curzio in 1753.[102] PSS can occur in any race and at any age. The youngest described patient was a 15-month-old female.[103] The overwhelming majority of affected patients are female.[69] The disease clinically is quite similar to adult progressive systemic sclerosis. This is in contrast to localized scleroderma (morphea), which is common in childhood and is described fully in Chapter 18, Sclerosing and Atrophying Conditions.

Patients generally seek medical attention because of sclerotic changes in the skin or Raynaud phenomenon. Skin complaints are tightening, firmness, and occasional pruritus. Only rarely does an erythematous phase occur; however, edema may precede tissue induration and sclerosis.[104] Raynaud phenomenon occurs in as many as 75% of PSS patients.[99] Raynaud phenomenon may precede PSS by months to years.[99,100]

The acrosclerotic type of PSS is the most common type of PSS seen in children. It is characterized by sclerodactyly and Raynaud phenomenon (Fig. 23.4). The "diffuse" scleroderma pattern of PSS is characterized by centrifugal rapidly advancing cutaneous sclerosis. Characteristic features

90. Press J, Uziel Y, Laxer R et al. (1996) Long-term outcome of mothers of infants with complete congenital heart block. **Am J Med** 100:328.
91. Provost TT, Watson R (1993) Anti-Ro(SSA) HLA-DR3-positive women: the interrelationship between some ANA negative, SS, SCLE and NLE mothers and SS/LE ovelap female patients. **J Invest Dermatol** 100:14s.
92. Reveille JD, Macleod MJ, Whitington K, Arnett FC (1991) Specific amino acid residues in the second hypervariable region of HLA-DQA1 and DQB1 chain genes promote the Ro(SSA)/La(SS-B) autoantibody responses. **J Immunol** 146:3871.
93. Lee LA (1993) Neonatal lupus erythematosus. **J Invest Dermatol** 100:9s.
94. LeFeber WP, Norris DA, Ryan SS (1984) Ultraviolet light induces expression of selected nuclear antigens on cultured human keratinocytes. **J Clin Invest** 74:1545.
95. Norris DA, Lee LA (1985) Antibody dependent cellular cytotoxicity and skin disease. **J Invest Dermatol** 85:165s.
96. Buyon JP, Swersky SH, Fox HE et al. (1987) Intrauterine therapy for presumptive fetal myocarditis with acquired heart block due to systemic lupus erythematosus. **Arthritis Rheum** 30:44.

97. Buyon JP, Waltuck J, Kleinmaan C, Copel J (1995) In utero identification and therapy of congenital heart block (CHB). **Lupus** 4:116.
98. McCuiston CH, Schoch EP (1964) Possible discoid lupus erythematosus in a newborn infant. **Arch Dermatol** 70:782.
99. Cassidy JT, Sullivan DB, Dabich L et al. (1977) Scleroderma in children. **Arthritis Rheum** 20(Suppl. 2):31.
100. Kornreich HK, Hanson V (1974) The rheumatic diseases of childhood. **Curr Probl Pediatr** 4:3.
101. Levine BW (1979) Case 43-1979. **N Engl J Med** 301:929.
102. Rodnan GP, Benedek TG (1962) A historical account of the study of progressive systemic sclerosis (diffuse scleroderma). **Ann Intern Med** 57:305.
103. Urano J, Kohno H, Watanabe T (1981) Unusual case of progressive systemic sclerosis with onset in early childhood and following infectious mononucleosis. **Eur J Pediatr** 136:285.
104. Dabich L (1982) Scleroderma. In: Textbook of Pediatric Rheumatology, Cassidy JT, ed. New York: John Wiley & Sons, p. 433.

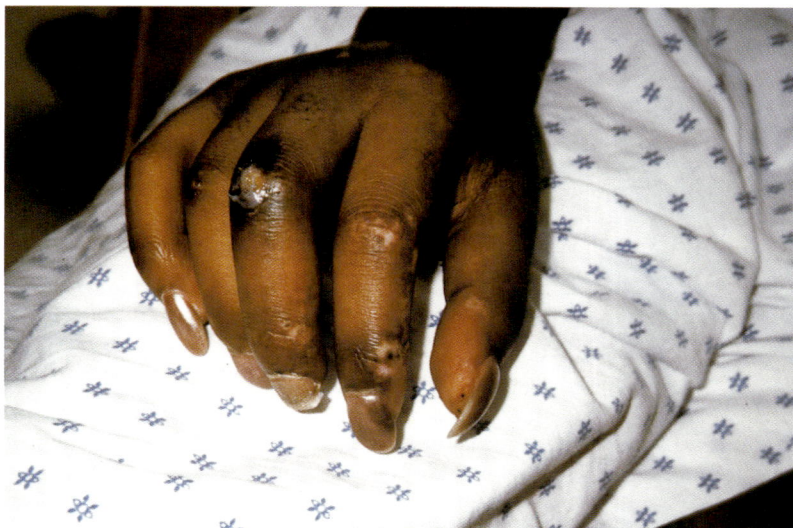

Fig. 23.4 Sclerodactyly, ulceration, and pigmentation abnormalities in progressive systemic sclerosis.

include sparing of the fingertips and absence of Raynaud phenomenon.[103] The rapid evolution of this latter type of PSS when associated with visceral involvement invariably leads to a poor prognosis.[105] At present, however, the strict separation of these two forms of PSS no longer appears clear-cut or especially beneficial prognostically.

It does appear beneficial, however, to identify scleroderma patients having the CREST syndrome. The name signifies the clinical features: *c*alcinosis, *R*aynaud phenomenon, *e*sophageal dysmotility, *s*clerodactyly, and *t*elangiectasia. Initially, this entity appeared to be more benign. However, mortality for CREST syndrome, although less than patients with PSS, is substantial, with a 10-year survival of approximately 75%.[106] The CREST syndrome is not common among children. Cutaneous sclerosis is universally found in PSS but calcinosis and telangiectatic mats occur in only 25 to 30% of patients. Other PSS skin findings are ulcerations (fingertip presumably secondary to vasospasm and overlying calcium deposits especially at pressure points) and pigmentary changes. Cassidy *et al*.[99] reported ulceration in 11 of their 15 patients with PSS and pigmentation abnormalities in three. In addition to skin sclerosis, other organ systems commonly involved in childhood PSS include the musculoskeletal, gastrointestinal, pulmonary, cardiac, and renal systems. Arthralgias, arthritis, myalgias, proximal muscle weakness, and muscle atrophy may be seen in children with PSS. Diarrhea, constipation,[104] abdominal pain,[100] and esophagitis[99] are rare symptoms of intestinal sclerosis. Pulmonary, cardiac, and renal disease involvement is usually silent except when far advanced.

LABORATORY FINDINGS

The laboratory findings in systemic scleroderma are nonspecific. The complete blood count and ESR are often normal.[107,108] Abnormal urinary sediment, albuminuria, blood urea nitrogen (BUN) and creatinine alterations can be detected with renal involvement.[100] Pulmonary function testing including carbon monoxide diffusion capacity and vital capacities should be obtained to establish baseline determinations. These tests were abnormal in two-thirds of the patients reported by Cassidy *et al*.[99] Myocardial sclerosis can

produce electrocardiogram (ECG) abnormalities (i.e., conduction defects, ectopic beats, etc).[99]

Radiologic examinations are of benefit in evaluating the child with PSS. For example, chest X-rays may reveal cardiomegaly or congestive heart failure, and barium swallow cine-esophagograms, small bowel series, and barium enemas should be considered in evaluating potential intestinal involvement. Approximately two-thirds of patients will demonstrate abnormal esophageal motility.[99,109] Rarely, intestinal sclerosis will produce duodenal dilatation or colonic sacculations.[99]

Hand X-rays may demonstrate several soft tissue and bony abnormalities. Soft tissue atrophy and osteopenia of the terminal portion of phalanges are frequently seen. Digital calcification may be prominent, but flexion contractures and erosive arthropathy appear to be rare in children.[109]

The pathologic findings in PSS involve many organs. The skin changes resemble morphea but there is generally less inflammatory infiltrate. Additionally, obliterative vessel changes in the subcutaneous tissue are more prominent; epidermal atrophy is common and calcium deposition is a late finding.[110] Other organs may reveal collagen hyalinization and deposition and/or precapillary arteriolitis with subsequent luminal narrowing. Additional findings include intestinal arteriolitis, smooth muscle fibrosis, and obliterative disease in renal interlobular arteries.[110] The pathogenic significance of vascular endothelial proliferation and intimal fibrosis with eventual luminal narrowing or obliteration in various organs in PSS is unclear at present. However, these findings plus collagen proliferation suggest that endothelial cells and fibroblasts are targets of pathologic significance in scleroderma.

PATHOGENESIS

The pathogenesis of scleroderma is unknown. There has been an accumulation of evidence to indicate that immunologic mechanisms are involved. Deep biopsies of early sclerodermatous lesions demonstrate that mononuclear cells are prominent in the inflammatory infiltrate. This inflammatory infiltrate may be responsible via cytokine release for induction of new collagen formation and the resultant fibrosis. These cytokines, especially transforming growth factor-β (TGF-β) may also be responsible for the small vessel vasculopathy seen in these lesions.

The most compelling evidence suggesting a role for immunologic mechanisms in the pathogenesis of scleroderma, however, has been obtained from ANA studies. With the introduction of tissue culture lines as substrates for ANA determination, it has been found by numerous investigators that greater than 90% of patients with scleroderma demonstrate ANAs.[111] These ANAs are directed against various nuclear and nucleolar macromolecules. Approximately 15% of patients with progressive systemic sclerosis demonstrate antinucleolar antibodies. These ANAs are directed against U3RNP (fibrillin), RNA polymerase I, and PM/ScL antigens. In addition, approximately 20% of patients with progressive systemic sclerosis demonstrate a precipitin antibody against a basic nucleoprotein of approximately 70kDa molecular weight termed SCL-70. This antigen has been identified as a breakdown product of topoisomerase I. Also, 5 to 10% of scleroderma patients have anti-nRNP (U1RNP) antibodies. ANA studies have also determined that patients with the CREST syndrome frequently possess antibodies against the inner and outer plates of the chromosomal centromere (anticentromere antibodies). Patients with anticentromere antibodies, as compared to scleroderma patients with other ANAs, appear to have a statistically significant increased duration of their disease, are almost always women, and have a statistically significant increased prevalence of calcinosis. They also have an absence of diffuse

105. Doyle JA, Connolly SM, Winkelmann RK (1982) Cutaneous and subcutaneous inflammatory sclerosis syndromes. **Arch Dermatol** 118:886.
106. Rodan GP, Jablonska S (1985) Classification of systemic and localized scleroderma. In: Systemic Sclerosis (Scleroderma), Black CM, Myers AR, eds. New York: Gower Medical, p. 3.
107. Kang B, Veres-Thorner C, Neredia R et al. (1982) Successful treatment of far advanced progressive systemic sclerosis by D-penicillamine. **J Allergy Clin Immunol** 69:297.
108. Kornreich H, Koster K, Hanson V (1973) The rheumatic diseases in adolescence. **Pediatr Clin North Am** 20:922.
109. Shanks MJ, Blane CE, Adler DD et al. (1983) Radiographic findings of scleroderma in childhood. **Am J Radiol** 141:657.
110. Lever WF, Schaumburg-Lever G (1975) Histopathology of the Skin, 5th edn. Philadelphia: JB Lippincott.
111. Tan EM (1989) Antinuclear antibodies: diagnostic markers for autoimmune diseases and probes for cell biology. **Adv Immunol** 44:93.

scleroderma, a very low prevalence of renal disease, and a statistically significant lower mortality. A genetic predisposition for PSS is seen in the association with HLA-DR11, DR5*0102, and DRB1*0802 in both Japanese and white patients with PSS.[112–115] A multifactorial hypothesis for the pathogenesis of PSS has recently been proposed.[116] This hypothesis suggests that in the correct genetic background, a cycle of immune activation, endothelial cell damage and subsequent fibrolast proliferation and collagen synthesis can result in PSS.

DIFFERENTIAL DIAGNOSIS

The diagnosis of scleroderma is usually not difficult. Scleredema (of Buschke), which in children may follow a streptococcal pharyngitis, can be distinguished histologically from scleroderma because the thickened collagen is not hyalinized. Eosinophilic fasciitis may be confused with scleroderma (see below). Perhaps the entity most difficult to distinguish from scleroderma is the mixed connective tissue disease (MCTD). This is an overlap syndrome having features of SLE, PSS, and dermatomyositis and the anti-nRNP (U1RNP) antibody. Studies of the original MCTD patients indicate that most have evolved into progressive systemic sclerosis. A few have developed classic SLE.[117] The designation mixed connective tissue disease is employed less and less since it has been realized that the overwhelming majority of anti-nRNP (U1RNP) antibody positive patients satisfy the American College of Rheumatology criteria for the diagnosis of SLE. These patients do, however, have an increased frequency of Raynaud phenomenon, sclerodactyly, esophageal dysmotility, pulmonary disease, and a decreased frequency of renal disease.

TREATMENT

There is no cure for scleroderma. In general, it is a slowly progressive disorder. General measures to forestall skin breakdown include lubrication with bland emollients, avoidance of temperature extremes to prevent ulceration from vasospasm and xerosis, and range of motion physiotherapy to prevent debilitating contractures. Arthralgias and arthritis may respond to NSAIDs or aspirin. Elevation of the head of the bed, antacids, and bethanechol are helpful in treating reflux esophagitis. Acute myositis and rapid pulmonary deterioration secondary to fibrosis may respond to systemic corticosteroids. Renal scleroderma may rarely result in malignant hypertension requiring captopril (angiotensin converting enzyme inhibitor) and/or hemodialysis for control. Oxygen, antibiotics, and diuretics may aid the patient with pulmonary fibrosis and congestive heart failure.[104]

There is some evidence to suggest that D-penicillamine may be effective in treating some progressive systemic sclerosis patients. Use of this drug has been rarely associated with the development of pancytopenia, glomerulonephritis, myasthenia gravis, SLE, and pemphigus. This mildly immunosuppressive drug, which inhibits collagen synthesis *in vitro*, may be tried in PSS to forestall internal involvement, lengthen survival, and decrease sclerosis. Kang et al.[107] refer to two successful reports of the use of D-penicillamine in children with progressive systemic sclerosis. The increasing numbers of uncontrolled reports of the efficacy of D-penicillamine suggest that this may, indeed, be beneficial. There is no good evidence to support the use of methotrexate for the treatment of PSS. Calcium channel blockers (e.g., nifedipine) are effective in controlling Raynaud phenomenon associated with PSS. In a recent study, recombinant human relaxin (the hormone responsible

for loosening of pelvic tissues in preparation for parturition) seemed to improve global assessment measures, but standard measures of scleroderma were unchanged.[118]

PROGNOSIS

Children with scleroderma generally survive for years with slow progression of their disease. Young males apparently have the worst prognosis,[99] as do patients with significant cardiac, pulmonary, or renal disease.

EOSINOPHILIC FASCIITIS

In 1975, Shulman described a scleroderma-like syndrome characterized by diffuse fasciitis with eosinophilia that has since been designated eosinophilic fasciitis (EF).[119] This entity, although rare, has been reported in children.[120] There is no apparent sex or racial predisposition. Patients usually complain of the rapid onset of swollen, tight skin frequently following strenuous physical exertion. Rarely these cutaneous changes have been associated with polyarthritis[121] and can progress to significant flexion contractures. The skin lesions typically begin on the extremities with relative sparing of the face, trunk, fingers, and toes. The skin thickening can occasionally be distinguished by an irregular puckered pattern. This can be especially prominent on the inner aspect of the upper arms. In contradistinction to PSS, the normal skin lines are preserved and Raynaud phenomenon is rare. Periungual telangiectasias and digital ulcers are unusual.[121]

Generally, systemic manifestations are unusual. However, a significant number of these EF patients have subsequently developed aplastic anemia. The sera of some of these patients have demonstrated the presence of humoral factors (probably antibodies) capable (*in vitro*) of inhibiting hemato- and myelopoiesis.[122]

LABORATORY FINDINGS

The laboratory findings typical of EF are transient peripheral eosinophilia, elevated ESR with disease activity, and hypergammaglobulinemia. Bone marrow biopsy may reveal plasmacytosis and eosinophilia.[121] The skin biopsy for diagnosis of EF must be full thickness to include the muscular fascia. The muscular fascia is characteristically thickened due to collagenous hypertrophy and contains a lymphocytic and plasmacytic infiltrate. Scattered or perivascular eosinophils may be seen in the thickened fascia. A similar, but less intense process may be seen in the subcutaneous tissue but the dermis may only exhibit a minimal cellular infiltrate. Occasionally dermal edema is prominent when skin swelling is initially noted. The early lack of new collagen deposition in the dermis and subcutaneous tissue distinguishes EF from scleroderma histologically. However, late EF biopsies may be indistinguishable from scleroderma.

PATHOGENESIS

The pathogenesis of EF is unknown as is the relationship of this entity to classic scleroderma. EF seems to be a distinct entity possessing many cutaneous features in common with scleroderma. This is supported by the facts that EF patients frequently respond to corticosteroids, that the onset of EF may be abrupt and is often associated with strenuous exercise. EF patients may also develop thrombocytopenia or a fatal aplastic anemia. Several EF patients have

112. Dunckley H, Jazwoniska EC, Gatenby PA, Serjentson W (1989) DNA-DR typing shows HLA-DRw11 RFLPs are increased in frequency in PSS and CREST variants of scleroderma. **Tissue Antigens** 33:418.

113. Livingstone JZ, Scott TE, Wigley FM et al. (1987) Systemic sclerosis (scleroderma), clinical genetic, and serologic subsets. **J Rheumatol** 14:512.

114. Gladman DD, Keystone EC, Baron M et al. (1981) Increased frequency of HLA-DR5 in scleroderma. **Arthritis Rheum** 24:854.

115. Takeuchi F, Nakono K, Yamada H et al. (1994) Association of HLA-DR with PSS in Japanese. **J Rheumatol** 21:857.

116. Furst DE, Clements PJ (1997) Hypothesis for the pathogenesis of systemic sclerosis. **J Rheumatol** 24(Suppl 48):53.

117. Nimelstein SH, Brody S, McShane D et al. (1980) Mixed connective tissue disease: a subsequent evaluation of the original 25 patients. **Medicine** (Baltimore) 59:239.

118. Seibold JR, Clements PJ, Furst DE et al. (1998) Safety and pharmacokinetics of recombinant human relaxin in systemic sclerosis. **J Rheumatol** 25:302.

119. Shulman LE (1975) Diffuse fasciitis with eosinophilia: a new syndrome. **Trans Assoc Am Phys** 88:70.

120. Britt WJ, Duray PH, Dahl MV et al. (1980) Diffuse fasciitis with eosinophilia: a steroid responsive variant of scleroderma. **J Pediatr** 97:432.

121. Shulman LE (1981) Eosinophilic fasciitis. **Johns Hopkins Med J** 148:81.

122. Michaels RM (1982) Eosinophilic fasciitis complicated by Hodgkin's disease. **J Rheumatol** 9:3.

been found to possess a serum factor (probably an autoantibody) that suppresses *in vitro* myeloid and erythrocyte precursors. These hematologic abnormalities have, thus far, not been reported in children with EF. Some but not all of these EF patients dramatically respond to systemic steroid therapy. Other patients have been treated with combinations including azathioprine or hydroxychloroquine with variable response.[123] Physical therapy can also be used to mobilize joint contractures.

TOXIC OIL SYNDROME AND EOSINOPHILIA MYALGIA SYNDROME

In the past, two additional syndromes characterized by sclerosis of the skin have been described. One of these syndromes occurred in epidemic proportions in Spain and its etiology was traced to the use of adulterated rapeseed oil. In addition to patchy areas of cutaneous sclerosis, many of these patients developed severe muscle weakness especially of the pulmonary accessory muscles. Unfortunately, prolonged muscle weakness secondary to a neuropathy was associated with a significant mortality.[124]

A similar condition termed the eosinophilia myalgia syndrome occurred in the United States secondary to ingestion of adulterated L-tryptophan obtained from a single manufacturer. The manifestations of this syndrome (patches of cutaneous sclerosis, myopathy, and pulmonary insufficiency associated with a significant mortality) was reminiscent of the toxic syndrome reported from Spain.[125]

JUVENILE DERMATOMYOSITIS

Juvenile dermatomyositis (JDM) is a rare, multisystem idiopathic inflammatory vasculopathy primarily affecting muscle and skin. The changes in small blood vessels include necrotizing vasculitis with intimal proliferation, thrombosis, and infarction. This microvascular angiopathy is the primary clinical and pathologic feature of JDM. The clinical presentation involves symmetric proximal muscle weakness caused by a nonsuppurative myositis, rash, occasional involvement of the myocardium and the gastrointestinal tract, and late emergence of calcinosis in severe cases. As differentiated from adult-onset disease, the childhood form has only rarely been associated with malignancy.[126]

INCIDENCE

Although JDM is a rare disease, it is the most common pediatric inflammatory myopathy, with an incidence of at least 2 cases per million children per year.[127,128] There are two age of onset peaks in childhood: between 5 and 9 years with equal race and gender distribution and early teenage with a 10:1 predominance of females. The group with onset after age 10 has a striking racial difference with blacks involved 10 times more frequently. This predominance of black women is described in adult cases as well.[129]

PRESENTING COMPLAINT

Disease onset is variable. Approximately 30% of children with JDM experience rapid appearance of rash, weakness, and pain. Another 50% have insidious development of muscle pain and progressive weakness associated with rash, limb edema with diffuse muscle induration, and dysphagia. The remainder (about 20%) have a subacute onset with skin rash often long antedating the appearance of muscular or constitutional symptoms. A portion of this group includes children with amyopathic dermatomyositis (dermatomyositis sine myositis).[130,131] Medical attention is sought for a variety of reasons. Easy fatigue is seen early in the course for most youngsters. Fever, weight loss, or fatigue may prompt the initial visit to the physician. The children with subacute onset may present with rash. They may then develop progressive muscle weakness and/or finger joint contractures because of tenosynovitis. These children often have subtle (more easily palpated than visualized) nodules over flexor tendons or over extensor aspects of the elbows. Approximately 20% percent of children with dermatomyositis have tenosynovitis (mainly hands and fingers) or arthritis (mainly knees) during the first year of illness.[132]

In those instances of rapid onset of muscle involvement, difficulty climbing or descending stairs or inclines, arising from bed, rising from the floor, and/or raising the upper extremities and reaching will be noted. Muscle pain or tenderness, although a common component of the syndrome, is usually not a cause of complaint early in its course. Similarly, although dysphagia and/or nasal speech due to palatal weakness with or without esophageal dysfunction occur fairly often, this is rarely an initial presenting complaint. Dyspnea, due to either myocarditis (with heart block) or to involvement of respiratory muscles, is also often seen in the chronic stages but rarely, if ever, at onset of the disease. When rash comprises all or part of the chief complaint, there is often a history of worsening noted after sun exposure. A recurrent, photosensitive, diffuse, widespread dermatitis can often precede the myopathy by extended periods.[133] Although cutaneous involvement is obvious in most cases within several weeks of onset of muscle disease, dermatitis of the knuckles and eyelids can be the first manifestation, sometimes antedating the rest of the syndrome by weeks or months.[130] Recently, the presenting clinical characteristics of 79 children with JDM were evaluated. At diagnosis, all the children had rash (100%), and proximal muscle weakness (100%); 73% had muscle pain; 65% fever; 44% dysphagia; 43% hoarseness; 37% abdominal pain; 35% arthritis; 23% calcinosis; and 13% melena.[134]

PHYSICAL FINDINGS

Skin

In the majority of children the rash is pathognomonic. It is manifest by findings as variable as minimal erythema over eyelids (Fig. 23.5) and extensor surfaces of joints to severe desquamating and ulcerating lesions over the entire body. Early on, there is edema and induration of structures on the face, especially the eyelids, with pink to violet (heliotrope) discoloration of the upper eyelids, often associated with a malar rash. Gottron's papules appear symmetrically over extensor surfaces of joints, especially over proximal interphalangeal (PIP) and metacarpophalangeal (MCP) and less over distal interphalangeal (DIP) finger joints (Fig. 23.6). These are scaly, erythematous, often atrophic and shiny, well-circumscribed papules and plaques. Knee and elbow extensor surfaces can also be involved, as can extensor surfaces of whole extremities and the trunk. The areas with extensive involvement include subcutaneous and intradermal edema. Edema and ulceration tend to occur not only in periorbital areas and the corners of the eyes as well as the digits, but also in the skin folds of the axillary and inguinal regions. Extensive cutaneous ulceration tends to be associated with a poor outcome.[135] The vascular

123. Lakhanpal S, Ginsburg WW, Michet CJ et al. (1988) Eosinophilic fasciitis: clinical spectrum and therapeutic response in 52 cases. **Semin Arthritis Rheum** 17(4):221.
124. Iglesias JL, DeMorazes JM (1983) The cutaneous lesions of the Spanish toxic oil syndrome. **J Am Acad Dermatol** 9:159.
125. Silver RM, Heyes HP, Maize JC et al. (1990) Scleroderma, fasciitis, and eosinophilia associated with the ingestion of tryptophan. **N Engl J Med** 322:874.
126. Falcini F, Taccetti G, Trapani S et al. (1993) Acute lymphocytic leukemia with dermatomyositis-like onset in childhood. **J Rheumatol** 20(7):1260.
127. Malleson PN, Fung MY, Rosenberg AM (1996) The incidence pediatric rheumatic diseases: results from the Canadian Pediatric Rheumatology Association Disease Registry. **J Rheumatol** 23:1981.
128. Mecsgar TA Jr, Dawson WN, Masi AT (1970) The epidemiology of polymyositis. **Am J Med** 48:715.

129. Oddis CV, Carter CG (1990) Incidence of polymyositis-dermatomyositis: a 20 year study of hospital diagnosed cases in Allegheny Country, PA 1963–1982. **J Rheumatol** 17:1329.
130. Euwer RL, Sontheimer RD (1991) Amyopathic dermatomyositis. **J Am Acad Dermatol** 24:959.
131. Eisenstein DM, Paller AS, Pachman LM (1997) Juvenile dermatomyositis presenting with rash alone. **Pediatrics** 100(3 Pt 1):391.
132. Ansell BA (1991) Juvenile dermatomyositis. **Rheum Clin North Am** 17:931.
133. Woo TR, Rasmussen J, Callen JP (1985) Recurrent photosensitive dermatitis preceding juvenile dermatomyositis. **Pediatr Dermatol** 2:207.
134. Pachman LM, Hayford JR, Chung A et al. (1998) Juvenile dermatomyositis at diagnosis: clinical characteristics of 79 children. **J Rheum** 25(6):1198.
135. Crowe WE, Bove KE, Levinson JE et al. (1982) Clinical and pathogenetic implications of histopathology in childhood polydermatomyositis. **Arthritis Rheum** 25:126.

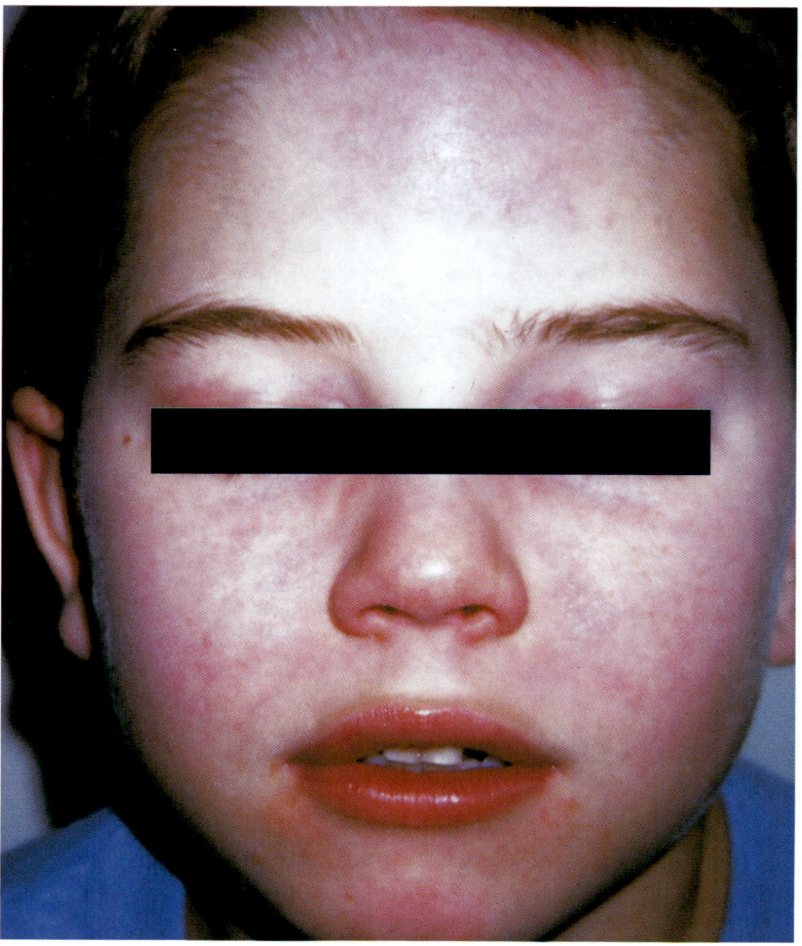

Fig. 23.5   Heliotrope and facial photodermatitis of juvenile dermatomyositis.

changes include telangiectasia of the upper eyelids and the cuticular nail beds. The periungual areas usually become erythematous. Nail fold capillaroscopy reveals capillary dilation with dropout of capillary loops. These capillary findings may require a high plus ophthalmoscope setting or dermatoscope for satisfactory visualization, but can frequently be identified with the unaided eye or hand magnifier. The severity of changes tends to correlate with chronic severity of the disease. Later on in the chronic stages, poikiloderma characterized by atrophy, telangiectasia, and hypo- and hyperpigmentation occurs (Fig. 23.7). Multifocal lipoatrophy has been seen in association with the panniculitis of this disorder.[136] Mucosal ulcerations can occur throughout the gastrointestinal tract. As many as 40% of children get oral lesions that can cause dysphagia.[137] Both scarring and nonscarring alopecia may be seen in JDM.

Prior to the aggressive use of multiple anti-inflammatory agents in the treatment of JDM, as many as 40–70% of the children developed one or another form of calcinosis late in the course of the disease (Figs 23.8 and 23.9). This is a finding that clinically differentiates childhood from adult onset dermatomyositis, where calcinosis occurs in fewer than 5%.[138] There are rare instances of initial presentation of JDM with calcinosis, but the usual experience is that it appears late in the course, from 6 months to 12 years after the onset. Those youngsters with chronic unremittive inflammation tend to get the calcinosis, and the more severe the initial inflammation, the more severe the calcinosis tends to be. With aggressive treatment, calcinosis is now seen only infrequently. There is a subgroup of youngsters who do poorly despite optimal therapeutic regimens. They have a severe disease course responding minimally to steroid therapy and manifested by persistent muscle weakness, generalized cutaneous vasculitis with ulcerations, telangiectasia, and poikiloderma. They are at high risk for developing exoskeleton-like calcification.[139,140] In many youngsters, the disabilities imposed by the calcinosis far exceed the impairments of the actual myositis. It is believed that the calcinosis is dystrophic and represents the end result of a scarring process produced by muscle micro-vasculature destruction and subsequent tissue necrosis.[139] The five patterns of calcinosis[139] include the following:

- Superficial plaques or nodules usually on extremities
- Calcinosis circumscripta: deep, large, tumorous deposits in proximal muscles

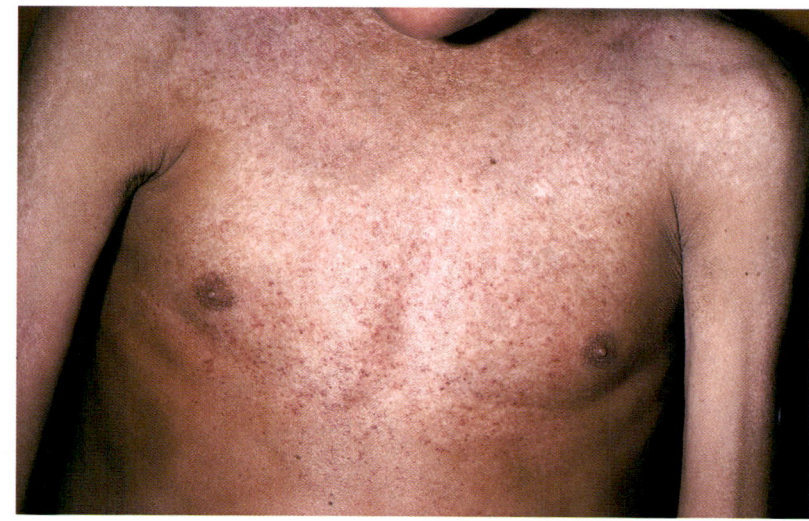

Fig. 23.6   Gottron's papules and nail bed capillary telangectasias of juvenile dermatomyositis.

Fig. 23.7   Poikiloderma in dermatomyositis.

136. Commens C, O'Neill P, Walker G (1990) Dermatomyositis associated with multifocal atrophy. **J Am Acad Dermatol** 22:966.
137. Hamlin C, Shelton JE (1984) Management of oral findings in a child with an advanced case of dermatomyositis. **Pediatr Dent** 6:46.
138. Kornreich HK, Hanson V (1974) Rheumatic diseases of childhood. **Curr Probl Pediatr** 4:3.

139. Bowyer SL, Blane CE, Sullivan DB, Cassidy JT (1983) Childhood dermatomyositis: factors predicting functional outcome and development of dystrophic calcification. **J Pediatr** 103:882.
140. Bowyer SL, Clark RAF, Ragsdale CG et al. (1986) Juvenile dermatomyositis: histological findings and pathogenetic hypothesis for associated skin changes. **J Rheumatol** 13:753.

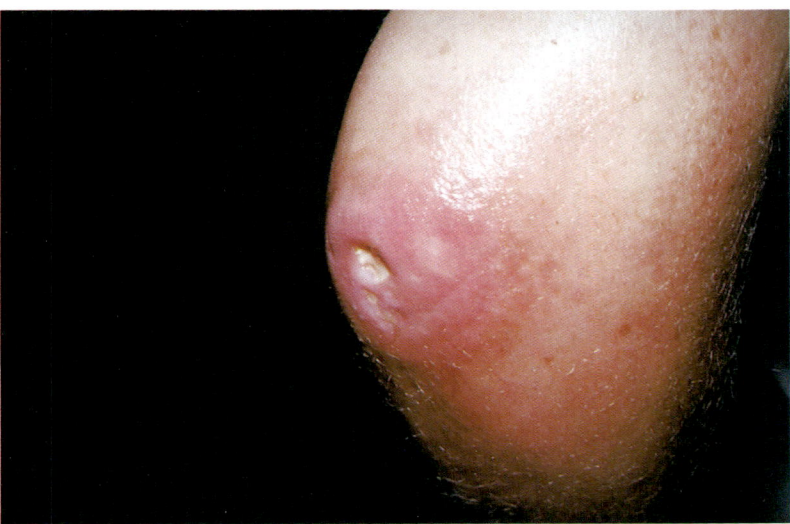

Fig. 23.8   Nodular calcinosis with ulceration in juvenile dermatomyositis.

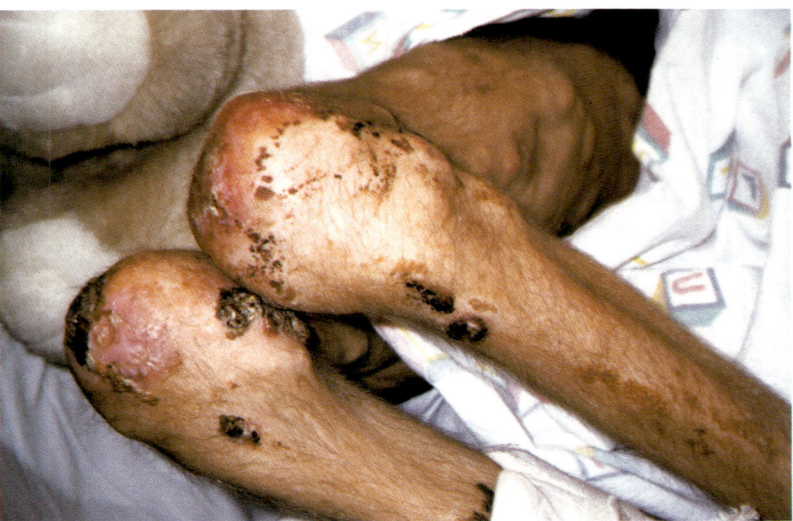

Fig. 23.9   Extensive tumorous calcium deposits in late-stage untreated juvenile dermatomyositis.

- Calcinosis universalis: intermuscular fascial plane deposition
- Severe, extensive subcutaneous reticular exoskeleton-like deposits
- Mixed forms.

These clinical patterns have corresponding radiologic findings.[141]

Speculation on the etiology of the calcinosis has included a provocative long-term study of 15 children with JDM, nine of whom developed calcinosis. Granulocyte chemotaxis to *Staphylococcus aureus* was severely depressed in those who developed calcinosis, whereas those without calcinosis did not differ from controls. The nine children with calcinosis had higher IgE concentrations than nonatopic controls. These IgE findings antedated the calcinosis as did the occurrence of staphylococcal infections. Those without calcinosis had findings similar to controls.[142] This suggests preceding immunologic differences in patients with dermatomyositis who do, compared to those who do not, develop calcinosis.

Muscles

Early muscle involvement includes proximal limb groups and anterior neck flexors with weakness of limb girdle function and impaired walking, rising, squatting, and reaching. Gower's sign is usually present, where on arising from the floor, the child rolls to the prone position, kneels, then pushes the hands against the shins, knees, and then the thighs to assist achievement of a standing position. Neck, trunk, paraspinal, and abdominal muscles are also involved but appear to have fewer implications as to functional disability except in advanced cases. Pain is moderate and is usually described as stiffness or tenderness. Other sites of involvement of striated muscle include palatal, pharyngeal, or hypopharyngeal groups that can cause nasal speech, dysphonia, choking, aspiration, dysphagia, or drooling. Dysphagia can also be provoked by upper esophageal involvement. Distal extremity weakness is a late phenomenon in severe cases and is, at times, very severe. Respiratory muscle involvement can cause restrictive pulmonary disease in the more severe chronic cases.

The arteritis can also involve the myocardium with heart block, the pericardium with pericarditis, the gastrointestinal tract with mucosal ulceration that can lead to perforation, the retina with small vessel occlusion causing cytoid bodies, and, rarely, the kidneys with glomerular cellular proliferation and microscopic hematuria that does not progress to insufficiency.

TECHNIQUES OF DIAGNOSIS

This disorder is diagnosed clinically by the pathognomonic rash and proximal muscle findings. Bohan and Peter[143] described diagnostic criteria that are helpful in establishing a correct diagnosis. These include characteristic rash, symmetric weakness of proximal muscles and anterior neck flexors, elevated skeletal muscle enzymes, and confirmation with either characteristic muscle biopsy findings and/or characteristic electromyography (EMG). More recently EMG and muscle biopsy have been deferred in the classic onset of JDM (see below). When a muscle biopsy is performed, it is often guided by MRI findings of inflammation, because muscle involvement is often spotty and unguided biopsies may miss sites of active inflammation.

Measurement of serum skeletal muscle enzymes helps with both initial diagnosis and monitoring of therapeutic intervention. The four most useful measurements include asparatate aminotransferase (AST), creatine phos-phokinase (CPK), lactic dehydrogenase (LDH) and aldolase. There is individual variation in how these enzymes elevate and it is useful to monitor all four. Any or all of the enzymes may be normal early in the course or during a chronic phase. Some authors have noted elevated neopterin and von Willebrand factor as markers of disease activity.[144,145]

EMG shows the characteristic findings of myopathy and denervation. Evidence of membrane instability and random fiber destruction are often found.

MRI is an alternative confirmatory procedure that has proven very useful in identifying areas of muscle edema and inflammation. MRI may also be employed to choose the site for muscle biopsy. MRI was used to follow the course of JDM from the onset of disease through resolution of a primary relapse. The signal intensity of the T2-weighted image of involved muscles was elevated during periods of disease activity and returned to normal levels with effective suppression of disease activity. T1-weighted images remained normal despite disease activity.[146] The same authors demonstrated similar usefulness of the technique in assessing the upper legs and lower pelvis of four other children.[147] The authors note that these T2-weighted images are related to accumulated extracellular water and that the abnormalities would exist in any inflammatory or infectious myopathy and in rhabdomyolysis. This differs from the fatty replacement of muscles seen in toxic myopathies and muscular dystrophies.

141. Blane CE, White SJ, Braunstein EM et al. (1984) Patterns of calcification in childhood dermatomyositis. **Am J Radiol** 142:397.
142. Moore EC, Cohen F (1992) Staphylococcal infections in childhood dermatomyositis. **Ann Rheum Dis** 51:378.
143. Bohan A, Peter JB (1975) Polymyositis and dermatomyositis. **N Engl J Med** 292 344.
144. Bloom BJ, Tucker LBL, Miller LC et al. (1995) von Willebrand factor in juvenile dermatomyositis. **J Rheumatol** 22:230.
145. Pachman LM (1995) An update on juvenile dermatomyositis. **Curr Opin Rheumatol** 7:437.
146. Keim DR, Hernandez RJ, Sullivan DB (1991) Serial magnetic resonance imaging in juvenile dermatomyositis. **Arthritis Rheum** 34:1580.
147. Hernandez RJ, Keim DR, Sullivan DB et al. (1990) Magnetic resonance imaging appearance of muscles in childhood dermatomyositis. **J Pediatr** 117:546.

Muscle biopsy is useful if the skin changes are not classical and muscle enzyme levels are not clearly abnormal (e.g., 20-fold increase in CPK). It provides histologic reassurance that another type of myopathy is not present. Not all pediatric rheumatologists concur on its usefulness.[148] A biopsy can provide useful prognostic information.[135,149] It is customary to perform open biopsies but needle biopsy may be useful in attempts at sequential monitoring. On biopsy one typically finds evidence of vasculitis, inflammatory cell infiltrates, and focal necrosis and phagocytosis of muscle fibers, as well as evidence of regeneration with basophilia, endomysial proliferation, random fiber atrophy, and perifascicular atrophy.

The histology of the skin lesions is nondiagnostic. The pathologic features are similar to the findings of LE. During later phases, calcinosis, accumulation of hydroxyapatite, and fibrosis occur.

ETIOLOGY AND PATHOGENESIS

Various infectious agents have been proposed as etiologically related to childhood onset dermatomyositis. Acute transient inflammatory myositis can occur in children in association with various viral infections such as influenza A and B.[150] This led to suggestions of possible viral etiology of JDM. It has been observed that sera from recently diagnosed children with JDM have a significantly increased titer of both complement-fixing antibody and neutralizing antibody to Coxsackie B, but further studies failed to confirm the presence of the virus in muscle tissue.[151] Toxoplasma may also cause significant myositis.[152] Other environmental agents, in addition to infectious agents, have been associated with chronic inflammatory myopathies. Numerous drugs and toxins have been implicated in chronic inflammatory myopathies.[153–155] An autoimmune pathogenesis is presumed based on observations of immune mechanisms of altered cell-mediated immunity, immune complex phenomena, and the association of dermatomyositis with immunodeficiency.

Abnormalities of cell-mediated autoimmunity

Lymphocyte infiltration is prominent in muscle biopsies from patients with dermatomyositis. Most of the infiltrate is made up of $CD4^+$ cells around blood vessels. Supernatants of peripheral lymphocytes (lymphokines) of children with dermatomyositis have been shown to impair protein synthesis and induce necrosis of monolayers of human fetal muscle in the presence of autologous muscle homogenates.[156] Lymphocytes of patients have been shown, *in vitro*, to proliferate and transform in the presence of allogeneic or autologous muscle extracts.[157] Lymphocytes from children with JDM are cytotoxic *in vitro* to human fetal or animal cells.[158,159] It has also been shown that a combination of sera and leukocytes produces cell-mediated toxicity

against endothelium, in addition to what is seen with muscle cells, in JDM.[160] Recently, the rise is the percentage of B cells was found to significantly correlate with increased disease activity.[161]

Immune complex disease and humoral immunity

Immune deposition in the vessels with a concomitant relative lack of inflammatory cells at sites of fiber atrophy tends to affirm the concept that immune complex vasculitis initiates or sustains the process. Immunoglobulin (IgG and IgM) and complement (C3) have been found in skeletal muscle blood vessel walls.[162] Endothelial injury is demonstrable in vasculitis in children, including the vasculitis of dermatomyositis, by the finding of circulating von Willebrand factor and C3d (a degradation product of C3), along with evidence of thrombin generation (elevation of fibrinopeptide A).[163] Further evidence of a complement-mediated vasculopathy is the demonstration of a C5-9 membrane attack complex in the muscle microvasculature. No IgG or IgA was present in these vessels.[164] The same investigators subsequently demonstrated that this complement-mediated vasculopathy is an early, primary immunopathogenic event in the evolution of muscle lesions in dermatomyositis.[165] The role of humoral-mediated immunity in dermatomyositis (as opposed to other inflammatory myopathies) is further supported by observations that as one moves from perivascular to endomysial sites, B cells become fewer and T cells more numerous. There is a higher proportion of B cells, a higher CD4:CD8 ratio, and a close proximity of $CD4^+$ cells to B cells and macrophages with a relative absence of invasion of non-necrotic muscle cells by lymphocytes.[166]

Many researchers have investigated the issue of an immunogenetic predisposition to this disorder. There is an increased prevalence of HLA-DRB1*0301, DQA1*0501, and DQB1*0201 haplotypes in JDM. The increased incidence of DQA1*0501 haplotype was consistent across racial lines and within families.[167,168] Recently, a familial dermatomyositis was identified and the two patients were shown to share the DQA1*0501 allele.[169] Polymorphisms in the HLA-DMA*0103 and HLA-DMB*0102 were shown to be associated with increased relative risk ratios of 5.7 and 8-fold, respectively.[170]

There has been some evidence that childhood and adult onset myositis are separate disease entities. In one study, a myositis specific antibody (anti-Jo-1) was found only in adults and not in children or adolescents evaluated in a study of ANA and arthropathy in polymyositis and dermatomyositis.[171] On the other hand, ANAs do occur in a significant percentage of first-degree relatives of patients with dermatomyositis, a finding that seems to be genetically conditioned.[172] Despite these observations, which strongly support immunogenetic predisposition, a familial incidence is very rare. It should be noted that of the five reported instances of familial occurrence,[169,173–176] two

148. Malleson PN (1990) Controversies in juvenile dermatomyositis. **J Rheumatol** 17(Suppl 22):1.
149. Banker BQ, Victor M (1966) Dermatomyositis (systemic angiopathy) of childhood. **Medicine** 45:261.
150. Dietzmann DE, Schaller JG, Ray CG et al. (1976) Acute myositis associated with influenza B infection. **Pediatrics** 57:255.
151. Christensen ML, Pachman LM, Schneiderman R et al. (1986) Prevalence of Coxsackie B virus antibodies in patients with dermatomyositis. **Arthritis Rheum** 29:1265.
152. Magid SK, Kagen LJ (1983) Serologic evidence for acute toxoplasmosis in polymyositis-dermatomyositis. **Am J Med** 75:313.
153. Mastaglia FL, Ojeda VJ (1985) Inflammatory myopathies: Part 1. **Ann Neurol** 17:215.
154. Belongia EA, Hedberg CW (1990) An investigation of the cause of the eosinophilia-myalgia syndrome associated with tryptophan use. **N Engl J Med** 323:357.
155. Kilbourne EM, Rigau-Perez JG, Heath CW Jr et al. (1983) Clinical epidemiology of toxic-oil syndrome: manifestations of a new illness. **N Engl J Med** 309:1408.
156. Johnson RL, Fink CW, Zink M (1972) Lymphotoxin formation by lymphocytes and muscle in polymyositis. **J Clin Invest** 51:2435.
157. Mastaglia FL, Currie S (1971) Immunologic and ultrastructural observations on the role of lymphoid cells in the pathogenesis of polymyositis. **Acta Neuropathol** 18:1.
158. Currie S (1970) Destruction of muscle cultures by lymphocytes from cases of polymyositis. **Acta Neuropathol** 15:11.
159. Miller ML, Lanter R, Pachman LM (1983) Natural and antibody dependent cellular cytotoxicity in children with SLE and dermatomyositis. **J Rheumatol** 10:640.
160. Iannaccone ST, Bowen D, Yarom A et al. (1984) In vitro study of cytotoxic factors against endothelium in childhood dermatomyositis. **Arch Neurol** 41:862.
161. Eisenstein DM, O'Gorman MRG, Pachman LM (1997) Correlations between change in disease activity and changes in peripheral blood lymphocyte subsets in patients with juvenile dermatomyositis. **J Rheumatol** 24:1830.

162. Whitaker JN, Engel WK (1971) Vascular deposits of immunoglobulin and complement in inflammatory myopathy. **N Engl J Med** 286:333.
163. Scott JP, Arroyave C (1986) Activation of complement and coagulation in juvenile dermatomyositis. **Arthritis Rheum** 30:572.
164. Kissel JT, Mendell JR, Rammohan KW (1986) Microvascular deposition of complement membrane attack complex in dermatomyositis. **N Engl J Med** 314:329.
165. Kissel JT, Halterman RK, Rammohan KW, Mendell JR (1991) Relationship of complement-mediated microvasculopathy to the histologic features and clinical duration of disease in dermatomyositis. **Arch Neurol** 48:26.
166. Engel AG, Arahata K (1986) Mononuclear cells in myopathies. **Hum Pathol** 17:704.
167. Reed AM, Stirling JD (1995) Association of the HLA-DQA*0501 allele in multiple racial groups with juvenile dermatomyositis. **Hum Immunol** 44:131.
168. Reed AM, Pachman LM, Hayford J et al. (1998) Immunogenetic studies in families of children with juvenile dermatomyositis. **J Rheumatol** 25(5):1000.
169. Plamondon S, Dent PB, Reed AM (1999) Familial dermatomyositis. **J Rheumatol** 26:2691.
170. West JE, Reed AM (1999) Analysis of HLA-DM polymorphism in juvenile dermatomyositis (JDM) patients. **Hum Immunol** 60(3):255.
171. Oddis CV, Medsgar TA Jr, Cooperstein LA (1990) Subluxing arthropathy associated with the anti-Jo-1 antibody in polymyositis/dermatomyositis. **Arthritis Rheum** 33:1640.
172. Valantini G, Improta RD (1991) ANA in first degree relatives of patients with polymyositis-dermatomyositis. **Br J Rheumatol** 30:429.
173. Lambie JA, Duff IF (1963) Familial occurrence of dermatomyositis. **Ann Intern Med** 59:839.
174. Lewkonia RM, Buxton PH (1973) Myositis in father and daughter. **J Neurol Neurosurg Psychiatr** 36:820.
175. Harati Y, Niakan E, Bergman EW (1986) Childhood dermatomyositis in monozygotic twins. **Neurology** 36:721.
176. Wedgwood RJP, Cook CD, Cohen J (1953) Dermatomyositis. **Pediatrics** 12:447.

coincidences[175,176] were seen in monozygotic twins, further strengthening the case for a genetic influence.

Specific autoantibodies have been detected commonly in adult patients with polymyositis/dermatomyositis.[177,178] The myositis-specific antibodies define rather homogeneous subsets of adult patients.[179] The most common of these antibodies are directed against aminoacyl-tRNA synthetases. Anti-Jo-1 (anti-histidyl-tRNA synthetase) is the most common antisynthetase antibody, occurring in 15 to 20% of adult polymyositis/dermatomyositis patients. The clinical picture associated with antisynthetase antibodies is characterized by a myositis more resistant to therapy, a high frequency of interstitial lung disease (50–70%), arthritis (greater than 90%), and Raynaud phenomenon (approximately 60%). Dermatologically, these patients may have a peculiar involvement of the hands, "mechanic's hand," characterized by hyperkeratosis with hyperpigmentation and fissuring along the sides of the fingers appearing as dirty horizontal lines.[180]

Another antibody commonly detected in myositis patients, anti-PM/Scl, is directed against non-RNA containing proteins (predominantly 100kD and 75kD) residing in the nucleolus. This antibody is found in a group of myositis patients who frequently demonstrate cutaneous features of scleroderma.[181] Most of the patients in whom this antibody has been described have been adults, but this antibody has also been detected in children.[182]

Anti-Mi-2 antibodies have been detected in dermatomyositis patients, including juveniles. This antibody is directed against a complex of non-nucleic acid containing five nuclear proteins.[177,183] Children with anti-Mi-2 have mild disease, which is readily controlled by corticosteroids.

Association with immune deficiency

A dermatomyositis syndrome has been seen in patients with X-linked hypogammaglobulinemia. ECHO virus (usually type II) has been grown from cerebrospinal fluid and muscle.[184] This syndrome has also been seen in patients with C2 complement component deficiency[185] and in children with selective IgA deficiency.[186]

DIFFERENTIAL DIAGNOSIS

The combination of the characteristic skin rash, proximal muscle weakness and elevated muscle enzymes usually makes the diagnosis reasonably simple. The alternative diagnoses that sometimes require consideration include postinfectious myositis (e.g., influenza A and B, Coxsackievirus B and trichinosis), inflammatory myopathy associated with another collagen vascular disorder, and the large group of congenital myopathies.

The postviral myositis disorders usually persist for 3 to 5 days and do not have the accompanying characteristic rash.[150] The myopathy associated with *Trichinella spiralis* infestation is related to the presence of the larval cysts of the nematode in the affected muscle. It involves muscles of the face, neck, and chest and is usually accompanied by significant peripheral blood eosinophilia.[187]

The malar rash of dermatomyositis often resembles the SLE "butterfly rash" but lacks the well-defined borders and extension to the forehead. Children with scleroderma do not have the typical Gottron's patches over extensor surfaces of elbows, knees, and knuckles. Children with myositis associated with SLE rarely have the significant elevation of muscle enzymes seen in dermatomyositis. When there is no rash, a broad variety of neuromuscular diseases requires consideration. Family history, age at onset, site of muscle involvement, and type of onset should be considered.[188]

THERAPY

JDM remains a serious disease despite many therapeutic advances. Prior to the widespread use of corticosteroids for this entity, approximately one-third of the children completely recovered, one-third had residual significant disability, and one-third died, usually of a perforated viscus or aspiration pneumonia.[189] In mild cases or with subacute onset, many rheumatologists begin with prednisone at 2mg/kg/day and taper that quickly to no more than 1mg/kg/day when there is adequate clinical (afebrile, increased muscle strength, improved well being) and laboratory (normalization of muscle enzymes) response. The dose is then tapered slowly over 6 months to one year, with careful monitoring of the clinical and laboratory response. The fever usually falls to normal within the first days, followed by a normal pattern of muscle enzymes within weeks and a resumption of normal muscle strength within 2 to 3 months. The cutaneous features often do not resolve and can persist for years despite total resolution of all other indicators of disease. The dermatitis appears to follow a course relatively independent of the myopathy.

In order to minimize the hazards of long-term use of systemic corticosteroids, an attempt has been made to use steroid-pulse iv therapy in doses from 30mg/kg up to 1.5g at 24- to 48-h intervals until laboratory markers have returned to normal.[190,191] Recently, Pachman et al., in a retrospective comparison of oral versus pulse steroids found that pulse steroids followed by low daily prednisone dosing, after disease control, resulted in shorter duration of rash and less functional impairment.[192] More importantly, 36% of the patients treated with oral steroids alone developed calcinosis, while none of the patients in the pulse steroid group developed any calcifications.

In children with inflammatory skin disease, low-dose hydroxychloroquine (5mg/kg/day) is often used. Its usefulness is primarily for treating the skin, but some have found it to be an effective steroid-sparing agent.[193,194]

Although most children can be successfully treated with corticosteroids alone, some relapse after initial improvement, some have incomplete responses, and others develop intolerable adverse effects of the drug. In cases that are steroid resistant, severe or prolonged, methotrexate, cyclosporin A, azathioprine, cyclophosphamide, and intravenous gammaglobulin (IVIG) have all been used.

Methotrexate has been successfully used to treat recalcitrant JDM and is often the second-line agent of choice.[195,196] One study has suggested that the recurrence of disease after withdrawal of methotrexate indicates that it has a

177. Targoff I (1993) Humoral immunity in polymyositis/dermatomyositis. **J Invest Dermatol** 100:116S.
178. Reichlin M, Arnett FC (1984) Multiplicity of antibodies in myositis sera. **Arthritis. Rheum** 27:1150.
179. Love LA (1991) A new approach to the classification of idiopathic inflammatory myopathy: myositis specific autoantibodies define useful homogeneous patients groups. **Medicine** 70:360.
180. Stahl NI (1979) A cutaneous lesion associated with myositis. **Ann Intern Med** 91:577.
181. Reichlin M (1984) Antibodies to a nuclear/nucleolar antigen in patients with polymyositis overlap syndrome. **J Clin Immunol** 4:40.
182. Blaszczyk M (1991) Childhood sclero-myositis: an overlap syndrome associated with PM/Scl antibodies. **Pediatr Dermatol** 8:1.
183. Targoff I, Reichlin M (1985) The association between Mi-2 antibodies and dermatomyositis. **Arthritis Rheum** 28:796.
184. Webster ADB (1984) Echovirus disease in hypogammaglobulinemic patients. **Clin Rheum Dis** 10:189.
185. Leddy JP, Griggs RC (1975) Hereditary complement (C2) deficiency with dermatomyositis. **Am J Med** 58:83.
186. Carroll JE, Silverman A (1984) Inflammatory myopathy, IgA deficiency and intestinal malabsorption. **J Pediatr** 89:216.

187. Baker JP, Goldstein M (1987) Myositis (post-influenza, Coxsackie virus, *Trichinella spiralis*). In: Textbook of Pediatric Infectious Diseases, 2nd edn. Feigin RD, Cherry JD, eds. Philadelphia: WB Saunders, p. 783.
188. Dubowitz V (1978) Muscle Disorders in Childhood. Philadelphia: WB Saunders.
189. Bitnum S, Daeschner CW Jr, Travis LB et al. (1964) Dermatomyositis. **J Pediatr** 64:101.
190. Miller JJ III (1980) Prolonged use of large intravenous steroid pulses in the rheumatic diseases of children. **Pediatrics** 65:989.
191. Laxer RM, Stein LD, Petty RE (1987) Intravenous pulse methylprednisolone treatment of juvenile dermatomyositis. **Arthritis Rheum** 30:328.
192. Pachman LM, Callen AM, Hayford J et al. (1994) Juvenile dermatomyositis: Decreased calcinosis with intermittent high-dose intravenous methylprednisolone therapy. **Arthritis Rheum** 37:S429.
193. Woo TY, Callen JP, Voorhees JJ et al. (1984) Cutaneous lesions of dermatomyositis are improved by hydroxychloroquine. **J Am Acad Dermatol** 10:592.
194. Olson NY, Lindsley CB (1988) Adjunctive use of hydroxychloroquine in childhood dermatomyositis. **J Rheumatol** 16:1545.
195. Malyaviya AN (1968) Treatment of dermatomyositis with methotrexate. **Lancet** 2:485.
196. Fischer TJ (1979) Childhood dermatomyositis and polymyositis: treatment with methotrexate and prednisone. **Am J Dis Child** 133:386.

suppressive, rather than remittive, effect.[197] Oral azathioprine at 2.5mg/kg/day has been used with varied success.[198] In severe vasculitis, Ansell[199] has used pulse iv cyclophosphamide covered by sodium-2-mercaptoethane sulfonate (MESNA) in order to avoid bladder wall toxicity.

Cyclosporin A has been effective when introduced early in severely involved children who have significant muscle weakness and skin ulceration.[200–202] The usual initial dosage is 5–8mg/kg/day. Hypertension and increased serum creatinine are risks accompanying the use of this agent. A recent study indicated that cyclosporin A was an effective agent in the treatment of refractory JDM and could be used in combination with methotrexate for added efficacy.[203]

An uncontrolled pilot study using high-dose IVIG was undertaken as a means of dealing with the long-term and short-term toxicities of traditional corticosteroid therapy, as well as treating clinical abnormalities that were not responding to glucocorticoid medication.[204] The use of this agent permitted lowering or discontinuation of steroid dosage with improvement of muscle weakness and amelioration of rash in many of those studied. A controlled study of this costly therapy has been reported and supports its use for refractory dermatomyositis.[205] More recently, the use of IVIG for the treatment of children with JDM was evaluated and found to be beneficial in improving the muscle strength and skin manifestations, as seen previously in adults.[206]

Claims of efficacy of both plasma exchange and leukapheresis in patients poorly responsive to corticosteroids have been made based on anecdotal reports and uncontrolled trials. A well-controlled study[207] concluded that neither leukapheresis nor plasma exchange was more effective than sham apheresis as treatments for corticosteroid-resistant inflammatory myositis.

OUTCOME

The long-term survival rate of children with JDM is greater than 90%. The greatest causes of mortality are myocarditis, progressive myositis, bowel perforation, and aspiration pneumonia.[208] Most children have a single course and, in a period of from 6 months to as long as 5 years, will completely recover. About a quarter of the children have either repeated acute exacerbations and remissions or have smoldering persistence of activity despite all interventions. Those with the chronic courses are at highest risk for development of calcinosis, and/or cutaneous and gastrointestinal ulcerations, progressive functional loss, severe disability, and risk of death due to gastrointestinal ulceration with acute perforation or, more commonly, respiratory failure. There has been increasing recognition of development of lipodystrophy associated with JDM.[209] Finally, panniculitis has been reported as a clinical finding in JDM.[210]

MIXED CONNECTIVE TISSUE DISEASE

In 1972 Sharp, *et al.*[211] described a group of patients with signs and symptoms that overlapped SLE, PSS, and dermatomyositis. In addition to displaying an "overlap" syndrome, these patients possessed high titers of antibodies directed against an RNAase sensitive extractable nuclear antigen (ENA), called nRNP.

This autoantigen is a uridylate-rich ribonuclear protein now termed U1RNP. Many of the original patients with mixed connective tissue disease (MCTD), however, subsequently developed progressive systemic sclerosis. Other patients have developed classic SLE.[212] Because of these observations, many investigators believe that MCTD is not, in fact, a distinct homogeneous entity but represents a heterogeneous group of collagen vascular disease patients in evolution. Furthermore, extensive serologic studies indicate that anti-nRNP (U1RNP) is not specific for MCTD; most anti-nRNP (U1RNP) patients satisfy the American College of Rheumatology criteria for the diagnosis of SLE. As with most of the other collagen vascular disorders, MCTD is usually described in female patients. Childhood cases of MCTD are rare, but seem to follow the same course as the adult form.[212] The majority of affected individuals are whites, although blacks are also affected.[214] Joint pain and/or Raynaud phenomenon are the most common presenting complaints, occurring in 50 to 70% of patients. A lupus-like dermatitis is seen in 50% of patients. The physical findings in MCTD are detailed in Table 23.3.

The arthritis of MCTD occurs in three-fourths of all patients and can be confused with juvenile rheumatoid arthritis. The arthritis is generally a

TABLE 23.3 Findings in mixed connective tissue disease

Cutaneous
  Lupuslike dermatitis
  Photosensitivity
  Periungual telangiectasia
  Hypo- and/or hyperpigmentation
  Heliotrope eyelid rash
  Sclerodactyly/sclerosis
  Alopecia

Musculoskeletal
  Arthralgia/arthritis
  Proximal muscle weakness
  Raynaud phenomenon

Gastrointestinal
  Abnormal esophageal motility

Pulmonary
  Abnormal pulmonary function tests
  Pulmonary fibrosis

Cardiac
  Pericarditis/myocarditis
  Aortic insufficiency
  Congestive heart failure

Renal
  Glomerulonephritis

Neurologic
  Seizures
  Headache
  Peripheral neuropathy

197. Miller LC (1992) Methotrexate treatment of recalcitrant childhood dermatomyositis. **Arthritis Rheum** 35:1143.
198. Jacobs JC (1977) Methotrexate and azathioprine treatment of childhood dermatomyositis. **Pediatrics** 59:212.
199. Ansell BM (1984) Inflammatory disorders of muscle. **Clin Rheum Dis** 10:205.
200. Heckmatt J (1989) Effectiveness of cyclosporin for dermatomyositis. **Lancet** 1:1063.
201. Dantzig P (1990) Juvenile dermatomyositis treated with cyclosporine. **J Am Acad Dermatol** 22 (part 1):310.
202. Giardin E (1988) Cyclosporine for juvenile dermatomyositis. **J Pediatr** 112:165.
203. Reiff A, Rawlings DJ, Shaham B et al. (1997) Preliminary evidence for cyclosporine A as an alternative in the treatment of recalcitrant juvenile rheumatoid arthritis and juvenile dermatomyositis. **J Rheumatol** 24(12):2436.
204. Lang BA, Laxer RM (1991) Treatment of dermatomyositis with intravenous gamma globulin. **Am J Med** 91:189.
205. Dalakas MC, Illa I, Dambrosia JM et al. (1993) A controlled trial of high-dose intravenous immune globulin infusions as treatment of dermatomyositis. **N Engl J Med** 329:1993.
206. Roifman CM (1995) Use of intravenous immune globulin in the therapy of children with rheumatological diseases. **J Clin Immunol** 15(6):42S.

207. Miller FW (1992) Controlled trial of plasma exchange and leukapheresis in polymyositis and dermatomyositis. **N Engl J Med** 326:1380.
208. Ansell BM (1992) Juvenile dermatomyositis. **J Rheumatol** 19:60.
209. Tucker LB (1990) The association of acquired lipodystrophy with juvenile dermatomyositis. **Arthritis Rheum** 33:D76.
210. Ghali FE, Reed AM, Groben PA et al. (1999) Panniculitis in juvenile dermatomyositis. **Ped Derm** 16(4):270.
211. Sharp GC, Irvin WS, Tan EM et al. (1972) Mixed connective tissue disease: an apparently distinct rheumatic disease syndrome associated with a specific antibody to extractable nuclear antigen (ENA). **Am J Med** 52:148.
212. Nimelstein SG, Brody S, McShane D et al. (1980) Mixed connective tissue disease: a subsequent evaluation of the original 25 patients. **Medicine** (Baltimore) 59:239.
213. Singsen BH, Bernstein BH, Kornreich HK et al. (1977) Mixed connective tissue disease in childhood: a clinical and serological survey. **J Pediatr** 90:893.
214. Bennett RM, O'Connell DJ (1978) The arthritis of mixed connective tissue disease. **Ann Rheum Dis** 37:397.

symmetric, nondeforming polyarthritis involving the PIP and MCP joints. Other extremity joints are involved in less than 25% of cases and arthritis mutilans occurs rarely.[213] Bone X-rays show relatively mild arthritic changes consisting of a few, small, asymmetric periarticular erosions that do not significantly progress over time. These changes are not unique. They are consistent with early but not late rheumatoid arthritis and the mild erosive arthritides of PSS, polymyositis,[213] and SLE.[215]

The presence of the anti-nRNP (U1RNP) antibody at high titer is required to make the diagnosis of MCTD. No other laboratory findings are significant. It is important to identify these anti-nRNP (U1RNP) patients whether or not they are considered to have MCTD because these patients do stand apart prognostically and therapeutically. These individuals typically have a rather benign course with slow progression of their disease and are usually responsive to relatively low doses of corticosteroids and/or NSAIDs. Renal disease can occur in these anti-nRNP (U1RNP) antibody positive patients but much less frequently than that seen in anti-nDNA antibody positive SLE patients.

SJÖGREN SYNDROME

Sjögren syndrome is a symptom complex of dry mouth (xerostomia) and dry eyes (keratoconjunctivitis sicca) resulting from a chronic lymphocytic and plasma cell infiltration of the salivary and lacrimal glands. It may be a primary process or found in association with such autoimmune diseases as lupus erythematosus, progressive systemic sclerosis, and rheumatoid arthritis.

The majority of patients are females over 50 years of age. Females outnumber males 3 to 1 in reported childhood cases.[216,217] The mean age at diagnosis in the pediatric population is 11 years.[216,217] Symptoms have occurred in patients as young as 30 months of age.[217]

The usual complaints are excessive water ingestion, lack of saliva, decreased tearing, or irritated eyes. Occasionally recurrent parotid swelling is a feature. The symptoms usually occur simultaneously or within a year of each other. However, there are reports of either dry mouth or dry eyes occurring alone or in the presence of other autoimmune phenomena.

Physical examination reveals a relatively dry oral mucosa with minimal saliva production, conjunctival injection and decreased tearing, and perhaps, parotid enlargement.

In addition to the physical findings of xerostomia and xerophthalmia, patients with Sjögren syndrome may demonstrate features of extraglandular manifestations such as arthritis and cutaneous vasculitis. Cutaneous vasculitis manifesting as palpable purpura of the lower extremities and urticarial vasculitis are found in 25% of adult primary Sjögren syndrome patients. Whether or not such a strong relationship exists between primary Sjögren syndrome and cutaneous vasculitis in childhood is unknown at present. In a large study including children a subset of patients with adverse predictors for mortality of purpura, decreased C4 complement levels and mixed cryoglobulinemia at intial presentation emerged.[218] Without these adverse prognostic factors the overall prognosis was the same as the general population.

LABORATORY FINDINGS

Minor salivary gland biopsy from the lip demonstrates a lymphocytic and plasma cell infiltrate. Eye findings can be evaluated by tear break-up time, the Schirmer's test, and Rose Bengal dye staining of the cornea and conjunctiva.[217]

Chudwin et al. reported a positive ANA in six of eight children with Sjögren syndrome,[217] whereas Bernstein et al. noted a negative ANA in all four of their patients with Sjögren syndrome.[216] Rheumatoid factor (RF) is found in approximately 90% of adult Sjögren syndrome patients.[219] Chudwin et al.[217] found a significant RF titer in five of eight Sjögren syndrome patients, whereas Bernstein et al.[216] failed to demonstrate RF activity in their four Sjögren syndrome patients. The ESR may be elevated. Hypergammaglobulinemia, leukopenia, thrombocytopenia, and anemia have been found in patients with Sjögren syndrome.

Serum should be examined for the presence of Ro(Sjögren syndrome-A or SSA) antibody, which is found in approximately 45% of adult Sjögren syndrome patients.[220] La antibody, which is identical to SS-B (Sjögren syndrome-B) antibody, should also be sought. The La(SS-B) antibody is found in a variable number of Sjögren syndrome patients. Approximately 50 to 60% of those Sjögren syndrome patients with Ro antibody[220] also have La(SS-B) antibodies. These Ro-positive Sjögren syndrome patients appear to be at risk of developing more extraglandular features than Ro-negative Sjögren syndrome patients. Three of four children with Sjögren syndrome followed at Johns Hopkins Hospital Rheumatology Clinic demonstrated anti-Ro(SSA) antibody.

Recent analysis of sera of patients with primary Sjögren syndrome including adolescents revealed 12.6% with anti CD4 antibodies.[221] The significance of this finding is unknown at present and did not correlate with CD4 and T lymphocyte depletion but the authors suggest that as in HIV these anti-CD4 antibodies lend support to a possible viral role in Sjögren's syndrome.[221]

Magnetic resonance imaging of enlarged parotid glands has been reported as characteristic in patients with the sicca syndrome and hyperlipidemia.[222] This technology could come to be used in children.

DIFFERENTIAL DIAGNOSIS

Sjögren syndrome has been reported in children with hypergammaglobulinemia, autoimmune hematologic abnormalities, juvenile rheumatoid arthritis (JRA), scleroderma, MCTD, lupus erythematosus, and dermatomyositis.[216,217] Sjögren syndrome needs to be distinguished from idiopathic xerostomia and salivary gland disorders, which also produce dry mouth (i.e., vitamin C deficiency and drug therapy). The sicca syndrome must be differentiated from eyelid, lacrimal gland, or duct abnormalities that cause keratoconjunctivitis sicca symptoms.

A recent study of twenty-three children recommends that Sjögren syndrome be assumed or confirmed when oral and ocular symptoms are present with recurrent salivary gland enlargement even in the absence of diagnostic criteria which are less reliable.[223]

TREATMENT

Treatment for Sjögren syndrome is presently symptomatic. Numerous water rinses alleviate xerostomia and the use of sour, sugarless hard candies induces saliva formation.[217] The frequent application of artificial tears will prevent ulcerations and scarring seen in keratoconjunctivitis sicca. A persistent conjunctivitis should suggest secondary infection in these individuals and requires a culture with subsequent use of topical or systemic antibiotics. Dental cavities are frequent and are caused by the decrease in salivation. This as well as early tooth decay was recently confirmed in a large study of Sjögren syndrome in

215. Hurwitz S (ed.) (1981) Clinical Pediatric Dermatology. Philadelphia: WB Saunders.
216. Berstein B, Koster-King K, Singsen B et al. (1977) Sjögren's syndrome in childhood. **Arthritis Rheum**, 20 suppl.:361.
217. Chudwin DS, Daniels TE, Wara DW et al. (1981) Spectrum of Sjögren's syndrome in children. **J Pediatr** 98:213.
218. Skopouli FN, Dafni U, Ioannidis JP, Moutsopoulos HM (2000) Clinical evolution and morbidity and mortality of primary Sjögren's syndrome. **Semin Arthritis Rheum** 29(5) 296.
219. Bloch KJ, Buchanan WW, Wohl MJ et al. (1965) Sjögren's syndrome. A clinical, pathological and serological study of sixty-two cases. **Medicine** 44:187.
220. Alexander EL, Arnett FC, Provost TT et al. (1983) Sjögren's syndrome: association of anti-Ro(SSA) antibodies with vasculitis, hematologic abnormalities and serologic hyperreactivity. **Ann Intern Med** 98:155.
221. Henriksson G, Manthorpe R, Bredberg A (2000) Antibodies to CD4 in primary Sjögren's syndrome. **Rheum** 39:142.
222. Izumi M, Hida A, Takagi Y et al. (2000) MR imaging of the salivary glands in sicca syndrome: comparison of lipid profiles and imaging in patients with hyperlipidemia and patients with Sjögren's syndrome. **Am J Roentgenol** 175(3):829.
223. Stiller M, Golder W, Doring E (2000) Primary and secondary Sjögren's syndrome in children-a comparative study. **Clin Oral Investig** 4(3):176.

childhood.[223] Dental health must be monitored regularly. Topical fluoride treatments may help to prevent cavities. Systemic steroids should be considered to treat extraglandular manifestations of Sjögren syndrome, such as vasculitis, arthritis, or associated autoimmune diseases.

JUVENILE IDIOPATHIC ARTHRITIS (JIA)

Juvenile arthritis is one of the most frequent chronic illnesses of children. The majority of children with JIA have syndromes that are unique to childhood. Even in those types of JIA which have an adult equivalent, such as ankylosing spondylitis and psoriatic arthritis, children often have a different pattern of onset and course than adults. There have been two major sets of criteria for the diagnosis and classification for juvenile arthritis. The diagnostic criteria for juvenile chronic arthritis (JCA) were defined by the European League Against Rheumatism (EULAR).[224] In North America, the most frequently used criteria have been those of the American College of Rheumatology (ACR) for juvenile rheumatoid arthritis (JRA).[225] These criteria, although similar, do not identify identical populations or spectra of disease, but have often been used interchangeably. This has led to confusion in interpretation of studies of the epidemiology, treatment and outcome of juvenile arthritis. Recently, the International League of Associations of Rheumatologists (ILAR) has proposed,[226] and revised[227] criteria for the diagnosis and classification of juvenile arthritis as the "Durban Criteria" (Table 23.4). The

term juvenile idiopathic arthritis (JIA) has been proposed to replace both JRA and JCA and will encompass all juvenile arthritides lasting longer than 6 weeks that are of unknown cause. This international compromise will allow uniform interpretation of clinical and therapeutic data. Recent studies have validated the ILAR criteria.[228,229] Despite our best attempts to categorize children with idiopathic arthritis, there will inevitably be children who do not fit into any known category. This group of children with JIA will be considered to have undifferentiated or overlap arthritis. This category of other arthritis is defined as children with arthritis of unknown cause that persists for at least 6 weeks but that either does not fulfill criteria for any other category or fulfills criteria for more than one of the other categories. The majority of children categorized as "other" have been shown to have a family history of psoriasis, which excludes them from all categories other than psoriatic arthritis, but they do not yet meet criteria for the diagnosis of psoriatic arthritis.[228,229] In the remainder of this chapter, the term juvenile arthritis will be used to denote any type of arthritis in childhood, JIA will be used as defined above, and the terms JRA and JCA will be used only when referring to specific epidemiologic, therapeutic or outcome data.

EPIDEMIOLOGY

Juvenile arthritis is the most common rheumatic disease of childhood. The worldwide incidence ranges from 7 to 20 cases per 100 000 children at risk

---

TABLE 23.4   Criteria for classification of juvenile idiopathic arthritis

Age of onset: less than 16 years	Arthritis in 1 or more joints for greater than 6 weeks
Systemic arthritis Arthritis with or preceded by daily fever of at least 2 weeks in duration, accompanied by one or more of the following: 1. Evanescent, nonfixed erythematous rash 2. Generalized lymph node enlargement 3. Hepatomegaly or splenomegaly 4. Serositis	*Oligoarthritis* 1. Persistent oligoarthritis: no more than 4 joints involved 2. Extended oligoarthritis: affects a cumulative total of 5 or more joints *after* the first 6 months of disease
Polyarthritis (RF negative) Arthritis affecting 5 or more joints during the first 6 months of disease. Tests for RF are negative	*Polyarthritis (RF positive)* Arthritis affecting 5 or more joints during the first 6 months of disease, associated with positive RF tests on 2 occasions at least 3 months apart.
Psoriatic arthritis 1. Arthritis and psoriasis, or 2. Arthritis and at least 2 of: 　(a) dactylitis 　(b) nail abnormalities (pitting or onycholysis) 　(c) family history of psoriasis confirmed by a dermatologist in at least one first degree relative	*Enthesitis-related arthritis* Arthritis and enthesitis, or arthritis or enthesitis with at least 2 of: 1. Sacroiliac joint tenderness and/or inflammatory spinal pain 2. Presence of HLA-B27 3. Family history of HLA-B27 associated disease in at least one first or second degree relative 4. Anterior uveitis that is usually associated with pain, redness, or photophobia 5. Onset of arthritis in a boy after the age of 8 years of age
Other arthritis Children with arthritis of unknown cause that persists for at least 6 weeks but that either 1. does not fulfill criteria for any of the other categories, or 2. fulfills criteria for more than one of the other categories	

RF, rheumatoid factor.

224. Nomenclature and classification of arthritis in children. European League Against Rheumatism (EULAR), Bulletin 4. Basel, National Zeitung AG, 1997.

225. Cassidy JT, Levinson JE, Bass JC et al. (1986) A study of classification criteria for a diagnosis of juvenile rheumatoid arthritis. **Arthritis Rheum** 29:274–281.

226. Fink CW (1995) Proposal for the development of classification criteria for idiopathic arthritides of childhood [published erratum appears in J Rheumatol 1995 22(11):2195]. **J Rheumatol** 22(8):1566–1569.

227. Petty RE, Southwood TR, Baum J et al. (1998) Revision of the proposed classification criteria for juvenile idiopathic arthritis: Durban, 1997. **J Rheumatol** 25(10):1991–1994.

228. Ramsey SE, Bolaria RK, Cabral DA et al. (2000) Comparison of criteria for the classification of childhood arthritis. **J Rheumatol** 27(5):1283–1286.

229. Foeldvari I, Bidde M (2000) Validation of the proposed ILAR classification criteria for juvenile idiopathic arthritis. International League of Associations for Rheumatology. **Rheumatol** 27(4):1069–1072.

per year.[230–233] Recent studies have suggested that the incidence of JRA may be decreasing.[233] Alternatively, the improved recognition of Lyme disease and the exclusion of psoriatic arthritis and juvenile spondyloarthropathies may be a contributing factor.

The overall prevalence of JRA in the United States has been estimated to be between 57 and 113 per 100 000 children younger than 16 years old.[234] The prevalence of juvenile ankylosing spondylitis is reported to be 2–10 per 100 000, while juvenile psoriatic arthritis has a prevalence of 2–12 per 100 000.[235]

In a study of the relative prevalence of each of the individual subtypes of juvenile arthritis, utilizing the ACR criteria, 11% had systemic onset, 24% polyarticular (RF−), 1% polyarticular (RF+), 38% pauciarticular, 24% spondyloarthritis (11% JAS) and 3% psoriatic arthritis.[236] Each subtype of juvenile arthritis has individual characteristics and each type can have widely different courses and outcomes, which further emphasizes the heterogeneity of JIA.

ETIOLOGY AND PATHOGENESIS

There are many reported associations between HLA types and juvenile arthritis. Other than HLA-B27, the majority of the associations of JIA have been with the HLA class II antigens, which are restricted to cells of lymphoid origin.[237] In oligoarticular arthritis, there is an increased association with HLA-DR8, HLA-DR6 and HLA-DR5, with relative risks of 2 to 27. The presence of uveitis is correlated with HLA-DR5, while protection from uveitis is correlated with HLA-DR1.[238] Chronic uveitis has also been associated with HLA-DRB1 and HLA-DQA1.[239] Polyarticular onset with positive rheumatoid factor is associated with HLA-DR4, which parallels the association with adult rheumatoid arthritis, while HLA-DR7 seems protective. Rheumatoid factor negative polyarticular disease is associated with HLA-DR8, HLA-DPw3, and HLA-DQw4 with relative risk factors of 3 to 10. Systemic onset disease has overlapping risk factors, showing an association with HLA-DR4, HLA-DR5 and HLA-DR8 with relative risks of ranging from around 2 to 7.[237]

Juvenile ankylosing spondylitis (JAS) and related diseases show a striking familial occurrence. The only immunogenic factor in common in this class of diseases has been shown to be HLA-B27. Data from multiple immunogenetic studies have shown that 90% of patients with JAS express the HLA-B27 antigen.[240,241] These data are supported by an animal model where spontaneous inflammatory disease of the gastrointestinal tract, peripheral and vertebral joints, male genital tract, skin, nails and heart were seen in transgenic rats expressing a functional human HLA-B27 allele.[242]

Imbalances in levels of proinflammatory and anti-inflammatory cytokines may be associated with chronic inflammation. A polymorphism in the interleukin (II)-1α gene was found to be associated with uveitis and pauciarticular arthritis in Norwegians.[243] Children who have an IL-6 genotype that has a relatively higher transcription rate when stimulated may be at greater risk for systemic arthritis.[244]

LABORATORY FINDINGS

The ANA titer is a measure of serum antibodies that can bind to one of many potential antigens present in the nucleus of normal human cells. ANA titers are usually considered to be elevated when they can be identified at a dilution of 1:40 or with an absolute value of 7.5 IU/ml. The presence of an elevated ANA should never be used to diagnose arthritis. However, the ANA does have some utility as a screening test for JIA.[245,246] The frequency of ANA positivity is greatest in younger girls with oligoarticular disease and represents an increased risk for anterior uveitis.[247] It is known that elevated ANA titers can be present in up to 20% of normal children (typically at titers of 1:40 to 1:80), can be induced by recent illness, or be present in first- or second-degree relatives of patients with SLE.[248,249] Children who have an elevated ANA to any level, with no evidence of systemic inflammation, and no arthritis on examination by a pediatric rheumatologist are extremely unlikely to subsequently develop a significant autoimmune disease.[248,250]

The rheumatoid factor (RF) is an autoreactive antibody, usually IgM, recognizing IgG that has bound to antigen. RF positivity is infrequent in children with arthritis and rarely occurs in children younger than 7 years of age. When present in children with arthritis, the RF signifies a chronic inflammatory state and has been associated with a higher frequency of erosive synovitis and poor prognosis.[251,252] Studies in children and adults demonstrated that a positive RF is as likely to be present in children with diseases other than JIA as it is in those with JIA.[253,254] Thus, there is no role for RF testing in the office evaluation of children with possible arthritis.

230. Symmons DP, Jones M, Osborne J et al. (1996) Pediatric rheumatology in the United Kingdom: data from the British Pediatric Rheumatology Group National Diagnostic Register. **J Rheumatol** 23(11):1975–1980.
231. Towner SR, Michet CJJ, O'Fallen WM, Nelson AM (1983) The epidemiology of juvenile arthritis in Rochester, Minnesota. **Arthritis Rheum** 26:1208–1213.
232. Kunnamo I, Kallio P, Pelkonen P (1986) Incidence of arthritis in urban Finnish children: A prospective study. **Arthritis Rheum** 29:2132–1238.
233. Peterson LS, Mason T, Nelson AMO et al. (1996) Juvenile rheumatoid arthritis in Rochester, Minnesota 1960–1993. Is the epidemiology changing? **Arthritis Rheum** 39(8):1385–1390.
234. Singsen BH (1990) Rheumatic diseases of childhood. **Rheum Dis Clin North Am** 16:581–599.
235. Cabral DA, Malleson PN, Petty RE (1995) Spondyloarthropathies of childhood. **Ped Clin North Am** 42(5):1051–1070.
236. Bowyer S, Roettcher P (1996) Pediatric rheumatology clinic populations in the United States: results of a 3 year survey. Pediatric Rheumatology Database Research Group. **J Rheumatol** 23(11):1968–1974.
237. De Inocencio J, Giannini EH, Glass DN (1993) Can genetic markers contribute to the classification of juvenile rheumatoid arthritis? **J Rheumatol** 40(Suppl):12–18.
238. Malagon C, Van Kerckhove C, Giannini EH (1992) The iridocyclitis of early onset pauciarticular juvenile rheumatoid arthritis: outcome in immunogenetically characterized patients. **J Rheumatol** 19:160–166.
239. Ploski R, Vinje O, Ronningen KS et al. (1993) HLA class II alleles and heterogeneity of juvenile rheumatoid arthritis. **Arthritis Rheum** 36(4):465–472.
240. Rubin LA, Amos CI, Wade JA et al. (1994) Investigating the genetic basis for ankylosing spondylitis. Linkage studies with the major histocompatibility complex region. **Arthritis Rheum** 37(8):1212–1220.
241. Burgos-Vargas R, Pacheco-Tena C, Vazquez-Mellado J (1997) Juvenile-onset spondyloarthropathies. **Rheum Dis Clin North Am** 23(3):569–598.

242. Hammer RE, Maika SD, Richardson JA et al. (1990) Spontaneous inflammatory disease in transgenic rats expressing HLA-B27 and human β₂m: an animal model of HLA-B27-associated human disorders. **Cell** 63:1099–1112.
243. McDowell TL, Symons JA, Ploski R et al. (1995) A genetic association between juvenile rheumatoid arthritis and a novel interleukin-1 alpha polymorphism. **Arthritis Rheum** 38(2):221–228.
244. Martin K, Woo P (1999) Juvenile idiopathic arthritides. In: Adolescent Rheumatology, Isenberg DA, Miller JJ, eds. London: Martin Dunitz Ltd, p. 78.
245. Haynes DC, Gershwin ME, Robbins DL (1986) Autoantibody profiles in juvenile arthritis. **J Rheumatol** 13:358–362.
246. Petty RE, Cassidy JT, Sullivan DB (1977) Serologic studies in juvenile rheumatoid arthritis. A review. **Arthritis Rheum** 20(Suppl):260–269.
247. Rosenberg AM (1987) Uveitis associated with juvenile rheumatoid arthritis. **Semin Arthritis Rheum** 16:158–162.
248. Cabral DA, Petty RE, Fung M, Malleson PN (1992) Persistent antinuclear antibodies in children without identifiable inflammatory, rheumatic or autoimmune disease. **Pediatrics** 89:441–448.
249. Allen RC, Dewez P, Stuart L (1991) Antinuclear antibodies using HEp-2 cells in normal children and in children with common infections. **J Paediatr Child Health** 27:39–44.
250. Deane PMG, Liard G, Siegel DM, Baum J (1995) The outcome of children referred to a pediatric rheumatology clinic with a positive antinuclear antibody test but without an autoimmune disease. **Pediatrics** 95:892–895.
251. Stillman JS, Barry PE (1977) Juvenile rheumatoid arthritis: Series 2. **Arthritis Rheum** 20(Suppl):171–175.
252. Schaller JG (1977) Juvenile rheumatoid arthritis: Series 1. **Arthritis Rheum** 20(Suppl):165–170.
253. Eichenfield AH, Athreya BH, Boughty RA (1986) Utility of rheumatoid factor in the diagnosis of juvenile rheumatoid arthritis. **Pediatrics** 78:480–487.
254. Shmerling RH, Delbanco TL (1992) How useful is the rheumatoid factor? **Arch Intern Med** 152:2417–2420.

CLINICAL SYNDROMES OF JIA

Systemic arthritis

Systemic onset juvenile arthritis[255] was first completely described by Still in 1897 and systemic arthritis has often been called Still's disease. His classic article was reprinted in 1978.[256] Systemic arthritis is characterized by the presence of daily or twice daily spiking fevers usually to 39°C or higher.[257] Children with systemic arthritis are frequently quite ill-appearing while febrile. The fever often responds poorly to nonsteroidal anti-inflammatory drugs, but will typically respond well to corticosteroids. In most children the fever is accompanied by a characteristic rash (Fig. 23.10).[258] The rash consists of discrete, erythematous macules, which are blanching, transient, and frequently nonpruritic. The rash is often more pronounced on the trunk, but is often present on the extremities and may occur on the face. Many children with systemic arthritis will have extra-articular manifestations including hepatosplenomegaly, pericarditis, pleuritis, lymphadenopathy and abdominal pain. The extra-articular features may be present for weeks, months and occasionally years prior to the onset of arthritis. Systemic arthritis can occur at any age but is slightly more common before the age of 6[230] and can occur rarely in adulthood, where it is referred to as adult-onset Still's disease. There is an equal ratio of males to females, which may support the premise that there is an infectious trigger for systemic arthritis.[259]

The laboratory features of systemic arthritis are notable for elevated acute phase reactants. The ESR and CRP are greatly elevated. The disease is often accompanied by anemia of chronic disease,[260–262] a leukocytosis, and a marked thrombocytosis, which may exceed 1 000 000/mm[3]. Elevation of serum ferritin has been correlated with active inflammation in some children with

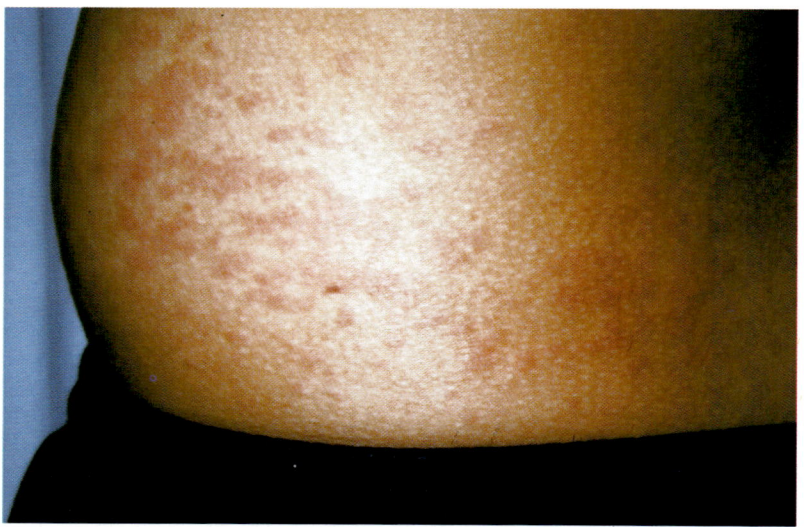

Fig. 23.10 Exanthem of systemic arthritis.

systemic arthritis.[263] Patients with systemic arthritis can have coagulation abnormalities with generation of fibrin split products, which have also been correlated with active disease.[264] Children with systemic arthritis are rarely ANA or RF positive.

Clinical course

One striking feature of systemic arthritis is arrest of linear growth during periods of active disease.[265,266] The use of glucocorticoids also may result in growth retardation, as well as Cushing's syndrome, in this same group of patients. The prognosis of systemic arthritis is determined predominantly by the course of arthritis. Nearly 50% of children with systemic arthritis will have an oligoarticular course, which is typically mild, and in the majority of these children the arthritis will ultimately remit. The remaining half of the children with systemic onset will develop a polyarticular arthritis which can remit but progresses in approximately 50% of cases (25% of all systemic onset JIA) to a severe, unrelenting, and destructive course despite all current therapeutic interventions.[267,268] Chronic anterior uveitis is extremely rare in systemic arthritis.

Macrophage activation syndrome (MAS) is a severe, potentially life-threatening complication seen nearly exclusively in systemic arthritis. It is characterized by macrophage activation with hemophagocytosis and is associated with hepatic dysfunction, disseminated intravascular coagulation with a precipitous fall in the ESR secondary to hypofibrinogenemia, and encephalopathy.[269] It has been suggested that anti-inflammatory medications and viral infections can induce this syndrome. High-dose corticosteroids and cyclosporin A have been shown to improve the outcome of MAS.[270,271]

Oligoarthritis

Oligoarthritis is the most common subtype of JIA and is characterized by arthritis in four or fewer joints during the first 6 months of disease. These children rarely have complaints of pain, do not have associated fever, and are not systemically ill. The knee is the most common joint affected, followed by ankles and elbows. The hips are only rarely affected. Small joints of the hands and feet are seldom affected in oligoarthritis. Asymmetric oligoarticular involvement of small joints, with or without large joint arthritis, is most characteristic of psoriatic arthritis. The majority of children with oligoarthritis present before 6 years of age and girls predominate (four to one).

Most children with oligoarthritis will have a mild elevation of the ESR (rarely above 80mm/h), but it can be normal. The CRP is usually normal or mildly elevated. Antinuclear antibodies are found in 40–80% of children with oligoarthritis and are associated with increased risk for anterior uveitis. A RF is generally absent in oligoarthritis. However, when a RF is present in children with chronic oligoarthritis, it has been associated with aggressive and erosive disease.[272]

Clinical course

The majority of children with oligoarthritis have a mild and remitting course. However, in children with long-standing unilateral knee arthritis there

255. Schneider R, Laxer RM (1998) Systemic onset juvenile rheumatoid arthritis. **Baillieres Clin Rheum** 12(2):245–271.
256. Still GF (1978) On a form of chronic joint disease in children. **Am J Dis Child** 132:195–200.
257. Calabro JJ, Marchesano JM (1967) Fever associated with juvenile rheumatoid arthritis. **N Engl J Med** 276:11–18.
258. Calabro JJ, Marchesano JM (1968) Rash associated with juvenile rheumatoid arthritis. **J Pediatr** 72(No. 5):611–619.
259. Lang B, Shore A (1990) A review of current concepts on the pathogenesis of juvenile rheumatoid arthritis. **J Rheumatol** 17(Suppl 21):1–15.
260. Vreugdenhil G, Baltus CAM, Van Eijk HG, Swakk AJG (1990) Anaemia of chronic disease: Diagnostic significance of erythrocyte and serological parameters in iron deficient rheumatoid arthritis. **Hum Nutr Clin Nutr** 40C:57–67.
261. Prouse PJ, Harvey AR, Bonner B (1986) Anaemia in juvenile chronic arthritis: serum inhibition of normal erythropoiesis *in vitro*. **Ann Rheum Dis** 36:127–132.
262. Koerper MA, Stempel DA, Dallman PR (1980) Anemia in patients with juvenile rheumatoid arthritis. **J Pediatr** 92:930–933.
263. Pelkonen P, Swanljung K, Siimes MA (1986) Ferritinemia as an indicator of systemic disease activity in children with systemic juvenile rheumatoid arthritis. **Acta Paediatr Scand** 75:64–69.
264. Bloom BJ, Tucker LB, Miller LC, Schaller JG (1998) Fibrin D-dimer as a marker of disease activity in systemic onset juvenile rheumatoid arthritis. **J Rheumatol** 25(8):1620–1625.
265. Bernstein BH, Stobie D, Singsen BH et al. (1977) Growth retardation in juvenile rheumatoid arthritis (JRA). **Arth Rheum** 20(Suppl):212–216.
266. Woo PM (1994) Growth retardation and osteoporosis in juvenile chronic arthritis. **Clin Exp Rheum** 12(Suppl 10):S87–90.
267. Schneider R, Lang BA, Reilly BJ (1992) Prognostic indicators of joint destruction in systemic-onset juvenile rheumatoid arthritis. **J Pediatr** 120:200–205.
268. Lomater C, Gerloni V, Gattinara M et al. (2000) Systemic onset juvenile idiopathic arthritis: a retrospective study of 80 consecutive patients followed for 10 years. **J Rheumatol** 27(2):491–496.
269. Prieur AM, Stephan JL (1994) Macrophage activation syndrome in children with joint diseases. **Rev Rheum Engl Ed** 61:385–388.
270. Ravelli A, De Benedetti F, Viola S, Martini A (1996) Macrophage activation syndrome in systemic juvenile rheumatoid arthritis successfully treated with cyclosporine. **J Pediatr** 128(2):275–278.
271. Mouy R, Stephan JL, Pillet P et al. (1996) Efficacy of cyclosporine A in the treatment of macrophage activation syndrome in juvenile arthritis: report of five cases. **J Pediatr** 129(5):750–754.
272. Sailer M, Cabral D, Petty RE, Malleson PN (1997) Rheumatoid factor positive, oligoarticular onset juvenile rheumatoid arthritis. **J Rheumatol** 24(3):586–588.

can be overgrowth of the affected limb resulting in a marked leg length discrepancy.[273,274]

Chronic uveitis is the most serious complication seen in oligoarthritis and occurs in 13 to 34% of all patients with juvenile arthritis. Nearly 80% of all cases of anterior uveitis in childhood are associated with JIA.[275] Initially, the eyes of most patients with JIA-associated uveitis appear normal and are asymptomatic. Of those children who will ultimately develop uveitis, it is already present in 6% of patients at onset of arthritis, but develops in a majority of children within 4 to 7 years after diagnosis. Although the overall incidence and severity of uveitis seems to be decreasing,[276,277] even a low-grade chronic uveitis can result in a poor visual outcome.[278]

Polyarthritis

Polyarticular onset JIA is characterized by the insidious, but occasionally acute, onset of a generally symmetric arthritis in five or more joints. It can involve both large and small joints and frequently affects the cervical spine and temporomandibular joints. Typically girls outnumber boys three to one. Mild systemic features can be present in children with polyarthritis. They may have low-grade fevers, lymphadenopathy, and hepatosplenomegaly. The fevers are not typically the high quotidian temperature spikes, which are diagnostic of systemic arthritis, and rash is rarely seen.[225] There are at least two distinct subgroups of polyarthritis: those with and without the presence of RF.

RF-negative polyarthritis can occur at any age, with the median age of onset at 6.5 years.[230] This subgroup can be ANA positive (40–50%) and this is associated with an increased incidence of uveitis (5%).[275]

The second subgroup of children with polyarthritis is those with a positive RF. This subtype occurs predominantly in older girls (>8 years) who are HLA-DR4 positive, and is indistinguishable from adult rheumatoid arthritis. These children are more likely to have a symmetric small joint arthritis, rheumatoid nodules, and early erosive synovitis with a chronic course. However, these children rarely develop chronic uveitis.

Most patients with active polyarthritis will have an elevated ESR, typically 20–80 mm/h. The ESR is often a useful measure of disease activity in children with polyarthritis.[246,279] Children with significant joint disease will often develop anemia of chronic disease with hemoglobin in the range of 7 to 10 g/dl, although this is more marked in systemic arthritis.[260,261]

Clinical course

Children with RF + polyarthritis are at risk for a prolonged and destructive course. These children are typically older girls with multiple joints involved (20 or greater), including the small joints of the hands and feet, early erosions, and rheumatoid nodules. The presence of hip arthritis has been shown to be a poor prognostic sign and may lead to destruction of the femoral heads.[280] The onset of puberty seems to have no relation to disease activity or remission.[281] Severe polyarticular (polyarticular and systemic JIA) disease with involvement of the temporomandibular joints prior to 5 years of age can result in micrognathia.[282]

Psoriatic arthritis

The diagnosis of juvenile psoriatic arthritis was considered to be rare in children. Prior to 1982 there were fewer than 80 cases described in the English literature, when Shore and Ansell[283] published the first large collection of 60 children with psoriatic arthritis. The rarity of juvenile psoriatic arthritis was unusual due to the relatively large number of children with psoriasis and the fact that 7% of adults with psoriasis have arthritis.[284] Juvenile psoriatic arthritis was historically considered a juvenile spondyloarthropathy. However, recent studies have shown the juvenile psoriatic arthritis is a distinct entity, which has been underdiagnosed, often due to the long period from onset of arthritis to onset of psoriasis.[284,285]

Psoriatic arthritis may account for up to 7% of JIA. There is a slight female predominance (1.6 to 2.3 girls to 1 boy) and often affects young children with a median onset age of 5.9 to 10.1 years. The arthritis is often an asymmetric oligo- or polyarthritis affecting both large and small joints. At onset, the majority have nail pitting (67%), a family history of psoriasis (69%), or dactylitis (39%), and less than half of the children have the rash of psoriasis (13 to 43%).[230,284,285] Current criteria do not require the development of psoriasis to confirm a diagnosis of psoriatic arthritis.[227]

Children with psoriatic arthritis usually do not develop a RF, but a positive ANA can be seen in 50% and is a risk factor for uveitis. HLA-DR1 and HLA-DR6 were statistically significant risk factors for development of juvenile psoriatic arthritis.[285] There is a mild but not statistically significant increase in the presence of HLA-B27 in children with psoriatic arthritis and these children are more likely to have axial arthritis.[283–285] The presentation of children under 5 years of age is often heralded by the involvement of a small number of fingers or toes which are relatively asymptomatic but result in marked overgrowth of the digit(s).

Clinical course

Children with psoriatic arthritis can have a chronic lifelong arthritis that may follow a relapsing and remitting course. Arthritis mutilans and predominant DIP joint disease are unusual in childhood. However, many of the children will have prolonged polyarthritis that may result in irreversible joint damage.[283] Chronic anterior uveitis has been observed in up to 17% of children,[284,285] is associated with a positive ANA titer, and is clinically indistinguishable from the uveitis in oligo- and polyarthritis. The uveitis associated with psoriatic arthritis may be more resistant to treatment than the other forms of chronic uveitis associated with childhood arthritis.[281]

Enthesitis-related arthritis

The criteria for classification of enthesitis-related arthritis (ERA) describes a group of arthritides, which includes undifferentiated spondyloarthritis, ankylosing spondylitis, and inflammatory bowel disease associated arthritis. At the onset, juvenile spondyloarthropathies are often undifferentiated, preventing the application of adult-onset criteria for diagnosis. The addition of criteria for the presence of HLA-B27, a family history of HLA-B27 associated disease, and the onset of arthritis in a boy after the age of 8, will increase the number of children included in this category.[227]

ERA is often associated with enthesitis and arthralgias or arthritis, long before any axial skeletal involvement is identified.[286] Enthesitis is identified when marked tenderness is noted at the 10, 2 and 6 o'clock positions on the patella, at the tibial tuberosity, iliac crest, or the attachments of the Achilles tendon or plantar fascia.[281] In some children, the only manifestation of ERA may be severe enthesopathy of the heel(s).[287]

273. Bunger C, Bulow J, Tondebold E (1986) Microcirculation of the juvenile knee in chronic arthritis. **Clin Orthop** 204:294–299.
274. Vostrejs M, Hollister JR (1988) Muscle atrophy and leg length discrepancies in pauciarticular juvenile rheumatoid arthritis. **Am J Dis Child** 142:343–349.
275. Kansk JJ (1988) Uveitis in juvenile chronic arthritis. **Eye** 2:641–645.
276. Sherry DD, Mellins ED, Wedgewood RJ (1991) Decreasing severity of chronic uveitis in children with pauciarticular arthritis. **Am J Dis Child** 145:1026–1028.
277. Chalom EC, Goldsmith DP, Koehler MA et al. (1997) Prevalence and outcome of uveitis in a regional cohort of patients with juvenile rheumatoid arthritis. **J Rheumatol** 24(10):2031–2034.
278. Nguyen QD, Foster S (1998) Saving the vision of children with juvenile rheumatoid arthritis-associated uveitis. **JAMA** 280(13):1132–1133.
279. Olshaker JS, Jerrard DA (1997) The erythrocyte sedimentation rate. **J Emerg Med** 15(6):869–874.
280. Blane CE, Ragsdale CG, Hensinger RN (1987) Late effects of JRA on the hip. **J Pediatr Orthop** 7:677–701.
281. Cassidy JT, Petty RE (1995) Textbood of Pediatric Rheumatology, 3rd edn. Philidelphia: WB Saunders.
282. Olson L, Echerdal O, Hallonsten AL (1991) Craniomandibular function in juvenile chronic arthritis. A clinical and radiographic study. **Swed Dent J** 15:71–76.
283. Shore A, Ansell BM (1982) Juvenile psoriatic arthritis-an analysis of 60 cases. **J Pediatr** 100(4):529–535.
284. Southwood TR, Petty RE, Malleson PN et al. (1989) Psoriatic arthritis in children. **Arthritis Rheum** 32(8):1007–1013.
285. Roberton DM, Cabral DA, Malleson PN, Petty RE (1996) Juvenile psoriatic arthritis: followup and evaluation of diagnostic criteria. **J Rheumatol** 23(1):166–170.
286. Cabral DA, Oen KG, Petty RE (1992) SEA syndrome revisited: a longterm followup of children with a syndrome of seronegative enthesopathy and arthropathy. **J Rheumatol** 19:1282–1285.
287. Gerster JC, Piccinin P (1984) Enthesopathy of the heels in juvenile onset seronegative B-27 positive spondyloarthropathy. **J Rheumatol** 12:310–314.

Laboratory evaluation of children with ERA is relatively unremarkable. There is often systemic inflammation with thrombocytosis and an elevated ESR. A highly elevated ESR (>100) is more likely to be associated with inflammatory bowel disease in a child who meets the criteria for ERA. The RF is uniformly negative, but ANAs can be present in the same proportion as the childhood population.[248,249,281]

The primary extra-articular manifestation of ERA is acute anterior uveitis (AAU), which can occur in up to 27% of children with ankylosing spondylitis.[288] AAU is highly associated with the presence of HLA-B27 (50%).[289] It typically presents with an acute, painful, red, photophobic eye. Although AAU may resolve with no ocular residua, some children will have a persistent uveitis that is relatively resistant to therapy and can result in blindness.[290,291]

Juvenile ankylosing spondylitis

Children with juvenile ankylosing spondylitis (JAS) have often been diagnosed based on adult criteria that require radiographic evidence of sacroiliitis. JAS most often presents in late childhood or adolescence. Children with JAS and sacroiliac involvement are often HLA-B27 positive (82–95%) and the male-to-female ratio is 6:1.[235] Most children ultimately diagnosed with JAS will initially have an episodic arthritis of large joints of the lower extremities and the tarsal bones. Regardless of axial disease, the most reliable predictors to differentiate JAS from oligo- or polyarticular JIA are the presence of enthesitis and tarsal disease in children who have arthritis of the lower but not of the upper extremities.[292]

The presentation of JAS is most remarkable for the absence of axial involvement. Only 12.8 to 24% of children with JAS have pain, stiffness or limitation of motion of the sacroiliac or lumbosacral spine at onset. A peripheral arthropathy or enthesopathy affecting predominantly the lower limb joints and entheses is seen in 79 to 89.4%. These children tend to have fewer than five joints involved and rarely more than 10. At presentation, the joint involvement is usually asymmetric or even unilateral.[293]

Clinical course

The initial course of JAS is characterized by remitting and relapsing symptoms, which are frequently mild. This can not be differentiated from the child who seems to have recurrent bouts of reactive arthritis. However, the pattern of joint disease often progresses to become polyarticular and axial disease is usually evident after the third year of illness.[293] Children with long-standing JAS have been shown to develop tarsal bone coalition, which has been termed ankylosing tarsitis.[294]

Outcome data for JAS are incomplete and at times contradictory. The prognosis of JAS has been reported as both worse and better than adult-onset ankylosing spondylitis.[295,296] Peripheral joint arthritis tends to be more common than that seen in adults.[281] Hip disease has been associated with a poor functional outcome,[295,297] and may require total hip arthroplasty.

Inflammatory bowel disease-associated arthritis

The prevalence of arthritis in children with inflammatory bowel disease (IBD) has been reported to be 7 to 21%, and usually occurs after the diagnosis of the bowel disease.[298–300] There are two different patterns of arthritis seen.[281] The most common type is an oligo- or polyarticular arthritis of the lower limbs. This group is less likely to meet the criteria for ERA. This arthritis is often episodic with exacerbation's lasting 4 to 6 weeks and rarely for months. The activity of the peripheral arthritis often reflects the underlying activity of the IBD. The less common type of IBD-associated arthritis is a HLA-B27 associated oligoarticular arthritis of the lower limbs, with sacroiliitis and enthesitis, and no relationship to bowel inflammation.[281] This form is more likely to persist and progress despite control of the bowel disease and seems identical to other ERA.

TREATMENT OF JIA

The fundamental purpose of pharmacologic therapy is to achieve pain control, decrease inflammation, promote and then maintain remission. The medications used are individualized for each patient, depending on their subtype of arthritis, degree of inflammation, and previous response to medications.

Nonsteroidal anti-inflammatory drugs (NSAIDs)

The mechanism of action of NSAIDs is by inhibition of the biosynthesis of prostaglandins by direct action on the enzyme cyclo-oxygenase (COX).[301] The discovery of a second COX enzyme (COX-2), which is induced in the proinflammatory cascade, and the differential inhibition of the two COX isoforms (COX-1 and COX-2) by individual NSAIDs, has provided the basis for the development of safer NSAIDs.[302] At this time, no COX-2-specific NSAID is approved for use in children. However, this exciting scientific advance will likely change NSAID use in children in the near future.

NSAIDs are the initial therapeutic intervention in most children with JIA. NSAIDs provide both analgesia and an anti-inflammatory effect. The average time course for response to NSAIDs is 4 to 12 weeks.[303] Thus, a NSAID is usually given for 4 to 8 weeks before substituting another if there has not been sufficient improvement. NSAIDs are generally safe and well tolerated in most children. Abdominal pain, nausea and vomiting are common side effects, but gastrointestinal hemorrhage is rare.[304] However, gastroduodenal injury is more frequent in children receiving high doses or more than one NSAID.[305] The use of aspirin for JIA is no longer recommended, due to the risk of Reye syndrome, increased hepatotoxicity, bleeding, and 4 times per day dosing.

In the United States, the most commonly used NSAID for JIA is naproxen (10–20mg/kg/day divided bid). In children with fevers and serositis associated with systemic arthritis and with JAS, indomethacin is often the most effective NSAID.[281]

288. Ansell BM (1980) Ankylosing spondylitis. In: Juvenile Spondylitis and Related Disorders, Moll JMH, ed. Edinburgh: Churchill Livingstone, pp. 120–125.
289. Derhaag PJFM, Feltkamp TEW (1990) Acute anterior uveitis and HLA-B27. **Int Opthalmol** 14:19–23.
290. Rosenbaum JT (1992) Acute anterior uveitis and spondyloarthropathies. **Rheum Dis Clin North Am** 18:143–151.
291. Power WJ, Rodriguez A, Pedroza-Seres M, Foster CS (1998) Outcomes in anterior uveitis associated with the HLA-B27 haplotype. **Ophthalmology** 105(9):1646–1651.
292. Burgos-Vargas R, Vazquez-Mellado J (1995) The early clinical recognition of juvenile-onset ankylosing spondylitis and its differentiation from juvenile rheumatoid arthritis. **Arthritis Rheum** 38(6):835–844.
293. Burgos-Vargas R, Petty RE (1992) Juvenile ankylosing spondylitis. **Rheum Dis Clin North Am** 18:123–142.
294. Burgos-Vargas R (1993) Spondyloarthropathies and psoriatic arthritis in children. **Curr Opin Rheumatol** 5(5):634–643.
295. Garcia-Morteo O, Maldonado-Cocco JA, Suarez-Almazor ME, Garay E (1983) Ankylosing spondylitis of juvenile onset: comparison with adult onset disease. **Scand J Rheumatol** 12:246–248.
296. Calin A, Elswood J (1988) The natural history of juvenile-onset ankylosing spondylitis: a 24-year retrospective case–control study. **Br J Rheumatol** 27:91–93.
297. Marks SH, Barnett M, Calin A (1982) A case–control study of juvenile- and adult-onset ankylosing spondylitis. **J Rheumatol** 9:739–747.
298. Farmer RG, Michener WM (1979) Prognosis of Crohn's disease with onset in childhood and adolescence. **Dig Dis Sci** 24:752–757.
299. Lindsley C, Schaller J (1974) Arthritis associated with inflammatory bowel disease in children. **J Pediatr** 84:16–20.
300. Hamilton JR, Bruce MD, Abdourhamam M (1979) Inflammatory bowel disease in children and adolescents. **Adv Pediatr** 26:311–322.
301. Vane JR (1971) Inhibition of prostaglandin synthesis as a mechanism of action for aspirin-like drugs. **Nat New Biol** 231:232–235.
302. Vane J (1994) Towards a better aspirin. **Nature** 367:215–216.
303. Lovell D, Giannini E, Brewer E (1984) Time course of response to nonsteroidal anti-inflammatory drugs in patients with juvenile rheumatoid arthritis. **Arthritis Rheum** 27:1433–1437.
304. Lindsley C (1993) Uses of nonsteroidal anti-inflammatory drugs in pediatrics. **Am J Dis Child** 147:229–236.
305. Mulberg AE, Linz C, Bern E et al. (1993) Identification of nonsteroidal antiinflammatory drug-induced gastroduodenal injury in children with juvenile rheumatoid arthritis. **J Pediatr** 122:647–649.

Nearly two-thirds of children with juvenile arthritis are inadequately treated with NSAIDs alone.[306] These children require additional pharmacologic interventions.

Corticosteroids

Intra-articular corticosteroid injections had been shown to be safe and effective in controlling the synovitis in JIA.[307,308] Triamcinolone hexacetonide (1mg/kg for large joints and 0.5mg/kg medium joints) is the most commonly used agent and often provides long-term control of inflammation. The most frequent adverse consequence of intra-articular corticosteroids is development of subcutaneous atrophy at the site of injection. Systemic corticosteroids can be used for rapid control of severe arthritis. However, long-term use should be restricted to those children with severe arthritis or systemic features that do not respond to other interventions.

Methotrexate

Methotrexate is the most commonly used second-line agent for treatment of juvenile arthritis. It is typically given at 0.5–1mg/kg (with a maximum of 20–30mg) once weekly by mouth or subcutaneous injection. It has been shown to be superior to placebo in polyarticular and extended oligoarticular, but not systemic arthritis[309,310] and can produce radiologic improvement of erosions.[311] Methotrexate has been shown to decrease the severity of uveitis in children with JIA who were dependent on topical corticosteroids.[312]

The major side effects with methotrexate use are nausea, diarrhea and oral ulcers. Supplementation with folic acid (1mg/day) can usually prevent gastrointestinal complications. One of the most significant long-term side effects of methotrexate use is the development of liver fibrosis and cirrhosis.[313–315] Serial abnormalities of hepatic enzymes were significantly associated with liver fibrosis in children taking methotrexate for juvenile arthritis,[316] suggesting that the current guidelines for patients with rheumatoid arthritis are applicable to patients with JIA.[317]

Sulfasalazine

Sulfasalazine has been used extensively in Europe, and increasingly in North America, for treatment of both spondyloarthropathies and JRA/JCA.[318,319] It is typically given in the enteric-coated form at a dose of 50mg/kg/day in two divided doses. Recently, a randomized, double-blind, placebo-controlled trial showed that sulfasalazine is both safe and effective for the treatment of oligo- and polyarticular JCA.[320] Serious side effects have been noted in children with systemic arthritis and the routine use of sulfasalazine is not recommended for this subgroup.[321,322]

Biologic agents

A new category of therapeutic agents, biologic response modifiers, are now available for the treatment of juvenile arthritis. Two of these agents are etanercept (Enbrel) and infliximab (Remicade), both of which bind tumor necrosis factor-α and decrease the activity of this important proinflammatory cytokine. Etanercept is the only agent approved for the treatment of juvenile arthritis at this time. Etanercept has been shown to be safe and effective in the treatment of juvenile arthritis.[323] A significant response was seen in children who received etanercept at a dose of 0.4mg/kg/dose, up to a maximum dose of 25mg, twice weekly.

NOMID

A *n*eonatal *o*nset *m*ultisystem *i*nflammatory *d*isease (NOMID) with chronic arthropathy has been described.[324–327] The rash seen in NOMID can resemble that of systemic arthritis, but is usually omnipresent, and there is often lymphadenopathy and hepatosplenomegaly.[328] However, the associated findings of distinctive epiphysitis (and even metaphysitis) with a predilection for the lower extremities, frontal bossing, head enlargement, occasional uveitis, and mental retardation set this syndrome apart. These children do poorly, are in constant pain, have diffuse wasting, and usually die in the first decade, although a few have survived into the late teenage years.

FAMILIAL MEDITERRANEAN FEVER

Familial Mediterranean fever (FMF) was first recognized as a separate disease entity by Siegal in 1945.[329] It is a genetic disorder with autosomal-recessive inheritance characterized by episodic febrile attacks of peritonitis, synovitis, pleuritis, and skin lesions. Rarely, episodic fevers occur alone. Those affected are predominantly Sephardic Jews, although Turks, Armenians, Ashkenazi Jews, and Levantine Arabs are also affected. Three male patients are affected for every two females.[330] FMF is truly a childhood rheumatic disorder in that 90% of cases have their onset before 20 years of age.[330]

The most frequent presentations are fever, abdominal pain, and synovitis. Abdominal discomfort may range from slight tenderness to severe pain with abdominal distention, rebound tenderness, and rigidity. Synovial attacks can vary from short typical monoarthritis or oligoarthritis, principally involving the large joints of the lower extremities and lasting up to a week, to a chronic monoarthritis with joint effusion and arthralgia, persisting for several months. Surprisingly, complete anatomic and functional recovery is to be expected. Acute febrile pleuritis with a sterile effusion is another frequent manifestation

306. Giannini EH, Cawkwell GD (1995) Drug treatment in children with juvenile rheumatoid arthritis. Past, present, and future. **Ped Clin North Am** 42(5):1099–1125.
307. Huppertz HI, Tschammler A, Horwitz AE, Schwab KO (1995) Intraarticular corticosteroids for chronic arthritis in children: efficacy and effects on cartilage and growth. **J Pediatr** 127(2):317–321.
308. Padeh S, Passwell JH (1998) Intraarticular corticosteroid injection in the management of children with chronic arthritis. **Arthritis Rheum** 41(7):1210–1214.
309. Giannini EH, Brewer EJ, Kuzmina N et al. (1992) Methotrexate in resistant juvenile rheumatoid arthritis. Results of the USA–USSR double-blind, placebo-controlled trial. **N Engl J Med** 326:1043–1049.
310. Woo P, Wilkes H, Southwood T, Prieur A-M (1997) Low dose methotrexate is effective in extended oligoarticular arthritis but not in systemic arthritis of children. **Arthritis Rheum** 40:S47.
311. Ravelli A, Viola S, Ramenghi B et al. (1998) Radiologic progression in patients with juvenile chronic arthritis treated with methotrexate. **J Pediatr** 133(2):262–265.
312. Weiss AH, Wallace CA, Sherry DD (1998) Methotrexate for resistant chronic uveitis in children with juvenile rheumatoid arthritis. **J Pediatr** 133(2):266–268.
313. Wallace CA, Sherry DD (1995) A practical approach to avoidance of methotrexate toxicity. **J Rheumatol** 22:1009–1011.
314. Hashkes PJ, Balistreri WF, Bove KE et al. (1997) The long-term effect of methotrexate therapy on the liver in patients with juvenile rheumatoid arthritis. **Arthritis Rheum** 40(12):2226–2234.
315. Kugathasan S, Newman AJ, Dahms BB, Boyle JT (1996) Liver biopsy findings in patients with juvenile rheumatoid arthritis receiving long-term, weekly methotrexate therapy. **J Pediatr** 128(1):149–151.
316. Hashkes PJ, Balistreri WF, Bove KE et al. (1999) The relationship of hepatotoxic risk factors and liver histology in methotrexate therapy for juvenile rheumatoid arthritis. **J Pediatr** 131(1):47–52.

317. Kremer JM, Alarcon GS, Lightfoot RW et al. (1994) Methotrexate for rheumatoid arthritis. Suggested guidelines for monitoring liver toxicity. **Arthritis Rheum** 37:316–328.
318. Huang JL, Chen LC (1998) Sulphasalazine in the treatment of children with chronic arthritis. **Clinical Rheumatology** 17(5):359–363.
319. Imundo LF, Jacobs JC (1996) Sulfasalazine therapy for juvenile rheumatoid arthritis. **J Rheum** 23(2):360–366.
320. van Rossum MA, Fiselier TJ, Franssen MJ et al. (1998) Sulfasalazine in the treatment of juvenile chronic arthritis: a randomized, double-blind, placebo-controlled, multicenter study. Dutch Juvenile Chronic Arthritis Study Group. **Arthritis Rheum** 41(5):808–816.
321. Ansell BM, Hall MA, Loftus JK et al. (1991) A multicenter pilot study of sulphasalazine in juvenile chronic arthritis. **Clin Exp Rheumatol** 9:201–203.
322. Hertzberger-ten Cate R, Cats A (1991) Toxicity of sulfasalazine in systemic juvenile chronic arthritis. **Clin Exp Rheumatol** 9:85–88.
323. Lovell DJ, Giannini EH, Reiff A et al. (2000) Etanercept in children with polyarticular juvenile rheumatoid arthritis. Pediatric Rheumatology Collaborative Study Group [see comments]. Comment in: **N Engl J Med** 342(11):810–861. **N Engl J Med** 342(11):763–769.
324. Ansell BM (1975) Familial arthropathy with rash, uveitis and mental retardation. **Proc R Soc Med** 68:584.
325. Prieur AM, Griscelli C (1981) Arthropathy with rash, chronic meningitis, eye lesions and mental retardation. **J Pediatr** 99:79.
326. Kaufman RA, Lovell DJ (1986) Infantile onset multisystem inflammatory disease; radiologic findings. **Radiology** 160:741.
327. Yarom A (1985) Infantile multisystem disease: a specific syndrome? **J Pediatr** 106:390.
328. De Cunto CL, Liberatore DI, San Roman JL et al. (1997) Infantile-onset multisystem inflammatory disease: A differntial diagnosis of systemic juvenile rheumatoid arthritis. **J Pediatr** 130:551.
329. Siegal S (1945) Begin paroxysmal peritonitis. **Ann Intern Med** 22:1.
330. Sohar E, Gofni J, Pras M et al. (1967) Familial Mediterranean fever. **Am J Med** 43:227.

of FMF. Patients display dyspnea, altered respiratory rate, and decreased breath sounds. Peritoneal and pleural attacks usually resolve in 48 hours.

An unusual but well-known sign of FMF is an erysipelas-like, well-demarcated, erythematous plaque that may occur anywhere, but particularly around the ankles. This finding may not be accompanied by fever, but can occasionally be precipitated by local trauma such as marching. Rarely, tender skin nodules, histologically reminiscent of polyarteritis nodosa, are seen.[223]

LABORATORY FINDINGS

Laboratory findings in FMF vary with the organ systems involved. Leukocytosis can occur with peritonitis. Urine sediment and BUN/creatinine abnormalities may occur with the onset of amyloid nephropathy, which develops in approximately 25% of all untreated FMF patients. Increased IgG and IgM levels have been occasionally noted.[330,331] The ESR, serum haptoglobin, and C-reactive protein may all be elevated. RF determinations, however, are consistently negative in FMF.

Radiologic studies are useful in the evaluation of FMF patients. Air fluid levels on abdominal films and pleural effusions on chest X-rays help to distinguish FMF from JRA, with which it is often confused. Joint findings are usually minimal except in protracted disease where mild osteoporosis or reversible lytic changes can occur. No digital spindling such as seen in JRA is noted clinically or radiologically. Other disorders confused with FMF include surgical abdominal emergencies, pleurisy, connective tissue disorders, and fever of unknown origin.

PATHOGENESIS

The FMF gene, *MEFV*, encodes a putative transcription factor.[332,333] Multiple mutations in this gene have been identified in patients with FMF and account for at least 95% of patents who meet clinical criteria for the diagnosis of FMF.

TREATMENT

Several studies have shown that daily colchicine is an effective prophylaxis to decrease the number of acute attacks in FMF.[334,335] The prognosis for this disease is good providing that amyloidosis does not occur. Some investigators believe that amyloidosis is inevitable in all FMF patients but only one-quarter develop significant morbidity secondary to amyloidosis. Death from renal failure due to amyloidosis is a real possibility and has been reported in a 5-year-old child.[330] Hemodialysis may forestall renal death and has been reported to decrease FMF attacks but the mechanism responsible is unknown.[336] Zemer et al.[337] have reported successful prevention of amyloidosis in a population of FMF patients with proteinuria who were compliant with the use of colchicine over nine years but the drug was not useful in those with nephrotic syndrome.

MULTICENTRIC RETICULOHISTIOCYTOSIS

Probably the first well-documented case of this rare disorder was by Weber and Freudenthal in 1937. It is a destructive polyarthritis with accompanying

mucocutaneous nodules, most often seen in middle-aged women. However, it is relevant to pediatric dermatology because it may be seen in childhood[338,339] as well as adolescence.[340,341] The majority of reported cases have been in white individuals although blacks and Asians have also been known to contract this disorder.

Either the arthritis or the nodules may appear first. Both processes initially progress rapidly but then seem to wax and wane until they burn themselves out over a period of years. Unfortunately, approximately 50% of patients have a disfiguring disease with arthritis mutilans or secondary hypertrophic osteoarthropathy. Occasionally systemic involvement (e.g., lymphatic, pulmonary, or cardiac[342]) has been noted.

Patients usually present with DIP joint swelling and arthralgias and develop a skin-colored to erythematous, papulonodular eruption, primarily on the face and hands[340] as well as the mucosa in 50%.[339] Fever, weight loss, and weakness are common. Approximately one-third of the patients also complain of pruritus.

LABORATORY FINDINGS

The skin or synovial biopsy is diagnostic. The biopsy shows well defined, nonencapsulated, histiocytic infiltrates containing characteristic multinucleated giant cells with an eosinophilic cytoplasm, described as "ground glass" in appearance. An admixture of lymphocytes and eosinophils compose the infiltrate. No other laboratory test is specific for this disorder; however, an elevated ESR and anemia may be found in about 50% of patients.

Radiologic findings are significant. Radiographs of the hands generally demonstrate a rapidly progressive, symmetric, erosive process involving subarticular bone extending from the margins centrally, primarily affecting the DIP joints. There is no subchondral sclerosis or periosteal new bone formation. MRI and CT have also been useful in evaluating bony and soft tissue involvement.[343,344]

PATHOGENESIS

The etiology of multicentric reticulohistiocytosis is unclear at present. Presumably, an unknown stimulus causes lipid-laden histiocytic proliferation primarily in the dermis and synovium. Some have speculated on the possibility of a rare infectious initiating factor because of the granulomatous nature of the infiltrate and the finding of positive tuberculin reactivity in approximately 50% of patients.[336] Recent studies focusing on cytokine and immunohistochemical analyses suggest evidence of monocyte/macrophage disease origin and pathogenesis.[345]

DIFFERENTIAL DIAGNOSIS

Multicentric reticulohistiocytosis is rarely confused with any other disorder when the clinical picture is correlated with biopsy and radiographic findings. Clinically it is most often confused with rheumatoid arthritis. However, rheumatoid arthritis usually involves the PIP rather than DIP joints. A complete differential diagnosis can be found in the reviews by Lesher and Allen[342] and Liang and Granston.[346] Multicentric reticulohistiocytosis is considered a marker

331. Schwabe AD, Lehman TJA (1984) C5a inhibitor deficiency-a role in familial Mediterranean fever? **N Engl J Med** 311:325.
332. International FMF Consortium (1997) Ancient missense mutations in a new member of the RoRet gene family are likely to cause familial Mediterranean fever. **Cell** 90:797.
333. The French FMF Consortium (1997) A candidate gene for familial Mediterranean fever. **Nat Genet** 17:25.
334. Zemer D, Revach M, Pras M et al. (1974) A controlled trial of colchicine in preventing attacks of familial Mediterranean fever. **N Engl J Med** 291:934.
335. Dinarello CA, Wolff SM, Goldfinger ES et al. (1974) Colchicine therapy for familial Mediterranean fever. A double-blind trial. **N Engl J Med** 291:934.
336. Ilfeld D, Weil S, Kuperman O (1982) Correction of a suppressor cell deficiency and amelioration of familial Mediterranean fever by hemodialysis. **Arthritis Rheum** 25:38.
337. Zemer D, Pras M, Schar E et al. (1986) Colchicine in the prevention and treatment of the amyloidosis of familial Mediterranean fever. **N Engl J Med** 314:1001.
338. Candell CE, Elenitsas R, Rosenstein ED, Kramer N (1998) A case of multicentric reticulohistiocytosis in a 6 year old child. **J Rheumatol** 25(4):794.

339. Havill, DuffillM, Rademaker M (1999) Multicentric reticulohistiocytosis in a child. **Aus J Dermatol** 40(1):44.
340. Barrow MV, Holubar K (1969) Multicentric reticulohistiocytosis. **Medicine** 48:287.
341. Raphael SA, Crowdery SL, Faerber EN et al. (1989) Multicentric reticulohistiocytosis in a child. **J Pediatr** 114:266.
342. Lesher JL, Allen BS (1984) Multicentric reticulohistiocytosis. **J Am Acad Dermatol** 11:713.
343. Yamada T, Kurohari YN, Kashiwazaki S et al. (1996) MRI of multicentric reticulohistiocytosis. **J Comput Assist Tomogr** 20(5):838.
344. Kamel H, Gibson G, Cassidy M (1996) Case report: The CT demonstration of soft tissue involvement in multicentric reticulohistiocytosis. **Clin Radiol** 51(6):440.
345. Gorman JD, Danning C, Schumacher HR et al. (2000) Multicentric reticulohistiocytosis: Case report with immunohistochemical analysis and literature review. **Arthritis Rheum** 43(4):930.
346. Liang GC, Granston AS (1996) Complete remission of multicentic reticulohistiocytosis with combination of therapy of steroid, cyclophosphamide and low dose pulse methotrexate. Case report, review of literature and proposal for treatment. **Arthritis Rheum** 39(1):171.

for malignancy but this has not been reported in childhood as of yet.[347,348] It has also been noted to coexist with other rheumatologic disorders such as Sjögren syndrome and scleroderma in adults.[349]

TREATMENT

No single treatment regimen, including systemic steroids, has been effective in preventing the appearance of nodules or the erosive arthritis. Reports have suggested that cyclophosphamide may control the arthritis and that topical nitrogen mustard can improve the skin nodules.[341,350] Joint symptoms only improved in a child on methotrexate.[339] Combination therapy with steroid, cyclophosphamide and low-dose pulse methotrexate purportedly induced remission in an older patient.[346] Aspirin has been used for symptomatic relief of pain.[340]

RELAPSING POLYCHONDRITIS

Relapsing polychondritis (RP) has been reported in all ages but occurs most frequently in the fourth decade. Both sexes are affected equally. In an early review of the literature of 159 patients with RP,[351] four cases occurred during the first decade of life and six cases occurred during the second decade of life. There is an interesting report of a pregnant woman with RP who delivered an infant who was similarly affected.[352]

The entity was first reported in 1923 as polychondropathia by Jaksch-Wartenhorst.[353] The signs and symptoms of RP are varied. Auricular chondritis is present in approximately 90% and arthritis occurs in approximately 50–60% of RP patients. Nasal chondritis and ocular inflammation occurs in about 50% each, and respiratory tract involvement also occurs in 30% of patients with RP.[354,355] Some patients with RP have audiovestibular damages accounting for approximately 38% in children.[355]

The arthritis of RP is a mild inflammatory oligo- or polyarthritis. It usually involves the large joints of the upper extremities, hips, and knees, but may also involve small joints as well as the costochondral, sternomandibular, and sternoclavicular joints.

The auricular chondritis typically begins with the sudden onset of redness, swelling, and pain limited to the cartilaginous portion of the external ear (helix, antihelix, tragus, and sometimes the external auditory canal; Fig. 23.11). This may be accompanied by lymphadenopathy, fever, headache, and malaise.[353] The acute auricular chondritis characteristically subsides within 5 to 10 days with or without treatment. A smoldering course has also been rarely described.

Respiratory tract involvement is a relatively unusual presenting or complicating feature of RP.[355] It is important because of its potential lethality. Laryngeal manifestations include hoarseness and, at times, aphonia. In some instances, these findings are accompanied by tenderness over the thyroid cartilage and anterior trachea. Some patients present with an asthma-like picture and/or a severe inspiratory stridor. Many have an associated cough and a minority of patients have hemoptysis. Most of the patients presenting the respiratory tract involvement require tracheostomy. The reason for tracheostomy is usually severe laryngeal, glottic, and subglottic inflammation and edema leading to airway obstruction. Recently, successful treatment of endobronchial obstruction by laser and silicon stent was reported in a child.[356]

Approximately 16% of patients will develop cutaneous lesions. The overwhelming majority of these are nonspecific, inflammatory lesions including

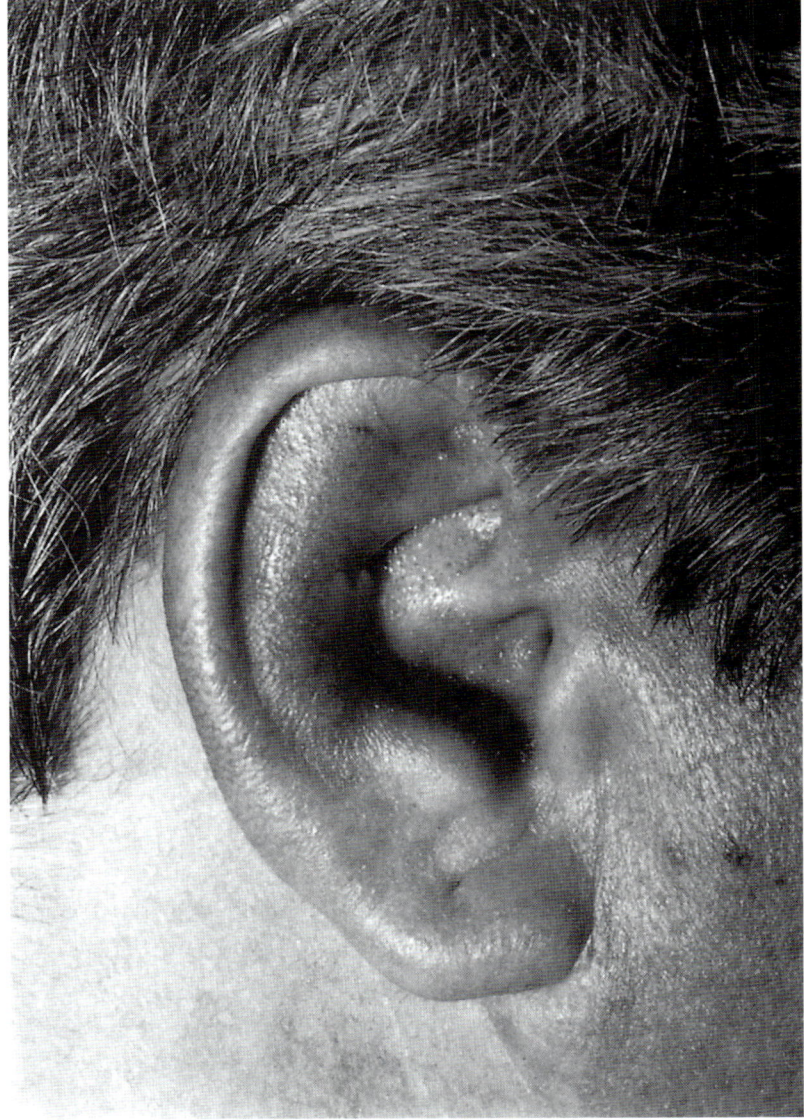

Fig. 23.11   Redness and swelling in auricular chondritis in a child with relapsing polychondritis.

erythematous nodules, and hyperpigmentation over involved joints and alopecia.[357] Mucosal lesions are rarely noted.[357] Some 25 to 35% of RP patients have an associated autoimmune disease.

LABORATORY FINDINGS

The only consistent laboratory findings occurring in RP are an elevated ESR and often a moderate leukocytosis with mild to moderate anemia. The diagnosis of RP is confirmed by biopsy of the involved cartilage. Chrondrolysis characterized by the loss of normal basophilia is noted. The chrondrolysis can be of such intensity that during the active phase of this

347. Valencia IC, Colsky A, Berman B (1998) Multicentric reticulohistiocytosis associated with recurrent breast carcinoma. **J Am Acad Dermatol** 39 (5, part 2):864.
348. Mody GM, Cassim B (1997) Rheumatologic manifestations of malignancy. **Curr Opin Rheumatol** 9(1):75.
349. Morris-Jones R, Walker M, Hardman C (2000) Multicentric reticulohistiocytosis associated with Sjogren's syndrome. **Br J Dermatol** 143(3):649.
350. Chalom E, Rosenstein ED, Kramer N (2000) Cyclosporine as a treatment for multicentric reticulohistiocytosis. **J Rheumatol** 27(2):556.
351. McAdam LP, O'Hanlan MA, Bluestone R et al. (1976) Relapsing polychondritis: prospective study of 23 patients and a review of the literature. **Medicine** 55:193.
352. Arundell FW, Haserick JR (1960) Familial chronic atrophic polychondritis. **Arch Dermatol** 82:439.
353. Ridgway HB, Hansotia PL, Schorr WFL (1979) Relapsing polychondritis. Unusual neurological findings and therapeutic efficacy of dapsone. **Arch Dermatol** 115:43.
354. Zeuner M, Straub RH, Rauh G et al. (1997) Relapsing polychondritis: clinical and immunogenetic analysis of 62 patients. **J Rheumatol** 24(1):966.
355. Knipp S, Bier H, Horneff G et al. (2000) Relapsing polychondritis in childhood – case report and short review. **Rheumatol Int** 19(6):231.
356. Sacco O, Fregonese B, Oddone M et al. (1997) Severe endobronchial obstruction in a girl with relapsing polychondritis: treatment with NdYAG laser and endobronchial silicon stent. **Eur Respir J** 10(2):494.
357. Dolan DL, Lemmon GB Jr, Teitelbaum SL (1966) Relapsing polychondritis. **Am J Med** 41:285.

disease acid mucopolysaccharides are recoverable in urine.[357] In addition to chondrolysis, biopsy reveals pyknotic chondrocytes, destruction of cartilaginous elastic fibers, a normal overlying dermis, and an inflammatory infiltrate of monocytes, macrophages, lymphocytes, and plasma cells.[358] Consideration must be given to the absolute necessity for biopsy as secondary infection of the site may cause death.[359]

Tc-99m MDP bone scintigraphy and Ga-67 citrate scintigraphy have recently been employed to diagnose and identify biopsy sites in an adult with relapsing polychondritis.[360]

PATHOGENESIS

The etiology of RP is unknown. The process appears to be an inflammatory-mediated degeneration of cartilage with subsequent replacement by fibrous tissue. There is evidence indicating that immunologic mechanisms may have a role in the pathogenesis. Foidart et al.[361] have found antibodies to native type II collagen in the sera of 5 of 15 patients with active disease and the antibody level appeared to correlate with disease activity. The remaining 10 patients were in a quiescent disease state, receiving prednisone or immunosuppressive therapy. These authors speculated, based on the fact that an experimentally induced autoimmunity to type II collagen produced arthritis in rats, that the type II collagen autoantibody may be pathogenic. Also, the transplacental passage of such an antibody might explain the occurrence of relapsing polychondritis in an infant of a mother with active disease.

Cellular immunity, however, cannot be excluded from the pathogenesis of this disorder because *in vitro* studies have demonstrated positive responses of patients' lymphocytes to unpurified cartilage or chondrocyte preparations[362] and the production of potentially destructive lymphokine(s).[363]

DIFFERENTIAL DIAGNOSIS

The differential diagnosis of RP primarily includes localized or systemic vasculitis and rheumatoid arthritis. Wegener's granulomatosis and polyarteritis nodosa can produce necrotizing scleritis, keratitis, polyarthritis, mastoiditis, and otitis media with sudden hearing loss, vertigo, and tinnitus. Also, Wegener's granulomatosis can result in granulomatous nasal chondritis with subsequent saddlenose deformity. Unlike relapsing polychondritis, both Wegener's granulomatosis and polyarteritis nodosa produce significant renal, pulmonary, parenchymal and central and peripheral nervous system damage.

Midline lethal granulomatosis, tuberculomas, and gummata can also produce this appearance. Cogan syndrome can also be confused with RP. This syndrome consists of interstitial keratitis, deafness, and vertigo but has no other features of RP. The arthritis of RP can also sometimes be confused with rheumatoid arthritis because rheumatoid arthritis may occasionally be associated with scleritis, keratitis, and rarely aortic insufficiency.

TREATMENT

Treatment of RP generally consists of systemic corticosteroids. The average dose of prednisone in one series was 25mg/day. The range was between 7.5

and 40mg/day. Most doctors believe that steroids produce resolution of an attack of chondritis and decrease the frequency and severity of recurrence. Methotrexate can be useful as a steroid–sparing agent.[364] Diaminodiphenylsulfone (dapsone) has also been shown to be effective in controlling RP.[342,365] Physical therapy for rehabilitation of affected joints is also an essential part of treatment for the patient with RP and NSAIDs have been used in several childhood cases.[355]

PROGNOSIS

The mortality figure for RP is between 22 and 30%. The most common causes of death are related to airway collapse, rupture of an aortic aneurysm, vasculitis, cardiac valvular disease, and pneumonia. It has been reported that relapsing polychondritis is associated with HLA-DR4 and the extent of organ involvement negatively with HLA-DR6.[354] Additionally, some 30% of patients have or develop associated rheumatic diseases such as lupus or rheumatoid arthritis.[354,355]

CRYOPROTEINEMIA

Cold insoluble proteins that precipitate reversibly at low temperatures include cryofibrinogen and cryoglobulin. Cryofibrinogen is produced by chilling plasma and is composed primarily of a complex of fibrinogen, fibrin, and fibrin–split products. Cryoglobulin is found by chilling serum, and is mostly composed of immunoglobulin(s). Cryoglobulins are classified into three types. Type 1 cryglobulins are of a single immunoglobulin or light chain group. Type 2 cryoglobulins consist of a homogeneous immunoglobulin component with anti-IgG activity, and one or more heterogeneous components, usually IgM rheumatoid factor and IgG. Type 3 cryoglobulin is a mixture of polyclonal immunoglobulins.

Cryofibrinogenemia is most commonly found in adults in association with thromboembolic disease or malignancy. It may occur alone or in association with cryoglobulinemia.[366] A few pediatric patients with cryofibrinogenemia have been reported.[367,368] The majority of children have had antecedent upper respiratory tract infections or gastroenteritis. Cryofibrinogens have also been associated with chronic inflammatory conditions, such as FMF (see above). An autosomal dominant familial form of cryofibrinogenemia has been triggered by exposure to anesthesia and hypothermia.[369]

Cryoglobulinemia is also more commonly described in adults, especially in patients with myeloma, macroglobulinemia, and other lymphoproliferative disorders.[370] In children with cryoglobulinemia, the pattern of cryoglobulins is usually mixed, types 2 or 3, and is generally due to underlying connective tissue disease, such as systemic lupus erythematosus or juvenile rheumatoid arthritis. In SLE the cryoglobulins contain immunoglobulins IgG and IgM and complement components. In a recent large series of SLE patients there was a prevalence of low-level cryoglobulinemia of 25% and some were children.[371] This study found that cutaneous vasculitis, rheumatoid factor positivity, hypocomplementemia and hepatitis C virus are associated with cryoglobulinemia in SLE patients. Type 3 cryoglobulinemia is seen with various infectious diseases, such as mycoplasma, infectious mononucleosis, cytomegalovirus, hepatitis B, subacute bacterial endocarditis, syphilis, leprosy, and toxoplasmosis. It has been described in children with cystic fibrosis[372] and

358. Lever WF, Schaumburg-Lever G (1975) Histopathology of the Skin, 5th edn. Philadelphia: JB Lippincott.
359. O'Connor RC, Garcia Iriarte MT, Barron Reyes FJ et al. (1999) When is a biopsy justified in a case of relapsing polychondritis? J Laryngol Otol 113(7):663.
360. Imanishi Y, Mitogawa Y, Takizawa M et al. (1999) Relapsing polychondritis diagnosed by Tc-99 MDP bone scintigraphy. Clin Nucl Med 24(7):511.
361. Foidart JM, Abe S, Martin GR et al. (1978) Antibodies to types II collagen in relapsing polychondritis. N Engl J Med 299:1203.
362. Herman JH, Dennis MV (1973) Immunologic studies in relapsing polychondritis. J Clin Invest 52:549.
363. Herman JH, Musgrave DS, Dennis MV (1977) Phytomitogen-induced lymphokine-mediated cartilage proteoglycan degradation. Arthritis Rheum 20:922.
364. Gowin PJ, Schumacher HR JR (1996) Steroid sparing effect of methotrexate in relapsing polychondritis. J Rheumatol 23(5):937–938.

365. Szermeta W, Dohar JE (1995) Dapsone-induced methemoglobinemia: an anesthetic risk. Int J Pediatr Otorhinolaryngol 33(1):75.
366. Blain H, Cacoub P, Musset L et al. (2000) Cryofibrinogenaemia. Clin Exp Immunol 120(2):253.
367. Ireland TA, Werner DA, Rietschel RL et al. (1984) Cutaneous lesions in cryofibrinogenemia. J Pediatr 105:67.
368. Robinson MG, Troiano G, Cohen H, Foadi M (1966) Acute transient cryofibrinogenemia in infants. J Pediatr 69:35.
369. Lolin Y, Razis PA, O'Gorman P et al. (1989) Transient nephrotic syndrome after anesthesia resulting from a familial cryofibrinogen precipitating at 35 degrees C. J Med Genet 26:631.
370. Winfield JB (1983) Cryoglobulinemia. Hum Pathol 14:350.
371. Garcia-Carrasco M, Ranes-Casab M, Cervera R et al. (2001) Cryoglobulinemia in systemic lupus erythematosus: prevalence and clinical characteristics in a series of 122 patients. Semin Arthritis Rheum 30(5):366.
372. Garty BZ, Scanlin T, Goldsmith DP et al. (1989) Cutaneous manifestations of cystic fibrosis: possible role of cryoglobulins. Br J Dermatol 121:655.

cirrhosis.[373] Some children have essential mixed cryoglobulinemia (usually type 2), in which no underlying etiology is found.

CLINICAL PRESENTATION

Patients with either cryofibrinogenemia or cryoglobulinemia may be asymptomatic. However, some patients with cryoglobulinemia may have life-threatening complications. Children with cryofibrinogenemia complain of pain of the involved extremities and arthralgias. The fingers, toes, legs, and buttocks may be involved in cryofibrinogenemia with purpura, ecchymoses, edema, cyanosis, vesicles, and ulcerations. Petechiae are absent and pulses are adequate.

Cutaneous changes are reported in 80% of patients with cryoglobulinemia. They are most commonly palpable purpura, especially of the legs, and less frequently, Raynaud phenomenon (Table 23.5).[374] Other cutaneous changes include distal necrosis, bullae, livedo, acrocyanosis, and leg ulcers. Cold urticaria occasionally results.[375] Arthralgias and arthritis are the most common noncutaneous complaints. The most common neurologic manifestation is peripheral neuropathy, but patients have been reported with CNS involvement as well. The syndrome of essential mixed cryoglobulinemia consists of palpable purpura,[376] Raynaud phenomenon, and leg ulcers, as well as weakness, polyarthralgias, peripheral neuropathy, immune-complex glomerulonephritis, abdominal pain, and hepatitis and most cases are associated with hepatitis C virus.[375]

LABORATORY FINDINGS

The temperature at which cryoproteins begin to precipitate varies considerably and may be as high as 35°C. Therefore, it is imperative that the blood for testing be kept at 37°C. For detection of cryofibrinogen and cryoglobulin, plasma and serum must be examined, respectively. The separated plasma or serum is chilled at 4°C for 48–72h. The cryoprecipitate is expressed as a percentage of the total plasma or serum volume. The cryoprecipitate must be dissolved on rewarming. Other laboratory parameters in cryofibrinogenemia are normal, except those that reflect an associated infection. In cryoglobulinemia, rheumatoid factor may be present as well as anemia, hypogammaglobulinemia, a positive ANA test, and hypocomplementemia. In addition, laboratory parameters that reflect an underlying disorder may be abnormal.

TABLE 23.5   Common signs and symptoms in patients with cryoglobulinemia

Entity	Incidence (%)
Cutaneous	80
Vasculitis, purpura	60
Raynaud phenomenon	50
Distal necrosis	14
Urticaria, especially cold	10
Livedo	10
Acrocyanosis	10
Leg ulcers	5
Arthralgias/arthritis	35
Nephritis	20
Neurologic findings	17

A biopsy of involved skin often demonstrates leukocytoclastic vasculitis. Immunofluorescence microscopy of skin sections in patients with cryoglobulinemia often demonstrates deposition of immune complexes with complement along vessel walls.

PATHOPHYSIOLOGY AND HISTOGENESIS

The presumed mechanism in cryoproteinemia is hyperviscosity with resultant sludging and thrombosis. It is assumed that a conformational change in protein structure that promotes self-association is produced by cold temperature. The mechanism for this change is unclear. The visceral manifestations of cryoglobulinemia may reflect immune-complex-mediated vascular injury.

DIFFERENTIAL DIAGNOSIS

The skin lesions and organ involvement may be confused with Henoch–Schöenlein purpura or other causes of leukocytoclastic vasculitis in children. Other conditions that should be distinguished are disseminated intravascular coagulation, especially due to such infections as Rocky Mountain spotted fever or meningococcus, septic emboli, the vascular thrombosis of sickle cell disease, or persistent vasospasm, such as in neonates with umbilical artery catheters.

TREATMENT

Cryofibrinogen levels associated with infection tend to normalize with resolution of the infection. There are conflicting reports as to whether cryoproteinemia due to connective tissue disease or chronic infection follows the course of the underlying disorder.[366,371,376] Symptomatic treatment and avoidance of cold are helpful. Treatment of the underlying condition is essential in patients with cryoglobulinemia. Cyproheptadine has been helpful for the cold urticaria associated with mixed cryoglobulinemia. Plasmapheresis and chemotherapeutic agents, especially cyclophosphamide, have been helpful in cases with life-threatening complications.[377]

KAWASAKI DISEASE

Tomisaku Kawasaki

Kawasaki disease (KD) is an acute febrile mucocutaneous lymph node syndrome with multisystem vasculitis mainly affecting infants and small children under 5 years of age.

It is an unique clinical symptom complex, originally reported in 1967,[378] and is characterized by persistent high fever, conjunctival injection, mucosal changes to the oropharynx, erythematous rash, changes in peripheral extremities, and cervical lymphadenopathy. Although KD originally was believed to be a benign syndrome,[379] approximately 25% of untreated patients with KD develop cardiovascular involvement, especially coronary artery changes[380] with a range of severity from asymptomatic ectasia or small aneurysms to giant aneurysms on echocardiogram. Because of the availability of the treatment with high-dose intravenous immunoglobulin (IVIG) since 1984, KD patients have shown rapid resolution of the fever and other clinical symptoms, in addition to the reduction in the frequency and severity of coronary artery abnormalities.

373. Ray D, Kalra V (1988) Indian childhood cirrhosis and cryoglobulinemia. **Indian Pediatr** 25:417.
374. Brouet JC, Clauvel JP, Danon F et al. (1974) Biologic and clinical significance of cryoglobulins. **Am J Med** 57:775.
375. Doutre MS (1993) Urticaria and angioedema associated with cryoglobulinemia in children. **Allerg Immunol** (Paris) 25(8):343.
376. Blanco R, Martinez-Taboada VM, Rodriguez-Valverde V, Garcia-Fuentes M (1998) Cutaneous vasculitis in children and adults. Associated diseases and etiologic factors in 303 patients. **Medicine** 77(6):403.
377. Wallace DJ (2001) Apheresis for lupus erythematosus. State of the art. **Lupus** 10(3):193.

378. Kawasaki T (1983) Clinical features of Kawasaki syndrome. **Acta Paediatr Jpn** 25:79–90. (overseas edition)
379. Kawasaki T (1967) Acute febrile mucocutaneous syndrome with lymphoid involvement with specific desquamation of the fingers and toes in children. **Japan J Allerg** 16:178–222. (in Japanese)
380. Kawasaki T, Kosaki F, Okawa S et al. (1974) A new infantile acute febrile mucocutaneous lymph node syndrome (MCLS) prevailing in Japan. **Pediatrics** 54:271–276.

KD is now known to have worldwide distribution, having been observed on all continents and in all ethnic groups.[381] At present, KD appears now to have replaced acute rheumatic fever as the leading cause of acquired heart disease in the USA and Japan.

EPIDEMIOLOGY

Kawasaki disease has been found on all continents, in numerous countries and in all races. The greatest number of patients have been found in Japan and as of 2000, where the total reported number of cases was more than 160 000. There were three nationwide outbreaks in 1979, 1982, and 1986 in Japan. All those outbreaks started from the early winter and ended by the early summer. The 1998 annual incidence rate in Japan per 100 000 children under 5 years old was 111.7.[382] The age distribution shows a peak at 10 to 11 months old and 80–85% are under 5 years old. Cases over 11 years old are rare. Adult cases are extremely rare. The male/female ratio is 1.4/1.

Nationwide surveys of countries other than Japan are less accurate. No conclusion can be reached about incidence in races and the relationship between industrialization and incidence.

CLINICAL FEATURES

In the absence of a diagnostic test for KD, the diagnosis is established by the presence of six principal symptoms.

1. *Fever of unknown etiology lasting 5 days or more (95%).* In general, the onset of the disease is usually with an abrupt and high fever, but without prodromal symptoms such as coughing, sneezing, or rhinorrhea. There is usually remittent or continuous fever ranging from 38 to 40°C for 1–2 weeks. High fever lasting for 30 days is rarely seen, while high fever lasting any longer may indicate another disease. The fever subsides more rapidly when IVIG is administered with aspirin, as compared to therapy with aspirin alone. The duration of fever usually depends on IVIG therapy and seems to be dose dependent. In KD the longer the fever continues, the higher the possibility of formation of coronary artery aneurysms. Although not included as a diagnostic criterion, typical patients with KD, particularly younger ones, are extremely irritable to a much greater degree than is commonly seen with other febrile illnesses.

2. *Bilateral congestion of ocular conjunctivae (87–90%).* Conjunctival injection occurs within 2 to 4 days from the onset of the disease. Upon close examination, each capillary vessel is clear because of individual dilatation. There is usually no purulent discharge, so the term "conjunctivitis" is not appropriate. The degree of redness of the eye is variable; in most cases, the redness can be seen at a glance, but in some cases it can be seen only upon close examination. Pseudomembrane formation, corneal ulceration, adhesion of the iris, or visual disturbance or damage has never been found. If there is careful slit-lamp examination early in the course of the disease, anterior uveitis[383] can frequently be discovered. Conjunctival injection usually subsides within one week, but persists for 1–2 weeks in some patients not treated with IVIG.

3. *Changes of the lips and the oral cavity (85–95%).* Dryness, redness, and fissuring of lips can be seen 3–5 days after the onset. In some cases, there is bleeding and formation of crust. At a glance, it seems as if there is lipstick on the lips. The membrane of the oral cavity and the pharyngeal mucosa are diffusely red (85–90%). There are no vesicles, aphthae, or pseudomembrane formations. Frequently, however, there is the so-called "strawberry tongue" (80%), which is similar to that seen in scarlet fever. The changes subside within two weeks after the onset of the disease, but sometimes the reddening of the lips will continue for 3–4 weeks. The disease can be recognized by

the characteristic appearance of the face with red eyes and red lips, which is the so-called "KD appearance" (Figs 23.12 and 23.13).

4. *Acute nonpurulent swelling of cervical lymph nodes (60–70%).* One can often notice swelling of the cervical lymph nodes for at least 1 day before the onset of fever or concomitant with the fever. The patient complains of pain, and often suffers wry neck. In some cases there is swelling several days after the onset of fever. The size of the swelling ranges from 1.5 to 5cm in diameter and is always a firm mass. Cervical lymphadenopathy is seen in about two-thirds of the cases in Japan, but less than 50% in the United States. The swelling usually disappears with defervescence. There are some patients, usually over the age of 3 years, in whom cervical lymphadenopathy is the most striking clinical sign of KD. In these patients, a unilateral, markedly enlarged, tender and erythematous cervical lymph node fails to improve following intravenous antibiotic therapy. Therefore, KD should be considered in patients with cervical adenitis, particularly if unresponsive to antibiotic treatment.

5. *Polymorphous exanthema of the body without vesicles or crusts (85–90%).* From the first to the fifth day after the onset of fever, a polymorphous

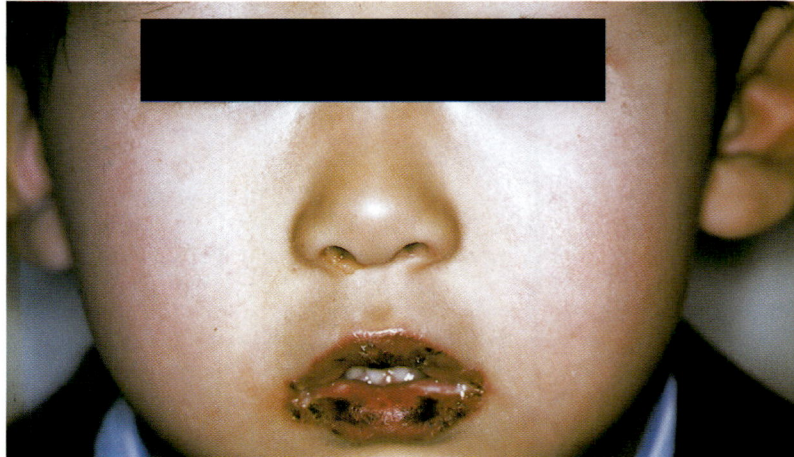

Fig. 23.12 Typical KD appearance of 7-year-old boy with bilateral conjunctival hyperemia and red, crusted lips at the fifth day of illness.

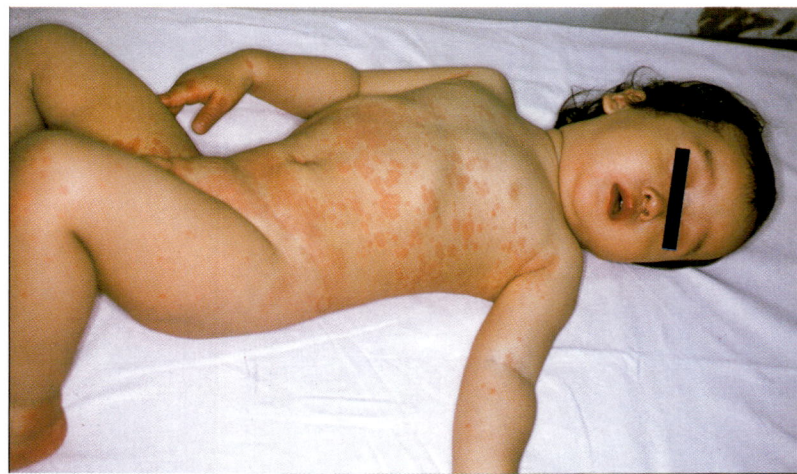

Fig. 23.13 Typical KD appearance with polymorphous erythema and red palms and soles at the fourth day of illness (18 month-old girl).

381. Melish ME, Hicks RV, Larson EJ (1976) Mucocutaneous lymph node syndrome in the United States. **Am J Dis Child** 130:599–607.
382. Yanagawa H, Nakamura Y, Yashiro M et al. (2001) Incidence survey of Kawasaki disease in 1997 and 1998 in Japan. **Pediatrics** 107:3. URL:http://www.pediatrics.org/cgi/content/full/107/3/e33

383. Burns JC, Joffe L, Sargent RA et al. (1985) Anterior uveitis associated with Kawasaki syndrome. **Pediatr Infect Dis J** 4:258–261.

exanthem appears on the body and/or the extremities (Figs 23.13 and 23.14), and may be morbilliform, maculopapular, scarlatiniform, urticarial with large erythematous plaques, or erythema multiforme-like with targetoid central clearing, or iris lesions; the exanthem may present as a combination of these forms. The individual lesions measure 5–30mm in diameter and spread over the body and extremities within several days. Each lesion becomes increasingly larger and often coalescent. They are not accompanied by vesicles or crusts, but sometimes small aseptic pustules are found on the knees, elbows, buttocks or other sites of the body. Erythema is variable and transient in nature. The rash disappears within 1 day at the earliest, and may continue for 1 week or more at the most. Sometimes it is recurrent in nature. Desquamation in the perineal region often occurs. Histopathologically, the lesion reveals marked edema of dermal papillae, focal intercellular edema of the basal cell layer, and very slight perivascular infiltration of mononuclear cells in the dermis. There is no evidence of vasculitis. These findings are identical to those for nonspecific exudative inflammation of the skin.

6. *Changes of the peripheral extremities (90–95%).* Approximately 2–5 days after the onset of the illness, when the polymorphous exanthem of the body has appeared, there is reddening of palms (Fig. 23.15) and soles (85–90%), at which time indurative edema (75%) also occurs. The degree of swelling is sometimes remarkable and the skin is shiny and appears to be about to burst. After the fever resolves, the swelling also disappears in most cases.

From 10–15 days after the onset, there is desquamation and fissuring (Fig. 23.16) between the nails and the tips of the fingers, after which membranous desquamation (90–95%) spreads over the palm up to the wrist. For the toes, membranous desquamation occurs several days after the appearance of desquamation of the fingers. Membranous desquamation spreads over the soles up to the ankles. There are cases that have only fingertip desquamation. From a month and a half to 2 months after the onset of the illness, transverse furrows frequently appear in the nails of both the fingers and toes (Beau's lines). Some cases have the five principal signs, but no red palms or indurative edema in the initial stage. If the fingertips are observed carefully in the stage of convalescence, desquamation at the fingertips can be seen in most cases. Fingertip desquamation is one of the most important features of this disease.

KD has been reported to recur in 3–4% of patients in Japan, although the recurrence rate in the United States appears to be lower.

DIAGNOSIS

If five or six of the principal signs are present, the diagnosis of KD can be established after other diseases with similar findings are excluded. However, patients with only four or less of the six principal signs can be diagnosed as KD when coronary artery aneurysm is recognized by two-dimensional echocardiography (2-DE). Since the introduction of IVIG treatment, patients

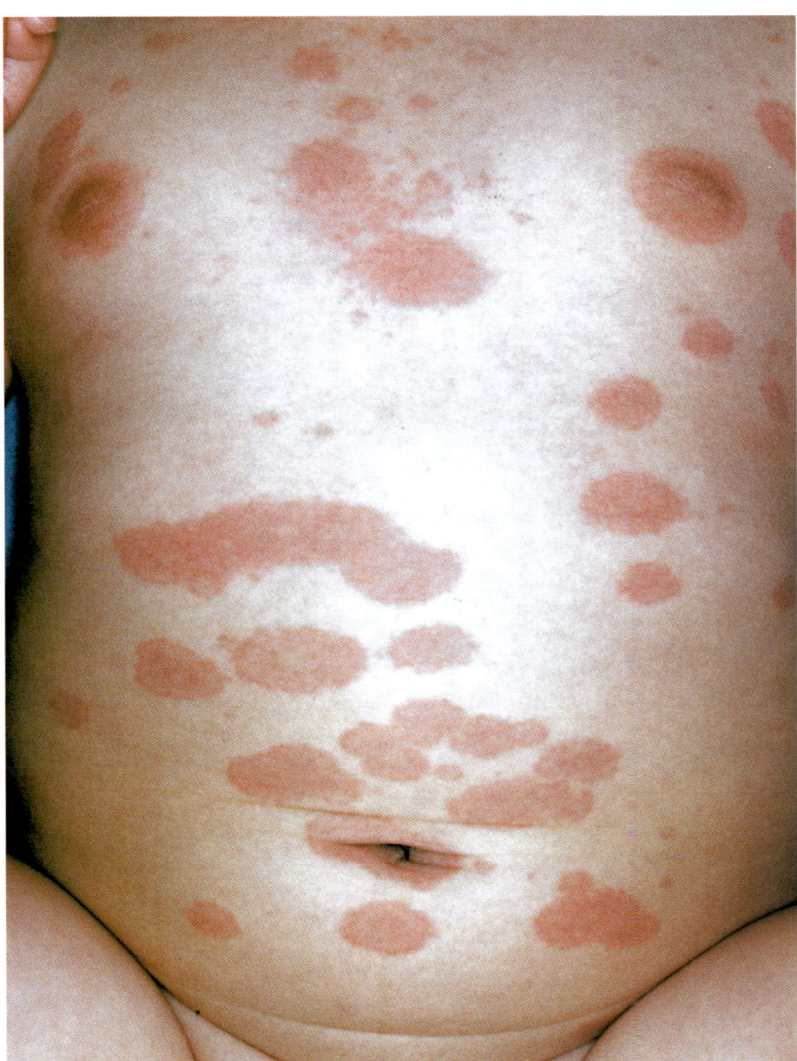

Fig. 23.14   Polymorphous erythema at the fifth day of illness (5-month-old boy).

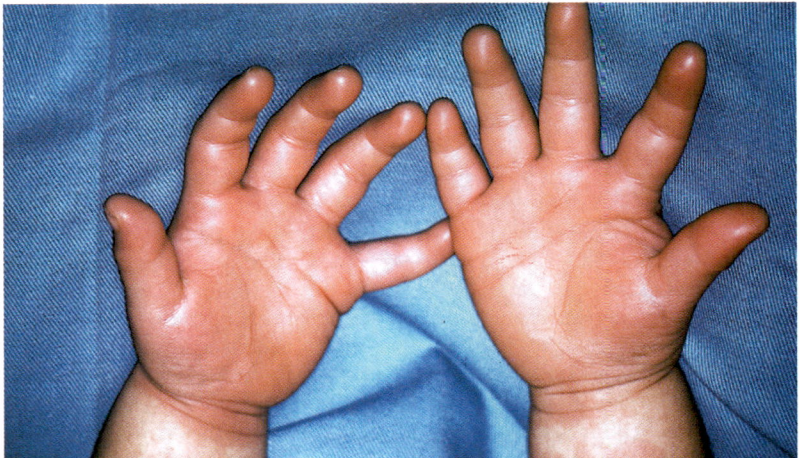

Fig. 23.15   Red palms and indurative edema of hands of 2-year-old boy at the 4th day of illness.

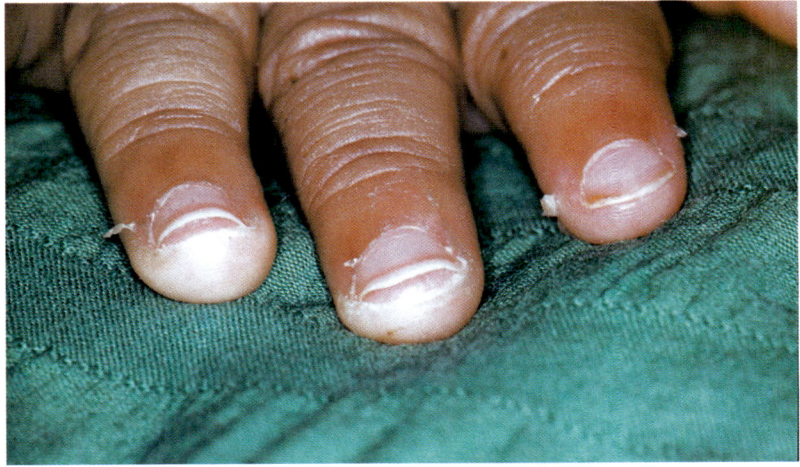

Fig. 23.16   The beginning of desquamation at the tip of fingers at the 11th day of illness (9-month-old boy).

are often diagnosed and treated before the full expression of the clinical features. In these patients, some of the principal signs may be obscured by therapy.

ATYPICAL KAWASAKI DISEASE

Diagnosis can be made easily for typical cases, but atypical cases with coronary complications that are either fatal or with remaining aneurysms can be found and these are difficult cases to diagnose.[384] Atypical cases may be more common in younger patients under 6 months of age. Prolonged high fever of more than seven days is an important sign that can be seen in atypical cases. Consequently, cases with fever of unknown origin can be considered as possible KD patients.[385] In such cases, if fingertip desquamation is present, even if other principal symptoms are not detected, KD is a strong possibility, especially in infants and small children. Mild bilateral conjunctival hyperemia with prolonged fever can also be KD and possible coronary complications should be checked by 2-DE. A third example of atypical KD is pale face and red lips with prolonged fever. A fourth example is polymorphous exanthem with prolonged fever. A fifth example is cervical adenopathy with prolonged fever. These prolonged fever cases with one of the principal signs should be considered possible KD and checked for coronary artery complications. Thus, KD should be considered in any infant with prolonged, unexplained fever and signs of mucocutaneous hyperemia. IVIG treatment should be considered as soon as possible.

OTHER FINDINGS

In addition to the physical findings associated with clinical criteria for KD, patients may present with other organ system involvement presumed to result from the systemic vasculitis. Right upper quadrant pain, nausea, and vomiting may be associated with tenderness and fullness on examination of the right upper quadrant. These signs and symptoms suggest hydrops of the gallbladder which can be confirmed by abdominal ultrasonography and resolves without surgical intervention. Other gastrointestinal manifestations are diarrhea, small bowel obstruction, ileus, hepatitis, and pancreatitis. Arthralgia and/or arthritis can be seen in up to 30% of patients. Arthritis can occur in the first week of illness and is usually polyarticular, involving the knees, ankles and hands. The arthritis usually persists for about three weeks. More common is a late-onset arthritis in the second to third week of illness, which is usually particular, involving the knees, ankles, and hips. The mean duration is approximately 2 weeks. The arthritis and arthralgias are self-limited, rarely persist beyond the fourth week of illness, but may be confused with Perthes' disease. Patients may complain of photophobia during the acute illness. Mild anterior uveitis is common in acute KD and has been reported in approximately 70% of the patients examined with a stationary slit-lamp during the first 10 days of illness.

Sterile pyuria with monocytes in the acute phase is common. Dysuria may be associated with urethral meatitis and cystitis during acute KD. Evidence of an aseptic meningitis is seen in at least one-half of patients who undergo lumbar puncture, with mild pleocytosis, but normal glucose and protein values in the cerebrospinal fluid.

Hepatic dysfunction with mild obstructive jaundice and mildly to moderately elevated levels of serum transaminases occurs occasionally. The localized erythema at the site of bacille Calmette–Guérin (BCG) inoculation is common in Japanese patients. Takayama et al.[386] reported erythema at the BCG inoculation site in 88% of patients who develop KD within 4–6 months following BCG vaccination, but was never seen in patients who developed KD beyond 36 months after vaccination.

A rare but serious complication of KD is the development of peripheral ischemia with resultant gangrene.[387] The peripheral gangrene may result in autoamputation.

Laboratory findings are nonspecific and nondiagnostic in KD. Most characteristic is a moderate to marked leukocytosis with shift to the left in the first week of illness. Other acute phase reactants such as increased ESR and elevated CRP are present with the onset of fever and persist for 3–4 weeks, usually in IVIG untreated cases. The platelet count, which is generally normal in the first week of illness, begins to rise in the second week, peaking at about three weeks at a mean count of 800 000/mm³, although it may rise as high as 2×10^6/mm³. Serum immunoglobulin levels may also increase, but ASO titers tend to be low.

CARDIOVASCULAR COMPLICATIONS

The most important clinical problem in KD is the cardiovascular lesion, which may lead to coronary artery disease, myocardial ischemia and sudden death. The important evaluation of the coronary artery in KD is performed using 2-DE and/or coronary angiography. It is now known through 2-DE and angiographic findings that, before the development of IVIG, approximately 25% of untreated patients with KD developed coronary artery abnormalities, such as dilatation and/or aneurysms. The earliest cardiac changes occur within the first 10 days from onset and include endocarditis, myocarditis and pericarditis. From studies employing daily echocardiograms,[388] it is known that increasing echodensity of the coronary artery wall usually occurs as early as 7 days after the onset of fever.

It becomes evident that coronary dilatation appears on approximately the tenth day of illness, and more than half of the patients have mild coronary dilatation. However, this is mainly transient and regresses within 3–5 weeks from onset. In Japan, the latest figures reveal that coronary aneurysms develop in about 15% of all KD patients and giant coronary aneurysms (diameter >8mm) in about 1% (Fig. 23.17).

One to 3 months after the onset of KD, about 20% of all patients have coronary aneurysms angiographically. Repeat angiography 6–18 months after

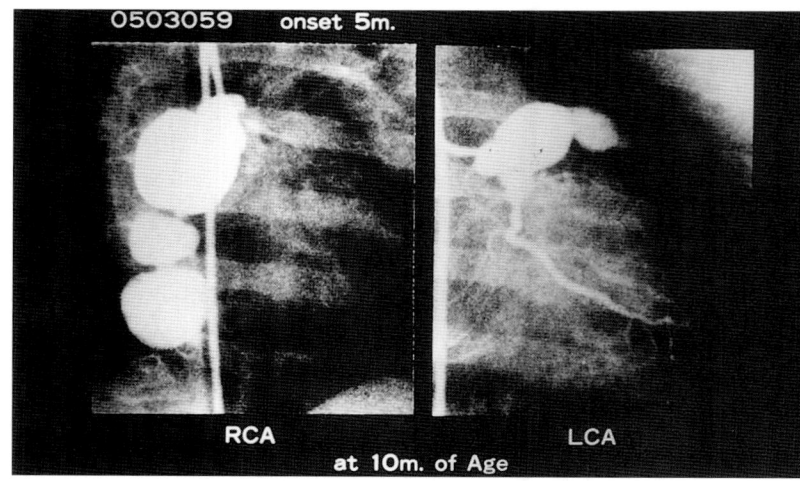

Fig. 23.17 Right and left giant coronary artery aneurysms. This 5-month-old boy with typical KD was treated with IVIG (400mg/kg/day for 5 days) and coronary angiography was performed 5 months after onset. (Courtesy of Dr. Atsuko Suzuki, Tokyo Teishin Hospital, Tokyo.)

384. Rowley AH, Gonzaliz-Grussi F, Gidding SS et al. (1987) Incomplete Kawasaki disease with coronary artery involvement. **J Pediatr** 110:409–413.

385. Kawasaki T (1989) Comment & Discussion: Atypical cases. In: Proceedings of the Third International Kawasaki disease Symposium, Kawasaki T, ed. Tokyo, Japan Heart Foundation, p. 294.

386. Takayama J, Yanase Y, Kawasaki T (1982) A study on erythematous changes at the site of BCG inoculation in Kawasaki disease. **Acta Pediatr Jap** 86:567–572. (in Japanese)

387. Tomita S, Chung K, Mas M et al. (1992) Peripheral gangrene associated with Kawasaki disease. **Clinical Infect Dis** 14:121–126.

388. Kamiya T, Suzuki A, Kijima Y et al. (1982) Coronary arterial lesion in Kawasaki disease – occurrence and prognosis. **Recent Adv Cardiovasc Dis** III:19–27 (in Japanese).

the first study in those with coronary aneurysms showed that about half of the patients had resolution of the aneurysms. This suggests that coronary aneurysms in KD show a strong tendency to regress. Of those with persistent abnormalities, approximately one-fourth showed minimal changes such as milder dilatation and a more irregular wall, but less than half showed persistent aneurysms; about two-thirds showed aneurysms plus stenoses and/or obstruction. Some of these latter patients had cardiac signs, such as cardiac dysfunction or myocardial infarction and sudden death.[389,390] The pathologic mechanism of aneurysm regression is a marked proliferation of intima without massive thrombus formation, consisting of smooth muscle cells and regenerated endothelium covering a superficial thrombus. Hemodynamic forces may regulate such arteries to maintain adequate lumina.[391]

Giant coronary aneurysms are a serious problem because they are likely to produce massive thrombus formation and develop into ischemic heart disease. Myocardial infarction occurs, in less than 1% of all KD patients. Aneurysms in other arteries, such as the axillary, iliac, renal, and mesenteric arteries, are observed in about 2% of patients, who invariably have coronary artery aneurysms also. The axillary aneurysms are recognized by palpation on daily physical examination.

Pericarditis or pericardial effusion in the acute phase is mostly subclinical and disappears within one to two weeks. Massive pericardial effusion or cardiac tamponade is rare. There have been no reports of its progression to chronic or constrictive pericarditis. Relatively mild myocarditis is observed in many patients in the acute phase, especially in the first and second weeks of illness, regardless of the presence of coronary aneurysms. Gallop rhythm, distant heart sounds, ST-T segment changes and low voltage on ECG suggest myocarditis.

TREATMENT AND MANAGEMENT

It is now clear that IVIG and aspirin combined therapy results in a markedly more rapid anti-inflammatory effect and reduces coronary artery abnormalities more than does aspirin alone. It is recommended that patients with acute KD be treated with a single 2g/kg infusion of IVIG and aspirin (30–50mg/kg) within the first 10 days from onset, and that the aspirin dose be reduced to 3–5mg/kg/day given as a single daily dose after defervescence.

Aspirin is discontinued if no coronary artery abnormalities have been detected by 2-DE by 6 weeks after onset. Aspirin is continued if coronary artery abnormalities are persistent. Aspirin should be discontinued if the patient develops an illness suspected to be varicella or influenza in order to reduce the risk of Reye syndrome. The use of an alternative antiplatelet agent such as flurbiprofen should be considered.

In 1984, high-dose immunoglobulin treatment for acute KD was reported to be effective by Furusho et al.[392] This was confirmed by the US multi-center randomized trial in 1986.[393] Both studies indicated that 400mg/kg/day for 4–5 days with aspirin effectively prevents coronary aneurysms. In the American second trial, published in 1991,[394] children were randomly assigned to receive either the four-dose IVIG regimen or a single-dose of 2g/kg of IVIG infused over 8–12h. All patients were treated with aspirin. The single-dose regimen accelerated the resolution of systemic inflammation and tended to lower the prevalence of coronary artery abnormalities.

For maximum efficacy, therapy with IVIG should be initiated within the first 10 days and ideally within the first week of the illness, even if coronary changes already exist. Early administration of IVIG usually causes rapid defervescence and dramatic resolution of the mucocutaneous features of KD. When the diagnosis of KD is made after the tenth day of illness, IVIG treatment should be administered if the patient is still febrile, and has signs of ongoing inflammation. Approximately 10% of patients with KD are resistant to IVIG therapy.[395] These patients are at greatest risk for development of coronary artery aneurysms and long-term sequelae of the disease. In KD as in other vasculitides, blood vessel damage appears to result from an aberrant immune response leading to endothelial cell injury and vessel wall damage. Steroids such as prednisolone or methylprednisolone are the treatment of choice in other forms of vasculitis, yet they have been considered to be unsafe in KD. However, it has been reported that at least some patients with severe KD who are resistant to IVIG therapy may be treated safely with intravenous pulse steroid therapy and that these patients may benefit from this therapy.[396]

The management of patients with severe obstruction of coronary artery who may develop ischemic heart disease is an important issue. When myocardial infarction occurs, patients must be hospitalized immediately. Vasodilators and nitroglycerin, as well as catecholamines such as dopamine and dobutamine for cardiogenic shock and heart failure, can be used. Anticoagulant therapy (heparin or urokinase) is given. Massive thrombus formation can be visualized by serial echocardiographic studies. Patients with complications or sequelae, such as ventricular dysfunction, heart failure, severe arrhythmias, or postinfarction angina, are managed by medical or surgical treatment.

According to Kitamura et al.,[397] 167 patients with KD in Japan have undergone coronary artery bypass surgery. The intrathoracic artery is recommended for left coronary artery bypass because the long-term patency is much more favorable than saphenous vein grafting. The gastroepiploic artery is suitable for right coronary artery bypass graft because it is usually large enough and has sufficient blood flow even in younger children.

Such surgery is technically difficult in infants and children under 4 years of age. Detailed coronary angiography is essential. Viability of the myocardium should be evaluated by thallium myocardial scintigraphy. The long-term results and prognosis after surgery need further investigation. Approximately 15 heart transplants have been performed on KD patients worldwide.[398]

PATHOLOGY

According to Amano et al.,[399,400] the arterial lesions of KD are categorized with regard to the degree of inflammatory changes and to the duration of the disease. They are divided into six characteristic types of lesions identified in the arterial system: type 1, endothelial degeneration and increased vascular permeability; type 2, edema and degeneration of the media; type 3, necrotizing panarteritis; type 4, granulation formation; type 5, scar formation; type 6, aneurysm formation. It is characteristic that these six types of lesions are simultaneously observed, not only in various areas of the arterial tree in the same patient, but also in different portions of one artery. The transition from type 1 to type 5 or 6 is thought to reflect the morphogenesis of the arteritis.

389. Kato H, Ichinose E, Yoshioka F et al. (1982) Fate of coronary aneurysms in Kawasaki disease: serial coronary angiography and long-term follow-up study. Am J Cardiol 49:1758–1766.
390. Kato H, Sugimura T, Akagi T et al. (1996) Long-term consequences of Kawasaki disease: a 10-to-21 year follow-up study of 594 patients. Circulation 94:1379–1385.
391. Sasaguri Y, Kato H (1982) Regression of aneurysms in Kawasaki disease: a pathologic study. J Pediatr 100:225–231.
392. Furusho K, Kamiya T, Nakano H et al. (1984) High-dose intravenous gammaglobulin for Kawasaki disease. Lancet 2:1055–1058.
393. Newburger JW, Takahashi M, Burns JC et al. (1986) The treatment of Kawasaki syndrome with intravenous gamma globulin. N Engl J Med 315:341–347.
394. Newburger JW, Takahashi M, Beiser AS et al. (1991) A single intravenous infusion of gamma globulin as compared with four infusions in the treatment of acute Kawasaki syndrome. N Engl J Med 324:1633–1639.
395. Sundel RP, Burns JC, Baker A et al. (1993) Gamma globulin re-treatment in Kawasaki disease. J Pediatr 123:657–659.
396. Wright DA, Newburger JW, Baker A et al. (1996) Treatment of immune globulin-resistant Kawasaki disease with pulsed doses of corticosteroids. J Pediatr 128:146–149.
397. Kitamura S, Kameda Y, Seki T et al. (1994) Long-term outcome of myocardial revascularization in patients with Kawasaki coronary artery disease. A multi-center cooperative study. J Thorac Cardiovasc Surg 107:663–674.
398. Checchia PA, Pahl E, Shaddy RE et al. (1997) Cardiac transplantation for Kawasaki disease. Pediatrics 100:695–699.
399. Amano S, Hazama F, Hamashima Y (1979) Pathology of Kawasaki disease: I. Pathology and morphogenesis of the vascular changes. Jpn Circ J 43:633–643.
400. Amano S, Hazama F, Hamashima Y (1979) Pathology of Kawasaki disease: II. Distribution and incidence of the vascular lesions. Jpn Circ J 43:633–643.

Aneurysm formation in the coronary artery is present in approximately 90% of autopsied cases. Aneurysm formation is rarely seen, except in the main coronary and iliac arteries. These six types of arteritic changes are not equally distributed throughout the entire arterial system. Severe lesions such as necrotizing panarteritis are usually localized in arteries such as the main coronary, iliac, mesenteric and renal arteries which directly branch from the aorta. Inflammatory lesions (phlebitis) are also observed in the venous system. Amano *et al.* thus suggested that the vascular lesions of KD should be termed systemic vasculitis rather than systemic arteritis.

DIFFERENTIAL DIAGNOSIS

Typical KD cases can be identified using the principal signs as a guideline. However, differentiation between KD and other diseases[401] such as Stevens–Johnson syndrome, toxic shock syndrome, scarlet fever and measles may be difficult in some patients.

Fever and rash (exanthema) are common in all of these disorders; desquamation of hands and feet are seen in all the other diseases except measles. Shock is seen in only toxic shock syndrome. In Stevens–Johnson syndrome, the exanthem often shows bullae. In the oral cavity, ulcer, erosions and pseudo-membrane formation can be frequently seen, and in the eyes, pus or pseudo-membrane formation is usual. Patients with toxic shock syndrome show diffuse erythroderma (sunburn-like) over the whole body with reddening of the eyes, lips and oral pharynx that resembles KD. When shock occurs, the exanthema disappears.

The specific scarlatiniform erythema (red, punctate, or finely papular) of scarlet fever is not associated with injection of the eyes and lips. The pharyngitis, however, is brightly erythematous and exudative. Cultures show group A streptococcus, and penicillin therapy is effective. In measles the exanthem is morbilliform, and associated with conjunctival injection with discharge. The oropharynx shows Koplik spots transiently.

The fever and exanthem of early KD can be confused with those of viral infections, particularly Epstein–Barr virus, adenovirus, enterovirus and parvovirus. The fever and exanthem of leptospirosis is also associated with bilateral hyperemia of the eye. Cases of *Yersinia pseudotuberculosis* infection (so-called Izumi fever)[402] also resemble KD, and have been described in Japan.

The prolonged fever with arthralgia or arthritis of KD and response to aspirin or, if ineffective, to systemic steroids may raise the misdiagnosis of JRA. However, KD cases recover with treatment, while JRA cases show recurrence of fever and arthralgia. Until 6 months from onset, cases should be followed with caution so that differential diagnosis can be made.

ETIOLOGY

Although numerous etiological hypotheses[403] such as *Propionibacterium acnes*,[404] retrovirus,[405,406] superantigens,[407] etc., have been proposed since Kawasaki disease was first reported in 1967, as of 2001 none of them has been confirmed by other investigators. Consequently the etiology of Kawasaki disease remains unknown.

SELECTED SYSTEMIC DISEASES WITH SKIN MANIFESTATIONS

Patricia Treadwell

CUTANEOUS MANIFESTATIONS OF INFLAMMATORY BOWEL DISEASE

Inflammatory bowel disease is a term used to describe chronic inflammation of the gastrointestinal tract in the absence of a detectable pathogenic agent. The two most well-described examples of inflammatory bowel disease are ulcerative colitis and Crohn's disease.

This discussion begins with those cutaneous manifestations associated with both ulcerative colitis and Crohn's disease, with particular emphasis on pyoderma gangrenosum. Skin findings associated more specifically with either ulcerative colitis or Crohn's disease are then addressed, followed by a commentary regarding the bowel-associated dermatosis/arthritis syndrome.

PYODERMA GANGRENOSUM

Pyoderma gangrenosum is a skin disorder that is rare in childhood. It was originally described by Brunsting *et al.*[408] in 1930. A typical lesion consists of an enlarging necrotic ulceration, usually on the lower limbs, with a mucopurulent base and a violaceous undermined border. Erythema is evident at the periphery of the lesion. The lesions often heal with cribriform scars. Classification into four different clinical variants (ulcerative, pustular, bullous, vegetative) has been proposed.[409]

Epidemiology

There appears to be no specific pattern of inheritance among patients with pyoderma gangrenosum. The average age of onset is 40 years; no sex predominance has been noted.[409] Powell and Perry[410] found that only 4% of 180 patients examined in a 50-year period had onset before 15 years of age. Pyoderma gangrenosum has been reported in infants, with two cases aged 1 and 9 months, respectively.[410,411]

As many as 78 to 100% of children with pyoderma gangrenosum are found to have associated systemic disease.[409,410] Diseases reported in association with pyoderma gangrenosum include the following:

- Arthritis[409,410]
- Inflammatory bowel disease (ulcerative colitis and Crohn's disease)[409,410]
- Blood dyscrasias (leukemia and polycythemia vera)[412–414]
- Cardiovascular disease (Takayasu's arteritis and congenital heart malformation)[410]
- Chronic active hepatitis[409,412]
- Sarcoidosis[409,412]
- Monoclonal gammopathy[409,412]
- Myeloma[412]
- SLE[409,412]
- Diabetes mellitus[409,412]

401. Mason WH, Burns JC (1997) Clinical presentation of Kawasaki disease. **Progr Pediatr Cardiol** 6:193–201.
402. Sato K, Ouchi K, Taki M (1983) Yersinia pseudotuberculosis infection in children resembling Izumi fever and Kawasaki syndrome. **Pediatr Infect Dis** 2(2):123–126.
403. Shulman ST, Rowley AH (1997) Etiology and pathogenesis of Kawasaki disease. **Progr Pediatr Cardiol** 6:187–192.
404. Kato H, Fujimoto T, Inoue O et al. (1983) Variant strain of propionibacterium acnes: a clue to the aetiology of Kawasaki disease. **Lancet** 2:1383–1388.
405. Shulman ST, Rowley AH (1986) Does Kawasaki disease have a retroviral etiology? **Lancet** 2:545–546.
406. Burns JC, Geha RS, Scheenberger EE et al. (1986) Polymerase activity in lymphocyte culture supernatants from patients with Kawasaki disease. **Nature** 323:814–816.
407. Leung DYM, Meissner HC, Fulton DR et al. (1993) Toxic shock syndrome toxin-secreting *Staphylococcus aureus* in Kawasaki syndrome. **Lancet** 342:1385–1388.

408. Brunsting L, Goeckerman W, O'Leary P (1930) Pyoderma (ecthyma) gangrenosum: clinical and experimental observations in five cases occurring in adults. **Arch Derm Syph** 22:655.
409. Powell FC, Su WPD, Perry HO (1996) Pyoderma gangrenosum: Classification and management. **J Am Acad Dermatol** 34:395–409.
410. Powell F, Perry H (1984) Pyoderma gangrenosum in childhood. **Arch Dermatol** 120:757–761.
411. Dick D, Mackie R, Patrick W et al. (1982) Pyoderma gangrenosum in infancy. **Acta Derm Venereol** (Stockh) 62:348–350.
412. Blitz NM, Rudikoff D (2001) Pyoderma gangrenosum. **Mt Sinai J Med** 68:287–297.
413. Ko CB, Walton S, Wyatt EH (1992) Pyoderma gangrenosum: associations revisited. **Int J Dermatol** 31:574–577.
414. Ho KK, Otridge BW, Vandenberg E et al. (1992) Pyoderma gangrenosum, polycythemia rubra vera, and the development of leukemia. **J Am Acad Dermatol** 27:804–808.

- Lymphoma[409]
- Immunodeficiency, immunosupression, and human immunodeficiency virus (HIV)[409]
- Other internal malignancies.[409]

Of these, the most important associations in children in terms of frequency are inflammatory bowel disease and arthritis.

PRESENTING HISTORY

Patients with pyoderma gangrenosum usually present with a skin lesion having the typical clinical appearance. The lesions frequently have evolved from a small pustule that can be considered the primary lesions of this disease. The lesions are generally painful. A history of preceding minor trauma is obtained in approximately 25–40% of cases.[412] A careful history may document the presence of symptoms, such as joint pain or swelling, bloody diarrhea, abdominal cramping, weight loss, fever, or malaise. Exacerbation of activity of the skin lesions may occur with or without exacerbation of the systemic symptoms.[410,412,415,416] The natural history of pyoderma gangrenosum follows one of two courses: an acute, rapidly progressive course or a chronic indolent progression.[412]

Lesions may occur simultaneously with the associated systemic disease or may develop later. Less commonly, skin lesions may precede the onset of the systemic symptoms.[410]

PHYSICAL EXAMINATION

A typical lesion consists of an ulceration with a necrotic center, mucopurulent exudate, and a violaceous undermined border (Fig. 23.18). Erythema is noted at the periphery. When healing occurs, a scar with a cribriform pattern is often evident (Fig. 23.19).

Lesions most commonly arise on the lower legs but not uncommonly may occur on the trunk, abdomen, and in the perineum (Figs 23.20 and 23.21). Less frequently, lesions are seen on the upper extremities and in the head and neck areas. Although mucous membrane lesions are uncommon, they have been noted in the oral cavity and genital region.[409,417] Bullous pyoderma gangrenosum lesions are least common (Fig. 23.22).

Arthritis, if associated, usually affects the large joints, especially the ankles, knees, and elbows. A few patients have been described with arthritis deformans[410] and ankylosing arthritis.[412]

Pathergy (the development of lesions at sites of minor trauma) has been reported, with lesions of pyoderma gangrenosum occurring at sites of penicillin injection and venipuncture.[410] Pathergy is apparently more common in childhood disease than in adult pyoderma gangrenosum.[410] The fact that the pathergy phenomenon may also occur at a biopsy site has dissuaded some clinicians from performing routine biopsies in cases of pyoderma gangrenosum. It is recommended that a biopsy be performed, especially in ambiguous cases, to rule out other entities. Biopsy from the edge of the ulcer can help rule out vasculitis; biopsy from the ulcer itself can be submitted for culture.

LABORATORY FINDINGS

Bacterial culture from the lesions of pyoderma gangrenosum may be sterile or, more usually, may show growth of multiple saprophytic organisms.[409,412] Other findings include elevated ESR and a mild anemia.[411] Various immune defects have been described in patients with this disease including cell-

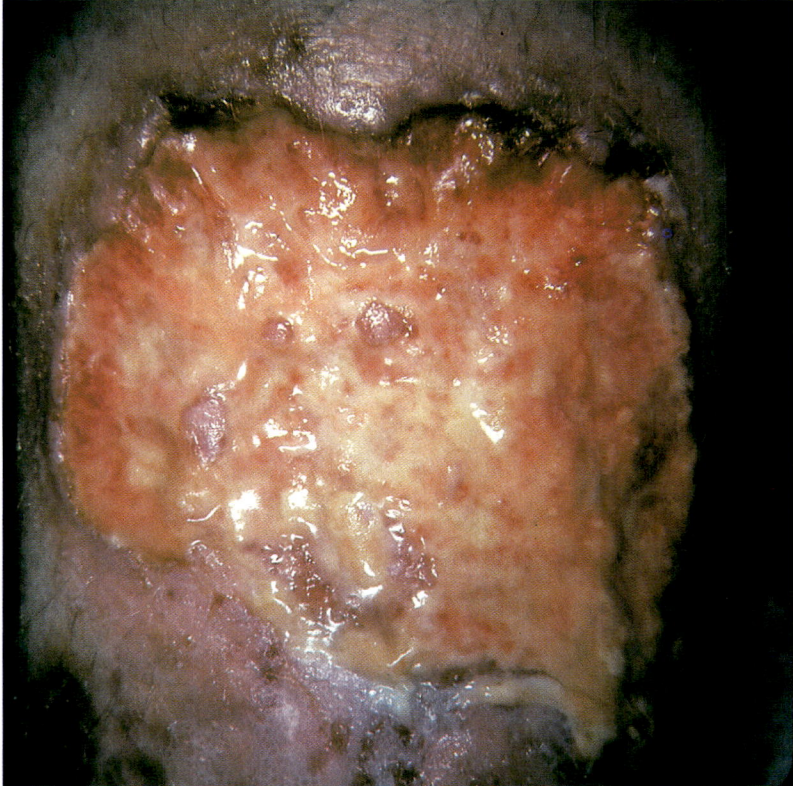

Fig. 23.18   A pyoderma gangrenosum lesion of the lower leg.

mediated, humoral and complement abnormalities, immune complex deposition, and T-lymphocyte activation.[412] Patients have also been noted to have abnormal immunoglubulins.[411,412]

PATHOPHYSIOLOGY AND HISTOGENESIS

A single pathogenic mechanism in pyoderma gangrenosum has not been identified. The variability in presentation, course, response to therapy, and multiple associated systemic diseases may indicate that different mechanisms are operating in different cases. Autoantibodies to skin and intestinal antigens have been demonstrated[409] in addition to antiphospholipid antibodies.[418]

Histologic findings are variable and dependent on the specific classification. Powell et al.[409] and Hurwitz et al.[419] described the following:

- *ulcerative*: neutrophilic abscess formation (centrally) and a lymphocytic angiocentric infiltrate (distally)
- *pustular*: subcorneal pustule, perifollicular neutrophilic infiltrate, dense dermal infiltrate with subepidermal edema
- *bullous*: subepidermal bulla formation, intraepidermal vesicle formation and neutrophilic dermal infiltrate
- *vegetative*: pseudoepitheliomatous hyperplasia, dermal neutrophilic abscesses, sinus tracts, and palisading granulomatous reaction.

It has been reported that PGM1 (a macrophage marker) + histiocytic giant cells within a pyoderma gangrenosum lesion may be indicative of associated inflammatory bowel disease, especially Crohn's disease.[420]

415. Katz SK, Gordon KB, Roenigk HH (1996) The cutaneous manifestations of gastrointestinal disease. **Prim Care** 23:455–476.
416. Gasparini G, Cantu AM, Rigoni C et al. (1993) Unusual features of pyoderma gangrenosum: Two atypical cases. **Cutis** 51:359–364.
417. Lebbe C, Moulonguet-Michau I, Perrin P et al. (1992) Steroid-responsive pyoderma gangrenosum with vulvar and pulmonary involvement. **J Am Acad Dermatol** 27:623–625.

418. Babe KS, Gross AS, Leyva WH et al. (1992) Pyoderma gangrenosum associated with antiphospholipid antibodies. **Int J Dermatol** 31:588–590.
419. Hurwitz RM, Haseman JH (1993) The evolution of pyoderma gangrenosum. A clinicopathologic correlation. **Am J Dermatopathol** 15:28–33.
420. Sanders S, Tahan SR, Kwan T et al. (2001) Giant cells in pyoderma gangrenosum. **J Cutan Pathol** 28:97–100.

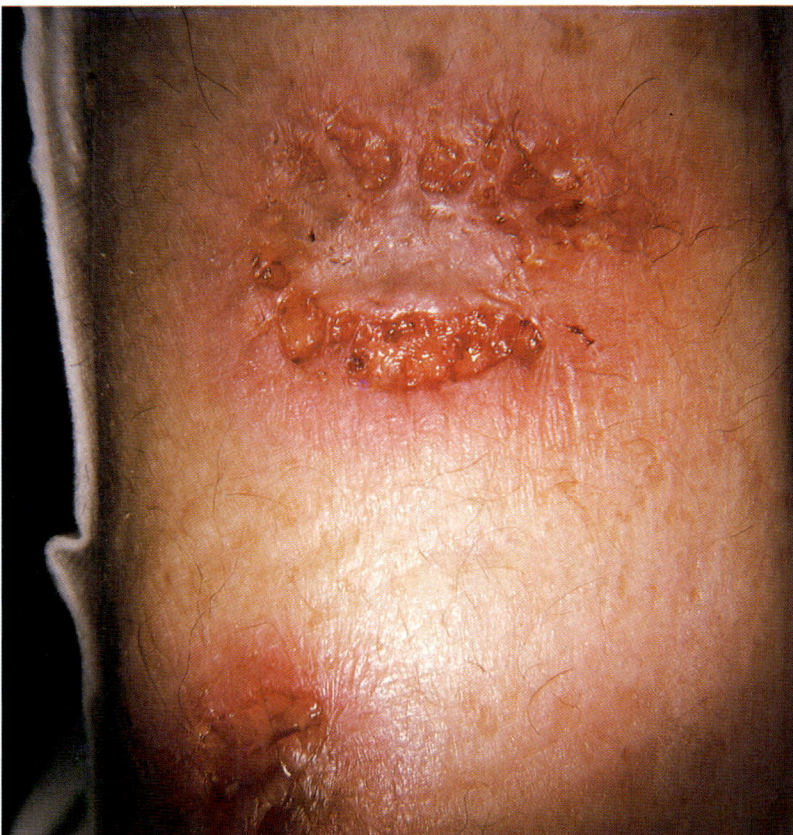

Fig. 23.19 Cribriform scar noted in healing lesion of pyoderma gangrenosum.

DIFFERENTIAL DIAGNOSIS

The differential diagnoses include halogenodermas, systemic vasculitis, factitious lesions, necrotizing fasciitis, periarteritis nodosa, mycobacterial and atypical mycobacterial infections, gummatous syphilis, brown recluse spider bites, and deep fungal infections, including blastomycosis, sporotorichosis, coccidioidomycosis, and cryptococcosis.[409]

MANAGEMENT AND PROGNOSIS

In some patients with inflammatory bowel disease, successful treatment of the bowel disease may result in clearing of the pyoderma gangrenosum.[415] Local care of the lesions of pyoderma gangrenosum consists of soaks or lavage with sterile saline, whirlpool therapy for debridement, and wet compresses. Biologic dressings may be useful in diminishing pain.[409] Most skin grafts placed have been rejected.[409] Intralesional corticosteroids may result in some improvement; however, they typically are not well tolerated because of the pain. Topical tacrolimus 0.1% may lead to rapid involvement if application is tolerated.

Systemic therapy is generally required (Fig. 23.23). Corticosteroids (oral or pulse intravenous) may be used initially.[409,410] If the response is inadequate or if there are contraindications to the use of cortico-

steroids, other immunomodulatory drugs are substituted or combined with the corticosteroids. These include dapsone, cyclosporin, tacrolimus, azathioprine, thalidomide, cyclophosphamide, and mycophenolate mofetil.[409,411,421]

Sulfapyridine, minocycline, and other antibiotics have been used with variable success.[409] Other treatment modalities include clofazimine,[422] mercaptopurine,[410] potassium iodide,[423] chlorambucil,[424] and plasmapheresis.[409] Limited success has been reported with the use of infliximab (an antitumor necrosis factor-α monoclonal antibody).[425]

PEDIATRIC ASPECTS

In pyoderma gangrenosum, limitation of physical activity and school attendance is mainly dependent on the activity of the associated systemic disease. Nutrition and its relationship to growth and development are particularly important in patients with inflammatory bowel disease, leukemias, and those receiving antimetabolites.

CUTANEOUS MANIFESTATIONS OF BOTH ULCERATIVE COLITIS AND CROHN'S DISEASE

The cutaneous manifestations seen in both ulcerative colitis and Crohn's disease are as follows:

- erythema nodosum
- pyoderma gangrenosum
- aphthous stomatitis
- finger clubbing
- pyostomatitis vegetans
- vesiculopustular eruptions.

Cutaneous findings are noted most often associated with ulcerative colitis, less often with Crohn's disease involving the colon, and least often with Crohn's disease involving the small bowel only.[426] The presence of one extraintestinal manifestation in inflammatory bowel disease increases the risk of other extraintestinal manifestations developing.[427]

ERYTHEMA NODOSUM

A common cutaneous manifestation is erythema nodosum, which is reported to occur in approximately 5–10% of pediatric patients with inflammatory bowel disease.[428] The presence of these lesions does not correlate with the extent or severity of the disease, but there is some correlation with the occurrence of arthritis. Erythema nodosum is a somewhat nonspecific finding. Because of the association with multiple diseases, we do not recommend an extensive gastrointestinal workup for every child with erythema nodosum. However, if the erythema nodosum is chronic or recurrent or if it is associated with arthralgias, arthritis, or linear growth deceleration, such a workup should be considered.

PYODERMA GANGRENOSUM

The next most common cutaneous finding is pyoderma gangrenosum. It occurs in 0.5–5% of patients with ulcerative colitis and 0.6–1.2% of those

421. Goldberg NS, Ottuso P, Petro J (1993) Cyclosporine for pyoderma gangrenosum. **Plast Reconstr Surg** 91:91–93.

422. Kaplan B, Trau H, Sofer E et al. (1992) Treatment of pyoderma gangrenosum with clofazimine. **Int J Dermatol** 31:591–593.

423. Richardson JB, Callen JP (1993) Pyoderma gangrenosum treated successfully with potassium iodide. **J Am Acad Dermatol** 28:1005–1007.

424. Resnik BI, Rendon M, Kerdel FA (1992) Successful treatment of aggressive pyoderma gangrenosum with pulse steroids and chlorambucil. **J Am Acad Dermatol** 27:635–636.

425. Tan M-H, Gordon M, Lebwohl O et al. (2001) Improvement of pyoderma gangrenosum and psoriasis associated with Crohn's disease with anti-tumor necrosis factor alpha monoclonal antibody. **Arch Dermatol** 137:930–933.

426. Bernstein CN, Blanchard JF, Rawsthorne P et al. (2001) The prevalence of extraintestinal diseases in inflammatory bowel disease: A population-based study. **Am J Gastroenterol** 96:1116–1122.

427. Rankin GB (1990) Extraintestinal and systemic manifestations of inflammatory bowel disease. **Med Clin North Am** 74:39–50.

428. Hofley PM, Piccoli DA (1994) Inflammatory bowel disease in children. **Med Clin North Am** 78:1281–1302.

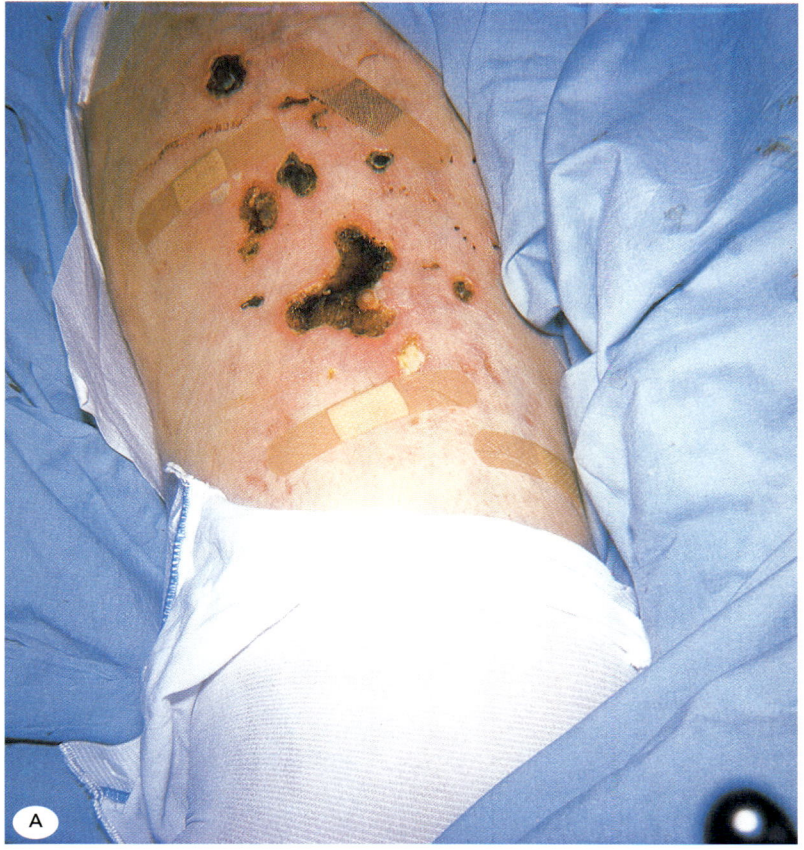
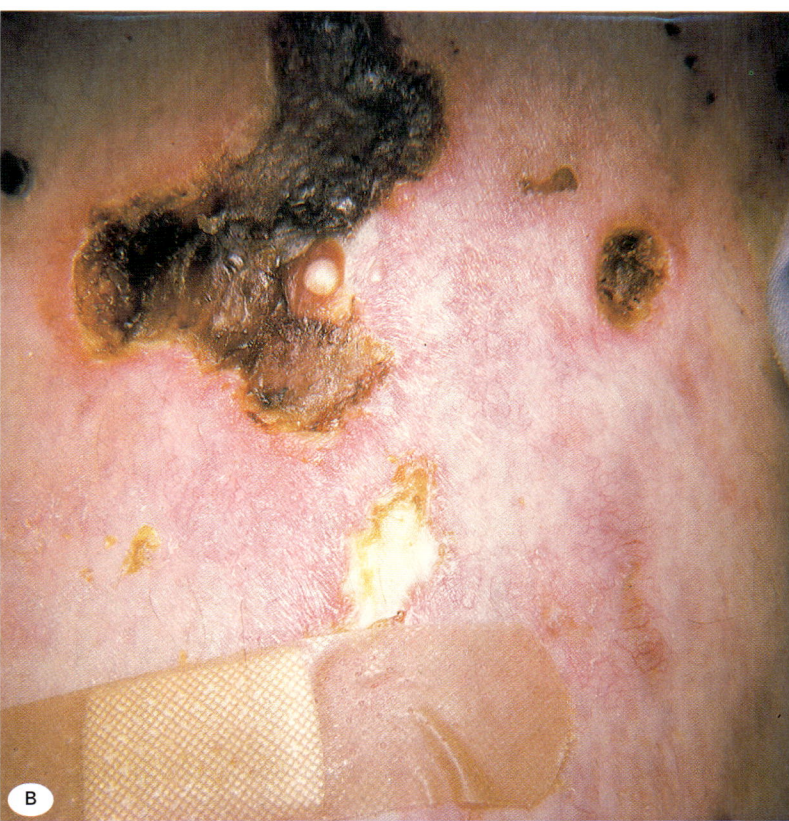

Fig. 23.20   (A) Multiple lesions of pyoderma gangrenosum on the trunk of a patient with ulcerative colitis. (B) Close-up of lesion on trunk of same patient.

with Crohn's disease.[426] Pyoderma gangrenosum has previously been discussed extensively.

APHTHOUS ULCERS

Superficial ulcerations of the oral cavity occur in 6–20% of adult patients with ulcerative colitis and Crohn's disease.[427,428] Pittock *et al.*[429] report that oral manifestations are more common in children than the literature would suggest (in their study >50%). They recommend an expert oral examination at the initial diagnostic evaluation when inflammatory bowel disease is suspected.

FINGER CLUBBING

Finger clubbing has been reported to occur in up to 33% of patients with Crohn's disease.[427] It is somewhat less common in patients with ulcerative colitis and is reported to be less common in children than in adults. The presence of clubbing correlates well with the duration, extent of involvement, and severity of the inflammatory bowel disease.

PYOSTOMATITIS VEGETANS

The term pyostomatitis vegetans was coined to describe a condition in patients with lesions that have a clinical and histologic resemblance to skin lesions in pyodermite vegetante of Hallopeau, a variant of pemphigus

vegetans.[430] Patients have erythema and edema of the oral mucosa. Multiple pustules stud the mucosa along with vegetating papillary projections. Erosions, ulcers, and fibrinopurulent membranes may also occur. Pyostomatitis vegetans is considered a highly specific mucosal marker for inflammatory disease of the gastrointestinal tract; the bowel should be thoroughly examined when this condition is present.[431]

VESICOPUSTULAR ERUPTIONS

Vesicopustular eruptions have been noted to occur in patients with ulcerative colitis and Crohn's colitis.[430] The course of the lesions parallels bowel disease activity. The eruptions may represent a variant of pyoderma gangrenosum.[432]

OTHER CUTANEOUS MANIFESTATIONS OF ULCERATIVE COLITIS

Other cutaneous manifestations of ulcerative colitis include thrombophlebitis and lichen planus. Thrombophlebitis occurs in 5–10% of adults with ulcerative colitis, but it is rare in children. Thrombophlebitis has been linked to a tendency for hypercoagulation in patients with ulcerative colitis.[427,428] Lichen planus has been reported in association with ulcerative colitis.[433] Other lichen planus–like eruptions have been noted and thought to be associated with the treatment rather than the inflammatory bowel disease itself.

429. Pittock S, Drumm B, Fleming P et al. (2001) The oral cavity in Crohn's disease. **J Pediatr** 138:767–771.
430. Bianchi L, Carrozzo AM, Orlandi A et al. (2001) Pyoderma vegetans and ulcerative colitis. **Br J Dermatol** 144:1224–1227.
431. Brinkmeier T, Frosch PJ (2001) Pyodermatitis-pyostomatitis vegetans: a clinical course of two decades with response to cyclosporine and low-dose prednisolone. **Acta Derm Venereol** 81:134–136.
432. Barnes L, Lucky AW, Bucuvalas JC et al. (1986) Pustular pyoderma gangrenosum associated with ulcerative colitis in childhood. **J Am Acad Dermatol** 15:608–614.
433. Gruppo Italiano Studi Epidemiologici in Dermatologia (1991) Epidemiological evidence of the association between lichen planus and two immune-related diseases. Alopecia areata and ulcerative colitis. **Arch Dermatol** 127:688–691.

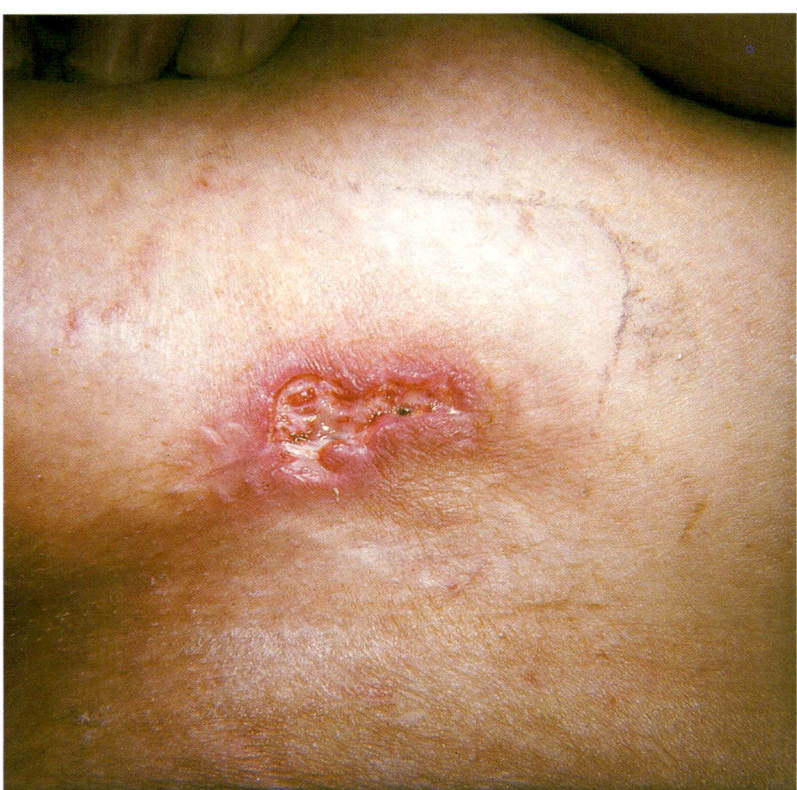

Fig. 23.21   Lesion of pyoderma gangrenosum present on thorax.

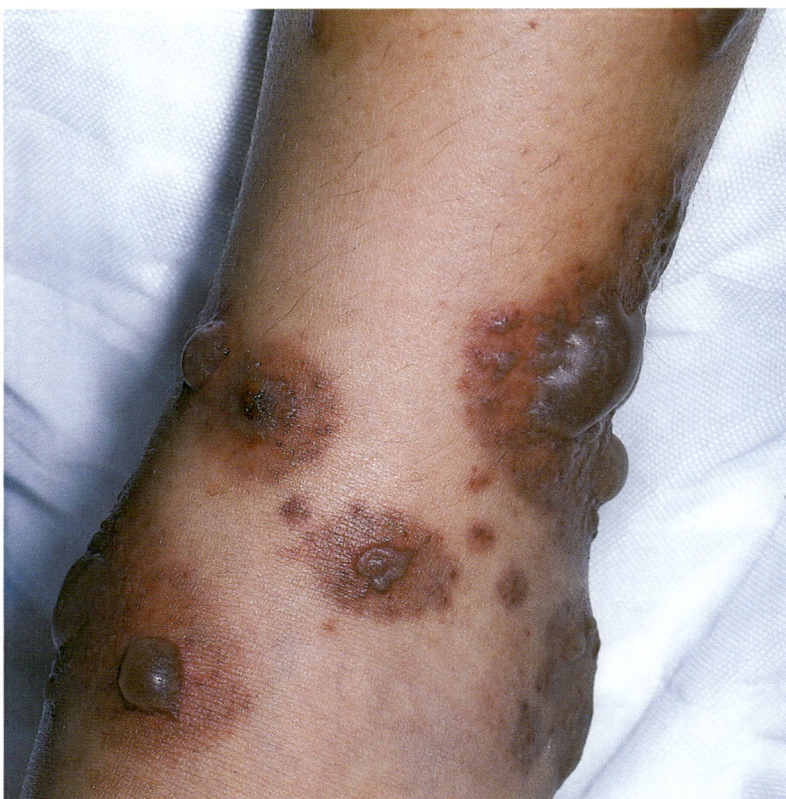

Fig. 23.22   Bullous pyoderma gangrenosum.

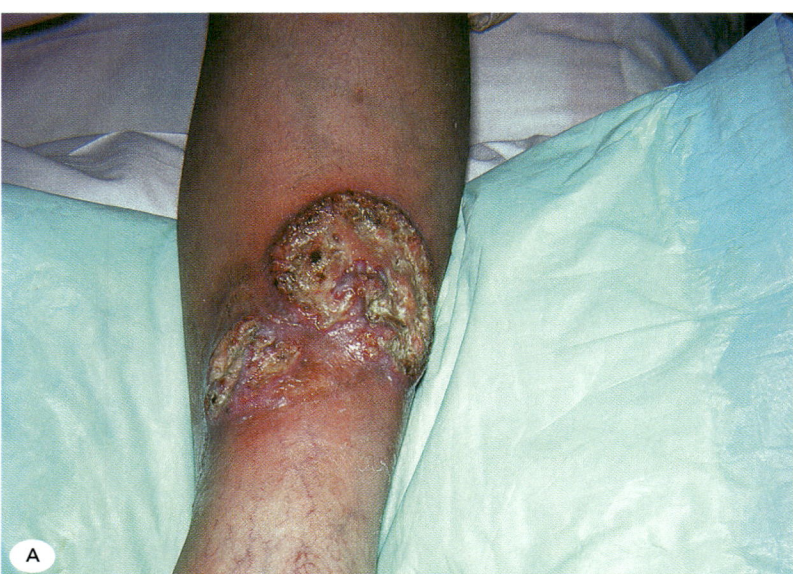

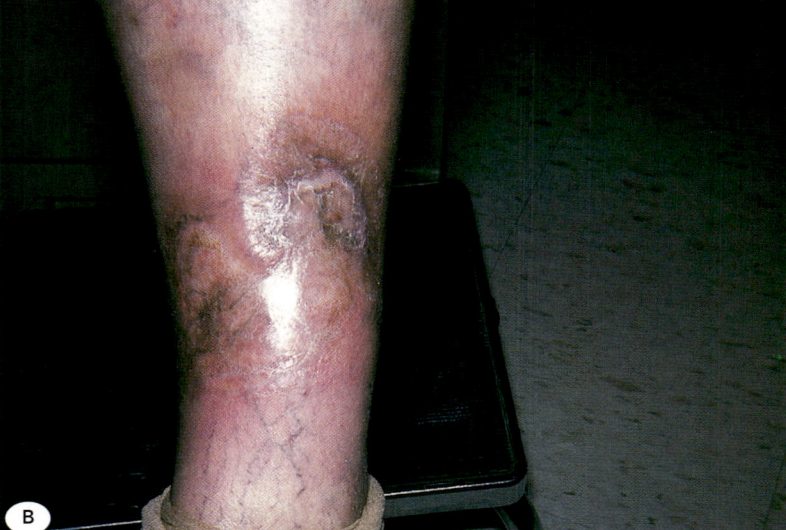

Fig. 23.23   (A) Pyoderma gangrenosum lesion on leg. (B) Well-healed lesion after successful 3-month therapy with dapsone and prednisone.

OTHER CUTANEOUS MANIFESTATIONS OF CROHN'S DISEASE

Other cutaneous manifestations of Crohn's disease are:

- perianal disease
- metastatic Crohn's disease
- perioral disease
- nutritional associations

- other cutaneous manifestations, such as polyarteritis nodosa, amyloidosis, acne fulminans, herpes zoster, and Hermansky–Pudlak syndrome.

PERIANAL DISEASE

Perianal disease, including anal fissures, fistulas, skin tags, and perianal abscesses, occurs in 36–60% of patients with Crohn's disease.[434] Twenty-five to 47% of patients have the perianal disease before the onset of intestinal

434. Palder SB, Shandling B, Bilik R et al. (1991) Perianal complications of pediatric Crohn's disease. J Pediatr Surg 26:513–515.

symptoms.[434] Abscesses and fistulae occur in approximately 20% of patients with Crohn's disease. Abscess formation is more common in patients with ileal disease than in those with purely colorectal disease.[435]

Anal fissures associated with Crohn's disease have a tendency not to occur in the midline, and they are usually painless. Fistulas that can occur are enterocutaneous, rectovaginal, and enterovesical.

METASTATIC CROHN'S DISEASE

Metastatic Crohn's disease is a term used to describe noncaseating granulomatous lesions of skin that are not contiguous to the gastrointestinal tract.[436] Most lesions of metastatic Crohn's disease are ulcerated, especially those in intertriginous areas. Those lesions that are nonulcerative may mimic erythema nodosum.

PERIORAL DISEASE

Four to 14% of patients have perioral disease that is distinctive for Crohn's disease.[437] The lesions may occur before, during, or after the onset of gastrointestinal disease. Nearly all patients with the characteristic perioral findings have perianal disease. The clinical findings include: (1) cobblestoning, especially of the buccal, gingival, and alveolar mucosae; (2) diffuse swelling of the lips and cheeks with fissuring; (3) angular cheilitis; (4) ulceration; (5) tags; and (6) pyostomatitis vegetans.[427,429] Histologically, noncaseating granulomas are seen.[427]

NUTRITIONAL ASSOCIATIONS

Malnutrition occurs in patients with inflammatory bowel disease.[428,457] Mucocutaneous diseases secondary to nutritional deficiencies include acrodermatitis-enteropathica-like syndrome,[438] cheilitis and glossitis.

OTHER CUTANEOUS MANIFESTATIONS

Other cutaneous manifestations noted in Crohn's disease are cutaneous necrotizing vasculitis,[439] necrotizing fasciitis,[440] and amyloidosis.[427]

BOWEL-ASSOCIATED DERMATOSIS/ARTHRITIS SYNDROME (BOWEL BYPASS SYNDROME)

The bowel bypass syndrome was initially described as a complication of jejunoileal bypass surgery. The syndrome consists of influenza-like episodes, with fever, chills, malaise, myalgia, polyarthralgia, and inflammatory papules (Fig. 23.24) and sterile pustules on the extremities and upper trunk. The proposed pathogenesis is thought to involve circulating immune complexes. The antigen may result from bacterial overgrowth in a blind loop in bowel bypass syndrome.

More recently, a bowel-associated dermatosis/arthritis syndrome in patients who have not had bypass surgery was described.[441,442] Patients with bowel-associated dermatosis/arthritis syndrome have been noted to have underlying gastrointestinal disease, some with inflammatory bowel disease. Several patients

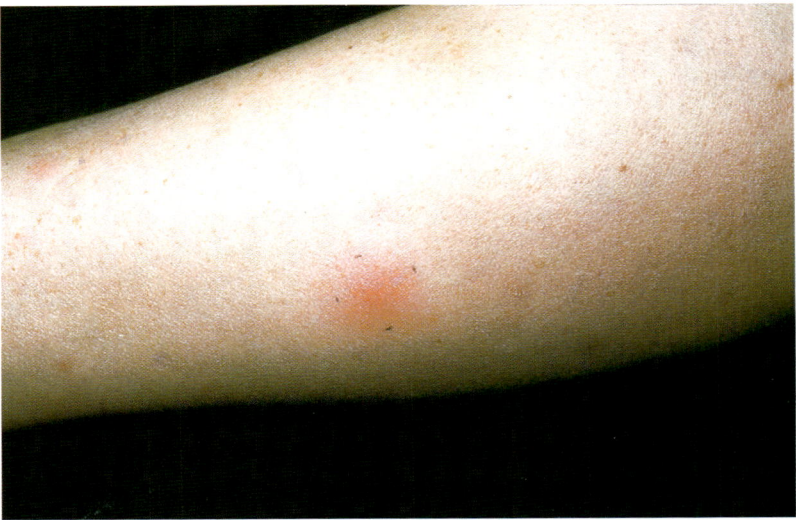

Fig. 23.24   Bowel bypass syndrome, showing an indurated, dusky, vasculitic lesion on leg. (Courtesy of R. Hansen.)

have noted clearing of the syndrome with treatment of the underlying inflammatory bowel disease.[441,442]

Biopsy of the skin lesions shows a diffuse and perivascular infiltrate consisting mainly of neutrophils in the superficial and mid-dermis.[442] Fully developed lesions may show marked dermal edema or a frank subepidermal pustule. Vasculitis (immune complex mediated) has also been noted.

GRAFT-VERSUS-HOST DISEASE

Graft-versus-host disease (GvHD) is an immunologic, multisystem disease which occurs primarily following bone marrow transplantation (BMT).[443,444] GvHD can also occur in neonates or infants with congenital immunodeficiencies who receive blood products. Less commonly, GvHD can be seen following solid organ transplantation.[445,446] The response may be early (acute) or late (chronic). Acute GvHD most commonly involves the skin, liver, and gastrointestinal tract. Chronic GvHD involves multiple organ systems and clinically is similar to a variety of autoimmune disorders.[447] Three conditions must be met for the development of GvHD:(1) immunocompetent cells must be transferred into the host; (2) there must exist a disparity between tissue antigens found in the host and those found in the donor; and (3) the host must be sufficiently immunocompromised so that the graft is not rejected.[448]

EPIDEMIOLOGY

Immunodeficient states in which GvHD have been reported include: (1) *in utero* GvHD, (2) congenital immunodeficiency, and (3) acquired immunodeficiency. The fetus is immunologically immature and cannot destroy viable maternal lymphocytes transfused by spontaneous maternal–fetal transfusion, or by intrauterine blood transfusion for hemolytic disease of the newborn.[449]

435. Hussien M, Mudd DG (2001) Crohn's disease presenting as left gluteal abscess. Int L Clin Pract 55:217–218.
436. Shum D, Guenther L (1990) Metastatic Crohn's disease. Case report and review of the literature. Arch Dermatol 126:645–648.
437. Stotland BR, Stein RB, Lichtenstein GR (2000) Advances in inflammatory bowel disease. Med Clin North Am 84:1107–1124.
438. Heimburger DC, Tamura T, Marks RD (1990) Rapid improvement in dermatitis after zinc supplementation in a patient with Crohn's disease. Am J Med 88:71–73.
439. Lotti TM, Comacchi C, Ghersetich I (1999) Cutaneous necrotizing vasculitis. Relation to systemic disease. Adv Exp Med Biol 455:115–125.
440. van der Merwe SW, Pretorius E, Elloitt E et al. (2001) Anaerobic bacteremia and necrotizing fasciitis in a patient with Crohn's disease. J Clin Gastroenterol 32:451–456.
441. Geary RJ, Long LL, Mutasim DF (1999) Bowel bypass syndrome without bowel bypass. Cutis 63:17–20.
442. Dicken CH (1986) Bowel-associated dermatosis-arthritis syndrome: Bowel bypass syndrome without bowel bypass. J Am Acad Dermatol 14:792–796.
443. Aractingi S, Chosidow O (1998) Cutaneous graft-versus-host disease. Arch Dermatol 134:602–612.
444. Rocha V, Wagner JE, Sobocinski KA et al. (2000) Graft-versus-host disease in children who have received a cord-blood or bone marrow transplant from an HLA-identical sibling. N Engl J Med 342:1846–1854.
445. Ohtsuka Y, Sakemi T, Ichigi Y et al. (1998) A case of chronic graft-versus-host disease following living-related donor kidney transplantation. Nephron 78:215–217.
446. Schmuth M, Vogel W, Weinlich G et al. (1999) Cutaneous lesions as the presenting sign of acute graft-versus-host disease following liver transplantation. Br J Dermatol 141:901–904.
447. Ratanatharathorn V, Ayash L, Lazarus, Fu J et al. (2001) Chronic graft-versus-host disease: clinical manifestation and therapy. Bone Marrow Transplantation 28:121–129.
448. Ferrara JLM, Cooke KR, Pan I et al. (1996) The immunopathophysiology of acute graft-versus-host-disease. Stem Cells 14:473–489.
449. Denianke KS, Frieden IJ, Cowan MJ et al. (2001) Cutaneous manifestations of maternal engraftment in patients with severe combined immunodeficiency: a clinicopathologic study. Bone Marrow Transplant 28:227–233.

Persistent maternal lymphocytes have been demonstrated by chimerism of fetal lymphocytes.[450] Because of the immunologic immaturity, GvHD has been known to occur in neonates without congenital immunodeficiencies. Neonates with GvHD that develops *in utero* may show features of chronic GvHD rather than acute GvHD.

In neonates or infants with congenital immunodeficiences, especially T-cell deficiencies and severe combined immunodeficiencies, the therapeutic transfusion of blood products can lead to transfusion associated GvHD. Irradiation of blood products can ameliorate the reaction by eliminating viable lymphocytes.[451] The reaction usually occurs 7–10 days after transfusion and in some cases is the initial indication of the diagnosis of immunodeficiency.

The largest group of children who develop GvHD are patients with acquired immunodeficiencies who receive bone marrow transplantations. It is estimated that GvHD occurs in 40–60% of allogeneic bone marrow transplant patients.[449]

CLINICAL PRESENTATION

Acute GvHD develops within the first 100 days, usually 2–6 weeks after the introduction of donor cells. The most common presenting feature is a pruritic morbilliform eruption with sudden onset.[443] The face, neck, palms, and soles are usually the initial areas of involvement, followed by a generalized exanthem. The early lesions may be desquamative (Fig. 23.25). During or following the onset of cutaneous manifestations, liver function tests abnormalities may be found. Gastrointestinal symptoms tend to begin with crampy pain or nausea, and often progress to watery or bloody diarrhea. It is not uncommon for patients to develop recurrent fevers, hepatomegaly and lymphadenopathy.

Mild acute GvHD may occur in patients who receive autologous transplants 1–3 weeks after transplantation. "Autologous GvHD" usually is limited to the skin and resolves spontaneously within a few weeks.[452]

Epidermal damage parallels the severity of the GvHD.[453] Early in the course of the disease, the erythema is reflected histologically as mild epidermal damage with few necrotic keratinocytes. Patients with more scaling and

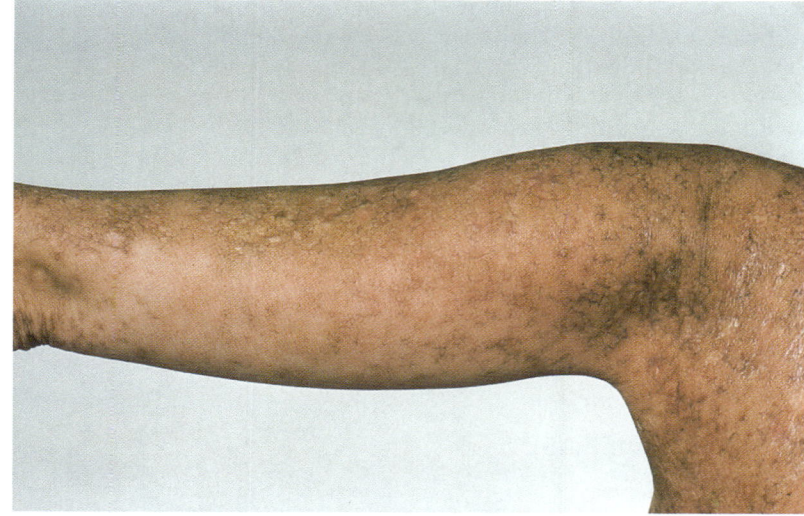

Fig. 23.26   Chronic lichenoid graft-versus-host disease.

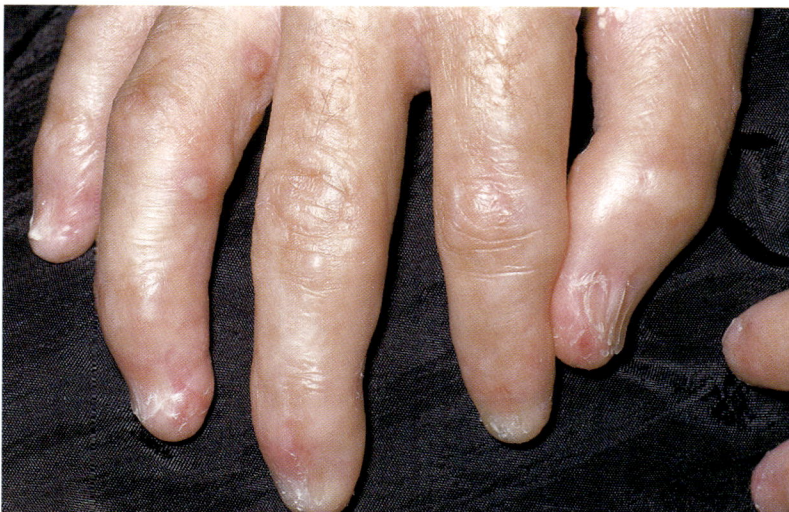

Fig. 23.27   Chronic graft-versus-host disease, sclerodermoid hand changes.

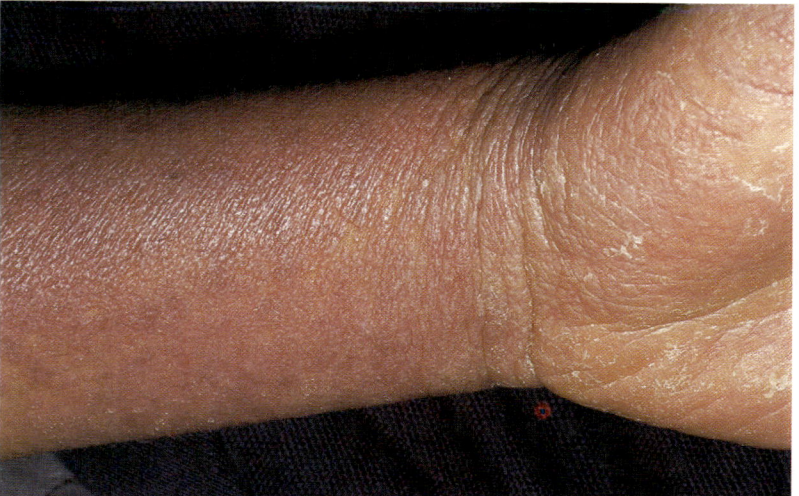

Fig. 23.25   Acute graft-versus-host disease, desquamative lesions.

superficial desquamation have moderate epidermal damage with more necrotic keratinocytes. The vesicobullous form of cutaneous GvHD shows severe epidermal damage with epidermal necrosis.

Chronic GvHD develops at least 30 days after donor cells are introduced. As opposed to the three target organ involvement of acute GvHD, the chronic form is a multiorgan autoimmune-like disorder. The skin is involved in almost all patients.[443] The majority of patients show generalized involvement, but occasional children with chronic GvHD have localized cutaneous lesions.[454,455] Patchy hyper- and hypopigmentation, flat-topped lichen planus–like violaceous papules, papulosquamous plaques, and malar erythema can be seen (Fig. 23.26). Other children have erythema and desquamation which resembles toxic epidermal necrolysis (TEN). After 6–18 months progressive poikiloderma, ulcerations, and sclerodermatous changes with joint contractures may develop (Fig. 23.27). Painful edema

450. Scaletti C, Vultaggio A, Maggi E et al. (2001) Microchimerism and systemic sclerosis. **Int Arch Allergy Immunol** 125:196–202.

451. Webb DK (1995) Irradiation in the prevention of transfusion associated graft-versus-host disease. **Arch Dis Child** 73:388–389.

452. Tokime K, Isoda K, Yamanaka K et al. (2000) A case of acute graft-versus-host disease following autologous peripheral blood stem cell transplantation. **J Dermatol** 446–449.

453. Zhou Y, Barnett MJ, Rivers JK (2000) Clinical significance of skin biopsies in the diagnosis and management of graft-versus-host disease in early postallogenic bone marrow transplantation. **Arch Dermatol** 136:717–721.

454. Beselga E, Drolet BA, Segura AD et al. (1996) Dermatomal lichenoid chronic graft-vs-host disease following varicella-zoster infection despite absence of viral genome. **J Cutan Pathol** 23:576–581.

455. Cordoba S, Fraga J, Bartolome B et al. (2000) Giant cell lichenoid dermatitis within herpes zoster scars in a bone marrow recipient. **J Cutan Pathol** 27:255–257.

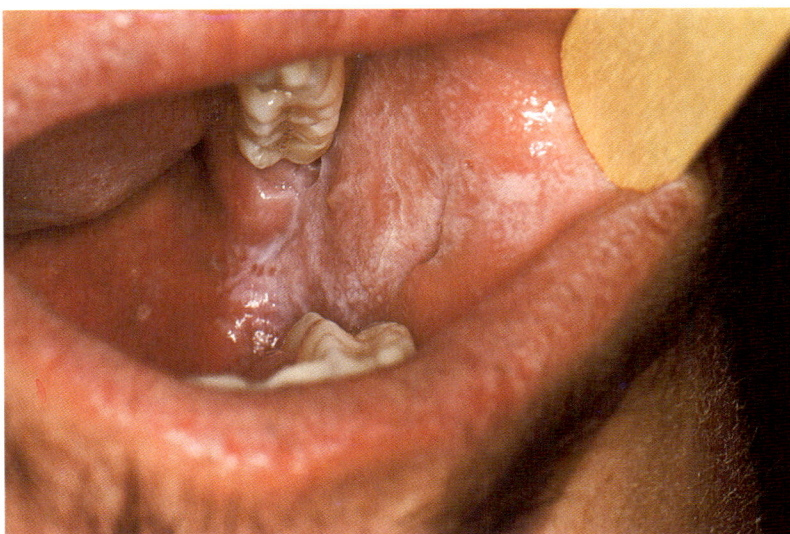

Fig. 23.28   Lichen planus-like mucosal features of chronic graft-versus-host disease. (Courtesy of R. Hansen.)

with overlying taut irregularly thickened skin on the proximal extremities or flanks is characteristic of GvHD- associated fasciitis. Other cutaneous features include: focal to diffuse scarring alopecia, vitiligo, and dystrophic nails. Mucosal lesions are found in 80 percent of patients, which can debilitating.[447] The oral lesions may resemble erosive lichen planus and can be very painful (Fig. 23.28). The lacrimal glands (ocular sicca) and esophagus (desquamative esophagitis with stricture) may be affected as well. Chronic diarrhea, lymphadenopathy, hepatomegaly, arthralgias, pleural and pericardial effusions, myositis, and pulmonary and hepatic insufficiencies are also manifested in chronic GvHD. Weight loss is common due to mucositis and dysphagia. Renal disease is not seen. Patients with chronic GvHD have had persistent immunologic impairment and suffer from recurrent infections.[447]

LABORATORY FINDINGS

In acute GvHD, the most common abnormal laboratory parameters are elevated hepatic function tests, including transaminases, alkaline phosphatase, and bilirubin. Eosinophilia is not unusual. The skin changes seen histologically in skin sections include degenerated keratinocytes with eosinophilic cytoplasm and a pyknotic nucleus, often surrounded by one or more satellite lymphocytes. This association is called *satellite cell necrosis*. In addition, basal cell vacuolar degeneration, spongiosis, and focal, or in severe cases extensive, areas of dermal–epidermal separation may be found.[456]

In acute GvHD, patients show hepatocellular enzyme elevation, whereas in later chronic GvHD the pattern reflects cholestasis. Patients commonly demonstrate eosinophilia (75%). A variety of autoantibodies, including positive ANAs (50%), polyclonal hyperglobulinemia (greater than 50%), and a positive Coombs test (almost 30%) are found. About 25% of patients have anemia, leukocytopenia, and thrombocytopenia. Chest radiographs often show interstitial fibrosis, and pulmonary function tests are abnormal in 50% of patients with chronic GvHD. The histopathologic picture of skin sections in chronic GvHD reflects the clinical appearance. The lichenoid lesions show hyperkeratosis, serrated degeneration of the dermal–epidermal junction (DEJ) with a bandlike infiltrate of lymphocytes, vacuolization of basal cells and

colloid bodies as well as dyskeratotic epidermal cells, often with satellite cell necrosis.[453] Direct immunofluorescence microscopy may show junctional deposits of IgM and C3. In the later poikilodermatous and sclerotic phase, the skin section is characterized by epidermal atrophy, a persistent band-like infiltrate at the DEJ, and dermal sclerosis beginning in the upper dermis. Direct immunofluorescence microscopy often demonstrates a pattern similar to a lupus band, with linear IgM, IgG, and C3 at the DEJ.

PATHOPHYSIOLOGY AND HISTOGENESIS

GvHD is an immunologic process that stems from a disparity between donor and host tissues.[457] The histocompatibility of cells is largely determined by the histocompatibility locus, human leukocyte antigens (HLA). Although the risk of GvHD is greatest in patients whose antigens are poorly matched, GvHD has been seen in recipients of graft whose donors have been HLA-A,B,C, and DRw identical with no stimulation in mixed lymphocyte culture assay. In cases of HLA-mismatched transplants, major histocompatibility antigens are likely responsible. However in HLA-matched transplants, minor histocompatibility antigens play a significant role.[458,459]

Damaged recipient tissues up-regulate HLA expression and intercellular adhesion molecules (ICAM-1) which serve to enhance host antigen presentation to immunocompetent donor T lymphocytes. Immunocompetent donor T lymphocytes recognize a subset of these antigens as foreign. Activated T lymphocytes produce numerous cytokines, including interleukin-2 (IL-2), that stimulate the proliferation and differentiation of T lymphocytes in an autocrine fashion.[448,460] Both CD4+ and CD8+ lymphocytes have been identified in lesional skin.[461]

Cytotoxicity to involved tissue occurs when T lymphocytes recruit monocytes and natural killer cells. A "cytokine storm" leads to local tissue damage. Tumor necrosis factor-α, interferon-γ, IL-1, IL-10, and others play a role. Cytokines may also stimulate fibroblasts that contribute to clinically sclerotic lesions. In addition, T lymphocytes can cause tissue damage through intrinsic cytopathic mechanisms.

The value of skin biopsies to confirm GvHD has been debated.[453,456] Zhou et al.[453] examined 51 patients with clinical findings suggestive of GvHD after allogeneic BMT. The percentage of positive biopsy results varied between 50 and 57% depending on the clinical stage of GvHD. Interestingly, the authors found that the biopsy results had no impact on the initiation of therapy.

DIFFERENTIAL DIAGNOSIS

Acute GvHD may be difficult to differentiate from drug-induced hypersensitivity or infections, especially viral. If the eruption is exfoliative, scarlet fever, staphylococcal scaled skin syndrome, or TEN may be suspected. GvHD in neonates or infants may be confused with ichthyosiform erythroderma, nutritional deficiencies of zinc, biotin, or essential fatty acids, severe seborrheic dermatitis, or Langerhans cell histocytosis. The histologic appearance of skin sections from involved and uninvolved skin often helps to make the diagnosis of GvHD. Occasionally, the histology of the cutaneous reaction to chemotherapy and irradiation can show features of GvHD, including satellite cell necrosis. Serial skin biopsies must be combined with other clinical and biopsy data to help make the diagnosis.

Chronic GvHD must be differentiated from lichen planus, TEN, SLE, dermatomyositis, progressive systemic sclerosis, and Sjögren syndrome. In contrast to progressive systemic sclerosis or LE, renal disease is not a feature of chronic GvHD. The late sclerotic lesions of GvHD can also be differentiated from scleroderma by the marked atrophy of the epidermis in GvHD, and by the

456. Kohler S, Hendrickson MR, Chao NJ et al. (1997) Value of skin biopsies in assessing prognosis and progression of acute graft-versus-host disease. **Am J Surg Pathol** 21:988–996.

457. Storb R (1991) Pathogenisis and recent therapeutic approaches to graft-versus-host disease. **J Pediatr** 118:S10–S13.

458. Tseng LH, Lin MT, Hansen JA et al. (1999) Correlation between disparity for the minor histocompatibility antigen HA-1 and the development of acute graft-versus-host disease after allogenic marrow transplantation. **Blood** 94:2911–2914.

459. Easaw SJ, Lake DE, Beer M et al. (1996) Graft-versus-host disease. Possible higher risk for African American patients. **Cancer** 78:1492–1497.

460. Antin JH (2001) Acute graft-versus-host disease: inflammation run amok? **J Clin Invest** 107:1497–1498.

461. Yamada H, Chihara J, Hamada K et al. (1997) Immunohistology of skin and oral biopsies in graft-versus-host disease after bone marrow transplantation and cytokine therapy. **J Allergy Clin Immunol** 100:S73–S76.

active collagen synthesis in the upper third of the dermis, as opposed to in the lower dermis and subcutaneous tissue in scleroderma.

TREATMENT

The prognosis of GvHD is excellent in patients with limited disease, but is extremely poor in patients with untreated extensive chronic GvHD.[457] The mortality from acute GvHD ranges from 12% (milder disease) to 55% (more extensive disease), and is usually related to infectious complications. Recurrent infections, malnutrition, and hepatic failure contribute to the 25% mortality in patients with chronic GvHD.

Prevention of GvHD in bone marrow transplant patients is extremely important, because acute GvHD itself is a major risk factor for the later development of the more devastating chronic GvHD. Two approaches to prevent GvHD have been used. The first involves the administration of immunosuppressive agents, usually cyclosporin, methotrexate, corticosteroids, or monoclonal antibodies for the first 100 days after transplantation.[462–464] The second approach involves elimination of T lymphocytes from donor bone marrow prior to treatment; this approach, however, is associated with an increased risk of engraftment failure and leukemic relapse. The confinement of patients to a protective environment decreases the risk of GvHD, as well as infection. In addition, any blood or blood product must be irradiated to eliminate viable noncompatible lymphocytes before transfusion into an immunocompromised individual, including a fetus or neonate.

In addition to prophylactic measures for acute GvHD, aggressive supportive care includes hyperalimentation and gastrointestinal rest as needed, and close attention to prevention and treatment of infection. Treatment of acute GvHD involves administration of immunosuppressive therapy, especially corticosteroids, cyclosporin, and/or antithymocyte globulin, thalidomide, and psoralen and ultraviolet radiation (PUVA).[465–467]

Supportive treatment for chronic GvHD includes artificial tears, sunscreens, and prophylaxis against *Pneumocystis carinii* with trimethoprim/sulfa. Early treatment with immunosuppressive drugs (prednisone, azathioprine, cyclosporin, and tacrolimus) given for periods up to a year has favorably affected the course of chronic GvHD.[468,469] Early treatment is important to prevent disability and joint contractures. More recent therapies include etretinate,[470] thalidomide,[465,466] and PUVA, UVB,[471] photochemotherapy,[472] and intravenous lidocaine[473] for the cutaneous involvement.

PEDIATRIC ASPECTS OF THE DISEASE

Patients and families undergoing transplantation require considerable psychosocial support. The isolation of the patient from family and friends can be emotionally difficult for any child. The transplant center is often quite a distance from the patient's home and the financial burden is heavy. Often the bone marrow transplantation is offered as the only hope of survival. The added burden of GvHD, rejection by the graft itself, often suggests failure to the

child. Chronic GvHD can not only be emotionally discouraging, but prolongs the period of removal from school and home, and can lead to extensive disability from sclerosis and contractures in 10% of surviving children.

NEUTROPHILIC DERMATOSES

HISTORICAL ASPECTS

The term acute febrile neutrophilic dermatosis (AFND) was initially used by Sweet[474] in 1964 to describe an uncommon skin condition characterized by painful plaques and associated with fever, arthralgias, myalgias, and leukocytosis.

EPIDEMIOLOGY

AFND is primarily noted to occur in patients in the mid-30s to mid-50s age range, although rare pediatric cases have been described in the literature.[475] Most series show a female predominance. However, the reported pediatric cases have not consistently demonstrated this trend.[475] The age range for the reported pediatric cases is 3 months to 12 years.

PRESENTING HISTORY

Patients with a diagnosis of AFND often present with a history of fever. The fever may be noted to precede the cutaneous findings by days or weeks. Many patients have a history of an upper respiratory tract illness 1 to 3 weeks before the onset of the skin lesions.[475] Patients may complain of headache and gastrointestinal upset.

PHYSICAL EXAMINATION

AFND is characterized by multiple painful erythematous papules, nodules, or plaques that are annular, dusky, infiltrated erythema multiforme-like or purple plum-like lesions (Fig. 23.29). The smaller lesions have a strong tendency to coalesce. The lesions are most commonly noted on the face, neck, and upper extremities. Lesions may be present on the lower extremities but tend to be uncommon on the trunk. The intense edema can produce a pseudovesicular appearance; however, the lesions are firm to palpation. Atypical cutaneous lesions that resemble cellulitis have been noted.[476,477] The lesions have a tendency to occur in crops.

Eye findings include conjunctivitis, episcleritis, and limbal nodules with similar histology to those of the skin lesions.[478]

ASSOCIATIONS

Approximately 15% of adults with AFND have an associated malignancy, with hematologic malignancies being the most common.[479] In pediatric cases, the most common associations are: osteomyelitis (20%), Fanconi

462. Kumar S, Chen MG, Gastineau DA et al. (2001) Prophylaxis of graft-versus-host disease with cyclosporine-prednisone is associated with increased risk of graft-versus-host disease. **Bone Marrow Transplant** 27:1133–1140.

463. Hiscott A, McLellan DS (2000) Graft-versus-host disease in allogeneic bone marrow transplantation: the role of monoclonal antibodies in prevention and treatment. **Br J Biomed Sci** 57:163–169.

464. Carlens S, Aschan J, Remberger M et al. (1999) Low-dose cyclosporine of short duration increases the risk of mild and moderate GVHD and reduces the risk of relapse in HLA-identical sibling marrow transplant recipients with leukaemia. **Bone Marrow Transplant** 24:629–635.

465. Mehta P, Kedar A, Graham-Poole J et al. (1999) Thalidomide in children undergoing bone marrow transplantation: series at a single institution and review of the literature. **Pediatrics** 103:e44.

466. Moraes M, Russo G (2001) Thalidomide and its dermatologic uses. **Am J Med Sci** 321:321–326.

467. Wiesmann A, Weller A, Lischka G et al. (1999) Treatment of acute graft-versus-host disease with PUVA (psoralen and ultraviolet irradiation): results of a pilot study. **Bone Marrow Transplant** 23:151–155.

468. Epstein JB, Nantel S, Sheoltch SM (2000) Topical azathioprine in the combined treatment of chronic oral graft-versus-host disease. **Bone Marrow Transplant** 25:683–687.

469. Choi CJ, Ngheim P (2001) Tacrolimus ointment in the treatment of graft-vs-host disease. A case series of 18 patients, **Arch Dermatol** 137:1202–1206.

470. Marcellus DC, Altomonte VL, Farmer ER et al. (1999) Etretinate therapy for refractory sclerodermatous chronic graft-versus-host disease. **Blood** 93:66–70.

471. Enk CD, Elad S, Vexler A et al. (1998) Chronic graft-versus-host disease treated with UVB phototherapy. **Bone Marrow Transplant** 22:1179–1183.

472. Alcindor T, Gorgun G, Miller K et al. (2001) Immunomodulatory effects of extracorporeal photochemotherapy in patients with extensive graft-versus-host disease. **Blood** 98:1622–1625.

473. Voltarelli JC, Ahmed H, Paton EJA et al. (2001) Beneficial effect of intravenous lidocaine in cutaneous chronic graft-versus host disease secondary to donor lymphocyte infusion. **Bone Marrow Transplant** 28:97–99.

474. Sweet RD (1964) An acute febrile neutrophilic dermatosis. **Br J Dermatol** 76:349.

475. Boatman B, Taylor R, Klein L et al. (1994) Sweet's syndrome in children. **South Med J** 87:193–196.

476. Dompmartin A, Troussard X, Lorier E et al. (1991) Sweet syndrome associated with acute myelogenous leukemia. Atypical form simulating facial erysipelas. **Int J Dermatol** 30:644–647.

477. Tercedor J, Rodenas J, Henraz MT et al. (1992) Facial cellulitis-like Sweet's syndrome in acute myelogenous leukemia. **Int J Dermatol** 31:598–599.

478. Davies R (1992) Limbal nodules in Sweet's syndrome. **Aust N Z J Ophthalmol** 20:263–265.

479. Yoon T-Y, Ahn G-B, Yang T-H et al. (2000) Sweet's syndrome with abscess-like lesions in a patient with acute myelogenous leukemia. **J Dermatol** 27:794–797.

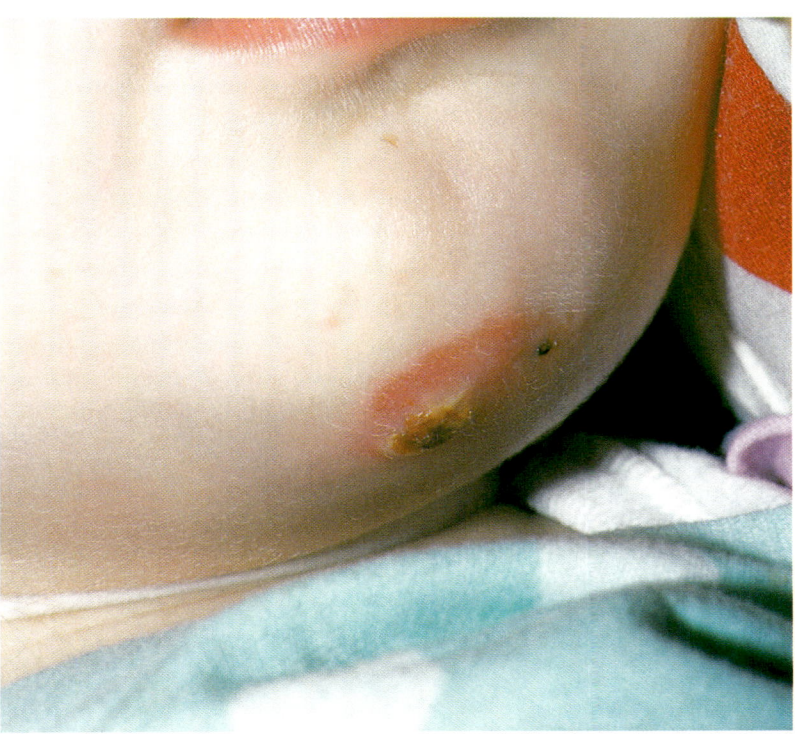

Fig. 23.29   Acute febrile neutrophilic dermatosis (Sweet syndrome) in an infant. (Courtesy of Libby Edwards.)

TABLE 23.6   Criteria for diagnosis of Sweet syndrome (AFND)

Major
    Abrupt onset of tender or painful erythematous or violaceous plaques or nodules
    Predominately neutrophilic infiltrate in the dermis without leukocytoclastic vasculitis
Minor
    Preceding fever or infection
    Accompanying fever, arthralgia, conjunctivitis, or underlying malignancy
    Leukocytosis
    Good response to systemic steroids and not to antibiotics

Adapted from Su and Lui,[490] with permission.

anemia (10%), leukemia (AML, CML) (10%) and coronary artery disease (5%).[475,480]

Acute myeloid leukemia is the disease most often reported in association with AFND in adults. In view of the fact that the lesions may be present for months to years preceding the onset of the leukemia, follow-up of the hematologic status of patients with AFND is recommended.

Other associations in adults include myelodysplastic syndrome,[481] solid tumors,[482] Sjögren syndrome, lupus erythematosus, Behçet's disease,[483] aseptic meningitis and encephalitis,[484] hepatitis B,[485] and inflammatory bowel disease.[486] There have also been reports associated with use of medications, including minocycline,[487] trimethoprim-sulfa-methoxazole, hydralazine, furosemide, celecoxib,[488] and diazepam.[489]

DIAGNOSIS

Major and minor criteria have been proposed by Su and Lui[490] to facilitate the diagnosis of AFND (Sweat syndrome). These are listed in Table 23.6.

LABORATORY FINDINGS

Peripheral leukocytosis is a minor criterion for diagnosis of AFND (Table 23.6). Neutrophils may be present in extracutaneous locations such as CSF, liver, and lungs. The ESR is usually elevated.

PATHOPHYSIOLOGY AND HISTOGENESIS

A dense neutrophilic infiltrate of the papillary and reticular dermis is characteristic of AFND. The infiltrate may be perivascular or diffuse with occasional eosinophils or lymphocytes. Edema of the papillary dermis is evident. Leukocytoclasia without frank vasculitis is considered one of the major criteria for diagnosis.[490] The infiltrate may extend into the subcutaneous tissue with more deeply seated lesions.

An upper respiratory tract illness may precede the cutaneous lesions. This has led to speculation that AFND is a hypersensitivity reaction to a bacterial, viral, or tumor antigen.[490] It has also been proposed that AFND is a response to inappropriate secretion of cytokines[476] and/or granulocyte colony-stimulating factor.[491–494]

DIFFERENTIAL DIAGNOSIS

The differential diagnoses for AFND include erythema multiforme, allergic or necrotizing vasculitis, Behçet's disease, granuloma faciale, erythema nodosum, periarteritis nodosa, erythema elevatum diutinum,[483] bowel-associated dermatosis/arthritis syndrome, and bullous pyoderma gangrenosum.

Lesions of erythema multiforme are characterized by a symmetrical distribution, iris-like morphology, and mucous membrane involvement without lesional pain as a prominent feature.

The absence of vasculitic features on histologic examination can help distinguish AFND from allergic or necrotizing vasculitis.

Behçet's disease is characterized by oral and genital aphthosis, synovitis, posterior uveitis, and meningoencephalitis. The cutaneous vasculitic lesions of Behçet's disease are typically pustular on a purpuric base. Histopathologic examination shows either fully developed leukocytoclastic vasculitis or a neutrophilic vascular reaction.

Granuloma faciale nodules are typically reddish-brown, located most often on the face, usually solitary, and not associated with fever. They have a slowly progressive course and can be distinguished histologically from the lesions in AFND. Nodules in erythema nodosum are located primarily on the leg and show a septal panniculitis on biopsy. Erythema elevatum diutinum plaques tend to be located over the elbows and knees and have characteristic

480. Mc Dermott MB, Corbally MT, O'Marcaigh AS (2001) Extracutaneous Sweet syndrome involving the gastrointestinal tract in a patient with Fanconi anemia. J Ped Hema Oncol 23:59–62.
481. Nogita T, Morioka N, Ishibashi Y et al. (1992) Pelgeroid-like anomalous cells in the diagnosis of neutrophilic dermatosis associated with myelodysplastic syndrome. Int J Dermatol 31:864–865.
482. Barnadas M, Sitjas D, Brunet S et al. (1992) Acute febrile neutrophilic dermatosis (Sweet's syndrome) associated with prostate adenocarcinoma and a myelodysplastic syndrome. Int J Dermatol 31:647–648.
483. Oguz O, Serdaroglu S, Tuzun Y et al. (1992) Acute febrile neutrophilic dermatosis (Sweet's syndrome) associated with Behçet's disease. Int J Dermatol 31:645–646.
484. Noda K, Okuma Y, Fukae J et al. (2001) Sweet's syndrome associated with encephalitis. J Neurol Sci 188:95–97.
485. Tan E, Yosipovitch G, Giam Y-C et al. (2000) Bullous Sweet's syndrome associated with acute hepatitis B infection: a new association. Br J Dermatol 143:892–918.
486. Petermann A, Tebbe B, Distler A et al. (1999) Sweet's syndrome in a patient with acute Crohn's colitis and longstanding anklosing spondylitis. Clin Exp Rheum 17:607–608.

487. Thibault MJ, Billick R, Srolovitz H (1992) Minocycline-induced Sweet's syndrome. J Am Acad Dermatol 27:801–804.
488. Fye KH, Crowley E, Berger T et al. (2001) Celecoxib-induced Sweet's syndrome. J Am Acad Dermatol 45:300–302.
489. Guimera FJ, Garcia-Bustinduy M, Noda A et al. (2000) Diazepam-associated Sweet's syndrome. Int J Dermatol 39:795–800.
490. Su WP, Lui H-N (1986) Diagnostic criteria for Sweet's syndrome. Cutis 37:167–174.
491. Park JW, Mehrotra B, Barnett B et al. (1992) The Sweet syndrome during therapy with granulocyte colony-stimulating factor. Ann Intern Med 116:996–998.
492. Garty BZ, Levy I, Nitzan M (1996) Sweet syndrome associated with GSF-treatment in a child with glycogen storage disease type 1B. Pediatrics 97:401–402.
493. Magro C, De Moraes E, Burns F (2001) Sweet's syndrome in the setting of CD34-positive acute myelogenous leukemia treated with granulocyte colony stimulating factor: evidence for a clonal neutrophilic dermatosis. J Cutan Pathol 28:90–96.
494. Karp DL (1992) The Sweet syndrome or GSF-reaction? Ann Int Med 117:875–876.

histologic features, including leukocytoclastic vasculitis. Although the lesions of bowel-associated dermatosis/arthritis syndrome have a similar histopathologic picture to those in AFND, the two entities are easily distinguishable clinically.

It has been stated previously in this chapter that AFND and bullous pyoderma gangrenosum have significant similarities clinically, histologically, and with regard to associated malignancies. This has prompted some authors to suggest they are indistinguishable neutrophilic dermatoses.

THERAPEUTICS AND PROGNOSIS

The prompt response of this disease to systemic corticosteroids is so characteristic that the response is included as a minor criterion. The recommended pediatric dose is 1–2mg/kg/day of prednisone or an equivalent preparation. The symptoms and signs resolve in 1–3 days. Some patients require a maintenance dose for 2–3 months.

Approximately 50% of patients with AFND experience recurrences. Spontaneous remission has been seen. Typically, there is no response to oral antibiotics. There are reports of improvement with indomethicin,[495] dapsone, and colchicine.

PEDIATRIC ASPECTS OF THE DISORDER

AFND itself is a benign disorder. With treatment, the lesions resolve without scarring. The long-term prognosis is affected by the presence of an underlying malignancy.

PRURITUS

Pruritus is defined as an unpleasant cutaneous sensation that provokes the desire to scratch.[496] It is one of the most common presenting symptoms in dermatologic practice.[497]

Dermatologists are familiar with the various cutaneous disorders that are associated with pruritus. Those patients with generalized pruritus without cutaneous disorders present an additional challenge in terms of evaluation for underlying systemic disease.[498] Estimates vary regarding the occurrence of systemic disease (10–50%) or occult malignancy (3–47%) associated with generalized pruritus.[496] Pruritus is a common complaint in patients with HIV infection.[499] Associations with pruritus are noted in Table 23.7.

TREATMENT

Treatment of the underlying associated disorder may relieve the pruritus. General measures can be instituted to minimize pruritus.[496] Patients are instructed to avoid excessive bathing, use cool or lukewarm water for bathing, and apply emollients while they are still damp. Cotton clothing tends to be less irritating than other fabrics, and use of a humidifier can reduce xerosis. Avoidance of hot foods, alcohol, and heat can be beneficial.

Topical application of preparations containing menthol or phenol can be soothing. Antihistamines are the mainstay for treatment of pruritus.[500] Trials of agents from different classes are recommended if the sedating side effects are not tolerated. H_2 blockers theoretically should be ineffective; however, in specific disorders (e.g., Hodgkin's disease), they can be useful.[496] Other therapies include aspirin, capsaicin, corticosteroids, thalidomide, and ultraviolet light therapy.[466,500]

CUTANEOUS SIGNS OF INTERNAL MALIGNANCY IN CHILDHOOD

There is less likelihood that cutaneous signs indicate internal malignancy in childhood for the following reasons: (1) malignancies are less common in children than adults;[501] (2) some malignancies associated with specific cutaneous disorders occur primarily in adults (e.g., migratory epidermal

---

TABLE 23.7   Associations with generalized pruritus

Renal	Myeloproliferative disorders	Miscellaneous
Chronic renal disease	Hodgkin's disease	Xerosis
	Lymphoma	
Obstructive biliary disease	Leukemia	Drugs
Primary biliary cirrhosis	Multiple myeloma	Aspirin
Extrahepatic biliary obstruction	Mycosis fungoides	Hormones
Intrahepatic cholestasis of pregnancy		Progestins
Drug-induced cholestasis	Visceral malignancies	Estrogens
	Breast carcinoma	Anabolic steroids
Endocrine	Gastric carcinoma	Oral contraceptives
Thyrotoxicosis	Lung carcinoma	Testosterone
Hypothyroidism		Opiates
Diabetes mellitus	Neurologic disorders	Cocaine
Carcinoid syndrome	Multiple sclerosis	Morphine
	Brain abscess	Vitamin B complex
Hematopoietic	Brain tumor	Phenothiazides
Iron-deficiency anemia		Tolbutamide
Polycythemia vera	Infestations	Quinidine
Mastocytosis	Scabies	Idiosyneratic drug reactions
Paraproteinemia	Trichinosis	
	Pediculosis corporis	
Psychiatric disorders	Onchocerciasis	
Emotional stress		
Anxiety, depression		

Adapted from Sher,[496] with permission.

---

495. Jeanfils S, Joly P, Young P et al. (1997) Indomethacin treatment of eighteen patient's with Sweet's syndrome. **J Am Acad Dermatol** 36:436–439.
496. Sher TH (1992) Clinical evaluation of generalized pruritus. **Compr Ther** 18:14–19.
497. Kantor GR (1990) Evaluation and treatment of generalized pruritus. **Cleve Clin J Med** 57:521–526.
498. O'Donnell B, Alton B, Carney D et al. (1993) Generalized pruritus: when to investigate further. **J Am Acad Dermatol** 28:117.
499. Gelfand JM, Rudikoff D (2001) Evaluation and treatment of itching in HIV-infected patients. **Mt Sinai J Med** 68:298–308.
500. Krajnik M, Zylicz Z (2001) Understanding pruritus in systemic disease. **J Pain Symptom Manage** 21:151–168.
501. Maher-Wiese VL, Wenner NP, Grant-Kels JM (1992) Metastatic cutaneous lesions in children and adolescents with a case report of metastatic neuroblastoma. **J Am Acad Dermatol** 26:620–628.

necrolysis and pancreatic glucagonoma); and (3) some disorders that are associated with malignancy in adults do not have that association in childhood (e.g., juvenile dermatomyositis, ichthyosis, and hypertrichosis lanuginosa).

Those signs that are of concern in the pediatric population include: (1) cutaneous metastases; (2) specific genodermatoses with increased incidence of malignancy; (3) specific dermatologic manifestations; and (4) nonspecific dermatologic conditions.

CUTANEOUS METASTASES

The neoplasms most frequently associated with cutaneous metastases in children and adolescents are neuroblastomas, leukemias, and lymphomas.[501] Metastatic cutaneous nodules have been reported in up to 32% of neonates with neuroblastomas. The nodules are firm and blue–gray and have a characteristic central blanching with stroking.

Leukemia cutis lesions are typically firm, reddish-brown, discrete dermal papules and nodules usually noted on the face, scalp, or extremities; they rarely ulcerate.

Cutaneous lesions in non-Hodgkin's lymphoma are characteristically dusky red to violaceous papules and nodules, which may coalesce. In Hodgkin's lymphoma, the lesions are pruritic red–brown to violaceous papules, nodules, and plaques with a predilection for the chest and a tendency to ulcerate. Prurigo nodularis has been reported as a presenting sign of Hodgkin's lymphoma.[502] Among the lymphomas, Ki-1 lymphomas have a particular affinity to metastasize to the skin (Fig. 23.30).[503]

GENODERMATOSES

Genodermatoses associated with an increased incidence of internal malignancy include Gardner syndrome, Cowden disease, Peutz–Jeghers syndrome, several genetic immunodeficiency disorders, basal cell nevus syndromes, tuberous sclerosis, and neurofibromatosis-1.[504] For further information, see Chapters 7 and 21.

SPECIFIC DERMATOLOGIC MANIFESTATIONS

Malignant acanthosis nigricans primarily affects elderly persons with only 10% occurrence in patients younger than 30 years of age.

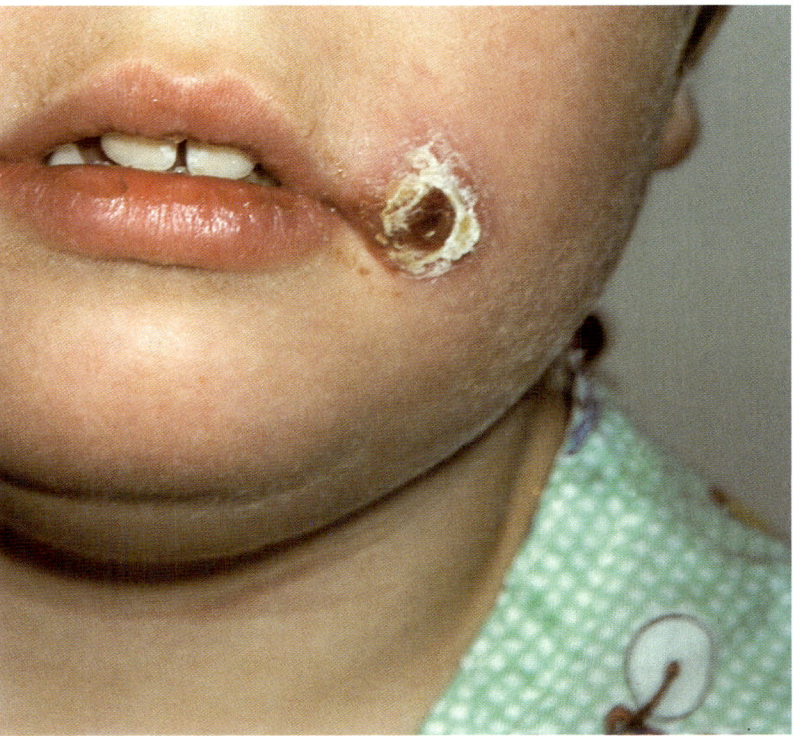

Fig. 23.30   Old large cell lymphoma. The crusted, indurated cutaneous lesion was present at the time of initial presentation.

NONSPECIFIC DERMATOLOGIC CONDITIONS

Several nonspecific conditions have been noted in association with internal malignancy. These include pruritus, AFND, clubbing, vasculitis,[505] erythroderma, and urticaria. Pruritus and AFND have already been discussed earlier in this section. The above signs occur in association with many benign disorders, and their transient occurrence alone does not warrant extensive workup in every patient.[481,506]

Clinicians who care for pediatric patients should be aware of cutaneous associations with malignancies. Although their occurrence is rare, early recognition of these associations can result in prompt therapeutic interventions.

502. Shelnitz L, Paller A (1990) Hodgkin's disease manifesting as prurigo nodularis. **Pediatr Dermatol** 7:136–139.

503. Meier F, Schaumburg-Lever G, Kaiserling E et al. (1992) Primary cutaneous large-cell anaplastic (Ki-1) lymphoma in a child. **J Am Acad Dermatol** 26:813–817.

504. Poole S, Fenske N (1993) Cutaneous markers of internal malignancy. **J Am Acad Dermatol** 28:1–13.

505. Mertz L, Conn D (1992) Vasculitis associated with malignancy. **Curr Opin Rheumatol** 4:39–46.

506. Sigurgeirsson G (1992) Skin disease and malignancy. An epidemiological study. **Acta Derm Venereol Suppl** (Stockh) 178:1–11.

Bacterial Infections

Gary L. Darmstadt, Wesley King Galen and Gayle Fischer

STREPTOCOCCAL AND STAPHYLOCOCCAL INFECTIONS

Gary L. Darmstadt

OVERVIEW

Bacterial skin infections are among the most common problems for which pediatric patients seek medical attention. Approximately one in five children who present for primary pediatric health care have a skin complaint, and among them, bacterial infections are the single most common diagnosis, accounting for up to 17% of visits for skin-related problems.[1,2]

Staphylococcus aureus and *Streptococcus pyogenes* (Group A β-hemolytic streptococci) are the primary pathogens of human cutaneous and subcutaneous tissues, and cause a wide variety of skin lesions through several pathogenetic mechanisms.[3–12] Primary infections develop in clinically normal skin, although minor breaks in the integrity of the skin barrier are required for either of these pathogens to initiate infection. Primary infections develop due to local bacterial replication accompanied by cutaneous inflammation, typically are small and cause little to no local tenderness or systemic manifestations, and remain superficially located in the epidermis and/or dermis. In many cases, these infections are self-limited, although antibiotic therapy may decrease the incidence of complications and hasten resolution. Some primary superficial infections, however (e.g., folliculitis, furunculosis, carbunculosis, paronychia), evolve into abscesses and/or extend from the epidermis and/or dermis to involve deeper subcutaneous tissues. Secondary infections occur in previously diseased or wounded skin. Examples include infection of dermatitis (e.g., atopic dermatitis), cysts (e.g., epidermal inclusion cyst), ulcers (e.g., decubitus ulcer), or wounds (e.g., surgical wound; burn; arthropod bite or burrow). Certain strains of *Staph. aureus* and *Strep. pyogenes* are capable of elaborating exotoxins from a site of primary or secondary skin infection and causing disease directly (e.g., proteolytic activity of staphylococcal epidermolytic toxin on desmoglein I within desmosomes) or through release of other biologically active mediators such as cytokines (e.g.,

toxic shock-like syndrome). Some strains of *Staph. aureus* and *Strep. pyogenes* also are capable, through expression of certain virulence factors, of invading the bloodstream or lymphatics to cause systemic manifestations of disease through bacterial dissemination and replication at tertiary sites, coagulopathy, or vasculopathy. The tertiary skin lesions can involve any of the deeper soft tissues, but spare direct involvement of the epidermis, due to its lack of vasculature. Finally, sterile skin lesions can form following postinfectious immunologic or idiopathic mechanisms (e.g., guttate psoriasis, Henoch–Schönlein purpura, rheumatic fever, erythema nodosum, erythema multiforme, erythema elevatum diutinum, polyarteritis nodosa, Sweet syndrome, scleredema). These latter lesions will not be reviewed here.[4]

Staph. aureus is isolated from approximately 70% of all skin and skin structure infections in children, whereas *Strep. pyogenes* is cultured from approximately 30% of lesions.[10] Notable exceptions to the predominance of *Staph. aureus* and *Strep. pyogenes* in skin lesions include complicated infections such as infected decubitus ulcers, particularly in the inguinal or perirectal regions or on the buttocks; certain bite wound infections; subcutaneous abscesses; and burns which are often polymicrobial and include Gram-negative enteric and anaerobic organisms, enterococci, and coagulase-negative staphylococci.[13–15]

MECHANISMS OF SKIN INFECTION

Development of skin infection due to *Staph. aureus* or *Strep. pyogenes* involves a complex interaction among environmental and local ecological factors; predisposing tissue factors such as local trauma; systemic and local tissue defense of the host; and bacterial factors regulating ability to attach, replicate locally and invade tissues (Table 24.1). Commensal bacterial flora normally play a protective role,[16] and recent evidence suggests that organisms such as *Staph. epidermidis* are capable of upregulating keratinocyte expression of certain cationic antimicrobial peptides (e.g., human β-defensin-2), and may play a role in priming the skin for challenge with pathogens.[17] Transient pathogenic flora are introduced from the environment onto exposed skin or mucosal surfaces and appear to attach only in the presence of a disturbance in the integrity of the skin. *Staph. aureus* and *Strep. pyogenes*, the most

1. Hayden GF (1985) Skin diseases encountered in a pediatric clinic. **Am J Dis Child** 139:36–38.
2. Tunnessen WW (1984) A survey of skin disorders seen in pediatric general and dermatology clinics. **Pediatr Dermatol** 1:219–222.
3. Darmstadt GL, Marcy SM (2001) Skin and soft tissue infection. In: Principles and Practice of Pediatric Infectious Disease, Long SS, Prober CG, Pickering LK, eds. New York: Churchill Livingstone.
4. Darmstadt GL (2000) The skin. In: Nelson Textbook of Pediatrics, 16th edn, Behrman RE, Kliegman RM, Jenson HB, eds. Philadelphia: WB Saunders, pp. 1965–2054.
5. Darmstadt GL, Dinulos JG (2000) Bacterial infections. In: Textbook of Neonatal Dermatology, Eichenfield LF, Frieden IJ, Esterly NB, eds. Philadelphia: WB Saunders, pp. 177–198.
6. Darmstadt GL (1999/2000) A guide to abscesses in the skin. **Contemp Pediatr** 16:135–145. Skin abscesses in children. **Patient Care** 30:1–12.
7. Darmstadt GL (1995) Scarlet fever and its relatives. **Contemp Pediatr** 15:44–63. **Patient Care** 15:109–133.
8. Darmstadt GL (1998) Antibiotics in the management of pediatric skin disease. **Dermatol Clin** 16:509–525.
9. Darmstadt GL (1997) Superficial strep and staph skin infections. **Contemp Pediatr** 14:95–116.
10. Darmstadt GL (1997) Oral antibiotic therapy for uncomplicated bacterial skin infections in children. **Pediatr Infect Dis J** 16:227–240.
11. Darmstadt GL (1997) Staphylococcal and streptococcal skin infections. In: Diagnosis and Treatment of Skin Infections, Harahap M, ed. Oxford: Blackwell Scientific pp. 7–115.
12. Darmstadt GL, Lane AT (1994) Impetigo: An overview. **Pediatr Dermatol** 11:293–303.
13. Brook I (1991) Microbiological studies of decubitus ulcers in children. **J Pediatr Surg** 26:207–209.
14. Brook I, Frazier EH (1990) Aerobic and anaerobic bacteriology of wounds and cutaneous abscesses. **Arch Surg** 125:1445–1451.
15. Brook I, Randolph JG (1981) Aerobic and anaerobic bacterial flora of burns in children. **J Trauma** 21:313–318.
16. Roth RR, James WD (1989) Microbiology of the skin: resident flora, ecology, infections. **J Am Acad Dermatol** 20:367–390.
17. Dinulos JG, Mentele L, Fredericks LP, Dale BA, Darmstadt GL. Keratinocyte expression of human beta-defensin-2 following bacterial infection: role in cutaneous host defense. **J Invest Dermatol**, in press.

TABLE 24.1   Primary factors regulating infection of human skin

Skin factors
Stratum corneum barrier integrity
   Inhospitable environment: dry, acidic pH
   Mechanical barrier: cell envelope
   Biochemical barrier: lipids. Corneocyte shedding removes attached
   bacteria
Skin trauma
Presence and balance of commensal flora
Production of antimicrobial substances
   Cationic antimicrobial peptides (e.g., LL-37, human beta defensin-2,
   secretory leukocyte protease inhibitor [SLPI; antileukoprotease], skin
   derived antileukoprotease [SKALP; elafin])
   Epidermal lipids: (e.g., free fatty acids, phospholipids,
   glycosphingolipids such as spingosine, sphinganine,
   hydroxysphinganine)
   Granzyme B
   Fas ligand proteins
   Hydrogen peroxide
   Nitric oxide
Production of primary epidermal cytokines (e.g., TNF-α, IL-1α, IL-6,
IL-8, IL-12)
   Inhibit group A streptococcal adherence (TNF-α, IL-1)
   Chemotaxis, immunoregulation
Langerhans cells: antigen presentation; elaboration of cytokines, cellular
adhesion molecules, chemotactic factors
Keratinocytes: elaboration of cytokines, cellular adhesion molecules,
chemotactic factors, cationic antimicrobial peptides

Host factors
Presence of chronic dermatoses (e.g., atopic dermatitis)
Corticosteroid therapy
Foreign body
Immunodeficiency disease (particularly involving neutrophils)
Malnutrition
Peripheral vascular disease
Skin trauma
Systemic disease, particularly diabetes mellitus

Environmental factors
Humidity
Temperature
Host exposure to antibiotics, immunosuppressive agents
(e.g., corticosteroids)

Bacterial factors
Inoculum size
Attachment
Virulence factor expression
Synergism with other bacteria

TNF, tumor necrosis factor; IL, interleukin.

important of the transient bacteria, encounter a high degree of natural resitance to colonization and infection of the skin. Although most body sites are free from colonization with *Staph. aureus*, persistent nasal carriage is detected in 20–40% of immunocompetent adults, and up to 20% of people may be colonized on the perineum.[18] This forms an important reservoir for infection of the skin, as staphylococci generally spread from the nose to normal skin prior to the initiation of lesions of impetigo.[19] Colonization of the skin with *Strep. pyogenes* occurs less frequently, but has been documented, particularly in areas with epidemics or a high endemic rate of impetigo. In these instances, in contrast to *Staph. aureus*, *Strep. pyogenes* colonizes the skin an average of 10 days before development of impetigo.[19,20]

Initiation of infection appears to require a break in the integrity of the barrier function of the skin or mucous membranes, although the injury often is trivial or inapparent. The mechanism whereby injury facilitates infection of the skin is unknown, but direct injury to keratinocytes did not alter adherence of *Strep. pyogenes*.[21] It appears that compromise of the epidermal barrier, located in the stratum corneum, may be the most important role of injury by facilitating access of the bacteria to subcorneal layers of skin.

Once pathogenic bacteria have adhered to the skin, they must overcome several avenues of host defense before infection can develop. Intact, overlapping cells of the stratum corneum provide the first and foremost mechanism of defense. Breakdown products of the stratum corneum, including free fatty acids, polar lipids, and glycosphingolipids have anti-staphylococcal and antistreptococcal activity.[22] Many of the resident flora, paticularly the lipophilic corynebacteria, release lipases and thus contribute to defense against *Strep. pyogenes* and *Staph. aureus* by liberating fatty acids from the triglycerides of sebum.[23] The acid mantle thus created favors growth of propionibacteria, which in turn produce propionic acid; this compound has relatively more antimicrobial activity against transient organisms than against resident flora. The skin's immune system, including antigen presentation by epidermal Langerhans cells and cytokine production by keratinocytes, plays a key role in defense from cutaneous infection.[24,25] On the other hand, compromise of immune defense is a primary predisposing factor for development of subcutaneous infections. This may occur locally through trauma or surgery that compromises the barrier function of the skin, or involve systemic immune deficiency, particularly defects in neutrophil response (e.g., insufficient numbers of neutrophils; defects in neutrophil chemotaxis, phagocytosis or intracellular killing; or lack of opsonization) (Table 24.1). Humoral or cell-mediated immunity are relatively less important for combating skin infections due to *Staph. aureus* or *Strep. pyogenes*.

Following attachment, bacterial virulence factors may facilitate invasion of host cells and penetration to deeper levels within tissues, act to evade host defenses, and mediate clinical symptoms of the disease. The bacterial adhesions and host cell surface receptors in the skin involved in initial attachment and infection of the skin with *Strep. pyogenes* or *Staph. aureus* are largely unknown, although insights have been gained recently.[26–30] Hyaluronic acid capsule appears to impede interaction of *Strep. pyogenes* with keratinocytes, whereas inhibition of capsule production is associated with markedly increased

18. Martin RR, Buttram V, Besch P, Kirkland JJ, Petty GP (1982) Nasal and vaginal *Staphylococcus aureus* in young women: quantitative studies. **Ann Intern Med** 96:951–953.
19. Dajani AS, Ferrieri P, Wannamaker LW (1972) Natural history of impetigo. II. Etiologic agents and bacterial interactions. **J Clin Invest** 51:2863–2871.
20. Ferrieri P, Dajani AS, Wannamaker LW, Chapman SS (1972) Natural history of impetigo. I. Site sequence of aquisition and familial patterns of spread of cutaneous streptococci. **J Clin Invest** 51:2851–2862.
21. Darmstadt GL, Fleckman P, Rubens CE (1999) Role of keratinocyte injury in adherence of *Streptococcus pyogenes*. **Infect Immun** 67:6707–6709.
22. Miller SJ, Aly R, Shinefield HR, Elias PM (1988) In vitro and in vivo antistaphylococcal activity of human stratum corneum lipids. **Arch Dermatol** 124:209–215.
23. Ushijima T, Takahashi M, Ozaki Y (1984) Acetic, propionic, and oleic acid as the possible factors influencing the predominant residence of some species of *Propionibacterium* and coagulase negative *Staphylococcus* on normal human skin. **Can J Microbiol** 30:647–652.
24. Nickoloff BJ, Griffiths CEM, Barker JNMN (1990) The role of adhesion molecules, chemotactic factors and cytokines in inflammatory and neoplastic skin disease–1990 update. **J Invest Dermatol** 94:151S–157S.

25. Darmstadt GL, Fleckman P, Rubens CE (1999) TNF-α and IL-1α decrease adherence of *Streptococcus pyogenes* to keratinocytes. **J Infect Dis** 180:1718–1721.
26. Darmstadt GL, Mentele L, Podbielski A, Rubens CE (2000) Role of group A streptococcal virulence factors in adherence to keratinocytes. **Infect Immun** 68:1215–1221.
27. Darmstadt GL, Fleckman P, Jonas M et al. (1998) Differentiation of cultured keratinocytes promotes adherence of *Streptococcus pyogenes*. **J Clin Invest** 101:128–136.
28. Mempel M, Schmidt T, Weidinger S et al. (1998) Role of *Staphyiococcus aureus* surface-associated proteins in the attachment to cultured HaCaT keratinocytes in a new adhesion assay. **J Invest Dermatol** 111:452–456.
29. Akiyama H, Yamasaki O, Tada J, Arata J (1999) Characteristics in adherence of streptococci and *Staphylococcus aureus* isolated from various infective skin lesions: serum IgA decreases adherence of *Streptococcus pyogenes* but not *Staphylococcus aureus*. **J Dermatol Sci** 21:165–169.
30. Akiyama H, Yamasaki O, Tada J, Arata J (1998) Adherence characteristics of *Staphylococcus aureus* and coagulase-negative staphylococci isolated from various skin lesions. **J Dermatol Sci** 18:132–136.

adherence to keratinocytes.[26] Thus, modulation of capsule expression by *Strep. pyogenes* may be important in the pathogenesis of skin infections. Expression of certain cell-surface proteins (e.g., M-protein)[31,32] as well as elaboration of extracellular products such as secreted cysteine protease (i.e., streptococcal pyrogenic exotoxin B, SpeB)[33] has also been associated with tropism for infection of the skin. Identification of the molecular mechanisms of attachment and the factors that facilitate initial bacterial replication in the skin will provide the foundation for development of novel preventative and, possibly, curative therapies.

Signs of infection in the skin may develop as a direct result of bacterial factors (e.g., cytotoxicity), the immunologic response to the presence of the bacteria,[34,35] or both. Invasion of *Strep. pyogenes* may be facilitated by a number of virulence factors.[36] For example, the presence of hyaluronic acid capsule as well as M-protein on the surface of *Strep. pyogenes* acts to impede phagocytosis by neutrophils.[37,38] Some strains of *Strep. pyogenes* produce a peptidase that cleaves the complement component C5a, abrogating its function as a chemotactic factor for neutrophils and thus allowing the bacterium to avoid detection by phagocytes.[39] Acquisition of surface-associated plasmin-like enzymatic activity also contributes to invasiveness,[40] as does streptolysin O, which has cell- and tissue-destructive activity.[41] Streptococcal pyrogenic exotoxins A (SpeA) and/or B (SpeB), as well as certain M-protein fragments of *Strep. pyogenes*, and the toxic shock syndrome toxin-1 (TSST-1) of *Staph. aureus* appear to have the ability to interact simultaneously with the major histocompatibility complex class II antigen on antigen presenting cells and specific Vβ regions of T-cell receptors, inducing massive synthesis and release of cytokines.[42] In hosts lacking toxin-neutralizing antibodies, production of cytokines may mediate systemic signs of toxicity seen in toxic shock syndrome, and tumor necrosis factor (TNF) may mediate, at least in part, the rapid, massive tissue destruction seen in streptococcal necrotizing fasciitis.[43,44] A central feature of the pathology in necrotizing fasciitis, as in many other necrotizing soft tissue infections, is vascular injury and thrombosis of arteries and veins passing through the fascia.[45] Possible mechanisms for the vascular injury leading to tissue ischemia and necrosis in streptococcal necrotizing fasciitis are direct cytolytic factors released from bacteria, immune mediated vascular damage due to the inflammatory infiltrate surrounding the blood vessels, and/or noninflammatory intravascular coagulation.

Skin defense against bacterial skin infection is poorly understood at the molecular level, but emerging evidence suggests that a variety of mechanisms are involved (Table 24.1).[46] Innate defenses include maintenance of an intact stratum corneum, including a dry, acidic environment, and elaboration of a variety of antimicrobial substances. Of particular interest is the role of cationic antimicrobial peptides (CAPs) produced in the skin, which assert direct antimicrobial activity on the bacterial cytoplasmic membrane, and also link innate assert and adaptive (specific, antigen-dependent) immune responses. Recent reports have demonstrated the functional importance of the cathelicidin family of antimicrobial peptides, including human LL-37, in innate cutaneous immunity against *Strep. pyogenes*.[47,48] It has also been suggested that cytokine production in the skin (i.e., TNF-α, interleukin (IL)-1) may serve directly in antimicrobial defense, for example by inhibiting adherence of *Strep. pyogenes*,[25] in addition to their role in activating inflammatory immune defenses.[49]

Some skin infections appear to be caused by two or more organisms that act synergistically. Synergism occurs when a mixture of organisms causes a more severe infection than the sum of the damage caused by each of the organisms acting alone. In these instances, therapy is most effective when directed against all the pathogenic organisms present. Synergism does not appear to be a factor in most superficial skin infections, and as a rule, superficial infections due to *Staph. aureus* and *Strep. pyogenes* can be treated with single antibiotics directed against them. In many instances of necrotizing soft tissue infection, however, synergism is operative,[50–52] and may involve a variety of anaerobic, aerobic and facultative bacteria. Mechanisms of synergy are not well understood, but may involve such factors as mutual protection from phagocytosis and intracellular killing; promotion of bacterial capsule formation; production of essential growth factors or energy sources; and utilization of oxygen by facultative bacteria, lowering host tissue oxidation-reduction potential and facilitating growth of anaerobes.[53,54]

DIAGNOSIS OF SKIN INFECTION

Identification of the pathogen(s) causing a particular skin infection may be enhanced through proper use and careful interpretation of diagnostic tests. If the surface of a wound or site of infection is swabbed and cultured, organisms that are colonizing but not infecting the skin may be identified. If an organism is found on both Gram stain, or special stains in the case of fungi, as well as culture, it increases the likelihood that it is playing a pathogenic role. Chances of identifying the true pathogen(s) are increased further if cultures are obtained by swabbing the exudate directly from the source of suppuration, by fine-needle aspiration, or by biopsy. Cultures from abscesses and subcutaneous tissue infections should be obtained for both aerobic and anaerobic organisms. Specimens should be cultured on blood agar, chocolate agar, and/or MacConkey's agar to identify the full range of pyogenic, fastidious, and Gram-negative enteric organisms that may infect the skin and subcutaneous tissues. Isolation of anaerobic organisms can be accomplished by

31. Bessen DE, Carapetis JR, Beall B et al. (2000) Contrasting molecular epidemiology of group A streptococci causing tropical and nontropical infections of skin and throat. **J Infect Dis** 182:1109–1116.
32. Bessen DE, Sotir CM, Readdy TL, Hollingshead SK (1996) Genetic correlates of throat and skin isolates of group A streptococci. **J Infect Dis** 173:896–900.
33. Svensson MD, Scaramuzzino DA, Sjobring U et al. (2000) Role for a secreted cysteine proteinase in the establishment of host tissue tropism by group A streptococci. **Mol Microbiol** 38:242–253.
34. Molne L, Verdrengh M, Tarkowski A (2000) Role of neutrophil leukocytes in cutaneous infection caused by *Staphylococcus aureus*. **Infect Immun** 68:6162–6167.
35. Molne L, Tarkowski A (2000) An experimental model of cutaneous infection induced by superantigen-producing *Staphylococcus aureus*. **J Invest Dermatol** 114:1120–1125.
36. Jonas M, Darmstadt GL, Rubens CE, Chi EY (1998) Ultrastructure of invasion of group A streptococcus into human keratinocytes. **Proc 14th Intl Congr Electron Microsc** 4:375–376.
37. Dale JB, Washburn RG, Marques MB, Wessels MR (1996) Hyaluronic acid capsule and surface M protein in resistance to phagocytosis of group A streptococci. **Infect Immun** 64:1495–1501.
38. Engleberg NC, Health A, Miller A et al. (2001) Spontaneous mutations in the CsrRS two-component regulatory system of Streptococcus pyogenes result in enhanced virulence in a murine model of skin and soft tissue infection. **J Infect Dis** 183:1043–1054.
39. Cleary P, Prabu U, Dale J et al. (1992) Streptococcal C5a peptidase is a highly specific endopeptidase. **Infect Immun** 60:5219–5223.
40. Li Z, Ploplis VA, French EL, Boyle MDP (1999) Interaction between group A streptococci and the plasmin(ogen) system promotes virulence in a mouse skin infection model. **J Infect Dis** 179:907–914.
41. Limbago B, Penumalli V, Weinrick B, Scott JR (2000) Role of streptolysin O in a mouse model of invasive group A streptococcal disease. **Infect Immun** 68:6384–6390.
42. Bisno AL, Stevens DL (1996) Streptococcal infections of skin and soft tissues. **N Engl J Med** 334:240–245.
43. Stevens DL (1994) Invasive group A streptococcal infections: the past, present and future. **Pediatr Infect Dis J** 13:561–566.
44. Eriksson BKG, Andersson J, Holm SE, Norgren M (1999) Invasive group A streptococcal infections: T1M1 isolates expressing pyrogenic exotoxins A and B in combination with selective lack of toxin-neutralizing antibodies are associated with increased risk of streptococcal toxic shock syndrome. **J Infect Dis** 180:410–418.
45. Stamenkovic I, Lew PD (1972) Early recognition of potentially fatal necrotizing fasciitis. **N Engl J Med** 310:1689–1693.
46. Gallo RL, Huttner KM (1998) Antimicrobial peptides: an emerging concept in cutaneous biology. **J Invest Dermatol** 111:739–743.
47. Nizet V, Ohtake T, Lauth X et al. (2001) Innate antimicrobial peptide protects the skin from invasive bacterial infection. **Nature** 414:454–457.
48. Dorschner RA, Pestonjamasp VK, Tamakuwala S et al. (2001) Cutaneous injury induces the release of cathelicidin anti-microbial peptides active against group A streptococcus. **J Invest Dermatol** 117:91–97.
49. Kupper TS, Groves RW (1995) The interleukin-1 axis and cutaneous inflammation. **J Invest Dermatol** 105:62S–66S.
50. Barker FG, Leppard BJ, Seal DV (1987) Streptococcal necrotizing fasciitis: comparison between histological and clinical features. **J Clin Pathol** 40:335–341.
51. Brook I, Frazier EH (1995) Clinical and microbiological features of necrotizing fasciitis. **J Clin Microbiol** 33:2382–2387.
52. Stevens DL (1992) Invasive group A streptococcus infections. **Clin Infect Dis** 14:2–13.
53. Brook I (1994) The role of encapsulated anaerobic bacteria in synergistic infections. **FEMS Microbiol Rev** 13:65–74.
54. Kingston D, Seal DV (1990) Current hypotheses on synergistic microbial gangrene. **Br J Surg** 77:260–264.

use of anaerobic media such as *Brucella* agar supplemented with vitamin K_1 and hemin, and brain heart infusion broth, or thioglycolate broth. Once the pathogen(s) has been identified, antibiotic susceptibility testing may aid in optimizing the antimicrobial regimen.

Some skin diseases caused by infectious agents have characteristic histopathologic findings (e.g., bullous impetigo) that may aid in reaching a diagnosis when such is unclear on clinical or microbiological grounds. Additional studies on biopsy material, such as immunofluorescence testing and electron microscopy may also be useful in certain situations, particularly in excluding noninfectious diseases that may closely mimic a given skin infection.

In some cases, in order to formulate a diagnosis and treatment plan, it may be imperative to define the depth of infection. For example, in the case of soft tissue infection, magnetic resonance imaging may be useful to distinguish cellulitis from necrotizing fasciitis or myositis.[55] In the case of necrotizing soft tissue infections, however, surgical exploration is necessary for definitive diagnosis and for effective treatment.

Antigen detection or immunologic tests have little utility in the management of skin infections. Antideoxyribonuclease B titers, however, may aid in confirming previous infection with *Strep. pyogenes* and may be useful in reaching a diagnosis of impetigo-associated poststreptococcal glomerulonephritis.[56]

TREATMENT OF SKIN INFECTIONS

Most superficial skin infections due to *Staph. aureus* or *Strep. pyogenes* can be treated effectively with local wound care and oral antibiotics. However, depending on the age and health of the patient; the rapidity, severity, and location of the infection; and the presence of constitutional signs of illness; parenteral antibiotic therapy may be necessary. In general, parenteral therapy is indicated for treatment of neonates.[5] Surgical drainage and tissue debridement, particularly for treatment of abscesses and necrotizing infections, may also be required.

ANTIBIOTIC RESISTANCE

Erythromycin resistance

Oral erythromycin has been a gold-standard therapy for uncomplicated skin infections for the past several decades. In recent years, however, resistance of *Strep. pyogenes* to erythromycin has emerged, although in North America the prevalence of erythromycin resistance among isolates of *Strep. pyogenes* has remained below 5%.[57] While resistance of *Strep. pyogenes* to erythromycin is not currently problematic, the threat of increased resistance exists, particularly if macrolide usage were to increase. The rate of erythromycin resistance among *Staph. aureus* strains isolated from sites of skin and soft tissue infection in children in the continental United States generally is 10 to 20%, although it is not yet clear whether *in vitro* erythromycin resistance is a clinically significant problem in the treatment of impetigo and other pyogenic skin infections.[10] Many experts, however, particularly in areas with relatively high resistance rates, choose to use other agents for empirical treatment.

Penicillin resistance

Classic resistance to penicillin among group A streptococci has not yet been documented, and the *in vitro* sensitivity of *Strep. pyogenes* to penicillin remains unchanged.[57] Apparent sensitivity of *Strep. pyogenes* to antibiotic therapy, however, may be affected by the inoculum (or Eagle) effect. This occurs when the clinical efficacy of penicillin is reduced in the presence of a large inoculum of bacteria due to their entry into a slower or stationary phase of growth,

rendering them less susceptible to β-lactam antibiotics that act by interrupting cell wall synthesis.[58] The inoculum effect may also be due to alterations in penicillin-binding proteins in slow-growing *Strep. pyogenes*, decreasing the target for the β-lactam antibiotics. Since clindamycin efficacy is not impacted, it is preferable to penicillin for treatment of deep-seated, serious soft tissue and exotoxin-elaborating group A streptococcal infections. The majority of skin isolates of *Staph. aureus* are resistant to penicillin. Consequently, penicillin or amoxicillin are unacceptable empiric choices for treatment of uncomplicated skin and skin structure infections, including impetigo.

Methicillin resistance

Methicillin resistance among isolates of *Staph. aureus* is associated with resistance to the semisynthetic penicillins cloxacillin and dicloxacillin, and most isolates of methicillin-resistant *Staph. aureus* (MRSA) also produce β-lactamase and may serve as reservoirs of transmissible resistance elements for a variety of other antimicrobial agents including erythromycin, clindamycin, tetracycline, sulfonamides, chloramphenicol, the cephalosporins and the quinolones.[59] Thus, the abbreviation MRSA in practice suggests the presence of "*multiply* resistant *Staph. aureus*." Currently, the only consistently reliable agent for treatment of MRSA is parenteral vancomycin, although each case needs to be evaluated individually and treated based on a consideration of the isolate's antibiotic susceptibility profile and the severity of the infection; alternatives, depending the isolate's specific resistance pattern, may include macrolides, tetracyclines, and the fluoroquinolones.[60,61] Newer or experimental agents that may play a role in the treatment of resistant *Staph. aureus* include streptogramins (quinopristin-dalfopristin), and oxazolidinones (linezolid).[62]

Mupirocin resistance

High-level resistance to mupirocin has emerged, but remains rare among isolates of MRSA, methicillin-sensitive *Staph. aureus*, and coagulase-negative staphylococci.[63] Mupirocin resistance has been reported primarily in patients with severe skin disease whose treatment was inappropriately prolonged or was intermittent. *In vitro* high-level resistance has clinical significance as it has been associated with failure to eradicate the organism from both colonized and infected adult patients.

ANTIBIOTIC TREATMENT

A number of oral antibiotics have been approved for treatment of skin and skin structure infections due to *Staph. aureus* and *Strep. pyogenes*, and have been reviewed previously (Table 24.2).[8,10] The first-line agents for treatment of skin infections during the past two decades have been erythromycin, dicloxacillin, cloxacillin, and cephalexin. Clindamycin has been used occasionally, particularly for treatment of recurrent, recalcitrant skin infections such as furunculosis due to *Staph. aureus*. Each of these agents, however, has important limitations to its use. Erythromycin commonly causes gastrointestinal intolerance; dicloxacillin suffers from an unpalatable taste; and all of the agents, including cephalexin, must be given three to four times daily to optimize their effectiveness. The relative risk of *Clostridium difficile* toxin-associated diarrhea is higher with clindamycin than with any other commonly used oral antibiotic. Fortunately, several new alternatives to these agents can be considered.

Topical agents

Mupirocin reversibly and selectively inhibits bacterial isoleucyl-tRNA synthetase relative to the human analog. Moreover, resident skin bacteria

55. Zittergruen M, Grose C (1993) Magnetic resonance imaging for early detection of necrotizing fasciitis. **Pediatr Emerg Care** 9:26–28.
56. Dillon HC, Reeves MSA (1974) Streptococcal immune responses in nephritis after skin infection. **Am J Med** 56:333–346.
57. Gerber MA (1995) Antibiotic resistance in group A streptococci. **Pediatr Clin N Am** 42:539–551.
58. Stevens DL, Yan S, Bryant AE (1993) Penicillin-binding protein expression at different growth stages determines penicillin efficacy in vitro and in vivo: An explanation for the inoculum effect. **J Infect Dis** 167:1401–1405.
59. Moreira BM, Daum RS (1995) Antimicrobial resistance in staphylococci. **Pediatr Clin N Am** 42:619–648.
60. Shetty N, Wilson AP (2000) Sitafloxacin in the treatment of patients with infections caused by vancomycin-resistant enterococci and methacillen-resistant *Staphylococcus aureus*. **J Antimicrob Chemother** 46:633–638.
61. Paradisi F, Corti G, Messeri D (2001) Antistaphylococcal (MSSA, MRSA, MSSE, MRSE) antibiotics. **Med Clin North Am** 85:1–17.
62. French G (2001) Linezolid. **Int J Clin Pract** 55:59–63.
63. Bradley SF, Ramsey MA, Morton TM, Kauffman CA (1995) Mupirocin resistance: Clinical and molecular epidemiology. **Infect Control Hosp Epidemiol** 16:354–358.

TABLE 24.2 Cutaneous and subcutaneous infections due to staphylococci and streptococci

Disease entity	Infectious agent(s)*
Superficial Infections	
Impetigo	Staph. aureus, Strep. pyogenes
Blastomycosis-like pyoderma	Staph. aureus, Strep. pyogenes
Ecthyma	Strep. pyogenes
Folliculitis	Staph. aureus, coagulase (−) staphylococci
Sycosis barbae	Staph. aureus
Blistering distal dactylitis	Strep. pyogenes, group B streptococcus, Staph. aureus
Perianal dermatitis	Strep. pyogenes, rarely Staph. aureus
Periocular infection	
Blepharitis	Staph. aureus
Internal hordeolum	Staph. aureus
External hordeolum	Staph. aureus
Dermatoblepharitis	Staph. aureus, Strep. pyogenes
Acute dacryocystitis	Staph. aureus, Strep. pyogenes
Dacryoadenitis	Staph. aureus, Strep. pyogenes
Abscesses	
Furuncle, carbuncle	Staph. aureus
Multiple sweat gland abscesses	Staph. aureus
Paronychia	Staph. aureus, Strep. pyogenes
Breast abscess	Staph. aureus, group B streptococcus
Perirectal abscess	Staph. aureus, Strep. pyogenes (generally mixed flora)
Scalp abscess	Staph. aureus, Strep. pyogenes, group B or D streptococci
Suppurative sialadenitis	Staph. aureus, Strep. pyogenes
Botyromycosis	Staph. aureus, α-hemolytic streptococci
Non-necrotizing subcutaneous tissue infections	
Cellulitis	Strep. pyogenes, Staph. aureus, group B, C or G streptococci, Strep. pneumoniae
Erysipelas	Strep. pyogenes, group B, C, D, or G streptococci; Staph. aureus; Strep. pneumoniae
Lymphangitis	Strep. pyogenes, group B or D streptococci; Staph. aureus
Necrotizing subcutaneous tissue infections	
Necrotizing fasciitis	Type I (mixed) infection: hemolytic or nonhemolytic nongroup A streptococcus, Staph. aureus
	Type II: Strep. pyogenes+/− Staph. aureus
	Rare monomicrobial infections: group B, C, F, or G streptococci; Staph. aureus, Strep. pneumoniae
Toxin-mediated diseases	
Scarlet fever	Strep. pyogenes
Scalded skin syndrome	Staph. aureus
Toxic shock syndrome	Staph. aureus, Strep. pyogenes

* See text for alternative causes of the diseases entities shown.

(e.g., *Micrococcus* spp., coryneforms, propionibacteria) generally are less sensitive than pathogenic *Strep. pyogenes* or *Staph. aureus* to mupirocin,[64] thus the natural skin flora is relatively undisturbed. Several studies have shown that mupirocin is equal in efficacy to erythromycin for treatment of impetigo (see Impetigo, below). A cream formulation has also shown excellent efficacy for treatment of common skin infections, and is less irritating to the nares than mupirocin ointment.[65]

Fusidic acid is also very effective in treating superficial infections, and appears comparable in efficacy to mupirocin.[66] Unfortunately, however, use in the United Kingdom has been associated with emergence of high-level resistant isolates of *Staph. aureus*.[67] The nonantibiotic agents, tacrolimus ointment and topical corticosteroids reduce skin colonization with *Staph. aureus* in patients with atopic dermatitis.[68]

Cephalosporins

The cephalosporins are bactericidal for most species through binding to penicillin-binding proteins and inhibition of mucopeptide synthesis in the bacterial cell wall. The risk of an allergic reaction to a cephalosporin in a patient with a history of penicillin sensitivity is low (2%).[69] Consequently, these agents generally are safe to administer to penicillin-allergic patients, although caution and appropriate supervision is advisable. Differences among the cephalosporins in their side-effect profile are minor, except that cefaclor appears to cause hypersensitivity reactions relatively more often (approximately 5%) than other cephalosporins or amoxicillin (approximately 3–4%).[69] It is important to consider that cephalosporins exhibit time-dependent or concentration-independent killing. Thus, the duration of time over which the drug concentration at its site of action (i.e., skin blister fluid) is above the minimum inhibitory concentration (MIC) or minimum bactericidal concentration of the pathogen is most closely correlated with ability to kill and with clinical outcome. Oral cephalosporins that remain equal to or more than 50% but less than 90% of their dosing interval over the MIC for 90% of *Staph. aureus* isolates include cefuroxime axetil, cephalexin, and cefadroxil.[70] This level of activity against *Strep. pyogenes* in skin and soft tissue is met by all cephalosporins tested (cephalexin, cefadroxil, cefaclor, cefprozil, cefuroxime axetil, loracarbef, cefpodoxime proxetil, cefixime). Although infrequent dosing intervals are convenient and associated with increased compliance, extending the dosing interval beyond that recommended for a given agent may increase the likelihood of clinical failure due to the time-dependence for killing.

First-generation cephalosporins

First-generation cephalosporins have excellent activity against methicillin-sensitive *Staph. aureus* and *Strep. pyogenes*. Among the first generation cephalosporins, cefadroxil has advantages of ease of administration (twice daily without regard to meals) and excellent tissue penetration. Cephalexin also has been shown to be effective for treatment of skin and skin structure infections with twice daily dosing,[10] but considering its pharmacokinetics and time-dependence for killing, twice daily dosing may not be adequate in some instances, and should be reserved for mild infections in postneonatal patients.

Second-generation cephalosporins

Cefprozil is the second-generation agent of choice for treatment of skin and skin structure infections. Its major advantage over first-generation cephalosporins, erythromycin, dicloxacillin, and amoxicillin/clavulanate for treatment of skin infections is the convenience and thus increased compliance associated with once-daily dosing. Its side effect profile also is more favorable.

64. Cookson BD (1990) Mupirocin resistance in staphylococci. **J Antimicrob Chemother** 25:497–503.
65. Gisby J, Bryant J (2000) Efficacy of a new cream formulation of mupirocin: comparison with oral and topical agents in experimental skin infections. **Antimicrob Agents Chemother** 44:255–260.
66. Sutton JB (1992) Efficacy and acceptibility of fusidic acid cream and mupirocin ointment in facial impetigo. **Curr Ther Res** 51:673–678.
67. Ravenscroft JC, Layton A, Barnham M (2000) Observations on high levels of fusidic acid resistant *Staphylococcus aureus* in Harrogate, North Yorkshire, UK. **Clin Exp Dermatol** 25:327–330.
68. Remitz A, Kyllonen H, Granlund H et al. (2001) Tacrolimus ointment reduces staphylococcus colonization of atopic dermatitis lesions. **J Allergy Clin Immunol** 107:196–197.
69. Anderson JA (1995) Cross-sensitivity to cephalosporins in patients allergic to penicillin. **Pediatr Infect Dis J** 15:557–561.
70. Quintiliani R, Nightingale CH, Freeman CD (1995) Pharmacokinetic and pharmacodynamic considerations in antibiotic selection, with particular attention to oral cephalosporins. **Infect Dis Clin Prac** 4(Suppl 2):S58–S63.

Cefuroxime axetil is a prodrug that is de-esterified to the active cefuroxime moeity in the intestinal mucosa. It is similar in activity to amoxicillin/clavulanate, but does not offer any distinct advantages over other cephalosporins for empiric treatment of uncomplicated skin and skin structure infections, and is relatively expensive.

Loracarbef is a carbacepham that has equivalent to slightly increased beta-lactamase stability relative to cefaclor, but less stability compared to cephalexin, cefadroxil or cefuroxime.[71] It spectrum of antimicrobial activity is similar to that of the second-generation cephalosporins and amoxicillin/clavulanate.

Third generation cephalosporins

Third-generation cephalosporins are active against most Gram-negative enteric organisms, but are variable in their activity against Gram-positive cocci, particularly methicillin-sensitive *Staph. aureus*. Cefixime, for example, has the best Gram-negative activity of the oral cephalosporins, and has excellent activity against *Strep. pyogenes*,[72] but has essentially no activity against methicillin-sensitive *Staph. aureus* due to low affinity for its β-lactam binding proteins. Thus, cefixime should not be used for treatment of primary skin and skin structure infections. Cefdinir is similar to cefixime in its spectrum of activity, but has improved yet marginal staphylococcal coverage.[72] Likewise, ceftibuten, cefetamet and cefteram lack sufficient activity against *Staph. aureus*. Cefpodoxime axetil is the third-generation cephalosporin of choice, but there are no inherent advantages to its broader spectrum of activity. To the contrary, the broad spectrum of activity tends to exert increased selective pressure for emergence of antibiotic resistance.

Macrolides

The macrolides are bacteriostatic, but may be bactericidal in high concentrations or against susceptible organisms. They inhibit bacterial RNA-dependent protein synthesis by binding to the 50S-subunit of the 70S-ribosome in the organism. Although erythromycin has been a front-line therapy for treatment of skin and skin structure infections, its use is limited by gastrointestinal side effects, erratic bioavailability, the need for three- to four-times dosing, and increasing resistance among isolates of *Staph. aureus*. Clarithromycin and azithromycin have a lower incidence of gastrointestinal side effects, improved pharmacokinetic properties, and broader *in vitro* antimicrobial activity, and are safe for use in patients with penicillin or sulfa allergies. Activity of clarithromycin and azithromycin is excellent against *Strep. pyogenes*, but no better than erythromycin against methicillin-sensitive *Staph. aureus*, although they are concentrated within neutrophils that have phagocytized *Staph. aureus*, and can be dosed less frequently. Thus, the same concerns regarding resistance among isolates of *Staph. aureus* applies to these newer agents, and like erythromycin, clarithromycin, and azithromycin should not be used to treat severe staphylococcal infections. For treatment of uncomplicated skin and skin structure infections, the primary advantages of clarithromycin compared to erythromycin are less frequent dosing and fewer gastrointestinal side effects. Compared to cephalexin and cefadroxil, both of which are well tolerated and can be dosed twice daily, there is little advantage to use of clarithromycin except less selective pressure for emergence of β-lactamase resistance.

Azithromycin is highly concentrated in tissues (10–100-fold, compared to 5–10-fold for erythromycin), within macrophages and neutrophils (up to 26-fold greater than erythromycin),[73] and may be transported within phagocytes to areas of inflammation. Due to its slow release from tissues, azithromycin can be dosed once daily for a relatively short period of time (5 days) for treatment of skin and skin structure infections.

Quinolones

Flouroquinolones are rapidly acting, concentration-dependent bacteriocidal antibiotics that are not FDA-approved for use in children less than 12 years of age. Ciprofloxacin, however, is increasingly being used in pediatric patients. Several quinolones have shown excellent efficacy for treatment of skin and skin structure infections in adults.[8] Their use, however, has been complicated by superinfection and the rapid development of resistance, particularly among isolates of *Staph. aureus*. Moreover, the quinolones ciprofloxacin and norfloxacin are active primarily against Gram-negative bacteria, and have limited activity against *Strep. pyogenes*. Newer quinolones have improved Gram-positive coverage, potentially expanding their role in treating skin infections.[74] In a recent trial in adults with uncomplicated skin infections, moxifloxacin given once daily had equivalent efficacy compared to cephalexin for treatment of *Staph. aureus* and superior eradication of *Strep. pyogenes*.[75] Although not standard of care, the once daily dosing afforded by the long half-life of moxifloxacin (11–14h) may be advantageous for children with compliance issues.

Systemic antibiotic therapy

The β-lactamase-resistant penicillin, nafcillin, is first-line for treatment of serious skin and soft tissue infections due to *Staph. aureus* or *Strep. pyogenes*. Treatment of *Strep. pyogenes* may be achieved with penicillin. A first-generation cephalosporin (e.g., cefazolin) is a suitable alternative. For more serious, deep-seated infections, however, particularly those due to exotoxin-producing isolates, clindamycin may be advantageous. In all serious infections and for treatment of infections in neonates,[5] the susceptibility profile of the isolate(s) should be determined and the results used to optimize antibiotic selection.

SUPERFICIAL SKIN INFECTIONS

IMPETIGO

Epidemiology

Impetigo is a superficial infection localized to the subcorneal epidermis.[12] It accounts for 1 to 2% of all visits to pediatricians,[76] and comprises approximately 10% of all skin problems in children and 50 to 60% of all bacterial skin infections,[1,2] making it the most common bacterial skin infection in children.

Nonbullous impetigo accounts for more than 70% of cases of impetigo,[10] and occurs most commonly in regions with a warm, humid climate. Among indigent schoolchildren in the southern United States, for example, most (approximately 80%) will become infected over the course of a summer.[77] Studies during epidemics in the 1960s suggested that colonization of skin preceded development of skin infection with *Strep. pyogenes*, whereas staphylococci generally spread from the nose to normal skin, and hence are able to infect the skin.[19,78] This has important implications for management of these infections (see below).

Since the early 1980s, *Staph. aureus* has been the predominant organism of nonbullous impetigo. Staphylococci can now be cultured from approximately 85% of lesions of impetigo and is the sole pathogen in approximately 50 to 60% of cases, whereas *Strep. pyogenes* can be cultured from approximately 30% of lesions and is the sole pathogen in only about 5% of cases; occasionally, group B, C, G, or F streptococci are present.[10] The lesions caused by these various organisms are indistinguishable. Several serotypes of *Strep. pyogenes*, termed "impetigo strains" are found most frequently in lesions of nonbullous impetigo, and are distinct from those which cause pharyngitis.[27,32] The *Staph. aureus* types which cause nonbullous impetigo are variable, but generally are not from phage

71. Doern G (1992) In vitro activity of loracarbef and effects of susceptibility test methods. **Am J Med** 92(Suppl 6A):7S–15S.
72. Neu HC (1995) Oral β-lactam antibiotics from 1960 to 1994. **Infect Dis Clin Prac** 4(Suppl 2): S39–S49.
73. Foulds G, Shepard RM, Johnson RB (1990) The pharmacokinetics of azithromycin in human serum and tissues. **J Antimicrob Chemother** 25(Suppl A):73–82.
74. Bush K, Goldschmidt R (2000) Effectiveness of fluoroquinolones against gram-positive bacteria. **Curr Opin Invest Drugs** 1:22–30.

75. Parish LC, Routh HB, Miskin B et al. (2000) Moxifloxacin versus cephalexin in the treatment of uncomplicated skin infections. **Int J Clin Pract** 54(8):497–503.
76. Lookingbill DP (1985) Impetigo. **Pediatr Rev** 7:177–181.
77. Nelson KE, Bisno AL, Waytz P et al. (1976) The epidemiology and natural history of streptococcal pyoderma. An endemic disease of rural southern United States. **Am J Epidemiol** 103:270–283.
78. Dillon HC (1968) Impetigo contagiosa: suppurative and non-suppurative complications. **Am J Dis Child** 115:530–541.

group 2, the group associated with toxin production and bullous impetigo.[78] *Staph. aureus* can be cultured from lesions of impetigo on individuals of all ages, while *Strep. pyogenes* is most common in children of preschool age, and is unusual before 2 years of age except in highly endemic areas.[79]

Bullous impetigo usually occurs sporadically, most often in neonates, infants and young children. A warm, humid climate favors its development, and consequently, like nonbullous impetigo, it is most common in the summer months in temperate climates. Unlike nonbullous impetigo, it is always caused by coagulase-positive *Staph. aureus*; approximately 80% are from phage group 2, as also seen in staphylococcal scalded skin syndrome (SSSS).[78] Lesions of bullous impetigo develop on grossly intact skin as a manifestation of localized toxin production (exfoliatin or epidermolytic toxins A or B), and represent a localized form of SSSS.[80]

Infection with nephritogenic strains of *Strep. pyogenes* can result in acute poststreptococcal glomerulonephritis, most commonly during epidemics in children 3 to 7 years old, 18 to 21 days after onset of impetigo.[81] Impetigo-associated epidemics are caused by M-serotypes (e.g., 2, 49, 53, 55, 56, 57, 60) distinct from those following pharyngitis (e.g., 1, 12). Strains of *Strep. pyogenes* that are associated with endemic impetigo in the United States have little or no nephritogenic potential. Acute rheumatic fever does not occur following impetigo.

Presenting history

Lesions of nonbullous impetigo form on skin which has been traumatized, such as at varicella lesions, insect bites, abrasions, lacerations, and burns. It appears that either colonization of normal-appearing skin followed by a break in its barrier function, or direct inoculation of pathogens concurrently with or soon after a skin wound can lead to the infection. Nonbullous impetigo also develops secondarily on previously diseased skin with a compromised skin barrier. Secondary infection, or "impetiginization" of atopic dermatitis, the most common form of secondary impetigo, almost uniformly involves *Staph. aureus*, although *Strep. pyogenes* can be cultured occasionally.[82]

Physical examination

Nonbullous impetigo begins as a tiny vesicle or pustule, and rapidly develops into a honey-color crusted plaque generally less than 2cm in diameter (Fig. 24.1). Lesions are associated with little to no pain or surrounding erythema, and constitutional symptoms generally are absent. Regional adenopathy is found in up to 90% of cases and leukocytosis is present in about half of patients.[56,78]

When impetigo develops secondarily on previously diseased skin, it may be more difficult to recognize, as clinical signs of the infection are superimposed on those of the primary disease process. In atopic dermatitis, impetiginization may present with little more than a mild exacerbation of the dermatitis, with increased pruritus, erythema, and superficial crusted erosions (Fig. 24.2). As the infection worsens, fissures develop and the dermatitis may become frankly exudative and malodorous. While impetigo tends to be localized in primary infections, it may generalize rapidly when superimposed on skin affected with a primary disease such as atopic dermatitis, chickenpox, or insect bites.

Bullous impetigo presents with flaccid, transparent bullae most commonly on skin of moist, intertriginous areas in the groin of neonates, sometimes with extension to the abdomen. Bullae may occur singly or clustered regionally, (Fig. 24.3). In bullous varicella, generalized bullae may develop when an exotoxin-producing strain of *Staph. aureus* infects lesions of chickenpox, producing moist, mildly tender, denuded areas that extend from the chickenpox vesicles. Due to the superficial location of the subcorneal bullae, they rupture easily, leaving a narrow rim of scale at the edge of a shallow, moist, erythematous erosion. The erosion does not penetrate below the epidermal–dermal junction,

and thus it heals without scarring. Postinflammatory pigmentary changes, however, may be present for weeks to months.

Laboratory findings

Diagnosis generally can be made on clinical criteria. When in doubt, however, swabbing the blister fluid or beneath the lifted edge of a crusted plaque generally yields reliable culture results.

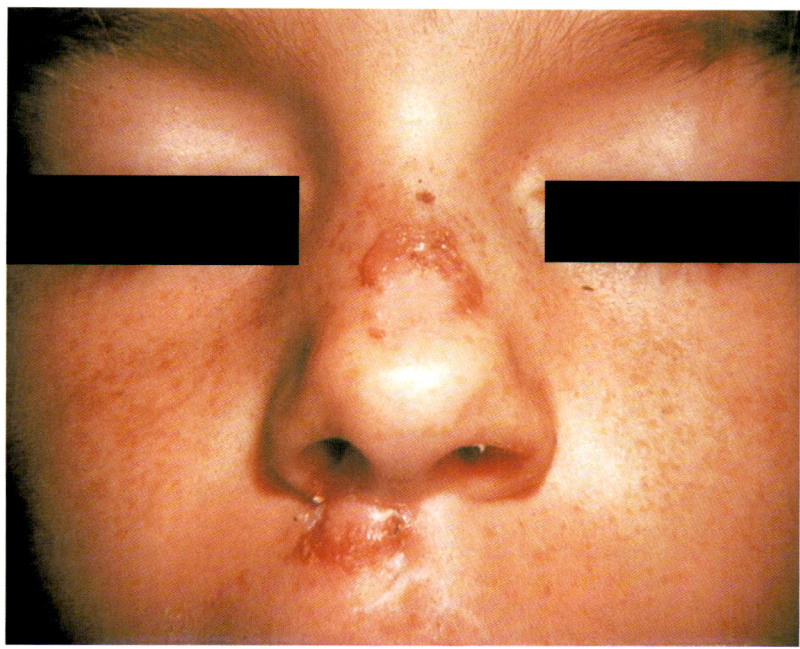

Fig. 24.1   Nonbullous impetigo. Honey-colored, crusted plaques of impetigo due to *Staphylococcus aureus* on the face of a child. Nasal carriage of *Staph. aureus* was also present.

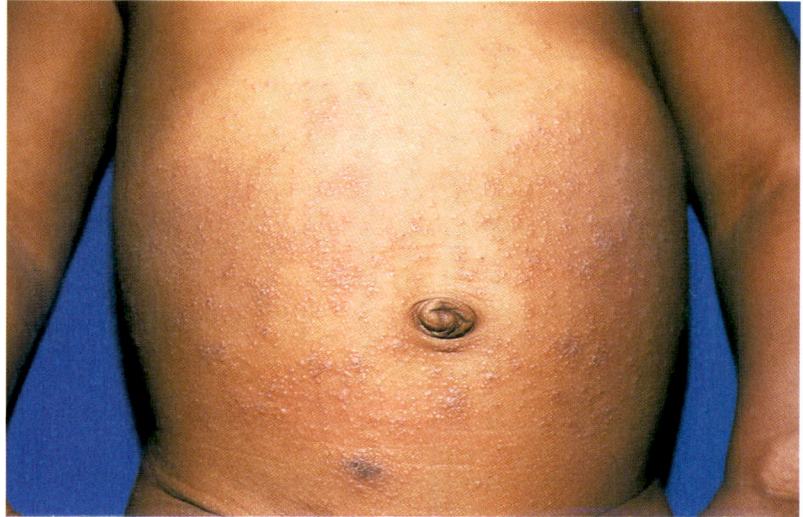

Fig. 24.2   Secondary nonbullous impetigo. Excoriated, lichenified, erythematous plaques of atopic dermatitis on the abdomen of a child secondarily infected ("impetiginized") with *Staphylococcus aureus*.

79. Dagan R (1993) Impetigo in childhood: changing epidemiology and new treatments. **Pediatr Ann** 22:235–240.
80. Elias PM, Levy W (1976) Bullous impetigo: occurrence of localized scalded skin syndrome in an adult. **Arch Dermatol** 112:856–858.
81. Dillon HC Jr (1972) Streptococcal infections of the skin and its complications: Impetigo and nephritis. In: Streptococci and Streptococcal Disease, Wannamaker LW, Masten P, eds. New York: Academic Press, pp. 571–587.
82. Dhar S, Kanwar AJ, Kaur S et al. (1992) Role of bacterial flora in the pathogenesis and management of atopic dermatitis. **Ind J Med Res** 95:234–238.

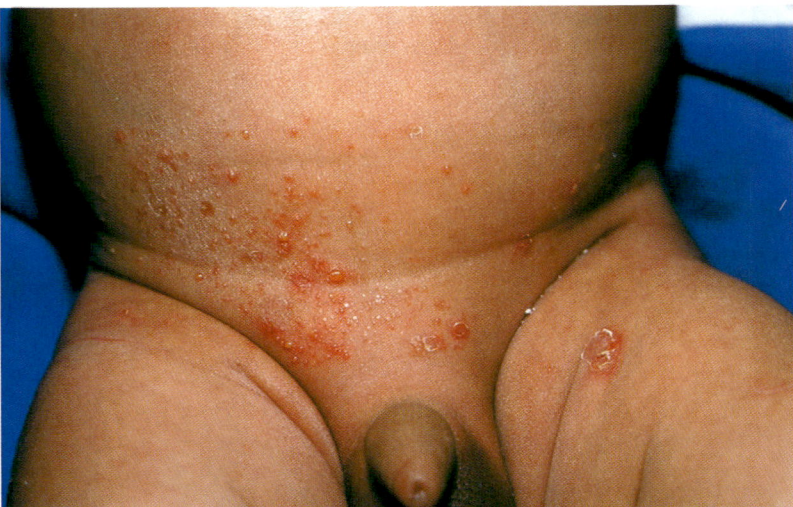

Fig. 24.3 Staphylococcal putulosis on the adomen and inguinal region of an infant.

Histopathologic examination of an early lesion of impetigo shows vesico-pustule formation in the subcorneal or granular region of the epidermis. The blister cavity is larger in the bullous form. Neutrophils are generally visible within the cavity of the blister, and often in the underlying epidermis as they migrate from dermal blood vessels. The underlying stratum malpighii and/or papillary dermis is spongiotic, and a mixed infiltrate of lymphocytes and neutrophils surrounds the blood vessels of the superficial dermal plexus. Biopsy of lesions in later stages may reveal serous crust and neutrophilic debris overlying a superficially eroded epidermis.

Pathophysiology
See above, Mechanisms of Skin Infection.

Differential diagnosis
The common infectious causes of lesions resembling impetigo include the enteroviruses, varicella-zoster and herpes simplex viruses. Bullous impetigo, occurring independently or as a superinfection of varicella lesions, is probably the most common cause of bullae in young children. Other bullous eruptions, such as SSSS, erythema multiforme (with herpes simplex virus or *Mycoplasma pneumoniae* infection), and the hemorrhagic bullae associated with Gram-negative sepsis, particularly *Pseudomonas aeruginosa* (ecthyma gangrenosum) and *Neisseria meningitides* (purpura fulminans), fortunately, are relatively infrequent. Several noninfectious conditions, however, may closely mimic impetigo. The appearance of bullae caused by thermal injury or a hypersensitivity response to insect bites is virtually identical to that seen with bullous impetigo. Similarly, nummular eczema may closely resemble nonbullous impetigo. Nevertheless, consideration of the season; the patient's age; history of exposure to infectious agents or recent ingestion of medications, prior disease and concurrent symptoms; and morphology, distribution, and evolution of the eruption will routinely allow one to make a diagnosis of impetigo on an empirical basis.

Unless Gram-positive cocci can be cultured from the vesicle, it may be impossible to differentiate impetigo from pemphigus foliaceus histopathologically. Pemphigus foliaceus tends to have more acantholysis and fewer neutrophils within the subcorneal blister, and may have dyskeratotic changes in cells of the granular layer. Clinically, pemphigus foliaceus differs from impetigo in its presentation with multiple small flaccid blisters that easily rupture, leaving erythematous, crusted erosions. Recent evidence has shown that bullous impetigo/SSSS and pemphigus foliaceus share a common target antigen, the cell–cell adhesion molecule desmoglein-1, which is damaged by interaction with epidermolytic toxin-induced serine protease activity or by autoantibodies, respectively, accounting for the similar clinical and histopathological presentation of these two diseases.[83,84] Subcorneal pustular dermatosis may also be indistinguishable histopathologically from impetigo but its clinical presentation is that of crops of grouped pustules in a serpiginous outline, generally on the abdomen or in the axillary and inguinal folds, sparing the face. Scabies with or without secondary infection may also be misdiagnosed as a bacterial infection alone.

Therapeutics and prognosis
In areas with a high prevalence of erythromycin resistant strains of *Staph. aureus*, superficial, localized, nonbullous impetigo located away from the mouth might be best treated topically with mupirocin, as mupirocin applied three times daily for 7 to 10 days is equal to or greater in effectiveness than oral erythromycin ethylsuccinate, with fewer side effects, at similar cost.[10]

A patient with recurrent impetigo should be evaluated for carriage of *Staph. aureus*, particularly in the nares as this is the site where the colonizing strains reside three-fourths of the time.[85] Nasal carriage of both methicillin-susceptible and methicillin-resistant strains of *Staph. aureus* has been eliminated in greater than 90% of individuals within 2–4 days through use of topical mupirocin three times daily,[86] and has resulted in a reduction in recurrences in children with atopic dermatitis.[82] In weeks to months after treatment, however, the nares become recolonized; thus, retreatment may be necessary if recurrences ensue, especially if the patient had a relatively disease-free period following eradication of colonizing strains.

An oral antibiotic active against β-lactamase producing strains of *Staph. aureus* should be prescribed for treatment of impetigo that is more widespread or has become complicated by involvement of deeper tissues or development of constitutional symptoms. Although dicloxacillin is a first-line oral agent for treatment of staphylococcal infections, its usefulness, particularly in infants and young children who cannot swallow a pill, is limited by poor taste and gastrointestinal complaints. Erythromycin and cephalexin also remain first-line agents for treatment of skin and skin structure infections in children. The clinical significance of *in vitro* erythromycin resisitance in the treatment of skin infections in children is unclear, and must be assessed on a local basis.[10] Cephalexin is the cephalosporin of choice in many regions due to its superior taste and adverse events profile, lack of resistance among isolates of *Staph. aureus* and *Strep. pyogenes*, and potential for twice daily dosing. If bid dosing of cephalexin proves to be ineffective, and tid or qid dosing around meals is unmanageable, then either cefadroxil (qd or bid dosing) or cefprozil (qd dosing) may be prefered. Either erythromycin or cephalexin are suitable for penicillin-allergic patients. Parenteral treatment is recommened for neonates with bullous impetigo.[5]

Without treatment, individual lesions of impetigo may progress slowly for several weeks, but in most cases will resolve spontaneously without scarring or complications within approximately 2 weeks. The disease often lasts several weeks, however, with new lesions developing, probably following auto-inoculation, as older lesions resolve. Cellulitis occurs on occasion, but is unusual. Lymphangitis, suppurative lymphadenitis, guttate psoriasis, and scarlet fever may be associated with streptococcal disease. Possible complications of impetigo due to hematogenous spread include osteomyelitis, septic arthritis, pneumonia, and septicemia. Positive blood cultures, however, are found rarely.

ECTHYMA
Epidemiology
The causative agent is usually *Strep. pyogenes*; *Staph. aureus* is also cultured from most lesions, but is probably a secondary invader, and may be a copathogen.

83. Amagai M, Matsuyoshi N, Wang ZH et al. (2000) Toxin in bullous impetigo and staphylococcal scalded skin syndrome targets desmoglein 1. **Nat Med** 6:1275–1277.

84. Ladhani S, Poston SM, Joannou CL, Evans RW (1999) Staphylococcal scalded skin syndrome: exfoliative toxin (ETA) induces serine protease activity when combined with A431 cells. **Acta Paediatr** 88:776–779.

85. Dancer SJ, Noble WC (1991) Nasal, axillary, and perineal carriage of *Staphylococcus aureus* among women: identification of strains producing epidermolytic toxin. **J Clin Pathol** 44:681–684.

86. Doebbeling BN, Breneman DL, Neu HC et al. (1993) Elimination of *Staphylococcus aureus* nasal carriage in health care workers: analysis of six clinical trials with calcium mupirocin ointment. **Clin Infect Dis** 17:466–474.

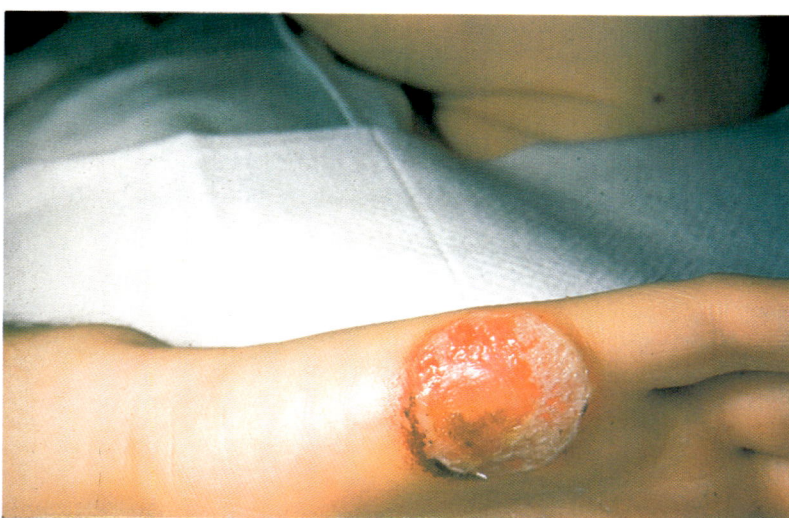

Fig. 24.4 **Ecthyma.** Well-defined ulcer of ecthyma due to *Streptococcus pyogenes* on the hand.

Presenting history

Ecthyma occur most frequently on the legs, particularly in the setting of poor hygiene and malnutrition, and at pruritic sites that are scratched, such as insect bites, scabies, or pediculosis.[87]

Physical examination

The initial lesion is a vesicle or vesicopustule with an erythematous base that erodes through the epidermis into the dermis to form a well-defined crusted ulcer with elevated margins up to 4cm in diameter surrounding by a rim of erythema (Fig. 24.4). Ecthyma resembles nonbullous impetigo in onset and appearance but gradually evolves into a deeper, more chronic infection. Because the lesion extends into the dermis, healing is frequently accompanied by scar formation. Complications include lymphadentitis, lymphangitis, cellulitis, and, rarely, post-streptococcal glomerulonephritis.

Pathophysiology

See above, Mechanisms of Skin Infection.

Differential diagnosis

Diagnosis of ecthyma can generally be made by visual inspection, although clinical distinction from impetigo may not be possible. Treatment for these two entities, however, is the same. Other unusual infections such as anthrax, cutaneous diphtheria, and ecthyma gangrenosum can closely resemble ecthyma.

Ecthyma gangrenosa is a necrotic ulcer covered with a gray–black eschar that generally is a sign of *Pseudomonas aeruginosa* bacteremia in neutropenic patients with leukemia or aplastic anemia. It also occurs rarely as a primary cutaneous infection by inoculation.

Therapeutics and prognosis

Systemic antibiotic therapy active against *Strep. pyogenes* and *Staph. aureus*, as for impetigo, is recommended. Local wound care, including removal of eschar, cleansing and application of occlusive ointment may aid healing.

FOLLICULITIS
Epidemiology

This superficial infection of the hair follicle is due predominantly to *Staph. aureus*, although coagulase negative staphylococci are involved occasionally.

Presenting history

Predisposing factors include a moist environment, maceration, poor hygiene, application of an occlusive emollient, and drainage from adjacent wounds and abscesses.

Physical examination

Folliculitis presents as discrete, dome-shaped pustules with an erythematous base, located at the ostium of the pilosebaceous canals. The lesions are asymptomatic to mildly tender. Occasionally, a lesion may extend to involve deeper tissues and form an abscess. Human immunodeficiency virus (HIV)-infected patients may develop confluent erythematous patches with satellite pustules in intertriginous areas, and violaceous plaques composed of superficial follicular pustules in the scalp, axillae or groin.[88]

Laboratory findings

The causative organism of folliculitis can be identified by Gram stain and culture of purulent material from the follicular orifice.

Differential diagnosis

Sycosis barbae is a deeper, more severe, inflammatory form of folliculitis due to *Staph. aureus* involving the entire depth of the follicle. Erythematous, follicular papules and pustules develop on the chin, upper lip, and angle of the jaw, primarily in young black males. Papules may coalesce into plaques, and healing may occur with scarring. Affected individuals frequently have recurrences, and are found to be *Staph. aureus* nasal carriers. Treatment includes warm saline compresses, topical antibiotics such as mupirocin in mild cases, or in more extensive, recalcitrant cases, systemic beta–lactamase resistant antibiotics, as well as elimination of *Staph. aureus* from sites of carriage using mupirocin.

Candida spp. cause satellite follicular papules and/or pustules surrounding patches of candidal intertrigo, particularly in patients on long-term corticosteroid or antibiotic therapy. *Malassezia furfur* can also produce pruritic, 2- to 3-mm, erythematous, perifollicular papules and papulopustules on the back, chest and extremities, particularly in patients with diabetes mellitus, or on long-term systemic corticosteroids or antibiotics. Diagnosis is made by potassium hydroxide examination of scrapings from a lesion. A skin biopsy may be necessary to identify grape-like clusters of yeast, and short, septate branching hyphal fragments ("spaghetti and meatballs") in widened follicular ostia, mixed with keratinous debris.

Gram-negative folliculitis occurs primarily in patients with acne vulgaris who have received long-term therapy with broad-spectrum systemic antibiotics, and may be caused by a variety of bacteria, including *Klebsiella* spp., *Enterobacter* spp., *Escherichia coli*, or *P. aeruginosa*, and *Proteus* spp. Culture of infected follicles is necessary to establish the diagnosis.

Hot tub folliculitis is attributable to *P. aeruginosa*, predominantly serotype O-11. The lesions are pruritic papules and pustules or deeply erythematous to violaceous nodules that develop 8 to 48h after exposure and are most dense in areas covered by a bathing suit. Patients occasionally develop fever, malaise, and lymphadenopathy. The organism is cultured from pus.

Therapeutics and prognosis

An attempt should be made to identify and eliminate predisposing factors. Topical antibiotic cleansers such as chlorhexidine usually are effective for mild cases, but more severe cases may require use of penicillinase-resistant systemic antibiotics such as cephalexin, dicloxacillin or cloxacillin. In chronic recurrent folliculitis, daily application of a benzoyl peroxide lotion or gel can facilitate resolution.

BLISTERING DACTYLITIS
Epidemiology

Blistering dactylitis is a superficial blistering infection, most commonly of of school-aged children, and, occasionally, infants. The causal organism nearly

87. Kelly C, Taplin D, Allen AM (1971) Streptococcal ecthyma. **Arch Dermatol** 103:306.

88. Becker BA, Frieden IJ, Odom RB, Berger TG (1989) Atypical plaquelike staphylococcal folliculitis in human immunodeficiency virus-infected persons. **J Am Acad Dermatol** 21:1024–1026.

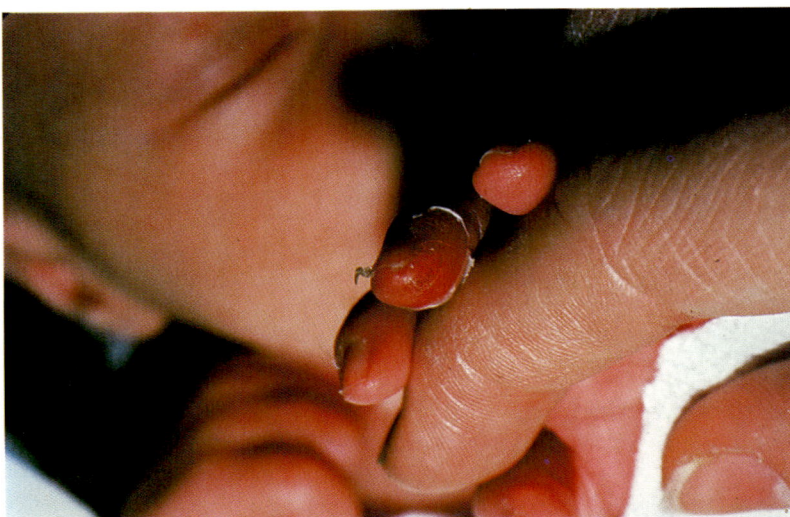

Fig. 24.5 Blistering dactylitis. Erythematous erosion with a rim of scale following rupture of a bulla of blistering dactylitis due to *Streptococcus pyogenes* on the distal finger of an infant (photograph courtesy of Alfred T. Lane).

always is *Strep. pyogenes*, although blistering dactylitis has occurred as a result of infection with *Staph. aureus* or group B streptococci.[89,90]

Physical examination

Bullae up to approximately 2cm in diameter develop on an erythematous base on the distal volar fat pad of the phalanges (Fig. 24.5). More than one digit may be involved, as may other surfaces with a thickened stratum corneum such as the volar surfaces of the proximal phalanges, the toes, and the palm. Lesions are asymptomatic to mildly tender; systemic symptoms generally are absent. If left untreated, blisters may continue to enlarge and extend to the paronychial area.

Laboratory findings

Blisters are filled with a purulent fluid containing polymorphonuclear leukocytes and infecting organisms. Diagnosis can be confirmed by Gram stain and culture.

Differential diagnosis

Herpetic whitlow presents most commonly on the terminal phalanges, particularly at a site of damaged cuticle on the fingers, or less often on the thumb, and frequently in a patient with herpetic gingivostomatitis that has been sucking on the finger. Presence of HSV in lesions (e.g., DFA, culture) confirms this diagnosis.

Therapeutics and prognosis

The infection responds to incision and drainage and a 10-day day course of systemic therapy with a beta-lactamase resistant penicillin or cephalosporin such as cephalexin, dicloxacillin or cloxacillin. Penicillin allergic patients can be treated with erythromycin or clindamycin.

PERIANAL DERMATITIS

Epidemiology

Perianal dermatitis is a superficial form of *Strep. pyogenes* infection localized to the perianal area; the infection has also been caused by *Staph. aureus*. It presents most commonly in boys (70% of cases) between the ages of 6 months to 10 years. Among children with perianal dermatitis, more than 50% have

concurrent positive perianal and pharyngeal cultures with an identical *Strep. pyogenes* type, and approximately 10% have symptomatic pharyngitis.[91] Rarely, perianal dermatitis has been preceded by streptococcal impetigo, suggesting that *Strep. pyogenes* may have spread from the impetigo lesion to the perianal skin.[91] Familial spread of perianal dermatitis is common, particularly when family members share the same bathwater.

Presenting history

Presentation most commonly includes perianal dermatitis (90% of cases) and pruritus (80% of cases).[92] Approximately half of patients have rectal pain or burning, especially during defecation, and one-third have blood-streaked stools. Fecal hoarding is a frequent behavioral response to the infection.

Physical examination

The rash is superficial, erythematous, well-marginated, nonindurated, and confluent from the anus outward (Fig. 24.6). Acutely (<6 weeks duration), the rash tends to be bright red, moist, and tender. Local induration or edema may occur. With time, painful fissures, a dried mucoid discharge, or psoriasiform plaques with yellow, peripheral crusts become more prominent and the erythema subsides. In girls, the perianal rash may be associated with vulvovaginitis.[91] Patients also may present with guttate psoriasis, emphasizing that the anus should be examined in all cases of guttate psoriasis.

Laboratory findings

A moderate to heavy growth of *Strep. pyogenes* is recovered from perianal swabs on blood agar. Individuals with asymptomatic perianal colonization tend to have a lighter growth of *Strep. pyogenes*. Direct antigen studies for *Strep. pyogenes* are also very sensitive (89%), but may be falsely negative early in the course of the disease.[91,92] The index case and family members should be cultured initially, and follow-up cultures to document bacteriologic cure after a course of treatment are recommended.

Differential diagnosis

The differential diagnosis of perianal dermatitis includes psoriasis, seborrheic dermatitis, candidosis, pinworm infestation, sexual abuse, essential pruritus, and inflammatory bowel disease. Differentiation from these other conditions can be accomplished by culture.

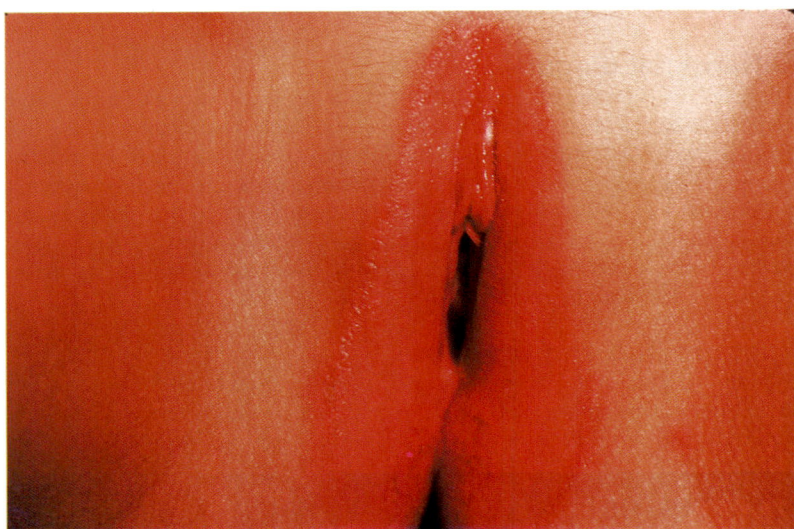

Fig. 24.6 Perianal dermatitis. Bright-red plaque of perianal dermatitis due to *Streptococcus pyogenes* (photograph courtesy of Alfred T. Lane).

89. Schneider JA, Parlette HL (1983) Blistering distal dactylitis: a manifestation of group A β-hemolytic streptococcal infection. **Arch Dermatol** 118:879–880.
90. Norcross MC, Mitchell DF (1993) Blistering distal dactylitis caused by *Staphylococcus aureus*. **Cutis** 51:353–354.
91. Kokx NP, Comstock JA, Facklam RR (1987) Streptococcal perianal disease in children. **Pediatrics** 80:659–663.
92. Amren DP, Anderson AS, Wannamaker LW (1966) Perianal cellulitis associated with group A streptococci. **Am J Dis Child** 112:546–552.

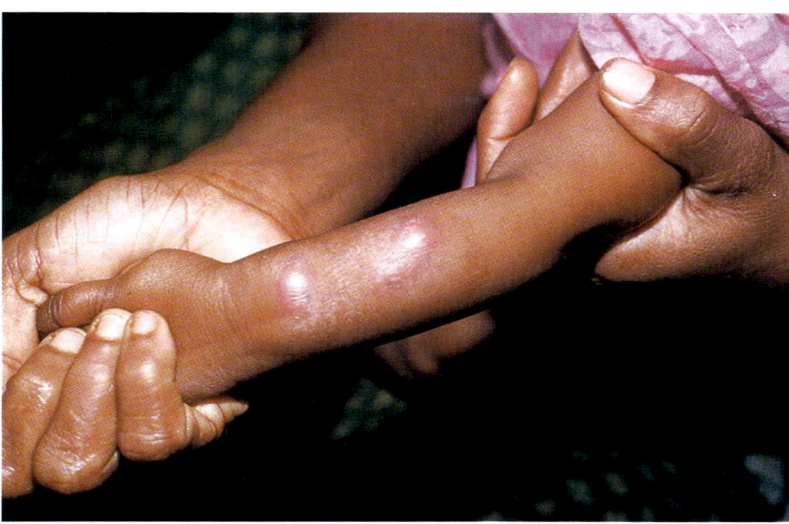

Fig. 24.7 Abscess. Tender erythematous indurated nodules on the arm of a malnourished child.

Therapeutics and prognosis

A single 10-day course of oral penicillin will resolve the condition; however, recurrence rates of 40 to 50% have been reported, emphasizing the need for close follow-up. Erythromycin is an alternative for persons who are allergic to penicillin, who have failed a course of penicillin, or who are infected with *Staph. aureus*. Clindamycin also has been used successfully to treat persons with recurrent perianal dermatitis. Given that the infection is relatively superficial, extending into the dermis but not the subcutaneous tissues, mupirocin has been used topically in conjunction with oral antibiotics to treat recurrences; however, it has not been evaluated as a single-drug therapy.

ABSCESSES

An abscess is a localized collection of pus in a cavity formed by disintegration or necrosis of tissue.[6] It is recognized clinically by the presence of a firm,

tender, erythematous nodule that becomes fluctuant (Fig. 24.7). Constitutional symptoms generally are absent unless the process has extended into deeper tissues or the bloodstream. Histopathologically, a cutaneous abscess is covered by normal epidermis but the dermis contains a dense infiltrate of acute inflammatory cells surrounded by a fibrinoid wall. Cutaneous and subcutaneous abscesses most commonly evolve by local extension of a primary infectious process in the epidermis and/or dermis, such as a cutaneous abscess originating from a skin appendage (e.g., furuncle, carbuncle, infected infundibular cyst) or from a secondarily infected skin tumor or site of skin disease or injury. An abscess can also arise by direct traumatic implantation or invasion of pathogens into subcutaneous tissue or, occasionally, by hematogenous spread. A number of conditions that disrupt the integrity of skin barrier function or local immunologic processes, particularly neutrophil function, are associated with abscess formation (Table 24.1), although most individuals with recurrent abscess formation (e.g., furunculosis) lack evidence of immunodeficiency.

Staph. aureus is the single most common pathogen of cutaneous and subcutaneous abscesses.[14] In general, cultures from perineal or perioral abscesses and ulcers contain organisms that originated from adjacent mucous membranes rather than skin, whereas lesions remote from the rectum or mouth contain primarily organisms which reside normally on skin at that site.[13,14]

FURUNCLE AND CARBUNCLE

Epidemiology

The causative agent of these lesions is almost always *Staph. aureus*, particularly phage type 80/81, which has a predilection for binding to abraded perifollicular skin. The lesions are more common in males than females. Recurrent funculosis frequently is associated with carriage of *Staph. aureus* in the nares, axillae, or perineum, or sustained close contact with someone who is a carrier.

Presenting history

Sites of predilection are hair-bearing areas on the face, neck, axillae, buttocks, and groin. Conditions that predispose to furuncle formation include a warm, humid environment; obesity; hyperhidrosis; maceration; friction; and preexisting dermatitis. Furunculosis is also more common in individuals with low serum iron, diabetes mellitus, malnutrition, HIV infection, or other immunodeficiency states, particularly those involving defects in neutrophil function.

TABLE 24.3 Oral antibiotics for treatment of skin infections due to *Staphylococcus aureus* or *Streptococcus pyogenes**

Antibiotic	Proprietary name	Pediatric dose (mg/kg/day)	Dosing interval	Length of therapy	Activity
Amoxicillin/clav.	Augmentin	20–40	tid	10	++++
Azithromycin†	Zithromax	10	qd	5	++
Cephalexin	Keflex	25–50	bid/qid	10	+++
Cefaclor	Ceclor	20–40	tid	10	++
Cefadroxil	Duricef	30	bid	10	+++
Cefpodoxime†	Vantin	10	bid	7–14	++
Cefprozil	Cefzil	20	qd/bid	10	+++
Cefuroxime†	Ceftin	30	bid	10	+++
Cephradine	Velocef	25–50	bid/qid	10	+++
Clarithromycin	Biaxin	15	bid	10	++
Clindamycin	Generic	15	tid/qid	10	+++
Cloxacillin	Generic	50	qid	10	+++
Dicloxacillin	Generic	12.5–50	qid	10	+++
Erythromycin					
ethylsuccinate	Generic	40	tid/qid	10	++
estolate	Generic	30	tid/qid	10	++
Loracarbef	Lorabid	15	bid	7	++

* Adapted from reference 11.
† Approved for use in individuals older than 12 years.

Physical examination

Furuncle presents as a deep-seated, tender, erythematous, perifollicular papule that evolves into a nodule. Surrounding cellulitis may develop. Pain may be intense if the lesion is situated in an area where the skin is relatively fixed, such as in the external auditory canal or over nasal cartilage. Patients with furuncles usually have no constitutional symptoms, although bacteremia may occur, particularly in association with malnutrition or manipulation of the lesion. Rarely, severe lesions on the upper lip or cheek may lead to cavernous sinus thrombosis.

Carbuncle is an infection of a group of contiguous follicles, with multiple drainage points, and inflammatory changes in surrounding connective tissue. Carbuncles may be accompanied by fever, leukocytosis, and bacteremia.

Pathophysiology

Influx of neutrophils, followed by vessel thrombosis, suppuration, and central tissue necrosis leads to rupture and discharge of a central core of necrotic tissue, destruction of the follicle, and scarring.

Laboratory findings

A variety of bacteria besides *Staph. aureus*, or fungi, may occasionally cause furuncles or carbuncles; therefore, Gram stain and culture of the pus are indicated.

Differential diagnosis

Hidradenitis suppurativa is a chronic, inflammatory, suppurative disorder of the apocrine glands that usually presents during puberty or early adulthood. The disease probably is initiated by plugging of apocrine gland ducts with keratinous debris. Bacterial infection, particularly with *Staph. aureus*, *Strep. milleri* (Anginosus group), *E. coli*, and possibly anerobic streptococci, appears to be important secondarily in contributing to progressive dilatation below the obstruction. Solitary or multiple painful, erythematous nodules, deep abscesses, and contracted scars are sharply confined to areas of skin containing apocrine glands (e.g., axillae, anogenital region; occasionally the scalp, posterior aspect of the ears, female breasts, around the umbilicus). Sinus tracts, ulcers, and thick, linear fibrotic bands may develop. The condition tends to persist for many years, punctuated by relapses and partial remissions. Complications include cellulitis, ulceration, or burrowing abscesses that may perforate adjacent structures in the anogenital region, forming fistulae to the urethra, bladder, rectum, or peritoneum. A minority of patients have the follicular occlusion triad, which includes acne conglobata and perifolliculitis capitis (dissecting cellulitis of the scalp); a tetrad with pilonidal sinus has also been described. Patients should be counseled to avoid tight-fitting clothes, as occlusion may exacerbate the condition. Systemic antibiotics, chosen on the basis of bacterial culture and susceptibility tests, may be helpful in the acute phase. Empiric therapy may be initiated with tetracycline, doxycycline, or minocycline (provided the patient is older than 8 years); clindamycin or cephalosporins also may be effective. Some patients require long-term treatment with tetracycline or erythromycin. Intralesional triamcinolone acetonide (5–10mg/ml) is often helpful in early disease. The addition of prednisone 40 to 60mg/day for 7 to 10 days, tapering gradually as inflammation subsides, to the regimen of patients who respond poorly to antibiotics may decrease fibrosis and scarring. Ultimately, surgical measures may be required.

Therapeutics and prognosis

Treatment includes frequent application of a hot, moist compress to facilitate drainage of lesions. Large lesions may require surgical drainage. Carbuncles and large or multiple furuncles, particularly those located on the central face, should be treated with oral penicillinase-resistant systemic antibiotics such as cephalexin, dicloxacillin or cloxacillin. The penicillin-allergic patient can be treated with clindamycin.

The carriage state may be eliminated temporarily by application of mupirocin ointment three times daily for 5 days to the anterior nares. Attention to personal hygiene, use of an antibacterial soap, and prophylactic low-dose oral antistaphylococcal penicillin or clindamycin also may be beneficial.

PARONYCHIA
Epidemiology

Staph. aureus and *Strep. pyogenes* are the most common causative organisms. Anaerobes and occasionally Gram-negative organisms (*Pseudomonas* spp., *Proteus* spp., *E. coli*) may be pathogenic.[93] *Candida albicans* is implicated in chronic infection.

Presenting history

Paronychia occurs most commonly in children who suck their fingers, or in individuals who bite their nails, have poor hygiene, or engage in activities that cause maceration and/or trauma to the nail fold.

Physical examination

The lateral nail fold becomes warm, erythematous, edematous and painful (Fig. 24.8). A purulent exudate may develop. Dermatitis often occurs around the affected area, and may contribute to initiation and/or perpetuation of the problem.

Laboratory findings

Acute paronychia usually can be diagnosed by clinical inspection. However, both aerobic and anaerobic cultures of purulent material are recommended.

Pathophysiology

Acute paronychia involves localized inflammation and infection of the nail fold, usually following local injury. The primary disorder is separation of the eponychium from the nail plate, followed by secondary invasion of the space by pathogens.

Differential diagnosis

Herpetic whitlow may also occur in the paronychial area. It typically is preceded by a prodrome of pain and present with vesicles on an erythematous base. The lesion may become purulent or necrotic. Due to the thickness of the stratum corneum on the fingers, the vesicles may appear to be more deeply set than is generally observed with herpes simplex virus infections. Occasionally, it may be necessary to perform a Tzanck smear, direct fluorescent antibody test and/or culture to identify the virus.

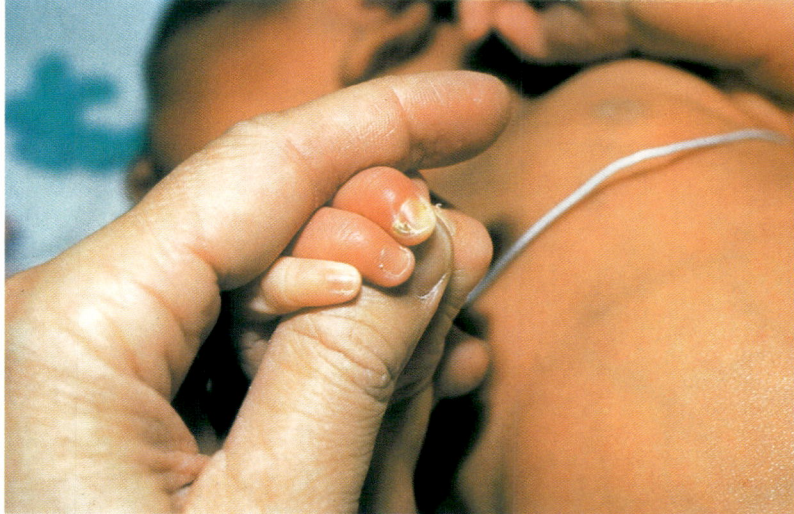

Fig. 24.8 Paronychia presenting with erythema and edema of the nail fold due to *Staphylococcus aureus*.

93. Brook I (1990) Aerobic and anaerobic microbiology of paronychia. **Ann Emerg Med** 19:994–996.

Therapeutics and prognosis

Attention must be directed toward eliminating or reducing predisposing factors of nail fold maceration and trauma. Warm compresses generally are curative for superficial lesions. Drainage of the abscess may be facilitated by gently pushing the nail fold away from the nail plate. Antibiotics, in addition to incision and drainage, are needed for treatment of deeper lesions. Dicloxacillin, cloxacillin, or cephalexin are the antibiotics of choice for treatment of infections caused by *Staph. aureus*, while amoxicillin plus clavulanic acid is preferred for empiric treatment. Chronic paronychia sometimes preceeds acute bacterial superinfection, and may require management after the acute infection has been cleared.

BREAST ABSCESS

Epidemiology

Breast abscess develops in full-term neonates during the first 1–6 weeks of life, most commonly during the second to third weeks of life.[94,95] Incidence is approximately equal in males and females during the first 2 weeks of life, but thereafter the incidence in girls is approximately twice that of boys.[95]

Breast abscess in neonates is usually due to *Staph. aureus*.[96] Infection is occasionally due to group B streptococcus, *E. coli*, *Salmonella* spp., *P. mirabilis*, or *P. aeruginosa*. Although anaerobic organisms can be isolated from up to 40% of infections, their pathogenic role in neonates is questionable and therapy directed specifically against them is unnecessary.

Physical examination

Breast abscess presents initially with breast enlargement, accompanied by varying degrees of erythema, induration, and tenderness. Progression to fluctuance may or may not occur, depending in part on how early antibiotic therapy is initiated. Bilateral infection occurs in less than 5% of cases.[94] Affected infants usually lack fever (present in approximately one-third) or constitutional symptoms such as irritability or toxicity; leukocytosis ($>15\,000/mm^3$) is found in approximately half to two-thirds of patients.[94] Breast abscess due to *Staph. aureus* is accompanied by cutaneous pustules or bullae on the trunk, particularly in the perineal region in 25 to 50% of patients,[94,95] and infants infected with *Salmonella* spp. generally also have gastrointestinal illness.[94,96]

Laboratory findings

Gram stain of material expressed from the nipple or obtained by needle aspiration or incision and drainage can help to guide initial antibiotic therapy. Blood cultures should be obtained.

Pathophysiology

The fact that physiologic breast enlargement and breast abscess is more common in infant girls than boys after, but not before, 2 weeks of age, suggests that breast enlargement may be a factor in the pathogenesis of breast abscess.[95] Breast manipulation has also been suggested as a predisposing factor.[95] Infants with *Staph. aureus* breast abscess, as a rule, are also colonized with the same organism on nasal or pharyngeal mucous membranes.[94] It seems likely that *Staph. aureus* spreads from the nasopharynx to colonize the skin of the nipple, and may move from there up the ducts of the physiologically enlarged, predisposed breast in a retrograde fashion, perhaps facilitated by breast manipulation, to infect deeper tissues.

Therapeutics and prognosis

If fluctuance is present, the abscess must be drained surgically; antibiotic therapy then is adjunctive. If fluctuance is absent, early antibiotic therapy alone may be curative and prevent abscess development. In general, a β-lactamase-resistant anti-staphylococcal antibiotic (e.g., nafcillin) should be given parenterally. If Gram-negative bacilli are seen on Gram stain or the infant appears systemically ill, initial therapy should include an aminoglycoside or cefotaxime. If no organisms are seen on Gram stain, antibiotics for control of both *Staph. aureus* and Gram-negative bacilli (e.g., nafcillin, gentamicin) should be started while awaiting culture results. Once infection has begun to subside and constitutional signs are absent, therapy may be completed orally with cloxacillin, dicloxacillin or cephalexin if the infection was due to *Staph. aureus* alone. In most instances, a total of 5 to 7 days of therapy is sufficient, although many experts continue treatment for 10 to 14 days.[94]

The most common complication of breast abscess is cellulitis, which develops in approximately 5 to 10% of affected infants.[94,95] Cellulitis is generally localized, but can extend rapidly to involve the shoulder and/or abdomen. Other complications such as bacteremia, pneumonia, osteomyelitis, or sepsis are unusual. Scar formation leading to decreased breast size following puberty can occur as a late complication.[95]

PERIRECTAL ABSCESS

Epidemiology

The organisms in perirectal abscesses are predominantly mixed anaerobic and aerobic flora of the intestine and skin of the anal verge.

Presenting history

Perirectal abscess may occur in healthy neonates and infants, more often boys than girls, with no apparent predisposing factor, although the abscess may develop following minor abrasions or fissures, particularly in association with diarrhea or constipation. Older children who develop perirectal abscess, however, usually have a predisposing condition such as neutropenia in association with neoplastic disease, autoimmunity, or chemotherapy administration; neutrophil dysfunction due to immunodeficiency disease such as chronic granulomatous disease; acquired immunodeficiency syndrome; diabetes mellitus; corticosteroid therapy; ulcerative colitis or Crohn's disease; or rectal surgery. In those with granulocytopenia, the risk for development of an abscess or perirectal cellulitis increases with perirectal mucositis, hemorrhoids, rectal fissure or manipulation. Superficial abscess in the infant usually presents with signs of pain on defecation, sitting or walking.

Physical examination

Onset is characterized by presence of redness, swelling and tenderness in the perianal region. Children with granulocytopenia may have absence or delayed development of erythema, induration and fluctuance. Extension of infection can occur in several directions: inferiorly along the anal sphincter to exit next to the anus on the buttock (fistula-in-ano); laterally through the external sphincter to the ischiorectal fossa to form a deep abscess; or superiorly to the deep space between the internal sphincter and the levator ani muscles.[97] An abscess in deeper tissues may be accompanied by poorly localized, deep pain, and constitutional signs. An anorectal abscess may not be apparent externally, but pain is generally elicited upon rectal examination. Complications, which occur more commonly in children with underlying disease (see Presenting History), include anorectal fistula, abscess recurrence, bacteremia, and necrotizing fasciitis.

Therapeutics and prognosis

In immunocompetent infants, a superficial perianal abscess can drain spontaneously and be self-limiting. Recommended management, however, includes prompt drainage and exploration of the abscess and fistulae, and Sitz baths. Administration of antibiotics such as clindamycin and an aminoglycoside may prevent regional spread of the infection and decrease the incidence of complications.[98] In the absence of fluctuance, extensive soft tissue disease, or evidence of sepsis, a trial of parenteral antimicrobial therapy may be initiated alone, without surgical intervention. A 7- to 10-day course of

94. Walsh M, McIntosh K (1986) Neonatal mastitis. **Clin Pediatr** 25:395–399.
95. Rudoy RC, Nelson JD (1975) Breast abscess during the neonatal period. **Am J Dis Child** 129:1031–1034.
96. Brook I (1991) The aerobic and anaerobic microbiology of neonatal breast abscess. **Pediatr Infect Dis J** 10:785–786.
97. Longo WE, Touloukian RJ, Seashore JN (1991) Fistula in ano in infants and children: implications and management. **Pediatrics** 87:737–739.
98. Kreiger RW, Chusid MJ (1979) Perirectal abscess in childhood: review of 29 cases. **Am J Dis Child** 133:411–412.

antibiotics is recommended. If fluctuance or progression of disease becomes apparent, surgery should be undertaken.

SCALP ABSCESS
Epidemiology
Scalp abscess develops at the insertion site of a fetal scalp monitoring electrode, and typically is a polymicrobial infection.

Presenting history
Presentation occurs most commonly on the third or fourth days of life, but may be as early as the first day and as late as 3 weeks of life.[99]

Physical examination
The lesion appears initially as a localized, erythematous area of induration 0.5–2cm in diameter. The site may become fluctuant or pustular. Regional lymphadenopathy may be present, but other more serious complications such as cranial osteomyelitis, subgaleal abscess, necrotizing fasciitis of the scalp, bacteremia, and sepsis are rare.

Laboratory findings
Culture for both aerobic and anaerobic organisms can be obtained by needle aspiration or swabbing the exudate from the puncture site.

Pathophysiology
Procedures which increase access of vaginal flora to the infant and cause trauma to the scalp may increase the risk for development of scalp abscess. The condition likely occurs through ascension of normal cervical flora into the uterus following rupture of membranes, aided by procedures that access the uterine cavity (e.g., electrode placement) and break the skin barrier.

Differential diagnosis
The primary differential diagnostic concern is HSV infection. The time of appearance of these lesions (peak incidence 4 to 10 days) overlaps with that for scalp abscess, and they may be indistinguishable clinically. If suspicion of HSV exists, therapy with acyclovir should be initiated while awaiting diagnostic test results (e.g., DFA, culture).

Therapeutics and prognosis
Many lesions resolve spontaneously, but if fluctuance develops without spontaneous suppuration, incision and drainage is necessary although extensive debridement should not be performed. If surrounding cellulitis is present, a 5- to 7-day course of parenteral antibiotic therapy is usually sufficient, with culture results guiding antibiotic choice.

BOTRYOMYCOSIS
Epidemiology
Cutaneous botryomycosis is an unusual, chronic, suppurative disease, most commonly associated with *Staph. aureus* infection, characterized by the presence of granules formed by clusters of bacteria within a suppurative focus. It can also result from infection with a variety of other bacteria.[100]

Presenting history
Although most patients are otherwise healthy, predisposing conditions appear to include cutaneous trauma, presence of a foreign body, malnutrition, systemic corticosteroid therapy, diabetes mellitus, alcoholism, HIV infection, and cell-mediated immunodeficiency.[101,102]

Physical examination
Cutaneous infection presents with firm, nontender subcutaneous nodules, sometimes associated with purulent sinus tracts, or with verrucous plaques associated with purulent exudate. Occasionally, the exudate appears granular to the naked eye. Exposed surfaces, particularly on the extremities, are affected most commonly, although intertriginous and gluteal areas are also frequently involved.[101] Occasionally, the infection extends to underlying muscle and bone. A patient with immunodeficiency due to HIV infection presented with papulonodular lesions of botryomycosis resembling prurigo nodularis.[102]

Laboratory findings
Histopathologic examination of biopsy specimens reveals either acute inflammation or mixed acute, chronic and granulomatous inflammation and central suppuration or microabscesses containing granules similar to those seen in actinomycosis and the mycetomas. The characteristic granules consist of clusters of swollen basophilic-staining bacterial cells surrounded by an eosinophilic matrix. With use of special stains, the cocci of *Staph. aureus* can be distinguished from the filaments of *Actinomyces*.[103] The amorphous matrix of the granules contains IgG produced by the host.

Pathogenesis
Pathogenesis of this condition is unclear, but it is most widely regarded as a symbiotic balance between a pathogen of relatively low virulence and the tissue resistance of the host, which may be attenuated.[103]

Therapeutics and prognosis
The lesions of botryomycosis are indolent and often refractory to antibacterial therapy. Antibacterial therapy must be tailored according to the susceptibility profile of the pathogen. The treatment of choice in refractory cases is often excision. Carbon dioxide laser therapy has been shown to also be effective.[104]

SUBCUTANEOUS TISSUE INFECTIONS

When managing patients with soft tissue infection, it is of paramount important to determine whether the infection is non-necrotizing or necrotizing. The former are managed with antibiotics alone, while the latter also require prompt surgical removal of all devitalized tissue.

NON-NECROTIZING SUBCUTANEOUS INFECTIONS
Cellulitis
Epidemiology
Cellulitis is characterized by infection and inflammation of loose connective tissue, with limited involvment of the dermis and relative sparing of the epidermis. *Strep. pyogenes* and *Staph. aureus* are the most common etiologic agents. Occasionally, *Strep. pneumoniae*, group G or C streptococci, and in neonates, group B streptococci or rarely *E. coli* are the causal organism. *Haemophilus influenzae* type b (HiB) remains an important cause of cellultis in developing countries without routine HiB immunization. In patients who are immunocompromised or have diabetes mellitus, a number of other bacterial or fungal agents may be involved.[3]

Presenting history
A break in the skin barrier predisposes to cellulitis. Cellulitis is also more common in individuals with lymphatic stasis as well as diabetes mellitus or immunosuppression.

99. Cordero L, Anderson CW, Zuspan FP (1983) Scalp abscess: a benign and infrequent complication of fetal monitoring. **Am J Obstet Gynecol** 146:126–130.
100. Mehregan DA, Su WPD, Anhalt JP (1991) Cutaneous botryomycosis. **J Am Acad Dermatol** 24:393–396.
101. Buescher ES, Hebert A, Rapini RP (1988) Staphylococcal botryomycosis in a patient with hyperimmunoglobulin-E-recurrent infection (Job's) syndrome. **Pediatr Infect Dis J** 7:431–433.
102. Patterson JW, Kitces EN, Neafie RC (1987) Cutaneous botryomycosis in a patient with acquired immunodeficiency syndrome. **J Am Acad Dermatol** 16:238–242.
103. Winslow DJ (1959) Botryomycosis. **Am J Pathol** 35:153–167.
104. Leffell DJ, Brown MD, Swanson NA (1989) Laser vaporization: a novel treatment of botryomycosis. **J Dermatol Surg Oncol** 15:703–705.

Physical examination

Cellulitis presents clinically as an area of edema, warmth, erythema and tenderness. The lateral margins tend to be indistinct because the process is deep in the skin, primarily involving the subcutaneous tissues in addition to the dermis. Application of pressure may produce pitting. Regional adenopathy and constitutional signs and symptoms of fever, chills, and malaise are common. Complications of cellulitis include subcutaneous abscess, osteomyelitis, septic arthritis, thrombophlebitis, bacteremia, and necrotizing fasciitis. Lymphangitis or glomerulonephritis also can follow infection with *Strep. pyogenes*.

Laboratory findings

Due to relatively low numbers of organisms in cellulitic tissue, aspirates from the leading edge of inflammation, skin biopsy, and blood cultures collectively allow identification of the causal organism in about 25% of cases of cellulitis.[105] An aspirate taken from the point of maximum inflammation yields the causal organism more often than does a leading-edge aspirate.[106]

Differential diagnosis

Facial cellulitis associated with a portal of entry such as a tooth abscess or cutaneous injury generally is due, respectively, to mouth anaerobes or to either *Strep. pyogenes* or *Staph. aureus*.[107] If facial cellulitis occurs without an apparent portal of entry, antibiotic therapy should include coverage for *Strep. pneumoniae*.

Periorbital or preseptal cellulitis develops anterior or superficial to an intact orbital septum. When the infection is associated with trauma to the periorbital skin or extension of infection from adjacent skin (e.g., dermatoblepharitis) or eyelid structures (e.g., hordeolum, dacryocystitis, dacryoadenitis), the most common pathogens are *Staph. aureus* or *Strep. pyogenes*. Additional potential agents include *Strep. pneumoniae*, particularly in infants and young children less than 5 years of age, which generally causes the infection following bacteremic spread. Periorbital cellulitis presents with erythema and swelling of the eyelid. Systemic signs of toxicity are variable in degree. Rapidly progressive, nonsuppurative cellulitis of the eyelid, which may progress to eyelid gangrene, can be caused by *Strep. pyogenes*.[108]

Orbital cellulitis involves structures behind the septum in the orbital space. *Staph. aureus* is the most common cause, particularly following trauma. *Strep. pyogenes*, nontypable *H. influenzae*, and *Strep. pneumoniae* may cause the disease in association with contiguous infection of the sinuses or oral cavity. Orbital cellulitis presents with eyelid erythema and edema, conjunctival hyperemia, chemosis, proptosis, decreased and painful extraocular movements, decreased visual acuity, fever and constitutional signs. As the infection progresses, an abscess of the orbital tissue and subperiosteum develops. Computed tomography is necessary to define the extent of infection.

Therapeutics and prognosis

Empiric therapy for cellulitis should be directed by the history of the illness, the location and character of the cellulitis, and the age and immune status of the patient. Cellulitis in the neonate should prompt a full sepsis workup, followed by initiation of empiric therapy intravenously with a beta-lactamase stable antistaphylococcal antibiotic and an aminoglycoside such as gentamicin or a cephalosporin such as cefotaxime.

Treatment of cellulitis in the infant or child younger than about 5 years of age should provide coverage for *Strep. pyogenes* and *Staph. aureus* as well as *Strep. pneumoniae*. The workup should include a blood culture and, if the infant is younger than 1 year of age or signs of systemic toxicity are present, a lumbar puncture should also be performed. In most cases of cellulitis on an extremity, regardless of age, *Staph. aureus* and *Strep. pyogenes* are the cause, and bacteremia is unlikely. Nevertheless, blood cultures should be obtained. If fever, lymphadenopathy and other constitutional signs are absent (e.g., white blood cell count <15 000), treatment of cellulitis on an extremity may be initiated orally on an outpatient basis with a penicillinase-resistant penicillin such as dicloxacillin or cloxacillin or a first-generation cephalosporin such as cephalexin. If improvement is not noted or the disease progresses significantly within the first 24 to 48h of therapy, parenteral therapy becomes necessary. If fever, lymphadenopathy and/or constitutional signs are present, therapy should be initiated parenterally. Nafcillin is effective in most cases, although if systemic toxicity is significant, consideration should be given to the addition of penicillin or clindamycin. Once the erythema, warmth, edema and fever have decreased significantly, a 10-day course of treatment may be completed on an outpatient basis. Immobilization and elevation of an affected limb, particularly early in the course of therapy, may help to reduce swelling and pain.

Children younger than 1 year of age who develop facial or periorbital cellulitis should receive antibiotics intravenously, regardless of the severity of the infection. A lumbar puncture should be included to rule out meningitis. Therapy can be initiated with a third-generation cephalosporin such as ceftriaxone or cefotaxime; or with cefuroxime provided that meningitis has been ruled out. Individuals older than 1 year of age with mild localized signs of infection and lack of all signs of systemic disease can be considered for outpatient management with an agent such as amoxicillin/clavulanate or possibly cefuroxime axetil. If a purulent wound was present adjacent to the inflamed eyelid, an antistaphylococcal agent such as dicloxacillin, cephalexin, or clindamycin should suffice. In most cases, however, therapy in patients with facial or periorbital cellulitis should be initiated parenterally. If an adequate response is achieved within 2 to 5 days of parenteral therapy, a 7–10-day course of therapy can be completed with an oral agent. Culture and antibiotic susceptibility results, when available, should be used to guide the choice of oral antibiotic. Orbital cellulitis is a medical emergency and should be managed as such by pediatric specialists well versed in care of these patients.

Erysipelas

Epidemiology

Erysipelas is a superficial form of cellulitis involving the dermis and upper subcutaneous tissue, with prominent lymphatic involvement, usually due to *Strep. pyogenes*. Group G as well as groups B, C, or D streptococci are involved occasionally, particularly in hosts who have been compromised by surgery or other illness. Other organisms (e.g., *Staph. aureus*, *Strep. pneumoniae*, *Klebsiella pneumoniae*, *Yersinia enterocolitica*) rarely are implicated.

Presenting history

Erysipelas usually begins at a break in the skin. Common portals of entry include leg ulcers; sites of local trauma; dermatoses, particularly intertrigo or tinea pedis; insect bites; and heel fissures. In neonates, infection may originate in the umbilical stump and spread to the abdominal wall, or on the external genitalia at an infected circumcision site. Predisposing host factors include a history of venous or lymphatic obstruction, nephrotic syndrome, and diabetes mellitus. The most common site of erysipelas is the lower extremities; in the past, the face was the favored site.[109] Onset of erysipelas is abrupt, with fever, chills and malaise, followed within a day or two by cutaneous signs.

Physical examination

A small area of burning and redness develops into a warm, shiny, bright-red, confluent, indurated, tender plaque with a brawny, *peau d'orange* appearance and elevated margins (Fig. 24.9). Vesicles, hemorrhagic bullae, petechiae and ecchymoses may develop in the plaque, and regional adenopathy may be present. Fine desquamation and sometimes residual pigmentation accompanies resolution of the plaque. Complications include bacteremia (5%), abscess, gangrene, thrombophlebitis, and glomerulonephritis.

105. Hook EW III, Hooton TM, Horton CA et al. (1986) Microbiologic evaluation of cutaneous cellulitis in adults. **Arch Intern Med** 146:295–297.
106. Howe FM, Fajardo JE, Orcutt MA (1987) Etiologic diagnosis of cellulitis: comparison of aspirates obtained from the leading edge and the point of maximal inflammation. **Pediatr Infect Dis J** 6:685–686.
107. Carter S, Feldman WE (1983) Etiology and treatment of facial cellulitis in pediatric patients. **Pediatr Infect Dis J** 2:222–224.
108. Stone L, Codere F, Ma SA (1991) Streptococcal lid necrosis in previously healthy children. **Can J Ophthalmol** 26:386–390.
109. Chartier C, Grosshans E (1990) Erysipelas. **Int J Dermatol** 29:459–467.

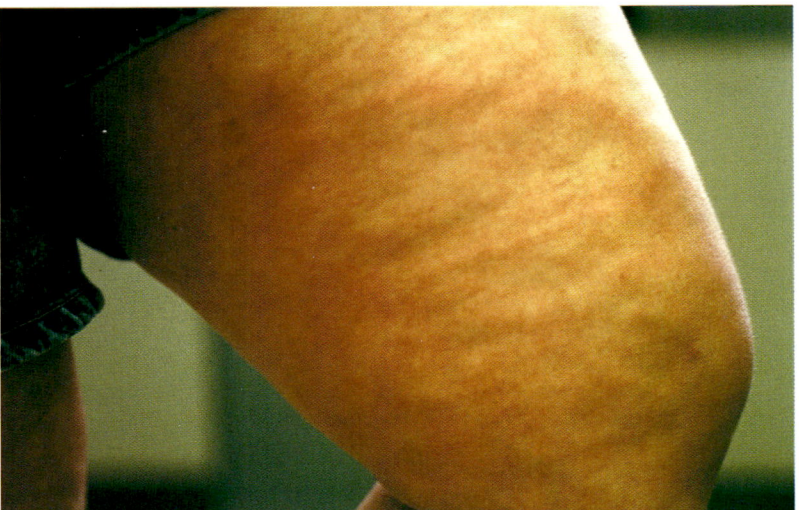

Fig. 24.9 **Erysipelas.** Erythematous, raised border of a plaque of erysipelas due to *Streptococcus pyogenes*.

Laboratory findings

Diagnosis of erysipelas is made primarily on clinical grounds. Skin culture from the portal of entry may be helpful in identifying the causal organism, although latex particle agglutination tests for streptococcal antigens in skin biopsy specimens can be more sensitive than skin culture.[110] Serologic tests for ASO and antiDNAase B titers can be conclusive in approximately 40% of cases, but are only helpful in retrospect.[111]

Skin biopsy shows edema and vascular dilatation in the dermis and upper subcutis; occasionally, organisms can be seen within lymphatic vessels, particularly early in the course of infection. Neutrophils are often seen infiltrating the tissues and lymphatic channels.

Therapeutics and prognosis

Parenteral penicillin is the mainstay of treatment, although a β-lactamase resistant antibiotic often is recommended for initial empiric treatment. In more indolent cases, oral therapy alone may be sufficient. Although in most cases therapy for 10 days is effective, patients with recurrent disease or who are immunocompromised may need to remain on therapy for prolonged periods with penicillin, erythromycin, or an alternative antistreptococcal drug.[109] Use of support stockings and maintenance of hygienic skin care may also aid in the prevention of recurrences.

Lymphangitis

Epidemiology

Lymphangitis occurs when a local skin infection with *Strep. pyogenes* is not fully contained, and spreads to cause inflammation in the walls and soft tissue surrounding dilated lymphatic vessels. Group B and D streptococci and *Staph. aureus* cause lymphangitis on occasion. Other rare infectious agents of acute lymphangitis include *Pasteurella multocida* and *Spirillium minus* (rat bite fever). Following the bite of a mosquito in an area endemic for filariasis, such as Africa, Southeast Asia, and South America, acute lymphangitis and/or lymphadenitis may be caused by *Wuchereria bancrofti* or *Brugia malayi*.

Presenting history

Primary predisposing factors are local trauma to skin on an extremity with lymphatic stasis due to congenital malformation, trauma or surgery, previous infection, chronic inflammation, associated venous disease, or tumor infiltration.

Physical examination

Acute lymphangitis presents most commonly on an extremity with an erythematous, tender, linear streak measuring millimeters to a few centimeters in width. The streak extends proximally from the portal of entry, which may or may not be visible as a site of local infection (e.g., impetigo, ecthyma, cellulitis, paronychia). The regional lymph nodes are enlarged and tender, and the distal extremity may become edematous.

Systemic manifestations of infection including fever, chills, malaise, and headache tend to develop quickly, and are often out of proportion to the degree of local signs. Following infection, some individuals develop chronic distal extremity lymphedema that worsens with subsequent infections and progressive lymphatic fibrosis. Ultimately, the epidermis may become hyperkeratotic, warty, and studded with vesicles and bullae containing lymphatic fluid.

Lymphangitis originating at the interdigital web of the thumb can present particular problems, as the lymphatic drainage from this site may bypass the epitrochlear and axillary nodes and enter the subpectoral nodes. Complications can include subpectoral abscess, chest wall cellulitis, and pleural effusion.

Laboratory findings

Leukocytosis is often present, and bacteremia may ensue. Gram stain and culture of the initial skin lesion or culture of the blood may reveal the causative organism.

Differential diagnosis

Thrombophlebitis on the leg may also present with a tender, swollen, red streak, but tender lymphadenopathy and a focal, distal skin infection are absent. Nodular lymphangitis, due most commonly to *Sporothrix schenckii* or *Mycobacterium marinum*, generally is not associated with significant tenderness, regional lymphadenopathy, or systemic signs of illness.

Therapeutics and prognosis

The affected limb should be elevated, and a search made for the portal of entry of the causative organism. In some instances, a treatable process such as tinea pedis may create the minor breaks in the skin.

Penicillin is the empiric treatment of choice, although suspicion of infection due to *Staph. aureus* should prompt use of a penicillinase-resistant antistaphylococcal penicillin. Patients with systemic signs of illness should be hospitalized and treated parenterally. Occasionally, early, mild disease can be managed initially with procaine penicillin G followed by oral penicillin V. As in the management of erysipelas, patients with recurrent disease and predisposing factors such as chronic lymphedema may need to remain on prophylactic therapy for prolonged periods with penicillin, erythromycin or an alternative antistreptococcal drug. In those with recurrent disease, attention should be given to conservative measures such as exercise, local skin care, and pressure gradient bandages or hosiery.

NECROTIZING SUBCUTANEOUS INFECTIONS

Necrotizing soft tissue infections form a continuum of diseases, some of which develop primarily in the more superficial layer(s) of the subcutaneous tissues, while others typically extend to the deep fascia and muscle. Although the rapidity and extent of tissue destruction and the etiologic agent(s) vary, these conditions characteristically present with a paucity of early cutaneous signs relative to the rapidity and degree of destruction of the subcutaneous tissues. In distinction to cellulitis, pain, tenderness and constitutional signs tend to be out of proportion to the cutaneous findings. This is particularly true with involvement of the fascia and muscle. In general, patients with involvement of the superficial or deep fascia and muscle tend to be more acutely and systemically ill and have more rapidly advancing disease than those with infection confined solely to subcutaneous tissues above the fascia. Tissue necrosis distinguishes these conditions from cellulitis, in which an inflammatory

110. Bernard P, Toty L, Mounier M et al. (1987) Early detection of streptococcal group antigens in skin samples by latex particle agglutination. **Arch Dermatol** 123:468–470.

111. Leppard BJ, Seal DV, Colman G et al. (1985) The value of bacteriology and serology in the diagnosis of cellulitis and erysipelas. **Br J Dermatol** 112:559–567.

infectious process involves, but does not destroy, subcutaneous tissue. Unlike an abscess, necrotizing soft tissue infections involve relatively diffuse tissue necrosis and lack localized purulence.

Necrotizing fasciitis

Necrotizing fasciitis is a subcutaneous tissue infection that involves the deep layer of superficial fascia but largely spares adjacent epidermis, deep fascia and muscle.

Epidemiology

Relatively few organisms possess sufficient virulence to cause necrotizing fasciitis when acting alone. The most fulminant infections, associated with toxic shock syndrome and a high case-fatality rate, are caused by *Strep. pyogenes*.[52,112] Streptococcal necrotizing fasciitis has a variety of presentations; a subacute form of the disease manifests with slowly advancing tissue necrosis and eschar formation, and a lesser degree of blood vessel thrombosis in histopathologic sections.[50]

Necrotizing fasciitis can occasionally be caused by a wide variety of organisms, most notably *Staph. aureus, Clostridium perfringens, C. septicum, P. aeruginosa, Vibrio* spp., particularly *V. vulnificus*, and fungi of the order Mucorales, particularly *Rhizopus* spp., *Mucor* spp., and *Absidia* spp.[3,52] Necrotizing fasciitis may be a polymicrobial infection due to a mixture of anaerobic, aerobic and/or facultative bacteria. Infections due to any one organism or combination of organisms cannot be distinguished clinically from one another, although development of crepitance signals the presence of *Clostridium* spp. or Gram-negative bacilli such as *E. coli, Klebsiella, Proteus*, and *Aeromonas*.

Presenting history

Necrotizing fasciitis may occur anywhere on the body; the most common locations, however, are the extremities, abdomen, and perineal region. The incidence is highest in hosts with systemic or local tissue immunocompromise, such as those with diabetes mellitus, neoplasia, peripheral vascular disease, recent surgery, intravenous drug abuse, or on immunosuppressive treatment, particularly corticosteroids. The infection also can occur in healthy individuals following minor puncture wounds, abrasions or lacerations; blunt trauma; surgical procedures, particularly of the abdomen, gastrointestinal or genitourinary tracts, or the perineum; or hypodermic needle injection. Since the mid-1980s, there has been a resurgence of fulminant necrotizing soft tissue infections due to *Strep. pyogenes*, which may occur in previously healthy individuals with little or no apparent compromise of immunologic or skin integrity.[52,112] Recent cases in children have highlighted its occurrence following streptococcal superinfection of varicella lesions.[113] Children with varicella and invasive *Strep. pyogenes* infection have tended to display onset, recrudescence or persistence of high fever and signs of toxicity after the third to fourth day of varicella.

Physical examination

Necrotizing fasciitis begins with acute onset of local swelling, erythema, tenderness and warmth (Fig. 24.10). Fever is usually present, and pain is out of proportion to cutaneous signs. Skin changes may appear over 24 to 48h as the infection advances along the superficial fascial plane and nutrient vessels are thrombosed, resulting in cutaneous ischemia. Cutaneous signs include formation of bullae filled initially with straw-colored and later bluish to hemorrhagic fluid, and darkening of affected tissues from red to purple to blue. Skin anesthesia and finally frank tissue gangrene and slough develop due to the ischemia and necrosis. Children with varicella lesions initially may show no cutaneous signs of superinfection with invasive *Strep. pyogenes* such as erythema or swelling.[113] Significant systemic toxicity may accompany necrotizing fasciitis, including shock, organ failure and death. Advance of the infection in this setting can be rapid, progressing to death within hours. The combined case fatality rate among children and adults with necrotizing fasciitis

and toxic-shock-like syndrome due to *Strep. pyogenes* has been approximately 60%.[43] Death is less common, however, in children and in cases not complicated by toxic-shock-like syndrome.[113] Fournier's gangrene is a form of necrotizing fasciitis that occurs in the male genital area, sometimes confined to the scrotum, but involving the perineum, penis and/or abdominal wall in other cases.

Laboratory findings

Histopathologically, necrotizing fasciitis involves necrosis and suppuration of the superficial fascia; edema and an acute inflammatory infiltrate in the deep dermis, subcutaneous fat and fascia; microorganisms present within destroyed tissue; and thrombosis of arteries and veins at all levels of tissue.[45,50] Some thrombosed vessels are surrounded by an inflammatory infiltrate and/or microorganisms, others may be vasculitic, while noninflammatory intravascular coagulation may be present in others. Early in infections due to *Strep. pyogenes* or *Clostridium* spp., inflammatory cells may be lacking at sites of tissue damage.

Definitive diagnosis is made by surgical exploration, which must be undertaken as soon as the diagnosis is suspected. Although magnetic resonance imaging may aid in delineating the extent and tissue planes of involvment, this procedure should not delay surgical intervention.[55] Frozen section incisional biopsy taken early in the course of the infection can aid management by decreasing the time to diagnosis and helping to establishing margins of involvement.[45] Gram-stain of tissue can be particularly useful if chains of Gram-positive cocci, indicative of infection with *Strep. pyogenes*, are seen.

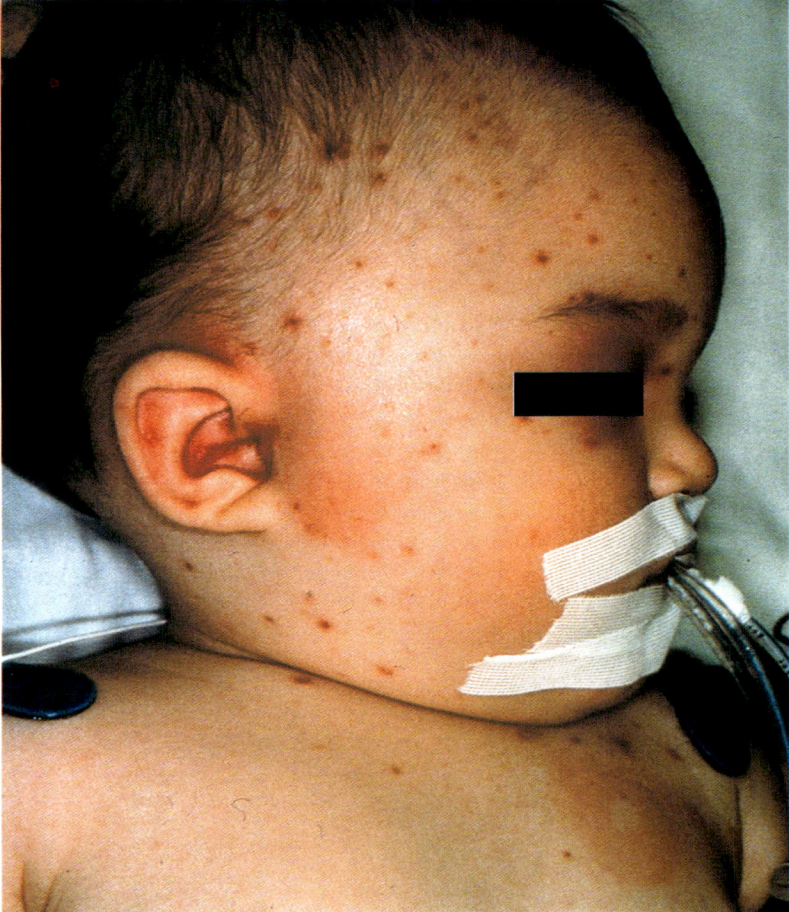

Fig. 24.10 Necrotizing fasciitis. Swelling and erythema early in the development of necrotizing fasciitis on the face of an infant with chickenpox, which provided the portal of entry for *Streptococcus pyogenes*.

112. Finegold DS, Weinberg AN (1996) Group A streptococcal infections. An old adversary reemerging with new tricks? Arch Dermatol 132:67–70.

113. Brogan TV, Nizet V, Waldhausen JHT et al. (1995) Group A streptococcal necrotizing fasciitis complicating varicella: a series of ten patients. Pediatr Infect Dis J 14:588–594.

Therapeutics and prognosis

Early supportive care, surgical debridement, and parenteral antibiotic administration are mandatory. All devitalized tissue must be removed to freely bleeding edges, and repeat exploration is generally indicated within 24 to 36h to confirm that no necrotic tissue remains. Surgery may need to be repeated on several occasions until devitalized tissue has ceased to form. Daily, meticulous wound care is also paramount. The testes can generally be saved in Fournier's gangrene because they have a separate blood supply from the adjacent fascia and skin.

Antibiotic therapy must be initiated parenterally as soon as possible with broad-spectrum agents against all potential pathogens. Most experts recommend initial empiric therapy with penicillin, ampicillin, or nafcillin; clindamycin; and an aminoglycoside.[42,43,52,114] Due to the inoculum effect in fulminant infections due to *Strep. pyogenes*, β-lactam antibiotics such as penicillin and the cephalosporins may become less effective (see Overview: Penicillin resistance).[58] Since efficacy of the protein synthesis inhibitor clindamycin is not adversely altered by the inoculum effect, it is preferred over penicillin by many experts for treatment of deep-seated, serious soft tissue infections due to *Strep. pyogenes*. Adjunctive therapies include hyperbaric oxygen and intravenous administration of intravenous pooled γ-globulin.[112–116]

DISEASES MEDIATED BY EXOTOXINS

Exotoxin-mediated diseases caused by *Staph. aureus* or *Strep. pyogenes* are due to the effects of extracellular toxin(s) produced at a focus of infection or colonization.[7] The site of bacterial replication is typically inconspicuous in relation to the clinical effects of the toxin(s). Toxins can act locally, as in bullous impetigo, or as with the diseases discussed in this section, can cause widespread clinical signs of disease due to hematogenous spread. To exert their effects, toxins may act directly as when staphylococcal epidermolytic toxin binds to and disrupts desmosomes to cause bullous impetigo or SSSS. Alternatively, toxins may act indirectly as when staphylococcal TSST-1 activates T lymphocytes to secrete massive amounts of cytokines; the cytokines, in turn, trigger the multisystem dysfunction that constitutes staphylococcal toxic shock syndrome. In most instances, however, both direct and indirect toxicity are responsible for the disease manifestations, as in scarlet fever where cytotoxicity and Arthus and delayed hypersensitivity skin reactions cause the rash.

SCARLET FEVER (SCARLATINA)
Epidemiology

Scarlet fever is characterized by fever, oral mucous membrane changes, and an exanthem associated with elaboration of streptococcal pyrogenic exotoxin(s) (SPE) from a focus of infection or colonization.[7] Most cases of scarlet fever appear to be due to SPE-A-producing strains, although all three of the SPEs (i.e., A, B, C) are capable of causing the clinical features of scarlet fever, and some isolates express more than one type.[117–119] Scarlet fever is occasionally caused by strains of group C or G streptococci that produce exotoxins that are anigenically distinct from the SPEs of group A streptococci.

During the course of scarlet fever, protective antibody is generated against SPE. Antibody to exotoxin does not provide protection against future infection with *Strep. pyogenes*, but by age 10 years, 80% of children have developed lifelong protective antibodies against the toxins. Consequently, the disease primarily affects children between 4 and 8 years old. Recurrent attacks

of scarlet fever are exceptional, due to protective cross-reactivity of antibody against the SPEs. Disease is also rare in children younger than 2 years of age, apparently due to the presence of maternal antiexotoxin antibodies, and the lack of prior hypersensitization to the exotoxins, which is necessary for development of the exanthem.

Presenting history

The most common infection that leads to scarlet fever is tonsillopharyngitis due to *Strep. pyogenes*. Rash develops, however, in less than 10% of individuals with streptococcal tonsillopharyngitis.[120] Scarlet fever also occurs following streptococcal skin and soft tissue infection, infection of surgical wounds (surgical scarlet fever) or the uterus (puerperal scarlet fever). The incubation period generally is 1 to 4 days. Mild to moderate scarlet fever associated with tonsillopharyngitis typically presents abruptly with fever and sore throat, followed within 1 to 2 days by appearance of rash. The illness may be accompanied by headache, nausea, vomiting, abdominal pain, myalgias, and malaise.

Physical examination

Exudative tonsillopharyngitis is accompanied by erythematous oral mucous membranes, and petechiae and punctate erythematous macules on the hard and soft palate and uvula (Forschheimer's spots). The tongue is covered initially by a yellowish white coat; protruding red papillae give the appearance of a "white strawberry tongue." Within approximately 2 to 4 days, disappearance of the white coating reveals a beefy red tongue with engorged papillae known as a "red strawberry tongue."

Rash generally appears first on the base of the neck, the face and upper trunk, and generalizes over the next 1 to 2 days (Fig. 24.11). The lower legs are involved last and least, and the palms and soles are usually spared. Generalized, blanchable erythroderma is puncuated by numerous pinpoint, erythematous, blanchable papules, imparting a sandpaper-like texture. Occlusion of sweat glands is apparently responsible for producing the papular rash. Erythema tends to be accentuated in the skin folds, and may develop into linear arrays of petechiae called Pastia's lines due to capillary fragility. Circumoral pallor may be prominent. Generalized lymphadenopathy and/or splenomegaly occur occasionally.

The rash fades over approximately 5 to 7 days, followed approximately 7 to 10 days later by fine superficial desquamation on the face and trunk, particularly in the axillae and groin (Fig. 24.12). Sheets of scale peel off the hands and feet; this may be most marked on the distal digits and base of the nails. Desquamation and peeling may continue for weeks. Months after the acute illness, transverse grooves (Beau's lines) may become apparent on the nails and telogen effluvium can develop. Toxin-mediated complications of the acute illness such as myocarditis may occur, but most complications are the result of direct bacterial invasion of tissues and are no more common than with other streptococcal infections of the pharynx or skin.[7] Late complications include rheumatic fever and acute poststreptococcal glomerulonephritis.

Toxic cases of scarlet fever begin with severe sore throat and painful cervical lymphadenopathy; high fever, greater than 40°C; delirium; and rash. Progression to convulsions, coma and death may occur within approximately 24h. Septic cases involve bacterial invasion of local soft tissues of the neck with suppuration, leading to otitis media with perforation, mucopurulent sinusitis, bronchopneumonia, upper airway obstruction, sepsis and death. Necrotizing fasciitis or myositis are not present in even the most severe forms of scarlet fever.

114. Stevens DL, Tanner MH, Winship J et al. (1989) Severe group A streptococcal infections associated with a toxic shock-like syndrome and scarlet fever toxin. **N Engl J Med** 321:1–8.
115. Shupak A, Shoshani O, Goldenberg I et al. (1995) Necrotizing fasciitis: an indication for hyperbaric oxygen therapy? **Surgery** 118:873–878.
116. Kaul R, McGeer A, Noirby-Teglund A et al. (1999) Intravenous immunoglobulin therapy for streptococcal toxic shock syndrome – a comparative observational study. **Clin Infect Dis** 28:300–807.
117. Knoll H, Sramek J, Vrbova K et al. (1991) Scarlet fever and the types of erythrogenic toxins produced by the infecting streptococcal strains. **Int J Med Microbiol** 276:94–106.
118. Belani K, Schlievert PM, Kaplan EL, Ferrieri P (1991) Association of exotoxin-producing group A streptococci and severe disease in children. **Pediatr Infect Dis J** 10:351–354.
119. Yu C, Ferretti JJ (1989) Molecular epidemiologic analysis of the type A streptococcal exotoxin (erythrogenic toxin) gene (speA) in clinical *Streptococcus pyogenes* strains. **Infect Immun** 57:3715–3719.
120. Breese BB (1960) Beta hemolytic streptococcal infections in children. **Pediatr Clin N Am** 7:843–867.

Laboratory findings

Leukocytosis (e.g., 12 to 16 000/mm³) with a left shift is common; eosinophilia (e.g., 10–20%) can also occur after a few days of illness. Diagnosis is generally made on clinical grounds, and can be confirmed by culture of *Strep. pyogenes* from a focal site of infection such as the throat or skin.

Highly specific rapid antigen detection technology is available for detection of tonsillopharyngeal infection and some cases of skin infection. False negative results can occur, however, particularly with low-level infection. Furthermore, antigen detection tests fail to identify infection due to nongroup A streptococci. Consequently, a negative antigen detection test result should be followed up with a confirmatory throat culture.

Histopathogically, dermal blood and lymphatic vessels show diffuse vaso-dilatation, which is most prominent around hair foillicles. Perivascular edema,

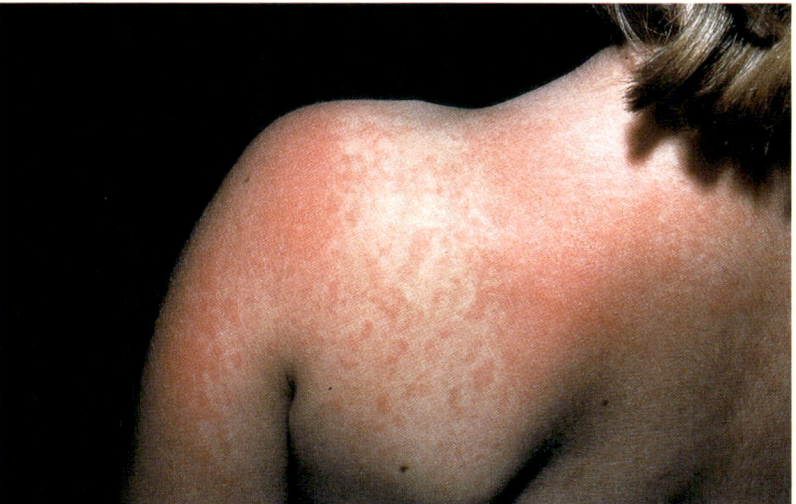

Fig. 24.11   Scarlet fever. Multiple erythematous, blanchable papules and patches of erythroderma, forming the "sandpaper" eruption of scarlet fever due to *Streptococcus pyogenes* (photograph courtesy of Alfred T. Lane).

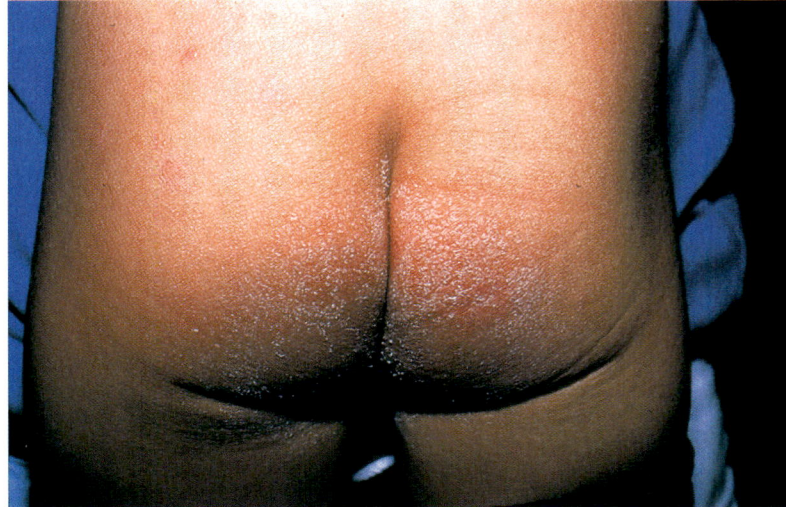

Fig. 24.12   Scarlet fever. Fine desquamating erythematous plaque on the buttocks of a child with resolving scarlet fever due to *Streptococcus pyogenes*.

mononuclear cell infiltrates, and occasional hemorrhage are also noted, but there is no evidence of vasculitis.

Differential diagnosis

An eruption virtually identical to that of streptococcal scarlet fever is caused by toxin-producing strains of *Staph. aureus*. Exudative tonsillopharyngitis, strawberry tongue and palatal petechiae are lacking in staphylococcal scarlet fever, however, and this entity is typically associated with focal infection such as an abscess, septic arthritis, osteomyelitis, or wound infection. Staphylococcal scarlet fever may be an abortive form of SSSS. Other cases share features with toxic shock syndrome, and may be mediated by other staphylococcal toxins such as TSST-1, enterotoxin B or enterotoxin C.

Exudative pharyngitis and a rash similar to that of scarlet fever have also been associated with infection caused by *Arcanobacterium haemolyticum*.[121,122] The infection is commonly accompanied by pruritus, anterior cervical or submandibular lymphadenopathy, low-grade fever, and a nonproductive cough. Most patients are between 10 and 25 years of age, and in this age group, pharyngitis with scarlatina is as likely to be due to *A. haemolyticum* as to *Strep. pyogenes*.[121] The scarlatiniform eruption appears 1–4 days after onset of pharyngitis, and unlike scarlet fever, develops first on the distal extremities and spreads centrally over the next 2 to 3 days. Rash may also involve the neck, chest and back, but the face, palms and soles are spared. Desquamation frequently occurs as the rash resolves, often on the hands and feet, but it is generally less prominent than that seen following scarlet fever. The organism does not produce significant β-hemolysis on sheep blood agar plates before 24–36h, when throat cultures for *Strep. pyogenes* typically are read for the final time. Growth and β-hemolysis are enhanced, however, when the organism is cultured on rabbit or human blood agar. Thus, sheep blood agar plates should be incubated for at least 48h, or these alternative media should be used when the diagnosis is suspected (i.e., scarlatiniform rash in a teenager). Within 48h on rabbit or human blood agar, hemolysis is prominent and a black opaque dot at the center of each colony is visible and remains if the colony is scraped aside. As with scarlet fever, the exanthem is presumably due to an extracellular toxin.

Kawasaki disease can also present with oral mucous membrane changes and a scarlatiniform rash virtually indistinguishable clinically from scarlet fever. Features that may be helpful in diagnosing Kawasaki disease, however, include prominent conjunctivitis, occasionally sparing the limbus; uveitis on slit-lamp examination; marked elevation of the erythrocyte sedimentation rate and C-reactive protein; sterile pyuria; and prolonged fever. Fever tends to resolve within 5 to 6 days in scarlet fever, whereas fever for more than 5 days is a diagnostic criterion for Kawasaki disease.

Additional infectious diseases that must be considered in the differential diagnosis of scarlet fever include SSSS and toxic shock syndrome (see below), rubella, measles, infectious mononucleosis, and parvovirus B19 or echovirus 14 infection. Cutaneous eruptions caused by drug hypersensitivity reactions can also closely mimic scarlet fever.

Therapeutics and prognosis

Early treatment of scarlet fever is associated with reduced infectivity, more rapid resolution of disease, and prevention of acute complications as well as rheumatic fever.[123] The drug of choice for treatment of scarlet fever is penicillin, which must be continued for 10 days to eradicate *Strep. pyogenes* from the pharynx. Patients who are acutely ill may benefit from an intramuscular injection of benzathine penicillin G, 1.2 million units in adults or 600 000 units for children who weigh less than 27kg. The dose of orally administered penicillin V is 250mg tid for 10 days. Narrow-spectrum oral cephalosporins are also effective, acceptable alternatives.[124] In penicillin-allergic patients, erythromycin, clarithromycin, and azithromycin appear to be effective.

121. Miller RA, Branzato F, Holmes KK (1986) *Corynebacterium haemolyticum* as a cause of pharyngitis and scarlatiniform rash in young adults. **Ann Int Med** 105:867–872.
122. Gaston DA, Zurowski SM (1996) *Arcanobacterium haemolyticum* pharyngitis and exanthem. **Arch Dermatol** 132:61–64.
123. Randolph MF, Gerber MA, DeMeo KK et al. (1985) Effect of antibiotic therapy on the clinical course of streptococcal pharyngitis. **J Pediatr** 106:870–875.
124. Pichichero ME (1993) Cephalosporins are superior to penicillin for treatment of streptococcal tonsillopharyngitis: is the difference worth it? **Pediatr Infect Dis J** 12:268–274.

STAPHYLOCOCCAL SCALDED SKIN SYNDROME

Introduction

Staphylococcal scalded skin syndrome (SSSS) is a staphylococcal epidermolytic toxin-mediated disease characterized by cutaneous tenderness and superficial, widespread blistering and/or desquamation.[125]

Epidemiology

SSSS occurs predominantly in infants and children under 5 years of age, apparently due to reduced renal clearance and lack of immunity to the toxins in this younger age group. It is caused predominantly by phage group II staphylococci, particularly strains 71 and 55, which are present at localized sites of infection.[126]

Presenting history

Foci of infection from which toxins are elaborated include the nasopharynx, or less commonly, the umbilicus in neonates, the urinary tract, a cutaneous wound, conjunctivae, or the blood. Onset of the rash may be preceded by malaise, fever, irritability, and exquisite tenderness of the skin.

Physical examination

Generalized macular erythema evolves rapidly into a scarlatiniform eruption that is accentuated in flexural and periorificial areas (Fig. 24.13). There may be pharyngitis, conjunctivitis, and superficial erosions of the lips, but intraoral mucosal surfaces are spared. Characteristically, circumoral erythema is prominent, and the brightly erythematous skin may acquire a wrinkled appearance, leading to thick flaky desquamation, particularly in the flexures, over approximately 2 to 5 days (Fig. 24.14). In severe cases, the erythrodermic phase is followed by the development of diffuse, sterile, flaccid blisters and erosions. At this stage, the superficial epidermis may separate in response to gentle shear force (Nikolski sign). Bullous desquamation of large sheets in the neonate is known as Ritter disease. As large sheets peel away, glistening areas become apparent, initially in the flexures and subsequently over much of the body surface. As the exposed skin dries, it develops a crusted, flaky appearance. Distinctive radial crusting and fissuring around the eyes, mouth, and nose develop approximately 2 to 5 days after the onset of erythroderma in all forms of the disease. Healing occurs without scarring in 10 to 14 days. Although some patients appear ill, many are reasonably comfortable except for the marked skin tenderness.

Laboratory findings

Intact bullae are consistently sterile, unlike those of bullous impetigo, but cultures should be obtained from all suspected sites of localized infection and from the blood in an attempt to identify the source for elaboration of the epidermolytic toxins. Histopathologically, the site of blister cleavage is subcorneal, through the granular layer. Absence of an inflammatory infiltrate is characteristic. In cases requiring a rapid diagnosis, a frozen biopsy specimen of the desquamating epidermis reveals the exfoliated corneal layer. Scattered acantholytic cells, which are evident histopathologically in the cleft-like bullae, can also be seen in a Tzanck preparation.

Pathophysiology

Severity of the disease is related to the toxin load in the blood, rather than the nature of the focal infection, since the clinical manifestations are mediated by hematogenous spread of epidermolytic toxins A or B in the absence of specific antitoxin antibody.[126] The epidermolytic toxins produce the granular layer split by binding to and exerting serine protease activity to cleave desmoglein I within desmosomes.[83,84]

Differential diagnosis

Staphylococcal scalded skin syndrome may be mistaken for a number of other blistering and exfoliating disorders, including scarlet fever, bullous impetigo, epidermolysis bullosa, epidermolytic hyperkeratosis, pemphigus foliaceus, drug eruption, erythema multiforme, and drug-induced toxic epidermal necrolysis (TEN). The latter can often be distinguished by a history of drug ingestion, presence of the Nikolski sign only at sites of erythema, and absence of perioral crusting. Distinction between the skin lesions of TEN and SSSS, however, may require histopathologic examination of a skin biopsy specimen; TEN results in full-thickness epidermal necrosis, with a blister cleavage plane in the lowermost epidermis, while the cleavage plane in SSSS is subcorneal. Distinguishing between these conditions is particularly important given the mortality (up to 30%) associated with TEN and the need to avoid the offending drug to prevent a recurrence.

Therapeutics and prognosis

Systemic therapy with a semisynthetic penicillinase-resistant penicillin should be administered promptly. Healing may be hastened by gentle cleansing of

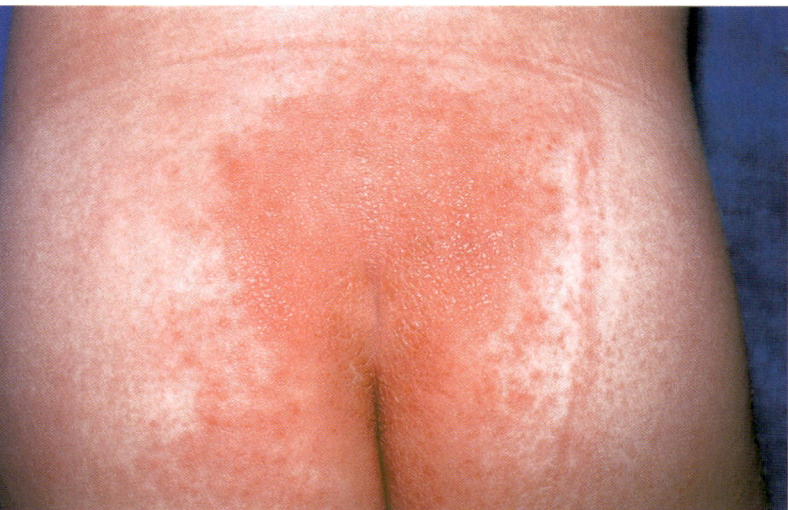

Fig. 24.13 **Staphylococcal scalded skin syndrome.** Erythematous, wrinkled plaque of mild SSSS in a child with pneumonia due to *Staphylococcus aureus*.

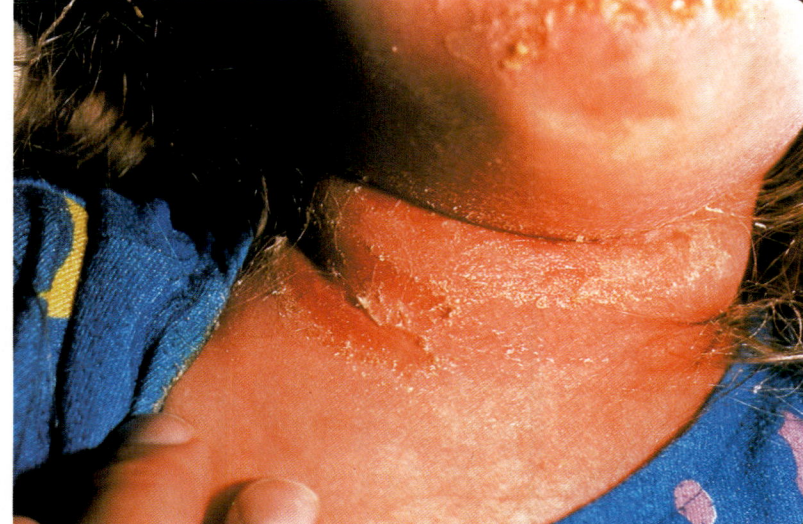

Fig. 24.14 **Staphylococcal scalded skin syndrome.** Crusted exfoliating plaques on the neck, and crusted perioral plaque on a child with SSSS due to *Staphylococcus aureus*.

125. Elias PM, Fritsch P, Epstein EH (1977) Staphylococcal scalded skin syndrome. Clinical features, pathogenesis, and recent microbiological and biochemical developments. **Arch Dermatol** 113:207–219.

126. Melish ME, Glasgow LA (1971) Staphylococcal scalded skin syndrome: the expanded clinical syndrome. **J Pediatr** 78:958–967.

crusted areas, although handling of the patient should be minimized, particularly early in the course of the disease. Application of an emollient will provide lubrication and may decrease discomfort in the resolution phase. Corticosteroids are detrimental and should be avoided.

Recovery from SSSS is usually rapid, but complications such as excessive fluid and heat loss, electrolyte imbalance, secondary cutaneous infection, pneumonia, septicemia, and cellulitis may cause increased morbidity. Mortality is rare, due predominantly to sepsis, but is higher in infants with Ritter disease.

STAPHYLOCOCCAL TOXIC SHOCK SYNDROME
Introduction
Staphyloccocal toxic shock syndrome (TSS) is characterized by acute onset of high fever; erythrodermic, scarlatiniform rash followed by desquamation, particularly on the hands and feet; hyperemic mucous membranes; hypotension; and multiorgan compromise.

Epidemiology
Staphylococcal toxic shock syndrome is due to infection or colonization with a toxin–producing strain of *Staph. aureus* in a susceptible host with low to absent levels of specific antitoxin antibody.[127] It was first described in 1978 in children who were colonized or infected on a mucosal surface (e.g., vaginal, nasopharyngeal, tracheal) or in a focal, sequestered site (e.g., empyema, cutaneous abscess) with phage group I *Staph. aureus*.[128] Disease occurs rarely in children, however, and half or more of cases worldwide occur in women who are vaginally colonized or infected during menstruation.

Toxic shock syndrome is caused by toxin–producing strains of *Staph. aureus*, particularly phage types 29, 52 and 29/52 of phage group I, although a significant proportion of isolates (30–40%) cannot be typed.[129] Manifestations of disease are mediated by one or more staphylococcal toxins, (e.g., TSST-1; also enterotoxins B, A, C_1) acting alone or in concert. Toxic shock syndrome has occurred in individuals from whom only coagulase negative staphylococci have been isolated, suggesting that these bacteria rarely can cause the syndrome.[130]

Presenting history
The most common nonmenstrual settings for TSS are upper airway infections such as sinusitis or tracheitis, burns, minor skin infections, and as a complication of a variety of surgical procedures, especially when nasal packing is involved.[131] Toxic shock syndrome encompasses a range of relatively mild to rapidly fatal disease. Characteristically, however, patients develop a well-defined constellation of signs involving multiple organ systems over a brief period of time. Some patients experience a prodrome of malaise, myalgias, low-grade fever, or vomiting during the week before acute onset of illness.[132] The average interval from precipating event to onset of symptoms of TSS is approximately 7 days for cases unrelated to menstruation.[133] Local signs of inflammation and infection typically are trivial to absent.

Physical examination
Onset of disease is marked by abrupt development of high fever, associated with chills, abdominal pain, headache, nausea, emesis, diarrhea, myalgias, and weakness. Hypotension ensues rapidly, leading to tissue ischemia and multiorgan

injury.[134] Patients typically present without focal neurologic or meningeal signs, but confusion and disorientation rapidly may ensue and progress to seizures and coma. Renal failure, respiratory distress syndrome, myocardial dysfunction, and disseminated intravascular coagulation may be life threatening.

Rash develops in virtually all patients within 1 to 3 days of onset of disease.[133] A diffuse, macular, erythrodermic, scarlatiniform eruption is most common, sometimes developing first on the trunk and spreading to the extremities or consisting of scattered erythematous papules.[135] The eruption often is accentuated in flexural areas, and may be patchy. Typically, the rash fades over a few days; on occasion it becomes petechial, purpuric, vesicular, and/or bullous.

Pharyngitis and hyperemia of conjunctival and mucosal membranes may be prominent, and may progress to oral, esophageal, vaginal, and/or bladder mucosal ulcerations or subconjunctival hemorrhage. Strawberry tongue is present in more than half of patients, and palatal petechiae may be present occasionally.[136] Edema of the hands and feet is characteristic. One to 2 weeks after onset of illness, approximately half of patients develop a pruritic, diffuse, maculopapular, sometimes urticarial eruption, typically involving the palms and soles but sparing the face.[137] This secondary eruption generally lasts 2 to 7 days, and may be accompanied by edema of the face and extremities. Full-thickness desquamation of the skin, particularly of the subungual areas of the digits, the palms and soles generally occurs 10 to 21 days after onset of the disease.

Toxic shock syndrome manifests in a similar manner, regardless of age, sex, and association with menses. Children, however, are more apt to suffer respiratory embarrassment.[138] A variant of TSS has presented in individuals with AIDS with prolonged, diffuse, cutaneous erythema; desquamation; conjunctival injection; hypotension; and multiorgan involvement.[139] Mean duration of the recalcitrant illness was 50 days.

Diagnosis is based on clinical recognition of the syndrome, and requires the presence of high fever, rash followed by desquamation, hypotension, and involvement of three or more organ systems. While recovery of *Staph. aureus* from a normally sterile site provides supportive evidence, the initial focus of infection may occur at a site that is frequently colonized, such as the upper respiratory or genital tract, making culture results difficult to interpret. Demonstration of toxin production by the isolate also supports its role in pathogenesis of the disease.

Laboratory findings
Laboratory abnormalities reflect the multisystem injury, and include low serum protein and albumin, leukocytosis with a predominance of immature forms, thrombocytopenia, and evidence of disseminated intravascular coagulation. Renal abnormalities include reduced urine output, pyuria, proteinuria, and elevated blood urea nitrogen (BUN) and creatinine; electrolyte abnormalities include hypocalcemia, hypophosphatemia, and hypomagnesemia; and hepatic enzymes and bilirubin and muscle creatine phosphokinase are elevated.[132]

Histopathologic examination shows a superficial, perivascular infiltrate of neutrophils, lymphocytes and a few eosinophils; epidermal spongiosis; individually necrotic keratinocytes; and papillary edema.[135,140] Vasculitis is lacking. When blisters form, they are located subepidermally, and ulcerations involve the full thickness of the epidermis. Biopsy generally permits differentiation from TEN or other drug eruptions.

127. Vergeront JM, Stolz SJ, Crass BA et al. (1983) Prevalence of serum antibody to staphylococcal enterotoxin F among Wisconsin residents: implications for toxic shock syndrome. J Infect Dis 148:692–698.
128. Todd J, Fishaut M, Kapral F, Welch T (1978) Toxic-shock syndrome associated with phage-group-I staphylococci. Lancet 2:1116–1118.
129. Ejlertsen T, Jensen A, Lester A, Rosdahl VT (1994) Epidemiology of toxic shock syndrome toxin-1 production in Staphylococcus aureus strains isolated in Denmark between 1959–1990. Scand J Infect Dis 26:599–604.
130. Crass BA, Bergdoll MS (1986) Involvement of coagulase-negative staphylococci in toxic shock syndrome. J Clin Microbiol 23:43–45.
131. Resnick SD (1990) Toxic shock syndrome: recent developments in pathogenesis. J Pediatr 116:321–328.
132. Chesney PJ, Davis JP, Purdy WK, Wand PJ, Chesney RW (1981) Clinical manifestations of toxic shock syndrome. JAMA 246:741–748.
133. Kain KC, Schulzer M, Chow AW (1993) Clinical spectrum of nonmenstrual toxic shock syndrome (TSS): comparison with menstrual TSS by multivariate discriminant analyses. Clin Infect Dis 16:100–106.
134. Chesney PJ (1989) Clinical aspects and spectrum of illness of toxic shock syndrome: overview. Rev Infect Dis 11(Suppl 1):S1–S7.
135. Hurwitz RM, Rivera HP, Gooch MH et al. (1982) Toxic shock syndrome or toxic epidermal necrolysis? J Am Acad Dermatol 7:246–254.
136. Bach MC (1983) Dermatologic signs in toxic shock syndrome – clues to diagnosis. J Am Acad Dermatol 8:343–347.
137. Chesney PJ, Crass BA, Polyak MB et al. (1982) Toxic shock syndrome: management and long-term sequellae. Ann Int Med 96:847–851.
138. Wiesenthal AM, Todd JK (1984) Toxic shock syndrome in children aged 10 years or less. Pediatrics 74:112–117.
139. Cone LA, Woddard DR, Byrd RG et al. (1992) A recalcitrant, erythematous, desquamating disorder associated with toxin-producing staphylococci in patients with AIDS. J Infect Dis 165:638–643.
140. Hurwitz RM, Ackerman AB (1985) Cutaneous pathology of the toxic shock syndrome. Am J Dermatopathol 7:563–578.

Pathophysiology

Colonization or infection with a toxigenic strain of *Staph. aureus* is not sufficient for production of TSS, even in a host lacking protective antitoxin antibody. It appears that the conditions present locally (e.g., neutral pH, aerobic environment, slightly elevated CO_2 level, high protein level) must favor expression of toxin.[141]

Approximately 80% of infants less than 1 year of age have levels of transplacentally acquired anti-TSST-1 antibody that are considered protective. Half or less of children aged 1 to 4 years, however, have protective levels of antibody;[142] nevertheless, their incidence of TSS is exceedingly low, emphasizing the importance of local conditions at the site of infection in facilitating toxin production.[141,142] The prevalence of protective antibody levels rises to 80–90% or more in the general population over age 20 years,[127,142] yet this is the age group most frequently affected. Women who develop menstrual TSS, however, lack protective levels of antibody and tend to develop antibody slowly, if at all, often only after several episodes over 1 to 2 years.

Once staphylococcal exotoxins have been produced and released into the circulation, they mediate manifestations of TSS predominantly through superantigen stimulation of massive cytokine release.[35,143,144] Direct cytotoxic action of the staphylococcal enterotoxins may also play a role in pathogenesis, as may enhancement by TSST-1 of susceptibility to endotoxin, or synergistic action of staphylococcal enterotoxins with streptococcal exotoxins.[131,143,145]

Differential diagnosis

The differential diagnosis of TSS is broad, due to its wide variety and spectrum of presentation. Initially, based on cutaneous and mucosal signs, it may be most easily confused with streptococcal scarlet fever, Kawasaki disease/infantile polyarteritis nodosa, SSSS, atypical measles, leptospirosis, Rocky Mountain spotted fever, viral exanthematous diseases, and drug-induced syndromes including Stevens–Johnson syndrome and TEN. Development of shock and multiorgan involvement are not characteristic of these other entities, except perhaps in severe cases of infantile polyarteritis nodosa or TEN. Toxic epidermal necrolysis generally can be distinguished from TSS on the basis of its histopathologic findings of interface dermatitis and subepidermal vesiculation.[135,140] Furthermore, development of exquisite skin tenderness, bullae, and full-thickness epidermal erosions characterize TEN but are unusual in TSS. Toxic epidermal necrolysis may be particularly difficult to distinguish from Kawasaki disease. Prominent crusting and fissuring of the lips, morbilliform or erythema multiforme-like rash, lymphadenopathy, coronary aneurysm, thrombocytosis, and marked elevation of C-reactive protein and the erythrocyte sedimentation rate favor a diagnosis of Kawasaki disease (see Chapter 23).[146]

Therapeutics and prognosis

Treatment of TSS centers on intensive supportive management of shock and multiorgan failure, identification and drainage of infection, and prompt institution of antibacterial therapy. Antibiotic therapy is necessary to eliminate bacterial toxin production, but is unlikely to alter the acute course of the disease unless given early, before significant amounts of toxin reach the circulation. A penicillinase-resistant antistaphylococcal antibiotic, such as oxacillin or nafcillin, or a first- or possibly second-generation cephalosporin should be administered intravenously at the maximal recommended dose for weight and age. In the event that the patient may have acquired a methicillin resistant isolate nosocomially or has an indwelling catheter, therapy may be initiated with vancomycin. Antibiotic choice can be tailored once the susceptibility profile of the isolate is known. A 10-day course of therapy may be completed with an oral agent (e.g., dicloxacillin, cephalexin) once the patient has defervesced, stabilized, and is taking fluids by mouth. Administration of intravenous immunoglobulin (IVIG) may be considered for treatment of TSS with unrelenting shock and organ failure despite optimal management,[134,147] since high levels of antibody to TSST-1 have been found in intramuscular and IVIG preparations.[137]

Most patients with TSS improve after approximately 3–5 days of therapy. Mortality is low (3%), although potential sequelae are numerous, involving the major organ systems affected during acute disease. Relatively more common sequelae include prolonged fatigue, weakness or myalgia; reversible hair loss consistent with telogen effluvium or possibly toxin-induced anagen effluvium; shedding of nails or appearance of Beau's lines; vocal cord paralysis; limb paresthesia; amenorrhea; prolonged renal failure; carpal tunnel syndrome; cognitive difficulties; and impaired capillary refilling leading to cyanotic extremities.[131,132,134]

STREPTOCOCCAL TOXIC SHOCK SYNDROME

Epidemiology

Streptococcal toxic shock syndrome (STSS) is characterized by acute onset of shock and multisystem organ failure due to *Strep. pyogenes* infection.[148,149] Children appear to be less apt than adults to develop STSS.[150] Unlike staphylococcal TSS, STSS is associated with invasion of *Strep. pyogenes*; thus, most patients are bacteremic and/or have focal tissue infection at the time of presentation.[52,113,149] Most isolates of *Strep. pyogenes* that cause STSS are M protein types 1, 3, 12 and 28 that produce SPE-A or SPE-B.[52,113,117,151] Lack of antibody against streptococcal exotoxins appears to be a risk factor for severe, invasive disease and STSS.[152]

Presenting history

Streptococcal toxic shock syndrome develops most often in a healthy host in the setting of a minor, focal skin and/or soft tissue[41,42,52,113,117,152–154] or mucosal[113,155,156] infection that provides a portal of entry.[52,117,149] Recent cases of STSS in children with varicella have highlighted the role of these lesions as a potential portal for *Strep. pyogenes* invasion.[113]

An influenza-like prodromal illness of fever, chills, myalgia and diarrhea heralds STSS in one-fifth of patients.[113] A cardinal distinguishing feature, and the most common (85%) initial symptom of STSS is abrupt onset of severe, localized pain out of proportion to physical findings, which may even be

141. Todd JK, Todd BH, Franco-Buff A et al. (1987) Influence of focal growth conditions on the pathogenesis of toxic shock syndrome. **J Infect Dis** 155:673–681.
142. Jacobson JA, Kasworm EM, Reiser RF, Bergdoll MS (1987) Low incidence of toxic shock syndrome in children with staphylococcal infection. **Am J Med Sci** 294:403–407.
143. Parsonnet J (1989) Mediators in the pathogenesis of toxic shock syndrome: overview. **Rev Infect Dis** 11(Suppl 1):S263–269.
144. Miethke T, Duschek K, Wahl C et al. (1993) Pathogenesis of the toxic shock syndrome: T cell mediated lethal shock caused by the superantigen TSST-1. **Eur J Immunol** 23:1494–1500.
145. Smith RJ, Schlievert PM, Himelright IM, Baddour LM (1994) Dual infections with *Staphylococcus aureus* and *Streptococcus pyogenes* causing toxic shock syndrome. Possible synergistic effects of toxic shock syndrome toxin 1 and streptococcal pyrogenic exotoxin C. **Diagn Microbiol Infect Dis** 19:245–247.
146. Hansen RC (1983) Staphylococcal scalded skin syndrome, toxic shock syndrome, and Kawasaki disease. **Pediatr Clin N Am** 30:533–544.
147. Todd JK (1990) Therapy of toxic shock syndrome. **Drugs** 39:856–861.
148. The Working Group on Severe Streptococcal Infections (1993) Defining the group A streptococcal toxic shock syndrome: rationale and consensus definition. **JAMA** 269:390–391.
149. Stevens DL (1995) Streptococcal toxic-shock syndrome: spectrum of disease, pathogenesis, and new concepts in treatment. **Emerg Infect Dis** 1:69–78.
150. Davies HD, Matlow A, Scriver SR et al. (1994) Apparent lower rates of streptococcal toxic shock syndrome and lower mortality in children with invasive group A streptococcal infections compared with adults. **Pediatr Infect Dis J** 13:49–56.
151. Forni AL, Kaplan EL, Schlievert PM, Roberts RB (1995) Clinical and microbiological characteristics of severe group A streptococcus infections and streptococcal toxic shock syndrome. **Clin Infect Dis** 21:333–340.
152. Mahieu LM, Holm SE, Goossens HJ, Acker KJV (1995) Congenital streptococcal toxic shock syndrome with absence of antibodies against streptococcal pyrogenic exotoxins. **J Pediatr** 127:987–989.
153. Cone LA, Woodland DR, Schlievert PM et al. (1987) Clinical and bacteriologic observations of a toxic shock-like syndrome due to *Streptococcus pyogenes*. **N Engl J Med** 317:146–149.
154. Torres-Martinez C, Mehta D et al. (1992) Streptococcus-associated toxic shock. **Arch Dis Child** 67:126–130.
155. Bradley JS, Schlievert PM, Peterson BM (1991) Toxic shock-like syndrome, a complication of strep throat. **Pediatr Infect Dis J** 10:790.
156. Silver RM, Heddleston LN, McGregor JA et al. (1992) Life-threatening puerperal infection due to group A streptococci. **Obstet Gynecol** 79:894–896.

absent. Pain most commonly involves an extremity, but may originate from the abdomen, chest, or pelvis. Most patients have localized swelling and erythema at the site of pain.

Physical examination

Patients rapidly develop hypotensive shock, accompanied in most by early renal impairment and onset of respiratory distress syndrome. Soft tissue infection becomes apparent in 80% of patients and evolves in the majority of cases (70%) into severe subcutaneous infections (e.g., necrotizing fasciitis, myositis) that require surgical debridement. Development of vesicles and bullae (5%) (Fig. 24.15) is a late, ominous sign of tissue devitalization.[113,157] Patients without soft tissue infection have a variety of focal infections including endophthalmitis, osteomyelitis, myositis, pneumonia, perihepatitis, peritonitis, myocarditis, and sepsis.[113,151]

Early in the course of STSS, conjunctival and/or oropharyngeal mucous membrane hyperemia may be present, but strawberry tongue is uncommon.[153,154] Other cutaneous signs in a minority of patients include a petechial, maculopapular, or diffuse scarlatiniform eruption.[154] Rarely, eruptions may appear several days into the course of the illness, and may even develop concurrently with the desquamation that develops in some patients (20–30%) 1 to 2 weeks after onset of illness.[149,154,157]

Laboratory findings

Laboratory abnormalities reflect the multiorgan system dysfunction. Hemoglobinuria, elevation of serum creatinine, and leukocytosis with a marked left shift develop early. As the disease progresses, the majority of patients display hypoalbuminemia, hypocalcemia, anemia, thrombocytopenia, and elevated creatine phosphokinase.[42,114]

Pathophysiology

Streptococcal pyrogenic exotoxins stimulate cytokine release from monocytes in a manner similar to TSST-1, suggesting parallels in pathogenesis of streptococcal and staphylococcal TSS.[158–160] Streptococcal pyrogenic exotoxin-B has protease activity, and may be capable of damaging tissue directly.[161] Due to an association reported between use of nonsteroidal anti-inflammatory agents and progression of infection to STSS, these agents are best avoided.[162,163]

Differential diagnosis

Definitive diagnosis of STSS requires isolation of *Strep. pyogenes* from a normally sterile site on a patient with hypotension and multiorgan failure. Features of STSS overlap with staphylococcal TSS, possibly due to similarities in their molecular pathogenesis, and with streptococcal necrotizing fasciitis because most cases of STSS originate from a focus of infection involving skin and/or soft tissue. In general, however, STSS is a more fulminant disease that is associated more often with bacteremia, an identifiable focal site of infection, bullae formation, extensive soft tissue devitalization and disfiguring morbidity, and a more lethal outcome than staphylococcal TSS. Scarlatiniform eruption, conjunctival or mucous membrane hyperemia, strawberry tongue, and late desquamation are present less frequently in STSS than staphylococcal TSS.

Therapeutics and prognosis

Patients suspected of having STSS should be managed in an intensive care setting, due to the rapidly progressive, fulminant nature of the syndrome. Early

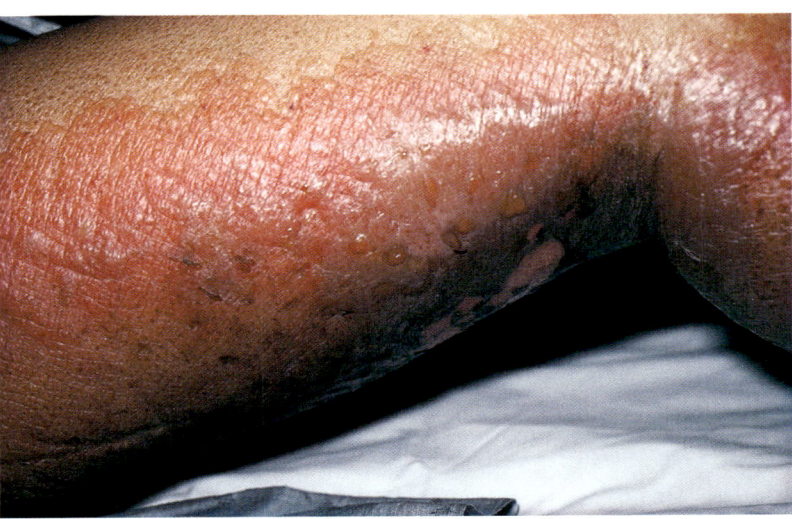

Fig. 24.15 Streptococcal toxic shock syndrome in a 19-year-old woman with severe sepsis. Bullae are prominent on day 5.

management consists of aggressive intravenous fluid resuscitation, culture of potential sites of infection, early surgical exploration of suspected deep-seated infections and debridement of devitalized tissue, and prompt administration of antibiotics. Broad-spectrum antimicrobial therapy should be initiated as discussed for necrotizing fasciitis. Once a diagnosis of STSS is made, therapy can be tailored. Clindamycin has advantages over penicillin (see Necrotizing Fasciitis), although many experts recommend use of both agents concurrently for treatment of STSS.[41,112,149]

OTHER BACTERIAL INFECTIONS

Wesley Galen

SALMONELLA

Salmonella spp. cause a broad spectrum of diseases. These include enteric fever, gastroenteritis, bacteremia, focal infections such as pneumonia, osteomyelitis, or cutaneous abcesses, and a chronic asymptomatic carrier state.[164–166] Patients may also suffer from a combination of the above, as in typhoid fever with sepsis and pneumonia.

Enteric fever, also known as typhoid or paratyphoid fever, is a severe multisystem illness with prolonged abdominal symptoms, bacteremia, fever, and significant complications if left untreated. It is associated with the development of rose spots which are classically noted during the second week of the illness. The presence of these skin lesions may help in separating the diagnosis of salmonellosis from other causes of systemic illness and gastroenteritis such as amebiasis, malaria, enteroviral infection, leishmaniasis or other causes of bacterial enteritis such as *Shigella*.

Salmonellae are extremely hardy bacteria and enjoy a worldwide distribution. They are pathogens for both humans and animals.[164] They are Gram-negative, flagellated, motile, nonencapsulated bacteria that grow on

157. Wolf JE, Rabinowitz LG (1995) Streptococcal toxic shock-like syndrome **Arch Dermatol** 131:73–77.
158. Hackett SP, Stevens DL (1993) Superantigens associated with staphylococcal and streptococcal toxic shock syndrome are potent inducers of tumor necrosis factor-β synthesis. **J Infect Dis** 168:232–235.
159. Hackett SP, Stevens DL (1992) Streptococcal toxic shock syndrome: synthesis of tumor necrosis factor and interleukin-1 by monocytes stimulated with pyrogenic exotoxin A and streptolysin O **J Infect Dis** 165:879–885.
160. Stevens DL, Bryant AE, Hackett SP et al. (1996) Group A streptococcal bacteremia: the role of tumor necrosis factor in shock and organ failure. **J Infect Dis** 173:619–626.
161. Musser JM (1992) Clinical relevance of streptococcal pyrogenic exotoxins in streptococcal toxic shock-like syndrome and other severe infections. **Pediatr Ann** 21:821–828.

162. Stevens DL (1995) Could nonsteroidal antiinflammatory drugs (NSAIDs) enhance the progression of bacterial infection to toxic shock syndrome? **Clin Infect Dis** 21:977–980.
163. Zerr DM, Alexander ER, Duchin JS et al. (1999) A case–control study of necrotizing fasciitis during primary varicella. **Pediatrics** 103:783–790.
164. Hohmann EL (1997) Pathogenesis of Salmonella gastroenteritis, 2001 Up To Date@www.uptodate.com, Vol 9, No. 2, 1–8.
165. Hohmann EL (1998) Approach to the patient with typhoid fever, 2001 Up To Date@www.uptodate.com.
166. Gomez HF, Cleary TG (1998) Salmonella. In: Textbook of Pediatric Infectious Disease, 4th edn, Feigin RD, Cherry JD, eds. Philadelphia: WB Saunders, pp. 1321–1334.

routine laboratory agar in aerobic and anaerobic conditions. Cultures from normally sterile sources such as blood, bone marrow, CSF, or joint fluid can be plated on ordinary media (i.e., blood or chocolate agar). Selective or differential media (i.e., SS-agar, bismuth sulfur or eosin-methylene blue agar) must be used to isolate it from feces.[164]

Salmonella classification is confusing because multiple overlapping nomenclature systems have been used.[164–166] *Salmonella* spp. can be separated biochemically or by various serum agglutination tests directed at surface antigens including lipopolysaccharide or somatic (0) antigens, the virulence or Vi antigen, and the flagellar or H antigen.[166] Serotypes can be further characterized by plasmid identification, outer membrane polypeptide analysis, bacteriophage typing, biochemical phenotype, and by antibiotic sensitivity.[164] This testing may help to establish common source outbreaks for epidemiologic purposes. A newer proposed classification that recognizes six subgroups is based on DNA similarities. Most pathogens important in human and animal disease fall under subgroup 1. Those affecting cold-blooded animals are in subgroups 2 to 5.[164]

Although typing is a very useful epidemiologic tool, it may not be especially helpful clinically[165,166] as many species affecting humans can cause a spectrum of mild to severe illness. Most cases of enteric fever, both typhoidal and paratyphoidal, which exhibit cutaneous manifestations are caused by (*S. typhi*, *S. paratyphi* A, *S. schottmulleri* (formerly *S. paratyphi* B) or *S. hirshfeldii* (formerly *S. paratyphi* C).

S. typhi causes an estimated 12.5 million cases of typhoid fever annually worldwide, particularly in developing countries where the incidence may vary from 10 to 540 cases per 100 000 population. The incidence is less in developed countries such as the United States, where 400 cases were reported in 1988 (0.018 cases per 100 000 population), although a high of 1700 cases was described in 1955 (1 case per 100 000 people). In the USA, only 28% of *S. typhi* infected patients are 19 years old or younger, in contrast to developing countries where the incidence is highest in patients between 5 to 25 years of age.[166] The occurrence of disease in infants in developing countries, however, has been highlighted recently.[167] Infections in the USA are frequently related to foreign travel (62–70%), especially to India and Mexico.[168–170] Paratyphoid fever is caused by *Salmonella* spp. now known as *S. paratyphi* A, *S. schottmulleri*, or *S. hirshfeldii*.

The primary reservoir for the salmonellae responsible for enteric fever (both typhoid and paratyphoid fever) is humans. Food and water contaminated by human feces is the most common source of transmission. Perinatal transmission has been attributed to the fecal–oral route, especially due to handling of neonates with contaminated hands or objects or rare transplacental transmission from a bacteremic mother.[171] Salmonella outbreaks in nurseries are usually traced back to an infected mother and also contaminated instruments and equipment. Nursery epidemics may spread rapidly to involve many infants and staff and take months to years to control.[172,173]

Adult infection can develop with an inoculum of 10^3 to 10^9 bacteria.[165,174] The incubation period is usually 7–14 days but illness may develop in as few as 3 days and as late as 60 days after ingestion of the bacteria. The more rapidly developing and severe infections follow larger inocula. Presumably the inoculum size causing illness in children is smaller.[175]

"Nontyphoidal" salmonellosis, illnesses caused by *salmonella* spp. other than *S. typhi*, has increased in incidence steadily during the last 40 years (50 000 cases annually),[176] probably due to the widespread use or misuse of antibiotics in humans and agriculture, altering gastrointestinal flora and increasing animal and human susceptibility to infection[177] and as well as increasing microbial resistance.[177,178]

Major reservoirs for nontyphoidal salmonella include animals, livestock, poultry, pets (especially turtles), birds, animal products including dairy products, eggs, and meats, and contaminated water, food, and infected humans. Certain serotypes are associated with particular reservoirs, i.e., *S. choleraesuis* with pigs, *S. marina* with pet iguanas, *S. dublin* with dairy cattle and raw meat, *S. typhimurium* and *S. java* with pet turtles and *S. arizona* with reptiles.[166]

Infections with nontyphoidal salmonellae result in fecal excretion of the bacteria for an average period of 5 weeks with prolonged excretion noted in children less than 5 years of age and rare chronic carrier states. *S. typhi* infections may result in a chronic carrier state in 1 to 4% of patients, with shedding of organisms in urine or stool for more than a year, posing a serious risk to the community, especially if present in food handlers. Salmonellae are hardy bacteria and may persist for months in food such as frozen milk, cheese, and ice cream in spite of refrigeration.

CLINICAL PRESENTATION

Enteric fever presents as a febrile illness 5 to 21 days after ingestion of the bacterial source. The initial manifestations are nonsepcific and include fever, abdominal pain, chills, anorexia, myalgias, and headaches. In untreated individuals, the classic reports of illness describe a first week with an incrementally rising fever and bacteremia. During the second week of illness the fever becomes unremitting and is often associated with a relative bradycardia. Increased abdominal pain, nausea, and transient diarrhea and then profound constipation are noted. Vomiting may occur but is usually not severe. Cough and sore throat may be present. A continuous dull headache is noted in 75% of patients. Children are often drowsy and irritable. Dizziness, confusion, seizures, psychosis, delerium and or coma may develop in both children and adults. Arthralgia and backpain are seen in 60% of patients.[164–166]

Rose spots may appear during the second week of illness.[166,179] These are pink to salmon-colored lesions, which usually occur in crops of 10 to 20 on the upper abdomen and trunk, especially between the nipples and umbilicus. They are 2- to 4-mm pink blanchable maculopapules which may be fleeting and fade over hours or persist to become purpuric, brown and then fade in 2 to 3 days. They usually resolve without a scar. These lesions are present in 50–60% of adult patients who are carefully examined, but are seen less frequently in children and are difficult to detect in dark-skinned patients. Rose spots occur less often in enteric fever caused by nontyphoidal species of salmonellae, but are more numerous and widespread when present. The appearance of rose spots has decreased dramatically since the advent of antibiotic therapy.

Another rash described during the acute early phase of enteric fever is "erythema typhosum," a confluent erythematous and diffusely scattered rash appearing during the 1st week of illness. Urticaria as well as erythema nodosum have been noted and attributed to hypersensitivity to the infection or its treatment. Skin abcesses and erosions have also been described in patients from the Indian subcontinent following bacteremia.[180] Rare patients with ulcerative vulvitis or vulvovaginitis due to salmonella infection have been

167. Saha SK, Begni AH, Hanif M et al. (2001) Epidermiology of typhoid fever in Bangladesh: implications for vaccine use. **Pediatr Dis J** 20:521–524.
168. Anonymous (1990) Centers for Disease Control and Prevention: typhoid immunization: Recommendations of the Immunization Practices Advisory Committee (ACID) **MMWR Morb Mortal Wkly Rep** 39:15.
169. Edelman R, Levine MM (1986) Summary of an international workshop on typhoid fever. **Rev Infect Dis** 8:329–349.
170. Ryan CA, Hargrett-Bean NT, Blake PA (1989) *Salmonella typhi* infections in the United States, 1975–1984: Increasing role of foreign travel. **Rev Infect Dis** 11:1–8.
171. Chin KC, Simmons EJ, Tarlow MJ (1986) Neonatal typhoid fever. **Arch Dis Child** 61:1228–1230.
172. Puri V, Therupuram S, Khalil A, et al. (1990) Nosocomial *S. typhimurium* epidemic in neonatal special care unit. **Indian Pediatr** 17:233–239.
173. Reed RP, Klugman KP (1994) Neonatal typhoid fever. **Pediatr Infect Dis J** 13:774–777.
174. Hornick RB, Gruesman SE, Woodward TE et al. (1970) Typhoid fever pathogenesis: Immunologic control Parts 1 and 2. **N Engl J Med** 283:686–691 and 739–746.

175. Taylor DN, Bopp C, Birkness K et al. (1984) An outbreak of Salmonellosis associated with a fatality in a healthy child. A large dose and severe illness. **Am J Epidemiol** 119:907–912.
176. Anonymous (1991) Centers for Disease Control and Prevention Multistate outbreak of Salmonella poona infections: United States and Canada. **MMWR Morb Mortal Wkly Rep** 40:549.
177. Pavia A, Shipman B, Wells J et al. (1990) Epidemiological evidence that prior antimicrobial exposure decreases resistance to infection by antimicrobial sensitive Salmonella. **J Infect Dis** 161:255.
178. Gruenewald R, Blum S, Chan J (1994) Relationship between HIV infection and salmonellosis in 20 to 50 year-old residents of New York City. **Clin Infect Dis** 18:358.
179. Litwack KD, Hoke AW, Borchardt KA (1972) Rose spots in typhoid fever. **Arch Dermatol** 105:1068–1070.
180. Gremillion DH, Geckler R, Ellenbogen C (1977) Salmonella abscess: a potential noscomial hazard. **Arch Surg** 112:843–846.

documented.[181] Late skin changes include nail dystrophies, hair loss, and post-salmonella hypohidrosis.[182]

During the second and by the third week of illness, hepatomegaly and splenomegaly are noted in 50% of patients. Complications may occur in severe cases, including overwhelming sepsis, intestinal bleeding or perforation with bacteremia and secondary peritonitis. Other complications include cholecystitis, pancreatitis, hepatitis, hyperpyrexia, pneumonia, myocarditis, endocarditis, pyelonephritis, orchitis, lymphadenitis, tonsilitis, bone marrow suppression, osteomyelitis, arthritis, suppurative parotitis, and death. These complications occur more frequently in neonates, young infants and children than adults.[164–166]

Typhoid fever has a variable clinical course and patients may lack some of the expected features. Toddlers and infants may present with a vague illness with low-grade temperatures mimicking a viral illness or may develop high spiking fever from the onset. They may present with pneumonitis or nephritis rather than gastroenteritis as a focal presentation. Though very ill, some debilitated patients may be afebrile throughout the course of illness. Infants, especially neonates, are at increased risk for complications, especially massive hepatosplenomegaly and thrombocytopenia, hypothermia and death.[173] Maternal typhoid is associated with an increased risk for fetal abortion, premature birth, and an 83% death rate in untreated congenitally infected newborns.[183,184]

In most uncomplicated patients, enteric fever resolves during weeks to months. Even the response to therapy is gradual with defervescence of fever noted only after 3–6 days of appropriate therapy. Despite institution of antibiotic and supportive therapy, rare complications such as relapsing infection, intestinal perforation, septic shock, and death may occur.

In the USA the mortality rate of enteric fever was 15% prior to the antibiotic era, but was reduced to 1.5% by 1990 with appropriate therapy.[183,185]

DIAGNOSIS

Diagnosis of enteric fever is confirmed when the organism is isolated from blood or other sterile sites. This is particularly useful during the 1st week of the illness when 50–60% of cultures may be positive. Additional techniques include culture of bone marrow aspirates.[186] Skin biopsy of rose spots for culture or histopathology proves most helpful during the second week of illness. During the later stages of illness the percentage of positive blood and bone marrow cultures becomes lower, but there is an increase in positive cultures from the duodenum (via string capsules),[187] urine, and stool.[164] Histologic examination of the rose spot demonstrates dermal edema, capillary dilitation and a perivascular infiltrate of macrophages.[179] The organisms may be seen in the tissues and intracellularly in macrophages. In a patient with a typical clinical course, isolation of organisms from stool may be helpful but not diagnostic of enteric fever.[187]

A fourfold rise in titer to typhoid antigens O and H, the Widal Test, though not seen in all patients, is said to be diagnostic.[188] It is less useful than positive cultures due to cross-reactions with antigens from other Gram-negative bacteria, yeilding false positive results. False negative results are also relatively common. Other nonspecific laboratory findings include an early leukocytosis and later a leukopenia or neutropenia. Abnormal electrolytes as well as abnormal liver functions and proteinuria may be seen in children with diarrhea.

Several new diagnostic serologic kits have been developed which are assays of passive bacterial agglutination, passive hemagglutination, and latex particle agglutination. Others utilize monoclonal antibody enzyme-linked immu-nosorbent assay (ELISA), radioimmunoassay and counter immunoelectrophoresis techniques to aid in diagnosis. These, as well as other tests for detection of salmonella in feces, are not yet widely used or available.

PATHOGENESIS OF ENTERIC FEVER

The incubation of and severity of the illness depends on many factors including the virulence of and the size of inoculum, the age and immunologic status of the host and the presence or absence of gastric acid. The illness tends to be more virulent in neonates, infants, children, and in adult patients with achlorhydria or those who are post-vagotomy, gastrectomy, or gastro-enterostomy, or those using gastric buffering agents or drugs which alter gastric emptying time.[189] Infections are more common and severe in patients pretreated with prophylactic antibiotics, because commensal flora maintain a low luminal gut pH, compete for nutrients, and produce compounds that inhibit growth of salmonellae.[177] Immunocompromised patients treated with corticosteroids or chemotherapeutic agent, and those with HIV infection, leukemia, lymphoma, hemolysis, or sickle cell hemoglobinopathy suffer more frequent and severe infections. Other chronic infectious diseases that may predispose patients to develop salmonella infections include amebiasis, bartonellosis, malaria, and schistosomiasis.

After ingestion of the bacteria and passage through the stomach, a latent asymptomatic period of 3 to 21 days occurs. During this period, organisms increase in number, colonize the intestinal mucosae, selectively attach to specialized epithelial cells known as M cells, which overlie Peyer's patches, and penetrate the mucosa. Thus, they gain entrance to intestinal lymphatics and lymph nodes where they continue to survive and multiply intracellularly in mononuclear cells. From lymph nodes the organisms spread to the blood, reticuloendothelial system, and may spread to further to involve other organs including the liver, spleen, bone marrow, and skin.[164–166]

DIFFERENTIAL DIAGNOSIS

Salmonella gastroenteritis and enteric fever must be distinguished from other infectious causes of diarrhea, especially bloody diarrhea. These include: staphylococcal food poisoning, shigella, enteroinvasive E. coli, enterohemorrhagic E. coli, enteroviral infections, rotavirus, campylobacter, Yersinia enterocolitica, Clostridium difficile, Entamoeba histoytica, Giardia lamblia, cholera, and malaria. Enteric fever can also mimic illnesses of the reticuloendothelial system, including Epstein–Barr virus, tuberculosis, ehrlichiosis, brucellosis, leptospirosis, tularemia, plague, malaria, systemic Bartonella hensellea infection, and typhus. Noninfectious illnesses with prolonged fever that can be confused with typhoid include lymphoma, juvenile rheumatoid arthritis and other collagen vascular diseases, and Kawasaki syndrome.

TREATMENT OF ENTERIC FEVER

The cornerstone of treatment of gastroenteritis due to typhoidal or non-typhoidal stains of salmonella is support with fluids and electrolytes. It is important to determine the species and antibiotic sensitivities of salmonella in directing antibiotic therapy.

Therapy of typhoid fever has become complicated because of the development and rapid spread of salmonellae resistant to ampicillin, chloramphenicol and trimethoprim–sulfamethaxazole (TMP/SMZ). These three antibiotics were considered the drugs of choice for many years. Multidrug resistant salmonella (MDRS) strains have caused numerous outbreaks in

181. Black PH, Kunz LJ, Swarez MN (1962) Salmonellosis – a review of some unusual aspects. **New Engl J Med** 262:811–814.
182. Cohen JL, Bartlett JA, Corey GR (1987) Extraintestinal manifestations of Salmonella. **Infect Med** 66:349–388.
183. Matieu JJ, Henning KJ, Bell E et al. (1994) Typhoid fever in New York City 1980 through 1990. **Arch Intern Med** 154:1713.
184. Diddle AW, Stephens RL (1939) Typhoid fever in pregnancy. **Am J Obstet Gynecol** 38:300–305.
185. Stuart BM, Pullen RL (1946) Typhoid clinical analysis of 360 cases. **Arch Intern Med** 78:269.

186. Gilman RH, Terminel MM et al. (1975) Relative efficacy of blood, urine, rectal swabs, bone marrow and rose spots cultures for recovery of Salmonella typhi in typhoid fever, **Lancet** 1:1211.
187. Hoffman S, Punjali N, Rockhill RC et al. (1986) Duodenal string-capsule culture compared with bone marrow, blood, and rectal swab cultures for diagnosing typhoid and paratyphoid fever. **J Infect Dis** 149:157.
188. Shukla S, Patel B, Chetnis PS (1997) 100 years of Widal test and its reappraisal in an endemic area. **Indian J Med Res** 105:53.
189. Gianella RA, Broctman SA, Zamcheck IV (1971) Salmonella enteritis. Role of reduced gastric secretion in pathogenesis. **Am J Dig Dis** 16:1000.

regions where salmonella infections are endemic, including Mexico, the Indian subcontinent, the Arabian Gulf, Southeast Asia, and Africa.[190] Multiresistant *S. typhi* is less of a problem in the USA, but MDRS must be considered if patients have a history of travel to endemic areas.

As a rule, enteric or typhoid fever is treated with a single antibiotic. Choice of antibiotic and duration of therapy are determined by clinical setting and available resources.

In adults and older adolescents, the antibiotics of choice for treatment of enteric fever include fluoroquinolones such as ciprofloxacin 500mg bid or ofloxacin 400mg bid, either orally or parenterally, for 7 to 10 days.[191–193] Alternative regimens include 3rd generation cephalosporins, such as ceftriaxone (2–3g daily),[194,195] given for 7 to 14 days; cefixime (20–30mg/kg divided bid) for 7 to 14 days; or azithromycin 1g orally followed by 500mg daily for 7 to 14 days.[196–199] Early parenteral therapy followed by a switch to oral medications when symptoms allow is reasonable.

Because MDRS are less common in the USA, the child with enteric fever may be treated with intravenous ampicillin 200mg/kg/day in four divided doses for 14 days; chloramphenicol 75mg/kg/day orally or intravenously in four divided doses;[197] or a third-generation cephalosporin for 14 days (e.g., ceftriaxone, 50–70mg/kg once daily or cefixime 10–30mg/kg/day divided bid). Short courses (5 days) of third-generation cephalosporins are associated with higher rates of relapse.

Therapy may also begin with a combination of medications such as ampicillin and TMP/SMZ 5–10mg/kg/day divided into two doses and is completed with the least toxic or least expensive regimen available as dictated by sensitivity studies. Currently, fluoroquinolones appear to be therapeutically superior to beta lactams for the treatment of uncomplicated typhoid fever, with virtually 100% efficacy if used for 7 to 10 days.[193,194]

Although the use of fluoroquinolones in children raises concern about cartilage toxicity,[200,201] no evidence of acute adverse bone, joint, or growth effects[202–204] have been reported. Thus, a fluoroquinolone may be reasonably used in children with enteric fever due to MDRS or when less toxic agents are not appropriate. Ciprofloxacin is given in doses of 10mg/kg/day and ofloxacin is administered at 15mg/kg/day to younger children. Fluoroquinolones have been successful in treating enteric fever, reducing relapse rates, as well as treating relapses (1–6% of cases).[205] They also significantly reduce the development of chronic carrier states because they concentrate in bile.[206,207] When the gall bladder is diseased, complete therapy may require cholecystectomy.[208,209] Rare chronic urinary carriage of *S. typhi* is usually associated with anatomic abnormalities of the urinary tract, and requires attention to underlying problems, such as kidney or bladder stone ablation.[210]

Patients with rare intestinal perforation often present with increased abdominal pain, distension, and signs of enteric peritonitis, including guarding and evidence of sepsis. Prompt recognition and surgical intervention with resection of the involved intestine and broad antibiotic coverage are required.[211]

Supportive treatment including rest, intravenous fluids, and electrolytes or hyperalimentation may be required for the severely ill patient. Antipyretics may lead to precipitous temperature drops, and should be avoided. Transient coagulation difficulties may occur, and treatment with heparin should be avoided in all but the most severe cases. Judicious use of intravenous corticosteroids in patients with shock, delerium, stupor, or coma may be life-saving, although associated with an increased rate of relapse.[211] Dexamethasone 3mg/kg iv bolus followed by several doses of 1mg/kg/day every 6h for 2 to 3 days has been helpful in severely ill children. The use of IVIG, especially in premature infants, has also been reported as helpful.[212,213]

BRUCELLOSIS

Brucellosis, also called Malta fever, Mediterranean remittent fever, or undulant fever, is a zoonotic infection which humans acquire from various animals or animal products. Worldwide it accounts for more than 500 000 cases each year,[214] but the disease is rare in the United States due to effective vaccination and eradication programs.[215] It largely affects men and is associated with occupational exposure (livestock handlers, slaughterhouse or abattoir workers)[216] and ingestion of contaminated raw milk or cheese.[217] Children comprise only 2.3 to 10.3% of cases reported worldwide.[217] It is still prevalent in the Mediterranean basin, Indian subcontinent, Arabian peninsula and in parts of Mexico, Central and South America.[218]

Brucellosis is an ancient disease but was first described accurately by J.A. Marston, who served as a British Army surgeon during the Crimean War and described an illness affecting troops stationed in Malta in 1863.[219] The bacteria is named in honor of David Bruce, another Royal Army surgeon, who isolated a microorganism from the spleen, blood, urine and feces of victims of Malta fever which he called *Micrococcus melitensis*.[219] Bruce later became the head of a commission to investigate the disease in Malta. A Maltese physician, Themistostocle Zamit, identified native goat and goat's milk as the source of this bacterium. The incidence of the illness in English troops declined dramatically when fresh goat's milk was removed from the

190. Rowe B, Ward LR, Threlfall EJ (1992) Multidrug-resistant *Salmonella typhi*: A worldwide epidemic. **Clin Infect Dis** 24(Suppl 1) S106.
191. Karamat KA, Malik AZ, Hashmi A et al. (1989) Efficacy of oxfloxacin in typhoid fever, particularly in drug resistant cases. **Rev Infect Dis** 11(Suppl. 5): S1193.
192. Lemson BM (1995) Short course quinolone therapy of typhoid fever in developing countries. **Drugs** 49S2:136.
193. Alam MM, Hag SA, Das KK et al. (1995) Efficacy of ciprofloxacin in enteric fever: Comparison of treatment duration in sensitive and multidrug resistant Salmonella. **Am J Trop Med Hyg** 53:306.
194. Rastegar LA, Validle N, Chaffarzadeh K et al. (1997) In vitro activity of cefixime vs. ceftizoxime against *Salmonella typhi*. **Pathol Biol** (Paris) 45:415.
195. Smith MD, Duong NM, Hoa NT et al. (1994) Comparison of ofloxacin and ceftriaxone for short course treatment of enteric fever. Antimicrob. **Agents Chemother** 38:1716.
196. Girgis NI, Butler T, French RW et al. (1999) Azithromycin vs. ciprofloxacin for treatment of uncomplicated typhoid fever in a randomized trial in Egypt that included patients with multidrug resistance. **Antimicrob Agents Chemother** 43:1441.
197. Butler T, Sridhar CB, Daga MK et al. (1999) Treatment of typhoid fever with azithromycin versus chloramphenicol in a randomized multicentre trial in India. **J Antimicrob Chemother** 44:243.
198. Rowe B, Ward L, Threlfall EJ (1995) Ciprofloxacin-resistant Salmonella typhi in the U.K. **Lancet** 346:1302.
199. Brown JC, Shanahan PM, Jesudason MW et al. (1996) Mutations responsible for reduced susceptibilty to quinolones in clinical isolates of multi-resistant *Salmonella typhi* in India. **J Antimicrob Chemother** 37:891.
200. Schaad V (1992) Toxicity of quinolones in pediatric patients. **Adv Antimicrob Antineoplast Chemother** 11:259.
201. Burkhart JE, Walterspiel JN, Schaad VB (1996) Quinolone arthropathy in animals versus children. **Clinical Infect Dis** 25:1997.
202. Bethell DB, Hien TT, Phi LT et al. (1996) The effects on growth of single short courses of fluoroquinolones. **Arch Dis Child** 74:44.
203. White NJ, Dung NM, Vinh H et al. (1996) Fluoroquinolone antibiotics in children with multidrug resistant typhoid. **Lancet** 348:547.
204. Tran TH, Bethell DB, Njuuyen TT et al. (1995) Short course ofloxacin for treatment of multi-drug resistant typhoid. **Clin Infect Dis** 20:917.
205. Vinh H, Wain J, Nga UT et al. (1996) Two or three days of oxfloxacin treatment for uncomplicated multidrug resistant typhoid fever in children. **Antimicrob Agents Chemother** 40:958.
206. Gotuzzo G, Guerra JG, Benavente L et al. (1988) Use of nonfloxacin to treat chronic typhoid carriers. **J Infect Dis** 157:1221.
207. Trujillo TZ, Aurroz CQ, Guiterrez MA et al. (1991) Fluoroquinolones in the treatment of typhoid fever and the carrier state. **Eur J Clin Microbiol Infect Dis** 10:334.
208. Munnich D, Bekesi S (1975) Curing of typhoid carriers by cholecystectomy combined with amoxicillin and probenecid treatment. **Chemotherapy** 25:362.
209. Mathai E, John TJ, Rani M et al. (1995) Significance of *Salmonella typhi* bacteria. **J Clin Microbiol** 33:1791.
210. Bilar R, Tarpley J (1985) Intestinal perforation in typhoid fever: a historical and state of the art review. **Rev Infect Dis** 7:257.
211. McGowen JE, Chesney PJ, Cossley KB, LaForce M (1992) Guidelines for the use of systemic glucocorticoids in the management of selected infections. **J Infect Dis** 165:1.
212. Gokalp AS, Toksoy HB, Turkay S et al. (1994) Intravenous immunoglobulin in the treatment of *Salmonella typhimurium* infections in preterm neonates. **Clin Pediatr** 33:349.
213. Geme JW 3rd, Hodes HL, Marcy SM et al. (1988) Consensus: Management of Salmonella infection in the first year of life. **Pediatr Infect Dis J** 7:615.
214. Havas L (1980) Problems and new developments in the treatment of acute and chronic brucellosis in man. **Acta Trop** (Basel) 37:281.
215. Centers for Disease Control (1979) Brucellosis surveillance. In: Annual Survey, 1978. Atlanta: Centers for Disease Control.
216. Fox MD, Kaufmann AF (1977) Brucellosis in the United States, 1965–1974. **J Infect Dis** 136:312.
217. Street L, Grant WW, Alva JD (1975) Brucellosis in childhood. **Pediatrics** 55:416.
218. Young EJ, Corbel MJ (1989) Brucellosis: epidemiology and prevalence worldwide, In: Brucellosis: Clinical and Laboratory Aspects, Young EJ, Corbel MJ, eds. Boca Raton: CRC Press, pp. 26–40.
219. Vassallo DJ (1992) The Corps disease: Brucellosis and its historical association with the Royal Army Medical Corps. **J R Army Med Corps** 138–150.

military dining halls. Since that time several other species of the bacterium have been identified and associated with particular animal hosts in whom they usually cause urinary tract disease.

Brucellosis has worldwide distribution in domestic and wild animals and nearly all human infections are due directly or indirectly to animal sources. Each species has a preferred or principal host and may have several biovars. *Brucella abortus* primarily affects cattle, *B. melitensis* affects goats, *B. suis* affects swine, and *B. canis* affects dogs. These four species are known to cause disease in humans.[220]

The organism is a small, fastidious, nonmotile, nonspore-forming, Gram-negative coccobacillus. All strains are aerobic but *B. abortus* requires 10% carbon dioxide for growth. They are successfully cultured on a variety of agars including chocolate serum dextrose and trypticase soy agars, except when cultured from stool or contaminated sources, which requires selective media. They are extremely slow growing. The laboratory must be informed if *Brucella* are suspected so that specimens are not discarded before 35 days or before growth appears. Special handling of specimens is required to avoid the risk of laboratory-acquired brucellosis.

Brucellosis is an occupational risk for farmers, ranchers, veterinarians, abattoir workers, butchers, meat inspectors, and laboratory personnel. Transmission may result from direct contact with diseased animals, (including cattle, swine, and goats) or their carcasses, blood or products such as raw milk.[221] Infection may be acquired through the skin, respiratory tract, gastrointestinal tract, or eyes. Live vaccinations pose some risk to veterinarians due to accidental self inoculation or ocular exposure.[222] *B. melitensis* is most often transmitted by the ingestion of unpasteurized goat's milk or cheese. In California and Texas, the incidence of food-borne brucellosis has increased, although occupational exposures have decreased.[223,224] Childhood brucellosis, though not common in the United States, is more common where brucellosis is enzootic and where the prevalent species is *B. melitensis*.[225] Human to human contagion is not thought to occur with the exception of extremely rare venereal transmission.[226,227] The bacteria has been recovered from banked sperm[228] and very rare *in utero* transmission to neonates from bacteremic mothers has been documented.[229]

CLINICAL FINDINGS

The clinical expression of brucellosis in humans is protean. It can be divided for convenience into subclinical, acute and subacute, relapsing and chronic illness. Subclinical cases have been documented by serologic surveillance of abattoir workers, 50% of whom had immunologic evidence of but no clinical history of exposure to brucella.

Acute and subacute infections may appear explosively, or gradually during several weeks. Common symptoms include fever, chills, drenching sweats, fatigue, malaise, backache, headache, and weakness. Less frequent symptoms include myalgia, anorexia, nausea, vomiting, abdominal discomfort, arthralgia, weight loss, and nonproductive cough. Fever is a consistent finding and brucellosis should be considered in the evaluation of any fever of unknown origin. The fever may assume an undulating pattern and may be associated with hepatomegaly and splenomegaly in 10–15% of symptomatic patients. When symptoms appear to be related to one organ, the disease is called localized.[230] Almost a third of patients developed localized complications in one report of 530 prospectively studied cases,[230] including joints (20–39%), testes (2–40%), brain (1–2%), heart (1%), and liver (10%). The most common localized lesions are osteoarticular, especially sacroileitis. In the genitourinary tract, epididymoorchitis is common.[230,231] Neurobrucellosis includes meningoencephalitis or less common neurologic complications, such as myelitis, stroke, cranial or peripheral neuropathies,[230,232,233] and psychiatric problems have been reported. Liver abscesses, and endocarditis,[234] especially affecting previously damaged valves, have also been reported. Less common complications include abscesses of the spleen, epidural space, and thyroid. Pneumonitis,[235] pleural effusion, empyema, ileus, colitis, spontaneous peritonitis, and uveitis are rarely reported. In the absence of localizing signs, the diagnosis may be extremely difficult as physical findings are often sparse and nonspecific, especially when compared to patient complaints. Brucella infections may recur with relapses months or even years after initial infection, especially if localized chronic infections are overlooked or incompletely treated.

Chronic brucellosis can be an insidious disease with nonspecific symptoms resembling chronic fatigue syndrome, persisting for more than a year. Symptoms may include headaches, lassitude, depression, anxiety, insomnia, and emotional lability. Fever is often less in evidence, but patients are likely to have hepatomegaly, splenomegaly and arthritis.

The cutaneous manifestations of brucellosis are protean but occur in only 5 to 10% of cases. In nearly all are caused by *B. melitensis*,[236–238] the lesions range from papulovesicles, pustules, abscesses, and ulcers. A hypersensitivity reaction consists of fever and discrete elevated 2–10mm violet–red papulonodules on the arms, legs, trunk, thighs, and hands. The rash is nonpruritic, spares the face, and varies from sparse to more than 100 lesions. Rarely lesions ulcerate or become purpuric, sometimes with accompanying thrombocytopenia and septicemia. Patients may also show erythema nodosum-like lesions; a 29-month-old child had small subcutaneous papules.[239] Examination of biopsied papulonodular skin lesions often reveals perivascular and periadenexal lymphohistiocytic infiltrates with some epithelioid histiocytes and occasional multinucleated giant cells. Biopsies may also reveal noncaseating granulomas and septal panniculitis consistent with erythema nodosum.[237] Skin cultures and cultures of biopsied skin may yield the organisms.[238,239] Generally, rashes reflect hematogenous spread of the bacteria to the skin. Lesions disappear with antibiotic treatment, but may recur with relapsing illness.[238] In addition, cutaneous features include malar erythema, bronzing of the skin in sun-exposed areas, crusted eschars, and disseminated abscesses.[214]

DIAGNOSIS

Because the symptoms of brucellosis are nonspecific, the importance of a detailed and careful history, including food exposure and work patterns cannot be overemphasized, especially in a patient with fever of unknown origin. Routine laboratory tests may reveal hemolytic anemia (75%) with thrombocytopenia (40%); white blood cell counts may be normal or low. Pancytopenia is more commonly seen in children (6%). Liver function tests may be abnormal. Radiographic studies such as X-ray, bone scan, magnetic resonance imaging

220. Young EJ (1998) Brucellosis. In: Textbook of Pediatric Infectious Disease, 4th edn, Feigin RD, Cherry JD, eds. Philadelphia: WB Saunders, pp. 1415–1423.
221. Arnow PM, Smaron M, Ormiste V (1984) Brucellosis in a group of travelers to Spain. JAMA 251:505–507.
222. Sadusk JF, Browne AS, Born JL (1957) Brucellosis in man, resulting from *Brucella abortus* (strain 19) vaccine. JAMA 164:1325–1328.
223. Chomel BB, DeBess EE, Mangiamele DM et al. (1994) Changing trends in the epidemiology of human brucellosis in California from 1973–1992: A shift toward foodborne transmission. J Infect Dis 170:1216–1223.
224. Taylor PM, Perdue JN (1989) The changing epidemiology of human brucellosis in Texas, 1977–1986. Am J Epidemiol 130:160–165.
225. Feiz J, Sabbaghain H, Mirali M (1978) Brucellosis due to *B. melitensis* in children. Clin Pediatr 12:904–907.
226. Rubin B, Band JD, Wong P et al. (1991) In vitro susceptibility of *Brucella melitensis*. Lancet 337:14–15.
227. Stantic-Pavlinic M, Cec V, Mehk J (1983) Brucellosis in spouses and the possibility of interhuman infection. Infection 11:313–314.
228. Vandercam B, Zech F, de Cooman S et al. (1990) Isolation of *Brucella tensis* from banked sperm. Eur J Clin Microbiol Infect Dis 9:303.
229. Lubani MM, Dudin KI, Sharda DC et al. (1988) Neonatal brucellosis. Eur J Pediatr 147:520–522.
230. Colmenero JD, Regnera JM, Martos F et al. (1996) Complications associated with *Brucella melitensis* infection: A study of 530 cases, Medicine (Baltimore) 75:195.
231. Afsar H, Baydar I, Sirmatel F (1993) Epididymo-orchitis due to brucellosis. Br J Urol 72:104.
232. McLean DR, Russell N, Kahn MY (1992) Neurobrucellosis: Clinical and therapeutic features. Clin Infect Dis 15:582.
233. Bouza E, de la Torre MG, Parras F et al. (1987) Brucella meningitis. Rev Infect Dis 9:810.
234. Ferandez Guerrero ML (1993) Zoonotic endocarditis. Infect Dis Clin North America 7:135.
235. Lubani MM, Dudin KI, Sharda DC et al. (1989) Pulmonary brucellosis. Q J Med 71:319–324.
236. Rigatos GA, Kappos-Rigatou I (1977) Cutaneous manifestations of brucellosis. Br J Clin Pract 11:167.
237. Berger TG, Guill MA, Goette DK (1981) Cutaneous lesions in brucellosis. Arch Dermatol 117:40.
238. Ariza J, Servitje O, Palleres R et al. (1989) Characteristic cutaneous lesions in patients with brucellosis. Arch Dermatol 125:380.
239. Gee Lew BM, Nicholas EA, Hirose FM et al. (1983) Unusual skin manifestations of brucellosis. Arch Dermatol 119:56.

(MRI), computerized tomography (CT) scan, and echocardiogram may be helpful in delineating localized disease but are not diagnostic of brucellosis. Definitive diagnosis is made by recovering brucella in cultures from blood, bone marrow, or other normally sterile tissue (e.g., liver). Depending on methods used and the length of incubation, cultures may be positive in 15 to 80% of cases.[240] In the abscence of a positive culture, the diagnosis can be made by measuring the titer of acute and convalescent specific antibodies in serum.

A number of serologic test have been developed for the diagnosis of brucellosis. These include serum agglutination, standard tube agglutination, complement fixation, Rose Bengal agglutination, anti-brucella Coombs' and enzyme-linked immunosorbent assay (ELISA).[241] The gold standard remains the serum agglutination test (SAT) to *B. abortus* strain 1119, which is widely available. This is useful for *B. abortus*, *B. melitensis*, and *B. suis*, but will not detect antibodies to *B. canis*. For diagnosis of *B. canis*, antigens from this species or *B. ovis* must be prepared for SAT testing.[241] The SAT, which measures both IgM and IgG agglutination, is considered diagnostic in patients with a titer of 1:160.[214,241] Although one test may not be diagnostic, a four-fold increase in titer over 4 to 12 weeks is diagnostic of acute disease.[214,241] Measuring IgM and IgG titers separately and following their levels may be useful clinically. The IgG titer usually declines with successful therapy whereas IgM levels to *Brucella* may persist for years. A resurgent rise in the IgG titers to *Brucella* may presage a clinical relapse.[242]

A new ELISA assay for *Brucella* antigens, described in 1998,[243] had 99% specificity. This test is not expected to replace the well-established SAT but may supplant blood cultures.[241,243] Newer tests utilizing polymerase chain reaction (PCR) techniques to rapidly detect *Brucella* antigens in blood specimens show promise.[244]

DIFFERENTIAL DIAGNOSIS

The differential diagnosis should include other bacterial diseases of the reticuloendothelial system, such as salmonellosis, tuberculosis, and listeriosis. Childhood lymphoreticular malignancy may need to be ruled out as well.

TREATMENT

Several antibiotic regimens have been useful in treating brucellosis. Unfortunately, none is 100% effective as some patients will relapse after therapy. Almost all relapses occur within 6 months of cessation of therapy, the majority within 3 months.[241]

Recently recommended regimens for adults, adolescents and children over 8 years of age include doxycycline 10mg twice daily for 6 weeks. Either streptomycin (1g im daily for the first 14–21 days) or rifampin (600–900mg [15mg/kg/day]) is added for the full 6 weeks;[241] nevertheless, relapses occur in 4–5% of patients. The combination of rifampin and doxycycline is preferred because of the well-known otoxicity of streptomycin.[245] Patients with localized disease or complications are more likely to suffer therapeutic failure, relapse, or death than those without focal disease (10.6 vs. 3.6%). Fifteen percent of patients with focal disease require surgical treatment[230] and may require a second course of therapy with the same or a modified regimen.

Other antibiotics useful in the treatment of brucellosis include fluoroquinolones, particularly ofloxacin 400mg orally twice daily combined with rifampin 600mg once daily for 6 weeks.[246] Ceftriaxone has been used but is not considered first-line because of variable clinical results.[247] Monotherapy with any of the preferred drugs is not recommended.

In children less than 8 years old and pregnant women, tetracyclines are avoided if possible due to staining of tooth enamel.[248] Children with brucellosis receive a 6-week course of trimethoprim (10–12mg/kg/day) and sulfamethoxazole (50mg/kg/day) (TMP/SMZ) in two divided doses plus rifampin (15–20mg/kg/day to a maximum of 600mg po daily) in two divided doses. Alternative regimens have substituted a 5-day course of im gentamicin 5mg/kg/day for rifampin. Pregnant women also may be treated for 6 weeks with rifampin (800mg daily) and, SMX/TMP, if therapy is required in the weeks just prior to delivery,[214,249] although this treatment increases the risk of neonatal kernicterus.

If infected children or pregnant women develop intolerance to sulfonamide or rifampin, then use of a tetracycline should be reconsidered if informed consent is obtained, given the severity and potential complications of brucellosis.

Neurobrucellosis requires prolonged therapy for up to 19 months with three drugs that cross the blood–brain barrier, and should be continued until the CSF analysis normalizes. Endocarditis requires both prolonged antibiotic therapy and surgical replacement of the affected heart valve. Accidental inoculation with attenuated live brucella strains used for vaccinating animals requires a two-drug theraputic regimen for 6 weeks.

PREVENTION

Prevention of brucellosis is directly related to control of the disease in domesticated herds and flocks. This requires serologic testing of animals, elimination of infected animals, and quarantine and immunization of exposed herds. Vaccination of cattle with attenuated live vaccine (*B. abortus* strain 19), and vaccination of goats and sheep with *B. melitensis* (Rev-1) are effective, but these methods must be part of a sustained program to be successful. Unfortunately, there is no vaccine for swine.[241]

Workers in abattoirs or slaughterhouses should wear protective clothing and glasses. Special care should be taken in treating wounds obtained in processing meats. Infected animals should not be slaughtered or processed in areas close to other animals. The pasteurization of both cow's and goat's milk is also very important in reducing transmission to humans. These methods have been highly successful in the United States, resulting in a dramatic drop from 6321 cases in 1947 to fewer than 200 cases per year in recent years.

TULAREMIA

INTRODUCTION

Tularemia is a zoonosis seen rarely in the United States and throughout the northern hemisphere between 30° and 70°N. In 1912, McCoy and Chapin isolated an organism causing a plague-like illness in rodents in Tulare County, California.[250,251] They named this organism *Bacterium tularense*. The first human case was reported in 1914 by Wherry and Lamb.[252] The association of deerflies and ticks as vectors was made by several investigators during the next 10 years.[252,253] Since then, the organism has been reclassified several times

240. Ariza J, Corredoira J, Pallares R et al. (1995) Characteristics of and risk factors for relapse of brucellosis in humans. **Clin Infect Dis** 20:1241.
241. Everett ED (2001) Brucellosis, clinical manifestations, diagnosis, treatment and prevention in 2001. Up to Date@www.uptodate.com. Vol 9:No 2 pp. 1–5.
242. Ariza J, Pellicer T, Pallares R et al. (1992) Specific antibody profile in human brucellosis. **Clin Infect Dis** 14:131.
243. Al-Shamahy HA, Wright SG (1998) Enzyme-linked immunosorbent assay for brucella antigen detection in human sera. **J Med Microbiol** 47:169.
244. Matar GM, Khneisser IA, Abdelnoor AM (1996) Rapid laboratory confirmation of human brucellosis by PCR analysis of a target sequence on the 31-kilodalton Brucella antigen DNA. **J Clin Microbiol** 43:447.
245. Ariza J, Guidiol F, Pallares R et al. (1992) Treatment of human brucellosis with doxycycline plus rifampin or doxyciline plus streptomycin. A randomized, double-blind study. **Ann Intern Med** 117:25–30.
246. Akova M, Uzun O, Akalin HE et al. (1993) Quinolones in treatment of human brucellosis: comparative trial of ofloxacin-rifampin versus doxycycline-rifampin. **Antimicrob Agents Chemother** 37:1831.
247. Lang R, Dagan R, Potasman I et al. (1992) Failure of ceftriaxone in the treatment of acute brucellosis. **Clin Infect Dis** 14:506.
248. Lubani MM, Dudin KI, Sherda DC et al. (1989) A multicenter therapeutic study of 1100 children with brucellosis. **Pediatr Infect Dis J** 8:75.
249. Sharda DC, Lubani M (1986) A study of brucellosis in childhood. **Clin Pediatr** 25:492–495.
250. Mc Coy GW (1911) A plague-like disease in rodents. **Public Health Bull** 43:53.
251. Mc Coy GW, Chapin CW (1912) Further observations on a plague-like disease of rodents with a preliminary note on the causative agent. **J Infect Dis** 10:61.
252. Wherry WB, Lamb B (1914) Infection of man with *Bacterium tularense*. **J Infect Dis** 15:331.
253. Francis E (1921) The occurence of tularemia in nature as a disease of man. **Public Health Rep** 36:1731.

and has been included in the genera *Bacterium*, *Bacillus*, *Brucella*, and *Pasteurella* before the genus *Francisella* was created. This designation honors Dr. Edward Francis who made great contributions to our knowledge about and understanding of tularemia.[254,255]

MICROBIOLOGY

F. tularensis is a small, singly occuring, nonmobile, nonencapsulated, poorly staining, bipolar, aerobic, pleomorphic, Gram-negative coccobacillus. They are slow-growing, fastidious organisms and most require cysteine or cystine for growth, but the bacteria will grow on coagulated egg yolk medium, cysteine–glucose–blood agar, enriched thioglycolate broth, or enriched chocolate agar. Growth in culture does not require incubation with CO_2, but is stimulated by it. The organism can be killed by heating to 56°C for 10 min, or adequate cooking, but it is resistant to freezing and can remain viable for up to 3 years in frozen animal carcasses.[256] Although it is difficult to grow in the laboratory, *F. tularensis* is hardy in nature; under normal conditions it can also persist in water or mud for weeks.[257]

All strains of *F. tularensis* appear serologically identical but three biovars exist which exhibit differential virulence.[258] *F. tularensis*, bv. *tularensis* (Group A, or Jellison Type A) accounts for 90% of isolates in North America and is more virulent in humans and rabbits. Group B, also known as Jellison Type B or *F. tularensis* bv. *palaearctica*, is primarily found in Europe and Asia. This strain appears to be ubiquitous and can coexist in the same ecosystem with Type A. It also appears to be less virulent for humans and rabbits and may be found in aquatic mammals and water. *F. tularensis* bv. *novicida* and the separate species *F. philomiraga* have been associated rarely with human disease.[257,259] Species identification can be done with antisera, biochemical testing or 16S rRNA sequencing.[259] Most human disease is caused by types A and B with more severe illness associated with type A.

F. tularensis is a virulent organism with experimental infections produced using only 10 organisms intradermally and 25 organisms if given by aerosol.[259] It may infect more than 100 species of vertebrate animals, both wild and domestic, especially rabbits, rodents, muskrats, deers voles and sheep. It can also infect a variety of invertebrates, especially ticks, biting flies (e.g., deerflies, horseflies), mosquitos, and lice.[256] It can be transmitted transovarially by ticks, bypassing the need for an infected animal reservoir. Some animals appear less susceptible to the illness, especially cats, cattle, dogs and horses; rare reported cases follow cat bites in which mechanical spread from contaminated teeth or claws is blamed.[260] Humans are terminal hosts and do not transmit the disease.

Humans usually acquire tularemia as a result of contact with tissue or body fluid of infected mammals or from the bite of an infected anthropod or diseased animal. Less commonly, *F. tularensis* is acquired when either undercooked infected meat or a water source contaminated by rodents or muskrats is ingested. Rarely, inhalation of aerosolized bacteria can occur in laboratory and farm workers. Epidemics are rare and most cases are sporadic. The incidence is less than 1 per 1 000 000 population in the United States with the highest attack rate in agricultural workers,[255] followed by rural housewives, preschool and school-age children.[261,262]

Although tularemia can occur year round, it has two seasonal peaks. Winter cases predominate in hunting season. Spring and summer cases predominate in vector-borne disease when ticks are more prevalent and people are outdoors. The presence of vector-borne disease has increased as fur trapping and the hunting and cleaning of rabbits has decreased. The disease is now most common in the south-central United States with most cases reported from Arkansas, Missouri and Oklahoma.[255,256,263] In European countries mosquito-borne as well as tick-borne disease is prevalent.[257,264,265]

INVASION AND PATHOGENESIS

The organism may gain entry to the human body through several routes including the skin, eye, oropharynx, respiratory, and gastrointestinal tracts. An intercellular parasite, it is thought to multiply locally and then spread by means of the blood or lymphatics to regional lymph nodes within 48 to 96h. There it multiplies and spreads further to involve the reticuloendothelial system. Primary inoculation sites may become necrotic and granulomatous as may the parenchema of the liver and spleen. Lymph nodes from nonfatal cases reveal caseating granulomas indistinguishable from those of tuberculosis, as well as follicular hyperplasia and numerous macrophages.

CLINICAL FINDINGS

The intensity and pace of the illness depend on the virulence of the strain, portal of entry, size of the inoculum, and immune status of the host. If organisms gain entry to the blood, typical endotoxemia may result which is occasionally associated with acute rhabdomyolysis and renal failure.[266] Disease associated with *F. tularensis* can be divided into six clinical syndromes which are defined by the portal of entry: ulceroglandular, glandular, oropharyngeal, oculoglandular, typhoidal, and pneumonic.

The ulcerograndular presentation is the most common form of tularemia (75%).[254,267,268] Following inoculation into the skin, a regional lymph node becomes enlarged, tender, and inflamed (Fig. 24.16). Soon after, the cutaneous portal of injury becomes swollen, tender, and may ulcerate, leaving a punched-out sore with raised edges. Untreated, these lesions may last for a month or more. The lymph nodes may suppurate in 50% of cases or remain indurated, firm, and tender. There may be associated generalized lymphadenopathy and hepatosplenomegaly. Tick-borne cases typically involve the lower extremities, whereas disease acquired from rabbits generally affects the hands. Ulcerations may be found on any location in small children.

Glandular tularemia occurs in 5–15% of patients and resembles the ulceroglandular form except for the absence of an obvious skin portal of entry. The oculoglandular presentation occurs in 1–2% of cases and follows inoculation of the conjunctival sac. The eyelid becomes swollen in association with a unilateral purulent painful conjunctivitis, (Fig. 24.17). The preauricular, submaxillary lymph nodes, and occasionally the axillary lymph nodes are swollen, tender, and may suppurate. Tiny nodules and ulcers may be present on the palpebral conjunctivae.[269]

Oropharyngeal tularemia is seen in 1–4% of patients and may follow ingestion of undercooked meat.[257,270,271] Patients may present with acute ton-

254. Parker RR, Spencer RR, Francis E (1924) Tularemia infection in ticks of the species *Dermacentor andersoni* Stiles in the Bitterroot Valley, Montana. **Public Health Rep** 39:1057.
255. Boyce JM (1992) *Francisella tularensis* (tularemia). In: Principles and Practice of Infectious Diseases, 3rd edn, Mandell GL, Douglas RG, Bennett JE, eds. New York: Churchhill Livingstone, p. 1742.
256. Lau CC, Feigin RD (1998) Tularemia. In: Textbook of Pediatric Infectious Disease, 4th edn, Feigin RD, Cherry JD, eds. Philadelphia: WB Saunders, pp. 1458–1464.
257. Everett ED (2001) Microbiology, pathogenisis and epidemiology of *Francisella tularensis*. Up to date @ www.uptodate.com. vol 9, no. 2 pp. 1–5.
258. Jaslaw S, Eigelsback HT, Prior JA et al. (1961) Tularemia vaccine study intracutaneous challenge. **Arch Intern Med** 107:689–701.
259. Hollis DG, Weaver RE, Steigerwalt AG et al. (1989) *Francisella phelomirgia* comb. Nov (formerly *Yersinia philomiragia*) and *Francisella tularensis* biogroup novocida (formerly *Francisella novocida*) associated with human disease. **J Clin Microbial** 27:1601.
260. Capellan J, Fong IW (1993) Tularemia from a cat bite. Case report and review of feline associated tularemia. **Clin Infect Dis** 16:472.

261. Uhari M, Syrjala H, Salminen A (1990) Tularemia in children caused by *Francisella tularensis* biovar palaearctica. **Pediatr Infect Dis J** 9:80–83.
262. Brooks GF, Buchanan TM (1970) Tularemia in the United States: epidemiology aspects in the 1960's and follow-up of the outbreak of tularemia in Vermont. **J Infect Dis** 121:357.
263. Callaway GD, Peterson SS, Good JT (1954) Tularemia in southwest Missouri. **Missouri Med** 51:906–909.
264. Markwife LE, Hymes NA, de la Crees P et al. (1985) Tick borne tularemia: An outbreak of lymphadenopathy in children **JAMA** 254:2922–2925.
265. Hubalek Z, Halouzka J (1997) Mosquitoes (Diptera: Culicidae), in contrast to ticks (Akari. Ixodidae), do not carry *Francisella tularensis* in natural focus of tularemia in the Czech Republic. **J Med Entomol** 34:660.
266. Kaiser AB, Rieves O, Price AH et al. (1985) Tularemia and rhabdomyolysis. **JAMA** 253:241–243.
267. Francis E (1928) A summary of present knowledge of tularemia. **Medicine** (Baltimore) 7:411.
268. Sanders CV, Hahn R (1968) Analysis of 106 cases of tularemia. **J La State Med Soc** 120:391.
269. Evans ME (1985) *Francisella tularensis*. **Infect Control** 6:381–383.
270. Hughs WT Jr, Etteldorf JN (1957) Oropharyngeal tularemia. **J Pediatr** 51:363.
271. Everett ED, Templer JW (1980) Oropharyngeal tularemia. **Arch Otolaryngol** 106:237.

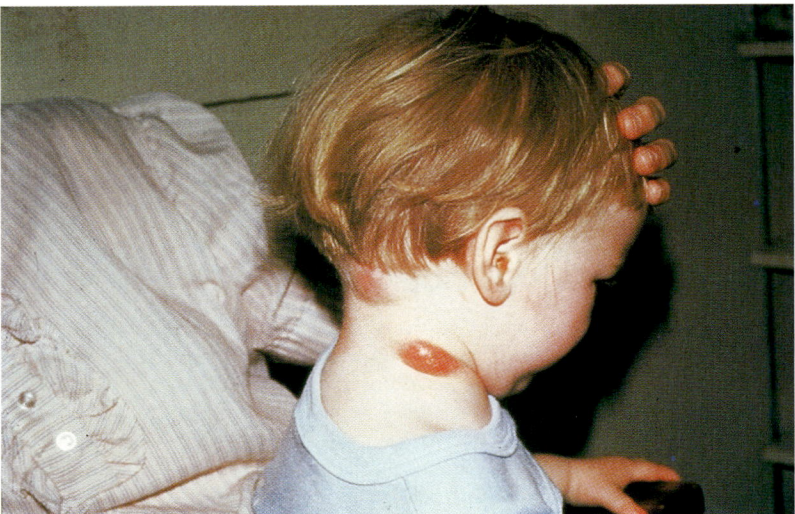

Fig. 24.16   Tularemia. Ulceroglandular form in a child (courtesy Dr Russell Steele).

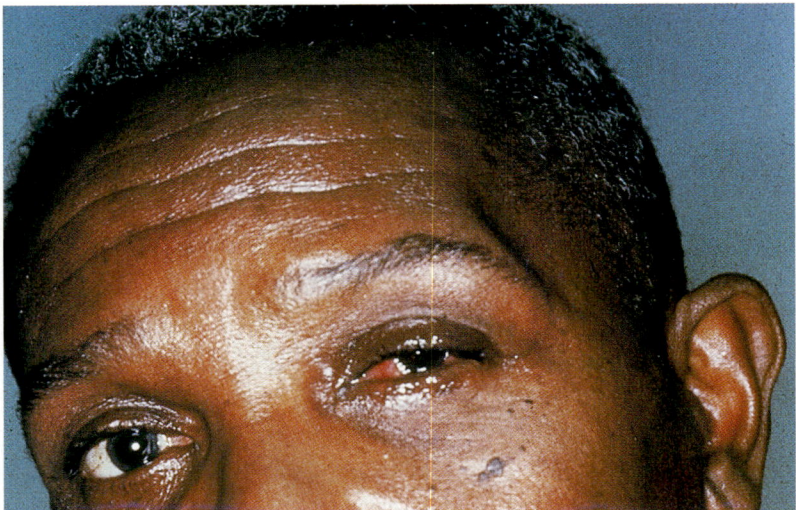

Fig. 24.17   Tularemia. Oculoglandular presentation in an adult (courtesy Dr Russell Steele).

sillitis and cervical adenitis. The pharyngeal exudate may be extensive and mimic a diphtheritic membrane. Small ulcerations of the tonsils and pharynx may be present and cervical lymph nodes may suppurate.[270,271] The bacteria may spread via saliva to the lower gastrointestinal tract, resulting in an associated typhoidal-like illness.

Typhoidal tularemia is a severe illness and the most difficult to diagnose. It often presents as a fever of unknown origin. Patients may complain of pharyngeal pain, but display few if any pharyngeal lesions. Signs include, diarrhea, dry cough, retrosternal pain, lymphadenopathy, weight loss, delerium, myalgias, headache, and unremitting fever. Toxemia, prostration and multiorganism sepsis may follow the development of necrotic bowel lesions.[256]

Pneumonic tularemia is the most severe and lethal form. It is acquired through inhalation of aerosolized bacteria and may be associated with other forms of tularemia, especially the typhoidal syndrome. This is the most frequent presentation of laboratory-acquired cases. Unfortunately, the patients often present with nonspecific and varying respiratory signs and symptoms depending on the degree and location of lung involvement, which may include pleural effusion. The nonspecific clinical and X-ray findings require that other illnesses be ruled out, including tuberculosis, bacterial pneumonias, mycotic infections, lymphoma and lung cancer.[256]

In certain aspects, the clinical presentation of the disease is similar without regard to portal of entry. The onset of symptoms is abrupt after an incubation of 3–4 days (range 1–21 days). These symptoms include high fevers, chills, fatigue, headache, vomiting, myalgia, and occasional photophobia. The fever, which may be unremitting or biphasic, may persist for 3 weeks in untreated cases. Other physical finding may include pharyngitis, skin lesions, lymphadenopathy, hepatomegaly, and often a relative bradycardia in spite of high fever.

CUTANEOUS LESIONS

Besides the primary ulcerations, a variety of skin lesions have been described in approximately 25% of patients with this illness. The primary skin lesion is often a vesiculopapule that evolves into a papulopustule and then a necrotic chancriform ulcer or eschar, associated with enlarged regional lymph nodes[272,273] in 70–80% of patients with the ulceroglandular presentation. Sporotrichoid

nodules ascending from the inoculation site have been noted, especially during the second week of illness. Macular, papular, vesicular, and pustular rashes, and rashes described as "blotchy" or "urticarial" have been seen several days after the onset of fever. Erythema nodosum and erythema multiforme[256] have been reported, and rarely a diffuse petechial exathem is seen.

Unusual complications of tularemia include: meningitis, encephalitis, pericarditis, peritonitis, osteomyelitis, acute respiratory distress syndrome, rhabdomyolysis with associated renal failure, and venous thombosis. Death occurs in 4% of patients.[269,274,275]

DIAGNOSIS

The diagnosis of tularemia requires a high index of suspicion. Often, early routine laboratory results are nonspecific. The complete blood count may be normal. Elevated liver enzymes are present in 50% of reported cases. The diagnosis is rarely made from culture as the bacteria is fastidious and many laboratories are reluctant to work with *F. tularensis* because of the risk of aerosolization. The gold standard of diagnosis remains a four-fold rise in titer of serum agglutinating antibodies, or the ELISA test. Unfortunately, antibodies may take from 2 to 6 weeks to develop. A single titer of 1:160 during a suspicious illness is sufficient to make a presumptive diagnosis of tularemia and initiate empiric therapy, but may not appear until or after the second week of illness; serum agglutinating antibodies may persist for years at high levels. The newer tests using ELISA assays to bacterial sonicate (ELISA-S) may confirm the presence of IgM, IgA, and/or IgG antibodies to *F. tularensis* earlier in the course of illness, but are not commercially or widely available. PCR has been applied successfully to human specimens to establish an early diagnosis but this test is not available for general use.[272]

The differential diagnosis of tularemia is vast, depending on clinical presentation. It most frequently includes other diseases producing chancriform lymph node complexes, such as cat scratch disease, extragenital syphilis, staphylococcal ecthyma with lymphadenitis, lymphogranuloma venereum, granuloma inguinale, and nocardia. Other disease to rule out include sporotrichosis, other causes of bacterial and or viral conjunctivitis, Rocky Mountain spotted fever, typhoid and enteric fever, mononucleosis, brucellosis, pulmonary tuberculosis, mycoplasma, Legionnaire's disease, psittacosis, viral pneumonia, fungal infection, and chemical pneumonitis.[256]

272. Jostedt SA, Eriksson V, Berglund L et al. (1997) Detection of *Francisella tularensis* in ulcers of patients with tularemia by PCR. **J Clin Microbial** 35:1045.
273. Markwitl LE, Hynes NA, de la Cruz P et al. (1985) Tick-borne tularemia: An outbreak of lymphadenopathy in children. **JAMA** 254:2922–2925.
274. Sunderrajan E, Hutton J, Marianfeld D (1983) Adult respiratory distress syndrome secondary to tularemia pnuemonia. **Arch Intern Med** 145:1435.
275. Yow MD (1992) Tularemia. In: Textbook of Pediatric Infectious Diseases, 3rd edn, Feigen RD, Cherry JD, eds. Philadelphia: WB Saunders, p. 1316.

THERAPY FOR TULAREMIA

The antibiotic treatment of choice for tularemia remains streptomycin. In adults, the dose should not exceed 2g/day. Regimens in children include 30–40mg/kg/day divided in two doses im for 7 days, or alternatively, the full dose for 3 days followed by 4 days of half the dose. These regimens have resulted in 97% cure with rare relapses. Alternative therapy includes gentamicin 3–5mg/kg im or iv q8h for 7 to 10 days. This requires more injections and has a reduced, 86% cure rate, with a 6% relapse rate.

In adults and adolescents, tetracycline HCl 500mg po four times a day or doxycycline 100mg po or iv twice daily for 14 days are also successful in curing 88% of patients but their use is associated with a 12% relapse rate. Tetracyclines are avoided in pregnant women and children less than 8 years old due to staining of tooth enamel. Chloramphenicol was used when streptomycin was in short supply but is associated with a 21% relapse rate. However, it has been used in doses of 25–60mg/kg/day iv in four divided doses for 14 days and may have special utility in tularemic meningitis. Other drugs reported to have beneficial results include erythromycin[276] and fluoroquinolones (e.g., ciprofloxacin).[277] Erythromycin, though rarely used, may have special utility in mild disease and in pregnant women. β-lactams, including ceftriaxone, are not recommended.[278]

Supportive care includes bed rest and hospitalization when dictated. Drainage of suppurative lymph nodes may reduce pain. Children on streptomycin should be monitored for ototoxicity and switched to an alternative antibiotic if preexisting or progressive hearing loss is noted. Intravenous fluids, hyperalimentation, and or intensive care for the severely ill patient is appropriate.

In the preantibiotic era, tularemia was a protracted illness requiring months of convalescence. The mortality rate varied from 5 to 30%. Antibiotic therapy, especially with streptomycin, has reduced the rate of mortality to 2 to 4% in the United States.

Prevention is difficult because the bacteria cannot be completely eradicated in wild hosts and insect reservoirs. It requires avoidance of sick or dead animals, especially those in the wild, use of insect repellants and protective clothing, and prompt and careful removal of ticks. Other preventive measures include drinking only potable water and the thorough cooking of wild meats. At present, there are no commercially available vaccines in the United States.

RAT-BITE FEVER

Rat-bite fever is caused by infection with either *Streptobacillus moniliformis* or *Spirillum minus*, typically after the bite or scratch of a rat or other small rodent. These bacteria are commonly found as normal oropharyngeal flora of rodents. Rat-bite fever due to either organism is found worldwide, but the major cause in the United States is *S. moniliformis*.

STREPTOBACILLUS MONILIFORMIS

S. moniliformis is a nonmotile, pleomorphic, Gram-negative, microaerophilic, nonencapsulated bacillus that appears in puffball colonies when growth in broth culture. It is fastidious and needs special care for isolation. Optimal growth is seen under 8–10% CO_2 in trypticase soy agar or broth supplemented with 20% horse or rabbit serum or panmede-supplemented brain infusion agar incubated at 35–37°C with humidity. Special blood culture bottles without sodium polyanethol sulfonate should be used when rat-bite fever is suspected.[279] L-forms resistant to penicillin have been recovered from isolates of human and rat blood and develop spontaneously upon transfer to solid media.[280]

Infection is typically associated with the bite of a rat, mouse, or other small rodent. The organism can be isolated from 50% of healthy rats but has also been isolated as the cause of pneumonia and arthritis in mice and from infected turkeys, gerbils, wood squirrels, and guinea pigs.[279] It may also be transmitted from bites of rodent-eating animals including cats, dogs, and pigs. *S. moniliformis* has been isolated from raw milk (Haverhill fever)[281] and other food and water products.

Rat-bite fever is seen most frequently in urban areas with poor sanitation and large rat populations. Children are more frequently infected than adults, and infants in cribs are at particular risk of being bitten. Because of its prevalence as normal flora in rat colonies, laboratory personnel who handle rats are also at risk.[282]

The incubation period after exposure or bite is usually 3–10 days, but can be up to about 21 days. High fever and shaking chills are followed by headache, vomiting, and myalgias. A rash develops 1–8 days after the onset of illness in most patients (75%). This generalized morbilliform rash can become petechial (Fig. 24.18), confluent, or purpuric and may involve the palms and soles (20% desquamate).[283] More than half of patients have arthralgias that can progress to arthritis with effusion.[279,284] The knees, wrists, and elbows are most frequently involved, and polyarticular arthritis is not infrequent.[279,284] Seven to 10 days after the onset of illness, the fever falls, and symptoms resolve within 2 weeks.

Streptobacillary rat-bite fever is a rare disease in the United States with fewer than 200 cases reported.[285,286] During the 1950s and early 1960s, rat-bite fever was commonly seen at Charity Hospital in New Orleans, but rat control programs have almost eliminated the problem. This illness may be seriously underdiagnosed.

In the absence of treatment, the disease may develop a pattern of relapsing fever lasting intermittently for several months, although the rash does not recur. Laboratory findings are not diagnostic but occasionally coagulopathy with thrombocytopenia develops.[283] Complications include anemia, pneumonia, endocarditis,[287] pericarditis,[288] myocarditis, abscesses of soft tissue

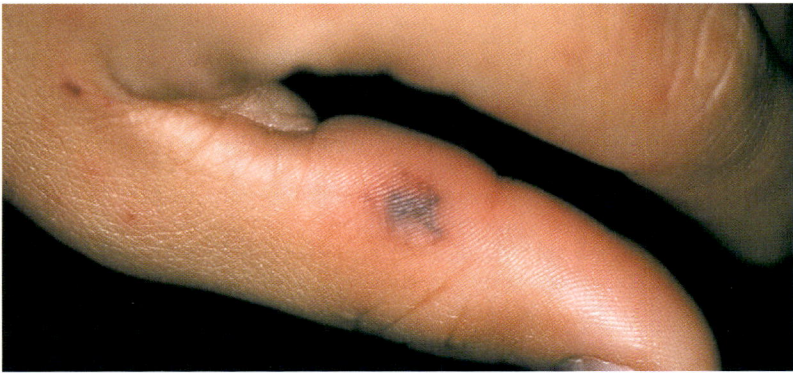

Fig. 24.18 Rat bite fever. Morbilliform purpuric eruption in a child (courtesy Dr Sean Elliott).

276. Harrell RE Jr, Simmons HF (1990) Pleuropulmonary tularemia: Successful treatment with erythromycin. **South Med J** 83:1363.
277. Russell P, Eley SM, Fulop MJ et al. (1998) The efficacy of ciprofloxacin against experimental tularemia. **J Antimicrob Chemother** 41:461.
278. Cross JT, Jacobs RF (1993) Tularemia: treatment failure with outpatient use of ceftriaxone. **Clin Infect Dis** 17:976.
279. Byington CL, Basoeo RD (1998) *Strepobacillus moniliformis.* In: Textbook of Pediatric Infectious Disease, 4th edn, Feigin RD, Cherry JD, eds. Philadelphia: WB Saunders, pp. 1509–1512.
280. Buchman RE, Gibbons NE (eds) (1974) Bergey's Manual of Determinative Bacteriology. Baltimore: William and Williams.
281. Parker F, Hudson NP (1926) The etiology of Haverhill fever (erythema arthriticum epidemicum). **Am J Pathol** 2:357.
282. Anderson LC, Leary SL, Manning P (1983) Rat bite fever in laboratory personnel. **Lab Anim Sci** 33:292–294.
283. Portnoy BL, Satterwhite TK, Dyclman JD (1979) Rat-bite fever misdiagnosed as Rocky Mountain spotted fever. **South Med J** 72:607.
284. Holroyd KJ, Reiner AP, Dick JD (1988) *Streptobacillus moniliformis* polyarthritis mimicking rheumatoid arthritis: an urban case of rat bite fever. **Am J Med** 85:711.
285. Raffin BJ, Freemark M (1979) Streptobacillary rat-bite fever: a pediatric problem. **Pediatrics** 64:214.
286. Azimi P (1990) Pets can be dangerous, your diagnosis, please. **Pediatr Infect Dis J** 9:670.
287. Mc Cormack RC, Kaye D, Hook EW (1967) Endocarditis due to *Streptobacillus moniliformis* **JAMA** 200:77.
288. Carbeck RB, Murphy TF, Britt EM (1967) Streptobacillary rat-bite fever with massive pericardial effusion. **JAMA** 201:703.

and solid organs including brain,[289] meningitis, pancreatitis, and periarteritis nodosa.[290] Children may have severe weight loss, failure to thrive, and diarrhea.[281] Untreated, streptobacillary rat-bite fever had a 10% mortality rate. This has been reduced to less than 1.5% with treatment.[279,291] Most deaths are due to complications of endocarditis.

Haverhill fever, which is transmitted by the ingestion of food or water contaminated by rat urine and the bacterium *S. moniliformis*, is similar to rat-bite fever. This illness follows a 1–3-day incubation period and is followed by the abrupt onset of fever and chills (100%), arthritis (97%), and rash (95%). Gastrointestinal and respiratory complaints are also often present. Its only reported complication is iron deficiency anemia, and the prognosis for complete recovery from Haverhill fever is excellent.[292] Diagnosis of streptobacillary illness is generally made by recovering the organism from cultures of blood, joint, or abscess fluid.[279,281] Confirmation of the culture can be obtained rapidly by gas liquid chromotography as *S. moniliformis* has a classic fatty acid profile.[293] Without an appropriate history, most patients will be evaluated for viral infections, febrile drug reactions, meningococcemia, syphilis, rickettsial infection, especially Rocky Mountain spotted fever, and even Henoch–Schönlein purpura. Causes of relapsing fevers such as typhoid and malaria should be considered, as should Lyme disease, brucellosis, leptospirosis, and disseminated gonococcal infection. Many older textbooks report that 25% of patients with *S. moniliformis* infections have biologic false positive tests for syphilis, but these probably represent confusion with *S. minus* infections in which greater than 50% of sera give a positive Wassermann reaction.[279]

Serologic diagnosis is frequently helpful, especially in patients treated before cultures are obtained *S. moniliformis*-specific agglutination antibody titers develop as early as 10 days, peak at 1 to 3 months, and remain elevated for several years. An agglutination titer of 1:80 or more is considered diagnostic of recent infection. Fluorescent antibody and complement fixation tests are available but do not represent any advantage. A recent ELISA assay has been developed for monitoring rodent colony infections, and may be helpful for detection of human disease in the future.[294]

SPIRILLUM MINUS

Rat-bite fever caused by *S. minus* is known as *sodoku* in Japan and is found worldwide, predominantly in Asia. *S. minus* is a short, 2 to 5mm, Gram-negative, tightly coiled, aerobic, flagellated spirochete. The organism, which is thicker than *Treponema pallidum*,[295] is recognized by its characteristic darting motility on dark-field examination. Like other spirochetes, as a rule *S. minus* cannot be grown on artificial media[296–298] and requires animal inoculation to confirm the diagnosis.[298,299] Serologic tests are not available but 50% of patients with *S. minus* have a false positive syphilis test.

The infection is usually acquired after a rat bite. Approximately 25% of rats carry *S. minus* in the nasopharynx or conjunctiva.[300] There are no reports of oral ingestion of the spirochete resulting in an illness like Haverhill fever. Theoretically, it might be transmitted by transfusion.[295]

Some 14 to 18 days following the rodent bite (range 1–36 days) a local reaction characterized as an indurated lesion develops at the site of the bite.[301] Histologically the bite reveals edema, mononuclear cell infiltrates, and local necrosis.[298] This "chancre-like lesion" may ulcerate or almost heal and is often associated with significant regional lymphadenopathy or lymphangitis. Patients abruptly develop fever and chills which may resolve, then recur during several weeks if diagnosed.[299] The relapsing symptoms are often associated with hematogenous spirella. Hemorrhagic, toxic, or necrotic changes may develop in the kidneys and liver.[295] Patients may also suffer headaches, myalgia, and vomiting when febrile and 50% develop a rash. The rash may consist of purple to red–brown macules and patches, indurated papules and plaques, and/or urticarial lesions. Joint manifestations are rare in contrast to streptobacillary rat-bite fever.

Diagnosis is difficult and is made with the isolation and identification of the spirochete. Rarely, a smear of the patient's blood will reveal the spirochete, but more often animal inoculation, which is time consuming, expensive and not widely available, is required. Nonspecific findings include anemia and leukocytosis.

Left untreated, the illness usually spontaneously resolves after several relapses during a 3–8-week course but the illness may persist for more than a year.[302–304]

S. minus is sensitive to penicillin, but due to the difficulty in separating the spirillary from the streptobacillary form of disease and the coexistence of both infections in some patients, therapy should be provided in doses that would be adequate for both *S. monilliformis* and *S. minus*.[295]

Common complications in children include weight loss, anemia, and severe diarrhea.[299,303] Other complications may include endocarditis, hepatitis, meningitis, myocarditis, nephritis,[298,302] splenomegaly, headache, nuchal rigidity, pleurisy, pleural effusion and epididymitis.[301]

Mortality in untreated cases is 6.5%,[279,302] whereas treated cases generally have a good prognosis. Control of rodent populations is the only effective means of disease prevention.

LEPTOSPIROSIS

Leptospirosis is a zoonotic infection caused by the spirochete, *Leptospira interrogens*.[305] It is primarily a disease of wild and domestic animals and only occasionally infects humans; it is rarely seen in children. The clinical syndrome of leptospirosis was first described by Weil in 1886[306] and the bacterium was first isolated in culture by Inada in 1915.[307] The illness produced, which has protean manifestations, has numerous synonyms including: Weil's, Swineherd's, and Stuttgart disease; it is also known as variously termed fevers including canicola, rice field, autumnal, seven-day, mud, swamp, Wycon, Bushy Creek, and Fort Bragg, as well as by the term hemorrhagic jaundice.[308]

MICROBIOLOGY

The genus *Leptospira* consists of two species: *L. bifexia* and *L. interrogens*. Only serovars or serotypes of *L. interrogens* are known to cause disease in

289. Oedig P, Alarson H (1950) *Streptothrix muris ratti* (*Streptobacillus moniliformis*) isolated from brain abscess. **Arch Pathol Microbiol Scand** 27:436.
290. Cole JS, Stroll RW, Bulger RJ (1969) Rat-bite fever. **Ann Intern Med** 71:979.
291. Roughgarden JM (1965) Antimicrobial therapy of rat bite fever. **Arch Intern Med** 116:39–53.
292. McEvoey M, Noah N, and Pilsworth R (1987) Outbreak of fever caused by *Streptobacillus moniliformis*. **Lancet** 2:1362–1367.
293. Rowbotham T (1983) Rapid identification of *Streptobacillus moniliformis*. **Lancet** 2:567.
294. Boot R, Bakker RHG, Thuis H et al. (1993) An enzyme immunosorbent assay (ELISA) for monitoring rodent colonies for *Streptobacillus moniliformis* antibodies. **Lab Anim** 27:350.
295. Byington CL, Basow RD (1988) *Spirillum minus* (rat-bite fever). In: Textbook of Pediatric Infectious Disease, 4th edn, Feigen RD, Cherry JD, eds. Philadelphia: WB Saunders, pp. 1542–1543.
296. Hitzig WM, Liebman A (1944) Subacute endocarditis associated with spirillum: Report of a case with repeated isolation of the organism from the blood. **Arch Int Med** 73:415.
297. Schwartzman G, Flonman AL, Bass MH et al. (1951) Repeated recovery of a spirillum by blood culture from two children with prolonged and recurrent fevers. **Pediatrics** 8:227.
298. Lennette EH, Balows A, Hausler JW, Jr et al. (eds) (1985) Manual of Clinical Microbiology, 4th edn. Washington, DC: American Society of Microbiology.

299. Taber L, Feigin RD (1979) Spirochetal infections. **Pediatr Clin N Am** 26:377–413.
300. Mc Dermott E (1928) Rat-bite fever: Study of experimental disease with critical review of literature. **Q J Med** 21:433–458.
301. Brown T, Nunnemaker J (1942) Rat-bite fever: review of American cases with reevaluation of its etiology and report of cases. **Bull Johns Hopkins Hosp** 70:201–302.
302. Gunning J (1976) Rat-bite fever In: Tropical Medicine, 5th edn, Hunter GW, Swartzwelder JC, Clyde DF, eds. Philadelphia: WB Saunders, pp. 245–247.
303. Roughgarden J (1965) Antimicrobial therapy of rat-bite fever. **Arch Intern Med** 116:39–53.
304. Robertson A (1930) *Spirillum minus*: etiological agent of rat-bite fever. **Ann Trop Med** 24:367.
305. Everett ED (2001) Leptospirosis. In: Up To Date www.Uptodate.com Vol.9 No. 2, 1–4.
306. Weil A (1886) Ueber eine Eigenthumliche, mit milztumor, icterus, and nephritis einhergehende, acute infectionskrankheit. **Dtsch Arch Klin Med** 39:209–232.
307. Inada R, Ido Y, Hoki R et al. (1916) The etiology, mode of infection and specific therapy of Weil's disease, Spirochietosis icterohemorrhaigna. **Exper Med** 23:377–402.
308. Feigin RD, Anderson DC (1998) Leptospirosis. In: Textbook of Pediatric Infectious Disease, 4th edn, Feigin RD, and Cherry JD, eds. Philadelphia: WB Saunders, pp. 1529–1542.

humans.[305] The serovars most found commonly in human infection include icterohemorrhagiae, autumnalis, pomona, grippotyphosa, hebdomdis and australis.[309–311]

Leptospires are spiral-shaped, flexible, aerobic, motile organisms with 18 or more coils per cell and semicircular hooked ends. They are best visualized by dark-field microscopy, fluorescent microscopy, or stained with silver, as they stain poorly with common laboratory stains.[308] They can be grown *in vitro* from clinical specimens such as blood, CSF, or urine on special media such as Ellinghausen's, Fletcher's or polysorbate 80 media. They are slow-growing and may take from 2 to 12 weeks to emerge.[308] Therefore, laboratories need to be notified if an attempt to grow *Leptospira* is initiated.[312,313]

EPIDEMIOLOGY

This zoonosis has a worldwide distribution except for the polar regions, and tends to be most prevalent in the tropics. Most cases in the United States are reported from the Pacific and Southern coastal states, especially Hawaii.[305] Natural hosts for the organism are various mammals, especially rodents, dogs, cattle, swine, foxes, horse, sheep and goats, in which it can produce a spectrum of diseases from asymptomatic infection to severe infection and death. A 10% mortality rate is estimated in dogs. Many farm animals, such as cattle, sheep, goats, and swine, suffer spontaneous abortions when infected. Cats are rarely infected.

Following infection, surviving animals shed the organism in their urine, from weeks to months, resulting in contamination of the environment. The leptospires spread to water and soil where, again, they may remain viable for weeks to months. Humans may become infected after exposure to infected animal urine, water, or soil contaminated by this urine, or infected animal tissue. Usually, the bacteria gain entry to humans through abraded or injured skin, mucous membranes, or the conjunctivae. Ingestion of contaminated food is an extremely rare source of infection.[305] Human-to-human transmission is exceptional but transmission from an infected mother to an infant through breast milk has been documented.[314]

Most human cases are sporadic but common source outbreaks have been reported. Competitive swimmers, 90 in Illinois and 70 in Borneo, Malaysia, who swam in contaminated lake or river water where the illness was endemic, met the CDC clinical case definition for leptospirosis.[315,316] Because travelers often participate in water-based recreational activities, they are at increased risk for infection especially if returning from the tropics.[312,313]

Major risk factors for this illness include occupational exposure to infected animals as seen in farmers, ranchers, veterinarians, trappers, and abattoir workers. Other at-risk occupations with exposure to contaminated soil and/or water include sewer workers, rice field workers, or military personnel. Recreational activities that may increase exposure to leptospires include swimming and boating, and sporting activities in or near fresh water. Household risk factors that have been associated with leptospirosis include exposure to infected pet dogs or rodent infestations, as well as exposure to rainwater catchment systems.[305,308,317]

CLINICAL PRESENTATION

Leptospires invade the bloodstream and spread throughout the body after penetration of the skin or mucous membranes. The resultant disease, although protean in expression, can be best described as an extensive vasculitis.

The disease is biphasic in 50% of patients. The early septicemic stage lasting 4 to 7 days, is followed by a period of improved symptoms and defervescence. This stage coincides with the development of antibodies to and the disappearance of leptospires in the blood and organs, except the kidneys and eyes. This second or immune stage lasts 4 to 30 days and is the period when serious renal, hepatic, or biphasic central nervous system manifestations may develop. Severity of illness depends on the inoculum and virulence of the organism, as well as portal of entry and host immune status.

After an incubation period of 2 to 20 days (average 10 days), most patients (75–100%) present with the abrupt onset of fever, myalgias, headaches, and rigor. Approximately 50% experience nausea, vomiting and diarrhea, and 25% to 35% have an associated nonproductive cough.[305,316] During the early septicemic stage of the illness, the spirochete becomes widespread and rash commonly develops. Rashes described include macules, papules, urticaria, and petechiae, which commonly appear on the trunk. Pretibial or Fort Bragg fever is associated with *L. autumnalis* and has a distinctive rash which appears on the fourth or fifth day of the illness and lasts for 4 to 5 days. It consists of 1- to 5-cm erythematous, raised papules and plaques located most commonly on the shins. Less common symptoms include abdominal pain, arthralgias, bone pain, and sore throat.

Physical examination reveals muscle tenderness or rigidity, lymphadenopathy, splenomegaly, hepatomegaly, and abnormal chest auscultation in 7–40% of patients. Conjunctival suffusion is common, and should raise the suspicion of leptospirosis in patients with fever of unknown origin.[305]

Most cases are mild and easily overlooked.[318] Less than 10% of cases present with classical Weil's disease (severe leptospirosis and jaundice). The illness, though classically defined as biphasic, is not biphasic in 50% of patients and may be asymptomatic or continuous.[305,316] The second or immune phase of the disease may last for 1–4 weeks. Aseptic meningitis, present in 50–55% of patients whose CSF is examined after 7 days of illness, is thought to be due to host immune responses to the leptospires rather than direct infection.[305,319]

Leptospirosis can also cause uveitis,[320] pneumonia, hepatic dysfunction, jaundice, severe anemia, thrombocytopenia, renal hemorrhage and/or renal failure,[321] myocarditis and rhabdomyolysis.[322,323] Hepatic dysfunction and failures are usually reversible.

LABORATORY FINDINGS

Routine laboratory tests are frequently nondiagnostic. The WBC count may be normal or raised, with a left shift noted in 65% of patients. Rare patients have low platelets and/or anemia. Urinalysis may reveal proteinuria, pyuria, granular casts and occasional hematuria.[317] Some 50% of patients have a raised

309. Farrar WE (1990) Leptospirosis species (Leptospirosis) In: Principals and Practice of Infectious Diseases, 3rd edn, Mandell GL, Douglas RG Jr, Benett JE, eds. New York: Churchill Livingstone p. 1813.
310. Heath CW Jr, Alexander AD, Galton MM (1965) Leptospirosis in the United States: analysis of 483 cases in man 1949–1961. **N Engl J Med** 273:857.
311. Kaufman AF (1976) Epidemiologic trends of leptospirosis in the United States 1965–1974. In: The Biology of Parasitic Spirochetes, Johnson RC, ed. New York: Academic Press, p. 177.
312. Kaufman AF, Weyant RS (1995) Leptospiraceae In: Manual of Clinical Microbiology, 6th ecn. Washington, DC: ASM Press, p. 621.
313. Acha PN, Szyfres B (1987) Leptospirosis In: Zoonoses and Communicable Disease Commcn to Man and Animals, 2nd Pan American Health Organization, Washington, DC p. 97.
314. Bolin CA, and Koellner P (1988) Human-to-human transmission of *Leptospira interrogens* by milk. **J Infect Dis** 158:246–247.
315. Update (1998) Leptospirosis an unexplained acute febrile illness among athletes participating in triathlons-Illinois and Wisconsin, 1998. **MMWR Morb Mortal Wkly Rep** 47:673.

316. Bovet P, Yersin C, Merier F et al. (1999) Factors associated with clinical leptospirosis: A population based case-control study in the Seychelles (Indian Ocean) **Int J Epidemiol** 28:583.
317. Faar RW (1995) Leptosporosis. **Clin Infect Dis** 21:1.
318. Berman SJ, Tsai C, Holmes K et al. (1973) Sporadic anicteric leptospirosis in South Vietnam. **Ann Intern Med** 79:167.
319. Bertherat E, Renaut A, Nabias R et al. (1995) Leptospirosis and Ebola virus infection in f ve gold-panning villages in northeastern Gabon. **Am J Trop Med Hyg** 60:610.
320. Dupont H, Dupont-Perdrizet D, Pere JL et al. (1997) Leptospirosis: prognostic factors associated with mortality. **Clin Infect Dis** 25:720.
321. Im JG, Yeon KM, Han MC et al. (1989) Leptospirosis of the lung: radiographic findings in 58 patients. **Am J Roentgenol** 152:955.
322. Watt G, Tuazon ML, Santiago E et al. (1988) Placebo-controlled trial of intraverous penicillin for severe and late leptospirosis. **Lancet** 1:433.
323. Emmanouilides CE, Kohn OF, Giribaldi R (1994) Leptospirosis complicated by a Jarisch-Herxheimer reaction and adult respiratory distress syndrome: A case report. **Clin Infect Dis** 18:1004.

creatinine kinase level and approximately 40% show elevated hepatic transaminases.

Severely affected patients may have high bilirubin levels, some as high as 60 to 80mg/dl. Examination of the cerebrospinal fluid may reveal elevated protein and normal glucose levels with some neutrophils or lymphocytes. Chest radiograph may reveal changes from small nodular densities to confluent consolidation or a ground glass appearance reflecting a hemorrhagic pneumonitis.[321]

DIAGNOSIS

The diagnosis is frequently missed because of the nondiagnostic characteristics of the illness and laboratory findings. The organism can be, but is infrequently, cultured.

Culture of blood and CSF may be positive during the first 10 days of illness and is successful in approximately 50% of cases.[305] Urine cultures become positive after 14 days of illness and may remain so for up to 4 weeks after symptoms resolve.[308]

The diagnosis is most commonly made by serologic testing. Serologic tests available for the diagnosis of leptospirosis include the microscopic agglutination test (MAT), macroscopic agglutination test, the indirect hemagglutination, a leptospiral ELISA, and a recently described PCR test.[324–326] All these assays are helpful but the current gold standard remains the MAT, which is performed only by reference laboratories such as the CDC.[305] A fourfold or greater rise in titer between acute and convalescent serum is diagnostic of infection as is a single high titer of 1:800. Cross-reactivity with leptospiral antibodies has been associated with other spirochetal diseases including syphilis, Lyme disease, legionellosis and relapsing fever.[305,312]

Apparently the ELISA test is more sensitive than the MAT at several points during the illness.[324–328] The CDC has reported that a commercial enzyme-linked dot immunoassay (Dip-S-Ticks) may have the best sensitivity for detection of early infection.[315,328] This test plus new PCR techniques show considerable promise for a quick and accurate diagnosis of leptospirosis in the future,[325,326] but are not yet widely available.

THERAPY

Many antibiotics have good antileptospiral activity, including penicillins, tetracyclines, erythromycin, and cephalosporins. While antibiotic therapy (e.g., doxycycline, penicillin) is best initiated early in the course of illness, resulting in fewer days of fever and hospitalization and reduction or elimination of leptospiruria, therapeutic benefit may be derived even if started late in the course of serious illness.[310,322,329]

Rare cases of penicillin-induced Jarisch–Herxheimer reactions have been reported.[323] Supportive care for severe cases may include iv fluids, transfusion, dialysis and ventilatory support.

Adverse outcomes appear to be associated with dyspnea, oliguria, cardiac repolarization abnormalities and high white blood cell counts.[305,308,323] Mortality rates have ranged from 4 to 50% of reported cases and probably overrepresents the severely affected cases.

PREVENTION

Vaccination of domestic animals may reduce but not totally protect a community from leptospirosis. Prophylactic use of doxycycline significantly reduced the incidence of disease among 940 US soldiers deployed in jungle training in Panama.[330] Antibiotic prophylaxis may be considered for known exposures to infected animals. Avoidance of stagnant water or water from farm run-off as well as control of rodent populations remain the main means for control of this disease. No human immunization is available.

BARTONELLA

Four *Bartonella* species have been shown to be pathogenic for humans. *B. bacilliformis* causes Oroya fever and verruga peruana; *B. henselae* and *B. clarridgeae* cause cat scratch disease; *B. henselae* and *B. quintana* can produce bacillary angiomatosis; and *B. quintana* causes Trench fever.[331]

BARTONELLOSIS

Bartonellosis (Carrion's disease, Oroya fever, or verruga peruana), due to *B. bacilliformis*, is an endemic infection found only in the mountain valleys of the Andes Mountains. Verruga peruana has been known since earliest records, and Inca carvings demonstrate lesions with a similar appearance at least 1000 years before the arrival of Europeans to the New World. Oroya fever was first recognized during an epidemic of fever and anemia in railway workers building the Trans-Andean Railway.[332] In 1885, a Peruvian medical student, Daniel Carrion, fatally inoculated himself with blood from the lesions of a child with verruga peruana and, while dying of Oroya fever, recognized and reported the connection between Oroya fever and verruga peruana.[332,333] Barton isolated the causative organism *B. bacilliformis* from blood in 1909.[331]

B. bacilliformis is a small, Gram-negative flagellate, motile, pleomorphic bacillus that grows best aerobically at 28°C on semisolid nutrient agar containing 10% fresh rabbit and 0.5% hemoglobin. Growth is subsurface and seen in 7–10 days. Although they stain poorly with Gram stains these intracellular pathogens can frequently be demonstrated by Giemsa staining within the erythrocytes of infected patients.[333,334] There is only one antigenic form of the organism and it is pathogenic only for humans and other primates.[334]

Endemic infection is limited to the mountain valleys of the Andes Mountains of Columbia, Ecuador, and Peru. This is due to the limited range of the sandfly vector, *Phlebotomus verrucarum*, which is killed by the dry arid winds of the desert below an altitude of 2500feet (760m) and by the cold above elevation of 8000 feet (2500m).[335] The sandfly feeds and transmits the agent principally at dusk. Human reservoirs for infection include asymptomatic cases and long-term carriers.

Pathogenesis

After the bite of the sandfly, *Bartonella* organisms enter and proliferate in the endothelial cells of blood vessels during the incubation period. Masses of organisms may be noted on microscopic examination of endothelial cells in both blood vessels and lymphatic channels. The organisms spread to involve cells within the reticuloendothelial system including lymph nodes, liver, spleen, bone marrow, as well as the kidneys, pancreas, adrenal glands, and on occasion the heart, lungs, and skin. The organisms proliferate in these locations and then bind to, enter, and parasitize up to 90% of red blood cells when they re-enter the blood stream. Destruction of infected erythrocytes and decreased bone marrow function results in a profound and rapidly developing anemia.

Patients who survive the acute illness, known as Oroya fever, may or may not develop eruptive skin lesions.[335] When the skin is involved, heman-

324. Winslow WE, Merry DJ et al. (1997) Evaluation of a commercial enzyme-linked immunosorbent assay for detection of immunoglobulin M antibody in human leptospiral infection. **J Clin Microbiol** 35:1938.

325. Levett PN, Whittington CU (1998) Evaluation of the indirect hemagglutination assay for diagnosis of acute leptospirosis. **J Clin Microbiol** 36:11.

326. Cumberland P, Everard COR, Levett PN (1999) Assessment of the efficacy of an IgM-ELISA and microscopic agglutination test (MAT) in the diagnosis of acute leptospirosis. **Am J Trop Med Hyg** 61:731.

327. Romero EC, Billerbeck AE, Lando VS et al. (1998) Detection of leptospira DNA in patients with aseptic meningitis by PCR. **J Clin Microbiol** 36:1453.

328. Merion F, Baranlon G, Perolate P (1995) Comparison of polymerase chain reaction with microagglutination test and culture for diagnosis of leptospirosis. **J Infect Dis** 172:281.

329. McClain JB, Ballou WR, Harrison SM, Steinweg DL (1984) Doxycycline therapy for leptospirosis. **Ann Intern Med** 100:696.

330. Takafujii ET, Kirkpatrick JW, Miller RN et al. (1984) An efficacy trial of doxycycline chemoprophylaxis against leptospirosis. **N Engl J Med** 310:497.

331. Spach DH, Kochlen JE (1998) Bartonella-associated infections. **Infect Dis Clin North Am** 12:137.

332. Schultz MG (1968) A history of bartonellosis (Carrion's disease). **Am J Trop Med Hyg** 17:503.

333. Schultz MG (1968) Daniel Carrion's experiment. **N Engl J Med** 278:1323.

334. Stechenberg BW (1998) Bartonellosis. In: Textbook of Pediatric Infectious Disease, 4th edn, Feigin RD, Cherry JD, eds. Philadelphia: WB Saunders, pp. 1415–1419.

335. Stechenberg BW (1992) Bartonellosis. In: Textbook of Pediatric Infectious Disease, Feigin RD, Cherry JD, eds. Philadelphia: WB Saunders, p. 1056.

giomatous nodules develop in the skin and subcutaneous tissue; older lesions can become fibrotic.

Clinical findings

Clinically, there are two forms of bartonellosis: the septicemic acute stage known as Oroya fever and the chronic stage with eruptive skin lesions known as verruga peruana. The incubation period is 18 to 21 days but can take up to 3 months. Asymptomatic cases have been documented and can have persistently positive blood cultures.

Oroya fever is seen when *B. bacilliformis* infects the nonimmune person. It may have an abrupt onset, but often the onset can be more insidious with anorexia, headache, malaise, and slight fever. The abrupt onset may present as high fever, chills, diaphoresis, headache, and change in mentation. Some patients experience vertigo, restlessness, tinnitus, angina pectoris, tachycardia and heart murmurs. A peculiar coloring characterized by extreme pallor and slight jaundice heralds a rapidly developing anemia. The anemia is characterized by macrocytosis, hypochromia, polychromasia, poikilocytes, Howell–Jolly bodies, basophilic granulation, nucleated erythrocytes, and many immature red blood cell forms. The leukocyte count usually has a left shift.

As the illness progresses, the patient develops muscle and joint pain. Ominous signs include the onset of dyspnea, angina, insomnia, delirium, coma, and/or vascular collapse, or shock. Thrombocytopenic purpura can be seen in more severe cases. Recovery is heralded by the appearance of antibodies to the organism. Nearly one-half of patients become secondarily infected during the acute stage of illness with salmonellosis, amebiasis, malaria, and/or tuberculosis.[336–338]

The cutaneous eruptions of verruga peruana appear as the Oroya fever resolves, or in some cases without any recognized preceding illness. Cutaneous lesions appear in crops often after a pre-eruptive phase characterized by joint pain and low-grade fever from 2 to 8 weeks following the acute stage. These lesions may last several months to years. The most common eruption is forma miliar, which consists of many small hemangioma-like lesions. Forma nodular consists of larger and deeper but less numerous lesions and appears mainly on the extensor surfaces of the arms and legs. These forms are usually nontender. Occasionally, a patient may develop one to two large ulcerated, forma mular lesions: pustular, blood-tinged lesions that are tender and generally secondarily infected. Lesions may regress as new ones appear concurrently.

Diagnosis is made on the basis of clinical presentation and typical blood smears demonstrating organisms, or cultures of the organism from blood or tissue. Blood cultures are rarely positive in patients with verruga peruana. Giemsa-stained skin biopsy specimens reveal pathognomonic endothelial cell intracytoplasmic organisms. Report of successful utilization of PCR techniques to identify bartonellosis in blood cultures and skin biopsies specimens has been described and may be useful in the future.[339]

Therapy

Several antibiotics are useful in treating *B. bacilliformis* infection including penicillin, streptomycin, tetracyclines, and chloramphenicol. Chloramphenicol (50–100mg/kg/day iv or po divided into four equal doses for 10 days) is usually the drug of choice because it may also treat secondary salmonella infection.[337] Blood transfusions are life-saving in severely anemic patients. Surgical treatment of verruga peruana is not usually necessary unless lesions are extremely large or interfere with vital functions because of location. Oral tetracycline usually helps to accelerate the healing of cutaneous lesions, but antibiotic therapy for verruga peruana also is not generally necessary.[334]

The prognosis of bartonellosis is greatly improved with antibiotic therapy. Untreated bartonellosis has a 40% mortality rate, which rises to 90% if associated with a concurrent salmonella infection. Most patients develop permanent immunity.

Prevention is dependent on eliminating or avoiding the sandfly vector. Spraying dwellings with insecticides, the use of insect repellents, use of bed-netting and protective clothing, and staying in at dusk are helpful. It is important to note, however, that this disease still causes epidemics in spite of these measures.

CAT-SCRATCH DISEASE

Cat-scratch disease, also known as benign lymphoreticulosis or cat-scratch fever, is an uncommon but by no means rare diagnosis. It affects approximately 22 000 people in the United States per year.[340,341] It is primarily a disease of the young, with more than 80% of patients being 21 years of age or younger.[340,341] It affects all races and both sexes equally.[342–344] Usually a benign disease, it is characterized by an inoculation-site lesion, usually of the skin but occasionally affecting the eye or mucous membrane, followed by regional lymphadenitis that often persists for weeks to months before resolving, but generally is self-limiting. In approximately 4% of cases, cat-scratch disease can develop into more severe illness and involve other organ systems.[343]

Etiology

Cat-scratch disease is due in most cases to a Rickettsia-like, Gram-negative organism, *Bartonella henselae*.[340,345–347] This organism was first isolated from cutaneous and bony lesions of patients with AIDS, bacillary (epithelioid) angiomatosis, and peliosis hepatis.[348–351] Recent cat scratches was a common feature in these patients.[345] This organism is closely related to *B. quintana*.[352]

For years, an infectious agent for this disease was proposed but defied identification until Wear *et al.* discovered an organism present in the lymph nodes of affected children.[353] This tiny organism stained positively with Warthin–Starry silver stain, and fulfilled Koch's postulates. Initially, the organism cultured from affected lymph nodes was thought to be *Afipia*

336. Ricketts WE (1949) Clinical manifestations of Carrion's disease. Arch Intern Med 84:751.
337. Urteaga BO, Payne EH (1955) Treatment of the acute febrile phase of Carrion's disease with chloramphenicol. Am J Trop Med 4:507.
338. Gray CG, Johnson AA, Thornton SA et al. (1990) An epidemic of Oroya fever in the Peruvian Andes. Am J Trop Hyg 42:215.
339. Maass M, Schriber M, Knobloch J (1992) Detection of *Bartonella bacilliformis* in cultures, blood and formalin-preserved skin biopsies by use of the polymerase chain reaction. Trop Med Parasitol 43:191.
340. Jackson LA, Perkins BA, Wenger JD (1993) Cat scratch disease in the United States: An analysis of three national databases. Am J Pub Health 83:1707.
341. Hamilton DH, Zangwill KM, Hadler JL et al. (1995) Cat-scratch disease – Connecticut, 1992–1993. J Infec Dis 172:570.
342. Margileth AM, Hadfield T (1985) Could the infection be cat-scratch disease? Contem Pediatr 1:62.
343. Margileth AM (1988) Dermatologic manifestations and update of cat scratch disease. Pediatr Dermatol 5:1.
344. Margileth AM, Wear DJ, English CK (1987) Systemic cat scratch disease: report of 23 patients with prolonged or recurrent severe bacterial infection. J Infect Dis 155:390.
345. Leboit PE, Berger TG, Egleat BM et al. (1988) Epithelioid hemangioma-like vascular proliferation in AIDS: manifestation of cat scratch disease bacillus infection. Lancet 1:960.

346. Welch DF, Pickett DA, Slater LN et al. (1992) *Rochalimaea henselae* sp nov-s: a cause of septicemia, bacillary angiomatosis, and parenchymal bacillary peliosis. J Clin Microbiol 30:275.
347. Dolan MJ, Wong MT, Regnery RL et al. (1993) Syndrome of *Rochalimaea henselae* adenitis suggesting cat scratch disease. Ann Intern Med 118:331.
348. Kochler JS, Quinn FD, Berger TG et al. (1992) Isolation of *Rochalimaea* species from cutaneous and osseous lesions of bacillary angiomatosis. N Engl J Med 327:1625.
349. Perkocha LA, Geaghan SM, Yen B et al. (1990) Clinical and pathological features of bacillary peliosis hepatis in association with human immunodeficiency virus infection. N Engl J Med 323:1581.
350. Slater LN, Welch DF, Hensel D et al. (1990) A newly recognized fastidious gram-negative pathogen as a cause of fever and bacteremia. N Engl J Med 323:1587.
351. Kochler JE, Leboit PE, Egbert BM, Bergert G (1988) Cutaneous vascular lesions and disseminated cat scratch disease in patients with the acquired immunodeficiency (AIDS) and AIDS-related complex. Ann Intern Med 109:449.
352. Relman DA, Lowitt JS, Schmidt TM et al. (1990) The organism causing bacillary angiomatosis, peliosis hepatis, and fever and bacteremia in immunocompromised patients. N Engl J Med 3223:1573.
353. Wear DJ, Margileth AM, Hadfield TI et al. (1983) Cat scratch disease: a bacterial infection. Science 221:1403.

felis.[353,354] Studies with serologic, PCR and genetic sequencing methods, however, have not supported this organism as the cause of most cases of cat-scratch disease.[345,355–357] The possibility remains that certain cases of cat-scratch disease may be caused by other pathogens, however, such as *R. quintana*, *A. felis*, or *B. clarridgeiae*.[347,358–360]

Clinical findings

In immunocompetent patients, the condition is characterized by chronic, asymptomatic or tender lymphadenopathy persisting beyond 3 weeks with evidence or history of a preceding local cat scratch. Affected patients generally are healthy children. A primary scratch or other contact with a cat, especially a kitten younger than 6 months old, has been documented in 93% of cases. In one study, 77% of cats and 90% of kittens showed positive serologic reactions to *B. henselae*.[361,362] In 6% of cases, the condition follows contact with a dog.[342] Fleas are also implicated in the transmission of cat-scratch disease as flea infestations are more prevalent in affected animals than in controls.

Most primary lesions occur on the arms or hands but may occur anywhere on the skin, including the trunk and face. The lesion usually appears 3–10 days after the initial scratch, and may take many forms, beginning as a macule and evolving into a maculopapule, vesiculopapule, or pustule and then a papule. Although nonpruritic, it may resemble an insect bite and may resolve in one to two weeks or persist for as long as five months. It usually resolves without a scar.[363] Seven percent of cases follow inoculation in the eye, with a resultant ocular granuloma or conjunctivitis.[342]

Regional lymphadenopathy follows this lesion in 3–50 days, developing in most cases about 2 weeks after the scratch. This lymphadenopathy generally is tender (80%) and seen in the axilla or head and neck distribution (80%). The skin overlying the node may be erythematous; occasionally, cellulitis is present, and resolves slowly along with the lymphadenopathy. Involvement of other areas such as the epitrochlear or inguinal nodes occurs less commonly. Multiple areas of nodal involvement are seen in 40% of cases.[364,365] Gross node enlargement up to 8cm may occur; in 12% of patients nodal suppuration may develop. The lymphadenopathy may persist for 6–24 months, but generally resolves within four months.[366]

Other symptoms reported include fever, malaise, and/or fatigue in approximately one-third of patients, and 10% may demonstrate one or more of the following: headache, anorexia, emesis, weight loss, sore throat, and/or splenomegaly. Other unusual mainfestations include Parinaud's oculoglandular syndrome, in which an ocular granuloma, polyps, or conjunctivitis is associated with parotid or preauricular lymphadenopathy. Other still rarer presentations include osteomyelitis, thrombocytopenic purpura, primary atypical pneumonia, hypercalcemia, endocarditis and septic shock.

Skin eruptions can be seen in 4–5% of patients, and include morbilliform, petechial, macular, maculopapular, granuloma annulare-like, vesiculopapular, and urticarial lesions. Erythema multiforme and/or erythema nodosum have also been reported.[366,367]

Rare cases have a more severe course. Some manifest generalized lymphadenopathy. CNS involvement, although seen in only 1–2% of cases, is a serious occurrence. Patients may have encephalopathy, meningitis, radiculitis, polyneuritis, and even myelitis with paraplegia.[368] Steady recovery over 6 months is seen in 90% of these cases.[369] In general, the prognosis for this illness is excellent in patients with normal immune function.[370,371] A few have residual neurologic sequelae.[369]

In immunocompromised patients, such as those with AIDS or bone marrow transplantation, the illness takes a more aggressive course known as bacillary (epithelioid) angiomatosis. These patients have vascular cutaneous lesions which may resemble pyogenic granuloma, Kaposi's sarcoma, bartonellosis, or angiosarcoma. Lesions can be solitary or multiple (with up to hundreds of lesions) and may be tiny papules of 0.1cm to nodules of up to 5cm in diameter. Histologically, the lesions consist of a proliferation of blood vessels lined by pale-staining endothelial cells. The proliferating cells have markers for both endothelial (factor III antigen) and macrophage (alpha-antichymotrypsin) lineages. The bacillus found in the lesions of bacillary angiomatosis has been found to be *B. henselae*, the cat-scratch disease bacillus. Skin lesions of bacillary angiomatosis may involve underlying bone. On occasion, these lesions may resolve spontaneously, but widespread dissemination of the organism with resultant disseminated intravascular coagulation, shock, and death is well documented.

Diagnostic features

In the past, diagnosis of cat-scratch disease was primarily clinical and minimally supported by laboratory proof. It was suspected if a patient had lymphadenopathy of 3 or more weeks' duration and a history of a scratch or primary skin lesion after animal contact (especially with kittens). The development of regional lymphadenopathy 2 weeks after this contact was also suggestive, and a positive skin test result was confirmatory, although these are now rarely done, as improved diagnostic methods are available.

Biopsy specimens from affected skin at sites of inoculation reveal a central acellular zone of dermal necrosis surrounded by a mantle of lymphocytes, giant cells, and histiocytes. Lymph node biopsy reveals multiple abscesses with necrotic centers surrounded by epithelioid cells, some giant cells, and eosinophilla. Warthin–Starry silver stains reveal small pleomorphic rods in the tissue which are Gram-negative on Brown–Hopps tissue Gram stain.

Isolation of *B. henselae* provides definitive diagnosis, but it is very difficult to isolate from tissues or blood. Blood cultures should be incubated in pediatric or adult isolater tubes or in blood culture tubes containing EDTA to increase the probability of isolation.[340] Subcultures may enhance the chance of isolation and should be plated onto fresh chocolate agar or heart infusion agar supplemented with 5% rabbit blood and incubated with 5% CO_2 at 35–37°C for at least 21 days. Yields are poor, however, as few patients have bacteremia.[372]

Serologic tests available for diagnosis of *B. henselae* infections include the indirect fluorescence assay (IFA), for which a titer of 1:64 is supportive of the diagnosis, and enzyme immunosorbent assay (EIA). Problems exist with both tests, however, due to cross-reactivity with other species of *Bartonella*. False positive results may be due to past infection.

354. Boyer KM, Cherry JD (1992) Cat scratch disease. In: Textbook of Pediatric Infectious Disease, 3rd edn, Feigin RD, Cherry JD, eds. Philadelphia: WB Saunders, p. 1084.
355. Regenery RC, Olson DG, Perkins BA et al. (1992) Serologic response to *Rochalimaea hensalae* antigen in suspected cat-scratch disease. **Lancet** 339:1443.
356. Perkins BA, Swaminathan B, Jackson LA et al. (1992) Pathogenesis of cat scratch disease (letter). **N Engl J Med** 327:1599.
357. Andrewa DM, Karnick JT, Ruoff KL (1992) Pathogenisis of cat scratch disease (letter) **N Engl J Med** 327:1600.
358. Bass JW, Vincent JM, Person DA (1997) The expanding spectrum of *Bartonella* infections: II. Cat-scratch disease. **Pediatr Infect Dis J** 16:163.
359. Szelc-Kelly CM, Goral S, Perez-Perez GI et al. (1995) Serologic responses to Bartonella and Afipia antigens in patients with cat scratch disease. **Pediatrics** 96:1137.
360. Kordick DL, Hilyard EJ, Hadfield TL et al. (1997) *Bartonella clarridgeiae*, a newly recognized zoonotic pathogen causing inoculation papules, fever, and lymphadenopathy (cat scratch disease). **J Clin Microbiol** 35:1813.
361. Koechler JE, Glaser CA, Tappero JW (1994) *Rochalimaea henselae* infection: A new zoonosis with the domestic cat as reservoir. **JAMA** 271:531.
362. Chomel BB, Abbott RC, Kasten RW et al. (1995) *Bartonella henselae* prevalence in domestic cats in California: Risk factors and association between bacteremia and antibody titer. **J Clin Microbiol** 33:2445.
363. Shinall EA (1990) Cat scratch disease: a review of the literature. **Pediatr Dermatol** 7:11.
364. Carithers HA (1970) Cat scratch disease. Notes on its history. **Am J Dis Child** 119:200.
365. Carithers HA, Carithers CM, Edwards RO Jr (1969) Cat-scratch disease—its natural history. **JAMA** 207:312.
366. Margileth AM (1985) Cat scratch disease. In: Cecil Textbook of Medicine, 17th edn, Wyngarden JB, Smith JH Jr, eds. Philadelphia: WB Saunders, p. 1618.
367. Moriarty RA, Margileth AM (1987) Cat-scratch disease. **Infect Dis Clin North Am** 1:575.
368. Miller P, Bell W (1980) Cat scratch disease with encephalopathy. **Clin Pediatr** (Phila) 19:233.
369. Margileth AM, Wear DJ, Hadfield TL et al. (1984) Cat scratch disease: bacteria in skin at the primary inoculation site. **JAMA** 252:928.
370. Marra CM (1995) Neurologic complications of *Bartonella henselae* infection. **Curr Opin Neurol** 8:164.
371. Johnson WT, Helwig EB (1969) Cat scratch disease. **Arch Dermatol** 100:148.
372. Spach DH, Meyers SA (2001) Cat scratch disease 1998; Up to Date, Vol. 9, No. 2 in www.uptodate.com.

A new PCR probe is available in some commercial laboratories. Skin testing is not widely available, not standardized, not FDA-approved, and now rarely done.[372]

The differential diagnosis of cat-scratch disease includes bacterial lymphadenitis caused by group A streptococcus or *Staph. aureus*; viral lymphadenopathy, such as from EBV, cytomegalovirus and/or HIV; toxoplasmosis; other infectious disorders associated with lymphadenopathy such as nocardia, atypical mycobacteria, tularemia, anthrax, or syphilis; lymphoreticular malignancy, sarcoidosis, histoplasmosis, and sporotrichosis.

Treatment

Because cat-scratch disease generally is self-limited in immunocompetent hosts, resolving spontaneously in 1 to 3 months, treatment of routine cases is controversial. One randomized, double-blind, placebo-controlled antibiotic trial showed that azithromycin-treated patients had more consistent and more rapid resolution of lymphadenopathy compared to placebo-treated controls.[373] Other uncontrolled clinical trials have also suggested that three antibiotics, rifampin, ciprofloxacin, and trimethoprim/sulfamethoxazole (Table 24.4), given within 3–5 days lead to absence or decrease in malaise, fatigue, fever, headaches and anorexia, and resolution of lymphadenopathy. Limited studies in cases of hepatosplenic and other invasive forms of the disease have demonstrated that therapy with rifampin initiated alone or in combination with gentamicin[372] or trimethoprim/sulfamethoxazole provides improvement within 1–5 days in patients who have had prolonged fever.

On the basis of limited clinical trials it appears appropriate to consider azithromycin for children with early presumed or proven cat-scratch disease adenopathy and to begin rifampin with or without gentamicin for severe, atypical cases (Table 24.4).[373]

Warm compresses may help to relieve the pain of enlarged nodes. Late in the course of cat-scratch disease, approximately 10% of lymph nodes will become fluctuant and likely suppurate and drain spontaneously if the abscess is not controlled by planned surgical intervention. Because of the risk of chronic fistulous tracts after needle aspiration or incision, some experts recommend that these procedures not be undertaken. However, if needle aspiration is accomplished using a "Z tract" technique where the skin is pulled tightly to one side prior to needle entry, continued drainage rarely occurs. If incision and drainage is necessary, the incision site should be left open, allowing closure by secondary intention and granulation formulation. The latter approach almost always results in complete healing without fistula formation.

TABLE 24.4 Antibiotics for cat-scratch disease

Adenopathy
Azithromycin 10mg/kg as an initial single dose followed by 5mg/kg/day divided q24h × 4 days
or
Rifampin 10–20mg/kg/day divided q12h × 10 days
or
Ciprofloxacin 20–30mg/kg/day divided q12h × 10 days
or
Trimethoprim/sulfamethoxazole 8–12mg TMP/40–60mg SMX/kg/day divided q12h × 10 days
Hepatosplenic and atypical disease
Rifampin 15–20mg/kg/day divided q12h × 14 days and/or
Gentamicin 7.5mg/kg/day divided q8h × 14 days

Prevention

The cornerstone of prevention is to avoid exposure to young cats, particularly flea-infested kittens. However, elimination of household animals is not always practical as the love and affection shared between children and their pets is an important quality-of-life issue. Flea control in cats is essential. It is recommended that immunocompromised hosts, particularly children and adults with AIDS, only obtain pet cats that are over 1 year of age since older animals are rarely infected. Indoor kittens could be declawed to prevent transmission of *B. henselae*.

It is common for a single kitten to cause cat-scratch disease in multiple family members or in other contacts who have been scratched. The family must, therefore, decide whether an infected kitten should remain in the household. It is not presently known whether antibiotic treatment of cats might eliminate the carrier state. Testing of cats for *Bartonella* infection is not recommended.

TRENCH FEVER

Trench fever was unknown until 1915; it came into prominence during World War I and reappeared in epidemic proportions on the Russian front in World War II. It is caused by *Bartonella quintana*, which is closely related to and was formerly considered to be a rickettsia.[374] It is spread by the human body louse; it is unusually resistant to destructive environmental conditions, and remains infective in louse feces for weeks.[375,376] The pathology appears to be very similar to that of the spotted fever group of rickettsial infections.[376]

Clinical findings

The clinical presentation is variable. The incubation period ranges from 10 to 30 days. Headache, malaise, and body pains may appear as a prodrome. Onset of illness can be sudden, with chills, headache, conjunctivitis, nystagmus, dizziness, back and leg pain, and fever. The fever usually lasts for 2 weeks but may be relapsing. A typhus-like rash is a common finding, although the time of its appearance is irregular. It is accentuated by the fever. This small, red, maculopapular rash blanches on pressure and chiefly involves the trunk. It may also be sparse and transitory.[376] The illness is rarely fatal, but latent disease states may last for years.[377] Influenza, dengue, malaria, rickettsial infections and brucellosis should be considered in the differential diagnosis. Treatment is similar to that for rickettsial illness.

RICKETTSIAL INFECTION

Rickettsial diseases are caused by bacteria that are obligate intracellular parasites that cannot be cultured on ordinary media. Furthermore, they are extraordinarily sensitive to heat, drying, and sunlight when passing from host to host (except for *Coxiella burnetii*, the agent of Q fever).[378] These small, nonmotile, Gram-negative coccobacilli usually multiply in the cytoplasm of host cells, except for the spotted fever group, which are also found in the nuclei. Special stains must be used to demonstrate their presence in cell smears. The cell membranes of rickettsiae are usually permeable to nuclei acids; it may be leakage of nucleotides that makes these organisms labile and unable to replicate outside the host cell.[379] They are named in honor of Dr. H.T. Ricketts who recognized and described Rocky Mountain spotted fever and its lifecycle in 1910 and went on to die of typhus while investigating this illness in Mexico.[380]

Mammals usually are infected only via such blood-sucking arthropods as the body louse, flea, tick, and mite, which can serve as both vector and

---

373. American Academy of Pediatrics, cat scratch disease (2000) In: 2000 Red Book of the Comittee on Infectous Diseases, 25th edn, Pickering LK, ed. Elk Grove Village, IL: American Academy of Pediatrics, pp. 201–203.
374. Spach DH, Kochler JE (1998) Bartonella-associated infections: Infect Clin North Am 12:137.
375. Riley HD Jr (1982) Trench fever In: Infections in Children, Wedgewood RJ, David SD, Ray CG, Kelley JC, eds. Philadelphia: Harper and Row, p. 1089.
376. Warren J (1965) Trench fever rickettsia. In: Viral and Rickettsial Infections of Man, 4th edn, Horsfall EL Jr, Tamm I, eds. Philadelphia: JB Lippincott, p. 1161.

377. Phillip CB (1967) Trench fever. In: A Manual of Laboratory Medicine, 4th edn, Hunter GW, Frye WW, Schwartzwelder JC, eds. Philadelphia: WB Saunders. p. 112.
378. Riley HD Jr (1982) Rickettsial diseases. In: Infections in Children, Wedgewood RJ, Davis SD, Ray CG, Kelley VC, eds. Philadelphia: Harper & Row, p. 1027.
379. Rapmund G (1986) Rickettsia. In: Infectious Diseases and Medical Microbiology, 2nd edn, Braude AL, Davis CE, Fierer J, eds. Philadelphia: WB Saunders, p. 433.
380. Feigin RD, Snider RL, Edwards MS (1998) Rickettsial disease. In: Textbook of Pediatric Infectious Disease, 4th edn, Feigin RD, Cherry JD, eds. Philadelphia: WB Saunders, op. 1847–1865.

reservoir. Rickettsioses are more common in temperate and tropical climates and where humans live closely with blood-sucking arthropods.[379]

At least ten species of rickettsia are pathogenic for humans, although, with the exception of epidemic typhus, the infections are not part of the natural cycle. Thus, humans are only incidental and terminal hosts and do not contribute to rickettsial survival. Rickettsial infection is virtually synonymous with disease. The illnesses they cause, which are discussed here, include epidemic typhus, Brill–Zinsser disease, endemic typhus, Rocky Mountain spotted fever, Mediterranean spotted fever, rickettsialpox, scrub typhus, Queensland tick typhus, Siberian tick-borne typhus, and Q fever. Only murine typhus, rickettsialpox, Rocky Mountain spotted fever, and Q fever are currently acquired in the United States.[381]

Rickettsial infections fall into four major groups: the typhus group, the spotted fever group, scrub typhus, and Q fever. Ehrlichia also produce infections but are part of a separate Rickettsial tribe, Ehrlichieae.[380]

Rickettsiae have a predilection for the endothelial cells of small blood vessels, in which they replicate. They cause the host cell to swell and divide, producing a microangiitis and widespread vasculitis.[379] All rickettsia produce acute infections characterized by fever, headache and a rash, except for Ehrlichiosis, which rarely produces a rash and Q fever which has no rash.[380,382] They vary enormously in severity from benign self-limiting illnesses to fulminant infections with high mortality rates.[380]

Diagnosis of human rickettsial disease is generally made by the detection of newly acquired specific agglutinating, complement-fixing, or immunofluorescent antibodies. New PCR techniques have recently aided in the diagnosis, although their availability is limited.

Treatment of the various rickettsial diseases is similar (e.g., doxycycline, tetracycline) (see Table 24.5). Therapy usually includes the use of either a tetracycline or chloramphenicol. Both antibiotics have been associated with serious side effects in children. The choice is, in part, determined by the patient's age and the severity of the illness. Although tetracycline antibiotics are not normally recommended for children younger than 8 years of age, the benefits and risks of antibiotic side effects must be weighed against prognosis for untreated disease. Most experts favor doxycycline over chloramphenicol in this context. Treatment should be continued until the patient is afebrile for 48h, generally 5 to 9 days after therapy is begun. Fluoroquinolones are also effective, but are not recommended for children younger than 18 years of age.

Early diagnosis and the proper use of antimicrobial agents are the most important factors in the management of rickettsial infections. Given the proper medical history, physical signs, and epidemiologic factors, antibiotic therapy should be instituted when a presumptive diagnosis is made. Vigorous supportive therapy may be necessary for the severely ill patient. Corticosteroids have not been beneficial.

TABLE 24.5 Antimicrobial therapy for rickettsial diseases

Organism	Disease	Antibiotic and daily dosage
Coxiella burnetti	Q fever	Doxycycline 5mg/kg/po (max 20mg/day) divided bid × 7–14 days or Tetracycline iv × 7–14 days or Chloramphenicol iv or po × 7–14 days or TMP-SMX: 6–12mg TMP/30–60mg SMX/kg po divided bid × 7–14 days
Ehrlichia chaffeensis	Ehrlichiosis	Chloramphenicol iv or doxycycline 5mg/kg po (max 200mg/day) divided bid until improved and afebrile
R. akari	Rickettsialpox	Tetracycline iv or po × 10 days Chloramphenicol iv or po × 10 days
R. australis	Queensland tick typhus	Doxycycline 4.4mg/kg po divided bid × 1 day then 2.2mg/kg divided bid until afebrile for 24h Adults: doxycycline po 400mg total dose, given as two 200mg doses 12h apart Tetracycline po × 10 days or until improved and afebrile for 24h (adults) ciprofloxacin 400mg iv divided bid × 2 days followed by po 1500mg divided bid × 8d
R. canada	Canadian typhus	No treatment necessary
R. conori	(Many common names)	(Same options as *R. australis*)
R. mooseri (*typhi*)	Murine typhus	Doxycycline 5mg/kg po (max 200mg) as a single dose
R. prowazekii	Epidemic typhus	Tetracycline iv or po × 10 days or Chloramphenicol iv or po × 7 days
R. prowazekii	Brill–Zinsser disease	Tetracycline or chloramphenicol iv or po until afebrile × 24h

381. Krugman S, Katz SL (1981) Rickettsial infections. In: Infectious Diseases of Children and Adults, 7th Edn. St. Louis: CV Mosby.

382. Murray ES (1981) Rickettsial diseases. In: Textbook of Pediatric Infectious Diseases, Feigin RD, Cherry JD, eds. Philadelphia: WB Saunders, p. 1437.

THE TYPHUS GROUP

EPIDEMIC TYPHUS, BRILL–ZINSSER, AND ENDEMIC TYPHUS

Epidemic typhus is worldwide in distribution. Currently, its highest prevalence is in Africa, South America, and in Asia, in Afghanistan.[383] Isolated cases but no epidemics have been noted in the United States in recent years.[384] Typhus flourishes during wars and periods of social upheaval, especially in poor, crowded, and cold conditions, where bathing and the changing of clothes are infrequent.[385] This situation facilitates the transfer of the causative agent, *R. prowazekii* from person to person by the human body louse, *Pediculus humanus* var. *corporis*.

The organism, which is excreted in the feces of the infected louse, gains entry through an abrasion made by scratching the site of the louse bite. Some infections may be acquired by inhalation or by conjunctival absorption of dried infective louse feces made airborne when contaminated clothes are shaken.[381] Typhus affects all ages, but mortality rates increase with age. The fatality rate ranges from less than 10% of young adults to up to 60% in patients over 50.[380] It is rarely lethal in children.[380] Infection usually results in long-lasting immunity; survivors are also immune to murine typhus.

Pathology

The typical lesions begin in the endothelial cells of small blood vessels. Infection results in cellular edema, causing obstruction, thrombosis, and hemorrhage. Perivascular accumulations (Fraenkel's nodules) of neutrophils, macrophages, and lymphocytes are seen, and areas of necrosis may develop.[381] The lesions are found widely but are most numerous in the skin, myocardium, and CNS.

Clinical findings

The incubation period ranges from 10 to 14 days. There are usually no prodromal symptoms. Illness begins with an abrupt, explosive onset of fever, flushing of the face and neck, chills, severe intractable headache, photophobia, conjunctivitis, malaise, and myalgias. The symptoms are indistinguishable from influenza. A centripetal pinhead maculopapular, blanchable rash usually begins on the fourth to sixth day of illness. The rash may be so slight as to be overlooked; in about 10% of cases, it does not occur. It appears on the trunk near the axillae, spreads to the abdomen and then the arms and legs, and coalesces but does not become confluent. The face, palms, and soles are usually not involved. During the second week, lesions become petechial or purpuric and finally adopt a brownish pigmentation. Desquamation occurs during convalescence.

Splenomegaly, anemia, and leukopenia are usually present. Severe illness may be marked by periods of altered states of awareness, weakness, prostration, and temporary deafness. Mortality rates vary with age.

Diagnosis, treatment, and prevention

The diagnosis of typhus can be confirmed through isolation of *R. prowazekii* from guinea pigs, adult white mice, or embryonated eggs injected with infected blood or by specific serologic tests.[386] The antibody titer usually reaches its peak by the end of the second week of illness. The agglutination reaction to Proteus OX19 antigen is often positive, and is greater than that to OX2.[380] Complement fixation and immunofluorescent tests using *R. prowazekii* strains are available. An ELISA assay and a latex agglutination test were found to be reproducible and sensitive.[380] A new PCR assay that may allow earlier detection by 48h of illness of due to *R. prowazekii* as well as several other important rickettsial strains shows great promise. During an epidemic, the diagnosis is relatively easy. For sporadic cases, early in the illness, before the appearance of the rash, an accurate diagnosis is virtually impossible. The differential diagnosis should include murine typhus, relapsing fever, typhoid fever, malaria, meningococcal and other forms of meningitis, measles, toxoplasmosis, yellow fever, and Rocky Mountain spotted fever. Treatment is similar to other rickettsial infections. Most survivors experience complete recovery except for those suffering from Brill–Zinssner disease.[378,381,383]

Patients should be thoroughly deloused with soap and water and a delousing agent such as malathion. Health care personnel who handle epidemic typhus cases should be immunized and should protect themselves with gloves and gowns while delousing patients. After the delousing of patients and contacts, no isolation is necessary. The early institution of appropriate antibiotic therapy is mandatory.[387] Typhus vaccines are not readily available and do not fully protect.[388]

BRILL–ZINSSER DISEASE

This is a recrudescent form of epidemic typhus due to reactivation of dormant *R. prowazekii* which proliferates following some stress or provocation. The clinical presentation is similar to epidemic typhus, except it is milder and of shorter duration and carries a better prognosis. Rash is often absent. The diagnosis should be suspected in a patient with fever, headache, and rash who has lived in an area endemic for typhus fever. Such patients can infect lice and can serve as a nidus for an epidemic.[389] The treatment is the same as for classic epidemic typhus.

ENDEMIC TYPHUS (MURINE TYPHUS)

Endemic typhus is a worldwide, relatively mild, acute illness occurring at all ages in both sexes and caused by *R. mooseri*, also known as, *R. typhi*. It is characterized by headache, fever, malaise, and a maculopapular rash. It is a natural infection of rats, mice, and opossums[380] and is spread to humans by the rat flea *Xenopsylla cheopis*. Humans can be infected by scratching and self-inoculating infected flea feces through the skin, deposited on the skin during biting and rarely by conjunctival absorption, inhalation, and ingestion of contaminated food.[390,391]

Typhus in the United States is almost exclusively murine typhus. Most cases are reported from areas along the Gulf of Mexico, but it is a potential hazard wherever rats are found, especially cities and around granaries where rats abound.[380,392] The incidence of infection has dropped from 2000 to 5000 cases a year reported in the 1940s, to fewer than 80 cases in recent years, most of which (80%) are from Texas.[391]

Clinical findings

The clinical picture is indistinguishable from mild epidemic typhus. After an incubation of 6–14 days, the onset may be gradual. The rash is usually centripetal, but in some instances it is first seen on the face and extremities. Edema is rarely present, and multisystem complications are rare. The illness typically lasts 9–13 days. An estimated 10% of cases occur in children. As with epidemic typhus, the illness is milder in children, and under-reporting is suspected. It may be a cause of mild fever of undetermined origin in the pediatric age group.

383. Brezina R (1986) Epidemic (louse borne) typhus. In: Infectious Diseases and Medical Microbiology, 2nd edn, Braude AI, Davis CE, Fierer J, eds. Philadelphia: WB Saunders, p. 1231.
384. Duma RJ, Sonenshine DE, Bozeman FM et al. (1981) Epidemic typhus in the United States associated with flying squirrels. JAMA 245:2318.
385. Zinsser H (1943) Rats, Lice and History. New York: Blue Ribbon Books.
386. Hechemy KE, Osterman JV, Eiseman CS et al. (1981) Detection of typhus antibodies by latex agglutination. J Clin Microbiol 13:24.
387. Riley HD Jr (1982) Typhus fevers. In: Infections in Children, Wedgewood RJ, Davis SD, Ray GG et al. eds. Philadelphia: Harper & Row, p. 1032.
388. Wisseman CL Jr (1983) Typhus fevers. In: Infectious Diseases, 3rd edn, Hoeprich PD, ed. Philadelphia: Harper & Row, p. 908.
389. Murray ES, Baehr G, Schwartzman G et al. (1950) Brill's disease. I. Clinical and laboratory diagnosis. JAMA 142:1059.
390. Brezina R (1986) Endemic (murine) typhus. In: Infectious Diseases and Medical Microbiology, 2nd edn, Braude AI, Davis CE, Fierer J, eds. Philadelphia: WB Saunders, p. 1235.
391. Anonymous (1983) Current trends, outbreak of murine typhus–Texas, MMWR Morb Mortal Wkly Rep 32:131–132.
392. Peterson JC, Overall JC, Shapiro JL (1947) Rickettsial disease of childhood. J Pediatr 30:495.

Diagnosis, treatment, and prevention

The diagnosis is confirmed by detection of rising convalescent titers of complement-fixing or microagglutinating antibodies. These tests are more specific than detection of agglutinating antibodies to *Proteus* antigens.[393] Complement fixation and immunofluoresent tests to *R. mooseri* are also positive. PCR assays are described but not readily available. More severe cases can be confused with meningoccemia or Rocky Mountain spotted fever. Complications are rare.

Untreated, murine typhus has a mortality rate of less than 1%.[380] The treatment is the same as for epidemic typhus. Control should be achieved through the systematic eradication of rat and rat flea populations. Isolation of cases is not necessary because the disease does not spread human-to-human. A vaccine is available, but its use is not routinely recommended because effective therapy exists and the illness is mild. Infection produces cross-protection against murine and epidemic typhus.[387]

SCRUB TYPHUS GROUP

Scrub typhus is a mite or chigger-borne illness caused by *R. tsutsugamushi*. It is a disease of the southwest Pacific area, especially Japan and Taiwan. It has not occurred in the Western hemisphere, except in rare patients who traveled to endemic areas.

It is transmitted to humans by chiggers or mites which serve as both vectors and reservoirs of infection. Rare transplacental transmission to neonates has been documented.[380]

Pathology

The pathologic hallmark of the disease is a disseminated focal perivasculitis with endothelial damage. Various organs develop interstitial edema, endothelial swelling, and infiltration by lymphocytes and macrophages. Arteritis, thrombosis, and gangrene, which are seen with other rickettsial diseases, are rare.

Clinical findings

The clinical features are similar to other rickettsial infections. Fever, headache, and occasionally anorexia and vomiting begin abruptly, 12 to 18 days after the mite or chigger bite. A nonpruritic pink papule is usually present at the site of the bite, which increases in size, becoming an eschar or shallow ulcer about 5mm in diameter, surrounded by a flat red margin. The base of the ulcer is yellowish-gray, lacks exudate, and is painless by the time symptoms begin. Before the end of the first week of illness, a black eschar develops, which slowly regresses, leaving a pinpoint scar. Eschars may not develop in more than 50% of cases and occasionally multiple lesions may be found with associated regional lymphadenopathy. Eschars may develop on all parts of the body, especially the lower legs. At the end of the first week of illness, a pink, nonpruritic, maculopapular, nonconfluent rash develops on the chest and abdomen that spreads to involve the entire body, usually sparing the hands and face. However, rash or eschar is lacking in up to one-fifth of cases. Generalized tender lymphadenopathy, usually greater in the region of the bite, is frequently found. Meningitis is almost always present. Conjunctival injection is common as is hepatosplenomegaly. Tinnitus and transient deafness may occur. Complications, though not common, include atypical or severe pneumonia, respiratory distress, myocarditis and disseminated intravascular coagulation. The clinical severity may vary widely and is attributed to the differing virulence of *R. tsutsugamushi* strains.[380] In severe cases, pulmonary and cardiac complications may develop during the second week of illness and be fatal. Otherwise, improvement usually begins by the second week.

Without a rash, the diagnosis of scrub typhus is difficult. With a rash, it can be confused with typhoid fever, infectious mononucleosis, dengue fever, leptospirosis, and arboviral illnesses.[394]

Diagnosis, treatment, and prevention

The diagnosis is confirmed by detecting rising titers of specific antibodies or by isolating rickettsiae from inoculated mice. The immunofluorescent (IF) technique is useful, but the complement-fixation test has not been satisfactory. More recently, ELISA and indirect immunoperoxidase tests have been used successfully. Agglutinating antibody to Proteus OXK antigen is an insensitive indicator of scrub typhus infection as it is positive in only 50% of cases.[380,395] When the titer to OXK is 1:320 or higher and associated with an IF titer of 1:400 or greater, however, the diagnosis is very likely.[381] Dot immunoassays are reported as helpful in the serodiagnosis of scrub typhus.[380]

Antibiotic and supportive management is the same as for other typhus diseases, and is effective. However, patients treated with antibiotics only during the first week of illness are likely to experience a relapse. Thus, such patients should receive a single dose of an appropriate antibiotic 8 days after the original course is completed. Relapses usually respond well to therapy.[394]

Measures to eliminate the arthropod vector and attempts to control the illness by vaccines have not been successful.[396] Protective personal measures and early antibiotic therapy appear to be the best ways to control the illness.

THE SPOTTED FEVER GROUP

ROCKY MOUNTAIN SPOTTED FEVER (RMSF)

Rocky Mountain spotted fever (RMSF) caused by *R. rickettsii*, can serve as a prototype of all tick-borne spotted fevers which, taken together, have a worldwide distribution. *R. conorii* causes Mediterranean spotted fever or boutonneuse fever in the Mediterranean basin and the spotted fever of India, the Near East, and all of Africa. *R. sibirica* causes spotted fever in central Asia, Armenia, Siberia, and Mongolia. *R. australis* causes tick-borne typhus in Australia. Illness attributable to *R. rickettsii* is generally more severe than that caused by the other agents. Also, *R. conorii* and *R. sibirica* usually leave an eschar or ulcer at the primary inoculation site, whereas *R. rickettsii*, and *R. australis* do not.

Organism and epidemiology

Rocky Mountain spotted fever, although primarily a disease of the southeastern and south central United States, has been reported from every state except Vermont. Additional cases have been reported from Canada and several Central and South American countries (San Paulo Disease).[397,398] Less severe spotted fevers or tick typhus forms are described in Europe, Asia, Africa and Australia and are due to other species.[396] Rickettsiae are maintained in nature by ticks and the animals on which they feed. Many animals including field mice, birds, and dogs can serve as accidental or intermediate hosts and reservoirs for the infection. Humans are incidental victims.[382]

In the United States, ticks of four genera serve as vectors and reservoirs. *Dermacentor variabilis* (American dog tick), *D. andersoni* (wood tick), and *Amblyomma americanum* are the most important.[397] The adults are active feeders from early spring until autumn. The rickettsiae can be transmitted by a bite of an infected tick or by contamination of the skin when the infected arthropod vector is being crushed. Occasionally, the disease is transmitted by transfusion, and clinical and epidemiologic evidence of laboratory-acquired illness suggests that person-to-person transmission may be possible.[399,400]

Persons of all ages are susceptible to the disease but two-thirds of cases occur in children less than 15 years of age.[401] Both sexes are equally affected. In

393. Fiset P, Ormsbee RA, Silberman R et al. (1969) A microagglutination technique for detection and measurement of rickettsial antibodies. **Acta Virol** (Praha) 13:60.
394. Murray ES (1977) Scrub typhus. In: Infectious Diseases, 2nd edn, Hoeprich PD, ed. Hagerton, MD: Harper & Row, p. 782.
395. Rapmund G (1986) Scrub typhus. In: Infectious Diseases and Medical Microbiology, 2nd edn, Braude AI, Davis CE, Fierer J, eds. Philadelphia: WB Saunders, p. 1239.
396. Gear JHS (1969) Rickettsial vaccines. **Br Med Bull** 25:171.

397. Aikawa JK (1966) Rocky Mountain Spotted Fever. Springfield, IL: Charles C. Thomas.
398. Peters AH (1971) Tick-borne typhus (Rocky Mountain spotted fever). **JAMA** 216:1003.
399. Oster CN, Burke DS, Kenyon RH et al. (1977) Laboratory acquired Rocky Mountain spotted fever. The hazard of aerosol transmission. **N Engl J Med** 297:859.
400. Wells GM, Woodward TE, Fiset P et al. (1978) Rocky Mountain spotted fever caused by blood transfusion. **JAMA** 239:2763.
401. Walker DH (1989) Rocky Mountain spotted fever: A disease in need of microbiological concern. **Clin Microbiol Rev** 2:227–240.

some areas, occupational and recreational activities can influence the risk of illness. In the southeast, infection is most often seen in children who play in vacant fields or open lots in either suburban or rural areas. Throughout the United States, the incidence is highest in July and lowest in December through February.[402]

Pathology

Following inoculation, *R. rickettsii* multiplies in the endothelial cells of small blood vessels and disseminates widely via the bloodstream. The essential pathologic lesion is an inflammatory reaction of the endothelium and smooth muscle of the arterioles and endothelia of capillaries. The infiltrating cells are usually mononuclear, and the reaction includes the formation of fibrin, thrombi, and edema. This may give rise to infarction and necrosis. It is usually possible to demonstrate the rickettsiae in the arteriolar lesions, which are most prominent in the testes and skin.[392,400] Although parenchymal lesions of most body organs are not extensive, abnormalities in the brain, heart, skeletal muscles, lungs, knees, adrenal glands, kidneys, and skin are usually present. Of all the rickettsial diseases, Rocky Mountain spotted fever causes the most damage to the brain.

Clinical findings

A history of a tick bite can be elicited in 80% of cases. The longer the infected tick feeds, the greater the chance of infection. The incubation period ranges from 2 to 12 days. There is usually no tenderness or lesion at the bite site, nor does local lymphadenopathy develop. The symptoms of the prodromal period may be marked by headache, malaise, anorexia, photophobia, chills, low-grade fever, and joint and muscle pain, especially of the gastrocnemius.

Onset of illness may be explosive, with prostration, sweating, shaking chills, severe aches and pains, vomiting, and diarrhea dominating the picture. As the illness progresses, myalgia, hyperesthesia, and mental status changes dominate. However, conjunctivitis, papilledema, photophobia, transient deafness, cough, nose bleeds, constipation, splenomegaly, abdominal distention, thrombocytopenia, and hyponatremia may also be seen. Azotemia and jaundice are rare and carry a poor prognosis.[402]

The most common clinical findings are rash, edema, and fever. The rash, present in 90% of cases, is the earliest dependable and most diagnostic sign. It may appear the day after the onset of symptoms, but it may be delayed until the fourth febrile day. It is usually noticed first on the ankles and feet, spreads within hours to the wrists and hands and then toward the head and trunk. No matter where it is first noticed, however, it becomes marked on the extremities and involves the soles and palms. At first, the rash is small, discrete, macular, and rose-colored, with blanching on pressure. It soon becomes papular and assumes a darker hue. In 2 to 3 days, it develops a petechial or purpuric character (Fig. 24.19). Gangrene may develop on parts of the body, such as the scrotum, fingers, toes, and ear lobes. The resolving rash may desquamate and may leave longstanding hyperpigmented areas.

Generalized nonpitting, nondependent edema frequently occurs. Periorbital edema is especially common in children and is a frequent presenting sign.[392,402–407] The illness appears to be worse in patients with glucose-6-phosphate dehydrogenase deficiency. It can be confused with many other illnesses, among them the other rickettsial diseases, meningococcemia, measles, enteroviral disease, typhoid fever, Kawasaki disease, juvenile rheumatoid arthritis, systemic lupus erythematosus, and anaphylactoid purpura.

Diagnosis, treatment, and prevention

Several serologic tests are available, but generally no rise in antibody titer is detected until late in the second week of the illness. The Weil–Felix test though nonspecific is useful for making a presumptive diagnosis. Its advantages include ready availability in diagnostic laboratories and its presence early in the illness. Agglutinating antibodies may develop against Proteus OX19, OX2, and OXK antigens. However, specific serologic procedures using rickettsial antigens are more reliable.[408] Rapid testing of the patient's serum for the development of IgM and IgG to *R. rickettsii* antigens has recently become available by indirect immunofluorescent techniques. An ELISA assay of IgM and IgG to *R. rickettsii* is both sensitive and specific. It shares the flaw of most tests in that the immune response it reveals is delayed and can only be demonstrated after 6 days of illness.

More rapid diagnoses are possible by identification of rickettsiae in monocytes of a buffy coat preparation[409] or in tissue by direct and indirect immunofluorescence.[410] Newer tests include frequency pulsed electron capture-gas liquid chomatography (FPEC-GLC). This test, in experienced hands, results in a unique profile for RMSF which may be detected as early as one day into the illness, and shows future promise once reliable result parameters are established and the technique is more widely available.[380] Also, a new PCR assay has been developed which recognizes DNA sequences common to several important rickettsia, including *R. rickettsii*, *R. prowazekii*, and *R. typhi*.[411] It is sensitive to as few as 30 organisms per sample and is positive as early as 48 hours into the illness, but is not yet broadly available.

Antimicrobial therapy is the same as for other rickettsial diseases and, as with the others, markedly improves the prognosis if begun early. Supportive therapy is necessary for patients with cardiac failure, shock, and disseminated intravascular coagulation.

The mortality rate of RMSF is reduced from 25% to 5–7% with treatment. Delay in diagnosis beyond the first week accounts for most deaths. Death usually occurs between the ninth and twelfth days of illness and is associated with renal or heart failure, thrombocytopenia, disseminated intravascular coaglutopathy, CNS involvement and/or vascular collapse.[380] Although a

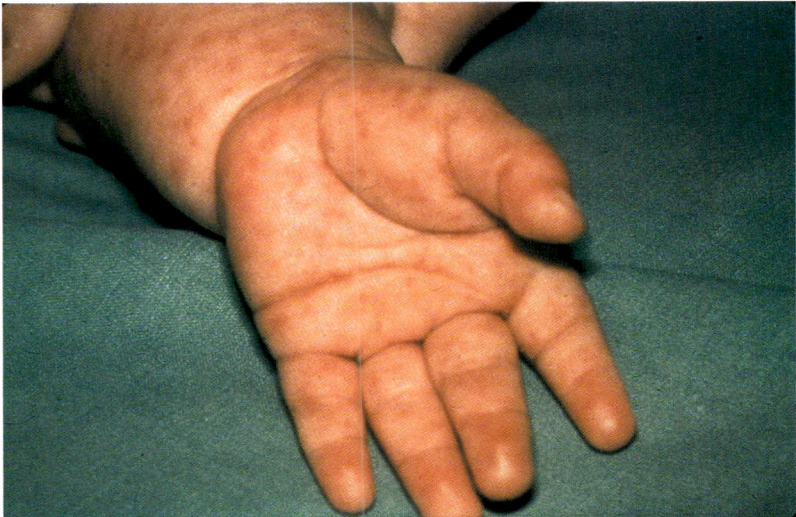

Fig. 24.19   Rocky Mountain spotted fever. RMSF, acral dusky oval purpuric lesions (courtesy Dr Russell Steele).

402. McMurray JF Jr (1966) Review of Rocky Mountain spotted fever. **J Okla State Med Assoc** 59:165.
403. Wolbach SB (1948) The pathology of rickettsial diseases of man. In: The Rickettsial Diseases of Man, Moulton, FR ed. American Association for the Advancement of Science: Washington, DC.
404. Harrell GT (1949) Rocky Mountain spotted fever. **Medicine** (Baltimore) 28:333.
405. Kelsey DS (1979) Rocky Mountain spotted fever. **Pediatr Clin North Am** 26:367.
406. Bradford WD, Hawkins HK (1978) Rocky Mountain spotted fever in children. **AM J Dis Child** 131:228.
407. Haynes RE, Sancers DY, Cramblett HG (1970) Rocky Mountain spotted fever in children. **J Pediatr** 76:685.
408. Philip RN, Casper EA, MacCormack JN et al. (1977) A comparison of serologic methods for diagnosis of Rocky Mountain spotted fever. **Am J Epidemiol** 105:56.
409. De Shazo RD, Boyce JR, Osterman JV et al. (1976) Early diagnosis of Rocky Mountain spotted fever: use of primary monocyte culture technique. **JAMA** 235:1353.
410. Walker DH, Cain BG, Olmstead PM (1978) Laboratory diagnosis of Rocky Mountain spotted fever by immunofluorescent demonstration of *Rickettsia rickettsii* in cutaneous lesions. **Am J Clin Pathol** 69:619.
411. Carl M, Tibbs CW, Dobson ME et al. (1990) Diagnosis of acute typhus infections using the polymerase chain reaction. **J Infect Dis** 161:791–793.

killed vaccine is available, it is unable to prevent the infection but may help ameliorate the severity of the infection. The most effective method of prevention is avoidance of attachment of a tick to the skin or, failing this, its prompt removal. In endemic tick-infested areas, children should be examined twice daily.[412]

MEDITERRANEAN SPOTTED FEVER

Mediterranean spotted fever (MSF) is caused by *R. conorii* and was first described by Connor in 1910.[380] It is also a tick-borne infection, seen predominantly in Spain, Italy, Israel and in Africa. Several names have been given to this illness, including Bottonneuse fever, Kenyan tick bite fever, African tick typhus, India tick typhus, and Marseille fever. The illness is most common from June to mid-October.

R. conorii is an intracellular parasite of mites and ticks, which act as both reservoirs and vectors of the illness. Intermediate hosts for the infection include dogs, rodents, and birds. Humans are accidental terminal hosts and do not transmit the disease. The illness affects all ages and both sexes, especially those with habitual contact with dogs.[413]

Clinical presentation and pathogenesis

Six to 10 days after an infecting bite, a *tache noire* or "black spot" develops at the bite site in 60 to 90% of patients. Rarely painful or pruritic, it develops a necrotic surface and obvious eschar associated with regional lymphadenopathy. Over time, it heals with pigmentation but no scarring, and is most often found on the legs of adults and the head of children. Scratches and conjunctivae may provide alternate routes of infection.

The disease has an abrupt onset with fatigue, malaise, fever, a severe headache, and myalgia. Rash appears on the third to fifth febrile day. Lesions first appear on the arms and legs and spread to the trunk, neck, face, buttocks, palms, and soles. The lesions evolve from macules to papules of 1–4mm in size. They persist for approximately 10–21 days and may become pruritic and purpuric. Rarely, patients develop nodular lesions or red patches reminiscent of the rash of murine typhus.[380]

The disease follows the invasion of endothelial cells of capillaries, arterioles, and venules. The vasculitis produced is similar to that seen in RMSF. As it disappears, the rash fades, leaving brown discoloration.[380]

The illness is generally milder than RMSF. Respiratory and cardiovascular changes typically are nonspecific and transient. Rarely, patients develop myocarditis, pericarditis, or heart failure. Phlebitis or deep vein thrombosis of the lower limbs are the main vascular complications.

Severe headaches are characteristic. Other CNS involvement may include impaired consciousness, rare seizures, delirium, stupor, or rarer still, permanent neurologic sequellae. Renal involvement is rare but occasionally serious with nephritis or renal failure. Hepatomegaly is present in one of three patients and splenomegaly in one of five. Photophobia, conjunctivitis, uveitis, retinal artery occlusion or other eye problems are rare but reported. Some cases of anemia, cryoglobulinemia and rare leukocytoclastic vasculitis have also been reported.

Diagnosis and differential diagnosis

The diagnosis of MSF can be accelerated if the *tache noire* is biopsied, as rickettsial organisms can then be detected by immunofluorescence.[414,415] The diagnosis is also supported by positive antibody responses to OX19, OX2 and OXK, which appear 7 to 10 days into the illness and peak at 21 days.[380]

MSF must be differentiated from other rickettsial diseases, meningococcemia, leukocytoclastic vasculitis, secondary syphilis, and drug reactions.[380]

Treatment and prevention

Treatment for this illness is similar to that for RMSF.[380] Treatment duration is usually 15 days but shorter therapy has been successful in some infections. In general MSF causes few fatalities and runs a benign course.[380]

The major method of control includes avoidance of tick bites and prompt removal of ticks. Infection confers long-term immunity. No vaccine is available.[416]

OTHER SPOTTED FEVERS

Other tick typhus fevers or spotted fevers are described. Siberian tick typhus is seen throughout central Asia and Queensland tick typhus is diagnosed in eastern Australia. Both are due to rickettsial species closely related to but not identical to *R. rickettsii*. The major mammalian reservoir for both infections is dogs and their ticks, which are both vectors and reservoirs. The diseases they produce are generally mild, like MSF. As with RMSF they appear to produce more complications in patients with glucose-6-phosphate dehydrogenase deficiency.[417] Treatment is also similar to the other spotted fevers.

RICKETTSIALPOX

Rickettsialpox was first described in New York City in 1946.[418,419] Since that time, incidence of the illness has decreased to only a few reported cases per year. It is caused by *R. akari*, which is transmitted from infected house mice to humans by a mouse mite. Because of the worldwide distribution of the vector mite, it is likely that the disease is widespread but underreported. All ages and both sexes are equally susceptible.[420]

Pathology

The pathology of the early maculopapular rash includes perivascular infiltration of monocytes in the dermis. The vesicles contain fibrin deposits and necrotic epithelial cells.[421]

Clinical findings

The incubation period ranges from 1 to 2 weeks. Illness is characterized by an initial cutaneous lesion, a grippe-like syndrome, and a generalized papulovesicular rash, appearing in that order, after the infected mite bite.

The initial lesion appears at the bite site after about 7 to 10 days. It is a firm, red papule about 1cm in diameter. Soon the papule is surrounded by an area of erythema, and the center vesiculates. Regional lymphadenopathy may develop as the papule becomes crusted. The crust usually falls off by the third week, leaving an eschar. Fever occurs about 1 week after the bite, accompanied by headache, rhinorrhea, cough, sore throat, chills, sweating, myalgia, anorexia, nausea, vomiting, abdominal pains, and photophobia.

The exanthem appears as a single crop of erythematous, discrete macules and papules several days after the onset of symptoms. The vesicles that develop in many of these lesions make this illness unique among the rickettsioses. They may involve the oral cavity but rarely the palms and soles. Lesions last about 1 week and leave no scar.[419,422] No deaths as a result of rickettsialpox have been reported in the United States. The illness can be confused with varicella and primary cutaneous herpes simplex, as well as various other viral exanthems.

412. Riley HD Jr (1982) Rocky Mountain spotted fever. In: Infections in Children, Wedgwood RJ, Davis SD, Ray CG, Kelley JC, eds. Philadelphia: Harper & Row, p. 1045.
413. Moraga FA, Martinez-Roig A, Alonzo JL et al. (1982) Boutonneuse fever. Arch Dis Child 57:149–151.
414. Walker DA, Occhino C, Tringali GR et al. (1988) Pathogenesis of rickettsial eschars; the tache noire of boutonneuse fever. Aum Pathol 19:1449–1454.
415. Montenegro MR, Mansueto S, Hegarty BC et al. The history of "taches noires" of boutonneuse fever and demonstration of Rickettsia conorii in them by immunofluorescence. Virchous Arch 900:309–317.
416. Mansueto S, Vitale G, Bentinegra M et al. (1985) Persistance of antibodies to Rickettsia conorri after an acute attack of boutonneuse fever. J Infect Dis 157:377.

417. Prias MA, Calia G, Saba F et al. (1983) Glucose 6-phosphate dehydrogenase deficiency in male patients with Mediterranean spotted fever in Sardinia. J Infect Dis 147:607–608.
418. Sussman LN (1946) Kew Garden's spotted fever. New York State J Med 2:27.
419. Shankman B (1946) Report of an outbreak of endemic febrile illness, not yet identified, occurring in New York City. New York State J Med 46:2156.
420. Brettman LR, Lewin S, Holzman S et al. (1981) Rickettsialpox: report of an outbreak and a contemporary review. Medicine (Baltimore) 60:363.
421. Dolgopol VB (1948) Histologic changes in rickettsialpox. Am J Pathol 24:119.
422. Patterson PY, Taylor W (1966) Rickettsialpox. Bull New York Acad Med 42:579.

The diagnosis can be confirmed by isolation of the organism from blood and its subsequent growth in white mice or embryonated eggs.[380] Skin biopsies of lesions reveal necrosis of capillaries with mononuclear cells and an angiitis. Organisms are not evident. Complement-fixing antibodies can be detected in convalescent serum, although there may be some cross-reactivity with RMSF antigens.[380]

Prevention and treatment

Treatment with tetracycline or chloramphenicol is effective, although not required, especially in young infants, because of its usually benign, self-limiting course. Deaths have not been reported. Prevention is most effective when activities are directed toward the control of mice and mites.[423]

Q FEVER GROUP

Q fever is an acute rickettsial infection characterized by fever, headache and pneumonia in 50% of patients. It does not produce a rash or vasculitis, and thus is not further reviewed.

EHRLICHIOSIS

Human ehrlichiosis has been recently recognized in the United States. Sennetsu fever, a disease with distinct, mononucleosis-like symptoms that is caused by a different *Ehrlichia* species, has been well known in Japan for some time. The first report of human ehrlichiosis in the US was published in 1987, and the infection was thought to be caused by an *Ehrlichia* species closely related to *E. canis*. In 1991 this pathogen was named *Ehrlichia chaffeenis*.[424]

Cases are clustered along the eastern seaboard, and throughout the southern USA. A history of tick bite or presence in a tick-infested area is present in almost 75% of cases. This disease occurs most often between March and October. Although most cases occur in middle-aged adults, increasing numbers are being reported in children.

This disease has a broad spectrum of clinical manifestations, with severity ranging from mild disease to life threatening illness. Fever, myalgia and headache are the most common features. Gastrointestinal symptoms including nausea, anorexia, vomiting and diarrhea are often present. A rash occurs in 35% and can vary from erythematous macules to petechial lesions resembling RMSF. Abdominal pain and tenderness, arthralgia, conjunctival injection, meningitis and pharyngitis are less commonly seen. As with RMSF, 85% of patients exhibit thrombocytopenia and, with severe disease, hyponatremia. Most have leukopenia, lymphopenia, elevated liver enzymes, elevated BUN and creatinine, hematuria, proteinuria, and 14% of patients are anemic.

Diagnosis

Because the Weil–Felix reaction is not positive, specific serologic testing must be requested. A fourfold or greater rise in antibody titer to *E. chaffeenis* (minimum titer 1:64) by indirect immunofluorescent antibody assay is diagnostic.

Treatment

Antibiotics of choice are doxycycline and chloramphenizol, as for the rickettsia (Table 24.5).

INFECTIONS CAUSED BY GRAM-POSITIVE BACTERIA

Gayle Fischer

NOCARDIOSIS

Nocardiosis refers to acute and chronic infection caused by three species of *Nocardia*, which are partially acid fast true bacteria and aerobic actinomycetes. The organism forms delicate branching Gram-positive filaments that may be seen in the exudate of various lesions. The two species most often implicated are *N. asteroides* and *N. brasiliensis*. They are natural soil saprophytes and may be found in decaying organic matter. They may infect humans, cattle and other mammals such as cats and dogs.

CLINICAL FINDINGS

Nocardial involvement of the skin is uncommon in both children and adults, but is important to recognize because of its potential for serious consequences. The most common and most ominous cutaneous presentation is lesions arising following dissemination from a primary pulmonary origin. The second most prevalent pattern is an actinomycoma or chronic cutaneous nocardiosis. A final cutaneous form is acute primary cutaneous nocardiosis.[424–426]

Acute primary cutaneous nocardiosis usually follows acute inoculation into the skin as a result of superficial injury with soil contamination, such as a cat scratch or thorn scratch, or as a result of an insect bite.[427,428] The lesions may present as pyoderma, cellulitis, subcutaneous abscess, or lymphocutaneous syndrome[429] (Fig. 24.20), in which a cutaneous lesion or nodule is associated with regional lymphadenopathy or suppurative lymphadenitis, or may mimic sporotrichosis. Systemic dissemination is unusual, but significant scarring may follow healing.[430]

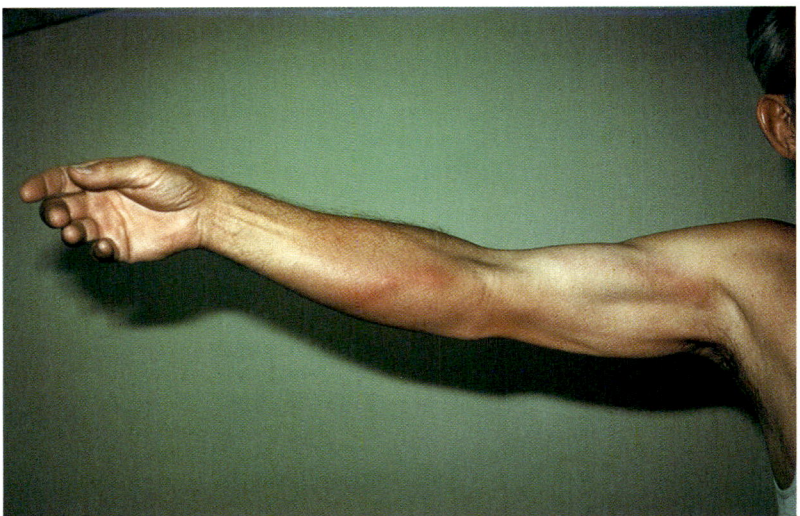

Fig. 24.20   Sporotrichoid *Nocardia* infection. Digital inoculation followed by multinodular sporotrichoid arm pattern.

423. Riley HD Jr (1982) Rickettsialpox. In: Infections in Children, Wedgwood RJ, David SD, Ray CG, Kelley JC, eds. Philadelphia: Harper & Row, p. 1077.
424. Schiff TA, Goldman R, Sanchez M et al. (1993) Primary lymphocutaneous nocardiosis caused by an unusual species of nocardia: *N. transvelensisi*. **J Am Acad Dermatol** 28:336.
425. Beckmeyer WJ (1959) Nocardiosis: report of a sucessfully treated case of cutaneous granuloma. **Pediatrics** 23:331.
426. Idriss ZH, Cunningham RJ, Wilfert CM (1975) Nocardiosis in children: report of three cases and review of the literature. **Pediatrics** 55:135.
427. O'Connor PT, Dire DJ (1992) Cutaneous nocardios is associated with insect bites. **Cutis** 50:301.
428. Angelika J, Hans-Jurgen G, Uwe-Frithjof FH (1999) Primary cutaneous nocardiosis in a husband and wife. **J Am Acad Dermatol** 41:338.
429. Lampe RM, Baker DJ, Septimus EJ, Wallace RJ (1981) Cervicofacial nocardiosis in children. **J Pediatr** 99:593.
430. Kannon GA, Kuechle MK, Garrett AB (1996) Superficial cutaneous *N. asteroides* infection in an immunocompetent pregnant woman. **J Am Acad Dermatol** 35:1000.

LABORATORY DIAGNOSIS

The diagnosis of nocardial infection is critical because of its potential for distant spread and lethal CNS involvement, which may occur in up to one-third of all cases. Diagnosis is usually based on cultures of biopsied tissue. Media without inhibitory antibiotics should be used, and incubation times of up to 4 weeks may be required. *Nocardia* species grow well at temperatures greater than 37°C; thus culturing at 40–50°C may successfully reduce the number of competitors while avoiding the use of inhibitory antibiotics in the media. Gram stain may reveal filamentous, slightly beaded, partially acid-fast Gram-positive organisms. Serological testing[431] and PCR have resulted in the identification of new species.[432] Leukocytosis with a shift to the left is common. Skin testing for *Nocardia* has been attempted but has not been successful due to cross-reaction between antigens of nocardia and tuberculosis.

DIFFERENTIAL DIAGNOSIS

Primary cutaneous nocardiosis can be clinically indistinguishable from the cutaneous mycetomas caused by actinomycetes or streptomycetes and mycetomas caused by true fungi. The lymphocutaneous form can resemble several other organisms, including *Staph. aureus*, *Strep. pyogenes*, atypical mycobacteria, *Yersinia pestis*, cat-scratch disease, cervicofacial actinomycosis, sporotrichosis, tularemia, cutaneous diphtheria, brucellosis, and syphilis.

MANAGEMENT

The current recommended therapy is trimethoprim-sulfamethoxazole 120–150mg/kg/day, or in sulfonamide-sensitive patients, amikacin 15–20mg/kg/day plus cefotaxime.[433] Treatment should be based on antibiotic sensitivity testing when available,[434] but *in vitro* results do not always correlate with clinical response. Therapy duration ranges from six weeks to six months for relatively minor infections to more than 1 year for severe cases. Patients should be observed for any sign of relapse and further cultures carried out if this occurs. Therapy may need to be carried on indefinitely for patients with concurrent HIV infection. Incision and drainage of abscesses or surgical debridement, where necessary, is helpful, as are supportive measures, including good nutrition and the treatment of concomitant infections.

ACTINOMYCOSIS

Actinomycosis is a chronic, suppurative and granulomatous disease of the skin, lungs, and gastrointestinal tract. It produces abscesses, which discharge characteristic sulfur granules through multiple draining sinuses found in the lesions; these are composed of small, tangled masses of Gram-positive branching filamentous anaerobic to microaerophilic organisms of the genus *Actinomyces*. Although "ray fungus" is the Greek origin of its name, this genus of pathogens is more closely related to bacteria than higher fungi. This claim is supported by the observations that actinomycetes lack a nuclear membrane, have chitin and muramic acid in their cell walls, reproduce by bacterial fission rather than by spore or formation filamentous budding, and are inhibited by antibacterial, not antifungal, antibiotics.

Actinomyces israelii is the most common species implicated in human disease. Other species include *A. naeslundii*, *A. viscosus*, *A. odontolyticus*, and *A. propionica*. All of these organisms are normal flora of the mouth and large intestine, and are found in dental plaque and cause periapical disease and gingivitis. Clinical disease is thought to follow trauma, aspiration into the lungs, or ingestion of the organisms.

Found worldwide, the disease is more common in males than in females (1.5–3:1), probably reflecting the increased incidence of maxillofacial trauma in males. More frequently seen in lower socio-economic groups, actinomycosis affects all races equally. Congenital actinomycosis has been reported. The age group most affected, however, is adults between the age of 30 and 60 years. Children account for only 3% of cases.[435–438] The increased incidence in middle-aged adults and lesser incidence in children and elderly patients is thought to parallel the presence of carious teeth. The shedding of teeth, seen in the very young and very old, appears to make them less vulnerable to this infection.

CLINICAL FINDINGS

Actinomycosis usually occurs as one of three distinct clinical patterns. The most common presentation is cervicofacial, which account for 41–55% of cases. The next most common presentations are pulmonothoracic (15–34%) and abdominopelvic (13–20%).[439] Other sites of involvement have also been reported and a rare disseminated form accounts for 5–6% of reported cases. Actinomycotic osteomyelitis has been reported in immunosuppressed children on chemotherapy.[440] The cervicofacial form of actinomycosis is usually associated with minor oral trauma and carious teeth. The disease may be painful initially but more often presents as a painless "wooden" brawny mass or pseudotumor. The overlying skin progressively becomes dark red to purple in color, and the surface becomes uneven. These woody nodules soften and develop sinus tracts that may drain the abscessed material. Trismus is a frequent symptom. Spread is by direct extension and does not follow lymphatic or hematogenous routes. Thus, lymph nodes may be involved late, if at all. Left untreated, the sinuses may drain and close intermittently. Extension to involve periosteum and bone with resultant bone destruction may occur. Cranial, vertebral, orbital, and otic invasion have occurred, as have deaths as a result of extension into, and involvement of, the CNS. On occasion, cervical disease spreading first to the base of the neck has extended directly to involve the pleura and upper chest. Focal infections have involved the mandible, cheek, paranasal sinuses, scalp, parotid and lacrimal glands, tongue, larynx, thyroid, and maxilla.

Aspiration of saliva that contains the actinomycete is believed to be responsible for the pulmonothoracic expression of actinomycosis. This is found to involve the basilar parenchym[441] in most cases in contrast to tuberculosis, which more often involves the apices of the lung. Low-grade fever, malaise, and cough are noted, in addition to signs of pneumonitis. Later, a more serious necrotizing pneumonitis develops, in which abscesses form, rupture, and fibrose, sometimes with empyema. Extension to the chest wall and fistula formation may follow. Pleural and pericardial involvement may also occur, as can rare extension of the disease into the abdomen. Although most pulmonary cases do not drain to the skin, extension to thoracic skin has been described in a child.[441] The characteristic radiographic triad of chronic lower lobe pulmonary consolidation, empyema, and wavy periostitis of the ribs may also support this diagnosis. Abdominal involvement is believed to represent actinomycotic superinfection of another gastrointestinal process. Signs of the latter usually include swelling and tenderness in and around the appendix or ileocecal valve and later development of an indistinct irregular mass. Sinuses

431. Hornef MW, Gandorfer A, Heeseman J, Roggenkamp A (2000) Humoral response in a patient with cutaneous nocardiosis. **Dermatology** 200:78.

432. Conville PS, Fischer SH, Cartwright CP, Witesby FG (2000) Identification of nocardia species by restriction endonuclease analysis of an amplified portion of the 16S rRNA gene. **J Clin Microbiol** 38:158.

433. Threlkeld SC, Hooper DC (1997) Update on the management of patients with Nocardia infection. **Curr Clin Top Infect Dis** 17:1.

434. Sakai C, Takagi T, Satoh Y (1999) *N. asteroides* pneumonia, subcutaneous abscess and meningitis in a patient with advanced lymphoma: successful treatment based on in vitro antimicrobial susceptibility. **Int Med** 38:683.

435. Benammar S, Helardot PG, Sapin E et al. (1995) Childhood actinomycosis: report of two cases. **Eur J Pediatr Surg** 5:180.

436. Drake DP, Holt PJ (1976) Childhood actinomycosis: report of 3 recent cases. **Arch Dis Child** 51:979.

437. Friduss ME, Maceri NR (1990) Cervicofacial actinomycosis in children. **Henry Ford Hosp Med J** 38:28.

438. Stewart MG, Sulek M (1993) Pediatric actinomycosis of the head and neck. **Ear Nose Throat J** 72:614.

439. Weese WC, Smith IM (1975) A study of 57 cases of actinomycosis over a 36 year period. **Arch Intern Med** 135:1562.

440. Houi L, Saarinen UM, Donner V, Lindqvist (1996) Opportunistic osteomyelitis in the jaws in children on immunosuppressive chemotherapy. **J Pediatr Hematol/Oncol** 18:90.

441. Stanley TV (1980) Deep actinomycosis in childhood. **Acta Pediatr Scand** 69:173.

may ultimately extend to involve the abdominal wall, liver, or kidney. A new form of the disease associated with the use of intrauterine devices was recently described involving the cervix and uterus.

LABORATORY DIAGNOSIS

The definitive diagnosis of actinomycosis depends on bacterial cultures in anaerobic brain-heart or blood agar in 5% CO_2 for 4–6 days at 37°C. More than 50% of biopsy-proven cases have negative cultures, attributed in part to overgrowth by other bacteria, suppression of growth by previous antibiotic treatment, and difficulty in anaerobic culturing. Diagnosis is often based on the presence of sulfur granules in the exudate obtained from sinus tracts or on histologic preparations of excised tissues, although similar granules have rarely been seen in nocardiosis and staphylococcal botryomycosis.

DIFFERENTIAL DIAGNOSIS

Differential diagnosis of the cervicofacial lesions includes malignant or benign neoplasm, abscess, or other fungal or bacterial granulomatous processes. Pulmonary and abdominal lesions are equally difficult, especially because they rarely penetrate to the chest or abdominal walls and frequently require surgical exploration and excision for diagnosis. Abdominal actinomycosis may simulate carcinoma of the colon and be associated with weight loss, malaise, fever, cramping, pain, nausea, and vomiting.

THERAPY

The treatment of choice is high-dose parenteral penicillin G 100 000 to 250 000 units/kg/day for 2–4 weeks, then penicillin V 25 to 50mg/kg/day for 3–6 months. Penicillinase-resistant penicillins are less effective than penicillin. Rifampin and isoniazid have been effective. Persistent or resistant cases should prompt a search for abscesses requiring surgical drainage.[442] If repeated cultures show mixed infections with bacteria, broader-spectrum antibiotics in combination with penicillin may be required.

ANTHRAX

Anthrax probably was first described as the "fifth plague" in the Book of Genesis in the Bible as the probable cause of death of Egyptian cattle. The disease entered the United States through Louisiana and was first recognized in animals in the early 1700s. Due to development of an effective vaccine in animals and more recently in humans,[443] the disease almost disappeared from the United States, Central Europe, and Australia before September 2001, but it persisted in semiarid Third World countries. Anthrax is a disease of herbivores; humans become infected primarily by contact with infected animals or infected animal products. Men are most frequently infected because of their increased occupational or recreational exposure. Anthrax is exceedingly rare in children, but persists in developing nations. The cases of both cutaneous and pulmonary anthrax in the United States at the end of 2001 (Fig. 24.21) were thought to be related to bioterrorism or a hoax to simulate bioterrorism.

Bacillus anthracis is a large Gram-positive rod with flattened ends that usually appears as short chains in clinical specimens. Spores are found in culture and environmental specimens. The organism grows well on blood agar without hemolysis. Most bacillus species are not pathogenic. Routine clinical laboratories often are not able to identify *B. anthracis* and may either discard it as a contaminant or report it as *Bacillus* species.

CLINICAL FINDINGS

The cutaneous form of anthrax is the major manifestation of disease in humans. The incubation period is usually 2 to 5 days but may be up to 8 days.[444] The initial lesion is a small painless papule that rapidly develops into a vesicle which contains serous or serosanguinous fluid. As the lesion enlarges, the center becomes hemorrhagic and necrotic, and the characteristic black eschar develops. The eschar is frequently surrounded by vesicles. The typical malignant pustule in children is frequently associated with fever and extensive edema. Evolution of the lesion to a dark brown eschar and later separation of the eschar generally takes 2 weeks. The nontender lesions are most frequently located on exposed areas of the head, neck, or upper extremities. Cutaneous anthrax of the eyelids results in cicatricial ectropion and corneal scarring,[445,446] despite response to antibiotic therapy. This childhood presentation raises the possibility of transmission by an insect vector.

Cutaneous anthrax can occasionally disseminate and, in its septic form, is associated with high fever, tachycardia, hypotension and significant mortality.[447] Pulmonary anthrax is seen among wool sorters and other people exposed to aerosolized organisms. Pulmonary manifestations include tachypnea, stridor, and progressive cyanosis. Meningitis can complicate septicemic and pulmonary anthrax.

Histologic examination of skin sections from lesions of cutaneous anthrax demonstrates perivascular and perilymphatic collections of the bacillus. Vessels are dilated with stasis and macro- and microthrombi, leading to tissue necrosis. The tissue planes are disrupted by interstitial edema and hemorrhage, and inflammation tends to be minimal and patchy. The organism spreads through the lymphatics to regional lymph nodes. The lymph nodes show proliferative changes followed by hemorrhage that is initially restricted to the subcapsular areas but can obliterate the lymph node.

LABORATORY DIAGNOSIS

Diagnosis of anthrax is usually suspected on the basis of a history of exposure and the characteristic skin lesion. Although rare, clinicians in developed countries must maintain a high index of suspicion, especially with the specter

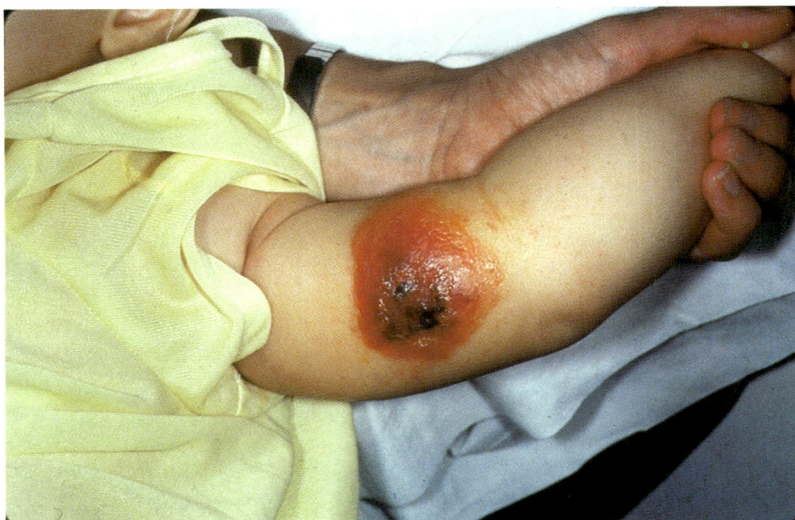

Fig. 24.21   Anthrax. Cutaneous anthrax in a child (courtesy Dr Mary W. Chang; case reported in N Engl J Med 345:1611, 2001).

442. Alad J, Hollak M, Sharm A et al. (1999) Pelvic actinomycosis: is longterm antibiotic therapy necessary? **J Reprod Med** 44:939.

443. Jefferson T, Demicheli V, Deeks J et al. (2000) Vaccines for preventing anthrax. Cochrane Database of Systemic Reviews 2 CD000975.

444. Singh RS, Sridhar MS, Sekhar PC et al. (1992) Cutaneous anthrax: a report of ten cases. **J Assoc Physicians India** 40:46.

445. Daboue A, Traore W, Nacro B, Sawadago A (2000) Suspected palpebral anthrax in children. **Bull Soc Pathol Exot** 93:20.

446. Manios S, Kavaliotis I (1979) Anthrax in children: a long forgotten potentially fatal infection. **Scand J Infect Dis** 11:203.

447. Doganay M, Baker M, Dokmetals I (1987) A case of cutaneous anthrax with toxaemic shock. **Br J Dermatol** 117:659.

of bioterrorism. Gram stains of vesicular fluid or scrapings from beneath the eschar demonstrate the characteristic Gram-positive rods. Cultures of the lesions grow a bacillus, which, if nonmotile and nonhemolytic, is usually sent off by most clinical laboratories to a reference laboratory for definitive identification. Serologic diagnosis can be performed with a sensitive and specific hemagglutination test. ELISA tests and immunoblotting techniques have been developed that test for titers to anthrax edema toxin, lethal toxin, and protective antigen. These may be helpful in establishing a retrospective diagnosis and for epidemiologic purposes.

THERAPY

High-dose penicillin given iv or oral doxycycline are the agents of choice. Intravenous penicillin is usually continued for 4 or 5 days until the patient shows steady improvement, at which time oral penicillin V 50mg/kg/day can be given to complete therapy. High-dose penicillin plus streptomycin or parenteral ciprofloxacin are recommended for treating inhalational anthrax or meningitis. Although ciprofloxacin and doxycycline are not recommended for patients under 18 and 8 years, respectively, they may be considered if the possible benefits are deemed to outweigh the potential risks. Erythromycin, clindamycin, aminoglycosides, chloramphenicol, or possibly first-generation cephalosporins are effective alternatives for the penicillin-sensitive patient.

Prevention of this disease in humans is dependent primarily on the control of anthrax in animals. Vaccines are used to prevent disease in animals and active surveillance prevents importation or spread of the disease. All animals that die of anthrax should be buried or cremated. Anthrax vaccination in a six-dose series is available for humans with frequent exposure to anthrax. No data are available on the safety or efficacy of the vaccine in children. In the event of biological terrorism, recommendations such as those from the American Academy of Pediatrics for diagnostic work-up, prophylaxis, and treatment should be considered.[448]

LISTERIOSIS

Listeria monocytogenes is a small mobile Gram-positive microaerophilic coccobacillus responsible for rare but severe perinatal infections and sporadic illness in adults and children, especially those with HIV infection or who are otherwise immunosuppressed.[449] Worldwide in distribution, it has been isolated from numerous sources, including soil, vegetation, insects, fish, and domestic and wild animals and from milk, cheese, and cabbage.[450,451] It is resistant to freezing, desiccation, and salt. Most human cases occur in the late summer and autumn.

CLINICAL FINDINGS

The spectrum of diseases produced by *Listeria* is broad. It tends to attack the vulnerable, with elderly people, pregnant women, children, and neonates most susceptible. The precise mode of transmission from animal reservoirs to humans is not clear, but epidemic listeriosis caused by oral ingestion of contaminated foods has been increasingly reported in the last decade.[450,451] Transplacental transmission from mother to fetus is well established.[452] Ascending vaginal infection, possibly from fecal contamination, may also lead to fetal infection.

In pregnancy, listeriosis is described as a febrile flu-like illness.[453] Major clinical symptoms include malaise, coryza, and abdominal pain. This may pass unmentioned by the mother or otherwise go unrecognized, with resultant

transplacental transmission to the fetus. A major cause of chorioamnionitis and placental abscesses, listeriosis is associated with a high incidence of fetal sepsis, premature delivery, and perinatal death. Proof of the maternal diagnosis is supported by cultures that have been reported as positive from various sources, including amniotic fluid (from amniocentesis) and cervical, vaginal, and blood cultures. Aggressive antibiotic therapy of affected pregnant women with listeriosis has significantly improved perinatal mortality and morbidity rates.[454,455]

Neonatal listeriosis may be early or delayed. The early form is a septicemic form that produces disseminated miliary granulomatous lesions. This often-fatal form, which has been called granulomatosis infantiseptica, is thought to be acquired transplacentally. Infants may be stillborn or severely ill at birth. Examination of the placenta often reveals multiple small abscesses on the fetal side. Despite aggressive diagnosis and treatment the mortality rate in this early form is approximately 30%.

The late form presents approximately 1 week after delivery with meningitis, meningoencephalitis, or sepsis, and probably is transmitted during delivery from the maternal genital tract.[449] In both the early and late forms, infected infants appear irritable and febrile with poor feeding, vomiting, and diarrhea, often with either a bulging or full fontanelle, respiratory distress, or both. In a small percentage of these infants, a characteristic skin eruption of small grayish-white papules or papulopustules is seen. These pustules, which resemble miliary abscesses, may contain the organism and are concentrated on the back and lumbar area, although they may be widespread, involving the conjunctivae, mouth, and pharynx. The mortality rate of late-onset sepsis is now less than 10%. Most infants who survive *L. monocytogenes*-induced sepsis appear to be normal except for complications associated with prematurity, which may include hydrocephalus, cerebral palsy, and mental retardation. Other skin lesions of neonatal listeriosis, including petchiae and purpura ("blueberry muffin" babies), morbilliform and roseola-like rashes, and localized and generalized erythema.[449]

Cultures from the neonate to support the diagnosis have been obtained from skin, cerebrospinal or amniotic fluid, gastric aspirates, meconium, and blood. *Listeria* grows well on many standard culture media and is sensitive to many antibiotics given intravenously. Therapy with ampicillin and gentamicin or penicillin and kanamycin has reduced the incidence of mortality and sequelae. Listeria is resistant to all cephalosporins, including third-generation agents. Adults who are penicillin-sensitive and children with *Listeria*-induced meningitis have been successfully treated with oral trimethoprim-sulfamethoxazole.[456]

CUTANEOUS DIPHTHERIA

Although rare today in the United States, diphtheria still occurs among people in the United States living in poor and unsanitary conditions.[457] Significant illness may be seen among those who have been inadequately immunized.

ETIOLOGY

Diphtheria is caused by *Corynebacterium diphtheriae*. These organims are Gram-positive rods 2-to 4μm in length that are broader at one end than the other, with a resultant club shape. On Gram stain they may have a beaded or banded appearance, producing the characteristic "Chinese letters" on smear. The bacterium is best grown on selective tellurite media, which allows differentiation of the three types of *C. diphtheriae*: *C. mitis*, *C. intermedius*, and *C. gravis*.

448. American Academy of Pediatrics (2000) Recommendations for care of children in special circumstances: chemical–biological terrorism. In: 2000 Red Book: Report of the Committee on Infectious Diseases, 25th edn, Pickering CK, ed. Elk Grove Village, IL: American Academy of Pediatrics, pp. 83–87.
449. Ahlfors CE, Goetzman BW, Halsted CC et al. (1977) Neonatal listeriosis. Am J Dis Child 131:405.
450. Dalton CB, Austin CC, Sobel J et al. (1997) Swaminatham An outbreak of gastroenteritis and fever due to *L. monocytogenes* in milk. N Engl J Med 336:100.
451. Aureli P, Fiorucci GC, Caroli D et al. (2000) An outbreak of febrile gastroenteritis associated with corn contaminated by *L. monocytogenes*. N Engl J Med 342:1236.

452. Smith KJ, Skelton HG 3d, Angritt P et al. (1991) Cutaneous lesions of listeriosis in a newborn. J Cutan Pathol 18:474.
453. Anderson G (1975) *Listeria monocytogenes* septicemia in pregnancy. Obstet Gynecol 46:102.
454. Lennon D, Lewis B, Mantell C et al. (1984) Epidemic perinatal listeriosis. Pediatr Infect Dis J 3:30.
455. Katz OL, Weinstein L (1982) Antepartum treatment of *Listeria monocytogenes* septicemia. South Med J 75:1353.
456. Scheer MS, Hirschman SZ (1982) Oral and ambulatory therapy of *Listeria* bacteremia and meningitis with trimethoprim-sulfamethoxazole. Mt Sinai J Med 49:311.
457. Harnish JP, Tronea, Nolan CM et al. (1982) Diphtheria among alcoholic urban adults: a decade of experience in Seattle. Ann Intern Med 111:71.

The exotoxin produced by toxigenic strains of *C. diphtheriae* is responsible for the serious clinical manifestations of the disease. The ability to produce toxin is conferred by the presence of a bacteriophage. Once synthesized by the virally infected bacteria, the toxin is released as an inactive polypeptide chain that becomes activated when cleaved into two fragments. Fragment B, although unstable, binds to cells and permits penetration of fragment A. Once in the cell, fragment A, which is enzymatically active and stable, produces toxic effects by inhibiting cellular protein synthesis. Although all human eukaryotic cells have receptor sites for fragment B, damage is most severe in the nervous tissue and heart muscle. As a result, the most serious clinical manifestations are severe myocardiopathy or neuropathy, including palatal paralysis, ocular and diaphragmatic or limb paralysis.

Although very rare, cutaneous diphtheria may be seen alone or in association with diphtheria of the nasopharynx or pharynx.[458] It is most prevalent in warm climates, both in desert and in tropical environments. It was thus labeled both tropical ulcer and desert ulcer during World War II, when it caused significant morbidity and deaths among American and European soldiers stationed in the Middle East, Mediterranean area, and South Pacific. Factors favoring its development include hot climates with high humidity, lower socio-economic status, poor hygiene, and frequent skin abrasions or insect bites. Spread of diphtheria from the respiratory tract to the skin and vice versa has been documented. Skin infections can be caused by both toxigenic and nontoxigenic *C. diphtheriae*.

CLINICAL FINDINGS

The earliest lesion of cutaneous diphtheria is a pustule that evolves into a fairly distinctive, sharply demarcated ulcer with a grayish-blue membrane as its base (Fig. 24.22). Its edge is frequently raised, indurated, and distinct. Healed ulcers leave depressed or smooth atrophic scars. *C. diphtheriae* has been reported to infect secondarily lesions of atopic dermatitis. Before the use of antibiotics, lesions healed in 30 to 40 days with slower healing noted with toxogenic strains of bacteria. In lesions caused by nontoxogenic diphtheria and those found in patients who have been adequately immunized by diphtheria toxoid, these sores are milder. They do require treatment with antibiotics to avoid the carrier state, however. The differential diagnosis of cutaneous diphtheria includes other causes of severe pyodermas, ecthyma, pyoderma gangrenosum, granulomatous infections, and ulcerations. Cases of purely cutaneous diphtheria may be associated with both cardiac and neurologic sequelae produced by the absorption of the diphtheria toxin, especially if the patient has not been immunized by diphtheria toxoid.

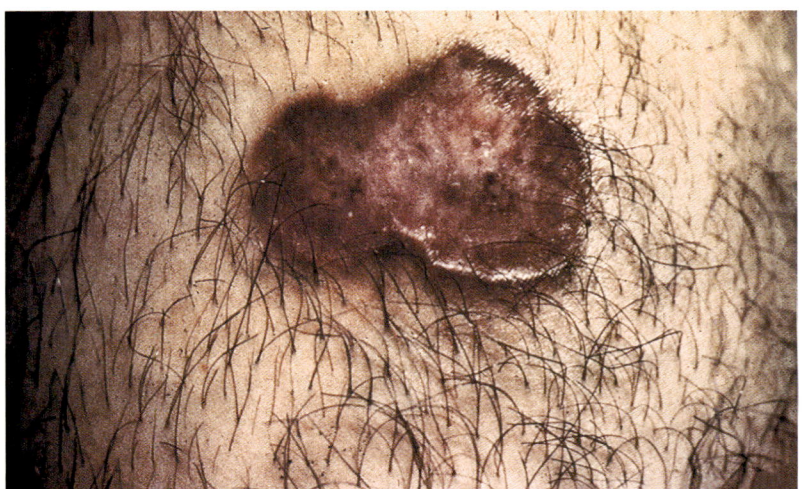

Fig. 24.22   Cutaneous diphtheria. Classic grayish blue membranous charge overlying an ulcer.

Neurologic sequelae, which occur in up to one-third of affected patients, vary from early parasthesias to significant weakness of the extremities and diminished or lost positional sense and deep tendon reflexes. Unlike pharyngeal diphtheria, cranial nerves are not usually involved. The illness can mimic Guillain–Barré syndrome and progress to quadriplegia. Cardiac sequelae, including heart block and diphtheric myocarditis, are not as common, but are serious complications frequently causing death in an otherwise recovering patient.

MANAGEMENT

Immunization with diphtheria toxoid to prevent vulnerability to the toxin is the mainstay of diphtheria prevention and has resulted in a drop of reported cases from 5800 in 1950 to less than 100 cases annually in the United States. The mainstay of diphtheria therapy remains prompt and adequate doses of antitoxin. The antitoxin neutralizes circulating exotoxin and exotoxin loosely bound to tissues. Unfortunately, exotoxin firmly bound to tissue is not affected. Institution of therapy with this horse serum antitoxin requires baseline testing for hypersensitivity to horse serum and careful monitoring during therapy. The dose varies with the site and duration of the diphtheritic ulcer from 20 000 to 60 000 units/kg/day im or iv. Treatment also includes antibiotics, preferably parenteral penicillin G 100 000 to 250 000 units/kg/day iv or erythromycin 50 mg/kg/day po in penicillin-sensitive patients. Rapid institution of antibiotics may reduce exotoxin production and its consequences. Oxygen and bedrest to minimize strain on the heart, and other supportive measures, such as adequate hydration and diet, are necessary. Depending on the extent of neurologic deficit, other supportive measures include assisted ventilation for diaphragmatic paralysis and nasogastric tube feeding to reduce aspiration from palatal paralysis.

The prognosis for acute diphtheria is guarded because of the possible respiratory compromise or heart failure. Complete neurologic and cardiac recovery is common in survivors, on rare occasions, although permanent myocardial damage may persist.

ERYSIPELOID OF ROSENBACH

Erysipeloid is an uncommon infection of the skin caused by *Erysipelothrix insidiosa*. This Gram-positive, filamentous, nonmotile, pleomorphic bacillus parasitizes numerous animals and is found in soil. Lesions are most commonly seen on exposed surfaces, especially on the hands and arms of persons who handle animals, birds, and fish (e.g., veterinarians, fishermen, crabbers, and meat handlers). Clinically, the disease may be confused with erysipelas, as its name implies. Infection is rare in children.[459]

CLINICAL FINDINGS

Human infections due to *Erysipelothrix* usually fall into one of three categories: localized skin infections, diffuse skin infections, and generalized infections with or without cutaneous features. Localized skin infections are by far the most common. More common in the warm summer months and in males, infection by direct inoculation usually follows minor trauma while handling infected animals or animals products. Erysipeloid has also occurred postoperatively without known exposure to animals.

One to 7 days after inoculation, clinical evidence of the disease occurs with onset of lilac pink or purplish-red, sharply demarcated, diamond-shaped patches (Fig. 24.23). Lesions are most prevalent on the hand but may occur on any exposed surface. In contrast to erysipelas, patches may spread peripherally and tend to clear centrally, and symptoms are usually not severe but may include burning, pain, or itching. Lymphangitis and constitutional symptoms are rare (<10%) but do occur. Before the availability of antibiotics, lesions would subside spontaneously after weeks but might recur or develop elsewhere, weeks to months later. In the diffuse cutaneous form, lesions appear

458. Belsey MA (1975) Skin infections and the epidemiology of diphtheria: acquisition and persistence of *C. diphtheriae* infections. Am J Epidemiol 102:179.

459. LaCroix J, DeLarge G, Mitchelle G et al. (1981) Erysipeloid of an infant. **J Pediatr** 99:745.

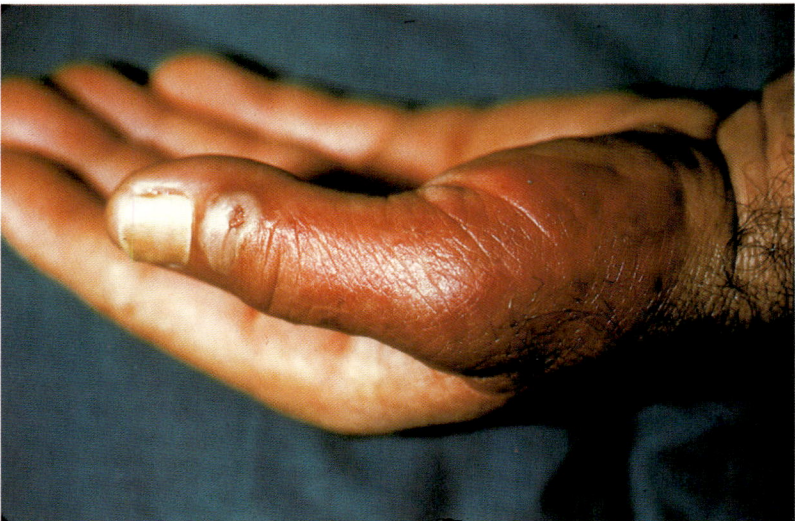

Fig. 24.23   Erysipeloid: dusky red hand lesion.

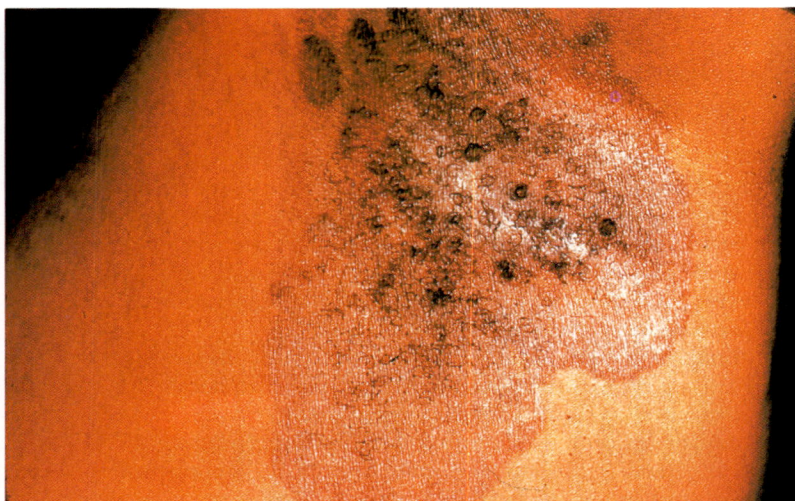

Fig. 24.24   **Erythrasma.** Sharply marginated axillary patch (courtesy W.K. Galen).

on several areas of the body in addition to the site of inoculation. Patients have more symptoms than in the localized form, including fever and malaise, but these cases, too, may be self-limited after a longer course, some lasting up to 9 months. The systemic form, which may or may not have associated skin lesions, may include septic arthritis, bacterial endocarditis, cerebral infarction, osseous necrosis, and pulmonary effusion. These patients are very ill, and constitutional symptoms are prominent. Cutaneous lesions, if present, may be necrotic with raised edges or scattered, red, raised perifollicular papules. Blood cultures are often positive in this form.

LABORATORY FINDINGS

Laboratory support of the diagnosis is limited, as culture is difficult. Material is inoculated in a brain-heart infusion broth with 1% glucose, at 35–37°C with 5–10% to CO_2. After 48h, a search is made for the tiny colonies of Gram-positive bacilli.[460] Histopathologic analysis may be helpful if it demonstrates the bacteria, but is not pathognomonic. Biopsy findings described by Barnett *et al.*[460] include spongiosis and intraepidermal vesiculation and rare bullae that contain sera, fibrin, erythrocytes, and neutrophils. Papillary dermal edema with engorged capillaries and lymphangitis are also seen. Gram stains of tissue are not helpful.

THERAPY

Both parenteral penicillin G 100 000 to 250 000units/kg/day in divided doses every 6h and oral penicillin V 25–50mg/kg/day for 4–10 days have been useful, as has erythromycin 40mg/kg/day, and doxycyline 100mg twice daily for 14 days. Clindamycin and some cephalosporms have been used successful. Some cases require therapy for 6 weeks or longer.[461]

ERYTHRASMA

Erythrasma is a superficial infection of the intertriginous skin by *Corynebacterium minutissimum*. This condition is characterized by dry, tan to

brown, slightly scaling patches with sharp margins (Fig. 24.24). The condition usually occurs in the axillae, inframammary areas, groin, or gluteal crease and may be found beneath an obese abdominal apron. A less common presentation is circular, scaling patches in a generalized distribution that may be confused with pityriasis rotunda, parapsoriasis en plaque, psoriasis, or tinea versicolor. This latter uncommon form, also known as tropical erythrasma, is seen predominantly in black women living in hot humid climates.

The lesions are usually asymptomatic, although some irritation may be noted in the groin, particularly in extensive cases seen in obese patients with diabetes mellitus or other chronic or debilitating illnesses. This condition affects both sexes equally and has been reported in all age groups, although its incidence increases with age. It is more common during or after hot months and in warm humid climates. It is rare in childhood.[462] *C. minutissimum* rarely causes recurrent breast abscesses,[463] subacute bacterial endocarditis,[464] and fatal sepsis.[465]

DIAGNOSIS

The diagnosis is usually made by examining the suspected patches with a Wood's light for dramatic coral red fluorescence due to a porphyrin produced by the bacteria. If the lesions are washed with antibiotic soaps before Wood's lamp examination, fluorescence may be transiently absent. Scapings of the lesions stained with methylene blue show coccoid and rod-like organisms when examined under oil immersion. Biopsy may also demonstrate the organism in the keratin layer. Culture is difficult and rarely necessary but may be accomplished with a special medium. The resultant growth fluoresces under a Wood's lamp for up to 4 days.

THERAPY

Topical regimens reported to be successful include topical 2% erythromycin, 2% clindamycin, 2% fucidin cream,[467] Whitfield's ointment, miconazole cream, econazole and tioconazole. Effective oral antibiotic regimens include erythromycin 40mg/kg/day every 6h for 5–12 days, single-dose clar-

460. Barnett JH, Estes SA, Wirman JA et al. (1983) Erysipeloid. **J Am Acad Dermatol** 9:116.
461. Razsi L, Sanchez MR (1994) Progressively enlarging painful annular plaque on the hand. **Arch Dermatol** 130:1311.
462. Sindhuphak W, MacDonald E, Smith EB (1985) Erythrasma: overlooked or misdiagnosed? **Int J Dermatol** 25:95.
463. Berger SA, Gorea A, Stadler J et al. (1984) Recurrent breast abscesses caused by *Corynebacterium minutissimum*. **J Clin Microbiol** 20:1219.

464. Herschorn BJ, Brucker AJ (1985) Embolic retinopathy due to *Corynebacterium minutissimum* endocarditis. **Br J Ophthalmol** 69:29.
465. Guarderas J, Kornad A, Alvarez S et al. (1986) *Corynebacterium minutissimum* bacteremia in a patient with chronic myeloid leukemia in a blast crisis. **Diagn Microbiol Infect Dis** 5:327.
466. Wharton JR, Wilson PL, Kincannon JM (1998) Erythrasma treated with single dose clarithromycin **Arch Dermatol** 134:671.
467. Hamann K, Thorn P (1991) Systemic or local treatment of erythrasma? A comparison between erythromycin tablets and fucidin cream in general practice. **Scand J Primary Health Care** 9:35.

ithromycin,[466,467] or oral tetracycline in adults and children 8 years of age or older.

TRICHOMYCOSIS AXILLARIS (TRICHOMYCOSIS PUBIS)

Trichomycosis axillaris is a infection of the axillary and pubic hairs caused by several variants of *Corynebacterium tenuis*. It is characterized by the development of yellow (flava), red (rubra), or black (nigra) concretions surrounding the hair shaft that are resistant to normal hygenic or simple mechanical removal.

CLINICAL FINDINGS

Yellow concretions are the most common; black are the rarest.[468] These concretions consist of tightly packed bacterial colonies and a glucan-like substance with cementing properties. The bacteria usually adhere to and grow between cells of the hair cuticle although they invade the cortex. Factors influencing the pigmentation of the lesions are not well established, but McBride *et al*.[469] demonstrated the production of a black pigment when tellurium was added to the medium. The adjacent skin is normal, but sweat may be malodorous and discolored by the growth.

The disease affects healthy people and usually begins during teenage and adult years. It is more prevalent in hot humid tropical areas, although cases are also described in temperate climates. The diagnosis is confirmed by treating affected hairs with potassium hydroxide and demonstrating the organisms surrounding the hair; this enables distinction from tinea, piedra, and the nits of pediculosis pubis. Gram stain reveals mats of Gram-positive threadlike bacteria. The organisms do not fluoresce under a Wood's lamp. Culture of the organisms is usually unnecessary and difficult, but may be accomplished on blood agar or brain–heart infusion agar at 30°C.

THERAPY

Treatment includes cutting the hair and application of topical clindamycin solution twice a day for 2 weeks.

PITTED KERATOLYSIS

Pitted keratolysis refers to a superficial infection of the plantar stratum corneum in which shallow, discrete, 1–7-mm pits are present, especially on weight-bearing areas and in between the toes.[470] In rare cases, it may involve the hands.[471] The condition, though malodorous, is usually asymptomatic. It may develop into painful erosions that require hospitalization in patients who wear occlusive boots or undergo prolonged immersion. Recently, a painful plaque-like variant characterized by tender erythematous or violaceous plaques with shallow erosions (Fig. 24.25) was described in children.[472]

The disease has a worldwide distribution but occurs most frequently in humid tropical and semitropical climates. It is most commonly seen in males, especially those whose feet are kept wet for long periods. Conditions favorable to its development include hot humid climates, hyperhidrosis, immersion of the feet, long-term wearing of boots (as seen in military personnel), and going barefoot in wet or muddy environments.

ETIOLOGY

The condition is caused by Gram-positive filamentous and branching organisms currently classified as *Dermatophilus*. These microorganisms produce

proteolytic enzymes that digest the keratin layer, resulting in the characteristic honeycombed appearance. These are best demonstrated by a Gram stain from a thin-shaved specimen of stratum corneum. Alternatively, hematoxylin and eosin or methenamine–silver stains may be used.

The differential diagnosis includes tinea pedis and plantar warts. These may be ruled out by potassium hydroxide preparations and paring the lesions, respectively. Culture is rarely indicated and requires special medium.

THERAPY

A number of topical antibiotics have been reported to successfully treat this condition, including mupirocin, erythromycin, and clindamycin applied twice daily for 3 weeks.[473,474] The lesions can also be treated with 40% formaldehyde in Aquaphor ointment or painting with 5% formaldehyde or 2% buffered glutaraldehyde and aluminum chloride.

INFECTIONS CAUSED BY GRAM-NEGATIVE BACTERIA

MELIOIDOSIS

Until recently, melioidosis has been considered a rare disease. It is endemic in tropical countries with poor access to health care, however, where it may have been underreported. It is now recognized as being an important cause of morbidity and mortality in Thailand, and has been increasingly reported throughout Southeast Asia and Northern Australia.[475] Cases have also been reported in India, Africa and Central America, and international travel and adoption has resulted in cases being diagnosed in nonendemic countries.[476] At present, melioidosis is considered an emerging tropical disease.[477]

The organism *Burkholderia pseudomallei* is a small, Gram-negative, motile, aerobic bacillus also known as Whitmore's bacillus. The bacillus grows well on all clinical media and is frequently resistant to multiple antibiotics. *B. pseudomallei* can be isolated from soil, stagnant water, rice paddies, and market produce. It causes disease in sheep, goats, swine, horses, seals, cows,

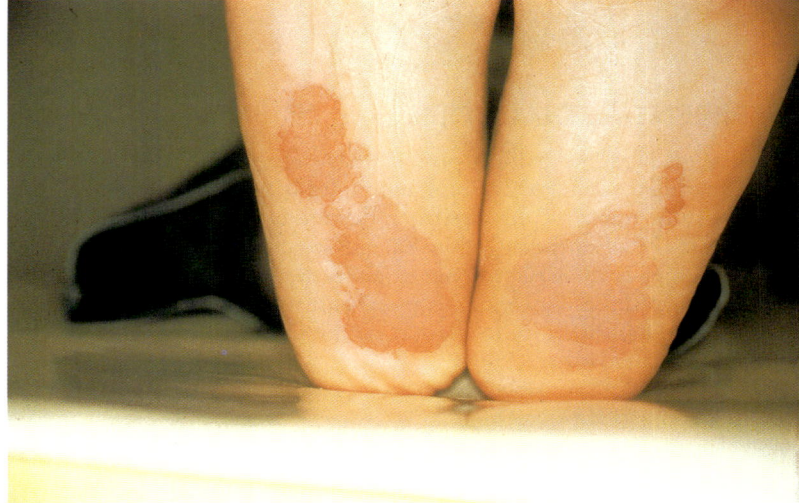

Fig. 24.25 Pitted keratolysis. Dusky plaques with erosions in a child (courtesy Maureen Rogers).

468. White SW, Smith J (1979) Trichomycosis pubis. **Arch Dermatol** 115:444.
469. McBride ME, Duncan WC, Knox JM (1970) The effects of selenium and tellurium compounds on pigmentation of granules of trichomycosis axillaris. **Int J Dermatol** 9:226.
470. Takama H, Yamada Y, Yano K et al. (1997) Pitted keratolysis: clinical manifestations in 53 cases. **Br J Dermatol** 131:282.
471. Lee HJ, Roh KY, Ha SJ, Kim JW (1999) Pitted keratolysis of the palm arising after herpes zoster. **Br J Dermatol** 140:974.
472. Shah AS, Kamino H, Prose NS (1992) Painful, plaque-like pitted keratolysis occurring in childhood. **Pediatr Dermatol** 9:251.

473. Vazquez-Lopez F, Perez-Oliva N (1996) Mupirocin ointment for symptomatic pitted keratolysis (letter). **Infection** 24:55.
474. Burkhart CG (1980) Pitted keratolysis: a new form of treatment (letter). **Arch Dermatol** 116:1104.
475. Thummakul T, Wilde H, Tantawichien T (1999) Melioidosis, an environmental and occupational hazard in Thailand. **Military Med** 164:658.
476. Dance DA (2000) Meilioidosis as an emerging global problem. **Acta Tropica** 74:115.
477. Dance DAB, Smith MD, Auchen HM, Pitt TL (1999) Imported melioidosis in England and Wales. **Lancet** 353:208.

rodents, and cats, but animals are not considered a reservoir for human disease. Although experimentally transmitted to guinea pigs by means of mosquitoes and fleas, arthropod-borne transmission has never been known to occur in humans. In endemic areas of Southeast Asia, humans become infected when they come in contact with soil through an abrasion of the skin, ingestion of the organism, or inhalation. Risk factors for disease include diabetes mellitus and renal insufficiency.

Mild inapparent infections are common, and recurrences after years of dormancy or treatment are not uncommon. Serologic surveys revealed exposure to the microbe in 1–2% of healthy nonwounded Vietnam veterans and 6–20% of indigenous persons living in Southeast Asia, which implies a high rate of mild unrecognized or inapparent infection. Seroconversion rates are highest in children between 6 and 42 months of age. After the war in Vietnam, the disease was seen in servicemen long after their return home, and in Vietnam refugees with sepsis or meningitis. It is now rarely seen in the United States and is particularly rare in children. Neonatal cases with sepsis and meningitis have been reported in Hawaii and Thailand.

CLINICAL FINDINGS

Melioidosis has an incubation period of 2 days to 26 years and can be acute, subacute, or chronic.[478] The acute suppurative form begins as a vesicle, pustule, bulla, urticarial lesion, or nodule at the site of inoculation and on occasion progresses to lymphangitis and regional lymphadenitis. Fever and general malaise are frequent with widespread abscesses. The most common form of the disease is the acute or subacute pulmonary form, which can vary from mild bronchitis to necrotizing pneumonia. Onset can be abrupt but generally begins gradually with headache, anorexia, myalgia, and fever, sometimes with rigors. The formation of lung cavities similar to tuberculosis is occasionally seen. A chronic suppurative form of the disease with dissemination of the organism to the skin, as well as the brain, lung, myocardium, liver, spleen, bones, and joints, results in the formation of multiple abscesses. This chronic form may become dormant for months to years only to recur when the host's defenses are impaired. Dance et al.[479] reported that parotitis was present in 38% of 126 children from Thailand with melioidosis. In children with the localized form, suppurative parotitis together with skin and subcutaneous abscesses are common manifestations.[479] Although children with the localized form tend to survive, the septicemic form has a mortality rate of 60%; hepatic and splenic abscesses may occur in the disseminated form.

DIFFERENTIAL DIAGNOSIS

The diagnosis is suspected in a patient with a history of travel to endemic areas, fulminant respiratory failure and multiple pustular or necrotic skin lesions. Radiographs of the chest demonstrate a pattern consistent with tuberculosis. Proof of the infection depends on culturing the bacteria from infected tissues or fluids. Cutaneous exudates demonstrate the characteristic safety pin-shaped organism with methylene blue staining. *B. pseudomallei* grows on most routine laboratory media and can be identified relatively easily by most clinical laboratories.

Serologic tests are available but are most useful as epidemiologic tools. The agglutination tests have problems with cross-reactivity, but fourfold increases in titer suggest active disease. Complement fixation titers of greater than 1:160 also suggest active disease but a negative complement fixation test finding does not exclude the presence of disease. Because the sensitivity of these tests is variable, both should be done in cases in which the diagnosis is suspected. These may be especially helpful when the illness appears to be dormant. A monoclonal antibody–based latex agglutination test is now available for rapid

diagnosis of acute melioidosis.[480] Newer tests using PCR, immunofluorescent techniques and latex agglutination are being developed but at present are considered experimental.[481]

MANAGEMENT

Treatment of melioidosis should be based on susceptibility test results. Isolates are frequently sensitive to tetracycline, doxycycline, chloramphenicol, amoxicillin-clavulanic acid, piperacillin third-generation cephalosporins (e.g., ceftazidime), sulfadiazine, sulfisoxazole, and trimethoprim–sulfamethoxazole. Resistance to aminoglycosides, fluoroquinolones and many beta-lactam antibiotics is typical.[476] The current treatment of choice for severe melioidosis is parenteral ceftazidime 150mg/kg per day, followed by amoxicillin-clavulanic acid.[482] Susceptibility testing should be carried out. Recent cases of treatment failure with ceftazidime have responded to imipenem.[483] Therapy must be continued for 6 months to 1 year, preferably with sulfamethoxazole.

GLANDERS

Glanders is a disease of equine animals caused by *Burkholderia mallei*. Horses, mules, donkeys, goats, sheep, cats, and dogs can be infected. Rare infections in humans are related to contact with infected animals. Sporadic cases occur in Africa, Asia, and South America. Men between 20 and 40 years of age constitute most cases, and children are only rarely infected. No cases had been reported in humans in the United States since 1945 until a recent report of a laboratory-aquired infection.[484] The severity of the occasional infections accounts for its medical importance.

B. mallei is a nonmotile Gram-negative organism that stains irregularly with methylene blue and optimally grows on media that contain glycerol. Care must be taken by laboratory personnel because of the potential hazard of acquiring the disease from aerosols created in processing the specimen.

CLINICAL FINDINGS

Infection most often occurs by inoculation of the bacteria from contaminated animal discharge through broken skin or nasal mucosae. Clinical presentation includes localized suppurative infection (acute or chronic), acute pulmonary infection, or acute septicemic infections. After an incubation period of 1 to 5 days, infection usually starts as a nodule with acute lymphangitis at the site of an abrasion or scratch of the skin. Local swelling and suppuration precede the development of a painful ulcer. The ulcer is irregular with a gray to yellow base. Multiple nodules may develop along the lymphatics and evolve into necrotic ulcers. Regional lymphadenopathy is common. Dissemination can occur and is followed by the development of multiple nodular lesions, which become necrotic abscesses. Infection of the mucous membranes is associated with mucopurulent discharge from the eyes, nose, or lips, followed by an ulcerating granulomatous lesion. Systemic involvement is associated with headache, malaise, chills, high fever, nausea, vomiting, and marked prostration. A generalized papular eruption that can become pustular is seen with systemic involvement. Septicemia is uniformly fatal in 7 to 10 days.

The chronic form of glanders has a gradual onset with the development of malaise, headache, muscle pains, arthralgias, and low-grade fever. It may follow infection by cutaneous inoculation or by inhalation of the bacteria and has an incubation period of 10 to 14 days. Cutaneous lesions appear only after weeks or months and consist of multiple cutaneous, subcutaneous, and intramuscular abscesses. The chronic skin lesions present as subcutaneous nodules on the extremities and occasionally on the face. The nodules ulcerate and become chronic draining sinuses. Lesions continue to form and eventually

478. Lumbiganon P, Viengnondha S (1995) Clinical manifestations of melioidosis in children. **Pediatr Infect Dis J** 14:36.
479. Dance DAB, Davis TME, Wattanogoonu Y et al. (1989) Acute suppurative parotitis caused by *Pseudomonas pseudomallei* in children. **J Infect Dis** 159:654.
480. Samosornsuk N, Lulitanond A, Saenla N et al. (1999) Short report: evaluation of monoclonal antibody based latex-agglutination test for rapid diagnosis of septicaemic melioidosis. **Am J Trop Med H** 61:735.
481. Vadivelu J, Puthucheay SD (2000) Diagnostic and prognostic value of an immunofluorescent assay for melioidosis. **Am J Trop Med Hyg** 62:297.
482. Supputtamagol Y, Dance DA, Chaowagul Wattanagoon Y et al. (1991) Amoxycillin-Clavulanic acid treatment of melioidosis. **Trans Royal Soc Med Hyg** 85:672.
483. Minassian MA, Gage A, Price E, Sefton AM (1999) Imipenem for the treatment of melioidosis **Int J Antimicrob Agents** 12:263.
484. Anon (2000) MMWR. **Morb Mortal Wkly Rep** 49:532.

break down. They may remain localized to the skin, or become disseminated and cause fatal disease in about one-fourth of cases without treatment. Dissemination may involve the lung, pleura, eyes, liver, spleen, CNS, and skeleton. The prognosis for recovery is much better in the localized or chronic forms of the disease.

DIAGNOSIS

The diagnosis is dependent on a high degree of suspicion based on a history of exposure. The organisms are not always easily identified in cutaneous lesions because of the scant numbers present. Cultures are positive from the skin lesions, but blood cultures do not become positive until late in the course. Routine clinical laboratory methods can isolate and identify the organism. Serologic tests are available but do not have any advantage and are difficult to evaluate.

THERAPY

The mainstay of therapy is sulfadiazine 150mg/kg/day for 3–4 weeks. In the seriously ill patient with glanders, initial therapy may include trimethoprim-sulfamethoxazole and ceftazidime, similar to that for melioidosis.[485] Supportive therapy is essential, including surgical drainage of the multiple abscesses. Prevention is based on care of the disease in animals to prevent spread to humans. Cases in humans should be isolated because person-to-person transmission of human glanders has been reported.

PSEUDOMONAS AERUGINOSA

P. aeruginosa is widely distributed and can be isolated from soil, water, plants, and animals. It is an opportunistic pathogen and infections acquired in hospitals are frequently secondary to this organism. Pseudomonal infections are becoming more common for a number of reasons: antimicrobial selection pressures, the more widespread use of immunosuppressive treatment, and lifestyle changes such as the use of spas and saunas.[486] Recent reports have described *P. aeruginosa* infections in neonates born in water baths.[487–489] Hospital reservoirs are another common source of infection, and may include respiratory equipment, cleaning solution, disinfectants, medications, sinks, cleaning equipment, food processors, vegetables, cut flower arrangements, and any other area where moisture is found. The use of false nails in nursing staff has resulted in nosocomial infection in neonatal intensive care units.[490,491]

Infections are frequently seen in debilitated or immunocompromised patients. Children with cystic fibrosis, HIV infection, chronic granulomatous disease, and acrodermatitis enteropathica[492,493] are particularly susceptible. However, *P. aeruginosa* can also be part of the normal flora of the axillae, anogenital region, and external auditory canals and infection can involve healthy individuals.[486] Infections caused by *P. aeruginosa* include endocarditis; bacteremia; and respiratory, CNS, ear, eye, bone and joint, urinary tract, gastrointestinal, and skin infections. This discussion is limited to cutaneous manifestations.

P. aeruginosa is a Gram-negative aerobic rod that frequently produces diffusible pigments, such as the soluble phenazine pigment called pyocyanin which appears blue or green and is the source of the name aeruginosa. Growth requirements are minimal because the organism grows on all routinely used media. A presumptive identification is based on production of green pigment, colony morphology, and the characteristic sweet, grape-like odor.

CLINICAL FINDINGS AND TREATMENT

The most common infection associated with *Pseudomonas* infections of the external auditory canal can be secondary to maceration of the canal from the drainage of perforated otitis media or failure to dry the ear canal after swimming or showering. The initial sign is frequently pain followed by drainage, swelling, and maceration around the opening of the external canal. Excruciating pain can be caused by movement of the pinna. If not treated at this stage, the infection can spread to involve the pinna and surrounding tissue. In diabetic and immunocompromised patients, a severe infection can develop known as malignant external otitis, which may involve invasion of the cartilage, bone, and nerves, and extend along soft tissue planes. Osteomyelitis and labyrinthitis are common complications, with a mortality rate as high as 50%.

Treatment of external otitis in the normal host can frequently be accomplished with topical therapy. The use of gentamicin; the combination of neomycin, polymyxin B and bacitracin; tobramycin otic or ophthalmic drops; or ciprofloxacin otic drops[494] applied with a cotton wick four times a day is usually adequate therapy. Patients with recurrent episodes of *P. aeruginosa*-caused external otitis may be treated with 2% acetic acid solutions for weeks to months. Malignant external otitis requires hospitalization for administration of intravenous gentamicin plus ticarcillin–clavulanate for 10–14 days. Ceftazidime iv is an alternative regimen; oral ciprofloxacin or ofloxacin have been administered for serious skin infections in older teens and adults.

Green nail syndrome is seen in persons who immerse their hands in water for prolonged periods or in those with previously traumatized or fungally infected nails. It is common in adults with occupational exposure such as housewives, dishwashers, bakers, barbers, and medical personnel but is unusual in children.[488] The nail is usually nontender with a greenish-gray discoloration of the nailfold, associated with paronychia.[486] The most effective therapy is avoidance of exposure. Soaking the infected fingernail in 2% acetic acid solution two to three times a day may be helpful. Topical applications of bacitracin-polymycin B–neomycin or gentamicin ointment two to four times a day cures most patients in 1 to 6 months. Therapy is less successful when the nail is initially dystrophic because of trauma or preceding fungal infection.

Toe web intertrigo with *P. aeruginosa* has been seen most frequently in soldiers in swampy conditions for prolonged periods. Although it is only rarely seen in children, it may develop in those with plantar hyperhidrosis. The toe web areas are macerated, boggy, and thickened. Lesions can be white to green with a fruity odour and often fluoresce a bright green–white under a Wood's light. This infection can be confused with interdigital tinea, with which it may coexist, leading to failure to respond to antifungal therapy alone. Topical therapies, including separation of the toes with cotton, lamb's wool, or gauze; application of silver nitrate solution, silver sulfadiazine cream, or gentamicin cream have been successful in treating this condition. Oral ciprofloxacin or ofloxacin, or even aminoglycoside intravenous therapy may be necessary in cases in which the infection becomes invasive and spreads beyond the skin.

Since the first reports of "Hot tub folliculitis" in persons using jacuzzis and whirlpools, pseudomonal folliculitis has been increasingly reported in children.[495–498] Children become infected as a result of prolonged contact in

485. Russell P, Eley SM, Ellis J et al. (2000) Comparison of efficacy of ciprofloxacin and doxycycline against experimental melioidosis and glanders. **J Antimicrob Chemother** 45:813.
486. Silvestre JF, Betlloch MI (1999) Cutaneous manifestations due to Pseudomonas infection. **Int J Dermatol** 38:419.
487. Parker P, Boles RG (1997) Pseudomonas otitis media and bacteremia following a water birth **Pediatrics** 99:653.
488. LeFeber WP, Golitz LE (1984) Green foot. **Pediatr Dermatol** 2:38.
489. Rawal J, Shah A, Stirk F, Mentar S (1994) Water birth and infection in babies. **Br Med J** 309:511.
490. Moolenaar RL, Crutcher JM, San Joaquin VH et al. (2000) A prolonged outbreak of *P. aeruginosa* in a neonatal Intensive Care Unit: did staff fingernails play a role in disease transmission? **Infect Control Hosp Epidemiol** 21:77.
491. Foca M, Jakob K, Whittier S et al. (2000) Endemic *P. aeruginosa* infection in a neonatal intensve care unit. **N Engl J Med** 343:695.

492. Ozkan S, Ozkan H, Fetil E et al. (1999) Acrodermatitis enteropathica with *P. aeruginosa* sepsis. **Pediatr Dermatol** 16:444.
493. Ozkan S, Ozkan H, Fetil E et al. (1999) Acrodermatitis enteropathica with *P. aeruginosa* sepsis. **Pediatr Dermatol** 16:444.
494. Wintermeyer SM, Hart ML, Nahata MC (1997) Efficacy of ototopical ciprofloxacin in pediatric patients with otorrhea. **Otolaryngol Head Neck Surg** 116:450.
495. Stahelin-Massik J, Gnehm ME, Itin PH (2000) Pseudomonas folliculitis in a young child. **Pediatr Inf Dis J** 19:362.
496. Trueb RM, Gloor M, Wuthrich B (1994) Recurrent pseudomonas folliculitis. **Pediatr Dermatol** 11:35.
497. Zichichi L, Asta G, Noto G (2000) *Pseudomonas aeruginosa* folliculitis after shower/bath exposure. **Int J Dermatol** 39:279.
498. Buttery JP, Alabaster SJ, Heine RG et al. (1998) Multiresistant *Pseudomonas aeruginosa* outbreak in a pediatric oncology ward related to bath toys. **Pediatr Inf Dis J** 17:509.

heated swimming pools or hot tubs. Contaminated water supplies, bath toys and sponges are also recognized sources of infection and the condition can become recurerrent and chronic unless such environmental sources are found and eliminated.[498] Patients with *P. aeruginosa*-caused folliculitis usually present 8–48h after exposure with superficial pruritic papules, pustules, and/or deep violaceous nodules that are most dense in the areas covered by the bathing suit. The head and neck are usually spared. Some patients may develop fever, malaise, and lymphadenopathy. Serotype O-11 appears to be the predominant type of *P. aeruginosa* found in hot tub folliculitis. Treatment is not always necessary because most cases resolve without therapy in 1 to 2 weeks. Conservative topical treatment with antipseudomonal agents (e.g., acetic acid, potassium permanganate, Neosporin, or gentamicin cream) may be used, but efficacy of these agents is unproven. Drying agents may be helpful. Topical steroids should be avoided because they may exacerbate the condition and cause the infection to spread. *P. aeruginosa*-related folliculitis in the immuno-suppressed patient is much more serious and may progress to ecthyma gangrenosum. In these cases, oral or intravenous fluoroquinolones or intravenous aminoglycosides and a semisynthetic penicillin are indicated. Prevention is best accomplished by maintaining the minimum chlorine level of the water within the desired range of 0.4 to 1.0ppm and a pH level of 7.2–7.4 and by changing the water at least every 6–8 weeks (more often if heavily used). Immunocompromised individuals should be advised to avoid hot tubs.

Pseudomonas-induced pyoderma is a secondary infection of the skin that is often indistinguishable from similar infections caused by other organisms. These infections occur in areas of previously traumatized skin, such as atopic dermatitis, areas of ulceration or umbilical stumps.[489] Although it may be difficult to differentiate between colonization and true infection, infected lesions tend to have a moth-eaten appearance with a macerated and eroded border. Pustules and vesicles with necrotic centers may appear at the periphery and may be surrounded by localized cellulitis. Local therapy for the underlying skin condition and an intravenous aminoglycoside and semisynthetic peni-cillin, or oral ciprofloxacin usually results in prompt improvement. Relapses are common if the underlying problem cannot be controlled or if frequent use of broad-spectrum antibiotics is needed.

Pseudomonas-associated burn wound sepsis is a very serious complication in children. It is characterized by black, dark brown, or violaceous dis-coloration of the eschar, followed by degeneration of the underlying granulation tissue. Subsequently, one sees separation of the eschar, hemorrhage into the subcutaneous tissue, and spread of the infection to the healthy skin, causing erythematous nodular lesions. Early diagnosis is critical. At the first signs of change in the burn surface, a biopsy that includes both burn and adjacent unburned tissues should be performed for histopathology and quan-titative culture. A bacterial count of more than 105 organisms/g of tissue, plus histologic changes that include the presence of organisms in the unburned tissue and subeschar space, vasculitis with perivascular cuffing, focal hemor-rhage, and intense inflammatory reaction at the burn margin require immediate therapy. Adolescents may be successfully treated with ciprofloxacin 15mg/kg iv bid, oral ciprofloxacin 500mg bid or ofloxacin 400mg bid.[499,500] The use of these agents in children has been controversial in all but the most serious infections because of possible adverse effects on rapidly growing cartilage and bone. However, a recent safety evaluation using ultrasound and magnetic resonance imaging failed to detect these adverse effects.[500]

P. aeruginosa has been reported to cause a blastomycosis-like pyoderma in adults.[501] These lesions may be misdiagnosed as North American blastomycosis or squamous cell carcinoma and present as large verrucous plaques with multiple pustules and elevated borders. Histologic findings include pseu-doepitheliomatous hyperplasia with abscesses that lack giant cells or fungal elements. Treatment based on local susceptibility patterns with an intravenous

aminoglycoside and semisynthetic penicillin plus topical therapy usually results in rapid cure.

Erysipelas-like lesions due to *P. aeruginosa* have be described in children.[502] The lesions are hyperesthestic, producing severe pain. The indurated erythematous lesions have sharply defined margins and frequently des-quamate. Therapy requires intravenous antibiotics, generally an amino-glycoside and semisynthetic penicillin.

Ecthyma gangrenosum is the most serious cutaneous manifestation of *P. aeruginosa*. These lesions are a characteristic skin manifestation of potentially fatal *P. aeruginosa* sepsis.[503,504] Nonspecific signs of septicaemia such as a truncal maculopapular eruption, vesicles, petechiae and purpura may also occur. Patients are likely to have some underlying immunosuppressive condition, such as cancer, chemotherapy, primary immunodeficiency syndromes, diabetes mellitus, extensive burns, and/or malnutrition.

Lesions may appear on any part of the body but are only rarely seen on the palms and soles. Characteristically, the ecthyma gangrenosum lesion starts as a central area of hemorrhage surrounded by a halo of uninvolved skin with a pink to violaceous rim. The central hemorrhagic vesicle ruptures, resulting in a punched-out ulcer with a necrotic base. The ulcer develops raised edges with a tense, black, depressed center. Lesions are usually discrete, but multiple lesions at different stages of evolution may be seen. The lesions may initially begin as bullous and/or erythema multiforme-like lesions. Nonulcerating cutaeous nodules (deep abscesses), with bullae, both yielding *Pseudomonas* on biopsy and aspiration, have been described and have been associated with cavitary pneumonia and sepsis.[505]

Histologically, lesions show involvement of the dermal veins and not the arteries. Bacterial invasion of the media and adventitia of the vein walls deep

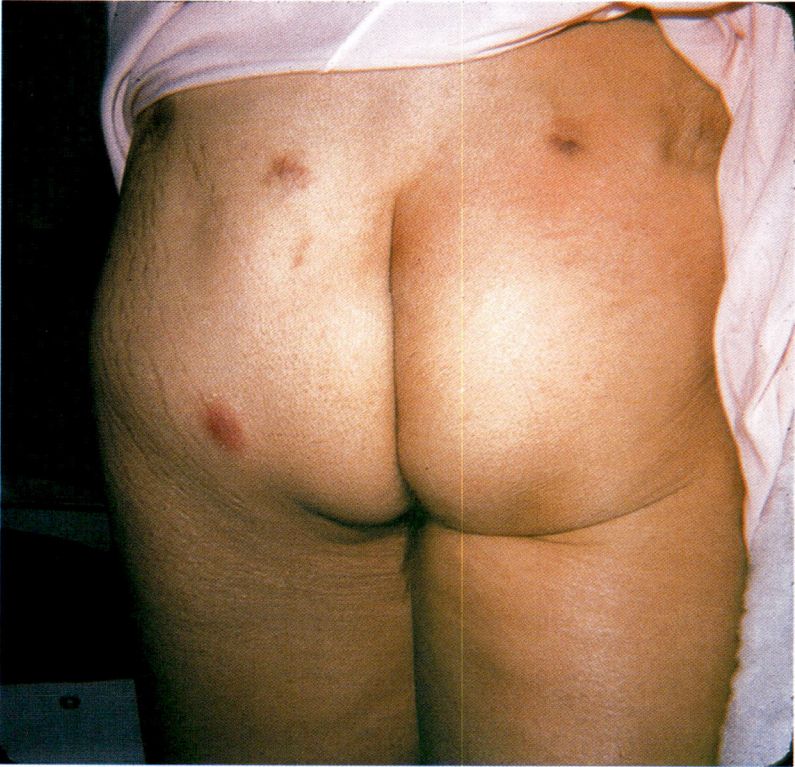

Fig. 24.26 Ecthyma gangrenosum. Multiple purpuric nodules in an immunocompromized host with lymphoma (courtesy W.K. Galen).

499. Gentry LO, Rodriguez-Gomez G (1993) Ofloxacin treatment of difficult infections of the skin and skin structure. **Cutis** 51:55.
500. Richard DA, Nousia-Arvanitakis S, Sollich V et al. (1997) Cystic Fibrosis Study Group. Oral ciprofloxacin vs intravenous ceftazidime plus tobramycin in pediatric cystic fibrosis patients: comparisons of anti-pseudomonal efficacy and assessment of safety with ultraonography and magnetic resonance imaging. **Ped Inf Dis J** 16:572.
501. Su DWP, Duncan SC, Perry HO (1979) Blastomycosis-like pyoderma. **Arch Dermatol** 115:170.
502. Roberts R, Tarpay MM, Marks MI et al. (1982) Erysipelas-like lesions and hyperesthesia as manifestations of *Pseudomonas aeruginosa* sepsis. **JAMA** 248:2156.
503. Sevinsky LD, Viecens C, Ballesteros DO, Stengel F (1993) Ecthyma gangrenosum: a cutaneous manifestation of *Pseudomonas aeruginosa* sepsis. **J Am Acad Dermatol** 29:104.
504. Gucluer H, Ergun T, Demircay A (2000) Ecthyma gangrenosum. **Int J Dermatol** 38:299.
505. Fleming MG, Milburn PB, Prose NS (1987) Pseudomonas septicemia with nodules and bullae. **Pediatr Dermatol** 4:18.

in the dermis is seen, but the lumen and intima are spared. Bullae are formed by the disruption of the dermis by fibrin exudates, hemorrhage, and engorgement of lymphatics. Necrosis of the dermis follows. Inflammation is minimal, and neutrophils are only rarely seen even in patients without neutropenia. Other Gram-negative organisms and disseminated *Candida* can cause similar lesions.

A "benign" form of ecthyma gangrenosum has been described in healthy children, usually in the axillary or anogenital regions.[506] It appears to be the result of a modification of the bowel microflora following antibiotic treatment, in conjunction with local skin maceration. In contrast to the septicemic form, blood cultures are negative. Affected children should be monitored for the possibility, however, of eventual emergence of underlying immunodeficiency.

Diagnosis is suggested by the characteristic lesions, which are painful and tender. Gram stains of scrapings from the base of the lesion frequently demonstrate the Gram-negative rods. Cultures of the lesions and blood cultures are positive. Aggressive therapy should be initiated as soon as cultures have been obtained. Treatment should be based on the pattern of antibiotic sensitivity seen in each hospital. Initial therapy should include an aminoglycoside such as tobramicin or gentamicin and a synthetic penicillin such as piperacillin. In penicillin-allergic patients, ceftazidime, cefepime, or aztreonam can be substituted for piperacillin. Aztreonam may be used in penicillin-allergic patients.[507] Supportive therapy is extremely important, and the patient should receive intensive care. Because of the shock and renal failure frequently seen in these patients, aminoglycoside concentrations should be monitored closely to prevent toxicity. In children with a chronic illness such as cystic fibrosis who suffer from repeated *P. aeruginosa* infections, immunization with a new anti-pseudomonal conjugate vaccine promises to be a useful adjunct to therapy.[508,509]

GRAM-NEGATIVE FOLLICULITIS IN ACNE VULGARIS

Gram-negative folliculitis usually develops in patients with acne who have received long-term broad-spectrum topical and/or systemic antibiotics.[510] Two major clinical varieties exist: the superficial form (type I) and the deep nodular form (type II).

CLINICAL FINDINGS

In type I, superficial pustules develop around and below the nostrils, later spreading to involve the cheeks or chin. A number of organisms are associated with the presentation, and these include species of *E. coli*, *Klebsiella*, *Enterobacter*, and *P. aeruginosa*.[511] The nares is most often the reservoir for infection of patients with *E. coli*, *Klebsiella*, and *Enterobacter*. Those with *Pseudomonas* were often found to have an associated external otitis. The presentation is of a sudden acute exacerbation of acne, unresponsive to therapy.

Type II Gram-negative overgrowth is associated with deep, often tender, nodular cysts of the face and trunk that may mimic severe nodular acne. *Proteus* species are most commonly recovered from these lesions, although *Pseudomonas* may also be found.

THERAPY

Treatment of Gram-negative folliculitis depends on its type and the specific bacteria that causes it. Cessation of antibiotics that alter Gram-positive flora

is important, and appropriate cultures should be taken. Superficial pustules are treated with 1% acetic acid or dilute povidone-iodine compressess. Although topical therapy may be effective, patients usually respond best to systemic antibiotics that are not usually used for acne. These include oral ampicillin, amoxicillin, trimethoprim-sulfamethoxazole or, in adolescents who have completed skeletal growth, ciprofloxacin or ofloxacin. Incision and drainage of deep cysts may also be helpful in unresolving cases. For patients with significant acne who acquire Gram-negative folliculitis, a 5-month course of oral isotretinoin (0.5–1.0mg/kg/day) is the treatment of choice. In one study, clearing was noted in most patients by 3 months of therapy.[512] Success was attributed to successful reduction of sebum production by isotretinoin, along with moisturization of dry skin, as isotretinoin has no direct antibacterial effect.

PASTEURELLA MULTOCIDA INFECTIONS

Pasteurella spp. are primarily animal pathogens, but they can cause disease in humans ranging from focal abscesses to septicemia and endocarditis. They are nonspore-forming, nonmotile, bipolar-staining, Gram-negative coccobacilli. Most strains grow on standard media at 37°C, but growth is facilitated by using enriched media (i.e., blood) under increased CO_2 tension.

EPIDEMIOLOGY

P. multocida is distributed worldwide and is recovered from the nasopharynx and gastrointestinal tract of many domestic and wild animals and birds. It is commonly found in the mouths of cats and dogs.[513] Human *P. multocida* infections may occur after exposure to animals, with or without a bite.[514] Most infections are related to animal bites, and young children (up to 4 years) have the greatest risk; however, in some cases there is no known animal exposure. Approximately 7 to 17% of people who report to hospitals for treatment of animal bites or scratches develop a *P. multocida* infection. Although most bites seen in the emergency room are inflicted by dogs, two-thirds of bites infected with *P. multocida* are caused by cats.[514] This may be explained by a higher colonization rate in cats, a greater degree of virulence exhibited by feline strains, or the type of wound.

PATHOGENESIS

Virulence is apparently related to the degree of encapsulation; strains with large capsules are more resistant to phagocytosis. Most infections in humans caused by *P. multocida* are localized, and are characterized by erythema, edema, infiltration by polymorphonuclear leukocytes, and occasionally, abscess formation. Septicemia and hematogenous dissemination are rare, usually occurring in a relatively immunocompromised host. Such events may give rise to microabscesses and hemorrhagic lesions in many tissues.

DERMATOLOGIC MANIFESTATIONS

P. multocida infections in humans usually manifest as focal soft tissue swellings after animal contact. The patient may have an acute onset of pain, erythema and swelling consistent with a diagnosis of cellulitis (Fig. 24.27), frequently within hours of the incident, but symptoms may occur as late as 3 days later. A gray serous or serosanguinous drainage is usually noted within 24 to 48 hours after the onset of symptoms. Infections are usually located on the

506. Boisseau AM, Sarlangue J, Perel Y et al. (1992) Perineal ecthyma gangrenosum in infancy and early childhood: septicaemic and non-septicaemic forms. **J Am Acad Dermatol** 27:415.

507. Boso JA, Black PG (1991) The use of aztreonam in pediatric patients: a review. **Pharmacotherapy** 11:20.

508. Cryz SJ, Lang A, Rudeberg A et al. (1997) Immunization of cystic fibrosis patients with a pseudomonas A O-polysaccharide-toxin A conjugate vaccine. **Behring Institute Mitteilungen** 98:345.

509. Lang AB, Schaad UB, Rudeberg A et al. (1995) Effect of a high-affinity anti-*Pseudomonas aeruginosa* lipopolysaccharide antibodies induced by immunization on the rate of *Pseudomonas aeruginosa* infections in patients with cystic fibrosis. **J Pediatr** 127:711.

510. Leyden JJ, Marples RR, Mills OH Jr et al. (1973) Gram-negative folliculitis – a complication of antibiotic therapy in acne vulgaris. **Br J Dermatol** 88:533.

511. Neubert V, Jansen T, Plewig G (1999) Bacteriologic and immunologic aspects of gram-negative folliculitis: a study of 46 patients. **Int J Dermatol** 38:270.

512. James WD, Leyden JJ (1985) Treatment of gram-negative folliculitis with isotretinoin: positive clinical and microbiologic response. **J Am Acad Dermatol** 12:319.

513. Francis DP, Holmes HA, Brandon G (1975) *Pasteurella multocida* infections after domestic animal bites and scratches. **JAMA** 233:42.

514. Hubbert WT, Rosen MN (1970) *Pasteurella multocida* infection in man unrelated to animal bite. **Am J Public Health** 60:1109.

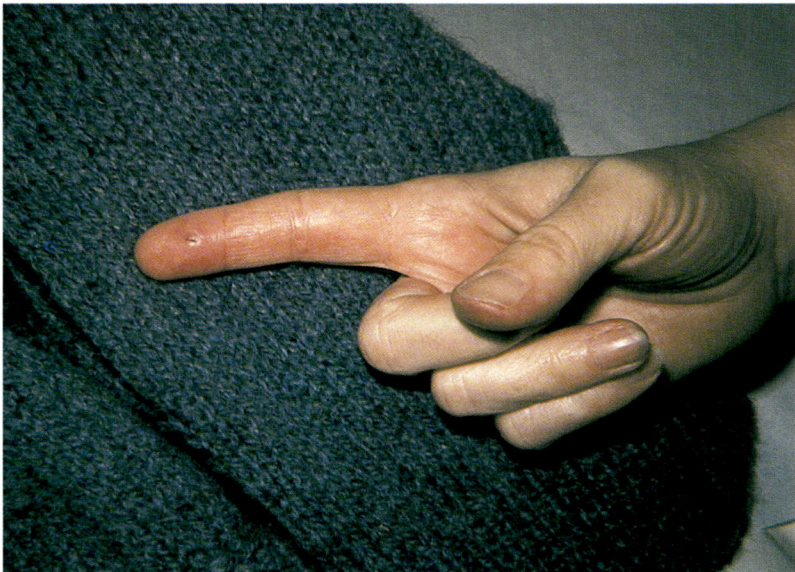

Fig. 24.27   *P. multocida* infection. Cellulitis-like digital infection after cat bite (courtesy Dr Carl Craft).

EPIDEMIOLOGY

Plague has been almost entirely limited to the southwestern states of the USA. It primarily occurs in the summer and autumn when outdoor activity increases exposure to animal fleas. Sixty percent of the cases occur in people younger than 20 years of age. Both sexes are equally affected.

ORGANISM AND PATHOGENESIS

Y. pestis belongs to the family Enterobacteriaceae. The organism is an aerobic or facultatively anaerobic, nonspore-forming, nonmotile, Gram-negative coccobacillus. It grows best at 28°C in blood or infusion broth or on MacConkey agar.[516] Presumptive cultures should be carefully handled and sent to the Plague Branch of the Centers for Disease Control and Prevention (Fort Collins, CO).

Y. pestis multiplies rapidly in tissue, which in part explains its high pathogenicity. This growth may be facilitated by an anti-phagocytic envelope.[516] The bacterial growth stimulates an intense inflammatory response. The resulting bubo consists of lymph nodes infiltrated by polymorphonuclear leukocytes with surrounding thrombosis, hemorrhage, edema, and necrosis. Bacteria subsequently may gain access to the blood stream, and it is probably the organism's biologically active endotoxin that causes the symptoms of sepsis in untreated cases. Septicemia leads quickly to shock, disseminated intravascular coagulation and coma.[517]

DERMATOLOGIC AND CLINICAL MANIFESTATIONS

Virtually every organ and tissue may be involved, and abscesses may form.[518] Because humans usually become infected through flea bites, the site of penetration of the bacterium is most commonly the legs and is occasionally marked by a pustule or ulcer. The incubation period varies from 2 to 8 days. After 1 to 2 days of symptoms, including anorexia, headache, fatigue, diffuse extremity pain, fever, and chills, prostration occurs. The organisms then migrate to regional lymph nodes, causing painful adenitis but no lymphangitis. In uncomplicated bubonic plague, the typical patient presents with lethargy, fever, tachycardia, and hypotension and may exhibit restlessness and agitation or occasional delirium and seizures. Careful examination may reveal the site of the insect bite, with various lesions such as a pustule, vesicle, eschar, or papule in as many as 25% of cases. Rarely, these initial skin sores may progress to cellulitis or an abscess. The skin lesions, if present, are often located near the lymphatic buboes.

The bubonic form, is present in 80 to 90% of patients, is characterized by lymphanopathy.[520] About 20–30% of victims experience pain in the inguinal or axillary region before a swelling is noted. The lymph nodes most commonly involved (in order of decreasing frequency) are inguinal-femoral, axillary, cervical, and epitrochlear. Lymphadenopathy in multiple areas occurs in 15% of cases.[519] The lymphadenitis is marked by severe tenderness with or without erythema and increased warmth. Over a period of days to weeks, suppuration and induration of the buboes may develop. Left untreated, dissemination to any tissue can occur, with sepsis, shock, and a 60% morality rate within 2 to 4 days after onset.[521] In some patients, no buboes form, and the clinical picture is of sepsis alone.[517]

Because plague can affect lymph nodes in any location, retroperitoneal lymphadenitis, for example, has erroneously led to exploratory laparotomy. These errors may be avoided if a history of animal exposure and a clinical picture of a skin pustule or ulcer followed by headache, myalgia, malaise, nausea, and

hands, arms, legs, neck, or head because these are the areas most frequently bitten. Lymphangitis and regional lymphadenopathy occur in one-third of cases. Less commonly, an indolent infection may result in a chronic skin ulcer. Extensive soft and hard tissue damage caused by the bite may lead to contiguous extension of the infection to tendons, bones, joints, and brain.

DIAGNOSIS, PREVENTION, AND THERAPY

P. multocida infection can be prevented by avoiding contact with wild and domestic animals. Bite wounds should be cleansed and debrided, and surgical closure should be avoided when possible. The use of prophylactic antibiotics is unproven. When infection occurs, a Gram stain and culture should be done. If the stain is unrevealing, empiric antibiotic coverage should always include *P. multocida* because it is the most common infecting organism.[513] Penicillin is the antibiotic treatment of choice although amoxicillin-clavulanate orally or intravenous ampicillin-sulbactam or ticorcillin-clavulanate for severe infection typically are given for empiric therapy of bite wound infections while culture results are pending. Other agents effective against *P. multocida* include ampicillin, amoxicillin-clavulanate, cefuroxime, celpodoxine, trimethoprim–sultamethoxazole, and tetracycline. Abscesses should be surgically drained. In general, children with such infections should be hospitalized and treated with parenteral preparations of penicillin (50 000 to 100 000units/kg/day). With appropriate treatment, resolution can be expected but may be slow.[515]

PLAGUE

Plague is a zoonotic infection caused by *Yersinia pestis*, which occasionally infects humans, producing fever and lymphadenitis. It is one of the few diseases endemic in the United States that requires quarantine.

515. Goldstein CJ, Reinhardt JF, Murray PM et al. (1987) Outpatient therapy of bite wounds. Dermographic data, bacteriology and a prospective, randomized trial of amoxicillin/clavulanic acid versus penicillin/dicloxacillin. **Int J Dermatol** 26:123.
516. Perry RD, Fetherston JD (1997) *Yersinia pestis* – etiologic agent of plague. **Clin Microbiol Review** 10:35.
517. Inglesby TV, Dennis DT, Henderson DA et al. (2000) Plague as a biological weapon: medical and public health management. **JAMA** 283:2281.

518. Crook LD, Tempest B (1992) Plague: a clinical review of 27 cases. **Arch Int Med** 152:1253.
519. Finegold MJ (1966) Pathogenesis of plague. A review of plague deaths in the United States during the last decade. **Am J Med** 45:549.
520. Butler T (1979) Plague and tularemia. **Pediatr Clin North Am** 26:355.
521. Butler T, Bell WR, Link NN et al. (1974) *Yersinia pestis* infection in Vietnam I. Clinical and hematologic aspects. **J Infect Dis** 129:578.

prostration and then lymphadenitis is appreciated. Other cutaneous lesions, although rare, include purpura, that may evolve into purple or black skin necrosis. Both are ominous lesions usually associated with disseminated intravascular coagulation and severe systemic disease and imply a poor prognosis. These lesions may be the basis of the term "Black Death" applied to plague since the Middle Ages.

Children frequently show signs of CNS toxicity, including delirium, coma, and seizures. Meningitis characteristically occurs during the second week of illness. When meningitis is present, 60% of these patients have axillary buboes. One of the most feared complications of bubonic plague is plague pneumonia, not only because of its high mortality rate, but also because it is highly contagious by airborne transmission. Thus, all patients with bubonic plague and cough must be kept in strict isolation.[522]

DIAGNOSIS, THERAPY, AND PREVENTION

Plague should be suspected in all febrile children with or without lymphadenopathy who have been exposed to animal reservoirs or vectors. Acute and convalescent serology, including IgM, immunoassay and PCR are available through the CDC and some government health and military laboratories.[517] Giemsa stain and culture should be done on material aspirated from a bubo. Intense leukocytosis and even leukemoid reactions in children, abnormal liver function tests, and abnormal renal function, are often seen. Because the lymph node does not contain pus early in the illness, nonbacteriostatic sterile saline must be injected and aspirated until blood-tinged fluid is returned. Cultures should be obtained from blood, sputum, the affected lymph node, and when appropriate the cerebrospinal fluid. Otherwise, excision or incision and drainage of the bubo should not be done because excessive manipulation may result in massive hematogenous seeding of Y. pestis.

Appropriate antibiotic therapy should be instituted immediately after the diagnostic procedures, since the mortality rate of untreated plague exceeds 50%. Streptomycin is still the antibiotic of choice for actually ill patients.[522] It should be administered intramuscularly for at least 10 days in two divided doses, totaling 30mg/kg/day. Gentamicin in standard doses is equally effective as streptomycin. For patients with meningitis, chloramphenicol, because of its excellent cerebrospinal fluid penetration, should be administered intravenously every 6h, totaling 50 to 100mg/kg/day for at least 10 to 14 days. Chloramphenicol and gentamicin, as well as tetracycline, may be used in penicillin-allergic patients. After clinical improvement is noted, the course can be completed with an oral agent. Serum levels of streptomycin must again be established during oral therapy because the palmitate ester, in general, gives higher serum levels of the active drug than does the intravenous, succinate preparation. Therapy with streptomycin has reduced mortality rates to less than 5%. If streptomycin is not available, gentamicin is an acceptable alternative, and ciprofloxacin has recently been shown to be effective.

All patients with suspected plague should be reported to local health departments. Those with cough should be placed in strict isolation for at least 48h after the start of antibiotic therapy. All infected material must be handled with gloves, and aerosolization of fluids and secretions must be avoided.

All contacts of patients with pulmonary involvement should be quarantined and treated propylactically with tetracyclines or a sulfonamide for 10 days. Contacts of patients with bubonic plague should be kept under surveillance for 10 days. A vaccine was available for persons with high-risk occupations but is not available at present.[517] Effective control requires a knowledge of the epidemiology of infected animals, vectors, and their possible contacts with humans.

NEISSERIA MENINGITIDIS

Most people have a profound dread of infections caused by N. meningitidis because of the rapid onset and fulminant course of the infection.[523] The high mortality rate of N. meningitidis, even with appropriate antibiotic and supportive therapy, has recently stimulated research aimed at controlling this disease with immunization. Such programs in closed populations such as the military have resulted in significant reductions in infection rates.[524]

ETIOLOGIC AGENT

N. meningitidis is a nonmotile, Gram-negative coccus that is usually arranged in pairs or diplococci, the opposing edges of which are flattened. In smears of infected blood or cerebrospinal fluid, they are commonly seen intracellularly. It is best grown on chocolate agar under increased CO_2 tension at a temperature of 35–37°C. Attempts at isolating the organism from nonsterile sites require selective media (Thayer–Martin medium). Meningococci can be subdivided into serogroups, subtypes and immunotypes[525] based on specific antisera and capsular polysaccharides.

EPIDEMIOLOGY

Meningococcal disease is a major world health problem with children younger than 5 years of age accounting for more than 50% of reported cases of meningitis. The disease is endemic in temperate climates with seasonal clusters in winter and spring. In sub-Saharan Africa, the so-called "meningitis belt," epidemics occur every 2–3 years. Serogroups A and C are the main causes of epidemics, with group B being responsible for sporadic cases.[526] The case fatality rate varies widely from 8% in major medical centers to 70% in developing countries. In survivors, sequelae rates are as high as 11 to 19%.[527]

CLINICAL FINDINGS

Transmission of infection is by direct contact and droplet spread, with an incubation period of two to ten days. Clinically, N. meningitidis may take one of several forms: benign nasopharyngeal carriage, bacteremia without sepsis, fulminant meningococcemia without meningitis, meningitis with or without meningococcemia, or chronic meningococcemia.

The frequency of meningococcal carriage in the nasopharynx during the first 4 years of life ranges from 0 to 1.2%.[528] No significant difference in prevalence was noted between 3 months and 4 years of age; however, the meningococcal carrier rate increased progressively in older children. Children with older siblings at home are also more likely to acquire N. meningitidis carriage. The duration of carriage is 3–4 months in most children, but carriage as long as 2 years has been seen. Meningococcal bacteremia without sepsis has not been reported in infants and children under age 2 years but has been seen in older children and adults.[529]

Meningococcemia is frequently preceded by a prodrome similar to a mild upper respiratory tract infection. This is followed within 2–8h by high fever, headache, nausea, and often diarrhea. A petechial rash on the skin and mucous membranes and, occasionally, bright pink tender macules or papules over the extremities and trunk are seen. They may develop hemorrhagic centers. The more fulminant form of meningococcemia associated with Waterhouse–Friderichsen syndrome is seen after a prodrome similar to the more benign form but compressed into less than 2h. It is characterized by the appearance of massive skin and mucosal hemorrhage, with shock within

522. Martin AR, Hurtado FP, Plessala RA (1967) Plague meningitis: a report of 3 cases in children and review of the problem. **Pediatrics** 40:610.
523. Darmstadt GL (1998) Acute infectious purpura fulminans: pathogenesis and management. **Pediatr Dermatol** 15:169–183.
524. American Academy of Pediatrics Policy Statement (2000) Meningococcal disease prevention and control strategies for practice-based physicians. **Pediatrics** 106:1500.
525. Caugant DA (1998) Population genetics and molecular epidemiology of Neisseria meningitidis **APMIS** 106:505.
526. Tzeng YL, Stephens DS (2000) Epidemiology and pathogenesis of Neisseria meningitidis. **Microbes and Infection** 2:687.
527. Erickson L, DeWals P (1998) Complications and sequelae of meningococcal disease in Quebec, Canada, 1990–1994. **Clin Inf Dis** 26:1159.
528. Gold R, Goldschneider I, Lepow ML et al. (1975) Carriage of Neisseria meningitidis and Neisseria lactamica in infants and children. **J Infect Dis** 137:112.
529. Teele DW, Pelton SI, Grant MJA et al. (1975) Bacteremia in febrile children under 2 years of age: results of cultures of blood of 600 consecutive febrile children seen in a walk-in clinic. **J Pediatr** 87:227.

hours. The blood pressure falls rapidly as massive bleeding into the body's tissues occurs. In those who survive, marked renal impairment and/or extensive skin necrosis may result in prolonged hospitalization. The fatality rate for this form of the disease exceeds 50%.

In most children in whom meningitis develops, meningococcal bacteremia precedes the seeding of the meninges. The typical prodrome, which is similar to the prodrome of meningococcemia, is followed by severe headache, stiff neck, nausea, vomiting, stupor, and coma. Some patients do not clear the organism from their blood and have a disease that appears to be a combination of meningococcemia and meningitis.

Chronic meningococcemia is characterized by periodic episodes of fever, arthralgia or arthritis, and recurrent petechial lesions. Splenomegaly is often present. The patient is relatively free of symptoms between episodes. Chronic meningococcemia is rare in children. Neonatal meningococcal disease is a rare occurrence and is not distinctive from other causes of sepsis and meningitis in infants. The mortality rate in neonates is extremely high.

The cutaneous manifestations of meningococcal disease are some of the most important clues in the diagnosis of this life-threatening infection. Skin lesions are common in *N. meningitidis*, but similar findings can be seen in patients with other severe forms of sepsis.[530–534] Symmetric peripheral gangrene, purpura fulminans, localized gangrene, and acrocyanosis describe the severe manifestations seen with *N. meningitidis*.[523] The earliest finding may be a grayish cyanosis (acrocyanosis) that does not blanch on pressure and that occurs on the legs, lips, nose, earlobes, and genitalia. This can be followed by purpura (Fig. 24.28) progressing to large confluent ecchymoses that subsequently blister, necrose, and develop eschars (Fig. 24.29). A consumption coagulopathy is seen in most patients. The ischemic necrosis involving the distal portions of the extremities can result in loss of digits and extremities in patients who survive. The histologic findings include a Shwartzmann-like reaction, diffuse perivascular hemorrhage, perivascular cuffing, and intravascular thrombosis in venous capillaries. Bacteria are not present in these large necrotic lesions. A component of vasospasm can occasionally be seen, but large vessel obstruction is not seen in symmetrical peripheral gangrene. Shock is generally present and may play a major role in the pathogenesis of symmetrical peripheral gangrene.

Purpura associated with sepsis can be seen in meningococcal, pneumococcal, and *H. influenzae*-caused sepsis and in viral infections. Local vascular inflammation, deposition of antigen-antibody complexes with complement activation, and subsequent increased permeability may lead to the development of purpura. Vascular invasion by bacteria is frequent with *N. meningitidis*. Demonstration of Gram-negative diplococci in smears of isolated purpuric skin lesions of meningococcemia is a helpful diagnostic clue in most cases.

Skin lesions of chronic meningococcemia generally develop 7–10 days after the onset of illness and are often associated with arthritis, nephritis, carditis, or episcleritis. The macular lesions may be discrete or multiple, occurring on the trunk and extremities. Occasionally, purpuric, nodular, pustular, and polymorphous lesions may develop. The lesions may appear in crops with clearing between episodes. Dark-skinned persons may have only an area of darkened skin with a blistered edge. Lesions in lighter-skinned patients start as an erythematous macule that becomes papular, then vesicular, and later hemorrhagic. Histologic examination of the lesions shows dilated small blood vessels, vascular and perivascular infiltration with mononuclear cells and neutrophils. Luminal thrombosis and necrosis of the vascular wall may be associated with disruption of the vessel and hemorrhage. Organisms are seldom seen in late-onset lesions, but antigen–antibody complexes can be demonstrated in the vessel walls. This finding suggests that the cutaneous lesions in chronic meningococcemia are usually related to the immune response and not to direct bacterial invasion.

Certain groups with immunodeficiency involving either the terminal complement system (C5–9) or properdin, or those with anatomic or functional asplenia, are more susceptible to *N. meningitidis*. Families with a low innate production of the cytokines tumor necrosis factor and interleukin-10 may be also more susceptible to meningococcal disease.[535] Bactericidal activity in serum is inversely proportional to the incidence of meningococcal disease during the first 12 years of life, and correlates well with the presence of specific IgG antibodies in serum. Specific and cross-reactive serum bactericidal activity can develop within 2 weeks after induction of the carrier state. The development of cross-reacting antibodies to group A, B, and C meningococci occurs frequently in children carrying *N. lactamica* and may provide some natural protection. Carriage of serogroups A, B or C meningococci is uncommon in early childhood, however, and unlikely to be responsible for induction of natural immunity. Children, on the other hand, do not develop lasting protective immunity from the presently available vaccines. Thus, chemoprophylaxis for exposed children is recommended. The usual recommended agent is rifampin 10mg/kg up to 600mg bid for 2 days in children over 1 year old, and 5mg/kg bid for 2 days in children less than 1 year old. Ceftriaxone 125mg for children under 12 and 250mg for those

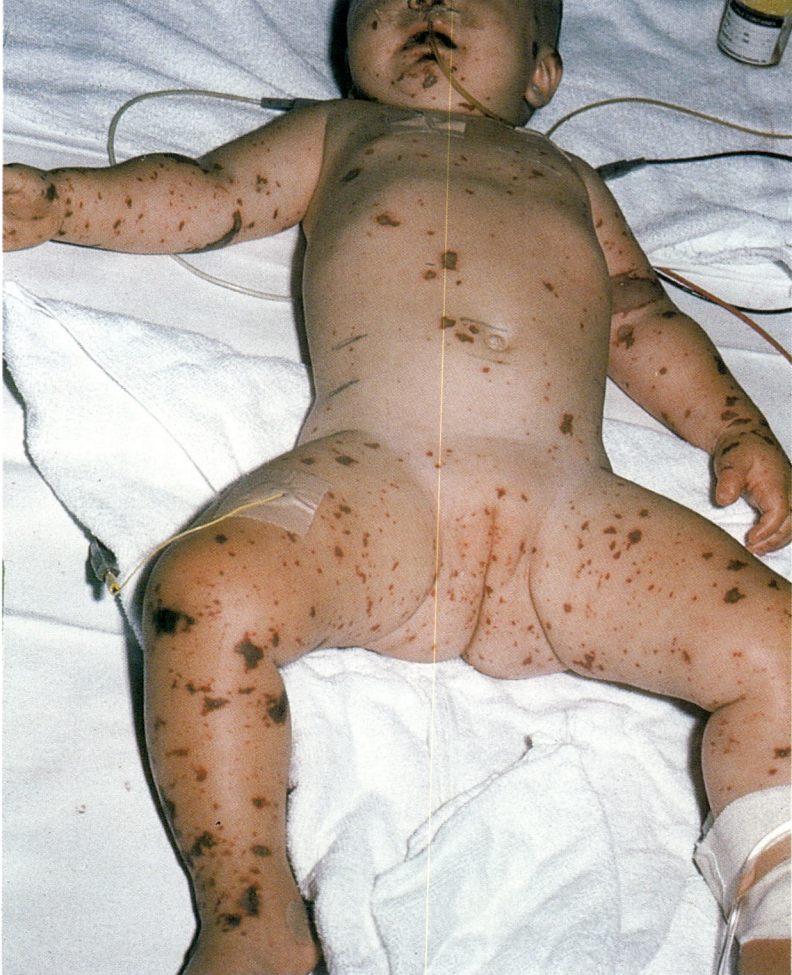

Fig. 24.28 Multiple purpuric papulescent plaques in an infant with meningococcal septicemia (courtesy Maureen Rogers).

530. Goodwin JN, Berne TV (1974) Symmetrical peripheral gangrene. **Arch Surg** 108:780.
531. Chu DZJ, Glaisdell FW (1982) Purpura fulminans. **Am J Surg** 143:356.
532. Spicer TE, Rau JM (1976) Purpura fulminans. **Am J Med** 61:566.
533. Hill WR, Dinney TD (1947) The cutaneous lesion in acute meningococcemia: a clinical and pathologic study. **JAMA** 134:513.
534. Bernhard WG, Jordan AC (1944) Purpuric lesions in meningococcemia infections: diagnosis from smears and cultures of the purpuric lesions. **J Lab Clin Med** 29:273.
535. Westendorp RGJ, Langermans JAM, Huizinga TWJ et al. (1997) Genetic influence on cytokine production and fatal meningococcal disease. **Lancet** 349:170.

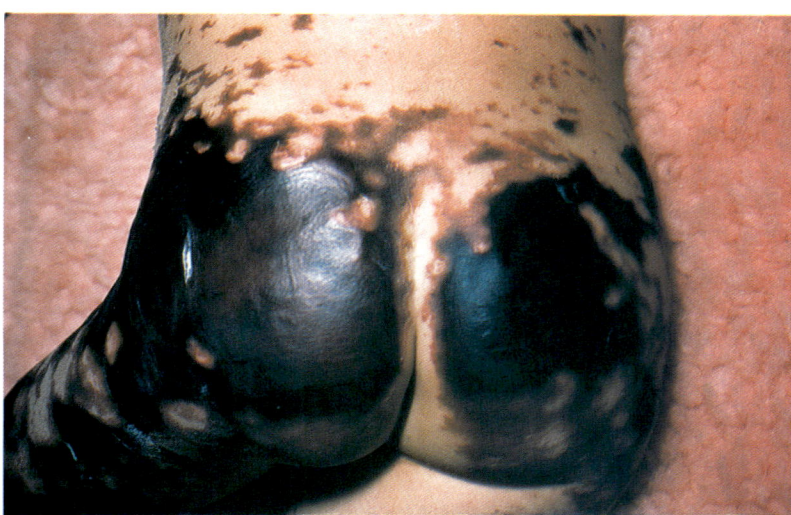

Fig. 24.29   Meningococcal septicemia. Large plaque necrosis with purpura fulminans (courtesy Maureen Rogers).

over 12 as a single im dose is an alternative, and ciprofloxacin 500mg or ofloxacin 400mg may be given as a single dose to children over 12 years.

Complications associated with infections caused by *N. meningitidis* include myocarditis, nephritis, pneumonia, subdural effusions, seizures, septic joints, skin necrosis, and neurologic manifestations.

DIFFERENTIAL DIAGNOSIS

The diagnosis is dependent on demonstrating the organism in the blood or cerebrospinal fluid. Gram stains of blood leukocytes (buffy coat), cutaneous lesions, and cerebrospinal fluid may demonstrate the characteristic Gram-negative diplococci but are frequently misinterpreted by inexperienced observers. Skin aspirates and skin biopsies of hemorrhagic or purpuric lesions examined with Gram stain and culture were found to provide rapid support of the diagnosis in 63–72% of patients with meningococcal meningitis and meningococcal sepsis in a recent study.[536] Cultures of blood and cerebrospinal fluid are generally positive during the acute illness but are frequently negative in chronic meningococcemia or in partially treated patients. Latex agglutination for antigen in cerebrospinal fluid is sometimes helpful when cultures do not demonstrate the organism, but false-positive and -negative results may occur. Techniques using PCR promise to become useful in rapid diagnosis particularly when antibiotic treatment has been commenced prior to investigation in hospital.[537–539] Differential diagnosis includes other acute bacteremias, other acute bacterial meningitides, endocarditis, hypersensitivity vasculitis, enteroviral infections, rheumatic fever, Henoch–Schönlein purpura, rat-bite fever, erythema multiforme, atypical measles, Rocky Mountain spotted fever, and ehrlichiosis.

MANAGEMENT

The treatment of meningococcal disease is based on penicillin, but initial therapy in children can never be limited to penicillin alone. Sepsis and meningitis in childhood can be caused by several different organisms; thus, initial therapy must be directed against the most common pathogens based on local antibiotic susceptibility patterns. Initial treatment in hospital should consist of ampicillin 50mg/kg iv every 4h plus cefotraxime 50mg/kg up to 2g iv every 6h or ceftriaxone 50mg/kg up to 2g iv every 12h. Doxycycline may also be considered if Rocky Mountain spotted fever or ehrlichiosis are in the differential diagnosis. When the culture results return and *N. meningitidis* has been isolated, the treatment can be changed to benzylpenicillin 60mg/kg up to 1.8/g iv every 4h for 7–10 days. In penicillin-sensitive patients cefotaxime 50mg/kg up to 2g iv qid or ceftriaxone 50mg/kg up to 2g iv bid may be used. Supportive therapy is important to the survival of the severely ill child with meningococcemia and to reduce complications. Patients should receive intensive care, with central venous pressure, blood pressure, and urine output monitored continuously. Aggressive treatment of shock associated with meningococcemia is essential. The treatment of complications such as renal failure and cutaneous necrosis may require extensive therapy long after the initial illness has resolved. Recent studies reveal that levels of various cytokines correlated with the severity of meningococcemia in children, suggesting that modulation these cytokines may ameliorate the shock and purpura fulminans often present in these cases.[523,540]

The appearance of even a single fulminant case of meningococcal disease in a community frequently generates considerable anxiety. The risk of secondary cases in household contacts in epidemic and endemic circumstances has been shown to be significantly greater than the risk in the general population. The risk of secondary contacts outside the family is not well understood but is probably similar to that of the general population. Hospital personnel are at no increased risk unless they have had direct contact with the patient's secretions before therapy was started. Day–care centers require special attention. Preschool-aged children are in general more susceptible than are older children and adults. The day–care setting puts the most susceptible population in conditions that most favor the transmission of the organism.

Immunization with polysaccharide vaccines has been used in adults with success. Polyvalent vaccines are commercially available for groups A, C, Y, and W-135. At present there is no effective vaccine for Group B. Efficacy is about 90% after a single dose in children over 2 years of age. The vaccines are well tolerated with low rates of adverse effects.

At present, routine immunization is not recommended because of the low rate of infection in the general population, the limited duration of protection, the fact that the most common group causing disease in children is group B, to which there is no vaccine, and that children younger than 2 years of age do not respond well to any of the currently available meningococcal vaccines. Nevertheless, vaccination is now recommended for travelers to endemic areas, patients with splenic dysfunction, complement or properdin deficiency, household contacts of cases, and persons in closed communities such as college dormitories and military personnel. Since the routine introduction of vaccination of military recruits, no large outbreaks have occurred. In the United Kingdom, where rates of infection, particularly with group C, are higher than in the USA, routine immunization for children 2 months to 17 years of age and for college students has recently been introduced.[541] Immunoprophylaxis promises to be the most effective way to reduce the toll of this serious infection.[542]

HAEMOPHILUS INFLUENZAE

H. influenzae was first isolated by Richard Pfeiffer in 1892 during the influenza pandemic. He mistakenly took it to be the cause of influenza, hence the name influenzae bacillus. *H. influenzae* can be divided into pathogenic groups by the presence or absence of a polysaccharide capsule. The nonencapsulated strains are commonly found colonizing the upper respiratory tracts

536. Van Deuren M, van Dijke BJ, Koopman RJ et al. (1993) Rapid diagnosis of the acute meningococcal infections by needle aspiration or biopsy of skin lesions. **Br Med J** 306:1729.

537. Gray SJ, Sobanski MA, Kaczmarski EB et al. (1999) Ultrasound-enhanced latex immunoagglutination and PCR as complementary methods for non-culture-based confirmation of meningococcal disease. **J Clin Microbiol** 37:1797.

538. Atobe JH, Hirata MH, Hoshino-Shimizu S et al. (2000) One-step hemi-nested PCR or amplification of *Neisseria meningitidis* DNA in cerebrospinal fluid. **J Clin Lab Analysis** 14:193.

539. Seward RJ, Towner KJ (2000) Evaluation of a PCR-immunoassay technique for detection of *N. meningitides* in cerebrospinal fluid and peripheral blood. **J Med Microbiol** 49:451.

540. Girardin E, Grou GE, Dayr JM et al. (1987) Tumor necrosis factor and interleukin-1 in the serum of children with severe infectious purpura. **N Engl J Med** 319:397.

541. Public Health Laboratory Service (1999) Vaccination program for Group C meningococcus infections is launched. **Common Dis Rep Weekly** 9:261.

542. Stephens DS (1999) Uncloaking the meningococcus dynamics of carriage and disease. **Lancet** 353:941.

and usually cause local infections: chronic bronchitis, otitis media, sinusitis, and conjunctivitis.[543] Encapsulated *H. influenzae* types a, c, d, e, and f are rarely the cause of local or invasive infection. *H. influenzae* type b has a carriage rate of 2–4% in the normal population[544] but is responsible for most of the serious illness seen in humans. Cutaneous manifestations are seen frequently with type b and not with the other strains.

Invasive *H. influenzae* disease has now been virtually eliminated in industrialized countries in North America, Northern Europe, Australia and New Zealand since the introduction of vaccination in the early 1990s.[545] The present vaccines have an excellent safety record and a high degree of efficacy in every environment in which they have been tested. These vaccines promise to bring the same benefits to less developed countries.[546]

Prior to effective vaccination, however, no pathogen had caused more concern for pediatricians seeing ill children than *H. influenzae* type b. It is primarily a disease of the child younger than 5 years of age who lacks immunity to the organism, and may result in meningitis, pneumonia and empyema, septic arthritis, cellulitis, osteomyelitis, pericarditis, endocarditis, tenosynovitis, peritonitis, glossitis, and epiglottitis. Transmission of the organism from person to person can occur by airborne droplets but mainly by direct contact with secretions or fomites. A carrier rate of 2–4% was seen in the general population before the vaccine became available and could be as high as 50% in closed populations such as day-care centers. Type b was the major cause of meningitis in most regions of the United States and exceeded the number of cases caused by all other bacterial pathogens combined until recent years. Peak attack rate was in 6 to 7 months of age, and occurred more frequently in males, blacks, poor families living in crowded conditions, and in the winter months. Epiglottitis is an illness of older children (2 to 6 years of age).

MICROBIOLOGY

H. influenzae is a small, nonmotile, pleomorphic Gram-negative coccobacillus that requires two supplements known as X and V factors for aerobic growth. These growth factors are present in erythrocytes and account for the generic name *Haemophilus*, meaning "blood loving." X factor is supplied by heat-stable iron-containing pigments in the blood and is used to distinguish *H. influenzae* from *H. parainfluenzae*. V factor is a heat-labile coenzyme that may be supplied by coenzyme I (nicotinamide adenine dinucleotide), by coenzyme II (nicotinamide adenine dinucleotide phosphate), or by nicotinamide nucleoside. Chocolate agar is the medium of choice for its growth. Cultures grow best if incubated at 35–37°C in the presence of 5–10% CO_2. The production of indole by most pathogenic strains produces a characteristically pungent odor. The production of capsular polysaccharides by *H. influenzae* is the basis of serologic typing. Strains that produce a linear polymer of ribosylribitol phosphate are designated type b and are responsible for most invasive disease.

CLINICAL FINDINGS

After colonization of the nasopharynx of the susceptible host, *H. influenzae* type b penetrates the submucosa of the nasopharynx and rapidly enters the bloodstream. Hematogenous spread accounts for the widespread manifestations of the disease. Bacteremia without focal signs (unsuspected bacteremia) is occasionally seen in this disease. Patients are seen in emergency rooms and doctors' offices with temperatures of 38.8°C or more and an elevated peripheral neutrophil count. If untreated, they can progress to more serious manifestations of the disease.

The cutaneous manifestations of this disease can be variable and difficult to differentiate from those of other pathogens that cause sepsis and/or cellulitis. Patients with fulminant sepsis may have a petechial rash on the skin and mucous membranes similar to that of meningococcemia. Occasionally, bright pink tender macules or papules can be seen over the extremities and trunk. The severe manifestations of symmetric peripheral gangrene are rare but can occur and are frequently confused with meningococcemia. Less common infections include osteomyelitis, pericarditis, preseptal or orbital cellulitis, urinary tract infections, epididymitis, soft tissue abscesses, lung abscesses, endocarditis, endophthalmitis, peritonitis, and bacteremia or neonatal sepsis.

The cellulitis of *H. influenzae* type b is classically a raised, warm tender area on the cheek or periorbital region with a reddish-blue to purple color[547,548] (Fig. 24.30), but the lesion may also occur on other parts of the body.[549] Other pathogens can cause bluish cellulitis but not as frequently.[550] *H. influenzae* type b has also caused an erysipelas-like scalp cellulitis. These cellulitic lesions are hematogenously spread and may be associated with underlying ethmoid sinusitis or otitis media. *H. influenzae* type b-associated cellulitis may precede other more serious manifestations, such as meningitis. Thus, the workup for suspected cases should include a spinal tap.

DIFFERENTIAL DIAGNOSIS

The diagnosis is dependent on culturing the organism from normally sterile sites such as blood, cerebrospinal or joint fluid, pleural effusion, or percutaneous lung aspirates, and from the leading edge of cellulitis.[549] The latex agglutination test for the detection of antigen to *H. influenzae* type b in serum, cerebrospinal fluid, and urine is a useful diagnostic test but has limitations and is costly. The differential diagnosis of this disease includes all bacterial causes of sepsis, pneumonia, arthritis, and meningitis seen in childhood. The cellulitis can be confused with streptococcal cellulitis, erysipelas, and occasionally staphylococcal disease.

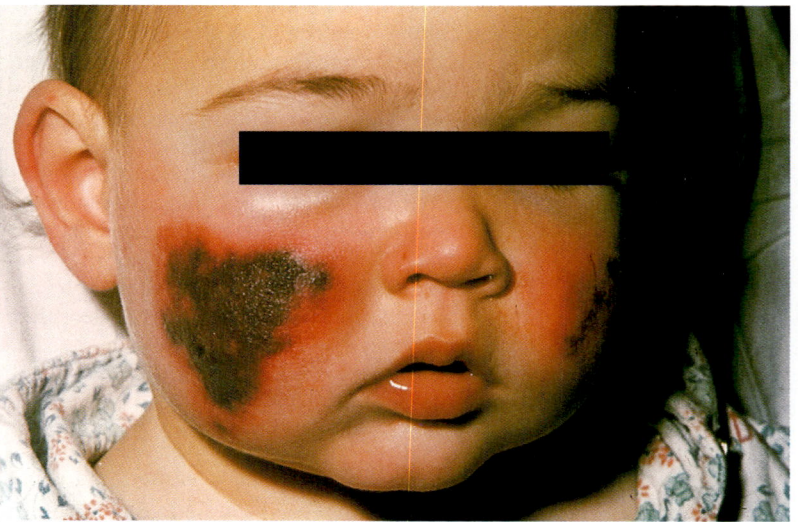

Fig. 24.30 *H. influenzae* infection. Bilateral cheek cellulitis with extreme purpura of right cheek plaque (courtesy Maureen Rogers).

543. Michaels RH, Poziviak CS, Stonebraker FE, Norden CW (1976) Factors affecting pharyngeal *Haemophilus influenzae* type b colonization rates in children. **J Clin Microbiol** 4:413.
544. Fothergill LD, Wright J (1993) Influenzal meningitis: the relation of age incidence to the bactericidal power of blood against the causal orgains. **J Immunol** 24:273.
545. Bisgard KM, Kao A, Leake J et al. (1998) *Haemophilus influenzae* invasive disease in the United States 1994–1995: near disappearance of a vaccine preventable childhood disease. **Emerg Infect Dis** 4:229.
546. Steinhoff MC (1997) *Haemophilus influenzae* type b infections are preventable everywhere. **Lancet** 349:1186.
547. Granoff DM, Narkervis GA (1976) Cellulitis due to *Haemophilus influenzae* type b. **Am J Dis Child** 130:1211.
548. Landwirth J (1977) Bilateral cellulitis of cheeks in an infant due to *Haemophilus influenzae*. **Clin Pediatr** (Phila) 16:182.
549. Rudoy RC, Nakashima G (1979) Diagnostic value of needle aspiration in *Haemophilus influenzae* type b cellulitis. **J Pediatr** 94:924.
550. Thirumoorthi MC, Asmar BI, Dajani AS et al. (1978) Violaceous discoloration in pneumococcal cellulitis. **Pediatrics** 62:492.

THERAPY

The treatment of *H. influenzae* type b has become more difficult in recent years because of the increasing incidence of resistant organisms. In the mid-1970s, the first cases of β-lactamase producing ampicillin-resistant *H. influenzae* type b were reported and a recent study indicates a present resistance rate of 36%.[551] Thus, ampicillin should not be used alone as initial therapy. Because the prevalence of resistant strains and mechanisms of resistance vary in different countries and regions within countries, standard initial therapy must be decided after reviewing local antibiograms. In general, treatment should be commenced with cefotaxime 50mg/kg iv tid or ceftriaxone 50mg/kg iv daily for 7–10 days. Ampicillin in combination with chloramphenicol may also be used. The erratic pharmacokinetic properties of chloramphenicol require monitoring of the serum concentration to avoid adverse effects and to ensure therapeutic concentrations. Drug therapy should be reevaluated at 48 hours after the results of antibiotic susceptibility testing are completed and the most appropriate and cost-effective therapy chosen for the remainder of the 10-day course. If the organism is susceptible, ampicillin or amoxicillin 50mg/kg up to 2–3g iv qid for 7 to 10 days can be used. Carriage can be eliminated by 4 days of rifampin 20mg/kg up to 600mg/day in children and 10mg/kg per day in neonates.

PREVENTATIVE APPROACHES

In the late 1970s, several investigators recognized that children exposed to a sibling or child in a day-care center with the disease were at increased risk. Several trials of prophylactic antibiotic therapy in these situations were conducted with limited success. From these data have come the most recent recommendations for rifampin prophylaxis in nonimmunized household and day-care center exposures.[552] Rifampin, 20mg/kg/dose, is given once a day for 4 days (maximum dose 600mg/dose).

Prevention of invasive disease with *H. influenzae* type b by immunization has been one of the most significant medical successes of the last decade. These vaccines are based on the observation that anticapsular polysaccharide antibodies provide effective protection against infection. The present conjugate vaccines are now in widespread use in developed countries, and most cases of *H. influenzae* infection now occur in unvaccinated or incompletely vaccinated children. Less than 300 cases of invasive disease now occur in the United States annually. An unexpected positive result of vaccination has been a reduction in carriage rates in the community and increased herd immunity.[542]

Three conjugate vaccines are licensed for use in infants: HbOC (HibTITER), PRP-OMP (PedvaxHIB) and PRP-T (ActHIB and Omni-HIB). A fourth conjugate vaccine, PRP-D (ProHIBIT), is licensed only for children 12–59 months of age. The present recommendation is that all infants should receive a primary series of vaccinations beginning at 2 months of age for a total of two to three doses two months apart depending on the vaccine used. A booster is given at 12–15 months regardless of which vaccine was used for the primary series. Vaccines should not be given before 6 weeks of age as this may induce immunologic tolerance and render the child non-immunizable. In children aged 15–59 months a single dose of vaccine is sufficient, and children over 59 months do not require vaccination unless they are asplenic. Adverse effects from the vaccines are uncommon and consist mainly of local reactions.

INFECTIONS CAUSED BY MYCOBACTERIA

More than 50 species of the genus *Mycobacterium* have been identified, and approximately one-half of these are capable of causing disease.[553] Mycobacteria, which are classified in the order Actinomycetales and the family Mycobacteriaceae, are true bacteria. They are nonmobile slender pleomorphic rods 1–5μm in length, which have variable amounts of lipid and mycolic acid in their walls. The constituents of the cell wall result in their distinctive ability to stain with the Ziehl–Neelsen stain and resist discoloration with alcohol and hydrochloric acid, thus remaining acid-fast. Runyon's classical method of separating mycobacteria into four groups, depending on their speed of growth and pigmentation, has been updated with the recognition of new species. Traditional methods used biochemical and nutritive requirements for species differentiation, while newer methods utilizing DNA or ribosomal RNA probes specific for certain species have increased the speed of mycobacterial diagnosis.

CUTANEOUS TUBERCULOSIS

Cutaneous tuberculosis was first recognized in 1826 by Laennec, who described his own "prosector's wart."[554] Extensive tuberculosis of the skin, with a great variety of clinical presentations, is not uncommon in adults in developing countries. In the United States, cutaneous tuberculosis has always been rare in both adults and children. Lincoln and Sewell,[555] with their vast experience of tuberculosis during many years at the Children's Chest Service of Bellevue Hospital in New York City, found that only 3% of the patients initially had tuberculous skin lesions. In the past, it was assumed that tuberculous skin lesions were always due to *Mycobacterium tuberculosis*. We know now that this is not the case, and recent evidence suggests that there is also a significant proportion of cases of cutaneous tuberculosis that may be due to environmental (i.e., atypical) tubercle bacilli.[556]

Classification schemes for cutaneous lesions vary, but for children the modification of the relatively simple outlines proposed by Platou and Lennox,[557] by Miller *et al.*,[558] and by Beyt *et al.*[559] is useful.

- Lesions caused by inoculation from an exogenous source
    In a previously uninfected child
    In a previously infected child
    Caused by inoculation with bacillus Calmette–Guérin (BCG) vaccine
- Lesions caused by hematogenous source
- Erythema nodosum.

CUTANEOUS TUBERCULOSIS LESIONS CAUSED BY INOCULATION FROM AN EXOGENOUS SOURCE

Infection of the skin can be caused by direct contact with mycobacteria, almost always in a traumatized area.[560,561] In a previously uninfected child, primary inoculation usually takes place in a wound, such as an abrasion on the sole of the foot or of the elbow, a mosquito bite, an ear puncture for earrings, or the foreskin at the time of ritual circumcision.[562] Primary mucous membrane lesions of the eye, mouth, and throat are also seen. The primary inoculation focus is usually both inconspicuous and painless and often goes unnoticed. It is apt to start as a red–brown papule that erodes centrally, developing into a dry crater or dell. Sometimes, there are adherent dry, silvery

551. Jones RN, Jacobs MR, Washington JA, Pfaller MA (1997b) A 1994–95 survey of *Haemophilus influenzae* susceptibility to ten orally administered agents. A 187 clinical laboratory center sample in the United States. **Diagn Microbiol Infect Dis** 27:75.
552. Committee on Infectious Diseases (1992) Ampicillin-resistant stains of *Haemophilus influenzae* type b. **Pediatrics** 55:145.
553. Wayne L (1986) The atypical mycobacteria: recognition and disease association. **Crit Rev Microbiol** 12:184.
554. Marmelzat WL (1962) Laennec and the "prosector's wart." **Arch Dermatol** 86:122.
555. Lincoln EMM, Sewell EM (1963) Tuberculosis in Children. New York: McGraw-Hill.
556. Sharma RC, Singh R, Bhatia VN (1975) Microbiology of cutaneous tuberculosis. **Tubercle** 56:324.
557. Platou RV, Lennox RH (1956) Tuberculosis cutaneous complexes in children. **AM Rev Respir Dis** 74:160.
558. Miller FJW, Seal RME, Taylor MD (1963) Tuberculosis in Children. Boston: Little, Brown.
559. Beyt BE Jr, Ortbals DW, Santa Cruz DJ (1980) Cutaneous mycobacteriosis: analysis of 34 cases with a new classification of the disease. **Medicine** (Baltimore) 60:95.
560. O'Leary PA, Harrison MW (1941) Inoculation tuberculosis. **Arch Dermatol Syphilol** 44:371.
561. Stoke JH (1925) Primary inoculation tuberculosis of the skin with metastasis to regional lymph nodes. **Am J Med Sci** 169:722.
562. Miller FJW, Cashman JM (1955) Natural history of peripheral tuberculous lymphadenitis associated with a visible primary focus. **Lancet** 1:1286.

scales in the center of lesions, which under pressure with a glass slide have an "apple jelly" translucence. Small satellite lesions on occasion surround the main one, which is sometimes large enough to appear umbilicated as it heals. The resemblance to a syphilitic chancre can be striking. A string-like lymphangitis sometimes appears, with clusters of "primary lesions" along the course. Three to 4 weeks after the appearance of the lesion at the site of inoculation, the regional lymph nodes enlarge, usually massively, and remain so for many months. At first firm but nontender, they later soften, possibly developing a sinus tract to the exterior. Granulomatous lesions may form around the stoma. This is called scrofula or scrofuloderma, a term applied to the skin lesion overlying a tuberculous lymph node, or arising adjacent to a tuberculous bone or joint process. In the semiliquid caseum oozing from the stoma, *M. tuberculosis* can readily be identified by stain and culture, especially early in the course; later, the granulomatous complex, is similar pathologically to the primary pulmonary complex, consisting of the primary focus, lymphangitis and regional lymphadenitis, except the portal of entry is through the skin instead of the lung.

In an individual previously infected with tubercle bacilli, skin lesions can also arise by inoculation, producing what might be called "reinfection" tuberculosis. In adults, these tend to be occupational lesions of pathologists ("prosector's wart") or butchers ("butcher's wart") and are referred to as tuberculosis verrucosa cutis or "warty tuberculosis" (Fig. 24.31). They are extraordinarily rare in children in the United States. Characteristically, the lesion is localized to the area of inoculation, usually the wrist or hand. It presents as a purplish wart, 2–5cm in diameter, is self-limited, unaccompanied by lymphangitis or lymphadenitis, and takes several months to heal.

A special form of inoculation tuberculosis is that produced by BCG vaccination.[563] Normally, 2 weeks after intracutaneous administration of the vaccine, a papule develops, continues to enlarge for another month, reaches a diameter of about 10mm, breaks down to form a small ulcer, and then heals spontaneously. Regional lymphadenitis may occur due to tuberculin sensitivity (Fig. 24.32). In 1 to 100 000 vaccinations or less, skin complications are seen, including excessive ulceration, subcutaneous abscesses, scrofuloderma, generalized tuberculid-like eruption, and even lupus vulgaris. In general, post-BCG cutaneous lesions resemble those caused by *M. tuberculosis* but are milder. Reaction at a BCC site is not uncommonly seen in children with Kawasaki disease.

CUTANEOUS TUBERCULOUS LESIONS CAUSED BY HEMATOGENOUS SPREAD

These usually occur during the early phase of dissemination. Papulonecrotic tuberculids, although rarely seen in the United States today, are still the most common tuberculous skin lesions seen in children. They were so common in infants with tuberculosis at the turn of the 20th century that Boeck considered them to be "the exanthem of tuberculosis." The lesions appear as small nodules (Fig. 24.33), some with a central nodule of semitranslucent "apple jelly" and some with scale that is easily scraped off, leaving a crater. Papulonecrotic tuberculids resemble chickenpox, both in appearance and in their distribution on the face, thighs, and abdomen. They eventually heal, leaving small, narrow, deep pits. Histologic examination is variously described as showing vasculitis followed by mononuclear infiltrates or scanty tubercle bacilli and giant cells. Tuberculids may, in fact, represent an Arthrus phenomenon in the skin. They respond promptly to appropriate antituberculosis chemotherapy.

Single or multiple metastatic ulcers or abscesses sometimes develop in the deep layers of the skin within 2 years of primary tuberculous infection; they are thought to represent a late manifestation of mycobacterial dissemination, particularly because they are apt to occur in immunosuppressed children with other metastatic lesions.[563] They can erode the skin and discharge pus, often blood-stained or brown, in which tubercle bacilli can be demonstrated. These abscesses sometimes develop at the site of trauma or intercurrent nontuberculous infection. They mainly need to be differentiated by stain and culture from staphylococcal abscesses, where the pus is usually white or yellow rather than brown or red.

True congenital tuberculosis, acquired in uterine life by the fetus from an infected placenta through the portal circulation has, on rare occasions, been accompanied by discrete, sparse, erythematous papules with crusted centers, distributed on the abdomen, extremities, and face.[564] They occur at 4–8 weeks of age. In one patient, granulomata with central necrosis yielded *M. tuberculosis*

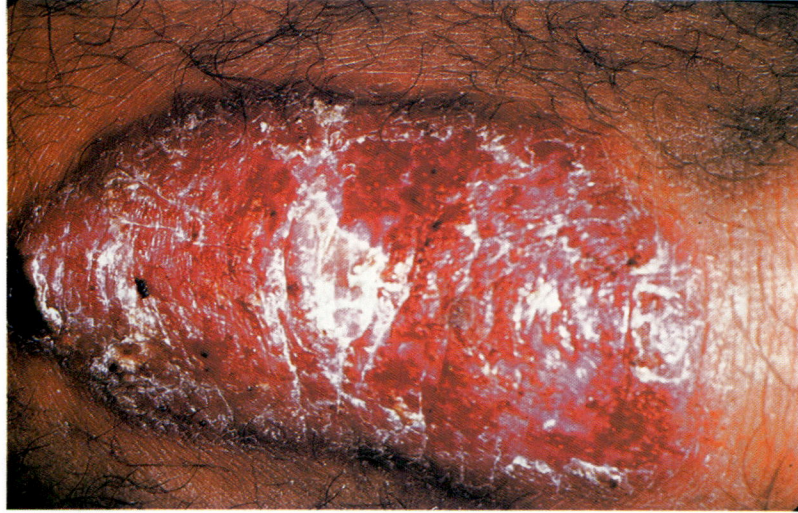

Fig. 24.31   Tuberculosis verrucosa cutis.

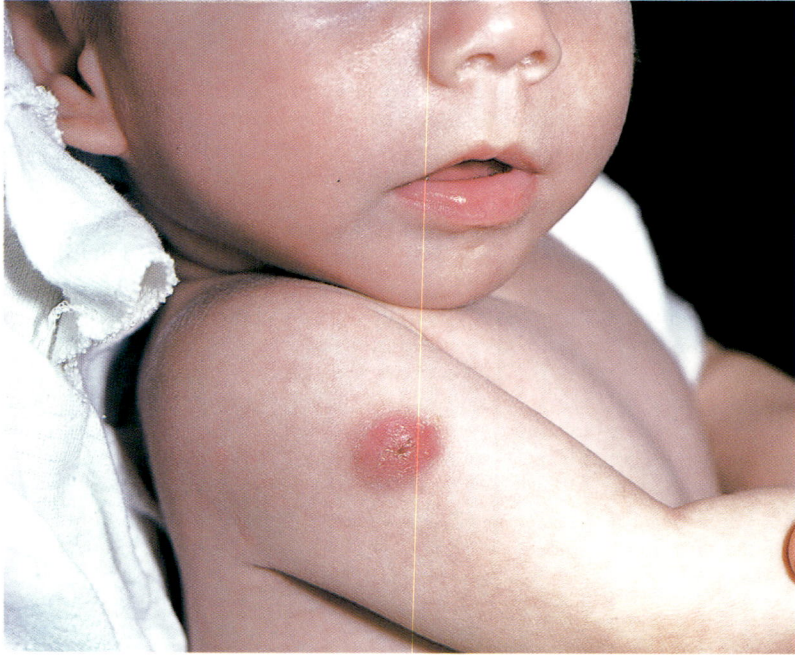

Fig. 24.32   BCG reaction with adenopathy 3½ months after inoculation.

563. Jorgensen BB, Horwitz O (1956) Dermatological complications of BCG vaccination. **Acta Tuberc Scand** 32:179.

564. Mc Cray MK, Esterly NB (1981) Cutaneous eruptions in congenital tuberculosis. **Arch Dermatol** 117:460.

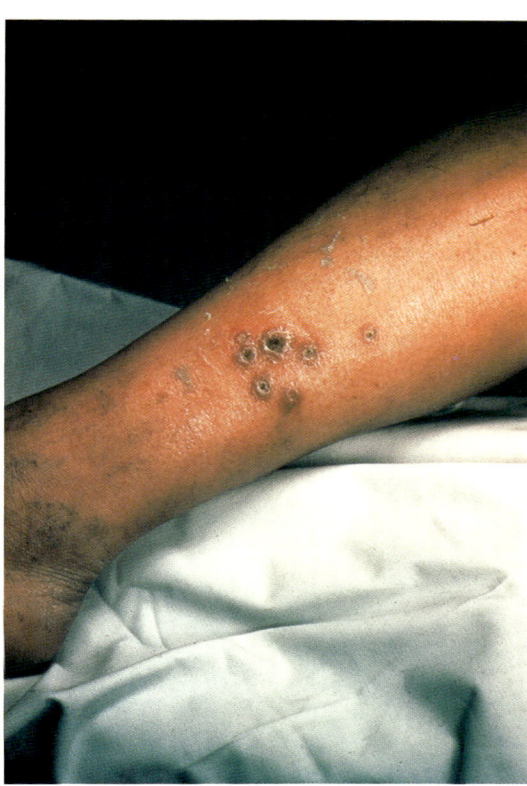

Fig. 24.33 Papulonecrotic tuberculid (courtesy Dr John Mosely).

bruises, which are distributed over the shins, less often on the thighs or extensor surface of the arm. Biopsy reveals only nonspecific change. The tuberculin reaction is always strongly positive when tuberculosis is the cause. Other evidence of tuberculosis should be appropriately sought and treated.

Differential diagnosis

The differential diagnosis of cutaneous tuberculosis includes analogous lesions caused by environmental mycobacteria of Runyon group I, that is, *M. marinum* or *M. kansasii*, or, more rarely in children, mycobacteria of Runyon group IV, that is, *M. fortuitum* or *M. chelonei*, both of which have been reported to be complications of diphtheria–tetanus–pertussis inoculations[565] or histamine injections.[566] *M. bovis* infection is so rare in any form anywhere in the world today that it hardly needs to be considered;[567] on the other hand, its derivative, BCG, is responsible for skin lesions in children wherever BCG vaccination is practiced.[563] Also to be considered in the differential diagnosis of skin tuberculosis, depending on circumstances, are impetigo, syphilitic chancre, cat-scratch disease, cutaneous diphtheria, sporotrichosis, nocardiosis, tularemia, and, in endemic areas, cutaneous leishmaniasis and even leprosy. Prompt recognition of papulonecrotic tuberculids is particularly important because they indicate recent dissemination of tubercle bacilli through the bloodstream, a mandatory indication for immediate chemotherapy.

Diagnostic procedures include appropriate smears, stains, and cultures of material obtained by swabbing, aspiration, or biopsy, using special stains, media, and incubation temperatures appropriate for the organisms in question. The intradermal tuberculin test (Mantoux), which uses 5 tuberculin units of purified protein derivative (PPD_1) is crucial because it is essentially always positive in cutaneous tuberculosis. Exceptions include poor technique of administration, outdated test material, or very young age (i.e., younger than

on culture. These could be considered papulonecrotic tuberlids in a child prenatally infected with *M. tuberculosis*.

CUTANEOUS TUBERCULOSIS FROM AN ENDOGENOUS SOURCE

Orofacial tuberculosis may occur by direct extension from adjacent, injected tissue in a manner similar to that of scrofula. Autoinoculation appears to take place from tubercle bacilli passed in secretions from the nose, mouth, rectum, or genitalia. Erythema induratum (Bazin's disease) consists of large, deep nodules and ulcerations on the posterior aspect of the lower legs.[555] It usually occurs in adolescents or older women, often after papulonecrotic tuberculids, and responds quickly to antituberculosis drugs.

Lupus vulagis is a rare form of chronic, indolent tuberculosis, usually seen on the face in adults (Fig. 24.34) who often give a history of its having started in a different form in childhood. Tubercle bacilli are difficult to demonstrate in the lesions, and response to antituberculosis chemotherapy is very slow.

Erythema nodosum

This puzzling clinical entity can be a manifestation of tuberculous infection but likewise of streptococcal, meningococcal, *Yersinia*, *Histoplasma* or coccidioidomycosis infections. It can also be due to sensitivity to certain drugs, including sulfonamides, or can arise in the setting of disorders such as inflammatory bowel disease or sarcoidosis. Frequently seen in northern countries in the early 20th century, particularly in older girls, it was often thought to presage severe tuberculosis in later years. Fever and malaise usually precede the appearance of large, indurated, painful nodules, resembling deep

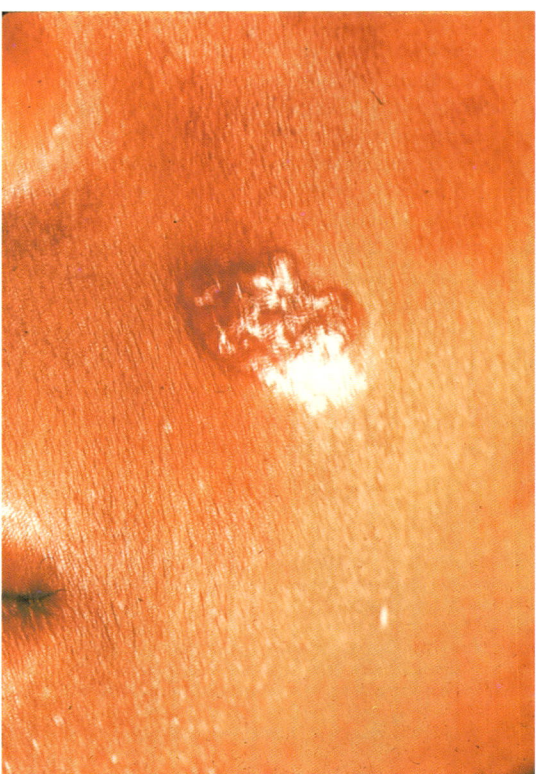

Fig. 24.34 Lupus vulgaris (courtesy Dr John Mosely).

565. Borhans JGA, Stanford JL (1973) *Mycobacterium chelonei* in abscesses after injection of diphtheria-pertussis-tetanus-polio vaccine. **Am Rev Respir Dis** 107:1.
566. Inman PM, Beck A, Brown AE et al. (1969) Outbreak of injection abscesses due to *Mycobacterium* abscesses. **Arch Dermatol** 100:141.
567. Iden DL, Rogers RS III, Schroeter AI (1978) Papulonecrotic tuberculid secondary to *Mycobacterium bovis*. **Arch Dermatol** 114:564.

3 months). Serologic tests for syphilis, cat-scratch disease, and tularemia would be helpful when these diseases are under consideration.

Treatment

Therapy for cutaneous tuberculosis should follow the recommendations for standard chemotherapy, as outlined by the American Academy of Pediatrics,[568] that is, either a 9-month regimen of isoniazid (10–15mg/kg/day in a single dose) and rifampin (10–20mg/kg/day in a single dose), with pyrazinamide, ethambutol, or streptomycin added the first 2 months if initial drug resistance is likely (as in Hispanic and Asian patients or when the duration of treatment is to be shortened to 6 months). Chemotherapy should be started as soon as the diagnosis seems reasonably certain on the basis of history, tuberculin test, and perhaps smear and biopsy findings, without waiting for culture results. If it is impossible, as it often is, to be sure whether the clinical picture is due to *M. tuberculosis* or to environmental mycobacteria, then it may be wise to treat with isoniazid and rifampin to cover *M. tuberculosis* and to add erythromycin, clarithromycin, and sulfonamides, which are effective against many of the environmental isolates (doxycycline is preferred in adults but should be avoided in children younger than age 8 years). Cefoxitin and amikacin are useful in severe infections caused by environmental mycobacteria.[567] The emergence of strains resistant to multiple drugs is a modern medical crisis. This is thought to be due to lack of compliance in taking medication, and may be addressed by institutions directly observing administration of therapy, when appropriate.[568]

NONTUBERCULOSIS MYCOBACTERIAL INFECTIONS

Infections due to nontuberculous or "atypical" mycobacteria (NTM), i.e., including infections due to any mycobacterium except *M. tuberculosis*, *M. bovis* and *M. africanum*,[569] have increased dramatically since the 1980s. Cases of disease due to these organisms have increased as the prevalence of immuno-compromised patients (with AIDS, transplants, or on chemotherapy, etc.) has increased.[570] In children, most infections involve cervical adenopathy, followed by infections of the skin and or soft tissues.[570] The most common presentation in adults is a chronic pulmonary disease similar to pulmonary tuberculosis.[570] Occasional patients, especially those with compromised immunity, may develop disseminated infections.[571] One survey by the Centers for Disease Control revealed that 35% of isolates of mycobacteria in American laboratories were nontuberculous.[572]

Atypical mycobacteria are found in soil, animals, food, milk, water, and even tap water. Unlike infections due to *M. tuberculosis*, infections with NTM are not, in general, transmitted person-to-person. They are due instead to environmental exposure, especially to soil and water. Those associated with soil and water include: *M. scrofulaceum*, *M. flavescens*, *M. avium intracellulare*,

M. gastri, *M. terrae*, *M. fortuitum*, and *M. chelonei*. Those primarily associated with water include: *M. marinum*, *M. kansasii*, *M. gordonae*, and *M. xenopi*.[570]

All NTM infections tend to be more common in males and in rural residents.[573] Geography appears to affect NTM infections, with *M. avium intracellulare* (MAI) complex being most commonly reported along coastal areas of the United States (especially Hawaii, Connecticut and Florida) and the midwest (Kansas). *M. marinum* is also most prevalent in coastal states,[570] while *M. kansasii* is most common in the midwest. These infections are fairly common in children.[574] Most skin infections are caused by the following members of the NTM: *M. marinum*, *M. ulcerans*, *M. fortuitum*, *M. chelonei*, *M. smegmatis*, *M. avium intracelluare*, and *M. szulgai*. The latter three species account for a few rare but well-documented case reports.

MYCOBACTERIUM MARINUM

By far the most common cutaneous infection caused by a NTM is the swimming pool granuloma caused by *M. marinum*.[574–577] This acid-fast microbe, formerly known as *M. balnei*,[576] is an opportunistic pathogen that affects aquatic animals and humans. It is worldwide in distribution, occurring in open seas and natural pools in warm areas, and in heated pools in temperate areas. It may become saprophytic in warm waters, where conditions favor its growth and existence outside such hosts as fish.[577]

This infection affects males more than females and all races equally. It is more common among fishermen and those playing in and working around water. It affects adolescents and children who frequent certain heated pools[578] and young and old caretakers of aquariums and tropical fish.[578–590] On rare occasions, cases have followed abrasions when no obvious exposure to a water source could be substantiated.[580]

M. marinum is a group I photochromogen in Runyon's classification.[578] It grows in most media but best at 30°C in Lownstein-Jensen medium, and it produces a whitish shiny colony when grown in the dark. These colonies, which are slow growing, develop a yellow pigment within a few days after exposure to light. They grow poorly at 37°C.[576,577]

Clinical findings

Most infections caused by *M. marinum* occur on exposed, injured surfaces, especially the fingers, hands, elbows, knees, feet, and occasionally the face. Typically, lesions appear 3 weeks after injury as purplish pink papules and nodules that spread slowly to involve adjacent skin (Fig. 24.35). The lesions may ulcerate, crust and scar and may occasionally develop a verrucous surface or resemble lupus vulgaris. More often, they present as chronic lilac pink papules and atrophic plaques. Most patients have solitary lesions, but multiple lesions have been reported. Swimming pool granuloma may also manifest a sporotrichoid pattern with pink to lilac nodules ascending the hand and arm.[576,579,584] These lesions need careful differentiation from sporotrichosis

568. American Academy of Pediatrics (2000) Tuberculosis. In: 2000 Red Book: Report of the Committee on Infectious Diseases, 25th edn, Pickering LK, ed. Elk Grove Village, IL: American Academy of Pediatrics, pp. 593–618.
569. Runyon EH (1981) Mycobacteria: an overview. **Rev Infect Dis** 3:819–821.
570. Cros TN, Jacobs RF (1998) Other Mycobacteria. In: Textbook of Pediatric Infectious Disease, 4th edn, Feigin RD, Cherry JD, eds. Philadelphia: WB Saunders, pp. 1237–1247.
571. O'Brian RJ (1989) The epidemiology of nontuberculous mycobacterial disease. **Chest Med** 10:407–418.
572. Good RC, Snider DE Jr (1982) Isolation of nontuberculous mycobacteria in the United States 1980. **J Infect Dis** 146:829–833.
573. Schaefer WB (1968) Incidence of the serotypes of *Mycobacterium avium* and atypical mycobacteria in human and animal disease. **Am Rev Resp Dis** 97:18–23.
574. Starke JR (1992) Non-tuberculosis mycobacterial infections in children. **Adv Pediatr Infect Dis** 7:123.
575. Street ML, Millet JU, Roberts GD et al. (1991) Nontuberculous mycobacterial infections of the skin. **J Am Acad Dermatol** 24:208.
576. Cartex LM, Pankey GA (1983) *Mycobacterium marinum* infections of the hand. **J Bone Joint Surg (AM)** 55A:363.
577. Runyon EH, Kubrea GP, Morse WC (1970) *Mycobacterium*. In: Manual of Clinical Microbiology, Blair HG, Lennette EH, Truant JP, eds. Bethesda, MD: American Society of Microbiology, p. 112.
578. Philpott JA Jr, Woodburne AR, Philpott OS et al. (1968) Swimming pool granuloma: a study of 290 cases. **Arch Dermatol** 88:158.

579. Jolly HW, Seabury JH (1972) Infections with *Mycobacterium marinum*. **Arch Dermatol** 106:32.
580. Black MM, Evky SJ (1977) The successful treatment of tropical fish tank granuloma with cotrimoxazole. **Br J Dermatol** 97:689.
581. Swift S, Cohen H (1962) Granulomas of the skin due to *Mycobacterium balnei* after abrasions from a fish tank. **N Engl J Med** 267:1244.
582. Black H, Rush-Munro FM, Woods G (1971) *Mycobacterium marinum* infections acquired from tropical fish tanks. **Aust J Dermatol** 12:155.
583. Barrow GI, Hewitt M (1971) Skin infections with *Mycobacterium marinum* from a tropical fish tank. **Br Med J** 2:505.
584. Glickman F (1983) Sporotrichoid mycobacterial infections. **J Am Acad Dermatol** 8:703.
585. Lacaille F, Blanche S, Bodimer C et al. (1990) Persistent *Mycobacterium marinum* infection in a child with probable visceral involvement. **Pediatr Infect Dis** 9:58.
586. Runyon EH (1965) Pathogenic mycobacteria. **Adv Tuberc Res** 14:235.
587. Shaefer WB, Davis CI (1961) A bacteriologic and histopathologic study of skin granulomas due to *Mycobacterium marinum*. **Am Rev Respir Dis** 84:837.
588. Schaffer WB, Blatman S, Bravo L (1962) Tuberculin sensitivity in children infected with *Mycobacterium balnei*. **Pediatrics** 29:404.
589. Van Dyke JJ, Lake KB (1975) Chemotherapy for aquarium granuloma. **JAMA** 233:1380.
590. Izumi AK, Hanke W, Higaki M (1977) *Mycobacterium marinum* infections treated with tetracycline. **Arch Dermatol** 113:1067.

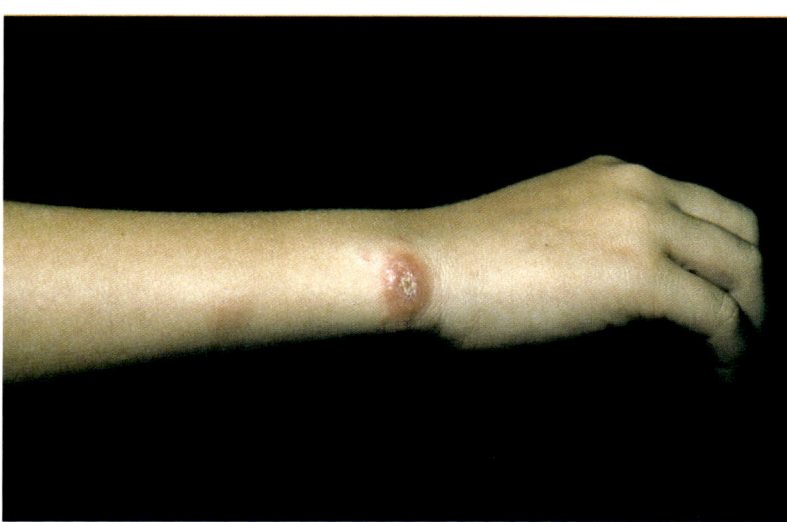

Fig. 24.35   *M. marinum* infection. Swimming pool granuloma (courtesy R. Hansen).

because saturated potassium iodide solution, which treats sporotrichosis effectively, will worsen *M. marinum* infections. Most lesions are minimally tender or asymptomatic.

Left untreated, lesions usually heal with scarring in 1 to 3 years, but rare cases have persisted for as long as 17 years. It is important to avoid incision and drainage of lesions to avoid deeper inoculation of the microbe.[580] Infections, although generally limited to skin, have extended more deeply, producing synovitis, bursitis, arthritis, draining sinuses, and osteomyelitis.[576,579] Disseminated cutaneous *M. marinum* infection is exceedingly rare, and may respond to aggressive therapy.[585]

Differential diagnosis

Lupus vulgaris, primary inoculation tuberculosis, and sporotrichosis may need to be excluded. The diagnosis is supported by histopathology but is best established by positive culture.

Histologic examination reveals a granulomatous dermatitis with diffuse epithelioid cell reaction and tubercle formation, with fibrinoid changes present more often than caseation necrosis. Langerhans giant cells are often but not always present.[586,587]

Sparse intracellular acid-fast bacilli are larger and longer than typical *M. tuberculosis*.[576] Increased sensitivity may be obtained with auramine-rhodamine stain, which causes acid-fast organisms to fluoresce under ultraviolet light. In some series, a positive culture was obtained in 70% of cases. Intradermal testing with PPD may be positive, especially if PPD-S (derived from *M. tuberculosis*) or PPD-Y (derived from photochromogens) is used. Considerable cross-reaction occurs; thus, this test can only be supportive but not diagnostic of infection.[579,588]

Management

Historically, treatment modalities have included curettage and excision to debulk infections, and warm compresses or heating pad application, because of the known inhibition of cultures of *M. marinum* by heating to 35–37°C. Traditional antituberculosis therapy with isoniazid, para-aminosalicylic acid, and streptomycin is ineffective.[577,589] Other antibiotic therapy which enjoyed some success included use of tetracycline,[580,591,592] minocycline,[592] doxycycline (in children age 8 years or older), rifampin, and ethambutol.[582,593]

Sulfamethoxazole, cotrimoxazole, trimethoprim-sulfamethoxazole,[583] or clarithromycin may also be used. All are known to have been successful if used for 2 to 3 months. When cases are unresponsive to antibiotic therapy, surgical excision can still be helpful.[579] In general, the prognosis for resolution of the lesions, particularly with proper treatment, is good, although rare reports of disseminated disease exist.[585]

If cases can be attributed to a specific swimming pool, public health authorities should be notified. The pool should be drained, cleaned, and then adequately chlorinated.

MYCOBACTERIA ULCERANS

Although extremely rare in the United States, cutaneous infections as a result of *M. ulcerans* are endemic in parts of Mexico, Africa, Asia and Australia.[594] The exact mode of transmission and the reservoir of this infection are not known[594–596] but Muelder and Nonrou[595] suggest that person-to-person transmission is possible, given the high prevalence of familial infections. Their observations suggest that this may, however, reflect common familial environmental exposures including trauma and scratches from prickly grass.

Clinical findings

M. ulcerans most frequently affects children aged 5–8 years in Africa and Australia and presents initially as a pruritic, firm, subcutaneous nodule or a painless boil on an exposed area, especially the leg or head and neck. It usually follows a thorn or grass scrape by about 3 weeks.[570] The preulcerative or nodular stage is followed by resolution, or the lesion develops into an abscess and breaks down, resulting in a shallow ulcer with a necrotic base and deep undermined edge. These are often called a Buruli ulcer in Africa or a Bairnsdale ulcer in Australia. The ulcers usually enlarge and deepen, involve fat, and are slow to heal, taking 6 to 9 months as a rule. The organism is plentiful in ulcerative lesions and easily isolated from tissues. Many relapse and develop ulcerations intermittently over a 3–4-year period. Affected patients may display satellite lesions and multiple cutaneous lesions in varying concurrent states of evolution. Lymphadenopathy typically is absent and patients are nonreactive to the Burulin *M. ulcerans* skin reagent test. The skin adjacent to the lesions is often hyperpigmented and shiny. The ulcer may slowly resolve during the third or reactive stage of the illness, and anergy to the Burulin test resolves. On biopsy, organisms are found to decrease in number in the lesions, and granulomas and mononuclear cell infiltrates increase in the lesions. Finally, the ulcers may heal with fibrosis and dense scarring, which may result in limb contractures.

Histologic changes vary with the clinical progress of the lesion. Early lesions display epidermal and dermal necrosis, with abundant organisms known as globi, but little cellular reaction. There is epidermal thinning at the edge of the ulcer as the process extends. Later, biopsies show destruction and fragmentation of dermal collagen and elastin, septal panniculitis, and a leukocytoclastic vasculitis of small and medium-sized vessels; a histiocytic infiltrate with Langerhans giant cells is also reported. Multiple organisms may still be present.[594]

The diagnosis should be suspected in any patient with an abscess or slow-healing ulcer who has traveled to endemic areas. Biopsies revealing clusters of acid-fast bacteria are helpful, but culture of the organism, although difficult, is the "gold standard" of diagnosis.

Treatment

Enthusiasm for antibiotic and surgical therapy varies widely in different reports.[595–598] Therapy may include hyperthermia to take advantage of the

591. Kim R (1974) Tetracycline therapy for atypical mycobacterial granuloma. **Arch Dermatol** 110:299.
592. Loria PO (1976) Minocycline hydrochloride treatment for atypical acid-fast infections. **Arch Dermatol** 112:517.
593. Wolinsky E, Gomez F, Zimpfer F (1972) Sporotrichoid *Mycobacterium marinum* infections treated with rifampin-ethambutol. **Am Rev Respir Dis** 105:964.
594. Hayman J, Mc Queen A (1985) The pathology of *Mycobacterium ulcerans* infection. **Pathology** 17:594.

595. Muelder K, Nourou A (1990) Buruli ulcer in Benin. **Lancet** 336:1109.
596. Van der Werf TS, Van der graat WT, Groutuis DG et al. (1989) Buruli ulcer in West Africa, *Mycobacterium ulcerans* infection in Ashanti Region, Ghana. **Trans R Soc Trop Med Hyg** 83:410.
597. Alsop D (1972) The Bairnsdale ulcer. **NZ J Surg** 41:317.
598. Song M, Vinke G, Vanachler H et al. (1985) Treatment of cutaneous infection due to *Mycobacterium ulcerans*. **Dermatologica** 171:197.

heat sensitivity of *M. ulcerans*. Surgical debridement or excision of nodules or ulcers and grafting has aided in the treatment, especially of early lesions. Antibiotics utilized include rifampin, trimethoprim-sulfamethoxazole, and minocycline INH, streptomycin, dapsone, and ethambutal and clofazamine, in various combinations, have also been reported to be helpful.

A certain therapeutic nihilism is evidenced by some clinicians dealing with this illness in Africa because they allege that therapeutic optimism is due to a lack of adequate follow-up.[595] The disease causes great morbidity in endemic areas, as most ulcerations heal with significant scarring within 9 to 12 months. Serious complications, however, including limb contractures, invasion of the orbit and loss of an eye, osteomyelitis, and dissemination, appear to be rare.[570,595]

CUTANEOUS INFECTIONS CAUSED BY RAPIDLY GROWING NONTUBERCULOSIS MYCOBACTERIA: *M. CHELONEI*, *M. FORTUITUM*, *M. SMEGMATIS* AND *M. ABSCESSUS*

Cutaneous infections caused by the rapidly growing NTM, *M. chelonei*, *M. fortuitum*, and *M. smegmatis*, often follow accidental or iatrogenic trauma.[599,600] Most of the lesions reported have been localized and have followed minor or severe skin trauma, such as puncture wounds. Outbreaks of several cases have followed immunizations and even plastic surgery where the marking liquid, gentian violet, was contaminated by *M. chelonei*.[601] The incubation period between the injury and the appearance of skin lesions is usually from 4 to 6 weeks but may be as long as 12 months.[570]

CLINICAL FINDINGS

Skin infections are varied and include single or multiple abscesses, which may or may not drain, tender nodules, localized cellulitis, granulomatous nodules, sporotrichoid lesions, and scrofuloderma.[602–605] Postsurgical infections have been reported after augmentation mammoplasty, median sternotomy, and even the placement of intravenous catheters. In these cases, poor wound healing was noted and followed by the development of sinus tracts and persistent seropurulent drainage. Dissemination and systemic illness are rare, but reported complications of skin infections caused by these rapidly growing species include osteomyelitis, mediastinitis, pericarditis, endocarditis, postoperative vasculitis, and disseminated disease.[606]

THERAPY

Treatment includes surgical debridement of lesions when appropriate, especially incision and drainage and packing of abscesses. Isolates should be tested for susceptibility to antituberculous agents. Other antibiotics reported to be successful include concurrent amikacin and cefoxitin with probenecid followed by erythromycin, ciprofloxacin, oral sulfonamide,[606] clarithromycin, doxycycline or minocycline for 4–6 weeks after wound healing is accomplished. The latter agents are appropriate only in children older than 8 years of age and in adult patients. Imipenim may be effective, and clari-

thromycin and orofloxin both have been successful in long-term monotherapy for these skin infections;[570] however, clarithromycin plus at least one other agent is the treatment of choice for cutaneous infection due to *M. chelonei*.

MYCOBACTERIUM KANSASII

M. kansasii, like *M. marinum*, is a photochromogen. Its major reservoir is thought to be soil, but it may also be water- or milk-borne.[607] It has, on rare occasions, been recovered from cattle and swine. Distributed worldwide, it is an important opportunistic infection in temperate regions. It primarily causes lung disease, which mimics tuberculosis in older male patients with underlying pulmonary problems.

Involvement of children, although rare, does occur. It has been recovered from a wide range of cutaneous lesions, including those resembling cellulitis. It has also been recovered from verrucous papules and nodules and indurated plaques, crusted papules and ulcerations, crusted pyodermatous plaques of the scalp (which resembled a kerion), necrotic papulopustules, and sporotrichoid infections. Immunocompromised patients appear more vulnerable to these infections.[608–610]

The diagnosis of this pathogen requires skin biopsy and culture of the organism from the affected tissue, preferably more than once. It has been successfully treated with a variety of antibiotics, although cure has usually required high doses of isoniazid, rifampin, and ethambutol for 12–24 months or amikacin, sulfonamides, and/or minocycline in children older than age 8 years.[611]

M. AVIUM COMPLEX

M. avium and *M. intracellulare* compose the *Mycobacterium avium* complex (MAC). These mycobacteria have been isolated from soil, water, birds, animals, and foods, are distributed worldwide and apparently colonize large segments of many populations. For example they are commonly recovered from adolescents and young adults with cystic fibrosis. In the United States, the greatest number of symptomatic infections occur in the southeast. Most common in men and in rural settings, they are a common cause of bronchopulmonary disease and may be a cause of lymphadenitis and osteomyelitis in children and adults. Cutaneous lesions, although very uncommon in the past, have been seen more frequently, especially in immunosuppressed individuals, as MAC has emerged as an important opportunistic infection in patients with AIDS,[612] in whom severe pulmonary disease and dissemination may occur.

CLINICAL FINDINGS

Cutaneous MAC lesions include rare primary inoculation papules or ulcers, are disseminated maculopapules and nodules, which are somewhat reminiscent of miliary lesions,[613] abscesses, ulcers, panniculitis,[585] and sporotrichoid lesions (Fig. 24.36). Cutaneous dissemination is most often associated with underlying pulmonary disease.

599. Hamrick HJ, Maddeix DW, Lowrey EK et al. (1984) *Mycobacterium chelonei*: facial abscess. **Pediatr Infect Dis** 3:335.
600. Subbarao EK, Tarpay MM, Marks MI (1987) Soft tissue infections caused by *Mycobacterium fortuitum* complex following penetrating injury. **Am J Dis Child** 141:1018.
601. Safranck TJ, Jarvis WR, Carson LA et al. (1987) *Mycobacterium chelonei* wound infections after plastic surgery, employing contaminated gentian violet solution. **N Engl J Med** 317:197.
602. Wallace RJ Jr, Swenson JM, Silcox VA et al. (1983) Spectrum of disease due to rapidly growing mycobacteria. **Rev Infect Dis** 5:657.
603. Greer KE, Gross GP, Marlensen SH (1979) Sporotrichoid cutaneous infection due to *M. chelonei*. **Arch Dermatol** 115:738.
604. Wallace RJ Jr, Nash DR, Tsukamura M et al. (1988) Human disease due to *Mycobacterium smegmatis*. **J Infect Dis** 158:52.
605. Hand WL, Sandford JP (1970) *Mycobacterium fortuitum*: a human pathogen. **Ann Intern Med** 73:971.

606. Tice AD, Soloman RJ (1979) Disseminated *Mycobacterium chelonei* infection. **Am Rev Respir Dis** 205:97.
607. Chapman JS, Speight M (1968) Isolation of Mycobacteria from pasteurized milk. **Am Rev Resp Dis** 98:1052.
608. Hanke CW, Temofew RK, Slama SL (1987) *Mycobacterium kansasii* infection with multiple cutaneous lesions. **J Am Acad Dermatol** 16:1122.
609. Mayberry JD, Mullins JF, Slone OJ (1963) Cutaneous infection due to *Mycobacterium kansasii*. **JAMA** 194:1135.
610. Owens DW, Mc Bride ME (1969) Sporotrichoid cutaneous infection with *Mycobacterium kansasii*. **Arch Dermatol** 100:54.
611. Dore N, Collins JP, Manliewiez E (1979) A sporotrichoid like *M. kansasii* infection of the skin treated with minocycline hydrochloride. **Br J Dermatol** 101:75.
612. Kaplan MH, Sadik N, McNutt NS et al. (1987) Dermatologic findings and manifestations of acquired immunodeficiency. **J Am Acad Dermatol** 16:485.
613. Lugo-James G, Curz A, Sanchez JL (1990) Disseminated cutaneous infection caused by *Mycobacterium avium* complex (letter). **Arch Dermatol** 126:1108.

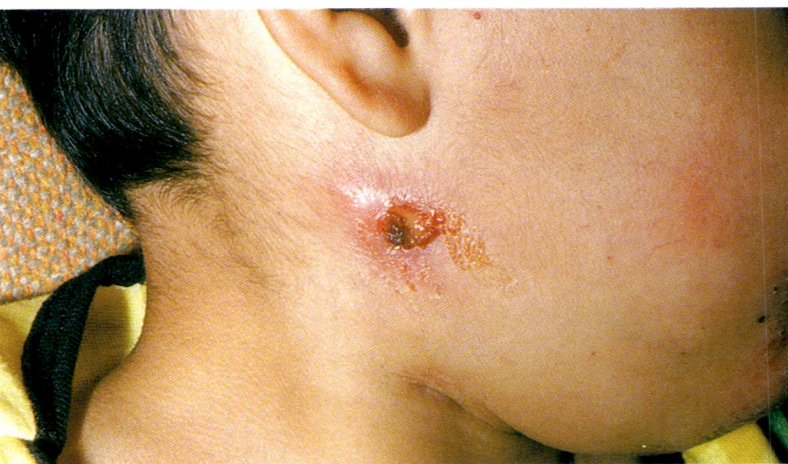

Fig. 24.36   Atypical mycobacterial infection due to *M. avium* complex organism.

THERAPY

Complete excision of lesions of MAC lymphadenitis is generally effective. Treatment of MAC infections, even with multiple drugs, was notoriously difficult in the past. Combinations including INH, ethambutol, rifampin and clofazimine, streptomycin, and amikacin have enjoyed some successes. The armamentarium for MAC has been greatly strengthened by the development of the new macrolide antibiotics clarithromycin and azithromycin. Clarithromycin is effective in doses of 100 to 200mg po bid over weeks to months in suppressing and or curing these infections.[570] It is also used as effective prophylaxis in immunosuppressed patients.[570]

MISCELLANEOUS NONTUBERCULOSIS MYCOBACTERIAL INFECTIONS

Reports of cutaneous infections from other mycobacteria exist. *M. gordonaie* caused an indurated nodular lesion of the dorsum of the hand in a case reported by Shelley et al.[614] Gross et al. reported cutaneous ulcerations and underlying osteomyelitis in an immunosuppressed man due to *M. szulzai*.[615]

To deal with these infections requires a thorough workup including biopsy, cultures and antituberculous drug sensitivity testing where possible. Many cases require a multiple-drug regimen for cure.

Many NTM are relatively resistant *in vitro* to antituberculosis drugs. *In vitro* resistance, however, does not necessarily correlate with clinical response. Only limited controlled therapeutic trials have been performed in patients with NTM infections. The approach to therapy should be dictated by the following: (1) the species causing the infection; (2) the results of drug susceptibility testing; (3) the site(s) of infection; (4) the patient's underlying disease (if any); and (5) the need to treat a patient presumptively for tuberculosis while awaiting culture reports that subsequently reveal NTM.

Isolates of rapid-growing mycobacteria (*M. fortuitum*, *M. abscessus*, and *M. chelonei*) should be tested *in vitro* against antituberculosis agents, as well as against other drugs (such as amikacin, imipinem, cefoxitin, ciprofloxacin, clarithromycin, and doxycycline) to which they frequently are susceptible and that have been used with some success. Details about choice of drugs, dosages, and duration should be reviewed with a consultant experienced in the management of these infections.

HANSEN'S DISEASE (LEPROSY)

HISTORY

History tells us that those afflicted with Hansen's disease have been inhumanely treated for many centuries. People with this illness have suffered exclusion from society, school, work, and family; once the diagnosis was made, these people carried it with them until they died. Unfortunately, many of the misunderstandings that precipitated this ostracism persist today.

Works by Dharmendra in India and Hua in China dating from about 500 BC yield authentic descriptions of the illness. Experts doubt that recorded descriptions of Hansen's disease existed in the Middle East before this period. The illness may have been brought west by the Persian conquerors of Greece in the 4th century BC and by the soldiers of Alexander the Great one century later. By contrast, experts believe that neither Aristotle nor Hippocrates encountered the illness. The disease was clearly prevalent in Europe between AD 1000 and AD 1400, and it may have been brought to the New World by sailors with Columbus, and later by slaves from West Africa. Worldwide distribution was achieved through the travels of explorers and immigrants.[616]

EPIDEMIOLOGY

Currently, the World Health Organization estimates that there are 5.5 million cases of Hansen's disease in the world,[617] a considerable reduction from the fairly constant global estimate of 10 to 12 million from the mid-1960s to the mid-1980s. This downward trend is ascribed to a reduced prevalence as a result of multidrug therapy. It is possible that there may be some reversal, however, with the appearance of leprosy in the setting of AIDS.[618]

Hansen's disease is found in almost every country but is most prevalent in India, Southeast Asia, and China (73%); it is also found, however, in Central and East Africa (12%) and the Americas (8%).[618,619] Although it is mainly a tropical disease today, it has flourished in temperate climates in the past and still exists in the colder areas of Japan and China. The areas of greatest prevalence are also those where the standard of living is low. Crowding, poor sanitation, and malnutrition all appear to increase the risk of contracting the disease.[620]

In the United States, there are at present more than 6000 known cases; 241 new cases were detected in 1989, considerably fewer than the 445 new cases reported in 1985.[621] Only 12% of these 241 patients were born in the United States. New cases are primarily seen in recent arrivals from Mexico, the Philippines, and Southeast Asia. Most cases in the United States are found in Hawaii, California, Texas, Louisiana, Florida, and New York City. A few indigenous cases are regularly diagnosed in gulf coast states including Louisiana and Texas.

The gender incidence depends on the type of disease. The lepromatous form is almost twice as common in males as in females, whereas tuberculoid leprosy occurs equally in males and females. In children, in whom lepromatous leprosy is rare, the gender incidence is approximately equal.

Some experts believe that children are more susceptible to Hansen's disease than adults with similar exposure. Overall, the spouse of a patient with leprosy appears to be less likely to contract the disease than the children. The number of cases found in children aged 0 to 14 years depends in large part on the degree of exposure to people with multibacillary disease; however, Hansen's disease is rare in children younger than 2 years of age in most areas.[622] Where the gross prevalence rate of the disease is high, however, the age-specific prevalence rate in children 0 to 14 years of age can exceed 4.0%.[623]

614. Shelley WB, Folkens AJ (1984) *Mycobacterium gordonae* infection of the hand. **Arch Dermatol** 120:1064.
615. Gross GM, Cecil MA, Aton JK (1985) Cutaneous *Mycobacterium szulgai* infection. **Arch Dermatol** 121:247.
616. Trautman JR (1984) A brief history of Hansen's disease. **Bull NY Acad Med** 60:659.
617. Noordeen SK, Lopez Bravo L, Sundaresan TK (1992) Estimated number of leprosy cases in the world. **Bull World Health Organ** 70:7.
618. Miller RA (1991) Leprosy and AIDS: a review of the literature and speculations on the impact of CD4+ lymphocyte depletion on immunity to *Mycobacterium leprae* (editorial). **Int J Lepr Other Mycobact Dis** 59:639.
619. Meyers WM (1998) Leprosy. In: Textbook of Pediatric Infectious Disease, 4th edn. Feigin RD, Cherry JD, eds. Philadelphia: WB Saunders, pp. 1149–1166.
620. Trautman JR (1984) Epidemiologic aspects of Hansen's disease. **Bull New York Acad Med** 60:722.
621. Jacobsen RR (1990) The face of leprosy in the United States today (editorial). **Arch Dermatol** 126:1627.
622. Kaur I, Kaur S, Sharma VK et al. (1991) Childhood leprosy in Northern India. **Pediatr Dermatol** 8:21.
623. Nossitou FM, Sansarrica H, Walter J (1976) Leprosy in children. Geneva: World Health Organization.

ETIOLOGY AND PATHOGENESIS

Hansen's disease is caused by *Mycobacterium leprae*, an acid-fast bacillus which is more weakly acid-fast than other mycobacteria so that pyridine can extract the stain.[619] Although Koch's postulates have not been fulfilled for the bacillus, the work of Shepard[624] with mouse footpads, the armadillo experiments of Kirchheimer and Storrs,[625] and more recent work with primates[626] leave few doubts. The bacillus multiplies slowly and tends to localize in cooler parts of the body. It produces a chronic infectious disease primarily affecting the skin, superficial segments of the peripheral nerves, the upper respiratory tract, and the testes.[619]

The usual mode of transmission of Hansen's disease is uncertain, but current theory supports an upper respiratory route of entry into the body.[621] Rare instances of accidental transmission during surgical procedures and tattooing have been reported.[627] In areas in which Hansen's disease is endemic, skin lesions may follow trauma, impetigo, or insect bites.[628] Transplacental infection is also possible,[629] and infected breast milk may be a source for some infants.[630]

Hansen's disease may also be a zoonosis, as naturally occuring infection, histologically indistinguishable from human Hansen's, has been found in monkeys[631] in West Africa and chimpanzees in Sierra Leone.[632] Though there has been no evidence of transmission from these two species, there is evidence to support transmission from infected armadillos to humans in both Texas and Louisiana.[631]

More than 90% of the world's population is believed to be immune to Hansen's disease, but it appears that pockets of people with increased susceptibility exist. Experience at The Gillis W. Long Hansen's Disease Center at Carville, LA, suggests that clinical disease seldom occurs in health care workers assigned to Hansen's disease hospitals or in family contacts of infected patients in the United States.[620] A contrary experience has been noted, however, in Hawaii and on the island of Malulu off the coast of New Guinea.[633]

The role of host immunity in the pathogenesis of Hansen's disease remains unclear. *M. leprae* causes disease by surviving and multiplying in macrophages. Susceptibility seems to depend on the individual having a relatively specific defect in their cell-mediated immune response to *M. leprae*, but the exact nature of this defect and whether its origin is acquired or genetic remain to be clarified.[621] Whether genetic or acquired, there are significant differences in the immune response to *M. leprae* among those least affected with the tuberculoid form of the disease compared to those most severely affected with lepromatous disease. Patients with tuberculoid leprosy develop positive skin reactions of 5mm or larger to the lepromin skin test at three to four weeks. They retain normal circulating T cells and suppressor T cells, and granulomas tend to have central helper cells and peripheral or marginal suppressor cells. They have normal B-cell levels and only slight increases in immunoglobulins, and are able to clear leprae bacilli from macrophages.[619]

In contrast, patients with the more severe lepromatous expression of Hansen's disease have a negative or minimal reaction to the Mitsuda test of 2mm or less in diameter. They have decreased helper T-cell lymphocytes and increased suppressor lymphocytes. Their circulating B cells are often increased as are their immunoglobulin levels, and they clear *M. leprae* infected macrophages poorly. Their macrophages may become activated and their function partially restored if exposed to interleukin-2 and/or interferon-γ.[619]

There is evidence that, once infection has occurred, expression of disease may be genetically controlled. This is supported by observations of the disease in identical and fraternal twins, showing that disease was similar in the former.[634]

CLINICAL FINDINGS

The duration of the latent period of infection is unknown. Most experts believe it is, on average, 3 to 5 years. Recently, however, Brubaker *et al.*[635] reported on 91 infants younger than 1 year of age in whom leprosy had been diagnosed. In other unusual instances, the latency period appeared to be more than 15 years. Prodromal symptoms are rarely identifiable and are of no diagnostic significance.

Ridley and Jopling[236] have classified the disease into five groups along a spectrum of declining cell-mediated immune responsiveness to the infecting organism. These groups are tuberculoid, borderline tuberculoid, mid-borderline, borderline lepromatous, and lepromatous. Although classification in the field is often limited to "paucibacillary" and "multibacillary" categories, this original schema remains very useful. An initial transient indeterminate stage is also described in those whose immunologic status has not yet been determined.

INDETERMINATE LEPROSY

This presents as one or a small number of macules which are hypopigmented and erythematous (Fig. 24.37). They are rarely larger than 12cm, and most often are oval with poorly defined margins and a smooth surface. There is no sensory impairment, there are no thickened nerves, and hair growth is intact. Lesions occur most commonly on the face and limbs.

TUBERCULOID LEPROSY

In tuberculoid disease, lesions are few in number or, more often, solitary. The lesion is usually an infiltrated plaque, erythematous or violaceous in color, with raised and well-demarcated edges and a flatter center. Later, lesions may be hyperpigmented (Fig. 24.38). Satelite lichenoid papules occasionally occur nearby. Hair growth and sensation (except on the face) are lost within the lesion because of damage to nerves. The surface is dry and sometimes scaly.

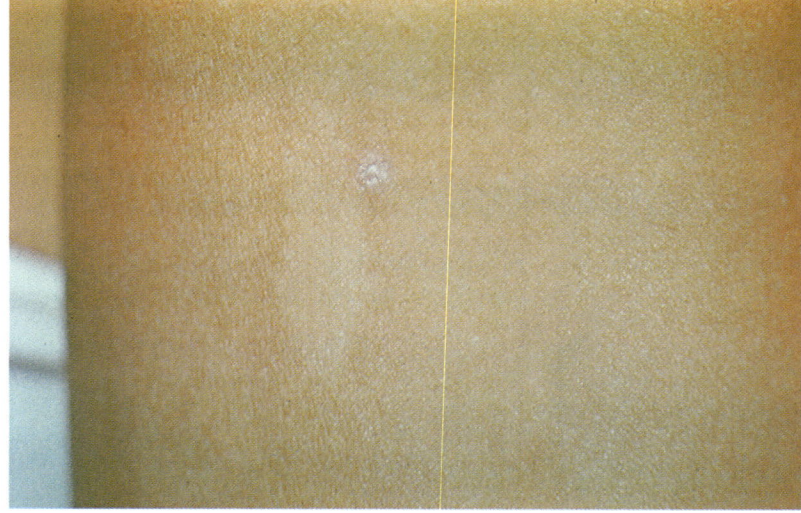

Fig. 24.37 **Indeterminate leprosy** (courtesy US Public Health Service Hospital, Carville, LA).

624. Shepard CC (1960) The experimental disease that follows the injection of human leprosy bacilli into the foot pads of mice. **J Exp Med** 112:445.
625. Kirchheimer WF, Storrs EE (1971) Attempts to establish the armadillo (*Dasypus novemcintus*) as a model for the study of leprosy. Report of lepromatoid leprosy in an experimentally infected armadillo. **Int J Lepr Other Mycobct Dis** 39:692.
626. Meyers WM, Walsh GP, Brown HL et al. (1980) Naturally acquired leprosy in a mangabay monkey. **Int J Lepr Other Mycobact Dis** 48:495.
627. Porritt RJ, Olsen RE (1947) Two simultaneous cases of leprosy developing in tattoos. **Am J Pathol** 23:805.
628. Kirchheimer WF (1073) The role of arthropods in the transmission of leprosy. **Lepr India** 45:29.
629. Meyer WM (1992) **Leprosy. Dermatol Clin** 10:73.
630. Pedley JC (1967) The presence of *M. leprae* in human milk. **Lepr Rev** 38:239–242.

631. Walsh GD, Meyers WM, Binford CH et al. (1988) Leprosy as a zoonosis: an update. **Acta Leprol** 6:51–60.
632. Donham KJ, Leuriger JR (1977) Spontaneous leprosy-like disease in a chimpanzee. **J Infect Dis** 136:132–136.
633. Spickett SG (1964) Genetic mechanisms in leprosy. In: Leprosy in Theory and Practice, 2nd ed, Cochrane RG, Davey TF, eds. Baltimore: Williams & Wilkins, p. 98.
634. Ali PM, Ramanujam K (1964) Genetics and leprosy: a study of leprosy in twins. **Lepr India** 37:77.
635. Brubaker ML, Meyers MW, Bourland J (1985) Leprosy in children one year of age and under. **Int J Lepr Other Mycobact Dis** 53:517.
636. Ridley DS, Jopling WH (1966) Classification of leprosy according to immunity: a five group system. **Int J Lepr Other Mycobact Dis** 34:255.

COMPLICATIONS

Leprosy reactions are episodes of immunologically mediated inflammation, which are acute in onset and can lead to considerable tissue damage. Reactions are much less frequent in childhood than in adults. The type I or lepra reaction occurs in borderline disease and may be associated with upgrading (improvement) or downgrading (worsening) of the patient's cell-mediated immune status. Serious acute-onset nerve damage is a major complication, particularly associated with upgrading or reversal reactions occurring during therapy. Type II reactions, of which erythema nodosum leprosum is the most common manifestation, occur in multibacillary disease, usually in response to treatment, and produce tissue injury more insidiously.[621] Paresis, paralysis, and neurotropic changes are rare in childhood leprosy.

PREVENTION

While the search for a specific and effective vaccine against Hansen's disease continues, preventive efforts are at present largely based on the effective use of chemotherapy to render multibacillary cases noninfectious.

PEDIATRIC PROBLEMS

Because children often lack the conspicious signs popularly associated with Hansen's disease, it is often difficult for parents and physician alike to accept the diagnosis. Such a diagnosis carries profound psychosocial impact. Adequate periods must be allotted for discussions of the ramifications of the disease, and with the family, treatment should be arranged at facilities where separate sites are used for people with advanced disease and those in the early stages of disease. Health education should stress that well-looking children may have Hansen's disease, that few children suffer from contagious forms, that the prognosis is excellent, and that there is a need to examine household contacts of children with the disease. Because childhood Hansen's disease is difficult to detect, regular examination of school children should be considered in those countries where the prevalence is greater than 5 per 1000.[623]

TREATMENT

Therapy for patients with leprosy should be undertaken in consultation with an expert in leprosy. The Gillis W. Long Hansen's Disease Center, Carville, LA (800-642-2477), provides consultation on clinical and pathologic issues and can provide information about local Hansen's disease clinics and clinicians who have experience with the disease.

Dapsone, one of the primary drugs used in the treatment of leprosy, usually is administered in a dosage of 100mg/day for adults and 1mg/kg/day for children. Persons in high-risk groups for glucose-6-phosphate dehydrogenase deficiency should be tested for this disorder before administration. To reduce the risk of drug resistance and possibly shorten the duration of therapy, multidrug therapy is necessary for all patients. Rifampin (600mg/day for adults or 10mg/kg/day for children) should be given with dapsone for 1 year for paucibacillary (indeterminate, tuberculoid, and borderline tuberculoid) disease, with close follow-up to detect relapses. Clofazimine (50mg/day for adults or 1mg/kg/day for children) should be added for multibacillary (borderline, borderline lepromatous, and lepromatous) disease and continued for at least 2 years. Other drugs, including ofloxacin, sparfloxacin, minocycline, and clarithromycin, have activity against *M. leprae* and could be considered for therapy for patients with intolerance to routine drugs or with drug-resistant infections. All clinically compatible patients with demonstrable acid-fast bacilli on skin biopsy specimens or smears should be treated for presumptive multibacillary leprosy.

Corticosteroids are used to treat erythema nodosum leprosum (ENL), which commonly occurs in patients with multibacillary disease after drug therapy is initiated. Occasionally, ENL occurs in untreated patients as well. Treatment with short-term, high-dose corticosteroids followed by maintenance thalidomide, often is useful for managing severe or recurrent ENL reactions. Thalidomide should never be given to a woman of childbearing age unless she is using a reliable means of contraception. Other agents, including clofazimine, also can be used to treat ENL.

The reversal reaction, seen primarily in patients with borderline disease, is characterized by delayed-type hypersensitivity reactions at the site of current or former leprosy lesions and acute neuropathies. These conditions require aggressive treatment with corticosteroids to avoid permanent neurologic sequelae.

Most patients can be treated as outpatients. Rehabilitative measures, including surgery and physical therapy, may be necessary for some patients.

Viral Infections

Anthony J. Mancini and Christine Bodemer

VIRAL EXANTHEMS

Anthony J. Mancini

An "exanthem" is defined as a skin eruption occurring as a symptom of a general disease, usually an infectious process.[1] Viral exanthems in children can present a diagnostic challenge for even the most seasoned of clinicians. In the early 1900s, exanthems were assigned and referred to by number, in the order in which they were clinically characterized. The initial six diseases named according to this system have been termed the "classic childhood exanthems." In this nomenclature, measles (rubeola) and scarlet fever were designated as "first" and "second" disease, and rubella as "third" disease. "Fourth" disease, also known as Dukes disease, has lost acceptance as a distinct entity and may have represented cases of misdiagnosed scarlet fever or rubella.[2] Erythema infectiosum became known as "fifth" disease and roseola infantum as "sixth" disease.[3] This numerical classification system eventually became obsolete with the advent of tissue culture techniques, which permitted the identification of many "new" viral agents as causes of exanthematous illnesses.[4] Recognition and clarification of the childhood exanthems continues to be an evolving field, with advances and recent developments the main focus of several recent review articles.[5-7]

Exanthems in children are extremely common, and their expression ranges from nonspecific rashes to eruptions with distinct lesional morphology and/or distribution. The large number of potential agents and the morphologic similarities of many exanthems can make specific etiologic diagnoses difficult, if not impossible, in some cases. Although the majority of viral exanthems are part of a self-limited illness, they may be associated with disorders of potentially serious consequence to the patient or exposed contacts, and thus rapid recognition and accurate diagnosis are vital. This may include such settings as evaluation of an exanthem in the contact of a pregnant female or an immunocompromised individual, or situations in which isolation of patients or immunization of exposed individuals might be necessary to prevent epidemic outbreaks. It is also important to distinguish viral exanthems from other more potentially severe and treatable infections, such as bacterial or rickettsial processes, and from exanthematous illnesses requiring the immediate institution of therapy, such as Kawasaki disease. Finally, in children who are taking one or more oral medications, differentiation of a viral exanthem from a drug reaction can be very difficult, and can lead to uncertainty in terms of appropriate counselling regarding future administration of the potentially offending agent(s).

TABLE 25.1 Assessment of the child with an exanthem
History
Season
Exposure history
Local epidemiology
Incubation history
Age of the patient
Past medical history
Immunization history
History of prodromal symptoms
Progression of exanthem
Associated enanthem
Medication history
Associated symptoms/review of systems
Physical examination
Vital signs, especially temperature
Rash: morphology, distribution
Mucous membranes (enanthem)
Eyes, ears, nose and pharynx
Lymph nodes
Neck (meningismus)
Heart, lungs, liver and spleen
Edema (facial or extremities)
Neurologic examination

Adapted from Cherry JD, 1983,[412] Esterly NB, 1984.[413]

Evaluation of the child presenting with an exanthem should include a thorough history and physical examination, with a focus on variables that are most likely to be useful in narrowing the differential diagnosis (Table 25.1). Examination for an associated "enanthem," or eruption of the mucous membranes, should always be performed and may guide the clinician toward a specific diagnosis (i.e., Koplik's spots in measles or Forschheimer's spots in rubella). Certain laboratory examinations, such as cultures of the throat and blood, complete blood cell count with differential, and urine or cerebrospinal fluid testing for bacterial antigens, may help to exclude bacterial disease. Viral cultures, fluorescent antibody tests, and specific viral serologic examinations may be useful in some cases. Skin biopsy is, in most cases, nonspecific and of little value in the evaluation of an exanthem.

1. Stedman's Medical Dictionary, 22nd ed. (1972) Baltimore: Williams & Wilkins.
2. Morens DM, Katz AR (1991) The "fourth disease" of childhood: reevaluation of a non-existent disease. Am J Epidemiol 134:628–640.
3. Bialecki C, Feder HM, Grant-Kels JM (1989) The six classic childhood exanthems: a review and update. J Am Acad Dermatol 21:891–903.
4. Cherry JD (1993) Contemporary infectious exanthems. Clin Infect Dis 16:199–207.
5. Resnick SD (1997) New aspects of exanthematous diseases of childhood. Dermatol Clin 15:257–266.
6. Mancini AJ (2000) Childhood exanthems: a primer and update for the dermatologist. Adv Dermatol 16:3–37.
7. Nelson JSB, Stone MS (2000) Update on selected viral exanthems. Curr Opin Pediatr 12:359–364.

While the exact pathogenesis of viral exanthems remains unclear, at least three mechanisms appear to play a role. First, direct invasion of the skin by way of the bloodstream may produce a rash, even in the absence of host immune factors. This mechanism typically results in vesicular or ulcerative lesions, such as those seen in varicella, herpes simplex, variola, vaccinia, and certain enteroviral infections. Second, viruses present in skin may react with circulating or cell-mediated immune factors, resulting in an exanthem. This mechanism is likely to account for the majority of viral rashes. Third, circulating immune factors may cause cutaneous abnormalities without the actual presence of virus or viral antigens in the skin. This mechanism may be at play in some cases of urticaria, erythema multiforme, and Stevens–Johnson syndrome.

Some features of childhood exanthems remain poorly understood. These include host susceptibility patterns, distinct morphologic characteristics of some exanthematous lesions, and the propensity for the lesions associated with some disorders to localize to certain anatomic locations (i.e., the palms and soles in hand-foot-and-mouth disease). Another frequently observed but poorly understood pattern is that of localization of viral exanthem (i.e., acute varicella) lesions to sites of inflammation or skin injury, including sunburn, casting, arthropod stings, trauma, and dermatitis.[8,9]

NONSPECIFIC VIRAL EXANTHEMS

A majority of childhood exanthems are nonspecific and cannot be accurately assigned to a discrete etiological diagnosis. These eruptions lack unique defining characteristics, such as specific lesional morphology, natural course, distribution, and associated enanthema or symptom complex. These exanthems are usually self-limited, resolving spontaneously over one week without long-term sequelae, and require only symptomatic therapy. Exanthems have been divided on the basis of morphology into erythematous, vesicular and papular types, with occasional pustular or petechial variants.[10] The erythematous type is most common, and nonspecific exanthems usually fall into this category, presenting with blanchable erythematous macules and papules, distributed diffusely on the trunk (Fig. 25.1) and extremities. Nonspecific associated symptoms may include low-grade fever, headache, myalgias, fatigue, and respiratory or gastrointestinal complaints.[11]

Multiple viral agents are capable of causing a nonspecific exanthem, including the nonpolio enteroviruses (i.e., coxsackievirus, echovirus, and enterovirus) and respiratory viruses (including rhinovirus, adenovirus, parainfluenza virus, respiratory syncytial virus, and influenza virus).[10,11] Epstein–Barr virus, human herpesvirus-6 (HHV-6) and human herpesvirus-7 (HHV-7), and parvovirus B19 may all result in nonspecific exanthems, but they are more frequently associated with specific exanthematous diseases as discussed subsequently in this chapter. In general, most nonspecific exanthems occurring during winter months are caused by respiratory viruses, and those occurring in the warmer months by the enteroviruses. Exanthems caused by the latter may at times mimic more serious bacterial exanthematous illnesses, and are discussed in more detail in the Enterovirus section.

MEASLES (RUBEOLA)

Measles, once a common childhood exanthem, is caused by a paramyxovirus, an RNA virus that is closely related to the canine distemper virus.[12] Humans are the natural hosts and only reservoir of the infection. Vaccination trials of

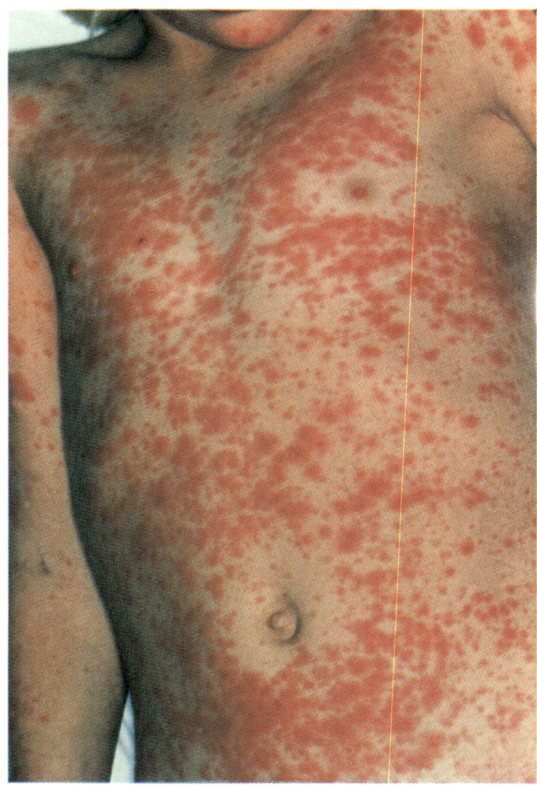

Fig. 25.1   Maculopapular exanthem due to adenovirus.

inactivated vaccine began in 1958, and attenuated measles vaccine became available for general use in 1963.[13]

EPIDEMIOLOGY

Despite the availability of an effective vaccine for over 35 years, measles continues to be a worldwide health burden, especially in developing countries. In the United States, where over 500 000 cases were reported annually in the prevaccine era,[14] the number of cases of measles infection decreased greatly after the introduction of a live-virus vaccine in 1963. However, a major resurgence of disease occurred in 1989–1990, and was associated with the highest morbidity and mortality since 1977.[14,15] Sixty percent of the reported deaths during this epidemic were among children < 5 years of age.[14] The most vulnerable populations during this resurgence were preschool-aged children from inner city regions, primarily unvaccinated, low-income patients, as well as vaccinated school-aged children and college students. Factors contributing to the vulnerability of these populations included low vaccine coverage (due to barriers to health care and immunization access) and lack of public awareness.[16] Insufficiency of a single dose of vaccine and waning immunity were other factors that increased the risk of infection.

A reevaluation of the measles immunization strategy, which at that time consisted of a single immunization at 15 months of age, was eventually performed. In December 1989, the US Public Health Service Advisory Committee on Immunization Practices (ACIP) recommended a routine two-

8. Belhorn TH, Lucky AW (1994) Atypical varicella exanthems associated with skin injury. Pediatr Dermatol 11:129–132.
9. Messner J, Miller JJ, James WD et al. (1999) Accentuated viral exanthems in areas of inflammation. J Am Acad Dermatol 40:345–346.
10. Hogan PA (1996) Viral exanthems in childhood. Aust J Dermatol 37:S14–S16.
11. Cherry JD, Jahn CL (1966) Virologic studies of exanthems. J Pediatr 68:204–214.
12. Gershon AA (2000) Measles virus (rubeola). In: Principles and Practice of Infectious Diseases, 5th ed, Mandell GL, Bennett JE, Dolin R, eds. Philadelphia: Churchill Livingstone, pp. 1801–1809.

13. Cherry JD (1998) Measles. In: Textbook of Pediatric Infectious Diseases, 4th ed, Feigin RD, Cherry JD, eds. Philadelphia: WB Saunders, pp. 2054–2074.
14. Atkinson WL, Orenstein WA, Krugman S (1992) The resurgence of measles in the United States, 1989–1990. Annu Rev Med 43:451–463.
15. Hutchins S, Markowitz L, Atkinson W et al. (1996) Measles outbreaks in the United States, 1987 through 1990. Pediatr Infect Dis J 15:31–38.
16. The National Vaccine Advisory Committee (1991) The measles epidemic. The problems, barriers and recommendations. JAMA 266:1547–1552.

dose vaccination schedule, and a change in the recommended age for the first dose from 15 months to 12 months in areas with significant measles morbidity in preschool-aged children.[17] The Committee on Infectious Diseases of the American Academy of Pediatrics (AAP) similarly adopted these recommendations, and the current recommended measles immunization strategy is a two-dose schedule with the first dose at 12–15 months and the second dose at 4–6 years of age.[18] These modified recommendations have clearly influenced the incidence of measles in the US, with a total of only 100 confirmed cases in 1998,[19] and again in 1999.[20] Cases continue to occur in the United States from importation of the virus from other countries, and of the 100 cases reported in 1999, 33% were imported. It should be remembered that measles reporting is incomplete.

Measles is highly contagious, and is spread by direct contact with infectious droplets or less commonly by airborne spread. It is most prevalent in winter and spring, and contagion is highest in the late prodromal phase. The incubation period is usually 8–12 days.[18]

PRESENTING HISTORY

Measles infection classically presents with a prodrome of fever (≥101°F), nasal congestion, cough and rhinoconjunctivitis. The cough is often brassy in quality, and is nearly always present.[12,13] The conjunctivitis is characterized by severe lacrimation and a transverse marginal line of conjunctival injection across the lower lids.[21] Photophobia is more common in adolescent and adult patients. A transient macular or urticarial rash has been described early in the prodrome as well.

PHYSICAL EXAMINATION

The characteristic enanthem of measles, Koplik's spots, usually presents during the prodromal phase and appears as punctate white-gray papules on a red background (Fig. 25.2). They begin on the buccal mucosa, opposite the lower molars, and often spread to involve other parts of the mucosa.

The exanthem occurs over 2–4 days, appearing approximately 14 days after viral exposure. It begins at the hairline and behind the ears (Fig. 25.3), and

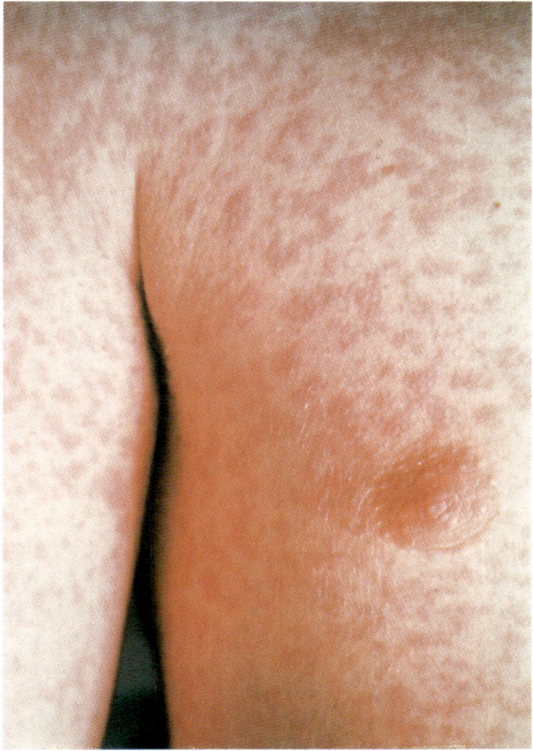

Fig. 25.3   Erythematous lesions of the measles exanthem.

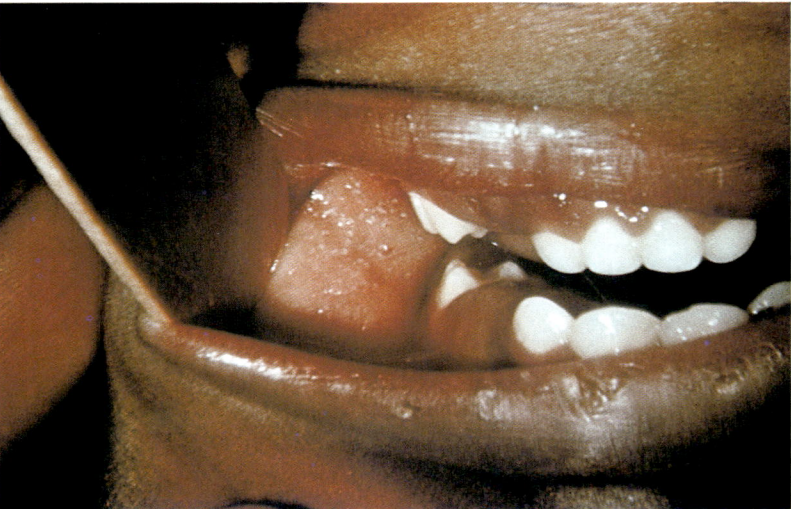

Fig. 25.2   An example of Koplic's spots (Courtesy of H. Blank, MD, University of Miami School of Medicine).

spreads centrifugally and in a cephalocaudad direction. Lesions begin as discrete, erythematous macules and papules, and gradually coalesce. By the third day of rash, the entire body is involved and the lesions are intensely erythematous, and at times purpuric. Pruritus is not a prominent symptom. Usually by the fourth day, the rash begins to fade, with a coppery-brown discoloration and desquamation, in the same order as it appeared. Fever persists through the second or third day of the rash and then falls. Persistent fever after the onset of exanthem may suggest complications. Other findings during the exanthematous period include generalized adenopathy and splenomegaly.[13]

Modified measles may occur in infants young enough to have residual maternal antibody, children who recently have received gamma globulin, or individuals immunized previously who posses levels of antibody insufficient to prevent infection but adequate to modify its course.[22] In these patients the prodrome may be shortened, and cough, congestion, and fever may be less severe. The presence of Koplik's spots is variable, and the skin eruption is usually less confluent.[13,23]

Atypical measles has been reported in previously immunized patients after infection with natural measles virus. Most cases have been in individuals immunized with killed measles vaccine, but a few cases have followed immunization with live, attenuated vaccine.[24] Killed measles vaccine was used in the US from 1963 to 1968, and until 1970 in Canada, and therefore if the condition is seen now, it tends to be in adults. Atypical measles is characterized by high fever, myalgias, cough, headache, and abdominal pain. Coryza and conjunctivitis are usually absent, and Koplik's spots are rarely present. The rash begins more distally, concentrated on the ankles and wrists and in creases. It spreads over a 3–5 day period to involve the more proximal extremities, trunk, and face. The morphology of the exanthem is variable, including vesicular,

17. Centers for Disease Control (1989) Measles prevention: recommendations of the Immunization Practices Advisory Committee (ACIP). **MMWR** 38:1–18.
18. American Academy of Pediatrics (2000) Measles. In: Red Book: Report of the Committee on Infectious Diseases, 25th ed, Pickering LK, ed. Elk Grove Village, IL: American Academy of Pediatrics, pp. 385–396.
19. Centers for Disease Control (1999) Final 1998 Reports of Notifiable Diseases. **MMWR** 48:749–753.
20. Centers for Disease Control (2000) Measles – United States, 1999. **MMWR** 49:557–560.

21. Mason WH (1995) Measles. **Adol Med** 6:1–14.
22. Gold E (1996) Almost extinct diseases: measles, mumps, rubella and pertussis. **Pediatr Rev** 17:120–127.
23. Cherry JD, Feigin RD, Shackelford PG et al. (1973) A clinical and serologic study of 103 children with measles vaccine failure. **J Pediatr** 82:802–808.
24. Cherry JD, Feigin RD, Lobes LA et al. (1972) Atypical measles in children previously immunized with attenuated measles virus vaccines. **Pediatrics** 50:712–717.

purpuric, petechial, and scarlatiniform lesions.[21] Swelling and pain in the hands and feet is common.[25,26] Pneumonia occurs in most patients, and marked hepatosplenomegaly, hyperesthesia or paresthesia may occur.

A *measles vaccination exanthem* may occur in approximately 5% of vaccine recipients,[18] and is usually a transient maculopapular eruption. Transient thrombocytopenia with thrombocytopenic purpura may also occasionally occur.

Complications of measles occur less frequently in the current era, but do still occur and may at times be life threatening, especially in the very young (<1 year), the elderly, and the immunosuppressed.[21] The major ones are otitis, pneumonia, bronchitis, encephalitis, and myocarditis. Otitis media is the most common complication of measles. Pneumonia accounts for many hospitalizations in affected children, especially those with previous cardiorespiratory disease.[27] Secondary bacterial infection may occur, most commonly with *Staphylococcus aureus, Streptococcus pneumoniae*, or *Streptococcus pyogenes*. Mild pulmonic changes such as rales or wheezes may be found in up to 50% of patients.[21] Encephalitis occurs in approximately 1 in 1000 cases, and is marked by the return of fever and changes in mental status as the rash begins to fade.[22] Clinically significant myocarditis and pericarditis are rare, but electrocardiographic (ECG) changes may be present in more than one-half of affected children.[13] Other rarely reported complications include thrombocytopenia, Stevens–Johnson syndrome, appendicitis, hepatitis, and lymphadenitis. An increased risk of the development of inflammatory bowel disease following early (<5 years) measles infection has recently been suggested.[28]

Subacute sclerosing panencephalitis (SSPE) is a rare neurodegenerative disease characterized by personality changes, seizures, coma, and death. It may occur many years following initial measles infection and occurs in 1 in 100 000 cases.[22] Widespread measles immunization has led to its virtual disappearance in the United States.

Infection with measles during pregnancy is associated with increased fetal loss and prematurity,[29] but no consistent pattern of congenital malformations has been associated with transplacentally acquired disease.[30] Complication rates from measles infection are substantially higher in developing countries, as well as in immunocompromised hosts. In the United States, death occurs in 1 to 3 of every 1000 cases reported, with higher case–fatality rates in children younger than 5 years of age.[18]

LABORATORY FINDINGS

Typical measles is usually diagnosed based on clinical findings, and laboratory evaluations are rarely necessary. The white count may be decreased, with an absolute lymphopenia, and there may be elevated liver function studies, cardiac conduction abnormalities and, in cases complicated by pneumonia, occasional persistent chest radiographic findings.[31] Laboratory diagnosis of measles can be accomplished by virus isolation and serologic assays, including complement fixation (CF), hemagglutination-inhibition (HAI), direct immunofluorescence (DIF), and enzyme-linked immunosorbent assay (ELISA).[32] The latter is the most commonly employed method for diagnosis. Evaluation of acute and convalescent (paired) sera is performed, and a fourfold rise in antibody titer is usually seen during infection.

PATHOPHYSIOLOGY

Typical measles begins with replication of the virus in the epithelial cells of the respiratory tract, followed by spread to lymphoid tissue and, eventually, a primary viremia. The virus then disseminates to multiple sites, including skin, liver, and the gastrointestinal tract.[33] The viremia occurs around days 5 to 7, and infection in the skin is established by days 7 to 11. Immune activation occurs during the period of acute measles infection and consists both of specific T cell and humoral immune responses, which are responsible for overcoming acute infection and preventing reinfection, respectively.[33]

The most characteristic cytopathic effect observed in tissue culture during the course of infection is syncytia formation with multinucleated giant cells, and infected cells may show nuclear and cytoplasmic inclusions. The multinucleated giant cells may be of two different types: Warthin–Finkeldey cells, which are found in lymphoid tissue, and epithelial giant cells, which are present in the skin, mucosa, and respiratory epithelium. Biopsies of lesional skin, which are nonspecific, show focal parakeratosis, dyskeratosis, and spongiosis.

DIFFERENTIAL DIAGNOSIS

Typical measles, especially if early in the course when the patient still has Koplik's spots, is usually a fairly straightforward diagnosis and unlikely to be confused with other childhood exanthems. However, at times, the exanthem can be confused with other viral exanthems, drug reactions, or Kawasaki disease. In one study of measles- and rubella-like illnesses in children who had already received MMR (measles, mumps, and rubella) vaccination, various viral etiologies were found, including parvovirus, enterovirus, adenovirus, and HHV-6.[34] Atypical measles may occasionally be confused with Rocky Mountain spotted fever or Henoch Schonlein purpura, as well.

THERAPEUTICS AND PROGNOSIS

No specific antiviral therapy is available for measles, and treatment is usually supportive. While *in vitro* studies have demonstrated sensitivity of the measles virus to ribavirin, controlled studies are lacking and this drug does not currently have US Food and Drug Administration (FDA) approval for this indication.

Vitamin A, which has been recommended by the World Health Organization and the United Nations International Children's Emergency Fund (UNICEF) for children diagnosed with measles in communities where vitamin A deficiency exists, is now recommended by the AAP for patients 6 months to 2 years of age hospitalized with the disease or any patient older than 6 months with risk factors for severe involvement (i.e., immunodeficiency, evidence of vitamin A deficiency, impaired intestinal absorption, or malnutrition).[18] This supplementation may reduce measles mortality in hospitalized children by up to 60%.[35] Isolation with airborne precautions should be followed for four days following onset of the rash and for the duration of illness in immunocompromised patients.

The live attenuated MMR vaccine is recommended for universal immunization, as noted above. Postexposure prophylaxis in susceptible individuals includes measles vaccine (if given within 72 hours of exposure), and immune globulin, which can be given up to six days following exposure to prevent infection or modify the course.

The prognosis for typical uncomplicated measles is generally good, but meticulous management of complicated cases is vital to decrease the risk of mortality.[36] The prognosis tends to be worse in patients with predisposing conditions such as malnutrition or immunodeficiency, as well as very young infants. Patients who develop SSPE have a poor prognosis, with loss of

25. Fulginiti VA, Eller JJ, Downie AW et al. (1967) Altered reactivity to measles virus. Atypical measles in children previously immunized with inactivated measles virus vaccines. JAMA 202:1075–1080.
26. Rauh LW, Schmidt R (2000) Measles immunization with killed virus vaccine. Serum antibody titers and experience with exposure to measles epidemic. 1965. Bull World Health Organ 78:226–231.
27. Cherry JD, Feigin RD, Lobes LA et al. (1972) Urban measles in the vaccine era: a clinical, epidemiologic and serologic study. J Pediatr 81:217–230.
28. Pardi DS, Tremaine WJ, Sandborn WJ et al. (2000) Early measles virus infection is associated with the development of inflammatory bowel disease. Am J Gastroenterol 95:1480–1485.
29. Eberhart-Phillips JE, Frederick PD, Baron RC et al. (1993) Measles in pregnancy: a descriptive study of 58 cases. Obstet Gynecol 82:797–801.
30. Rosa C (1998) Rubella and Rubeola. Sem Perinatol 22:318–322.

31. Mitnick J (1980) Nodular lung lesions of atypical measles pneumonia. Am J Roentgenol 134:257–260.
32. Boyd AS (1994) Laboratory testing in patients with morbilliform viral eruptions. Dermatol Clin 12:69–82.
33. Schneider-Schaulies S, Meulen VT (1999) Pathogenic aspects of measles virus infections. Arch Virol (S15):139–158.
34. Davidkin I, Valle M, Peltola H et al. (1998) Etiology of measles and rubella-like illnesses in measles, mumps, and rubella-vaccinated children. J Infect Dis 178:1567–1570.
35. Villamor E, Fawzi WW (2000) Vitamin A supplementation: implications for morbidity and mortality in children. J Infect Dis 182(S1):S122–S133.
36. Marufu T, Siziya S, Murugasampillay S et al. (1997) Measles complications: the importance of their management in reducing mortality attributed to measles. Cent Afr J Med 43:162–165.

cognitive functioning and, usually, death within one to three years following the diagnosis.

The risks of mass campaigns to avoid vaccination were demonstrated in a large measles outbreak which occurred in Philadelphia in 1990–1991, among two church groups not accepting of vaccination. In this epidemic, six childhood deaths occurred, five of them in children who had not received medical care.[37]

RUBELLA

Rubella, or German measles, is an exanthematous illness caused by an RNA virus in the Togaviridae family. Humans are the only known natural host for the virus. Rubella is generally a benign, self-limited disease except when it is transmitted *in utero*, in which case it may produce severe congenital infection. Congenital rubella is discussed in Chapter 6.

EPIDEMIOLOGY

Rubella was once a common childhood exanthematous disease, but since licensure of the rubella vaccine in 1969 and its widespread use, the incidence in the United States has declined by 99% from the prevaccine era.[38] A resurgence of disease, however, was seen in 1989–1990, with the greatest proportion of cases seen in adolescents and adults >15 years of age, and was believed to be due to failure of vaccination of susceptible individuals.[39] The risk of acquiring rubella has again declined in all age groups, and the total number of reported US cases in 1999 was 267.[40] Before 1969, epidemics of rubella occurred in six to nine year intervals, and the majority of cases occurred in children 5 to 9 years of age.[41] Recent serologic surveys indicate that approximately 10% of young adults in the US are susceptible to rubella.[38] Epidemics of the disease occasionally occur in developed countries, and rubella infection continues to be common in countries where vaccinations are not widely available. The rubella vaccine is very effective, inducing serum antibody in 95% or more of the recipients after a single dose at 12 months of age.

Rubella occurs most commonly in the spring, and the incubation period is usually between 16 and 18 days. Droplet precautions are recommended for seven days after the onset of the rash, after which time the patient is no longer considered contagious.

PRESENTING HISTORY

A majority of patients with rubella may be asymptomatic, and up to half of the primary infections in children may be subclinical.[41] The disease otherwise presents insidiously, with mild prodromal symptoms including headache, low-grade fever, malaise, conjunctivitis, and upper respiratory symptoms sometimes occurring 1–5 days prior to onset of the rash. Prodromal symptoms are more common in adolescents and young adults, and fairly uncommon in children. Lymphadenopathy may also present prior to the onset of rash, during the prodromal period.

PHYSICAL EXAMINATION

The rubella exanthem is a generalized, erythematous macular and papular eruption, with a variable progression, extent, and duration. It usually starts on the face and progresses downward to the trunk and then the extremities.

The full expression of the exanthem is usually apparent by 24 hours after its onset, and it begins to fade on day two in the same order of distribution in which it appeared. The eruption is usually completely absent by the third day, but may persist in some patients for four to five days.[42] Generally, the rash consists of discrete pink macules and papules, which may become confluent with a morbilliform (measles-like) appearance or it may at times appear scarlatiniform (scarlet fever-like). An erythema infectiosum-like exanthem has been reported in children in whom rubella virus was recovered.[43,44] An enanthem characterized by erythematous and petechial macules on the soft palate (Forschheimer's spots) may also be present.[32]

A consistent finding in patients with rubella is tender lymphadenopathy, most frequently in the occipital, posterior auricular, and posterior cervical regions, which may have its onset during the prodromal period. It tends to be most pronounced during the period of the exanthem.[30] Generalized adenopathy may also occur. The presence of fever is variable, but marked temperature elevation is rare.

The most common complication of rubella is joint involvement, including both arthralgias and arthritis, which occurs especially in postpubertal females, 70% of whom may have such complaints.[45] The fingers, wrists, and knees are most often affected, and the complaints are usually transient with resolution by one month following the infection. Other less common complications include encephalitis, myocarditis, pericarditis, hemolytic anemia, thrombocytopenic purpura, and hepatitis.

LABORATORY FINDINGS

Clinical diagnosis of rubella may be difficult except in classic cases occurring during an epidemic, given the phenotypic overlap with other exanthematous illnesses. Conventional laboratory examinations may reveal neutropenia or thrombocytopenia, but most of the routine studies are usually normal.

Virus isolation is possible from blood, urine, cerebrospinal fluid, and nasopharyngeal specimens, but these studies are tedious and time consuming and have been supplanted by serologic diagnostics. The hemagglutination inhibition test was at one time the most frequently used method for serologic screening, but other equally or more sensitive assays are now in use, including latex agglutination, direct immunofluorescence, enzyme immunoassay (EIA) and antibody capture techniques.[32,38] A four fold or greater rise in antibody titer or seroconversion between acute and convalescent serum titers indicates infection. False positive results may occur from cross-reactivity with rheumatoid factor, Epstein–Barr virus, and cytomegalovirus.[30] Congenital rubella is diagnosed by the presence of rubella-specific immunoglobulin (Ig)M antibody or increasing serum concentrations of rubella-specific IgG.

PATHOPHYSIOLOGY

The primary site of infection in rubella is the nasopharynx, followed by spread to regional lymphatics and, eventually, a viremia. Rash appears as the serum antibody titer is rising, suggesting a potential contribution of antigen-antibody interactions in the skin. Virus has also been demonstrated in both involved and uninvolved skin during the course of infection, and therefore widespread distribution of the agent is another factor which may play a role in the pathogenesis of the exanthem.[46] The HAI antibody peaks 12 to 14 days after the onset of the rash, and reaches stable lifelong levels approximately two weeks later. The rubella virus has three major polypeptides, including the capsid protein and two envelope glycoproteins,

37. Rodgers DV, Gindler JS, Atkinson WL et al. (1993) High attack rates and case fatality during a measles outbreak in groups with religious exemption to vaccination. **Pediatr Infect Dis J** 12:238–292.
38. American Academy of Pediatrics (2000) Rubella. In: Red Book: Report of the Committee on Infectious Diseases. 25th ed, Pickering LK, ed. 2000 Elk Grove Village, IL: American Academy of Pediatrics, pp. 495–500.
39. Lindegren ML, Fehrs LJ, Hadler SC et al. (1991) Update: rubella and congenital rubella syndrome, 1980–1990. **Epidemiol Rev** 13:341–348.
40. Centers for Disease Control (2000) Measles, rubella and congenital rubella syndrome – United States and Mexico, 1997–1999. **MMWR** 49:1048–1050.
41. Kimberlin DW (1997) Rubella immunization. **Pediatr Ann** 26:366–370.

42. Leissa B, Sever JL (1992) Rubella (German measles). In: Infectious Diseases Gorbach SL, Bartlett JG, Blacklow NR, eds. Philadelphia: WB Saunders, pp. 1093–1101.
43. Balfour HH, May DB, Rottee TC et al. (1972) A study of erythema infectiosum: recovery of rubella virus and echovirus 12. **Pediatrics** 50:285–290.
44. Cherry JD (1998) Rubella. In: Textbook of Pediatric Infectious Diseases, 4th ed, Feigin RD, Cherry JD, eds Philadelphia: WB Saunders, pp. 1922–1949.
45. Murph JR (1994) Rubella and syphilis: continuing causes of congenital infection in the 1990s. **Sem Pediatr Neurol** 1:26–35.
46. Heggie AD (1978) Pathogenesis of the rubella exanthem: distribution of rubella virus in the skin during rubella with and without rash. **J Infect Dis** 137:74–77.

E_1, and E_2.[47] Anti-E_1 antibodies probably play the predominant role in the serologic response.[48]

DIFFERENTIAL DIAGNOSIS

Rubella may present in a nonspecific fashion, and the exanthem may resemble that of several other exanthematous illnesses, including enteroviruses, reoviruses, adenoviruses, measles, and streptococcal scarlet fever. In a Finnish study, a significant number of children who had had MMR vaccination and presented with measles- and rubella-like illnesses were found to have other viral infections, including parvovirus, enterovirus, adenovirus, and HHV-6,[34] confirming the common overlap in clinical presentations of these infections. Prominent suboccipital adenopathy may be a useful clinical feature, but may be found in other infections and therefore is not pathognomonic for rubella. Although the occurrence of rubella is now rare, clinicians should include it in the differential of an acute exanthematous illness, especially in adolescents and young adults.

THERAPEUTICS AND PROGNOSIS

Therapy of rubella is supportive, and the prognosis is excellent. Children should be kept away from school for seven days following onset of the rash, and hospitalized patients should be in respiratory isolation for the same period of time. Exposed hospital personnel who may come into contact with pregnant females should be screened for rubella immunity. Live-virus vaccination given after exposure has not been demonstrated to prevent illness, whereas the use of immune globulin for postexposure prophylaxis, although not routinely recommended, may decrease the incidence of clinically apparent infection from 87% to 18%.[38] Prevention of rubella is best accomplished by timely vaccination. The live-virus vaccine is recommended as part of the combined MMR vaccine, and should be given at 12–15 months of age and again at school entry at 4–6 years. All susceptible adolescents and adults should be immunized, as well, to eliminate the virus reservoir.

ERYTHEMA INFECTIOSUM (FIFTH DISEASE)

Erythema infectiosum (EI), fifth disease, and "slapped cheek" disease all refer to the same exanthematous illness, caused by human parvovirus B19 (B19). The latter name stems from the bright erythema of the cheeks seen early in the illness. B19 was discovered in 1974 by Cossart *et al.* during a study of hepatitis B virus laboratory assays, and was named from the well from which she identified the particles, row "B" panel "19".[49] It was identified as the etiologic agent of EI in 1983,[50] and since that time has been implicated as a potential cause of numerous other conditions (Table 25.2). B19 is a single-stranded DNA virus with trophism for erythroid progenitor cells. In addition to EI, the B19-associated conditions most clinically relevant to pediatrics include hematologic disease, fetal hydrops, and the papular-purpuric gloves and socks syndrome (discussed in a separate section below).

EPIDEMIOLOGY

B19 virus infection has a distinct seasonal pattern, with most community outbreaks occurring in the winter and spring. There appears to be a cyclic pattern, with peaks occurring every six years and lasting for about three years.[51]

TABLE 25.2 Clinical associations with parvovirus B19

Asymptomatic disease
Erythema infectiosum
Arthropathy/arthritis
Transient aplastic crisis
Chronic anemia
Hydrops fetalis
Neurologic disease
Rheumatologic disease
Vasculitis

Reprinted, with permission, from Mancini AJ, **Adv Dermatol** 2000; 16:3–38.

B19 infection occurs worldwide and at any age, although it is most common in school-aged children. Girls are affected more frequently than boys. The seroprevalence of antibodies against parvovirus ranges 2–15% in children 1–5 years old, 15–60% between 5 and 19 years of age, and 30–80% in adults.[52,53] The attack rate during an epidemic is high, with up to 60% of susceptible school children and 30% of susceptible adults acquiring infection.[54] Transmission of B19 is via respiratory droplets, blood products, or vertically from mother to fetus. The appearance of the characteristic rash coincides with the appearance of antibody and disappearance of B19 DNA in respiratory secretions and serum, hence patients with the skin eruption of EI are no longer considered contagious. The incubation period is 4–14 days, and the rash and joint symptoms occur two to three weeks after acquisition of infection.[55]

PRESENTING HISTORY

In most patients, the first reported manifestation of EI is the characteristic rash. Prodromal symptoms may occasionally occur, and include low-grade fever, headache, chills, myalgias, and malaise. Frequently, however, these symptoms are so mild that they go unnoticed by the patient.

PHYSICAL EXAMINATION

The exanthem of EI is divided into three stages. Initially, a bright, fiery red macular erythema appears on the cheeks (Fig. 25.4). This "slapped cheek" appearance is often associated with a rim of sparing around the mouth, or "circumoral pallor." This eruption may be confused with the rash of scarlet fever, a photosensitive drug reaction, or the rash of systemic lupus erythematosus.[51] A more generalized eruption marks the second stage, which occurs 1–4 days after the onset of facial erythema, and is more prominent initially on the proximal extremities with subsequent spread to the trunk. This eruption evolves from a maculopapular erythematous rash to one marked by a lacy, reticulate pattern (Fig. 25.5). The palms and soles are spared. Pruritus is noted in up to 15% of children.[56] The third stage of the exanthem varies in duration from one to several weeks, and is marked by a waxing and waning intensity of the eruption. Factors that may lead to an exacerbation of the rash include sun exposure, hot baths, physical exertion, and emotional lability.

Arthralgias and arthritis are common findings in adult patients with B19 infection, but occur in only 8–10% of pediatric patients with EI. Joint symptoms may occur with or without the characteristic rash of EI, or concomitant with a different type of exanthem. Nocton *et al.*[57] described 22

47. Cradock-Watson JE (1991) Laboratory diagnosis of rubella: past, present and future. **Epidemiol Infect** 107:1–15.
48. Katow S, Sigiura A (1985) Antibody response to individual rubella virus proteins in congenital and other rubella virus infection. **J Clin Microbiol** 21:449–451.
49. Cossart YE, Cant B, Field AM et al. (1975) Parvovirus-like particles in human sera. **Lancet** 1:72–73.
50. Anderson MJ, Jones SE, Fisher-Hoch SP et al. (1983) Human parvovirus, the cause of erythema infectiosum (fifth disease)? **Lancet** 1:1378.
51. Cherry JD (1999) Parvovirus infections in children and adults. **Adv Pediatr** 46:245–269.
52. Anderson LJ (1987) Role of parvovirus B19 in human disease. **Pediatr Infect Dis J** 6:711–718.
53. Torok TJ (1992) Parvovirus B19 and human disease. **Adv Intern Med** 37:431–455.

54. Gillespie SM, Cartter NL, Asch S (1990) Occupational risk of human parvovirus B19 infection for school and day-care personnel during an outbreak of erythema infectiosum. **JAMA** 263:2061–2065.
55. American Academy of Pediatrics (2000) Parvovirus B19. In: 2000 Red Book: Report of the Committee on Infectious Diseases, 25th ed, Pickering LK, ed. Elk Grove Village, IL: American Academy of Pediatrics; 423–425.
56. Stiefel L (1995) Erythema infectiosum (fifth disease). **Pediatr Rev** 16:474–475.
57. Nocton JJ, Miller LC, Tucker LB et al. (1993) Human parvovirus B19-associated arthritis in children. **J Pediatr** 122:186–190.

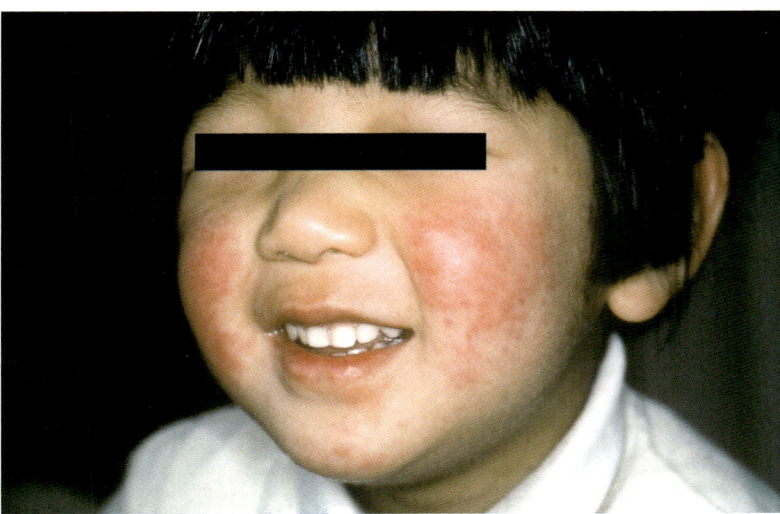

Fig. 25.4 Bright red erythema of the cheeks in the initial stage of erythema infectiosum (Fifth Disease).

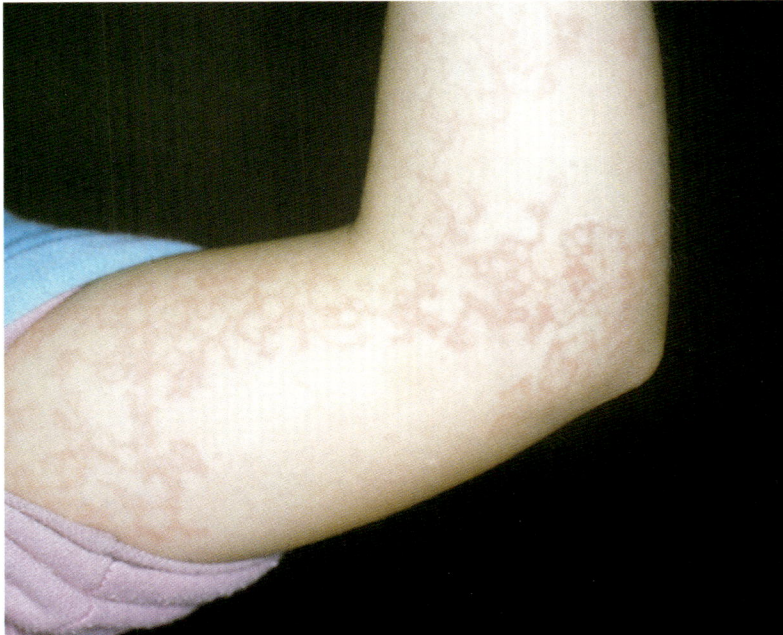

Fig. 25.5 Lacy, reticulate erythema of the arm in erythema infecticsum.

children from a rheumatology practice who presented with joint complaints in association with serologic evidence of recent B19 infection. In this group, 20 children had arthritis, and two had arthralgias. Sixteen were female and six were male, with an age range of 2–19 years. Seven of the patients had an EI rash by history or at the time of presentation for the joint complaints, and seven others had different eruptions, including one patient with petechiae and one with a history of urticaria. Joint involvement was polyarticular in 10

patients and pauciarticular in 12 patients, and the joints involved (in order of descending frequency) were the knees, ankles and wrists, elbows, neck, hands and feet, hip, shoulder, and sternoclavicular joints.[57] The duration of joint symptoms was under six weeks in 11 children, with an additional four experiencing resolution within four months. Eight children continued to have persistent joint symptoms, and six of them fulfilled criteria for the diagnosis of juvenile rheumatoid arthritis (JRA). While it is established that B19 infection may result in a pattern of joint involvement similar to autoimmune arthritis, the exact relationship between this agent and JRA remains unclear.

Fetal infection with B19 may result in fetal anemia, high output cardiac failure, pleural effusions, polyhydramnios, generalized edema and ascites (nonimmune hydrops fetalis), and intrauterine fetal demise.[6,58] Although up to 60% of pregnant females may be seropositive for B19 (and therefore immune),[59,60] only 30–44% of those with acute infection report signs or symptoms, including arthralgias or rash.[61,62] The risk of fetal loss in pregnancies complicated by acute parvovirus B19 infection is around 8–10%.[61,63] The greatest risk appears to be when infection is acquired before 20 weeks' gestation, and the majority of fetal losses occur between 20 and 28 weeks of gestation. The majority of infants born to B19-infected mothers, however, are delivered asymptomatic and at term and have normal developmental outcomes.[61,63,64] Sporadic reports of fetal anomalies in association with B19 infection appear in the literature,[65,66] but a definitive association remains to be conclusively demonstrated.

LABORATORY FINDINGS

Laboratory evaluation is rarely necessary in typical cases of EI in an otherwise healthy child. In cases where diagnostic confirmation is indicated, detection of serum B19-specific IgM via EIA is the preferred study, although in the immunocompromised host, the optimal and most sensitive methods for diagnosis are demonstration of the virus by nucleic acid hybridization or polymerase chain reaction (PCR) assay.[51,55]

Anemia with reticulocytopenia are occasionally seen, due to the tropism of B19 for erythroid precursor cells in the bone marrow. These changes are usually inconsequential in the normal host, but in patients with hemolysis or any condition that results in red blood cell destruction (i.e., hereditary spherocytosis, sickle cell disease, glucose-6-phosphate dehydrogenase deficiency, pyruvate kinase deficiency) or decreased red blood cell production (i.e., iron deficiency anemia or thalassemias), transient aplastic crises (TAC) may result.[58,67] Although usually a pure red cell aplasia, thrombocytopenia, neutropenia, or pancytopenia may infrequently occur. TAC episodes are accompanied by symptoms of anemia, and usually last 10–15 days.

In the early-gestation gravid female with a known history of B19 exposure or symptoms suggesting possible acute infection, serologic evaluation for anti-B19 IgM antibody should be performed. Other reported detection methods include B19 DNA measurement via polymerase chain reaction (PCR) studies of fetal or maternal blood[68] and assaying for B19 capsid antigens (VP1 and VP2) in amniotic fluid samples.[69]

PATHOPHYSIOLOGY

One week after viral inoculation, a viremia appears and persists for several days.[67] Anti-B19 IgM antibody appears 10 days after inoculation, followed by the production of IgG antibody one week later, and they are directed primarily against the VP2 protein early on and, later in the course, against the

58. Heegaard ED, Hornsleth A (1995) Parvovirus: the expanding spectrum of disease. **Acta Paediatr** 84:109–117.
59. Adler SP, Manganello AA, Koch WC et al. (1993) Risk of human parvovirus B19 infections among school and hospital employees during endemic periods. **J Infect Dis** 168:361–368.
60. Anderson LJ, Hurwitz ES (1988) Human parvovirus B19 and pregnancy. **Clin Perinatol** 15:273–286.
61. Gratacos E, Torres PJ, Vidal J et al. (1995) The incidence of human parvovirus B19 infection during pregnancy and its impact on perinatal outcome. **J Infect Dis** 171:1360–1363.
62. Koch WC, Harger JH, Barnstein B et al. (1998) Serologic and virologic evidence for frequent intrauterine transmission of human parvovirus B19 with a primary maternal infection during pregnancy. **Pediatr Infect Dis J** 17:489–494.
63. Miller E, Fairley CK, Cohen BJ et al. (1998) Immediate and long term outcome of human parvovirus B19 infection in pregnancy. **Br J Obstet Gynecol** 105:174–178.
64. Rodis JF, Rodner C, Hansen AA et al. (1998) Long-term outcome of children following maternal human parvovirus B19 infection. **Obstet Gynecol** 91:125–128.
65. Katz VL, McCoy MC, Kuller JA et al. (1996) An association between fetal parvovirus B19 infection and fetal anomalies: a report of two cases. **Am J Perinatol** 13:43–45.
66. Tiessen RG, van Elsacker-Niele AMW, Vermeij-Keers C et al. (1994) A fetus with a parvovirus B19 infection and congenital anomalies. **Prenat Diagn** 14:173–176.
67. Balkhy HH, Sabella C, Goldfarb J (1998) Parvovirus: a review. **Bull Rheum Dis** 47:4–9.
68. Dieck D, Schild RL, Hansmann M et al. (1999) Prenatal diagnosis of congenital parvovirus B19 infection: value of serological and PCR techniques in maternal and fetal serum. **Prenat Diagn** 19:1119–1123.
69. Gentilomi G, Zerbini M, Gallinella G et al. (1998) B19 parvovirus induced fetal hydrops: rapid and simple diagnosis by detection of B19 antigens in amniotic fluids. **Prenat Diagn** 18:363–368.

VP1 protein. The appearance of IgG antibody coincides with the appearance of rash and arthralgia,[51] suggesting an immune-mediated pathogenesis, although a report of viral capsid proteins and viral DNA in the skin biopsy of a patient with EI suggests a possible direct effect of the virus.[70] During the viremic phase, infection of erythrocyte precursors with B19 causes lysis of these progenitor cells, resulting in reticulocytopenia.

Recent studies have demonstrated that erythrocyte "P antigen" (globoside) is the major receptor for B19, and the virus gains entry into the cell via binding of capsid proteins to this receptor.[71] Preincubation of erythrocytes with monoclonal antibodies to globoside prevents cellular infection by B19.[71] Individuals with "P phenotype" blood (lacking P antigen) have been shown to be naturally immune to infection with B19.[72]

DIFFERENTIAL DIAGNOSIS

When all three phases of EI are present in an otherwise well or only mildly ill child, the diagnosis is quite straightforward. Other helpful features in confirming the clinical diagnosis are occurrence in the spring and spread of disease in an epidemic fashion. Other exanthematous diseases occasionally confused with EI include scarlet fever, enterovirus infection, and rubella. The evanescent rash of JRA can be confused with the eruption of EI, but the former usually occurs in conjunction with temperature elevation and has a more chronic, relapsing course.

THERAPEUTICS AND PROGNOSIS

No specific therapy is available for EI, but fortunately most infections in the normal host are self-limited and without sequelae. In patients with significant arthralgias or arthritis, non-steroidal anti-inflammatory agents are useful. Parents should be educated about the third phase of the eruption, with the possibility of a waxing and waning rash and potential exacerbating factors (i.e., sunlight, overheating). Children with the classic EI rash may return to school or day care and are no longer considered infectious.[55]

Hospitalization and red blood cell transfusions may be required in children with TAC. Immunodeficient patients with B19 infection may develop chronic bone marrow suppression, and intravenous immune globulin (IVIG) therapy has been demonstrated to be useful in this setting.[51,73] Exposed pregnant females should have the risks explained to them and be offered serologic (or other diagnostic) testing. If acute infection is confirmed, serial fetal ultrasonography should be performed, assessing for congestive heart failure, IUGR, or fetal hydrops. Management of severely afflicted fetuses has included digitalization and *in utero* blood transfusions.

PAPULAR-PURPURIC GLOVES AND SOCKS SYNDROME

In 1990, an acute and self-limiting condition comprising pruritic, edematous plaques with petechial purpura over the palms and soles was described by

Harms *et al.*[74] Papular-purpuric gloves and socks syndrome (PPGSS) was subsequently demonstrated to be associated with B19 infection in several, but not all, cases.[75–81] Other infectious agents that have been proposed in association with PPGSS include human herpesvirus-6 (HHV-6),[82] human herpesvirus-7 (HHV-7),[83] measles virus,[84,85] and cytomegalovirus.[86] Most of the described cases in the literature involve young adults, although pediatric cases also occur. The exanthem usually presents in the spring and summer months.

Patients with PPGSS may complain of low-grade fever, myalgias, fatigue, anorexia, or arthralgias.[80] The most distinctive clinical findings are rapidly progressive erythema and edema of the palms and soles (Fig. 25.6), which progress to petechiae or purpura with a sharp demarcation at the wrists and ankles. Involvement of the dorsal surfaces of the hands and feet may occur, as may involvement of the elbows, knees, and buttocks. Patients usually complain of pruritus, burning, or pain of involved areas of skin. An associated enanthem may be present, consisting of vesicles and small erosions on the hard and soft palates, pharynx, tongue, and inner aspects of the lips. Lymphadenopathy occurs in up to 16% of patients.[80]

Laboratory findings are variable, and probably depend on the etiologic agent for each specific case. Hematologic abnormalities including leukopenia, thrombocytopenia, eosinophilia, and neutropenia have been reported, as have mild elevations in hepatic transaminases, C-reactive protein and erythrocyte sedimentation rate.[77,84,87] Histologic evaluation of lesional skin has demonstrated perivascular-predominant, lymphocytic dermal infiltrates, dermal edema, basal layer vacuolar degeneration, and extravasation of red blood cells.[78,81,88] Direct immunofluorescence has shown deposits of immuno-

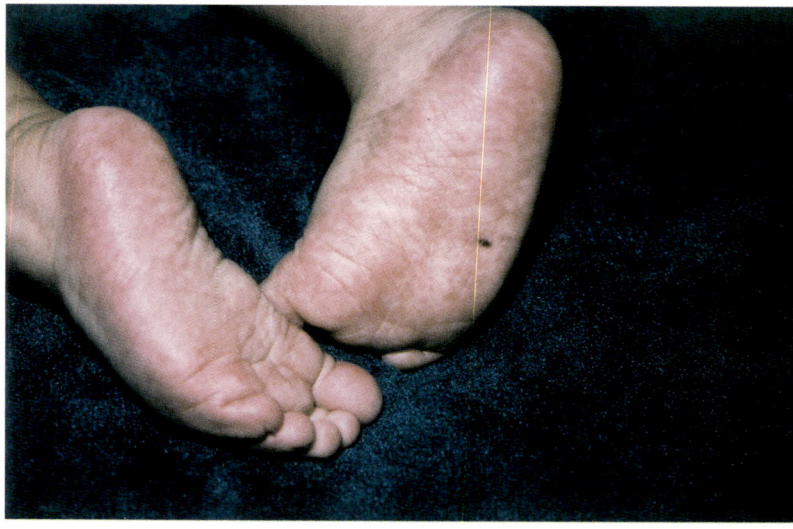

Fig. 25.6 Petechial erythema of the soles in papular-purpuric gloves and socks syndrome.

70. Schwartz TF, Wiersbitzky S, Pambor M (1994) Case report: detection of parvovirus B19 in a skin biopsy of a patient with erythema infectiosum. **J Med Virol** 43:171–174.
71. Brown KE, Anderson SM, Young NS (1993) Erythrocyte P antigen: cellular receptor for B19 parvovirus. **Science** 262:114–117.
72. Brown KE, Hibbs JR, Gallinella G et al. (1994) Resistance to parvovirus B19 infection due to lack of virus receptor (erythrocyte P antigen). **N Engl J Med** 330:1192–1196.
73. Koch WC, Massey G, Russell CE et al. (1990) Manifestations and treatment of human parvovirus B19 infection in immunocompromised patients. **J Pediatr** 116:355–359.
74. Harms M, Feldmann R, Saurat JH (1990) Papular-purpuric "gloves and socks" syndrome. **J Am Acad Dermatol** 23:850–854.
75. Bagot M, Revuz J (1991) Papular-purpuric "gloves and socks" syndrome: primary infection with parvovirus B19? **J Am Acad Dermatol** 25:341.
76. Feldmann R, Harms M, Saurat JH (1994) Papular-purpuric "gloves and socks" syndrome: not only parvovirus B19. **Dermatol** 188:85–87.
77. Vargas-Diez E, Buezo GF, Aragues M et al. (1996) Papular-purpuric gloves-and-socks syndrome. **Int J Dermatol** 35:626–632.
78. Aractingi S, Bakhos D, Flageul B et al. (1996) Immunohistochemical and virological study of skin in the papular-purpuric gloves and socks syndrome. **Br J Dermatol** 135:599–602.
79. Larralde M, Enz PA, Gomez AS et al. (1998) Papular-purpuric "gloves-and-socks" syndrome due to parvovirus B19 infection in childhood. **Pediatr Dermatol** 15:413–414.
80. Smith PT, Landry ML. Carey H et al. (1998) Papular-purpuric gloves and socks syndrome associated with acute parvovirus B19 infection: case report and review. **Clin Infect Dis** 27:164–168.
81. Grilli R, Izquierdo MJ, Farina MC et al. (1994) Papular-purpuric "gloves and socks" syndrome: polymerase chain reaction demonstration of parvovirus B19 DNA in cutaneous lesions and sera. **J Am Acad Dermatol** 41:793–796.
82. Ruzicka T, Kalka K, Diercks K et al. (1998) Papular-purpuric "gloves and socks" syndrome associated with human herpesvirus 6 infection. **Arch Dermatol** 134:242–244.
83. Ongradi J, Becker K, Horvath A et al. (2000) Simultaneous infection by human herpesvirus 7 and human parvovirus B19 in papular-purpuric gloves-and-socks syndrome. **Arch Dermatol** 136:672.
84. Veraldi S, Rizzitelli G, Scarabelli G et al. (1996) Papular-purpuric "gloves and socks" syndrome. **Arch Dermatol** 132:975–977.
85. Perez-Ferriols A, Martinez-Aparicio A, Aliaga-Boniche A (1994) Papular-purpuric "gloves and socks" syndrome caused by measles virus. **J Am Acad Dermatol** 30:291–292.
86. Carrascosa JM, Bielsa I, Ribera M et al. (1995) Papular-purpuric gloves-and-socks syndrome related to cytomegalovirus infection. **Dermatol** 191:269–270.
87. Halasz CL, Cormier D, Den M (1992) Petechial glove and sock syndrome caused by parvovirus B19. **J Am Acad Dermatol** 27:835–838.
88. Trattner A, David M (1994) Purpuric "gloves-and-socks" syndrome: histologic, immunofluorescence, and polymerase chain reaction study. **J Am Acad Dermatol** 30:267–268.

globulin and C3 in a granular pattern within papillary dermal vessel walls,[78,88] and B19 DNA has been demonstrated in skin biopsy specimens by PCR analysis.[78,81] These results suggest that the pathogenesis of PPGSS may involve both a direct viral effect and an immune-mediated vascular reaction to infection.

Based on limited studies, the timing of the antibody response to B19 in PPGSS appears to differ from that in EI. While symptoms coincide with the appearance of antibody and disappearance of viremia in EI, patients with PPGSS develop mucocutaneous lesions during the period of viremia, and subsequently develop a humoral immune response.[77,78,80] These preliminary observations prompt important epidemiologic considerations, especially regarding the counseling of patients with the rash of PPGSS or their caretakers regarding the ongoing risks to susceptible exposed contacts.

The distribution of lesions in PPGSS, the limited involvement, and the generally healthy status of most patients help in differentiating the process from other disorders with clinical overlap, such as Rocky Mountain spotted fever, vasculitis, and meningococcemia. Hand-foot-and-mouth disease has a similar distribution, but a different morphology with deep-seated blisters and lack of a petechial component. Other enteroviral exanthems may be petechial and acrally accentuated but such eruptions tend to extend beyond the gloves and socks distribution.

Therapy of PPGSS is supportive, and the syndrome usually clears spontaneously over 1–2 weeks.

ROSEOLA (EXANTHEM SUBITUM)

Roseola, or exanthem subitum, is a common exanthematous illness of infancy, characterized by high fever and the appearance of a skin rash after defervescence, which was first described by Zahorsky in 1910.[89] Yamanishi et al. in 1988[90] discovered that roseola is caused by infection with HHV-6, a double-stranded DNA virus that is a relative of the other human herpesviruses: herpes simplex 1 and 2, varicella-zoster virus, EBV, and cytomegalovirus. It may also be caused by HHV-7, a closely related virus.[91] As with all herpesviruses, HHV-6 and HHV-7 establish latency after primary infection in childhood, and sites of latency may vary.[92]

EPIDEMIOLOGY

The vast majority of cases of roseola occur in patients 6 months to 3 years of age, with a peak age of 6–7 months.[93] This correlates with the epidemiology of the etiologic agents, as most HHV-6 and -7 infections occur early in life. While 80–100% of newborns have maternally derived antibodies, by 4 to 6 months of life these levels decline[92,94] and the infant is thus susceptible to infection. Acquisition of HHV-6 is common, with 50–60% of children becoming seropositive by 12 months and nearly all with evidence of past infection by 3 years of age. HHV-7 is also a ubiquitous virus, but infection tends to occur later in life than with HHV-6.[95–97] By adulthood, around 85% of individuals have serologic evidence of HHV-7 infection.[98]

Roseola may occur at any time throughout the year, although cases may be more common during the spring.[93] The incubation period is around 9–10 days. Transmission of HHV-6 and -7 is airborne, most often via saliva. Suga et al. demonstrated HHV-6 DNA persistently or intermittently in

TABLE 25.3 Clinical associations with HHV-6 and/or -7 infection in children

Roseola (exanthem subitum)
Fever without rash
Febrile seizures
Encephalitis/encephalopathy
Hemiplegia
Aseptic meningitis
Posttransplantation reactivation
Disseminated organ involvement in AIDS patients

saliva both during and after the disease,[99] and molecular epidemiologic studies have suggested that in many cases the route of transmission may be via salivary secretions from mother to child.[100,101] HHV-7 transmission to young children is also likely to occur from contact with infected respiratory tract secretions.

Table 25.3 summarizes the clinical disease associations with HHV-6 and -7 infections in children.

PRESENTING HISTORY

The hallmark of classic roseola is a high fever (101°F to 106°F) for 3–5 days in an infant or young child who otherwise appears well. A prodrome other than fever is rarely present, including mild catarrhal inflammation of the pharyngeal mucosa and otitis media.[94] Mild cough, coryza, or abdominal pain may be present, and irritability or malaise occur in up to 14% of patients.[93] The rash of roseola characteristically occurs following abrupt defervescence of the patient.

PHYSICAL EXAMINATION

The majority of patients with roseola look well. Occipital, posterior cervical, and postauricular adenopathy are common. An enanthem of erythematous papules on the mucosa of the soft palate and the uvula may be present in up to 65% of patients, and is termed Nagayama's spots in Japan.[93] Pharyngitis, tonsillitis, and injection of tympanic membranes may be present, and bulging of the anterior fontanelle may be seen in young infants.

The rash of roseola usually coincides with loss of fever, or may follow it by 1–2 days. It is characterized by rose-pink macules and papules, and occurs predominantly on the neck and trunk, although it may involve the proximal extremities and the face. The lesions are typically discrete, 2–5mm in diameter and blanchable, and the eruption is not pruritic. Edema of the eyelids was appreciated in 30% of patients with virologically confirmed roseola in one large series.[93] Mild pigmentation may be seen with resolution of the rash, but desquamation usually does not occur.[93,94] The eruption usually fades over a few days, rarely persisting for up to one week.

Neurologic complications associated with HHV-6 and -7 infection include febrile seizures and, rarely, encephalitis or encephalopathy. These associations have been suggested by confirmation of infection via virus isolation from peripheral blood mononuclear cells, evidence of

89. Zahorsky J (1910) Roseola infantilis. **Pediatrics** 22:60.
90. Yamanishi K, Okuno T, Shiraki K et al. (1988) Identification of human herpesvirus 6 as a causal agent for exanthem subitum. **Lancet** 1:1065–1067.
91. Tanaka K, Kondo T, Torigoe S et al. (1994) Human herpesvirus 7: another causal agent for roseola (exanthem subitum). **J Pediatr** 125:1–5.
92. Leach CT (2000) Human herpesvirus 6 and -7 infections in children: agents of roseola and other syndromes. **Curr Opin Pediatr** 12:269–274.
93. Asano Y, Yoshikawa T, Suga S et al. (1994) Clinical features of infants with primary human herpesvirus 6 infection (exanthem subitum, roseola infantum). **Pediatrics** 93:104–108.
94. Kimberlin DW (1998) Human herpesviruses 6 and 7: identification of newly recognized viral pathogens and their association with human disease. **Pediatr Infect Dis J** 17:59–68.
95. Yoshikawa T, Asano Y, Kobayashi I et al. (1993) Seroepidemiology of human herpesvirus 7 in healthy children and adults in Japan. **J Med Virol** 41:319–323.
96. Wyatt LS, Rodriguez WJ, Balachandran N et al. (1999) Human herpesvirus 7: antigenic properties and prevalence in children and adults. **J Virol** 65:6260–6265.
97. Tanaka-Taya K, Kondo T, Mukai T et al. (1996) Seroepidemiological study of human herpesvirus-6 and -7 in children of different ages and detection of these two viruses in throat swabs by polymerase chain reaction. **J Med Virol** 48:88–94.
98. American Academy of Pediatrics (2000) Human Herpesvirus 6 (including Roseola) and 7. In: 2000 Red Book: Report of the Committee on Infectious Diseases, 25th ed, Pickering LK, ed. Elk Grove Village, IL: American Academy of Pediatrics, pp. 322–324.
99. Suga S, Yoshikawa T, Kajita Y et al. (1998) Prospective study of persistence and excretion of human herpesvirus-6 in patients with exanthem subitum and their parents. **Pediatrics** 102:900–904.
100. Mukai T, Yamamoto T, Kondo T et al. (1994) Molecular epidemiological studies of human herpesvirus 6 in families. **J Med Virol** 42:224–227.
101. van Loon NM, Gummuluru S, Sherwood DJ et al. (1995) Direct sequence analysis of human herpesvirus 6 (HHV-6) sequences from infants and comparison of HHV-6 sequences from mother/infant pairs. **Clin Infect Dis** 21:1017–1019.

seroconversion, or detection of viral DNA in cerebrospinal fluid via PCR.[102–105] The neuroinvasive capability of HHV-6 and -7 is well established,[102–104,106] and HHV-6 DNA persistence in the central nervous system (CNS) following acute infection has been demonstrated.[102] In one study initial febrile seizures were associated with evidence of HHV-6 infection in up to 25% of patients;[107] the exact causal relationship has not been clearly established. Suga et al. demonstrated that primary infection with HHV-6 may be associated with severe or atypical patterns of convulsions, including partial, prolonged, or recurrent seizures and possibly a risk for the subsequent development of epilepsy.[108] Caserta et al. found that children with primary HHV-7 infection were even more likely than those with primary HHV-6 infection to have seizures associated with the illness.[109] Some studies have refuted this association with seizures. In a case-control study of a group of children 6 months to 2 years old presenting with a first or second febrile seizure, there was no significant difference in incidence of primary HHV-6 infection from control patients without a seizure history.[110] The exact relation between HHV-6 or -7 infection and febrile seizures in children remains a focus of ongoing investigation.

LABORATORY FINDINGS

Except in complicated cases, laboratory confirmation is rarely performed and usually unnecessary. Routine laboratory testing is nonspecific and generally unhelpful. Specific testing is available in some laboratories and includes serology, antigen detection, PCR, and immunofluorescence studies. Serologic evidence of infection is usually defined as development of IgM antibody or a fourfold (or greater) rise in the IgG titer. Virus isolation in cell culture utilizes peripheral blood mononuclear cells (PBMC) and reveals "balloon-like" cytopathic effect, but is costly and time consuming and therefore is primarily used as an investigational tool.[32] In interpreting the results of diagnostic tests for HHV-6 or -7, the latent nature of these agents must be considered, as these examinations have varying abilities in differentiating active infection from non-replicating latency.[92]

PATHOPHYSIOLOGY

Humans are the only known natural hosts for HHV-6 and HHV-7. HHV-6 has two viral subtypes, type A (HHV-6A) and type B (HHV-6B), which are differentiated on the basis of antigenic specificity and restriction site polymorphisms.[94,111] HHV-6B is associated with the majority of childhood HHV-6 infections. Upon entry into the host, HHV-6 replicates actively inside CD4+ T cells, although there is a broad cellular tropism, including into neurologic tissues.[111,112] Mononuclear cell-associated viremia is present 1–2 days prior to the onset of fever, and resolves around five days after the onset of fever, coincident with an increase in circulating anti-HHV-6 neutralizing antibodies.[111] Extensive viral spread is possible, and has been demonstrated in various sites including lung, liver, brain, salivary glands, bronchial glands, and the genital tract. Latency is eventually established, with the primary sites being salivary glands and peripheral blood mononuclear cells.[92] The incubation period for HHV-6 is around 9–10 days.[111]

DIFFERENTIAL DIAGNOSIS

Enteroviruses, adenovirus, parvovirus B19, rubella, and parainfluenza virus may cause clinically similar syndromes.

THERAPEUTICS AND PROGNOSIS

Most cases of roseola require no therapy apart from antipyretics. In immunosuppressed patients or those with a complicated course, however, therapy may be a consideration. Although there exist no well-established treatment recommendations for patients with HHV-6 or -7 infection, in vitro studies have demonstrated sensitivity of HHV-6 to ganciclovir and foscarnet, and relatively decreased sensitivity to acyclovir.[113,114] Susceptibility patterns of HHV-6 seem similar to those for cytomegalovirus.[115] Early studies have also suggested that cidofovir may be useful for treatment of both HHV-6 and -7 infections.[115,116]

ENTEROVIRUS INFECTION

Enteroviruses are a subgroup of the picornaviruses, and cause a wide array of clinical syndromes with associated exanthems. In the United States alone, they are estimated to cause 10 to 15 million symptomatic infections annually.[117] These viruses consist of a single-stranded RNA genome enclosed in an unenveloped capsid. Members of this family include poliovirus, echovirus, Coxsackievirus, and the newer numbered enteroviruses. There are currently 31 serotypes of echovirus, 23 serotypes of Coxsackievirus A, 6 serotypes of Coxsackievirus B, and 4 other enteroviruses (types 68 to 71).

EPIDEMIOLOGY

Enteroviruses are found worldwide, and they are spread from person to person predominantly via the fecal-oral route, although water exposures such as swimming pools may be a source of some infections.[118] They may also be spread via the respiratory route and from mother to infant in the peripartum period.[98]

Attack rates from enteroviral infection are highest in young children, especially in settings of low socio-economic status or poor hygiene. The prevalence of specific antibodies rises with age. Enteroviral infections are most common in the summer and fall, although sporadic cases may occur throughout the year. In tropical climates, there is no seasonal pattern noted.

There is tremendous overlap and variation in the cutaneous and systemic manifestations of enteroviral infection. Most enteroviral exanthems are not specific enough to allow for an etiologic diagnosis, although the time of year, morphology, and associated symptoms may greatly increase the clinician's index of suspicion.

102. Caserta MT, Hall CB, Schnabel K et al. (1994) Neuroinvasion and persistence of human herpesvirus 6 in children. **J Infect Dis** 170:1586–1589.
103. Yoshikawa T, Nakashima T, Suga S et al. (1992) Human herpesvirus-6 DNA in cerebrospinal fluid of a child with exanthem subitum and meningoencephalitis. **Pediatrics** 89:888–890.
104. Suga S, Yoshikawa T, Asano Y et al. (1993) Clinical and virological analyses of 21 infants with exanthem subitum (roseola infantum) and central nervous system complications. **Ann Neurol** 33:597–603.
105. Torigoe S, Koide W, Yamada M et al. (1996) Human herpesvirus 7 infection associated with central nervous system manifestations. **J Pediatr** 129:301–305.
106. Yoshikawa T, Ihira M, Suzuki K et al. (2000) Invasion by human herpesvirus 6 and human herpesvirus 7 of the central nervous system in patients with neurological signs and symptoms. **Arch Dis Child** 83:170–171.
107. Barone SR, Kaplan MH, Krilov LR (1995) Human herpesvirus-6 infection in children with first febrile seizures. **J Pediatr** 127:95–97.
108. Suga S, Suzuki K, Ihira M et al. (2000) Clinical characteristics of febrile convulsions during primary HHV-6 infection. **Arch Dis Child** 82:62–66.
109. Caserta MT, Hall CB, Schnabel K et al. (1998) Primary human herpesvirus 7 infection: a comparison of human herpesvirus 7 and human herpesvirus 6 infections in children. **J Pediatr** 133:386–389.
110. Hukin J, Farrell K, MacWilliam LM et al. (1998) Case-control study of primary human herpesvirus 6 infection in children with febrile seizures. **Pediatrics** 101:E3.
111. Yoshikawa T, Asano Y (2000) Central nervous system complications in human herpesvirus-6 infection. **Brain Develop** 22:307–314.
112. Huang LM, Pfeiffer BD, Cho CT (1997) Human herpesvirus 6 infection. **Acta Paed Sin** 38:1–7.
113. Agut H, Collandre H, Aubin JT et al. (1989) In vitro sensitivity of human herpesvirus-6 to antiviral drugs. **Res Virol** 140:219–228.
114. Burns WH, Sandford GR (1990) Susceptibility of human herpesvirus 6 to antivirals in vitro. **J Infect Dis** 162:634–637.
115. Reyman D, Naesens L, Balzarini J et al. (1995) Antiviral activity of selected acyclic nucleoside analogues against human herpesvirus 6. **Antiviral Res** 28:343–357.
116. Safrin S, Cherrington J, Jaffe HS (1997) Clinical uses of cidofovir. **Rev Med Virol** 7:145–156.
117. Strikas RA, Anderson LJ, Parker RA (1986) Temporal and geographic patterns of isolates of nonpolio enterovirus in the United States, 1970–83. **J Infect Dis** 153:346–351.
118. Keswick BH, Gerba CP, Goyal SM (1981) Occurrence of enteroviruses in community swimming pools. **Am J Public Health** 71:1026–1030.

COMMON EXANTHEMS

Hand-foot-and-mouth disease

Hand-foot-and-mouth disease (HFMD) is the most distinctive and well-recognized enteroviral exanthem. It is caused most often by Coxsackievirus A16 infection, but may be due to a variety of other enteroviruses, including Coxsackievirus A5, A7, A9, A10, B1, B2, B3, B5, and enterovirus 71.[4,119]

HFMD occurs most commonly during the late summer or early fall. The incubation period is 4–6 days, and it is highly contagious, hence the frequent occurrence of epidemics. A brief prodrome may occur, characterized by low-grade fever and malaise, followed by the appearance of the characteristic enanthem, which is then followed shortly by the appearance of the exanthem. Fever is present in less than one-half of cases, and cough or diarrhea occur infrequently.

The enanthem of HFMD is the most consistent finding, and consists of vesicles that rapidly rupture to leave behind erosions and ulcers superimposed on an erythematous base. They are usually 4–8mm in size, and occur most commonly over the buccal mucosa and tongue, as well as the palate, uvula, and anterior tonsillar pillars. The lesions are quite painful and lead to anorexia and, occasionally, dehydration.

The exanthem of HFMD occurs as gray-white vesiculopustules ranging in size between 3 and 7mm, with variable amounts of associated erythema. They are most common on the palms (Fig. 25.7) and soles, and are less often seen on the dorsal or lateral surfaces of the hands and feet. Another common area of involvement in young children is the buttocks and perineum. Maculopapular or vesicular lesions of a more diffuse distribution are less common. Other findings include occasional lymphadenopathy in the submandibular and cervical regions.

Herpangina

Herpangina is a characteristic enanthem caused by several enteroviruses, most notably Coxsackievirus group A, but also group B and echoviruses.[120–122] Herpes simplex virus may result in a similar clinical pattern of infection.

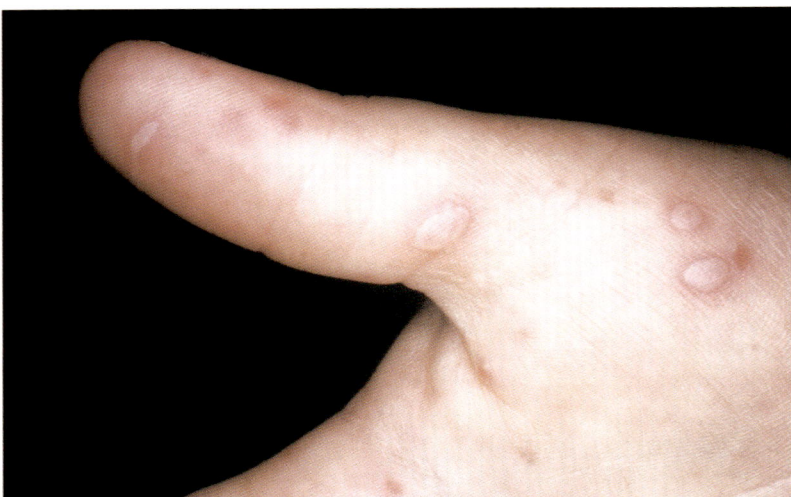

Fig. 25.7   Vesicular palm lesions in hand-foot-and-mouth disease.

Herpangina most often occurs in children between 3 and 10 years of age. The hallmark of infection is painful tiny vesicles and punched-out erosions distributed on the soft palate, uvula, anterior pillars of the fauces, and pharynx. Tonsillar and buccal mucosl involvement may also be present. The shallow erosions usually have a rim or erythema, and may reveal a yellow-gray coating. A quarter of affected patients have abdominal pain and vomiting, and fever is very common. The ulcers of herpangina may last for up to one week.

Other enteroviral exanthems and associated illnesses

Enteroviral exanthems are diverse in their manifestations, and may be quite nonspecific. A variety of eruption patterns have been reported, including rubelliform, morbilliform, roseola-like, vesicular, urticarial, scarlatiniform, pustular, and petechial eruptions. The most common type of enteroviral exanthem is that consisting of erythematous macules and papules in a diffuse distribution. Petechiae may also be present (Fig. 25.8), especially in the setting of echovirus 9 infection, and at times the clinical presentation may mimic meningococcemia.[123] Table 25.4 lists some less common exanthem associations with several of the nonpolio enteroviruses.

Echovirus 16 is an important enteroviral agent more for its historical significance than for its epidemiologic importance. The exanthem resulting from echovirus 16 infection, the so-called Boston exanthem, was the first of a series of new viral exanthems to be described and virologically confirmed in the 1950s. This infection now occurs infrequently.

Enteroviral infection may result in a variety of organ involvement, ranging from a mild, self-limited illness to severe, life-threatening disease. In addition to the aforementioned exanthems and enanthems, other benign illnesses include pleurodynia, pharyngitis, conjunctivitis, and croup. More severe manifestations of enterovirus infection include viral meningitis and encephalitis, myocarditis, pulmonary disease, neonatal sepsis, and severe infection in immunocompromised hosts. Neonatal enteroviral sepsis is a very serious condition, most often associated with echovirus 6 and 11. Transmission from mother to infant may occur at the time of birth, and nursery epidemics have been reported, including a recent nursery outbreak of severe neonatal echovirus 17 infection.[124,125]

One of the most common sites of serious nonpolio enteroviral infections is the CNS, and potential manifestations include meningitis, encephalitis, and flaccid paralysis. The most common neurologic complications in children during a recent epidemic of enteroviral infection were rhombencephalitis, aseptic meningitis, and acute flaccid paralysis.[126] The majority of these patients presented with HFMD or herpangina. Younger children seem to be more susceptible to the CNS manifestations of enteroviral infection. During two separate outbreaks of aseptic meningitis caused by echovirus 9, the peak age of incidence for this finding was 4 years, with an age range of 1 month to 15 years.[127,128]

The recent epidemic of enterovirus 71 infection in Taiwan demonstrates the potential morbidity and mortality associated with these illnesses in children. During this outbreak, of the reported 129 106 of HFMD or herpangina, 405 had severe disease and the majority of these were children less than 5 years of age.[129] Seventy-one of 78 patients who died were 5 years of age or younger, with the majority of deaths related to pulmonary edema or pulmonary hemorrhage.[129] In a small sampling of pediatric patients in the Tainan and Chiayi areas, the spectrum of involvement was noted to include aseptic meningitis, encephalitis, and acute flaccid paralysis, with

119. Lindenbaum JE, Van Dyck PC, Allen RG (1975) Hand, foot and mouth disease associated with Coxsackievirus group B. **Scand J Infect Dis** 7:161–163.
120. Yamadera S, Yamashita K, Kato N et al. (1991) Herpangina surveillance in Japan, 1982–1989. A report of the national epidemiological surveillance of infectious agents in Japan. **Jpn J Med Sci Biol** 44:29–39.
121. Nakayama T, Urano T, Osano M et al. (1989) Outbreak of herpangina associated with Coxsackievirus B3 infection. **Pediatr Infect Dis J** 8:495–498.
122. Zavate O, Avram G, Pavlov E et al. (1984) Coxsackie A virus-associated herpetiform angina. **Virologie** 35:49–53.
123. Frothingham TE (1958) Echovirus type 9 associated with three cases simulating meningococcemia. **N Engl J Med** 259:484.
124. Sawyer MH (1999) Enterovirus infections: diagnosis and treatment. **Pediatr Infect Dis J** 18:1033–1044.
125. Jankovic B, Pasic S, Kanjuh B et al. (1999) Severe neonatal echovirus 17 infection during a nursery outbreak. **Pediatr Infect Dis J** 18:393–394.
126. Huang CC, Liu CC, Chang YC et al. (1999) Neurologic complications in children with enterovirus 71 infection. **N Engl J Med** 341:936–942.
127. Akasu Y (1997) Outbreak of aseptic meningitis due to ECHO-9 in northern Kyushu island in the summer of 1997. **Kurume Med J** 46:97–104.
128. Gondo K, Kusuhara K, Take H et al. (1995) Echovirus type 9 epidemic in Kagoshima, southern Japan: seroepidemiology and clinical observation of aseptic meningitis. **Pediatr Infect Dis J** 14:787–791.
129. Ho M, Chen ER, Hsu KH et al. (1999) An epidemic of enterovirus 71 infection in Taiwan. Taiwan Enterovirus Epidemic Working Group. **N Engl J Med** 341:929–935.

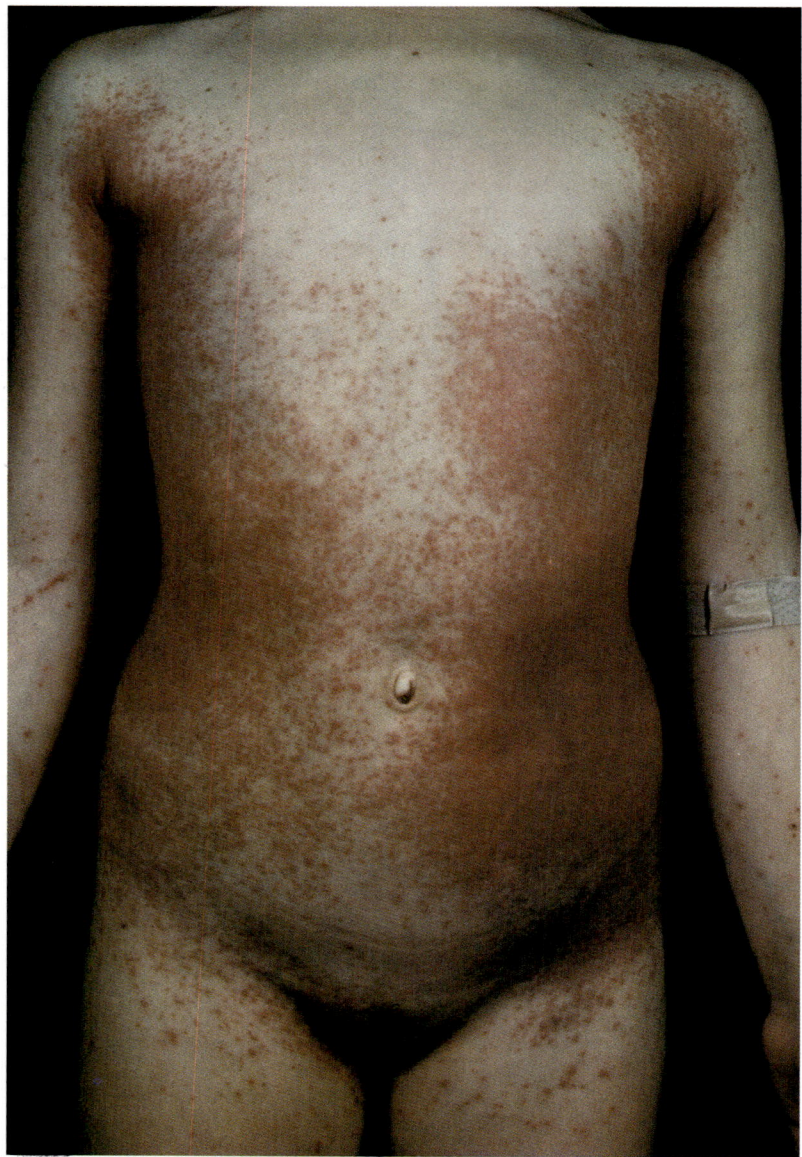

Fig. 25.8 Petechial rash in a child with echoviral infection.

TABLE 25.4 Some less common exanthem associations with enteroviruses

Agent	Association(s)	Reference no.
Coxsackie A4	Generalized vesicular exanthem	414
Coxsackie A16	Measles-like illness	415
	Gianotti-Crosti eruption	416
Coxsackie B1	Henoch-Schonlein purpura	417
Coxsackie B3	Congenital skin lesions	418
Coxsackie B4	Stills-like disease (evanescent rash, arthritis, fever)	419
	AGEPD	420
Echovirus 6	Zoster-like eruption	421
Echovirus 9	Illness simulating meningococcemia	123
Echovirus 11	Herpes-like vesicular exanthem/enanthem	422
Echovirus 12	EI-like eruption	423
Echovirus 25, 32	Hemangioma-like lesions	424
Enterovirus	AGEPD	425
Not specified (patients with HFMD)	Nail matrix arrest	426

EI, erythema infectiosum; AGEPD, acute generalized exanthematous pustular dermatitis; HFMD, hand-foot-mouth disease

isolation of virus from a stool sample must be interpreted cautiously and in the clinical context.[131] An advantage of culture is the ability to isolate and identify the serologic subtype.

Serologic diagnosis is difficult because of the multiple enteroviral subtypes, and generally has little role in clinical practice. Enterovirus PCR is now available, and has the advantages of being rapid, sensitive, and specific. While PCR-based diagnosis may be applicable to several types of samples, it is best established for use with CSF.[124] Skin biopsies are generally not clinically useful in diagnosing enteroviral infections. In HFMD, histologic evaluation of early vesicles reveals intraepidermal blistering, whereas old vesicles reveal a subepidermal location.[132] Pronounced reticular degeneration of the epidermis occurs, resulting in a multilocular process, and there are no inclusion bodies or multinucleated giant cells. The dermal inflammatory infiltrate is nonspecific.[132]

PATHOPHYSIOLOGY

Enteroviruses are acquired by the oral or respiratory route, infect epithelial surfaces, replicate in lymphoid tissues and then disseminate in a hematogenous fashion. Viral replication may occur at multiple anatomic sites, including the CNS, heart, liver, lungs, skin, and mucous membranes.[133]

DIFFERENTIAL DIAGNOSIS

Because of the relatively nonspecific nature of many enteroviral exanthems, the differential diagnosis is broad. The seasonal pattern of enteroviral infections and a history of exposure, however, may help distinguish them from other viral exanthems.

HFMD is generally a straightforward diagnosis owing to the distinct distribution of vesicular lesions. The presentations of herpangina and herpetic gingivostomatitis may be quite similar, but the frequent concomitant involvement of perioral skin, revealing clustered vesicles on an erythematous base,

myoclonus and sleep disturbance the most important early sign of CNS involvement.[130]

LABORATORY FINDINGS

There are no specific laboratory aberrations in patients with enteroviral illnesses. When meningitis is present, the typical cerebrospinal fluid (CSF) profile is that of a mononuclear pleocytosis, a normal or slightly elevated protein level, and a normal glucose concentration.[124]

Specific diagnosis of enteroviral infections may be accomplished by viral culture, serologic studies, or PCR-based diagnosis. These agents grow readily in cell culture, and can be recovered from the oropharynx, stool, blood, urine, CSF, and other tissues. However, the delay in diagnosis makes this method less useful clinically. In addition, prolonged shedding of enteroviruses in the stool following acute infection may occur for up to 12 weeks, and therefore

130. Liu CC, Tseng HW, Wang SM et al. (2000) An outbreak of enterovirus 71 infection in Taiwan, 1998: epidemiologic and clinical manifestations. **J Clin Virol** 17(1):23–30.
131. American Academy of Pediatrics (2000) Enterovirus (Nonpolio) Infections. In: 2000 Red Book: Report of the Committee on Infectious Diseases, 25th ed, Pickering LK, ed. Elk Grove Village, IL: American Academy of Pediatrics, pp. 236–38.
132. Lever WF, Schaumburg-Lever G (1990) Diseases caused by viruses. In: Histopathology of the Skin, 7th ed, Lever WF, Schaumburg-Lever G. Philadelphia: JB Lippincott, pp. 399–425.
133. Cherry JD (1998) Enteroviruses: Coxsackieviruses, echoviruses, and polioviruses. In: Textbook of Pediatric Infectious Diseases, 4th ed, Feigin RD, Cherry JD, eds. Philadelphia: WB Saunders, pp. 1787–1839.

helps to distinguish infection due to herpes simplex virus (HSV). In cases where there is a question, Tzanck preparation or direct fluorescent examination may be useful.

Measles and rubella-like illnesses may also be confused with enteroviral infection. In one study, 993 acutely ill Finnish children with fever and such rashes were tested for a variety of viral agents, and 9% had a significant change in acute and convalescent enterovirus antibody levels.[34] Bacterial infections may also be in the differential diagnosis of enteroviral infection, most notably meningococcemia when the patient presents with a petechial exanthem and nuchal rigidity. In a study of children evaluated during the summer–autumn season who required blood culture and/or lumbar puncture to rule out bacterial sepsis/meningitis, 46% tested positive for enteroviral infection via viral culture or PCR.[134] 28% of the enterovirus-infected patients had an exanthem, but details of the cutaneous findings were not specifically addressed.

THERAPEUTICS AND PROGNOSIS

The prognosis for mild enteroviral exanthematous illnesses such as HFMD or herpangina is excellent, and full recovery is the norm. For more disseminated or serious infections, especially in immunocompromised individuals or neonates, the possibility of significant morbidity or even mortality exists. Until recently, specific therapy of these infections did not exist, and treatment was supportive. Newer pharmacologic agents with anti-enteroviral activity, the first of which is pleconaril, have shown promise both *in vitro* and in clinical studies of patients with enteroviral meningitis and other life-threatening infections.[124,134,135]

EPSTEIN–BARR VIRUS (EBV) INFECTIONS

Christine Bodemer

EBV, a member of the herpesvirus family, was discovered 37 years ago by electron microscopy of cells, cultured from Burkitt's lymphoma tissue by Epstein, Achong, and Barr.[135] In 1968, EBV was shown to be the etiologic agent of infectious mononucleosis.[136] In 1970, EBV DNA was detected in tissues from patients with nasopharyngeal carcinoma.[137] In the 1980s, EBV was found to be associated with non-Hodgkin's lymphoma and oral hairy leukoplakia in patients with the acquired immunodeficiency syndrome (AIDS).[138,139] More recently, EBV was found to be associated with several lymphoproliferative diseases in patients with congenital or acquired immunodeficiency, smooth-muscle tumors in transplants recipients[140,141] and with nasal T-cell/natural killer-cell lymphomas, lymphomatoid granulomatosis, angioimmunoblastic lymphadenopathy, central nervous system lymphomas,[142] and gastric carcinoma[143] in nonimmunocompromised patients. Viral DNA or proteins have also been found in peripheral T-cell lymphomas which can be accompanied by virus-associated hemophagocytic syndrome.[144,145]

EPIDEMIOLOGY

EBV is one of the most successful viruses, infecting over 90% of humans and persisting for a life-time.[146] Infection of humans with EBV usually occurs by contact with oral secretions. The incubation period varies from 10 to 60 days.[147] The virus replicates in cells of the oropharynx and seropositive individuals actively shed virus in the saliva.[148] Infection with the virus is worldwide, but the type of infection acquired appears to be related to the age of the individual at the time of the primary infection. Warm climates and lower socio-economic level favor earlier acquisition of infection. EBV infections are usually asymptomatic or nonspecific in infants and young children, but in adolescents and young adults infection results in infectious mononucleosis.

PRESENTING HISTORY AND PHYSICAL EXAMINATION

Infectious mononucleosis

The classical manifestations of infectious mononucleosis are fever, sore throat, and lymphadenopathy. In 85% of cases, patients present with erythema of the pharynx, and in 20% a grayish-white pharyngeal exudate. A palatal enanthem consisting of multiple petechiae that sometimes coalesce into large plaques has been reported in 3–13% of cases.[149]

Other frequent manifestations include malaise, headache, anorexia, myalgias, splenomegaly and hepatomegaly. Nausea, abdominal pain, jaundice and rash can also be observed. A rare but very serious complication is splenic rupture. The disease is usually self-limiting after being symptomatic for 2–4 weeks but in some cases fatigue can persist for months.

A morbilliform or papular rash is present in 5–15% of cases. The rash is sometimes very atypical, being scarlatiniform, urticarial vesicular or petechial.[149] It is usually present during the first week of the disease, and may persist during the second week. This rash is more frequent in young children. Periorbital edema is present in up to 35% of patients with infectious mononucleosis.[149] Ninety to one hundred percent of patients treated with ampicillin during the course of primary EBV infection develop a macular-papular eruption.[150,151] A similar eruption has also been observed in patients treated with amoxicillin (amoxycillan), but it is less frequent with other beta-lactam antibiotics.

The eruption associated with antibiotics differs somewhat from the eruption observed in untreated patients. It begins 1–2 days after the administration of antibiotics and is more severe. It is characterized by erythematous or copper-colored macules and papules beginning on the trunk and gradually spreading over the entire body, including the palms and soles. It is variably pruritic and in some cases is accompanied by edema of the face and extremities.[152] It is important to appreciate that skin reactions to ampicillin may be observed even in patients who have never been previously treated with this antibiotic and that the eruption is not predictive of future adverse reactions to ampicillin or penicillin.[153]

134. Rotbart HA, McCracken GH, Whitley RJ et al. (1999) Clinical significance of enteroviruses in serious summer febrile illnesses of children. Pediatr Infect Dis J 18:869–874.
135. Espstein MA, Achong BG, Barr YM (1964) Virus particles in cultured lymphoblast from Burkitt's lymphoma. Lancet 1:702–703.
136. Henle G, Henle W, Diehl V (1968) Relation of Burkitt's tumor-associated herpes type virus to infectious mononucleosis. Proc Natl Acad Sci USA 59:94–101.
137. Zur Hausen H, Schulte-Holthausen H, Klein G et al. (1970) EBV DNA in biopsies of Burkitt tumours and anaplastic carcinomas of the nasopharynx. Nature 228:1056–1058.
138. Ziegler JL, Drew WL Miner RC et al. (1982) Outbreak of Burkitt's-like lymphoma in homosexual men. Lancet 2:631–633.
139. Greenspan JS, Greenspan D, Lennette ET et al. (1985) Replication of Epstein-Barr virus within the epithelial cells of oral "hairy" leukoplakia, an AIDS-associated lesion. N Engl J Med 313:1564–1571.
140. Lee ES, Locker J, Nalesnik M et al. (1995) The association of Epstein-Barr virus with smooth-muscle tumors occuring after organ transplantation. N Engl J Med 332:19–25.
141. Reyes C, Abuzaitoun O, De Jong A (2002) Epstein-barr virus associated smooth muscle tumors in ataxia telangiectasia: A case report and review. Human Pathol 33:133–136.
142. Hochberg FH, Miller G, Schooley RT et al. (1983) Central-nervous-system lymphoma related to Epstein-Barr virus. N Engl J Med 309:745–748.
143. Imai S, Koizumi S, Sugiura M et al. (1994) Gastric carcinoma, monoclonal epithelial malignant cells expressing Epstein-barr virus latent infection protein. Proc Natl Acad Sci USA 91:9131–9135.
144. Pallessen G, Hamilton-Dutoit SJ, Zhou X (1993) The association of Epstein-Barr virus (EBV) with T cell lymphoproliferations and Hodgkin's disease: two new developments in the EBV field. Adv Cancer Res 62:179–239.
145. Michalek J, Horvath R (2002) High incidence of Epstein-Barr virus, cytomegalovirus and human herpes virus 6 infections in children with cancer. BMC Pediatr 2:1.
146. Cohen JI (2000) Epstein-Barr virus infection. N Engl J Med 343:481–492.
147. Sumaya CV (1992) Epstein-Barr virus. In: Textbook of Pediatric Infectious Disease, 3rd ed, Feigin RD, Cherry JD, eds. Philadelphia: WB Saunders, p. 1547.
148. Yao QY, Rickinson AB, Epstein MA (1985) A re-examination of the Epstein-Barr virus carrier state in healthy seropositive individuals. Int J Cancer 35:35–42.
149. McCarthy JT, Hoagland RJ (1964) Cutaneous manifestations of infectious mononucleosis. JAMA 187:153.
150. Weary PE et al. (1970) Eruptions from ampicillin in patients with infectious mononucleosis. Arch Dermatol 101:86.
151. Patel BM (1967) Skin rash with infectious mononucleosis and ampicillin. Paediatrics 40:910.
152. Pullen H et al. (1967) Hypersensitivity reaction to antibacterial drugs in infectious mononucleosis. Lancet 2:1176.
153. Nazareth I et al. (1972) Ampicillin sensitivity in infectious mononucleosis – temporary or permanent. Scand J Infest Dis 4:229.

Some less frequent cutaneous manifestations in patients with infectious mononucleosis are acrocyanosis and cold urticaria associated with cryoglobulinemia or cold agglutinins,[154–156] palmar papules and erythema,[157] erythema nodosum,[158] erythema multiforme,[159] and painful genital ulcerations.[160] Recently, the association of hydroa vacciniforme and EBV has been discussed. Some authors consider that the disease of Epstein–Barr virus–associated recurrent necrotic papulo-vesicles is a distinct clinicopathologic entity different from classic hydroa vacciniforme.[161] Hydroa vacciniforme-like lesions may be the presenting cutaneous symptoms of Epstein–Barr virus-associated peripheral T-cell lymphoma,[162] and so children with these lesions require biopsy and close follow-up.

Infants and young children

Some cases of infantile papular acrodermatitis have been associated with acute EBV infections.[163–166] Kawasaki disease[167] and a granuloma annulare–like eruption have also been reported in young patients with EBV infections.[168] Children with X-linked lymphoproliferation, Wiskott–Aldrich syndrome, on immunosupression following transplants and with acquired immune deficiency syndrome (AIDS) are at particular risk of developing EBV-associated lymphomas.

LABORATORY FINDINGS AND DIAGNOSIS

In infectious mononucleosis, the lymphocyte count usually rises during the second or third week of illness with the presence of more than 10% of atypical and vacuolated lymphocytes. Most of the atypical lymphocytes are T cells, responding to the EBV-infected B cells, and most symptoms of infectious mononucleosis are due to the primary immune response to the virus.[146] Occasionally, a "leukemoid" reaction, with 30 000 to 50 000μl/ml may occur. Neutropenia, thrombocytopenia, and elevated levels of transaminases and alkaline phosphatase are frequent during the first month of illness. Acute EBV infection is usually confirmed by a positive monospot test (heterophile antibody test). However, heterophile antibodies may not become elevated until the third week of the illness, and they are less frequent in patients who have atypical disease. The heterophile antibody test is very sensitive, except in children younger than 4 years of age, in whom a high proportion of false-negative results occur. In these cases EBV-specific antibody tests can be helpful for the diagnosis. IgM antibody to the viral capsid antigen (VCA) is only elevated during the acute phase of the infection. Antibody to the early antigens (EA) are elevated in less than 70% of patients with infectious mononucleosis. Seroconversion to IgG VCA and EBV nuclear antigen (EBNA) antibody positivity are useful for the diagnosis of acute EBV infection. IgG VCA and EBNA antibodies persist for life. In some particular cases, such as EBV-associated lymphoproliferative diseases and EBV-associated malignancies, EBV DNA, RNA and proteins can be detected in tissues.

DIFFERENTIAL DIAGNOSIS

Cutaneous manifestations of EBV acute infections are nonspecific, and may be confused with other childhood exanthems, when the characteristic triad of infectious mononucleosis (fever, lymphadenopathy and pharyngitis) is not present. In older children and in adolescents, EBV infection must be differentiated from streptococcal, and sometimes gonococcal pharyngitis and also arcanobacterium hemolyticum infection, another cause of pharyngitis and rash.[169] In some cases, the clinical findings may be confused with Kawasaki disease, and in other cases the periorbital edema could be evocative of dermatomyositis.

TREATMENT

Treatment is generally supportive. Acyclovir inhibits EBV replication and reduces viral shedding, but no specific treatment is indicated for most patients with acute EBV infection because manifestations of infectious mononucleosis are not related to replication of viral genomes, but are secondary to the immune response to the virus.[170] Corticosteroids are not indicated for uncomplicated disease and should be considered only in severe infectious mononucleosis with major visceral complications.[171]

ACQUIRED CYTOMEGALOVIRUS INFECTIONS

Cytomegaloviruses (CMV) are DNA viruses that are members of the herpesvirus family. Although rash is a common manifestation of congenital CMV infection, cutaneous involvement is rare in acquired CMV infections.[172–174]

EPIDEMIOLOGY

The prevalence of CMV infection varies, depending on the clinical setting. In the United States, 20–80% of adults have antibodies to CMV. Viruria is present in up to 40% of children living in institutions.[174] Infection is usually spread by respiratory droplets but may involve the urine-oral or fecal-oral route. Virus is also present in breast milk, semen, cervical secretions, and blood.[172] Persistent viral shedding has made it difficult to evaluate the role of CMV in causing specific clinical infections. Early acquisition of virus, including congenital infection, is frequently followed by persistent shedding of virus and may contribute to a high prevalence of infection

154. Tyson CJ, Czarny D (1981) Cold-induced urticaria in infectious mononucleosis. **Med J Aust** 1:33.
155. Lemanske EF, Bushe RK (1982) Cold urticaria in infectious mononucleosis. **JAMA** 247:1604.
156. Dickerman JD, Howard P, Dopp S et al. (1980) Infectious mononucleosis initially seen as cold-induced acrocyanosis. **Am J Dis Child** 134:159.
157. Petrozzi JW (1971) Infectious mononucleosis manifesting as a palmar dermatitis. **Arch Dermatol** 104:207.
158. Bodansky HJ (1979) Erythema nodosum and infectious mononucleosis. **Br Med J** 2:1263.
159. Williamson DM (1974) Erythema multiforme in infectious mononucleosis. **Br J Dermatol** 91:345.
160. McKenna G, Edwards S, Cleland H (1994) Genital ulceration secondary to Epstein-Barr virus infection. **Genitourin Med** 70:356.
161. Yoon TY, Yang TH, Hahn YS et al. (2001) Epstein-Barr virus-associated recurrent necrotic papulovesicles with repeated bacterial infections ending in sepsis and death: consideration of the relationship between Epstein-Barr virus and immune defect. **J Dermatol** 28:442–447.
162. Cho KH, Kim CW, Heo DS et al. (2001) Epstein-Barr virus associated peripheral T-cell lymphoma in adults with hydroa vacciniforme-like lesions. **Clin Exp Dermatol** 26:242–247.
163. Konno M, Kikuta H, Ishikawa M et al. (1982) A possible association between hepatitis-B antigen negative infantile papular acrodermatitis and Epstein-Barr virus infection. **J Pediatr** 101:222.
164. Lowe L, Hebert AA, Duvic M (1989) Gianotti-Crosti syndrome associated with Epstein-Barr virus infection. **J Am Acad Dermatol** 201:336.
165. Iosub S, Santos C, Gromisch DS (1984) Papular acrodermatitis with Epstein-Barr virus infection. **Clin Pediatr** 23:33.
166. Baldari U, Monti A, Righini MG (1994) An epidemic of infantile papular acrodermatitis (Gianotti-Crosti syndrome) due to Epstein-Barr virus. **Dermatology** 188:203.
167. Kikuta H, Matsumoto S, Osato T (1991) Kawasaki disease and Epstein-Barr virus. **Acta Paediatr Jpn** 33:765–770.
168. Spencer SA, Fenske NA, Espinoza CZ et al. (1988) Granuloma annulare-like eruption due to chronic Epstein-Barr infection. **Arch Dermatol** 124:250.
169. Kain KC, Noble MA, Barteluk RL et al. (1991) Arcanobacterium hemolyticum infection: confused with scarlet fever and diphtheria. **J Emerg Med** 9:33–35.
170. Van der Horst C, Joncas J, Ahronheim G et al. (1991) Lack of effect of per oral acyclovir for the treatment of acute infectious mononucleosis. **J Infect Dis** 164:778–792.
171. Tynell E, Aurelius E, Brandell A et al. (1996) Acyclovir and prednisolone treatment of acute infectious mononucleosis a multicenter, double-blind, placebo-controlled study. **J Infect Dis** 174:324–331.
172. Weller TH (1971) The cytomegaloviruses: ubiquitous agents with protean clinical manifestations. **N Engl J Med** 285:203.
173. Sullivan JL, Hanshaw JB (1982) Human cytomegalovirus infections. In: Human Herpesvirus Infections: Clinical Aspects, Glaser R, Gotlieb-Stematsky T, eds. New York: Marcel Dekker, p. 57.
174. Demmler GJ (1992) Acquired cytomegalovirus infections. In: Textbook of Pediatric Infectious Diseases, 3rd ed, Feigin RD, Cherry JD, eds. Philadelphia: WB Saunders, p. 1532.

in a community. Severe infections with CMV are common in patients with leukemia, in bone marrow, stem cell and organ transplant recipients, in patients with HIV infection and after pump perfusion in cardiac surgery.[175–178]

CLINICAL MANIFESTATIONS

Congenital CMV infection is discussed in Chapter 6. Cutaneous manifestations of acquired CMV infection are uncommon. Rubelliform or maculopapular rashes have been reported in CMV-induced infectious mononucleosis, either with or without ampicillin exposure.[179] A papular acrodermatitis has been reported in an infant with CMV hepatitis.[180] Virtually all other cutaneous eruptions associated with acquired CMV infection occur in immunocompromised individuals, usually adults. Two main types of lesions occur: cutaneous ulcers and generalized exanthematous eruptions. Morbilliform, urticarial, and petechial eruptions have also been described.

CMV may cause a wide variety of clinical illnesses. An EBV-like mononucleosis with fever, malaise, mild hepatitis, and atypical lymphocytosis may occur, usually in young, healthy individuals. Exudative pharyngitis and cervical adenopathy are less prominent in CMV-induced mononucleosis.[173] A similar syndrome may occur 3–5 weeks after transfusion or cardiopulmonary bypass[174] and with reactivation of CMV infection in renal transplant patients. In immunocompromised patients, CMV may cause an often fatal interstitial pneumonia.[173] Other clinical manifestations of acquired CMV infection include the Guillain–Barré syndrome, chorioretinitis, and widespread gastrointestinal ulcerations.

LABORATORY FINDINGS

In CMV-induced mononucleosis, an atypical lymphocytosis and abnormal liver function test findings may be present. The heterophile and specific EBV test results are negative. Viral isolation is the best method for diagnosing CMV infection. A fresh urine specimen is an excellent method because systemic CMV infections are nearly always accompanied by viruria.[173,174] A virus-specific cytopathic effect may be present as early as 24 hours but usually occurs 7–21 days after inoculation. CMV may also be recovered from the throat, CSF, and many other secretions. When virus is cultured, serologic confirmation may be required to demonstrate acute infection, because persistent viral shedding occurs in many settings. This can be demonstrated by a fourfold rise in complement fixation titers, drawn in the acute period and 4–5 weeks later, or by demonstration of CMV-specific IgM.

PATHOPHYSIOLOGY AND HISTOGENESIS

The skin lesions of disseminated CMV infection have demonstrated cytomegalic nuclear inclusions in the endothelial cells of cutaneous blood vessels.[181,182]

TREATMENT

CMV lacks the thymidine kinase necessary for efficient drug phosphorylation. The drugs used to treat severe CMV infections target the DNA polymerase. Ganciclovir is the drug most utilized.[183,184] Ganciclovir is similar in structure to acyclovir, but is more active than acyclovir against CMV. Viruses resistant to acyclovir because of DNA polymerase mutation may remain sensitive to ganciclovir, because mutations leading to aciclovir-resistance differ from those leading to ganciclovir resistance. The major side effects of ganciclovir are thrombocytopenia and neutropenia. Ganciclovir is widely used for treatment and for prophylaxis of CMV infections in immunosuppressed patients. It is also used for the treatment of CMV retinitis. Foscarnet, which does not require phosphorylation for its antiviral activity, is an alternative for ganciclovir-resistant strains.[185] Its major side effect is renal toxicity. The major use of foscarnet is in the treatment of CMV retinitis. Cidofovir is effective against CMV *in vitro*; however, there is limited data on its use in severe infection. Cidofovir has recently been evaluated as primary pre-emptive therapy for cytomegalovirus infections following allogenic stem cell transplantation.[186] In this indication, cidofovir has the practical advantage of weekly administration rather than daily as for ganciclovir and foscarnet.

PAPULAR ACRODERMATITIS OF CHILDHOOD

Papular acrodermatitis of childhood (PAC), or Gianotti–Crosti syndrome, is a unique childhood viral exanthem, characterized by papular or papulovesicular lesions that are most prominent on the extremities, face, and buttocks. Another name is papulovesicular acrolocated syndrome.

HISTORY AND EPIDEMIOLOGY

The first cases were described in 1955 by Gianotti[187] in Italy. Cases have now been reported from most parts of the world. Most cases are sporadic but small family outbreaks have occured. It tends to occur in childhood, though it has also been reported in adults. Possibly some adult cases are misdiagnosed and some authors suggest that the syndrome may not be as uncommon as previously supposed beyond the childhood age group.[188] The age of onset is usually between 6 months and 14 years (mean 2 years) and the eruption is more frequent in spring and early summer. The role of hepatitis B virus in some cases was confirmed in the 1970s.[189–191] In these cases, acute anicteric hepatitis was always present. However, further studies did not demonstrate the constant presence of Australia antigen, the surface antigen of hepatitis B, and underlined the role of a variety of other viruses. Initially it was suggested that there were clinical differences between those cases with and those without an association with hepatitis B, but finally in 1992 a review of 308 cases proved that it was not possible to make a clinical distinction.[192]

175. Borkowky W (1984) Viral infections in immunocompromised children. **Pediatr Ann** 13:682.
176. Tsinontides AC, Bechtel TP (1996) Cytomegalovirus prophylaxis and treatment following bone marrow transplantation. **Ann Pharmacol** 30:1277–1290.
177. Dini D, Castagnola E, Comoli P et al. (2001) Infections after stem cell transplantation in children: state of the art and recommendations. **Bone Marrow Transplantation** 28(Suppl 1):S18–S21.
178. Slifkin M, Tempesti P, Poutsiaka DD (2001) Late and atypical cytomegalovirus disease in solid organ transplant recipients. **Clin Infect Dis** 33:E62–E68.
179. Ho M (1995) Cytomegalovirus. In: Principles and Practice of Infectious Diseases, 4th ed, Mandell GL, Douglas RG, Bennett JE, eds. New York: Churchill Livingstone, p. 1351.
180. Berant M, Naveh Y. Weissman I (1983) Papular acrodermatitis with cytomegaiovirus hepatitis. **Arch Dis Child** 58:1024.
181. Pariser RJ (1983) Histologically specific skin lesions in disseminated cytomegalovirus infection. **J Am Acad Dermatol** 9:937.
182. Lin C, Penha PD, Krishnan MN, Zak FG (1981) Cytomegalic inclusion disease of the skin. **Arch Dermatol** 117:282.
183. Mobberley MA, Rycer TA, Hart H et al. (1987) Fine structure of cells infected with human cytomegalovirus after treatment with 9-(1,3-dihydroxy-2-propoxymethyl) guanine. **J Gen Virol** 68:1553–1562.
184. Crumpackers CS (1995) Drug therapy: Ganciclovir. **N Engl J Med** 335:721–729.
185. Drobyski WR et al. (1991) Foscarnet therapy for ganciclovir-resistant cytomegalovirus in marrow-transplantation. **Transplantation** 52:155.
186. Chakrabarti S et al. (2001) Cidofovir as primary pre-emptive therapy for post transplant cytomegalovirus infections. **Bone Marrow Transplant** 28:879–881.
187. Gianotti F (1955) Rilievi di una particolare casistica tossinfettiva caratterizzata da eruzione eritemato-infiltrativa desquamativa a focolai lenticolari, a sede elettiva acroesposta. **Giorn Ital Dermatol Sifilol** 96:678–697.
188. Gibbs S, Burrows N (2000) Gianotti-Crosti syndrome in two unrelated adults. **Clin Exp Dermatol** 25:594–596.
189. Gianotti F (1973) Papular acrodermatitis of childhood. An Australia antigen disease. **Arch Dis Child** 48:794–795.
190. Gianotti F (1979) Papular acrodermatitis of childhood and other papulovesicular acrolocated syndromes. **Br J Dermatol** 100:49–59.
191. De Gasperi G, Bardare M, Costantino D (1970) An antigen in Crosti-Gianotti acrodermatitis. **Lancet** i:1116.
192. Caputo R, Gelmetti C, Ermacora E et al. (1992) Gianotti-Crosti syndrome: a retrospective analysis of 308 cases. **J Am Acad Dermatol** 26:207–210.

PATHOPHYSIOLOGY

PAC is clearly a nonspecific cutaneous reaction to several viruses. Hepatitis B virus and Epstein–Barr virus are now considered as the most frequent causes of Gianotti–Crosti syndrome, and worldwide Epstein–Barr virus appears to be the commonest cause of the syndrome.[192–201] Epidemic cases due to hepatitis B virus and Epstein–Barr virus have been reported.[193,195,202] Epstein–Barr virus is the commonest cause in the United States. The role of several other viruses have been reported and those implicated include enteroviruses,[203,204] which are the commonest cause in Australia, hepatitis A,[205] hepatitis non A-non B,[206] cytomegalovirus,[207–210] adenovirus, rotavirus, rubella, polio virus, parainfluenzae, and respiratory syncitial virus.[211–218] A similar eruption has been reported with toxoplasmosis.[219] The possible causative role of immunization to diphteria, pertussis, tetanus and polio, and bacille Calmette–Guérin (BCG) vaccination has been discussed by some authors.[215,220–222]

LABORATORY FINDINGS AND HISTOPATHOLOGY

The histologic features of cutaneous lesions of Gianotti–Crosti are nonspecific. These include parakeratosis, focal spongiosis, hyperkeratosis, and mild acanthosis. Liquefactive degeneration of the basal cell layer may be seen, along with a band-like lymphohistiocytic infiltration in the upper dermis, with extensive exocytosis of mononuclear cells. Similar features could be seen in other inflammatory diseases. In more severe cases, a lymphocytic vasculitis may be noted.[194]

Other laboratory abnormalities may be demonstrated, depending on the causative agent and the degree of systemic disease associated.

PRESENTING HISTORY

PAC is characterized by the abrupt onset of symmetric flat-topped (lichenoid) skin-colored or erythematous papules, localized to the face, limbs, and buttocks. Itching may or may not be present, and occasionally mild consti-tutional symptoms such as malaise, general lymphadenopathy, low-grade fever, and diarrhea may occur.

PHYSICAL EXAMINATION

The eruption is monomorphic and symmetrically distributed with firm papules that are usually pink or violaceous but sometimes are very pale, especially in dark-skinned individuals. Less frequently, papulovesicles or purpuric lesions occur. The size of the papules is variable from case to case – from 1 to 10mm, but usually fairly constant in an individual case. The lesions may be asymptomatic or quite pruritic. They usually begin on the extremities and then may spread to the buttocks and face. They may coalesce in oedematous plaques over the elbows and the knees (Figs 25.9, 25.10). The trunk is usually spared and the mucous membranes are not affected. The rash usually develops over a week, but sometimes all areas become involved at once. Lymphadenopathy is frequent, particularly in the axillary and inguinal area, and in the hepatitis B form the liver may be enlarged. Systemic symptoms are variable, depending on the causative organism, but often these children are completely well. In most cases the syndrome is self-limiting and resoves within 3–6 weeks, exceptionally lasting for up to eight weeks. There is no desquamation. Chronic active hepatitis, with persistent HbsAg and persistent abnormal liver function studies, has been reported in two children.[223,224]

DIFFERENTIAL DIAGNOSIS

Papular acrodermatitis may be confused with insect bites, micropapular eczema, frictional lichenoid dermatitis, micropapular psoriasis, lichen planus, and lichenoid drug eruption.

THERAPY

Most cases do not require treatment. Antihistamines may relieve itch in very pruritic cases. Topical steroids are usually ineffective.[225]

193. Ishimaru Y, Ishimaru H, Toda G et al. (1976) An epidemic of infantile papular acrodermatitis (Gianotti's disease) in Japan associated with hepatitis B surface antigen subtype ayw. Lancet i:707–709.
194. Spear KL, Winkelmann RK (1984) Gianotti-Crosti syndrome. A review of ten cases not associated with hepatitis B. Arch Dermatol 120:891–896.
195. Gianotti F (1978) HbsAg and papular acrodermatitis of childhood. N Engl J Med 298:460.
196. Labbe A, Gouney J, Peyrot P et al. (1981) Syndrome acropapulo-vésiculeux de Gianotti-Crosti en cours d'une primo-infection à virus Epstein-Barr. Nouv Presse Med 36:2993.
197. Konno M, Kikuta S, Ishikawa N et al. (1982) A possible relationship between hepatitis B antigen negative infantile papular acrodermatitis and Epstein-Barr virus. J Pediatr 101:2224.
198. Iosub S, Santos C, Gromisch DS (1984) Papular acrodermatitis with Epstein-Barr virus infection. Clin Pediatr Phila 23:334.
199. Timar L, Budai J, Gero A et al. (1985) Rare complications and unusual syndromes associated with Epstein-Barr virus. Pediatr Infect Dis 4:212–213.
200. Lowe L, Hebert AA, Duvic M (1989) Gianotti-Crosti syndrome associated with Epstein-Barr virus infection. J Am Acad Dermatol 20:336–338.
201. Maeda S, Tsuda H, Haruki S, Mitsuto I (1999) Atypical Epstein-Barr virus infection associated with Gianotti-Crosti syndrome and Bell's palsy. Pediatr Int 41:315–317.
202. Baldari U, Monti A, Righini MG (1994) An epidemic of infantile papular acrodermatitis (Gianotti-Crosti syndrome) due to Epstein-Barr virus. Dermatology 188:203–204.
203. James WD, Odom RB, Hatch MH (1982) Gianotti-Crosti like eruption associated with coxsackie virus A-16 infection. J Am Acad Dermatol 6:862–866.
204. Taïeb A, Plantin P, du Pasquier P et al. (1986) Gianotti-Crosti syndrome: a study of 26 cases. Br J Dermatol 15:4959.
205. Sagi EF, Linden N, Shonval D (1985) Papular acrodermatitis of childhood associated with hepatitis A virus infection. Pediatr Dermatol 3:31–3.
206. Schiuma A, Pierini AM, Galimberti R, Gelmetti C (1990) Papular acrodermatitis of childhood: a review. In: Pediatric Dermatology Proceeding of the Fifth International Congress of Pediatric Dermatology, Caputo R, Gelmetti C, eds. Milano.
207. Berant M, Naveh Y, Weismann I (1983) Papular acrodermatitis with cytomegalovirus hepatitis. Arch Dis Child 58:1024–1025.
208. Ramelet AA (1984) Mononucléose infectieuse avec manifestations cutanées. A type d'acrosyndrome de Gianotti-Crosti. Dermatologica 168:19–24.
209. Haki M, Tsuchida M, Kotsuji M et al. (1997) Gianotti-Crosti syndrome associated with cytomegalovirus antigenemia after bone marrow transplantation. Bone Marrow Transplant 20:691–693.
210. Baleviciene G, Maciuleviciene R, Schwartz RA (2001) Papular acrodermatitis of childhood: the Gianotti-Crosti syndrome. Cutis 67:291–294.
211. Rogers S, Connolly JH (1974) Gianotti-Crosti syndrome and viral infection. Br Med J 3:529.
212. Labbe A, Peyrot J, Goumot P et al. (1982) Syndrome acropapulovésiculeux de l'enfant et maladie de Gianotti-Crosti. Pédiatrie 37:467.
213. Patrizi A, Balducci A, Varotti A et al. (1987) Sindrome di Gianotti-Crosti riferita a infezione da rotavirus. Pediatr Dermatol News (Bari) 6:60–62.
214. Patrizi A, Di Lemia V, Neri I, Ricci G (1994) An unusual case of recurrent Gianotti-Crosti syndrome. Pediatr Dermatol 11:283–284.
215. Draelos ZK, Hansen RC, James WD (1986) Gianotti-Crosti syndrome associated with infections other than hepatitis B. JAMA 256:2386–2388.
216. Carton FX, Daniel P, Denoeux JP (1974) Isolement de poliovirus à l'occasion d'une éruption papuleuse infantile. Bull Soc Fran Dermatol Syph 81:201.
217. Blauvelt A, Turner NE (1994) Gianotti-Crosti syndrome and human immunodeficiency virus infection. Arch Dermatol 130:481–483.
218. Stratte EG, Esterly NB (1995) Human immunodeficiency virus infection and Gianotti-Crosti syndrome. Arch Dermatol 131:108–109.
219. Blancher G, Sugier J, Pringuet G et al. (1962) Acrodermatite érythémato-papuleuse infantile (syndrome de Gianotti-Crosti). Contribution à la discussion de l'étiologie. La Semaine des Hôpitaux. Ann Pédiatr 38:669–673.
220. Duperrat B, Puissant A (1958) Syndrome de Gianotti-Crosti. Presse Med 66:1862–1863.
221. Boyanov L, Boyanov B, Dimitrova I (1963) The clinical picture and pathogenesis of the Gianotti-Crosti syndrome. Vest Derm 37:14–17.
222. Murphy LA, Buckley C (2000) Gianotti-Crosti syndrome in an infant following immunization. Pediatr Dermatol 17:225–226.
223. Colombo M, Gerber MA, Vernace SJ et al. (1977) Immune response to hepatitis B virus in children with papular acrodermatitis. Gastroenterology 73:1103.
224. Chuang TY, Ilstrup DM, Perry HO et al. (1982) Pityriasis rosea in Rochester, Minnesota 1969 to 1978. J Am Acad Dermatol 7:80.
225. Hjorth N, Kopp H, Osmunden PE (1967) Gianotti Crosti syndrome – papular eruption of infancy. Trans St John's Hosp Derm Soc 53:46.

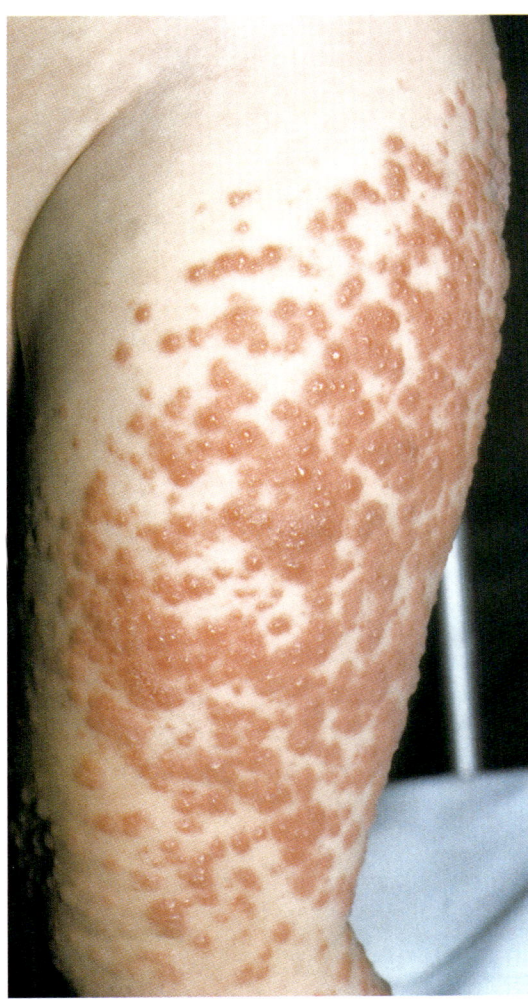

Fig. 25.9   Papular acrodermatitis of childhood (Gianotti–Crosti syndrome); coalescent leg lesions.

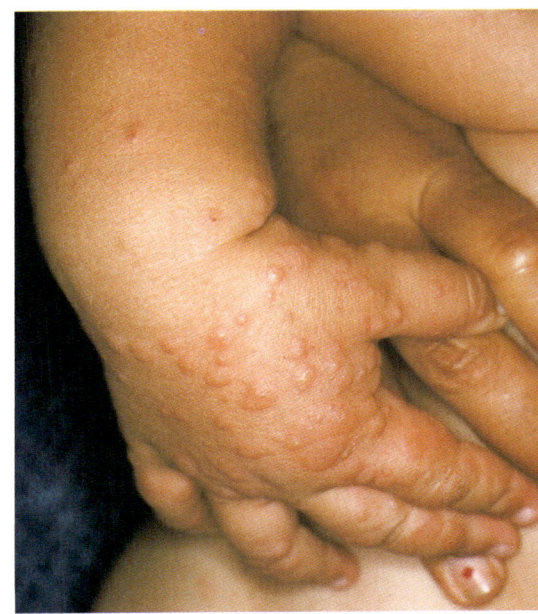

Fig. 25.10   Papular acrodermatitis of childhood (Gianotti–Crosti syndrome); discrete hand lesions.

was proposed.[226] In 1993, the series was expanded to include 30 cases of ULE, with the same clinical characteristics.[227] In the same year, another series of 21 cases from southwest France was published, and the authors proposed the term of "asymmetric periflexural exanthem of childhood" (APEC).[228] This entity had been described previously in the literature in 1986 as "a localized erythema with regional lymphadenopathy"[229] and in 1962 as "a new papular erythema of childhood."[230,231] More recently there have been many publications regarding further cases of this distinctive condition,[232–249] showing that this rediscovered exanthem is not so rare, occurs worldwide, and probably has often been misdiagnosed in the past.

EPIDEMIOLOGY AND PATHOPHYSIOLOGY

A slight increase in incidence in the spring has been observed in some studies but no significant associated environmental factor has been clearly defined. A family history including the typical rash, or a localized eruption has been rarely reported.[226,231,238] In these cases, the rash develops in the second member of the family at the same time or with a delay of 10 to 14 days. In large series there has been a female preponderance.[231,238]

The mean age of patients is around 24 months.

The etiology of this exanthem remains unknown, despite active research.[226,237,238,249] It has not been possible to implicate influenza, rubella,

UNILATERAL LATEROTHORACIC EXANTHEM

HISTORY

In 1992 a series of 18 children, living in or near Paris, with a distinctive childhood exanthem was reported. Because of the characteristics of this particular skin eruption, beginning unilaterally close to the axilla, with secondary centrifugal spreading, the term of "unilateral laterothoracic exanthem" (ULE)

226. Bodemer C, de Prost Y (1992) Unilateral laterothoracic exanthem in children: a new disease? **J Am Acad Dermatol** 27:693–696.
227. de Prost Y, Bodemer C (1993) L'exantheme unilateral laterothoracique de l'enfant: Une nouvelle maladie? **Nouv Dermatol** 12:19–20.
228. Taieb A, Megraud F, Legrain V et al. (1993) Asymmetric periflexural exanthem of childhood. **J Am Acad Dermatol** 29:391–393.
229. Taieb A, Megraud F, le Roy JM et al. (1986) Erytheme localize avec adenopathie regionale de l'enfant; Une maladie d'inoculation? **Ann Dermatol Venereol** 113:1023–1024.
230. Brunner MJ, Rubin L, Dunlop F (1962) A new papular erythema of childhood. **Arch Dermatol** 85:539–540.
231. Laur WE (1993) Unilateral laterothoracic exanthem in children. **J Am Acad Dermatol** 29:799–800.
232. Melski JW (1993) Unilateral laterothoracic exanthem. **J Am Acad Dermatol** 29:130.
233. Maroon M, Billingsley EM (1994) Unilateral laterothoracic exanthem. **J Am Acad Dermatol** 30:1045.
234. Gelmetti C, Grimalt R, Cambiaghi S et al. (1994) Asymmetric periflexural exanthem of childhood: report of two new cases. **Pediatr Dermatol** 11:42–45.
235. Mendelsohn SS, Verbov JL (1994) Asymmetric periflexural exanthem of childhood. **Clin Exp Dermatol** 19:421.
236. Frieden IJ (1995) Childhood exanthems. **Curr Opin Pediatr** 7:411–414.
237. Harangi F, Varszegi D, Szucs G (1995) Asymmetrical periflexural exanthem of childhood and viral examinations. **Pediatr Dermatol** 12:112–115.
238. McCuaig CC, Russo P, Powell J et al. (1996) Unilateral laterothoracic exanthem. A clinicopathologic study of forty-eight patients. **J Am Acad Dermatol** 34:979–984.
239. Resnick SD (1997) New aspects of exanthematous diseases of childhood. **Dermatol Clin** 15:257–266.
240. Adams SP (1997) Unilateral laterothoracic exanthem. **Can Fam Physician** 43:1355–1363.
241. Corazza M, Virgili A (1997) Asymmetric periflexural exanthem in an adult. **Acta Derma Venereol** 77:79–80.
242. Gutzmer R, Herbst RA, Kiehl P et al. (1997) Unilateral laterothoracic exanthem (asymmetrical periflexural exanthem of childhood): report of an adult patient. **J Am Acad Dermatol** 37:484–485.
243. Bauza I, Redondo P, Fernandez J (2000) Asymetric periflexural exanthem in adults. **Br J Dermatol** 143:224–226.
244. Fort DW, Greer KE (1998) Unilateral laterothoracic exanthem in a child with acute lymphoblastic leu. **Pediatr Dermatol** 15:51–52.
245. Strom K, Mempel M, Folster-Holst R et al. (1999) Unilateral laterothoracic exanthema in childhood. Clinical characteristic diagnostic criteria in 5 patients. **Hautarzt** 5:39–41.
246. Peker S, Hoger PH, Moll I (2000) Unilateral laterothoracic exanthema. Case report and review of the literature. **Hautarzt** 51:505–508.
247. Coustou D, Leaute-Labreze C, Bioulac-Sage P et al. (1999) Asymmetric periflexural exanthem of childhood: a clinical, pathologic, and epidemiologic prospective study. **Arch Dermatol** 135:799–803.
248. Mortz CG, Bygum A (2000) Asymmetric periflexural exanthema of childhood. **Ugeskr Laeger** 162:2050–2051.
249. Coustou D, Masquelier B, Lafon ME et al. (2000) Asymmetric periflexural exanthem of childhood: microbiologic case-control study. **Pediatr Dermatol** 17:169–173.

parvovirus B19, EBV, CMV, HSV, HHV-6, HHV-7, HHV-8, picornavirus, adenovirus, enterovirus, hepatitis B virus, borrelia, coxsackieviruses, rickettsia, spiroplasma, or mycoplasma. The possibility of an infectious etiology is tenable, but the responsible microorganism has yet to be identified.

LABORATORY FINDINGS AND HISTOPATHOLOGY

Laboratory investigations have been unremarkable in almost all reported cases, with normal leukocyte count, occasional relative lymphocytocis but without atypical lymphocytes, no rise in inflammatory markers and normal liver enzymes. The results of throat and stool cultures, when performed, have not been significant. Histologic findings are variable,[226,228,231,238] and the histologic pattern observed depends on the time at which the skin biopsy has been performed. In one patient a skin biopsy, performed 15 days after onset of the rash, showed a nonspecific superficial dermatitis; in another patient the biopsy was performed at the beginning of the eruption and showed a perivascular and periappendageal lymphocytic infiltrate with epidermal spongiosis and mononuclear cell exocytosis.[226] Laur[231] described a superficial and focally lichenoid infiltrate with parakeratosis. McCuaig[238] described a prominent lymphocytic infiltration of the eccrine glands and ducts, including the terminal intraepidermal portion.

PRESENTING HISTORY

The onset of the eruption is frequently preceded from a few days to three weeks by a low-grade fever or mild gastrointestinal or upper respiratory tract symptoms. The earliest sign of the exanthem in over 95% of cases is an erythematous patch, unilateral and localized on the thorax, usually around the axillary region. In the other cases the eruption occurs close to other periflexural areas, often the inguinal area. The evolution of this remarkable unilateral laterothoracic exanthem is characteristic, and consists of two phases. The first is a centrifugal extension of the initial lesions and the second is a frequent, but inconstant, dissemination of the eruption.

PHYSICAL EXAMINATION

The initial localized eruption is very variable in morphology, and patterns include a group of small, pink papules, very often surrounded by a pale halo,[231,238] a poorly demarcated eczematous patch and less frequently urticarial, vesicular or even purpuric lesions occur.[238] A purpuric spot suggestive of an inoculation site, but without history of a bite, was observed in two cases.[226] Pruritus is noticed in more than 50% of patient but excoriations are uncommon.

During the first week of the evolution there is centrifugal extension of the initial lesion, sometimes separated by intervals of normal skin. As the lesions progress they become more inflammatory, and sometimes annular patterns emerge. Around the eighth day, the patients demonstrate a morbilliform or eczematous exanthem with a hemicorporal distribution involving the inner surface of the arm, the flank, and the thigh (Fig. 25.11). Even when the eruption originates at another site, it will almost invariably later involve the thorax.

The second phase of the eruption is characterized by varying degrees of dissemination between the eighth and fifteenth day, with new patches appearing on the opposite side of the body and at distal sites. Even after dissemination, the exanthem often retains a markedly asymmetrical distribution with predominant involvement of the half of the body which was initially affected. In a few cases involvement of the face, hands, and feet has been observed but this is rare. There is no enanthem.

The general health remains good although there may be a mild regional lymphadenopathy and a low-grade fever.

The lesions start to improve spontaneously, during the third week with older plaques developing a central dusky gray discoloration. Usually, only residual skin dryness remains during the fourth or fifth week, and all signs have disappeared by six weeks.

Recurrence appears exceptional. However, Laur[231] reported two cases with recurrences, one with three episodes over a six-year period and the other with with two episodes within four months. The age of onset, the lack of recurrence in the majority of cases, and the fact that adolescents and adults are generally not affected by ULE suggest the development of immunity. Nevertheless, it is possible that ULE is misdiagnosed in adults, and new cases have been recently reported in this population.[241–243]

DIFFERENTIAL DIAGNOSIS

This includes papular eczema, contact dermatitis, tinea corporis, Gianotti–Crosti syndrome, and atypical pityriasis rosea. Indeed, as ULE, Gianotti–Crosti syndrome, and pityriasis rosea all have a sudden onset in a child, a localized initial distribution and spontaneous resolution in 4–6 weeks, they have been compared.[231,232,234] However, there are distinctive clinical features: none of the infectious agents related to the Gianotti–Crosti syndrome has been found in ULE; ULE presents with small papules with a unilateral predominence, whereas pityriasis rosea has oval scaly plaques in a bilateral "Chrismas-tree" distribution.

TREATMENT

No treatment is necessary, as spontaneous resolution is the rule. Topical corticosteroids have sometimes been prescribed, but their efficacy is variable.

ERUPTIVE PSEUDOANGIOMATOSIS

Anthony J. Mancini

In 1969, Cherry *et al.* described four children who presented with fever and transitory hemangioma-like lesions, and who were confirmed to have

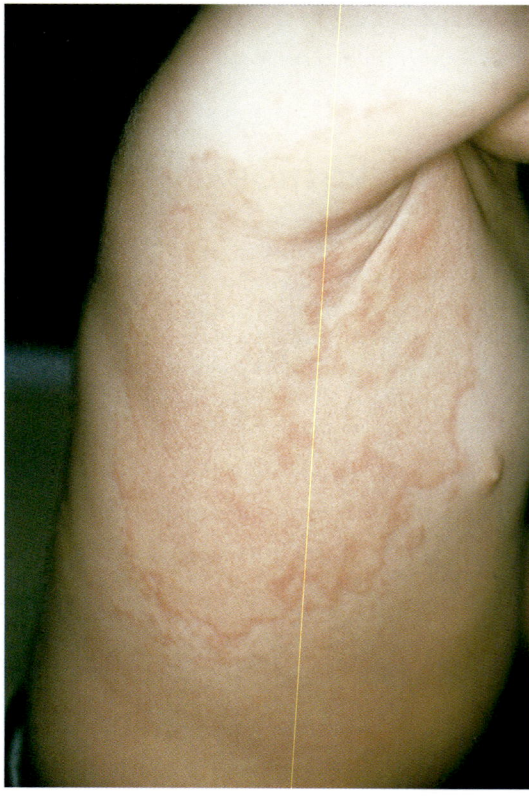

Fig. 25.11 Unilateral laterothoracic exanthem (asymmetric periflexural exanthem).

echovirus 25 (two patients) or echovirus 32 (2 patients) infection via virus isolation and/or serologic studies.[250] The skin lesions in these patients were described as blanchable angiomatous papules, 2–8mm in diameter, with a peripheral halo of blanching and, in some, a central dilated vessel and radiating branches, similar to spider telangiectasia. The authors hypothesized either a direct viral effect in endothelial cells or an antigen–antibody phenomenon as the possible cause of these findings. All of the patients experienced spontaneous involution of the skin lesions over 2–6 days.

In a subsequent report, three children were described with the acute onset and spontaneous resolution of similar angiomatous papules during an apparent viral illness.[251] Two of the patients had symptoms of upper respiratory tract infection, and the third had fever, headache, vomiting, and malaise. Skin biopsy revealed dilated capillaries with plump endothelial cells in the upper dermis, and electron microscopy showed swollen endothelial cells without viral particles. Based on these histologic findings, the authors proposed the name *eruptive pseudoangiomatosis* to describe this condition. Examinations for specific viral agents were not performed in this series. Similar lesions have also been reported in adults, where the association with viral symptoms was noted to be less common, and the lesions lasted 1–3 months before spontaneously involuting.[252]

It appears likely that eruptive pseudoangiomatosis represents a distinct vascular reaction pattern to infection, although the etiologic agent in most cases remains speculative. Observations of this disorder, in conjunction with the recognition of *Bartonella* species causing bacillary angiomatosis and the association of human herpesvirus-8 (HHV-8) and Kaposi's sarcoma, highlight the association between vascular eruptions and infectious organisms.

HERPES SIMPLEX INFECTION

The Herpesviridae family includes herpes simplex virus 1 (HSV-1) and 2 (HSV-2), varicella zoster virus, EBV, cytomegalovirus (CMV), and HHV-6, HHV-7, and HHV-8. These double-stranded DNA viruses have a central nucleic acid core surrounded by an icosahedral capsid and containing several viral-encoded glycoproteins. Herpesviruses are further classified into three subfamilies, with HSV-1 and HSV-2 belonging to the Alphaherpesvirinae subfamily and the genus *Simplexvirus*. Although these viruses are structurally similar, there is considerable variation in their biochemical characteristics and in their response to antiviral drugs. In this section, HSV-1 and HSV-2 infections are discussed. The reader is also referred to Chapter 6 (Neonatal Skin and Skin Disorders) and Chapter 28 (Sexually Transmitted Diseases).

EPIDEMIOLOGY

Primary infection with HSV-1 is generally a childhood disease involving the mouth, lips, and eyes. Seroprevalence data for HSV-1 infections varies according to several factors, including socio-economic background and geographic location. The prevalence of HSV-1 infection increases steadily with increasing age, and a direct correlation seems to exist between age at acquisition of infection and socio-economic status. It is estimated that 18–35% of children are infected with HSV-1 by the age of 5 years, and 90% of adults have antibodies against the virus.[253] HSV-1 infections are ubiquitous and most often result from direct contact with infected oral secretions or skin lesions.

HSV-2 infection is most commonly acquired via intimate sexual contact, although an increasing proportion of genital herpes infection is being caused by HSV-1. The frequency of HSV-2 infection correlates with the number of sexual partners and with the acquisition of other sexually transmitted diseases.[254] It is estimated that 45 million Americans are infected with HSV-2,[255] and this infection is often subclinical. In the National Health and Nutrition Examination Survey (NHANES) III, 1988–1994, the seroprevalence of HSV-2 in persons 12 years or older in the US was 22%, with a dramatic increase of fivefold in white teenagers and twofold among whites in their 20s.[256] Lifetime number of sexual partners seems to be the strongest predictive factor of HSV-2 infection. While genital infection with HSV-1 can result from autoinoculation of virus from the mouth, sexual abuse should always be considered in prepubertal children with genital HSV-2 infection. Therefore, when genital herpes is diagnosed in a prepubertal patient, viral typing should be performed to differentiate between HSV-1 and HSV-2.

Neonatal HSV infection occurs in approximately 1 per 3000 deliveries in the United States, and is most often caused by HSV-2. It is usually transmitted during birth through an infected maternal genital tract. Ascending *in utero* infection acquired transplacentally may result in congenital HSV, which is diagnosed when the findings present within the first week of life. Postpartum transmission via close contact with infected skin or secretions occurs in only 5% of cases.[257] The risk of neonatal HSV infection is significantly higher in infants born to mothers with primary infection as opposed to those born to mothers shedding HSV as a result of reactivated infection,[254] but the latter can still transmit disease. Subclinical shedding of genital HSV is common.[258] Acquisition of HSV infection during pregnancy has been associated with spontaneous abortion, prematurity, and congenital or neonatal disease. HSV infection may be acquired by up to 2% of susceptible women during pregnancy, and the risk of neonatal infection in this setting is greatest when infection is acquired at or near the time of labor.[259] It is important to remember that skin lesions due to neonatal HSV infection may be seen both in the more benign form of disease as well as with disseminated infection.

CLINICAL MANIFESTATIONS
Primary herpetic gingivostomatitis
In this primary infection, most often seen in infants and young children, fever is accompanied by irritability, refusal to eat or drink, and malaise. Examination reveals erythema, superficial ulcerations and exudate of the oral mucous membranes, and there are frequently perioral cutaneous lesions as well (Fig. 25.12). Tender submandibular lymphadenopathy may also be present. Dehydration, in some cases requiring hospitalization, is the most common complication.[260]

Primary herpetic lesions on the skin
Primary cutaneous HSV infection in children is probably more common than is appreciated and may be misdiagnosed due to unfamiliarity with its occurrence. Lesions can occur over any skin surface, but are most common on the face and extremities. They may be associated with systemic symptoms and a prolonged time to healing. As with most cutaneous HSV infections, lesions are characterized by clustered vesicles or erosions on an erythematous

250. Cherry JD, Bobinski JE, Horvath FL et al. (1969) Acute hemangioma-like lesions associated with ECHO viral infections. **Pediatrics** 44:498–502.
251. Prose NS, Tope W, Miller SE et al. (1993) Eruptive pseudoangiomatosis: A unique childhood exanthem? **J Am Acad Dermatol** 29:857–859.
252. Guillot B, Dandurand M (2000) Eruptive pseudoangiomatosis arising in adulthood: 9 cases. **Eur J Dermatol** 10:455–458.
253. Desselberger U (1998) Herpes simplex virus infection in pregnancy: diagnosis and significance. **Intervirol** 41:185–190.
254. American Academy of Pediatrics (2000) Herpex simplex. In: 2000 Red Book: Report of the Committee on Infectious Disease. 25th ed, Pickering LK, ed. Elk Grove Village, IL: American Academy of Pediatrics, pp. 309–318.

255. Marques AR, Straus SE (2000) Herpes simplex type 2 infections – An update **Adv Int Med** 45:175–208.
256. Fleming DT, McQuillan GM, Johnson RE et al. (1997) Herpex simplex virus type 2 in the United States, 1976 to 1994. **N Engl J Med** 337:1105–1111.
257. Riley LE (1998) Herpes simplex virus. **Sem Perinatol** 22:284–292.
258. Wald A, Zeh J, Selke S et al. (1995) Virologic characteristics of subclinical and symptomatic genital herpes infections. **N Engl J Med** 333:770–775.
259. Brown ZA, Selke S, Zeh J et al. (1997) The acquisition of herpes simplex virus during pregnancy. **N Engl J Med** 337:509–515.
260. Amir J, Harel L, Smetana Z et al. (1999) The natural history of primary herpes simplex type 1 gingivostomatitis in children. **Pediatr Dermatol** 16:259–263.

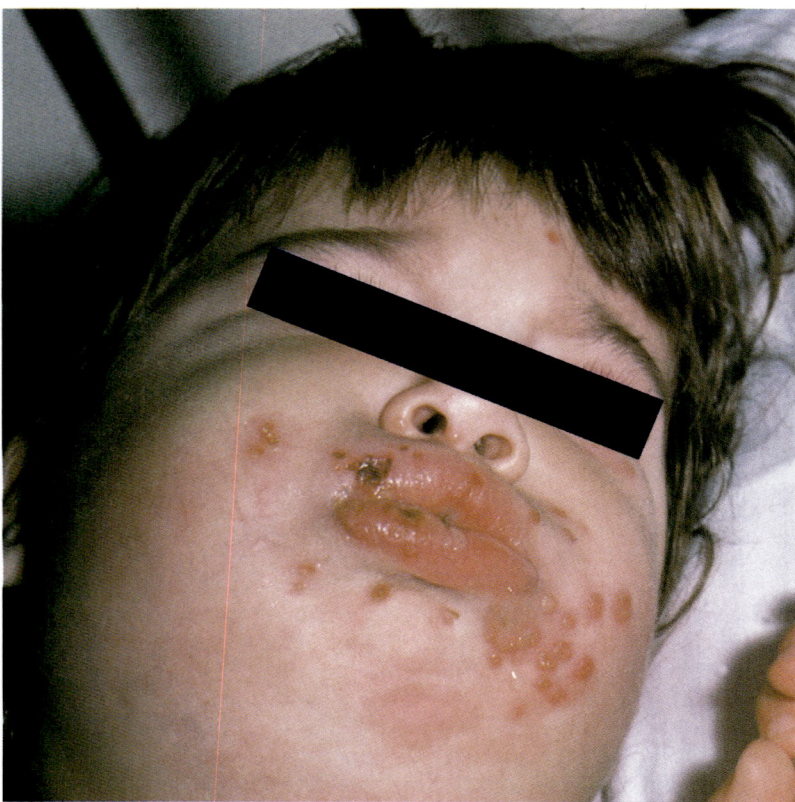

Fig. 25.12   Clustered perioral vesicles and erosions in an infant with primary herpetic gingivostomatitis.

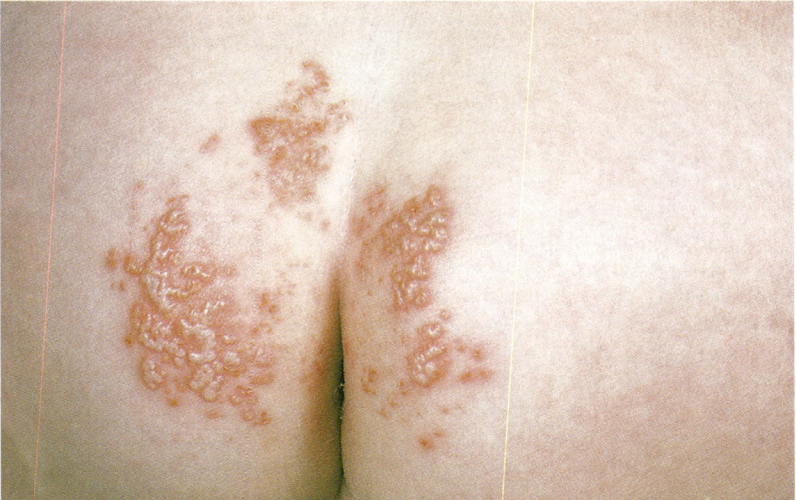

Fig. 25.13   Grouped vesicles and pustules on an erythematous base in cutaneous herpes simplex virus infection.

base (Fig. 25.13). The lesions often coalesce to produce geographic-shaped lesions with a scalloped edge. While bacterial superinfection may be present, nonculture-proven impetigo is generally overdiagnosed given overlap in the clinical presentation. Infection acquired during wrestling (herpes gladiatorum) may result in endemic spread of HSV, with lesions most commonly located on the head, neck, and shoulders.[261]

Primary neonatal herpetic infection
Three characteristic patterns of neonatal HSV infection are classically described: skin, eye and mouth (SEM) disease; central nervous system disease; and disseminated disease. All three forms of disease may have skin involvement, or skin lesions may be completely absent. Neonatal HSV infection tends to be manifest within the first four weeks of life, and most commonly within the first week.[262] Up to 30% of infected newborns will have symptoms on the first day of life.[257] Skin lesions include grouped vesicles, herpes zoster-like eruptions, disseminated vesicles, or erosions and ulcers, especially in areas of trauma such as fetal scalp electrode sites. Pustular, bullous, or necrotic lesions may also occur.[262]

Children with SEM disease present with cutaneous lesions and lesions of eye and mouth. Oral mucous membrane involvement may manifest as vesicles, erosions or ulcers, and ocular involvement with conjunctivitis and/or keratitis. In those infants presenting with apparent SEM disease, careful evaluation and follow-up for CNS or disseminated involvement is vital, as these findings may be delayed. The delay in CNS symptoms has been attributed to possible dormancy of the virus followed by later reactivation in the brain. Recent data has suggested an increasing frequency in

SEM disease relative to disseminated disease possibly related to increased recognition and early institution of therapy for SEM infection before it progresses.[263]

Neonates with CNS infection with HSV may develop focal encephalitis or meningoencephalitis. They often present with fever, changes in sensorium, seizures, lethargy or coma.[264] Cerebrospinal fluid analysis usually shows a lymphocytic pleocytosis. Skin manifestations are often absent in infants with CNS infection. Disseminated infection may involve multiple organs, including liver, lung, brain, and adrenals. The disease in these infants typically presents in a similar fashion to neonatal sepsis with features including jaundice, fever, respiratory insufficiency, evidence of disseminated intravascular coagulopathy, and neurologic deterioration.

Primary herpetic infection of the genital region
Primary infection with HSV in the genital region leads to similar signs and symptoms as does infection in other locations. Vesicles, pustules and erosions or ulcers occur in a grouped configuration on an erythematous base. They may occur on the genitalia, perineum, or perianal areas. Females may have severe pain associated with vulvovaginitis, urethritis, cervicitis, and cystitis. In males, there may be severe genital edema, ulceration, and pain. Lesions in the anal or perirectal region are seen primarily in homosexual males, may progress to large necrotic ulcers, and may result in proctitis associated with pain, tenesmus, and discharge. Inguinal lymphadenopathy may be present in the setting of genital HSV infection. Inoculation with HSV-2 in a patient with a history of previous exposure to HSV-1 may result in a more mild primary HSV-2 infection.

Herpetic eye infection
HSV, most commonly HSV-1, is a leading cause of recurrent keratoconjunctivitis with associated corneal opacification and visual loss.[255] Blepharitis, conjunctivitis, superficial or deep keratitis, and anterior uveitis may all occur. Patients present with pain, blurred vision, eyelid swelling, and conjunctivitis. Dendritic ulcers seen on corneal examination are a classic finding and subsequent scarring may result in significant visual loss. Acute retinal necrosis is another serious complication, and is usually associated with HSV-2.[265] Chorioretinitis may occur in infants.

261. Dworkin MS, Shoemaker PC, Spitters C et al. (1999) Endemic spread of herpes simplex virus type 1 among adolescent wrestlers and their coaches. **Pediatr Infect Dis J** 18:1108–1109.
262. Kohl S (1997) Neonatal herpes simplex virus infection. **Clin Perinatol** 24:129–150.
263. Whitley RJ, Corey L, Arvin A et al. (1988) Changing presentation of herpes simplex virus infection in neonates. **J Infect Dis** 158:109–116.
264. Jacobs RF (1998) Neonatal herpes simplex virus infections. **Sem Perinatol** 22:64–71.
265. Liesegang TJ (2001) Herpes simplex virus epidemiology and ocular importance. **Cornea** 20:1–13.

Herpetic infection in immunocompromised patients

Severe mucocutaneous manifestations may be seen with HSV infections in the setting of immunocompromise. In addition to typical grouped vesicles, large non-healing ulcerative and necrotic lesions may occur. There may also be disseminated HSV infection with visceral involvement. Patients with defects of T-cell immunity are at particular risk, and these infections tend to be more difficult to treat and more prone to recurrence.[255] HSV infection is one of the most common infections seen in patients with human immunodeficiency virus (HIV) infection or AIDS. Oropharyngeal involvement in this setting may progress to painful esophagitis.

Eczema herpeticum

Eczema herpeticum, also known as Kaposi's varicelliform eruption, refers to widespread cutaneous infection with HSV in sites affected by eczema or another pre-existing skin disease. Other predisposing conditions include Darier's disease, burns, and contact dermatitis. The disruption of epidermal integrity in these conditions decreases the host's ability to localize infection, and it appears that replication of HSV occurs more readily on eczematous skin when compared to normal skin.[266] Primary herpetic infections in the areas of abnormal skin results in a rapidly progressive, vesicular and erosive eruption (Fig. 25.14) that may be accompanied by fever and malaise. Examination may reveal lesions in different stages, including vesicles, crusts, and superficial ulcerations. Eczema herpeticum occurs most often in infants and young children, and is associated with significant pain and irritability.

Herpetic whitlow

Herpetic whitlow is a term used for infection of the fingertip by HSV. Patients present with erythema and tenderness, usually over the distal phalanx. Grouped and often coalescing vesicles (Fig. 25.15), bullae, and pustules occur and ipsilateral regional lymphadenopathy may be present. Because the skin is thick in this area the lesions tend to remain intact and erosions are rarely seen. The intact pustules may simulate a bacterial infection. Whitlow is an occupational hazard for medical professionals with frequent exposure to oral mucous membranes (i.e., dentists, dental hygienists, and oral surgeons), and may also be transmitted via digital-genital contact with an infected partner. In children, it usually occurs as a result of digital contact with the mouth of an affected parent.

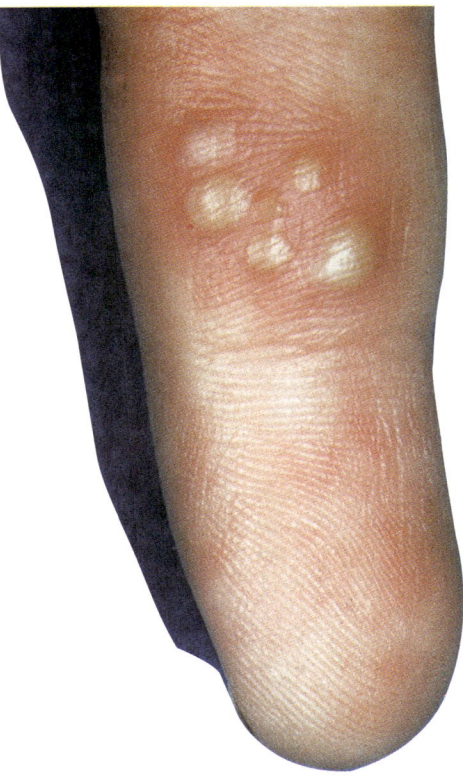

Fig. 25.15   Herpes simplex infection of fingertip (Whitlow).

Recurrent herpetic lesions

Reactivation of herpetic infection may occur at any site of primary infection. Patients often report an abnormal sensation or aura in the area to be affected prior to the appearance of the eruption. Lesions are similar to those seen in primary infection, although there may be fewer and they tend to heal more rapidly, usually within one week. Reactivation with viral shedding may occur in the absence of visible lesions, and this subclinical shedding is instrumental in transmitting HSV infection to contacts and neonates. Recurrences are less frequent with HSV-1 than HSV-2.

LABORATORY FINDINGS

Isolation of HSV in viral culture is the gold standard for diagnosis. Standard cultures become positive 2–3 days after inoculation, but with the rapid shell vial technique combined with viral antigen detection methods, a culture may be positive in 18–24 hours.[262] Skin lesions have the highest yield for viral culture, but other suitable sites for obtaining specimens include conjunctivae, nasopharynx, rectum, urine, CSF, and blood.[264]

Relatively rapid techniques that can be utilized when skin lesions are present include Tzanck smears and direct fluorescent antibody (DFA) examinations. In the Tzanck smear, scrapings from the base of an intact blister are smeared onto a glass slide and stained with Giemsa's or Wright's stain. Infected keratinocytes reveal multinucleation, molding of nuclear borders, and nuclear inclusions. Unfortunately, this study has low sensitivity and is dependent on the experience of the operator. DFA examination of skin lesion scrapings may give an answer in hours, but, again, sensitivity is dependent on technique. Skin biopsy of lesions demonstrates characteristic findings within the epidermis, identical to those of herpes zoster. Biopsy in general is not a practical diagnostic technique.

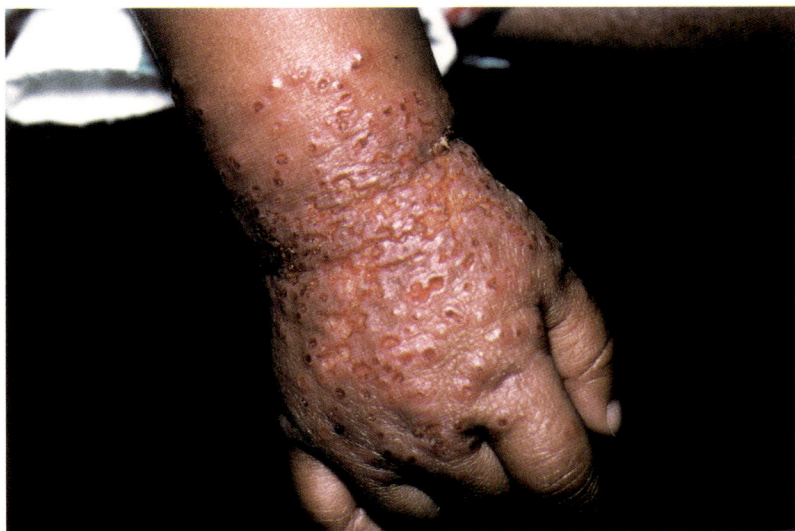

Fig. 25.14   Numerous clustered vesicles and erosions in eczema herpeticum.

266. Goodyear HM, Davies JA, McLeish P et al. (1996) Growth of herpes simplex type 1 on skin explants of atopic eczema. **Clin Exp Dermatol** 21:185–189.

The application of PCR techniques for the detection of HSV DNA is being utilized more frequently, especially in the setting of CNS infection in neonates or infants. This method offers the potential advantages of high sensitivity and specificity,[267] and when positive for HSV DNA in the CSF at the completion of therapy, may be a marker for poorer neurologic outcome.[268] PCR-based diagnosis of HSV is best utilized in combination with other diagnostic modalities and needs to be performed by experienced laboratory personnel.

Serologic studies are generally not useful for the diagnosis of HSV infection, due to cross-reactivity between HSV-1 and HSV-2 antibodies and altered titers as a result of prior infections. These studies are even less useful in neonatal HSV infection, as newborns may have a delayed or undetectable serologic response and there may be a confounding factor of transplacentally derived maternal antibody.[262,264]

PATHOPHYSIOLOGY

Initial infection of the nonimmune host with HSV is characterized by viral replication at the initial site of contact such as skin, mucous membranes, or eyes. The virus then travels along the regional nerves to the regional nerve ganglia and establishes a latent infection, where it apparently remains for life. During this latent infection, viral DNA and a few RNA transcripts are detectable, but no viral-encoded proteins are produced.[257] These RNA transcripts may be important for subsequent viral reactivation. The incubation period ranges from two days to two weeks. Initial infection with HSV is termed "primary infection" if it occurs in a host with no prior HSV infection, or as an "initial nonprimary infection" in a host previously infected with the heterologous HSV. Initial primary infections tend to be clinically less severe than true primary infections.[262]

DIFFERENTIAL DIAGNOSIS

Recognition is quite simple when the characteristic grouped vesicles are present on an erythematous base or when coalescing erosions are seen. Differentiation between HSV-1 and HSV-2 may be accomplished via viral culture or fluorescent antibody studies. Herpes zoster due to varicella zoster reactivation may reveal a similar morphology, and if not present in a clearly dermatomal pattern, may require differentiation from HSV infection.

The differential diagnosis varies according to the type and location of infection. Other disorders that cause vesicular skin eruptions may need to be considered, including allergic contact dermatitis, bullous impetigo, other viral infections such as HFMD, and vesicular hypersensitivity reactions. Similar eye lesions can be caused by herpes zoster, vaccinia, and *Chlamydia*. Herpetic whitlow may be confused with streptococcal blistering distal dactylitis, staphylococcal pustules, accidental burns and child abuse. In the genital region, other sexually transmitted diseases must be excluded, including syphilis, chancroid, and granuloma inguinale. In the neonate with cutaneous HSV, considerations might include bacterial or candidal infections, congenital syphilis or varicella, aplasia cutis congenital, Langerhans cell histiocytosis, bullous mastocytosis, incontinentia pigmenti, neonatal pemphigus, or other blistering diseases.

THERAPEUTICS AND PROGNOSIS

In many instances, supportive therapy suffices. Local measures are useful to suppress secondary bacterial infection and to minimize discomfort. Treatment is desired by most patients with a history of severe outbreaks or frequently recurrent infection. In addition, therapy is indicated in neonates with HSV infection or in individuals at risk for significant morbidity. Table 25.5 is a summary of available therapies for HSV infections. Treatment of cutaneous HSV infections may accelerate healing and decrease the rate of viral shedding. It should be noted that neither valacyclovir nor famciclovir is approved by the United States Federal Drug Administration for use in children.

Primary herpetic gingivostomatitis is generally self-limiting with low morbidity. However, in severe cases, systemic antiviral therapy may be useful to shorten the duration of clinical symptoms and decrease viral shedding. A randomized placebo-controlled study of 61 children with culture-proven herpetic gingivostomatitis compared treatment with acyclovir (15mg/kg five times a day for seven days) to no therapy.[269] Children treated with acyclovir had a shorter duration of lesions, fever, and drinking difficulties, and as well demonstrated a shortened duration of viral shedding. The use of chlorhexidine mouth washes is also useful in reducing pain.

Hospitalized patients with HSV infection should be roomed privately and managed with contact precautions. Women with active genital HSV lesions during labor may have a reduced risk of transmission to the infant if delivered by cesarean section, especially if performed within 4–6 hours of membrane rupture. Fetal scalp electrodes should be avoided when possible if the mother has active genital herpes infection. Patients with genital herpes should be counseled to refrain from sexual intercourse during outbreaks and for several days after, and to use condoms between outbreaks.

The overall prognosis for mucocutaneous HSV infection in older children and adults is excellent, although the frequency of reactivation may range from none to very high. Recurrences tend to be most common in the first months to years following the acquisition of infection. In neonates, untreated CNS or disseminated HSV infection results invariably in death or severe neurologic consequences. Overall, the outcome is dependent on the extent of involvement. Whitley *et al.* described outcomes in a prospective multicenter collaborative study of infants less than one month with virologically confirmed HSV infection, and found no deaths among infants with localized (SEM) disease, and mortality rates of 15% and 57% in those with encephalitis or disseminated infection, respectively.[270] Morbidity was most common in infants with encephalitis, seizures, or disseminated infection, and included psychomotor retardation, blindness, and learning disabilities. Although SEM disease most often results in a good outcome, neurologic impairment can result and a direct correlation exists between the development of neurologic deficit and the frequency of recurrent skin lesions. One study has demonstrated a decreased frequency of such cutaneous recurrences in infants treated with suppressive oral acyclovir therapy for six months following neonatal HSV infection.[271]

VARICELLA-ZOSTER INFECTIONS

Christine Bodemer

Primary infection with varicella-zoster virus causes the common childhood disease, chickenpox. Chickenpox was apparently distinguished from smallpox in 1802 by William Herberden.[272] Nearly one century later, von Bokay described the relationship between zoster and varicella after observing cases of varicella that occurred after household cases of zoster. We now recognize that varicella and zoster are caused by the same virus, with the former representing primary infection and the latter caused by reactivation of virus, which had remained present in a latent state in nerve root ganglia. Varicella-zoster virus is a member of the herpesvirus family and is a double-stranded DNA virus. It was first grown in tissue culture in 1952. Humans are the only known hosts for the virus.

267. Troendle-Atkins J, Demmler GJ, Buffone GJ (1993) Rapid diagnosis of herpes simplex virus encephalitis by using the polymerase chain reaction. **J Pediatr** 123:376–380.

268. Atkins JT (1999) HSV PCR for CNS infections: pearls and pitfalls. **Pediatr Infect Dis J** 18:823–824.

269. Amir J, Harel L, Smetana Z et al. (1997) Treatment of herpes simplex gingivostomatitis with aciclovir in children: a randomized double blind placebo controlled study. **Br Med J** 314:1800–1803.

270. Whitley R, Arvin A, Prober C et al. (1991) Predictors of morbidity and mortality in neonates with herpes simplex virus infections. The National Institute of Allergy and Infectious Diseases Collaborative Antiviral Study Group. **N Engl J Med** 324:450–454.

271. Kimberlin D, Powell D, Gruber W et al. (1996) Administration of oral acyclovir suppressive therapy after neonatal herpex simplex virus disease limited to the skin, eyes and mouth: results of a phase I/II trial. **Pediatr Infect Dis J** 15:247–254.

272. Brunell PA (1985) Varicella-zoster virus. In: Principles and Practice of Infectious Diseases, 2nd ed, Mandell GL, Douglas RG, Bennett JE, eds. New York: John Wiley & Sons, p. 952.

TABLE 25.5   Treatment of HSV infections

Drug	Formulations
Acyclovir (ACV)	200mg capsule; 400, 800mg tablet; 200mg/5ml suspension; 5% ointment
Famciclovir (FAM)	125, 250, 500mg tablet (safety not established < 18 years)
Valacyclovir (VAL)	500mg, 1gm caplets (safety not established < 18 years)
Penciclovir (PEN)	1% cream

Condition	Drug	Regimen[1]	Comment
Orolabial/Skin			
Primary	ACV	200mg 5x/d for 7–10 d	Less than 2 years[2]
		100mg 5x/d for 7–10 d	
	ACV ointment	Apply 6x/d for 7 d	
Recurrent	ACV	200mg 5x/d for 5 d	Start within 48h of onset
	PEN	Apply q 2 hr during waking hours for 4 d	
Suppression	ACV	400mg bid or 200mg tid	
Genital			
Primary	ACV	200mg 5/d for 7–10 d	
	ACV ointment	Apply 6x/d for 7 d	
	FAM	250mg tid for 7–10 d	
	VAL	1gm bid for 10 d	
Recurrent	ACV	200mg 5x/d for 5 d	Start within 48h of onset
	FAM	125–250mg bid for 5–7 d	Start within 48h of onset
	VAL	500mg bid for 5 d	Start within 48h of onset
Suppression	ACV	400mg bid or 200mg tid	
	FAM	250mg bid	
	VAL	1gm q d	
Neonatal	ACV	30–60mg/kg/d divide q 8 hr for 21 d	Also consider vidarabine
Immunocompromised	ACV	80mg/kg/d divide qid	
		15mg/kg/d iv divide q 8 h	For severe infection

[1]Oral, unless otherwise stated.

[2]Orally administered acyclovir in children less than 2yr of age has not been fully studied.

bid, two times per day; tid, three times per day; qid, four times per day; iv, intravenous

VARICELLA EPIDEMIOLOGY

Varicella is a highly contagious disease of childhood. Ninety-six percent of susceptible children will have varicella within one month (two incubation periods) of exposure to an index case.[272] The average incubation period is 14 to 16 days, and 99% of cases occur between 11 and 20 days after exposure. Varicella infections generally occur in late winter and early spring. In colder climates, the disease is often present in the community for longer periods than it is in temperate or tropical climates.

More than 90% of cases occur in children aged 1 to 14 years. Infection in children aged 5 to 9 accounts for 60% of reported cases, whereas infection in infants younger than 1 year of age, combined with that of adults older than 19 years of age, accounts for only 3% of reported cases.[273] The number of susceptible adults is somewhat greater in tropical and temperate climates.[274]

The disease is spread through person-to-person contact. Airborne spread of infection has been documented and can occur from two days before the onset of rash to five days after its onset. There is no evidence that the disease is spread by inanimate objects. Unless progressive varicella is present, children are no longer contagious, even with direct skin-to-skin contact, eight days after the onset of rash.[272,274] Transplacental infection may occur. Congenital and neonatal varicella are discussed in Chapter X (Neonatal skin and skin disorders).

CLINICAL MANIFESTATIONS

A vesicular exanthem is the most striking manifestation of primary varicella infection in normal children. Other systemic symptoms are usually mild. There may be a low-grade fever (37.5–38.5°C) for the first few days of illness, and malaise may be present. Occasionally, a group of one to three lesions appears on the trunk, one to two days before the generalized eruption. Usually the exanthem begins on the scalp or trunk. Lesions occur in crops and may first appear as erythematous macules, which rapidly develop into vesicles. The erythematous base of these vesicles gives rise to the characteristic appearance of a "dewdrop on a rose petal" in early lesions. The lesions usually form crusts within a few hours to 1–2 days and then gradually begin to heal. They spread

273. Preblud SR, Orenstein WA, Bart KJ (1984) Varicella: Clinical manifestations, epidemiology and health impact in children. **Pediatr Infect Dis** 3:505.

274. Brunnell PA (1992) Varicella-zoster infections. In: Textbook of Pediatric Infectious Diseases. 3rd ed, Feigin RD, Cherry JD, eds. Philadelphia: WB Saunders, p. 1206.

centrifugally and as the disease progresses. Fresh lesions can often be found on the extremities with crusted lesions present on the trunk. They may be found in increased concentration in areas of skin injury or irritation, such as grazes, eczema, or sunburn (Fig. 25.16).[272] The number of lesions may vary considerably from a few to several hundred. Generally, younger children have fewer lesions, with the exception of children younger than 1 year of age, who may have a more severe course.[273] A more severe course is also often seen in adolescents and adults. In contrast to typical childhood disease, in which lesions of all stages of development are present, lesions may be monomorphous in appearance. Pruritus is variable but may be severe. In rare instances, skin lesions other than vesicles may occur. Bullous lesions have been reported.[275,276] In some cases, bullae are due to supervening infection with *Staphylococcus aureus* but may occur in the absence of such infection.[277] Most patients with bullous varicella recover without incident.[275] In patients with thrombocytopenia, lesions may appear hemorrhagic.[278] The mucous membranes are frequently affected. Vesicles rapidly erode to form one or more sharply marginated, superficial ulcerations, with a surrounding halo of erythema. These occur most

frequently on the hard palate, uvula, and tonsillar pillars, but they also may occur on the palpebral conjunctiva, vulva, and other mucosal sites.

Recurrent varicella–zoster infections occur in immunosuppressed patients but are thought to be extremely rare in healthy individuals. However, a recent report of 14 previously healthy children with two episodes of chickenpox suggests that this condition may be more common than generally recognized.[279] Severe, life-threatening, and progressive varicella may occur in children who are immunocompromised in situations such as leukemia, treatment with high-dose corticosteroids, congenital immunodeficiency syndromes and AIDS.[272,280,281] In this form of varicella, lesions may continue to occur for two weeks or longer after the onset of rash. The lesions tend to be somewhat larger, more deep-seated, monomorphous, and umbilicated. The palms and soles often are affected. Visceral involvement is common.

Continuous varicella

Long-lasting varicella–zoster infection associated with acyclovir resistance and human immunodeficiency virus (HIV) infection has been described in children.[282]

Complications of varicella infection

A hospital-based survey in 1935[283] found that 5.2% of children with varicella had complications. Of these, 57% had skin infections, 28% had otitis media, 16% had pneumonia, and 4% had encephalitis. The overall mortality rate was 0.4%.[283] Another survey of children hospitalized with varicella found 27% with bacterial infections, 25% percent with encephalitis, 21% with Reye syndrome, and 7% with pneumonia.[276] Virtually all cases with CNS involvement occured in normal children, whereas cases of pneumonia were evenly divided between normal and immunocompromised children. In a recent study, the authors examined varicella deaths in the United States during the 25 years before vaccine licencure (1970–1994) and identified 2262 people who died with varicella as the primary cause of death.[284] Adults had a risk 25 times greater and infants had a risk 4 times greater of dying from varicella than did children 1–4 years old. Most people who died of varicella were previously healthy. A marked decline in deaths due to encephalitis was noticed in this most recent study. This may be due to the awareness of the association between Reye syndrome and the use of aspirin in common viral illnesses such as varicella and influenza. Since CNS complications have declined, pneumonia has become the most common lethal complication among healthy children and adults, followed by secondary infections, especially invasive group A streptococcal infections.

The most common complication of varicella infection is bacterial infection of the skin, either with *S. aureus* or group A beta-hemolytic streptococci. Staphylocci may cause impetigo or staphylococcal scalded skin syndrome. Group A streptococci may cause impetigo or cellulitis, which may be mild or deep and severe. The presence of fever after four or five days of illness or unusually indurated skin lesions should alert the clinician to the possibility of bacterial cellulitis. Life-threatening gangrenous cellulitis has been a rare complication,[285] but recently an increasing number of reports of primary varicella complicated by serious infections with group A streptococcus including gangrenous cellulitis and necrotizing fasciitis have appeared in the literature. In a case-controlled study, ibuprofen use was associated with necrotizing fasciitis, and additional studies are necessary to establish the role of ibuprofen in the development of necrotizing fasciitis.[286]

Purpura fulminans may also occur as a very serious complication of varicella infection (Fig. 25.17).[273,287]

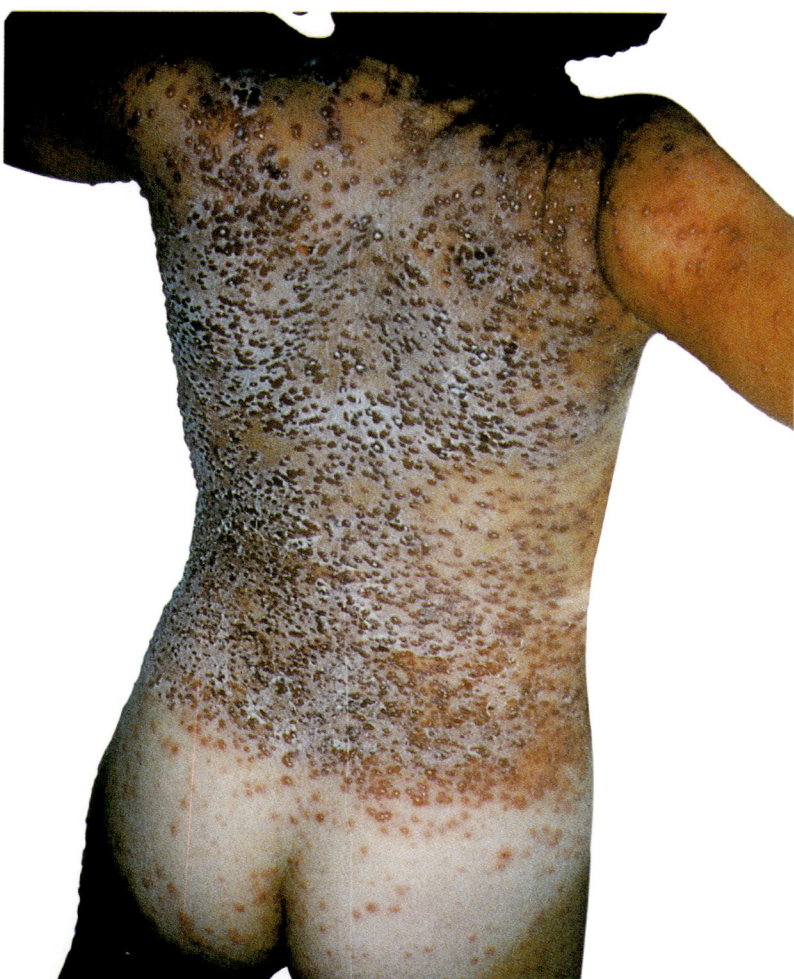

Fig. 25.16   Severe varicella, with accentuation in area of sunburn.

275. Saslaw S, Kluck C, Prior JA (1960) Varicella bullosa. **JAMA** 173:118.
276. Fleisher G, Henry W, McSorley M et al. (1981) Life-threatening complications of varicella. **Am J Dis Child** 135:896.
277. Wald ER, Levine MM, Togo Y (1973) Concomitant varicella and staphylococcal scalded skin syndrome. **J Pediatr** 83:1017.
278. Charkes ND (1961) Purpuric chickenpox: report of a case, review of the literature and classification by clinical features. **Ann Intern Med** 54:745.
279. Junker AK, Angus E, Thomas EE (1991) Recurrent varicella-zoster virus infections in apparently immunocompetent children. **Pediatr Infect Dis** 10:569.
280. Pryles CV, Gellis SS (1958) Further warning. **N Engl J Med** 259:842.
281. Gershon A, Brunnell PA, Doyle EF (1972) Steroid therapy and varicella. **J Pediatr** 81:1034.

282. Pahva S, Biron K, Lim W et al. (1988) Continuous varicella-zoster infection associated with acyclovir resistance in a child with AIDS. **JAMA** 260:2879.
283. Bullowa JGM, Wishik SM (1935) Complications of varicella. I. Their occurrence among 2,534 patients. **Am J Dis Child** 49:923.
284. Meyer P, Seward J, Jumaan A et al. (2000) Varicella-mortality: trends before vaccine licensure in the United States 1970–1994. **J Infect Dis** 182:383–390.
285. Smith EWP, Garson A, Boyleston JA et al. (1976) Varicella gangrenosa due to group A beta-hemolytic *Streptococcus*. **Pediatrics** 57:306.
286. Zerr DM, Alexander ER, Duchin JS et al. (1999) A case-control study of necrotizing fasciitis during primary varicella. **Pediatrics** 103:783–790.
287. Phua HK, Chong CY, Lim KW et al. (1998) Complicated varicella zoster infection in 8 patients and review of the literature. **Sing Med J** 39:115–120.

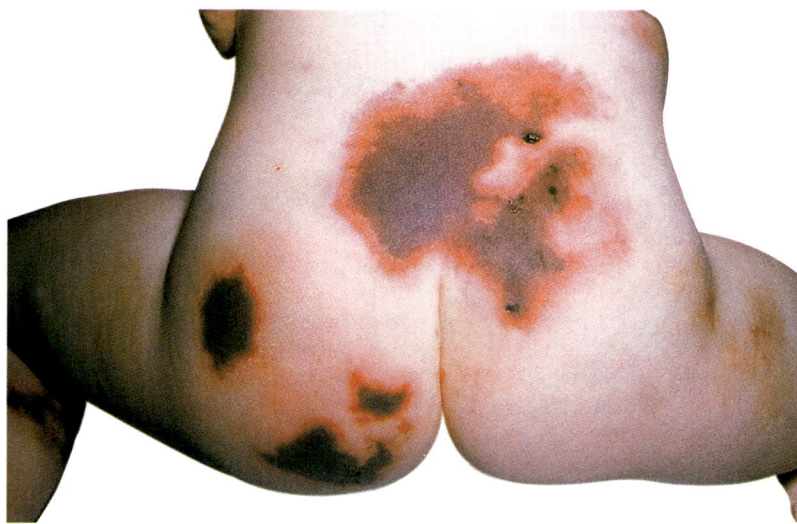

Fig. 25.17 Purpura fulminans following varicella.

Pneumonia usually occurs between one and six days after the onset of rash. It is characterized by tachypnea, dyspnea, cough, and occasionally hemoptysis. Pulmonary abnormalities may persist for months to years after the illness.[272]

CNS manifestations of varicella include encephalitis, cerebellar ataxia, aseptic meningitis, transverse myelitis, Guillain–Barré syndrome, and Reye syndrome.[272,273] Cerebellar ataxia occurs about one week after the onset of illness and lasts from a few days to weeks. The prognosis is good. Reye syndrome also occurs during the convalescent period of illness. The explosive onset of vomiting, confusion, delirium, and coma may be present in association with hepatic abnormalities and elevated serum ammonia levels.[288]

Thrombocytopenia may occur one week or more after varicella infection and arthritis, nephritis, carditis, and myositis are rare complications of varicella.[273]

Pneumonia, hepatitis, and meningoencephalitis are the most common complications of progressive varicella. The mortality rate of progressive varicella, if untreated, is about 20%.[274]

LABORATORY FINDINGS

Laboratory tests are rarely necessary in uncomplicated varicella. The white blood cell count may be slightly elevated, normal or slightly decreased during the first few days of infection.[272] Mild elevations of hepatic enzymes occur frequently but appear to have little clinical significance.[289] Direct fluorescent antibody examination using a swab taken from the base of a freshly opened lesion is a very useful investigation; it has a high sensitivity and can differentiate between HSV and VZV. A Tzanck preparation demonstrates balloon cells and mutinucleated giant cells, but it is not specific for varicella because herpes simplex produces identical findings. Viral cultures of vesicular fluid are frequently positive during the first three days of illness, but virus is rarely recovered from other sites. Acute and convalescent serum may be tested for complement-fixing antibodies to confirm infection, but the test is not sensitive enough to use in determining immune status. For this purpose, antibodies to membrane antigen (FAMA) may be measured. Varicella-zoster DNA can be demonstrated directly in equivocal Tzanck preparations, tissue, or body fluids by molecular diagnostic methods if warranted clinically.[290]

PATHOGENESIS

Primary infection with varicella-zoster virus probably occurs by way of the respiratory route, followed by viremia and the transmission of virus into the skin. Biopsy of the skin demonstrates intraepidermal vesicles with acantholysis and necrotic keratinocytes. Epidermal cells are greatly enlarged, with large steel-gray nuclei, and peripheral accentuation of the nuclear contents. Multinucleated epithelial giant cells, papillary dermal edema, a variable degree of dermal inflammation and extravasated erythrocytes may also be present.[291]

DIFFERENTIAL DIAGNOSIS

The differential diagnosis of primary varicella infection includes other vesicular viral exanthems, such as generalized herpes simplex infections, hand-foot-and-mouth disease, and other enteroviral exanthems. In the past, variola and vaccinia were important in differential diagnosis, but these infections are at present virtually nonexistent. Herpes simplex infection can be differentiated by the grouping of vesicles, location, and by immunofluorescent testing or viral cultures, if necessary. Hand-foot-and-mouth disease has a more acral distribution, more prominent mucosal involvement and lacks multinucleated giant cells in the Tzanck preparation. Other enteroviral exanthems usually occur during the summer and early autumn but may be difficult to distinguish clinically. A Tzanck preparation may help because it will not show multinucleated giant cells in enteroviral exanthems. Vesicular exanthems caused by enteroviruses probably account for most anecdotal reports of children who get chickenpox twice. Vesicular reactions to insect bites may resemble varicella, but they are often clustered and acral in distribution and usually have a central punctum and an underlying wheal. In contrast to varicella, they rarely occur on the scalp. Dermatitis herpetiformis, pityriasis lichenoides and varioliformis acuta, scabies, molluscum contagiosum, and bullous impetigo may occasionally mimic varicella infection.

THERAPY

In normal children in whom disease is limited to the skin, treatment is supportive and aimed at decreasing pruritus and minimizing the risk of infection. Bland shake lotions, such as calamine or 0.25% menthol in calamine lotion may be soothing. Topical antihistamines, containing diphenhydramine, should be avoided because of a potential for toxicity or sensitization. Oral antihistamines may be used to control pruritus. Under no circumstances should aspirin or other salicylates be used because their use appears to increase the risk of Reye syndrome. Oral antibiotics, such as erythromycin or dicloxacillin, may be used if superficial cutaneous infection occurs.

The use of systemic antiviral agents in the treatment of varicella has been studied in immunocompromised patients. Both vidarabine and acyclovir given intravenously appear to be effective in preventing progressive varicella complications, if started early in the course of illness. No study to date has compared their efficacy, but intravenous acyclovir is generally considered to be the treatment of choice.[292–294] Oral acyclovir (20mg/kg four times a day for five days) reduces the duration and severity of chickenpox in normal children when therapy is initiated during the first 24 hours of the rash, but the recommended use of this therapy for healthy children remains controversial.[292,295]

Passive immunization with varicella-zoster hyperimmune globulin has been shown to modify or prevent illness in high-risk individuals. Its use is recommended for patients with immunodeficiencies, leukemia, or lymphoma

288. DeLong GR. Reye's syndrome. In: Smith's The Critically Ill Child: Diagnosis and Medical Management, 3rd ed, Dickerman JD, Lucey JF, eds. Philadelphia: WB Saunders, p. 173.

289. Pitel PA, McCormick KL, Fitzgerald E et al. (1980) Subclinical hepatic changes in varicella infection. **Pediatrics** 65:631.

290. Nahass GT, Goldstein BA, Zhu W-Y et al. (1992) Comparison of Tzanck smear, viral culture, and DNA diagnostic methods in detection of herpes simplex and varicella-zoster infection. **JAMA** 268:2541.

291. Ackerman AB (1978) Histologic Diagnosis of Inflammatory Skin Diseases: A Method by Pattern Analysis. Philadelphia: Lea & Febiger.

292. Committee on Infectious Diseases, American Academy of Pediatrics (1993) The use of oral acyclovir in otherwise healthy children with varicella. **Pediatrics** 91:674.

293. White R, Hilty M, Haynes R et al. (1982) Vidarabine therapy of varicella in immunosuppressed patients. **J Pediatr** 101:125.

294. Prober CG, Kirk LE, Keeney RE (1982) Acyclovir therapy of chickenpox in immunosuppressed children – a collaborative study. **J Pediatr** 101:622.

295. Dunkle LM, Arvin AM, Whitley RJ et al. (1991) A controlled trial of acyclovir for chickenpox in normal children. **N Engl J Med** 325:1539.

and in those patients receiving chemotherapy or other immunosuppressive agents. It is also recommended for newborns whose mothers have developed primary varicella within five days before or two days after delivery. It should be given within 72 hours of exposure.[296,297] Thousands of children have now been vaccinated with a live, attenuated varicella vaccine. It has been administered safely to normal children and to children with leukemia; it appears to provide adequate immunity. Varicella vaccine was developed in Japan in the early 1970s,[298] and has been approved in USA by the Food and drug Administration in 1995, and is recommended for persons 12 months of age or older, who are susceptible to chickenpox.[299] A case-control study was recently conducted to assess the effectiveness of the varicella vaccine.[300] Varicella vaccine appeared highly effective as used in clinical practice.

Children with varicella infection may return to school one week after the onset of rash or when all vesicular lesions have become dry and crusted. Immunosuppressed patients should be isolated for the duration of the illness.[297] Cutaneous scarring, although infrequently mentioned, is a common, and at times distressing, sequela of varicella infection. Keloidal scarring may be treated with intralesional corticosteroids. Generally, no surgical revision of scars should be attempted for the first 6–12 months after infection because the appearance may improve during this time.

Varicella infections in hospitalized patients can create monumental problems for hospital infection control personnel. Children with varicella and those susceptible individuals who have been exposed to varicella need strict respiratory isolation from other children in the hospital. Health care personnel who care for hospitalized children and have no known history of varicella infection should be tested for immunity.

Herpes zoster

Herpes zoster represents an acute reactivation of an endogenous infection in the sensory root ganglia by varicella–zoster virus that has persisted in latent form after a preceding infection.

EPIDEMIOLOGY

There are no racial, sexual, or seasonal preferences for herpes zoster. The incidence of herpes zoster increases with age, although it may occur at all ages.[301–303] The incidence in children is low. Hope-Simpson[304] reported a rate of infection of 0.74 per 1000 subjects per year in the age group under 9. Guess *et al.*[305] noted that the rate increased from 20 cases per 100 000 person-years in the age group younger than 5 years, to 63 cases per 100 000 person-years in the group aged 15 to 19 years. These authors also noted that the incidence of herpes zoster was 122 times higher in children with acute lymphocytic leukemia than in children who did not have an underlying malignancy. Herpes zoster in neonates and children may represent the result of an attenuated response to intrauterine or neonatal infection. Baba *et al.*[306] reported that children who had varicella before 2 months of age had lower varicella–zoster antibody titers and diminished skin test reactions; thus, reactivation in these cases may be secondary to an abnormal immune response to the primary infection. There is little evidence that the development of herpes zoster follows re-exposure to varicella or herpes zoster.[307] Herpes zoster can be a manifestation of HIV infection in children.[308,309]

CLINICAL CHARACTERISTICS

The development of herpes zoster is often preceded by radicular pain. Pain and paresthesia, which is less common in children than in adults, may occur before the development of skin changes and the discomfort may be confused with pleurisy, myocardial infarction, and a variety of other internal catastrophes. Malaise, headache, and fever may precede the rash, particularly in younger patients. Herpes zoster is chiefly a unilateral eruption that can involve from one to three dermatomes. The most commonly involved dermatomes are the thoracic dermatomes (Fig. 25.18) and the ophthalmic branch of the trigeminal nerve. Involvement of the nasociliary branch of the ophthalmic branch of the trigeminal nerve leads to Hutchinson's sign, herpetic lesions on the tip of the nose. Recognition is important because involvement of this branch is associated with keratitis, scleritis, conjunctivitis, and a variety of other ocular manifestations. Involvement of the facial and auditory nerves produces the Ramsey Hunt syndrome, which is facial palsy coupled with herpes zoster and associated signs and symptoms of otic involvement. Vesicles develop over several days in the affected dermatomes. Early lesions may be

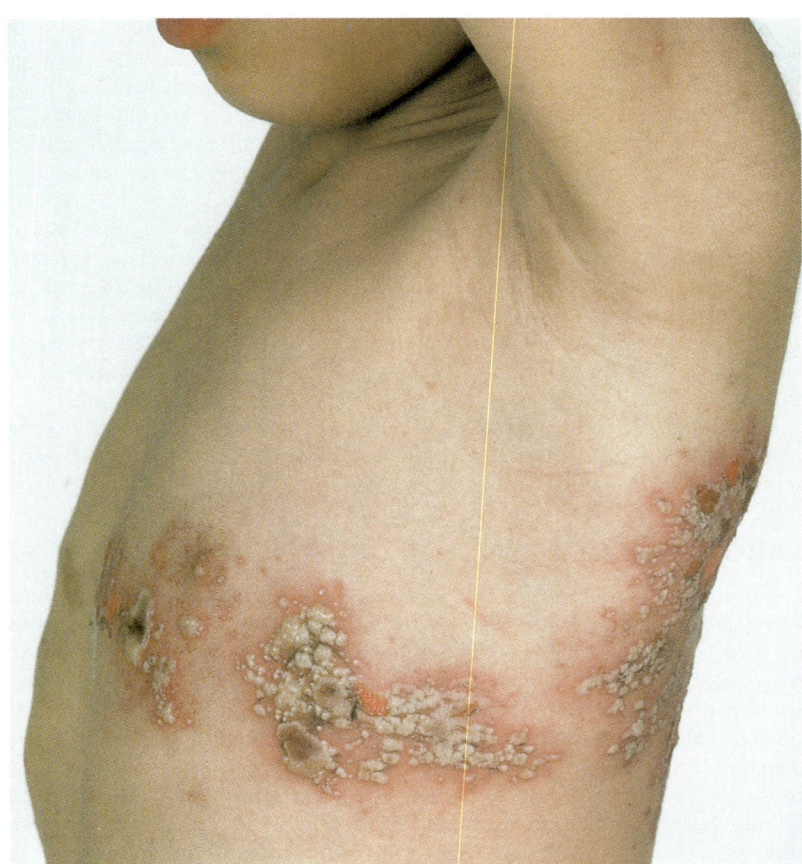

Fig. 25.18   Herpes zoster infection.

296. Cherry JD (1992) Enteroviruses: polioviruses (poliomyelitis), Coxsackieviruses, echoviruses, and enteroviruses. In: Textbook of Pediatric Infectious Diseases, 3rd ed, Fei RD, Cherry JD, eds. Philadelphia: WB Saunders, p. 1705.

297. Committee on Infectious Diseases (1994) Report of the Committee on Infectious Diseases, 23rd ed. Elk Grove, IL: American Academy of Pediatrics.

298. Takahashi M, Otsuka T, Okuno Y et al. (1974) Live vaccine used to prevent the spread of varicella in children in hospital. Lancet 2:1288–1290.

299. Prevention of varicella (1996) Recommendation of Advisory Commitee of Immunization Practices (ACIP). MMWR Morb Mortal Wkly Rep 45:(RR-11):1–36.

300. Vazquez M, Larussa PS, Gershon AA et al. (2001) The effectiveness of the varicella vaccine in clinical practice. N Engl J Med 344:955–960.

301. Elmer KB, George RM (1999) Herpes zoster in a seven month old infant. Cutis 63:217–218.

302. Petursson G, Helgason S, Gudmundsson S et al. (1998) Herpes zoster in children and adolescents. Pediatr Infect Dis 17:905–908.

303. Kakourou T, Theodoridou M, Mostrou G et al. (1998) Herpes zoster in children. J Am Acad Dermatol 38:207–210.

304. Hope-Simpson RE (1965) The nature of herpes zoster. A long term study and a new hypothesis. Proc R Soc Med 58:9.

305. Guess HA, Broughton DD, Melton LJ et al. (1985) Epidemiology of herpes zoster in children and adolescents: a population-based study. Pediatrics 76:512.

306. Baba K, Yabuuchi H, Takahashi M et al. (1986) Increased incidence of herpes zoster in normal children infectec with varicella zoster virus (VZV) during infancy: community-based follow-up study. J Pediatr 108:372.

307. Miller LH, Brunell PA (1970) Zoster, reinfection or activation of latent virus? Am J Med 49:480.

308. Prose NS (1992) Cutaneous manifestations of pediatric HIV infection. Pediatr Dermatol 9:326.

309. Eyster ME, Rabkin CS, Hilgartner MW et al. (1993) Human immunodeficiency virus-related conditions in children and adults with hemophilia: Rates, relationship to CD4 counts, and predictive value. Blood 81:828.

urticarial, and incompletely developed cases in which the skin lesions are mainly urticarial plaques have been observed. Morphologically, individual lesions are similar to those found in varicella. As the eruption resolves, vesicles break, become crusted, and slowly heal. The entire process usually lasts from one to three weeks. Both normal and immunosuppressed patients may have generalization of herpes zoster. Generalization usually occurs within one week of the onset of the eruption and may be associated with internal involvement, including pulmonary, hepatic, and CNS findings. Serious complications are for the most part limited to patients who are immunosuppressed. Rogers and Tindall[310] noted that painless herpes zoster occasionally may disseminate in children and resemble varicella.

One of the most feared complications of herpes zoster is postherpeutic pain, but this is rare in children. The risk of this problem increases with the age of the patient and is frequently resistant to treatment but usually slowly remits over time. Severe eruptions can be associated with scarring and persistent local anesthesia.

DIFFERENTIAL DIAGNOSIS

The recognition of dermatomal herpes zoster is usually straightforward. Occasionally, herpes simplex infection simulates the pattern of herpes zoster.

LABORATORY FINDINGS

In most cases, little supportive data are needed to confirm the diagnosis of herpes zoster. Direct fluorescent antibody examination using a swab taken from the base of a freshly opened lesion is a very useful investigation; it has a high sensitivity and can differentiate between HSV and VZV. As with herpes simplex and varicella infections, a Tzanck smear taken from the base of an intact blister reveals the characteristic cytopathic effects of herpetic infection, and a skin biopsy shows similar changes within keratinocytes. Virus can be grown from vesicle fluid early in the course of the disease. Molecular diagnostic methods can be used to demonstrate varicella-zoster DNA when the diagnosis is suspected and other techniques fail.

THERAPY

Therapy in most cases is supportive. In immunosuppressed patients with severe or disseminated herpes zoster, oral or intravenous acyclovir therapy can be administered at standard doses to prevent or control dissemination.[311] In most cases, local wound care coupled with analgesics is sufficient treatment for herpes zoster. When the ophthalmic branch of the trigeminal nerve is involved, consultation with an ophthalmologist should be obtained.

VARIOLA AND VACCINIA

SMALLPOX (VARIOLA)

Variola is an orthopox virus affecting only humans.[312] Global eradication of smallpox was officially declared in 1980, and any further cases of the disease will likely result from laboratory spread or bioterrorism.[312] Vaccination of US military personnel continued until 1990 but since 1984 there has been no smallpox vaccination of the general population in any country. Hence, the majority of individuals under 30 are not immune to this disease. This large non-immune population, the lack of effective treatment, the high secondary attack rate and the case fatality rate of 25% make smallpox a potentially very dangerous agent of terrorism.[312]

After a seven to 17-day incubation period, a prodrome of high fever, malaise, and myalgia occurrs.[312,313] The most characteristic cutaneous eruption consists of a maculopapular eruption appearing on the face and scalp and spreading to the trunk and centrifugally to the extremities. Lesion density is increased over the bony prominences of the limbs. Within a 24–48-hour period, the lesions become vesicular with deep firm vesicles, then pustular, then crusted and finally resolve, leaving pitted scars. Lesions are mostly in the same stage of development at any one time. The total duration is two to three weeks. Several other clinical forms exist, including "flat" smallpox, with a petechial and vesicular eruption, and hemorrhagic smallpox, in which fever and myalgias are followed by widespread hemorrhage of mucous membranes, skin, and other sites. Vaccine-modified cases of smallpox may resemble varicella. Outbreaks of monkeypox, which resembles smallpox, have recently been reported in Africa.[314]

VACCINIA

Vaccinia is an orthopox virus affecting a wide range of vertebrate hosts.[312] Vaccinia infections are now rare. There is no natural host for this virus, and infections are nearly always the result of vaccination. With the worldwide eradication of smallpox, the need for vaccinia inoculation appeared to have been eliminated, although there was still some interest in using the virus as a vehicle for administering other viral vaccines.[312,315] Recent events have led to a discussion about the potential requirement for the reintroduction of mass vaccination programs.

Clinical manifestations

Vaccinia inoculation produces a vesicle in 3–5 days in primary vaccinations and in 1–2 days in repeat vaccinations. The lesion evolves from a vesicle to a pustule and usually reaches its maximum size about nine days after inoculation. Primary vaccinations usually result in a scar about 1cm in diameter, whereas revaccination generally does not result in scar formation.[315] Secondary lesions may occur on other parts of the skin through physical transfer of infection.[316]

Several cutaneous complications may result from vaccinia inoculation. The most serious of these is progressive vaccinia (vaccinia necrosum), which occurs in immunodeficient patients. There is a normal vaccine "take," but the lesion does not heal. The area of necrosis gradually enlarges. New vesicles begin to occur in both adjacent and distant skin sites and may spread to the mouth, larynx, pharynx, and other organs. Viremia may be present for several weeks, and the infection often leads to death.[315,316] Individuals with atopic dermatitis may have "eczema vaccinatum," characterized by extensive local or disseminated cutaneous infection with vaccinia after inoculation or close contact with a recently vaccinated individual. Umbilicated vesicles usually occur in areas of pre-existing dermatitis, but they may occur on normal skin. Fever and adenitis are common.[316]

Two types of generalized eruptions may occur 7–14 days after immunization with vaccinia. The first is a generalized vesicular eruption, most commonly seen in children younger than 1 year of age. Lesions may occur in crops over 2–3 days. Virus cannot be cultured from the vesicles. Other systemic symptoms are usually not present. Generalized erythematous eruptions resembling roseola or enteroviral exanthems may also occur 7–12 days after inoculation. Bullous erythema multiforme has been reported.[315,316]

Pathophysiology

Eczema vaccinatum and progressive vaccinia are due to direct viral invasion of the skin. The generalized eruptions occurring one week or more after inoculation coincide with the rise in delayed antibody response to vaccination and probably have a pathogenesis similar to that of many other viral exanthems.

310. Rogers RS, Tindall JF (1972) Herpes zoster in children. Arch Dermatol 106:204.
311. Eaglestein WH, Katz R, Brown JA (1970) The effects of early corticosteroid therapy on the skin eruption and pain of herpes zoster. JAMA 211:1681.
312. Diven D (2001) An overview of poxviruses. J Am Acad Dermatol 44:1–14.
313. Wehrle PF (1992) Smallpox (variola). In: Textbook of Pediatric Infectious Diseases, 3rd ed, Feigin RD, Cherry JD, eds. Philadelphia: WB Saunders, p. 1666.
314. Neff JM (1985) Variola virus (smallpox). In: Principles and Practice of Infectious Disease, 2nd ed, Mandell GL, Douglas RG, Bennett JE, eds. New York: John Wiley & Sons, p. 985.
315. Neff JM (1995) Vaccinia virus (cowpox). In: Principles and Practice of Infectious Disease, 4th ed, Mandell GL, Douglas RG, Bennett JE, eds. New York: Churchill Livingstone, p. 1325.
316. Downie AW (1965) Poxvirus group. In: Viral and Rickettsial Infections of Man, 4th ed, Horsfall FL, Tamm I, eds. Philadelphia: JB Lippincott, p. 932.

Skin biopsy of primary vaccinia infection demonstrates intraepidermal vesicles caused by intracellular edema. The epithelial cells are ballooned, and intracytoplasmic inclusions (Guarnieri bodies) may be present. The upper dermis has an inflammatory infiltrate consisting primarily of large histiocytes and occasional polymorphonuclear leukocytes.

Differential diagnosis

In the post-smallpox era, the differential diagnosis of vaccinia infection includes herpes simplex infection, varicella, monkeypox, and other vesicular viral exanthems. A history of vaccination or exposure to vaccination is helpful in distinguishing vaccinia from other conditions.

Therapy

Vaccinia immune globulin 0.4mg/kg per day may be used to treat eczema vaccinatum and should be given daily until no new lesions occur.[315] Massive doses of intravenous gamma-globulin have been used with some success in treating progressive vaccinia.[316]

Individuals who receive vaccinia inoculation should not have close contact with immunosuppressed or atopic individuals until the vaccination site has healed.

MILKER'S NODULES (PSEUDOCOWPOX)

Anthony J. Mancini

Milker's nodules, also known as pseudocowpox, are caused by infection with paravaccinia, a parapoxvirus that infects the teats of cattle. This virus is a DNA virus that duplicates in the cytoplasm of infected cells.[317] Infection of the bovine mouth with the same agent results in *bovine papular stomatitis*.

Milker's nodules are found worldwide, most commonly in new milkers, but also in stock handlers and veterinary students. Transmission is via direct contact with the udder or mouth of an infected cow. However, transmission of the virus to sites of first- and second-degree burns in patients without a history of direct contact with infected animals has been reported,[318] suggesting the potential for indirect viral transmission.

The skin lesion is characterized by an early erythematous macule that progresses into a papule or nodule, usually on a digit or extremity. The nodule may break down and weep, followed by crusting. Most often the lesions are solitary. Secondary bacterial infection occasionally occurs. The differential diagnosis includes orf (see below) and a variety of other primary inoculation infections, including primary inoculation tuberculosis, anthrax, tularemia, atypical mycobacterial infection, and deep fungal infection, particularly sporotrichosis. Pyogenic granuloma or a solitary neoplasm may also be considered. A history of exposure to livestock, if present, helps narrow the differential diagnosis.

Histopathologic examination of a skin biopsy specimen is often nonspecific, but early lesions may reveal intracytoplasmic eosinophilic inclusions.[319] Electron microscopy shows characteristic brick-shaped viral particles.[319] Cell culture and serologic studies may also be useful for confirming the diagnosis. There is no specific therapy for milker's nodules, and lesions generally resolve spontaneously over several weeks. Superficial epidermal subsection has been described as a simple, rapid, and effective therapy.[320] Human infection confers lasting immunity.

ORF (SHEEPPOX)

Orf, also known as sheeppox or ecthyma contagiosum, is caused by a parapoxvirus that infects sheeps and goats. This agent is identical to that which

produces milker's nodules. Infected animals have papillomatous lesions on the mucous membranes, which has been termed *scabby mouth* or *sore mouth*.

Transmission of orf to humans is via direct contact with infected lesions in animals or from fomites, including fences, barn doors, and feeding troughs.[319] Infection is seen most commonly in professional workers who have direct contact with sheeps and goats, including shepherds, sheep shearers, butchers, abbatoir workers, and veterinary surgeons.[321] Frequent contact with dogs was positively associated with a self-reported history of orf in farmers in one study,[322] but the significance of this finding is unclear, and orf infection in dogs is not well established.

The lesions of orf begin as a red maculopapule, which progresses through several stages, including target lesion, acute weeping nodule, regenerative dry stage, papillomatous stage, and resolution with a dry crust. Involvement is most common on the hands and fingers (Fig. 25.19) but the face may be involved in children with close contact with pet sheep. Associated lymphadenopathy or lymphadenitis can be seen. The differential diagnosis and

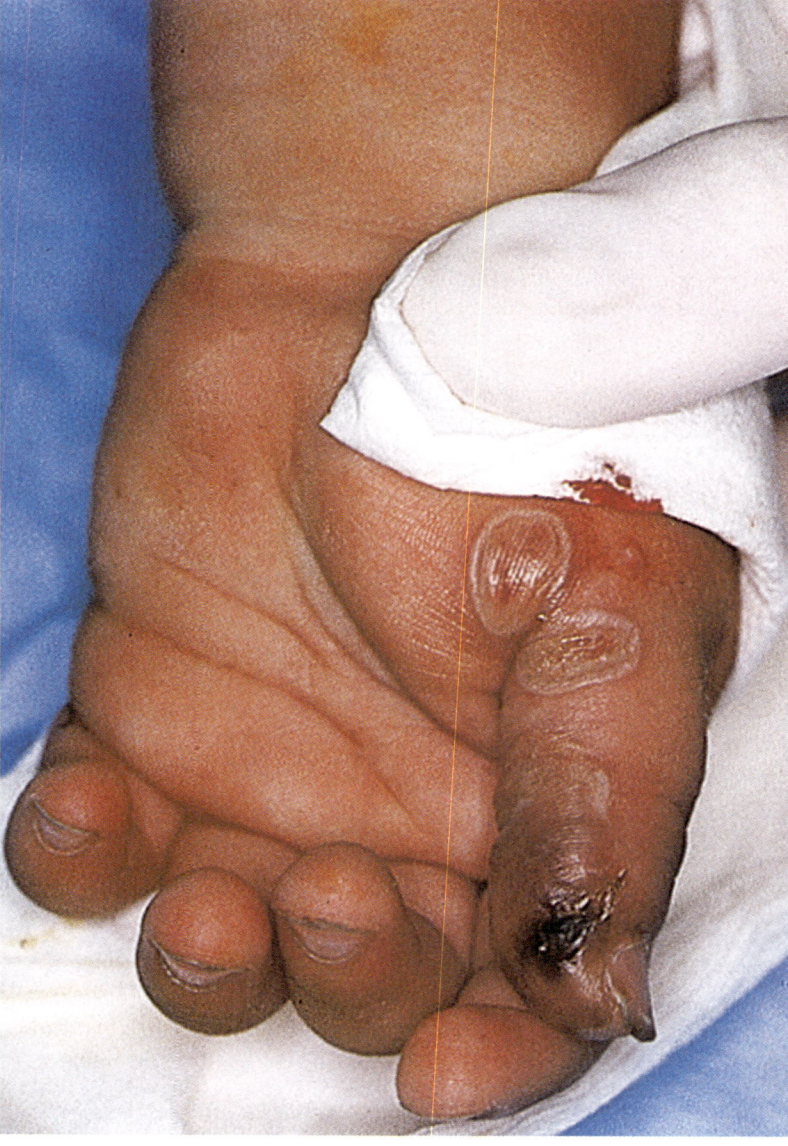

Fig. 25.19   Vesicular and necrotic lesions of orf infection on a finger.

317. Thomas V, Flores L, Holowczak JA (1980) Biochemical and electron microscopic studies of the replication and composition of milker's nodule virus. **J Virol** 34:244–255.
318. Schuler G, Honigsmann H, Wolff K (1982) The syndrome of milker's nodules in burn injury: evidence for indirect viral transmission. **J Am Acad Dermatol** 6:334–339.
319. Diven DG (2001) An overview of poxviruses. **J Am Acad Dermatol** 44:1–14.
320. Shelley WB, Shelley ED (1983) Surgical treatment of farmyard pox. Orf, milker's nodules, bovine papular stomatitis pox. **Cutis** 31:191–192.
321. Chahidi N, deFontaine S, Lacotte B (1993) Human orf. **Br J Plast Surg** 46:532–534.
322. Paiba GA, Thomas DR, Morgan KL et al. (1999) Orf (contagious pustular dermatitis) in farmworkers: prevalence and risk factors in three areas of England. **Vet Record** 145:7–11.

the histopathologic and electron microscopic examinations are similar, as noted above for milker's nodules. Treatment is supportive, and lesions usually subside over 4–6 weeks. Antibiotics are indicated if secondary bacterial infection is present. As with milker's nodules, infection confers long-lasting immunity.

HUMAN PAPILLOMAVIRUS

Christine Bodemer

Human papillomaviruses are a subgroup of the Papovaviridae family and are DNA viruses that are host specific and infect a wide variety of mammalian species. These viruses are fastidious and have resisted culture attempts *in vitro* until recently.[323] Advances in molecular biology have permitted characterization of viral types by direct examination of the viral genome, using Southern blot techniques. During the last decade, as many as 76 types and subtypes of human papillomaviruses have been identified.[323,324] In many cases, these subtypes have become associated with specific types of cutaneous and mucous membrane infection (Table 25.6).[325–339]

TABLE 25.6   Pattern of disease course in human papillomavirus

Human papillomavirus Type	Pattern of disease
1, 2, 4, 7	Plantar, palmar, periungual (verruca vulgaris)
7, 10	Butcher's warts
3, 10, 28	Verrucae planae
13	Oral focal epithelial hyperplasia (Heck)
6, 11, 16, 30, 31, 37, 47	Condyloma acuminatum
16, 18, 30	Bowenoid papulosis
6, 11	Giant condyloma of Buschke–Löwenstein
16, 18, 31, 33, 42	Penile cancer
9, 37	Keratoacanthoma
17a, 38	Melanoma
One-third of all known types	Epidermodysplasia verruciformis
11, 16	Anal cancer
2, 16, 18	Carcinoma of the tongue
6, 11, 16, 18	Leukoplakia and oral carcinoma
16, 18, 31, 33, 47	Invasive carcinoma of the cervix
6, 11, 16, 18, 30	Laryngeal papillomas

EPIDEMIOLOGY

In all types of papillomavirus infection, transmission is apparently by direct contact. Infection can be autoinoculated (i.e., kissing warts), particularly in intertriginous regions and, most likely, indirectly from inanimate objects. Condylomata acuminata and laryngeal papillomas can be acquired at the time of delivery from infective lesions in the maternal birth canal.[339] Tang *et al.*[340] reported a case in which condylomata acuminata were present at the time of birth, which suggests either ascending infection or hematogenous dissemination before delivery. Because of a variable incubation period, the mode of acquisition is usually not obvious (other than in direct sexual contact, as for condyloma acuminatum). A certain element of "receptivity" is involved. Patients who are immunocompromised either iatrogenically, such as in renal transplant patients, or as part of AIDS have increased chances of having widespread infection develop as a result of papillomavirus infection.

Each characteristic papillomavirus lesion is discussed separately, including the differential diagnosis and therapy.

Common warts (verruca vulgaris)

Common warts are found on all body surfaces and are associated with infection by human papillomavirus types 1, 2, 4, and 7.

Clinical characteristics

These lesions are skin colored and sessile. Occasionally, common warts are filiform, characterized by a slender stalk on which there is a papule with numerous projections. Filiform warts may be found in any location but are most common on mucous membranes and in the hairy regions. Common warts may be found as solitary lesions but also tend to form groups and, occasionally, variably sized plaques. Autoinoculation may be apparent when warts are found in a linear array in an apparent scratch mark.

Laboratory findings

Generally, laboratory tests are not needed to identify common verrucae. A skin biopsy, if performed, reveals hyperkeratosis, focal vertical parakeratosis, papillomatosis, koilocytosis, and benign acanthosis. Typing of papillomavirus may be obtained through the use of molecular diagnostic methods, such as the polymerase chain reaction or DNA probes.[341]

Therapy

A wide range of therapies is advocated for the treatment of verrucae and there is a spectrum of views as to what is the most appropriate and likely successful treatment in an individual situation.[342–345] Warts frequently resolve spontaneously, leaving no evidence of prior infection. This fact must be kept in

323. Mayers C, Frattini MG, Hudson JB et al. (1992) Biosynthesis of human papillomavirus from a continuous cell line upon epithelial differentiation. **Science** 257:971.
324. Chan SY, Bernard HV, Ong CK et al. (1992) Phylogenetic analysis of 48 papillomavirus types and 28 subtypes and variants: a showcase for the molecular evolution of DNA viruses. **J Virol** 66:5714.
325. Pfister H (1983) Biology and biochemistry and papillomaviruses. **Rev Physiol Biochem Pharmacol** 99:111.
326. Gissmann L, De Villiers EM, zur Hausen H (1982) Analysis of human genital warts (condylomata acuminata) and other genital tumors for human papilloma virus type 6 DNA. **Int J Cancer** 29:143.
327. Gissmann L, Diehl V, Schultz-Coulon HJ et al. (1982) Molecular cloning and characterization of human papillomavirus DNA derived from a laryngeal papilloma. **J Virol** 44:393.
328. Gissmann L (1984) Papillomaviruses and their association with cancer in animals and man. **Cancer Surv** 3:161.
329. Gassenmaier A, Lammel M, Prister H (1984) Molecular cloning of the DNAs of human papillomaviruses 19, 20, and 25 from a patient with epidermodysplasia verruciformis. **J Virol** 52:1019.
330. Ostrow RS, Bender M, Niimura M et al. (1982) Human papillomavirus DNA in cutaneous primary and metastasized squamous cell carcinomas from patients with epidermodysplasia verruciformis. **Proc Natl Acad Sci USA** 79:1634.
331. Kremsdorf D, Jablonska S, Favre M et al. (1982) Biochemical characterization of human papillomaviruses associated with epidermodysplasia verruciformis. **J Virol** 43:436.
332. Kremsdorf D, Jablonska S, Favre M et al. (1983) Human papillomaviruses associated with epidermodysplasia verruciformis. II. Molecular cloning and biochemical characterization of HPV-3a, -8, -10, and -12 genomes. **J Virol** 48:340.
333. Lutzner M (1978) Epidermodysplasia verruciformis. An autosomal recessive disease characterized by viral warts and skin cancer. A model for viral oncogenesis. **Bull Cancer** (Paris) 65:169.
334. De Villiers EM, Weidauer H, Otto H, zur Hausen H (1985) Papillomavirus DNA in human tongue carcinomas. **Int J Cancer** 36:575.
335. Scheurlen W, Gissmann L, Gross G, zur Hausen H (1986) Molecular cloning of two new HPV types (HPV 37 and HPV 38) from a keratoacanthoma and a malignant melanoma. **Int J Cancer** 37:505.
336. Villa LL, Lopes A (1986) Human papillomavirus DNA sequences in penile carcinomas in Brazil. **Int J Cancer** 37:853.
337. Loning T, Ikenberg H, Becker J et al. (1985) Analysis of oral papillomas, leukoplakias and invasive carcinomas for human papillomavirus-type related DNA. **J Invest Dermatol** 84:417.
338. Kremsdorf D, Favre M, Jablonska S et al. (1984) Molecular cloning and characterization of the genomes of nine newly recognized human papillomavirus types associated with epidermodysplasia verruciformis. **J Virol** 52:1013.
339. Hajek E (1956) Contribution to the etiology of laryngeal papilloma in children. **J Laryngol Otol** 70:166.
340. Tang CK, Shermeta DW, Wood C (1978) Congenital condylomata acuminata. **Am J Obstet Gynecol** 131:912.
341. Manos MM, Ting Y, Wright DR et al. (1989) Use of polymerase chain reaction amplification for the detection of genital human papillomavirus. **Cancer Cells** 7:209.
342. Sterling JC, Handfield-Jones S, Hudson PM (2001) Guidelines for the management of cutaneous warts. **Br J Dermatol** 144:4–11.
343. Allen AL, Siegfried EC (2000) What's new in human papillomavirus infection. **Curr Opin Pediatr** 12:365–369.
344. Allen AL, Siegfried EC (2001) Management of warts and molluscum in adolescents. **Adol Med** 12:229–242.
345. Verbov J (1999) How to manage warts. **Arch Dis Child** 80:97–99.

mind when considering various therapies. In children who have limited wart infection that is not disabling physically or cosmetically, it seems appropriate to use the least traumatic forms of therapy, either reassurance and observation or the application of a topical placebo. If treatment is indicated, a number of ablative therapies exist, including cryosurgery, chemovesicants, electrodesiccation, and laser therapy. Usually, simple cryotherapy is sufficient for resolution. The possible therapeutic benefits of ablative forms of treatment that may produce scarring should be weighed against the fact that many verrucae resolve spontaneously. Before the use of ablative therapy, the repeated topical application of salicyclic acid-containing substances, coupled with soaking and the use of abrasives, can be tried as a relatively nontraumatic approach to removal of the verrucae; the major drawback with this approach is that it is lengthy and not always successful. Other topical agents that may be successful for common warts are cidofovir 3% cream and imiquimod although the latter is more effective for condylomata than for common warts.[343]

Contact immunotherapy is a novel treatment for which there are many reports of success. The patient is sensitized by the application of a man-made allergen to normal skin and then a contact allergic dermatitis is elicited in the area of the warts by the weekly application of the sensitizer to them. The favored agents are diphencyprone and squaric acid dibutylester and cure rates of 50–80% are reported in children.[343,347–349] There are reports of success using high-dose oral cimetidine, 30–40mg/kg per day for six weeks or more in treating multiple recalcitrant warts in children.[343,350,351] This treatment is most effective in younger children and much less so in adolescents and adults[352] and the inclusion of older patients may account for less favorable reports.[353] The combination of cimetidine and levamisole may be more effective than cimetidine alone.[354]

Flat warts (verruca plana)

Flat warts follow infection by human papillomavirus types 3, 10, and 28.

Clinical characteristics

These lesions may be found on all body surfaces but are most common on the face. In adults, autoinoculation appears to be secondary to the trauma of shaving. The lesions are broad based and flat topped, with little scale.

Laboratory findings

Generally, laboratory tests are not needed to confirm the diagnosis of verrucae planae. Skin biopsy reveals a mildly acanthotic epidermis with a prominent granular zone. Koilocytotic cells are present in the granular zone, a finding typical of papillomavirus infection.

Differential diagnosis

A solitary verruca plana may not be clinically diagnostic. The diagnostic possibilities may include other viral lesions, such as molluscum contagiosum, folliculitis, acne, juvenile xanthogranuloma, benign cephalic histiocytosis, and granuloma annulare. When these lesions are grouped, other processes to consider include epidermal nevus; lichenoid processes, such as lichen nitidus and lichen planus; and superficial infections, such as tinea versicolor.

Therapy

Topical tretinoin is often effective in treating flat warts. Otherwise, the treatment approaches are similar to those described above

Condyloma acuminatum

Condylomata acuminata are papillomavirus-induced lesions associated primarily with types 6 and 11 and, occasionally, with types 16, 18, and 30. In children, human papillomavirus types 2 and 4 have also been isolated. A most important sequel of infection by some types of human papillomavirus is the oncogenic risk associated with their presence. There is strong evidence that human papillomavirus infection by oncogenic types is an important etiologic agent of intraepithelial neoplasia of the cervix, vulva, nasopharynx, penis, and rectum.[355] Most anogenital papillomas are produced by infection with human papillomavirus types 6 and 11, both of which are of low oncogenic potential. However, similar clinical lesions may be produced by infection with types 16 and 18, both of which are associated with the development of dysplasia. Cervical and vulvar dysplasias associated with this viral infection have been reported in adolescent females.[356,357]

Clinical characteristics

These lesions are mainly found in the anogenital region, the external genitalia, and contiguous mucous membranes. Warts associated with the same human papillomavirus types may also be found on other mucous membranes, such as that in the oral cavity, nasopharynx,[358] and conjunctiva.[359,360] These papillomavirus types are a frequent cause of laryngeal papillomatosis, transmitted vertically from the mother during delivery. Chronic friction in the anogenital area results in papules that are less verrucous and vary in color from pink to brown (Fig. 25.20). Condylomata acuminata may be solitary and scattered or multiple and confluent. In children who are immunosuppressed, condylomata may be very extensive and grow to large sizes. Although not usually an immediate concern in children, condylomata acuminata have malignant potential.

The mechanisms of transmission of HPV to the anogenital area in children have been clearly identified as vertical or perinatal transmission from an HPV-infected maternal genital tract, horizontal transmission by auto- or hetero-inoculation from cutaneous or mucosal warts elsewhere, and transmission by sexual abuse.[361] Vertical transmission is most likely in children under 3 years of age.[362,363] When anogenital warts appear in children over 3 years of age, vertical transmission is an unlikely explanation.[364,365]

In 1985, Schachner and Hankin[366] defined criteria for assessing the sensitive areas that surround the evaluation of children with these lesions. When these

346. Buckley DA, Keane FM, Munn SE et al. (1999) Recalcitrant viral warts treated with diphencyprone immunotherapy **Br J Dermatol** 26:162–165.
347. Lee AN, Mallory SB (1999) Contact immunotherapy with squaric acid dibutylester for the treatment of recalcitrant warts. **J Am Acad Dermatol** 41:595–599.
348. Micali G, Nasca MR, Tedeschi A et al. (2000) Use of squaric acid dibutylester (SADBE) for cutaneous warts in children. **Pediatr Dermatol** 17:315–318.
349. Silverberg NB, Lim JK, Paller AS et al. (2000) Squaric acid immunotherapy for warts in children. **J Am Acad Dermatol** 42:803–808.
350. Orlow S, Paller AS (1993) Cimetidine therapy for multiple viral warts in children. **J Am Acad Dermatol** 28:794.
351. Fischer G, Rogers M (1997) Cimetidine therapy for warts in children. **J Am Acad Dermatol** 37:289–290.
352. Gooptu C, Higgins CR, James MP (2000) Treatment of viral warts with cimetidine: an open label study. **Clin Exp Dermatol** 25:183–185.
353. Yilmaz E, Alpsoy E, Basaran E (1996) Cimetidine therapy for warts: a placebo controlled double blind study. **J Am Acad Dermatol** 34:1005–1007.
354. Parsad D, Pandhi R, Juneja A et al. (2001) Cimetidine and levamisole versus cimetidine for recalcitrant warts in children. **Pediatr Dermatol** 18:349–352.
355. Kurman RJ, Jenson AB, Lancaster WD (1983) Papillomavirus infection of the cervix. II. Relationship to intraepithelial neoplasia based on the presence of specific viral structural proteins. **Am J Surg Pathol** 7:39.

356. Lister UM, Akinla O (1972) Carcinoma of the vulva in childhood. **Br J Obstet Gynaecol** 79:470.
357. Boutselis G (1972) Intraepithelial neoplasia of the vulva. **Am J Obstet Gynecol** 113:733.
358. Wu T-C, Trujillo JM, Kashima HK, Mounts P (1993) Association of human papillomavirus with nasal neoplasia. **Lancet** 341:522.
359. Naghashfar Z, Sawada E, Kutcher MJ et al. (1985) Identification of genital tract papillomaviruses HPV-6 and HPV-16 in warts of the oral cavity. **J Med Virol** 17:313.
360. Lass JH, Grove AS, Papale JJ et al. (1983) Detection of human papilloma-virus DNA sequences in conjunctival papilloma. **Am J Ophthalmol** 96:670.
361. Armstrong DKB, Bingham EA, Dinsmore WW et al. (1998) Anogenital warts in pre-pubertal children: a follow-up study. **Br J Dermatol** 138:544–545.
362. Boyd AS (1990) Condylomata acuminata in the pediatric population. **Am J Dis Child** 144:817.
363. Cohen BA, Honig P, Androphy E (1990) Anogenital warts in children. **Arch Dermatol** 126:1575.
364. Gutman LT, Herman-Giddens ME, Phelps WC (1993) Transmission of human genital papillomavirus disease: comparison of data from adults and children. **Pediatrics** 91:31.
365. Ingram DL, Everett VD, Lyna PR et al. (1992) Epidemiology of adult sexually transmitted disease agents in children being evaluated for sexual abuse. **Pediatr Infect Dis J** 11:945.
366. Schachner L, Hankin DE (1985) Assessing child abuse in childhood condyloma acuminatum. **J Am Acad Dermatol** 12:157.

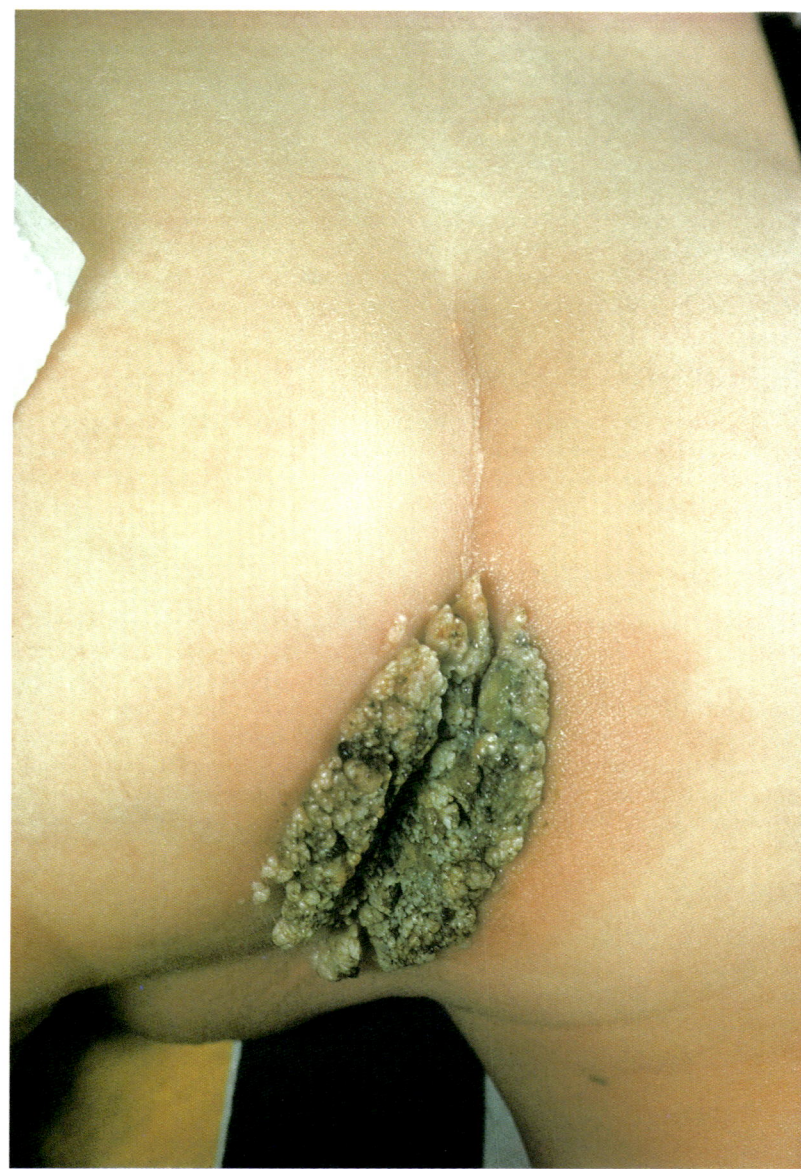

Fig. 25.20 Perianal warts occurring as a result of sexual abuse.

lesions are present, a careful and discreet history must be obtained from the child and the parents. The child should also be evaluated for other signs of abuse. Oral condylomata in children may also be sexually transmitted and this issue must always be considered when presented with such a case.[367]

Differential diagnosis

Pseudoverrucous papules and nodules, a condition that may be seen in association with ureterostomies and in the perianal area in association with chronic fecal incontinence, may closely mimic condyloma acuminatum.[368] Lesions of condylomata acuminata must also be separated from condylomata in which bowenoid changes have developed, from condylomata lata, the moist papules of secondary syphilis, which occur commonly in the anogenital region, from agminated mollusca, and from skin tags. Although rare, benign and malignant neoplasms need to be considered as possibilities, particularly when condylomata acuminata are solitary.

Laboratory findings

Appropriate dark-field examination and serologic tests exclude condylomata lata. If performed, skin biopsy shows papillomatosis, focal parakeratosis, and acanthosis. Koilocytosis is seen focally in the granular zone. Papillomavirus common antigen can be detected by immunohistochemical means overlying the nuclei of infected cells in the granular zone in many cases. Other diagnostic possibilities have their characteristic histologic pictures, which are not present if the lesions are condylomata acuminata. A skin biopsy of a lesion that clinically is a condyloma acuminatum may show focal or diffuse dysplasia characterized by disorderly maturation, nuclear atypia, and parakeratosis. These changes indicate that the lesion is a bowenoid papule; in these histologically atypical lesions, papillomavirus common antigen can routinely be demonstrated.[369] Lesions with dysplasia are most frequently associated with human papillomavirus types 16 and 18; lesions with no atypical features (simple anogenital condylomata acuminata) are produced most commonly by infection with types 6 and 11. Differentiating these two entities is of great importance. It is unclear whether bowenoid papulosis represents a significant cancer risk on the male genitalia; it is clear, however, that these types are significantly associated with invasive carcinoma of the cervix and anorectal carcinoma and cervical and labial dysplasias.[370,371] Determination of papillomavirus type by molecular diagnostic methods is not helpful in the evaluation of anogenital condylomata in cases where sexual abuse is a possibility. Transmission of any virus type can occur by abuse, digital or genital-to-genital transmission, vertical transmission, or innocent contact. However, papillomavirus typing may be useful to define patients at high risk for oncogenic change and also for medicolegal reasons. Podophyllin resin may induce histologic atypia in condyloma acuminata that resemble bowenoid changes. A pathologist should be informed if a podophyllin-treated lesion has been sampled.

Therapy

While spontaneous resolution of condylomata may occur in over 50% of cases over a period of a few years,[372] the discomfort of these lesions and the understandable distress of the parents usually lead to a preference for prompt treatment.

The treatment of condylomata acuminata in children usually rests on ablative or chemical methods. Excision, cryotherapy, cauterisation, electrodesiccation, and laser techniques have all been used but require general anesthesia.[373] Newer topical agents for which success is reported include podophilox gel 5% (the biologically active component of podophyllin resin),[374] imiquimod 5% cream,[374] and cidofovir topical gel.[375] These agents are either applied by the physician or by the parents after very careful instruction. Repeated applications are required and the almost inevitable side effect of irritation can be managed by titrating the frequency of application.

Patients in whom extensive condyloma acuminata develop while they are immunosuppressed may have spontaneous resolution if the immunosuppression is reversed. Spontaneous regression may also occur in immunologically intact individuals; therefore, conservative approaches to therapy are often elected in treating these lesions in children.

367. Squires J, Persaud D., Simon P et al. (1999) Oral condylomata in children. **Arch Pediatr Adol Med** 153:651–654.
368. Goldberg NS, Esterly NB, Rothman KF et al. (1992) Perianal pseudo verrucous papules and nodules in children. **Arch Dermatol** 128:240.
369. Penneys NS, Mogollon RJ, Nadiji M et al. (1984) Papillomavirus common antigens. Papillomavirus antigen in verruca, benign papillomatous lesions, trichilemmoma, and bowenod papulosis: an immunoperoxidase study. **Arch Dermatol** 120:859.
370. Campion MJ, Singer A, Clarkson PK et al. (1985) Increased risk of cervical neoplasia in consorts of men with penile condylomata acuminata. **Lancet** 1:943.
371. Crum CP, Ikenberg H, Richart RM et al. (1984) Human papillomavirus type 16 and early cervical neoplasia. **N Engl J Med** 310:880.
372. Allen AL, Siegfried EC (1998) The natural history of condyloma in children. **J Am Acad Dermatol** 39:951–955.
373. Handley JM, Maw RD, Horner T et al. (1991) Scissor excision plus electrocautery of anogenital warts in prepubertal children. **Pediatr Dermatol** 8:243.
374. Moresi JM, Herbert CR, Cohen BA (2001) Treatment of anogenital warts in children with topical 0.05% podophilox gel and 5% imiquimod cream. **Pediatr Dermatol** 18:448–452.
375. Snoeck R, Bossens M, Parent D (2001) Phase II double-blind, placebo-controlled study of the safety and efficacy of cidofovir topical gel for the treatment of patients with human papillomavirus infection. **Clin Infect Dis** 33:597–602.

Plantar warts

Clinical characteristics

Plantar warts are endophytic lesions on the sole of the foot. As a result of their location, these lesions are flat topped and hyperkeratotic. Plantar warts can be extensive (and specially named, mosaic warts) and frequently painful.

Differential diagnosis

Plantar warts, corns, and calluses may be clinically similar. Removing the superficial layers of the stratum corneum overlying the lesion reveals bleeding points or brown flecks, which represent extravasated erythrocytes or thrombosed superficial capillaries; these findings are typical of wart infection and serve to separate plantar warts from other lesions found on the sole.

Laboratory findings

Generally, laboratory studies are not needed to identify plantar warts. If a skin biopsy is performed, it reveals the typical histology of verruca vulgaris with papillomatosis, koilcytosis, and acanthosis.

Therapy

The most common form of treatment for plantar warts is repeated paring of the thickened stratum corneum followed by the application of salicylic acid. This is in the form of salicyclic acid plaster or as a liquid in a volatile vehicle, both used as home treatments. Softening of the keratinous plantar lesion by the application of salicylic acid–containing substances and soaking allows removal of the outermost layers by abrasion with an emery board or pumice stone. Another approach is to harden the surface with the daily application of a 20% formalin (3% formaldehyde) preparation followed by regular paring with a scalpel blade. More aggressive ablative methods of treatment are usually avoided because of the risk of scar formation in this weight-bearing region.

EPIDERMODYSPLASIA VERRUCIFORMIS

EPIDEMIOLOGY

The skin lesions in epidermodysplasia verruciformis have been associated with infection by human papillomavirus types 3, 5, 8 through 10, 12, 14, 15, 17, 19 through 25, and 30. These virus types represent an evolutionary cluster.[376] Many EV patients are infected with multiple HPV-types. Epidermodysplasia verruciformis is most likely an autosomal-recessive genodermatosis. Data supporting this conclusion derive from the high incidence of consanguinity in families in which there is an affected individual and from the observation that more than one family member may be involved.[377] Evidence for a nonallelic heterogeneity of EV has been demonstrated, with two susceptibility loci mapped to chromosomes 2 and 17.[378]

CLINICAL CHARACTERISTICS

Rarely, warty lesions are present at birth; most lesions develop during childhood and puberty. Warty lesions tend to develop confluence and be present over bony prominences. Some lesions have the appearance of flat warts, other present as flat scaly red–brown macules, and look like lesions of pityriasis rosea or tinea versicolor. Despite treatment, warts in EV always recur, suggesting a specific immune deficiency. In most of cases, EV patients do not suffer from other viral infections or from recurrent bacterial infections.

This papillomavirus infection spares the oral cavity. The lesions persist, and a large percentage of the lesions evolve into cutaneous malignancies. Cutaneous squamous cell carcinomas usually arise on sun-exposed areas and remain local, but regional and distant metastases may occur. The risk of developing malignant lesions appears greater with HPV-5 and -8, as lesions with these two HPV types account for the majority of malignancies.

DIFFERENTIAL DIAGNOSIS

Patients have characteristic warty lesions in a distribution that is suggestive of this entity. Extensive common wart infection should be excluded. Epidermodysplasia verruciformis-like presentations can be observed in patients who have HIV infection.[379]

LABORATORY FINDINGS

A skin biopsy in helpful in many cases. The warty lesions present in these individuals may have a characteristic change in the upper layers of the epidermis composed of swollen keratinocytes, which contain basophilic granules. The nuclei are pale and enlarged. Dysplastic changes may be found within keratinocytes in these lesions. Exophytic lesions may show the changes of squamous cell carcinoma. Immunohistochemical staining for bovine papillomavirus common antigen may be positive. Viral genomic studies may be performed. Many EV patients have defects of cellular immunity.

THERAPY

No effective treatment is available. No apparent effect of cidofovir has been reported in EV patients, despite the previously demonstrated effectiveness against a range of different papillomavirus-associated conditions.[380] Some improvement has been observed in an adult case with topical 5-aminolaevulinic acid photodynamic therapy.[381] Systemic retinoids may be of some use.[382,383] Cutaneous malignancies must be surgically removed.

MOLLUSCUM CONTAGIOSUM

Molluscum contagiosum is a common cutaneous viral infection in children. It is caused by infection with a DNA virus of the Molluscipox genus.[384] Four subtypes of the virus have been identified with type I being the main one affecting immunocompetent children.[385,386]

EPIDEMIOLOGY

Although the disease is worldwide in distribution and can occur at any age, infection is most common in young children, sexually active adults, and persons of all ages with impaired cellular immunity.[384]

376. Chan SY, Bernard HV, Ong CK et al. (1992) Phylogenetic analysis of 48 papillomavirus types and 28 subtypes and variants: a showcase for the molecular evolution of DNA viruses. J Virol 66:5714.
377. Lutzner M (1978) Epidermodysplasia verruciformis. An autosomal recessive disease characterized by viral warts and skin cancer. A model for viral oncogenesis. Bull Cancer (Paris) 65:169.
378. Ramoz N, Taieb A, Rueda LA et al. (2000) Evidence of nonallelic heterogeneity of epidermodysplasia verruciformis with two susceptibility loci mapped to chromosomes regions 2p21-p22 and 17q25. J Invest Dermatol 114:1148–1153.
379. Berger TG, Sawchuk WS, Leonardi C et al. (2001) Epidermodysplasia verruciformis-associated papillomavirus infection complicating human immunodeficiency virus disease. Br J Dermatol 124:79–83.
380. Preiser W, Kapur N, Snoeck R, Groves RW, Brink NS (2000) No apparent effect of cidofovir in epidermodysplasia verruciformis. J Clin Virol 16:55–57.
381. Karrer S, Szeimies RM, Abels C et al. (1999) Epidermodysplasia verruciformis treated using topical 5-aminolaevulinic acid photodynamic therapy. Br J Dermatol 140:935–938.
382. Jablonska S, Obalek S, Wolska H et al. (1981) RO 10-9359 in epidermodysplasia verruciformis. In: Retinoids: Advances in Basic Research and Therapy, Orfanos CE, Braun-Falco O, Farber EM et al. eds. New York: Springer-Verlag, p. 401.
383. Lutzner MA, Blanchet-Bardon C, Puissant A (1981) Oral aromatic retinoid (RO 10-9359) treatment of two patients suffering with the severe form of epidermodysplasia verruciformis. In: Retinoids: Advances in Basic Research and Therapy, Orfanos CE, Braun-Falco O, Farber EM et al., eds. New York: Springer-Verlag, p. 410.
384. Diven DG (2001) An overview of poxviruses. J Am Acad Dermatol 44:1–14.
385. Porter CD, Blake NW, Archard LC et al. (1989) Molluscum contagiosum virus types in genital and non-genital lesions. Br J Dermatol 120:37–41.
386. Yamashita H, Uemura T, Kawashima M (1996) Molecular epidemiologic analysis of Japanese patients with molluscum contagiosum. Int J Dermatol 35:99–105.

It is usually postulated that infection is spread by skin-to-skin contact, fomites, or autoinoculation. However, the observation that the incidence of molluscum contagiosum was found to be twice as high in children exposed to swimming pools than children who were not[387] and the reports of epidemics related to public pools[388] point to the importance of spread of the virus through water. The spread of lesions is enhanced in warm water and outbreaks occur particularly among children who swim together in heated pools or share baths or spas. Further spread of mollusca within a single individual is also encouraged by being in warm water of these types. The spread seems to be minimal in cold water.

The incubation period has been estimated to be from two to eight weeks, although a case in a 1-week-old child has been reported.[389]

PRESENTING HISTORY

Children present to the physician most frequently because of the presence of visible bumps, but pruritus or soreness occasionally may be prominent symptoms.

PHYSICAL EXAMINATION

The typical lesions of molluscum contagiosum are discrete, dome-shaped, umbilicated waxy papules.[384] They vary in color and may be skin colored, pink, or white. A small central punctum frequently is visible. Lesions may appear to be vesicular because of a translucent quality. They also may appear as tiny, pinpoint papules simulating milia or as pedunculated tag-like lesions. Lesions usually vary in size 1–5mm, although lesions as large as 10–15mm (so-called giant molluscum) can occur. Secondary bacterial infection may occur producing crusting, redness, and pus formation. However, these same changes may be seen during spontaneous resolution.

Lesions may occur on any part of the body but, in young children, are found most commonly on the axilla, side of trunk (Fig. 25.21), lower abdomen, thighs, and face. Lesions in the genital area that occur in adolescents or young adults are usually sexually transmitted.[384] The presence of lesions in the genital areas of young children is not usually a consequence of sexual abuse, but this possibility should be considered by the examining physician.

An eczematous eruption on the skin adjacent to molluscum, so-called "molluscum dermatitis" is present in approximately 10% of cases.[390] The dermatitis may be associated with pre-existing atopic dermatitis but may also occur de novo. It usually disappears spontaneously when the molluscum is treated or regresses.

Widespread cutaneous infection, with hundreds of lesions present, has been reported in individuals with atopic dermatitis and in immunosuppressed individuals.[391,392] In patients with HIV infection the lesions may be extremely numerous, large and sometimes almost confluent, and lesions confined to the hair follicles, so-called molluscum folliculitis, are also reported.[393]

Periocular molluscum may be associated with conjunctival molluscum and with a "toxic" conjunctivitis. Ocular infection rarely causes permanent structural damage.[394] Lesions may rarely also occur on other mucous membranes. Individual lesions last for several weeks or occasionally months but the spread of lesions often accounts for a very prolonged course for the infection.

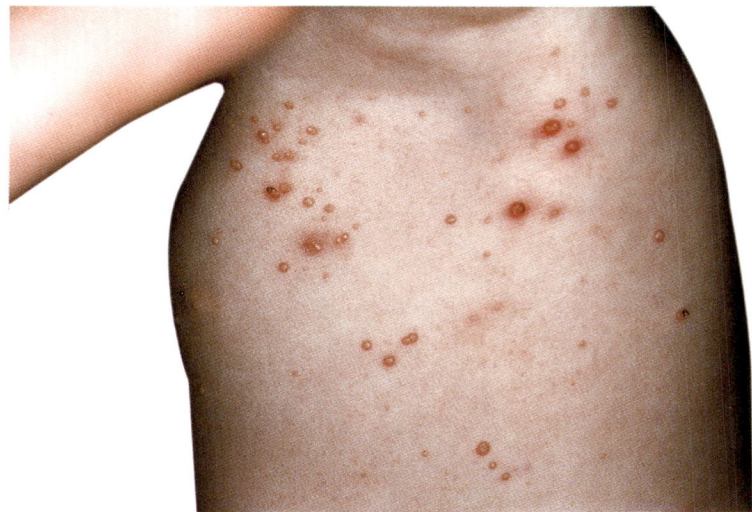

Fig. 25.21 Mollusca contagiosa.

LABORATORY FINDINGS

The molluscum contagiosum virus has not been successfully cultured in vitro. Using an ELISA for molluscum contagiosum, virus specific antibodies have been demonstrated in the sera in individuals both with and without clinical lesions. In one study, antibodies against the virus were found in 58% of patients with active disease, 6% of healthy controls, 9% of patients with atopic dermatitis without mollusca and 2% of patients with HIV infection without mollusca.[395] In another study, the antibody was demonstrated in 77% of patients with obvious lesions.[396] In a population study of 357 persons aged 1 week to 69 years without clinical lesions, the overall seropositivity rate was 23% the lowest antibody prevalence was in children aged 6–24 months (3%) and it increased with age to reach 39% in the group of individuals over 50.[396] Detection of the virus in skin lesions has been achieved using PCR.[397]

Histologically, molluscum lesions are acanthomas consisting of hyperplastic and hypertrophied epidermal cells, which proliferate in a downward fashion into the dermis. The basement membrane remains intact. Cells are filled with intracytoplasmic inclusion bodies, so-called Henderson-Paterson bodies, which are eosinophilic ovoid structures in the lower Malpighian layer. In the upper epidermis, they become more basophilic and may be as large as 35µm in diameter, far larger than the size of epidermal cells.[398,399] These homogeneous molluscum inclusion bodies may also be demonstrated by smearing the cheesy contents from a lesion onto a slide and staining with Gram, Giemsa, or Wright's stain.[400]

Inflammation is rarely present histologically unless a lesion ruptures into the dermis, causing a foreign body or immune reaction.[398] Lesions of molluscum eczema show spongiosis, dermal edema, and a perivascular round cell infiltrate.

Studies of cellular kinetics demonstrate three distinct stages of evolution in growth: an early stage, in which epithelial nuclei divide; a middle stage, in which epithelial division diminishes; and a late stage, in which dermal

387. Niizeki K, Kano O, Kondo Y (1984) An epidemic study of molluscum contagiosum. Dermatologica 169:197–198.
388. Oren B, Wende SO (1991) An outbreak of molluscum contagiosum in a kibbutz: relationship to swimming. Infection 19:159–161.
389. Mandel MJ, Lewis RJ (1970) Molluscum contagiosum of the newborn. Br J Dermatol 84:370.
390. Kipping HF (1971) Molluscum dermatitis. Arch Dermatol 03:106.
391. Rosenberg EW, Yusk JW (1970) Molluscum contagiosum. Eruption following treatment with prednisone and methotrexate. Arch Dermatol 101:439.
392. Pauly CR, Artis WM, Jones HE (1978) Atopic dermatitis, impaired cellular immunity, and molluscum contagiosum. Arch Dermatol 114:391.
393. Jang KA, Kim SH, Choi JH et al. (2000) Viral folliculitis on the face. Br J Dermatol 142:555–559.
394. Margo C, Katz NNK (1983) Management of periocular molluscum contagiosum in children. J Pediatr Ophthalmol Strabismus 20:19.

395. Wantanabe T, Nakamura K, Wakugwa M et al. (2000) Antibodies to molluscum contagiosum virus in the general population and susceptible patients. Arch Dermatol 136:1518–1522.
396. Konya J, Thompson CH (1999) Molluscum contagiosum virus: antibody responses in persons with clinical lesions and seroepidemiology in a representative Australian population. J Infect Dis 179:701–704.
397. Thompson CH (1997) Identification and typing of molluscum contagiosum virus in clinical specimens by polymerase chain reaction. J Med Virol 53:205–211.
398. Landau JW, Gurevitch AW (1992) Molluscum contagiosum. In: Textbook of Pediatric Infectious Diseases, 3rd ed, Feigin RD, Cherry JD, eds. Philadelphia: WB Saunders, p. 818.
399. Postlethwaite R (1970) Molluscum contagiosum: a review. Arch Environ Health 21:432.
400. Brown ST, Nalley JF, Krause SJ (1981) Molluscum contagiosum. Sex Transm Dis 18:227.

endothelial cells and fibroblasts become activated.[401] The precise mechanism of spontaneous regression of lesions is unknown, but cellular immunity is probably involved.[401]

DIFFERENTIAL DIAGNOSIS

In typical cases, the diagnosis is usually obvious, but lesions may resemble verrucae, varicella, folliculitis, furunculosis, milia, juvenile xanthogranuloma, Spitz nevi, and skin tags. A smear of the contents of a lesion should demonstrate characteristic molluscum bodies.

THERAPY

Molluscum infection left untreated nearly always resolves spontaneously, but this may take from a few weeks to a few years. However, individual lesions usually last for no more than a few weeks. With this natural history in mind, consideration should always be given to opting for no treatment.[402] If the child is kept out of heated pools and spas and has showers rather than baths at home the proliferation is curbed in most cases and the number of lesions usually decreases quickly. If these measures are rigidly adhered to, treatment is rarely required.

In some patients, however, the lesions appear to be persistent and therapy needs to be considered. A large variety of topical treatments have been reported to have some success, including tretinoin cream, benzoyl peroxide, podophyllum resin in tincture of benzoin, cantharidin, and silver nitrate.[384,403–405] Prepared cantharadin preparations are banned from sale in some countries but can be made made up from available pure cantharadin in hospital pharmacies. A preparation of 0.9% cantharadin in flexible collodion is carefully applied by the physician to individual lesions and washed off after 2–4 hours;[403,404] it often causes a small blister and enough inflammation to eradicate lesions and is usually very well tolerated, but occasionally very large blisters occur despite careful application. A 97% success rate without residual scarring is reported in a very large series of patients with 1–3 applications of a 40% silver nitrate paste.[405] There has been some success reported with the use of imiquimod 1–5% cream,[406,407] but in some cases the irritation caused led to a spread of new lesions.[408] Topical 3% cidofovir has been used successfully in childhood patients immunodeficient as a result of HIV infection[409] and Wiskott–Aldrich syndrome.[410] Oral cidofovir, which has been used in adult patients in this setting,[411] has not been approved for use in children.

Physical therapies include incision with a cutting edged needle or #11 blade and wiping out the contents or superficial curettage. Application of a eutectic mixture of prilocaine and lidocaine cream (EMLA) for one to two hours before treatment may help diminish the discomfort in ablative forms of treatments or, if available, nitrous oxide sedation makes the procedure very much easier. In immunodeficient patients with very extensive disease, curettage or superficial surgical excision under general anesthesia may be the only practical approach.

Treatment of periocular molluscum contagiosum is especially difficult because the use of vesicants, liquid nitrogen, or sharp instruments near the eye of a young child is fraught with danger. In this situation, observation without treatment is usually justified unless symptomatic conjunctivitis is present, in which case removal of the lesion while the patient is under a general anesthetic may be necessary.[394]

Spread to other children is only likely through sharing a bath or spa or swimming together in the same heated pool. Therefore, these activities should be avoided not only to prevent spread to other children but to prevent further proliferation on the infected individual.

401. Pierard-Franchimont C, Legrain A, Pierard GE (1983) Growth and regression of molluscum contagiosum. **J Am Acad Dermatol** 9:669.
402. Weston WL, Lane AT (1980) Should molluscum be treated? **Pediatrics** 65:865.
403. Silverberg NB, Sidbury R, Mancini AJ (2000) Childhood molluscum contagiosum: experience with cantharadin therapy in 300 patients. **J Am Acad Dermatol** 43:503–507.
404. Moed L, Shwayder TA, Chang MW (2001) Cantharadin revisited. **Arch Dermatol** 137:1357–1360.
405. Niizeki K, Hashimoto K (1999) Treatment of molluscum contagiosum with silver nitrate paste. **Pediatr Dermatol** 16:395–397.
406. Syed TA, Goswami J, Ahmadpoir OA et al. (1998) Treatment of molluscum contagiosum in males with an analog of imiquimod 1% in cream: a placebo-controlled, double-blind study. **J Dermatol** 25:309–313.
407. Skinner RB, Ray S, Talanin NY (2000) Treatment of molluscum contagiosum with topical 5% imiquimod cream. **Pediatr Dermatol** 17:420.
408. Liota E, Smith KG, Buckley R et al. (2000) Imiquimod cream for molluscum contagiosum. **J Cut Med Surg** 4:76–82.
409. Toro JR, Wood LV, Patel NK (2000) Topical cidofovir: a novel treatment for recalcitrant molluscum contagiosum in children infected with human immunodeficiency virus 1. **Arch Dermatol** 136:983–985.
410. Davies EG, Thrasher A, Lacey K et al. (1999) Topical cidofovir for severe molluscum contagiosum. **Lancet** 353:2042.
411. Meadows KP, Tyring SK, Pavia AT et al. (1997) Resolution of recalcitrant molluscum contagiosum virus lesions in human immunodeficiency virus infected patients treated with cidofovir. **Arch Dermatol** 133:987–990.
412. Cherry JD (1983) Viral exanthems. **Curr Probl Pediatr** 13:1–44.
413. Esterly NB (1984) Viral exanthems: diagnosis and management. **Semin Dermatol** 3:140–145.
414. Forman ML, Cherry JD (1968) Enanthems associated with uncommon viral syndromes. **Pediatrics** 41:873–882.
415. Gohd RS, Faigel HC (1966) Hand-foot-and-mouth disease resembling measles a life threatening disease: case report. **Pediatrics** 37:644–648.
416. James WD, Odom RB, Hatch MH (1982) Gianotti–Crosti-like eruption associated with Coxsackie virus A-16 infection. **J Am Acad Dermatol** 6:862–866.
417. Costa MM, Lisboa M, Romeu JC et al. (1995) Henoch-Schonlein purpura associated with Coxsackie-virus B1 infection. **Clin Rheumatol** 14:488–490.
418. Sauerbrei A, Gluck B, Jung K et al. (2000) Congenital skin lesions caused by intrauterine infection with Coxsackievirus B3. **Infection** 28:326–328.
419. Roberts-Thomson PJ, Southwood TR, Moore BW et al. (1986) Adult onset Still's disease or coxsackie polyarthritis? **Aust N Z J Med** 16:509–511.
420. Feio AB, Apetato M, Costa MM et al. (1997) Acute generalized exanthematous pustulosis due to Coxsackie B4 virus. **Acta Med Port** 10:487–491.
421. Meade RH, Chang T-W (1979) Zoster-like eruption due to echovirus 6. **Am J Dis Child** 133:283–284.
422. Deseda-Tous J, Byatt PH, Cherry JD (1977) Vesicular lesions in adults due to echovirus 11 infections. **Arch Dermatol** 113:1705–1706.
423. Balfour HH, May DB, Rottee TC et al. (1972) A study of erythema infectiosum: recovery of rubella virus and echovirus-12. **Pediatrics** 50:285–290.
424. Cherry CD (1969) Newer viral exanthems. [Review] [303 refs] **Adv Pediatr** 16:233–286.
425. Rouchouse B, Bonnefoy M, Pallot B et al. (1986) Acute generalized exanthematous pustular dermatitis and viral infection. **Dermatologica** 173:180–184.
426. Clementz GC, Mancini AJ (2000) Nail matrix arrest following hand-foot-mouth disease: A report of five children. **Pediatr Dermatol** 17:7–11.

Fungal, Protozoal, and Helminthic Infections

Sheila F. Friedlander, Monica Rueda, Bryan K. Chen and Hector W. Caceres-Rios

This chapter reviews a diverse group of organisms that all possess the ability to infect humans and produce cutaneous lesions. These infections are extremely common and occur worldwide. Fungal infections do not usually pose a threat to life in normal hosts, but serious and life-threatening complications can occur, particularly in premature infants and immunocompromised individuals. Protozoal and helminthic infections are more likely to produce significant morbidity, as is illustrated by the fact that the helminthic infection onchocerciasis is the second most common cause of blindness worldwide. The medical, economic, and social burden imposed by this diverse group of infections is enormous, and continues to mount as the prevalence of fungal and protozoal infections in immunocompromised individuals continues to increase. Protozoal infections such as amebiasis and leishmaniasis are escalating causes of morbidity in immunocompentent hosts as well in many parts of the world.

Fungi, protozoa, and helminths are largely accidental pathogens that do not normally depend on humans for their growth. Serious infection is most likely when the patient's defenses are compromised through disruption of the skin's normal barrier function, colonization of damaged tissue, immune dysfunction, or nutritional deficiency. Many organisms discussed in this chapter regularly infect healthy individuals and may cause debilitating illness, but subclinical or mild disease with spontaneous resolution is fortunately the more common outcome.

FUNGAL INFECTIONS

Sheila F. Friedlander

Fungal infections are responsible for significant morbidity in the pediatric population and may account for up to 15% of all pediatric outpatient visits in the USA.[1,2] In a recent prospective study evaluating over 32 000 patients in a pediatric service in Lima, Peru, the prevalence rate of superficial mycoses was 4.42%, and the most frequent diagnosis tinea capitis.[3] The three major classes of fungus capable of causing cutaneous infections in humans are yeasts, dermatophytes and molds (Table 26.1). Cutaneous yeast infections of clinical importance commonly result from infections secondary to Candida and Malassezia. The dermatophytes most likely to infect man are found in the genera Microsporum, Trichophyton, and Epidermophyton.

Yeasts and dermatophytes are common pathogens in normal hosts. In contrast, molds do not usually cause disease in immunocompetent hosts or tissues, and are more likely to be found as secondary invaders in previously damaged tissue (e.g., dystrophic or onychomycotic nails) or immunocompromised hosts. The particular type of fungal infection that is most prevalent varies with age. Candida yeast infections are common in the diaper area in infancy, while dermatophyte infections of the scalp are most common in early school-age children. Dermatophyte infections of the feet, groin, and nails become more prevalent in adolescence, as does cutaneous yeast infection pityriasis versicolor.

In addition to the above classification scheme, pathogenic fungal infections in humans are traditionally divided into superficial, subcutaneous, and deep forms. The superficial forms include those that are limited to skin, hair, nails, and mucous membranes. Deep infections penetrate the skin and are capable of infecting subcutaneous tissue, blood, and/or other organs. However, this customary distinction between superficial disease and infection that invades beyond the skin or mucosa continues to blur as new and unusual manifestations of these infections occur, particularly in association with prematurity, immunosuppression and AIDS.

SUPERFICIAL FUNGAL INFECTIONS

DERMATOPHYTOSES

Historical background and introduction

The term "tinea" is frequently used to identify dermatophyte infections. This label has probably been in use for more than 1500 years, as references can be found as far back as AD 400. The Romans thought the "moth-eaten" appearance of afflicted scalps resulted from the work of the tinea moth worm, and so the term was born. All diseases of the scalp subsequently became known as "tinea." It appears that the British first utilized the term "ringworm" in the 16th century.

Dermatophytoses are infections caused by fungi belonging to the genera Trichophyton, Microsporum, and Epidermophyton. These organisms digest and invade keratin, and their growth is normally confined to the epidermis, nails, and hair. Although dermatophytes are found throughout our environment and cause appreciable disease worldwide, most skin inoculations are eliminated without producing lasting or symptomatic manifestations, and

TABLE 26.1   Major pathogens causing superficial fungal infections

Dermatophytes	Yeasts	Molds
Trichophyton	Candida	Scytalidium
Microsporum	Malassezia	Fusarium
Epidermophyton	Trichosporon	Scopulariopsis
	Hendersonula	Aspergillus
	Phaeoannelomyces	Cephalosporium

1. Tunnessen WW (1984) A survey of skin disorders seen in pediatric general and dermatology clinics. Pediatr Dermatol 1:219.
2. Schachner L, Ling NS, Press S (1983) A statistical analysis of a pediatric dermatology clinic. Pediatr Dermatol 1:157.
3. Grandez N, Caceres H (2001) Prevalence of superficial mycoses in children at Instituto de Salud del Nino, Lima, Peru. Pediatr Derm 18:109–110.

only a minority of exposures produce clinical changes. Infections of the scalp are most frequent during childhood. Although fungal disease of the hands, feet, or nails can be seen before puberty, it is much more common in adolescence and adult life.

Epidemiology

Currently, at least 40 species of dermatophytes have been well described; 22 members of the genus Trichophyton, 16 in the genus Microsporum, and two species of Epidermophyton. The dermatophytes have also been grouped into three categories based on natural habitat and host preference: anthropophilic, geophilic and zoophilic (Table 26.2). Anthropophilic species generally infect only humans; geophilic organisms reside in the soil and infect humans and animals, and zoophilic species are usually pathogenic for animals, though transmission to humans may occur.

At least 16 species affect man, but the five of major importance in the continental United States are *T. rubrum*, *T. tonsurans*, *T. mentagrophytes*, *M. canis*, and *E. floccosum*.[4,5] The epidemiology of fungal species differs according to age, geography, and other demographic factors (Table 26.3). Environmental conditions and sampling methods may also affect epidemiologic data. In addition, the prevalent species tends to change over time.[5,6] While *T. rubrum* was previously the most common pathogen in human disease, a recent US survey of human dermatophyte isolates documented that in 1995 *Trichophyton tonsurans* was present in 48% of samples and the most commonly isolated genus.[6] The second most common organism was *T. rubrum*, with a distant third comprising *T. mentagrophytes*. An epidemiologic study from Japan for the year 1992 revealed that *T. rubrum* was the most frequent isolate there (70.5%), followed by *T. mentagrophytes*.[7] In Melbourne, a marked increase in *T. rubrum* isolates was noted in 1995/6 as compared to the early 1960s.[8] In southern Europe, *M. canis* and *T. mentagrophytes* appear to be more common.

Etiology/pathogenesis

Slight trauma or an abrasion is required for dermatophyte infections to occur in immunocompetent individuals. Other optimizing factors include moisture, warmth, and increased carbon dioxide tension. Under the right circumstances fungal spores (arthroconidia) attach to the skin, germinate and then penetrate the stratum corneum. Fungal elements produce keratinases that facilitate this invasion. The infected keratin is eventually desquamated, but successful fungi infect new keratin fast enough to persist within the stratum corneum or hair.

Several factors are important in preventing or overcoming dermatophyte infections. Inhibitory factors in both serum and sebum may play a role in mediating infection. Unsaturated fatty acids in sebum may be the inhibitory factors responsible for the decreased incidence of tinea capitis when sebum production increases in adolescence. It is thought that the T helper 1 (Th1) response plays a role in host immune response, as does interferon-gamma production.

Host immune response to dermatophytes is a critical determinant of the likelihood of infection and of the clinical presentation.[9,10] Direct dermal invasion of dermatophytes has been documented in immunocompromised

---

TABLE 26.2 Host preference and natural habitat of dermatophytes

Anthropophilic	Zoophilic	Geophilic
Trichophyton concentricum	Microsporum canis	Microsporum boullardii
T. gourvilii	M. equinum	M. fulvum
T. kanei	M. gallinae	M. gypseum
T. krajdenii	M. persicolor	M. praecox
T. megninii		M. racemosum
T. mentagrophytes (pro parte)		M. nanum
T. raubitschekii		M. vanbreuseghemii
T. rubrum	Trichophyton mentagrophytes	
T. soundanense	T. equinum	
T. schoenleinii	T. verrucosum	
T. tonsurans	T. sarkisovii	T. longifusum
T. violaceum	T. simii	T. vanbreuseghemii
T. yaoundei		T. simii
		M. cookei
Microsporum audouinii		
M. ferrugineum		
Epidermophyton floccosum		

TABLE 26.3 Fungal species specific to geographic location

T. concentricum	T. megninii	M. persicolor	M. distortum	M. ferrugineum	T. gourvilii, T. soudanense, T. yaoundei
W. Pacific, S. America, S.E. Asia	W. Europe, North Africa	Europe, USA	New Zealand, USA	Africa, Far East	Africa

---

4. Sinski JT, Kelly LM (1991) A survey of dermatophytes from human patients in the United States from 1985 to 1987. **Mycopathologia** 114:117.
5. Sinski JT, Flouras K (1984) A survey of dermatophytes isolated from human patients in the United States from 1979 to 1981 with chronological listings of worldwide incidence of five dermatophytes often isolated in the United States. **Mycopathologia.** 85:97–120.
6. Weitzman I et al. (1998) A survey of dermatophytes isolated from human patients in the US from 1993–1995. **J Am Acad Dermatol** 39:255–261.
7. Hishimoto K (1993) The presence of dermatophytes in the environment and on healthy looking skin: their significance as a cause of disease in Japan. **Curr Top Med Mycol** 5:201–214.
8. Coloe SV, Baird RW (1999) Dermatophyte infections in Melbourne: trends from 1961/64 to 1995/96. **Pathology** 31(4):395–397.
9. Martinez Roig A, Torres Rodriquez JM (1987) The immune response in childhood dermatophytes. **Mykosen** 30:574.
10. Jones HE (1993) Immune response and host resistance of humans to dermatophyte infection. **J Am Acad Dermatol** 28:S12–S18.

hosts. The prevalence and severity of dermatophytosis are probably increased in association with AIDS.[11] However, some investigators have found that overall prevalence of infection in patients with AIDS was not "substantially" increased over that in patients without AIDS.[12] Infections in those patients with AIDS often involve multiple species, and are more extensive and refractory to treatment.[12]

Infection with dermatophytes is commonly referred to as tinea, followed by a reference to the affected body area (Table 26.4). The pattern of infection depends on the involved anatomic site, the organism and quantity of fungal inoculum, and the host immune response.

TINEA CAPITIS

Historical note

Microsporum species were the most frequent causes of tinea capitis in the United States in the 19th and early 20th century. *Microsporum audouinii* reached epidemic proportions in the 1940s, declining in importance as *T. tonsurans* became predominant. Presumably *T. tonsurans*-infected immigrants from Central America brought the disease to the southwestern US in the early 20th century. Initial reports came from Texas in the late 1920s. By the 1970s and 1980s, *T. tonsurans* was the major agent causing tinea capitis in the United States.[6,13–15]

Epidemiology

Tinea capitis is the most common fungal infection in young children. The prevalence varies with the geographical setting, socio-ecomic group, and type of population studied. A large US sample survey of office-based physicians found 172 000 new cases of tinea capitis in the USA in 1996.[16] As most cases of disease go unreported, the true prevalence is much higher. Most cases occur in children aged 4–7 years, but all ages are susceptible, and affected neonates less than a month of age, as well as adult females have been reported. Williams *et al*.[17] documented a prevalence of 2.5% in early school-age African-American children attending an urban school, but rates of less than 1% are the norm in nonurban, mainly Caucasian populations. The predilection for higher incidence of disease in inner city populations has also been documented in London.[18] An epidemiologic study of the incidence of tinea capitis in California from 1984 to 1993 found an overall increase in incidence of 84% with the most dramatic change occurring in African-Americans, in whom there was a greater than 200% increase in incidence of disease.[19] Tack *et al*. found the relative risk of infection for tinea capitis in African-Americans to be 29.4 times greater than in the general US population.[16] It has been speculated that grooming and hair care practices such as tight braiding may put African-American patients at higher risk for tinea capitis; however, a case-controlled study of 66 patients with tinea capitis failed to document an association of hairstyling, frequency of washing, or use of greases with an increased incidence of tinea infections.[20]

T. capitis is generally uncommon in adults, presumably because of the antifungal characteristics of sebum. Postmenopausal women and immunocompromised patients appear to be at higher risk for tinea capitis.[21]

The predominant species varies with geographic locale, with *T. tonsurans* currently accounting for for more than 90% of tinea capitis in the USA (Table 26.5). *T. tonsurans* is anthropophilic and is readily transmitted by person-to-person contact, especially in schools, day care, or similar social settings, often leading to infection of an entire group.[22] In contrast, *M. canis* is a zoophilic agent transmitted from cats or dogs. Epidemics of *M. canis* tinea capitis have been reported in association with infections in kittens. This form of tinea capitis is often quite inflammatory. Outbreaks of both tinea capitis and corporis transmitted by rabbits infected with *T. mentagrophytes* have also been documented.

Favus is a form of tinea capitis with specific clinical and histologic findings which is most commonly caused by *T. schoenleinii*. The disease is rare in the US but endemic in certain areas of Europe, the Middle East, South Africa, and South America. Small pockets of favus also exist in parts of Quebec and Kentucky.

Etiology/pathogenesis/transmission

Fungal infections of the scalp occur when hyphae invade the stratum corneum and then grow down a follicular wall between the wall and hair until they reach the mid-follicle. At this point they directly invade the hair itself and continue downward invasion of the hair until they reach Adamson's fringe, where keratinization first occurs within the hair. If the infection is

---

TABLE 26.4   Nomenclature for dermatophyte infections by location

Scalp	T. capitis
Skin – general	T. corporis
Hands	T. manuum
Feet	T. pedis
Groin	T. cruris
Nails	T. unguium
Face	T. facei
Beard	T. barbae

TABLE 26.5   Epidemiology of tinea capitis

North America	South America	Europe	Africa	Australia
Trichophyton tonsurans	M. canis	M. canis	M. canis	M. canis
Microsporum canis	T. violaceum	M. andouinii	M. audouinii	T. tonsurans
	T. tonsurans	T. tonsurans	T. violaceum	
		T. violaceum	T. soudanense	
		T. mentagrophytes	T. mentagrophytes	
		T. schoenleinii	T. yaoundei	
			T. gourvilii	

---

11. Coopman SA, Johnson RA, Platt R, Stern RS (1993) Cutaneous disease and drug reactions in HIV infection. **N Engl J Med** 328:1670.
12. Lowinger-Seoane M, Torres-Rodriquez JM, Madrenys-Brunet N et al. (1992) Extensive dermatophytosis caused by *Trichophyton mentagrophytes* and *Microsporum canis* in a patient with AIDS. **Mycopathologia** 120:143.
13. Prevost E (1983) The rise and fall of fluorescent tinea capitis. **Pediatr Dermatol** 1:127.
14. Philpot C (1978) Geographical distribution of dermatophytes: a review. **J Hyg** (Lond) 80:301.
15. Hebert AA (1988) Tinea capitis. Current concepts. **Arch Dermatol** 124:1554.
16. Tack DA (1999) The epidemic of tinea capitis disproportionately affects school-aged African Americans. **Pediatr Dermatol** 16:75.
17. Williams JV, Honig PJ, McGinley KJ, Leyden JJ (1995) Semiquantitative study of tinea capitis and the asymptomatic carrier state in inner-city school children. **Pediatrics** 96:265–267.
18. Hay RJ, Clayton YM, DeSilva N et al. (1996) Tinea capitis in south-east London – a new pattern of infection with public health implications. **Br J Dermatol** 135:955–958.
19. Lobato MN, Vugia DJ, Frieden IJ (1997) Tinea capitis in California children: a population-based study of a growing epidemic. **Pediatrics** 99:551–554.
20. Sharma V, Silverberg NB, Howard R et al. (2001) Do hair care practices affect the acquisition of tinea capitis? A case-control study. **Arch Pediatr Adolesc Med** 155:818–821.
21. Silverberg NB, Weinberg JM, DeLeo VA (2002) Tinea capitis: Focus on African American women. **J Am Acad Dermatol** 46:S120–S124.
22. Philpot C (1977) Some aspects of the epidemiology of tinea. **Mycopathologia** 62:3–13.

TABLE 26.6 **Hair invasion by dermatophytes**

Organism	Diameter of spore	Pattern
Ectothrix		
M. audouinii	1–3μm	Mosaic sheath around the hair
M. canis	1–3μm	
M. ferrugineum	1–3μm	
M. gypseum	3–4μm	Arthroconidia scattered around the outside of the hair
M. fulvum	3–4μm	
T. mentagrophytes	3–4μm	Chains on surface of hair
T. verrucosum	8–12μm	Large dense chains around hair
Endothrix		
T. tonsurans	3–4μm	Arthroconidia present within the shortened hair stubs
T. violaceum	3–4μm	
T. gourvilii	3–4μm	
T. schoenleinii	none within hair	Air spaces and hyphae within hair

endothrix in nature (Table 26.6), the hyphal elements segment into arthrocondidia inside the hair, which becomes full of these spores. These hairs are severely damaged, and tend to break off close to the scalp because of their fragility. In an ectothrix infection the hyphae fragment into spores on the surface of the hair shaft, rather than within it. In favus-type infections arthroconidia are not prominent, but but hyphal elements may be visualized and air spaces develop within the hair shaft.

Transmission may be direct through person-to-person or animal-to-person contact, but usually occurs through contact with infected spores present in shed scales, hairs, or fomites (inanimate objects). Presence of viable spores has been documented on toys, brushes, theater seats, bedsheets and instruments used by barbers.[23] The organism is quite hardy, as spores from *T. tonsurans*-infected hairs stored in bottles in the dark can remain viable for up to two years.

The carrier state

Individuals colonized with dermatophytes but lacking symptoms (carriers) are a particular source of concern regarding transmission of disease. The prevalence of this condition is variable, but can be quite high in families of infected children and classrooms of index cases. Pomeranz *et al.* found that 32% of families with an infected child had at least one carrier, and overall 16% of household contacts were asymptomatic carriers. Thirteen percent of the carriers were still positive six months later, and one of the carriers developed overt disease.[24] Williams *et al.* noted an asymptomatic carrier rate of 14% in an African-American parochial school in Philadelphia where the incidence of overt disease was 3%.[17] Other investigators have found that if at least two children in a classroom are infected, there is a higher rate of asymptomatic carriage in the classroom.[18] In addition, if the index case is

removed, the prevalence of the asymptomatic carriage state decreases. The role that asymptomatic carriers play in the pathogenesis of tinea capitis is unclear, but it appears that they contribute to transmission and persistence of infection in the home and classroom environment.

Clinical findings

Most patients present complaining of patchy hair loss with associated scale (Table 26.7). Those with inflammatory disease may have significant pruritus, and occaisionally develop marked tenderness and swelling at the affected site (kerion). "Gray patch" involvement can occur, where affected hair has a dull gray appearance close to the scalp. An extensive pruritic eacazema-like eruption on the trunk and extremities (id reaction) may also develop, particularly after institution of antifungal therapy. This reaction occurred in almost one-third of tinea patients followed in one study.[25] Rarely, a patient may complain of tender "knots in the neck" (posterior occipital nodes). Non-inflammatory disease may be quite insidious in nature, and patients may only note an increased amount of dandruff, with little or no hair loss.

Tinea capitis more commonly involves the scalp, and rarely the eyebrows or eyelashes.

TABLE 26.7 **Clinical presentations of tinea capitis**

Patchy alopecia
"Black dot" hairs
"Gray patch" hairs
Follicular pustules and papules
Scale with or without subtle diffuse hair loss
Boggy masses, draining sinuses (kerion)
Lymphadenopathy – cervical, post auricular, posterior occipital
Id (auto-sensitization) reaction

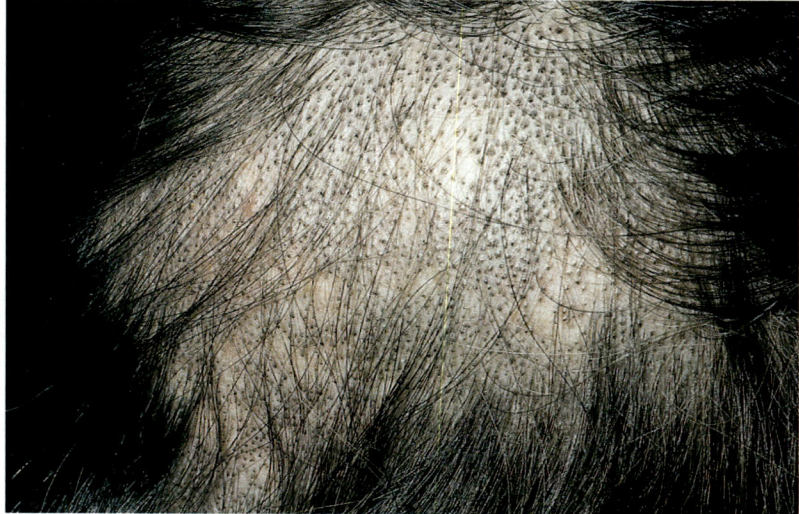

Fig. 26.1 Black dot tinea.

23. Hebert AA, Head ES, MacDonald EM (1985) Tinea capitis caused by Trichophyton tonsurans. **Pediatr Dermatol** 2:219–223.
24. Pomeranz AJ, Sabnis SS, McGrath GJ, Esterly NB (1999) Asymptomatic dermatophyte carriers in the households of children with tinea capitis. **Arch Pediatr Adolesc Med** 153:483–486.
25. Honig PJ, Caputo GL, Leyden JJ et al. (1994) Treatment of kerions. **Pediatr Dermatol** 11:69–71.

Noninflammatory disease

This pattern is characterized by scaling and patchy hair loss. "Black dots," which are short, 1–3mm, broken-off hairs, may be noted within areas of alopecia (Fig. 26.1). In some patients, no discrete hair loss is noted, and such cases may be misdiagnosed as seborrheic dermatitis. In other instances, particularly with disease caused by Micorsporum, patches of hair may be tinged gray, which is the result of spores coating the outside of the hair shaft. Scale is almost always present.

Asymptomatic posterior auricular and occipital adenopathy is often present in tinea capitis, even in the absence of inflammatory findings. Hubbard *et al.* found that alopecia or scaling in association with adenopathy was highly predictive of tinea capitis.[26]

Inflammatory disease

Papules, pustules, erythema, and significant crusting are often present in this form of disease. An initial cluster of small follicular papules or pustules may gradually expand and coalesce. Hair loss follows, which may be discrete and patchy or confluent. The most severe reaction consists of a tender, red, sometimes oozing, boggy mass known as a kerion (Figs 26.2, 26.3). Significant alopecia with loose hairs is present, and draining sinuses may develop. Such cases are frequently misdiagnosed as bacterial abscesses. Severe scarring and permanent hair loss (Fig. 26.4) may occur even if appropriate therapy is introduced, but is more likely if therapy is delayed.

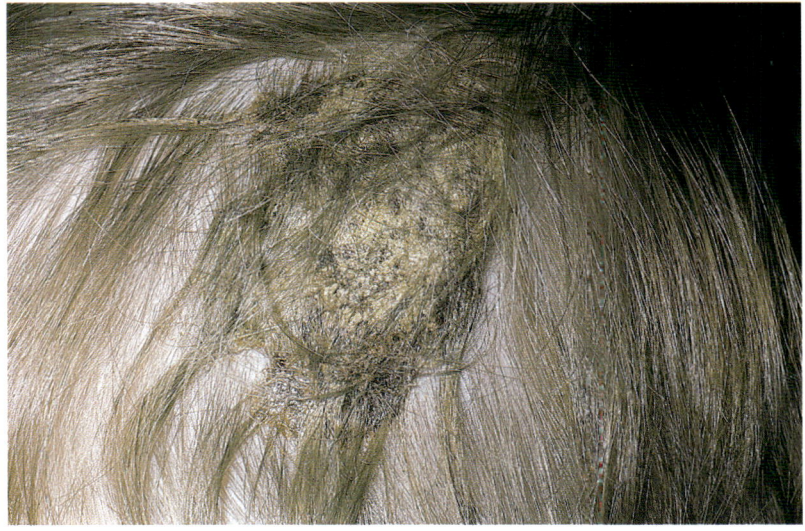

Fig. 26.3   Kerion: heavily crusted, hairless plaque.

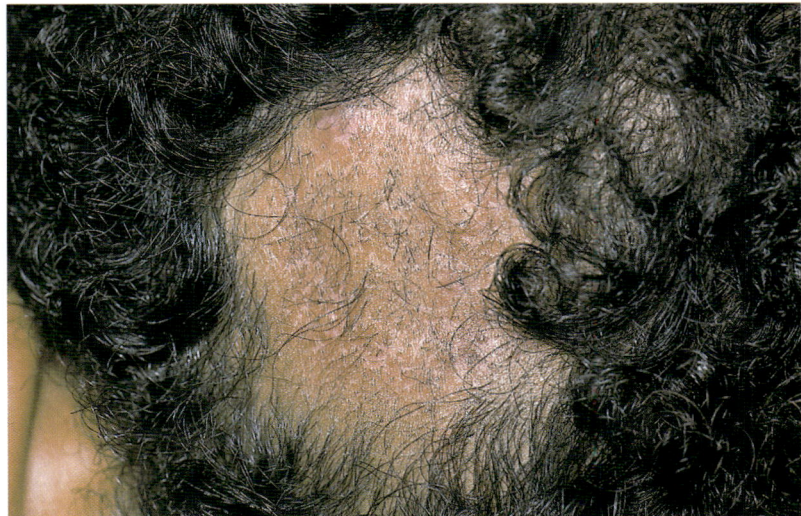

Fig. 26.4   Permanent scarring alopecia post kerion.

Favus is an inflammatory pattern typically due to *T. schoenleinii*. The first manifestation of infection is single or multiple small areas of yellow-red perifollicular scaling, which may progress to papules. Eventually, the hair becomes gray and matted together. Yellow cup-shaped concretions of fungal mycelia called *scutula* form with one or more hairs at the center of each. Destruction of the hair follicle with atrophy and progression of the disease outward to new areas of the scalp can occur. The process is sometimes accompanied by a "mousy" odor and purulent discharge, as seen with a kerion.

Dermatophytid or "id" reactions

A vigorous immune response to fungi may cause manifestations distant from the site of infection. These frequently pruritic skin findings are thought to result from an interaction between the host and fungal antigens. Termed dermatophytid, or "-id" reactions, they usually develop on the trunk and extremities, but may involve the face, particularly the forehead and postauricular areas.[27] Autosensitization dermatitis is another term for "id" reactions.

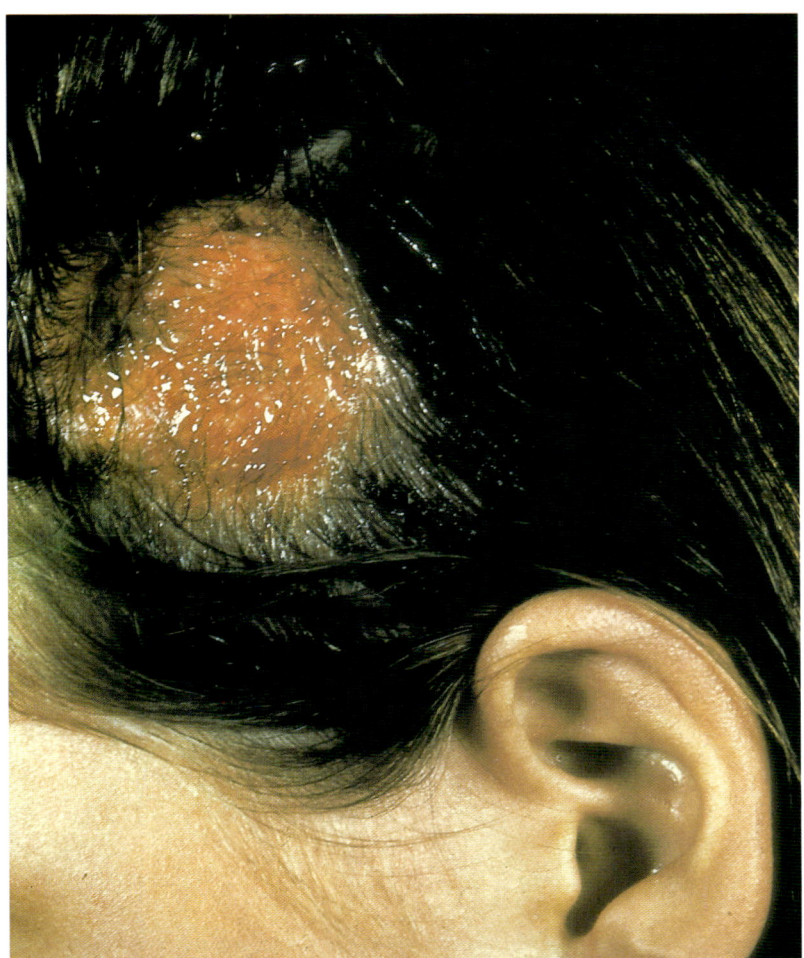

Fig. 26.2   Kerion: red, oozing, hairless plaque.

26. Hubbard TW (2000) The predictive value of symptoms in diagnosing childhood tinea capitis. Arch Pediatr and Adol Med 153:1150–1153.

27. Kaaman T, Torssander J (1983) Dermatophytid—a misdiagnosed entity? **Acta Derm Venereol** (Stockh) 63:404.

On examination, a symmetrical eczematous fine papular eruption, or a follicular rash or one resembling pityriasis rosea is seen. The rash may be present on the palms and soles, especially in patients beyond the first decade of life. Erythema nodosum[28] or erythema annulare centrifugum can rarely develop, as can systemic signs such as fever or leukocytosis. A dermatophytid reaction may develop when therapy is intiated and should not be interpreted as a drug reaction.

Diagnosis/laboratory findings

Any child with scalp scaling, erythema, or hair loss should be evaluated for the possibility of this infection. Culture is the gold standard for diagnosis.

Infection can be quickly, though less reliably diagnosed using KOH evaluation of hair. Hairs are placed on a microscope slide, then covered with one or two drops of 10–30% KOH and a coverslip. With time or heat, sufficient keratin dissolves to allow visualization of spores and hyphae within and around the hair. This may take 30 to 90 minutes or more. Gentle warming will hasten the process, but excessive heat will cause crystallization of the KOH, rendering the material useless. The slide should be examined under low-power magnification initially, with a low-light setting and the condenser adjusted down to enhance contrast. Gentle pressure on the coverslip will thin the material and ease observation. When DMSO reagent (40% dimethyl sulfoxide) is added to KOH, heating of the speciman is unnecessary and not recommended. Special stains, such as Schwartz Lampkin and Chlorazo black are also helpful to better identify hyphal elements. Calcofluor white (0.1%) may be utilized for better visualization, but this analysis requires examination with a fluorescence microscope. False negative results may occur, and a fungal culture should always be obtained when in doubt.[29,30]

Several patterns of hair invasion can be appreciated microscopically, which may provide a clue as to the specific pathogen present. (Table 26.6) Arthroconidia and/or hyphae are noted within (endothrix) (Fig. 26.5A,B) or around (ectothrix) the hair, with air spaces present in the case of favus.

Wood's light inspection of the scalp for fluorescence may be helpful if *Microsporum* or *T. schoenleinii* infection is suspected. Green-fluorescent pteridines are produced by these species and apparent when long-wave (300–400nm) UV light examination is performed. Wood's light examination will be negative in patients with *T. tonsurans* infection.

Culture confirmation is the gold standard for diagnosis of tinea capitis. Samples can be obtained using a variety of methods, including hair plucking,

scalp scraping, and swabbing of the scalp with a toothbrush. The least expensive, simplest method appears to be the cotton-tip swab technique, in which a cotton swab is moistened with tap water, then rolled quickly over affected sites and all four quadrants of the scalp. The swab is then inoculated onto fungal culture media, or transported to the lab in routine transport medium. This method has been documented to be both sensitive and specific for the diagnosis of scalp fungal infections.[31]

Several culture media may be used for diagnosis. Sabouraud's agar is a standard mycologic media that allows reliable examination of colony morphology. Cycloheximide is frequently added to inhibit the growth of saprophytic fungi and chloramphenicol to impede bacterial growth. Sabouraud's cycloheximide-chloramphenicol agar is sold commercially as Mycosel, Mycobiotic agar, or other brand names.

Dermatophyte test media (DTM) is an inexpensive office culture technique, and is extremely useful because of its selectivity and ability to change to a deep red color on exposure to growing dermatophytes. Metabolites released by the growth of a dermatophyte turn DTM from the natural tan of agar to a deep led by causing alkalinization of the media and a change in the color of the phenol red (Fig. 26.6). The media should be incubated at room temperature without being tightly capped, allowing free gas exchange. Colonies normally begin to grow out in approximately one week at room temperature, but cultures should be incubated for at least two weeks. Color change will occur within 14 days of inoculation. If cultures incubate over a period longer than two weeks, other organisms, such as Candida, may eventually produce a red color change. In addition, color change alone should not be interpreted as

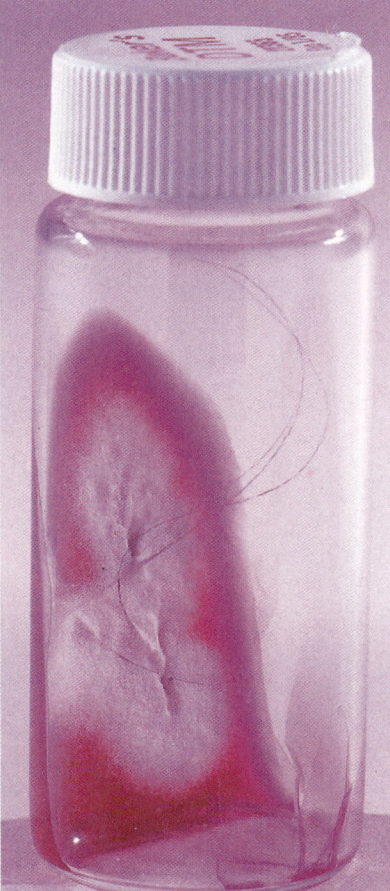

Fig. 26.6 Positive DTM culture. Red color change indicates dermatophyte growth.

TABLE 26.8 Differential diagnosis of tinea capitis	
Alopecia areata	Psoriasis
Trichotillomania	Folliculitis – bacterial/yeast
Traction alopecia	Seborrheic dermatitis
Lichen planopilaris	Lupus erythematosus

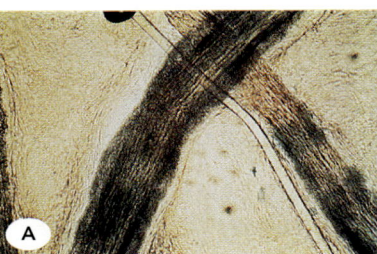
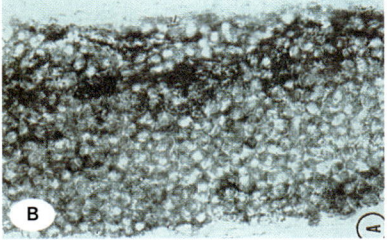

Fig. 26.5 **(A)** Endothrix infection, (low-power KOH mount): arthroconidia noted within hair shaft (courtesy Maureen Rogers); **(B)** Endothrix infection (high-power KOH mount) showing total hair shaft involvement.

28. Martinez-Roig A, Llorens-Terol J, Torres J (1982) Erythema nodosum and kerion of the scalp. **Am J Dis Child** 136:440.
29. Haldane DJM, Robart E (1990) A comparison of calcofluor white, potassium hydroxide and culture for the laboratory diagnosis of superficial fungal infection. **Diagn Microbiol Infect Dis** 13:337.
30. Miller MA, Hodgson Y (1993) Sensitivity and specificity of potassium hydroxide smears of skin scrapings for the diagnosis of tinea pedis. **Arch Dermatol** 129:510.
31. Friedlander SF, Pickering B, Cunningham BB et al. (1999) Use of the cotton swab method in diagnosing Tinea capitis. **Pediatrics** 104:276–279.

indicative of dermatophyte growth; some examination of colony morphology is essential. Dermatophytes produce fluffy, furry, wooly, cottony, or powdery colonies. In contrast, Candida tends to grow as white to off-white or yellowish, creamy, smooth-surfaced colonies. Speciation of dermatophyte type based on colony morphology is difficult when the organism is grown on DTM, as classic morphologic features may not develop. Such speciation is easier when colonies are grown on Sabouraud's agar.

Biopsy is usually not necessary, but if tissue is obtained, it should be stained with periodic acid–Schiff or another appropriate stain. Such staining reveals fungal elements in the stratum corneum and hair follicle, accompanied by a mixed cellular infiltrate.

Polymerase chain reaction techniques have been utilized in the identification of dermatophyte fungi with some success.[32] This may prove a faster and more specific means of identification in the future.

Differential diagnosis

Alopecia areata and trichotillomania present with hair loss, but scale is usually absent. Traction alopecia usually localizes to peripheral borders, and erythematous follicular papules and pustules may be evident. Seborrheic dermatitis and psoriasis may be confused with tinea, but in these conditions hair loss and adenopathy are rarely present. Bacterial or yeast folliculitis and bacterial abscesses should be kept in mind in inflammatory presentations, and less common causes of hair loss and scarring such as lichen plano-pilaris and discoid lupus erythematosus should also be considered (Table 26.8).

Therapeutics

Treatment should begin immediately after obtaining a culture, if the index of suspicion is high. Oral therapy in combination with appropriate measures to reduce spread as discussed below will allow children to return to school shortly after institution of therapy. Delayed treatment may result in additional cases or more severe scarring.

Topical therapy may be helpful in the treatment of tinea capitis but systemic treatment is essential for optimal outcome (Table 26.9). Griseofulvin has served as first line therapy for tinea capitis for more than 40 years because of its efficacy, safety profile, and cost. However, a decrease in sensitivity to this agent appears to have developed. This has been corroborated by a change in both the initial response rate and the cure rate at follow-up evaluation. Abdel-Rahman et al.[33] recently reported a 60.7% initial response rate to a course of griseofulvin therapy in tinea capitis patients in the midwestern US; this contrasts with the 96 to 100% cure rates noted in studies conducted a decade previously. A small retrospective study of patients with tinea capitis[34]

documented that the griseofulvin cure rate for tinea capitis was directly related to dosing, with a significant number of failures in those treated with 10mg/kg per day, better response rates in those treated with 20mg/kg per day, and complete cure in the small number of patients treated with 25mg/kg per day. Laboratory documentation of such resistance is difficult to obtain, as no reliable sensitivity standards exist for antifungal agents.

Most practitioners currently use griseofulvin, 20–25mg/kg per day (maximum 1gr) microsize formulation as first-line therapy for the treatment of tinea capitis. Treatment usually consists of 6–8 weeks of therapy, and most experts recommend continuing therapy for at least two weeks beyond clinical resolution. Higher doses generally have a higher incidence of adverse side effects, particularly gastrointestinal symptoms. Several other therapeutic options exist, which may become first-line therapy in the future. One of these agents (see below) should be substituted if griseofulvin is poorly tolerated or appears to be ineffective at adequate doses (see Table 26.9).

Accumulating experience with systemic terbinafine, itraconazole, and fluconazole indicates that they may be more effective short-course therapies for the treatment of tinea infections. Gupta et al. recently conducted a multicenter, prospective, parallel group study of tinea capitis caused by trichophyton species.[35] The majority of patients were infected with T. tonsurans. Griseofulvin (20mg/kg per day for six weeks) was compared with short course terbinafine, itraconazole, or fluconazole therapy. The newer antifungals were administered for two weeks, and a third week of treatment was given at week four if clinically indicated. At week 12, 185 children were evaluable, and the mycological and clinical cure rate following six weeks of griseofulvin therapy was 92%, while the rate following 2–3 weeks of terbinafine therapy was 94%. The cure rate for itraconazole was 86%, and for fluconazole 84%. Other studies have also confirmed that terbinafine, fluconazole, and itraconazole are reasonable therapeutic options for the treatment of tinea capitis. However, these agents are not yet FDA approved for this purpose in the United States.

Wide variability in response rate may occur, depending on the offending organism, and the time and manner in which follow-up evaluation occurs. M. canis appears more resistant to treatment, regardless of the type of agent used, and prolonged therapy is often required with this organism.

Rapid elimination of contagion risk is best achieved through systemic treatment in conjunction with twice-weekly use of a spore-inhibiting shampoo containing selenium sulfide, ketoconazole, or zinc pyrithione. Various studies have documented the utility of these agents, as well as povidone-iodine solution to decrease spore counts and therefore hypothetically minimize infectivity.[36,37] Others, however, have not found a

TABLE 26.9   Systemic therapies for tinea capitis

Griseofulvin	Terbinafine	Itraconazole	Fluconazole
20–25mg/kg per d micro, max 1g, × 6–8 weeks; continue 2 weeks after cessation of symptoms	3–6mg/kg per d <20kg = 62.5mg/d 20–40kg = 125mg/d >40kg = 250mg/d Duration of therapy varies with organism. Efficacy has been noted with treatment courses as short as 2 weeks. M. canis infection may require 8 weeks of therapy	5mg/kg per d Duration of therapy varies. 2–4 weeks continuous therapy or pulse dosing (one week of therapy per month for 1–3 pulses as needed clinically)	6mg/kg per d × 20 days 8mg/kg per week × 4–8 wks

Some of the therapies listed above may not be FDA approved for this purpose. All patients should utilize topical therapy c/o an antifungal agent (e.g., ketroconazole shampoo or selenium sulphide shampoo) twice weekly. Symptomatic family members or contacts should be evaluated and treated as appropriate.

32. Harmsen D, Schwinn A, Brocker EB, Frosch M (1994) Molecular differentiation of dermatophyte fungi. Mycoses 2:67–70.
33. Abdel-Rahman SM, Nahata MC, Powell DA (1997) Response to initial griseofulvin therapy in pediatric patients with tinea capitis. Ann Pharmacother 31:406–410.
34. Sharpe, BA (2000) Investigation into the efficacy of conventional dose griseofulvin for treatment of tinea capitis. Poster Presentation. Society for Pediatric Dermatology Annual Meeting. Santa Fe, NM, July 12–15.
35. Gupta AK, Adam P, Dlova N et al. (2001) Therapeutic options for the treatment of tinea capitis caused by Trichophyton species: griseofulvin versus the new oral antifungal agents, terbinafine, itraconazole, and fluconazole. Pediatr Dermatol 18:433–438.
36. Allen H, Honig PJ, Leyden JJ, McGinley KJ (1982) Selenium sulfide: adjunctive therapy for tinea capitis. Pediatrics 69:81–83.
37. McGinley KJ, Leyden JJ (1982) Antifungal activity of dermatological shampoos. Arch Dermatol Res 272:339–342.

significant effect of selenium sulfide shampoo 2.5% in eradicating asymptomatic carriers, nor a significant difference in relapse rate among tinea capitis patients who used adjunctive topical therapy versus those who did not.[33] Such studies had design flaws and therefore it remains unclear whether topical therapy is efficacious. In addition, the likelihood of compliance with use of these topical agents is low in those ethnic groups whose hair grooming practices preclude frequent washing, and study results may reflect this fact.

Contaminated hairbrushes, towels, pillowcases, or other fomites may spread infection. Therefore, scalp grooming items and hats should not be shared with infected individuals. Symptomatic family members and contacts should be evaluated and cultured as appropriate. Some experts recommend topical therapy (use of an antifungal shampoo twice a week) for all family members, as the likelihood of familial carriers is high (see pathology above).

Symptomatic dermatophytid reactions are more likely to develop as antifungal treatment commences and often require either topical or systemic corticosteroid therapy. Mild cases respond to medium- to high-potency topical corticosteroids applied twice daily in conjunction with oral anti-histamines; otherwise 1mg/kg per day of systemic prednisone for 10–14 days can be used.

In some instances kerions will not respond to systemic antifungal agents. Given that the marked edema and erythema noted in kerions is a severe inflammatory response, some practitioners believe it is beneficial to add oral prednisone, 1–2mg/kg per day for 10 to 14 days to the therapeutic regimen. At least two studies have documented that the addition of systemic steroids does not significantly affect outcome, and for this reason most practitioners reserve systemic coricosteroid therapy for those patients who fail to respond after two weeks of systemic antifungal therapy.[38] Similarly, the addition of antibacterial agents does not appear to alter the course of illness, and therefore oral or topical antibacterial agents are not indicated, except in the rare instance in which bacterial infection is clearly demonstrated and there is failure to respond to antifungal therapy at adequate doses, despite good compliance.

TINEA CORPORIS

Tinea corporis is a dermatophyte infection of body surfaces, not otherwise designated as to specific area. Although worldwide in distribution, tinea corporis is more prevalent in warm or moist climates.[39] Any species of dermatophyte that infects humans can cause tinea corporis. One predominant species in a geographic area is less likely with tinea corporis than it is with tinea capitis. However, in recent years, as *T. tonsurans*-related tinea capitis has become predominant, increasing amounts of *T. tonsurans* tinea corporis have been identified. In one Chicago survey, *T. tonsurans* accounted for 96% of tinea capitis and 75% of tinea corporis.[40] Most cases of tinea corporis were in adults, predominantly young women who had contact with children, but cases did occur in infants and children. Hospital-based outbreaks of *T. tonsurans* have also been reported. In one instance, a 7-year-old child was the index patient.[41] Another cluster of cases was attributable to *M. canis* and appeared to be spread by a nursery employee. Infections were superficial and involved a variety of body areas.[42] Zoophilic species of dermatophyte, such as *M. canis*, are common, and acute cases of tinea corporis in children are often due to contact with dogs or cats that carry *M. canis* on their fur.

Clinical presentation

Tinea corporis most often presents as one or more red scaly papules which may be follicular. These papules spread and eventually coalesce into plaques that become scaly (Fig. 26.7). The center of these plaques tends to clear,

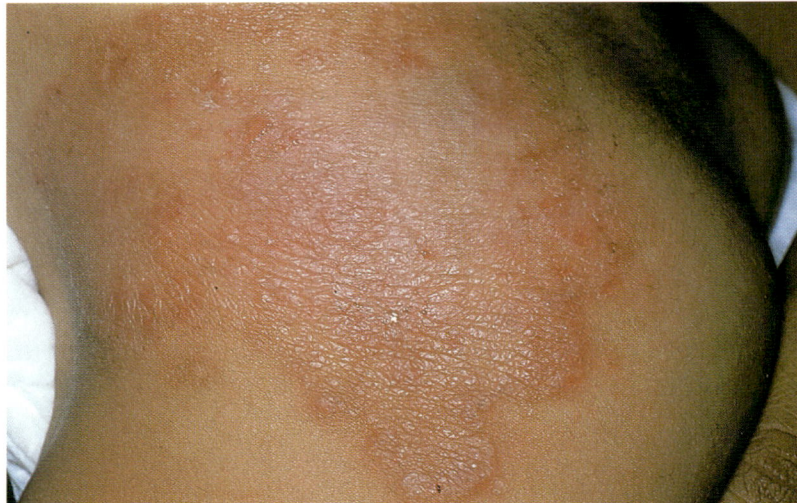

Fig. 26.7 Tinea corporis: large gyrate plaque with advancing border, perhaps worsened by diapering.

producing annular configurations and occasionally concentric rings. Mild erythema, edema, vesicles, pustules, or even bulla formation may occur. If extensive crusting develops, the resulting plaques can resemble psoriasis. Infection is ordinarily confined to a small number of sites and is often unilateral. Itching may be prominent with inflammatory infections. As in tinea capitis, the greater the immune response of the host, the greater the amount of inflammation that is evident clinically. Highly inflammatory tinea corporis is more likely to resolve spontaneously. Unusual presentations include verrucous or vegetating tumor-like growths, and a boggy mass resembling a kerion termed tinea profunda.[43] Pustules and inflammation are more often associated with infection by zoophilic species such as *M. canis*. The cup-shaped scutula of non-scalp favus is another uncommon finding.

A marked perifollicular or follicular granulomatous inflammatory response may occur, particularly in patients inadvertently treated with topical corticosteroids. This disorder is termed Majocchi's granuloma. Trauma may play a role in this disorder, perhaps by disrupting the integrity of the hair follicle. Shaving of the legs or immunologic deficits may also put patients at risk. *Trichophyton rubrum* is principally responsible for persistent follicular and perifollicular dermatophyte infection, but various other species of Trichophyton and Microsporum have been implicated. Eradication of a follicular infection often requires oral antifungals.[44]

Wrestlers are at particular risk for tinea corporis infections, and in this setting the disease is referred to as tinea gladiatorum. A midwestern US study of high school wrestlers and runners found that the increased risk was limited to wrestlers, presumably on the basis of close body contact during matches.[45] The lesions tended to be located on the neck and upper arms, and *T. tonsurans* was identified in all isolates

Diagnosis

The diagnosis of tinea corporis is made by demonstration of the infecting organism on KOH examination or culture, as described for tinea capitis. Material for these procedures should be obtained from scale found just inside the advancing edge of an infected site. False-negative KOH test or culture results are less frequent than with tinea capitis but may occur. PCR evaluation may prove useful in the future.

38. Laude TA, Shah BR, Lynfield Y (1982) Tinea capitis in Brooklyn. **Am J Dis Child** 136:1047–1050.
39. Allen AM, Taplin D (1973) Epidemic *Trichophyton mentagorphytes* infections in servicemen. **JAMA** 226:864.
40. Bronson DM, Desai DR, Barsky S et al. (1983) An epidemic of infection with *Trichophyton tonsurans* revealed in a 20-year survey of fungal infections in Chicago. **J Am Acad Dermatol** 8:322.
41. Arnow PM, Houchins SG, Pugliese G (1991) An outbreak of tinea corporis in hospital personnel caused by a patient with *Trichophyton tonsurans* infection. **Pediatr Infect Dis J** 10:355.
42. Snider R, Landers S, Levy ML (1993) The ringworm riddle: an outbreak of *Microsporum canis* in the nursery. **Pediatr Infect Dis J** 12:145.
43. Powell FC, Muller SA (1982) Kerion of the glabrous skin. **J Am Acad Dermatol** 7:490–494.
44. Smith KJ, Neafie RC, Skelton HG 3rd et al. (1991) Majocchi's granuloma. **J Cutan Pathol** 18:28–35.
45. Adams BB (2000) Tinea corporis gladiatorum: a cross-sectional study. **J Am Acad Dermatol** 43:1039–1041.

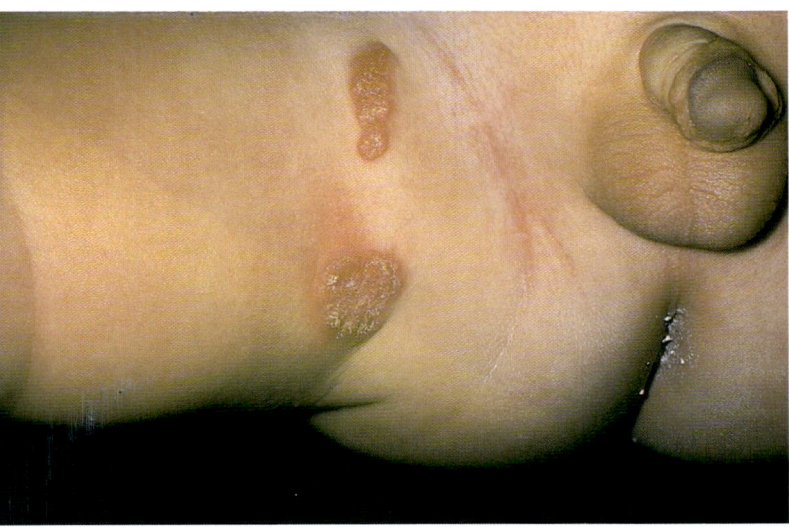

Fig. 26.8 Tinea in diapered area.

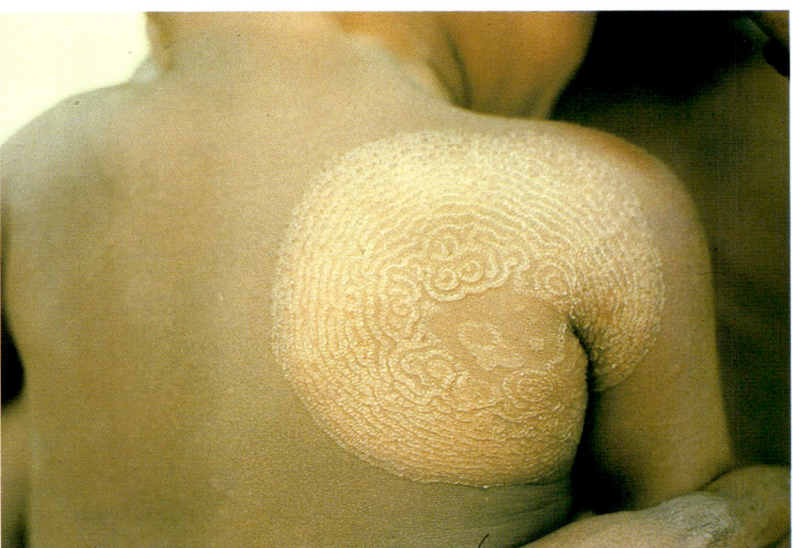

Fig. 26.9 Tinea imbricata: concentric rings of scale caused by *T. concentricum* (Courtesy Maureen Rogers).

Differential diagnosis

Nummular eczema and granuloma annulare are frequently mistaken for tinea corporis. Other disorders in the differential diagnosis of tinea corporis are candidiasis, erythema annulare centrifugum, psoriasis, pityriasis rosea, and subacute cutaneous or discoid lupus. Tinea corporis in the diaper area may be mistaken for diaper dermatitis (Fig. 26.8).

Therapeutics

Children with treated tinea corporis do not need to be excluded from school, especially when the affected area is covered. Wrestlers with tinea are a special case due to the close contact that occurs in matches; infected individuals should be removed from competition unless such lesions are completely covered and undergoing treatment. Some practitioners are now treating infected wrestlers or at-risk team members with systemic antifungals such as fluconazole and itraconazole; however, this is not currently the standard of care.

Many cases of tinea corporis resolve spontaneously;[46] however, contagion is still an issue that compels the recognition and treatment of these infections. Topical treatment alone is usually effective in those patients with limited disease. Ordinarily, application once or twice daily is sufficient, but a more frequent schedule may be needed if there is a great deal of perspiration or the drug is otherwise washed away. Treatment that involves the lesion and surrounding borders should be continued for about one week after apparent eradication. Dermatophytes grow more readily in warm or humid conditions, so the surface of the skin should be kept as cool and dry as possible. High-potency topical corticosteroids, even in combination with topical antifungals, are likely to worsen the infection, induce chronicity, and are associated with substantial adverse effects.[47] In cases in which the response to treatment is poor, oral antifungals are sometimes helpful. The newer oral antifungals are also therapeutic options in recalcitrant cases.[48,49]

TINEA IMBRICATA

Tinea imbricata is a distinctive form of tinea corporis found primarily among Indonesians and Polynesians. It is seen principally in Southeast Asia, in the Pacific, and in Central and South America. Most exposed individuals do not acquire infection, even after chronic exposure. Also called Tokelau ringworm, it is caused by *T. concentricum*, which invades skin or nails but not hair. It is more common in rural than in urban areas. The sexes are affected equally, and infection is often lifelong, beginning at any age.

Brown papules develop, then enlarge, coalesce, and spread peripherally, leaving annular plaques with scale attached along the outer edge, with a trailing margin of scale detached. Erythema is minimal or absent, but itching may be severe. New involved sites form continuously, and outwardly migrating rings result in extensive rings of concentric scales (Fig. 26.9). These exotic geographic patterns are considered marks of beauty in some cultures.

The relapse rate following griseofulvin therapy is extremely high. Recurrences are often more inflammatory and symptomatic than chronic infections.

TINEA FACIEI

The causative organisms and clinical presentations of tinea affecting the face are similar to those associated with tinea corporis. However, tinea faciei is often more acute with significant erythema (Fig. 26.10). Beard involvement is referred to as tinea barbae, a condition which often presents with vesicles, pustules, and crusting. Culture or KOH examination confirms the diagnosis. Tinea barbae may necessitate treatment with oral antifungals because of follicular involvement. Topical treatment generally suffices in other forms of tinea faciei.

TINEA CRURIS

More common in men and less common before puberty, this groin infection is especially prevalent in warm or humid environments. Epidemics have been described among military troops, athletic teams, and in other settings in which there is close personal contact. Infection is transmitted by clothing, sheets or towels, and by direct interpersonal contact. Dermatophyte infection of the axillae or other intertriginous sites produces a clinical pattern similar to that seen with groin infection. Patients who have tinea cruris may also have tinea pedis, with the same organism responsible for involvement in both areas. The

46. Jones HE, Reinhardt JH, Rinaldi MG (1974) Acquired immunity to dermatophytes. **Arch Dermatol** 109:840–848.
47. Reynolds RD, Boiko S, Lucky AW (1991) Exacerbation of tinea corporis during treatment with 1% clotrimazole/0.05% betamethasone diproprionate (Lotrisone). **Am J Dis Child** 145:1224–1225.
48. Robertson MH, Rich P, Parker F, Hanifin JM (1982) Ketoconazole in griseofulvin-resistant dermatophytosis. **J Am Acad Dermatol** 6:224–229.
49. Jones HE, Ketoconazole (1984) In: Progress in Diseases of the Skin, Fleischmajer R, ed. New York: Grune & Stratton, p. 217.

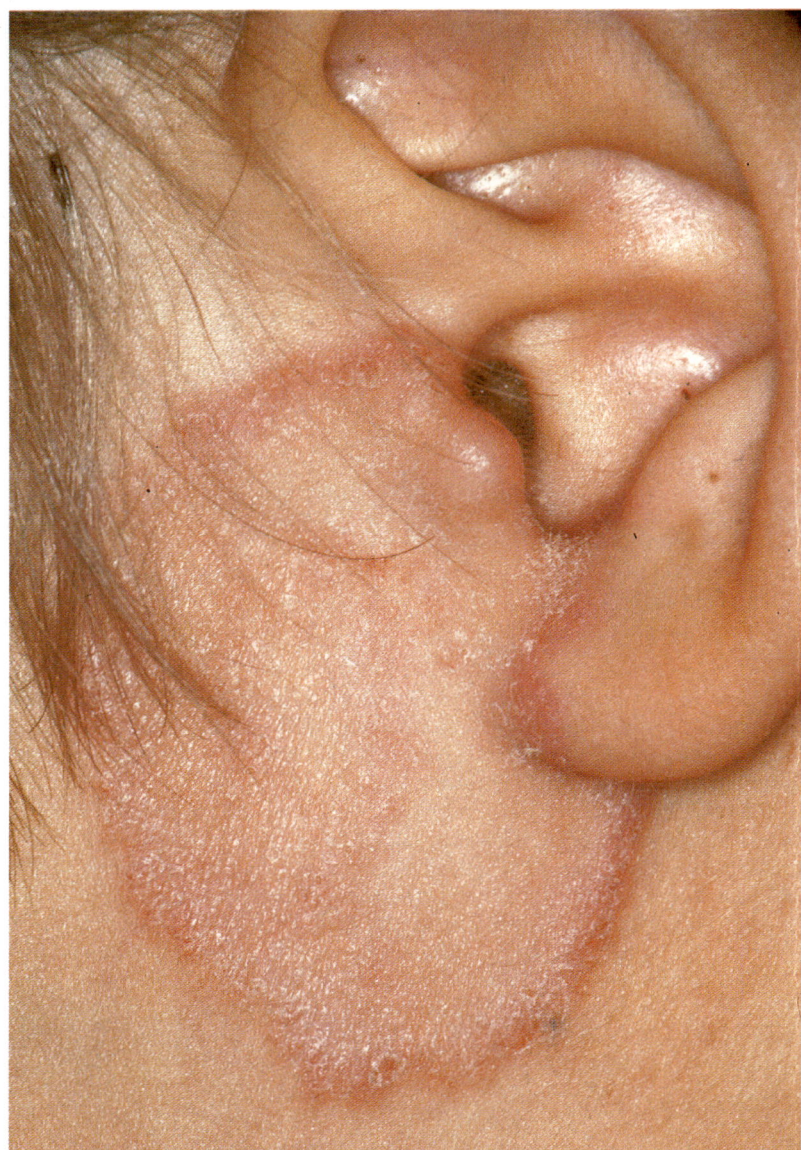

Fig. 26.10 Tinea corporis involving the face (tinea faciei).

predominant pathogen in the United States is *T. rubrum*,[50,51] but *E. floccosum* is also common, especially in other countries. The incidence of *T. tonsurans*-caused tinea cruris may be increasing.[52]

Clinical presentation

The upper medial portions of the thighs develop edematous, erythematous, skin-colored or hyperpigmented scaling papules or plaques that can evolve into vesicles or pustules. Areas of involvement tend to coalesce with well-defined borders that advance outward. Maceration and scaling are frequent, and there is less tendency for central clearing and usually less inflammation than is seen with tinea corporis. Infection may extend posteriorly onto the buttocks and gluteal cleft and superiorly up beyond the waistline. Tinea cruris is often associated with intense pruritus, and scratching can result in lichenification of the skin. Tinea cruris ordinarily spares the scrotum, unless there is accompanying candidiasis, but because the patient scratches, the scrotal skin often becomes thickened and falsely appears infected, despite a lack of

inflammation or actual fungal growth. Injudicious use of topical medications may complicate the situation by causing an irritant or allergic contact dermatitis that can also involve the scrotum.

Differential diagnosis

Erythrasma may resemble tinea cruris, but unlike tinea fluoresces coral-red under Wood's light evaluation. Candidiasis, psoriasis, seborrheic dermatitis, and contact dermatitis are all diagnostic considerations.

Treatment

The approach to treatment is similar to that for tinea corporis. Antifungal powders and attempts to keep the area aerated and dry are particularly important in this disorder.

TINEA PEDIS AND TINEA MANUM

Dermatophyte infection of the hands (t. manum) and feet (t. pedis) are discussed together because their clinical presentations are similar. *T. rubrum* is the most common cause and, along with *T. mentagrophytes* and *E. floccosum*, accounts for most cases of tinea pedis and manum. These disorders are less likely to occur before puberty.

Tinea pedis is extremely prevalent worldwide and is probably the most common form of fungal disease in the twentieth century. The disease appears more prevalent in societies where occlusive footwear is used.

Clinical presentation

There are several clinical presentations, any of which can itch (Table 26.10). More than one presentation can be found in the same patient at various times or even simultaneously (Fig. 26.11).

Tinea manum is often noted with tinea pedis and is commonly of the dry scaly variety with varying degrees of hyperkeratosis. It is likely to affect only one hand. Scaling of the hand tends to be finer than that seen on the foot and is white or silvery. Although often localized to the creases of the palm, tinea manum can be diffuse and form scattered rings of scale approximately 1–4mm in diameter. Mild erythema and less commonly vesicles, pustules, or bullae may develop. Interdigital involvement tends to be absent unless there are predisposing risk factors.

Dermatophytid reactions ("-id" reactions) may also develop on the hands and feet. They present as small deep-seated vesicles, resulting in a clinical presentation similar in appearance to dyshidrotic eczema (pompholyx). There may also be a less acute dermatitis consisting of erythema, edema, weeping, crusting, scaling, and itching of the hands, arms, legs, or other body areas. Most patients with id reactions have a positive intradermal skin test finding to the antigen trichophytin.[27]

Differential diagnosis

Erythrasma may mimic interdigital tinea pedis and Wood's light is helpful in distinguishing the two disorders. Various forms of dermatitis, including

TABLE 26.10 Tinea pedis – clinical presentations		
Interdigital	**Moccasin**	**Vesicular**
Erythema, scale maceration usually in interdigital web spaces; Secondary findings: fissures, cellulitis, lymphangitis	Dry scaly, hyperkeratotic papules; minimal erythema, primarily plantar or lateral aspects	Vesicles, pustules, bullae in any location

50. Todaro F, Germano D, Criseo G (1983) An outbreak of Tinea pedis and Tinea cruris in a tire factory in Messina, Italy. **Mycopathologia** 83:25–27.
51. Chakrabarti A, Sharma S, Talwar P (1992) Isolation of dermatophytes from clinically normal sites in patients with tinea cruris. **Mycopathologia** 120:139–141.

52. Arnow PM, Houchins SG, Pugliese G (1991) An outbreak of tinea corporis in hospital personnel caused by a patient with Trichophyton tonsurans infection. **Pediatr Infect Dis J** 10:355–359.

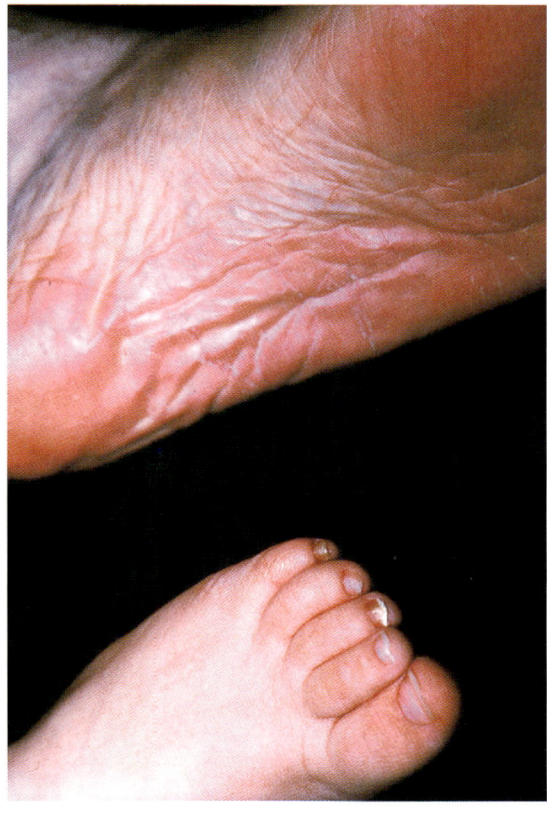

Fig. 26.11 Tinea pedis and onychomycosis in father/son pair. Father shows classic moccasin distribution of tinea pedis and son shows distal subungual onychomycosis

contact or atopic dermatitis, should also be considered. Dyshidrotic foot eczema is frequently mistaken for tinea pedis. Such disorders are often extremely pruritic, and small deep-seated tapioca-like papulovesicles are often present. The lesions generally spare the web spaces, but may involve the lateral aspects of the digits. Juvenile plantar dermatitis is a consideration, especially in young children. In such cases, shiny dry, scaly, hyperkeratotic, fissured areas classically involve the plantar aspects of the medial and anterior portions of the foot, especially the great toe, but may spread to involve the entire foot.

Diagnostic procedures for tinea pedis and manum are similar to those described above for tinea corporis. When vesicles are present, the roof of the blister should be removed and cultured or examined with KOH.

Therapeutics

Topical antifungals are often effective if the feet are kept cool and dry. Where feasible, sandals should be worn and the patient allowed to aerate his feet as much as possible. Socks should contain as much cotton as possible and should be changed frequently, and shoes should be allowed to air one day or more between wearings. Topical antiperspirants, such as aluminum chloride are useful adjunctive measures when hyperhidrosis is present. Badly macerated interdigital tinea pedis is best treated with a combination of antifungal and antibacterial agents, with the latter used topically or systemically. When these measures fail, consideration should be given to the use of griseofulvin or other systemic antifungals. Some experts add topical or systemic corticosteroids briefly to reduce extreme inflammation and pruritus, but this is not generally required in children. Cool tap water or Burow's solution soaks help to cleanse and relieve discomfort. The area should then be thoroughly dried before topical medications are applied. Once-daily application of a topical antifungal powder may help to prevent reinfection or reactivation of disease.

NONDERMATOPHYTE CAUSES OF "TINEA"

Hendersonula toruloidea and *Scytalidium hyalinum* are nondermatophyte molds with pigmented cell walls that have been reported as a cause of tinea pedis, tinea manus, and onychomycosis in human.[53] Findings are clinically indistinguishable from those caused by dermatophytes. These organisms grow on Sabouraud's dextrose agar, but the addition of cycloheximide inhibits the growth of *H. toruloidea*. These fungi are not sensitive to griseofulvin or the imidazoles, and it is therefore important to exclude them as etiologic agents before utilizing those agents. Topical agents such as salicylic acid that cause desquamation may be effective in some cases. Species of Fusarium and Allescheria also cause superficial infection.[54–57] Tinea capitis caused by *Scopulariopsis brevicaulis*, a cause of onychomycosis, has recently been reported.[58] Oral antifungal agents such as itraconazole have shown some efficacy in the treatment of these disorders

ONYCHOMYCOSIS

Onychomycosis is a generic term referring to infection of the nail by any fungus. More specifically, dermatophyte infection of the nail plate is called tinea unguium. Onychomycosis is unusual before puberty but becomes increasingly common with advancing age. The incidence may be increasing in childhood, presumably on the basis of urban cultural habits including the prolonged use of occlusive shoeware such as sneakers. The results of a multicenter North American survey of 2500 children revealed an overall prevalence of onychomycosis of 0.4%.[59] In a recent British survey, the prevalence of onychomycosis was 1.3% in the 16- to 34-year-old age group, 2.4% in 35- to 50-year-old patients, and 4.7% in those 55 or older.[60] Tinea unguium is usually associated with tinea pedis. Toenails are affected more frequently than fingernails.

Clinical findings

Zaias[61] and, more recently, Haneke[62] reviewed the four classical types of onychomycosis, which are listed in Table 26.11. Figure 26.12A, B depicts the distal subungual and superficial white variants.

Diagnosis

Material obtained from nail edges frequently lacks viable organisms. KOH evaluation is optimized by the use of high concentrations, and digestion of the nail keratin usually takes a lengthy period of time. A sample of subungual debris can yield a positive culture, but it is best to scrape into the substance of the nail plate or take fine clippings or filings through the entire thickness

---

TABLE 26.11 Onychomycosis variants

Distal and lateral subungal
Proximal subungal
Superficial white
Total dystrophic
Mycotic paronychia with onycholysis

---

53. Gupta AK, Elewski BE (1996) Nondermatophyte causes of onychomycosis and superficial mycoses [Review]. **Curr Top Med Mycol** 7:87–97.
54. Elewski BE, Greer DL (1991) *Hendersonula toruloidea* and *Scytalidium hyalinum*. Review and update. **Arch Dermatol** 127:1041–1044.
55. Kong BHP, Kapica L, Lee R (1984) Keratin invasion by *Hendersonula toruloidea*. **Int J Dermatol** 23:65.
56. Eady R, Moore M (1974) *Hendersonula toruloidea*. Infection of the skin and nails. **Trans St John's Hosp Dermatol Soc** 60:104.
57. Moore M (1978) Skin and nail infections by non-dermatophyte filamentous fungi. **Mykosen** (Suppl) 1:128.
58. Cox NH, Irving B (1993) Cutaneous "ringworm" lesions of *Scopulariopsis brevicaulis*. **Br J Dermatol** 129:726–728.
59. Ghannoum MA, Hajjeh RA, Scher R et al. (2000) A large-scale North American study of fungal isolates from nails: the frequency of onychomycosis, fungal distribution, and antifungal susceptibility patterns. **J Am Acad Dermatol** 43:641–648.
60. Williams HC (1993) The epidemiology of onychomycosis in Britain. **Br J Dermatol** 129:101–109.
61. Zaias N (1972) Onychomycosis. **Arch Dermatol** 105:263–274.
62. Haneke E (1991) Fungal infections of the nail. **Semin Dermatol** 10:41–53.

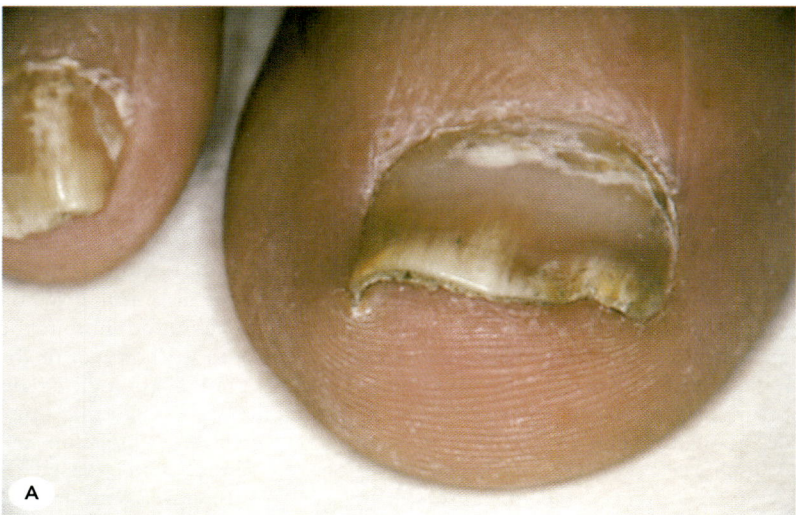
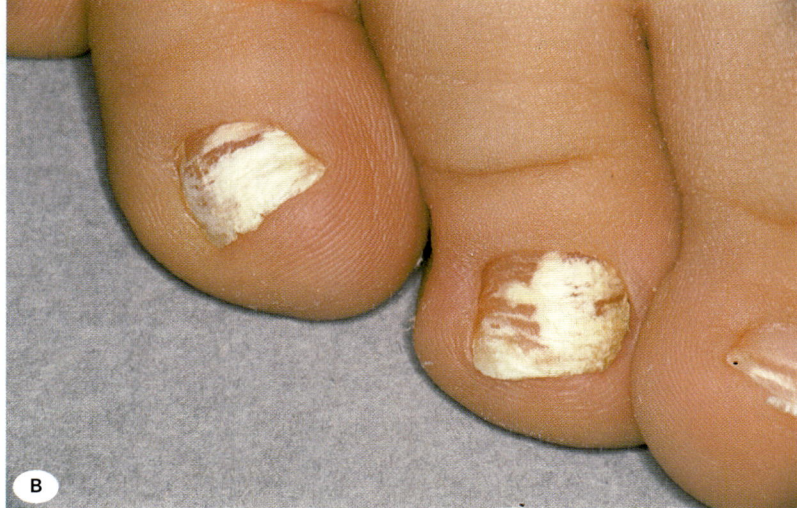

Fig. 26.12 (A) Distal subungual, onchomycosis occurring simultaneously with superficial white onchomycosis. (B) Superficial white onchomycosis.

of the nail. A small curette is often useful for this purpose. Histologic evaluation with PAS staining of nail clippings may be used to diagnose disease as well; most pathology departments can process and evaluate such samples. PCR evaluation and subtyping of *T. rubrum* is helpful but is not yet widely available.[32]

Differential diagnosis

Psoriasis may mimic onychomycosis and should be considered in the differential diagnosis. Lichen planus, trauma, and 20-nail dystrophy can all cause distortion of the finger and toenails. Onychomycosis may result from yeasts or molds rather than dermatophytes, and proper identification is therefore important before instituting therapy.

Therapeutics

Onychomycosis usually requires systemic therapy, particularly in adults. However, young children appear to respond somewhat faster than adults, and topical therapy or observation alone should be options offered to parents, particularly in cases where the patient has asymptomatic superficial disease that does not involve the matrix. Topical therapies currently available include ciclopirox 8% lacquer, amorolfine 5%, and urea 40% plus bifonazole. Cure rates with topical therapy alone are low in adults, and rates of 29–36% are typical for ciclopirox lacquer monotherapy. However, children empirically appear to respond better, and such therapy may be preferred by families because there is no risk of systemic toxicity.

Oral therapeutic options for onychomycosis include griseofulvin, itraconazole, terbinafine and fluconazole (Table 26.12).

SUBCUTANEOUS DERMATOPHYTES

Dermatophytes sometimes invade the dermis and subcutaneous tissue in immunosuppressed patients, especially those with hematologic malignancies. *T. rubrum* is the most commonly identified pathogen.[63,64] Erythematous papules, nodules, tumors, or abscesses develop that may be hemorrhagic and tender. Involved areas can ulcerate or become vegetating, taking on the characteristics of a mycetoma (see below). Biopsy reveals hyphae in the dermis and subcutaneous tissue, sometimes resembling Majocchi's granuloma. Oral therapy is mandatory in such cases and the newer antifungal agents are probably more efficacious for such infections.

GENERAL THERAPEUTIC CONSIDERATIONS FOR DERMATOPHYTES

A large number of new topical and oral agents are now available, facilitating the treatment of dermatophytoses as well as other fungal infections. With the exception of infections affecting hair or nails, topical therapy is appropriate first-line intervention.

Topical agents

Many highly effective topical agents are currently available for the treatment of dermatophytosis (Table 26.13). These include the imidazoles, which interfere with cell wall ergosterol synthesis by inhibiting lanosterol demethylation. Imidazole action depends on inhibition of fungal cytochrome P450. Imidazoles include compounds such as econazole, miconazole, oxiconazole, and clotrimazole; all are broad-spectrum antifungal agents that have good activity against dermatophytes, Candida, and various other yeasts. A second class of antifungals includes ciclopirox olamine, a pyridone-ethanolamine salt that interferes with the synthesis of cell membrane proteins. The allylamines are a third class of agents, which include naftifine and terbinafine. Allylamines interfere with ergosterol synthesis through inhibition of squalene oxidase and are fungicidal *in vitro*. In addition, naftifine has anti-inflammatory properties and may be particularly useful in severe inflammatory disease.[65] This class of agents can also be effective when used for a short five-

TABLE 26.12 Oral therapeutic options for onychomycosis

Griseofulvin 15–20mg/kg per d micro, max 1g	Fingernails 3–9 months	Toenails 4–12 months
Itraconazole 5mg/kg per d continuous or 5mg/kg per d 1 week/month	Fingernails 6 weeks 2 pulses	Toenails 12 weeks 3 pulses
Terbinafine 3–6mg/kg per d	Fingernails 6 weeks	Toenails 12 weeks
Fluconazole 6mg/kg weekly	Fingernails 12–16 weeks	Toenails 18–26 weeks

Some therapies may not be FDA approved.

63. Roseuw D, De Doncker P (1993) New approaches to the treatment of onychomycosis. J Am Acad Dermatol 29:S45–S50.
64. Faergemann J, Gisslen H, Dahlberg E et al. (1989) Trichophyton rubrum abscesses in immunocompromised patients. A case report. Acta Derm Venereol 69:244–247.
65. Solomon BA, Lee WL, Geen SC et al. (1993) Modification of neutrophil functions by naftifine. Br J Dermatol 128:393–398.

TABLE 26.13   Topical drugs for superficial fungal infections

Drug	Strength	Formulation*	Application(s) per day
Amphotericin B	3%	C, O	2–4
Butenafine	1%	C	1
Ciclopirox	1%	C	2
Clotrimazole	1%	C, L, S, Su	2
Econazole	1%	C	1
Halopirogin	1%	C, S	2
Ketoconazole	2%	C, Sh	2
Miconazole	2%	C, P, S, Su	2
Naftifine	1%	C, gel	2
Nystatin	100 000U/ml or 100 000U/g	C, L, P, O, Su	2–3
Oxiconazole	1%	C, L	1–2
Sulconazole	1%	C, S	1–2
Terbinafine	1%	C	2
Tolnaftate	1%	C, P, S	2
Triacetin	% varies	C, O	3
Undecylenate	10%–25%	P, C, O, L	2–3
Other remedies			
Gentian violet	1%–2%	S	2
Selenium sulfide	2.5%	L, Sh	1
	1%	Sh	1
Sodium thiosulfate	25%	L	1–2

* C indicates cream; L, lotion; O, ointment; P, powder, S, solution; Sh, shampoo; Su, suppositories

day treatment course under some circumstances. The older topical antifungal compounds, undecylenic acid and tolnaftate, are of limited value and have no activity against Candida. Haloprogin, another older antifungal agent, is somewhat useful against Candida and dermatophytes but, like undecylenic acid, has been supplanted by newer topical antifungals.

Topical antifungals are generally applied once or twice daily but may need to be applied more often if removed by washing or perspiration. Miconazole, clotrimazole, and terbinafine are available over the counter in topical formulations, and are acceptable first-line agents for most uncomplicated fungal infections.

Oral agents in the treatment of dermatophytes

Griseofulvin

When griseofulvin became available in 1959, it constituted an important breakthrough in the treatment of dermatophyte infections, especially tinea capitis.[66–69] Griseofulvin is produced by various species of Penicillium and is active against dermatophytes through inhibition of the microtubules necessary for mitosis. Its clinical efficacy is somewhat limited by the fact that it is water insoluble and erratically absorbed. Poor absorption or noncompliance may account for many treatment failures seen with this drug. Absorption is enhanced by dispersion of ultramicrosize particles of the drug in polyethylene glycol or in a corn oil-in-water emulsion. Therefore, the dosage of these ultramicrosized preparations can be reduced by one half to one third (7.5 to 10mg/kg per day) of that used for other dosage forms. Unfortunately, ultramicrosize formulations are available only in tablet form. Older microsize tablet preparations tend to be erratically and incompletely absorbed; although absorption is improved through administration with fatty foods.

Liquid griseofulvin is a microsize rather than an ultramicrosize preparation. The recommended dose for tinea capitis is currently 20mg/kg per day with milk or other lipids to enhance absorption. Griseofulvin is detectable in stratum corneum after 4–8 hours, but it gradually accumulates in the skin and hair, reaching steady-state concentrations over several days. The dose of drug may be increased to 25mg/kg per day if response is not evident after 2–3 weeks, and compliance is not an issue; however gastrointestinal side effects may increase with this dose.

Griseofulvin has a long history of safety and efficacy. Adverse reactions are generally minimal and include headache and gastrointestinal upset. Such symptoms often resolve with continued therapy. Occasional hypersensitivity reactions to the drug may present as urticaria or a morbilliform rash sometimes accompanied by low-grade fever. Hepatotoxicity is possible but appears to be rare; however, the drug is contraindicated in patients with hepatic porphyria or hepatocellular failure. Laboratory monitoring of liver function tests is unnecessary during routine use of griseofulvin for periods of less than eight weeks. Photosensitivity and exacerbation or induction of lupus erythematosus have been observed but are unusual. Tumorigenicity, teratogenicity, and embryotoxicity have been shown in rodents but never in humans or other animals. Drug interactions may occur with warfarin and phenobarbitol.

Ketoconazole

Ketoconazole was the first of the imidazole antifungals to become available for oral use. It is not generally recommended for treatment of dermatophytes because of its adverse hepatic reaction profile with long-term use and its lack of superiority over griseofulvin.

66. Ginsburg CM, McCracken GH, Petruska M, Olsen K (1983) Effect of feeding on bioavailability of griseofulvin in children. **J Pediatr** 102:309–311.
67. Gupta AK, Sauder DN, Shear NH (1994) Antifungal agents: an overview. Part I. **J Am Acad Dermatol** 30:677–698.
68. Artis WM, Odle BM, Jones HE (1981) Griseofulvin-resistant dermatophytosis correlates with in vitro resistance. **Arch Dermatol** 117:16–19.
69. Hay RJ, Clayton YM, Griffiths WA, Dowd PM (1985) A comparative double blind study of ketoconazole and griseofulvin in dermatophytosis. **Br J Dermatol** 112:691–696.

Fluconazole

Fluconazole, a triazole, has been used successfully in the treatment of dermatophyte infections.[70–74] It is highly water soluble and accumulates in the skin. In addition, it is readily absorbed and has been shown to be effective, even with once-weekly dosing for conditions such as onychomycosis. The duration of therapy depends on the clinical response, but less frequent and shorter courses of therapy have been shown effective in a number of dermatophyte conditions including tinea capitis.[35] However, pediatric experience with fluconazole is limited, apart from treatment for candidiasis, for which it is FDA approved.

The most frequent adverse reactions to fluconazole are gastrointestinal. Headaches have been reported with some regularity. It can rarely cause acute hepatic necrosis and abnormal aminotransferase activity; thus, liver function should be monitored. Fluconazole is largely excreted unchanged by the kidney and its dosage must be therefore be reduced and carefully monitored in the face of impaired renal function. Cutaneous reactions include urticaria, Stevens–Johnson syndrome, or toxic epidermal necrolysis. Drug interactions are a concern with this drug, and it increases serum concentrations of cyclosporine, phenytoin, tolbutamide, and oral anticoagulants.

Itraconazole

Itraconazole, a second oral triazole, accumulates in the skin, clearing more slowly than it does from plasma.[75,76] It disrupts fungal cell membrane formation through interference with cytochrome P450-dependent ergosterol synthase. Because of this, it can be effective after administration for durations shorter than those required for griseofulvin and may offer a treatment advantage over that agent. Its accumulation in skin and a tissue half-life measured in weeks to months allow for initial administration over two to three weeks with continued improvement of the patient even after therapy is discontinued. Optimum pediatric treatment schedules are not established. Pediatric experience is accumulating with this drug, and doses of approximately 5mg/kg per day are usually used. Itraconazole is well absorbed after oral administration if taken with food, and is 99% protein bound. An oral suspension is available, but is not a pediatric formulation and is intended to treat esophageal candidosis used where oral absorption is required.

Itraconazole's side effect profile is similar to that of fluconazole. Gastrointestinal upset is the most common adverse effect. Headache is next in frequency, followed by dizziness and itching. Itraconazole's propensity to cause serious liver disease appears low, but 1–2% of patients have serum transaminase concentration elevations. Some experts obtain baseline liver function tests on children before instituting therapy, and repeat this screen two to four weeks following institution of therapy. However, if short-course therapy is expected, such evaluation is often deferred, or performed only if underlying health conditions or clinical status warrants such. The drug can elevate cyclosporine levels, and concomitant administration of both drugs should be carefully monitored. It can also increase digoxin, terfenadine, and astemizole concentrations. Interference with testosterone and cortisol synthesis (a problem with ketoconazole) appears to be minimal.

Terbinafine

Terbinafine is the first of the allylamines to become available in an oral preparation and is currently the drug of choice for the treatment of adult onychomycosis. It inhibits squalene oxidase, with subsequent inhibition of ergosterol and cell wall synthesis. This drug is well absorbed from the gastrointestinal tract, and absorption is unaffected by food. It is extensively metabolized by the liver, and dosage adjustment may be required in those with hepatic or renal disease. Terbinafine is stongly lipophilic, and drug is detected in the skin for at least 55 days following discontinuation of therapy. Adverse effects are uncommon. These include anorexia, gastrointestinal disturbance, taste disturbance, and vesicopustular eruption. Rare cases of liver toxicity, neutropenia, and lupus-like reactions have been reported. Drug interactions are uncommon but can occur with cyclosporine, cimetidine, theophylline, nortriptyline, and rifampin. Dosing has traditionally been 3–6mg/kg in rounded doses (Table 26.9), but recent data suggests that higher cure rates may occur with doses greater than 4.5mg/kg per dose.[77] Short-course therapy of two weeks appears to be effective in the majority of cases of tinea capitis caused by trichophyton species, but *microsporum canis* infections often require prolonged courses of therapy.[77,78]

YEAST INFECTIONS

MALASSEZIA (PITYROSPORUM) INFECTIONS

Introduction and historical note

Pityriasis (tinea) versicolor is a condition caused by proliferation of pityrosporum filamentous yeast forms within the stratum corneum of human skin. The term tinea is inappropriate since this infection is caused by a yeast rather than a dermatophyte. Pityriasis versicolor is the most common infection caused by malassezia, but a number of other disorders have been attributed to this fungus.[79] Malassezia is a dimorphic lipophilic yeast that usually resides on the skin as a member of the normal skin flora. However, it can also be an opportunistic pathogen, and under appropriate conditions, the benign yeast form can transform into an invasive hyphal phase. It is the definitive pathogenic agent in pityriasis versicolor and pityrosporum folliculitis. It has also been identified as a cause of catheter-associated septicemia in the immunocompromised and in those receiving intralipid hyperalimentation.[80] This organism has been implicated in the pathogenesis of seborrheic dermatitis,[81] confluent and reticulate papillomatosis of Gougerot–Carteaud,[82] rare cases of onychomycosis and peritonitis,[83,84] and some flares of atopic dermatitis.[85] Most recently, it has also been mentioned as a pathogen in neonatal cephalic pustulosis, a form of neonatal acne.[86]

Controversy exists regarding the name of this genus of dimorphic yeasts. The terms pityrosporum ovale and orbiculare, as well as furfur, have now been discarded. In the mid-1980s this group was officially reduced to Malassezia as the valid name for the genus.[86] Subsequently, Gueho *et al.* using molecular biology techniques, confirmed the existence of six lipophilic and one non-lipohilic species of Malassezia[87] (Table 26.14). The

70. Terrell CL, Hughes CE (1992) Antifungal agents used for deep-seated mycotic infections. **Mayo Clin Proc** 67:69–91.
71. Como JA, Dismukes W (1994) Oral azole drugs as systemic antifungal therapy. **N Engl J Med** 330:263–272.
72. Montero-Gei F, Perera A (1992) Therapy with fluconazole for tinea corporis, tinea cruris, and tinea pedis. **Clin Infect Dis** (14 Suppl) 1:S77–S81.
73. Suchil P, Gei FM, Robles M et al. (1992) Once-weekly oral doses of fluconazole 150mg in the treatment of tinea corporis/cruris and cutaneous candidiasis. **Clin Exp Dermatol** 17:397–401.
74. Anonymous (1994) Systemic antifungal drugs. **Med Letter, Drugs Ther** 36:16.
75. Terrell CL, Hughes CE (1992) Antifungal agents used for deep-seated mycotic infections. **Mayo Clin Proc** 67:69–91.
76. Como JA, Dismukes W (1994) Oral azole drugs as systemic antifungal therapy. **N Engl J Med** 330:263–272.
77. Friedlander SF, Aly R, Krafchik B et al. Terbinafine in the treatment of Trichophyton tinea capitis: a randomized, double-blind parallel group, duration-finding study. **Pediatrics** In press.
78. Krafchik B, Pelletier J (1999) An open study of tinea capitis in 50 childen treated with a 2 week course of oral terbinafine. **J Am Acad Dermatol** 41:60–63.
79. Marcon MJ, Powell DA (1992) Human infections due to Malassezia spp. **Clin Microbiol Rev** 5:101–119.

80. Powell DA, Aungst J, Snedden S et al. (1984) Broviac catheter-related Malassezia furfur sepsis in five infants receiving intravenous fat emulsions. **J Pediatr** 105:987–990.
81. Bergbrant I, Faergemann J (1990) The role of Pityrosporum ovale in seborrheic dermatitis. **Semin Dermatol** 9:262–268.
82. Hamilton D, Tavafoghi V, Shafer JC, Hambrick GW Jr (1980) Confluent and reticulated papillomatosis of Gougerot and Carteaud. Its relation to other papillomatoses. **J Am Acad Dermatol** 2:401–410.
83. Wallace M, Bagnall H, Glen D, Averill S (1979) Isolation of lipophilic yeast in "sterile" peritonitis. **Lancet** 2(8149):956.
84. Crozier WJ, Wise KA (1993) Onychomycosis due to Pityrosporum. **Australas J Dermatol** 34:109–112.
85. Kieffer M, Bergbrant I-M, Faergemann J et al. (1990) Immune reactions to Pityrosporum ovale in adult patients with atopic dermatitis and seborrhoeic dermatitis. **J Am Acad Dermatol** 22:739–742.
86. Niamba P et al. (1998) Is common neonatal cephalic pustulosis triggered by Malassezia sympodialis? **Arch Dermatol** 134:995–998.
87. Gueho E, Midgley G, Guillot J (1996) The genus Malassezia with description of four new species. **Antonia van Leeuwenhoek** 69:337–355.

TABLE 26.14   Malasezzia species

M. sympodialis*+^
M. obtuse*
M. globosa*^
M. slooffiae
M. furfur*+
M. restricta
M. pachydermatis**

* Commonly isolated from normal skin
\+ Suspected pathogen for neonatal cephalic pustulosis
** Non-liphilic, usually found in animals
^ Suspected pathogen – P. versicolor

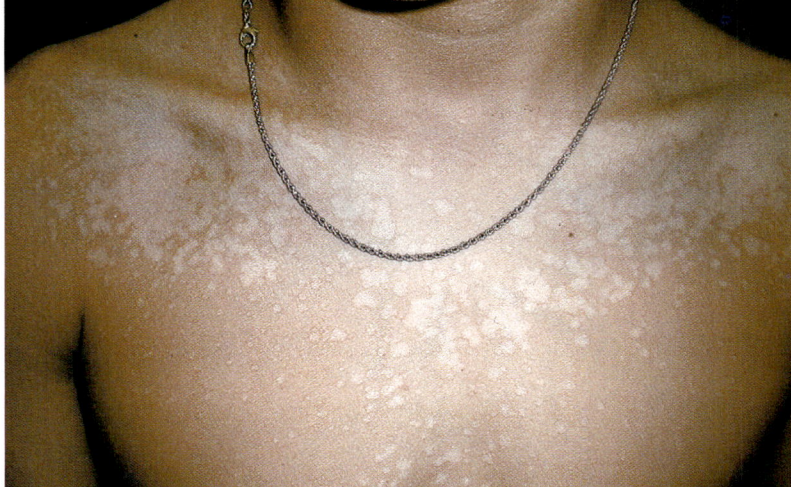

Fig. 26.14   Tinea versicolor, upper chest in teenage (Courtesy Jon Alexander).

sole non-lipophilic species, *M. pachydermatis*, is mainly found on the skin of animals, especially dogs.

Epidemiology

Malassezia infections are found worldwide, but are more common in areas of high heat and humidity. Thirty to forty percent of the population in tropical climates may be affected; however, the incidence in temperate climates approaches 1–4%.[88] The majority of cases occur in healthy adolescents and affect cutaneous areas where sebaceous glands are active. One study found that 5–7% of confirmed cases occurred in children under the age of 13, and approximately one-third of children manifested lesions on the face.[89] Heredity may play a role, as a positive family history is often obtained from patients. Pityriasis versicolor tends to be a chronic disease, and even with treatment, recurrence is common, with 80% of those treated relapsing after two years.[88] Pityrosporum folliculitis is also more common in tropical countries and more common in teenagers or young adult males. Both diseases are more common in immunosuppressed patients, those on systemic corticosteroids, and those with Cushing's disease. Hyperhidrosis also appears to place patients at risk of pityrosporum infection.

Presenting history/clinical findings

Pityriasis versicolor

Patients usually present for cosmetic reasons and may complain of pruritus. Children, and those in a tropical climate, frequently have facial lesions which

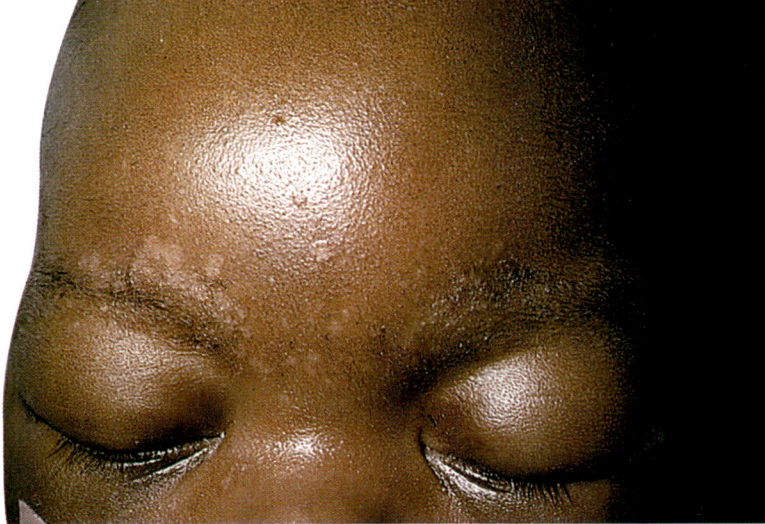

Fig. 26.13   Tinea versicolor infant.

usually involve the forehead and temple (Fig. 26.13). Adolescents and adults commonly have lesions on the upper back, chest and arms (Fig. 26.14). Other sites of involvement include the neck and less commonly the axillae, legs, popliteal fossae and forearms, penis/genitalia, or a radiotherapy field.[90] Even tinea versicolor of the ear canal has been reported, where colonization of earwax plays an important role.[91]

Lesions on the face are usually hypopigmented, faintly scaling ovoid lesions. Lesions at other sites, as the name "versicolor" implies, can vary in color. Hypopigmented, faint pink, red, or tan to darker brown lesions may be present. They consist of discrete and coalescent ovoid macules of varying size that possess a fine, faint scale that is more noticeable upon scraping the area. They are often concentrated symmetrically over areas of high sebum content such as the upper chest and back. Papules and annular plaques are sometimes also seen.

Pityrosporum folliculitis

This disorder is characterized by follicular papules and pustules most commonly located on the back, chest, and upper arms (Fig. 26.15). The lesion may itch or rarely sting. This condition is frequently confused with acne vulgaris, but lacks comedones. Involvement of the scalp, neck, and rarely the trunk and extremities can occur, particularly in the immunocompromised.

Confluent and reticulate papillomatosis

Also known as Gougerot–Carteaud syndrome, this disorder consists of greyish-brown verrucous papules that coalesce into confluent plaques with a reticulated pattern. It usually involves the central chest and back, but extension to the shoulders and abdomen or groin can be seen. Some consider this a disorder of keratinazation, with pityrosporum functioning as a secondary invader.[92]

Pityrosporum septicemia/catheter-associated infection

Malessezia sepsis is most common in premature infants who receive intralipid alimentation through intravenous lines. Contamination of the indwelling catheter from organisms present on the skin is the presumed mode of infection. Initial studies suggested that low-birth-weight infants in neonatal intensive care units (NICUs) were at higher risk for colonization with pityrosporum, and thus more susceptible to this infection.[93] More recently, a high prevalence of colonization has been documented in neonates that is age rather

88. Faergemann J (1999) Pityrosporum species as a cause of allergy and infection. **Allergy** 54:413–419.
89. Terragni L, Lasagni A, Oriani A (1991) Pityriasis versicolor of the face. **Mycoses** 34:345–347.
90. Conill C, Azon-Masoliver A, Verger E, Lecha V (1990) Pityriasis versicolor confined to the radiation therapy field. **Acta Oncol** 29:949–950.
91. Sykes N (1994) Earwax and tinea versicolor. **Int J Dermatol** 33:543–544.
92. Yamamoto A et al. (2000) Two cases of confluent and reticulate papillomatosis: successful treatments of one case with cefdinir and another with minocycline. **J Dermatol** 27:598–603.
93. Powell DA, Hayes J, Durrell E et al. (1987) Malassezia furfur skin colonization of infants hospitalized in intensive care units. **J Pediatr** 111:217–220.

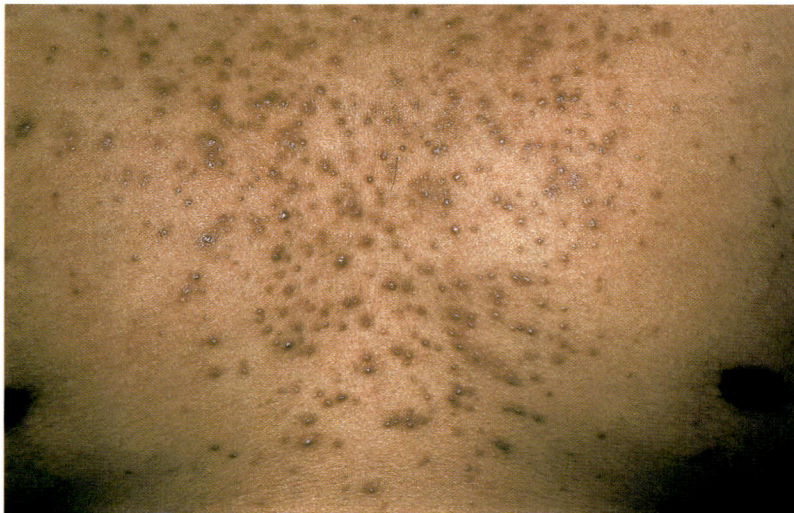

Fig. 26.15   Pityrosporum folliculitis in a teenager.

than weight related; in one study 100% of infants older than 40 days were colonized.[94] *M. furfur* is most commonly isolated in pityrosporum fungemia, but multiple cases of *M. pachydermatis* sepsis have been reported in a neonatal ICU.[95] The organism was presumably transmitted by a nurse who owned a dog. The clinical signs of yeast sepsis are similar to those of bacterial sepsis, which include fever, temperature instability, respiratory distress, and hepatosplenomegaly.

Etiology/pathogenesis
Malassezia yeasts are a normal part of the normal flora of most individuals. More than 90% of normal adults harbor this yeast on their scalp and trunk. Although initial studies failed to culture the organism from children less than one year of age, a recent study noted positive cultures from normal skin in approximately one-third of infants by 19 days of age, with 100% colonized by 40 days of life.[94]

Why this usually benign commensal sometimes converts into a pathogenic form is unclear. Certain endogenous and exogenous factors appear to play a role. High temperatures and humidity predispose to infection, and disease has been experimentally induced by occluding skin with a dressing.[95] Endogenous factors that play a role may include hyperhidrosis, increased sebum production, corticosteroid therapy, immunodeficiency, Cushing's disease, and hereditary factors.

Depressed or altered cellular immunity may be a factor in development of the disease. Lymphocytes from patients with pityriasis versicolor appear to show decreased transformation processing, and produce less leukocyte stimulation factor when stimulated with Malassezia extract.[96] Humoral responses do not appear to be important in pityriasis versicolor, since antibody titers appear similar in normal and uninfected individuals. In contrast, patients with pityrosporum folliculitis do have higher circulating antibodies against Malassezia organisms than do healthy controls, perhaps explaining the increased inflammation seen in this form of pityrosporum infection.[97]

Dicarboxylic acids, such as azaleic acid, produced by Malassezia species can inhibit melanogenesis, and there is also evidence that azaleic acid can cause direct damage to melanocytes, which may account for the prolonged hypopigmentation that occurs following infection.

The role of Malassezia in the pathogenesis of classic seborrheic dermatitis is less well understood, but pityrosporum may play an important role in the pathogenesis of this disorder. Disease may result from an abnormal immunologic reaction to the organism.[88] Some studies have shown an increased concentration of pityrosporum organisms in areas affected with seborrheic dermatitis, while others have not. A response to topical and systemic antifungal therapy, with concomitant decrease in spore counts while on therapy, has been documented, as has a subsequent increase in spore counts when patients relapse.[98] Cytokine profiles also support this association; IL-2 and interferon-gamma production is markedly depressed, while interleukin 10 synthesis is increased in lymphocytes from patients with seborrheic dermatitis after they are stimulated with yeast extract antigens.[99]

The relationship between Malassezia and the infantile form of seborrheic dermatitis is also unclear. Broberg[100] found that 90% of children with seborrheic dermatitis were culture positive for the yeast, while only 20% of heathy children harbored the organism. Response to 20% ketoconazole cream has also been reported in infantile seborrheic dermatitis.[101]

Pityrosporum has been implicated in flares of atopic dermatitis, particularly in the head and neck area.[102] A positive response to systemic ketoconazole, and a higher proportion of positive pityrosporum skin prick tests in patients with active head and neck eczema support the possible association between pityrosporum disease and flaring atopic dermatitis.[103] Increased anti-pityrosporum IgE synthesis and cytokine profiles have also been noted in some flaring atopics.[104]

There are conflicting results regarding which subtype of pityrosporum is most common in normal individuals, as well as those with disease. *M. globosa* and *M. sympodialis* tend to be the predominant species isolated from normal skin, while *M. furfur* and *M. globosa* are more common in seborrheic dermatitis.[105] In the case of tinea versicolor, the predominant species appears to vary with geographic location. *M. sympodialis* has been most frequently isolated in Canada, while in Spain and Japan *M. globosa* appears more common.[106,107]

Histopathologic findings
Nonspecific, common findings include mild hyperkeratosis and epidermal acanthosis. Lymphocytes, plasma cells, and histiocytes are usually present in the dermis in a perivascular location. PAS and silver methenamine stains are helpful, and demonstrate short hyphae and round budding yeast forms. In pityriasis versicolor the organisms will be located in the stratum corneum, and occasionally the keratinocytes themselves, while in pityrosporum folliculitis yeast forms will be noted within a dilated follicular ostium. Tissue sections from sites other than the skin will show only unipolar budding yeast forms; hyphae or pseudohyphae are not seen, which is helpful in distinguishing the organism from candida or other deep fungal infections.

94. Leeming JP, Sutton TM, Fleming PJ (1995) Neonatal skin as a reservoir of Malassezia species. **Pediatr Inf Dis J** 14:719–721.
95. Chang HJ, Miller HL, Watkins N et al. (1998) An epidemic of Malassezia pachydermatis in an intensive care nursery associated with colonization of health care workers' pet dogs. **New England J Med** 338:706–711.
96. Shonle PG, Collins-Lech C (1982) Analysis of the lymphjocyte transformation response to Pityrosporum orbiculare in patients with tinea versicolor. **Clin Exp Immunol** 49:559–564.
97. Faergemann J, Johansson S, Back O, Scheynius A (1986) An immunologic and cultural study of Pityrosporum folliculitis. **J Am Acad Dermatol** 14:429–433.
98. Shuster S (1984) The aetiology of dandruff and the mode of action of therapeutic agents. **Br J Dermatol** 111:235–242.
99. Neuber K et al. (1996) Effects of Pityrosporum ovale on proliferation, immunoglobulin synthesis, and cytokine production of peripheral blood mononuclear cells from patients with seborrhoeic dermatitis. **Arch Dermatol Res** 288:532–536.
100. Broberg A (1994) Pityrosporum ovale in healthy children, infantile seborrhoeic dermatitis and atopic dermatitis [Review]. **Acta Derm Venereol Suppl** (Stockh) 191:1–47.
101. Taieb A, Legrain V, Palmier C et al. (1990) Topical ketoconazole for infantile seborrhoeic dermatitis. **Dermatologica** 181:26–32.
102. Clemmensen OJ, Hjorth N (1983) Treatment of dermatitis of the head and neck with ketoconazole in patients with a type I sensitivity to Pityrosporum orbiculare. **Semin Dermatol** 2:26–29.
103. Waersted A, Hjorth N (1998) Pityroporum orbiculare – a pathogenic factor in atopic dermatitis of the face, scalp and neck? **Acta Derm Venereol** (Suppl) 114:146–148.
104. Kroger S, Neuber K, Gruseck E et al. (1995) Pityrosporum ovale extracts increase interleukin-4, interleukin-10 and IgE synthesis inpatients with atopic eczema. **Acta Derm Venereol** 75:357–360.
105. Nakabayashi A, Sei Y, Guillot J (2000) Identification of Malassezia species isolated from patients with seborrheic dermatitis, atopic dermatitis, pityriasis versicolor and normal subjects. **Med Mycol** 38:337–341.
106. Gupta AK, Kohli Y, Faergemann J, Summerbell RC (2001) Epidemiology of Malassezia yeasts associated with pityriasis versicolor in Ontario, Canada. **Med Mycol** 39:199–206.
107. Crespo Erchiga V et al. (2000) Malassezia globosa as the causative agent of pityriasis versicolor. **Br J Dermatol** 143:799–803.

Laboratory findings

Microscopic examination of skin scrapings mounted in 10% KOH reveals both budding yeast and short, stubby hyphal forms, frequently referred to as "spaghetti and meatballs." The budding yeast forms have a broader base than that seen with other yeast forms such as Candida. Some clinicians utililize a blade or glass slide to obtain scale, while other experts prefer to use the "Scotch-tape" method, which involves applying clear adhesive tape to the affected skin, then stripping this from the site and applying the tape to a glass slide upon which a drop of 1% methylene blue has been placed.[108] Chlorazol Black E, Paragon stain or Albert's solution can also be used to identify the organism. Wood's lamp evaluation of affected areas will often show a yellow-green fluorescence.

Culture is usually not helpful, because pityrosporum is a normal commensal organism on the skin, and would be expected to grow from skin samples. In addition, the culture medium must be modified because the pityrosporum organism is fastidious and requires an enriched lipid medium. When culture is required (blood, pustules, peritoneal fluid), the laboratory should be notified regarding the clinical suspicion, and a medium such as SDA covered with sterile olive oil should be used and incubated at 30°C. Molecular biolgy techniques utilizing rRNA sequence analysis and nDNA comparisons are now available at some research institutions when speciation of Malassezia is necessary.

Differential diagnosis

The hypopigmented lesions of pityriasis versicolor may be confused with vitilgo, but vitiligo lesions are usually symmetrical or segmental, commonly involve acral areas, and do not scale. Pityriasis alba lesions are generally larger and KOH evaluation will be negative. Pityriasis rosea, seborrheic dermatitis, and tinea are other scaling lesions to consider, as is hypopigmented pityriasis lichenoides chronica and the rare disorder hypopigmented mycosis fungoides.

Pityrosporum folliculitis may be confused with acne vulgaris, but is usually more pruritic than acne, and does not possess comedones. Other causes of folliculitis, including staphylococcus, pseudomonas, and candida must also be considered in the differential diagnosis.

Therapeutics and prognosis

A number of topical agents are effective in the treatment of pityriasis versicolor and folliculitis (Table 26.15). Topical agents should be applied to the whole trunk, neck, arms, legs, and scalp if possible to decrease the spore count and minimize the possibility of relapse. Although selenium sulfide lotion 2.5% applied for 5–10 minutes for seven days is commonly utilized, the cosmetic problems and prolonged therapy required with this agent have led to the increasing use of other therapeutic alternatives in the last decade (Table 26.15).

Ketoconazole shampoo is an attractive therapy for this often chronic disorder. In a large multicenter study, the shampoo was applied to wet skin, lathered in and washed off 3–5 minutes later.[109] This was performed for for

---

TABLE 26.15 Therapy of pityrasis versicolor

Ketoconazole shampoo daily × 3 days
Selenium sulfide shampoo daily × 7 days
Terbinafine solution bid × 5–7 days
Ketoconazole 200–400mg po × 3 days
Itraconazole 200mg po x 5–7 days
Fluconazole 400mg × 1, repeat prn

1–3 days in a row. Cure rates as assessed by the Scotch tape method and clinical response were quite high, even when only one treatment was utilized. Use of this shampoo is an easy, cosmetically acceptable treatment for this common disease. Prophylactic monthly treatments are sometimes required, as relapse rates of 60% at one year and 80% at 2 years have been documented following a variety of therapeutic interventions, including systemic therapy. Multiple systemic therapeutic options are available; the easiest and probably most efficacious is one 400mg dose of fluconazole. Regardless of treatment modality, patients must be counseled regarding the high risk of relapse and the often prolonged (months) period required for normalization of pigment at the affected sites.

Systemic therapy is generally indicated for extensive lesions resistant to topical treatment, or those with frequent relapse. Ketoconazole, itraconazole, and fluconazole have all been used for this purpose with good results. Varying regimens have been utilized, as listed in Table 26.15. The risk of drug interactions, and the lack of FDA approval for such use in children at the present time should be kept in mind when prescribing oral agents, as well as the small risk of systemic toxicities such as hepatitis. Patients should be instructed to exercise after ingesting ketoconazole or fluconazole, as the drugs are preferentially excreted in sweat. Oral terbinafine is not effective for the treatment of pityriasis versicolor, but a topical 1% solution is available and has proven efficacious when used twice a day for seven days.[110]

Pityrosporum folliculitis may respond to the topical agents listed above. Benzoyl peroxide formulations may also be helpful. Systemic therapy is recommended for immunocompromised patients and those who do not respond to topical agents.

Reticulated papillomatosis may respond to topical tretinoin, or any of the topical formulations mentioned above. Calcipitriol cream may also be efficacious.[111] However, the unique efficacy of minocycline[92] in treating confluent of reticulated papillomatosis suggests that the yeast component may be less important in many cases. Systemic Malassezia infections and peritonitis require systemic antifungal therapy.

Catheter-associated Malassezia sepsis may respond to removal of the infected line with discontinuation of intralipid therapy. However, systemic antifungal therapy should be considered if rapid improvement is not noted.

CANDIDAL INFECTIONS

Introduction and historical note

Thrush (oral candidiasis) has been recognized since the time of Hippocrates. Bergin in 1841 and Bennett in 1844 demonstrated that the agent responsible for thrush was a fungus. Subsequently, Zenker described systemic candidiasis in 1861.

Candida albicans is part of the normal flora of the gastrointestinal tract and mucocutaneous areas of humans and virtually all other mammals. It is transmitted predominantly through person-to-person contact.

Candida is ordinarily noninvasive, with infection limited to the skin and mucous membranes when barrier function is disrupted or compromised. Macerated, inflamed, or otherwise damaged skin is at particular risk for infection with Candida. The incidence of both superficial and invasive candidal infections has increased substantially. This is due to an increasing population of patients who are chronically immunosuppressed following premature birth, organ transplantation, chemotherapy, or infection with HIV.[112,113] Candidiasis is increasingly noted as the presenting sign of HIV infection or AIDS.

Numerous factors influence the degree of oral and intestinal Candida colonization, as well as the propensity for overgrowth and invasion of mucosal or

108. Rogers CJ, Cook TF, Glaser DA (2000) Diagnosing Tinea versicolor: Don't scrape, just tape. **Pediatric Dermatol** 17:68–69.

109. Lange DS, Richards HM, Guarnieri J, Humeniuk JM et al. (1998) Ketoconazole 2% shampoo in the treatment of tinea versicolor: a multicenter, randomised, double-blind, placebo-controlled trial. **J Am Acad Dermatol** 39:944–950.

110. Vermeer BJ, Staats CC (1997) The efficacy of a topical application of terbinafine 1% solution in subjects with pityriasis versicolor: a placebo-controlled study. **Dermatology** 194 Suppl 1:22–24.

111. Schwartzberg JB, Schwartzberg HA (2000) Response of confluent and reticulate papillomatosis of Gougerot and Carteaud to topical tretinoin. **Cutis** 66:291–293.

112. McCarthy GM (1992) Host factors associated with HIV-related oral candidiasis. A review. **Oral Surg Oral Med Oral Pathol** 73:181–186.

113. Carpenter CC, Mayer KH, Stein MD et al. (1991) Human immunodeficiency virus infection in North American women: experience with 200 cases and a review of the literature. **Medicine** (Baltimore) 70:307–325.

cutaneous surfaces. Age, endocrine dysfunction, resident flora, malnutrition, trauma, prematurity, and the use of antibiotics or other medical interventions are all important risk factors. *C. albicans* is responsible for most infections, but *C. glabrata*, *C. tropicalis*, *C. Iusitaniae* and *C. parapsilis* have assumed increasing pathogenic importance in the past decade, particularly in the HIV-infected population. More than 20 additional and generally less virulent species of Candida have been identified.

Epidemiology

C. albicans colonizes the oral cavity of most newborns by the end of the second week of life, and can be cultured from the mouths of approximately 80% of infants by 4 weeks of age. If the yeast proliferates, the clinical findings of acute pseudomembranous candidiasis (thrush) develop. The prevalence of thrush varies with the population examined; approximately 0.5–20% of normal infants are affected.[114] More than 50% of HIV-infected individuals have oral candidiasis at some point in the course of their illness, and persistent thrush in a patient without other risk factors suggests HIV infection.[115]

Pathology

Infants born to mothers with symptomatic vaginal candidiasis appear to have an increased chance of developing thrush. If the maternal vagina is not infected, then the risk is as low as 1%. Prolonged length of stay in the hospital after birth is another risk factor for thrush. Treatment in a special care unit, such as an intensive care nursery, results in rapid colonization by Candida.[114] Infants born to HIV-positive mothers are at greatly increased risk of oral candidiasis.[115] Despite high colonization rates, only a fraction of infants with positive candidal cultures have clinical thrush, and the disease is temporary in most. It is thought that the establishment of normal oral flora eventually impedes the continued overgrowth of *C. albicans*, though proof is lacking.[116] Immunosuppression or changes in the oropharyngeal ecology induced by the use of steroid aerosols, antibiotics, or dental appliances can lead to recurrent oropharyngeal candidiasis.

Candida cannot ordinarily be cultured from most areas of the skin. The organism is, however, a common inhabitant of the perianal region and frequently causes infection when diapers are worn.[117] Candida dermatitis may occur in 4–6% of term infants, and peaks in incidence at 3 to 4 months of age. The increased warmth and moisture of the skin, and the presence of maceration and inflammation are important predisposing factors. Candida regularly colonizes areas of diaper dermatitis leading to prolonged and often more severe symptoms in affected infants. In one study, skin cultures from the diaper area of normal infants did not grow candida albicans, but 92% of infants with diaper dermatitis grew *C. albicans* from skin cultures.[118]

Several virulence factors have been identified as contributing to the pathogenicity of specific Candida strains. Resistance to neutrophil ingestion, increased adherence to epithelial cell walls, and specific fungal proteinases all play a role in the pathogenicity of a specific strain. Phospholipase B1 has been implicated as an important factor in candidal invasiveness. A candidal strain with a deletion of the gene encoding PLBI was found to possess decreased ability to invade gastric mucosa in a murine model. Reintroduction of the gene restored invasiveness and pathogenicity of the strain.[119] An intact immune system is crucial in preventing infection, and patients with deficiencies of secretory IgA or other immunodeficiencies are at particular risk for recurrent or severe infection.

Clinical findings

These are summarised in Table 26.16.

TABLE 26.16   Clinical presentations of candida infections
1. Thrush (oral candidiasis)
2. Paronychia
3. Onychia
4. Folliculitis
5. Vaginitis and vulvovaginitis
6. Intertriginous candidiasis
7. Esophagitis
8. Laryngitis
9. Line sepsis
10. Candidemia
11. Candiduria
12. Chronic mucocutaneous candidiasis

Thrush

On examination, thrush appears as white to gray, often "cheesy"-looking colonies that form "pseudomembranous" patches in the mouth (Fig. 26.16). When this material is gently removed with a tongue depressor, a raw red base is exposed. A KOH preparation from this pseudomembrane reveals abundant mycelial forms consisting of pseudohyphae often mixed with ovoid yeast forms (Fig. 26.17). A smear demonstrating only yeast forms is considered a normal finding and is not diagnostic.[116] Cultures of the oral cavity are often positive even in the absence of disease and are not helpful.

Other forms of oral candidiasis

Candida sometimes overgrows areas of leukoplakia, angular cheilitis, or black hairy tongue; in the latter a "fur" develops on the tongue. Some forms of oral inflammation with erosions or atrophy, including cases of erosive (atrophic) glossitis, are secondary to candidal overgrowth without formation of a pseudomembrane. One example is the erosive glossitis seen with antibiotic treatment.[120] Angular cheilosis, also called perlèche, is an inflammatory process caused by irritation at the angles of the mouth secondary to repeated licking or other irritants. These areas become secondarily infected with Candida,

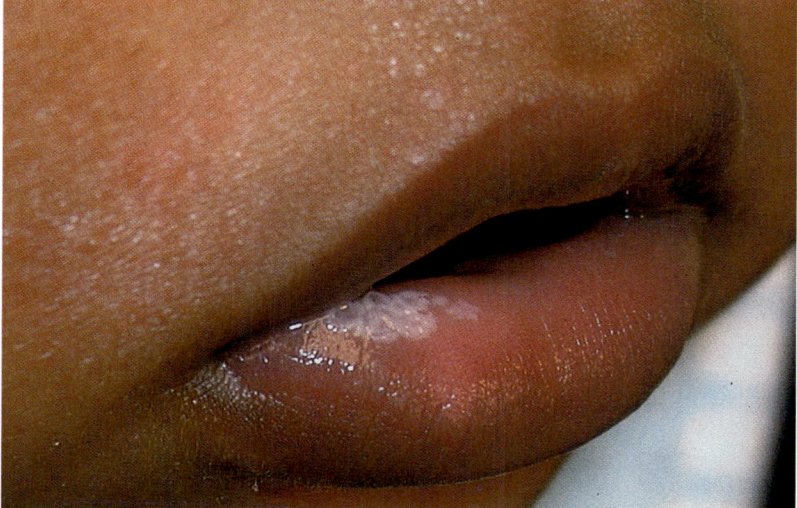

Fig. 26.16 Thrush with extension to the vermilion border (Courtesy Jon Alexander).

114. Jennison RF (1977) Thrush in infancy. **Arch Dis Child** 52:747–749.
115. Samaranayake LP, Holmstrup P (1989) Oral candidiasis and human immunodeficiency virus infection. **J Oral Pathol Med** 18:554–564.
116. Smith SMB, Meech RJ (1984) The polymicrobial nature of oropharyngeal thrush. **N Z Med J** 97:335–336.
117. Reboral A, Leyden JJ (1981) Napkin (diaper) dermatitis and gastrointestinal carriage of Candida albicans. **Br J Dermatol** 105:551–555.
118. Gokalp AS, Aldirmaz C, Oguz A et al. (1990) Relation between the intestinal flora and diaper dermatitis in infancy. **Trop Geogr Med** 42:238–240.
119. Mukherjee PK, Seshan KR, Leidich DS, Chandra J et al. (2001) Reintroduction of the PLB1 gene into Candida albicans restores virulence in vivo. **Microbiology** 147:2585–2597.
120. Dreizen S (1984) Oral candidiasis. **Am J Med** 77:28–33.

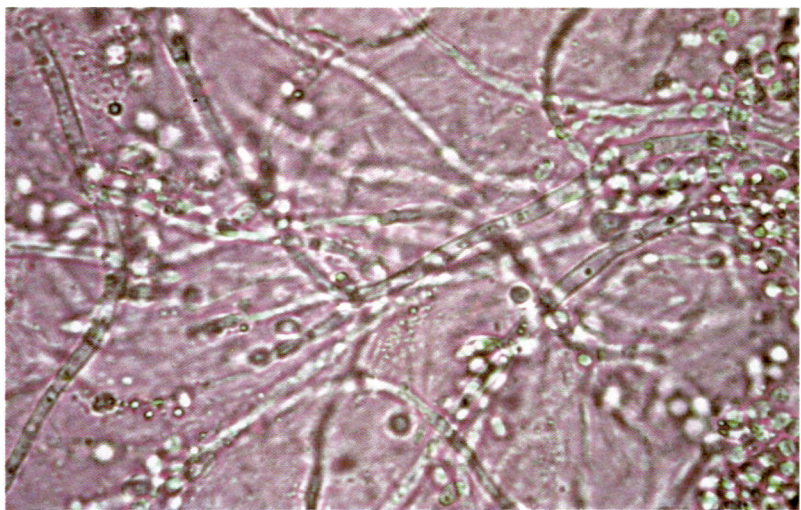

Fig. 26.17 KOH mount from infant with thrush (Fig. 26.16) showing pseudohyphae and yeast forms (Courtesy of Jon Alexander).

sometimes in combination with bacterial species. Median rhomboid glossitis may also represent a form of chronic oral candidiasis.[121]

Cutaneous candidiasis

Infected skin takes on a deep red color, similar to that of uncooked beef, with edema and "weeping." Crusting and tiny pustules, along with small rings of scale (collarettes), are often found, especially at the edge or periphery of the affected area; hence the name "satellite lesions." On occasion, plaques that closely resemble psoriasis are present. In candidiasis of the diaper area, the recessed areas of the inguinal folds are usually involved. The scrotum and penile shaft are commonly inflamed and oozing, and the vulva may become diffusely inflamed and tender. Involvement of the axillae, intragluteal cleft, or other intertriginous areas is more likely in obese or diabetic individuals. Changes in these intertriginous regions are identical to those seen with candidiasis of the groin. Itching is more common in intertriginous areas. Cutaneous candidiasis can be extremely tender, particularly in the diaper area, where periodic urine and stool deposition may lead to extreme burning. On rare occasions, Candida causes a highly inflammatory infection of the scalp that is accompanied by hair loss and closely resembles a kerion caused by dermatophytes. This process is associated with mucocutaneous candidiasis, as described below. Neonatal candidiasis developing after the first week of life, as opposed to congenital candidiasis (discussed below), tends to be more pustular.[122]

Paronychia

Chronic inflammation of the skin surrounding the nails is most often due to Candida; acute reactions are more commonly of bacterial origin. Candidal paronychia frequently follows chronic finger or thumb sucking and presents with periungual erythema, edema, and separation of the skin of the nail fold from the nail plate. Purulent discharge and nail dystrophy are frequent complications.

Infection of the web spaces between the fingers or toes (interdigital candidiasis or erosio interdigitale blastomycetica) is especially likely in individuals whose hands or feet remain moist for prolonged periods. In this disorder, erythema, scale and maceration occur at the involved sites. Occasionally the initial site of infection occurs underneath a ring. New mothers who frequently wash their hands following diaper changes are a high-risk group for this condition.

Vulvovaginal candidiasis is more common in adults than children, but can occur in childhood and adolescence, particularly when risk factors such as diabetes, immunosuppression, or prolonged antibiotic therapy are present. Clinical findings consist of tender or pruritic beefy red erythema, sometimes surrounded by small satellite papules and/or pustules. Yellow–white or cheesy discharge may also be present. The possibility of HIV infection must be considered in children with persistent or severe disease.

Diagnosis

A diagnosis of cutaneous candidiasis is confirmed by identifying mycelial forms, with pseudohyphae and budding yeast on KOH examination. Culture on Sabouraud's agar can be helpful but may be misleading because Candida can be cultured from noninfected skin, especially in the diaper area. Histopathologic examination may show subcorneal spongiform pustules with ovoid spores and branching septate hyphae present within the stratum corneum.

Differential diagnosis

Thrush

Food in the mouth may be mistaken for candida, but easily rubs away, revealing normal underlying mucosa. Lichen planus, squamous cell carcinoma, "leukoplakia," and the mucous patches of secondary syphilis are diagnostic considerations. None of these is ordinarily found in infancy or early childhood. Species of the yeast Trichosporon can cause an infection that imitates thrush (see below).[123]

Cutaneous candidiasis

Alternative diagnoses that should be considered in cutaneous candidiasis depend on the site involved (Table 26.17). Contact dermatitis and rarely psoriasis may be confused with candidiasis, particularly in the intertriginous

---

TABLE 26.17   Differential diagnosis of cutaneous candidiasis

Candida diaper dermatitis	Intertrigenous candida	Vulvovaginitis
Contact dermatitis	Erythrasma	Bacterial infection (staph, strep)
Seborrheic dermatitis	Psoriasis	Contact dermatitis
Psoriasis	Contact dermatitis	Pinworms
Tinea	Seborrheic dermatitis	Psoriasis
Metabolic deficiencies		Lichen sclerosus et atrophicus
Staph scalded skin		Foreign body
		Sexual abuse

121. Cooke BED (1975) Median rhomboid glossitis: candidiasis and not a developmental anomaly. **Br J Dermatol** 93:399.
122. Resnick SD, Greenberg RA (1989) Autoinoculated palmar pustules in neonatal candidiasis. **Pediatr Dermatol** 6:206.
123. Oelz O, Schaffner A, Frick P, Schaer G (1983) Trichosporon capitatum: thrush-like oral infection, local invasion, fungaemia and metastatic abscess formation in a leukaemic patient. **J Infect** 6:183–185.

areas. A reaction to wipes, cleansing agents, or creams being used for therapy may occur. Paronychia, particularly acute lesions, may represent a bacterial infection or herpetic whitlow.

Therapeutics

Oral thrush

Most oral candidiasis in immunocompetent hosts will respond to oral nystatin suspension (100 000 units/ml, four times a day) or clotrimazole troches. Questions have arisen regarding the efficacy and potential carcinogenicity of Gentian violet, which was utilized in the past for this purpose.[124] For persistent cases, clotrimazole troches can be administered one to three times daily and allowed to dissolve in the mouth. In young children it can be inserted into a pacifier or may be crushed, mixed into a viscous material such as methylcellulose, and applied to the inside of the mouth.[125] Oral fluconazole or intraconazole may be beneficial when the patient's immune status is compromised or there is otherwise an increased risk of complications from oral candidiasis.[126,127] However, itraconazole is not yet FDA approved for this use. An important part of treatment is elimination or reduction of predisposing factors, such as antibiotic use or immunosuppression.

Cutaneous, diaper dermatitis and vulvovaginal candidiasis

An essential component of the treatment of cutaneous candidiasis is elimination of predisposing factors. Frequent diaper changes are crucial in those with diaper dermatitis, and the introduction of superabsorbant disposable diapers has been a useful adjunct in the treatment of candida diaper dermatitis, and diaper dermatitis in general.

Predisposing factors such as antibiotic therapy, immunologic or endocrine disorders should be identified. Topical nystatin or topical antifungal creams such as clotrimazole, econazole, naftifine, or terbinafine may be used, and the addition of oral nystatin is sometimes helpful in cases of candida diaper dermatitis.[128] As necessary, topical agents should be reapplied sparingly after washing or diaper change. Protective barrier ointments containing zinc oxide can be applied over the antifungal agent once the skin is thoroughly dry. Sulcralfate, a bile acid and pepsin neutralizer, has been used effectively in paste form for severe diaper dermatitis. One oral dose of fluconazole 150mg is also effective for the treatment of candida vulvovaginitis in adolescents and adults.

GRANULOMATOUS CANDIDIASIS (GRANULOMA GLUTEALE INFANTUM)

The etiology of this disorder is unknown, but many consider it a form of candidal infection. Clinical findings consist of deep purplish red smooth, firm nodules usually present in the genital area, buttocks, and inner thighs. It generally presents in the first year of life, though cases have been reported in incontinent adults. Granulomas are not present on histopathology. Many believe it is a complication of diaper dermatitis treated with topical steroids, while others consider it an unusual response to candidal infection. This disorder can occur in the absence of prior topical steroid therapy. Treatment consists of good hygiene in the area, and topical antifungal therapy if candidal infection is documented. Topical corticosteroids have been used by some experts, but flare may occur. Differential diagnosis includes mastocytoma, juvenile xanthogranuloma, Langerhans cell histiocytosis, and cutaneous

TABLE 26.18	Manifestations of candida infections in infancy

Congenital candidiasis
Neonatal candidiasis
Thrush
Candida diaper dermatitis
Candidemia

leukemic infiltrates. Most cases usually resolve within one to two months, but if lesions are refractory or atypical, biopsy should be considered.

CONGENITAL CUTANEOUS CANDIDIASIS

Epidemiology

Congenital cutaneous candidiasis is an uncommon and ordinarily benign infection, presenting at birth or within the first six days of life in neonates exposed to candida *in utero* (Table 26.18).[129–133] Although 20–25% of all pregnant women develop candidal vulvovaginitis, only a small number of infants born to infected women develop congenital candidiasis. Risk factors for congenital disease include early preterm birth, the presence of a maternal foreign body such as an IUD or cervical sutures, and diagnostic amniocentesis.

Pathogenesis

Congenital candidiasis presumably occurs when candidal organisms within an infected vagina ascend and penetrate the uterine cavity. Infection can occur despite the presence of intact membranes, and infected babies have been born following cesarean section in the absence of ruptured membranes.[134] The organisms spread from infected chorioallantoic membranes to the amniotic fluid which surrounds and bathes the fetus. Contamination of the gastrointestinal and pulmonary tract theoretically results from swallowing and aspiration of infected amniotic fluid.

Risk of invasive disseminated disease is highest in very low birth weight pre-term infants. Their incompletely developed epidermal barrier, as well as the immature immune system of such neonates, increases the risk of invasive systemic disease. Neonates weighing <1000 grams are at greater risk for the development of systemic infection and death.[135]

Clinical findings

Skin lesions characteristically develop within the first few days of life and consist of a generalized erythematous 2–4mm macular eruption which quickly progresses to small papules and pustules superimposed on an erythematous base. The back, skin folds and extensor surfaces are most frequently involved, and pustular lesions on the palms and soles are usually present. A burn-like dermatitis, ecchymotic areas, onychia and paronychia have also been reported.[135] Very premature infants may present with a variety of findings. The majority of infants weighing <1000 grams present with diffuse erythematous patches which then desquamate or erode. White to yellow papules and plaques may stud the surface of the umbilical cord (funisitis) or placenta. Thrush is not usually seen.

Full-term infants usually have a benign course with disease limited to the cutaneous surface. Premature, and especially very low birth weight infants are

124. Littlefield NA, Gayler DW, Blackwell BN, Allen RR (1989) Chronic toxicity/carcinogenicity studies of gentian violet in Fisher 311 rats: two-generation exposure. Food Chem Toxicol 27:239.
125. Quintilliani R, Owens NJ, Quercia RA et al. (1984) Treatment and prevention of oropharyngeal candidiasis. Am J Med 77(4D):44–48.
126. Dhondt F, Ninane J, De Beule K et al. (1992) Oral candidosis: treatment with absorbable and nonabsorbable antifungal agents in children. Mycoses 35:1.
127. Blatchford NR (1990) Treatment of oral candidosis with itraconazole: a review. J Am Acad Dermatol 23:565–567.
128. Munz D, Powell KR, Pai CH (1982) Treatment of candidal diaper dermatitis: a double-blind placebo-controlled comparison of topical nystatin with topical plus oral nystatin. J Pediatr 101:1022.

129. Kam LA, Giacoia GP (1975) Congenital cutaneous candidiasis. Am J Dis Child 129:1215.
130. Chapel TA, Gagliardi C, Nichols W (1982) Congenital cutaneous candidiasis. J Am Acad Dermatol 6:926.
131. Almeida Santos L, Beceiro J, Hernandez R et al. (1991) Congenital cutaneous candidiasis: report of four cases and review of the literature. Eur J Pediatr 150:336–338.
132. Whyte RK, Hussain Z, de SA D (1982) Antenatal infections with Candida species. Arch Dis Child 57:528.
133. Faix RG, Naglie RA, Barr M (1986) Intrapleural inoculation of Candida in the infant with congenital cutaneous candidiasis. Am J Perinatol 3:119.
134. Dvorak AM, Gavaller B (1966) Congenital systemic candidiasis. N Engl J Med 274:540–543.
135. Darmstadt GL, Dinulos JG, Miller Z (2000) Congenital Cutaneous Candidiasis: Clinical Presentation, Pathogenesis, and Management Guidelines. Pediatrics 105:438–444.

at higher risk for pneumonia, hepatitis, and sepsis. Many reports have documented a high morbidity and mortality in such children. The death rate in neonates with burn-like dermatitis appears higher than in those with the typical papulo-pustular presentation.[136]

Diagnosis/laboratory findings

KOH preparation of an unroofed vesicle reveals pseudohyphae and budding yeast forms. KOH and culture of suspicious lesions on the skin, umbilical cord, or placenta should be obtained. Children with systemic disease may have positive blood, urine, and cerebrospinal fluid cultures. Elevated white blood cell counts, hepatitis, hyperglycemia, and glucosuria may also develop.

Treatment

Full-term infants who lack systemic symptoms generally have a benign course and do not require any therapy. Topical antifungal agents can be applied twice a day to affected areas, and the infant should be observed for pulmonary distress or other signs of systemic disease, as more severe involvement can rarely occur in full-term infants. Any child with respiratory distress or signs of systemic illness should receive systemic antifungal therapy. Amphotericin B is first-line therapy, but fluconazole has been used successfully in some instances, when the organism is sensitive and significant concern regarding the toxicity of Amphotericin B exists. Additional therapy with 5-flucytosine is sometimes utilized. Liposomal formulations of amphotericin are currently under investigation, and appear as efficacious with less toxicity; they are therefore often substituted if toxicity develops while on stardard amphotericin therapy.

Premature and low-birth-weight infants are at higher risk for systemic involvement and warrant full evaluation and systemic antifungal therapy.

Differential diagnosis

A variety of other infections need to be considered in the differential diagnosis of CCC. These include staphylococcal disease, listeria, syphilis, herpes simplex, varicella zoster, and enteroviral infections. Other considerations are benign pustular disorders such as erythema toxicum and transient neonatal pustular melanosis. Langerhans cell histiocytosis must also enter the differential diagnosis.

Invasive fungal dermatitis

This condition is seen in very low birth weight infants and consists of erosive crusting lesions. Candida, Aspergillus, and Trichosporum have all been cultured from skin biopsies of this disorder. Histopathological exam shows hyphal elements extending from the stratum corneum to the epithelium, and occasionally the dermis. It is distinguished from typical congenital candidiasis by its onset after birth, and its classic erosive, crusting lesions.

NEONATAL CANDIDIASIS
Epidemiology/pathogenesis

This disorder is not contracted *in utero*, but instead is usually acquired during passage of the fetus through an infected birth canal, with ingestion of contaminated fluids. Premature and low-birth-weight infants are at higher risk for disseminated disease, and must be monitored for this possibility. One multicenter study of late-onset sepsis in neonates documented that Candida

species accounted for 7% of bloodstream infections[137] while another indicated that Candida species were second in frequency among blood culture isolates from neonates in high-risk nurseries.[138] Risk factors for systemic neonatal candidiasis include prematurity, broad-spectrum antibiotics, steroids, prolonged endotracheal intubation, parenteral alimentation, and central venous catheter placement. Most infants with *Candida albicans* infections acquire them vertically, while those with *C. parapsilis* are more often associated with nosocornial acquistion.[139] An increased incidence of systemic candidiasis in extremely low birth weight infants was noted in one series when a neonatal nursery instituted treatment of premature infants with topical petrolatum ointment for skin care.[140]

Clinical findings

Neonatal candidiasis generally presents after the first week of life, and consists of oropharyngeal involvement and perianal erythema with pustules and satellite lesions. The genital area is often involved as well. If disseminated disease occurs, signs of sepsis develop, including temperature instability, fever, and pneumonia.

Treatment

The use of agents such as topical antifungals and barrier creams in the perianal and genital area, and oral nystatin are usually sufficient to resolve cutaneous manifestations in full-term healthy children. Short-term use of a weak topical corticosteroid agent such as hydrocortisone ointment 2.5% may be helpful initially to decrease severe erythema in the diaper area. Refractory or severe cases are occasionally the result of coexistent candidal infection in the mother, and examination of her nipples and queries regarding moniliasis should be undertaken. Pacifiers should also be thoroughly cleansed. Rarely, treatment with a systemic fluconazole for a short course of therapy may be required to treat particularly severe cases.

Amphotericin B is the treatment of choice for premature infants and those who have systemic findings; liposomal formulations are utilized when toxicity develops during standard amphotericin therapy. Fluconazole may be used in those cases where the organism is susceptible.

Candida esophagitis

Gastrointestinal overgrowth and invasion by Candida species has become an increasing health problem in both very low birth weight infants, and in the ever-growing numbers of immunocompromised patients. Symptoms of candidal esophagitis include dysphagia, chronic pain, and bleeding. Many of these patients do not have thrush. Gastric and intestinal infections are less common than esophagitis. Although radiographs may be diagnostically helpful, endoscopy along with culture or biopsy is superior. Gastrointestinal candidiasis is treated similarly to oral candidiasis, but medications are swallowed and given in higher doses, when indicated. Useful regimens include oral nystatin, 5–10ml or clotrimazole troches four or more times daily. Fluconazole and itraconazole have been used for therapy of such patients. Fluconazole-resistant species are being increasingly identified, and species identification and sensitivity patterns should be obtained in appropriate cases.

SYSTEMIC CANDIDIASIS
Pathogenesis

Disseminated candidiasis continues to increase in prevalence with increasingly intensive medical care and immunosuppression. Systemic candidiasis, which

136. Pradeepkuma VK, Rajaurai VS, Tan KW (1998) Congenital candidiasis: varied presentations. **J Perinatol** 18:311–316.
137. Stoll BJ, Gordon T et al. (1996) Late-onset sepsis in very low birth weight neonates: a report from the National Institute of Child Health and Human Development Neonatal Research Network. **J Pediatr** 129:63–71.
138. Gaynes RP, Edwards JR, Jarvis WR et al. (1996) Nosocomial infections among neonates in high-risk nurscries in the United States. **Pediatrics** 98:357–361.
139. Melville C, Kempley S, Graham J, Berry CL (1996) Early onset systemic Candida infection in extremely preterm neonates. **Eur J Pediatr** 155:904–906.
140. Campbell JR, Zaccaria E Baker CJ (2000) Systemic candidiasis in extremely low birth weight infants receiving topical petrolatum ointment for skin care: A case-control study. **Pediatrics** 105:1041–1045.

consists of Candida infection in an otherwise sterile site such as urine, blood, or cerebrospinal fluid, occurs in 2–4% of very low birth weight infants. Long-term hospitalization, especially in an intensive care nursery, is associated with a substantial risk of candidal sepsis, and its common sequelae of renal or central nervous system (CNS) involvement.[141,142] Invasive measures such as catheters greatly increase the risk of systemic candida infection.

Clinical findings

Macules and papules are the more common cutaneous findings. Nodules occasionally develop, and in such cases Candida is often found in the dermis. These lesions may sometimes possess pale centers. Abscesses or areas of necrotic skin may also develop.[143,144] *Candida tropicalis* may be more likely to cause cutaneous manifestations in association with sepsis than *C. albicans*.[145] *C. krusei* appears especially likely to cause nodules of the skin.[146] Systemic signs associated with Candida sepsis are similar to bacteremia, and include termperature instability, respiratory distress, seizures, and hypotension. Ophthalmologic examination may reveal retinal lesions.

Diagnosis

A KOH or Gram stain of material from an involved area of skin in a patient with systemic candidiasis usually reveals a mixture of mycelia and yeast-phase organisms that is characteristic of Candida. Biopsy, with or without the aid of fungal stains, shows mycelia and spores in a pustule, dermis or deep epidermis, sometimes accompanied by a polymorphonuclear cell infiltrate. Buffy coat smear microscopy may be performed at the bedside, is 100% specific, and confirms the diagnosis rapidly. A frozen section of a biopsy or snip of skin sometimes allows rapid identification of organisms. Recovery of the organism is optimized by the use of biphasic or lysis-centrifugation systems. Germ tube formation within culture supports the diagnosis of *Candida albicans*. Opthalmologic evaluation may be useful if retinal lesions are noted.

Treatment

Early institution of treatment is critical. Because cultures can take several days to grow, it is necessary to treat on the basis of clinical suspicion. An imidazole agent such as fluconazole is indicated in cases where involvement is limited to the esophagus or stomach, but intravenous amphotericin B is still generally recommended for disseminated disease. Intravenous treatment with 0.5–1.0mg/kg per day is recommended, and usually administered for 14–21 days in severe systemic disease. Liposome formulations of amphotericin have also been used successfully. Nephrotoxicity and hepatotoxicity are possible complications of therapy. *In vitro* and clinical studies support synergism of flucytosine and amphotericin against *C. albicans*; therefore 5-fluorocystosine is sometimes added to the therapeutic regimen. Systemic fluconazole has also been used for treatment, but resistant forms of Candida have been identified, particularly in the non-albicans species.

CHRONIC MUCOCUTANEOUS CANDIDIASIS

Chronic mucocutaneous candidiasis is (CMC) a rare disorder of unknown cause characterized by recurrent or severe infections of the mouth, nails, or other skin surfaces with Candida. It is usually recognized in infancy or childhood, and is often associated with genetic, immunologic, or endocrinologic defects. Autosomal recessive and dominant forms occur, which are associated with long-term infection with Candida and other fungi.[147–150] Though T-cell defects are

TABLE 26.19 Forms of chronic mucocutaneous candidiasis

Autosomal recessive – otherwise healthy, early onset
Autosomal dominant – usually more severe skin involvement, early onset
CMC with endocrinopathy – AR and AD forms, early onset
Diffuse granulomatous – early onset
Late onset – may be associated with thymoma/myasthenia gravis
Associated with immunologic disorders (T-cell deficiency, DiGeorge, Nezelof thymic dysplasia, Swiss-type agammaglobulinemia, AIDS)
Associated with zinc deficiency

most common, defects in cell lines other than lymphocytes may be present.[149] Patients with CMC are also susceptible to infections with encapsulated bacteria, and may have associated IgG2 and IgG4 deficiency. Recurrent or severe infections with organisms other than Candida can be seen in 80% of patients, and may result in serious morbidity or death. There is some tendency for the condition to improve in adulthood. Several distinct syndromes are collectively referred to as chronic mucocutaneous candidiasis, as defined by clinical characteristics and associated features (Table 26.19).

Clinical findings

The early-onset syndrome usually presents with yeast infections of the mouth, skin, vagina, and fingernails in early childhood. Thrush, paronychia, diaper dermatitis, and nail involvement are persistent and unresponsive to traditional topical therapies. The distal fingers become bulbous, with swelling and erythema of the nail folds. Crusted, massive hyperkeratotic masses (Candida granulomas) with sharp borders may develop on the scalp. Brown plaques may appear on the dorsa of the hands and feet, in the perioral area and on intertriginous skin. Late-onset syndromes develop similar, but less severe findings.

Diagnosis

Early onset of recalcitrant and recurrent candidal infections should raise suspicion for this disorder. Children should be evaluated for underlying autoimmune and endocrine disorders.

Treatment

Antifungal therapy is the mainstay of treatment. Systemic therapy with fluconazole, itraconazole, or ketoconazole is often necessary. Attempts to restore T-cell function utilizing transfer factor are usually associated with temporary improvements. As drug resistance may occur, the use of maintenance therapy is not recommended. The possibility of concurrent dermatophytosis or bacterial infections must be kept in mind.

TRICHOSPORON INFECTIONS

Trichosporon is a yeast which is found in soil and water, as well as on human skin, hair, nails, mucocutaneous surfaces and the respiratory tract. Usually a commensal, it can cause superficial hair and skin conditions, as well as invasive and disseminated disease. Superficial infections are more common in tropical and subtropical regions, but this yeast is associated with a number of disorders (Table 26.20). The yeast shares many clinical and histopathological features with Candida, and is frequently confused with that organism.

141. Faix RG (1984) Systemic Candida infections in infants in intensive care nurseries: high incidence of central nervous system involvement. J Pediatr 105:616–622.
142. Pappu LD, Purohit DM, Bradford BF et al. (1984) Primary renal candidiasis in two preterm neonates. Report of cases and review of literature on renal candidiasis in infancy. Am J Dis Child 138:923–926.
143. File TM, Jr, Marina OA, Flowers FP (1979) Necrotic skin lesions associated with disseminated candidiasis. Arch Dermatol 15:214.
144. Baley JE, Kliegman RM, Fanaroff AA (1984) Disseminated fungal infections in very-low-birth-weight infants: clinical manifestations and epidemiology. Pediatrics 73:144.
145. Leibovitz E, Iuster-Reicher A, Amitai M, Mogilner B (1992) Systemic candidal infections associated with use of peripheral venous catheters in neonates; a 9 year experience. Clin Infect Dis 14:485.

146. McQuillen DP, Zingman BS, Meunier F, Levitz SM (1992) Invasive infections due to Candida krusei: report of 10 cases of fungemia that include three cases of endophthalmitis. Clin Infect Dis 14:472.
147. Kirkpatrick CH (1989) Chronic mucocutaneous candidiasis. Eur J Clin Microbiol Infect Dis 8:448.
148. Kirkpatrick CH (1984) Host factors in defense against fungal infections. Am J Med (suppl.)77,4D:1–12.
149. Yamazaki M, Yasui K, Kawai H et al. (1984) A monocyte disorder in siblings with chronic candidiasis. A combined abnormality of monocyte mobility and phagocytosis-killing ability. Am J Dis Child 138:192–196.
150. Dwyer JM (1981) Chronic mucocutaneous candidiasis. Annu Rev Med 32:491.

TABLE 26.20 Trichosporon infections

White piedra
Sepsis
Onychomycosis
Pneumonia
Meningitis
Arthritis
Endophthalmitis

Epidemiology

Up to 27% of normal individuals are colonized with *T. beigelii* in the perigenital area.[151] The prevalence of colonization varies with the population examined. On average, 12% of a population is colonized, with the lowest frequency in women.[151] In tropical climates, colonization of the perianal or other intertriginous areas can produce intertrigo with itching and burning.[152] At least seven human pathogenic subtypes of Trichosporon have been identified using molecular biology techniques. White piedra, also called trichosporosis, is found sporadically in the USA and Europe, especially among children and young adults.

Clinical findings

White piedra presents as asymptomatic white to tan elongated nodules that are loosely adherent to the hair of the scalp, eyelashes, beard, axillae, or groin. Scalp involvement is less common. The nodules may be mistaken for the nits of pediculosis or for hair shaft abnormalities; however, they completely encircle the hair shaft, and on KOH examination, yeast-like cells can be identified (Fig. 26.18A, B).

Individuals with systemic infection may have nonspecific findings consistent with sepsis. Cutaneous findings in infected neonates may include peeling, oozing, and erosions. Pustules and erythema are not usually present. Lesions in older children and adults can consist of papules, erythema, or pigmented scaling. Similar to Malassezia, trichosporon may be found as an asymptomatic colonizer of catheters in very low birth weight infants, as well as a pathogen which can lead to sepsis and death.[153] *T. beigelii* sepsis can cause localized or multifocal infection of the kidneys, spleen, lungs, liver, bone marrow, eyes, or CNS, especially in patients undergoing chemotherapy or those with neutropenia.[154] Cutaneous findings in older children or adults with disseminated disease include erythematous papules or necrotic areas. Biopsy reveals perivascular budding yeast forms. Treatment is difficult, and the mortality rate is high.[153]

Diagnosis

KOH examination reveals small nodules containing arthroconidia that encircle the shaft. KOH evaluation of scales from infected skin shows arthrocondia arranged in a tightly packed fashion, which resembles a cluster of pomegranate seeds. Fungal culture is positive for white creamy colonies, which may be mistaken for candida species.

Differential diagnosis

Differential diagnosis of hair lesions includes black piedra, which will be dark. Combined infections with both *P. hortae* and *T. beigelii* have been documented and result in clinical manifestations of both black and white piedra. Other considerations in the differential diagnosis include scabies, nits, dandruff, and hair casts. Trichomycosis axillaris, an infection caused by corynebacterium species, may also resemble piedra. This condition involves the axillary or pubic hairs. White, yellow, red, or black concretions may be present in this condition.

Treatment

Clipping or shaving the infected hair is often recommended, as no highly efficacious topical agent exists. Mercuric bichloride has been used successfully for scalp infections in India, as has topical dequalinium chloride.

Systemic infection has a high mortality rate, and systemic antifungal therapy is not always effective. Although Amphotericin B is the usual treatment, intolerance to this therapy has been documented.[153] 5-flucytosine, fluconazole, itraconazole, miconazole, and voriconazole are active against trichosporon *in vitro*, and are considered therapeutic alternatives by many experts.[154]

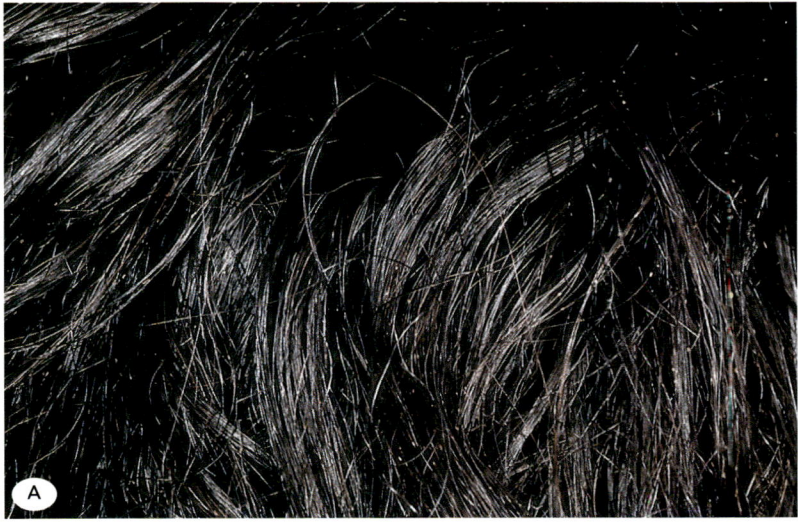
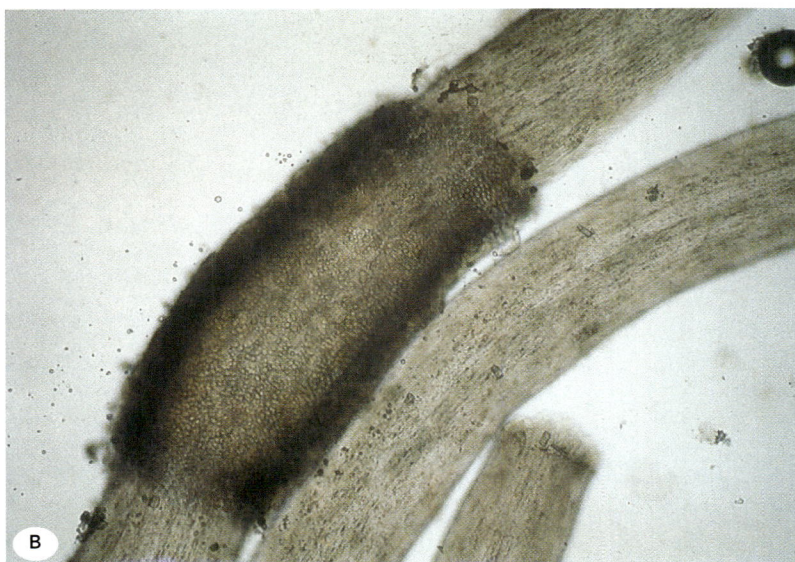

Fig. 26.18 White piedra. (A) Numerous white nodules on the hair of a 7-year-old girl, resembling nits. (B) Encircling nodule of white piedra (Courtesy of Julie Schaffer MD and Richard Antaya MD).

151. Ellner K, McBride ME, Rosen T, Berman D (1991) Prevalence of *Trichosporon beigelii*. Colonization of normal perigenital skin. **J Med Vet Mycol** 29:99.
152. Kamalem A, Senithamilselvi G, Ajithadas K, Thambiah AS (1988) Cutaneous trichosporosis. **Mycopathologia** 101:167.
153. Fisher DJ, Christy C, Spafford P et al. (1993) Neonatal Trichosporon beigelii infection: report of a cluster of cases in a neonatal intensive care unit. **Pediatr Infect Dis J** 12:149–155.
154. Erer B, Galimbert M, Lucarelli G et al. (2000) Trichosporon beigelii: a life-threatening pathogen in immunocompromised hosts. **Bone Marrow Transplantation** 25:745–749.

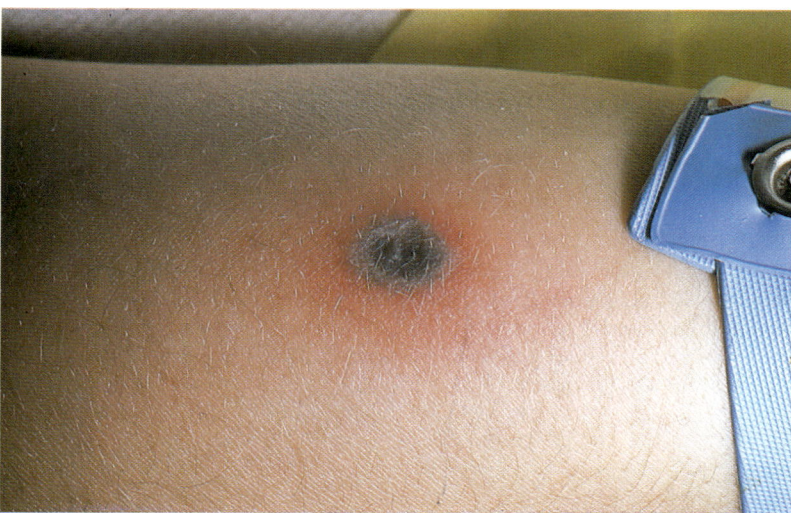

Fig. 26.19 Fusarium: necrotic nodule of Fusarium sepsis.

PATHOGENIC MOLDS

A number of molds have been identified as cutaneous pathogens in humans. These include Aspergillus, Zygomycosis and Fusarium. They frequently infect immunocompromised individuals, including premature infants, at sites where a break in the skin has occurred. Typical appearance includes blisters, purpura, necrosis, or nodules (Fig. 26.19). Crusted erosions are another common lesion, and may occur at sites of intravenous taping. Contamination of dressings and tongue depressors used as splints with zygomyces has been reported. Penicillium marniffei, an organism which produces a characteristic red pigment in culture, has also been isolated in immunosuppressed individuals.

Diagnosis and treatment
Skin biopsy with culture should be obtained and evaluated for the presence of hyphal elements. Amphotericin B is currently the treatment of choice for most mold infections, and lipid formulations are often utilized. Concurrent therapy with 5-flucytosine is sometimes used. Debridement and more aggressive surgical excision is often required in infected neonates.

TINEA NIGRA

Tinea nigra is caused by a dermatiaceous fungus, not by a dermatophyte; therefore, like pityriasis versicolor (tinea versicolor), it is misnamed.[155–157] *Phaeoannellomyces werneckii*, previously classified as Cladosporium or Exophiala, is responsible. Although usually a tropical disease, it is sometimes seen in the United States and Europe. Increasingly, cases develop after travel to tropical or subtropical regions.

Infection is confined to the stratum corneum. The palms are affected most frequently, but other body areas, particularly the dorsum of the hands or the plantar aspect of the feet may be involved. There is usually no itching or inflammation. Characteristically, light brown, dark brown, or black macules with sharp borders develop and enlarge peripherally. The edges tend to be more darkly pigmented, and visible scale is minimal to absent. Tinea nigra is easily confused with talon noir, malignant melanoma, or melanocytic nevus.[155,156]

KOH examination reveals abundant gray-brown to olive branching mycelia. A superficial shave biopsy of the stratum corneum, examined with KOH, may increase the yield of visualized fungi. *P. werneckii* can be cultured on Sabouraud's glucose agar. Colonies tend to be dark green with gray to black areas. Biopsy shows branching or nonbranching hyphae in the outermost portions of a thickened stratum corneum. Hyphae may be present in large quantities, forming clusters, but ordinarily there is only a scant superficial perivascular infiltrate. Miconazole cream,[157] newer topical antifungals, keratolytic agents such as salicylic acid, or 10% thiabendazole suspension applied topically are effective treatments. The organism is not sensitive to griseofulvin.

DEEP FUNGAL INFECTIONS

Hector W. Caceres-Rios

Fungal infections involving structures apart from the epidermis include many uncommon "tropical" and chronic disorders classified unclearly as deep mycosis, subcutaneous mycosis or systemic mycosis. Classifications based on taxonomical, clinical or immunological criteria are of limited value for clinicians. In this chapter we propose a classification based on clinical hallmarks, under the heading of "Deep fungal infections" (Table 26.21).

The term *subcutaneous mycosis* will refer to fungal infections affecting subcutaneous tissue and skin, *systemic mycosis* will refer to to infections caused by dimorphic fungi with primary inner organ involvement and a tendency to dissemination, and *opportunistic mycosis* to infections caused by usually low pathogenic agents in immunocompromised hosts.

SUBCUTANEOUS MYCOSIS
Mycetoma

Introduction and historical note
Mycetoma is a chronic granulomatous infection caused by true fungi (maduromycotic mycetoma or eumycetoma) and anaerobic bacteria (actinomycotic mycetoma or actinomycetoma). The main characteristics are striking swelling, multiple fistulae, and grain-filled discharge.

The first description is attributed to missionaries working in Madura, India, in 1714 and therefore Colebrook in 1842 called the disease "Madura foot." In 1861, Carter proposed the term mycetoma.

Etiology and pathogenesis
The organisms conglomerate into compact colonies that are discharged from fistulae as grains with characteristics varying according to species (Table 26.22).

Actinomycotic mycetomas have been named exogenous actinomycotic mycetoma in order to differentiate them from the endogenous actinomycotic mycetoma, which corresponds to actinomycosis, a chronic suppurative infection produced by other Actinomyces species.[158]

TABLE 26.21 Deep fungal infections: clinical classification		
Subcutaneous	**Systemic**	**Opportunistic**
Mycetoma	Blastomycosis	Cryptococcosis
Sporotrichosis	Paracoccidioidomycosis	Aspergillosis
Chromoblastomycosis	Coccidiodomycosis	Zygomycosis
Lobomycosis	Histoplasmosis	
Rhinosporidiosis		

155. Palmer SR, Bass JW, Mandojana R, Wittler RR (1989) Tinea nigra palmaris and plantaris: a black fungus producing black spots on the palms and soles. **Pediatr Infect Dis J** 8:48.
156. Vaffee AS (1970) Tinea nigra palmaris resembling malignant melanoma. **N Engl J Med** 238:1112.
157. Marks JG, King RD, Davis BM (1980) Treatment of tinea nigra palmaris with miconazole **Arch Dermatol** 116:321–322.
158. De Souza V, Zaitz C (1998) Actinomicetos, micetomas actinomicóticos e outras doenças causadas por actinomicetos. In: Compêndio de Micologia Médica, Zaitz C, Campbell I, Marques S, et al. eds. Rio de Janeiro: Editora Médica e Científica, pp. 21–34.

TABLE 26.22 Etiological agents of mycetomas

		Species	Characteristics of grains
Actinomycetes	Nocardia	brasiliensis	White microscopic
		asteroides	White microscopic
		caviae	White microscopic
	Streptomyces	somaliensis	White small
	Actinomadura	madurae	White yellowish large (Fig. 26.20)
		pelletieri	Red microscopic
Eumycetes	Madurella	mycetomatis	Dark
		grisea	Dark
	Pyrenochaeta	romeroi	Dark
		mackinnonii	Dark
	Leptosphaeria	senegalensis	Dark
		tompkinsii	Dark
	Exophiala	jeanselmei	Dark
	Curvularia	lunata	Dark
		geniculata	Dark
	Phialophora	verrucosa	Dark
	Pseudoallescheria	boydii	White or yellow
	Acremonium	falciforme	White or yellow
		recifei	White or yellow
		kiliensi	White or yellow
	Fusarium		White or yellow
	Neotestudina	rosatii	White or yellow

Fungal walls become thickened into grains, making the fungus less penetrable by antifungals. Immunoglobulin M (IgM) may contribute to the formation of the grain periphery. Fungi like *Madurella mycetomatis* and *M. grisea* produce 1,8-dihydroxynaphthalene melanin, an extracellular cement that combines with host tissue debris and proteins, providing extra protection.[159]

Epidemiology

The distribution is predominantly in tropical and subtropical climates, between latitudes 15°S and 30°N, with temperatures of 30°–37°C, relative humidity of 60–80% and 200–1000mm of rain. The highest frequencies occur in Africa[160] and India. In America, the most important series come from Mexico, Venezuela, and Brazil.[161,162]

Actinomycotic mycetoma is the most frequent; Nocardia causes 97.8% of cases in Central America[161] and in West Africa *A. pelletieri* is the usual pathogen.[163]

In general, eumycetomas constitute the minority of mycetomas. In Mexico they account for 2.2% of cases.[161] However, in Africa they represent the most frequent form.[164] The responsible agents are largely *M. mycetomatis* and *M. grisea*. A case of maduromycotic mycetoma associated with human immunodeficiency virus (HIV) infection has been recently reported.[165]

Cutaneous inoculation occurs through minor injuries with thorns or splinters or from animal bites.

The disease appears mainly in men in 3rd to 5th decades of life, although a large survey in Mexico showed 35% of cases between 16 and 30 years old.[164] Isolated cases have been reported in children.[166,167]

Clinical features

Incubation ranges from weeks to months and even years and the course is chronic. The lower extremities are affected in 70%, mainly the feet (50%).

Clinical features are similar in actinomycetomas and eumycetomas, although certain differences have been claimed. *N. brasiliensis* and *A. pelletieri* cause more inflammation and fistulae, while *A. madurae* and *S. somaliensis* produce lesions with a woody consistency with fewer fistulae.[164]

Mycetoma starts with a papule, nodule or localized subcutaneous inflammation that progressively enlarges to form abscesses and draining sinuses. Purulent drainage contains grains of varying size (Fig. 26.20) and color depending on the causative organism. Crusting scarring and exuberant granulation tissue may develop (Fig. 26.21). The infection may spread to fascia, muscle, bones, and viscera.

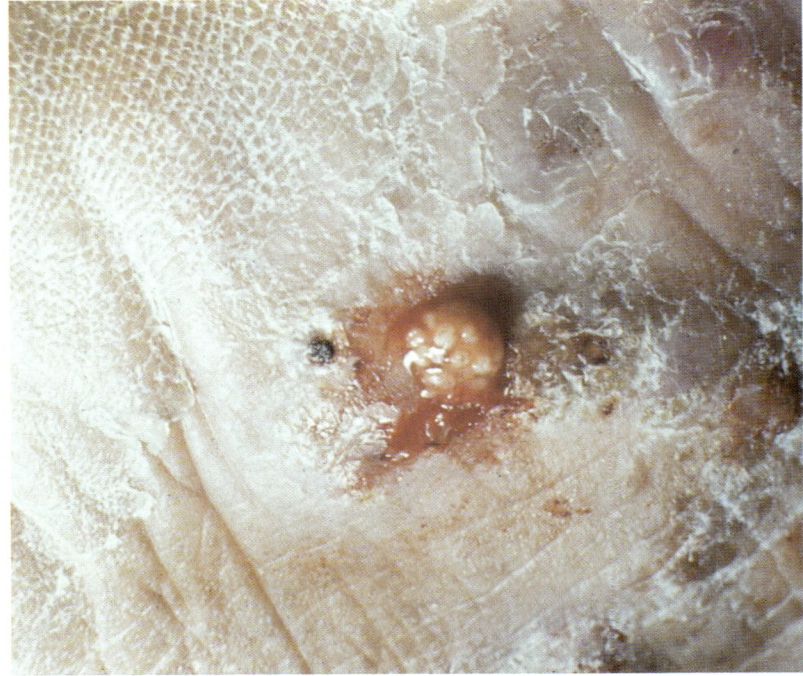

Fig. 26.20 Mycetoma: grains of purulent discharge. (Courtesy of Prof. Oscar Romero).

159. Mc Ginnis M (1996) Mycetoma. **Dermatol Clin** 14:97–104.
160. Develoux M, Ndiaye B, Dieng MT (1995) Les mycetomes en Afrique. **Sante** 5:211–217.
161. Lopez-Martínez R, Mendez-Tovar LJ, Lavalle P et al. (1992) Epidemiología del micetoma en México: Estudio de 2105 casos. **Gac Med Mex** 128:477–481.
162. Castro LG, Belda W, Salebian A et al. (1993) Mycetoma: A retrospective study of 41 cases seen in Sao Paulo, Brazil, from 1978 to 1989. **Mycosis** 36:89–95.
163. Arenas R, Lavalle P (2001) Mycetoma (Madura foot). In: Tropical Dermatology Vademecum, Arenas R, Estrada R, eds. Georgetown: Landes Bioscience, pp. 51–61.
164. Bonifaz A (2000) Micologia médica básica, 2nd edn. México: Mendez Editores.

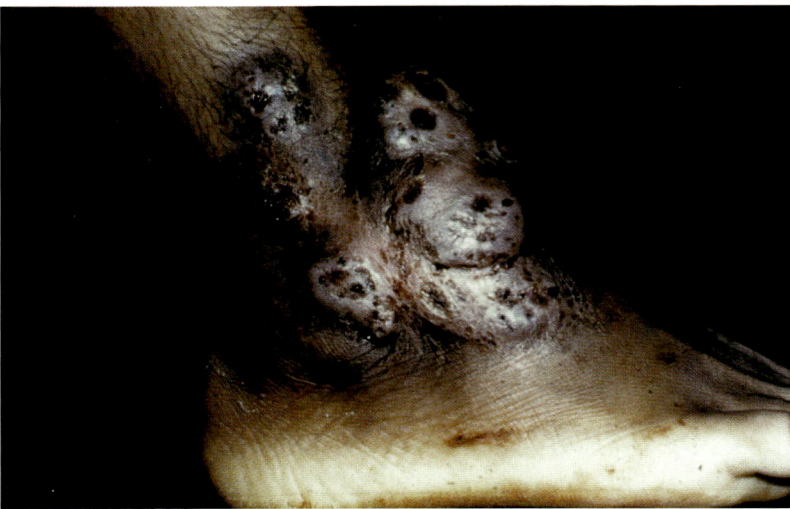

Fig. 26.21   Mycetoma: exuberant granulation tissue and scarring. (Courtesy of Prof. Oscar Romero).

Occasionally multiple mycetomas can be seen as a result of several inoculations or lymphatic spread. A form with minimal swelling and scant small fistulae has been called mini-mycetoma, commonly reported in children and young adults.[163]

The disease is usually oligosymptomatic; pain and general illness are related to secondary bacterial infection. Eumycotic mycetoma develops more slowly than actinomycotic mycetoma in all age groups.

Diagnosis

Direct examination of grains may disclose the etiologic agents. Culture is performed on blood agar containing chloramphenicol and Sabouraud's glucose peptone agar at room temperature for eumycetes and on chocolate agar and brain–heart infusion for actinomycetes. Histopathology discloses a nonspecific suppurative granulomatous pattern. The fungi may be identified with Gram, periodic acid–Schiff (PAS), and Gomori stains.

Random amplified polymorphic deoxyribonucleic acid (RAPD) and restriction endonuclease analysis (REA) allow discrimination and characterization of Madurella mycetomatis strains.[168]

Differential diagnosis

Sporotrichosis, chromoblastomycosis, botryomycosis, osteomyelitis, colliquative tuberculosis, hidradenitis, keloids, furunculosis.

Therapeutics

EUMYCOTIC MYCETOMA

Both medical treatment and surgery are used. Complete excision eliminates small lesions with no risk of recurrence.[169] Ketoconazole 3–5mg/kg per day and itraconazole 5–8mg/kg per day, for months or years, are useful.

Liposomal amphotericin B has produced an overall cure rate of 86% in immunocompromised children.[170]

ACTINOMYCOTIC MYCETOMA

Recommendations include streptomycin 20–40mg/kg per day im in divided doses every 12 hours with sulfamethoxazole/trimethoprim (SMX/TMP) 30/6mg/kg per day for six months to two years, or dapsone 2mg/kg per day. Addition of amikacin cures about 95% of resistant cases.[171]

Sporotrichosis

Introduction and historical note

This is a granulomatous subacute or chronic mycosis characterized by involvement mainly of cutaneous tissues and lymphatics.

In 1898, Schenck described the first case of sporotrichosis, in Baltimore, USA, and recovered the organism.[172] After this report, several cases were described in USA, France, and worldwide, particularly in Latin America and Japan.[173]

Etiology and pathogenesis

Sporothrix schenckii is a dimorphic fungus with a mycelial saprophytic form at 25°C, and a yeast parasitic form at 37°C. After inoculation, an interaction with the immune system produces cutaneous lesions and regional lymphatic involvement constituting the cutaneous lymphatic complex.

The initial polymorphonuclear (PMN) response does not stop the disease. Subsequent granuloma formation seemed ineffectual in laboratory mice, unless there was previous macrophage T-cell activation. Both CD4+ T cells and macrophages are required for cellular immunity against *S. schenckii*. On the other hand, IgG- and IgA-secreting plasmacytes have been identified in granulomas, but immune serum does not enhance resistance.[174]

Epidemiology

Mexico, Guatemala, Brazil, Colombia, and Peru are considered major endemic regions.

Optimal conditions include temperatures of 26°C, 92–100% humidity, and a location 900–1200m above sea level.

Infection usually follows injury with contaminated material or animal bites. The condition predominates in adults of both sexes, but in some hyperendemic areas 60% of cases occur in children under 15 years.[175]

Clinical features

Three clinical subtypes are recognized: lymphocutaneous, fixed and disseminated.

LYMPHOCUTANEOUS

This is the most frequent form (46–92%),[176] commonly located on upper (53%) and lower (18%) extremities, or face (21%).[177] The incubation period varies from 1 to 3 weeks.

Early lesions are small, firm, subcutaneous, violaceous, asymptomatic nodules or gummata, with regional lymphadenopathy. During the first two weeks, secondary lesions erupt following the course of lymphatics (Fig. 26.22). The initial lesion typically heals with scarring after several weeks.

Facial localization is extremely frequent in children and may be unilateral or bilateral, and sometimes keloidal[176] (Fig. 26.23).

165. Castro LG, Valente NY, Germano JA et al. (1999) Mycetoma in an HIV-infected patient. **Rev Hosp Clin Fac Med Sao Paulo** 54:169–171.
166. Anim JT, El-Gaali NO (1986) Mycetoma of the scalp: report of a case. **Trans R Soc Trop Med Hyg** 80:412–414.
167. Welsh O (1975) Mycetoma in children. **Mod Probl Paediatr** 17:248–253.
168. Lopes MM, Freitas G, Boiron P (2000) Potential utility of random amplified polymorphic DNA(RAPD) and restriction endonuclease assay (REA) as typing systems for Madurella mycetomatis. **Curr Microbiol** 40:1–5.
169. Welsh O, Salinas MC, Rodriguez MA (1995) Treatment of eumycetoma and actinomycetoma. **Curr Trop Med Mycol** 6:47–71.
170. Ringden O, Tollemar J (1993) Liposomal amphotericin B (AmBisome) treatment of invasive fungal infections in immunocompromised children. **Mycoses** 36:187–192.

171. Welsh O (1993) Mycetoma. **Semin Dermatol** 12:290–295.
172. Davis B (1996) Sporotrichosis. **Dermatol Clin** 14:69–76.
173. Rippon JW (1982) Sporotrichosis. In: Medical Mycology. The Pathogenic Fungi and the Pathogenic Actinomycetes, 2nd edn. Philadelphia: WB Saunders, pp. 277–302.
174. Tachibana T, Matsuyama T, Mitsuyama M (1999) Involvement of CD4+ T cells and macrophages in acquired protection against infection with Sporothrix schenckii in mice. **Med Mycol** 37:397–404.
175. Pappas PG, Tellez I, Deep A et al. (2000) Sporotrichosis in Peru: Description of an area of hyperendemicity. **Clin Infect Dis** 30:65–70.
176. Bustamante B, Campos P (2001) Endemic sporotrichosis. **Curr Opin Infect Dis** 14:145–149.
177. Arenas R. Sporotrichosis (2001) In: Tropical Dermatology Vademecum, Arenas R, Estrada R, eds. Georgetown: Landes Bioscience, pp. 62–67.

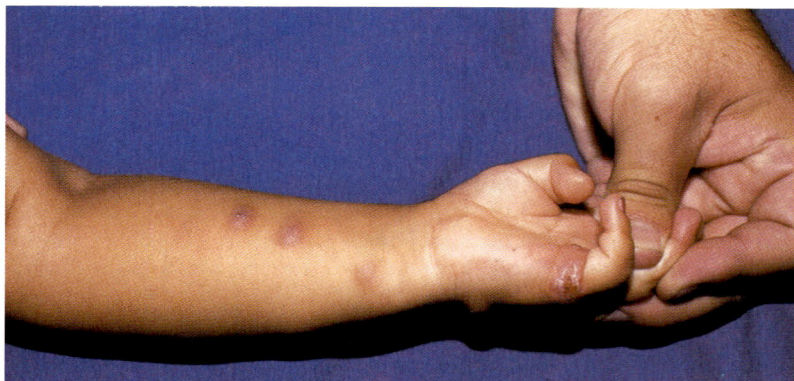

Fig. 26.22   Sporotrichosis: lymphocutaneous presentation.

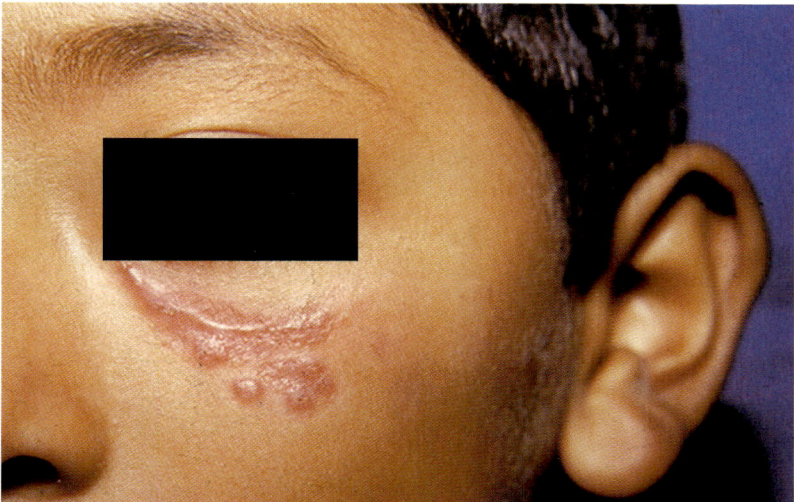

Fig. 26.23   Sporotrichosis: keloidal scarring on the face.

FIXED CUTANEOUS

This is a localized sporotrichosis that accounts for 25% of cases. Lesions generally appear on face, neck, trunk, and legs. Initial chancres appear as erythematous papules, nodules, or verrucous plaques, sometimes ulcerated, covered with scale or crust and surrounded by a violaceous halo. Scaly rashes, vesicles, pustules, or acneiform papules may be associated.[178] Small satellite lesions may appear, but additional involvement distant from the point of inoculation does not occur. Depending on the immunocompetence of the host, spontaneous resolution may occur. Some forms in children are verrucous or ulcerative, and nasal obstruction may occur.[179-181]

Cutaneous superficial   Considered a dermo–epidermic variant of the fixed sporotrichosis, this is characterized by violaceous plaques on the face that spread superficially without involvement of lymphatics.

Cutaneous hematogenous   This is a rare form (1–2%) associated with anergic conditions, which may result from multiple inoculations or autoinoculations of skin or mucous membranes. There is a poor response to treatment and a tendency to dissemination.[164]

SYSTEMIC OR DISSEMINATED

This is prevalent in the immunocompromised, resulting from hematogenous spread from the primary focus or foci. Features include weight loss, fever, malaise, pyelonephritis, orchitis, mastitis, osteitis, and arthritis.

Cutaneous manifestations are similar to those of lymphocutaneous sporotrichosis but less localized, with widespread deep subcutaneous nodules as well as more superficial nodules, verrucous or crusted plaques and ulcers.

Disseminated disease in AIDS presents with widespread cutaneous nodules, polyarthritis, eye disease or CNS involvement,[182] and may be the initial presentation of HIV infection.[183]

The late association with squamous cell carcinoma is known as sporotrichosis recurrens cicatrisans.[177]

Diagnosis

Direct mycologic examination is of limited value. Culture is considered the gold standard for definitive diagnosis and is obtained within 3–6 days on Sabouraud glucose agar at 25–27°C. Dimorphism is demonstrated by inoculation on blood agar at 37°C.

Histopathology discloses a nonspecific combined granulomatous and suppurative pattern. Yeasts surrounded by radiating eosinophilic material, known as asteroid bodies, may be seen. Immunohistochemical staining can reach 83% sensitivity.[184]

Latex agglutination, immunodiffusion (ID), complement fixation (CF), immunoelectrophoresis, enzyme-linked immunosorbent assay (ELISA), Western blot, direct immunofluorescence (DIF), and fluorescent antibody tests are available for diagnosis.

Differential diagnosis

Cutaneous tuberculosis, atypical mycobacterial infection, tularemia, nocardiosis, leishmaniasis, tertiary syphilis, mycetoma, blastomycosis, chromoblastomycosis, pyoderma gangrenosum.

Therapeutics

Itraconazole 200–300mg/day for 4–6 months is the treatment of choice for cutaneous or lymphocutaneous sporotrichosis in adults.[176,185] There have been few reports of successful treatment in children with itraconazole.[179] We have used itraconazole in children, 5mg/kg per day for 16 weeks at least, with complete cure without recurrences.

Saturated solution of potassium iodide (KI) remains an acceptable, effective, and inexpensive alternative. The adult dose is 3–6g/day orally with an initial dose of 1g/day, taken with milk in three doses, increased slowly by 1–1.5g/week. In children, the dose should be 33–50% of the adult dose. Improvement should be seen within three months, but treatment must be continued for 4–6 weeks after resolution to prevent relapses.

Severe and systemic infections require amphotericin B 0.25–1mg/kg per day.

Chromoblastomycosis

Introduction and historical note

Chromoblastomycosis is a chronic and polymorphic cutaneous disease caused by certain dematiaceous fungi.

178. Dellatore D, Lattanand A, Buckley HL et al. (1982) Fixed cutaneous sporotrichosis of the face: successful treatment of a case and review of the literature. **J Am Acad Dermatol** 6:97–100.
179. Kwon KS, Yim CS, Jang HS et al. (1998) Verrucous sporotrichosis in an infant treated with itraconazole. **J Am Acad Dermatol** 38:112–114.
180. Tran CT (1994) Chronic buttock ulcer in a young girl. **Pediatr Infect Dis J** 13:836, 841–842.
181. Clay BM, Anand VK (1996) Sporotrichosis: Nasal obstruction in an infant. **Am J Otolaryngol** 17:75–77.
182. Heller HM, Fuhrer J (1991) Disseminated sporotrichosis in patients with AIDS: case report and review of the literature. **AIDS** 5:1243–1246.

183. Al Tawfiq JA, Wools KK (1998) Disseminated sporotrichosis and Sporothrix schenckii fungemia as the initial presentation of human immunodeficiency virus infection. **Clin Infect Dis** 26:1403–1406.
184. Marquez MEA, Coelho KIR, Sotto MN et al. (1992) Comparison between histochemical and immunohistochemical methods for diagnosis of sporotrichosis. **J Clin Pathol** 45:1089–1093.
185. Sharkey-Mathis PK, Kauffman CA, Graybill JR et al. (1993) Treatment of sporotrichosis with itraconazole. NIAID Mycoses Study Group. **Am J Med** 95:279–285.

Although unpublished, the initial description was made by Pedroso in 1911 in Brazil as "blastomycosis negra." Years later, Brumpt classified the fungus as Hormodentrum pedrosoi.[164] Historically many names have been used, but at present the accepted terminology is chromoblastomycosis.

Etiology and pathogenesis

Agents of chromoblastomycosis belong to the pigmented dematiaceous or "dark fungi" family or chromomycetes, like agents of phaeohyphomycosis and some mycetomas. Species reported as etiological agents of chromoblastomycosis include *Fonsecaea pedrosoi*, *Fonsecaea compacta*, *Cladosporium carrionii*, *Phialophora verrucosa*, *Rhinocladella aquaspersa*, *Wangiella dermatitidis*, *Cladosporium bantianum*, *Exophiala gougerotti*, and *Taeniolella boppii*,[164] *P. Verrucosa* is the prototypic agent, though *F. pedrosoi* is the most commonly isolated. In a recent review in Brazil, *F. pedrosoi* was found in 96% of the cases.[186]

All fungi generate dark, spherical, thick-walled yeasts that are reproduced by binary fission. The spherical shape of the parasitic forms, known as sclerotic or fumagoid cells or Medlar bodies, allows differentiation from phaeophomycosis and eumycetomas.

Some species produce either mycetoma or chromoblastomycosis, depending on the conditions in which the infection develops.

Lesions appear at inoculation sites and progress over years, leading to a granulomatous reaction with dermal fibrosis. The epidermis eliminates 10%–20% of the organisms in the lesions, a phenomenon known as transepithelial elimination.

Epidemiology

The disease is prevalent in American and African tropical and subtropical regions. The biggest series come from Brazil and Madagascar. Other reports have come from Caribbean, Central America regions, and South America.

Optimal conditions are moderate humidity, temperatures of 20°–25°C, and 800–1500mm of rain precipitation.

Infection follows cutaneous trauma and predominates in men (M:F 4:1) 30–50 years old,[186] however, onset before age 20[187] and childhood infection[188,189] have been reported.

Clinical features

Five different clinical forms have been described: nodular, tumoral, verrucous, plaque-like, and scar. The verrucous type is the most frequently reported lesion in adults (53%)[186] (Fig. 26.24). In children lesions are mainly of the nodular and plaque-like type (Fig. 26.25).

After an undetermined incubation period, a pink scaly papule appears and expands to form a warty plaque spreading by contiguity without lymphatic involvement, developing satellite lesions that may coalesce into large vegetating tumors. Because of their friable surface, lesions become easily ulcerated. Patients sometimes complain of itch, and scratching may inoculate organisms into new sites. A common localization is on feet and legs (85%).[186] The process can be extremely indolent, lasting for 20 years or more. Eventually, lesions may partially resolve with scarring, producing secondary lymphedema due to lymphatic involvement.

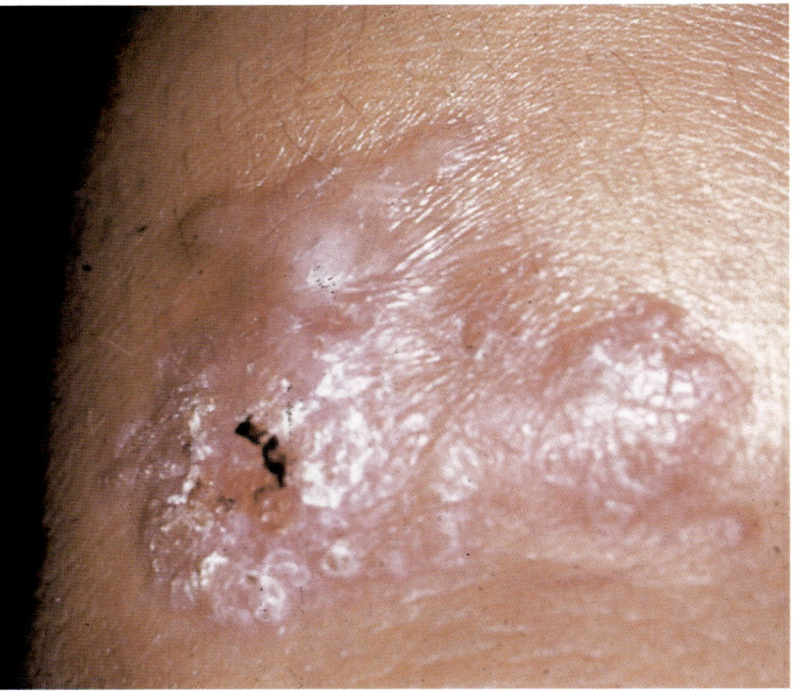

Fig. 26.25 Chromoblastomycosis: nodular and plaque lesions in a child. (Courtesy of Prof. Segundo Barroeta)

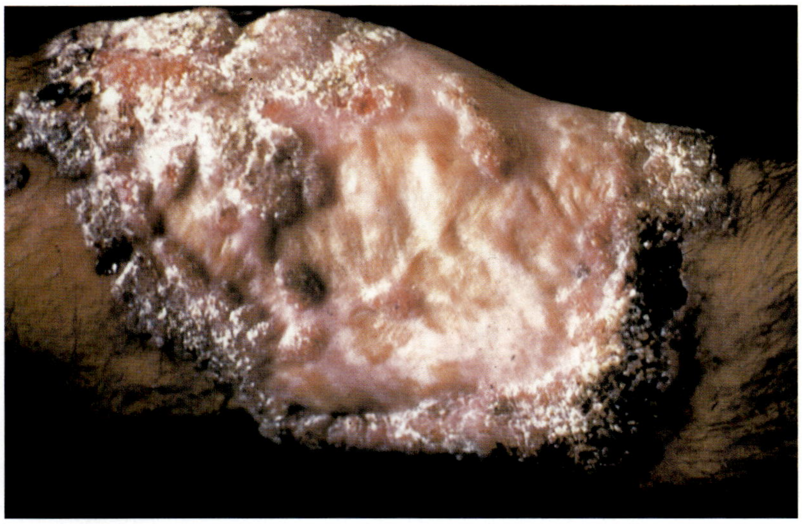

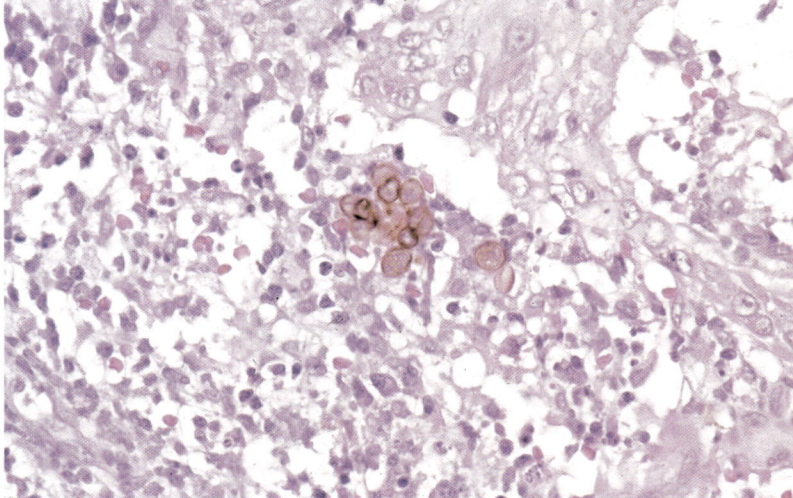

Fig. 26.26 Chromoblastomycosis: "copper penny" bodies seen on routine H & E staining. (Courtesy of Yhomtom Alegre MD)

Fig. 26.24 Chromoblastomycosis: verrucous presentation in an adult. (Courtesy of Yhomtom Alegre MD)

186. Minotto R, Varejão C, Mallman L, et al. (2001) Chromoblastomycosis: A review of 100 cases in the state of Rio Grande do Sul, Brazil. **J Am Acad Dermatol** 44:585–592.
187. Sharma NL, Sharma RC, Grover PS et al. (1999) Chromoblastomycosis in India. **Int J Dermatol** 38:846–851.
188. Mohamed KN (1990) Verrucous lesions in children in the tropics. **Ann Trop Paediatr** 10:273–277.
189. Hughes WT (1967) Chromoblastomycosis: Successful treatment with topical amphotericin B. **J Pediatr** 71:351–356.

Diagnosis

Direct potassium hydroxide (KOH) examination shows fumagoid cells as 4–10μm, double-walled, brown structures.

Culture requires Sabouraud's agar alone or with antibiotics at 25°–30°C and should be maintained for four weeks at least.

Histopathology demonstrates hyperkeratotic pseudoepitheliomatous hyperplasia and granulomatous inflammation. Fumagoid bodies (often referred as "copper pennies"[190]) are found without special stains (Fig. 26.26).

Differential diagnosis

Verrucous tuberculosis, sporotrichosis, paracoccidioidomycosis, leishmaniasis, squamous cell carcinoma.

Therapeutics

Excisional surgery is the first alternative for limited early lesions. Electrodesiccation, radiotherapy and cryosurgery should be considered. Curettage can spread the infection, and thus must be avoided.

Due to specific resistance, amphotericin B appears ineffective when used alone. A schedule of 5-flucytosine 50–150mg/kg per day alone or combined with amphotericin B 0.25–1mg/kg per day should be used in extensive disease for at least 3–9 months.

Other alternatives are thiabendazole 50mg/kg per day orally, ketoconazole 3–5mg/kg per day[191] and itraconazole 5–8mg/kg per day.[192]

In adults, terbinafine 500mg/day for up to 12 months has been used with 85.7% of mycological cure.[193] Suggested dosage in children is 5–10mg/kg per day. Besides its antifungal action, terbinafine decreases type I collagen synthesis and leads to a partial reversal of the fibrotic lesions.[194]

Lobomycosis
Introduction and historical note

This is an exclusively cutaneous chronic granulomatous infection caused by a microorganism of uncertain classification.

Jorge Lobo described the first case in Brazil, in 1913. Fialho performed a histologic study of the same case in 1938, and introduced the name "Lobo's disease." In 1971, practically identical lesions were described in a dolphin in Miami, US, and subsequently several cases have been reported in this species.[164]

Etiology and pathogenesis

The causal agent is Lobomyces, currently known as *Lacazia loboi*,[195] which is inoculated through traumatic cutaneous injuries with plants, snakes, or insect bites. The disease remains localized with no involvement of mucous membranes or internal organs.

Epidemiology

It is distributed in Amazonian tropical forests, particularly in Brazil. Other cases have been reported in other Latin American countries.[196–198]

Favourable conditions probably consists of temperatures of 26–30°C, and 2000mm of annual rain precipitation. Soil and water are suspected as sources of infection, the latter due to cases reported in dolphins.[199]

The condition is most frequent in males between 21 and 40 years old, but some cases have been reported in adolescents.[200]

Clinical features

The incubation period can be extremely long and the disease is characteristically chronic, slowly progressive, and long standing, lasting even up to 30 or 40 years.[198] The initial lesion is a small papule or plaque with slow peripheral extension. Later lesions turn into solid, pink or dark brown, shiny nodules of different sizes with a typical keloidal appearance, sometimes with small scales, crusts, and telangiectases. The confluence of individual lesions separated by gaps leads to a cobblestone appearance.[201] The preferred locations are upper and lower limbs and ears.

New lesions arise by contiguity or by lymphatic dissemination, but are restricted to skin and subcutaneous tissue. Lymph node enlargement has been found in 10–25% of cases.[198]

Although the condition is usually asymptomatic, some patients complain about intense pruritus and pain.

Diagnosis

Direct examination shows ovoid 9–10μm doubly refractile, thick-walled, multiple budding cells, in chains of 20 or more microorganisms. Culture has never been attained.

Histopathology reveals epidermal atrophy, pseudoepitheliomatous hyperplasia or ulceration. In the dermis there are newly formed vessels, fibrosis, and a mixed infiltrate with numerous giant cells. Intracytoplasmatic asteroid bodies, unrelated to those of sporotrichosis have been observed.[202] Large numbers of single or budding fungi arranged in chains are observed within these, especially with PAS, Gridley or Gomori methenamine silver stains.

Differential diagnosis

Xanthomatosis, lepromatous leprosy, anergic leishmaniasis, keloids, fibromas, dermatofibrosarcoma protuberans, verrucous tuberculosis, chromoblastomycosis, paracoccidioidomycosis, fixed sporotrichosis.

Therapeutics

Complete surgical excision, cryosurgery or electrofulguration of small lesions is curative. Lobomycosis is often resistant to chemotherapy, but favorable results have been reported with clofazimine 1mg/kg per day for 1–2 years.[196] Ketoconazole, 5-fluorocytosine, TMP-SMX, itraconazole and amphotericin B, have yielded variable results.

SYSTEMIC MYCOSIS
Blastomycosis

Introduction and historical note

Blastomycosis is a subacute and chronic mycosis caused by *Blastomyces dermatitidis*, characterized by granulomatous suppurative lesions, primarily pulmonary, with later dissemination to skin, subcutaneous tissue and bone. First described in 1894 by Gilchrist, the disease was mistakenly considered to have two forms, cutaneous and pulmonary, until 1951, when Schwartz and Baum demonstrated that these were stages of the same disease.[203]

190. Zaias N, Rebell G (1973) A simple and accurate diagnostic method in chromoblastomycosis. **Arch Dermatol** 108:545–546.
191. Tuffanelli L, Milburn PB (1990) Treatment of chromoblastomycosis. **J Am Acad Dermatol** 23:728–732.
192. Queiroz-Telles F, Purim KS, Fillus JN et al. (1992) Intraconazole in the treatment of chromoblastomycosis due to Fonsecaea pedrosoi. **Int J Dermatol** 31:805–812.
193. Hay RJ (1999) Therapeutic potential of terbinafine in subcutaneous and systemic mycoses. **Br J Dermatol** 141(supp 56):36–40.
194. Esterre P, Risteli L, Ricard-Blum S (1998) Immunohistochemical study of type I collagen turn-over and of matrix metalloproteinases in chromoblastomycosis before and after treatment by terbinafine. **Pathol Res Pract** 194:847–853.
195. Taborda P, Taborda V, McGinnis M (1999) Lacazia loboi gen. nov. comb nov., the etiologic agent of lobomycosis. **J Clin Microbiol** 37:2031–2033.
196. Zaitz C (2001) Lobomycosis (Jorge Lobo's disease). In: Tropical Dermatology Vademecum, Arenas R, Estrada R, eds. Georgetown: Landes Bioscience, pp. 72–76.
197. Rodriguez-Toro G, Tellez N (1992) Lobomycosis in Colombian Amer Indian patients. **Mycopathologia** 120:5–9.
198. Brun A (1999) Lobomycosis in three Venezuelan patients. **Int J Dermatol** 38:302–305.
199. Elgart M (1996) Unusual subcutaneous infections. **Dermatol Clin** 14:105–111.
200. Pierini A (2000) Deep mycosis and opportunistic infections. In: Textbook of Pediatric Dermatology, Harper J, Oranje A, Prose N, eds. Oxford: Blackwell Science, pp. 473–496.
201. Romero O (1972) Enfermedad de Jorge Lobo (Blastomicosis queloidiana) Primer caso diagnosticado en el Perú. **Arch Per Pat Clin** 26:63–86.
202. Rodriguez G, Barrera GP (1996–1997) The asteroid body of lobomycosis. **Mycopathologia** 136:71–74.
203. Body BA (1996) Cutaneous manifestations of systemic mycoses. **Dermatol Clin** 14:125–135.

Etiology and pathogenesis

The agent is *Blastomyces dermatitidis*, a thermally dimorphic fungus. Inhaled spores differentiate into yeasts that initially cause a suppurative reaction followed by granuloma formation; from this primary pulmonary focus, dissemination occurs, especially to skin and bone. The fungal cell surface adhesine WI-1 triggers both humoral and cellular responses.[204,205]

Epidemiology

The condition is endemic in North America. The annual incidence in central and south-central Mississippi is 1.3 cases per 100 000 inhabitants.[206]

The ideal habitat consists of moist acidic soil with decaying organic material.[207] The routes of infection are via the airway and accidentally by cutaneous inoculation.

The condition predominates in men (M:F 4:1), in the 3rd–6th decade of life, but also occurs in children.[208–211]

Clinical features

The clinical spectrum is varied, including asymptomatic infection, acute or chronic pneumonia, and disseminated disease. Symptomatic disease develops after an incubation period ranging from 3 to 6 weeks. However, symptomatic disease occurs only in 50% of infected persons.[212]

Primary pulmonary blastomycosis is self-limiting and usually asymptomatic in adults with only 1–5%[164] presenting with fever, dyspnea, chest pain, cough, and purulent or blood-stained sputum mimicking tuberculosis. However, almost 50% of children develop symptomatic pulmonary disease. These cases may progress to chronic disease. Dissemination may occur to skin, bone, joints and other organs.

Primary cutaneous blastomycosis produces a self-healing primary complex after direct inoculation, generally on the face and limbs.[213]

Secondary cutaneous blastomycosis presents as papules, papulovesicles (Fig. 26.27) or nodules which may ulcerate or develop into verrucous plaques with central scarring. The presence of subcutaneous abscesses and draining sinuses usually portends a fulminant course. Systemic disease involves mainly the lungs but extrapulmonary disease was found in 25% of patients in one series.[214] Periosteitis, osteofibrosis, osteolysis, monoarthritis, and polyarthritis may occur.[215]

In the presence of AIDS almost 40% of patients develop meningoencephalitis or cerebral lesions.[216]

Diagnosis

Direct examination shows thick double-walled, 8–15μm yeasts with broad-based single buds. Culture on Sabouraud's agar at 28°C produces filamentous colonies in 2–8 weeks, while yeast colonies grow in 2–4 weeks on blood or chocolate gelose agar at 35–37°C.

Histopathology reveals pseudoepitheliomatous hyperplasia, granulomas and microabscesses. Fungal stains are often not helpful, but can show typical organisms as illustrated (Fig. 26.28). CF and ID are limited by cross-reactivity with other fungi, especially *Histoplasma capsulatum*.

Chest X-ray may show pulmonary infiltrates, nodules and consolidation, the latter a common finding in children.[211]

Differential diagnosis

Pulmonary: tuberculosis, coccidioidomycosis, histoplasmosis, paracoccidioidomycosis, bronchial carcinoma.

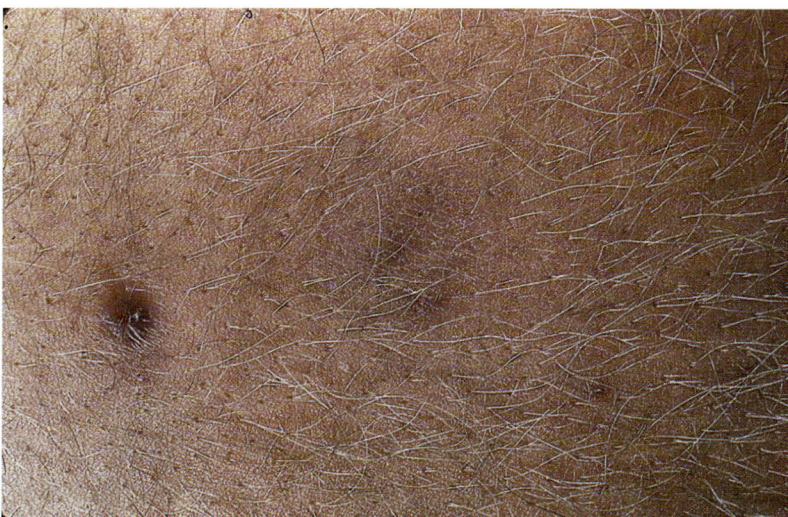

Fig. 26.27 Blastomycosis: two innocuous appearing papulovesicles on leg of 18-year-old farm boy.

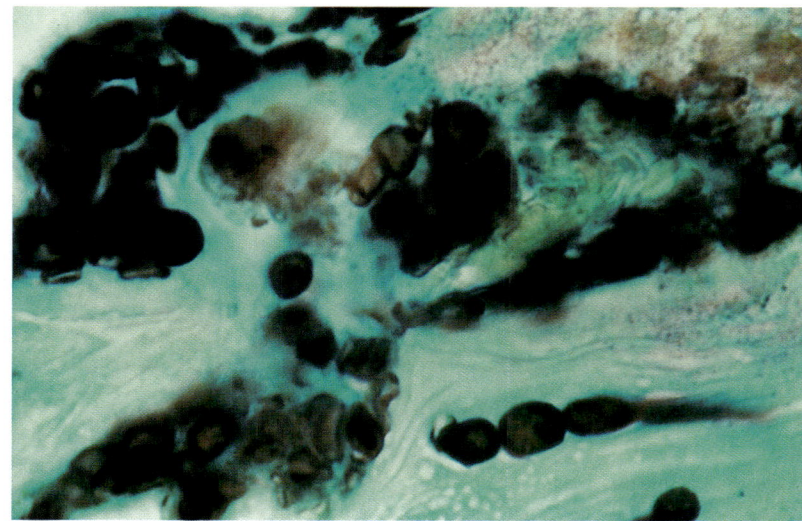

Fig. 26.28 Biopsy of lesion in Fig. 26.27, showing broad-based budding forms (Silver stain 1000 power/year).

204. Wutrich M, Chang WL, Klein BS (1998) Immunogenicity and protective efficacy of the WI-1 adhesin of Blastomyces dermatitidis. **Infect Immun** 66:5443–5449.
205. Klein BS (1997) Role of cell surface molecules of Blastomyces dermatitidis in the pathogenesis and immunobiology of blastomycosis. **Semin Respir Infect** 12:198–205.
206. Patel RG, Patel B, Petrini MF et al. (1999) Clinical presentation, radiographic findings, and diagnostic methods of pulmonary blastomycosis: a review of 100 consecutive cases. **South Med J** 92:289–295.
207. Bradsher RW (1992) Blastomycosis. **Clin Infect Dis** 14 (suppl 1):S82–S90.
208. Dismukes WE (1986) Blastomycosis: leave it to a beaver [editorial]. **N Engl J Med** 314:575–577.
209. Varkey B (1997) Blastomycosis in children. **Semin Respir Infect** 12:235–242.
210. Schutze GE, Hickerson SL, Fortin EM et al. (1996) Blastomycosis in children. **Clin Infect Dis** 22:496–502.

211. Alkrinawi S, Reed MH, Pasterkamp H (1995) Pulmonary blastomycosis in children: findings on chest radiographs. **Am J Roentgenol** 165:615–654.
212. Klein BS, Vergeront JM, Weeks RJ (1986) Isolation of Blastomyces dermatitides in soil associated with a large outbreak of blastomycosis in Wisconsin. **N Engl J Med** 314:529–534.
213. Graham WR Jr, Callaway JL (1982) Primary inoculation blastomycosis in a veterinarian. **J Am Acad Dermatol** 7:785–786.
214. Chapman SW, Lin AC, Hendricks KA et al. (1997) Endemic blastomycosis in Mississippi: epidemiological and clinical studies. **Semin Respir Infect** 12:219–228.
215. Abril A, Campbell MD, Cotten VR Jr et al. (1998) Polyarticular blastomycotic arthritis. **J Rheumatol** 25:1019–1021.
216. Pappas PG, Pottage JC, Powderly WG et al. (1992) Blastomycosis in patients with acquired immunodeficiency syndrome. **Ann Intern Med** 116:847–853.

Cutaneous: sporotrichosis, coccidioidomycosis, paracoccidioidomycosis, tuberculosis, chromomycosis, lupus vulgaris, tertiary syphilis.
Osseous: osteomyelitis, coccidioidomycosis, tuberculosis, osteoarticular sporotrichosis.
Disseminated: histoplasmosis, coccidioidomycosis and tuberculosis.

Therapeutics

Amphotericin B 0.3–0.6mg/kg per day or its liposomal equivalent results in cure without relapse in 70–91%.[217]

In adults, ketoconazole 400mg/day may be effective in mild to moderate disease, fluconazole 200–400mg/day has 65% efficacy,[218] and fluconazole 400–800mg/day has 87% efficacy in non-life-threatening disease.[62] Itraconazole 200–400mg/day for 2 months has shown 95% efficacy.[219]

In children, amphotericin B 0.25–1mg/kg per day with a total dose of 30mg/kg is useful for life-threatening cases. Itraconazole 5–7mg/kg per day has been used successfully for limited number of patients with non-life-threatening disease.[220]

Paracoccidioidomycosis (PCM)

Introduction and historical note

Paracoccidioidomycosis represents the most important systemic mycosis in Latin America.[221,222] First reports by Lutz in 1908, calling it "hyphoblastomycosis pseudococcidioidal" identified a budding parasitic fungus. Splendore and Carini in 1912 classified the agent as *Zymonema brasiliensis* and described the histopathology. In 1930, Almeida clarified the etiology, establishing a new fungal genus, and coined the name *Paracoccidioides brasiliensis*.

Etiology and pathogenesis

Paracoccidioides brasiliensis is a thermally dimorphic fungus with a mycelial phase at 25°C and a pathogenic yeast phase at 36°C. The "mariner's wheel" which describes multiple budding yeasts with narrow points of attachment, is considered a typical characteristic. When spores reach the lungs, an inflammatory reaction starts, followed by a pyogenic reaction, and subsequent granuloma formation.

Phagocytosis requires tumoral necrosis factor (TNF) and interleukins (IL), found only if previous immunization has occurred. Chronic disease has been associated with lymphocyte T-helper subset 1 (Th1) response and acute disease with lymphocyte T-helper subset 2 (Th2) response.[223]

Dissemination to skin, lymphatics, and other organs may occur, depending on immunocompetence, inoculum size, and virulence.

Epidemiology

The main endemic countries are Brazil, Venezuela, Colombia, Argentina, Peru, and Mexico.[224,225]

The ideal conditions are temperatures of 15–30°C, altitude of 400–1500m and annual rain fall of 800–2000mm.

Infection is mainly via the airway and uncommonly by cutaneous inoculation.[223]

TABLE 26.23 Clinical classification of paracoccidioidomycosis

Paracoccidioidomycosis – infection	Paracoccidioidomycosis – disease

• Primary pulmonary
• Primary cutaneous
	• Acute – subacute forms
	• Chronic form
	  Unifocal
	    Pulmonary
	    Cutaneous
	    Lymphatic
	  Multifocal or disseminated
	  Sequelae

The disease predominates in 30–60-year-old males (M:F 15:1), but a survey in Brazil reported 5.5% of cases in individuals under 14 years.[224]

Clinical features

PCM shows a wide spectrum of clinical manifestations as shown in Table 26.23.

PARACOCCIDIOIDOMYCOSIS – INFECTION
This is characterized by a self-healing and even silent processes,[226] either pulmonary or cutaneous.

PARACOCCIDIOIDOMYCOSIS – DISEASE
This is an acute, rapidly spreading and sometimes fulminant form in immuno-suppressed patients that accounts for 5% of cases,[227] with primary involvement of reticuloendothelial system (RES) organs.[228] Because its predominance in individual between 3 and 20 years old it is commonly called the juvenile form but its but association with malnutrition and HIV infection, independent of age, has made this adjective inappropriate.

Generalized prominent lymphadenopathy, especially remarkable in children,[224] long-standing fever, intestinal ulceration, osteoarticular symptoms, hepatosplenomegaly, malaise, and weight loss are usual.

Pulmonary involvement presents as an infiltrative pneumonic disease or "primary pulmonary complex" that is clinically nonspecific. Eventually an acute pleuropulmonary disease with fever, thoracic pain, hemoptysis, and severe respiratory insufficiency may develop.

Cutaneous involvement includes widely distributed papules or ulcerated nodules, destructive centrofacial granulomatous plaques, and, rarely, an acneiform rash.[229]

Chronic form

UNIFOCAL
Pulmonary: This results from reactivation of latent pulmonary foci. The features are productive cough, hemoptysis, dyspnea, weight loss, and fatigue.
Cutaneous: This is rarely seen as a single manifestation and clinically presents as nonspecific erythematous or violaceous nodules and cutaneous ulcers.

217. Bradsher RW (1996) Histoplasmosis and blastomycosis. **Clin Infect Dis** 22(suppl 2):S102–S111.
218. Pappas PG, Bradsher RW, Chapman SW et al. (1995) Treatment of blastomycosis with fluconazole: a pilot study. **Clin Infect Dis** 20:267–271.
219. Pappas PG, Bradsher RW, Kauffman CA et al. (1997) Treatment of blastomycosis with higher doses of fluconazole. The National Institute of Allergy and Infectious Diseases Mycoses Study Group. **Clin Infect Dis** 25:200–205.
220. Chapman SW, Bradsher RW Jr, Campbell GD Jr et al. (2000) Practice guidelines for the management of patients with blastomycosis. **Clin Infect Dis** 30:679–683.
221. Londero AT, Mello IS (1983) Paracoccidioidomycosis in childhood. A critical review. **Mycopathologia** 82:49–55.
222. Brummer E, Castañeda E, Restrepo A (1993) Paracoccidioidomycosis: an update. **Clin Microbiol Rev** 6:89–117.
223. Zaitz C (2001) Paracoccidioidomycosis. In: Tropical Dermatology Vademecum, Arenas R, Estrada R, eds. Georgetown: Landes Bioscience, pp. 92–98.

224. Blotta M, Mamoni R, Oliveira S et al. (1999) Endemic regions of paracoccidioidomycosis in Brazil: A clinical and epidemiologic study of 584 cases in the southeast region. **Am J Trop Med Hyg** 61:390–394.
225. Rueda M, Romero O, Galarza C (1999) Clinical and epidemiological aspects of South American Blastomycosis. Poster Exhibit of the 57th American Academy of Dermatology Annual Meeting, March 19–24, New Orleans.
226. Carrada-Bravo T (1996) La infección pulmonar y sistémica causada por el Paracoccidioides brasiliensis. Avances recientes y perspectivas terapéuticas. **Rev Inst Nal Enf Resp Mex** 9:288–314.
227. Manns BJ, Baylis BW, Urbanski SJ et al. (1996) Paracoccidioidomycosis: Case report and review. **Clin Inf Dis** 23:1026–1032.
228. San Blas G (1993) Paracoccidioidomycosis and its etiologic agent Paracoccidioides braziliensis. **J Med Vet Mycol** 31:99–113.
229. De Almeida OP, Jorge J, Scully C et al. (1991) Oral manifestations of paracoccidioidomycosis (South American blastomycosis). **Oral Surg Oral Med Oral Pathol** 72:430–435.

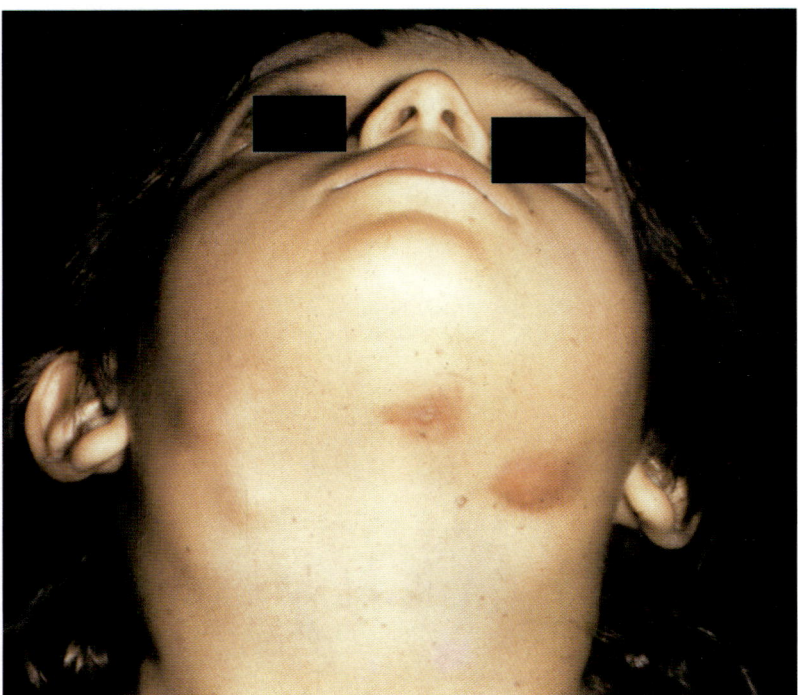

Fig. 26.29 Paracoccidioidomycosis: adenopathy with suppuration.

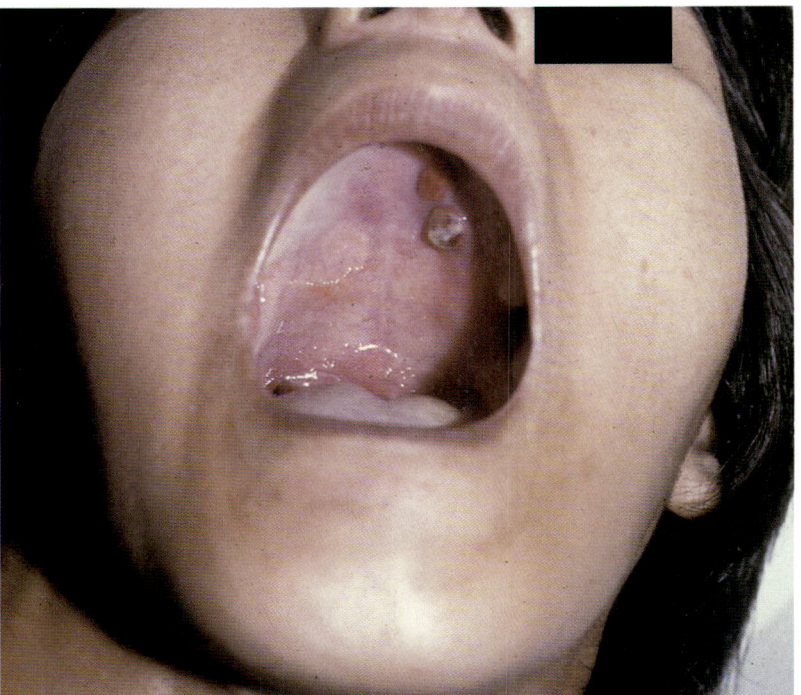

Fig. 26.30 Paracoccidioidomycosis: palatal involvement.

Lymphatic: Enlargement, induration, tenderness or cold abscesses develop, involving particularly the cervical, supraclavicular, axillary and inguinal lymph nodes (Fig. 26.29).

MULTIFOCAL OR DISSEMINATED
This is the most frequent form. It initially involves the lungs and is characterized by a triad of pneumonitis, mucocutaneous, and lymphatic involvement.

Typically, mucocutaneous lesions surround the mouth and nose. Oral cavity involvement (Fig. 26.30) occurs in 80%, particularly in the elderly, affecting lips, gums, dental alveoli, tongue, pharynx, and larynx. Initial mucosal lesions are papules that enlarge into red or violaceous granular plaques producing the so-called "moriform granulomas," because of resemblance to "mora," a Spanish word for blackberry. These lead to pain, dysphagia, toothache, looseness, and loss of teeth. Cutaneous lesions are painful ulcerative or verrucous plaques similar to oral moriform granuloma,[230] but erythematous papules, pustules, gummata and subcutaneous abscesses have been described also.

Submaxillary and cervical lymphadenopathy is a regular feature that eventually progresses to a periadenitis and fistula formation.

Adrenal involvement may produce Addison disease.[222,231] Cases of orchitis, epididimitis, and prostatitis, as well as osseous, renal, and palpebral lesions have been reported.[226] Liver, spleen, intestines, and CNS may also be affected.

Sequelae
Pulmonary disease leads to fibrosis, cor pulmonare, and emphysema. A characteristic serious limitation in mouth opening due to scarring of the lips[225,232] results from perioral lesions.

Diagnosis
Direct examination reveals typical "mariner's wheel" yeasts. Cultures are performed on Sabouraud agar for 2–4 weeks at 25°C and on enriched blood agar at 37°C.

Histopathology discloses a suppurative and granulomatous pattern. Budding cells are seen with PAS or Grocott stains.

A polymerase chain reaction (PCR) assay has been developed for *P. brasiliensis*.[233]

Differential diagnosis
Cutaneous: blastomycosis, tuberculosis, yaws, tertiary syphilis, sporotrichosis, leishmaniasis, coccidioidomycosis, histoplasmosis, chromoblastomycosis, prototothecosis, oral carcinoma.
Pulmonary: abscesses, bronchiectasis, Wegener granulomatosis.

Therapeutics
Amphotericin-B 0.25–1mg/kg per day is effective in severe cases. Alternatively, itraconazole 5–8mg/kg per day,[234] or fluconazole 5–8mg/kg per day[235] may be used.

Coccidioidomycosis
Introduction and historical note
Coccidioidomycosis is a polymorphic disease caused by *Coccidioides immitis*. The first descriptions appear in 1892 in Argentina and 1894 in San Joaquin valley, California. Stiles called the agent *Coccidioides immitis*, but considered it a protozoan. In 1900, Ophüls and Moffitt realized its fungal dimorphic nature and reproduced the disease experimentally.

230. Carrada-Bravo T, Rivera-Carrada LP, Corona-Sanchez AL et al. (1992) Lesiones bucales de paracoccidioidomycosis: Avances recientes y perspectivas. **Practica Odontol Mex** 13:23–27.
231. Faical S, Borri ML, Hauache OM et al. (1996) Addison's disease caused by Paracoccidioices brasiliensis: diagnosis by needle aspiration biopsy of the adrenal gland. [letter] **Am J Roentgenol** 166:461–462.
232. Romero O (1961) Blastomicosis sudamericana. Estudio clínico y terapéutico de 15 nuevos casos. **Anales de la Facultad de Medicina** 44:487–530.

233. Gomes GM, Cisalpino PS, Taborda CP et al. (2000) PCR for diagnosis of paracoccidioidomycosis. **J Clin Microbiol** 38:3478–3480.
234. Borgia G, Reynaud L, Cerini R et al. (2000) A case of paracoccidioidomycosis: experience with long-term therapy. **Infection** 28:119–120.
235. Martinez R, Malta MH, Verceze AV et al. (1999) Comparative study of fluconazole and amphotericin B in the parenteral treatment of experimental paracoccidioidomycosis in the rat. **Mycopathologia** 146:131–134.

Etiology and pathogenesis

This is a thermally dimorphic fungus, with saprophytic arthrosporated mycelia and parasitic spherules containing endospores, known as *Coccidioides immitis*. After inhalation the spores in the lungs are usually phagocyted by PMNs, but sometimes differentiate into spherules with a secondary inflammatory response. The cellular response limits the infection; thus, dissemination is related to immunodeficiency.

Epidemiology

Three endemic regions are recognized: San Joaquin valley and South Western deserts of the USA Guatemala, Nicaragua, Honduras, Venezuela and Colombia; and El Chaco territories in Argentina, Paraguay, and Uruguay. The ideal habitat has includes semi-arid areas with low annual rainfall, rapidly variable temperatures of 7–28°C and dry, alkaline, clay or sandy soil.

Usually, infection is via the airway but accidental cases have been reported from skin wounds. Occurrence in nonendemic areas results from prior travelling to endemic areas and immunosuppression due to medications and AIDS.[236] This is of particular significance in children.[237]

Clinical features

PRIMARY COCCIDIOIDOMYCOSIS

Acute pulmonary coccidioidomycosis accounts for 98% of cases. It is usually self-limiting and asymptomatic. Less commonly, a mild or moderate disease with flu-like features occurs. This form is frequently associated with morbilliform or erythema modosum eruptions in adults, and erythema multiforme-like eruptions in children. Generalized arthealgias ("desert rheumatism") are commonly associated. Rarely, there is a severe form presenting as a brochopneumonia.[164]

Primary cutaneous coccidioidomycosis occurs in 2%,[164] involving head, neck or limbs, as a primary complex similar to sporotrichosis.

SYSTEMIC OR DISSEMINATED COCCIDIOIDOMYCOSIS

This occurs in less than 1%,[238] usually in the immunosuppressed and mainly involves CNS, bones, joints, and skin.[236] The usual cutaneous features are granulomatous plaques on the head and neck[239] (Fig. 26.31) but also subcutaneous draining abscesses, acneiform papules and pustules. Because of this striking polymorphism, coccidioidomycosis has been considered "a great imitator."[236]

Diagnosis

Direct examination demonstrates double-membraned 20–70μm spherules. Culture is performed on Sabouraud's or Mycosel agar at room temperature and thermal dimorphism should be demonstrated. Extreme care must be applied in proper facilities in handling this organism as it is extremely dangerous.

Histopathology reveals pseudoepitheliomatous hyperplasia, abscesses, necrosis, and vasculitis. Spherules of 10–100μm containing endospores can be found. The coccidioidin test is useful for epidemiological detection. CF and ID are closely related to the activity of disease.

Differential diagnosis

Pulmonary: influenza, atypical bronchopneumonia, bronchitis, colliquative tuberculosis, histoplasmosis, blastomycosis, mycoplasma, rickettsial diseases, aspergillosis, malignancies.
Cutaneous: verrucous tuberculosis, sporotrichosis, mycetoma, chromoblastomycosis, osteomyelitis, atypical mycobacteriosis, contact dermatitis, actinic keratosis, mycosis fungoides, verrucous carcinoma.[236]
Disseminated: blastomycosis, sporotrichosis, histoplasmosis, cryptococcosis.

Therapeutics

Amphotericin B 0.25–1mg/kg per day, or its liposomal form 3–5mg/kg per day are effective. Itraconazole 5–8mg/kg per day and fluconazole 5–8mg/kg per day have proven effectiveness and can be added to amphotericin B. The treatment must be continued for at least six months after the disease has become inactive.[240]

Histoplasmosis

Introduction and historical note

Histoplasmosis is a severe mycosis caused by *Histoplasma capsulatum*, first detected by Darling in 1905 during a postmortem. Rocha-Lima, in 1913, recognized a fungal etiology and in 1929 Dood and De Mombreum isolated *H. capsulatum* from a patient.[241]

Etiology and pathogenesis

It is produced by the dimorphic fungus *Histoplasma capsulatum* var. *capsulatum* that reaches the alveoli by inhalation, generating a primary complex and inducing an interstitial inflammatory response with macrophages, lymphocytes, and PMNs, sometimes so severe as to produce massive exudate, alveolar tamponade, respiratory failure, and death. It eventually disseminates, with yeasts released by macrophages invading new ones and spreading thus to RES, bone marrow, and other organs.

Epidemiology

The highest incidence is in Panama, Nicaragua, Honduras, Venezuela, Colombia, Brazil, and the Caribbean islands. It is endemic in Ohio and the Mississippi River valley. In general, the positivity to histoplasmin in the USA is about 80%.[242]

Important sources are feathers and droppings from birds and bats. Optimal growth conditions include temperatures of 20–30°C, humidity of 70–90%, and limestone soil.

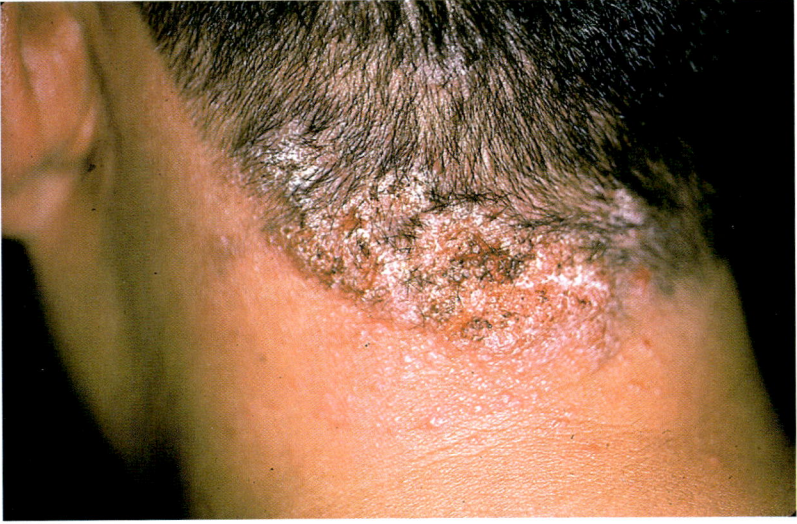

Fig. 26.31 Verrucous neck lesions of cutaneous coccidioidomycosis (Courtesy of A. Petropolis, MD).

236. Quimby SR, Connolly SM, Winkelmann RK et al. (1992) Clinicopathologic spectrum of specific cutaneous lesions of disseminated coccidioidomycosis. Am Acad Dermatol 26:79–85.
237. Grigoriu D, Delacrétaz J, Borelli D (1987) Coccidiodomycosis. In: Medical Mycology. Switzerland: Hans Huber Publishers, pp. 311–317.
238. Diógenes MJ, Sidrim JJ (1998) Coccidioidomicose. In: Compêndio de Micologia Médica. Zaitz C, Campbell I, Marques S, et al., eds. Rio de Janeiro: Editora Médica e Cientifica, pp. 277–288.
239. Choon SE, Khoo JJ (1999) Coccidiodomycosis in Malaysia [letter]. Br J Dermatol 140 557–558.
240. Tucker RM, Denning DW, Aratoon EG et al. (1990) Itraconazole therapy for non-meningeal coccidioidomycosis: clinical and laboratory observations. J Am Acad Dermatol 23:593–601.
241. Marques SA, Pires RM (1998) Histoplasmose. In: Compêndio de Micologia Médica. Zaitz C, Campbell I, Marques S, et al., eds. Rio de Janeiro: Editora Médica e Cientifica, pp. 265–276.
242. Lopex-Martinez R (2001) Histoplasmosis In: Tropical Dermatology Vademecum, Arenas R, Estrada R, eds. Georgetown: Landes Bioscience, pp. 99–106.

Infection is via the airway. The frequency peaks in the 3rd and 4th decades of life, particularly in males (M:F 4:1). Positivity to histoplasmin has been found in 9.2% of children 4–14 years old.[243] Before the AIDS epidemic, most cases occurred in children under 2 years old.[244]

Clinical features

The clinical spectrum includes several primary or secondary forms affecting mainly lungs, RES, and skin.

PRIMARY HISTOPLASMOSIS

Pulmonary   This is asymptomatic in 60–95% of cases.[164] Symptomatic disease is mild, moderate, or severe. The mild form resembles influenza and the moderate form simulates atypical pneumonia. During these infections, erythema multiforme, erythema nodosum, lymphadenopathy, and, rarely, exfoliative dermatitis may appear. Severe cases appear as outbreaks in individuals who have inhaled a massive inoculum in bat caves or abandoned mine shafts. The disease resembles hematogenous tuberculosis or other severe bacterial or viral infections.

Children commonly show hilar and mediastinal lymphadenopathy without radiological evidence of pulmonary disease.

Cutaneous   This is extremely uncommon (0.5%)[164] and follows direct inoculation. Immunocompetent individuals develop a self-limiting cutaneous complex. Widespread disease is possible in the immunocompromised,[245] presenting as nodules, gummata or vegetative lesions.

SECONDARY HISTOPLASMOSIS

This is a disseminated form occurring mainly in immunocompromised patients and may be acute or chronic.

Acute disseminated   This is a rare form found especially in the immuno-compromised and also in the very young and the very old.[246] Is usually fulminant in childhood, especially during the first year. The features include fever, persistent non-productive cough, adenopathy, hepatosplenomegaly, diarrhea, weight loss, anemia, and leukopenia.

Chronic disseminated   This usually occurs in adults presenting with weakness, weight loss, and chronic cough with scant expectoration, resembling chronic tuberculosis. Severe cases have mucocutaneous and lymphatic involvement.

Dissemination of histoplasmosis may be a sign of progression to AIDS,[247,248] with cutaneous involvement in 5–25%, including lesions resembling molluscum contagiosum.[203] In children from endemic regions, disseminated histoplasmosis is associated with primary immunodeficiency.[249,250]

Diagnosis

Direct examination is of limited value. Culture on Sabouraud's with antibiotics at 28°C may take as long as three months and subcultures on blood agar at 37°C are necessary.

Biopsy discloses a variety of patterns including histiocytic, granulomatous, leukocytoclastic vasculitis, and a sparse inflammatory infiltrate.[251] Giemsa, PAS, and Grocott stains reveal 1–2μm, budding yeasts with refrigent halos.

Differential diagnosis

Pulmonary: influenza, atypical pneumonia, tuberculosis.

Mucocutaneous: sporotrichosis, coccidioidomycosis, aphthae, leishmaniasis, PCM.
Disseminated: Hodgkin's disease, tuberculosis.

Therapeutics

Itraconazole 5–8mg/kg per day for 6–12 months is the treatment of choice in moderate and chronic pulmonary disease. Fluconazole 5–8mg/kg per day is also effective for mild or moderate forms.[252] Severe disease requires amphotericin B 0.5–1mg/kg per day, to a total dose 2.5g.

OPPORTUNISTIC MYCOSIS

Advances in transplantation, immunosuppresive therapy, and intensive care, in addition to the worldwide spreading of AIDS, have lead to the emergence of special patients with serious immunodeficiency who are vulnerable to usually non-pathogenic fungi, which may produce disseminated and fatal infections, currently known as opportunistic mycoses.

Cryptococcosis

Introduction and historical note

Cryptococcosis is a chronic or subacute systemic mycosis, produced by the encapsulated yeast Cryptococcus neoformans. In 1894, Sanfelice named this fungi *Saccharomyces neoformans*, and in 1901 Vullemin renamed it Cryptoccocus.

Etiology and pathogenesis

Cryptococcus neoformans is a dimorphic fungus with an unencapsulated environmental form, and a pathogenic yeast form with a broad polysaccharide and glycopeptide capsule[164] that masks opsonic antibodies.[253]

C. neoformans proliferates in mononuclear cells and disseminates through bloodstream or lymphatics but is essentially neurophilic, probably related to growth stimulating substances and the absence of an anti-cryptococcal factor in cerebrospinal fluid (CSF).[164]

In immunocompetent hosts, *C. neoformans* causes mild transitory diseases,[254] but in the immunocompromised it behaves pathogenically. It is one of the most common opportunistic infections in AIDS.

Epidemiology

Cryptococcosis predominates in Europe and the USA. The main sources are pigeon or hen droppings; hence, subclinical infection is common in cities with large pigeon populations.[254] Infection is via the airway, mainly affecting women (F:M 2:1) 30–60 years old. AIDS has become the main predisposing factor worldwide, with the incidence of cryptococcosis in these patients varying from 3–8% in the USA to 12% in Zaire,[255,256] constituting the 4th most common opportunistic infection.[257]

Clinical features

Common clinical patterns are neurological, pulmonary, cutaneous, osseous, and disseminated. Neurological disease is the most frequent (65–85%),[164] presenting commonly as chronic basal meningitis, meningoencephalitis or cryptococcoma. Pulmonary disease is unusual (5%), and may be asymptomatic, mild or severe. Mild disease presents with cough, fever and pleural pain and

243. Mangiaterra M, Alonso J, Galvan M et al. (1996) Histoplasmin and paracoccidioidin skin reactivity in infantile population of northern Argentina (1). **Rev Inst Trop Sao Paulo** 38:394–353.
244. Leggiadro RL, Barrett FF, Hughes WT (1988) Disseminated histoplasmosis of infancy. **Pediatr Infect Dis J** 7:799–805.
245. Cott GR, Smith TW, Hinthorn DR et al. (1979) Primary cutaneous histoplasmosis in an immunosuppressed patient. **JAMA** 242:456–457.
246. Hughes WT (1984) Hematogenous histoplasmosis in the immunocompromised child. **J Pediatr** 105:569–575.
247. Bonifaz A, Cansela R, Novales J et al. (2000) Cutaneous histoplasmosis associated with acquired immunodeficiency syndrome (AIDS). **Int J Dermatol** 39:35–38.
248. Orozco-Topete RL, Reyes E (1998) Histoplasmosis cutanea en nueve pacientes con SIDA. **Rev Invest Clin** 50:525–528.
249. Odio CM, Navarrete M, Carrillo JM et al. (1999) Disseminated histoplasmosis in infants. **Pediatr Infect Dis J** 18:1065–1068.
250. Yilmaz GG, Yilmaz E, Coskun M et al. (1995) Cutaneous histoplasmosis in a child with hyper-IgM. **Pediatr Dermatol** 12:235–238.

251. D'Avila SC, Chapadeiro E (1998) Caracteristicas histopatologicas e imunohistoquimicas das lesoes cutaneas e da mucosa oral na histoplasmose disseminada de portadores da sindrome da imunodeficiencia adquirida (AIDS). **Rev Soc Bras Med Trop** 31:539–547.
252. Wheat J, MaWhinney S, Hafner R et al. (1997) Treatment of histoplasmosis with fluconazole in patients with acquired immunodeficiency syndrome. National Institute of Allergy and Infectious Diseases Acquired Immunodeficiency Syndrome Clinical Trials Group and Mycoses Study Group. **Am J Med** 103:223–232.
253. Dimino-Emme L, Gurevith AW (1995) Cutaneous manifestations of disseminated cryptococcosis. **J Am Acad Dermatol** 32:844–850.
254. Levitz SM (1991) The ecology of Cryptococcus neoformans and the epidemiology of cryptococcosis. **Rev Infect Dis** 13:1163–1169.
255. Fischman O, Zaror L (1998) Criptococose e outras levaduroses. In: Compêndio de Micologia Médica, Zaitz C, Campbell I, Marques S, et al. eds. Rio de Janeiro: Editora Médica e Cientifica, pp. 297–308.
256. Hay RJ (1996) Yeast infections. **Dermatol Clin** 14:113–124.
257. Grant IH, Armstrong D (1988) Fungal infections in AIDS – cryptococcosis. **Infect Dis Clin North Am** 2:457–462.

the severe form with fever, weakness, productive cough, and hemoptysis, simulating Gram-negative pneumonia or miliary tuberculosis. Primary cutaneous cryptococcosis occurs rarely in immunodeficient individuals and exceptionally in immunocompetent ones after traumatic inoculation.[258] A case in a 6-year-old girl recovering from varicella has been reported.[259] A primary complex appears, with a chancre that may involute or progress to a nodule or an ulcerated plaque.[260] Secondary cutaneous cryptococcosis is most common, usually associated with neurological or disseminated disease.[253] Lesions are widely distributed and very polymorphic, including lesions mimicking acne and mollusca contagiosa.[253,261] Osseous cryptococcosis occurs in 5–10%,[255] secondary to pulmonary or meningeal foci. Osteitis, osteofibrosis, osteolysis and draining fistulae may appear. Dissemination and generalized illness occurs in severe immunosuppression, with multiple organ failure.

Diagnosis

Direct KOH or Indian ink mounts disclose large, budding, encapsulated cells. Culture is performed on Sabouraud's glucose agar at 37°C, and is usually positive in 24–48 hours. Biochemical characteristics allow identification. Biopsy shows little inflammation or a granulomatous reaction with the presence of medium-sized encapsulated yeasts that stain bright pink with Mayer's mucicarmine. Differentiation from other dimorphic fungi can be difficult. Latex agglutination tests can be performed[262] as well as ELISA.

Differential diagnosis

Pulmonary tuberculosis, gram-negative pneumonia, coccidioidomycosis, histoplasmosis, North American blastomycosis, paracoccidioidomycosis, candidosis and carcinoma.
Neurological: tuberculosis, neoplasia, toxoplasmosis, bacterial meningitis, and degenerative diseases.
Cutaneous: molluscum contagiosum, sporotrichosis, acne, atypical mycobacterial infection, pyoderma gangrenosum, tuberculosis, coccidioidomycosis, and paracoccidioidomycosis.
Osseous: osteomyelitis, osteosarcomas, sporotrichosis, coccidioidomycosis, and paracoccidioidomycosis.
Disseminated: tuberculosis, coccidioidomycosis, paracoccidioidomycosis, and histoplasmosis.

Therapeutics

Intravenous amphotericin B 0.25–0.75mg/kg per day, with a total dose of 1–3g, alone or with oral 5-flucytosine 75–150mg/kg per day for six weeks is recommended.[253] Pulmonary and cutaneous infections may respond to ketoconazole 3–5mg/kg per day, or itraconazole 5–8mg/kg per day for 4–6 months; fluconazole 8mg/kg per day and maintenance dosages of 5mg/kg per day are preferred in neurological disease.

In AIDS, amphotericin B alone or with flucytosine or fluconazole for two to three weeks, followed by long-term maintenance with fluconazole or itraconazole, is recommended.

Aspergillosis

Introduction and historical note

Aspergillosis is one of the most frequent opportunistic respiratory fungal infections. Its definition dates from 1720, when Micheli noticed the resemblance of the agent to the aspergillum, an instrument used to sprinkle holy water. Aspergillus was noticed as a human pathogen in 1844 by Bennett. Subsequently, many species have been described.[263]

Etiology and pathogenesis

Aspergillus species belong to the Deuteromycetes class. Common agents are *A. fumigatus* and *A. flavus*. The fungus demonstrates specialized club-shaped hyphae with globular appendages, topped with multiple small branches, constituting the typical "aspergillar head."[164]

Aspergillus induces respiratory illness due to hypersensitivity and also by invasive proliferation, behaving as a saprophyte or pathogen respectively.

Saprophytic species induce a type I hypersensitivity response with eosinophilia, bronchial plugging, and collapse,[263] and, exceptionally, tissue damage. This is allergic aspergillosis, usually related to *A. fumigatus* and *A. niger*.[164,263] These species may also produce compact mycelial "balls" or aspergillomas that colonize existing pulmonary cavities.[164]

Invasive disease and hematogenous spread may occur as a result of host immunodeficiency and the hydrolytic enzymes of *A. fumigatus*. Because of the tendency of the fungus to reach blood vessels, thrombotic phenomena, angiitis, and subsequent hemorrhagic infarction occur.

Cutaneous aspergillosis is usually produced by *A. flavus*, *A. fumigatus*, and *A. niger*,[164] and has been reported in patients with hematologic malignancies, intravenous catheters, arm boards, or skin wounds that have been covered with occlusive dressings.[263]

Epidemiology

Aspergillus is distributed worldwide and is easily recovered from air, soil, and vegetation, and especially from carbohydrate and fiber-rich food. Infection occurs through inhalation, characteristically in immunosuppressed hosts, including those with hematological disorders, diabetes, or immunosuppressive therapies, and in also neonates.[264,265]

Clinical features

The respiratory system is the most common localization, accounting for up to 94% of cases,[266] and the condition presents as a hypersensitivity syndrome, localized colonization or pulmonary invasive disease.

Hypersensitivity syndromes or allergic aspergillosis are clinically nonspecific and indistinguishable from other allergic processes, such as rhinitis, asthma, or alveolitis. Individuals exposed to massive inhalation can develop extrinsic allergic alveolitis, commonly known as "farmer's lung," which presents with dyspnea, fever and rigors. Continued exposure may induce pulmonary fibrosis.

Localized pulmonary colonization or aspergilloma is usually initially asymptomatic but later cough, mucopurulent sputum, recurrent hemoptysis, and dyspnea may occur. Pulmonary invasive aspergillosis is an unusual necrotizing and fulminant disease. The clinical picture is of a severe infection with eventual dissemination to gastrointestinal tract and CNS in 20–50% of patients.[263]

Cutaneous aspergillosis is a rare condition with polymorphic manifestations. Chronic granulomatous disease, AIDS and underlying hematological or lymphoreticular malignancies have been reported as predisposing factors in children.[264,267,268] However, it has been ocassionally reported in immunocompetent individuals.[269]

The primary cutaneous form is related to direct inoculation and use of occlusive dressings or adhesive tape.[270] Initial lesions are erythematous papules or nodules that turn into purpuric plaques with hemorrhagic bullae and finally into dark eschar-covered ulcers. Underlying structures can become

258. Patel P, Ramanathan J, Kayser M et al. (2000) Primary cutaneous cryptococcosis of the nose in an immunocompetent woman. **J Am Acad Dermatol** 43:344–345.
259. Erdem G, Connelly BL (2000) Isolated cutaneous cryptococcosis in an otherwise healthy girl. **Pediatr Infect Dis J** 19:85–86.
260. Haight DO, Esperanza LE, Greene JN et al. (1994) Case report: cutaneous manifestations of cryptococcosis. **Am J Med Sci** 308:192–195.
261. Blanco P, Viallard JF, Beylot-Barry M et al. (1999) Cutaneous cryptococcosis resembling molluscum contagiosum in a patient with non-Hodgkin's lymphoma. **Clin Infect Dis** 29:683–684.
262. De Repentigny L (1992) Serodiagnosis of Candidiasis, aspergillosis, and cryptococcosis. **Clin Infect Dis** 14 (suppl 1):S11–S22.
263. Isaac M (1996) Cutaneous aspergillosis. **Dermatol Clin** 14:137–140.
264. Galimberti R, Kowalczuk A, Hidalgo I et al. (1998) Cutaneous aspergillosis: a report of six cases. **Br J Dermatol** 139:522–526.
265. Gupta M, Weinberger B, Whitley-Williams PN (1996) Cutaneous aspergillosis in a neonate. **Pediatr Infect Dis J** 15:464–465.
266. Kaiser L, Huguenin T, Lew PD et al. (1998) Invasive aspergillosis. Clinical features of 35 proven cases at a single institution. **Medicine** Baltimore 77:188–194.
267. Murakawa GJ, Harvell JD, Lubitz P et al. (2000) Cutaneous aspergillosis and acquired immunodeficiency syndrome. **Arch Dermatol** 136:365–369.
268. Grossman ME, Fithian EC, Behrens C et al. (1985) Primary cutaneous aspergillosis in six leukemic children. **J Am Acad Dermatol** 12:313–318.
269. Mowad CM, Nguyen TV, Jaworsky C et al. (1995) Primary cutaneous aspergillosis in an immunocompetent child. **J Am Acad Dermatol** 33:136–137.
270. Romero LS, Hunt SJ (1995) Hickman catheter associated primary cutaneous aspergillosis in a patient with the acquired immunodeficiency syndrome. **Int J Dermatol** 34:551–553.

involved and hematogenous dissemination is usual. Secondary cutaneous aspergillosis follows hematogenous dissemination.

Diagnosis

Direct mycological examination may show conidia, septate hyphae, and aspergillar heads. Repeated cultures should be performed on Sabouraud's agar without antibiotics at 28°C for 1–3 days, because Aspergillus is usually considered a contaminant. Skin tests, immunoglobulin levels, and eosinophil count in nasal discharge are helpful in hypersensitivity syndromes. Histopathology reveals sepatate and branching hyphae, remarkable edema, necrotic areas and a granulomatous infiltrate.

Differential diagnosis

Cutaneous aspergillosis: mucormycosis, cryptococcosis, phaeohyphomycosis, ecthyma gangrenosum, candidiasis, and atypical mycobacteriosis.
Pulmonary aspergillosis: other allergic reactions, histoplasmomas, cryptococcomas, coccidioidomycosis, histoplasmosis, mucormycosis, and miliary tuberculosis.
Disseminated: kala-azar, histoplasmosis, blastomycosis, and coccidioidomycosis.

Therapeutics

Allergic aspergillosis requires antihistamines, desensitization, and corticosteroids. Amphotericin B 0.25–0.75mg/kg per day is the choice for pulmonary disease and its liposomal form has been used safely in children with severe aspergillosis.[271]

Itraconazole 5–8mg/kg per day is an alternative. Terbinafine 5–15mg/kg per day for 12–38 weeks is comparable to amphotericin B or itraconazole.[193] Another alternative is KI-saturated solution 3–6gr/day orally (1–3gr/day for children). Aspergillomas may require surgery.

Zygomycosis

This term encompasses entities caused by molds of the class Zygomyces, namely mucormycosis and entomophthoromycosis, contrasting disorders except for some histopathological similarities.

Mucormycosis

Mucormycosis is an acute, rapidly progressive, and lethal disease caused by opportunistic fungi in immunocompromised patients.

Etiology and pathogenesis

It is caused by genus Mucor, Rhizomucor, Rhizopus and Absidia. Opportunistic infection develops when macrophage and PMN mechanisms to arrest fungi are suppressed.[272] Hyphae invade the mucosa of oropharynx, nasopharynx or sinuses and underlying structures, due to the well-recognized ability to invade blood vessels. Secondary thrombosis and necrosis lead to fulminant disease.

Enzymatic mechanisms that perform optimally in acidic and hyperglycemic conditions and in the presence of iron overload and ferrioxamine

enhance the growth and virulence of certain species.[273–276] Cutaneous disease has been commonly associated with immunodeficiency, but immunocompetent trauma patients may develop a serious disease secondary to wound colonization.[277,278]

Epidemiology

This is distributed worldwide, especially in warm and humid climates. Fungi can be found as saprophytes in soil, decaying vegetation, fruits, wheat, rye bread, and even in the air, and can be part of the normal flora of skin, gastrointestinal, respiratory, and urinary tracts.[279]

The disease can affect all age groups. Around 25 cases have been reported in children in the last 35 years, including in some premature newborns.[280–284] Presentation in the 2nd and 3rd decade of life occurs in young diabetics.[164]

The disease is acquired predominantly via the airway with predisposition by diabetes mellitus in 85% of cases,[164] and also by neutropenia of various causes, leukaemia, and lymphoma. Predisposing factors in premature infants are bandages and perinatal complications.[281,282]

Clinical features

The disease may be rhinocerebral, pulmonary, cutaneous, gastrointestinal and disseminated.

Rhinocerebral mucormycosis is an aggressive, fulminant, and fatal disease, frequently found in uncontrolled diabetics,[285] which begins in nasal sinus or pharyngeal mucosa, spreading to paranasal sinuses and finally to the frontal or retro-orbital brain. Early features include visual loss, periorbital swelling (Fig. 26.32), mucosal congestion, epistaxis and nasal and palatal necrotic eschars. Thereafter, severe headache, necrosis of nasal septum, fever and lethargy appear. Finally, all features become strikingly severe, with extensive secondary necrosis of skin, septum or palate, cranial nerve involvement, unconsciousness and convulsions. Widespread dissemination may follow.

Pulmonary mucormycosis is more frequent in patients with granulocytopenia, lymphatic malignancies, in intensive care, and following organ transplantation. The features are nonspecific, with productive cough, fever, hemoptysis, dyspnea, and thoracic pain. Mucormycomas resembling aspergillomas may occur.

Gastrointestinal disease is infrequent and affects especially children and patients with peptic ulceration, post-traumatic peritonitis, or bowel disease. Black ulcers appear on any segment of gastrointestinal tract. Common symptoms are severe abdominal pain, moderate fever, and melena.

Cutaneous mucormycosis is rarely primary and presents two variants. The first is a benign subacute superficial form with initial vesicles or pustules and late eschars limited to the skin in otherwise normal adults and children, almost always related to bandages. The second is a rapidly progressive gangrenous form with red, indurated necrotic plaques, surrounded by a violaceous area, occurring in immunosuppressed patients and with the potential to disseminate, especially in children.[280,283,284,286–291]

271. Ringden O, Tollemar J (1993) Liposomal amphotericin B (AmBisome) treatment of invasive fungal infections in immunocompromised children. **Mycoses** 36:187–192.
272. Diamond RD, Krzesicki R, Epstein B et al. (1978) Damage to hyphal forms of fungi by human leukocytes in vitro: a possible host defense mechanism in aspergillosis and mucormycosis. **Am J Pathol** 91:313–328.
273. Abramson E, Wilson D (1967) Rhinocerebral phycomycosis in association with ketoacidosis. **Ann Int Med** 66:737–742.
274. McMulty J (1982) Rhinocerebral mucormycosis. Predisposing factors. **Laryngoscope** 92:1140–1143.
275. McDonald ML, Weiss PJ, Deloach-Banta LJ et al. (1994) Primary cutaneous mucormycosis with Mucor species: is iron overload a factor? **Cutis** 54:275–278.
276. Verdonck AK (1993) Effect of ferrioxamine on the growth of Rhizopus. **Mycoses** 36:2–12.
277. Song WK, Park HJ, Cinn YW et al. (1999) Primary mucormycosis in a trauma patient. **J Dermatol** 26:825–828.
278. Seguin P, Musellec H, Le Gall F et al. (1999) Post traumatic course complicated by cutaneous infection with Absidia corymbifera. **Eur J Clin Microbiol Infect Dis** 18:737–739.
279. Sugar AM (1995) Agents of mucormycosis and related species. In: Principles and Practice of Infectious Diseases, 4th ed, Mandell GHL, Bennet JE, Dolin R, eds. New York: Churchill Livingstone, pp. 2311–2321.
280. Wirth F, Perry R, Eskenazi A et al. (1997) Cutaneous mucormycosis with subsequent visceral dissemination in a child with neutropenia: A case report and review of the pediatric literature. **J Am Acad Dermatol** 36:336–341.
281. Linder N, Keller N, Huri C et al. (1998) Primary cutaneous mucormycosis in a premature infant: case report and review of the literature. **Am J Perinatol** 15:35–38.
282. Du Plessis PJ, Wentzel LF, Delport SD et al. (1997) Zygomycotic necrotizing cellulitis in a premature infant. **Dermatology** 195:179–181.
283. Hughes C, Driver SJ, Alexander KA (1995) Successful treatment of abdominal wall Rhizopus necrotizing cellulitis in a preterm infant [letter]. **Pediatr Infect Dis** 14:336.
284. Craig NM, Lueder FL, Pensler JM et al. (1994) Disseminated Rhizopus infection in a premature infant. **Pediatr Dermatol** 11:346–350.
285. Karmeh DS, Gonzales OR, Pearl GS et al. (1997) Fatal rhino-orbital-cerebral zygomycosis. **South Med J** 90:1133–1135.
286. Ryan ME, Ochs J (1982) Primary cutaneous mucormycosis: superficial and gangrenous infections. **Pediatr Infect Dis** 1:110–114.
287. Kline MW (1985) Mucormycosis in children: review of the literature and report of cases. **Pediatr Infect Dis** 4:672–676.
288. Ryan-Poirier K, Eiseman RM, Beaty JH et al. (1988) Post-traumatic cutaneous mucormycosis in diabetes mellitus. Shorth-term antifungal therapy. **Clin Pediatr** (Phila) 27:609–612.
289. Dennis JE, Rhodes KH, Cooney DR et al. (1980) Nosocomial Rhizopus infection (zygomycosis) in children. **J Pediatr** 96:824–828.
290. Arisoy AE, Arisoy ES, Correa-Calderon A et al. (1993) Rhizopus necrotizing cellulitis in a preterm infant: a case report and review of the literature. **Pediatr Infect Dis J** 12:1029–1031.
291. White CB, Barcia PJ, Bass JW (1986) Neonatal zygomycotic necrotizing cellulitis. **Pediatrics** 78:100–102.

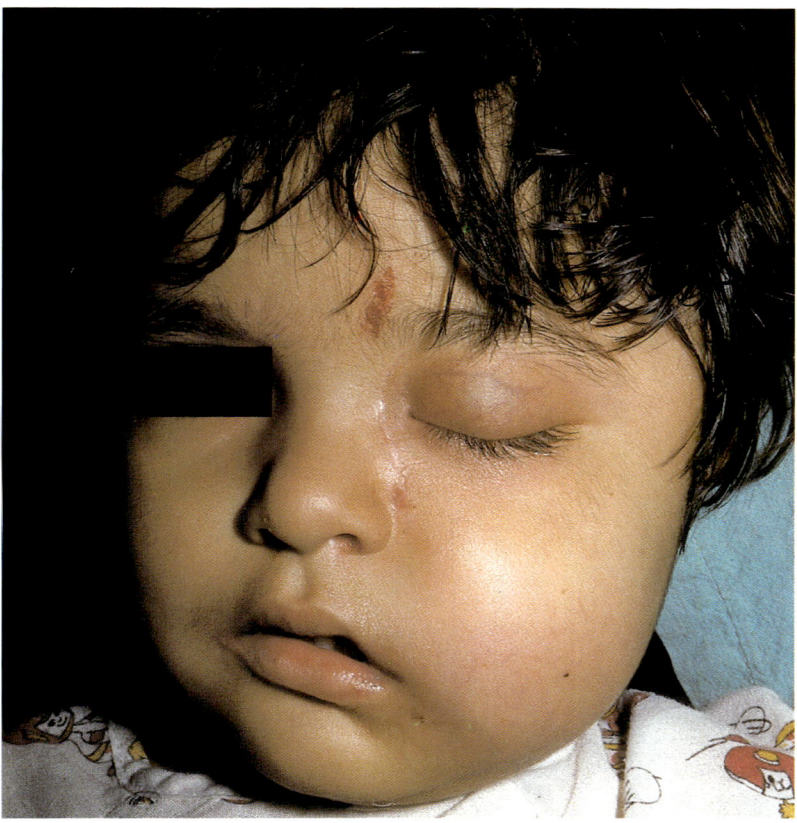

Fig. 26.32 Mucormycosis: rhinocerebral involvement with facial distortion, and 'closed' eye.

Diagnosis

Direct examination discloses broad, thick-walled, non-septate, $5\times20\mu m$ hyphae, branching at right angles. The value of culture is limited to identification of the species because these organisms are ubiquitous. These fungi grow rapidly on Sabouraud's agar at $25-37°C$ in 1–3 days and cultures must be repeated. Histopathologic findings include edema, PMN infiltrate, hyphae invading blood vessels, and necrosis. X-rays and CT scan show blurred paranasal sinuses, fistulae, and osteolytic changes. Chest X-rays show the picture of nonspecific pneumonia, and sometimes fungal masses.

Differential diagnosis

Ecthyma-like lesions, bacterial periorbital cellulitis, aspergillosis, atypical mycobacterial infection, osteomyelitis.

Therapeutics

Amphotericin B 0.25–0.75mg/kg per day, or its liposomal presentation, is the first-line therapy. Fluconazole 5–8mg/kg per day can be added to amphotericin B.[292] Alternatives are hyperbaric oxygen, iodides and trimethoprim-sulfmethoxazole. Surgical management may be indicated in some cases.

PROTOZOAL INFECTIONS

Hector W. Caceres-Rios

LEISHMANIASIS
Introduction and historical note

Leishmaniasis is a chronic parasitic infestation caused by species of intracellular protozoan of the genus Leishmania that may involve skin, mucous membranes, or viscera. The severity depends both on the species of Leishmania and the immune response of the host.

The first description of leishmaniasis can be attributed to Russell in 1756, who describe the "Aleppo evil" from Turkey. In 1898, Borovsky discovered the protozoan nature of the agent, but it was not until 1903 that Leishman described the parasite in a soldier who died from the systemic disease known as kala-azar. Evidence of the disease in the New World dates from the beginning of the Christian era. Pottery from the Mochica culture in Peru (AD 200–800) illustrates faces afflicted with mucocutaneous disease. Native words "uta" and "espundia" are still used in endemic areas of Peru to refer to cutaneous or mucocutaneous forms of leishmaniasis, respectively.

Etiology and pathogenesis

Parasites belong to order Kinetoplastida, family Trypanosomatidae and genus Leishmania. There has been recent acceptance of the existence of two subgenera, leishmania and viannia, each subclassified into complexes, which in turn are subdivided into species (Table 26.24).

The organisms are dimorphic during their life cycle. In humans and other vertebrate hosts, they live inside macrophages as $2-3\mu m$ oval or round, nonflagellated parasites known as amastigotes. In arthropod vectors or cultures, they turn into $15-25 \times 3\mu m$ elongated and flagellated organisms called promastigotes. Both forms have a nucleus and a smaller rod-shaped portion of mitochondrial DNA named a kinetoplast, which is at the base of the flagellum.

Following inoculation by vectors, promastigotes are exposed to a hostile medium, with different temperature and factors like PMN cells and complement that may damage the parasites and facilitate their phagocytosis by macrophages.[293] Once phagocytozed and supported by the host cell, promastigotes transform into and survive within phagolysosomes as "aflagellated" amastigotes, that replicate unrestrictedly.[294] The full macrophage finally bursts and amastigotes are freed into the extracellular space and are taken up by other macrophages, repeating this cycle.

Once inside the macrophage, the parasite induces the production of TNF-alpha, which potentiates the action of interferon (IFN) gamma and promotes macrophage activation due to its capacity to produce toxic oxygen and nitrogen radicals.[295,296] On the other hand, Leishmania induces transforming growth factor beta,[297] which is associated with inhibition of IFN-gamma, and macrophage deactivation.[298,299] The initial survival of the parasite is critically dependent on which of these opposing cytokines predominate in the microenvironment of the infection.[300]

Th-1 type cellular immune response is associated clinically with localized cutaneous forms and with a role in protection against Leishmania, while the Th-2 type response results in anergic, diffuse nodular, and progressive forms.[301,302]

292. Woods SG, Elewski BE (1995) Zosteriform zygomycosis. **J Am Acad Dermatol** 32:357–361.
293. Mosser DM, Edelson PJ (1984) Activation of the alternative complement pathway by Leishmania promastigotes: parasites lysis and attachment to macrophages. **J Immunol** 132:1501–1505.
294. Rittig MG, Bogdan C (2000) Leishmania-host-cell interaction: complexities and alternative views. **Parasitol Today** 16:292–297.
295. Bittencourt A, Barral-Netto M (1995) Leishmaniasis. In: Tropical Pathology. Doerr W, Seifert G. Heidelberg: Springer, pp. 597–651.
296. Titus RG, Sherry B, Cerami A (1989) Tumor necrosis factor plays a protective role in experimental murine cutaneous leishmaniasis. **J Exp Med** 6:2097–2104.
297. Barral-Netto M, Barral A, Brownell CE et al. (1992) Transforming growth factor-β in leishmanial infection: a parasite escape mechanism. **Science** 257:545–548.

298. Barral A, Barral-Netto M, Yong EC et al. (1993) Transforming growth factor-β as a virulence mechanism for Leishmania braziliensis. **Proc Natl Acad Sci USA** 90:3442–3446.
299. Ding A, Natham CF, Graycar J et al. (1990) Macrophage deactivating factor and transforming growth factors-betal, beta2, and beta3 inhibit induction of macrophage nitrogen oxide syntesis by IFN-gamma. **J Immunol** 145:940–944.
300. Bittencourt A, Barral A, Costa J (1996) Tegumentary leishmaniasis in childhood. **Pediatric Dermatol** 13:455–463.
301. Tapia FJ, Cáceres-Dittmar G, Sánchez MA et al. (1993) The cutaneous lesion in American leishmaniasis: leukocyte subsets, cellular interaction and cytokine production. **Biol Res** 26:239–247.
302. Ajdary S, Alimohammadian MH, Eslami MB et al. (2000) Comparison of the immune profile of nonhealing cutaneous leishmaniasis patients with those with active lesions and those who have recovered from infection. **Infect Immun** 68:1760–1764.

TABLE 26.24   Etiologic agents and clinical forms of leishmaniasis

Family	Genus	Subgenus	Complex	Species	Usual clinical form
Trypanosomatida	Leishmania	Leishmania	L. major	L. major	LCL
			L. tropica	L. tropica	LR
			L. aethiopica	L. aethiopica	DCL
			L. donovani	L. donovani	VL, PKDL
				L. infantum	VL5
			L. mexicana	L. chagasi	VL
				L. venezuelensis	LCL, MCL
				L. amazonensis	DCL, MCL
				L. mexicana	LCL, DCL
				L. pifanoi	DCL
		Viannia	L. braziliensis	L. braziliensis	LCL, MCL, LR
				L. peruviana	LCL
			L. guyanensis	L. guyanensis	MCL
				L. panamensis	MCL

☐ OLD WORLD LEISHMANIASIS   ☐ NEW WORLD LEISHMANIASIS

LCL: localized cutaneous leishmaniasis   VL: visceral leishmaniasis
PKDL: post-kala-azar dermal leishmaniasis
MCL: mucocutaneous leishmaniasis   LR: leishmaniasis recidivans

Parasitized circulating macrophages have been seen in chronic *L. braziliensis* infections,[303] and Villela showed macrophages with amastigotes present in apparently normal nasal mucosa from patients with cutaneous disease.[304] This finding suggests that these circulating cells carry the parasite to nasal and other mucosae.

Epidemiology

The condition occurs predominantly in tropical and subtropical regions, and is endemic in 88 countries worldwide. It does not occur in Australia and Antarctica.[305] There are 400 millions individuals estimated at risk of infection, 500 000 annual new cases of the visceral form, and about 1.5 million of cutaneous disease. Over 90% of tegumentary (cutaneous and mucocutaneous) leishmaniasis occurs in Afghanistan, Iran, Iraq, Saudi Arabia, Syria, Brazil, and Peru.[306–308] The disease is found in rain forests and damp regions, but also in arid and dry zones like western Asia and the western slopes of the highlands in Peru. Leishmaniasis may occur in both rural and suburban areas.

Humans are accidental hosts and transmission requires both infected vectors and reservoirs. The arthropod vector of leishmaniasis is the female of more than 30 species of sand flies, in the Old World the genus Phlebotomus, and in the New World Lutzomyia and rarely Psychodopygus.[309] Only the females are blood suckers and blood meals may be a stimulus for egg deposition.

The sand flies are infected when biting the reservoir animals, a variety of native wild or domestic animals like sloths, anteaters, rodents, foxes, and dogs.

Infection may rarely occur through direct contact and Leishmaniasis on the upper lip has been reported in a 3-month-old baby who was breast-feeding from by a mother with a nipple lesion.[310] Several cases of congenital transmission have been observed, from mothers with the active visceral form during pregnancy.[311,312]

Different reports reveal that in some hyperendemic areas between 19% and 66% of cases are in children.[299,313,314] All activities that increase the risk of sand fly bites are predisposing.[315] Unlike other parasitic diseases, association with AIDS seems infrequent.

Clinical forms

This includes a polymorphic spectrum of diseases. The traditional classification into Old World and New World cutaneous leishmaniasis according to its geographic presentation has been substituted by clinical classifications that have resulted in some confusion. The most useful classification for dermatologists is based on division by clinical aspects into two broad forms: cutaneous and visceral.

Cutaneous forms

LOCALIZED CUTANEOUS LEISHMANIASIS (LCL)

This is the most frequent clinical presentation in children and adults, and is widespread throughout the world. It usually affects unclothed areas of the body particularly, face, neck, and limbs, but may involve any exposed area. In children, lesions are most frequently located on the head (67.6%) and upper limbs (26%)[316] (Fig. 26.33).

303. Palau MT, Corredor A (1993) Aislamiento de Leishmania de monocitos circulantes. Resumenes Cuarto Congreso Latinoamericano de Medicina Tropical. Guayaquil, Ecuador: Sociedad Latinoamericana de Medicina Tropical y Parasitología.
304. Villela F, Pestana B, Pessoa SB (1939) Presença da "Leishmania braziliensis" na mucosa nasal sem lesao aparente, em casos recentes de leishmaniose cutanea. O Hospital 16:953–960.
305. Kalter DC (1989) Cutaneous and mucocutaneous leishmaniasis. Prog Dermatol 23:1–11.
306. Herwaldt BL (1999) Leishmaniasis. Lancet 354:1191–1199.
307. Lucas CM, Franke ED, Cachay MI et al. (1998) Geographic distribution and clinical description of leishmaniasis in Peru. Am J Trop Med Hyg 59:312–317.
308. Costa JM, Balby IT, Rocha EJ et al. (1998) Comparative study of American tegumentary leishmaniasis between childhood and teenagers from the endemic areas Buriticupu, Maranhao and Corte de Pedra, Bahia, Brazil. Rev Soc Bras Med Trop 31:279–288.
309. Ashford RW (1997) The leishmaniasis as model zoonosis. Ann Trop Med Parasitol 91:693–701.

310. Nanji AA, Greenway DC (1985) Leishmania braziliensis infection of the nipple. Br Med J 290:433–434.
311. Yadav TP, Gupta H, Satteya U et al. (1989) Congenital kala-azar. Ann Trop Med Parasitol 83:535–537.
312. Nyakundi PM, Muigai R, Were JB et al. (1988) Congenital visceral leishmanisis: a case report. Trans R Soc Trop Med Hyg 82:564.
313. Bonfante-Garrido R, Meléndez E, Barroeta S et al. (1992) Cutaneous leishmaniasis in western Venezuela caused by infection with L. venezuelensis and L. braziliensis variants. Trans R Soc Trop Med Hyg 86:141–148.
314. Al-Gindan Y, Abdul-Azia O, Kubba R (1984) Cutaneous leishmaniasis in Al-Hassa, Saudi Arabia. Int J Dermatol 23:194–197.
315. Kerdel-Vegas F (1982) American leishmaniasis. Int J Dermatol 21:291–303.
316. Cucé LC, Belda W Jr, Zolli CA (1990) Leishmaniose tegumentar na infância. An Bras Dermatol 65:185–195.

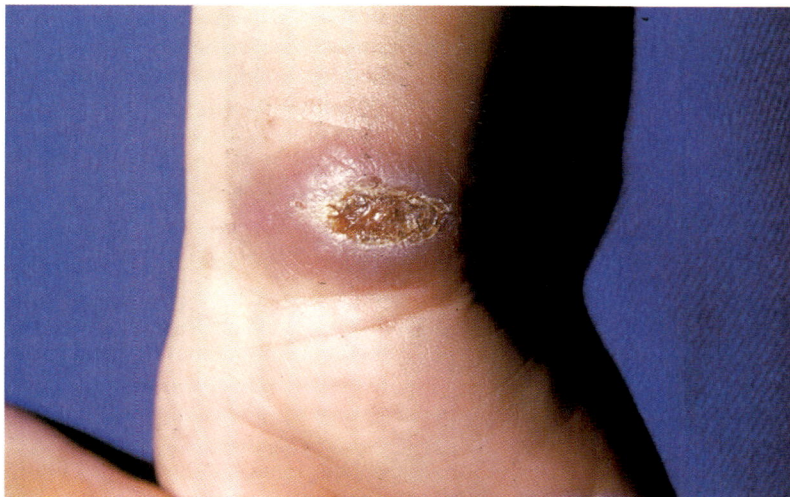

Fig. 26.33   Leishmaniasis in a child.

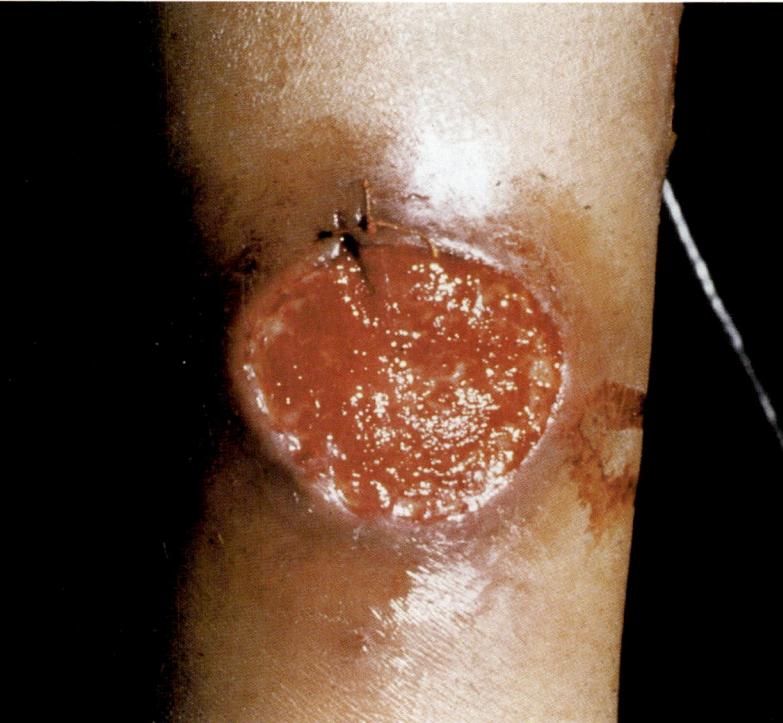

Fig. 26.34   Leishmaniasis: larger ulcerated lesion simulating pyoderma gangrenosum. (Courtesy of Evelyne Halpert MD)

The initial lesion develops in the inoculation site as a slightly firm erythematous papule that gradually enlarges peripherally. The center of the lesion may be covered by a serosanguinous scab and often ulcerates. Established lesions may be ulcerated, vegetative or nodular with the ulcerated form by far the most common. Single lesions are the rule and are found in 60% of children. Nevertheless, multiple simultaneous lesions may occur.[317] The classical ulcer is painless and well circumscribed, with thick, raised and violaceous borders surrounding a granulomatous base covered with a crust or a yellow membrane (Fig. 26.34). Regional lymphadenopathy can appear even without active skin or mucosal lesions.

There are differences in the clinical picture depending on the endemic area. Old World cutaneous leishmaniasis heals spontaneously in 90% to 95%.[300] New World leishmaniasis has some peculiarities. The so-called chiclero's ulcer of southeastern Mexico and Central America is produced by *L. mexicana* complex, and is characterized by single, painless, ulcerated lesions without adenopathy, located on the ear, with a tendency to slow destruction of the pinna with resultant disfigurement. "Uta" is another special form characterized by round, clean ulcerated lesions with spontaneous healing after 6–12 months, which occur in individuals of all ages, leaving a permanent atrophic pigmented or achromic scar.

MUCOCUTANEOUS LEISHMANIASIS (MCL)

This is usually caused by *L. braziliensis*, but also *L. panamensis*, *L. guyanensis*, and *L. amazonensis*.[306] MCL results from hematogenous or lymphatic dissemination of amastigotes from the skin to the nasal and oropharyngeal mucosa. Fifty percent of patients develop mucosal lesions within two years of the initial cutaneous involvement, and 90% within 10 years,[318] but it may occur when lesions are present or long after healing.

Initial features are nasal obstruction, serosanguinous discharge and epistaxis. The nasal septum appears swollen and infiltrated, and is covered with crusted papules and nodules. Subsequently, ulceration and even perforation may occur. Due to a propensity to involve the distal nasal cartilage and columella, disfiguring destruction of the tip of the nose can occur producing the so-called "tapir's nose," or "camel's nose". Mutilating lesions may involve palate, pharynx, tonsils, gums and lips, while bones usually remain unaffected. Invasion of the respiratory tract, including the larynx, trachea, and bronchi, may occasionally

occur. Sporadic cases of MCL have been described in children (3.5%),[319] probably due to the long latent period after the initial cutaneous lesions.

DIFFUSE CUTANEOUS LEISHMANIASIS (DCL)

This is a rare anergic variant, with no more than 500 reports worldwide. It occurs as a result of a specific cellular immune deficiency against *L. mexicana*, *L. amazonensis*, and *L. pifanoi* in America and *L. aethiopica* in Africa.[320] A case of cutaneous dissemination of *L. infantum*, the agent of Mediterranean visceral leishmaniasis, has been described in a child with no evidence of immunosuppression.[321]

This form occurs predominantly in children older than 5 years and in young adults.[322] It usually begins with a single papule or nodule that takes from three months to 20 years to disseminate to other areas of the skin, but not to internal organs. Established disease resembles lepromatous leprosy, with multiple lesions scattered specially over the face, ears, and limbs.

LEISHMANIASIS RECIDIVANS (LR)

This is a chronic relapsing cutaneous variant characterized by the development of new active confluent lesions inside or surrounding the scar of a healed lesion of LCL. It probably represents a reactivation of "dormant" organisms in scarred tissue after 1–15 years. Lesions have an indolent course and are resistant to treatment; papules and nodules are the usual forms, but ulcers, psoriasiform, and verrucous lesions have also been described.[323]

DISSEMINATED LEISHMANIASIS (DL)

DL is due to hematogenous dissemination, presenting as multiple simultaneous acneiform papules that may turn into small ulcers. This form is

317. Halpert E, Rodriguez G, Hernandez CA (2000) Leishmaniasis. In: Textbook of Pediatric Dermatology, Harper J, Oranje A, Prose N, eds. Oxford: Blackwell Science, pp. 514–526.
318. Marsden PD, Llanos-Cuentos EA, Lago EL et al. (1984) Human mucocutaneous leishmaniasis in Três Braços, Bahia-Brazil: an area of Leishmaniasis braziliensis braziliensis transmission. III. Mucosal disease, presentation and initial evolution. Rev Soc Bras Med Trop 17:179–186.
319. Marsdon PD (1986) Mucosal leishmaniasis ("espundia" Escomel, 1911). Trans R Soc Trop Med Hyg 80:859–876

320. Rodriguez G (2000) Leishmaniasis difusa. Revista Asociaón Colombiana de Dermatología y Cirugia Dermatologica 8:33–40.
321. Nuwayri-Salti N, Salman S, Shanin NM et al. (1999) Leishmania donovani invasion of the blood in a child with dermal leishmaniasis. Ann Trop Paediatr 19:61–64.
322. Belli A, García D, Palacios X et al. (1999) Widespread atypical cutaneous leishmaniasis caused by Leishmania (1.) chagasi in Nicaragua. Am J Trop Med Hyg 61:380–385.
323. Grevelink S, Lerner E (1996) Leishmaniasis Part I. J Am Acad Dermatol 34:257–272.

completely different from DCL which is characterized by disseminated nodular nonulcerated lesions.[324,325]

Visceral leishmaniasis

Commonly known as kala-azar, this is a severe and sometimes fatal systemic disease caused by *L. donovani* complex, usually in malnourished children younger than 5 years old and in young adults.[322] The infection may be asymptomatic, or have an acute, subacute, or chronic course.

The classic form is a severe life-threatening disease that develops after an incubation period of weeks to months, and is characterized by high fever, malaise, wasting, lymphadenopathy, hepatosplenomegaly, pancytopenia, and hyperglobulinemia. Intestinal or pulmonary involvement is usually fatal. An unusual case of bronchopulmonary and mediastinal leishmaniasis has been described.[326]

During the disease, patchy cutaneous hyperpigmentation may appear, probably as a result of increased melanoblastic activity as well as an enhancement of the natural skin color because of xerosis,[323] which is the origin of the term "kala-azar," a Sanskrit world meaning "black fever."

VISCERAL LEISHMANIASIS (VL)

This was described in soldiers who served in the Middle East as part of Operation Desert Storm in 1991.[327] The etiology was attributed to *L. tropica*, an agent previously thought to cause cutaneous disease exclusively. Clinical features were different from those of VL caused by *L. donovani* and included high fever, malaise, intermittent diarrhea, and abdominal pain, but no cutaneous lesions.

POST KALA-AZAR DERMAL LEISHMANIASIS (PKDL)

This is a clinical variant of CL caused by *L. donovani* that occurs after VL, particularly in long-standing or inadequately treated cases. It is very common in India, where almost 20% of patients develop the disease 1–2 years after recovery.[328] PKDL affects mainly individuals under 20 years of age.[329]

The first cutaneous manifestations are hypopigmented macules, which progress to large, irregular, erythematous patches which are later replaced by soft, painless, non-ulcerated, yellow-pink papules, nodules or plaques. Involvement of the face with numerous nodules and plaques following skin folds can mimic lepromatous leprosy.

Diagnosis

Tissue smears stained with Giemsa, Wright or Leishman stains reveal amastigotes. Culture can be performed on Nicolle–Novy–McNeal medium and promastigotes grow between two days and four weeks.

Immunodiagnostic methods include tests for antibody or antigen detection and assays for Leishmania-specific cell-mediated immunity.

The intradermal hypersensitivity or Montenegro test constitutes a diagnostic tool in non-endemic areas and a survey test in endemic regions. It is particularly important in children, because a positive reaction could mean not only infection but also disease.

Isoenzyme analysis on cultured amastigotes is presently considered the gold standard technique for Leishmania identification.[330] Other methods include detection of monoclonal antibodies to parasite surface antigens,[331] molecular techniques that involve analysis of kinetoplast DNA (kDNA) by restriction endonuclease digestion[332] or DNA hybridization,[333] as well as PCR.[334]

Histopathology shows different patterns depending on the type and stage of the disease. A diffuse lymphohistiocytic infiltrate is seen in cutaneous forms. A granulomatous pattern with well-organized granulomas and Langhans giant cells may be observed in PKDL and LR.

Vacuolated histiocytes filled with amastigotes, known as Leishman-Donovan bodies, are numerous in DCL, and many are seen in early lesions of LCL (Fig. 26.35) and PKDL but they are scant in MCL, VL, and LR.[323]

Differential diagnosis

LCL: tropical and traumatic ulcerative lesions, foreign-body reactions, infected insect bites, myiasis, impetigo, fungal and mycobacterial infections, sarcoidosis, and neoplasms.
MCL: paracoccidioidomycosis, rhinoscleroma, rhinosporidiosis, midline granuloma, mucormycosis, entomophtoromycosis, and cutaneous free living amoebiasis.
VL: malaria, schistosomiasis, African trypanosomiasis, miliary tuberculosis, brucellosis, typhoid fever, bacterial endocarditis, histoplasmosis, malnutrition, lymphoma, and leukaemia.
PKDL: leprosy

Treatment

The natural course of the illness should be considered when deciding on treatment, as Old World LCL is usually self-healing in one month to three years, whereas lesions of MCL and VL rarely heal without treatment.

The first therapeutic alternative is sodium stibogluconate, a pentavalent antimony compound, 10–20mg/kg per day im or iv is administered for 20 days in cutaneous disease and for 28 days in mucosal or visceral disease.[335] Side effects of stibogluconate include phlebitis, arthralgias, myalgias, abdominal upset and, more rarely, cardiotoxicity, nephrotoxicity, hepatotoxicity, and

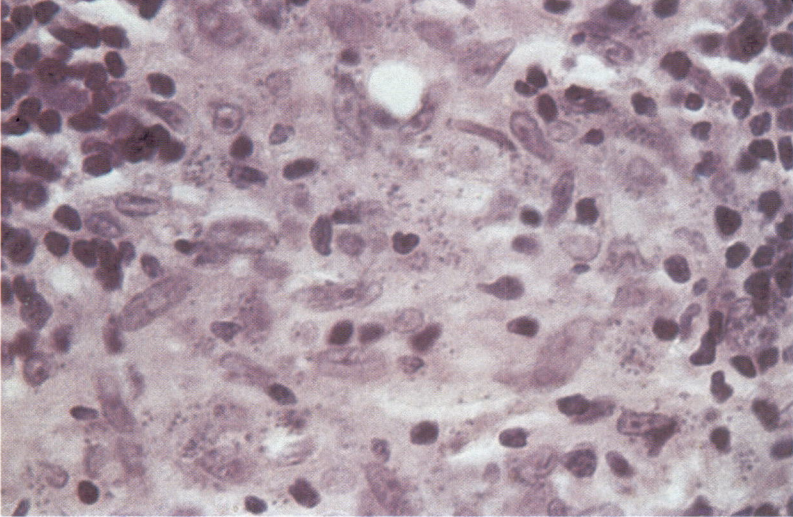

Fig. 26.35 Localized cutaneous leishmaniasis child: photomicrograph, H & E stain x 400. Numerous tiny amastigotes within histiocytes (Courtesy Dr Gerald Goldberg).

324. Kubba R, El-Hassan AM, Al-Gindan Y et al. (1987) Dissemination in cutaneous leishmaniasis: I. Subcutaneous nodules. **Int J Dermatol** 26:300–304.
325. Carvalho EM, Barral A, Costa JML et al. (1994) Clinical and immunological aspects in disseminated cutaneous leishmaniasis. **Acta Tropica** 56:315–325.
326. Marshall BG, Kropf P, Murray K et al. (2000) Bronchopulmonary and mediastinal leishmaniasis: an unusual clinical presentation of Leishmania donovani infection. **Clin Infect Dis** 30(5):764–769.
327. Magill AJ, Grogl M, Gasser RA Jr et al. (1993) Visceral infection caused by Leishmania tropica in veterans of Operation Desert Storm. **N Engl J Med** 328:1383–1387.
328. Rees PH, Kager PA (1987) Visceral leishmaniasis and post kala-azar dermal leishmaniasis. In: The Leishmaniases in Biology and Medicine, Peters W, Killick-Kendrick R, eds. London: Academic Press, pp. 848–907.
329. Zijlstra EE, Khalil EA, Kager PA et al. (2000) Post kala-azar dermal leishmaniasis in the Sudan: clinical presentation and differential diagnosis. **Br J Dermatol** 143:136–143.

330. Evans D (1989) Handbook on Isolation, Characterization and Cryopreservation of Leishmania. Geneva: UNDP/World Bank/WHO (TDR).
331. McMahon-Pratt D, Bennett E, David JR (1982) Monoclonal antibodies that distinguish subspecies of Leishmaniasis braziliensis. **J Immunol** 129:926–927.
332. Jackson PR, Wohlieter JA, Jackson JE et al. (1984) Restriction endonuclease analysis of Leishmania kinetoplast DNA characterizes parasites responsible for visceral and cutaneous disease. **Am J Trop Med Hyg** 33:808–819.
333. Wirth DF, Pratt DM (1982) Rapid identification of Leishmania species by specific hybridization of kinetoplast DNA in cutaneous lesions. **Proc Natl Acad Sci USA** 38:6999–7003.
334. Blackwell JM (1992) Leishmaniasis epidemiology: all down to the DNA. **Parasitology** 104(suppl):S19–S34.
335. Aronson NE, Wortmann GW, Johnson SC et al. (1998) Safety and efficacy of intravenous sodium stibogluconate in the treatment of leishmaniasis: recent US military experience. **Clin Infect Dis** 27:1457–1464.

hemolytic anemia. Electrocardiogram (ECG) changes, such as T-wave inversion, ST segment elevation or depression, and QT prolongation, may occur.

Amphotericin B 0.5–1.0mg/kg per day to a total dose of 20–30mg/kg has been used successfully as second-line agent, especially in MCL.[336] Pentamidine 2mg/kg should be administered on alternate days for one week in LCL or five weeks in MCL and DCL. Some studies, predominantly in the viannia subgenus, have shown that short-course pentamidine therapy is effective and acceptably tolerated.[337] Ketoconazole[338] and itraconazole[339] have been effective in some cases.

Immunotherapy with live bacille Calmette–Guérin (BCG) combined with killed Leishmania promastigotes is considered comparable to standard antimony therapy in LCL.[340] Systemic monotherapy with IFN-gamma can be an effective treatment of complicated cases of CL without the side effects of pentavalent antimony.[341] Combination of antimony and IFN-gamma has been used in refractory VL in Brazil.[342]

FREE LIVING-AMOEBIASIS (FLA)
Introduction and historical note
This is a protozoan disease caused by free-living amoebae belonging to genera Naegleria, Acanthamoeba and Balamuthia, which usually produces severe CNS involvement, sometimes associated with cutaneous involvement.

The first human case of cerebral FLA was reported in 1960 by Kernohan, who attributed the disease to Acanthamoeba.[343] In 1965, Fowler and Carter reported another cerebral case initially thought to be of acanthamoebic origin,[344] years later it was proved to be caused by Naegleria fowleri.

Some cases of cerebral FLA, initially ascribed to Acanthamoeba, later were thought to be produced by members of the order Leptomyxida.[345] However, the organism has now been reclassified into the genus Balamuthia, to honor William Balamuth. Balamuthia mandrillaris denotes the origin of the species isolated from a pregnant baboon that died at the San Diego Zoo.[346]

The first case of cutaneous acantamoebiasis was reported in 1986 in an AIDS patient.[347] It is now appreciated that B. mandrillaris may cause cutaneous and mucosal disease preceding CNS involvement.[348] In Peru, about 25 cases with cutaneous involvement related to Balamuthia have been described.[349]

Etiology and pathogenesis
Free-living amoebae that produce infection in humans include *Naegleria fowleri*, *Acanthamoeba* species and *Balamuthia mandrillaris*.

Naegleria fowleri is a thermophilic, aerobic, and highly invasive amoeba that has been isolated from the CNS of humans. The agent enters through nasal mucosa, initially involving the olfactory neuroepithelium, and subsequently reaches the CNS by active phagocytosis of sustentacular cells. Due to the contiguity with subarachnoid membranes, amoebas may easily disseminate to other areas of the CNS,[350] producing an acute and fulminating primary amoebic meningoencephalitis (PAM).

Acanthamoeba species have 15–40μ trophozoites with finely granular cytoplasm and star-shaped cysts. This agent enters through skin or respiratory tract and thereafter spreads to the CNS, producing the so-called granulomatous amoebic encephalitis (GAE), and eventually spreads through the bloodstream.[351] Acanthamoeba infections usually occur in immunocompromised patients.

B. mandrillaris is a newly described free-living amoeba. The trophozoites measure 15–60μ and its double-walled cyst 15–30μ. The pathogenic mechanisms of *B. mandrillaris* have not been well established.

Epidemiology
Most cases of FLA have been reported in Mexico, Peru, Venezuela, Argentina, Canada, USA, and Australia.[345] At present, more than 200 cases of PAM produced by *N. fowleri* have been reported; around 100 cases of GAE are related to *Acanthamoeba*; and approximately 66 human *Balamuthia* cases have been recognized worldwide.[352]

Amoebae are usually found in fresh water lakes, thermal discharge of power plants, hot springs, ponds, streams with still water, sewage, and even in the nasal cavity of healthy persons.[350] The organisms enter the nasal cavity by inhalation of dust, through contaminated water, or in air that contains trophozoites or cysts.[353]

Although the disease may occur in any age, most reported cases are in children and adolescents, especially those produced by *B. mandrillaris*.[354–358]

Immersion in swimming pools, freshwater lakes or ponds and any form of immunodeficiency are predisposing factors for Acanthamoeba species.[359] There are no identified predisposing factors for Balamuthia infections, particularly in pediatric patients.[355]

Clinical features
FLA produces mainly CNS disease, but also may involve other organs such as eyes, nasal mucosa or skin.

Neurological FLA
PAM is a disease with an abrupt onset and fulminant course produced by *N. fowleri* that usually affects children and young adults, and is characterized by signs and symptoms of meningeal irritation and encephalitis. Sudden onset of bifrontal or bitemporal headache, fever, nausea, vomiting, and stiff neck may progress rapidly to lethargy, confusion, coma, and death in 48–72 hours.[353]

336. Barral-Netto M, Machado P, Barral A (1995) Human cutaneous leishmaniasis: recent advances in physiopathology and treatment. **Eur J Dermatol** 5:104–113.
337. Berman JD (1997) Human leishmaniasis: clinical, diagnostic, and chemotherapeutic developments in the last 10 years. **Clin Infect Dis** 24:684–703.
338. Wali JP, Aggarwal P, Gupta U et al. (1990) Ketoconazole in treatment of visceral leishmaniasis. **Lancet** 336:810–811.
339. Dogra J, Saxena VN (1996) Itraconazole and leishmaniasis: a randomised double-blind trial in cutaneous disease. **Int J Parasitol** 26:1413–1415.
340. Convit J, Rondon A, Ulrich M et al. (1987) Immunotherapy versus chemotherapy in localised cutaneous leishmaniasis. **Lancet** 1:401–405.
341. Kolde G, Luger T, Sorg C et al. (1996) Successful treatment of cutaneous leishmaniasis using systemic interferon-gamma. **Dermatology** 192:56–60.
342. Harms G, Zwingenberger K, Sandkamp B et al. (1993) Immunotherapy of visceral leishmaniasis: a pilot trial of sequential treatment with recombinant interferon-gamma and pentavalent antimony. **J Interferon Res** 13:39–41.
343. Kernohan JW, Magath TB, Schloss GT (1960) Granuloma of the brain probably due to Endolimax williamsi (Iodamoeba butschlii). **Arch Pathol** 70:576–580.
344. Fowler M, Carter RF (1965) Acute pyogenic meningitis probably due to Acanthamoeba sp. a preliminary report. **Br Med J** 2:740.
345. Visvesvara GS, Martinez AJ, Schuster FL et al. (1990) Leptomyxyd amoeba, a new agent of amoebic meningoencephalitis in humans and animals. **J Clin Microbiol** 28:2750–2756.
346. Visvesvara GS, Schuster FL, Martinez AJ (1993) Balamuthia mandrillaris, agent of amebic meningoencephalitis in humans and other animals. **J Eukariot Microbiol** 40:504–514.
347. Gonzalez MM, Gould E, Dickinson G et al. (1986) Acquired immunodeficiency syndrome associated with Acanthamoeba infection and other opportunistic organisms. **Arch Pathol Lab Med** 110:749–751.
348. Bravo F, Delgado W, Sacsaquispe S et al. (1995) Infections by the free-living amoeba Balamuthia mandrillaris: the clinical and histopathological findings of the skin and mucous membrane

involvement. Abstract presented at American Society of Dermatopathology 32nd Annual Meeting, USA.
349. Bravo F, Torres C, Delgado W et al. (1999) Hallazgos histopatologicos de la infección de la piel y mucosas por Balamuthia mandrillaris. Poster Exhibit at XXII Congreso de la Sociedad Latinoamericana de Patologia; Octubre; Lima, Peru.
350. Ma P, Visvesvara GS, Martinez J et al. (1990) Naegleria and Acanthamoeba infections: Review. **Rev Infect Dis** 12:490–513.
351. Martinez J (1993) Free living amoebas: Infection of the central nervous system. **Mount Sinai J Med** 60:271–278.
352. Martinez AJ, Visvesvara GS (1997) Free-living amphizoic and opportunistic amebas. **Brain Pathol** 7:583–598.
353. Martinez AJ, Visvesvara GS (1991) Laboratory diagnosis of pathogenic free-living amoebas: Naegleria, Acanthamoeba, and Leptomyxid. **Clin Lab Med** 11:861–872.
354. Recavarren-Arce S, Velarde C, Gotuzzo E et al. (1999) Amoeba angeitic lesions of the central nervous system in Balamuthia mandrillaris amoebiasis. **Hum Pathol** 30:269–273.
355. Rowen JL, Doerr CA, Vogel H et al. (1995) Balamuthia mandrillaris: a newly recognized agent for amebic meningoencephalitis. **Pediatr Inf Dis** 14:705–710.
356. Popek EJ, Neafie RC (1992) Granulomatous meningoencephalitis due to Leptomyxid ameba. **Pediatr Pathol** 12:871–881.
357. Lowichik A, Rollins N, Delgado R et al. (1995) Leptomyxid amebic meningoencephalitis mimicking brain stem glioma. **Am J Neuroradiol** 16:926–929.
358. Reed RP, Cooke-Yarborough CM, Jaquiery AL et al. (1997) Fatal granulomatous amoebic encephalitis caused by Balamuthia mandrillaris. **MJA** 167:82–84.
359. Seijo Martinez M, Gonzales-Mediero G, Santiago P et al. (2000) Granulomatous amebic encephalitis in a patient with AIDS: Isolation of Acanthamoeba sp. Group II from brain tissue and successful treatment with sulfadiazine and fluconazole. **J Clin Microbiol** 38:3892–3895.

GAE is a chronic and fatal disease characterized by neurological signs depending on multifocal hemorrhagic and necrotic of areas of the brain. The disease may be caused by Acanthamoeba or Balamuthia species in debilitated or immunosuppressed patients,[360] but the latter also affects immunocompetent children.[361] Symptoms resemble those of single or multiple space-occupying lesions. Hemiparesis, drowsiness, personality changes, and seizures appear early in the clinical course; insidious headache, low-grade fever, stiff neck, nausea, vomiting, and lethargy may be present. Death occurs from one week to several months after onset.

Cutaneous FLA

Disease due to *B. mandrillaris* occurs in otherwise healthy children. The primary cutaneous lesion occurs in the nasal pyramid and rarely in other areas of the skin, such as gluteal or lumbar areas.[354] The centrofacial plaque has a granulomatous appearance with typical elevated and serpiginous borders that slowly spread peripherally. GAE symptoms may develop months later, with progressive deterioration and death.

Primary cutaneous lesions produced by Acanthamoeba species are multiple chronic nodules or ulcers usually presenting in immunocompromised patients.

Disseminated FLA

This occurs especially in the immunosuppressed. Granulomas and amoebae have been found in adrenal gland, kidney, liver, lungs, pancreas, spleen, thyroid gland, and uterus.[362]

Diagnosis

Direct examination of CSF in PAM and GAE using a phase-contrast microscope discloses pear-shaped biflagellated motile amoebae. Smears stained with Giemsa, Wright or hematoxylin and eosin (H&E) disclose the morphology of the amoebae.

N. fowleri and *Acanthamoeba* species can be cultured easily in agar seeded with bacteria like *E. coli* at 37°C. Cultures of *B. mandrillaris* require monkey kidney cells but are often unsuccessful;[358] a new axenic (cell-free) medium may be more suitable.[363]

Gel diffusion, immunoelectrophoresis, indirect immunofluorescence, and immunoblotting may be useful. Isoenzyme analysis of cell-free extracts can differentiate pathogenic species.[353]

Histopathology of the brain demonstrates clusters of trophozoites and cysts around blood vessels and resultant hemorrhagic necrosis of the meninges and brain.[355]

Skin biopsies disclose a granulomatous reaction, with multinucleated giant cells, and a mixed inflammatory infiltrate. The amoebae can be seen using routine H&E stains.[348]

Differential diagnosis

Neurologic FLA: bacterial meningitis, viral encephalitis, tuberculosis, cysticercosis, coccidioidomycosis, and any other intracerebral masses. Cutaneous FLA: MCL, rhinosporidiosis, rhinoscleroma, conidiobolomycosis, Wegener's granulomatosis, sarcoidosis, Melkersson Rosenthal syndrome, mid-line granuloma, and cutaneous T cell lymphoma.

Therapeutics and prognosis

Successful treatment of Naegleria encephalitis with intravenous and intrathecal amphotericin B has been reported.[364] There is no known effective therapy for Balamuthia infection. Miconazole, 5-fluorocytosine, pentamidine, sulfadiazine, fluconazole, itraconazole, amphotericine-B, azithromycin, and clarithromycin have been used with variable results.

Long-term albendazole 20mg/kg per day and itraconazole 10mg/kg per day have been used as a therapeutic alternatives in some of our patients with promising results.

HELMINTHIC INFECTIONS AND OTHER PARASITIC ERUPTIONS

Sheila F. Friedlander

Parasitic worms that are capable of causing disease in humans fall into three broad categories: nematodes or roundworms, trematodes or flukes, and cestodes or tapeworms. Flukes and tapeworms possess a flat morphology, and are members of the phylum Platyhelminthes, while nematodes are members of the class Nematoda. Though infestations by these parasites are mostly endemic to tropical and subtropical regions, certain parasites such as *Enterobius vermicularis* have a worldwide distribution. With the modern increase of travel to different countries, tourists can contract parasitic infections that are not endemic to their place of residence. Clinicians everywhere should therefore be familiar with common presentations of these disorders. Worldwide, the burden of helminths in humans is staggering and accounts for significant morbidity and mortality in hundreds of millions of people.

Helminthic infections are often multisystem infestations that may lack cutaneous findings. Infections with helminths that are limited to the skin do occur, but are less frequent. Common signs of systemic infestation include eosinophilia and pruritus. Cutaneous findings are highly variable and depend upon the parasite involved, but the range of manifestations includes a localized papular rash, the serpiginous meandering track of larva migrans, subcutaneous nodules and migratory angioedema. Though there are increasingly sophisticated serologic means of diagnosing these diseases, helminthic infections can largely be diagnosed on the basis of signs, symptoms, and a good history. When a helminthic infection is suspected, the patient's recent and occasionally remote travel history is crucial. Because the cells of mammals and helminths are quite similar, the effective antihelminthics frequently carry a high level of human toxicity. The parasites' often complicated life-cycles may require therapy targeted at multiple stages of their development in order to eradicate the organism. In certain cases, systemic corticosteroids may reduce inflammation and treat symptoms, but their use may also increase the worm burden as a result of their immunosuppressive effect. As treatment recommendations are frequently revised, the treating clinician is encouraged to consult an experienced practitioner and the current literature to help guide therapy. The Centers for Disease Control in Atlanta may serve as a reliable source for medications and current treatment guidelines.

SCHISTOSOMIASIS

Introduction

Schistosomiasis is the most common and important trematode infection of mankind. These flatworms are capable of undergoing a portion of their life cycle in humans, causing significant morbidity and pathology. Of historical interest, calcified *Schistosoma hematobium* eggs have been discovered in the kidneys of ancient Egyptian mummies, dating back to 1200 BC.

360. Di Gregorio F, Rivasi N, Mongiardo B et al. (1992) Acanthamoeba meningoencephalitis in a patient with acquired immunodeficiency syndrome. **Arch Pathol Lab** 116:1363–1365.
361. Grieserner DA, Barton LL, Reese CM et al. (1994) Amebic meningoencephalitis caused by Balamuthia mandrillaris. **Pediatr Neurol** 10:249–254.
362. Gullet J, Mills J, Hadley K et al. (1979) Disseminated granulomatous acanthamoeba infection presenting as an unusual skin lesion. **Am J Med** 67:891–895.
363. Schuster FL, Visvesvara GS (1996) Axenic growth and drug sensitivity studies of Balamuthia mandrillaris, an agent of amebic meningoencephalitis in humans and other animals. **J Clin Microbiol** 34:385–388.
364. Seidel JS, Harmatz P, Visvesvara GS et al. (1982) Successful treatment of primary amebic meningoencephalitis. **N Engl J Med** 306:346–348.

Epidemiology

The disease affects an estimated 200 million people, with 80 million cases in Africa. The disease is also endemic in the Middle East, Brazil, China, and certain parts of Southeast Asia. According to the World Health Organization, 120 million of the individuals harboring the parasite are symptomatic, while 20 million have severe disease. Schistosomiasis kills an estimated 800 000 persons annually.

Presenting history

There are four species of *Schistosoma* that cause disease in humans, their definitive hosts. In the infected individual, eggs of the parasite are discharged into the environment through urine or feces. In fresh water, the eggs hatch, releasing motile miracidium that enter the intermediate host (the snail), and transform into cercariae that are then released from the snail after six weeks. It is this stage of schistosomal development that is infectious. After cercariae are released from the snail, they enter the human host by penetrating the skin, causing an urticarial, macular, papular or less commonly purpuric eruption at the site of entry. Following entry into the body, the adult flukes of *S. hematobium* establish residence in the pelvic veins surrounding the urinary bladder, causing a urinary tract infection or obstruction. Resulting symptoms include dysuria, hematuria, and anemia. The primary target organs of the other species *S. japonicum*, *S. mansoni* and *S. mekongi* are the liver and intestine.[365] All schistosomal species can affect the lung vasculature and cause pulmonary hypertension. During the acute phase of infection, migration of the organism in the body cause a granulomatous inflammation, with damage to the adjacent tissue.

Physical examination

Two distinctive cutaneous syndromes are recognized with systemic *Schistosoma* infection, depending on the developmental stage of the parasite and whether the disease is acute or chronic.[366] The first syndrome known as bilharzides, most commonly due to *S. japonicum*, occurs in two phases. Early bilharzides describes the febrile syndrome during early migratory invasion of the parasite. Generalized urticarial eruptions and edema are often present, with occasional purpura. These allergic effects frequently resolve weeks later when eggs are detectable in the urine and stool. Late bilharzides may occur with the eventual production and deposition of a large egg burden and resultant immune response. It is characterized by urticaria, excoriations, generalized pruritus, and often by lichenified and hyperpigmented plaques. Bilharzides should be suspected in any febrile individual with urticaria from an endemic area, and a recent history of contact with fresh water where snails may have existed. The second systemic syndrome, bilharziasis cutanea tarda presents with granulomatous anogenital papules, nodules or tumors. Ova that reach the skin through the portosystemic circulation explain the location of the granulomatous lesions, though extragenital sites of cutaneous involvement have also been reported. Furthermore, several cases of cutaneous schistosomiasis involving the genital area, in the apparent absence of systemic involvement, have also been described in the literature.[367,368]

Diagnosis and laboratory findings

The diagnosis of schistosomiasis is suggested by the presence of symptoms and by eosinophilia. Confirmation can be established with serologic tests including complement fixation and immunofluorescence earlier in the course of infection. Assaying for the presence of eggs in the feces and urine continues to be the most common means of diagnosis and is both sensitive and cost-effective.

Pathophysiology and histogenesis

The primary pathologic lesion is the result of an immunologic response to deposited eggs. The ova secrete soluble glycoprotein antigens that elicit an exuberant host granulomatous response in the acute phase of the disease, resulting in significant tissue inflammation and injury. During chronic infections, the immune response is down-regulated, with less proximal tissue injury. The inflammation and resultant scar are reversible during the early stages of schistosomiasis, whereas the dense, fibrotic scarring that occurs with chronic infestations may be permanent.

Therapeutics and prognosis

Standard therapy for systemic schistosomiasis is praziquantel. A recent cost reduction has made the medication more widely available. The recommended treatment for *S. hematobium* and *S. mansoni* is a single 40mg/kg dose. The less sensitive species *S. japonicum* and *S. mekongi* require a total of 60mg/kg that is administered in divided doses, to achieve comparable cure rates of 75–100%. Recent data suggest that individuals with greater intensity of infection, as evidenced by a greater number of eggs per gram of stool, have lower cure rates than those with light infections.[369] The side effects of Praziquantel are mild and include dizziness, headaches, and abdominal pain. The cutaneous manifestations of schistosomiasis can be treated symptomatically with antihistamines and antipruritic lotions for itching. Systemic treatment with praziquantal induces the resolution of small lesions, while larger lesions may require weekly intralesional triamcinolone injections or surgical excision.

CYSTICERCOSIS

Introduction

This disorder results from human infection with the larval stage *Cysticercus cellulosae* of the pork tapeworm, *Taenia solium*. This disease is associated with poverty and with poor hygiene. Cutaneous manifestations of this disease are common, but the most alarming form of *Taenia solium* infection occurs with central nervous system involvement. Untreated neurocysticercosis carries a fatality rate of 50%.

Epidemiology

Cysticercosis occurs worldwide, but is endemic in parts of South America, Asia, sub-Saharan Africa, and Mexico. An estimated 1000 new cases are diagnosed each year in the United States, primarily in the southwestern region. Worldwide, 50 million people are affected.[370]

Presenting history and physical examination

Neurocysticercosis may be asymptomatic or present with seizures. In one study involving 500 pediatric patients with neurocysticercosis, seizures were present in nearly 95% of cases.[371] Chronic headache, nausea and vomiting, visual changes, mental status changes, and focal neurologic deficits may develop. Recent-onset seizures in an otherwise healthy child is suggestive, particularly in combination with a history of residence or travel in an endemic area. Physical findings may include papilledema, nystagmus, intraocular larvae, muscle pseudohypertrophy, and subcutaneous nodules. These lesions are painless, usually asymptomatic, and similar in appearance to benign subcutaneous tumors and epidermoid cysts. The trunk, extremities, and chest are more common locations, but eyelid lesions have rarely been known to occur. In an early study of 450 cases of cysticercosis, 54% of the study group presented with cutaneous lesions.[372] The time interval from the initial infection to the appearance of cutaneous nodules ranged greatly from one month to 27 years.

365. Olds GR, Dasarathy S (2001) Recent advances in schistosomiasis. **Curr Infect Dis Rep** 3:59–67.
366. Amer M (1994) Cutaneous schistosomiasis. **Dermatol Clin** 12:713–717.
367. Davis-Reed L, Theis JH (2000) Cutaneous schistosomiasis: Report of a case and review of the literature. **J Am Acad Dermatol** 42:678–680.
368. Farrel AM et al. (1996) Ectopic cutaneous schistosomiasis: extragenital involvement with progressive upward spread. **Br J Dermatol** 135:110–112.

369. Utzinger J et al. (2000) Efficacy of praziquantel against Schistosoma mansoni with particular consideration for intensity of infection. **Trop Med Int Health** 5:771–778.
370. Tenzer R, Blumstein H (2001) E-medicine: Cysticercosis from Emergency Medicine/Infectious Diseases [online]. http://www.emedicine.com/emerg/topic119.htm
371. Singhi P, Ray M, Singhi S, Khandelwal N (2000) Clinical spectrum of 500 children with neurocysticercosis and response to albendazole therapy. **J Child Neurol** 15:207–213.
372. Dixon HBF, Lipscomb FM (1961) Cysticercosis: An analysis and follow-up of 450 cases. **Med Res Spec Rep London**:1–58.

Laboratory findings

The presence of subcutaneous nodules in an individual from an area endemic for cysticercosis should prompt a skin biopsy, particularly if neurologic signs are present. CT scan or MRI may demonstrate calcification with inactive disease or a ring-enhanced lesion showing an active cysticercus with surrounding edema. Eosinophilia is present in only 15% of patients with systemic cysticercosis.[373] The most useful and sensitive laboratory studies are the serologic assays, though checking stool for proglottids and ova may yield a diagnosis. Biopsy of a nodule will reveal an inflammatory response surrounding recognizable parts of the larvae, including the head or scolex.

Pathophysiology and histogenesis

Humans may serve as either the definitive or intermediate host in this disorder. When humans are the intermediate host, severe disease involving the skin and central nervous system may occur (Table 26.25).

Differential diagnosis

Because the clinical manifestations of neurocysticercosis are nonspecific, the differential is quite broad, including toxoplasmosis, brain abscess, and viral encephalitides as well as stroke, hemorrhage, and migraine. Subcutaneous cysticercosis may be confused with lymphadenopathy and a variety of benign skin tumors or cysts.

Therapeutics and prognosis

Albendazole, administered at 10 mg/kg in children for a 2-week course is a more affordable medication and probably more efficacious than other options such as praziquantel. Controversy exists as to the need to treat patients with cysticercosis who are symptomatic, since such symptoms are produced by pericystic inflammation that precedes involution of the parasite. Within a few days of the start of antihelminthic therapy, an exacerbation of symptoms occurs secondary to a local inflammatory reaction occurring upon death of the larvae. To minimize the inflammation that occurs with treatment, prednisolone is usually administered concurrently. The neurologic sequelae are highly variable and depend in part on the location(s) of the encysted larvae. The surgical excision of remnant subcutaneous cysticerci over cosmetically sensitive areas should be considered.

SPARGANOSIS

Sparganosis is a rare infection caused by the migration of larval tapeworms of the genus Spirometra, most commonly *Spirometra mansoni*. The dog and cat are the definitive hosts while the snake, fish, and amphibians serve as intermediate hosts. There are three routes of human infection. The most common is by drinking water contaminated with microscopic crustaceans (Cyclops) infected with larvae of the tapeworm. Other routes include the ingestion of an infected intermediate host and transmission through wounds that have been treated with the application of poultices of raw meat, a common practice in certain Asian countries. There have been some 63 cases reported in the United States and only three cases of patients under the age of 15 are described in the literature.[374] A subcutaneous, mobile, often migratory mass is the most common manifestation of the infection. Peripheral eosinophilia is not a feature of cutaneous sparganosis. The larvae may encyst themselves or migrate through certain tissues to involve other sites, including the eye and central nervous system. Several fatal cases of infection with a particularly aggressive larval form called *Sparganum proliferum* have been described.[375] No current antihelminthic or steroid medications have demonstrated efficacy in the treatment of sparganosis. Both the diagnosis and treatment of cutaneous sparganosis are accomplished by surgical excision of the entire sparganum.

ECHINOCOCCUS (HYATID DISEASE)

The larvae of *Echinococcus granulosus*, or the dog tapeworm, is the cause of unilocular hyatid cyst disease. Infection with *Echinococcus multilocularis*, a cestode that infects certain wild animals including rodents and foxes, is the cause of alveolar hyatid disease. The former condition carries a worldwide distribution, whereas the latter is limited to the northern hemisphere. Dogs are the definitive host for both species, while *E. multilocularis* has also been found in cats. Sheep are the usual intermediate hosts, while humans serve as dead-end intermediate hosts. In the dog's intestine, the tapeworm releases thousands of eggs that are passed in the feces. When humans ingest these eggs, oncosphere embryos invade the intestinal wall and migrate to virtually all organs of the body, including the liver, lungs, bones, brain, and skin, though extrahepatic and extrapulmonary involvement are rare. *E. granulosus* usually forms one large fluid-filled hyatid cyst while *E. multilocularis* larvae form multiloculated cysts. Cutaneous lesions, found in 3.4% of infected children, resemble subcutaneous cysts that may be elevated and palpable.[376] Skin involvement in most cases is the result of extension of infection from the liver via the falciform ligament to cause supraumbilical lesions or by the presence of communicating fistulae between the skin and affected internal organs, following hepatic surgery.[377] Subcutaneous hyatid disease is diagnosed and, in part, treated by surgical excision. Care should be taken, however, to remove the entire cyst without rupture or leakage of the infectious contents. Recent studies suggest that albendazole in combination with praziquantel may be more effective than albendazole alone in the treatment of hyatid disease.[378]

CUTANEOUS LARVA MIGRANS

Introduction

Cutaneous larva migrans or creeping eruption describes a cutaneous syndrome caused by the nematode larvae of several species that all have the ability to penetrate the skin. The usual etiologic agent of this unique eruption

---

TABLE 26.25   Distinctive infectious sequences with *Taenia solium*

Primary mode of transmission	Intermediate host	Primary sites of involvement	Diagnosis	Treatment
Ingest larvae in raw or undercooked pork	Pigs	Intestine	Proglottids in stool	Albendazole, praziquantal
Ingest eggs in contaminated food or water	Humans	Brain, eyes, skin, muscle	Biopsy CT scan	Albendazole, praziquantal, surgical excision

---

373. Raimer S, Wolf JE (1978) Subcutaneous cysticercosis. **Arch Dermatol** 114:107–108.
374. Kim CY et al. (1997) Cerebral sparganosis in a child. **Pediatr Neurosurg** 26:103–106.
375. Nakamura T, Hara M, Matsuoka M et al. (1990) Human proliferative sparganosis. **Am J Clin Pathol** 94:224–228.
376. Basaklar AC (1991) Hyatid cysts in children: report of 88 cases. **J R Coll Surg Edinb** 36:166–169.
377. Ambo M, Adachi K, Ohkawara A (1999) Postoperative alveolar hyatid disease with cutaneous-subcutaneous involvement. **J Dermatol** 26:343–347.
378. Mohamed AE, Yasawy MI, Al Karawi MA (1998) Combined albendazole and praziquantel versus albendazole alone in the treatment of hyatid disease. **Hepatogastroenterology** 45:1690–1694.

in the USA is the dog or cat hookworm, *Ancylostoma braziliense*.[379] Less common causes include the dog hookworm, *Ancylostoma caninum*, and the human hookworms, *Ancylostoma duodenale* and *Necator americanus*. Other bovine, feline, canine, and porcine species of hookworm are rare causes of cutaneous larva migrans.

Epidemiology
The disease occurs worldwide, but most commonly in tropical and subtropical environments such as Africa, South America, the Caribbean, and Southeast Asia. In the USA, creeping eruption is endemic in the southeastern region and the gulf coast.

Presenting history
The infection is frequently acquired where dogs and cats routinely defecate, including children's sand boxes, parks, and beaches. The eggs of *A. braziliense* are passed in the feces of the dog or cat. The eggs hatch, develop initially into noninfective rhabditiform larvae, molt, and develop into infectious filariform larvae, capable of penetrating intact skin. Often a tingling sensation accompanies entrance of the larvae through the skin. A prolonged contact time increases the likelihood of infection. Though all exposed areas of the skin are at risk, the feet are most commonly affected, while the knees, hands, buttocks, and the perianal area are occasionally affected. Because of the mode of infection, cutaneous larva migrans frequently occurs in the foot as a result of the tendency of children to play without shoes in sand containing hookworm eggs.

Physical examination and laboratory findings
Within a few hours of the initial penetration by filariform larvae, an erythematous, pruritic papule develops at the site. Larval migration begins several days to weeks later at a rate of up to several centimeters per day. The rash appears as intensely pruritic, linear, erythematous, raised, serpiginous tracts (Fig. 26.36). The larva is usually located 1–2cm distal to the advancing border of the lesion. An associated papular folliculitis may occur in the same area. If untreated, the migration usually spontaneously ceases with the death of the larvae over 2–8 weeks. In a study of 98 patients with cutaneous larva migrans, 73.4% of all involved locations were on the lower extremities, while 28.9% of them had symptoms for longer than one month.[380] It is often difficult to determine the responsible etiologic species of hookworm, though there are some subtle differences in presentation. The feline hookworm *Gnathostoma spinigerum*, for example, causes deep, broad tunnels and, untreated, may last for years. Diagnosis is largely based on the presence of the characteristic serpiginous lesions in combination with an exposure history including play in a sandbox or on a beach. Extraction of the offending larvae generally is not feasible, since the larvae are always in advance of the eruption. Eosinophilia is present in only 20% of patients.

Pathophysiology and histogenesis
Following penetration of the skin, filariform larvae are confined to the epidermis and almost always remain above the basal layer due to a lack of collagenases to penetrate through the basement membrane. It is this tunneling migration in the epidermis that causes the characteristic appearance of the lesion.

Therapeutics and prognosis
The standard treatment at this time for cutaneous larva migrans is topical thiabendazole. It is applied as a 10–15% solution or ointment to the affected area. Cure rates of 98% can be achieved with twice-daily therapy for 10 days. A lipophilic vehicle may allow for greater skin absorption and efficacy.[381] Thiabendazole can also be administered orally for a 5–7 day course of twice-

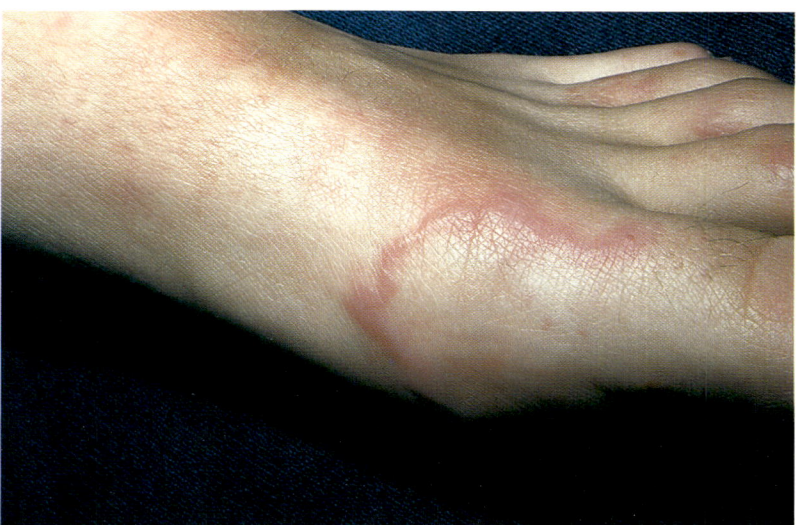

Fig. 26.36 Cutaneous larva migrans: creeping eruption in a teenager.

daily dosing, though topical therapy obviates the problem of systemic side effects, including anorexia, nausea, vomiting, diarrhea, and headache. Alternative systemic therapies include albendazole and ivermectin, drugs that appear to be promising because of their superior side effect profiles and convenient single-dose regimens. Oral ivermectin may be more effective than albendazole in the treatment of cutaneous larva migrans. A small comparative study involving 21 patients demonstrated a cure rate of 100% in patients receiving single doses (12mg) of ivermectin, while the cure rate for albendazole in single doses was only 46% with a high relapse rate. Ivermectin also appears to be well tolerated, with no reported adverse effects. A now-abandoned treatment involved freezing the leading edge of the developing lesion with liquid nitrogen, carbon dioxide, or ethylene chloride. This imprecise approach was largely unsuccessful, due in part to difficulty in localizing the larva, which lies 1–2cm beyond the edge of the rash. Furthermore, it has been demonstrated that the larvae are capable of surviving temperatures as low as −21°C for longer than five minutes.[382]

STRONGYLOIDIASIS AND LARVA CURRENS
Introduction
Larva currens is a cutaneous manifestation of infection with *Strongyloides stercoralis*, the intestinal nematode that is clinically distinguishable from cutaneous larva migrans. Arthur and Shelley originally proposed the term larva currens (racing larva) for this disease to emphasize the rapid cutaneous migration of the filariform larvae.

Epidemiology
Strongyloidiasis is widely distributed, affecting nearly all tropical and subtropical countries of the world, but is most prevalent in Southeast Asia. *Strongyloides fulleborni*, a species that usually affects Old World monkeys, is an uncommon cause of human strongyloidiasis in certain areas of Africa. In the USA, strongyloidiasis is endemic in the southern states where prevalence rates as high as 4% have been observed.

Presenting history
Strongyloidiasis primarily affects the skin, lungs, and GI tract, though nearly half of infected individuals are asymptomatic. Acute stongyloidiasis most

379. Chaudhry AZ, Longworth DL (1989) Cutaneous manifestations of intestinal helminthic infections. **Dermatol Clin** 7:275–289.
380. Jelinek T, Maiwald H, Nothdurft HD, Loscher T (1994) Cutaneous larva migrans in travelers: synopsis of histories, symptoms, and treatment of 98 patients. **Clin Infect Dis** 19:1062–1066.
381. Chatel G et al. (2000) Efficacy and tolerability of thiabendazole in a lipophil vehicle for cutaneous larva migrans. **Arch Dermatol** 136:1174–1175.
382. Elliot DL, Tolle SW, Goldberg L, Miller JB (1985) Pet-associated illness. **N Eng J Med** 313:985–995.

frequently presents with GI manifestations, including epigastric pain and diarrhea accompanied by a peripheral eosinophilia. Cutaneous involvement occurs in up to 92% of patients with chronic strongyloidiasis and is considered a sign of intestinal disease.[383] Cases of strongyloidiasis acquired in the USA are rarely associated with larva currens.

Physical examination

Though the presence of a serpiginous urticarial lesion is characteristic, the rash commonly appears as a papular or urticarial eruption. After the filariform larva burrows into the skin, it is capable of migrating at a rate of 10–15cm/hour. Each episode of the rash is usually transient, lasting a few hours to days, with intervening symptom-free periods lasting weeks to months. The buttocks, perineum, thighs, and trunk are the most frequent sites of involvement. A rare cutaneous manifestation of strongyloidiasis occurs in the immunocompromised host. The massive migration of filariform larvae to the skin associated with accelerated autoinfection and migration of the larvae through blood vessel walls in the superficial dermis result in a petechial and purpuric eruption.[384]

Laboratory findings

The diagnosis of strongyloidiasis is established by the detection of rhabditiform larvae in concentrated stool specimens that carries a sensitivity of up to 86% per single concentrated stool sample.[385] A new agar plate method may be more sensitive than the direct smear method for the detection of the parasite in the stool.[386] Skin biopsy is neither sensitive nor helpful except in the case of disseminated strongyloidiasis. In patients with negative stool specimens in whom strongyloidiasis is still suspected, use of the string test to obtain duodenal aspirates is the diagnostic procedure of choice because it is relatively noninvasive and sensitive. When GI studies are negative in the face of a strong clinical suspicion of infection, serologic assays can be performed. Peripheral eosinophilia is present in approximately 85% of patients with strongyloidiasis.

Pathophysiology

The life-cycle in humans begins with penetration of the skin by filariform larvae in a moist soil environment, followed by their migration in the blood to the lungs. When they reach the trachea via the alveoli and bronchial tree, the larvae are swallowed, and mature in the small intestine. In the mucosa of the gut, the worms produce eggs that hatch into rhabditiform larvae that are passed and develop into the infectious filariform larvae to repeat the life cycle once again. This intestinal parasite is unique in that it is capable of undergoing a complete life cycle as a free-living worm in the soil or in humans without exogenous reinfection. Autoinfection occurs when rhabditiform larvae still in the gut molt to form filariform larvae that penetrate the intestinal wall and migrate to the lungs. Autoinfection enables the parasite to persist for several decades in infected individuals. Another unfortunate consequence of autoinfection pertains to immunocompromised patients, in whom accelerated autoinfection can occur with the rapid transformation of rhabditiform to infective filariform larvae, resulting in a heavy parasite burden and disseminated strongyloidiasis.

Therapeutics and prognosis

The treatment of choice for uncomplicated larva currens is oral thiabendazole 25mg/kg twice daily for two days, with cure rates approaching 100%. Previously listed side effects, mostly gastrointestinal, are common.

For the hyperinfection syndrome in the immunocompromised patient, the same dose of thiabendazole is given for a minimum of one week. Albendazole is less effective. Ivermectin appears to be safe and efficacious in the treatment of strongyloidiasis, with few side effects and reported cure rates of up to 100%.[387]

HOOKWORM DISEASE

Introduction and epidemiology

Hookworm disease in humans is the symptomatic infection of the small intestine with the Old World hookworm *Ancylostoma duodenale* or the New World hookworm *Necator americanus*. The presence of symptoms correlates with worm burden, and since most infected individuals have a low parasite burden, the prevalence of hookworm infection is far greater than that of hookworm disease. The worldwide prevalence of hookworm infection is estimated at one billion with a widespread distribution in nearly all subtropical and tropical countries.[388] The etiologic agent of hookworm disease in the United States is *Necator americanus*. The optimal environmental conditions for the infection of humans with filariform larvae is the moist soil of locales with 1.27m or more of annual rainfall.

Presenting history

The gastrointestinal manifestations of hookworm disease include abdominal discomfort, diarrhea, weight loss, and an iron deficiency anemia.[389] Pulmonary symptoms including cough, bronchitis, and a pneumonitis characterized radiographically by localized fluffy infiltrates are uncommon. The dermatitis associated with penetration by the infective filariform larvae is termed "ground itch" or "coolie itch" and consists of erythematous papules that persist for 7–10 days in individuals with primary infections. Reinfection may result in vesiculation and localized edema with regional lymphadenopathy that last two weeks or more. Creeping eruption, as previously mentioned, is another cutaneous manifestation of hookworm disease. Signs of chronic infection include malaise, shortness of breath, dizziness, and pallor and edema of the lower extremities as a result of hypoproteinemia. Cutaneous depigmentation, involving primarily the face, extremities, and perineum, is the result of both iron deficiency and hypoalbuminemia.

Diagnosis and laboratory findings

Hookworm disease should be suspected in a patient with symptoms consistent with a chronic iron deficiency anemia and a history of possible exposure to filariform larvae, such as walking barefoot in moist soil in an endemic area. The diagnosis is made by detecting characteristic eggs in the stool. With light infections, stool concentration techniques may be necessary.

Pathophysiology

The life cycle of the two hookworm species parallels that of *Strongyloides stercoralis*, except that in hookworm disease autoinfection does not occur. Blood ingestion, following attachment of the adult worm to the intestinal mucosa, results in clinically significant blood losses.

Therapeutics

Mebendazole is the treatment of choice for this infection. The dose of 100mg twice daily for three days in children greater than 2 years of age, has been effective in 95% of infected individuals. Patients with heavy worm burdens often require several courses of therapy for cure. In the USA, the recom-

383. Amer M, Attia M, Ramadan AS, Matout K (1984) Larva currens and systemic disease. **Int J Dermatol** 23:402–403.
384. Kalb RE, Grossman ME (1987) Periumbilical purpura in disseminated strongyloidiasis. **JAMA** 256:1170–1171.
385. Beal CB, Viens P, Grant RGL et al. (1970) A new technique for sampling duodenal contents: Demonstration of upper small bowel pathogens. **Am J Trop Med Hyg** 19:349–352.
386. Iwamoto T, Kitoh M, Kayashima K, Ono T (1998) Larva currens: The usefulness of the agar plate method. **Dermatology** 196:343–345.
387. Toma H, Sato Y, Shiroma Y et al. (2000) Comparative studies on the efficacy of three antihelminthics on treatment of human strongyloidiasis in Okinawa, Japan. **Southeast Asian J Trop Med Public Health** 31:147–151.
388. Georgiev VS (2000) Necatoriasis: treatment and developmental therapeutics. **Expert Opin Investig Drugs** 9:1065–1078.
389. Georgiev VS (1999) Parasitic infections. Treatment and developmental therapeutics. I. Necatoriasis. **Curr Pharm Des** 5:545–554.

mended alternative to mebendazole is pyrantel pamoate, administered as a single 11mg/kg dose.

TOXOCARIASIS

Toxocara canis, for which the dog is the definitive host, is the major cause of toxocariasis or visceral larva migrans.[390] *T. cati* can also cause this disease. The disease is prevalent in temperate climates where there are dogs, including the USA. Young children are primarily affected because they are most likely to ingest contaminated soil. Humans are infected when they ingest eggs that are produced by the adult parasite in the dog intestine and passed into their feces. In the human intestine, eggs hatch into larvae that migrate primarily to the liver, brain, eyes, and muscles to cause disease. The most serious complication of *toxocara* infection is blindness, resulting from ocular larva migrans.

The cutaneous findings related to toxocariasis include urticaria, papular eruptions, and tender subcutaneous nodules. In a recent case-control investigation of the skin manifestations thought to be associated with toxocariasis, a statistically significant excess risk of having a positive *Toxocarai* ELISA was found in patients with urticaria and prurigo.[391] The authors suggest a role of *T. canis* infection as a co-factor in the etiology of these common skin conditions. The diagnosis of toxocariasis is based on serologic tests. The sensitivity and specificity of these antibody-based assays, however, vary considerably, and a definitive diagnosis requires visualization of the larvae in tissue. Eosinophilia and hypergammaglobulinemia support the diagnosis. The standard treatment for toxocariasis is diethylcarbamazine, administered at a dose of 2mg/kg three times a day for 7–10 days. Thiabendazole, albendazole, and mebendazole are alternative treatments.

ENTEROBIASIS

Introduction and epidemiology

Enterobius vermicularis is the causative agent of enterobiasis. Commonly known as pinworm, it is the most prevalent and widespread human helminthic infection in the world, with greater than 1 billion cases. Twenty to thirty percent of the population may be infected in the USA.[392] Enterobiasis is more common in temperate climates, and is most prevalent in children under 12 years of age, particularly those with poor personal hygiene in crowded living conditions.[393] The only natural hosts of *E. vermicularis* are humans. The most common route of transmission is fecal-oral spread, though the infection may also be transmitted through contact with formites and the ingestion of infected food and drink. Acquisition of the disease by the inhalation of contaminated dust particles has also been suggested. The intense pruritus ani that usually occurs with infection facilitates both reinfection of the host and transmission to uninfected individuals.

Presenting history and clinical findings

Pruritus ani is the most common presentation, and may lead to insomnia and irritability in children. Scratching may result in an eczematous dermatitis and secondary bacterial infection. There have been several reports of perianal abscesses or granulomas containing *E. vermicularis* eggs.[394] The mechanism appears to be entry of worms into the anal crypts at the dentate line.

E. vermicularis rarely migrates to other internal organs, including the vermiform appendix, to cause lymphoid hyperplasia, the liver to cause hepatic granulomas, the lung to cause coin lesions, and the female reproductive tract to cause tubo-ovarian abscesses.[395–398] Pinworm infestation should be suspected in all cases of perianal scratching in children. The organisms resemble pieces of white thread and are often visible to the naked eye in the perianal area.

Diagnosis and laboratory findings

The Scotch tape test is the diagnostic method of choice. A clear adhesive tape is applied to the perianal area at night. The tape is placed on a glass slide and examined by light microscopy for pinworm eggs. Eggs can also be found under the fingernails. Infection of multiple family members is common. Eosinophilia is uncommon, and stool examination is of little diagnostic value since eggs are found in the stool in only 5% of cases.

Pathophysiology

Ingestion of eggs is followed by the emergence of rhabditiform larvae in the duodenum. The mature adult forms migrate to the cecum where they mate. For unknown reasons the female migrates to the anus, deposits approximately 11 000 eggs on the perianal skin, and dies. Intense itching leads to scratching, and facilitates the subsequent ingestion of eggs.

Therapeutics

A single dose of mebendazole 100mg in children greater than 2 years of age is usually effective. Side effects are rare, and cure rates of 90–100% have been obtained with this regimen. Pyrantel pamoate, given as a single 11mg/kg dose is an alternative therapy. Conscientious hand washing after use of the toilet and before meals, and frequent fingernail clipping are effective measures against fecal-oral transmission. In certain populations, including long-term care facilities, the mass medication of residents may be an effective approach to the control of this extremely common affliction.[399]

TRICHINOSIS

Introduction

Trichinosis is caused by the intestinal nematode *Trichinella spiralis*. Most infections are asymptomatic, and only an estimated 1 in 2000 infections are brought to medical attention.[400]

Epidemiology

The infection occurs worldwide in tropical and subtropical locales. The disease is endemic in the USA and prevalence is highest in the northeastern and mid-Atlantic states where transmission is related to eating home-prepared sausage. Prevalence is declining, and only 38 cases per year were reported from 1991 to 1996.[401] Inadequately cooked pork, or less commonly bear or walrus meat, is the source of infection. The disease has a predilection for ethnic groups including Laotians, Cambodians, German, Italians, and Poles who tend to consume undercooked pork.

390. Gillespie SH (1993) Human toxocariasis. **CDR Review** 3:R140–143.
391. Humbert P, Niezborala M, Salembier R, Aubin F et al. (2000) Skin manifestations associated with toxocariasis: a case-control study. **Dermatology** 201:230–234.
392. Wagner ED, Eby WC (1983) Pinworm prevalence in California elementary school children, and diagnostic methods. **Am J Trop Med Hyg** 32:998–1001.
393. Grencis R, Cooper E (1996) Enterobius, trichuris, capillaria, and hookworm. **Gastroenterol Clin North Am** 25:579–596.
394. Avolio L, Avoltini V, Ceffa F, Bragheri R (1998) Perianal granuloma caused by Enterobius vermicularis: Report of a new observation and review of the literature. **J Pediatr** 132:1055–1056.
395. Dorfman S et al. (1995) Parasitic infestation in acute appendicitis. **Ann Trop Med Parasitol** 89:99–101.
396. Beaver PC, Kriz JJ, Lau TJ (1973) Pulmonary nodule caused by Enterobius vermicularis. **Am J Trop Med Hyg** 22:711–713.
397. Mondou EN, Gnepp DR (1989) Hepatic granuloma resulting from Enterobius vermicularis. **Am J Clin Pathol** 91:97–100.
398. Vazquez Piloto A, Cruz Robaina JC, Nunez Fernandez F, Sanchez Diaz JM (1994) Bilateral tubo-ovarian abscess caused by Enterobius vermicularis. Presentation of a case. **Rev Cubana Med Trop** 46:65–67.
399. Lohiya GS, Tan-Figueroa L, Crinella FM, Lohiya S (2000) Epidemiology and control of enterobiasis in a developmental center. **West J Med** 172:305–308.
400. Kasper DK (1987) Headache, fever, and periorbital edema – I.D. Rounds. **Rev Infect Dis** 9:804–809.
401. Moorhead A, Grunenwald PE, Dietz VJ, Schantz PM (1999) Trichinellosis in the United States, 1991–1996: declining but not gone. **Am J Trop Med Hyg** 60:66–69.

Presenting history

The initial enteric phase of infection carries symptoms of diarrhea, abdominal pain, nausea, and vomiting, lasting one week. Fever, periorbital edema, and myalgias subsequently develop in over 80% of symptomatic individuals.

Physical examination

Pruritus in association with a diffuse macular, papular rash is common. Subconjunctival hemorrhages, splinter hemorrhages of the nail beds, cardiac, and CNS involvement may occur. Symptoms tend to diminish after several weeks. Trichinosis should be suspected in patients who present with the clinical triad of fever, myalgias, and periorbital swelling.

Laboratory findings

Eosinophilia is present in over 90% of individuals with the clinical signs and symptoms of trichinosis.[402] Sensitive and specific serologic assays, including a new immunoenzymatic test, are available to establish the diagnosis, though seroconversion frequently does not occur until three weeks after the initial infection.[403] The most expedient and definitive means of diagnosing trichinosis is by demonstrating encysted Trichinella larvae in a muscle biopsy. Tissue is best obtained near the tendinous insertion of the gastrocnemius or deltoid muscles.

Pathophysiology

Human trichinosis begins with the ingestion of raw or undercooked pork containing encysted larvae. These larvae are liberated by the action of stomach acid and digestive enzymes in the intestine, where they burrow into the intestinal mucosa and mature. The adult worms mate, releasing larvae via the bloodstream to other organs. The larvae have a predilection for dissemination to the skeletal muscle, where they encyst and calcify. Humans are dead-end hosts.

Therapeutics

Therapy in most instances is supportive and includes bedrest and salicylates to treat constitutional and musculoskeletal complaints. Thiabendazole given at a dose of 25mg/kg twice daily for one week is only effective during the initial enteric phase of the infection.

DRACUNCULIASIS

Dracunculiasis results from infection with the nematode *Dracunculus medinensis*, or guinea worm. The disease is endemic in India and parts of Africa, particularly Ghana and Nigeria. The worldwide prevalence of dracunculiasis in 1998 was less than 80 000 cases, due to the dracunculiasis eradication program and improved water supplies in endemic areas.[404]

Presenting history and clinical findings

Fever, urticaria, periorbital edema, and pruritus commonly occur. As the head of the worm penetrates the skin, an erythematous papule develops with burning, itching, and progression into a blister.[405] When the blister ruptures, the head of the worm is frequently exposed. The head of the gravid female nematode may explode, resulting in the extrusion of microfilariae from her uterus. Diagnosis is usually clinically apparent. The condition can be quite debilitating. Any area of the skin can be affected including the eyelid, and multiple infection is not unusual.

Pathophysiology

Following the ingestion of tiny Cyclops crustaceans harboring the infectious organism, larvae are subsequently released in the small intestine and migrate via the lymphatics to subcutaneous tissues. Meter-long females cause ulceration in the skin and release larvae into fresh water where they are ingested by crustaceans to complete the life cycle.

Therapeutics

The usual treatment in native endemic populations involves wrapping the worm around a stick and gradually extracting it over the course of several days. If this method is employed, care should be taken not to break the body of the worm. The administration of oral medication expedites the physical extraction process, and the drug of choice is metronidazole, 35mg/kg daily in four divided doses for 5–7 days. Thiabendazole in a dose of 50mg/kg twice a day for three days is also effective. A simple and effective preventive measure consists of boiling drinking water.

LOIASIS
Introduction

Loiasis, caused by the nematode *Loa loa*, is transmitted to humans by deer flies of the genus *Chrysops*. The disease is limited to tropical central and West Africa.[406] The bite of the larvae-infested deer fly deposits infectious larvae on the skin that then enter the bite wound, migrate in the body and develop into adults. The parasite lives in the connective tissues of humans. Females release microfilariae into the blood during the day.

Presenting history and clinical findings

Migratory angioedema (Calabar swellings) have been reported in approximately half of patients with loiasis. Seventy percent of them report the presence of eyeworm in which migration of the adult worm through the subconjunctiva of the eyelid is visible to the patient.[407] Pruritus and localized papular or vesicular skin rashes are also present in more than 50% of patients, most commonly over the arms. The less common occurrence of subcutaneous migration of the worms lasts only minutes, leaving no visible trace.

Laboratory findings

The diagnosis of loiasis is based on the detection of microfiliariae in peripheral blood smears. Eosinophilia and elevated IgE levels aid in diagnosis.

Therapeutics and prognosis

The standard therapy for loiasis is diethylcarbamazine, though the recurrence rate is high and multiple courses of medication are often required. Single annual doses of ivermectin may reduce the transmission of loiasis.[408]

402. Grove DI, Warren KS, Mahmous AAF (1975) Algorithms in the diagnosis and management of exotic diseases. VII. Trichinosis. **J Infect Dis** 132:485–488.
403. Gomez-Priego A, Crecencio-Rosales L, De-La-Rosa JL (2000) Serological evaluation of thin-layer immunoassay-enzyme-linked immunosorbent assay for antibody detection in human trichinellosis. **Clin Diagn Lab Immunol** 7:810–812.
404. Hopkins DR et al. (2000) Dracunculiasis eradication: delayed, not denied. **Am J Trop Med Hyg** 62:163–168.
405. Elgart ML (1989) Onchocerciasis and dracunculosis. **Dermatol Clin** 7:323–330.

406. Nutman TB, Mulligan M, Ottesen EA (1987) Loa loa infection in temporary residents of endemic regions: recognition of a hyperresponsive syndrome with characteristic clinical manifestations. **J Infect Dis** 154:10–18.
407. Noireau F, Apembet JD, Nzoulani A, Carme B (1990) Clinical manifestations of loiasis in an endemic area in the Congo. **Trop Med Parasit** 41:37–39.
408. Duong TH et al. (1997) Reduced loa loa microfilaria count ten to twelve months after a single dose of ivermectin. **Trans R Soc Trop Med Hyg** 91:592–593.

Infestations

Terri Meinking and David Taplin

LICE

HISTORY

Pediculosis, the infestation of humans by lice, has been documented for thousands of years.[1] The insects themselves have been in existence for several million years, long enough to enable a wide range of species differentiation.[2] Today, some 560 species of bloodsucking lice, which are found only on mammals,[3] are recognized.

These insects of the order Phthiraptera include only two genera that infest humans: *Pthirus* and *Pediculus*. Both of these genera are also found on gorillas and chimpanzees. Species of *Pediculus* are known to infest spider monkeys (*Ateles*) in the New World. The fur of *Ateles* is much like human hair and their blood is physiologically similar to our own. This led Buxton to speculate that at least in the New World, lice may have been transmitted from human to monkey.[4]

Today, only three species of lice infest humans: *Pediculus humanus humanus*, the body, or more accurately, the clothing louse; *Pediculus humanus capitis*, the head louse; and *Pthirus pubis*, the crab louse. Our observations lead us to the conclusion that the distinct differences in habitat, feeding habits, and metabolism between body lice and head lice merit their separation into two distinct species: *Pediculus humanus* and *Pediculus capitis*.

The most widely quoted early reference to lice is contained in Exodus 8:17, which records that Aaron, "stretched out his hand with his rod and smote the dust of the earth, and it became lice in men and beast."

In ancient Egypt, the priests shaved their bodies every three days to keep lice away.[5] The 20m-long papyrus from the 16th century BC obtained by the German Egyptologist, George Moritz Ebers, proved, on translation, to be a one-volume reference library for the practicing physician.[6,7] It contained the following instructions for the eradication of lice: "One part of date flour and one part of water shall be cooked to a volume of two hennu jars (450ml). Sip up a mouthful while warm and then spray it out on the parts of the body infected by the vermin."

Desiccated head lice and their eggs have been found on the hair and scalps of Egyptian mummies, and crab lice have been recovered from the genital area.[8] Ivory nit combs carved in the Phoenician style date back to the 13th to 12th centuries BC.[8] Pharaohs had shaved heads, and it has long been thought that head shaving was part of the burial ritual. It wouldn't be surprising to find that under those elaborate headdresses, pharaohs kept their heads shaved to prevent infestation.

Christian hermits and monks considered lousiness as a sign of humility and a saintly way of life.[8] Muslim and Jewish traditions also addressed the issue of pediculosis. The Muslim tradition prohibits killing of lice in mosques or other holy places, whereas the Jewish tradition forbids killing of lice on the Sabbath.[8]

There is no doubt that head lice were present in the New World long before Columbus. They have been identified on the scalps of prehistoric North American Indian mummies.[2] One of the more interesting accounts concerns the "Prince of El Plomo." In 1954, three fortune seekers in search of the legends of gold in Chile discovered the undisturbed tomb of a 9-year-old Inca prince on Cerro el Plomo, a dominant peak of the Andes, east of Santiago. The young prince apparently had been sacrificed to the Sun God, and at this altitude of 17 712 feet (5400m), above the permafrost line, his body remained frozen and perfectly preserved for 500 years.[9,10] During a later detailed examination, nits, or eggs of head lice, were found on his hair and were photographed by scanning electron microscopy (SEM).[10]

The Aztecs offered lice to Montezuma as a token of respect. Because the poor had little else to offer, they collected their lice daily until they had sufficient numbers to fill small bags, which they laid at the foot of their king. Cortez, who witnessed the scene, was horrified, since he had mistakenly assumed that the bags contained gold dust.[2,11]

Not all civilizations consider lice in a negative light. Young women in northern Siberia once threw lice at men as a sign of affection. This expression of love was based on the thought that "my louse is thy louse."[2]

In a medieval Swedish town, candidates for mayor gathered around the council table, on which they laid their beards. A live louse was placed in the center of the table. The owner of the beard that attracted the louse first was proclaimed the new mayor.[2,11]

For many, lice are considered an oral delicacy. In Tonga, the catching and eating of lice of one's parents was a sign of filial duty.[12] The eating of lice has been noted in the Budini nomads of the Middle Volga river and in their descendants, the Kirghiz and the Kazaks.[11,13] Frequently, we have observed this practice among Indian tribes in Central and South America, where the daily search for head lice forms an important part of social grooming. Similar grooming behavior is observed in both Old and New World monkeys. These practices may play a role in social development and rank within the troop or community.[14,15]

Unlike the examples given above, in which cultures have accepted lice as part of their normal ecosystem, most westernized countries consider these parasites undesirable. In most European and British societies, they have long

1. Pernet G (1918) An historical note on the nits of the body-louse. Br J Dermatol 30:208.
2. Zinsser H (1935) Rats, Lice and History. Boston: Little Brown.
3. Maunder JW (1983) The appreciation of lice. Proc R Inst Gr Brit 55:1.
4. Buxton PA (1946) The Louse, 2nd edn. Baltimore: Williams & Wilkins.
5. Driver GR (1974) Lice in the Old Testament. Palestine Explor Q 159.
6. Fagan BM (1975) The Rape of the Nile. New York: Scribner's.
7. Mertz B (1978) Red Land, Black Land. Daily Life in Ancient Egypt. New York: Dodd, Mead.
8. Mumcuoglu KY, Zias J (1989) How the ancients deloused themselves. Bibl Archaeol Rev XV(6):66.
9. McIntyre L (1973) The lost empire of the incas. National Geographic 144:729.
10. Horne RT, Kawasaki SQ (1984) The prince of El Plomo. A paleopathological study. Bull NY Acad Med 60:925–931.
11. Orkin M, Maibach HI (1985) Cutaneous Infestations and Insect Bites. New York: Marcel Dekker.
12. Andrews M (1976) The Life that Lives on Man. New York: Taplinger.
13. Orkin M, Maibach HI, Parish LC et al. (1977) Scabies and Pediculosis. Philadelphia: JB Lippincott.
14. Harcourt A (1985) All's fair in play and politics. New Scientist 1486:35.
15. Ghigliere M (1985) The social ecology of chimpanzees. Sci Am 252:102.

been considered disgusting. England raged with lousiness in the 1600s. Bathing was an infrequent practice, and many individuals shaved their heads to avoid lice. This did not prevent their elaborate wigs from becoming infested. Samuel Pepys (1633–1703) was most offended to find that his newly acquired periwig contained nits.[11]

In 1634, Thomas Mouffet, the father of the arachnophobic "Little Miss Muffet" of the nursery rhyme, published an encyclopedia of current knowledge of insects of the time entitled *Theatrum Insectorum*.[12] He described body lice as beastly creatures, common in armies and prisons. He theorized that "sweat became corrupted by wearing always the same clothes, which gives rise to matter for their origin by the mediation of heat." Although he was supporting the theory of spontaneous generation, his epidemiologic observations of body lice in the dispossessed and less fortunate members of society still remain valid today.

The naturalist Francesco Redi (1626–1697) gave the first scientific description of the "crab" or "pubic louse" in 1668. In the final year of his life, Carl De Geer (1720–1778) assigned the terms *capitis* and *corporis* to the head and body louse. Today, older terms for *Pediculus humanus*, including *Pediculus corporis* and *Pediculus vestimenti*, have been declared invalid by the International Commission on Zoological Nomenclature and should not be used.[3]

More deaths have occurred due to the louse than from any other insect apart from the malaria mosquito.[3] Since the early 1900s, the body louse has been the subject of intense scientific investigation, primarily due to its role as the vector of epidemic or louse-borne typhus. The disease was well recognized in the 15th century. Don Fernando lost 20 000 of his soldiers from typhus during the siege of Granada in 1489 to 1490, compared with 3000 from enemy action. Forty years later, the French army of 25 000 men was reduced by typhus to only 4000 within one month. Their siege of Naples turned to defeat and Charles V became the new ruler of the Holy Roman empire.[12]

By the mid-1700s, typhus had become a significant problem aboard ships of the Royal Navy, killing up to one-third of the crew after a call in port. James Lind, a physician to the Royal Naval Hospital at Haslar in England, became convinced that typhus was in some manner spread by clothing and close body contact. He noted that 17 of 23 persons who had been fitting out tents for typhus patients had died. Dr Lind ordered fumigation with smoke and, more important, the thorough cleaning and airing on deck of clothes and bedding. He also instituted the changing of clothes by nurses and physicians before leaving the hospital. Although he was ignorant of the role of the louse, his preventative measures were appropriate.[12]

It was not until the early 1900s that the associations between typhus, lice, and the causative pathogen *Rickettsia prowazekii* were made. Charles Nicolle in 1909 successfully transferred typhus to monkeys by injecting blood from an infected human, and he later demonstrated that lice could transmit the disease.[12]

Unfortunately, these early workers believed the disease to be transmitted by the bite of the louse, which they were careful to avoid. It is now established that the mechanism of transmission is through the infected feces of the louse, which enter the circulation through the puncture wounds created when they feed, or more likely the excoriations made by the host. Failure to recognize this fact probably led to the death from typhus of several pioneers in the field, including Bacot, Ricketts, and Prowazek.

DEFINITIONS: EFFECTS OF PEDICULOSIS ON THE HOST

The clinical signs and symptoms of pediculosis arise from host reactions to louse saliva injected at the time of feeding. Depending on the degree of sensitization and the number of previous exposures, sites of feeding may produce small 2–3mm erythematous macules, papules, or acute hive-like reactions with typical flare and wheal formations. These eruptions may occur within minutes to days after feeding.

The hallmark of all types of pediculosis is pruritus. Intense itching at the site of the bite compels the host to scratch, often excoriating the skin. The excoriations, in turn, create an entry point for germs and lice feces and the possibility of secondary infection. A low-grade fever, lymphadenopathy and, in severe cases, anemia may be present. Because lice prefer the dark and are more active at night, the infested individual may also feel tired and irritable due to lack of sleep, hence the term "feeling lousy."

Pediculosis corporis

Pediculosis corporis is the condition brought about by infestation of humans and their clothing by *P. humanus*, the body louse. Body lice spend most of their lives in clothing and go to the body only to feed. Therefore, they are most commonly found among homeless individuals, refugees, victims of natural disaster or war, and others who lack the ability to wash or change their clothes.

The bites of body lice are relatively painless to some and quite annoying to others. Several years ago, one of the authors was awakened by a fierce pain in her neck. Grasping at the source of this piercing sensation, she removed an engorged body louse that had escaped from a laboratory colony that day.

Pediculosis corporis may result in chronic excoriation and a condition known as "vagabond's skin," which is characterized by lichenification and brownish hyperpigmentation. It is most common on the trunk and abdomen, but may be present in any area that can be scratched by the host.

Pediculosis capitis

Pediculosis capitis is the term applied to infestation of the scalp by the human head louse *P. capitis*. Individual sites of feeding are difficult to see. There may be signs of irritation in the form of erythema and scaling, and the periphery of the hairy areas may exhibit linear excoriations. Pruritus is a common symptom in subjects who have had head lice for several weeks, but first-time infestations may not produce any symptoms whatsoever. Individuals who have had previous episodes usually develop pruritus within 48 hours of exposure.

Most cases of head louse infestation in United States schools are first detected by observations of one or more children scratching their heads. Closer scrutiny may reveal nits adherent to the hairs. Usually, these are the whitish to sandy-colored empty shells of eggs that have hatched. Newly laid or viable intact eggs are more difficult to see, and may be tan to coffee-colored or darker (Figs 27.1, 27.2). The cap or operculum of the egg always faces away from the skin or scalp. Other conditions that can give a false diagnosis of pediculus capitis include contact or seborrheic dermatitis, insect bites, eczema, psoriasis, or piedra. It is common for desquamated epithelial cells (DEC) or pseudonits (commonly known as "hair muffs" or hair casts) to be mistaken for eggs (Fig. 27.3).

Pediculosis pubis

Pediculosis pubis refers to infestation with the crab or pubic louse (Fig. 27.4). In adults, the pubic and perianal areas are most often affected, but occasionally

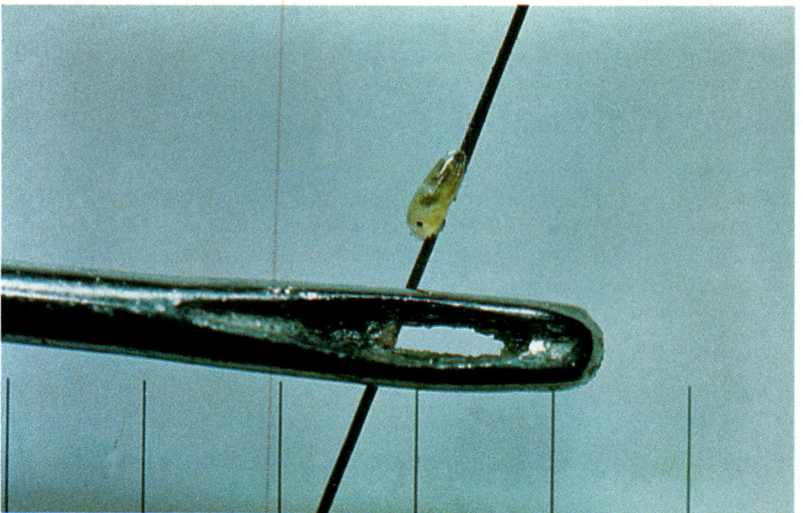

Fig. 27.1 Head louse nit (approximately 0.8mm) attached to child's hair seen next to the eye of a sewing needle.

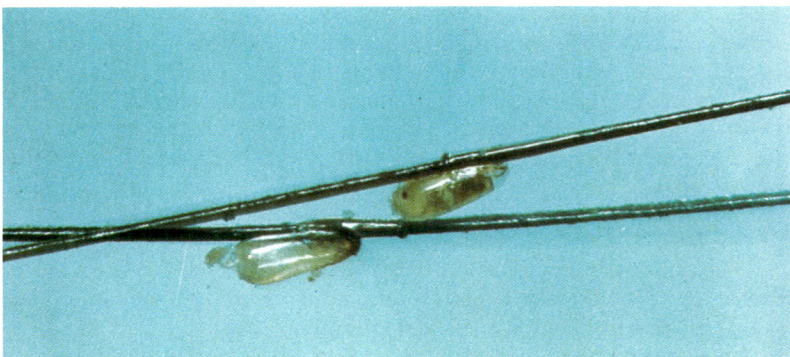

Fig. 27.2   Viable head louse egg (right) and hatched empty nit (left), attached to child's hair.

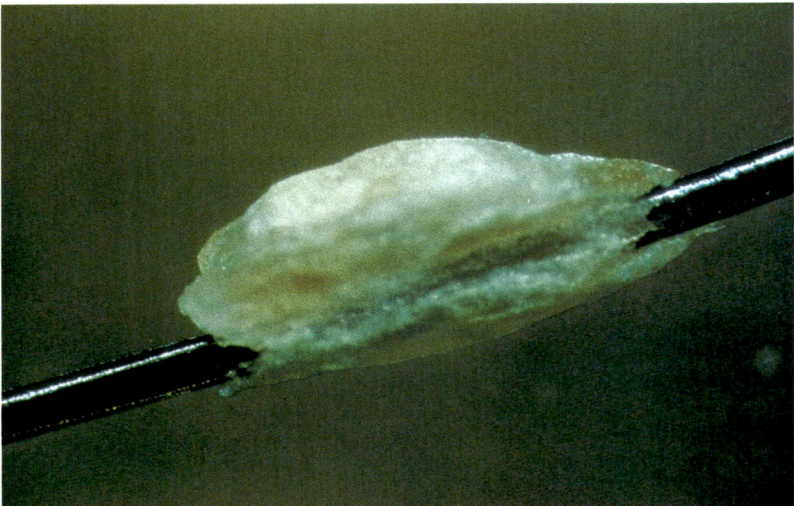

Fig. 27.3   A pseudonit or "hair muff," a sebaceous plug attached to the hair is often mistaken for a nit.

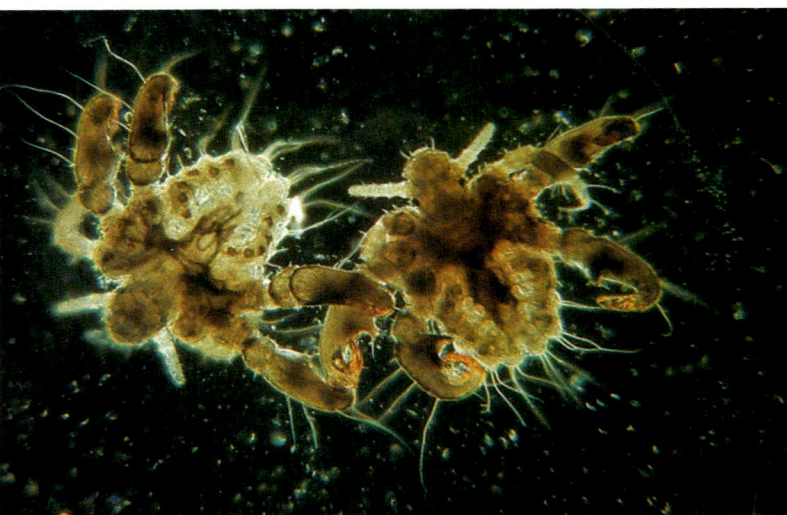

Fig. 27.4   Dorsal and ventral view of two adult crab lice recently removed from their host (dark field).

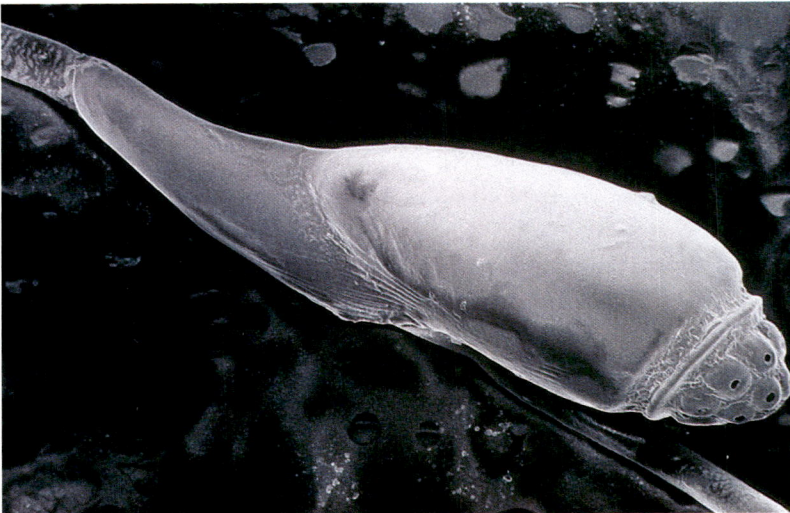

Fig. 27.5   Scanning electron microscopy of a crab louse egg. Notice that the cap or operculum is domed and the nit is firmly attached to the hair and coated with cement from the mother louse.

the lice may spread to the mustache, beard, axillae, eyelashes, or scalp hair. In 1991, Meinking conducted a study of 45 homeless individuals suffering from *P. pubis* infestations. Twenty-seven subjects (60%) were infested not only in the pubic and perianal regions, but also in other hairy parts of the body. Commonly affected sites included the legs, axillae, scalp, eyelashes, and in hairy individuals, the chest and back. One woman with very long, thick, straight hair had crab lice on her scalp with at least 60 adult lice at the nape of the neck. No other part of her body was infested. Over half (53%) of the subjects had severe infestations with over 10 visible adult lice. Because *P. pubis* can affect any hairy area of the body, the term "crab" lice may be more appropriate than "pubic" lice.

Crab lice firmly attach their mouthparts to the skin like a tick and feed for longer periods of time than other lice. They are often mistaken for a scab, or blend in with the skin color, making them difficult to detect. Pediculosis pubis is traditionally associated with sexual activity and is often listed with sexually transmitted diseases (STDs). Undoubtedly, intimate body contact is the most efficient way in which these bloodsucking insects may be acquired, but other modes of transmission are possible (see Epidemiology). Adult crab lice can remain alive for 1 1/2 days without feeding, and viable eggs cemented to public hairs shed into the environment remain viable for up to 10 days in suitable temperature and humidity.

The nits of crab lice, like those of head lice, are firmly cemented to the hair and are less than 1mm long. Unlike the flat cap or operculum of the body or head louse egg, the nit of a crab louse is shaped like an ice cream cone (Fig. 27.5). The egg may appear cream to tan or brown when viable and unhatched. The empty egg cases are sandy-colored to white and may resemble

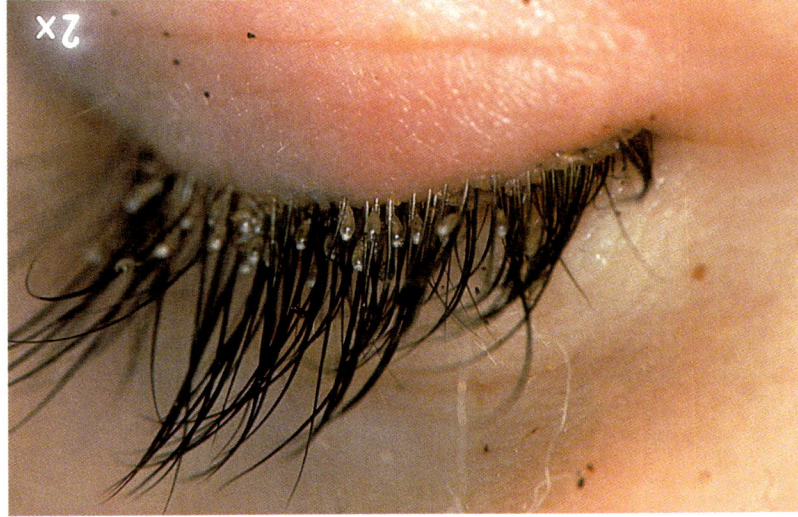

Fig. 27.6   Infestation of a child's eyelashes with crab lice. Note the erythema and edema. (Courtesy of Tony Burns, MD)

dandruff. Unlike dandruff, textile fibers, or hair casts (pseudonits), the egg cases are difficult to remove from the hair with the fingers.

Very rarely in adults, skin lesions may be seen that are peculiar to pediculosis pubis. These are 0.5–1.0cm slate-gray to bluish macules, often irregular in shape, and known as *maculae caeruleae*. From 1991 to 1993, we saw none of these lesions in repeated examination of 150 cases of *P. pubis* infestations.

Pediculosis palpebrarum

Pediculosis palpebrarum is the infestation of the eyelashes with *P. pubis* (Fig. 27.6). This condition, which is also termed phthiriasis palpebrarum, may be complicated by bacterial infections with painful edema and erythema of the eyelids. *P. pubis* on the eyelashes or hair of children should alert the physician to the possibility of sexual abuse, but other modes of transmission, such as sharing a bed with an infested parent or sibling, should also be considered.

EPIDEMIOLOGY

Body lice

In most industrialized nations today, body lice are encountered primarily among persons forced by their economic circumstances to live on the streets or in crowded substandard dwellings, where personal hygiene is difficult to maintain. Although pediculosis corporis is rarely encountered in private medical practice, it may be found in the emergency departments of major hospitals that serve indigent patients. Health providers and others who have close contact with these cases may acquire body lice, but their ability to wash, and most important, change their clothes, make them unlikely hosts for continued infestation.

While little information is available on the prevalence of body lice in most countries, recent reports suggest that infestation is on the rise. In Russia, social and economic upheavals following the collapse of the Soviet Union have led to an increase in the number of homeless people, among whom *P. humanus* is reportedly widespread.[16] In the Netherlands, where infestation with body lice is normally rare, pediculosis corporis was diagnosed 41 times in 31 homeless patients during 1993 and 1994.[17] In 1991, a finding of *P. humanus* was reported in Czechoslovakia for the first time since 1945.[18]

No current prevalence or incidence data for body lice are available in the United States. However, in the last decade, trench fever, which is normally louse-borne, has emerged among the homeless population in Seattle.[19] Further research is necessary to determine the association, if any, between the re-emergence of this disease and the prevalence of *P. humanus* (see Lice as disease vectors).

In Miami during 1991 and 1992, Meinking *et al.* screened more than 300 homeless individuals with complaints of pruritus. Of these individuals, 130 were infested with crab lice, but only one case of body lice was found. This experience suggests that, at least in southern Florida where the temperature is warm year round, the body louse is becoming an endangered species, while crab lice seem to be thriving.

The prevalence of *P. humanus* may rise rapidly in situations where war, famine, or natural disaster force large numbers of people into crowded, unsanitary living conditions. In the last decade, overcrowding and lack of hygiene lead to widespread body louse infestation among refugees in Burundi, Rwanda and Zaire.[20,21] Evidence of infestation was also reported among refugees in the former Yugoslavia, but the magnitude of the problem could not be assessed.[22]

Head lice

In contrast to body lice, head lice prefer clean, healthy hosts. They are not linked to poverty or poor living conditions and are most commonly found in individuals with good hygiene and grooming habits.

In many countries, the erroneous assumption that head lice are an indication of poor hygiene or parental neglect tends to discourage the reporting of cases. Therefore, official prevalence reports almost always underestimate actual prevalence rates. Nevertheless, official reports show pediculosis capitis to be a significant problem throughout the world. High rates of infestation can be found in developed as well as developing countries and in both temperate and tropical regions.[22] In many developed countries, including the United States and England, head lice prevalence is believed to be on the rise, despite the expenditure of billions of dollars for treatment and control.[23,24] In less developed countries, where pediculosis capitis may be a lower priority than other, more serious health problems, it is not uncommon to find head lice among 90% or more of all children.[22]

In the United States, head lice infest all levels of society and most ethnic groups. They can be found among whites, Asians, Hispanics, and North, Central, and South American Indians. The notable exception is the African-American population, where prevalence is so low that it is recommended that African-Americans be excluded from prevalence estimates. In a 1977 study, Juranek found pediculosis capitis in only 0.3% (6/1853) of African-American children, compared with 10.4% (573/5513) of children of other races.[25] It is believed that the head louse indigenous to this part of the world is not well adapted to grip the oval-shaped hair shaft characteristic of the hair found in the African-American population.[26] In Africa, where the head lice have claws adapted to tightly curled, oval-shaped hair, pediculosis capitis is a serious problem among blacks.[22]

Despite the relatively low incidence of head lice among North American blacks, such cases occasionally do occur and may even be on the rise. In Miami in recent years, North American-type head lice have been noted in Haitians, Jamaicans, and African-Americans, while African-type lice have been found on blonde, straight-haired whites.

Although people of all ages are susceptible to head lice, infestation is most common in children age 3 to 11 years.[24,27] The relatively high incidence of head lice in this group is probably related to head-to-head and body contact during play and the sharing of objects to which lice cling (e.g., combs, brushes, hats, barrettes, helmets, head phones, and other head gear).

Numerous surveys, including our own studies in the United States, show infestation to be more common in girls than in boys.[25,28–33] Other studies,

16. Rydkina EB, Roux V, Gagua EM et al. (1999) *Bartonella quintana* in body lice collected from homeless persons in Russia. **Emerg Infect Dis** 5:176–178.
17. Van der Laan JR, Smit RB (1996) [Back again: the clothes louse]. **Ned Tijdschr Geneeskd** 140:1912–1915.
18. Rupes V, Chmela J, Kapoun S (1992) [Findings of body lice (*Pediculus humanus* L.) in Czechoslovakia]. **Cesk Epidemiol Mikrobiol Imunol** 41:362–365.
19. Spach DH, Kanter AS, Dougherty MJ et al. (1995) *Bartonella* (*Rochalimaea*) *quintana* bacteremia in inner-city patients with chronic alcoholism. **N Engl J Med** 332:424–428.
20. Raoult D, Ndihokubwayo JB, Tissot-Dupont H et al. (1998) Outbreak of epidemic typhus associated with trench fever in Burundi. **Lancet** 352:353–358.
21. World Health Organization (1997) A large outbreak of epidemic louse-borne typhus in Burundi. **Wkly Epidemiol Rec** 72:152–153.
22. Gratz NG (1997) Human lice: their prevalence, control and resistance to insecticides. A review 1985–1997. Document WHO/CTD/WHOPES/97.8. Geneva: World Health Organization.
23. Downs AMR, Stafford KA, Coles GC (1999) Head lice: prevalence in schoolchildren and insecticide resistance. **Parasitol Today** 15:1–4.
24. Meinking TL (1999) Infestations. **Curr Probl Dermatol** 11:73–120.
25. Juranek DD (1977) Epidemiologic investigations of pediculosis capitis in school children. In: Scabies and pediculosis, Orkin M, Maibach HI, Parish LC, Schwartzman RM, eds. Philadelphia: JB Lippincott. pp. 168–173.
26. Maunder JW (1974) The Louse. In: Head Infestation: A Community Problem. Proceedings of a Symposium held at the Royal Society of Medicine. London: Sponsored by Napp Laboratories.
27. Mumcuoglu KY, Klaus S, Kafka D et al. (1991) Clinical observation related to head lice infestation. **J Am Acad Dermatol** 25:248–251.
28. Childs ND (1998) Head lice from hell aren't going away. **Pediatr News** 26.
29. Maguire J, McNally AJ (1972) Head lice infestation in school children: extent of the problem and treatment. **Commun Med** 128:374–375.
30. Sarov B, Neumann L, Herman Y (1988) Evaluation of an intervention program for head lice infestation in school children. **Pediatr Infect Dis** 7:176–179.
31. Mumcuoglu KY, Hemingway J, Miller J et al. (1995) Permethrin resistance in the head louse *Pediculus capitis* from Israel. **Med Vet Entomol** 9:427–432, 447.
32. Mumcuoglu KY, Miller J, Gofin R et al. (1990) Epidemiological studies on head lice infestations in Israel. I. Parasitological examinations of children. **Int J Dermatol** 29:502–506.
33. DeFelice J, Wagner D (1985) Head lice outbreaks and their impact on the community; a public health perspective. Ft. Lauderdale, FL: World Health Communications Symposium.

including our studies in Panama, show no association between infestation and gender.[24,27,34] The relatively high rate of infestation among girls reported in many studies may reflect girls' greater tendency to share brushes, combs, and hair accessories.

Length of hair has not been shown to be a significant factor in host preference among head lice. Although investigators in Israel[32] have reported an association between hair length and infestation, we believe that this association may be attributable to other confounding factors, such as gender. When controlling for gender, we could not establish a correlation between hair length and infestation in any of 15 studies conducted over 10 years.

Anecdotal evidence suggests that head lice may have a preference for certain blood types. Many years ago, we noticed that the head lice living on the indigenous Indian population with which we were working actually avoided one of us. Nymphs and adult lice plucked from the scalps of infested children and placed on the arm of the investigator often refused to feed or even tried to get away. Newly hatched nymphs would readily take their first bloodmeal from the investigator and continued to take subsequent meals. However, adult lice that had been starved for at least eight hours were finicky, and lice that still retained some of their previous bloodmeal refused to feed altogether. This clear host preference might have been attributable to blood type; while everyone in the study population had type O-positive blood, the investigator's blood type was O-negative. When a starving louse that had fed briefly on an O-positive volunteer did finish feeding on an O-negative individual, the gut of the louse would rupture, killing the louse within a few minutes. This phenomenon, called a "red louse," is usually associated with the causative agent in typhus, which multiplies so rapidly in the gut of the louse that the gut finally ruptures.

Blood type preferences in bloodsucking insects are not unknown. In a study conducted in 1974,[35] the malaria mosquito, *Anopheles gambiae*, showed a preference for hosts with type-O blood. Sholdt *et al.*,[36] found blood type to be significantly associated with body lice infestations in Ethiopia. Further research is needed to determine the relationship between blood type, Rh factor, and infestation with head lice. The existence of such an association might help explain why, within a family or classroom, some children are more prone to infestation than others.

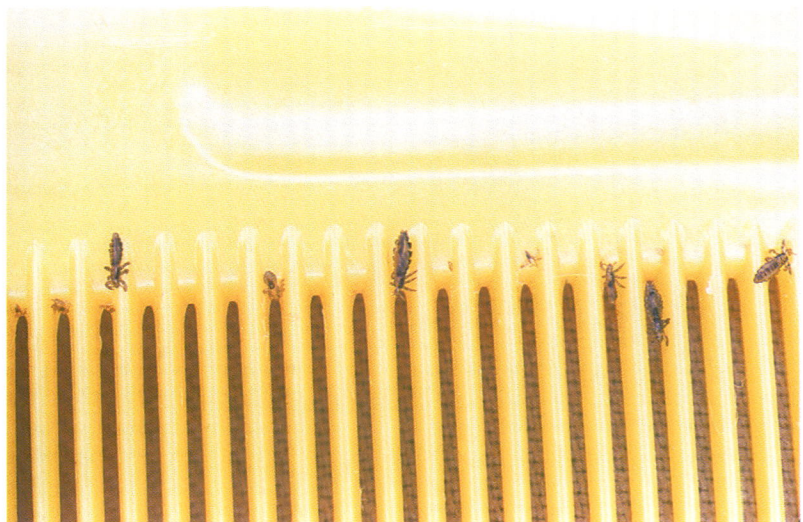

Fig. 27.7   Head lice transmission by fomites (comb).

The mechanisms of head lice transmission differ between cool and warm climates. In cool and temperate regions, where lice are hesitant to leave the warm protective environment of the human head, direct head-to-head contact is the most common mode of transmission. In the tropics and over most of the United States in the summer months, head lice are often transmitted by shared inanimate objects, such as towels, brushes, combs, and head gear (Fig. 27.7). Although lice cannot survive for long on such objects, they can more readily from them to another scalp. Thus, it is not uncommon to trace an outbreak of head lice to a single, shared object such as a batting helmet or a set of language lab headphones.

Crab lice

Few statistics exist on the incidence or prevalence of crab lice, perhaps because infested individuals are reluctant to take part in prevalence surveys. However, infestation is believed to be widespread, with incidence fluctuating over long periods of time.[37] Most cases occur in young, single, sexually active individuals,[38] but virtually anyone can become infested. Crab lice have been reported on the scalp of elderly persons with no history of sexual exposure and on the eyelashes of children. Unlike head lice, which are rarely seen in the African-American population, crab lice affect all races and ethnic groups. They are relatively uncommon among Asians, however, perhaps because genital hair is sparse in this group.[24]

Crab lice are transmitted by close physical contact, usually sexual intercourse, and by the sharing of infested clothing, towels or beds. Toilets may also play a role in transmission. Children usually contract *P. pubis* by sharing a bed or towel with an infested family member.[24,37,39]

Transmission of crab lice without bodily contact might occur more frequently than previously recognized, especially in warm, humid climates. In Miami in 1991, Meinking surveyed 45 homeless individuals with crab lice. Twenty-two respondents (49%) reported no sexual contact for several months or years and were convinced that they had obtained their undesirable arthropods from clothing, towels, or bedding recently used by infested individuals. Many recalled a specific homeless shelter, blanket, sleeping bag, or mattress as the source. The fact that clusters of patients who did not know each other identified the same homeless shelter and time frame gave some credence to these claims. Live crab lice collected from towels used by the infested patients stayed alive for up to 36 hours at laboratory temperature (22°C, 72°F). Viable eggs on pubic hairs clipped from the patients or collected from the towels hatched up to 10 days later when incubated at outdoor Miami temperatures (29° to 31°C; 85° to 87°F) and relative humidity of 70% to 80%. At the implicated homeless shelter, bedding was changed once per week, while the inhabitants of the beds changed every night.

BIOLOGY

Body lice and head lice are similar in appearance. They are easily distinguished when examined side by side, but considerable experience is required to identify individual specimens. The differential characteristics are listed in Table 27.1. In general, body lice are longer and wider across the abdomen than head lice. Pubic lice have wide, short bodies resembling a tiny crab and look quite different from *Pediculus* (Fig. 27.8).

In 1946, Culpepper successfully reared a laboratory colony of body lice adapted to feed on rabbits.[40] Descendants from this original colony still exist in a few laboratories around the world. After 60 years and thousands of generations they have become attenuated by an artificial laboratory existence.[41,42] They differ in feeding habits, lifestyle, and appearance from body lice obtained

34. Slonka GF, Fleissner ML, Berlin J et al. (1977) An epidemic of pediculosis capitis. **J Parasitol** 63:377–383.
35. Wood CS (1974) Preferential feeding of *Anopheles gambiae* mosquitoes on human subjects of blood group O: A relationship between the ABO polymorphism and malaria vectors. **Hum Biol** 46:385–404.
36. Sholdt LL, Holoway ML, Fronk WD (1979) The Epidemiology of Human Pediculosis in Ethiopia. Jacksonville, FL: Navy Disease Vector Ecology and Control Center, Naval Air Station.
37. Robinson AJ, Ridgway GL (1994) Sexually transmitted diseases in children: non viral including bacterial vaginosis, *Gardnerella vaginalis*, mycoplasms, *Trichomonas vaginalis*, *Candida albicans*, scabies and pubic lice. **Genitourin Med** 70:208–214.
38. Brown TJ, Yen-Moore A, Tyring SK (1999) An overview of sexually transmitted diseases. Part II. **J Am Acad Dermatol** 41:661–677.
39. Klaus S, Shvil Y, Mumcuoglu KY (1994) Generalized infestation of a 3 1/2-year-old girl with the pubic louse. **Pediatr Dermatol** 11:26–28.
40. Culpepper GH (1944) The rearing and maintenance of a laboratory colony of the body louse. **Am J Trop Med Hyg** 39:472.
41. Cole M (1966) Body Lice. In: Insect Colonization and Mass Production, Smith CN, ed. New York: Academic Press, pp. 15–24.
42. Meinking TL, Taplin D, Kalter DC, Eberle MW (1986) Comparative efficacy of treatments for pediculosis capitis infestations. **Arch Dermatol** 122:267–271.

TABLE 27.1 The facts of lice			
	Pediculus humanus	**Pediculus capitis**	**Pthirus pubis**
Size (mm)			
Female	2.4–4.0	2.4–3.3	1.0–1.2
Male	2.3–3.0	2.1–2.6	0.8–1.0
Egg incubation period (days)	7–10	10–12	9–11
Size of nit (mm)	0.7–0.8	0.8	0.8
1st nymphal stage (days)	3–4	3–4	3–6
2nd nymphal stage (days)	3–4	3–4	3–6
3rd nymphal stage (days)	3–4	3–4	3–5
Adult female to gravid female (days)	1/2–2	1/2–2	1–2
Egg to adult (days)	17–25	17–25	22–27
Adult longevity (days)			
Female	23–25	23–30	17–28
Male	23–32	23–30	17–28
Total egg output	275–300	110–400	30–50
Survival away from host	1–7 days	6–20 hours	6–36 hours
Adult mobility	6–30cm/min	6–30cm/min	10cm/day
Habitat	Body and clothing	Head	Pubic area, beard, axillae, eyelashes, any hairy area

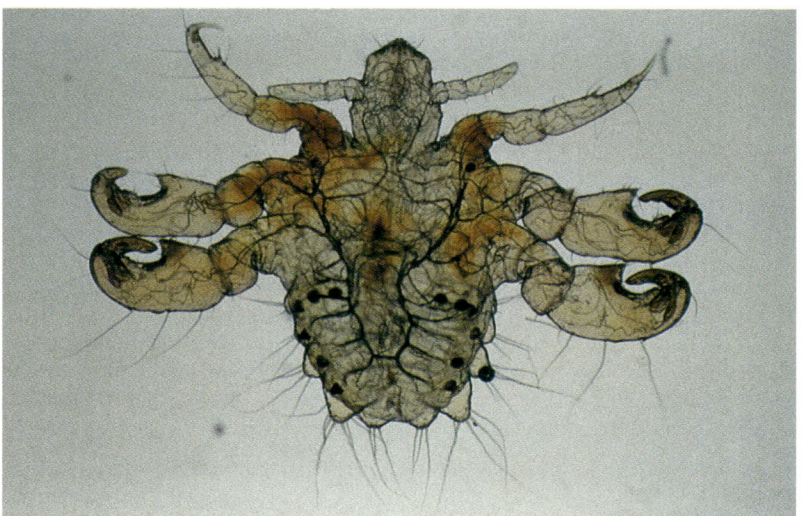

Fig. 27.8   Adult crab louse. Respiratory spiracles and circulatory system are easily seen. (Courtesy of Tony Burns, MD)

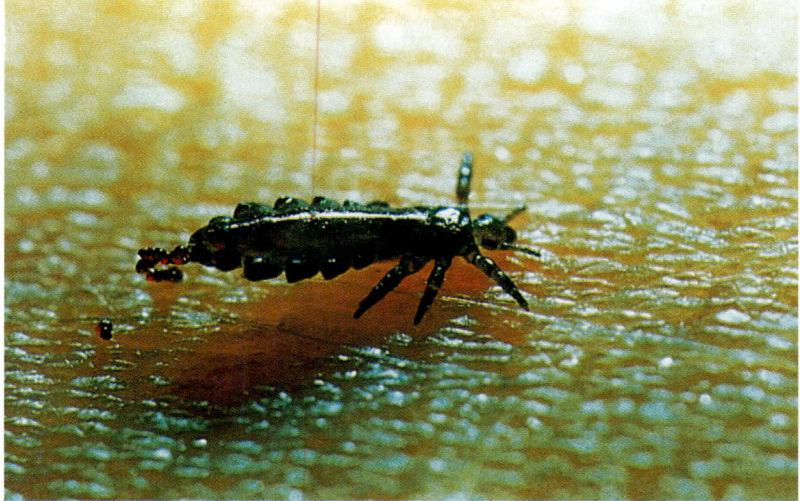

Fig. 27.9   Female louse feeding and defecating on author's arm.

from infested humans.[42] So far, all attempts to establish laboratory colonies of head and crab lice have failed. However, encouraging progress is being made.

Body and head lice have nine body segments. The first two are fused into a thoracic plate, which supports three pairs of short, segmented legs. Each leg terminates in a single grasping claw (Fig. 27.9). A respiratory spiracle is located between the first and second leg on each side of the thorax (Figs 27.10, 27.11). The remaining seven segments are bilaterally lobed, with all but the final segment containing a pair of breathing spiracles. The eyes of *Pediculus* are located posterior to the antennae and are simple eyes or ocelli.[43] The antennae of *Pediculus* have five segments in the adult, but only three in the nymphal form. These segments, each of which serves a specific function, are sparsely covered with tactile sensory hairs, with the last one appearing hollow with sensory hairs inside. The antennae of the head louse are shorter and wider than those of the body or crab louse.

Like *Pediculus*, the crab louse has six respiratory spiracles on each side of the abdomen, but the plates are fused into one. Of the three pairs of legs, the first pair terminates in a slender claw. The second and third pairs have well-developed claws resembling those of stone crabs. This anatomic configuration is perfectly adapted to grasping the coarse, widely spaced hairs of the pubis, axilla, beard, and, occasionally, the eyelashes of the host (Fig. 27.12). According to Marples,[44] *P. pubis* tolerates higher levels of humidity than other lice and is unaffected by sweat. Nuttall[45] reported that pubic lice exhibit an extremely marked aversion to light.

Unlike head lice and body lice, which may travel up to 23cm per minute, pubic lice are sluggish, traveling a maximum of 10cm per day. They may remain in one location for hours or days at a time and may attach themselves to the host, a behavior more typical of ticks than of body or head lice. This may explain why the bite of *P. pubis* produces a more severe cutaneous reaction than that of *Pediculus*. When the pubic louse decides to relocate, it

43. Alexander JO (1984) Arthropods and Human Skin. Berlin: Springer-Verlag.
44. Marples MJ (1965) The Ecology of the Skin. Springfield, IL: Charles C. Thomas.
45. Nuttall GHF (1917) The biology of *Phthirus pubis*. Parasitology 10:383.

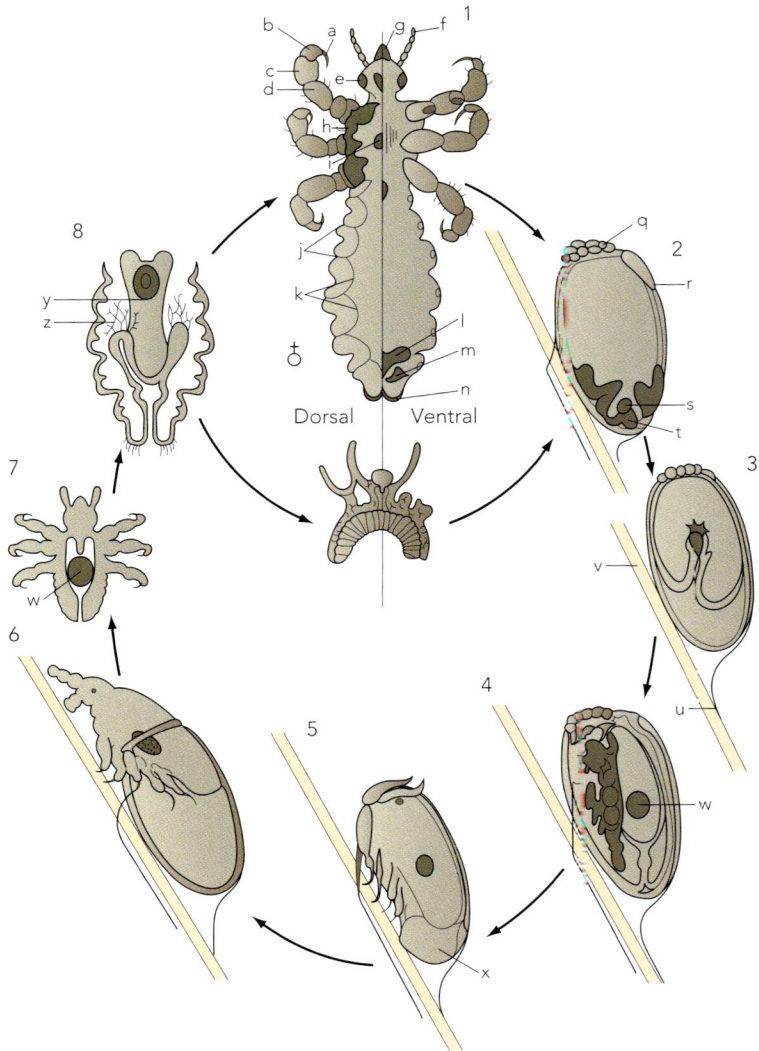

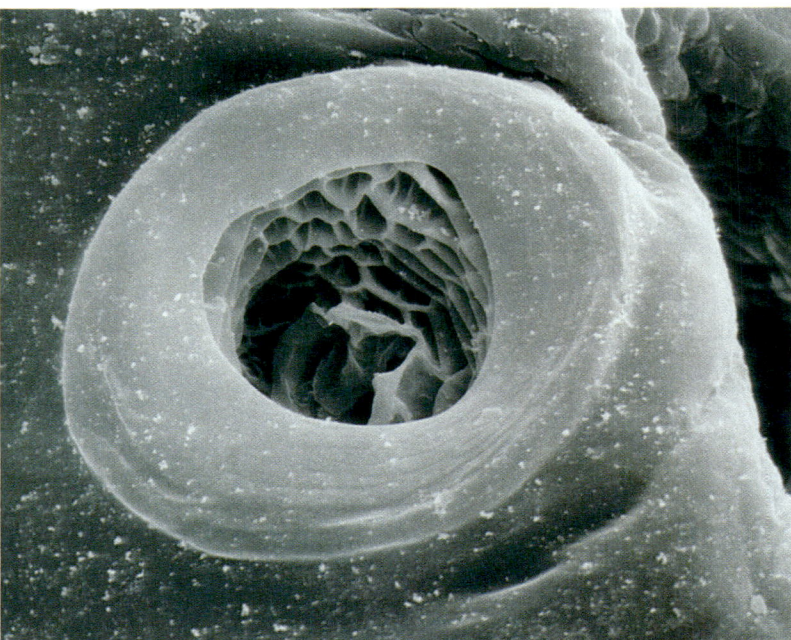

Fig. 27.11 Scanning electron microscopy of head louse respiratory spiracle (thoracic). This honeycomb structure creates maximum surface area and efficient exchange of air and moisture.

Fig. 27.10 Life cycle of the *Pediculus capitis*. Respiratory spiracle is apparent between stages 3 and 4 Stage 1: Adult female head louse. Stage 2: Egg at first day of development of embryo. Stage 3: Invagination of germ band. Stage 4: Transitory mycetome in embryonic gut of louse. Stage 5: Larva taking in air to expel itself from egg. Stage 6: Emerging nymph or first instar stage. Stage 7: Second instar stage of nymph. Stage 8: Third instar stage showing nymph molting to adult female as symbiotes migrate to ovarian ampullae. Stage 9: Enlargement of ovarian ampullae with symbiotes *a*, claw; *b*, tarsus; *c*, tibia; *d*, femur; *e*, ocellar eye; *f*, antenna; *g*, labrum; *h*, thoracic spiracle; *i*, notal pit; *j*, abdominal spiracles; *k*, respiratory system; *l*, shield plate or central shield; *m*, gonopod for grasping hair during egg laying; *n*, claspers brace female on the hair during egg laying and aid in spreading cement; *o*, vaginal orifice; *p*, oviduct epithelium; *q*, operculum or cap; *r*, egg or nit; *s*, chromosomes; *t*, symbiotic bacteria; *u*, cement or glue secreted; *v*, hair shaft; *w*, mycetome; *x*, air pocket; *y*, migrating symbiotes; *z*, ovarian ampulla.

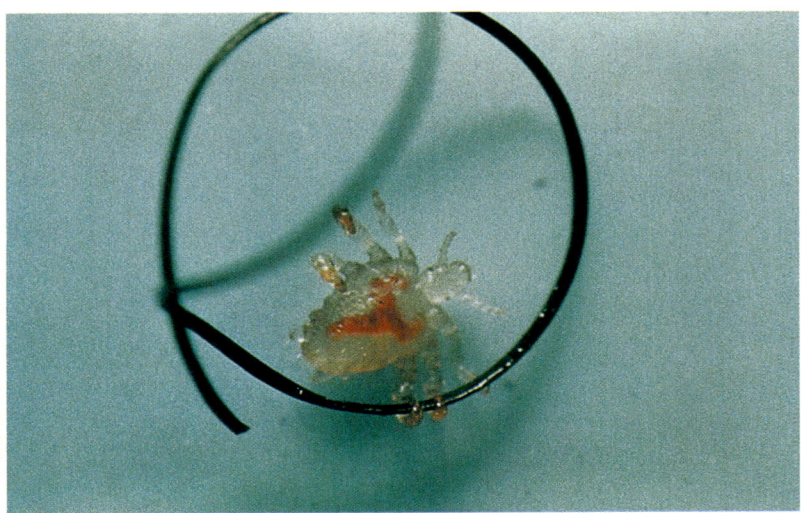

Fig. 27.12 Crab louse nymph with blood meal.

does so cautiously, retaining its grasp on one hair until it is assured of a secure hold on the next.

Lice tend to adapt their color to their surroundings. Therefore, lice found on dark-skinned, dark-haired individuals are normally darker than those found on people with lighter skin or blond hair.[3,24] *P. humanus* is generally lighter in color than *P. capitis*, presumably because it lives in the dark recesses of clothing and has little need for protective coloration.[46]

The brown color of lice is due to melanin formation in the cuticle, a process closely allied to quinone tanning of proteins responsible for hardening of the cuticle or chitinous shell. According to Wigglesworth,[47] this mechanism is temperature-dependent. Therefore, lice in warmer climates tend to be darker than those found in cooler regions. The dark pigmentation of head lice found in the tropics may be related to the higher ambient temperatures in addition to the need for camouflage.

When the head louse is newly hatched, its only pigmented areas are the claws and eyes. Within minutes of the first bloodmeal, brown shoulder patches appear at the junction of each leg and the thorax. As adults, the abdomen of females is uniformly pigmented. Males have readily distinguishable brown bands that traverse the abdomen at the edge of each overlapping abdominal plate (Fig. 27.13).

With the aid of a 10x hand lens, one can easily distinguish a female from a male, regardless of genus and species (Fig. 27.14). In general, females are

46. Nuttall GHF (1917) Notes on the biology of *Pediculus humanus*. Parasitology 9:259.

47. Wigglesworth VB (1984) Insect Physiology, 8th edn. New York: Chapman & Hall.

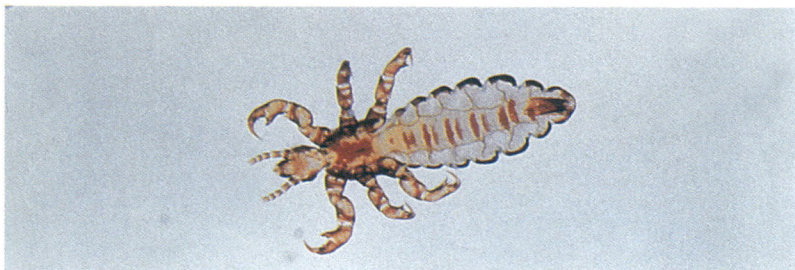

Fig. 27.13 Adult male head louse with dark pigmented bands.

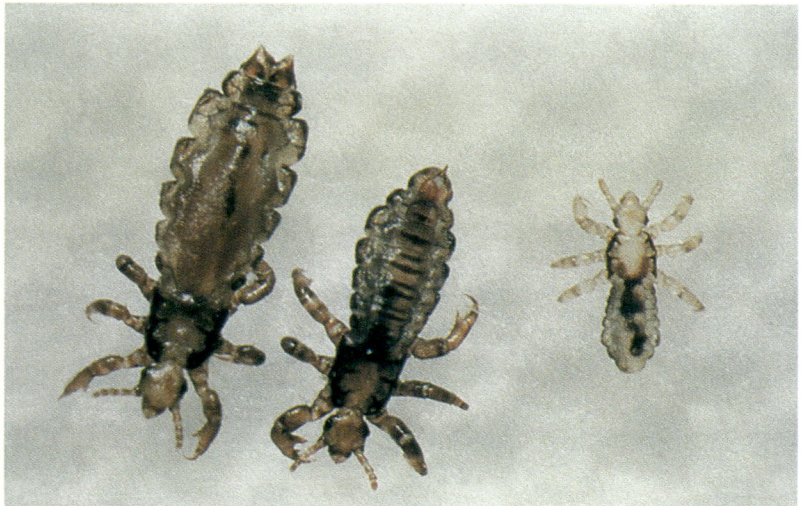

Fig. 27.14 A family of head lice; an adult female, adult male (center), and a second instar nymph.

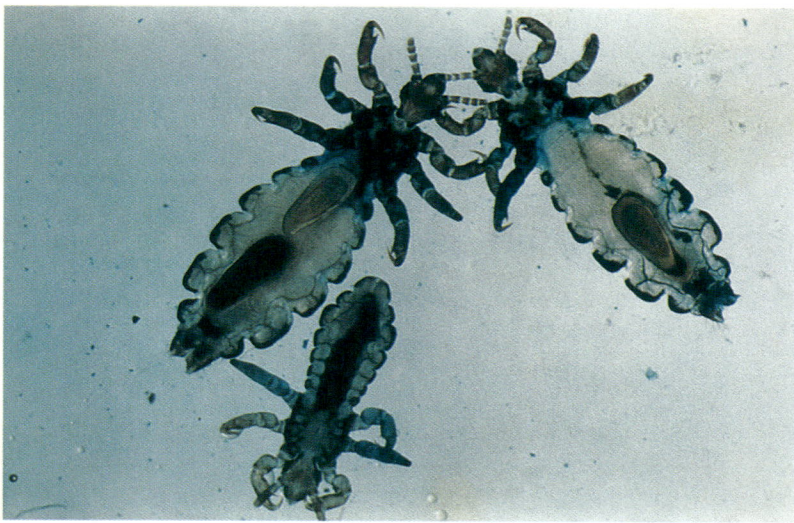

Fig. 27.15 Cleared female head lice reveal fully formed eggs inside abdomen. The body tapers to form an invaginated V.

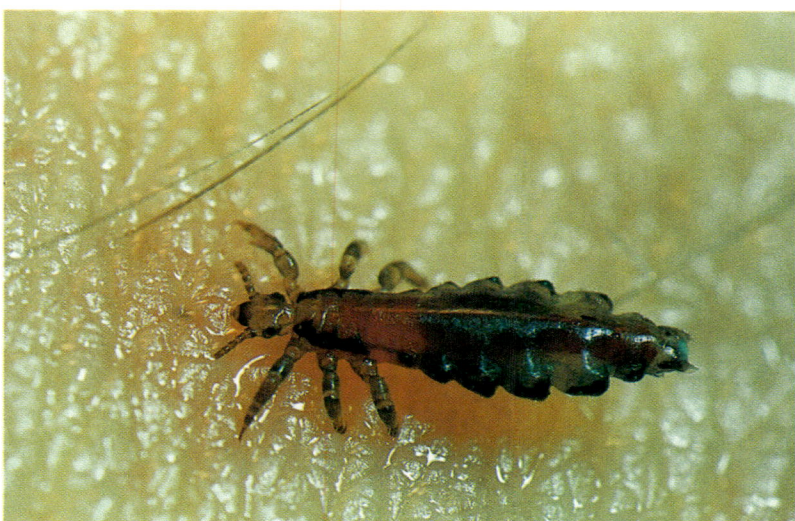

Fig. 27.16 An adult female head louse with bloodmeal. Note that the exoskeleton terminates in an invaginated V-shape.

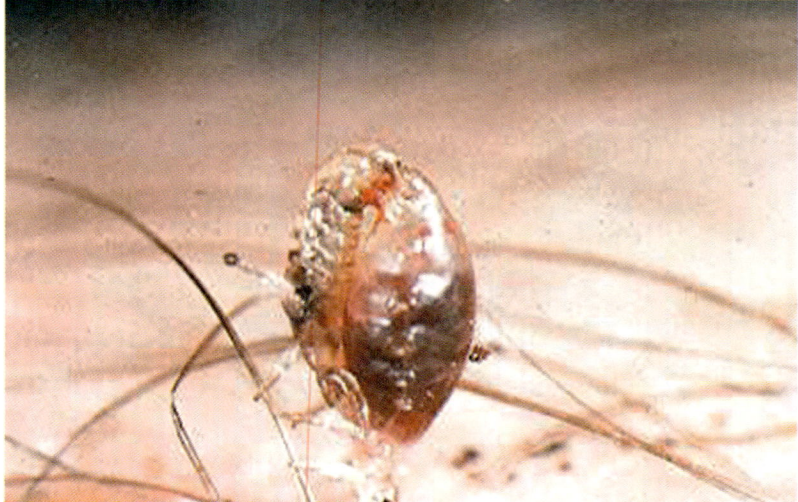

Fig. 27.17 Male and female laboratory body lice copulating and feeding.

20% larger than males of the corresponding species, but there is considerable variation and some overlap occurs. Females are longer and wider, and the dorsal and ventral abdominal surfaces have a more rounded and full appearance. Using a special clearing technique, one can see that females are basically "egg factories" and that the eggs are formed full size (Fig. 27.15). The posterior portion of the female exoskeleton terminates in two protrusions with gonopods, creating an invaginated V-shape the width of an egg[3,48] (Figs 27.15, 27.16). The gonopods are supportive structures that enable the female louse to grasp the hair shaft while laying eggs. The male exoskeleton or epicuticle tilts upward at the rounded posterior end with the anal and sexual apparatus on the dorsal surface. This arrangement enables the male to crawl beneath the female for the purpose of copulation. The epicuticle of the male is stronger and more developed, with an armored thoracic plate. While copulating, the female grasps the male around the thorax, placing each of her legs between his. This position enables both lice to feed while copulating (Fig. 27.17).

The mouthparts of lice are developed to enable piercing of the skin and sucking of the capillary blood of the host. The haustellum, a tube-like structure complete with teeth, remains invaginated when not in use. When feeding, the mouth is pressed against the host's skin and the chitinous haustellum is thrust through the skin's surface, enabling the averted teeth to anchor the head of the louse to the epidermis of the host (Fig. 27.18). Three

48. Busvine JR (1980) Insects and Hygiene, 3rd edn. London: Chapman & Hall.

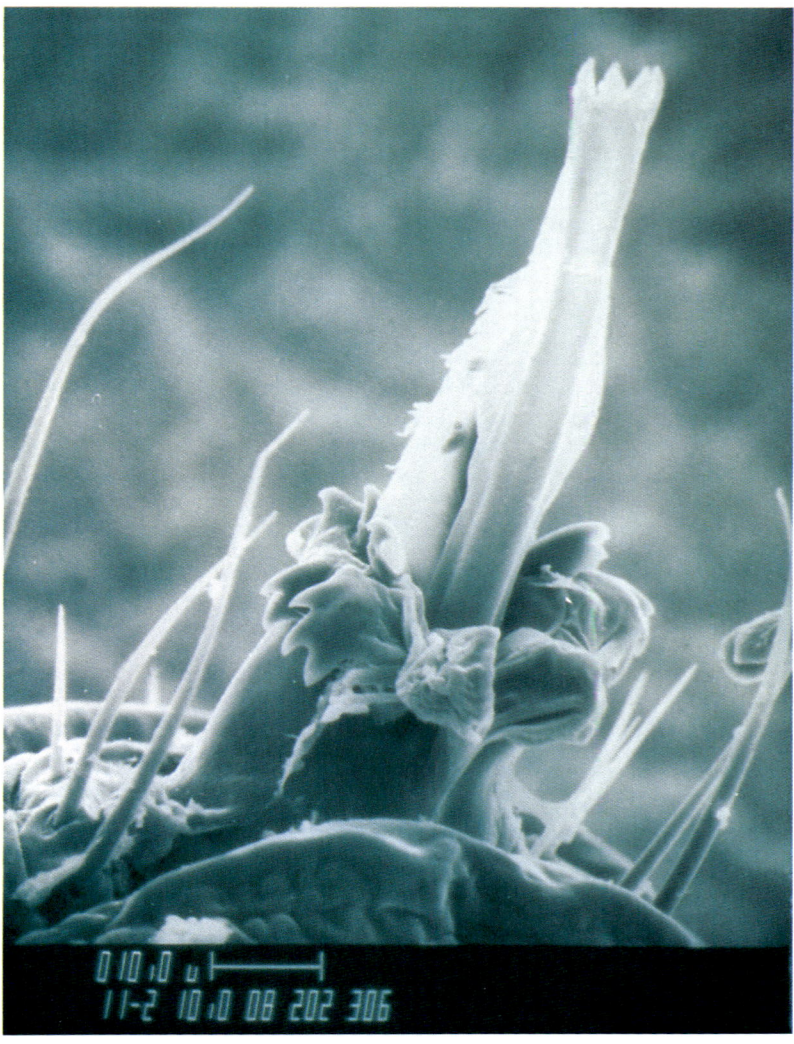

Fig. 27.18 Scanning electron microscopy of extruded haustellum of a body louse, preparing to pierce the skin. (Courtesy of Mark Eberle, PhD)

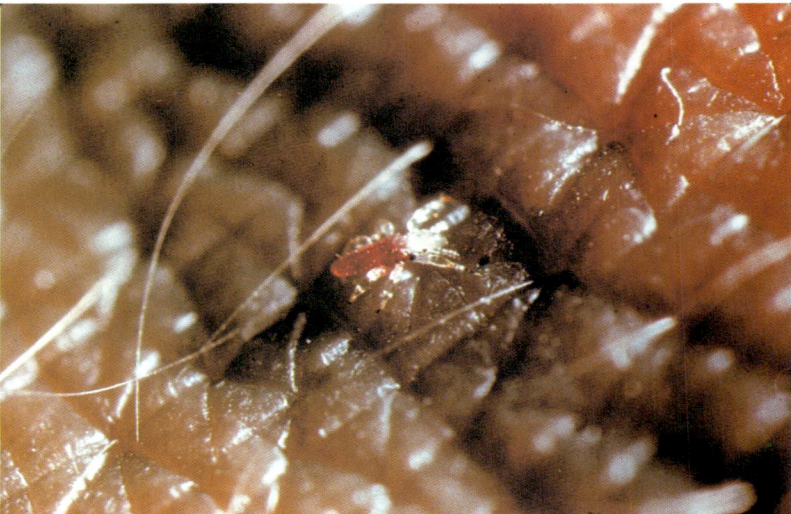

Fig. 27.19 Blood-engorged head louse nymph after taking its first bloodmeal from the investigator's arm (TLM).

stylets housed within the haustellum draw up the bloodmeal by use of a cibarial pump in the insect's head. The intermediate stylet or hypopharynx delivers the anticoagulant, probably antithrombin,[47] as well as a vasodilator responsible for erythema around the bite site. There are two pairs of salivary glands, the reniform and the tubular, both located in the thorax. The glands unite at their introduction to the hypopharynx. Their salivary contents produce irritation when injected into the host. When these glands were dissected out and injected separately into volunteers, only the reniform gland produced a cutaneous reaction.[4] Buxton noted that neither he, his colleagues, nor volunteers became tolerant to louse bites after repeated feedings.[4] Our personal experience suggests that we have become more sensitized over several years as a result of feeding experiments.

There is some evidence that the saliva of body and head lice may have different antigenic constituents. One of us had fed wild head lice on herself on many occasions over a period of 4 years. She became increasingly sensitized. Eventually, the bite of a single head louse was sufficient to elicit a highly pruritic reaction in all other sites previously used, including ones that had been quiescent for a few years. In contrast, when she later allowed laboratory body lice to feed on her, she noted a 48-hour delayed reaction at the feeding site, but no reactivation of the previous head louse bites.

LIFE CYCLE

Lice are hemimetabolic in development; that is, they do not go through a complete metamorphosis. The larval stage of the louse merely looks like a baby adult, unlike the larva of a mosquito or pupa of a flea, which bears no resemblance to the adult form. The louse larva, more commonly referred to as a nymph or "instar," must feed on human blood shortly after hatching from the egg. This first instar undergoes two more molts before it becomes an adult. After the first feeding, the almost transparent nymph takes on the appearance of a tiny ruby (Fig. 27.19). The nymph must take a bloodmeal between each molt. Several feedings occur between the shed of each exoskeleton, since each instar stage lasts about three days, and often longer in the case of *P. pubis*.[43]

Approximately 9–12 days after hatching, the third instar casts aside its chitinous shell and becomes an adult louse. It is only at this point that the sexual identity of this creature is unmasked. Mating can occur as soon as 10 hours after the third molt; however, 24 hours is closer to the average.[44] One day after the first copulation, the female slides down the hair or clothing fiber that she has clasped between her gonopods. Special glands secrete a cement into the uterus. This cement then flows out of the genital opening in advance of the egg extrusion, cementing the egg to the hair or clothing fiber. This rapid process is completed in about 17 seconds. Because the cement hardens on contact with the air, the adult female occasionally becomes fatally entangled in it.[43] There is no known solvent for this adhesive. There are a few products on the market that claim to loosen or dissolve the glue, but in our experience, and that of colleagues, they have not proven to be highly effective. Although the exact composition of this cement remains a mystery, preliminary analysis suggests that it is a proteinaceous matrix, which closely resembles the amino acid composition of the hair shaft.[49]

The female louse repeats the egg-laying process three to ten times per day. Under ideal laboratory conditions, she can lay as many as 300 eggs in her lifetime, although there is some variation among species (Table 27.1). Therefore, in a child harboring a few dozen head lice for several weeks, one could find, theoretically, many thousands of viable eggs and empty nit. In practice, one rarely finds more than a few hundred eggs and usually far less. An interesting exception concerns individuals with mental disabilities, who may lack the capability, or perhaps desire, for self-grooming and the benefit of daily social grooming. On these individuals, we may find many hundreds of large, well-nourished head lice and many thousands of eggs. This

49. Burkhart CN, Slankiewicz BA, Pchalek I et al. (1999) Molecular composition of the louse sheath. J Parasitol 85:559–561.

observation has been recorded for centuries and is thought to be the origin of the term "nit wit." At the other end of the spectrum, well-groomed children in economically advanced societies usually have only one or two dozen eggs and rarely more than 10 adult lice. These low numbers are largely due to awareness among school health officials and parents and also grooming and the availability of pediculicides to treat the condition before it gets out of hand.

In cool and temperate climates, head lice lay eggs close to the scalp and rarely lay more than one egg per hair. However, in the tropics or in warm months in the United States, eggs may be laid six or more inches down the hair shaft, and as many as six viable eggs may be found on one hair. Crab lice commonly lay more than one egg per hair due to their limited motility. Maximum egg production occurs at optimum temperatures of 29° to 30°C (84° to 86°F) with an ample food supply.[43] Nuttall found that this process ceases at temperatures over 39°C (102°F).[46] An average nit measures 0.8mm by 0.3mm and incubates most successfully at temperatures of 28° to 32°C (82° to 90°F) and relative humidity of 70% to 90%. In a drier atmosphere, there is an increased chance that the nymph will pop the operculum but not completely emerge from the egg, a phenomenon best described as a "stillbirth." Stillbirths are common after treatment with lindane and natural pyrethrins.[42] Nymphs that are stillborn are considered nonviable for practical purposes, but this phenomenon indicates that the pediculicide did not kill the nymph *in situ*. Prolonged temperatures lower than 22°C (72°F) and higher than 45°C (113°F) are also fatal to eggs.[43] Under favorable conditions, the nit hatches in approximately 10 days.

Our observations suggest that an egg containing a fully developed embryo is more likely to succumb to a pediculicide than is a freshly laid egg. We believe that pediculicides enter the egg through the doughnut-shaped holes in the operculum,[42] which supply air and humidity to the embryo (Fig. 27.20). Upon hatching, the prominent thoracic spiracles of the louse are the first body part to emerge. SEM shows them to possess an elaborate honeycomb structure, which is perfectly designed for maximum surface area and efficient exchange of air and moisture (Fig. 27.11).

The hatching process is interesting. The young louse uses its haustellum teeth to cut a circular hole in the operculum. It then sucks in outside air and expels it from its posterior end. The accumulated air pressure inside the egg causes the nymph to pop out like a cork from a bottle of champagne. The newly emerged nymph is immediately active and highly mobile. Within 30 seconds, it seeks out a suitable host, thrusts its stylets through the skin, and enjoys its first bloodmeal (Fig. 27.19). If the first instar nymph does not feed within the first hour after hatching, it will soon die of starvation and desiccation.

SYMBIOTIC BACTERIA

It is a common occurrence in the world of entomology for insects to harbor symbiotic bacteria. Lice are no exception, for they possess a mycetome or stomach disc containing symbiotic, Gram-positive rods. For over two centuries, investigators have been observing the mycetome, oblivious to its significance to the louse.[50] Robert Hooke[51] was the first to describe the mycetome of the human louse. He thought it was the liver. In 1934, Aschner[52] described this organ, noting that it could be easily recognized in living nymphs with the aid of a hand lens because of its color, which stands out against the dark red background of the blood-filled stomach (Fig. 27.21). This 12- to 16-chambered structure is derived from the midgut or stomach lumen during embryonic development in the egg, but by the time the nymph hatches, although the mycetome is still attached to the stomach, it has no opening to it. One misconception is that these symbiotic bacteria harbored in the mycetome aid in digestion of the bloodmeal. Although this is a function of symbiotes in many insects, it is not the case in *Pediculus*.[53]

The general consensus among investigators is that the gut is sterile. In our experience, we have repeatedly cultured *Escherichia coli* from louse feces and from homogenized lice. The potential role of lice in the transmission of pathogens from bacteremic infants to others deserves closer study.

The mycetome of *Pthirus* is larger than that of *Pediculus* and consists of 20 to 24 chambers. Besides symbiotic sausage-shaped rods in the mycetome, *Pthirus* also has a *Rickettsia*-like organism in the intestines or hindgut.[53] Little is known about these symbiotics organism or their role in the crab louse.

The symbiotes of Anoplura are passed on to their progeny by indirectly infecting the ovarial ampullae, special organs between the ovaries and oviducts. Changes in the mycetome begin with the approach of the third molt.[50] The symbiotes of the female begin to flourish, while those of the male

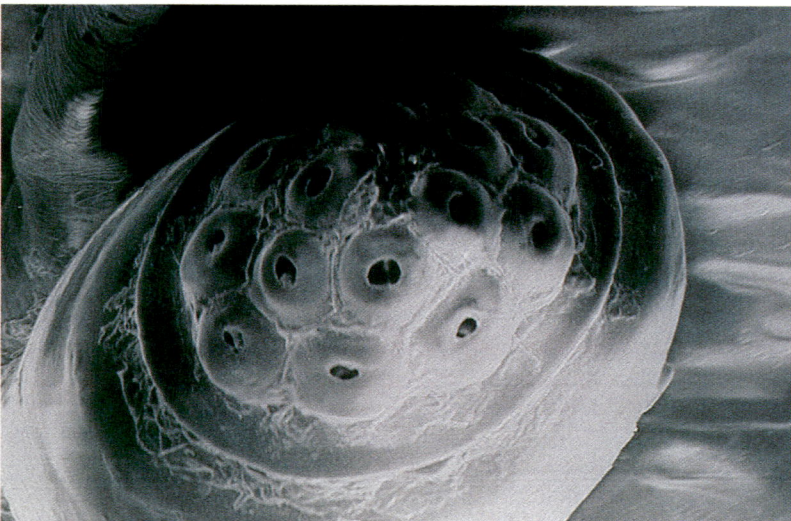

Fig. 27.20 Scanning electron microscopy of head louse nit operculum. Pediculicides enter through these doughnut-shaped holes to kill the developing embryo.

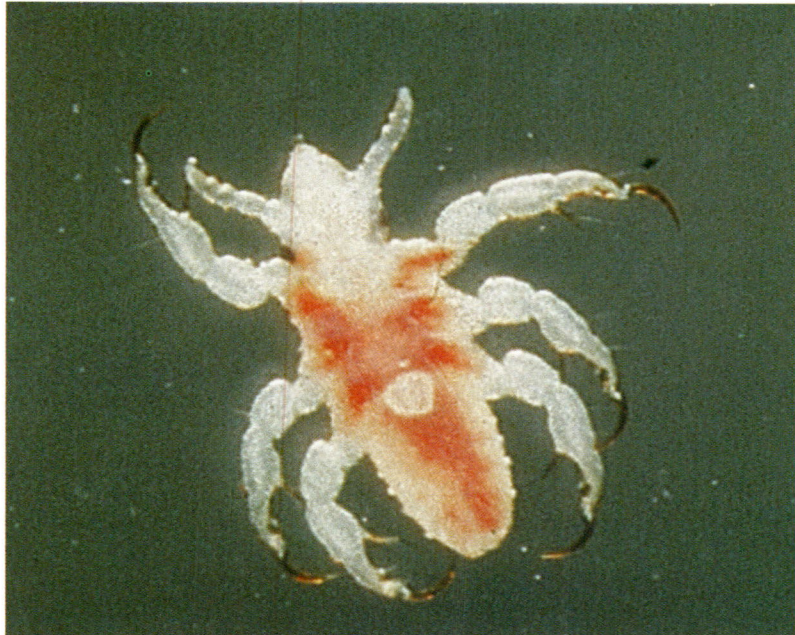

Fig. 27.21 Adult crab louse after recent bloodmeal. Note mycetome in center.

50. Buchner P (1965) Endosymbiosis of Animals with Plant Microorganisms. New York: Wiley.
51. Hooke R (1665) Micrographia. London.

52. Aschner M (1934) Studies on the symbiosis of the body louse. 1. Elimination of the symbiotes by centrifugalisation of the eggs. **Parasitology** 26:309.
53. Steinhaus EA (1946) Insect Microbiology. Ithaca, NY: Comstock.

degenerate. Although the male retains his mycetome and symbiotes, they soon begin to clump and become irregular in shape, finally degenerating into "symbiote debris."[53] In the female louse the symbiotes migrate down the ventral side of the stomach and deposit themselves in the oviduct epithelium. The mycetome is now symbiote-free, and is no longer visible or functional. The above sequence of events is much the same in *Pthirus*.

It has been shown that *P. humanus*, the body louse, cannot survive without symbiotes unless its bloodmeal is supplemented with B vitamins (nicotinic acid, pantothenic acid, and biotin).[50] Similar work has not been applied to the head or crab louse. These human lice prefer to feed on healthy, well-nourished individuals. The body louse, however, feeds on malnourished hosts that are nutritionally deficient.

This preference of head lice for a well-balanced diet was demonstrated in 1976. For several weeks, our team attempted to reach a small coastal village in Panama, which had been cut off from its normal supplies of food and fortified flour by exceptionally high seas. This also prevented fishing, which was the population's main source of protein. When we finally reached the community, we found the people in extremely poor health. Virtually all children had some degree of protein calorie malnutrition, and many showed the unmistakable flag sign of dull, stiff, multicolored hair associated with kwashiorkor. In addition, there was a critical shortage of fresh water, and none could be spared for bathing. We mistakenly assumed that this deprived population would provide a perfect haven for head lice, which we were interested in studying. To our surprise, we found only 10 light infestations, in a population of 382 that normally has a prevalence of over 90% among the children. The presence of many empty egg cases, some 10 cm from the scalp in long-haired girls, but none closer to the head, further suggested that there had been a severe depletion in the louse population over the previous two months. We believe this was due to the poor nutritional state of the hosts. When conditions improved, the head lice reestablished themselves within months.

Body lice require little cement to attach their eggs to the seams of clothing. The head louse and crab louse, however, elaborately coat the egg and hair with a glue-like cement that quickly hardens on exposure to air. Since some areas of the oviduct epithelium function as a cement gland,[50] it is possible

that the symbiotes of *P. capitis* and *P. pubis* may play a role in the manufacturing of this glue.

Prior to laying an egg, the female injects some symbiotes into the apex of the nit. The symbiotes are situated opposite from the operculum in a tight bundle along with the chromosomes. As the embryo develops, this packet moves up the center of the embryo and becomes the mycetome (Figs 27.10, 27.22).

LICE AS DISEASE VECTORS

It has been well documented that body lice are capable of transmitting epidemic typhus, murine typhus, trench fever, and relapsing fever. Louse-borne typhus has not been reported in the United States since 1921.[54] Endemic foci exist in Central and South America, Africa, and Asia, requiring only the conditions of squalor, overcrowding, war or refugee camps to initiate an outbreak. Between January and September 1997, more than 45 000 cases of epidemic louse-borne typhus occurred among refugees and prisoners in Burundi.[20] Other countries reporting outbreaks in the last decade include Russia, Peru, Nigeria, Ethiopia, Rwanda, and the Democratic Republic of Congo (Zaire).[20,21,55] Physicians, other health providers, and military personnel who may be called upon to work in these countries or who volunteer for foreign assistance programs should be familiar with this potentially fatal disease.

Lice also play a role in the transmission of murine typhus (endemic or flea-borne typhus). The course of murine typhus resembles that of epidemic typhus but is less severe, with a shorter duration and a lower case fatality rate. The causative agent, *Rickettsia typhi* (*mooseri*), is transmitted to humans by rat lice or fleas, and from human to human by the human body louse, *P. humanus*.[3] While murine typhus continues to occur in the United States, most cases are associated with close contact with rats or mice.[54]

Louse-borne trench fever, caused by *Bartonella quintana* (formerly *Rochalimaea quintana* and *Rickettsia quintana*) was responsible for much disability among troops in World Wars I and II.[2,54] More recently, a large outbreak of trench fever associated with epidemic typhus was reported in Burundi,[20] and sporadic cases have emerged in Russia, France, and the United States.[16,19,56,57] In industrialized countries, infection with *B. quintana*, also known as "urban trench fever," is found mainly among persons of low socioeconomic standing, particularly homeless or alcoholic individuals.[58] In France, *B. quintana* infections are also significantly associated with the presence of body lice.[56,59] In other reported cases, the role of ectoparasitic vectors remains unclear. However, in Russia, 12.3% of lice collected from 57 homeless individuals tested positive for *B. quintana*, thus confirming the role of *P. humanus* in the contemporary life cycle of this disease agent.[16] Because infection with *B. quintana* produces a broad array of nonspecific clinical manifestations, health professionals should have a heightened awareness of this disease and a knowledge of appropriate diagnostic kits and laboratories that are capable of conducting rapid diagnostic tests.[60]

The fourth disease known to be transmitted by body lice is European or louse-borne relapsing fever (LBRF), an acute febrile illness caused by the spirochete *Borrelia recurrentis*. Transmission of LBRF occurs when a body louse is crushed against abraded or excoriated skin. In the last century, LBRF caused devastating epidemics with mortality rates of 30% to 70% in Africa, Asia, and South America.[61,62] Sporadic cases continue to appear in each of these regions, although antibiotic treatment has greatly reduced the case fatality rate. In Ethiopia, where infestation with body lice is widespread, an estimated 10 000 cases of LBRF occur each year.[22]

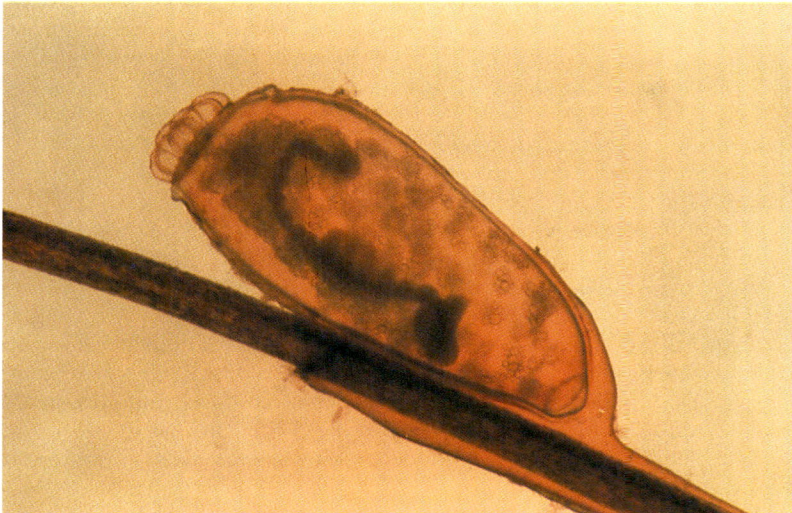

Fig. 27.22   Developing head louse embryo about 4 days old.

54. Chin J, ed. (2000) Control of Communicable Diseases Manual. 17th edn. Washington, DC: American Public Health Association.
55. Tarasevich I, Rydkina E, Raoult D (1998) Outbreak of epidemic typhus in Russia. **Lancet** 352:1151.
56. Brouqui P, Lascola B, Roux V et al. (1999) Chronic *Bartonella quintana* bacteremia in homeless patients. **N Engl J Med** 340:184–189.
57. Comer JA, Flynn C, Regnery RL et al. (1996) Antibodies to *Bartonella* species in inner-city intravenous drug users in Baltimore, Md. **Arch Intern Med** 156:2491–2495.
58. Ohl ME, Spach DH (2000) Bartonella quintana and urban trench fever. **Clin Infect Dis** 31:131–135.

59. Brouqui P, Houpikian P, Dupont H et al. (1996) Survey of seroprevalence of *Bartonella quintana* in homeless people. **Clin Infect Dis** 23:756–759.
60. Jackson LA, Spach DH (1996) Emergence of *Bartonella quintana* infection among homeless persons. **Emerg Infect Dis** 2:141–144.
61. Rahelenbeck SI, Gebre-Yohannes A (1995) Louse-borne relapsing fever and its treatment. **Trop Geograph Med** 47:49–52.
62. Bryceson AD, Parry EH, Perine PL et al. (1970) Louse-borne relapsing fever. **Q J Med** 39:129–170.

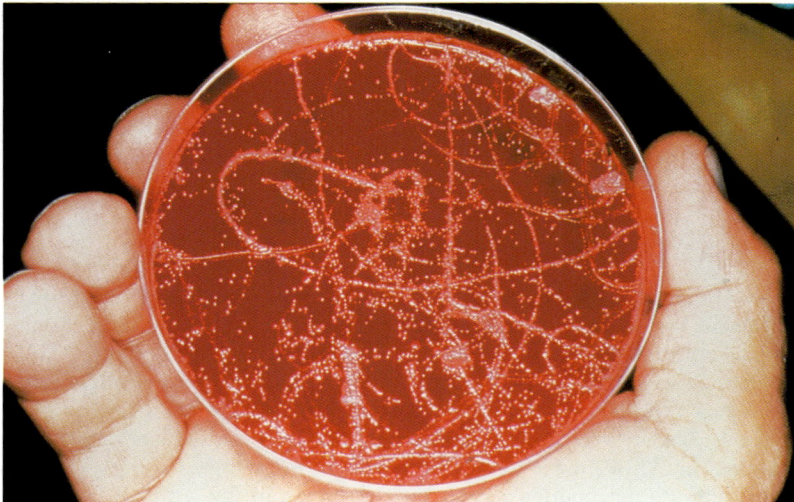

Fig. 27.23 Bacterial growth on a blood agar plate where head lice, recently obtained from children, have walked.

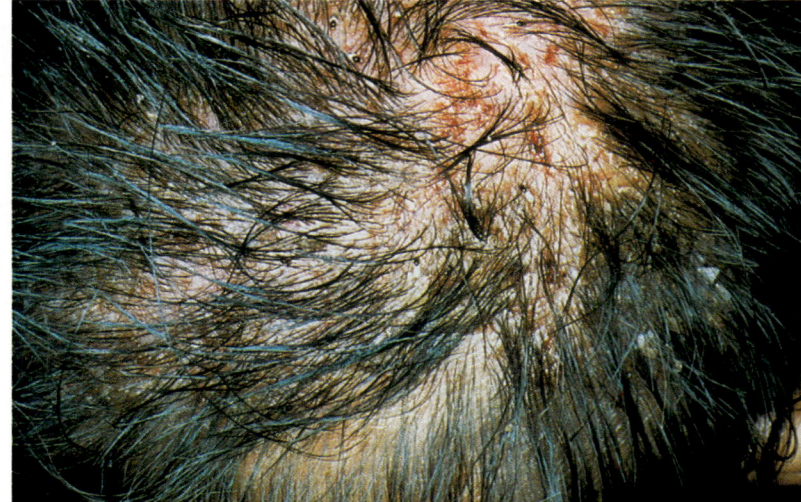

Fig. 27.24 Streptococcal/staphylococcal pyoderma of the scalp secondary to head louse infestation. Note small wound-feeding eye gnats (*Hippelates*) on scalp; these are known vectors of skin infections.

Head and crab lice have not been firmly established as vectors of blood-borne disease, perhaps because they have received less attention from microbiologists and entomologists. Also, unlike body lice, there is no laboratory colony of head or crab lice to study transmission of louse-borne diseases. Maunder states that body, head, and crab lice can transmit epidemic typhus, murine typhus, and trench fever with equal effectiveness in the laboratory.[3] In 1975, Murray and Torrey[63] showed that head lice collected from Boston children were susceptible to *R. prowazeki*, although there are no known reports of head louse-borne typhus. Another important consideration is that head and crab lice have a much narrower temperature range than body lice, and will leave a host that has a fever or dies. Individuals that arrive at emergency rooms with high fever, common with louse-borne diseases, no longer have lice. The type of louse transmitting the disease is therefore unknown.

Head lice are known to carry a variety of bacteria on their exterior surfaces. Figure 27.23 shows the trails of bacterial colonies deposited by three head lice allowed to walk over a blood plate for five minutes. Included in this flora are group A *Streptococcus pyogenes* and coagulase-positive *Staphylococcus aureus*. Transmission of these bacteria by head lice is a major, and perhaps the only, cause of the common multiple streptococcal/staphylococcal pyodermas of the scalp in many areas of the world, particularly in the tropics (Fig. 27.24). The multiple puncture wounds, pruritus, and excoriations associated with pediculosis capitis provide an ideal setting for chronic scalp pyoderma, particularly in populations where daily hygiene is difficult to maintain. Treatments with oral antibiotics are only temporary cures. However, we have consistently noted decreases in the prevalence and severity of scalp pyoderma following treatment for head lice, often without the use of antibiotics.

The viable bacilli of bubonic plague, *Yersinia pestis*, have been found in both body and head lice taken from disease victims.[64] Both species have been able to transmit plague from rodent to rodent experimentally. Lice can also harbor and transmit *Yersinia tularensis*, a related bacillus that causes tularemia.[64] Salmonellae, including species that cause typhoid and other diseases, multiply rapidly in human lice, but like typhus are also fatal to the lice, killing them within 48 hours.[64] The bacilli have been known to remain alive in dead lice and their fecal pellets for at least one year.[64] As with other louse-born diseases, the mechanism of transmission is not the bite of the louse, but rather contamination of excoriated skin or bite sites with lice feces or by crushing the insect.

In a collaborative effort with the FBI Forensic Science Unit, human mitochondrial DNA was successfully isolated, amplified, and sequenced from adult human crab lice fed on human volunteers. The resulting mitochondrial DNA sequences matched those obtained from the volunteers' saliva, effectively linking each louse to its host.[65] The ability to identify individual human hosts may be invaluable in rape, child abuse, and homicide cases. In the future, similar techniques could also aid in diagnosis of diseases transmitted by lice or rule them out in infections for which they are suspect.

In one of our studies of homeless individuals with *P. pubis* infestations, lice from volunteers were deep-frozen at −70°C while alive and then tested by the polymerase chain reaction (PCR) for the human immunodeficiency virus (HIV). All specimens obtained from HIV-positive individuals were found positive by use of ethidium bromide gel with confirmation on Southern blot. Lice specimens from known HIV-negative individuals recently tested at a local clinic were confirmed negative with use of the above method. One individual who had had prior STDs and three *P. pubis* infestations in two years had not been tested for HIV, but her lice specimens were strongly positive on both the gel and Southern blot. Future studies should assess the possibility of HIV transmission by crab lice and determine whether there is a correlation between the viral burden of HIV and the number of lice needed to show a positive confirmation with PCR. In the future, PCR may also be useful in determining whether lice can transmit other diseases.

In 1986, the National Pediculosis Association (NPA) raised the question of whether head lice are capable of transmitting HIV.[66] No evidence is available to suggest that this occurs. On the other hand, the role of head lice as vectors of blood-borne viruses has not been extensively studied. On epidemiologic grounds, and by mathematical probability, the transmission of HIV in US public schools through the mediation of head lice must be so small as to escape detection, even if this mode of transmission were possible (see Epidemiology).

The situation may well be different in parts of Africa, where head, crab, and body lice are highly endemic, and the opportunities for transfer of lice between individuals are constantly present. It is evident that a concerning proportion of AIDS cases in Africa and other countries cannot be explained by sexual exposure.

63. Murray ES, Torrey SB (1975) Virulence of *Rickettsia prowazekii* for head lice. **Ann NY Acad Sci** 266:25–34.
64. Chandler AC, Read CP (1961) Introduction to Parasitology, 10th edn. New York: Wiley.
65. Lord WD, DiZinno JA, Wilson MR et al. (1998) Isolation, amplification, and sequencing of human mitochondrial DNA obtained from human crab louse. *Pthirus pubis* (L.), blood meals. **J Forensic Sci** 43:1097–1100.
66. Altschuler DZ, Kenney LR (1986) Pediculicide performance, profit and the public health. **Arch Dermatol** 122:259–261.

The potential for the transmission of blood-borne diseases deserves more thorough investigation than has been applied in the past. Although pediculosis capitis does not usually produce anemia, head lice are capable of extracting considerable quantities of blood. Based on Buxton's figure of 1mg of blood extracted per feeding by a single louse,[4] we estimate that as much as 200mg of blood may be extracted daily and disseminated as fecal pellets on a heavily infested child. It is not uncommon to find thousands of fecal pellets on the scalp and in the hair of children with limited opportunities to shampoo, and without treatment, this situation may continue for years. Furthermore, because there is no reservoir for head or crab lice other than humans, newly acquired lice are always derived from another individual, creating the risk of disease transmission from the sick to the healthy.

In summary, body lice have been clearly identified as vectors of typhus, trench fever, and relapsing fever. Head and crab lice have not been positively incriminated in the transmission of blood-borne infections, but this may reflect the paucity of investigation. None of the three species of lice that infest humans has been closely studied as vectors of viral infections. Further research is needed in this area.

THERAPY

Body lice

Because body lice are usually found on individuals who cannot wash or change their clothing, the most important treatment for pediculosis corporis consists of disinfestation of all contaminated clothing and linens. In dealing with individual cases seen in, for example, a hospital emergency room, the clothing is treated like infectious material, bagged in appropriately labeled and tightly sealed plastic bags, and handled separately from other hospital trash until incineration. Where this is not possible, clothing may be fumigated with methyl bromide, steam fumigated, dry cleaned, or simply machine washed in hot water and dried on high heat. Any means of applying uniform heat, wet or dry, that maintains a temperature of 65°C (149°F) for 15 to 30 minutes is sufficient to kill all lice and their eggs.

Because body lice have been known to lay eggs on the piping or seams of bedding and sofas, mattresses and furniture should either be sprayed with agents specifically approved for such use or, if this is not possible, be burned. Household or agricultural sprays, powders, and other commercial insecticides intended for environmental use should never be used on people, clothing, bedding or furniture. Products approved for use in the home may be used to treat living quarters, provided that the labeling instructions are followed and not exceeded. Caution should be used to avoid inhalation of the sprays.

Following appropriate disposition of clothing, the patient should be treated from head to toe with a pediculicide. This will ensure that any louse or viable egg that may happen to be on the body cannot continue its life cycle. Permethrin 5% topical cream is the safest and most effective therapy available, although it is not specifically indicated as a treatment for body lice. The patient should be treated head to toe for 8–14 hours, as indicated for the treatment of scabies (see Scabies therapy), and repeated in one week to ensure that any eggs that survived treatment cannot survive. Oral ivermectin (200–400µg/kg) would probably also be effective, but dosage requirements are not available for its use in pediculosis. In a laboratory study, Mumcuoglu et al.[67] reported a high mortality rate among body lice fed on rabbits treated with ivermectin at 200µg/kg. The effect lasted 2–3 days after feeding and declined thereafter.

In large populations, mass delousing may be accomplished with the use of insecticidal dusting powders. In general, dusting powder tends to be a good vehicle for pediculicides because powder has abrasive properties and passes through the breathing spiracles of the louse. Active agents in insecticidal dusts include permethrin, malathion, temephos, propoxur, and carbaryl. Although DDT powder has been used since the 1940s, worldwide resistance and environmental contamination have prevented further use of this organochlorine pesticide.[20,68] The first studies on permethrin dusting powder were conducted by Nassif et al. in Egypt, showing that permethrin was highly effective even in DDT- and malathion-resistant body lice.[69,70] Standard treatments with permethrin powder were employed in the immediate control of epidemic typhus among prisoners and refugees in Burundi during 1996 and 1997.[20,68] While permethrin is a safe and effective treatment, the emergence of permethrin-resistant body lice in some countries suggests that this agent may be of limited use in the future.[31,71]

In many parts of the world, especially those affected by war, civil unrest, or natural disaster, limitations on distribution and communication infrastructures may prevent the widespread dissemination of large quantities of insecticidal dust. Therefore, overreliance on permethrin or any other insecticidal agent should be avoided. The optimum strategy for the control of body lice in large populations includes not only mass delousing, but also improvements in access to washing facilities and clean clothing.

Emergency room personnel, disaster relief teams, and goodwill medical groups working overseas should take extreme precautions in working with body lice infestations, especially if louse-borne diseases are suspected. Medical personnel who have been exposed to body lice or their eggs might consider prophylactic treatment with 5% permethrin topical cream or oral ivermectin (200–400µg/kg).

Head lice

Common measures to remove lice and nits mechanically from the hair, such as brushing, combing with a good nit comb, shampooing and towel- or blow-drying, play a role in reducing the number of viable lice and eggs on the head, but are insufficient to cure an active infestation. Effective treatment involves the application of a pediculicide to kill lice and nits followed by manual nit removal (see Nit-picking).

Most pediculicide products currently available in the United States kill lice but not their eggs. Therefore, all topical treatments should be applied twice, one week apart. The second application is necessary to kill any nymphs that may have hatched from eggs that survived the first treatment. The rise in head lice resistant to lindane and over-the-counter products currently makes treatment options difficult.

There has been a continuing struggle to find new pediculicidal agents ever since head lice developed resistance to DDT in England in 1949. In the past, it seemed as though investigators were always one step ahead of the louse with a new treatment, but now it appears that lice are developing resistance to lice-killing products faster than new ones are being developed. The active ingredients of the pediculicidal products currently available in the United States include lindane, natural pyrethrins, permethrin, and malathion. These and other alternative head lice treatments are discussed in detail below.

Lindane

Currently, 1% lindane (GBHC) is one of two prescription products that have been approved by the Food and Drug Administration (FDA) for the treatment of pediculosis (the other, 0.5% malathion, is discussed below). Lindane has been available as a 1% shampoo for the treatment of head lice and a 1% lotion and cream for the overnight treatment of scabies for more than 50 years. The lotion is FDA-approved for scabies only and is potentially toxic if used for head lice, due to increased percutaneous absorption.

Lindane shampoo is simple to use, with a recommended treatment time of only four minutes, but it also has some significant drawbacks. First, lindane belongs to the class of chemical insecticides called organochlorines, which

67. Mumcuoglu KY, Miller J, Rosen LJ et al. (1990) Systemic activity of ivermectin on the human body louse *Pediculus humanus humanus*. **J Med Entomol** 27:7275.
68. Bise G, Coninx R (1997) Epidemic typhus in a prison in Burundi. **Trans R Soc Trop Med Hyg** 91:133–134.
69. Nassif M, Kamel O (1977) A field trial with permethrin against body lice, *Pediculus humanus humanus* in Egypt, 1976. **Pestic Sci** 8:301–304.
70. Nassif M, Brooke JP, Hutchinson DBA et al. (1980) Studies with permethrin against body lice in Egypt. **Pestic Sci** 11:679–684.
71. Rupes V, Moravec J, Chmela J et al. (1995) A resistance of head lice (*Pediculus capitis*) to permethrin in Czech Republic. **Cent Eur J Public Health** 3:30–32.

also includes DDT. These insecticides do not degrade and thus persist in the environment for decades. Lindane rinsed off after use passes through the sewer system into creeks, rivers, lakes and oceans, where it can contaminate the tissues of fish and other wildlife. In 2000, evidence of lindane pollution in Los Angeles drinking water prompted California to ban the sale of all lindane products in that state beginning in 2002.

Lindane not only persists in the environment but also accumulates in the body with repeated use. Studies have shown that this pediculicide can be stored in human adipose and nerve tissue, creating the potential for central nervous system (CNS) toxicity.[72,73] When lindane shampoo is used as directed, the likelihood of convulsions or clinical signs of CNS toxicity following a single treatment is remote.[74] Most reports of CNS toxicity have been related to accidental ingestion or overuse. Precautions against accidental ingestion include the usual care exercised in a household to keep toxic or corrosive liquids away from children. It would seem obvious that pesticides should not be stored in the medicine cabinet, but this is often where pediculicides or scabiecides are placed, since they are, after all, "medicines." We know of two instances in which lindane lotion was given orally to children with scabies, due to the lack of communication in one case, and a language barrier in the other. Warning instructions on smaller bottles of products are displayed in fine print and are difficult to read, often requiring a magnifying glass. Safety precautions and instructions may be obscured by the pharmacy, which places a typed label stating "Use as directed" over the original. Often the doctor has not explained the directions in much detail. The patient or parent must understand that this is a pesticide that can be toxic if misused.

We recall an incident that occurred several years ago in a busy emergency room of a general hospital in midwestern USA. A resident working in the hospital saw a poor, uneducated woman with crab lice in the pubic area. He prescribed 1% lindane shampoo. Four days later she returned much worse, with all hairy areas infested, including the eyelashes. This time she brought her three small children, ages 3 to 7, who also had phthiriasis palpebrarum. When she was asked why she had not used the medicine, she replied, "I took one tablespoonful and it tasted so bad I couldn't drink any more." Despite the controversy surrounding lindane toxicity, there is one issue on which all authorities agree: this product is not safe to drink! In this scenario, the doctor assumed that the pharmacist would type simple directions on the label or that the patient would read and understand the tiny printed directions on the bottle. The pharmacist assumed the doctor had explained the directions. Luckily, the mother had tested it first and therefore did not give it to her children.

Often patients will claim they understand directions, when in fact they do not. Regardless of the treatment, it is always advisable to have the patient repeat the instructions verbally to ensure that they do understand. All health care providers and pharmacists should warn patients and parents of the potential hazards of lindane.

Regardless of warnings given in good faith, the potential for abuse and overuse of lindane products exists. Parents may conclude that if the treatment is effective, more treatments will be even more so. This is particularly true when children are sent home from school several times with a diagnosis of head lice. However, repeated applications of this pediculicide are not recommended, given its potential to accumulate in the body. Because percutaneous absorption is greater in the scalp than most other parts of the body, lindane shampoo should not be left on for longer than the prescribed time and should not be used more than two times one week apart.

A third major disadvantage of lindane is its slow killing time. Chlorinated hydrocarbons are slow-acting pediculicides and lindane is no exception. Those with a concern for the welfare of creatures great and small would be disturbed to watch the suffering of the poor head louse following exposure to lindane. First, they begin to twitch and become disoriented. They frantically cling to each other in a final embrace, during which the adult male suffers complete extrusion of the sexual organs. Violent peristalsis ensues, followed by seizure-like convulsions. After several hours of suffering, only the twitching antennae betray the last signs of life. Finally, this too ceases, and the creature dies. Many of our patients have complained that their lice "held a discotheque on their head" after the shampoo. In our experience, patients prefer a product that rapidly kills the lice. The appearance or feeling of twitching lice is sometimes a cause of emotional distress.

Finally and, perhaps, most importantly, lindane has a relatively high treatment failure rate, due in large part to tolerance or resistance in lice. Reports of lindane-resistant head lice emerged in the early 1970s in the UK,[75] followed by similar accounts from the Netherlands.[76,77] In 1986, on an island in Panama where lindane products had been used extensively, Taplin et al.[78] found that 57% (17/30) of children with head lice failed to respond to 1% lindane shampoo (Kwell). By comparison, when the same research team treated 49 subjects with the same lot of Kwell in a nearby village with no previous lindane exposure, 90% (44/49) of cases responded to treatment. These results strongly suggest that there were lindane-resistant head lice developing in Panama in areas with a history of extensive lindane use.

Lindane resistance was observed in the United States as early as 1986. We recall a case in Miami involving a young girl who had been repeatedly treated with 1% lindane shampoo (Kwell) to no avail. We removed the live lice from her hair and immersed them in undiluted Kwell shampoo. The lice were not affected by the lindane for over six hours. After six hours away from the host, lice normally succumb to starvation and begin to die. These lice were alive for over eight hours, demonstrating, we believe, true lindane resistance.

Florida, Texas, and California are considered "hot spots" of lindane resistance in the United States. This may be partly due to the large number of immigrants coming to these states from countries in Central and South America, where organochlorines such as DDT and lindane have been used extensively for agricultural, veterinary and medicinal purposes for over four decades. Bars of DDT soap for human ectoparasitic infestations are still available in the local tiendas (shops) and pharmacies in Ecuador.

Even in sensitive populations with no history of extensive lindane use, 1% lindane shampoo is less effective than several pediculicides available over the counter. In 1984 and again in 2000, Meinking et al.[42,79] tested the comparative efficacy of a number of leading pediculicides, using head lice collected from a sensitive population to control for the formulation's changes over the years. Lindane was by far the slowest-killing and least ovicidal product tested under continual exposure in either study. In their most recent Panama study, only 61% of lice were dead after three hours of continual, direct contact with undiluted 1% lindane shampoo, and this product was only 24% ovicidal.[79] In the US study, only 17% of lice were dead after three hours of continuous exposure to undiluted lindane, demonstrating lindane-resistant lice in the USA[80] (Tables 27.2, 27.3).

In view of the many negative aspects of this pediculicide, it is difficult to see the advantage of future lindane use, particularly when several other less toxic and equally or more effective treatments are available.

72. Ginsberg CM, Lowry W (1983) Absorption of gamma benzene hexachloride following application of Kwell shampoo. **Pediatr Dermatol** 1:74–76.

73. Pramanik AK, Hansen RC (1979) Transcutaneous gamma benzene hexachloride absorption and toxicity in infants and children. **Arch Dermatol** 115:1224–1225.

74. Kramer MS, Hutchinson TA, Rudnick SA et al. (1980) Operational criteria for adverse drug reactions in evaluating suspected toxicity of a popular scabiecide. **Clin Pharmacol Ther** 27:149–155.

75. Maunder JW (1971) Resistance to organochlorine insecticides in head lice and trials using alternative compounds. **Med Officer** 125:27–29.

76. Blommers L, van Lennep M (1978) Head lice in the Netherlands: susceptibility for insecticides in field samples. **Entomol Exp** 23:243–251.

77. Blommers L (1979) Insecticidal tests on immature head lice, *Pediculus capitis*: a new technique. **Med Entomol** 16:82–83.

78. Taplin D, Meinking TL, Castillero PM et al. (1986) Permethrin 1% Creme Rinse (NIX) for treatment of *Pediculus humanus* var *capitis* infestation. **Pediatr Dermatol** 3:344–348.

79. Meinking TL, Entzel P, Villar ME et al. (2001) Comparative efficacy of treatments for pediculosis capitis infestations: Update 2000. **Arch Dermatol** 137:287–292.

80. Meinking TL, Serrano L, Hard B et al. (2002) Comparative *in vitro* pediculicidal efficacy of treatments in a resistant head lice population in the United States. **Arch Dermatol** (forthcoming).

TABLE 27.2   Comparative pediculicidal activity as determined by *in vitro* method

Product	Rank 1984	Rank 2000	% dead @ 10 minutes, 2000 Panama	% dead @ 10 minutes, 2000 S. Florida	% dead @ 1 hour, 2000 Panama	% dead @ 1 hour, 2000 S. Florida	% dead @ 3 hours, 2000 Panama	% dead @ 3 hours, 2000 S. Florida
Lindane	4	6	17	2	15	8	61	17
0.5% Malathion (Ovide)	1	1	100	100	100	100	100	100
RID	2	5	73	8	50	21	53	34
A-200	3	4	97	60	99	82	100	100
Undiluted Nix	NA[a]	2	90	10	100	49	100	74
Diluted Nix (90% Nix)	NA[a]	3	73	8	94	18	100	46

[a] NA indicates not applicable because product was not on the market at the time of the study.
(Adapted from Meinking et al.[79] and Meinking et al.[80] with permission.)

TABLE 27.3   Comparative ovicidal activity in a sensitive population (Panama) as determined by a 10-minute dip *in vitro* method

Product	Ovicidal activity, % of nits nonviable 1984	Ovicidal activity, % of nits nonviable 2000
Lindane K well brand (1984) vs generic (2000)	70	24[b]
0.5% Malathion Prioderm lotion (1984) vs Ovide (2000)	95	100
RID	74	69
A-200	77	33
Undiluted Nix	NA[a]	89
Diluted Nix (90% Nix)	NA[a]	81

[a] NA indicates not applicable because product was not on the market at the time of the study.
[b] Significance level p<0.001
(From Meinking et al.,[79] with permission.)

Pyrethrins (natural plant extracts)

Extracts of the flower heads of *Chrysanthemum cinerariaefolium* contain a mixture of active agents called natural pyrethrins, which include pyrethrin I, pyrethrin II, jasmolin I, jasmolin II, cinerin I, and cinerin II. These extracts are available in lotion, shampoo, foam mousse, and gel formulations that also contain the synergist piperonyl butoxide (PBO; Butacide). Trade named include RID; A-200 shampoo; R&C shampoo; Paratrol; Pronto; Clear shampoo; and generic formulations.

The insecticidal properties of extracts of certain species of chrysanthemums have been known in Europe for well over a century and in Persia for much longer.[81,82] All natural pyrethrin products manufactured since 1950 are combined with piperonyl butoxide (PBO), which has insecticidal properties of its own, greatly enhances the activity of pyrethrins and reduces the amount necessary but provides the same activity. Originally, it was added purely for financial reasons but it has been found to block the mixed function oxidase (MFO) pathway of resistance. The active agents in the pyrethrum flowers are extracted with kerosene or petroleum distillates, which may cause eye irritation. As with any pediculicide, care must be exercised in the use of these products to avoid contact with the eyes. Wash the eyes thoroughly with tap water if accidental contact occurs.

The natural pyrethrins demonstrate low mammalian toxicity (600–900mg/kg oral, 1500mg/kg dermal calculated as LD_{50}) (Table 27.4). They suffer, however, from poor stability to heat and light and have no residual activity.

None of the natural pyrethrin pediculicides are totally ovicidal. Twenty to 30 percent of the eggs of the head lice remain viable after treatment.[42,79] This necessitates a second treatment 7–10 days later in order to kill newly emerged nymphs hatched from eggs that survived the first treatment.

Apart from the inconvenience and expense of having to treat twice, there is no evidence that multiple treatments with pyrethrins are hazardous. As with all topical agents, repeated use invites the development of cutaneous allergic reactions (contact dermatitis) and dry itchy scalp, which may be mistaken as a treatment failure. These reactions are probably due to a component in the vehicle and not from an active agent.

Much has been made of the alleged cross-reaction between ragweed pollen and natural pyrethrins. Undoubtedly, the early crude flower extracts contained components of other plants and weeds from the chrysanthemum fields. Since 1950, modern refining techniques have produced an extract that is cleaner and quality controlled, and there is no theoretical reason to suspect cross-reactions. Nevertheless, all pyrethrin pediculicides carry a warning of possible allergic reaction in patients who are sensitive to ragweed. We believe such reactions are rare. We know of one authenticated case of severe allergic reaction with anaphylaxis in a child sensitive to chrysanthemums and roses, which is entirely logical in view of the origin of natural pyrethrins.

Although there is no published documentation of pyrethrin resistance in the United States, there has recently been an increase in reports of treatment failures. Since pyrethrins are the natural molecular formulations from which permethrin, a synthetic version, was developed, it would not be surprising to have pyrethrin-resistant lice in the United States and worldwide.

Permethrin (a synthetic pyrethroid)

By synthesizing and modifying the molecular structure of natural pyrethrins, chemists were able to develop compounds called pyrethroids. Permethrin (3-phenoxybenzyl(+, −)-3-(2,2-dichlorovinyl)-2-2 dimethyl cyclopropane carboxylate), one of the first heat-stable and photostable synthetic pyrethroids, has even lower mammalian toxicity than natural pyrethrins. Based on oral studies in animals, this compound is about three times less toxic than natural pyrethrins and approximately 36 times less toxic than lindane (Table 27.4).

In the US, permethrin is available by prescription as a 5% cream (Elimite/Acticin) for scabies or over the counter (OTC) as a 1% cream rinse (Nix, generics). In some other countries, preparations of both strengths are available OTC. The 5% permethrin cream is FDA-approved for scabies but not for the treatment of head lice, although it is recommended by some doctors. It is safe for an 8–14-hour application in children as young as 2

81. Casida JE (1973) Pyrethrum: The Natural Insecticide. New York: Academic Press.

82. Meinking TL, Taplin D (1990) Advances in pediculosis, scabies and other mite infestations. **Adv Dermatol** 5:131–150.

TABLE 27.4 Approved therapy for head lice infestations

Approved therapy	1% lindane[b]	0.5% carbaryl[a]	0.5% malathion[b]	Natural pyrethrins with piperonyl butoxide	1% permethrin	Coconut oil, alcohol, anise, and ylang ylang oil[c]
Pediculicide Classification	Organochlorine	Carbamate	Organophosphate	Plant extract with synergist	Synthetic pyrethroid	Non-pesticide essential oil
Recommended Application time	4–10 minutes	8–12 hours	8–12 hours	10 minutes	10 minutes	15 minutes (3 treatments every 5 days)
Killing Time	6–24 hours	Unknown	10 minutes	3–28 hours	3–28 hours	15–60 minutes
% Ovicidal activity	10–24	90	98–100	30–80	30–80	Unknown
Residual activity	No	Yes	Yes	No	Yes	Unknown
Cosmetic Acceptability	Good	Fair	Poor	Good	Good	Fair–Good
LD$_{50}$ mg/kg (rats) Oral	88	850	2800	584–900	3185	Has not been determined
Dermal	1000	4000	4400	1500	Over 5000	Has not been determined
Adverse properties	Slow killing time, CNS toxicity, seizures, abuse, accidental ingestion, delusions of parasitosis	Reversible cholinesterase inhibitor, long application time	Irreversible cholinesterase inhibitor, flammable, unpleasant odor	Possible allergic reaction in hay fever suffers	No substantiated reports	Flammable, strong licorice scent
Resistance reported	UK, Panama, US, Netherlands, Egypt, other countries worldwide	No	UK, Egypt, Burundi (body lice only)	USA, reported in other countries worldwide	Israel, Czecholslovakia, UK, US, France	
Trade names	Kwell, Kwellada shampoo, Gammexane, Gammexol, generic	Sevin, Derbac, Caryldera lotion and shampoo, New Suleo	Prioderm, Ovide	RID, A-200 shampoo, R&C shampoo, Barc, Pronto, Paratrol, Clear, other generics	Nix creme rinse, Lyclear, generic	

a Not available in the United States.
b Available only by prescription in the United States.
c FDA-approved as lice removal system with comb (device).

months. The 1% permethrin creme rinse (Nix) has been approved by the FDA for the treatment of pediculosis since 1986. This product has undergone more clinical trials and toxicology studies than any other pediculicide on the US market. Clinical trials conducted for FDA approval of Nix involved over 2000 subjects enrolled at 10 centers in three different countries.

Like the natural pyrethrin products, Nix is not completely ovicidal; approximately 20–50% of viable eggs hatch after treatment. Also, although residual permethrin on the hair once killed nymphs soon after they hatched, this is no longer the case. The decline in the residual activity of Nix suggests that permethrin levels that were lethal in the past may be sublethal today.

When Nix was first introduced, a single application of this product was sufficient to cure most cases. In controlled studies conducted in 1987 with no nit combing or removal, a single 10-minute application of Nix showed a treatment failure rate of less than 1% (4/709), compared with 29% (50/172) for RID and 11% (40/376) for lindane shampoo (Kwell).[82]

However, since 1994, it has become clear that permethrin is no longer as effective against head lice as it had been previously. Data from researchers in the UK, France, the Czech Republic, Israel, and Argentina show that head lice have become resistant to permethrin.[31,69,83–85] Recent studies in the USA have not only confirmed the existence of permethrin resistance,[86] but also traced this resistance to specific genetic mutations in lice.[87]

With resistance to permethrin on the rise, it has become necessary to apply Nix two times, one week apart. In studies conducted in South Florida in 1998, 39% of children treated with Nix applied to dry hair for 15 minutes had live lice one week later. The majority of the lice were newly-hatched nymphs that were not affected by the residual permethrin on the hair. When a second treatment was administered one week after the first application, all children were cured; however, this was not according to the labeling instructions. In another population in South Florida, composed mainly of farmworkers and their children, we found that lice collected in the rinse water and on the towel after a 15-minute treatment of Nix on dry hair were alive and walking 12 hours later. Although in the past 5% permethrin cream applied overnight under a shower cap often worked when Nix had failed, we now occasionally find live lice after treatment with 5% permethrin cream as well. Therefore, permethrin resistance is a current and increasing problem in the USA as well as worldwide.

Malathion

Used successfully for many years in the UK and continental Europe, 0.5% malathion lotion (Prioderm/Ovide) is the quickest acting and most ovicidal of any pediculicide developed in the last 30 years.[42,88] This product was approved by the FDA around 20 years ago but has been marketed in the USA only intermittently. In 1999, it became available in the USA by prescription under the brand name Ovide.

Ironically, despite its quick action, Ovide has a relatively long recommended application time. Because the original malathion studies for FDA approval involved an 8–12-hour application, this became the recommended treatment protocol. There is evidence, however, that Ovide is highly effective against lice and nits in less than 10 minutes.[79] Clinical trials should be conducted to establish the optimum application time.

Malathion is an organophosphate and an irreversible cholinesterase inhibitor. Illnesses linked to agricultural use of this pesticide have raised concerns about its toxicity in humans. However, the high grade of malathion used for the treatment of human pediculosis is very different from the grade used for agricultural or veterinary purposes. Based on extensive toxicity studies for an 8–12-hour application time, the FDA has approved 0.5% malathion alcoholic lotion for pediculosis treatment, and this product is believed to be safe when used as directed.

The high content of isopropyl alcohol (78%), pine needle oil, and turpineol in this product make it quite flammable if accidentally ignited. Also, the odor is quite objectionable and when the product is applied for the recommended 8–12 hours, the fumes can cause severe headaches. A 10-minute application does not have this drawback.

Malathion resistance in head lice has been documented in England,[23] but so far there are no documented cases of resistance in the United States. Lice in the USA may have remained sensitive to malathion because this product is not as readily available here as it is in the UK, where it can be purchased over the counter. Also, the formula available in the US is different than in other countries and incorporates a resistance strategy component.

Ivermectin

Ivermectin is perhaps best known as a safe and effective treatment for onchocerciasis, or "river blindness," caused by the parasitic worm *Onchocerca volvulus*. A single oral dose of 150–200µg/kg body weight given semiannually in a 6mg tablet is effective against this disfiguring and blinding disease. Worldwide, an estimated 18 million children and adults are treated with ivermectin each year.

In the early 1990s, anecdotal reports that ivermectin cured ectoparasitic infections in patients with onchocerciasis prompted studies of the effectiveness of this drug for the treatment of scabies and head lice. In studies using ivermectin against onchocerciasis, individuals who had received ivermectin tended to have significantly fewer head lice than individuals who had not received this drug.[89]

While the FDA has approved ivermectin for the treatment of onchocerciasis and strongyloides, another internal parasitic infection, this drug does not have an FDA-approved indication for the treatment of head lice. However, ivermectin has been used "off label" for pediculosis treatment when all other treatments have failed. A public health official in the US prescribed this treatment for pediculosis when grade schools in parts of Washington state closed due to outbreaks of "resistant head lice." Ivermectin delivered orally at 200µg/kg seemed to cure most individuals, but follow-up was difficult, and some people required a second dose the next day to kill surviving lice.[90] Since the half-life of ivermectin in the bloodstream is only 16 hours, it is necessary to give another dose a week later in order to kill nymphs that hatched from the eggs. Although clinical trials are needed to determine the optimum dose, ivermectin has an excellent safety profile from not only the Onchocerciasis Eradication Program but also from the US Poison Control database, where toddlers have consumed their dogs' heartworm pills with no side effects.

Carbaryl

Carbaryl (1-naphthyl *N*-methylcarbamate) is used for the treatment of pediculosis capitis in the United Kingdom, where it is available in both a 0.5% lotion and a shampoo formulation (Sevin, Carylderm, New Suleo, Derbac). It is not available in the United States.

In clinical trials reported by Maunder,[91] the lotion form appeared to be more effective than the shampoo but required a 24-hour treatment time. The

83. Burgess IF, Peock S, Brown CM et al. (1995) Head lice resistant to pyrethroid insecticides in Britain. **BMJ** 311:752.
84. Chosidow O, Chastang C, Brue C et al. (1994) Controlled study of malathion and D-phenothrin lotions for *Pediculus humanus* var *capitis*-infested children. **Lancet** 344:1724–1727.
85. Picollo MI, Vassena CV, Mougabure Cueto GA et al. (2000) Resistance to insecticides and effects of synergists on permethrin toxicity in *Pediculus capitis* (Anoplura: Pediculidae) from Buenos Aires. **J Med Entomol** 37:721–725.
86. Pollack RJ, Kiszewski A, Armstrong P et al. (1999) Differential permethrin susceptibility of head lice sampled in the United States and Borneo. **Arch Pediatr Adolesc Med** 153:969–973.
87. Lee SH, Yoon KS, Williamson MS et al. (2000) Molecular analysis of *kdr*-like resistance in permethrin-resistant strains of head lice, *Pediculus capitis*. **Pesticide Biochem & Physiol** 66:130–143.

88. Taplin D, Castillero PM, Spiegel J et al. (1982) Malathion for treatment of *Pediculus humanus* var *capitis* infestation. **JAMA** 247:3103–3105.
89. Dunne CL, Malone CJ, Whitworth JAG (1991) A field study of the effects of ivermectin on ectoparasites of man. **Trans R Soc Trop Med Hyg** 85:550–551.
90. Brettman A (1997) Untested pill kills lice fast, dozens of local parents say. **The Daily News** (Longview, WA) Jul 10.
91. Maunder JW (1981) Clinical and laboratory trials employing carbaryl against the human head louse, *Pediculus humanus capitis* (De Geer). **Clin Exp Dermatol** 6:605–612.

recommended application time for the shampoo is only 3–10 minutes, but it requires a second treatment. Carbaryl products are reported to have good ovicidal properties, but this has been demonstrated in laboratory body lice only, which are quite different from head lice.

Like malathion, carbaryl is a cholinesterase inhibitor and has an objectionable odor. However, it has low mammalian toxicity similar to that of natural pyrethrins. Carbaryl also appears to have some residual activity. Unfortunately, the residual activity diminishes upon exposure to heat or chlorine (i.e., hair dryers and swimming pools). At present, this product is still effective against permethrin- and malathion-resistant lice.

Cotrimoxazole

Reports have appeared suggesting that oral administration of cotrimoxazole (sulfamethoxazole/trimethoprim, TMPX, Septra, Septrin, Bactrim) is an effective treatment for pediculosis capitis.[92,93] Because lice are obligate blood feeders and are dependent on their symbiotic bacteria for survival, these reports may indeed have merit. However, additional research is needed in this area. In particular, there is a need for studies to either confirm or rule out a direct toxic effect on the lice.

This form of therapy, even if confirmed by adequate controlled studies, is unlikely to gain acceptance. Cotrimoxazole is a valuable antibiotic combination that should be reserved for significant infections. Also, in rare cases, this drug may produce harmful side effects, including allergic reactions, aplastic anemia, toxic epidermal necrolysis (TEN), and blood dyscrasias. The use of such an agent for the treatment of pediculosis capitis is not suggested unless the patient also has secondary bacterial infections of the scalp or another infection such as otitis media that would warrant its use.

Non-pesticide products

Reluctant to apply pesticides to children's heads, many desperate and frustrated parents and health professionals are turning to alternative therapies to battle head lice. HairClean 1-2-3, an all-natural lice removal product consisting of anise oil, ylang ylang oil, coconut oil, and isopropyl alcohol (40%), is a particularly attractive alternative. In studies conducted in South Florida,[24] HairClean 1-2-3 appeared to be a safe and highly-effective pediculicide. This product killed all lice and nits in 98% (51/52) of study participants. No adverse experiences were reported. By comparison, Nix showed a treatment success rate of 89% (17/19) when used on clean, dry hair for 15 minutes and repeated. In our experience over the last 20 years, current Nix used according to labeling is ineffective.

Many individuals claim to have successfully cured their infestations by using inexpensive, readily-available products such as petroleum jelly, hair pomade, olive oil, mayonnaise, vegetable shortening, vinegar, mineral oil, and essential oils sold at health food stores. There is no doubt that oily alternatives such as petroleum jelly, olive oil, or mayonnaise slow down the lice, making them easier to find and comb out, and even killing some. In our experience, when these alternatives are rinsed off the next morning, the lice usually survive. Unfortunately, because these therapies are not as effective as the currently available pesticide products, they usually require repeated overnight treatments and many hours of painstaking combing. The need for repeated overnight treatments can in turn delay a child's return to school.

Nit picking

It is common practice to comb or "nit pick" through the hair after treatment to remove lice and nits. Nit removal is important for two main reasons. First, it removes an outwardly visible sign of head lice infestation, thus preventing stigmatization. Second, because no pediculicide product kills 100% of eggs, manual nit removal is recommended to eliminate any nits that may have survived treatment.

Many school authorities in the United States insist on a "no nit" policy to ensure freedom from infestation and proof of adequate treatment. Under this policy, parents or others must remove all nits from infested children's hair before the children can return to school. Although time consuming, manual nit-removal relieves school authorities, nurses, and physicians of the difficulty of deciding whether or not eggs are viable.

Nit removal is a slow and careful process of examining individual hairs from root to tip and dislodging all nits with a special fine-toothed comb. Plastic nit combs that come with pediculicide products often are not as good as metal combs purchased separately. The use of a detangler or hair conditioner may facilitate combing, and the process is made easier when the hair is parted and combed in sections. We have not found vinegar solution to be useful.

It is not necessary to cut long hair or shave the head to manage a head lice infestation. While such measures may ease the task of looking for and removing nits, the possible psychological damage done by such shearing should override any potential benefits.

Additional therapeutic recommendations

Other measures that may be necessary for management of pediculosis capitis include appropriate antibiotics for the treatment of pyoderma of the scalp (Fig. 27.25). Cultures are recommended to identify the presence of *Streptococcus pyogenes* and *Staphylococcus aureus*. Antibiotic sensitivity tests are recommended. When these are not available, one should assume that the *S. aureus* is resistant to penicillin and frequently erythromycin and other antibiotics (see Ch. 24).

Antihistamines may be administered to reduce itching and facilitate sleeping. Pruritus is a difficult parameter to measure in children and we have no definitive data on the value of antihistamines, which appear to offer relief in some cases, but certainly not all.

On the family level, all members of the household should be treated for head lice at the same time. In theory, it should be necessary to treat other contacts only where active infestation is revealed by the presence of viable nits or live lice. In practice, it is often difficult to detect early infestation. Newly hatched nymphs are only 0.5mm in length, and a single gravid female louse is sufficient to initiate a new infestation. Also, head lice have excellent camouflage and are capable of taking evasive action. Thus, one never can be certain that another family member or contact is louse free. If treatment of the entire family is not possible, parents should be advised that new infestations may occur.

The NPA and some other authorities believe that a "pesticide" should not be used on a child who does not have clinically proven pediculosis. We have conducted extensive studies over 15 years that confirm that it is better to treat everyone once than have to treat the same children over and over.

A final step in controlling pediculosis and preventing reinfestation is to thoroughly clean all objects of potential transmission. It should be emphasized that direct contact, particularly head-to-head contact, is the most common and efficient form of transmission. However, inanimate objects do play a role, and it is worthwhile to decontaminate them.

Floors, play areas, and furniture should be thoroughly vacuumed to remove hairs that have been shed with viable eggs attached. Bedding, clothing, and headgear should be washed on a hot cycle and dried in a domestic dryer. Items that cannot be washed may be dry cleaned. Pyrethrin and pyrethroid-based sprays approved for the control of lice on household items are sold in pharmacies and some grocery stores. Household sprays designed for the control of cockroaches, ants, and other pests are not recommended. Children should not be present during spraying, and unused cans must be kept out of their reach.

Combs, brushes, grooming aids, towels, facial cloths, and other items that actually come into contact with the head should not be shared.

92. Shashindran CH, Gandhi IS, Krishnasamy S et al. (1978) Oral therapy of pediculosis capitis with cotrimoxazole. **Br J Dermatol** 98:699–700.

93. Hipolito RB, Mallorca FG, Zuniga-Macaraig ZO et al. (2001) Head lice infestation: single drug versus combination therapy with one percent permethrin and trimethoprim/sulfamethoxazole. **Pediatrics** 107:E30.

Combs and brushes can be coated with a pediculicide for at least 15 minutes, followed by washing in hot water. The use of microwave ovens for decontamination is not always effective and can melt many types of combs and brushes.

Items that can be taken out of use may be stored in plastic bags and left in a warm place (24° to 29°C; 75° to 85°F) for two weeks. This is adequate time for eggs to hatch and for nymphs to starve. In cold climates, items may be bagged and placed outside for two weeks provided that the temperature is freezing. In planning preventative measures, it is helpful to recall that head lice cannot live more than 20 hours off of the host at normal room temperatures (21° to 27°C; 70° to 80°F) or higher. Eggs attached to hairs may remain viable for up to 10 days after treatment, but the nymph must find a bloodmeal within hours of hatching.

To summarize the current status of therapy of pediculosis capitis in 2000, we believe that a cosmetically elegant, rapid acting, completely ovicidal single treatment pediculicide has yet to be developed. Therefore, no single approach is likely to be effective in eradicating the head louse from modern society. Successful control measures require an integrated approach that involves the medical profession, the pharmaceutical industry, school and public health authorities, and most of all, the education and cooperation of parents.

Crab lice

Lindane lotion, once the treatment of choice for crab lice infestations, is no longer indicated for the treatment of *P. pubis* due to concerns about its toxicity. Undiluted lindane shampoo, which requires only a 4-minute application, is approved for this infestation. However, as previously discussed (see Head lice therapy), lindane is less effective and potentially more toxic than treatments available over the counter. Also, sale of lindane shampoo in the state of California will be prohibited beginning in 2002. Malathion and carbaryl formulations, also discussed above (see Head lice therapy), are too irritating for use in the pubic area.

In 1990, Meinking executed an investigator-blinded *P. pubis* study designed to compare two treatments one week apart using 1% permethrin cream rinse (Nix) versus 1% lindane shampoo (Kwell) applied to all hairy areas. Twenty-four out of 28 volunteers (86%) were louse-free at one week after a single treatment of 1% permethrin, whereas only 21 out of 29 subjects (72%) treated with 1% lindane were free of lice. All volunteers were given a second treatment at one week whether or not they still had lice. This was designed to kill any nymphs recently hatched but too small to be noticed. At two weeks, 27 of the 28 subjects (96%) treated with Nix were cured and 24 of 29 (83%) treated twice with Kwell were treatment successes. The six treatment failures were again treated head to toe with 5% permethrin cream (Elimite) overnight and were all cured when they returned the following week.[24]

Meinking and colleagues conducted a similar investigator-blinded study the following year comparing a single treatment of 5% permethrin cream (Elimite) with a single treatment of 1% lindane shampoo (Kwell) when each product was used as directed. After a single total body treatment, 93% of the permethrin group were cured and the lindane group had a disappointing 59% cure rate. The treatment failures received an 8–14-hour application of Elimite and they were cured a week later. The combined results of both studies after

a single treatment are shown in Table 27.5. Note that one-third of the volunteers still had live crab lice and newly laid eggs one week after a supervised head-to-toe 10-minute treatment with Kwell shampoo.[24]

In view of the fact that approximately one half of the subjects in our studies had lice in hairy areas other than the genital region, we recommend treatment of all hairy parts of the body including the scalp. Our recommended therapy for crab lice is an overnight treatment of the entire body with 5% permethrin cream (Elimite/Acticin). Instructions to the patient are simple. Before retiring, apply the cream from the crown of the scalp to the toes. Avoid the eyes. Shower or bathe the next morning with soap and water.

Because pediculicides and scabicides are merely adjunct therapies to the body's own defense mechanisms, crab lice infestations may be especially difficult to treat in immunocompromised hosts. In 1986 Kalter *et al.*[94] conducted an investigator-blinded comparison of 1% permethrin cream rinse (Nix) vs. 1% lindane shampoo (Kwell) as a single treatment for pediculosis pubis. The study was conducted in a largely homosexual population living in Houston. Both products achieved an unsatisfactory cure rate of 60% for lindane and 57% for permethrin as a single treatment. Although the investigators did not know the HIV status of the volunteers, it has been suggested that the poor response to therapy may have been due to immunodeficiencies in some individuals. Further research is needed on the role of the host's immune system in resistance and susceptibility to lice infestations.

A 1996 study conducted in Egypt[95] analyzed the association between infestation with crab or head lice and the presence of certain human leukocytic antigens (HLA) in the host. HLA status, which plays an important function in the development of the immune response, was analyzed for 14 adult patients with crab lice and 25 healthy controls. Results showed a significant association between the presence of crab lice and the frequency of HLA A11, B5, and B27, with the frequency of these antigens increasing in lousy patients. From this association, the authors conclude that the genetic background of the host can influence the pathogenic mechanism of phthiriasis.

In order to prevent reinfestation after treatment, all contaminated bedding and clothing should be either removed from body contact for 72 hours or machine-washed and dried using the high heat cycle.[38]

Phthiriasis palpebrarum (infestation of the eyelashes with *Pthirus pubis*)

All products available for head and pubic lice are too irritating or dangerous to use in the sensitive eye area. Although Klaus *et al.*[39] found 1% permethrin cream rinse safe and effective when applied to the eyelashes with a cotton swab, the 20% isopropyl alcohol in the US product together with the contraindication for use in the eye area make this course of treatment difficult to justify.

The safest and most effective treatment for *P. pubis* infestations of the eyelashes is petrolatum (Vaseline) without additives. This non-wettable substance is thought to clog the breathing spiracles, causing the lice to die of suffocation and desiccation. The ointment is applied to the eyelashes 3–5 times a day, using a clean cotton swab or finger. Treatment should be continued for eight to 10 days to kill all hatching nymphs and viable eggs. Since nymphs and adult lice may try to migrate to the scalp or other suitable region, the scalp and other hairy areas should be treated with a permethrin product to avoid infestation.

A course of 10 days with trimethoprim/sulfamethoxazole or tetracycline can be useful in killing the lice sooner and also in preventing secondary bacterial infections. The physician should consider the possible side effects of these antibiotics and the benefit-to-risk ratio when treating such patients.

Physostigmine 0.25% (eserine), a pupillary dilator, has also been successfully used when applied to the eyelashes frequently over a three-day period. Its major drawback is inhibition of the dark adaptation of the eye.[43]

For severe cases or cases that have failed to respond to other treatments, oral ivermectin might offer a safe and effective alternative. Burkhart and

TABLE 27.5   *Pthirus pubis* therapy. 1990: cure rates 1 week after supervised total body treatment

	No. cured/No. treated	% Cured
K well shampoo (10 min)	38/58	66
Nix cream rinse (10 min)	24/28	86
Elimite 5% cream (8–14hr)	26/28	93

94. Kalter DC, Sperber J, Rosen T et al. (1987) Treatment of pediculosis pubis. Clinical comparison of efficacy and tolerance of 1% lindane shampoo vs. 1% permethrin creme rinse. Arch Dermatol 123:1315–1319.

95. Morsy TA, Alalfy MS, Sabry AH et al. (1996) Abnormal distribution of the histocompatibility antigens (HLA) in lousy patients. J Egypt Soc Parasitol 26:227–235.

Burkhart[96] reported the use of ivermectin therapy for phthiriasis palpebrarum in four children ranging in age from 3 to 10 years. Three of the four patients had previously been unsuccessfully treated with 1% lindane shampoo and topical physostigmine. Each patient was treated with two 200μg/kg doses of oral ivermectin administered one week apart. All cases were successfully cured, and no adverse effects were reported.

SCABIES

INTRODUCTION AND HISTORICAL NOTE

Human scabies is caused by the release of toxic or antigenic secretions of the female mite *Sarcoptes scabiei* var *hominis* (Hering), family Sarcoptidae, class Arachnida. Sometimes erroneously referred to as an insect, the scabies mite is appropriately classed with spiders. Like them, adult mites have eight legs but no wings. The clinical expression in humans is that of a contagious, papular, pustulovesicular and occasionally crusting, pruritic eruption of the skin.

Humans have suffered from "the itch" for at least 3000 years. Descriptions may be found in ancient texts from China, India, and the Middle East.[97] One of the earliest descriptions of the mite is that of the Arab physician Abou-mezzan Avenzoar (1070–1162), who lived in Spain but died in Morocco. He described something called "soab," which bores into the skin where it lives until scratched, emerging as a tiny animal hardly visible to the naked eye.[98] He did not, however, link this little creature with the associated skin eruption.

Most historians credit Giovanni Cosimo Bonomo (1663–1696) for making the connection between the mite and the itch. When he was 24 years old, he witnessed the manner in which poor women, using needles, extracted "little bladders of water" from the scabby skin of their itchy children.[99,100] On asking a pruritic person where he itched the most, Bonomo himself extracted, with a fine needle, a very small white globule, which under the microscope turned out to be a "very minute living creature, in shape resembling a tortoise, of whitish color, a little dark on the back, with some thin and long hairs and with two little horns at the end of the snout." Bonomo described his little animal as having six legs and two horns on the snout. We believe he confused the two pediculate suckers on the anterior legs as horns, and that he did in fact retrieve an eight-legged adult *Sarcoptes scabiei*.

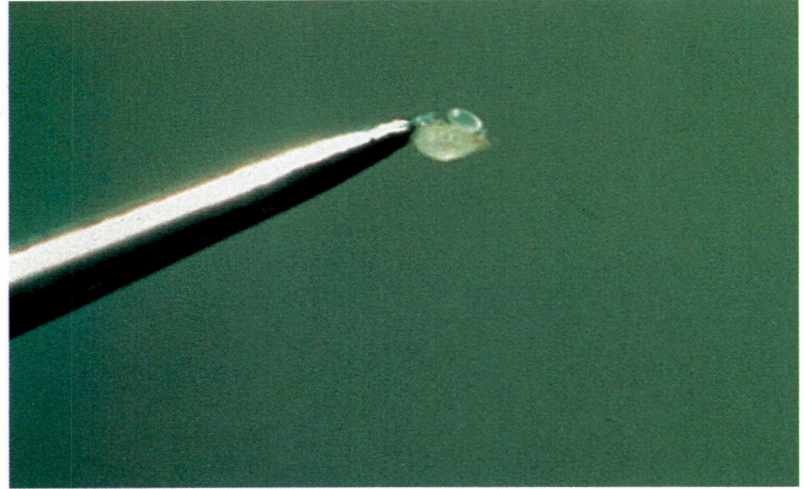

Fig. 27.25 Female scabies mite extracted from a burrow with a sewing needle. Notice the recently laid egg on her abdomen.

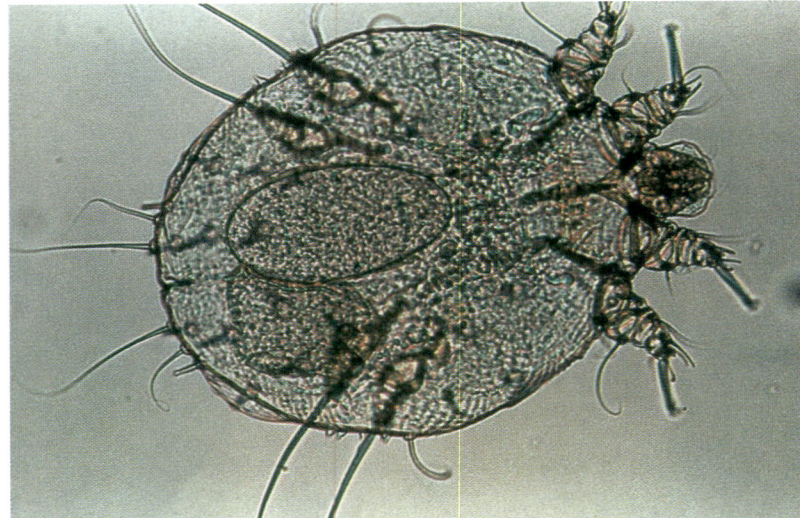

Fig. 27.26 Microscopic view of female scabies mite with ovum.

Our own experiences, over 300 years later, closely duplicated that of Bonomo. We had great difficulty in finding the cause of the itch among the Kuna Indians in Panama until we noticed mothers picking on their children with sewing needles (Figs 27.25, 27.26). Since that day in 1982, when we realized that their skills far outmatched our own, our success in finding mites jumped from 5% of suspected cases to over 95%, and new teams of mothers recruited in 2001 from other islands continue to exercise these skills with the same degree of dexterity. We, on the other hand, maintain the same level of incompetence, which we described in a 1990 publication[101] as follows: "In addition, the remarkable ability of our assistants to extract mites with sewing needles enabled us to confirm that the papular rashes on the scalps of infants and the scaling dermatitis behind the ears were due to scabies. They (the local mothers) were also able to extract mites from areas not normally described as susceptible to scabies, such as the perianal area, umbilicus, and face, and were able to accomplish this feat without waking sleeping infants. We have been unable to master this skill ourselves. . . . With no burrows to guide us, our personal attempts to find the mites were successful in less than 10% of active cases. This was due in some measure to the difficulty of scraping small, highly mobile and sweating babies with a scalpel."

Unlike head lice, scabies was probably not present in the Americas prior to Columbus. No records exist to determine whether the disease was first brought by the English, Dutch, Swedes, Spanish, or French. It may be assumed that the scabies mite made the trans-Atlantic journey on the Mayflower, Susan Constant, Godspeed, or Discovery, and probably on all of them.[98] The itch was a constant aggravation among the early settlers of Jamestown, Plymouth, and Philadelphia. By 1731, the Widow Read was making a tidy living from her well-known ointment for the itch (two shillings for a gallypot containing an ounce). The fact that she was the mother-in-law of Benjamin Franklin may well have been related to the appearance of her advertisement for four separate weeks in the *Pennsylvania Gazette* of 1731, of which Franklin was the publisher. Since poor Ben had only recently married her daughter, and her mother lived with them, he probably had little choice.[98]

In times of war, famine, and natural disasters, scabies may reach epidemic proportions. Sokoloff,[102] describing Napoleon's Italian campaign (1796–1797), stated that whole regiments of soldiers, the moment they encamped at night, threw off their knapsacks and scratched en masse. Their commander-in-chief

96. Burkhart CN, Burkhart CG (2000) Oral ivermectin therapy for phthiriasis palpebrum. **Arch Ophthalmol** 118:134–135.
97. Green MS (1989) Epidemiology of scabies. **Epidemiol Rev** 111:126–150.
98. Friedman R (1941) Scabies—Civil and Military. New York: Froben Press.
99. Beeson BB (1927) Acarus scabiei: Study of its history. **Arch Dermatol Syphilol** 16:294.
100. Lane JE (1928) Bonomo's letter to Redi. **Arch Dermatol Syphilol** 18:1.
101. Taplin D, Meinking TL, Chen JA et al. (1990) Comparison of crotamiton 10% cream (Eurax) and permethrin 5% cream (Elimite) for the treatment of scabies in children. **Pediatr Dermatol** 7:67–73.
102. Sokoloff B (1937) Napoleon. A doctor's biography. New York: Prentice Hall.

was no exception, scratching himself with a vengeance until blood appeared. Napoleon was usually portrayed with his hand inside his uniform, leading some to believe that he was scratching his scabies.

No account of the history of scabies would be complete without a mention of Kenneth Mellanby, MD. He and his team, working in the early years of World War II in England, conducted exhaustive studies on the life cycle and modes of transmission of the scabies mite that form the basis of our current knowledge. Published as one of the *Oxford War Manuals* in 1943, it was subsequently reprinted in 1972 as a small paperback, and is highly recommended.[103] Difficult to find now, but to be treasured and guarded if you do, is *Scabies—Civil and Military* by R. Friedman.[98]

As we begin the 21st century, population increases, migration, climate change, crop failures, floods and drought, wars, and natural disasters ensure that scabies will continue to inflict a heavy toll. In economically stressed countries in which we have worked for more than 25 years, we see little change in the prevalence of the disease. The highest incidence continues to occur in communities that can least afford treatment. Far from being a rare condition seen mainly by dermatologists or pediatricians, in many areas of the world scabies and the secondary infections that frequently accompany it are a major public health problem, draining 50% or more of local medical resources and time of clinic personnel.

Two events have occurred for the first time in history. First, the diagnosis and management of scabies have been further complicated by the arrival of the human immunodeficiency virus (HIV) and the subsequent debilitating effects of AIDS. It is now evident, from our own and other studies, that HIV-positive and AIDS patients are more likely to become infested and develop more severe manifestations, up to and including the highly infectious crusted form. There are now several reports indicating that HIV/AIDS patients are less responsive to therapy. On the positive side, the second unique event has been the introduction of ivermectin, the first effective oral medication for the treatment of scabies. These new milestones in the history of scabies are discussed further in the relevant sections of this chapter.

SCABIES AND SEXUALLY TRANSMITTED DISEASES

Older literature frequently classifies scabies together with sexually transmitted diseases (STDs). We have had difficulty over the last 10 to 15 years in confirming this connection.

This classification is unfair to the millions of people worldwide who acquire their infestations innocently and usually unknowingly. Unlike the scabies mite, our lifestyles and habits have changed dramatically over the millennia and as recently as the last 25 years. Where people join together in close proximity, whether by choice or unfortunate circumstances, the opportunities for scabies transmission are directly related to the degree and frequency of close body contact.

Thus, scabies flourished among families and strangers huddled together in London's underground during World War II. Similarly, during the "sexual revolution" of the 1960s, when drugs, multiple casual bedmates, and increased body contact was common, scabies was often seen in adolescents and young adults attending clinics for treatment of STDs.

SCABIES IN THE NEW MILLENNIUM

Unlike the reported intervals between epidemics, scabies in the United States never really went away. Dermatologists nationwide report that they continue to see cases, although not at the same frequency as in the 1970s, except in patients with AIDS or the elderly in nursing homes. We believe that the incidence of scabies in nursing homes and extended-care facilities has actually increased. This is partly due to the increasing number of elderly. Of greater concern is the fact that the incidence is on the increase within these institutions. In those we have investigated, we have been astonished to find prevalence as high as 48% in the residents and over 20% in the nursing staff and their aides. This is similar to some of the worst villages we have studied in the least developed areas of South and Central America.

Another reason, we believe, that scabies continues in the United States is the constant priming of the system by immigrant families from highly endemic areas. In approximately one-half of the cases in which we have been called concerning a new cluster or outbreak, we have been able to trace the origin to newly arrived individuals, families, or children adopted from other countries. No single country heads the list, but we have identified imported cases from most of the Central and South American countries and from the Pacific rim countries.

We do not foresee a drop in the incidence in the United States in the foreseeable future. In 2001, the disease was rampant in rural areas of the developing world and we feel certain that scabies must be on the increase among the victims of the armed conflicts now in progress.

EPIDEMIOLOGY

Genetics (inheritance)

"The *acarus scabiei* is notorious for its lack of respect for person, age, sex, or race. Whether it be in the epidermis of an emperor or a slave, a centurion or a nursling, it makes itself perfectly at home with undiscriminating impudence and equal obnoxiousness."[98] At the turn of the millennium, we know of no reason to dispute this statement. All ages, sexes, races, and nationalities appear to be equally susceptible.

Statistics

Published statistics have little value except in bringing the emergence of an epidemic to more widespread attention. Statistics based on clinical visits are notoriously inaccurate as a guide to community prevalence, but the simultaneous increase of scabies at several medical facilities in a city or community usually represents an increase in the general population. Orkin, in 1971,[104] published the results of a questionnaire mailed to 86 American and 71 foreign dermatologists that correctly identified an increase in Europe that had not, at that time, reached the United States. In 1979, Andrews cautioned against the acceptance of published statistics at face value.[105] In terms of population at risk worldwide, children are more likely to have scabies than adults, mothers of young infants more so than fathers, elderly residents of nursing homes more so than those at home. HIV-positive individuals and AIDS victims are more likely to be infested. A single person living in an apartment is less susceptible than one living in crowded conditions. The most practical guide to transmission, and one that is often of value in family or community management, is to estimate the degree and frequency of close body contact. Family size and sleeping arrangements are also significant factors.

The perception of the frequency of scabies is strongly influenced by the degree of exposure to cases by observers. A physician practicing in an affluent suburb of a major city may see four or five cases in a year, while health care providers serving homeless shelters in the same city may deal with the same number in a day. Arfi *et al.*, in a study published in 1999,[106] reported that 56% of all patients attending the Dermatology Clinic for the Socioeconomically Disadvantaged at Hôpital Saint-Louis in Paris were seeking treatment for their scabies. These authors stated the problem succinctly: "Poverty leads to a deterioration in general health, and skin disorders are very common among patients with limited means." Of interest is the fact that exactly 100 years ago, most of the beds in Saint-Louis hospital were occupied by scabies patients.[107]

Our own experiences during 35 years of studies in rural areas of Central and South America, Africa, and Southeast Asia are similar. We see little change in prevalence among economically stressed populations. We were privileged to witness the introduction of scabies into a population in which the disease

103. Mellanby K (1972) Scabies, 2nd ed. Middlesex: EW Classey.
104. Orkin M (1971) Resurgence of scabies. **JAMA** 217:593–597.
105. Andrews JRH (1979) Scabies in New Zealand. **Int J Dermatol** 18:545–552.
106. Arfi C, Dehen L, Benassaia E et al. (1999) [Dermatologic consultation and poverty: Prospective sociomedical study at Saint-Louis Hospital, Paris]. **Ann Dermatol Venereol** 126:682–696.
107. Ghesquier D (1999) A Gallic affair: The case of the missing itch-mite in French medicine in the early 19th century. **Med Hist** 43:26–54.

had never occurred in living memory, records, or folklore, although other infestations such as head lice and bedbugs had been known and recorded for centuries. Our Field Epidemiology Survey Team from the University of Miami has lived and worked in this population almost continuously since 1965. We offer this account because we believe it is instructive and typical of many similar situations worldwide.

We were in an excellent position to observe the increase in scabies that began in Venezuela in 1967, swept through Colombia, Panama, Costa Rica, and further north, reaching the Caribbean around 1970 and South Florida in 1971–1972, and peaking throughout the United States in 1975. At first, the mite appeared to have spared the Kuna Indians, who live on 66 of the approximately 360 islands forming the Archipelago of San Blas, off the Caribbean coast of Panama. In 1975, we saw an explosive outbreak of scabies in this population, which lives on small, densely inhabited islands, with a mean household size of 13 or more. The Kunas believed that this pruritic affliction had been brought on by the evil spirits from the underworld. Unlike the head louse, this new, obviously contagious problem was not familiar. When we showed them the little spider-like animal under the microscope, they understood the cause of their itching, but still insisted that the "evil spirits" sent the little mite.

In our first surveys, we found a prevalence of 28% in one community and 42% in another. Forty-two to 50 percent of all persons under 18 years of age were infested. These figures were based only on clearly evident clinical disease, and undoubtedly were an underestimate. Two years later, in 1977, on a larger island of over 2000 persons, 90% of 207 individuals in randomly selected households were found to be infested.

In July 1986, a survey of another island village of 756 persons revealed that 61% of all children 1 to 10 years of age had scabies, as did 84% of infants less than 1 year old. Over the previous 10 years, treatment in this village was available in the local clinic to individual patients in the form of lindane lotion or crotamiton cream. We were able to demonstrate that mass therapy with 5% permethrin cream (Elimite) applied to every inhabitant at the same time was effective in controlling the epidemic.[108] Continued surveillance and treatment of new or imported cases kept the prevalence below 2% for the next four years on this island, while the prevalence remained high in 18 other communities in which cases continued to be treated one at a time in clinics or health posts.

Certainly, thousands of patients obtained temporary relief from their itch, but scabies in epidemic proportions provides a perfect example of the need for community-based control methods. Since our model for controlling epidemics was published and editorialized in *The Lancet* in 1991,[108] it has been successfully applied, or is being planned for similar populations, in Australia, New Zealand, Canada, Fiji, and India. The plan, which is based on the active participation by the entire community, has also proven valuable in the management of nursing home epidemics in the United States.[109]

In 2000–2001, we conducted house-to-house surveys on five islands in the San Blas archipelago. In four of them prevalence remains high more than 25 years after scabies was introduced. Many women on whom we have records from 20 years ago when they were infants are now mothers of children with scabies. These were communities in which patients continue to be treated one by one. On our "model" island the prevalence was below 10%, which was once again quickly reduced to less than 2% by treating all scabies subjects and contacts and reinstituting house-to-house scabies examinations by a dedicated survey team.

Thus, we have had a unique opportunity to observe the beginning of a large epidemic that started in 1975, and its propagation in a population of over 40 000 left for the most part untreated. Spending much of the last 25 years with these people has led us to the following conclusions that do not necessarily reflect new concepts, but serve to confirm the observation of many authors over the last 200 years.

1. In these types of communities, treatment of individual cases in a clinic setting is wasteful of time and resources and has no effect on the community problem.
2. "Herd immunity" or individual immunity plays little if any role in reducing incidence or prevalence, or modifying or shortening an epidemic. Chronicity is the rule, and reinfestation after treatment is usual.
3. Age and sex have no bearing on susceptibility. The degree of personal contact is the predominant factor, resulting in the following order of risk: young infants, nursing mothers, older children, female adolescents, male adolescents, and adult males.
4. In warm climates, burrowing of the mite is rare. Small erythematous papules are the rule.
5. Scabies frequently occurs above the neck, and in young infants may involve the entire body surface, including the scalp. The intergluteal cleft is a favorite hiding place of the mite.
6. Scabies is the predominant underlying cause of Streptococcal/Staphylococcal pyoderma in tropical climates.
7. Hypersensitivity may develop in some individuals, producing lichenification from chronic excoriation, nodular lesions, and papular urticaria.

In the United States we have examined and treated several cases of scabies in patients who were HIV positive, suffering from full-blown AIDS, or immunocompromised due to other diseases or therapy. The epidemiology among these individuals is markedly different from that seen in the normal population. They appear to have an increased likelihood of becoming infested. We base this observation on the fact that unlike immunologically competent individuals, we have only rarely been able to identify a source or contact with another case. In situations where other individuals share the same lifestyle, living facilities, and furniture, the person or persons with AIDS are often the only ones to contract scabies. In normal situations, we can usually identify other individuals in the household or social group. Relapses or reinfestation are common in immunocompromised hosts, with weeks or months between apparently successful treatments and another mite-positive eruption.

In a few instances, when normal contacts have contracted scabies from an immunocompromised patient, the normal individuals promptly responded to a single application of topical therapy. Most of those who deal with scabies in HIV-positive, AIDS, or otherwise immunocompromised subjects share the opinion that they are extremely difficult to treat. A single treatment with any topical therapy is rarely effective. We, like others, have found live mites in scrapings after three or four treatments that have included lindane lotion and permethrin cream. This suggests that a competent immune system plays an important role in the effectiveness of topical therapy.

Persistent or recurrent scabies in which the degree of pruritus is more severe than the skin lesions would indicate, and cases not responding well to repeated therapy, should alert the clinician to the possibility of immunodeficiency such as AIDS. When all contacts have been treated and easily cured, or have always been asymptomatic, further credence is given to the underlying reason for treatment failure.

Among Australian Aborigines, crusted scabies has been associated with human T-lymphotropic virus type I (HTLV-I).[110] This severe and often chronic form of scabies may also be associated with Down's syndrome, lymphoma, cerebrovascular accident, organ transplantation, use of topical corticosteroids, and leprosy.[111] Because AIDS/HIV-positive persons with scabies may not conform to classic descriptions of the disease, the diagnosis is often

108. Taplin D, Porcelain SL, Meinking TL et al. (1991) Community control of scabies: A model based on the use of permethrin cream. **Lancet** 337:1016–1018.
109. Yonkosky D, Ladia L, Gackenheimer L et al. (1990) Scabies in nursing homes: An eradication program with permethrin 5% cream. **J Am Acad Dermatol** 23:1133–1136.
110. Mollison LC, Lo STH, Marning G (1993) HTLV-I and scabies in Australian Aborigines. **Lancet** 341:1281–1282.
111. Schlesinger I, Oelrich M, Tyring SK (1994) Crusted (Norwegian) scabies in patients with AIDS: The range of clinical presentations. **South Med J** 87:352–356.

missed. In several instances these cases have been the focus of institutional outbreaks. A typical example was provided by Portu *et al* from Bilbao, Spain, in 1996.[112] They described the case of a 28-year-old HIV-positive man, initially diagnosed with seborrheic dermatitis and psoriasis, who was admitted to a hospital, resulting in 72 cases of scabies among healthcare workers and other patients.

PRESENTING HISTORY

The earliest and most common symptom of scabies is that of itching, particularly at night. These symptoms may be present before any overt physical signs of erythematous papules or burrows. Exposure may have occurred a month or more previously, during which period there may be no discomfort or clinical signs, so that a careful retrospective history is often revealing.

The sites of itching are also valuable clues. In women, nipples and areolae, elbows, wrists, finger webs, belt line, intergluteal cleft, and axillae often itch early and intensely. In men, the penis is frequently an early site of pruritus in addition to the other areas mentioned above. The skin underneath watch bands, rings, and frequently worn occlusive bracelets are also favorite hiding places for the mites.

In young children and infants, the hands, palms, wrists, buttocks, intergluteal cleft, feet (including soles [Figs 27.27, 27.28]), behind the ears, in and around the umbilicus, and skin folds around the neck are the most common sites. In infants, particularly in warm weather, scabies may occur anywhere on the body, including the scalp and face (Figs 27.29, 27.30). The scalp may also be involved in older children, but is difficult to diagnose because of the hair. Human scabies is almost always contracted from another person. The chain of transmission may be in the family, from a friend, a visit to a nursing home, a kindergarten or school daycare, summer camp, or very rarely from fomites.[113] In our experience, fomite transmission has only been associated with cases of crusted scabies.

Epidemiologic history, the occurrence of itching, and the distributions of lesions and pruritus form the basis of diagnosis. Parents and guardians should always be questioned and examined when possible. Siblings should be examined for scabies. We have, on several occasions, clinched the diagnosis of an infant by examining and recovering mites from the mother. Demonstration of the mite, eggs, or fecal pellets, known as scybala, is confirmatory, but often difficult or impossible. *Failure to find the mite does not rule out scabies.* It is often difficult to get a scraping from a crying, moving, frightened child or infant.

If the parent, other family members, or contacts itch, and the child has clinical signs and symptoms, it is safer to treat the child overnight with 5% permethrin cream (Elimite, Acticin) than to traumatize the infant or youngster with a scalpel or curette.

Scabies should always be considered as a possible cause of skin eruptions in HIV-positive subjects, regardless of whether the clinical presentation resembles scabies. Often it does not. AIDS patients frequently suffer from other chronic pruritic skin conditions, including pruritic papular eruption (PPE).[114] Scabies may mimic this condition, and patients may have both.

PHYSICAL EXAMINATION

Skin

Small 1–2mm red papules in the areas of the body most attractive to the mites are the earliest physical signs. Because of the intense itching, excoriations from

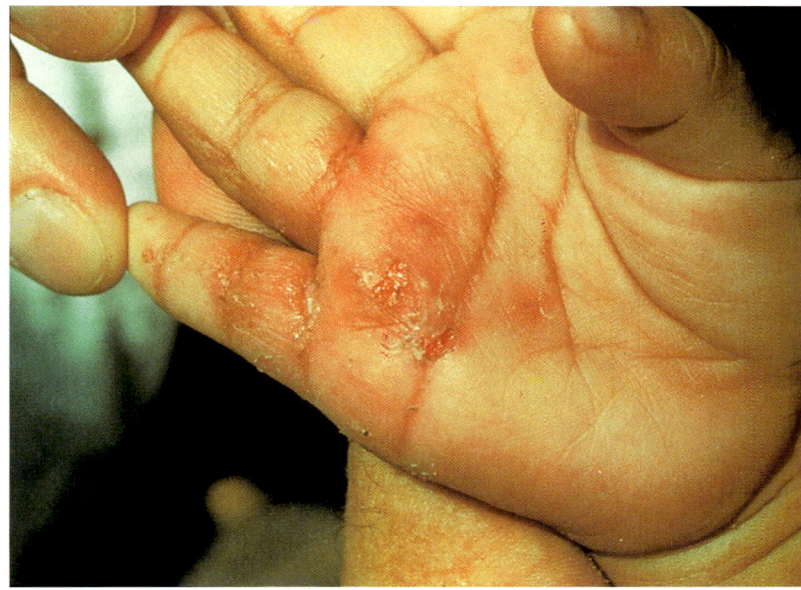

Fig. 27.28   Scabies lesions on the hand of an infant.

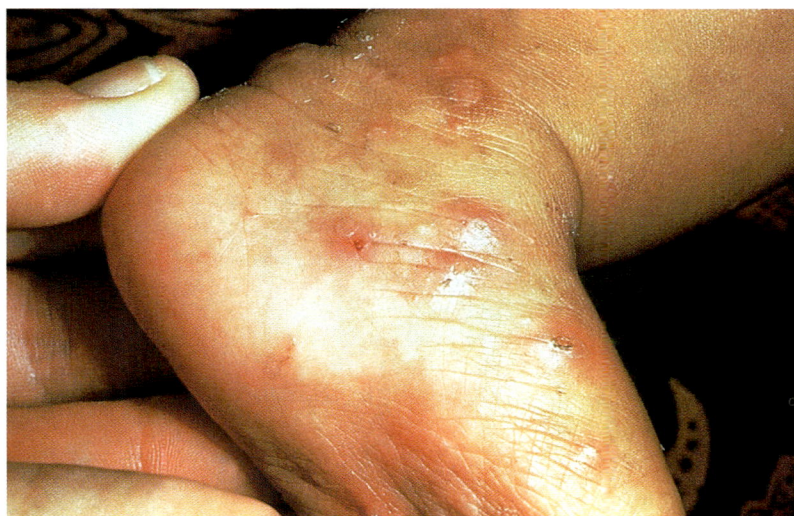

Fig. 27.27   Scabies lesions on the foot of an infant.

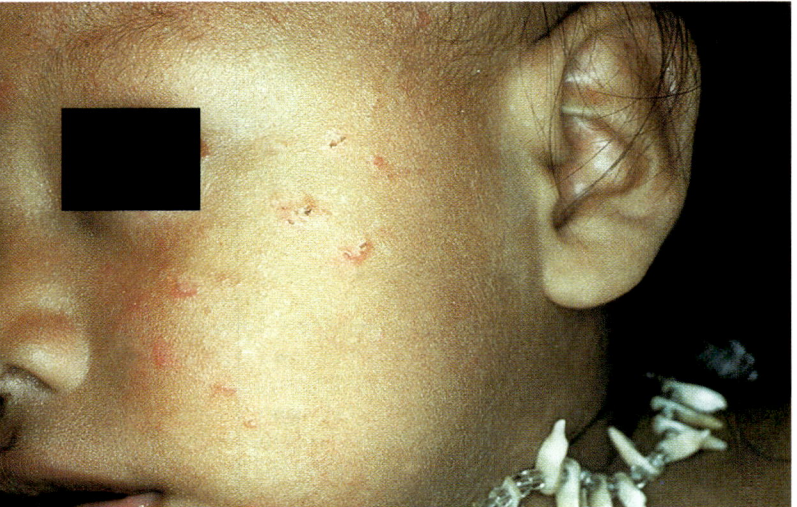

Fig. 27.29   Scabies on the face of a toddler.

112. Portu JJ, Santamaria JM, Zubero Z et al. (1996) Atypical scabies in HIV-positive patients. **J Am Acad Dermatol** 34:915–917.
113. Arlian LG, Estes SA, Vyszenski-Moher DL (1988) Prevalence of *Sarcoptes scabiei* in the homes and nursing homes of scabietic patients. **J Am Acad Dermatol** 19:806–811.
114. Pardo RJ, Bogaert MA, Penneys NS et al. (1992) UVB phototherapy of the pruritic papular eruption of the acquired immunodeficiency syndrome. **J Am Acad Dermatol** 26:423–428.

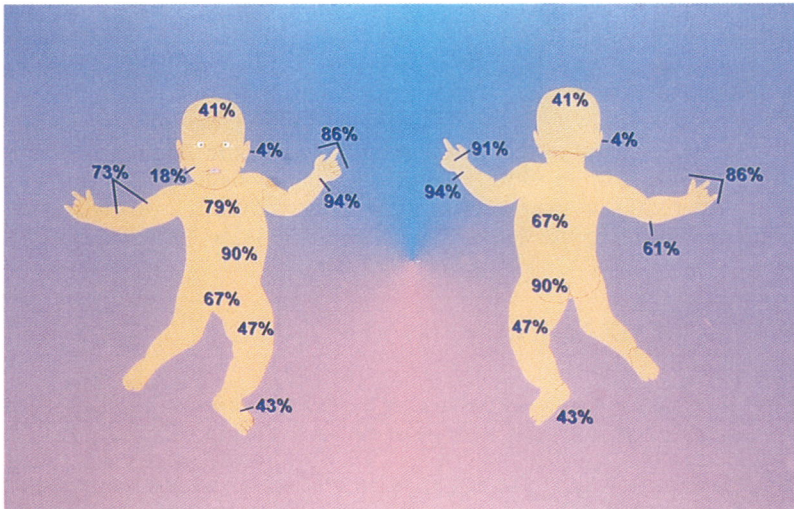

Fig. 27.30 Distribution of scabies lesions in infants. (Adapted from Taplin et al.,[101] with permission.)

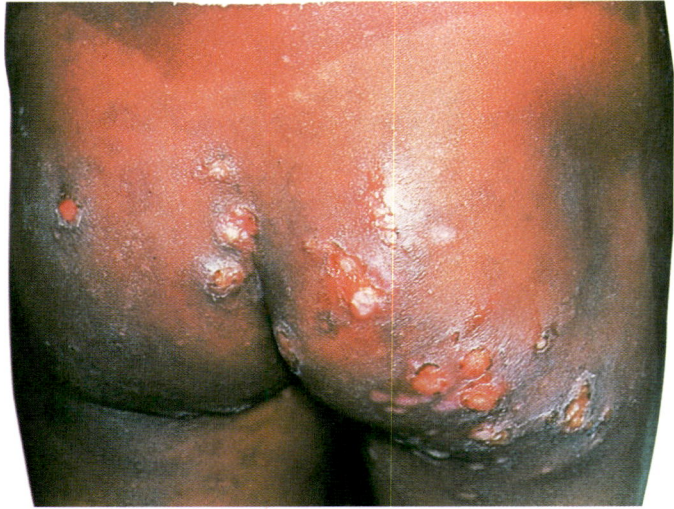

Fig. 27.32 Secondary bacterial infection in scabies.

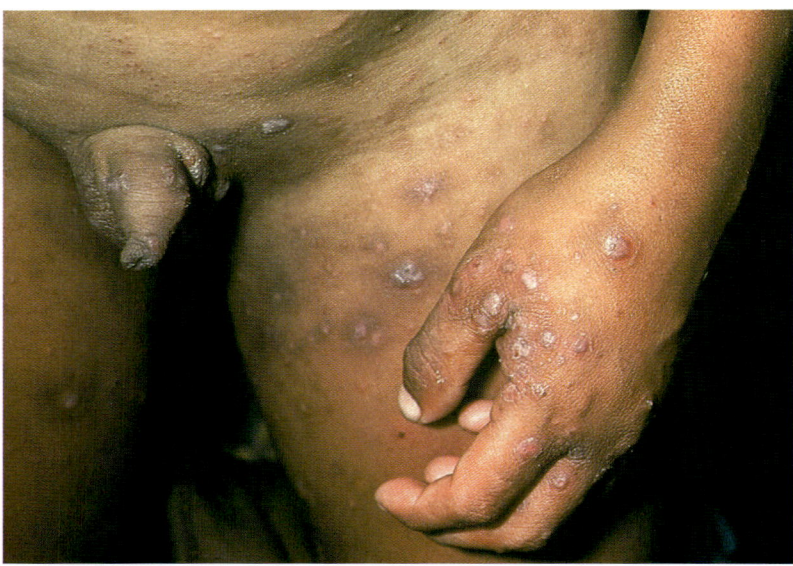

Fig. 27.31 Chronic nodular scabies with pyoderma and crusting.

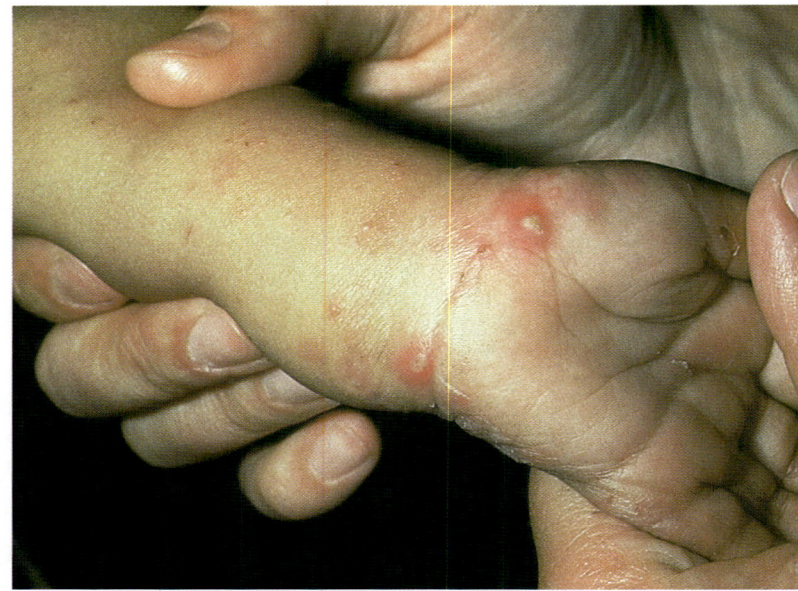

Fig. 27.33 Pyodermatous sequelae of scabies.

the nails may be evident, with various degrees of crusting or scaling. In chronic cases the skin may be thickened (lichenified), or exhibit small 2–4mm granulomatous nodules (Fig. 27.31). Hyperpigmentation resulting from chronic irritation may be present.

In addition to the small erythematous papules of early scabies, one may often observe 1–2mm noninflammatory papules, which are skin-colored or lighter. These may persist for weeks after successful treatment, and represent a granulomatous reaction to the dead remains of mites or their feces. They do not indicate active scabies. Particularly in warm climates, and in families or communities where good hygiene is difficult to maintain, secondary bacterial infection is common. In these cases, there may be hundreds of crusted, purulent sores (ecthyma) clustered in the scabies' susceptible sites (Fig. 27.32). These are usually the result of secondary infection by group A *Streptococcus pyogenes*, often accompanied by coagulase-positive *Staphylococcus aureus*. Occasionally, bullous, pustular infections occur, due to exfoliatin-producing *S. aureus* strains (Fig. 27.33) (see Ch. 24).

The scabies mite is, for practical purposes, never found in purulent lesions. Typical burrows are often rare or absent. This is particularly true in infants, and in all ages in warm climates. Hair, teeth, and mucous membranes offer no clues to diagnosis. Nails are important as the principal tools for scratching, and may also act as a reservoir for mites and their eggs.[115]

Nodular scabies has several unique presentations in infancy and childhood. In the early weeks and months of life scabies may provoke a nodular inflammatory response in the skin of babies with scabies. The lesions are frequently present in intertriginous areas, such as the axilla and groin, but may be found in a generalized distribution. The highly infiltrated nature of the lesions may suggest a disorder such as histiocytosis. In older infants it is not unusual to see nodular scabies of the male genitalia as part of the acute picture. In older children the characteristic chronic prurigo nodularis-like lesions may be seen.

The clinical appearance of scabies in immunocompromised, HIV-positive, or AIDS patients varies widely. Cases of severe crusted (previously called

115. Witkowski JA, Parish LC (1984) Scabies. Subungal areas harbor mites. *JAMA* 252:1318–1319.

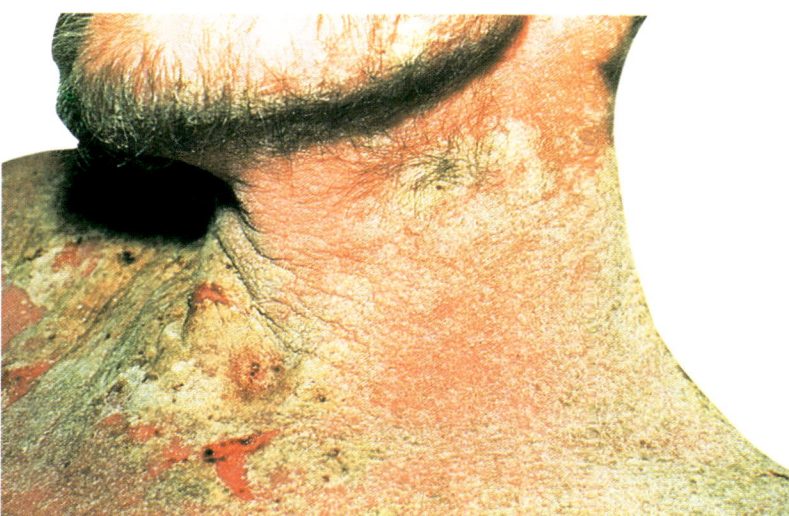

Fig. 27.34   Crusted scabies in AIDS patient.

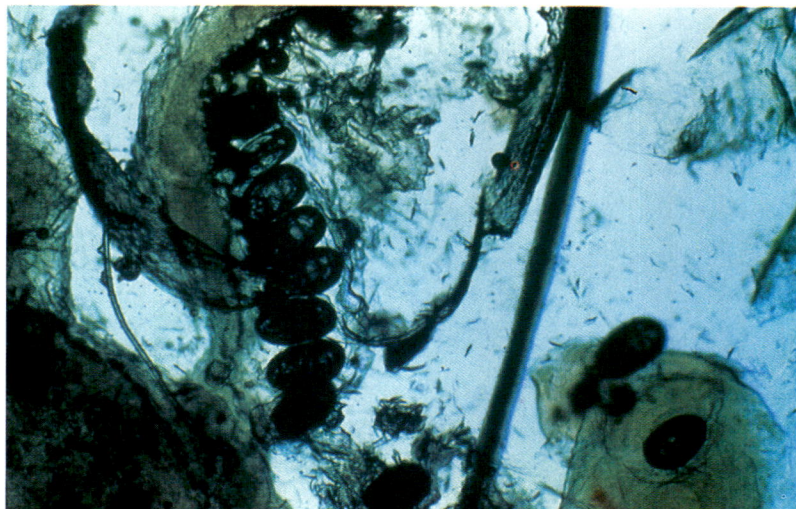

Fig. 27.36   Mineral oil scraping under light microscope.

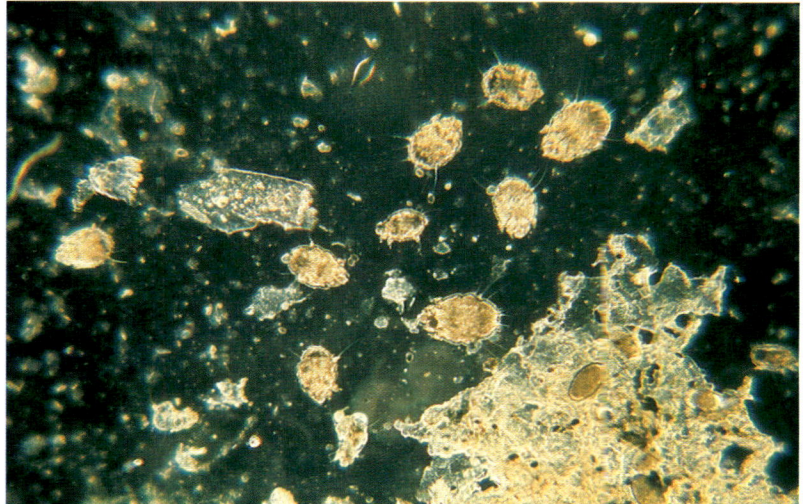

Fig. 27.35   Mineral oil scraping showing scabies, mites, eggs, and scybala under dark field microscopy.

Norwegian) scabies are found in AIDS patients of both sexes and all ages (Fig. 27.34). Crusted lesions may occur on the scalp, face, ears, neck, chest, elbows, hands, and knees. The crusts and shedding skin scales are teeming with mites. These individuals should be considered highly infectious. Scabies preparations from these patients are usually overwhelmingly positive (Figs 27.35, 27.36).

We have also seen scabies in AIDS patients in which the only signs were multiple erythematous papules over large areas of the body, including the back and chest. This also commonly occurs in the elderly, especially in nursing homes, an observation confirmed by other observers. Mites have been easy to recover, even from areas with no visible lesions. This leads us to believe that these cases have many mites freely roaming the body surface. Patients claim they can sense them "running all over" or that "bugs are crawling all over them." Pruritus can be severe in AIDS and elderly patients, and we believe that it is worse than in normal individuals with scabies. This is backed up by the aggressive, even mutilating excoriation produced by these subjects. We have also noted that the body distribution of scabies in the elderly and immunocompromised adults is very similar to that seen in infants.

Other situations in which unusual forms of scabies may occur include severe, often crusted, infestations in subjects with spinal cord injuries and associated paralysis. They may neither feel the pruritus, nor be able to scratch. The mites are therefore free to multiply at will. The patient may harbor millions of mites and be a focus of infestation of medical staff, caregivers, and other patients. This is made more likely by the fact that many patients are not ambulatory and need physical assistance from others, with frequent body contact.

Patients on systemic or topical glucocorticosteroids or immunosuppressive drugs for organ transplants or rheumatoid arthritis may also display bizarre forms of scabies, ranging from pruritic or nonpruritic skin rashes to explosive exacerbations when their drugs are discontinued or reduced.

Systemic manifestations

Children may be tired and irritable as a result of sleep deprivation due to nocturnal pruritus, which in turn may affect feeding habits. Fever and lymphadenopathy may accompany secondary infections. Acute glomerulonephritis (AGN) may reach endemic proportions when widespread scabies is infected by nephritogenic strains of Group A *Streptococcus pyogenes* (GAS).

Nausea and vomiting, twitching and tremors, disorientation, apprehension or excitability, weakness, paresthesia, or convulsions should alert the physician to the possibility of overexposure to lindane scabicides.[116] In some instances, the previous use of such products may not be voluntarily reported by the patient, parent, or guardian. Similarly, signs of generalized erythema, scaling, vesicles, or denudation should invite inquiry into the use of home remedies, which in our experience have included scrubbing with laundry detergent or hard soaps, or application of kerosene, used automobile engine oil, and even battery acid.

It cannot be stressed too often that a patient may have two or more skin problems. Scabies may coexist with psoriasis, atopic dermatitis, contact dermatitis, papular urticaria from insect bites, and pruritic papular eruption of AIDS. Many cases of scabies referred to our clinics as resistant to the standard treatments turn out to have had two diseases. Likewise, once a diagnosis is confirmed, for example as psoriasis, additional causes for the patient's pruritic rash may not be considered.

LABORATORY FINDINGS

The demonstration of *S. scabiei* mites, eggs, or scybala is diagnostic (Figs 27.35, 27.36). The age-old practice, in use for over 300 years, of picking the mite

116. Diaz JE (1998) Lindane toxicity is preventable. **Acad Emerg Med** 5:1126–1128.

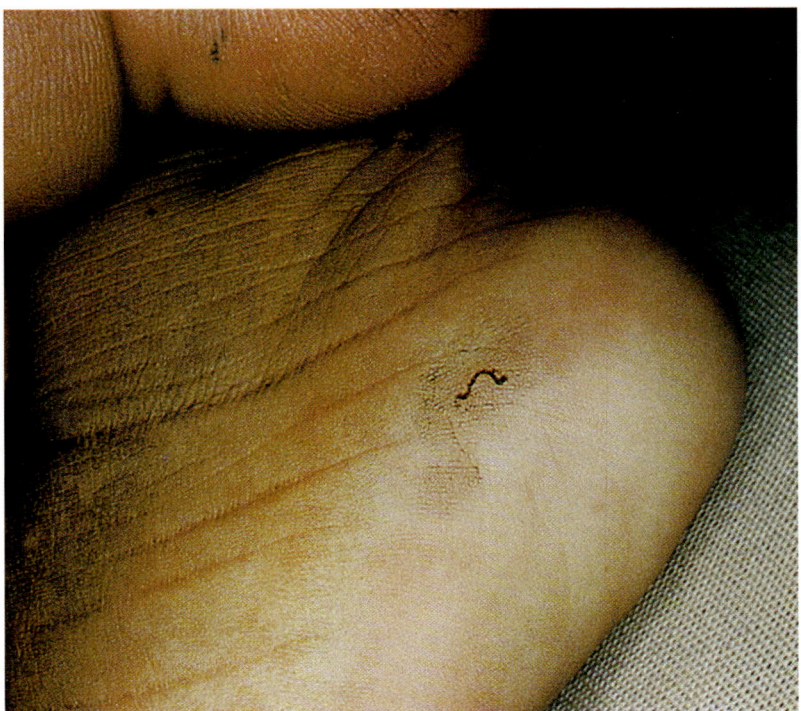

Fig. 27.37 Burrows Ink Test on an infant's foot indicating a scabies mite burrow.

from the skin with a needle is still valid, but requires skill and experience (Fig. 27.25). Where burrows are present, they are usually tortuous, and rarely more than 2–3mm in length. At the end of this burrow there may be seen a speck, or minute globule. By "threading" the point of a sharp needle along the burrow, and rupturing its roof, it is possible to lift out the mite on the tip of a needle. It is white or cream color, and just barely visible to those with excellent vision. Under a 10× hand lens it is seen to posses tiny hairs, and the two stumpy anterior legs that are usually in motion.

A diagnostic test using a sewing needle has been developed by Kuna women, who paint their nails with red nail polish. This provides a convenient surface on which to watch the mites run before they are put to death by crushing, and is proof that the mite is alive.

Two methods have been introduced to enhance the detection of burrows. The Burrow Ink Test[117] employs a fountain pen or a felt-tipped marker that is rubbed over the suspected burrow and wiped with an alcohol pad to remove most of the ink. The ink that remains indicates the location of the burrow (Fig. 27.37). According to Estes, blue and green markers work best because they do not obscure the microscopic finding.[117] We often use black markers and still have success with this method but the black ink may leave residue that can be mistaken for scybala by the less experienced eye. Working in a tropical climate in 1985, we used the Burrow Ink Test to diagnosis scabies but found only two tracts in about 100 attempts, confirming our previous suspicions that burrows are rare in the tropics. Topicycline, a topical tetracycline solution used for acne, may be used in the same way, but requires an ultraviolet (Woods) lamp for detection.[117] Dermatoscopes with epilumi-nescence allow direct visualization of the female mite, her stools, and eggs.[118]

Most dermatologists use a drop of mineral oil or microscope immersion oil placed on a suspected burrow. The area is scraped with a no. 10 or no. 15 scalpel, and the scrapings and oil placed on a slide and coverslipped for microscopic examination. When scraping children or HIV-positive individuals, we use either a 4mm or 7mm disposable curette, with almost equally effective

results. A more aggressive approach uses a superficial shave biopsy technique, in which the skin is pinched up and the superficial epidermis sawn off with a no. 15 scalpel. The authors[119] claim positive findings in suspected scabies cases as high as 95%.

No serologic or other specific tests have been developed for the diagnosis of scabies.

PATHOPHYSIOLOGY AND HISTOGENESIS
Biology of the mite

The adult female mite is most commonly found. The description given by Mellanby is excellent:[103] "Her body is rounded, and is approximately 400 microns (about 1/60 of an inch) in length. She has no distinct head, but her mouth parts or 'jaws', which protrude beyond the anterior edge of the body, are often erroneously identified as the 'head.' There are four pairs of legs, the front two pairs ending in 'suckers,' the hind two pairs in 'trailing bristles.' " (Fig. 27.26).

Arlian *et al.*,[120] in a creative series of experiments, demonstrated that a female mite, when placed on the skin, exudes a fluid that dissolves the skin surface, forming a well, into which she sinks. Again we refer to Mellanby: "when just below the surface of the horny layer, she begins to dig with the jaws and sharp elbows of the first two pairs of limbs." At least in cool climates, she may form a tunnel, or burrow, which may extend a distance of 0.5–5mm per day.[103] Gravid females lay their first egg within a few hours of burrowing. Thereafter, she remains in her burrow for the rest of her life, which may exceed 30 days. In relation to body size, the eggs of *S. scabiei* are enormous and occupy about one-third to one-half of the body. The female lays two to three eggs a day, which require only 3–4 days to hatch.

The newly hatched mites, called larvae, have only six legs, and are about one-third the size of the adult female. About one day later, these larvae leave the burrow and move to the skin surface to roam freely for a short time until they burrow or "sink" back into the stratum corneum to seek food and shelter. After four days, the larva molts to produce a six-legged nymph. It molts again after three more days to become an eight-legged adult. Only at this stage can the sexes be determined. Males are half the size of females and may be mistaken for baby mites. Mating occurs once. The female constructs a short burrow in which she awaits a wandering male. Copulation takes place in the burrow, after which the male departs, leaving her gravid for the rest of her life. The time from egg laying to the adult form is 10 to 14 days. In warm environments, the female can walk at speeds up to one inch (2.5cm) per minute when on the skin surface.[103] Depending on environmental conditions, a female mite may live away from the host for 24 to 36 hours, but we have observed live mites from crusted cases up to five days at laboratory temperatures (22°C; 72°F). We believe that there is sufficient moisture and nutrition in the crusts to enable them to survive. *Sarcoptes* are not blood feeders, but are thought to feed on intercellular fluid.

IMMUNOLOGY

Epidemiology of scabies indicates that most people are susceptible to infestation. It is also well established that the individual host responses may vary. Mellanby[103] noted that first infestations may proceed for weeks without the slightest signs of itching or erythema. He observed that most published photographs of scabies depict the host reaction or secondary infection, and that it is almost impossible to illustrate early uncomplicated lesions. He goes further to state that clinical diagnosis is almost never made until sensitization has occurred.

Unlike first infestations, those who have been cured of the disease and are subsequently reinfested exhibit immediate reactions, often within 48 hours. These are manifest by the usual symptoms of cutaneous hypersensitivity,

117. Estes SA (1982) Diagnosis and management of scabies. **Med Clin North Am** 66:955–963.
118. Argenziano G, Fabbrocini G, Delfino M (1997) Epiluminescence microscopy: A new approach to *in vivo* detection of *Sarcoptes scabiei*. **Arch Dermatol** 133:751–753.
119. Martin WE, Wheeler CE (1979) Diagnosis of human scabies by epidermal shave biopsy. **J Am Acad Dermatol** 1:335–337.
120. Arlian LG, Runyan RA, Achar S et al. (1984) Survival and infestivity of *Sarcoptes scabiei* var *canis* and var *hominis*. **J Am Acad Dermatol** 11:210–215.

including erythema, vesicles, and edema. An excellent account of current knowledge relating to the immunology of scabies is that of Cabrera *et al.* from the University of Chile, in collaboration with colleagues at the University of Minnesota.[121] In this scholarly review, they explain once again that first encounters with the mite elicit immune responses to antigens in the saliva, and probably the fecal pellets, but the cutaneous signs and symptoms may take 2–6 weeks to manifest themselves. This information is important to the physician attempting to reconstruct a patient history, or infection control personnel faced with the task of identifying the source or sources of an outbreak.

Nodular scabies probably represents an ongoing or chronic cell-mediated response to antigens or mite remnants that have not been degraded. The number of mites on the skin is related to the integrity of the cell-mediated response. Crusted scabies harboring many thousands of mites occurs in AIDS patients and has also been described in patients undergoing iatrogenic cell-mediated immunosuppression, patients with HTLV-I infections, malignancies, and those with congenitally impaired cell-mediated immunity.[110,111,121] Treatment with systemic or topical corticosteroids may produce a spectrum of manifestations from attenuated to severe crusted scabies.

Histologic findings

The histopathology of tissue sections is not specifically diagnostic unless the mite or parts of it can be identified. The cytology is that of acute or chronic allergic dermatitis. The histology of the red papule is that of delayed hypersensitivity to insects (arthropods), with superficial and deep perivascular inflammatory mononuclear cell infiltrate with numerous eosinophils, papillary edema, and epidermal spongiosis. Biopsies of nodular scabies show the pattern of ongoing and chronic inflammation with reactive lymphocytes indicative of cell-mediated immune response. The infiltrate of lymphocytes may be so intense as to mimic cutaneous lymphoma.[121]

THERAPEUTICS AND PROGNOSIS

Topical therapy

Permethrin

Permethrin 5% dermal cream (Elimite and Acticin/United States; Nix 5% cream/Canada; Lyclear cream/worldwide) is today considered the treatment of choice for scabies. We briefly describe the history of the research and development behind this highly successful agent.

Five percent permethrin cream was developed by Burroughs Wellcome, United Kingdom, in the late 1970s and early 1980s. Following extensive animal and human toxicologic studies, we conducted the first clinical trial in 1984 in collaboration with the Ministry of Health of the Republic of Panama. We compared the permethrin cream against 1% lindane lotion (Kwell), which at that time was the most widely prescribed scabies treatment in the United States. The study was a randomized, investigator-blinded trial.[122]

There was an excellent response after a single "head-to-toe" treatment with Elimite. Twenty-one of 23 completed cases (91%) were cured. In contrast, and to our surprise, only 15 of 23 (65%) were cured with lindane lotion (Kwell). Hernandez-Perez reported in 1983 that scabies in El Salvador was no longer responding to lindane therapy.[123] We related our own failures in Panama to the extensive use of lindane products in this island community during the previous five years.

Encouraged by the results of our first Elimite trial, we conducted a similar investigator-blinded, controlled study in 1985 on younger patients ranging in age from 2 months to 5 years. Because of the severe infestation in infants, their age, and presence of secondary infection, excoriation, and already "damaged" skin, we chose not to use lindane lotion based on the clinical failures of the first trial and the concern of local physicians over the potential for CNS toxicity. Instead, we compared a single application of 5% permethrin cream (Elimite) with a single treatment with 10% crotamiton cream (Eurax).[101] In this study, 42 of 47 (89%) of infants were completely cured one month after a single treatment with permethrin. The other five patients were much improved, but still had a few lesions and live mites on their hands or feet. Reinfestation could not be excluded. These five cases were promptly cured with a second permethrin treatment. The 10% crotamiton cream was significantly less effective.

There was no evidence of irritation, allergic reactions, or other adverse effects relating to treatment with permethrin 5% topical cream, lindane, or crotamiton in any of the 145 patients treated in these studies. As noted above, 10 subjects became worse after Eurax with increased numbers of lesions and inflammation, but we recorded this as an exacerbation of the disease rather than a direct effect of the crotamiton cream. Results of the combined studies are shown in Table 27.6.[124]

Following our trials in Central America, a multicenter, investigator-blinded, clinical study was conducted in the United States and Mexico in which 199 scabies patients treated with permethrin cream (Elimite) were compared with 205 subjects who received 1% lindane lotion (Kwell). Of the permethrin group 91% were cured at one month, compared with 85% in the lindane-treated cases, which was not a significant difference.[125] In 1986, our teams treated 99% of the 756 persons in a community severely afflicted with scabies using Elimite. This reduced the prevalence from 245 cases (33%) to 19 (2.5%) one month later.[108]

It is now well established that 5% permethrin cream is more effective than 1% lindane lotion, and considerably more so in areas of the world where lindane-resistant scabies is prevalent. We occasionally receive reports of cases not responding completely to a single treatment with 5% permethrin cream. This is not surprising. Note in Table 27.7 that in several studies by competent investigators under strictly controlled conditions, the clinical response is around 90% cured after a single treatment.[126] Thus, we should expect one of every 10 patients to require further treatments, even under the best conditions.

TABLE 27.6   Efficacy of Elimite for scabies

	Elimite cream	Kwell lotion	Eurax cream
Active ingredient(s)	5% permethrin	1% lindane	10% crotamiton
No. cured/no. treated	64/70	15/23	28/47
% cured[a]	91	65	60

[a] No mites, eggs, scybala, or new lesions one month after treatment.

TABLE 27.7   Results of a single treatment with permethrin 5% cream for scabies

Source	No. of subjects	% cured at 1 month
Taplin et al.[127]	23	91
Schultz et al.[125]	199	91
Taplin et al.[a]	47	89
Taplin et al.[b]	252	92
Total	521	91

[a] Infants 2 months to 5 years of age; double-blind study.
[b] Community eradication project; subjects ranged in age from 2 months to more than 60 years, open label. (Adapted from Taplin and Meinking,[126] with permission.)

121. Cabrera R, Agar A, Dahl MV (1993) The immunology of scabies. Semin Dermatol 12:15–21.
122. Taplin D, Meinking TL, Porcelain SL et al. (1986) Permethrin 5% dermal cream: a new treatment for scabies. J Am Acad Dermatol 15:995–1001.
123. Hernandez-Perez E (1983) Resistance to antiscabietic drugs (Letter). J Am Acad Dermato 8:121–123.
124. Taplin D, Meinking TL (1989) Scabies, lice, and fungal infections. Primary Care 16:551–576.
125. Schultz MW, Gomez M, Hansen RC et al. (1990) Comparative study of permethrin 5% cream and 1% lindane lotion for the treatment of scabies. Arch Dermatol 126:167–170.
126. Taplin D, Meinking TL (1990) Pyrethrins and pyrethroids in dermatology. Arch Dermatol 126:213–221.

In the real world, with lower standards of control and patient compliance, we would expect the number to be higher; perhaps every fifth patient or so. The situation was made more confusing in the United States by a statement in the package insert that stated, "one treatment is curative." This has now been modified to indicate that a second or even third treatment may be indicated in some cases. Unlike lindane, permethrin is rapidly metabolized and does not accumulate in adipose or CNS tissues.

TOXICOLOGY AND SAFETY OF PERMETHRIN

Permethrin is the generic name for 3-phenoxybenzyl (±)-cistrans-3-(2,2-dichlorovinyl)-2,2-dimethylcyclopropane-carboxylate. In the Glaxo Wellcome and Allergan/Herbert product, it is a mixture of 25% cis isomer to 75% trans. In mammals, including man, the cis-isomer has a higher potential for toxicity than the trans-isomer, which is more rapidly metabolized and excreted. The 25:75 cis:trans ratio is, therefore, preferred for human use.[126]

Widely used in agriculture, animal husbandry, and veterinary practice for the control of arthropod pests and ectoparasites, permethrin is also extensively used to impregnate bed nets, fly screens, and clothing for protection against vector and pestiferous arthropods (flies, mosquitoes, biting midges, ticks, and chigger mites).[126] The 5% permethrin cream for scabies has an excellent record of safety. The rare adverse reactions have been associated with localized burning, irritation, or tingling sensations, but these should be considered in light of the fact that the product is often applied to skin already damaged by the scabies mite. The preservative in Elimite is formaldehyde, and we might expect to encounter cases of allergic contact dermatitis. In practice, the reported incidence of allergic skin reactions has been extremely low: about two patient reports for every 500 000 units distributed. Formaldehyde has been specifically mentioned only one time. Unlike lindane, permethrin has not been shown to accumulate in adipose or brain tissue after topical application. In the 12 years since permethrin 5% cream (Elimite) was introduced in the United States, no incidents of CNS toxicity related to use of the medication have been found.

In view of the high level of efficacy compared with other products and the rare incidence of side effects, we consider permethrin 5% cream to be the drug of choice for scabies. In Central America we have seen local physicians treat several 2- to 4-week-old, malnourished infants suffering from total body scabies, with only positive results. Quarterman & Lesher, from Augusta, Georgia, described in 1994 the case of a 9-day-old boy with erythematous papules and pustules of the lower abdomen, perineum, and thighs which was thought to be a *Staphylococcal* dermatitis.[127] Twelve days later the diagnosis was confirmed as scabies based on skin scrapings, which showed adult mites, eggs, and scybala. A 10-hour treatment with permethrin 5% cream from scalp to toes and 1% hydrocortisone lotion was prescribed to control pruritis. The child was completely cured at one month, and had no recurrence. The authors provide sound justifications for choosing permethrin over other remedies.

LACK OF RESISTANCE TO PERMETHRIN

In our own studies, our teams apply the medications head-to-toe, paying particular attention to intertriginous sites. We have found no evidence that *S. scabiei* has developed resistance to permethrin. In a project completed in July 2001, we continued to achieve 93% cures following a single supervised permethrin treatment of 170 cases of scabies in populations in which permethrin products for head lice and scabies have been used frequently over a period of 15 years. We do receive communications from physicians who prescribe a single treatment with permethrin and later find evidence of active scabies, although most cases are improved. As noted, a single treatment with Elimite or Acticin may not be curative, but this is often due to poor compliance, failure to treat all body surfaces, or reinfestation from an untreated contact.

Infants and children are more difficult to treat because the feet and palms are often involved, and because the medication may be removed when the child is cleaned after urination or defecation. Parents should be advised to reapply Elimite or Acticin if this occurs, or if children get their hands or feet wet. We recommend applying the treatment at bedtime and washing it off in the morning. Socks or mittens are also of value to prevent finger and foot sucking.

Lindane (γ-benzene hexachloride)

The following are products for scabies containing γ-benzene hexachloride (GBHC, BHC, BHCH, hexachlorocyclohexane, lindane): Gammexane, Scabene, Lorexane, Gammene, Gammexol, Bio-Well™, G-well™, GBH™, and Kildane™.

Lotions and creams containing 1% GBHC have been used since 1948 for the treatment of scabies. Cannon and McCrae achieved a successful cure of 100 cases using three applications of lindane in a vanishing cream base.[128] One percent became the standard concentration when Kornblee and Combes reported in 1950 that a 0.5% concentration produced only a 55% cure rate.[129] For 20 years thereafter, 1% lindane lotion was considered a safe and effective treatment of scabies.

During scabies control efforts in Central America between 1972 and 1979, our teams personally treated over 2000 scabies patients. More than half were over 10 years of age, and more than 200 were younger than 6 months. Only one treatment was applied, except in rare cases when a second treatment was given one month later. We applied the lotion from the scalp to the soles of the feet to prevent self-reinfestation from untreated areas. Our teams maintained possession of all lotion containers. During the seven years' conduct of this project, we encountered no overt cases of CNS toxicity.

In spite of extensive experience of safe clinical use, reports began to accumulate of CNS toxicity, convulsions, and death following accidental ingestion or overexposure to lindane, and it became clear that young children and infants were at greatest risk. Considerable concern was generated by Lee and Groth in 1977, when they published reports of nine cases of CNS toxicity following exposure to lindane.[130] Three of these involved accidental ingestion, but the other six patients developed neurologic symptoms due to percutaneous absorption.

There is little doubt that overexposure to lindane products applied topically can cause CNS toxicity, convulsions, and, rarely, death. In view of the millions of cases of scabies treated over 50 years, and in many instances overtreated with these products, the incidence of severe adverse reactions is rare. Nevertheless, these reports have provoked apprehension related to the safety of lindane applied to the skin, particularly when it is damaged by excoriations and infections associated with scabies. These concerns were further increased by the report by Solomon et al. that lindane concentrated in brain tissue of guinea pigs following topical application.[131] That this selective absorption also occurred in humans was confirmed in 1983 by Davies et al., who described a fatal outcome in a 2-month-old infant treated excessively with topical 1% GBHC lotion. They found brain levels of lindane three times higher than blood levels.[132]

Clinical signs of CNS toxicity following lindane poisoning may include headache, nausea, dizziness, amblyopia, vomiting, restlessness or hyperactive behavior, increased excitability, apprehension, tremors, disorientation, hallucinations, weakness, twitching of eyelids, stupor, convulsions, respiratory failure, coma, and death.[24]

Reports of CNS toxicity following lindane exposure continue to surface, most commonly in medical journals concerned with disciplines other than dermatology. We offer two of them here that we considered particularly informative. In December 1999, Hall et al. described the ordeal of a 37-year-old nurse who contracted scabies and applied three topical applications of

127. Quarterman MJ, Lesher JL (1994) Neonatal scabies treated with 5% permethrin cream. **Pediatr Dermatol** 11:264–266.
128. Cannon AB, McCrae ME (1948) Treatment of scabies; report of one hundred patients treated with hexachlorocyclohexane in vanishing cream base. **JAMA** 138:557.
129. Kornblee LV, Combes EC (1950) Gammexane in the treatment of scabies. **Arch Dermatol** 61:407.
130. Lee B, Groth P (1977) Scabies transcutaneous poisoning during treatment. **Pediatrics** 59:643.
131. Solomon LM, West DP, Fitzloff JF, Becker AM (1977) Gamma benzene hexachloride in guinea-pig brain after topical application. **J Invest Dermatol** 68:310–312.
132. Davies JE, Dadhia HW, Morgade C et al. (1983) Lindane poisoning. **Arch Dermatol** 119:142–144.

lindane lotion over a period of three weeks.[133] She spent the next 20 months suffering from symptoms ranging from speech and thought difficulties, hallucinations, painful urinary and bowel spasms, and other problems that required hospitalization and heavy sedation. The article includes a comprehensive explanation of the pathophysiology of chlorinated hydrocarbon poisoning, of which lindane is one. The second recommended reference is that of Dr José Eric Diaz, Director of the University Medical Center in Camden, New Jersey.[116] This article includes and excellent review and recommendations for the management of lindane intoxication. He also describes one of the symptoms with which most dermatologists are familiar; that of visual hallucinations of "bugs crawling all over." These delusions are often confined to visual hallucinations. Patients may claim that they see the tiny creatures but do not feel them. The possibility of lindane toxicity should always be considered in such cases. In the United States, the general public may be more aware of the danger of lindane, thanks to television coverage of poisoning cases and the work of the National Pediculosis Association (NPA) in the United States.

In view of the above limitations, it is becoming increasingly difficult to justify the continued use of lindane for scabies now that a safe alternative (permethrin 5% cream) is available. The cost of 1% lindane lotion, particularly in generic form, is low compared with the permethrin cream, but this should be weighed against the risk of accidental ingestion, CNS damage, and treatment failures due to lindane-resistant mites. In some instances, such as treatment of large numbers of indigent patients on limited funds, costs may represent the difference between available therapy to all or expensive therapy for a few. In addition, permethrin cream is not available in many countries. For those who have no alternative to lindane, we offer the following safety tips based on our own experiences and other data.

1. Apply to cool dry skin. Skin hydrated by sweat or warm soapy baths has a greater potential for absorption. Soap may react with lindane, rendering it less effective.
2. Six to eight hours application time is sufficient. Two hours is not adequate.[134] The medication should be washed off at six to eight hours with soap and tepid water and the skin thoroughly rinsed.
3. Do not use on infants less than 2 years of age, or on underweight or malnourished children or adults, particularly strict vegetarians. Lack of adipose tissue may result in higher blood and possibly brain levels of lindane. Do not use excessively on the genital area in young boys. Scrotal skin has increased permeability.
4. Do not use on sick children with pre-existing CNS complications. Symptoms or complications of common pediatric illnesses may mimic CNS toxicity and may have no relationship to lindane therapy.
5. Do not use excessively on inflamed, secondarily infected, heavily excoriated, or denuded skin, since absorption will be increased.
6. Do not repeat treatment within seven days.
7. Do not use in concentration other than 1%. Lower concentrations are less effective.
8. Use as little as possible, avoiding the eyes and mouth. Pay particular attention to body crevices, intergluteal cleft, toe webs. and postauricular folds. Remove rings, tight bracelets, and watch bands. Avoid bathing for six hours. Adequate total body first-time treatment prevents self-reinfestation and need for retreatment. For bedtime use in babies, cover hands and feet with mittens or socks.
9. Treat all other family and close contacts such as babysitters, nursing staff, and visiting family members. Many failures are actually reinfestations from other cases who may be incubating scabies without clinical signs. Proper treatment of contacts prevents "ping-pong" effects, which may last for months or years. Adequate treatment of contacts lessens need for retreatment.

10. Make sure patient, parents, and guardians can read and understand instructions *in their own language*. Ensure they are told that all lindane products are poisonous to drink and must be kept away from children or elderly, infirm persons. Insist that multiple treatments are unnecessary and potentially toxic. Dispensing pharmacists should not obscure warning labels with additional labels and should offer instructional leaflets in the appropriate language.
11. When possible, treat children in the clinic or office under supervision.
12. Prescribe no more than necessary, with no refills.
13. Remind patients that itching may persist for several weeks. Most patients are comfortable by the fifth week.

Sulfur ointment

No treatment for scabies has a longer history than that of sulfur. Around AD 25, Celsus[135] stated that sulfur mixed with liquid pitch afforded relief to the human species as well as cattle suffering from scabies. Friedman,[98] in his landmark book, *Scabies—Civil and Military*, devotes an entire chapter to sulfur remedies. When he wrote this in 1941, sulfur had been considered the specific treatment for scabies for over 100 years, although its mechanism of action against the mite was, as it is today, unknown.

The recommended method at that time was to take a hot bath for 30 minutes, scrub the crusts off all sores with a handbrush, and apply 15% sulfur ointment over the entire body, except the face and scalp. This was reapplied morning and evening for three days, without bathing or changing pyjamas, which were worn day and night. This cumbersome procedure often produced primary irritant dermatitis, leading Friedman to advise reducing the level of sulfur to 10% for children. Even at these concentrations, primary irritancy may occur, particularly in hot, humid environments. This may produce red, dry, cracked skin or frank denudation, particularly in the flexures and inguinal folds. Topical sulfur ointment is messy, malodorous, stains clothing, and requires several applications over two or three days. It has the advantage of being cheap, and may be the only choice in areas of the world where the need for mass therapy or economy dictate the choice of scabicide.

In recent years in the United States, sulfur therapy has come into vogue again for the treatment of infants and pregnant women because of concern over the potential CNS toxicity of lindane. It should be recognized that no controlled trials on the efficacy and safety of topical sulfur have been published in recent years. In 1926, Basch applied 25% sulfur in petrolatum to abraded skin of guinea pigs. After only three to five daily applications, all animals developed paralysis and died within seven days. Older German literature records deaths in infants treated with high concentrations of sulfur for scabies.[136] Today, sulfur ointment is used in concentrations of 6% or less, and we know of no recent reports of severe toxicity. Because permethrin cream is approved for use on infants 2 months old or older, it has largely replaced sulfur in pediatric practice.

Benzyl benzoate

A volatile oil originally obtained from balsam of Peru and Tolu but now made synthetically, benzyl benzoate was first used in 1932 at the Kommune Hospital in Copenhagen by Kissmeyer.[137] It was applied to patients as a lotion consisting of equal parts of benzyl benzoate, isopropyl alcohol, and soft soap, and left on for 24 hours. Several formulations have been used since then, the usual concentration of the active agent being 10% to 25% in a lotion to be applied for three alternate or consecutive nights. There are insufficient animal and human toxicologic data available to consider it safe to use by current US federal standards. Benzyl benzoate is no longer available in the United States.

In the warm climates of Costa Rica, Venezuela, and Colombia we have seen several cases of irritant dermatitis following the use of benzyl benzoate lotion,

133. Hall RCW, Hall RCW (1999) Long-term psychological and neurological complications of lindane poisoning. **Psychosomatics** 40:513–517.
134. Taplin D, Rivera A, Walker JG et al. (1983) A comparative trial of three treatment schedules for the eradication of scabies. **J Am Acad Dermatol** 9:550–554.
135. Celsus AC (1831) A Translation of the Eighth Book of Aurl. Corn. Celsus on Medicine (de re Medicine), 2nd ed. London: GF Collier, Simpkin and Marshall.
136. Basch F (1925) Uber schwefelwasserstaffvergiftung bei auss Berlicker Application von elementarem Schwefel in Salbenform, Naunyn Schmiedebergs. **Arch Exp Path Pharmacol** 11:126.
137. Kissmeyer A (1937) Rapid ambulatory treatment of scabies with a benzyl benzoate lotion. **Lancet** 1:21.

and we have received reports from physicians who encounter similar problems. The effects are sometimes severe. Scrotal irritation, burning and stinging, and allergic dermatitis have also been reported. It is a conjunctival irritant and should not be used on children and infants. The excellent textbook by Alexander contains a good summary of adverse effects.[43]

In addition to the problems of irritation and poor compliance, the product does not appear to be highly effective, at least as a single treatment. Schmeller, in 1998,[138] described the difficulties in trying to reduce the prevalence of scabies among rural communities in the tropics. They offered treatment with 25% benzyl benzoate emulsion to 478 cases of scabies and their families. Forty-six percent did not return for refills of their medication even though it was free, and in follow-up examinations five weeks later, 82% still had scabies and 59% were unchanged from their baseline states. Two years later the prevalence of scabies was higher than before. The author includes the statement: "The treatment of individuals, or even entire families, is not sufficient. For the eradication of such a highly contagious disease, a more complex control and treatment program is necessary." We agree.[108]

In 2001, Nnoruka & Agu[139] published the results of a study in Nigeria in which 29 patients were treated with a single 72-hour application of 25% benzyl benzoate and compared with 29 similar patients given a single oral dose of ivermectin (200μg/kg of body weight). Twenty-seven (93.1%) of those given ivermectin were cured 30 days later, compared with only 14 (48.3%) of the benzyl benzoate group. In situations where benzyl benzoate may be the only choice due to cost and availability, we suggest the methods employed by Terry and colleagues in and around Freetown, Sierra Leone.[140] Scabies in the refugee camps set up as a result of the rebel war had reached alarming proportions, and was identified in 77% of children under five and 86% of those aged 5 to 9 years! In order to minimize the irritant effects of the treatment, it was applied as a 10% lotion, left on overnight, and washed off the next day. This was repeated three times on alternate days, a process which requires a week of patient compliance. The authors reported a cure rate of 85%, with no reports of irritation from the treatment.

Crotamiton (crotonyl-N-ethyl-O-toluidine)

Shortly after World War II, several newly synthesized compounds were screened for scabicidal activity using an *in vitro* method against *Psoroptes cuniculi*, a mite that infests rabbits. The results were reported by Domenjoz in 1946.[141] The first clinical trial was reported by Burckhardt and Rymarowicz in the same year.[142]

Between March 1975 and June 1977, V. Cubela MD, a dermatologist in Mostar, Yugoslavia, and S.J. Yawalkar MD, a dermatologist with the CIBA-Geigy Company in Switzerland, treated 50 infants and small children aged 2 months to 2 years suffering from scabies. The trial was open (i.e., unblinded and uncontrolled). In the first 16 children, three applications on consecutive nights resulted in only a 44% cure rate. Five nightly treatments of the next 34 subjects resulted in a 69% cure rate.[143] These infants were treated on an outpatient basis, and therapy was presumably administered by the parents. In a study conducted a year later in Skopje, Yugoslavia,[144] different investigators observed a 100% response following five daily applications of crotamiton (Eurax) lotion or cream in 50 hospitalized infants and small children. Bathing was not permitted during the 5-day treatment period.

These two studies are worthy of closer scrutiny in the light of modern dermatologic and pediatric practice and the need for the fuller knowledge of the toxicology of medications. The first study, based on outpatient treatments, clearly demonstrated inadequate efficacy, even after five consecutive treatments. The second trial required hospitalization of the children, a practice that would today be considered unnecessary and expensive.

Much has been made of the reputed antipruritic properties of crotamiton. In the Skopje study, pruritus was measured on a scale of 0 to 4, although the patients were aged 2 months to 24 months. We have been unable to elicit such accurate reports on itching from our subjects of the same age. The only parameter we have been able to measure is that of increased scratching, obvious discomfort, and loss of sleep in babies whose lesions became more severe after Eurax treatment. Greaves *et al.*[145] pointed out in 1982 that no study of percutaneous absorption of crotamiton in children or adults has been conducted. Short- and long-term toxicity in humans have not been studied. The mammalian oral LD_{50} is 10 times greater than lindane in animals. It is compounded at 10 times the concentration, and is recommended to be used daily for five days without bathing.

In a study conducted in 1985, we compared 10% crotamiton cream (Eurax) against 5% permethrin cream (Elimite) in an investigator-blinded study. Forty-two of 47 infants (89%) were completely cured after a single treatment with permethrin. In contrast, 19 of 47 (40%) of the crotamiton cases were judged as treatment failures, and 10 of them (21%) became worse after treatment.[101]

In summary, we do not recommend crotamiton for the treatment of scabies due to lack of efficacy and lack of toxicity data. Permethrin 5% topical cream is significantly more effective and has been subjected to exhaustive animal and human toxicologic studies over several years.

Systemic management

Ivermectin

In the 1970s the Kitasato Institute in Japan, in collaboration with the Merck Institute for Therapeutic Research in the United States, screened over 40 000 cultures of actinomycetes in a search for substances with antihelminthic properties. Only one soil organism, *Streptomyces avermitilis*, isolated from a Japanese golf course, produced a class of compounds known as avermectins. One of these, avermectin B (abamectin), was later chemically modified to form ivermectin, a name coined to reflect its broad-spectrum activity as a vermicide and antiectoparasitic agent.[146] Ivermectin is a macrocyclic lactone, similar in structure to the macrolide antibiotics but devoid of antibacterial activity. It is a highly effective antiparasitic agent against a wide variety of nematodes (roundworms) and arthropods, including lice, mites, and ticks.[147]

Ivermectin was introduced in veterinary medicine in 1981, and is registered in 77 countries for use in dogs, horses, cattle, pigs, sheep, goats, swine, camels, reindeer, llamas, and farm foxes. In the United States, it is the most widely prescribed veterinary nematocide, and is used for the prophylaxis of *Dirofilaria immitis* (heartworm) in dogs. Human experience with ivermectin is also extensive. It has become the strategy of choice for community-based control of onchocerciasis (river blindness), which is caused by the filarial worm *Onchocerca volvulus*. In 1987, Merck and Co. introduced a plan to donate oral ivermectin (Mectizan) for prevention and treatment of onchocerciasis wherever it was needed. During the next ten years, 96 million treatments were given to approximately 19–20 million people in 34 countries in Africa, the Middle East, and Latin America.[148] During such large-scale programs it was inevitable that some pregnant women would receive ivermectin, giving

138. Schmeller W (1998) Community health workers reduce skin diseases in East African children. **Int J Dermatol** 37:370–377.
139. Nnoruka EN, Agu CE (2001) Successful treatment of scabies with oral ivermectin in Nigeria. **Trop Doct** 31:15–18.
140. Terry BC, Kanjah F, Sahr F et al. (2001) Sarcoptes scabiei infestation among children in a displacement camp in Sierra Leone. **Public Health** 115:208–211.
141. Domenjoz R (1946) Veber ein neves antiscabiosum. **Schweiz Med Wochenschr** 76:1210.
142. Burckhardt W, Rymarowicz R (1946) Ehrfahrunge mit dem neuen antiscabiosum Eurax. **Schweiz Med Wochenschr** 47:213.
143. Cubela V, Yawalkar SJ (1978) Clinical experience with crotamiton cream and lotion in treatment of infants with scabies. **Br J Clin Pract** 32:229–231.
144. Konstantinov D, Stanoeva I, Yawalkar SJ (1979) Crotamiton cream and lotion in treatment of infants and young children with scabies. **J Int Med Res** 7:443–448.
145. Greaves WL, Juranek DD, Washington AE (1962) Treatment of scabies and pediculosis. **Rev Infect Dis** 4(Suppl):857.
146. Campbell WC (1985) Ivermectin: An update. **Parasitol Today** 1:10–16.
147. Campbell WC, Fisher MH, Stapley EO et al. (1983) Ivermectin: A potent new antiparasitic agent. **Science** 221:823–828.
148. Dull HB, Meredith SEO (1998) The Mectizan Donation Programme—A 10-year report. **Ann Trop Med Parasitol** 92(Supp.1):S69–S71.

rise to concerns over the effect on their unborn children. Extensive studies in Liberia,[149] Mali,[150] and Cameroon[151] could uncover no evidence of adverse pregnancy outcomes, stillbirths, birth defects, or developmental problems. A later report from Ecuador[152] stated that the rates of spontaneous abortion in onchocerciasis-endemic areas declined significantly after treatment with ivermectin was introduced. At the end of three years, rates were approximately the same in endemic and nonendemic areas. Oral ivermectin has also been used for the treatment and chemoprophylaxis of loiasis and Bancroftian filariasis. Based on a limited number of reports, it appears to be effective in human infestations by masonella ozzardi, Loa loa microfilaremia, ascaris, trichuris, enterobius, cutaneous larva migrans, chronic intestinal strongyloidiasis, scabies, and lice.[153]

Ivermectin binds selectively to receptors of neurotransmitters that function in the peripheral motor synapses of invertebrates. Specifically, it blocks chemical transmission across nerve synapses that use glutamate-gated anion channels or gamma aminobutyric acid (GABA)-gated channels. The reason that ivermectin has an excellent safety record in humans, but is toxic to invertebrates, relates to the fact that GABA- and glutamate-mediated nerves in mammals are found only in the central nervous system, whereas in many invertebrates such nerves regulate peripheral muscles.[154] This is why ivermectin causes selective paralysis in certain worms, insects, mites, and ticks. Although the drug does not readily cross the blood–brain barrier in humans, Burkhart and Burkhart point out that this barrier may be deficient in young animals.[155] A more detailed account of the pharmacology and mechanisms of action against parasites of man and animals can be found in the February 2000 publication by Burkhart.[153]

The current recommendation in the United States is that oral ivermectin should not be given to children under 5 years of age. This excludes the largest section of the population that is afflicted with scabies worldwide.[108,140] This age restriction dictates that community-based control programs utilizing oral ivermectin for scabies must be backed up by appropriate treatment of those under 5 years of age.

HISTORY OF IVERMECTIN FOR HUMAN SCABIES

During a placebo-controlled study of oral ivermectin for onchocerciasis in villages in southern Sierra Leone, investigators from the Liverpool School of Tropical Medicine took the opportunity to observe the effects of oral ivermectin on human head lice and scabies.[89] In their account, published in 1991, they reported significantly fewer children with head lice in the ivermectin group (12 of 74 subjects) than those given placebo (25 of 84). They found no difference in the number of children with clinical scabies; six had scabies in the placebo group versus seven in the ivermectin-treated subjects. These observations were made two months after a single dose of oral ivermectin, allowing ample time for reinfestations. In addition, some of the subjects received only 100μg/kg, which we now consider insufficient. In 1992, Glaziou et al. conducted an investigator-blinded trial in French Polynesia in which a single oral dose of ivermectin (100μg/kg of body weight) was compared with topical therapy using 10% benzyl benzoate preparation. One month later 70% of patients given ivermectin were cured, compared with only 48% of those treated with benzyl benzoate.[156]

At the same time as the studies in Polynesia, trials were underway in Mexico, where Dr Macotela-Ruiz et al. were conducting the first placebo-

controlled study of oral ivermectin on 45 patients with scabies.[157] Twenty-six of 29 (79%) were considered cured one week after a single dose of 200μg/kg, compared with only four of 16 patients (25%) given the placebo. The authors concluded that ivermectin is a safe and effective treatment for scabies. The same investigators conducted a larger study in a closed rural community from January 1993 until December 1995.[158] This study compared the efficacy of a single dose of 250μg/kg with three doses of 250μg/kg at days 1, 3, and 10 in 273 subjects. The investigators report that all subjects were cured of scabies at 45 days, and that scabies had been "eradicated" from the community three years later.

Marty et al.,[159] also in 1993, were able to eliminate scabies in a nursing home in Nice, France, by treating all 53 persons residing or working in the facility with two 6mg tablets of ivermectin on day one and two more a week later. These authors made the observation, which later reports by others have confirmed, that pruritis may increase within 24 hours of taking the drug, presumably due to the sudden release of irritant components of the dying mites. Prompted by the earlier reports from French Polynesia and Nice, Aubin et al. successfully treated two cases of crusted scabies in Bensancon, France. They employed single doses of 12mg oral ivermectin combined with topical 3% salicylic acid ointment.[160]

Unaware of the ongoing studies in French Polynesia, Mexico, and France, in June 1992 Meinking et al.[161] began treating scabies patients in Miami, Florida, using oral doses of 200μg/kg. All of 11 otherwise healthy patients were free of signs and symptoms one month after a single dose. Also included in the trial were another 11 cases of scabies in HIV-positive or AIDS patients. Eight of these 11 were cured one month after a single 200μg/kg dose. Two of the HIV-infected subjects required two doses, and a third case suffering from crusted scabies and AIDS needed three doses over six weeks and topical therapy with 5% permethrin cream (Figs 27.38, 27.39). In their report, the authors offered guidelines for the treatment of scabies with oral ivermectin. First, they

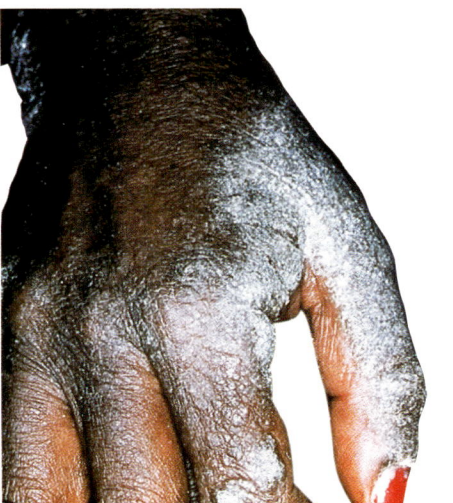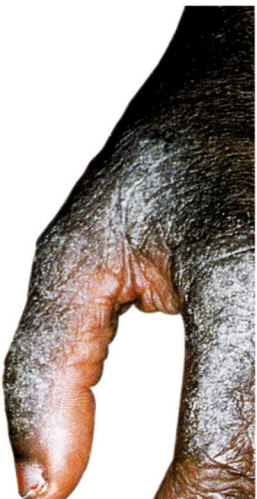

Fig. 27.38   Crusted scabies in an AIDS patient before treatment. (Reprinted from Meinking et al.,[161] with permission.)

149. Pacque M, Muñoz B, Poetschke G et al. (1990) Pregnancy outcome after inadvertent ivermectin treatment during community-based distribution. Lancet 336:1486–1489.
150. Doumbo O, Soula G, Kodio B et al. (1992) [Ivermectin and pregnancy in mass treatment in Mali.] Bull Soc Pathol Exot 85:247–251.
151. Chippaux JP, Gardon-Wendel N, Gardon J et al. (1993) Absence of any adverse effect of inadvertent ivermectin treatment during pregnancy. Trans R Soc Trop Med Hyg 87:318.
152. Guderian RH, Lovato R, Anselmi M et al. (1997) Onchocerciasis and reproductive health in Ecuador. Trans R Soc Trop Med Hyg 91:315–317.
153. Burkhart CN (2000) Ivermectin: An assessment of its pharmacology, microbiology, and safety. Vet Human Toxicol 42:30–35.
154. Elmogy M, Fayed H, Marzok H et al. (1999) Oral ivermectin in the treatment of scabies. Int J Dermatol 38:926–928.

155. Burkhart CN, Burkhart CG (1999) Ivermectin: A few caveats are warranted before initiating therapy for scabies. Arch Dermatol 135:1549–1550.
156. Glaziou P, Cartel JL, Alzieu P et al. (1993) Comparison of ivermectin and benzyl benzoate for the treatment of scabies. Trop Med Parasitol 44:331–332.
157. Macotela-Ruiz E, Peña-Gonzalez G (1993) Tratamiento de la escabiasis con ivermectina por via oral. Gac Med Mex 129:201–205.
158. Macotela-Ruiz E, Peña-Gonzalez G (1996) Tratamiento de la escabiasis con ivermectina por via oral en una comunidad rural cerrado. Dermatol Rev Mex 40:179–184.
159. Marty P, Gari-Toussaint M, Le-Fichoux Y et al. (1994) Efficacy of ivermectin in the treatment of an epidemic of sarcoptic scabies. Ann Trop Med Parasitol 88:453.
160. Aubin F, Humbert P (1995) Ivermectin for crusted (Norwegian) scabies. N Engl J Med 332:612.
161. Meinking TL, Taplin D, Hermida J et al. (1995) The treatment of scabies with ivermectin. N Engl J Med 333:26–30.

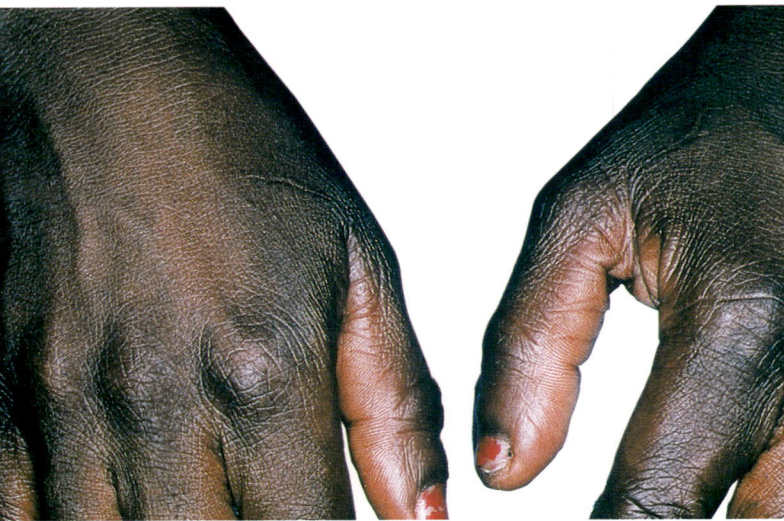

Fig. 27.39 Same patient one month after two oral doses of 200µg/kg ivermectin. (Reprinted from Meinking et al.,[161] with permission.)

emphasized that final evaluations of any form of therapy should not be made until four weeks after the initiation of treatment since, in many cases, it takes that long for all cutaneous signs and symptoms to resolve. Evaluation of clinical response too soon after treatment may have been a factor in apparent failures reported in early studies.[89,156,157] A second observation indicated that ivermectin has limited residual activity, at least at the level of epidermal tissues in which the female mite and her eggs reside, thus allowing some eggs to survive, hatch and continue the infestation. The third guideline offered was that crusted scabies requires multiple doses of ivermectin combined with topical therapy and, in severe cases, keratolytic agents.

Currie and colleagues in Darwin, Australia, eloquently confirmed these observations.[162] They report that scabies is endemic in remote Aboriginal communities, and many cases are crusted, chronic, and refractory to standard topical therapies. Oral ivermectin has become a useful addition to their regimen, but some cases require months of combination therapy, relapses are common, and reinfection usual. One patient required 11 doses of ivermectin over 11 months, and another received nine doses over 24 months. They also report finding live mites up to 19 days after the start of ivermectin therapy.

Our literature searches revealed over 50 publications in English relating to the treatment of scabies with ivermectin since 1995. Space does not permit an exhaustive review. Instead, we have selected those citations that we feel add new knowledge or particularly interesting information.

In 1997, a letter to the journal *Lancet* reported an apparent statistical association between the administration of ivermectin to residents of a nursing home in Canada and an increase in the number of deaths over time.[163] Subsequent reports refuted these findings,[164,165] and ivermectin continues to enjoy an excellent safety record. The letter from Canada did stimulate a reply from Norway reminding readers that certain breeds of herding dogs, including collies, may exhibit a peculiar sensitivity to ivermectin.[166] Fatal reactions may occur within hours of administration, possibly due to a genetic defect in the integrity of the blood–brain barrier in these breeds. A review of ivermectin and other antiparasitic macrolides and their properties in relation to blood–brain transport mechanisms in animals and man was published by Burkhart & Burkhart in 1999.[167]

A particularly informative report by Dourmishev *et al.* from Sofia, Bulgaria, describes a clinical study conducted between September 1995 and February 1998, in which 10 otherwise healthy outpatients with scabies and nine inpatients with scabies and another skin disease were treated with 200µg/kg of oral ivermectin on days 1 and 8. Patients were followed for four weeks, diagnosis and response to therapy were confirmed by microscopic examination of scrapings, and appropriate physical and biochemical parameters were measured. All patients were cured. Seven cases reported an increase in pruritis 24–72 hours after the first dose. At eight days the itching had disappeared. This publication could well serve as a model of how to conduct and report a clinical trial of this type.[168]

IVERMECTIN FOR CONTROL OF SCABIES IN INSTITUTIONS

In the year 2000, Leppard & Naburi reported the largest study to date in which oral ivermectin was used specifically to control scabies in an institution, in this case in a prison near Kilamanjaro in Tanzania.[169] Eight hundred and eighteen of 1153 prisoners (70.9%) were found to have scabies, as did 65 of the 251 (25.9%) of the prison staff. Under close supervision, all inmates were given a dose of ivermectin (150µg/kg) with a cup of water, whether or not they showed evidence of scabies. The prison staff and their families were treated with topical 1% lindane lotion. Two months later, 95.5% of the prisoners were cured. None of the subjects in the study had scabies 12 weeks after treatment. All newly admitted prisoners were given a single oral dose of ivermectin if they showed signs of scabies, and there were no outbreaks during the next two years.

Oral ivermectin has also proven valuable in the management of endemic scabies in nursing homes and extended-care facilities. From Germany comes a report of the successful management of long-standing problems with scabies in three residences for the elderly in a district of Saxony.[170] In one facility, 91.5% of the patients, 54.1% of the staff and 7% of their family members had clinical evidence of scabies that had been endemic in the nursing home for over a year. Previous attempts to handle the problem using only topical treatments such as crotamiton, lindane, allethrin, and permethrin had failed to stem the outbreak, which was apparently started and propagated by a case of severe crusted scabies. The investigators were able to control and end the epidemic by treating all 252 patients in the three residences with topical pyrethroid cream or spray. In addition, 12 cases were treated once with oral ivermectin, and seven cases with two doses.

A different approach was adopted by dermatologists in New South Wales, Australia.[171] For three years, patients in a lock-up ward for elderly, demented males had suffered from scabies. They were described as mobile, aggressive, difficult to manage, frequently involved in skirmishes, and confrontational towards staff members. Previous attempts to cure them using repeated applications of permethrin, lindane, benzyl benzoate, and precipitated sulfur in white soft paraffin had proved ineffectual and difficult to apply. Several of the residents had crusted scabies. Staff morale had become very low. All residents were given 200µg/kg of oral ivermectin, which was repeated two weeks later in all subjects. No topical treatments were given. Four weeks after the first dose there were no active cases, and all rashes were resolved by six weeks. As noted in previous reports by others, several subjects were seen to be scratching more in the days immediately following the treatment, presumably due to increased pruritis.

In 1995, the treatment of all residents of a nursing home in Lyon, France, using topical 1% lindane and careful disinfection of bedding and furniture failed to eliminate scabies.[172] Eight months later in 1996, all residents were treated with 12mg of ivermectin, whether or not they were symptomatic. A

162. Currie B, Huffam S, O'Brien D, Walton S (1997) Ivermectin for scabies. **Lancet** 350:1551.
163. Barkwell R, Shields S (1997) Deaths associated with ivermectin for scabies. **Lancet** 349:1144–1145.
164. Reintjes R, Hoek C (1997) Deaths associated with ivermectin for scabies (reply). **Lancet** 350:215.
165. Coyne PE, Addiss DG (1997) Deaths associated with ivermectin for scabies (reply). **Lancet** 350:215–216.
166. Bredal WP (1997) Deaths associated with ivermectin for scabies (reply). **Lancet** 350:216.
167. Burkhart CN, Burkhart CG (1999) Before using ivermectin therapy for scabies. **Pediatr Dermatol** 16:478–480.
168. Dourmishev A, Serafimova D, Dourmishev L (1998) Efficacy and tolerance of oral ivermectin in scabies. **J Eur Acad Dermatol & Venereol** 11:247–251.

169. Leppard B, Naburi AE (2000) The use of ivermectin in controlling an outbreak of scabies in a prison. **Br J Dermatol** 143:520–523.
170. Paasch V, Hausstein UF (2000) Management of endemic outbreaks of scabies with allethrin, permethrin, and ivermectin. **Int J Dermatol** 39:463–470.
171. Sullivan JR, Watt G, Barker B (1997) Successful use of ivermectin in the treatment of endemic scabies in a nursing home. **Australas J Dermatol** 58:137–140.
172. Dannaoui E, Kiazand A, Piens MA et al. (1999) Use of ivermectin for the management of scabies in a nursing home. **Eur J Dermatol** 9:443–445.

second dose was administered 14 days later. The outbreak was successfully contained with only one case experiencing a recurrence four weeks after treatment. As in many similar reports, the outbreak was believed to have originated with a case of crusted scabies. The authors noted that the clinical appearance and distribution of lesions in their nursing home patients was atypical. Burrows were uncommon, and the rashes were papular or vesicular in more than half of these cases. We have noted similar findings in nursing homes in Florida.

Elderly persons in nursing homes are often incontinent, necessitating plastic covers over mattresses. This creates a tropical, humid microclimate between the individual and the bed. As noted previously, burrowing of the mite is rare under these conditions. We have seen cases in which the lower extremities are cold due to vascular insufficiency, but warm between the back and the mattress. Burrows were confined to the lower legs, but we were able to collect several scabies mites from the papular rash on the back.

GUIDELINES FOR USE OF IVERMECTIN FOR SCABIES IN HUMANS

In spite of more than 10 years' experience in the use of oral ivermectin for scabies, including over 50 published reports, the drug has not been approved for this use in any country as of November 2001, nor for any reason in children under 5 years. Although many uncomplicated cases are successfully treated with a single dose of 200μg/kg of ivermectin, experience clearly shows that a second dose at 10–14 days results in a significantly higher cure rate. Meinking and Elgart offered an explanation for this in April 2000.[173] The scabicidal effect of ivermectin depends on the levels achieved in cellular fluids, since the scabies mite is not a blood feeder. The half-life in humans is about 16 hours, so little if any remains in the patient's system one week later, at which time eggs, not affected by the ivermectin, will have hatched into nymphs, which will evolve into adults able to continue the infestation. Other recommendations by these authors form the basis of the following guidelines:

1. Uncomplicated cases are best treated with two doses of oral ivermectin 10–14 days apart using 200–250μg/kg. All patients should be weighed to ensure that the dose is sufficient to achieve adequate tissue levels.[174]
2. Oral dosing allows for complete body treatments and avoids the problem of failure to apply topical agents to all body areas including intertriginous sites such as toe webs, intergluteal cleft, and postauricular creases.
3. As in all forms of therapy, a month or more may be required before all signs and symptoms of scabies are resolved, particularly in severe cases with secondary infection or excoriations.
4. Close contacts should be treated whether or not they exhibit symptoms. Our surveys indicate that up to 50% of individuals in populations in which scabies is endemic may be incubating infestations without clinical signs.[174] This is particularly important in crowded communities such as prisons, nursing homes, refugee centers, and similar situations. Failure to adopt these prevention measures is almost certain to thwart control efforts.[171] In conditions such as those described above, treatment of patients one at a time in a clinic setting is a waste of valuable professional time, medications, and resources,[174] and has little effect on community prevalence.
5. Whether treating single patients, families, or communities in which scabies is endemic or epidemic, two doses of ivermectin of 200 or 250μg/kg results in higher cure rates than single doses. In large-scale control programs, this is essential because single treatments leave sufficient active cases to maintain the epidemic or endemic levels. Community control must include head-to-toe treatment for children under 5 and pregnant women, preferably with 5% permethrin cream.
6. Crusted scabies in patients with HIV, AIDS, or HTLV-1 infection and patients with other immunological impairments should be treated with

two doses of ivermectin two weeks apart, plus topical therapy and keratolytic agents in severely crusted patients. Finger and toe nails should be clipped before topical treatments, since they are favorite hiding places for mites and their eggs.[115] Crusted scabies cases are particularly likely to infest others, including caregivers. To prevent institutional epidemics, early diagnosis, isolation, and environmental control measures are strongly advised, and are well worth the financial costs.

Summary of therapies for scabies

Table 27.8 summarizes the available scabies therapies.

ENVIRONMENTAL DECONTAMINATION

There is little evidence that clothing, bedding, or other articles play a significant role in the spread of scabies except in crusted forms. Mellanby[103] conducted exhaustive studies during the war years in England. In all but a few instances, he failed to infest volunteers by the interchange of clothing or by placing men in beds recently vacated by active cases. We were able to eliminate or reduce the prevalence of scabies to very low levels in island populations by treating all inhabitants at the same time.[108,174] We made no attempt to treat or wash clothing, hammocks, or bedding. Patients or parents may on occasion present a convincing story of a motel bed, borrowed sleeping bag, or article of clothing as the originating source. We have usually been unable to incriminate such items because often evidence of person-to-person contact was also present. On one occasion, however, a mattress used by a 3-year-old child with scabies appeared to have introduced the mites into another household without direct human contact. In another instance, a borrowed flannel shirt was identified as the mode of transfer between two campers who had no physical contact. Blumenthal *et al.*[175] studied an outbreak of scabies in a Florida school in 1976, and determined that contact in the school was not a likely environment for transmission. In contrast, children who visited and slept in other houses were more likely to have scabies than those who did not.

We do not recommend environmental insecticidal sprays. They are unlikely to play any role in management, and such a recommendation reinforces the erroneous concept of an environmental reservoir of *S. scabiei*. Parents should be advised that the usual mode of transmission is close body contact and that heroic efforts to decontaminate clothing, environment, or bedding are unnecessary. Normal laundering of clothing or dry cleaning is sufficient to prevent this mode of spread, and should be recommended.

Patients with crusted scabies represent an exception to the above scenario. Their crusts are teeming with mites and viable eggs that are constantly shed into the environment. These patients should be treated as a hazard to others and appropriate isolation procedures should be instituted. Their crusts may also contaminate furniture.[113,120]

In the home setting, good cleaning practices and vacuuming is recommended. The use of household insecticide sprays approved for bedding and mattresses should be considered but no studies have been published to indicate their effectiveness in the prevention of scabies. Safety precautions on the labels should be strictly followed and the amounts recommended should not be exceeded.

COMPLICATIONS

Streptococcal/staphylococcal infections superimposed on scabies are common. In warmer climates, and particularly in overcrowded conditions, secondary infection is almost universal. Taplin *et al.*,[176] working in Colombia, showed a direct correlation between altitude and the prevalence of streptococcal pyoderma. As might be expected, these infections were more

173. Meinking TL, Elgart GW (2000) Scabies therapy for the millennium. **Pediatr Dermatol** 17:154–156.
174. Taplin D, Arrue C, Walker JG et al. (1983) Eradication of scabies with a single treatment schedule. J **Am Acad Dermatol** 9:546–550.
175. Blumenthal DS, Taplin D, Schultz MG (1976) A community outbreak of scabies. **Am J Epidemiol** 104:667–672.
176. Taplin D, Lansdell L, Allen AM et al. (1973) A prevalence of streptococcal pyoderma in relation to climate and hygiene. **Lancet** 1:501–503.

TABLE 27.8   Summary of therapies for scabies

Acaricide	Dosage	Pros	Cons
Permethrin 5% cream • Elimite, Acticin (United States) • Nix (Canada) • Lyclear (Other countries)	Single overnight application of cream. Second treatment may be necessary.	Little toxicity. Low absorption. Rapid metabolite excretion. Cosmetically elegant. Approved for infants as young as 2 months of age.	Second or third treatment may be required, particularly for crusted scabies.
Lindane 1% cream and lotion • Bio-Well, GBH, G-well, Kildane, Kwildane, Scabene, Thionex (United States) • GBH, Hexit, Kwellada, PMS Lindane (Canada) • Gamma benzene hexachloride • Generics	Single overnight treatment, not less than 6 hours or more than 12 hours. Do not repeat in less that 1 week. No more than 2 doses.	Generic forms inexpensive.	Potential CNS toxicity. Absorbed through skin. Lindane resistance reported worldwide in pediculosis and scabies.
Crotamiton 10% lotion and cream • Eurax	Overnight may require several treatments.	Not recommended.	Poor efficacy. Repeated treatments needed to obtain higher success rates. Safety and efficacy have not been evaluated by current standards.
Sulfur 3%–10% ointment • 6% Ointment	Application of cream each night for 3 nights.	Extensive use in young infants and pregnant women.	Safety and efficacy have not been evaluated by current standards. Animal studies suggest caution. Requires several treatments. Malodorous. Stains clothing. May cause irritant dermatitis in hot climates.
Benzyl Benzoate 10%–25% • Not available in the United States or Canada • Ascabiol (Other countries)	Three applications of 10% lotion on alternate nights, wash off each morning.	Used in developing countries. Inexpensive.	Adequate animal and human toxicological studies have not been performed. Requires several treatments. May cause stinging, dermatitis, and allergic reactions. Eye irritant. Poor efficacy reported.
Ivermectin • Stromectol (United States) • Mectizan (Canada, Africa, Europe, South America)	Single oral dose of 200μg/kg.	Few side effects. Approved for use in children 5 years old.	Not as yet approved for scabies. Not approved for children under 5 years old.

common at lower altitudes, where higher temperatures and biting insects favor skin infections. At all altitudes, however, there were more infections in children from environments or families where good daily hygiene was difficult to maintain or was nonexistent. Overcrowding, poor hygiene, and a warm climate produce the ideal setting for pyoderma and transmission of scabies. In the populations in which we have worked in the tropics, it is unusual to find scabies that is not infected. *S. pyogenes* is the initial pathogen in most lesions, but they quickly become colonized by *S. aureus*, which also may be pathogenic.[177] Occasionally, we have noted scabies secondarily infected with exfoliatin-producing *S. aureus*, leading to multiple lesions of staphylococcal bullous impetigo.

A review of the literature at the turn of the millennium reveals that the combination of poverty, overcrowding, poor hygiene, scabies, streptococcal pyoderma, and nephritis still exacts an enormous toll on health services in many countries. In Aboriginal communities in northern Australia, the

prevalence of streptococcal pyoderma may exceed 70% in children. These communities also have the highest published incidence of acute rheumatic fever in the world, in spite of very low throat carriage rates for Group A *Streptococcus*. This suggests that where scabies and streptococcal skin infections are rampant, the sequellae may include acute glomerulonephritis and rheumatic fever. Further examination of these factors can be found in the excellent publication by Carapetis *et al.*[178] It is now well established that scabies treatment of individual patients in medical facilities has little, if any, effect on the prevalence of scabies in a community. In contrast, well-conducted community-control projects have dramatic beneficial effects that are long-lasting if surveillance for new cases is included in the planning. We have noted in three scabies management programs conducted in Panama that the prevalence of streptococcal skin infections is also greatly diminished without antibiotic intervention once the scabies infestations are controlled. This phenomenon has been confirmed in several studies in Australia.[178,179]

177. Schachner L, Taplin D, Scott GB et al. (1983) A therapeutic update of superficial skin infections. **Pediatr Clin North Am** 30:397–404.

178. Carapetis JR, Currie BJ, Kaplan EL (1999) Epidemiology and prevention of Group A streptococcal infections: Acute respiratory tract infections, and their sequelae at the close of the twentieth century. **Clin Infect Dis** 28:205–210.

179. Currie BJ, Carapetis JR (2000) Skin infections and infestations in Aboriginal communities in northern Australia. **Australas J Dermatol** 41:139–145.

DEMODEX: THE HAIR FOLLICLE MITE

HISTORY

In 1841, *Demodex folliculorum* was discovered by Henle.[43] The following year Simon independently gave a detailed account of the morphology and habitat of this pilosebaceous follicle mite.[180]

Although most dermatologists considered it a harmless saprophyte, Erasmus Wilson in 1843 discussed its role as a possible pathogen. In that year, Owen named the genus *Demodex*.[181] It had been known for quite some time, however, that *Demodex* caused serious skin lesions in domestic animals and a pustular mange in dogs that can be fatal.[182] Investigators throughout the world have attributed and described the skin changes associated with this mite. Early investigators include Dubreuilh (1901),[183] Lawrence (1916),[180] De Amicis (1918),[184] Majocchi (1918),[185] and Ayres (1930).[186] Although most physicians still consider *Demodex* as normal flora of the ecosystem of the skin, a growing opinion seems to indicate that it can be pathogenic to some individuals under certain conditions.[43]

MORPHOLOGY AND BIOLOGY

Demodex is unlike any other mite in appearance. It has adapted very well to living in a hair follicle by assuming the shape of a short hair with a root-like broad head, followed by four pairs of tubercle-like, stumpy, three-jointed legs. It is somewhat worm-like in appearance.[43] It has been speculated that *Demodex* is phylogenetically related to the cheyletiellid fur mites.[181]

In the original work by Simon in 1842, he mentions two forms, a long and a short. Lawrence (1921),[187] Fuss,[188] and Norn[189] agreed that there were indeed two forms, or perhaps two distinct species. In 1931, Lawrence and Brodie[190] isolated mites from scrapings from a patient with pityriasis folliculorum, which were all short forms, unlike the long slender version found in hair follicles of normal skin of the same individual. It was not until 1963 that Akbulatova suggested the two subspecies be named *Demodex folliculorum* for the long form and *Demodex brevis* for its shorter counterpart.[191] Desch and Nutting[191] convincingly confirmed that these were distinct species, both morphologically and biologically (Table 27.9).

According to Spickett,[192] Demodex eggs have an incubation period of 2 1/2 days, with the first molt occurring about 2 1/2 days later. The second nymphal stage lasts less than two days, and the third stage consists of three days. The six-legged larva emerges into an eight-legged adult, but lives only four to six more days. Thus the entire life span is complete in 14 to 16 days. Two methods of reproduction may occur: viviparous or oviparous.

Demodex are extremely mobile.[193] They travel from follicle to follicle at 8–16mm per hour and tend to be most active at night. They are most commonly found on the forehead, cheeks, nose and nasolabial folds, but may be found anywhere on the face, eyelids, lashes, ears, or their surrounding area.

TABLE 27.9   Demodex

	D. folliculorum	D. brevis
Morphology of an adult E, ventral magnified 200×		
Ovum (length × width)[a]	105 × 42	60 × 34
Larva (length × width)	283 × 34	105 × 34
Protonymph (length × width)	365 × 36	148 × 34
Nymph (length × width)	392 × 42	165 × 41
Male adult		
(length)	280	166
(width)	24–45	17–46
Female adult		
(length)	294	208
(width)	27–52	19–50
Male to female ratio	1:4.5	1:3.4
Habitat	Hair follicle	Sebaceous gland

[a] Measurements of all sizes in μm. (From Desch and Nutting,[191] with permission.)

The number and prevalence of *Demodex* in healthy individuals seems to have a seasonal variation, being highest in spring and lowest in winter.[191,194] Prevalence also depends on the age of the host, reaching 100% among older people.[195] Forton and Seys[196] reported a prevalence rate of 33.3% in a group of 45 individuals with a mean age of 41 years. Aydingoz, Mansur, and Dervent[197] found an infestation rate of 26.6% in a group of 30 subjects with a mean age of 28.5 years. Infestation in children is rare, perhaps due to their low sebum.[195] Ku Quizun[198] was unable to recover any *Demodex* from 150 neonates examined.

Infestation most likely occurs from close family contacts. During the nymphal stage the mites reside closer to or on the skin surface, thus facilitating transfer among hosts.[198] A few cases of adults and children with pustular lesions on the chest, abdomen, forearms, and hands have been reported after sleeping with a mangy pet goat.[199] *Demodex* was found in high numbers in the lesions of the patients. To our knowledge, no other accounts of pustular lesions from animal contact have been reported.

DEMODICIDOSIS

Two to six mites, on average, occupy one hair follicle and are considered harmless. Ten or more is considered abnormal and can elicit a response in the host.[200,201] The terms demodicidosis or demodicosis designate a high-density infestation giving rise to clinical signs and symptoms.

An unusually high density of *Demodex* mites has been suggested as a causative agent in rosacea.[194,196,202,203] The lesions of rosacea are 1–4mm in

180. Lawrence H (1916) On a skin eruption association with the presence of great numbers of *Demodex folliculorum*. **Med J Aust** 2:555.
181. Hirst S (1919) Studies on Acari No 1. The genus *Demodex* (Owen). London: The Trustees of the British Museum (Natural History).
182. Martin A (1913) La gale demodecique des herbivores. **Rev Vet** 38:321, 389.
183. Dubreuilh W (1901) (1925) Referenced by Kaufman-Wolf M: Uber regehmassiges Vorkommen von *Demodex folliculorum* in der Pusteln von Rosacea pustulosa. **Dermatol Wochenschr** 81:1095.
184. De Amicis T (1918) *Demodex folliculorum* e ipercromia cutanea. **G Ital Malatta Venereol Pelle** 33:205.
185. Majocchi (1918) In discussion of De Amicis (1918). **G Ital Maltta Venereol Pelle** 33:205.
186. Ayres S (1930) *Pityriasis folliculorum (Demodex)*. **Arch Dermatol Syphilo** 21:19.
187. Lawrence H (1921) The pathogenicity of the *Demodex* (Owen) in the human being. **Med J Aust** 2:39.
188. Fuss F (1933) La vie parasitaire du *Demodex folliculorum hominis*. **Ann Dermatol Syphiligr** (Paris) 74:1053.
189. Norn MS (1970) *Demodex folliculorum*: incidence and possible pathogenic role in the human eyelid. **Acta Ophthalmol** 108(Suppl.):7–85.
190. Lawrence H, Brodie R (1961) *Pityriasis folliculorum Demodex*. **Med J Aust** 1:529.
191. Desch C, Nutting WB (1972) *Demodex folliculorum* (Simon) and *Demodex* and *D. brevis* Akbulatova of man: re-description and re-evaluation. **J Parasitol** 58(1):169–177.
192. Spickett SG (1961) Studies of *Demodex folliculorum* Simon (1842). **Parasitol** 51:181.
193. Norn MS (1971) *Demodex folliculorum*: incidence, regional distribution, pathogenicity. **Dan Med Bull** 18:14–17.
194. Bonnar E, Eustace P, Powell FC (1993) The *Demodex* mite population in rosacea. **J Am Acad Dermatol** 28:443–448.
195. Rufli T, Mumcuoglu Y (1981) The hair follicle mites *Demodex folliculorum* and *Demodex brevis*: biology and medical importance. **Dermatologica** 162:1–11.
196. Forton F, Seys B (1993) Density of *Demodex folliculorum* in rosacea: a case-control study using standardized skin-surface biopsy. **Br J Dermatol** 128:650–659.
197. Aydingoz IE, Mansur T, Dervent, B (1997) *Demodex folliculorum* in renal transplant patients. **Dermatology** 195:232–234.
198. Ku Quizun (1982) An epidermiological investigation of human demodicidosis. **Clin J Dermatol** 15:89.
199. Kaufman-Wolf M (1925) Uber regelmassiges Vorkommen von *Demodex folliculorum* in der Pusteln von Rosacea pustulosa. **Dermatol Wochenschr** 81:1095.
200. Agostini A (1939) La questione del *Demodex folliculorum* in dermatologia: a proposito di un caso pigmentazioni circoscritte del volto. Il **Dermosifilografo** 14:421.
201. Nutting WB, Beerman H (1983) Demodicosis and symbiophobia status terminology and treatment. **Int J Dermatol** 22:13–17.
202. Abd-el-al AM, Bayoumy AMS, Abou Salem, EA (1997) A study on *Demodex folliculorum* in rosacea. **J Egypt Soc Parasitol** 27:183–195.
203. Erbagci Z, Ozgoztasi O (1998) The significance of *Demodex folliculorum* density in rosacea. **Int J Dermatol** 37:421–425.

diameter, often with a central pustule. The surrounding skin is erythematous. Rosacea may be found anywhere on the face, but is usually located in the oily skin areas. Rosacea-like dermatitis producing a firm red papule with a yellowish-white head is also attributed to these mites.[204]

An overabundance of mites in the hair follicle may cause it to rupture, producing an inflammatory response.[43] Demodex in the dermis may produce an immunologic reaction resulting in inflammation and granulation.

Patients may complain of skin irritation, or a hot or burning sensation of the face. The skin may appear dry, scaly, and rough. Scaly, circinate eruptions on the face caused by an overabundance of these mites is known as pityriasis folliculorum.[205]

Demodex has also been implicated in histologic folliculitis,[206] pustular folliculitis,[207] and blepharitis.[208,209] Although Demodex can cause severe mange in animals, it seldom appears to play a devastating pathogenic role in humans.[64]

Reports of demodicidosis in young children are rare and tend to involve patients with impaired immune systems. Patrizi et al.[210] described eight cases of demodicidosis in immunocompetent children ranging in age from 10 months to 5 years. Most other reported pediatric cases were associated with HIV[211,212] or chemotherapy for malignant diseases.[213–215] Children receiving maintenance therapy for acute leukemia might be especially predisposed to Demodex proliferation and subsequent disease.[213–215]

Reports of demodicidosis in association with HIV or chemotherapy suggest that immune defense mechanisms might play a protective role by limiting mite numbers. However, studies of the association between immune function and Demodex density show conflicting results. While an overabundance of mites has been implicated in skin lesions of immunosuppressed patients,[213,215–217] Forton and Seys[196] found no increased Demodex density in a group of patients with HIV. Aydingoz, Mansur, and Dervent[197] failed to find any Demodex in a group of renal transplant patients, although the mite was present in healthy controls. These studies suggest that there may be factors other than immunosuppressive therapy influencing Demodex density.

TREATMENT

Good hygiene is among the best recommendations for treatment of Demodex in healthy patients. Soap and water and sulfur preparations are sufficient treatments to cure most conditions associated with these mites. Cosmetic creams and cleansers should be avoided.

In cases that do not respond to washing with soap and water, permethrin 5% cream is a safe and effective alternative. Overnight applications of permethrin 5% cream resulted in complete resolution of skin eruptions in several reported cases,[214,215] although multiple applications often were required.[214] Antibiotics, in particular metronidazole, have been reported to decrease the population of Demodex,[210,218] but are often insufficient to cure active cases of demodicidosis.[208,213]

Forton et al.[219] tested the comparative efficacy of metronidazole 2%, permethrin 1%, sublimed sulphur 10%, lindane 1%, crotamiton 10% and benzyl benzoate 10% in 34 patients suffering from skin conditions with high Demodex density. Of the six topical treatments tested, only crotamiton and benzyl benzoate demonstrated an acaricidal effect.

Other promising treatments include ivermectin and pilocarpine gel. A single oral dose of 200μg/kg ivermectin with subsequent weekly topical 5% permethrin cream led to substantial clinical improvement within one month in a case that had failed to respond to conventional treatments, including metronidazole.[208] Pilocarpine gel applied to the base of the eyelashes was reported to significantly reduce mite density in the eyelash follicles, with a subsequent reduction in eye irritation.[220,221] Further study of these treatments is needed.

DERMANYSSIDAE OR GAMASIDAE (BLOODSUCKING MITES)

The members of the family Dermanyssidae, taxonomically revised to Gamasidae[43] (suborder Mesostigmata) consist of several species of mites that are parasites of animals such as birds, rodents, and snakes.[64] Attacks on humans by the Gamasidae family have been reported and documented throughout the world.[43] They commonly cause pruritus, irritation, and sometimes painful skin eruptions. The feeding sites of these bloodsucking mites may present with lesions that resemble papular urticaria.[222] Due to the varying distribution of bites, gamasid infestations have also been misdiagnosed as miliaria (prickly heat).[222] Members of this family are known vectors of several viral and rickettsial diseases and are prime suspects in others.[43]

Anyone, regardless of age, ethnic background, social status, or sex may be attacked by members of this family of mites. Children, however, tend to have a more severe reaction to the bites of these bloodsucking parasites.[43] The following culprits are most commonly recognized as deviating from their natural host and affecting humans: the chicken or poultry mite (Dermanyssus gallinae), the tropical rat mite (Ornithonyssus bacoti), the tropical fowl mite (O. bursa), the northern fowl mite (O. sylviarum), the house mouse mite (Liponyssoides sanguineus), and the snake mite (Ophionyssus natricis).

D. gallinae (De Geer 1779), the chicken mite, is also known as the red mite, especially among poultry handlers, who find this red, blood-engorged parasite to be a common but severely irritating problem. It is important to recognize and understand that the gamasid red mite is different from the red bug or chigger, which is the six-legged larvae of the trombiculid mites (or harvest mite; see family Trombiculidae).

Although D. gallinae is associated with infestations of poultry, it is not uncommon for this mite to parasitize both wild and domestic birds, from pigeons to parakeets. The host versatility of this mite was noted by Hirst,[223] when he found horses and other domestic animals occasionally infested. Of all the Gamasidae mites, D. gallinae is the species most associated with attacks on humans and has, therefore, been more extensively studied. D. gallinae is a nocturnal feeder, allowing only an hour or less from the time the victim goes to bed until the mite begins to dine. It is common for patients to complain of itching upon awakening in the morning, and skin eruptions are noticed within 24 hours.[43] The feeding habits of the Gamasidae may vary among

204. Ayers S Jr, Ayers S 3rd (1961) Demodectic eruptions (demodiciosis) in the human. **Arch Dermatol** 83:816.
205. Dominey A, Tschen J, Rosen T (1989) Pityriasis folliculorum revisited. **J Am Acad Dermatol** 21:81–84.
206. Vollmer RT (1996) *Demodex*-associated folliculitis. **Am J Dermatopathol** 18:589–591.
207. Purcell SM, Captain MC, Hayes TJ (1986) Pustular folliculitis associated with *Demodex folliculorum*. **J Am Acad Dermatol** 15:1159–1162.
208. Forstinger C, Kittler H, Binder M (1999) Treatment of rosacea-like demodicidosis with oral ivermectin and topical permethrin cream. **J Am Acad Dermatol** 41:775–777.
209. Roth AM (1979) *Demodex folliculorum* in hair follicles of eyelid skin. **Ann Ophthalmol** 11:37–40.
210. Patrizi A, Neri I, Chieregato C et al. (1997) Demodicidosis in immunocompetent young children: report of eight cases. **Dermatology** 195:239–242.
211. Barrio J, Lecona M, Hernanz JM et al. (1996) Rosacea-like demodicosis in an HIV-positive child. **Dermatology** 192:143–145.
212. Sanchez-Viera M, Hernanz JM, Sampelayo T et al. (1992) Granulomatous rosacea in a child infected with the human immunodeficiency virus. **J Am Acad Dermatol** 27:1010–1011.
213. Castanet J, Monpoux F, Mariani R et al. (1997) Demodicidosis in an immunodeficient child. **Pediatr Dermatol** 14:219–220.
214. Ivy SP, Mackall CL, Gore L et al. (1995) Demodicidosis in childhood acute lymphoblastic leukemia: an opportunistic infection occurring with immunosuppression. **J Pediatr** 127:751–754.
215. Sahn EE, Sheridan DM (1992) Demodicidosis in a child with leukemia. **J Am Acad Dermatol** 27:799–801.
216. Ashack R, Frost M, Norins A (1989) Papular pruritic eruption of Demodex folliculitis in patients with acquired immunodeficiency syndrome. **J Am Acad Dermatol** 21:306–307.
217. Dominey A, Rosen T, Tschen J (1989) Papulonodular demodicidosis associated with acquired immunodeficiency syndrome. **J Am Acad Dermatol** 20:197–201.
218. Persi A, Rebora A (1981) Metronidazole and *Demodex folliculorum*. **Acta Dermatol Venereol** (Stockh) 61:182–183.
219. Forton F, Seys B, Marchal JL, Song M (1998) *Demodex folliculorum* and topical treatment: acaricidal action evaluated by standardized skin surface biopsy. **Br J Dermatol** 138:461–466.
220. Celorio J, Fariza-Guttmann E, Morales V (1989) Pilocarpine as a coadjuvant treatment of blepharioconjunctivitis caused by *Demodex folliculorum*. **Invest Opthalmol Vis Sci** 30:40.
221. Fulk GW, Murphy B, Robins MD (1996) Pilocarpine gel for the treatment of demodicosis – a case series. **Optom Vis Sci** 73:742–745.
222. Theis T, Lavoipierre MM, Lapierre R et al. (1981) Tropical rat mite dermatitis. Report of six cases and review of mite infestations. **Arch Dermatol** 117:341–343.
223. Hirst S (1922) Mites injurious to domestic animals. **Econ Ser Br Museum** 13:1.

species and even within species, just as the response of the patient to the bite of the mite manifests itself in different ways. While some patients describe the gamasid attacks as painful with no pruritus, others have itching with or without a rash, and still others have neither itching nor pain. Therefore, the number of mites attacking and the immunologic response of the host both probably play a role in the pathogenicity of an infestation.

All mites in the family Gamasidae or Dermanyssidae produce similar lesions. Diagnosis of these infestations must be determined in large part from the history of onset, environmental location, distribution of clothing, animal contacts, occupational exposure, recent outdoor activities, hobbies, knowledge of similar cases among co-workers or personal contacts, and any other clues to determine the source of the infestation. Occasionally, mites may be found on the skin or clothing, but they do not burrow. Transmission by person-to-person contact is not possible, but unless the source is identified and treated or disposed of, the patient may suffer from repeated reinfestations for several months or more.

Unlike scabies, there is no classic or generally preferred distribution of gamasid lesions. Often there is a cluster of about two to six lesions,[224] with the neck, back, and shoulders frequently involved.

Although exposed areas are usually attacked more often and more severely, this is not always the case. Areas covered by clothing, especially tight-fitting clothing, are sometimes affected. The arms, abdomen, axillae, and groin are common sites of attack. It is interesting, however, that the hands (interdigital webs and palms), soles of feet, and head are almost always spared.[43,225–229]

The life cycle of Gamasidae averages about nine days, under optimum conditions, from ovipositing to adult,[43] although this varies slightly among species. Eggs hatch in about two days and there are three molts before the adult stage is reached. The nymphs must engorge with blood before molting. Adults may, under certain conditions, live for several months and are able to survive without a bloodmeal for considerable periods of time. A female *D. gallinae* has been known to live for 113 days without a blood meal;[223] however, a fresh bloodmeal is required before each batch of eggs (three to seven) is laid. Usually an adult female lays between 25 and 35 eggs during her lifetime.[43] While *D. gallinae* can survive for months if the microclimate is suitable, they do not thrive at low relative humidities or at temperature extremes.[230]

The tropical fowl mite, *O. bursa*, is increasingly gaining notoriety (Fig. 27.40). In tropical climates it has replaced *D. gallinae* and, because it is so closely related to *O. sylviarum*, the northern fowl mite, it has extended its distribution during summer months. The tropical fowl mite was reported to infest humans on an Air Force base in Puerto Rico.[231] The source was traced back to a nearby nesting grackle that was heavily infested. A report from India describes a case of a boy with severe pruritus and rash in the axillae and groin area. *O. bursa* mites were isolated from the affected areas, and an infested sparrow's nest was found in the boy's room.[232] A patient in Cairo presented with a classic distribution of lesions of scabies. Scraping of the patient revealed the culprit to be the tropical fowl mite. When Lodha[232] examined infested tropical birds, the mites migrated directly to his axillae and began to bite fiercely. Unlike the other gamasid mites, *O. bursa* appears to have a preference in choosing human body areas, and these sites also happen to be among the favorites of *S. scabiei*. If no mites of any kind are found on the patient, epidemiologic questions should be asked about pets, nesting birds, etc.

A 5-month history of pruritic papular eruptions tormented several members of a family with a pet python.[233] *Ophionyssus natricis*, the snake mite,

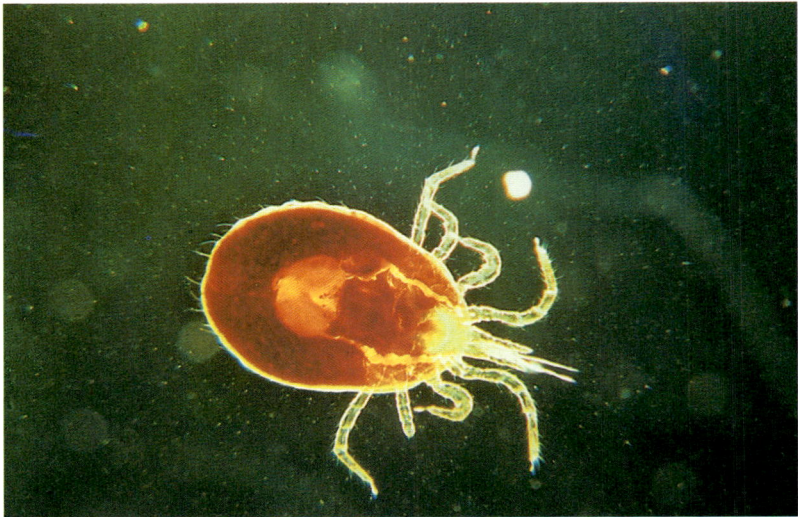

Fig. 27.40 Blood-filled tropical fowl mite (*Ornithonyssus bursa*) obtained from a patient in Miami.

was found attached to the snake and the skin of the infested family members. Mites were also harbored in the python's favorite chair. After treating the snake, his cage, and, of course, his favorite chair, with pyrethrins, the problem was solved. Since the sources of infestation were treated, there was no need to treat the family members and they had no further problems.

TREATMENT

Although some members of the family Gamasidae or Dermanyssidae prefer to eat and run, like the tropical rat mite, *O. bacoti*, others may remain on the skin or clothes even though they may escape detection during examination. A single treatment of permethrin 5% topical cream should be used to treat the infestation (see Scabies, treatment). If no new lesions have developed since the onset, treatment should consist merely of an antipruritic lotion. Oral antihistamines are helpful in relieving itching, and may provide more restful sleep. Clothing, bedding, and other articles of potential infestation should be washed in a hot water cycle and dried thoroughly in a hot dryer.

If the patient becomes reinfested after treatment, the source must be located. The source may be anything from a bird's nest in the roof gutter, a dead mouse the cat brought home, to even an exotic pet parrot. Depending on the source, the patient can treat the natural host and the infested area or dispose of it. Since domestic animals vary widely in their susceptibility, referral to a veterinarian is always advisable. Likewise, disinfestation of living quarters should not exceed recommended labeling for consumers or should be conducted by professional exterminators. Once the origin of the mite infestation is eliminated, the patient will have no new lesions, the biting will cease, and the itching should stop within a week. There are various means to eliminate the mites without harming the hosts. Alexander[43] offers control measures that eliminate the parasites and are non-toxic to the infested animal. In chicken roosts, 40% nicotine sulfate rapidly kills the mites, leaving the poultry and eggs unaffected. In fact, eradication of the mites increases the health of the poultry and increases egg laying.

224. Shelmire B, Dove WE (1931) The tropical rat mite *Liponyssus bacoti* Hirst 1914. The cause of a skin eruption of man and a possible vector of endemic typhus fever. **JAMA** 96:579.
225. Sulzberger MB, Kamenstein I (1936) Avian itch mites as a cause of human dermatoses. Canary birds' mites responsible for two groups of cases in New York. **Arch Dermatol Syphilol** 33:60.
226. Anderson CR (1944) Rat mite dermatitis; acariasis caused by the tropical rat mite *Liponyssus bacoti* Hirst 1914. **Arch Dermatol Syphilol** 50:90.
227. Shaw JW, Pommerening RA (1950) Avian mite dermatitis (gamasoidosis). **Arch Dermatol** 61:466.
228. Frenken JH (1962) *Dermanyssus gallinae* (*D. avium*) *Strophulus* or insect bites, diet or D.D.T. **Dermatologica** 125:322.
229. Hidano A, Asanuma K (1976) Acariasis caused by bird mites. **Arch Dermatol** 112:882.
230. Nordenfors H, Hoglund J, Uggla A (1999) Effects of temperature and humidity on oviposting, molting and longevity of *Dermanyssus gallinae* (Acari: Dermanyssidae). **J Med Entomol** 36:68–72.
231. Fox I (1957) Ornithonyssus bursa (Berlese) attacking man in Puerto Rico. **J Econ Entomol** 50:838.
232. Lodha KR (1969) The occurrence of tropical fowl mites *Ornithonyssus* (*Bdellonyssus, Liponyssus*) bursa on a man in Ragasthan (India). **Vet Rec** 84:363–365.
233. Schultz H (1975) Human infestation by *Ophionyssus natricis* snake mite. **Br J Dermatol** 93:695–697.

DISEASE VECTORS

The gamasid mites are known transmitters of viral and rickettsial diseases. We tend to view the insect world as a democracy in which the individuals are innocent until proven guilty. Unfortunately, the list of the guilty continues to expand as researchers provide more proof of their role as disease vectors. Table 27.10 provides a list of the family Gamasidae and their role as vectors of disease.[234]

PYEMOTES (GRAIN MITES)

The itching associated with the family Pyemotidae has been recognized for almost 300 years.[235] The species that is associated with attacks on humans was named *Pediculoides ventricosus* in 1878;[236] however, the proper nomenclature at present is *Pyemotes ventricosus*. No other species in this family has been incriminated in attacks on people. Infestation with *P. ventricosus* has been reported from North America, Australia, Asia, Africa, and Europe.

TABLE 27.10   Dermanyssidae or Gamasidae: bloodsucking mites

Name	Mite morphology	Habitats, hosts, pathology, and symptomatology	Role as disease vectors
Dermanyssus gallinae (DeGeer) (chicken mite)		A common parasite of domestic and wild birds. Often infests animals and humans. A nocturnal feeder found predominantly in temperate climates; in humans severe cutaneous eruptions appear within 24 hours of exposure; primary lesion: 1–6mm urticated papule, may have vesicles, crusts, an erythematous halo; wheals, macules, papules can be present in a variable distribution. The eruption may be accompanied by pain and/or itching.	Fowl tick fever; endemic typhus; St Louis encephalitis; Eastern encephalitis
Ornithonyssus bursa (Berlese) (tropical fowl mite)		Similar in host and habitat to *D. gallinae*, but restricted to warm and tropical locations; human case reports suggest a more "scabieslike" distribution of lesions; groin and axillae are most common sites with severe pruritic rash; bites are painful.	Western equine encephalitis; Q fever (suspected only)
Ornithonyssus sylviarum (Canestrini and Franzago) (northern fowl mite or feather mite)		A parasite of wild and domestic birds in temperate climates; also infests a wide variety of animals from cockroaches to kangaroos; attacks on humans cause intense pruritus but no rash; source of infestation must be found and treated or destroyed; most cases tracked to birds' nests near windows, eaves of house, or in garage.	Western equine encephalitis; St Louis encephalitis; rickettsialpox
Ornithonyssus bacoti (Hirst) (tropical rat mite)		With a worldwide distribution "tropical rat mite" is a deceiving name; rarely found on examination; "an eat and run" mite, always in search of a fresh host; bites can be found on all parts of the body presenting as small urticarial papules, often clustered; swelling and erythema last a week or more.	Endemic typhus; relapsing fever; St Louis encephalitis; murine typhus (suspected only). Western equine encephalitis. Rickettsialpox; Q fever, tularemia, plague, also serves as an intermediate host to filaria of cotton rats.
Dermanyssus sanguineus (house mouse mite) *Allodermanyssus sanguineus*; (Hirst) *Liponyssoides sanguineus*		A common parasite of the house mouse, but often infests rats and other mammals; found wherever mice are found; very common throughout the USA and other parts of the world; frequently attacks humans, causing a severe eruption.	Rickettsialpox (*Rickettsia akari*), tularemia
Ophionyssus natricis (Gervais) (snake mite)		Associated with all types of snakes raised in captivity; found in zoos and pet shops in the USA and worldwide; also infests rats, various other animals, and humans; a common problem for zookeepers and pet snake owners; presents with papular eruptions; mites attach firmly to the hosts' skin; pruritic lesions will persist for months until source is treated.	*Pseudomonas hydrophilus* (which causes hemorrhagic septicemia – a fatal disease in reptiles); transmits haemogregarina of snakes

(Adapted from McDaniel,[234] with permission.)

234. McDaniel B (1979) How to Know the Mites and Ticks. Dubuque, IA: William C. Brown.
235. Glass FA (1948) Grain itch. A report of the first outbreak in the city of Baltimore. Ind Med 17:95.
236. Oudemans AC (1937) Oven de Veelhard der sorten van Pediculoiden. Tijdschr Entomol 80:4.

Pyemotes infestations are generally associated with the grain industry and are often referred to as "grain itch," "straw itch," "hay itch," "cereal itch," "miller's itch," "copra itch," "barley itch," and "prairie itch." Dock workers, farmers, packers and storers of grain, or even people sleeping on straw mats or mattresses can be victims.[43,64,201,234,237] An outbreak among nursing home patients and staff in rural Australia was traced to nearby grain storage facilities.[238] Dust containing mites was presumably blown from the storage facilities into the hospital. Recently, investigators in Spain[239] reported 126 cases of *Pyemotes* dermatitis in orange pickers whose only risk factor was exposure to orange trees where *Pyemotes* was found.

Pyemotes has a seasonal distribution that directly correlates to the harvesting and processing of grain, usually late summer and fall. The pupal form may remain dormant in hay or straw over the winter.[43] Adult *Pyemotes* measure about 160 to 223µm for male and female, respectively.[43] They are long and slender and look somewhat like a formula one race car. This family of mites possesses external diastase enzymes that are injected into the host to liquefy the body materials. The mite remains attached to the host while it proceeds to suck the body fluid into its mouth parts, which contain a tube-like structure.[43] The usual host of *Pyemotes* is, however, another insect, to which the digestive toxin of this mite can often be fatal. If grain heavily infested with *Pyemotes* is fed to chickens or other animals, the animals may soon die, presumably due to ingestion of a large dose of *Pyemotes* toxin.[234]

Human host preference of *Pyemotes* is much like that of the bloodsucking mites in that they will attack anyone. The first symptoms are unbearable itching at the sites of attack, with heat and sweat intensifying this pruritic reaction.[43]

A rash appears a few hours after exposure, but it may take up to 16 hours to become fully manifest. The appearance is that of papular urticaria, with small papules developing into vesicles. In some cases, hemorrhagic punctae may occur prior to vesiculation. The vesicles rupture easily, often due to excoriation, or friction from clothing or bedding. The broken vesicles result in lesions that may become crusted, bloody or purulent. Systemic symptoms are common in severe cases. A fever of 39°C (102°F) or higher, nausea, vomiting, rapid pulse, headache, backache, dizziness, malaise, anorexia, and asthmatic attacks have all been associated with *P. ventricosus* infestations.[43,64,161,240]

Diagnosis can be difficult in severe cases. The presence of 10 000 or more lesions is not uncommon[241] and may mimic measles[242] or scarlatiniform rash.[243] Although *Pyemotes* are transient irritating visitors, diagnosis occasionally can be made by scraping lesions or using cellophane tape[43] to capture a suspect that has yet to leave the area of infestation. Because *Pyemotes* are only rarely found in skin scrapings, it is important to investigate the immediate environment for ectoparasites.[238] Without further exposure, the patient usually recovers from symptoms in a week or less. In two weeks, there may be no signs of the previous attack.

THERAPY

The treatment is the same as that of the gamasid mites (see Dermanyssidae or Gamasidae). Occasionally patients infested with *P. ventricosus* have secondary infections that should be treated with oral antibiotics, and in very rare, extremely serious cases, a short course of oral corticosteroids may be warranted.[43]

CHEYLETIELLIDAE AND/OR CHEYLETIDAE (PET OR FUR MITES)

At present, the family Cheyletidae has 186 known species.[234] These mites are predators of small invertebrates and feed off of other insects, including parasitic mites. Cheyletidae are sometimes referred to as "fur mites" because some species are associated with infestations of furry animals. Cheyletidae mites prey on members of the family Listrophoridae, which are actually the true fur mites and parasites of mammals, but which apparently do not infest humans.[234]

There appears to be some confusion between the Cheyletidae and the closely related Cheyletiellidae. Some investigators do not recognize the family Cheyletiellidae and vice versa, or consider it to be synonymous with Cheyletidae.[43,64,234,244–246]

The morphologic difference between Cheyletidae and Cheyletiellidae is in the shape of the claws. The former has a strong tibial claw to grasp prey, whereas the latter has claws that are ventrally curved to grasp fur.[43,247] Regardless, both are free-living mites that prey on ectoparasites of mammals.[244,245,248] Cheyletiellidae have been known to have a symbiotic relationship with dogs by feeding on the *Demodex* infesting the animal. Bart[249] observed that Cheyletiellidae were found in large numbers on animals that were not harboring another food source or infestation. The mites were finally caught in the act of engorging themselves on bodily fluids from the furry animal host.[249,250] In some cases, these mites can be beneficial to the animal host, since they eat other animal ectoparasites. They are always, however, unwanted visitors of humans.

The following three species are known to attack humans and are all associated with animal infestations: *Cheyletiella parasitovorax* (the rabbit mite), *C. yasguri*, (the dog mite), and *C. blakei*, (the cat mite).[250] Human infestations with cheyletiellid mites have been reported worldwide.[251–255] The handling of furry domestic animals is the major means of transmission. Children often carry their pets around with them, or allow the animal to sleep on their bed at night.[256–258] As with the other mites, children have a more severe reaction to the bites than do adults. Younger animals also have a more intense reaction to infestation by Cheyletiellidae than do adults of the same species.[43,259] Some adult animals harbor mites but are asymptomatic or perhaps carriers.[260] This suggests that immunity may develop in some animals. To our knowledge, this aspect has not been investigated.

237. Fine RM, Scott HG (1963) Straw itch mite dermatitis caused by *Pyemotes ventricosus*. **J Med Assoc Ga** 52:162.
238. Letchford J, Strungs I, Farrell D (1994) *Pyemotes* species strongly implicated in an outbreak of dermatitis in a Queensland country hospital. **Pathology** 26:330–332.
239. Bellido-Blasco JB, Arnedo-Pena A, Gonzalez-Moran F et al. (2000) [Dermatitis outbreaks caused by *Pyemotes*]. **Med Clin** (Barc) 114:294–296.
240. Ancona G (1923) Asma epidemicoda *Pediculoides ventricosus*. **Policlinico** 30:45.
241. Schamberg JF (1910) Grain itch. **J Cutan Genitourin Dis Syphilol** 28:67.
242. Thompson AGG (1925) Barley itch. **BMJ** 1:71.
243. Pascal (1900) Erytheme scarlatiniforme desquamitif generalise d'origine parasitaire. **Ann Dermatol Syphiligr** (Paris) 1:947.
244. Cooper KW (1946) The occurrence of the mite *Cheyletiella parasitovorax* (Megnin) in North America with notes on its synonymy and parasitic habit. 32:480.
245. Rothschild M (1969) *Cheyletiella parasitovorax* feeding upon the rabbit flea. **Entomol Monthly Mag** 105:1262.
246. Megnin P (1878) Memoires sur les cheyletides parasites. **J Anat Physiol** (Paris) 14:416.
247. Smiley RL (1970) A review of the family Cheyletiellidae (Acarina). **Ann Entomol Soc Am** 63:1056.
248. Kuscher A (1940) Raumilben beim Hund (*Cheyletiella parasitovorax*). **Wein Tierarzt Monatsschr** 27:10.
249. Barr AR (1955) A case of mange of the domestic rabbit due to *Cheyletiella parasitovorax* (Megnin). **J Parasitol** 41:323.
250. Smiley RL (1965) Two new species of the genus *Cheyletiella* (Acarina: Cheyletidae). **Proc Entomol Soc Washington** 67:75.
251. Moxham JW, Goldfinch TJ, Heath ACG (1967) *Cheyletiella parasitovorax* infestation of cats associated with skin lesions of man. **NZ Vet J** 16:50–52.
252. Dodd K (1970) Skin lesions associated with *Cheyletiella yasguri* infestation. **J Ir Med Assoc** 63:413–414.
253. Rack G (1971) *Cheylitiella yasguri*. Smiley, 1965 (Acarina: Cheyletiellidae) ein fakultatine menschen pathogene Parasit des Hundes. **Z Parasitenkt** 36:321–334.
254. Shelley ED, Shelley WB, Pula JF et al. (1984) The diagnostic challenge of nonburrowing mite bites, *Cheyletiella yasguri*. **JAMA** 251:2690–2691.
255. Davies JHT (1938) Another acarine disease. **Br J Dermatol** 50:243.
256. Cohen SR (1980) *Cheyletiella* dermatitis, a mite infestation of rabbit, cat, dog and man. **Arch Dermatol** 116:435–437.
257. Foxx TS, Ewing SA (1969) Morphologic features, behavior and life history of *Cheyletiella yasguri*. **Am J Vet Res** 30:269–285.
258. Reed CM (1961) Infestation of pups. **J Am Vet Med Assoc** 138:306.
259. Michener CD (1946) Observation on the habits and life history of a chigger mite, *Eutrombicula batatas* (Acarinae Trombiculinae). **Ann Entomol Soc Am** 39:101.
260. Jenkins DW (1948) Trombiculid mites affecting man. I. Bionomics with reference to epidemiology in the United States. **Am J Hyg** 48:22.

The pet must be treated and animal contacts of the same species should be examined for infestation and treated if necessary. Kennels can often be a source of infestation. Household sprays used for lice, such as R&C spray or Liban, are safe and effective for spraying animal bedding, chairs, carpets, and even children's blankets and beds. With the elimination of the source, the human patient simply needs a topical antipruritic and oral antihistamines to reduce pruritus and increase the quality of sleep.

TROMBICULIDAE (CHIGGERS)

The family Trombiculidae has well over a hundred members with a worldwide distribution. New species have recently been discovered in Argentina,[261] Kenya,[262] Russia,[263] Thailand,[264] and the United States.[265] In the adult form, the body colors range from reds and browns to golden depending on species. The eight-legged adults are not parasites of humans; the six-legged larval forms are human parasites (Fig. 27.41). The female lays her eggs each month in the soil where they incubate for about seven to 14 days.[260] Trombiculids have been known to lay 7–15 eggs per day[261,266] in the laboratory, each averaging about 150μm in diameter, although 30–40 eggs per month is thought to be more realistic in the wild.[267] The eggs hatch into six-legged larvae, which are quite successfully capable of attacking humans and also surviving 30 days of starvation.[186] These larvae are known as chiggers or red bugs because of their color. Several species of this family, during the larval stage, are known to attack vertebrate hosts; however, the best known is *Trombicula autumnalis*, the harvest mite or berry bug.[268]

The larvae climb onto grass in search of a vertebrate meal, and drop off into the soil after this has been fulfilled. They develop into an eight-legged adult and never need or desire a vertebrate meal again.

Chiggers prefer a warm, moist environment both on the ground and on the host. They are most common in wet or damp grass or weeds, and commonly attack the ankles right above the shoes.[250] Bites are also common

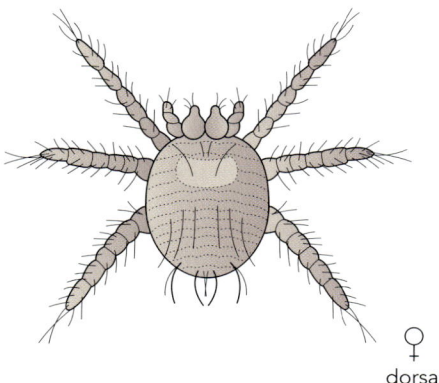

Fig. 27.41 Trombiculid or "chigger." (Adapted from McDaniel,[234] with permission.)

♀

dorsal

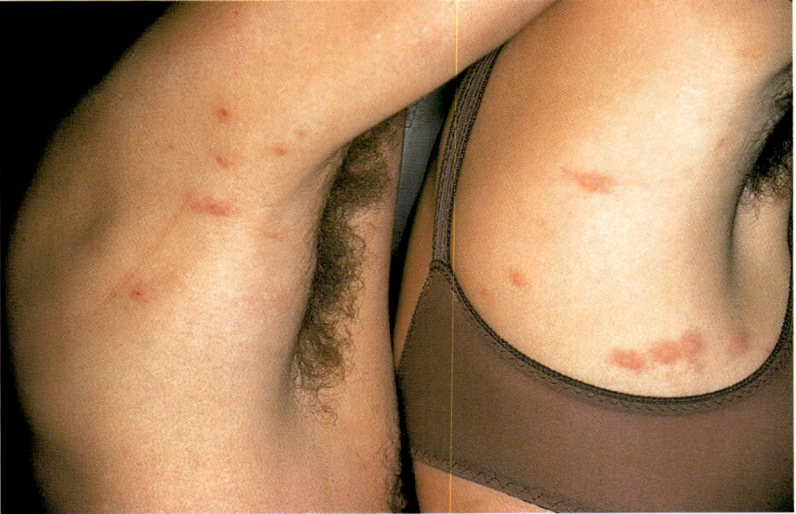

Fig. 27.42 Chigger bites.

in the moist areas of the host's body such as the axillae, genitalia, and the popliteal and antecubital fossae,[269] or wherever clothing fits snuggly, such as waistbands.[248] It has been noted that the areas most commonly attacked have generally thinner skin. The trombiculids appear to be "habitat specific rather than host specific."[43]

Within a few hours after the attack, the patient develops 2–3mm pale macules.[43] In the center of some lesions, the mites still may be present, and appear as tiny red points. The lesions increase in size for the following 10- to 16-hour period until they resemble dome-shaped papules (Fig. 27.42).[43] These papules or urticarial lesions may become hemorrhagic, and the pruritus is often intense. The shape and size of the lesions may vary. This is thought to be due to the location of the papule rather than the species of mite that initiated the lesion.[268] The itching subsides in a few days and the lesions are generally healed in seven to 14 days. However, there may be residual hyperpigmentation at the lesion sites.[270]

There are possible complications that may arise following Trombiculidae infestations. In the Far East, certain species are known vectors of Japanese river fever (scrub typhus, rickettsial typhus, tsutsugamushi fever).[43] The most common problem, however, is that of secondary infection of excoriations. Lymphangitis and lymphadenopathy,[271,272] erysipelas,[273] and streptococcal or staphylococcal pyodermas may follow.

Treatment of trombiculid infestations is the same as that of the gamasid mite previously discussed. Prevention of infestation consists of avoidance of warm, moist, grassy or overgrown areas of land when possible. Insect repellents should be used, especially on the body areas where this mite is likely to bite.

261. Goff ML, Gettinger D (1995) New genus and six new species of chiggers (Acari: Trombiculidae and Leeuwenhoekiidae) collected from small mammals in Argentina. **J Med Entomol** 32:439–448.
262. Goff ML (1995) New species of *Neotrombicula* (Acari: Trombiculidae) from African primates (Galagidae and Cercopithecidae). **J Med Entomol** 32:12–15.
263. Kadosaka T, Tamura A, Tarasevich I (1995) New species of *Neotrombicula* (Acari: Trombiculidae) from the southern Primorye territory, Russian Far East. **J Med Entomol** 32:381–383.
264. Tanskul P, Linthicum K (1997) A new species of *Leptotrombidium* (Acari: Trombiculidae) collected in active rice fields in northern Thailand. **J Med Entomol** 34:368–371.
265. Goff ML, McKown RD (1997) The genus *Hexidionis* (Acari: Trombiculidae) with the description of a new species from Texas. **J Med Entomol** 34:438–440.

266. Jenkins DW (1949) Trombiculid mites affecting man. III. Trombicula (*Eutrombicula Splendens*) Ewing in North America. **J Parasitol** 35:201.
267. Gordon RM, Lavoipierre MMJ (1962) Entomology for Students of Medicine. Oxford: Blackwell.
268. Gordon RM, Lavoipierre MMJ (1960) Annotations, The harvest mite. **Lancet** 625:1395.
269. Hirst S (1925) On a harvest bug (*Leeuwenhoekia australiensis* sp n) attacking human beings at Sydney, New South Wales. **Trans R Soc Ther Med Hyg** 19:150.
270. Frazier CA (1969) Insect allergy. In: Allergic Reactions to Bites of Insects and Other Arthropods. St. Louis: Warren H. Green.
271. Parkhurst HJ (1937) Trombidiosis (infestation with chiggers). **Arch Dermatol Syphilol** 35:1011.
272. Andrews GC, Domonkos A (1971) Diseases of the Skin, 6th ed. Philadelphia: WB Saunders.
273. Chittenden FH (1915) Harvest mites or chiggers. Washington, DC: U.S. Dept of Agriculture Farmers Bulletin 671, US Government Printing Office.

Sexually Transmitted Diseases

Gail Todd and Walter Krause

Sexually transmitted diseases (STDs) are infectious diseases in which (1) the infection is mainly mediated by genital contact or (2) the signs and symptoms of the disease are mainly found on the genital regions. Formerly, only the classical venereal diseases syphilis, gonorrhea, granuloma inguinale, chancroid, and lymphogranuloma venereum were emphasized in venereal disease training. During the past three decades the spectrum of these diseases has broadened. Table 28.1 gives an overview of the wide range of STDs as presently encountered. Infections caused by the human immunodeficiency virus (HIV) are also STDs according to this definition.

As a consequence, the spectrum of STDs observed in children has likewise expanded. Obviously, other infectious diseases such as a common cold may be transmitted by sexual contact. Nobody, however, would consider this disease to be a STD. There are some other diseases that are usually transmitted non-sexually, but sexual transmission may also occur, as is observed in hepatitis B. Other examples include herpes simplex, in which the genital form is sexually transmitted but the labial form is not. Candidosis may be transmitted by sexual contact, but is usually nonsexually acquired. Thus, physicians who care for children should be aware of the entire spectrum of STDs presently known.

In principle, children acquire STDs in three different ways, although only two of these ways fulfill the criteria outlined in the first paragraph. First, sexually active adolescents are at risk of acquiring any of the STDs seen in adults. Second, STDs observed in prepubertal children often result from sexual abuse, a problem that only recently has become a focus of medical attention. In young children, several STDs such as condyloma acuminatum or gonorrhea are highly suggestive of sexual abuse if there is no other plausible explanation with regard to their origin. A third mode of transmission of STDs in childhood is transplacental infection or contact with infectious agents present in the birth canal. Such "innocent bystander" diseases include congenital syphilis, neonatal herpes simplex infections, papillomavirus infections, and diseases caused by HIV.

SYPHILIS

Gail Todd

Syphilis (or lues) is caused by *Treponema pallidum*. With the exception of a transplacental infection, syphilis is virtually always acquired by sexual contact. There are several stages of the infection. At the first stage, a chancre develops at the site of inoculation. The second stage includes generalized symptoms with adenopathy and a cutaneous eruption. The late stages are characterized by destructive lesions present in the central nervous system (CNS), cardiovascular system, bones, skin, and other organs.[1,2]

T. pallidum belongs to the order Spirochetales including treponemas that are pathogenic for humans. The bacterium contains three axial fibrils inserted at each end of the protoplasmic cylinder. The ends may be used for attachment to host cells. Possibly a "slime" of bound host macromolecules sometimes covers the bacteria and alters their antigenicity. Unravelling the antigenicity of *T. pallidum* has been hampered due to the inability to grow pathogenic bacteria in cultures free of animal cells or tissue. However, recent developments in genome sequencing have led to new diagnostic tools for the diagnosis of syphilis.[3–6]

T. pallidum measures approximately 12μm in length and 0.15μm in width; it is tightly coiled, with 8 to 10 coils on average, and as it moves it both spins in a rotary fashion and flexes centrally. This rotary and back-and-forth motion typifies the organism and separates it from saprophytic, nonpathogenic treponemas frequently obtained on specimens taken from mucous membranes. *In vitro* culturing has suggested a replication time of 33 hours, approximating *in vivo* estimates. Very small numbers of organisms suffice to cause active infection in rabbits, suggesting that only limited inoculum size is needed in humans as well. Although disease states equivalent to primary and secondary syphilis can be produced in rabbits, tertiary syphilis has not been created in laboratory animals.

TABLE 28.1   Spectrum of sexually transmitted diseases in children and adolescents

Bacterial diseases
   Syphilis
   Diseases caused by *N. gonorrhoeae*
   Diseases caused by *C. trachomatis*
   Granuloma inguinale
   Chancroid
Viral diseases
   Herpes simplex
   Condylomata acuminata
   Mollusca contagiosa
   Diseases caused by HIV
   Diseases caused by human cytomegalovirus
Mycotic diseases
   Candidosis
Other diseases
   Diseases caused by *T. vaginalis*
   Diseases caused by arthropods

1. Fiumara NJ (1985) The treponematoses. In: Dermatology, 2nd ed, Moschella SL, Hurley HJ, eds. Philadelphia: WB Saunders, p. 817.
2. Swartz MN (1984) Syphilis and nonvenereal treponematoses. In: Scientific American Medicine, vol. 7, Rubenstein E, Federman DE, eds. New York: Scientific American, p 1.
3. Egglestone SI, Turner AJ (2000) Serological diagnosis of syphilis. PHLS Syphilis Serology Working Group. **Commun Dis Public Health** 3:158.
4. Wicher K, Horowitz HW, Wicher V (1999) Laboratory methods of diagnosis of syphilis for the beginning of the third millennium. **Microbes Infect** 1:1035.
5. Bruisten SM, Cairo I, Fennema H et al. (2001) Diagnosing genital ulcer disease in a clinic for sexually transmitted diseases in Amsterdam, The Netherlands. **J Clin Microbiol** 39:601.
6. Backhouse JL, Nesteroff SI (2001) Treponema pallidum western blot; comparison with the FTA-ABS test as a confirmatory test for syphilis. **Diagn Microbiol Infect Dis** 39:9.

EPIDEMIOLOGY

Distribution of syphilis is worldwide, in contrast with the nonvenereal treponematoses that are endemic in certain geographic regions. Syphilis tends to be a disease of metropolitan areas, although it is observed in rural populations as well. No absolute natural immunity to syphilis exists, and all races and both sexes are equally susceptible. For obvious reasons, syphilis is most frequent in age groups with a high sexual activity. Although early syphilis (primary and secondary) remain a problem, the numbers of reported cases of tertiary and congenital syphilis have markedly decreased in the United States and other industrialized countries. By contrast, in certain underdeveloped countries[7] and specific population subgroups,[8–12] congenital syphilis may contribute significantly to the prevailing perinatal mortality rate.

With respect to the general modes of transmission of the diseases discussed herein, we can estimate that transmission of syphilis in the sexually active teenager or preteen child abuse victim will be as frequent as in the adult. The reported rates of syphilis in adult rape victims range from 0% to 3%.[13–15] Amongst adolescents, substance abuse is a risk factor for syphilis.[16]

The association of syphilis with other STDs is high. For example, an association with seropositivity for hepatitis virus antigens B and C was found in 67.5% of patients evaluated for other STDs.[17] Likewise, genital ulcer disease, including syphilis, is a risk factor for HIV disease.[18–22] Special attention should be given to these problems.

The true incidence of "innocent bystander" syphilitic infections of children is unknown.[12] They occur mainly by transplacental transmission. Infections during labor are not proven. Diagnosis and treatment during pregnancy are in principle the same as in nonpregnant women and it should therefore be possible to avoid congenital syphilis by routine maternal serologic testing.[23,24] Syphilis still contributes significantly to perinatal mortality.[7–12]

CLINICAL FEATURES

The patient or parent may complain of one or more of the lesions or symptoms of syphilis. Cutaneous manifestations will be emphasized throughout, and tertiary syphilis will be minimally covered because of its rarity in pediatric cases. Congenital syphilis will be emphasized because of its importance in pediatrics and dermatology. For diagnosis, serologic screening and physical findings are far more important than a case history, although sometimes a history of sexual contact with a person having lesions suggestive of syphilis may help to establish the correct diagnosis.

Primary syphilis

The classical chancre appears three weeks after inoculation. The time of incubation, however, may vary from 10 days to three months. Starting as a papule, the syphilitic chancre quickly erodes and appears as an indurated, punched-out, "clean," nontender ulcer with a granular tissue base. The induration and the rolled border confer its classical buttonlike consistency on palpation. The size and the depth of the chancre as well as the induration of the surrounding tissue tend to increase during the first two weeks. In males, the site of predilection is the penis (Fig. 28.1) and in particular the prepuce,

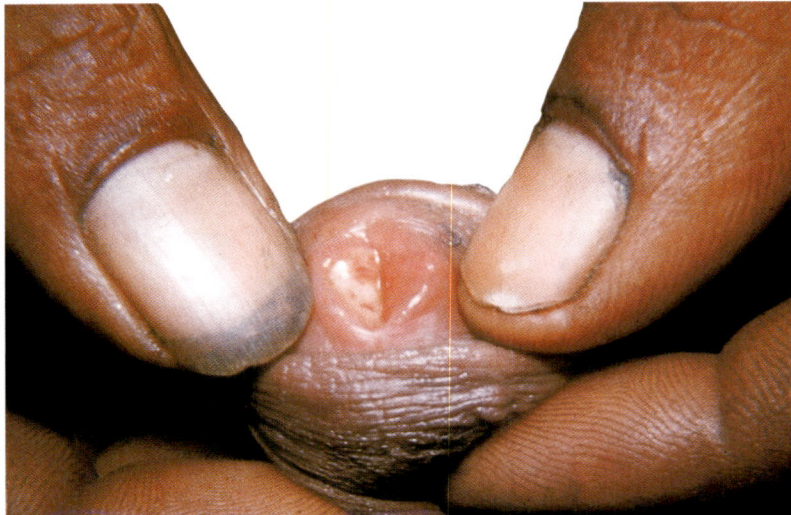

Fig. 28.1 Primary syphilis. Perimeatal chancre in a young male. (Courtesy of Cape Town University)

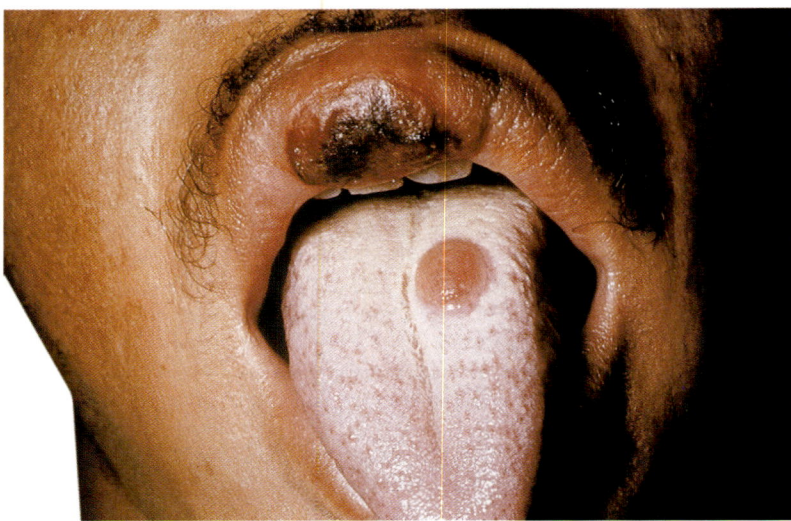

Fig. 28.2 Primary syphilis. Extragenital chancres on the lip and tongue in a young male. (Courtesy of Cape Town University)

coronary sulcus, frenulum, or glans. In women, labial chancres are common, but lesions are frequently found internally as well, especially on the cervix.

Extragenital primary lesions may also occur and are most often seen on the lips, tongue, nipples, or hands (Fig. 28.2). Specific attention should be given

7. Gerbase AC, Rowley JT, Heymann DH et al. (1998) Global prevalence and incidence estimates of selected curable STDS. **Sex Transm Infect** 74:1S12.
8. Ballot DE, Rothberg AD (1993) Congenital syphilis as a notifiable disease. **S Afr Med J** 83:721.
9. Nakashima AK, Rolfs RT, Flock ML et al. (1996) Epidemiology of syphilis in the United States, 1941–1993. **Sex Transm Dis** 23:16.
10. Klass PE, Brown ER, Pelton SI (1994) The incidence of prenatal syphilis at the Boston City Hopital: a comparison across four decades. **Pediatrics** 94:24.
11. Rawstron SA, Jenkins S, Blanchard S et al. (1993) Maternal and congenital syphilis in Brooklyn, NY. Epidemiology transmission and diagnosis. **Am J Dis Child** 147:727.
12. Finelli L, Crayne EM, Spitalny KC (1998) Treatment of infants with reactive syphilis serology, New Jersey: 1992 to 1996. **Pediatrics** 102:e27.
13. Schwarcz SK, Whittington WL (1990) Sexual assault and sexually transmitted diseases: detection and management in adults and children. **Rev Infect Dis** 12:S682.
14. de Villiers FP, Prentice MA, Bergh AM et al. (1992) Sexually transmitted disease surveillance in a child abuse clinic. **S Afr Med J** 81:84.
15. Ingram DL, Everett VD, Lyna PR et al. (1992) Epidemiology of adult sexually transmitted disease agents in children being evaluated for sexual abuse. **Pediatr Infect Dis J** 11:945.

16. Cox JM, D'Angelo LJ, Silber TJ (1992) Substance abuse and syphilis in urban adolescents: a new risk factor for an old disease. **J Adolesc Health** 13:483.
17. Petersen EE, Clemens R, Bocks HL et al. (1992) Hepatitis B and C in heterosexual patients with various sexually transmitted diseases. **Infection** 20:128.
18. Blocker ME, Levine WC, St Louis ME (2000) HIV prevalence in patients with syphilis, United States. **Sex Transm Dis** 27:53.
19. Pham-Kanter GB, Steinberg MH, Ballard RC (1996) Sexually transmitted diseases in South Africa. **Genitourin Med** 72:160.
20. Schofer H, Imhof M, Thoma-Greber E et al. (1996) Active syphilis in HIV infection: a multicentre retrospective survey. The German AIDS Study Group (GASG). **Genitourin Med** 72:176.
21. McCabe E, Jaffe LR, Diaz A (1993) Human immunodeficiency virus seropositivity in adolescents with syphilis. **Pediatrics** 92:695.
22. Tramont EC (1993) Syphilis in HIV-infected persons. **AIDS Clin Rev** 94:61.
23. Wendel GD Jr (1990) Sexually transmitted diseases in pregnancy. **Semin Perinatol** 14:171.
24. Rawstron SA, Bromberg K (1991) Comparison of maternal and newborn serologic tests for syphilis. **Am J Dis Child** 145:1383.

to anal chancres, indicating anal coitus. There is accumulating evidence that genital ulcers facilitate the transmission of HIV, and they may also be markers of high-risk behaviour for acquisition of HIV. Patients with genital ulcers, particularly those with syphilis or chancroid, should be encouraged to undergo testing for HIV infection.

Atypical presentations are increasingly recognized. For example, multiplicity of lesions, tenderness, crusting, and shagginess of the ulcers, and other deviations from the normal appearance do not exclude the presence of syphilis. Because multiple STDs are often seen in the same patient, syphilitic ulcers may coexist with the lesions of herpes simplex, chancroid, or other STDs.

Another important symptom of the first stage of syphilis is a firm and nontender enlargement of the regional lymph nodes. In the case of genital chancres these involve the inguinal lymph nodes. When the chancre is located on the lips or the tongue, the submandibular or submental lymph nodes are affected.

Spontaneous resolution of the chancre usually occurs within four to six weeks although exact figures are unknown. In about 60–70% of immuno-competent primary syphilis cases this means spontaneous healing of the disease.[25]

Secondary syphilis

In about 30–40% of untreated patients, a secondary phase begins about six weeks after healing of the primary chancre and results from hematogenous dissemination of the spirochetes. However, secondary signs and symptoms may overlap with primary syphilis, or they may develop as late as six months after the primary lesion has healed. Secondary syphilis affects virtually all organs, including liver, lung, and meninges. Three major features, however, determine the clinical picture: lymphadenopathy, influenza-like symptoms, and mucocutaneous eruptions.

The lymphadenopathy of secondary syphilis is generalized, nontender, and may be long-standing. Nodes are easily palpable in the cervical and axillary chains or in the epitrochlear area. The latter finding makes possible the "dermatologist's handshake" of previous times wherein the epitrochlear node is palpated with the opposite hand while the patient's hand is being shaken.

The presence of influenza-like symptoms underscores the fact that secondary syphilis is a systemic disorder. Headache and upper respiratory symptoms occur early. Signs of pharyngeal irritation, lacrimation, and generalized aching ensue. Fever, malaise, and weight loss may be noticed. Invasion of the reticuloendothelial system may give rise to hepatosplenomegaly.

Eruptions of secondary syphilis may involve the skin, the mucous membranes, and the scalp, and may last for two weeks to one year. In about a quarter of the patients the exanthems wax and wane. A generalized asymptomatic, macular eruption ("roseola") is seen early. The faint pink, blanching, vascular reaction does not have visible scale (Fig. 28.3) and lasts for one to three weeks. It is seen mainly on the trunk and flexures of the limbs and closely resembles a drug eruption or urticaria. It may be difficult to identify on a dark skin. It fades after several days leaving no trace or faint pigmentation. Some lesions may progress to papular syphilides.

The later appearing papular and papulosquamous lesions frequently involve the entire body and have a predilection for the palms and soles (Fig. 28.4). These eruptions are more intensely red than the preceding macular rash, and are often described as copper-colored. Scaling, sharp margination, and dusky redness reminiscent of psoriasis (Fig. 28.5) or lichen planus is seen. Truncal lesions may resemble pityriasis rosea, showing a Christmas tree-like or fernlike array of papules on the back. Lesions at this stage often show residual pigmentary changes after healing. When these lesions involve moist intertrigenous areas of the body they appear as hypertrophic moist papules and plaques, known as condyloma lata, which are highly infectious (Figs 28.6–28.9). The mucosal surfaces are frequently involved in secondary

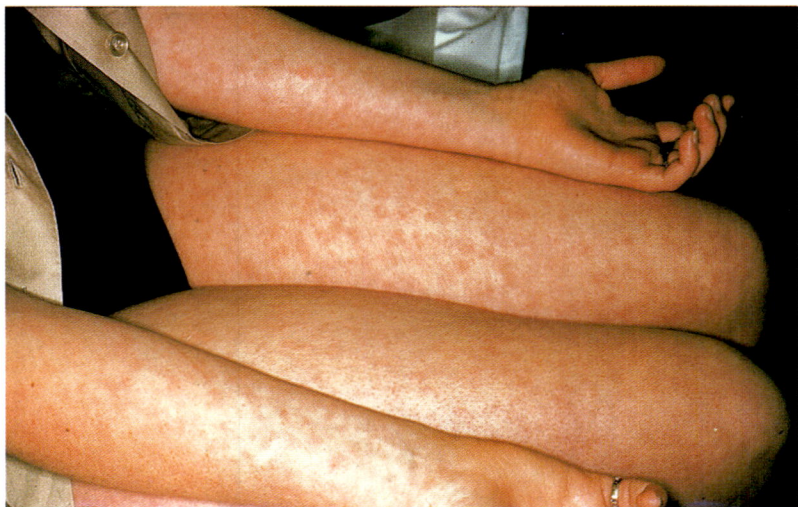

Fig. 28.3 Secondary syphilis: unusual extensive vascular reaction (luetic livedo). (Courtesy J. Moseley, MD)

syphilis either alone or coincidentally with other skin lesions. The mucous patches have a slightly raised, grayish–white margin, and may be eroded or ulcerated centrally (Fig. 28.10). These asymptomatic, highly infectious enanthems can occur on all mucous membranes. A patchy or "moth eaten" alopecia is a characteristic symptom of secondary syphilis (Figs 28.11, 28.12). Hair regrowth occurs with resolution of the secondary stage.

Less common lesions of secondary syphilis include the somewhat linear arrays of papular lesions over the forehead or neck, referred to as either the "crown of Venus" or the "collar of Venus," respectively. Pustular and acneiform lesions may also be seen, especially in debilitated individuals. Necrotic pustular lesions (Fig. 28.13) associated with ulceration and systemic symptoms are described as malignant syphilis. These are seen more frequently in HIV-coinfected individuals.[20] Annular lesions of secondary syphilis are more prevalent in black patients (Fig. 28.14) and are seen most commonly in the midface (Fig. 28.15).

After untreated secondary syphilis heals, about one out of every four patients develops a clinical relapse with secondary features. There is no evidence that a relapse is of prognostic importance with respect to development of late syphilis.[25]

Late syphilis (tertiary disease)

As we learned from the Oslo study, tertiary syphilis occurs in about 1 of 6 patients with untreated secondary syphilis, affecting organs with a different frequency: neurosyphilis 6.5%; cardiovascular disease 10.5%; other forms 2%. In 10.8% of patients, syphilis was the primary cause of death.[25]

Penicillin therapy has produced a dramatic decline in the incidence of all types of tertiary syphilis in developed countries. Neurosyphilis and cardiovascular syphilis have become much less frequent and are virtually absent in the pediatric age group. The recent HIV epidemic has been associated with increased neurosyphilis.[26] Accordingly, the interested reader should consult other texts for a review of tertiary syphilis, including neurosyphilis, cardiovascular syphilis, and late benign syphilis.[1,2,27]

SYPHILIS AND HIV INFECTION

In HIV-infected patients, a concomitant infection with *T. pallidum* is frequently found. The epidemiology of HIV infection varies in different parts of the world. In the United States and Europe heterosexual and mother-to-

25. Gjestland T (1955) The Oslo study of untreated syphilis. **Acta Derm Venereol**, suppl. 34:35.
26. Musher DM, Hamill RJ, Baughn RE (1990) Effect of human immunodeficiency virus (HIV) infection on the course of syphilis and on the response to treatment. **Ann Intern Med** 113:872.

27. Swartz MN (1984) Neurosyphilis. In: Sexually Transmitted Diseases, Holmes KK, Mardh PA, Sparling PF et al. eds. New York: McGraw-Hill, p. 318.

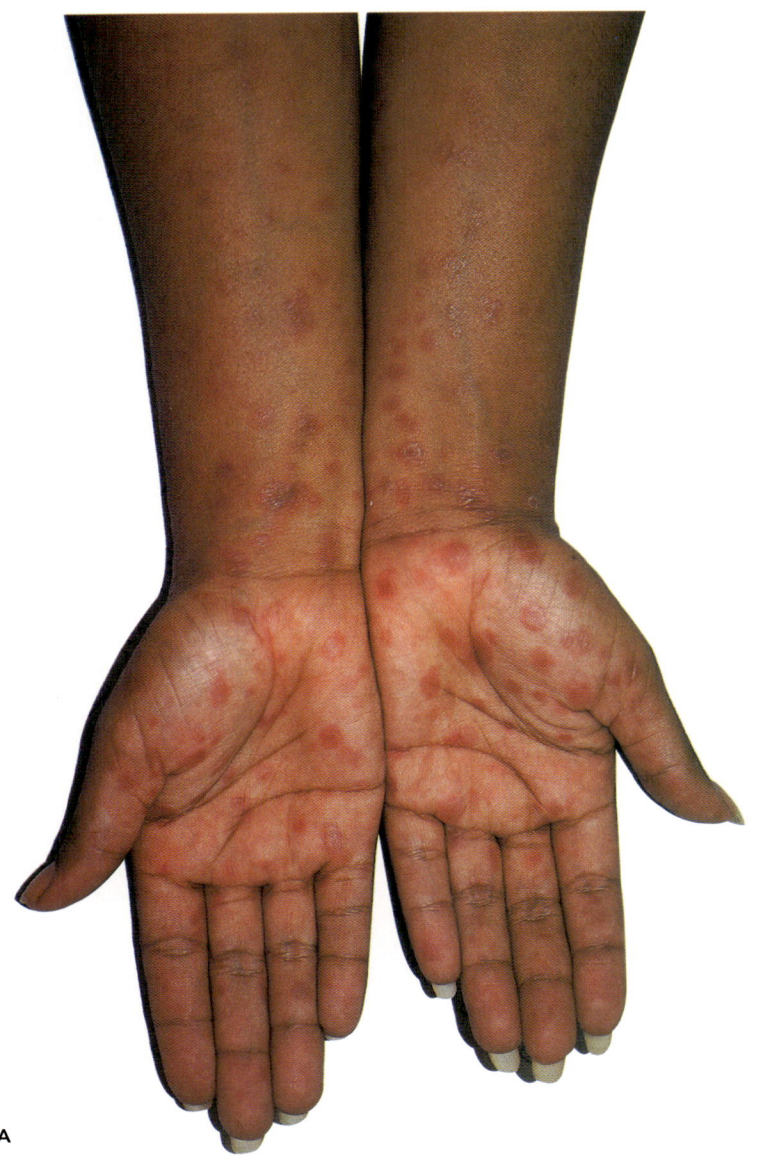
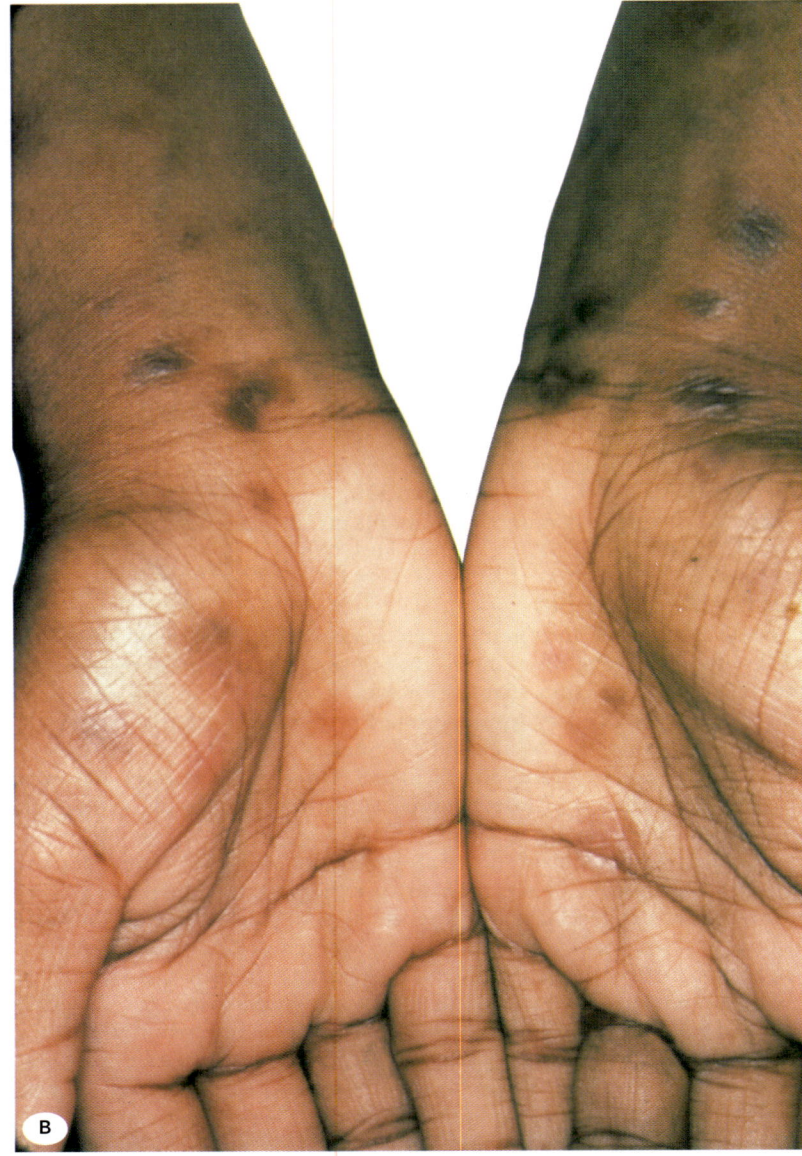

A   **B**

Fig. 28.4A,B   Secondary syphilis. Palmar papulosquamous lesions. (Courtesy of Cape Town University)

child transmission of HIV is increasing while in a large part of the developing world it is the main mode of transmission. The control of STDs, particularly in those populations that are at a high risk for HIV infection, should be of high priority and should be an integral component of AIDS control programs.[28] Among 4863 patients attending two inner-city STD clinics, 24.3% of those with a reactive syphilis serologic test result were HIV infected, whereas 3.5% of patients with a nonreactive test for syphilis were HIV positive. In multivariate analysis, a reactive scrologic test for syphilis was significantly associated with HIV infection in all major risk behaviour categories.[29] Eighty percent of the patients with colorectal syphilis are homosexuals.[30] There is accumulating evidence that genital ulcers facilitate

the transmission of HIV, and they are therefore a marker of high-risk behaviour for acquisition of HIV. Appropriate therapy of patients with genital ulcers (as well as their sexual partners) is mandatory.[19,31]

In HIV-positive women, the frequency of syphilis and *Chlamydia* infection was found to be significantly increased.[32] STD patients were unlikely to know whether they had had sex with an HIV-positive person.[33]

HIV infection is also of increasing significance for children. For example, in one series 28 victims of sexual abuse were infected with HIV. Coinfection with another STD occurred in nine (33%) cases.[34]

The clinical appearance of syphilis in HIV disease is similar to the symptoms described above, but the lesions tend to be larger, more inflammatory, eroded,

28. Moss GB, Kreiss JK (1990) The interrelationship between human immunodeficiency virus infection and other sexually transmitted diseases. **Med Clin North Am** 74:1647.
29. Quinn TC, Cannon RO, Glasser D et al. (1990) The association of syphilis with risk of human immunodeficiency virus infection in patients attending sexually transmitted disease clinics. **Arch Intern Med** 150:1297.
30. Wexner SD (1990) Sexually transmitted diseases of the colon, rectum, and anus. The challenges of the nineties. **Dis Colon Rectum** 33:1048.
31. Schmid GP (1990) Approach to the patient with genital ulcer disease. **Med Clin North Am** 74:1559.
32. Kell PD, Barton SE, Summerbell CD et al. (1991) Sexually transmitted diseases in HIV 1 seropositive women at presentation. **Int J STD AIDS** 2:204.
33. Holtedahl KA, Doumenc M, Steinert S et al. (1991) Patients with sexually transmitted disease: a well-defined HIV risk group in general practice? **Fam Pract** 8:42.
34. Gellert GA, Durfee MJ, Berkowitz CD et al. (1993) Situational and sociodemographic characteristics of children infected with human immunodeficiency virus from pediatric sexual abuse. **Pediatrics** 91:39.

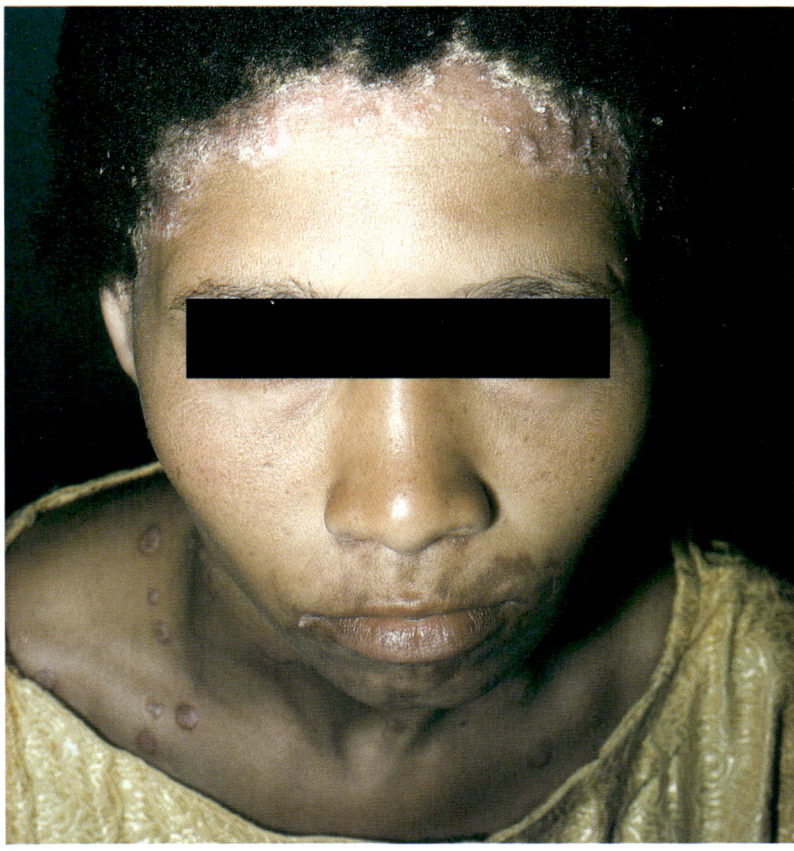

Fig. 28.5 Secondary syphilis. Papulosquamous lesions in a young girl's scalp. (Courtesy of Cape Town University)

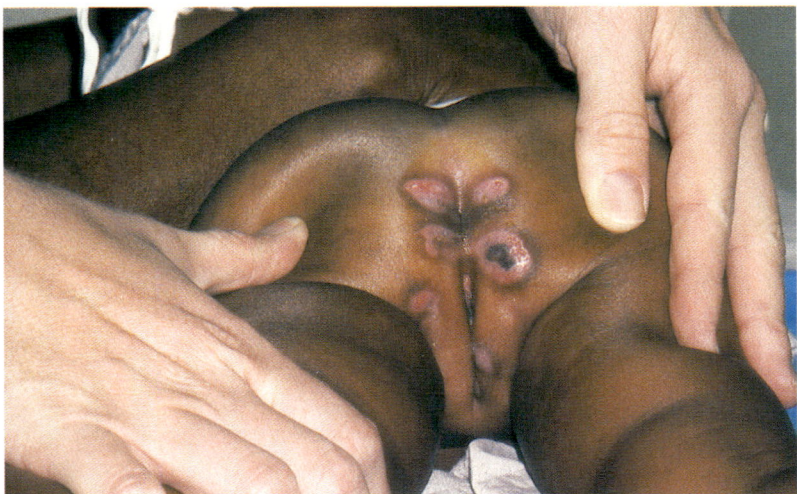

Fig. 28.6 Secondary syphilis. Multiple flat-topped syphilis condylomata (condylomata lata) of the perineum. (Courtesy of Cape Town University)

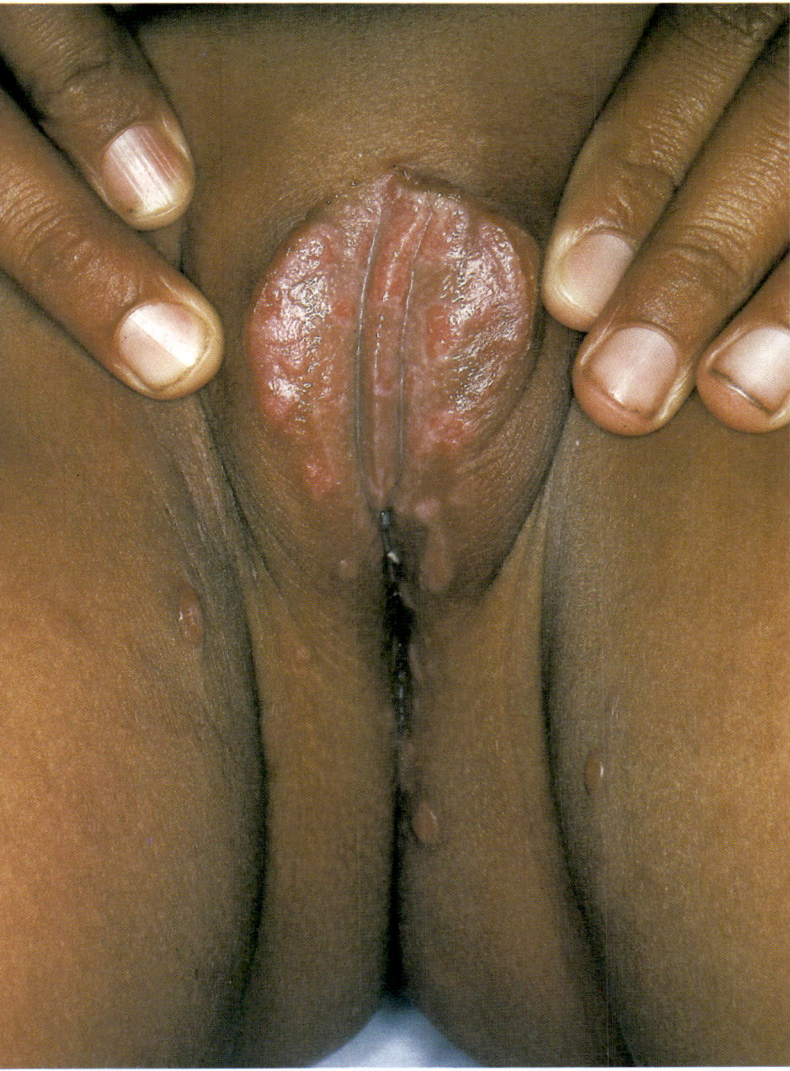

Fig. 28.7 Secondary syphilis. Multiple flat-topped syphilis condylomata (condylomata lata) of the genitalia. (Courtesy of Cape Town University)

CONGENITAL SYPHILIS (PRENATAL SYPHILIS)

A pregnant woman with untreated or inadequately treated syphilis can transmit the infection to her fetus via the placenta. Formerly, it was believed that infection of the fetus could not occur prior to the 16th week of pregnancy. However, studies during the 1970s on abortuses from syphilitic women infected with syphilis showed that transplacental transmission of spirochetes does occur prior to the fourth month of gestation. A study from Kenya compared the role of STDs as risk factors for spontaneous abortion in a case-controlled study. The result of the study demonstrated spontaneous abortion to be independently associated with maternal HIV-1 antibody (odds ratio: 2.3), and with maternal syphilis seroreactivity (odds ratio: 4.3), whereas no association was found with maternal gonococcal infection.[35] Most of the fetal damage in congenital syphilis occurs after the fourth month of gestation. Therefore, early treatment should diminish the risk of severe defects of the newborn.

When compared with the disease of the adult, prenatally acquired syphilis can be taken as analogous to severe secondary syphilis, because many clinical

and scaling, and are similar to "malignant syphilis." This occurs not only in the stage of acquired immunodeficiency syndrome (AIDS) but also in earlier stages of HIV disease.

35. Temmerman M, Lopita MI, Sanghvi HC et al. (1992) The role of maternal syphilis, gonorrhoea and HIV-1 infections in spontaneous abortion. Int J STD AIDS 3:418.

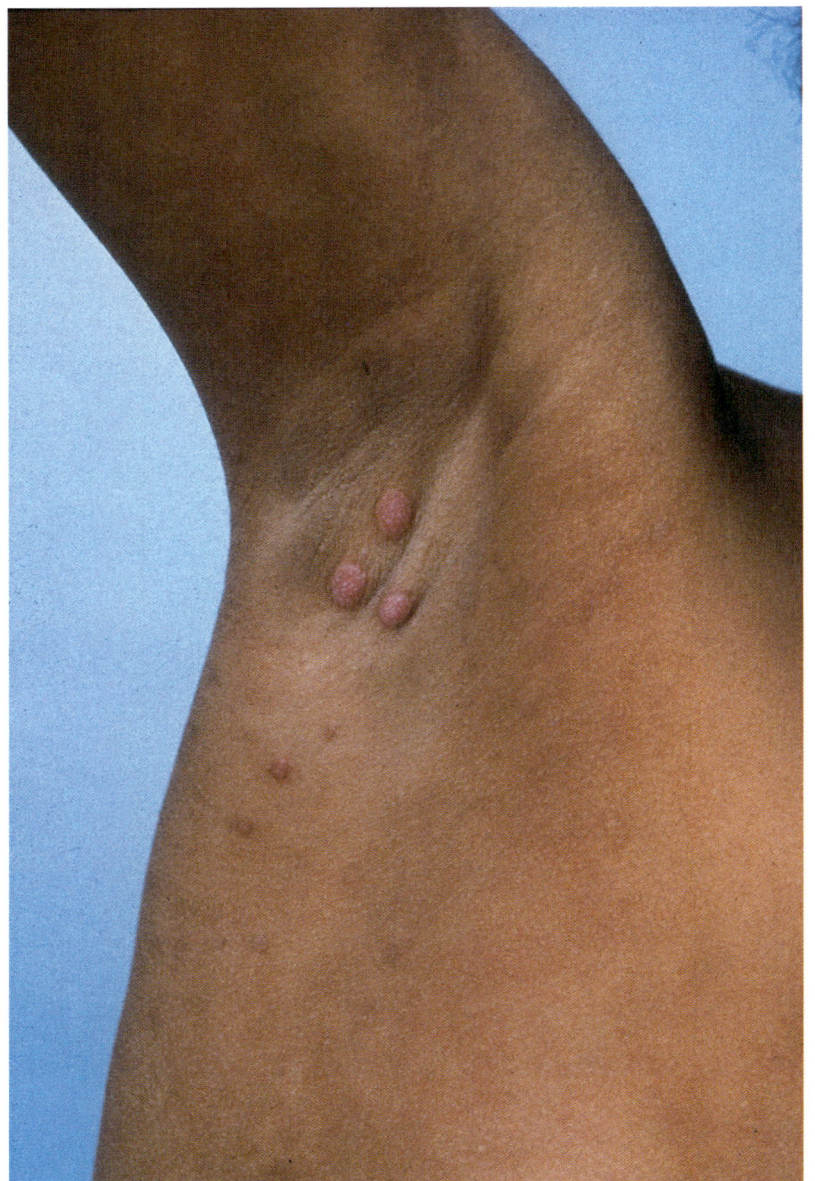

Fig. 28.8 Secondary syphilis. Multiple flat-topped syphilis condylomata (condylomata lata) of the axilla. (Courtesy of Cape Town University)

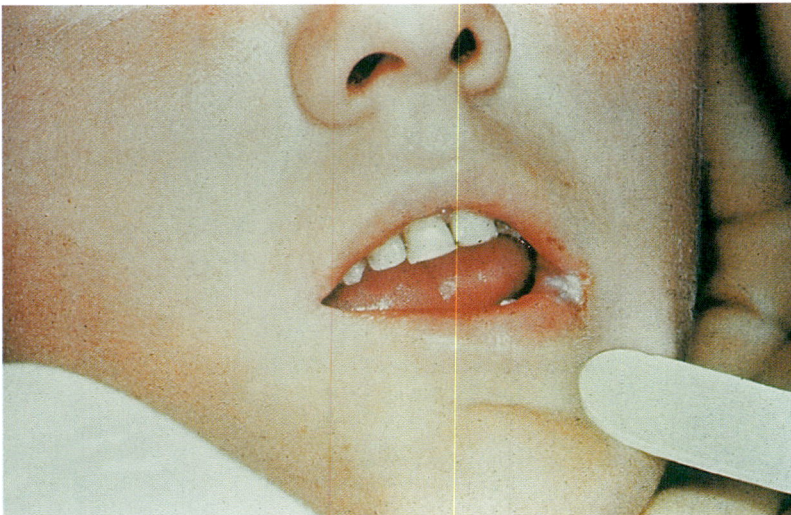

Fig. 28.9 Secondary syphilis. Split papules (condylomata lata) of the lip.

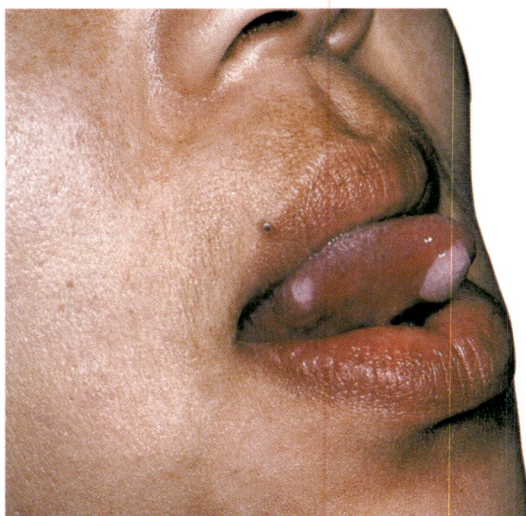

Fig. 28.10 Secondary syphilis. Mucous patches in a young woman. (Courtesy of Cape Town University)

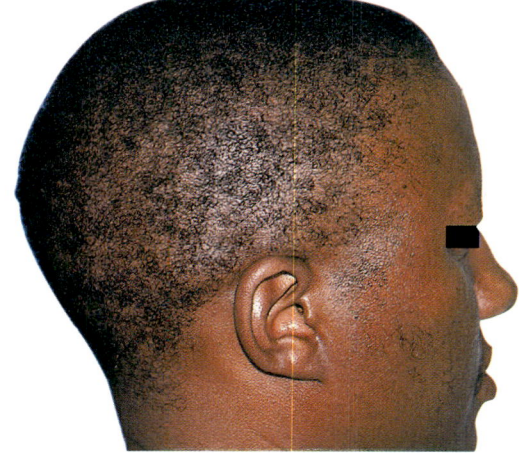

Fig. 28.11 Secondary syphilis. Patchy (moth-eaten) alopecia in an adolescent. (Courtesy of Cape Town University)

findings seen in early congenital syphilis represent an exaggeration of the findings of secondary syphilis in an adult. Severe effects may be noted in organogenesis and growth, resulting in fetal wastage.

Early congenital syphilis

Early congenital syphilis presents in the first two years of life. Clinical features observed in a series of 206 consecutive cases are shown in Table 28.2.[36,37] No generally accepted diagnostic criteria for early congenital syphilis have been established. Table 28.3 is a modification of those suggested by Rathbun.[37] Influenza-like (respiratory) features, generalized involvement of the reticuloendothelial system, and mucocutaneous findings are common. In the developing fetus, however, severe multisystem involvement may occur, resulting in an extremely small-for-date newborn. Such infants with marasmic syphilis have a particularly poor prognosis. The influenza-like features include irritability, poor feeding, lacrimation, rhinitis (so-called snuffles) (Fig. 28.16A, B), hoarse crying, and fever. Generalized lymphadenopathy and hepato-

36. Lowy G (1979) Syphilis in a children's hospital. Presented at the International Congress of Pediatric Dermatology, Chicago.

37. Rathbun KC (1983) Congenital syphilis: a proposal for improved surveillance, diagnosis, and treatment. **Sex Transm Dis** 10:102.

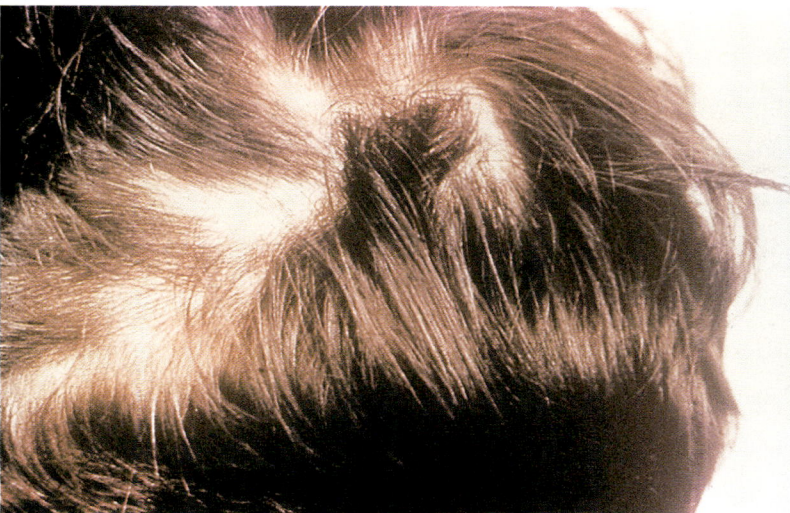

Fig. 28.12 Secondary syphilis. Patchy (moth-eaten) alopecia in an adolescent.

splenomegaly are frequently present. All of these features may be absent at birth but subsequently develop during the first 2–4 weeks of life.

Similarly, mucocutaneous lesions are not always present at birth, but may develop during the neonatal period. These lesions are mostly morbilliform or papulosquamous in appearance (Figs 28.16A, 28.17), but two distinctive patterns in congenital syphilis deserve emphasis. Vesiculobullous lesions and eroded lesions (Figs 28.18, 28.19), sometimes hemorrhagic, can be seen especially on the distal parts of arms and legs. In other cases, a dry scaly desquamation can be seen (Figs 28.19, 28.20) either as a generalized phenomenon, or as a localized change in the periungual areas. This dry, desquamating eruption may occur as a major feature or as a sequela of the vesiculobullous phase. Living treponemas are present in any of these lesions that are therefore highly contagious. Less common lesions are the mucous membrane changes and large papules of the anogenital region. Purpura and petechiae may be seen when severe thrombocytopenia is present (Fig. 28.21). In cases of severe anemia, "blueberry muffin" nodules may be seen (Fig. 28.22), representing cutaneous islands of extramedullary hematopoiesis.

Systemic involvement is more frequent and prominent in early congenital syphilis when compared with the disease in adulthood. Hepatomegaly is common and florid hepatitis is frequently seen. Hemolytic anemia, sometimes associated with a cold hemolysin phenomenon, is often seen, as is thrombo-cytopenia. On X-rays, signs of osteochondritis or periostitis of the proximal tibia or distal fibula are observed in most infected infants (Fig. 28.23). Clinical features of dactylitis are less frequent. Periosteal lesions of other bones, in particular of the skull, may likewise be part of late congenital syphilis. Involvement of the CNS is common. Abnormal findings in the cerebrospinal fluid (lymphocytes, elevated protein, and nontreponemal antibodies) may be seen in 50% of affected infants, but a manifest neurosyphilis is less common.[38] Accordingly, treatment should be sufficient to clear a CNS infection (see Treatment). Because meningovascular involvement is often present in congenital syphilis, ultimate neurologic prognosis should be regarded as doubtful.

Late congenital syphilis

A certain number of stigmata of late congenital syphilis have been summarized.[39,40] According to definition, late congenital syphilis begins at age 2 years. The number of treponemata surviving in the tissue has decreased when this stage has been reached, and thus patients with late congenital syphilis are usually noninfectious.

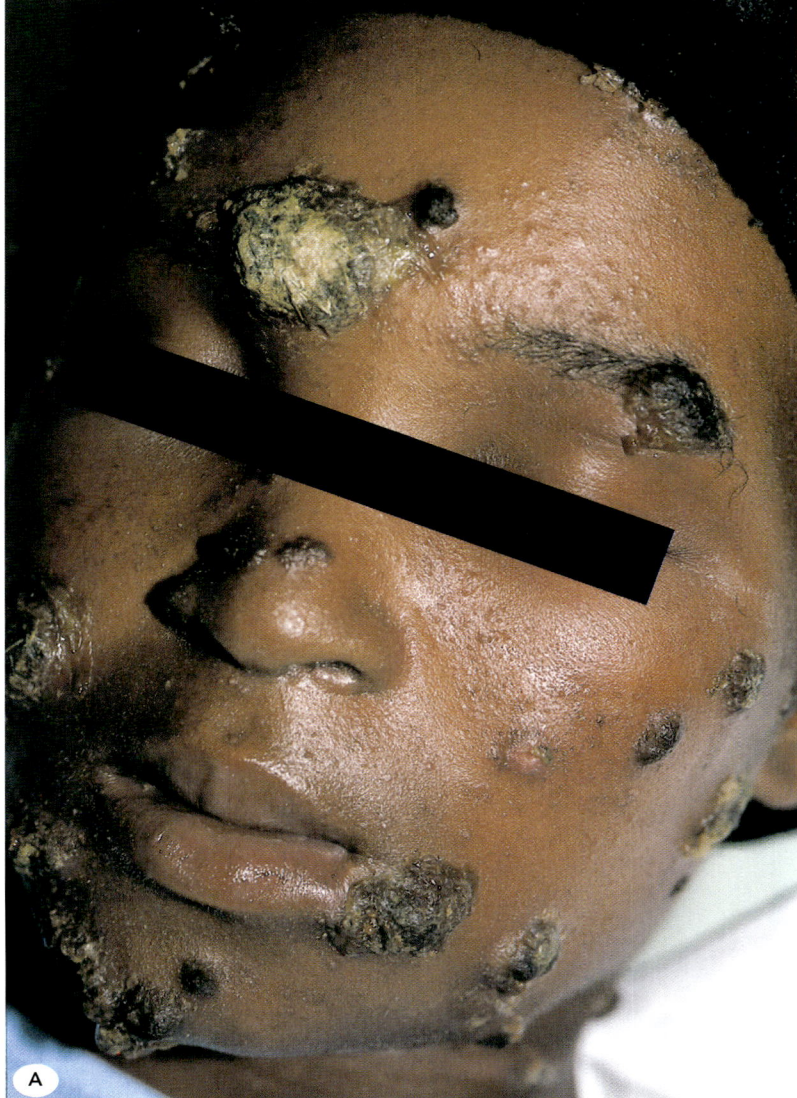

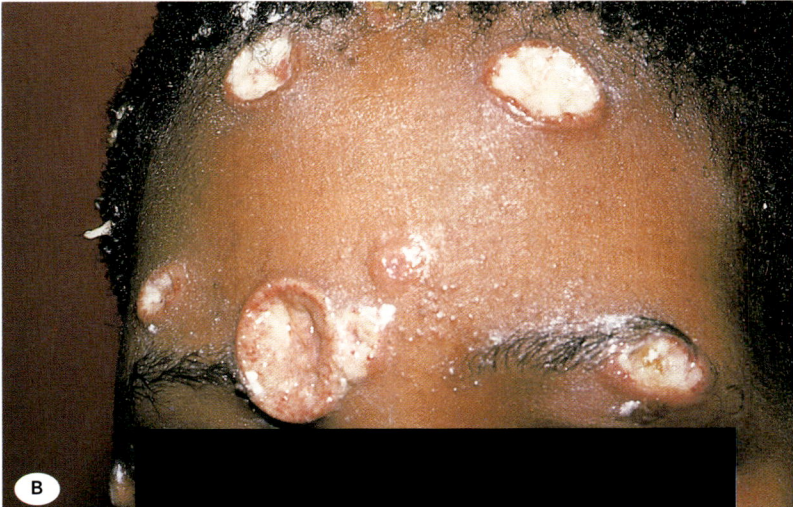

Fig. 28.13 Secondary syphilis. Nodular ulcerative lesions (**A**) before and (**B**) after crust removal in a young girl. (Courtesy of Cape Town University)

38. Murphy KF, Patamasucon P (1984) Congenital syphilis. In: Sexually Transmitted Diseases, Holmes KK, Mardth P-A. Sparling PF et al. eds. New York: McGraw-Hill, p. 352.

39. Albright RE Jr, Christenson RH, Emlet JL et al. (1991) Issues in cerebrospinal fluid management. CSF Venereal Disease Research Laboratory testing. **Am J Clin Pathol** 95:397.

40. Fiumara NJ, Lessel S (1983) The stigmata of late congenital syphilis: an analysis of 100 patients. **Sex Transm Dis** 10:126.

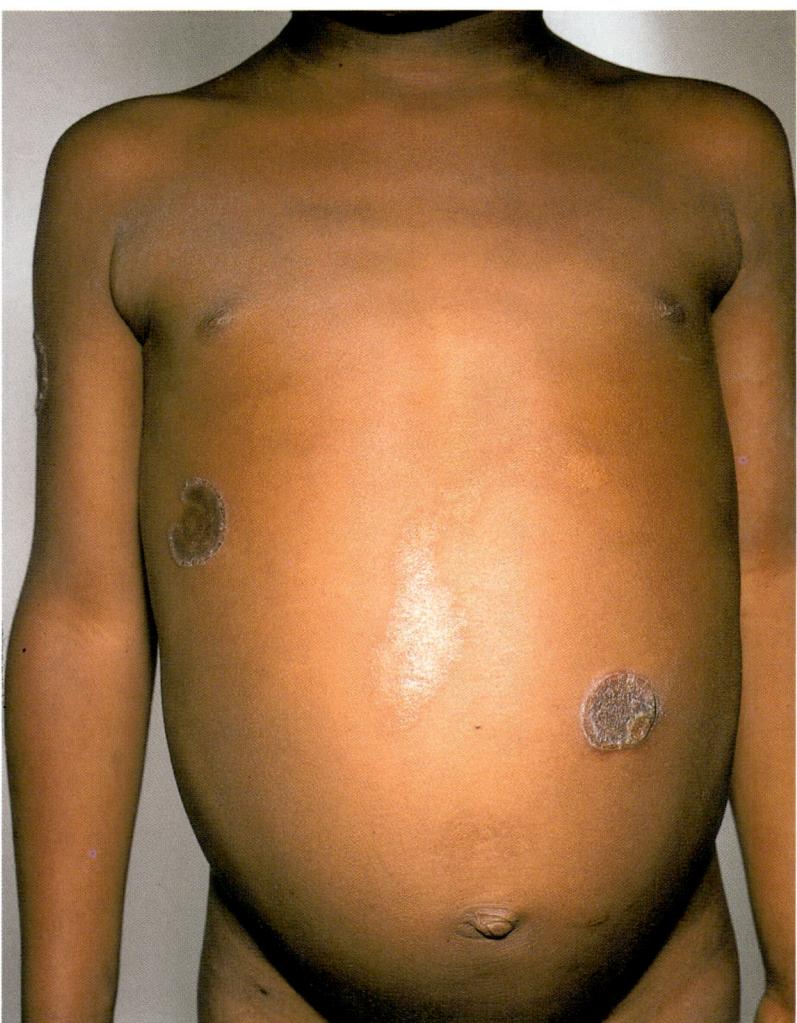

Fig. 28.14 Secondary syphilis. Annular lesions in a young boy with lymphadenopathy and hepatosplenomegaly. (Courtesy of Cape Town University)

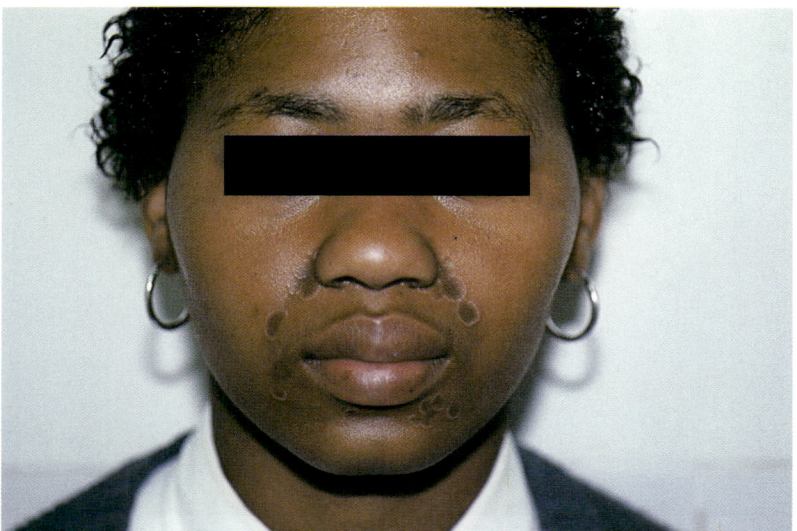

Fig. 28.15 Secondary syphilis. Annular lesions of the face in a young woman. (Courtesy of Cape Town University)

Today, late congenital syphilis has become a rare condition. If infants born to serologically positive mothers are managed as potential cases of congenital syphilis, these late sequelae of prenatal syphilis could be eliminated. Because

TABLE 28.2   Manifestations of early congenital syphilis based on 206 consecutive cases

	Percentage
Onset of clinical signs	
At birth	32
By 4 weeks	64
Specific manifestations	
Pain on handling (pseudoparalysis of Parrot)	38
Nasal congestion (snuffles)	18
Persistent irritability	11
Organomegaly	
Hepatosplenomegaly	48
Hepatomegaly	17
Splenomegaly	5
Skin lesions	51
Palmoplantar scaling	44
Maculopapular and papulosquamous	14
Eroded intertriginous papules	17
Periorificial rhagades	14
Seborrheic-like dermatitis	2
Palmoplantar bullae, hemorrhagic	0
Bone lesions (osteochondritis, periostitis)	80

Other potential findings: anemia, thrombocytopenia, disseminated intravascular coagulation, nephrotic syndrome, generalized lymphadenopathy, peritonitis, pneumonia alba, uveitis, chorioretinitis, glaucoma, pancreatitis, enteritis, placental inflammation.

(Data from Lowy,[36] and Rathbun.[37])

the clinical findings may be subtle in an individual patient, most children or young adults with this disease are ascertained and treated because of positive serologic findings that were obtained for routine or other reasons. As in early congenital syphilis no definite, generally accepted diagnostic criteria have so far been established. Table 28.4 presents an approach that combines the criteria of Rathbun[37] with the diagnostic features proposed by Fiumara and Lessel.[40]

The stigmata of late congenital syphilis will be discussed in decreasing order of incidence. Percentages listed are those of Fiumara and Lessel.[40]

1. Frontal bossing of Parrot (87%). Persistent periostitis of the frontal and parietal bones results in an overhanging deformity of the forehead. Although this is present in most patients, the finding may not be dramatic in individual cases, and is readily overlooked.

2. Shortening of the maxillary bones (83%). Syphilitic infection of the bones of the midface gives rise to underdeveloped maxillae. In fact, the predilection for visible changes due to syphilis in the midface is responsible for several other listed features, including the saddle nose, high palatal arch, and a relative protuberance of the mandible (see below).

3. High palatal arch (76%). Underdevelopment of the maxillae causes a heightening of the palatal arch, and this is seen most patients with late congenital syphilis. Palatal perforation may also occur.

4. Saddle nose (73%). Underdevelopment of the nasal bones and cartilage results in this proximal deformity, depression of the base of the nose. Septal perforation may also result from the chronic, ulcerative rhinitis. A saddle nose is often the first recognized sign of congenital syphilis.

5. Mulberry molars (65%). The sixth-year molar, or first lower molar, normally has four well-defined cusps. The mulberry molars of late congenital syphilis have numerous poorly formed cusps, surmounting a rather dome-shaped tooth, which is considerably narrower on the grinding surface than it is at the base (gingival surface). Like Hutchinson's teeth, these molars have a poor enamel structure and are easily injured and subject to caries. Consequently, one may retrospectively identify patients with late congenital syphilis who have had these teeth extracted, or fitted with crowns. Only 71% of Fiumara and Lessel's second series

TABLE 28.3 Suggested diagnostic criteria for early congenital syphilis (patients younger than 2 years of age)[a]

Clinical criteria

Absolute
Specimen from skin or genital lesions showing *Treponema pallidum* on dark-field examination.

Major
Positive VDRL[b] of CSF
"Condylomata lata"
Osteochondritis, periostitis
Snuffles, hemorrhagic rhinitis, rhagades
Vesiculobullous lesions, typical papulosquamous pa moplantar rash, or diffuse acral scaling

Minor
Mucous patches
Hepatomegaly, splenomegaly
Generalized lymphadenopathy
Central nervous system signs
Hemolytic anemia, diffuse intravascular coagulation, thrombocytopenia
Elevated cell count or protein in CSF
Pneumonitis
Edema, ascites
Placental villitis or vasculitis
Intrauterine growth retardation

Serologic criteria

Major
Fourfold rise in VDRL[b] over 3 months and positive FTA-ABS[c] after birth

Minor
Positive VDRL[b] after 4 months of age
Positive FTA-ABS[c] after 1 year of age

Epidemiologic criteria

Major
Untreated early maternal syphilis (within 4 weeks of delivery)

Minor
Untreated late latent maternal syphilis
Early maternal syphilis within 3 months of delivery
Maternal contact with early syphilis during pregnancy
Maternal syphilis treatment during pregnancy with a drug other than penicillin
Maternal treatment for syphilis during pregnancy but not followed serologically to delivery

[a] Diagnose with certainty when patient meets: (1) absolute criterion; (2) one major criterion plus one major or minor criterion from another category; or (3) one minor criterion from each of the three categories.
[b] VDRL, generic designation for all nontreponemal or reaginic tests to include RPR, etc.
[c] FTA-ABS designates all treponemal tests to include TPI, MHA-TP, etc.
(Modified from Rathbun[37])

showed mulberry molars, but the remainder were edentulous and presumably likewise affected.[40]

6. Hutchinson's teeth (63%). These abnormal upper central incisors erupt at about age 6 years, similar in time to the appearance of mulberry molars. Hutchinson's teeth tend to be tapered, or peg-shaped, and a central enamel defect allows for the characteristic notched appearance (Fig. 28.24). Because of the poor vitality of these teeth, similar to the mulberry molars, extraction and various stages of restorative work may obscure the nature of Hutchinson's teeth. Alert pediatric dentists may well suspect congenital syphilis in patients showing carious changes in poorly formed central incisors, or lower first molars. Both mulberry molars and Hutchinson's teeth are so specific for late congenital syphilis that these two signs should be considered major or even absolute diagnostic criteria (Table 28.4).

7. Proximal clavicular thickening or Higoumenakis's sign (39%). Periostitis of the proximal portion of the clavicle, near the sternal attachment, gives

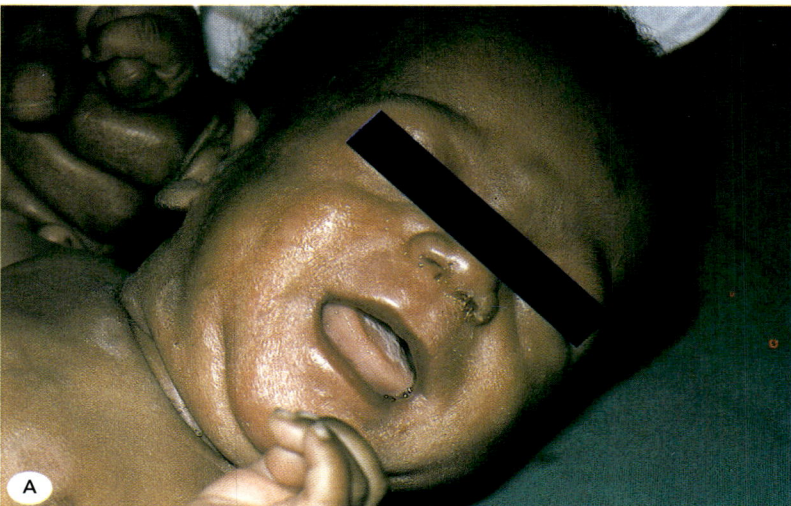
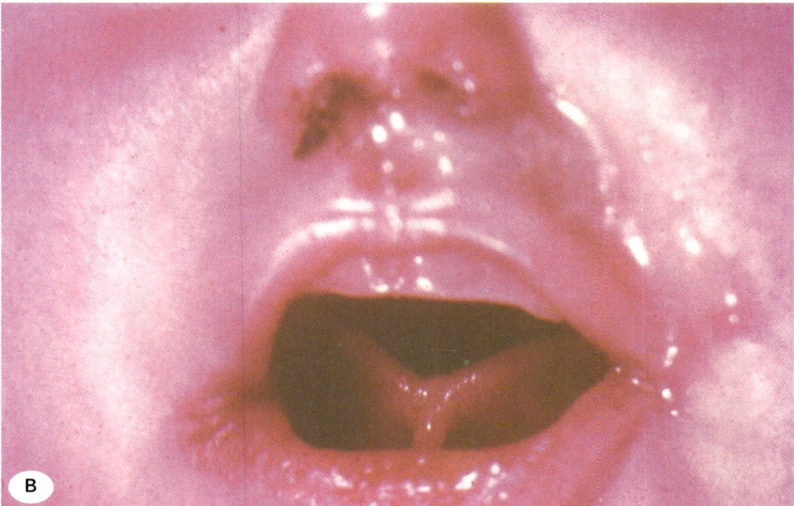

Fig. 28.16A,B Early congenital syphilis. Rhinitis (snuffles), (A) psoriasiform lesions and (B) mucous patches. (A, Courtesy of Cape Town University)

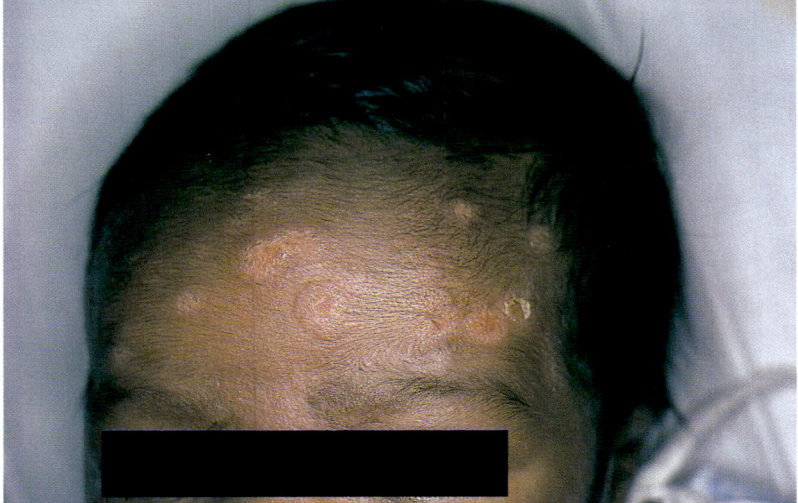

Fig. 28.17 Early congenital syphilis. Psoriasiform lesions of the face. (Courtesy of Cape Town University)

rise to a clinically visible and palpable thickening. Because of the frequency of clavicular injuries in children and specifically clavicular

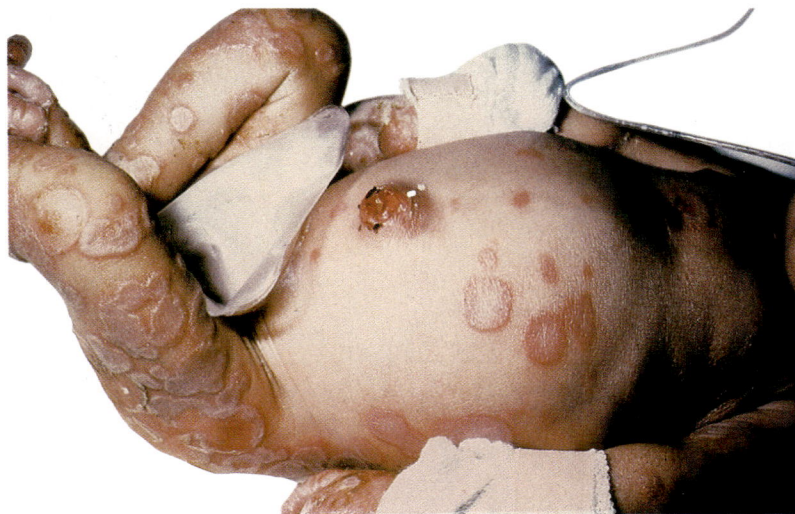

Fig. 28.18 Early congenital syphilis. Erosive vesiculobullous lesions. (Courtesy of Cape Town University)

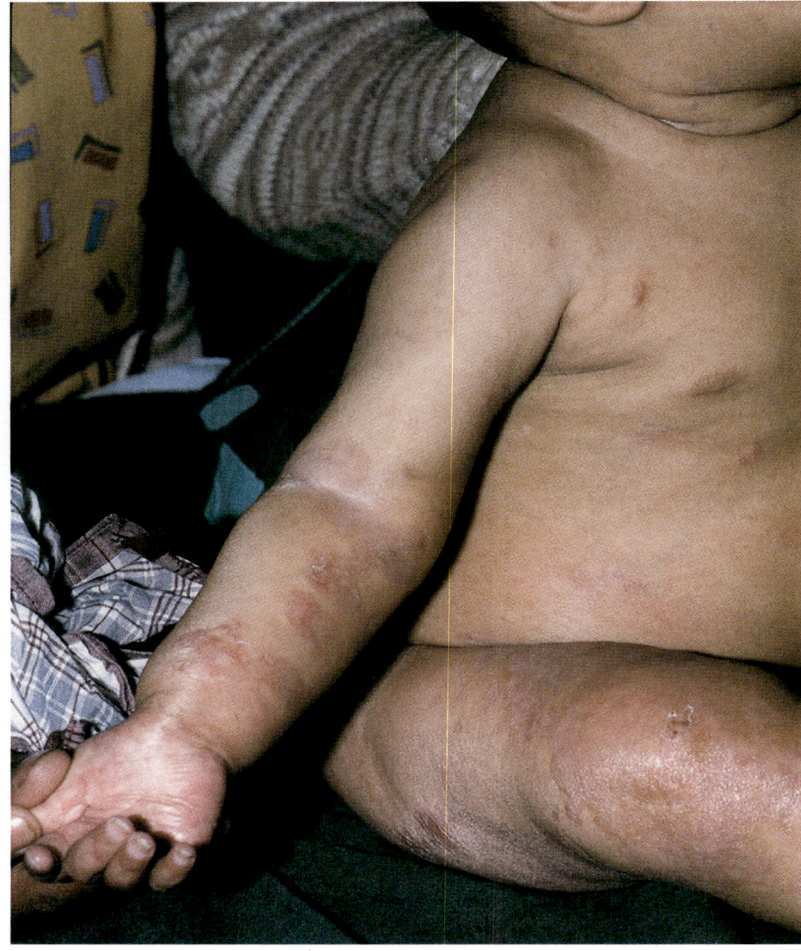

Fig. 28.20 Early congenital syphilis. Generalized flaky desquamation with acral accentuation. (Courtesy of Cape Town University)

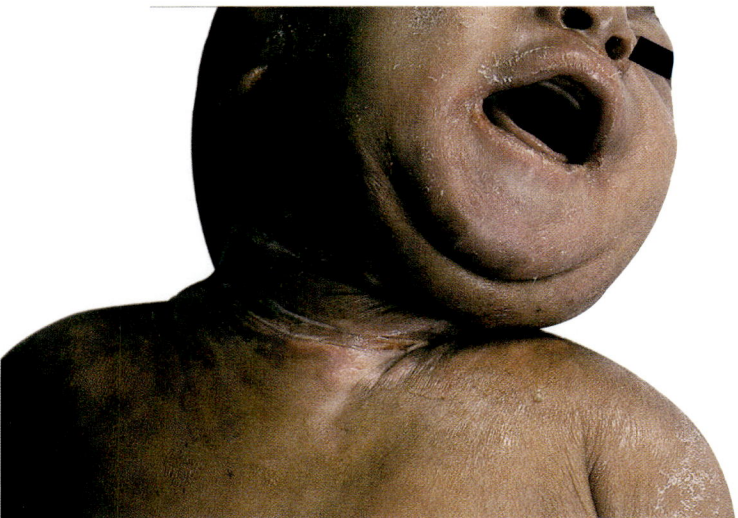

Fig. 28.19 Early congenital syphilis. Erosive vesiculobullous lesions with flaky desquamation of the face. (Courtesy of Cape Town University)

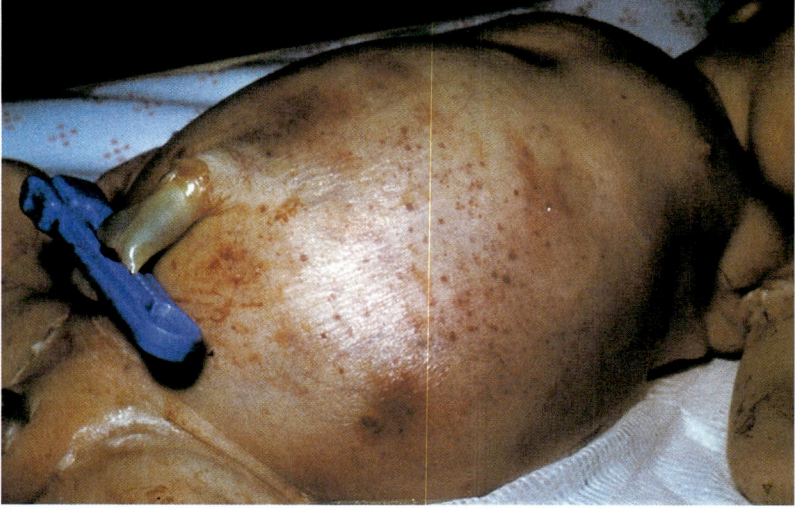

Fig. 28.21 Early congenital syphilis. Thrombocytopenia with petechiae and purpura. (Courtesy of Cape Town University)

fractures in the newborn, this may be a less reliable sign than some of the other stigmata. However, it was present in a high percentage of the series studied by Fiumara.

8. Relative protuberance of the mandible (26%). This change is apparent only because of the under development of the maxillae, giving the illusion of a large jaw. Therefore it fits into the spectrum of midfacial underdevelopment.

9. Interstitial keratitis (9%). Once considered a classical feature of congenital syphilis, interstitial keratitis now is an uncommon finding (Fig. 28.25). It tends to appear in later childhood, or even past the teenage years. Lacrimation, blepharospasm, and photophobia accompany clinical inflammation. Ultimately, corneal erosion and neovascularization may occur and blindness may result. The condition is usually bilateral. Aggressive ophthalmologic treatment with anti-inflammatory agents is needed, since this problem is not penicillin-responsive. It is presumably a late, immunologically mediated reactive inflammatory condition.

10. Rhagades (7%). This finding usually overlaps with the early congenital syphilis stigmata. Rhagades persist into childhood and adult life as fine linear scars, especially seen periorifically. These can occur as radiating lines around the eyes, nose, mouth, and anal orifices. In the child or teenager, this might be mistaken as a premature, actinically induced wrinkling of the skin. As indicated in Table 28.4, rhagades are uncommon in congenital syphilis today.

11. Saber shin (4%). Periostitis seems to weaken the mid- and anterior portions of the tibiae, causing an anterior bowing. Much less common today, this

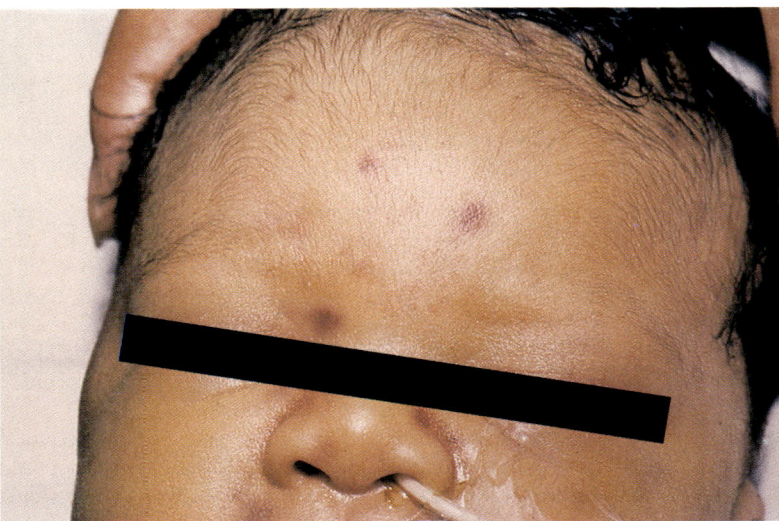

Fig. 28.22 Early congenital syphilis. Extramedullary hematopoiesis, "blueberry muffin" spots. (Courtesy of Cape Town University)

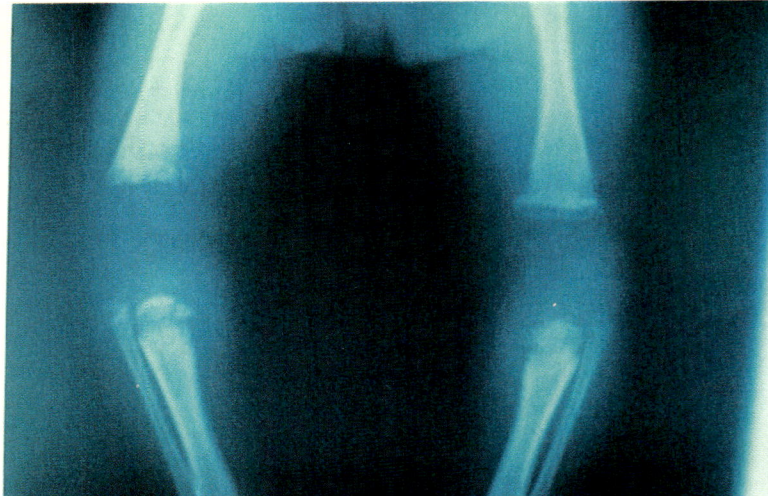

Fig. 28.23 Early congenital syphilis. Prominent proximal tibial lesions may be seen. (Courtesy of Cape Town University)

TABLE 28.4 Suggested diagnostic criteria for late congenital syphilis (patient older than two years)[a]
Absolute criteria[b]
Mulberry molars (65%)
Notched incisors (Hutchinson's teeth) (63%)
Epidemiologic criteria
Untreated maternal syphilis
Positive maternal FTA-ABS
Sibling with congenital syphilis
Serologic Criteria
Positive VDRL test[c]
Positive FTA-ABS[c] (VDRL and FTA-ABS are used in a generic sense for nontreponemal and treponemal tests)
Clinical criteria[b]
Frontal bossae (Parrot) (87%)
Shortened maxilla (83%)
High palatal arch (76%), perforation (73%)
Sternoclavicular thickening (Higoumenakis's sign) (39%)
Relative mandibular prominence (26%)
Interstitial keratitis (96%)
Rhagades (7%)
Saber shin (4%)
Nerve deafness[c] (3%)
Scaphoid scapula (1%)
Clutton's joints (0.3%)
Gummas[c]
Paresis, paralysis[c]
Delayed mental development, seizures, hydrocephalus[†]

[a] Diagnose with certainty when patient meets: (1) any absolute criterion; or (2) one criterion from at least two categories.
[b] Where percentages appear next to clinical stigmata these are based on Fiumara and Lessel.[40]
[c] These criteria should be considered only when it is unlikely that they could be caused by acquired syphilis.
[†] These criteria should be considered only when other diagnoses have been excluded. (Modified from Rathbun[37])

sign may have required the presence of vitamin D deficiency rickets as a cofactor to have reached the 40% prevalence levels previously cited.[41]

12. Deafness (3%). Unilateral or bilateral 8th nerve deafness develops somewhere between early childhood and the teenage years. Symptoms of labyrinthitis may precede the high-frequency hearing loss. Because of its unilaterality, patients may well escape detection. Along with mumps and rubella, syphilis should be considered in the infectious etiologies of hearing loss in childhood. The classical Hutchinson's triad consists of Hutchinson's teeth, interstitial keratitis, and 8th nerve deafness. Since both nerve deafness and interstitial keratitis are currently seen in fewer than 10% of patients with late congenital syphilis, this classical triad is no longer a significant clinical complex.

13. Scaphoid scapula (1%). Syphilitic involvement of the scapulae results in a dished-out appearance of the vertebral border of the scapulae bilaterally. This is an uncommon manifestation of late congenital syphilis.

14. Clutton's joint. Not found in early childhood, bilateral knee swelling occurs sometimes during the second decade of life. This is a painful synovitis, causing cartilage destruction. It eventually subsides. Serologic

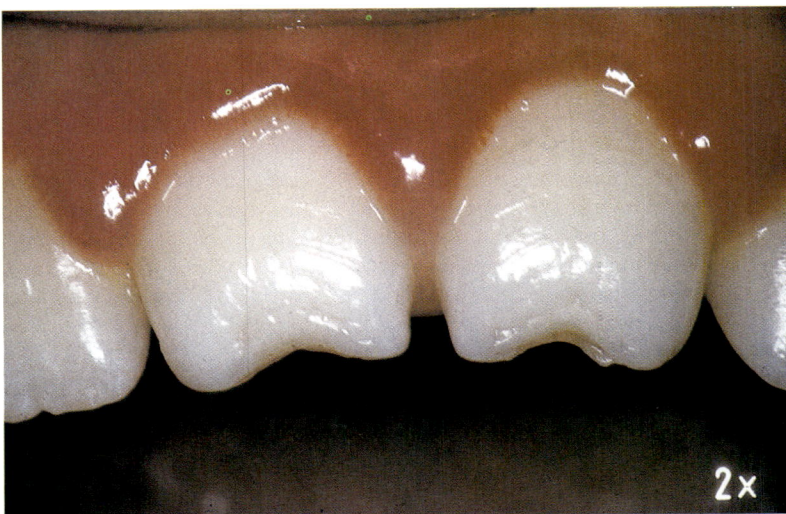

Fig. 28.24 Late congenital syphilis. Hutchinson's teeth are shown. (Courtesy of Cape Town University)

testing of synovial fluid will be positive, but the condition is not improved by penicillin therapy. It is seen rarely today in late congenital syphilis, and

41. Fulkerson AR (1981) Congenital syphilis. J Assoc Military Dermatol 3:7.

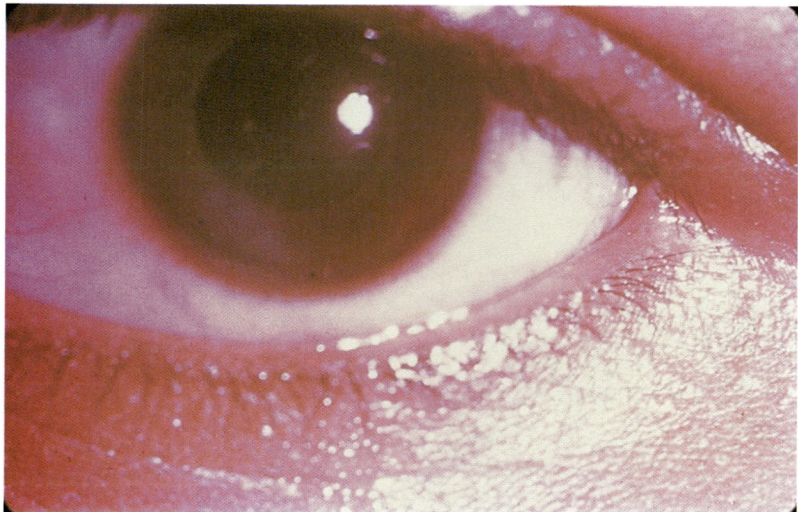

Fig. 28.25 Late congenital syphilis. Interstitial keratitis. (Courtesy of J. Moseley, MD)

was present in only 1 of 271 patients in Fiumara's initial series, and in none of 100 patients in his second series.[40]

Untreated meningovascular syphilis (early congenital syphilis) can be inferred from the presence of seizures, mental retardation, or hydrocephalus persisting into the later childhood years. On the other hand, symptomatic neurosyphilis due to late congenital syphilis is quite rare and usually delayed until adolescence. When it occurs, it may be more severe than the corresponding acquired disease. Juvenile paresis is the most common form. This syphilitic encephalopathy may present with predominantly psychotic symptoms of emotional lability, and bizarre behavior.[38]

DIAGNOSIS OF SYPHILIS

As clinical signs and symptoms of syphilis may not allow one to establish a diagnosis, it is important to have objective instruments to confirm the infection.[1,3,4,42] These include the demonstration of (1) treponema, (2) antibodies in serum, and (3) characteristic histologic features. The value of these investigations varies with the stage of the disease. The Centers for Disease Control and Prevention (CDC) Guidelines[43] provides full details for the diagnosis of syphilis.

Dark field examination and direct fluorescent antibody tests of lesion exudate or tissue are definitive methods for diagnosing early syphilis. The cleaned exudating surface of a lesion is pressed against a microscope slide. Desiccation, which immobilizes the spirochetes, is prevented by the addition of a few drops of warm saline and immediate occlusion of the specimen under a coverslip. Motile spirochetes are identified using dark-field or phase contrast microscopy. Alternately, *dried* smears can be stained with antibodies specific for *T. pallidum* providing for a permanent record. This technique is time consuming but requires less expertise.

Three consecutive negative examinations are required to exclude syphilis from the differential diagnosis. Saprophytic spirochetes may cause great confusion on material collected from mouth or vaginal mucosa. Characteristically, however, *T. pallidum* is tightly coiled, rotates continuously, and alternately bends in the middle and extends as it is viewed in the microscope.

A presumptive diagnosis is possible with the use of two types of serologic tests:

a. nontreponemal (e.g., Venereal Disease Research Laboratory {VDRL} and rapid plasma reagin RPR)
b. treponemal (e.g., fluorescent treponemal antibody absorbed {FTA-ABS} and microhemagglutination assay for antibody to *T. pallidum* {MHA-TP}).

Nontreponemal test antibody titers correlate with disease activity and are quantitatively expressed. The nontreponemal tests usually become nonreactive after treatment; however, in some patients, nontreponemal antibodies can persist at a low titer for prolonged periods, possibly for life. Treponemal test antibody titers correlate poorly with disease activity and should not be used to assess treatment response. Most patients who have reactive treponemal tests will have reactive tests for life. However, up to 25% of patients treated during the primary stage might revert to being serologically nonreactive after a few years.

Sequential serologic tests should be performed by using the same testing method (e.g., VDRL or RPR), preferably by the same laboratory. A four-fold change in titer (equivalent to a change of two dilutions) for the same serologic test is considered clinically significant.

HIV-infected patients can have abnormal serologic test results[22,27] but for most HIV-infected patients, serologic tests appear to be accurate and reliable for the diagnosis of syphilis and for evaluation of treatment response.

No single test can be used to diagnose all cases of neurosyphilis, which is best made using various combinations of reactive serologic test results, cellular or protein abnormalities of cerebrospinal fluid (CSF), or a reactive VDRL-CSF with or without clinical manifestations.

Effective prevention and detection of congenital syphilis depends on the identification of the infection in the pregnant woman and thus on routine screening for syphilis at the first antenatal visit. The diagnosis of early congenital syphilis is often difficult in the newborn as the presence of antibodies may reflect passive maternal levels, and clinical signs may be absent or unconvincing. Routine serologic screening of newborn is not recommended, except for infants born to seropositive mothers. A serum nontreponemal test titer that is fourfold greater than the mother's titre should be managed as congenital syphilis. Umbilical cord blood may be contaminated by maternal blood and should not be used. Discriminating between IgG and IgM specific antibodies may assist in diagnosis, as IgM proteins do not cross the placental barrier, but tests are not always reliable. Failure to adequately document cases prior to therapy may produce an underestimation of the actual incidence of this disease. In the United States, state health departments do not record poorly documented cases[12,37,38] and in large parts of the world notification is absent or incomplete.[7,19]

The serologic tests will show falling titers correlating with adequate treatment. When observing the VDRL or RPR tests, adequate treatment for primary syphilis should result in a seronegative patient within 12 months and in secondary syphilis the patient should become seronegative within two years. The TPHA and FTA-ABS decline to low titers that may remain constant indefinitely. Likewise, early congenital syphilis usually converts to seronegativity after adequate treatment, whereas late congenital syphilis may manifest stable seropositivity in spite of adequate therapy. Serologic test titers may decline more slowly for patients who previously had syphilis or are immunocompromised.[22,27] Information is lacking with regard to follow-up of patients treated for late syphilis. The clinical response depends partially on the nature of the lesions.

Some medical conditions can cause short- or long-term seroreactivity against nontreponemal antigens.[44] Acute false-positive tests of importance for pediatricians may be seen with immunizations (diphtheria and pertussis), mycoplasma pneumonia, infectious mononucleosis, measles, mumps, varicella,

42. Rudolph AW, Duncan WC (1975) Syphilis diagnosis and treatment. **Clin Obstet Gynecol** 18:1.
43. Centers for Disease Control and Prevention (1998) Guidelines for treatment of sexually transmitted diseases. **Morb Mortal Wkly Rep**:47.
44. Nandwani R, Evans DT (1995) Are you sure it's syphilis? A review of false positive serology. **Int J STD AIDS** 6:241.

and pneumococcal pneumonia. Chronic false-positive reactivity may occur in patients with any of the autoimmune or rheumatic conditions, especially systemic lupus erythematosus (SLE), as well as in hepatitis B, leprosy, and malaria. The use of tests based on treponemal antigens minimizes the problem of false-positive nontreponemal test results. In endemic areas, yaws, pinta, or bejel will give positive serologic tests for syphilis since the treponemas involved in these infections are immunologically indistinguishable from *T. pallidum*. Infections caused by *Borrelia burgdorferi* may result in reactive treponemal tests in about 20% of cases.[45]

HISTOGENESIS AND PATHOLOGY

The intact epithelium of the mucous membranes and skin offer some protection against *T. pallidum*, since the stratum corneum cannot be penetrated by the treponemata. When microscopic defects due to the trauma of sexual activity are present, the spirochete can migrate through the epithelium. Polymorphonuclear leukocytes (PMNs) are attracted to the site of inoculation, appear to actively ingest the organisms but do not readily kill them. Although the mechanisms for its survival are unclear, it is evident that this very slowly replicating treponema escapes the initial barriers offered by the PMN influx.[46]

During the incubation period, the accumulated PMNs are rapidly replaced by T lymphocytes, plasma cells, and macrophages. In experimental syphilis, both humoral and cell-mediated mechanisms of immunity have been activated when primary syphilitic lesions appear.[46] Histopathologically, the initial lesions show epidermal edema with central thinning, and a mixed inflammatory infiltrate. Dermal changes include a dense central infiltrate of lymphoid and plasma cells as well as a marked endothelial cell proliferation of the dermal capillaries. Silver stains (Warthin-Starry) can usually demonstrate the treponemas.[47]

Secondary syphilis indicates the hematogenous dissemination of treponemas throughout the body. Paradoxically, it represents control of the exuberant local lesion (chancre) while the ability to control systemic infection is impaired. Although the immunologic basis for this discrepancy is not understood, immune complex deposition may be responsible for some of the features of secondary syphilis[48] and loss of cell-mediated immunity against treponemal antigens may favour the dissemination.[49]

Secondary syphilis may present varied histologic features.[47] As in primary syphilis, one sees perivascular infiltrate containing plasma cells, and vascular prominence with large endothelial cells. Acanthosis may be seen as well, associated with influx of PMNs. This picture can resemble psoriasis microscopically and clinically. Silver stains may demonstrate the organism in about one-third of cases.

Tertiary syphilis is characterized by granulomatous lesions (gummata) in connective tissue, bone, or viscera, but a diffuse interstitial inflammation occurs as well. Organisms are usually not demonstrable, except in brain material from patients with general paresis. The granulomatous reaction is presumed to represent a cellular immune response to recurrence of the spirochetal activity.

DIFFERENTIAL DIAGNOSIS

Equipped with the proper diagnostic instruments it is possible to exclude other diseases having similar symptoms. When primary syphilis is considered, other major ulcerative disorders in the differential diagnosis include herpes simplex, chancroid, and granuloma inguinale. Repeated dark field microscopy and serologic tests, appropriate cultures to detect other infectious agents, and occasionally lesional biopsy should distinguish these disorders.

On genital sites, the chancre is often diagnosed by the patient. Differential diagnosis includes herpes simplex, chancroid, and granuloma inguinale and may be problematic with atypical presentations and mixed infections. Studies conducted in the United States and Kenya[13,14] have previously demonstrated the unreliability of clinical findings alone in the diagnoses of genital ulcerative disease. The clinical diagnosis of primary syphilis was confirmed by antibody tests in only 55% of cases. This means that the probability of syphilitic chancre is overestimated on the basis of clinical inspection.[50]

On extragenital sites, even skilled physicians may make an erroneous diagnosis. Differential diagnosis includes deep fungal infections, mycobacterial disease, chancriform bacterial infections such as *Nocardia* infection and tularemia, as well as noninfectious ulcerative conditions, such as pyoderma gangrenosum.

The clinical diagnosis of secondary syphilis is even more complex, but facilitated by the spectrum of laboratory tests. When the diagnosis of syphilis is considered in patients presenting with unexplained rashes, papulosquamous lesions, alopecia, mucosal white patches, or unexplained lymphadenopathy, a positive serologic test confirms the diagnosis and a negative test usually rules it out.

As an important differential diagnosis, nonvenereal treponematoses must be considered (Table 28.5). They are unknown in North America or Western Europe, but may be imported by immigrants coming from endemic areas where these treponematoses are extremely common. Yaws, pinta, and bejel (endemic syphilis) are infectious diseases caused by closely related spirochetes, which are morphologically inseparable from *T. pallidum*. The precise relationships among these disorders have not been defined, nor has the relationship between venereal syphilis and the nonvenereal treponematoses been clarified. The conditions tend to begin in childhood and hence are a significant pediatric dermatologic problem. Since syphilis is likewise endemic in the same geographic areas, clinical and serologic diagnosis may be difficult at times. Table 28.5 presents the comparative features of the nonvenereal treponematoses.

TREATMENT OF SYPHILIS, INCLUDING FOLLOW-UP

The following section is modified from the detailed guidelines for the management of syphilis as compiled by the Centers for Disease Control (CDC).[43] Additional guidelines on the management of syphilis in childhood are available from the American Academy of Pediatrics.[51]

Parenteral penicillin G (benzathine, aqueous procaine, or aqueous crystalline), is the preferred drug for treatment of all stages of syphilis. Its efficacy was well established through clinical experience before the value of randomized controlled clinical trials was recognized. Parenteral penicillin G is the only therapy with documented efficacy for neurosyphilis or for treating syphilis during pregnancy. The dosage and the length of treatment depend on the stage and clinical manifestations of disease (Table 28.6).

The Jarisch–Herxheimer reaction is an acute febrile reaction that may occur within the first 24 hours after any therapy for syphilis. All patients should be advised of this possible adverse reaction which is more common among patients who have early syphilis. There are no proven methods to prevent this reaction, which can be treated with antipyretics. The Jarisch–Herxheimer reaction may induce early labor or cause fetal distress among pregnant women, but this should not prevent or delay therapy.

Other management considerations

All patients who have syphilis should be tested for HIV infection, and in geographic areas in which the prevalence of HIV is high, patients who have primary syphilis should be retested for HIV after three months if the first HIV test result was negative.

45. Hunter EF, Russell H, Farshy CE (1986) Evaluation of sera from patients with Lyme disease in the fluorescent treponemal antibody absorption test for syphilis. **Sex Transm Dis** 13:232.
46. Musher DM (1984) Biology of *Treponema pallidum*. In: Sexually Transmitted Diseases, Holmes KK, Mardh P-A, Sparling PF et al. eds. New York: McGraw-Hill, p. 352.
47. Lever W, Schaumburg-Lever G (1997) Histopathology of the Skin, 8th ed. Philadelphia: JB Lippincott.
48. Engel S, Dietzel W (1980) Persistent immune complex in syphilis. **Br J Venereol Dis** 56:221.
49. Marshak LC, Rothman S (1951) Skin testing with a purified suspension of *Treponema pallidum*. **Am J Syph Gon Venereol Dis** 35:35.
50. Dangor Y, Ballard RC, da L Exposto F et al. (1990) Accuracy of clinical diagnosis of genital ulcer disease. **Sex Transm Dis** 17:184.
51. American Academy of Pediatrics (1994) Syphilis. In: 1994 Red Book: Report of The Committee on Infectious Diseases. 23rd ed, Peter G, ed. Elk Grove, Il: American Academy of Pediatrics, p. 445.

TABLE 28.5 The nonvenereal treponematoses

Disease and organism	Endemic areas	Primary stage (1°)	Secondary stage (2°)	Tertiary stage (3°)	Serology/dark-field	Pathology	Therapy/prognosis/comment
Yaws (Frambesia Tropica) caused by T. pertenue	Worldwide in tropics	Transmitted by direct contact with 1° or 2° lesions after 3–5 weeks incubation. A small papule may be verrucous or papillomatous, becoming crusted and possibly ulcerated as it enlarges (Mother yaw). Most common site is buttock or lower extremity of child. Heals with atrophic scars.	After 2–6 months disseminated papillomata are seen (frambesiform means raspberry like). These resemble the 1° lesion except they are smaller and multiple. Macular and nodular lesions also seen. Mucous membrane and periorificial lesions also common. Painful periostitis occurs.	After latent period of months to years, gummatous lesions develop in skin, joints, and bones. The cardiovascular system and CNS are not involved.	Dark field positive in mother yaws and early 2° lesions. Serologies positive to all treponemal and nontreponemal tests.	1° and 2° lesions show acanthosis, papillomatosis, neutrophilic epidermal infiltrate, and a mixed dermal infiltrate with numerous plasma cells. 3° lesions resemble those of late syphilis. Silver stains demonstrate organisms in 1° and early 2° lesions (in epidermis).	Benzathine penicillin 1.2 to 2.4 million units im (depending on age). Late stages can be very deforming and bone/joint involvement can produce dysfunction.
Pinta (carate, malde-pinto) caused by T. carateum	Central America and northern parts of South America	After 1–2 week incubation period, multiple pink papules appear on exposed skin. Tendency to become confluent forming large patches and plaques. Scaling occurs but no ulceration.	Disseminated lesions (pentides) appear months to years later. Color varies from red to purple to slaty, and some may be papulosquamous or psoriasislike.	The burned out phase of dyspigmentation shows variable depigmentation and slate-colored dyschromia. Symmetric hyperkeratotic lesions may also persist on the extremities.	Dark field positive in all three stages except achromic area. Treponemal and nontreponemal tests positive after 2 months.	1° and 2° stages show acanthosis and spongiosis. Basal layer liquifaction even in 1° stage. Dense upper dermal infiltrate is mixed but prominent macrophages and plasma cells. 3° stage shows progressive loss of basal melanin, and variable melanophages as well as organisms in early phases.	Same treatment as for yaws above. This is a skin disease only with chiefly cosmetic sequelae. The dyschromic phase can be confused with the ashy dermatosis (erythema dyschromicum perstans of Ramirez) which coexists in same locale as pinta.
Bejel (endemic syphilis) caused by T. pallidum	Middle Eastern and North African desert areas	Short incubation period (3–5 weeks) after exposure to infected person. Usual onset in childhood. Nonvenereal transmission is rule, although organism can penetrate mucous membranes. Proliferation of organism at inoculation site but primary lesions are uncommon.	Disseminated 2° lesions are usually first sign of disease. Mucous membrane plaques and periorificial papillomatous lesions most common. Intertriginous lesions resembling condylomata lata are common (axilla, perineum, etc.). Painful periostitis occurs.	Gummatous lesions progress in small fraction of patients. These cause skin and bone destruction similar to yaws, but do not involve cardiovascular system or CNS.	Dark field positive in 2° stage or in the rarely seen 1° stage. Seropositivity analogous to venereal syphilis.	Histologic features comparable with similar stages of venereal syphilis.	Same treatment as for above disorders. Periostitis of 2° stage can be disabling, and ulcerodestructive 3° lesions can be deforming, similar to yaws.

TABLE 28.6   Treatment regimens for syphilis in patients not allergic to penicillin

	Adult regimens	Pediatric regimens
Primary and secondary syphilis*	Benzathine penicillin G 2.4 million units im as a single dose.	Benzathine penicillin G 50 000 units/kg im, up to the adult dose of 2.4 million units in a single dose.
Early latent syphilis*	Benzathine penicillin G 2.4 million units im in a single dose.	Benzathine penicillin G 50 000 units/kg im, up to the adult dose of 2.4 million units in a single dose.
Late latent syphilis or latent syphilis of unknown duration*	Benzathine penicillin G 7.2 million units total, administered as three doses of 2.4 million units im each at 1-week intervals.	Benzathine penicillin G 50 000 units/kg im, up to the adult dose of 2.4 million units, administered as three doses at 1-week intervals (total 150 000 units/kg up to the adult total dose of 7.2 million units).
Tertiary syphilis*	Benzathine penicillin G 7.2 million units total, administered as three doses of 2.4 million units im at 1-week intervals.	
Neurosyphilis	Aqueous crystalline penicillin G (recommended)# 18–24 million units a day, administered as 3–4 million units iv every 4 hours for 10–14 days. Procaine penicillin (alternate)+ 2.4 million units im a day, PLUS Probenecid 500mg orally four times a day, both for 10–14 days.	Aqueous crystalline penicillin G 200 000–300 000 units/kg/day iv (administered as 50 000 units/kg every 4–6 hours) for 10 days.

* Regimens recommended for patients who are not allergic to penicillin and who have normal CSF examinations.

Regimen for patients who have neurosyphilis or syphilitic eye disease and are not allergic to penicillin.

+ If compliance with therapy can be ensured, patients may be treated with this alternative regimen.

#+ The durations of the recommended and alternative regimens for neurosyphilis are shorter than that of the regimen used for late syphilis in the absence of neurosyphilis. Therefore, some experts administer benzathine penicillin, 2.4 million units im, after completion of these neurosyphilis treatment regimens to provide a comparable total duration of therapy.

Patients who have syphilis and who also have symptoms or signs suggesting neurologic disease or ophthalmic disease should be evaluated fully for neurosyphilis and syphilitic eye disease; this evaluation should include CSF analysis and ocular slit-lamp examination. Such patients should be treated appropriately according to the results of this evaluation.

Children who have reactive serologic tests for syphilis after the neonatal period could have congenital or acquired syphilis. Any child who possibly has congenital syphilis or who has neurologic involvement should be treated with aqueous crystalline penicillin G, 200 000–300 000 units/kg per day iv (administered as 50 000 units/kg every 4–6 hours) for 10 days.

All children should be evaluated for neurosyphilis and sexual abuse should be excluded.

All patients who have latent syphilis of unknown duration should be managed as if they had late latent syphilis. All patients who have latent syphilis should be evaluated clinically for evidence of tertiary disease (e.g., aortitis, neurosyphilis, gumma, and iritis). Patients who have symptomatic late syphilis should have a CSF examination before therapy is initiated. Some experts treat all patients who have cardiovascular syphilis with a neurosyphilis regimen.

Following appropriate treatment, patients should be examined clinically and serologically to ensure resolution of signs and symptoms and decreasing nontreponemal titers. Re-treatment recommendations are for three weekly injections of benzathine penicillin G 2.4 million units im, unless CSF examination indicates that neurosyphilis is present.

Special considerations

Penicillin allergy

Recommended regimens

> Doxycycline 100mg orally twice a day,
> OR
> Tetracycline 500mg orally four times a day.

Both drugs should be administered for two weeks if the duration of infection is known to have been less than one year, otherwise, they should be administered for four weeks.

There is less clinical experience with doxycycline than with tetracycline, but compliance is likely to be better with doxycycline. The use of tetracyclines in children less than 8 years of age is associated with dental discoloration. Data concerning ceftriaxone are limited and clinical experience is insufficient to enable identification of late failures.

For patients whose compliance with therapy and follow-up can be ensured, an alternative regimen is erythromycin 500mg orally four times a day for two weeks. However, erythromycin is less effective than the other recommended regimens and macrolide resistance has been described.[52]

Reliable data are not available for evaluation of therapeutic alternatives to penicillin for the treatment of neurosyphilis.

HIV-infected persons

Penicillin regimens should be used to treat all stages of syphilis in HIV-infected patients. Treatment with benzathine penicillin G, 2.4 million units im, as for HIV-negative patients, is recommended for early and early latent syphilis. Some experts recommend additional treatments (e.g., three weekly doses of benzathine penicillin G as suggested for late syphilis) or other supplemental antibiotics in addition to benzathine penicillin G 2.4 million units im. A patient with late latent syphilis or syphilis of unknown duration and a normal CSF examination can be treated with 7.2 million units of benzathine penicillin G (as three weekly doses of 2.4 million units each). Patients who have CSF findings consistent with neurosyphilis should be treated and managed as described for neurosyphilis.

HIV-infected patients who have early syphilis may be at increased risk for neurologic complications and may have higher rates of treatment failure with currently recommended regimens.[22,26,52] Most HIV-infected patients respond appropriately to the currently recommended penicillin therapy; however,

52. Goldmeier D, Hay P (1993) A review and update on adult syphilis, with particular reference to its treatment. Int J STD AIDS 4:70.

some experts recommend CSF examination before therapy and modification of treatment accordingly.

HIV-infected patients who meet the criteria for treatment failure should be managed the same as HIV-negative patients.

Pregnancy

Pregnant patients who are allergic to penicillin should be desensitized and treated with penicillin. Treatment during pregnancy should be the penicillin regimen appropriate for the stage of syphilis. Penicillin is effective for preventing mother-to-child transmission and for treating fetal-established infection. Some experts recommend additional therapy in some settings. A second dose of benzathine penicillin 2.4 million units im may be administered one week after the initial dose for women who have primary, secondary, or early latent syphilis. Ultrasonographic signs of fetal syphilis (i.e., hepatomegaly and hydrops) indicate a greater risk for fetal treatment failure.

No infant should leave the hospital without the maternal serologic status having been determined at least once during pregnancy. Seropositive pregnant women should be considered infected unless an adequate treatment history is documented clearly in the medical records and sequential serologic antibody titers have declined. Any woman who delivers a stillborn infant after 20 weeks of gestation should be tested for syphilis.

Congenital syphilis

Infants should be treated for presumed congenital syphilis if they were born to mothers who met any of the following criteria:

● Had untreated syphilis at delivery;*
● Had serologic evidence of relapse or reinfection after treatment (i.e., a fourfold or greater increase in nontreponemal antibody titer);
● Was treated with erythromycin or other nonpenicillin regimen for syphilis during pregnancy;†
● Was treated for syphilis less than or equal to one month before delivery;
● Did not have a well-documented history of treatment for syphilis;
● Was treated for early syphilis during pregnancy with the appropriate penicillin regimen, but nontreponemal antibody titers did not decrease at least fourfold; or
● Was treated appropriately before pregnancy but had insufficient serologic follow-up to ensure an adequate treatment response and lack of current infection (i.e., an appropriate response includes a) at least a fourfold decrease in nontreponemal antibody titers for patients treated for early syphilis and b) stable or declining nontreponemal titers of less than or equal to 1:4 for other patients).

Recommended Regimens

> Aqueous crystalline penicillin G 100 000–150 000 units/kg/day, administered as 50 000 units/kg/dose iv every 12 hours during the first 7 days of life, and every 8 hours thereafter for a total of 10 days;
>
> OR
>
> Procaine penicillin G 50 000 units/kg/dose im a day in a single dose for 10 days.

If more than 1 day of therapy is missed, the entire course should be restarted. When possible, a full 10-day course of penicillin is preferred. There is insufficient data on the use of other antimicrobial agents (e.g., ampicillin). The use of agents other than penicillin requires close serologic follow-up to assess adequacy of therapy.

---

* A woman treated with a regimen other than those recommended in these guidelines for treatment of syphilis should be considered untreated.

† The absence of a fourfold greater titer for an infant does not exclude congenital syphilis.

PROGNOSIS AND PEDIATRIC ASPECTS OF THE DISEASE

The primary and secondary stages of syphilis are cured by appropriate therapy, and such therapy will prevent progression from latency to tertiary syphilis. The prognosis for congenital syphilis may be more guarded, depending on the extent of involvement and timing of therapy. CNS involvement may be arrested with penicillin therapy, but neurodevelopmental defects may persist. The mucocutaneous lesions of congenital syphilis heal rapidly with therapy, but the osseous lesions heal more slowly. Interstitial keratitis and Clutton's joints do not respond to penicillin, and 8th nerve deafness is not cured by treatment, although its progression is arrested.[38] Obviously, the fixed stigmata of late congenital syphilis caused by midfacial underdevelopment do not change with therapy.

Acquired syphilis in prepubertal children is usually a consequence of sexual abuse, and hence investigation of that possibility is of great importance for the protection of the child. In sexually active adolescents, it is important to screen for other STDs and to have public health workers do the appropriate epidemiologic tracing so that all sexual contacts are treated. For children with persistent handicaps related to congenital syphilis, individual programs should be tailored to assist them with their visual, auditory, dental, or neurodevelopmental problems.

DISEASES CAUSED BY *NEISSERIA GONORRHOEAE*

Walter Krause

EPIDEMIOLOGY

Gonorrhea is a common infectious disease transmitted by genital sexual contact. In the prepubertal child the presence of this organism strongly suggests child abuse. In the sexually active teenager gonorrhea has become a common infection. Diseases caused by *Neisseria gonorrhoeae* have been the most common infectious disease reported to the CDC in the United States. With more than one million cases reported per year in the United States the prevalence rate may reach as high as 5% in certain parts of the population. Fear of AIDS has had a powerful motivating effect on sexual behavior, and in the United States has been associated with an overall reduction of over 95% in the incidence of gonorrhea in homosexual men. After peaking in 1985, the incidence of gonorrhea in white heterosexual men and women has declined as well. A diagnosis of gonorrhea in 1990 implied recent high-risk behavior for acquiring HIV infection. The gonorrhea epidemic in the United States involves mainly poor urban minorities, suggesting these populations as an appropriate target for screening resources.[53]

The tracing of gonorrhea transmission is difficult, because sexual partners are frequently difficult or impossible to identify. Even if an interview gives apparently reliable results, gonococcal opa-typing is a superior method to identify transmitting patients. The 11 opa genes are amplified with a single pair of primers by the polymerase chain reaction. The method appears to be highly discriminatory as the opa-types of gonococci, isolated world-wide over the last 30 years, showed well-characterized differences. Opa-typing is possible within the same auxotype class or serovars, thus increasing the discriminatory power. The identification of gonococci with identical opa-types is believed to be a good indicator that the individuals from which they were recovered were sexual partners, or part of a short chain of disease transmission.

The overall incidence of diseases caused by *N. gonorrhoeae* is decreasing worldwide. The transmission between homosexual men is more pronounced than between heterosexual partners, thus giving higher rates in men than in women. On the other hand, the number of strains, which develop clinically important antimicrobial resistance, increases continuously. Resistance against

53. Judson FN (1990) Gonorrhea. **Med Clin North Am** 74:1353.

cephalosporins or fluoroquinolones now has to be taken in account even in industrialized countries.

Gonococcal infections in the child are usually the consequence of sexual abuse. When children were able to give answers to questions regarding sexual contact, 89% with *N. gonorrhoeae* (and 100% with *Chlamydia trachomatis*) had a history of sexual contact. Reported rates of gonorrhea in adult rape victims range from 6% to 12%.[54] Although healthy children do not harbor *N. gonorrhoeae*, 25 of 33 children were infected in a group of 532 sexual abuse victims.[55,56] The rates of gonococcal infection were nearly twofold higher for children with multiple episodes of abuse, and also higher for children evaluated for "suspicion of abuse" without a specific history. An important message from that study is that gonococcal infections may be discovered at sites not reportedly involved in the abuse. Hence, routine microbiologic examination of oropharyngeal and anogenital sites is necessary in sexually abused children even without a specific history. A thorough microbiologic diagnosis of *N. gonorrhoeae* is important in these cases, because an incorrect identification of the bacteria may have severe medicolegal implications.[57,58] Gonorrhea is found in juvenile prostitutes more often than in adult ones.[59]

Gonorrhea and chlamydia infection lead to few maternal problems during pregnancy but may be more important as a cause of puerperal endometritis-myometritis, which constitutes one of the leading causes of maternal death in many underdeveloped countries. Hence, neonatal and infant morbidity may be affected by gonorrhea and chlamydia infection in those developing countries.[60] The indirect threat to the neonatal child in underdeveloped countries, when the mother suffers from severe gonorrhea, is also noted in other publications.[61]

MICROBIOLOGY

N. gonorrhoeae are nonmotile, small, Gram-negative cocci that grow in pairs with adjacent sides characteristically flattened, thus the name diplococci. As with all *neisseriae*, they carry pili on their cell surfaces, which facilitate the attachment to epithelial cells. The major subunit, PilE, displays homology to similar systems of type-4 pili currently being identified on an increasing number of pathogenic bacteria. The type-4 pili are essential for DNA uptake and transformation. This is one of the factors explaining the population structure and genetic flexibility of *N. gonorrhoeae*. The bacteria may posses more than 15 gene copies of a silent pilin gene, which enable a single strain to produce theoretically more than 10^7 different variants. In culture, some gonococci have the ability to produce pili. The cell membrane contains distinct proteins, which show antigenic variations allowing serotyping of the bacteria. They secrete an IgA protease that cleaves the heavy chain of human IgA. The outer membrane also contains a lipopolysaccharide (LPS), which may be associated with resistance to killing and to type and severity of disease.[62,63] There are six known serotypes of LPS. The bacteria contain plasmids, of which one causes the production of β-lactamase, the molecular basis of penicillin resistance.

The only natural host of *N. gonorrhoeae* is man. In culture, the organisms do not grow well at reduced temperatures or on simple nutrient agar. They do not tolerate drying and care must be taken to immediately place the samples onto appropriate media. Chocolate agar containing vancomycin, colistin, and nystatin (Thayer–Martin medium) has been used to inhibit the normal flora from the pharynx, rectum, and cervix, which would otherwise overgrow the less hardy *Neisseria*.[64] Some strains of *N. gonorrhoeae* are sensitive to vancomycin, may not grow on selective media, and cannot be grown from sites with indigenous flora.[65,66]

The gonococcus has been extensively studied for virulence factors but the significance of these factors has not been determined. Piliated strains (T1 and T2) are better able to adhere to the human mucosal surface,[67] are resistant to killing by neutrophils,[68] and are more virulent in animal models.[69] The outer membrane protein of *N. gonorrhoeae* has been used to serotype gonococci. The protein I serotypes are strongly associated with serum resistance[70] and dissemination of infection. Protein II serotypes are associated with colony opacity, virulence in the chick embryo,[71] adherence to a wide variety of eukaryotic cell types,[72] attachment to phagocytes, serum and antibiotic resistance, and with specific sites of isolation.[73] Auxotyping of gonococci has shown that strains requiring arginine, hypoxanthine, and uracil (AHU) for growth are much more likely to be found in asymptomatic infection in males[63] and disseminated infection in females.[74] Gonococci containing the 24 MDa conjugal plasmid are able to conjugally transfer small, non-self-transferable penicillinase plasmids with high efficiency.[75]

Penicillinase-producing *N. gonorrhoeae* (PPNG) were first reported in 1976 in patients in the United States. The penicillin resistance is mediated by a 3.2 Mda and a 4.4 Mda plasmid.[76] The incidence of resistant strains has demonstrated a steady increase since 1976 with a rise from 350 cases to 4457 cases in 1982.[55] In 1983, higher-level antibiotic resistance was recognized as chromosomally mediated (CMRNG). These bacteria lack penicillinase. In 1984, 446 cases of CMRNG were reported to the CDC.[59] In 1994, 15% of the isolated strains were CMRNG, while also 155 were PPNG. In 1985, plasmid-mediated resistance to tetracycline was reported. This plasmid can move between bacteria of different genera. It may, therefore, spread more quickly than the penicillinase-plasmids.[76]

PHYSICAL EXAMINATION

In pubertal children the features are similar to those seen in adults (Table 28.7). In the prepubertal girl, the primary complaint is a purulent vulvovaginitis. The incubation period is 2–7 days in symptomatic patients.

54. Schwarcz SK, Whittington WL (1990) Sexual assault and sexually transmitted diseases: detection and management in adults and children. **Rev Infect Dis** (12 suppl) 6:S682.
55. Gardner JJ (1992) Comparison of the vaginal flora in sexually abused and nonabused girls. **J Pediatr** 120:872.
56. De-Jong AR (1986) Sexually transmitted disease in sexually abused children. **Sex Transm Dis** 13:123.
57. Whittington WL, Rice RJ, Biddle JW et al. (1988) Incorrect identification of *Neisseria gonorrhoeae* from infants and children. **Pediatr Infect Dis J** 7:3.
58. Alexander ER (1988) Misidentification of sexually transmitted organisms in children: medicolegal implications. **Pediatr Infect Dis J** 7:1.
59. Bell Ta, Farrow JA, Stamm WE et al. (1985) Sexually transmitted diseases in females in a juvenile detention center. **Sex Transm Dis** 12:140.
60. Bergstrom S (1990) Genital infections and reproductive health: infertility and morbidity of mother and child in developing countries. **Scand J Infect Dis** (Suppl) 69:99.
61. Goeman J, Meheus A, Piot P (1991) L'epidemiologie des maladies sexuellement transmissibles dans les pays en development a l'ere du SIDA. **Ann Soc Belg Med Trop** 71:81.
62. Rice PA, McCormack WM, Kasper DL (1980) Natural serum bactericidal activity against *Neisseria gonorrhoeae* isolates from disseminated, locally invasive, and uncomplicated disease. **J Immunol** 124:105.
63. Crawford G, Knapp JS, Hale J et al. (1977) Asymptomatic gonorrhea in men: caused by gonococci with unique nutritional requirements. **Science** 196:1352.
64. Thayer JD, Martin JE Jr (1966) Improved medium selective for the cultivation of *Neisseria gonorrhoeae* and *Neisseria meningitidis*. **Public Health Rep** 81:559.
65. Minnett S, Reller LB, Knapp JS (1981) *Neisseria gonorrhoeae* stains inhibited by vancomycin in selective media and correlation with auxotype. **J Clin Microbiol** 14:94.
66. Windall JJ, Hall MM, Washington JA et al. (1980) Inhibitory effects of vancomycin on *Neisseria gonorrhoeae* in Thayer Martin medium. **J Infect Dis** 142:775.
67. Watt PF, Ward ME (1980) Adherences of *Neisseria gonorrhoeae* and other *Neisseria* species to mammalian cells. In: Bacterial Adherence, Beachey EH, ed. New York: Chapman & Hall, p. 253.
68. Ofek I, Beachey EH, Bisno AL (1974) Resistance of *Neisseria gonorrhoeae* to phagocytosis: relationship to colonial morphology and surface pili. **J Infect Dis** 129:413.
69. McGee ZA, Johnson AP, Taylor-Robinson D (1974) Pathogenic mechanism of *Neisseria gonorrhoeae*: observations on damage to human fallopian tubes in organ culture by gonococci of colony type I or type IV. **J Infect Dis** 129:310.
70. Tam MR, Buchanan TM, Sandstrom EG et al. (1982) Serologic classification of *Neisseria gonorrhoeae* with monoclonal antibodies. **Infect Immunol** 38:1042.
71. Salit IE, Gotschlich EC (1978) Gonococcal color and opacity variants: virulence for chicken embryos. **Infect Immunol** 22:359.
72. Heckels JE, James LT (1980) The structural organization of the gonococcal cell envelope and its influence on pathogenesis. In: Genetics and Immunobiology of Pathogenic Neisseria, Danielsson D, Normark S, eds. Sweden: University of Umea, p. 75.
73. Draper DL, James JF, Brooks FG et al. (1980) Comparison of virulence markers of peritoneal and fallopian tube isolates with endocervical *Neisseria gonorrhoeae* isolates from women with acute salpingitis. **Infect Immunol** 27:882.
74. Knapp JS, Holmes KK (1975) Disseminated gonococcal infection caused by *Neisseria gonorrhoeae* with unique nutritional requirements. **J Infect Dis** 132:204.
75. Biswis GD, Blackman EY, Sparling PF (1980) High-frequency conjugal transfer of a gonococcal penicillinase plasmid. **J Bacteriol** 143:1318.
76. Peterson BH, Lee TJ, Snyderman R et al. (1979) *Neisseria meningitidis* and *Neisseria gonorrhoeae* bacteremia associated with C6, C7, or C8 deficiency. **Ann Intern Med** 90:917.

TABLE 28.7   Clinical spectrum of infections with *N. gonorrhoeae*

Male genitalia
Urethritis
Cowperitis
Prostatitis
Vesiculitis
Epididymitis
Orchitis
Tysonitis
Infertility (?)

Female genitalia
Urethritis
Bartholinitis
Vaginitis (only in prepubertal children)
Cervicitis
Endometritis
Salpingitis
Oophoritis
Pelviperitonitis
Curtis–Fitz–Hughes syndrome
Infertility

Both sexes
Proctitis
Conjunctivitis
Ophthalmia neonatorum
Pharyngitis

Disseminated gonococcal infection
Tendosynovitis
Septic arthritis
Cutaneous metastatic infection
Septicemia

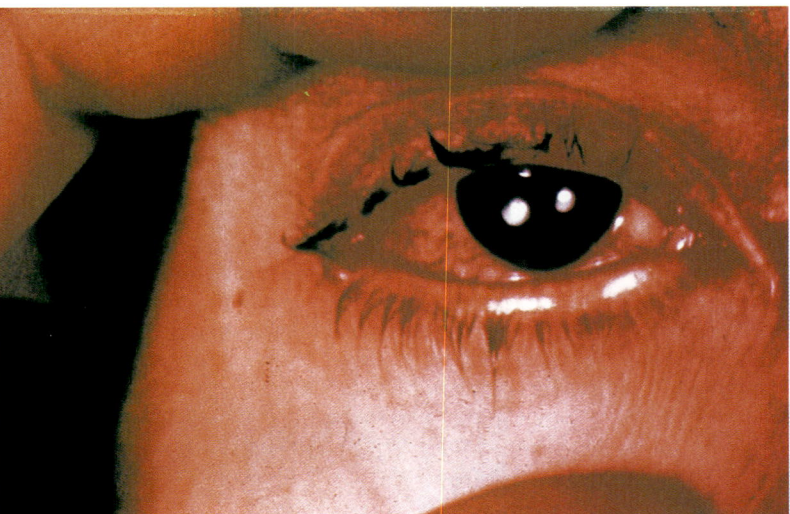

Fig. 28.26   Gonococcal conjunctivitis. (Courtesy of J. Moseley, MD)

Asymptomatic infections occur frequently and account for the high rate of this infection in sexually active teenagers. Genital infections in males begin with purulent urethral discharge, dysuria, or both. Complications include epididymitis, prostatitis, periurethral abscess, penile lymphangitis, and urethral stricture. All but epididymitis are now rare. Symptoms in genital infections in females include vaginal discharge, dysuria, urinary frequency, menstrual abnormalities, and abdominal pain. Spread of infection in women can result in salpingitis, tubo-ovarian abscesses, and pelvic peritonitis. The symptoms of pelvic inflammatory disease (PID) include abdominal pain, dysuria, increased vaginal discharge, increased uterine bleeding, fever, chills, nausea, vomiting, and toxicity. PID frequently follows the onset of menses, suggesting an association. Perihepatitis (Fitz–Hugh–Curtis syndrome) caused by the spread of gonococci from the fallopian tubes to the surface of the liver, or bacteremia can complicate genital infections. Pharyngeal gonorrhea can present as sore throat or cervical adenitis but frequently is asymptomatic. Anorectal gonorrhea is associated with proctitis, pruritus, tenesmus, purulent discharge, and rectal bleeding. Purulent conjunctivitis in adults and older children is seen occasionally (Fig. 28.26). Ophthalmia neonatorum is still seen despite the effectiveness of prophylaxis with 1% silver nitrate, 0.5% erythromycin, or 1% tetracycline given into the conjunctival sac immediately after birth. Sepsis and arthritis can also occur in the infant.

Disseminated gonococcal infection (DGI) occurs infrequently in children and adults (less than 1–3% of infections in adults). Specific factors in the host and the bacteria are involved in pathogenesis of DGI. Gonococci associated with DGI are resistant to bactericidal action of serum,[70] demonstrate AHU-auxotype[63,74] on transparent colony phenotype,[71] show specific serotypes of protein I, and are markedly susceptible to penicillin.[72] Increased host suscep-

tibility to gonococcal bacterial infection may be due to homozygous deficiency of complement components C5, C6, C7, or C8.[76] Women are affected more frequently with DGI than men, and are more likely to have asymptomatic infection. Infection frequently begins 7–30 days before dissemination. Disseminated *N. gonorrhoeae* infection may lead to septic arthritis, which may be rapidly destructive but responds promptly to appropriate antibiotic therapy.[77] Both gonococcal and nongonococcal infections may lead to aseptic "reactive" arthritis or Reiter's syndrome. Inheritance of HLA B27 confers an increased relative risk of 30–50 times for the development of this condition.

Cutaneous manifestations in DGI are late-onset immune mediated lesions. As a rule, the lesions usually appear with the fever and consist of red macules. The erythematous macule becomes papular and a central pustule develops. The characteristic red papule with a gray umbilicated center, frequently has a hemorrhagic base[78] (Fig. 28.27). These lesions last 3–4 days and are often tender. Papules, bullae, pustules, petechiae, and hemorrhagic lesions may occur at the same time. The lesions usually consist of one or two discrete lesions on the extremities or face, but numerous lesions are occasionally seen. The trunk and mucous membranes usually are spared. Histologic examination of the lesions demonstrates focal vasculitis, fibrin deposition, necrosis, and neutrophil infiltration. Organisms are rarely seen on Gram staining, but antigen can be demonstrated by immunofluorescent techniques in most lesions.[79,80]

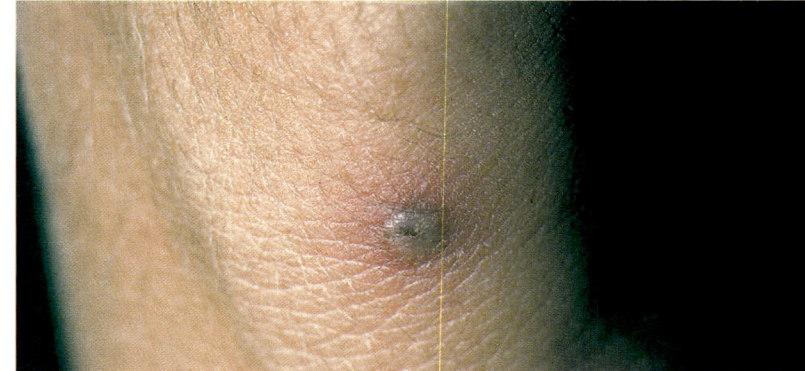

Fig. 28.27   Disseminated gonococcal infection. Typical purpuric pustule on the wrist of a teenager.

77. Keat A (1990) Sexually transmitted arthritis syndromes. **Med Clin North Am** 74:1617.
78. Holmes KK, Counts GW, Beaty HN (1971) Disseminated gonococcal infection. **Ann Intern Med** 74:979.
79. Barr J, Danielsson D (1971) Septic gonococcal dermatitis. **Br Med J** 1:482.
80. Tronca E, Handsfield HH, Weisner PJ et al. (1974) Demonstration of *Neisseria gonorrhoeae* with fluorescent antibody in patients with disseminated gonococcal infection. **J Infect Dis** 129:583.

GONORRHEA AND HIV INFECTIONS

Especially in homosexual men, it is important to be aware of gonococcal infections of the rectum and colon.[81] HIV infection may coexist in these cases. Little is known, however, about the incidence of gonorrhea in HIV-infected men, because the combined infection appears to be a rare event. Diagnosis and treatment are similar to other cases of gonorrhea. In prepubescent children, a culture must be performed to identify the organism. This is particularly true because of the medicolegal consequence of *N. gonorrhoeae* in the prepubertal child. Immunofluorescent antibody assays are now available and can be useful. Susceptibility testing should be done on all isolates.

LABORATORY FINDINGS

Diagnosis of infection with *N. gonorrhoeae* is impossible without proof of the presence of bacteria in the biological material concerned. In acute disease the bacteria are easily to demonstrate in Gram-stained smears as diplococci within leukocytes. The sensitivity and specificity of this method are near 100%. In subacute infections, this method is less helpful. Especially in children, it is necessary to perform culture and/or DNA amplification methods for *N. gonorrhoeae* in order to obtain a correct diagnosis. Sophisticated methods like auxotyping, serotyping or typing of OPA genes are not necessary in order to allow the diagnosis, but are of interest in epidemiological investigations. The use of serological testing for antibodies is of no benefit in the diagnosis. Special problems of diagnosis are discussed in the next section.

THERAPY

The following section is adopted from the 1998 STD treatment guidelines published by the CDC.[43]

Dual therapy for gonococcal and chlamydial infection

"Patients infected with *N. gonorrhoeae* often are coinfected with *C. trachomatis*. A routine dual therapy without testing for chlamydiae may be cost-effective, because the cost of therapy for chlamydiae (e.g., with doxycycline) is less than the cost of testing. Because most gonococci are susceptible to doxycycline and azithromycin, routine co-treatment might also hinder the development of resistant strains of *N. gonorrhoeae*."

Uncomplicated gonococcal infections

RECOMMENDED REGIMENS (Table 28.8)
The antibiotics listed are safe and effective for treating gonorrhea, eradicating *N. gonorrhoeae*, ending the possibility of further transmission, relieving symptoms, and reducing the changes of sequelae. In clinical trials, these recommended regimens cured more than 95% of anal and genital infections; any of the regimens may be used for uncomplicated anal or genital infection.

TABLE 28.8 Recommended treatment regimens for uncomplicated gonococcal infections

Drug	Dose	Route
Cefixime	400mg single dose	po
Ceftriaxone**	125mg single dose	im
Ciprofloxacin*	500mg single dose	po
Ofloxacin	400mg single dose	po
Azithromycin	1g single dose	po
Alternative regimes		
Spectinomycin**	2g single dose	im

* Not approved for the use in children.
** Recommended regimen for children.

Published studies indicate that ceftriaxone 125mg and ciprofloxacin 500mg can cure 90% or more of pharyngeal infections. If pharyngeal infection is a concern, one of these two regimens should be used.

Cefixime has an antimicrobial spectrum similar to that of ceftriaxone, but the 400mg oral dose does not provide as high nor as sustained a bactericidal level as does 125mg of ceftriaxone. In published clinical trials, Cefixime appears to be effective against pharyngeal gonococcal infection, but few patients with pharyngeal infection have been included in studies. No gonococcal strains resistant to cefixime have been reported. The advantage of cefixime is that it can be administered orally. It is not known if the 400mg dose can cure incubating syphilis.

Ceftriaxone in a single dose of either 125mg or 250mg provides sustained, high bactericidal levels in the blood. Extensive clinical experience indicates that both doses are safe and effective for the treatment of uncomplicated gonorrhea at all sites, curing 99.1% of uncomplicated urogenital and anorectal infections in published clinical trials.

Single-dose cephalosporin regimens other than ceftriaxone 125mg and cefixime 400mg orally that are safe and highly effective against uncomplicated anorectal or urogenital gonococcal infections include (a) ceftizoxime 500mg im, (b) cefotetan 1g im, (c) cefoxitin 2g im with probenicid 1g orally. None of these injectable cephalosporins offers any advantage compared with ceftriaxone, and clinical experience with them for the treatment of uncomplicated gonorrhea is limited.

Ciprofloxacin is effective against most strains of *N. gonorrhoeae*. At a dose of 500mg it provides sustained bactericidal levels in the blood. In published clinical trials it has cured 99.8% of uncomplicated gonorrhea. Ciprofloxacin is safe, relatively inexpensive, and can be administered orally. However, the most recent reports on antibiotic resistance against flouroquinolones have to be considered.[82] Ciprofloxacin is not approved for the treatment of gonococcal infection in children.

Ofloxacin is also effective against most strains of *N. gonorrhoeae*, and it has favorable pharmacokinetics. The 400mg oral dose has been effective for the treatment of uncomplicated anorectal infections, curing 98.4% of infections in published trials.

Single-dose quinolone regimens include enoxacin 400mg orally, lomefloxacin 400mg orally, and norfloxacin 800mg orally. These regimes appear to be safe and effective for the treatment of uncomplicated gonorrhea, but data regarding their use are limited.

ALTERNATIVE REGIMENS
Spectinomycin is expensive and must be injected; however, it has been effective in published clinical trials, curing 98.2% of uncomplicated urogenital and anorectal gonococcal infections. Spectinomycin is useful for the treatment of patients who cannot tolerate cephalosporins and quinolones.

Many other antimicrobials are active against *N. gonorrhoeae*. However, these guidelines are not intended to be a comprehensive list of all effective treatment regimens. Azithromycin 2g orally is effective, but it is expensive and causes gastrointestinal distress.

Uncomplicated gonococcal infection of the pharynx

These infections are more difficult to eradicate than infections at urogenital or anorectal sites. Few antigonococcal regimens can reliably cure such infection >90% of the time. Recommended regimens: Ceftriaxone 125mg im in a single dose; ciprofloxacin 500mg orally in a single dose; ofloxacin 400mg orally in a single dose; azithromycin 1g orally in a single dose; or doxycycline 100mg orally twice a day for seven days.

FOLLOW-UP
Persons who have uncomplicated gonorrhea and who are treated with any of the regimens in these guidelines need not return for a test of cure. Patients who have symptoms that persist after treatment should be evaluated by culture for *N. gonorrhoeae*, and any gonococci isolated should be tested for

81. Wexner SD (1990) Sexually transmitted diseases of the colon, rectum, and anus. The challenge of the nineties. **Dis Colon Rectum** 33:1048.

82. Peerbooms PG, Spaargaren J, Fennema JS et al. (2001) [Increased Neisseria gonorrhoeae quinolone resistance in Amsterdam] [Article in Dutch]. **Ned Tijdschr Geneeskd** 145:1899.

antimicrobial susceptibility. Infections identified after treatment with one of the recommended regimens usually result from reinfection rather than treatment failure, indicating a need for improved patient education and sex partner referral. *C. trachomatis* and other organisms also may cause persistent urethritis, cervicitis, or proctitis.

MANAGEMENT OF SEX PARTNERS

Patients should be instructed to refer sex partners for evaluation and treatment. All sex partners of patients who have *N. gonorrhoeae* infection should be evaluated and treated for *N. gonorrhoeae* and *C. trachomatis* infections if their last sexual contact with the patient was within 60 days of onset of symptoms or diagnosis of infection in the patient. If a patient's last sexual intercourse was >60 days before onset of symptoms or diagnosis, the patient's most recent sex partner should be treated. Patients should be instructed to avoid sexual intercourse until therapy is completed and they and their sex partners no longer have symptoms.

SPECIAL CONSIDERATIONS

Allergy, intolerance, or adverse reactions Persons who cannot tolerate cephalosporins or quinolones should be treated with spectinomycin. Because spectinomycin is unreliable (only 52% effective) against pharyngeal infection, patients who have suspected or known pharyngeal infection should have pharyngeal culture evaluated 3–5 days after treatment to verify eradication of infection.
Pregnancy Pregnant women should not be treated with quinolones or tetracyclines. Those infected with *N. gonorrhoeae* should be treated with a recommended or alternate cephalosporin. Women who cannot tolerate a cephalosporin should be administered a single dose of 2g of spectinomycin im. Erythromycin is the recommended treatment for presumptive or diagnosed *C. trachomatis* infection during pregnancy (see Chlamydial infections).

HIV INFECTION

Persons with HIV infection and gonococcal infection should receive the same treatment as those who are HIV negative.

Gonococcal conjunctivitis

Only one North American study of the treatment of gonococcal conjunctivitis among adults has been published in recent years. In that study, 12 of 12 patients responded favorably to a single 1g im injection of ceftriaxone. The recommendations that follow reflect the opinions of expert consultants.

TREATMENT

Recommended regimen Ceftriaxone 1g im in a single dose and lavage of the infected eye with saline solution once.

Disseminated gonococcal infection

No studies of the treatment of DGI among persons in North America have been published recently. The recommendations that follow reflect the opinions of expert consultants. No treatment failures have been reported.

TREATMENT

Hospitalization is recommended for initial therapy, especially for patients who cannot be relied on to comply with treatment, for those for whom the diagnosis is uncertain, and for those who have purulent synovial effusions or other complications. Patients should be examined for clinical evidence of endocarditis and meningitis. Patients treated for DGI should be treated presumptively for concurrent *C. trachomatis* infection unless appropriate testing excludes this infection.

RECOMMENDED INITIAL REGIMEN (Table 28.9)

All regimens should be continued for 24 to 48 hours after improvement begins; at which time therapy may be switched to one of the following regimens to complete a full week of antimicrobial therapy: cefixime 400mg orally twice a day, ciprofloxacin 500mg orally twice a day or ofloxacin 400mg orally twice a day.

TABLE 28.9 Initial treatment for DGI in adults and children >45kg

First choice treatment	Alternative regimens
Ceftriaxone 1g im or iv every 24 hours	Cefotaxime 1g iv every 8 hours ceftizoxime 1g iv every 8 hours ciprofloxacin 500mg iv revery 12 hours* ofloxacin 400mg iv every 12 hours* spectinomycin 2g im every 12 hours

* For persons allergic to β-lactam drugs; quinolones are not approved for the use in children. However, investigations of ciprofloxacin in children who have cystic fibrosis demonstrated no adverse effects.

Gonococcal meningitis and endocarditis

RECOMMENDED INITIAL REGIMEN

1–2g of ceftriaxone iv every 12 hours. Therapy for meningitis should be continued for 10 to 14 days and for endocarditis for at least four weeks. Treatment of complicated DGI should be undertaken in consultation with an expert.

GONOCOCCAL INFECTIONS AMONG INFANTS

Gonococcal infection among neonates usually results from peripartum exposure to infected cervical exudate at birth. It is usually an acute illness beginning 2–5 days after birth. The prevalence of infection among neonates depends on the prevalence of infection among pregnant women, on whether pregnant women are screened for gonorrhea, and on whether newborns receive ophthalmic prophylaxis.

The most serious manifestation of *N. gonorrhoeae* infection in newborns are ophthalmia neonatorum and sepsis, including arthritis and meningitis. Less serious manifestations at sites of infection include rhinitis, vaginitis, urethritis, and inflammation at sites of intrauterine fetal monitoring.

Ophthalmia neonatorum

Although *N. gonorrhoeae* is a less frequent cause of ophthalmia neonatorium in the United States than *C. trachomatis* and nonsexually transmitted agents, it is especially important because it may result in perforation of the globe and in blindness.

Diagnostic considerations

Infants at increased risk for gonococcal ophthalmia in the United States are those who do not receive ophthalmia prophylaxis and those whose mothers have had no prenatal care or whose mothers have a history of STDs or substance abuse. Gonococcal ophthalmia is strongly suggested when typical Gram-negative diplococci are identified in conjunctival exudate, justifying presumptive treatment after appropriate cultures for *N. gonorrhoeae* are obtained. Appropriate chlamydial testing should be done simultaneously. Presumptive treatment for *N. gonorrhoeae* may be indicated for newborns who are at increased risk for gonococcal ophthalmia and who have conjunctivitis but do not have gonococcae in a Gram-stained smear of conjunctival exudate.

In all cases of neonatal conjunctivitis, conjunctival exudate should be cultured for *N. gonorrhoeae* and tested for antibiotic susceptibility before a definitive diagnosis is made. A definitive diagnosis is important because of the public health and social consequences for the infant of a diagnosis of gonorrhea. Nongonococcal causes of neonatal ophthalmia include *Moraxella catarrhalis* and other *Neisseria* species that are indistinguishable from *N. gonorrhoeae* on Gram-stained smear, but can be differentiated in the microbiologic laboratory.

Recommended regimen

The recommended regimen is ceftriaxone 25–50mg/kg iv or im in a single dose, not to exceed 125mg. Topical antibiotic therapy alone is inadequate and is unnecessary if systemic treatment is administered.

Other management considerations

Simultaneous infection with *C. trachomatis* should be considered when a patients does not respond satisfactorily to treatment. Both mother and infant should be tested for chlamydial infection at the same time that gonorrhea testing is done (see Ophthalmia neonatorum caused by *C. trachomatis*). Ceftriaxone should be administered cautiously to hyperbilirubinemic infants, especially those born prematurely.

Follow-up

Infants should be hospitalized and evaluated for signs of disseminated infection (e.g., sepsis, arthritis, meningitis). One dose of ceftriaxone is adequate for gonococcal conjunctivitis, but many pediatricians prefer to continue antibiotics until cultures are negative at 48 to 72 hours. The duration of therapy should be decided in consultation with experienced physicians.

Management of mothers and their sex partners

The mothers of infants who have gonococcal infection and the mother's sex partners should be evaluated and treated following the recommendations for treatment of gonococcal infections in adults (see Gonococcal infections among adolescents and adults).

Disseminated gonococcal infection

Sepsis, arthritis, meningitis, or any combination thereof, are rare complications of neonatal gonococcal infection. Localized gonococcal infection of the scalp might result from fetal monitoring through scalp electrodes. Detection of gonococcal infection in neonates who have sepsis, arthritis, meningitis, or scalp abscesses requires cultures of blood, CSF, and joint aspirate on chocolate agar. Specimens obtained from the conjunctiva, vagina, oropharynx, and rectum that are cultured on gonococcal selective medium are useful for identifying sites of primary infection, especially if inflammation is present. Positive Gram-stained smears of exudate, CSF, or joint aspirate provide a presumptive basis for initiating treatment for *N. gonorrhoeae*. Diagnoses based on positive Gram-stained smears or presumptive isolation by cultures should be confirmed with definitive tests on culture isolates.

Recommended regimen

Other management considerations

Infants born to mothers who have untreated gonorrhea are at high risk for infection. Mother and infant should be tested for chlamydial infection (Table 28.10).

Follow-up

A follow-up examination is not required.

Management of mothers and their sex partners

The mothers of infants with gonococcal infection and the mother's sex partners should be evaluated and treated following the recommendations for treatment of gonococcal infections among adults (see Gonococcal infections).

TABLE 28.10   Recommended treatment for DGI in infants

Infants with DGI	Prophylactic treatment for infants whose mothers have gonococcal infection
Ceftriaxone 25–50mg/kg per day iv or im in a single daily dose for 7 days	Ceftriaxone 25–50mg/kg iv or im, not to exceed 125mg, in a single dose
Cefotaxime 25mg/kg iv or im every 12 hour for 7 days duration of 10 to 14 days, if meningitis is documented	

GONOCOCCAL INFECTIONS AMONG CHILDREN

After the neonatal period, sexual abuse is the most common cause of gonococcal infection among pre-adolescent children. Vaginitis is the most common manifestation of gonococcal infection among pre-adolescent children. PID following vaginal infection appears to be less common than among adults. Among sexually abused children, anorectal and pharyngeal infections with *N. gonorrhoeae* are common and frequently asymptomatic.

Diagnostic considerations

Because of the potential medicolegal use of the test results for *N. gonorrhoeae* among children, only standard culture systems for the isolation of *N. gonorrhoeae* should be used for children. Nonculture gonococcal tests, including Gram-stained smear, DNA probes, or EIA tests should not be used alone; none of these tests have been approved by the Food and Drug Administration (FDA) for use with specimens obtained from the oropharynx, rectum, or genital tract of children. Specimens from the vagina, urethra, pharynx, or rectum should be streaked onto selective media for isolation of *N. gonorrhoeae*, and all presumptive isolates of *N. gonorrhoeae* should be confirmed by at least two tests that involve different principles (e.g., biochemical, enzyme substrate, or serologic). Isolates should be preserved to permit additional or repeated analysis.

Follow-up

Follow-up cultures are unnecessary if ceftriaxone is used. If spectinomycin is used to treat pharyngitis, a follow-up culture is necessary to ensure that treatment was effective.

Other management considerations

Only parenteral cephalosporins are recommended for use among children. Ceftriaxone is approved for all gonococcal indications among children; cefotaxime is approved for gonococcal ophthalmia only. Oral cephalosporins used for treatment of gonococcal infections in children have not been evaluated adequately.

All children who have gonococcal infections should be evaluated for co-infection with syphilis and *C. trachomatis*. For a discussion of issues regarding sexual assault, refer to Sexual Assault or Abuse of Children.

Ophthalmia neonatorum prophylaxis

Instillation of a prophylactic agent into the eyes of all newborn infants is recommended to prevent gonococcal ophthalmia neonatorum; this procedure is required by law in many locations. All the recommended prophylactic regimens in this section prevent gonococcal ophthalmia. However, the efficacy of these preparations in preventing chlamydial ophthalmia is less clear, and they do not eliminate nasopharyngeal colonization with *C. trachomatis*. The diagnosis and treatment of gonococcal and chlamydial infections in pregnant women is the best method for preventing neonatal gonococcal and chlamydial disease. Not all women, however, receive prenatal care; and ocular prophylaxis is warranted because it can prevent sight-threatening gonococcal ophthalmia and is safe, easy to administer, and inexpensive.

Recommended preparations

Silver nitrate (1%) aqueous solution in a single application, or erythromycin (0.5%) ophthalmic ointment in a single application, or tetracycline ophthalmic ointment (1%) in a single application.

One of these recommended preparations should be instilled in both eyes of every neonate as soon as possible after delivery. If prophylaxis is delayed (i.e., not administered in the delivery room), a monitoring system should be established to ensure that all infants receive prophylaxis. All infants should be administered ocular prophylaxis, regardless whether delivery is vaginal or cesarean. Single-use tubes or ampoules are preferable to multiple-use tubes. Bacitracin is *not* effective. Povidone iodine has not been studied adequately.

CHANCROID

Chancroid is characterized by painful, ragged, undermined ulcerations of the genital or anogenital skin associated with enlarged regional lymph nodes in 50% of cases. Suppurative lymphadenopathy evolves in approximately 25% of cases.[83,84]

The disease is endemic worldwide but is more common in tropical and semitropical regions and in underdeveloped countries.[83,85] Its incidence increases in times of war and population migration. Previously observed mainly around sea harbors, today chancroid is frequently seen in the vicinity of international airports. In 1988, 5000 cases of this disease were reported in the United States.[83,85] Although rare among children, it may occur in sexually active teens or in cases of child abuse and, therefore, deserves the attention of pediatricians and dermatologists.

The causative agent is a bacterium called *Haemophilus ducreyi*. The Gram-negative, nonmotile, non-acid-fast streptobacillus was already discovered in 1889; however, even today it is difficult to culture. On the other hand, culture of *Haemophilus ducreyi* remains the definitive way to diagnose chancroid. Highest cultural yields are obtained (in a local chancroid epidemic in the US in 1991) using enriched gonococcal agar base and enriched Mueller–Hinton agar in a biplate fashion. Immunodiagnostic and DNA probe tests are not available routinely. Special culture media are not widely available from commercial sources. Even using these media, sensitivity is below 80%.[43]

HISTORY AND PHYSICAL EXAMINATION

The incubation period for chancroid varies from one to 14 days, but most cases begin within 2–6 days following coitus with a carrier or infected partner. The first lesion is usually an inflammatory macule, which rapidly evolves into a vesiculopustule, and then into a shallow ulcer. The ulcer is not indurated and has a shaggy irregular border that may be undermined. Ulcers may be covered by an exudate and may spread or multiply as a result of auto-inoculation (Fig. 28.28). Chancroidal ulcers vary in size from 3mm to over 2cm and are often, but not always, painful. They may be present anywhere on the anogenital skin of both sexes. In addition, on rare occasions extragenital sites have been reported including breasts, lips, tongue, eyelids, and

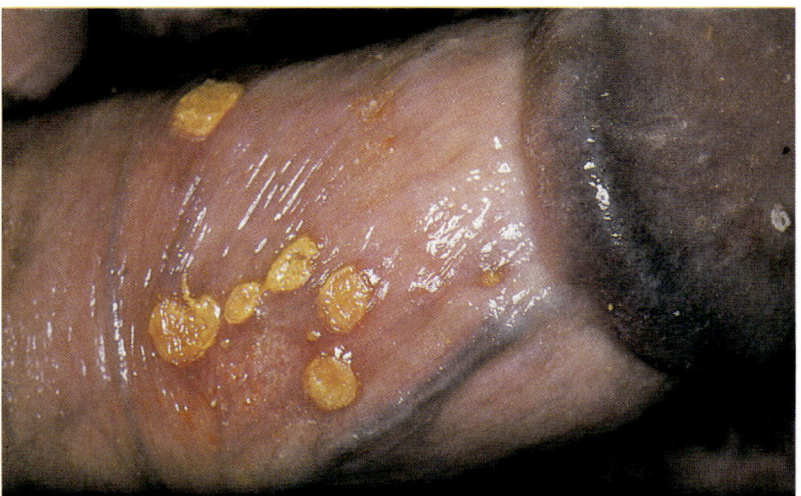

Fig. 28.28 Chaneroid. Multiple ulcers are shown.

oropharynx.[86] One case of conjunctivitis due to *H. ducreyi* has als been reported following accidental inoculation of the bacteria to the eye of a health care worker.[87] Unusual presentations, including cases with lesions resembling granuloma inguinale, have been reported by Kraus *et al*.[88] and Olansky.[89] Occasional cases of suppurative lymphadenopathy in the absence of genital ulceration have also been reported.[90] The mechanisms for protective immunity in chancroid are unclear, but both humoral and cell-mediated mechanisms may be involved.

Chancroid has been associated with increased rates of HIV infection outside the United States or Western Europe, making its diagnosis even more important. As with other genital ulcerations, epithelial disruption presumably allows more ready transmission of the HIV infection. Dickerson *et al*.[91] in 1996 performed a meta-analysis of case-controlled, cross-sectional, and cohort studies that examined the association between HIV seroconversion and genital ulcers cited in the literature. They found twenty-seven epidemiologic studies eligible for analysis. Approximately two-thirds of the analyses reported a statistically significant association between genital ulcer disorder (GUD) and HIV infection; a significant negative association was never reported. The temporal association between pre-existing GUD and subsequent HIV acquisition, however, is unclear.

LABORATORY FINDINGS

The diagnosis of chancroid is based on clinical presentation and Gram stains showing Gram-negative "school of fish," that is, chains of bacilli. This procedure has a sensitivity of 62% and a specificity of 99%.[31] *H. ducreyi* can also be cultured by means of special selective culture media, containing hemin derived from enriched chocolate agar or heart infusion rabbit blood agar, and vancomycin hydrochloride to inhibit overgrowth of contaminants.[92] The organism is best grown at 33°–35°C with high humidity.[83] Colonies are yellow-gray and nonmucoid. They produce chains when grown in solid or liquid media. Confirmation of the identity of the culture is possible by monoclonal antibodies. It is recovered from about 80% of the suspected ulcers.[31]

DIFFERENTIAL DIAGNOSIS

The differential diagnosis of chancroid includes a variety of lesions. Zipper and other traumatic injuries to the penile skin, especially if secondarily infected, can produce ulceration mimicking chancroid. Other diseases producing genital sores should also be considered. These include the primary chancre of syphilis, herpes simplex genitalis, granuloma inguinale, and lymphogranuloma venereum (LGV). All of these may be associated with lymphadenopathy, although suppurative lymphadenopathy is usually seen only in LGV.

THERAPY

Successful treatment cures infection, resolves clinical symptoms, and prevents transmission to others. In extensive cases, scarring may result despite successful therapy. Treatment of chancroid has been successful with several antibiotics; however, resistance to a variety of compounds has become clinically important. The 1998 CDC recommendations[43] are listed in Table 28.11.

All three regimens are effective for the treatment of chancroid among patients without HIV infection. Azithromycin and ceftiaxone offer the advantage of single-dose therapy. Antimicrobial resistance to ceftriaxone and

83. Felman YM, Nikitas JA (1983) Update on chancroid. **Cutis** 31:602.
84. Felman YM, Nikitas JA (1980) Chancroid. **Cutis** 25:464.
85. Margolis RJ, Hood AF (1982) Chancroid: diagnosis and treatment. **J Am Acad Dermatol** 6:493.
86. Kinghorn GR, Hafiz S, McEntegart MG (1983) Oropharyngeal *Haemophilus ducreyi* infection. **Br Med J** 287:650.
87. Gregory JE, Henderson RW, Smith R (1980) Conjunctivitis due to *Haemophilus ducreyi* infection. **Br J Venereal Dis** 56:414.
88. Kraus SJ, Werman BS, Biddle JW et al. (1982) Pseudogranuloma inguinale caused by *Haemophilus ducreyi*. **Arch Dermatol** 118:494.

89. Olansky S (1982) A new sexually transmitted disease or an old disease uncovered? **Arch Dermatol** 118:449.
90. Himmelstein R, Ravits M (1982) An unusual case of chancroid. **Cutis** 29:463.
91. Dickerson MC, Johnston J, Delea TE et al. (1996) The causal role for genital ulcer disease as a risk factor for transmission of human immunodeficiency virus. An application of the Bradford Hill criteria. **Sex Transm Dis** 23:429.
92. Salzman RS, Kraus SJ, Miller RG et al. (1984) Chancroidal ulcers that are not chancroid. **Arch Dermatol** 120:636.

TABLE 28.11   Recommended treatment regimens for chancroid

Drug	Dose	Route
Azithromycin	1g single dose	po
Ceftriaxone	250mg in a single dose	im
Erythromycin base	500mg 4 times a day for 7 days	po

azithromycin has not been reported. Although two isolates resistant to erythromycin were reported from Asia a decade ago, similar isolates have not been reported.

Alternative regimens

Alternative regimens include amoxicillin 500mg plus clavulanic acid 125mg orally three times a day for seven days, or ciprofloxacin 500mg orally two times a day for three days. Note: ciprofloxacin is contraindicated for pregnant and lactating women, children, and adolescents 17 years of age or younger.

These regimens have not been evaluated as extensively as the recommended regimens; neither has been studied in the United States.

GRANULOMA INGUINALE (DONOVANOSIS)

Granuloma inguinale (GI) manifests as a chronic, ulcerative, granulomatous process involving the skin and subcutaneous tissues. It is found almost exclusively in the Far East. Schmid[31] reports 11 cases for 1988 in the United States. Its general incidence has dramatically fallen over the past decades.[93] In one study its prevalence was as high as 4% in children in New Guinea, and nonvenereal transmission was suggested for its occurrence in that age group.[94] Neonatal occurrence has been recorded.[95]

Its predilection for genital skin, frequent coexistence in sexual partners, and perianal location in anal-receptive homosexual males offer circumstantial support for the sexual transmission route. However, it appears to be inefficiently transmitted, and multiple contacts may be required.[95] Because of difficulty in culturing the putative organism, *Calymmatobacterium granulomatis*, research is limited on this disease, and Koch's postulates have never been satisfied.

C. granulomatis is a Gram-negative rod that will not grow on artificial media, but has been isolated on the yolk sac of the chick embryo.[96] In lesional smears stained with Giemsa or Wright stain, the characteristic Donovan bodies are seen. These are large encapsulated bacillary forms, with a bluish-purple safety-pin configuration. This appearance is due to the bipolar condensation of the nuclear chromatin.

The lesions begin as genital or perianal papules or nodules, which subsequently ulcerate. Although the ulcer may be clean-based, its border is irregular and often indurated. As it enlarges, this ulcerodestructive process can be very mutilating. If it invades vital structures, or becomes superinfected, it can cause dysfunction or, rarely, become life threatening. An occasional deep granuloma may clinically resemble a fluctuant node (pseudobubo).

Differential diagnosis includes the other ulcerative STDs, such as syphilis, chancroid, and chronic herpes simplex. One must occasionally rule out mycobacterial or deep fungal processes when considering the diagnosis of

TABLE 28.12   Therapeutic recommendations for granuloma inguinale

Drug	Dose	Route
Trimethoprim-sulfamethoxazole	double strength twice a day for three weeks	po
Doxycycline	100mg per day for three weeks	po
Alternative regimens		
Ciprofloxacin*	750mg twice daily for three weeks	po
Erythromycin base	500mg four times daily for three weeks	po

* Not approved for the use in children.

GI. In children and adults, extraintestinal Crohn's disease may produce chronic ulcerating granulomas resembling GI. Destructive processes should be distinguished from Fournier's gangrene.

Diagnosis is best made by crush preparations of lesional material, stained and examined for Donovan bodies as previously noted. Lesional biopsy may also be diagnostic, although perhaps less frequently than with stained tissue smears.[93,97] Characteristic features include pseudoepitheliomatous hyperplasia of the epidermis, microabscesses composed of neutrophils, and large mononuclear cells with abundant cytoplasm in which the pathognomonic Donovan bodies may be seen. Failure to see the Donovan bodies on a single biopsy or smear does not rule out the diagnosis of GI, and multiple studies may be required.

THERAPY

Patients should be followed clinically until signs and symptoms have resolved. Sex partners of patients who have granuloma inguinale should be examined and treated if they a) had sexual contact with the patient during the 60 days preceding the onset of symptoms in the patient and b) have clinical signs and symptoms of the diseases (Table 28.12).

INFECTION CAUSED BY *CHLAMYDIA TRACHOMATIS*

EPIDEMIOLOGY

Infections caused by *C. trachomatis* are now recognized as the most prevalent and are among the most damaging STDs seen in North America and Europe.[98] An estimated 3 to 4 million Americans suffer from a chlamydial infection each year.[99] Men, women, and infants are affected, but women bear an inordinate burden because of their increased risk for adverse reproductive consequences. These include ectopic pregnancy, infertility, and neonatal morbidity. Today, STDs caused by *C. trachomatis* constitute a severe socio-economic and medical problem.[100]

C. trachomatis causes approximately 30–70% of the reported cases of non-gonococcal (NGU) or postgonococcal urethritis among men. This STD has an estimated incidence 2.5 times that of gonococcal urethritis.[98] Chlamydiae are also responsible for approximately 50% of the estimated 500 000 cases of acute epididymitis seen each year in the United States.[99]

93. Hart G (1984) Donovanosis. In: Sexually Transmitted Diseases, Holmes KK, Mardh PA, Sparling PF et al. eds. New York: McGraw-Hill, p. 393.
94. Zigas V (1971) Medicine from the past: Donovanosis project in Goilala (1951–1954). Papua New Guinea Med J 14:148.
95. Scott CW, Harper D, Jason RS et al. (1953) Neonatal granuloma inguinale. Am J Dis Child 45:308.
96. Anderson K (1943) The cultivation from granuloma inguinale of a micro-organism having the characteristics of Donovan bodies in the yolk sac of chick embryos. Science 97:560.
97. Felman YM, Nikitas JA (1981) Granuloma inguinale. Cutis 27:364.
98. Thompson SE, Washington AE (1983) Epidemiology of sexually transmitted *Chlamydia* infections. Epidemiol Rev 5:96.
99. National Institutes of Health NIAID Study Group on Sexually Transmitted Diseases: 1980 status report (1981) Summaries and panel recommendations. Washington, DO: US Government Printing Office.
100. Millar MI (1987) Genital chlamydial infection: a role for social scientists. Soc Sci Med 25:1289.

TABLE 28.13   Clinical spectrum of *C. trachomatis* infections (excluding trachoma)

Male genitalia
  Urethritis
  Prostatitis (?)
  Epididymitis
  Infertility (?)
  LGV
Female genitalia
  Urethritis
  Cervicitis
  Endometritis
  Salpingitis
  Oophoritis
  Pelviperitonitis
  Curtis–Fitz–Hugh syndrome
  Infertility
  LGV
Both sexes
  Proctitis
  Pharyngitis (?)
  Conjunctivitis
  Pneumonia
  Otitis media
Disseminated infections
  Reiter syndrome

In men and women most, chlamydial infections are asymptomatic, but *C. trachomatis* also plays an important role in causing urethral syndrome (dysuria-pyuria syndrome), mucopurulent cervicitis (MPC),[101] acute PID,[102] consequent periappendicitis, perihepatitis (Fitz–Hugh–Curtis syndrome),[103] and maternal and infant infections during pregnancy and following delivery.[104] Chlamydia accounts for one-quarter to one-half of the one million recognized cases of PID in the United States each year. These infections, in addition to *C. trachomatis* infections of the fallopian tube not clinically recognized as PID, contribute significantly to the increasing number of women who experience ectopic pregnancy or involuntary infertility (Table 28.13).

Maternal infection during pregnancy has been associated with postpartum endometritis and, in some studies, with an increased perinatal mortality; the latter relationship requires further study. Infants with infected mothers can acquire a chlamydial infection at birth from contact with infected cervicovaginal secretions. Each year more than 155 000 infants are born to *Chlamydia*-infected mothers. These newborns are at high risk of developing inclusion conjunctivitis and pneumonia and are at slightly elevated risk of having otitis media and bronchiolitis. In fact, *Chlamydia* is the most common cause of neonatal eye infections and of afebrile interstitial pneumonia in infants less than 6 months of age.

Urogenital infection with *Chlamydia trachomatis* can also lead to development of an acute inflammatory arthritis, and this acute disease becomes chronic in some individuals. Metabolic and other characteristics of intra-articular chlamydia differ from those of actively growing bacteria. The interaction of chlamydiae and the synovium is not completely understood.[105]

Enormous cost is associated with chlamydial infections. Many of these costs result from the management of women with PID and its complications[106] and from the management of infants hospitalized with chlamydial pneumonia. This estimated cost does not reflect the human suffering experienced by those with chlamydial disease. Further growth in the economic burden of chlamydial infections will occur as these infections become more prevalent.

To reduce the morbidity and subsequent complications associated with *C. trachomatis* infection in North America and Europe, effective prevention and control strategies must be followed. Comprehensive guidelines for the formulation of such control programs, as well as diagnostic and therapeutic approaches to infected individuals, are provided in the following sections.

RISK ASSESSMENT

Establishing a profile for patients at increased risk of having a genital infection caused by *C. trachomatis* can be based on multiple criteria.

Individual characteristics and practices

Age, number of sex partners, socio-economic status, and sexual preference are predictors of *C. trachomatis* infection. Genital infection rates appear to be inversely related to age and positively correlated with number of sex partners. Sexually active women younger than 20 years of age have chlamydial infection rates two to three times higher than those for women 20 years of age or older, and the rates for women ages 20 to 29 are considerably higher than those for women 30 years of age or older.[107]

Similarly, the rates of urethral infection among teenage males are higher than those for adults.[108] Risk of infection increases with the number of sex partners.[109,110] In some studies, lower socio-economic status has been correlated with an increased risk of chlamydial infections.[107,109] The prevalence of urethral chlamydial infection among homosexual men is approximately one-third the prevalence among heterosexual men,[108,111] but 4–8% of homosexual men seen in STD clinics have rectal chlamydial infection.

Method of contraception

Although applying for all STDs, it was demonstrated in particular for chlamydial infections that persons who use barrier methods of contraception (condom, diaphragm, diaphragm and foam) are at reduced risk for chlamydial infection relative to those who use other methods or no form of contraception.[109] Use of intrauterine devices has not yet been investigated for its effect on rates of *C. trachomatis* infection.[112]

Pregnancy

In the United States, the prevalence of reported cervical chlamydial infection among pregnant women has varied from 2% to 37%, with most studies reporting infection rates of approximately 8 to 12%.[99,110,113] In general, infection has been most prevalent in the youngest age group, among unmarried women, and among inner-city, lower socio-economic status women.

101. Bruham RC, Paavonen J, Stevens CE et al. (1984) Mucopurulent cervicitis—the ignored counterpart in women of urethritis in men. **N Engl J Med** 311:1.
102. Sweet RL, Schachter J, Robbie MO (1983) Failure of beta-lactam antibiotics to eradicate *Chlamydia trachomatis* in the endometrium despite apparent clinical cure of acute salpingitis. **J Am Med Assoc** 250:2641.
103. Schachter J, Dawson CR (1978) Human Chlamdial Infections. Littleton, MA: PSG Publishing.
104. Alexander ER, Harrison HR (1983) Role of *Chlamydia trachomatis* in perinatal infection. **Rev Infect Dis** 5:713.
105. Villareal C, Whittum-Hudson JA, Hudson AP (2002) Persistent Chlamydiae and chronic arthritis. **Arthritis Res** 4:5.
106. Washington AE, Arno PS (1985) Economic cost of pelvic inflammatory disease 1984–1990: including associated ectopic pregnancy and infertility, abstracted. Presented at the 6th International Meeting of International Society for Sexually Transmitted Diseases, Brighton, England, August.
107. Schacter J, Stoner E, Moncada J (1983) Screening for chlamydial infections in women attending family planning clinics. Evaluation of presumptive indicators for therapy. **West J Med** 138:375.
108. Stamm WE, Koutsky LA, Benedetti JK et al. (1984) *Chlamydia trachomatis* urethral infections in men. Prevalence, risk factors, and clinical manifestations. **Ann Intern Med** 100:47.
109. McCormack WM, Rosner B, McComb DE et al. (1985) Infection with *Chlamydia trachomatis* in female college students. **Am J Epidemiol** 121:107.
110. Chacko MR, Lovchik JC (1984) *Chlamydia trachomatis* infection in sexually active adolescents: prevalence and risk factors. **Pediatrics** 73:836.
111. Judson FN (1981) Epidemiology and control of nongonococcal urethritis and genital chlamydial infections: a review. **Sex Transm Dis** 8:117.
112. Washington AE, Gove S, Schachter J et al. (1985) Oral contraceptives. *Chlamydia trachomatis* infection, and pelvic inflammatory disease. A word of caution about protection. **J Am Med Assoc** 253:2246.
113. Harrison HR, Alexander ER, Weinstein L et al. (1983) Cervical *Chlamydia trachomatis* and mycoplasmal infections in pregnancy. Epidermiology and outcomes. **J Am Med Assoc** 250:172.

Health care facility

Various types of health care facilities will report different expected infection rates among women attendees. Not surprisingly, STD clinics report the highest rates of *C. trachomatis* infection (an average of 20–30% of all patients tested).[98,114] The next highest isolation rates are reported from clinics for adolescent patients (8–20%),[110,115,116] and from family planning clinics (6–23%).[107] Insufficient data are available to estimate expected rates in private practices, community health centers, and hospital emergency rooms.

Contact with an STD patient

Individuals with a history of sexual exposure to persons with a chlamydial or gonococcal infection are at high risk of chlamydial infection. Female sex partners of men with confirmed chlamydial urethritis, or confirmed gonococcal urethritis, have *Chlamydia* isolated from the endocervical tract in 70% and 36% of cases, respectively. Of all the women whose sex partners are reported to have NGU, 30–40% harbor cervical chlamydial infection. Of men who are the sex partners of women with confirmed chlamydia mucopurulent cervicitis (MPC) PID, 25–50% have *Chlamydia* isolated from the urethra. Many of these contacts are asymptomatic.

MICROBIOLOGY

Chlamydiae are obligate intracellular bacteria that have been placed in their own order and family. They share a common group antigen, and a unique developmental cycle involving two morphologic forms: one adapted to extracellular survival, the elementary body (EB), and the other to intracellular multiplication, the reticular body (RB).

The first step in the infectious process involves attachment of the EB to a susceptible host cell. Next, the EB penetrates the host cell by a unique mechanism. It appears that the chlamydiae induce nonphagocytic host cells to specifically phagocytize the organism by means of "parasite specified" endocytosis. The EB then enters the cell within a phagosome. Within a few hours after entry, the EB undergoes profound changes in the cell envelope. The resulting RB continues to grow and in 10 to 15 hours after infection binary fission begins. At 20 to 30 hours, some of the RBs become typical EBs, which leave the cell. The mechanism of release is not well understood.

The EB envelope is rigid and is characterized by a major outer membrane protein (MOMP). Parts of this molecule moderate the serotype specificity. The genes encoding for the MOMP of several serovars have been cloned and sequenced. *C. trachomatis* can be divided into 15 serovars by the means of specific antibodies. All chlamydiae contain a serologically identical LPS, which is quite similar to the LPS of some Gram-negative bacteria.[117]

C. trachomatis expresses a heat-shock protein of 60 kDa. This protein exhibits about 50% homology with human heat-shock proteins. Thus, part of the immune responses may be explained by the shared antigens. Some studies demonstrated antibodies to the heat-shock proteins in women with PID in a high prevalence. It is unclear, however, whether these antibodies are directly involved in the pathological process of PID or whether they only indicate the persistent chlamydial infection. Other authors found antibodies in infertile men binding to this protein as well as to their own spermatozoa.[118]

PHYSICAL EXAMINATION

Several clinical syndromes are associated with *C. trachomatis* infection. Although they are always indistinguishable from those caused by other bacteria, the clinical features often provide the most suitable basis for initiating treatment, especially if complete bacteriologic evaluation is not possible, or while the practitioner awaits the results of specific laboratory tests. However, it cannot be overemphasized that there are also "silent" infections in men and women, from which infections of a sexual partner may result. Clinical signs of STD do not correlate with chlamydial serovars.[119]

CHLAMYDIA-ASSOCIATED SYNDROMES IN POST-PUBERTAL MALES

The typical clinical syndrome following the infection of male genital organs is a mild, late-developing urethritis, formerly, when positive diagnosis of chlamydia was impossible, called NGU. The incubation period of urethritis is about 10 days and it disappears spontaneously within three weeks in about 80% of the males. Prostatitis may follow in 20% of urethritis cases appearing with the typical symptoms of acute prostatitis: dysuria, perineal or abdominal pain, and symptoms of general infection. With and without urethritis or prostatitis, acute epididymo-orchitis may occur. Although it is not possible to culture chlamydiae from the affected epididymis (even not from the ejaculate), it is generally accepted that *C. trachomatis* is found in the urethra of 30–50% of patients with acute epididymitis. Thus, the organism is the leading known cause of epididymitis among men younger than 35 years of age.[98] Approximately 15–30% of heterosexual men with gonococcal urethritis have simultaneous urethral infection caused by *C. trachomatis*.[98,114,120] An even higher proportion (25–50%) of women with *N. gonorrhoeae* infection also have *C. trachomatis* infection of the cervix.[98,114,121] Women who have other STDs, such as trichomoniasis and bacterial vaginosis, are also at increased risk of having chlamydial infection.

Male chlamydial diseases often resolves spontaneously. However, there are insufficient data to describe the mean duration of an untreated infection. The duration of chlamydial infection is reduced in animals previously exposed to chlamydiae and in older humans, suggesting that partial immunity may result from exposure.[122]

CHLAMYDIA-ASSOCIATED SYNDROMES IN POST-PUBERTAL FEMALES

Women may also develop a urethral syndrome or urethritis, the clinical signs and symptoms being milder than those in men. The "counterpart" to the male urethritis is the mucopurulent cervicitis (MPC) (Fig. 28.29). This may be followed by ascension of chlamydiae, resulting in the most severe complication, PID. *C. trachomatis* has been isolated from 30–50% of women examined who have mucopurulent endocervical exudate.[101] Similarly, *C. trachomatis* has been isolated from female patients with acute dysuria, particularly those with pyuria and a negative Gram stain of unspun urine.[105] Among women with PID, the *Chlamydia* recovery rate is approximately 25–50% with optimal technique, but serologic data suggest that as many as 50% of acute PID cases may be associated with *C. trachomatis*.

114. Stamm WE, Guinan ME, Johnson C et al. (1984) Effect of treatment regimens for *Neisseria gonorrhoeae* on simultaneous infection with *Chlamydia trachomatis*. **N Engl J Med** 310:545.

115. Shafer MA, Beck A, Blain B et al. (1984) *Chlamydia trachomatis*: important relationships to race, contraception, lower genital tract infection, and Papanicolaou smear. **J Pediatr** 104:141.

116. Anglin TM, Brown RF, Kumar ML (1981) *Chlamydia trachomatis* in adolescent females [Abstracted]. **Pediatr Res** 15:440.

117. Schachter J (1984) Biology of *Chlamydia trachomatis*. In: Sexually Transmitted Diseases, Holmes KK, Mardh P-A, Sparling PF, eds. New York: McGraw-Hill, p. 243.

118. Witkin SS, Toth A (1983) Relationship between genital tract infections, sperm antibodies in seminal fluid and infertility. **Fertil Steril** 40:805.

119. Näher H, Petzoldt D (1991) Chlamydia-trachomatis-Serovars und das klinische Bild der urogenitalen Infektionen. **Hautarzt** 42:298.

120. Washington AE (1982) Update on treatment recommendations for gonococcal infections. **Rev Infect Dis** (Suppl) 4:S758.

121. Bruham RC, Kuo CC, Stevens CE et al. (1982) Treatment of concomitant *Neisseria gonorrhoeae* and *Chlamydia trachomatis* infections in women: comparison of trimethoprim-sulfamethoxazole with ampicillin-probenecid. **Rev Infect Dis** 4:491.

122. Golden MR, Schillinger JA, Markowitz L, St Louis ME (2000) Duration of untreated genital infections with chlamydia trachomatis: a review of the literature. **Sex Transm Dis** 27:329.

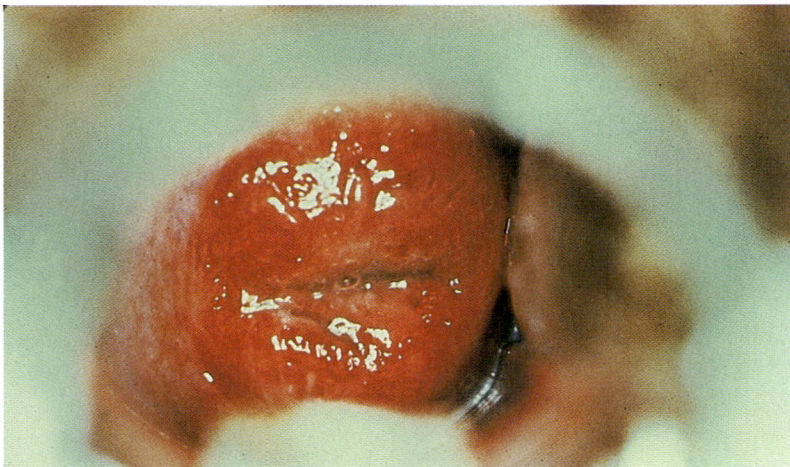

Fig. 28.29 Mucopurulent cervicitis due to chlamydia trachomatis. (Courtesy of ER Alexander, MD)

Severe consequences of PID include female infertility, ectopic pregnancy, chronic pelvic pain, complications during pregnancies, and neonatal diseases. There is a significant association between chlamydial infection and chorioamnionitis, birth weight, and severe neonatal infection.[123]

C. trachomatis may cause arthritis syndromes.[124] The term "sexually acquired reactive arthritis" (SARA) was proposed for that condition. Inheritance of HLA B27 confers an increased relative risk of 30 to 50 times for the development of this condition, which may be part of Reiter syndrome. In joint material of patients with SARA, *C. trachomatis* antigen and *C. trachomatis* DNA were demonstrated, suggesting that direct interaction between microbial components and class I HLA antigens in the joint may be central to the pathogenesis of this disease.[125]

CHLAMYDIA-ASSOCIATED SYNDROMES IN INFANTS

Initial *C. trachomatis* perinatal infection involves mucous membranes of the eye, oropharynx, urogenital tract, and rectum. *C. trachomatis* infection among neonates can most often be recognized by conjunctivitis that develops 5–12 days after birth. Chlamydia is the most frequent identifiable infectious cause of ophthalmia neonatorum. *C. trachomatis* also is a common cause of subacute, afebrile pneumonia with onset from 1 to 3 months of age. Asymptomatic infections can also occur in the oropharynx, genital tract, and rectum among neonates. *C. trachomatis* infection of neonates results from perinatal exposure to the mother's infected cervix. The prevalence of *C. trachomatis* infection among pregnant women is usually >5%, regardless of race/ethnicity or socio-economic status. Neonatal ocular prophylaxis with silver nitrate solution or antibiotic ointments does not prevent perinatal transmission of *C. trachomatis* from mother to infant. However, ocular prophylaxis with those agents does prevent gonococcal ophthalmia and should be continued for that reason (see Prevention of ophthalmia neonatorum).

DIAGNOSIS

There are no typical signs and symptoms that allow the diagnosis without laboratory confirmations. Näher *et al.*[126] investigated the frequency of symptoms in the case histories of 68 female patients with, and of 313 without, *C. trachomatis* infections. Dysuria, vaginal discharge, and burning or itching in the genital region were reported by 50% of chlamydia-positive

TABLE 28.14   Statistics on *C. trachomatis* (review of recent publications)

Epidemiology	
Women:	
Annualized incidence rates	1.5%
<25 years	5.4%
>25 years	0.3%
Family planning clinics	3.9–12.3%
STD clinic	2.5–14%
With genital symptoms	7.2%
Positive for *N. gonorrhoeae*	1.0%
Abortion seekers	4.6–14.5%
Sterility	5.4%
General practice	3.9–7.1%
Laboratories	2.8–5.5%
Men:	10–14.4%
Male partners of PID	43.7%
Presenting with condylomata	44%
Risk factors	
Age <25 years	
Relationship <1 year	
More than one sexual partner	
Hormonal or no contraception	
Nulliparity	
No history of genital infection	
Past chlamydial or gonococcal infection	
Having vaginal discharge or dysuria	
Being an STD contact	
None of the risk factors has a high sensitivity and a high positive predictive value for infection	
Obtaining material	
Cytobrush is superior to Ayre's spatula	
positive when samples are adequately taken	7.2%
positive when samples are inadequately taken	0.78%
Direct antigen test (compared with cell culture)	
Sensitivity (irrespective symptomatic/asymptomatic)	25.0–92.0%
Specificity	89.0–99.1%
Positive predictive values	32.1–93.0%
Negative predictive values	96.4–98.6%
ELISA (compared with cell culture)	
Sensitivity (higher in women, lower in urine)	29.0–100%
Specificity	92.0–100%
Positive predictive value	63.3–100%
Negative predictive value	95.7–100%
DNA-Probes and PCR	
Sensitivity (more sensitive than cell culture)	68.0–90.9%
Specificity	75.0–100%
Positive predictive value	96.2–100%
Negative predictive value	97.2%
Serology	
Differences in antibody prevalence to specific chlamydial antigens were not related to the site of chlamydial isolation	
Costs	
Identification of each positive case:	
Routine EIA confirmed by DFA (1995)	$434
PMNs followed by EIA confirmed by DFA (1995)	$199
Hospital admissions more than double the costs of a routine screening program and prophylactic treatment. (1995)	

123. Donders GG, Moerman P, De-Wet GH et al. (1991) The association between *Chlamydia* cervicitis, chorioamnionitis and neonatal complications. **Arch Gynecol Obstet** 249:79.

124. Keat A (1990) Sexually transmitted arthritis syndromes. **Med Clin North Am** 74:1617.

125. Taylor-Robinson D, Gilroy CB, Thomas BJ et al. (1992) Detection of *Chlamydia trachomatis* DNA in joints of reactive arthritis patients by polymerase chain reaction. **Lancet** 340:81.

126. Näher H, Lamminger C, Zimmerman J et al. (1991) Die Aussagekraft von Symptomen und Befunden bei der zervikalen Chlamydia trachomatis Infektion. **Hautarzt** 42:687.

women and 53.7% ($n = 168$) of Chlamydia-negative women. In the chlamydia-positive patients, vaginal discharge was observed in 83.8%, whereas in chlamydia-negative women discharge occurred in 72.8%. Leukocytosis (more than 4 per high-power field) was found in 52.9% of the chlamydia-positive women, as compared to 23% of the chlamydia-negative women. Therefore, microbiologic detection of the infectious agent is essential for a diagnosis of *C. trachomatis* cervicitis.

Until now, the absence of an inexpensive, rapid, simple, and reliable diagnostic test for chlamydial infection has limited control efforts. In recent years, antigen detection methods and DNA probes have offered steps toward this goal. Despite encouraging improvements in diagnostic capability, current tests are not ideal. They are relatively difficult to perform, the reagents are expensive, the test procedures require considerable experience, and have limited application. The search for new diagnostic methods for *C. trachomatis* continues. An overview of the current diagnostic methods for chlamydiae is given in Table 28.14.

Cultures

Tissue culture is the gold standard for laboratory diagnosis.[103]

Two major components are needed to culture *C. trachomatis*: (1) a cell-culture system, and (2) a method to identify inclusions growing in cell culture. The cell line of choice is McCoy. Alternatively, a particular strain of HeLa cells (HeLa 229)[127] can be used, but is usually restricted to research laboratories. The incubation requires 2–3 days in medium containing cycloheximide.[128,129] For identification, fluorescent or otherwise stained antibodies are usually used.[130]

Culturing also has the following disadvantages: (1) the cost and complexity of laboratory requirements can be prohibitive; (2) viability of cells in specimens is limited, Specimens can be kept at 4°C only up to 24 hours before processing, or frozen at −70°C if they cannot be inoculated within 24 hours, but both methods reduce the number of cell-infecting units; (3) specimens must be placed in specially prepared transport media; (4) the cell monolayer may be contaminated with other bacteria or viruses, particularly in vaginal or rectal specimens; and (5) the results are not available until 48 hours after incubation.

Cytologic methods for the detection of chlamydiae are of limited value. They have a low level of sensitivity and are thus inadequate in modern diagnostic efforts.

Antigen detection

Methods of antigen detection are widely used. Two kinds of methods are available: (1) examination of a direct smear with specific antibody, either stained by FITC or with peroxidase; and (2) EIA. Kits of both methods have undergone considerable evaluation.

Direct-smear fluorescent antibody test

With this procedure, specimen material is obtained by swab and applied directly to a slide, which is fixed and then incubated with fluorescein-conjugated monoclonal antibody before being examined under a fluorescent microscope. Total processing time is usually 30 to 40 minutes. Critical steps include: (1) obtaining a satisfactory specimen and preparing a satisfactory smear (this can be checked before or after staining); (2) drying the specimen properly before fixing it; (3) using a high-quality fluorescent microscope; and (4) obtaining and maintaining an experienced microscopist who can recognize elementary bodies and artifacts.

The major advantages of the direct smear test are: (1) the uncomplicated transport and storage of specimens; (2) rapid processing time compared with that required for other methods;[131] (3) a high specificity; and (4) the ability to check on adequacy of specimen collection (i.e., cells on the slide). Disadvantages of the method are: (1) the requirement for precise specimen collection; (2) the need for a high-quality fluorescent microscope equipment; (3) the need for an experienced microscopist; and (4) the relatively labor-intensive nature of the process.

In principle, direct antibody tests are rapid and easy to handle. They have sensitivities that range from 70–100% for men and 68–100% for women, and specificities that range from 87% to 99% for men and 82% to 100% for women; if the tests are read by competent observers the values are at the top end of the ranges.[132]

Other authors report on similar rates of sensitivity, specificity, as well as positive and negative predictive values (73.1%, 93.8%, 63.3%, and 96% for men and 80%, 95.6%, 71.4%, and 97.2% for women, respectively.[133] The same rates were found in patients with low prevalence of infection.[134]

Enzyme immunoassay

Enzyme immunoassay[135] measures antigen-antibody reactions through an enzyme-linked immunoabsorbent assay (ELISA) and requires a spectrophotometer. Processing time for specimens is approximately one hour in modern test kits.[136]

The advantages of the ELISA are: (1) the uncomplicated transport and storage of specimens; (2) the objective method of measurement in the laboratory, which involves standard equipment and does not depend on a specially trained observer; and (3) the ability to test large numbers of specimens at a time.

Skilled reading is not a feature of ELISAs, which according to the literature have sensitivities that range from 62 to 97% for men and 64 to 100% for women, and specificities that range from 92 to 100% for men and 89 to 100% for women. However, the cut-off point for detection of positive results is critical and influences the given rates of sensitivity and specificity.[137,138] A strong association between the number of chlamydial inclusions in cell culture and a positive ELISA outcome is noted.[139]

The disadvantages of ELISAs are: (1) the adequacy of the specimen cannot be checked; and (2) the test cannot be performed while the patient is waiting (although this is also true for the direct smear test if no fluorescence microscope is available).

Chlamydial antigen is restricted to infected cells; since these are discharged with the urine, it was suggested to use voided urine as test material for ELISA. However, this gives lower rates of specificity and sensitivity and does not add advantages to the direct antigen detection, other than ease of specimen collection.[140]

127. Kuo CC, Wang SS, Wentworth BB et al. (1972) Primary isolation of TRIC organisms in HeLa 229 cells treated with DEAE Dextran. *J Infect Dis* 125:665.

128. Ripa KT, Mardh PA (1977) Cultivation of *Chlamydia trachomatis* in cycloheximide treated McCoy cells. *J Clin M crobiol* 6:328.

129. Yoder BL, Stamm WE, Koester CM et al. (1981) Microtest procedure for isolation of *Chlamydia trachomatis*. *J Clin Microbiol* 13:1036.

130. Stamm WE, Tam M, Koester M et al. (1983) Detection of *Chlamydia trachomatis* inclusions in McCoy cell cultures with fluorescein-conjugated monoclonal antibodies. *J Clin Microbiol* 17:666.

131. Lossick JG, Smeltzer M (1984) Direct smear diagnosis of chlamydia infections. XI International Congress for Tropical Medicine and Malaria. Abstract and Poster. vol. 87.

132. Taylor-Robinson D, Thomas BJ (1991) Laboratory techniques for the diagnosis of chlamydial infections. *Genitourin Med* 67:256.

133. Mumtaz G, Ridgway GL, Nayagam AT et al. (1990) Comparison of an enzyme immunoassay (Ortho) with cell culture and immunofluorescence for the detection of genital chlamydial infection. *Int J STD AIDS* 1:187.

134. Skulnick M, Small GW, Simor AE et al. (1991) Comparison of the Clearview *Chlamydia* test, Chlamydiazyme, and cell culture for detection of *Chlamydia trachomatis* in women with a low prevalence of infection. *J Clin Microbiol* 29:2086.

135. Dowda HE, Parker EK, Redden SE et al. (1983) Evaluation of the chlamydiazyme EIA for the detection of *Chlamydia trachomatis* in genital specimens. Abstract No. 54. Interscience Conference on Antimicrobial Agents and Chemotherapy Proceedings 88, October 24.

136. Reichart CA, Gaydos CA, Brady WE et al. (1990) Evaluation of Abbott Testpack Chlamydia for detection of *Chlamydia trachomatis* in patients attending sexually transmitted diseases clinics. **Sex Transm Dis** 17:147.

137. Taylor-Robinson D, Thomas BJ (1991) Laboratory techniques for the diagnosis of chlamydial infections. **Genitourin Med** 67:256.

138. Clark A, Stamm WE, Gaydos C et al. (1992) Multicenter evaluation of the AntigEnz Chlamydia enzyme immunoassay for diagnosis of *Chlamydia trachomatis* genital infection. **J Clin Microbiol** 30:2762.

139. Magder LS, Klontz KC, Bush LH et al. (1990) Effect of patient characteristics on performance of an enzyme immunoassay for detecting cervical *Chlamydia trachomatis* infection. **J Clin Microbiol** 28:781.

140. Sellors JW, Mahony JB, Jang D et al. (1991) Comparison of cervical, urethral, and urine specimens for the detection of *Chlamydia trachomatis* in women. **J Infect Dis** 164:205.

This technique may be useful in symptomatic men, but not in symptomatic women.[141] Other studies describe converse results. In a group with low prevalence of chlamydia, the urinary ELISA sample had a sensitivity of 84% whereas the urethral ELISA sample had a sensitivity of 57%. The authors concluded that the urinary sample is superior to the urethral sample, and that the urinary sample could be used for screening programs to detect chlamydia infection among women.[142]

Immunoassays with antigens labeled by a chemoluminescent agent are also available.[143]

DNA probes

The introduction of DNA amplification tests such as the polymerase chain reaction (PCR) and the ligase chain reaction (LCR) allowed a higher sensitivity and specificity than tissue culture. The association with the results of the culture is excellent, even in populations with low prevalence of infection. In the next five years, the newly developed technique of multiplex PCR that allows for the detection of DNA of several bacteria in one assay will improve the diagnostic capabilities of the STD laboratory.

Serology

Chlamydia serology has little value in routine clinical management and basically remains a tool in epidemiologic reasearch. Although some serologic tests are commercially available, they have not been shown to be useful in routine diagnosis. High antibody titers may be suggestive of an etiologic association in deep-seated chlamydial infections (epididymitis, arthritis, salpingitis, etc.), but interpretation is difficult, since the distinction between a current and past infection is problematic.[144]

Diagnostic considerations

The value of diagnostic tests for detecting *C. trachomatis* infection depends mainly on the prevalence of disease in the population tested. For low-risk groups, the predictive value of a positive test is lower than for high-prevalence populations, even if the test is highly sensitive and specific. For example, in a population with a 5% prevalence, a rapid test with a 95% specificity and sensitivity will have a predictive positive value of 50% (meaning that there is only a 50% chance that an individual who is diagnosed as having disease actually has it). If an increase in the predictive value of a positive test is desired, in order to lower risks of incorrectly labeling persons as having an STD, positive screening tests have to be confirmed by other tests (with an accompanying rise in cost). The significance of new tests, such as DNA probes, has to be viewed in this respect.

Laboratory quality control assumes increasing importance when tests are widely used. The test kits that are distributed by manufacturers should include positive and negative reference samples. Their sensitivity, specificity, and positive and negative predictive values should be indicated with respect to the population tested.

THERAPY

High-risk groups

High-risk groups should be defined using demographic profiles and the estimated or established prevalence of chlamydial infection in a particular community or patient population. Although the criteria described under Risk assessment can be used as a guide to establishing a high-risk profile, local determinants of risk are more precise and should be identified if possible. Local data also provide more accurate baseline prevalences, against which the success of prevention and control strategies can be measured.

Patients in the following groups should immediately receive a regimen that includes effective treatment against *C. trachomatis* infection, unless local or individual circumstances dictate otherwise. Although highly desirable, methods for vaccination against *C. trachomatis* are not yet beyond the experimental status.

Asymptomatic contacts of patients with syndromes associated with chlamydia

Individuals exposed through sexual contact with patients who have any of the above symptomatic syndromes (within 30 days of the onset of their symptoms or clinical evaluation) should be evaluated for STD and treated for presumptive chlamydial infection. Since PID is a frequent cause of female infertility, all patients in whom a tubal factor is demonstrated have to be examined for chlamydia infections.

Gonococcal infection

Women with confirmed *N. gonorrhoeae* infection of the endocervix, heterosexual men with diagnosed gonococcal infection of the urethra, and sex partners of members of both of these groups of patients should be treated with an antimicrobial regimen that is effective against both *N. gonorrhoeae* and *C. trachomatis* infection.

In particular, in patients of high risk groups and when the diagnostic equipment is insufficient, the "syndromic therapy" is advised. In these cases, when urethritis, cervicitis or adnexitis is present, an antibiotic therapy covering both *C. trachomatis* and *N. gonorrhoeae* should be used.[145,146]

Screening

Selective screening to detect asymptomatic infection is an essential component of a successful control program. Whenever possible, criteria for routine screening should be based on local determinants of risk. An appropriate diagnostic method must be selected. Diagnostic considerations for current testing methods are discussed above. The following guidelines are provided to assist in determining which test to use.

SCREENING CRITERIA

No single individual characteristic or practice is in itself a sufficient criterion to define which person should be screened. However, a composite of individual factors, in conjunction with a community factor, such as type of health care facility, will help to maximize yield from screening. Consequently, available evidence leads to the recommendation that the priorities for routine screening shown below be used.

STD clinic   At a clinic, the following steps should be taken: (1) individuals attending STD clinics who otherwise would not be offered antichlamydial treatment should be screened first (The screening of asymptomatic, high-risk women should be accorded the highest priority. In general, the screening of heterosexual men should have a higher priority than screening homosexual men.); and (2) individuals with symptomatic syndromes associated with *Chlamydia* should be screened next. (Screening of women should be accorded higher priority than screening of men.)

Other high-risk health care facilities   Health care facilities other than STD clinics may also have a high prevalence of chlamydial infections. In particular, many adolescent and family palnning clinics are categorized as high-risk centers, but a wide disparity in rates of chlamydial infection may be observed in different populations. Facilities that serve high-risk populations should follow the order of screening priority for STD clinics above; those serving undetermined or low-risk populations should follow the priority below for Undetermined/low-risk health care facility.

141. Gene M, Stary A, Bergman S et al. (1991) Detection of *Chlamydia trachomatis* in first-void urine collected from men and women attending a venereal clinic. **Acta Pathol Microbiol Immunol Scand** 99:455.
142. Svensson LO, Mares I, Olsson SE (1991) Detection of *Chlamydia trachomatis* in urinary samples from women. **Genitourin Med** 67:117.
143. Scieux C, Bianchi A, Henry S et al. (1992) Evaluation of a chemiluminometric immunoassay for detection of *Chlamydia trachomatis* in the urine of male and female patients. **Eur J Clin Microbiol Infect Dis** 11:704.
144. Gardner JJ (1992) Comparison of the vaginal flora in sexually abused and nonabused girls. **J Pediatr** 120:872.
145. Uuskula A, Plank T, Lassus A, Bingham JS (2001) Sexually transmitted infections in Estonial–syndromic management of urethritis in a European country? **Int J STD AIDS** 12:493.
146. Behets FM, Miller WC, Cohen MS (2001) Syndromic treatment of gonococcal and chlamydial infections in women seeking primary care for the genital discharge syndrome: decision-making. **Bull World Health Organ** 79:1070.

Undetermined/low-risk health care facilities   Patients should be screened in the following manner: (1) persons in urban settings who are younger, have lower socio-economic status, and have multiple sex partners, and who otherwise would not be offered antichlamydial treatment, should be screened first (In this category of high-risk patients, women should be accorded highest priority for screening.); and (2) individuals with symptomatic syndromes associated with *Chlamydia* should also be screened. Screening of women should be accorded higher priority than screening of men.

PREGNANT PATIENTS

Certain groups of pregnant women are at high risk of chlamydial infections. Transmission to the newborn is a well-established consequence of these infections. The precise effects of chlamydial infection on pregnancy outcome are uncertain, and studies are under way to resolve this issue.
Recommendation   Screening is suggested at the first prenatal visit for the following groups of pregnant women:

1. Adolescents (younger than 20 years of age)
2. Unmarried women
3. Married women who may be at high risk because of multiple sex partners or a history of other STD.

Screening of pregnant women who fall into any of these high-risk categories in inner-city hospitals is particularly important because of the high prevalence of asymptomatic infections among the patients served by these facilities. Although tubal infertility is often related to chlamydial infection, it is unknown whether the infection of the newborn is more frequent in pregnancies following *in vitro* fertilization for tubal infertility.

NEONATES

Ophthalmia prophylaxis   None of the presently recommended approaches for prophylaxis against gonococcal and chlamydial ophthalmia neonatorum is completely effective. Silver nitrate is effective in preventing gonococcal infections, but it does not prevent chlamydial disease and frequently causes chemical conjunctivitis. Erythromycin is effective in preventing both gonococcal and chlamydial ophthalmia and does not cause chemical conjunctivitis, but the topical use of this drug does not prevent nasopharyngeal chlamydial infection or pneumonia. Furthermore, erythromycin prophylaxis is considerably more expensive than silver nitrate prophylaxis. Tetracycline ointment has not been as extensively evaluated as has erythromycin but appears to be as effective. Whichever type of prophylaxis is used, it should be implemented no later than one hour after birth and preferably immediately after delivery since delayed application may reduce efficacy.
Recommendation   Erythromycin (0.5%) ophthalmic ointment, tetracycline (1%) ointment, or aqueous solution (1%) of silver nitrate should be instilled into the eyes of all neonates as soon as possible after delivery and never later than one hour after birth. Single-use tubes or ampoules are preferable to multiple-use tubes.

NEONATAL INFECTION

Eighteen to 50% of infants born to infected mothers will have conjunctivitis between one and three weeks after birth.[104] The symptoms are often mild, and the disease may be missed unless looked for carefully. Although considerable morbidity results acutely from the severe form of this disease, it is usually self-limited and does not appear to result in loss of vision. Three to 18% of infants born to infected mothers will develop chlamydial pneumonia/bronchiolitis, usually at 1 to 4 months of age. In most cases this is a mild disease, but it can be severe and require hospitalization.
Recommendation   Screening for neonatal infection is not indicated. Newborns with conjunctivitis and afebrile pneumonia/bronchiolitis should have specimens culture-tested for *C. trachomatis* and be appropriately treated as recommended below. If cultures are positive, mothers (and their sex partners) of the infected children should also be treated.
The following sections are adopted from the 1998 CDC recommendations.[43]

TABLE 28.15   Recommended treatment regimens for *C. trachomatis* infection

Drug	Dose	Route
Azithromycin	1g in a single dose	po
Doxycycline	100mg 2 times a day for 7 days	po
Alternatives		
Erythromycin base	500mg four times a day for 7 days	po
Erythromycin ethylsuccinate	800mg four times a day for 7 days	po
Ofloxacin	300mg twice a day for 7 days	po

Chlamydial infections among adolescents and adults

Treatment of infected patients prevents transmission to sex partners, and, for infected pregnant women treatment might prevent transmission of *C. trachomatis* to infants during birth. Treatment of sex partners helps to prevent reinfection of the index patient and infection of other partners. Recommended regimens are listed in Table 28.15.

The results of clinical trials indicate that azithromycin and doxycycline are equally efficacious. These investigations were conducted primarily in populations in which follow-up was encouraged and the adherence to a 7-day regimen was good. Azithromycin should always be available to health care providers to treat at least those patients for whom compliance is a question.

To maximize compliance with recommended therapies, medication for chlamydial infections should be dispensed on site, and the first dose should be directly observed. To minimize further transmission of infection, patients treated for chlamydia should be instructed to abstain from sexual intercourse for seven days after single-dose therapy or until completion of a 7-day regimen. Patients also should be instructed to abstain from sexual intercourse until all of their sex partners are cured to minimize the risk of reinfection.

Follow-up

Patients do not need to be retested for chlamydia after completing treatment with doxycycline or azithromycin unless symptoms persist or reinfection is suspected, because these therapies are highly efficacious. A test of cure may be considered three weeks after completion of treatment with erythromycin. The validity of chlamydial culture testing performed at less than three weeks following completion of therapy among patients failing therapy has not been established. False-negative results may occur because of small numbers of chlamydial organisms. In addition, nonculture tests conducted at more than three weeks following completion of therapy for patients successfully treated may sometimes be false-positive because of the continued excretion of dead organisms.

Some studies have demonstrated high rates of infection among women retested several months following treatment, presumably because of reinfection. In some populations, rescreening women several months following treatment may be an effective strategy for detecting further morbidity.

Special considerations

PREGNANCY

Doxycycline and ofloxacin are contraindicated for pregnant women. The safety and efficacy of azithromycin among pregnant and lactating women have not been established. Repeat testing, preferably by culture, three weeks after completion of therapy with the following regimens is recommended because a) none of these regimens are highly efficacious and b) the frequent side effects of erythromycin may discourage patient compliance with the prescribed treatment. The recommended regimens are listed in Table 28.16.

HIV INFECTION

Persons with HIV infection and chlamydial infection should receive the same treatment as patients without HIV infection.

TABLE 28.16 Recommended treatment regimens for *C. trachomatis* infection in pregnant women

Drug	Dose	Route
Erythromycin base	500mg four times a day for 7 days	po
Amoxicillin	500mg three times a day for 7 days	po
Alternative regimen		
Erythromycin base	250mg four times a day for 14 days	
Erythromycin ethylsuccinate	800mg four times a day for 7 days	po
Erythromycin ethylsuccinate	400mg four times a day for 14 days	po
Azithromycin	1g in a single dose	po

Chlamydial infections in infants

Prenatal screening of pregnant women can prevent chlamydial infection among neonates. Pregnant women <25 years of age or who have new or multiple sex partners should be targeted for screening. Periodic prevalence surveys of chlamydial infection can be conducted to confirm the validity of using these recommendations in specific clinical settings.

Ophthalmia neonatorum caused by C. trachomatis

A chlamydial etiology should be considered for all infants aged ≤30 days, who have conjunctivitis.

DIAGNOSTIC CONSIDERATIONS
Chlamydial ophthalmia in the neonate may be diagnosed using the methods described above. Giemsa-stained smears are not sensitive enough. Specimens must contain conjunctival cells, not exudate alone. Specimens should be obtained from the everted eyelid. A specific diagnosis of *C. trachomatis* infection confirms the need for chlamydial treatment not only for the neonate, but also for the mother and her sex partner(s). Ocular exudate from infants being evaluated for chlamydial conjunctivitis should also be tested for *N. gonorrhoeae*.

RECOMMENDED REGIMEN
Erythromycin base 50mg/kg per day orally divided into four doses for 10 to 14 days. Topical antibiotic therapy alone is inadequate for treatment of chlamydial infection and is unnecessary when systemic treatment is administered.

FOLLOW-UP
The efficacy of erythromycin treatment is approximately 80%; a second course of therapy may be required. Follow-up of infants to determine resolution is recommended. The possibility of chlamydial pneumonia should be considered.

MANAGEMENT OF MOTHERS AND THEIR SEX PARTNERS
The mothers of infants who have chlamydial infection and the mother's sex partner should be evaluated and treated (see Chlamydial infections among adolescents and adults).

Infant pneumonia caused by C. trachomatis

Characteristic signs of chlamydial pneumonia among infants include (a) a repetitive staccato cough with tachypnea, and hyperinflation, and (b) bilateral diffuse infiltrates on a chest radiograph. Wheezing is rare, and infants are typically afebrile. Peripheral eosinophilia sometimes occurs in infants who have chlamydial pneumonia. Because clinical presentations differ, initial treatment and diagnostic tests should encompass *C. trachomatis* for all infants 1 to 3 months of age who have possible pneumonia.

DIAGNOSTIC CONSIDERATIONS
Specimens for chlamydial testing should be collected from the nasopharynx. Tissue culture remains the definitive standard for chlamydial pneumonia;

nonculture tests can be used with the knowledge that nonculture tests of nasopharyngeal specimens produce lower sensitivity and specificity than nonculture tests of ocular specimens. Tracheal aspirates and lung biopsy specimens, if collected, should be tested for *C. trachomatis*.

The microimmunofluorescence test for *C. trachomatis* antibody may be helpful. An acute IgM antibody titer 1:32 or greater is strongly suggestive of *C. trachomatis* pneumonia.

Because of the delay in obtaining test results for chlamydia, the decision to include an agent in the antibiotic regimen that is active against *C. trachomatis* must frequently be based on the clinical and radiologic findings. The results of tests for chlamydial infection assist in the management of an infant's illness and determine the need for treatment of the mother and her sex partners.

RECOMMENDED REGIMEN
Erythromycin 50mg/kg per day orally divided into four doses for 10 to 14 days.

FOLLOW-UP
The effectiveness of erythromycin treatment is approximately 80%; a second course of therapy may be required. Follow-up of infants is recommended to determine that the pneumonia has resolved. Some infants with chlamydial pneumonia have had abnormal pulmonary function tests later in childhood.

MANAGEMENT OF MOTHERS AND THEIR SEX PARTNERS
Mothers of infants who have chlamydial infection and the mother's sex partners should be evaluated and treated according to the recommended treatment of adults with chlamydial infections.

Infants born to mothers who have chlamydial infection

Infants born to mothers who have untreated chlamydia are at high risk for infection; however, prophylactic antibiotic regimen is not indicated, and the efficacy of such treatment is unknown. Infants should be monitored to ensure appropriate treatment if infection develops.

Chlamydial infections among children

Sexual abuse must be considered a cause of chlamydial infection among pre-adolescent children, although perinatally transmitted *C. trachomatis* infection of the nasopharynx, urogenital tract, and rectum may persist for >1 year. Because of the potential for a criminal investigation and legal proceedings for sexual abuse, a diagnosis of *C. trachomatis* in a pre-adolescent children requires the high specificity provided by isolation in cell culture. The cultures should be confirmed by microscopic identification of the characteristic intracytoplasmic inclusions, preferably by fluorescein-conjugated monoclonal antibodies specific for *C. trachomatis*.

Diagnostic considerations

Nonculture chlamydia tests should not be used because of the possibility of false-positive test results. With respiratory tract specimens, false-positive test results can occur because of cross-reaction of test reagents with *Chlamydia pneumoniae*; with genital and anal specimens, false-positive test results occur because of cross-reaction with fecal flora.

Treatment regimens are listed in Table 28.17.

Follow-up

Follow-up cultures are necessary to ensure that treatment has been effective.

LYMPHOGRANULOMA VENEREUM (LGV)

LGV is caused by serotypes (serovars) L1, L2, L3 of *C. trachomatis*. These serotypes may proliferate within lymphoid tissue and macrophages, and have an inherent tendency toward systemic infection, whereas the non-LGV serotypes (D through K) almost exclusively infect squamous and columnar epithelial tissue. Indeed, LGV can mimic lymphoproliferative disorders.

TABLE 28.17　Recommended treatment regimens for chlamydial infections in children

Children <45kg age	Children >45kg and <8 years of age	Children >8 years of age
Erythromycin* 50 mg/kg/day divided into four doses for 10 to 14 days	Azithromycin 1g orally in a single dose.	Azithromycin 1g orally in a single does
		Doxycycline 100mg orally twice a day for 7 days

* The effectiveness of erythromycin treatment is approximately 80%; a second course of therapy may be required.

LGV is a major health problem only in less–developed countries, whereas the number of reported cases remains low in North America and Europe.[147] It is rarely reported in children or adolescents, but since its peak incidence coincides with peak sexual activity, occurrence in the teenager should not be a surprise. Sexual transmission is the only known mode of spread.

The pathogenesis and clinical findings of LGV have been extensively reviewed elsewhere.[147] The course of LGV may be divided as comprising early and late lesions. The early lesions comprise eroding papules at the site of infection, a lymphangitis leading to the regional lymph nodes, and the swelling of the regional lymph nodes (buboes) (Fig. 28.30), which are usually the inguinal nodes in anogenital infections. The late findings are unique for

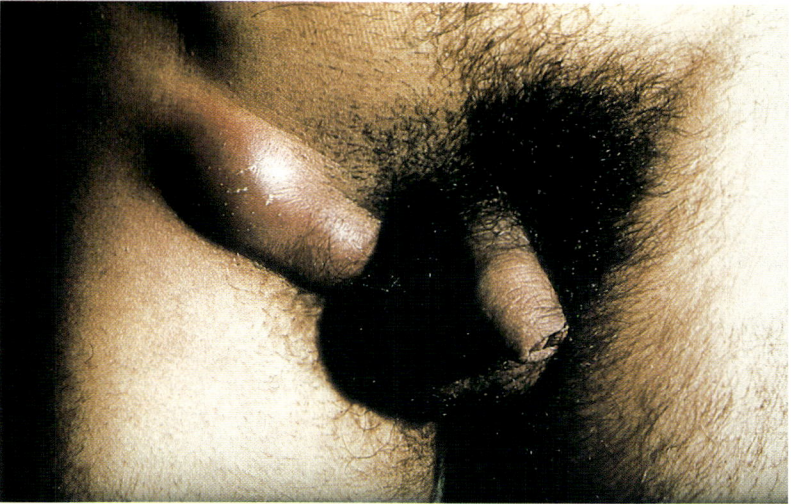

Fig. 28.30　Lymphogranuloma venereum. An ascending inguinal bubo.

TABLE 28.18　Lymphogranuloma venereum (LGV)

	Clinical description	Diagnostic studies Culture/PCR or LCR	Serology	Comments
Early LGV				
Primary infection	Seven-day incubation period. Four types of lesions: papules, eroded nodules, herpetiform coalescent lesions, and urethritis. Lesions are frequently asymptomatic and heal without trace. Not diagnosed in the majority of cases. Site: penis, vulva, anterior urethra, anoderm	Positive with material from lesion	Negative	Patients present mostly only with inguinal syndrome
Inguinal syndrome (secondary)	Follows primary lesion. Average incubation 20 days, longer period possible. Inguinal bubo usually unilateral and slightly painful. Bubo may become fluctuant, but most heal without rupture. 20% show enlarged femoral node as well, separated by inguinal ligament from inguinal bubo (Groove sign).	Positive in secretion or pus from bubo	Positive usually – >1:64 (IgA, IgG)	Histopathology: necrotizing granuloma with stellate abscesses
Anogenitorectal syndrome (secondary)	In the male: resulting from posterior urethral or rectal primary lesion. In the female: resulting from anal intercourse, or spread from vaginal secretions, or translymphatic spread from cervical. Early symptoms are proctocolitis and lymphatic proliferation	Positive as above	Positive as above	Inflammatory bowel disease must be separated clinically and serologically.
Late LGV	Typically the inguinal adenopathy resolves after 2–3 months. Inflammation persists in more proximal lymph nodes. Consequences may be elephantiasis of penis and scrotum or the vulva with chronic fistulations, rectal stricture and perineal ulceration.	Positive	Persistently positive but titer falls as disease subsides	Anogenitorectal involvement is of importance in homosexual males. Differential diagnosis: granulomatous infections, schistosomiasis, and cancer.

147. Perine PL, Osoba AO (1984) Lymphogranuloma venereum. In: Sexually Transmittec Diseases, Holmes KK, Mardh P-A, Sparling PF, eds. New York: McGraw-Hill, p. 281.

STDs in terms of scarring, stricture, fistulae, and elephantiasis–like lymphatic obstruction. See Table 28.18 for a summary for the clinical and histologic features of LGV.

THERAPY

Treatment cures infection and prevents ongoing tissue damage, although tissue reaction can result in scarring. Buboes may require aspiration or incision and drainage through intact skin. Doxycycline is the preferred treatment (CDC Guidelines 1998).[43]

Recommended regimen

The recommended regimen for adults is doxycycline 100mg orally twice a day for 21 days.

Alternative regimens

Alternative regimens (preferable in children): erythromycin 500mg orally four times a day for 21 days. The activity of azithromycin against *C. trachomatis* suggest that it may be effective, but clinical data are lacking.

FOLLOW-UP

Patients should be followed clinically until signs and symptoms have resolved.

MANAGEMENT OF SEX PARTNERS

Sex partners of patients who have LGV should be examined, tested for urethral or cervical chlamydial infection, and treated if they had sexual contact with the patient during the 30 days preceding onset symptoms in the patient.

SPECIAL CONSIDERATIONS

Pregnancy

Pregnant and lactating women should be treated with the erythromycin regimen.

HIV infection

HIV-infected persons who have LGV should be treated according to the regimens cited previously. Anecdotal evidence suggests that LGV infection in HIV-positive patients may require prolonged therapy and that resolution might be delayed.

GENITAL AND ANAL WARTS (CONDYLOMATA ACUMINATA)

EPIDEMIOLOGY

Human papillomaviruses (HPV) are the most common sexually transmitted diseases. More than half of men are infected with HPV during a lifetime. However, only 1% of them develop the manifest disease of genital warts, while in about 10% of them, HPV-DNA is demonstrable in the epithelium of the lower genital tract.[148]

Virions consist of a central core of DNA, enclosed with an outer capsid of viral protein arranged in a symmetrical 20–sided pattern. The virion does not have an outer membrane, which may, in part, account for the antigenicity of the infection. This hinders the use of serum antibodies in the diagnosis of HPV infections as well as the development of a useful vaccination.

TABLE 28.19   Pattern of diseases caused by human papillomavirus

Human papillomavirus type	Pattern of disease
1, 2, 4, 7	Plantar, palmar, periungual (verrucae vulgares)
7, 10	Butcher's warts
3, 10, 28	Verrucae planae
13	Oral focal epithelial hyperplasia (Heck)
6, 11, 16, 30	Condyloma acuminatum
16, 18, 30	Bowenoid papulosis
6, 11	Giant condyloma of Buschke–Lowenstein
11, 18	Penile cancer
9, 37	Keratoacanthoma
1–5, 7–10, 12, 14, 17–20, 23–25	Epidermodysplasia verruciformis
11, 16	Anal cancer
2, 16	Carcinoma of the tongue
11, 16	Leukoplakia and oral carcinoma
16, 18, 31, 33	Invasive carcinoma of the cervix
6, 11, 16, 30	Laryngeal papillomas

There are now over 100 HPV types, based on the techniques of restriction endonuclease cleavage followed by DNA hybridization. Table 28.19 shows the major HPV types that were isolated. Very few genital warts in childhood have been studied for HPV types. In principle, the reported types are similar to those seen in adults.

Based on the presence of virus types in genital warts, one can discriminate types with low risk of malignancy, such as type 6 and 11, and high risk types, such as 16, 18, 31, 33, the presence of which increases the relative risk of the development of invasive squamous cell cancer up to 296! If HPV is not sufficient for cervical carcinogenesis, it represents, however, a necessary factor. Nearly 100% of cervical cancers are indeed positive for HPV DNA.[149] The mechanisms of transformation of keratinocytes depend fundamentally on the expression of the E6-E7 region of the HPV-DNA. The gene products of these regions interact with tumor suppressor genes such as p53. Also, loss of heterozygosity was observed at different chromosomal regions in most genital cancers associated with HPV infection.

The current epidemic of genital warts is most manifest in teenagers and adults. However, numerous reports point to an increase in prepubertal children as well.[150,151] Teenagers acquire their warts by sexual contact. Innocent transmission of HPV from mother to child postnatally probably also occurs, but the major concern in acquired condyloma in childhood is often sexual abuse. Although the only means of transmission of genital HPV diseases supported by observations in adults is direct sexual contact, the mode of transmission in the child is controversial. The rate of perinatal transmission from genital HPV-positive mothers in the pharyngeal mucosa of the infant is about 50% The rates of transmission to the genital skin, however, are not known and seem to be substantially lower. Nevertheless, lesions that are recognized within the first year after birth may be considered perinatally acquired. A longer incubation period is possible, but a child over age 3 should be suspected for having sustained sexual abuse. However, the most recent studies suggest that sexual abuse as a cause of HPV infections in children was overestimated. It has to be taken into account that the long incubation period makes it difficult to determine the mode of transmission.

Another mode of transmission to be discussed is through inoculation – from a caring family member – or through autoinoculation from the child him or herself. Virus types of genital warts have been described to be identical

148. Koutsky L (1997) Epidemiology of genital human papilloma infection. **Am J Med** 102:3.
149. Riethmuller D, Schaal JP, Mougin C (2002) Epidemiology and natural history of genital infection by human papillomavirus. **Gynecol Obstet Fertil** 30:139.
150. Grace DA, Ochsner JA, McLain CR et al. (1967) Vulvar condylomata acuminata in prepubertal females. **J Am Med Assoc** 201:151.
151. Stumpf PG (1980) Increasing occurrence of condylomata acuminata in premenarchal children. **Obstet Gynecol** 56:262.

to those occurring in hand warts in several studies. A third way of transmission would be by social "benign" contact, which has, however, not yet been proven and remains conjectural.[152] An underestimated route of infection is the transmission by surgical instruments, e.g., on cryoprobe tips, where HPV DNA could be detected in 4.5%.

Papillomaviruses can be transmitted to the fetus before or during birth; they are also a risk to the infant born to an infected woman. Laryngeal HPV infections, while presumably much less prevalent than genital tract infections, are associated with a high degree of morbidity and a significant degree of mortality when they cause laryngeal papillomas.[153]

The viral clearance average is eight months. The clearance is the consequence of host immunity intervention that leads to spontaneous regression of infection. Interestingly, also the majority of low-grade squamous intraepithelial lesions (more than 80% within a period of two years) regress spontaneously without any treatment.[149]

PHYSICAL EXAMINATION

Typical condylomata acuminata are raised, papillomatous, often slightly pointed lesions with a rugose surface. The warts are localized predominantly on the glans penis and the prepuce in the male, and on the vulva and the vaginal introitus in the female. In both sexes, the perianal skin may be involved when sexually transmitted. It is generally assumed that the site of condylomata is also the site of infection (i.e., anal condylomata indicate a history of anal coitus). The incidence of urethral or cervical condylomata is low[154] (Figs 28.31–28.33).

Genital papillomas do not uniformly correspond to the description of condyloma acuminatum, hence the more general term "genital warts" may be preferable. There are four morphological types of genital warts: cauliflower-shaped condylomata, dome-shaped skin colored papules, keratotic warts, and

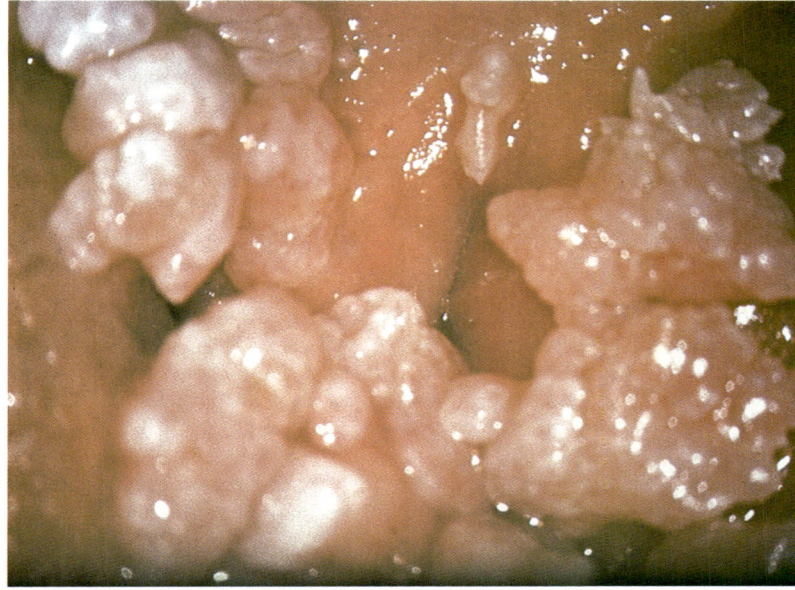

Fig. 28.32 Condylomata acuminata. Cauliflower-like, violaceous lesions in the vaginal introitus.

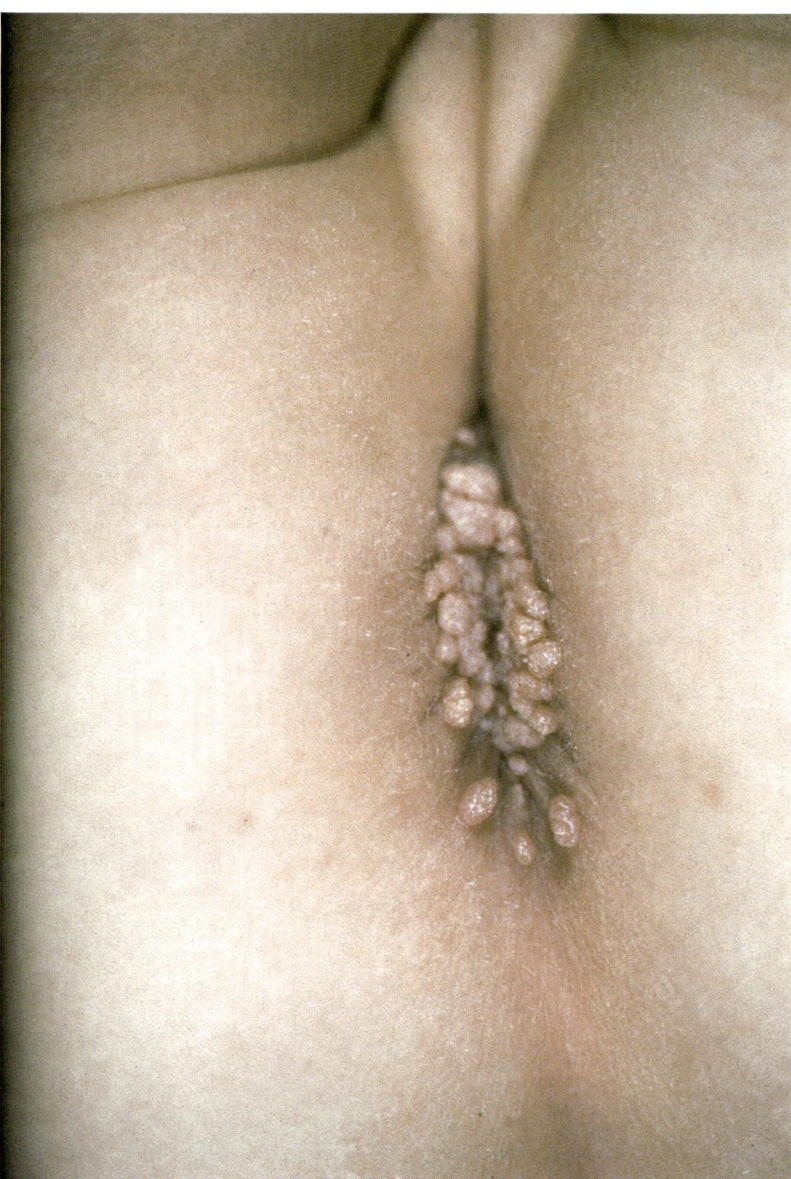

Fig. 28.31 Condylomata acuminata. Perianal papules allegedly present at birth. These persisted until age 2 in spite of multiple therapies.

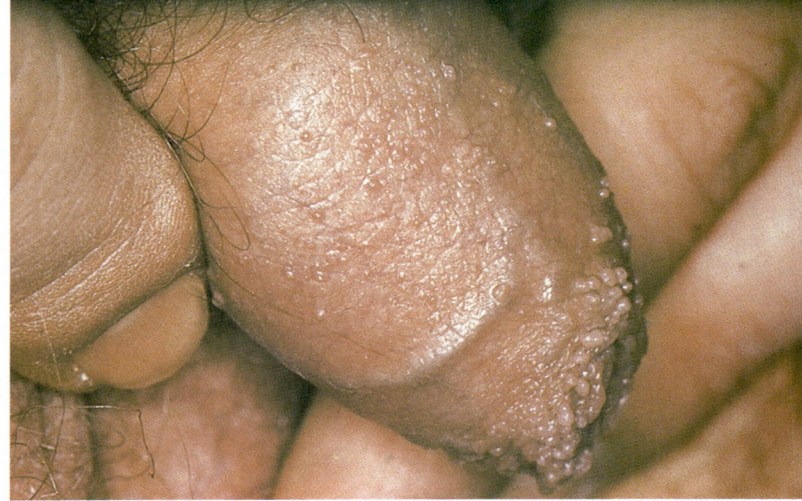

Fig. 28.33 Condylomata acuminata, Multiple pinhead-like, waxy transparent lesions.

152. Gutman LT, Herman-Giddens ME, Phelps WC (1993) Transmission of human genital papillomavirus disease: comparison of data from adults and children. **Pediatrics** 91:31.
153. Steinberg BM (1988) Papillomavirus. Effects upon mother and child. **Ann NY Acad Sci** 549:118.
154. Gross G, Ikenberg H, Gissman L et al. (1985) Papillomavirus infection of the anogenital region: correlation between histology, clinical picture, and virus type. Proposal of a new nomenclature. **J Invest Dermatol** 85:147.

flat-topped papules. A special feature is Bowenoid papulosis, representing dome-shaped or flat, hyperpigmented papules, which shows histologically high-grade intraepithelial neoplasia. The association of flat cervical warts with varying degrees of dysplasia, and ultimately cervical cancer, is a rather newly recognized phenomenon. These cervical warts may be barely perceived by the naked eye, necessitating acetic acid application and colposcopy for evaluation and treatment. Although treatment approaches vary, it is agreed that such women need frequent pap smears, biopsies of suspicious lesions, and treatment of their cervical warts.

Giant condyloma acuminatum are rare in childhood. The mean age at presentation is 43.9 years, but there seems to be a recent trend toward a younger presentation. The most common presenting symptoms are perianal mass (47%), pain (32%), abscess or fistula (32%), and bleeding (18%). Foci of invasive carcinoma are noted in 50% of the reports, "carcinoma in situ" in 8%.[155]

Of the other conditions listed under anogenital and mucosal warts, only laryngeal papillomatosis is a specifically pediatric entity. A cause of weak cry, hoarseness, and stridor in childhood, this condition is now clearly associated with HPV, usually transmitted at birth from the mother.[156] Bowenoid papulosis manifests as flat-topped pigmented papules of the vulva, groin, or penis, showing full-thickness epithelial atypia on biopsy. It is common in young adults and has also been reported in childhood.[157] The atypia does not seem to progress to carcinoma in males, but this may be more likely in females.

THERAPY

The primary goal of treating visible genital warts is the removal of symptomatic warts. Treatment can induce wart-free periods in most patients. Genital warts often are asymptomatic. No evidence indicates that currently available treatments eradicate or affect the natural history of HPV infection. The removal of warts may or may not decrease infectivity. If left untreated, visible genital warts may resolve on their own, remain unchanged, or increase in size or number. No evidence indicates that treatment of visible warts affect the development of cervical cancer (CDC Guidelines 1998).[43]

Regimens

Treatment of visible warts should be guided by the preference of the patient, the available resources, and the experience of the health-care provider. No one of the available treatments is superior to other treatments, and no single treatment is ideal for all patients and all warts.

Many factors might influence selection of treatment. Having a treatment plan or protocol is important, because many patients will require a course of therapy rather than a single treatment. In general, warts located on moist surfaces and/or in intertriginous areas respond better to topical treatment than do warts on drier surfaces.

The treatment modalities should be changed if a patient has not improved substantially after three provider-administered treatments or if warts have not completely cleared after six treatments. The risk-benefit ratio of treatment should be evaluated throughout the course of therapy to avoid overtreatment. Providers should be knowledgeable about, and have available to them, at least one patient-applied and one provider-administered treatment.

Complications rarely occur if treatments for warts are employed properly.

External genital warts, recommended treatments

PATIENT APPLIED
1. Podofilox 0.5% solution or gel. Patients may apply podofilox solution with a cotton swab, or podofilox gel with a finger, to visible genital warts twice a day for three days, followed by four days of no therapy. This cycle may be

repeated for a total of four cycles. The total wart area treated should not exceed 10cm², and a total volume of podofilox should not exceed 0.5ml. The use of podofilox during pregnancy has not been established.
2. Imiquimod 5% cream. Imiquimod is a topically active immune enhancer that stimulates production of interferon and other cytokines. Patients should apply imiquimod cream with a finger at bedtime, three times a week for as long as 16 weeks. The treatment area should be washed with mild soap and water 6–10 hours after the application. Many patients may be clear of warts by 8–10 weeks or sooner. The safety of imiquimod during pregnancy has not been established.

PROVIDER-ADMINISTERED
1. Cryotherapy with liquid nitrogen or cryoprobe.
2. Podophyllin resin 10–25% in compound tincture of benzoin. To avoid the possibility of complications associated with systemic absorption and toxicity, some experts recommend that application be limited to 0.5ml <10cm² of warts per session. Repeat weekly if necessary. The safety of podophyllin during pregnancy has not been established. Please observe that some experts suggest that podophyllin office therapy should be abandoned.[158]
3. Trichloracetic acid (TCA) 80–90%. Apply a small amount only to warts, at which time a white frosting develops; powder with talc or sodium bicarbonate to remove unreacted acid. Repeat weekly if necessary. Although these preparations are widely used, they have not been investigated thoroughly.
4. Surgical removal either by tangential scissors excision, tangential shave excision, curettage, or electrosurgery. Surgical removal of warts has an advantage over other treatment modalities in that it renders the patient wart-free, usually with a single visit.
5. Interferons have been administered systemically or intralesionally. Systemic interferon is not effective. The efficacy and recurrence rates of intralesional interferon are comparable to other treatment modalities.
6. Laser surgery.

Cervical warts

For women who have exophytic cervical warts, high-grade squamous intraepithelial lesions must be excluded before treatment is begun. Management should include consultation with an expert (gynecologist).

Vaginal warts (for details see External genital warts)

1. Cryotherapy. The use of a cryoprobe in the vagina is not recommended because of the risk for vaginal perforation and fistula formation.
2. TCA 80–90%.
3. Podophyllin.

Urethral meatus warts

1. Cryotherapy with liquid nitrogen.
2. Podophyllin 10–25% in compound tincture of benzoin. The treatment area must be dry before contact with normal mucosa. Podophyllin must be applied weekly if necessary. *The safety of podophyllin during pregnancy has not been established.*

Anal warts

1. Cryotherapy with liquid nitrogen; OR
2. TCA 80–90% applied to warts; OR
3. Surgical removal.

Follow-up

After visible genital warts have cleared, a follow-up evaluation is not mandatory.[43] Patients should be cautioned to watch for recurrences, which occur most frequently during the first three months. Women should be counseled regarding the need for regular cytologic screening, as recommended

155. Trombetta LJ, Place RJ (2001) Giant condyloma acuminatum of the anorectum: trends in epidemiology and management: report of a case and review of the literature. **Dis Colon Rectum** 44:1878.
156. Kaufman RS, Balogh K (1969) Verrucas and juvenile laryngeal papilloma. **Arch Otolaryngol** 89:90.
157. Breneman DL, Lucky AW, Ostrous RS et al. (1985) Bowenoid papulosis of the genitalia associated with human papillomavirus DNA Type 16 in an infant with atopic dermatitis. **Pediatr Dermatol** 2:297.
158. von Krogh G, Longstaff E (2001) Podophyllin office therapy against condyloma should be abandoned. **Sex Transm Infect** 77:409.

for women without genital warts. The presence of genital warts is not an indication for colposcopy.

Management of sex partners

Examination of sex partners is not necessary for management of genital warts because the role of reinfection is probably minimal, and, in the absence of curative therapy, treatment to reduce transmission is not realistic (CDC guidelines 1998).[43] Because treatment of genital warts does not eliminate the HPV infections, patients should be cautioned that they might remain infectious even though the warts are gone.

SPECIAL CONSIDERATIONS

Pregnancy

Imiquimod, podophyllin, and podofilox should not be used during pregnancy. Because genital warts can proliferate during pregnancy, many experts advocate their removal during pregnancy. HPV type 6 and 11 can cause laryngeal papillomatosis among infants. The route of transmission (transplacental, birth canal, or postnatal) is not completely understood. The preventive value of cesarean delivery is unknown; thus, cesarean delivery should not be performed solely to prevent transmission of HPV infection to the newborn.

Immunosuppressed patients

Persons who are immunosuppressed because of HIV or other reasons may not respond as well a immunocompetent persons to therapy for genital warts, and they may have more frequent recurrences.

GENITAL HERPES SIMPLEX INFECTIONS

The basic features of herpes simplex virus (HSV) infections are detailed in Chapter 25. Neonatal HSV and its prevention by examining and treating the pregnant woman is discussed in Chapter 25. This section will deal with some special issues of genital HSV infection, and the role of acyclovir in treating and preventing episodes of genital HSV infection. Other recent sources cover the topic of HSV infections in great detail.[159,160]

Herpes genitalis is an important sexually transmitted disease affecting about 20% of sexually active people; up to 80% of cases are undiagnosed.[161] There are, however, no exact data on prevalence and infection rates. Today, genital herpes is a risk factor for infections with HIV.[162] A case-control study demonstrated that HIV-positive men and women had a higher prevalence of HSV-2 antibodies than HIV-negative men. The data suggested that the genital ulcerative disease caused by herpes virus may contribute to increased risk for HIV-1 infection among heterosexuals.

Herpes genitalis threatens the newborn infant by infection from the maternal birth channel. This does not only concern symptomatic women but asymptomatic shedding of HSV occurs in all women with genital herpes. Neonatal herpes is a rare but serious disease. In an 18-month hospital-based surveillance study by the CDC, 184 cases of neonatal herpes were reported. Only 22% of mothers had a history of herpes infections and only 9% had lesions at the time of delivery.[163] Fifteen neonates had herpes infections although they were delivered by cesarean section. This suggests that intrauterine infection may also be an important route of transmission of late third trimester HSV infection.

Newborn children are "innocent" victims of herpes simplex infections. In older children, herpes is a symptom of sexual abuse as often as in other sexually transmitted diseases. Adolescents may be infected during their active sexual contacts.

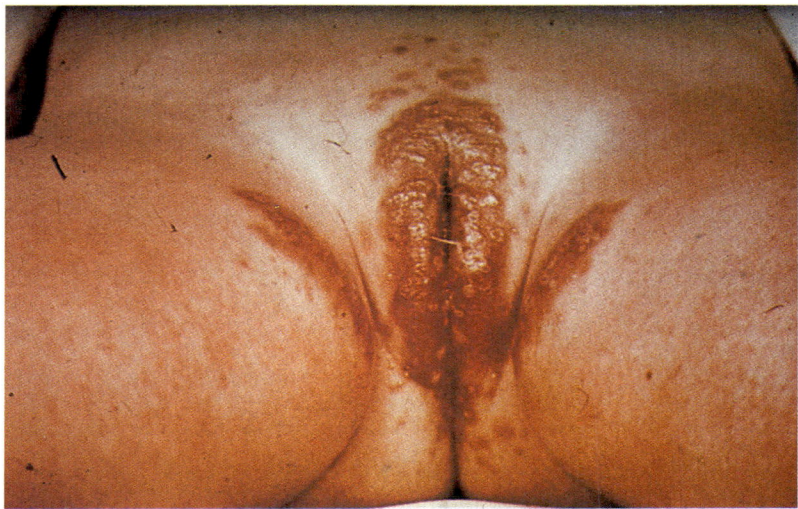

Fig. 28.34 Genital herpes simplex virus (HSV) infection involving vulva and adjacent skin.

GENITAL HSV INFECTIONS IN THE PREPUBERTAL CHILD

These infections are rare, and the literature is limited.[163,164] Lesional morphology is usually similar to that of older patients (Fig. 28.34). Our policy is to investigate each case as suspicious for sexual abuse unless there is a compelling alternative explanation.

The recommended treatment regimen in the first clinical episode of genital herpes in adolescents or adults is acyclovir 200mg orally five times a day for seven to 10 days or until resolution occurs. Children older than 2 years receive the same dose as adults; for younger children it is divided in half.

In frequently recurrent genital HSV infection (more than six per year), a daily suppressive therapy with acyclovir, 200mg orally 2–5 times a day is recommended. After one year it should be discontinued so that the recurrence rate can be reassessed.

THERAPY

Systemic antiviral drugs partially control the symptoms and signs of herpes episodes when used to treat first clinical episodes or recurrent episodes or when used as daily suppressive therapy. However, these drugs neither eradicate latent virus nor affect the risk, frequency, or severity of recurrences after the drug is discontinued. Randomized trials indicate that three antiviral medications provide clinical benefit for genital herpes: acyclovir, valacyclovir, and famciclovir. Valacyclovir is a valine ester of acyclovir with enhanced absorption after oral administration. Famciclovir, a prodrug of pencyclovir, also has high oral bioavailability. Both famciclovir and valacyclovir are not approved for the use in children, although they are effective. Topical therapy with acyclovir is substantially less effective than the systemic drug, and its use is discouraged (CDC Guidelines 1998).[43]

First clinical episode of genital herpes

Management of patients with first clinical episode of genital herpes includes antiviral therapy and counseling regarding the natural history of genital herpes, sexual and perinatal transmission, and methods to reduce such transmission. Therapy is listed in Table 28.20.

159. Rapp F (1984) Herpes simplex viruses. In: Sexually Transmitted Diseases, Holmes KK, Mardh P-A, Sparling PF et al. ecs. New York: McGraw-Hill, p. 438.
160. Rooney JF, Felser JM, Ostrove JM et al. (1986) Acquisition of genital herpes from an asymptomatic sexual partner. N Engl J Med 314:1561.
161. Tetrault I, Boivin G (2000) Recent advances in management of genital herpes. Can Fam Physician 46:1622.
162. Hook EW 3rd, Cannon RO, Nahmias AJ et al. (1992) Herpes simplex virus infection as a risk factor for human immunodeficiency virus infection in heterosexuals. J Infect Dis 165:251.
163. Nahmias AJ, Dowdle WR, Naib ZM et al. (1968) Genital infection with Herpesvirus hominis types 1 and 2 in children. Pediatrics 42:659.
164. Gardner M, Jones JG (1984) Genital herpes acquired by sexual abuse of children. J Pediatr 104:243.

TABLE 28.20   Recommended treatment regimens for herpes genitalis

Drug	Dose	Route
Acyclovir	400mg three times a day for 7–10 days	po
Acyclovir	200mg five times a day for 7–10 days	po
Famciclovir*	250mg three times a day for 7–10 days	po
Valacyclovir*	1g twice a day for 7–10 days	po

* Not approved for the use in children.

Treatment may be extended if healing is incomplete after 10 days of therapy.

Counseling is an important aspect of managing patients who have genital herpes. Although initial counseling can be provided at the first visit, many patients benefit from learning about the chronic aspects of the disease after the acute illness subsides. Counseling of these patients should include the following:

- the natural history of genital herpes;
- advise to abstain from sexual activity when lesions are present and to inform their sex partners; the use of condoms may also prevent infection of the partner, but does not offer complete protection;
- sexual transmission can occur during asymptomatic periods;
- the risk of neonatal infections should be explained to all patients, including men. Child-bearing women who have herpes should be advised to inform health care providers who care for them during pregnancy about the HSV infection;
- patients having a first episode of genital herpes should be advised that (a) episodic antiviral therapy during recurrent episodes might shorten the duration of lesions and (b) suppressive antiviral therapy can ameliorate or prevent recurrent outbreaks.

Recurrent episodes of HSV disease

When treatment is started during the prodrome or within one day after onset of lesions, many patients who have recurrent disease benefit from episodic therapy. If episodic treatment of recurrences is chosen, the patient should be provided with antiviral therapy, or a prescription for the medication, so that treatment can be initiated at the first sign of prodrome or genital lesions. Therapeutic options are listed in Table 28.21.

Daily suppressive therapy reduces the frequency of genital herpes recurrences by >75%. Suppressive therapy has not been associated with emergence of clinically significant acyclovir resistance. After one year of continuous suppressive therapy, discontinuation should be discussed with the patient. Suppressive treatment with acyclovir reduces but does not eliminate asymptomatic viral shedding. Therefore, the extent to which suppressive therapy may prevent HSV transmission is unknown.

TABLE 28.21   Recommended treatment regimens for recurrent herpes genitalis

Drug	Dose	Route
Acute lesion		
Acyclovir	400mg three times a day for 5 days	po
Acyclovir	200mg five times a day for 5 days	po
Acyclovir	800mg twice a day for 5 days	po
Famciclovir*	125mg twice a day for 5 days	po
Valacyclovir*	500mg twice a day for 5 days	po
Suppressive therapy		
Acyclovir	400mg orally twice a day	po
Famciclovir*	250mg orally twice a day	po
Valacyclovir*	500mg orally once a day	po

* Not approved for the use in childhood.

Severe disease

IV therapy should be provided for patients who have severe disease or complications necessitating hospitalization, such as disseminated infection, pneumonitis, hepatitis, or complications of the central nervous system (e.g., meningitis or encephalitis).

Recommended regimen

Acyclovir 5–10mg/kg body weight iv every eight hours for 5–7 days or until clinical resolution is attained.

Special considerations

HIV infection

Immunocompromised patients might have prolonged and/or severe episodes of genital or perianal herpes. Lesions caused by HSV are relatively common among HIV infected patients.

The dosage of antiviral drugs for HIV-infected patients is controversial, but clinical experience strongly suggests that immunocompromised patients benefit from increased doses of antiviral drugs. Therapy should be continued until clinical resolution is attained. In the doses recommended for treatment of genital herpes, valacyclovir, acyclovir, and famciclovir are safe. For severe cases, acyclovir 5mg/kg iv every eight hours may be required.

If lesions persist in a patient receiving acyclovir treatment, resistance of the HSV strain to acyclovir should be suspected. All acyclovir-resistant strains are resistant to valacyclovir, and most are resistant to famciclovir. Foscarnet, 40mg/kg body weight iv every eight hours until clinical resolution is attained, is often effective. Topical cidofovir gel 1% applied to the lesions once daily for five consecutive days also might be effective.

Pregnancy

The safety of systemic acyclovir or valacyclovir therapy in pregnant women has not been established. Glaxo-Wellcome, Inc., in cooperation with CDC, maintains a registry. Women who receive acyclovir or valacyclovir during pregnancy should be reported to this registry (telephone in the USA (888) 825-5249, extension 39441). Current registry findings do not indicate an increased risk for major birth defects after acyclovir treatment.

The first clinical episode of genital herpes during pregnancy may be treated with oral acyclovir. In the presence of life-threatening maternal HSV infection acyclovir administered iv is indicated. However, routine administration of acyclovir to pregnant women who have a history of recurrent genital herpes is not recommended at this time.

Perinatal infection

Most mothers of infants who acquire neonatal herpes lack histories of clinically evident genital herpes. The risk of transmission to the neonate from an infected mother is high among women who acquire genital herpes near the time of delivery (30%–50%) and is low among women who have a history of recurrent herpes at term and women who acquire genital HSV during the first half of pregnancy (3%). Therefore, prevention of neonatal herpes should emphasize prevention of acquisition of genital HSV infection during late pregnancy. Susceptible women whose partners have oral or genital HSV infection, or those whose sex partners' infection status is unknown, should be counseled to avoid unprotected genital or oral sexual contact during late pregnancy. The results of viral cultures during pregnancy do not predict viral shedding at the time of delivery, and such cultures are not indicated routinely.

At the onset of labor, all women should be examined and carefully questioned regarding whether they have symptoms of genital herpes. Cesarean section does not completely eliminate the risk for HSV infection in the neonate.

Infants exposed to HSV during birth, as proven by virus isolation or presumed by observation of lesions, should be followed carefully. Available data do not support the routine use of acyclovir for asymptomatic infants exposed during birth, because the risk for infection is low. However, infants born to women who acquired herpes near term are at high risk for neonatal herpes, and some experts recommend acyclovir therapy for these infants. All infants who have evidence of neonatal herpes should be promptly evaluated and treated with systemic acyclovir. Thirty to sixty mg/kg per day for 10–21 days is the regimen of choice.

MOLLUSCUM CONTAGIOSUM

Molluscum contagiosum is a disease caused by a poxvirus. The molluscum body, a large cytoplasmatic inclusion, can be observed by light microscopy; the observation by electron microscope shows this inclusion to be composed of virions indistinguishable from other poxviruses. Mature viral particles develop by a process reminiscent of vaccinia virus. The direct detection of molluscum contagiosum virus (MCV) DNA in clinical specimens submitted for virus isolation by a dot blot hybridization protocol was described.[165] The MCV DNA was distinguishable from herpes simplex virus or orf virus.

Experimental transmission to humans has been shown in HeLa cells, and other cell cultures could be infected. DNA analysis from mollusca has recently identified two separate subtypes. Recently, the DNA sequence of the 190 kbp MCV genome was reported.[166] MCV was predicted to encode 163 proteins of which 103 were clearly related to those of smallpox virus. In contrast, it was found that MCV lacks 83 genes of VAR, including those involved in the suppression of the host response to infection, nucleotide biosynthesis, and cell proliferation. However, MCV possesses 59 genes predicted to code for novel proteins including MHC-class I, chemokine and glutathione peroxidase homologs not found in other poxviruses.[166] The virus does not induce antibody reaction by inhibiting the immunologic response of the host and increasing the resistance of infected host cells to apoptosis. A viral MHC peptide interferes with human MHC proteins in presentation of MCV-specific peptides. An analog to the human macrophage inflammatory protein binds to the receptor but lacks activity. Another protein coded by the MCV genome is a homolog of the epidermal growth factor.[157]

The incidence has increased nearly fourfold during the past 20 years. Although mollusca appear in all skin regions, a predominance in the genital area is obvious. Literature on the incidence of sexually transmitted molluscum, however, is lacking. It is questionable whether each case of perigenital mollusca requires the suggestion of sexual abuse.

Following an incubation period of two weeks to several months the mollusca are seen as umbilicated papules of 2–5mm pearly appearance (Figs 28.35, 28.36). Giant mollusca, with a halo, mollusca inflamed abscess-like lesions, and those resembling cutaneous cryptococcosis[168] are rare. The lesions are mostly asymptomatic, but pruritus and a dermatitis may occur. The natural history of mollusca is spontaneous involution within 6–12 months, or sometimes longer.

In HIV-infected patients of different stage, mollusca may appear in extensive distribution all over the skin.

THERAPY

The disease is self-limiting within some months in the immunocompetent patient, but may have a prolonged course in immunosuppressed patients.[169] The recurrence rate is low.

Usually, mollusca are treated surgically by scraping out with a lancet, by curettage by vesicants or by cryosurgery with liquid nitrogen. These procedures are not painless and are therefore more difficult in younger children. Pretreatment with EMLA cream may diminish the discomfort.

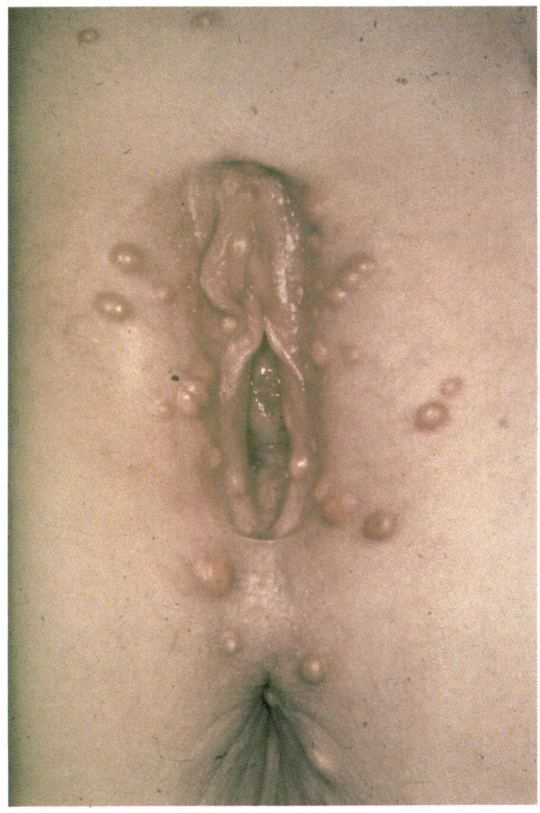

Fig. 28.35   Genital lesions of molluscum contagiosum in a five-year-old girl.

As a topical chemotherapy, cidofovir was administered. In treatment of three patients for two months, all molluscum lesions cleared. The conduction of a multicenter trial is quoted.[170] There are also some trials of treatment with Imiquimod.[171] Conclusive statements on the value of the treatments proposed are impossible, for there are virtually no controlled trials on the different treatment modalities

HUMAN IMMUNODEFIENCY VIRUS (HIV) INFECTION, INCLUDING ACQUIRED IMMUNODEFICIENCY SYNDROME (AIDS), IN CHILDREN

HIV, a cytopathic RNA retrovirus with specific affinity for the CD4 surface antigen,[172] causes AIDS. HIV infection is characterized by T-cell immunodeficiency and recurrent or opportunistic infections, although it has the potential to affect all organ systems.[173] HIV infection in children is associated with a variety of dermatological conditions, particularly muco-cutaneous infections and inflammatory disorders.[174–180]

Because the clinical characteristics of HIV infection in children are different from those in adults, a separate classification system was devised in 1987. The

165. Hurst JW, Forghani B, Chan CS et al. (1991) Direct detection of molluscum contagiosum virus in clinical specimens by dot blot hybridization. **J Clin Microbiol** 29:1959.

166. Lewis EJ, Lam M, Crutchfield CE (1997) An update on molluscum contagiosum. **Cutis** 60:29.

167. Bugert JJ, Darai G (1997) Recent advances in molluscum contagiosum virus research. **Arch Virol** (Suppl) 13:35.

168. Ghigliotti GC, Varrega G, Farris A et al. (1992) Cutaneous cryptococcosis resembling molluscum contagiosum in a homosexual man with AIDS. **Acta Derm Venereol** 72:182.

169. Smith KJ, Yeager J, Skelton H (1999) Molluscum contagiosum: its clinical, histopathologic, and immunohistochemical spectrum. **Int J Dermatol** 38:664.

170. Zabawski EJ, Cockerell CJ (1998) Topical and intralesional cidofovir: a review of pharmacology and therapeutic effects. **J Am Acad Dermatol** 39:741.

171. Edwards L (2000) Imiquimod in clinical practice. **J Am Acad Dermatol** 43:S12.

172. Rabson AB (1990) HIV virology: Implications for the pathogenesis of HIV infection. **J Am Acad Dermatol** 22:1196.

173. Domachowske JB (1996) Pediatric human immunodeficiency virus infection. **Clin Microbiol Rev** 9:448.

174. Prose NS (1991) Mucocutaneous disease in pediatric human immunodeficiency virus infection **Pediatr Clin N Am** 38:977.

175. Torre D, Zeroli C, Fiori GP et al. (1991) Dermatologic manifestations of AIDS in children. **Pediatrician** 18:195.

176. Nance KV, Smith ML, Joshi VV (1991) Cutaneous manifestations of acquired immunodeficiency syndrome in children. **Int J Dermatol** 30:531.

177. Prose NS (1990) HIV infection in children. **J Am Acad Dermatol** 22:1223.

178. Straka BF, Whitaker DL, Morrison SH et al. (1988) Cutaneous manifestations of the acquired immunodeficiency syndrome in children. **J Am Acad Dermatol** 18:1089.

179. Prose NS, Mendez H, Menikoff H et al. (1987) Pediatric human immunodeficiency virus and its cutaneous manifestation. **Pediatr Dermatol** 4:67.

180. Kline WM (1996) Oral manifestations of pediatric human immunodeficiency virus infection: A review of the literature. **Pediatrics** 97:380.

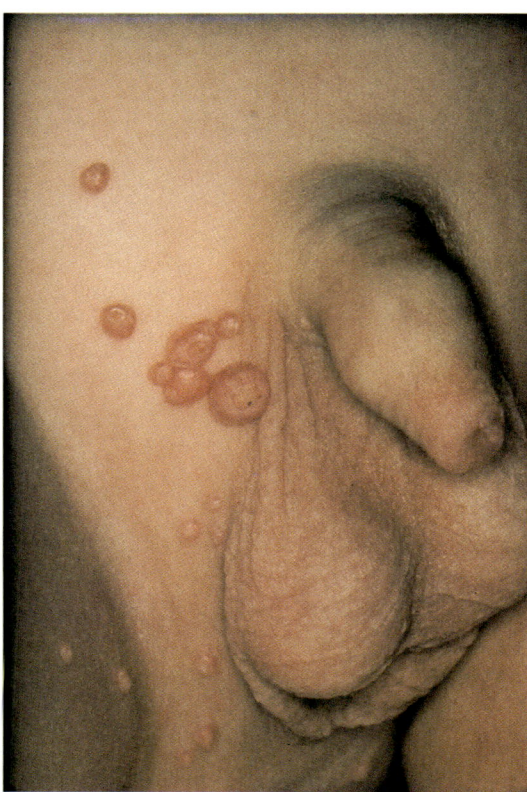

Fig. 28.36 Large lesions of molluscum contagiosum in a six-year-old boy.

current classification for HIV infection in infants and children separates infected individuals into mutually exclusive categories based on infective (HIV serology or detection), clinical (presence of signs, symptoms or diagnoses) (Table 28.22), and immunological (CD4 T-lymphocyte count or CD4 percentage of total lymphocytes) status.[181] Exact criteria can be obtained from the Centers for Disease Control and Prevention at http://www.cdc.gov. At any one time, the number of children infected with HIV is greater than those with AIDS.

DIAGNOSIS

The serologic confirmation of HIV infection in children is similar to that in adults once children have reached the age of 18 months.[173,181] The best currently available assays for detection of serum antibodies involve a screening assay with high sensitivity, such as an enzyme-linked immunoassay, and confirmatory testing by a high-specificity assay, such as by Western blot or indirect immunofluorescence.

Recognition of infection in the neonate is difficult because of contamination by maternal antibodies. At the present time, a reliable way to detect all infected infants at birth is not available. HIV culture appears to have the best sensitivity, specificity, and positive and negative predictive value of HIV

infection.[182] No currently available HIV antibody test distinguishes between passively acquired maternal antibodies and those produced by the infant.

Repeated serologic testing is the most reliable way to confirm the presence of HIV infection in all children, including those less than 18 months of age. A persistently positive titer beyond 18 months of age indicates infection. Seropositive newborn babies that become seronegative by 18 months of age and have no evidence of HIV infection are uninfected and are referred to as seroreverters.[173,181]

EPIDEMIOLOGY

HIV infection and AIDS is a global problem, with the epicenter of the pandemic centered in sub-Saharan Africa where 80% of those infected with the virus are found.[173,183] Broad global patterns of HIV infection have become evident.[183,184] These are influenced by the time of entry and spread of the virus in a population, the relative frequency of the various modes of transmission in the population (sexual, parental or perinatal), local factors (poverty, associated disease burden, education, access to appropriate medical care, traditions and beliefs, etc.) and viral characteristics (virulence, subtypes, resistance, etc.). Although one pattern may predominate in any one region at any one time, sub-populations within the region may reflect a totally different pattern, which may predominate with time. North America's epidemic began amongst homosexual men and intravenous drug users in the 1970s, but current data suggest that this has shifted to include women and children, especially in urban areas, amongst African-American and Hispanic cohorts.[173] HIV infections are not randomly distributed in any population, and in many cohorts and populations epidemiology data are inadequate, unreliable or totally lacking. Worldwide, the number of women and children with new disease is expanding at a rate greater than the rest of the population.[173,183–185]

The majority of pediatric patients come from families in which one or both parents had AIDS or were at risk for developing AIDS. In children younger than 13 years of age, most HIV infections are acquired by vertical, mother-to-child transmission. This mode of transmission is relatively efficient, but not absolute, with transmission rates of up to 39% recorded in certain studies.[173] The identification of factors that increase or decrease transmission risk is becoming more important than overall mother-to-child transmission rates as potential targets for intervention are revealed. Perinatal transmission is affected by the mother's disease status, the route of delivery, the duration of membrane rupture, obstetric complications, including maternal hemorrhage and infection, and perinatal feeding practices. Research has suggested that antibodies against the V3 loop of the envelope protein gp120 may protect the fetus from vertical transmission.[185]

Other routes of transmission may have more significance in certain population groups. Parenteral transmission from blood or tissue products is important in hemophiliacs and intravenous drug users. The adolescent population is at high risk for acquiring HIV infection via sexual exposure or the use of injected drugs. This group represents a special growth area needing specific attention.[173,186] Children can acquire HIV infection after sexual abuse[173,187,188] and this should be considered especially in the older child where vertical transmission is less likely. Household transmission is exceptionally rare.[173]

181. Caldwell MB, Oxtoby MJ, Simonds RJ et al. (1994) Revised classification system for human immunodeficiency virus infection in children less than 13 years of age. **Morb Mortal Wkly Rep** 43(RR-12):1, (http:// www.cdc.gov/mmwr)

182. Kline MW, Hollinger FB, Rosenblatt HM et al. (1993) Sensitivity, specificity and predictive value of physical examination, culture and other laboratory studies in the diagnosis during early infancy of vertically acquired human immunodeficiency virus infection. **Pediatr Infect Dis J** 12:33.

183. Chin J (1990) Current and future dimensions of the HIV/AIDS pandemic in women and children. **Lancet** 6:221.

184. UNAIDS: Aids epidemic update. December 2001 (http://www.unaids.org/epidemic)

185. Peckham C, Gibb D (1995) Mother-to-child transmission of the human immunodeficiency virus. **N Engl J Med** 333:298.

186. Kann L, Kinchen SA, Williams BI et al. (2000) Youth risk behavior surveillance – United States, 1999. State and local YRBSS Coordinators. **J Sch Health** 70:271.

187. Gellert GA, Durfee MJ, Berkowitz CD et al. (1993) Situational and sociodemographic characteristics of children infected with human immunodeficiency virus from pediatric sexual abuse. **Pediatrics** 91:39.

188. Gutman LT, St. Claire KK, Weedy C et al. (1991) Human immunodeficiency virus transmission by child sexual abuse. **Am J Dis Child** 145:137.

TABLE 28.22   Clinical categories for children with HIV infection[181]

Category N – not symptomatic
Children who have no signs or symptoms considered to be the result of HIV infection or who have only one of the conditions listed in Category A

Category A – mildly symptomatic
Children with two or more of the conditions listed below but none of the conditions listed in Categories B and C
    Lymphadenopathy (≥0.5cm at more than two sites, bilateral = one site)
    Hepatomegaly
    Splenomegaly
    Dermatitis
    Parotitis
    Recurrent or persistent upper respiratory infection, sinusitis, or otitis media

Category B – moderately symptomatic
Children who have symptomatic conditions other than those listed for Category A or C that are attributed to HIV infection. Examples of conditions in clinical Category B include but are not limited to:
    Anemia (<8gm/dL), neutropenia (<1000/mm^3), or thrombocytopenia (100 000/mm^3) persisting
    Bacterial meningitis, pneumonia, or sepsis (single episode)
    Candidiasis, oropharyngeal (thrush), persisting (>2 months) in children >6 months of age
    Cardiomyopathy
    Cytomegalovirus infection, with onset before 1 month of age
    Diarrhea, recurrent or chronic
    Hepatitis
    Herpes simplex virus (HSV) stomatitis, recurrent (more than 2 episodes within 1 year)
    HSV bronchitis, pneumonitis, or esophagitis with onset before 1 month of age
    Herpes zoster (shingles) involving at least two distinct episodes or more than one dermatome
    Leiomyosarcoma
    Lymphoid interstitial pneumonia (LIP) or pulmonary lymphoid hyperplasia complex
    Nephropathy
    Nocardiosis
    Persistent fever (lasting >1 month)
    Toxoplasmosis, onset before 1 month of age
    Varicella, disseminated (complicated chickenpox)

Category C – severely symptomatic
    Serious bacterial infections, multiple or recurrent (i.e., any combination of at least two culture-confirmed infections within a 2-year period), of the following
        types: septicemia, pneumonia, meningitis, bone or joint infection, or abscess of an internal organ or body cavity (excluding otitis media, superficial skin
        or mucosal abscesses, and indwelling catheter-related infections)
    Candidiasis, esophageal or pulmonary (bronchi, trachea, lungs)
    Coccidioidomycosis, disseminated (at site other than or in addition to lungs or cervical or hilar lymph nodes)
    Cryptococcosis, extrapulmonary
    Cryptosporidiosis or isosporiasis with diarrhea persisting >1 month
    Cytomegalovirus disease with onset of symptoms at age >1 month (at a site other than liver, spleen or lymph nodes)
    Encephalopathy (at least one of the following progressive findings present for at least 2 months in the absence of a concurrent illness other than HIV
        infection that could explain the findings: (a) failure to attain or loss of developmental milestones or loss of intellectual ability, verified by standard
        developmental scale or neuropsychological tests; (b) impaired brain growth or acquired microcephaly demonstrated by head circumference
        measurements or brain atrophy demonstrated by computerized tomography or magnetic resonance imaging (serial imaging is required for children
        <2 years of age); (c) acquired symmetric motor deficit manifested by two or more of the following; paresis, pathologic reflexes, ataxia, or gait disturbances
    Herpes simplex virus infection causing a mucocutaneous ulcer that persists for >1 month; or bronchitis, pneumonitis, or esophagitis for any duration
        affecting a child >1 month of age
    Histoplasmosis, disseminated (at a site other than or in addition to lungs or cervical or hilar lymph nodes)
    Kaposi's sarcoma
    Lymphoma, primary, in brain
    Lymphoma, small, noncleaved cell (Burkitt's), or immunoblastic or large cell lymphoma of B cell or unknown immunologic phenotype
    Mycobacterium tuberculosis, disseminated or extrapulmonary
    Mycobacterium, other species or unidentified species, disseminated (at a site other than or in addition to lungs, skin, or cervical or hilar lymph nodes)
    Mycobacterium avium complex or *Mycobacterium kansasii*, disseminated (at site other than or in addition to lungs, skin, or cervical or hilar lymph nodes)
    Pneumocystis carinii pneumonia
    Progressive multifocal leukoencephalopathy
    Salmonella (nontyphoid) septicemia, recurrent
    Toxoplasmosis of the brain with onset at >1 month of age
    Wasting syndrome in the absence of a concurrent illness other than HIV infection that could explain the following findings: (a) persistent weight loss
    >10% of baseline, OR (b) downward crossing of at least two of the following percentile lines on the weight-for-age chart (e.g., 95th, 75th, 50th, 25th, 5th)
    in a child ≥1 year of age OR, (c) <5th percentile on weight-for-height chart on two consecutive measurements, ≥30 days apart PLUS a) chronic diarrhea
    (i.e., at least two loose stools per day for ≥30 days), OR d) documented fever (for ≥30 days, intermittent or constant)

PROGNOSIS

The natural history and prognosis of HIV infection is influenced by many confounding variables, including viral load, immune response, timing of the infection and, importantly, advances in supportive and antiretroviral strategies. Two general patterns of progression occur in children.[173,187,189] Up to 25% develop symptoms in the first year of life. Early symptoms of opportunist infections, in particular *Pneumocystis carinii* (PCP), or progressive neurodevelopment disease are associated with rapid progression. In the remaining group, progression is more gradual and features supporting a lymphoproliferative response to the virus, such as lymphadenopathy, hepatosplenomegaly, parotitis and lymphoid interstitial pneumonitis/pulmonary lymphoid hyperplasia complex (LIP), impart a more favorable prognosis.

Identifying infected children early in the disease process and supplying them with regular support, appropriate prophylactic care, and antiviral therapy can improve survival and quality of life for the affected children. In large parts of the world at the center of the pandemic, even basic care is often not available, and child mortality figures are expected to increase 30% due to rampant AIDS.[183]

CLINICAL FEATURES

The symptoms in younger children with AIDS usually start by 3 to 6 months of age.[173,185,189] Some affected children are small for gestational age at birth. A wide variety of clinical manifestations characterize pediatric HIV infection as the virus has the potential to affect all organ systems. Early signs may be nonspecific (Table 28.22).

Dermatological manifestations

Skin diseases are common amongst children infected with HIV. Whilst the literature is full of case reports and case series which have been extensively reviewed,[174–179] good prevalence studies highlighting real differences between affected and unaffected children in various parts of the world are rare.[190,191] Compounding this lack of prevalence data is the variation in disease prevalence in different populations and geographic locations making extrapolation from one area to another unreliable. Opportunist infection with *Penicillium marneffei*, a dimorphic fungus endemic in Southeast Asia and southern China, has been included as an AIDS-defining illness in Thailand.[191] Pruritic papular eruption (PPE) is found with equal frequency in adults and children with HIV infection in Africa,[192] whereas in Italy it was not found[190] and in Thailand it was 80% less common than in adults.[191]

Although most of the dermatological manifestations in children with HIV infection are skin disorders common to children in general, in the immunocompromised child these conditions tend to be more severe, persistent, recurrent, and resistant, despite appropriate conventional therapy. They may also manifest with unusual presentations. In general, cutaneous manifestations worsen as the CD4 T-helper cell numbers decrease.[190,191,193] The cutaneous findings in children with AIDS are similar to those found in other immunocompromised children, with few exceptions.

The macular exanthem and influenza-like illness that marks seroconversion in adults has not been described in children, probably because most infections occur *in utero*.

Infections and infestations

Mucocutaneous *Candida* infections (Fig. 28.37) are the most common skin manifestations of HIV/AIDS in children.[180,190,191,193,194] Oral pseudo-membranous *Candida* infection predominates with its creamy plaques and underlying erythematous mucosa, but angular cheilitis, chronic hyperplastic candidiasis, and atrophic candidiasis may also occur. Oral thrush may be severe and associated with *Candida* esophagitis. Severe, erosive *Candida* diaper dermatitis or intertrigo may be present early in the course of HIV infection. In older children, chronic *Candida* paronychia may occur. Unusual presentations or subtypes of *Candida* may be present (Fig. 28.38).

Atypical, severe dermatophyte infections have been described (Fig. 28.39). Rarely, local or systemic infections due to other fungal organisms may occur, including *Cryptococcus*[195] and *Penicillium*[191] presenting with umbilicated, molluscum-like papules. Infections with *Sporothrix* and *Histoplasma*, as seen in adults, have not been described in children.

Cutaneous bacterial infections are most commonly caused by *Staphylococcus* or *Streptococcus* species and result in impetigo, cellulitis, folliculitis, furunculosis, and abscesses (Fig. 28.40).[174–179,190,191,196] Despite pulmonary mycobacterial infections having a high association with HIV infection, cases of cutaneous infection in children are rare.[197,198] Cutaneous bacillary angiomatosis has been described in a child, presenting as an erythematous nodule.[199] Isolated reports of uncommon and unusual bacterial skin infections (*Listeria monocytogenes*)[200] serve to heighten the dermatologist's awareness when dealing with children infected with HIV.

Viral infections, particularly molluscum contagiosum (Fig. 28.41), herpes simplex virus, varicella-zoster virus, and papillomaviruses, are very common and may be severe.[174–179,190,191] Primary varicella-zoster infection may be prolonged, recurrent, extensive, and complicated by secondary bacterial infections, especially in children with low CD4 counts.[201] The incidence of

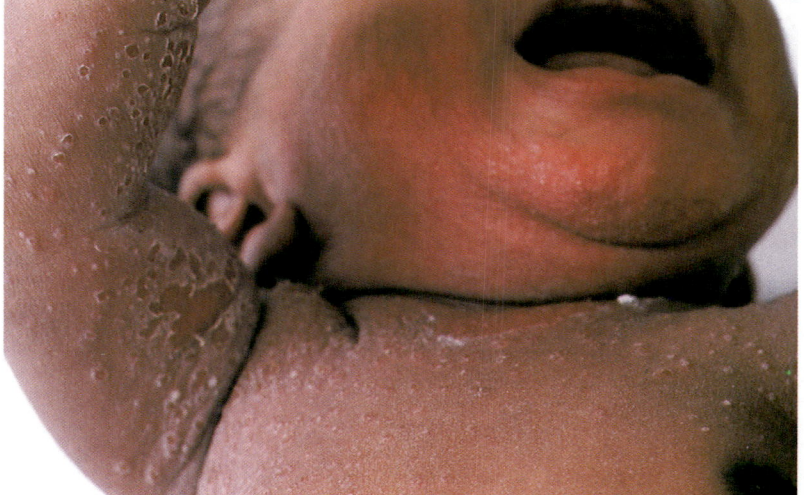

Fig. 28.37 Mucocutaneous candidiasis in an HIV-infected infant. (Courtesy of Cape Town University)

189. Tovo PA, de Martino M, Gabiano C et al. (1992) Prognostic factors and survival in children with perinatal HIV-1 infection. **Lancet** 339:1249.
190. Hachem ME, Bernardi S, Pianosi G et al. (1998) Mucocutaneous manifestations in children with HIV infection and AIDS. **Pediatr Dermatol** 15:429.
191. Wananukul S, Thisyakorn U (1999) Mucocutaneous manifestations of HIV infection in 91 children born to HIV-seropositive women. **Pediatr Dermatol** 16:359.
192. Colebunders R, Mann JM, Francis H et al. (1987) Generalized papular pruritic eruption in African patients with human immunodeficiency virus infection. **AIDS** 1:117.
193. Lim W. Sadick N, Gupta A et al. (1990) Skin diseases in children with HIV infection and their association with degree of immunosuppression. **Int J Dermatol** 29:24.
194. Emodi IJ, Okafor GO (1998) Clinical manifestations of HIV infection in children at Enugu, Nigeria. **J Trop Pediatr** 44:73.
195. Tuerlinckx D, Bodart E, Garrino MG et al. (2001) Cutaneous lesions of disseminated cryptococcosis as the presenting manifestation of human immunodeficiency virus infection in a twenty-two-month-old child. **Pediatr Infect Dis J** 20:463.
196. Bernstein LJ, Krieger BZ, Novick B et al. (1985) Bacterial infection in the acquired immunodeficiency syndrome of children. **Pediatr Infect Dis J** 4:472.
197. Madhi SA, Huebner RE, Doedens L et al. (2000) HIV-1 co-infection in children hospitalized with tuberculosis in South Africa. **Int J Tuberc Lung Dis** 4:448.
198. Mukadi YD, Wiktor SZ, Coulibaly IM et al. (1997) Impact of HIV infection on the development, clinical presentation, and outcome of tuberculosis among children in Abidjan, Cote d'Ivoire. **AIDS** 11:1151.
199. Malane MS, Laude TA, Chen C-K, Fikrig S (1995) An HIV positive child with fever and a scalp nodule. **Lancet** 346:1466.
200. Smith KJ, Skelton HG, Angritt P et al. (1991) Cutaneous lesions of listeriosis in a newborn. **J Cutan Pathol** 18:474.
201. Jura E, Chadwick EG, Josephs SH et al. (1989) Varicella-zoster virus infections in children infected with human immunodeficiency virus. **Pediatr Infect Dis J** 8:586.

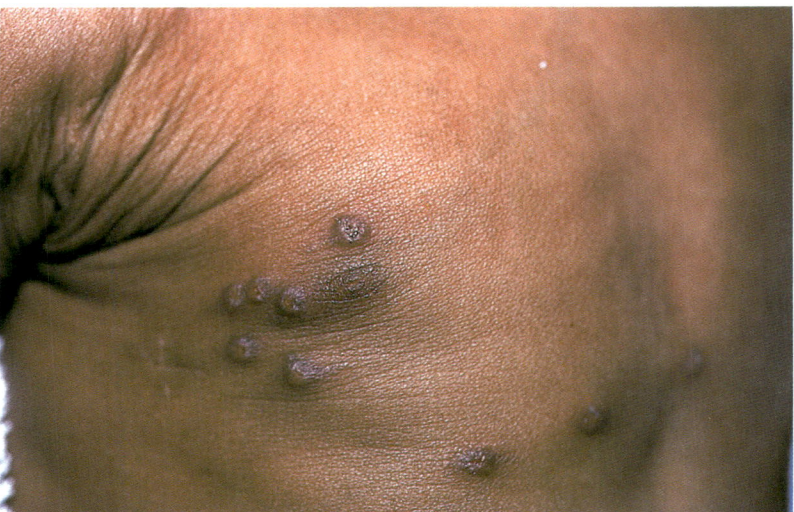

Fig. 28.38 Disseminated unidentified *Candida* septicemia presenting as papular necrotic lesions in an HIV-infected infant. (Courtesy of Cape Town University)

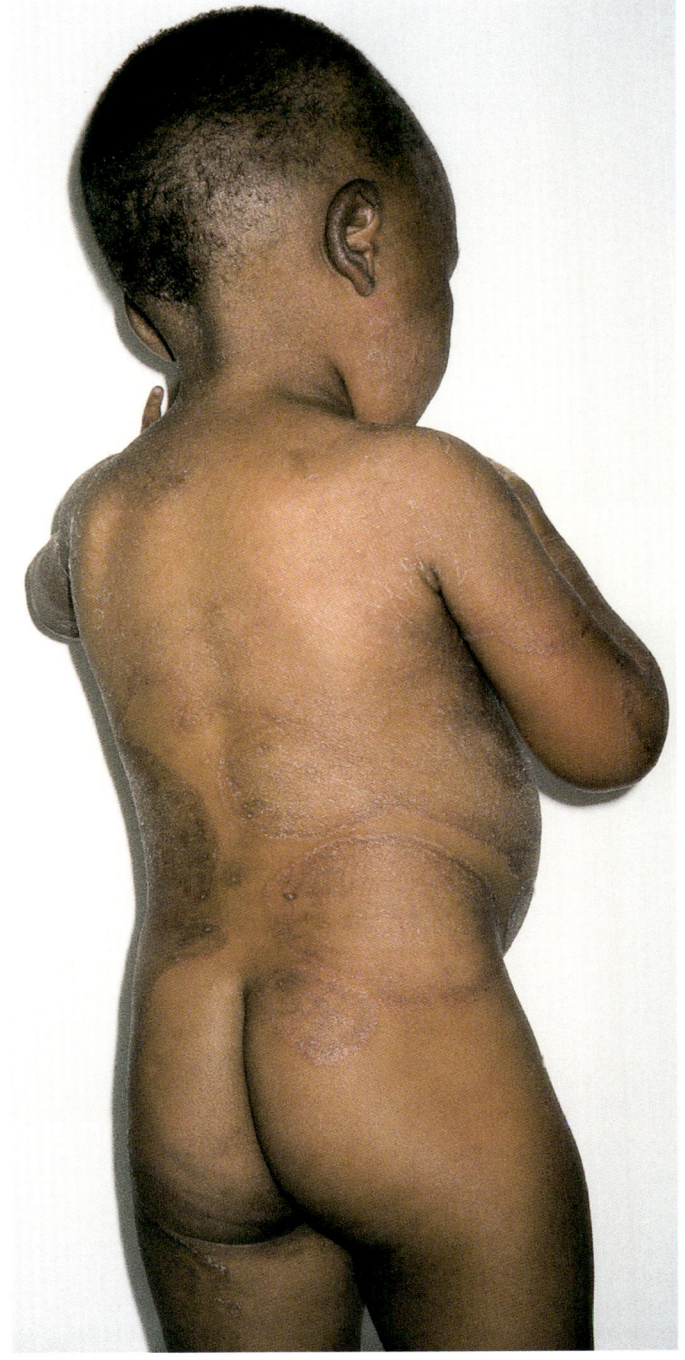

Fig. 28.39 Extensive *Trichophytum violaceum* infection. (Courtesy of Cape Town University)

herpes zoster (Fig. 28.42) is significantly increased in children with AIDS.[202–204] Chronic varicella–zoster or herpes simplex infection, characterized by hyperkeratotic lesions and ulcerations (Fig. 28.43) may develop in children with AIDS.[202,205] Although evidence of cytomegalovirus co-infection occurs frequently in children infected by HIV,[206] skin lesions caused by this virus are rare. An erosive, bullous diaper (napkin) dermatitis due to a cytomegalovirus infection has been described.[207] In addition to numerous, recalcitrant warts, condylomata acuminata have been reported[208] and may reflect the tendency of some children with AIDS to be sexually abused.[188] Oral hairy leukoplakia, thought to be related to Epstein–Barr infection, is rare in infected children.[188,209] Measles can be associated with a higher case fatality rate in HIV-infected children,[210–213] and, in up to 30% of reported cases, is not associated with an exanthem.[213] Some chronic skin lesions (verrucous and nodular lesions) in HIV-infected children have grown mixed cultures, including viruses (varicella zoster) and bacteria (*Listeria*)[201] or fungi (*Alternaria*).[214] Many patients with HIV infection, including several children, have been noted to have crusted (Norwegian) scabies.[193,215,216] Scrapings demonstrate large numbers of infesting mites, and several courses of treatment or systemic therapy with invermectin may be required to eradicate scabies.

Inflammatory skin conditions

Several common childhood inflammatory skin conditions have been reported to be associated with HIV infection. It is the severity, extent, persistence, and resistance to adequate conventional treatment that should alert the physician to underlying immunocompromise.

Severe seborrheic dermatitis (Fig. 28.44), similar to that described as "Leiner's disease," may occur in affected infants, and significant scaling and erythroderma that resembles psoriasis has been described in older children

202. Strugo I, Israele V, Wittek AE et al. (1993) Clinical manifestations of varicella-zoster virus infections in human immunodeficiency virus-infected children. **Am J Dis Child** 147:742.
203. Verroust F, Lemay D, Laurian Y (1987) High frequency of herpes zoster in young hemophiliacs. **N Eng J Med** 316:166.
204. Naburi AE, Leppard B (2000) Herpes zoster and HIV infection in Tanzania. **Int J STD AIDS** 11:254.
205. Gilson IH, Barnett JH, Conant MA et al. (1989) Disseminated ecthymatous herpes varicella-zoster infection in patients with acquired immunodeficiency syndrome. **J Am Acad Dermatol** 20:637.
206. Chandwani S, Kaul A, Bebenroth D et al. (1996) Cytomegalovirus infection in human immunodeficiency virus type 1-infected children. **Pediatr Infect Dis J** 15:310.
207. Thiboutot DM, Beckford A, Mart CR et al. (1991) Cytomegalovirus diaper dermatitis. **Arch Dermatol** 127:396.
208. Forman A, Prendiville J (1988) Association of human immunodeficiency virus seropositivity and extensive perineal condylomata acuminata in a child. **Arch Dermatol** 124:1010.
209. Greenspan JS, Mastrucci MT, Leggott PJ et al. (1988) Hairy leukoplakia in a child. **AIDS** 2:143.

210. Centers for Disease Control and Prevention (1988) Measles in HIV-infected children. **Mor Mortal Wkly Rep** 37:183.
211. Lucas SB, Peacock CS, Hounnou A et al. (1996) Disease in children infected with HIV in Abidjan, Cote d'Ivoire. **Br Med J** 312:335.
212. Embree JE, Datta P, Stackiw W et al. (1992) Increased risk of early measles in infants of human immunodeficiency virus type 1-seropositive mothers. **J Infect Dis** 165:262.
213. Kaplan LJ, Daum RS, Smaron M, McCarthy CA (1992) Severe measles in immunocompromised patients. **J Am Med Assoc** 267:1237.
214. Fisher BK, Warner LC (1987) Cutaneous manifestations of the acquired immunodeficiency syndrome. Update 1987. **Int J Dermatol** 26:615.
215. Jucowics P, Ramon ME, Don PC et al. (1989) Norwegian scabies in an infant with acquired immunodeficiency syndrome. **Arch Dermatol** 125:1670.
216. Sadick N, Kaplan MH, Pahwa SG et al. (1986) Unusual features of scabies complicating human T-lymphotrophic type III infection. **J Am Acad Dermatol** 15:482.

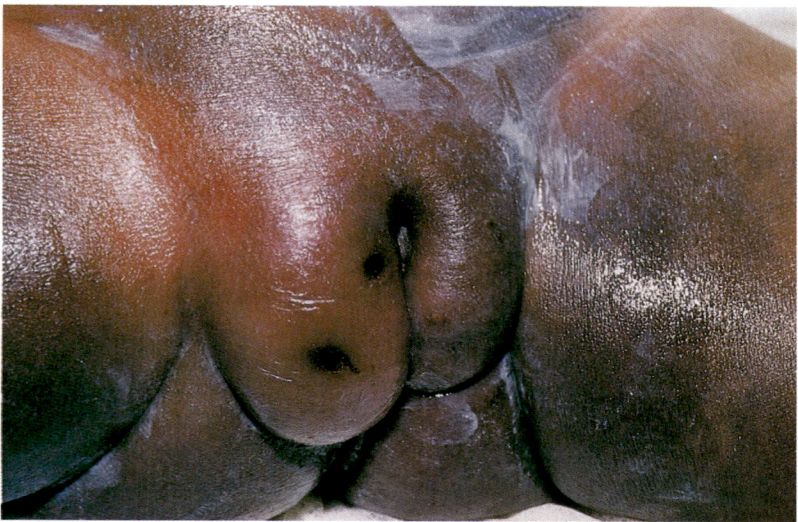

Fig. 28.40 Labial abscess due to *Staphylococcus aureus*. (Courtesy of Cape Town University)

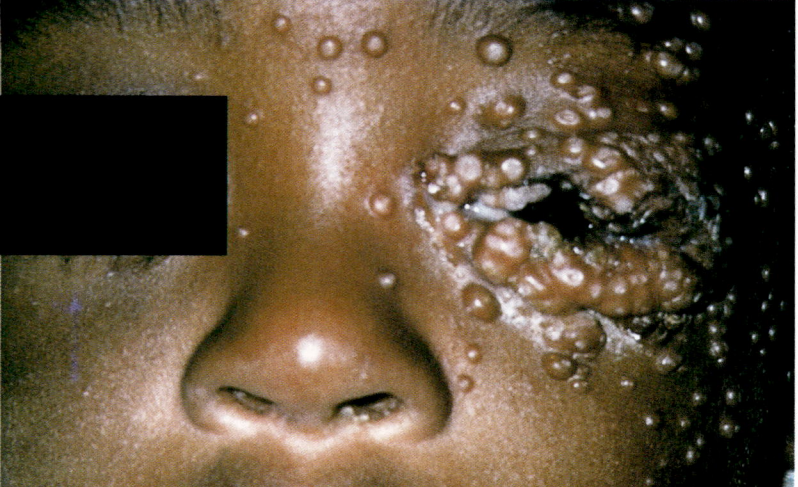

Fig. 28.41 Severe, recalcitrant molluscum contagiosum. (Courtesy of Cape Town University)

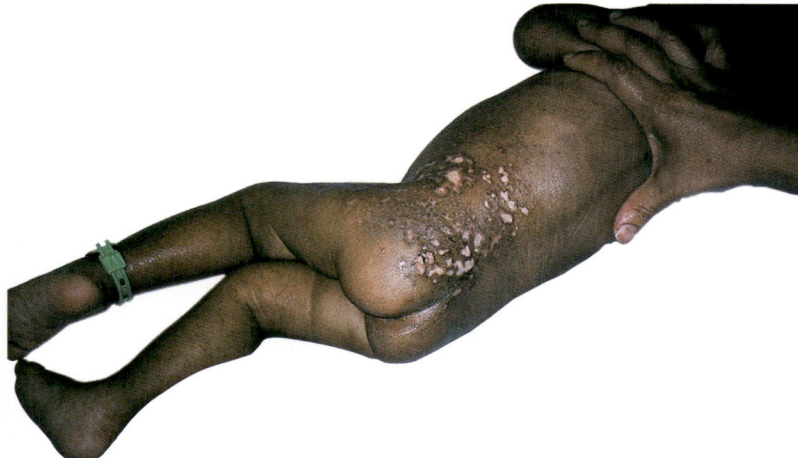

Fig. 28.42 Severe ulcerating herpes zoster in an HIV-infected infant. (Courtesy of Cape Town University)

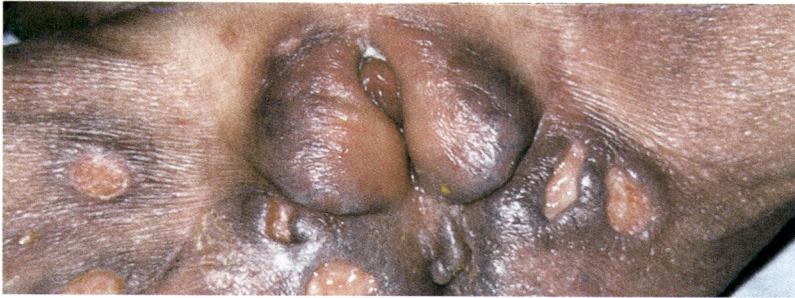

Fig. 28.43 Persistent, deep, painful ulcers of herpes simplex in a wasted HIV-infected infant. (Courtesy of Cape Town University)

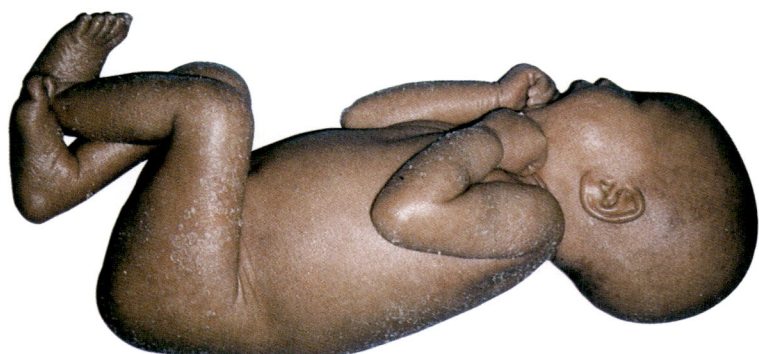

Fig. 28.44 Severe seborrheic dermatitis. (Courtesy of Cape Town University)

with AIDS. Although the strong association of onset or exacerbation of psoriasis that has been described in adults with AIDS has not been noted in childhood, children and adolescents may have psoriasis and be HIV infected. Atopic dermatitis may increase in severity in the context of HIV infection.[217] However, the prevalence does not appear to be greater than in those children that are not infected.[190]

As in adults with AIDS, children with HIV infection are at increased risk of developing drug eruptions, particularly to trimethoprim-sulfamethoxazole (TMP/SMX),[191,193] although the reactions occur less frequently in children[178] than in adults. Toxic epidermal necrolysis (Fig. 28.45) has been reported in HIV-infected children administered antituberculous drugs,[218] TMP/SMX,[219] and anticonvulsants.[220]

Pruritic papular eruption (PPE) (Fig. 28.46) occurs variably in different parts of the world and probably represents a variety of different conditions including eosinophilic folliculitis,[221] which has been described in HIV-infected children.[222,223] The initial itchy lesion is a discrete, urticarial, vesico-

217. Ball LM, Harper JI (1987) Atopic eczema in HIV-seropositive hemophiliacs. **Lancet** 2:627.
218. Hira SK, Wadhawan D, Kamanga J et al. (1988) Cutaneous manifestations in human immunodeficiency virus in Lusaka, Zambia. **J Am Acad Dermatol** 19:451.
219. Revuz J (1986) Necrolysé epidermique toxique par les sulfamides au cours du SIDA; a propós de 3 cas. **J Dermatol Paris** 72:153.
220. Salomon D, Saurat J-H (1990) Erythema multiforme major in a 2-month-old child with human immunodeficiency virus (HIV) infection. **Br J Med** 123:797.
221. Basson MM, Berger TG, Nesbitt LT (1993) Pruritic papular eruption of HIV-disease. **Int J Dermatol** 32:784.
222. Ramdial PK, Morar N, Dlova NC, Aboobaker J (1999) HIV-associated eosinophilic folliculitis in an infant. **Am J Dermatopathol** 21:241.
223. Lucky AW, Esterley NB, Heskel N et al. (1984) Eosinophilic pustular folliculitis in infancy. **Pediatr Dermatol** 1:202.

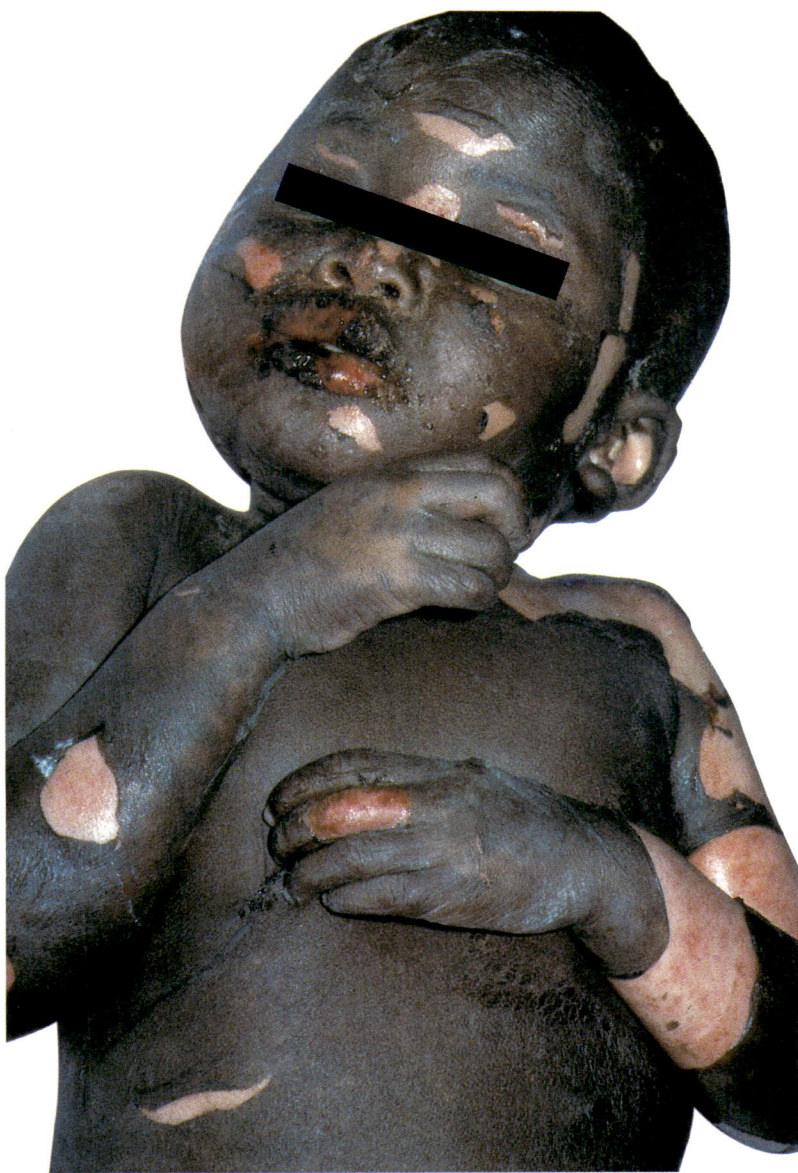

Fig. 28.45   Toxic epidermal necrolysis in an infant receiving antituberculosis therapy for pulmonary disease. (Courtesy of Cape Town University)

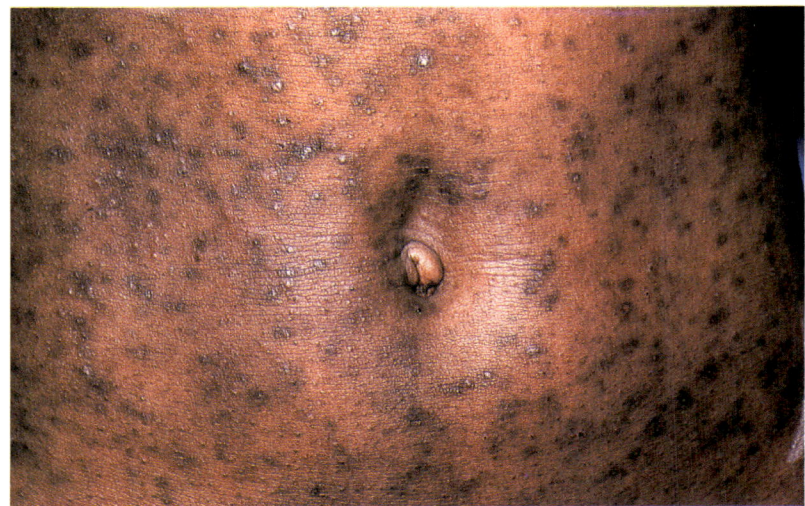

Fig. 28.46   Pruritic papular eruption of HIV. (Courtesy of Cape Town University)

papule. These are found on the limbs, trunk, and face. Excoriations and secondary infection complicate the picture. The lesions occur chronically, often in crops, and heal with postinflammatory hyper- or hypopigmentation and scarring. Response to a variety of treatments is poor. A hypersensitivity reaction to a spectrum of antigens, including insect bites[221] or a follicular antigen,[224] has been proposed as the etiology for some lesions,[191,221] occurring on a background of immune dysregulation.[225]

Gianotti–Crosti syndrome[226] has been described in children with HIV infection presenting with symmetrical monomorphous vesico-papules of the acral areas (Fig. 28.47).

Malignancies

Unlike infected adults, HIV-associated malignancies are rare in children but particularly lymphomas and Kaposi's sarcoma (KS) have been reported to the CDC as AIDS-identifying illnesses. B-cell lymphoproliferative disorders commonly involving the brain are most often reported.[227] KS been reported in a number of children with AIDS,[228–232] especially from Africa.[232] The lymph nodes and viscera, but not the skin, are primarily affected in perinatally acquired AIDS.[229] In children infected postnatally, skin lesions of KS are more common.[229] Increased life expectancy due to the use of antiretroviral agents and appropriate prophylactic and supportive care may be associated with an increase in childhood malignancies in the future.

General features

A wide range of clinical manifestations and nonspecific signs and symptoms herald symptomatic HIV infection in children (Table 28.22).

A variety of clinical neurodevelopment disorders are seen. Commonly, a progressive encephalopathy manifests with impaired brain growth, loss of development milestones, and motor dysfunction.[173] Infection *in utero* can be associated with a dysmorphic syndrome that includes microcephaly and craniofacial abnormalities.[233]

Chronic parotid swelling is common in children with AIDS compared to their adult counterparts and appears to be associated with a better prognosis.

Lymphoid interstitial pneumonia is one of the most common forms of pulmonary involvement associated with HIV infections in children. It is of unknown etiology and virtually unique to children with HIV infection.[173] The onset is usually insidious, but cough and, less commonly, wheezing may

224. Fearfield LA, Rowe A, Francis N et al. (1999) Itchy folliculitis and human immunodeficiency virus infection: clinicopathological and immunological features, pathogenesis and treatment. **Br J Dermatol** 141:3.
225. Magro CM, Crowson AN (1994) Eosinophilic pustular follicular reaction: a paradigm of immune dysregulation. **Int J Dermatol** 33:172.
226. Blauvelt A, Turner ML (1994) Gianotti-Crosti syndrome and human immunodeficiency virus infection. **Arch Dermatol** 130:481.
227. Gandemer V, Verkarre V, Quartier P et al. (2000) Lymphomes chez l'enfant infecte par le VIH-1. **Arch Pediatr** 7:738.
228. Malekzadeh MH, Church J, Siegel SE et al. (1987) Human immunodeficiency virus-associated Kaposi's sarcoma in a pediatric renal transplant recipient. **Nephron** 42:62.

229. Orlow SJ, Cooper D, Petrea S et al. (1993) AIDS-associated Kaposi's sarcoma in Romanian children. **J Am Acad Dermatol** 28:449.
230. Connor E, Boccon-Gibod L, Joshi V et al. (1990) Cutaneous acquired immunodeficiency syndrome-associated Kaposi's sarcoma in pediatric patients. **Arch Dermatol** 126:791.
231. Gutierrez-Ortega P, Hierro-Orozco S, Sanchez-Cisneros R et al. (1989) Kaposi's sarcoma in a 6-day-old infant with human immunodeficiency virus. **Arch Dermatol** 125:432.
232. Ziegler JL, Katongole-Mbidde E. (1996) Kaposi's sarcoma in childhood: an analysis of 100 cases from Uganda and relationship to HIV infection. **Int J Cancer** 65:200.
233. Marion RW, Wiznia AA, Hutcheon RG, Rubinstein A (1986) Human T-cell lymphotropic virus type III (HTLV-III) embryopathy. **Am J Dis Child** 140:638.

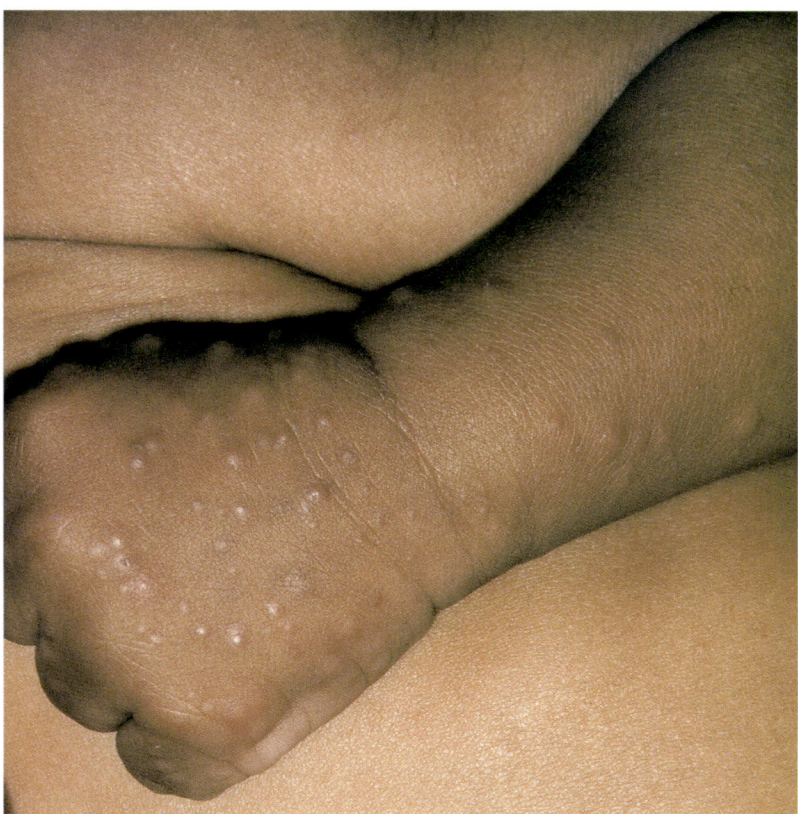

Fig. 28.47 Gianotti–Crosti syndrome in an HIV-infected infant. (Courtesy of Cape Town University)

present early in the course. It is generally associated with a better disease prognosis. *Pneumocystis carinii* pneumonia (PCP) is the most frequent serious opportunistic pulmonary infection, and occurs most commonly during the first year of life in young children with AIDS. Pulmonary infections with opportunist organism such as PCP are associated with a worse prognosis.[211] Pulmonary tuberculosis in some studies is associated with a worse prognosis,[197,234] while in others it is not.[235]

Hematological manifestations of symptomatic HIV infection are common,[236] especially anemia. Thrombocytopenia and leukopenia are less common. The lymphopenia, common in adult cases, is rare, although decreased CD4 counts with elevated CD8 counts and functional T-cell defects are seen regularly. Immunoglobulins are elevated in most affected children, but decreased to absent IgG_2 levels[236] may account for increased risk of infection, especially with encapsulated bacteria. Hypogammaglobulinemia occurs rarely and infants are at high risk for bacterial infections.

Failure to thrive is a universal feature of symptomatic HIV infection[173] and carries a poor prognosis. Gastrointestinal dysfunction, in particular chronic diarrhea (usually infective), significantly affects clinical outcome and contributes to nutritional deficiencies (Fig. 28.48) and weight loss.

DIFFERENTIAL DIAGNOSIS

AIDS should be suspected in any child, especially of a high-risk group, who develops an opportunistic infection or shows any of the features that characterize AIDS. The most easily confused disorders are the primary immuno-

deficiencies, such as Nezelof combined immunodeficiency syndrome, Wiskott–Aldrich syndrome, severe combined immunodeficiency, ataxia-telangiectasia, and the hypogammaglobulinemias. Secondary immuno-deficiency states, including graft-versus-host disease, starvation, lymphoreticular neoplasias, and the side effects of immunosuppressive therapy must also be distinguished from AIDS. These disorders all lack laboratory evidence of HIV infection.

TREATMENT
Prevention

Prevention of HIV infection is the cornerstone of management. Behavior modification, education, and the use of infection protection devices should be encouraged. Although not yet available, the search for an effective vaccine dominates HIV research. Encouraging results in reducing vertical, mother-to-child transmission have been achieved by the use of antiretroviral agents during pregnancy and the immediate postnatal period.[173,183,185,237] Interventions found to be successful should be sustainable and affordable.

Supportive and prophylactic therapy

Death in children with AIDS is usually due to opportunistic infections. Chemoprophylaxis with TMP/SMX is useful in preventing PCP and also decreases the risk of serious bacterial infection. Aerosolized pentamidine or dapsone are alternative prophylactic agents for PCP. Intravenous immuno-globulin (IVIG) has been suggested for infection prophylaxis but results are conflicting, although it is recommended in combination with antiretroviral agents for children with humoral immunodeficiencies. Mucocutaneous candidiasis is generally unresponsive to topical therapy and a systemic azole should be considered, especially in severe infections or when it interferes with the ability of the child to eat. Amphotericin B is the drug of choice for invasive fungal infections. Multiple-organism prophylactic regimens using combinations of antimicrobial and antiparasitic regimens are being evaluated in children.

Herpetic infections should be treated with the appropriate dosages of acyclovir. Prophylactic daily suppression may be needed for severe recurrent infections, but should be used with increased vigilance for the emergence of resistant strains. Although symptomatic, HIV-infected children have poor immunological responses to vaccines, routine immunizations, other than with live or attenuated organisms, should be given.

Some patients with LIP respond to systemic corticosteroid therapy. Nutrition is a critical aspect of care for the child with symptomatic HIV infection or AIDS. The increased metabolic rate usually related to infectious complications, malabsorption secondary to chronic diarrhea and decreased food intake (due to poor appetite, inability to eat due to mucocutaneous lesions or lack of food) may result in growth failure. The poor growth of a child may inhibit physical interactions and the social acceptance of the affected child. Diets that are acceptable to the child and maximize caloric intake among the various food groups are best developed with the assistance of a dietician.

Primary antiretroviral therapy

Significant advances have been made in the use of antiretroviral agents for infected children since Zidovudine (AZT) was approved for use in 1990. Currently, 13 of the 15 medications licensed for use in HIV-infected individuals have been approved for use in children and adolescents. Full management recommendations for children with HIV infection are available from the hivartis website http://www.hivartis.org that is regularly updated on current trends. Ongoing research on mother-to-child transmission

234. Kawo G, Karlsson K, Lyamuya E et al. (2000) Prevalence of HIV type I infection, associated clinical features and mortality among hospitalized children in Dar es Salaam, Tanzania. **Scand J Infect Dis** 32:357.

235. Chintu C, Luo C, Bhat G et al. (1995) Impact of the human immunodeficiency virus type-1 on common pediatric illnesses in Zambia. **J Trop Pediatr** 41:348.

236. de Martino M, Tovo P-A, Galli L et al. (1991) Prognostic significance of immunologic changes in 675 infants perinatally exposed to human immunodeficiency virus. **J Pediatr** 119:702.

237. Bulterys M (2001) Preventing vertical HIV transmission in the year 2000: progress and prospects – a review. **Placenta** 22(Suppl A):S5.

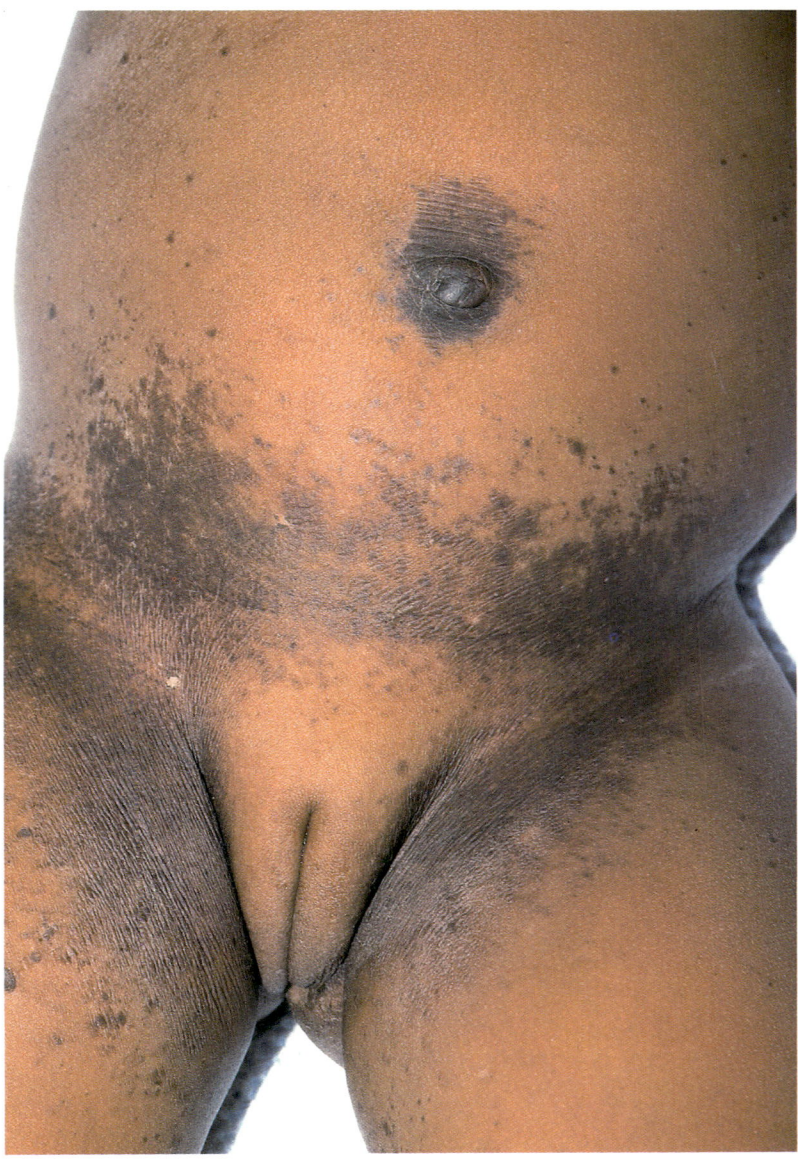

Fig. 28.48   Pellagra-like skin lesions in a child with HIV infection complicated by diarrhea and malnutrition. (Courtesy of Cape Town University)

prevention,[237] post-exposure prophylaxis,[238] and new therapeutic approaches continues.

Comprehensive, multidisciplinary care, and psychosocial support must be coupled with antiretroviral therapy to maximize the pharmaceutical advances made in this field that have lead to improved and prolonged life in those infected with HIV.

PSYCHOLOGICAL AND SOCIAL CONSIDERATIONS

AIDS can be a devastating chronic disease and is currently almost uniformly fatal.[239] Some children who have developed AIDS have subsequently been rejected by family, friends, and medical practitioners who fear contracting this devastating disease even though there is little evidence of horizontal transmission among household contacts.[173] Children should be encouraged to attend school and should not be restricted in their physical activities unless complications require their curtailment. Negative stressful life events aggravate immune suppression in HIV-infected children.[240]

In large parts of the world, children are left destitute with no income and no means of support as parents and supporting family members die of AIDS. Many of these children are not infected with the virus that caused the death of their parents. The lack of provision for this vulnerable group means that they have to resort to crime, prostitution, and violence to survive,[241] putting them at great risk of becoming infected. This forgotten group represents the second devastating pandemic due to HIV.

238. Merchant RC, Keshavarz R (2001) Human immunodeficiency virus postexposure prophylaxis for adolescents and children. **Pediatrics** 108:E38.

239. Meyers A, Weitzman M (1991) Pediatric HIV disease. The newest chronic illness of childhood. **Pediatr Clin N Am** 38:169.

240. Howland LC, Gortmaker SL, Mofenson LM et al. (2000) Effects of negative life events on immune suppression in children and youth infected with human immunodeficiency virus type I. **Pediatrics** 106:540.

241. Schönteich M (2002) The coming crime wave? AIDS orphans and crime in South Africa. **S Afr J HIV Med** 7:30.

Physical Injury and Environmental Hazards

Sharon S. Raimer, Ben G. Raimer, Ana M. Duarte, Chulabhorn Pruksachatkunakorn,

and Lesley Boyer

PHYSICAL INJURY

**Sharon S. Raimer
and Ben G. Raimer**

The skin acts as an effective barrier to limit invasion by outside chemicals and microbes while retaining internal fluids, electrolytes, and molecules that are important in homeostasis. As a membrane, the skin is neither impermeable nor freely permeable. The intact skin may show 10 000-fold differences in rates of penetration of different substances, depending on molecular charge and configuration of the substance. In addition, regional variations exist in that the palms and soles are far more resistant to penetration than are other body surface areas. The major barrier of the skin is the stratum corneum, which, when injured, may lose its ability to function effectively.

The dermal portion of the skin is effective in rendering it durable and flexible. In addition, the dermal vessels act as thermal regulators to control internal temperature in response to changing environmental temperature. The dermal vessels also supply nutrients to the skin; when injury occurs, they respond with cells of inflammation that assist in the process of wound healing. The combination of epidermis and dermis offers a protective cover over the body, which is extremely effective but not totally indestructible. The purpose of this chapter is to review many of the external agents that can injure the skin, the body's response, and the therapeutic approaches designed to promote healing. Preventive measures to avoid injury (e.g., photoprotection and insect repellents) are also discussed.

SOLAR RADIATION

Photobiology is the scientific study of the interaction of nonionizing electromagnetic radiation with living matter. People are exposed daily to the effects of radiation through the products of photosynthesis, photoexposure, and occasionally phototherapy. Understanding the principles of electromagnetic radiation is helpful in approaching light-related conditions.

Electromagnetic radiation has the properties of both waves and particles. All electromagnetic radiation is propagated at the same velocity through space. The equation

$$c = \nu \times \lambda$$

where c is the velocity of radiation that expresses the relationship between ν (frequency of oscillations per second) and λ (wavelength in meters); C is a constant for the speed of light (186 500miles/s or 3×10^8m/s). This formula establishes the precise inverse relationship between ν and λ. Electromagnetic

radiation can also be described as streams of discrete packets of energy called photons, which have no mass. When photons are absorbed, they impart energy to the absorbing matter and cease to exist. Plancks' law

$$E = h\nu = hc/\lambda$$

where E is the energy of the photons in Joules and h is Planck's constant $(6.625 \times 10-34\text{J/s})$, which establishes the directly proportional relationship between the energy in photons and the frequency of the radiation ν. Because an inverse relationship exists between ν and λ, radiation of higher frequency has greater photon energy and a shorter wavelength. Light is divided into various types according to the wavelengths. Ultraviolet (UV) radiation (wavelength, 100–400nm) is composed of the following wavebands: UVC (100–290nm), UVB (290–320nm), and UVA (320–400nm). Visible light has a 400 to 700-nm wavelength.[1]

Responses of the skin to light are initiated when photons are absorbed by endogenous or exogenous molecules called chromophores. Action spectra show which wavelengths of the UV and visible spectra are absorbed by a particular chromophore. Less unsaturated molecules such as DNA absorb in the UVC and UVB ranges, and many photosensitizing drugs absorb in the UVA range. In general, molecules with many conjugated double bonds such as β-carotene or unsaturated ring systems such as porphyrins absorb in the visible range. When a molecule absorbs the energy of a photon, it transfers into an excited state, which can undergo new chemical reactions.

EFFECTS OF ULTRAVIOLET LIGHT IRRADIATION ON SKIN

Early effects

Sunburn

Sunburn is a delayed inflammatory reaction resulting from molecular and cellular damage caused by the absorption of UV light by skin chromophores (Fig. 29.1). Wavelengths of light from the sun shorter than 290nm are absorbed by ozone in the stratosphere. Sunburn is mainly due to exposure to UVB radiation. Approximately 20 to 70mJ/cm of UVB energy is required to produce minimally perceptible erythema.[2] The UVA energy is required to produce a sunburn is 800 to 1000 times higher than that of UVB radiation. For fair-skinned, untanned persons, a sunburn would occur after approximately 20min in midday summer daylight at a latitude of 44°N, but less than 10 minutes may be required in areas of high UV intensity in the southern United States.[3] Radiation intensity is increased by reflection from snow (85%), sand (25%), and water (5%).[1]

After exposure to UVB radiation, bright red erythema begins in 3 to 5h and reaches a maximum between 12 and 24h, occasionally resulting in

1. Hawk JLM (1992) Cutaneous photobiology. In: Rook/Wilkinson/Ebling Textbook of Dermatology, 5th edn, Vol 2, Champion RH, Burton JL, Ebling FJG, eds. Oxford: Blackwell Scientific Publications, p. 849.
2. Pathak MA (1982) Sunscreens: topical and systemic approaches for protection of human skin against harmful effects of solar radiation. **J Am Acad Dermatol** 7:285.
3. Parrish JA, White HAD, Pathak MA (1979) Photomedicine. In: Dermatology in General Medicine, 2nd edn, Fitzpatrick TB, Eisen AZ, Wolff K et al., eds. New York: McGraw-Hill, p. 942.

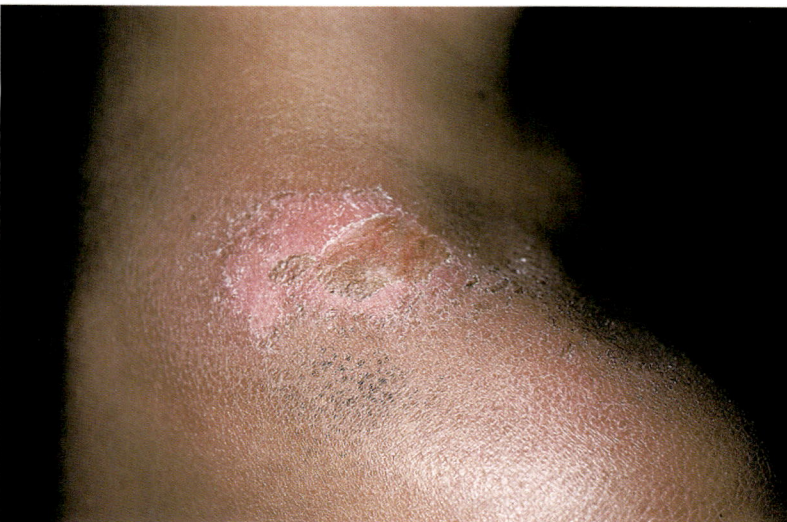

Fig. 29.1 Sunburn resulting in blistering and desquamation in a teenage boy. (Photo courtesy of Anne W. Lucky.)

blistering; then it gradually subsides over 72h.[4] Histologically, epidermal spongiosis, sunburn cells, dermal vasodilation, edema, and a neutrophil and mononuclear cell infiltration are present. Damage to the epidermis that occurs after UVC and UVB exposure appears to be largely due to biochemical mediators such as prostaglandins and histamines.[5] Sunburn from UVA results in a painful violaceous delayed erythema, which is more persistent than that caused by UVB, but blistering and epidermal injury are less prominent, suggesting that the depth of injury and inflammation correlates with the greater depth of penetration of UVA radiation into skin.

The symptoms of sunburn include pain and tenderness in the skin and occasional constitutional complaints including headache, fever, chills, malaise, and even prostration. An attempt should be made to prevent sunburn by UV avoidance, protective clothing, and sunscreens. Treatment once a sunburn has occurred is mainly to decrease symptoms. The patient should have an adequate intake of oral fluids. Nonsteroidal anti-inflammatory agents, cool soaks and baths, and low to midpotency topical steroids (to nonblistered skin only) may give minimal relief.

Tanning

Immediate pigment darkening. An immediate grayish-brown darkening occurs within seconds of exposure to UVA radiation and is most prominent in more pigmented individuals. This darkening appears to result from direct photo-oxidative changes in preformed melanin or melanin precursors and the transfer of melanosomes from melanocytes to keratinocytes.

Delayed tanning. Delayed tanning occurs within 48h of sufficient UV exposure and persists for weeks to months. The size and enzyme activity of melanocytes are increased, and new melanocytes result from cell division. Tanning results from increased synthesis and transfer of melanosomes from melanocytes to keratinocytes. Most epidermal melanin is carried in basal keratinocytes and is frequently found in the cytoplasm of these cells above the nucleus.

Hyperplasia. Skin hyperplasia occurs after UVB and UVC exposure and may persist for up to 2 months. The epidermis, particularly the stratum corneum, and dermis thicken by two to four times or more, giving a sev-

eralfold protection against UV erythema.[1] This combines with tanning to protect individuals from further UV exposure and may be even more important than tanning for protection in very fair-skinned individuals.

Immunologic changes

UV irradiation of human skin has been shown to cause several biologic effects on the immune system. Among these are the suppression of induction of contact allergy;[6] suppression of delayed-type hypersensitivity reactions, including those designed to eradicate infectious organisms such as herpes simplex;[7] and suppression of immunosurveillance against nonmelanoma, UV-induced skin cancer.[8] The effect of light on the immune system may be due in part to the decrease in the number of resident Langerhans cells seen on histologic examination after UVB exposure. One hour after exposure, the number of detectable cells has been reported to decrease by 25%; by 24 to 72h, only 10% of the Langerhans cell population remains or fully expresses surface markers.[4] Also, whole-body erythemogenic UV radiation has been shown to decrease peripheral T cells, to alter the proportion of circulating helper lymphocytes, and to increase nonspecific suppressor cell activity.[9] Although the impact of UV irradiation on the immune system appears to have more negative than positive effects, the downregulation of immune responses can have a beneficial effect on several skin disorders.

Vitamin D synthesis

A major nutritional effect of solar radiation is the conversion of 7-dehydrocholesterol to the metabolically active, hydroxylated form of vitamin D_3.[10] The cutaneous photochemical product is important in calcium hemostasis because very little vitamin D exists in the normal, unsupplemented diet; therefore, endogenous vitamin D_3 production in the skin is crucial.

Late effects

Photoaging (dermatoheliosis)

Photoaging appears to occur from the long-term cumulative effects of UV irradiation of the skin. The epidermis is affected mainly by UVB and the dermis, by both UVA and UVB. With sufficient UV exposure, the skin develops fine and coarse wrinkling, laxity, mottled pigmentation, telangiectasias, and comedones.

Histologically, there is elastosis, which may result in an accumulation of amorphous material composed primarily of abnormal elastic fibers in the upper dermis. In addition, elastin, microfibrillar proteins, fibronectin, glycosaminoglycans, and type III collagen have been reported to be increased by UVB radiation.[11,12]

Photocarcinogenesis

Human epidemiologic and animal irradiation studies indicate that chronic UVB, and to a lesser extent UVA, exposures are largely responsible for the induction of actinic keratoses, actinic cheilitis, and nonmelanoma skin cancer.[13] These types of lesions may occur in normal adolescents with fair skin who have had excessive sun exposure and in children with photosensitive genodermatoses. Incomplete repair of UV-induced DNA damage and impaired immunosurveillance may be of etiologic importance.[12] Ultraviolet irradiation appears to contribute to the induction of melanoma in some individuals, especially fair-skinned individuals who receive intense intermittent sun exposure of certain anatomic sites.[14] Epidemiologic studies suggest that ultraviolet radiation (UVR) exposure in childhood and early adolescence may be of greater importance in promoting melanoma development

4. Hruza LL, Pentland AP (1993) Mechanisms of UV-induced inflammation. **J Invest Dermatol** 100:35s.
5. Soter NA (1990) Acute effects of ultraviolet radiation on the skin. **Semin Dermatol** 9:11.
6. Cruz PD, Jr, Bergstresser PR (1990) Antigen processing and presentation by epidermal Langerhans cells: induction of immunity or unresponsiveness. **Dermatol Clin** 8:633.
7. Howie SEM, Norval M, Maingay J (1986) Exposure to low dose ultraviolet radiation suppresses delayed-type hypersensitivity to herpes simplex virus in mice. **J Invest Dermatol** 86:125.
8. Baadsgaard O (1991) *In vivo* ultraviolet irradiation of human skin results in profound perturbation of the immune system: revelence to ultraviolet-induced skin cancer. **Arch Dermatol** 127:99.
9. Granstein RD (1990) Photoimmunology. **Semin Dermatol** 9:16.

10. Holeck MF, Smith E, Pincers S (1987) Skin as the site of vitamin D synthesis and target tissue for 1,25 dihydroxyvitamin D_3. **Arch Dermatol** 123:1677a.
11. Schwartz E (1988) Connective tissue alterations in the skin of ultraviolet irradiated hairless mice. **J Invest Dermatol** 91:158.
12. Young AR (1990) Cumulative effects of ultraviolet radiation of the skin: cancer and photoageing. **Semin Dermatol** 9:25.
13. Green A, Battistutta D (1990) Incidences of determinants of skin cancer in a high risk Australian population. **Int J Cancer** 46:356.
14. Stevens RG, Moolgavkar SH (1984) Malignant melanoma: dependence of site-specific risk on age. **Am J Epidemiol** 119:880.

than that received later in life.[15,16] Sunlight also appears to promote the development of both normal, acquired, and atypical nevi.[17,18] The incidence of melanoma appears to be higher in patients with large numbers of acquired nevi.[19] In certain individuals, atypical nevi may be both markers for and precursors of melanoma.

PHOTOPROTECTION

Human skin has several natural defenses against radiation. The outermost layer of the epidermis, the stratum corneum, absorbs photons in the UVC and UVB range, thereby protecting against sunburn. Melanin is generally regarded as the major defense of the skin against the acute and chronic effects of sun exposure.[1] The number of melanocytes in black skin is essentially identical to that in white skin, but the melanocytes in black skin synthesize larger melanosomes that have a diffuse nonaggregated appearance.[2] Increased melanin in the skin produces increased pigment and protection against UV damage. Children who lack adequate skin pigmentation to prevent sunburn from moderate sun exposure need additional protection to prevent acute and chronic skin damage.

Protective clothing

The use of hats (children and teenagers should be reminded to wear their caps bill forward during sun exposure) and protective clothing should be encouraged. Sun-protective clothing, which is lightweight and designed to shield the skin maximally from sun is now being marketed and thus may be of benefit for the photosensitive child. For the average child, however, tightly woven fabrics appear to give adequate protection, and the additional expense of buying specialized clothing seems unwarranted.

In vitro testing measuring UV transmission through clothing with a spectrophotometer has led to the introduction of the concept of UV protective factor (UPF) which is analogous to the sun protective factor (SPF) of sunscreens. This UPF standard has been officially adopted in Australia and New Zealand to access UV protection of fabrics *in vitro*.

A recent study analysed the effects of shrinkage, dyeing and the use of a UV-absorbing chemical on the UPF of white cotton T-shirt fabrics with low UPF values.[20] Washing with hot water or water plus detergent increased the UPF approximately 50%. Adding a UV-absorbing agent to the wash, which was a stilbene disulfonic acid triazine derivative (Tinosorb by Ciba Speciality Chemicals), increased the UPF by 400% after five treatments of the fabric without producing noticeable changes in the whiteness or texture of the fabric.

The color of fabrics is known to affect UPF with dark colors most effectively blocking UV light. The study described above noted that dyeing T-shirt fabric yellow increased the UPF 212%, while dyeing it navy blue increased the UPF 544%. It was also noted in the study that more UVA is transmitted through fabrics than UVB.

Sunscreens

Sunscreens, which reduce the consequences of UV radiation through reflection, absorption, or scattering of light,[21] have been improved significantly in recent years. Topical sunscreens are divided into the two general categories: physical and chemical agents. Sunscreens are characterized by their sun protection factor (SPF). SPF is a measure of their efficacy against sunburning:

$$SPF = \frac{\text{Minimal erythema dosage of light for sun-protected skin}}{\text{Minimal erythema dosage of light for unprotected skin}}$$

SPF is measured under highly controlled circumstances, with the sunscreen applied to an internationally established thickness of $2mg/cm.^2$ With actual use much less sunscreen generally is applied, which results in a markedly reduced SPF of the product.[22]

The four major physical sunblocks are zinc oxide, talc, titanium dioxide, and red veterinary petroleum.[23] These opaque agents scatter, reflect, and physically block UV light throughout the UV spectrum. They are particularly valuable for patients who have photosensitive diseases or who are very sun sensitive. Cosmetic unacceptability, occlusiveness, and the fact that they easily rub off the skin have limited patient compliance in the past. Recently, cosmetically elegant products containing a microsize or ultrafine grade of titanium dioxide and zinc oxide have become available. These products eliminate the worry of applying potentially absorbable chemicals to the skin of young children and appear not to sting if the sunscreen accidentally gets into the eyes. Physical sunscreens may be useful in the first 6 months of life as well.

Chemical sunscreens are nonopaque and maintain a thin invisible film on the skin. Most products contain one or more UV radiation-absorbing chemicals. At the present time, chemical sunscreens are not recommended for use in infants less than 6 months of age. Compounds available in the past absorbed light principally in the UVB range; however, some newer commercial sunscreens contain UVA- and UVB-absorbing chemicals. Most sunscreen products available in the United States do not provide broad-spectrum UV protection, even though the majority of products claim UVA protection. Broad-spectrum claims, including claims of UVA protection may presently be made for sunscreen products simply on the basis of the inclusion of a UVA 1 or UVA 2 filter, regardless of the amplitude or breadth of wavelength protection.[24] Table 29.1 contains some of the more commonly used chemicals and the wavelengths of light absorbed by each

The compound para-aminobenzoic acid (PABA) was one of the first chemical sunscreens to be widely available and offer good protection against UVB. Both PABA and the PABA esters have the advantage of binding with the epidermis, thus resisting easy removal by perspiration or water. The major disadvantage of PABA is its ability to cause both contact and photocontact dermatitis. Ester derivatives, mainly Padimate O (octyldimethyl PABA) which is the most potent UVB absorber available, came into greater use because of a lower potential for adverse effects.[25] The demand for higher SPF products led to the incorporation of multiple active ingredients into a single product. Presently octyl methoxycinnamate is the most frequently used sunscreen ingredient.

The most widely used UVA screening agents have been the benzophenones. Avobenzone or Parsol 1789 4-*tert*-butyl-methoxydibenzoylmethane has been approved for use and is the most broad-spectrum UVA screen currently available in the United States. This chemical may benefit patients with UVA photosensitivity. Concerns have been raised regarding its photostability and potential to degrade other sunscreen ingredients in products where it is used.[25]

In addition to products marketed as sunscreens, numerous makeup bases, facial moisturizers, and moisturizing lotions contain chemical sunscreens. Also, although not advertised as sunscreens, many makeup bases contain ingredients such as zinc oxide and therefore function as physical sunblocks.

15. Khlat M, Vail A, Parkin M et al. (1992) Mortality from melanoma in migrants to Australia: variation by age at arrival and duration of stay. **Am J Epidemiol** 135:1103.
16. Weinstock MA, Colditz GA, Willett WC et al. (1989) Nonfamilial cutaneous melanoma incidence in women in associated with sun exposure before age 20. **Pediatrics** 84:199.
17. Gallagher RP, Rivers JK, Yang CP et al. (1991) Melanocytic nevus density in Asian, Indo-Pakistani, and white children. The Vancouver Mole Study. **J Am Acad Dermatol** 25:507.
18. Weinstock MA, Stampfer MJ, Willett WC (1991) Sunlight and dysplastic nevus risk. **Cancer** 67:1701.
19. Kruger S, Garbe C, Buttner P et al. (1992) Epidemiologic evidence for the role of melanocytic nevi as risk markers and direct precursors of cutaneous malignant melanoma. **J Am Acad Dermatol** 26:920.
20. Wang SQ, Kopf AW, Marks J et al. (2001) Reduction of ultraviolet transmission through cotton T-shirt fabrics with low ultraviolet protection by various laundering methods and dyeing: Clinical implications. **J Am Acad Dermatol** 44:767.
21. Luftman DB, Lowe NJ, May RL (1991) Sunscreens. Update and review. **Dermatol Surg Oncol** 17:744.
22. Autier P (2001) Quantity of sunscreen used by European students. **Br J Dermatol** 144:288.
23. O'Donoghue MN (1991) Sunscreen: one weapon against melanoma. **Dermatol Clin** 9:789.
24. Diffey BL, Tanner PR, Matts PJ et al. (2000) In vitro assessment of the broad spectrum ultraviolet protection of sunscreen products. **J Am Acad Dermatol** 43:1024.
25. Levy SB (2001) Sunscreen In: Comprehensive Dermatologic Drug Therapy, Wolverton SE, ed. Philadelphia: WB Saunders, p. 632.

TABLE 29.1   Wavelength protection of chemical sunscreens

Sunscreen	Range of protection (nm)	Maximal effect of protection (nm)
PABA and PABA Esters		
PABA	260–313	283
Padimate A	290–315	309
Padimate O	290–315	311
Glycerol aminobenzoate	260–313	297
Cinnamates		
Octyl methoxycinnamate	280–310	310
Cinoxate	270–328	290
Salicylates		
Homosalicylate	290–315	306
Octyl salicylate	260–310	307
Triethanolamine salicylate	269–320	298
Octocrylene	287–323	303
Etrocrylene	296–383	303
Benzophenones		
Oxybenzone	270–350	290, 325
Dioxybenzone	206–380	284, 327
Sulisobenzone	250–380	286, 324
Avobenzone (Parsol 1789)	310–400	358
Methylanthranilate	200–380	336

PABA, para-aminobenzoic acid.
Modified from O'Donoghue,[21] with permission.

Regular use of sunscreen has been shown to reduce actinic keratosis,[26] solar elastosis, cutaneous immunosuppression[27] and in children with freckles, new nevi.[28] Most dermatologists recommend use of sunscreen with a SPF of 15 or greater. The SPF number is correlated with the proportion of ultraviolet radiation (UVR), which is filtered out. An SPF 2 product prevents 50% of UVR from penetrating while SPF 15 filters out 93.3% and SPF 30.96.1%.[25] Erythema, the key measurement in the SPF assay, is not a boundary between no biological effect and biological effect, rather it is a boundary between effect and severe effect. Many significant consequences, including mutations and tumor formation, can and do occur with suberythemal UV exposure.[26] Comparison of an SPF 15 with a SPF 30 sunscreen showed the SPF 30 product provided significantly greater protection with regard to sunburn cell production, even though no visible erythema was seen in either group.[29]

Concerns that higher SPF products with greater concentrations of chemicals would be associated with a higher incidence of side effects do not appear to be well founded. Objective irritation appears unrelated to SPF levels in formulations.[25]

Since for most individuals the majority of ones lifetime exposure to sunlight occurs before age 18, regular use of sunscreens as well as use of protective clothing in children should be emphasized to parents. Parents who regularly apply sunscreen to their children at an early age will find that as adolescents they are more likely to continue this practice.[30]

In addition to the SPF rating, many sunscreens carry a designation of "water resistant" or "waterproof," which is a measure of substantivity.[31] A sunscreen is considered water resistant if it maintains SPF after two 20-minute immersions with moderate activity in a swimming pool. It is waterproof if it survives four such immersions.

Self-tanning products

The number of self-tanning or sunless tanning lotions available has increased dramatically in recent years in response to a demand for a safer or more convenient way to tan. Presently available products contain dihydroxyacetone ($C_3H_6O_3$), DHA, a three-carbon sugar that, when reacted with the amino group of amino acids, peptides, or proteins, results in a "browning reaction" known as the Maillard reaction.[32] The brown products formed have been referred to as melanoidins. When creams or lotions that contain DHA are applied to the skin, this browning reaction occurs in the stratum corneum where the amino groups are supplied by keratin and sweat. The brown pigment formed remains until the stratum corneum is sloughed.

Self-tanning products appear to be safe. The incidence of contact sensitization to DHA appears to be extremely low, and this compound does not appear to be mutagenic. Patients need to be informed, however, that these products offer no protection against UVB. If they are formulated with standard sunscreens, the duration of UV protection is more short-lived than the skin color change. The combination of 3% DHA and 0.035 to 0.13% lawsone has been shown to provide protection to patients sensitive to UVA and visible radiation and may be beneficial as adjunctive therapy for these patients.[33] Lawsone is the principal dye component of henna, a vegetable dye from which the naphthquinone is derived from the dried plant leaves.

PHOTOSENSITIVITY DISORDERS

Photosensitivity disorders are those in which abnormal cutaneous responses occur after exposure to nonionizing radiation. These disorders can be classified according to cause into four main groups: genetic/metabolic, photoaggravated, idiopathic, and exogenous chemical. The genetic/metabolic group of diseases would include the porphyrias, xeroderma pigmentosum, Cockayne syndrome, Bloom syndrome, Rothmund–Thomson syndrome (poikiloderma congenitale), pellagra, kwashiorkor, and Hartnup disease. These diseases have been discussed previously in this textbook. Diseases that are aggravated by sunlight, such as the collagen vascular diseases, have also been previously discussed. Idiopathic photosensitivity disorders that are acquired disorders with a possible immunologic basis, and photoreactions to exogenous chemicals, are discussed below.

Acquired disorders with a possible immunologic basis

Polymorphic light eruption (PMLE), actinic prurigo, and hydroa vacciniforme are discussed below as separate entities because of some distinguishing clinical and prognostic features. However, a great deal of overlap of clinical features occurs, and these entities may represent a spectrum of findings of a single disease process.

Polymorphic light eruption (PMLE)

PMLE is a common, intermittent, UV radiation-induced eruption of generally nonscarring, pruritic, skin-colored to erythematosus papules, plaques, and occasionally vesicles or prurigolike lesions on sun-exposed skin. The disease occurs principally in the spring and summer.

Epidemiology

PMLE is seen most commonly in women younger than 30 years of age, and a familial incidence is recognized.[34] It is also the most common of the childhood-onset photodermatoses, which constituted 82% of cases in a study

26. Naylor MF, Farmer KC (1997) The case for sunscreens: a review of their use in preventing actinic damage and neoplasia. **Arch Dermatol** 133:1146.
27. Whitmore SD, Morison WL (1995) Prevention of UVB-induced immunosuppression in humans by a high sun protection factor sunscreen. **Arch Dermatol** 131:1128.
28. Gallagher RP, Rivers JK, Lee TK et al. (2000) Broad-spectrum sunscreen use and the development of new nevi in white children. A randomized controlled trial. **JAMA** 283:2955.
29. Kaidbey KH (1990) The photoprotective potential of the new superpotent sunscreens. **J Am Acad Dermatol** 22:449.
30. Banks BA, Silverman RA, Schwartz RM et al. (1992) Attitudes of teenagers toward sun exposure and sunscreen use. **Pediatrics** 89:40.
31. Lowe NJ (1990) Photoprotection. **Semin Dermatol** 9:78.
32. Levy SB (1992) Dihydroxyacetone-containing sunless or self-tanning lotions. **J Am Acad Dermatol** 27:989.
33. Johnson JA, Fusaro RM (1993) Therapeutic potential of dihydroxyacetone. **J Am Acad Dermatol** 29:284.
34. Ros A, Wennersten G (1986) Current aspects of polymorphous light eruptions in Sweden. **Photodermatology** 3:298.

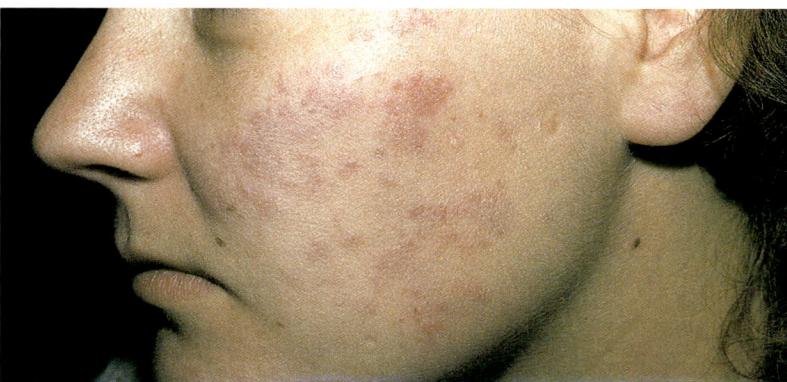

Fig. 29.2 Erythematous papules and plaques of PMLE.

of 95 children with photoinduced skin eruptions.[35] All ethnic groups are affected. The clustering of PMLE among first-degree relatives of subacute cutaneous and discoid lupus probands suggests that there may be a shared pathogenic basis for PMLE and cutaneous lupus.[36]

History and physical examination

The eruption of PMLE has an acute onset hours to days after exposure to sunlight and generally persists for 1 to 6 days and, rarely, for weeks if exposure continues. It occurs most commonly in the spring, typically recurring but gradually diminishing during the summer months. Fifteen minutes to several hours of sun exposure are required to induce the eruption.

The lesions of PMLE are usually pruritic, often grouped, skin-colored or erythematosus papules and plaques (Fig. 29.2). Vesicles and papulovesicles or nodules occur occasionally. Lesions tend to occur symmetrically, and the distribution of recurrent lesions generally remains fairly consistent in any one patient. Only some exposed sites, particularly those normally covered in the winter, such as the V of the neck and arms, are affected by PMLE.[37] In children, however, the face and ears are more commonly affected than in adults. A probable variant of PMLE, which is known as juvenile spring eruption of the ears, occurs mainly in boys aged 5 to 12 years.[38] The eruption consists of erythematosus papules that affect the ears, which may progress to vesicles and then crust and heal with little or no scarring. Rarely, systemic symptoms, including chills, headache, fever, and nausea, accompany PMLE.

Laboratory findings

There are no specific laboratory findings in this disease. Circulating antinuclear antibody, anti-Ro, and anti-LA titers for lupus erythematosus are negative, and urinary, stool, and blood porphyrin concentrations are normal.

Pathophysiology and histogenesis

The eruption of PMLE is best induced by bright summer sunlight. Artificial induction is difficult, and evoking wavelengths vary among patients, generally requiring broad-band exposure rather than monochromatic irradiation. The eruption may be elicited by UVA, UVB, and/or UVA and UVB wavelengths of light.[39]

Epstein[40] postulated several years ago that PMLE was due to a delayed-type hypersensitivity response to a UV radiation–induced cutaneous antigen. More recently, sequential biopsies after low-dose, solar-simulated irradiation have demonstrated dermal, perivascular T cells of predominately CD4 type at 5h and CD8 type at 72h along with increased dermal and epidermal antigen-presenting cells.[41] These changes suggest a delayed-type hypersensitivity reaction.

Histologically, there is variable epidermal spongiosis with a dermal perivascular lymphocytic infiltrate. The histologic findings are suggestive rather than diagnostic of this entity.

Differential diagnosis

The diagnosis of PMLE is suggested by the history and clinical appearance of the lesions. Lupus erythematosus can be ruled out by negative serologic findings and the porphyrias, by the clinical appearance and negative porphyrin studies. Solar urticaria is distinguished by its short evolution and different morphology. Drug and chemical photosensitivites should be excluded.

Therapy and prognosis

Milder cases of PMLE may be controlled satisfactorily by limiting UV light exposure, protective clothing, and the use of broad-spectrum sunscreens. Topical corticosteroids may be of some benefit. Prophylaxis by using gradually increasing low-dose UVA or psoralen and UVA (PUVA) therapy two to three times a week for several weeks is safe and usually effective.[42] Hydroxychloroquine in a dosage of 5–6mg/kg/day for short-term therapy in the spring and early summer may be effective. A guideline for the use of antimalarials in children has been published.[43] Ocular toxicity is highly unlikely with short-term use and appropriate dosage of medication,[44] however, great care should be taken to avoid acute overdosage, which may result in respiratory and cardiac arrest. Severe PMLE may respond to a brief course of systemic steroids.[45] PMLE tends to persist but frequently becomes less severe with time and occasionally remits.[46]

Actinic prurigo

Actinic prurigo (AP), previously designated Hutchinson's summer prurigo, may be a variant of PMLE.[47] Actinic prurigo usually begins by 10 years of age, more commonly in girls, and may resolve in adolescence or early adult life. A family history can be obtained from approximately 50 percent of patients,[37] particularly from those of Native American extraction, in whom the condition has sometimes been called hereditary or familial PMLE.[48] There is evidence for simple dominant inheritance with incomplete penetrance among North American Indians in Saskatchewan.[49]

The eruption of actinic prurigo consists of pruritic papules and nodules, which are frequently excoriated. Eczematization, lichenification, crusting, and secondary infection are often present (Fig. 29.3). All exposed skin is generally affected, and covered skin on the limbs and buttocks may occasionally be involved. Cheilitis is common, as is bulbar conjunctival inflammation. The condition worsens in the summer and tends to diminish in winter.

35. Jansen CT (1981) Photosensitivity in childhood. **Acta Derm Venereol** (Stockh) S95:54.
36. Millard TP, Lewis CM, Khamashta MA et al. (2001) Familial clustering of polymorphic light eruption in relatives of patients with lupus erythematosus: evidence of shared pathogenesis. **Brit J Dermatol** 144:334.
37. Norris PG, Hawk JLM (1990) The acute idiopathic photodermatoses. **Semin Dermatol** 9:32.
38. Berth-Jones J, Norris PG, Graham-Brown RAC et al. (1991) Juvenile spring eruption of the ears: a probable variant of polymorphic light eruption. **Br J Dermatol** 124:375.
39. Ortel B, Tanew A, Wolff K et al. (1986) Polymorphous light eruption: action spectrum and photoprotection. **J Am Acad Dermatol** 14:748.
40. Epstein JH (1962) Polymorphous light eruptions. Phototest technique studies. **Arch Dermatol** 85:502.
41. Morris PG, Morris J, McGibbon DM et al. (1989) Polymorphic light eruption: an immunopathological study of evolving lesions. **Br J Dermatol** 120:173.
42. Murphy GM, Logan RA, Lovell CR et al. (1987) Prophylactic PUVA and UVB therapy in polymorphic light eruption – a controlled trial. **Br J Dermatol** 116:531.
43. Ziering CL, Rabinowitz LG, Esterly NB (1993) Antimalarials for children: indications toxicities, and guidelines. **J Am Acad Dermatol** 28:764.
44. Bernstein HN (1992) Ocular safety of hydroxychloroquine sulfate (Plaquenil). **South Med J** 85:274.
45. Patel DC, Bellaney GJ, Seed PT et al. (2000) Efficacy of short-course prednisolne in polymorphic light eruption: a randomised controlled trial. **Br J Dermatol** 143:828.
46. Jansen CT, Kravonen J (1984) Polymorphous light eruption. A seven-year-follow-up evaluation of 114 patients. **Arch Dermatol** 120:862.
47. McGregor JM, Grabczynxka S, Vaughan R et al. (2000) Genetic modeling of abnormal photosensitivity in families with polymorphic light eruption and actinic prurigo. **J Invest Dermatol** 115:471.
48. Brit AR, Davis RA (1971) Photodermatitis in North American Indians: familial actinic prurigo. **Am J Dermatol** 10:107.
49. Schnell AH, Elston RC, Hull et al. (2000) Major gene segregation of actinic prurigo among North American Indians in Saskatchewan. **Am J Med Genetics** 92:212.

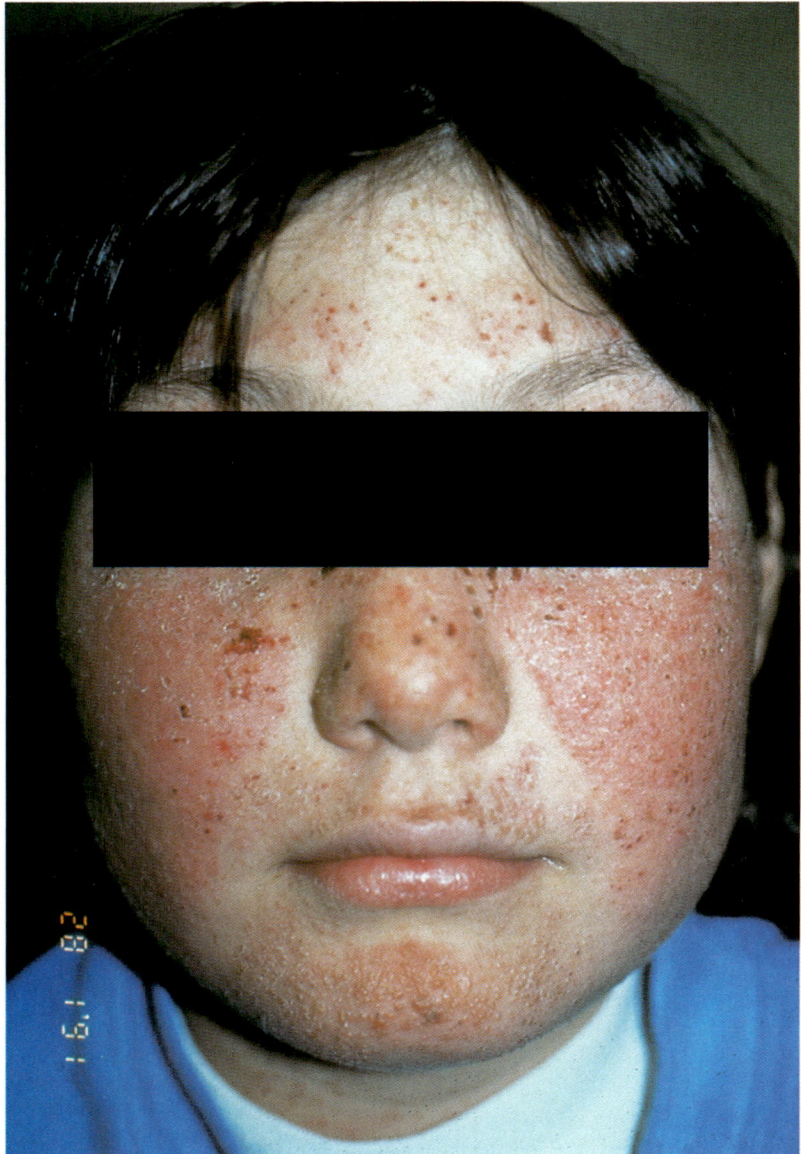

Fig. 29.3   Actinic prurigo in a 12-year-old girl of American Indian extraction.

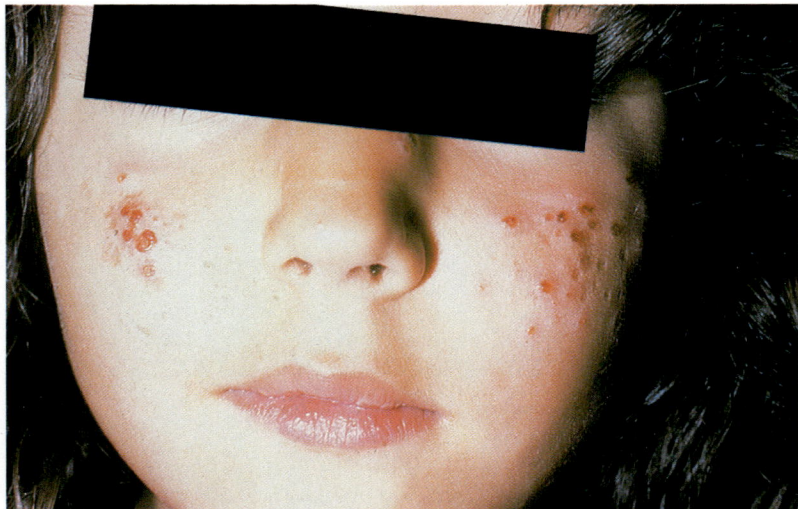

Fig. 29.4   Hydroa vacciniforme in an 8-year-old girl. Note vacciniforme lesions and scarring.

Actinic prurigo has been found to be strongly associated with HLA–DR4, DRB1 0407 subtype, whereas no HLA association has been found with PMLE.[50,51] The pathogenesis of AP is yet to be determined. It has been noted that transforming growth factor (TGF)-β and interleukin (IL)-13 genes are found in most AP skin lesions and that the number of Langerhan cells in the skin of AP patients does not decrease with sunlight exposure as it does in normal controls.[52]

Management of the disease should include an attempt to restrict sunlight and the use of protective clothing and broad-spectrum sunscreens. Emollients, topical steroids, and antihistamines help to control symptoms. Topical macrolides such as tacrolimus ointment would be expected to be of benefit in this condition, particularly for eczematous lesions. Cyclosporin 2% eyedrops may be effective treatment for the conjunctival manifestations of AP.[53] Secondary infection should be treated with appropriate antibiotics. Unresponsive cases have responded to prophylactic low-dose UVB or PUVA therapy.[37] PUVA often is the superior therapy. Intermittent therapy with low-dose thalidomide has been reported to be effective,[54] however many of the patients are young women of child bearing age. Its risk of teratogenicity and of neuropathy require careful monitoring. Tetracycline and vitamin E have been reported to be efficacous in relieving the pruritis of actinic prurigo.[55]

Hydroa vacciniforme

Hydroa vacciniforme (HV) is a rare photodermatosis of childhood characterized by recurrent crops of vesicles on sun-exposed skin that develop within hours of sun exposure and heal with vacciniform scarring (Fig. 29.4). The eruption usually only occurs during the summer months and generally improves or resolves in adolescence.[56] HV has an equal sex ratio, however boys have been reported to have a later onset and longer duration of the disease than girls.[57] Lesions have been reproduced by exposure to broad-spectrum UVA[56,58] and UVB[37] irradiation. Latent Epstein–Barr virus infection has been reported to be associated with the development of cutaneous lesions of HV.[59]

Histopathologic studies show early epidermal spongiosis followed by focal keratinocyte degeneration with epidermal and upper dermal necrosis. There is an early monocytic perivascular infiltrate that later includes neutrophils. Direct immunofluorescence findings are nonspecific.

The diagnosis is suggested by history, clinical findings, histologic appearance, and if necessary cutaneous phototesting. Porphyrin concentrations are normal, and viral cultures are negative.

Symptoms are often controlled by regular and frequent use of broad-spectrum sunscreens and by wearing protective clothing.[56] Antimalarials have been reported occasionally to be beneficial,[56,60] as have prophylactic UVB, narrow band UVB, and PUVA. The latter may precipitate an exacerbation.[56]

50. Grabczynska SA, Hawk JL (1997) What is actinic prurigo in Britain? **Photodermatol, Photoimmunrnol and Photomed** 13:85.

51. Haojyo-Tomoka T, Granados J, Vargos-Alarcon G et al. (1997) Further evidence of the role of HLA-DR4 in the genetic susceptibility to actinic prurigo. **J Am Acad Dermatol** 36:935–937.

52. Torres-Alverez B, Baronda L, Fuentes C et al. (1998) An immunohistochemical study of UV-induced skin lesions in actinic prurigo. Resistance of Langerhans cells to UV light. **Eur J Dermatol** 8:24.

53. McCombes JA, Hirst LW, Green WR (2000) Use of topical cyclosporin for conjuctional manifestations of actinic prurigo. **Am J Opthalmol** 130:830.

54. Lovell CR, Hawk JLM, Calmar CD et al. (1983) Thalidomide in actinic prurigo. **Br J Dermatol** 108:467.

55. Duran MM, Ordonez CP, Prieto JC et al. (1996) Treatment of actinic prurigo in Chimila Indians. **Int J Dermatol** 35:413.

56. Sonnex TS, Hawk JLM (1988) Hydroa vacciniforme: a review of ten cases. **Br J Dermatol** 118:101.

57. Gupta G, Man I, Kemmett D (2000) Hydroa vacciniforme: A clinical and follow-up study of 17 cases. **J Am Acad Dermatol** 42:208.

58. Hann SK, Im S, Park Y et al. (1991) Hydroa vacciniforme with unusually severe scar formation: diagnosis by repetitive UVA phototesting. **J Am Acad Dermatol** 25:401.

59. Iwatsuki K, Xw Z, Takata M et al. (1998) The association of latent Epstein–Barr virus infection with hydroa vacciniforme. **Br J Dermatol** 138:173.

60. Goldgeier MH, Nordlund JJ, Lucky AW et al. (1982) Hydroa vacciniforme. Diagnosis and therapy. **Arch Dermatol** 118:588.

TABLE 29.2 Exogenous photosensitizers

Drugs	Antibiotics, tranquilizers, antidepressants, anti-inflammatory, diuretics, antiarrhythmic/antihypertensives
Plant materials	Furocoumarins, α-terthienyl, polyacetylenes
Dyestuffs	Thiazides, methylene blue, toluidine blue, xanthenes, fluorescein, eosin, erythrosin, rose bengal, anthraquinone based, Disperse Blue 35, benzathrone
Polycyclic hydrocarbons	Pitch, coal tars, anthracene, acridine, fluoranthrene
Perfumes and cosmetics	Bergamot oil, musk ambrette, 6-methylcoumarin
Sunscreens, inks	PABA, benzophenones, benzoylmethanes, cinnamates, amylodimethylaminobenzoic acid
Tatoos	Cadmium sulfide
Miscellaneous	Cyclamate sweetener, blankophore fabric whitener, quinoxaline-n-dioxide

PABA, para-aminobenzoic acid.
Modified from Johnson and Ferguson,[45] with permission.

Dietary fish oil rich in omega-3 polyunsaturated fatty acids have been reported to benefit some children.[61]

Solar urticaria

Exposure to the sun or artificial light may be followed within 5 to 10min by pruritus, erythema, wheals, and occasionally by angioedema with bronchospasm and syncope. Skin that is normally uncovered such as the face may be spared. With sun avoidance, lesions resolve within 1 to 2h. Rarely solar urticaria is drug induced.

Solar urticaria is a rare disorder that occurs somewhat more commonly in women. The onset is usually between the ages of 10 and 50 years[1] with the majority of cases occurring between ages 20 and 30.[62] It is occasionally associated with systemic lupus erythematosus or erythropoietic protoporphyria but is usually idiopathic. Skin lesions may be elicited by UVB, UVA, or visible light ranges or by a combination of these.[37]

Avoidance of exposure to the precipitating wavelengths, wearing of protective clothing, and use of broad-spectrum sunscreens may be helpful. Nonsedating H$_1$ antihistamines may be beneficial in reducing symptoms and are well tolerated. Careful use of low-dose PUVA may induce tolerance to light.[63,64] Rapid induction of tolerance by exposure to multiple UVA irradiations at one hour intervals over three days has also been reported to be successful.[65]

Drug and chemical photosensitivity

Chemicals and drugs, either topical or systemic, coupled with light exposure, can produce four types of reactions: phototoxicity from a topical agent, photoallergic contact dermatitis, phototoxicity from a systemic agent, and photoallergy from a systemic agent. Because the latter two groups are difficult to distinguish, the more general term, photosensitivity from a systemic agent, is used for both. Most chemical and drug sensitivity occurs with exposure to UVA and visible light; therefore, light penetrating window glass may elicit the eruption. Table 29.2 lists a number of common photosensitizing agents.

Phototoxic reactions occur in any subjects with sufficient cutaneous photosensitizer exposed to enough appropriate radiation.[66] Topical phototoxic reactions occur uniformly on the areas of skin exposed to the photosensitizing chemical. The eruption develops several hours after exposure as erythema,

edema, and occasionally blistering and may resolve, leaving hyperpigmentation often in a bizarre configuration (Fig. 29.5), which fades slowly over time. Phytophotodermatitis is the most common topical phototoxic reaction occurring in children and is due to exposure to plants or plant products that contain psoralens. Limes, which contain about 10 times as much oil of bergamot (containing 5-methoxy psoralen) as other citrus fruits, are common offenders (Fig. 29.6).

Photoallergic reactions are less commonly seen because they are immunologic and thus occur only in sensitized individuals. The eruption is eczematous and often patchy in sun-exposed areas. The major groups of chemicals that produce this disorder are antibacterials, fragrances, and sunscreens. The fragrances include sandalwood oil, 6-methylcoumarin, and musk ambrette. The latter was formerly the most common cause of this eruption, but this fragrance has now been removed from cosmetics in the United States. Presently, sunscreens that contain PABA esters or oxybenzone are the leading cause of photoallergic reactions in the United States.

The diagnosis of a topical photoallergic reaction may be confirmed by photopatch testing. Identifying and removing the offending agent is the most important step in treatment. Topical steroids and antihistamines may also be beneficial.

Most photosensitivity reactions to systemic agents are phototoxic in nature and caused by a combination of a drug and UVA light. Photoallergic reactions are rare in children. Sulfonamides are a common cause of systemic phototoxic reactions in this age group. In adolescents who are receiving treatment for acne tetracycline, and doxycycline or systemic retinoids may induce phototoxicity (Fig. 29.7).

Photosensitivity reactions to systemic agents occur in sun-exposed areas and most commonly mimic a sunburn, but occasionally they may resemble lichen planus, lupus erythematosus, porphyrias, or the photodermatoses previously discussed in this chapter. Photoallergic reactions usually simulate allergic contact dermatitis with small papules and vesicles. Drug light reactions generally spare the upper eyelids, submental, and retroauricular areas. Unlike phototoxic reactions, photoallergic reactions may spread beyond irradiated areas. Phototoxicity may present as photo- onycholysis, not all cases of which exhibit obvious skin phototoxicity.[67] Photo-onycholysis has been reported with tetracyclines, psoralens, and other photoactive drugs. The diagnosis of systemic photosensitivity reactions is made by physical examination and

61. Rhodes LE, White SI (1998) Dietary fish oil as a photoprotective agent in hydroa vacciniforme. **Br J Dermatol** 138:173.
62. Monfrecola G, Masturzo E, Riccardo AM et al. (2000) Solar urticaria: a report on 57 cases. **Am J Contact Dermatitis** 11:89.
63. Parrish JA, Jaenicke KF, Morrison WL et al. (1982) Solar urticaria, treatment with PUVA and mediator inhibitors. **Br J Dermatol** 106:575.
64. Armstrong RB (1986) Solar urticartia. **Dermatol Clin** 4:253.
65. Beissert S, Stander H, Schwarz T (2000) UVA rush hardening for the treatment of solar urticaria. **J Am Acad Dermatol** 42:1030.
66. Johnson BE, Ferguson J (1990) Drug and chemical photosensitivity. **Semin Dermatol** 9:39.
67. Rothstein MS (1977) Onycholysis through phototoxicity. **Arch Dermatol** 113:520.

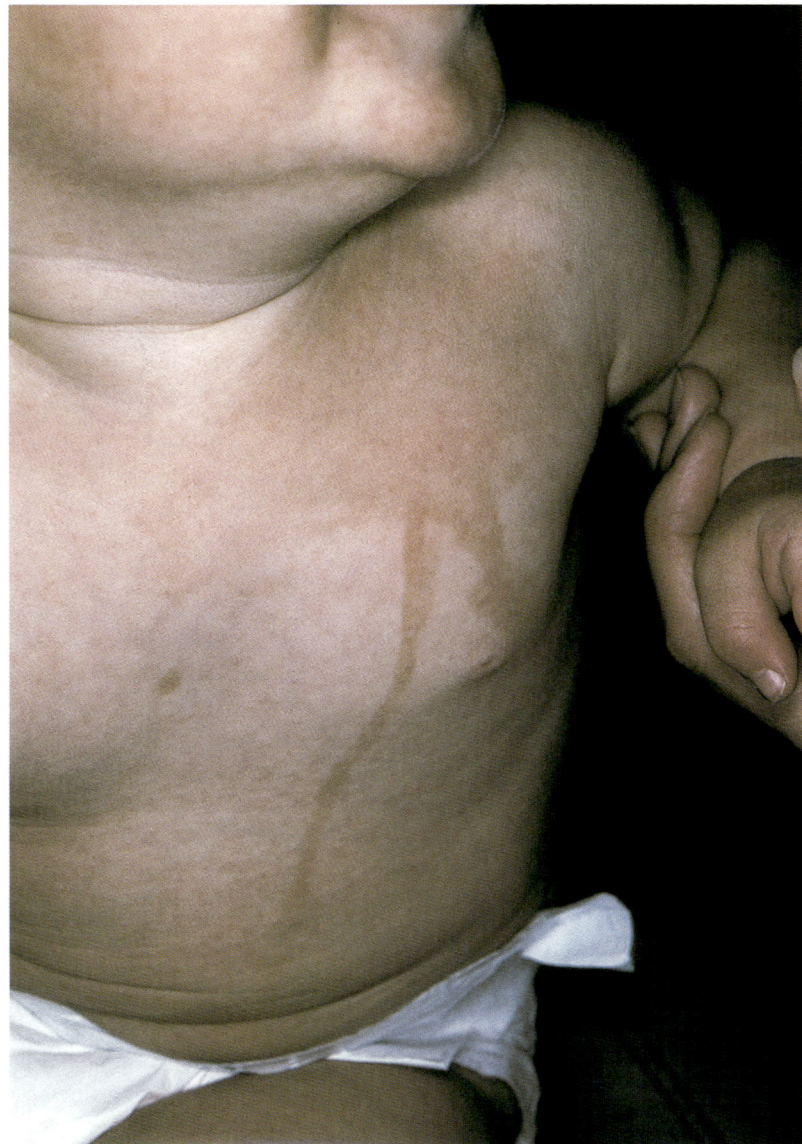

Fig. 29.5 Phototoxic reaction on the chest of a child after spilling mixed fruit juice before sun exposure. (Photo courtesy of Anne W. Lucky.)

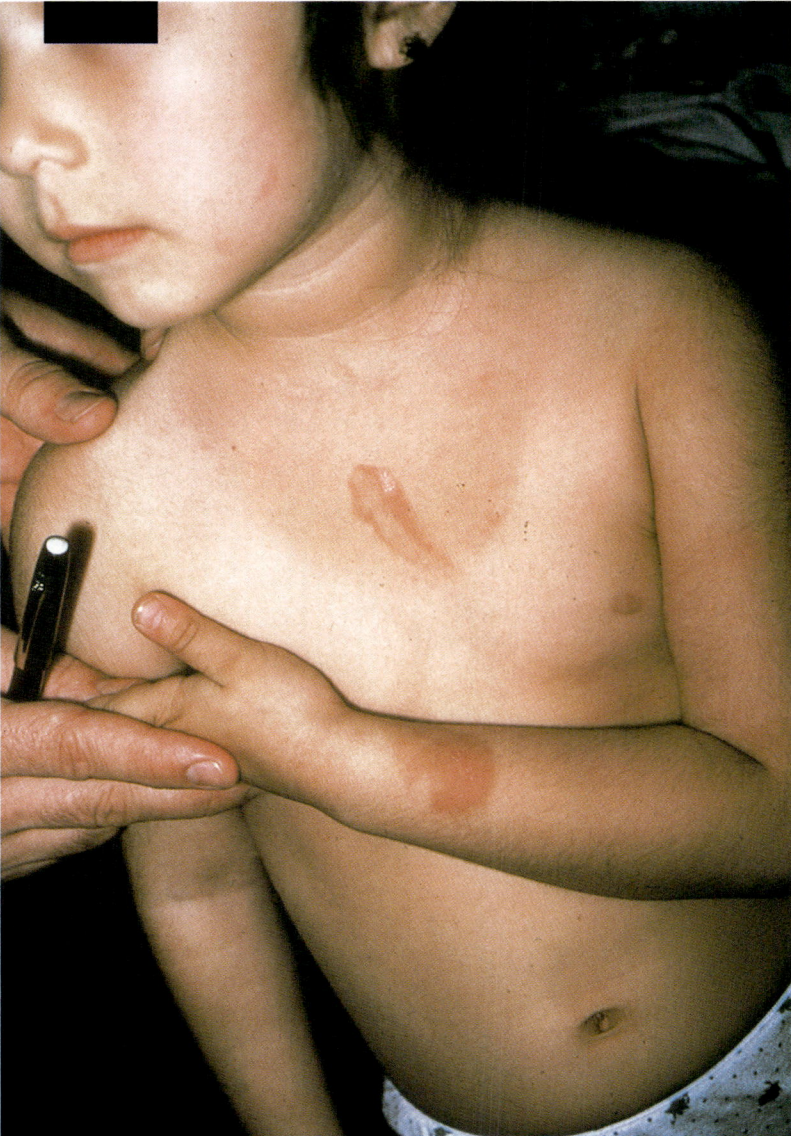

Fig. 29.6 Phyto photodermatitis. Dermatitis and pigmentation following sun exposure to lime juice on skin may be confused with bruises of child abuse.

history. Photopatch testing of systemic agents is not recommended. Treatment consists of discontinuing the eliciting drug or of protecting the patient from UVA exposure while the eliciting drug is being given. Antihistamines and topical steroids may provide symptomatic relief.

COLD INJURIES

FROSTNIP AND FROSTBITE

Acute cold injuries can be divided according to the severity of the insult. Frostnip is a very superficial frostbite that involves only the skin and causes no significant damage. It usually occurs on the exposed areas of face, nose, cheek, chin, and ears and is secondary to temperatures below freezing and rapid motion of surrounding wind. The lesions are identified as white patches on the face that are numb and insensitive. With rewarming, erythema develops, but no edema or superficial blistering is identified.

Frostbite may be either superficial or deep. As the temperatures continue to cool past the frostnip stage, an initial erythema may be followed by areas of white, waxlike skin. The sensation of real cold may progress to numbness followed by pain, or a sensation of warmth may follow burning or hypoesthesia. Eventually, immobility of the joints and extremities may occur. As with frostnip, exposed areas of the face, the nose, chin, cheeks, ears, and the distal extremities are the most likely sites of injury. Frost bite may also occur from the therapeutic application, in excess, of ice to the skin.[68]

Therapy for frostnip or frostbite should begin immediately on noticing the injury. For frostnip, the therapy is simply removing the individual to a warmer environment by going indoors. Frostbite requires more aggressive therapy. Initially, the frostbitten area should be rapidly thawed in a warm bath 40–42°C (104–108°F) for 15–30min.[69] If there is a possibility that the tissue could be refrozen before definitive therapy, it is better to seek out definitive therapy before thawing the tissue because repeated episodes of freezing and thawing may be more destructive than prolonged freezing.[70] As the lesions are thawed,

68. Graham CA, Stevenson J (2000) Frozen chips: an unusual cause of severe frostbite injury. **Br J Sports Med** 34:382.
69. Bracker MD (1992) Environmental and thermal injury. **Clin Sports Med** 11:419.
70. Colbett DW (1982) Cold injuries. **J Assoc Mil Dermatol** 8:34.

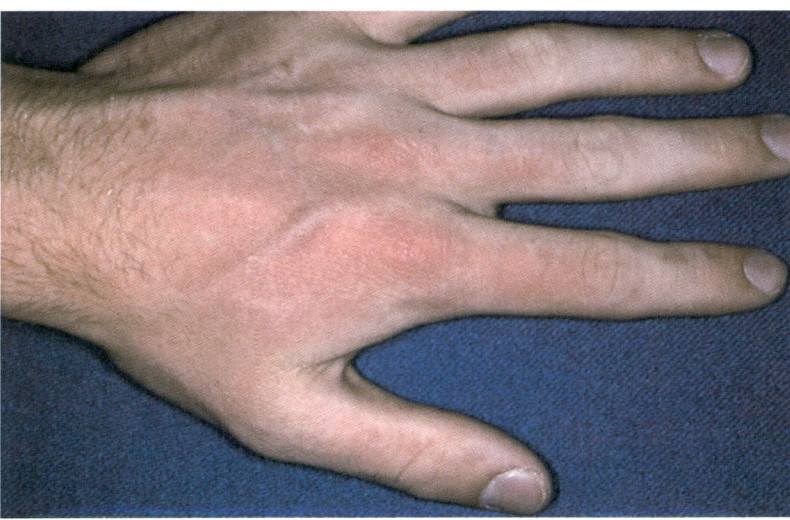

Fig. 29.7 Phototoxicity reaction (sunburn) on the back of the hand of a teenage boy taking doxycycline for acne. (Photo courtesy of Anne W. Lucky.)

the skin should become pink, and movement should return to the extremities. In addition to thawing the lesions, evaluation and therapy for hypothermia may also be required. With thawing, severe pain may occur, and analgesia may be necessary. In addition to analgesia, aspirin or ibuprofen may be indicated to inhibit the local production of prostaglandins that may increase damage after severe thermal injury.[71] Pentoxifylline which increases red blood cell flexibility resulting in increased perfusion[72] and hyperbaric oxygen, may help to preserve tissue.[73] Vasodilators have also been reported to be beneficial in a large series of patients.[74] The blisters that may occur once thawing is initiated may be left intact as long as they do not become infected. The affected area should be elevated to decrease edema, and the wound should be kept clean to prevent secondary infection. The status of tetanus prophylaxis should be determined, and reimmunization should be given if required. In children, distal epiphyses may be severely injured with frostbite, resulting in digital deformity and absence of continued digital growth.[75] Traditionally, observation and delayed amputation have been employed to manage frostbite. More recently triple-phase bone scans have been used to distinguish tissue that is irreversibly destined for necrosis from tissue that is potentially salvageable allowing for earlier surgery. Early surgical intervention may provide at-risk tissue with a new blood supply and preserve both tissue and function.[76]

Prevention is the best defense against cold injury. Small children are potentially at high risk in cold climates because of their inability to recognize and express the severity of their cold injury. Very importantly, layered, warm clothing should be worn when prolonged exposure to cold is anticipated.

IMMERSION FOOT

Prolonged exposure to a cold, wet environment may induce the characteristics of immersion foot, which appear clinically as pale, swollen feet that may exhibit vesiculobullous or purpuric lesions, suggesting impending gangrene. Usually, the history concurs with the prolonged exposure to a cold wet environment. In severe cases, gangrene can occur, requiring extensive reconstructive surgery

or may result in loss of limbs. Therapy for immersion foot is similar to therapy for frostbite injuries and may require prolonged rehabilitative care.[77]

PERNIO

Pernio and chilblain are terms commonly used in describing acute or chronic forms of cold induced lesions. *Pernio* is derived from the Latin, meaning "frostbite," *chilblain* is of Anglo-Saxon origin and means "cold sore." The lesions of pernio may occur at any age but appear to be more common in childhood. The cause of pernio is not clear, but a vasospastic response of arterioles from exposure to cold may play a significant role. Humidity along with cold also appears to be important because this entity is more common in the humid climate of northwestern Europe and less common in dry cold climates.

Pernio lesions occur predominately on the distal aspects of the hands and feet. The lesions are generally bilateral and symmetrical, although they may be single or asymmetrical. The lesions usually occur 12 to 24h after cold exposure and initially are often erythematous to purplish edematous plaques and nodules, but pernio may present as digital cyanosis only.[78] Blister formation and ulceration are rare in children. Involved areas may be pruritic, or patients may experience a burning sensation. Individual lesions can be very painful and tender. Lesions may persist for days or occasionally weeks but slowly resolve once exposure to the cold is removed and do not reappear unless reexposure to cold occurs. Similar cold induced lesions in patients with underlying diseases such as systemic lupus erythematosus, primary antiphospholipid antibody syndrome, and rheumatoid arthritis have been referred to as secondary perniosis.[79]

Shoe-boot pernio has been associated with the wearing of wet or damp shoes or boots at the time of cold exposure.[80] Lesions develop that are localized to the plantar and lateral surfaces of the feet.

The histologic appearance of the lesion of pernio is characterized by a marked superficial and deep perivascular mononuclear cell infiltrate and a peculiar edema and vacuolated thickening of the blood vessel walls.[81] Intense edema of the papillary dermis may be present. Lymphocytic exocytosis to retia or acrosyringia may be present. Lesions of secondary perniosis may be distinguishable histologically.[79]

Recurrence of pernio usually can be prevented by avoiding exposure of the extremities to damp cold, and by keeping the body warm to prevent vasoconstriction. Prazosin has been reported to be effective in the acute management and prophylaxis against recurrence of chronic pernio in adolescents and adults,[78] as has nifedipine in one individual.[82]

COLD PANNICULITIS

Cold panniculitis is a localized injury to fat tissue that results from cold exposure; infants appear to be particularly susceptible. Cold panniculitis in infancy most commonly follows exposure of the cheeks to extremely cold air, chin straps on hats in the snow, or to ice cubes or popsicles.[83] In older individuals, thin, tight-fitting clothing during cold exposure may promote this injury on the thighs and buttocks, particularly in horseback riders.[84]

Indurated, erythematous subcutaneous plaques develop hours to days after cold exposure. Histologically, early lesions show a lymphohistiocytic infiltrate around blood vessels at the junction of the dermis and subcutaneous fat.[83] Later, cystic cavities surrounded by a marked inflammatory infiltrate can be seen in the subcutaneous fat.

71. Robson MC, Heggers JP (1981) Evaluation of hand frostbite blister fluid as a clue to pathogenesis. **J Hand Surg** 6:43.
72. Hayes DW Jr, Mandracchia VJ, Considine C, Webb GE (2000) Pentoxiflylline Adjunctive therapy in the treatment of pedal frostbite. **Clin Podiatr Med Surg** 17:715.
73. Murphy JV, Banwell PE, Roberts AH et al. (2000) Frostbite: pathogenesis and treatment. **J Trauma Injury Infect J Critical Care** 48:171.
74. Foray S (1992) Mountain frostbite, current trends in prognosis and treatment (from results concerning 1261 cases). **Int J Sports Med** 13:S193.
75. Brown FE, Speigel PK, Boyle WE (1983) Digital deformity: an effect of frostbite in children. **Pediatrics** 71:955.
76. Su CW, Lohman R, Gottlieb LJ (2000) Frostbite of the upper extremity. **Hand Clinics** 16:235.
77. Adnot J, Lewis CW (1995) Immersion foot syndromes. **J Assoc Mil Dermatol** 11:87.
78. Spittell JA, Jr, Spittell PC (1992) Chronic pernio: another cause of blue toes. **Int Angiol** 11:46.
79. Crowson AN, Magro CM (1997) Idiopathic perniosis and its mimics: a clinical and histological study of 38 cases. **Human Pathol** 28:478.
80. Coskey RJ, Mehregan AH (1974) Shoe boot pernio. **Arch Dermatol** 109:56.
81. Herman DW, Keyes JS, Silvers DN (1981) A distinct variant of pernio: clinical and histopathological study of nine cases. **Arch Dermatol** 117:26.
82. Parlette EC, Parlett HL (2000) Erythocyanostic discoloration of the toes. **Cutis** 65:223.
83. Duncan WC, Freeman RG, Heaton CL (1966) Cold panniculitis. **Arch Dermatol** 94:722.
84. Beachman BE, Cooper PH, Buchanan CS et al. (1980) Equestrian cold panniculitis in women. **Arch Dermatol** 116:1025.

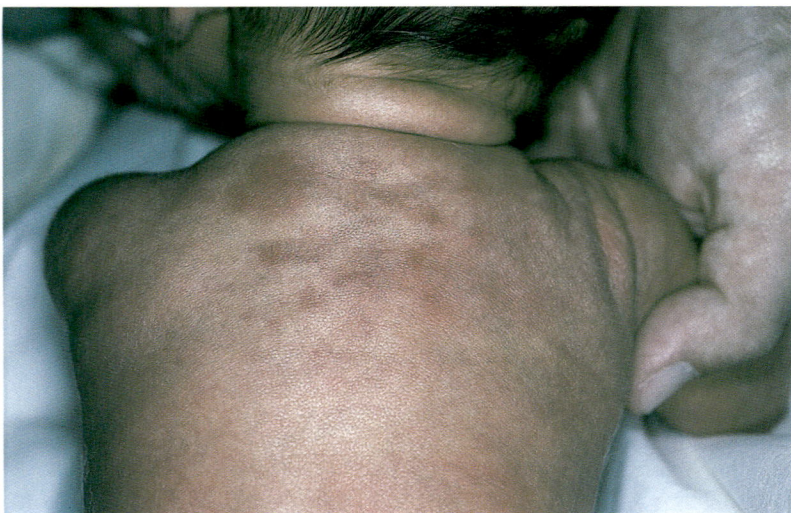

Fig. 29.8 The typical erythematous nodules over the upper back of a 3-day-old boy with acute subcutaneous fat necrosis of the newborn. (Photo courtesy of Anne W. Lucky.)

No treatment is necessary because the condition resolves spontaneously without scarring. Avoidance of cold exposure of the type that precipitated the panniculitis is advisable.

SUBCUTANEOUS FAT NECROSIS OF THE NEWBORN

This rare entity is seen most commonly in full-term or post-term infants of normal birthweight. A history of obstetric trauma frequently can be obtained. Lesions occur most commonly between days 2 and 21 of life as firm subcutaneous plaques that may vary in diameter from a few millimeters to several centimeters. (Fig. 29.8) The overlying skin is frequently erythematous. The sites most commonly involved are the buttocks, thighs, shoulders, back, cheeks, and arms. The plaques or nodules generally resolve within a few months without residue but occasionally leave slight atrophy (Fig. 29.9).

Biopsies of affected tissue show patchy fat necrosis with a granulomatous inflammatory reaction of the foreign body type. Fat cells contain needle-shaped clefts that, on frozen section analysis, are seen to contain doubly refractile crystals when examined with polarized light.[85] Rarely, liquified fat may be noted. Calcium deposits occur frequently in areas of fat necrosis.

The cause of subcutaneous fat necrosis of the newborn is unclear. Cold has been implicated as an eliciting factor. Infants undergoing hypothermic cardiac surgery have developed similar lesions, principally at the sites subjected to the greatest cold exposure.[86] Tissue hypoxia has also been suggested as an etiologic factor.[87]

Specific treatment of the lesions is usually unnecessary because they gradually spontaneously resolve. A number of infants, however, have been reported with associated hypercalcemia.[88] In a series of II patients with subcutaneous fat necrosis of the newborn reported by Burden and Krafchik, four infants with extensive involvement developed hypercalcemia between days 23 and 60 of life. They recommended weekly calcium levels be obtained for the first 3–4 months of life unless involvement is limited.[89]

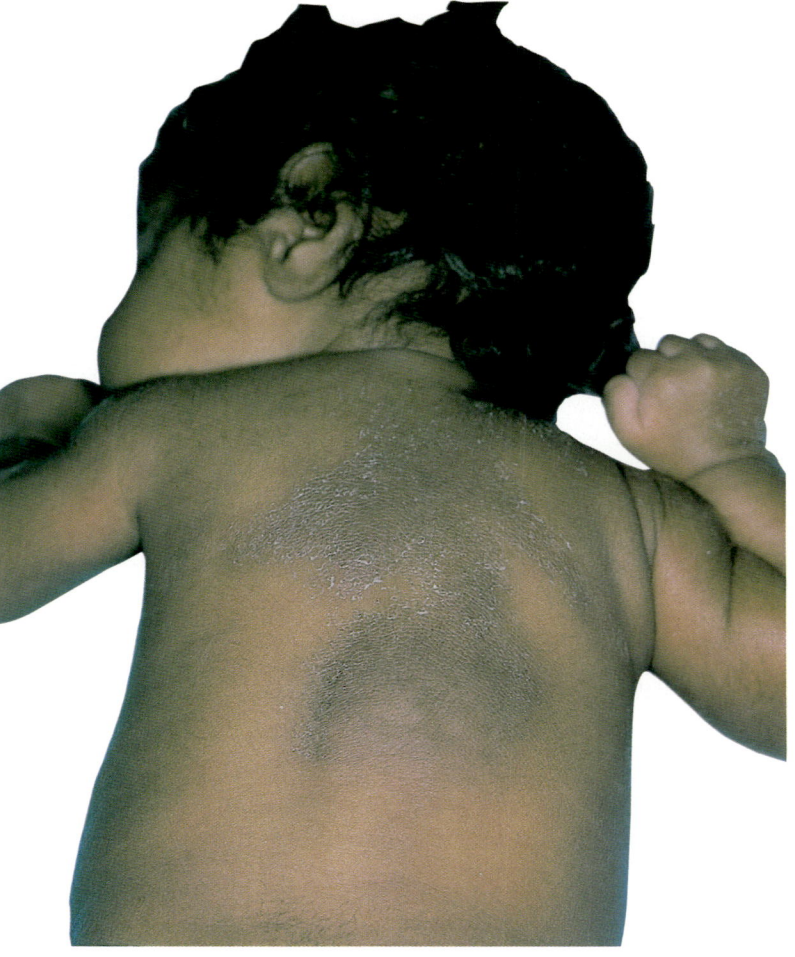

Fig. 29.9 Hyperpigmented, desquamating nodules of a child with subcutaneous fat necrosis of the newborn several weeks after the acute episode. (Photo courtesy of Anne W. Lucky.)

NEONATAL COLD INJURY

Neonatal cold injury is a disorder in which cold exposure of a small-for-gestational-dates neonate results in hypothermia associated with generalized pitting edema and lethargy.[90] The entity is clinically and pathologically distinct from sclerema neonatorum. This condition is now rare in developed countries because of improved home heating and the decreased frequency of home delivery.

Most cases occur within the first 4 days of life, usually during the first 24h.[91] Intense erythema or cyanosis occurs on the face and extremities, and firm pitting edema occurs, beginning on the extremities and spreading centrally. The skin feels cold, and the infant is usually hypothermic. Associated features of hypothermia, including immobility, drowsiness, poor feeding, and vomiting, are frequently present. The condition is associated with a mortality rate of about 25%. At autopsy, massive pulmonary hemorrhage is the predominant postmortem finding. The occurrence of this condition in

85. Balogs M (1987) Subcutaneous fat necrosis of the newborn with emphasis on ultrastructural studies. **Int J Dermatol** 26:227.
86. Silverman AK, Michels EH, Rasmussen JE (1986) Subcutaneous fat necrosis in an infant occurring after hypothermic cardiac surgery. **J Am Acad Dermatol** 15:331.
87. Chen TH, Shewmake SW, Hansen DD et al. (1981) Subcutaneous fat necrosis of the newborn: a case report. **Arch Dermatol** 11:36.
88. Fernandez-Lopez E, Garcia-Dorado J, De Unamundo P et al. (1990) Subcutaneous fat necrosis of the newborn and idiopathic hypercalcemia. **Dermatologica** 180:250.

89. Burden AD, Krafhik BR (1999) Subcutaneous fat necrosis of the newborn – 11 cases. **Pediatr Dermatol** 16:384.
90. Atherton DJ (1992) The neonate. In: Rook/Wilkinson/Ebling Textbook of Dermatology, 5th ed. Vol 1, Champion RH, Burton JL, Ebling FJG, eds. Oxford: Blackwell Scientific Publications, p. 381.
91. Bower RD, Jones LF, Weeks MM (1960) Cold injury in the newborn: a study of 70 cases. **Br Med J** 1:303.

otherwise healthy infants, the pitting nature of the edema, a history of cold exposure, and a low rectal temperature help to distinguish this disorder from sclerema neonatorum.

COLD URTICARIA

Cold urticaria should be considered in the child who presents with a history of urticarial papules and plaques after exposure to cold. Cold urticaria can occur as a rare familial dominant trait or in an acquired form. In familial cold urticaria, the symptoms begin early in life and may persist indefinitely. Prolonged edematous swellings follow cold exposure and may be accompanied by headache, fever, arthralgias, and leukocytosis. Linkage to chromosome 1q44 has recently been identified.[92]

Acquired cold urticaria starts in childhood or may appear for the first time in adult life. Whealing of the skin occurs with cold exposure. Cold wind is a particularly effective stimulus. The symptoms may range from mild to disabling. Symptoms that resemble histamine shock have been responsible for loss of consciousness, or even death, while swimming in cold water.[93] Cold urticaria may occur in association with dermographism or cholinergic urticaria.[94]

The diagnosis of cold urticaria is based on history. This diagnosis can frequently be confirmed by placing an ice cube wrapped in a plastic bag on the forearm for 30s to 10min. Wheals form on warming. Water at 7°C may be even more effective than ice in provoking symptoms.

Acquired cold urticaria may remit after a few weeks, or the symptoms may persist for months or years. Occasionally, increasing exposure time to cold may induce tolerance. Treatment with the antihistamine cyproheptadine may lessen symptoms. Improvement has also been reported with treatment with the leukotriene receptor antagonist montelukest.[95] Stanozolol has been reported occasionally to be beneficial in treating familial cold urticaria.[96] Awareness of possible severe anaphylaxis should alert patients with cold urticaria to avoid sudden exposure to cold water such as in showers or when swimming.

BURNS

Thermal burns are generally classified by the depth of skin injury. First-degree or superficial partial thickness burns involve the epidermis and are pink or red in appearance, blanch on pressure, and are painful to touch. Second-degree burns or deep partial-thickness burns are those that involve the entire epidermis but leave intact the deeper portions of the sweat glands and hair follicles. The skin is red and blistered, and may be moist with exudate. The tissue is painful to the touch. The individual lesions heal with regeneration from the epidermal appendages. Third-degree burns are identified as full-thickness burns that destroy the epidermis and the epidermal appendages in the dermis and, occasionally, the bone or muscle beneath. The skin is white, dry, or charred, and painless.

The principles of burn wound management are the same for minor or major burns. Prevention of secondary infection and maintenance of a local environment conducive to wound healing must be accomplished. For the minor burn, this may require only cool water applied to the burn initially, followed by topical antibiotic care with silver sulfadiazine 1% cream, polymixin B/bacitracin ointment, or mupirocin. The latter should not be applied to large denuded surfaces because absorption of the polyethylene glycol base may cause systemic toxicity in burn patients. Many of the newer wound dressings, particularly the hydrogel dressings, may promote re-epithelialization and decrease pain associated with first- and second-degree burns. Superficial partial thickness burns generally heal spontaneously in 3–10 days with skin which is elastic, supple, and of excellent quality and which in time may be indistinguishable from normal skin.[97] Deep partial thickness burns (second degree) generally heal in 10–14 days with scarring which is often hypertrophic. Third-degree burns generally require skin grafting to facilitate healing. Autologous cultured keratinocytes may be valuable when donor skin available is insufficient. For the major burn, hospitalization and treatment in a surgical burn unit is generally required.

Initially, the burn size should be evaluated and expressed as a percentage of the body surface area. As an initial evaluation, the rule of nines is frequently used for adolescents and older children. The head and the entire upper extremity are each given the value of 9% of the body surface. The anterior and posterior trunk are each valued at 18%, as is each leg. The total of these parts is 99%, and the perineum is valued at 1%, to make 100%. In young children, the head and trunk account for a relatively higher percentage of body surface, making this method of evaluation less accurate. Children with greater than 10% surface area burns or greater than 2% full-thickness burns should be hospitalized.

AIR BAG INJURY TO THE SKIN

Most new car models have driver-side air bags and many also have passenger-side and side-impact air bags which may deploy even with low impact collisions.[98] The airbag explosion produces strong forces that may injure small children; it therefore follows that small children should not sit in seats where air bags may deploy. In addition to death and serious injuries such as fractures and cerebral spinal injury, severe lower extremity burns have been reported.[99] Shearing forces during the rapid inflation of the air bags are thought to abrade the epidermis.[98] During deflation the abraded skin is exposed to sodium hydroxide and sodium agide. Dry sodium hydroxide is not very damaging, but once the sodium hydroxide becomes wet it produces chemical burns. If such an injury occurs, any powder present should be brushed away first and then copious amounts of water should be used to thoroughly rinse the affected area.

PRESSURE ULCERS

Pressure ulcers may occur in children whose mobility is severely restricted and from other sources of pressure such as appliances or improperly fitting prostheses. The lesions initially arise secondary to anoxia of dermal tissues, with subsequent ischemia and irreversible tissue damage. Evaluation and therapy of pressure sores are dependent on the severity of the injury. Initially, injury from pressure may be identified as blanchable erythema. As the trauma continues and increased injury occurs, the vessels begin to leak blood into the tissue, giving a nonblanchable erythema, which may eventually develop overlying scales, vesicles, and bullae, signaling the onset of true epidermal necrosis. With increased severity, superficial ulcers may develop into or through the dermis. As the lesions become more severe, deeper ulcers may progress, going through the muscle to the tendons or joints.

Deep pressure ulcers are characterized by deep tissue necrosis and loss of volume that are disproportionately greater than the overlying skin defect.[100] The preferential muscle and subcutaneous injury may be due to pressure on the segmental arteries that perfuse the tissue or may be due to the fact that muscle fibers show degenerative changes after as little as 60mmHg of contact pressure applied over a 1-h period. On the other hand, it requires as much as

92. Hoffman HM, Wright FA, Biode DH et al. (2000) Identification of a locus on chromosome 1q44 for familial cold urticaria. **Am J Human Genetics**. 66:1693.
93. Wanderer AA, Grancel KE, Wasserman SI et al. (1986) Clinical characteristics of cold-induced systemic reactions in acquired cold urticartia syndrome. **J Allergy Clin Immunol** 78:417.
94. Neitaanmaki H (1985) Cold urticaria. Clinical findings in 220 patients. **J Am Acad Dermatol** 13:636.
95. Hani N, Hortmann K, Casper C et al. (2000) Improvement of cold uticaria by treatment with leukotriene receptor antagonist montelukast. **Acta Dermol Venereol** 80:229.
96. Ormerod AD, Smart L, Reid TMS et al. (1993) Familial cold urticaria. Investigation of a family and response to stanozolol. **Arch Dermatol** 129:343.
97. Calvin M (1995) Theraml burns: Classification and pathophysiology. **Wounds.** 4:122.
98. Foley E, Helm TN (2000) Air bag injury and the dermatologist. **Cutis** 66:251.
99. Pudpud AA, Linares M, Raffaele R (1998) Airbag-related lower extremity burns in a pediatric patient [letter]. **Am Acad Emerg Med** 16:438.
100. Falanga V (1992) Chronic wounds: pathophysiologic and experimental considerations. **Prog Dermatol** 26:1.

600mmHg over 11h before full-thickness necrosis develops in pig skin.[101] Ischemia from pressure is closely linked to anatomic location. Although the midcapillary pressure is only about 20mmHg, the forces of the compression over the body are not uniform and can reach as much as 2600mmHg over bony prominences. Intermittent pressure appears to cause little, if any, tissue damage. Tissue damage appears to depend on both the duration and magnitude of pressure. Other factors responsible for tissue damage include shearing forces, friction, and moisture. Shearing forces may result in stretching and angulation of vessels and eventual thrombosis with resulting necrosis of overlying tissue. The effect of friction is twofold. Friction is important in increasing shearing forces, and it may injure the stratum corneum of the epidermis. Another critical causative factor is moisture, generally caused by fecal or urinary soilage or perspiration. This hyperhydration of the epidermis weakens the adhesive bonds of the stratum corneum.

In approaching the therapy of pressure sores, one should first consider prevention. Frequent rotation of the patient, to decrease the duration of pressure in any one area, is extremely important. Air mattresses and soft cushion surfaces and properly positioning the patient may help to reduce pressure on tissue. An air suspension bed or low-air loss bed has been shown to an aid in the prevention of pressure ulcers.[102] This bed provides a smooth, low-friction, low-shear surface with a high moisture vapor transmission rate. Each section of the bed has separate air-controlled settings to redistribute body weight away from bony prominences, resulting in interface pressure of less than 30mmHg. Additional methods to reduce pressure would be to reduce spasticity in patients who are very tonic by the use of such drugs as diazepam; in very severe cases, partial amputation of limbs may be necessary. Reduction of shearing forces to decrease pressure sores is very important. Keeping a patient in a horizontal or vertical position may help prevent sliding and can reduce shearing forces.

To reduce friction, soft bedclothes and loose sheets should always be used. When a patient is to be moved, the patient should not be dragged; instead, the patient should be carefully lifted so as not to abrade the skin. To reduce moisture against the skin, it is important that, once patients have become soiled, they should be cleaned quickly and the skin dried. Sheepskin placed against the skin absorbs perspiration and serves to decrease some of the moisture caused by sweating. Frequent lubrication of the skin with a moisturizing lotion helps prevent the skin from becoming chapped and abraded.

Treatment of ulcers begins with elimination of the detrimental physical factors mentioned above. Ulcers cannot heal when they are chronically contaminated and infected; therefore, control of infection is necessary. Initially, the ulcers should be cultured for routine pathologic bacteria, and topical or systemic antibiotics should be used when necessary.

All ulcer therapy involves the removal of debris and devitalized tissue. Wet to dry dressings and whirlpool are frequently beneficial. Enzymatic or surgical débridement are occasionally necessary. Burows solution compresses and dextran beads may be useful in treating exudative wounds.

Topical negative pressure applied to pressure ulcers has been reported to be beneficial, although no controlled trials comparing this to conventional therapy have been done.[103] Topical negative pressure is achieved by placing an open cell foam into the wound and covering the site with an adhesive polyurethane dressing to provide a seal. A length of drainage tubing is inserted into the foam and connected to a vacuum pump. Intermittent negative pressure is applied and is felt to increase blood flow in and around the wound, reduce edema, effectively remove exudate and reduce bacterial counts, all of which may contribute to wound healing.

Many specific wound dressings have been developed that may facilitate re-epithelialization of the overlying defect and can also decrease the pain and discomfort associated with the ulcer. Because of the occlusive moist nature of the dressings, the physician must be aware that a potential problem, although relatively infrequent, associated with occlusive dressings is wound infection. Other methods of treating ulcers include the use of benzoyl peroxide and hyperbaric oxygen.

Pressure bullae may develop from prolonged pressure from lying in one position during surgery or occasionally from other sources of prolonged pressure such as adhesive tape applied too tightly when taping an extremity to a board used to protect an intravenous line. Lesions generally heal with local wound care.

ARTIFACTUAL DISEASE

Artifactual disease should be considered when clinical lesions are not consistent with the history. Factitial skin lesions most frequently present as nonhealing wounds, recurrent purpura,[104] or bizarre recurring cellulitis. When such lesions are present in young children, they may be produced by a parent or caregiver (usually female) and would be considered a manifestation of the Münchhausen syndrome by proxy.[105] When this syndrome occurs, repeated requests for evaluation are usually made by the perpetrator who denies any knowledge of the cause of the lesions. Lesions begin to heal and no new lesions develop when the child and perpetrator are separated.

Artifactual lesions often have a bizarre appearance with a linear (Fig. 29.10) or geometric outline (Fig. 29.11) that is clearly demarcated from normal skin. Often, the lesions are in different stages of healing as the patient continues to produce new lesions as other lesions heal.

Exogenously induced purpura in children may be self-inflicted, or a site of external trauma associated with child abuse.[106] Purpura across the knuckles or proximal and dorsal aspects of the fingers of adolescents may be a sign of bulimia and is created by pressure of the teeth against the fingers as vomiting is intentionally induced. Occasionally, cultural practices such as coin rubbing (cao gio) (Fig. 29.12),[107] or burns from folk medicine can be mistaken for factitial disease or child abuse.[108]

Evaluation of the child should take into account historical information related to the appearance of the lesion. In addition to examining the areas presenting with lesions, a total body examination should be accomplished to look for other lesions associated with possible child abuse or other signs of self-inflicted injury, such as trichotillomania.

The differential diagnosis and management of a child with artifactual disease is often difficult and complicated. The most difficult period of management is when the factitial disorder is suspected but not proved.[104] The nature and diagnosis of the lesions are occasionally confirmed by secure application of occlusive dressings that prevent continued manipulations of the lesions. Often, this needs to be done in a hospital setting, where the patient can be closely observed and supervised. In addition, close observation of the patient includes obsearches for possible needles, syringes, or objects that may be used to manipulate the lesions. If Münchhausen syndrome by proxy is suspected, all parent or caretaker visits with the child should be supervised. Once other pathologic conditions have been disproved and the lesions are most likely artifactual, confrontation with the patient may be the most effective start to future therapy. Occasionally, when confronted, the patient may admit to the nature of the lesion, the lesions may heal spontaneously, or the lesions may persist and the patient may seek medical care elsewhere. Often, confrontation is not as traumatic as expected, and actual or tacit admission of the self-inflicted nature of the disease may be followed by clinical improvement. The psychological aspects of this disease cannot be dismissed, and intensive psychiatric follow-up is required.

101. Allman RM (1989) Pressure ulcers among the elderly. **N Engl J Med** 320:850.
102. Inman KJ, Sibbald WJ, Rutledge FS et al. (1993) Clinical utility and cost-effectiveness of an air suspension bed in the prevention of pressure ulcers. **JAMA** 269:1139.
103. Cooper SM, Young E (2000) Topical negative pressure. **Int J Dermatol** 39:892.
104. Reich P, Gottfried LA (1983) Factitious disorders in a teaching hospital. **Ann Intern Med** 99:240.
105. Mercer SO, Perdue JD (1993) Munchhausen syndrome by proxy: social work's role. **Soc Work** 38:74.
106. Rasmussen JE (1982) Puzzling purpuras in children and young adults. **J Am Acad Dermatol** 6:67.
107. Yateman GW, Duang VB (1980) Cao gio (coin rubbing): Vietnamese attitudes toward health care. **JAMA** 244:2748.
108. Feldman KW (1984) Pseudo-abusive burns in Asian refugees. **Am J Dis Child** 138:769.

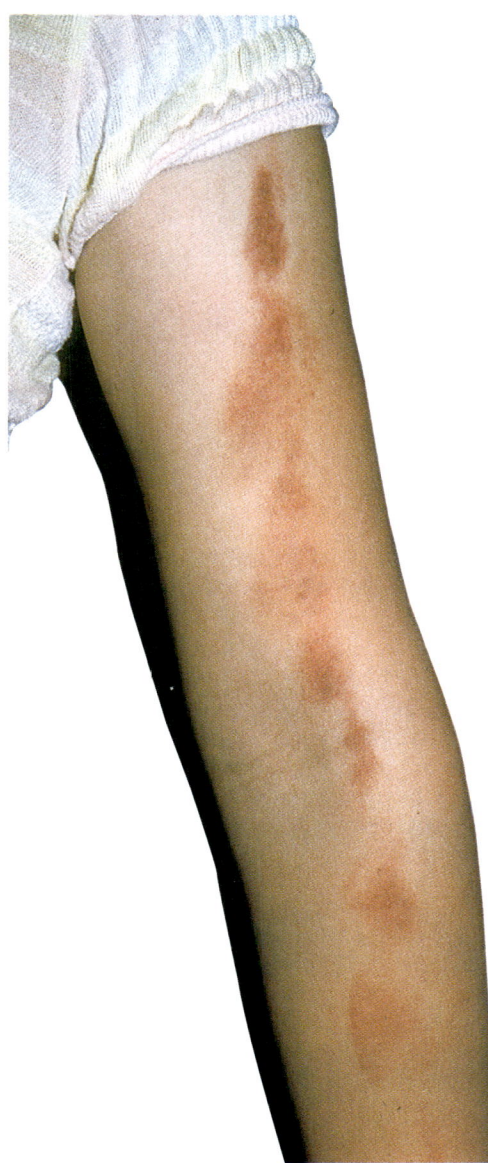

Fig. 29.10   Linear lesions, characteristic of factitial injury.

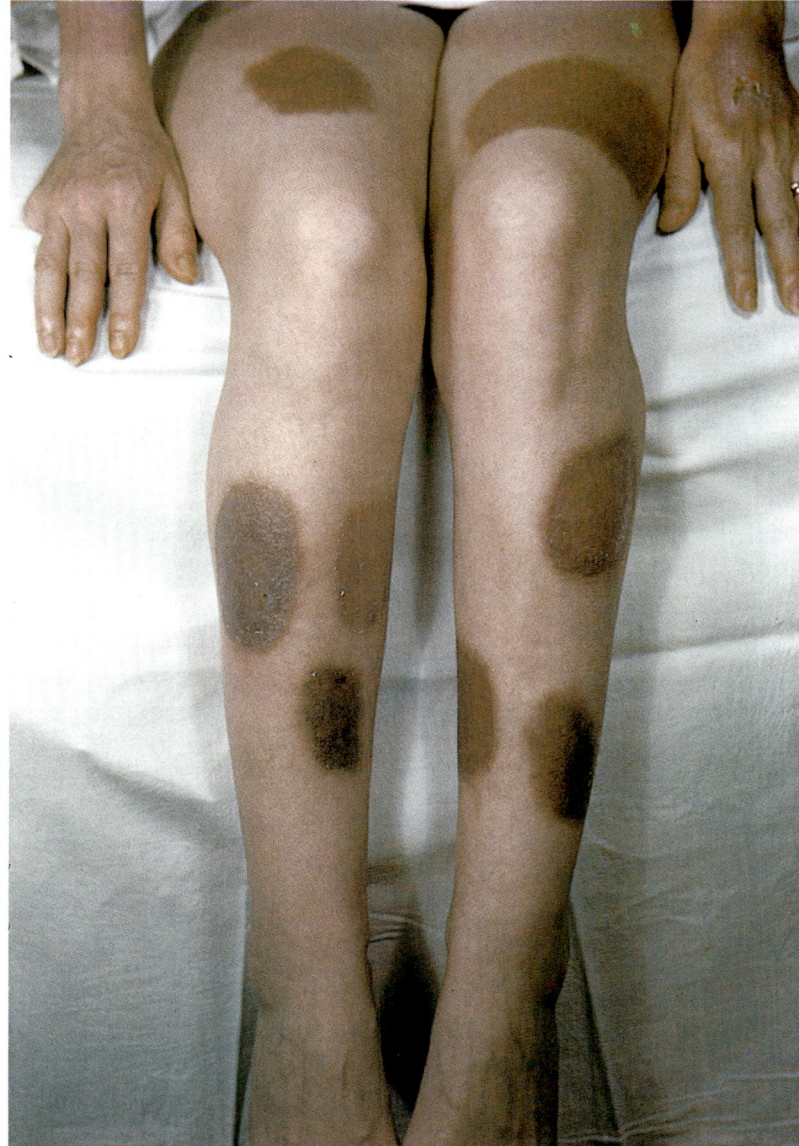

Fig. 29.11   Facticial injury showing suction-induced purpura.

SPORTS-RELATED INJURIES TO THE SKIN

Participating in sports may expose the skin to certain infections such as tinea corporis and herpes gladiatorium in wrestlers or Gram-negative bacterial infections from mud wrestling.[109] Sports activities may also aggravate pre-existing dermatologic problems. The discussion below, however, concentrates on injury, other than minor bruises, abrasions, and lacerations, that results from direct stress on the skin, which follows participation in a sport.[110,111]

Friction blisters are produced by excessive or prolonged rubbing and result from the accumulation of tissue exudate or blood at sites of dyshesion within the epidermis or between the epidermis and dermis.[110] The macerating effects of heat and sweating may promote blister formation. Powders to reduce friction and absorbant socks for the feet may have some preventative value. Friction blisters should be drained, and the overlying epidermal roof should be allowed to remain in place as a natural protective membrane. Soaking of the affected area may be of some benefit.

Chafing from the friction of clothing or equipment rubbing on the skin is a common problem. Powders or heavy lubrication may decrease friction and help prevent chafing. Chafing may progress to actual erosions. This is particularly a problem on the buttocks of bikers, which is related to the rocking motion the rider may make when the seat is too high or angled too much upward.[112] Shallow erosions that may occur on the areolae and nipples of long distance runners has been referred to as *jogger's nipples* and can be prevented by wearing soft shirts or actually bandaging the tender area before running.

Patients may seek medical attention for minor sports-related hemorrhages generally because of the concern that they might represent pigmented neoplasms. *Black heel* or *talon noir* (Fig. 29.13) presents as a blue-to-black discoloration on the posterior or posterolateral aspect of the heel that results from a mild ecchymosis caused by the sheering force from sudden turns made in basketball or racket sports. A similar lesion referred to as *black palm* can occasionally be seen in weightlifters, golfers, tennis players, and mountain climbers. The diagnosis of black heel or black palm can be confirmed by gently paring the surface of the epidermis, which yields tiny black dots that are pared away with the horny layer.

109. Adler AI, Altman J (1993) An outbreak of mud-wrestling-induced pustular dermatitis in college students. JAMA 269:502.
110. Basler RSW (1989) Skin injuries in sports medicine. J Am Acad Dermatol 21:257.
111. Adams BA (2001) Sports dermatology. In: Adolescent dermatology, Krowchuk DP, Lucky AW, eds. Adolescent Medicine: State of the Art Reviews 12:305–322.
112. Million MB (1991) Common cycling injuries. Management and prevention. Sports Med 11:52.

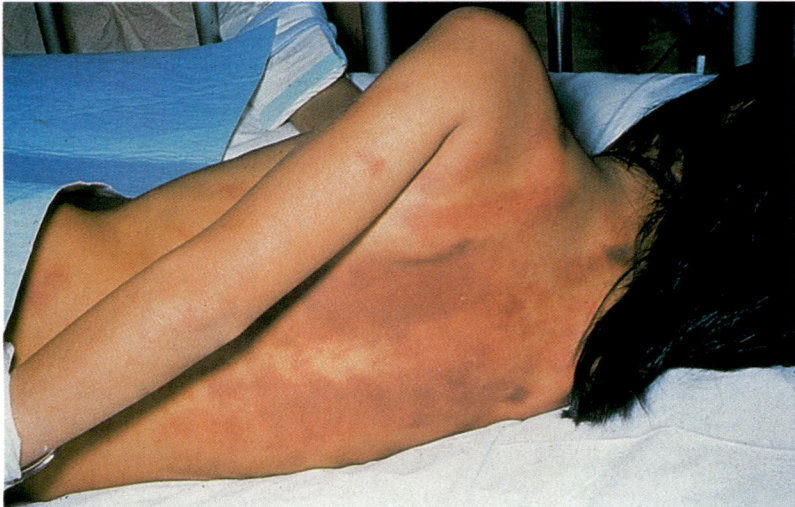

Fig. 29.12 Linear lesions induced by coining in a child with meningitis were initially thought to represent child abuse.

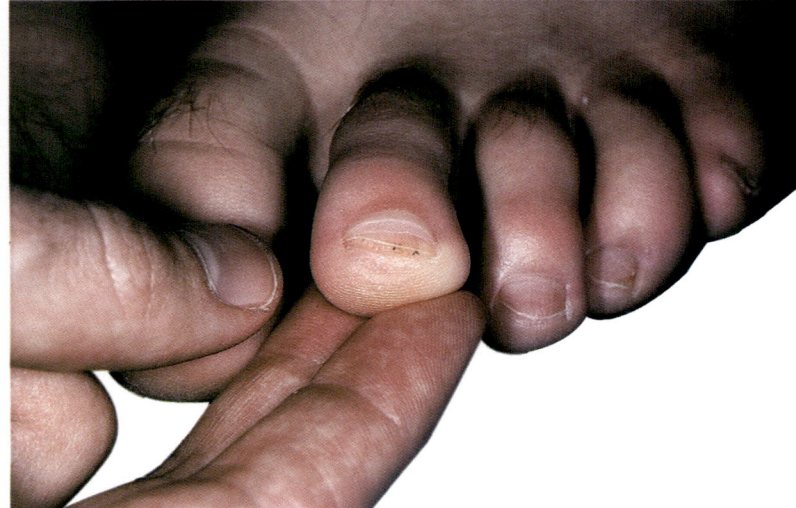

Fig. 29.14 Subungual hemorrhages and callus on the 2nd (and longest) toe of a basketball player. (Photo courtesy of Anne W. Lucky.)

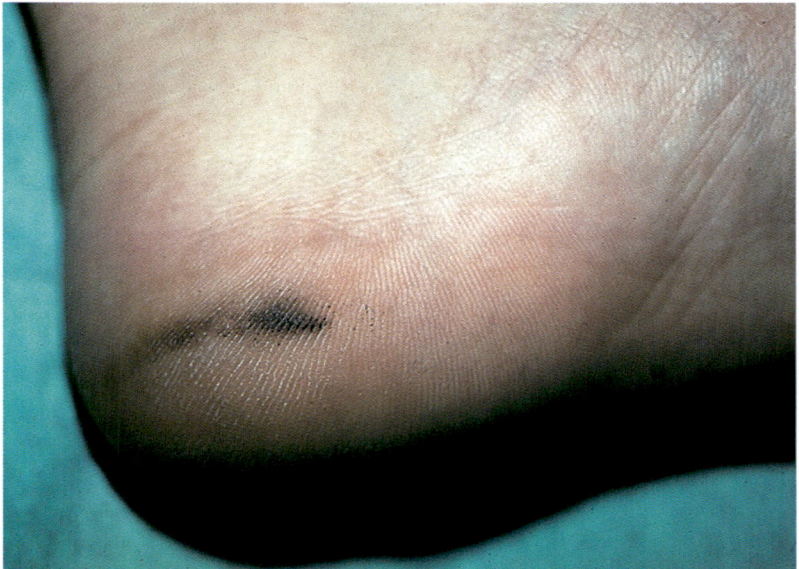

Fig. 29.13 Black heel, acquired in this patient while playing basketball.

Hemorrhages under the plates of the great toenails are usually the result of repeated abrupt contact of the distal end of the nail plate with the anterior part of the shoe (Fig. 29.14). Because it is most commonly seen in racquet sports, it is usually referred to as *tennis toe*, but the terms *jogger's toe* and *skier's toe* are also used. Nail trauma may also be seen in avid hikers. Properly fitting shoes or boots, along with trimming of the toenails, may be preventative. Generally, no treatment is indicated, but occasionally draining of the pooled blood from under the nail plate may be needed for pain relief after an acute injury.

Female cyclists may develop hematomas of the vulva, which may have the clinical appearance of a thrombophlebitis; however, thrombophlebitis does not occur in this area because there is no major vein that could be clotted.[112] A more chronic condition resulting from small ecchymosis on the superior portion of the gluteal cleft in long distance runners has been referred to as *runner's rump*.[110] The ecchymoses are apparently produced by the contact between the cheeks of the buttocks that occurs with every stride in running

and tends to resolve during periods of diminished running. Patients may benefit from sitz baths or local heat.

Callus formation represents a protective response to chronic friction; although located most commonly on the feet, any area where there is contact between the body and an athletic uniform, equipment, or appliance may be affected. On the feet they occasionally may be misdiagnosed as plantar warts. *Hand calluses* develop frequently in oarsmen, devotees of racket sports, and serious golfers.[110] In gymnasts, calloused palms are considered a competitive advantage. However, these calluses need to be pared when they become too thick; otherwise high friction causes skin tears and bleeding.[113] Keeping the hands dry and thoroughly chalked helps to reduce friction and the likelihood of skin tears. In many other instances, treatment of calluses is not necessary. If they interfere with normal function, however, then careful paring, abrasive reduction after soaking, or the regular application of salicylic acid plasters may be valuable.

Other lesions may also develop in athletes from chronic rubbing and pressure. Lichenified plaques on the buttocks have been reported from the friction of a metal seat of a rowing machine rubbing against the skin. These patches have been termed *rower's rump*.[114] Surfers may develop a fibrotic nontender lump on the anterior tibial prominence known as a *surfer's nodule*. Histologically, fibrosis is present within the dermis and subcutaneous tissue and results from chronic injury of the skin from pressure occurring between the underlying bone and the surfboard. Racers and other serious bike riders may have *perineal nodules*, which generally have a cystic quality and may appear like "accessory testicles" posterior to the testicles.[112] Histologically, these lesions represent areas of aseptic necrosis of the connective tissue with pseudocyst formation.

Piezogenic papules are protrusions of subcutaneous fat through the collagen matrix of the reticular dermis, generally on the lateral aspects of the feet or hands. The individual papules are soft, 2–7mm in size, and easily compressible. Lesions are generally asymptomatic but may be painful, particularly in endurance event competitors such as long distance runners and triathletes.[110] Discomfort from the lesions occasionally is reduced by wearing specially constructed orthotic appliances resembling heel caps.

Acne mechanica, a superficial occlusive folliculitis that produces a chronic acneiform eruption in athletes, is the result of heat, occlusion, friction, and pressure on skin underlying athletic apparel. Football players seem most affected because of the pressure of chin straps of helmets and the shoulder pads on acne-prone areas of the body. Individuals who wear occlusive leotards for aerobic dance or exercise, hockey players, weight-lifters in contact with a plastic-covered weight bench, and golfers who carry a golf bag over the

113. Weiker GG (1992) Hand and wrist problems in the gymnast. **Clin Sports Med** 11:189.

114. Tomecki KJ, Mikesell JF (1987) Rower's rump. **Am Acad Dermatol** 16:890.

shoulder may also be prone to acne mechanica.[110] Keratolytic agents, benzyl peroxides, and tretinoin may be of benefit in treatment. Systemic antibiotics appear to be of less value than in acne vulgaris.

Although not an actual injury, cosmetically unacceptable *green hair* may develop from long-term exposure to pool water in swimmers with natural or tinted blond, gray, or white hair. The pigmentary change is the result of copper ions being assimilated into the hair matrix. Bleaching with 3% hydrogen peroxide for 2–3h or treating with a commercial chelating agent[115] is usually effective in removing the green color. Swimmers may develop a periorbital contact dermatitis from wearing rubber swim goggles.[116] Allergic contact dermatitis may also be seen in swimmers and divers from bathing caps, nose clips, ear plugs, fins, fin straps, diving suits, and underwater masks and mouthpieces. Occasionally swimmers may present may with periocular purpura, which has been denoted *purpura gogglelorum*.[117] The purpura results from mechanical trauma such as direct collision forces, or goggles snapping back onto the eye, suction trauma from repeated pulling away of goggles under negative pressure, or a progressive pressure which is usually seen in children with poorly fitting goggles who gradually tighten the strap to compensate for a leaking seal. Contact dermatitis from protective gear containing latex such as shin guards and knee pads or from dyes in uniforms may occur in sensitized individuals.

Injuries from sunlight and cold exposure have been discussed previously in this chapter. All children participating in outdoors sports should be adequately protected from the sun. Individuals participating in high-altitude winter sports are particularly prone to cold injury because of the combined effects of increased oxygen needs produced by exercise in the decreased oxygen tension of the high atmosphere potentiating peripheral vasoconstriction and cutaneous anoxia. Layered clothing and adequate protection of the face and anterior neck are beneficial in preventing injury.

EXERCISE-INDUCED ANAPHYLAXIS AND URTICARIA

Exercise is one of several physical stimuli that can provoke urticaria or anaphylaxis.[118] The clinical features of exercise-induced changes range from generalized warmth, flushing, and pruritus to urticaria and angioedema and often to laryngeal edema, bronchospasm, and hypotension. Exercise may also induce cholinergic urticaria in which small punctuate lesions 2–4mm in diameter develop in response to an increase in core body temperature. Pulmonary function may be impaired during attacks, but progression to anaphylaxis is rare.

Individuals with classic exercised-induced anaphylaxis have larger urticarial lesions measuring 1.0–2.5cm in diameter.[118] The symptoms frequently progress to angioedema or anaphylaxis. Exercise is the necessary stimulus for an attack; passive body warming does not cause symptoms. Females appear to be more commonly affected than males.[119] Jogging is the most frequently reported provoking activity, although aerobics, walking, dancing, tennis, bicycling, racquetball, swimming, cross-country skiing, and downhill skiing are not rare initiators. Most symptoms are brought on by moderate or fast-paced exercise. The onset of an attack typically occurs approximately 5min into the exercise and resolves spontaneously within 30min to 4h. The diagnosis can often be made on the basis of the patient's history. Documentation of an elevated plasma histamine level during exercise strongly suggests the diagnosis.

Antihistamines, particularly diphenhydramine and hydroxyzine, may be effective in preventing symptoms and helpful in treatment once symptoms have developed.[118] The newer nonsedating antihistamines may be effective in some individuals. Cromolyn sodium insufflation may be helpful in preventing the pulmonary symptoms of exercise-induced anaphylactic attacks. Individuals

with known disease should not exercise alone and should always have epinephrine kits such as EpiPen available for emergency use. The wearing of a MedicAlert is also advisable. A form of exercise-induced anaphylaxis, which is caused by ingestion of a specific food before exercise has been recognized. Neither the ingested food nor the exercise alone induces symptoms. Wheat is a frequent cause of food-dependent, exercise induced anaphylaxis, and a gluten-free diet is recommended when wheat is the cause.[120]

CHILD ABUSE AND NEGLECT

BATTERED CHILD SYNDROME

The reported incidence of child abuse and neglect in the United States has increased yearly over the last several years and has been referred to as America's "hidden epidemic." The immense importance of this problem was not generally recognized until 1962, when Kempe *et al.*[121] coined the term "battered child syndrome." Essential to the diagnosis of battered child syndrome are unexplained or inadequately explained signs of trauma, multiple fracture at different stages of healing, and/or failure to thrive that responds to either nutritional therapy or to placing the child in an emotionally supportive environment.

The abused child is often an infant. Younger children are at greater risk because they are demanding, nonverbal, and defenseless. As many as 90% of abused children are younger than 10 years of age and more than 70% are 3 years of age or younger.[122] Besides physical abuse, many of these children suffer from nutritional deprivation, emotional abuse, medical care neglect, and occasionally deliberate assault with intent to murder. Child abuse is rarely an isolated incident; once children have been battered, they are at high risk of again being abused if they are returned to the abusive adult without active intervention.[123] Often the child has frequent medical contacts with evidence of neglect of basic health maintenance activities and absence of the appropriate immunizations.

The parent may describe the child as a difficult child, which may in fact be true; however, the parents may attempt to intervene in a manner that is excessive and inappropriate. Many parents themselves were not well parented and were abused as children. They are often lonely, immature people who are socially isolated, do not trust others, and have unrealistic expectations of their own children. The parents may have poor impulse control, particularly in a stressful situation or when an incident triggers an inappropriate response. Also, the family may live in a culture where corporal punishment is sanctioned or encouraged. All parents have the potential to abuse their children, but most parents do not exercise that potential because of adequate impulse control, inner resources, and adequate support systems.[124] Child abuse may occur in any social background but appears to occur more frequently when other problems such as unemployment, substance abuse, unplanned pregnancies, or discord between the parents increase stress.

Physical abuse is frequently identified by bruises, which may be multiple, and in areas such as the genitalia or buttocks, which are not commonly accidentally injured.[125] Bruises may be in different stages of healing, suggesting different temporal sequences of injury. The figurate characteristics of the bruises may identify the object with which the child was hit. *Linear bruising* is produced by an object such as a rod, stick, plate, or strap. Hematomas and traumatic fracture of underlying bone may be present. *Loop marks* are perhaps the single most characteristic finding in child abuse (Fig. 29.15).[126] Such curvilinear marks are produced by small ropes, cords, electrical cords, and belts and may appear randomly over the child's body. *Buckles* from belts leave a characteristic imprint, which can often be matched to the belt buckle used (Fig. 29.16).

115. Goldschmidt H (1979) Green hair. **Arch Dermatol** 115:1288.
116. Basler RS, Basler GC, Pazlmer AH et al. (2000) Special skin symptoms seen in swimmers. **J Am Acad Dermatol** 43:299.
117. Jowett NI, Jowett SG (1997) Ocular purpura in a swimmer. **Postgrad Med J** 73:819.
118. Nichols AW (1992) Exercise-induced anaphylaxis and urticaria. **Clin Sports Med** 11:303.
119. Wade JP, Liang MH, Sheffer AL (1989) Biochemistry of the acute Allergic Reactions. Fifth International Symposium. New York: Alan R Liss.
120. Palosui K, Alenius H, Varjomen E et al. (1999) A novel wheat gliadin as a cause of exercise induced anaphylaxis. **J Allergy Clin Immunol** 103:912.
121. Kempe CH, Silverman FN, Steele BF et al. (1962) The battered child syndrome. **JAMA** 181:17.
122. Wilcox K (1979) Child abuse: an approach for early diagnosis. **J Fam Pract** 9:801.
123. Morse CW, Sahler OJ, Friedman SB (1970) A 3 year follow up study of abused and neglected children. **Am J Dis Child** 120:439.
124. Heins M (1984) The battered child revisited. **JAMA** 251:3295.
125. Pascoe JM, Hildebrant HM, Tarrier A, Murphy M (1979) Patterns of skin injury in nonaccidential and accidental injury. **Pediatrics** 64:245.
126. Raimer BG Raimer SS, Hebeler JR (1981) Cutaneous signs of child abuse. **J Am Acad Dermatol** 5:203.

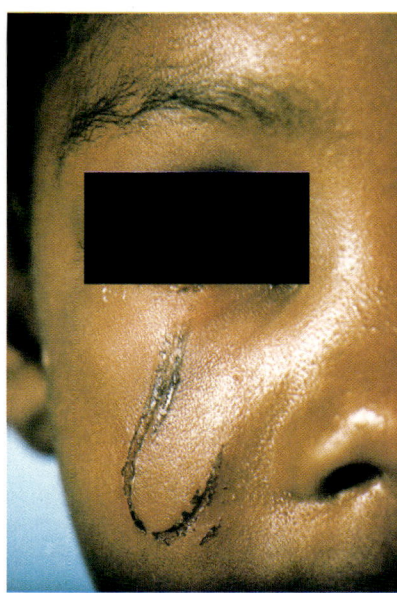

Fig. 29.15 **Child abuse.** Loop marks from an electrical cord on the cheek of a child.

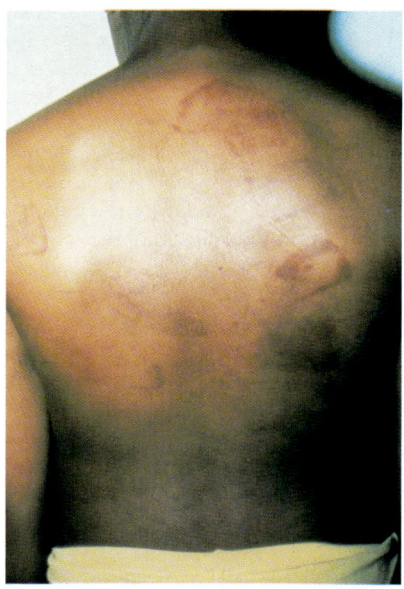

Fig. 29.16 **Child abuse.** Bruises in the shape of a belt buckle.

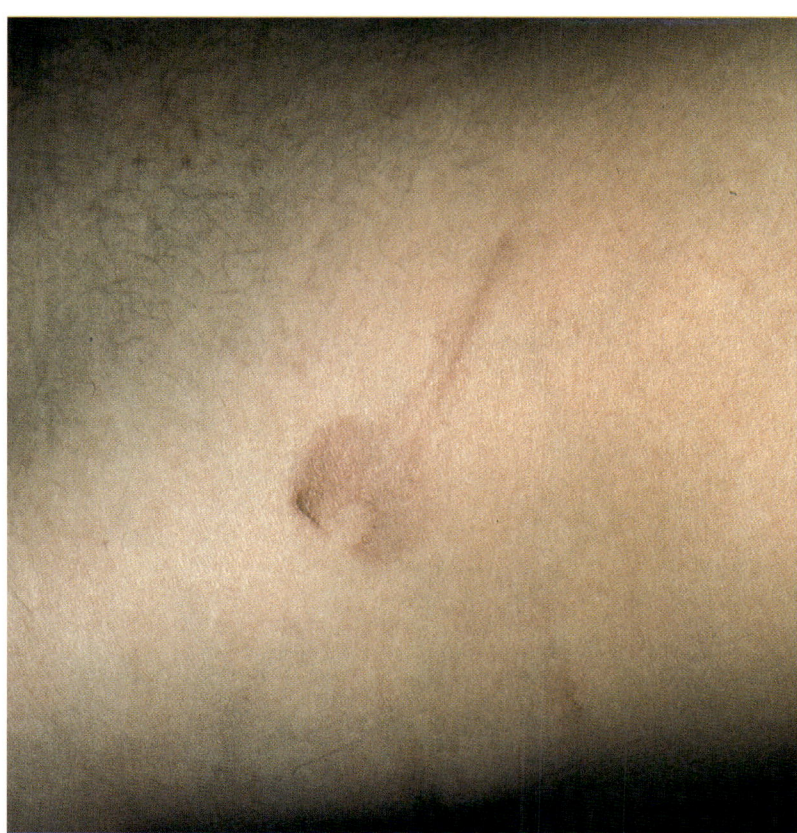

Fig. 29.17 Burn showing the outline of hot metallic key used to injure a child.

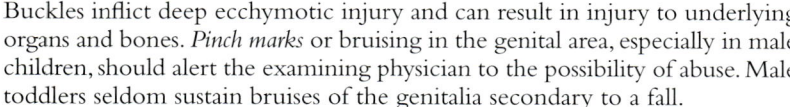

Buckles inflict deep ecchymotic injury and can result in injury to underlying organs and bones. *Pinch marks* or bruising in the genital area, especially in male children, should alert the examining physician to the possibility of abuse. Male toddlers seldom sustain bruises of the genitalia secondary to a fall.

Blunt trauma can be a very severe form of abuse that may or may or may not result in cutaneous lesions. Blunt trauma to the abdomen can result in severe injury, even death, to the child. Soft intra-abdominal organs are injured when they are slammed against the vertebral column by a kick or severe blow delivered to the abdomen. Blunt trauma in the form of slapping injuries often leaves the imprint of the perpetrator's hand across the child. Capillaries break between the fingers, producing linear bruises outlining the blunt object (fingers).

Binding injuries are more likely to occur when the perpetrator is emotionally disturbed or psychotic. Acute binding injuries cause edema of tissue around the wrists and ankles; they may also resemble rope burns with redness and warmth or abrasions. Chronic binding injuries may result in bands of postinflammatory hyperpigmentation.

Traumatic alopecia results from the forceful pulling of the hair out of the scalp. The occipital region is the most common location for traumatic alopecia. Acutely, when a large tuft of hair is pulled out, the underlying scalp may hemorrhage, with subsequent hematoma formation.

Human bite marks leave the indelible mark of the perpetrator and may serve to identify the abuser. Adult human bite marks must be distinguished from those of a child because the healthy toddler may have numerous bite marks from peers. Adult bites can be identified by the width of the dental arch (greater than 4cm).[127] Human bite marks differ from animal bites in that they produce a crushing type of injury, whereas typical animal bites result in puncture of the skin.

Thermal burns constitute an especially traumatic form of injury to the young child, and the abuser in such cases is likely to be suffering from a severe psychiatric disturbance. Cigarette burns represent a frequent form of thermal injury and tend to be randomly distributed. Branding injuries are also common, taking the shape of the heated object (Fig. 29.17). Dunking scald injuries occur most often in the infant and toddler age groups, and scalds on the buttocks may be associated with attempts to toilet train the infant. "Donut-type sparing" may occur on a child's buttocks when the buttocks are held against a cooler tub or basin while the surrounding hot water scalds the remaining immersed skin. Dunking scalds of the extremities leave a characteristic "stocking and glove" distribution with very sharp demarcation of the burn (Fig. 29.18).

The distribution of injuries can suggest child abuse. In one study that compared abuse versus accidental injury, children with suspected child abuse had significantly more soft tissue injuries over the cheek, trunk, genitalia, and upper legs.[125] In a retrospective review of medical records submitted to the National Pediatric Trauma Registry over a 10-year period child abuse accounted for 10.6% of all blunt trauma to all patients younger than 5 years.[128]

127. Levine LJ (1973) The solution of a battered child homicide by dental evidence: report of case. **J Am Dent Assoc** 87:1234.

128. DiScala C, Sege R, Li G et al. (2000) Child abuse and unintentional junjuries. A 10-year retrospective. **Arch Pediatr Adolesc Med** 154:16.

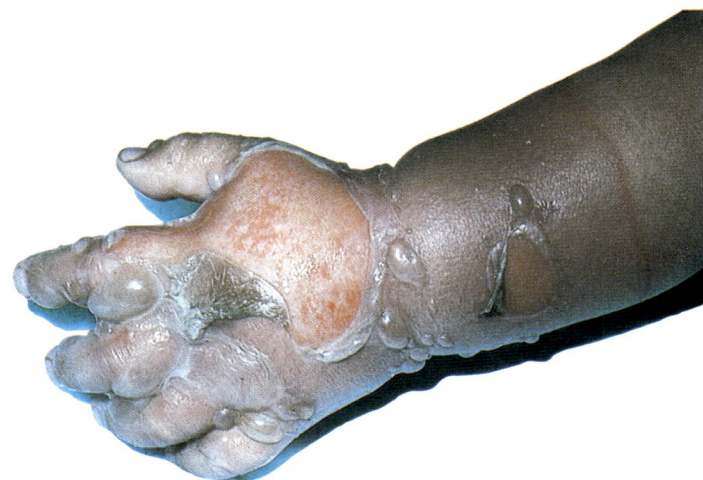

Fig. 29.18   Child abuse. Well-demarcated burn caused by dipping the extremity in hot water.

TABLE 29.3   Evaluation and acute management of the abused child

Detailed history (medical/social)
Physical examination
Laboratory data (complete blood count, serology, appropriate cultures, etc.)
Treatment of acute injuries or infections
Radiographs
Photographs, diagrams, videos as indicated
Documentation in case records
Reporting to a local child protective service agency by telephone followed by a detailed written report.
Protection of the child

Children injured by abuse were significantly younger and were more likely to have a preinjury medical hisory, retinal hemorrhages, intraabdominal and very severe injuries than children with unintentional injuries. A child may present with skin signs of multiple types of physical abuse. Such a child may be severely injured at the time of presentation or, if not, should be considered at high risk for the future occurrence of a severe injury. Both acute and healing injuries are frequently present in chronically abused children.

If individual lesions are present, leading to suspicion of abuse, the entire cutaneous surface of the child should be examined, including the oral, rectal, and genital mucosa. Detailed records of the observed lesions should be made. If possible, photographs should be taken to characterize the physical findings more precisely. During the examination, an attempt should be made to age the temporal development of the individual lesions, which may suggest a sequence of repeated injuries. Identification of possibly associated injuries, such as subdural hematomas or previous fractures, should be evaluated. A good funduscopic examination should be done to look for retinal hemorrhages, which occasionally can be seen secondary to head trauma or after severe shaking of the child, and an otoscopic examination of the ears to rule out hemotympanum. Skeletal surveys are usually recommended to evaluate for other sites of trauma, but their benefit has been questioned.[129] Awareness of possible head trauma, blunt abdominal trauma, fractures, dislocations, and malnutrition may require additional testing to identify these associated conditions. The child should be protected from further injury if abuse is suspected. Suggestions for the evaluation and acute management of the abused child are summarized in Table 29.3.

Occasionally, other diseases or nonabusive skin injuries may mimic child abuse. Conditions that have been confused with child battering include clotting and platelet abnormalities, erythema multiforme,[130] Ehlers–Danlos syndrome,[131] cupping lesions,[132] cao gio (coin rubbing),[133] Mongolian spots,[134] phytophotodermatitis (Fig. 23.6),[135] and the bone lesions of osteogenesis imperfecta and Menke syndrome.

SEXUAL ABUSE

Sexual abuse of children can be considered as part of the overall spectrum of child abuse. It can be defined as the engaging of a child in sexual activities that the child cannot comprehend, for which the child is developmentally unprepared, for which the child cannot give informed consent, and/or that violate the social and legal taboos of society.[136] Sexual abuse in children includes intercourse, fondling of the genitalia, sodomy, orogenital contact, incest, exhibitionism, and using the child in the production of pornography. The child's involvement is either coerced through physical threats or rewarded through bribes or misrepresentations of moral values. In a study of 311 children evaluated for sexual abuse, only 18% of the victims were assaulted by strangers.[137] Girls are more frequently reported abused than boys.[137,138] However, a great deal of sexual abuse of boys may go undetected or unreported (Fig. 29.19).[138–140] Epidemiologic studies have shown that the risk for sexual abuse rises in preadolescence.[100] Features related to family structure that have been associated with a small but statistically significant increased risk for abuse are the presence of a stepfather in the household; children living without one or both of their natural parents; or children whose mother is disabled, ill, or extensively out of the home.[138] Paternal violence has been reported to be a risk factor for father–daughter child sexual abuse.[141]

The diagnosis of child sexual abuse is based on the patient's history, the physical examination, and, when appropriate, laboratory tests. Children rarely fabricate reports of sexual abuse, and any such report by a child should be thoroughly investigated. Unfortunately, false accusations by parents involved in custody disputes have become increasingly common in recent years and are a burden to the system.

After an extensive review of the literature, Bays and Chadwick[139] described findings that are specific or consistent with child sexual abuse (Tables 29.4 and 29.5). Physical findings may be absent after sexual abuse. Many types of sexual molestation such as fondling or oral sodomy may not leave physical findings. Even when injury occurs, healing in the genital area is rapid and may result in very subtle or undetectable physical findings.[142]

129. Ellerstein NS, Norris KJ (1984) Value of radiological skeletal survey in assessment of abused children. **Pediatrics** 74:1075.
130. Adler R, Kane-Nussen D (1983) Erythema multiforme: confusion with child battering syndrome. **Pediatrics** 72:718.
131. Roberts DLL, Pope FM, Nicholls AC, Narcisi P (1984) Ehlers–Danlos syndrome type IV mimicking non-accidental injury in the child. **Br J Dermatol** 111:341.
132. Asnes RS, Wisotsky DH (1981) Cupping lesions simulating child abuse. **J Pediatr** 99:267.
133. Silfen E, Wyre HW (1981) Factitial dermatitis – cao gio. **Cutis** 28:399.
134. Bungy CI (1982) Mongolian spots, day care centers, and child abuse. **Pediatrics** 69:672.
135. Coffman K, Boyce WT, Hansen RC (1985) Phytophotodermatitis simulating child abuse. **Am J Dis Child** 139:239.
136. Committee on Child Abuse and Neglect of the American Academy of Pediatrics (1991) Guidelines for the evaluation of sexual abuse of children. **Pediatrics** 87:254.

137. Rimsza ME, Niggemann EH (1982) Medical evaluation of sexually abused children: a review of 311 cases. **Pediatrics** 69:8.
138. Finkelhor D (1993) Epidemiological factors in the clinical identification of child sexual abuse. **Child Abuse Negl** 17:67.
139. Bays J, Chadwick D (1993) Medical diagnosis of the sexually abused child. **Child Abuse Negl** 17:91.
140. Spencer MJ, Dunklee P (1986) Sexual abuse of boys. **Pediatrics** 78:133.
141. Paveza G (1988) Risk factors in father–daughter child sexual abuse: a case–control study. **J Interpersonal Violence** 3:290.
142. McCann J, Voris J, Simon M (1992) Genital injuries resulting from sexual abuse: a longitudinal study. **Pediatrics** 89:307.

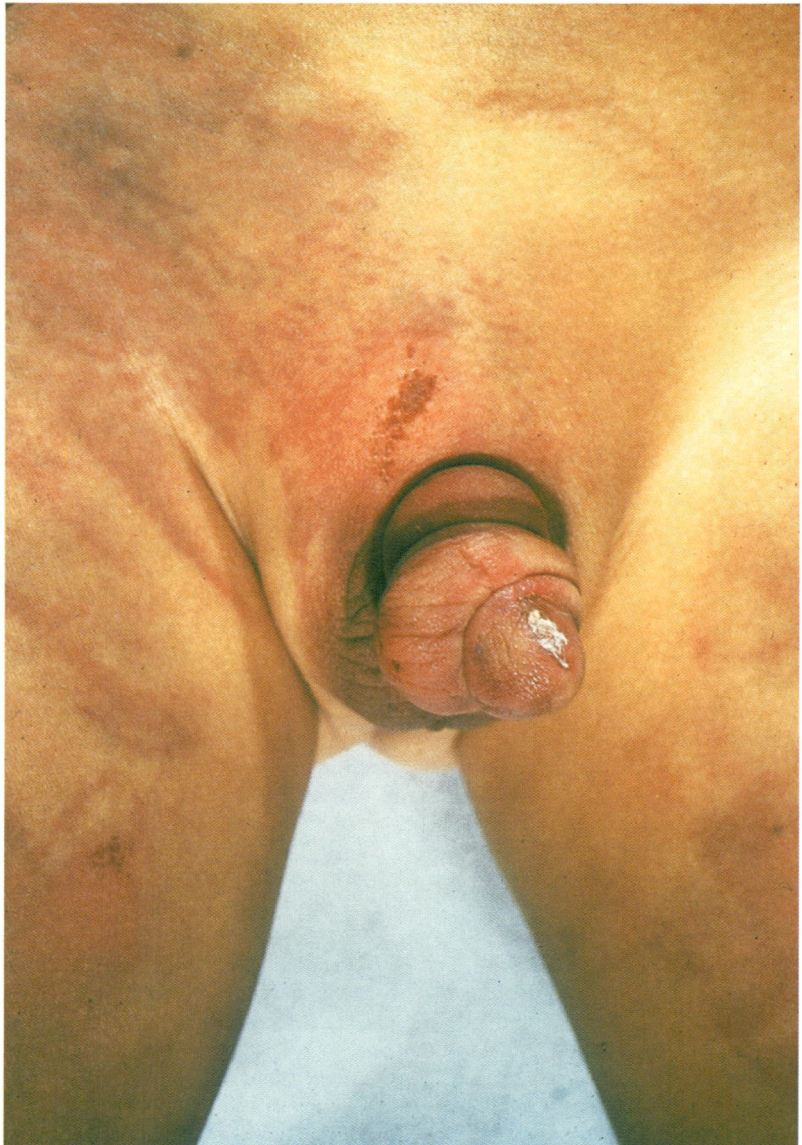

Fig. 29.19 **Sexual child abuse.** Genital and soft tissue trauma document abuse.

TABLE 29.4 **Findings specific for sexual abuse even in the absence of a history of abuse**

Presence of semen, sperm, or acid phosphatase
Pregnancy
Fresh genital or anal injuries (lacerations, abrasions, contusions, transections, avulsions, hematomas, ecchymoses, petechiae, and bite marks) in the absence of an adequate accidental explanation
Positive test or culture for syphilis or gonorrhea (not perinatally acquired)
Human immunodeficiency virus infection (if not acquired perinatally or through intravenous routes)
A markedly enlarged hymenal opening for age with associated findings of hymen disruption, including absent hymen, hymenal remnants, healed transections, or scars in the absence of an adequate accidental or surgical explanation

TABLE 29.5 **Findings consistent with sexual abuse: history and other investigations may be important in diagnosing abuse**

Genital or anal *Trichomonas, Chlamydia,* condyloma acuminatum, herpes type II, if not perinatally acquired
Disruptions of hymen tissue, including posterior or lateral angular concavities (also termed clefts or notches), transections, absence, decrease in amount, and scars
Anal scars outside the midline
Anal skin tags outside the midline
Anal dilation >15–20mm without stool in the ampulla
Irregularity of the anal orifice after complete dilation
Marked dilation of the hymenal opening, persisting in different examination positions

of the child and the degree of separation or traction on the labia majora influences the size of the orifice, and thus the way in which the examination is performed should be recorded in the chart.[136] Whenever possible, the physical examination of a child suspected of being sexually abused should be done by a pediatrician or gynecologist experienced in evaluating children for possible abuse. Examination by multiple physicians should be avoided if possible because this may be traumatic to the child.

The American Academy of Child and Adolescent Psychiatry has published guidelines for interviewing sexually abused children.[149] Such interviews are preferably conducted by experienced personnel. The use of line drawings and dolls may be helpful in interviewing young children. Because children who have been sexually abused are generally coerced into secrecy, a high index of suspicion may be required to recognize the problem. Presenting symptoms may be very general, such as sleep disturbance, enuresis, encopresis, or phobias, or more specific, such as rectal or genital pain, bleeding, sexually transmitted diseases, or precocious sexual behavior.[136]

When the history and/or physical findings suggest the possibility of oral, genital, or rectal contact, appropriate cultures and serologic tests should be obtained.[136] The presence of semen, sperm, or acid phosphatase is indicative of abuse as is the presence of nonperinatally acquired syphilis, gonorrhea,[136] or human immunodeficiency virus not acquired perinatally or through intravenous routes.[139] Natal infections with *Chlamydia trachomatis* have been documented to persist as long as 28 months; therefore, infection with this organism in young children is not conclusive evidence of abuse.[150] Present evidence suggests that anogenital warts in children may be perinatally acquired,

The amount of data regarding normal physical findings in nonabused children is increasing rapidly.[143–146] There is no documented case in the literature of an infant girl being born without a hymen.[139] Studies of newborns indicate that anterior hymenal clefts are common, but posterior clefts are not seen normally. Thus, when they are present they are likely acquired.[144] Twenty-five percent of newborns have a white line or linear vestibularis in the posterior vestibule, which could be confused with scar tissue produced by sexual abuse.[147] It has also been noted that the hymenal opening increases with age. Woodling[148] proposed a general "rule of thumb" that, after 5 years of age, the normal transhymenal diameter equals the child's age expressed in millimeters. An enlarged hymenal opening is suggestive of abuse but may not be present after a single episode of sexual assault. The position

143. McCann J, Wells R, Simon M et al. (1990) Genital findings in prepubertal girls selected for non-abuse: a descriptive study. **Pediatrics** 86:428.
144. Berenson AB (1993) Appearance of the hymen at birth and one year of age: a longitudinal study. **Pediatrics** 91:820.
145. McCann J, Voris J, Simon M et al. (1989) Perianal findings in prepubertal children selected for nonabuse: a descriptive study. **Child Abuse Negl** 13:179.
146. Berenson AB, Somma-Garcia A, Barnett S (1993) Perianal findings in infants 18 months of age or younger. **Pediatrics** 91:838.
147. Kellogg ND, Parra JM (1991) Linear vestibularis: a previously undescribed normal genital structure in female neonates. **Pediatrics** 87:926.
148. Woodling BA (1986) Sexual abuse and the child. **Emerg Med Services** 15:17.
149. American Academy of Child and Adolescent Psychiatry (1988) Guidelines for the clinical evaluation of child and adolescent sexual abuse: position statement of the American Academy of Child and Adolescent Psychiatry. **J Am Acad Child Adolesc Psychiatry** 27:655.
150. Bell TA, Stamm WE, Wag S et al. (1992) Chronic *Chlamydia trachomatis* infections in infants. **JAMA** 267:400.

transmitted during the routine care of children, autoinoculated from other sites of infection, or acquired as the result of sexual abuse.[151] Great variation exists in the incidence of documented or strongly suspected sexual abuse in recent studies,[152–155] ranging from a low of 11%[153] of 75 children to a high of 91% of 11 children with anogenital warts.[155] Two recent studies of 40 children with anogenital warts in whom adequate evaluation for abuse was documented yielded an approximate 50% incidence of sexual abuse. In most studies, proven abuse is rare in children who are younger than 3 years of age. Conversely, in a study of girls 11 years of age and younger known to have been abused, 5 of 15 or 33% were found to have human papillomavirus infection in intravaginal washes.[156] If the examining physician is not experienced in evaluating children for sexual abuse, the child with genital warts should be referred in a non-accusatory fashion to a physician with such experience or to a child abuse evaluation team, which is often composed of a cooperating group of medical personnel, including physicians, psychologists, nurses, and social workers. If such a referral is not possible, Schachner and Hankin's[157] article on assessing sexual abuse in childhood condyloma acuminatum may be helpful in determining whether or not a referral to child protective services is indicated.

Other conditions in the anogenital area have been confused with sexual abuse. These conditions include congenital anomalies, accidental injury, streptococcal cellulitis, lichen sclerosus et atrophicus,[158] localized vulvar pemphigoid,[159] and Crohn's disease. The perianal papillomatous lesions of Goltz syndrome may be misdiagnosed as perianal warts. Definite child abuse is required by law to be reported to the local child protective service agency. Referral to a child abuse expert is desirable when the diagnosis is uncertain because the negative impact on the family structure of misdiagnosis is substantial.[160]

Victims of all types of abuse may suffer long-term psychological consequences. Some children withdraw and develop feelings of worthlessness, helplessness, hopelessness, and depression. Others exhibit aggressive and impulsive behavior and are at risk for delinquency, substance abuse, absenteeism from school or work, adolescent pregnancy, and prostitution. Abused children are more likely as adults to be abusive to their own children and spouses. Long-term psychological support for abused children is therefore desirable.

ENVIRONMENTAL HAZARDS

Ana M. Duarte

AQUATIC ENVIRONMENT

NATURAL HAZARDS

Marine injuries
Marine injuries are caused by a wide variety of organisms and range from self-limited dermatoses to life-threatening conditions often with confusing symptoms. Skin exposures are by far the most common type of aquatic injury.[161]

Coelenterates
Coelenterate stings are the most common type of marine envenomation.[162] Phylum Coelenterata is divided into four classes: Scyphozoa, the true jellyfish; Hydrozoa, the Cubozoa, the box jellyfish; the Portuguese man-of-war (*Physalia physalis*); and Anthozoa, the sea anemones and soft corals.

Portuguese Man-of-War. Portuguese man-of-war stings are common in the coastal waters of the southern United States. These coelenterates are distinguished by their long tentacles, each containing thousands of nematocysts (stinging cells).[161] Envenomation occurs by injection from nematocysts, which contain venom within cnidoblasts. The toxin is proteinaceous and induces histamine release and prostaglandin-induced vasodilatation. The venom induces calcium influx into the cells by making plasma cell membranes more permeable.[163] Even detached tentacles, which may be found laying on the beach, remain potent for days. The severity of envenomation is dependent on season, species, number of nematocysts triggered, size, age, general health of the victim, and location of the sting.[161,164,165]

Signs and symptoms are usually immediate but may be delayed.[161,164] These include pain; paresthesias; intense burning; and a linear, red, papular eruption at the contact site (Fig. 29.20).[161,164,166] Systemic symptoms such as nausea, myalgias, headaches, chills, and pallor may occur.[161,164,165] In the most severe cases, envenomation may induce cardiovascular collapse and death. Drowning secondary to limb paralysis has been reported.[169] Small children may also pick up tentacles found laying on the beach and place them in their mouth, resulting in rapid intraoral swelling and potential airway obstruction.[164] Therefore, cutaneous lesions should be sought in cases of unexplained water-related death and near drowning. Chronic cutaneous findings include keloids, hyperpigmentation, fat atrophy, contractures, gangrene and erythema nodosum.[167,168]

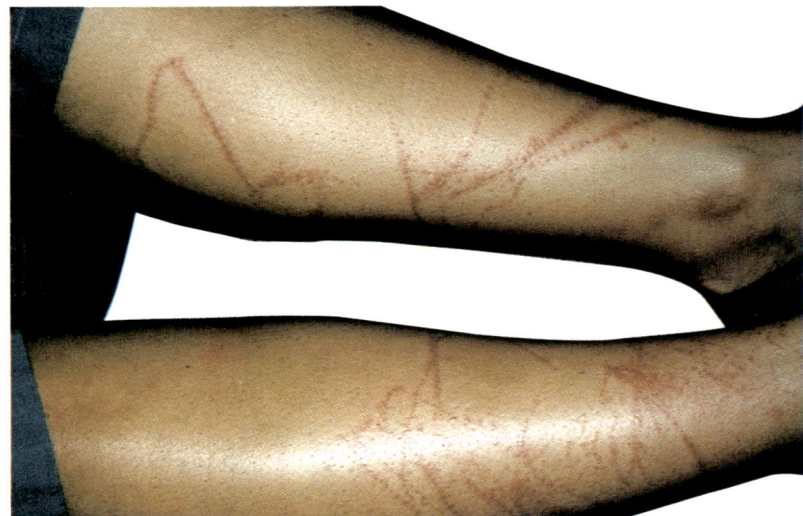

Fig. 29.20　Portuguese man-of-war stings.

151. Raimer SS, Raimer BG (1992) Family violence, child abuse, and anogenital warts. Arch Dermatol 128:842.
152. Gibson PE, Gardner SD, Best SJ (1990) Human papillomavirus types in anogenital warts of children. J Med Virol 30:142.
153. Cohen BA, Honig P, Androphy E (1990) Anogenital warts in children: clinical and virologic evaluation for sexual abuse. Arch Dermatol 126:1575.
154. Hanson RM, Glasson M, McCrossin I et al. (1989) Anogenital warts in childhood. Child Abuse Negl 13:225.
155. Herman-Giddens ME, Gutman LT, Berson NL (1988) Association of coexisting vaginal infections and multiple abuses in female children with genital warts. Sex Transm Dis 15:63.
156. Gutman LT, St. Claire K, Herman-Giddens ME et al. (1992) Evaluation of sexually abused and nonabused young girls for intravaginal human papillomavirus infection. Am J Dis Child 146:306.
157. Schachner L, Hankin ED (1985) Assessing child abuse in childhood condyloma acuminatum. J Am Acad Dermatol 12:157.
158. Bays J, Jenny C (1990) Genital and anal conditions confused with child sexual abuse trauma. Am J Dis Child 144:1319.
159. Levine V, Sanchex M, Nestor MS (1992) Localized vulvar pemphigoid in a child misdiagnosed as sexual abuse. Arch Dermatol 128:804.
160. Vorenberg E (1992) Diagnosing child abuse: the cost of getting it wrong. Arch Dermatol 128:844.
161. Kizer KW (1983–1984) Marine envenomations. J Toxicol Clin Toxicol 21:527.
162. Soppe GG (1989) Marine envenomations and aquatic dermatology. Am Fam Physician 40:97.
163. Edwards L, Hessinger DA. Portuguese Man of war (*Physalia physalis*) venom induces calcium influx into cells by permeabilizing plasma membranes. Toxicon 200 Aug; 38(8): 1015–1028.
164. Auerbach PS, Halstead BW (1989) Hazardous aquatic life. In: Management of Wilderness and Environmental Emergencies, Auerbach PS, Geehr EC, eds. St. Louis: CV Mosby, p. 933.
165. Matusow RJ (1980) Oral inflammatory response to a sting from a Portuguese man-of-war. J Am Dent Assoc 100:73.
166. Gonzaga RAF (1985) Venomous fish stings on the European seashore. Postgrad Med 77:146.
167. Auerbach PS, Hays JT (1987) Erythema nodosum following a jellyfish sting. J Emerg Med Nov-Dec; 5(6):487–.
168. Burnett JW, Calton GJ (1987) Venomous pelagic coelenterates: chemistry, toxicology, immunology and treatment of their stings. Toxicon 25:581.

Therapy consists of first removing any adherent tentacles with a gloved hand or forceps.[164] After this, the treatment of choice is 5% acetic acid (vinegar) soaks, which functions by deactivating the venom.[161,164,169,171–173] These soaks should be applied continuously for 30min, or until there is no pain.[164] Proteolytic meat tenderizers are also useful; however, papain may cause secondary exfoliation of the epidermis. Baking soda also aids in dissolving tentacle debris.[162,164,174–176] Wound care consists of Burow's solution compresses, mild topical corticosteroids, oral antihistamines, and topical anesthetics (however, paradoxical reactions to benzocaine have been reported).[164] Topical agents should only be used after the toxin has been completely inactivated. If anaphylaxis occurs, appropriate supportive therapy should be instituted. In severe cases, systemic corticosteroids, epinephrine ephedrine, atropine, and methysergide may be administered; however, there are no data that they are beneficial. Verapamil has been shown to be effective against jellyfish cardiotoxins in some animal models.[177] The symptoms of Portuguese man-of-war envenomation resolve in approximately 3 days. However, post inflammatory changes may last for months. Tetanus prophylaxis should be current.[170] Preventive measures include avoiding infested waters or wearing a body suit made of thin nylon or Lycra.[178]

The Irukandji syndrome is a group of delayed severe systemic symptoms occurring after an initial mild skin sting by the box jellyfish. It is well known in tropical Australian waters, and is notable for the unusually high numbers of victims with severe toxic heart failure and other systemic problems. Frequently, these patients require intensive care, but to date there have been no deaths reported. There may be more than one species of jellyfish causing this syndrome.[179]

Venomous Fish

Bony fish. Venomous bony fish include the lion fish, scorpion fish, cat fish, weaverfish, and stone fish. These fish inject their venom by a dorsal spine, and their toxin may remain potent for up to 24 hours after death.[170] The most poisonous bony fish are found in the Indo-Pacific ocean.[162]

Cutaneous reactions are characterized by local redness, ecchymosis, severe pain, weakness, and paralysis.[162]

Because the venom is heat labile, hot water immersion is therapeutically beneficial.[162] The wound should be irrigated with warm saline; all slime and debris should be removed, and it should be left open. Prophylaxis with imipenem-cilastatin, trimethoprim-sulfamethoxazole, cefoperazone, or tetracycline is recommended if the lesions are deep and present on the hands or feet.[180] Antivenom may be required when reactions are severe and is available through Sea World in San Diego, Sharp Cabrillo Hospital in San Diego, and the Steinhart Aquarium in San Francisco.[181]

Sea snakes. Sea snakes are found in the Indo-Pacific Ocean and in the Gulf of California. There are no sea snakes in the Atlantic Ocean or the Caribbean.[161,182] The venom of the sea snake is a neurotoxin that is injected through short fangs. This toxin is more potent than any found in terrestrial snakes.[161,182]

Signs and symptoms of envenomation occur within 5 to 10min after the bite.[170] One to four hypodermic punctures are found. Painful, stiff muscles and myoglobinuria are characteristically seen.[161] An ascending paralysis, which may cause death, may result.[162]

Therapy consists of immobilizing the affected limb and maintaining it in a dependent position while keeping the patient quiet and warm.[161,164,183,184] This helps to localize the venom and decrease its systemic distribution until it is less potent.[161,183,184] Polyvalent antivenom is available from the Commonwealth Serum Laboratory in Australia and is indicated for envenomation.[178] Incision and suction therapy for snake bites remains controversial.

Stingrays. Stingrays are the most commonly encountered venomous fish.[162] Approximately 2000 stings are reported annually.[170] They usually burrow in the sand and inject their venom through a serrated, barbed tail. The resulting wound is a laceration usually to the lower extremities.[170]

These stings are best prevented by shuffling feet when walking, allowing the fish to swim away.[162] Once envenomation has occurred, cold water should be applied immediately along with a constriction band followed by soaking in hot water for 30–90min to deactivate the toxin.[170] Pain may be controlled using topical lidocaine. The wound should be packed open, and antibiotic prophylaxis with trimethoprim-sulfamethoxazole or cefoperazone should be given. Corticosteroids have not been found to be efficacious.[180]

Sponges

At least 13 species of sponges cause dermatitis on contact.[162] These sponges have tiny spicules containing silica and calcium and a chemical irritant (crinotoxin), which may cause an acute burning sensation and eczematous lesions.[168] Papules and plaques may remain for months. Erythema multiforme and anaphylaxis have been reported after contact with the *Fibula* species.[161]

Treatment consists of removal of foreign spicules with adhesive tape.[170] Topical acetic acid (vinegar) soaks or isopropyl alcohol should be applied three times daily.[163,185] Erythema multiforme and severe allergic reactions may require systemic corticosteroids.[163] Tetanus immunization should be current.

Echinoderms

Sea urchins. There are 6000 species of sea urchins; 80 are known to be poisonous or venomous.[161] These spiny animals passively deliver a mild toxin. Penetration of spines into the skin produces major injury and may result in infections by marine organisms or lacerations of deeper structures.[186] Hand lesions are serious.[187] In general, these injuries are painful. Irritation from residual fragments may ultimately result in a granulomatous reaction.[170] In severe cases, cellulitis, and synovitis may occur.

Treatment consists of immediate hot water immersion, careful removal of embedded spines, and prevention of cellulitis or synovitis by debridement.[161] Infection is common, and prophylactic antibiotic therapy is recommended.[161,180] Wearing shoes while walking/wading in shallow water is the best preventive measure.[162]

Starfish. Only a few starfish are venomous.[162] These echinoderms inject their toxin through dorsal spines, resulting in a painful penetrating injury and mild systemic signs and symptoms. Envenomation responds to hot water immersion soaks.[163] The puncture wound should be irrigated and thouroughly explored to remove all foreign material. A contact dermatitis from handling the starfish may occur. This responds to topical agents such as calamine and 0.5% menthol or corticosteroids.[163,164,180] Systemic therapy, if required, is supportive.[164]

169. Burnett JW, Gable WD (1989) A fatal jellyfish envenomation by the Portuguese man-of-war. **Toxicon** 27:823.
170. Brown CK, Shepherd SM (1992) Marine trauma, envenomations and intoxications. **Emerg Med Clin North Am** 10:385.
171. Fisher AA (1984) Toxic versus allergic reactions to jellyfish. **Cutis** 34:450.
172. Turner B, Sullivan P (1983) Disarming the bluebottle: treatment of *Physalia* envenomation. **South Med J** 76:870.
173. Kaufman M (1992) Portuguese man-of-war envenomations. **Pediatr Emerg Care** 8:27.
174. Auerbach PS, Halstead B (1982) Marine hazards: attacks and envenomations. **J Emerg Nurs** 8:115.
175. Burnett JW, Rubinstein H, Calton GJ (1983) First aid for jellyfish envenomation. **South Med J** 76:870.
176. Hartwick R, Callanan V, Williamson J (1980) Disarming the box jellyfish: nematocyst inhibition in chronic fleckeri. **Med J Aust** 1:15.
177. Burnett JW, Gean CJ, Calton GJ, Warnick JE (1985) The effect of verapamil on the cardiotoxic activity of Portuguese Man o'War (*Physalia physalis*) and sea nettle (*Chrysaora quinquecirrha*) venoms. **Toxicom** 23(4):681–689.

178. Fenner P (1987) Marine envenomations. **Aust Fam Physician** 16:93.
179. Fenner P, Carney I (1999) The Irukandji syndrome. A devastating syndrome caused by an Australian jellyfish. **Aust Fam Physician** 26(11):1131–1137.
180. Auerbach PS (1989) Stings of the deep. **Emerg Med** 30:27.
181. Kizer KW, McKinney HE, Auerbach PS (1985) Scorpaenidae envenomations: a five year poison center experience. **JAMA** 253:807.
182. Johnson L (1980) A review of bites and stings by venomol animals of southern California. Part II. Arthropods and marine animals. **STAT** 2:16.
183. Tu AT (1987) Biotoxicology of sea snake venoms. **Ann Emerg Med** 16:1023.
184. Burnett JW, Calton GJ, Burnett HW (1986) Jellyfish envenomation syndromes. **J Am Acad Dermatol** 14:100.
185. Burnett JW, Calton GJ, Morgan RJ (1987) Dermatitis due to stinging sponges. **Cutis** 39:476.
186. Fenner PJ, Williamson JA, Burnett JW et al. (1988) The "Irukandji syndrome" and acute pulmonary edema. **Med J Aust** 149:150.

Sea cucumber. Handling a sea cucumber may result in a dermatitis and conjunctivitis caused by the holothurin compound on the surface of the echinoderm.[164,180] Even swimming near sea cucumbers may cause symptoms as a result of high concentrations of the holothurin compound in the water.[170] Blindness can occur if the cornea is contacted and injured.[163,164,178] Ingestion of the sea cucumber may cause death because holothurin is a potent cardiac glycoside.[180] Immediate washing with soap and hot water and topical 5% acetic acid (vinegar) or 40–70% isopropyl alcohol diminishes symptoms.[164,178] Topical or systemic corticosteroids may be needed in severe reactions.[164] If eye involvement has occurred, copious irrigation and referral to an ophthalmologist are required.[178]

Coral

Coral cuts are probably the most commonly sustained underwater injury.[164] These wounds are often complicated by the presence of foreign material, envenomation from small nematocysts, and inoculation with abundant microorganisms.[186] As a result, these wounds tend to heal poorly, may result in granulomas, and may scar.[163] Treatment consists of thorough cleansing with hydrogen peroxide, debridement, and topical chloramphenicol or tetracycline. Wounds that appear infected should be cultured and treated with oral antibiotics.

Seaweed and algae

Seaweed and algae may produce a dermatitis caused by contact with an, as yet, unidentified toxin.[163] Seaweed dermatitis occurs most commonly while the patient is swimming near beaches with an unusually large amount of seaweed both on the beach and in the water.[187] As in seabather's eruption, pruritic vesicles occur in the bathing suit distribution.[187,188] Vigorous washing and cool compresses are useful therapeutic measures.[163] Severe dermatitis may require systemic corticosteroids.[187] Prevention involves immediate showering with soap and water and washing the swimsuit after swimming in seaweed-laden water.

Aquatic dermatitis

Cercarial dermatitis (swimmer's itch)

Swimmer's itch occurs in a worldwide distribution. In the United States, it is found most frequently in the north central region and occurs most commonly in fresh waters and during the warmer months.[189,190] This condition is also known as clam digger's itch, bather's itch,[191] paddy field dermatitis and Cardiff's tropical disease.[192]

Cercarial dermatitis occurs as a result of an infestation by avian cercariae, a larval form of animal schistosomes, which has a two-host cercariae life cycle.[189,190] The snail is the intermediate host, and most cercariae complete their life cycle in animals: ducks, cows, sheep, or rodents. Human beings become dead-end hosts when they are accidentally penetrated. Once the cercariae penetrate the human host, they die, but their presence results in a dermatitis.

Clinically, a transient pruritic dermatitis develops (Fig. 29.21). In contrast to seabathers' eruption, this reaction usually involves exposed skin.[162,190] In previously unaffected hosts, there is an irritant reaction consisting of 1- to 2-mm macules, lasting approximately 10h.[193] The reaction is often so mild it goes unnoticed. In sensitized hosts, the cutaneous eruption is striking and presents with intense pruritus, vesicles, bullae, and eczematous changes and frequently becomes secondarily infected. There are usually 10 to 30 lesions, with as many as 200 occasionally present. Cercarial dermatitis appears to be a sensitization phenomenon, with accelerated and more intense reactions occurring with each subsequent exposure.[194,195] The differential diagnosis includes impetigo, chickenpox, mosquito or chigger bites, algae-related dermatitis, and scabies.[192]

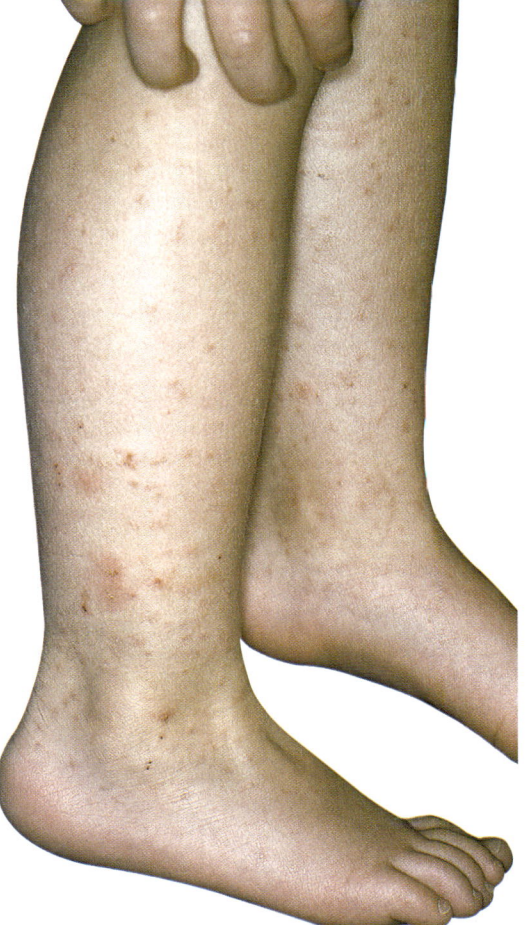

Fig. 29.21   Red papules of swimmer's itch on the exposed skin of the legs of a 6-year-old girl who was swimming in a freshwater lake in Michigan. (Photo courtesy of Anne W. Lucky.)

Treatment consists of antipruritic and anti-inflammatory medications and antibiotics if there is a secondary infection.[189,190] Brisk toweling after swimming may prevent symptoms.[192,196]

Estuary dermatitis

The avian blood fluke, *Austrobilharzia terrigalensis* (Trematoda: Schistosomatidae), has been implicated as the cause of dermatitis among users of the Swan River estuary in Perth, Australia. Most cases are contracted around 12 noon when terrigalensis cercariae emerged from the intermediate host, *Velacumantus australis*, with the resulting dermatitis appearing 12 to 24h later. The lesions, which are sometimes widespread over the body and itch severely, persist for 1–2 weeks systemic finding such as malaise. Somnolence and confusion have been reported in North American Estuary dermatitis. Treatment is similar to that of cercarial dermatitis.

Seabather's eruption

The term "sea lice" has been used synonomously with seabather's eruption by lay persons. This is incorrect as sea lice are parasites of fish and have no relationship to seabather's eruption. Although contact with marine plants, hydroids,

187. Baden DG, Bikhazi G, Decker SJ (1984) Neuromuscular blocking action of two brevitoxins from the Florida red tide organism *Ptychodiscus brevis*. **Toxicon** 22:75.
188. Cooper MA (1981) Treatment of coral cuts in Hawaii. **Hawaii Med J** 40:73.
189. Auerbach PS (1989) Aquatic skin disorders. In: Management of Wilderness and Environmental Emergencies, Auerbach PA, Geehr EC, eds. St. Louis: CV Mosby, p. 933.
190. Izumi AK, Moore RE (1987) Seaweed (*Lyngbya majuscula*) dermatitis. **Clin Dermatol** 5:92.
191. Gonzalez E (1989) Schistosomiasis, cercarial dermatitis, and marine dermatitis. **Dermatol Clin** 7:291.
192. Mulvihill CA, Burnett JW (1990) Swimmer's itch: a cercarial dermatitis. **Cutis** 46:211.
193. Anonymous (1982) Cercarial dermatitis among bathers in California; Katayama syndrome among travelers to Ethiopia. **MMWR Morb Mortal Wkly Rep** 31:435.
194. Narain K, Mahanta J, Dutta R, Dutta P (1994) Paddy field dermatitis in Assam: a cercarial dermatitis. **J Comm Dis** 26(1):26–30.
195. Harding JR (1978) Cardiff's tropical disease: cercarial dermatitis. **Med Hist** 22:83.
196. Cort WW (1928) Schistosome dermatitis in the United States (Michigan). **JAMA** 90:1027.

and corals have all been implicated, more recent studies have identified the etiologic agent of this eruption to be the cnidarian larvae of the sea anemone or Portuguese man-of-war.[202–204] In south Florida and the Caribbean, the thimble jellyfish (*Linuche ungucalata*) is the etiologic organism.[203,204] It was recently found that all three swimming stages of *Linuche* can cause the eruption.[205] In New York, seabather's eruption is caused by *Edwarsiella lineata*, a cnidarian that does not inhabit the waters south of North Carolina.[202] Therefore, the specific cnidarian larval organism seems to vary geographically.[203,204]

Cutaneous lesions are usually limited to areas covered by the swimsuit, bathing cap, wet suit, and/or fins.[202–206] Uncovered areas subject to friction such as the chest of surfers have also been involved.[203,204] The eruption consists of severely pruritic macules and papules that appear up to 2h after exposure (Fig. 29.22).[203,204] These lesions may evolve into vesicles and pustules.[203] Systemic symptoms, including fatigue, malaise, and lymphadenopathy, are experienced.[206–208] High fever is most often seen in the pediatric population. An increased severity of eruption in patients with underlying atopic dermatitis remains uncertain.[203,209] The differential diagnoses include insect bites, varicella, other viral exanthems, syphilis, or urticaria from other sources.[204] The high fever seen in children may lead to inappropriate and unnecessary diagnostic evaluations to rule out meningitis.

Treatment with high-potency topical and oral corticosteroids and antihistamines has yielded variable results.[203,204] The dermatitis usually resolves spontaneously within 2 weeks. Precautions swimmers may take to avoid acquiring this eruption include not wearing a T-shirt and, for women, wearing a two-piece suit. In addition, the swimsuit should be changed as soon as possible after exiting the water, and once an infection has occurred the

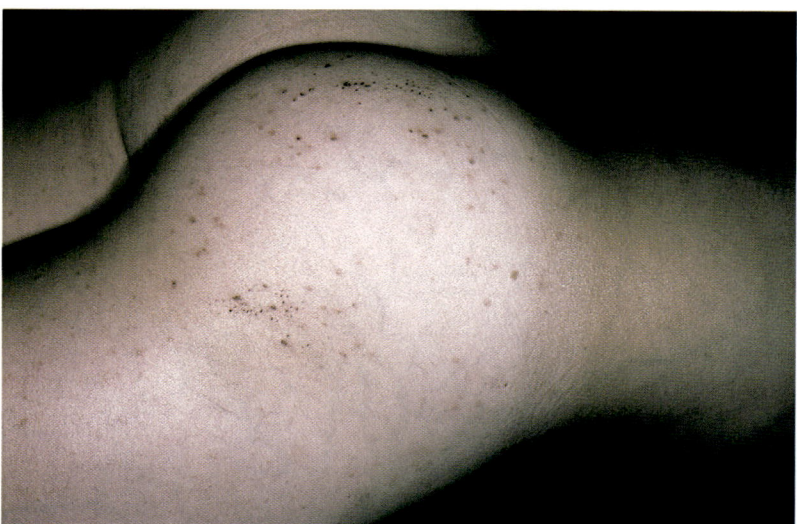

Fig. 29.22 Erythematous papules located under the bathing suit of a 13-year-old boy who was swimming in Florida, typical of seabather's eruption. (Photo courtesy of Anne W. Lucky.)

affected swimming attire should be discarded. Children and persons with allergies, autoimmune diseases, or other immune-mediated conditions may be at risk for severe or unusual reactions and should therefore exercise caution when there are outbreaks.[204]

Dogger Bank itch (coral dermatitis)

Dogger Bank itch, also known as coral dermatitis, is an allergic eczematous eruption secondary to a marine bryozoan *Alcyonidium gelatinosum* or *A. hirsutum*, which grow in spongelike or coraline colonies along the rocks and shells in the shallow waters of the North Sea and the Mediterranean Sea.[191,210–212]

A chronic eczematous dermatitis may develop that evolves through four stages: an acute urticarial phase, followed by a vesiculobullous dermatitis, a subacute granulomatous dermatitis, and lastly a lichenoid dermatitis.[210] This results from a cell-mediated hypersensitivity reaction to a hapten identified as (2-hydroxyethyl) dimethylsufoxonium ion, a metabolite isolated from these organisms.

Therapy with oral or topical corticosteroids and antihistamines has been successful in relieving the associated symptoms of acute lesions.[210] The lichenoid eruption runs a prolonged course in spite of therapy.

Red tide dermatitis

Red tide is a worldwide natural phenomenon caused by dinoflagellates.[213,214] These are flagellated protozoans that belong to the order Mastigophora. When conditions are right, their numbers can be so great they discolor the water red. Red tides have been associated with paralytic shellfish poisoning in humans.[212] *Gonyaulax breve* red tides result in respiratory paralysis in fish and, consequently, massive fish kills. *G. breve* also causes a syndrome consisting of severe conjunctivitis and upper respiratory irritation in persons living on or visiting the beach during a red tide.[213] This is thought to be due to aerosolization of the *G. breve* toxins in the ocean spray.[214] The symptoms resolve once exposure is stopped, and there are no lasting effects. Outbreaks of red tide may also be associated with an acute urticarial and papular eruption. Treatment is symptomatic with topical corticosteroids and oral antihistamines.[215]

AQUATIC INFECTIONS

Vibrio species

Vibrio are part of the United States coastal flora and are an established source of extraintestinal infection.[170] These organisms are endemic to the Gulf of Mexico and are potential pathogens for severe wound infections, bacteremia, and sepsis.[216] Infections are contracted by swimming in brackish water, sustaining lacerations while swimming, and/or handling seafood during the warmer months of April through October.

Vibrio vulnificus may produce a pustular bullous eruption, which may progress to a life-threatening necrotizing invasive wound infection, with rapidly progressive fasciitis and septicemia.[216,217] Persons with underlying chronic diseases such as diabetes, leukemia, chronic renal failure, steroid-dependent asthma, and especially chronic liver disease are at an increased risk

197. Cort WW (1950) Studies on schistosome dermatitis: status of knowledge after more than twenty years. **Am J Hyg** 52:251.
198. Brackett S (1940) Pathology of schistosome dermatitis. **Arch Derm Syph** 42:410.
199. Baired JK, Wear DJ (1987) Cercarial dermatitis: the swimmer's itch. **Clin Dermatol** 5:88.
200. Appleton CC, Lethbridge RC (1979) Schistosome dermatitis in the Swan Estuary, Western Australia. **Med J Aust** 1(5):141–145.
201. Pike AW (1989) Sea lice – major pathogens of farmed Atlantic salmon. **Parasitol Today** 5:291.
202. Freudental AR (1991) Seabather's eruption: range extended northward and a causative organism identified. **Rev Int Oceanograph Med** 101:137.
203. Wong DE, Meinking TL, Rosen LB et al. (1994) Seabather's eruption: clinical, histological and immunological features. **J Am Acad Dermatol** 30:399.
204. Tomchik RS, Russell MT, Szmant AM, Black NA (1993) Clinical perspectives on seabather's eruption, also known as sea lice. **JAMA** 269:1669.
205. Segura-Puertas L, Ramos ME et al. (2001) One *Linuche* mystery solved: All three stages of the coronate syphomedusa *Linuche unguiclata* cause seabather's eruption. **J Am Acad Dermatol** 44(4):624–628.

206. Sams WM (1949) Seabather's eruption. **Arch Dermatol** 60:227.
207. Strauss JS (1956) Seabather's eruption. **Arch Dermatol** 74:293.
208. Moschella SL (1951) Further clinical observations on seabather's eruption. **Arch Dermatol** 64:55.
209. Diepgen TL, Fartasch M (1992) Recent epidemiological and genetic studies in atopic dermatitis. **Acta Derm Venereol Suppl (Stockh)** 176:13.
210. Addy JH (1991) Red sea coral contact dermatitis. **Int J Dermatol** 30:271.
211. Seville RH (1957) Dogger Bank itch: report of a case. **BMJ** 69:92.
212. Levin OL, Behrman HT (1941) Coral dermatitis. **Arch Derm Syph** 44:600.
213. Bureau of Research, Division of Health (1972) Red Tide, Dinoflagellates, Toxic Shellfish.
214. Music SI, Howell JT, Brumback CL (1973) Red tide: its public health implications. **J Fla Med Assoc** 60:27.
215. Mandojana RM, Sims JK (1987) Miscellaneous dermatoses associated with the aquatic environment. **Clin Dermatol** 5:134.
216. Bonner JR, Coker AS, Berryman CR, Pollock HM (1983) Spectrum of *Vibrio* infections in a Gulf Coast community. **Ann Intern Med** 99:464.
217. Johnson JM, Becker SF, McFarland LM (1985) *Vibrio vulnificus*: man and the sea. **JAMA** 253:2850.

of sepsis,[170,218,219] possibly as a result of decreased phagocytic function.[216] The other *Vibrio* species, *V. alginolyticus* and *V. damsela*, may produce moderate to severe wound and ear infections.[220,221]

Therapy involves aggressive wound care, including débridement to remove foreign bodies, drainage of abscesses, irrigation with saline and/or antiseptic solution, and systemic antibiotics such as chloramphenicol or tetracycline plus an aminoglycoside.[218,222] Tetanus immunization status should be current.

Chromobacterium violaceum

C. violaceum is a saprophyte of soil and water in the tropics and subtropics and only rarely causes human infection.[223] This Gram-negative anaerobic bacillus is considered a potential etiologic agent in wound infections of patients exposed to environmental sources of stagnant water (i.e., drainage ditches or ponds).

The organism gains entry through lesions present on the skin (e.g., insect bites).[223] Although rare, this infection is potentially rapidly progressive and life threatening. Interestingly, an association between *C. violaceum* infection and chronic granulomatous disease has been made.[224]

Patients present with fever, abdominal pain, nausea, vomiting, and diarrhea. Liver, spleen, and lung abscesses and osteomyelitis may occur. The skin manifestations are due to systemic involvement and include vesicles, pustules, ulcers, lymphangitis, and digital gangrene.[189]

C. violaceum may be cultured from both the blood and pustules.[189] Treatment involves intravenous aminoglycosides followed by at least 4 weeks of tetracycline or trimethoprim-sulfamethoxazole.[223]

Aeromonas hydrophila

A. hydrophila is a Gram-negative organism that is found in water and soil.[225] Water-associated *Aeromonas* infections have been reported in fresh waters after puncture by a fish bone or scale, crustacean shells, and other immersion injuries.[225–227]

Signs of infection occur within 8 to 48h after the injury. Infection is rapidly progressive with the development of a myositis, tendonitis, osteomyelitis, and/or fasciitis.[225,228–230]

Appropriate therapy includes a third-generation cephalosporin or aminoglycosides, chloramphenicol, trimethoprim-sulfamethoxazole, aztreonam, tetracycline, or ciprofloxacin.[225,231–233] Because of the microbiologic similarity of *Aeromonas* to the Enterobacteriaceae family, the laboratory should be alerted as to the clinical setting.[189]

Pseudomonas species

Swimmer's ear, otherwise known as otitis externa, is an inflammation of the auricle, external ear canal, and/or the outer surface of the tympanic membrane.[234] Otitis externa results from the combination of moisture, warmth, excess cerumen,[234] and *Pseudomonas* species, the most common etiologic organisms.[234,235] However, *Achromobacter xylosoxidans* has been identified as the causative organism in a large number of cases of otitis externa in Hawaii.[236]

Clinically, the external auditory canal is red and painful and may have a pustular exudate.[237] Therapy consists of a solution of polymyxin B, neomycin, and hydrocortisone.[162] Acetic acid (7% solution) and ethanol (93% solution) may also be useful and are associated with fewer side effects. Pain relief may be achieved through topical lidocaine or benzocaine.[237] Swimmer's ear may be prevented by using a hair dryer and ethanol (93% solution) drops after swimming to dry any moisture that may be present.[162]

Pseudomonal folliculitis (hot tub folliculitis) is most commonly acquired through the use of hot tubs and whirlpools[238] and, to a lesser extent, swimming pools,[239,240] home showers,[241] contaminated sponges,[242] diving suits,[243] after depilation,[244] and water slides.[245] The largest reported outbreak to date was in a water park in Salt Lake City, Utah, where 265 persons were infected in association with the use of a water slide.[245] Pseudomonal folliculitis that is recreationally acquired is most commonly caused by serotype 0:11.[193] Other serotypes include 0:1, 0:4, 0:6, 0:7, 0:9, and 0:10. Factors that contribute to the infection include high water temperature, turbulence, aeration, heavy bather load, the ubiquitous distribution of *Pseudomonas aeruginosa*, and the ability of this organism to withstand low concentration of chlorine and to multiply rapidly in water at high temperatures.[240,246–248] Occlusion promotes pseudomonal infection.[247] Thus, tight-fitting bathing suits and one-piece suits are associated with a greater risk of infection.[247,248] In addition, swim suits worn for long periods after infection may increase severity.[239] Topical occlusive oils are not considered to be a factor.[248]

Clinically, the dermatosis is characterized by follicular papules and pustules, which are usually in the bathing suit distribution (Fig. 29.23).[240] Associated symptoms include otitis externa, pharyngitis, conjunctivitis, lymphadenopathy, rhinitis, mastitis, headaches, chills, and low-grade fevers.[239,240,245,246]

There is no specific treatment for pseudomonal folliculitis.[249] This is usually a self-limited dermatosis, however, symptoms may persist for weeks, and can be recurrent. Topical and systemic corticosteroids are to be avoided because they may worsen the eruption.[249] Disorders such as otitis externa, otitis media,

218. Klontz KC, Lieb S, Schreiber M et al. (1988) Syndromes of *Vibrio vulnificans* infection: clinical and epidemiological features in Florida cases, 1981–1987. **Ann Intern Med** 109:318.

219. Morris JG Jr (1988) *Vibrio vulnificans* – a new monster of the deep (editorial)? **Ann Intern Med** 109:261.

220. Pien FD, Lee K, Higa H (1977) *Vibrio alginolyticus* infections in Hawaii. **J Clin Microbiol** 5:670.

221. Morris JG, Jr, Miller HG, Wilson R et al. (1982) Illness caused by *Vibrio damsela* and *Vibrio hollisae*. **Lancet** 1:1294.

222. Morris JG, Jr, Black RE (1985) Cholera and other vibrioses in the United States. **N Engl J Med** 312:343.

223. Ponte R, Jenkins SG (1992) Fatal *Chromobacterium violaceum* infections associated with exposure to stagnant waters. **Pediatr Infect Dis J** 11:583.

224. Machler AM, Casale TB, Fauci AS (1982) Chronic granulomatous disease of childhood and *Chromobacterium violaceum* infections in the southeastern United States. **Ann Intern Med** 97:51.

225. Semel JD, Trenholme G (1990) *Aeromonas hydrophila* water associated traumatic wound infections: a review. **J Trauma** 30:324.

226. Winslow DL, Jones R (1984) Severe cellulitis due to *Aeromonas hydrophila* following immersion injury. **Del Med J** 56:361.

227. Deepe GS, Coonrod JD (1980) Fulminant wound infection with *Aeromonas hydrophila*. **South Med J** 73:1546.

228. Champagne KJ, Sanders CV, Hastings PR (1989) *Aeromonas hydrophila* in water and soil contaminated injuries. **Infect Surg** 8:139.

229. Karam GH, Ackley AM, Dismukes WE (1983) Post traumatic *Aeromonas hydrophila* osteomyelitis. **Arch Intern Med** 143:2073.

230. Smith JA (1980) *Aeromonas hydrophila*: analysis of 11 cases. **Can Med Assoc J** 122:1270.

231. Fainstein V, Weaver S, Bodey GP (1982) In vitro susceptibilities of *Aeromonas hydrophila* against new antibiotics. **Antimicrob Agents Chemother** 22:513.

232. Motyl MR, McKinley G, Janda JM (1985) In vitro susceptibilities of *Aeromonas hydrophila*, *Aeromonas sobria* and *Aeromonas caviae* to 23 antimicrobial agents. **Antimicrob Agents Chemother** 28:151.

233. Reinhardt JF, George WL (1985) Comparative in vitro activities of selected antimicrobial agents against *Aeromonas* species and *Plesiomonas shingelloides*. **Antimicrob Agents Chemother** 27:643.

234. Marcy SM (1985) Infections of the external ear. **Pediatr Infect Dis** 4:192.

235. Hoadley AW, Knight DE (1975) External otitis among swimmers and non-swimmers. **Arch Environ Health** 30:445.

236. Pien FD, Higa HY (1978) *Achromobacter xylosoxidans* isolates in Hawaii. **J Clin Microbiol** 7:239.

237. Chang WJ, Pien FD (1986) Marine-acquired infections: hazards of the ocean environment. **Marine Infect** 80:30.

238. Ratnam S, Hogan K, March S, Butler R (1986) Whirlpool associated folliculitis caused by *Pseudomonas aeruginosa*: report of an outbreak and review. **J Clin Microbiol** 23:655.

239. Fox AB, Hambrick GW (1984) Recreationally associated *Pseudomonas aeruginosa* folliculitis: report of an epidemic. **Arch Dermatol** 120:1304.

240. Gustafson TL, Band JD, Hutcheson RH, Jr, Schaffner W (1983) Pseudomonas folliculitis: an outbreak and review. **Rev Infect Dis** 5:1.

241. Huminer D, Shmuely H, Block C, Pitlik SD (1989) Home shower-bath *Pseudomonas* folliculitis. **Isr J Med Sci** 25:44.

242. Kitamua M, Kawai S, Horio T (1998) *Pseudomonas aeruginosa* folliculitis: a sporadic case from use of a contaminated sponge. **Br J Dermatol** 139(2):359–360.

243. Saltzer KR, Schutzer PJ, Weinberg JM et al. (1997) Diving suit dermatitis: a manifestation of Pseudomonas folliculitis. **Cutis** 50(5):245–246.

244. De La Cuadra J, Gil-Mateo P, Llucian R (1996) *Pseudomonas aeruginosa* folliculitis after depilation. **Ann Dermatol Benereol** 123(4):268–270.

245. Perrotta DM, Johns RE, Jr, Bradley R et al. (1983) An outbreak of Pseudomonas folliculitis associated with a waterslide – Utah. **JAMA** 250:1259.

246. McCutchan J, Rutala WA, Holdway R et al. (1983) Otitis due to *Pseudomonas aeruginosa* serotype 0:10 associated with a mobile redwood hot tub system – North Carolina. **MMWR** 31:541.

247. Salem P, Dwyer DM, Vorse H, Kruse W (1983) Whirlpool-associated *Pseudomonas aeruginosa* urinary tract infections. **JAMA** 250:2025.

248. Vogt RD, LaRue D, Parry MF et al. (1982) *Pseudomonas aeruginosa* skin infections in persons using a whirlpool in Vermont. **J Clin Microbiol** 15:571.

249. Gregory DW, Schaffner W (1987) Pseudomonas infections associated with hot tubs and other environments. **Infect Dis Clin North Am** 1:635.

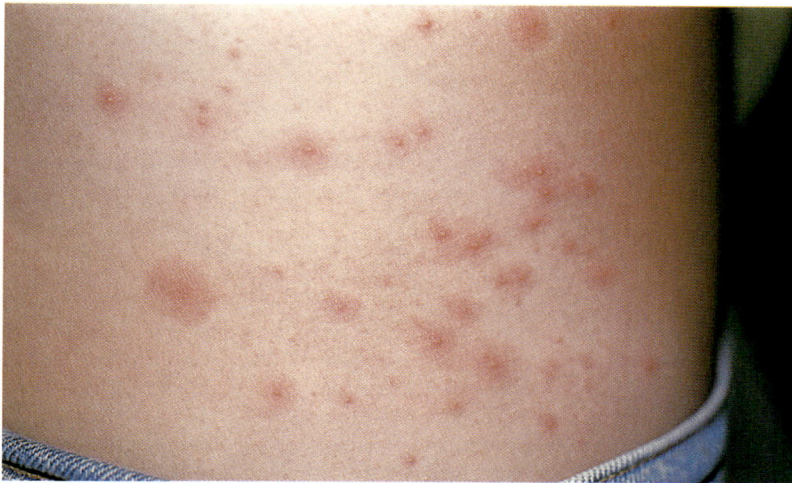

Fig. 29.23 Pseudomonas folliculitis. Note erythema surrounding follicular papules.

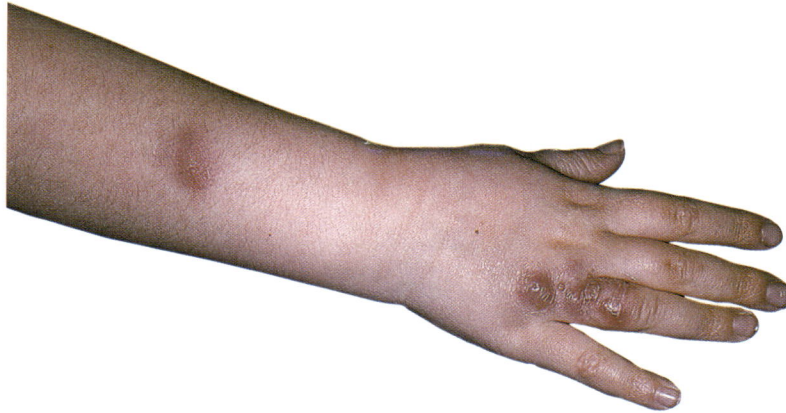

Fig. 29.24 Sporotrichoid spread of *Mycobacterium marinum* on the arm of a 6-year-old girl who cleaned her fish tank. (Photo courtesy of Anne W. Lucky.)

urinary tract infections, and pneumonia may also be acquired through the use of whirlpools and should be treated appropriately.

Prevention may be accomplished through unflagging attention to chlorination (levels should be 0.5mg/l) or bromination and maintaining the pH between 7.2 and 7.8.[250] Some authors advocate the need to culture water for *P. aeruginosa* routinely.[238]

Mycobacterium marinum

Swimming pool granuloma is caused by *M. marinum*, which may inhabit fresh or salt water, including fish tanks and swimming pools. This organism gains entry through open wounds and may be associated with ascending sporotrichoidlike lesions or disseminated infection (Fig. 29.24).[162] Activation of cutaneous sarcoidosis following mycobacterium marinum of the skin has been reported.[251] The diagnosis is best made histologically and by culture. Treatment involves surgical wound debridement and antibiotic therapy with minocycline for 2 to 4 months.[162]

WATER-INDUCED PRURITUS

Aquagenic urticaria, a rarely encountered physical urticaria,[252,253] provokes follicular pruritic wheals with surrounding redness in skin areas in contact with water of any temperature.[252,254] The mechanism may involve acetylcholinesterase because scopolamine applied topically abolishes wheal formation.[251] Another hypothesis suggests wet sebum may act as an inciting allergen.

Treatment may include the application of inert skin oils, or barrier creams before contact with water and/or oral antihistamines.[252,253] PUVA and astemizole have been used as treatments.[255] Cyproheptadine and promethazine hydrochloride have been reported to be more efficacious than chlorpheniramine maleate and hydroxyzine hydrochloride.[252]

Aquagenic pruritus is a disorder of water-induced itching without signs of urticaria, eczema, or other skin lesions.[256] The pathophysiology is unknown; however, cutaneous fibrinolytic activity is elevated in these patients, and acetylcholine release may also play a role.[257,258] Aquagenic pruritus may be the presenting symptom of idiopathic hypereosinophila,[259] juvenile xanthgranuloma,[260] acute lymphoblastic leukemia,[261] myelodysplastic syndrome,[262] metastatic squamous cell,[263] or polycythemia rubra vera.[264,265]

There is no consistently effective treatment for aquagenic pruritus.[258] Complete avoidance of water is the best therapy but is impractical. Antihistamines are only marginally effective. UVB, topical capsaicin,[266] alcohol,[267] PUVA,[268] and propanalol[269] have been used with some success.[256] Scopolamine has reduced symptoms but has undesirable side effects.[258] Sodium bicarbonate (25–200g) added to the bath water has relieved symptoms in many patients and remains the most effective and safe treatment for patients to date.[270–272]

HUMAN-MADE AQUATIC HAZARDS
Contact dermatitis

Masks, wet suits, goggles, snorkels, bathing caps, and other articles may produce an allergic contact dermatitis in rubber sensitive individuals.[273–276] Irritant

250. David BJ (1985) Whirlpool operation and the prevention of infection. **Infect Control Hosp Epidomiol** 6:394.
251. Gudit VS, Campbell SM, Gould D, Marshall R, Winterton MC (2000) Activation of cutaneous sarcoidosis following *Mycobacterium marinum* infection of skin. **J Eur Acad Dermatol Verereol** 14(4):296–297.
252. Burrall BA, Halpern GM, Huntley AC (1990) Chronic urticaria. **West J Med** 152:268.
253. Horan RF, Sheffer AL, Briner WW (1992) Physical allergies. **Med Sci Sports Exerc** 24:845.
254. Greaves MW (1981) Urticaria: new approaches of investigation and management. **Aust J Dermatol** 22:47.
255. Martinez-Escribano JA, Quecedo E, De la Cuadra J et al. (1997) Treatment of aquagenic urticaria with PUVA and astemizole. **J Am Acad Dermatol** 36(1):118–119.
256. Steinman HK, Greaves MD (1985) Aquagenic pruritus. **J Am Acad Dermatol** 13:91.
257. Lotti T, Steinman H, Greaves M et al. (1986) Increased cutaneous fibrinolytic activity in aquagenic pruritus. **Int J Dermatol** 25:508.
258. Bircher A, Meier-Ruge W (1988) Aquagenic pruritus. Water induced activation of acetylcholinesterase. **Arch Dermatol** 124:84.
259. Newton JA, Singh AK, Greaves et al. (1990) Aquagenic pruritus associated with the idiopathic hypereosinophilic syndrome. **Br J Dermatol** 122(1):103–106.
260. Handfield-Jones SE, Hills RJ et al. (1993) Aquagenic pruritus associated with juvenile xanthogranulomas. **Clin Exp Dermatol** 18(3):253–255.
261. Ratnaval RC, Burrows NP et al. (1993) Aquagenic pruritus and acute lymphoblastic leukaemia. **Br J Dermatol** 129(3):348–349.
262. McGrath JA, Greaves MW (1990) Aquagenic pruritus and the myelodysplastic syndrome. **Br J Dermatol** 123(3):414–415.

263. Ferguson JE, August PJ, Guy AJ (1994) Aquagenic pruritus associated with metastatic squamous cell carcinoma of the cervix. **Clin Exp Dermatol** 19(3):257–258.
264. Fjellner B, Hagermark O (1979) Pruritus in polycythemia vera: treatment with aspirin and possibility of platelet involvement. **Acta Derm Venerol** (Stockh) 59:505.
265. Archer C, Camp R, Greaves M (1988) Polycythaemia vera can present with aquagenic pruritus. **Lancet** 1:1451.
266. Lotti T, Teofoli P, Tsampau D (1994) Treatment of aquagenic pruritus with topical capsaicin cream. **J Am Acad Dermatol** 30:232–235.
267. Norris JF (1998) Treatment of aquagenic pruritus with alcohol. **Br J Dermatol** 139(5):927.
268. Holme SA, Anstey AV (2001) Aquagenic pruritus responding to intermittent photochemotherapy. **Clin Exp Dermatol** 26(1):40–41.
269. Thomsen K (1990) Aquagenic pruritus responds to propanolol. **J Am Acad Dermatol** 22(4):697.
270. Bayoumi A, Highet A (1986) Baking soda baths for aquagenic pruritus. **Lancet** 2:464.
271. Wolf R, Krakowsly A (1988) Variations in aquagenic pruritus and treatment alternatives. **J Am Acad Dermatol** 18:1081.
272. Meunier L, Levy A, Costes Y, Maeynadier J (1988) Idiopathic aquagenic pruritus treated with the addition of sodium bicarbonate to bath water (letter). **Presse Med** 17:962.
273. Maibach H (1975) Scuba diver facial dermatitis: allergic contact dermatitis to *N*-isopropyl-*N*- phenylparaphenylenediamine. **Contact Dermatitis** 1:330.
274. Tuyp E, Mitchell JC (1983) Scuba diver facial dermatitis. **Contact Dermatitis** 9:334.
275. Taylor J (1984) Contact dermatitis from goggles. Presented at the Patch Test Symposium, American Academy of Dermatology Meeting, Washington, DC, December, 1984.
276. Fisher AA (1986) Contact Dermatitis, 3rd edn. Philadelphia: Lea & Febiger.

reactions are also described. Defogging agents may produce conjunctivitis if the mask is not allowed to dry before wearing. The pattern and distribution of the lesions help in making the correct diagnosis. However, patch testing is necessary to make a definitive diagnosis.[277] Treatment includes topical corticosteroids, antihistamines, and Burow's solution soaks.[162] Oral corticosteroids may be required in severe reactions. Preventive measures include the use of silicone gear and nylon substitutes.[162]

Pool palms is a recently described clinical entity in which children present with red to violaceous macules and patches on the palmar aspect of the hands and usually limited to the distal fingerpads after coming into contact with the swimming pool surfaces. (Fig. 29.25).[278] Blisters may occur. This self-limiting condition, which is thought to be a consequence of friction and possibly an irritant contact dermatitis, resolves within a few weeks once contact with these surfaces is eliminated.[278]

Decompression sickness

The cutaneous manifestations of decompression sickness are known as the "skin bends." Symptoms usually present on surfacing or within 4h and consist of intense pruritus[162,279] and the presence of a livedo pattern which may herald systemic symptoms.[279] These cutaneous findings are caused by nitrogen

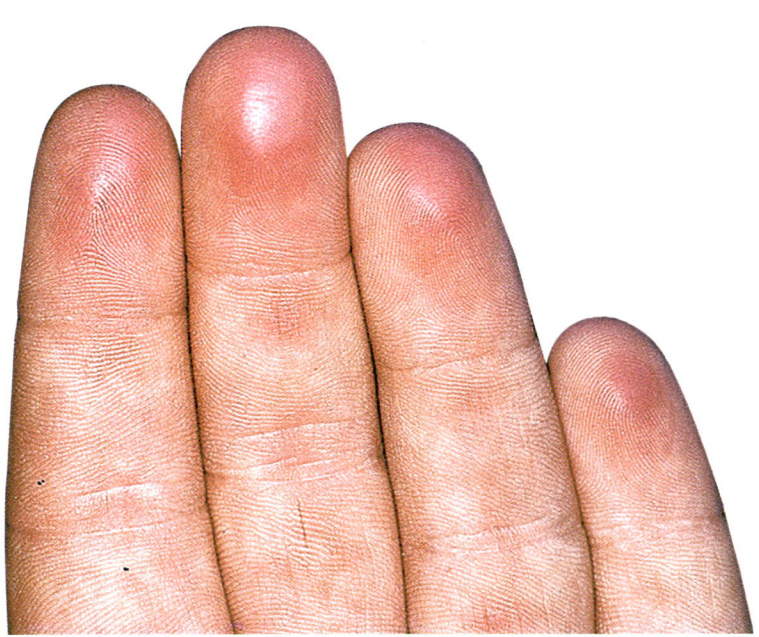

Fig. 29.25   Red, shiny finger pads in a teenage swimmer who had rubbed her fingertips against the pool wall for several hours practicing flip turns (pool palms). (Photo courtesy of Anne W. Lucky.)

oversaturation and usually resolve over time, although recompression in a hyperbaric recompression chamber may be required.[162]

Aquatic pollutants

The infectious risks of swimming in heavily polluted water are undisputed,[280–283] with typhoid,[284] shigellosis,[285] leptospirosis,[286] and hepatitis A[287] all being well documented, as are other skin, gastrointestinal, ear, eye, and respiratory infections.[288,289] The most commonly seen illness is an acute benign gastroenteritis,[290] which may be associated with Norwalk virus,[291] rotavirus,[292] or coxsackievirus.[293]

The microbiologic criteria used for establishing the safety of recreational marine waters varies. *Escherichia coli* remains the best indicator of overall health effects of swimming in polluted beaches in Hong Kong and Egypt.[280] *Staphylococcus* is used as a second indicator. In the United States, enterococci are the best indicators of overall illness. Staphylococci highly correlate with total illness and eye and skin disorders.[283]

In fresh water lakes, *Streptococcus faecalis* is best correlated with gastrointestinal morbidity. Fresh water swimmers have skin ailments associated with the concentration of fecal coliform bacteria, *Aeromonas* and *Pseudomonas*.[280] In swimming pools, microorganisms of the mouth, nose, and skin are more relevant.[294]

OTHER SELECTED NATURALLY OCCURRING HAZARDS

Chulabhorn Pruksachatkunakorn

PLANT-INDUCED CONTACT DERMATITIS

Poison ivy, poison oak, and poison sumac are the plants most commonly associated with allergic contact dermatitis.[295] *Compositae dermatitis* is an allergic contact dermatitis related to the Compositae family of plants (daisy, artichoke, burweed, blackeyed Susan, dandelion, chrysanthemum, sunflower, etc.),[296] and is most often seen in persons who repeatedly come in contact with the plants such as florists or home gardeners.[297] The symptoms usually start in summer and disappear in autumn or winter. An airborne pattern of dermatitis affecting the face, "V" of the neck, hands and forearms is a common presentation. In children, it may present with a localized dermatitis mainly on a dominant hand.[298] Therapy requires thorough washing of the involved area, cool compresses, antihistamines, topical corticosteroids, and, in severe reactions, systemic corticosteroids.

Other plant-induced irritant contact dermatitis usually present with mild pruritus or red, linear wheals that are excoriated.[297] The plants most commonly involved include Euphorbiaceae (Spurge): poinsettia, beach apple,

277. Foussereau J, Tomb R, Cavelier C (1990) Allergic contact dermatitis from safety clothes and individual protective devices. **Dermatol Clin** 8:127.
278. Blauvelt A, Duarte AM, Schachner LA (1992) Pool palms. **J Am Acad Dermatol** 27:111.
279. Jerrard DA (1992) Diving medicine. **Emerg Clin North Am** 10:329.
280. Cheung WHS, Chang KCK, Hung RPS (1990) Health effects of beach water pollution in Hong Kong. **Epidemiol Infect** 105:139.
281. Ferley JP, Zmirou D, Balducci F et al. (1989) Epidemiological significance of microbiological pollution criteria for recreational waters. **Int J Epidemiol** 18:198.
282. Seyfried PL, Tobin RS, Brown NE, Ness PF (1985) A prospective study of swimming-related illness. I. Swimming-associated health risk. **Am J Public Health** 75:1068.
283. Seyfried PL, Tobin RS, Brown NE, Ness PF (1985) A prospective study of swimming-related illness. II. Morbidity and the microbiological quality of water. **Am J Public Health** 75:1071.
284. Craun GF (1992) Waterborne disease outbreaks in the United States of America: causes and prevention. **World Health Stat** 45:192.
285. Rosenberg ML, Hazlet KK, Schaafer J et al. (1976) Shigellosis from swimming. **JAMA** 236:1849.
286. Jackson LA, Kaufman AF, Adams WG et al. (1993) Outbreak of leptospirosis associated with swimming. **Pediatr Infect Dis J** 12:48.
287. Bryan JA, Lehmann JD, Setiady IF, Hatch MH (1974) An outbreak of hepatitis A associated with recreational lake water. **Am J Epidemiol** 99:145.
288. Baron RC, Murphy FD, Greenberg HB et al. (1982) Norwalk gastrointestinal disease: an outbreak associated with swimming in a recreational lake and secondary person-to-person transmission. **Am J Epidemiol** 115:163.
289. Koopman JS, Eckert EA, Greenberg HB et al. (1982) Norwalk virus: enteric illness acquired by swimming exposure. **Am J Epidemiol** 115:173.
290. Cabelli VJ (1977) Indicators of recreational water quality. In: Bacterial Indicators/Health Hazards Associated with Water, Hoadley AW, Dutka BJ, eds. ASTM STP 635. Philadelphia: American Society for Testing and Materials.
291. Cabelli VJ (1983) Health Effects Criteria for Marine Recreational Waters (publication no. EPA-600/1–80–031). Washington DC: US Environmental Protection Agency.
292. Cabelli VJ (1981) Epidemiology of enteric viral infections. In: Viruses and Wastewater Treatment, Goddard M, Butler M, eds. London: Pergamon Press, p. 291.
293. White DO, Fenner F (1986) Medical Virology, 3rd edn. London: Academic Press.
294. Mallmann WL (1962) Cocci test for detecting mouth and nose pollution of swimming pool. **Am J Public Health** 52:2001.
295. Epstein WL, Epstein JH (1989) Emergency treatment of plant-induced dermatitis. In: Management of Wilderness and Environmental Emergencies, Auerbach PS, Geehr EC, eds. St. Louis: CV Mosby, p. 617.
296. Epstein WL (1987) Plant induced dermatitis. **Ann Emerg Med** 16(9):950–955.
297. Perpall A (1992) Selected environmental skin disorders. **Emerg Clin North Am** 10(2):437–448.
298. Wakelin SH, Marren P, Young E et al. (1997) Compositae sensitivity and chronic hand dermatitis in seven-year old boy. **Br J Dermatol** 137(2):289–291.

noseburn, coral plant, milkweed, wolfmilk, croton bush; Ranunculaceae; buttercup, wolfbane, windflower, meadow rue; and Brassicaceae; mustard seed and radishes. Irritation is caused directly by chemicals and/or thorns. The involved chemicals include terpenes, phorbol esters, terpinoids, and thioglycosides.[295]

Treatment includes avoiding the irritating plant, antihistamines, and topical and systemic corticosteroids.[297] An uncomplicated dermatitis usually resolves in a few days.

ARTHROPODS

Bees, wasps, and hornets

The Hymenoptera order of insects consists of two superfamilies: the apids (honeybees) and the vespids (yellow jackets, hornets, and wasps).[299] Approximately 1 to 3% of the population has had a systemic reaction, urticaria, obstruction of the upper or lower airway, and/or hypotension from stings by these insects. Persons who experience such reactions have an increased risk of future systemic reactions. Symptoms of anaphylaxis usually develop within 10min after a sting.[300] It takes more than 50 bees to inflict a lethal dose of venom in a child; however, one sting may cause a fatal anaphylactic reaction in a hypersensitive person. In the United States, there are 25 to 40 deaths yearly attributed to insect sting anaphylaxis.[301]

The major allergenic constituents of honeybee venom are phospholipase A_2, hyaluronidase, and acid phosphatase.[302] The major allergens in vespid venom include phospholipase, hyaluronidase, and antigen 5.[303]

The usual local reaction to the insect sting is mild redness and edema associated with pain at the site. These symptoms usually resolve within hours.[304]

The stingers of many Hymenoptera may remain in the skin and should be removed by teasing or scraping rather than pulling.[304] A cold compress application over the sting area is usually effective in reducing pain. Oral corticosteroids may be required in severe local reactions. The treatment of systemic reactions is identical to the treatment of anaphylaxis and should include epinephrine. Prevention of stings includes avoiding perfumes and bright colored clothing. Repellents are not effective in preventing stings.

Persons with known hypersensitivity to stings should carry an epinephrine kit, ("EpiPen" or "EpiPen Jr." or "Ana-Kit", etc.) be familiar with its use, and wear a bracelet that identifies them as allergic to insect stings.[305] Furthermore, patients who have had a reaction should be assessed by an allergist and evaluated for immune therapy.[299] Desensitization may be carried out using venom immunotherapy, which is 98–99% effective in conferring protection to patients with previous systemic reactions to insect stings.[306] The decision to desensitize is based on the patient's desires, reaction severity, and risk of subsequent stings. Fortunately sting-sensitive individuals tend to lose their sensitivity over time.[299,307]

Fire ants

Fire ants were imported on board ships to the United States in the early 1900s.[304] These ants, the *Solenopsis* species, belong to the order Hymenoptera, and like other ants, live in large colonies. Their mounds may extend 3 ft in diameter, and most are found on soil in fields and playgrounds.

Fire ants inflict their injury in two phases.[304,308,309] First, they bite the victim, and then they swivel their body around their head and sting with their ovipositor aparatus. This results in the characteristic fire ant bite lesion: a circular sting with two central hemorrhagic puncta. These circularly arranged red papules and wheals evolve into vesicles and then pustules (Fig. 29.26). The ants attack in swarms, with as many as 5000 bites reported in one victim. Fatal outcomes are rare, but disfiguring scars, secondary infection, delayed onset of seizures and anaphylaxis have been reported.[310,311]

Local therapy for these bites is symptomatic. Systemic reactions require glucocorticoids and antihistamines. Desensitization may be helpful.[312] The best therapy is avoidance and pest control.[313]

Ticks and mites

Ticks may transmit a variety of human pathogens and are second only to mosquitoes as a vector of human disease.[313] Spotted fever, ehrlichiosis and Lyme disease are known worldwide to be caused by the transmission of infectious agents to humans through the bite of an infected tick.[314–317] Tick bites cause a local vesiculation, pustulation, rupture, ulceration, and eschar, with varying degrees of local swelling and pain. Dermatologic manifestations of arthropod-borne rickettsiosis include maculopapular rash, petechiae, purpura and desquamation. Systemic symptoms including fever, headache and regional lymphadenopathy may also occur.

Mite infestations are common and are responsible for chiggers (an intensely pruritic dermatitis caused by the mite larva or chigger), scabies, demodicidosis, and a number of other diseases. The bites produce varying degrees of local tissue reaction and may transmit scrub typhus.

Avian mite dermatitis has been reported under a variety of names, including gamasoidosis, fowl or bird mite dermatitis and acariasis.[318] *Ornithonyssus sylviarum* and *Dermanyssus gallinae* have been the most commonly identified mites. Avian mites frequently infest domestic poultry or birds nesting in or near human habitation. Most commonly patients had contact with birds, chickens and pigeons. Contact with canaries, sparrows, robins, swallows, tiger finches, parakeets, starlings and white wagtails have been also reported. At night avian mites suck their host blood and leave the host extremely rapidly. During the day they reside in the bedding of nests, in cages or in cracks and crevices of buildings. Humans frequently acquire their infestation from nests found outside the windows and air-conditioners of the houses and offices. Lucky *et al.*[319] recently reported two children with persistent pruritic erythematous papules and identified the mites, *Dermanyssus gallinae* and *Ornithonyssus sylviarum* on pet gerbils, the latter acquired from the chickens kept in the science classroom. Mite infestations most commonly manifest as pruritic papules, with or without a hemorrhagic or punctate center. Vesicles, urticaria and dermatitis may be seen. The lesions occur predominantly on the exposed surfaces in a linear array or in a widespread distribution (Fig. 29.27). The diagnosis is confirmed by identifying the mites on the host animals, cages and the bedding of nests at night. Avian mite bites may have been unrecognized or misdiagnosed as bites from other arthropods such as fleas and scabies mites.

299. Li JT, Yunginger JW (1992) Management of insect sting hypersensitivity. **Mayo Clin Proc** 67(2):188–194.
300. Lockey RF, Turkeltaub PC, Baird-Warren IA et al. (1988) The Hymenoptera venom study I, 1979–1982: demographics and history-sting data. **J Allergy Clin Immunol** 82(3 pt 1):370–381.
301. Barnard JH (1973) Studies of 400 Hymenoptera sting deaths in the United States. **J Allergy Clin Immunol** 52(5):259–264.
302. Franklin R, Baer H (1975) Comparison of honeybee venoms and their components from various sources. **J Allergy Clin Immunol** 55(5):285–298.
303. King TP, Sobotka AK, Alagon A et al. (1978) Protein allergens of white-faced hornet, yellow, hornet, and yellow jacket venoms. **Biochemistry** 17(24):5165–5174.
304. Elgart GW (1990) Ant, bee and wasp stings. **Dermatol Clin** 8(2):229–236.
305. Portnoy JM, Moffitt JE, Golden DB et al. (1999) Stinging insect hypersensitivity: a practice parameter. **J Allergy Clin Immunol** 103 (5 pt 1):963–980.
306. Valentine MD, Lichtenstein LM (1987) Anaphylaxis and stinging insect hypersensitivity. **JAMA** 258(20):2881–2885.
307. Savliwala MN, Reisman RE (1987) Studies of the natural history of stinging-insect allergy: long term follow-up of patients without immunotherapy. **J Allergy Clin Immunol** 80(5):741–745.
308. Ward RA (1976) Fire ants. In: Pathology of Tropical and Extraordinary Diseases, Binford CH, Connor DH, eds. Washington, DC: Armed Forces Institutes of Pathology.

309. Paull BR (1984) Imported fire ant allergy. **Postgrad Med** 76(1):155–162.
310. Ginsburg CM (1984) Fire ant envenomation in children. **Pediatrics** 73(5):689–692.
311. Candiotti KA, Lamos AM (1993) Adverse neurologic reactions to the sting of the imported fire ant. **Int Arch Allergy Immunol** 102(4):417–420.
312. Graft DF (1996) Stinging insect hypersensitivity in children. **Curr Opin Pediatr** 8(6):597–600.
313. Doan-Wiggins L (1991) Tick-borne disease. **Emerg Clin North Am** 9(2): 303–325.
314. Brouqui P, Harle JR, Delmont J et al. (1997) African tick-bite fever. An imported spotless rickettsiosis. **Arch Intern Med** 157(1):119–124.
315. Mahara F (1997) Japanese spotted fever: report of 31 cases and review of the literature. **Emerg Infect Dis** 3(2):105–111.
316. Fournier PE, Roux V, Caumes E et al. (1998) Outbreak of Rickettsia africae infections in participants of an adventure race in South Africa. **Clin Infect Dis** 27(2):316–323.
317. Carpenter CF, Gandhi TK, Kong LK et al. (1999) The incidence of ehrlichial and rickettsial infection in patients with unexplained fever and recent history of tick bite in central North Carolina. **J Infect Dis** 180(3):900–903.
318. Kowalska M, Kupis B (1976) Gamasoidosis (gamasoidosis) – not infrequent skin reactions, frequently unrecognized. **Pol Med Sci Hist Bull** 15–16:391–394.
319. Lucky AW, Sayers CP, Argus JD, Lucky A (2001) Avian mite bites acquired from a new source – pet gerbils: report of 2 cases and review of the literature. **Arch Dermatol** 137(2):167–170.

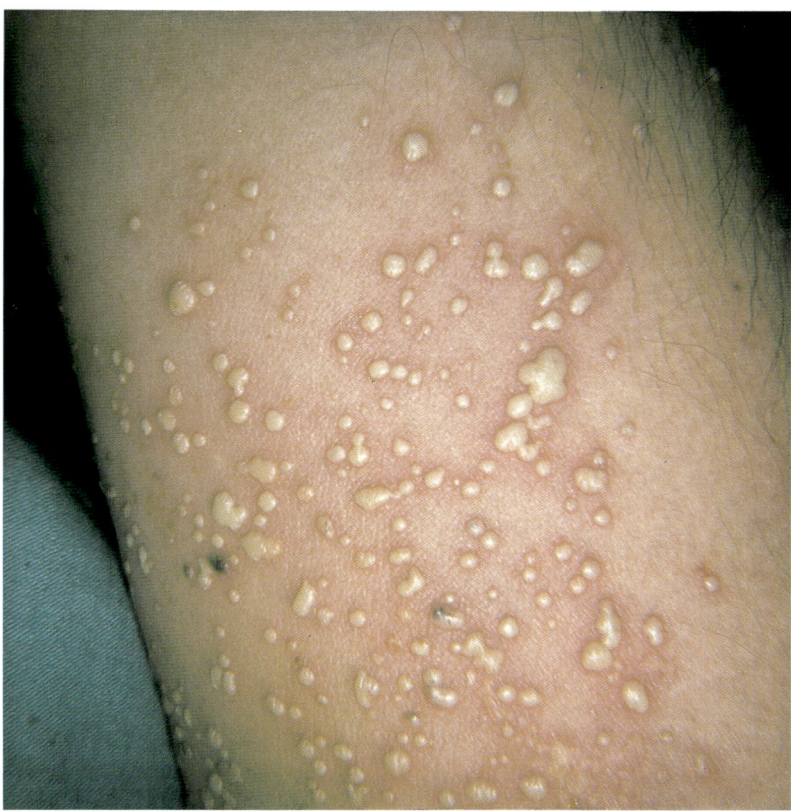

Fig. 29.26   Fire ant stings.

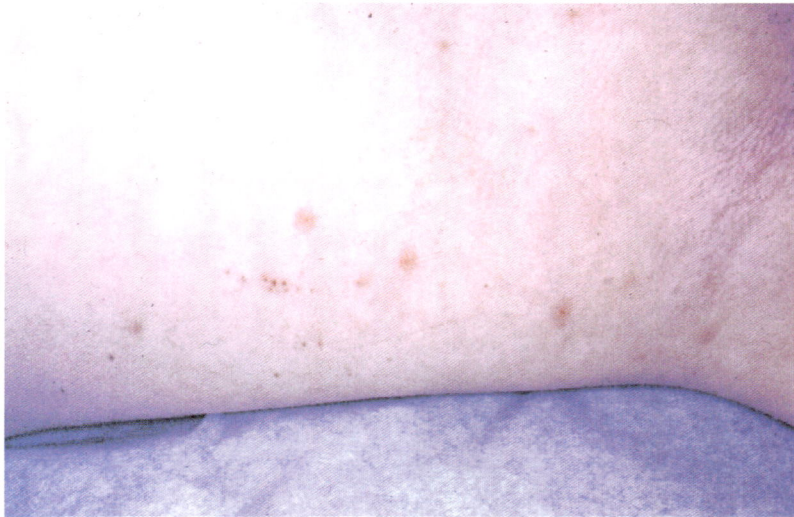

Fig. 29.27   Avian mite bites, in this case acquired from a pet gerbil, in the axilla of a 10 year old boy. (Photo courtesy of Anne W. Lucky.)

There are no burrows associated with avian mite bites. Treatment of avian mite dermatitis requires removing the source of the mites including the pets, their cages and nests. House cleaning and fumigation are helpful.

If a tick should become attached, it should be removed promptly and completely with fine tweezers, forceps or with fingers protected with gloves or facial tissues[313] (see below). Local cleansing is required. Topical steroids may be helpful for local reactions. Infections are not uncommon and rarely require more than local antibacterial measures. Should one of the rickettsioses be transmitted, use of doxycycline, tetracycline or chloramphenicol would be required. Doxycycline is recommended for children because its risk of dental staining is less than with other tetracyclines.[320] Amoxicillin, erythromycin or cefuroxime are recommended should a child become infected with the spirochetes of Lyme disease from a tick bite.[321]

The best way to prevent tick-borne diseases is to avoid tick-infested areas.[313] Persons who must enter these areas should wear protective clothing, use a tick repellent, and wear permethrin-impregnated clothing (Table 29.6).[322,323]

Mosquito bites

In tropical climates, mosquitoes are well known vectors of diseases such as malaria, yellow fever and dengue hemorrhagic fever.[324–326] The inflammatory response to the bite results from sensitization to the mosquito saliva which is injected into the skin during feeding.[327,328] There is usually an immediate reaction consisting of a wheal and flare 2–10mm in diameter.[324] There are a few case reports of anaphylaxis to mosquito bites.[329,330] Some reactions are delayed and last 1–3 days. In addition, cutaneous manifestations of an Arthus-type reaction, erythema multiforme, and anaphylactoid purpura have been reported.[329,331] Pediatric patients who develop chronic lymphocytic leukemia may exhibit severe delayed bite reactions, which commonly appear before the manifestations of the disease.[332] Altered reactions to mosquito bites have also been reported in patients with acquired immunodeficiency syndrome.[333]

Symptomatic treatments with antipruritic lotions and low potency topical steroids are of variable efficacy.[324] Suspensions, lotions, or creams containing diphenhydramine should not be used topically because sensitization and severe systemic reactions may occur.[334] Repellents containing DEET are effective; however, they need to be used cautiously because of their potential for toxicity. DEET products with 10% or less concentration are recommended pediatric use (e.g., Skintastic, Skeedaddle). Desensitization may be helpful.[335]

Caterpillar dermatitis

The order Lepidoptera consists of the butterflies and moths. There are many such insects, most of which are harmless.[336] However, up to 12 families of moths and one family of butterflies (i.e., 0.1% of all known butterflies and moths) contain members that can induce inflammatory lesions of the eyes, respiratory system, and skin.[337] These include conjunctivitis, keratitis, iridocyclitis, rhinitis, wheezing, and dermatitis.[336] Tachycardia, arrhythmias, chest pain, dyspnea, generalized bleeding diatheses, peripheral neuropathy, limb paralysis, shock, and convulsions are rarely seen. Most cases of lepidopterism involve the skin. Cutaneous lepidopterism is also known as "caterpillar dermatitis."

320. Dumler JS (2000) Rickettsial infections. In: Nelson Textbook of Pediatrics, 16th edn. Behrman RE, Kliegman RM, Jenson HB, eds. Philadelphia: WB Saunders, 922–932.
321. Shapiro ED (2000) Lyme disease (*Borrelia burgdorferi*). In: Nelson Textbook of Pediatrics, 16th edn, Behrman RE, Kliegman RM, Jenson HB, eds. Philadelphia: WB Saunders, 910–914.
322. Schreck CE, Snoddy EL, Spielman A (1986) Pressurized sprays of permethrin or DEET on military clothing for personal protection against *Ixodes dammini* (Acari: Ixodidae). **J Med Entomol** 23(4):396–399.
323. Young GD, Evans S (1998) Safety and efficacy of DEET and permethrin in the prevention of arthropod attack. **Mil Med** 163(5):324–330.
324. Reunala T, Brummer-Korvenkontio H, Lappalainen P (1990) Immunology and treatment of mosquito bites. **Clin Exp Allergy** 20 suppl 4:19–24.
325. Chareonsook O, Foy HM, Teeraratkul A et al. (1999) Changing epidemiology of dengue hemorrhagic fever in Thailand. **Epidemiol Infect** 122(1):161–166.
326. Vaughn DW (2000) Invited commentary: Dengue lessions from Cuba. **Am J Epidemiol** 152(9):800–803.
327. Hudson A, Bowmand L, Orr CWM (1960) Effects of absence of saliva on blood feeding by mosquitos. **Science** 131:1730–1731.
328. Nelson WA (1987) Other blood sucking and myiasis producing arthropods. In: Immune Responses in Parasitic Infections: Immunology, Immunopathology and Immunoprophylaxis, Vol. IV, Soulsby EJL, ed. Boca Raton, FL: CRC Press, p.175.
329. Frazier CA (1984) Insect allergy, 2nd edn. St. Louis: WH Green.
330. McCormack DR, Salata KF, Hershey JN et al. (1995) Mosquito bite anaphylaxis: immunotherapy with whole body extracts. **Ann Allergy Asthma Immunol** 74(1):39–44.
331. Suzuki S, Negishi K, Tomizawa S et al. (1976) A case of mosquito allergy: Immunological studies. **Acta Allergol** 31(6):428–441.
332. Weed RI (1965) Exaggerated delayed hypersensitivity to mosquito bites in chronic lymphocytic leukemia. **Blood** 26(3):257–268.
333. Diven DB, Newton RC, Ramsey KM (1988) Heightened cutaneous reactions to mosquito bites in patients with acquired immunodeficiency syndrome receiving zidovudine. **Arch Intern Med** 148(10):2296.
334. Bernhardt DT (1991) Topical diphenhydramine toxicity. **Wis Med J** 90(8):469–471.
335. Peng Z, Simons FER (1998) A prospective study of naturally acquired sensitization and subsequent desensitization to mosquito bites and concurrent antibody responses. **J Allergy Clin Immunol** 101 (2 pt 1):284–286.
336. Rosen T (1990) Caterpillar dermatitis. **Dermatol Clin** 8(2):245–252.
337. Henwood BP, MacDonald DM (1983) Caterpillar dermatitis. **Clin Exp Dermatol** 8(1):77–93.

TABLE 29.6   Insect avoidance and environmental approaches to prevention

Mosquito	Protective clothing Eliminate breeding sites Avoid outdoor activity during late afternoons and early evening Outdoor sprays Personal insect repellents (DEET) to skin and clothing Protective clothing
Fleas	Identify and treat animal source (dips, powders, collars, etc, for cats and dogs) Treat and eliminate infested outdoor areas (e.g., sand boxes) Professional extermination or equivalent "do-it-yourself" aerosol approach to home Personal insect repellent (DEET) to skin and clothes
Bedbug	Protective nightwear Professional extermination Personal insect repellent (DEET) to exposed skin surface
Kissing bug (Southwestern United States)	Same as bedbug Remove packrat nests, where feasible, as these are frequent nesting sites of kissing bugs
Flies	Protective clothing Cleanup of breeding sites Simple avoidance Personal insect repellents (DEET)
Ticks	Protective clothing Inspect and treat (dip) dogs regularly Personal insect repellents (DEET)

DEET, N, N-diethyl-*m*-totuamide.

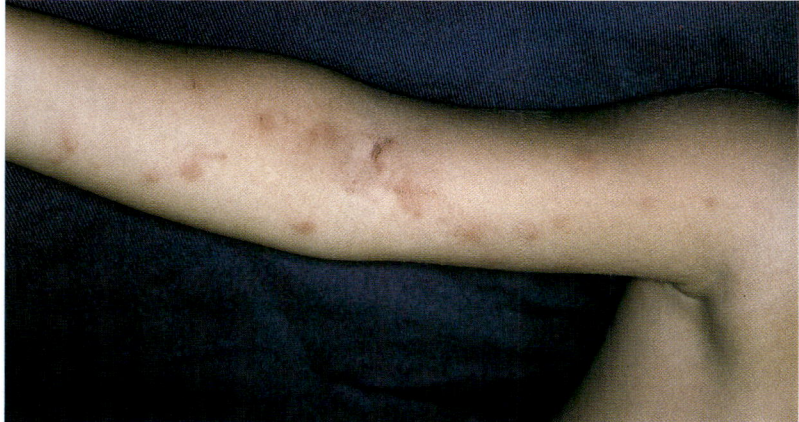

Fig. 29.28   Caterpillar dermatitis in a 4-year-old boy who played with them on his arm. (Photo courtesy of Anne W. Lucky.)

Most cases of lepidopterism result from incidental contact with insect larvae after recreational activities.[338] Pets may also bring caterpillar remnants attached to their fur into homes.[339] Contact with caterpillars causes lesions due to histamine contained in the hairs.[340]

Caterpillar dermatitis presents locally or with widespread red macules and urticarial wheals (Fig. 29.28).[341] These wheals become infiltrated papules and then vesicles.[336] Chronic cutaneous lesions include lichen simplex chronicus, postinflammatory hyperpigmentation, and bruising.[339]

Treatment involves symptomatic care, including antihistamines, antipruritic lotions, and low-potency topical corticosteroids.[336] Rarely, systemic cortiosteroids may be indicated.[342] Stripping the skin with adhesive tape to remove lingering hairs is advocated by some.[343,344] Symptoms resolve within hours to 10 days.[336]

Centipedes and millipedes

Some of the larger centipedes of the genus *Scolopendra* can inflict a painful bite, with some localized swelling and erythema. Lymphangitis and lymphadenitis are not uncommon. Necrosis is rare, and infections almost unknown. Symptoms and signs seldom persist for more than 48h. The millipedes do not bite but, when handled, may discharge a toxic secretion that can cause local skin irritation and, in severe cases, some necrosis. Some species outside the United States can spray a highly irritating repugnant secretion that may cause severe conjunctival reactions.

An ice cube controls the pain of most centipede bites. However, systemic analgesics may be required in more severe cases. Corticosteroids have been used as anti-inflammatory agents. The toxic secretions of millipedes should be washed from the skin with copious amounts of soap and water. Cleansing with alcohol should be avoided. Eye injuries require immediate irrigation and the application of a corticosteroid–analgesic ointment.

Other biting and stinging arthropods

In the United States, a number of biting arthropods possess salivary secretions that can produce various reactions and lesions. Among the more common biting and sometimes blood-sucking arthropods are the ticks and mites; sand, horse, and deer flies; lice and bedbugs; kissing bugs; and certain waterbugs. The saliva of these arthropods varies considerably in composition, their vasodilator effect and anticoagulant activity.[345] The lesions produced by their bites can vary from a small papule to a large ulcerating wound with swelling and acute pain. Dermatitis may also occur. Most serious bites are complicated by sensitivity reactions or infection. In hypersensitive children, these injuries can be fatal.

The offending arthropod should be quickly removed. For ticks and some of the bugs, this is best accomplished by direct application of a petroleum product or by grasping the animal with broad forceps and slowly pulling it from the wound. Other techniques include application of gasoline and chloroform or burning the tick with a match or other hot object. Turning it slightly may facilitate removal, but care should be taken not to leave the capitulum in the wound because it may induce chronic inflammation or may migrate into deeper tissues and give rise to a granuloma. The bite should be cleaned and dressed. A piece of ice placed on the wound usually reduces the pain. Serious hypersensitivity reactions should be treated and has been reviewed elsewhere.[346,347]

PREVENTION OF INSECT BITES

Methods for preventing the bites, which include the use of insect repellents, are important strategies for reducing insect-borne diseases. There are two categories of insect repellents which are currently marketed: chemical

338. deJong MC, Bleumink E, Nater JP (1975) Investigative studies of the dermatitis caused by the larvae of the brown tail moth (*Euproctis chrysorrhoea*). I. Clinical and experimental findings. **Arch Dermatol Res** 253(3):287–300.
339. Blair CP (1979) The browntail moth, its caterpillar and their rash. **Clin Exp Dermatol** 4(2):215–222.
340. Shama SK, Etkind PH, Odell TM et al. (1982) Gypsy-moth caterpillar dermatitis. **N Engl J Med** 306(21):1300–1301.
341. Werno J, Lamy M, Vincendeau P (1993) Caterpillar hairs as allergens. **Lancet** 342(8876):936–937.
342. Ducombs G, Lamy M, Mollard S et al. (1981) Contact dermatitis from processional pine caterpillar. **Contact Dermatitis** 7(5):287–288.

343. Burnett JW, Calton GJ, Morgan RJ (1986) Caterpillar and moth dermatitis. **Cutis** 37(5):320.
344. Dunlop K, Freeman S (1997) Caterpillar dermatitis. **Aust J Dermatol** 38(4):193–195.
345. Jones D (1998) The neglected saliva: medically important toxins in the saliva of human lice. **Parasitology** 116(Suppl.):S73–S81.
346. Heng MCY, Kloss SG, Haberfelde GC (1984) Pathogenesis of papular urticaria. **J Am Acad Dermatol** 10(6):1030–1034.
347. Honig PJ (1986) Arthropod bites, stings and infestation: their prevention and treatment. **Pediatr Dermatol** 3(3):189–197.

repellents and plant-derived repellents.[348,349] Among the chemical group, *N,N*-diethyl-3-methylbenzamide (previously called *N,N*-diethyl-*m*toluamide; DEET) is the most effective repellent. DEET has been shown to be effective against fleas, mosquitoes, biting flies, chiggers, and ticks. The concentrations range from 5 to 100% in multiple formulations, including lotions, creams, aerosol and pump sprays, and impregnated towelettes.[349] The American Academy of Pediatrics recommends that DEET-containing repellent used on children should not contain more than 10% DEET.[350,351]

Permethrin acts primarily as an insecticide rather than a repellent. The combination of skin application of DEET-based repellent and permethrin-treated clothing provides an effective barrier against bites.[352] Newer agents, including pyridines and piperidines, are being developed and tested for their acaricidal and repellent activity.[353]

Non-DEET plant extracts have been used worldwide as traditional repellents. These include citronella oil, which is the most popular ingredient, eucalyptus oil, soybean oil and garlic.[349] Unlike DEET, plant-derived repellents provide shorter protection times (usually less than 2h), and their safety, especially in young children, has yet to be determined. Specific environmental approaches can also help prevent insect bites (Table 29.6). Unfortunately, stinging insects (Hymenoptera) are not deterred by the usual repellents and require special precautions for prophylaxis (Table 29.7).[354]

MAN-MADE ENVIRONMENTAL HAZARDS

SICK BUILDING SYNDROME

The sick building syndrome is characterized by the presence of multiple complaints of occupants of a "sick" building involving the eyes, skin, and upper airway. Headaches and fatigue are frequent.[355–360] In most normal buildings, about 10–20% of the occupants complain of such symptoms.[361] Symptoms reported by 30% or more of occupants are indicative of conditions in the building that warrant attention.[361] However, the symptoms are generally not traceable to a specific substance, but are attributed to exposure to a combination of substances or to an individual's increased susceptibility, e.g., due to atopy or pre-existing asthma with low concentrations of contaminants.

Reported symptoms include eye irritation and swelling, nasal catarrh and blockage, dryness and soreness of the throat, cough, headache, abnormal tiredness, sensation of "getting a cold", and nausea.[356] Cutaneous symptoms include facial rashes, facial and hand pruritus, and eczema.[362]

TABLE 29.7 Avoidance of stinging insects

Always wear shoes when outdoors
Avoid wearing brightly colored clothes or flowery prints
Do not wear loose-fitting clothing, which may entrap a bee
Avoid hair tonics, hair spray, deodorants, perfumes, and scented soaps with strong odors, which may attract bees
Avoid insect feeding grounds such as flower beds, clover, garbage, wasp or hornet nests, yellow jacket burrows, or any hills. Wasp or hornet nests or bee hives near the patient's home should be destroyed by a professional exterminator
Do not leave food or garbage uncovered. It may attract ants or wasps
Avoid rapid movements when near stinging insects unless being pursued
Keep automobile windows closed
Keep windows and doors at patient's home closed unless protected with screens
Keep a fast-acting insecticide aerosol in the kitchen, glove compartment of the automobile, and someplace readily accessible from outdoors such as the garage (out of reach of small children)

Most studies have been performed in office buildings; however, schools and day care centers may also be affected.[358–359] The concentration of volatile organic hydrocarbons,[360] wall-to-wall carpets,[359] fleecy material in buildings,[363] age of the building,[364] ambient temperature,[365] ventilation system,[366] video display units,[367] static electricity,[368] passive smoking,[365] degree of crowding,[369] molds,[370] and moisture[371] have all been associated with the aforementioned symptoms. In addition, personal factors such as a history of atopy, allergy to nickel, proneness to infection, and hyper-reactivity are related to an increase in symptoms.[372] Remedial action involves removal of all contaminated wallboard, paneling, and carpeting in the water-damaged area of the home. An approved disinfectant and cleaning of the heating, ventilation and air-conditioning systems are also required.[373]

ENVIRONMENTAL CARCINOGENS

ARSENIC

Exposure to arsenic may result from environmental sources such as well water in areas where there are high arsenic concentrations in the soil. Foods;[374]

348. Brown M, Hebert AA (1997) Insect repellents: an overview. **J Am Acad Dermatol** 36(2 pt 1):243–249.
349. Fradin M (1998) Mosquitoes and mosquito repellents: a clinician's guide. **Ann Intern Med** 128(11):931–940.
350. Shelov SP, ed. (1991) Caring for Your Baby and Young Child: Birth to Age 5. New York: Bantam Books.
351. Garrettson LK (1997) Commentary-DEET: caution for children still needed. **J Toxicol Clin Toxicol** 35(5):443–445.
352. Gupta RK, Sweeney AW, Rutledge LC et al. (1987) Effectiveness of controlled-release personal-use arthropod repellents and permethrine-impregnated clothing in the field. **J Am Mosq Control Assoc** 3(4):556–560.
353. Schreck CE, Fish D, McGovern TP (1995) Activity of repellents applied to skin for protection against *Amblyomma americanum* and *Ixodes scapularis* ticks (Acari: Ixodidae). **J Am Mosq Control Assoc** 11(1):136–140.
354. Golden DBK (1983) Insect sting allergy in adults. In: Current Therapy in Allergy and Immunology, 1983–84, Lichtenstein LM, Fauci AS, eds. Barbington, Ontario: BC Decker, p. 70.
355. Finnegan MJ, Pickering CAC, Burge PS (1984) The sick building syndrome: prevalence studies. **Br Med J (Clin Res Ed)** 289(6458):1573–1575.
356. Akimenko VV, Andersen I, Lebowitz MD, Lindvall T (1986) The "sick" building syndrome. In: Indoor Air, Vol. 6. Stockholm: Swedish Council for Building Research, p. 87.
357. Burge S, Hedge A, Wilson S et al. (1987) Sick building syndrome: a study of 4373 office workers. **Ann Occup Hyg** 31(4A):493–504.
358. Widstrom J, Norback D (1988) An inventory of sick buildings among workplaces connected to occupational health centers in the counties of Gavleborg, Kopparberg and Uppsala. In Proceedings of the 37th Nordic Meeting of Work Environment, Gothenberg, Stockholm: National Institute of Occupational Health, p. 292.
359. Norback D, Torgen M (1989) A longitudinal study relating carpeting with sick building syndrome. **Environ Int** 15:129.
360. Norback D, Michel I, Widstrom J (1990) Indoor air quality and personal factors related to the sick building syndrome. **Scand J Work Environ Health** 16(2):121–128.
361. Stolwijk JA (1991) Sick-building syndrome. **Environ Health Perspect** 95:99–100.
362. Norback D, Torgen M, Edling C (1990) Volatile organic compounds, respirable dust, and personal factors related to prevalence and incidence of sick building syndrome in primary schools. **Br J Ind Med** 47(11):733–741.
363. Valbjorn O, Skov P (1987) Danish indoor climate study group. Influence of indoor climate on the sick building syndrome prevalence. In: Indoor Air '87, Vol. 2. Proceedings of the Fourth International Conference on Indoor Air Quality and Climate. Institute for Water, Soil and Air Hygiene, Berlin (West), p. 593.
364. Skov P, Valbjorn O (1987) Danish indoor climate study group. The "Sick" building syndrome in the office environment: The Danish town hall study. **Environ Int** 13:339.
365. Laakkola JJK, Heinonen OP, Seppanen O (1989) Sick building syndrome, sensation of dryness and thermal comfort in relation to room temperature in an office building: need for individual control of temperature. **Environ Int** 15:163.
366. Berblund B, Lindvall T (1986) Sensory reaction to "sick" buildings. **Environ Int** 12:147.
367. Linden V, Rolfsen S (1981) Video computer terminals and occupational dermatitis. **Scand J Work Environ Health** 7(1):62–64.
368. Michel I, Norback D, Edling C (1989) An epidemiologic study of the relationship between symptoms of fatigue, dental amalgam and other factors. **Swed Dental J** 13(1–2):33–38.
369. Taylor PR, Dell' Acqua BJ, Baptiste MS et al. (1984) Illness in an office building with limited fresh air access. **J Environ Health** 47:24.
370. Cooley JD, Wong WC, Jumper CA et al. (1998) Correlation between the prevalence of certain fungi and sick building syndrome. **Occup Environ Med** 55(9):579–584.
371. Waegemackers M, Van Wageningen N, Brunekreef B et al. (1989) Respiratory symptoms in damp houses. A pilot study. **Allergy** 44(3):192–198.
372. Norback D, Edling C (1991) Environmental, occupational, and personal factors related to the prevalence of sick building syndrome in the general population. **Br J Ind Med** 48(7):451–462.
373. Vesper S, Dearborn DG, Yike I et al. (2000) Evaluation of *Stachybotrys chartarum* in the house of an infant with pulmonary hemorrhage: quantitative assessment before, during, and after remediation. **J Urban Health** 77(1):68–85.
374. Tao SS, Bolger PM (1999) Dietary arsenic intakes in the United States: FDA total diet study, September 1991–December 1996. **Food Addit Contam** 16(11):465–472.

industrial sources (such as pesticides, sheep dips, copper and other ores, and fabric dyes), or medicinal sources (such as Fowler's solution (potassium arsenite), Asiatic pills, Donovan's solution, and DeValagin's solution) have all been implicated.[375–378]

Arsenic toxicity results in the development of internal and cutaneous malignancies.[377,379–381] Cancer of the skin lungs, mouth, esophagus, liver, and urinary bladder have been reported.[381] Cutaneous changes include hyperpigmentation, the most frequently encountered skin alteration in chronic arsenic toxicity.[382–384] These dark brown patches may contain hypopigmented macules.[383] Other cutaneous signs include small wartlike keratoses on the palms, soles, and ears; Bowen's disease; invasive squamous cell carcinoma; and, rarely, basal cell carcinoma.[385] The squamous cell carcinomas that arise from Bowen's disease tend to be of higher grade and very aggressive.[383] Metastases with resultant death are also more common with arsenic-induced than with sun-induced squamous cell carcinomas. The occurrence of multiple skin cancers on exposed and unexposed areas at a relatively young age should raise suspicion of arsenic toxicity.[382–383]

It is important to prevent arsenic toxicity by awareness of these environmental hazards and vigilance in assuring that adequate laws protecting the public are enforced. Severe acute intoxication with arsenic responds to therapy with dimercaprol or penicillamine.[386]

VINYL CHLORIDE

Vinyl chloride is a human-made chemical.[387] Its primary use is in the production of polyvinyl chloride, a plastic that is used to make a wide variety of products including electrical wire coating, flooring, home furnishings, toys, packaging, apparel, and automobile parts and upholstery. Those at greatest risk of exposure are persons involved in its manufacture, transportation, storage, and disposal.[387] However, consumers are exposed in small amounts to vinyl chloride from the plastic in new car interiors, packaging of certain foods and beverages, and pipes for drinking water. Exposure to vinyl chloride either in the prenatal period or in early childhood may result in an increased risk of cancer. Exposure to 20 000ppm for 5min may cause dizziness, lightheadedness, nausea, and dulling of vision and auditory acuity.[386] Epidemiologic data suggests that chronic exposure to very high doses (500–1000ppm) often leads to hepatotoxicity. Exposure to lower doses (100ppm) is more often associated with carcinogenicity. Chronic exposure has led to "vinyl chloride disease."[387] The signs of this disorder include scleroderma-like changes of the fingers, acro-osteolysis, Raynaud's phenomenon, and liver disease.[387–389] Vinyl chloride is known to cause hepatic angiosarcomas.[377,387–389] In addition, authors have suggested an increased risk of brain, breast, lung, thyroid, skin (melanoma),[390] lymphatic, and hematopoietic cancer; however, there is insufficient evidence to establish a causal relationship.[377,387]

RADIATION

The greatest exposure to ionizing radiation results from natural background sources. Other sources include medical diagnostic and therapeutic procedures and fallout of radionuclides. The cutaneous effects of ionizing radiation depend on the intensity and duration of exposure.[377] Acutely painful redness and edema may develop, sometimes progressing to vesiculation and ulceration.[391] Long-term effects include atrophy, telangiectasias, dyspigmentation, sclerosis, alopecia, and chronic ulceration.[391] In more severe cases, development of cutaneous squamous cell and basal cell carcinomas may be observed.[392] Importantly, skin cancers arising in areas of radiodermatitis are more malignant in behavior than skin cancer that is actinically induced.[391,393]

Artificial tanning is a rapidly growing, human-made cutaneous environmental hazard, and the use of artificial tanning has become very popular among adolescents. Such radiation results in skin and eye burns, photosensitivity, alteration of immune function and DNA damage associated with photocarcinogenesis in human cells.[394,395] Counseling adolescents seen for other reasons regarding the dangers of artificial tanning, and working with state legislatures to promote laws requiring parental permission for tanning in underaged individuals is encouraged.

PERCUTANEOUS ABSORPTION AND TOXICITY

PESTICIDES

Pesticides are chemicals used in agriculture for the control of pests, weeds, or plant diseases.[396] Children can be exposed to pesticides from multiple sources including food, drinking water, toys, and residential pesticide and by living in agricultural communities.[397,398] These chemicals may be extracted from plants or may be synthetic. Pesticides are the most important chemicals that cause acute or chronic systemic toxicity from percutaneous absorption.[390] Sores and abrasions may facilitate uptake.[396] Pesticides usually cause an irritant contact dermatitis.[390] The most common sensitizing pesticides include the thiocarbamates, formaldehyde, nitrofurazone, organic mercury compounds, thiuram sulfides, hexachlorocyclohexane, and pyrethrum.[399] Reactions

375. Stolman LP, Kopf AW, Garfinkel L (1970) Are palmar keratoses a sign of internal malignancy? Arch Dermatol 101(1):52–55.
376. Cuzick J, Evans S, Gillman M, Price Evans DA (1982) Medicinal arsenic and internal malignancies. Br J Cancer 45(6):904–911.
377. Poole S, Fenske NA (1993) Cutaneous markers of internal malignancy. II. Paraneoplastic dermatoses and environmental carcinogens J Am Acad Dermatol 28(2 pt 1):147–164.
378. Smith AH, Arroyo AP, Mazumder DN et al. (2000) Arsenic-induced skin lesions among Atacameno people in Northern Chile despite good nutrition and centuries of exposure. Environ Health Perspect 108(7):617–620.
379. Ott MG, Holder BB, Gordon HL (1974) Respiratory cancer and occupational exposure to arsenicals. Arch Environ Health 29(5):250–255.
380. Mabuchi K, Lillienfield AM, Snell LM (1980) Cancer and occupational exposure to arsenic: a study of pesticide workers. Prevent Med 9(1):51–77.
381. Smith AH, Hopenhayn-Rich C, Bates MN et al. (1992) Cancer risks from arsenic in drinking water. Environ Health Perspect 97:259–267.
382. Tseng WP, Chu HM, How SW et al. (1968) Prevalence of skin cancer in an endemic area of chronic arsenicism in Taiwan. J Natl Cancer Inst 40(3):453–463.
383. Shannon RL, Strayer DS (1989) Arsenic-induced skin toxicity. Hum Toxicol 8(2):99–104.
384. Kurokawa M, Ogata K, Idemori M et al. (2001) Investigation of skin manifestations of arsenicism due to intake of arsenic-contaminated ground water in residents of Samta, Jessore, Bangladesh. Arch Dermatol 137(1):102–103.
385. Sanderson KV (1976) Arsenic and skin cancer. In: Cancer of the Skin, Rafael A, ed. Philadelphia: WB Saunders, p. 473.
386. Hathaway GW, Proctor NH, Hughes JP et al. (1991) The chemical hazards. In: Chemical Hazards of the Workplace, 3rd edn, Hathaway GJ, Proctor NH, Hughes JP et al., eds. New York: Van Nostrand Reinhold, p. 55.
387. ASTDR (1990) Case studies in environmental medicine – vinyl chloride toxicity. J Toxicol Clin Toxicol 28(3):267–286.
388. Nicholson WJ, Henneberger PK, Seidman H (1984) Occupational hazards in the VC-PVC industry. Prog Clin Biol Res 141:155–175.
389. Doll R (1988) Effects of exposure to vinyl chloride: an assessment of the evidence. Scand J Work Environ Health 14(2):61–78.
390. American Academy of Dermatology (1992) Comprehensive position statement. Presented at National Conference on Environmental Hazards to the Skin, Washington DC, October 15–16.
391. Goldschmidt H, Sherwin WK (1980) Reactions to ionizing radiation. J Am Acad Dermatol 3(6):551–579.
392. Traenkle HL (1979) Late radiation injury and cutaneous neoplasia. In: Cancer Dermatology, Helm F, ed. Philadelphia: Lea & Febiger.
393. Shore RE (1990) Overview of radiation-induced skin cancer in humans. Int J Radiat Biol 57(4):809–827.
394. Burnett JW (1993) National American Academy of Dermatology Conference on Environmental Hazards. Cutis 51(4):223–224.
395. Woolens A, Clingen PH, Price ML et al. (1997) Induction of mutagenic DNA damage in human fibroblasts after exposure to artificial tanning lamps. Br J Dermatol 137(5):687–692.
396. World Health Organization/United Nations Environment Programme (1990) Public Health Impact of Pesticides Used in Agriculture. Macmillan/Clays, UK.
397. Gurunathan S, Robson M, Freeman N et al. (1998) Accumulation of chlorpyrifos on residential surfaces and toys accessible to children. Environ Health Perspect 106(1):9–16.
398. Fenske RA, Lu C, Simcox NJ et al. (2000) Strategies for assessing children's organophosphorus pesticide exposures in agricultural communities. J Exp Anal Environ Epidemiol 10(6 Pt 2):662–671.
399. Rycroft RJG, Wilkinson JD (1992) Irritants and sensitizers. In: Rook, Wilkinson, Ebling Textbook of Dermatology, 5th edn, Champion RH, Burton JL, Ebling FJG, eds. Oxford: Blackwell Scientific Publications, p. 739.

including allergic contact dermatitis, photoallergic reactions, and porphyria cutanea tarda have been described.[396] Chloracne, although rare, may indicate exposure to highly toxic herbicide chemicals found in agricultural and industrial settings.[390,400] Chloracne appeared after the accidental spread of 2,3,7,8-tetrachlorodibenzo-*p*-dioxin (TCDD).[401]

Acute anticholinergic effects of pesticide exposure consist of headache, abdominal pain, vomiting, sweating, miosis, and muscular twitching.[402] These may be controlled with atropine or pralidoxime. Convulsions, coma, and death may result from acute severe poisoning.[402] Chronic exposure has been implicated in various disorders, including impaired immune function, neurobehavioral disorders, neuropathies, and cancer.[396,403] Recent reports suggest that there may be an increased risk for the development of acute monoblastic leukemia in children whose parents have occupational exposure to pesticides and solvents. The highest relative risk was in children younger than 5 years of age.[404] Household exposures to pesticides and petroleum products were also associated with a significantly elevated risk of acute monoblastic leukemia and lymphoma.[404,405]

Precautions to avoid nonoccupational, accidental exposure include keeping pesticides in clearly marked containers in a locked cabinet and away from bulk foodstuffs.[396] When pesticides are used, protective clothing is critical to prevent systemic absorption.

INSECT REPELLENTS

DEET is the most commonly used insect repellent. Few cases of local or systemic effect have been reported. In the United States, of 3098 exposures to DEET studied between 1985 and 1990, five had serious adverse reactions, which were mostly from inhalation or ocular contact.[406] In the United Kingdom, of the 25 adverse reports in 1996, most were from ingestion by children and all resulted in mild symptoms.[407] Even though only a small amount of topical DEET is absorbed through the skin, a number of adverse reactions have been reported, both dermatologic and systemic.[408–411] Local dermatologic reactions have included a tingling sensation, mild desquamation, contact dermatitis, a bullous eruption with a predilection for flexural areas and generalized urticaria.

Systemic effects may occur either from ingestion or skin exposure. *N,N*-diethyl-*m*-toluamide is absorbed through intact skin and, being lipid soluble, could accumulate in the brain.[412,413] The signs and symptoms in children include crying spells, disorientation, ataxia, involuntary movement, behavior changes, opisthotonic posture, convulsion, coma and death.[409,414–420] Toxic encephalopathy from DEET was first reported in children in 1961. One case developed after the bedding, night clothes and skin of a 3 1/2 year-old girl were sprayed daily for 2 weeks, with an amount equal to 0.14ml/kg/day of a 15%

DEET product.[421] Another occurred in a 6-year-old girl who died after dermal exposure to 15% DEET and who had an underlying ornithine carbamoyl transferase (OCT) deficiency.[415] Ornithine is involved in urea biosynthesis. DEET can increase ammonia levels in normal mice. Individuals with defects in OTC may develop severe encephalopathy in response to DEET exposure. OCT deficiency is a sex-linked dominant condition, which is fatal in males during the neonatal period, but affects females with variable severity. This enzyme deficiency may account for encephalopathy which has been reported more in girls.[415,422] Brain edema and congestion of the meninges are common pathologic findings in fatal cases with severe toxic encephalopathy.[414,415]

In children with toxic encephalopathy, gradual, uneventful improvement usually occurs after vigorous medical treatment that includes skin decontamination, intravenous fluid and anticonvulsants. Charcoal slurry and a saline cathartic may be needed in cases of ingestion.

ANILINE, CYANIDE SALTS, AND BENZENE

Skin exposure to aniline, cyanide salts, and benzene may occur directly with either raw materials or toxins generated during the manufacturing process.

Aniline is used in the synthesis of synthetic dyes. Its absorption causes anoxia as a result of the formation of methemoglobin.[386] Rapid absorption through intact skin is the main route of entry. Human exposure of 7 to 53 ppm causes slight symptoms. Concentrations of 100–160ppm may cause serious disturbances. A small amount absorbed through clothing or shoes may cause significant disease.

The signs of methemoglobinemia include headache, cyanosis, ataxia, dyspnea, tachycardia, and coma.[386] Therapy includes removing all the aniline from the skin by thorough washing with soap and water. Oxygen should be administered, and a methemoglobin level should be ascertained. Skin cleansing should be repeated if the methemoglobin level continues to rise. Levels in patients normalize within 24 hours if further absorption is eliminated

Cyanide is used in the extraction of gold and silver, electroplating, hardening of metals, manufacture of mirrors, and the reclamation of silver from photographic film.[386] Cyanide salts result in acute cellular asphyxia and cell death by an inhibitory action on cytochrome oxidase, the enzyme involved in the ultimate transfer of electrons to molecular oxygen.[386,390] It is estimated that the lethal dose for 50% of humans for a 1-min exposure is 3404ppm[386] A dose of 270ppm is fatal after 6–8min of exposure and 135ppm after 30min.

If large amounts are absorbed, collapse is instantaneous.[386] Less severe intoxications are characterized by headache, weakness, confusion, nausea, and vomiting. Hydrogen cyanide has been found in the combustion products of

400. Zugerman C (1990) Chloracne: clinical manifestations and etiology. **Dermatol Clin** 8(1):209–213.
401. Caputo R, Monti M, Ermacora E et al. (1988) Cutaneous manifestations of tetrachlorodibenzo-*p*-dioxin in children and adolescents. Follow-up 10 years after the Seveso, Italy, accident. **J Am Acad Dermatol** 19(5 pt 1):812–819.
402. Jacobs JM, LeQuesne PM (1992) Toxic disorders. In: Greenfield's Neuropathology, 5th edn, Adams JH, Duchen LW, eds. New York: Oxford University Press, p. 293.
403. van Wendel de Joode B, Wesseling C, Kromhout H et al. (2001) Chronic nervous-system effects of long-term occupational exposure to DDT. **Lancet** 357(9261):1014–1016.
404. Odom LF, Lampkin BC, Tannous R et al. (1990) Acute monoblastic leukemia: a unique subtype – a review from the Childrens Cancer Study Group. **Leuk Res** 14(1):1–10.
405. Meinert R, Schuz J, Kaletsch U et al. (2000) Leukemia and non-Hodgkin's lymphoma in childhood and exposure to pesticides: results of a register-based case-control study in Germany. **Am J Epidemiol** 151(7):639–646.
406. Veltri JC, Osimitiz TG, Branford DC et al. (1994) Retrospective analysis of calls to poison control centers resulting from exposure to the insect repellent DEET from 1985–1989. **J Toxicol Clin Toxicol** 32:1–16.
407. Goodyear L, Behrens RH (1998) Short report: The safety and toxicity of insect repellents. **Am J Trop Med Hyg** 59(2):323–324.
408. Lamberg SI, Mulrennan JA Jr (1969) Bullous reaction to diethyltoluamide (DEET) resembling a blistering insect eruption. **Arch Dermatol** 100(5):582–586.
409. Lipscomb JW, Kramer JE, Leikin JB (1992) Seizure following brief exposure to the insect repellent *N,N*-diethyl-*m*-toluamide. **Ann Emerg Med** 21(3):315–317.
410. Selim S, Hartnagel RE Jr, Osimitz TG et al. (1995) Absorption. Metabolism, and excretion of *N,N*-diethyl-*m*-toluamide following dermal application to human volunteers. **Fundam Appl Toxicol** 25(1):95–100.
411. Wantke F, Focke M, Hemmer W et al. (1996) Generalized urticaria induced by a diethyltoluamide-containing insect repellent in a child. **Contact Dermatitis** 35(3):186–187.

412. Feldman RJ, Maibach HI (1970) Absorption of some organic compounds through the skin in man. **J Invest Dermatol** 54(5):399–404.
413. Blomquist L, Thorsell W (1977) Distribution and fate of the insect repellent ¹⁴C-*N,N*-diethyl-*m*-toluamide in the animal body: II. Distribution and excretion after cutaneous application. **Acta Pharmacol Toxicol (Copenh)** 41(3):235–243.
414. Zadikoff CM (1979) Toxic encephalopathy associated with the use of insect repellent. **J Pediatr** 95(1):140–142.
415. Heick HMC, Shipman RT, Norman MG et al. (1980) Reye-like syndrome associated with the use of insect repellent in a presumed heterozygote for ornithine carbamoyl transferase deficiency. **J Pediatr** 97(3):471–473.
416. de Garbino JP, Laborde A (1983) Toxicity of an insect repellent *N,N*-diethyltoluamide. **Vet Hum Toxicol** 25(6):422–423.
417. Roland EH, Jan JE, Riggs JM (1985) Toxic encephalopathy in a child after brief exposure to insect repellents. **Can Med Assoc J** 132(2):155–156.
418. Edwards DL, Johnson CE (1987) Insect-repellent-induced toxic encephalopathy in a child. **Clin Pharm** 6(6):496–498.
419. Tenenbein M (1987) Severe toxic reactions and death following the ingestion of diethyltoluamide-containing insect repellents. **JAMA** 258(11):1509–1511.
420. Petrucci N, Sardini S (2000) Severe neurotoxic reaction associated with oral ingestion of low-dose diethyltoluamide-containing insect repellent in a child. **Ped Emerg Care** 16(5):341–342.
421. Gryboski J, Weinstein D, Ordway NK (1961) Toxic encephalopathy apparently related to the use of an insect repellent. **N Engl J Med** 264(6):289–291.
422. Dhont JL, Farriaux JP (1975) Trial of detection of female carriers for ornithine-carbamoyltransferase deficiency by the urine assay of orotic acid. Apropos of a family study. **Ann Genet** 18(3):197–202.

wool, silk, and synthetic polymers and may play a role in toxicity and death from smoke inhalation.

Skin contact results in pruritus and hypopigmentation.[386] Solutions as weak as 0.5% have resulted in caustic burns. Treatment requires vigilance and prompt action. Cardiopulmonary resuscitation should be administered as needed, the patient's skin should be decontaminated thoroughly by washing with water, and amyl nitrite followed by sodium nitrite and sodium thiosulfate should be administered.

Benzene is a common industrial chemical used in the manufacture of organic chemicals, detergents, pesticides, solvents, and paint thinners.[386] It is also found in gasoline, engine emissions, and tobacco smoke.[422] It is a widely distributed environmental contaminant in water, food and air. Percutaneous absorption has been reported.[418] Acute benzene exposure causes central nervous system depression.[386] Chronic exposure results in aplastic anemia, pancytopenia, multiple myeloma, leukemia, diabetes, kidney diseases, respiratory allergies and skin rashes.[386,390,425–427] Chronic occupational exposure has resulted in porokeratosis on genitoanocrural areas which can be successfully treated by CO_2 laser.[428] Human exposure to benzene in very high concentrations of 20 000 ppm is fatal in 5–10min.[386] Hematotoxicity in humans has been associated with a benzene concentration in the work place of more than 50ppm. Direct contact with the liquid may cause redness and vesiculation. If the contact persists, a dry scaly dermatitis may occur.

MERCURY

Acrodynia, or pink disease, is a form of childhood mercury poisoning. It is a result of prolonged exposure to mercury. Inhalation of household products, such as latex paint or of mercury spilled on the floor, is a major source of poisoning.[429–435] Animal studies also indicate that elemental, mercury as a liquid or vapor may be absorbed percutaneously.[435] Direct skin contact was reported in children exposed to a mercurial antibacterial agents such as 1% ammoniated mercury.[436,437]

Other infrequent sources include calomel-containing teething and diaper powders, repeated gamma-globulin injections, anthelmintics, termite-protected wood (mercury bichloride), ingestion of watch batteries, and laxative use.[438–442] (The Mad Hatter in *Alice's Adventures in Wonderland* supposedly had mercury poisoning because of the mercury in felt used for hat making.) The mechanisms of disease involve adrenocortical hyperfunction and catecholamine excess.[443] Mercury blocks the action of catechol methyl transferase leading to increased amount of vanillylmandelic and homovanillic acid in the urine.[440] Clinical manifestations initially are anorexia, lethargy, hypotonia, and irritability.[437] Older children may have personality changes which include declining school performance and inability to think clearly.[444] Leg cramps and weakness of the pelvic and pectoral girdles are noted.[432] Increased drooling and profuse perspiration are common.[431,440] Blood pressure and heart rate increase. An intermittent low-grade fever may accompany other symptoms.[432] Early cutaneous changes are pink color on tips of the fingers, toes and nose and significant pain of the hands and feet (Fig. 29.29). Pruritus can lead to excoriation and lichenification as children constantly rub and scratch at their skin. This will disturb their sleep. Scalp hair is often pulled out. Later, the hands and feet swell and become a dusky pink. Eventually the palms and soles desquamate. Gums are swollen, erythematous and erode focally. Teeth and nail loss may occur. Photophobia is seen.[442] Death may ensue rapidly in children.[439]

Accurate diagnosis requires analysis of 24-h urine mercury by atomic absorption.[431,432,444] Treatment involves the use of chelating agents such as dimercaprol or its newer derivatives: dimercaptosuccinic acid or 2,3-di-mercaptopropane-1-sulfonate.[434–435] Removal of the source and decontamination efforts are necessary to prevent further exposure.

ELECTRICAL INJURIES AND LIGHTNING INJURIES

Electrical injuries are the result of contact with high or low voltage electricity. Low voltage (<1000) injuries generally occur in the home caused by children inserting metallic objects into electrical sockets or biting electrical wires. High voltage (>1000) injuries usually occur in children who play near high-voltage power lines or in those with job-related activities. Both forms may be fatal. There are four classes of electrical injuries.[445] The first is the true electrical injury in which the patient becomes part of the circuit. This injury reflects the passage of current through the body and is usually demarcated by entrance and exit wounds. The second also has flash burns that occur when the current strikes the skin but it does not enter the body. These may result in first-degree through third-degree burns. The third class, flame injuries, occur by the spontaneous combustion of the patient's clothing. In the fourth class, electrical injuries are caused by lightning which has the equivalent to a direct current of around 1 million volts.[446]

In United States, nearly 52 000 people each year sustain electrical injuries and require hospitalization. In Europe, electrical injuries account for 3 to 8% of the total trauma admissions to burn units.[447–449] Electrical injuries requiring hospitalization are potentially devastating, with a mortality rate of 90 percent in children, usually from prehospital cardiac arrest.[450]

Lightning strikes are responsible for more deaths per year in the United States than hurricanes and floods combined.[451] Although the incidence of lightning-related deaths has decreased since the 1950s, 1,318 persons died of

423. Kalf GF (1987) Recent advances in the metabolism and toxicity of benzene. **Crit Rev Toxicol** 18(2):141–159.
424. Wester RC, Maibach HI (2000) Benzene percutaneous absorption: dermal exposure relative to other benzene sources. **Int J Occup Environ Health** 6(2):122–126.
425. Aksoy M (1989) Hematotoxicity and carcinogenicity of benzene. **Environ Health Perspect** 82:193–197.
426. Subrahmanyam VV, Ross D, Eastmond DA, Smith MT (1991) Potential role of free radical in benzene-induced myelotoxicity and leukemia. **Free Radic Biol Med** 11(5):495–515.
427. Gist GL, Burg JR (1997) Benzene: a review of the literature from a health effects perspective. **Toxicol Ind Health** 13(6):661–714.
428. Trcka J, Pettke-Rank CV, Brocker EB et al. (1998) Genitoanocrural porokeratosis following chronic exposure to benzene. **Clin Exp Dermatol** 23(1):28–31.
429. Curtis HA, Ferguson SD, Kell RL et al. (1987) Mercury as a health hazard. **Arch Dis Child** 62(3):293–295.
430. Tunnessen WW Jr, McMahon KJ, Baser M (1987) Acrodynia: exposure to mercury from fluorescent light bulbs. **Pediatrics** 79(5):786–789.
431. Dinehart SM, Dillard R, Raimer SS et al. (1988) Cutaneous manifestations of acrodynia (Pink disease). **Arch Dermatol** 124(1):107–109.
432. Agocs MM, Etzel RA, Parrish RG et al. (1990) Mercury exposure from interior latex paint. **N Engl J Med** 323(16):1096–1101.
433. Zelman M, Camfield P, Moss M et al. (1991) Toxicity from vacuumed mercury: a household hazard. **Clin Pediatr** (Phila) 30(2):121–123.
434. Schwartz JG, Snider TE, Montiel MM (1992) Toxicity of a family from vacuumed mercury. **Am J Emerg Med** 10(3):258–261.
435. Anonymous (1992) Mercury toxicity. Agency for Toxic Substances and Disease registry. **Am Fam Physician** 46(6):1731–1741.
436. Astalfi A, Goelli C (1981) Monitereo Biologico: Proceedings of Academia Nacional de Medicino de Buenos Aires Conference, Nov 3, 1981, Buenos Aires, Argentina.
437. Mucklow ES (1988) Mercury as a health hazard. **Arch Dis Child** 63(11):1416–1417.
438. Dathan JG (1954) Acrodynia associated with excessive intake of mercury. **Br Med J** 1:247–249.
439. Warkany J (1966) Acrodynia: postmortem of a disease. **Am J Dis Child** 112(2):146–156.
440. Ellenhorn MJ, Schonwold S, Ordag G, Wasserberger J, ed (1997) Metal and related compounds. In: Ellenhorn's Medical Toxicology, 2nd edn. Baltimore: Williams & Wilkins, pp. 1532–1613.
441. Graeme KA, Pollack CV (1998) Heavy metal toxicity, part I: arsenic and mercury. **J Emerg Med** 16(1):45–56.
442. Boyd AS, Seger D, Vannucci S et al. (2000) Mercury exposure and cutaneous disease. **J Am Acad Dermatol** 43(1 pt 1):81–90.
443. Cheek DB, Wu F (1959) The effect of calomel on plasma epinephrine in the rate and the relationship to mechanisms in pink disease. **Arch Dis Child** 34:501–504.
444. Anonymous (1990) Elemental mercury poisoning in a household – Ohio, 1989. **MMWR Morb Mortal Wkly Rep** 39(25):424–425.
445. Browne BJ, Gaasch WR (1992) Electrical injuries and lightning. **Emerg Clin North Am** 10(2):211–229.
446. Fahmy FS, Brinsden MD, Smith J et al. (1999) Lightning: the multisystem group injuries. **J Trauma** 46(5):937–940.
447. Haberal MA (1995) An eleven-year survey of electrical burn injuries. **J Burn Care Rehabil** 16(1):43–48.
448. Hulsbergen-Kruger S, Pitzler D, Partecke BD (1995) High voltage accidents, characteristics and treatment. **Unfallchirurg** 98(4):218–223.
449. Caneira E, Serafim Z, Duarte R et al. (1996) Electrical burns in children. 3 years of case histories. **Acta Med Port** 9(10–12):325–330.
450. Zaritsky A, Nadkarni V, Getson P et al. (1987) CPR in children. **Ann Emerg Med** 16(10):1107–1111.
451. Ghezzi KT (1989) Lightning injuries. **Postgrad Med** 85(8):197–198, 201–203, 207–208.

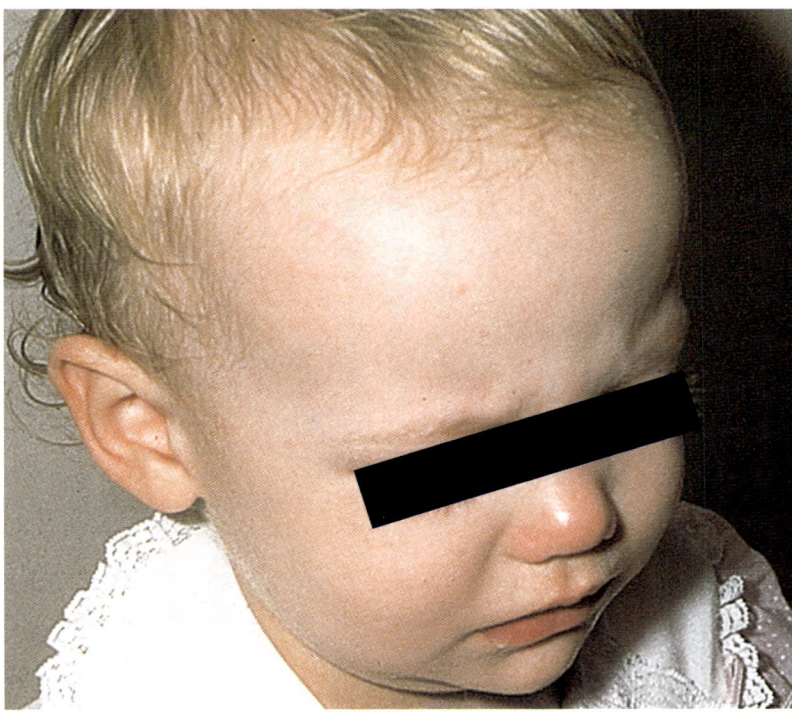
Fig. 29.29   A pink nose in a child with acrodynia.

gastrointestinal, renal, and ophthalmologic injuries.[445] Among these, the most important complication is cardiac disturbance: cardiac arrest is the main cause of death. A major complication is deep muscle injury. Tympanic membrane rupture caused by lightning can be detected in patients with severe ear pain, tinnitus and hearing impairment.[457] Patients with localized pain and swelling, even in the absence of other associated trauma, require radiographic assessment for fracture from prolonged tetanic contraction.[458]

Cutaneous burns resulting from lightning strikes include feathering, linear, punctuate, and thermal burns. Any combination of these burns may occur when a patient is struck by lightning. Feathering burns appear as a fern pattern on the skin within several hours of the injury and resolve 24h later; they are pathognomonic for lightning injury.[451] This may represent electron showering over the surface of the patient. Linear burns occur over areas where there is an abundance of sweat, e.g., the axillae, under the breasts and in the middle of the chest.[445] Punctate burns present as small circular burns and may occur in groups. Small circular full-thickness thickness burns, so-called "tip-toe sign", and the linear burns on the tips of the toes and the side of the soles may be the exit points of the current and can help physicians to diagnose lightning injuries especially in the unconscious patient.[456,446] Thermal burns occur as a result of the combustion of the patient's clothing.[459]

Mouth commissure burns are most commonly seen among children who either bite into an electrical cord or suck on the end of an extension cord.[445] Injury involving the mouth, mucosa, lips, and face occurs. Staining of the teeth is seen.[460] No hemorrhage is identified immediately, but delayed hemorrhage from the labial artery, when the child dislodges the eschar overlying the damaged artery, may be observed.[461,462]

TREATMENT
High-voltage electrical injuries
Whenever possible, the electricity must be turned off. Otherwise, the patient should be removed from the vicinity of the electrical source using well-insulated rubber tools (although these are not always reliable).[445] Aggressive resuscitative efforts should be instituted. The patient should be treated like any trauma patient. Careful cardiac monitoring for arrhythmias that may occur within 1h of the injury is indicated. Massive fluid replacement is needed in cases of severe injury. Electrical injuries are considered major burn injuries, and patients should be transferred to a burn center.

Wound care consists of standard cleansing, débridement, and topical dressings. Topical antibiotics such as silver sulfadiazine are also used in wound care.[463,464] In severe burns, prophylactic antibiotics are recommended. Tetanus immunization should be current. Deeper involvement may result in limb edema, which may evolve into a compartment syndrome requiring fasciotomy or escharotomy in circumferential wounds.[465,466]

Lightning injuries
As with any trauma patient, victims require assessment and stabilization of breathing, and circulation.[445,455] The cervical spine should be immobilized. Intravenous access should be obtained; however, volume resuscitation is usually not required. When lightning strikes involve several people, the rule is "resuscitate the dead" because those who show signs of life will, in all

lightning injuries from 1980 through 1995.[452] Most fatalities are among young outdoor enthusiasts.[446,453]

The age distribution for electrical burns is bimodal: Children younger than 5 years of age are at greatest risk for low-voltage burns, with the largest proportion from electrical contact. High voltage injuries are a problem particularly in males ages 11 to 18 years.[454]

Entrance and exit wounds mark locations where electric current enters and exits the body.[445] Typically, these are small circumscribed third-degree burns. The skin surface is depressed and appears "blown out". There is surrounding hyperemia. Flexoral crease burns occur when electrical current traverses the body along a limb, then changes direction, and jumps across a flexed joint.[445] The severity of lightning injuries depends on the nature of the strike and the pathway of the current inside the victim.[455] The most dangerous way is a direct strike in which the current travels through the victim. Entrance, exit and path lesions are seen. Internal organ injury along the path is common. The most common type of lightning injury is a "splash" or side flash, in which the current initially strikes a high resistance object and then flashes over the victim's body instead of going through. Step voltage is observed when the current strikes the ground and travels up one leg and down the other leg. Contact voltage occurs when the lightning hits an object in direct contact with the victim.[456]

The clinical involvement of electrical and lightning injuries can range from superficial wounds to multisystem, complex disorders. These include cutaneous wounds, cardiovascular, musculoskeletal, neurologic, pulmonary,

452. Anonymous (1998) Lightning-associated deaths – United States, 1980–1995. **MMWR Morb Mortal Wkly Rep** 47(19):391–394.
453. Craig SR (1986) When lightning strikes. Pathophysiology and treatment of lightning injuries. **Postgrad Med** 79(4):109–112, 121–124.
454. Rai J, Jeschke MG, Barrow RE et al. (1999) Electrical injuries: a 30-review. **J Trauma** 46(5):933–936.
455. Cooper MA (1989) Lightning injuries. In: Management of Wilderness and Environmental Emergencies, Auerbach PS, Geehr EC, eds. St. Louis: CV Mosby, pp. 173–193.
456. Volinsky JB, Hanson JB, Lustig JV (1994) Picture of the month. Lightning burns. **Arch Pediatr Adolesc Med** 148(5):529–530.
457. Gluncic I, Roje Z, Gluncic V et al. (2001) Ear injuries caused by lightning: report of 18 cases. **J Laryngol Otol** 115(1):4–8.
458. Hostetler MA, Davis CO (2000) Galeazzi fracture resulting from electrical shock. **Pediatr Emerg Care** 16(4):258–259.
459. Bartholome CW, Jacoby WD, Ramchand SC (1975) Cutaneous manifestations of lightning injury. **Arch Dermatol** 111(11):1466–1468.

460. Neiburger EJ (1978) Tooth stain due to electric burn. **Oral Surg Oral Med Oral Path** 45(2):178.
461. Orgel MG, Brown HC, Woolhouse FM (1975) Electrical burns of the mouth in children; a method for assessing results. **J Trauma** 15(4):285–289.
462. Canady JW, Thompson SA, Bardach J (1996) Oral commissure burns in children. **Plast Reconstr Surg** 97(4):738–744.
463. Kucan JO, Smoot EC (1993) Five percent mafenide acetate solution in the treatment of thermal injuries. **J Burn Care Rehabil** 14(2Pt1):158–163.
464. Klasen HJ (2000) A historical review of the use of silver in the treatment of burns. II. Renewed interest for silver. **Burn** 26(2):131–138.
465. Kunkle R (1988) Electrical injuries. In: Emergency Medicine, 2nd edn, Rosen P, Baker FJ, Barkin RM et al., eds. St. Louis: CV Mosby, p. 621.
466. Wong L, Spence RJ (2000) Escharotomy and fasciotomy of the burned upper extremity. **Hand Clin** 16(2):165–174, vii.

probability, recover. Prolonged cardiopulmonary resuscitation is the key to the resuscitation of lightning strike victims.

Lightning burns are generally superficial, requiring only minimal topical care.[445,455] In the absence of cardiac arrest or serious secondary injury, the care of lightning victims is generally supportive. Tetanus prophylaxis is recommended.

LONG-TERM PROBLEMS

Patients receiving both electrical and lightning burns may experience sleep disturbances, anxiety, chronic pain syndromes, peripheral nerve damage, fear of storms (for lightning victims), and neuropsychiatric damages. The neurologic sequelae include seizures, severe brain damage and spinal artery syndrome which is the result of vascular spasm.[467] Cataracts are a possible sequelae even in children without skin burns on the face.[468]

PEDIATRIC ASPECTS

The most common places of lightning injuries in children are on sports playing fields, swimming pools, and in tents.[469] Children should be educated to abandon outdoor activities during a storm. Whenever they are caught in a thunderstorm, they should avoid high ground, tall trees, bodies of water, and isolated structures. They should avoid contacting, or being in proximity to, metal structures; and remain in a crouching or sitting position to avoid being the tallest object in the immediate vicinity. Electrical burn and lightning survivors require emotional and psychological support. The prognosis depends on the age and severity of the organ involvement. Younger children with more severe burns have a less favourable outcome.[462]

VENOMOUS REPTILE AND ARTHROPOD BITES AND STINGS

Lesley Boyer

INTRODUCTION

Venomous animals are found in all oceans and continents of the world. These include members of every vertebrate class, arthropods, and countless marine invertebrates, most of which species rarely pose a risk to humans. In the United States, clinically significant effects are commonly recognized following envenomation by pit vipers, certain spiders and one scorpion species.

In nature, venom delivery may serve any of several functions, including prey immobilization, prey digestion, and defense. Target animals for these purposes are occasionally mammalian, but frequently they are not; and the complex mixture of chemicals found in any particular animal's venom reflects the ecology and evolutionary biology involved. Depending on the source, venoms may contain a variety of enzymes, low molecular weight polypeptides, lipids, mucopolysaccharides, kinins, and other substances.[470–476]

Effects on human victims, not surprisingly, are widely varied across the spectrum of venomous creatures. Depending on the quantity, composition, and tissue depth of venom injected, patients may present with local trauma, hypersensitivity reactions, direct chemical injury to local tissues, or systemic effects ranging from generalized capillary leak and shock to specific receptor-mediated neurotoxicity. Differential diagnosis accordingly varies with the specific envenomation pattern, and treatment ranges from simple and supportive (e.g., for uncomplicated local inflammation following an insect bite) to intensive care and specific antivenom administration (e.g. for management of complex coagulopathy from rattlesnake bite).

The role of the dermatologist in recognition and management of venomous injury also varies depending on the creature involved. After a bark scorpion sting, for example, there may be little or no recognizable skin abnormality despite severe neurotoxicity. A brown spider bite, on the other hand, may result in dramatic local findings requiring differentiation from other vesiculo-bullous or necrotizing disorders.

Physiology, diagnosis, and treatment will be described separately for snake, scorpion and spider venom poisoning.

SNAKES

In North America, snakes from two native families, Viperidae and Elapidae, are dangerous to humans. Among the vipers, subfamily Crotalinae alone is represented. This subfamily, the pit vipers, includes rattlesnakes, pygmy rattlesnakes, cottonmouths, copperheads, and massasaugas. American elapids include the coral snakes of genera *Micrurus* in the southeast and *Micruroides* in Arizona. Coral snake envenomation, although notorious for its neurotoxicity, provokes very little local tissue injury except that from the direct trauma of the bite. This chapter will accordingly focus on the effects of pit viper envenomation.

The venom apparatus of pit vipers consists of two venom glands, two venom ducts, and two or more upper maxillary teeth. The venom glands lie posterior to the eyes and near the outer edge of the upper jaw.

North American pit viper venoms are rich in enzymatic activity, which is associated with marked tissue destruction. Enzymes may include collagenases, proteases, lipases, and hyaluronidase. Hyaluronidase catalyzes the cleavage of internal glycoside bonds of mucopolysaccharides, resulting in decreased integrity of connective tissue and facilitating the local spread of edema fluid and venom components. Within the region of local spread, a pattern of dramatic capillary leak ensues. This is promoted by the spread of low-molecular-weight venom polypeptides, accompanied in some cases by direct injury to soft tissues, presumably by the degradative actions of larger enzymes.[470,475]

In addition to locally-acting components, crotaline venom may contain a variety of hematologic toxins, including thrombinlike enzymes.[470,475,477] *In vivo*, the net result of actions of these toxins may be severe hypofibrinogenemia, thrombocytopenia, or both. Commonly, this is accompanied by extensive ecchymosis, particularly in the injured tissues near the bite site.

Clinical presentation

Acute pit viper envenomation is a true medical emergency. Although almost all cases begin with relatively simple fang marks and pain at the puncture site, most continue to evolve over the course of many hours. This characteristically involves a mainly proximal progression of dermal and subcutaneous injury, with some combination of tenderness, edema, erythema, lymphangitis, ecchymosis, and bullae (Figs 29.30–29.32). In mild cases, these local manifestations are confined to the tissues immediately surrounding the inoculation site. Severe cases may involve an entire extremity, with edema and ecchymosis spreading across the adjacent trunk; in such cases the loss of blood volume to local edema and extravasation may be sufficient to result in life-threatening anemia or hypovolemic shock.

467. Cooper MA (1995) Emergent care of lightning and electrical injuries. **Semin Neurol** 15(3):268–278.
468. Reddy SC (1999) Electric cataract: a case report and review of the literature. **Eur J Ophthalmol** 9(12):134–138.
469. Cherington M, Martorano FJ, Siebuhr LV et al. (1994) Childhood lightning injuries on the playing field. **J Emerg Med** 12(1):39–41.
470. Dart RC, Russell FE (1992) Animal poisonings. In: Principles of Critical Care, Hall JB, Schmidt GA, Wood LD, eds. New York: McGraw-Hill, p. 2163.
471. Maretić Z, Lebez D (1979) Araneism. Nolit, Belgrade.
472. Sutherland SK (1983) Australian Animal Toxins. Melbourne: Oxford University Press.
473. Russell FE (1965) Marine toxins and venomous and poisonous marine animals. In: Advances in Marine Biology, Vol. 3, Russell FS, ed. London: Academic Press, p. 255.
474. Russell FE (1971) Marine Toxins and Venomous and Poisonous Marine Animals. Neptune City, NJ: TFH Publishers.
475. Russell FE (1980) Snake Venom Poisoning. Philadelphia: JB Lippincott.
476. Russell FE (1988) Venomous arthropods. In: Pediatric Dermatology, Schachner LA, Hansen R, eds. New York: Churchill Livingstone.
477. Kitchen CS, Van Mierop LHS (1983) Mechanism of defibrination in humans after envenomation by the eastern diamondback rattlesnake. **Am J Hermatol** 14:345.

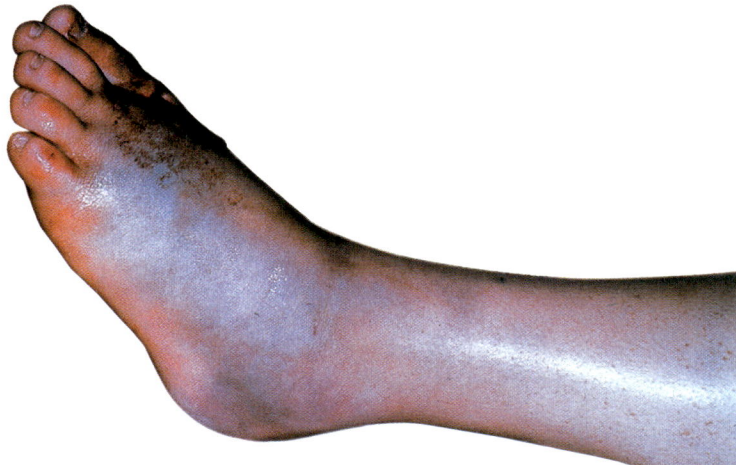

Fig. 29.30   Ecchymosis of foot and leg with minimal swelling 6h following bite by red diamond rattlesnake.

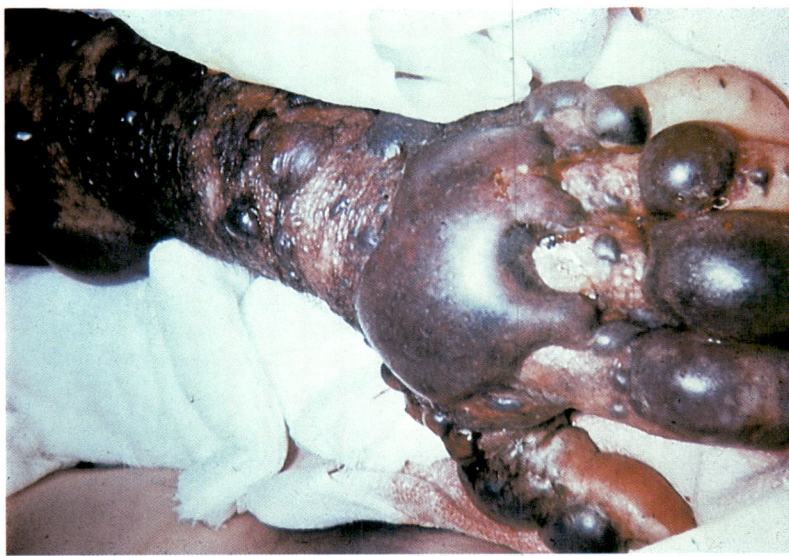

Fig. 29.32   Untreated timber rattlesnake bite at 4 days.

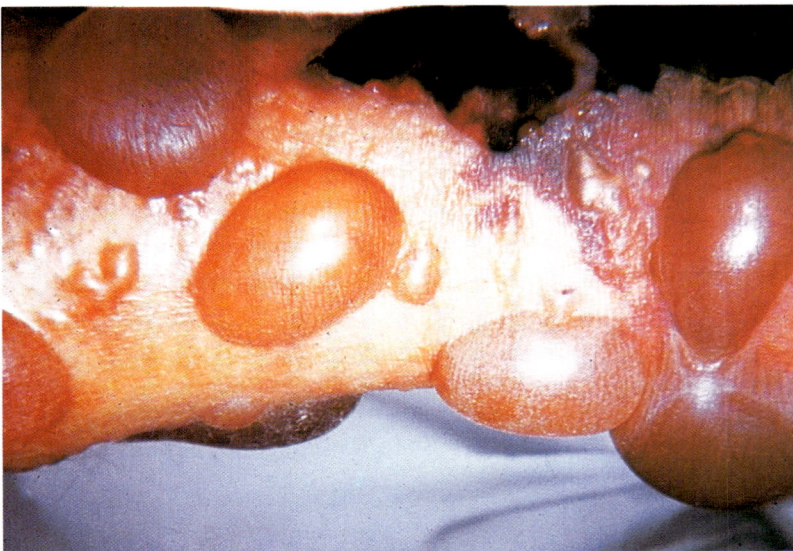

Fig. 29.31   Hemorrhagic bullae 24h following bite by large black-tailed rattlesnake.

Edema and tenderness may be profound enough to mimic compartment syndrome, which although rare in snakebite must be ruled out in equivocal cases by intracompartmental pressure measurement. Depending on the anatomic location of the bite, frank tissue necrosis may become evident days to weeks after the injury; this is commonly observed in bites to the finger or thumb and may require debridement or, rarely, partial amputation. Local injury may be compounded by the damage from "first aid" practices including tourniquet placement, wound incision, cryotherapy, and electric shock.

Systemic signs and symptoms of pit viper envenomation are common, particularly in the first hours following the bite. These may include weakness, sweating, chills, nausea, vomiting, paresthesias, dysgeusia, fasciculations, and central nervous system depression. The best understood systemic effects of pit viper envenomation are hematologic, with thrombocytopenia, hypofibrinogenemia, prolonged prothrombin time and prolonged partial thrombo-plastin time that may occur separately or may combine to mimic disseminated intravascular coagulation (DIC). True DIC is rare but may also occur in severe cases. Acute signs and symptoms associated with snakebite coagulopathy most commonly involve hemorrhage in the bitten limb; but hematemesis, melena, hematuria, and generalized petechiae and ecchymoses have been observed. Coagulopathy may persist for weeks following snakebite, or it may recur after initial normalization with antivenom therapy.[477,478]

Treatment

Initial management of pit viper bite is nonspecific and supportive, including establishment of intravenous access, wound cleansing, tetanus prophylaxis, laboratory assessment, and close observation for local and systemic signs of envenomation. Laboratory work at this time should include a complete blood count, fibrinogen, prothrombin time, partial thromboplastin time, fibrin degradation products, and ethanol level. Formal monitoring of local wound progress should commence immediately and continue for at least 6–12h; this may involve marking the leading edge of the affected area every 15–30min in an effort to recognize ongoing wound progression suggestive of active venom effect.

Although the diagnosis of snakebite is seldom in doubt, there are occasions when the vagaries of intoxicated, farsighted, or very young historians leave the source of a puncture wound uncertain; or an injury may have occurred out of the victim's direct line of sight during rock-climbing or gardening. On such occasions, where the differential diagnosis may include non-venomous animal bite, cactus spine puncture, or necrotizing fasciitis, it is best to observe for at least 6 to 12h and to treat as soon as the diagnosis is manifest.

Once it is clear, on the basis of coagulopathy or of local wound progression, that envenomation is active, the mainstay of pit viper bite treatment is prompt initiation of specific antivenom administration. At present there are two FDA-approved pit viper antivenoms on the US market. One (Wyeth polyvalent anticrotalid) is an equine whole-immunoglobulin product; the other (CroFab®, Protherics) is an ovine affinity-purified Fab-fragment preparation. Product selection, dose, frequency, and duration of treatment depend on product availability and on patient-specific factors such as severity of envenomation and type of coagulopathy involved.[479,480] Precautions are

478. Boyer LV, Seifert SA, Clark RF et al. (1999) Recurrent and persistent coagulopathy following pit viper envenomation. **Arch Int Med** 159:706–710.

479. Seifert SA, Boyer LV (2001) Recurrence phenomena following immunoglobulin therapy of snake envenomations. Part 1: Pharmacokinetics and pharmacodynamics of immunoglobulin antivenoms and related antibodies. **Ann Emerg Med** 37(2):189–195.

480. Boyer LV, Seifert SA, Cain JS (2001) Recurrence phenomena following immunoglobulin therapy of snake envenomations. Part II: Guidelines for clinical management with Crotaline Fab Antivenom. **Ann Emerg Med** 37(2):196–201.

necessary to minimize the risk of acute anaphylactic or anaphylactoid reaction to serum product administration. Physicians not familiar with antivenom dosing and precautions are advised to consult a medical toxicologist before initiating therapy. In the US, 24h access to regional poison information and medical toxicology consultation is available through the American Association of Poison Control Centers by calling 1 (800) 222–1222.

Cutaneous injury from snakebite usually does not require specific topical therapy. Tense bullae sometimes require decompression to relieve distal ischemia, particularly on finger bites. Necrotic tissue may require debridement one to two weeks following the event. Damage from "first aid" such as incision, cryotherapy, tourniquet or electric shock may contribute to local tissue loss and may require surgical intervention.

SCORPIONS

Scorpions are found worldwide, native to every continent but Antarctica. All are predators, most with predominantly arthropod prey. Depending on the species and on the circumstances of prey capture, they rely on a combination of physical restraint and chemical paralysis, with venom, to subdue prey animals. Scorpion venom, which is stored in the final segment of the tail, typically contains neurotoxins specific to arthropod prey. Scorpion venom does *not* typically contain digestive enzymes or other necrotizing factors. Stings by most scorpion species, consequently, have minimal human clinical significance outside of immediate local pain. Very rarely, apparent hypersensitivity to scorpion venom may cause allergic reactions analogous to those seen with hymenoptera stings;[481]

One scorpion family, the Buthidae, includes various species whose venoms contain mammalian neurotoxins of potential hazard to humans. One representative of this family, *Centruroides exilicauda* (a.k.a. *C. sculpturatus*) is native to the southwestern United States.[482] It is found from western New Mexico throughout Arizona and in selected areas along the basin of the Colorado river in California. Isolated colonies have been reported in Clark County Nevada, and in Texas.

These *Centruroides* scorpions contain several ion channel toxins, principally directed against neuronal sodium channels, which disrupt the normal signal-carrying capacity of mammalian axons. Potentiation or aberrant initiation of axonal signals results in a generalized peripheral nervous syndrome, with sympathetic, parasympathetic, and neuromotor hyperactivity.

Clinical presentation

The great majority of adults stung by *Centruroides* scorpions complain of local symptoms only. Pain at the sting site may be severe, although the sting site itself may exhibit little or no objective evidence of inflammation. A small red wheal is sometimes observed around the punctum, but this appearance clears within minutes to hours whereas complaints of exquisite tenderness and shooting pains may continue for hours to days.

In small children, rarely in adults, *Centruroides* envenomation results in a dramatic and characteristic syndrome of neuronal hyperactivity. Symptoms in such cases involve onset within 15 to 30min of agitation, restlessness, abnormal eye movements, hypersalivation, diaphoresis, hypertension, tachycardia, dysphasia, dysphagia, fasciculations, gastrointestinal complaints, and occasionally pulmonary edema. Agitated motor activity includes erratic

twitching, thrashing, and bizarre eye movements that are commonly mistaken for seizure. Without specific antivenom, most patients will show significant neurological and cardiorespiratory improvement by 12–30h,[483,484] however some numbness and tingling may persist for days to weeks.[485]

Treatment

Adults complaining of local pain find some relief in the intermittent application of ice to the sting site. Ongoing or more severe pain can be reduced with non-steroidal anti-inflammatory drugs or with narcotic analgesics.

In the United States, treatment of severe *Centruroides* envenomation has been controversial. A non-FDA-approved caprine whole IgG antivenom has been available, within the state of Arizona only, since 1965. The effectiveness of this antivenom in the control of systemic symptoms of envenomation has been well described, although its use (like that of all serum products) carries risks of acute and delayed serum reactions.[483,485] In 2000, however, production of this antivenom was discontinued. At the current rate of use, a shortage should be seen in the year 2004.[486]

Without specific antivenom, treatment of the systemic *Centruroides* syndrome is supportive for the duration of toxicity, which is usually less than 24h. Short-acting benzodiazepines, such as midazolam, may be administered in the intensive care setting, with supplemental intravenous fluids, oxygen, and ventilatory management as needed. Although there have been no reported deaths using this management approach, mild hypoxemia has been reported in 12% of cases.[484]

In Mexico, Centruroides envenomation is routinely treated with an equine F(ab)$_2$ antivenom. This product (Alacramyn®, Instituto Bioclon) has potential utility against the Arizona species, but it has not yet undergone testing under US INDA.

SPIDERS

The spiders number approximately 34 000 described species and are found in all habitats except for the open sea.[487,488]

Like ticks, mites, scorpions, and other arachnids, spiders have a body consisting of an abdomen and an unsegmented cephalothorax (prosoma) with chelicerate jaws, pedipalps, and four pairs of legs. Spider venom is produced in a gland in the anterior prosoma and delivered through a cheliceral fang.

The primary function of venom in spiders is prey capture or, rarely, defense. Venoms are complex mixtures of neurotoxic and proteolytic peptides, proteins and biogenic amines.[489–492] Most of these toxins are target-specific, acting selectively on arthropods, vertebrates or other groups including some with mammalian-specific activity.[493,494] Venom composition varies widely across spider species and there is evidence of variation within species, between sexes and among geographically isolated populations. In the USA, only a few spider species are considered harmful to people, because in most others the quantity of venom is insufficient, the toxins do not affect mammals, or the fangs cannot penetrate beneath the superficial layers of human epidermis. Of greatest interest in dermatology are spiders of genus *Loxosceles*, the brown or recluse spider group.

The *Loxosceles* genus contains over 100 species that are distributed world-wide, with centers of diversity in central America and around the Mediterranean.[495–497] These spiders are 8–15mm in adult body length, are light

481. Demain G(1995) J Aller Clin Immunol 95(1):135–137.
482. Dehesa-Davila M, Alagon AC, Possani LD (1995) Clinical toxicology of scorpion stings. In: Clinical Toxicology of Animal Venoms and Poisons, Meier J, White J, eds. Boca Raton, FL: CRC Press, pp. 221–238.
483. LoVecchio F, Welch S, Klemens J et al. (1999) Incidence of immediate and delayed hypersensitivity to *Centruroides* antivenom, 34:615–619.
484. Gibley R, Williams M, Walter FG et al. (1999) Continuous intravenous midazolam infusion for *Centruroides exilicauda* scorpion envenomation, 34:620–625.
485. Curry SC, Vance MV, Ryan PJ, Kunkel DB, Northey WT (1983) Envenomation by the scorpion *Centruroides sculpturatus*. J Tox Clin Toxicol 21(4&5):417–449.
486. Bloom, M (2000) Personal communication.
487. Coddington JA, Levi HW (1991) Systematics and evolution of spiders (Araneae). Ann Rev Col Sys 22:565–592.
488. Peters W (1992) Zoology of the arthropods: a colour atlas of arthropods in clinical medicine, London, Wolfe.

489. Atkinson RK, Wright LG (1991) Studies of the necrotic actions of the venoms of several Australian spiders. Comp Biochem Physiol 98C:441.
490. Geren CR, Chan TK, Howell DE, Odell GV (1976) Isolation and characterization of toxins from brown spider venom (*Loxosceles reclusa*). Arch Biochem Biophys 174:90.
491. Misler S, Falke L (1987) Dependence on multivalent cations of quantal release of transmitter induced by black widow spider venom. Am J Physiol 253:C469.
492. Shultz S (1997) The chemistry of spider toxins and spider silk. Angew Chem Int Ed Engl 36:314–326.
493. Grishin EV (1998) Black widow spider toxins: the present and the future. Toxicon 36:1693–1701.
494. Olivera BM, Miljanich GP, Ramachandran J, Adams M (1994) Calcium channel diversity and neurotransmitter release: the w-conotoxins and the w-agatoxins. Annu Rev Biochem 63:823–867.
495. Duffey PH, Limbacher HP (1971) Brown spider bites in Arizona. Ariz Med 28:89.
496. Majeski JA, Durst GG (1976) Necrotic arachnidism. South Med J 69:887.
497. Schenone H, Rojas A, Reyes H et al. (1970) Prevalence of *Loxosceles laeta* in houses in central Chile, Am J Trop Med Hyg 19(3):564.

to dark brown, and have a dark, violin-shaped spot centered anterodorsally, such that the neck of the fiddle extends backward across the cephalothorax.[497,498]

At least five species in the genus have been associated with necrotic arachnidism in the United States, including *L. reclusa* (the true "brown recluse" spider), *L. refuscens*, *L. arizonica*, *L. unicolor*, and *L. laeta*. These spiders are native to all of the southernmost states of the United States. In the Mississippi River valley, their territory extends as far north as southern Wisconsin.[499]

Like pit viper venom, fractionated *Loxosceles* venom contains hyaluronidase, which probably plays a facilitating role in lesion development, encouraging the spread of other venom components.

The most important dermonecrotic factor in *L. reclusa* venom appears to be sphingomyelinase D, a protein fraction of molecular weight 32 000. Sphingomyelinase D is postulated to operate by a variety of mechanisms, among them cell membrane binding and polymorphonuclear leukocyte chemotaxis.[500–502]

Clinical presentation

Necrotic arachnidism, or "loxoscelism" in the case of bite by spiders of the genus *Loxosceles*, is a term applied to the clinical syndrome that follows envenomation by a variety of spiders for which *Loxosceles reclhusa*, the brown recluse spider, is the prototype. The bites of these spiders may result in serious cutaneous injuries, with subsequent necrosis and tissue loss. Less often, there may be severe systemic reactions with hemolysis, coagulopathy, renal failure, and even death.[503]

Venom from *L. reclusa* has been shown to have a direct hemolytic effect on human erythrocytes; this process depends on the presence of serum components that include C-reactive protein and calcium.[504,505] Platelet aggregation, also calcium dependent, can also be induced *in vitro* with sphingomyelinase D; this process may activate the prostaglandin cascade.[506,505]

The clinical spectrum of loxoscelism runs from mild and transient skin irritation to severe local necrosis accompanied by dramatic hematologic and renal injury. Isolated cutaneous lesions are the most common presentation, and it has been suggested that most bites resolve spontaneously without the need for medical intervention.[507] Many authors distinguish between simple local presentation and more severe systemic, or "viscerocutaneous," loxoscelism.

Local symptoms usually begin at the moment of the bite, with a sharp stinging sensation, although it is not uncommon for a patient to report no awareness of having been bitten. Frequently the bite site corresponds to a portal of entry or a region of constriction of clothing, such as cuff, collar, waistband, or groin. The stinging usually subsides over 6–8h and is replaced by aching and pruritus as the site becomes ischemic from local vasospasm. The site then becomes edematous, with an erythematous halo surrounding an irregular violaceous center of "incipient necrosis" (actually hemorrhage and thrombosis)[505,508] (Figs 29.33 and 29.34). A white ring of vasospasm and ischemia may be discernible between the central lesion and the halo. Often the erythematous margin spreads irregularly, in a gravitationally influenced pattern that leaves the original center eccentrically placed near the top of the lesion. In more severe cases, serous or hemorrhagic bullae may arise at the center within 24 to 72h and an eschar forms beneath. Skin biopsy material 4 days following an *L. arizonica* bite shows necrosis of the epidermis as well as fibrinoid necrosis around vessels, necrosis of follicles and eccrine units, and inflammatory infiltrate (color image of skin biopsy).[509] After 2 to 5 weeks the eschar sloughs, leaving an ulcer of variable size and depth through skin and adipose tissue, but sparing muscle.[510] Lesions involving adipose tissue may be extensive, perhaps as a result of lipolytic action of the venom.[511] The ulcer may persist for many months, leaving a deep scar.[512,513]

Systemic involvement is less common but may occur in combination with cutaneous injury from any *Loxosceles* species.[514,515] Systemic reaction may develop in cases with minor-appearing local findings, making diagnosis difficult.[505] When there is systemic involvement, hemolytic anemia with hemoglobinuria is commonly the prominent feature, usually beginning within 24 hours of envenomation and resolving within 1 week.[516] Fever, chills, maculopapular rash, weakness, leukocytosis, arthralgias, nausea, vomiting, thrombocytopenia, disseminated intravascular coagulation, hemoglobinuria, proteinuria, renal failure and death have been reported.[503,517–520]

The diagnosis of loxoscelism is based on spider observation and identification, typical history, and local and systemic signs. The differential diagnosis of the local injury includes bacterial and mycobacterial infection, herpes simplex, decubitus ulcer, burn, embolism, thrombosis, direct trauma, vasculitis, and pyoderma gangrenosum.[521–523] An ELISA assay, developed for the detection of circulating venom antigen, has the potential to develop into a tool for clinicians and epidemiologists.[524,525]

Because *Loxosceles* venom is known to provoke an immune response in experimental animals, efforts have been made to develop diagnostic tests based on antigen or antibody detection in human blood. In 1973, Berger reported an *in vitro* lymphocyte transformation assay for *L. reclusa* venom, which turned positive in the lymphocytes of exposed individuals within 4 to 6 weeks of initial exposure. This test may help to document prior exposure, but not to diagnose envenomation at the time of the initial bite.[526] Barrett and coworkers reported a passive hemagglutination inhibition test using rabbit antibody and human erythrocytes incubated *in vitro* with venom from *L. reclusa*.[527] Cardoso

498. Horen WP (1963) Arachnidism in the United States. **JAMA** 185:839.
499. Waldron WG, Madon MB, Suddarth T (1975) Observations on the occurrence and ecology of *Loxosceles laeta* (Araneae: Scytodidae) in Los Angeles County, California, California Vector Views 22(4):29.
501. Rees RS, Naney LB, Yates RA, King LE (1984) Interaction of brown recluse spider venom on cell membranes: the inciting mechanism? **J Investig Derm** 83:270.
502. Smith CW, Micks DW (1976) The role of polymorphonuclear leukocytes in the lesion caused by the venom of the brown spider, *Loxosceles reclusa*. **Lab Invest** 22:90.
503. Vorse H, Seccareccio P, Woodruff K, Humphrey GB (1972) Disseminated intravascular coagulopathy following fatal brown spider bite (necrotic arachnidism). **J Pediatr** 80:1035.
504. Hufford DC, Morgan PH (1981) C-reactive protein as a mediator in the lysis of human erythrocytes sensitized by brown recluse spider venom. **Proc Soc Exp Biol Med** 167:493.
505. Truett AP III, King LE (1993) Sphingomyelinase D: a pathogenic agent produced by bacteria and arthropods. **Adv Lipid Res** 26:275.
506. Gates CA, Rees RS (1990) Serum amyloid P component: its role in platelet activation stimulated by sphingomyelinase D purified from venom of the brown recluse spider (Loxosceles reclusa). **Toxicon** 28:1303.
507. Berger RS (1973) The unremarkable brown recluse spider bite. **JAMA** 225:109.
508. Butz WC (1971) Envenomation by the brown recluse spider (Aranae, Scytodidae) and related species: a public health problem in the United States. **Clin Toxicol** 4:515.
509. Boyer LV, Theodorou AA, Gomez HF, Binford GJ (2000) Spider on the headboard, child in the unit: severe *Loxosceles arizonica* envenomation confirmed by delayed spider identification and tissue antigen detection. (abstract) Clin Tox.
510. Hershey FB, Aulenbacher CE (1969) Surgical treatment of brown spider bites. **Ann Surg** 170:300.
511. Jong Y-S, Norment BR, Heitz JR (1979) Separation and characterization of venom components in *Loxosceles reclusa*. III. Hydrolytic enzyme activity. **Toxicon** 17:539.
512. Alario A, Price G, Stahl R, Bancoft P (1987) Cutaneous necrosis following a spider bite: a case report and review. **Pediatrics** 79:618.
513. Wasserman GS, Anderson PC (1983) Loxoscelism and necrotic arachnidism. **J Toxicol Clin Toxicol** 21:451.
514. Prince GE (1956) Arachnidism in children. **J Pediatr** 49:101.
515. Taylor EH, Denny WF (1966) Hemolysis, renal failure and death, presumed secondary to the bite of brown recluse spider. **South Med J** 59:1209.
516. Eichner ER (1984) Spider bite hemolytic anemia: positive Coombs' test, erythrophagocytosis, and leukoerythroblastic smear. **Am J Clin Pathol** 81(5):683.
517. Bey TA, Walter FG, Lober W et al. (1997) *Loxosceles arizonica* bite associated with shock. **Ann Emerg Med** 30(5):701–703.
518. Denny WF, Dillaha CJ, Morgan PN (1964) Hemotoxic effect of *Loxosceles reclusa* venom: in vivo and *in vitro* studies. **J Lab Clin Med** 64:291.
519. Ginsburg CM, Weinberg AG (1988) Hemolytic anemia and multiorgan failure associated with localized cutaneous lesion. **J Pediatr** 112:496.
520. Nance WE (1961) Hemolytic anemia of necrotic arachnidism. **Am J Med** 31:801.
521. Kemp DR (1990) Inappropriate diagnosis of necrotizing arachnidism: watch out Miss Muffet but don't get paranoid. **Med J Aust** 152:669.
522. Rand RP, Brown GL, Bostwick J 3rd (1988) Pyoderma gangrenosum and progressive cutaneous ulceration. **Ann Plastic Surg** 20:280.
523. Rees R, Campbell D, Reeger E, King LE (1987) The diagnosis and treatment of brown recluse spider bites. **Ann Emerg Med** 16:9.
524. Chávez-Olórtegui C, Zanetti VC, Ferreira AP et al. (1998) ELISA for the detection of venom antigens in experimental and clinical envenoming by *Loxosceles intermedia* spiders. **Toxicon** 36(4):563–569.
525. Gomez HF, Miller MJ, Warren JS (1999) Antigenic cross-reactivity of venoms from medically important North American *Loxosceles* spider species. **Acad Emerg Med** 6:378 (abs 028).
526. Berger RS, Millikan LE, Conway F (1973) An *in vitro* test for *Loxosceles reclusa* spider bite. **Toxicon** 11:465.
527. Barrett SM et al. (1989) Passive hemagglutination inhibition test for diagnosis of brown recluse spider bite envenomation, poster presentation at the Society for Academic Emergency Medicine, San Diego, CA.

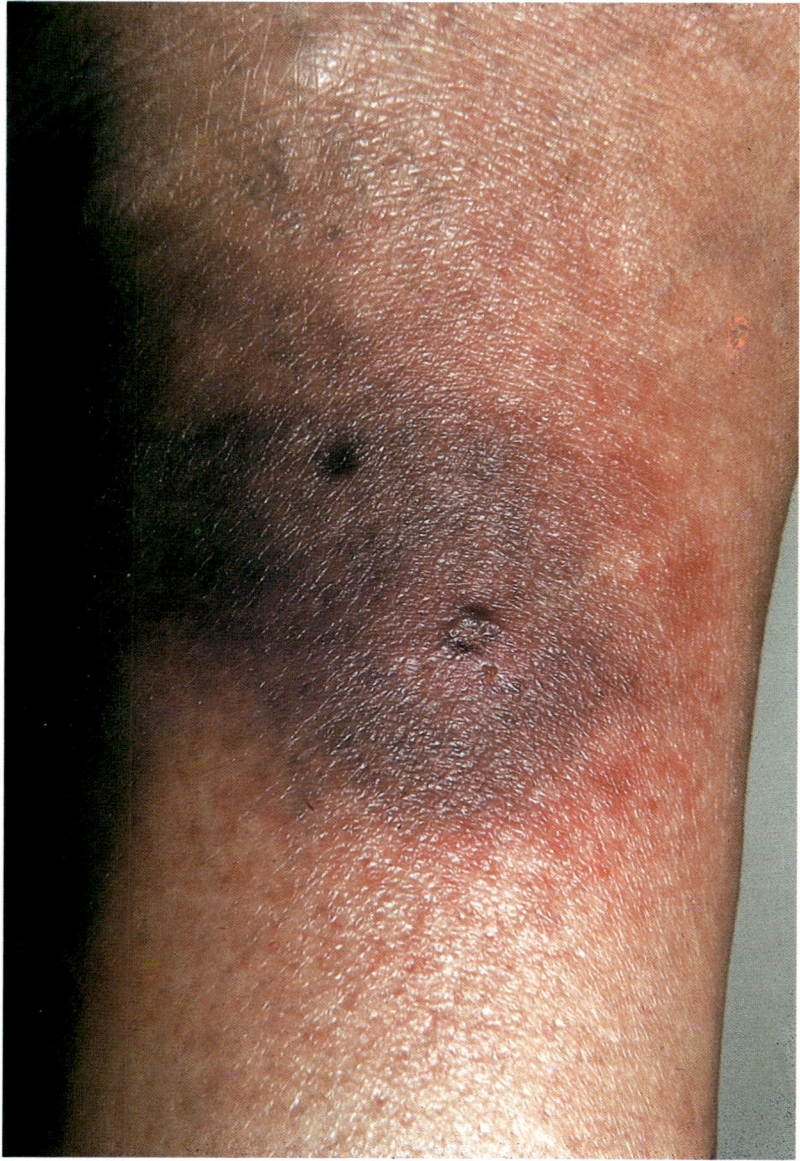

Fig. 29.33 Brown spider bite showing ruptured vesicle and hemorrhogic area. (Courtesy of R. Moser.)

and associates, observing that efforts to detect antigen in human serum may fail because of insufficient antigenemia, have demonstrated the presence of *L. gaucho* venom in biopsy homogenate using enzyme-linked immunosorbent assay. More recently, Barbaro and colleagues have demonstrated circulating IgG against *L. gaucho* venom in 4 out of 20 patients, detectable between 9 and 120 days after the bite.[528]

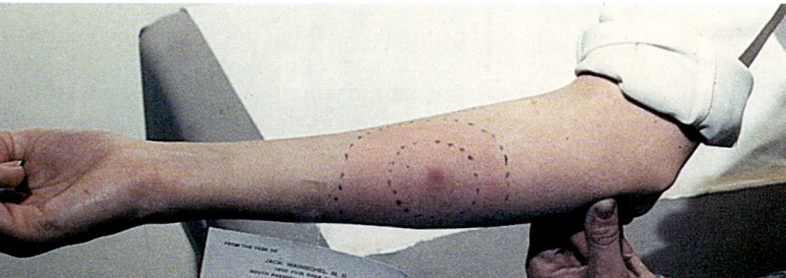

Fig. 29.34 Bull's eye lesion following brown or violin spider (*Loxosceles devi*) bite.

Treatment

Treatment of loxoscelism depends on its severity. Cutaneous loxoscelism can usually be managed on an outpatient basis. Most mild cutaneous envenomations respond symptomatically to application of local cold compresses,[529] elevation of the affected extremity, and loose immobilization. Tetanus prophylaxis should be provided where indicated. Necrotic lesions may need debridement after erythema has subsided to define the margins of the central eschar. This commonly involves significant debridement 1 or 2 weeks after the bite, with close follow-up for several weeks thereafter. In severe cases this can be followed with skin grafting or plastic surgery when the wound is stable. Severe necrotic or infected lesions may lead to hospitalization.

The use of dapsone has been proposed for the prevention of lesion progression in potentially necrotic wounds seen within 48 to 72h of a bite.[530,531] Dapsone is a leukocyte inhibitor that in theory can minimize the local inflammatory component of cutaneous loxoscelism, thereby preventing or lessening subsequent skin necrosis.[532] No prospective, controlled human trial has proved dapsone efficacy, but a variety of case reports and series have been put forward in support of its use in the treatment of potentially necrotic wounds treated in the first days after envenomation.[512,533–535] Typical dosage recommendations are for 50–100mg orally, twice daily. Risks of dapsone therapy include hypersensitivity,[536] methemoglobinemia, and hemolysis in the presence of glucose-6-phosphate dehydrogenase (G6PD) deficiency.

Patients with systemic symptoms should be considered for admission when there is evidence of coagulopathy, hemolysis and hemoglobinuria, or rapid progression of other systemic signs. Care is mainly supportive, commonly involving wound care, fluid management, presumptive treatment for bacterial superinfection, and occasionally blood transfusion. Rarely, hemodialysis has been required for oliguric renal failure.[537] Discharge is appropriate when renal and hematologic statuses are stable.

In patients with significant local or systemic signs or symptoms, laboratory evaluation should include peripheral blood cell count, basic coagulation screening, and urinalysis. Liver and renal function tests are indicated in severe poisonings. When use of dapsone is considered, a screening test for G6PD deficiency may be indicated. The frequency of follow-up testing depends on the course and severity of envenomation. Hospitalized patients may need close follow-up of anemia and renal function over the course of several days.

528. Barbaro KC, Cardoso JL, Eickstedt VR, Mora I (1992) Dermonecrotic and lethal components of *Loxosceles gaucho* spider venom, **Toxicon** 30:331.
529. King LE, Rees RS (1986) Brown recluse spider bites: stay cool. **JAMA** 254:2895.
530. Futrell JM (1992) Loxoscelism. **Am J Med Sci** 304:261.
531. Gendron BP (1990) *Loxosceles reclusa* envenomation. **Am J Emerg Med** 8:51.
532. King LE, Rees RS (1983) Dapsone treatment of a brown recluse bite. **JAMA** 250:648.
533. Benavides MI, Moncada X (1990) Tratamiento de loxocelismo cutaneo con dapsona. **Rev Med Chile** 118:1247.
534. Mack RB (1992) The bite of the spider woman, **NC Med J** 53(5):200.
535. Wesley RE, Ballinger WH, Close LW, Lay AM (1985) Dapsone in the treatment of presumed brown recluse spider bite of the eyelid. **Ophthalmic Surg** 16(2):116.
536. Wille RC, Morrow JD (1988) Case report: dapsone hypersensitivity syndrome associated with treatment of the bite of a brown recluse spider. **Am J Med Sci** 296(4):270. 473.
537. Gonzalez C et al. (1986) Insuficiencia renal aguda en loxocelismo cutaneo-visceral: 11 casos. **Rev Med Chile** 114:1155.

In the past, several authors have reported the use of corticosteroids injected either at the wound site or systemically[538-541] but this remains of questionable benefit.[507] Antihistamines may help control itching but do not change the lesion.[542] Early surgical excision of the wound site has been advocated by some,[543-545] but others have demonstrated that outcomes are better with early medical management in human patients,[546,547] as well as in experimental animals. Hyperbaric oxygen (HBO) treatment has been tried empirically in uncontrolled human trials with reports of good outcome.[548] Comparison of HBO with no treatment in rabbits showed enhanced recovery at 24 days at the histologic level, but there was no apparent clinical difference between the two groups.[549]

There is currently no commercially available *Loxosceles* antivenom in the United States.

SUMMARY

Presentation of venom injury depends on a combination of animal and host factors and ranges from transient epidermal disruption to life-threatening systemic disease. Differential diagnosis, assessment tools, therapies, and prognosis vary with the type of venomous creature involved or suspected. In most cases with skin findings, the dermatologist's primary role is diagnostic. Therapy of systemic envenomation may involve intravenous administration of specific antivenom. Most dermatologic manifestations are managed symptomatically and supportively.

ACKNOWLEDGMENTS

The editors gratefully acknowledge contributions by Alfred T. Lane and Dr. Findlay E. Russell, which were retained from the first edition of *Pediatric Dermatology*.

538. Dillaha CJ et al. (1964) North American loxoscelism – necrotic bite of the brown recluse spider. **JAMA** 188:153.
539. Ingber A, Trattner A, Cleper R, Sandbank M (1991) Morbidity of brown recluse spider bites: clinical picture, treatment and prognosis. **Acta Derm Venereol** (Stockh) 71:337.
540. Jansen GT, Morgan PN, McQueen JN, Bennett WE (1971) The brown recluse spider bite: controlled evaluation of treatment using the white rabbit as an animal model. **South Med J** 64(10):1194.
541. Mara JE, Myers BS (1977) Brown spider bites: treatment with hydrocortisone. **Rocky Mt Med J** 74:257.
542. Lessenden CM Jr, Zimmer LK (1960) Brown spider bites: a survey of the current problem, **J Kans Med Soc** 61:379.
543. Auer AI, Hershey FB (1974) Surgery for necrotic bites of the brown spider. **Arch Surg** 108:612.
544. Fardon DW, Wingo CW, Robinson DW, Masters FW (1967) The treatment of brown spider bite. **Plast Reconst Surg** 40(5):482.
545. Hollabaugh RS, Fernandes ET (1989) Management of the brown recluse spider bite. **J Pediatr Surg** 24(1):126.
546. DeLozier JB, Reaves L, King LE Jr, Rees RS (1988) Brown recluse spider bites of the upper extremity. **South Med J** 81(2):181.
547. Rees R, King LE (1981) Management of the brown recluse spider bite, **Plast Reconstr Surg** 68(5):768.
548. Svendsen FJ (1986) Treatment of clinically diagnosed brown recluse spider bites with hyperbaric oxygen: a clinical observation. **J Ark Med Soc** 83:199.
549. Strain GM, Snider TG, Tedford BL, Cohn GW (1991) Hyperbaric oxygen effects on brown recluse spider (*Loxosceles reclusa*) envenomation in rabbits. **Toxicon** 29(8):989.

Drug Eruptions

Sandra R. Knowles, Lori E. Shapiro and Neil H. Shear

There is limited information available on the incidence of adverse drug reactions (ADRs) in children. A meta-analysis of prospective studies showed that the overall incidence of ADRs in hospitalized children was 9.5%. The rate of pediatric hospital admissions due to ADRs was 2.1%; of these, 39.3% were considered to be life-threatening reactions. For children in outpatient settings, the overall incidence of ADRs was 1.5%.[1] In adults, ADRS have been reported to occur in 10–20% of all hospitalized patients and are thought to be the fourth leading cause of death.[2,3]

Cutaneous eruptions are one of the most frequent presentations of ADRs. The results of a voluntary reporting system in the Netherlands showed that in the 15-year period spanning 1973 to 1988, 4.5% of reported ADRs had occurred in the pediatric population. Of these, 40% had cutaneous manifestations.[4] In a study of pediatric outpatients, ADRs were documented in 4.7% of separate drug courses taken by children and antibiotic-associated rashes were among the most commonly reported reactions.[5] Adverse reactions in children treated as outpatients vary from 1.5 to 4.7%, but drug-induced rashes are at or close to the most common manifestations of drug toxicity.

Drug reactions in the skin range from common mild eruptions, such as an exanthematous eruption, to rare life-threatening drug-induced diseases, such as toxic epidermal necrolysis (TEN). Early recognition of these severe reactions and appropriate management of patients can save lives and reduce morbidity. Problems, other than toxicity, can arise when drug eruptions occur. Patients may be improperly labeled as drug allergic or a drug cause may be missed. A structured approach to drug eruptions is very useful. The focus should be on the drug-induced disease and the process should be organized.

APPROACH TO THE PATIENT WITH A SUSPECTED ADVERSE DRUG REACTION

DIAGNOSIS

The approach to diagnosing drug eruptions is the same as that used for ADRs in general (Table 30.1)[6] The first step in managing an ADR is to make the proper diagnosis. Drug eruptions are distinct disease entities that must be approached as one would any other cutaneous disease. A more precise diagnosis of the reaction pattern will help shorten the list of possible causes, as different drugs are more commonly associated with specific types of reactions.

The morphology of a drug eruption is usually exanthematous, urticarial, blistering or pustular. Exanthematous and urticarial eruptions (with or without angioedema) are the most common types of cutaneous eruptions.[7] Once the morphology of the reaction has been documented, then a more precise differential can be made (e.g., fixed drug eruption, acute generalized exanthematous pustulosis). Fever associated with a cutaneous drug eruption heralds a more serious adverse reaction. This has led us to classify eruptions as simple (no fever or systemic symptoms) or complex (with fever and possibly other systemic manifestations). Most eruptions can be seen in isolation (simple) or in the presence of symptoms or signs (especially fever). This difference can lead to different diagnoses (for example simple urticaria compared with the more complex serum sickness-like reaction).

DIFFERENTIAL DIAGNOSIS

The second step in diagnosing a drug eruption involves an evaluation of the differential diagnosis of the eruption, which often includes viral exanthems (e.g., infectious mononucleosis, parvovirus B19 infection), bacterial infections, Kawasaki disease, collagen vascular disease, and neoplasia. In addition, although the reaction is believed to be caused by a medication, it is not clear which one drug is involved.

Active viral infection and concurrent medications may alter the frequency of drug-associated eruptions. A prime example of this is the ampicillin-induced eruption associated with infectious mononucleosis. Sixty to 100% of patients with this combination will develop a typical exanthematous eruption. However, rechallenge with the ampicillin once the infectious process has cleared does not result in an eruption.[8]

TABLE 30.1 Approach to a suspected adverse reaction

Bedside management
   Clinical diagnosis
   Analysis of drug exposure
   Differential diagnosis

Treatment
   Initiation of treatment strategies

Future management
   Literature search
   Confirmation
   Advice to the patient
   Reporting to licensing authorities and/or manufacturer

1. Impicciatore P, Choonara I, Clarkson A et al. (2001) Incidence of adverse drug reactions in paediatric in/out-patients: a systematic review and meta-analysis of prospective studies. **Br J Clin Pharmacol** 52:77–83.
2. Miller R (1973) Drug surveillance utilizing epidemiological methods: a report from the Boston collaborative drug surveillance program. **Am J Hosp Pharm** 30:584–592.
3. Lazarou J, Pomeranz B, Corey P (1998) Incidence of adverse drug reactions in hospitalized patients: a meta-analysis of prospective studies. **JAMA** 279:1200–1205.
4. Meyboom R (1991) Adverse drug reaction to drugs in children, experiences with "spontaneous monitoring" in Netherlands. **Bratisl Lek Listy** 92:554–559.
5. Kramer M, Hutchinson T, Flegel K et al. (1985) Adverse drug reactions in general pediatric outpatients. **J Pediatr** 106:305–310.
6. Shear N (1990) Diagnosing cutaneous adverse reactions to drugs. **Arch Dermatol** 126:94–97.
7. Roujeau J, Kelly J, Naldi L et al. (1995) Medication use and the risk of Stevens–Johnson syndrome or toxic epidermal necrolysis. **N Engl J Med** 333:1600–1607.
8. Kerns D, Shira J, Go S (1973) Ampicillin rash in children. **Am J Dis Child** 125:187–190.

DRUG EXPOSURE

Drug reactions often occur in complicated clinical scenarios that include exposures to multiple agents. Although most drug eruptions occur within 1 to 6 weeks after initiation of drug therapy, some drug syndromes (e.g., drug-induced lupus) may take up to 3 years to manifest. One should also inquire about drugs that are used intermittently, including over-the-counter preparations and herbal/naturopathic remedies. In patients previously sensitized to a drug, re-administration of the drug may cause symptoms that are typical of an IgE-mediated reaction occurring within 1h. For complex medication histories, it is recommended that a timeline be developed for drug-exposure analysis.

Many patients are unable to remember specific details regarding their reaction. In these cases, especially when the adverse reaction was severe, efforts should be made to obtain original notes from hospitals to correctly document details regarding the timing of the reaction, the names of drugs, the signs, symptoms, laboratory abnormalities, and the treatment of the reaction.

LITERATURE SEARCH

Literature review may include information on onset and duration of the reaction, use of diagnostic tests (skin testing, in-vitro tests) and use of alternative non-crossreacting drugs. Various sources should be consulted including textbooks, medical journals and the pharmaceutical manufacturers.

CONFIRMATION

Skin biopsy should be considered in all severe reactions, particularly those with systemic symptoms, erythroderma, blistering, skin tenderness, purpura and pustulation, or where the diagnosis is uncertain. Certain cutaneous reactions are always due to drug therapy including fixed drug eruptions, and approximately 90% of TEN-cases.[7] For many patients with a drug-induced skin eruption, no laboratory tests are necessary. The diagnosis is based on the morphology and distribution of the eruption.

In vivo or *in vitro* testing can aid in the diagnosis of some drug-induced eruptions. The *in vivo* diagnostic tests that are available include oral rechallenge, skin testing, and patch testing.

An oral provocation test is used when the drug is deemed essential, the risk of eliciting a reaction is known, is considered manageable, and does not exceed the perceived benefit of subsequent treatment with the drug. A drug rechallenge should not be used if a serious reaction such as TEN or a hypersensitivity syndrome reaction occurred to the drug.

Skin tests, usually composed of both prick and intradermal tests, are used primarily for confirmation of IgE-mediated allergic reactions. High-molecular weight drugs, such as vaccines and insulin, are complete antigens and are reliable skin testing materials. However, for most low-molecular weight compounds, reactive metabolites or drug–antigen complexes have not been identified, and skin testing is generally not helpful as a diagnostic test. The exceptions to this include penicillin and local anesthetics. Patch testing can be used to confirm contact dermatitis, fixed drug eruptions, and other delayed dermatologic eruptions such as acute generalized exanthematous pustulosis.[9]

In vitro testing, although posing less risk for the patient, is only used for research purposes. Examples include a radioallergosorbent assay (RAST), a lymphocyte transformation test, and a lymphocyte cytotoxicity assay.[10]

MORPHOLOGIC APPROACH TO DRUG ERUPTIONS

The major presenting morphologies of drug-induced rashes are exanthematous, urticarial, pustular, and blistering. Each of these can be seen alone (simple eruptions) or associated with fever or other systemic symptoms (complex eruptions) and may be seen in viral and complex drug eruptions. Other morphologies exist, such as ichthyosiform, nail changes, hair loss, and psoriasiform eruptions. Because of the rarities of these morphologies in children, they will not be discussed further.

EXANTHEMATOUS ERUPTIONS ("DRUG RASH")

SIMPLE ERUPTION

Simple exanthematous eruptions, are the most common form of drug eruptions, accounting for approximately 95% of skin reactions.[11] These eruptions manifest as generalized erythematous changes in the skin without evidence of blistering or pustulation (Fig. 30.1). They are traditionally call "maculopapular." The term has limited utility since it is nonspecific and is contradictory. Other classic terms are morbilliform or scarlatiniform eruptions, but the diseases these are based on (measles and scarlet fever) are not common enough nowadays to be a true standard for comparison. Amazingly, the most common drug eruption has no name. We use the term exanthematous. These eruptions are usually self-limited but may require symptomatic treatment. Pruritus is the most frequently associated symptom, though it is not a specific symptom, since it is seen in viral or complex drug eruptions. In general, these eruptions are observed within the first ten days of therapy.

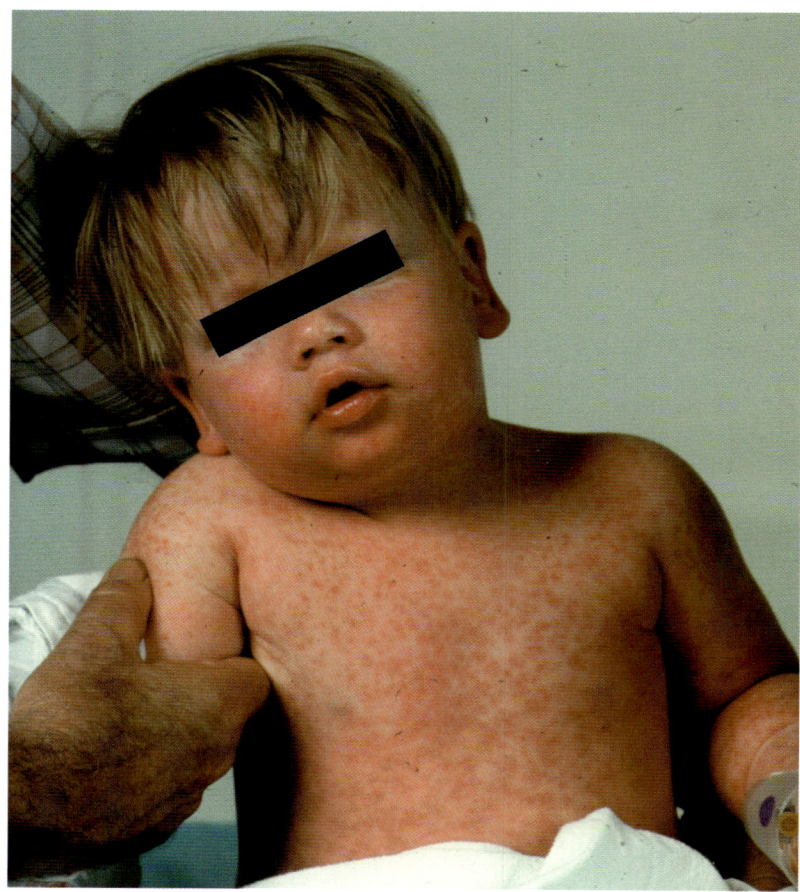

Fig. 30.1   Typical exanthem in an afebrile child after 7 days of amoxicillin therapy.

9. Vicente-Calleja J, Aguirre AN, Crespo V, Gonzalez-Perez R, Diaz-Perez J (1997) Acute generalized exanthematous pustulosis due to diltiazem: confirmation by patch testing. **Br J Dermatol** 137:825–841.

10. Rieder M (1997) In vivo and in vitro testing for adverse drug reactions. **Pediatr Clin North Am** 44:93–111.

11. Bigby M, Jick S, Jick H, Arndt K (1986) Drug-induced cutaneous reactions: a report from the Boston Collaborative Drug Surveillance Program on 15,438 consecutive inpatients, 1975 to 1982. **JAMA** 256:3358–3363.

Resolution occurs with a change in color from bright to a brownish red within 7 to 14 days of discontinuing the offending drug. Scaling or desquamation may follow the colour change. Repeated administration of the same drug is most likely to cause a similar response, or no response at all, rather than a more accelerated or severe reaction.

Exanthematous eruptions can be caused by many drugs including the penicillins, sulfonamides, barbiturates and antiepileptic medications.[11] The histology consists of a mononuclear cell infiltrate of variable intensity, presence of eosinophils and an interface dermatitis, which is characterized by the accumulation of lymphocytes at the dermal–epidermal junction in association with hydropic degeneration of keratinocytes in the basal layer.[12]

COMPLEX ERUPTION: DRUG HYPERSENSITIVITY SYNDROME

When an exanthematous rash occurs in combination with fever, the drug hypersensitivity syndrome (DHS) should be suspected (Fig. 30.2). This is a potentially life-threatening syndrome that presents as a triad of fever, skin eruption and internal organ involvement (Table 30.2).[13] DHS occurs most frequently on first exposure to the offending agent, with initial symptoms starting 1 to 6 weeks after exposure. The rash may appear first at the site of previous radiotherapy (Fig. 30.3). The reaction occurs in approximately 1:3000 exposures with drugs such as aromatic anticonvulsants (phenytoin, carbamazepine, phenobarbital). Other drugs that cause DHS include lamotrigine, sulfonamide antibiotics, dapsone, minocycline and allopurinol.[7,14,15]

Fever and malaise are the first symptoms, but because of the non-specific nature of these events in children, the initial diagnosis, as well as the subsequent discontinuation of the offending agent, may be delayed. Pharyngitis and cervical lymphadenopathy may also be early manifestations. The first signs of the eruption are edema and swelling of the face; followed by erythema and pruritus on the face, with subsequent spread of the erythema caudally. Atypical lymphocytosis eosinophilia may occur during the initial phases of the reaction in a subset of patients.

Approximately 85% of patients will develop an eruption, that ranges from exanthematous to Stevens–Johnson syndrome (SJS) and TEN.

Internal organ involvement most often results in hepatitis, other organs such as the kidney (e.g., interstitial nephritis, vasculitis), CNS (e.g., encephalitis, aseptic meningitis), or the lungs (e.g., interstitial pneumonitis) may be involved. The internal organ involvement can be asymptomatic with only abnormal laboratory tests. Other involvement can include aplastic anemia (or agranulocytosis alone), hypogammaglobulinemia, a syndrome of inappropriate antidiuretic hormone (SIADH), pancreatitis, epididymitis, myositis, carditis, and colitis. Thyroiditis occurs in a subgroup of patients with DHS and may be missed because of the fever, tachycardia and malaise. Thyroid-

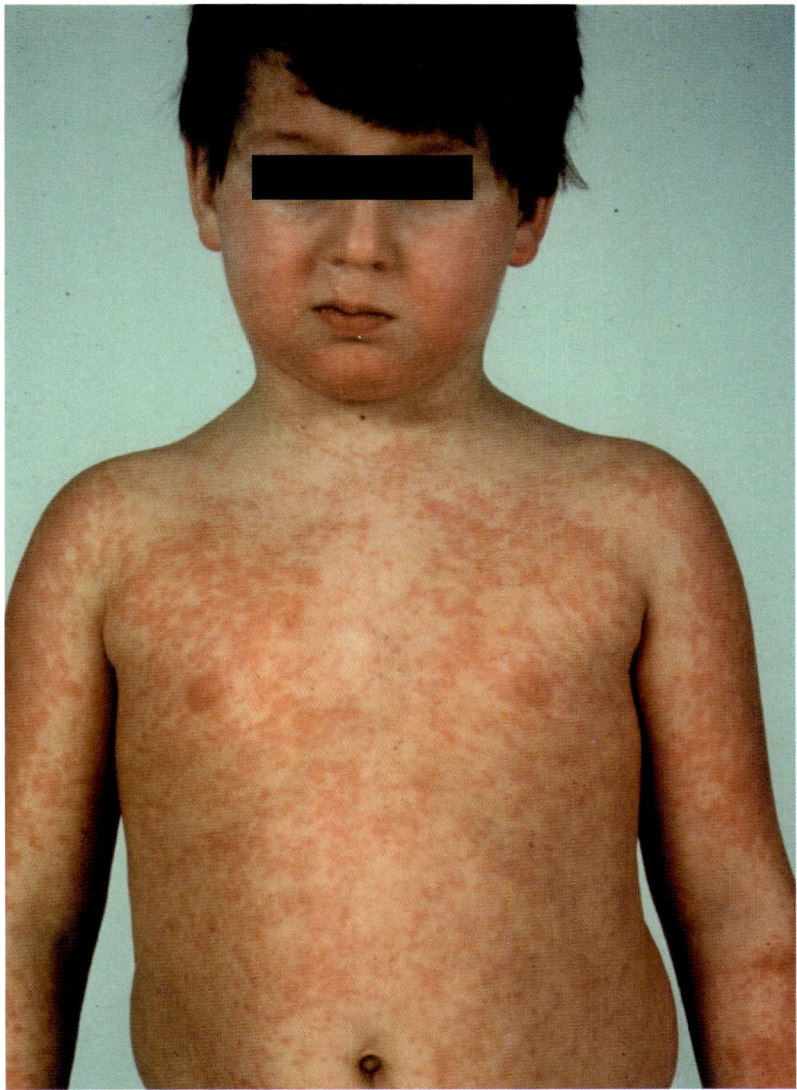

Fig. 30.2   Nine-year-old boy with cerebral palsy and seizures was treated with carbamazepine. Seventeen days after start of therapy he developed fever, rash (exanthematous), lymphadenopathy and nephritis, all part of a drug-induced hypersensitivity syndrome.

TABLE 30.2   Clinical features of drug-hypersensitivity syndrome, drug-induced lupus and serum sickness-like reaction

	Drug hypersensitivity syndrome	Serum sickness-like reaction	Drug-induced lupus
Symptoms	Fever, cutaneous eruption, internal organ involvement	Fever, cutaneous eruption, arthralgias	Musculoskeletal complaints, fever, weight loss
Laboratory abnormalities	Atypical lymphocytosis with prominent eosinophilia; laboratory abnormalities dependent on the organ involved	Mild leukocytosis with eosinophilia	Antinuclear antibodies with homogeneous pattern
Onset of symptoms	2–8 weeks	7–14 days	Up to 2 years
Implicated drugs	Aromatic anticonvulsants (phenytoin, phenobarbital, carbamazepine), lamotrigine, allopurinol, dapsone, sulfonamide, antimicrobials	β-Lactam antibiotics (especially cefaclor), sulfonamide antimicrobials, minocycline	Procainamide, hydralazine, chlorpromazine, isoniazid, methyldopa, penicillamine, minocycline

12. Crowson A, Magro C (1999) Recent advances in the pathology of cutaneous drug eruptions. **Dermatol Clin** 17:537–560.
13. Carroll M, Yueng-Yue K, Esterly N, Drolet B (2001) Drug-induced hypersensitivity syndrome in pediatric patients. **Pediatrics** 108:485–493.
14. Schlienger R, Knowles S, Shear N (1998) Lamotrigine-associated anticonvulsant hypersensitivity syndrome. **Neurology** 51:1172–1175.
15. Knowles S, Shapiro L, Shear N (1996) Serious adverse reactions induced by minocycline: a report of 13 patients and review of the literature. **Arch Dermatol** 132 934–939.

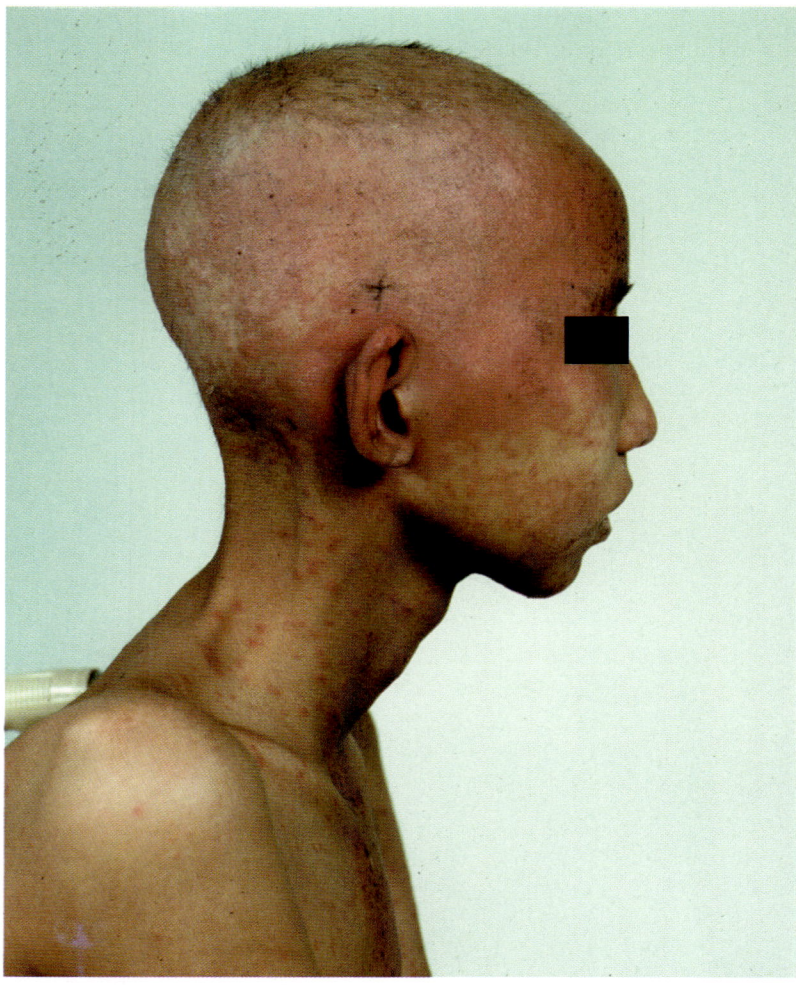

Fig. 30.3   Fourteen-year-old boy with a pinealoma who received radiotherapy followed by phenytoin and dexamethasone. He developed generalized exanthem with fever and neutropenia (anticonvulsant hypersensitivity syndrome.)

When DHS is associated with aromatic anticonvulsants, namely phenytoin, phenobarbital and carbamazepine,[17,18] the formation of toxic metabolites by the anticonvulsants play a pivotal role in the development of DHS.[19–20] Phenytoin, carbamazepine and phenobarbital are metabolized by the cytochrome P450 system to chemically reactive metabolites, although the specific metabolite is unknown. This metabolite is theoretically detoxified by epoxide hydrolases; if detoxification is defective, the toxic metabolite may act as a hapten and initiate an immune response, causing cell necrosis or apoptosis.

In one study,[19] 75% of a series of patients with anticonvulsant DHS to one aromatic anticonvulsant showed *in vitro* cross-reactivity to the other two. Clinically, this correlated with a cross-reactivity rate of 70%. In addition, since primidone is metabolized to phenobarbital, it would be expected to have a high rate of cross-reactivity. Although some reports have indicated that oxcarbazepine may be an alternative to carbamazepine,[21] the reports are conflicting[22] and therefore oxcarbazepine should be considered potentially cross-reactive with carbamazepine. Alternate medications such as benzodiazepines, valproic acid (not in the acute phase because of the risk of hepatitis), or one of the newer anticonvulsants (gabapentin, topiramate, vigabatrin, zonisamide) should be used for seizure control. There is no evidence that lamotrigine cross-reacts with the aromatic anticonvulsants, but it can also cause hypersensitivity reactions[23] including SJS/TEN.

In vitro testing has shown that there is a familial occurrence of hypersensitivity to anticonvulsants, with an autosomal recessive pattern of inheritance.[19,24] This suggests that a patient's siblings risk of having a reaction to an aromatic anticonvulsant may be as high as 1 in 4. In one study, three siblings from a family of 12 siblings, of which eight were available for study, developed hypersensitivity reactions to phenytoin, characterized by fever, rash, lymphadenopathy, and hepatitis.[24] Using the lymphocyte toxicity assay, cells from each of the patients who had experienced an anticonvulsant hypersensitivity syndrome exhibited increased toxicity from metabolites of phenytoin and carbamazepine, while the response to phenobarbital was within normal limits. Of the other five siblings, four showed an abnormal response to phenytoin metabolites, whereas one sibling detoxified phenytoin metabolites normally.[24] In another report of four children who manifested symptoms of anticonvulsant DHS with carbamazepine, three patients had an exacerbation after conversion to another aromatic anticonvulsant. Discontinuation of treatment with the aromatic anticonvulsants resulted in resolution of symptoms; valproic acid was well tolerated in three patients who required continued anticonvulsant therapy.[25]

DHS has also been associated with minocycline,[15,26] usually occurring 2–4 weeks after initiation of therapy. Neither tetracycline nor doxycycline is associated with DHS.[27] The pathogenesis of minocycline-induced DHS is unknown; it has been theorized that a reactive metabolite may be generated during the metabolism of minocycline.[28] Cross-reactivity between minocycline and other tetracyclines has not been described; despite this caution is advised regarding administration of other tetracyclines in the context of DHS due to minocycline.

Sulfonamide antibiotics such as sulfamethoxazole and sulfadiazine are frequently associated with DHS. The primary metabolic pathway for sulfonamides involves renal excretion after acetylation to a nontoxic metabolite. An alternative metabolic pathway, quantitatively more important in slow

stimulating hormone (TSH) levels are extremely low early in this reaction but chemical hypothyroidism may take 2 months to develop after initiation of the reaction.[16] Antimicrosomal antibodies are often positive. Antibody-positive hemolytic anemia has been seen.

In managing patients with DHS, it is not uncommon for the disease to initially improve and then flare 3–4 weeks after the start of the reaction. Patients will redevelop an eruption, fever, malaise and may have a recurrence of internal organ involvement; the recurrence generally results in much milder symptoms than the original presentation. In patients who are re-exposed to the drug, the usual reaction is development of fever and erythroderma within hours. This lasts for up to a week, but patients generally recover without sequelae.

16. Gupta A, Eggo M, Uetrecht J et al. (1992) Drug-induced hypothyroidism: The thyroid as a target organ in hypersensitivity reactions to anticonvulsants and sulfonamides. **Clin Pharmacol Ther** 51:56–67.
17. Vittorio C, Muglia J (1995) Anticonvulsant hypersensitivity syndrome. **Arch Intern Med** 155:2285–2290.
18. Konishi T, Naganuma Y, Hongo K et al. (1993) Carbamazepine-induced skin rash in children with epilepsy. **Eur J Pediatr** 152:605–608.
19. Shear N, Spielberg S (1988) Anticonvulsant hypersensitivity syndrome, in vitro assessment of risk. **J Clin Invest** 82:1826–1832.
20. Spielberg S, Gordon G, Blake D et al. (1981) Anticonvulsant toxicity in vitro: possible role of arene oxides. **J Pharmacol Exp Ther** 217:386–389.
21. Zakrzewska J, Ivanyi L (1988) In vitro lymphocyte proliferation by carbamazepine, carbamazepin-10 11 epoxide, and oxcarbazepine in the diagnosis of drug-induced hypersensitivity. **J Allergy Clin Immunol** 82:110–115.
22. Pirmohamed M, Graham AP, Smith D et al. (1991) Carbamazepine-hypersensitivity: assessment of clinical and in vitro chemical cross-reactivity with phenytoin and oxcarbazepine. **Br J Clin Pharmacol** 32:741–749.
23. Chattergoon D, McGuigan M, Koren G et al. (1997) Multiorgan dysfunction and disseminated intravascular coagulopathy in children receiving lamotrigine and valproic acid. **Neurology** 49.
24. Gennis M, Vemuri R, Burns E et al. (1991) Familial occurrence of hypersensitivity to phenytoin. **Am J Med** 91:631–634.
25. Alldredge B, Knutsen A, Ferriero D (1994) Antiepileptic drug hypersensitivity syndrome: in vitro and clinical observations. **Pediatr Neurol** 10:169–171.
26. Colvin J, Sheth A (2001) Minocycline hypersensitivity syndrome with hypotension mimicking septic shock. **Pediatr Dermatol** 18:295–298.
27. Shapiro L, Knowles S, Shear N (1997) Comparative safety and risk management of tetracycline, doxycline and minocycline. **Arch Dermatol** 133:1224–1230.
28. Shapiro L, Uetrecht J, Shear N (2001) Minocycline, perinuclear antibody, and pigment. The biochemical basis. **J Am Acad Dermatol** 45:787–789.

acetylators, involves the cytochrome P450 mixed function oxide system (CYP2C9). These enzymes can transform the parent compound to reactive metabolites, namely hydroxylamine and nitroso compounds that produce cytotoxicity independent of preformed drug-specific antibody. In most individuals, detoxification of the metabolite occurs. In susceptible patients who are unable to detoxify this metabolite, accumulation of the toxic metabolite occurs, resulting in the development of DHS.[29] Other aromatic amines, such as procainamide, dapsone and acebutolol, are metabolized to similar compounds and should be avoided in patients who develop DHS.[30] Cross-reactivity does not occur with sulfonamides that are not aromatic amines (e.g., sulfonylureas, thiazide diuretics, furosemide, acetazolamide).[31]

After DHS has been identified, there are laboratory tests that will help in evaluating internal organ involvement that is asymptomatic. Liver transaminase levels, complete blood cell count (CBC), urinalysis, and serum creatinine level should be obtained; in addition, the clinician should be guided by the presence of symptoms that may suggest specific internal organ involvement. Thyroid function tests should be measured and repeated after 2–3 months. A skin biopsy may be helpful if the patient has a blistering or a pustular eruption. There are no readily available diagnostic or confirmatory tests, although an *in vitro* test has been used to identify abnormalities in detoxification.[32]

The role of corticosteroids is controversial, but most clinicians elect to start prednisone at a dose of 1–2mg/kg/day if symptoms are severe for 3–4 weeks with a gradual taper to avoid rebound of symptoms. Antihistamines and topical corticosteroids can also be used to alleviate symptoms. Intravenous immunoglobulin (1g/kg/day for 2 days) was used in a 6-year-old boy with phenytoin-induced DHS.[33] The risk of DHS in first-degree relatives of patients with this reaction is substantially higher than the general population; counseling of family members is a crucial part of management.

URTICARIAL ERUPTIONS

Urticaria is characterized by pruritic red wheals of varying sizes. Individual lesions generally last for less than 24–48h, although new lesions can continually develop. When deep dermal and subcutaneous tissues are involved, the reaction is known as angioedema. Angioedema is frequently nonpruritic and typically lasts for 1–2h, although it may persist for 2–5 days. Urticaria and angioedema, when associated with drug use, are usually indicative of an IgE-mediated (immediate) hypersensitivity reaction; this mechanism is typified by immediate reactions to penicillin and other antibiotics. Combinations of the drug or metabolites with IgE bound to the surfaces of cutaneous mast cells lead to activation, degranulation and release of vasoactive mediators including histamine, leukotrienes, and prostaglandins.[34] Nonimmunologic activation of inflammatory mediators may also result in urticarial reactions. For example, narcotic analgesics may directly cause release of histamine from mast cells independent of the IgE mechanism.[35] Other causes of nonimmunologic

reactions include radiocontrast media, acetylsalicylic acid, and nonsteroidal anti-inflammatory drugs (NSAIDS).

Latex allergy is a type I reaction to natural rubber latex proteins with clinical manifestations ranging from contact urticaria to fatal anaphylaxis.[36] Those at most risk of latex allergy include children with spina bifida; such children have frequent exposure to natural rubber latex products via catheters and multiple surgeries where latex products are used.[37] A 23-kDa polypeptide from natural rubber has been incriminated in causing latex allergy in children with spina bifida.[38] Other children at risk include those with an atopic diathesis.

The diagnosis of latex allergy is based on the history and clinical presentation. Symptoms include contact urticaria at sites of latex exposure, such as lip swelling after blowing up a balloon or sucking a pacifier; mucosal symptoms such as itchy, swollen eyes, runny nose, sneezing or wheezing after aerosolization of the powder from latex gloves, to which the latex protein adheres; and anaphylaxis.[39] Certain foods contain proteins that can cross-react with latex, such as banana, kiwi, avocado, and chestnuts, and can cause oral pruritus, edema, urticaria, and wheezing after ingestion. The best treatment for latex allergy is avoidance. Nonlatex substitutes are available for most commonly used natural rubber latex products. Skin testing with latex allergen utilizes the suspected product, and *in vivo* tests to detect specific IgE antibodies in sera are used for evaluation of the latex allergy.

SERUM SICKNESS-LIKE REACTION (SSLR)

It is important to differentiate between true serum sickness (which is seldom seen nowadays) and serum sickness-like reactions. True serum sickness is characterized by fever, lymphadenopathy, arthralgias, cutaneous eruptions, gastrointestinal disturbances and malaise, as well as proteinuria.[40] In contrast, serum sickness-like reaction is defined by fever, rash (either urticarial or erythema multiforme-like) and arthralgias occurring 1–3 weeks after drug exposure (Fig. 30.4). Lymphadenopathy and eosinophilia may also be present; however, immune complexes, hypocomplementemia, vasculitis, and renal lesions are usually absent in serum sickness-like reactions.

Epidemiological evidence in children suggest that the risk of SSLR is greatest with cefaclor than with other antibiotic therapy, including other cephalosporins.[41–43] The overall incidence rate of cefaclor SSLRs has been estimated to be approximately 0.024% to 0.2% per course of cefaclor prescribed. The data suggest that SSLR occurs more frequently with cefaclor than with amoxicillin, especially in children younger than 5 years of age who are exposed to multiple courses of cefaclor.[44] Although the pathogenesis is unknown, a reactive cefaclor metabolite is generated during its metabolism that may bind to tissue proteins and elicit an inflammatory response manifested as SSLR.[45] Other drugs that have been recently implicated in SSLRs include cefprozil,[46] minocycline,[47,48] and bupropion (especially as Zyban used for smoking cessation).[49]

29. Shear N, Spielberg S, Grant D et al. (1986) Differences in metabolism of sulfonamides predisposing to idiosyncratic toxicity. **Ann Int Med** 105:179–187.
30. Knowles S, Uetrecht J, Shear N (2000) Idiosyncratic drug reactions: the reactive metabolite syndromes. **Lancet**: in press.
31. Knowles S, Shapiro L, Shear N (2001) Should celecoxib be contraindicated in patients who are allergic to sulfonamides? Revisiting the meaning of "sulfa" allergy. **Drug Saf** 24:239–247.
32. Neuman M, Malkiewicz I, Shear N (2000) A novel lymphocyte toxicity assay to assess drug hypersensitivity syndromes. **Clin Biochem** 33:517–524.
33. Scheuerman O, Nofech-Moses Y, Rachmel A, Ashkenazi S (2001) Successful treatment of antiepileptic drug hypersensitivity syndrome with intravenous immune globulin. **Pediatrics** 107:E14.
34. Anderson J (1992) Allergic reactions to drugs and biologic agents. **JAMA** 268:2845–2857.
35. Fisher M, Harle D, Baldo B (1991) Anaphylactoid reactions to narcotic analgesics. **Clin Rev Allergy** 9:309–318.
36. Taylor J, Praditsuwan P (1996) Latex allergy: review of 44 cases including outcome and frequent association with allergic hand eczema. **Arch Dermatol** 132:265–271.
37. Porri F, Pradal M, Lemiere C et al. (1997) Association between latex sensitization and repeated latex exposure in children. **Anesthesiology** 86:599–602.
38. Lu L, Kurup V, Hoffman D et al. (1995) Characterization of a major latex allergen associated with hypersensitivity in spina bifida patients. **J Immunol** 155:2721–2728.
39. Sullivan T, Magera B (1995) Recurrent allergic reactions to latex in a hospitalized pediatric patient. **J Allergy Clin Immunol** 96:423–425.
40. Lawley T, Bielory L, Gascon P et al. (1984) A prospective clinical and immunologic analysis of patients with serum sickness. **N Engl J Med** 311:1407–1413.
41. Heckbert S, Stryker W, Coltin K et al. (1990) Serum sickness in children after antibiotic exposure: estimates of occurrence and morbidity in a Health Maintenance Organization population. **Am J Epidemiol** 132:336–342.
42. Stricker B, Tijssen J (1992) Serum sickness-like reactions to cefaclor. **J Clin Epidemiol** 45:1177–1184.
43. Isaacs D (2001) Serum sickness-like reaction to cefaclor. **J Paediatr Child Health** 37:298–299.
44. Vial T, Pont J, Pham E et al. (1992) Cefaclor-associated serum sickness-like disease: eight cases and review of the literature. **Ann Pharmacother** 26:910–914.
45. Kearns G, Wheeler J, Childress S, Letzig L (1994) Serum sickness-like reactions to cefaclor: role of hepatic metabolism and individual susceptibility. **J Pediatr** 125:805–811.
46. Lowery N, Kearns G, Young R, Wheeler J (1994) Serum sickness-like reactions associated with cefprozil therapy. **J Pediatr** 125:325–328.
47. Harel L, Amir J, Livni E et al. (1996) Serum sickness-like reaction associated with minocycline therapy in adolescents. **Ann Pharmacother** 30:481–483.
48. Malakar S (2001) Is serum sickness an uncommon adverse effect of minocycline treatment? **Arch Dermatol** 137:100–101.
49. McCollom R, Elbe DA (2000) Bupropion-induced serum sickness-like reaction. **Ann Pharmacother** 34:471–473.

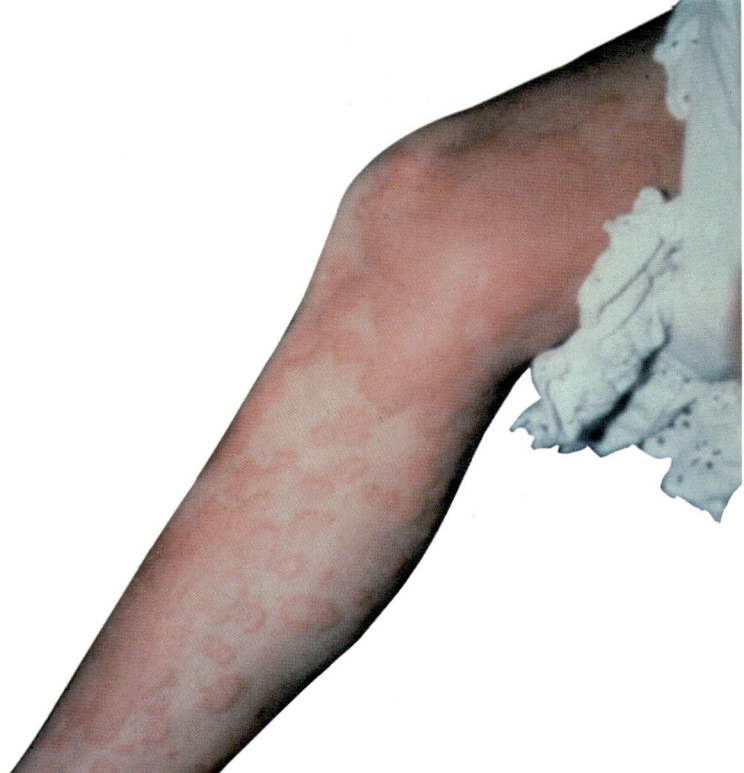

Fig. 30.4 Urticarial rash associated with fever and arthritis due to cefaclor (serum sickness-like reaction).

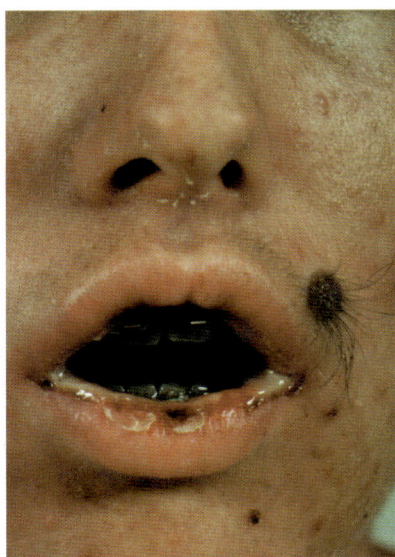

Fig. 30.5 Sixteen-year-old boy being treated with high dose methotrexate developed typical oral mucositis and an acneiform eruption.

portional to the dose and/or duration of therapy, and patients with a history of acne, particularly if severe, are predisposed. Topical medications or cosmetics, especially oil-based products, may also cause an acneiform eruption referred to as pomade acne. Acne fulminans has been induced by testosterone in 1–2% of adolescent boys treated for excessively tall stature.[54]

Discontinuation of the drug and symptomatic treatment with antihistamines and topical corticosteroids are recommended in patients with SSLR. A short course of oral corticosteroids may be required in patients with more severe symptoms. The drug causing the SSLR should be avoided in the future. For cefaclor and cefprozil, the risk of cross-reaction among β-lactam antibiotics is small, and further administration of another cephalosporin is usually well tolerated.[44] Some clinicians recommend that all beta-lactam drugs be avoided in patients who experience SSLR from cefaclor.[50]

PUSTULAR ERUPTIONS

ACNEIFORM ERUPTIONS

Drug-induced acne may appear in atypical areas such as the arms and legs, is usually monomorphous and generally heals without scarring.[51] Comedones are usually absent. Acneiform eruptions do not affect prepubertal children, indicating that prior hormonal priming is a necessary prerequisite. Topical tretinoin may be useful, if the drug cannot be discontinued.[52] Once the drug is discontinued, the eruption clears, over a period of weeks.

Acneiform eruptions occur with various drugs including iodides, bromides, ACTH, corticosteroids, isoniazid, androgens, lithium, actinomycin D, and phenytoin (Fig. 30.5). Corticosteroids can precipitate "steroid acne" within 2 weeks of starting the medication.[53] The risk appears to be directly pro-

ACUTE GENERALIZED EXANTHEMATOUS PUSTULOSIS (AGEP)

More commonly reported in adults, AGEP has been reported in children.[55,56] The reaction is characterized by an acute onset, with a temperature above 38°C, and a cutaneous eruption composed of nonfollicular sterile pustules on an edematous erythema.[57] In half the patients, additional cutaneous lesions are found, including edema of the face, target lesions, purpura, vasculitis, blisters, and mucosal erosions. Following discontinuation of the offending agent, generalized desquamation occurs after two weeks. Leukocytosis is a common finding, usually subsiding before the desquamation begins. Eosinophilia, hypocalcemia, and renal failure have been documented.

The exact pathogenesis of AGEP is not known; it is theorized that a circulating antigen-antibody complex produced by medication may be responsible for the skin eruption. Patch testing to the putative drug is often positive resulting in a localized pustular reaction.[58]

AGEP most commonly results from the use of β-lactam and macrolide antibiotics, and calcium channel blockers. The estimated incidence rate is approximately 1 to 5 cases per million per year.[59] Treatment consists of discontinuation of the offending drug, and the occasional use of prednisone in severe cases in a dose of 1–2mg/kg/day until resolution of the eruption. The differential diagnosis includes pustular psoriasis, DHS with pustulation, subcorneal pustular dermatosis (Sneddon–Wilkinson disease), pustular vasculitis and TEN, especially in severe cases of AGEP. A Tzanck-smear preparation of a pustule will show predominantly polymorphonuclear white blood cells. The typical histopathology shows spongiform subcorneal and/or intraepidermal pustules, marked edema of the papillary dermis and perivascular infiltrates with neutrophils and exocytosis of eosinophils.

50. Grammer L (1996) Cefaclor serum sickness. **JAMA** 275:1152–1153.
51. Heng C (1982) Cutaneous manifestation of lithium toxicity. **Br J Dermatol** 106:107–109.
52. Remmer H, Falk W (1986) Successful treatment of lithium-induced acne. **J Clin Psychiatry** 47:48.
53. Hurwitz R (1989) Steroid acne. **J Am Acad Dermatol** 21:1179–1181.
54. Traupe H, von Muhlendahl K, Bramswig J, Happle R (1988) Acne of the fulminans type following testosterone therapy in three excessively tall boys. **Arch Dermatol** 124:414–417.
55. Roujeau J, Bioulac-Sage P, Bourseau C et al. (1991) Acute generalized exanthematous pustulosis: analysis of 63 cases. **Arch Dermatol** 127:1333–1338.
56. Meadows K, Egan C, Vaderhooft S (2000) Acute generalized exanthematous pustulosis (AGEP), an uncommon condition in children: case report and review of the literature. **Pediatr Dermatol** 17:399–402.
57. Beylot C, Doutre M, Beylot-Barry M (1996) Acute generalized exanthematous pustulosis. **Semin Cutaneau Med Surg** 15:244–249.
58. Moreau A, Dompmartin A (1995) Drug-induced acute generalized exanthematous pustulosis with positive patch tests. **Int J Dermatol** 34:263–266.
59. Sidoroff A, Haleevy S, Bainck J et al. (2001) Acute generalized exanthematous pustulosis (AGEP): a clinical reaction pattern. **J Cutan Pathol** 28:113–119.

BULLOUS ERUPTIONS

PSEUDOPORPHYRIA

Pseudoporphyria is a cutaneous phototoxic disorder, which resembles either porphyria cutanea tarda (PCT) or erythropoietic protoporphyria (EPP). When the clinical picture resembles PCT it is characterized by skin fragility, blister formation, crusting and scarring, in a photodistribution, on the face and dorsa of the hands. The porphyrin levels are normal. When the eruption resembles EPP there is cutaneous burning, erythema, vesiculation, angular chicken-pox-like scars and waxy thickening of the skin.[60] Fair skin and light eye color are significant risk factors. The development of pseudoporphyria is not dose-dependent nor is it limited to geographic areas with excessive sun exposure. There was no difference in age or sex observed in a study in the juvenile rheumatoid arthritis population.[61] Other features of PCT such as milia, hypertrichosis, hyperpigmentation and sclerodermoid features are absent.[62]

Both clinical presentations are photosensitive drug reactions caused most frequently by chronic NSAID use, and most commonly in children with JRA. Approximately 12% of children receiving naproxen, a propionic acid derivative, for JRA developed pseudoporphyria in one series.[61] Other NSAIDs, particularly propionic acid derivatives such as oxaprozin and ketoprofen, have also been associated with pseudoporphyria.[60] Nonrelated drugs including furosemide, tetracycline, isotretinoin, and erythropoietin have also been reported to cause pseudoporphyria.

The mechanism of drug-induced pseudoporphyria is unknown; it is thought to result from a non-immunologic phototoxic effect. After absorption of ultraviolet radiation in the skin, a chemically reactive species such as singlet oxygen, may lead to cell membrane damage.[63] Naproxen and other propionic acid derivatives, have been shown to be phototoxic *in vitro*.[64]

A skin biopsy and a normal porphyrin level is needed to confirm the diagnosis of pseudoporphyria. Because of the risk of permanent facial scarring, the implicated drug should be discontinued when skin fragility and blistering is noted.[61] Despite discontinuation, blisters may continue to appear for weeks, and skin fragility may persist for months. Once naproxen is discontinued, resolution of all the cutaneous findings, except scarring occurs.[65] If the patient requires continued use of an NSAID, a medication should be chosen that is less photosensitizing (e.g., diclofenac, indomethacin, sulindac). Broad-spectrum sunscreen and protective clothing should be recommended for all children treated with naproxen.

ERYTHEMA MULTIFORME MAJOR, SJS, TEN

Erythema multiforme major (EMM), SJS and TEN may represent variants of the same disease process. The exact incidence of EMM, SJS and TEN is unknown since there is disagreement over the definition of each entity, as well as clinical and histopathological overlap.[66] Clinically, each of these reaction patterns is characterized by the presence of a triad of mucous membrane erosions, atypical target lesions and epidermal necrosis with skin detachment (Fig. 30.6A,B).

The most frequent drugs cited as causes for EMM, SJS or TEN are the anticonvulsants, antibiotics (especially sulfonamide antimicrobials and penicillins), allopurinol, and NSAIDs (e.g., piroxicam).[7] SJS and TEN have been reported with lamotrigine; the reaction rate may be as high as 1 in 1000 in adults and higher in children; the risk is even greater when coadministered with valproic acid.[67–69] The more severe the reaction, the more likely it is that is has been drug-induced. A large percentage of cases of EMM and SJS are not drug related and may develop as a result of a variety of other predisposing factors including infections, neoplasia and autoimmune disease. Drugs are implicated as the causative factor in 15 to 65% of pediatric patients.[70] Determining the etiology of SJS is difficult; of 51 children with SJS, 56% had an antecedent upper respiratory tract or nonspecific viral infection, and 67% had received a prescription medication in the 3 weeks before the onset of SJS.[71] In a review of 259 adult patients with TEN, 90% were associated with medication use.[72]

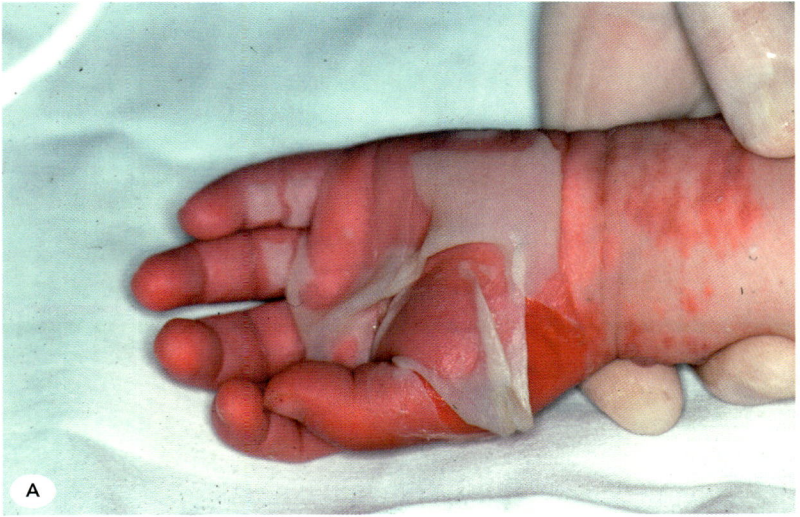 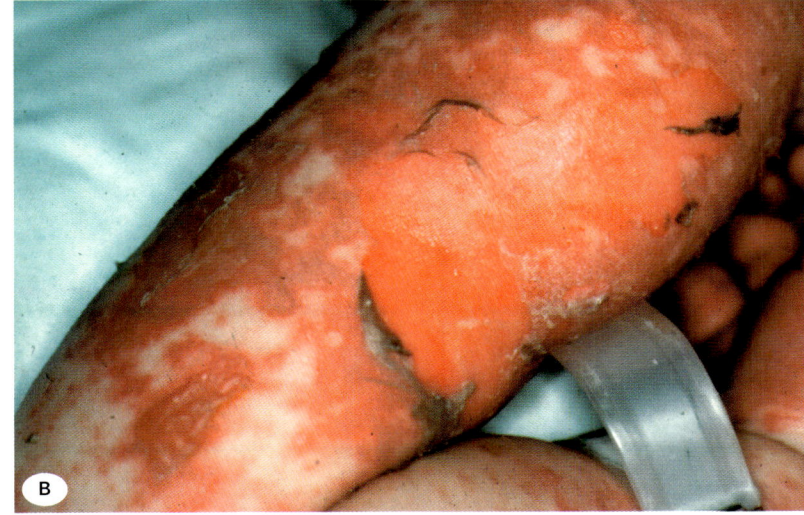

Fig. 30.6 (A, B) Both are photos of patient who had SJS/TEN overlap from phenobarbital. This is characterized by hemorrhagic mucositis, atypical targets and blisters.

60. Al-Kehnaizan S, Schechter J, Sasseville D (1999) Pseudoporphyria induced by propionic acid derivatives. **J Cutan Med Surg** 3:162–166.
61. Lang B, Finlayson L (1994) Naproxen-induced pseudoporphria in patients with juvenile rheumatoid arthritis. **J Pediatr** 124:639–642.
62. Bigby M, Stern R (1985) Cutaneous reactions to nonsteroidal anti-inflammatory drugs. **J Am Acad Dermatol** 12:866–876.
63. Kochevar I (1989) Photoxicity of nonsteroidal anti-inflammatory drugs. **Arch Dermatol** 125:824–826.
64. Ljunggren B (1985) Propionic acid-derived nonsteroidal anti-inflammatory drugs are phototoxic in vitro. **Photodermatol** 2:3–9.
65. Levy M, Barron K, Eichenfield A, Honig P (1990) Naproxen-induced pseudoporphyria: a distinctive photo dermatitis. **J Pediatr** 117:660–664.
66. Bastuji-Garin S, Rzany B, Stern R et al. (1993) Clinical classification of cases of toxic epidermal necrolysis, Stevens–Johnson syndrome, and erythema multiforme. **Arch Dermatol** 129:92–96.
67. Dooley J, Camfield P, Gordon K et al. (1996) Lamotrigine-induced rash in children. **Neurology** 46:240–242.
68. Mitchell P (1997) Paediatric lamotrigine use hit by rash reports. **Lancet** 349:1080.
69. Wadelius M, Karlsson T, Wadelius C et al. (1996) Lamotrigine and toxic epidermal necrolysis. **Lancet** 348:1041.
70. Rasmussen J (1976) Erythema multiforme in children. **Br J Dermatol** 95:181–186.
71. Ginsberg C (1982) Stevens–Johnson syndrome in children. **Pediatr Infect Dis** 1:155–158.
72. Schopf E, Stuhmer AB, Victor N et al. (1991) Toxic epidermal necrolysis and Stevens–Johnson syndrome: an epidemiologic study from West Germany. **Arch Dermatol** 127:839–842.

Children with SJS or TEN are acutely ill with nonspecific prodromal symptoms of malaise, anorexia and fever. Symptoms usually start within the first 2 months of drug initiation. In general, the prodromal period lasts approximately 1–2 days before the onset of skin lesions. Patients who have SJS develop mucosal lesions, preceding the onset of the eruption by 1 to 2 days. Extensive blisters with a gray–white membrane, hemorrhagic crusts, especially on the lips, and superficial erosions and ulcerations occur.[73] In patients with TEN, the initial lesions are morbilliform or a diffuse painful erythema that rapidly generalizes. Superficial bullae develop within the areas of erythema and rapidly enlarge. Extensive mucous membrane involvement is typified by conjunctivitis and rhinorrhea;[74] the trachea, bronchi and anogenital area can also be involved. Severe ocular complications include pseudomembrane formation that can lead to permanent visual impairment.[75–77]

Fluid and electrolyte imbalance and secondary bacterial infections lead to an overall mortality rate in TEN that ranges from 25 to 50%. Internal organ involvement includes pulmonary complications (e.g., pulmonary edema, atelectasis, pneumonitis, bronchiolitis obliterans, organizing pneumonia), hepatic and hematologic abnormalities (e.g., anemia, leukocytosis, lymphopenia, thrombocytopenia).

The pathogenesis of severe cutaneous adverse drug reactions is unknown, although a metabolic basis similar to that of DHS has been hypothesized.[19] Sulfonamides and aromatic anticonvulsants are metabolized to toxic metabolites that are subsequently detoxified in most individuals. However, in predisposed patients with a genetic defect, the metabolite may bind covalently to proteins. These metabolites may trigger apoptosis resulting in severe cutaneous adverse reactions.[78] In some of these patients, the metabolite-protein adducts may trigger an immune response that may lead to a cutaneous adverse drug reaction.[79]

Management of EMM, SJS and TEN includes discontinuation of the suspected drug and supportive measures, such as careful wound care, hydration and nutritional support. To rule out concurrent internal organ involvement, a complete blood cell count, liver enzyme analysis and chest radiograph should be performed. The patient should be treated in an intensive care or burn unit if skin involvement is severe or widespread. Intravenous immunoglobulin (IVIG), which contains naturally occurring FasL-blocking antibodies, has been shown to halt progression of TEN in 10 adult patients, and produce a favorable outcome in all patients within 48h of administration.[78] The current published maximum dose of IVIG used has been 0.75g/kg/day for 4 consecutive days. We now recommend a total of 2.5–3g/kg administered daily over 3 days. A limited number of adult patients have been treated with other drugs such as cyclophosphamide[80] and cyclosporin.[81] The use of corticosteroids in SJS and TEN is controversial. Some clinicians believe corticosteroids may be beneficial when administered early in the disease and at relatively high dosage.[82] Other clinicians suggest that corticosteroids do not shorten the recovery time and may increase the risk of complications including secondary infections and gastrointestinal bleeding.[83] Thalidomide was shown to be detrimental in the treatment of TEN, possibly because of paradoxical enhancement of tumor necrosis factor α production.[84] Patients

---

TABLE 30.3   Drug eruptions

Eruption	Pattern and distribution of skin lesions	Mucous membrane involvement	Key implicated drugs
Erythema multiforme major	Target lesions, limbs	Absent/present	Anticonvulsants, sulfonamide antibiotics, allopurinol, NSAIDs (e.g., piroxicam), dapsone
Stevens–Johnson syndrome	Atypical targets, widespread	Present	
Toxic epidermal necrolysis	Epidermal necrosis with skin detachment	Present	
Pseudoporphyria	Skin fragility, blister formation in photodistribution	Absent	Tetracycline, furosemide, naproxen
Exanthematous	Erythematous changes without blistering or pustulation, often generalized	Absent	Penicillins, sulfonamides, antiepileptic medications, non-nucleoside reverse transcriptase inhibitors
Urticaria	Pruritic red wheals, variable presentation	Absent	Penicillins, aspirin/NSAIDs, opiates, sulfonamides, radiocontrast media
Angioedema	Swollen deep dermal and subcutaneous tissues, frequently unilateral	Present or absent	ACE-inhibitors, aspirin/NSAIDs
Acneiform	Inflammatory lesions and comedones usually absent, atypical areas (e.g., arms, legs)	Absent	Iodides, corticosteroids, isoniazid, androgens, lithium, phenytoin
Fixed drug eruption	Solitary, erythematous, bright red or dusky red macules that may evolve into an edematous plaque, variable presentation	Present or absent	Phenolphthalein, ibuprofen, sulfonamides, tetracyclines, lamotrigine, barbiturates

ACE, angiotensin-converting enzyme; NSAID, nonsteroidal anti-inflammatory drug.

---

73. Leaute-Labreze C, Lamireau T et al. (2000) Diagnosis, classification and management of erythema multiforme and Stevens–Johnson syndrome. **Arch Dis Child** 83:347–352.

74. Rasmussen J (1975) Toxic epidermal necrolysis. A review of 75 cases in children. **Arch Dermatol** 111:1135–1139.

75. Ringheanu M, Laude T (2000) Toxic epidermal necrolysis in children – an update. **Clin Pediatr** 39:687–694.

76. Sheridan R, Schulz J, Ryan C et al. (2002) Long-term consequences of toxic epidermal necrolysis in children. **Pediatrics** 109:74–78.

77. Spies M, Sanford AJF, Wolf S, Herndon D (2001) Treatment of extensive toxic epidermal necrolysis in children. **Pediatrics** 108:1162–1168.

78. Viard I, Wehrli P, Bullani R et al. (1998) Inhibition of toxic epidermal necrolysis by blockade of CD95 with human immunoglobulin. **Science** 282:490–493.

79. Wolkenstein P, Charue D, Lawent P et al. (1995) Metabolic predisposition to cutaneous adverse drug reactions. **Arch Dermatol** 131:544–551.

80. Heng M, Allen S (1991) Efficacy of cyclophosphamide in toxic epidermal necrolysis. **J Am Acad Dermatol** 25:778–786.

81. Sullivan J, Watson A (1996) Lamotrigine-induced toxic epidermal necrolysis treated with intravenous cyclosporin: a discussion of pathogenesis and immunosuppressive management. **Aust J Dermatology** 37:208–212.

82. Patterson R, Miller M, Kaplan M et al. (1994) Effectiveness of early therapy with corticosteroids in Stevens-Johnson syndrome: experience with 41 cases and a hypothesis regarding pathogenesis. **Ann Allergy** 73:27–34.

83. Prendville J, Hebert A, Greenwald M, Esterly N (1989) Management of Stevens–Johnson syndrome and toxic epidermal necrolysis in children. **J Pediatr** 115:881–887.

84. Wolkenstein P, Latarjet J, Roujeau J et al. (1998) Randomised comparison of thalidomide versus placebo in toxic epidermal necrolysis. **Lancet** 352:1586–1589.

in whom a severe cutaneous adverse reaction has developed should not be rechallenged with the drug or undergo desensitization with the medication. Although SJS and TEN are usually seen as single organ reactions, they may coexist with DHS; it is prudent to investigate a patient with possible SJS/TEN for systemic involvement (Table 30.3).

MISCELLANEOUS DRUG REACTIONS

NEUTROPHILIC ECCRINE HIDRADENITIS (NEH)

There are numerous cases of NEH temporally linked to chemotherapy in both children and adults. The eruption generally begins 11 days after starting chemotherapy for acute myelogenous leukemia or lymphoma, and is associated with neutropenia and fever.[85] The most common clinical presentation is with erythematous and edematous papules and plaques on the face and trunk. Other manifestations include unilateral or bilateral periorbital edema and erythema. Although neutrophilic eccrine hidradenitis resolves spontaneously without treatment in most patients, corticosteroids and nonsteroidal antiinflammatories have been used for the treatment of the accompanying fever and tender skin lesions. Dapsone has been used to prevent recurrence when chemotherapy regimens are cyclical and has been successful in one case in preventing repeat attacks.[86]

FIXED DRUG ERUPTION

Fixed drug eruptions (FDE) are characterized by lesions that recur at the same sites, whenever the responsible drug is administered. The lesion of FDE is a well-circumscribed, oval edematous plaque, dusky brown or gray; it may be a large bulla in some cases[87] (Fig. 30.7). If exposure to the offending agent continues, the inflammation intensifies and the lesion turns dusky red or

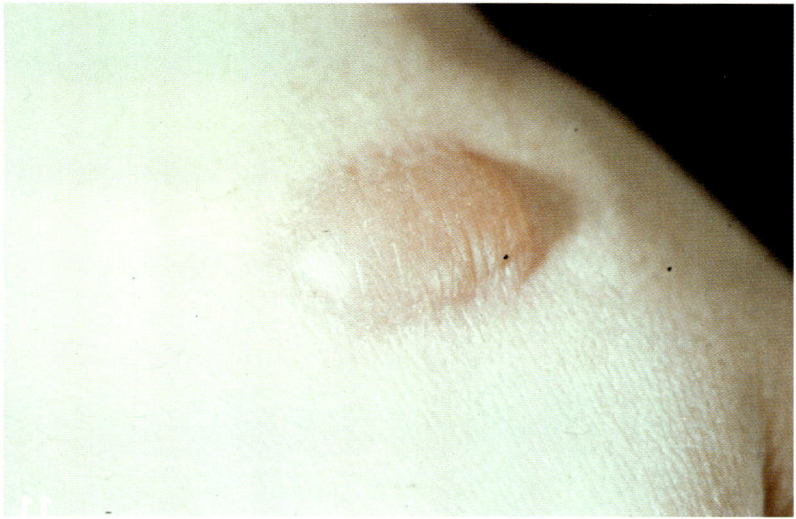

Fig. 30.7   Bullous fixed drug eruption on the dorsum of the hand in a patient who was taking tetracycline for acne.

violaceous. Local symptoms include pruritus and a burning sensation. Systemic symptoms are rare. The cardinal morphological feature is a persistent pigmentation following the acute stage. This highly typical hyperpigmentation makes the diagnosis obvious even weeks to months after the eruption subsides.

There are usually few lesions which vary in size. The sites include lips, trunk, legs, arms and genitals. The glans penis is often affected. Once the patient has acquired an FDE to a drug, rechallenge will always result in an immediate (within 30min to 8h) recurrence of the existing lesions and appearance of new lesions.

FDE is more commonly observed in adults than children. In one series, FDE was the second most common drug eruption, after exanthematous drug eruptions, in both children and adults. FDE was seen in 22% of children with cutaneous drug reactions.[88]

The drugs commonly associated with FDE are barbiturates, sulfonamides, phenolphthalein, tetracyclines, acetaminophen, salicylates, and NSAIDs.[89] Significantly higher frequencies of the A30 antigen and A30 B13 Cw6 haplotype were found in 42 patients with FDE induced by trimethoprim-sulfamethoxazole. HLA-B55 (a split of B22) was present exclusively in trimethoprim-sulfamethoxazole-induced FDE, and in a higher frequency than in control subjects. This is the first report that finds a haplotype linkage in the setting of trimethoprim-sulfamethoxazole-induced FDE.[90]

Histologically, FDE resembles erythema multiforme, with an interface dermatitis of lymphocytes at the dermal-epidermal junction and degenerative changes of the epithelium with dyskeratosis.[12] In addition, there is evidence of chronic injury in FDE manifested by acanthosis, hyperkeratosis, and hypergranulosis. Eosinophils and neutrophils are also present. An increased number of helper and suppressor T lymphocytes is observed in lesional skin. The T cells may persist within lesional skin and are believed to contribute to immunological "memory".[91]

Cases of FDE are asymptomatic and do not pose serious sequelae for the child. Discontinuation of the drug is key to the management of the reaction. FDE can be mistaken for insect bites, urticaria, or erythema multiforme; bullous FDE can be confused with SJS and TEN.

Although a challenge or provocation test with the suspected drug may be useful in establishing the diagnosis, the patient may be at risk for a more severe reaction. Patch testing at the site of a previous lesion yields a positive response in up to 30% of patients.[92] Prick and intradermal skin tests may be positive in 24 and 67% of patients, respectively.[93]

DRUG-INDUCED LUPUS

Drug-induced lupus (DIL) is defined by the development of antinuclear antibodies, at least one clinical symptom of lupus erythematosus (LE), symptom resolution on discontinuation of drug therapy, and absence of idiopathic LE.[94] Most patients have frequent musculoskeletal complaints, fever and weight loss, pleuropulmonary involvement in more than half of the patients, and rarely, renal, neurologic or vasculitic involvement. Cutaneous findings of LE are rare. DIL is a relatively uncommon event in children, since many of the drugs known to cause DIL (procainamide, hydralazine) are rarely used in children.

There have been several reports of DIL attributed to minocycline.[95–97] Most cases have been reported in young adult women who were using it for

85. Wenzel F, Horn T (1998) Nonneoplastic disorders of the eccrine glands. **J Am Acad Dermatol** 38:1–17.
86. Shear N, Knowles S, Shapiro L, Poldre P (1996) Dapsone in prevention of recurrent neutrophilic eccrine hidradenitis. **J Am Acad Dermatol** 35:819–822.
87. Baird B, DeVillez R (1988) Widespread bullous fixed drug eruption mimicking toxic epidermal necrolysis. In: **J Dermatol** 27:170–174.
88. Sharma V, Dhar S (1995) Clinical pattern of cutaneous drug eruption among children and adolescents in north India. **Pediatr Dermatol** 12:178–183.
89. Sehgal V, Gangwani O (1987) Fixed drug eruption: current concepts. **Int J Dermatol** 26:67–72.
90. Ozkaya-Bayazit E, Akar U (2001) Fixed drug eruption induced by trimethoprim-sulfamethoxazole: evidence for a link to HLA-A30 B13 Cw6 haplotype. **J Am Acad Dermatol** 45:712–717.
91. Breathnach S (1995) Mechanisms of drug eruptions: part 1. **Aust J Derm** 36:121–127.
92. Bork K (1988) Cutaneous side effects of drugs. Philadelphia: WB Saunders.
93. Barbaud A, Reichert-Penetrat S, Trechot P et al. (1998) The use of skin testing in the investigation of cutaneous adverse drug reactions. **Br J Dermatol** 49:139.
94. Price E, Venables P (1995) Drug-induced lupus. **Drug Saf** 12:283–290.
95. Gough A, Chapman S, Wagstaff K et al. (1996) Minocycline-induced autoimmune hepatitis and systemic lupus erythematosus-like syndrome. **Br Med J** 312:169–172.
96. Bryne P, Williams B, Pritchard M (1994) Minocycline-related lupus. **Br J Rheumatol** 33:674–676.
97. Akin E, Miller L, Tucker L (1997) Minocycline-induced lupus in adolescents. **Pediatrics** 926–928.

treatment of acne vulgaris. The drug eruption may occur after several weeks of usage, but may also occur 2 years after the initiation of drug therapy.[95,96] The common clinical findings are arthritis, hepatitis and positive antinuclear antibody. A rash, if present, can be urticarial as well as erythematous or vasculitic.[97] Unlike other drugs causing DIL, antihistone antibody is seldom present.[95–97] HLA-DR-4 or HLS-DR-2 were present in many of the patients when HLA class II alleles were investigated.[98,99] Treatment includes discontinuation of minocycline. There is fairly prompt resolution of arthritis in days to weeks with disappearance of the ANA within one year. Avoidance of tetracycline antibiotics is prudent.

PEDIATRIC ASPECTS OF THE DISEASE

Some complications arise in the diagnosis of drug eruptions in children. The most common issue is with the differential diagnosis between drug versus infection ("drug or bug"). Infectious exanthemata are common and confound the diagnostic process. Drug hypersensitivity syndrome is due to drugs that are often used for the first time in childhood, such as antiepileptic drugs or sulfonamide antimicrobials. The presence of fever and rash in a child has a large differential and with an assumed focus on infectious causes, a drug etiology can easily be missed. Despite some diagnostic issues, drug eruptions in children are similar to those seen in adults.

98. Dunphy, Oliver M, Rands A et al. (2000) Antineutrophil cytoplasmic antibodies and HLA class II alleles in minocycline-induced lupus-like syndrome. **Br J Dermatol** 142:461–467.

99. Ellkayam O, Levartovsky D, Bratubar C et al. (1998) Clinical and immunological study of 7 patients with minocycline-induced autoimmune phenomena. **Am J Med** 105:484–487.

INDEX

Page numbers in *italic* represent figures, those in **bold** represent tables.

ELSEVIER CD-ROM LICENSE AGREEMENT

PLEASE READ THE FOLLOWING AGREEMENT CAREFULLY BEFORE USING THIS CD-ROM PRODUCT. THIS CD-ROM PRODUCT IS LICENSED UNDER THE TERMS CONTAINED IN THIS CD-ROM LICENSE AGREEMENT ("Agreement"). BY USING THIS CD-ROM PRODUCT, YOU, AN INDIVIDUAL OR ENTITY INCLUDING EMPLOYEES, AGENTS AND REPRESENTATIVES ("You" or "Your"), ACKNOWLEDGE THAT YOU HAVE READ THIS AGREEMENT, THAT YOU UNDERSTAND IT, AND THAT YOU AGREE TO BE BOUND BY THE TERMS AND CONDITIONS OF THIS AGREEMENT. ELSEVIER INC. ("Elsevier") EXPRESSLY DOES NOT AGREE TO LICENSE THIS CD-ROM PRODUCT TO YOU UNLESS YOU ASSENT TO THIS AGREEMENT. IF YOU DO NOT AGREE WITH ANY OF THE FOLLOWING TERMS, YOU MAY, WITHIN THIRTY (30) DAYS AFTER YOUR RECEIPT OF THIS CD-ROM PRODUCT RETURN THE UNUSED CD-ROM PRODUCT, ALL ACCOMPANYING DOCUMENTATION TO ELSEVIER FOR A FULL REFUND.

DEFINITIONS As used in this Agreement, these terms shall have the following meanings:

"Proprietary Material" means the valuable and proprietary information content of this CD-ROM Product including all indexes and graphic materials and software used to access, index, search and retrieve the information content from this CD-ROM Product developed or licensed by Elsevier and/or its affiliates, suppliers and licensors.

"CD-ROM Product" means the copy of the Proprietary Material and any other material delivered on CD-ROM and any other human-readable or machine-readable materials enclosed with this Agreement, including without limitation documentation relating to the same.

OWNERSHIP This CD-ROM Product has been supplied by and is proprietary to Elsevier and/or its affiliates, suppliers and licensors. The copyright in the CD-ROM Product belongs to Elsevier and/or its affiliates, suppliers and licensors and is protected by the national and state copyright, trademark, trade secret and other intellectual property laws of the United States and international treaty provisions, including without limitation the Universal Copyright Convention and the Berne Copyright Convention. You have no ownership rights in this CD-ROM Product. Except as expressly set forth herein, no part of this CD-ROM Product, including without limitation the Proprietary Material, may be modified, copied or distributed in hardcopy or machine-readable form without prior written consent from Elsevier. All rights not expressly granted to You herein are expressly reserved. Any other use of this CD-ROM Product by any person or entity is strictly prohibited and a violation of this Agreement.

SCOPE OF RIGHTS LICENSED (PERMITTED USES) Elsevier is granting to You a limited, non-exclusive, non-transferable license to use this CD-ROM Product in accordance with the terms of this Agreement. You may use or provide access to this CD-ROM Product on a single computer or terminal physically located at Your premises and in a secure network or move this CD-ROM Product to and use it on another single computer or terminal at the same location for personal use only, but under no circumstances may You use or provide access to any part or parts of this CD-ROM Product on more than one computer or terminal simultaneously.

You shall not (a) copy, download, or otherwise reproduce the CD-ROM Product in any medium, including, without limitation, online transmissions, local area networks, wide area networks, intranets, extranets and the Internet, or in any way, in whole or in part, except for printing out or downloading nonsubstantial portions of the text and images in the CD-ROM Product for Your own personal use; (b) alter, modify, or adapt the CD-ROM Product, including but not limited to decompiling, disassembling, reverse engineering, or creating derivative works, without the prior written approval of Elsevier; (c) sell, license or otherwise distribute to third parties the CD-ROM Product or any part or parts thereof; or (d) alter, remove, obscure or obstruct the display of any copyright, trademark or other proprietary notice on or in the CD-ROM Product or on any printout or download of portions of the Proprietary Materials.

RESTRICTIONS ON TRANSFER This License is personal to You, and neither Your rights hereunder nor the tangible embodiments of this CD-ROM Product, including without limitation the Proprietary Material, may be sold, assigned, transferred or sublicensed to any other person, including without limitation by operation of law, without the prior written consent of Elsevier. Any purported sale, assignment, transfer or sublicense without the prior written consent of Elsevier will be void and will automatically terminate the License granted hereunder.

TERM This Agreement will remain in effect until terminated pursuant to the terms of this Agreement. You may terminate this Agreement at any time by removing from Your system and destroying the CD-ROM Product. Unauthorized copying of the CD-ROM Product, including without limitation, the Proprietary Material and documentation, or otherwise failing to comply with the terms and conditions of this Agreement shall result in automatic termination of this license and will make available to Elsevier legal remedies. Upon termination of this Agreement, the license granted herein will terminate and You must immediately destroy the CD-ROM Product and accompanying documentation. All provisions relating to proprietary rights shall survive termination of this Agreement.

LIMITED WARRANTY AND LIMITATION OF LIABILITY NEITHER ELSEVIER NOR ITS LICENSORS REPRESENT OR WARRANT THAT THE CD-ROM PRODUCT WILL MEET YOUR REQUIREMENTS OR THAT ITS OPERATION WILL BE UNINTERRUPTED OR ERROR-FREE. WE EXCLUDE AND EXPRESSLY DISCLAIM ALL EXPRESS AND IMPLIED WARRANTIES NOT STATED HEREIN, INCLUDING THE IMPLIED WARRANTIES OF MERCHANTABILITY AND FITNESS FOR A PARTICULAR PURPOSE. IN ADDITION, NEITHER ELSEVIER NOR ITS LICENSORS MAKE ANY REPRESENTATIONS OR WARRANTIES, EITHER EXPRESS OR IMPLIED, REGARDING THE PERFORMANCE OF YOUR NETWORK OR COMPUTER SYSTEM WHEN USED IN CONJUNCTION WITH THE CD-ROM PRODUCT. WE SHALL NOT BE LIABLE FOR ANY DAMAGE OR LOSS OF ANY KIND ARISING OUT OF OR RESULTING FROM YOUR POSSESSION OR USE OF THE SOFTWARE PRODUCT CAUSED BY ERRORS OR OMISSIONS, DATA LOSS OR CORRUPTION, ERRORS OR OMISSIONS IN THE PROPRIETARY MATERIAL, REGARDLESS OF WHETHER SUCH LIABILITY IS BASED IN TORT, CONTRACT OR OTHERWISE AND INCLUDING, BUT NOT LIMITED TO, ACTUAL, SPECIAL, INDIRECT, INCIDENTAL OR CONSEQUENTIAL DAMAGES. IF THE FOREGOING LIMITATION IS HELD TO BE UNENFORCEABLE, OUR MAXIMUM LIABILITY TO YOU SHALL NOT EXCEED THE AMOUNT OF THE LICENSE FEE PAID BY YOU FOR THE SOFTWARE PRODUCT. THE REMEDIES AVAILABLE TO YOU AGAINST US AND THE LICENSORS OF MATERIALS INCLUDED IN THE SOFTWARE PRODUCT ARE EXCLUSIVE.

If this CD-ROM Product is defective, Elsevier will replace it at no charge if the defective CD-ROM Product is returned to Elsevier within sixty (60) days (or the greatest period allowable by applicable law) from the date of shipment.

Elsevier warrants that the software embodied in this CD-ROM Product will perform in substantial compliance with the documentation supplied in this CD-ROM Product. If You report a significant defect in performance in writing to Elsevier, and Elsevier is not able to correct same within sixty (60) days after its receipt of Your notification, You may return this CD-ROM Product, including all copies and documentation, to Elsevier and Elsevier will refund Your money.

YOU UNDERSTAND THAT, EXCEPT FOR THE 60-DAY LIMITED WARRANTY RECITED ABOVE, ELSEVIER, ITS AFFILIATES, LICENSORS, SUPPLIERS AND AGENTS, MAKE NO WARRANTIES, EXPRESSED OR IMPLIED, WITH RESPECT TO THE CD-ROM PRODUCT, INCLUDING, WITHOUT LIMITATION THE PROPRIETARY MATERIAL, AND SPECIFICALLY DISCLAIM ANY WARRANTY OF MERCHANTABILITY OR FITNESS FOR A PARTICULAR PURPOSE.

If the information provided on this CD-ROM contains medical or health sciences information, it is intended for professional use within the medical field. Information about medical treatment or drug dosages is intended strictly for professional use, and because of rapid advances in the medical sciences, independent verification of diagnosis and drug dosages should be made.

IN NO EVENT WILL ELSEVIER, ITS AFFILIATES, LICENSORS, SUPPLIERS OR AGENTS, BE LIABLE TO YOU FOR ANY DAMAGES, INCLUDING, WITHOUT LIMITATION, ANY LOST PROFITS, LOST SAVINGS OR OTHER INCIDENTAL OR CONSEQUENTIAL DAMAGES, ARISING OUT OF YOUR USE OR INABILITY TO USE THE CD-ROM PRODUCT REGARDLESS OF WHETHER SUCH DAMAGES ARE FORESEEABLE OR WHETHER SUCH DAMAGES ARE DEEMED TO RESULT FROM THE FAILURE OR INADEQUACY OF ANY EXCLUSIVE OR OTHER REMEDY.

U.S. GOVERNMENT RESTRICTED RIGHTS The CD-ROM Product and documentation are provided with restricted rights. Use, duplication or disclosure by the U.S. Government is subject to restrictions as set forth in sub-paragraphs (a) through (d) of the Commercial Computer Restricted Rights clause at FAR 52.22719 or in subparagraph (c)(1)(ii) of the Rights in Technical Data and Computer Software clause at DFARS 252.2277013, or at 252.2117015, as applicable. Contractor/Manufacturer is Elsevier Inc., 360 Park Avenue South, New York, NY 10010 USA.

GOVERNING LAW This Agreement shall be governed by the laws of the State of New York, USA. In any dispute arising out of this Agreement, You and Elsevier each consent to the exclusive personal jurisdiction and venue in the state and federal courts within New York County, New York, USA.